# AVERY'S DISEASES OF THE NEWBORN

# AVERY'S DISEASES OF THE NEWBORN

EIGHTH EDITION

**H. William Taeusch, M.D.**
Professor and Vice Chair of Pediatrics
University of California, San Francisco
San Francisco General Hospital
San Francisco, California

**Roberta A. Ballard, M.D.**
Professor of Pediatrics and Obstetrics and Gynecology
University of Pennsylvania School of Medicine
The Children's Hospital of Philadelphia
Hospital of the University of Pennsylvania
Philadelphia, Pennsylvania

**Christine A. Gleason, M.D.**
W. Alan Hodson Professor of Pediatrics
Head, Division of Neonatology
University of Washington
Children's Hospital and Regional Medical Center
Seattle, Washington

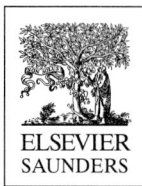

ELSEVIER
SAUNDERS

The Curtis Center
170 S Independence Mall W 300E
Philadelphia, Pennsylvania 19106

AVERY'S DISEASES OF THE NEWBORN ISBN 0-7216-9347-4


**NOTICE**

Neonatology is an ever-changing field. Standard safety precautions must be followed, but as new research and clinical experience broaden our knowledge, changes in treatment and drug therapy may become necessary or appropriate. Readers are advised to check the most current product information provided by the manufacturer of each drug to be administered to verify the recommended dose, the method and duration of administration, and contraindications. It is the responsibility of the treating physician, relying on experience and knowledge of the patient, to determine dosages and the best treatment for each individual patient. Neither the Publisher nor the editor assumes any liability for any injury and/or damage to persons or property arising from this publication.

The Publisher

Previous editions copyrighted 1998, 1991, 1984, 1977, 1971, 1965, 1960

**Library of Congress Cataloging-in-Publication Data**

Avery's diseases of the newborn. — 8th ed./[edited by] H. William Taeusch, Roberta A. Ballard, Christine A. Gleason.
p. ; cm.
Includes bibliographical references and index.
ISBN 0-7216-9347-4
1. Infants (Newborn)—Diseases. I. Title: Diseases of the newborn. II. Taeusch, H. William. III. Ballard, Roberta A. IV. Gleason, Christine A. V. Avery, Mary Ellen, 1927–
[DNLM: 1. Infant, Newborn, Diseases. WS 421 A955 2004]
RJ254.S3 2004
618.92′01—dc22

2003066852

*Executive Publisher*: Judith Fletcher
*Managing Editor, Developmental Editorial*: Deborah Thorp
*Publishing Services Manager*: Frank Polizzano
*Project Manager*: Jeff Gunning
*Design Coordinator*: Gene Harris

Printed in the United States of America

Last digit is the print number: 9 8 7 6 5 4 3 2 1

To the newborn
infants and parents
who challenge us
to get it right.

# Contributors

**Ira Adams-Chapman, M.D.**
Co-Director, Developmental Progress Clinic, Department of Pediatrics, Emory University School of Medicine, Atlanta, Georgia
*Nosocomial Infections in the Nursery*

**Anne M. Ades, M.D.**
Clinical Associate Professor of Neonatology, University of Pennsylvania School of Medicine; Neonatologist, The Children's Hospital of Philadelphia, Philadelphia, Pennsylvania
*Management of Congenital Heart Disease in the Low-Birth-Weight Infant*

**Amina Ahmed, M.D.**
Clinical Assistant Professor, University of North Carolina at Chapel Hill School of Medicine; Pediatric Infectious Disease, Carolinas Medical Center, Charlotte, North Carolina
*Toxoplasmosis, Syphilis, Malaria, and Tuberculosis*

**Simone Albers, M.D.**
Fellow in Pediatrics, Muenster University Faculty of Medicine and University Children's Hospital, Muenster, Germany
*Newborn Screening*

**Marilee C. Allen, M.D.**
Professor of Pediatrics, Johns Hopkins University School of Medicine; Associate Director of Neonatology, Johns Hopkins Hospital, and Co-Director, NICU Developmental Clinic, Kennedy Krieger Institute, Baltimore, Maryland
*Risk Assessment and Neurodevelopmental Outcomes*

**Maureen Andrew, M.D., F.R.C.P.**[†]
Formerly Professor of Pediatrics, McMaster University and Hamilton Civic Hospitals Research Centre, Hamilton, Ontario; Professor of Pediatrics, The Hospital for Sick Children, Toronto, Ontario, Canada
*Hemostatic Disorders of the Newborn*

**Stephen A. Back, M.D., Ph.D.**
Assistant Professor of Pediatrics and Neurology, Department of Pediatrics, Oregon Health Sciences University, Portland, Oregon
*Developmental Physiology of the Central Nervous System; Congenital Malformations of the Central Nervous System*

**H. Scott Baldwin, M.D.**
Katrina Overall Professor of Pediatrics, Professor of Cell and Developmental Biology, and Vice-Chair for Laboratory Sciences in Pediatrics, Department of Pediatrics, Vanderbilt University School of Medicine; Senior Cardiologist, Vanderbilt Children's Hospital, Nashville, Tennessee
*Embryology and Development of the Cardiovascular System*

**Philip L. Ballard, M.D., Ph.D.**
Gisela and Dennis Alter Professor of Pediatrics, Division of Neonatology, Department of Pediatrics, University of Pennsylvania School of Medicine; Director of Neonatal Research, The Children's Hospital of Philadelphia, Philadelphia, Pennsylvania
*Hormonal Influences on Fetal Development; Lung Development: Embryology, Growth, Maturation, and Developmental Biology*

**Roberta A. Ballard, M.D.**
Professor of Pediatrics, University of Pennsylvania School of Medicine; Neonatologist, The Children's Hospital of Philadelphia and Hospital of the University of Pennsylvania, Philadelphia, Pennsylvania
*Nonimmune Hydrops; Resuscitation in the Delivery Room; Respiratory Failure in the Term Infant; Bronchopulmonary Dysplasia; Disorders of the Chest Wall, Pleural Cavity, and Diaphragm*

**Beverly A. Banks-Randall, M.D., Ph.D., M.H.S.**
Director of Neonatology, Roy Lester Schneider Hospital, St. Thomas, U.S. Virgin Islands
*Bronchopulmonary Dysplasia*

**Stephen Baumgart, M.D.**
Professor of Pediatrics, State University of New York at Stony Brook School of Medicine; NICU Director, University Hospital at Stony Brook, Stony Brook, New York
*Temperature Regulation of the Premature Infant*

**Karen P. Beckerman, M.D.**
Clinical Associate Professor, Department of Obstetrics and Gynecology, New York University School of Medicine, New York, New York
*Identification, Evaluation, and Care of the Human Immunodeficiency Virus–Exposed Neonate*

**Thomas J. Benedetti, M.D., M.H.A.**
Vice Chair/Professor, Department of Obstetrics and Gynecology, University of Washington School of Medicine, Seattle, Washington
*Complicated Deliveries: Overview*

[†]Deceased.

**Gerard T. Berry, M.D.**
Professor of Pediatrics and Vice Dean for Research, Jefferson Medical College, Thomas Jefferson University, Philadelphia, Pennsylvania
*Introduction to the Metabolic and Biochemical Genetic Diseases; Inborn Errors of Carbohydrate, Ammonia, Amino Acid, and Organic Acid Metabolism*

**Carol Lynn Berseth, M.D.**
Director, Medical Affairs, Mead Johnson and Company, Evansville, Indiana
*Developmental Anatomy and Physiology of the Gastrointestinal Tract; Structural Anomalies of the Gastrointestinal Tract; Physiologic and Inflammatory Abnormalities of the Gastrointestinal Tract; Abdominal Wall Problems; Necrotizing Enterocolitis and Short Bowel Syndrome*

**Kathleen E. Bethin, M.D., Ph.D.**
Assistant Professor of Pediatrics, Division of Endocrinology and Diabetology, Indiana University School of Medicine, Indianapolis, Indiana
*Disorders of the Adrenal Gland*

**Diana W. Bianchi, M.D.**
Natalie V. Zucker Professor of Pediatrics, Obstetrics, and Gynecology, Tufts University School of Medicine; Chief, Division of Genetics, Tufts–New England Medical Center, Boston, Massachusetts
*Prenatal Genetic Diagnosis*

**Mitchell S. Cairo, M.D.**
Professor of Pediatrics, Medicine, and Pathology, Columbia University College of Physicians and Surgeons; Chief, Division of Pediatric Hematology and Bone Marrow Transplantation, Children's Hospital of New York–Presbyterian, New York, New York
*Neonatal Leukocyte Physiology and Disorders*

**Anthony Caldamone, M.D.**
Professor of Surgery (Urology) and Pediatrics, Brown School of Medicine; Director, Urology Residency Program, Rhode Island Hospital, Providence, Rhode Island
*Ambiguous Genitalia in the Newborn*

**Sudhish Chandra, M.D.**
Assistant Professor of Pediatrics, Case Western Reserve University School of Medicine; Attending Neonatologist, Rainbow Babies and Children's Hospital, Cleveland, Ohio
*Temperature Regulation of the Premature Infant*

**Ramen Chmait, M.D.**
Staff Physician, Florida Institute for Fetal Diagnosis and Therapy, Florida Perinatal Associates, Tampa, Florida
*Endocrine Disorders in Pregnancy*

**Ronald I. Clyman, M.D.**
Professor of Pediatrics, University of California, San Francisco, School of Medicine; Senior Staff, Cardiovascular Research Institute, San Francisco, California
*Patent Ductus Arteriosus in the Premature Infant*

**Bernard A. Cohen, M.D.**
Associate Professor of Pediatrics and Dermatology, Johns Hopkins University School of Medicine; Director, Pediatric Dermatology, Johns Hopkins Hospital, Baltimore, Maryland
*Newborn Skin: Development and Basic Concepts; Congenital and Hereditary Disorders of the Skin; Infections of the Skin; Common Newborn Dermatoses; Cutaneous Congenital Defects*

**Meryl S. Cohen, M.D.**
Interim Director of Echocardiography Laboratory, The Children's Hospital of Philadelphia, Philadelphia, Pennsylvania
*Echocardiography in the Neonatal Intensive Care Unit*

**Mitchell I. Cohen, M.D.**
Medical Director of Pediatric Cardiology and Director of Pacing and Electrophysiology, Phoenix Children's Hospital, Phoenix, Arizona
*Arrhythmias in the Fetus and Newborn*

**Robert M. Cohn, M.D.**
Associate Professor Emeritus, University of Pennsylvania School of Medicine, Philadelphia, Pennsylvania
*Lysosomal Storage, Peroxisomal, and Glycosylation Disorders and Smith-Lemli-Opitz Syndrome Presenting in the Neonate*

**F. Sessions Cole, M.D.**
Park J. White, M.D., Professor of Pediatrics, Professor of Cell Biology and Physiology, and Vice Chairman, Department of Pediatrics, Washington University School of Medicine; Director, Division of Newborn Medicine, St. Louis Children's Hospital, St. Louis, Missouri
*Immunology of the Fetus and Newborn; Viral Infections of the Fetus and Newborn*

**Anthony Corbet, M.B.**
Clinical Professor of Pediatrics, University of Texas Health Science Center at San Antonio; Partner, Magella Medical Associates (Pediatrix Medical Group); Staff Neonatologist, Christus Santa Rosa Children's Hospital, Methodist Children's Hospital, and St. Luke's Baptist Hospital, San Antonio, Texas
*Control of Breathing, Pulmonary Physiology of the Newborn; Principles of Respiratory Monitoring and Therapy; Respiratory Distress in the Preterm Infant; Respiratory Failure in the Term Infant; Anomalies of the Airways, Mediastinum, and Lung Parenchyma; Disorders of the Chest Wall, Pleural Cavity, and Diaphragm*

**Scott C. Denne, M.D.**
Professor of Pediatrics, Indiana University School of Medicine; Attending Neonatologist, James Whitcomb Riley Hospital for Children, Indianapolis, Indiana
*Parenteral Nutrition*

**Theresa J. Di Maggio, R.N., M.S.N., C.R.N.P.**
Pain Management Nurse Practitioner, Departments of Anesthesiology and Nursing, The Children's Hospital of Philadelphia, Philadelphia, Pennsylvania
*Neonatal Pain Management in the 21st Century*

**Eric C. Eichenwald, M.D.**
Assistant Professor of Pediatrics, Harvard Medical School; Associate Director, Newborn Intensive Care Unit, Brigham and Women's Hospital, Boston, Massachusetts
*Care of the Extremely Low-Birth-Weight Infant*

**Jacquelyn R. Evans, M.D.**
Clinical Professor, Department of Pediatrics, University of Pennsylvania School of Medicine; Clinical Director, Newborn Services, and Medical Director, Neonatal ECMO Program, The Children's Hospital of Philadelphia, Philadelphia, Pennsylvania
*Acid-Base, Fluid, and Electrolyte Management; Clinical Evaluation of Renal and Urinary Tract Disease; Acute and Chronic Renal Failure; Renal Vascular Disease in the Newborn*

**Nick Evans, D.M., M.R.C.P.Ch.**
Clinical Associate Professor of Pediatrics, University of Sydney Faculty of Medicine; Director, NICU, Royal Prince Alfred Hospital, Lamperdown, New South Wales, Australia
*Cardiovascular Compromise in the Newborn Infant*

**Avroy A. Fanaroff, M.D.**
Eliza Henry Barnes Professor in Neonatology and Interim Chair, Department of Pediatrics, and Professor of Reproductive Biology, Case Western Reserve University School of Medicine; Neonatologist, Rainbow Babies and Children's Hospital, Cleveland, Ohio
*Perinatal-Neonatal Epidemiology*

**Donna M. Ferriero, M.D.**
Professor of Neurology and Pediatrics, Division of Child Neurology, University of California, San Francisco, School of Medicine, San Francisco, California
*Central Nervous System Injury and Neuroprotection*

**Delbert A. Fisher, M.D.**
Vice President, Science & Innovation, Quest Diagnostics Nichols Institute, San Juan Capistrano, California
*Disorders of the Thyroid Gland*

**Laura Flores-Sarnat, M.D.**
Postdoctoral Research Fellow in Neuropathology, Cedars-Sinai Medical Center, Los Angeles, California
*Neonatal Neuromuscular Disorders*

**Philippe S. Friedlich, M.D.**
Assistant Professor of Clinical Pediatrics, University of Southern California Keck School of Medicine; Section Head, CHLA Operations, and Medical Director, Center for Newborn and Infant Critical Care, Children's Hospital Los Angeles, Los Angeles, California
*Clinical Evaluation of Renal and Urinary Tract Disease; Acute and Chronic Renal Failure*

**J. William Gaynor, M.D.**
Associate Professor of Surgery, University of Pennsylvania School of Medicine; Daniel M. Tabas Endowed Chair in Pediatric Cardiothoracic Surgery, The Children's Hospital of Philadelphia, Philadelphia, Pennsylvania
*Long-Term Neurologic Outcomes in Children with Congenital Heart Disease*

**Alfred L. Gest, M.D.**
Associate Professor of Clinical Pediatrics, Department of Pediatrics, The Ohio State University School of Medicine and Public Health; Neonatologist, Children's Hospital, Columbus, Ohio
*Principles of Respiratory Monitoring and Therapy*

**Tal Geva, M.D.**
Associate Professor of Pediatrics (Radiology), Department of Pediatrics, Harvard Medical School; Senior Associate in Cardiology, Children's Hospital Boston, Boston, Massachusetts
*Nomenclature and the Segmental Approach to Congenital Heart Disease*

**Mary Ann E. Gibbons, R.N., B.S.N.**
Clinical Nurse IV, Newborn/Infant Center, The Children's Hospital of Philadelphia, Philadelphia, Pennsylvania
*Neonatal Pain Management in the 21st Century*

**William M. Gilbert, M.D.**
Professor and Vice Chair, Department of Obstetrics and Gynecology, University of California, Davis, School of Medicine; Attending Physician, University of California, Davis, Medical Center, Sacramento, California
*Placental Function and Diseases: The Placenta, Fetal Membranes, and Umbilical Cord*

**Bertil E. Glader, M.D., Ph.D.**
Professor of Pediatrics, Stanford University School of Medicine; Attending Pediatrician, Stanford University Hospitals, Stanford, California
*Erythrocyte Disorders in Infancy*

**Christine A. Gleason, M.D.**
Professor of Pediatrics, University of Washington School of Medicine; Head, Division of Neonatology, Children's Hospital and Regional Medical Center, Seattle, Washington
*Developmental Physiology of the Central Nervous System; Appendix 2: Illustrative Forms and Normal Values*

**Michael J. Goldberg, M.D.**
Professor and Chairman, Department of Orthaepedics, Tufts University School of Medicine; Orthopaedist in Chief, Tufts–New England Medical Center, Boston, Massachusetts
*Common Neonatal Orthopedic Ailments*

**William V. Good, M.D.**
Senior Scientist, Smith-Kettlewell Eye Research Institute, San Francisco, California
*Disorders of the Eye*

**Gregory Goodwin, M.D.**
Assistant Professor of Pediatrics, Brown School of Medicine; Director, Pediatric Endocrine Clinic, Rhode Island Hospital, Providence, Rhode Island
*Ambiguous Genitalia in the Newborn*

**Sameer Gopalani, M.D., M.S.**
Acting Instructor and Fellow, Division of Perinatal Medicine, Department of Obstetrics and Gynecology, University of Washington School of Medicine, Seattle, Washington
*Complicated Deliveries: Overview*

**Carol L. Greene, M.D.**
Clinical Professor, George Washington University School of Medicine; Clinical Faculty, Division of Genetics and Metabolism, Department of Pediatrics, Children's National Medical Center, Washington, DC
*Lysosomal Storage, Peroxisomal, and Glycosylation Disorders and Smith-Lemli-Opitz Syndrome Presenting in the Neonate*

**Brian E. Grottkau, M.D.**
Chief of Pediatric Orthopaedics and Adult Spine Surgeon, Massachusetts General Hospital, Boston, Massachusetts
*Common Neonatal Orthopedic Ailments*

**Peter J. Gruber, M.D., Ph.D.**
Assistant Professor of Surgery, University of Pennsylvania School of Medicine; Pediatric Cardiologist, The Children's Hospital of Philadelphia, Philadelphia, Pennsylvania
*Common Congenital Heart Disease: Presentation, Management, and Outcomes*

**Jean-Pierre Guignard, M.D.**
Professor of Pediatric Nephrology, University of Lausanne Faculty of Medicine; Head, Division of Pediatric Nephrology, University Hospital Medical Center, Lausanne, France
*Renal Morphogenesis and Development of Renal Function*

**Susan Guttentag, M.D.**
Assistant Professor of Pediatrics, University of Pennsylvania School of Medicine; Neonatologist, The Children's Hospital of Philadelphia, Philadelphia, Pennsylvania
*Lung Development: Embryology, Growth, Maturation, and Developmental Biology*

**Shannon E. G. Hamrick, M.D.**
Clinical Instructor of Pediatrics, Division of Neonatology, University of California, San Francisco, School of Medicine, San Francisco, California
*Central Nervous System Injury and Neuroprotection*

**Thomas N. Hansen, M.D.**
Professor and Chairman, Department of Pediatrics, The Ohio State University School of Medicine and Public Health; Chief Executive Officer, Children's Hospital, Columbus, Ohio
*Control of Breathing; Pulmonary Physiology of the Newborn; Principles of Respiratory Monitoring and Therapy; Respiratory Distress in the Preterm Infant; Respiratory Failure in the Term Infant; Anomalies of the Airways, Mediastinum, and Lung Parenchyma; Disorders of the Chest Wall, Pleural Cavity, and Diaphragm*

**Margaret K. Hostetter, M.D.**
Professor of Pediatrics and Microbial Pathogenesis, Yale University School of Medicine; Physician-in-Chief, Yale–New Haven Children's Hospital, New Haven, Connecticut
*Fungal Infections in the Neonatal Intensive Care Unit*

**Samuel C. Hughes, M.D.**
Professor of Anesthesia, University of California, San Francisco, School of Medicine; Director, Obstetric Anesthesia, San Francisco General Hospital, San Francisco, California
*Maternal and Fetal Anesthesia and Analgesia*

**Andrew D. Hull, B.Med.Sci., B.M., B.S., F.R.C.O.G., F.A.C.O.G.**
Assistant Professor of Reproductive Medicine and Director of Research, University of California, San Diego, School of Medicine, San Diego, California
*Hypertensive Complications of Pregnancy; Antepartum Fetal Assessment*

**Roy Jedeikin, M.D.**
Medical Director of Pediatric Cardiology, St. Joseph's Hospital and Medical Center, Phoenix, Arizona
*Arrhythmias in the Fetus and Newborn*

**Sandra E. Juul, M.D., Ph.D.**
Associate Professor of Pediatrics, University of Washington School of Medicine, Seattle, Washington
*Developmental Biology of the Hematologic System*

**Bernard S. Kaplan, M.B., B.Ch.**
Professor of Pediatrics and Medicine, University of Pennsylvania School of Medicine; Director of Pediatric Nephrology, The Children's Hospital of Philadelphia, Philadelphia, Pennsylvania
*Developmental Abnormalities of the Kidneys; Glomerulonephropathies and Disorders of Tubular Function*

**Paige Kaplan, M.B., B.Ch.**
Professor of Pediatrics, University of Pennsylvania School of Medicine; Section Chief, Metabolic Diseases, Department of Pediatrics, The Children's Hospital of Philadelphia, Philadelphia, Pennsylvania
*Skeletal Dysplasias and Connective Tissue Disorders*

**Rebecca A. Kazin, M.D.**
Resident in Dermatology, Johns Hopkins Medical Institutions, Baltimore, Maryland
*Common Newborn Dermatoses*

**Thomas F. Kelly, M.D.**
Associate Clinical Professor of Reproductive Medicine, University of California, San Diego, School of Medicine, La Jolla; Director of Maternity Services, UCSD Medical Center, San Diego, California
*Maternal Medical Disorders of Fetal Significance: Seizure Disorders, Isoimmunization, Cancer, and Mental Disorders*

**Stefan Kuhle, M.D.**
Senior Registrar, Department of Neonatology, University Children's Hospital, Tübingen, Germany
*Hemostatic Disorders of the Newborn*

**Ian A. Laing, M.A. M.D., F.R.C.P.E., F.R.C.P.Ch.**
Senior Lecturer, Department of Reproductive and Developmental Sciences, University of Edinburgh Faculty of Medicine; Clinical Director, Neonatal Unit, Simpson Centre for Reproductive Health, Royal Infirmary of Edinburgh, Edinburgh, United Kingdom
*Surfactant Treatment of Respiratory Disorders*

**Harvey L. Levy, M.D.**
Associate Professor of Pediatrics, Harvard Medical School; Senior Associate in Medicine (Genetics), Children's Hospital Boston, Boston, Massachusetts
*Newborn Screening*

**Mignon L. Loh, M.D.**
Assistant Professor of Clinical Pediatrics, University of California, San Francisco, School of Medicine; Attending Physician, UCSF Children's Hospital, San Francisco, California
*Congenital Malignant Disorders*

**Scott A. Lorch, M.D., M.S.C.E.**
Assistant Professor, University of Pennsylvania School of Medicine; Clinical Associate, Division of Neonatology, The Children's Hospital of Philadelphia, Philadelphia, Pennsylvania
*Nonimmune Hydrops*

**Ralph A. Lugo, Pharm.D.**
Associate Professor, University of Utah College of Pharmacy, Salt Lake City, Utah
*Pharmacologic Principles and Practicalities*

**Geoffrey A. Machin, M.D., Ph.D.**
Fetal/Genetic Pathologist, The Permanente Medical Group, Department of Pathology, Kaiser Oakland, Oakland, California
*Placental Function and Diseases: The Placenta, Fetal Membranes, and Umbilical Cord; Multiple Birth*

**James R. MacMahon, M.D.**
Associate Professor of Pediatrics, Staff Physician, Maine Medical Center, Portland, Maine
*Neonatal Hyperbilirubinemia*

**George A. Macones, M.D., M.S.C.E.**
Associate Professor, Department of Obstetrics and Gynecology, University of Pennsylvania School of Medicine; Director, Maternal Fetal Medicine, Hospital of the University of Pennsylvania, Philadelphia, Pennsylvania
*Prematurity: Causes and Prevention*

**Ashima Madan, M.D.**
Associate Professor of Pediatrics, Stanford University School of Medicine; Staff Physician, Lucile Salter Packard Children's Hospital, Stanford, California
*Central Nervous System Injury and Neuroprotection; Neonatal Hyperbilirubinemia; Disorders of the Eye*

**Bradley S. Marino, M.D.**
Assistant Professor of Anesthesia and Pediatrics, University of Pennsylvania School of Medicine; Assistant Physician, Division of Cardiology and Division of Critical Care Medicine, The Children's Hospital of Philadelphia, Philadelphia, Pennsylvania
*Stabilization and Transport of the Neonate with Congenital Heart Disease*

**Alma Martinez, M.D., M.P.H.**
Associate Clinical Professor of Pediatrics, San Francisco General Hospital and University of California, San Francisco, School of Medicine, San Francisco, California
*Abnormalities of Fetal Growth; Perinatal Substance Abuse*

**Kathryn L. Maschoff, M.D., Ph.D.**
Clinical Associate Professor, Department of Pediatrics, University of Pennsylvania School of Medicine; Attending Neonatologist, The Children's Hospital of Philadelphia and Hospital of the University of Pennsylvania, Philadelphia, Pennsylvania
*Embryology and Development of the Cardiovascular System*

**Patricia Massicotte, M.D., M.Sc., F.R.C.P.C.**
Professor of Pediatrics, University of Alberta Faculty of Medicine; Attending Physician, Stollery Children's Hospital, Edmonton, Alberta, Canada
*Hemostatic Disorders of the Newborn*

**Katherine K. Matthay, M.D.**
Professor of Pediatrics, University of California, San Francisco, School of Medicine; Interim Chief, Pediatric Hematology-Oncology, and Director, Pediatric Oncology, UCSF Children's Hospital, San Francisco, California
*Congenital Malignant Disorders*

**William C. Mentzer, M.D.**
Professor of Pediatrics Emeritus, University of California, San Francisco, School of Medicine; Attending Pediatric Hematologist/Oncologist, University of California Medical Center, San Francisco, California
*Erythrocyte Disorders in Infancy*

**Jeffrey D. Merrill, M.D.**
Assistant Professor of Pediatrics, University of Pennsylvania School of Medicine; Medical Director, Intensive Care Nursery, Hospital of the University of Pennsylvania, Philadelphia, Pennsylvania
*Resuscitation in the Delivery Room*

**Carol A. Miller, M.D.**
Clinical Professor, Department of Pediatrics, University of California, San Francisco, School of Medicine, San Francisco, California
*Routine Newborn Care*

**Lesley Mitchell, A.R.T., M.Sc.**
Associate Professor of Pediatrics, University of Alberta Faculty of Medicine; Scientific Director, Pediatric Thrombosis Program, Stollery Children's Hospital, Edmonton, Alberta, Canada
*Hemostatic Disorders of the Newborn*

**Alicia A. Moise, M.D.**
Associate Professor of Clinical Pediatrics, Department of Pediatrics, The Ohio State University School of Medicine and Public Health; Neonatologist, Children's Hospital, Columbus, Ohio
*Principles of Respiratory Monitoring and Therapy*

**Thomas J. Mollen, M.D.**
Instructor, University of Pennsylvania School of Medicine; Clinical Associate, The Children's Hospital of Philadelphia, Philadelphia, Pennsylvania
*Nonimmune Hydrops*

**Timothy P. Monahan, M.A., M.D.**
Resident in Dermatology, Johns Hopkins Hospital, Baltimore, Maryland
*Congenital and Hereditary Disorders of the Skin*

**Thomas R. Moore, M.D.**
Professor and Chairman, Department of Reproductive Medicine, University of California, San Diego, School of Medicine; Faculty Physician, UCSD Medical Center, San Diego, California
*Endocrine Disorders in Pregnancy; Maternal Medical Disorders of Fetal Significance: Seizure Disorders, Isoimmunization, Cancer, and Mental Disorders; Hypertensive Complications of Pregnancy; Antepartum Fetal Assessment*

**Louis J. Muglia, M.D., Ph.D.**
Associate Professor of Pediatrics, Molecular Biology and Pharmacology, and Obstetrics and Gynecology, Washington University School of Medicine; Attending Physician, St. Louis Children's Hospital, St. Louis, Missouri
*Disorders of the Adrenal Gland*

**Robert M. Nelson, M.D., Ph.D.**
Associate Professor of Anesthesia and Pediatrics, University of Pennsylvania School of Medicine; Attending Physician, Anesthesiology and Critical Care Medicine, The Children's Hospital of Philadelphia, Philadelphia, Pennsylvania
*Ethical Decisions in the Neonatal-Perinatal Period*

**Thomas B. Newman, M.D., M.P.H.**
Professor of Epidemiology and Biostatistics, Departments of Epidemiology and Biostatistics and Pediatrics, University of California, San Francisco, School of Medicine; Attending Physician, Well Baby Nursery, UCSF Medical Center, San Francisco, California
*Routine Newborn Care*

**Eugenia K. Pallotto, M.D.**
Assistant Professor of Pediatrics, University of Missouri–Kansas City School of Medicine; Attending Physician, Section of Neonatology, Department of Pediatrics, Children's Mercy Hospitals and Clinics, Kansas City, Missouri
*Disorders of Carbohydrate Metabolism*

**Erica S. Pan, M.D., M.P.H.**
Clinical Instructor, University of California, San Francisco, School of Medicine; Director, Bioterrorism and Emerging Infections Unit, Community Health Epidemiology and Disease Control, San Francisco Department of Public Health, San Francisco, California
*Viral Infections of the Fetus and Newborn*

**Elvira Parravicini, M.D.**
Assistant Professor of Clinical Pediatrics, Columbia University College of Physicians and Surgeons; Assistant Clinical Attending, Children's Hospital of New York–Presbyterian, New York, New York
*Bacterial Sepsis and Meningitis; Neonatal Leukocyte Physiology and Disorders*

**J. Colin Partridge, M.D., M.P.H.**
Clinical Professor, University of California, San Francisco, School of Medicine; Attending Neonatologist, San Francisco General Hospital, San Francisco, California
*Perinatal Substance Abuse*

**Dan Poenaru, M.D., M.H.P.E., F.R.C.S.C., F.A.C.S., F.I.C.S.**
Adjunct Associate Professor of Surgery and Pediatrics, Queen's University Faculty of Health Sciences, Kingston, Ontario, Canada; Medical Education and Research Director, AIC Kijabe Hospital, Kijabe, Kenya
*Structural Anomalies of the Gastrointestinal Tract; Abdominal Wall Problems; Necrotizing Enterocolitis and Short Bowel Syndrome*

**Brenda B. Poindexter, M.D.**
Assistant Professor of Pediatrics, Indiana University School of Medicine; Attending Neonatologist, James Whitcomb Riley Hospital for Children, Indianapolis, Indiana
*Parenteral Nutrition*

**Richard A. Polin, M.D.**
Professor of Pediatrics, Columbia University College of Physicians and Surgeons; Director, Division of Neonatology, Children's Hospital of New York–Presbyterian, New York, New York
*Bacterial Sepsis and Meningitis*

**Daniel H. Polk, M.D.**
Professor of Pediatrics, Northwestern University Feinberg School of Medicine; Vice Chief, Division of Neonatology, Children's Memorial Hospital, Chicago, Illinois
*Disorders of the Thyroid Gland*

**DeWayne M. Pursley, M.D., M.P.H.**
Assistant Professor of Pediatrics, Harvard Medical School; Neonatologist in Chief, Beth Israel Deaconess Medical Center, Boston, Massachusetts
*Impact of the Human Genome Project on Neonatal Care*

**Rangasamy Ramanathan, M.D.**
Professor of Clinical Pediatrics, University of Southern California Keck School of Medicine; Associate Division Chief and Section Head, USC Division of Neonatology; Director, Neonatal-Perinatal Medicine Fellowship Program, and Director, NICU Women's and Children's Hospital, LAC + USC Women's and Children's Hospital and Children's Hospital Los Angeles, Los Angeles, California
*Acid-Base, Fluid, and Electrolyte Management; Renal Vascular Disease in the Newborn*

**Daniela Ramierez-Schrempp, M.D.**
Clinical Assistant Instructor in Pediatrics, State University of New York; Children's Hospital at Downstate Medical Center, Brooklyn, New York
*Surfactant Treatment of Respiratory Disorders*

**Joan A. Regan, M.D.**†
Formerly Associate Professor of Clinical Pediatrics, Columbia University College of Physicians and Surgeons, and Associate Clinical Attending, Children's Hospital of New York–Presbyterian, New York, New York
*Bacterial Sepsis and Meningitis*

**Elisabeth G. Richard, M.D.**
Resident in Dermatology, Johns Hopkins Medical Institutions, Baltimore, Maryland
*Infections of the Skin*

**Richard L. Robertson, M.D.**
Assistant Professor of Radiology, Harvard Medical School; Director of Neuroradiology, Children's Hospital Boston, Boston, Massachusetts
*Neonatal Neuroimaging*

**Mark A. Rosen, M.D.**
Professor of Anesthesia and Obstetrics, Gynecology, and Reproductive Sciences, University of California, San Francisco, School of Medicine; Director, Obstetric Anesthesia, University Hospitals (Moffitt-Long), San Francisco, California
*Maternal and Fetal Anesthesia and Analgesia*

**Lewis P. Rubin, M.Phil., M.D.**
Associate Professor of Pediatrics and Co-Director, Program in Fetal Medicine, Brown Medical School; Staff Neonatologist, Women and Infants Hospital of Rhode Island, Providence, Rhode Island
*Embryology, Developmental Biology, and Anatomy of the Endocrine System; Disorders of Calcium and Phosphorus Metabolism*

**Jack Rychik, M.D., F.A.C.C.**
Associate Professor of Pediatrics, University of Pennsylvania School of Medicine; Medical Director, The Fetal Heart Program, Division of Cardiology, The Children's Hospital of Philadelphia, Philadelphia, Pennsylvania
*Echocardiography in the Neonatal Intensive Care Unit*

**Sulagna C. Saitta, M.D., Ph.D.**
Assistant Professor of Pediatrics, University of Pennsylvania School of Medicine; Attending Physician, Division of Human Genetics, The Children's Hospital of Philadelphia, Philadelphia, Pennsylvania
*Evaluation of the Dysmorphic Infant; Specific Chromosome Disorders in Newborns*

†Deceased.

**Pablo J. Sánchez, M.D.**
Professor of Pediatrics, Division of Neonatal-Perinatal Medicine and Division of Pediatric Infectious Diseases, Department of Pediatrics, University of Texas Southwestern Medical Center; Attending Physician, Parkland Memorial Hospital and Children's Medical Center, Dallas, Texas
*Toxoplasmosis, Syphilis, Malaria, and Tuberculosis*

**Harvey B. Sarnat, M.D., F.R.C.P.C.**
Professor of Pediatrics (Neurology) and Pathology (Neuropathology), David Geffen School of Medicine at UCLA; Director, Division of Pediatric Neurology, Neuropathologist, and Director, Neuromuscular Pathology Laboratory, Cedars-Sinai Medical Center, Los Angeles, California
*Neonatal Neuromuscular Disorders*

**Richard J. Schanler, M.D.**
Professor of Pediatrics, Albert Einstein College of Medicine of Yeshiva University, Bronx; Chief, Neonatal-Perinatal Medicine, Schneider Children's Hospital at North Shore, North Shore University Hospital, Manhasset, New York
*Enteral Nutrition for the High-Risk Neonate*

**Mark S. Scher, M.D.**
Professor of Pediatrics and Neurology, Case Western Reserve University School of Medicine; Division Chief, Pediatric Neurology, and Director, Pediatric Sleep/Epilepsy and Fetal/Neonatal Neurology Programs, Rainbow Babies and Children's Hospital, University Hospitals of Cleveland, Cleveland, Ohio
*Neonatal Seizures*

**Istvan Seri, M.D., Ph.D.**
Professor of Pediatrics, University of Southern California Keck School of Medicine; Head, USC Division of Neonatal Medicine, and Medical Director, Institute of Maternal and Fetal Health, Children's Hospital Los Angeles and the LAC + USC Women's and Children's Hospital, Los Angeles, California
*Acid-Base, Fluid, and Electrolyte Management; Cardiovascular Compromise in the Newborn Infant; Clinical Evaluation of Renal and Urinary Tract Disease; Acute and Chronic Renal Failure; Renal Vascular Disease in the Newborn*

**Elaine C. Siegfried, M.D.**
Associate Clinical Professor of Pediatrics and Dermatology, Saint Louis University School of Medicine; Staff Physician, Cardinal Glennon Children's Hospital, St. Louis, Missouri
*Newborn Skin: Development and Basic Concepts; Congenital and Hereditary Disorders of the Skin; Infections of the Skin; Common Newborn Dermatoses; Cutaneous Congenital Defects*

**Gary A. Silverman, M.D., Ph.D.**
Associate Professor of Pediatrics, Harvard Medical School; Children's Hospital, Boston, Massachusetts
*Impact of the Human Genome Project on Neonatal Care*

**Rebecca Simmons, M.D.**
Assistant Professor of Pediatrics, University of Pennsylvania School of Medicine; Attending Neonatologist, The Children's Hospital of Philadelphia and Hospital of the University of Pennsylvania, Philadelphia, Pennsylvania
*Abnormalities of Fetal Growth*

**Susan Sniderman, M.D.**
Professor of Pediatrics, Chief, Neonatal Service, San Francisco General Hospital, University of California-San Francisco, San Francisco, California
*Initial Evaluation: History and Physical Examination of the Newborn*

**Thomas L. Spray, M.D.**
Alice Langdon Warner Professor of Surgery, University of Pennsylvania School of Medicine; Chief, Division of Cardiothoracic Surgery, The Children's Hospital of Philadelphia, Philadelphia, Pennsylvania
*Management of Congenital Heart Disease in the Low-Birth-Weight Infant*

**Charles A. Stanley, M.D.**
Chief, Division of Endocrinology/Diabetes, The Children's Hospital of Philadelphia, Philadelphia, Pennsylvania
*Disorders of Carbohydrate Metabolism*

**David K. Stevenson, M.D.**
Harold K. Faber Professor of Pediatrics and Senior Associate Dean for Academic Affairs, Stanford University School of Medicine; Director, Charles B. and Ann L. Johnson Center for Pregnancy and Newborn Services, and Chief, Division of Neonatal and Developmental Medicine, Lucile Salter Packard Children's Hospital, Stanford, California
*Neonatal Hyperbilirubinemia*

**Barbara J. Stoll, M.D.**
Professor of Pediatrics and Interim Chair, Department of Pediatrics, Emory University School of Medicine, Atlanta, Georgia
*Nosocomial Infections in the Nursery*

**H. William Taeusch, M.D.**
Professor and Vice Chair, Department of Pediatrics, University of California, San Francisco, School of Medicine; Chief, Pediatric Service, San Francisco General Hospital, San Francisco, California
*Perinatal Substance Abuse; Initial Evaluation: History and Physical Examination of the Newborn; Bacterial Sepsis and Meningitis; Surfactant Treatment of Respiratory Disorders*

**Peter Tarczy-Hornoch, M.D.**
Associate Professor, Division of Neonatology, Department of Pediatrics, and Associate Professor and Head, Division of Biomedical and Health Informatics, University of Washington School of Medicine, Seattle, Washington
*Evaluation of Therapeutic Recommendations, Database Management, and Information Retrieval*

**George A. Taylor, M.D.**
John A. Kirkpatrick Professor of Radiology, Harvard Medical School; Radiologist-in-Chief and Chairman, Department of Radiology, Children's Hospital Boston, Boston, Massachusetts
*Neonatal Neuroimaging*

**Janet A. Thomas, M.D.**
Assistant Professor of Pediatrics, University of Colorado School of Medicine; Director, Inherited Metabolic Diseases Clinic, University of Colorado Health Sciences Center and The Children's Hospital, Denver, Colorado
*Lysosomal Storage, Peroxisomal, and Glycosylation Disorders and Smith-Lemli-Opitz Syndrome Presenting in the Neonate*

**Tivadar Tulassay, M.D., D.Sc.**
President, Semmelweis University Budapest; Professor and Chair, Department of Pediatrics, Semmelweis University Budapest Faculty of Medicine, Budapest, Hungary
*Acute and Chronic Renal Failure; Renal Vascular Disease in the Newborn*

**Carmella van de Ven, M.A.**
Senior Staff Associate, Columbia University College of Physicians and Surgeons, New York, New York
*Neonatal Leukocyte Physiology and Disorders*

**Betty R. Vohr, M.D.**
Professor of Pediatrics, Brown Medical School; Director, Neonatal Follow-up Clinic, Women and Infants Hospital of Rhode Island, Providence, Rhode Island
*Perinatal-Neonatal Epidemiology*

**Robert M. Ward, M.D.**
Professor of Pediatrics, Department of Pediatrics, Division of Neonatology, University of Utah College of Medicine; Director, Pediatric Pharmacology Program, University of Utah Hospital, Salt Lake City, Utah
*Pharmacologic Principles and Practicalities; Appendix 1: Drugs*

**Peggy Sue Weintrub, M.D.**
Clinical Professor, Department of Pediatrics, University of California, San Francisco, School of Medicine; Chief, Division of Pediatric Infectious Diseases, USCF Medical Center, San Francisco, California
*Viral Infections of the Fetus and Newborn*

**Stephen Welty, M.D.**
Associate Professor, Department of Pediatrics, The Ohio State University School of Medicine and Public Health; Chief, Section of Neonatology, Department of Pediatrics, Children's Hospital, Columbus, Ohio
*Respiratory Distress in the Preterm Infant*

**Gil Wernovsky, M.D.**
Professor of Pediatrics, University of Pennsylvania School of Medicine; Director of Program Development, The Cardiac Center, The Children's Hospital of Philadelphia, Philadelphia, Pennsylvania
*Stabilization and Transport of the Neonate with Congenital Heart Disease; Common Congenital Heart Disease: Presentation, Management, and Outcomes; Management of Congenital Heart Disease in the Low-Birth-Weight Infant; Long-Term Neurologic Outcomes in Children with Congenital Heart Disease*

**Calvin B. Williams, M.D., Ph.D.**
Associate Professor of Pediatrics, Associate Professor of Microbiology and Molecular Genetics, Section Chief, Pediatric Rhenumatology, and D.B. and Marjorie Reinhart Family Foundation Chair in Rhenumatology, Medical College of Wisconsin; Attending Physician, Children's Hospital of Wisconsin, Milwaukee, Wisconsin
*Immunology of the Fetus and Newborn*

**Linda L. Wright, M.D.**
Pregnancy and Perinatology Branch, Center for Research for Mothers and Children, National Institute of Child Health and Human Development, Rockville, Maryland
*Perinatal-Neonatal Epidemiology*

**Alison Z. Young, M.D.**
Resident, Department of Dermatology, Johns Hopkins Hospital, Baltimore, Maryland
*Cutaneous Congenital Defects*

**Elaine H. Zackai, M.D.**
Director, Clinical Genetics, Department of Clinical Genetics, The Children's Hospital of Philadelphia, Philadelphia, Pennsylvania
*Evaluation of the Dysmorphic Infant; Specific Chromosome Disorders in Newborns*

**Stephen A. Zderic, M.D.**
Associate Professor of Urology, University of Pennsylvania School of Medicine; Associate Surgeon, Department of Urology, The Children's Hospital of Philadelphia, Philadelphia, Pennsylvania
*Developmental Abnormalities of the Genitourinary System; Urinary Tract Infections and Vesicoureteral Reflux*

# Preface

Dr. Alexander Shaffer, a noted Baltimore pediatrician and a former chief resident in pediatrics at Johns Hopkins Hospital, wrote the first edition of *Diseases of the Newborn*, which was published in 1960. At that time, he recognized that the care of newborns would become a subspecialty, which he termed *neonatology*. Composed from extensive case records, his book was of use mainly for diagnosis but included reference to the work of many who, with difficulty, studied the needs of newborns by applying techniques developed by such physiologists and biochemists as Barcroft and Gamble, who were fascinated by complexities of the fetus and newborn. The senior editor of this edition had the opportunity to see Dr. Shaffer diagnose the extent of an empyema in a 1-week-old infant by gentle percussion of the chest. This disease (thankfully) and this technique (regretfully) are now much less commonly observed. Many of the great names in pediatrics were contemporaries of Shaffer, and they, too, wed careful observation of newborns to clinical research in neonatology: Ethel Dunham, Warkany, Gamble, Gordon, Julius Hess, Levine, Clement Smith, Taussig, Diamond, Lubchenco, Rudolph, James, Apgar, and Silverman. With the use mainly of antibiotics, warmth, and attention to feeding techniques, the infant mortality rate in the United States dropped from 47/1000 live births in 1940 to 26/1000 in 1960.

Shaffer's book preceded the advent of ventilator management of newborn infants that, coupled with micro blood gas analysis and expertise in the use of umbilical artery catheterization, led to the development of neonatal intensive care for newborns in the 1960s on both sides of the Atlantic. Advances in neonatal surgery and cardiology and further developments in technology paralleled the rise of neonatal intensive care units (NICUs) and regionalization of care for sick newborn infants. Some of the leaders in North America were Stahlman in Nashville; Tooley and colleagues in San Francisco; Avery in Baltimore; Auld in New York; Usher and Stern in Montreal; Swyer in Toronto; Oh and Hodgman in Los Angeles; Battaglia, Meschia, and Butterfield in Denver; Sinclair in Hamilton; Sunshine in Palo Alto; and Lucey in Burlington.

Mary Ellen Avery joined Shaffer for the third edition of this book in 1971. A further drop in the infant mortality rate occurred by 1974, to 16.5/1000 live births. By 1977 and the fourth edition, the need for multiple contributors with subspecialty expertise was clear. In the preface for that edition, Shaffer wrote, "We have also seen the application of some fundamental advances in molecular biology to the management of our fetal and newborn patients." At that time he was referring to the new knowledge of hemoglobinopathies. In 1981, Shaffer died at the age of 79. Taeusch joined Avery for the fifth edition, and Ballard, for the sixth in 1991, with the addition of Gleason for this edition.

The need for updating and revision is constant. Despite the use of the Internet for the latest knowledge, textbooks of neonatology, along with even more "subspecialized" books, lie dog-eared, broken-spined, and coffee-stained on countless conference room tables where caregivers congregate in nurseries. In looking over past editions, we note not that what was said was wrong but that the right things were not said as extensively, or as insightfully, or as clearly, as we now understand them. This edition has been completely and often painfully revised by some of the best clinicians/investigators in the field. They did this despite the demands of their day jobs in the hopes that their syntheses could, as Ethel Dunham wrote, "spread more widely what is already known, . . . and make it possible to apply these facts," as well as stimulating the search for new knowledge.

This edition is notable for its breadth—from the classic history and physical examination of a full-term newborn to the details of tiny DNA perturbations that result in lethal problems after birth. There are new sections on genetics and prenatal diagnosis. Eighty-four new authors contributed to this edition, and every section of the book has been updated. New diagnostic and therapeutic techniques are included for virtually every organ system, along with countless other changes to this new edition. Thanks to the newest member of our editorial team, Christine Gleason, the neurology section has been thoroughly updated; Gil Wernovsky, working with Roberta Ballard, has done the same for the cardiology section. The discussion of eye disorders has been expanded to include structural defects, transient motility disorders, and infection, as well as retinopathy of prematurity. An excellent new section on nutrition has been added, as has a discussion of fetal origins of adult disease.

In the era of sudden infant death syndrome (SIDS) prevention, fetal diagnosis of anomalies and genetic disorders, surfactant therapy, and improved techniques for cardiorespiratory support, the infant mortality rate for 2002 was 6.9/1000. Huge areas remain frustratingly intractable, however. Premature birth rates have increased. The problems of fetal exposure to addicting drugs and intoxicants remain ever present. Common germs are brilliantly adaptable in the face of formidable anti-infectives. Garden-variety problems of the NICU such as chronic lung disease, recurrent apneas, retinopathy, necrotizing enterocolitis, intracranial bleeding, and hypoxic ischemic encephalopathy continue to impair the well-being of thousands of infants each year. Problems so simple they are almost silly remain unsolved (what's a safe level of bilirubin? of blood glucose?). Basic questions concerning the nature of growth and development remain, and the search for answers is underfunded, as resources are diverted in ways that hurt the children of the world. Many, if not most, of the neonatal medical problems that occur worldwide (like those of medicine in general) are rooted in poverty, a problem that can be markedly reduced if we do what is obvious.

As usual, we invite your comments and feedback, so that the next edition can correct any shortcomings or errors of this one.

We wish to thank key staff at Elsevier—Deborah Thorp, Managing Editor, Developmental Editorial, and Judith Fletcher, Executive Publisher, both of whom demonstrated endless patience and persistence, and Jeff Gunning, Project Manager for our book—and our colleagues, families, and academic institutions for their continued support of this effort. Last, we would like to thank Mary Ellen Avery for her wise influence on the field of pediatrics, on the lives of many children throughout the world, and on us, the editors of the eighth edition of this text.

H. William Taeusch
Roberta A. Ballard
Christine A. Gleason

# Contents

Color plate section follows page xxiii.

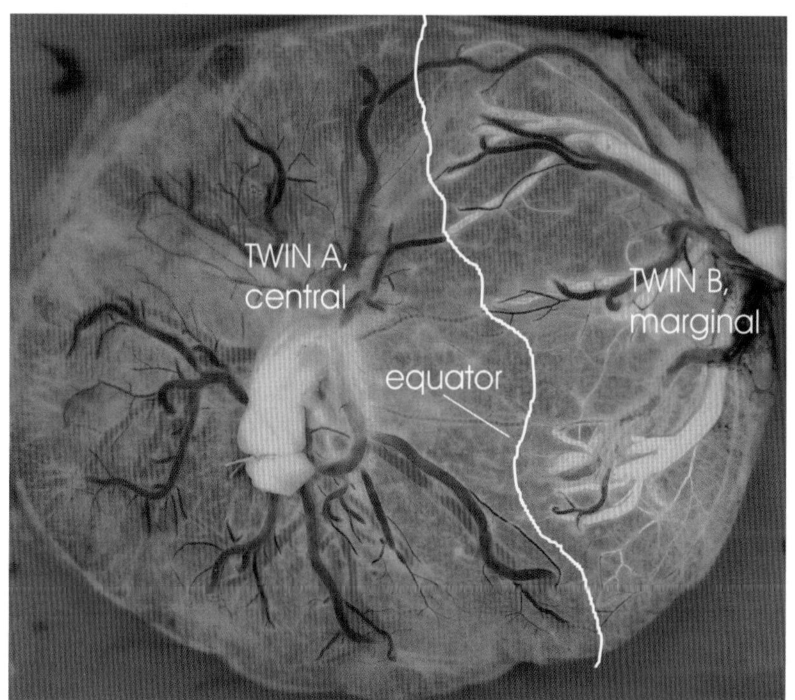


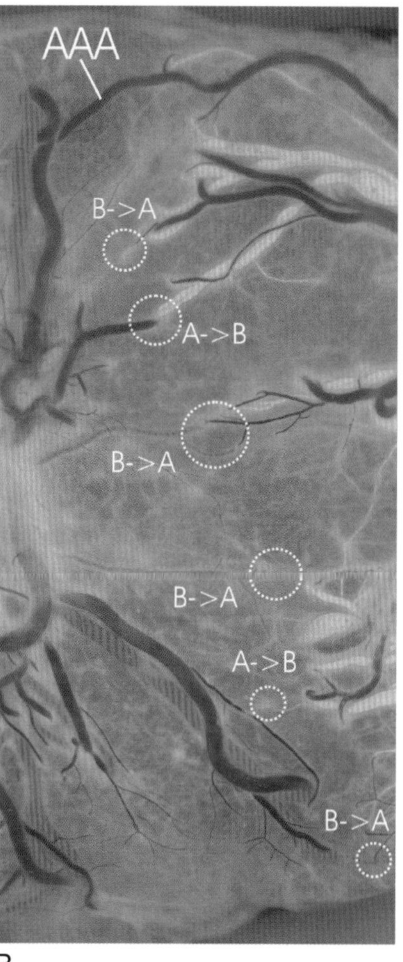


**COLOR PLATE 7–2. A,** Monochorionic twin placenta. Twin A (*left*) has a centrally inserted cord, whereas the cord of twin B (*right*) is marginally inserted. The *line* represents the vascular equatorial zone between the circulations of the twins. This is the region where intertwin vascular connections are found. There is markedly unequal sharing of the parenchyma, with growth discordance. **B,** Close-up view of the equator, showing a direct arterio-arterial connection (AAA) and multiple bidirectional arteriovenous connections (*circles*) from A to B and from B to A. This resulted in no net transfusion. Although twin-twin transfusion syndrome did not occur, there was growth discordance.

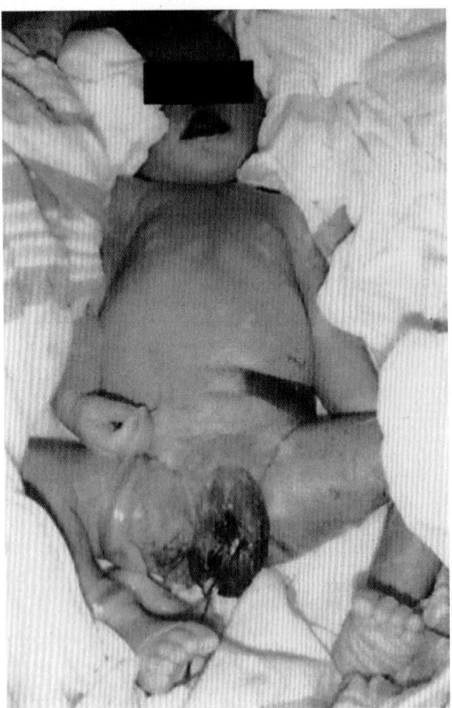

**COLOR PLATE 15–6.** A 28-year-old woman presented to the labor and delivery department with an intrauterine demise. Examination of the fetus shows the cord wrapped tightly around the torso, leg, and ankle, suggesting cord accident as a cause of death. No other pathologic abnormalities were found on autopsy. *(Photo courtesy of Thomas R. Easterling, MD.)*

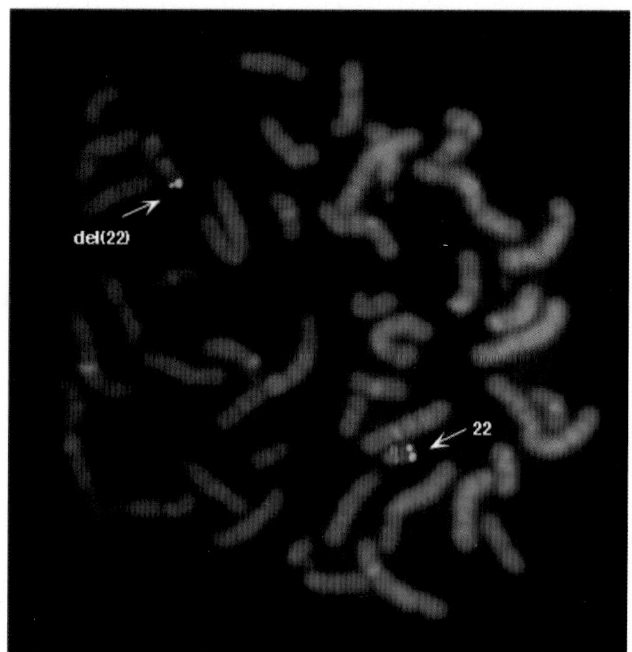


**COLOR PLATE 20–8.** FISH study of a 22q deletion. *(Photograph courtesy of Dr. Beverly S. Emanuel.)*

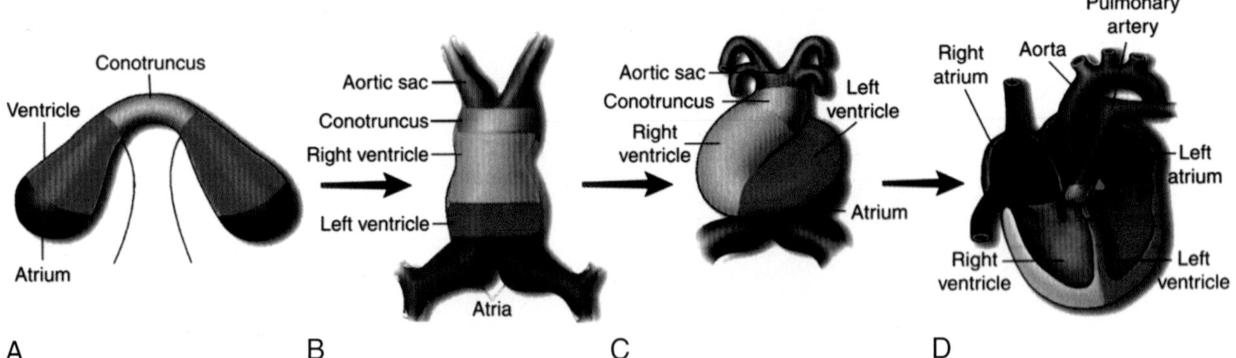


**COLOR PLATE 53–1.** Schematic diagram of cardiogenesis. Bilaterally symmetrical cardiac progenitor cells (**A**) are prepatterned to form distinct regions of the heart, as shown in color-coded fashion. The precardiac mesodermal cells give rise to a linear heart tube (**B**), which forms a rightward loop (**C**) and begins to establish the spatial orientation of the four-chambered mature heart (**D**). *(Adapted from Srivastava D, and Olson EN: Knowing in your heart what's right. Trends Cell Biol. 7:447, 1997.)*

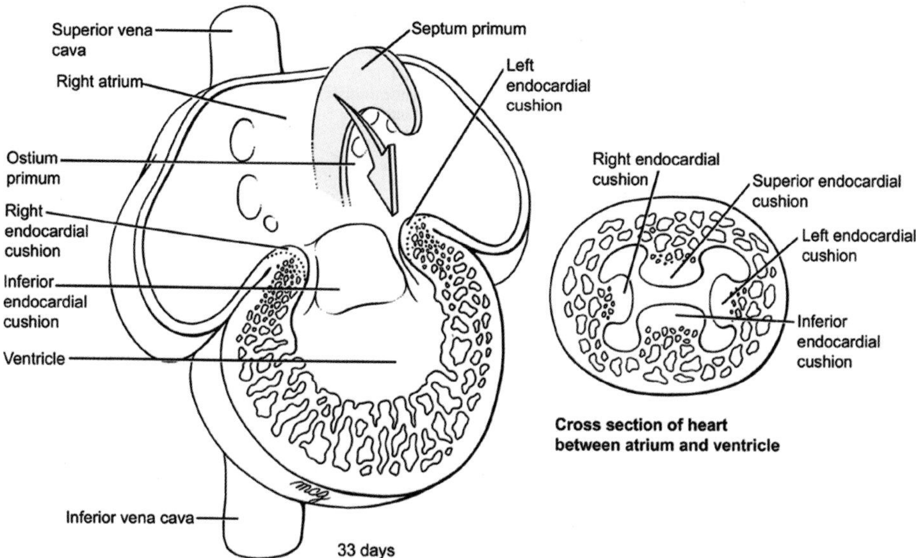


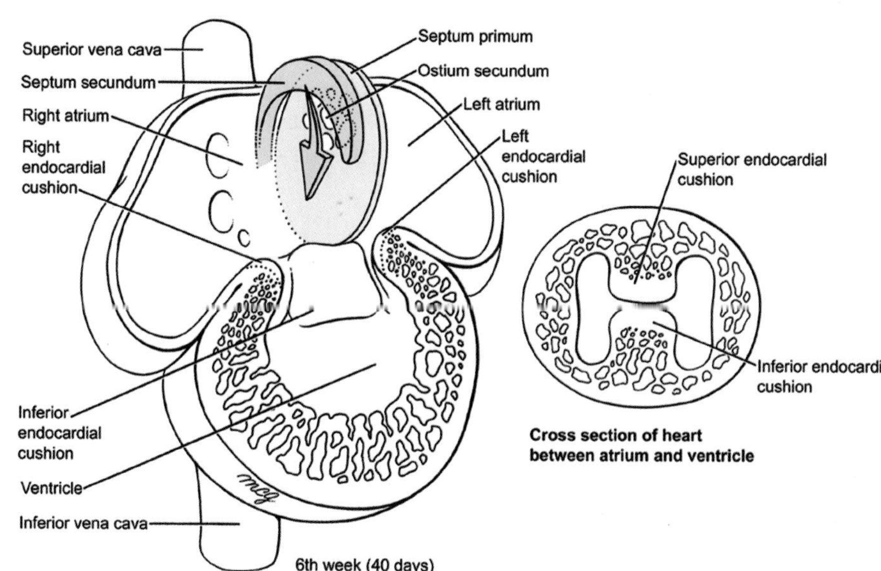


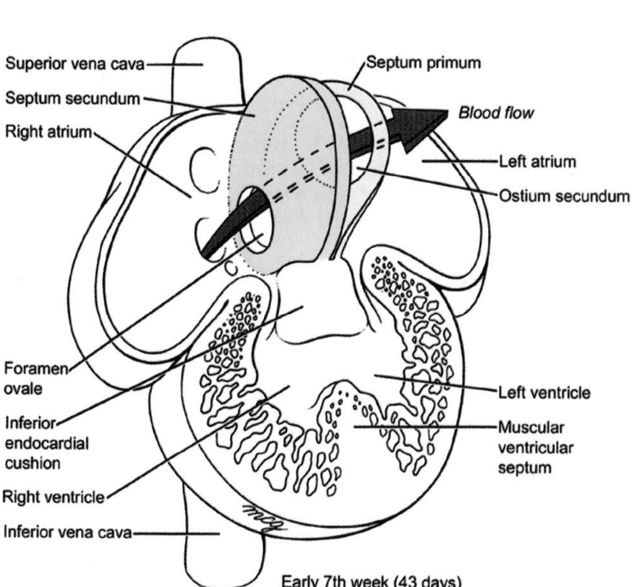


**COLOR PLATE 53–2.** Septation of the atria. **A,** Atrial septation begins during the fifth week, when the septum primum forms from the roof of the atrium and grows toward the atrioventricular canal, which is being divided into right and left orifices by the superior and inferior endocardial cushions. **B,** During the sixth week, the septum primum fuses with the superior and inferior endocardial cushions, and the septum secundum grows from the roof of the right ventricle. The ostium secundum forms when small openings in the septum primum coalesce. **C,** Definitive fetal separation of the atria. *(From Larsen WJ: Development of the human heart. In Larsen WJ [ed]: Human Embryology. New York, Churchill Livingstone, 1977, pp 151-188.)*

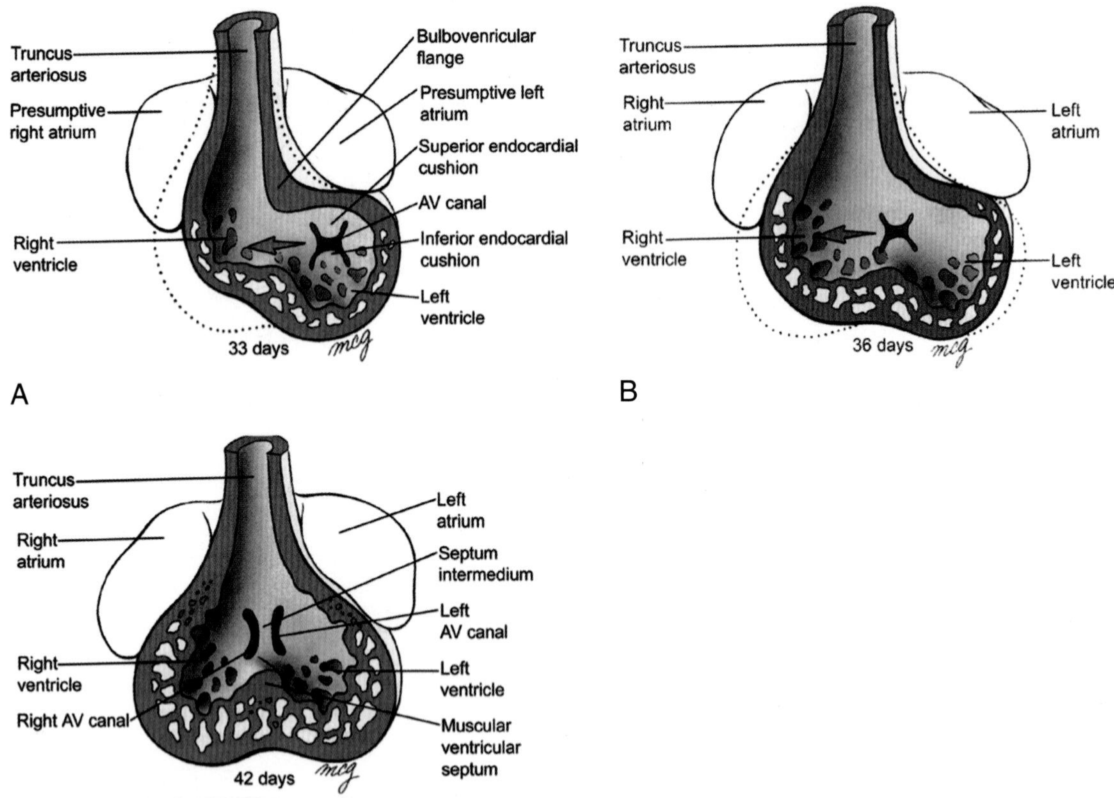


**COLOR PLATE 53–3.** Realignment of the heart from 33 days (**A**) through 36 days (**B**), and 42 days (**C**). Remodeling of the heart during the fifth and sixth week, results in progressive alignment of the developing left atrioventricular canal with the left atrium and ventricle and the right atrioventricular canal with the right atrium and ventricle. **A,** The atrioventricular canal initially opens into the presumptive left ventricle. **B,** The atrioventricular can shifts to the right, so that it will overlie the developing ventricular septum. **C,** The single atrioventricular canal is divided into right and left atrioventricular canals. *(From Larsen WJ: Development of the human heart. In Larsen WJ [ed]: Human Embryology. New York, Churchill Livingstone, 1977, pp 151-188.)*

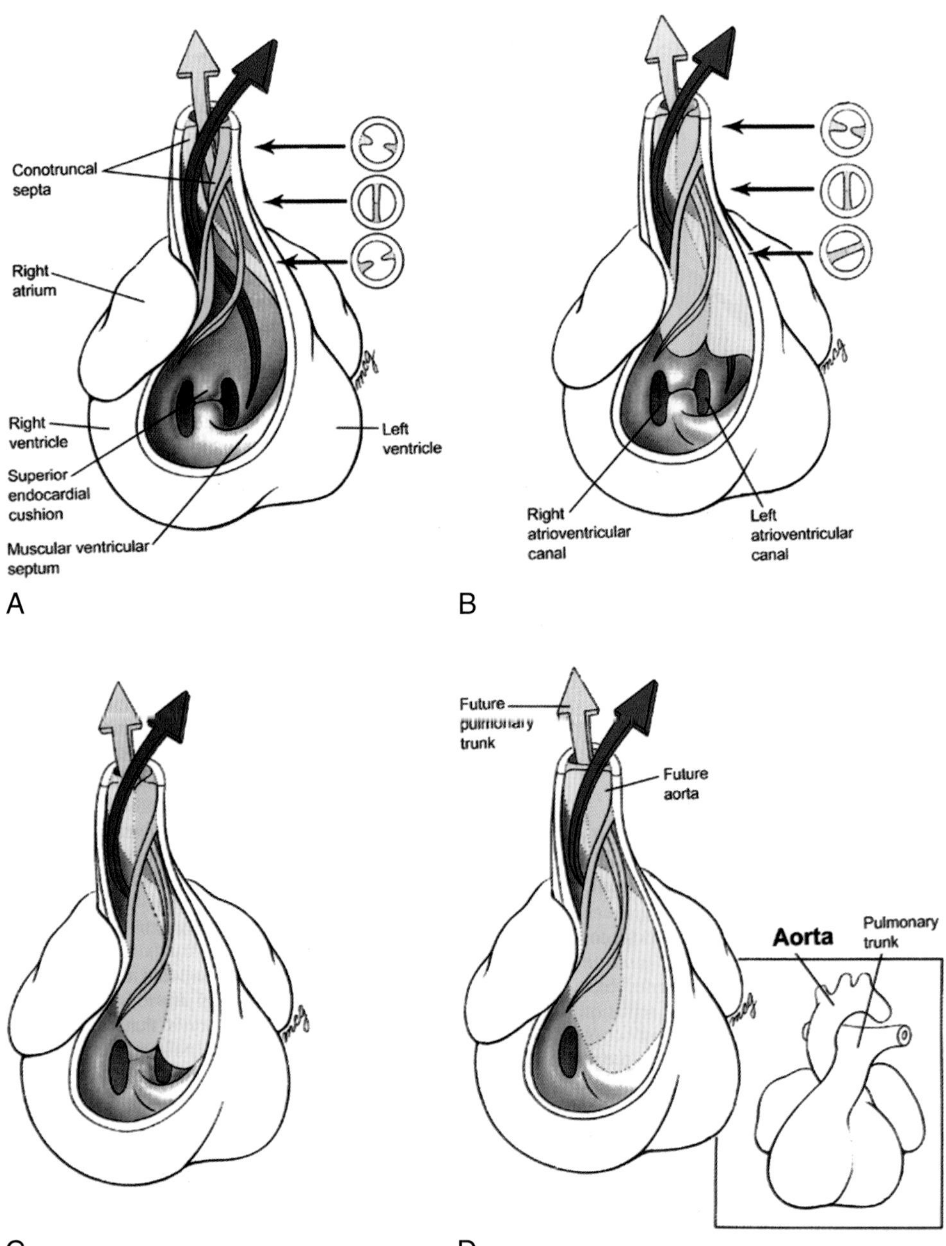


**COLOR PLATE 53–4.** Septation of the cardiac outflow tract. During the fifth week, the right and left conotruncal swellings grow out of the wall of the outflow tract in a spiral configuration (**A**), fusing where they meet (**B**). By the ninth week, the inferior portion of the conotruncal swellings has grown onto and fuses with the muscular ventricular septum and the inferior endocardial cushion (**C** and **D**). *(From Larsen WJ: Development of the human heart. In Larsen WJ [ed]: Human Embryology. New York, Churchill Livingstone, 1977, pp 151-188.)*

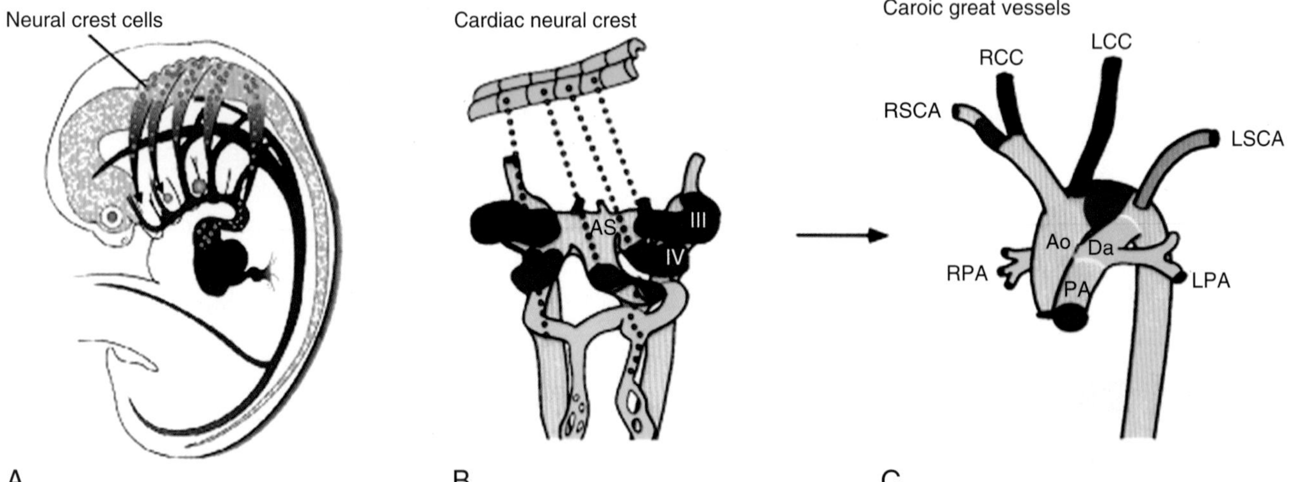


**COLOR PLATE 53–5.** Contribution of neural crest cells to aortic arch selection and conotruncal development. **A,** Between the fifth and sixth week, neural crest cells migrate from the hindbrain through pharyngeal arches 4 and 6, then invade the truncus arteriosus to form the conotruncal septa. **B,** Neural crest cells are required for normal remodeling of the pharyngeal arch arteries to the adult configuration (**C**). Ao, aorta; Da, ductus arteriosus; LCC, left common carotid artery; LPA, left pulmonary artery; LSCA, left subclavian artery; PA, pulmonary artery; RCC, right common carotid artery; RPA, right pulmonary artery; RSCA, right subclavian artery.

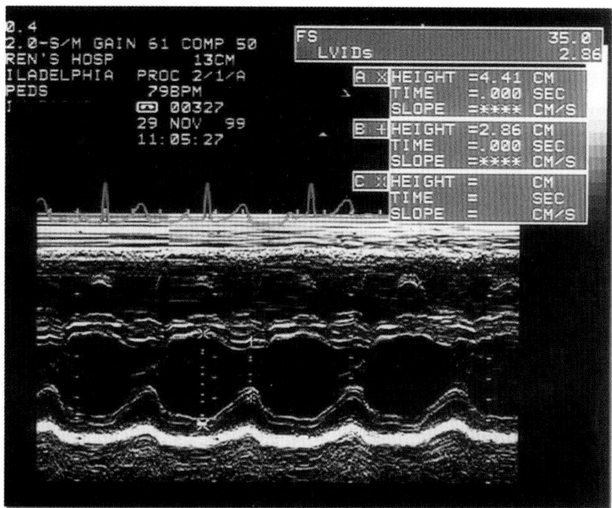


**COLOR PLATE 54–2.** M-mode tracing of the left ventricle dimensions over time obtained in the short-axis view. The electrocardiographic tracing helps identify the timing of the cardiac cycle as systolic or diastolic. Measurement A demonstrates the left ventricle end-diastolic dimension, and measurement B, the left ventricle end-systolic measurement. The shortening fraction is calculated at 35%.

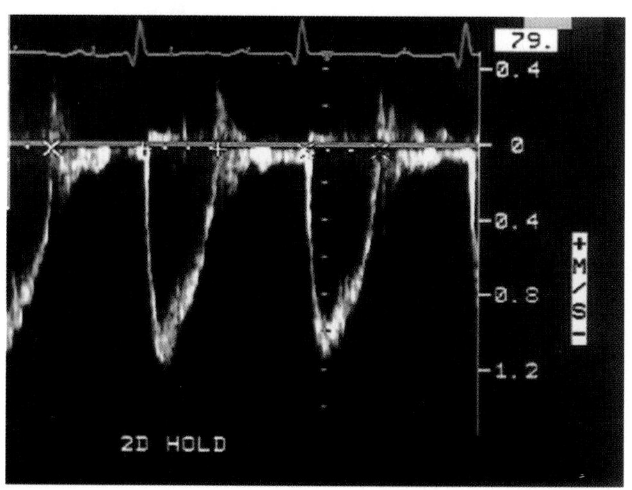


A

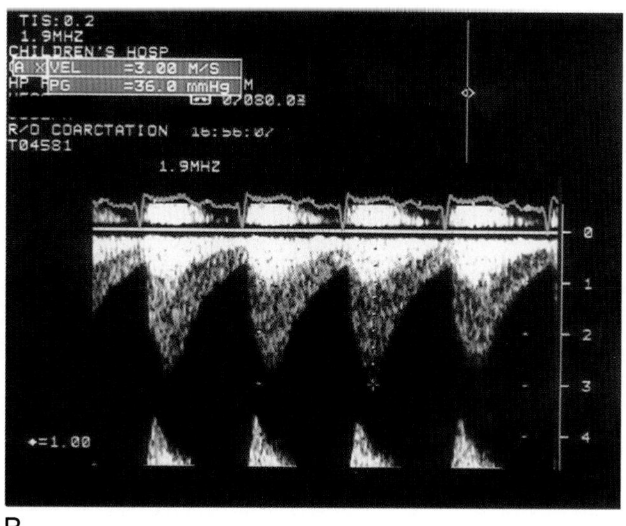


B

**COLOR PLATE 54–4.** **A,** Example of a pulsed wave Doppler signal. Time is on the *x*-axis, and velocity is in meters/second on the *y*-axis. Note the central clearing of the signal, with a fine envelope displayed. The maximal velocity is approximately 1 meter/second. **B,** Example of a continuous wave Doppler signal. Note the filling-in of the signal envelope. The peak velocity is 3 meters/second. This pattern is classic for coarctation of the aorta: There is a run-off of the Doppler signal into diastole, with a double-peak envelope (a smaller peak at 1 meter/second within the larger peak of 3 meters/second). This latter feature reflects the fact that continuous wave Doppler cannot distinguish between the lower velocities proximal to the coarctation from the elevated velocities just distal to the coarctation; hence, both velocities are displayed as a single signal, one overlaid on the other.

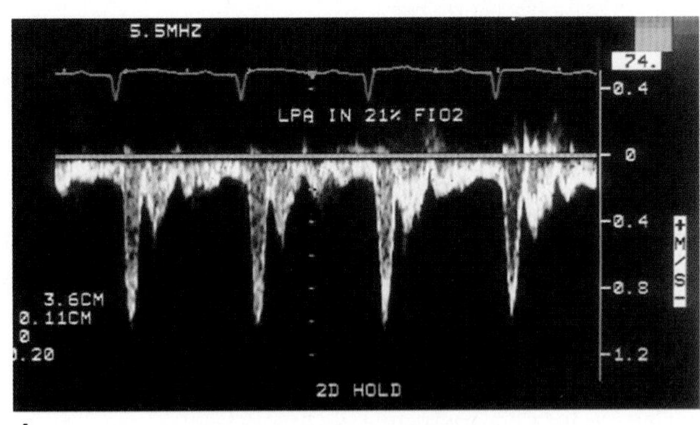


A

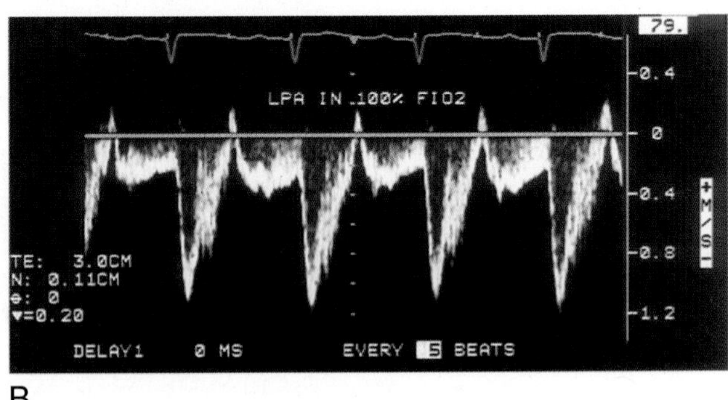


B

**COLOR PLATE 54–7.** **A,** Doppler flow pattern obtained in the left pulmonary artery of an infant with severe pulmonary hypertension breathing room air (21%). **B,** Doppler flow pattern obtained in the same left pulmonary artery after the addition of supplemental oxygen (100%). Note the increase in area under the Doppler flow envelope with increased flow in both systole and diastole, reflecting pulmonary vasodilatation.

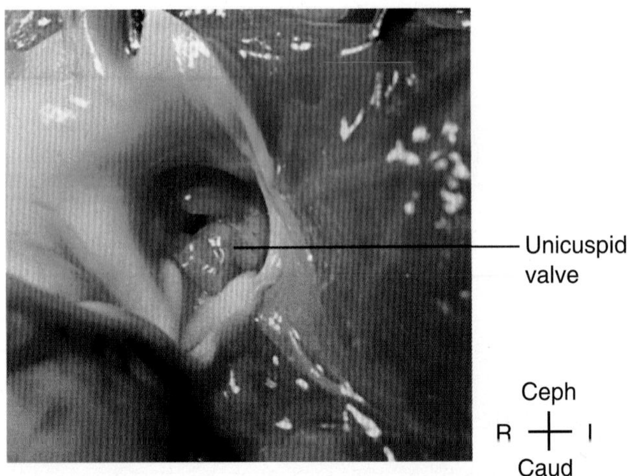


**COLOR PLATE 57–8.** Congenital aortic stenosis. Frontal view through opened aorta demonstrates stenotic and dysmorphic aortic valve with commissural fusion. *(From Litwin SB: Color Atlas of Congenital Heart Surgery. St. Louis, Mosby, 1996.)*

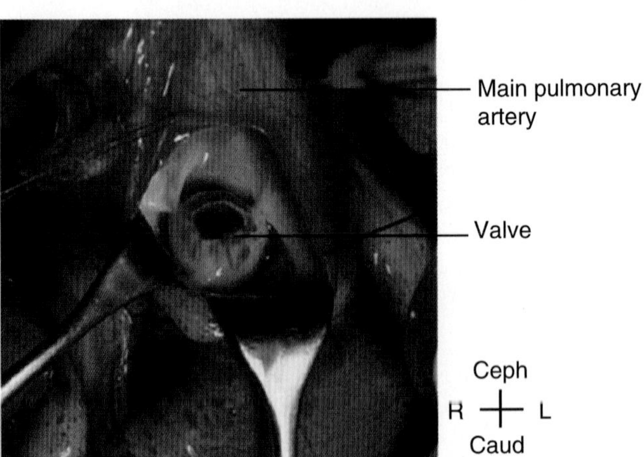


**COLOR PLATE 57–25.** Exposure of a severely stenotic pulmonary valve through a pulmonary arteriotomy. *(From Litwin SB: Color Atlas of Congenital Heart Surgery. St. Louis, Mosby, 1996.)*

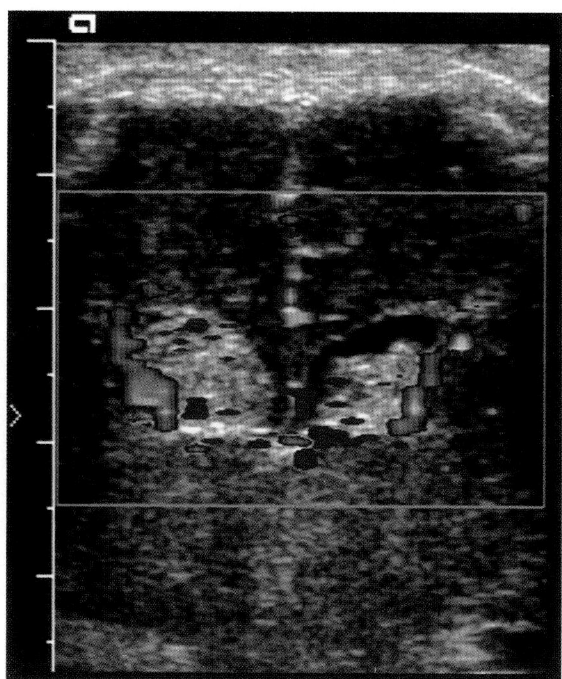

**COLOR PLATE 62–11.** Coronal color Doppler image of bilateral grade I germinal matrix hemorrhages. The hemorrhages are echogenic. Although flow is confirmed within the terminal veins *(blue)*, the veins are laterally displaced by the subependymal hemorrhages.

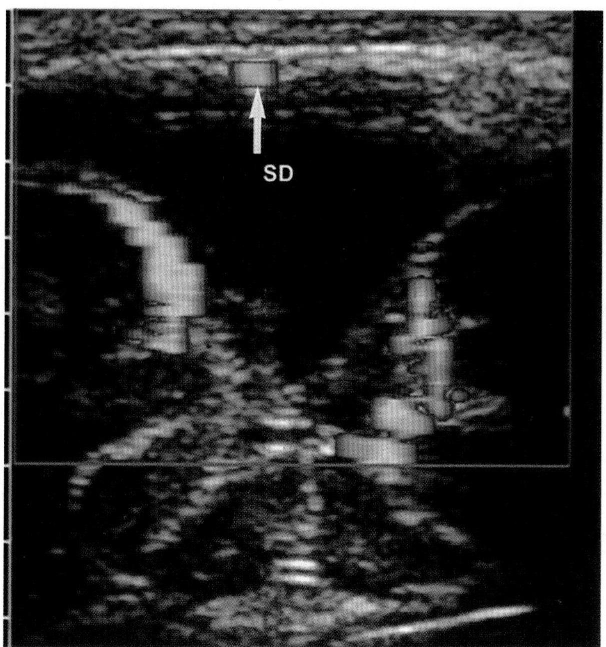


**COLOR PLATE 62–17.** Coronal color Doppler ultrasound study shows that the vessels (color) are displaced toward the brain parenchyma by the subdural fluid (SD). Note flow in the superior sagittal sinus *(arrow)*.

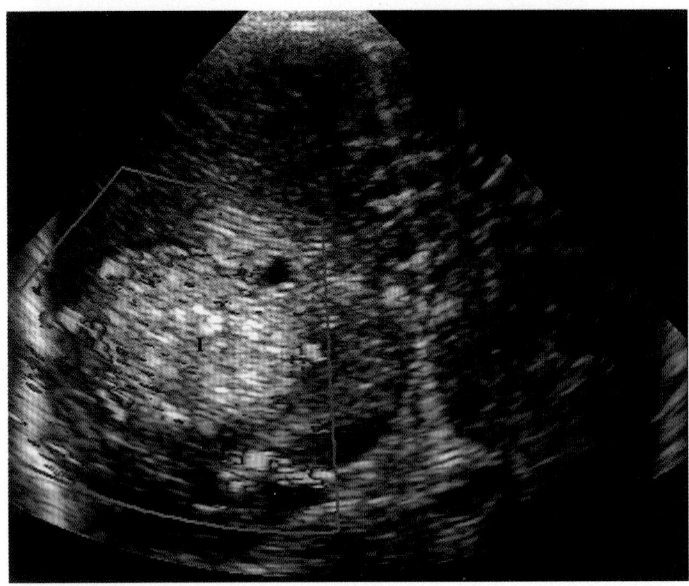

**COLOR PLATE 62–23.** The patient was a neonate with a focal right occipital infarction with surrounding "luxury perfusion." A coronal ultrasound image obtained through the anterior fontanel shows a hyperechoic right occipital infarction (I) surrounded by increased flow on color Doppler examination.

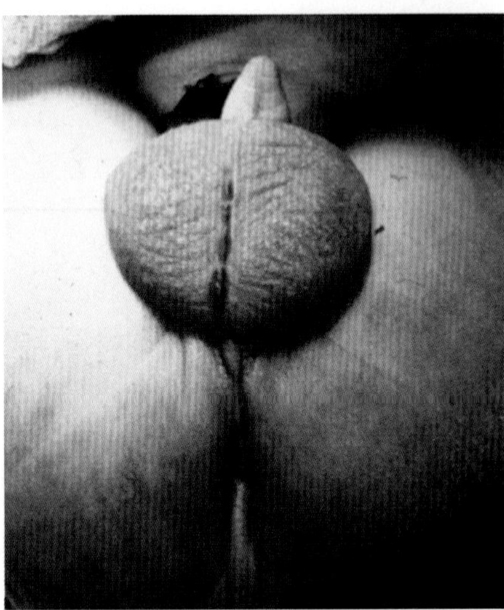

**COLOR PLATE 71–5.** Perineum of male newborn with low imperforate anus and anocutaneous fistula. The fistula is seen as a dark meconium-filled track along the median raphe of the scrotum.

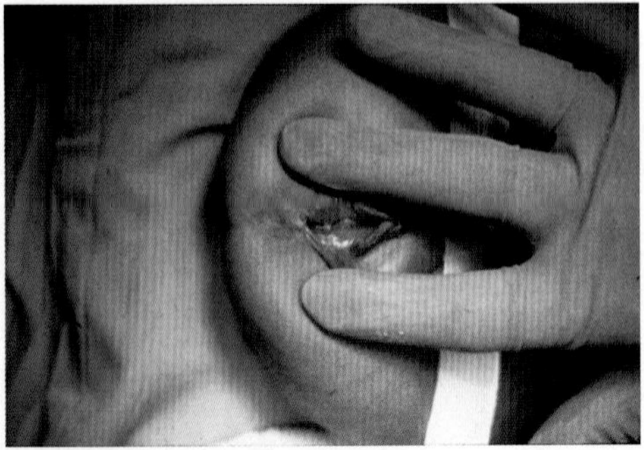

**COLOR PLATE 71–6.** Perineum of female newborn with low imperforate anus and rectovestibular fistula. The fistula is evident as the meconium-stained site within the posterior vestibule.

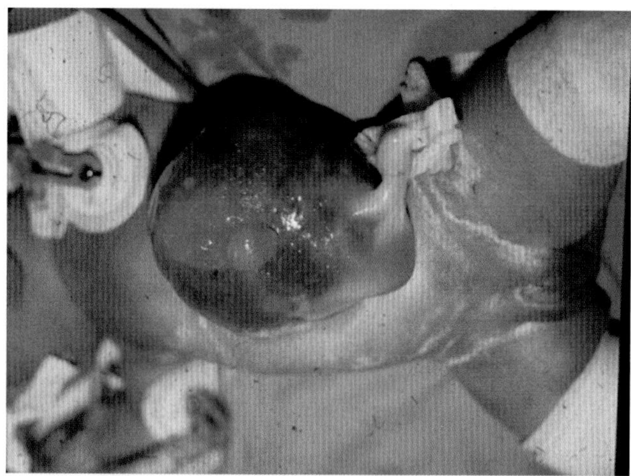

**COLOR PLATE 73–5.** Male newborn with omphalocele. The fascial defect is large, situated at the base of the umbilical cord, and covered by a glistening membrane and contains both liver and bowel.

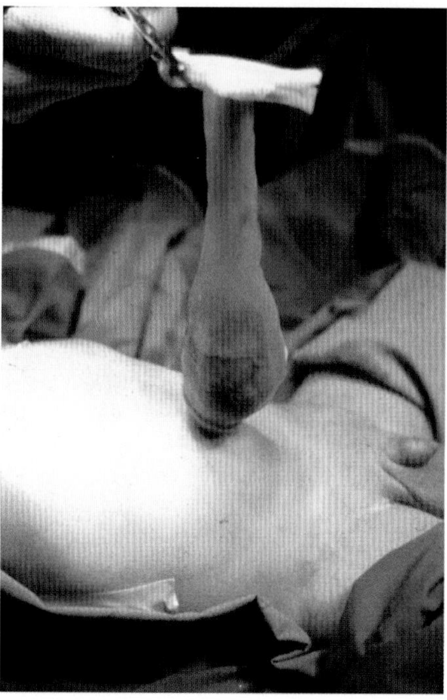

**COLOR PLATE 73–8.** Hernia of the umbilical cord. This is in fact a small omphalocele, containing only bowel loops in a small sac within the umbilical cord.

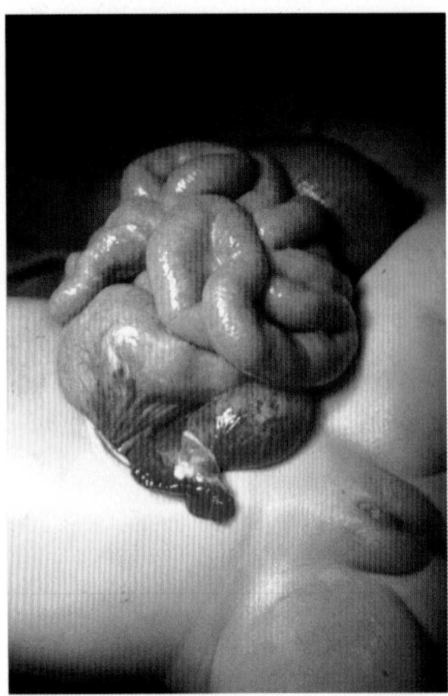

**COLOR PLATE 73–9.** Female newborn with gastroschisis. The fascial defect is relatively small and situated to the right of the umbilical cord and contains exposed bowel (as well as an ovary in this instance).

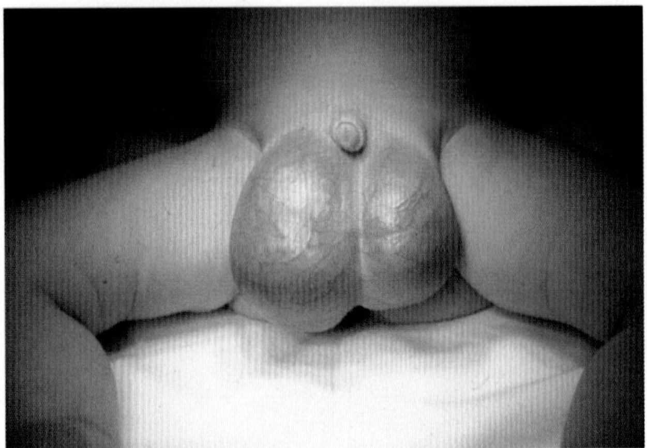

**COLOR PLATE 73–10.** Large bilateral inguinal hernias in a previously premature infant.

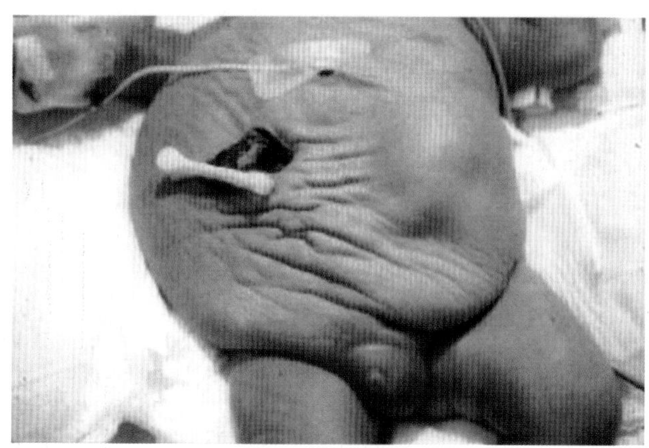

A

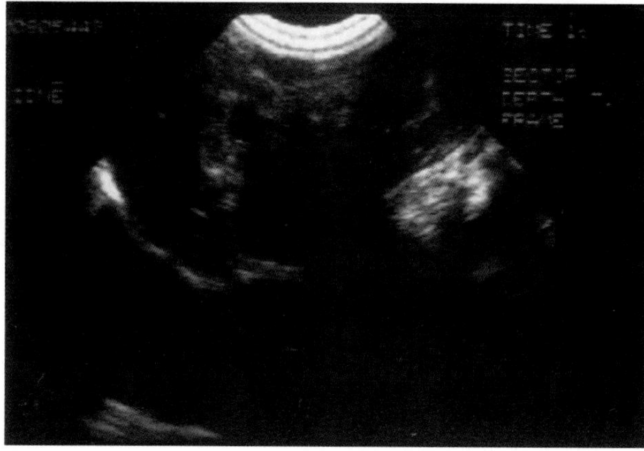

B

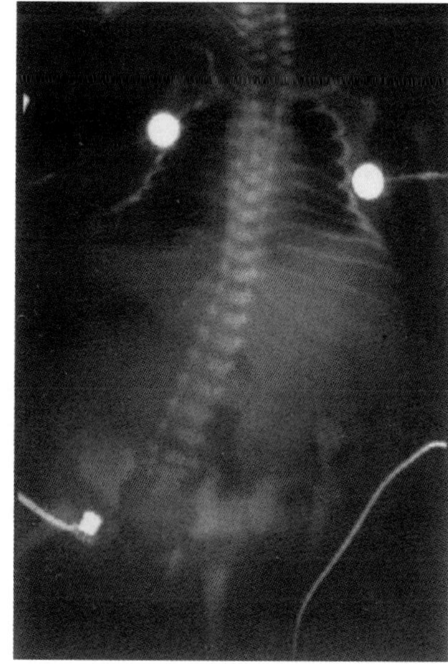

C

**COLOR PLATE 83–8.** The classic wrinkled abdominal wall seen in the prune-belly syndrome is accompanied by bilateral undescended testes (**A**). Affected patients will have marked hydronephrosis. In severe cases as illustrated here, these small kidneys may have a markedly dysmorphic sonographic appearance (**B**), and renal insufficiency may be present from the beginning. In cases with severe renal insufficiency, pulmonary development may be compromised, as evident on the radiograph (**C**); the patient required prolonged mechanical ventilation in the neonatal period.

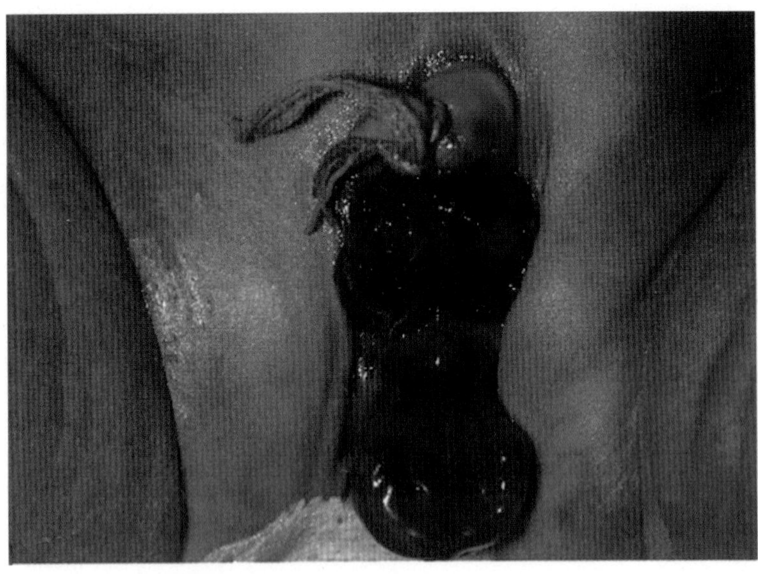

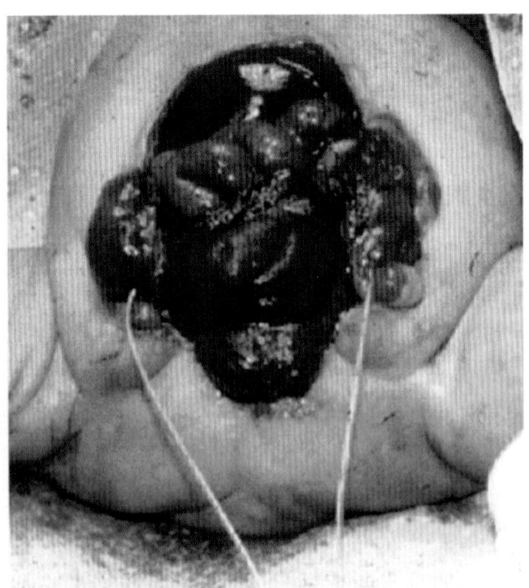

A B

**COLOR PLATE 83–9.** The appearance of classic bladder exstrophy (**A**), in contrast with the dramatic appearance of cloacal exstrophy (**B**). In cloacal exstrophy, the bladder halves are separated by the presence of a large cecal plate, and a protruding ileal stump. **B**, In this intraoperative photograph, the omphalocele has been removed to expose the small bowel and liver.

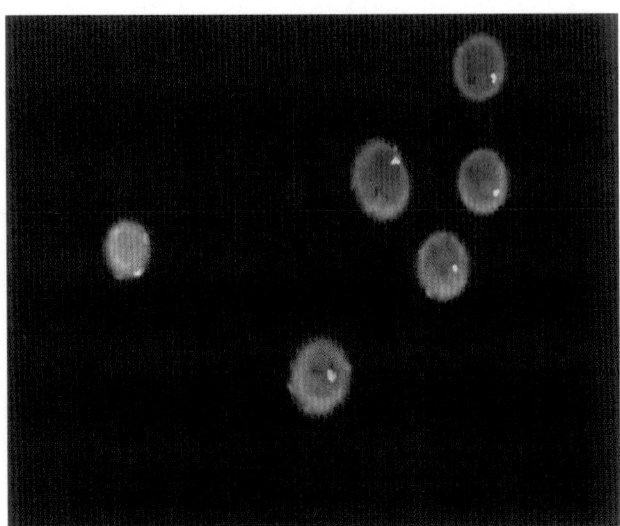

**COLOR PLATE 91–10.** Fluorescence in situ hybridization (FISH) technique demonstrating the sex chromosome constitution of peripheral blood leukocytes. Centromeric probes to the X and Y chromosomes are represented by green (X) and orange (Y) markers.

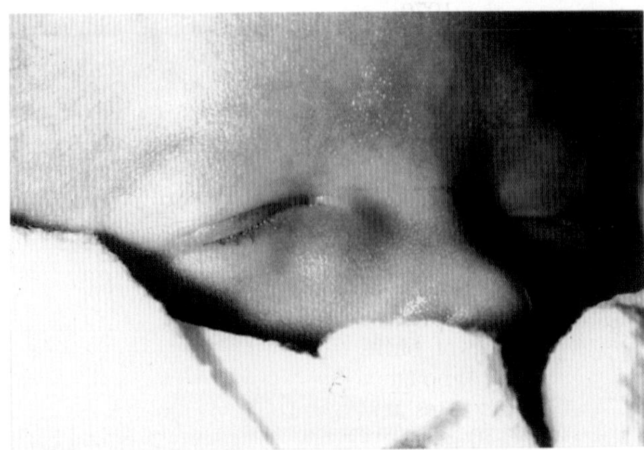

**COLOR PLATE 101–1.** One-week-old infant with dacryocele. Note the bump in the area of the medial canthus.

# INTRODUCTION

Editor: ROBERTA A. BALLARD

PART I

CHAPTER 1

# Perinatal-Neonatal Epidemiology

**Linda L. Wright, Betty R. Vohr, and Avroy A. Fanaroff**

Application of knowledge from biomedical research and improved public health have resulted in dramatic improvements in the health of Americans during the 20th century. During this period, the population has grown 2.7 fold, from 75,994,575 to 281,421,906. The increase in size and change in composition of the population during the last century reflect trends in the number of births and the fertility rate (births per 1000 women of childbearing age). Fertility rates declined steadily between 1900 and 1936 and then rose again between 1937 and 1957, peaking in the post-war baby boom, when 123 of every 1000 women of childbearing age gave birth. With the advent of more effective contraception in the 1960s and the legalization of abortion in the 1970s, fertility rates fell by nearly 50%. Since 1976, fertility rates have been relatively stable at approximately 65 per 1000. Trends in the number of births generally parallel trends in the fertility rate; however, there was a sharp rise in the number of births between 1975 and 1990 despite a stable fertility rate, reflecting childbearing of the baby-boom generation (Guyer et al, 2000).

The 1990s saw a steady decline in both the number of births and the fertility rates. This trend was interrupted between 1998 and 2000, when both increased (Martin et al, 2002a). However, preliminary data for 2001 suggest that the overall number of births and the fertility rates declined slightly again. Although they have differed historically, the current fertility rates among racial groups are quite similar (range 58 to 70 per 1000) except among Hispanic women (107 per 1000). Births to Hispanic women represented 21% of all U.S. births in 2001, an increase from 14% in 1989.

Other notable trends over the last decade include a continued dramatic decline in the teenage birth rate and a rise in birth rates among older women. In 2001, the teenage birth rate fell for the tenth consecutive year to a 60-year low of 49.5, a 5% decline from the 2000 rate and a 26% decrease from 1991. The 2001 decline in teenage birth rates was consistent for all racial groups but was largest among black teenagers (whose birth rate fell from 80 to 73 per 1000 in 1 year). The birth rate among women 20 to 24 years old decreased by 2%, whereas that in women 25 to 44 years old continued to increase. The birth rate for women 30 years and older was the highest seen in three decades, reflecting both a delay in childbearing and greater use of assisted reproduction. The number and rate of twin births also rose each year since 1980; the absolute number increased by 74% between 1980 and 2000 (from 68,339 to 118,916). In contrast, the number and rate of triplet and other higher-order multiple births declined between 1998 and 2000 after soaring between 1980 and 1998 (37.0 to 193.5 per 100,000 live births) (Martin et al, 2002a). The "plateauing" of higher-order multiples reflects a decrease in the aging baby-boomer generation and refinements in assisted reproductive technologies designed to prevent higher-order multiple pregnancies.

Age-adjusted death rates have declined steadily over the last century as the life expectancy has risen from 49.2 to 76.5 years. The largest reductions in mortality were among children and infants: Between 1915 and 1998, the infant mortality rate (IMR; deaths in the first year of life per 1000 live births) declined by 93%, the neonatal mortality rate (NNR; deaths in the first 28 days of life) fell by 89%, and the post-neonatal mortality rate (PNMR; deaths between 29 days and 1 year of age) dropped by 96%.

Approximately half of the decreases in infant, neonatal, and post-neonatal mortality rates achieved in the 20th century occurred between 1980 and 2000 (Table 1–1). These trends in mortality cannot be attributed to decreases in the rate of preterm (<37 weeks of gestation) or low-birth-weight babies (LBW, <2500 g): between 1981 and 1999, the percentage of preterm births rose steadily from 9.4% to 11.8%. The rate of very preterm births (<32 weeks of gestation) also rose between 1981 and 1999, increasing from 1.81% of live births to 1.92% in 1990 and remaining essentially unchanged in the subsequent years. The 11.6% preterm birth rate for 2000 represents the first decline since 1992.

Birth weight data over the last two decades reflect similar trends: both LBW and very low-birth-weight (VLBW, <1500 g) rates rose in the 1990s after declining during the 1970s and early 1980s (Fig. 1–1). In the mid-1980s the LBW rate was 6.8%, but it rose to 7.6% between 1998 and 2001. In 2000 and 2001, VLBW infants represented 1.43% of the annual live births, a rise from less than 1.15% in 1980 (Martin et al, 2002b).

The racial disparity in LBW births among black and white women remains a complex, persistent problem. Infant mortality dropped among all races between 1980

**TABLE 1-1**

**Infant, Neonatal, Postneonatal, Perinatal, and Fetal Mortality Rates by Race of Mother: Final 1980, 1998, and 1999 and Preliminary 2000 Data***

| | 2000 | 1999 | 1998 | 1980 | Percentage Change, 1980 to 2000 |
|---|---|---|---|---|---|
| Infant Mortality Rate (IMR)†‡ | 6.9 | 7.1 | 7.2 | 12.6 | −45.2 |
| White, total | 5.7 | 5.8 | 6.0 | 10.9 | −47.7 |
| White non-Hispanic | 5.7 | 5.8 | 6.0 | — | — |
| Black, total | 14.0 | 14.6 | 14.3 | 22.2 | −36.9 |
| Hispanic | 5.6 | 5.8 | 5.9 | — | — |
| Black/white ratio | 2.5 | 2.5 | 2.4 | 2.0 | — |
| Neonatal Mortality Rate (NMR)†‡ | 4.6 | 4.7 | 4.8 | 8.5 | −45.9 |
| White, total | 3.8 | 3.9 | 4.0 | 7.4 | −48.6 |
| White non-Hispanic | 3.8 | 3.9 | 3.9 | — | — |
| Black, total | 9.3 | 9.8 | 9.5 | 14.6 | −36.3 |
| Hispanic | 3.7 | 3.9 | 4.0 | — | — |
| Black/white ratio | 2.4 | 2.5 | 2.4 | 2.0 | — |
| Post-Neonatal Mortality Rate (PNMR)†‡ | 2.3 | 2.3 | 2.4 | 4.1 | −43.9 |
| White, total | 1.9 | 1.9 | 2.0 | 3.5 | −45.7 |
| White non-Hispanic | 1.9 | 1.9 | 2.0 | — | — |
| Black, total | 4.7 | 4.8 | 4.8 | 7.6 | −38.2 |
| Hispanic | 1.9 | 1.9 | 1.9 | — | — |
| Black/white ratio | 2.5 | 2.5 | 2.4 | 2.2 | — |
| Perinatal Mortality Rate†** | — | — | 7.2 | 13.2 | −45.5¶ |
| White, total | — | — | 6.2 | 11.8 | −47.5¶ |
| White non-Hispanic | — | — | 5.8 | — | — |
| Black, total | — | — | 12.9 | 21.3 | −39.4¶ |
| Hispanic§ | — | — | 6.2 | — | — |
| Black/white ratio | — | — | 2.1 | 1.8 | — |
| Fetal Mortality Rate†‖ | — | — | 6.7 | 9.1 | −26.4¶ |
| White, total | — | — | 5.7 | 8.1 | −29.6¶ |
| White non-Hispanic§ | — | — | 5.2 | — | — |
| Black, total | — | — | 12.3 | 14.7 | −16.3¶ |
| Hispanic§ | — | — | 5.6 | — | — |
| Black/white ratio | — | — | 2.2 | 1.8 | — |

*NOTE: Infant, fetal, and perinatal deaths are tabulated separately by race and Hispanic origin; persons of Hispanic origin may be of any race. IMRs, NMRs, and PNMRs by race from unlinked data may differ slightly from those based on the linked file. Source: Centers for Disease Control and Prevention/National Center for Health Statistics, National Vital Statistics System, natality, mortality (unlinked file) and fetal death files.

†Includes races other than white and black.

‡Rate per 1000 live births.

§States not reporting Hispanic origin for 1998 for fetal deaths are Maryland and Oklahoma.

‖Number of fetal deaths at ≥20 weeks of gestation per 1000 live births plus fetal deaths.

¶Percentage change is from 1980 to 1998 because data for 1999 and 2000 are not available.

**Number of fetal deaths at ≥28 weeks of gestation plus number of infant deaths at <7 days of age per 1000 live births plus fetal deaths.

—, Data not available.

Modified from Hoyert DL, Freedman A, Strobino DM, Guyer B: Annual summary of vital statistics: 2000. Pediatrics 108:1241-1255, 2001.

and 2000. The overall gap between black and white infant mortality rates widened because of (1) the two- to threefold greater risk for LBW and VLBW babies among black women, (2) the relatively smaller reductions in birth weight–specific mortality rates (BWSMRs) among black infants, and (3) a relatively greater increase in the percentage of LBW and VLBW births among whites (Infant, 2002). The historically lower BWSMRs among moderately LBW and VLBW black infants disappeared during the 1990s. The LBW rate among black women in 2000 and 2001 was 12.9%, a decrease from a 1991 high of 13.6%. The LBW rate was 6.5% over the same period among Hispanic mothers, and 6.7% among non-Hispanic white mothers. Multiple births, the rate of which has risen by one third since 1989, are a major factor in the increase in LBW babies among non-Hispanic white women in the

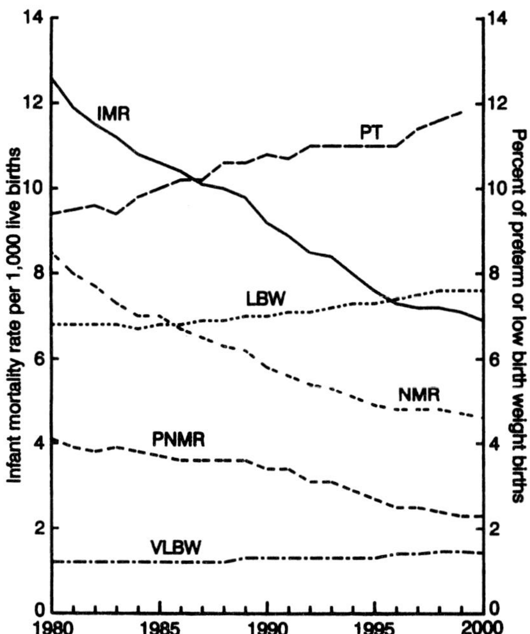


**FIGURE 1–1.** Infant mortality rate (IMR), neonatal mortality rate (NMR), and post-neonatal mortality rate (PNMR), and rates of low birth weight (LBW), very low birth weight (VLBW), and preterm delivery (PT), United States, 1980 to 2000. IMR is expressed as infant deaths per 1000 live births, and PNMR as post-neonatal deaths per 1000 live births. LBW rate is the percentage of babies born with low birth weight (<2500 g); VLBW rate is the percentage of babies born with VLBW (<1500 g); and PT rate is percentage of babies born preterm (<37 weeks of gestation). *(From Hoyert DL, Freedman A, Strobino DM, Guyer B: Annual summary of vital statistics: 2000. Pediatrics 108:1241-1255, 2001.)*

last two decades. Ten percent of singletons, 57% of twins, and 93% of triplets were born at less than 37 weeks of gestation in 2000. The risk of infant mortality is more than 6 times greater for multiple births than for singleton births (Mathews et al, 2002).

The dramatic decline in the infant mortality rate over the last two decades (from 12.6 to 6.9 deaths per 1000 live births) is directly attributable to decreases in BWSMRs. Between 1995 and 2000, the IMR decreased by nearly 17% for infants weighing 2500 g or more, by 8% for LBW infants, and by 9% for VLBW infants. In 2000, the IMR for infants weighing 2500 g or more at birth was 2.5 per 1000; it was 59.4 per 1000 for LBW infants, and 244.3 per 1000 for VLBW infants. Overall, more than 65% of all infant deaths occurred in LBW infants (7.6% of all births), and 51% of infant deaths occurred in VLBW infants (1.4% of births). Comparable gestational age–specific data from the 2000 linked birth/death data set document an IMR of 180.9 per 1000 for very preterm infants (<32 weeks of gestation), more than 69 times the rate of 2.6 per 1000 for term infants. Among moderately preterm infants (32 to 36 weeks), the IMR was 9.4 per 1000, more than 3.5 times the rate for term births (Mathews et al, 2002).

More than half of neonatal deaths in the United States still occur in the approximately 60,000 VLBW infants born each year, but advances in neonatal and perinatal care have improved the chances of survival for such infants. A number of research networks, including the National Institute of Child Health and Human Development (NICHD) Neonatal Research Network, the Vermont Oxford Network, and the Canadian NICU (Neonatal Intensive Care Unit) Network, have been developed to track changes in the morbidity and mortality of VLBW infants and to improve neonatal outcomes by conducting large randomized controlled trials, observational studies, and outcomes research. Although each infant's prognosis depends on individual risk factors as well as the organization and aggressiveness of care, data from these research networks suggest that approximately 85% of VLBW infants born in U.S. level III facilities survive to hospital discharge.

Established in 1986, the NICHD Neonatal Research Network reports morbidity and mortality rates to discharge for VLBW infants admitted to the participating tertiary care centers and neurodevelopmental outcome for the subset of extremely LBW (ELBW) infants (<1000 g at birth). Data from the 4438 VLBW infants born in 14 participating centers from 1995 to 1996 documented the dramatic improvements in VLBW morbidity and mortality achieved in the 1990s. In 1995 to 1996, 84% of the VLBW cohort survived to discharge, compared with 80% in 1991 and 74% in 1988 (Lemons et al, 2001).

Table 1–2 presents perinatal and survival data from 11,733 VLBW infants born in 16 Network centers between 1997 and 2000. The mean gestational age was 28 weeks, and the mean birth weight was 1038 g. Overall, 26% of the cohort were from multiple gestations, 80% received antenatal glucocorticoids for fetal maturation, 70% received antenatal antibiotics, 57% were delivered by cesarean section, and 53% were intubated in the delivery room. Eighty-five percent of the cohort survived until discharge to home or a long-term care facility. Survival rose with increasing birth weight and gestational age up to 1000 g and 27 weeks, respectively, leveling off thereafter. Only 17% of infants who weighed 401 to 500 g at birth survived; however, 56% of 501- to 750-g infants, 88% of 751- to 1000-g infants, and 95% of 1001- to 1500-g infants survived to hospital discharge. Survival nearly doubled between 23 and 24 weeks (32% vs. 61%, respectively), increased steadily between 25 and 27 weeks, and leveled off thereafter (78% at 25 weeks, 85% at 26 weeks, 90% at 27 weeks, and 92% at 28 weeks). More girls than boys survived at each birth weight and in each gestational age group.

In contrast to the dramatic improvements in VLBW survival observed between 1988 and 1995, there was not a significant increase in VLBW survival between 1997 and 2000. Birth weight–specific survival rose by 2% among the subsets of infants 501 to 750 g (from 54% to 56%) and 751 to 1000 g (from 86% to 88%), but there was no increase in survival among infants weighing 1001 to 1500 g at birth.

The most common neonatal disorders were growth failure (93%), bronchopulmonary dysplasia (BPD; 23%) and nosocomial infection (22%). The rate of early-onset sepsis was 1.5%, unchanged since the early 1990s, despite the greater use of antibiotics during labor to reduce the risk of neonatal group B streptococcal infection and neonatal illness after preterm rupture of the membranes (Stoll et al, 2002). Eight percent of the cohort was diagnosed with

TABLE 1–2

**Perinatal, Mortality, and Morbidity Information for Infants Born in the National Institute of Child Health and Human Development (NICHD) Neonatal Research Network from 1997 to 2000, According to Birth Weight***

| | 501 to 750 g (1997-2000) | 751 to 1000 g (1997-2000) | 1001 to 1250 g (1997-2000) | 1251 to 1500 g (1997-2000) | 501 to 1500 g (1997-2000) |
|---|---|---|---|---|---|
| No. | 2327 | 2787 | 2255 | 3477 | 11733 |
| **Perinatal Data** | | | | | |
| Mean birth weight (g) | 636 | 878 | 1128 | 1381 | 1038 |
| Mean gestational age (wks) | 25 | 27 | 29 | 31 | 28 |
| Antenatal steroids (%) | 74 | 83 | 83 | 78 | 80 |
| Antenatal antibiotics | 73 | 70 | 70 | 69 | 70 |
| Multiple births | 24 | 25 | 27 | 29 | 26 |
| Cesarean section | 46 | 64 | 61 | 56 | 57 |
| Endotracheal intubation in delivery room | 80 | 72 | 47 | 25 | 53 |
| Apgar score ≤3 at 5 min | 25 | 6 | 4 | 3 | 9 |
| **Morbidity (%)** | | | | | |
| Respiratory distress syndrome (RDS)† | 71 | 54 | 36 | 22 | 43 |
| Surfactant therapy | 88 | 74 | 51 | 31 | 57 |
| Postnatal steroids | 53 | 30 | 9 | 2 | 20 |
| Bronchopulmonary dysplasia ($O_2$ at 36 wks) | 47 | 33 | 15 | 6 | 22 |
| Growth failure | 99 | 94 | 91 | 89 | 93 |
| Sonogram done | 96 | 98 | 95 | 84 | 93 |
| Grade III intracranial hemorrhage (ICH) | 12 | 9 | 6 | 4 | 7 |
| Grade IV ICH | 13 | 5 | 3 | 1 | 5 |
| Preventricular leukomalacia (PVL) | 4 | 3 | 2 | 2 | 3 |
| Necrotizing enterocolitis (NEC) (proven) | 11 | 9 | 6 | 3 | 7 |
| Late-onset septicemia (>72 hrs) | 44 | 30 | 17 | 7 | 22 |
| **No. Survivors (%)** | 1412 (56) | 2455 (88) | 2756 (94) | 3344 (96) | 9967 (85) |
| Survived without morbidity‡ | 512 (36) | 1440 (59) | 2161 (79) | 2997 (90) | 7110 (71) |
| Survived with morbidity‡ | 900 (64) | 1015 (41) | 595 (22) | 347 (11) | 2857 (29) |

*Data to initial hospital discharge or 120 days for infants surviving at least 12 hours.

†An infant was determined to have RDS if he or she (1) required oxygen at 6 hours of life continuing to age 24 hours, (2) demonstrated clinical features within age 24 hours, (3) needed respiratory support to age 24 hours, and (4) had an abnormal chest x-ray within age 24 hours.

‡Morbidity defined as a diagnosis of BPD, grade III to IV ICH, or proven NEC.

severe intracranial hemorrhage (ICH), 3% had periventricular leukomalacia (PVL), and 7% experienced proven necrotizing enterocolitis (NEC).

Overall, 71% of the cohort survived without major neonatal morbidity, including bronchopulmonary dysplasia, severe intracranial hemorrhage, periventricular leukomalacia, and confirmed necrotizing enterocolitis. Survival without major neonatal morbidity was only 36% among infants 750 g or less, but approximately 60% of infants 751 to 1000 g, 80% of infants 1000 to 1250 g, and 90% of infants 1251 to 1500 g at birth survived without major neonatal morbidity.

A similar plateauing of VLBW neonatal survival between 1991 and 1999 was reported by the Vermont Oxford Network, a large voluntary network of international investigators (Horbar et al, 2002). The study documented the many changes in obstetric and neonatal management and associated outcomes among 31,219 VLBW infants cared for in the 39 institutions that participated in the Vermont Oxford Network between 1991 and 1999. Over the study period, the mean birth weight decreased significantly from 1061 to 1032 g. Changes in obstetric management included a three-fold increase in VLBW infants treated with antenatal steroids (from 23.8% to 71.6%), and significant rises in the proportion of mothers receiving prenatal care and cesarean delivery. Changes in neonatal management during the study period included increases in the proportions of infants treated with surfactant (from 54.5% to 63.4%), nasal continuous positive airway pressure (from 36.3% to 62.5%), high-frequency ventilation (from 6.7% to 26.2%), and postnatal steroids (from 19.1% to 28.1%). The proportion of infants treated with any assisted ventilation fell from 81.5% to 76.2%. Overall mortality diminished significantly, from approximately 18% in 1991 to approximately 15% in 1996, but did not decrease significantly after 1995. Mortality rates by 250-g birth weight categories reflected similar trends, decreasing in all categories from 1991 to 1995 but remaining stable from 1995 to 1999. These data from two major U.S. networks document that the decades-long trend of improving VLBW neonatal morbidity and mortality has slowed or stopped altogether after 1995.

Whether the dramatic improvements in survival of extremely preterm infants have resulted in higher rates and higher absolute numbers of disabled survivors has been a matter of much debate and concern for physicians caring for these infants. This is especially true in the United States, where care of extremely preterm neonates tends to be more aggressive than in Europe (Lorenz et al, 2001), New Zealand, and Australia. These differences in approach to support of the extremely preterm infant are reflected in differences in survival rates as well as rates of long-term neurodevelopmental disability. Interpretation of the literature on long-term outcome of extremely preterm infants is limited by small sample sizes, lack of samples based on population and gestational age, differing proportions of inborn infants, different ages at assessment and outcome measures, inconsistent classification of neurodevelopmental impairment, and excessive loss to follow-up (Lorenz et al, 1998).

Gestational age–specific survival of extremely preterm infants from large population-based or regional studies in the United Kingdom and Ireland, Australia, and the United States (North Carolina and Rhode Island) are compared with survival data from the NICHD Neonatal Research Network in Table 1–3. These data illustrate that the threshold of viability (defined as survival of at least 50% of infants) in the United States remains 24 weeks, with a stepwise increase in survival for each additional week of gestation. At 24 weeks, 50% to 60% survive; at 25 weeks, 70% to 80% survive; and at 26 weeks, approximately 85% survive.

The two large population-based studies from Australia and the United Kingdom and Ireland represent a similar approach to the support of extremely preterm infants, but survival without neurodevelopment impairment is nearly 1.5-fold higher at follow-up among Australian children than among the United Kingdom and Irish children of comparable gestational ages. In Australia, Doyle and colleagues (2001) studied a geographically determined sample of infants born between 23 and 27 weeks of gestation in 1991 to 1992. They compared these infants with matched controls of normal birth weight and examined neurodevelopmental outcomes at 5 years. Fifty-six percent of the preterm sample (n = 225) survived to 5 years of age. The survival rate for preterm infants born at level III centers was higher than for those born outside a level III center (odds ratio [OR], 3.1; 95% confidence interval [CI], 1.6 to 5.9, adjusted for gestational age). The rate of preterm survival without major sensorineural disability at 2 years, based on infants who had survived to initial hospital discharge, was 80%. Twenty percent of the children had a major sensorineural disability (bilateral blindness, deafness, or cerebral palsy of such severity that the child did not walk or walked with great difficulty or had an intelligence quotient greater than 2 standard deviations below the mean); 11% had cerebral palsy. Risk factors during the initial hospitalization for major disability at 5 years of age were grade 3 or 4 cerebroventricular hemorrhage, cystic periventricular leukomalacia, postnatal steroid therapy, and surgery before discharge. Among the nearly one half of the cohort that had none of these risk factors, the rate of survival without major sensorineural disability was 93%, similar to the rate among the controls with normal birth weight.

Wood and associates (2000) examined a population-based cohort of 283 infants born at 25 weeks or less in the United Kingdom and Ireland in 1995, and then evaluated them at a median corrected age of 30 months. Twenty-six percent of the cohort survived to initial hospital discharge; 2% died after discharge. Among infants who lived to discharge, the overall rate of disability was 49%; nearly half (23% of the sample) were severely disabled and required assistance for daily living. Thirty percent of survivors had developmental delay (Bayley Scales of Infant Development, Second Edition, Mental Developmental Index [Bayley II MDI] score <70); 10% had a severe neuromotor disability, 2% were blind, and 3% had severe hearing impairment.

Very few large population or gestational age-based studies of the long-term outcome of extremely preterm infants have been conducted in the United States. The NICHD Neonatal Research Network published a large prospective multicenter study of outcome among U.S. ELBW infants born from 1993 to 1994 (Vohr et al, 2000). Neurodevelopmental and functional outcomes at 18 months corrected age were reported for the 1151 ELBW survivors (401-1000 g at birth, 63% survival) who were cared for in 12 participating Network centers. The mean birth weight of the cohort was 796 gm ± 135 g and the mean gestational age was 26 ± 2 weeks. Forty nine percent of the cohort had one or more major neurodevelopmental and/or neurosensory abnormality (Bayley II MDI or physical developmental index [PDI] score <70, blindness, deafness requiring hearing aids, or cerebral palsy); 17% had cerebral palsy. Specific impairments of the 401- to 700-g survivors (mean gestational age 25 weeks) included a 53% rate of major impairment and a 20% rate of cerebral palsy; 6% were unable to sit. Forty-two percent of infants weighing 401 to 700 g at birth had significant developmental delay (a Bayley II MDI score <70); 4% had bilateral blindness; and 5% required a hearing aid. Risk factors for neurodevelopmental morbidity in the Network ELBW survivors included lower birth weight, bronchopulmonary dysplasia, severe intracranial hemorrhage, periventricular leukomalacia, postnatal administration of glucocorticoids for bronchopulmonary dysplasia, necrotizing enterocolitis, and male gender.

The results of large outcome studies of extremely preterm infants born in the early 1990s suggest that both survival to hospital discharge and neurodevelopmental outcome are variable. However, approximately half of extremely preterm infants born in 1990 to 1995 survived

**TABLE 1–3**

**Survival to Hospital Discharge and Survival Without Neurodevelopmental Impairment (NDI) Among Extremely Preterm Infants**

| | Australia (1991-1993)* | | UK and Ireland (1995)† | | North Carolina (1995-2000)‡ | | Rhode Island (1993-1997)§ | | NICHD Neonatal Research Network (1999-2000)‖ | |
|---|---|---|---|---|---|---|---|---|---|---|
| **Gestational Age (wks)** | **Survival to Discharge (%)** | **Survival w/o NDI (%)** | **Survival to Discharge (%)** | **Survival w/o NDI (%)** | **Survival to Discharge (%)** | **Survival w/o NDI (%)** | **Survival to Discharge (%)** | **Survival w/o NDI (%)** | **Survival to Discharge (%)** | **Survival w/o NDI (%)** |
| 22 | — | — | 1 | 50 | — | — | 5 | — | — | — |
| 23 | 10 | 60 | 11 | 42 | 24 | 37 | 46 | — | 32 | — |
| 24 | 33 | 67 | 26 | 45 | 57 | 81 | 59 | — | 61 | — |
| 25 | 58 | 75 | 44 | 53 | 66 | 95 | 82 | — | 78 | — |
| 26 | 72 | 75 | | — | 83 | 91 | | — | 85 | — |
| 27 | 77 | 92 | | — | 90 | 95 | | — | 90 | — |

*Data from Doyle LW: Victorian Infant Collaborative Study Group: Outcome at 5 years of age of children 23 to 27 weeks' gestation: Refining the prognosis. Pediatrics 108:134-141, 2001.

†Data from Wood NS, Marlow N, Costeloe K, et al: Neurologic and developmental disability after extremely preterm birth. N Engl J Med 343:378-384, 2000.

‡Data from Washburn LK, Dillard RG, Goldstein DJ, et al: Survival and developmental impairment in extremely low gestational age newborns born 1980-2000, Abstract. Pediatr Res 51:288, 2002.

§Data from El-Metally D, Vohr B, Tucker R: Survival and neonatal morbidity at the limits of viability in the mid 1990s: 22 to 25 weeks. J Pediatr 137:616-622, 2000.

‖Data from Fanaroff AA, Stoll BJ, Wright LL, et al: Very-low-birth-weight outcomes of the NICHD Neonatal Research Network, January 1997 through December 2000: Is further improvement possible? In press.

without neurodevelopmental impairment at follow-up (Vohr et al, 2000; Hack et al, 2000; Wood et al, 2000). The high rate of survival without neurodevelopmental impairment may be explained in part by the inclusion of more mature infants in the Australian and North Carolina studies and by differences in outcome definitions. The rates of specific disabilities among the Australian infants were comparable with those reported from the United Kingdom and Ireland and the Neonatal Research Network (Table 1–4).

Whether neurodevelopmental outcome is improving among ELBW infants born in the late 1990s has not been established. In the North Carolina geographic cohorts reported by Washburn and colleagues (2002), there were no differences in the rates of survival to discharge or survival without developmental impairment at 1-year follow-up between the early 1990s (1990 to 1995) and the late 1990s (1995 to 2000). However, outcome in the 1995 to 2000 North Carolina cohort is among the highest reported—68% of the cohort survived and 89% survived without developmental impairment. Data from the NICHD Neonatal Research Network demonstrate that neurodevelopmental outcome improved in the late 1990s: The overall rate of neurodevelopmental impairment in infants born between 22 and 32 weeks decreased from 49% in 1993 to 39% in 1998. Survival improved and disability diminished in 22- to 26-week survivors (Fig. 1–2) as well as in infants 28 to 32 weeks, among whom survival increased from 84% to 97%, the rate of cerebral palsy decreased from 18% to 11%, and the rate of developmental impairment (MDI score <70) dropped from 29% to 22% over the study period (Vohr et al, 2001).

**TABLE 1–4**

**Outcome of Extremely Preterm Infants: 401 to 700 g, 22 to 25 Weeks, and 23 to 27 Weeks**

| | Percentage Affected | | |
|---|---|---|---|
| **Outcome** | **401-700 g*** | **22-25 wks†** | **23-27 wks‡** |
| Bilateral blindness | 4 | 2 | 2 |
| Hearing aids | 5 | 2 | 1 |
| Bayley II MDI§ score <70 | 42 | 30 | 15 |
| Cerebral palsy | 18 | 18 | 11 |
| Inability to sit | 6 | 3 | — |
| Major impairment | 53 | 23-49 | 20 |

*Data from Vohr BR, Wright LL, Dusick AM, et al: Neurodevelopmental and functional outcomes of extremely low birth weight infants in the National Institute of Child Health and Human Development Neonatal Research Network, 1993-1994. Pediatrics 105:1216-1226, 2000.

†Data from Wood NS, Marlow N, Costeloe K, et al: Neurologic and developmental disability after extremely preterm birth. N Engl J Med 343:378-384, 2000.

‡Data from Doyle LW; Victorian Infant Collaborative Study Group: Outcome at 5 years of age of children 23 to 27 weeks' gestation: Refining the prognosis. Pediatrics 108:134-141, 2001.

§Bayley Scales of Infant Development, Second Edition, Mental Developmental Index.

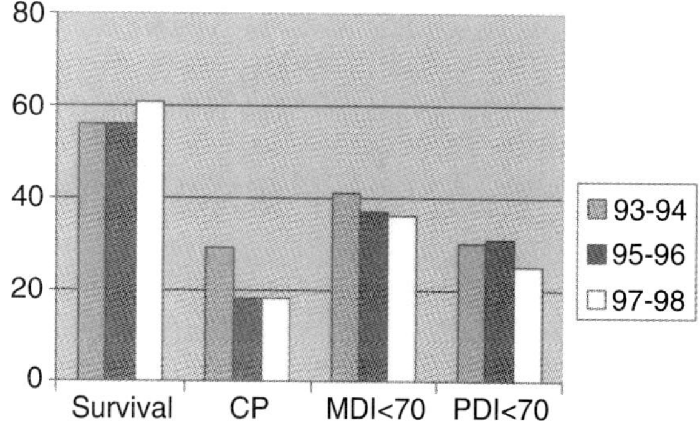


**FIGURE 1–2.** Neurodevelopmental outcome among 22- to 26-week survivors cared for in the National Institute of Child Health and Human Development (NICHD) Neonatal Research Network, 1993 to 1998. CP, cerebral palsy; MDI, Bayley Scales of Infant Development II, Mental Developmental Index; PDI, Bayley Scales of Infant Development II, Physical Developmental Index.

Parents and physicians of extremely preterm neonates require reliable information on their children's prognosis for survival and survival without disability in order to make informed decisions about how to best provide for their care. This information is, of necessity, offset in time from current practice and is often not specific to the institution caring for the infant or to the individual infant. Current estimates of survival without impairment (calculated from the product of the lowest survival and the lowest survival without impairment rates vs. the highest survival and highest survival without impairment rates), at 23 weeks range from 4% to 28%; at 24 weeks, from 12% to 49%; and at 25 weeks, from 23% to 78% (see Table 1–3). Given the limitations of the data, the estimated probability of survival without neurodevelopmental impairment for a 23-week neonate is 1/20 to 1/4; for a 24-week neonate, 1/5 to 1/2; and for a 25-week neonate, 1/4 to 4/5. Survival is rare with birth at 22 weeks of gestation.

Although preterm infants may not be neurodevelopmentally impaired at follow-up, they are at significant risk for academic difficulties. Studies of ELBW infants followed to school age report that 45% to 50% receive resource or special education services (Halsey et al, 1996; Saigal et al, 1990; Saigal et al, 1991). Bhutta and associates (2002), who performed a meta-analysis of case-control studies of 1556 preterm infants (<37 weeks) born between 1975 and 1988 and evaluated between 5 and 14 years of age, found that cognitive scores were directly proportional to birth weight and gestational age ($P < .001$) and significantly lower than those of the term controls (weighted mean difference, 10.9; 95% CI 9.2, 12.5). The preterm survivors were 50% more likely to be enrolled in special education classes and had a 2.64-fold higher risk for development of attention deficit hyperactivity disorder (ADHD) compared with the term controls. A subsequent report of the outcome at 20 years of age of 242 VLBW survivors born between 1977 and 1999 (mean birth weight 1179 g and gestational age 29.7 weeks) and 233 term controls reported similar findings (Hack et al, 2002). The VLBW participants had lower mean cognitive scores (87 vs. 92) and lower achievement scores than the term controls. They had significantly higher rates of neurosensory impairment (10% vs. <1%) and shorter stature than the controls. Fewer VLBW young adults had graduated from high school, and the VLBW males were less likely to be enrolled in post-secondary education (30% vs. 50%), after adjustment for maternal sociodemographic status. Of interest, the VLBW participants were also less likely to participate in risk-taking behavior (pregnancy, alcohol and drug use, and criminal activity) than the controls.

In summary, advances in perinatal care have led to the survival of growing numbers of children born at the lower limits of viability. Very low birth weight children have poorer outcomes compared with normal-birth-weight term controls in neurologic and health status, cognitive-neuropsychological skills, school performance, academic achievement, and behavior. Outcomes are highly variable but are related to medical risk factors, neonatal medical complications of prematurity, and social risk factors. Attention is increasingly focused on long-term outcome as an indicator of the individual infant's medical and social risk factors as well as the quality of the medical care the infant received. Systematic evaluation of risk factors (e.g., inflammatory exposures, nutritional status, brain injury on magnetic resonance imaging) and care practices (e.g., ventilatory management) may identify strategies and interventions needed to achieve further improvements in the outcome of babies born at the limits of viability.

## SELECTED READINGS

Bhutta AT, Cleves MA, Casey, PH, et al: Cognitive and behavioral outcomes of school-aged children who were born preterm: A meta-analysis. JAMA 288:728-737, 2002.

MacDonald H; American Academy of Pediatrics, Committee on Fetus and Newborn: Clinical report: Perinatal care at the threshold of viability. Pediatrics 110:1024-1027, 2002.

## REFERENCES

Doyle LW: Victorian Infant Collaborative Study Group: Outcome at 5 years of age of children 23 to 27 weeks of gestation: Refining the prognosis. Pediatrics 108:134-141, 2001.

Guyer B, Freedman MA, Strobino DM, Sondik EJ: Annual summary of vital statistics: Trends in the health of Americans during the 20th century. Pediatrics 106:1307-1317, 2000.

Hack M, Flannery DJ, Schluchter M: Outcomes in young adulthood for very-low-birth-weight infants. N Engl J Med 346:149-157, 2002.

Hack M, Wilson-Costello D, Friedman H, et al: Neurodevelopment and predictors of outcomes of children with birth weights of less than 1000 g. Arch Pediatr Adolesc Med 154:725-731, 2000.

Halsey CL, Collin MF, Anderson CL: Extremely low-birth-weight children and their peers: A comparison of school-age outcomes. Arch Pediatr Adolesc Med 150:790-794, 1996.

Horbar JD, Badger GJ, Carpenter JH, et al: Trends in mortality and morbidity for very low birth weight infants, 1991-1999. Pediatrics 110:143-151, 2002.

Hoyert DL, Freedman A, Strobino DM, Guyer B: Annual summary of vital statistics: 2000. Pediatrics 108:1241-1255, 2001.

Infant mortality and low birth weight among black and white infants—United States, 1980-2000. MMWR Morb Mortal Wkly Rep 51:589-592, 2002.

Lemons JA, Bauer CR, Oh W, et al: Very low birth weight outcomes of the National Institute of Child Health and Human Development Neonatal Research Network, January 1995 through December 1996. NICHD Neonatal Research Network. Pediatrics 107:E1, 2001.

Lorenz JL, Wooliever DE, Jetton JR, et al: A quantitative review of mortality and developmental disability in extremely premature newborns [review]. Arch Pediatr Adolesc Med 152:425-255, 1998.

Lorenz JL, Paneth N, Jetton JR, et al: Comparison of management strategies for extreme prematurity in New Jersey and the Netherlands: Outcomes and resource expenditure. Pediatrics 108:1269-1274, 2001.

Martin JA, Hamilton BE, Ventura SJ, et al: Births: Final data for 2000. Natl Vital Stat Rep 50(5):1-20, 2002a.

Martin JA, Park MM, Sutton PD: Births: Preliminary data for 2001. Natl Vital Stat Rep 50(10):1-20, 2002b.

Mathews TJ, Menacker F, MacDorman MF: Infant mortality statistics from the 2000 period linked birth/infant death data set. Natl Vital Stat Rep 50(12):1-28, 2002.

Saigal S, Szatmari P, Rosenbaum P, et al: Cognitive abilities and school performance of extremely low birth weight children and matched term control children at 8 years: A regional study. J Pediatr 118:751-760, 1991.

Saigal S, Szatmari P, Rosenbaum P, et al: Intellectual and functional status at school entry of children who weighed 1000 grams or less at birth. J Pediatr 116:409-416, 1990.

Stoll BJ, Hansen N, Fanaroff AA, et al: Changes in pathogens causing early-onset sepsis in very-low-birth-weight infants. N Engl J Med 347:240-247, 2002.

Vohr BR, Wright LL, Dusick AM, et al: Neurodevelopmental and functional outcomes of extremely low birth weight infants in the National Institute of Child Health and Human Development Neonatal Research Network, 1993-1994. Pediatrics 105:1216-1226, 2000.

Vohr BR, Wright LL, Poole, K et al: Neurodevelopmental outcome of ELBW infants <32 weeks gestation between 1993 and 1998, Abstract. Pediatr Res 49:339, 2001.

Washburn LK, Dillard RG, Goldstein DJ, et al: Survival and developmental impairment in extremely low gestational age newborns born 1980-2000, Abstract Pediatr Res 51:288, 2002.

Wood NS, Marlow N, Costeloe K, et al: Neurologic and developmental disability after extremely preterm birth. N Engl J Med 343:378-384, 2000.

CHAPTER 2

# Evaluation of Therapeutic Recommendations, Database Management, and Information Retrieval

Peter Tarczy-Hornoch

## BACKGROUND

At a fundamental level, the practice of neonatology can be considered an information management problem. The care provider is combining patient-specific information (history, findings of physical examination, and results of physiologic monitoring, laboratory tests, and radiologic evaluation) with generalized information (medical knowledge, practice guidelines, clinical trials, personal experience) to make medical decisions (diagnostic, therapeutic, and management). Though medicine remains a quintessentially human endeavor, computers are playing a growing role in information management in general and in neonatology in particular. Both patient-specific information and generalized information are becoming increasingly available in electronic form. In the United States, a growing number of hospitals are adopting electronic medical record systems to manage patient-specific information, the approaches ranging from electronic flow sheets in the intensive care unit (ICU) to paperless hospitals. Around the world, the Internet has made possible a revolution in the sharing and dissemination of knowledge in all fields, including medicine.

Parallel with and related to the adoption of information technology is the growth of societal pressures to improve the quality of medical care while controlling costs. These changes are beginning to affect the way in which medicine and neonatology are practiced. In turn, it is becoming important for neonatologists to understand basic principles related to biomedical and health informatics, databases and electronic medical record systems, evaluation of therapeutic recommendations, and online information retrieval.

This expansion of information technology in clinical practice and the concurrent growth of medical knowledge have great promise but also potential pitfalls. One pitfall that must not be underestimated, and which is as great a danger today as when Blois (1984) first cautioned against it, is the unquestioning adoption of information technology: "And, since the thing that computers do is frequently done by them more rapidly than it is by brains, there has been an irresistible urge to apply computers to medicine, but considerably less of an urge to attempt to understand where and how they can best be used." A present and very real challenge is information overload. Bero and Rennie (1995) observed, "Although well over 1 million clinical trials have been conducted, hundreds of thousands remain unpublished or are hard to find and may be in various languages. In the unlikely event that the physician finds all the relevant trials of a treatment, these are rarely accompanied by any comprehensive systematic review attempting to assess and make sense of the evidence." The potential of just-in-time information at the point of care is thus particularly appealing. "New information tools are needed: they are likely to be electronic, portable, fast, easy to use, connected to both a large valid database of medical knowledge and the patient record" (Smith, 1996).

## BIOMEDICAL AND HEALTH INFORMATICS

In the 1970s, clinicians with expertise in computers became intrigued by the potential that these tools had to help improve the practice of medicine, and the field of medical informatics was born. The importance of this field to address the issues of information management in health care is growing rapidly, as can be seen in the activities of the American Medical Informatics Association (AMIA) (American Medical, on line). *Medical informatics* can be concisely defined as "the rapidly developing scientific field that deals with the storage, retrieval, and optimal use of biomedical information, data, and knowledge for problem solving and decision making" (Blois and Shortliffe, 1990). Further definitions are available in the "Frequently Asked Questions" section of the AMIA's home page, in "About AMIA." The field includes both applied and basic research, with the focus here on the applied aspects. Examples of basic research are artificial intelligence in medicine, genome data analysis, and data mining (sorting through data to identify patterns and establish relationships). As our knowledge about the genetic mechanisms of disease expands and more data about patients and outcomes are available electronically, the role of informatics in medicine in general and neonatology in particular will expand.

The applied focus of the field in the 1960s and 1970s was data oriented, focusing on signal processing and statistical data analysis. In neonatology, the earliest applications of computers were for physiologic data monitoring in the neonatal ICU (NICU). As the field matured in the 1980s, applied work focused on systems to manage patient information and medical knowledge on a limited basis. Examples are laboratory systems, radiology systems, centralized transcription systems, and, probably the best-known medical knowledge management system, the database of published medical articles maintained by the National Library of Medicine known first as MEDLARS, then as Medline, and currently as PubMed (PubMed, on line). For instance, neonatologists began to develop tools to aid in the management of NICU patients, such as computer-assisted algorithms to help manage ventilators, although the algorithms have not been successfully deployed on a large scale in the clinical setting.

As computers and networking became mainstream in the workplace and home in the 1990s, informatics researchers began to develop integrated and networked systems (Fuller, 1992, 1997). With the explosion of information from the Human Genome Project, the intersection between bioinformatics and medical informatics began to blur, leading to the adoption of the term *biomedical informatics*. This decade saw the development of a number of important systems. In terms of patient-specific information retrieval, they included integrated electronic medical record systems that in their full implementation can encompass, in a single piece of easy-to-use software, interfaces to physiologic monitors, electronic flow sheets, access to laboratory and radiology data as well as tools for electronic documentation (charting), electronic order entry, integrated billing, and modules to help reduce medical errors. The Internet has permitted ready access and sharing of this information within health-care organizations and, in some instances, limited secured remote access to this information from home. In terms of patient population information retrieval, a number of tools were developed to help clinicians and researchers look at aggregate data in these electronic medical records to document outcomes and help improve quality of care. The Internet and particularly the World Wide Web have transformed access to medical knowledge (Fuller et al, 1999). Health sciences libraries are becoming digital as well as paper repositories. Journals are available on line. Knowledge is now available at the point of care in ways it never has been before (Tarczy-Hornoch et al, 1997).

Evidence-based medicine as an approach to the evaluation of therapeutic recommendations has increased in prominence (see later discussion). In 1988, neonatologists established and expanded the Vermont Oxford Network to improve the quality and safety of medical care for newborn infants and their families (Vermont, on line). As part of the activities, they established and maintain a nationwide database about the care and outcome of high-risk newborn infants. Duncan (on line) maintains an excellent bibliographic database on the literature about computer applications in neonatology.

## DATABASES

In broad terms, a *database* is an organized, structured collection of data designed for a particular purpose. Thus, a stack of 3 × 5 cards with patient information is a database, as is the typical paper prenatal record. Most frequently, the term is used to refer to an electronic collection of information, such as a database of clinical trial data for a group of patients in a study. Databases come in a variety of fundamental types, such as single-table, relational, and object-oriented.

A *simple database* can be set up using a single table by means of a spreadsheet program (such as Microsoft's Excel) or a database program (such as Microsoft's Access). The advantage of such a database is that it is very easy to set up and maintain. For an outcomes database in a neonatology unit, each row can represent a patient and each column represents information about the patients (for example name, medical record number, gestational age, birth date, length of stay, PDA [patent ductus arteriosus] yes/no, NEC [necrotizing enterocolitis] yes/no). The major limitation of such a database is that each time the researcher wants to track another outcome (e.g., maple syrup urine disease), a column must be added to store the information. This can result in tables with dozens to hundreds of columns, which then become difficult to fill out and maintain.

The vast majority of databases and electronic medical records in neonatology is built using *relational database software*. To set up a simple outcomes relational database that permits easy adding of new outcome measures, one could use a three-table database design (Fig. 2–1). The first table would contain all the information for each patient has (e.g., basic demographic information—name, medical record number, gestation, birth date, admit date, discharge date). The second table would be a dictionary that would assign a code number to each diagnosis or outcome one wanted to track (e.g., PDA = 1, NEC = 2, plus dozens of rare diagnoses, like maple syrup urine disease = 10234). The third table would be the diagnosis tracking table—it would tie a patient number to a particular code and assign a value to that code. Adding a new diagnosis to track would require adding an entry to the diagnosis dictionary table. To add a diagnosis to a patient, one would add an entry to the tracking table. For example, Girl Smith (medical record number 00-00-01) is diagnosed with NEC. To add the diagnosis, one would add to the diagnosis table an entry that has a value of 00-00-01 in the medical record column, a value of 2 (code for NEC) in the code column, and a value of 2 in the value column (code for surgical). Though relational databases are harder to set up, they provide much more flexibility for expansion and maintenance and thus are the preferred implementation for clinical databases.

The distinction between a NICU quality assessment/quality improvement (a.k.a., outcomes) database and an electronic medical record is largely a matter of degree. Some characteristics typical of a neonatal outcomes database are data collection and data entry after the fact, limited amount of data collected (a small subset of the information needed for daily care), lack of narrative text, lack of interfaces to laboratory and other information systems, and the episodic (e.g., quarterly) use of the system for report generation. Some characteristics typical of an electronic medical record are "real-time" (daily or more frequent) entry of data, a large amount of data collected (approximating all the information needed for daily care), narrative text (e.g., progress notes, radiology reports, pathology reports), interfaces to laboratory and other information systems, and, most importantly, the use of the system for daily patient care.

In the past, the majority of neonatal databases and first-generation NICU electronic medical record systems were developed locally by and for neonatologists. The literature describing these efforts is available on line (Duncan, on line). Unfortunately, the majority of these systems were never published or publicly documented, and thus, a number of important and useful innovations are lost or must be repeatedly rediscovered. Anybody thinking about building his or her own neonatology database would be well advised to review the existing literature and existing commercial products before embarking on this path. That said, there is room for improvement of the existing products, and neonatologists continue to develop their own databases today.

Tables in the database:

| DEMOGRAPHIC DATA |
|---|
| Name |
| Hospital_Number |
| Gestational_Age |
| Birthdate |
| Admit_Date |
| Discharge_Date |

| DIAGNOSES |
|---|
| Hospital_Number |
| Diagnosis_Code |
| Value |

| DIAGNOSIS DICTIONARY |
|---|
| Diagnosis_Code |
| Description |

Example Entries in the Tables:

DEMOGRAPHIC DATA

| Name | Hospital_Number | Gestational_Age | Birthdate | Admit_Date | Discharge_Date |
|---|---|---|---|---|---|
| John Smith | 00-00-01 | 27 | 1/1/2003 | 1/1/2003 | 3/21/2003 |
| Jane Doe | 00-00-02 | 24 | 1/2/2003 | 1/3/2003 | 4/15/2003 |

DIAGNOSES

| Hospital_Number | Diagnosis_Code | Value |
|---|---|---|
| 00-00-01 | 1 | 1 |
| 00-00-01 | 2 | 1 |
| 00-00-02 | 1 | 2 |
| 00-00-02 | 10234 | |

DIAGNOSIS DICTIONARY

| Diagnosis_Code | Description |
|---|---|
| 1 | PDA (1=small, 2=large) |
| 2 | NEC (1=medical, 2=surgical) |
| .... | |
| 10234 | Maple Syrup Urine Disease |

**FIGURE 2-1.** Example of a relational database.

The largest neonatal outcomes database is the centralized database maintained by the nonprofit organization Vermont Oxford Network (Vermont, on line), with the mission of improving the quality and safety of medical care for infants and their families. One of the key activities of the network is their outcomes database, which involves more than 400 participating intensive care nurseries. Other activities of the network are clinical trials, follow-up of extremely low birth weight (ELBW) infants, and NICU quality and safety studies. The focus of the database has been very low birth weight (VLBW) infants (401 to 1500 g). At present, the network collects data on more than 50% of the VLBW infants born in the United States (>30,000 infants per year). Participants in the network submit data and in return receive both outcome data for their own institution and comparative data from other nurseries nationwide. All data except their own are anonymous for all participants. The network does have access to both the individual and aggregate data. The network database is maintained centrally, and data quality monitoring and data entry are centralized. Initially, the process involved paper submission of data by participating nurseries. Now a number of the commercial and custom NICU databases and electronic medical record systems can export their data in the format required by the Vermont Oxford Network. Submissions of data today are thus a combination of paper forms and reports generated by commercial and custom software packages.

The data tracked in the database focuses on tracking outcomes. With the passage of the Health Insurance Portability and Accountability Act of 1996 (HIPAA), federal regulations governing the confidentiality of electronic patient data, some of the anonymous demographic data that was collected by the Network in the past has decreased. This change has grown from concerns that, in combination with identity of the referring center, these data could be used to uniquely identify patients, a violation of the HIPAA.

## ELECTRONIC MEDICAL RECORD

An electronic medical record is much more complex than an outcomes database, because the system is intended to be used continually on a daily basis to replace electronically some if not all of the record keeping, laboratory result review, and order writing that occur in a neonatal intensive care nursery. The complexity of this task becomes rapidly evident if one imagines that for a paperless medical record environment, every paper form in a nursery would need to be replaced with an electronic equivalent. Organizations are moving in this direction because of a combination of forces, of which the desires to reduce error in and to control the spiraling costs of health care are particularly important. These reasons are addressed at great length in two reports from the Institute of Medicine (Institute, 1997; Kohn et al, 2000). These benefits are typically achieved when information is not only available electronically (e.g., results of laboratory tests, radiology procedures, and transcription) but is also input into the system (e.g., problem lists, allergies) and when both sets of information are combined and checked against electronic orders. Only with electronic orders has it been shown that errors can be reduced and care provider behavior clearly changed. Combining just electronic laboratory results (e.g., creatinine level) and electronic order entry (e.g., a drug order), for example, enables one to verify drug dosages have been correctly adjusted for renal failure. This approach would work well in adults, but in neonates, whose renal function is more difficult to assess and for whom drug dosage norms depend on gestational age and post-delivery age, additional information must be entered into the system (e.g., urine output, gestational age).

Results review systems include basic demographic data, such as name, age, and address from the hospital registration system. These systems require a moderate amount of work to tie them to the various laboratory, radiology, and other systems and to train users. The benefits are hard to quantify, but users typically prefer them to the paper alternative because of the more rapid access to information. The challenge in moving beyond the results review level to the integrated system level is that the documentation level and order entry level are essentially prerequisites for the integrated system level but, in and of themselves, have marginal benefit, particularly given the human and financial costs. Integrated systems require significant work to implement, including the presence of computers virtually at each bedside, as well as significant work to train users. The benefits accrue mainly to the organization, in the form of reduced costs of filing, printing, and maintaining paper records and, if providers are forced to enter notes instead of dictate them, significant savings in transcription costs. The challenge is that the end users often find it takes much longer to do their daily work with electronic documentation. Without moving to at least electronic order entry, if not an integrated system, the users do not realize major day-to-day benefits.

The benefits start to clearly accrue to both providers and institutions at the next level, electronic order entry. The complexity of implementing and deploying an electronic order entry system cannot be overstated. Interfaces need to be built not only with all the systems that are part of results review but also with other systems. Furthermore, a huge database of possible orders must be created to allow users to pick the right orders. This database and the menu of choices are needed because computers are poor at recognizing and interpreting a narrative text typed by a human. Finally and most importantly, there is a huge training challenge, because writing orders electronically is more complex and time consuming than handwriting them. The change management issues become apparent when one considers that typically, these systems take the unit assistant out of the loop; thus, a lot of the oversight that can occur at the unit assistant level does not, or the burden of oversight is now borne by the person entering the orders.

Once one overcomes the barriers to electronic order entry, organizations can start to benefit from integrated systems. For this reason, the trend today is not a stepwise move from results review to documentation of integrated systems but, rather, a big leap from results review straight to integrated systems. Interestingly, the technical complexities and the training and usage complexities of integrated systems are not that much higher than those for order entry. Essentially, integrated systems add tools to make life easier for care providers using all the data in the system. An analogy might help one understand this issue. An integrated electronic medical record system is like an office software suite that encompasses a word processor, a spreadsheet, a slide presentation tool, a graphic drawing tool, and a database, all of which can "talk" to one another, making it easy to put a picture from the drawing tool or a graph from a spreadsheet into a slide show. Integrated systems include (1) error checking of orders, (2) alerts and reminders triggered by orders or by problems on the problem list or other data in the system, (3) care plans tied to patient-specific information, (4) charting modules customized to the problem list, (5) charting and progress notes that automatically pull in information from laboratory tests, flow sheets, and so on, and that help generate orders for the day as the documentation occurs, (6) modules to facilitate hyperalimentation ordering, and (7) modules to assist in management. For example one could imagine a system in which reminders for screening studies (e.g, for retinopathy of prematurity [ROP], intraventricular hemorrhage [IVH], and brainstem auditory evoked response [BAER]) were triggered by gestational age, problem list, and previous results of screening studies. Similarly, admission of a neonate at a particular gestational age with a particular set of problems could trigger pathways, orders, and reminders specific to that clinical scenario. An important caveat is that all such systems are only as good as the data and rules put into them. The issues raised in the section on evaluation of therapeutic recommendations are very important to consider in the context of electronic order entry and integrated systems.

The electronic medical record market is still relatively young and continually evolving. This is true of both products designed specifically for the neonatal intensive care unit and more generic products designed to be used throughout a hospital or health-care system. Order entry and documentation systems are in their adolescence, and integrated systems in their infancy. The major reason for this situation is that the needs of different health-care systems vary significantly, and the existing products are not flexible enough to meet all these needs in one system. Furthermore, there is a trend among health-care organizations and electronic medical record developers and vendors to move away from niche systems tailored to particular subsets of care providers, such as neonatology, and toward a focus on systems that are generically useful. There are two important drivers behind this trend.

The first and most important reason for adopting a single integrated system is that the benefits of an electronic medical record system begin to accrue only when an entire organization uses the same one. Consider the following scenario: A woman receives prenatal care in the clinic of an institution and then presents in preterm labor to the emergency department (ED). Her infant is delivered in the labor and delivery department, is hospitalized in the neonatal intensive care nursery, and is discharged to an affiliated pediatric follow-up clinic. In the current era of paper medical records, paper is used to convey information from one site to the other. In an integrated electronic medical record system, all the information for both mother and infant is in one place for all providers to see. If the institution were to adopt niche software tailored to the needs of each site, a provider caring for the infant might need to access an ED system, an obstetric system, an NICU system, and an outpatient pediatric system to gather all the pertinent information. Each system would require the user to learn a separate piece of software (for example, four different word processors). Learning a site-specific piece of software is a considerably greater burden on care providers than learning to use a site-specific paper form.

The second factor driving adoption of integrated systems is economies of scale. The ideal electronic medical record system contains electronic interfaces that automatically pull into the system data from laboratory, pharmacy, radiology, transcription as well as integrated electronic orders, error checking, and electronic documentation by care providers. Given that development of these interfaces and provision of training and maintenance of the system cost more than the purchase of the system itself, it is far more cost effective to install one system with one set of interfaces and one set of training and maintenance issues than to replicate the process multiple times.

The neonatal intensive care environment poses some unique challenges for electronic medical records. Thus, it is important to try to ensure that when health-care systems are making decisions about the purchase of an electronic medical record, neonatologists and other neonatal health-care providers are involved in the process. An excellent source of information about NICU medical record systems and databases is an article by Stavis (1999). Neonatologists in the position of helping select an electronic medical record system must acquire the necessary background through reading some basic introductory texts on medical informatics, focusing on electronic medical records. It is then critical that they survey other organizations similar to their own to find out what systems have worked in that environment and what systems have not. For example, the needs of a level III academic nursery that performs extracorporeal membrane oxygenation (ECMO) are very different from those of a community level II hospital that does not perform mechanical ventilation of infants. Most important, using a medical informatics framework, the neonatologists must develop a list of prioritized criteria specific to their institution and compare available products in the marketplace with this list.

All end user needs must also be considered; thus, if residents, nurse practitioners, nutritionists, pharmacists, and respiratory therapists are expected to use the system, their input must be solicited as well. Ensuring broad-based input is especially relevant if the goal is an electronic medical record system into which it is expected that a lot of data will be entered by health-care providers (i.e., electronic charting, note writing, medication administration records, order entry). The reason to ensure "buy-in" by all the users into systems that require data entry is that a significant percentage of systems requiring data entry has ultimately been unsuccessful because of lack of user acceptance. Unfortunately, there is little literature on this issue, because institutions rarely publicize and publish their failures in this arena, although the situation is beginning to change. Lack of adoption is rarely a problem when the system is a results review system.

The final step in evaluating a potential system is to develop a series of use scenarios and to have potential users sit down in front of the system and test the scenarios. Evaluating use scenarios typically involves visits to sites that have installed the electronic medical record system under consideration. An example of a use scenario might be for a nurse, a respiratory therapist, a resident, and an attending physician to try to electronically replicate, on a given system under consideration, the bedside charting, progress note charting, and order writing for a critically ill patient who undergoes ECMO and then decannulation. The reason for developing and testing such scenarios is that this approach is the best way to ensure that aspects of charting, note writing, and documentation unique to the NICU are supported by the system.

## EVALUATING THERAPEUTIC RECOMMENDATIONS

Once all the data about a patient, whether in electronic or paper form, is in hand, the clinician is faced with the challenge of medical decision-making and applying all that he or she knows to the problem at hand. This, in turn, means it is vital that the clinician understand what is known and what is still uncertain in terms of the validity of therapeutic recommendations. The evaluation of new recommendations arising from a variety of sources, including journal articles, meta-analyses, and systematic reviews, is thus a critical skill that all neonatologists must master. Broadly speaking, this approach has been termed *evidence-based medicine*. A full discussion of this approach to evaluation of new approaches in clinical medicine is beyond the scope of this discussion. Two outstanding sources of information are the works by Guyatt and colleagues (2002) and Sackett and associates (2000). An important caveat is that evidence-based medicine is not a panacea. It is not helpful when the primary literature does not address a particular clinical situation because of its rarity or complexity, for example. This approach also does not necessarily address broader concerns, such as clinical importance or cost effectiveness (although it sometimes does).

In the early days of medicine, the "gold standard" was observation of individual patients and subjective description of aggregate experiences from similar patients. As the science of medicine evolved, formal scientific methods were applied to help assess possible therapeutic and management interventions. Important tools in this effort are epidemiology, statistics, and clinical trial design. Today, medicine in general and neonatology in particular are faced with an interesting paradox. For some areas, there is a wealth of information in the form of the gold standard randomized controlled clinical trial, whereas for others, there is scant information to guide clinical practice. A wealth of well-designed clinical trials on the use of surfactant has been published, for example, but there are essentially none addressing the management of chylothorax. One might assume that the practice of medicine reflects the available evidence, but this is not the case. McDonald (1996) summarized the problem as follows: "Although we assume that medical decisions are driven by established scientific fact, even a cursory review of practice patterns shows that they are not." Investigators have examined medical practice (generally in the outpatient primary care setting) and have determined that of all medical interventions, roughly 50% are not adequately addressed by the medical literature, 30% continue despite evidence against their efficacy in the medical literature, and only about 20% are well supported by the literature. Thus, neonatologists have a responsibility to identify what knowledge is available in the literature and elsewhere and to critically evaluate this information before applying it to practice. Furthermore, because this information is constantly evolving, one must continually revisit the underlying literature as it expands; a good example is the recommendations regarding the use of steroids for chronic lung disease.

The evidence-based practice of medicine is an approach that addresses these issues. It is helpful to consider the process as involving two steps—the critical review of the primary literature and the synthesis of the information offered in the primary literature. Critical review of the primary literature is an area that most neonatologists have a lot of experience with through journal clubs and other similar forums. The approach involves systematically reviewing each section of an article (i.e., background, methods, results, discussion) and, for each section, asking critical questions (e.g., for the methods section: Is the statistical methodology valid? Were power calculations made? Was a hypothesis clearly stated? Do the methods address the hypothesis? Do the methods address alternative hypotheses? Do the methods address confounding variables?). The formal evaluation of each section must then be synthesized into some conclusions. A helpful question to ask is "Does this paper change my clinical practice, and if so, then how?" Further resources for systematic review of the primary literature are listed in the Selected Readings. It is important to note that guidelines for systematic review of a single article differ according to whether it describes (1) a preventive or therapeutic trial (e.g., use of nitrous oxide for chronic lung disease), (2) evaluation of a diagnostic study (e.g., use of C-reactive protein level for prediction of infection), or (3) prognosis (e.g., prediction of outcome from a Score for Neonatal Acute Physiology [SNAP] score).

The second, and arguably the more important, step is to determine not the affect of one article on one's practice but the overall impact of the body of relevant literature on one's practice. For example, if the preponderance of the literature favors one therapeutic recommendation, then a single article opposing the recommendation must be weighed against the other articles that favor it. This is a complex task, and the most complete and formal statistical approach to combining the results of multiple studies (meta-analysis) requires significant investment of time and effort. Part of the evidence-based practice of medicine approach therefore involves the collaborative development of evidence-based systematic reviews and meta-analyses by communities of care providers. Within the field of neonatology, Sinclair and associates (1992) laid the seminal groundwork for this approach. Their textbook, *Effective Care on the Newborn*, remains an important milestone but illustrates the problem of information currency. Because the textbook was published in 1992, none of the clinical trials in neonatology in the last decade are included. The Internet has permitted creation and continual maintenance of up-to-date information by a distributed group of collaborators, lending itself beautifully to the maintenance of a database of evidence-based medicine reviews of the literature. This international effort is termed the Cochrane Collaboration, and the *Cochrane Neonatal Review* is devoted to neonatology (Cochrane, on line). A limitation of the Cochrane approach is illustrated by the relatively restricted scope of topics covered at the National Institute of Child and Human Development (NICHD) Web site (www.nichd.nih.gov/cochrane/cochrane.htm)—existence of a review requires adequate literature on a topic and a dedicated and committed clinician to create and update the review.

It is important to distinguish between these formal approaches to reviewing the literature (systematic literature reviews and meta-analyses) that have specific methodologies and more ad hoc reviews of the literature. Evidence-based medicine aggregate resources such as the Cochrane Collaboration take a more systematic approach, but review articles published in the literature vary in their approach. Meta-analyses are easy to distinguish but systematic reviews versus ad hoc reviews are harder to distinguish. Systematic reviews focus on quality primary literature (e.g., controlled studies rather than case series or case reports) and must include (1) a methods section for the review article that explicitly specifies how articles were identified for possible inclusion and (2) what criteria were used to assess the validity of each study as well as to include or exclude primary literature articles in the systematic review. Systematic reviews also tend to present the literature in aggregate tabular form even when meta-analyses of statistics of all the articles cannot be done. One commonly used source of overview information in neonatology—the *Clinics in Perinatology* series—is a mix of opinion (written in the style of a book chapter), ad hoc literature review, systematic literature review, and meta-analysis. Guidelines (such as screening recommendations for group B streptococcal [GBS] infection), although based on primary literature review, are typically neither meta-analyses nor systematic reviews of the literature. Whereas formal methods are used to derive conclusions with meta-analyses and systematic review, guidelines are developed frequently instead by consensus among committee members (true of both national and local practice guidelines). General textbooks of neonatology are typically based on ad hoc literature review that includes both primary literature and systematic literature review. When one is reading overviews of the aggregate state of current knowledge on a given topic in neonatology, it is important to keep these distinctions in mind.

Anyone interested in developing his or her own evidence-based reviews on a particular topic should review some of the textbooks on evidence-based practice listed at the end of the chapter; initially, he or she should collaborate (in person or by e-mail and telephone) with someone who has experience in systematic review and meta-analyses. The process consists of the following steps: (1) identification of the relevant clinical question (e.g., management of bronchopulmonary dysplasia [BPD]), (2) narrowing of the question to a focus that enables one to determine whether a given article in the primary literature answers it or not (e.g., Does prophylactic high-frequency ventilation have positive or negative effects on acute and chronic morbidity—pulmonary and otherwise?), (3) extensively searching the primary literature (frequently in collaboration with a librarian with expertise searching the biomedical literature) and retrieving the articles, (4) critically, formally, and systematically reviewing each article for inclusion, validity, utility, and applicability, and (5) formally summarizing the results of the preceding process, including conclusions valid throughout the body of included primary literature.

## ONLINE INFORMATION RETRIEVAL

In the long run, because of the rapid growth of biomedical information and the fact it changes over time, both investigators in informatics and publishers believe that print (paper) media will soon no longer be the way that biomedical information is shared and distributed (Weatherall, 1995; Smith, 1996). Economic realities will dictate, however, that quality information will generally come at a price. The medical digital library at the University of Washington (available on line at www.healthlinks.washington.edu, then click on the Care Provider tab) serves to illustrate the current state of the art. The information available is a combination of locally developed material (e.g., University of Washington faculty writing practice guidelines), material developed by institutions elsewhere (faculty elsewhere writing such guidelines), material developed by organizations (e.g., the neonatal Cochrane Collaboration), and ever increasingly electronic forms of journals and textbooks and evidence-based medicine databases. The last (journals, textbooks, databases) are generally not free, and the University of Washington pays a "subscription fee" (termed a *site license*) to provide access to these resources for their faculty, staff, and students. Libraries will likely remain the pimary source of information but will shift their attention from paper to electronic materials. Health sciences libraries can provide invaluable training in the efficient use of online medical resources, and most offer training sessions and consultation.

A number of online resources are valuable for neonatologists. For accessing the primary literature, the most valuable resource is the National Library of Medicine's database of the published medical literature accessible (PubMed, on line) along with many other databases accessible from the Health Information Web site (National Library, on line). The PubMed system is continually being enhanced; thus, it is very useful to review the help documentation on line and to regularly look at the New/Noteworthy section to see what has changed. One of the most powerful and most frequently under-utilized tools is the "Find Related" link that appears next to each article listed on PubMed. This link locates articles that are related to the one selected (Liu and Altman, 1998). The PubMed system applies a powerful statistical algorithm with complex weightings to the article selected to each word in the title, to each author, to each major and minor keyword (Medical Subject heading [MeSH]), and to each word in the abstract and then finds statistically similar articles in the database. In general, this system outperforms the novice to advanced health-care provider performing a complex search and begins to approach the accuracy of an experience medical librarian. All the major pediatric journals are available on line either through a package at local hospital libraries or by subscription (instead of or in addition to a print/paper subscription). The value of having an electronic subscription to a journal is that it provides access not only to the current issue but also to past issues. The best online free source of information on evidence-based practice is the *Cochrane Neonatal Review* (Cochrane, on line). Subscriptions to the full Cochrane database can be purchased on line as well.

Given the growing role of genetics in health care and, in particular, the importance of genetic diseases in infants, one should consider accessing two genetics databases that are available free of charge on line. The first is Online Mendelian Inheritance in Man (OMIM), accessible at the National Library of Medicine through their menus or directly at the Web site (OMIM, on line). This database, a catalog of human genes and genetic disorders, is an online version of the textbook by the same name. It is a diachronic collection of information on genetic disorders, meaning that each disease entry chronologically cites and summarizes key papers in the field. The second is the GeneTests database (GeneTests, on line), which is both a yellow pages of genetic testing (what testing is available on a clinical and research basis, where, and how one sends a specimen) as well as a user manual (how to apply genetic testing). The user's manual section consists of entries for a growing number of diseases or clinical phenotypes of particular importance (>200). Entries are written by experts, peer reviewed both internally and externally, subject to a formal process similar to a systematic review, and updated regularly on line. An excellent site that maintains links to the majority of locally developed neonatology-specific content around the country is the site maintained by Duncan (on line). In addition to a database of links to clinical resources around the country, the site also has a jobs listing and a database of the literature on computer applications in medicine.

The clinician must realize that, unlike journals, textbooks, and guidelines, the material on the World Wide Web (whether accessed from Duncan's site or whether based on a search of the World Wide Web), is not necessarily subject to any editorial or other oversight as to what is published; thus, as Silberg and associates (1997), put it, "caveat lector" (reader beware). A number of articles and Web sites address criteria for assessing the validity and reliability of material on a Web site (Mitretek Systems, on line; Health, on line). If one keeps this caution in mind, a search on the entire World Wide Web using a sophisticated search engine (such as Google, available at www.google.com) can yield very valuable information, though with a lot of chaff for a little wheat. Google also has a sophisticated statistical algorithm that allows a user to find similar web pages once he or she has identified one of interest.

## SELECTED READINGS

Norris T, Fuller SL, Goldberg HI, Tarczy-Hornoch P: Informatics in Primary Care: Strategies in Information Management for the Healthcare Provider. New York, Springer-Verlag, 2002.

Shortliffe EH, Perreault LE, Wiederhold G, Fagan LM (eds): Medical Informatics: Computer Applications in Health Care. Reading, MA, Addison-Wesley, 1990.

## REFERENCES


American Medical Informatics Association: Home Page. At www.amia.org/

Bero L, Rennie D: The Cochrane Collaboration: Preparing, maintaining, and disseminating systematic reviews of the effects of health care. JAMA 274:1935-1938, 1995.

Blois M: Information and Medicine: The Nature of Medical Descriptions. Berkeley, CA, University of California Press, 1984, p xiii.

Blois M, Shortliffe E: The computer meets medicine: Emergence of a discipline. In Shortliffe EH, Perreault LE, Wiederhold G, Fagan LM (eds): Medical Informatics: Computer Applications in Healthcare. Reading, MA, Addison-Wesley, 1990.

Cochrane Neonatal Collaborative Review Group: Cochrane Neonatal Review. Available on line at http://www.nichd.nih.gov/cochrane/

Duncan R: Computers in neonatology. Available on line at http://www.neonatology.org/neo.computers.html/

Fuller S: Creating the future: IAIMS planning premises at the University of Washington. Bull Med Libr Assoc 80:288-293, 1992.

Fuller S: Regional health information systems: Applying the IAIMS model. J Am Med Inform Assoc 4:S47-S51, 1997.

Fuller SS, Ketchell DS, Tarczy-Hornoch P, Masuda D: Integrating knowledge resources at the point of care: Opportunities for librarians. Bull Med Libr Assoc 87:393-403, 1999.

GeneTests Web site. At www.genetests.org/

Guyatt GH, Rennie D (eds): Users' Guide to the Medical Literature: A Manual for Evidence-Based Clinical Practice. Chicago, American Medical Association, 2002.

Health on the Net Foundation: HON Code of Conduct (HONcode) for medical and health Web sites. Available on line at www.hon.ch/HONcode/Conduct.html/

Institute of Medicine Committee on Improving the Patient Record: The Computer-Based Patient Record: An Essential Technology for Health Care. Washington, DC, National Academy Press, 1997.

Kohn LT, Corrigan JM, Donaldson MS: To Err is Human: Building a Safer Health System. Washington, DC, National Academy Press, 2000.

Liu X, Altman R: Updating a bibliography using the related articles function within PubMed. Proc AMIA Symp 1998:750-754, 1998.

McDonald C: Medical heuristics: The silent adjudicators of clinical practice. Ann Intern Med 124:56-62, 1996.

Mitretek Systems: Working draft. White paper: Criteria for assessing the quality of health information on the Internet. Available on line at hitiweb.mitretek.org/docs/criteria.html/

National Institute of Child and Human Development (NICHD). Available on line at www.nichd.nih.gov/cochrane/cochrane.htm

National Library of Medicine: Health Information page. Available on line at www.nlm.nih.gov/hinfo.html/

OMIM (Online Mendelian Inheritance in Man). At www.ncbi.nlm.nih.gov/entrez/query.fcgi?db = OMIM/

PubMed: Available on line at http://www.ncbi.nlm.nih.gov/entrez/

Sackett DL, Richardson WS, Rosenberg W, Haynes RB: Evidence-based Medicine: How to Practice and Teach EBM, 2nd ed. London, Churchill Livingstone, 2000.

Silberg W, Lundberg G, Musacchio RA, et al: Assessing, controlling, and assuring the quality of medical information on the Internet. Caveat lector et viewor—Let the reader and viewer beware. JAMA 277:1244-1245, 1997.

Sinclair JC, Bracken BB, Silverman W (eds): Effective Care of the Newborn Infant. New York, Oxford University Press, 1992.

Smith R: What clinical information do doctors need? BMJ 313:1062-1068, 1996.

Stavis R: Neonatal databases. Part 3: Physicians' programs: Products and features. Perinatal Section News AAP 25:17-20, 1999.

Tarczy-Hornoch P, Kwan-Gett T, Fouche L, et al: Meeting clinician information needs by integrating access to the medical record and knowledge resources via the Web. Proc AMIA Annu Fall Symp 1997:809-813, 1997.

Vermont Oxford Network, Health Information Technology Institute: Home Page. Available on line at http://www.vtoxford.org/

Weatherall D: On dinosaurs and medical textbooks. Lancet 346:4-5, 1995.

CHAPTER 3

# Ethical Decisions in the Neonatal-Perinatal Period

**Robert M. Nelson**

In 1973, Duff and Campbell published a groundbreaking article supporting the withdrawal of life-sustaining medical treatment (LSMT) from 43 infants described as severely impaired from congenital disorders. One infant, who suffered from Down syndrome and intestinal atresia, died without surgical intervention at the request of his parents. Seven other infants had meningomyeloceles (spina bifida), which also were not surgically corrected (Duff and Campbell, 1973). A year earlier, Lorber (1972) had advocated the "selective non-treatment" of infants with spina bifida who met certain diagnostic criteria associated with a poor neurologic prognosis, functional prognosis, or both. The following decade saw a vigorous professional debate about the treatment of newborns with congenital disorders on the basis of their anticipated quality of life, with widespread support for withholding otherwise standard medical or surgical treatment from infants with either Down syndrome or spina bifida.

This debate burst onto the public stage with the 1982 birth of an infant known as "Baby Doe." Born with Down syndrome and a tracheoesophageal fistula, Baby Doe died at 6 days of age of a pulmonary hemorrhage while lawyers were seeking court-ordered treatment over the parents' objection. Aligned with disability rights and antiabortion activists, the Reagan Administration issued a regulation, based on section 504 of the Rehabilitation Act of 1973, that failure to treat disabled newborns was a violation of their rights to equal access. This version of the "Baby Doe" regulations was struck down in 1986 by the U.S. Supreme Court; however, the federal child abuse statutes had already been amended in 1984 to include "failure to provide medically necessary treatment" to disabled newborns under the definition of *child abuse*. The statute provided for only three exceptions; medically necessary treatment could be withheld from a disabled newborn if (1) the infant was irreversibly comatose, (2) the treatment was futile, or (3) providing treatment was inhumane because it would merely prolong suffering for an infant whose death was imminent. Enforcement of these statutes was tied to funding for state child abuse programs, resulting in a patchwork of responses from state legislators. Some states made no change (without any adverse funding consequences); other states simply made procedural changes, such as establishing a special office for disability rights; and yet other states incorporated the revised definition of *child abuse* into specific regulations guiding parent and provider conduct—a situation that remains true today. Thus, the political and legal effects of the "Baby Doe" regulations on parent and provider conduct vary tremendously from state to state.

Significant advances in the care of critically ill newborns were made during this time of social and political controversy. In the 1980s, improvements in technology led to high-profile innovations such as extracorporeal membrane oxygenation (ECMO) for infants with persistent pulmonary hypertension and surgical advances in the treatment of infants with hypoplastic left heart syndrome. As more and more premature infants began to survive, attention shifted to the extremely low birth weight (ELBW) infant. Surfactant replacement for hyaline membrane disease progressed, so that the routine use of surfactant in the 1990s significantly increased the overall survival for ELBW infants. At the same time, public attention shifted to the alleged overtreatment of ELBW premature infants who may have a poor prognosis for meaningful survival. Improvements in fetal imaging and surgical techniques have also made possible fetal surgical interventions both at mid-gestation and just before delivery. Although previously the debate had focused on "selective non-intervention" for infants born with spina bifida, controversy has shifted to the selection criteria for operating on unborn fetuses with spina bifida in hopes of improving neurologic and functional outcomes (Sutton et al, 1999).

## WORKING AT THE EDGES OF VIABILITY

The debate as to whether an ELBW infant should be resuscitated at birth has generally focused on the question of *viability*, defined as the lowest gestational age (GA) at which extrauterine biologic existence is possible. A related distinction between terminal and nonterminal is also used in some state legislation (such as that in Texas) to demarcate when a parent may or may not withhold LSMT (such as resuscitation). However, understanding viability as a biologic property that is either present or absent at birth reinforces the aggressive resuscitation of ELBW infants pending later resolution of the uncertainty by the infant's either living or dying. This simplistic concept of viability fails to capture the complex medical, ethical, and social considerations involved in treatment decisions for ELBW infants. Instead, ELBW infants should be divided into the following three groups (Lorenz and Paneth, 2000):

*Viable*: ELBW infants whom nearly all neonatal clinicians agree should be treated (e.g., GA ≥ 25 weeks)

*Nonviable*: ELBW infants whom nearly all neonatal clinicians agree should not be treated (e.g., GA ≤ 22 weeks)

*Viability uncertain*: ELBW infants about whom there is much disagreement about whether they should undergo resuscitation, intensive treatment, or both (e.g., GA 23 to 24 weeks).

Although surfactant replacement therapy has allowed survival at 23 to 24 weeks of gestation to approach 50% in a few centers, reports of neurodevelopmental outcomes suggest that a significant number of survivors will suffer major disabilities in later childhood (Vohr et al, 2000). The widespread professional disagreement over how to treat an ELBW infant of uncertain viability renders problematic the notion of an accepted standard of medical care for this population (Lorenz and Paneth, 2000). The argument that biologic survival regardless of neurodevelopmental outcome justifies, in retrospect, the resuscitation of an ELBW infant over parental objections dishonors the appropriate moral boundaries of parental discretion.

Grouping ELBW infants in this manner clarifies when a clinician may take unilateral action regardless of parental wishes, and when parental choice should prevail. First, resuscitating a nonviable ELBW infant born at or before 22 weeks of gestation is *strictly futile*, in that endotracheal intubation and ventilation will not be successful in reversing the premature infant's physiologic limitations. Given this restricted definition of futility, unilateral action by a clinician to withhold resuscitation is ethically appropriate and arguably mandatory. Second, for an ELBW infant of uncertain viability, born at 23 to 24 weeks of gestation, reasonable persons may disagree whether the burden of treatment is proportionate to the benefits that can reasonably be expected. The informed judgment of the parent or parents should prevail in this instance over the personal choice of the clinician, resuscitation being withheld if the treatment is judged to be *disproportionately burdensome*. Third, failure to resuscitate an ELBW infant born at 25 weeks of gestation or later may be considered *medical neglect*, in light of such an infant's more favorable chance of an acceptable long-term outcome, and may perhaps justify resuscitation regardless of parental wishes (depending on the presence or absence of other prognostic factors). The use of GA to distinguish these three groups does not imply that GA is a sufficient diagnostic criterion for determining the viability of any given ELBW infant.

## COUNSELING PARENTS AND INFORMED CONSENT

When faced with treatment decisions, new or prospective parents should be fully informed of all the relevant facts, helped to understand and appreciate the meaning of these facts in light of their own beliefs, values, and circumstances, and supported in acting on their choice (if a choice is available). At a minimum, the information that should be provided is as follows: (1) the probable morbidity and mortality associated with the infant's condition, (2) the interventions that are medically indicated, (3) the effect of intervention (and no intervention, if appropriate) on the morbidity and mortality, and (4) the level of uncertainty of these predictions (Harrison, 2001). If the prognosis is reasonably certain either with intervention (i.e., for a viable ELBW infant) or without intervention (i.e., for a nonviable ELBW infant), the clinician can be fairly directive with the parents. If no medical intervention can prevent the imminent death of the infant, counseling should be directed toward the provision of comfort and nurture for the infant and support for the bereaved family. If medical intervention is clearly in the infant's best interest, counseling should be directed to enhance parental understanding and appreciation of the infant's condition, the necessary intervention, and the continued importance of the parental role (Hulac, 2001).

Situations of prognostic uncertainty, such as the ELBW infant of uncertain viability, require a less directive and more collaborative approach to counseling. Sufficient time for such an approach may not be available, given the need for immediate intervention to preserve the possibility of parental choice. Even so, informed consent is not a moment but a process that requires helping the parent or parents understand and appreciate the importance and effect of various interventions (including the undoing of an intervention already performed).

Some clinicians argue that, in addition to information about anticipated morbidity and mortality, parents should be told that most physicians would not want intensive care for their own ELBW infant (Harrison, 2001). Consistently, however, health professionals have been found to value living with a severe disability at a much lower level compared with the reported views of children with disabilities and their parents (Saigal et al, 1999). These findings are often used to argue that medical professionals discriminate against the disabled by pressuring parents to forgo treatment (in spite of lack of evidence of such discrimination even at the height of the "Baby Doe" controversy). Other investigators interpret the positive outlook reported by disabled children and parents as the politically correct "brave face we instinctively offer to the public," contrasted with the private reality of guilt, shame, and regret (Harrison, 2001). Some researchers argue that parents of an ELBW infant of uncertain viability should be informed of the apparent conflict of interest created by financial and professional incentives to provide intensive care as well as the lack of properly conducted research studies for some "recommended" interventions (Harrison, 2001).

Because of the diversity of strongly held opinions, the use of a videotape may help clinicians give a consistent and balanced presentation of the alternatives to parents faced with the difficult choice between continued medical or surgical intervention and supportive care only (Hulac, 2001). Although it is difficult under these trying circumstances, a clinician should try to establish a relationship of trust based on open and honest communication about the various treatment options.

Conversations (and interventions) before birth introduce new complexities. First, there is the added uncertainty of estimating fetal weight and GA before a premature infant can actually be weighed or examined. As a result, most clinicians try to reserve some margin for clinical judgment after an infant's birth. If an infant may be of "uncertain viability," the clinician should discuss the upper and lower boundaries of the classification and seek input from the prospective parent or parents about preferences for resuscitation. Second, until an infant is delivered, clinical decision-making about interventions on behalf of the fetus must balance the best interests of the fetus with a pregnant woman's self-interest in health and freedom from unwanted bodily invasion. Pregnant women almost always accept a recommendation for fetal intervention that is of proven efficacy and low maternal risk. For procedures presenting greater maternal risk, the assessment and choice of the pregnant woman should be respected even if they place the fetus at risk of harm. Interventions of unproven efficacy should be performed only with the informed and voluntary consent of the pregnant woman and should be conducted according to an institutionally approved research protocol (Chervenak and McCullough, 2002). At times, neonatal clinicians may be drawn into situations of conflict when a pregnant woman refuses a recommended intervention.

The American Academy of Pediatrics proposes three conditions that must be met before a clinician opposes the woman's refusal: (1) there is reasonable certainty that the fetus will suffer irrevocable and substantial harm without the intervention, (2) the intervention has been shown to be effective, and (3) the risk to the health and well-being of the pregnant woman is negligible (AAP, 1999). All health care institutions should have a procedure in place for conflict resolution, such as consultation with other clinicians or a clinical ethics committee.

## THE FETUS AS PATIENT

Improvements in fetal diagnosis and imaging, anesthetic management, and surgical techniques provide new approaches for treating neonatal diseases that manifest during pregnancy. Generally, interventions that place the pregnant woman at risk of serious morbidity or mortality have been reserved for fetal conditions believed to have a high risk of mortality with postnatal treatment. Innovative approaches to surgical palliation or correction have been tried (and later abandoned) for severe hydrocephalus and congenital diaphragmatic hernia (CDH). Placement of ventriculoamniotic shunts for aqueductal stenosis did not improve outcome, resulting in a voluntary moratorium on such procedures. An open surgical approach to the repair of CDH failed to better the results of modern neonatal intensive care in one of the few randomized controlled trials of fetal surgery and so was abandoned in favor of clipping the trachea in hopes of improving fetal lung growth (Flake et al, 2000; Harrison et al, 1997). With the development of appropriate selection criteria, maternal-fetal surgical interventions for life-threatening malformations such as fetal urinary tract obstruction, congenital cystic adenomatoid malformation, and sacrococcygeal teratoma have been successful (Harrison, 1996). Amnioreduction and laser photocoagulation have both been used for treatment of twin-twin transfusion syndrome, with a randomized comparative trial currently under way (2004) to determine the optimal approach. Because improved care for the pregnant woman appears to have minimized the risks of fetal intervention, a willingness to develop surgical approaches to nonfatal and disabling conditions, such as myelomeningocele, is emerging (Sutton et al, 1999). A randomized controlled trial comparing prenatal maternal-fetal surgery with standard postnatal surgery for myelomeningocele is currently under way (2004).

The uncontrolled use of maternal-fetal surgery for the prenatal correction of fetal myelomeningocele has generated much controversy (Chervenak and McCullough, 1999; Flake, 2001; Lyerly et al, 2001). The decision for the performance of surgery on a pregnant woman and fetus in hopes of ameliorating the subsequent disability of a child with myelomeningocele involves a complex balancing of risks and benefits to two parties. Invariably, the fetus is delivered prematurely, with the subsequent risks of death and neurodevelopmental disability. The potential benefit is either a reduction in secondary hydrocephalus and the need for shunting or an (unlikely) improvement in lower extremity function. For what may be a marginal gain in neurodevelopmental outcome for the child, the pregnant woman places herself at risk of operative morbidity and mortality as well as the need for future deliveries by cesarean section (Lyerly et al, 2001). Prospective parents choose to risk the death of their unborn child in hopes of avoiding a nonfatal albeit serious disability. In the absence of properly controlled studies, passionate advocates exist on both sides of the debate, including parents convinced that maternal-fetal surgery saved the life and health of their children. Once the feasibility of a surgical innovation has been established, physicians are morally obligated to subject an innovation to the rigors of an appropriately designed research protocol (Chervenak and McCullough, 1999; Lyerly et al, 2001). Otherwise, we are unable to answer the parents' question, "Is the intervention going to help our child?"

## CONGENITAL HEART DISEASE: THE EXAMPLE OF HYPOPLASTIC LEFT HEART SYNDROME

The surgical treatment of infants born with hypoplastic left heart syndrome (HLHS) is a useful example of innovative approaches that evolved over the past 25 years despite the lack of concurrently controlled clinical trials. First reported in 1980, the initial Norwood operation served to prepare the infant for a subsequent modified Fontan procedure (Norwood et al, 1980). In 1991, Norwood described the currently used three-stage approach, in which a hemi-Fontan procedure is performed as an intermediate step to reduce the morbidity and mortality associated with the subsequent Fontan operation. In this report, the rate of survival through the first two stages was 64%, with no early mortality among the 27 patients who underwent the third stage, the Fontan procedure (Norwood et al, 1991).

With the introduction of cyclosporine to control rejection, cardiac transplantation became the treatment of choice at some centers, most notably Loma Linda Health Center. Of 111 infants with HLHS referred for transplant between 1985 and 1991 at Loma Linda, 27 infants died while waiting for a donor heart, and 84 infants underwent cardiac transplantation. Transplant recipients had a 5-year survival rate of 81%, yielding an overall 5-year actuarial survival rate of 61% when all infants are included (Chiavarelli et al, 1993). By the early 1990s, parents were usually offered one of three alternatives (weighed according to clinician and institutional preference): a three-stage surgical repair, cardiac transplantation, or nonoperative supportive care (Gutgesell and Massaro, 1995).

Compared with the mortality rate of historical controls, surgical intervention (whether staged repair or transplant) clearly improved overall survival; however, the perceived burden of treatment and doubts about neurodevelopmental outcomes lent support to nonsurgical supportive care as an acceptable option for parents to consider. However, the options presented to parents began to shift in the mid-1990s. A 1996 survey of 93 neonatology section chiefs indicated that 78% discussed and 24% recommended "comfort care only"; the remaining clinicians recommended either staged repair or transplantation. Although the clinicians perceived the surgical survival rate and subsequent quality of life to favor transplantation, the majority recommended the staged surgical repair, presumably reflecting the lack of availability of infant donor hearts (Caplan et al, 1996). As survival after staged surgical repair continued to improve, reports of neurodevelopmental outcome in children with HLHS were mixed. In one report, cognitive testing of school-age children who previously underwent staged repair of HLHS demonstrated a medial full scale IQ of 86, with one third of the children receiving some form of special education and 18% scoring below 70 (i.e., mental retardation) (Mahle et al, 2000). By comparison, patient actuarial survival for cardiac transplantation as a primary treatment for HLHS was 70% at both 7 years and 10 years, with late deaths occurring from rejection or graft vasculopathy. School-age children who underwent cardiac transplantation in infancy demonstrated average achievement and low average intelligence scores on testing (Fortuna et al, 1999).

Although a head-to-head comparison of staged surgical repair and cardiac transplantation has not been performed, decision analysis based on data from 1989 through 1994 suggests that staged surgical repair optimizes first-year survival in the presence of a low (<10%) organ donation rate and stage 1 mortality of less than 20% (Jenkins et al, 2001). Later reports suggest that a stage 1 survival rate of 80% is achievable at selected centers, a rate consistent with the finding that staged surgical repair has become the most common management strategy for infants born with HLHS (Gutgesell and Gibson, 2002).

The uncontrolled surgical experiment of the 1980s and 1990s demonstrates the efficacy of both staged surgical repair and cardiac transplantation for HLHS when compared with untreated nonsurgical historical controls. Even though questions remain about the comparative advantages of the two surgical approaches, should parents continue to be offered the option of "comfort care only" for an infant born with HLHS? In experienced centers, such an infant now has a greater than 50% chance of surviving through all three staged surgical procedures, and the majority of infants so treated have an acceptable neurodevelopmental outcome. Therefore, some (perhaps most) clinicians believe that parents should no longer have the option of "comfort care only." Others remain concerned that the overall burden of treatment for both child and family remains significant, arguing that parents should continue to have a choice whether to bear that burden. In addition, some infants are born at a significant distance from an experienced center, adding the burden of transfer and perhaps family relocation to the equation. Nevertheless, it is increasingly difficult to justify the withholding of surgical treatment from infants born with HLHS in the absence of new information about an unacceptable burden of treatment or poor neurodevelopmental outcomes.

## PALLIATIVE CARE AND THE NEONATAL INTENSIVE CARE UNIT

Recent years have seen a growing concern about limiting or withdrawing LSMT in favor of supportive or palliative care for infants whose prospects for meaningful survival are uncertain at best (Catlin and Carter, 2002; Fost, 1999). In general, there is no obligation to either initiate or continue to provide LSMT when doing so would be either futile or unduly burdensome. Although there may be widespread agreement with this principle, knowing when any given treatment is either futile or unduly burdensome for a particular infant may be difficult. Many neonatologists support the strategy of treating each infant on the basis of an individualized prognosis, but the ability to predict an unacceptable outcome to a reasonable degree of certainty is problematic (Meadow et al, 2002). Limitation or withdrawal of LSMT may be a consideration for ELBW newborns who are of uncertain viability or who suffer a life-limiting complication, newborns with complex or multiple congenital anomalies that are incompatible with prolonged life, and newborns who are not responding to intervention, are deteriorating despite all appropriate efforts, or suffer a life-threatening event (Catlin and Carter, 2002). Agreeing on an appropriate course of action requires a collaborative relationship with a family based on trust and open communication, supplemented as needed with an ethics or other consultation.

Clinicians may fear that once a treatment is started, it is more difficult to stop. Legally, there is no difference between not starting a treatment that is either futile or unduly burdensome and stopping it (Meisel et al, 2000). The general view is that there is no moral difference between starting and stopping treatment that is not medically indicated, and that the fear that there is a difference stems from the psychological difficulty of removing LSMT. This view, however, assumes that our technology is value-neutral. The application of current technology brings with it the moral and social values that shape it, as, for example, in the decision to perform a tracheostomy for long-term ventilator support. The moral and social landscape shifts in a way that is not value-neutral once the tracheostomy has been performed. Although a trial of therapy may be necessary before one decides to withdraw LSMT, it may be best to delay certain decisions (such as placement of a tracheostomy or a gastrostomy tube) until after the family has resolved any uncertainty about continuing LSMT.

The concept of futility has been proposed as a justification for physicians to unilaterally withhold or withdraw LSMT over the objections of family members. However, the concept of futility is subject to different interpretations, from the more restrictive "strictly futile"—meaning that a treatment simply will not work physiologically—to the broader "disproportionate burden"—meaning that the burden of treatment outweighs any potential benefit. Judgments about the disproportionate burden of treatment involve the relative value and risk (or probability) of different outcomes and should not be imposed unilaterally. Treatments that are strictly futile can be withdrawn or withheld unilaterally, but this label applies to an extremely limited set of interventions. For example, continued endotracheal intubation and mechanical ventilation are not strictly futile even for an anencephalic infant, because such support corrects the physiologic abnormality of respiratory insufficiency. Every institution should have a policy for conflict resolution that makes available to staff and parents a stepwise process consisting of enhanced communication, followed by negotiation, mediation, and, in instances of irresolvable conflict, court proceedings. The policy should emphasize the importance of communication in preventing differences of opinion escalating into conflict and should also support and empower parents as the primary decision-makers when an infant's prospects for meaningful survival are unavoidably uncertain.

Whether or not a parent agrees to a "do not attempt resuscitation" (DNAR) order should be placed in the context of the infant's overall care plan. A physician may decide not to perform cardiopulmonary resuscitation (CPR) in the absence of a DNAR order, on the basis of an assessment of strict futility. The details and duration of CPR should be tailored to the needs and condition of the infant, with CPR perhaps limited to a short but focused intervention. The presence of a DNAR order allows nursing and other ancillary personnel to not start CPR while waiting for a physician to arrive. Obtaining a DNAR order is often more important to the staff than to parents, relieving staff anxiety and serving as a "symbol" that the parents have accepted the infant's condition. However, prematurely pushing a parent to agree to a DNAR order without proper preparation through previous discussions of palliative care may precipitate a defensive posture (i.e., premature closure on the decision to "do everything" for the child). Parents also should be persuaded, through the actions of all medical personnel, of the truth of the oft-quoted cliché "*Do not resuscitate* does not mean *do not care*." A DNAR order can be consistent with continued treatment with the hope for recovery, however remote. Finally, the interventions associated with CPR have different effects on the perceived burden of care, lending support for customized DNAR orders, such as allowing for the use of bag-valve-mask ventilation or the administration of medication but not chest compressions.

Attention should always be paid to the relief of an infant's pain and agitation. Once a decision is made to either limit or withdraw LSMT, relieving an infant's pain and agitation should become a primary goal regardless of the risks of undesired consequences, such as hypotension and respiratory depression. Although an infant's life may be shortened by the appropriate administration of sedatives and analgesics, a clinician should not administer medications with the primary purpose of killing the infant. Neuromuscular blocking agents mask signs of distress and should not be administered when ventilatory support is being withdrawn. In addition, such medications should ideally be withdrawn to allow for the proper assessment and treatment of an infant's pain and agitation (Truog et al, 2000). In some limited circumstances, waiting for the effects of neuromuscular blockade to dissipate will impose an undue burden on the infant and family; the discussion with the family about this issue should be documented, and careful attention paid to providing adequate sedation and analgesia in light of the difficulty in assessment (Catlin and Carter, 2002). Finally, there may be other interventions that can and should be withdrawn, such as inotropic and other cardiovascular support, as part of a decision to withdraw LSMT. For a number of infants, limitation or withdrawal of cardiovascular support may be an acceptable option for parents who are reluctant to limit or withdraw mechanical ventilation.

## NEONATAL RESEARCH

Absent significant mortality in historical controls, advancements in neonatal care will require concurrently controlled clinical trials. The continued use of unproven or innovative therapies that have not been validated through properly designed clinical trials does little to advance our knowledge of those interventions that truly benefit critically ill neonates (Tyson, 1995). Recognizing the difficulty of obtaining informed and voluntary consent from the parents in situations of stress, we should nevertheless provide unproven treatments within the context of a clinical trial (Mason and Allmark, 2000; Tyson and Knudsen, 2000). Clinical trials usually involve a number of interventions, with the risks and benefits requiring individual consideration. Interventions or procedures that do not offer the prospect of direct benefit must present no more than a minor increase over minimal risk, assuming that the information to be obtained is vital to the understanding or amelioration of the infant's condition. Interventions or procedures that offer the prospect of direct benefit may present more than a minor increase over minimal risk but can only be offered if there is genuine uncertainty on the part of the expert medical community about the comparative therapeutic merits of the experimental interventions and standard medical care (Freedman, 1987).

## JUSTICE AND THE DISTRIBUTION OF HEALTH CARE

Ethnic and racial disparities continue to exist in the provision of prenatal and neonatal medical care, with subsequent differences in infant mortality. Improvements in infant mortality based on the provision of neonatal intensive care to premature infants appear to have leveled off since 1995, suggesting that further investments in such care will have limited impact. There have been isolated efforts to redistribute available health care resources away from extremely premature infants toward more effective services, most notably in Oregon (Demissie et al, 2001; Horbar et al, 2002; Merkens and Garland, 2001). These efforts have been unsuccessful in shifting resources away from the provision of neonatal intensive care to the prevention of the birth of premature infants through equalizing access to known effective interventions such as prenatal care. The continued racial disparity in the provision of appropriate and effective prenatal and neonatal medical care remains the most egregious ethical problem facing neonatology today.

## SELECTED READINGS

American Academy of Pediatrics (AAP), Committee on Bioethics and Committee on Hospital Care. Palliative care for children. Pediatrics 106:351-357, 2000.

American Academy of Pediatrics, Committee on Bioethics. Ethics and the care of critically ill infants and children. Pediatrics 98:149-152, 1996.

American College of Obstetricians and Gynecologists: ACO Practice Bulletin: Clinical Management Guidelines for Obstetrician-Gynecologists. Number 38, September 2002. Perinatal care at the threshold of viability. Obstet Gynecol 100:617-624, 2002.

Caplan AL, Blank RH, Merrick JC (eds): Compelled compassion: government intervention in the treatment of critically ill newborns. Contemporary issues in biomedicine, ethics, and society. Totowa, NJ, Humana Press, 1992, p 336.

Helft PR, Siegler M, Lantos J: The rise and fall of the futility movement. N Engl J Med 343:293-236, 2000.

## REFERENCES


American Academy of Pediatrics, Committee on Bioethics. Fetal therapy: Ethical considerations. Pediatrics 103:1061-1063, 1999.

Caplan WD, Cooper TR, Garcia-Prats JA, Brody BA: Diffusion of innovative approaches to managing hypoplastic left heart syndrome. Arch Pediatr Adolesc Med 150:487-490, 1996.

Catlin A, Carter B: Creation of a neonatal end-of-life palliative care protocol. J Perinatol 22:184-195, 2002.

Chervenak FA, McCullough LB: A comprehensive ethical framework for fetal research and its application to fetal surgery for spina bifida. Am J Obstet Gynecol 187:10-14, 2002.

Chiavarelli M, Grundy SR, Razzouk AJ, Bailey LL: Cardiac transplantation for infants with hypoplastic left-heart syndrome. JAMA 270:2944-2947, 1993.

Demissie K, Rhoads GG, Ananth CV, et al: Trends in preterm birth and neonatal mortality among blacks and whites in the United States from 1989 to 1997. Am J Epidemiol 154:307-315, 2001.

Duff RS, Campbell AG: Moral and ethical dilemmas in the special-care nursery. N Engl J Med 289: 890-894, 1973.

Flake AW: Prenatal intervention: Ethical considerations for life-threatening and non-life-threatening anomalies. Semin Pediatr Surg 10:212-221, 2001.

Flake AW, Cromblehome TM, Johnson MP, et al: Treatment of severe congenital diaphragmatic hernia by fetal tracheal occlusion: Clinical experience with fifteen cases. Am J Obstet Gynecol 183:1059-1066, 2000.

Fortuna RS, Chinnock RE, Bailey LL: Heart transplantation among 233 infants during the first six months of life: The Loma Linda experience. Loma Linda Pediatric Heart Transplant Group. Clin Transplants 1999:263-272, 1999.

Fost N: Decisions regarding treatment of seriously ill newborns. JAMA 281:2041-2043, 1999.

Freedman B: Equipoise and the ethics of clinical research. N Engl J Med 317:141-145, 1987.

Gutgesell HP, Gibson J: Management of hypoplastic left heart syndrome in the 1990s. Am J Cardiol 89:842-846, 2002.

Gutgesell HP, Massaro TA: Management of hypoplastic left heart syndrome in a consortium of university hospitals. Am J Cardiol 76:809-811, 1995.

Harrison H: Making lemonade: A parent's view of "quality of life" studies. J Clin Ethics 12:239-250, 2001.

Harrison MR: Fetal surgery. Am J Obstet Gynecol 174:1255-1264, 1996.

Harrison MR, Adzick NS, Bullard KM, et al: Correction of congenital diaphragmatic hernia in utero. VII: A prospective trial. J Pediatr Surg 32:1637-1642, 1997.

Horbar JD, Badger GJ, Carpenter JH, et al: Trends in mortality and morbidity for very low birth weight infants, 1991-1999. Pediatrics 110:143-151, 2002.

Hulac P: Creation and use of You Are Not Alone, a video for parents facing difficult decisions. J Clin Ethics 12:251-253, 2001.

Jenkins PC, Flanagan ME, Sargent JD, et al: A comparison of treatment strategies for hypoplastic left heart syndrome using decision analysis. J Am Coll Cardiol 38:1181-1187, 2001.

Lorber J: Spina bifida cystica: Results of treatment of 270 consecutive cases with criteria for selection for the future. Arch Dis Child 4:854-873, 1972.

Lorenz JM, Paneth N: Treatment decisions for the extremely premature infant. J Pediatr 137:593-595, 2000.

Lyerly AD, Cefalo RC, Socol M, et al: Toward the ethical evaluation and use of maternal-fetal surgery. Obstet Gynecol 98:689-697, 2001.

Mahle WT, Clancy RR, Moss EM, et al: Neurodevelopmental outcome and lifestyle assessment in school-aged and adolescent children with hypoplastic left heart syndrome. Pediatrics 105:1082-1089, 2000.

Mason SA, Allmark PJ: Obtaining informed consent to neonatal randomised controlled trials: Interviews with parents and clinicians in the Euricon study. Lancet 356(9247):2045-2051, 2000.

Meadow W, Frain L, Ren Y, et al: Serial assessment of mortality in the neonatal intensive care unit by algorithm and intuition: Certainty, uncertainty, and informed consent. Pediatrics 109:878-886. 2002.

Meisel A, Snyder L, Quill T, et al: Seven legal barriers to end-of-life care: Myths, realities, and grains of truth. JAMA 284:2495-2501, 2000.

Merkens MJ, Garland MJ: The Oregon Health Plan and the ethics of care for marginally viable newborns. J Clin Ethics 12:266-274, 2001.

Norwood WI Jr: Hypoplastic left heart syndrome. Ann Thorac Surg 52:688-695, 1991.

Norwood WI, Kirklin JK, Sanders SP: Hypoplastic left heart syndrome: Experience with palliative surgery. Am J Cardiol 45:87-91, 1980.

Saigal S, Stoskopf BL, Feeny D, et al: Differences in preferences for neonatal outcomes among health care professionals, parents, and adolescents. JAMA 281:1991-1997, 1999.

Sutton LN, Adzick NS, Bilaniuk LT, et al: Improvement in hindbrain herniation demonstrated by serial fetal magnetic resonance imaging following fetal surgery for myelomeningocele. JAMA 282:1826-1831, 1999.

Truog RD, Burns JP, Mitchell C, et al: Pharmacologic paralysis and withdrawal of mechanical ventilation at the end of life. N Engl J Med 342:508-511, 2000.

Tyson JE: Use of unproven therapies in clinical practice and research: How can we better serve our patients and their families? Semin Perinatol 19:98-111, 1995.

Tyson JE, Knudson PL: Views of neonatologists and parents on consent for clinical trials. Lancet 356(9247):2026-2027, 2000.

Vohr BR, Wright LL, Dusick AM, et al: Neurodevelopmental and functional outcomes of extremely low birth weight infants in the National Institute of Child Health and Human Development Neonatal Research Network, 1993-1994. Pediatrics 105:1216-1226, 2000.

# FETAL DEVELOPMENT

Editor: ROBERTA A. BALLARD

CHAPTER 4

## Placental Function and Diseases: The Placenta, Fetal Membranes, and Umbilical Cord

William M. Gilbert and Geoffrey A. Machin

In most normal pregnancies, the newborn is healthy and goes home in a day or two with the mother. If unexpected complications develop in the newborn period, the placenta has quite often been discarded and is therefore unavailable for examination for clues to help determine possible causes of these problems. Physicians involved in the delivery of high-risk pregnancies usually send the placenta to the pathology department for a pathologic examination. A detailed examination often yields clues helpful in the management of such high-risk pregnancies. The same is not necessarily true of the normal pregnancy. Thorough examination of the placenta at the time of birth may identify some abnormality that would be of assistance in explaining complications in the newborn. For this reason, anyone involved in the care of pregnant women or their newborns should be able to examine a placenta and know the basics of normal and abnormal architecture.

This chapter examines the normal development of the placenta and the development of particular disease states relating to it. In addition, placental hormones, the immunology of the placenta, and abnormalities of amniotic fluid volume are summarized. Finally, an extensive list of placental findings associated with disease conditions is presented in an easy-to-read table format.

### EMBRYOLOGIC DEVELOPMENT OF THE PLACENTA

Shortly after fertilization takes place in the ampullary portion of the fallopian tube, the fertilized ovum or zygote begins dividing into a ball of cells called a morula. As the morula enters the uterus (by the fourth day after fertilization), it forms a central cystic area and is called a blastocyst. The blastocyst implants within the endometrium by day 7 (Moore, 1988).

The blastocyst has two components, an inner cell mass, which becomes the developing embryo, and the outer cell layer, which becomes the placenta and fetal membranes (Hertig, 1968). The cells of the developing *blastocyst*, which eventually become the placenta, are differentiated quite early in gestation (within 7 days after fertilization). The outer cell layer, the *trophoblast*, invades the endometrium to the level of the decidua basalis. Maternal blood vessels are also invaded en route (Fig. 4–1). Once entered and controlled by the trophoblast, these maternal blood vessels form *lacunae*, which provide nutrition and substrates for the developing products of conception. The trophoblast differentiates into two cell types, the inner cytotrophoblast and the outer syncytiotrophoblast (see Fig. 4–1). The former has distinct cell walls and is thought to represent the more immature form of trophoblast. The syncytiotrophoblast, which is essentially acellular, is the site of most placental hormone and metabolic activity. Once the trophoblast has invaded the endometrium, it begins to form outpouchings called *villi*, which extend into the blood-filled maternal lacunae or further invade the endometrium to attach more solidly with the decidua, forming anchoring villi.

The three types of villi are related to the location and stage of development. Figure 4–2 shows primary, secondary, and tertiary villi; they are classified according to whether they contain cytotrophoblastic tissue with or without fetal blood vessels. In Figure 4–3, a scanning electron micrograph of terminal villi is shown.

### PLACENTAL CIRCULATION

With the formation of the tertiary villi (19 days after fertilization), a direct vascular connection is made between the developing embryo and the placenta (Moore, 1988). Umbilical circulation between the placenta and the embryo is evident by 5½ weeks of gestation. Figure 4–4 demonstrates aspects of the maternal and fetal circulation in the mature placenta. The umbilical arteries from the fetus reach the placenta and then divide repetitively to cover the fetal surface of the placenta. Terminal arteries then penetrate the individual cotyledons, forming capillary beds for substrate exchange within the tertiary villi. These capillaries then re-form into tributaries of the umbilical venous system, which carries oxygenated blood back to the fetus.

It is evident that the fetal circulatory system is a closed system having no direct connection with the maternal blood. Indeed, maternally delivered substrates must cross

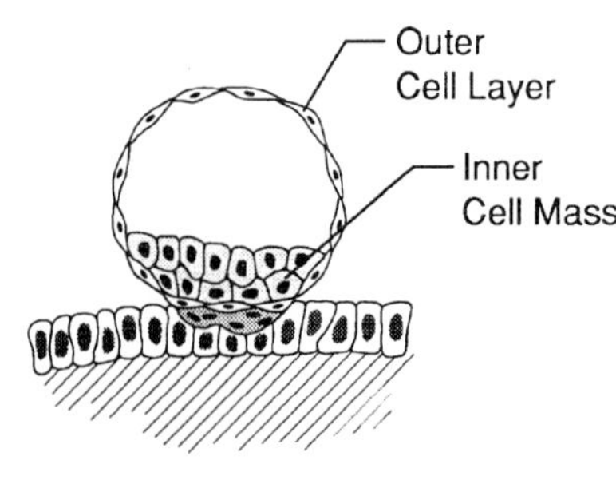


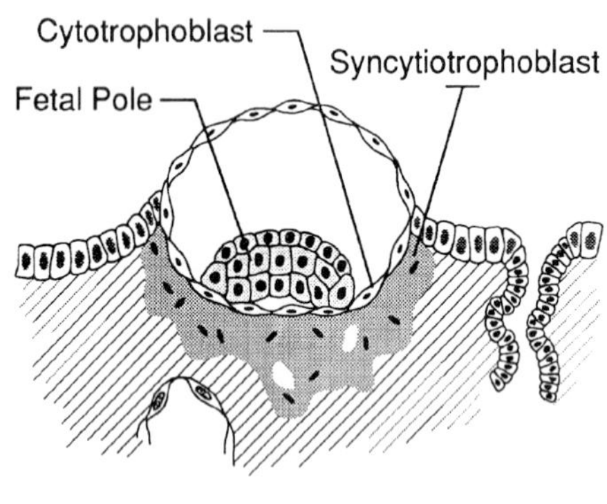


**FIGURE 4–1.** **A,** The human blastocyst contains two portions, an inner cell mass, which develops into the embryo, and an outer cell layer, which develops into the placenta and membranes. **B,** The outer acellular layer is the syncytiotrophoblast, and the inner cellular layer is the cytotrophoblast. *(In Moore TR, Reiter RC, Rebar RW, Baker VV [eds]: Gynecology and Obstetrics: A Longitudinal Approach. New York, Churchill Livingstone, 1993, p 209. From Gilbert WM: Anatomy and physiology of the placenta, fetal membranes, and amniotic fluid.)*

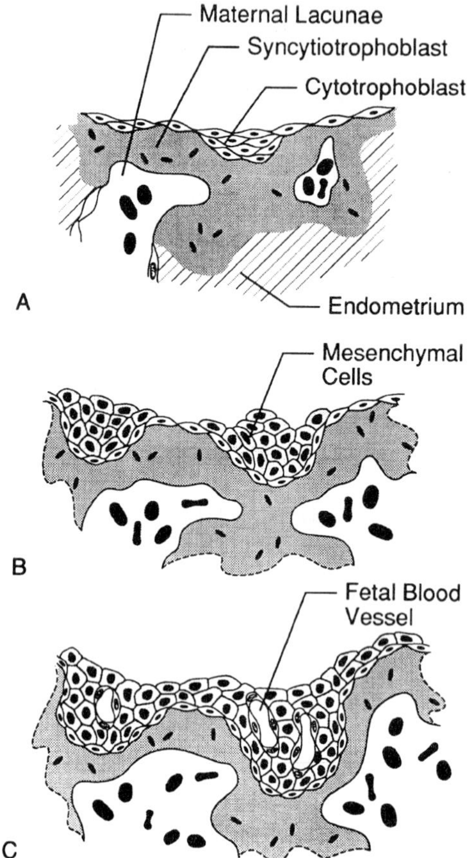


**FIGURE 4–2.** **A,** The cytotrophoblast indents the syncytiotrophoblast to form primary villi. **B,** Mesenchymal cells invade the cytotrophoblast 2 days after formation of the primary villi to form secondary villi. **C,** Blood vessels arise de novo and eventually connect with blood vessels from the embryo, forming tertiary villi. *(In Moore TR, Reiter RC, Rebar RW, Baker VV [eds]: Gynecology and Obstetrics: A Longitudinal Approach. New York, Churchill Livingstone, 1993, p 209. From Gilbert WM: Anatomy and physiology of the placenta, fetal membranes, and amniotic fluid.)*

three tissue layers within the villus in order to reach the fetal blood. Despite this barrier, however, fetal cells have been identified within the maternal circulation and vice versa. Research attempting to use these cells of fetal origin within the maternal circulation for prenatal diagnosis is under way (Steel et al, 1996).

Maternal blood enters the intervillous space in a pulsatile fashion with each maternal heartbeat, bathing the fetal villi with blood and providing a site for exchange of nutrients and waste products. The maternal blood then collects in sinuses at the basilar layer of the intervillous space and flows into the uterine vein. This type of placenta, in which the maternal blood is in contact only with the fetal trophoblast, is *hemochorial*.

## PLACENTAL ANATOMY

At term, the normal placenta covers roughly one third of the interior portion of the uterus and weighs approximately 500 g. The appearance is of a flat circular disc about 2 to 3 cm thick and 15 to 20 cm across (Benirschke and Kaufmann, 2000). Placental and fetal weights throughout gestation are presented in Table 4–1. During the first trimester and into the second, the placenta weighs more than the fetus; after that period, the fetus outweighs the placenta.

The umbilical cord normally inserts into the center of the placenta but may insert in other locations, such as the margin (*marginal* or battledore insertion) or onto the membranes (*velamentous* insertion) (Fig. 4–5) before they join the border of the placenta. In the case of a velamentous insertion, in which the umbilical cord inserts into the amnionic membrane and fetal blood vessels travel within the membranes for a distance, perinatal outcome may be poor (Case Study 1). If the fetal vessels cross the cervical os, a high-risk condition called vasa *previa* is present (Pent, 1979). Rupture of the amniotic membrane in labor may rupture fetal vessels near the cervical os, resulting in fatal hemorrhage. Most vaginal bleeding before and during labor is of maternal origin, but with new-onset vaginal bleeding and simultaneous evidence of fetal distress, the diagnosis of vasa previa must be considered if fetal death from exsanguination is to be prevented.

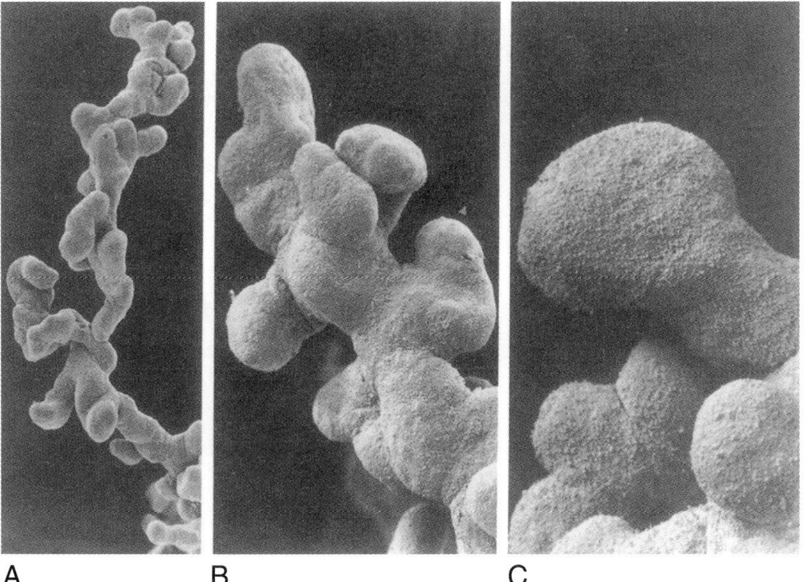


**FIGURE 4–3.** Scanning electron microscopic appearance of terminal villi. **A,** A single, long, mature intermediate villus shows the characteristic bends of its longitudinal axis and multiple grape-like terminal villi. Note the terminal villi largely have the same diameter as the mature intermediate villus from which they branch (×180). **B,** Tip of mature intermediate villus with rich final branching into terminal villi (×470). **C,** A group of terminal villi, the central one showing a typical constricted neck region and a dilated final portion (×500). *(From Kauffmann P, Sen DK, Schweikhart G: Classification of human placental villi. I: Histology and scanning electron microscopy. Cell Tissue Res 200:409, 1979.)*

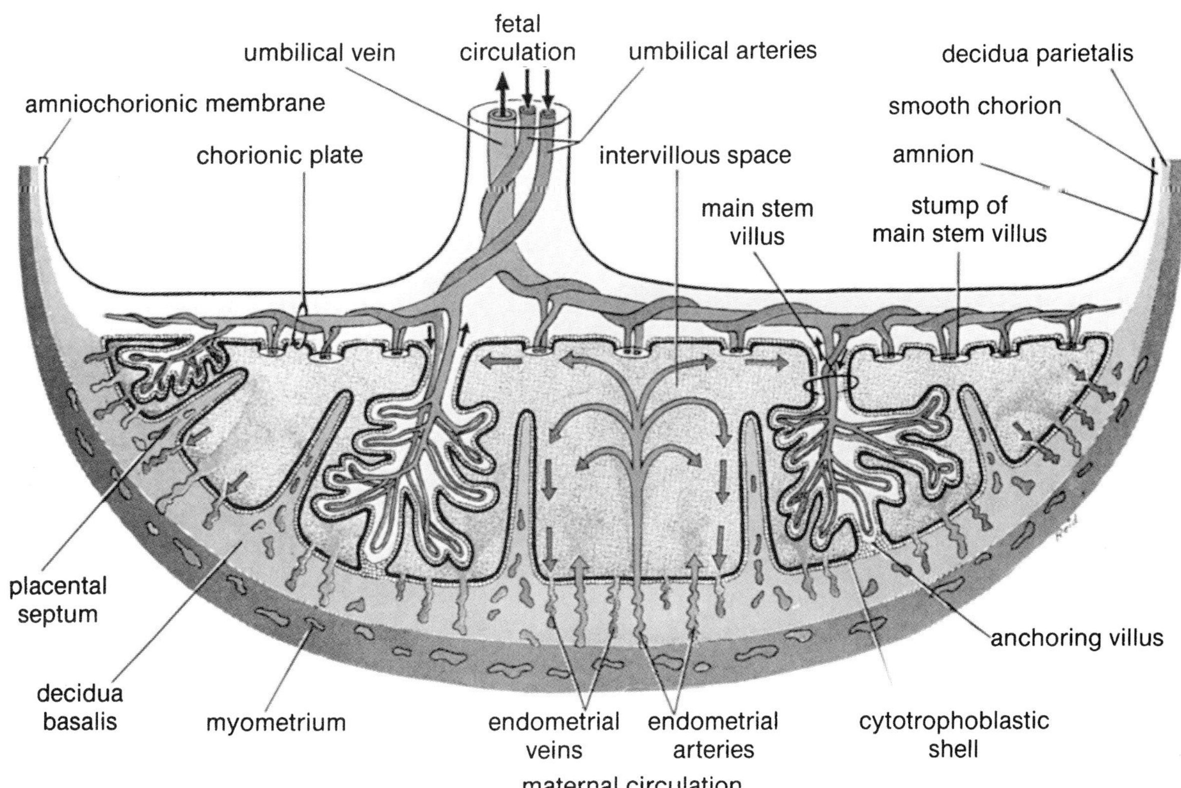


**FIGURE 4–4.** Schematic drawing of a section of a mature placenta showing (1) the relation of the villous chorion (fetal part of the placenta) to the decidua basalis (maternal part of the placenta), (2) the fetal placental circulation, and (3) the maternal placental circulation. Maternal blood flows into the intervillous spaces in funnel-shaped spurts, and exchanges occur with the fetal blood as the maternal blood flows around the villi. Note that the umbilical arteries carry deoxygenated fetal blood to the placenta, and the umbilical vein carries oxygenated blood to the fetus. Note also that the cotyledons are separated from each other by decidual septa of the maternal portion of the placenta. Each cotyledon consists of two or more main-stem villi and their main branches. In this drawing, only one main-stem villus is shown in each cotyledon, but the stumps of those that have been removed are shown. *(From Moore KL: The Developing Human: Clinically Oriented Embryology, 5th ed. Philadelphia, WB Saunders, 1993, p 117.)*

**TABLE 4–1**

**Fetal and Placental Weights Throughout Gestation**

| Gestational Age (wks) | Placental Weight (mg) | Fetal Weight (g) |
|---|---|---|
| 14 | 45 | — |
| 16 | 65 | 59 |
| 18 | 90 | 155 |
| 20 | 115 | 250 |
| 22 | 150 | 405 |
| 24 | 185 | 560 |
| 26 | 217 | 780 |
| 28 | 250 | 1000 |
| 30 | 282 | 1270 |
| 32 | 315 | 1550 |
| 34 | 352 | 1925 |
| 36 | 390 | 2300 |
| 38 | 430 | 2850 |
| 40 | 470 | 3400 |

Adapted from Benirschke K, Kaufmann P: Pathology of the Human Placenta, 4th ed. New York, Springer-Verlag, 2000.

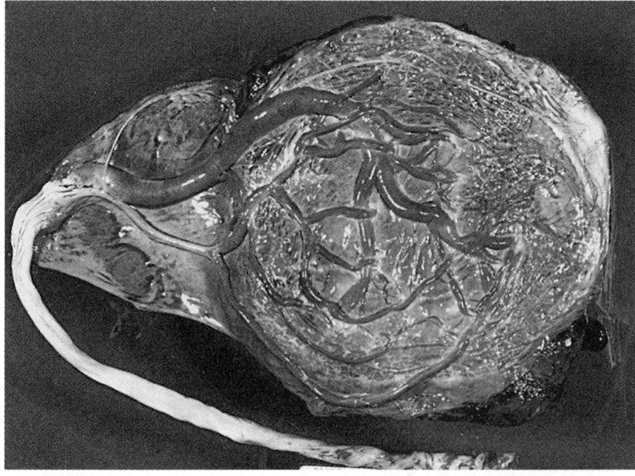

**FIGURE 4–5.** Velamentous insertion of the umbilical cord onto the membranes with fetal vessels running onto the placenta.

In early pregnancy the placenta covers most of the inside of the uterus. At 20 weeks of gestation, approximately 5% of placentas cover the cervix and thus are classified as *placenta previa* (Townsend et al, 1986). By 37 weeks, however, fewer than 1% are still "previa" (Newton et al, 1984). This apparent placental movement away from the cervical os is *placental migration*. The placenta does not actually migrate; further differential growth of the uterus and the placenta results in positioning of the placenta away from the cervix. When the placental tissue remains centrally placed over the cervix, a diagnosis of *complete placenta previa* is made. The complications of pregnancy associated with placenta previa derive from the risk of massive hemorrhage when the cervix begins to dilate. Patients with placenta previa almost always require a cesarean section, although rare cases of successful vaginal delivery through a complete placenta previa have been reported.

Other abnormalities of placental development include the presence of an accessory lobe of placenta, which may be connected to the main portion of the placenta by only a strand of fetal blood vessels and membranes. This condition, called succenturiate *placenta* (Fig. 4–6), may be problematic if the accessory lobe of placenta is inadvertently left within the uterus at the time of delivery. The retained placental tissue may cause postpartum hemorrhage or infection, requiring curettage for removal. For this reason, placental examination after delivery should include inspection of the placental edges to look for ragged portions suggestive of a succenturiate lobe.

In another recognized placental abnormality, the chorionic portion of the fetal membranes does not insert at the edge of the placenta but rather inserts some distance more centrally. This condition, called *circumvallate placenta*, occurs in about 5% of pregnancies (Fig. 4–7) and is associated with antepartum bleeding, preterm labor, intrauterine growth restriction (IUGR), and a single umbilical artery (Naftolin et al, 1973). The cause of this condition is largely unknown (Case Study 2).

**CASE STUDY 1**

A 29-year-old woman presented in her first pregnancy at 41 weeks of gestation with a stillbirth. The patient had noted good fetal movement until one day before admission, at which point she noted the sudden loss of movement. A nonstress test conducted 3 days before presentation demonstrated a reactive fetal heart rate tracing with one variable deceleration. The amniotic fluid index (AFI) was normal at 12 cm. An ultrasonographic examination on admission demonstrated no amniotic fluid and the stillbirth. The patient underwent induction of labor with the delivery of a 3100-g female fetus. An autopsy did not demonstrate any congenital defects, and there was no sign of chorioamnionitis. The only abnormal finding on placental examination was the presence of a velamentous insertion of the umbilical cord (see Fig. 4–5). A velamentous insertion of the umbilical cord often exposes the umbilical blood vessels to compression from fetal parts, because the vessels are not protected by Wharton's jelly within the normal umbilical cord.

**CASE STUDY 2**

A 2075-g newborn male infant was delivered by forceps because of increased vaginal bleeding during the second stage of labor. The Apgar scores were 6 at 1 minute and 8 at 5 minutes. The gestational age at delivery was 39 weeks, and the baby was given the diagnosis small for gestational age (SGA), with a birth weight below the 10th percentile for gestational age. The maternal history included continued bleeding and spotting throughout the second and third trimesters with increasing contractions but no cervical dilation. Ultrasonographic examinations had demonstrated a picture consistent with asymmetrical intrauterine growth restriction and low-normal amniotic fluid volume. The placental examination demonstrated a circumvallate placenta (see Fig. 4–7).

## FETAL MEMBRANES

After delivery, the placenta and membranes should be inspected for completeness. What appears at delivery to be a single membrane is actually made up of two closely

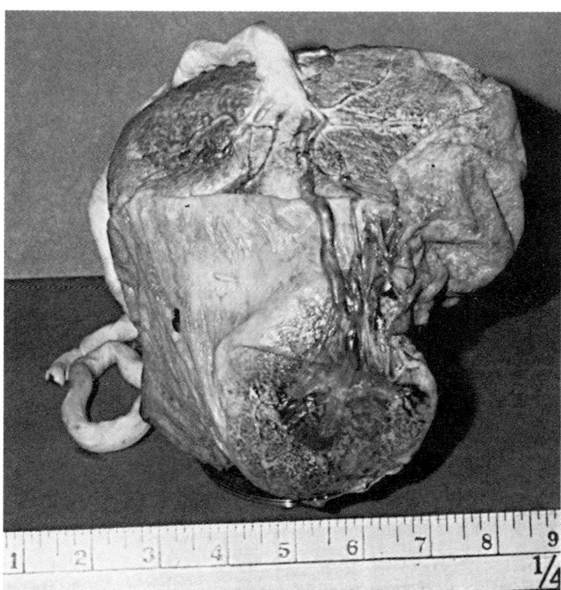

**FIGURE 4–6.** Succenturiate placenta, or accessory lobe. Note the membrane connecting the separate lobes of placental tissue.

applied membranes, an inner amnion and outer chorion. The chorion is covered with villi early in pregnancy. Later, the majority of the villi degenerate, except in the area where the placenta is located. The inner membrane is derived from the developing embryo and grows and expands to fill the extraembryonic coelom, which is the fluid filled area surrounding the early embryo. By 13 weeks of gestation, the amnion joins with the chorion. Before this time, the amnion may be seen on ultrasonographic examination as a thin inner membrane surrounding the embryo. The two membranes remain closely applied for the remainder of the pregnancy and can be manually separated after birth.

## UMBILICAL CORD

The umbilical cord averages 50 cm in length, although a wide range of normal lengths is recognized. The cord should be measured only if it is at one or the other extremes of length (Benirschke and Kaufmann, 2000). The overall length of the umbilical cord is determined by fetal activity in utero, cords being longer for more active fetuses and shorter in association with less activity. The umbilical cord usually contains two umbilical arteries and one umbilical vein. An umbilical cord with only two vessels (one artery, one vein) occurs about 1% of the time and is associated with an increase in fetal structural malformations and chromosomal abnormalities (Leung and Robson, 1989). If the diagnosis of a single umbilical artery is made either before or after birth, the fetus or newborn should undergo complete examination for other abnormalities, with particular attention to the fetal kidneys and heart. In some cases, a two-vessel cord should be an indication for an amniocentesis and chromosomal analysis (Nicolaides et al, 1993).

## EXAMINATION OF THE PLACENTA

A renaissance in placental pathology has led to a new relevance of the placenta to neonatology and early infant life, including issues of preterm birth, growth restriction, and cerebral, renal, and myocardial diseases. The placenta can give some clues to the timing and extent of important adverse prenatal or neonatal events as well as to the relative effects of sepsis and asphyxia on the causation of neonatal diseases. This section reviews placental disorders that can be noted immediately in the delivery room and others that are diagnosed through detailed gross and microscopic examinations over the ensuing 48 hours but that remain important for early childhood development and also have medical-legal significance. Every placenta should be examined at the time of birth regardless of whether the newborn has any immediate problems. Most placentas invert with traction at the time of delivery, and the fetal membranes cover the maternal surface. It is important to reinvert the membranes and examine all surfaces of the placenta and membranes, looking for abnormalities. Table 4–2 lists pregnancy complications or conditions diagnosable at birth through gross examination of the placenta.

The initial placental examination should include checking the edges for completeness. The membranes and fetal surface should be shiny and translucent. An odor may

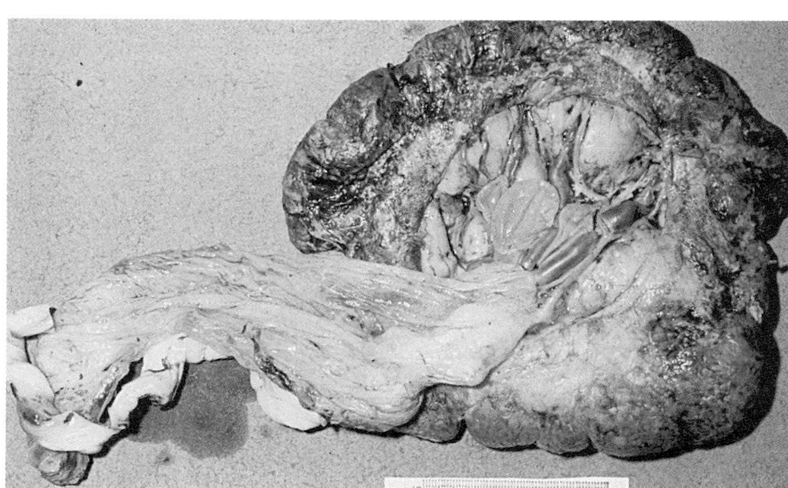

**FIGURE 4–7.** Circumvallate placenta. Note the insertion of the membranes into the placenta halfway between the edge of the placenta and the center.

**TABLE 4–2**

**Pregnancy Conditions Diagnosable at Birth by Gross Placental Examination and Associated Neonatal Outcomes**

| | |
|---|---|
| Monochorionic twinning | Twin-twin transfusion (TTT) syndrome donor/recipient status, pump twin in TRAP, survivor status after fetal demise, selective termination, severe growth discordance without TTT |
| Dichorionic twinning | Less likelihood of survivor brain disease in event of fetal demise of one |
| Purulent acute chorioamnionitis | Risk of fetal sepsis, fetal inflammatory response syndrome, cerebral palsy |
| Chorangioma | Hydrops, cardiac failure, consumptive coagulopathy |
| Abnormal cord coiling | IUGR, fetal intolerance of labor |
| Maternal floor infarction | IUGR, cerebral disease |
| Abruption | Asphyxial brain disease |
| Velamentous cord | IUGR, vasa previa |
| Cord knot | Asphyxia |
| Chronic abruption oligohydramnios syndrome (CAOS) | IUGR |
| Single umbilical artery | Malformation, IUGR |
| Umbilical vein thrombosis | Asphyxia |
| Amnion nodosum | Severe oligohydramnios leading to pulmonary hypoplasia |
| Meconium staining | Possible asphyxia, aspiration lung disease |
| Amniotic bands | Fetal limb reduction abnormalities |
| Chorionic plate vascular thrombosis | Asphyxia, possible thrombophilia |
| Breus mole | Asphyxia, ?IUGR |

IUGR, intrauterine growth retardation; TRAP, twin reversed arterial perfusion; TTT, twin-to-twin transfusion.

suggest infection, and cultures of the placenta may be beneficial (Benirschke and Kaufmann, 2000). Greenish discoloration may represent meconium staining or old blood; placentas with such discoloration should be sent to the pathologist for complete histologic examination. The finding of deep meconium staining of the membranes and umbilical cord suggests that the meconium was passed at least 2 hours before delivery; this fact may be helpful in cases of meconium aspiration syndrome, for which legal questions may arise as to whether or not the aspiration occurred before or during labor. If the membranes are deeply stained, the passage of meconium by the fetus may have predated onset of labor; thus, the aspiration could have occurred before labor.

The umbilical cord should also be examined for the number of vessels and their insertion into the placenta. Vessels on the fetal surface of the placenta should be examined for evidence of clot or thrombosis. Table 4–3 lists the gross placental lesions that can be seen in the pathology laboratory (mostly parenchymal in nature) and possible associated neonatal outcomes. Normally, the fetal arteries cross superficially over the veins. Clots or thrombosis may be firm, whitish knots on the placental surface.

Microscopic features of the placenta, which are discovered only after preparation by the pathologist, are listed in Table 4–4, along with their associated maternal and neonatal clinical conditions. Finally, Table 4–5 summarizes the placental findings associated with acquired or genetic thrombophilia, and Table 4–6 lists the tests that should be performed for further investigation.

**TABLE 4–3**

**Gross Placental Lesions Seen in the Pathology Laboratory (Mostly Parenchymal)**

| Lesion | Possible Neonatal Outcome(s) |
|---|---|
| Intervillous thrombosis | Fetomaternal hemorrhage |
| Massive perivillous fibrin deposition | Intrauterine growth retardation (IUGR), asphyxia |
| Standard infarcts | Maternal vascular disease, IUGR, asphyxia |
| Stem villous arterial thrombosis–induced infarction | Fetal thrombophilia and sequelae |

**TABLE 4–4**

**Microscopic Pathologic Findings in the Placenta**

| Finding | Associated Maternal or Neonatal Conditions |
|---|---|
| Funisitis | Fetal inflammation, cerebral palsy |
| Villitis | Transplacental (usually viral) infection, especially cytomegalovirus |
| Chorangiosis | Fetal stress or a nonspecific finding |
| Stem villous thrombosis | Fetal thrombophilia, cerebral disease |
| *Listeria* abscesses | Preterm labor, fetal demise |
| Abnormal villous maturation, especially acceleration | — |
| Maternal vascular disease (decidua) | Intrauterine growth retardation |

**TABLE 4-5**

**Lesions Associated with Acquired and Genetic Thrombophilia**

| | |
|---|---|
| Placental lesions | Chorionic plate vein thrombosis in absence of abnormal cord coiling<br>Maternal floor infarction/massive perivillous fibrin deposition<br>Stem villous arterial thrombosis–fetal induced infarction. |
| Clinical lesions | Porencephalic cysts<br>Perinatal stroke<br>Terminal transverse limb defects |

**TABLE 4-6**

**Parental and/or Neonatal Laboratory Investigations for Thrombophilia**

| | |
|---|---|
| Acquired thrombophilia | Anticardiolipin, lupus anticoagulant measurements |
| Genetic thrombophilia | Screening for protein S and protein C deficiencies, antithrombin III deficiency, factor V Leiden mutation, prothrombin 20121A mutation; fasting homocysteine evaluation (screen for MTHFR mutations) |

MTHFR, methyltetrahydrofolate reductase.

## PLACENTAL PHYSIOLOGY

### Placental Transport

The developing embryo obtains all of its nutrients from the mother during gestation. Initial transport of nutrients to the conceptus is via simple diffusion from the maternal blood in the decidua. The early primitive vitelline circulation, which circulates blood from the yolk sac to the embryo at 5 to 6 weeks, is replaced by a true umbilical circulation by 7 weeks. This circulation functions as the mature transport system throughout pregnancy until delivery.

The four main substrate transport mechanisms across the placenta are simple diffusion, facilitated diffusion, active transport, and pinocytosis. Examples of substances that are delivered to the fetus by each of these routes are shown in Table 4–7. The major osmotic ions of sodium, chloride, and free water move by simple diffusion. Fetal concentrations of amino acids may be 20 times the maternal concentrations as a result of active transport (Faber and Thornburg, 1985). Glucose moves by both simple and facilitated diffusion, resulting in fetal glucose levels that are about 80% of maternal levels.

**TABLE 4-7**

**Mechanisms of Placental Transport**

| Mechanism | Substance |
|---|---|
| Simple diffusion | Oxygen, carbon dioxide, sodium, chloride |
| Facilitated diffusion | Glucose |
| Active transport | Certain amino acids, calcium |
| Pinocytosis | Immunoglobulins |

### Water Transport

The fetus is capable of producing water as a byproduct of the breakdown of glucose and the formation of energy. This water, however, is insufficient for fetal requirements. Water is also driven into the fetal compartment by pure hydrostatic forces and osmotic forces, measured in milliosmole per kilogram (Schroder, 1989). Both forces are important for fluid movement, but the interplay between them in the human placenta is poorly understood.

In the past, the fluid homeostasis of the mother and that of the developing fetus were thought to be largely independent. However, mounting evidence indicates that they are intricately intertwined. With maternal dehydration in the sheep, for example, amniotic fluid is observed to decrease (*oligohydramnios*). With maternal rehydration, normal amniotic fluid volume returns. A study in humans demonstrated that maternal oral hydration in cases of decreased amniotic fluid volume resulted in a rise in amniotic fluid volume as measured ultrasonographically by the amniotic fluid index. These studies provide strong evidence of the interconnectedness of maternal and fetal fluid spaces across the membranes and placenta (Kilpatrick et al, 1991).

## HORMONE PRODUCTION

Shortly after fertilization, the blastocyst synthesizes and releases human chorionic gonadotropin (hCG) into the maternal circulation as it implants into the endometrium. This embryonic control of maternal hCG levels is vital to maintaining the corpus luteum and preventing ejection of the conceptus. The hCG molecule is very similar in structure to the luteinizing hormone released by the pituitary gland, with a primary difference in the hCG beta chain. Placental production of hCG peaks at 8 to 10 weeks of gestation, after which its levels drop markedly. The hCG maintains the production of progesterone from the corpus luteum until the placenta takes over at about 9 weeks of gestation. Progesterone, produced in the syncytiotrophoblast, is the primary hormone of pregnancy involved in maintaining uterine and other smooth muscle relaxation. It also functions in immune suppression. Many of the vasodilatory and gastrointestinal symptoms of pregnancy noted by the mother are due to the action of progesterone.

Several estrogens are produced by the placenta, with the greatest proportion secreted into the maternal compartment.

A primary role of estrogens is to increase uterine blood flow and help maintain the pregnancy (Resnik et al, 1974). The synthetic pathway of estriol involves both the fetal adrenal gland and the placenta. Measurement of this hormone in maternal urine or plasma was historically believed to be an effective method of fetal surveillance in high-risk pregnancies because the estriol concentration reflected both fetal and placental well-being. With a significant decrease in maternal estriol levels, placental function was supposed to be declining as well. However, studies have shown that measurement of estriol is not predictive of fetal jeopardy. Interestingly, other studies have shown that abrupt elevations of estriol in saliva may be predictive of preterm labor (Hedriana et al, 1996). In the future, a simple saliva test may predict the onset of labor either before term or at term.

The final major hormone of pregnancy is human chorionic somatomammotropin (hCS), which is also called human placental lactogen. This hormone is a growth factor primarily involved with mobilization of maternal stores of glucose, fatty acids, and ketones (Speroff et al, 1989). The level of hCS increases with placental mass, and the hormone is a major mediator of glucose intolerance in pregnancy. With the larger placental mass associated with multiple gestations, there is likewise a higher rate of glucose intolerance.

## IMMUNOLOGY

Pregnancy is a unique state in which the mother has a functionally intact immune system, able to eliminate infection and suppress neoplasia while allowing a genetically different "tumor" (the fetus) to grow relatively unchecked within the uterus. The uterus itself does not prevent rejection because intra-abdominal pregnancies are not immunologically rejected. Although the exact mechanisms that prevent maternal rejection are not completely clear, several key facts are known.

The invading trophoblast does not express the major histocompatibility complex (MHC) human leukocyte antigens (HLA-A, -B, and -C), which are expressed on almost all somatic cells and induce specific immune responses by presenting peptide antigens to T cells (Blaschitz et al, 2001). The nonclassic HLA antigens, HLA-G and HLA-E, are preferentially expressed in trophoblastic tissue and are thought to be involved in immune tolerance by acting as ligands for inhibitory receptors present on natural killer (NK) cells and macrophages (Blaschitz et al, 2001; Colbern and Main, 1991). The exact mechanisms by which HLA-G prevents rejection by the mother are still unknown or are debated (Bainbridge et al, 2001).

In addition, the trophoblast secretes a sialomucin coating over its outer surface, which shields the trophoblast from maternal recognition. Finally, the trophoblast produces extremely high levels of progesterone, which is known to effectively suppress mitogen activation, mixed lymphocyte reactions, and cytotoxic T-cell generation in human blood lymphocytes (Stites et al, 1985; Szekeres-Bartho et al, 1985).

Historically, one mechanism that was thought to prevent maternal rejection of the embryo was the development of "blocking antibodies" (Rocklin et al, 1976). These antibodies, produced by the mother in response to the antigenically foreign embryo, were thought to bind antigens that were found on the trophoblast. By blocking these fetal antigens, the mother would not reject the fetus. The follow-up studies examining these antibodies have not supported the initial studies, and further work in this area is needed (Neppert et al, 1989). It appears that the maternal-fetal immune interaction is largely a local one occurring at the placental interface and is not related to systemic factors.

## AMNIOTIC FLUID VOLUME

Amniotic fluid is an integral part of and is closely connected with the fetus, placenta, and membranes. All of these tissues contribute at one time or another to amniotic fluid formation and removal. Structural or physiologic abnormalities of either the fetus or the placenta may first manifest as too much (*polyhydramnios*) or too little (oligohydramnios) amniotic fluid. To understand the associations with abnormal amniotic fluid, one must conceptualize the mechanisms involved in formation and removal of amniotic fluid. However, the mechanisms that regulate amniotic fluid volume in the normal state are only rudimentarily understood.

It is known that the main contributor to the formation of amniotic fluid is fetal urination, and either absence or obstruction of the fetal urinary system results in severe oligohydramnios and fetal or neonatal death. With uteroplacental insufficiency, which is often associated with maternal conditions such as chronic hypertension and preeclampsia, oligohydramnios may be the first presenting sign of fetal compromise (Wladimiroff and Campbell, 1974). The fetal lung is another major source of amniotic fluid. (See also Chapter 45.)

Fetal swallowing is the main route by which amniotic fluid is removed, and any interruption in fetal swallowing, such as is found with duodenal atresia, may result in polyhydramnios. Whenever extremes of amniotic fluid volume are suspected, a detailed ultrasonographic examination of the fetus should be performed. Particular attention should be given to identifying structural abnormalities in the gastrointestinal and genitourinary systems. Under normal conditions, the fetus is able to maintain the amniotic fluid volume in a relatively narrow range of normal (800 to 1200 mL), as shown in Figure 4–8 (Brace and Wolf, 1989).

## SUMMARY

It is common for the importance of the placenta, membranes, and amniotic fluid to be underappreciated, because all attention is focused on the fetus during pregnancy and the newborn after birth. Abnormalities in amniotic fluid volume may suggest structural or developmental abnormalities in the growing fetus that require further examination. A simple but complete examination of the placenta and membranes at the time of delivery may provide important clues that may be helpful in the future care of the mother and newborn.

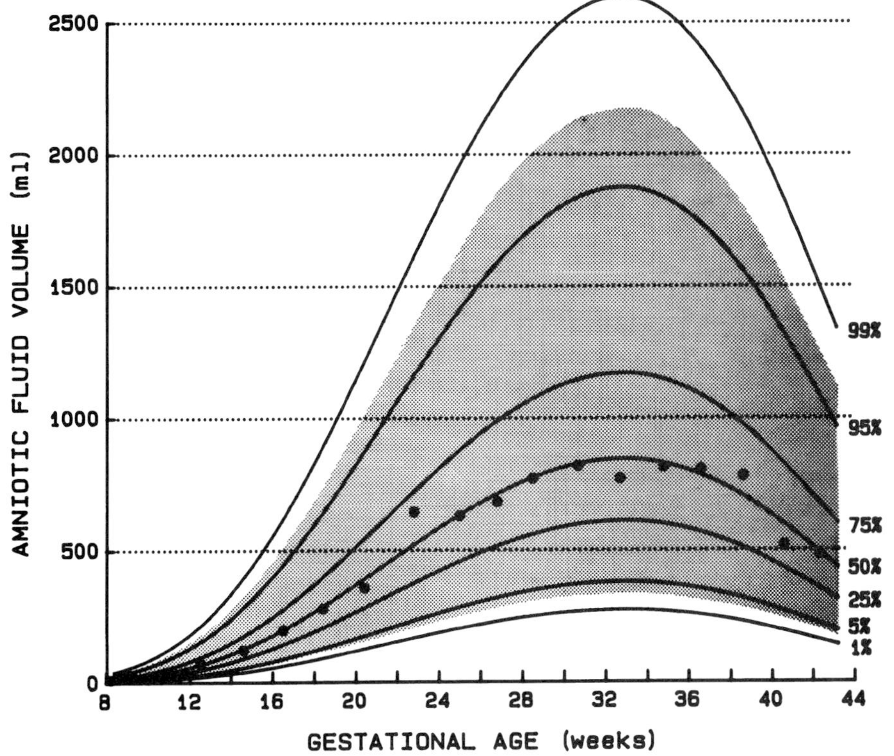


**FIGURE 4–8.** Nomogram showing amniotic fluid volumes as a function of gestational age. *Dots* indicate means for 2-week intervals. Percentiles are calculated from polynomial regression equation and standard deviation of residuals. The *shaded area* covers the 95% confidence interval. *(From Brace RA, Wolf EJ: Characterization of normal gestational changes in amniotic fluid volume. Am J Obstet Gynecol 161:382, 1989.)*

## REFERENCES

Bainbridge D, Ellis S, Le Bouteiller P, Sargent I: HLA-G remains a mystery. Trends Immunol 22:548, 2001.

Benirschke K, Kaufmann P: Pathology of the Human Placenta, 4th ed. New York, Springer-Verlag, 2000.

Blaschitz A, Hutter H, Dohr G: HLA Class I protein expression in the human placenta. Early Pregnancy 5:67, 2001.

Brace RA, Wolf EJ: Characterization of normal gestational changes in amniotic fluid volume. Am J Obstet Gynecol 161:382, 1989.

Colbern GT, Main EK: Immunology of the maternal-placental interface in normal pregnancy. Semin Perinatol 15:196, 1991.

Faber II, Thornburg KL: Placental Physiology. New York, Raven Press, 1985, p 151.

Hedriana HL, Monroe CJ, Eby-Wilkins EM, Lasley BL: Changes in rates of salivary estriol increase prior to parturition at term. J Soc Gynecol Invest 3:316A, 1996.

Hertig AT: Human Trophoblast. Springfield, IL, Charles C Thomas, 1968.

Kilpatrick SJ, Safford KL, Pomeroy T: Maternal hydration increases amniotic fluid index. Obstet Gynecol 78:1098, 1991.

Leung AKC, Robson WLM: Single umbilical artery: A report of 159 cases. Am J Dis Child 148:108, 1989.

Moore KI: The Developing Human, Philadelphia, WB Saunders, 1988.

Naftolin F, Khudr G, Benirschke K, Hutchinson D: The syndrome of chronic abruptio placentae, hydrorrhea, and circumvallate placenta. Am J Obstet Gynecol 116:347, 1973.

Neppert J, Mueller-Eckhardt G, Neumeyer H, et al: Pregnancy-maintaining antibodies: Workshop report (Giessen, 1988). J Reprod Immunol 15:159, 1989.

Newton ER, Barass V, Cetrulo CL: The epidemiology and clinical history of asymptomatic midtrimester placentae previa. Am J Obstet Gynecol 148:161, 1984.

Nicolaides K, Shawwa L, Brizot M, Snijders R: Ultrasonographically detectable markers of fetal chromosomal defects. Ultrasound Obstet Gynecol 2:56, 1993.

Pent D: Vasa previa. Am J Obstet Gynecol 134:151, 1979.

Resnik R, Killam AP, Battaglia FC, et al: The stimulation of uterine blood flow by various estrogens. Endocrinology 94:1192, 1974.

Rocklin RE, Kitzmiller JL, Carpenter CB, et al: Absence of an immunologic blocking factor from the serum of women with chronic abortions. N Engl J Med 295:1209, 1976.

Schroder HJ: Basics of placental structures and transfer functions. In Brace RA, Ross MG, Robillard JE (eds): Fetal and Neonatal Body Fluids: The Scientific Basis for Clinical Practice. Ithaca, NY, Perinatology Press, 1989, p 187.

Speroff L, Glass RH, Kase NG: Clinical Gynecologic Endocrinology and Infertility, 4th ed. Baltimore, Williams & Wilkins, 1989.

Steel CD, Wapner RJ, Smith JB, et al: Prenatal diagnosis using fetal cells isolated from maternal peripheral blood: A review. Clin Obstet Gynecol 39:801, 1996.

Stites DP, Bugbee S, Siiteri PK: Differential action of progesterone and cortisol on lymphocyte and monocyte interaction during lymphocyte activation: Relevance to immunosuppression in pregnancy. J Reprod Immunol 5:215, 1985.

Szekeres-Bartho J, Hadnagy J, Pacsa AS: The suppressive effect of progesterone on lymphocytic cytotoxicity: Unique progesterone sensitivity of pregnancy lymphocytes. J Reprod Immunol 7:121, 1985.

Townsend RR, Lainge FC, Nyberg DA, et al: Technical factors responsible for "placental migration": Sonographic assessment. Radiology 160:105, 1986.

Wladimiroff JW, Campbell S: Fetal urine-production rates in normal and complicated pregnancy. Lancet 2:151, 1974.

CHAPTER

# 5

# Abnormalities of Fetal Growth

Alma Martinez and Rebecca Simmons

Normal fetal growth pattern is determined by a number of factors, including genetic potential, the ability of the mother to provide sufficient nutrients, the ability of the placenta to transfer nutrients, and intrauterine hormones and growth factors. The pattern of normal fetal growth involves rapid increases in fetal weight, length, and head circumference during the last half of gestation, with leveling off toward term gestation. The birth weight for gestational measurements among populations have been shown to increase over time, and thus, standards for normal fetal growth require periodic reevaluation for clinical relevance. These increases in birth weight for gestational age over time are attributed to improvements in living conditions and maternal nutrition and changes in obstetric management. Variations in fetal growth have been identified in diverse populations and are associated with geographic locations (sea level versus high altitude), populations (white, African-American, Latino), maternal constitutional factors, parity, maternal nutrition, fetal gender, and multiple gestations. In this chapter, we discuss these factors in greater detail and critically review the long-term effects of abnormal fetal growth.

## INTRAUTERINE GROWTH RESTRICTION/RETARDATION AND INFANTS WHO ARE SMALL FOR GESTATIONAL AGE

There is an important distinction in identifying the fetus that suffers from IUGR or retardation (IUGR), and the fetus that is constitutionally small. IUGR represents deviation and reduction in the expected fetal growth pattern, complicates about 5% to 8% of all pregnancies, and is associated with higher perinatal mortality and morbidity rates. A large cohort study of 37,377 pregnancies found a fivefold to sixfold greater risk of perinatal death for both preterm and term fetuses that had IUGR (Lackman et al, 2001). Epidemiologic evidence shows that IUGR can lead to higher rates of complications such as stillbirth, prematurity, and perinatal morbidity (Cnattingius et al, 1998; Mongelli and Gardosi, 2000). Causes of fetal growth restriction are identified in less than 40% of cases in the United States, with the majority of cases labeled "idiopathic." Postnatal growth after IUGR depends on the cause of growth retardation, postnatal nutritional intake, and the infant's social environment.

Although the growth-restricted fetus may show symmetric or asymmetric growth at birth, it is unclear whether the proportionality of the fetus with IUGR truly affects outcomes or is related to the timing, the type, or the severity of the insult. Infants with symmetric IUGR have reduced weight, length, and head circumference at birth. Weight (and then length) of infants with asymmetric growth retardation is affected, with a relatively normal or "head-sparing" growth pattern. Historically, for infants with symmetric IUGR, higher rates of intrauterine infections, chromosomal abnormalities, dysmorphic syndromes, and intrauterine toxins (alcohol) were described as reasons for the growth restriction; and asymmetric IUGR was associated with maternal medical conditions such as preeclampsia, chronic hypertension, and uterine anomalies.

Lin and colleagues (1991) suggest that the timing of the risk factor is more important than the risk factor itself in determining whether symmetric or asymmetric growth restriction is seen. They report that asymmetric growth restriction is more commonly seen from effects on the fetus later in gestation. In their study, symmetric IUGR resulted in higher levels of prematurity and higher rates of neonatal morbidity. In contrast, Villar and associates (1990) have shown that infants with asymmetric IUGR have higher morbidity rates at birth. They found that infants with low ponderal index measurements (which they defined as weight/length$^3$) had higher risk for low Apgar scores, long hospitalization, hypoglycemia, and asphyxia at birth than infants with symmetric IUGR. There is evidence to suggest that infants with asymmetric IUGR show better gains in weight and length in the postnatal period than symmetrically restricted infants (May et al, 2001). Other investigators propose that IUGR represents a continuum, with asymmetric IUGR occurring as the severity of the growth retardation increases. Data also suggest that the more severe the growth restriction, the worse the neonatal outcomes, including risk of stillbirth, fetal distress, neonatal hypoglycemia, hypocalcemia, polycythemia, low Apgar scores, and mortality (Kramer et al, 1990; Spinillo et al, 1995).

A fetus with IUGR may be born small for gestational age (SGA) or appropriate for gestational age (AGA) according to population reference charts. There is no universal agreement in the definition of a SGA (or large for gestational age [LGA]) infant. Various definitions appear in the medical literature, making comparisons between studies difficult. Additionally, investigators have shown that the prevalence of fetal growth restriction varies according to the fetal growth curve used (Alexander et al, 1996). Historically, SGA infants were defined as those with measurements below the tenth percentile (Battaglia and Lubchenco, 1967). Some investigators, however, also use measurements below the third percentile, or two standard deviations below the mean derived from population charts, to define SGA. McIntire and colleagues (1999) reported a "threshold" of increased adverse outcomes in infants born with measurements below the third percentile and suggested that this level of restriction represents a clinically relevant measurement. Other researchers have found higher rates of neonatal complications when the 15th percentile of birth weight is used as a cutoff level (Seeds and Peng, 1998).

Similarly, AGA infants are defined as those with measurements between the 10th and 90th percentiles, or between the 3rd and 97th percentiles, or between two standard deviations below and standard deviations above the mean. LGA infants are defined as those with measurements greater than 90th percentile, greater than 97th percentile, or more than two standard deviations above the mean.

## Etiology

### National and International Perspectives

The epidemiology of fetal growth restriction varies internationally (Keirse, 2000). In developed countries, the most frequently identified cause of growth restriction is smoking, while in developing countries, maternal nutritional factors (pre-pregnancy weight, maternal stature) and infections (malaria) are the leading identified causes (Kramer, 2000; Robinson et al, 2000). Additionally, in developing countries, there is a direct correlation between the incidence of low birth weight (<2500 g) and IUGR. In developing countries, the high incidence of low-birth-weight (LBW) infants is almost exclusively due to the incidence of IUGR. Data from developed countries show the opposite, rates of low birth weight being explained almost exclusively by prematurity rates.

Numerous factors have been identified as influencing size at birth. In a simplified manner, these factors can be grouped as fetal, placental, or maternal in origin. Recognized causes of IUGR are listed in Table 5–1. In the United States, the cause of IUGR is identified in only about 40% of cases, with the remainder of cases labeled "idiopathic."

### Fetal Causes of Growth Restriction

Fetal factors affecting growth include fetal gender, familial genetic inheritance, and chromosomal abnormalities or dysmorphic syndromes. In one large population-based study, the frequency of IUGR among infants with congenital malformations was 22%. The majority of the infants affected had chromosomal abnormalities. Other studies have similarly found that fetal growth restriction is more common among infants with malformations. Fetal gender also influences size, with male infants showing greater intrauterine growth than female infants (Glinianaia et al, 2000; Skjaerven et al, 2000; Thomas et al, 2000).

### Placental Causes of Growth Restriction

Placental factors are known to influence fetal growth. The transfer of nutrients across the placenta depends on uterine blood flow, which normally increases throughout gestation. Maternal health conditions associated with chronic decreases in uteroplacental blood flow (maternal vascular diseases, preeclampsia, hypertension, maternal smoking) are associated with poor fetal growth and nutrition. Preeclampsia has been shown to be associated with fetal growth restriction (Ødegård et al, 2000; Spinillo et al, 1994; Xiong et al, 1999). Investigators have shown that the extent of growth restriction correlates with the severity and the onset during pregnancy of the preeclampsia. Ødegård et al, 2000, showed that fetuses exposed to preeclampsia from early in pregnancy had the most serious growth restriction, and more than half of these infants were born SGA. Chronic maternal diseases (cardiac, renal) may decrease the normal uteroplacental blood flow to the fetus and thus may also be associated with poor fetal growth (Spinillo et al, 1994).

Placental maturation at the end of pregnancy is associated with an increase in substrate transfer, a slowing (but not cessation) of placental growth, and a plateau in fetal growth near term (Fox, 1997). Abnormalities of placental growth, senescence, and infarction have been shown to affect fetal growth. The placentas from pregnancies complicated by poor fetal growth have a higher incidence of vascular damage and abnormalities (Pardi et al, 1997). Fetal size and placental growth are directly related, and placentas from pregnancies yielding growth-retarded infants demonstrate a higher incidence of smallness and abnormality than those from pregnancies with appropriately

**TABLE 5–1**

**Causes of Intrauterine Growth Restriction (IUGR)**

| | |
|---|---|
| Genetic | Inheritance, chromosomal abnormalities, fetal gender |
| Maternal constitutional effects | Low maternal pre-pregnancy weight, low pregnancy weight gain, ethnicity, socioeconomic status, history of IUGR |
| Nutrition | Low pre-pregnancy weight (body mass index), low pregnancy weight gain, malnutrition (macronutrients, micronutrients), maternal anemia |
| Infections | TORCH infections (toxoplasmosis, rubella, cytomegalovirus, syphilis) |
| Decreased $O_2$-carrying capacity | High altitude, maternal congenital heart disease, hemoglobinopathies, chronic anemia, maternal asthma |
| Uterine/placental anatomy | Abnormal uterine anatomy, uterine fibroid, vascular abnormalities (single umbilical artery, velamentous umbilical cord insertion, twin-twin transfusion), placenta previa, placental abruption |
| Uterine/placental function | Maternal vasculitis (system lupus erythematosus), decreased uteroplacental perfusion, maternal illness (preeclampsia, chronic hypertension, diabetes, renal disease) |
| Toxins | Tobacco, ethanol, lead, arsenic |

grown infants. The difference in size is seen even in a comparison of placentas associated with growth-restricted infants and those associated with AGA infants of the same birth weight (Heinonen et al, 2001). Placental growth in the second trimester correlates with placental weight and function and, thus, with weight at birth (Godfrey et al, 1996). Clinical conditions associated with reduced placental size (and subsequent reduced fetal weight) include maternal vascular disease, uterine anomalies (fibroids, abnormal uterine anatomy), placental infarctions, unusual cord insertions, and abnormalities of placentation.

Investigators have also shown fetal growth restriction in infants born with placental abruption. Abruption is increasingly common in older, multiparous women, smokers, and drug abusers (cocaine), with multiple births, and in women with hypertensive disorders. Using a large population-based study, Ananth and coworkers (2001) showed a downward shift of birth weight in infants with placental abruption from about 28 weeks of gestation through term gestation. These investigators speculate that although placental abruption is an acute peripartum event, the strong association between placental abruption and growth restriction suggests that chronic and underlying processes contribute to fetal outcome in abruption. Although associated with a small increase in fetal growth restriction, placenta previa appears to affect fetal growth more significantly through its association with prematurity.

Multiple gestations are associated with greater risk for fetal growth restriction. The higher risk stems from crowding and from abnormalities with placentation, vascular communications, and umbilical cord insertions. Divergence in fetal growth appears from about 30 to 32 weeks in twin gestation compared with singleton pregnancies (Alexander et al, 1996; Glinianaia et al, 2000; Skjaerven et al, 2000). Others have identified differences in fetal growth between twins and singletons as occurring earlier in gestation, at about 21 weeks (Devoe and Ware, 1995). Larger effects on fetal growth are seen with increasing number of fetal multiples. Abnormalities in placentation are also more common with multiple gestations (Benirschke, 1995). Monochorionic twins can share placental vascular communication (twin-twin transfusion), leading to fetal growth restriction during gestation. Fetal "competition" for placental transfer of nutrients raises the incidence of growth restriction and discordance in growth between fetuses. The rate of birth weights less than the fifth percentile is higher in monochorionic twins. Placental growth is restricted in utero because of limitation in space, leading to a higher incidence of placenta previa in multiple-gestation pregnancies. Additionally, abnormalities in cord insertions (marginal and velamentous cord insertions) and occurrence of a single umbilical artery are more frequently found in multiple gestations. The higher incidence of growth restriction in multiple gestation pregnancies is strongly associated with monochorionic gestations, the presence of vascular anastomoses, and discordant fetal growth (Hollier et al, 1999; Sonntag et al, 1996; Victoria et al, 2001). Placentas of smaller fetuses with discordant growth are significantly smaller than those of their larger twin counterparts (Victoria et al, 2001). (See also Chapter 7.)

Investigators have shown an effect of altitude on fetal growth, with infants born at high altitudes having lower birth weights (Galan et al, 2001). Differences in fetal growth are detected from about 25 weeks with pregnancies at 4000 meters. In these high-altitude pregnancies, the abdominal circumference is most affected (Krampl et al, 2000). At tremendously high altitudes, the incidence of LGA infant births is markedly reduced. In the United States (and at less severe altitudes), infants born at higher altitudes are lighter at birth, but those differences are not pronounced. Interestingly, investigators have shown that adaptation to high altitude during pregnancy is also possible. Tibetan infants have higher birth weights than infants of more recent immigrants of ethnic Chinese living at the same high-altitude (2700 to 4700 m) region of Tibet (Moore et al, 2001). Tibetan infants also have less IUGR than infants born to more recent immigrants to the area.

## Maternal Causes of Growth Restriction

Maternal constitutional factors have a significant effect on fetal growth. Maternal weight (pre-pregnancy), maternal stature, and maternal weight gain during pregnancy are directly associated with maternal nutrition and correlate with fetal growth (Clausson et al, 1998; Doctor et al, 2001; Goldenberg et al, 1997; Mongelli and Gardosi, 2000). Numerous studies show that these findings are often confounded by highly associated cultural and socioeconomic factors. The woman with a previous SGA infant has a higher risk of a subsequent small infant (Robinson et al, 2000). Investigators have shown a higher incidence of SGA infants to be associated with lower levels of maternal education (Clausson et al, 1998). Parity of the mother also affects fetal size, nulliparous women having a higher incidence of SGA infants (Cnattingius et al, 1998). A large population-based study in Sweden found that women who were older than 30 years, were nulliparous, or had hypertensive disease were at increased risk of preterm and term growth-restricted infants.

Studies have shown differential fetal growth for women of diverse ethnicities, with Latina and white women having higher rates of LGA infants, and African-American women having a higher incidence of SGA infants (Alexander et al, 1999; Fuentes-Afflick et al, 1998). These gender and ethnic differences in birth weight become pronounced after 30 weeks of gestation (Thomas et al, 2000). Investigators in California have shown that U.S.-born black women have higher rates of prematurity and LBW infants than foreign-born black women, the difference being associated with higher rates of tobacco use and inadequate prenatal care in the former group. Other researchers have found that even among women with very low risk of LBW infants (married, age 20 to 34 years, 13 or more years of education, adequate prenatal care, and absence of maternal health risk factors and of tobacco or alcohol use), the risk of delivering an SGA infant is still higher for African-American women than for white women (Alexander et al, 1999). It is unclear whether these differences in fetal growth are due to inherent differences or to differential exposure to environmental factors.

Maternal nutrition and supply of nutrients to the fetus affect fetal growth. Evidence shows a relationship between maternal nutrition during pregnancy and infant birth weight. Investigators have found a significant relation between maternal energy intake and placental and infant weights (Godfrey et al, 1996). Maternal nutritional status both before and during pregnancy is associated with fetal growth patterns (Doctor et al, 2001). Pre-pregnancy weight influences fetal size and may be a potential marker for intergenerational effects on infant weight in developing countries. A woman's birth weight has been shown to correlate with her infant's weight as well as the placental weight during pregnancy. Maternal nutrition and maternal weight gain during pregnancy are associated with infant weight (Neggers et al, 1997; Robinson et al, 2000; Zeitlin et al, 2001). Strauss and Dietz (1999) report that low maternal weight gains in the second and third trimesters are associated with double the risk of IUGR, whereas poor maternal weight gain in the first trimester has no such effect on fetal growth (Strauss and Dietz, 1999). These investigators also showed that older women (>35 years) as well as smokers were at increased risk of IUGR associated with lower weight gains in late pregnancy. Others have shown low intakes of meat protein in late pregnancy to be associated with lower birth weights.

Teen pregnancy represents a special condition in which fetal weight is highly influenced by maternal nutrition. Teen mothers (<15 years) have been shown to have a higher risk for delivering a growth-restricted infant (Ghidini, 1996). Teen pregnancies are complicated by the additional nutritional needs of a pregnant mother, who is still actively growing, as well as by socioeconomic status of pregnant teens in developed countries (Scholl and Hediger, 1995). Maternal nutrition and maternal weight gain are adversely affected by inadequate or poorly balanced intake in conditions such as alcoholism, drug abuse, and poverty.

The effects of micronutrients on pregnancy outcomes and fetal growth have been less well studied. Maternal intake of certain micronutrients has also been found to affect fetal growth. Zinc deficiency has been associated with fetal growth restriction as well as other abnormalities, such as infertility and spontaneous abortion (Jameson, 1993; Shah and Sachdev, 2001). Additionally, dietary intake of vitamin C during early pregnancy has been shown to be associated with an increase in birth weight (Mathews et al, 1999). Others have shown strong associations between maternal intake of folate and iron and infant and placental weights (Godfrey et al, 1996). In developing countries, the effects of nutritional deficiencies during pregnancy are more prevalent and easier to detect. For example, Rao and colleagues (2001) have estimated that one third of infants in India are born weighing less than 2500 g, mainly because of maternal malnutrition. These investigators have shown significant associations between infant birth weight and maternal intake of milk, leafy greens, fruits, and folate during pregnancy.

Although toxins such as cigarette smoke and alcohol have a direct effect on placental function, they may also affect fetal growth through an associated compromise in maternal nutrition. Other environmental toxins (lead, arsenic, mercury) are associated with IUGR and are believed to affect fetal growth by entering the food chain and depleting body stores of iron, vitamin C, and possibly other nutrients (Iynengar and Nair, 2000; Srivastava et al, 2001).

Numerous studies have shown associations between birth weight and maternal intake of macronutrients and micronutrients, but the effects of nutritional supplements used during pregnancy have not been proved to have a beneficial effect on fetal growth (de Onis et al, 1998; Jackson and Robinson, 2001; Rush, 2001; Say, Gülmezoglu and Hofmeyr, 2003). Studies of the effects of supplements during pregnancy have been undertaken in mainly developed countries and among women with adequate nutrition. It seems more likely that supplementation programs for pregnant women in developing countries or among women with severe nutritional imbalances may show benefit for their infants (Ladipo, 2000).

Maternal illness and conditions leading to decreased oxygen availability in the mother (e.g., maternal anemia, cyanotic heart disease, hemoglobinopathy, respiratory failure), as well as maternal hypertension, pre-eclampsia, and diabetes all have been shown to have adverse effects on fetal growth. Women with systemic lupus erythematosus (SLE) have a higher prevalence of fetal growth restriction (Yasmeen et al, 2001). Some researchers have shown that the majority of adverse fetal outcomes associated with SLE are related to maternal antiphospholipid antibodies (Khamashta and Hughes, 1996).

Maternal socioeconomic status and ethnicity have also been identified as risk factors for IUGR and poor health outcomes in infants. Numerous investigators have shown a significant effect of socioeconomic status on birth outcomes, including fetal growth restriction, in both developing and developed countries (Wilcox et al, 1995). In the United States, low levels of maternal and paternal education, certain maternal and paternal occupations, and low family income are associated with lower birth weights in children of both African-American and white women (Parker et al, 1994). In a large population-based study from Sweden, investigators have similarly shown a higher incidence of fetal growth restriction in association with low maternal education (Clausson et al, 1998). Researchers have also shown that rates of compromised birth outcome are higher among African-American women than among Mexican-American and non-Hispanic white women (Collins and Butler, 1997; Frisbie et al, 1997; Thomas et al, 2000). Some of these studies also show that the risk of IUGR is higher in women without medical insurance. In the United States, the incidence of IGUR is significantly higher among African-American women than among white women; this higher incidence is seen even among African-American women with higher socioeconomic status (Alexander et al, 1999).

In a study from Arizona, the incidence of IUGR was found to be lower in Mexican-American women than in white women (Balcazar, 1994). Other researchers have shown that Mexican-born immigrants in California have better perinatal outcomes (including birth weight) than both African Americans and U.S.-born women of Mexican descent (Fuentes-Afflick et al, 1998). The reasons for this apparent paradox are unclear, but one postulate is the tendency of recent immigrants to maintain the favorable nutritional and behavioral characteristics of their country of origin (Guendelman and English, 1995). These studies support the speculation that the differences in fetal growth between groups do not reflect inherent differences in fetal growth, but rather stem from inequalities in nutrition, health care, and other environmental factors (Keirse, 2000; Kramer et al, 2000).

### Smoking

Cigarette smoking is consistently found to adversely affect intrauterine growth in all studies in which this factor is considered. In developed countries, cigarette smoking is the single most important cause of poor fetal growth (Kramer et al, 2000). The incidence of IUGR in smokers is estimated to be 3 to 4.5 times higher than in nonsmokers (Nordentoft et al, 1996). Cigarette smoking has a significant effect on abdominal circumference and fetal weight but not on head circumference (Bernstein et al, 2000b). Lieberman and associates (1994) report that cigarette smoking also appears to have a dose-dependent effect on the incidence of IUGR, with this effect being seen especially with heavy smoking and smoking during the third trimester. These investigators have shown that if women stop smoking during the third trimester, their infants' birth weights are indistinguishable from those of infants born to the normal population. Other researchers have shown that even a reduction in smoking is associated with improved fetal growth (Li et al, 1993; Walsh et al, 2001). Numerous potential causes of the effects of smoking on fetal growth have been suggested, including direct effects of nicotine on placental vasoconstriction, decreased uterine blood flow, higher levels of fetal carboxyhemoglobin, fetal hypoxia, adverse maternal nutritional intake, and altered maternal and placental metabolism (Andres and Day, 2000; Pastrakuljic et al, 1999). See Chapter 12 for further discussion of the effects of cigarette smoking during pregnancy.

### Infections

A number of infections are associated with IUGR. They include viral infections from the TORCH (toxoplasmosis, rubella, cytomegalovirus, herpes simplex virus) group. Unless there are other findings on examination of the neonate suggestive of intrauterine TORCH infection, growth restriction alone may not justify an evaluation for these uncommon perinatal infections. Investigators have shown a low yield (and significant associated costs) in these evaluations for infants with growth restriction (Khan and Kazzi, 2000). See Chapter 37 for further discussion of intrauterine infections.

## Antenatal Diagnosis of Intrauterine Growth Restriction/Retardation

Despite the use of various screening techniques and fetal measurements to assess fetal growth, antenatal diagnosis of IUGR is difficult. Such a diagnosis relies on established fetal growth charts as an estimation of fetal growth. There are inherent difficulties with using established growth charts, including population variations and maternal constitutional factors (parity, pre-pregnancy weight, stature, multiple gestations). These factors must be considered by clinicians evaluating the adequacy of growth. The diagnosis of fetal growth restriction may vary according to the fetal growth curve used. Using U.S.-wide population data for more than 3 million births, Alexander and coworkers (1996) have published current national fetal growth curves. Others have done similar work for infants in Europe (Skjaerven et al, 2000). Investigators have recommended using customized growth charts that take maternal characteristics as well as fetal characteristics into consideration (Mongelli et al, 2000). Additionally, various researchers suggest that estimation of fetal growth rate or velocity in the third trimester may be a better predictor of fetal outcome than a calculation of fetal size (Owen and Khan, 1998), although others have not found this approach to be helpful (Williams and Nwebube, 2001).

With ultrasound measurement, it is possible to estimate fetal weight, brain size, and placental size and morphology. Prenatal ultrasound examinations are used to detect abnormalities in fetal growth and fetal structural abnormalities associated with chromosomal abnormalities, and to assess fetal well-being during gestation. Despite limitations, fetal ultrasonography remains the most widespread and most accurate method for detecting growth restriction. Ultrasound biometry is considered the most reliable method of assessing fetal growth (see also Chapter 13).

Investigators have shown that because the liver size of the fetus is affected profoundly by IUGR, the abdominal circumference is the earliest and most sensitive ultrasound biometric measurement for predicting fetal growth abnormalities (Degani, 2001; Hobbins, 1997; Jazayeri et al, 1999; Williams and Nwebube, 2001). In a large retrospective study, Smith and colleagues (1997) found a linear correlation between abdominal circumference and subsequent birth weight. These investigators estimated the error in predicting birth weight was close to 7% and was greatest for the largest infants. Others have shown that abdominal circumference measurement less than the fifth percentile was associated with higher incidence of fetal distress and the need for cesarean section. Owen and Kahn (1998) have suggested that measurement of abdominal circumference growth rate (but not a single measurement) may be a better predictor of the need for cesarean section or abnormal fetal growth.

Despite the growing use of the modalities discussed here and in Chapter 13, investigators have questioned whether current antenatal detection and surveillance of, and subsequent obstetric intervention for, growth-restricted fetuses improves infant outcomes (Jahn et al, 1998). These concerns are greater regarding management of the preterm infant with suspected IUGR. SGA preterm infants have a higher incidence of neonatal morbidities, and gestational age continues to be a significant determinant of perinatal mortality and neurologic outcomes for growth-restricted fetuses (Hershkovitz et al, 2001; Scherjon et al, 1998; Sung et al, 1993). These data suggest that the adverse effects of severe prematurity may outweigh the benefit of the early delivery of a growth-restricted fetus. Judicial use of measurement techniques and data from studies of fetal well-being, in addition to sound clinical judgment for each case of suspected fetal growth abnormality, is required.

## Medical Complications and Outcomes

Fetal growth restriction is associated with intrauterine demise. Almost 40% of term stillbirths and 63% of preterm stillbirths are SGA (Mongelli and Gardosi, 2000). Both short-term and long-term effects of abnormalities in SGA fetuses have been described. Perinatal mortality for intrauterine SGA infants is higher overall than that for appropriately grown term and preterm infants (Clausson et al, 1998). The risk of perinatal death is estimated to be fivefold to sixfold greater for both preterm and term fetuses with IUGR (Lackman et al, 2001). In a large population-based study in Sweden, the risk of fetal death for fetuses "mildly" SGA was double that for term LGA infants, and was 16 times greater for more severely affected SGA infants (Cnattingius et al, 1998). Overall, intrauterine death, perinatal asphyxia, and congenital anomalies are the main contributing factors to the higher mortality rate in SGA infants. The effects of acute fetal hypoxia may be superimposed on chronic fetal hypoxia, and placental insufficiency may be an important etiologic factor in these outcomes. Investigators have described higher incidences of low Apgar scores, umbilical artery acidosis, need for intubation at delivery, seizures on the first day of life, and sepsis in SGA infants (McIntire et al, 1999). The incidence of adverse perinatal effects correlates with the severity of the growth restriction, the highest rates of respiratory distress syndrome, metabolic abnormalities, and sepsis being found in the most severely growth-restricted infants (Spinillo et al, 1995). As previously described, Villar and associates (1990) reported that infants with asymmetric IUGR and low ponderal index measurements (weight/length$^3$) had higher risk of low Apgar scores, hypoglycemia, asphyxia, and long hospitalization.

Preterm infants with growth abnormalities also have higher risk of adverse outcomes. In a large multicountry study conducted in Europe, more than 40% of preterm infants whose births were induced were shown to be SGA (Zeitlin et al, 2000). Other researchers have similarly found a higher incidence of SGA infants among preterm deliveries than among term deliveries (Hershkovitz et al, 2001). Preterm SGA infants have been shown to have a higher incidence of a number of complications, including sepsis, severe intraventricular hemorrhage, respiratory distress syndrome, necrotizing enterocolitis, and death, than normally grown preterm infants (Gortner et al, 1999; McIntire et al, 1999; Simchen et al, 2000). In the United States, administration of antenatal steroids was found to be beneficial in reducing the incidence of respiratory distress syndrome, intraventricular hemorrhage, and mortality in SGA preterm infants (Bernstein et al, 2000a). These benefits were similar to those seen in normally grown preterm infants. Additionally, SGA infants have higher incidence of chronic lung disease at corrected gestational ages of 28 days and 36 weeks.

Neonatal hypoglycemia and hypothermia occur more frequently in growth-restricted infants (Doctor et al, 2001). These metabolic abnormalities presumably occur from decreased glycogen stores, inadequate lipid stores, and impaired gluconeogenesis in the growth-restricted neonate. Such infants are also more vulnerable to starvation. Growth-restricted neonates have inadequate fuel stores and are at increased risk for hypoglycemia during fasting, and these risks are increased in preterm SGA infants. Infants with IUGR also have a higher incidence of hypocalcemia, the incidence correlating strongly with the severity of the growth restriction (Spinillo et al, 1995).

### Developmental Outcomes: Early Childhood

Neurologic outcomes, including intellectual and neurologic function, are affected by growth restriction. Overall, neurologic morbidity is higher for SGA infants than for AGA infants.

Even without identified perinatal events, SGA infants have a higher incidence of long-term neurologic or developmental handicaps. Investigators have found the incidence of cerebral palsy to be greater in IUGR infants than in a population with normal fetal growth (Blair and Stanley, 1990; Spinillo et al, 1995; Uvebrant and Hagberg, 1992). SGA infants born at term appear to have double or triple the risk for cerebral palsy, between 1 to 2 per 1000 live births and 2 to 6 per 1000 live births (Goldenberg et al, 1998). The rate of cerebral palsy is also higher in preterm growth-restricted infants than in preterm infants with appropriate fetal growth (Gray et al, 2001). At 7 years of age, children whose birth was associated with hypoxia-related factors had a higher risk for adverse neurologic outcomes. Infants with symmetric IUGR (or perhaps more severe restriction) were at higher risk than infants with asymmetric IUGR. Other researchers have shown higher rates of learning deficits, lower IQ scores, and increased behavioral problems in children with a history of fetal growth restriction, even at 9 to 11 years of age (Low et al, 1992).

## Long-Term Consequences: The Fetal Origins of Adult Disease

### Programming

The period from conception to birth is a time of rapid growth, cellular replication and differentiation, and functional maturation of organ systems. These processes are very sensitive to alterations in the intrauterine milieu. *Programming* describes the mechanisms whereby a stimulus or insult at a critical period of development has lasting or lifelong effects. The "thrifty phenotype" hypothesis proposes that the fetus adapts to an adverse intrauterine milieu by optimizing the use of a reduced nutrient supply to ensure survival; but because this adaptation favors the development of certain organs over that of others, it leads to persistent alterations in the growth and function of developing tissues (Hales and Barker, 1992). Also, although the adaptations may aid in survival of the fetus, they become a liability in situations of nutritional abundance.

### Epidemiology

It has been recognized for nearly 70 years that the early environment in which a child grows and develops can have long-term effects on subsequent health and survival

(Kermack, 1934). The landmark cohort study of 300,000 men by Ravelli and colleagues (1976) showed that men who were exposed in utero to the effects of the Dutch famine of 1944 and 1945 during the first half of gestation had significantly higher obesity rates at age 19 years. Subsequent studies demonstrated a relation between low birth weight and the later development of cardiovascular disease (Barker et al, 1989) and impaired glucose tolerance (Fall et al, 1995) in men in England. Those men who were smallest at birth (2500 g) were nearly seven times more likely to have impaired glucose tolerance or type 2 diabetes than those who were largest at birth. Barker and colleagues (1993) also found a similar relationship between lower birth weight and higher systolic blood pressure and triglyceride levels.

Valdez and associates (1994) observed a similar association between birth weight and subsequent glucose intolerance, hypertension, and hyperlipidemia in a study of young adult Mexican-American and non-Hispanic white men and women participants in the San Antonio Heart Study. Normotensive, nondiabetic individuals whose birth weights were in the lowest tertile had significantly higher rates of insulin resistance, obesity, and hypertension than subjects whose birth weights were normal. In the Pima Indians, a population with extraordinarily high rates of type 2 diabetes, McCance and coworkers (1994) found that the development of diabetes in the offspring was related to both extremes of birth weight. In their study, the prevalence of diabetes in subjects 20 to 39 years old was 30% for those weighing less than 2500 g at birth, 17% for those weighing 2500 to 4499 g, and 32% for those weighing 4500 g or more. The risk for development of type 2 diabetes was nearly fourfold higher for those whose birth weight was less than 2500 grams. Other studies of populations in the United States (Curhan et al, 1996), Sweden (Lithell et al, 1996; McKeigue et al, 1998), France (Leger et al, 1997; Jaquet et al, 2000), Norway (Egeland et al, 2000), and Finland (Forsen et al, 2000) have all demonstrated a significant correlation between low birth weight and the later development of adult diseases.

Studies controlling for the confounding factors of socioeconomic status and lifestyle have further strengthened the association between low birth weight and higher risk of coronary heart disease, stroke, and type 2 diabetes. In 1976, the Nurses' Health Study was initiated, and a large cohort of American women born from 1921 to 1946 established. The association between low birth weight and increased risks of coronary heart disease, stroke, and type 2 diabetes remained strong even after adjustment for lifestyle factors such as smoking, physical activity, occupation, income, dietary habits, and childhood socioeconomic status (Rich-Edwards et al, 1999).

## The Role of Catch-up Growth

Many studies have suggested that the associations between birth size with later disease can be modified by body mass index (BMI) in childhood. The highest risk for the development of type 2 diabetes is among adults who were born small and become overweight during childhood (Eriksson et al, 2000). Insulin resistance is most prominent in Indian children who were SGA at birth but had a high fat mass at 8 years of age (Bavdekar et al, 1999). Similar findings were reported in 10-year-old children in the United Kingdom (Whincup et al, 1997). In a Finnish cohort, adult hypertension was associated with both lower birth weight and accelerated growth in the first 7 years of life. In contrast, in two preliminary studies from the UK, catch-up growth in the first 6 months of life was not clearly related to blood pressure in young adulthood, although birth weight was (McCarthy et al, 2001).

Interpretation of the findings of these studies is complicated by the vague definitions of *catch-up growth*. The term, which can encompass either the first 6 to 12 months only or as much as the first 2 years after birth, usually refers to realignment of one's genetic growth potential after IUGR. This definition allows for fetal growth retardation at any birth weight; even large fetuses can be growth retarded in relation to their genetic potential. However, postnatal factors can obviously affect infant growth in the first few months of life. For example, breast-feeding appears to protect against obesity later in childhood, yet breast-fed infants usually exhibit higher body mass during the first year of life than formula-fed infants. Although it is likely that accelerated growth confers an additional risk to the growth-retarded fetus, these conflicting results demonstrate the need for additional, carefully designed studies to determine just how childhood growth rates affect the later development of cardiovascular disease and type 2 diabetes.

## Size at Birth, Insulin Secretion, and Insulin Action

The mechanisms underlying the association between size at birth and impaired glucose tolerance or type 2 diabetes are unclear. A number of studies in children and adults have shown that nondiabetic or prediabetic subjects with low birth weight are insulin resistant and thus are predisposed to development of type 2 diabetes (Bavdekar et al, 1999; Clausen et al, 1997; Flanagan et al, 2000; Hoffman et al, 1997; Leger et al, 1997; Li et al, 2001; Lithell et al, 1996; McKeigue et al, 1998; Phillips et al, 1994; Yajnik et al, 1995). IUGR is known to alter the fetal development of adipose tissue, which is closely linked to the development of insulin resistance (Lapillonne et al, 1997; Widdowson et al, 1979). In a well-designed case-control study of 25 year-old-adults, Jaquet and colleagues (2000) demonstrated that individuals who were born SGA at 37 weeks or later had a significantly higher percentage of body fat (15%). Insulin sensitivity, even after adjustment for BMI or total fat mass, was markedly impaired in these SGA subjects. There were no significant differences between the SGA and control groups with respect to parental history of type 2 diabetes, cardiovascular disease, hypertension, or dyslipidemia. Of importance to generalization of the findings to other populations, the causes of IUGR in these subjects were gestational hypertension (50%), smoking (30%), maternal short stature (7%), congenital anomalies (7%), and unknown (6%).

The adverse effect of IUGR on glucose homeostasis was originally thought to be mediated through programming of the fetal endocrine pancreas. Growth-retarded fetuses and newborns have been shown to have a reduced population of pancreatic β-cells (Van Assche et al, 1977). Low birth weight has been associated with reduced insulin response after glucose ingestion in young nondiabetic men; however, a number of other studies have found no effect of low birth weight on insulin secretion in humans (Clausen et al, 1997; Flanagan et al, 2000; Lithell et al, 1996). However, none of these earlier studies had adjusted for the corresponding insulin sensitivity, which has a profound impact on insulin secretion. Therefore, Jensen and colleagues (2002) measured insulin secretion and insulin sensitivity in a well-matched population of 19-year-old, glucose-tolerant white men whose birth weights were either below the 10th percentile (SGA) or between the 50th and 75th percentiles (controls). To eliminate the major confounding factors, such as "diabetes genes," the researchers ensured that none of the participants had a family history of diabetes, hypertension, or ischemic heart disease. They found no differences between the groups with regard to current weight, BMI, body composition, and lipid profile. When data were controlled for insulin sensitivity, insulin secretion was found to be lower by 30%. However, insulin sensitivity was normal in the SGA subjects. These investigators hypothesized that defects in insulin secretion may precede defects in insulin action and that once SGA individuals accumulate body fat, they do demonstrate insulin resistance.

## Epidemiologic Challenges

The data described in the preceding section suggest that low birth weight is associated with glucose intolerance, type 2 diabetes, and cardiovascular disease. However, the question remains whether these associations reflect fetal nutrition or other factors that contribute to birth weight and the observed glucose intolerance. Because of the retrospective nature of the cohort identification, many confounding variables were not always recorded, such as lifestyle, socioeconomic status, education, maternal age, parental build, birth order, obstetric complications, smoking, and maternal health. Maternal nutritional status, either directly in the form of diet histories, or indirectly in the form of BMI, height, and pregnancy weight gain, were usually not recorded. Instead, birth anthropometric measures were used as proxies for presumed undernutrition in pregnancy.

## Size at Birth Cannot Be Used as a Proxy for Fetal Growth

Birth weight is determined by the sum of multiple known and unknown factors, including gestational age, maternal age, birth order, genetics, maternal pre-pregnancy BMI, and pregnancy weight gain, plus multiple environmental factors, such as smoking, drug use, infection, and maternal hypertension. Some of these determinants may be related to susceptibility to adult disease, and others may not. Conversely, some prenatal determinants of adult outcomes may not be related to fetal growth. A good example of how size at birth may potentially be a proxy for an underlying causal pathway is the hypothesis that essential hypertension in the adult is due to a congenital nephron deficit (Brenner et al, 1993). A study has now shown that kidney volume is smaller in adults who were thinner at birth, after adjustment for current body size. In contrast, maternal cigarette smoking is a good example of a prenatal exposure that restricts fetal growth, but to date, no association has been found between cigarette smoking and adverse long-term outcome in offspring.

## Genetics versus Environment

Several epidemiologic and metabolic studies of twins and first-degree relatives of patients with type 2 diabetes have demonstrated an important genetic component of diabetes (Vaag et al, 1995). The association between low birth weight and risk of type 2 diabetes in some studies could theoretically be explained by a genetically determined reduced fetal growth rate. In other words, the genotype responsible for type 2 diabetes may itself restrict fetal growth. This possibility forms the basis for the *fetal insulin hypothesis*, which suggests that genetically determined insulin resistance could result in insulin-mediated low growth rate in utero as well as insulin resistance in childhood and adulthood (Hattersley et al, 1999). Insulin is one of the major growth factors in fetal life, and monogenic disorders that affect the fetus's insulin secretion or insulin resistance also affect its growth (Elsas et al, 1985; Froguel et al, 1993; Hattersley et al, 1998; Stoffers et al, 1997). Mutations in the gene encoding glucokinase have been identified that result in low birth weight and maturity-onset diabetes of the young. However, such mutations are rare, and no analogous common allelic variation has yet been discovered, but it is likely that some variations exist that, once identified, will explain a proportion of the cases of diabetes in LBW subjects.

There is obviously a close relationship between genes and the environment. Not only can maternal gene expression alter the fetal environment, the maternal intrauterine environment also affects fetal gene expression. An adverse intrauterine milieu is likely to have profound long-term effects on the developing organism that may not be reflected in birth weight.

## Cellular Mechanisms

Fetal malnutrition has two main causes, poor maternal nutrition and placental insufficiency. In the extensive literature about the fetal origins hypothesis, these two concepts have not been clearly discerned. Such a distinction is necessary, however, because maternal nutrition has probably been adequate in the majority of populations in which the hypothesis has been tested. Only extreme maternal undernutrition, such as occurred in the Dutch famine, reduces the birth weight to an extent that could be expected to raise the risk of adult disease (Lumey et al, 1995). Thus, it is reasonable that placental insufficiency has been a main cause of low birth weight in these populations. The oxygen and nutrients that support fetal growth and development rely on the entire nutrient supply line, beginning with maternal consumption and body size but extending also to uterine perfusion, placental function, and fetal metabolism. Interruptions of the supply line at any point could result in programming of the fetus for the future risk of adult diseases.

The intrauterine environment influences development of the fetus by modifying gene expression in both pluripotential cells and terminally differentiated, poorly replicating cells. The long-range effects on the offspring (into adulthood) are determined by which cells are undergoing differentiation, proliferation, or functional maturation at the time of the disturbance in maternal fuel economy. The fetus also adapts to an inadequate supply of substrates (such as glucose, amino acids, fatty acids, and oxygen) through metabolic changes, redistribution of blood flow, and changes in the production of fetal and placental hormones that control growth.

The fetus's immediate metabolic response to placental insufficiency is catabolism, consuming its own substrates to provide energy. A more prolonged reduction in availability of substrates leads to a slowing in growth. This enhances the fetus's ability to survive by reducing the use of substrates and lowering the metabolic rate. Slowing of growth in late gestation leads to disproportion in organ size, because the organs and tissues that are growing rapidly at the time are affected the most. Placental insufficiency in late gestation may, for example, lead to reduced growth of the kidney, which is developing rapidly at that time. Reduced replication of kidney cells may permanently reduce cell numbers, because there seems to be no capacity for renal cell division to catch up after birth.

Substrate availability has profound effects on fetal hormones and on the hormonal and metabolic interactions between the fetus, placenta, and mother. These effects are most apparent in the fetus of the mother with diabetes. Higher maternal concentrations of glucose and amino acids stimulate the fetal pancreas to secrete exaggerated amounts of insulin, and the fetal liver to produce higher levels of insulin-like growth factors (IGFs). Fetal hyperinsulinism stimulates the growth of adipose tissue and of other insulin-responsive tissues in the fetus, often leading to macrosomia. However, many offspring of diabetic mothers with fetal hyperinsulinism are not overgrown by usual standards, and many with later obesity and glucose intolerance were not macrosomic at birth (Pettitt et al, 1987; Silverman et al, 1995). These observations suggest that birth weight is not a good indication of intrauterine nutrition.

## What Animal Models Can Tell Us

Animal models have a normal genetic background which environmental effects can be tested for their role in inducing diabetes. In the rat, maternal dietary protein restriction (approximately 40% to 50% of normal intake) throughout gestation and lactation has been reported to alter glucose homeostasis and cause hypertension in the adult offspring (Berney et al, 1997; Burns et al, 1997; Dahri et al, 1991; Langley-Evans et al, 1996; Ozanne et al, 1996; Snoeck et al, 1990; Wilson and Hughes, 1997). Offspring are significantly growth retarded, remain growth retarded throughout life, and demonstrate mild β-cell secretory abnormalities in some cases and insulin resistance in others. However, none of these animal models results in the development of type 2 diabetes.

To extend these experimental studies of growth retardation, a model of IUGR in the rat was developed that does in fact lead to diabetes in later life (Boloker et al, 2002; Simmons et al, 2001). This model of fetal growth retardation has the following advantages over other animal models: (1) bilateral uterine artery ligation induces uteroplacental insufficiency, one of the most common causes of human IUGR, (2) growth-retarded fetal rats have critical features of a metabolic profile characteristic of growth-retarded human fetuses—decreased levels of glucose, insulin, IGF-1, amino acids, and oxygen (Ogata et al, 1986; Simmons et al, 1991; Unterman et al, 1990)—and, most importantly, (3) the diabetes that develops in IUGR rats has a phenotype remarkably similar to that observed in the human with type 2 diabetes—progressive dysfunction in insulin secretion and insulin action. Because of this IUGR model's similarity to human growth retardation and subsequent disease states, the IUGR rat represents one of the best experimental tools for studying the effect of uteroplacental insufficiency on the evolution of diabetes.

Although insulin resistance is a critical component of human type 2 diabetes, it is the failure of β-cell function and growth that determines progression to the diabetic phenotype (Gerich, 1998). Most pancreatic islet growth takes place during the fetal and neonatal periods, but replication of existing β cells and neogenesis of precursor cells occur throughout life. Insufficient proliferation and neogenesis have been hypothesized to be the underlying cause of the lack of β-cell compensation that leads to type 2 diabetes. Thus, uteroplacental insufficiency during the last trimester in the fetus permanently impairs the processes of neogenesis, proliferation, and differentiation. If new β cells are not generated to replace the normal loss of existing β cells, β-cell mass will eventually be reduced, and diabetes will ensue.

β cells are particularly vulnerable to changes in substrate and hormone availability. Indeed, SGA infants have reduced plasma insulin concentrations (Economides et al, 1989) and pancreatic β-cell numbers, whereas β-cell growth is enhanced in the fetus exposed to excess nutrients and hormones in the diabetic milieu of diabetes in pregnancy.

A major consequence of uteroplacental insufficiency is oxidative stress in the fetus (Bowen et al, 2001; Ejima et al, 1999; Karowicz-Billinska et al, 2002; Kato et al, 1997; Myatt et al, 1997). Decreased substrate supply alters the redox state in susceptible tissues, leading to an imbalance between the production of reactive oxygen species (ROS) and antioxidant capacity that results in mitochondrial dysfunction and oxidative stress. The β cell is particularly vulnerable to oxidative stress because expression of antioxidant enzymes in the pancreatic islets is very low (Lenzen et al, 1996; Tiedge et al, 1997), and the pancreas has a high oxidative energy requirement. Animal studies in the IUGR rat support the concept that oxidative stress plays a major role in the impairment of β-cell function and maturation that is observed in the human growth-retarded fetus (Simmons and Gertz, 1998).

### Conclusions

The combined epidemiologic, clinical, and animal studies clearly demonstrate that the intrauterine environment influences both growth and development of the fetus and the subsequent development of adult diseases. There are specific, critical windows during development, often coincident with periods of rapid cell division, during which a stimulus or insult may have long-lasting consequences on tissue or organ function after birth. Birth weight is only one marker of an adverse fetal environment, and confining studies to the LBW population may lead to erroneous conclusions regarding etiology of growth retardation. Studies using animal models of uteroplacental insufficiency can provide some insights into possible mechanisms underlying the fetal origins hypothesis; however, much work remains to be done.

## MACROSOMIA

Excessive fetal growth (macrosomia, being large for gestational age) is found is 9% to 13% of all deliveries and can lead to significant complications in the perinatal period (Gregory et al, 1998; Wollschlaeger et al, 1999). Maternal factors associated with macrosomia during pregnancy include increasing parity, higher maternal age, and maternal height. Additionally, the previous delivery of a macrosomic infant, prolonged pregnancy, maternal glucose intolerance, high pre-pregnancy weight or obesity, and large pregnancy weight gain have all been found to raise the risk of delivering a macrosomic infant (Mocanu et al, 2000).

Maternal complications of macrosomia include morbidities related to labor and delivery. Prolonged labor, arrest of labor, and higher rates of cesarean section and instrumentation during labor have been reported. Also, the risks of maternal lacerations and trauma, delayed placental detachment, and postpartum hemorrhage are higher for the woman delivering a macrosomic infant (Lipscomb et al, 1995; Perlow et al, 1996). Complications of labor are more pronounced in primiparous women than in multiparous women (Mocanu et al, 2000). The neonatal complications of macrosomia include traumatic events such as shoulder dystocia, brachial nerve palsy, birth trauma, and associated perinatal asphyxia. Other complications for the neonate are elevated insulin levels and metabolic derangements, such as hypoglycemia and hypocalcemia (Wollschlaeger et al, 1999). In a large population-based study in the United States, macrosomia (defined as birth weight greater than 4000 g) was detected in 13% of births. Of these, shoulder dystocia was noted in 11% (Gregory et al, 1998).

Macrosomia is often not detected during pregnancy and labor. The clinical estimation of fetal size is difficult and has significant false-positive and false-negative rates. Ultrasonography estimates of fetal weight are not always accurate, and the literature reports a wide range of sensitivity estimates for the ultrasound detection of macrosomia. Additionally, there is controversy in how to define macrosomia and which ultrasound measurement is most sensitive in predicting macrosomia. Smith and colleagues (1997) have demonstrated a linear relation between abdominal circumference and birth weight. They showed that the equations commonly used for estimated fetal weight (EFW) have a median error rate of 7%, with greater errors seen with larger infants. Using receiver operating characteristics (ROC) curves to measure the diagnostic accuracy of ultrasound, O'Reilly-Green and Divon (1997) reported sensitivity and specificity rates of 85% and 72%, respectively, for estimation of birth weight exceeding 4000 g. In their study, the positive predictive value (i.e., a positive test result represents a truly macrosomic infant) is about 49%. Chauhan and associates (2000) found lower sensitivity for the use of ultrasound measurement of abdominal and head circumference and femur length (72% sensitivity), similar to the sensitivity of using clinical measurements alone (73%). Other investigators have shown that clinical estimation of fetal weight (43% sensitivity) had higher sensitivity and specificity than ultrasound evaluation in predicting macrosomia (Gonen et al, 1996). In a retrospective study, Jazayeri and coworkers (1999) showed that ultrasound measurement of abdominal circumference of greater than 35 cm predicts macrosomia in 93% of cases and is superior to measurements of biparietal diameter or femur. Other researchers have reported that an abdominal circumference of either more than 37 cm or more than 38 cm to be a better predictor (Al-Inany et al, 2001; Gilby et al, 2000).

Numerous investigators have also questioned whether antenatal diagnosis improves birth outcomes in macrosomic infants. Investigators point to the low rates of specificity of antenatal tests resulting in high rates of false-positive results (Bryant et al, 1998, O'Reilly-Green and Divon, 1997). Antenatal identification of macrosomia (or possible macrosomia) may lead to a higher rate of cesarean section performed for infants with normal birth weights (Gonen et al, 2000; Mocanu et al, 2000; Parry et al, 2000). Macrosomia is a risk factor for shoulder dystocia, but the majority of cases of shoulder dystocia and birth trauma occurs in nonmacrosomic infants (Gonen et al, 1996). A retrospective study of infants weighing more than 4200 g at birth showed a cesarean section rate of 52% in infants predicted antenatally to have macrosomia, compared with 30% in infants without such a antenatal prediction. The antenatal prediction of fetal macrosomia is also associated with a higher incidence of failed induction of labor and no reduction in the rate of shoulder dystocia (Zamorski and Biggs, 2001). Using retrospective data from a 12-year period, Bryant and colleagues (1998) estimated that a policy of routine cesarean section for all infants with estimated fetal weight greater than 4500 g would require between 155 and 588 cesarean sections to prevent a single case of permanent brachial nerve palsy.

## SUMMARY

We have described many identified biologic and genetic factors associated with fetal growth and with abnormalities of fetal growth. Physicians are limited in the ability to identify a causative agent in every case. Modification of fetal growth is possible and occurs from such diverse influences as socioeconomic status, maternal nutrition, and maternal constitutional factors. Abnormal fetal growth influences not only acute perinatal outcomes but also health during infancy, childhood, and, intriguingly, adulthood. In schools of public health, students are taught to search "up river" for solutions to health problems. Solutions for ill health in adulthood may lie in the identification of methods to improve the health of the fetus.

## SELECTED READINGS

Alexander GR, Himes JH, Kaufman R, et al: A United States national reference for fetal growth. Obstet Gynecol 87:163-168, 1996.

## REFERENCES

Alexander GR, Kogan MD, Himes JH, et al: Racial differences in birth weight for gestational age and infant mortality in extremely-low-risk US populations. Paediatr Perinat Epidemiol 13:205-217, 1999.

Al-Inany H, Allaa N, Momtaz M, Abdel B: Intrapartum prediction of macrosomia: Accuracy of abdominal circumference estimation. Gynecol Obstet Invest 51:116-119, 2001.

Ananth C, Wilcox A: Placental abruption and perinatal mortality in the United States. Am J Epidemiol 153:332-337, 2001.

Ananth C, Demissie K, Smulian J, Vintzileos A: Relationship among placenta previa, fetal growth restriction, and preterm delivery: A population-based study. Obstet Gynecol 98:299-306, 2001.

Andres R, Day M: Perinatal complications associated with maternal tobacco use. Semin Neonatol 5:231-241, 2000.

Balcazar H: The prevalence of intrauterine growth retardation in Mexican Americans. Am J Public Health 84:462-465, 1994.

Barker DJP, Winter PD, Osmond C, et al: Weight in infancy and death from ischaemic heart disease. Lancet 2:577-580, 1989.

Barker DJP, Hales CN, Fall CHD, et al: Type 2 diabetes mellitus, hypertension, and hyperlipidemia (syndrome X): Relation to reduced fetal growth. Diabetologia 36:62-67, 1993.

Battaglia F, Lubchenco L: A practical classification of newborn infants by weight and gestational age. J Pediatr 71:159-163, 1967.

Bavdekar A, Yajnik CS, Fall CH, et al: Insulin resistance syndrome in 8-year-old Indian children: Small at birth, big at 8 years, or both? Diabetes 48:2422-2429, 1999.

Benirschke K: The biology of the twinning process: How placentation influences outcomes. Semin Perinatol 19:342-350, 1995.

Berney DM, Desai M, Palmer DJ, et al: The effects of maternal protein deprivation on the fetal rat pancreas: Major structural changes and their recuperation. J Pathol 183:109-115, 1997.

Bernstein I, Horbar J, Badger C, et al: Morbidity and mortality among very-low-birth weight neonates with IUGR: The Vermont Oxford Network. Am J Obstet Gynecol 182:198-206, 2000a.

Bernstein I, Plociennik K, Stahle S, et al: Impact of maternal cigarette smoking on fetal growth and body composition. Am J Obstet Gynecol 183:883-886, 2000b.

Blair E, Stanley F: Intrauterine growth and spastic cerebral palsy. I: Association with birth weight for gestational age. Am J Obstet Gynecol 162:229-237, 1990.

Boloker J, Gertz S, Simmons RA: Offspring of diabetic rats develop obesity and type II diabetes in adulthood. Diabetes 51:1499-1506, 2002.

Bowen RS, Moodley J, Dutton MF, Theron AJ: Oxidative stress in pre-eclampsia. Acta Obstet Gynecol Scand. 80:719-725, 2001.

Brenner BM, Chertow GM: Congenital oligonephropathy: An inborn cause of adult hypertension and progressive renal injury? Curr Opin Nephrol Hypertens 2:691-695, 1993.

Bryant D, Leonardi M, Landwehr J, Bottoms S: Limited usefulness of fetal weight in predicting neonatal brachial plexus injury. Am J Obstet Gynecol 179:686-689, 1998.

Burns SP, Desai M, Cohen RD, et al: Gluconeogenesis, glucose handling, and structural changes in livers of the adult offspring of rats partially deprived of protein during pregnancy and lactation. J Clin Invest 100:1768-1774, 1997.

Chauhan S, West D, Scardo J, et al: Antepartum detection of macrosomic fetus: Clinical versus sonographic, including soft-tissue measurement. Obstetr Gynecol 95:639-642, 2000.

Clausen JO, Borch-Johnsen K, Pedersen O: Relation between birth weight and the insulin sensitivity index in a population sample of 331 young, healthy Caucasians. Am J Epidemiol 146:23-31, 1997.

Clausson B, Cnattingius S, Axelsson O: Preterm and term births of small for gestational age infants: A population-based study of risk factors among nulliparous women. Br J Obstet Gynaecol 105:1011-1017, 1998.

Cnattingius S, Haglund B, Kramer M: Differences in late fetal death rates in association with determinants of small for gestational age fetuses: Population based cohort study. BMJ 316:1483-1487, 1998.

Collins J, Butler A: Racial differences in the prevalence of small-for-dates infants among college-educated women. Epidemiology 8:315-317, 1997.

Curhan GC, Willett WC, Rimm EB, et al: Birth weight and adult hypertension, diabetes mellitus and obesity in US men. Circulation 94:3246-3250, 1996.

Dahri S, Snoeck A, Reusens-Billen B, et al: Islet function in offspring of mothers on low-protein diet during gestation. Diabetes 40:115-120, 1991.

de Onis M, Villar J, Gulmezoglu M: Nutritional interventions to prevent intrauterine growth retardation: Evidence from randomized controlled trials. Eur J Clin Nutr 52(Suppl 1):S83-S93, 1998.

Degani S: Fetal biometry: Clinical, pathological, and technical considerations. Obstet Gynecol Survey 56:159-167, 2001.

Devoe L, Ware D: Antenatal assessment of twin gestation. Semin Perinatol 19:413-423, 1995.

Doctor B, O'Riordan M, Kirchner H, et al: Perinatal correlates and neonatal outcomes of small for gestational age infants born at term gestation. Am J Obstet Gynecol 185:652-659, 2001.

Economides DL, Proudler A, Nicolaides KH: Plasma insulin in appropriate and small for gestatonal age fetuses. Am J Obestet Gynecol 160:1091-1094, 1989.

Egeland GM, Skjaerven R, Irgrens LM: Birth characteristics of women who develop gestational diabetes: Population based study. BMJ 321:546-547, 2000.

Ejima K, Nanri H, Toki N, et al: Localization of thioredoxin reductase and thioredoxin in normal human placenta and their protective effect against oxidative stress. Placenta. 20:95-101, 1999.

Elsas LJ, Endo F, Strumlauf E, et al: Leprechaunism: An inherited defect in a high-affinity insulin receptor. Am J Hum Genet 37:73-88, 1985.

Eriksson J, Forsen T, Tuomilehto J, et al: Fetal and childhood growth and hypertension in adult life. Hypertension. 36:790-794, 2000.

Fall CHD, Osmond C, Barker DJP, et al: Fetal and infant growth and cardiovascular risk factors in women. BMJ 310:428-432, 1995.

Flanagan DE, Moore VM, Godsland IF, et al: Fetal growth and the physiological control of glucose tolerance in adults: A minimal model analysis. Am J Physiol Endocrinol Metab 278:E700-E706, 2000.

Forsen T, Eriksson J, Tuomilehto J, et al: The fetal and childhood growth of persons who develop type 2 diabetes. Ann Intern Med 133:176-182, 2000.

Fox H: Aging of the placenta. Arch Dis Child Fetal Neonatal Ed 77:F171-F175, 1997.
Frisbie WP, Biegler M, deTurk P, et al: Racial and ethnic differences in determinants of intrauterine growth retardation and other compromised birth outcomes. Am J Public Health 87:1977-1983, 1997.
Froguel P, Zouali H, Vionnet N: Familial hyperglycemia due to mutations in glucokinase: Definition of a subtype of diabetes mellitus. N Engl J Med 328:697-702, 1993.
Fuentes-Afflick E, Hessol N, Perez-Stable E: Maternal birthplace, ethnicity, and low birth weight in California. Arch Pediatr Adolesc Med 152:1105-1112, 1998.
Galan H, Rigano S, Radaelli T, et al: Reduction of subcutaneous mass, but not lean mass, in normal fetuses in Denver, Colorado. Am J Obstet Gynecol 185:839-844, 2001.
Gerich JE: The genetic basis of type 2 diabetes mellitus: Impaired insulin secretion versus impaired insulin sensitivity. Endocr Rev 19:491-503, 1998.
Ghidini A: Idiopathic fetal growth restriction: A pathophysiologic approach. Obstet Gynecol Surv 51:376-382, 1996.
Gilby J, Williams M, Spellacy W: Fetal abdominal circumference measurements of 35 and 38 cm as predictors of macrosomia: A risk factor for shoulder dystocia. J Reprod Med 45:936-938, 2000.
Glinianaia S, Skjærven R, Magnus P: Birth weight percentiles by gestational age in multiple births: A population-based study of Norwegian twins and triplets. Acta Obstet Gynecol Scand 79: 450-458, 2000.
Godfrey K, Robinson S, Barker D, et al: Maternal nutrition in early and late pregnancy in relation to placental and fetal growth. BMJ 312:410-414, 1996.
Goldenberg R, Cliver S, Neggers Y, et al: The relationship between maternal characteristics and fetal and neonatal anthropometric measurements in women delivering at term: A summary. Acta Obstet Gynecol Scand Suppl 165:8-13, 1997.
Goldenberg R, Hoffman H, Cliver S: Neurodevelopmental outcome of small-for-gestational-age infants. Eur J Clinical Nutrition 52(Suppl 1): S54-S58, 1998.
Gonen R, Speigel D, Abend M: Is macrosomia predictable, and are shoulder dystocia and birth trauma preventable? Obstet Gynecol 88:526-529, 1996.
Gonen R, Bader D, Ajami M: Effects of a policy of elective cesarean delivery in cases of suspected fetal macrosomia on the incidence of brachial plexus injury and the rate of cesarean delivery. Am J Obstet Gynecol 183:1296-1300, 2000.
Gortner L, Wauer R, Stock G, et al: Neonatal outcome in small for gestational age infants: Do they really do better? J Perinat Med 27:484-489, 1999.
Gray P, Jones P, O'Callaghan M: Maternal antecedents for cerebral palsy in extremely preterm babies: A case-control study. Dev Med Child Neurol 43:580-585, 2001.
Gregory K, Henry O, Ramicone E, et al: Maternal and infant complications in high and normal weight infants by method of delivery. Obstet Gynecol 92:507-513, 1998.
Guendelman S, English P: Effect of United States residence on birth outcomes among Mexican immigrants: An exploratory study. Am J Epidemiol 142(Suppl):S30-S38, 1995.
Hales CN, Barker DJP: Type 2 diabetes mellitus: The thrifty phenotype hypothesis. Diabetologia. 35:595-601, 1992.
Hattersley AT, Beards F, Ballantyne E, et al: Mutations in the glucokinase gene of the fetus result in reduced birth weight. Nat Genet 19:268-270, 1998.
Hattersley AT, Tooke JE: The fetal insulin hypothesis: An alternative explanation of the association of low birth weight with diabetes and vascular disease. Lancet 353:1789-1792, 1999.
Heinonen S, Taipale P, Saarikoski S: Weights of placentae from small-for-gestational age infants revisited. Placenta 22:399-404, 2001.
Hershkovitz R, Erez O, Sheiner E, et al: Comparison study between induced and spontaneous term and preterm births of small-for-gestational-age neonates. Eur J Obstet Gynecol Reprod Biol 97:141-146, 2001.
Hobbins J: Morphometry of fetal growth. Acta Paediatr Suppl 423:165-168, 1997.
Hoffman PL, Cutfield WS, Robinson EM, et al: Insulin resistance in short children with intrauterine growth retardation. J Clin Endocrinol Metab 82:402-406, 1997.
Hollier L, McIntire D, Leveno K: Outcome of twin pregnancies according to intrapair birth weight differences. Obstet Gynecol 94:1006-1010, 1999.
Iyengar G, Nair P: Global outlook on nutrition and the environment: Meeting the challenges of the next millennium. Sci Total Environ 249:331-346, 2000.
Jackson A, Robinson S: Dietary guidelines for pregnancy: A review of current evidence. Public Health Nutr 4:625-630, 2001.
Jahn A, Razum O, Berle P: Routine screening for intrauterine growth retardation in Germany: Low sensitivity and questionable benefit for diagnosed cases. Acta Obstet Gynecol Scand 77:643-648, 1998.
Jameson S: Zinc status in pregnancy: The effect of zinc therapy on perinatal mortality, prematurity, and placental ablation. Ann N Y Acad Sci 678:178-192, 1993.
Jaquet D, Gaboriau P, Czernichow, Levy-Marchal C: Insulin resistance early in adulthood in subjects born with intrauterine growth retardation. J Clin Endocrinol Metab 85:1401-1406, 2000.
Jazayeri A, Heffron J, Phillips R, Spellacy W: Macrosomia prediction using ultrasound fetal abdominal circumference of 35 centimeters or more. Obstet Gynecol 93:523-526, 1999.
Jensen CB, Storgaard H, Dela F, et al: Early differential defects of insulin secretion and action in 19-year-old Caucasian men who had low birth weight. Diabetes 51:1271-1280, 2002.
Karowicz-Bilinska A, Suzin J, Sieroszewski P: Evaluation of oxidative stress indices during treatment in pregnant women with intrauterine growth retardation. Med Sci Monit 8:CR211-CR216, 2002.
Kato H, Yoneyama Y, Araki T: Fetal plasma lipid peroxide levels in pregnancies complicated by preeclampsia. Gynecol Obstet Invest 43:158-161, 1997.
Keirse M: International variation in intrauterine growth. Eur J Obstet Gynecol Reprod Biol 92:21-28, 2000.
Kermack WO: Death rates in Great Britain and Sweden. Lancet 1:698-703, 1934.
Khamashta M, Hughes G: Pregnancy in systemic lupus erythematosus. Curr Opin Rheumatol 8:424-429, 1996.
Khan N, Kazzi S: Yield and costs of screening growth-retarded infants for torch infections. Am J Perinatol 17:131-135, 2000.
Kramer M, Olivier M, McLean F, et al: Impact of intrauterine growth retardation and body proportionality on fetal and neonatal outcome. Pediatrics 86:707-713, 1990.
Kramer M, Seguin L, Lydon J, Goulet L: Socio-economic disparities in pregnancy outcome: Why do the poor fare so poorly? Paediatr Perinat Epidemiol 14:194-210, 2000.
Krampl E, Lees C, Bland J, et al: Fetal biometry at 4300 m compared to sea level in Peru. Utrasound Obstet Gynecol 16:9-18, 2000.
Lackman F, Capewell V, Richardson B, et al: The risk of spontaneous preterm delivery and perinatal mortality in relation to size at birth according to fetal versus neonatal growth standards. Am J Obstet Gynecol 184:946-953, 2001.
Ladipo O: Nutrition in pregnancy: Mineral and vitamin supplements. Am J Clin Nutr 72(Suppl):280S-290S, 2000.
Langley-Evans SC, Phillips GJ, Benediktsson R, et al: Protein intake in pregnancy, placental glucocorticoid metabolism and the programming of hypertension in the rat. Placenta 17:169-172, 1996.

Lapillonne A, Braillon P, Chatelain PG, et al: Body composition in appropriate and small for gestational age infants. Acta Paediatr 86:196-200, 1997.

Leger J, Levy-Marchal C, Bloch J, et al: Reduced final height and indications for insulin resistance in 20 year olds born small for gestational age: regional cohort study. BMJ 315:341-347, 1997.

Lenzen S, Drinkgern J, Tiedge M: Low antioxidant enzyme gene expression in pancreatic islets compared with various other mouse tissues. Free Radic Biol Med. 20:463-466, 1996.

Li C, Windsor R, Perkins L, et al: The impact on infant birth weight and gestational age of cotinine-validated smoking reduction during pregnancy. JAMA 269:1519-1524, 1993.

Li C, Johnson MS, Goran MI: Effects of low birth weight on insulin resistance syndrome in Caucasion and African-American children. Diabetes Care 24:2035-2042, 2001.

Lieberman E, Gremy F, Lang JM, Cohen AP: Low birth weight at term and the timing of fetal exposure to maternal smoking. Am J Public Health 84:1127-1131, 1994.

Lin C, Su S, River L: Comparison of associated high-risk factors and perinatal outcome between symmetric and asymmetric fetal intrauterine growth retardation. Am J Obstet Gynecol 164:1535-1541, 1991.

Lipscomb K, Gregory K, Shaw K: The outcome of macrosomic infants weighing at least 4500g: Los Angeles County and University of Southern California experience. Obstet Gynecol 85:558-564, 1995.

Lithell HO, McKeigue PM, Berglund L, et al: Relation of size at birth to non-insulin dependent diabetes and insulin concentrations in men aged 50-60 years. BMJ 312:406-410, 1996.

Low J, Handley-Derry M, Burke S, et al: Association of intrauterine fetal growth retardation and learning deficits at age 9 to 11 years. Am J Obstet Gynecol 167:1499-1505, 1992.

Lumey LH, Stein AD, Racelli ACJ: Timing of prenatal starvation in women and birth weight in their first and second offspring: The Dutch Famine Birth Cohort Study. Eur J Obstet Gynecol Reprod Biol. 61:25-30, 1995.

Mathews F, Yudkin P, Neil A: Influence of maternal nutrition on outcome of pregnancy: Prospective cohort study. BMJ 319:339-343, 1999.

May R, Tramp J, Bass K, et al: Early postnatal growth of low birth weight infants in the WIC program. Am J Human Biol 13:261-267, 2001.

McCance DR, Pettitt DJ, Hanson RL, et al:. Birth weight and non-insulin dependent diabetes: Thrifty genotype, thrifty phenotype, or surviving small baby genotype. BMJ 308:942-945, 1994.

McCarthy A, Ben-Schlomo Y, Elwood P, et al: The relationship between birth weight, catch-up growth in infancy, and blood pressure in young adulthood. Pediatr Res 50:45A, 2001.

McIntire D, Bloom S, Casey B, Leveno K: Birth weight in relation to morbidity and mortality among newborn infants. N Engl J Med 340:1234-1238, 1999.

McKeigue PM, Lithell HO, Leon DA: Glucose tolerance and resistance to insulin-stimulated glucose uptake in men aged 70 years in relation to size at birth. Diabetologia 41:1133-1138, 1998.

Mocanu E, Greene R, Byrne B, Turner M: Obstetric and neonatal outcome of babies weight more than 4.5 kg: An analysis by parity. Eur J Obstet Gynecol Reprod Biol 92:229-233, 2000.

Mongelli M, Gardosi J: Fetal growth. Curr Opin Obstet Gynecol 12:111-115, 2000.

Moore L, Young D, McCullough R, et al: Tibetan protection from IUGR (IUGR) and reproductive loss at high altitude. Am J Hum Biol 13:635-644, 2001.

Myatt L, Eis ALW, Brockman DE, et al: Differential localization of superoxide dismutase isoforms in placental villous tissue of normotensive, pre-eclamptic, and intrauterine growth-restricted pregnancies. J Histochem Cytochem 45:1433-1438, 1997.

Neggers Y, Goldenberg R, Tamura T, et al: The relationship between maternal dietary intake and infant birth weight. Acta Obstet Gynecol Scand Suppl 165:71-75, 1997.

Nordentoft M, Lou H, Hansen D, et al: Intrauterine growth retardation and premature delivery: The influence of maternal smoking and psychosocial factors. Am J Public Health 86:347-354, 1996.

O'Reilly-Green C, Divon M: Receiver operating characteristic curves and sonographic estimated fetal weight for prediction of macrosomia in prolonged pregnancies. Ultrasound Obstet Gynecol 9:403-408, 1997.

Ødegård R, Vatten L, Nilsen S, et al: Preeclampsia and fetal growth. Obstet Gynecol 96:950-955, 2000.

Ogata Es, Bussey M, Finley S: Altered gas exchange, limited glucose, branched chain amino acids, and hypoinsulinism retard fetal growth in the rat. Metabolism 35:950-977, 1986.

Owen P, Khan K: Fetal growth velocity in the prediction of intrauterine growth retardation in a low risk population. Br J Obstet Gynaecol 105:536-540, 1998.

Ozanne SE, Wang CL, Coleman N, Smith GD: Altered muscle insulin sensitivity in the male offspring of protein-malnourished rats. A J Physiol 271:E1128-E1134, 1996.

Pardi G, Marcon AM, Cetin I: Pathophysiology of intrauterine growth retardation: Role of the placenta. Acta Paediatr Suppl 423:170-172, 1997.

Parker J, Schoendorf K, Keily J: Associations between measures of socioeconomic status and low birth weight, small for gestational age, and premature delivery in the United States. Ann Epidemiol 4:271-278, 1994.

Parry S, Severs C, Sehdev H, et al: Ultrasonographic prediction of fetal macrosomia: Association with cesarean delivery. J Reprod Med 45:17-22, 2000.

Pastrakuljic A, Derewlany L, Koren G: Maternal cocaine use and cigarette smoking in pregnancy in relation to amino acid transport and fetal growth. Placenta 20: 499-512, 1999.

Perlow J, Wigton T, Hart J, et al: Birth trauma: A five-year review of incidence and associated perinatal factors. J Reprod Med 41:754-760, 1996.

Pettitt DJ, Knowler WC, Bennett PH, et al: Obesity in offspring of diabetic Pima Indian women despite normal birth weight. Diabetes Care 10:76-80, 1987.

Phillips DI, Barker DJ, Hales CN, et al: Thinness at birth and insulin resistance in adult life. Diabetologia 37:150-154, 1994.

Rao S, Yajnik C, Kanade A, et al: Intake of micronutrient-rich foods in rural Indian mothers is associated with the size of the babies at birth: Pune maternal nutrition study. J Nutr 131:1217-1224, 2001.

Ravelli GP, Stein ZA, Susser MW: Obesity in young men after famine exposure in utero and early infancy. N Engl J Med 295:349-353, 1976.

Rich-Edwards JW, Colditz GA, Stampfer MJ, et al: Birth weight and the risk for type 2 diabetes mellitus in adult women. Ann Intern Med 130:278-284, 1999.

Robinson J, Moore V, Owens J, McMillen C: Origins of fetal growth restriction. Eur J Obstet Gynecol Reprod Biol 92:13-19, 2000.

Rush D: Maternal nutrition and perinatal survival. Nutr Rev 59:315-26, 2001.

Say L, Gülmezoglu AM, Hofmeyr GJ, in Cochrane Database Syst Rev (1):CD0000148, 2003.

Scherjon S, Oosting H, Smolders-DeHaas H, et al: Neurodevelopmental outcome at three years of age after fetal "brain-sparing." Early Hum Dev 52:67-79, 1998.

Scholl T, Hediger M: Weight gain, nutrition, and pregnancy outcome: Findings from the Camden study of teenage and minority gravidas. Semin Perinatol 19:171-181, 1995.

Seeds J, Peng T: Impaired growth and risk of fetal death: Is the tenth percentile the appropriate standard? Am J Obstet Gynecol 178: 658-669, 1998.

Shah D, Sachdev H: Effect of gestational zinc deficiency on pregnancy outcomes: Summary of observation studies and zinc supplementation trials. Br J Nutr 85(Suppl 2):S101-S108, 2001.
Silverman BL, Metzger BE, Cho NH, Loeb CA: Impaired glucose tolerance in adolescent offspring of diabetic mothers. Diabetes Care 18:611-617, 1995.
Simchen M, Beiner M, Strauss-Liviathan N, et al: Neonatal outcome in growth-restricted versus appropriately grown preterm infants. Am J Perinatol 17:187-192, 2000.
Simmons RA, Gertz SJ: Intrauterine growth retardation induces diabetes in pregnancy producing obese offspring with glucose intolerance and impaired insulin secretion. Pediatr Res 43:486A, 1998.
Simmons RA, Gounis AS, Bangalore SA, Ogata ES: Intrauterine growth retardation: Fetal glucose transport is diminished in lung but spared in brain. Pediatr Res 31:59-63, 1991 .
Simmons RA, Templeton L, Gertz S, Niu H. Intrauterine growth retardation leads to type II diabetes in adulthood in the rat. Diabetes 50:2279-2286, 2001.
Skjærven R, Gjessing H, Bakketeig L: Birth weight by gestational age in Norway. Acta Obstet Gynecol Scand 79:440-449, 2000.
Smith GC, Smith MF, McNay MB, Fleming JE: The relation between fetal abdominal circumference and birth weight: Findings in 3512 pregnancies. Br J Obstet Gynaecol 104:186-190, 1997.
Snoeck A, Remacle C, Reusens B, Hoet JJ: Effect of a low protein diet during pregnancy on the fetal rat endocrine pancreas. Biol Neonate 57:107-118, 1990.
Sonntag J, Waltz S, Schollmeyer T, et al: Morbidity and mortality of discordant twins up to 34 weeks of gestational age. Eur J Pediatr 155:224-229, 1996.
Spinillo A, Capuzzo E, Piazzi G, et al: Maternal high-risk factors and severity of growth deficit in small for gestational age infants. Early Hum Dev 38:35-43, 1994.
Spinillo A, Capuzzo E, Egbe T, et al: Pregnancies complicated by idiopathic intrauterine growth retardation: Severity of growth failure, neonatal morbidity and two-year infant neurodevelopmental outcome. J Reprod Med 40:209-215, 1995.
Srivastava S, Mehrotra P, Srivastava SP, et al: Blood lead and zinc in pregnant women and their offspring in intrauterine growth retardation cases. J Anal Toxicol 25:461-465, 2001.
Stoffers DA, Zinkin NT, Stanojevic V, et al: Pancreatic agenesis attributable to a single nucleotide deletion in the human IPF1 gene coding sequence. Nat Genet 15:106-110, 1997.
Strauss R, Dietz W: Low maternal weight gain in the second or third trimester increases the risk for intrauterine growth retardation. J Nutr 129:988-993, 1999.
Sung I, Vohr B, Oh W: Growth and neurodevelopmental outcome for very low birth weight infants with intrauterine growth retardation: Comparison with controls subject matched by birth weight and gestational age. J Pediatr 123:618-624, 1993.
Thomas P, Peabody J, Turnier V, Clark R: A new look at intrauterine growth and the impact of race, altitude, and gender. Pediatrics 106:E21, 2000.
Tiedge M, Lortz S, Drinkgern J, Lenzen S: Relationship between antioxidant enzyme gene expression and antioxidant defense status of insulin-producing cells. Diabetes 46:1733-1742, 1997.
Unterman T, Lascon R, Gotway M, et al: Circulating levels of insulin-like growth factor binding protein-1 (IGFBP-1) and hepatic mRNA are increased in the small for gestational age fetal rat. Endocrinology 127:2035-2037, 1990.
Uvebrant P, Hagberg G: Intrauterine growth in children with cerebral palsy. Act Paediatr 81:407-412, 1992.
Vaag A, Henricksen JE, Madsbad S, et al: Insulin secretion, insulin action, and hepatic glucose production in identical twins discordant for NIDDM. J Clin Invest 95:690-698, 1995.
Valdez R, Athens MA, Thompson GH, et al: Birth weight and adult health outcomes in a biethnic population in the USA. Diabetologia 37:624-531, 1994.
Van Assche FA, De Prins F, Aerts L, Verjans F: The endocrine pancreas in small-for-dates infants. Br J Obstet Gynaecol 84: 751-753, 1977.
Victoria A, Mora G, Arias F: Perinatal outcome, placental pathology, and severity of discordance in monochorionic and dichorionic twins. Obstet Gynecol 97:310-315, 2001.
Villar J, de Onis M, Kestler E, et al: The differential neonatal morbidity of the intrauterine growth retardation syndrome. Am J Obstet Gynecol 163:151-157, 1990.
Walsh R, Lowe J, Hopkins P: Quitting smoking in pregnancy. Med J Aust 175:320-323, 2001.
Whincup PF, Cook DG, Adshead T, et al: Childhood size is more strongly related than size at birth to glucose and insulin levels in 10–11 year-old children. Diabetologia 40:319-326, 1997.
Widdowson EM, Southgate DAT, Hey EN: In Visser HKA (ed): Nutrition and Metabolism of the Fetus and Infant: Fifth Nutricia Symposium, Rotterdam, 11–13 October, 1978. The Hague, Martinus Nijhoff, 1979, pp 169-177.
Wilcox M, Smith S, Johnson I, et al: The effect of social deprivation on birth weight, excluding physiological and pathological effects. Br J Obstet Gynaecol 102:918-924, 1995.
Williams KP, Nwebube N: Abdominal circumference: A single measurement versus growth rate in the prediction of intrapartum cesarean section for fetal distress. Ultrasound Obstet Gynecol 17:493-495, 2001.
Wilson MR, Hughes SJ: The effect of maternal protein deficiency during pregnancy and lactation on glucose tolerance and pancreatic islet function in adult rat offspring. J Endocrinology 154:177-185, 1997.
Wollschlaeger K, Nieder J, Köppe I, Härtlein K: A study of fetal macrosomia. Arch Gynecol Obstet 263:51-55, 1999.
Xiong X, Mayes D, Demianczuk N, et al: Impact of pregnancy-induced hypertension on fetal growth. Am J Obstet Gynecol 180:207-213, 1999.
Yajnik CS, Fall CH, Vaidya U, et al: Fetal growth and glucose and insulin metabolism in four-year-old Indian children. Diabet Med 12:330-336, 1995.
Yasmeen S, Wilkins E, Field N, et al: Pregnancy outcomes in women with systemic lupus erythematosus. J Matern Fetal Med 10:91-96, 2001.
Zamorski M, Biggs W: Management of suspected fetal macrosomia. Am Fam Physician 63:302-306, 2001.
Zeitlin J, Ancel P, Saurel-Cubizolles M, Papiernik E: Are risk factors the same for small for gestational age versus other preterm births? Am J Obstet Gynecol 185:208-215, 2001.
Zeitlin J, Ancel P, Saurel-Cibizolles M, Papiernik E: The relationship between IUGR and preterm delivery: An empirical approach using data from a European case-control study. Brit J Obstet Gynecol 107:750-758, 2000.

CHAPTER 6

# Hormonal Influences on Fetal Development

**Philip L. Ballard**

The physiology of the fetal endocrine system differs from that of the adult endocrine system with regard to the hormonal milieu, production sites, plasma levels, rates and pathways of degradation, and biologic function. The unique endocrine environment of the fetus and placenta is important for both normal growth and differentiation of the fetus and timely parturition. Although there are major differences in endocrine physiology and regulated genes between the fetus and adult, the basic cellular mechanisms of hormone action do not change during development.

## SITES OF PRODUCTION AND ACTION

### Autocrine

Hormones in the autocrine system act primarily on the cells where they are synthesized. Hormones are synthesized within the cells, secreted at the cell surface into the extracellular domain, and then bind to specific cell surface receptors on the same cell. This interaction initiates a series of intracellular events, as described subsequently, that modify growth, differentiation, or function of the cell.

### Paracrine

In the paracrine system, hormones are secreted by one cell type and act on adjacent neighboring cells of another type. This mechanism provides for cell-cell communication within a tissue and is involved in regulating both growth and differentiation. In the fetal lung and other tissues, for example, insulin-like growth factors (IGFs) are produced and secreted by mesenchymal cells and influence the growth of adjacent epithelial cells.

### Endocrine

Most hormones are produced in a specific cell type of a tissue, are secreted into the circulation, and exert their regulatory effects on distant tissues. Included in this category, the endocrine system, are polypeptide hormones synthesized in the hypothalamus, pituitary, placenta, and other tissues as well as the steroid hormones (androgens, estrogens, progestins, mineralocorticoids, vitamin D, and glucocorticoids). The steroid hormones and many of the protein hormones are bound to specific binding proteins in the plasma, providing a hormone reservoir that is less susceptible to degradation. For most hormones, the plasma concentration of free (unbound) hormones represents the physiologically active hormones available to target cells. After secretion, the activity of hormones may be modified by metabolism in the circulation or tissues. For example, inactive cortisone may be converted to active cortisol by target tissues (e.g., lung and liver), and thyroxine ($T_4$) can undergo deiodination to either active triiodothyronine ($T_3$) or inactive reverse triiodothyronine ($rT_3$) in the adult or fetus, respectively.

## CELLULAR MECHANISMS

The signal inherent in a hormone is expressed through its binding to specific receptors, which initiates a series of biochemical events within the cell leading to altered replication or function. In general, the steps in this process of signal transduction are identical for adult and fetal cells, although different genes or proteins (or both) of a given cell type may be responsive during the developmental process. Furthermore, in the fetus, developmental immaturity or deficiency of specific components in the signal transduction system can alter hormone responsiveness.

### Membrane Receptors

The protein and peptide hormones as well as biogenic amines exert their effects on cells by binding to specific receptor proteins located on the cell membrane. The receptors are membrane-spanning proteins with an extracellular domain containing the binding site for the hormone and a cytoplasmic domain that transmits the hormonal signal to intracellular molecules. For many hormonal systems, binding of hormone to receptor results in higher intracellular levels of a second messenger, such as cyclic adenosine monophosphate (cAMP). Membrane receptors are capable of moving within the cell membrane and may aggregate and undergo endocytosis after binding of the hormone. Receptors are also substrates for various protein kinases, and in some cases, phosphorylation depends on the binding of hormones. These processes can produce a transient deficiency or inactivity of receptors (down-regulation) and relative unresponsiveness of the cells to continued hormonal exposure. For example, down-regulation and hormone refractoriness may be observed clinically with continued administration of a β-adrenergic agonist.

The membrane receptor system for β-adrenergic agonists has been well characterized. The cytoplasmic domain of the receptor is associated with G (GTP [guanosine triphosphate]–binding) proteins, which either activate or inhibit the catalytic component of adenyl cyclase. In the case of activation, binding of the hormone results within minutes in increased production of cAMP from adenosine triphosphate (ATP); the response is transient, and levels rapidly return to near baseline values through degradation by cAMP phosphodiesterase. This enzyme is inhibited by drugs such as methylxanthines. Cyclic AMP, in turn, binds to the regulatory subunit of protein kinase A, releasing and activating the catalytic subunit. This enzyme phosphorylates specific cellular proteins that contain the amino acid sequence Arg-Arg-*x*-Ser, resulting in either activation or inactivation with subsequent effects on enzyme activity (e.g., glycogen phosphorylase), intracellular structure (e.g., in the cytoskeleton), or gene expression in the nucleus. This sequence of events is summarized in Figure 6–1.

## Intracellular Receptors

Thyroid hormones, steroid hormones, and certain polypeptide hormones enter target cells and bind to specific receptors in the cytoplasm or within the nucleus. In the case of steroid hormones, interaction with a receptor protein modifies receptor structure and increases its affinity for specific binding sites (response elements) on regulated genes. This process alters the rate of gene transcription and, subsequently, the levels of the encoded protein. Hormones can also alter messenger RNA levels by influencing stability or efficiency of translation of the transcript. When the hormone is removed, steroid dissociates from the receptor through the law of mass action, and the response is reversed. Although binding of hormones to membrane receptors often produces responses within minutes (e.g., adrenocorticotropic hormone [ACTH] stimulation of cortisol production), steroid and other hormones that regulate gene expression require several hours to increase the content of specific messenger RNAs and the encoded proteins. The mechanism of steroid hormone action is depicted in Figure 6–2.

Hormonal responsiveness of a cell is determined by both the levels of circulating hormone and the concentration and activity of cellular receptors and other mediating proteins. In the undisturbed adult organism, for example, responsiveness is determined primarily by the level of circulating hormone that normally fluctuates over a relatively limited range (e.g., diurnal variation). As hormone levels rise, the percentage of receptors occupied by hormone also increases, often in a nearly linear fashion, resulting in a highly responsive and tightly regulated stimulus-response system. In the fetus, particularly early in gestation, hormonal responsiveness is limited by developmental deficiencies in hormone levels, number of receptors, necessary cofactors, or mediating proteins. In the adrenergic system, for example, low receptor number and altered ratio of G protein subunits result in relative insensitivity of fetal tissues to adrenergic stimulation. Furthermore, cells may be hormonally unresponsive at certain points in development owing to alterations in chromatin structure that prevent receptor-hormone binding.

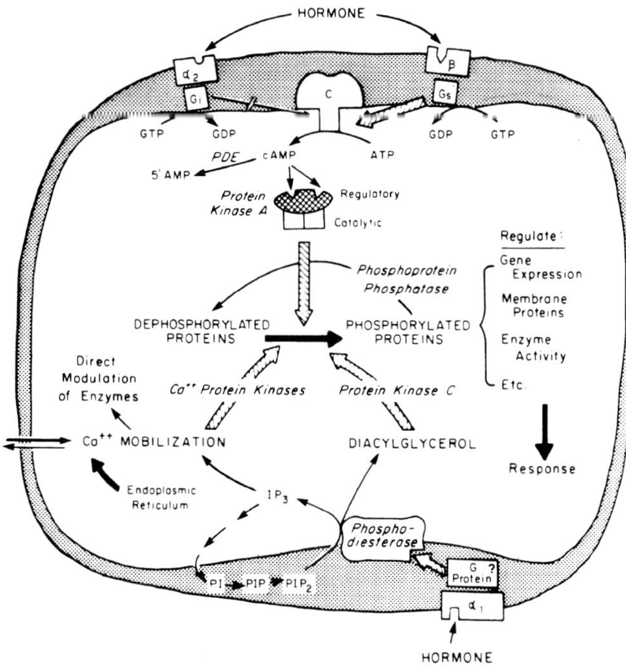


**FIGURE 6–1.** Molecular mechanism of catecholamine action. This model applies for a variety of hormones that act through either cyclic adenosine monophosphate (cAMP) or inositol trisphosphate ($IP_3$) as secondary messengers. 5′-AMP, adenosine-5′-monophosphate; ATP, adenosine triphosphate; C, catalytic subunit of adenylate cyclase; G, guanine nucleotide regulatory protein (stimulatory or inhibitory); GDP, guanosine-5′-diphosphate; GTP, guanosine-5′-triphosphate; PDE, phosphodiesterase; PI, phosphatidylinositol; PIP, phosphatidylinositol-4-phosphate; $PIP_2$, phosphatidylinositol-4,5-diphosphate. *(From Ballard PL: Mechanism of hormone action. In Rudolph AM, Hoffman JIE [eds]: Pediatrics, 18th ed. Norwalk, CT, Appleton & Lange, 1987, p 1450.)*

## Postreceptor Events

Hormones have diverse effects on cells, but their mechanism of action is in general limited to one of the following three categories: (1) direct modification of an enzyme or a protein and alteration of function (e.g., phosphorylation), (2) activation of specific genes that increase synthesis and content of the encoded protein, or (3) repression of the expression of a gene. All three processes occur during fetal life. Hormones that act via membrane receptors trigger a variety of different intracellular signaling cascades. The G proteins, which are composed of three subunits, are associated with the cytoplasmic side of the plasma membrane. There are a variety of alpha subunits, which mediate different hormonal responses, including cAMP-mediated effects. Both inositol triphosphate and diacylglycerol are generated through activation of phosphodiesterase and lipid kinase enzymes in the cell membrane. These agents cause phosphorylation of specific signaling proteins via mobilization of calcium and activation of protein kinase C, respectively. Initial phosphorylation events lead to activation of other major pathways of signal transduction, such as the mitogen-activated protein kinase (MAPK) pathway, the phosphatidylinositol 3-kinase–protein kinase B (PI3-Akt) pathway, the Janus-activated kinase–signal transducer and activator transcription factor (JAK-STAT) pathway, the Smad pathway for transforming growth factor-β (TGF-β), and production of ceramide from sphingomyelin in response to tumor necrosis factor-alpha (TNF-α).

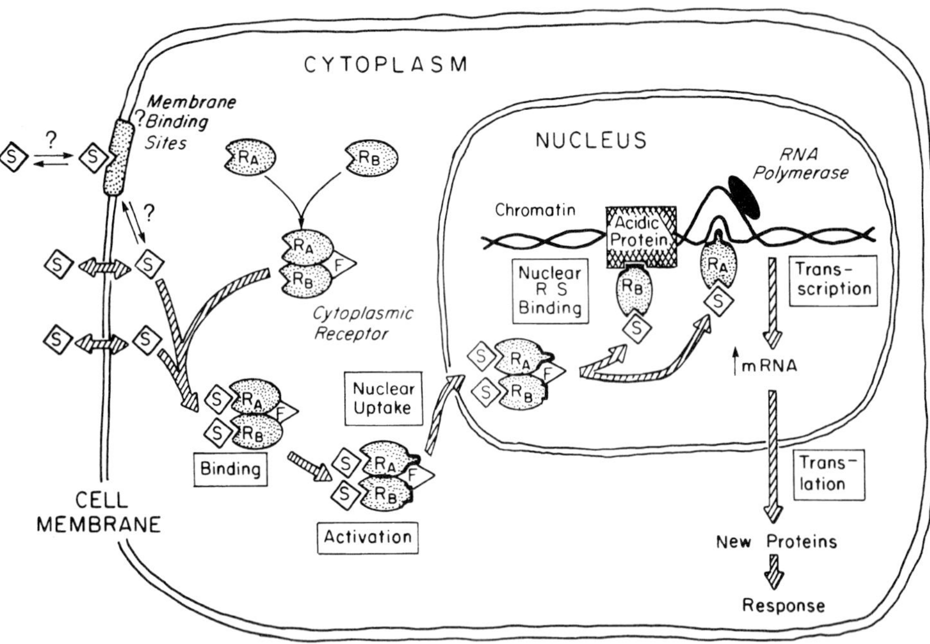


**FIGURE 6–2.** Molecular mechanism of action of steroid hormones in their target cells. This model applies in general to glucocorticoids, estrogens, androgens, progestins, mineralocorticoids, and vitamin D. F, heat shock proteins; $R_A$, subunit A of receptor; $R_B$, subunit B of receptor; RS, receptor-steroid complex; S, steroid. *(From Ballard PL: Mechanism of hormone action. In Rudolph AM, Hoffman JIE, Rudolph CE [eds]: Pediatrics, 20th ed. San Mateo, CA, Appleton & Lange, 1996, p 1678.)*

## UNIQUE FEATURES OF THE FETAL ENDOCRINE SYSTEM

The endocrine environment of the fetus is unique with regard to the endocrine organs, the presence of certain hormones, developmental regulation of circulating hormone concentration, hormone metabolism, and specialized responses related to in utero development. The pattern of fetal growth and development is not generally dependent on hormones, but with some important exceptions, the timing of these events is modulated by levels of endogenous hormones and by exposure to hormone treatment.

### Hormones and Sources

During pregnancy, various steroid hormones are produced through the complex interactions of mother, fetus, and placenta. Progesterone is initially synthesized by the maternal corpus luteum, whereas during the second and third trimesters, the placenta is the major source. Progesterone is synthesized from maternal low-density lipoprotein and occurs independent of the fetus. The high levels of progesterone appear to serve at least two functions, suppressing uterine activity and decreasing maternal immune responses against fetal antigens. One clinical trial indicates that weekly administration of progesterone reduces the rate of premature delivery in high-risk women (Brancazio et al, 2003).

The adult zone of the fetal adrenal gland produces cortisol (in increasing amounts during gestation), and the inner fetal zone acts in concert with the placenta to produce estrogens and their precursors. The fetal zone is deficient in δ-5,3-β-hydroxysteroid dehydrogenase and δ-4,5,3-ketosteroid isomerase and has considerable steroid sulfokinase activity, resulting in production of dehydroepiandrosterone sulfate (DHAS) from pregnenolone supplied by the placenta. DHAS undergoes 16-hydroxylation in the fetal liver and then is transported to the placenta, where 16-hydroxyDHAS as well as DHAS (of both fetal and maternal origins) are the major substrates for estrogen synthesis. Much of the estrogen, predominantly estriol, enters the maternal circulation and is subsequently excreted in the urine. High levels of estrogen also accumulate in the fetus and amniotic fluid, and appear to influence ovarian folliculogenesis and activation of the hypothalamic-pituitary-adrenal axis. Estrogen biosynthesis is greatly reduced in infants with steroid sulfatase deficiencies; development of the fetus under these circumstances, however, appears to be normal.

In addition to production of progesterone, the placenta synthesizes a number of polypeptide hormones throughout pregnancy. These include human chorionic somatomammotropin (hCS), human chorionic gonadotropin (hCG), human chorionic corticotropin (hCC), human chorionic thyrotropin (hCT), β-endorphin, α-melanocyte-stimulating hormone (α-MSH), and both β-lipoprotein and α-lipotropin. The placenta also produces most, if not all, of the releasing hormones synthesized by the hypothalamus. Thus, the placenta contributes to the circulating pool of pituitary and hypothalamic hormones in the fetus. Other fetal tissues in addition to the placenta, particularly the gut and pancreas, synthesize a number of the releasing hormones characteristic of the hypothalamus. The presence of extrahypothalamic peptides is established, but their role in fetal development is not certain.

Another unique source of hormone production in the fetus is the para-aortic chromaffin system. The extramedullary paraganglia of this system, the largest of which are referred to as the organs of Zuckerkandl, are located along the abdominal and pelvic sympathetic plexuses during fetal life and disappear completely in the first years after birth. By the second trimester of gestation, this tissue actively produces norepinephrine but relatively little epinephrine because of low levels of phenylethanolamine-*N*-methyl transferase. The chromaffin cells of the para-aortic system as well as the sympathetic nerve cells are derived from a neuroectodermal stem cell and are responsive to nerve growth factor.

The catecholamine responses at birth are due in part to the para-aortic chromaffin system as well as increased postganglionic sympathetic neuronal and adrenal medullary secretion of catecholamines. Levels of circulating catecholamines (norepinephrine, epinephrine, and dopamine) rise exponentially after delivery and cord cutting. In the newborn sheep, which lacks para-aortic chromaffin tissue, the increased circulating norepinephrine is derived predominantly from the spillover of postganglionic sympathetic neurons, whereas the increased epinephrine derives solely from adrenal medullary secretion. Lacking complete organ sympathetic innervation and maturation of adrenergic receptor mechanisms, the fetus and newborn exhibit profound dependence on circulating catecholamines for maintenance of cardiovascular and metabolic homeostasis in response to physiologic stress such as the transition to extrauterine life. Adrenalectomized animals, lacking the normally increased levels of circulating epinephrine in the newborn period, are impaired in the ability to increase cardiac output and myocardial contractility, secrete surfactant, and mobilize energy substrates for successful postnatal adaptation. It is not known precisely how long this dependence on circulating catecholamines persists postnatally, but basal myocardial function and the high resting cardiac output characteristic of the first weeks of life remain dependent on an intact sympathoadrenal system. Survival during hypoxic stress in newborn rats has been shown to depend on similar mechanisms.

In addition to the anterior and posterior lobes, the fetal pituitary gland has an intermediate lobe that regresses after birth and is not found in adults. In animals, however, the intermediate lobe is maintained throughout adult life. The intermediate lobe secretes primarily α-MSH and β-endorphin, which are derived from proopiomelanocortin (POMC). In the anterior lobe of the pituitary, POMC is cleaved primarily to β-lipotropin and ACTH. By the second trimester of gestation, the fetal neurohypophysis contains arginine vasopressin (AVP), oxytocin, and arginine vasotocin (AVT). The pituitary gland contains AVT throughout fetal life, but this hormone disappears after birth. AVT is also present in the pineal glands of both fetuses and adults.

## Ontogeny

The response to hormones in the fetus is determined primarily by the developmental patterns of hormone concentrations and functional receptor systems. In general, most endocrine systems of the fetus are functional by the end of the first trimester, although circulating levels of many hormones rise substantially only during the third trimester. One exception to this pattern is illustrated by the hypothalamus-pituitary-gonad axis. Secretion of hypothalamic gonadotropin-releasing hormone (GRH) becomes active in the first trimester, resulting in the pulsatile release of luteinizing hormone (LH) and follicle-stimulating hormone (FSH), which stimulates production of testosterone or estradiol by the fetal gonads. Throughout the rest of fetal life and childhood, until the onset of puberty, this hormonal axis remains quiescent. Control of this hormonal system is believed to reside in the central nervous system.

Hormones known to influence terminal *differentiation* (acquisition of specialized functions by cells) have developmental patterns consistent with this role. For example, cortisol is detected in fetal plasma at low levels during the second trimester and then increases exponentially during the third trimester (Murphy, 1982). Glucocorticoid receptors are detected relatively early in gestation in many fetal tissues and appear to be fully functional. The influence of endogenous cortisol on fetal development, therefore, is determined by the rate of adrenal production of cortisol and perhaps by postreceptor responsiveness in target tissues. Similarly, plasma levels of $T_3$ and $T_4$ increase only during the third trimester, whereas thyroid hormone receptors are present throughout the second trimester (Ballard, 1989).

Other hormones also display developmental patterns, but their roles in fetal growth and differentiation have not been defined. Prolactin levels in plasma and amniotic fluid rise throughout the third trimester to levels much greater than those found in the adult or in the mother. In pregnant animals, prolactin promotes olfactory neurogenesis and development of both pancreatic islets and mammary glands (Shingo et al, 2003). Effects of prolactin in the fetus are less well defined and may include chondrogenesis and development of pancreatic and adipose tissue (Freemark, 2001). Levels of growth hormone in the fetus increase during the first two thirds of gestation and then decline toward term; however, there are no known effects during most of gestation owing to the absence of functional receptors.

The adrenergic response system appears to be constrained throughout most of gestation. The catecholamine response to the stress of delivery is greater at term than in preterm deliveries, and in the fetal lung and heart, for example, the number of β-adrenergic receptors and the ability to provoke cAMP are low in the midgestation fetus compared with the adult.

## Metabolism

In the human fetus, the levels of circulating cortisol (an active glucocorticoid) and cortisone (inactive) are similar. Although most adult tissues, particularly the liver, readily convert cortisone to cortisol, fetal tissues generally lack this ability because of a deficiency of enzyme 17β-hydroxysteroid dehydrogenase or cofactors nicotinamide adenine dinucleotide phosphate (NADP) and its oxidized form, NADPH. The low enzymatic activity in most tissues reduces the possible contribution of cortisone to tissue glucocorticoid activity. In the fetal lung of animals, the ability to convert cortisone to cortisol increases markedly during the third trimester, coincident with lung maturation. Lung tissue from the second-trimester human fetus is similarly responsive to cortisone and cortisol during explant culture, reflecting rapid conversion of cortisone to cortisol (Ballard, 1989). In this tissue, therefore, cortisone contributes to the pool of circulating glucocorticoids. Administered corticosteroids are rapidly cleared from the fetal circulation by metabolism in the maternal liver, whereas similar doses administered to the newborn are metabolized slowly because of liver immaturity.

Thyroid hormone metabolism also varies markedly in the fetus compared with that of the adult (see Chapter 92). In the fetus, $T_4$ is deiodinated preferentially to inactive $rT_3$ rather than active $T_3$. This occurs in most fetal tissues but particularly the placenta. In fetal sheep, at least, the switch from production of $rT_3$ to $T_3$ is regulated by endogenous cortisol (levels increase greatly in late gestation) and is stimulated precociously by administered glucocorticoids. Compared with the mother, the fetus has relatively high levels of iodothyronine sulfates, which may represent a mechanism for reversible inactivation of circulating thyroid hormones. The generalized inactivation of $T_4$ during most of fetal life appears to have at least two beneficial effects in the fetus: (1) to protect most fetal tissues from the catabolic effects of thyroid hormone and (2) to provide a mechanism whereby selected tissues could increase their exposure to active $T_3$ by increasing local $T_3$ production. Moreover, several fetal tissues in animals are relatively unresponsive to administered $T_3$ with regard to thermogenesis, a function that is not needed by the fetus before birth.

## HORMONES AND TISSUE DEVELOPMENT

The developmental processes of organogenesis and subsequent maturation of tissue structure and function are, for the most part, programmed and occur in the absence of hormonal influences. Chapter 17 reviews the current understanding of the genetic control of tissue development, which involves coordination and interaction of multiple gene products. Maintenance of the differentiated state appears to be an active process requiring continued synthesis of specific regulatory proteins. Hormones and growth factors have three general roles in the process of differentiation. First, they modulate the rate of tissue development by virtue of increased concentrations or tissue responsiveness during normal gestation. Hormonal effects involve both enzyme induction, which results in differentiated tissue function (e.g., pulmonary surfactant production), and repression of specific genes (e.g., hepatic α-fetoprotein) with loss of a fetal-specific protein. Within a given tissue, the response to a particular hormone typically involves a specific subset of cellular proteins (e.g., glucose-metabolizing enzymes of the intestine), providing a coordinated maturational response. Second, hormones can accelerate the normal timetable of development, resulting in precocious organ maturation. This accelerating effect is observed with exogenous hormone treatment and at times of increased hormone production, such as during chronic in utero stress, during both premature and term labor and delivery, in the immediate postnatal period, and, in animals, around the time of weaning. The third area of hormonal influence relates to tumorigenesis, in which there is loss of growth control and dedifferentiation. A number of oncogenes have been described, the overexpression of which is associated with the genesis of cancer. The oncogenes of retroviruses represent slightly mutated cellular genes that have been obtained by the virus and that are constitutively expressed on viral infection. Many of the oncogenes encode growth factors, their receptors, other hormone receptors, or proteins involved in signal transduction. For example, oncogenes encode for proteins related to epidermal growth factor receptor (*erb*B), platelet-derived growth factor (*sis*), fibroblast growth factor (*int*-2), the G proteins of adenyl cyclase (*ras*), and thyroid hormone receptor (*erb*A). Thus, appropriate expression of hormones, growth factors, and receptors is important in both initial differentiation and maintenance of the differentiated state. Table 6–1 gives a partial listing of hormones that probably play a role in fetal development.

### Intrinsic Timetable

Experiments of nature, such as anencephaly with panhypopituitarism, indicate that fetal growth and development proceed in a near-normal fashion in the absence of hypothalamic and pituitary input. Such fetuses are still exposed to hormones from the mother and placenta. Circulating levels of many hormones are much lower than in normal fetuses but apparently sufficient to ensure organ maturity at term. In experimental animals with a genetically engineered knockout of corticotropin-releasing hormone, rendering homozygous fetuses deficient in both fetal-derived and maternal-derived corticosteroids, newborns died of respiratory failure because of inadequate surfactant and air space development (Muglia et al, 1995). Absence of corticosteroids, however, did not appear to interfere with organogenesis (e.g., airway branching in the lung). When fetal tissue is placed in explant culture in the absence of serum or added hormones, growth, structural development, and biochemical differentiation continue at a rate equal to or greater than the in vivo rate. Fetal lung, for example, undergoes airway branching, formation of peripheral air spaces, and cytodifferentiation of epithelial cells into surfactant-producing type II cells (Fig. 6–3). This process requires the presence of lung mesenchymal tissue and paracrine factors.

The findings in vivo and in vitro suggest that tissue growth and differentiation proceed even in the absence of circulating hormones as a result of gene expression that is apparently determined by cell lineage and cell interactions. It is likely that tissue interactions, which are essential for normal development, are mediated in part through the production of growth factors and possibly other regulators acting in an autocrine or a paracrine fashion. The primary role of circulating hormones in the fetus, therefore, is to modulate the rate of differentiation, in part as a response to changes in the fetal environment.

### Terminal Differentiation

In addition to modulating normal tissue development, circulating hormones accelerate the process in stressful conditions (e.g., placental insufficiency, prolonged rupture of mem-

**TABLE 6–1**

**Hormones of the Fetus that Influence Growth or Differentiation (in vitro and/or in vivo)**

| Hormone or Growth Factor | Sources | Fetal Effects |
|---|---|---|
| Adrenocorticotropic hormone (ACTH) | Pituitary, placenta | Activates fetal adrenal gland |
| Androgens (testosterone) | Testes, adrenal gland, liver | Produce male sexual differentiation<br>Delay lung maturation? |
| β-Endorphin | Pituitary, placenta | Maintains vasoregulation? |
| Calcitonin | Thyroid | Promotes bone mineralization and anabolism? |
| Catecholamines | Adrenal gland | Produce lung differentiation<br>Increase cardiac output, thermogenesis, and glycogen and fat mobilization |
| Human chorionic corticotropin (hCC) | Placenta | Regulates fetal adrenal cortex |
| Human chorionic gonadotropin (hCG) | Placenta | Luteotropic; stimulates steroid production by the fetal testes and adrenals |
| Human chorionic somatomammotropin (hCS), human placental lactogen (hPL) | Placenta | Promotes secretion of insulin-like growth factors (IGFs)? |
| Cortisol | Adrenal adult zone | Needed for parturition and differentiation of numerous tissues |
| Eicosanoids (prostaglandins, leukotrienes, and thromboxanes) | Most tissues | Initiate uterus contraction<br>Regulate vessel tone and lung maturation<br>Activate fetal adrenals |
| Epidermal growth factor (EGF) | Multiple tissues | Regulates epithelial cell division |
| Estrogens (estrone, estradiol, and estriol) | Placenta | Regulate lung differentiation?<br>Increase uteroplacental blood flow |
| Fibroblast growth factors (FGFs) | Fibroblasts | Regulate cell division |
| Insulin-like growth factors (IGFs) | Multiple tissues | Regulate cell division (and differentiation?) |
| α-Melanocyte-stimulating hormone (α-MSH) | Pituitary and placenta | Activates fetal adrenals |
| Müllerian-inhibiting factor (MIF) | Testes (Sertoli cells) | Activates involution müllerian ducts |
| Nerve growth factor (NGF) | | Needed for development and maintenance of neurons and Sertoli cells? |
| Parathyroid hormone | Parathyroids | Produce 1,25-vitamin D |
| Platelet-derived growth factor (PDGF) | Platelets, other tissues | Needed for cell replication |
| Progesterone | Placenta | Precursor for fetal steroids<br>Needed for pregnancy maintenance |
| Prolactin | Pituitary | Needed for water balance |
| Releasing hormones (TRH, SRIF, CRF, GRH) | Hypothalamus, placenta, gut | Augment output of fetal pituitary hormones and placental hormones? |
| Thyroid hormones (thyroxine [$T_4$], triiodothyronine [$T_3$]) | Thyroid, liver | Activate lung and heart differentiation |
| Transforming growth factor (TGF) | Multiple tissues | Regulates cell division, deposition of extracellular matrix, and differentiation |
| Vasopressin, vasotocin | Neurohypophysis, pineal gland | Maintain placental and lung water transport<br>Stimulate ACTH release from fetal pituitary? |
| Vitamin D | Maternal skin, liver, kidney | Placental calcium transport |

CRF, coagulase-reacting factor; GRH, gonadotropin-releasing hormone; SRIF, somatotropin-releasing inhibiting factor; TRH, thyroid-releasing hormone.

branes, premature labor), a process that has been described as preparation for birth. Several different hormones, as described subsequently, are involved in the stress response, and in several tissues there is an interaction between hormones to stimulate maturation. Many of the problems encountered by the premature infant may be thought of as developmental deficiencies or immaturity of critical functions in select tissues. Table 6–2 lists diseases that result from immaturity of hormonally regulated systems.

## Glucocorticoids

Endogenous cortisol—and in some tissues, cortisone—is the most important hormone regulating tissue maturation. Cortisol levels increase continually through the third trimester and are elevated in both acutely and chronically stressful situations. Glucocorticoids have maturational effects in a variety of fetal and newborn tissues of animals. Experimentally, the findings about glucocorticoids arise from studies of administered hormone, ablation procedures (e.g., hypophysectomy or adrenalectomy) that delay organ maturation, and temporal associations between circulating corticosteroids and inducible responses. A prepartum rise in circulating fetal corticosteroids occurs in all species that have been studied, and the experimental manipulations of steroid treatment or withdrawal provide consistent results in a variety of animal models.

In many tissues, the maturational effects of glucocorticoids require or are synergistic with effects of other

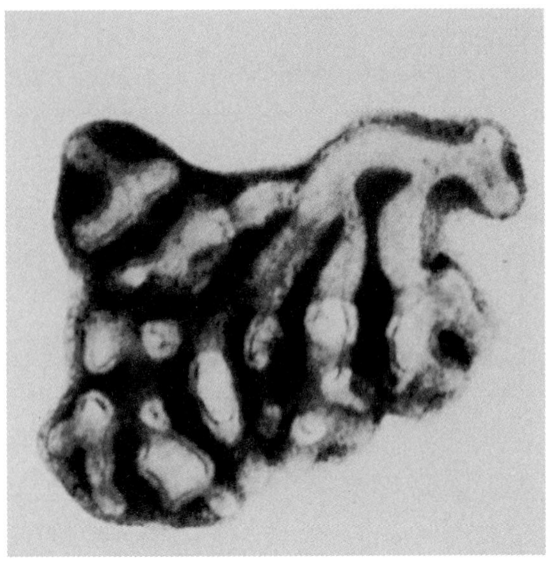
A

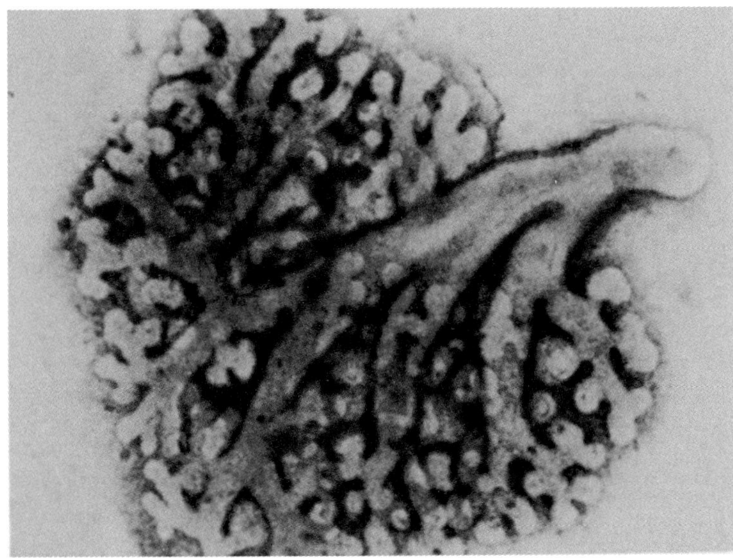
B

**FIGURE 6–3.** Development of the fetal lung in vitro. Intact lungs from 14-day rat fetuses were cultured as explants in medium without hormones for 1 day (**A**) and 4 days (**B**). Branching morphogenesis proceeds without the addition of hormones or growth factors but requires the presence of the mesenchymal tissue. *(From Gross I, Wilson CM: Fetal rat lung maturation: Initiation and modulation. J Appl Physiol 55:1725, 1731, 1983.)*

hormones, such as $T_3$ and catecholamines (cAMP). Although it is not possible to extrapolate all of the findings in animals to the human infant, a number of these regulatory events appear to occur in the human and has clinical implications (see Table 6–2).

The effects and physiologic role of glucocorticoids are best described with regard to maturation of the fetal lung. Studies with explant cultures of human tissue have established that glucocorticoids affect both lung structure and production of surfactant by type II cells (Ballard, 1989).

**TABLE 6–2**

**Abnormalities of the Newborn that may be Related to Hormonal Conditions**

| Abnormality | Hormone | Cause (Known or Postulated) |
|---|---|---|
| Male pseudohermaphroditism | Testosterone | Genetic defects in testosterone biosynthesis, metabolism (5α-reductase), or responsiveness (receptor deficiency or abnormality) |
| Testicular feminization | Dihydrotestosterone | Decreased receptors in androgen target tissues yield female phenotype in genetic male |
| Female pseudohermaphroditism (congenital hyperplasia) | Cortisol, insulin | Enzymatic defects in cortisol biosynthesis with excess androgen |
| Infant of diabetic mother | Insulin | Fetal hyperinsulinemia increases growth and fat deposition and delays lung development |
| Infant leprechaunism | Insulin | Decreased insulin receptors with intrauterine growth retardation |
| Congenital hypothyroidism | Thyroxine, triiodothyronine ($T_3$) | Hormone deficiency alters development of brain, heart, lung, and other tissues |
| Respiratory distress syndrome | Cortisol, $T_3$, catecholamines | Developmental deficiency in one or more hormones may delay lung development |
| Transient tachypnea of newborn | Cortisol, catecholamines, arginine vasopressin, and others? | Decreased hormone levels or responsiveness of lung epithelium for fluid clearance |
| Lung hypoplasia | Unknown growth factors | Presumed to be decreased production of lung factors |
| Persistent pulmonary hypertension of newborn | ? | Stress-related hormones may delay pulmonary vascular development in utero |
| Patent ductus arteriosus | Cortisol, prostaglandins? | Possible imbalance in levels and/or responsiveness for dilating and constricting prostaglandins |
| Necrotizing enterocolitis | Cortisol, glucagon? | Developmental deficiency in hormones may delay gut development |

Treatment accelerates differentiation of the epithelial cells into type II cells, reduces mesenchymal volume, narrows the intra-alveolar septal distance, and increases maximal lung volume and compliance. Surfactant production and secretion are increased, and the response includes all of the known components of pulmonary surfactant (saturated phosphatidylcholine and the three surfactant-associated proteins, SP-A, SP-B, and SP-C). The response to glucocorticoids in the fetal lung is mediated by glucocorticoid receptors and involves greater gene expression (i.e., higher content of messenger RNA) for SPs, SP-processing enzymes, (e.g., cathepsin H), lipogenic enzymes (e.g., fatty acid synthetase), and lipid transporters. It is likely that glucocorticoids have other maturational effects in the lung, because a number of as yet unidentified proteins are induced by glucocorticoid treatment of cultured lung cells (Gonzales et al, 2002). Glucocorticoids also act by receptor-mediated inactivation of the NF-κB (a transcription factor) system, decreasing synthesis of cytokines, but it is uncertain whether this mechanism contributes to enhanced organ maturation. The clinical effects of prenatal corticosteroid therapy are discussed in Chapters 42 and 45. The improved survival rates in treated infants result from precocious maturation of the lung as well as other organs.

## Thyroid Hormones

Levels of both $T_3$ and $T_4$ rise in the human fetus during the third trimester. Although thyroid hormones are important for normal postnatal growth, the athyroid human fetus grows normally (see Chapter 92). Thyroid hormones, however, contribute to fetal lung maturation and are important for development of other tissues. Surfactant production and structural pulmonary development are retarded in hypothyroid sheep fetuses. Treatment with thyroid hormone accelerates phospholipid synthesis in cultured lung, and thyroid hormones are necessary for maximal response to cortisol treatment in fetal sheep. These and other observations on the interactions of glucocorticoids and thyroid hormones led to clinical trials of prenatal therapy with betamethasone plus thyrotropin-releasing hormone (TRH) for prevention of respiratory distress syndrome (RDS). Initial results indicated benefit with regard to incidence of RDS and chronic lung disease for treated infants; however, later trials have not found benefit (Australian collaborative trial, 1995; Ballard et al, 1998).

Thyroid hormones are important for cardiac development. In the sheep fetus, thyroidectomy during late gestation blunts the increases in heart rate, cardiac output, and oxygen consumption normally seen after birth, and replacement $T_3$ therapy before birth is corrective. This $T_3$ effect appears to be mediated through β-adrenergic receptor concentration and responsiveness to endogenous catecholamines. The normal hypertrophic growth of the myocardium also depends on thyroid hormones but apparently does not involve the β-adrenergic system.

The role of thyroid hormones in normal postnatal brain development is well recognized. There is accumulating epidemiologic evidence that the level of maternal thyroxine in the first trimester of pregnancy influences fetal neurodevelopment. Maternal iodine deficiency and other causes of hypothyroidism reduce placental transfer of thyroxine, the primary source of intracellular $T_3$ in the fetus.

## Catecholamines

Circulating catecholamine concentrations increase dramatically with labor and delivery, and amniotic fluid levels, which probably reflect production by the fetus, are generally elevated in complicated pregnancies. A well-described effect of catecholamines on terminal differentiation occurs in the fetal lung. Treatment with β-adrenergic agonists causes a prompt increase in surfactant secretion both in vivo and in isolated type II cells, and endogenous catecholamines contribute to release of surfactant at the time of birth. For example, the amount of surfactant in airways of fetal animals is decreased by blockade of the β-adrenergic receptors with an irreversible antagonist, by treatment with an inhibitor of catecholamine biosynthesis, and by adrenalectomy.

A second effect of catecholamines is to stimulate the rate of surfactant synthesis. In cultured lung tissue, treatment with analogues of cAMP, inhibitors of cAMP phosphodiesterase, β-agonists, and other agents that induce cAMP increases synthesis of surfactant phospholipids, SP-A and SP-B. Alveolar structure in cultured lung explants is also modified by these treatments, probably as a result of altered ion and fluid transport.

A third effect of catecholamines is reduction of lung fluid. In fetal animals, β-agonists decrease fluid accumulation in the air spaces by inhibiting the chloride pump and promoting fluid reabsorption through a sodium pump in epithelial cells. The physiologic relevance of these responses has been demonstrated in the fetal lamb, in which there is a close correlation between fluid flux and endogenous levels of catecholamines during labor. Responsiveness to catecholamines normally increases during the third trimester; the response is markedly blunted in thyroidectomized fetuses but is restored by combined treatment with $T_3$ and hydrocortisone, although not by treatment with either hormone alone (Barker et al, 1989). These findings suggest that rising concentrations of cortisol and $T_3$ during development enhance the sensitivity of epithelial cells for responding to catecholamines. This system illustrates the interaction of hormones in regulating a developmental process important for successful adaptation to extrauterine life. Clinical aspects of lung fluid are discussed in Chapters 44 and 45.

Catecholamines are also involved in increasing myocardial contractility and systemic vascular resistance and in triggering the onset of thermogenesis through mobilization of energy substrates. Infants born prematurely are thus at greater risks with regard to cardiac function and thermal stability because of both decreased metabolic reserves and suboptimal catecholamine levels.

## Insulin

The infant of a diabetic mother is at increased risk for a number of abnormalities, including macrosomia with organomegaly, placental hypertrophy, polyhydramnios, congenital anomalies, and intrauterine death (see Chapter 7). On the basis of animal models of diabetes, it is generally believed that fetal hyperinsulinemia also delays the appearance of pulmonary surfactant and may alter surfactant composition (and therefore its function), alveolar structure, or both. One possible explanation for this effect relates to the mitogenic activity of insulin and the general biologic principle that cell differentiation (e.g., production of surfactant) is associated with decreased cell division. Thus, under the stimulation of increased circulating insulin, lung type II cells may remain in an active cell cycle, not entering the $G_0$ stage when specialized cell products are synthesized. Another possible explanation is an inhibitory effect of insulin on synthesis of surfactant per se. Experiments with cultured lung tissue found that insulin can inhibit synthesis of surfactant proteins A, B, and C, which are required for normal surfactant structure and function (Guttentag et al, 1992). A third possible explanation suggested by in vitro studies is that insulin blocks cortisol stimulation of lung structure and type II cell function. Infants of diabetic mothers also have a higher incidence of respiratory distress because of delayed fluid clearance. The mechanism of this abnormality is not known but could relate to either increased cell division or antagonism of glucocorticoid effects in the lung.

## Eicosanoids

Eicosanoids, which include prostaglandins, thromboxanes, and leukotrienes, are produced from arachidonic acid (released from phospholipids) in the placenta and various fetal tissues. Although many effects of prostaglandins are paracrine, these hormones are present in the circulation, and levels of some (e.g., prostaglandin $E_2$ [$PGE_2$]) are much higher in the fetus than the adult, reflecting in part the lower metabolic clearance by the poorly perfused fetal lung. Synthesis of prostaglandins is increased by a variety of stimuli, many of which involve perturbation of cell membrane integrity, and their production is inhibited by glucocorticoids (induction of lipocortin, which blocks phospholipase $A_2$) and drugs that block synthetic enzymes, such as xanthine derivatives. Effects of prostaglandins are mediated through membrane receptors (primarily on the cell surface) and, at least in part, by the generation of cAMP.

In addition to their important role in initiation of parturition, prostaglandins have several known effects in maturational events of the cardiopulmonary system. Prostaglandins, in particular $PGE_2$, maintain the patency of the ductus arteriosus in fetal life; in fetal sheep, sensitivity to $PGE_2$ decreases during late gestation and in response to glucocorticoid treatment, allowing greater responsiveness to the contracting influence of oxygen. The higher incidence of patent ductus arteriosus in premature infants (and closure with prenatal glucocorticoid and postnatal indomethacin treatment) probably results from changing prostaglandin levels and sensitivity. Prostaglandins also influence the tone of the pulmonary vessels in utero and after birth. Maintenance of pulmonary vasoconstriction in the fetus is due in part to leukotrienes produced within the lung. The rapid fall in pulmonary vascular resistance at the time of birth results in part from the vasodilating effects of prostacyclin as well as other agents (e.g., prostaglandin $D_2$, bradykinin, and histamine) that are released by stretching the lung. Thus, an alteration in prostaglandin production or responsiveness could conceivably contribute to the development of persistent pulmonary hypertension in some newborn infants.

Prostaglandins may also play physiologic roles in other aspects of lung development. Treatment of fetal sheep with inhibitors of prostaglandin synthesis increases fetal breathing movements and in some studies reduces both the rate of lung fluid production and its surfactant content. In newborn lambs, treatment with $PGE_2$ produces hyperventilation and apnea. In cultured lung tissue, $PGE_2$ and $PGE_1$, presumably acting through cAMP, stimulate syntheses of surfactant lipids and SP-A and promote the release of surfactant from type II cells. Thus, endogenous prostaglandins may contribute to lung growth (via fluid production and breathing movements) and maturation of the surfactant system in utero. Conceivably, the administration of inhibitors of prostaglandin synthesis such as tocolytics might adversely affect lung maturation in the human fetus.

## Arginine Vasopressin and Arginine Vasotocin

Although AVP and AVT are present in the pituitary gland of the human fetus, it is not known whether they have a unique physiologic role in the fetus. In addition to its role in conserving water for the fetus, vasopressin is increased in response to hypoxic stress to levels greater than those occurring with osmolar stimuli. As a stress response hormone, AVP may contribute to maintenance of fetal blood pressure during hemorrhage or hypoxia. Administration of AVP to fetal animals decreases production of fetal lung fluid without affecting fluid osmolarity. This response is greater in older fetuses, indicating developmental changes in responsiveness. Plasma AVP is higher in infants delivered vaginally than in those delivered by cesarean section, and exposure to labor reduces the incidence of respiratory distress after birth. It is possible, therefore, that the higher levels of endogenous AVP or AVT associated with labor and delivery contribute to the clearance of lung water.

## Atrial Natriuretic Peptide

Fluid production, and possibly other lung functions, may be influenced by atrial natriuretic peptide (ANP), which is secreted from atrial myocytes under glucocorticoid regulation. ANP is also synthesized in pulmonary type II cells of newborn rats, and high-affinity binding sites for this peptide occur within lung tissue. In fetal sheep, infusion of ANP or saline reduces production of lung fluid. In the human, plasma concentrations of ANP are higher in term newborns than in adults and are further elevated in infants with RDS. Thus, ANP, levels of which are regulated by cortisol, may have a developmental influence in fluid production by both the kidney and the lung. ANP also has vasodilatory properties and thus could have an effect on pulmonary blood flow and the occurrence of patent ductus arteriosus in the newborn.

Studies indicate that ANP is also synthesized in a number of extra-atrial tissues, such as adrenal, gut, pancreas, nerve, and endocrine cells of the adult animal. The presence of ANP receptors in many of these same tissues suggests possible autocrine or paracrine roles of ANP in addition to its regulation of water and salt homeostasis. Possible roles of ANP in developing tissues other than the lung have not yet been investigated.

## Neuropeptides

A variety of regulatory peptides are synthesized and secreted by a diffuse endocrine system of small granule cells of the intestine, pancreas, thyroid, lung, and other organs. Products of these cells are the biogenic amines and neuropeptides such as bombesin (gastrin-releasing peptide), bombesin-related compounds, calcitonin, calcitonin gene–related peptides, leucine enkephalin, somatostatin, and cholecystokinin. The neuroendocrine cells and their products are present in the fetus from early gestation, increase during fetal life, and then generally decline during childhood. The developmental pattern and distribution of these endocrine and paracrine systems suggest that the neuropeptides may have a role in fetal growth and development. At present, specific biologic functions have not been defined, although there is evidence for stimulatory effects on lung development.

## FETAL GROWTH

Growth of the fetus is determined primarily by genetic factors, the capacity of the mother to provide nutrients, and the ability of the placenta to transfer nutrients. Relatively little is known about the role of hormones and growth factors in the complex process of fetal growth. Although growth hormone and thyroid hormones are important for postnatal growth, they appear to have no growth-promoting role in utero. In fact, growth retardation is not a feature of anencephaly, which often involves complete absence of hypothalamic and pituitary hormones.

It is likely that tissue growth in the fetus is determined in large part by the interplay of locally produced growth factors. Studies in cell lines indicate that stimulation of cell division requires both competence factors (e.g., platelet-derived growth factor [PDGF] and fibroblast growth factor [FGF]), which render growth-arrested cells capable of entering the cell cycle ($G_0$ to $G_1$), and progression factors (e.g., IGFs) that promote entry into the DNA synthesis phase of the cell cycle.

One fetal hormone known to influence fetal growth is insulin. It is present in the human fetal pancreas and circulation by 10 weeks of gestation, and its levels are influenced by the blood glucose concentration. The rare condition of congenital absence of the pancreas is associated with marked reduction in birth length and weight. The syndrome of leprechaunism, which involves a genetic deficiency of insulin receptors and therefore lack of responsiveness, is also characterized by severe growth retardation. In animals, experimental hypoinsulinism leads to fetal growth retardation, and infusion of insulin increases fetal weight and causes organomegaly. Infants of diabetic mothers with poorly controlled disease are often macrosomic; this overgrowth is not observed when the diabetes is well controlled. In mothers with severe diabetes, with vascular disease and decreased uterine blood flow, fetuses are growth retarded because of nutrient deprivation. Infants with the Beckwith-Wiedemann syndrome are macrosomic with generalized organomegaly and appear to be hypersensitive to circulating insulin. The mechanism of insulin action in fetal growth is not fully defined but probably includes a direct stimulation of cell division through insulin receptors (insulin promotes cell division in culture), enhanced glucose and amino acid uptake into cells, and possible interactions with IGFs.

IGFs (or somatomedins) are a family of proteins that are structurally related to insulin, have some insulin-like metabolic activities, and mediate the action of growth hormone on postnatal growth. They circulate bound to specific binding proteins (IGF-binding proteins [IGF-BPs]) and act via cell membrane receptors. IGFs and their receptors are present in most fetal tissues (except the brain) and undoubtedly have a role in both organ and somatic growth. There is a correlation between size at birth and levels of IGFs in cord blood consistent with a physiologic role. Production of IGFs by tissues is developmentally controlled and cell specific. For example, in the lung, messenger RNA for IGF-II is high in the fetus, drops markedly by term, and is not detected in adult lung; by contrast, IGF-I messenger RNA is found in both fetal and adult tissue. IGF-II messenger RNA is found only in lung mesenchymal cells, indicating the cellular site of synthesis, whereas immunostaining occurs in epithelial cells but not mesenchymal fibroblasts. These and other findings suggest that IGFs are produced by certain cell types (e.g., fibroblasts), are secreted, and stimulate proliferation of neighboring cells after binding to cell surface receptors. Agents or hormones that influence either IGFs or their receptors could potentially influence the rate of fetal growth. The six different IGF binding proteins, for example, sequester IGFs from their receptors and inhibit IGF action. The binding proteins also have separate effects, independent of IGF receptors, on cell functions that are important in fetal development, such as adhesion, migration, proliferation, and apoptosis.

Epidermal growth factor (EGF) was first identified as a protein from the mouse submaxillary gland, which accelerated eruption of the incisors and eyelid opening in the newborn animal. EGF has generalized effects on epithelial growth and keratinization in several species and in a variety of cell types (mammary epithelial cells, chondrocytes, corneal cells, vascular smooth muscle cells, prostatic cells, glial cells, fibroblasts, and epithelial cells of the female reproductive organs). In vitro, EGF stimulates DNA synthesis in cultured cells. In explant culture of fetal lung, EGF stimulates both cell division and phospholipid biosynthesis. Infusion of EGF into fetuses stimulates epithelial growth in many tissues, with major effects on the weight of the placenta, intestine, kidneys, and adrenals, but does not affect general somatic growth. These observations suggest that endogenous EGF may have a role in growth and maturation of the kidney, adrenal cortex, intestine, and lung.

Nerve growth factor (NGF) was also first isolated from mouse salivary glands but has been detected in various tissues, including human placenta. Treatment of chick embryos with NGF increases the size of sensory and sympathetic ganglia owing to survival of neurons that normally degenerate. Sympathetic ganglia of newborn animals contain more NGF than adult ganglia and are more responsive in terms of transformation of sympathetic neuroblasts into differentiated neurons. It has been postulated that locally produced NGF is important in the maturation of adrenergic neurons, the sympathetic nervous system, and fetal brain development in general.

Basic FGF (B-FGF) and related proteins (A-FGF, K-FGF, int-2, and FGF-5) appear to play an important role in early embryonic induction, angiogenesis of myocardial and vascular disease, and wound healing. They are mitogenic for vascular endothelial cells through an autocrine mechanism, and they promote endothelial cell migration and invasion as well as production of plasminogen activator, which are all necessary features of angiogenesis in vivo. Acidic FGF appears to be essential for branching morphogenesis in embryonic lung, on the basis of observations in animals with FGF receptor knockout (Peters et al, 1994). PDGF, in combination with other growth factors, stimulates division of glial cells, muscle cells, ovarian granulosa cells, pancreatic beta cells, and certain cell types of the immune system.

The transforming growth factors, in particular TGF-β, have multiple effects on a variety of tissues. For example, TGF-β stimulates growth and extracellular matrix production by fibroblasts, promotes a switch from chondrocytic to osteoblastic phenotype, and inhibits the synthesis of surfactant components in cultured lung (Beers et al, 1998). Cardiac development is regulated at multiple developmental stages by members of the TGF-β superfamily. These findings indicate that TGF-β may act in early embryogenesis (e.g., heart) as a growth stimulator (e.g., of bone), and as a differentiation inhibitor (e.g., in the lung). It is also conceivable that TGF-β (and other growth factors) play a role in the disordered growth and repair process that is a part of bronchopulmonary dysplasia in infants.

## SELECTED READINGS

Albrecht ED, Pepe GJ: Placental steroid hormone biosynthesis in primate pregnancy. Endocr Rev 11:124, 1990.

Bauer MK, Harding JE, Bassett NS, et al: Fetal growth and placental function. Mol Cell Endocrinol 140:115, 1998.

Care AD: Development of endocrine pathways in the regulation of calcium homeostasis. Baillieres Clin Endocrinol Metab 3:671, 1989.

Handwerger S, Freemark M: The roles of placental growth hormone and placental lactogen in the regulation of human fetal growth and development. J Pediatr Endocrinol Metab 13:343, 2000.

Hertzog PJ, Hwang SY, Kola I: Role of interferons in the regulation of cell proliferation, differentiation, and development. Mol Reprod Dev 39:226, 1994.

Morreale de Escobar G: The role of thyroid hormone in fetal neurodevelopment. J Pediatr Endocrinol Metab 14(Suppl 6): 1453, 2001.

Pepe GJ, Albrecht ED: Actions of placental and fetal adrenal steroid hormones in primate pregnancy. Endocr Rev 16:608, 1995.

Reis FM, D'Antona D, Petraglia F: Predictive value of hormone measurements in maternal and fetal complications of pregnancy. Endocr Rev 23:230, 2002.

Zachos NC, Billiar RB, Albrecht ED, Pepe GJ: Developmental regulation of baboon fetal ovarian maturation by estrogen. Biol Reprod 67:1148, 2002.

## REFERENCES

Australian collaborative trial of antenatal thyrotropin-releasing hormone (ACTOBAT) for prevention of neonatal respiratory disease. Lancet 345:877, 1995.

Ballard PL: Hormonal regulation of pulmonary surfactant. Endocr Rev 10:165, 1989.

Ballard RA, Ballard PL, Cnaan A, et al: Antenatal thyrotropin-releasing hormone to prevent lung disease in preterm infants. North American Thyrotropin-Releasing Hormone Study Group. N Engl J Med 338:493, 1998.

Barker PM, Markiewicz M, Parker KA, et al: Induction of the adrenaline-dependent reabsorption of lung liquid in the fetal sheep by synergistic action of triiodothyronine and hydrocortisone. Proc Physiol Soc 146P:137, 1989.

Beers MF, Solarin KO, Guttentag SH, et al: TGF-beta1 inhibits surfactant component expression and epithelial cell maturation in cultured human fetal lung. Am J Physiol 275:L950, 1998.

Brancazio LR, Murtha AP, Heine RP: Prevention of recurrent preterm delivery by 17 alpha-hydroxyprogesterone caproate. N Engl J Med 349:1087, 2003.

Freemark M: Ontogenesis of prolactin receptors in the human fetus: Roles in fetal development. Biochem Soc Trans 29:38, 2001.

Gonzales LW, Guttentag SH, Wade KC, et al: Differentiation of human pulmonary type II cells in vitro by glucocorticoid plus cAMP. Am J Physiol Lung Cell Mol Physiol 283:L940, 2002.

Guttentag SH, Phelps DS, Floros J: Surfactant protein regulation and diabetic pregnancy. Semin Perinatol 16:122, 1992.

Muglia L, Jacobson L, Dikkes P, Majzoub JA: Corticotropin-releasing hormone deficiency reveals major fetal but not adult glucocorticoid need. Nature 373:427, 1995.

Murphy BEP: Human fetal serum cortisol levels related to gestational age: Evidence of a midgestational fall and a steep late gestational rise independent of sex or mode of delivery. Am J Obstet Gynecol 144:276, 1982.

Peters K, Werner S, Liao X, et al: Targeted expression of a dominant negative FGF receptor blocks branching morphogenesis and epithelial differentiation of the mouse lung. EMBO J 13:3296, 1994.

Shingo T, Gregg C, Enwere E, et al: Pregnancy-stimulated neurogenesis in the adult female forebrain mediated by prolactin. Science 299:117, 2003.

CHAPTER 7

# Multiple Birth

Geoffrey A. Machin

The present epidemic of twin and higher-order multiple births (multiple-fetus pregnancy [MFP]) brings many young patients to the neonatal intensive care nursery (NICU). Twin births occur at a rate of 1 per 45 gestations in the United States today (contribution of assisted reproductive technology, 2000). The frequency of preterm delivery increases from singletons through twins to quadruplets and quintuplets (Botting et al, 1990) (Fig 7–1). MFP neonates are over-represented in the NICU; 10 times as many MFP neonates as newborns from singleton births received NICU care. Preterm delivery and complications of preterm birth are caused not only by spontaneous preterm labor or preterm rupture of membranes but also by a higher frequency of interventions for gestational complications, such as severe pregnancy-induced hypertension. The impact on NICU occupation by preterm birth in MFPs cannot be underestimated, but this chapter concentrates on special issues and disorders that are found in MFPs and that must be considered in clinical care.

## SPONTANEOUSLY AND ARTIFICIALLY CONCEIVED MULTIPLE-FETUS PREGNANCIES

Spontaneously conceived MFPs vary in frequency by ethnic origin, maternal age, and maternal nutritional status. The prevalence of monozygotic (MZ) twins is virtually constant worldwide, at 4 in 1000 births. But the prevalence of dizygotic (DZ) twins varies widely, being common in parts of West Africa and rarer in Southeast Asia. Both MZ and DZ twins may occur with greater frequency in some families. Therefore, it is not possible to give an overall ratio of MZ and DZ twins, but 35:65 is a reasonable estimate in an ethnically mixed population. Very few sets of spontaneously conceived triplets are trizygotic. The majority contains at least a pair of MZ twins, and more than one third of triplet sets are totally MZ (Machin and Bamforth, 1996). Zygosity in quadruplets is not well documented, but several MZ sets are known. The Dionne quintuplets appear to have been MZ.

Artificially conceived MFPs contain MZ twins in 6% to 10% of cases. This rate may relate to mechanical factors, such as manipulation of the zona pellucida during in vitro fertilization (IVF) (Sheen et al, 2001). The high frequency of MZ twins in artificial reproduction is not widely known and can cause confusion for caregivers and parents alike. For instance, implantation of three IVF embryos may result in the birth of triplets. However, two of the triplets may be MZ twins from one embryo, and the third the singleton of the second embryo; the third IVF embryo in such a case has not survived. The prevalence of sex chromosome aneuploidy is higher in embryos produced by intracytoplasmic sperm injection for treatment of oligospermia. The two main reasons are (1) a greater prevalence of sex chromosome aneuploidy in the oligospermic fathers results in aneuploid sperm and (2) sex chromosomes in the sperm head are normally located in the subacrosomal region, and may not enter appropriately into the union of male and female pronuclei (Sbracia et al, 2002).

## CHORIONICITY IN MULTIPLE-FETUS PREGNANCIES

In prenatal life, the importance of chorion number is overwhelming in terms of mortality and morbidity. This fact has been known for several years, but unfortunately, chorionicity is not always diagnosed accurately by ultrasound in MFPs. This is partly due to the restriction on the number of ultrasound examinations in pregnancy. A dating ultrasound at 16 to 18 weeks is usually too late to determine chorionicity, because the septal membranes of dichorionic (DC) gestations will already have thinned out to resemble the septum of monochorionic (MC) twins. Ideally, chorionicity should be determined in the first trimester. DC twin placentas, whether separate or fused, show bright placental tissue in the septum, with a "twin peak," "lambda," or "delta" sign. The placentas of DC twins collide like tectonic plates, throwing ridges of placental tissue up into the septal area. This chorionic ridge effectively separates the two gestations, so that any adverse effect on the integrity of one DC twin will not affect the other because there are no interfetal vascular communications.

In MC twins, the chorion surrounds the whole gestation but is not present in the septal membranes which consist only of two layers of amnion in 95% of MC twins, who are diamniotic (DA). About 5% of MC twins are monoamniotic (MA). The cords of MC-MA twins are usually entwined from early in pregnancy, causing greater risks of vascular problems than in MC-DA twins. MC twin placentas are designed and developed for a singleton pregnancy and do not always adapt well to the demands of twin circulations. About 90% of MC twin placentas have connecting vessels between the twins that run on the surface of the placenta, into the parenchyma, or both. This is the main reason for higher rates of complications in MC than in DC twin pregnancies, because adverse events in one twin usually affect the other twin.

### Complications of Monochorionicity

Two vascular characteristics of MC twin placentas affect outcomes. First, the parenchyma of the single placenta is often not shared equally between the twins, usually because of asymmetric cord insertions. Velamentous cord insertion is found in about 10% of MC twins, compared with 1% of singletons. If one twin's cord is inserted more toward the center of the placenta, that twin will control a much larger proportion of the placenta than the twin with the velamentous cord. This is the usual cause of significant

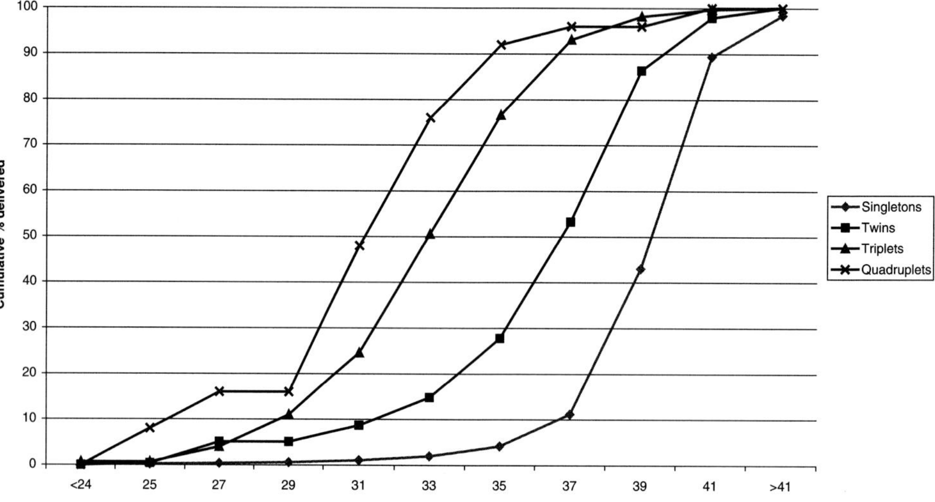


**FIGURE 7–1.** Cumulative percentages of singletons, twins, triplets, and quadruplets born at a given gestational age.

growth discordance in MC twins. Paradoxically, the growth rate of the twin with the central cord is often equal to or better than that of a singleton, because the MC twin placenta is larger than a singleton placenta.

Second, there are three kinds of intertwin vascular connections (anastomoses) in MC placentas, as follows: (1) direct arterio-arterial (AA), (2) direct venovenous (VV), and (3) indirect arteriovenous (AV). The characteristics of these anastomoses are shown in Table 7–1.

Blood in AV connections transfuses steadily from donor (arterial end) to recipient (venous end) down the pressure gradient. The artery and vein abut very closely on the fetal surface, but blood flow occurs in the underlying parenchyma. If not adequately compensated by other types of connections, unopposed arteriovenous flow inevitably leads to twin-twin transfusion (TTT). Blood shunts back and forth readily in direct, surface AA, and VV connections, but there is little net flow if the twin cardiac outputs are roughly equal. This has good effects (allows blood to flow back from recipient to donor) and bad effects (rapid transfer of blood to a twin if its circulation fails or the fetus dies). Thus, the outcomes in MC twins depend largely on the types and combinations of vascular connections. The more connections there are, the less likely are the twins to decompensate into TTT. Fortunately, most MC twins have several connections (usually a combination of AA and VV), and TTT does not develop.

Combinations of such connections are shown in Figure 7–2. This illustration shows the types and combinations of connections in those 90% of MC placentas that have connections. AA connections are found in three quarters of placentas, frequently in combination with other types of connections, especially AV. AV connections are also very common, but one third of them occur alone, without compensation, putting the twins at risk for TTT. VV connections are much less common (20%), but they are potentially dangerous, because large blood volumes at low pressure, can rapidly cross the placenta from twin to twin if the cardiovascular status of one twin deteriorates.

## Complications of Intertwin Vascular Connections in Monochorionic Twins

### Chronic Prenatal Twin-Twin Transfusion

Uncompensated AV connections allow steady blood transfusion, probably at the rate of a few milliliters every 24 hours. Diagnosis is signified by simultaneous oligohydramnios and

**TABLE 7–1**

**Types and Effects of Interfetal Vascular Anastomoses**

| | Type of Anastomosis | | |
|---|---|---|---|
| **Characteristic** | **Arterio-arterial** | **Venovenous** | **Arteriovenous** |
| Location | Fetal surface | Fetal surface | In underlying villi, but feeder vessels on fetal surface |
| Net flow | Little | Little | Arteriovenous transfusion |
| Pressure/resistance | High | Low | Intermediate |
| Flow | Low | High | Very low |
| Effect on twin-twin transfusion | Protective | ? | Causative |

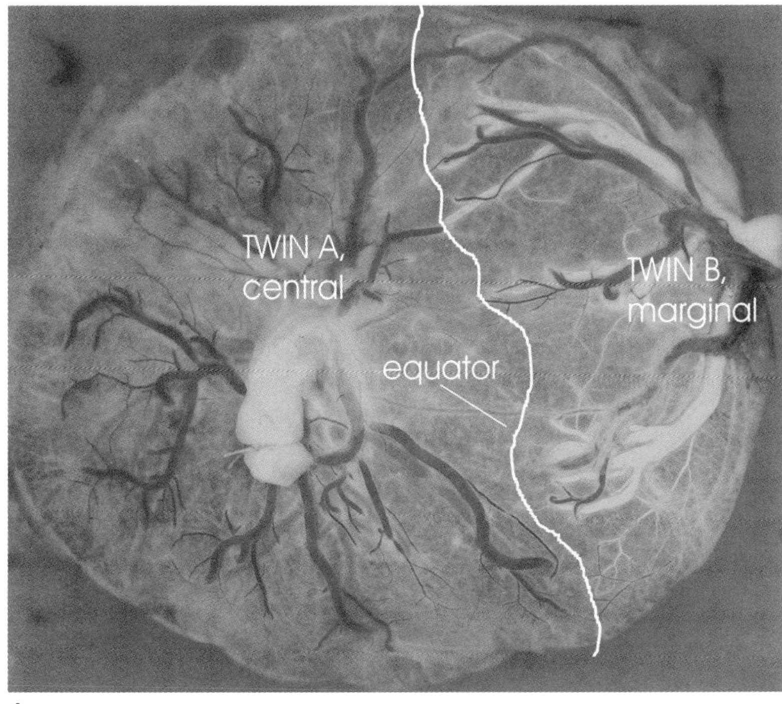


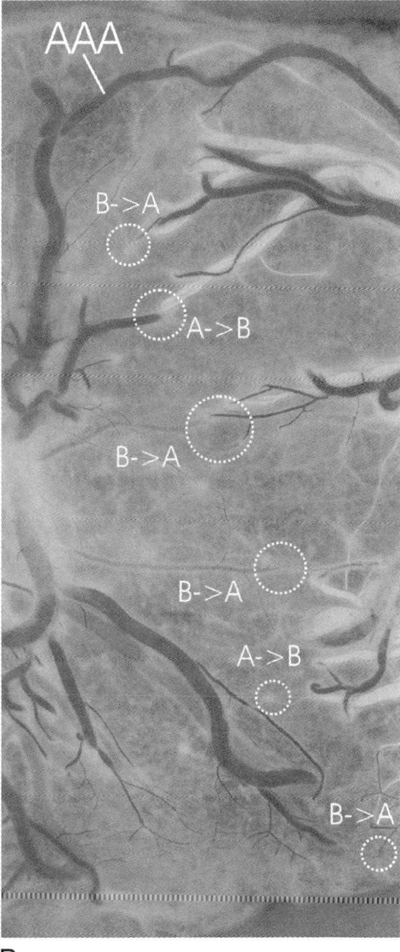


**FIGURE 7–2.** (See also Color Plate 7–2.) **A,** Monochorionic twin placenta. Twin A *(left)* has a centrally inserted cord, whereas the cord of twin B *(right)* is marginally inserted. The *line* represents the vascular equatorial zone between the circulations of the twins. This is the region where intertwin vascular connections are found. There is markedly unequal sharing of the parenchyma, with growth discordance. **B,** Close-up view of the equator, showing a direct arterio-arterial connection (AAA) and multiple bidirectional arteriovenous connections *(circles)* from A to B and from B to A. This resulted in no net transfusion. Although twin-twin transfusion syndrome did not occur, there was growth discordance.

polyhydramnios (oli/poly). The donor is often (but not always) growth restricted because of peripheral cord insertion. Severe growth restriction causes oligohydramnios. The recipient responds to transfusion with polyuria or polyhydramnios, and the blood becomes hyperviscous, leading to low cardiac output because of resistance to forward flow. Tricuspid valve regurgitation leads to pulsatile umbilical venous flow and, eventually, hydrops. Treatment options include amnioreduction and fetoscopic laser coagulation of connecting placental vessels. In survivors, early exchange transfusion and correction of metabolic disturbances may be necessary. However, there are also chronic sequelae of TTT, with typical patterns affecting each fetus (Table 7–2).

Long-term follow-up studies of TTT have been published. In a series of 17 twin pairs with antenatal TTT treated conservatively or by amnioreduction, there were five fetal deaths, and a further six neonatal deaths among the 29 surviving twins (neonatal death rate 21%) (Cincotta et al, 2000). Of the survivors, 14 were donors and 15 were recipients. The most significant morbidities were resolving oliguria (7 of 14 donors and 7 of 15 recipients), periventricular leukomalacia in three infants and cerebral atrophy in two infants. These five neurologic injuries were distributed in 3 donors and 2 recipients. At long-term follow-up, two infants had cerebral palsy (CP) with developmental delay (DD), one infant had CP only, and two infants had DD only. Thus, of the 29 newborns, 62% were intact survivors.

In another study of 33 TTT pairs treated with aggressive amnioreduction, there were 51 newborns, of whom 9 died in infancy (18% postnatal mortality) (Mari et al, 2000). Two survivors had CP. Ten recipients had resolving cardiomegaly. Seven other cases of recipient cardiomegaly occurred in newborns who died. In this series, the majority of neonatal deaths and complications occurred in recipients. In a third study, detailed neurologic analyses of

**TABLE 7-2**

**Chronic Sequelae of Twin-Twin Transfusion and Typical Patterns Affecting Each Fetus**

| Sequelae | Donor Affected | Recipient Affected |
|---|---|---|
| Cerebral hypoxia/hemorrhage | Yes | Yes |
| Cardiomyopathy | No | Yes |
| Acquired prenatal heart disease (flow defects) (Nizard et al, 2001) | Left | Right |
| Limb gangrene (Dawkins et al, 1995; Scott et al, 1995) | No | Yes |
| Arterial distensibility (Gardiner, 2001) | No | Yes |
| Oliguria (Genest et al, 1991)* | Yes | Yes |

*Renal tubular dysgenesis is a malformation of renal tubules in which convoluted tubules fail to differentiate. It occurs in an autosomal recessive form but is also associated with the donor fetus in twin-twin transfusion. The defect is one cause of postnatal oliguria and does not resolve.

40 survivors of TTT showed only 18 (45%) intact children (Haverkamp et al, 2001). Thirteen of the survivors had specific delayed language development, minor neurologic dysfunction, or both. Nine survivors had severe psychomotor retardation and CP; these major neurologic problems occurred in 6 of 19 recipients and 3 of 21 donors. One of the reported advantages of laser coagulation over amnioreduction is a lower prevalence of cerebral disease in survivors. However, it has been suggested that this lower prevalence arises from the demise of some severely affected fetuses during and after the more invasive procedure of laser therapy.

### Acute Perinatal Twin-Twin Transfusion

After the cord of the first-born twin is clamped, the second twin has full access to the whole MC placenta and may receive a significant boost transfusion before birth. Thus, the second-born MC twin frequently has a higher hematocrit than the first born. In the context of chronic prenatal TTT, the donor is often born second, but may be paradoxically plethoric because of acute perinatal transfusion. Exchange transfusion may be required.

### Fetal Death of One Twin

With or without TTT, there are serious potential sequelae if one MC twin fetus dies. The fetal body, cord, and portion of the placenta previously perfused by the dying fetus now have zero blood pressure, and the surviving twin may acutely hemorrhage into these zones via interfetal vascular connections, suffering catastrophic hypotension, and ischemia. In the second trimester, the skin and bowel are affected (aplasia cutis and jejunal atresia), whereas in the third trimester, cystic encephalomalacia is common (Weig et al, 1995). Similar considerations apply to ill-considered attempts at selective termination of an anomalous fetus of an MC pair; appropriate care must be taken to isolate the two circulations during the termination procedure.

### Twin Reversed Arterial Perfusion

In twin reversed arterial perfusion, a "pump twin" fetus maintains an "acardiac" fetus as a passive tissue culture. In so doing, the pump twin may develop high-output cardiac failure. In addition, the pump twin receives back from the acardiac fetus stale blood that has not been circulated through the placenta. This blood may be toxic to the brain of the pump twin. Blood flows slowly across VV connections between the cord insertion points, and there may be thrombosis in the vessels, with potential for thromboembolism to the brain of the pump twin. Selective termination of the acardiac fetus can be achieved through obliteration of cord vessels or aorta. Long-term survival characteristics of pump twins are not well documented.

## COMPLICATIONS OF MONOAMNIONICITY

Monoamniotic twins almost always have intertwined umbilical cords. Most investigators recommend early delivery of MA twins by cesarean section. TTT occurs in MC-MA twins but may be less common than in MC-DA twins, because the cords of MC-MA twins are often inserted close together, usually with large AA and VV anastomoses. Complications are usually asphyxial either because of tight cord intertwining or, during vaginal delivery, because the cord around the neck of twin A actually belongs to twin B.

## CONJOINED TWINNING

Many conjoined twins are prenatally diagnosed, and the parents opt for termination. Some anatomic subtypes (thoracopagus, omphalopagus) are potentially separable. Newborn care involves maintenance of pulmonary-cardiovascular status while imaging studies are performed to determine whether the extent of interpenetrance of the organ systems will permit surgical separation. In some subtypes, one twin is quite hypoplastic compared with the other. In these cases, separation may be considered in the hopes of saving one life. Several procedures, including "skin expansion," may be required before separation surgery.

## CHROMOSOME ABNORMALITIES AND CONGENITAL ANOMALIES IN TWINS

The maternal age effect in induction of DZ twins also affects the prevalence of Down syndrome. The risks of trisomy 21 in DZ twins, however, are higher per pregnancy than for singletons at any age (Rodis et al, 1990). Thus, separate risk figures for Down syndrome are required for DZ twins.

Several environmental and non-mendelian genetic events occurring soon after conception ensure that MZ twins are never "identical" (Rodis et al, 1990). MZ twins (whether MC or DC) may be discordant for chromosome status; this is a special form of mosaicism. Chromosomal discordance in MZ twins is the result of mitotic nondisjunction during early postzygotic cell divisions. Examples of discordant MZ twins are (1) one twin with Down syndrome and the other normal and (2) one twin with a 46,XX or 46,XY karyotype and the other with 45,X. When a 46,XY zygote loses a Y chromosome in one cell line at an early stage in cell division, the result may be MZ twins of different sexes. This is surely a good reason for never calling MZ twins "identical."

Because MC-MZ twins usually have interfetal vascular connections, they exchange hematopoietic stem cells throughout gestation. Therefore, results of blood lymphocyte chromosome analysis may not accurately reflect the distribution of normal and aneuploid cell lines in "fixed," somatic cells. Such results may adequately indicate the number and types of the cell lines derived from the single zygote but are not reliable in explaining discordant phenotypes caused by uneven distribution of somatic cell lines in different organs and tissues of the twins themselves.

MZ twins may also be discordant as the result of unequal X chromosome inactivation (lyonization) and gene imprinting (Machin, 1996).

In DZ twins, blood chimerism is well known but the mechanism is less clear. Male-female pairs may show blood chimerism for male and female cell lines (as well as blood group chimerism). Because DZ (DC) twins seldom if ever have interfetal vascular anastomoses, it seems likely that hematopoietic stem cells are exchanged when the placentas are disrupted at delivery. In one study, a fertile woman had a 46,XY karyotype in 99% of lymphocytes, but 100% of the cells in fibroblasts from skin, muscle, and ovary had 46,XX chromosomes. Her male co-twin had died early in the neonatal period (Sudik et al, 2001). In a series using a sensitive fluorescent antibody technique, blood group chimerism was found in 32 of 415 twins (8%) and 12 of 57 triplets (21%) (van Dijik et al, 1996). Unusual blood group results should therefore be anticipated in DZ newborn twins and triplets.

Both MZ and DZ twins are commonly discordant for congenital malformations. In fact, it is relatively rare for MZ twins to be concordant for major malformations, with a few exceptions (anencephaly and sacral agenesis). Discordant congenital heart disease in MC-MZ twins usually involves "flow" lesions, suggesting that interfetal vascular connections are already operating during cardiogenesis, allowing interfetal transfusion and transient alterations in blood volume that affect the growth and development of the cardiac outflow tracts. This is particularly true in twins with TTT. When malformations in MZ twins are caused by aneuploidy or single genes, phenotypic severity is usually discordant between the twins, suggesting that some modifying factors also exist.

## NEONATAL FOLLOW-UP CLINICS AND MULTIPLE-FETUS PREGNANCIES

A case can be made for following all products of MFPs in the perinatal clinic. MC-MZ twins have a number of problems that involve understanding of the embryology and genetics of MZ twinning as well as the complications of MC placentation. Parents may need education on these issues, which may not have been explored during the prenatal and postnatal periods. The terms *identical* and *fraternal* can be discarded in favor of *monozygotic* and *dizygotic*, and parents can easily learn the reasons why their MZ twins are not "identical." MC twins are at high risk for neurodevelopmental problems secondary to transfusional events, even in the absence of classic TTT. There is anecdotal evidence that TTT recipients may die of cardiomyopathy in infancy, but no statistics are available. Few studies have followed severely growth-discordant DZ and MZ twins to early childhood, and no good prognostic advice is available about growth potential. Long-term iron level monitoring may be needed in TTT survivors.

## PARENTAL CONCERNS ABOUT ZYGOSITY

Parents are often uninformed or misinformed by their health-care providers about zygosity issues. MC twins are definitely MZ, and parents can be strongly reassured about this at the time of the twins' birth or later at follow-up clinic. However, many parents are told that their DC twins are necessarily DZ, which is quite untrue. Like-sexed DC twins may be MZ or DZ. Screening tests could include simple blood typing. If the results fail to show dizygosity, formal DNA-based testing is needed; such testing is not, however, a medical benefit covered by most insurance carriers. About 1 in 4 like-sexed DC twin pairs is MZ. The majority of naturally conceived sets of triplets or quadruplets contain at least MZ twins. Zygosity is not just a matter of curiosity, and parents feel foolish when they do not know the zygosity of their twins. Concordance rates in MZ twins are high (on average, 60% to 70%) for a wide range of medical disorders that have at least one component of genetic predisposition. The availability of a rejection-free donor co-twin for solid organ transplantation and skin grafting is clearly important. However, the healthy member of an MZ twin pair cannot donate bone marrow for transplantation to his or her co-twin unless it is known that they are DC. If one MC-MZ twin demonstrates an early hematopoietic malignancy, the same disease will develop in the other twin sooner or later, because of prenatal transplacental transfusion of premutated blood stem cells (Wiemels et al, 1999).

## POTENTIAL FOR NEONATAL RESEARCH IN TWINS

Some suggested research topics in twins include:

- Longitudinal anthropometric studies in growth-discordant twins, according to zygosity-chorionicity and cause (if known)
- Studies of cerebral and physical lateralities ("mirroring") in MZ-DZ twins
- Long-term multidisciplinary studies of the natural history of MC twins surviving transplacental transfusional events, including TTT and its treatment, TRAP, fetal death, and selective termination
- Long-term studies of iron storage and utilization after TTT
- Long-term studies of chromosome mosaicism ratios in mosaic MZ twins
- Studies of the effects of fetal sex hormone secretions on brain and gonadal development in unlike-sexed DZ twin pairs

## REFERENCES


Botting BJ, Macfarlane AJ, Price, FV (eds): Three, Four and More: A Study of Triplet and Higher Order Births. London, HMSO, 1990, p 82.

Cincotta RB, Gray PH, Phythian G, et al: Long term outcome of twin-twin transfusion syndrome. Arch Dis Child Fetal Neonatal Ed 83:F171-F176, 2000.

Contribution of assisted reproductive technology and ovulation-inducing drugs to triplet and higher order multiple births—United States, 1980-1997. MMWR Morbid Mortal Wkly Rep 49:535-538, 2000.

Dawkins RR, Marshall TL, Rogers MS: Prenatal gangrene in association with twin-twin transfusion syndrome. Am J Obstet Gynecol 172:1055-1057, 1995.

Gardiner HM: Early changes in vascular dynamics in relation to twin-twin transfusion syndrome. Twin Res 4:371-377, 2001.

Genest DR, Lage JM: Absence of normal-appearing proximal tubules in the fetal and neonatal kidney: Prevalence and significance. Hum Pathol 22:147-153, 1991.

Haverkamp F, Lex C, Hanisch C, et al: Neurodevelopmental risks in twin-to-twin transfusion syndrome: Preliminary findings. Eur J Paediatr Neurol 5:21-27, 2001.

Machin GA, Bamforth F: Zygosity and placental anatomy of 15 consecutive sets of spontaneously conceived triplets. Am J Med Genet 61:247-252, 1996.

Machin GA: Some causes of genotypic and phenotypic discordance in monozygotic twin pairs. Am J Med Genet 61:216-228, 1996.

Mari G, Detti L, Oz U, Abuhamad AZ: Long-term outcome in twin-twin transfusion syndrome treated with serial aggressive amnioreduction. Am J Obstet Gynecol 183:211-217, 2000.

Nizard J, Bonnet D, Fermont L, Ville Y: Acquired right heart outflow tract anomaly without systemic hypertension in recipient twins with twin-twin transfusion syndrome. Ultrasound Obstet Gynecol 18:669-672, 2001.

Rodis JF, Egan JF, Craffey A, et al: Calculated risk of chromosomal abnormalities in twin gestations. Obstet Gynecol 76:1037-1041, 1990.

Sbracia M, Baldi M, Cao D, et al: Preferential location of sex chromosomes, their aneuploidy in human sperm, and their role in determining sex chromosome aneuploidy in embryos after ICSI. Hum Reprod 17:320-324, 2002.

Scott F, Evans M: Distal gangrene in a polycythemic recipient fetus in twin-twin transfusion. Obstet Gynecol 86:677-679, 1995.

Sheen TC, Chen SR, Au HK, et al: Herniated blastomere following chemically assisted hatching may result in monozygotic twins. Fertil Steril 75:442-444, 2001.

Sudik R, Jacubiczka S, Nawroth F, et al: Chimerism in a fertile woman with 46,XY karyotype and female phenotype. Hum Reprod 16:56-58, 2001.

van Dijk BA, Boomsma DI, de Man AJ: Blood group chimerism in human multiple births is not rare. Am J Med Genet 61:264-268, 1996.

Weig SG, Marshall PC, Abroms IF, Gauthier NS: Patterns of cerebral injury and clinical presentation in the vascular disruptive syndrome of monozygotic twins. Pediatr Neurol 13:279-285, 1995.

Wiemels JL, Cazzaniga G, Daniotti M, et al: Prenatal origin of acute lymphoblastic leukemia in children. Lancet 354:1499-1503, 1999.

CHAPTER 8

# Nonimmune Hydrops

**Scott A. Lorch, Thomas J. Mollen, and Roberta A. Ballard**

An infant with *hydrops* has abnormal accumulation of excess fluid. The condition varies from mild, generalized edema to massive edema, with effusions in multiple body cavities and with peripheral edema so severe that the extremities are fixed in extension. Severely hydropic fetuses may die in utero; if delivered alive, they may die in the neonatal period from the severity of their underlying disease or from severe cardiorespiratory failure.

The first description of a hydropic newborn, in a twin gestation, appeared in 1609. In 1892, Ballantyne suggested that the finding of hydrops was an outcome for many different causes, in contrast to the belief at that time that hydrops was a single entity. Potter (1943) first distinguished between hydrops secondary to erythroblastosis fetalis and nonimmune hydrops, by describing a group of infants with generalized body edema who did not have hepatosplenomegaly or abnormal erythropoiesis. His description of more than 100 cases of hydrops included two sets of twins in which one of the infants was hydropic and the other was not, thus presenting the first description of twin-twin transfusion syndrome. With the nearly universal use of anti-D globulin and refinement of the schedule and doses for its administration, the occurrence of immune-mediated hydrops has steadily declined. Later studies have suggested that immune-mediated causes account for only 6% to 10% of all cases of hydrops (Heinonen et al, 2000; Machin, 1989). The reported incidence of nonimmune hydrops in the general population has been highly variable, ranging from 6 per 1000 pregnancies in a high-risk referral clinic in the United Kingdom between 1993 and 1999 (Sohan et al, 2001) to 1 in 4000 pregnancies (Norton, 1994); other published rates are 6 per 1000 pregnancies (Santolaya et al, 1992), 1.3 per 1000 pregnancies (Wafelman et al, 1999), and 1 per 1700 pregnancies (Heinonen et al, 2000). However, all of the published studies come from single institutions, with the at-risk populations ranging from that of a high-risk pregnancy clinic to infants in a neonatal intensive care unit (NICU). No study yet published has monitored all pregnant women in one geographic area to calculate the true population incidence of nonimmune hydrops. Geography also affects the incidence; several causes of nonimmune hydrops, such as α-thalassemia, are more common in certain areas of the world. Finally, the incidence of nonimmune hydrops may be rising because of the more routine use of ultrasound investigation in the late first trimester of pregnancy (Iskaros et al, 1997).

## ETIOLOGY

Nonimmune hydrops has been associated with a wide range of conditions (Table 8–1). In many of these conditions, edema formation results from one of the following possible processes:

- Elevated central venous pressure, in which the cardiac output is less than the rate of venous return
- Anemia, resulting in high-output cardiac failure
- Decreased lymphatic flow
- Capillary leak

The actual pathophysiology of hydrops for many of the conditions in Table 8–1, however, is still not understood.

The most common causes of nonimmune hydrops are chromosomal, cardiovascular, thoracic, infectious, and related to twinning (Wilkins, 1999). As with reported incidence rates, the relative contribution of these causes varies from study to study. Those studies that focus on early fetal presentation of hydrops (postconceptual age of less than 24 weeks) have found that chromosomal abnormalities, such as Turner syndrome and trisomies 13, 18, and 21, are the causes of 32% to 78% of all cases of hydrops (Boyd and Keeling, 1992; Heinonen et al, 2000; Iskaros et al, 1997; McCoy et al, 1995; Sohan et al, 2001). For infants whose hydrops becomes evident after 24 weeks of postconceptual age, cardiovascular and thoracic causes are most prevalent, with rates ranging between 30% and 50% (Machin, 1989; McCoy et al, 1995; Sohan et al, 2001). Studies from Asia have noted a higher percentage of cases from hematologic causes, probably because of the higher rates of α-thalassemia in the population of that continent (Lin et al, 1991; Nakayama et al, 1999).

The percentage of infants with "idiopathic" hydrops, or hydrops of unknown etiology, varies from 5.2% to 50%, depending on the ability of the clinicians to complete their diagnostic evaluation (Heinonen et al, 2000; Iskaros et al, 1997; Machin, 1989; McCoy et al, 1995; Nakayama et al, 1999; Santolaya et al, 1992; Sohan et al, 2001; Wafelman et al, 1999; Wy et al, 1999). Yaegashi and associates (1998) used enzyme-linked immunosorbent assay (ELISA) and polymerase chain reaction (PCR) techniques to improve the detection of parvovirus infection. In both their own institution, and in eight other series of patients, these investigators found evidence of parvovirus infection in 15% to 19% of all infants previously diagnosed with "idiopathic" hydrops. It is likely that, as we improve the understanding of and testing for many of the conditions listed in Table 8–1, the number of infants diagnosed with "idiopathic" nonimmune hydrops will continue to decline.

## PATHOPHYSIOLOGY

### Normal Fluid Homeostasis

Abnormal body fluid homeostasis is the underlying cause of edema, whether local or generalized. To understand the pathogenesis of hydrops, the clinician must consider the forces underlying normal fluid homeostasis. The regulation of net fluid movement across a capillary membrane depends

**TABLE 8–1**

**Conditions Associated with Hydrops Fetalis**

| | |
|---|---|
| Hemolytic anemias | Alloimmune, Rh, Kell, c |
| | α-chain hemoglobinopathies (homozygous α-thalassemia) |
| | Red blood cell enzyme deficiencies (glucose phosphate isomerase deficiency, glucose-6-phosphate dehydrogenase) |
| Other anemias | Fetomaternal hemorrhage |
| | Twin-twin transfusion |
| Cardiac conditions | Premature closure of foramen ovale |
| | Ebstein anomaly |
| | Hypoplastic left or right heart |
| | Subaortic stenosis with fibroelastosis |
| | Cardiomyopathy, myocardial fibroelastosis |
| | Atrioventricular canal |
| | Myocarditis |
| | Right atrial hemangioma |
| | Intracardiac hamartoma or fibroma |
| | Tuberous sclerosis with cardiac rhabdomyoma |
| Cardiac arrhythmias | Supraventricular tachycardia |
| | Atrial flutter |
| | Congenital heart block |
| Vascular malformations | Hemangioma of the liver |
| | Any large arteriovenous malformation |
| | Klippel-Trenaunay syndrome |
| Vascular accidents | Thrombosis of umbilical vein or inferior vena cava |
| | Recipient in twin-twin transfusion |
| Infections | Cytomegalovirus, congenital hepatitis, human parvovirus, other viruses |
| | Toxoplasmosis, Chagas disease |
| | Coxsackie virus |
| | Syphilis |
| | Leptospirosis |
| Lymphatic abnormalities | Lymphangiectasia |
| | Cystic hygroma |
| | Noonan syndrome |
| | Multiple pterygium syndrome |
| Nervous system lesions | Absence of corpus callosum |
| | Encephalocele |
| | Cerebral arteriovenous malformation |
| | Intracranial hemorrhage (massive) |
| | Holoprosencephaly |
| | Fetal akinesia sequence |
| Pulmonary conditions | Cystic adenomatoid malformation of the lung |
| | Mediastinal teratoma |
| | Diaphragmatic hernia |
| | Lung sequestration syndrome |
| | Lymphangiectasia |
| Renal conditions | Urinary ascites |
| | Congenital nephrosis |
| | Renal vein thrombosis |
| | Invasive processes and storage disorders |
| | Tuberous sclerosis |
| | Gaucher disease |
| | Mucopolysaccharidosis |
| | Mucolipidosis |
| Chromosome abnormalities | Trisomy 13, trisomy 18, trisomy 21 |
| | Turner syndrome |
| | XX/XY |
| Bone diseases | Osteogenesis imperfecta |
| | Achondroplasia |
| | Asphyxiating thoracic dystrophy |
| Gastrointestinal conditions | Bowel obstruction with perforation and meconium peritonitis |
| | Small bowel volvulus |
| | Other intestinal obstructions |
| | Prune-belly syndrome |

**TABLE 8–1**

**Conditions Associated with Hydrops Fetalis—Cont'd**

| | |
|---|---|
| Tumors | Neuroblastoma |
| | Choriocarcinoma |
| | Sacrococcygeal teratoma |
| | Hemangioma of the liver |
| | Congenital leukemia |
| Maternal or placental conditions | Maternal diabetes |
| | Maternal therapy with indomethacin |
| | Multiple gestation with parasitic fetus |
| | Chorioangioma of placenta, chorionic vessels, or umbilical vessels |
| | Toxemia |
| | Systemic lupus erythematosus |
| Miscellaneous | Neu-Laxova syndrome |
| | Myotonic dystrophy |
| Idiopathic | |

on the Starling forces—first described by E.H. Starling in 1896. Flow between intravascular and interstitial fluid compartments is determined by the balance among (1) capillary hydrostatic pressure, (2) serum colloid oncotic pressure, (3) interstitial hydrostatic pressure or tissue turgor pressure, and (4) interstitial osmotic pressure, which depends on lymphatic flow. The Starling equation defines the relationship among these forces and their net effect on net fluid movement, or filtration, across a semipermeable membrane (such as the capillary membrane) as

$$\text{filtration} = K\,[(P_c - P_t) - R(O_p - O_t)]$$

where $K$ = capillary filtration coefficient, representing the extent of permeability of a membrane to water and thus describing capillary integrity; $P_c$ = capillary hydrostatic pressure; $P_t$ = interstitial hydrostatic pressure or tissue turgor pressure; $R$ = reflection coefficient for a solute, representing the extent of permeability of the capillary wall to that solute; $O_p$ = plasma oncotic pressure as determined by plasma proteins and other solutes; and $O_t$ = interstitial osmotic pressure (Fig. 8–1).

Although an abnormality of any of the components of this equation may, in theory, result in accumulation of edema fluid, the fetal-placental unit presents a unique physiologic condition that effectively eliminates two of the factors, assuming unimpeded fetal-placental flow and an appropriately functioning maternal-placental interface. Because approximately 40% of fetal cardiac output is allocated to the placenta, there is rapid transport of water between fetus and mother. Any condition resulting in elevated fetal capillary hydrostatic pressure or low plasma colloid oncotic pressure would likely cause the net flow of water from fetal villi in the placenta to the maternal blood stream, where it can be effectively eliminated. This elimination of fluid would counteract the accumulation of interstitial fluid by the fetus. Although the placenta of a hydropic fetus is also edematous, these changes are believed to occur along with, and not prior to, fetal fluid accumulation.

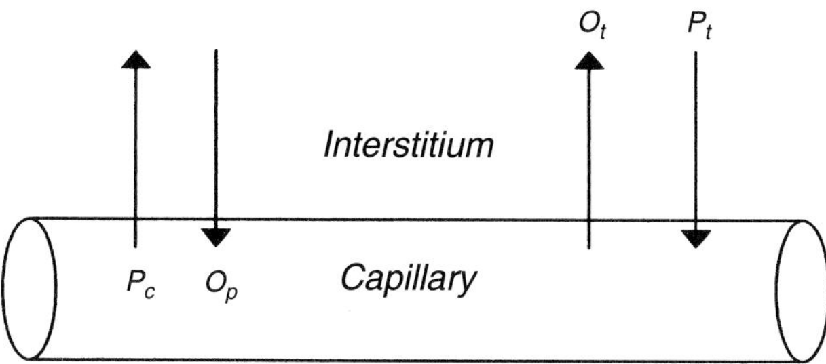


**FIGURE 8–1.** Starling forces and net effect on fluid homeostasis. *Arrows* represent net effect of movement of fluid across the capillary membrane for each factor under normal conditions. $P_c$ = capillary hydrostatic pressure; $P_t$ = interstitial hydrostatic pressure or tissue turgor pressure; $O_p$ = plasma oncotic pressure as determined by plasma proteins and other solutes; $O_t$ = interstitial osmotic pressure.

## Derangements in Fluid Homeostasis

Diamond and coworkers (1932) suggested three possible mechanisms that might be relevant in infants with hydrops: anemia, low colloid osmotic pressure with hypoproteinemia, and congestive heart failure with hypervolemia. Others have reviewed these potential mechanisms (Phibbs, 1998), which remain among the central hypotheses addressed by investigators in this area. The causes of hydrops appear to be multifactorial, however, with mechanisms that produce elevated central venous pressure (CVP), capillary leakage, and impaired lymphatic drainage all contributing to its development.

Infants with alloimmune hydrops (and several of the nonimmune hydrops conditions as well) have significant anemia. It has been proposed that anemia leads to congestive heart failure with increased hydrostatic pressure in the capillaries, causing vascular damage that results in edema. However, the hematocrit values of infants with and without hydrops overlap significantly, suggesting that anemia alone is not the complete explanation. A rapidly lowered hemoglobin concentration results in greater cardiac output to maintain adequate oxygen delivery. This results in higher oxygen demands by the myocardium, which may be difficult to meet because of the anemia.

The hypoxic myocardium may become less contractile and less compliant, with ventricular stiffness causing increased afterload to the atria. High-output congestive heart failure may then exist, resulting in elevated CVP. Raised CVP leads to increased capillary filtration pressures and impairment of lymphatic return (Weiner, 1993). Also, reduced compliance of a right ventricle may result in flow reversal in the inferior vena cava (IVC), which may in turn cause end-organ damage to the liver, with consequent hypoalbuminemia and portal hypertension enhancing formation of both edema and ascites. Hydrops has been produced in fetal lambs (Blair et al, 1994), in which the hemoglobin content was lowered in 12 fetuses through exchange transfusion using cell-free plasma; six became hydropic. Anemia developed more rapidly with a higher CVP in the hydropic fetuses than in the fetuses without hydrops. In the most severely anemic fetuses, it is probable that decreased oxygen transport causes tissue hypoxia, which in turn increases capillary permeability to both water and protein. These changes in capillary permeability also likely contribute to the development of hydrops.

Infants who have erythroblastosis and hydrops seem to demonstrate a correlation between serum albumin concentration and the severity of hydrops (Phibbs et al, 1974). Initial therapy after birth, however, tends to raise the serum albumin value toward normal rapidly, and with diuresis, the infants have normal albumin concentrations. This finding suggests that hypoalbuminemia may be the result of dilution rather than the cause of the hydrops.

To elucidate the role of isolated hypoproteinemia in the genesis of hydrops, Moise and colleagues (1991) have induced hypoproteinemia in sets of twin fetal lambs. One twin of each set underwent serum protein reduction through repeated removal of plasma and replacement with normal saline; the other twin served as the control. Over 3 days, plasma protein concentrations were reduced by an average of 41%, with a 44% reduction in colloid osmotic pressure, in the experimental subjects. No fetuses became edematous, and total body water content values were similar in experimental and control animals. Thus, hypoproteinemia alone was not sufficient to cause hydrops fetalis over the course of the study. Transcapillary filtration probably increased with hypoproteinemia but was compensated by lymphatic return. Human fetuses with hypoproteinemia due to nephrotic syndrome or analbuminemia rarely experience hydrops, further supporting the hypothesis that hypoproteinemia alone is not sufficient to cause hydrops. Hypoproteinemia may, however, lower the threshold for edema formation in the presence of impaired lymphatic return or increased intravascular hydrostatic pressures.

The most commonly diagnosed causes of nonimmune hydrops that appears in fetuses older than 24 weeks postconceptual age are cardiac disorders. Any state in which cardiac output is lower than the rate of venous return results in an elevated CVP. Increased CVP raises capillary filtration pressures and, if high enough, restricts lymphatic return. Both of these mechanisms may then contribute to interstitial accumulation of fluid. Structural cardiac causes of elevated CVP include right-sided obstructive lesions and valvular regurgitation. The most common single cause of nonimmune hydrops, and fortunately also the most easily reversible cause, is supraventricular tachycardia (SVT). In general, cardiac output rises with heart rate. At the increasingly high rates seen in SVT, however, cardiac output plateaus and then diminishes. The rates observed with SVT are often associated with decreased cardiac output. Impaired cardiac output results in elevated CVP, which may give rise to edema through mechanisms discussed previously (Gest, 1990). Myocardial hypoxia (most often due to severe anemia) and myocarditis (usually infectious) reduce both the contractility and compliance of the myocardium and can also cause an increase in CVP.

A fourth factor that contributes to hydrops is decreased lymph flow. If the rate of fluid filtration from plasma to tissues exceeds the rate of lymph return to the central venous system, edema and effusions may form. A structural impediment or increased CVP that opposes lymphatic return to the heart may impair lymph flow. To determine the effects of alterations in CVP on lymphatic return, Gest and colleagues (1992) applied an opposing hydrostatic pressure to the thoracic duct in fetal lambs. They inserted catheters into the thoracic ducts of 10 fetuses. Varying the height of the catheter altered the thoracic duct outflow pressure. Thoracic duct flow was nearly constant over the physiologic range of CVP, but sharply decreased at elevated pressures. Thus, lymphatic flow may be reduced or essentially blocked in pathologic states associated with elevated CVP.

## PRENATAL DIAGNOSIS

The initial presentation of fetal hydrops varies by report. Watson and Campbell (1986) found that two thirds of prenatally diagnosed cases were discovered on routine ultrasonographic examinations, and the other one third referred for evaluation because of suspected polyhydramnios. Graves and Baskett (1984) reported that hydrops was more commonly discovered after referral for polyhydramnios, fetus large for dates, fetal tachycardia, or pregnancy-induced hypertension. Despite the underlying etiology of hydrops or the clinical presentation, the prenatal diagnosis is made via the ultrasonographic finding of excess fluid in the form of ascites, pleural or pericardial effusions, skin edema, placental edema, or polyhydramnios. Several definitions for ultrasonographic diagnosis based on quantity and distribution of excess fluid have been proposed. One widely accepted set of criteria consists of the presence of excess fluid in any two of the previously listed compartments. Because this definition is based on the presence of excess fluid alone, the degree of severity is generally subjective.

Swain and colleagues (1999) outlined a multidisciplinary approach to the evaluation and management of the mother and fetus with hydrops. Table 8–2 provides recommendations for the investigation of fetal hydrops. Patient history should focus on ethnic background, familial history of consanguinity, genetic or congenital anomalies, and complications of pregnancy, including recent maternal illness and environmental exposures. Maternal disorders such as diabetes, systemic lupus erythematosus, myotonic

**TABLE 8–2**

**Antenatal Investigation of Fetal Hydrops**

| | |
|---|---|
| Maternal | History, including:<br>Age, parity, gestation<br>Medical and family histories<br>Recent illnesses or exposures<br>Medications<br>Complete blood count and indices<br>Blood typing and indirect Coombs antibody screening<br>Hemoglobin electrophoresis<br>Kleihauer-Betke stain of peripheral blood<br>Syphilis, TORCH (toxoplasmosis, other infections, rubella, cytomegalovirus, and herpes simplex), and parvovirus B19 titers<br>Anti-Ro and anti-La, systemic lupus erythematosus preparation<br>Oral glucose tolerance test<br>Glucose-6-phosphate dehydrogenase, pyruvate kinase deficiency screening |
| Fetal | Serial ultrasound evaluations<br>Limb length, fetal movement<br>Echocardiography |
| Amniocentesis | Karyotype<br>Alpha-fetoprotein<br>Viral cultures; polymerase chain reaction analysis for toxoplasmosis, parvovirus 19<br>Establishment of culture for appropriate metabolic or DNA testing<br>Lecithin-to-sphingomyelin ratio to assess lung maturity |
| Fetal blood sampling | Karyotype<br>Complete blood count<br>Hemoglobin analysis<br>Immunoglobulin M test; specific cultures<br>Albumin and total protein measurements<br>Measurement of umbilical venous pressure<br>Metabolic testing |

Adapted from Swain S, Cameron AD, McNay MB, Howatson AG: Prenatal diagnosis and management of nonimmune hydrops fetalis. Aust N Z J Obstet Gynaecol 39:285-290, 1999.

dystrophy, and any type of liver disease should also be noted. Initial laboratory investigation includes blood typing and Coombs test to rule out immune-mediated hydrops. Other blood tests are a screening for hemoglobinopathies, a Kleihauer-Betke test to eliminate fetal-maternal hemorrhage, and testing for the TORCH diseases (toxoplasmosis, other infections, rubella, cytomegalovirus infection, and herpes simplex), including syphilis and parvovirus B19.

Further evaluation is directed at identifying possible causes (Forouzan, 1997). Rapid evaluation is necessary to determine whether intervention is possible and to estimate the prognosis for the fetus. Many fetal conditions, such as arrhythmias, twin-twin transfusion, large vascular masses, and congenital diaphragmatic hernias and other chest-occupying lesions, are discovered during the initial ultrasonographic evaluation (Coleman, 2002). If the examination is not helpful in identifying a cause, ultrasonography should be repeated at a later date to reassess fetal anatomy, monitor progression of the hydrops, and evaluate the well-being of the fetus.

Fetal echocardiography should also be performed to evaluate for cardiac malformations and arrhythmia. Amniotic fluid can be obtained for fetal karyotyping, cultures, and lecithin to sphingomyelin ratio to assess lung maturity. Fetal blood sampling allows for other tests, such as a complete blood cell count, routine chemical analyses, karyotyping, bacterial and viral cultures, metabolic studies, and serum immunoglobulin measurements.

## PRENATAL MANAGEMENT

The goals of antenatal evaluation of fetal hydrops depend on the underlying cause. In diagnoses in which therapy is futile, the goal is to avoid unnecessary invasive testing and cesarean section. The prognosis should be discussed frankly with the parents, who should be given the option of terminating the pregnancy. If the underlying cause is amenable to fetal therapy, the risks and benefits of such therapy, as well as the warning that diagnostic error is possible, should be discussed with the family.

SVT is the most common known cause of nonimmune hydrops and is also the most amenable to treatment (Newburger, 1979). Usually, the mother is given antiarrhythmic agents, and the fetus is monitored closely for resolution of the SVT. Digoxin is most commonly administered, although quinidine, procainamide, or other drugs may be used. Transplacental transfer of digoxin may be impaired in the setting of hydrops. In extreme circumstances, such as fetal tachyarrhythmia refractory to maternal treatment, direct fetal administration of antiarrhythmic agents via percutaneous umbilical blood sampling (PUBS), although untested and highly risky, has met with some success.

If anemia is the cause of hydrops, transfusions of packed red blood cells may be administered to the fetus. Often a single transfusion reverses the edema, although serial transfusions may be necessary. Parvovirus B19 (Anand, 1987) and fetal-maternal hemorrhage are examples of diagnoses amenable to this therapy. Other diagnoses involving anemias that are refractory to transfusions, such as α-thalassemia, may require neonatal stem cell transplantation. Transfusions should be given, with the use of ultrasonographic guidance, into the intraperitoneal space or umbilical vein. Blood instilled into the abdominal cavity is taken up by lymphatics, but elevated CVPs present in hydropic fetuses may impair this uptake. If uptake of intraperitoneal blood is incomplete, treatment for the hydrops is less successful; degeneration of the remaining hemoglobin may create a substantial bilirubin load, necessitating phototherapy or exchange transfusion after the infant is delivered.

Fetal surgery is emerging as a promising therapy for select cases of fetal hydrops (Kitano, 1999). Fetal lung lesions such as congenital cystic adenomatoid malformation (CCAM) and pulmonary sequestration can, in the most extreme cases, result in mediastinal shift, pulmonary hypoplasia, cardiovascular compromise, and hydrops. Adzick and colleagues (1998) reported on the outcome of 175 cases of fetal lung masses, including 134 cases of CCAM and 41 of extralobar pulmonary sequestration. The 76 fetuses with CCAM lesions without associated hydrops were all managed expectantly (maternal transport to a high-risk center, planned delivery near term, and resection in the newborn period). CCAMs frequently involute and may disappear before delivery. Thus, there were no deaths in the nonhydropic group of fetuses in this study. Twenty-five fetuses with hydrops were managed expectantly, and all 25 died before or after preterm labor at 25 to 26 weeks of gestation. These results highlight the fact that fetuses with lung lesions leading to hydrops have high mortality rates. Thirteen fetuses with CCAM and associated hydrops underwent open fetal resection or lobectomy. Eight survived and were reported as healthy at 1 to 7 years of follow-up. Maternal morbidities related to fetal intervention ranged from uterine wound infection with dehiscence to mild postoperative interstitial pulmonary edema, which was treated with diuretics.

Fetal intervention has met with some success in other diagnoses with associated hydrops. Thoracoamniotic shunts for large unicystic lesions and pleuroamniotic shunts for hydrothorax have reportedly enhanced survival in extreme cases. Similarly, in cases of massive urinary ascites, urinary diversion via peritoneal shunts has been reported but with poor long-term prognosis (Crombleholme, 1990). Finally, laser coagulation of aberrant interfetal vascular connections has resulted in the resolution of hydrops in the recipient twin in twin-twin transfusion syndrome (Milner, 1999). These studies have been promising enough to warrant a randomized controlled trial, sponsored by the National Institutes of Health (NIH), comparing this intervention with conservative management strategies such as serial amnioreduction.

In cases in which the cause can be corrected by appropriate care at the time of delivery, such as elimination of a chorioangioma, and in cases in which no cause can be ascertained, close observation for fetal demise is the focus of prenatal management. Many cases of nonimmune hydrops manifest in the third trimester as preterm labor. It is difficult to decide whether to attempt tocolysis and delay delivery so as to allow the potentially beneficial administration of steroids before birth or to deliver the fetus immediately. If tocolysis is possible, expectant management should include usual biophysical testing, although fetal decompensation may be difficult to measure. Abnormal fetal heart tracings, oligohydramnios, decreased fetal movement, and poor fetal tone are all ominous signs. There is no indication to prolong pregnancy beyond attainment of a mature lung profile unless available evidence indicates improvement or resolution of the hydrops.

## NEONATAL EVALUATION

Table 8–3 summarizes the diagnostic evaluations recommended for newborn infants with nonimmune hydrops of unknown cause.

**TABLE 8–3**

**Diagnostic Evaluation of Newborns with Nonimmune Hydrops**

| System | Type of Evaluation |
|---|---|
| Cardiovascular | Echocardiogram, electrocardiogram |
| Pulmonary | Chest radiograph, pleural fluid examination |
| Hematologic | Complete blood cell count, differential platelet count, blood type and Coombs test, blood smear for morphologic analysis |
| Gastrointestinal | Abdominal radiograph, abdominal ultrasonography, liver function tests, peritoneal fluid examination, total protein and albumin levels |
| Renal | Urinalysis, blood urea nitrogen and creatinine measurements |
| Genetic | Chromosomal analysis, skeletal radiographs, genetic consultation |
| Congenital infections | Viral cultures or serologic testing, including TORCH (toxoplasmosis, other infections, rubella, cytomegalovirus, and herpes simplex) agents and parvovirus |
| Pathologic | Complete autopsy, placental examination |

Adapted from Carlton DP, McGillivray BC, Schreiber MD: Nonimmune hydrops fetalis: A multidisciplinary approach. Clin Perinatol 16:839-851, 1989.

## Intensive Care of the Infant with Hydrops Fetalis

After successful resuscitation, including intubation, administration of surfactant, and placement of umbilical catheters, the clinical management can address both the cause and the complications of hydrops. Morbidity and mortality may result from the hydropic state, the underlying conditions giving rise to hydrops, or both. A hydropic fetus who is delivered prematurely is subject to the additional complications of prematurity. If there is massive ascites or pleural effusions, initial resuscitation may require thoracentesis or tapping of the ascites. Because of pulmonary edema, hydropic infants are susceptible to pulmonary hemorrhage and require high levels of positive end-expiratory pressure (PEEP).

### Respiratory Management

Virtually all infants with hydrops require mechanical ventilation because of pleural and peritoneal effusions, pulmonary hypoplasia, surfactant deficiency, pulmonary edema, poor chest wall compliance due to edema, or persistent pulmonary hypertension of the newborn. The presence of persistent pleural effusions may necessitate placement of chest tubes. Ascites may also compress the diaphragm and impair lung expansion. Breath sounds, chest movement, blood gas levels, and radiographs must all be monitored frequently, so that ventilator support can be reduced in response to improvements in lung compliance and water clearance. Pneumothoraces and pulmonary interstitial emphysema remain potential complications as long as ventilator support is continued. Infants who need a prolonged course of ventilation, particularly those born prematurely, may have bronchopulmonary dysplasia. Chronic lung disease results in a longer and more complicated hospital course and contributes to the late mortality of hydrops.

### Fluid and Electrolyte Management

A primary goal of fluid management is resolution of the hydrops itself. Maintenance fluids should be restricted, with volume boluses given only in response to clear signs of inadequate intravascular volume. The hydropic newborn has not only an excess of free extracellular water but also an excess of sodium. Fluids given during resuscitation further increase the amount of water and sodium that must be removed during the immediate neonatal period. Initial maintenance fluids should not contain sodium. Serum and urine sodium levels, urine volume, and daily weights should be monitored carefully to guide administration of fluids and electrolytes. Urinary sodium levels may help differentiate between hyponatremia due to hemodilution and that due to urinary losses.

### Cardiovascular Management

Shock may be a prominent feature of patients with hydrops. Hydropic infants may have hypovolemia as a result of capillary leakage, poor vascular tone, and impaired myocardial contractility from hypoxia or infection, impaired venous return due to shifting or compression of mediastinal structures, or pericardial effusion. Adequate intravascular volume must be maintained, and correctable causes of impaired venous return should be addressed. Peripheral perfusion, heart rate, blood pressure, and acid-base status should be monitored carefully.

## CLINICAL COURSE AND OUTCOME

Despite improvements in diagnosis and management, mortality from nonimmune hydrops remains high. Reported survival rates for all fetuses diagnosed antenatally with hydrops range from 12% to 24% (Heinonen et al, 2000; McCoy et al, 1995; Negishi et al, 1997). Higher survival rates have been reported in infants born alive, but the highest rates are still only 40% to 50% (Wy et al, 1999). Improved ultrasonography techniques and earlier testing may actually lead to lower survival rates as more first-trimester infants are diagnosed with hydrops. These infants are more likely to have chromosomal abnormalities that are incompatible with survival, but were previously not included in populations of hydropic fetuses. The best predictor of survival is the cause of the hydrops. Highest survival rates are seen in infants with parvovirus infection, chylothorax, or SVT. The lowest survival rates are for hydrops from chromosomal cause, although the figures may be biased because a significant number of the pregnancies in such cases are terminated (Heinonen et al, 2000; Sohan et al, 2001).

Carlton and coworkers (1989) reported on a group of 36 infants with nonimmune hydrops and noted that 90% of the infants who died within 24 hours had pleural effusions, compared with only 50% of those who survived. More than one third of the infants in this study required thoracentesis in the delivery room to aid in lung expansion. All of the infants who lived more than 24 hours were treated with mechanical ventilation and received supplemental oxygen. They needed ventilation for an average of 11 days (range 2 to 48 days). Most hydropic infants lose a minimum of 15% of their birth weight, and some lose as much as 30%. Ordinarily, diuresis begins on the second or third day after birth and continues for a period of 2 to 4 days. Once the edema has resolved, the infants have normal levels of circulating protein and eventually recover from their apparent capillary leak syndrome. No specific management strategies during the neonatal period, such as the use of high-frequency oscillatory ventilation, have been shown to improve outcome, although the published studies are small and not powered sufficiently to detect small differences in survival (Wy et al, 1999).

For infants who survive the immediate neonatal period, long-term outcomes appear to be excellent. Nonimmune hydrops by itself does not seem to lead to residual developmental delay. A small study from Japan found that 13 of 19 surviving infants with nonimmune hydrops had normal development at 1 to 8 years of age (Nakayama et al, 1999). The six infants with mild or severe delays in this study had other morbidities, such as extreme prematurity, structural cardiac lesions, or chromosomal anomalies. Thus, long-term morbidities from nonimmune hydrops appear to result from the underlying cause of the hydrops as well as from complications arising immediately after delivery.

## REFERENCES

Adzick NS, Harrison MR, Cromblehome TM, et al: Fetal lung lesions: Management and outcome. Am J Obstet Gynecol 179:884-889, 1998.

Anand A, Gray ES, Brown T, et al: Human parvovirus infection in pregnancy and hydrops fetalis. N Engl J Med 316:183-186, 1987.

Ballantyne JW: The Diseases and Deformities of the Fetus. Edinburgh, Oliver and Boyd, 1892.

Blair DK, Vander Straten MC, Gest AL: Hydrops in fetal sheep from rapid induction of anemia. Pediatr Res 35:560-564, 1994.

Boyd PA, Keeling JW: Fetal hydrops. J Med Genet 29:91-97, 1992.

Carlton DP, McGillivray BC, Schreiber MD: Nonimmune hydrops fetalis: A multidisciplinary approach. Clin Perinatol 16:839-851, 1989.

Coleman BG, Adzick NS, Crombleholme TM, et al: Fetal therapy: State of the art. J Ultrasound Med 21:1257-1288, 2002.

Crombleholme TM, Harrison MR, Golbus MS, et al: Fetal intervention in obstructive uropathy: Prognostic indicators and efficacy of intervention. A J Obstet Gynecol 162:1239-1244, 1990.

Diamond LK, Blackfan KD, Baty JM: Erythroblastosis fetalis and its association with universal edema of the fetus, icterus gravis neonatorum and anemia of the newborn. J Pediatr 1:269, 1932.

Forouzan I: Hydrops fetalis: Recent advances. Obstet Gynecol Surg 52:130-138, 1997.

Gest AL, Hansen TN, Moise AA, Hartley CJ: Atrial tachycardia causes hydrops in fetal lambs. Am J Physiol 258:H1159-H1163, 1990.

Gest AL, Blair DK, Vander Straten MC: The effect of outflow pressure upon thoracic duct lymph flow rate in fetal sheep. Pediatr Res 32:385-388, 1992.

Graves GR, Baskett TF: Nonimmune hydrops fetalis: Antenatal diagnosis and management. Am J Obstet Gynecol 148: 563-565, 1984.

Heinonen S, Ryynanen M, Kirkinen P: Etiology and outcome of second trimester non-immunologic fetal hydrops. Acta Obstet Gynecol Scand 79:15-18, 2000.

Iskaros J, Jauniaux E, Rodeck C: Outcome of nonimmune hydrops fetalis diagnosed during the first half of pregnancy. Obstet Gynecol 90:321-325, 1997.

Kitano Y, Flake AW, Crombleholme TM, et al: Open fetal surgery for life-threatening fetal malformations. Semin Perinatol 23:448-461, 1999.

Lin CK, Lee SH, Wang CC, et al: Alpha-thalassemic traits are common in the Taiwanese population: Usefulness of a modified hemoglobin H preparation for prevalence studies. J Lab Clin Med 118:599-603, 1991.

Machin GA: Hydrops revisited: Literature review of 1414 cases published in the 1980s. Am J Med Genet 34:366-390, 1989.

McCoy MC, Katz VL, Gould N, Kuller JA: Non-immune hydrops after 20 weeks' gestation: Review of 10 years' experience with suggestions for management. Obstet Gynecol 85:578-582, 1995.

Milner R, Crombleholme TM: Troubles with twins: Fetoscopic therapy. Semin Perinatol 23:474-483, 1999.

Moise AA, Gest AL, Weickmann PH, McMicken HW: Reduction in plasma protein does not affect body water content in fetal sheep. Pediatr Res 29:623-626, 1991.

Nakayama H, Kukita J, Hikino S, et al: Long-term outcome of 51 liveborn neonates with non-immune hydrops fetalis. Acta Paediatr 88:24-28, 1999.

Negishi H, Yamada H, Okuyama K, et al: Outcome of nonimmune hydrops fetalis and a fetus with hydrothorax and/or ascites: With some trials of intrauterine treatment. J Perinat Med 25:71-77, 1997.

Newburger JW, Keane JF: Intrauterine supraventricular tachycardia. J Pediatr 95:780-786, 1979.

Norton ME: Nonimmune hydrops fetalis. Semin Perinatol 18:321-332, 1994.

Phibbs RH, Johnson P, Tooley WH: Cardiorespiratory status of erythroblastotic newborn infants. II: Blood volume, hematocrit and serum albumin concentrations in relation to hydrops fetalis. Pediatrics 53:13-23, 1974.

Potter EL: Universal edema of the fetus unassociated with erythroblastosis. Am J Obstet Gynecol 46:130, 1943.

Santolaya J, Alley D, Jaffe R, et al: Antenatal classification of hydrops fetalis. Obstet Gynecol 79:256-259, 1992.

Sohan K, Carroll SG, De la Fuente S, et al: Analysis of outcome in hydrops fetalis in relation to gestational age at diagnosis, cause, and treatment. Acta Obstet Gynecol Scand 80:726-730, 2001.

Starling EH: On the absorption of fluids from connective tissue spaces. J Physiol 19:312, 1896.

Swain S, Cameron AD, McNay MB, Howatson AG: Prenatal diagnosis and management of nonimmune hydrops fetalis. Aust N Z J Obstet Gynaecol 39:285-290, 1999.

Wafelman LS, Pollock BH, Kreutzer J, et al: Nonimmune hydrops fetalis: Fetal and neonatal outcome during 1983-1992. Biol Neonate 75:73-81, 1999.

Watson J, Campbell S: Antenatal evaluation and management in nonimmune hydrops fetalis. Obstet Gynecol 67:589-593, 1986.

Weiner CP: Umbilical pressure measurement in the evaluation of nonimmune hydrops fetalis. Am J Obstet Gynecol 168: 817-823, 1993.

Wilkins I: Nonimmune hydrops. In Creasy RK, Resnick R (eds): Maternal-Fetal Medicine. Philadelphia, WB Saunders, 1999, pp 769-782.

Wy CA, Sajous CH, Loberiza F, Weiss MG: Outcome of infants with a diagnosis of hydrops fetalis in the 1990s. Am J Perinatol 16:561-567, 1999.

Yaegashi N, Niinuma T, Chisaka H, et al: The incidence of, and factors leading to, parvovirus B19-related hydrops fetalis following maternal infection: Report of 10 cases and meta-analysis. J Infect 37:28-35, 1998.

# MATERNAL HEALTH AFFECTING NEONATAL OUTCOME

Editor: ROBERTA A. BALLARD

PART III

CHAPTER 9

# Endocrine Disorders in Pregnancy

Ramen Chmait and Thomas R. Moore

## DIABETES IN PREGNANCY

Currently, 17 million people in the United States have some form of diagnosed diabetes. Alarmingly, 2002 data indicate that new cases of type 2 diabetes are occurring at an increasing rate among American Indian, African American, and Hispanic and Latino children and adolescents (National Institute of Diabetes, 2002). Continued immigration among populations with high rates of type 2 diabetes and the effects of changes in diet (increases in number of calories and fat content) and lifestyle (sedentary) portend marked rises in the percentage of patients with preexisting diabetes who will become pregnant in the future. The epidemic of childhood obesity currently under way in the United States will lead to a sharp rise in childhood and adolescent diabetes over the next two decades. This trend will have a profound effect on obstetrics and pediatric practice in the future. Expanded efforts to reach the populations at risk are necessary if a significant increase in maternal and newborn morbidity is to be avoided (Persson and Hanson, 1998).

Depending on the population surveyed, abnormalities of glucose regulation occur in 3% to 8% of pregnant women. Although more than 80% of this glucose intolerance arises only during pregnancy (gestational diabetes) and involves relatively modest episodes of hyperglycemia, the attendant fetal and newborn morbidity is disproportionate. Compared with weight-matched controls, infants of diabetic mothers (IDMs) have double the risk of serious birth injury, triple the likelihood of cesarean section, and quadruple the incidence of admission to a newborn intensive care unit. Studies indicate that the magnitude of risk of these maloccurrences is proportional to the level of maternal hyperglycemia. Therefore, to some extent, the excessive fetal and neonatal morbidity of diabetes in pregnancy is preventable or at least reducible through meticulous prenatal and intrapartum care.

### Maternal-Fetal Metabolism in Normal Pregnancy and Diabetic Pregnancy

#### Normal Maternal Glucose Regulation

With each meal, a complex combination of maternal hormonal actions, including the secretion of pancreatic insulin, glucagon, somatomedins, and adrenal catecholamines, ensures an ample but not excessive supply of glucose to the mother and fetus during pregnancy. The key effects of pregnancy on maternal metabolic regulation are as follows:

- Because the fetus continues to draw glucose from the maternal blood stream across the placenta even during periods of fasting, the tendency to maternal hypoglycemia between meals becomes increasingly marked as pregnancy progresses and fetal glucose demand grows.
- Placental steroid and peptide hormone production (estrogens, progesterone, and chorionic somatomammotropin) rises linearly throughout the second and third trimesters, resulting in a progressively increasing tissue resistance to maternal insulin action.
- Progressive maternal *insulin resistance* requires a significant augmentation in pancreatic insulin production (more than twice nonpregnant levels) during feeding to maintain euglycemia. Twenty-four hour mean insulin levels are 30% higher in the third trimester than in the nonpregnant state.
- If pancreatic insulin output is not adequately augmented, maternal hyperglycemia and then fetal hyperglycemia result. The severity of hyperglycemia and its timing depend on the relative inadequacy of insulin production.

#### Fetal Effects of Maternal Hyperglycemia

##### *Congenital Anomalies*

A major threat to the IDM is the possibility of a life-threatening structural anomaly. In the normoglycemic pregnancy, the risk of a major birth defect is 1% to 2%. Among women with pregestational diabetes, the risk of a fetal structural anomaly is fourfold to eightfold higher (Fig. 9–1). The typical defects and their frequency of occurrence noted in a prospective study of infants with major malformations are listed in Table 9–1. The majority of lesions involve the central nervous and cardiovascular systems, although other series have reported an excess of genitourinary and limb defects as well (Cousins, 1991).

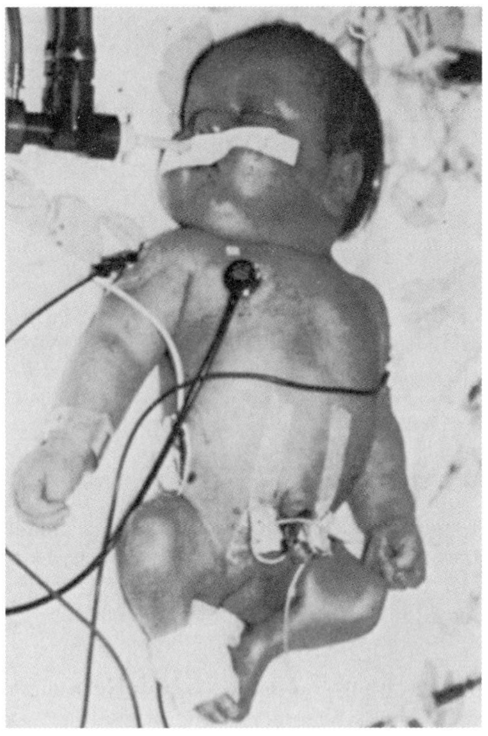

**FIGURE 9–1.** Newborn with caudal regression syndrome, macrosomia, and respiratory distress. The mother had type 1 diabetes and a glycosylated hemoglobin ($HbA_{1c}$) concentration of 13.5% when first seen for prenatal care at 12 weeks of gestation. *(From Creasy RK, Resnik R [eds]: Maternal-Fetal Medicine: Principles and Practice, 2nd ed. Philadelphia, WB Saunders, 1989.)*

There is no increase in birth defects among offspring of diabetic fathers, nondiabetic women, or women in whom gestational diabetes develops after the first trimester. These findings suggest that glycemic control during embryogenesis is a critical factor in the genesis of diabetes-associated birth defects. In a study by Miller and colleagues (1981), the frequency of congenital anomalies was proportional to the maternal glycohemoglobin ($HbA_{1c}$) value in the first trimester (rate of anomalies 3.4% with $HbA_{1c}$ <8.5%, and 22.4% with $HbA_{1c}$ >8.5%). Lucas and associates (1989) reported a similar experience with 105 diabetic patients, finding an overall malformation rate of 13.3%. The risk of delivering a malformed infant, however, was nil for a woman with an $HbA_{1c}$ value of less than 7.1%, 14% with an $HbA_{1c}$ value of 7.2% to 9.1%, 23% with an $HbA_{1c}$ value of 9.2% to 11.1%, and 25% with an $HbA_{1c}$ value of higher than 11.2%.

**TABLE 9–1**

**Congenital Malformations in Infants of Insulin-Dependent Diabetic Mothers**

| Anomaly | Appropriate Risk Ratio | Percent Risk |
|---|---|---|
| All cardiac defects | 18× | 8.5 |
| All central nervous system anomalies | 16× | 5.3 |
| Anencephaly | 13× | |
| Spina bifida | 20× | |
| All congenital anomalies | 8× | 18.4 |

Data from Becerra et al (1990).

### Pathogenesis

The specific mechanisms by which hyperglycemia disturbs embryonic development are incompletely elucidated, but reduced levels of arachidonic acid and *myo*-inositol and accumulation of sorbitol and trace metals in the embryo have been demonstrated in animal models (Pinter et al, 1986). Fetal hyperglycemia may promote excessive formation of oxygen radicals in the mitochondria of susceptible tissues, leading to the formation of hydroperoxides, which inhibit prostacyclin. The resulting overabundance of thromboxanes and other prostaglandins may then disrupt vascularization of developing tissues. In support of this theory, the addition of prostaglandin inhibitors to mouse embryos in culture medium prevents glucose-induced embryopathy.

### Prevention

Because the critical period for teratogenesis is the first 3 to 6 weeks after conception, normal glycemic control must be instituted before pregnancy to prevent these birth defects. Several clinical trials of meticulous preconception glycemic control in women with diabetes have demonstrated malformation rates equivalent to those in the general population (Fuhrmann et al, 1983). The threshold level of glycemic control, as evidenced by the $HbA_{1c}$ value, necessary to normalize a patient's risk of congenital anomalies appears to be a near-normal value. Any elevation of the $HbA_{1c}$ above normal increases the risk of teratogenesis proportionately.

## *Macrosomia*

Fetal overgrowth is a major problem in pregnancies complicated by diabetes, leading to unnecessary cesarean sections and potentially avoidable birth injuries. A 1992 study of birth weights in the previous 20 years indicated that 21% of infants with birth weights of 4540 g or greater were born to mothers who were glucose intolerant, a rate clearly disproportionate to the only 2% to 5% of gravidas with some form of diabetes (Shelley-Jones et al, 1992). Thus the problem of abnormal fetal growth in diabetic pregnancy remains an important clinical challenge.

Defined variously as birth weight above the 90th percentile for gestational age or birth weight greater than 4000 g, *macrosomia* occurs in 15% to 45% of diabetic pregnancies. Excessive fetal size contributes to a greater frequency of intrapartum injury (shoulder dystocia, brachial plexus palsy, and asphyxia). Macrosomia is also a major factor in the higher rate of cesarean delivery among diabetic women. Because the risk of macrosomia is fairly constant for all classes of diabetes, it is likely that first-trimester metabolic control has less effect on fetal growth than glycemic regulation in the second and third trimesters.

### Growth Dynamics

The macrosomic IDM does follow a unique pattern of in utero growth compared with fetuses in euglycemic pregnancies. During the first and second trimesters, differences in size between diabetic and nondiabetic fetuses are usually undetectable with ultrasound measurements. After 24 weeks, however, the growth velocity of the IDM fetus's abdominal circumference typically begins to rise above normal (Ogata et al, 1980). Reece and colleagues (1990) have demonstrated that the IDM fetus has normal head growth, despite even marked degrees of hyperglycemia. Landon and coworkers (1989) have reported that although head growth and femur growth of IDM fetuses were similar to those of normal fetuses, abdominal circumference growth significantly exceeded that of controls beginning at 32 weeks (abdominal circumference growth in IDM fetuses is 1.36 cm/week, versus 0.901 cm/week in normal subjects).

Morphometric studies of the IDM newborn indicate that the greater growth of the abdominal circumference is due to deposition of fat in the abdominal and interscapular areas. This central deposition of fat is a key characteristic of diabetic macrosomia and underlies the pathology associated with vaginal delivery in these pregnancies. Acker and colleagues (1986) showed that although the incidence of shoulder dystocia is 3% among infants weighing more than 4000 g, the incidence in infants from diabetic pregnancies who weigh more than 4000 g is 16%.

### Childhood Effects

Higher growth velocity, begun in fetal life during a pregnancy complicated by diabetes, may extend into childhood and adult life. Silverman and coworkers (1995) reported follow-up of IDMs through age 8 years in which half the infants weighed more than the 90th percentile for gestational age at birth. By age 8 years, approximately half of the IDMs weighed more than the heaviest 10% of the nondiabetic children. The asymmetry index was 30% higher in diabetic offspring than the controls by age 8 years. These investigators also showed that diabetic offspring have permanent derangement of glucose-insulin kinetics, resulting in a higher incidence of impaired glucose tolerance.

### Pathophysiology

The pathophysiology of excessive fetal growth is complex and reflects the delivery of an abnormal nutrient mixture to the fetoplacental unit, regulated by an abnormal confluence of growth factors. Pedersen (1952) hypothesized that maternal hyperglycemia stimulates fetal hyperinsulinemia, which in turn mediates acceleration of fuel utilization and growth. The features of the abnormal growth in diabetic pregnancy include excessive adipose deposition, visceral organ hypertrophy, and acceleration of body mass accretion (Ogata et al, 1980).

Data from the Diabetes in Early Pregnancy (DIEP) project suggest that maternal metabolic control is a critical factor leading to fetal macrosomia (Jovanovic-Peterson et al, 1991). In this study, in which meticulous glycemic care was maintained in early pregnancy and beyond, fetal weight did not correlate significantly with fasting glucose levels. During the second and third trimesters, however, *postprandial* blood glucose levels were strongly predictive of both birth weight and the overall percentage of macrosomic infants. With postprandial glucose values averaging 120 mg/dL, approximately 20% of infants were macrosomic; a 30% rise in postprandial levels to 160 mg/dL resulted in a predicted percentage of macrosomia of 35%.

The Pedersen hypothesis presumes that abnormal fuel milieu in the maternal blood stream is reflected contemporaneously in the fetal compartment:. *Maternal hyperglycemia = fetal hyperglycemia*. Studies by Hollingsworth and Cousins (1981) have confirmed much of Pedersen's hypothesis and note the following features of normal pregnancy:

- Maternal fasting blood glucose levels decline from about 85 mg/dL to about 75 mg/dL. Mean blood glucose also declines.
- At night, maternal glucose levels drop markedly as the fetus continues to draw glucose stores from the maternal circulation.
- Postprandial peaks in maternal blood glucose rarely exceed 120 mg/dL at 2 hours or 130 mg/dL at 1 hour.
- If maternal glucose levels surge excessively after a meal, the consequent fetal hyperglycemia is accompanied by fetal pancreatic beta-cell hyperplasia and hyperinsulinemia.
- Fetal hyperinsulinemia, lasting only episodically for 1 to 2 hours, has detrimental consequences to fetal growth and well-being, in that it (1) promotes storage of excess nutrients, resulting in macrosomia, and (2) drives catabolism of the oversupply of fuel, using energy and depleting fetal oxygen stores.
- Episodic fetal hypoxia stimulated by episodic maternal hyperglycemia leads to an outpouring of adrenal catecholamines, which in turn causes hypertension, cardiac remodeling, and cardiac hypertrophy.

### Prevention of Macrosomia

Because macrosomic fetuses are at an increased risk for immediate complications related to birth injury as well as for potential long-term consequences such as late childhood obesity and insulin resistance, measures for prevention of macrosomia have been recommended. As described previously, fetal hyperinsulinemia, which acts as a fetal growth factor, occurs in response to fetal hyperglycemia, which in turn reflects the maternal hyperglycemic condition. Therefore, measures that promote consistent maternal euglycemia may prevent macrosomia. Several prospective trials have shown that strict maternal glycemic control utilizing insulin and dietary therapy and fastidious blood glucose monitoring can reduce the incidence of macrosomia (Coustan and Lewis, 1978, Langer et al, 1994; Thompson et al, 1990). Langer and associates (1994) compared outcomes of conventional management (four blood glucose measurements a day) of intensely monitored pregnancies (seven blood glucose measurements a day) in which fasting blood glucose values were maintained between 60 and 90 mg/dL and 2-hour postprandial values at less than 120 mg/dL, and of control subjects without diabetes. The rate of infants born weighing more than 4000 g was 14% in the conventionally managed group, 7% in the intensely managed group, and 8% in nondiabetic controls. Similarly, the rate of shoulder dystocia was 1.4% in the conventionally managed group, 0.4% in the intensely managed group, and 0.5% in the control group. Thus, like the reduction of congenital anomalies in diabetic mothers by means of first-trimester euglycemia, strict glycemic control in the second and third trimesters may reduce the fetal macrosomia rate to near baseline.

### *Fetal Hypoxic Stress*

As previously noted, episodic maternal hyperglycemia promotes a fetal catabolic state in which oxygen depletion occurs. Several fetal metabolic adaptive responses to this episodic hypoxia occur. For example, the drop in fetal oxygen tension causes stimulation of erythropoietin, red cell hyperplasia, and elevation in fetal hematocrit. Polycythemia may lead to poor circulation and postnatal hyperbilirubinemia. Profound episodic hyperglycemia in the third trimester causing severe fetal hypoxic stress has been theorized as the cause of sudden intrauterine fetal demise in poorly controlled diabetic women.

## Classifying and Diagnosing Diabetes in Pregnancy

The classification system for diabetes in pregnancy recommended by White has been replaced by a scheme based on the pathophysiology of hyperglycemia and developed by the National Diabetes Data Group (NDDG) in 1979. The types are summarized in Table 9–2. This nomenclature is useful because it categorizes patients according to the underlying pathogenesis of their diabetes—insulin-deficient (type 1) and insulin-resistant (type 2 and gestational). One must remember that the diagnosis *gestational diabetes* applies to any woman who is found to have hyperglycemia during pregnancy. A certain percentage of such women actually have type 2 diabetes, but the diagnosis cannot be confirmed until postpartum testing.

**TABLE 9–2**

**Classification of Diabetes Mellitus**

| Type | Old Nomenclature | Clinical Features |
|---|---|---|
| Type I | Juvenile-onset diabetes | Insulin-deficient, ketosis-prone<br>Virtually all patients with type I diabetes are insulin-dependent |
| Type II | Adult-onset diabetes | Insulin-resistant, not ketosis-prone<br>Few patients with type II diabetes are truly insulin-dependent |
| Gestational | | Occurs in and resolves after pregnancy<br>Insulin-resistant, not ketosis-prone |

### Pregestational Diabetes

Patients with type 1 diabetes (formerly termed "juvenile-onset diabetes") typically present with hyperglycemia, ketosis, and dehydration in childhood or adolescence. Often the diagnosis is made during a hospital admission for diabetic ketoacidosis and coma. Rarely the diagnosis is first made during pregnancy. It is not unusual for women tentatively diagnosed with gestational diabetes to be found to have overt diabetes after delivery. The diagnosis of type 2 diabetes in nonpregnant subjects is made using the 75-g, 2-hour glucose tolerance test (GTT). Diagnostic criteria are listed in Table 9–3.

### Gestational Diabetes

*Gestational diabetes* (GDM) is defined as glucose intolerance that begins or is first recognized during pregnancy (American Diabetes Association, 2002). Almost uniformly, GDM arises from significant maternal insulin resistance, a state similar to type 2 diabetes. Indeed, and in many cases, GDM is simply preclinical type 2 diabetes unmasked by the hormonal stress imposed by the pregnancy. Although GDM complicates no more than 2.5% of pregnancies in the United States (>135,000 cases annually) (Engelgau et al, 1995), the prevalence of GDM in specific populations varies from 1% to 14% (American Diabetes Association, 2002). Clinical recognition of GDM is important because therapy—including medical nutrition therapy, insulin when necessary, and antepartum fetal surveillance—can reduce the well-described perinatal morbidity and mortality associated with GDM.

Traditionally, universal screening for GDM has been recommended (Metzger, 1991). However, both the Fourth International Workshop-Conference on Gestational Diabetes and the American College of Obstetricians and Gynecologists have now indicated that either a risk-factor approach or universal screening can be considered (American College of Obstetricians and Gynecologists,

**TABLE 9–3**

**Criteria for the Diagnosis of Type II Diabetes with 75-g Glucose Tolerance Test***

| Diagnosis | Venous Plasma Glucose Level (mg/dL) Fasting | 2-Hour |
|---|---|---|
| Normal | <140 | <200 |
| Impaired glucose tolerance | <140 | >140 and <200 |
| Diabetes | ≥140 | ≥140 |

*Note: Diagnosis of non–insulin-dependent diabetes mellitus after pregnancy requires a 1-hour value of >200 mg/dL in addition to abnormal fasting and 2-hour values.

2001; Metzger and Coustan, 1998). This recommendation is based on the findings of Sermer and colleagues (1994), who reported the results of screening Canadian women at 26 weeks of gestation with the 100-g, 3-hour GTT. They identified several risk factors as significantly increasing the likelihood of GDM, among which were maternal age of 35 years or more, body mass index (BMI) higher than 22 kg/m$^2$, and Asian or "other" ethnicity. Women with one or no risk factors had a 0.9% risk of GDM, whereas the risk for those with two to five factors who were diagnosed with GDM was 4% to 7%. By limiting screening for GDM to gravidas with more than one risk factor, these investigators were able to reduce testing by 34% while retaining a sensitivity rate of approximately 80% with a false-positive result rate of 13%. Thus, in patients meeting *all* of the criteria listed in Tables 9–4 and 9–5, it may be cost effective to avoid screening.

**TABLE 9–4**

**Oral Glucose Tolerance Test For Gestational Diabetes**

**Test Prerequisites**

1-hr 50-g glucose challenge result >135 mg/dL
Overnight fast of 8-14 hours
Carbohydrate loading for 3 days including >150 g carbohydrate
Seated, not smoking during the test
Two or more values must be met or exceeded
Either a 2-hr (75-g glucose) or 3-hr (100-g glucose) test can be performed

**Criteria for Gestational Diabetes: Venous Plasma Glucose Level**

| | With 100-g Glucose Load | | With 75-g Glucose Load | |
|---|---|---|---|---|
| | *mg/dL* | *mmol/L* | *mg/dL* | *mmol/L* |
| Fasting value | 95 | 5.3 | 95 | 5.3 |
| 1-hr value | 180 | 10.0 | 180 | 10.0 |
| 2-hr value | 155 | 8.6 | 155 | 8.6 |
| 3-hr value | 140 | 7.8 | — | — |

**TABLE 9–5**

**Criteria For "Low Risk" of Gestational Diabetes (GDM)***

Age <25 yr
Normal pre-pregnancy body weight
No first-degree relatives with diabetes
Not a member of an ethnic group at high risk for GDM
No history of GDM in prior pregnancy
No history of adverse pregnancy outcome

*Note: Screening for GDM may be omitted only if *all* criteria are met.

Data from Metzger BE, Coustan DR: Summary and Recommendations of the Fourth International Workshop-Conference on Gestational Diabetes Mellitus. The Organizing Committee. Diabetes Care 21(Suppl 2):B161, 1998.

Notwithstanding these findings, multiple studies from more heterogeneous U.S. populations have demonstrated the inadequacy of GDM screening of patients with risk factors. Lavin and coworkers (1981) noted that if only those with risk factors were screened, the percentage of GDM cases detected was similar to the detection rate in those without risk factors (1.4%). A later study (Weeks et al, 1995), which assessed the effect of screening only patients with risk factors, reported that selective screening would have failed to detect 43% of cases of GDM. Moreover, 28% of the women with undiagnosed GDM would have required insulin and had a several-fold higher risk of cesarean section due to macrosomia.

Therefore, universal screening should be performed in members of ethnic groups recognized to be at higher risk for glucose intolerance during pregnancy, namely women of Hispanic, African, Native American, South or East Asian, Pacific Islands, or Indigenous Australian ancestry. For simplicity of administration, universal screening, with the possible exception of the very lowest risk category, is probably best. The universal screening method for GDM has been shown to result in earlier diagnosis and improved pregnancy outcomes, including lower rates of macrosomia and a decrease in neonatal admissions to NICUs (Griffin et al, 2000).

The timing of screening for GDM is important. Because maternal insulin resistance rises progressively during pregnancy, screening too early may miss some patients who will become glucose intolerant later. Screening too late in the third trimester may limit the time during which metabolic interventions can take place. Thus, risk factors for GDM should be assessed at the initial prenatal visit. Factors that should lead to a first-trimester glucose challenge test are listed in Table 9–6. In the remaining patients, screening should be performed with the use of 50 g of glucose at 26 to 28 weeks of gestation.

Various threshold levels for the 50-g glucose challenge are in use, including 140 mg/dL, 135 mg/dL, and 130 mg/dL. The sensitivity of the GDM testing regimen depends on the threshold value used. The most commonly utilized threshold, 140 mg/dL, detects only 80% of patients with GDM and results in requirement for a 3-hour oral GTT in approximately 10% to 15% of patients. Using a challenge threshold of 135 mg/dL improves sensitivity to more than 90% but increases the number of 3-hour oral GTTs by 42% (Ray et al, 1996). Thus, the clinician encountering a newborn with multiple stigmata of an IDM yet whose

**TABLE 9–6**

**Indications for the First-Trimester 50-g Glucose Challenge**

Maternal age >25 yr
Previous infant >4 kg
Previous unexplained fetal demise
Previous pregnancy with gestational diabetes
Strong immediate family history of type II or gestational diabetes
Obesity (>90 kg)
Fasting glucose level >140 mg/dL (7.8 mmol) or random glucose reading >200 mg/dL (11.1 mmol)

mother had a "negative" diabetes screening test result during pregnancy does not rule out GDM. This is also why every patient who delivered a macrosomic infant in a prior pregnancy should be screened early in all subsequent pregnancies.

Definitive diagnosis of gestational diabetes is made with a GTT. Either 100 g of glucose and 3 hours of testing, or 75 g of glucose and 2 hours of testing can be utilized. The diagnostic criteria are shown in Table 9–3. Two or more values must be met or exceeded for the diagnosis of GDM to be made. A GTT should be performed after an overnight fast and with modest carbohydrate loading before the test.

## Perinatal Complications of Diabetes During Pregnancy

### Fetal Morbidity and Mortality

#### *Perinatal Mortality*

Perinatal mortality in diabetic pregnancy has decreased 30-fold since the discovery of insulin in 1922 and the advent of intensive obstetric and infant care in the 1970s (Fig. 9–2). Improved techniques for maintaining maternal euglycemia have led to later timing of delivery and reduced incidence of iatrogenic respiratory distress syndrome (RDS).

Nevertheless, the currently reported perinatal mortality rates among diabetic women remain approximately twice those observed in nondiabetic women (Table 9–7). Congenital malformations, RDS, and extreme prematurity account for most perinatal deaths in contemporary diabetic pregnancy. Figure 9–3 show the different rates of RDS in diabetic and euglycemic pregnancies. In the past decade, fewer intrauterine deaths have been reported, probably reflecting more careful fetal monitoring. Nevertheless, intrapartum asphyxia and fetal demise remain persistent problems.

**TABLE 9–7**

**Perinatal Mortality Rates (No. of Deaths per 100 Births) in Diabetic and Normal Pregnancies**

| | Mothers with Gestational Diabetes | Mothers with Preexisting Diabetes | Normal Mothers* |
|---|---|---|---|
| Fetal mortality | 4.7 | 10.4 | 5.7 |
| Neonatal mortality | 3.3 | 12.2 | 4.7 |
| Perinatal mortality | 8.0 | 11.6 | 10.4 |

*California data for 1986, corrected for birth weight, sex, and race.

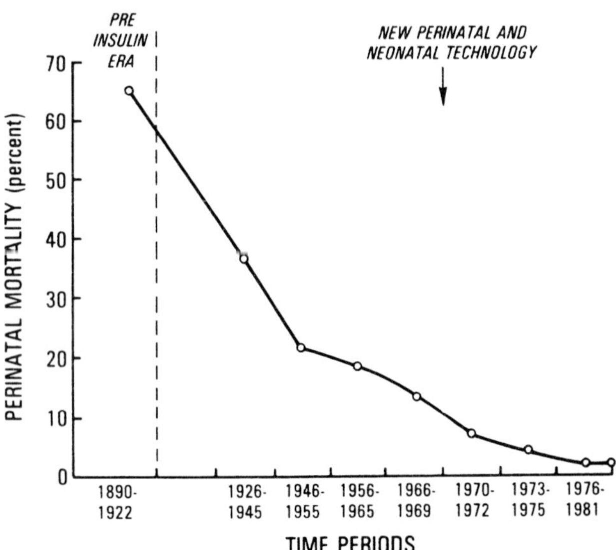


**FIGURE 9–2.** Perinatal mortality rate (percentage) among infants of diabetic mothers from 1890 to 1981. Data plotted from reports of Craigin and Ryder (1916), DeLee (1920), Williams (1925), Pedersen (1977), Gabbe et al (1978), and Jorge et al (1981). *(From Creasy RK, Resnik R [eds]: Maternal-Fetal Medicine: Principles and Practice, 2nd ed. Philadelphia, WB Saunders, 1989.)*

#### *Birth Injury*

Birth injury, including shoulder dystocia (Keller et al, 1991) and brachial plexus trauma, is more common among IDMs, and macrosomic fetuses are at the highest risk (Mimouni et al, 1992). *Shoulder dystocia*, defined as difficulty in delivering the fetal body after expulsion of the fetal head, is an obstetric emergency that places the fetus and mother at great risk. Shoulder dystocia occurs in 0.3% to 0.5% of vaginal deliveries among normal pregnant women; the incidence is twofold to fourfold higher in women with diabetes, probably because the hyperglycemia of diabetic pregnancy causes the fetal shoulder and abdominal widths to become massive (Nesbitt et al, 1998). Although half of shoulder dystocias occur in infants of normal birth weight (2500 to 4000 g), the incidence of shoulder dystocia is 10-fold higher (5% to 7%) among infants weighing 4000 g or more and rises to 31% for infants whose mothers are diabetic (Gilbert et al, 1999). (See also Chapter 15 for discussion of complicated deliveries and Chapter 64 for discussion of the neurologic consequences of birth injury.)

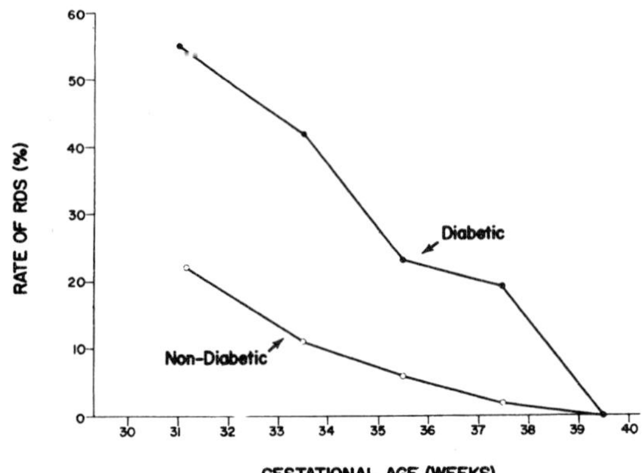


**FIGURE 9–3.** Rate of respiratory distress syndrome (RDS) versus gestational age. Improved management of maternal glycemic control permits delaying delivery until after 38 weeks of gestation, when the risk of RDS approaches that in nondiabetic pregnancy.

## Neonatal Morbidity and Mortality

(For complete discussion, see Chapter 93, on disorders of carbohydrate metabolism.)

### *Polycythemia and Hyperviscosity*

Polycythemia (defined as central venous hemoglobin concentration >20 g/dL or hematocrit >65%) is not uncommon in IDMs and is apparently related to glycemic control. Widness and associates (1990) demonstrated that hyperglycemia is a powerful stimulus to fetal erythropoietin production, probably mediated by decreased fetal oxygen tension. Untreated, neonatal polycythemia may promote vascular sludging, ischemia, and infarction of vital tissues, including the kidneys and central nervous system.

### *Neonatal Hypoglycemia*

The hyperinsulinemic IDM is at higher risk for low plasma glucose levels after birth. This complication is usually much milder and less common in the infant of the woman whose insulin-dependent diabetes is well controlled throughout the *entire* pregnancy and who is euglycemic during labor and delivery. Unrecognized postnatal hypoglycemia may lead to neonatal seizures, coma, and brain damage. Thus, it is imperative that the nursery receiving the IDM have a protocol for frequent monitoring of the infant's blood glucose level until metabolic stability is ensured.

### *Hyperbilirubinemia*

The risk of hyperbilirubinemia is higher in IDMs than in normal infants. There are multiple causes of hyperbilirubinemia in IDMs, but prematurity and polycythemia are the primary contributing factors. Increased destruction of red blood cells contributes to the risks of jaundice and kernicterus. This complication is usually treated with phototherapy, but exchange transfusions may be necessary for marked bilirubin elevations.

### *Hypertrophic and Congestive Cardiomyopathy*

In some macrosomic infants of mothers with poorly controlled diabetes, a thickened myocardium and significant septal hypertrophy have been described (Gutgesell et al, 1976). Although the prevalence of myocardial hypertrophy in IDMs may exceed 30% at birth, almost all cases have resolved by 1 year of age (Mace et al, 1979).

Hypertrophic cardiac dysfunction in a newborn IDM often leads to respiratory distress, which may be mistaken for hyaline membrane disease. IDMs with cardiomegaly may have either congestive or hypertrophic cardiomyopathy. Echocardiograms show a hypercontractile, thickened myocardium, often with septal hypertrophy disproportionate to the ventricular free walls. The ventricular chambers are often smaller than normal, and there may be anterior systolic motion of the mitral valve producing left ventricular outflow tract obstruction.

The pathogenesis of hypertrophic cardiomyopathy in IDMs is unclear, although it is recognized to be associated with poor maternal metabolic control. There is evidence that the fetal myocardium is particularly sensitive to insulin during gestation, and Susa and colleagues (1979) reported a doubling of cardiac mass in hyperinsulinemic fetal rhesus monkeys. The myocardium is known to be richly endowed with insulin receptors.

IDMs may also have *congestive* cardiomyopathy without hypertrophy. Echocardiography shows the myocardium to be overstretched and poorly contractile. This condition is often rapidly reversible with correction of neonatal hypoglycemia, hypocalcemia, and polycythemia; it responds to digoxin, diuretics, or both. In contrast, treatment of hypertrophic cardiomyopathy with an inotropic or diuretic agent tends to further decrease the size of the ventricular chambers and leads to obstruction of blood flow. Echocardiographic examination of IDMs with enlarged hearts is recommended to detect and treat clinically silent cardiomyopathy.

### *Respiratory Distress Syndrome*

Since the 1970s, improved maternal management and better protocols for timing of delivery have resulted in a dramatic decline in the incidence of RDS from 31% to 3%. Nevertheless, respiratory dysfunction in the newborn IDM continues to be an all too common complication of diabetic pregnancy. It may be due to surfactant deficiency or to some other form of pulmonary distress. Surfactant production occurs late in diabetic pregnancies. Studies of fetal lung ion transport in the diabetic rat by Pinter and coworkers (1991) demonstrated decreased fluid clearance and lack of thinning of the lung's connective tissue in diabetics compared with controls. In humans, Kjos and associates (1990) noted *respiratory distress* in 18 of 526 infants delivered of diabetic gestations (3.4%). Surfactant-deficient airway disease accounted for less than one third of cases, with transient tachypnea, hypertrophic cardiomyopathy, and pneumonia responsible for the majority.

Thus, the near-term infant of a mother with poorly controlled diabetes is more likely to have neonatal RDS than the infant of a nondiabetic mother at the same gestational age. This circumstance further compounds the diabetic infant's metabolic and cardiovascular difficulties after birth. The nondiabetic fetus achieves pulmonary maturity at a mean gestational age of 34 to 35 weeks. By 37 weeks, more than 99% of normal newborn infants have mature lung profiles as assessed by phospholipid assays. In a diabetic pregnancy, however, it is unwise to assume that the risk of respiratory distress has passed until after 38.5 weeks of gestation (Moore, 2002). Any delivery contemplated before 38.5 weeks for other than the most urgent fetal and maternal indications should be preceded by documentation of pulmonary maturity through amniocentesis.

## Obstetric Complications

Pregnancy complicated by diabetes is subject to a number of obstetric disorders, including ketoacidosis, preeclampsia, polyhydramnios, and abnormal labor, at higher rates than in nondiabetic pregnancy.

### Preeclampsia

Preeclampsia is an unpredictable multisystem disorder in which maternal neurologic, renal, and cardiovascular status can decline precipitously and that may threaten fetal health through placental ischemia and abruptio placentae. Preeclampsia is more common among women with diabetes, occurring two to three times more frequently in women with pregestational diabetes than in nondiabetic women (Moore et al, 1985; Sibai et al, 2000). However, the risk of developing preeclampsia is proportional to the duration of diabetes before pregnancy and the existence of nephropathy and hypertension; preeclampsia develops in more than one third of women who have had diabetes for more than 20 years. Patients with White's class B diabetes have a risk profile similar to that of nondiabetic patients, but the risk of hypertensive complications is 50% higher in women with evidence of renal or retinal vasculopathy (classes D, F, R) than in those with no hypertension. The rate of fetal death is higher in diabetic women with preeclampsia. In the diabetic patient with chronic hypertension, preeclampsia may be difficult to distinguish from near-term blood pressure elevations. The onset is typically insidious and not confidently recognized until severe.

When a patient with diabetes experiences preeclampsia, she should be evaluated for delivery. If signs of severe disease are present (e.g., blood pressure >160 mm Hg systolic/110 mm Hg diastolic, neurologic symptoms, or significant renal dysfunction), delivery should be performed promptly. In mild cases, the patient may be observed if the fetal lungs are immature. Preeclampsia after 38 weeks of gestation, however, is adequate grounds for initiating delivery.

### Polyhydramnios

*Polyhydramnios* is defined as excess amniotic fluid. The precise clinical definition varies, encompassing the recording of more than 2000 mL of amniotic fluid at delivery and various measures of amniotic fluid pocket depths as observed on ultrasonography. In practice, polyhydramnios is usually diagnosed when any single vertical pocket of amniotic fluid is deeper than 8 cm (equivalent to the 97th percentile) or when the sum of four pockets, one from each quadrant of the uterus (amniotic fluid index), exceeds approximately 24 cm (95th percentile) (Moore and Cayle, 1990). The principal causes of hydramnios in diabetic pregnancy are fetal gastrointestinal anomalies (e.g., esophageal atresia) and poor glycemic control. A rapid increase in fundal height should prompt a thorough ultrasound examination by a skilled examiner. The main clinical problems associated with hydramnios are fetal malposition and preterm labor.

Management of the patient with hydramnios is predominantly symptomatic, focused on improving glycemic control and preventing premature labor. Enhanced patient awareness of contractions and the signs and subtle sensations of preterm labor is essential.

## Management

### Preconception Management

Preconception counseling and a detailed medical risk assessment are recommended for all women with overt diabetes as well as for those with a history of gestational diabetes in a previous pregnancy. Significant impact on the maternal and neonatal complications of diabetic pregnancy cannot be realized until meticulous preconception metabolic control is achieved in all women contemplating pregnancy.

The important elements to be considered in preconception counseling of the diabetic patient are the patient's level of glycemic control; current status of the patient's retinal and renal health; and any medications being taken, especially antihypertensive or thyroid medications. A realistic assessment of the patient's risk of complications during pregnancy, including worsening of renal or ophthalmologic function, should be provided.

Preconception management should lead to a comprehensive program of glucose control. The major goals of the prepregnancy metabolic program are as follows:

- Establishing a regimen of frequent, regular monitoring of capillary blood glucose levels
- Adopting an insulin dosing regimen that results in smooth interprandial glucose profile (fasting blood glucose value 80 to 100 mg/dL, 2-hour postprandial glucose level <120 mg/dL, no reactions between meals or at night)
- Bringing $HbA_{1c}$ level into the normal range
- Developing family, financial, and personal resources to assist the patient if pregnancy complications require that she lose work time or assume total bed rest

This preconception care has been shown to decrease congenital anomalies and to result in fewer hospitalizations, fewer infants requiring intravenous glucose after delivery, and a substantial reduction in total costs (Herman et al, 1999).

### Prenatal Metabolic Management

The goals of glycemic monitoring, dietary regulation, and insulin therapy in diabetic pregnancy are to prevent the postnatal sequelae of diabetes in the newborn—macrosomia, shoulder dystocia, and postnatal metabolic instability. These measures must be instituted early and aggressively if they are to be effective.

#### *Principles of Dietary Therapy*

Because women with diabetes have inadequate insulin action after feeding, the goal of dietary therapy is to avoid single, large meals and foods with a large proportion of simple carbohydrates. Three major meals and three snacks are prescribed. The use of *nonglycemic foods* that release calories into the gut slowly also improves metabolic control.

Nutritional therapy should be supervised by a trained professional who performs formal dietary assessment and counseling at several points during the pregnancy. The dietary prescription should provide adequate quantity and distribution of calories and nutrients to meet the needs of the pregnancy and support achieving the plasma glucose targets that have been established. For obese women (BMI >30 kg/m$^2$), a 30% to 33% restriction in caloric intake (to 25 kcal per kg actual weight per day or less) has been shown to reduce hyperglycemia and plasma triglycerides with no increase in ketonuria. Moderate restriction of dietary carbohydrate intake to 35% to 40% of calories has been shown to reduce maternal glucose levels and improve maternal and fetal outcomes (Major et al, 1998). In a nonrandomized study, subjects with low carbohydrate intake (<42% of calories) led to lower requirements for insulin for glucose control as well as to significantly lower rates of macrosomia and cesarean deliveries for cephalopelvic disproportion and macrosomia.

### Principles of Glucose Monitoring

The availability of chemical test strips for capillary blood glucose measurements has revolutionized the management of diabetes, and their use should now be considered the standard of care for pregnancy monitoring. The discipline of measuring and recording blood glucose levels before and after meals may have the effect of improving glycemic control (Goldberg et al, 1986).

The frequency and timing of home glucose monitoring should be individualized, but *postprandial* values must be assessed because they have the strongest correlation with fetal growth (Jovanovic-Peterson et al, 1991). The Diabetes in Early Pregnancy Study found that *postprandial* glucose levels were strongly predictive of both birth weight and the overall percentage of macrosomic infants. With postprandial glucose values averaging 120 mg/dL, approximately 20% of infants were macrosomic; a 30% rise in postprandial levels to 160 mg/dL resulted in a predicted percentage of macrosomia of 35%.

Similar results were reported by de Veciana and associates (1995). Compared with the group who performed preprandial glucose monitoring, the group performing postprandial glucose monitoring demonstrated a greater mean change in the $HbA_{1c}$ value (3.0% vs. 0.6%; $P < .001$), lower birth weights (3469 g vs. 3848 g; $P = .01$), and lower rates of both neonatal hypoglycemia (3% vs. 21%, $P = .05$), and macrosomia (12% vs. 42%; $P = .01$).

A typical schedule involves performing blood glucose checks upon rising in the morning, 1 or 2 hours after breakfast, before and after lunch, before dinner, and before bedtime. The goal of *physiologic* glycemic control in pregnancy, however, is not met by simply avoiding hypoglycemia. The data summarized here regarding fetal macrosomia and postnatal morbidity emphasize the key role of excessive postprandial excursions in blood glucose values. Thus, close attention must be paid to both preprandial and postprandial glycemic profiles.

### Principles of Insulin Therapy

No available insulin delivery method approaches the precise secretion of the hormone from the human pancreas. The therapeutic goal of exogenous insulin therapy during pregnancy is to achieve diurnal glucose excursions similar to those of nondiabetic pregnant women. Normal pregnant women maintain postprandial blood glucose excursions within a relatively narrow range (70 to 120 mg/dL). As pregnancy progresses, the fasting and between-meal blood glucose levels drop progressively lower as a result of the continual uptake of glucose from the maternal circulation by the growing fetus. Any insulin regimen for pregnant women must be designed to avoid excessive unopposed insulin action during the fasting state.

Insulin type and dosage frequency should be individualized. Use of regular insulin before each major meal helps limit postprandial hyperglycemia. To provide basal insulin levels between feedings, a longer-acting preparation is necessary, such as isoprotane insulin (NPH) or insulin zinc (Lente). Typical subcutaneous insulin dosing regimens are 2/3 of total insulin in the morning, of which 2/3 as intermediate-acting and 1/3 as regular insulin. The remaining 1/3 of the total insulin dose is given in the evening, with 50% as short-acting insulin prior to dinner and 50% as intermediate-acting given at bedtime.

The use of an insulin pump for type 1 diabetes mellitus during pregnancy has become more widespread (Gabbe et al, 2000). An advantage of this approach is the more physiologic insulin release pattern that may be achieved with the pump.

Ultrasonography has also been utilized to direct insulin management (Rossi et al, 2000). Kjos and coworkers (2001) showed that serial normal fetal abdominal circumference measurements may be used to avoid insulin therapy without increasing neonatal morbidity.

### Oral Hypoglycemic Therapy

Historically, insulin has been the mainstay of therapy for gestational diabetes because of early reports that oral hypoglycemic drugs are a potential cause of fetal anomalies and neonatal hypoglycemia. Sulfonylurea compounds have been considered contraindicated during pregnancy due to a high level of transplacental penetration and clinical reports of prolonged and severe neonatal hypoglycemia (Zucker and Simon, 1968). An increased rate of congenital malformations, particularly ear anomalies, has been reported from a small case-control study (Piacquadio et al, 1991). However, when Towner and coworkers (1995) evaluated the frequency of birth defects in patients who took oral hypoglycemic agents during the periconception period, they noted that first-trimester $HbA_{1c}$ level and duration of diabetes were strongly associated with fetal congenital anomalies but that use of oral hypoglycemic medications was not.

Glyburide, a second-generation sulfonylurea, has been shown to cross the placenta minimally in both laboratory studies (Elliott et al, 1994) and a large clinical trial. The prospective randomized trial, conducted by Langer and associates (2000), compared glyburide and insulin in 404 women with gestational diabetes and showed equivalently excellent maternal glycemic control and perinatal outcomes.

However, beyond this single, encouraging study, experience with glyburide during pregnancy is limited (Coetzee and Jackson, 1985; Lim et al, 1997). Chmait and Moore

(2002), reporting experience with 69 patients with gestational diabetes who were given glyburide, found a failure rate of 19% (>10% glucose values above target). Glyburide failure rate was higher in women diagnosed earlier in pregnancy (20 vs. 27 weeks; $P < .003$) and whose average fasting glucose in the week prior to starting glyburide was higher (126 vs. 101 mg/dL). Until more studies of glyburide in pregnancy have been reported, the American College of Obstetricians and Gynecologists (2001) considers this agent to be experimental.

## Prenatal Obstetric Management

The overall strategy of the management of diabetic pregnancy in the third trimester involves preventing stillbirth and asphyxia and monitoring growth of the fetus to select the proper time and route of delivery to minimize maternal and infant morbidity. The first goal is accomplished by testing fetal well-being at frequent intervals, and the second through ultrasonographic monitoring of fetal size.

### *Periodic Biophysical Testing of the Fetus*

A variety of biophysical tests of the fetus are available to the clinician, including fetal heart rate testing, fetal movement assessment, ultrasound biophysical scoring, and fetal umbilical Doppler studies. Most of these tests, if applied properly, can be used with confidence to provide assurance of fetal well-being while awaiting fetal maturity. They are summarized in Table 9–8.

Testing should be initiated early enough to avoid significant risk of stillbirth but not so early that the risk of a false-positive result is high. In patients with poor glycemic control or significant hypertension, testing should begin as early as 28 weeks of gestation. In lower-risk patients, most centers begin formal fetal testing by 34 weeks. Counting of fetal movements is performed in all pregnancies from 28 weeks of gestation onward.

### *Assessing Fetal Growth*

Monitoring of fetal growth continues to be a challenging and highly inexact process. Although today's tools, consisting of serial plotting of fetal growth parameters, are superior to earlier clinical estimations, accuracy is still ±15%. Both single and multiple longitudinal assessments of fetal size have been attempted.

#### Calculation of Estimated Fetal Weight

Several polynomial formulas using combinations of head, abdominal, and limb measurements have been proposed to predict the weight of the macrosomic fetus from ultrasonography parameters (Ferrero et al, 1994; Tongsong et al, 1994). Unfortunately, in such formulas, small errors in individual measurements of the head, abdomen, and femur are typically multiplied together. In the obese fetus, the inaccuracies are further magnified. Bernstein and Catalano (1992) observed that a significant correlation exists between the degree of error in the ultrasonographically estimated fetal weight and the percentage of body fat on the fetus ($r = 0.28$; $P < .05$). Perhaps this problem explains why no single formula has proved to be adequate in identifying the macrosomic fetus (Tamura et al, 1985).

Shamley and Landon (1994) reviewed the relative accuracy of the various available formulas. Approximately 75% of the fetal weight predictions were within 10% of actual birth weight, with sensitivity for detecting macrosomia varying greatly (11% to 76%). In another study, McLaren and colleagues (1995) found that 65% of weight estimates based on a simple abdominal circumference and femur length formula were within 10% of actual weight. A similar accuracy was achieved with more complex models (53% to 66% of estimates within the range).

**TABLE 9–8**

**Tests of Fetal Well-Being**

| Test | How Often Performed | Reassuring Result | Comment |
|---|---|---|---|
| Counting of fetal movements | Every night from 28 wk | Ten movements in <60 min | Performed in all patients |
| Nonstress test | Twice weekly | Two heart rate accelerations in 20 min | Begin at: 28-34 wk in patients with insulin-dependent diabetes<br>36 wk in patients with diet-controlled gestational diabetes |
| Contraction stress test | Weekly | No heart rate decelerations in response to ≤3 contractions in 10 min | Same as for nonstress test |
| Ultrasound biophysical profile | Weekly | Score of 8 in 30 min | The following findings are given 2 points each:<br>3 movements<br>1 flexion<br>30 sec breathing<br>2 cm amniotic fluid |

The formula developed by Shepard and colleagues (1982), which uses biparietal diameter and abdominal circumference, is readily available in textbooks and is used most commonly in current ultrasonographic equipment software. It has accuracy levels similar to the statistics quoted.

#### Serial Estimated Fetal Weight Assessments

Because prediction of fetal weight from a single set of measurements is inaccurate, serial estimates showing the trend of ultrasonographic parameters (typically made every 1.5 to 3 weeks) might theoretically offer a better estimate of actual weight percentile. A comparison of the efficacy of serial estimated fetal weight calculations to a single measurement, however, did not show better predictive accuracy. Larsen and associates (1995) reported that predictions based on the average of repeated weight estimates, on linear extrapolation from two estimates, or on extrapolation by a second-order equation fitted to four estimates were no better than the prediction from the last estimate before delivery. Similar findings (that a single estimate is as accurate as multiple assessments) were reported by Hedriana and Moore (1994).

### *Choosing the Timing and Route of Delivery*

Timing of delivery should be selected to minimize maternal and neonatal morbidity and mortality. Delaying delivery to as near as possible to the estimated date of confinement helps maximize cervical ripeness and improve the chances of spontaneous labor and vaginal delivery. Yet the risks of fetal macrosomia, birth injury, and fetal death rise as the due date approaches (Rasmussen et al, 1992). Although earlier delivery at 37 weeks of gestation might reduce the risk of shoulder dystocia, the higher rates of failed labor inductions and poor neonatal pulmonary status at this time must be considered. Thus, an optimal time for delivery of most diabetic pregnancies is between 38.5 and 40 weeks.

Delivery of a diabetic patient before 38.5 weeks of gestation without documentation of fetal lung maturity should be performed only for compelling maternal or fetal reasons. Fetal lung maturity should be verified in such cases from the presence of more than 3% phosphatidyl glycerol or the equivalent in amniotic fluid as ascertained from an amniocentesis specimen. After 38.5 weeks, the obstetrician can await spontaneous labor if the fetus is not macrosomic and results of biophysical testing are reassuring. In patients with gestational diabetes and superb glycemic control, continued fetal testing and expectant management can be considered until 41 weeks (Lurie et al, 1992).

Kjos and associates (1993) compared the outcomes of labor induction in gestational diabetics at 38 weeks and those of expectant management combined with fetal testing. Expectant management increased the gestational age at delivery by 1 week, but the cesarean delivery rate was not significantly different. The prevalence of macrosomic infants in the expectantly managed group (23%) was significantly greater than that in the active induction group (10%). This finding suggests that routine induction of diabetic gravidas on or before 39 weeks of gestation does not raise the risk of cesarean section and may reduce the risk of macrosomia.

Given the previous data, the decision to attempt vaginal delivery or perform a cesarean section is inevitably based on limited data. The patient's obstetric history from previous pregnancies, the best estimation of fetal weight, the fetal adipose profile (abdomen larger than head), and results of clinical pelvimetry should all be considered. A policy of elective cesarean section for suspected fetal macrosomia (ultrasonographically estimated fetal weight of greater than 4500 g) would require 443 cesarean deliveries to avoid one permanent brachial plexus injury (Rouse et al, 1996). Most large series of diabetic pregnancies report a cesarean section rate of 30% to 50%. The best means by which this rate can be lowered is early and strict glycemic control in pregnancy. Conducting a long labor induction in the patient with a large fetus and marginal pelvis may increase rather than lower morbidity and costs.

## Intrapartum Glycemic Management

Maintenance of intrapartum metabolic homeostasis is essential to avoid fetal hypoxemia and promote a smooth postnatal transition. Strict maternal euglycemia during labor does not guarantee newborn euglycemia in infants with macrosomia and long-established islet cell hypertrophy. Nevertheless, the use of a combined insulin and glucose infusion during labor to maintain maternal blood glucose in a narrow range (80 to 110 mg/dL) during labor is common and reasonable practice. Typical infusion rates are 5% dextrose in lactated Ringer's solution at 100 mL/hr and regular insulin at 0.5 to 1.0 U/hr. Capillary blood glucose levels are monitored hourly in such patients.

For patients with diet-controlled gestational diabetes in labor, avoiding dextrose in all intravenous fluids normally maintains excellent blood glucose control. After 1 to 2 hours, no further assessments of capillary blood glucose are typically necessary.

## Neonatal Management

### *Neonatal Transitional Management*

One of the metabolic problems common to IDMs is hypoglycemia, which is related to the level of maternal glycemic control over the 6 to 12 weeks before birth. Neonatal hypoglycemia is most likely to occur between 1 and 5 hours after birth, as the rich supply of maternal glucose stops with ligation of the umbilical cord and the infant's levels of circulating insulin remain elevated. These infants therefore require close monitoring for blood glucose concentration during the first hours after birth. IDMs also appear to have disorders of both catecholamine and glucagon metabolism as well as diminished capability to mount normal compensatory responses to hypoglycemia.

In the past, IDMs were treated with glucagon; however, this treatment frequently results in high blood glucose levels that trigger insulin secretion and repeated cycles of hypoglycemia and hyperglycemia. Current recommendations, therefore, consist of early oral feeding, when possible, along with infusion of intravenous glucose.

Ordinarily, blood glucose levels can be controlled satisfactorily with an infusion of 10% glucose. If greater amounts of glucose are required, bolus administration of 5 mL/kg of 10% glucose is recommended, with gradually increasing concentrations of glucose administered every 30 to 60 minutes, if necessary. Close monitoring to correct hypoglycemia while avoiding hyperglycemia and consequent stimulation of insulin secretion is important.

#### *Breast-Feeding*

Most authorities prefer to maintain strict monitoring of newborn IDM glucose levels for at least 4 to 6 hours, which frequently necessitates admission to a newborn special care unit. IDMs delivered atraumatically and well oxygenated, however, can be kept with their mothers while undergoing close glycemic monitoring for the first 1 to 2 hours of life. This approach permits early breast-feeding, which may reduce the need for intravenous glucose therapy.

#### Summary

Intensive management of women with glucose intolerance during pregnancy has resulted in markedly improved outcomes. Despite these advances, care of the IDM continues to require vigilance and meticulous monitoring with a full understanding of the quality of the glycemic milieu in which the infant developed.

## DISORDERS OF THE THYROID

### Incidence

Thyroid disorders, in general, are more common in women than in men and represent a common endocrine abnormality during pregnancy. Both hyperthyroidism and hypothyroidism in the mother put the infant at risk and require careful management by the perinatal-neonatal team. Table 9–9 presents an overview of the approach to infants who are thought to be at risk for abnormal thyroid function because of maternal thyroid abnormalities. The most frequently described problem is the syndrome of postpartum thyroiditis, which has been reported to complicate as many as 5% of all pregnancies. The diagnosis of thyroid disease in pregnancy is complicated by the natural

**TABLE 9–9**

**Approaches for Infants Judged to be at Risk for Abnormal Thyroid Function**

| Possible Thyroid Abnormality | Cord Blood Analyses | Assessment at Birth | Assessment at 2-7 Days of Life |
|---|---|---|---|
| Congenital hyperthyroidism because mother has any of the following:<br>Graves disease with hyperthyroidism and may have been treated with PTU, methimazole, $^{131}$I, iodides, or surgery<br>History of Graves disease<br>History of Hashimoto disease | $T_4$, RSH, TSAb | Physical examination for intrauterine growth restriction, goiter, exophthalmos, tachycardia, bradycardia, size of anterior fontanel, synostosis, congenital anomalies<br>Determination of gestational age by dates, ultrasonography during pregnancy, or Dubovitz examination<br>Neurologic examination<br>Determination of bone age (knee)<br>For selected cases: electrocardiogram, auditory and visual evoked potentials, motor conduction, velocity tests, skull radiographs | $T_4$, TSH, TSAb (if available) determinations:<br>If results normal, give no treatment; observe and repeat $T_4$, $T_3$, TSH determinations at 7-10 days*<br>If results indicate hypothyroidism, repeat T4, TSH; if results abnormal, begin treatment at 7-10 days†<br>If results indicate hyperthyroidism, begin treatment with PTU (8 mg/kg) and propranolol |
| Congenital or early childhood hypothyroidism because mother has any of the following:<br>Graves disease with excessive PTU therapy<br>Hashimoto disease<br>?Acute (subacute) thyroiditis<br>Familial genetic defect in thyroxine synthesis<br>Treatment with iodides or lithium for nonthyroidal illness<br>Exposure to $^{131}$I while pregnant | $T_4$, RSH, ThyAb | Same as for suspected hyperthyroidism | $T_4$, TSH, ThyAb determinations:<br>If results indicate hypothyroidism, perform ultrasound scan to define presence, size, location of thyroid tissue<br>If hypothyroidism confirmed, begin treatment with levothyroxine sodium (Synthroid), 0.05 mg/day |

*Graves disease does not develop at 7-10 days in children whose mothers receive PTU.

$^{131}$I, radioactive iodine; PTU, propylthiouracil; $T_3$, triiodothyronine; T4, thyroxine; ThyAb, thyroid antibody; TSAb, thyroid-stimulating antibody; TSH, thyroid-stimulating hormone.

Adapted from Creasy RK, Resnik R (eds): Maternal-Fetal Medicine: Principles and Practice, 2nd ed. Philadelphia, WB Saunders, 1989.

changes that occur in immunologic status of the mother and fetus and that variously affect the assessment of any of the autoimmune thyroid disorders.

## Maternal-Fetal Thyroid Function in Pregnancy

### Maternal Thyroid Function

Several pregnancy-related physiologic conditions affect maternal thyroid function, and the appropriate interpretation of thyroid function test results during pregnancy must take these normal physiologic factors into account. One important modification that occurs during pregnancy is the estrogen-dependent increase in thyroid-binding globulin. This results in an increase in total thyroxine ($TT_4$) and total triiodothyronine ($TT_3$) levels throughout pregnancy. The levels of unbound (free) thyroxine ($FT_4$) and triiodothyronine ($FT_3$), as well as levels of thyroid-stimulating hormone (TSH), in general remain unchanged. However, human chorionic gonadotropin (hCG), a second factor in pregnancy that may modify thyroid function, has a stimulatory effect on the thyroid and may transiently effect the $FT_4$, $FT_3$, and TSH levels in the first trimester and early in the second trimester. This stimulatory effect of hCG rarely causes aberrations of the thyroid function parameters into the thyrotoxic range (American College of Obstetricians and Gynecologists, 2001).

### Fetal Thyroid Function

The fetal thyroid actively concentrates iodide after 10 weeks, releases $T_4$ after 12 weeks, and becomes responsive to pituitary TSH at 20 weeks of gestation. Although maternal TSH does not cross the placenta, maternal thyroid hormones and thyrotropin-releasing hormone (TRH) are transferred to the fetus throughout gestation. In one study, cord blood thyroid function testing of neonates with congenital thyroid agenesis revealed hormone levels that were 30% of normal (Vulsma et al, 1989), suggesting a maternal source. Transplacental transfer of thyroid-stimulating immunoglobulin (TSI) may occur, causing fetal thyrotoxicosis. Other substances that may be transferred from the maternal compartment to the fetal compartment and affect fetal thyroid function are iodine, a radioactive isotope of iodine, propylthiouracil (PTU), and methimazole. The fetal effects of these agents are reviewed later.

## Hyperthyroidism

Hyperthyroidism occurs in approximately 0.2% of pregnancies and results in a significant increase in the prevalence of both low-birth-weight delivery and a trend toward higher neonatal mortality. The most common cause of thyrotoxicosis (85% of cases) in women of childbearing age is Graves disease; other causes are acute (or subacute) thyroiditis (transient), Hashimoto disease, hydatidiform mole, choriocarcinoma, toxic nodular goiter, and toxic adenoma. Graves disease has a peak incidence during the reproductive years, but patients with the disorder may actually have remissions during pregnancy, followed by postpartum exacerbations. The unique feature of these pregnancies is that the fetus may also be affected, regardless of the mother's concurrent medical condition. Thyroid function is difficult to evaluate in the fetus, and the status of the fetus may not correlate with that of the mother.

### Diagnosis

The differential diagnosis of thyrotoxicosis becomes more difficult during pregnancy because normal pregnant women may have a variety of hyperdynamic signs and symptoms—intolerance to heat, nervousness, irritability, emotional lability, and increased perspiration, along with tachycardia and anxiety. Laboratory data are also difficult to evaluate because total serum thyroxin values are normally elevated during pregnancy as a result of estrogen-induced increases in thyroxine-binding globulin. Thus, if thyroxine-binding globulin is increased, $T_3$ resin uptake may be in the euthyroid to slightly increased range in a patient who has true hyperthyroidism.

Hollingsworth (1989) has reviewed the assessment of thyroid function tests in nonpregnant and pregnant women, along with the differential diagnosis of hyperthyroidism during pregnancy.

### Pathogenesis of Graves Disease

The pathogenesis of Graves disease is not completely understood, but it probably represents an overlapping spectrum of disorders that are characterized by production of polyclonal antibodies. It has been appreciated since the 1960s (Sunshine et al, 1965) that abnormal TSIs, which appear to be immunoglobulin G (IgG), are present in pregnant women with Graves disease and cross the placenta easily to cause neonatal hyperthyroidism in some infants (McKenzie and Zakarija, 1978). The clinical spectrum of Graves disease in utero is quite broad and may result in stillbirth or preterm delivery. Some affected infants have widespread evidence of autoimmune disease, including thrombocytopenic purpura and generalized hypertrophy of the lymphatic tissues. Thyroid storm can occur shortly after birth, or the infant may have disease that is transient in nature, lasting from 1 to 5 months. Infants born to mothers who have been treated with thioamides may appear normal at birth but demonstrate signs of thyrotoxicosis at 7 to 10 days of age, when the effect of thioamide suppression of thyroxine synthesis is no longer present. The measurement of thyroid-stimulating antibodies (TSAbs) is useful in predicting whether the fetus will be affected.

### Management of the Mother

Because radioactive iodine therapy is contraindicated during pregnancy, treatment of the pregnant woman with thyrotoxicosis involves a choice between antithyroid drugs and surgery. The therapeutic goal is to achieve a euthyroid, or perhaps slightly hyperthyroid, state in the mother while preventing hypothyroidism and hyperthyroidism in the fetus. Either PTU or methimazole may be used to treat thyrotoxicosis during pregnancy. Because methimazole therapy may be associated with aplasia cutis in the offspring of treated women and because PTU crosses the placenta more slowly than methimazole, PTU has become the drug of choice for use during pregnancy. Ordinarily, thyrotoxicosis can be controlled with doses of 300 mg per day. Once the disorder is under control, however, it is important to keep the dose as low as possible, preferably less than 100 mg daily, because this drug does cross the placenta and blocks fetal thyroid function, possibly producing hypothyroidism in the fetus.

In women with cardiovascular effects, the use of beta-blockers may be appropriate to achieve rapid control of thyrotoxicosis. Because administration of propranolol to pregnant women has been associated with intrauterine growth restriction and impaired responses of the fetus to anoxic stress as well as postnatal bradycardia and hypoglycemia, the dosages must be closely controlled. Iodides have also been used, particularly in combination with beta-blocking agents, to control thyrotoxicosis. Long-term iodide therapy, however, presents a risk to the fetus. Because of the inhibition of the incorporation of iodide into thyroglobulin, a large, obstructive goiter can develop in the fetus. Surgery during pregnancy is best reserved for cases in which the mother is hypersensitive to antithyroid drugs, compliance with medication is poor, or in rare cases in which drugs are ineffective in controlling the disease.

### Effects on the Newborn

Approximately 1% of infants born to mothers with some level of thyrotoxicosis themselves have thyrotoxicosis (Fig. 9–4). Assessment of fetal risk in utero includes measurement of TSIs, with expectation that if the titers are high, there is a higher risk of thyrotoxicosis. Additional assessment of the fetus should pay particular attention to elevated resting heart rate and poor fetal growth. Daneman and Howard (1980) reported on the outcome of nine infants with neonatal thyrotoxicosis and noted normal growth but a high incidence of craniosynostosis and intellectual impairment. It may, therefore, be necessary to treat the asymptomatic mother with thioamides and propranolol (and thyroid replacement) during pregnancy in order to treat the infant and prevent serious neonatal morbidity and long-term problems.

Mothers with thyrotoxicosis who are taking normal doses of thioamides may safely breast-feed their infants, although thioamides do appear in breast milk in low amounts. Currently, there does not appear to be any long-term adverse outcome for infants whose mothers have received PTU during pregnancy.

## Hypothyroidism

Treatment with replacement doses of thyroid hormone is usually well tolerated and easily titrated. The clinician must be aware of the fact that the increased TSI levels in maternal plasma may result in movement of thyroid hormone from the fetus to the mother, with a decrease in severity of her disease during the pregnancy. Hypothyroidism has occurred in fetuses whose mothers have inadvertently received radioactive iodine ($^{132}$I) during pregnancy. There is currently no reliable method for diagnosing hypothyroidism in utero.

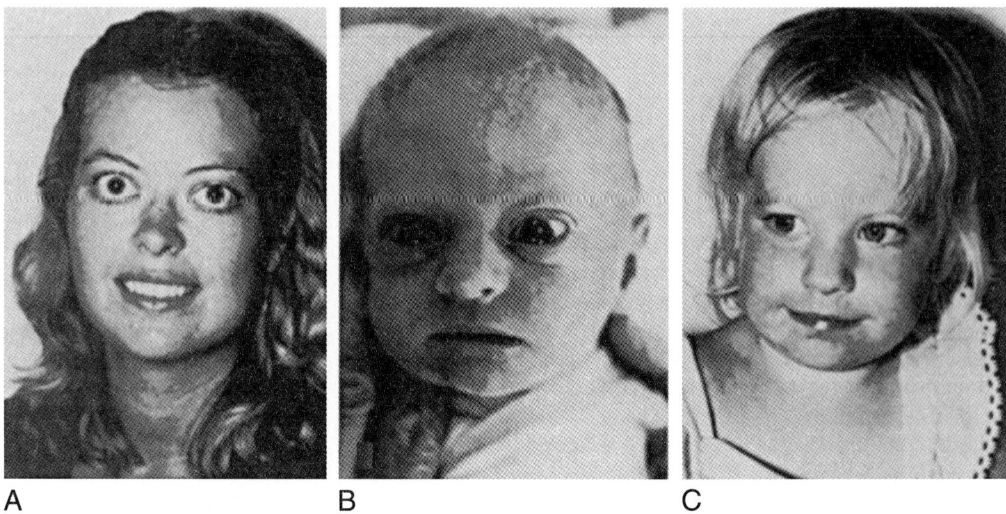


**FIGURE 9–4.** **A,** Hypothyroid 21-year-old mother who experienced Graves disease at age 7 and was treated by subtotal thyroidectomy. She was given maintenance therapy with daily levothyroxine sodium (Synthroid), 0.15 mg, throughout pregnancy. **B,** Her infant girl was born at term with severe Graves disease, goiter, and exophthalmos that persisted for 6 months. **C,** The child was normal at age 20 months. *(From Creasy RK, Resnik R [eds]: Maternal-Fetal Medicine: Principles and Practice, 2nd ed. Philadelphia, WB Saunders, 1989.)*

## REFERENCES


Acker DB, Sachs BP, Friedman EA: Risk factors for shoulder dystocia in the average-weight infant. Obstet Gynecol 67:614, 1986.

American College of Obstetricians and Gynecologists. ACOG Practice Bulletin: Thyroid disease in pregnancy. Obstet Gynecol 98:879, 2000.

American College of Obstetricians and Gynecologists: ACOG Practice Bulletin: Clinical Management Guidelines for Obstetrician-Gynecologists. Number 30, September 2001 (replaces Technical Bulletin Number 200, December 1994). Gestational diabetes. Obstet Gynecol 98:525, 2001.

American Diabetes Association: Expert Committee on the Diagnosis and Classification of Diabetes Mellitus: Report of the Expert Committee on the Diagnosis and Classification of Diabetes Mellitus. Diabetes Care 25(Suppl 1):S5, 2002.

Bernstein IM, Catalano PM: Influence of fetal fat on the ultrasound estimation of fetal weight in diabetic mothers. Obstet Gynecol 79:561, 1992.

Bevier WC, Fischer R, Jovanovic L: Treatment of women with an abnormal glucose challenge test (but normal oral glucose tolerance test) decreases the prevalence of macrosomia. Am J Perinatol 16:269, 1999.

Chmait R, Dinise T, Daneshmand S, et al: Prospective cohort study to establish predictors of glyburide success in women with gestational diabetes mellitus. Am J Obstet Gynecol 185:S197, 2002.

Coetzee EJ, Jackson WP: The management of non-insulin-dependent diabetes during pregnancy. Diabetes Res Clin Pract 1:281, 1985.

Cousins L: The California Diabetes and Pregnancy Programme: A statewide collaborative programme for the pre-conception and prenatal care of diabetic women. Balliere's Clin Obstet Gynecol 5:443, 1991.

Coustan DR, Lewis SB: Insulin therapy for gestational diabetes. Obstet Gynecol 51:306, 1978.

Craigin EB, Ryder GH: Obstetrics: A Practical Textbook for Students and Practitioners. Philadelphia, Lea & Febiger, 1916.

Daneman D, Howard NJ: Neonatal thyrotoxicosis: Intellectual impairment and craniosynostosis in later years. J Pediatr 97:257, 1980.

de Veciana M, Major CA, Morgan MA, et al: Postprandial versus preprandial blood glucose monitoring in women with gestational diabetes mellitus requiring insulin therapy [see comments]. N Engl J Med 333:1237, 1995.

DeLee JB: The Principles and Practice of Obstetrics, 3rd ed. Philadelphia, WB Saunders, 1920.

Elliott BD, Schenker S, Langer O, et al: Comparative placental transport of oral hypoglycemic agents in humans: A model of human placental drug transfer. Am J Obstet Gynecol 171:653, 1994.

Engelgau MM, Herman WH, Smith PJ, et al: The epidemiology of diabetes and pregnancy in the U.S., 1988. Diabetes Care 18:1029, 1995.

Ferrero A, Maggi E, Giancotti A, et al: Regression formula for estimation of fetal weight with use of abdominal circumference and femur length: A prospective study. J Ultrasound Med 13:823, 1994.

Fuhrmann K, Reiher H, Semmler K, et al: Prevention of congenital malformations in infants of insulin-dependent diabetic mothers. Diabetes Care 6:219, 1983.

Gabbe SG, Holing E, Temple P, et al: Benefits, risks, costs, and patient satisfaction associated with insulin pump therapy for the pregnancy complicated by type 1 diabetes mellitus. Am J Obstet Gynecol 182:1283, 2000.

Gilbert WM, Nesbitt TS, Danielsen B: Associated factors in 1611 cases of brachial plexus injury. Obstet Gynecol 93:536, 1999.

Goldberg JD, Franklin B, Lasser D, et al: Gestational diabetes: Impact of home glucose monitoring on neonatal birth weight. Am J Obstet Gynecol 154:546, 1986.

Griffin ME, Coffey M, Johnson H, et al: Universal vs. risk factor-based screening for gestational diabetes mellitus: Detection rates, gestation at diagnosis and outcome. Diabet Med 17:26, 2000.

Gutgesell HP, Mullins CE, Gillette PC, et al: Transient hypertrophic subaortic stenosis in infants of diabetic mothers. J Pediatr 89:120, 1976.

Hedriana H, Moore TR: Comparison of single vs multiple growth sonography in predicting birthweight. Am J Obstet Gynecol 170:1600, 1994.

Herman WH, Janz NK, Becker MP, et al: Diabetes and pregnancy: preconception care, pregnancy outcomes, resource utilization and costs. J Reprod Med 44:33, 1999.

Hollingsworth DR: Endocrine disorders in pregnancy. In Creasy RK, Resnik R (eds): Maternal-Fetal Medicine: Principles and Practice, 2nd ed. Philadelphia, WB Saunders, 1989.

Hollingsworth DR, Cousins L: Diabetes in pregnancy: A new perspective. In Milunsky A, Friedman E, Gluck L (eds): Advances in Perinatal Medicine, vol 2. New York, Plenum Press, 1981.

Jorge CS, Artal R, Paul RH, et al: Antepartum fetal surveillance in diabetic pregnant patients. Am J Obstet Gynecol 141:641, 1981.

Jovanovic-Peterson L, Peterson CM, Reed GF, et al: Maternal postprandial glucose levels and infant birth weight: The Diabetes in Early Pregnancy Study. The National Institute of Child Health and Human Development–Diabetes in Early Pregnancy Study. Am J Obstet Gynecol 164:103, 1991.

Keller JD, Lopez-Zeno JA, Dooley SL, Socol ML: Shoulder dystocia and birth trauma in gestational diabetes: A five-year experience. Am J Obstet Gynecol 165:928, 1991.

Kjos SL, Walther FJ, Montoro M, et al: Prevalence and etiology of respiratory distress in infants of diabetic mothers: Predictive value of fetal lung maturation tests. Am J Obstet Gynecol 163:898, 1990.

Kjos SL, Henry OA, Montoro M, et al: Insulin-requiring diabetes in pregnancy: A randomized trial of active induction of labor and expectant management. Am J Obstet Gynecol 169:611, 1993.

Kjos SL, Schaefer-Graf U, Sardesi S, et al: A randomized controlled trial using glycemic plus fetal ultrasound parameters versus glycemic parameters to determine insulin therapy in gestational diabetes with fasting hyperglycemia. Diabetes Care 24:1904, 2001.

Landon MB, Mintz MC, Gabbe SG: Sonographic evaluation of fetal abdominal growth: Predictor of the large for gestational age infant in pregnancies complicated by diabetes mellitus. Am J Obstet Gynecol 160:115, 1989.

Langer O, Rodriguez DA, Xenakis MJ, et al: Intensified versus conventional management of gestational diabetes. Am J Obstet Gynecol 170:1036, 1994.

Langer O, Conway D, Berkus M, et al: A comparison of glyburide and insulin in women with gestational diabetes mellitus. N Engl J Med 343:1134, 2000.

Larsen T, Greisen G, Petersen S: Prediction of birth weight by ultrasound-estimated fetal weight: A comparison between single and repeated estimates. Eur J Obstet Gynecol Reprod Biol 60:37, 1995.

Lavin JP, Barden TP, Miodovnik M, et al: Clinical experience with a screening program for gestational diabetes. Am J Obstet Gynecol 141:491, 1981.

Lim JM, Tayob Y, O'Brien PM, Shaw RW: A comparison between the pregnancy outcome of women with gestation diabetes treated with glibenclamide and those treated with insulin. Med J Malaysia 52:377, 1997.

Lucas MJ, Leveno KJ, Williams ML, et al: Early pregnancy glycosylated hemoglobin, severity of diabetes, and fetal malformations. Am J Obstet Gynecol 161:426, 1989.

Lurie S, Matzkel A, Weissman A, et al: Outcome of pregnancy in class A1 and A2 gestational diabetic patients delivered beyond 40 weeks' gestation. Am J Perinatol 9:484, 1992.

Mace S, Hirschfeld SS, Riggs T, et al: Echocardiographic abnormalities in infants of diabetic mothers. J Pediatr 95: 1013, 1979.

Major CA, Henry MJ, de Veciana M, Morgan MA: The effects of carbohydrate restriction in patients with diet-controlled gestational diabetes. Obstet Gynecol 91:600, 1998.

McKenzie JM, Zakarija M: Pathogenesis of neonatal Graves' disease. J Endocrinol Invest 2:183, 1978.

McLaren RA, Puckett JL, Chauhan SP: Estimators of birth weight in pregnant women requiring insulin: A comparison of seven sonographic models. Obstet Gynecol 85:565, 1995.

Metzger BE: Summary and recommendations of the Third International Workshop-Conference on Gestational Diabetes Mellitus. Diabetes 40(Suppl 2):197, 1991.

Metzger BE, Coustan DR: Summary and Recommendations of the Fourth International Workshop-Conference on Gestational Diabetes Mellitus. The Organizing Committee. Diabetes Care 21(Suppl 2):1, 1998.

Miller E, Hare JW, Cloherty JP, et al: Elevated maternal $HbA_{1c}$ in early pregnancy and major congenital anomalies in infants of diabetic mothers. N Engl J Med 304:1331, 1981.

Mimouni F, Miodovnik M, Rosenn B, et al: Birth trauma in insulin-dependent diabetic pregnancies. Am J Perinatol 9:205, 1992.

Moore TR: A comparison of amniotic fluid fetal pulmonary phospholipids in normal and diabetic pregnancy. Am J Obstet Gynecol 186:641, 2002.

Moore TR, Cayle JE: The amniotic fluid index in normal human pregnancy. Am J Obstet Gynecol 162:1168, 1990.

Moore TR, Key TC, Reisner LS, et al: Evaluation of the use of continuous lumbar epidural anesthesia for hypertensive pregnant women in labor. Am J Obstet Gynecol 152:85, 1985.

National Institute of Diabetes & Digestive & Kidney Diseases: Epidemiology of diabetes in the United States, 2002. Available online at http://diabetes.nddk.nih.gov/dm/pubs/statistics/index.htm#7

Nesbitt TS, Gilbert WM, Herrchen B, et al: Shoulder dystocia and associated risk factors with macrosomic infants born in California. Am J Obstet Gynecol 179:476, 1998.

Ogata ES, Sabbagha R, Metzger BE, et al: Serial ultrasonography to assess evolving fetal macrosomia: Studies in 23 pregnant diabetic women. JAMA 243:2405, 1980.

Pedersen J: Diabetes and Pregnancy: Blood Sugar of Newborn Infants. Copenhagen, Danish Science, 1952.

Pedersen J: The Pregnant Diabetic and Her Newborn, 2nd ed. Baltimore, Williams & Wilkins, 1977, p 9.

Persson B, Hanson U: Neonatal morbidities in gestational diabetes mellitus. Diabetes Care 21(Suppl 2):B79, 1998.

Piacquadio K, Hollingsworth DR, Murphy H: Effects of in-utero exposure to oral hypoglycaemic drugs. Lancet 338:866, 1991.

Pinter E, Reece EA, Leranth CZ, et al: Arachidonic acid prevents hyperglycemia-associated yolk sac damage and embryopathy. Am J Obstet Gynecol 155:691, 1986.

Pinter E, Peyman JA, Snow K, et al: Effects of maternal diabetes on fetal rat lung ion transport: Contribution of alveolar and bronchiolar epithelial cells. J Clin Invest 87:821, 1991.

Rasmussen MJ, Firth R, Foley M, Stronge JM: The timing of delivery in diabetic pregnancy: A 10-year review. Aust N Z J Obstet Gynaecol 32:313, 1992.

Ray R, Heng BH, Lim C, Ling SL: Gestational diabetes in Singaporean women: Use of the glucose challenge test as a screening test and identification of high risk factors. Ann Acad Med Singapore 25:504, 1996.

Reece EA, Winn HN, Smikle C, et al: Sonographic assessment of growth of the fetal head in diabetic pregnancies compared with normal gestations. Am J Perinatol 7:18, 1990.

Rossi G, Somigliana E, Moschetta M, et al: Adequate timing of fetal ultrasound to guide metabolic therapy in mild gestational diabetes mellitus—results from a randomized study. Acta Obstet Gynecol Scand 79:649, 2000.

Rouse DJ, Owen J, Goldenberg RL, et al: The effectiveness and costs of elective cesarean delivery for fetal macrosomia diagnosed by ultrasound. JAMA 276:1480, 1996.

Sermer M, Naylor CD, Gave DJ, et al: Impact of time since last meal on the gestational glucose challenge test: The Toronto Tri-Hospital Gestational Diabetes Project. Am J Obstet Gynecol 171:607, 1994.

Shamley KT, Landon MB: Accuracy and modifying factors for ultrasonographic determination of fetal weight at term. Obstet Gynecol 84:926, 1994.

Shepard MJ, Richards VA, Berkowitz RL, et al: An evaluation of two equations for predicting fetal weight by ultrasound. Am J Obstet Gynecol 142:47, 1982.

Shelley-Jones DC, Beischer NA, Sheedy MT, Walstab JE: Excessive birth weight and maternal glucose tolerance: A 19-year review. Aust N Z J Obstet Gynaecol 32:318, 1992.

Sibai BM, Caritis S, Hauth J, et al: Risks of preeclampsia and adverse neonatal outcomes among women with pregestational diabetes mellitus. National Institute of Child Health and Human Development Network of Maternal-Fetal Medicine Units. Am J Obstet Gynecol 182:364, 2000.

Silverman BL, Metzger BE, Cho NH, Loeb CA: Impaired glucose tolerance in adolescent offspring of diabetic mothers: Relationship to fetal hyperinsulinism. Diabetes Care 18:611, 1995.

Sunshine P, Kusomoto H, Kriss JP: Survival time of long-acting thyroid stimulator in neonatal thyrotoxicosis: Implications of diagnosis and therapy of the disorder. Pediatrics 36:869, 1965.

Susa JB, McCormick KL, Widness JA, et al: Chronic hyperinsulinemia in the fetal rhesus monkey: Effects of fetal growth and composition. Diabetes 25:1058, 1979.

Tamura RK, Sabbagha RE, Dooley SL, et al: Real-time ultrasound estimations of weight in fetuses of diabetic gravid women. Am J Obstet Gynecol 153:57, 1985.

Thompson DJ, Porter KB, Gunnells DJ, et al: Prophylactic insulin in the management of gestational diabetes. Obstet Gynecol 75:960, 1990.

Tongsong T, Piyamongkol W, Sreshthaputra O: Accuracy of ultrasonic fetal weight estimation: A comparison of three equations employed for estimating fetal weight. J Med Assoc Thai 77:373, 1994.

Towner D, Kjos SL, Leung B, et al: Congenital malformations in pregnancies complicated by NIDDM. Diabetes Care 18:1446, 1995.

Vulsma T, Gons MH, De Vijlder JJ: Maternal-fetal transfer of thyroxine in congenital hypothyroidism due to a total organification defect or thyroid agenesis. N Engl J Med 321:13, 1989.

Weeks JW, Pitman T, Spinnato JA 2nd, et al: Fetal macrosomia: Does antenatal prediction affect delivery route and birth outcome? Am J Obstet Gynecol 173:1215, 1995.

Widness JA, Teramo KA, Clemons GK, et al: Direct relationship of antepartum glucose control and fetal erythropoietin in human type 1 (insulin dependent) diabetic pregnancy. Diabetologia 33:378, 1990.

Williams JW: Obstetrics: A Textbook for the Use of Students and Practitioners. New York, D Appleton, 1925.

Zucker P, Simon G: Prolonged symptomatic neonatal hypoglycemia associated with maternal chlorpropamide therapy. Pediatrics 42:824, 1968.

CHAPTER 10

# Maternal Medical Disorders of Fetal Significance: Seizure Disorders, Isoimmunization, Cancer, and Mental Disorders

**Thomas F. Kelly and Thomas R. Moore**

A significant spectrum of medical complications may complicate pregnancy. Some of these, very manageable in the nonpregnant patient, can be lethal to the gravid woman. Thus, two basic questions arise for the obstetrician dealing with the pregnant female who is experiencing a medical complication. First, is the condition affected by the patient's normal adaptations to pregnancy? And second, how does the medical problem affect the woman and her fetus? Although many medical conditions during pregnancy can be managed much like they would be in the nonpregnant woman, there are usually nuances in care during gestation to which the obstetrician must be attuned and that will potentially affect the fetus and neonate.

During pregnancy, any potential medical therapy should be carefully considered so that fetal risks are minimized. For example, thalidomide and diethylstilbestrol were prescribed in the past for morning sickness and recurrent miscarriages, respectively, on the basis of reasonable hypotheses that maternal sedation would decrease nausea and increased estrogens would "support" the placenta and reduce the likelihood of first-trimester loss. Unfortunately, use of both of these agents led to significant and tragic congenital anomalies in the offspring. In view of the profusion of new drugs available today, the importance of assessing the expected risk-to-benefit ratio for each medication prescribed to a pregnant woman is more important than ever. An example is phenytoin treatment for maternal seizures. If there is a less teratogenic alternative, it should be prescribed if effective. However, for most women taking phenytoin, other agents are unable to control their seizures, and the risks to the fetus must be accepted.

The altered pharmacokinetics of many agents during pregnancy must be considered, because the dosage of familiar medications may have to be adjusted if toxicity is to be avoided. Classic examples are thyroid hormone replacement (a higher level of thyroid-binding globulin in pregnancy increases total thyroxin [$T_4$] but leaves the serum free thyroxin value unchanged) and aminoglycoside antibiotic therapy (increased glomerular filtration in pregnancy results in lower serum drug levels).

This chapter discusses four maternal conditions that may influence fetal growth, development, and outcome—seizure disorders, hypertensive states, and red blood cell isoimmunization. The basics of management, the potential effects of pregnancy on the condition, and the effects of the condition on the gravida and the fetus are considered.

## MATERNAL SEIZURE DISORDERS

Epilepsy is not uncommon, affecting more than 3 million people and approximately 1.1 million women of childbearing age in the United States, with a prevalence in pregnancy approximating 0.5%. The pattern of maternal seizures ranges from complex partial to generalized tonic clonic seizures and generalized absence (petit mal). Physiologically, seizures arise from paroxysmal episodes of abnormal brain electrical discharges, and when associated with motor activity, they are termed *convulsive*.

The effect of pregnancy on the frequency and severity of the seizure disorder is highly variable from patient to patient. Although the condition worsens in 25% of patients (Wilhelm et al, 1990), and many patients experience improvement, the disease remains the same in the majority. Neither the type of epilepsy nor a prior pregnancy experience reliably influences the seizure frequency (Yerby, 2001). In patients in whom higher numbers of seizures occur during gestation, decreased plasma concentrations of antiepileptic medications have been hypothesized as causative. The fall in plasma drug levels during pregnancy may be in part due to increased protein binding, reduced absorption, and increased drug clearance. Adequacy of prepregnancy seizure control may influence a patient's course during gestation; the patient whose disease was poorly controlled tends to have more frequent seizures during pregnancy, and the patient who was seizure free for 2 years before pregnancy has only a 10% chance of experiencing seizures during gestation (Schmidt et al, 1983).

### Perinatal Risk

For reasons that are not immediately clear, women with seizures have more obstetrical complications during pregnancy and a higher rate of poor perinatal outcomes. Rates of preeclampsia, preterm delivery, small-for-gestational-age infants, congenital malformations, cerebral palsy, and perinatal mortality have all been reported as higher in women with an antecedent seizure disorder (Nelson and Ellenberg, 1982). Pregnancy outcome is also greatly influenced by the mother's socioeconomic status and age as well as by the prenatal care received.

The well-documented increased frequency of congenital malformations among women with seizure disorders is curious, because it is observed irrespective of fetal exposure to anticonvulsant medications (Bjerkedal, 1982). The malformation risk is, however, correlated with the severity of epilepsy and the number of medications used. Overall, the risk is increased over baseline by 3.5% to 4.4%. Specific malformations reported include a fivefold rise in rate of orofacial clefts (Friis et al, 1986), an increase in rate of congenital heart disease, particularly with trimethadione

(Friis and Hauge, 1985), and a 1% to 2% incidence of neural tube defects in fetuses exposed to valproic acid (Lammer et al, 1987). Facial abnormalities (e.g., mid-face hypoplasia) are not specific to any particular antiepileptic drug, being seen with phenytoin, carbamazepine, and trimethadione.

The classic features of the hydantoin syndrome are facial clefting, broad nasal ridge, hypertelorism, epicanthal folds, distal phalangeal hypoplasia, and growth and mental deficiencies; however, these are features of the use of other antiseizure medications as well (Table 10–1). The postulated cause of this syndrome is the action of a common epoxide intermediate of these medications on a teratogen. The hydantoin syndrome was found to develop in fetuses with inadequate epoxide hydrolase activity (Buehler et al, 1990). This enzymatic deficiency appears to be recessively inherited.

### Management

Management of the pregnant patient with epilepsy is based on keeping her seizure free. Theoretically, this goal reduces maternal physical risk and lowers the incidence of fetal complications. Preconception counseling is preferable and should entail (1) adjustment of medication dosages into the therapeutic range, (2) attempting to limit the patient to one drug if possible, and (3) choosing an agent with the least risk of teratogenesis. Frank discussion of the various risks of each agent should be conducted, particularly the risks associated with valproic acid and trimethadione. Usually, if the patient's disease is adequately controlled with one agent, it rarely needs to be changed, because the risks of increasing seizure activity are believed to outweigh the potential for reducing congenital malformations.

**TABLE 10–1**

**Clinical Features of the Fetal Hydantoin Syndrome**

| | |
|---|---|
| Craniofacial abnormalities | Broad nasal ridge |
| | Wide fontanel |
| | Low-set hairline |
| | Broad alveolar ridge |
| | Metopic ridging |
| | Short neck |
| | Ocular hypertelorism |
| | Microcephaly |
| | Cleft lip and/or palate |
| | Abnormal or low-set ears |
| | Epicanthal folds |
| | Ptosis of eyelids |
| | Coloboma |
| | Coarse scalp hair |
| Limb abnormalities | Smallness or absence of nails |
| | Hypoplasia of distal phalanges |
| | Altered palmar crease |
| | Digital thumb |
| | Dislocated hip |

Data from Briggs GC, Freeman RK, Yaffe SJ: Drugs in Pregnancy and Lactation, 5th ed. Baltimore, Williams & Wilkins, 1998.

Patients taking antiepileptic medications should also take folic acid supplements (800 to 1000 μg) before conception, because inhibition of folate absorption has been proposed as a teratogenic mechanism, particularly with phenytoin. During gestation, the anticonvulsant levels should be checked monthly, and the dose adjusted accordingly. Medications should not be changed unless they prove ineffective at the optimal serum level. If a patient reports greater seizure activity, the drug serum level should be checked immediately. A common source of increased seizures is that the patient is not taking her medication, usually because she fears its teratogenicity.

Mothers taking phenytoin, phenobarbital, or primidone may have a higher incidence of neonatal coagulopathy due to vitamin K–dependent clotting factor deficiency. Maternal vitamin K supplementation in the third trimester is reasonable; a single parenteral dose of 10 mg can be given at 34 to 36 weeks of gestation.

## ISOIMMUNIZATION

Hydrops fetalis, a condition associated with abnormal fluid collections in various body cavities of the fetus, was first described in 1892. The causes are many but can be conceptualized in two categories, immune causes and nonimmune causes. In immune-mediated hydrops, circulating immunoglobulins lead to the destruction of fetal red blood cells and hemolytic anemia. Landsteiner and Weiner first elucidated the Rhesus factor in 1940. Levine and associates showed pathogenesis of erythroblastosis to be due to maternal isoimmunization in 1941. Rh immune globulin (RhIG) was developed in the mid-1960s. Prophylaxis protocols utilizing Rh immune globulin significantly reduced the incidence of D isoimmunization, increasing the relative frequency of alloimmunization against atypical red blood cell antigens such as E, Duffy, and Kell. The pathophysiology of immune-mediated fetal hemolytic disease is similar, irrespective of the blood group antigen involved; therefore, the bulk of the discussion here is on the Rh system.

### Genetics

The Rh blood group actually represents a number of antigens, designated D, Cc, and Ee. The genes for these antigens, located on the short arm of chromosome 1, are inherited in a set of three from each parent. The presence of D determines whether the individual is Rh positive, and the absence of D (there is no recessive allele, so "d" does not exist) yields the Rh-negative type. Rarely, a patient exhibits a Du variant and should be considered D positive. The combinations of these various antigens occur with different frequencies. For example, prevalence of Cde (41%) is higher than that of CDE (0.08%) (Lewis et al, 1971). Although the Rh phenotype is the result of D status, the various genotype combinations help predict the zygosity of an individual. About 45% of Rh-positive individuals are homozygous and therefore will always produce an Rh-positive offspring, and 55% are heterozygous and will have an Rh-negative child if paired with an Rh-negative partner.

There are no sex differences in the frequency of Rh negativity. However racial variations are striking. Rh negativity is common in the Basque population (30% to 35%), but rare in Chinese persons, Japanese persons, and North American Indians (1% to 2%). The average incidence in white populations is about 15%. North American blacks have a higher incidence (8%) than African blacks (4%).

## Pathogenesis

Before modern blood banking, the Rh-negative patient became immunized from the transfusion of Rh-positive blood. In the case of atypical red blood cell antigens (Duffy, Kidd, etc.), blood transfusion is still a significant cause of isoimmunization. Today, fetal transplacental hemorrhage is currently the primary cause of Rh isoimmunization. Rh immune globulin prophylaxis protocols have reduced but not eliminated this problem. Transplacental hemorrhage of fetal cells into the maternal circulation is surprisingly common, with 75% of women showing evidence of this event at some time during gestation (Bowman et al, 1986). The amount of fetal blood is usually small, but approximately 1% of women have 5 mL, and in 0.25% of women, 30 mL or more of fetal cells are noted at Kleihauer-Betke testing. Obstetrical events increase the chance of transplacental hemorrhage (Table 10–2), as do the incidence and amount of hemorrhage with advancing gestational age (from 12% in the first trimester to 45% in the third trimester). As little as 0.3 mL of Rh-positive blood produces immunization, and the risk is dose dependent. ABO blood group incompatibility between fetus and mother affords some protection, reducing the risk from 16% to 2%.

The primary maternal immune response is slow and may take as long as 6 months to develop. First appearance of immunoglobulin (Ig) M class anti-D antibodies is weak; they do not cross the placenta but are soon followed by smaller IgG antibodies that are capable of traversing the placental barrier. Therefore, the initial event causing sensitization rarely results in fetal hemolysis. A second transplacental hemorrhage then leads to the more rapid and abundant amnestic IgG response that, in the presence of fetal D-positive cells, may cause significant hemolysis and fetal anemia.

The severity of hemolytic disease is related to the maternal antibody titer, the affinity for the red blood cell membrane, and the ability of the fetus to compensate for the red blood cell destruction. Table 10–3 summarizes the levels of fetal and neonatal disease and their incidence. Most cases are mild and result in normal outcomes; the cord blood is strongly Coombs positive, but the babies do not become significantly anemic or hyperbilirubinemic. Moderate disease results from the red blood cell destruction and the greater production of indirect bilirubin; although the mother is able to clear this product for the fetus in utero, the neonate is deficient in the liver glucuronyl transferase enzyme, leading to the buildup of this water-insoluble molecule. Albumin carries the indirect bilirubin, but if the binding capacity is exceeded, diffusion of the bilirubin into the fatty tissues occurs. Neural tissue is high in lipid content. Ultimate destruction of neurons can occur, resulting in kernicterus. Treatment depends on the recognition of the hyperbilirubinemia and usually entails phototherapy and exchange transfusion in the nursery. (See also Chapter 79.)

Severe disease occurs when the fetus is unable to produce enough red blood cells to compensate for the increased destruction of these cells. Extramedullary hematopoiesis, prominent in the liver, ultimately leads to enlargement, hepatocellular damage, and portal hypertension. This process is believed to be the etiology of placental edema and ascites. Albumin production diminishes due to hepatocellular damage and results in anasarca, giving rise to hydrops fetalis. The theory that hydrops is due to fetal heart failure no longer holds, as a result of observations that these infants are neither hypervolemic or in failure. The relationship between fetal anemia and hydrops is variable, but most hydropic fetuses have hemoglobin levels below 60 g/L.

**TABLE 10-2**

**Clinical Conditions Associated with Increased Risk of Fetal-Maternal Hemorrhage**

Unexplained vaginal bleeding
Abruptio placentae
External breech version
Amniocentesis
Chorionic villus sampling/placental biopsy
Umbilical cord sampling
Manual removal of the placenta
Abdominal trauma
Ectopic pregnancy

**TABLE 10-3**

**Classification of the Severity of Hemolytic Disease**

| Severity | Description | Incidence (%) |
|---|---|---|
| Mild | Indirect bilirubin result 16-20 mg/dL | 45-50 |
| | No anemia | |
| | No treatment needed | |
| Moderate | Fetal hydrops does not develop | 25-30 |
| | Moderate anemia | |
| | Severe jaundice with risk of kernicterus unless treated after birth | |
| Severe | Fetal hydrops develops in utero | 20-25 |
| | Before 34 weeks of gestation | 10-12 |
| | After 34 weeks of gestation | 10-12 |

Data from Bowman JM: Maternal blood group immunization. In Creasy R, Resnik R (eds): Maternal-Fetal Medicine: Principles and Practice. Philadelphia, WB Saunders, 1984, pp 561-602.

## Management

Management of the sensitized patient, for both Rh and atypical red blood cell antigens, requires an understanding of the mechanism of disease and the skill and the experience to predict its severity. Although management schemes follow some very basic guidelines, successful management requires access to a blood bank with expertise in antibody typing and individuals skilled in prenatal diagnostic procedures (e.g., cordocentesis). Referral to experienced high-risk centers for the management of this problem is common in the United States.

### Monitoring

At their first visit, all pregnant patients should undergo a blood type and antibody screen (indirect Coombs test), which identifies the Rh-negative woman and screens for the presence of anti-D antibody and other immunoglobulins associated with atypical red blood cell antigens and capable of causing fetal hemolytic disease (Table 10–4). Any positive result on antibody screening should be evaluated aggressively so as to identify the antibody and quantify its amount by titer. Consulting a blood bank pathologist may be necessary for atypical antibodies.

The amount of the anti-D antibody present according to indirect antibody titer is important. For a titer that is less than 1:16 and remains at that level throughout the pregnancy, most centers consider the fetus to be at negligible risk of hydrops or stillbirth. Each blood bank sets different standards for this critical titer, which depend on the assay used. At a titer of 1:16, the risk is 10%; at 1:128, it is 75%. For a woman with a previously affected fetus, no titer is predictive, and therefore management based on its result may underestimate the severity of fetal disease.

Once the patient has been identified as isoimmunized, her obstetrical history is important. All of her prior pregnancies and their outcomes must be documented to attempt to elucidate the timing and cause of the sensitization as well as to assess the risk in her current pregnancy. In general, the condition is worse with each pregnancy. In a first sensitized pregnancy, the risk of hydrops is approximately 10%. More than 90% of patients who have delivered one hydropic baby will deliver another one subsequently.

Paternal blood typing and Rh genotyping should be performed to calculate the fetal risk of Rh positivity. For atypical blood group immunization, history of prior outcomes plus transfusions (a significant cause of such antibodies) and determination of the father's antigen status are of similar importance. For example, a woman with an anti-Kell antibody titer of 1:128 would be at moderate risk of hydrops—unless the father of the baby is found to be Kell-negative. No invasive procedures for isoimmunization should be performed until the father's antibody status is established, unless the fetus's paternity is in question or the partner is unavailable.

**TABLE 10–4**

**Examples of Atypical Red Blood Cell Antigens Associated with Fetal Hemolytic Disease**

| Blood Group System | Antigen | Severity of Hemolytic Disease |
|---|---|---|
| Kell | K | Mild to severe |
| Duffy | Fya | Mild to severe |
| Kidd | JKa | Mild to severe |
| | JKb | Mild to severe |
| MNSs | M | Mild to severe |
| | N | Mild |
| | S | Mild to severe |
| | s | Mild to severe |
| | U | Mild to severe |
| P | PP | Mild to severe |
| Public antigens | Yta | Moderate to severe |

Ultrasonographic screening to identify the prehydropic fetus is notoriously unreliable, in that significantly anemic fetuses may not be grossly hydropic. However, clues that have been proposed to suggest impending hydrops are polyhydramnios, skin thickening, early ascites (particularly around the fetal bladder), and placental thickening. Ultrasonographic measurements of the liver and spleen have been suggested as aids in predicting anemia in nonhydropic fetuses but lack sensitivity and specificity (Bahado-Singh, 1998; Vintzileos, 1986).

Doppler blood flow measurements in the umbilical vein (Iskarios et al, 1998) and in the middle cerebral artery have shown promise. Using reference ranged middle cerebral artery peak systolic velocities, Mari (2000) was able to predict which nonhydropic fetuses had moderate or severe anemia. Currently, a multicenter trial is evaluating this promising noninvasive technology, which has already shown utility in reducing the number of invasive tests (amniocentesis) needed for surveillance of an otherwise lower risk patient.

Antibody titers should be followed monthly to predict which fetus is at risk (in the absence of a history of a prior hydropic infant). If the indirect antibody titer value is less than 1:16, the development of hydrops is unlikely. Most centers consider the critical value to be 1:16, because at and above this level, one cannot ensure the absence of hydrops. When a patient's antibody titer value is at or above 1:16, more invasive testing is needed. Such testing is usually accomplished with amniocentesis and, less commonly, through direct fetal blood sampling.

Amniocentesis remains the primary screening technique for fetal anemia because amniotic fluid contains hemolytic products excreted from the kidneys and lungs, including bilirubin. The unconjugated form of bilirubin is secreted across the respiratory tree and therefore into the amniotic fluid. The supernatant is analyzed with a spectrophotometer, and the bilirubin peak corresponding to the level of absorbance (or optical density [OD]) of these hemoglobin products (450 nm) is quantified. The magnitude of the peak is calculated after subtracting the mean baseline value surrounding the peak. The difference from baseline to peak is the $\Delta OD_{450}$ value.

The amount of the increase in the $\Delta OD_{450}$ value correlates reasonably well with severity of hemolysis. In 1961, Liley developed a graph that has been used to predict the severity of fetal hemolytic disease using the $\Delta OD_{450}$ value. The graph is divided into three zones: Zone I represents the lowest risk and indicates an unaffected fetus, whereas zone III strongly suggests a severely affected fetus, in which fetal hydrops and death can ensue if disease is not treated within the next 7 to 10 days (Fig. 10–1). The Liley curve is authoritative in the third trimester, but its reliability before 26 weeks of gestation has been questioned (Queenan et al, 1993). At less than 20 weeks of gestation,

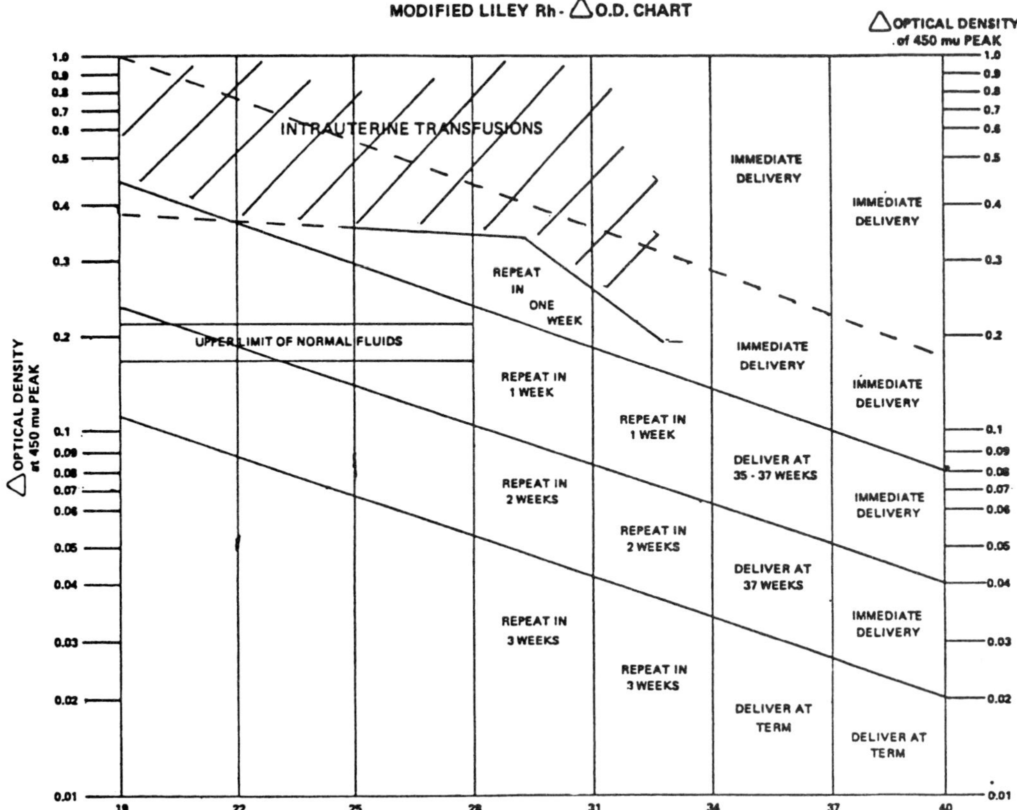


**FIGURE 10–1.** Liley graph used to assess severity of fetal hemolysis. *(From Liley AW: Liquor amnii analysis in management of pregnancy complicated by rhesus immunization. Am J Obstet Gynecol 82:1359, 1961.)*

the $\Delta OD_{450}$ value must be greater than 0.15 or less than 0.09 to be predictive of severe or mild disease, respectively, with a "gray zone" between the two values that is nonpredictive (Ananth and Queenan, 1989). Thus, the clinician must integrate clinical history and ultrasonography clues for possible impending hydrops or must consider fetal blood sampling in a fetus at risk between 18 and 25 weeks of gestation.

Amniocytes can be obtained at the amniocentesis, and through polymerase chain reaction (PCR) analysis, fetal D antigen typing can be obtained as early as 14 weeks (Dildy et al, 1996). This process allows the identification of the fetus at no risk for gestations in which the paternal status is heterozygous or unknown. Isoimmunization with atypical red blood cell antigens other than D can be detected similarly, reducing the amount of unnecessary invasive procedures on an otherwise unaffected fetus.

Direct ultrasound-guided fetal umbilical blood sampling provides valuable data for the fetus at risk, particularly after 18 weeks of gestation. Cordocentesis is used most often when the risk determined from history, indirect antibody titer values, Liley curve comparisons, or ultrasonographic clues are significant. It also provides vascular access if fetal transfusion becomes necessary. Although most obstetricians are skilled in amniocentesis, cordocentesis is usually performed in tertiary centers by perinatologists. The latter procedure carries a higher risk of fetal loss and morbidity and is associated with a more significant chance of worsening maternal sensitization (Bowman and Pollock, 1994).

## Therapy

Fetal transfusion therapy is the mainstay of treatment for the severely affected but premature fetus. In most centers, for pregnancies beyond 33 weeks of gestation with suspected fetal anemia, administration of steroids and delivery are preferable to an invasive procedure with significant morbidity and mortality. Intraperitoneal transfusions, the primary therapy in the past, are still a useful treatment. O-negative, tightly packed, irradiated blood is percutaneously infused into the fetal peritoneal cavity via an amniocentesis needle with real-time ultrasound guidance. Approximately 10 mL is transfused for each week of gestation beyond 20 weeks. Red blood cell absorption occurs quite promptly through the subdiaphragmatic lymphatics, although it may be erratic in the hydropic fetus. Fetal survival rates approaching 100% for nonhydropic fetuses and 75% in hydropic fetuses have been reported (Harman et al, 1983). Problems associated with intraperitoneal transfusions include injury to vascular or intra-abdominal organs and the inability to obtain fetal blood type and blood count. This procedure should be avoided if at all possible in the hydropic fetus, because the resulting higher abdominal pressure may precipitate venous compression and lead to circulatory collapse.

Direct intravascular transfusions are now the first line of treatment. The advantages of this procedure include assessing the severity of fetal anemia and documenting the fetal blood type. Ultimate success does not appear to be affected by the presence of hydrops (Ney et al, 1991). The overall success rate is about 85%. Limitations are usually procedure related. The most accessible site usually requires an anterior placenta, in which the cord root can be visualized; posterior placentation makes the technique more difficult. Also, risks include bleeding from the cord puncture site, fetal exsanguination, cord hematoma, rupture of membranes, and chorioamnionitis.

Further transfusions are required every 2 to 3 weeks to compensate for the falling hematocrit associated with fetal growth, the finite life of the transfused red blood cells, and ongoing hemolysis of the existing fetal erythrocytes. Ultimately, the entire fetal blood supply is replaced with Rh-negative blood by successive transfusions. A major neonatal side effect is bone marrow depression, which typically peaks at 3 to 6 weeks after birth.

As the pregnancy proceeds through the third trimester, frequent fetal testing is carried out either with nonstress tests and amniotic fluid index or with biophysical profiles. Delivery is planned for 3 to 6 weeks before term, usually after demonstration of a mature fetal lung profile. Preterm delivery may be indicated in the severely affected fetus, regardless of lung profile, if the risk of transfusion is deemed to exceed the morbidity of a delivery of a near-term yet premature baby.

## CANCER

### Principles

Cancer complicating pregnancy is rare, with an estimated frequency of 1 case per 1000 live births. The trend of delaying child-bearing to later maternal age may have influenced this rate. The sites or types of cancer in pregnancy, in descending order of frequency, are cervical, breast, ovarian, lymphoma, melanoma, brain, and leukemia (Haas, 1984; Jacob and Stringer, 1990) (Table 10–5). Finding a malignancy during gestation poses a unique set of issues that must be addressed with care. Will the pregnancy accelerate the malignant process? Are the accepted therapies appropriate for the gravida, and are they safe for the unborn fetus? Will delay of therapy adversely affect the mother? Should the pregnancy be terminated, or should the child be delivered prematurely so as to maximize treatment of the mother with no resultant risk to the child?

**TABLE 10–5**

**Cancers That Commonly Complicate Pregnancy**

| Site/Type | Cases per 1000 Pregnancies |
|---|---|
| Cervix | 0.8 |
| Breast | 0.3 |
| Melanoma | 0.2 |
| Ovary | 0.05 |
| Thyroid | <0.05 |
| Colorectal | 0.02 |
| Leukemia | 0.01 |
| Lymphoma | 0.01 |

Data from Jacob JH, Stringer AC: Diagnosis and management of cancer during pregnancy. Semin Perinatol 14:79-87, 1990.

Few conditions in pregnancy require as meticulous a multidisciplinary approach as cancer. Oncologists who are unaccustomed to interacting with a pregnant woman commonly wish to have the child delivered before giving definitive cancer therapy, for fear of the teratogenic risks to the fetus. Therefore, input regarding the situation must be acquired not only from an oncologist but also from the obstetrician, perinatologist, pediatrician, neonatologist, and dysmorphologist. The patient and her family must be involved in decision-making, being given information not only about the risks of the disease and its potential therapies but also about the limitations of current knowledge about cancer in pregnancy and the uncertainties of outcomes.

### Surgery in Pregnancy

Patients may undergo indicated surgery during pregnancy safely. The risk of fetal loss does not seem to rise with uncomplicated anesthesia and surgery. However, if there are any complications in either the anesthesia or the operation, the risk of not only fetal but also maternal mortality increases. For example, fetal loss is rarely related temporally to maternal appendectomy but is common when the mother's appendix has ruptured. The most comprehensive series of pregnant patients undergoing surgery was collected in Sweden (Mazze and Kallen, 1989). Although these researchers found a slight increase in rates of low birth weight and neonatal death by 7 days of life, the rates of stillbirth and congenital malformation were similar to the outcomes expected without surgery. Anesthetic agents are not believed to teratogenic.

A few management guidelines help optimize outcome for the pregnant patient undergoing surgery,. If general anesthesia is used, the maternal airway must be protected to avoid aspiration. Gastrointestinal motility is reduced during pregnancy, and even many after hours without eating, the stomach may contain significant residual contents. A left lateral decubitus position on the operating table is preferred in to maximize uteroplacental blood flow. If the fetus is viable, monitoring of the fetal heart rate should be performed to assist the anesthesia team in optimizing fetal status. Preoperative counseling of the patient is important to allow the surgical team to make appropriate choices with regard to any interventions for fetal distress.

### Chemotherapy

Administering agents that impair cell division in pregnancy is a concern for both the mother and the care team. Often the patient is more concerned about this issue than about the underlying cancer. Cytotoxic chemotherapy should be avoided in the first trimester due to the high incidence of spontaneous abortion and the potential teratogenic effects on the fetus (Table 10–6). For a few agents with confirmed teratogenic effects, such as methotrexate, amethopterin, and chlorambucil, chemotherapy must be avoided during organogenesis. The use of folic acid antagonists in first-trimester cancer treatment raises the specific problem of possible induction of neural tube defects, because these lesions are known to be folate sensitive.

The literature regarding most other chemotherapeutic agents is limited, consisting of a few collected series. Therefore, use of these agents should be cautious, their potential harm to the fetus balanced against their benefit to the maternal condition. Little is also known regarding the long-term outcomes of fetuses exposed to chemotherapeutic agents in utero. The National Cancer Institute in Bethesda, Maryland, maintains a registry in hopes of determining the delayed effects. Small series of fetuses exposed to chemotherapeutic agents for acute leukemia revealed normal mental development with follow-up between 4 and 22 years (Aviles and Niz, 1988).

**TABLE 10–6**

**Common Chemotherapy Agents and Uses**

| Class/Drug | Risk Category | Common Uses |
|---|---|---|
| **Alkylating Agents** | | |
| Busulfan | D | Leukemias |
| Chlorambucil | D | Lymphomas, leukemias |
| Cyclophosphamide | D | Breast, ovary, lymphomas, leukemias |
| Melphalan | D | Ovary, leukemia, myeloma |
| Procarbazine | D | Lymphomas |
| **Antimetabolites** | | |
| 5-Fluorouracil | D | Breast, gastrointestinal |
| 6-Mercaptopurine | D | Leukemias |
| Methotrexate | D | Trophoblastic disease, lymphomas, leukemias, breast |
| 6-Thioguanine | D | Leukemias |
| **Antibiotics** | | |
| Bleomycin | D | Cervix, lymphomas |
| Daunorubicin | D | Leukemias |
| Doxorubicin | D | Leukemias, lymphomas, breast |
| **Other Agents** | | |
| All-trans-retinoic acid | X | Leukemias |
| L-Asparaginase | C | Leukemias |
| Cisplatin | D | Ovary, cervix, sarcoma |
| Hydroxyurea | D | Leukemias |
| Prednisone | B | Lymphomas, leukemias, breast |
| Tamoxifen | D | Breast, uterus |
| Taxol | D | Breast, ovarian |
| Vinblastine | D | Breast, lymphomas, choriocarcinoma |
| Vincristine | D | Leukemias, lymphomas |

Data from Cunningham FG, MacDonald PC, Gant NF, et al: Neoplastic diseases. In Williams Obstetrics, 20th ed. Stamford, CT, Appleton & Lange, 1997, pp 1281-1296.

The risk of teratogenicity does not appear to be higher with combination chemotherapy than with single-agent therapy (Doll et al, 1989). Studies performed so far involve small numbers of patients, with power insufficient to show a statistic difference, but there seems not even to be a trend. Low birth weight is found in approximately 40% of babies whose mothers received cytotoxic drugs during pregnancy (Nicholson, 1968). Theoretical consequences, such as bone marrow suppression, immune suppression, and anemia, could occur in the fetus, and timing of chemotherapy should take the anticipated date of delivery into account. Data regarding safety for the breast-feeding neonate of a mother receiving cancer chemotherapy are limited, and for this reason, the majority of agents are contraindicated in the nursing mother.

### Radiation Therapy

The deleterious effects of irradiation on the fetus have been both theorized and actual. Fortunately, the amount of concern about the former far exceeds the incidence of the latter. Irradiation promotes genetic damage and thus the potential for congenital malformations. The risk depends on both dose and time. Less than 5 rad is believed to be of little consequence (Brent, 1989). If radiation exposure occurs before implantation, the adverse outcomes are usually a small increase in miscarriage.

The major concern is high-dose radiation (>10 rad) received during the period of organogenesis (embryonic weeks 1 to 10). The central nervous system is the most radiation-sensitive organ, and the complications most often observed are microcephaly and mental retardation. Cataracts and retinal degeneration are also seen. After organogenesis is complete, there is still a risk of central nervous system abnormalities. However, the sequelae most often seen are skin changes and anemia. Because of the highly variable, yet potentially grave consequences of irradiation of greater than 10 rad, patients should be counseled accordingly and termination of pregnancy should be offered as an alternative if exposure has occurred in the previable period (Orr and Shingleton, 1983).

There are several other considerations for a pregnant woman undergoing radiation therapy. First, the dose used in estimating risk should be the amount that the fetus actually receives. For example, axillary or neck irradiation for lymphoma involves a lower direct fetal exposure than direct pelvic irradiation for cervical cancer. The latter treatment, if given in the second trimester, will likely cause fetal demise. Second, the magnitude of radiation scatter to the pelvis must be considered. External shielding does not prevent internal reflection of the ion beam. Third, the advancing size of the uterus actually increases the amount of radiation exposure of the fetus because of the closer proximity of the nonpelvic irradiation. Therefore, an 8-week fetus may actually receive a smaller radiation dose from supraclavicular irradiation than a 30-week fetus. Fourth, will the fetus concentrate the radiation, and therefore increase its dosage? This is exemplified by the use of radioactive iodine ($^{131}I$) for maternal thyroid conditions. The actual rad dosage is markedly higher in the fetus because the fetal thyroid concentrates the iodine.

**TABLE 10–7**

**Estimated Radiation Dose to the Pelvis From Common Radiologic Procedures**

| Procedure | Pelvic Dose (millirads) |
|---|---|
| Chest x-ray | 8 |
| Abdominal series | 289 |
| Lumbar spine series | 275 |
| X-ray pelvimetry | 40 |
| Intravenous pyelogram | 407 |
| Barium enema (x-ray + fluoroscopy) | 805 |
| Upper gastrointestinal series (x-ray + fluoroscopy) | 558 |

Data from Pentel RL, Brown ML: Genetically significant dose to the United States population from diagnostic medical roentgenology. Radiology 90:209-216, 1968.

Diagnostic tests such as radiography may also be associated with radiation exposure for the fetus (Table 10–7). The doses involved are usually much smaller than those used for cancer therapy. Nonetheless, the practitioner should limit the amount of radiographic testing if at all possible. Inadvertent imaging of a patient who is not known to be pregnant continues to occur despite sensitive pregnancy tests, creating significant concerns. Indicated radiographs should never be withheld because of pregnancy, but lead shielding of the maternal abdomen and careful selection of the type of study should be performed to minimize the pelvic dose. Usually the amount of fetal exposure is well less than 5 rad, with no significantly greater risk of malformations. There does appear to be a slightly higher incidence of childhood leukemia, even with low-dose irradiation.

## Cervical Cancer

Cervical cancer is the most common malignancy found in pregnancy. The incidence is approximately 1 in 2500 gestations. A Papanicolaou ("Pap") smear should be obtained in all patients at their first prenatal visit. However, about 30% of cervical cancers can be associated with negative cytologic smear results. Although the evaluation for an abnormal Pap smear result should not be altered because of pregnancy, many physicians are reluctant for fear of cervical hemorrhage. Cervical biopsy remains the mainstay of diagnosis. The greater vascularity of the cervix during pregnancy predisposes to bleeding. An experienced colposcopist may be able to defer actual biopsy in cases of suspected visual findings of a noninvasive process. However, if cancerous invasion is suspected or the physician is uncertain of the visual findings, biopsy is necessary (Table 10–8). If microinvasive disease is confirmed by biopsy, cone biopsy is required to rule out frankly invasive disease. This procedure is undertaken with caution during pregnancy, because of the associated high rate of bleeding complications and miscarriage. Cervical conization may raise the risk of incompetence or preterm labor. The assistance of a gynecologic oncologist is preferred, given these unique sets of potential consequences. A shallow cone biopsy will reduce the risk of subsequent cervical weakness.

The therapy for invasive cervical cancer is based on the stage of disease and the gestational age of the fetus (Table 10–9). In most cases, delay of definitive therapy by 4 to 14 weeks may be acceptable. Pregnancy does not seem to accelerate the growth of the tumor. However, patient counseling is important. In the extremely previable gestation, the likelihood of achieving a safe gestational age for the fetus without worsening the stage or spread of the cancer in the mother must be balanced against parental desires based on ethical or religious beliefs. Conversely, it appears reasonable to delay definitive therapy until a time in pregnancy when delivery would not likely result in a handicapped infant.

## Breast Cancer

Breast cancer is the most common malignancy of women, with approximately 1 of every 10 women affected in their lifetimes. The incidence of breast cancer in pregnancy is estimated to be 10 to 30 per 100,000 pregnancies (Isaacs, 1995). Pregnancy does not seem to influence the actual course of the disease. However, there appears to be a higher risk of delay in diagnosis and a trend towards more advanced stages at diagnosis in pregnant women than in nonpregnant controls.

The diagnostic procedures for breast cancer should not be altered during pregnancy. Any suspicious mass should

**TABLE 10–8**

**Management of Cervical Abnormalities**

| Papanicolaou Test Result | Colposcopy/Biopsy Result | Management |
|---|---|---|
| Cervical intraepithelial neoplasia | Cervical intraepithelial neoplasia | Defer further evaluation and therapy until 6 weeks after delivery |
| Invasive cancer | Cervical intraepithelial neoplasia | Cone biopsy* |
| | Microinvasive cancer | Cone biopsy* |
| | Invasive cancer | Radical hysterectomy or radiotherapy |

*Proceed to radical hysterectomy or radiotherapy if invasive cancer is confirmed.

Data from Berman ML, Di Saia PJ, Brewster WR: Pelvic malignancies, gestational trophoblastic neoplasia and nonpelvic malignancies. In Creasy RK, Resnik R (eds): Maternal-Fetal Medicine, 4th ed. Philadelphia, WB Saunders, 1999, pp 1128-1150.

**TABLE 10-9**

**Treatment Options for Cervical Cancer in Pregnancy**

| Gestational Age | Stage I to IIa | Stage IIb to IIIb |
|---|---|---|
| <20 weeks | 4500 cGy<br>Wide pelvic irradiation<br>If no abortion: modified radical hysterectomy<br>If spontaneous abortion: brachytherapy<br>*or*<br>radical hysterectomy with lymphadenectomy | 5000 cGy<br>Wide pelvic irradiation<br>If no abortion: type II radical hysterectomy<br>If spontaneous abortion: brachytherapy<br>*or*<br>cesarean section at fetal viability<br>Subsequent wide pelvic radiation (±5000 cGy) and brachytherapy (±5000 cGY) |
| >20 weeks | Cesarean section at fetal viability<br>Subsequent wide pelvic radiation (5000 cGy) and brachytherapy (5000 cGy) *or* cesarean radical hysterectomy with lymphadenectomy | Cesarean section at fetal viability<br>Subsequent wide pelvic radiation (±5000 cGy) and brachytherapy (±5000 cGY) |

Data from Berman ML, Di Saia PJ, Brewster WR: Pelvic malignancies, gestational trophoblastic neoplasia and nonpelvic malignancies. In Creasy RK, Resnik R (eds): Maternal-Fetal Medicine, 4th ed. Philadelphia, WB Saunders, 1999, pp 1128-1150.

undergo biopsy. Mammography, although discouraged for routine screening in pregnancy, may be safely employed if indicated. The amount of radiation is negligible, approximately 0.01 cGy (Liberman et al, 1994). Metastatic evaluation may be hampered somewhat because of a reluctance to use bone and liver scans during pregnancy. However, magnetic resonance imaging appears to be a reasonable alternative.

Surgical therapy for breast cancer should not be delayed because of pregnancy. The risks of mastectomy and axillary node dissection appear very low (Isaacs, 1995). Radiation therapy is usually not recommended during pregnancy because of the risk of scatter. If the pregnancy is to continue and the patient has "positive" lymph nodes, adjuvant chemotherapy is often given. The timing of delivery should take into account the following factors:

- When would the fetus have a reasonable chance for survival with a low risk of severe permanent morbidity?
- Can the number of cycles of chemotherapy be minimized with an earlier delivery? Also, avoiding delivery just before or just after administration of chemotherapy is important to reduce the risk of immunosuppression and infection.
- How long could radiotherapy be delayed without increasing the risk of metastatic spread of the tumor?

About 10% of women treated for breast cancer become pregnant, the majority within 5 years of diagnosis. Small series suggest that pregnancy does not influence the rate of recurrences or of distant metastasis (Dow et al, 1994). However, women should be encouraged to delay childbearing for at least 2 to 3 years, the time of the highest rate of recurrence. Breast-feeding may be possible in women who have undergone conservative breast cancer surgery.

## Ovarian Cancer

Most ovarian cancer occurs in women older than 35 years. Because later child-bearing has been more widely accepted, it would not be surprising for the rate of ovarian cancer as well as other cancers during pregnancy to increase. However, the current estimate of actual ovarian malignancies in pregnancy is quite low, estimated at 1 in 25,000 deliveries (Jacob and Stringer, 1990). Although most ovarian cancers are epithelial in origin, borderline epithelial and germ cell tumors are more common in pregnancy.

The widespread use of ultrasonography, particularly in the first two trimesters, has been helpful in identifying adnexal masses. Fortunately, most are benign functional cysts. Actual malignancy is rare, estimated at 5% of the ovarian masses found. In the nonpregnant female, the risk is higher, approaching 15% to 20%. Surgery for a suspected ovarian mass occurs in about 1 per 1000 pregnancies. Most procedures are performed not for suspected malignancy, but rather because of concern about torsion and rupture. The maximal times of risk of these events are at the end of the first trimester, when the uterus elevates beyond the true pelvis, and at the time of delivery. The characterization of an ovarian process can be aided by ultrasonography as well as magnetic resonance imaging, but these modalities are not definitive. Although the patient can gain some reassurance that an ovarian cyst, particularly if it is simple in nature, is very likely not malignant, she must be cautioned that histologic diagnosis is more definitive. Any complex mass or persistent simple cyst 6 cm or larger should undergo surgical exploration and removal. The optimal time for laparotomy is in the second trimester. At that time, there is minimal interference from the gravid uterus and less of a risk of fetal loss, and the theoretical concerns of teratogenic exposure to anesthetic agents are avoided. Some patients opt for more conservative management. They should be counseled that they have a 40% chance of needing urgent intervention with either surgery or percutaneous drainage (Platek et al, 1995).

If a malignancy is confirmed at the time of laparotomy, treatment and staging are no different from those in the nonpregnant woman. Frozen-section diagnosis, peritoneal washings, omentectomy, and subdiaphragmatic biopsy are performed. Depending on the cell type and the stage, treatment may range from removal of the affected adnexa to complete hysterectomy and bilateral oophorectomy. Chemotherapy may be given during pregnancy if necessary.

Fortunately, most cancers found in pregnant women are usually of a lower stage and a lesser malignant potential than those found in nonpregnant women.

## MENTAL DISORDERS

Pregnancy can be a stressful process. At times, it may induce a psychotic event. Women experiencing a mental disorder during pregnancy who have no history of a mood disorder usually present with a milder constellation of symptoms. Serious disorders such as mania and schizophrenia that are antecedent to pregnancy may not be so benign. In women with all types of mental illness as well as in previously nonaffected women, the postpartum state is a time of greater maternal risk. Ten percent to 15% of newly delivered women experience a depressive disorder (Weissman and Olfson, 1995). Women with preexisting mental illness have a higher recurrence risk in the puerperium. Patients presenting with suspected mental illness should be assessed for substance abuse and thyroid dysfunction. A multidisciplinary approach is advantageous. If the patient's mental competency is an issue, the caregiver should obtain legal assistance so as to be able to make medical decisions for the patient.

### Depression

One of every eight individuals suffers from a depressive disorder during his or her lifetime. Women appear to have an increased risk. However, less than one fourth of depressed women are appropriately treated (American College of Obstetricians and Gynecologists, 1993). The diagnosis of depression requires the presence of at least five of the following symptoms for a 2-week period:

- Depressed mood
- Diminished pleasure in most activities
- Weight loss or gain, or alterations of appetite
- Sleep abnormalities
- Psychomotor retardation or agitation
- Fatigue
- Feelings of worthlessness or guilt
- Diminished ability to concentrate
- Thoughts of suicide

These symptoms are associated with significant distress or impairment in all areas of functioning. They are symptoms of depression only if they are not related to a medical or substance abuse condition and are not associated with a recent (2 months) loss of a loved one (Mood disorders, 2000). If the onset is within 3 to 6 months after delivery, postpartum depression is diagnosed.

The predisposing risk factors for depression include early childhood loss, physical or sexual abuse, socioeconomic deprivation, genetic predisposition, and lifestyle stress due to multiple roles (McGrath et al, 1990), These factors may exaggerate or prolong symptoms and, if not addressed, can lengthen the duration of depression. The obstetrician must be aware that life events such as miscarriage, infertility, and complicated pregnancy in patients with risk factors are likely to precipitate depression, and must maintain a low threshold for diagnosis and treatment of mood alterations in such patients. Alternatively, perinatal loss experienced by a woman without predisposing risk factors will probably lead to a grief reaction or adjustment disorder, which may be misdiagnosed as depression.

Chronic medical conditions that are associated with a high prevalence of depression and may occur in women of child-bearing age include renal failure, cancer, acquired immunodeficiency syndrome (AIDS), and chronic fatigue or pain. Antihypertensives, hormones, anticonvulsants, steroids, chemotherapeutics, and antibiotics can cause depression. Alcoholism and substance abuse may manifest as depression. Underlying personality disorders complicate the diagnosis of depression, not only by confusing the clinical situation but also secondary to many physicians' avoidance of patients suffering from the disorders.

Therapeutic interventions for depression include psychotherapy and medication. Electroconvulsive therapy has been shown to be an effective and relatively safe treatment in refractory cases (Rabheru, 2001). Treatment of depression is effective in about 70% of cases. Supportive treatment alone is rarely effective in major depressive episodes. Most antidepressant medications currently prescribed during pregnancy are serotonin reuptake inhibitors (SSRIs). Fluoxetine, paroxetine, and sertraline are class Bm according to the manufacturer (Briggs et al, 1998). SSRIs have the advantage over the tricyclic antidepressants in not causing orthostatic hypotension. Unfortunately, although limited series suggest that the SSRIs are relatively safe, little is known about long-term consequences for children exposed to them in utero (Altshuler et al, 1996; Chambers et al, 1996; Karasu et al, 2000). Currently, there is no consensus regarding use of SSRIs during breast-feeding. Although data suggests minimal passage of SSRI medications into the breast milk, the long-term side effects are currently listed as "unknown" (Briggs et al, 1998; Buist and Norman, 2000). The theoretical concerns are that such drugs may affect the developing central nervous system of the newborn and that abnormalities may not be readily apparent in the short term. Therefore, SSRIs should be prescribed for a nursing mother only if the benefit clearly exceeds the risk and after the patient has been counseled regarding the potential yet currently ill-defined risks. Given the current medical knowledge, bottle-feeding should be offered as an acceptable alternative if antidepressants must be used.

### Postpartum Psychosis

A severe disorder, postpartum psychosis is fortunately rare, occurring 1 to 4 per 1000 births (Weissman and Olfson, 1995). This condition is more worrisome than postpartum depression because of the patient's inability to discern reality and the periods of delirium. Patients at risk for postpartum psychosis may have underlying depression, mania, or schizophrenia. Other risks are younger age and family history. The recurrence rate is approximately 25%. The peak onset of symptoms is between 10 and 14 days after delivery. Recognition of this disorder is extremely important to the protection of the patient and her family.

## Schizophrenia

Schizophrenia is fairly common, with a prevalence of 1% (Myers et al, 1984). It is associated with delusions, hallucinations, and incoherence. Morbidity due to this mental illness is higher than that due to any other. There appears to be a genetic component to the etiology; schizophrenia develops in about 10% of offspring of an affected person. Concordance of schizophrenia in identical twins reaches 65%. There is some speculation and controversy as to whether low birth weight (Smith et al, 2001) and obstetric complications (Kendell et al, 2000) are associated with a higher rate of schizophrenia.

Because the peak age of incidence is around 20 years and females are more affected than males, it is unrealistic to assume that obstetricians will never encounter patients with schizophrenia. There appear to be higher rates of cesarean section and surgical vaginal delivery in affected patients (Bennedsen et al, 2001b). Children of women with schizophrenia may have a higher rate of sudden infant death syndrome and congenital malformations (Bennedsen et al, 2001a). However, it is difficult to ascertain whether these risks are independent of other factors, such as smoking, poor socioeconomic status, and use of certain medications.

Treatment is primarily achieved through the use of psychotropic medication. The potential for teratogenesis appears low with the older-generation medications in the phenothiazine class, but most data for this issue were derived from the use of lower doses given to patients with hyperemesis gravidarum. Antipsychotic medication does cross the placenta. Current recommendations include avoidance of their use in the first trimester if possible, the use of lower doses or higher-potency alternatives, and cessation of medication 5 to 10 days before delivery (Herz et al, 2000). The use of antipsychotics in breast-feeding is associated with an unknown risk (Briggs et al, 1998).

Lithium, used primarily in mania, is associated with a higher rate of Ebstein anomaly. Although the incidence of this consequence is low, either discontinuing the medication in the first trimester or continuing its use with careful counseling is a viable alternative. Fetal echocardiography should be performed in women who have used lithium in early pregnancy.

## SELECTED READING

Berman ML, Di Saia PJ, Brewster WR: Pelvic malignancies, gestational trophoblastic neoplasia and nonpelvic malignancies. In Creasy RK, Resnik R (eds): Maternal-Fetal Medicine, 4th ed. Philadelphia, WB Saunders, 1999, pp 1128-1150.

## REFERENCES

Ananth U, Queenan JT: Does midtrimester $\Delta OD_{450}$ of amniotic fluid reflect severity of Rh disease? Am J Obstet Gynecol 161:47-49, 1989.

American College of Obstetricians and Gynecologists: Depression in Women. Technical Bulletin No. 182. 1993.

Atshuler LL, Cohen L, Szuba MP, et al: Pharmacologic management of psychiatric illness during pregnancy: Dilemmas and guidelines. Am J Psychiatry 153:592-606, 1996.

Aviles A, Niz J: Long-term follow-up of children born to mothers with acute leukemia during pregnancy. Med Pediatr Oncol 16:3, 1988.

Bahado-Singh R, Oz U, Mari G, et al: Fetal splenic size in anemia due to Rh-alloimmunization. Obstet Gynecol 92:828-832, 1998.

Bennedsen BE, Mortensen PB, Olesen AV, Henriksen TB: Congenital malformations, stillbirths and infant deaths among children of women with schizophrenia. Arch Gen Psychiatry 58:674-679, 2001a.

Bennedsen BE, Mortensen PB, Olesen AV, et al: Obstetric complications in women with schizophrenia. Schizophrenia Res 47:167-175, 2001b.

Bjerkedal T: Outcome of pregnancy in women with epilepsy, Norway, 1966 to 1978: Congenital malformations. In Janz D, Dam M, Richens A (eds): Epilepsy, pregnancy, and the child. New York, Raven Press, 1982, p 289.

Bowman JM, Pollock JM: Fetomaternal hemorrhage following funipuncture: Increase in severity of maternal red-cell alloimmunization. Obstet Gynecol 84:839, 1994.

Bowman JM, Pollock JM, Penston LE: Fetomaternal transplacental hemorrhage during pregnancy and after delivery. Vox Sang 51:117-143, 1986.

Brent RC: The effect of embryonic and fetal exposure to x-ray, microwaves, and ultrasound: Counseling the pregnant and non-pregnant patient about these risks. Semin Oncol 16: 347-368, 1989.

Briggs GC, Freeman RK, Yaffe SJ: Drugs in Pregnancy and Lactation, 5th edition. Baltimore, Williams & Wilkins, 1998.

Buehler BA, Delimont D, van Waes M, Finnell RH: Prenatal prediction of risk of the fetal hydantoin syndrome. N Engl J Med 322:1567-1572, 1990.

Buist DS, Norman TR: Antidepressants and breast-feeding: A review of the literature. Paediatr Drugs 2:183-192, 2000.

Chambers CD, Johnson KA, Dick LM, et al: Birth outcomes in pregnant women taking fluoxetine. N Engl J Med 335: 1010-1015, 1996.

Dildy GA, Jackson GM, Ward K: Determination of fetal RhD status from uncultured amniocytes. Obstet Gynecol 88:207-210, 1996.

Doll DC, Ringenberg S, Yarbro JW: Antineoplastic agents and cancer. Semin Oncol 16:337-346, 1989.

Dow KH, Harris JR, Roy C: Pregnancy after breast-conserving surgery and radiation therapy for breast cancer. Monogr Natl Cancer Inst 16:131, 1994.

Friis ML, Hauge M: Congenital heart defects in liveborn children of epileptic patients. Arch Neurol 42:374-376, 1985.

Friis ML, Holm NV, Sindrop EH: Facial clefts in sibs and children of epileptic patients. Neurology 30:346-351, 1986.

Haas JF: Pregnancy in association with a newly diagnosed cancer: A population based epidemiologic assessment. Int J Cancer 1984; 34:229-235.

Harman CR, Manning FA, Bowman JM, Lange IR: Severe Rh disease: Poor outcome is not inevitable. Am J Obstet Gynecol 145:823-829, 1983.

Herz MI, Liberman RP, Liberman JA, et al: Treatment of patients with schizophrenia. In Practice Guidelines for the Treatment of Psychiatric Disorders: Compendium. Washington, DC, American Psychiatric Association, 2000, pp 299-411.

Isaacs JH: Cancer of the breast in pregnancy. Surg Clin North Am 75:47-51, 1995.

Iskarios J, Kingdom J, Morrison J, Rodeck CH: Prospective non-invasive monitoring of pregnancies complicated by red cell alloimmunization. Ultrasound Obstet Gynecol 11:432-437, 1998.

Jacob JH, Stringer AC: Diagnosis and management of cancer during pregnancy. Semin Perinatol 14:79-87, 1990.

Karasu TB, Gelenberg A, Merriam A, Wang P: Practice guideline for the treatment of patients with major depressive disorder. In Practice Guidelines for the Treatment of Psychiatric

Disorders: Compendium. Washington, DC, American Psychiatric Association, 2000, pp 413-495.

Kendell RE, McInneny K, Juszczak E, Bain M: Obstetric complications and schizophrenia: Two case-control studies based on structured obstetric records. Br J Psychiatry 176:516-522, 2000.

Lammer EJ, Sever LE, Oakley GP: Teratogen update: Valproic acid. Teratology 35:465-473, 1987.

Landsteiner K, Weiner AS: An agglutinable factor in human blood recognized by immune sera for rhesus blood. Proc Soc Exper Biol Med 43:223, 1940.

Levine P: Isoimmunization in pregnancy and the pathogenesis of erythroblastosis fetalis. In Karsner HT, Hooker SB (eds): 1941 Yearbook of Pathology and Immunology. Chicago, Yearbook Publishers, 1941, p 505.

Lewis M, Kaita H, Chown B: The inheritance of the Rh blood groups: Frequencies in 1000 unrelated Caucasian families consisting of 2000 parents and 2806 children. Vox Sang 20: 502-508, 1971.

Liberman L, Giess CS, Dershaw DD, et al: Imaging of pregnancy-associated breast cancer. Radiology 191:245, 1994.

Liley AW: Liquor amnii analysis in management of pregnancy complicated by rhesus immunization. Am J Obstet Gynecol 82:1359-1370, 1961.

Mari G: Noninvasive diagnosis by Doppler ultrasonography of fetal anemia due to maternal red-cell alloimmunization. N Engl J Med 342:9-14, 2000.

Mazze RI, Kallen B: Reproductive outcome after anesthesia and operation during pregnancy: A registry study of 5405 cases. Obstet Gynecol 161:1178, 1989.

McGrath E, Ketia GP, Strickland BR, Russo NF: Women and Depression: Risk Factors and Treatment Issues. Washington, DC, American Psychological Association, 1990.

Mood disorders. In American Psychiatric Association: Diagnosis and Statistical Manual of Mental Disorders, 4th ed, Text Revision. Washington, DC, American Psychiatric Association, 2000, pp 345-428.

Myers JK, Weissman MM, Tischler GL, et al: Six month prevalence of psychiatric disorders in three communities. Arch Gen Psychiatry 41:959, 1984.

Nelson KB, Ellenberg JH: Maternal seizure disorder, outcome of pregnancy, and neurologic abnormalities in the children. Neurology 32:1247-1254, 1982.

Ney JA, Socol ML, Dooley SN, et al: Perinatal outcome following intravascular transfusion in severely isoimmunized fetuses. Int J Gynaecol Obstet 35:41-46, 1991.

Nicholson HD: Cytotoxic drugs in pregnancy. J Obstet Gynecol Br Commonw 75:307-312, 1968.

Orr JW, Shingleton HM: Cancer in pregnancy. Curr Prob Cancer 8:1-50, 1983.

Pentel RL, Brown ML: Genetically significant dose to the United States population from diagnostic medical roentgenology. Radiology 90:209-216, 1968.

Platek DN, Henderson CE, Goldber GL: The management of a persistent adnexal mass in pregnancy. Am J Obstet Gynecol 173:1236-1240, 1995.

Queenan JT, Tomai TP, Ural SH, King JC: Deviation in amniotic fluid optical density at a wavelength of 450 nm in Rh isoimmunized pregnancies from 14 to 40 weeks gestation: A proposal for clinical management. Am J Obstet Gynecol 168:1370-1376, 1993.

Rabheru K: The use of electroconvulsive therapy in special patient populations. Can J Psychiatry 46:710-719, 2001.

Schmidt D, Canger R, Avanzini G, et al: Change of seizure frequency in pregnant epileptic women. J Neurol Neurosurg Psychiatry 46:751-755, 1983.

Smith GN, Flynn SW, McCarthy N, et al: Low birthweight in schizophrenia: Prematurity or poor fetal growth? Schizophrenia Res 47:177-184, 2001.

Vintzileos AM, Campbell WA, Storlazzi E, et al: Fetal liver ultrasound measurement in isoimmunized pregnancies. Obstet Gynecol 68:162-167, 1986.

Weissman MM, Olfson M: Depression in women: Implications for health care research. Science 269:799, 1995.

Wilhelm J, Morris D, Hotham N: Epilepsy and pregnancy: A review of 98 pregnancies. Aust N Z J Obstet Gynaecol 30: 290-295, 1990.

Yerby MS: The use of anticonvulsants during pregnancy. Semin Perinatol 25:153-158, 2001.

CHAPTER

# 11

# Hypertensive Complications of Pregnancy

Andrew D. Hull and Thomas R. Moore

Hypertension is the most common medical problem in pregnancy, affecting 10% to 15% of all women. The second most common cause of maternal mortality after thromboembolic disease, hypertension accounts for almost 18% of maternal deaths in the United States (Koonin et al, 1997). Complications arising from hypertensive disorders have profound effects on the fetus and neonate and thus are a major source of perinatal mortality and morbidity. Preeclampsia is the primary cause of iatrogenic prematurity.

## CLASSIFICATION OF HYPERTENSIVE DISORDERS OF PREGNANCY

Any discussion of hypertension and pregnancy must begin with a set of definitions. Although many classifications are in use worldwide, perhaps one of the more useful is that of the National High Blood Pressure Education Program Working Group on High Blood Pressure in Pregnancy (Report, 2000) (Table 11–1). Although this classification scheme appears to be somewhat pedantic, it is of paramount importance because pregnancy outcome varies according to the type of hypertension involved. For practical purposes, hypertension in pregnancy may be divided into the following categories: chronic hypertension, gestational hypertension, and preeclampsia.

*Hypertension* is defined as a blood pressure of 140 mm Hg or higher systolic or 90 mm Hg or higher diastolic measured on two separate occasions. Korotkoff phase V (disappearance of sound) is used rather than Korotkoff phase IV (muffling of sound) to define *diastolic pressure*, because Korotkoff IV is poorly reproducible in pregnancy. *Severe hypertension* arising from any cause is defined as a blood pressure of 160 to 180 mm Hg or higher systolic or 110 mm Hg or higher diastolic.

### Chronic Hypertension

Up to 5% of pregnant women have *chronic hypertension*, which is diagnosed when hypertension is present before pregnancy or recorded before 20 weeks of gestation. Typically, the patient with chronic hypertension has an elevated first-trimester blood pressure or is known to have hypertensive disease before her pregnancy begins. However, when hypertension is first noted in a patient after 20 weeks of gestation, it may be difficult to distinguish chronic hypertension from pregnancy-induced hypertension or preeclampsia. In such cases, the precise diagnosis may not be made until after delivery. Hypertension that is first diagnosed during the second half of pregnancy and persists more than 12 weeks postpartum is diagnosed as chronic hypertension.

Chronic hypertension has an adverse effect on pregnancy outcome. Women with the disorder are at higher risk for preterm delivery and placental abruption, and their fetuses for intrauterine growth restriction (IUGR) and demise (Ferrer et al, 2000). Superimposed preeclampsia complicates up to 50% of pregnancies in women with preexisting severe chronic hypertension (Sibai and Anderson, 1986) and may have a particularly early onset. The adverse effects on fetal and maternal perinatal outcomes are directly related to severity of the preexisting hypertension. When chronic hypertension is secondary to maternal renal disease, the risks of poor outcome are further increased, with up to a tenfold rise in fetal loss rate (Jungers et al, 1997). Women with untreated severe chronic hypertension are at increased risk of cardiovascular complications during pregnancy, including stroke (Brown and Whitworth, 1999).

The majority of cases of chronic hypertension seen in pregnancy are idiopathic (essential hypertension), but causes of secondary hypertension should always be sought because pregnancy outcome is worse in women with secondary hypertension. Renal disease (e.g., chronic renal failure, glomerulonephritis, renal artery stenosis), cardiovascular causes (coarctation of the aorta, Takayasu arteritis), and, rarely, Cushing disease, Conn syndrome, and pheochromocytoma should be excluded through physical examination, history, and more detailed testing if needed.

All patients with chronic hypertension should be evaluated periodically with serum urea, creatinine, and electrolyte measurements, urinalysis, and 24-hour urine collection for protein and creatinine clearance determinations. Typically, this assessment should be performed in each trimester and more frequently if the patient's condition deteriorates.

#### Antihypertensive Treatment of Chronic Hypertension in Pregnancy

Except in cases of severe hypertension, randomized trials have shown that antihypertensive treatment of chronic hypertension in pregnancy does not improve fetal outcome (Sibai and Anderson, 1986). Rates of preterm delivery, abruption, IUGR, and perinatal death are similar in treated and untreated women. Thus, treatment is usually reserved for patients whose hypertension places them at significant risk of stroke (blood pressure of 180 mm Hg or higher systolic or 110 mm Hg or higher diastolic). Patients with less severe hypertension who were taking medications before conception may be able to discontinue therapy with close surveillance. The risk of superimposed preeclampsia is not changed by antihypertensive therapy, so its development should be watched for carefully.

The choice of antihypertensive agent for use in pregnancy is governed by a desire to adjust blood pressure without having ill effects on the fetus. Because excessive lowering of maternal blood pressure below 140 mm Hg systolic or 90 mm Hg diastolic (140/90 mm Hg) can compromise uterine perfusion, with consequent slowing of

**TABLE 11-1**

**National High Blood Pressure Education Program Working Group on High Blood Pressure in Pregnancy Classification of Hypertensive Disorders of Pregnancy***

| | |
|---|---|
| Chronic hypertension | Hypertension present before pregnancy, *or* diagnosed before 20 wks of gestation, *or* diagnosed for the first time during pregnancy that persists postpartum |
| Gestational hypertension | *Transient* if blood pressure returns to normal by 12 wks after delivery and preeclampsia was not diagnosed before delivery<br>*Chronic* if blood pressure does not resolve by 12 wks after delivery |
| Preeclampsia-eclampsia | Usually occurs after 20 wks of gestation<br>Hypertension accompanied by proteinuria in a woman normotensive prior to 20 wks of gestation<br>Strongly suspected if nonproteinuric hypertension is accompanied by systemic symptoms such as headache, visual disturbance, abdominal pain, or laboratory abnormalities such as low platelet count and elevated liver enzyme values (HELLP [hemolysis, elevated liver enzymes, and low platelets] syndrome) |
| Preeclampsia superimposed on chronic hypertension | Preeclampsia occurring in a chronically hypertensive woman |

*Hypertension is defined as a blood pressure of ≥140 mm Hg systolic or ≥90 mm Hg diastolic.

Adapted from the Report of the National High Blood Pressure Education Program Working Group on High Blood Pressure in Pregnancy. Am J Obstet Gynecol 183:S1-S22, 2000.

fetal growth, fetal hypoxia, or both, the therapeutic goal is to maintain maternal pressures at 140 to 155 systolic and 90 to 105 diastolic. The drugs most commonly used in pregnancy are listed in Table 11–2.

Methyldopa is probably the most widely used drug in this setting. Obstetricians remain faithful to the use of this agent even though it has been largely abandoned by others, because of extensive clinical and research experience demonstrating its safety for both mother and fetus during pregnancy (Report, 2000). This agent does not impair uteroplacental perfusion and has a wide therapeutic margin before side effects are seen. However, methyldopa has the disadvantage of rather slow onset of action with prolonged time to therapeutic effect (days), and compliance with methyldopa therapy may be impeded by side effects such as sedation in some patients.

Labetalol is a mixed $alpha_1$-adrenergic and $beta_1$- and $beta_2$-adrenergic blocking agent. It is often used as an alternative to methyldopa or added as the second agent. Some pure beta-blockers have been associated with a significant increase in the risk of IUGR (e.g., atenolol), and the mixed adrenergic blockade produced by labetalol is thought to mitigate this unwanted effect (Pickles et al, 1989).

Calcium channel blockers (e.g., nifedipine) are used mainly as second-line drugs, usually in long-acting (extended-release) forms. Calcium channel blockers appear to be as effective as methyldopa and labetalol with minimal fetal side effects (Levin et al, 1994).

**TABLE 11-2**

**Drugs Commonly Used to Treat Chronic Hypertension in Pregnancy and Their Modes of Action**

| | |
|---|---|
| Methyldopa | Centrally acting antihypertensive |
| Labetalol | Mixed alpha- and beta-adrenergic blocker |
| Nifedipine | Calcium channel blocker |
| Hydralazine | Peripheral vasodilator |
| Prazosin | Alpha-blocker |

A potent peripheral vasodilator, hydralazine is often used as a first-line parenteral drug to treat acute hypertensive emergencies in pregnancy (blood pressure of >160/110 mm Hg). Its role as an oral agent in the management of chronic hypertension is limited to a second- or third-line choice. Long-term use of hydralazine may be associated with a lupus-like syndrome in some patients.

Prazosin has been used as a second- or third-line drug in pregnant women whose hypertension is difficult to control or is severe with an early onset. This agent appears to be similar in efficacy to nifedipine in such a setting (Hall et al, 2000).

Although diuretics are used extensively in hypertensive nonpregnant adults, there appears to be little role for them in the treatment of chronic hypertension. They have been alleged to reduce or prevent the normal plasma volume expansion seen in pregnancy (Sibai et al, 1984), an effect that theoretically might impede fetal growth, although the evidence for it is mixed. Most authorities restrict the use of diuretics to patients with a cardiac dysfunction or pulmonary edema.

Angiotensin-converting enzyme (ACE) inhibitors are not used in pregnancy. Their use in the second and third trimesters is associated with malformation of the fetal calvarium, fetal renal failure, oligohydramnios, pulmonary hypoplasia, and fetal and neonatal death (Buttar, 1997). These agents appear to be safe when taken in the first trimester (Steffensen et al, 1998), but a patient who conceives while taking an ACE inhibitor should be switched to a safer alternative as soon as possible. Similar precautions apply to the use of angiotensin receptor blockers in pregnancy.

### Antenatal Fetal Surveillance in Chronic Hypertension

As the third trimester progresses, patients with chronic hypertension are at growing risk of a slowing of fetal growth as well as superimposed preeclampsia. Antenatal surveillance in women with chronic hypertension should include careful screening for signs and symptoms of superadded preeclampsia, which constitutes the greatest perinatal risk. Fetal growth should be followed with serial ultrasonography evaluations (every 3 to 6 weeks). All patients should perform fetal kick counts from 28 weeks of gestation onward, and cases of suspected fetal growth impairment should be followed with nonstress tests as well as modified nonstress tests including an amniotic fluid index or biophysical profile determination. Although the optimum interval for these tests is controversial (every 3 to 7 days), and their role is unproven in the absence of fetal IUGR or other evidence of fetal compromise, most centers begin regular fetal biophysical testing at 32 to 34 weeks and continue until delivery.

Women with renal impairment and chronic hypertension have a markedly higher risk of poor perinatal outcome than normotensive women and women with hypertension without renal impairment. Additionally, moderate or severe renal disease (serum creatinine level ≥1.4 mg/dL) may accelerate the loss of renal function during pregnancy (Cunningham et al, 1990; Hou, 1999). Fetal growth is directly related to renal impairment, and women undergoing dialysis are at particular risk of fetal growth impairment, preterm delivery, and fetal death, even with optimal management. Those who start dialysis during pregnancy are at greatest risk, with only a 50% chance of a surviving infant (Hou, 1999).

## Gestational Hypertension

The diagnosis of gestational hypertension can be made with confidence only after delivery. It is defined as hypertension occurring in the second half of pregnancy in the absence of any other signs or symptoms of preeclampsia. Because a patient with what appears to be gestational hypertension at 36 weeks can finally evolve into full-blown preeclampsia at 39 weeks, the diagnosis of gestational hypertension should always evoke caution and vigilance. Only if the patient's blood pressure returns to normal postpartum without development of signs of preeclampsia should the final diagnosis of gestational hypertension be applied. During pregnancy, gestational hypertension is indistinguishable from preeclampsia-in-evolution. Thus, all patients with gestational hypertension should be regarded as being at risk for progression to preeclampsia.

The earlier gestational hypertension is evident, the greater the risk of preeclampsia. Of patients in whom the diagnosis is made before 30 weeks of gestation, more than one third will experience preeclampsia, whereas in those whose diagnosis is made after 38 weeks, the risk is less than 10%. Decisions to treat patients in this group with antihypertensives must be carefully considered, given the risk of subsequent preeclampsia and the lack of evidence supporting improved fetal outcome. Transient gestational hypertension tends to recur in subsequent pregnancies and predisposes women to hypertension in the future (Marin et al, 2000).

## Preeclampsia-Eclampsia

Preeclampsia is one of the most enigmatic diseases affecting human beings. It is unique to humans and has proved difficult to emulate in experimental animals. Despite years of effort, we have a relatively poor understanding of the underlying cause of the disease, although much of the pathophysiology is known. Underlying the clinical manifestations of the disorder is a pattern of vascular endothelial dysfunction that may involve the central nervous system, the renal and hepatic systems, and the cardiovascular system and may produce a coagulopathy. Preeclampsia has an enormous variety of presentations with a wide range of severity and timing during the pregnancy or immediately postpartum.

The classic symptom triad that defines preeclampsia consists of hypertension, proteinuria, and edema. Most classifications of preeclampsia now dispense with edema because it affects around 80% of all pregnant women at term. Preeclampsia may be divided into mild and severe forms (Table 11–3). This distinction is important, because in the presence of severe disease at any gestational age, the only treatment option is delivery, whereas conservative management may be acceptable for a patient who has mild disease and whose pregnancy is remote from term.

Although the precise cause of preeclampsia remains uncertain, numerous factors raise the risk of the disease (Table 11–4). These factors may be additive, producing a well-defined group of patients at greatly increased risk. Up to 10% of primigravid patients have mild preeclampsia, and about 1% have severe disease.

### Preeclampsia

#### Etiology

The most widely accepted theory for the pathophysiology of preeclampsia is based on a model of impaired placental implantation that results in placental hypoperfusion and hypoxia. The placenta then releases substances into the maternal circulation that adversely affect endothelial

**TABLE 11–3**

**Features of Mild and Severe Preeclampsia**

| | |
|---|---|
| Mild | Blood pressure ≥140 mm Hg systolic or 90 mm Hg diastolic<br>Proteinuria ≥300 mg/24 hr |
| Severe* | Blood pressure ≥160 mm Hg systolic or 100 mm Hg diastolic<br>Proteinuria ≥5 g/24 hr<br>Elevated serum creatinine value<br>Eclampsia<br>Pulmonary edema<br>Oliguria <500 mL/hr<br>HELLP (hemolysis, elevated liver enzymes, and low platelets) syndrome<br>Intrauterine growth restriction<br>Symptoms suggestive of end-organ involvement: headache, visual disturbance, epigastric or right upper quadrant pain |

*Any single feature in the severe definition satisfies the diagnosis of severe preeclampsia.

Modified from ACOG practice bulletin: Diagnosis and management of preeclampsia and eclampsia. Number 33, January 2002. American College of Obstetricians and Gynecologists. Int J Gynaecol Obstet 77:67-75, 2002.

**TABLE 11–4**

**Risk Factors for Development of Preeclampsia**

| Factor | Relative Risk |
|---|---|
| Primigravida | 3 |
| Age >40 yrs | 3 |
| African-American race | 1.5 |
| Family history | 5 |
| Chronic hypertension | 10 |
| Chronic renal disease | 20 |
| Antiphospholipid syndrome | 10 |
| Insulin dependent diabetes mellitus | 2 |
| Multiple gestation | 4 |

function, leading to the clinical syndrome of preeclampsia (Myers and Baker, 2002). Individual responses to this process vary in severity and timing in a manner that seems to have genetic, familial, and immunologic components. Thus, preeclampsia occurring in a first-degree relative confers a fourfold increase in risk of the disease (Chesley and Cooper, 1986), and women born to mothers with preeclampsia themselves have a higher risk. There is some evidence that the presence of certain genotypes, such as factor V Leiden and other thrombophilias (de Vries et al, 1997), or metabolic defects, such as hyperhomocystinemia secondary to methylenetetrahydrofolate reductase deficiency (Kupferminc et al, 1999), predispose women to preeclampsia, although a true "candidate gene" has yet to be established and will probably never be so. Population studies have suggested that women exposed to the antigenic effects of sperm before conception have a lower rate of preeclampsia than women who conceive with lesser degrees of exposure, although the evidence is inconclusive (Koelman et al, 2000).

The endothelial dysfunction that characterizes preeclampsia (Roberts, 1999) manifests as greater vascular reactivity to circulating vasoconstrictors such as angiotensin, reduced production of endogenous vasodilators such as prostacyclin and nitric oxide (Ashworth et al, 1997), and increases in both vascular permeability and a tendency toward platelet consumption and coagulopathy. The end result is hypertension, proteinuria secondary to glomerular injury, edema, and a tendency toward extravascular fluid overload with intravascular hemoconcentration.

### Predictors

Perhaps one of the most important contributions that prenatal care makes to maternal and fetal outcomes is the detection of preeclampsia and the prevention of eclampsia (Backe and Nakling, 1993; Karbhari et al, 1972). A wide variety of biochemical and physical tests has been proposed as screening tools for the early detection of preeclampsia (Dekker and Sibai, 1991). Most physical tests have been discredited, and even the most widely used biochemical tests have poor predictive values. Uric acid levels are elevated in many cases of preeclampsia, but the sensitivity of the measurement is low (Lim et al, 1998). Early detection of proteinuria is possible with the use of more sensitive tests, such as gel electrophoresis (Winkler et al, 1988), rather than conventional urinalysis but such tests do not lend themselves to routine use. Clinicians should be aware of the limitations of routine urine testing for detection of proteinuria, standard dipstick testing being notoriously inaccurate (Bell et al, 1999).

Doppler ultrasonographic assessment of the vascular dynamics in the uterine arteries during the second trimester has been proposed as a valuable screening tool in populations in which obstetric ultrasonography is routine (Kurdi et al, 1998). Up to 40% of women who go on to develop preeclampsia have abnormal waveforms, and this finding was reported to be associated with a six-fold rise in the risk of preeclampsia (Papageorghiou et al, 2002). Other researchers have obtained less impressive results (Goffinet et al, 2001). On balance, then, no effective screening test to predict preeclampsia currently exists, and clinicians are faced with the necessity of diagnosing the disease early and managing it as adroitly as possible.

### Prevention

If an accurate predictor of preeclampsia could be identified, the next logical step would be the application of a preventive or ameliorative treatment. Unfortunately, attempts to identify an effective treatment have proved equally difficult. Given the recognized association between vascular endothelial dysfunction and preeclampsia (in particular, vasoconstriction and excessive clotting in the maternal placental arteries), prostaglandin inhibitors have been viewed as a likely candidate for prophylaxis or treatment. Numerous trials have been conducted with low-dose aspirin, on the basis of the idea that aspirin's ability to irreversibly inhibit production of the vasoconstrictive prostaglandin thromboxane would promote greater activity of prostacyclin, a vasodilatory prostaglandin. This would help maintain patency in the maternal placental vascular bed and limit or prevent the evolution of preeclampsia. Unfortunately, although a modest reduction in the frequency of preeclampsia (≈15%) was documented, no improvement in key measures of perinatal outcome was demonstrable in a meta-analysis of the results of available studies (Duley et al, 2001).

Calcium supplementation was briefly in vogue as a preventive treatment in the 1990s, on the basis of the known vasodilatory effect of calcium and impressive results in early, small studies. However, its worth was not supported in a meta-analysis of studies (Atallah et al, 2000). Similarly, it has been suggested that antioxidants may have a role in preeclampsia prevention, but the only available trial to date showed mixed results, with improvements in biochemical indices in women receiving vitamins C and E, although perinatal outcomes were not different in treated and untreated groups (Chappell et al, 1999). Of concern was the finding that women in whom preeclampsia developed despite vitamin therapy had markedly worsened preeclampsia than controls in whom the disease developed. Thus, at present, an ideal preventive measure for preeclampsia does not exist.

### Antepartum Management

Given the current inability to predict or prevent preeclampsia, clinicians are left to deal with established disease and prevent maternal and fetal morbidity. The division of established preeclampsia into mild and severe forms is of great worth in determining management and minimizing morbidity (see Table 11–3). Mild disease is generally managed conservatively (bed rest and frequent fetal and maternal biophysical assessments) until term is reached or there is evidence of maternal or fetal compromise. The appearance of severe preeclampsia mandates delivery in all but highly selected cases regardless of gestational age.

Patients with a diagnosis of mild preeclampsia should be evaluated for signs of maternal or fetal compromise, which would make their disease severe. Evaluation should include a 24-hour urine collection to evaluate for proteinuria, full blood count and platelet measurements, determination of serum uric acid, blood urea nitrogen, and creatinine levels, and evaluation of liver transaminases. Fetal size should be estimated with ultrasonography; the presence of IUGR (<10$^{th}$ percentile) is a sign of severe preeclampsia. Patients with mild disease at 37 weeks or more of gestation should be delivered, because prolongation of pregnancy has no material benefit to be gained from and increases the risks of maternal and fetal morbidity. Patients at earlier gestational stages should be closely monitored with sequential clinical and laboratory evaluations. Such monitoring often begins in the hospital and may be continued in an outpatient or home setting with appropriate supervision. If the clinical picture deteriorates or term is reached, delivery should be effected. There is no evidence that antihypertensive therapy influences progression of preeclampsia, and its use may actually be dangerous by masking worsening hypertension. Fetal well-being should be evaluated until delivery by means of kick counts and regular nonstress tests or modified biophysical profiles.

Patients with severe disease should be delivered. The only exception to this approach is the diagnosis of severe preeclampsia, in a patient remote from term (<28 weeks), on the basis of proteinuria and transiently (unsustained) severe hypertension *alone*. Such patients may be managed conservatively under close supervision while antenatal corticosteroids are administered without adversely affecting maternal or fetal outcome (Sibai et al, 1990). There is no place for conservative management in any other circumstance. The patient with severe preeclampsia at less than 24 weeks of gestation should be offered termination of the pregnancy; all others should be delivered by the most expedient means. Cesarean section should be reserved for obstetric indications.

Severe hypertension requires treatment with fast-acting antihypertensive agents if stroke and placental abruption are to be avoided. Intravenous hydralazine is well established as a first-line drug for this purpose, although there is a growing experience with other agents, including intravenous labetalol and oral nifedipine (Duley and Henderson-Smart, 2000a) (Table 11–5). The aim of treatment is to lower blood pressure into the mild preeclampsia range (140/90 mm Hg) to reduce the risk of stroke and other maternal cardiovascular complications. There is good evidence to support the use of parenteral magnesium sulfate to prevent eclampsia in all cases of severe disease (Duley et al, 2003).

Severe preeclampsia may manifest as classic disease with severe proteinuric hypertension or may cause atypical findings, such as pulmonary edema or severe central nervous system symptoms, including blindness. More commonly, patients show evidence of microangiopathy leading to the HELLP syndrome. The full-blown clinical syndrome of HELLP carries a significant maternal risk. Early reports suggested that the disease carries a grave prognosis (Weinstein, 1982). This suggestion remains true for florid clinical cases, but most patients now have “laboratory” HELLP and never experience major clinical features of the syndrome because they are delivered before deteriorating to that point.

**TABLE 11-5**

**Drugs for Acute Treatment of Hypertension in Severe Preeclampsia**

| Drug | Dosage |
|---|---|
| Hydralazine | 1-2 mg test dose<br>5-10 mg IV followed by 5-10 mg q 20 min as required, to a total of 30 mg |
| Labetalol | 10-20 mg IV followed by 20-80 mg q 10 min to a total of 300 mg |
| Nifedipine | 10 mg PO q 10-30 min up to three doses |

### Preeclampsia and Fetal Risk

Because the only recourse in severe preeclampsia is delivery, the disease has a corresponding effect on prematurity and its attendant complications. IUGR is not uncommon in severe preeclampsia, and there may be evidence of progressive deterioration in fetal well-being with worsening disease. Infants delivered at less than 34 weeks of gestation will benefit from antenatal steroid therapy—even as little as 8 hours of therapy before delivery may have benefit. Many patients are able to deliver vaginally, but fetal compromise may preclude aggressive induction and mandate delivery by cesarean section. The incidence of respiratory distress syndrome is lower in infants of preeclamptic mothers delivered preterm than in those of age-matched controls without antenatal steroid exposure (Yoon et al, 1980). Nonetheless, the morbidity of such infants is greater because of hyoxemic insults received in utero. Infants born to preeclamptic mothers may have thrombocytopenia or neutropenia, which further complicates their newborn course (Fraser and Tudehope, 1996).

### Intrapartum Management

All laboring women with a diagnosis of preeclampsia should receive magnesium sulfate as seizure prophylaxis (Table 11–6). Although the absolute risk of seizure is low, the occurrence of seizures is unpredictable and the margin of safety of magnesium sulfate therapy is fairly wide. Blood pressure should be maintained in the mild preeclampsia range. Epidural anesthesia is indicated for pain control and to aid in blood pressure management. Vaginal delivery should be possible in most cases. Delivery by cesarean section should be reserved for obstetric indications. Careful attention to fluid balance should be maintained. After delivery, the preeclamptic process should begin to resolve rapidly.

**TABLE 11-6**

**Magnesium Sulfate Therapy for Prevention of Eclampsia**

1. Bolus 4-6 g IV over 20 min
2. Continuous infusion 1-2 g/hr
3. Follow up levels q 6-8 hr to target 4-6 mEq/L
4. Continue infusion 24 hr after delivery or 24 hr after seizure if seizure occurs despite magnesium therapy

### Eclampsia

*Eclampsia* is the occurrence of generalized tonic-clonic seizures in association with preeclampsia. It affects about 1 in 2500 deliveries in the United States and may be much more common in developing countries, affecting as many as 1% of parturients. Up to 10% of maternal deaths are due to eclampsia (Duley, 1992).

Most cases of eclampsia occur within 24 hours of delivery. Almost 50% of seizures occur before the patient's admission to labor and delivery, about 30% are intrapartum, and the remainder are postpartum. There is a considerable drop in the risk of eclampsia by 48 hours postpartum, seizures occurring in less than 3% of women beyond that time. Most patients have antecedent features suggestive of preeclampsia, although in some cases eclampsia may occur without warning. If eclampsia is left untreated, repetitive seizures become more frequent and of longer duration, and ultimately, status eclampticus develops. Maternal and fetal mortality may be as high as 50% in severe cases, especially if the seizures take place while the patient is far from medical care.

Randomized controlled trials have demonstrated the clear superiority of magnesium sulfate for the treatment of eclampsia over all other anticonvulsants (Duley and Gulmezoglu, 2002; Duley and Henderson-Smart, 2002b, 2002c). Intravenous magnesium sulfate is given as a 4-g bolus over 5 minutes followed by a maintenance infusion of 1 to 2 g/hr for 24 hours after delivery. Subsequent seizures may be treated by further bolus injections; in refractory cases, second-line treatment with other anticonvulsants may be required, or the patient may have to be paralyzed and ventilated.

Delivery after an eclamptic seizure should take place in a controlled, careful manner. There is little to be added by performing a "crash" cesarean section (Coppage and Polzin, 2002). The patient should be stabilized first. Vaginal delivery is possible in most cases, although cesarean delivery may be indicated if the status of the cervix is unfavorable or fetal compromise is ongoing despite control of seizures and maternal stabilization. Infants born to mothers after eclampsia require careful monitoring after birth.

## REFERENCES


Ashworth JR, et al: Loss of endothelium-dependent relaxation in myometrial resistance arteries in pre-eclampsia. Br J Obstet Gynaecol 104:1152-1158, 1997.

Atallah AN, Hofmeyr GJ, Duley L: Calcium supplementation during pregnancy for preventing hypertensive disorders and related problems. Cochrane Database Syst Rev (3):CD001059, 2000.

Backe B, Nakling J: Effectiveness of antenatal care: A population based study. Br J Obstet Gynaecol 100:727-732, 1993.

Bell SC, et al: The role of observer error in antenatal dipstick proteinuria analysis. Br J Obstet Gynaecol 106:1177-1180, 1999.

Brown MA, Whitworth JA: Management of hypertension in pregnancy. Clin Exp Hypertens 21:907-916, 1999.

Buttar HS: An overview of the influence of ACE inhibitors on fetal-placental circulation and perinatal development. Mol Cell Biochem 176:61-71, 1997.

Chappell LC, et al: Effect of antioxidants on the occurrence of pre-eclampsia in women at increased risk: A randomised trial. Lancet 354:810-816, 1999.

Chesley LC, Cooper DW: Genetics of hypertension in pregnancy: Possible single gene control of pre-eclampsia and eclampsia in the descendants of eclamptic women. Br J Obstet Gynaecol 93:898-908, 1986.

Coppage KH, Polzin WJ: Severe preeclampsia and delivery outcomes: Is immediate cesarean delivery beneficial? Am J Obstet Gynecol 186:921-923, 2002.

Cunningham FG, et al: Chronic renal disease and pregnancy outcome. Am J Obstet Gynecol 163:453-459, 1990.

Dekker GA, Sibai BM: Early detection of preeclampsia. Am J Obstet Gynecol 165:160-172, 1991.

de Vries JI, et al: Hyperhomocysteinaemia and protein S deficiency in complicated pregnancies. Br J Obstet Gynaecol 104:1248-1254, 1997.

Duley L: Maternal mortality associated with hypertensive disorders of pregnancy in Africa, Asia, Latin America and the Caribbean. Br J Obstet Gynaecol 99:547-553, 1992.

Duley L, Gulmezoglu AM: Magnesium sulfate compared with lytic cocktail for women with eclampsia. Int J Gynaecol Obstet 76:3-8, 2002.

Duley L, Henderson-Smart DJ: Drugs for rapid treatment of very high blood pressure during pregnancy. Cochrane Database Syst Rev (2):CD001449, 2000a.

Duley L, Henderson-Smart DJ: Magnesium sulphate versus diazepam for eclampsia. Cochrane Database Syst Rev (2): CD000127, 2000b.

Duley L, Henderson-Smart DJ: Magnesium sulphate versus phenytoin for eclampsia. Cochrane Database Syst Rev (2): CD000128, 2000c.

Duley L, Gulmezoglu AM, Henderson-Smart DJ: Magnesium sulphate and other anticonvulsants for women with pre-eclampsia. Cochrane Database Syst Rev (2):CD000025, 2003.

Duley L, et al: Antiplatelet drugs for prevention of pre-eclampsia and its consequences: Systematic review. BMJ 322:329-333, 2001.

Ferrer RL, et al: Management of mild chronic hypertension during pregnancy: A review. Obstet Gynecol 96:849-860, 2000.

Fraser SH, Tudehope DI: Neonatal neutropenia and thrombocytopenia following maternal hypertension. J Paediatr Child Health 32:31-34, 1996.

Goffinet F, et al: Screening with a uterine Doppler in low risk pregnant women followed by low dose aspirin in women with abnormal results: A multicenter randomised controlled trial. BJOG 108:510-518, 2001.

Hall DR, et al: Nifedipine or prazosin as a second agent to control early severe hypertension in pregnancy: A randomised controlled trial. BJOG 107:759-765, 2000.

Hou S: Pregnancy in chronic renal insufficiency and end-stage renal disease. Am J Kidney Dis 33:235-252, 1999.

Jungers P, et al: Pregnancy in women with impaired renal function. Clin Nephrol 47:281-288, 1997.

Karbhari DS, et al: Eclampsia—the influence of antenatal care. J Postgrad Med 18:175-180, 1972.

Koelman CA, et al: Correlation between oral sex and a low incidence of preeclampsia: A role for soluble HLA in seminal fluid? J Reprod Immunol 46:155-166, 2000.

Koonin LM, et al: Pregnancy-related mortality surveillance—United States, 1987-1990. MMWR CDC Surveill Summ 46:17-36, 1997.

Kupferminc MJ, et al: Increased frequency of genetic thrombophilia in women with complications of pregnancy. N Engl J Med 340:9-13. 1999.

Kurdi W, et al: The role of color Doppler imaging of the uterine arteries at 20 weeks' gestation in stratifying antenatal care. Ultrasound Obstet Gynecol 12:339-345, 1998.

Levin AC, Doering PL, Hatton RC: Use of nifedipine in the hypertensive diseases of pregnancy. Ann Pharmacother 28:1371-1378, 1994.

Lim KH, et al: The clinical utility of serum uric acid measurements in hypertensive diseases of pregnancy. Am J Obstet Gynecol 178:1067-1071 1998.

Marin R, et al: Long-term prognosis of hypertension in pregnancy. Hypertens Pregnancy 19:199-209, 2000.

Myers JE, Baker PN: Hypertensive diseases and eclampsia. Curr Opin Obstet Gynecol 14:119-125, 2002.

Papageorghiou AT, et al: Second-trimester uterine artery Doppler screening in unselected populations: A review. J Matern Fetal Neonatal Med, 12:78-88, 2002.

Pickles CJ, Symonds EM, Pipkin FB: The fetal outcome in a randomized double-blind controlled trial of labetalol versus placebo in pregnancy-induced hypertension. Br J Obstet Gynaecol 96:38-43, 1989.

Report of the National High Blood Pressure Education Program Working Group on High Blood Pressure in Pregnancy. Am J Obstet Gynecol 183:S1-S22, 2000.

Roberts JM: Objective evidence of endothelial dysfunction in preeclampsia. Am J Kidney Dis 33:992-997, 1999.

Sibai BM, Anderson GD: Pregnancy outcome of intensive therapy in severe hypertension in first trimester. Obstet Gynecol 67:517-522, 1986.

Sibai BM. Grossman RA, Grossman HG: Effects of diuretics on plasma volume in pregnancies with long-term hypertension. Am J Obstet Gynecol 150:831-835, 1984.

Sibai BM, et al: A protocol for managing severe preeclampsia in the second trimester. Am J Obstet Gynecol 163:733-738, 1990.

Steffensen FH, et al: Pregnancy outcome with ACE-inhibitor use in early pregnancy. Lancet 351:596, 1998.

Weinstein L: Syndrome of hemolysis, elevated liver enzymes, and low platelet count: A severe consequence of hypertension in pregnancy. Am J Obstet Gynecol 142:159-167, 1982.

Winkler U, et al: Urinary protein patterns for early detection of preeclampsia. Contrib Nephrol 68:227-229, 1988.

Yoon JJ, Kohl S, Harper RG: The relationship between maternal hypertensive disease of pregnancy and the incidence of idiopathic respiratory distress syndrome. Pediatrics 65:735-739, 1980.

CHAPTER

# 12

# Perinatal Substance Abuse

**Alma Martinez, J. Colin Partridge, and H. William Taeusch**

Substance abuse during pregnancy has been recognized for more than a century. Overall prevalence of cocaine or crack use has diminished since the epidemic of the late 1980s and early 1990s but has been followed by greater opiate use in pregnancy. Since the 1950s, awareness has also grown regarding the adverse effects of tobacco and ethanol on pregnancy.

Psychotropic substances, both legal (alcohol, cigarettes, and prescription drugs) and illegal (heroin, amphetamine, cocaine, and phencyclidine [PCP]), may cause obstetric complications and fetal injury. These substances have short-term and long-term consequences for the newborn infant. Although chronic or sporadic drug abuse can occur in a person in any socioeconomic class, several elements, such as lifestyle, health risks, poverty, and drug, tobacco, and alcohol abuse, often coexist. From this point of view, substance abuse, like many other health conditions, is a consequence of multiple societal, familial, psychological, medical, educational, and personal ills. Additionally, substance abuse often exacerbates disadvantageous medical and socioeconomic conditions (Table 12–1).

In general, the consequences of fetal exposure to drugs, alcohol, and tobacco smoking are poor intrauterine growth, prematurity, fetal distress, abortion, stillbirth, cerebral infarctions and other vascular accidents, malformations, and neurobehavioral dysfunction. It is often quite difficult to determine the effects of a single drug on the fetus and newborn, who are often exposed to multiple drugs during gestation. Multiple drug exposure, socioeconomic status of parents, and subsequent postnatal environmental factors typically confound studies of drug effects on the fetus and newborn. Nonetheless, established correlates of substance use during pregnancy are listed in Table 12–2.

Prevalence of drug use among pregnant women is less than among non-pregnant women, but about 3% of women use illicit drugs during pregnancy (HHS/Substance Abuse, 2001). Illicit drug use is estimated at nearly 13% among women aged 15 to 17 years, pregnant or not. Illicit drug use during pregnancy is more prevalent among black women (7%) than among white (3%) and Hispanic (2%) women. Additionally, as of 1999, 13% of pregnant women use alcohol, and nearly 3% report frequent or binge drinking, again substantially lower than nonpregnant women (53% and 12%, respectively) (Alcohol use, 2002). The largest gestational exposure rates are for smoking. About 19% of pregnant women between 15 and 44 years of age continue to smoke during pregnancy. Nationally, women make up approximately 30% of drug treatment admissions and 25% of alcohol treatment admissions.

One of the most comprehensive geographically based studies on substance abuse by pregnant women was undertaken by the Perinatal Substance Exposure Study Group (Vega et al, 1993). In the study, urine was collected from more than 30,000 women at the time of delivery in California in 1992. The state of California has approximately 600,000 deliveries per year, representing about 15% of all deliveries in the United States. The major results of this study are shown in Table 12–3. These prevalence rates of maternal drug use (except for the higher rates of alcohol in California) are similar to those of earlier statewide surveys from South Carolina and Rhode Island, and lower than a statewide survey in Georgia that was based on newborn bloodspot screening (Surveillance, 1997). If these results are extrapolated to the United States at large, an estimated 450,000 infants per year (11% of 4 million live births) are exposed to alcohol or drugs (or both) in the days before delivery.

Table 12–4 shows the distribution of exposure of neonates to drugs, alcohol, and tobacco by ethnic group. Prevalence rates of alcohol, smoking, and drugs are highest among blacks and lowest among Asians and Pacific Islanders. While at lower risk for substance use, white, non-Hispanic babies account for roughly half the newborns exposed to drugs, smoking, and alcohol. Parents with substance use have lower educational achievement and are less likely to be employed full time, less likely to be married, and more likely to receive welfare support than nonusing parents. Substance exposure is twofold higher in groups identified as "poor" on the basis of eligibility for Medicaid health insurance, indicating the expected association between substance abuse and poverty. As documented by investigators, smoking serves as a major risk for illicit substance exposure, with a 22-fold higher risk for cocaine use among those who reported that they smoke (Vega et al, 1993). In the California prevalence study, polydrug use was not common. The rate reported, 0.5%, may underestimate polydrug use, however, because women may use drugs sequentially according to preference and availability rather than simultaneously. Studies that attempt to detail true dose and duration of exposures throughout gestation are not available.

Drug withdrawal and drug effects are seen in exposed infants, related to the specific drug as well as the timing, dose, and duration of exposure. Other emotional, medical, legal, familial, financial, and societal consequences play important roles in the outcome of drug-exposed newborn infants. Hospital costs average approximately $7500 more for infants who have been exposed to drugs than for those who have not (Joyce et al, 1995). Frustrated by adverse consequences, some prosecutors have charged substance-abusing women with fetal or child abuse (Annas, 2001). For the most part, these efforts have been unsuccessful. The infant with a positive toxicology screen result has a 26% to 58% chance of being referred for foster care placement, compared with 1% to 2% for the infant with a negative result (U.S. General Accounting Office, 1990). Costs of foster care are roughly $5000 per year for a normal infant and $20,000 per year for an infant with special medical needs.

**TABLE 12–1**

**Associated Risks of Drug Use, Alcohol Use, and Smoking in Child-Bearing Women**

| |
|---|
| Suboptimal parenting |
| Physical, sexual, domestic violence |
| Poverty |
| Poor schooling, illiteracy, school dropout |
| Limited job skills, training |
| Limited jobs |
| Poor self-image, poor coping skills |
| Peer pressure |
| Ineffectuality of birth control and protection against sexually transmitted diseases (STDs) |
| Unplanned, unwanted pregnancy; teenage pregnancy |
| Poor nutrition and preconception health care |
| Poor access, receipt, and quality of prenatal care |
| Little family/father support |
| Stress |
| Psychological disorders, depression |
| Limited access to support services in community |
| Dependence/addiction |
| Pregnancy wastage |
| Increased risk of premature birth |
| Increased risk of fetal malformations |
| Fetal growth retardation |
| Fetal/neonatal death |
| Newborn assigned to foster care |
| Attempts at rehabilitation |
| Increased risk of human immunodeficiency virus, syphilis, hepatitis B or C, other STDs |
| Incarceration |
| Recapitulation in next generation |

## OPIATES

Opium derivatives have been used as analgesics for centuries and remain the most effective analgesics available. Opioids of clinical interest are morphine, heroin, methadone, meperidine, and codeine. Morphine's potential for abuse and addiction was documented in the mid-1800s, shortly after it began to be used extensively. Perinatal problems associated with opium were first reported in the late 1800s. Since the 1950s, heroin use has been endemic in most major American cities.

Specific opiate receptors ($\mu$, $\delta$, $\kappa$) have been identified in the nervous system and the bowel that are activated by endogenous opiates, such as the naturally occurring endorphins and enkephalins (Vaccarino and Kastin, 2000). Modulators of the sympathoadrenal system, endogenous opiates are important during periods of diverse forms of stress. Activation of these receptors by the endogenous opiates has physiologic effects, including analgesia, drowsiness, respiratory depression, decreased gastrointestinal motility, nausea, and vomiting as well as alterations in the endocrine and autonomic nervous systems. Activation of these same endogenous opiate receptors by exogenous opioid drugs has similar clinical effects.

The use of opioid drugs can result in the development of tolerance, physiologic dependence, and addiction. Tolerance leads to a shortened duration of the action of opioids and a decrease in the intensity of the drug action, followed by the need for a higher dose of drug to obtain the same clinical effect. Tolerance is believed to result from continued occupancy of the opioid receptor. Continuous administration of opioids, therefore, leads to more rapid onset of tolerance (Anand and Arnold, 1994; Suresh and Anand, 2001). With physiologic dependence, there is a need for further drug administration to prevent withdrawal symptoms (agitation, dysphoria, temperature instability). Addiction is a more severe form of dependence that involves a complex pattern of drug-seeking behavior.

### Epidemiology

Prevalence of opiate use among pregnant women is reported to range from 1% to 2% (Vega et al, 1993; Yawn et al, 1994) to as much as 21% in a highly selected group of women (Behnke and Eyler, 1993; Nair et al, 1994; Ostrea et al, 1992b). One multicenter study found that the

**TABLE 12–2**

**Enhanced Risk for Various Events or Processes after Substance Use During Pregnancy***

| Event or Process | Ethanol | Cigarettes | Cannabis | Opiates | Cocaine | Amphetamines | Barbiturates | Phencyclidine |
|---|---|---|---|---|---|---|---|---|
| Malformation | + | – | – | – | + | – | – | + |
| Abortion | – | + | ? | ? | + | + | – | + |
| Intrauterine growth restriction | + | + | ? | + | + | + | – | + |
| Prematurity | – | + | ? | + | + | + | – | ? |
| Withdrawal | ? | – | – | + | – | – | – | – |
| Central nervous system sequelae | + | ? | ? | ? | + | ? | – | ? |
| Sudden infant death syndrome | + | + | ? | + | + | ? | – | ? |
| Foster care | + | – | – | + | + | + | ± | + |

+, Causes event or process; –, does not cause event or process; ?, not known whether agent causes event or process.

*Although risk is increased, the risk ratio ranges for many from 1 to 2 for these associations.

**TABLE 12-3**

**Prevalence Rates of Substance Abuse at Delivery in California, 1992**

| Substance | Prevalence Rate (%)* |
|---|---|
| Amphetamines | 0.7 |
| Barbiturates | 0.3 |
| Benzodiazepines | 0.1 |
| Tetrahydrocannabinol/marijuana | 1.9 |
| Cocaine | 1.1 |
| Methadone | 0.2 |
| Opiates | 1.5 |
| PCP (phencyclidine) | 0.0 |
| Alcohol | 6.7 |
| Illicit drugs | 3.5 |
| Drugs and/or alcohol+ | 11.3 |
| Tobacco‡ | 8.8 |

*Percentages represent the positive urine test results obtained from 29,494 women delivering infants from March through October 1992.

+Includes alcohol and/or any drug; excludes tobacco.

‡Tobacco was self-reported and not based on urine testing.

Data from Vega W, Kolody B, Hwang J, Noble A: Prevalence and magnitude of prenatal substance exposures in California. N Engl J Med 329:850, 1993.

prevalence of opiate use varied by center and ranged from 1.6% to 4.5% at the different sites (Lester et al, 2001). Additionally, these centers reported higher rates of opiate use with low-birth-weight and very low-birth-weight infants. Rates for heroin use are higher in metropolitan areas and cities and are more concentrated in Northeast and West Coast cities. Opiate abuse is more common in groups of lower socioeconomic status. Studies of the distribution of opiate abuse among ethnic groups in the United States have shown inconsistencies and apparent contradictions. Reports showing blacks and Hispanics to be disproportionately represented (Hartnoll, 1994) can be contrasted with those showing a higher incidence among white women (Gillogley et al, 1990). In a population-based study in California, the prevalence of opiate use during pregnancy was highest in black women, followed by white women, and then Asian and Hispanic women (Vega et al, 1993).

Women using opiates during pregnancy are more likely to use other drugs (Bauer, 1999; Brown et al, 1998; van Baar et al, 1994a, 1994b). Investigators have also reported that 93% of women identified as using opiates and cocaine during pregnancy had also used a combination of alcohol, nicotine, or marijuana (Bauer, 1999). Women who smoke during pregnancy are more likely to use opiates, alcohol, cocaine, amphetamines, and cannabis during pregnancy than women who do not smoke (Vega et al, 1993). In a study from Amsterdam, only 7% of heroin-using and methadone-using women did not smoke during pregnancy (Boer et al, 1994).

Of the opiate drugs known to be abused during pregnancy, heroin has been the most extensively studied. Heroin can be ingested through smoking or by the intranasal or intravenous route. Intranasal use is common among women, especially in the western United States, whereas the intravenous route is more popular among users on the eastern seaboard. Reports from European countries suggest a trend away from intravenous injection of opiates (Hartnoll, 1994). The use of noninjectable heroin may reduce the risk of transmission of human immunodeficiency virus (HIV); however, its wider use ensures the emergence of new groups of heroin users for whom the risk of intravenous use is a major deterrent.

## Clinical Aspects

### Maternal Health

Many heroin-addicted pregnant women have poor general health with multiple medical problems associated with the drug abuse lifestyle. Intravenous drug use places the woman at risk for multiple infectious complications, including cellulitis, thrombophlebitis, hepatitis, endocarditis, syphilis, gonorrhea, and acquired immunodeficiency syndrome (AIDS). In a prospective study undertaken in

**TABLE 12-4**

**Race/Ethnicity and Substance Exposure at Term in California, 1992***

| Race/Ethnicity | Positive Screen Results: Alcohol Exposure | Illicit Drugs | Nonillicit Drugs | Any Drug† | Total Positive Results‡ | Tobacco Exposure§ |
|---|---|---|---|---|---|---|
| Asian/Pacific Islander | 5 | 0.4 | 1 | 2 | 7 | 2 |
| Black | 12 | 12 | 2 | 14 | 24 | 20 |
| Hispanic | 7 | 2 | 1 | 3 | 9 | 3 |
| White, non-Hispanic | 6 | 5 | 2 | 7 | 12 | 15 |
| Other | 4 | 2 | 1 | 3 | 7 | 5 |

*Numbers equal percentages of sample in which substance was identified through urine screen at delivery.

†Excludes alcohol and tobacco. Indicates percentage of women in whom one or more drugs was identified in urine.

‡Includes alcohol and/or any drug; excludes tobacco.

§Tobacco was self-reported and not based on urine testing.

Data from Vega W, Kolody B, Hwang J, Noble A: Prevalence and magnitude of prenatal substance exposures in California. N Engl J Med 329:850, 1993.

Canada, a 5-year incidence of HIV seroconversion was 13.4%; the rate of conversion associated with injection of heroin or cocaine was 40% higher in women than in men (Spittal et al, 2002). Opiate abusers are also less likely to receive prenatal care or to obtain late prenatal care (Bauer, 1999). Heroin-addicted mothers are often poorly nourished, and iron-deficiency anemia is more common in pregnant opiate users than nonusers. In studies throughout the world, women who use heroin have higher rates of maternal complications of pregnancy, such as prematurity, small-for-gestational-age infants, and antepartum hemorrhage, as well as a higher incidence of sexually transmitted diseases (Bauer, 1999; Lam et al, 1992; Little et al, 1990). Bauer (1999) found that maternal hepatitis infections were five times higher in opiate-using women than in a control group of non-users.

The rates of maternal complications of pregnancy are further increased when drug use is added to infection with HIV. Women infected with HIV who also use opiates (methadone) have higher rates of miscarriage, preterm deliveries, and small-for-gestational-age infants, and more vaginal and urinary tract infections than women who are HIV-positive but are not using drugs (Mauri et al, 1995). Domestic violence is also identified as a significant factor complicating perinatal outcomes for women using opiates (Bauer, 1999).

### *Maternal Methadone Maintenance*

The potential benefits of maternal methadone maintenance are numerous (Kandall and Doberczak, 1999; Ward et al, 1999). They include the prevention of opiate withdrawal symptoms in the mother, better medical and prenatal care, improved health and growth of the fetus, maintenance of opiate levels in the mother to decrease both the use of illicit drugs and the potential for perinatal infections. Methadone maintenance programs associated with comprehensive medical and psychosocial services for the pregnant woman are of additional benefit. Methadone maintenance has been shown to be associated with higher birth weight in some but not all studies (Brown et al, 1998; Kandall and Doberczak, 1999). Because maternal drug withdrawal is believed to be associated with subsequent fetal withdrawal, fetal asphyxia, and spontaneous abortions, detoxification of a pregnant heroin user is infrequently attempted (Barr and Jones, 1994). Dashe and colleagues (1998) reported on a small study of opiate-using pregnant women undergoing safe maternal detoxification. Close to 60% of the women completed detoxification, but almost 30% resumed opiate use. McCarthy and associates (1999) showed that women who reduced their methadone dose during pregnancy had infants with higher birth weights than a control group who continued on the same (or increased) methadone dose throughout pregnancy. In the United States, most pregnant women are treated with daily methadone. Some authorities, however, have urged reappraisal and reevaluation of the benefits of methadone maintenance in pregnancy (Brown et al, 1998; Hulse and O'Neil, 2001).

In the Netherlands, women enrolled in a methadone program had higher rates of prenatal care. In this study, higher rates of prenatal care were associated with higher birth weights and less prematurity in the offspring (Soepatmi, 1994). When women in a methadone maintenance program were enrolled in an enhanced prenatal care program, their infants' birth weights were significantly larger than those in the control group of women receiving regular methadone maintenance during pregnancy (Chang et al, 1992). Others have shown that higher methadone doses are associated with improved head circumference and increased gestational age at delivery (Hagopian et al, 1996). Using meta-analysis design, Hulse and coworkers (1997) found that infant birth weight was associated with heroin use and that birth weights were better with methadone treatment during pregnancy. These favorable outcomes are believed to be due to a stable intrauterine environment uncomplicated by periods of intoxication and withdrawal as well as less stress and better nutrition in the mother.

Several investigators have found that neonatal withdrawal symptoms, birth weight, length of pregnancy, and number of days infants require treatment for abstinence do not correlate with maternal methadone dosage (Brown et al, 1998; Finnegan, 1991; Madden et al, 1977; Rosen and Pippenger, 1976). In contrast, others have reported correlation between the severity of neonatal withdrawal and maternal methadone dose (Harper et al, 1977; Maas et al, 1990; Malpas et al, 1995). Studying maternal and neonatal serum levels of methadone does not help clarify this dilemma. Investigators have found no correlation between neonatal serum levels of methadone and the maternal methadone dose at delivery, the maternal serum levels, or the severity of withdrawal symptoms in the neonates (Harper et al, 1977; Mack et al, 1991). Other researchers have reported that neonatal signs of withdrawal correlate with the rate of decline of the neonatal plasma level during the first few days of life (Doberczak et al, 1993). Still others have suggested that neonatal withdrawal occurs after plasma methadone levels fall below a threshold level (Rosen and Pippenger, 1976).

There are no guidelines for methadone dosages during pregnancy. Controversy continues over the most appropriate dose of methadone maintenance during pregnancy. The divergent findings noted previously have been used to argue either for weaning a pregnant woman to a low methadone maintenance dose or for attempting complete maternal detoxification during pregnancy. Some authorities believe in maintaining high methadone doses to keep the mother from "chipping" with additional street drugs, which would put her at risk not only for greater complications of pregnancy but also for higher risk of infections transmitted by intravenous use of drugs (HIV, hepatitis) or of sexually transmitted disease. High-dose methadone maintenance ranges between 60 and 150 mg/day. Despite reports of the safe detoxification of pregnant women, there are still concerns that the fetus is placed at risk during maternal detoxification. The medical management of pregnant women who are addicted to opiates remains controversial.

### Fetal and Neonatal Health

Obstetric complications reported in the literature to be associated with use of opiates include higher incidences of spontaneous abortions, premature delivery and preterm labor, abruptio placentae, chorioamnionitis, increased risk of cesarean section associated with breech presentation, impaired fetal growth, and fetal distress. In women who use opiates during pregnancy, the incidence of preterm labor and premature delivery ranges between 25% and 41% (Chiriboga, 1993; Lam et al, 1992; Little et al, 1990). Infants exposed to opiates have a higher incidence of intrauterine growth restriction (IUGR) (Lam et al, 1992) and smaller head circumference (Bauer, 1999; Boer et al, 1994). Maternal opiate use is associated with higher rates of meconium staining, lower Apgar scores, and longer duration of membrane rupture (Gillogley et al, 1990). Others have also reported increased incidences of syphilis and HIV infection at birth (Bauer, 1999).

The higher risks for fetal loss, IUGR, prematurity, and low birth weight are multifactorial. Maternal lifestyle, malnutrition, and infections as well as polydrug affects are likely to result in poor perinatal outcomes, including poor intrauterine growth and prematurity. Finally, because the drug supply is often episodic, the pregnant addict is subject to episodes of withdrawal and overdose, thereby subjecting the fetus to intermittent episodes of hypoxia in utero, hindering growth and raise the risk of spontaneous abortion, stillbirth, fetal distress, and prematurity. Infants born to opiate addicts are more likely to be of low birth weight, to be premature, and to suffer from infection and perinatal asphyxia. The incidence of respiratory distress syndrome is reportedly lower in infants exposed to heroin in utero than in nonexposed infants. This difference may represent a direct effect of heroin on lung maturation, stress-induced accelerated lung maturation, or both (Taeusch et al, 1973).

### *Neonatal Withdrawal Syndrome*

The classic neonatal withdrawal or abstinence syndrome consists of a wide variety of central nervous system (CNS) signs of irritability, gastrointestinal and feeding problems (diarrhea, hyperphagia), autonomic signs of dysfunction, and respiratory symptoms (Table 12–5). The incidence of neonatal withdrawal syndrome in the infants of women using heroin or methadone is quite high, with wide ranges reported between 16% and 90% (Agarwal, et al, 1999; Boer et al, 1994; Maas et al, 1990; van Baar et al, 1994a).

The mortality rate for withdrawal infants was estimated as high as 10% for the years 1969 through 1979 in Amsterdam. Current estimates, however, show marked improvement, with perinatal mortality rates of less than 1% (Boer et al, 1994). Death is rarely associated with withdrawal alone but occurs as a consequence of prematurity, infection, and severe perinatal asphyxia.

A number of evaluation tools is used to assess the severity of opiate withdrawal after birth. The Neonatal Abstinence Score is a scale based on nursing observations of the severity of signs of withdrawal (Finnegan et al, 1975). Green and Suffet (1981) introduced the Neonatal Narcotic Withdrawal Index as a rapid physician-based evaluation for neonatal signs of withdrawal. Use of these scoring systems enables one to quantify the severity of the infant's withdrawal. The scores are used to guide the clinician's treatment of the withdrawing infant. It is important to not rely simply on an absolute score to either institute pharmacologic interventions or to wean the infant from such medications. Rather, a daily evaluation of the abnormal clinical elements observed in the scoring system is also critical. These methods have shown good interobserver reliability and can improve clinicians' ability to treat the withdrawing infant appropriately (Anand and Arnold, 1994; Franck and Vilardi, 1995). The goal of medical management of opiate withdrawal is to maintain infant comfort while enabling the infant to feed, sleep, and gain weight in an appropriate manner. Standard medical practice is to combine both developmental and behavioral methods with pharmacologic interventions as necessary to soothe the infant.

**TABLE 12-5**

**Clinical Signs of Neonatal Withdrawal Syndrome**

| | |
|---|---|
| Central nervous system dysfunction | Irritability, excessive crying |
| | Jitteriness, tremulousness |
| | Hyperactive reflexes |
| | Increased tone |
| | Sleep disturbance |
| | Seizures |
| Autonomic dysfunction | Excessive sweating |
| | Mottling |
| | Hyperthermia |
| | Hypertension |
| Respiratory symptoms | Tachypnea |
| | Nasal stuffiness |
| Gastrointestinal and feeding disturbances | Diarrhea |
| | Excessive sucking |
| | Hyperphagia |

#### Treatment

Treatment for opiate withdrawal consists of soothing (swaddling, rocking, decreased environmental stimulation) and pharmacologic management when necessary. Medications most commonly used for opiate withdrawal are dilute tincture of opium, benzodiazepines, and phenobarbital (Levy and Sino, 1993; Neonatal drug withdrawal, 1998). The mainstay of treatment for opiate withdrawal is the use of opiates, either alone or in combination with other medications. The medication is titrated according to the severity of the signs of withdrawal for each infant.

A usual standard starting dose of diluted tincture of opium (0.4 mg/mL of morphine equivalent) is 0.1 mL/kg given orally every 3 to 4 hours. This dose can be increased in increments of 0.05 to 0.1 mL until the symptoms are controlled. The usual dose for infants withdrawing at birth ranges from 0.2 to 0.5 mL every 3 to 4 hours (Anand and Arnold, 1994; Levy and Sino, 1993; Neonatal drug withdrawal, 1998). Higher doses may often be needed to control significant physiologic signs of withdrawal such as diarrhea, pyrexia, hypertension, and significant hypertonicity. Investigators suggest that the use of shorter dosing intervals and lower peak doses of tincture of opiate solution are associated with shorter hospital stays for infants withdrawing from opiates (Jones, 1999).

Phenobarbital has been used for signs of acute opiate withdrawal. Phenobarbital does not, however, reduce significant physiologic signs of withdrawal such as diarrhea and seizures. Studies comparing phenobarbital with paregoric (morphine equivalent) showed that 11% of infants treated with phenobarbital had clinical seizures, whereas none of the infants treated with paregoric had this complication (Kandall et al, 1983). At higher doses, phenobarbital has also been shown to impair infant sucking and cause excessive sedation. The therapeutic blood level of phenobarbital for control of opiate withdrawal signs is not known. In addition to the limitations just noted, phenobarbital levels must be monitored when this medication is used for treatment of withdrawal. Coyle and associates (2002) showed that combining deodorized tincture of opium (DTO) and phenobarbital was associated with decreases in hospitalization days, hospital costs, and severity of withdrawal signs in opiate-exposed term infants. In this study, however, the infants were discharged home on phenobarbital therapy, from which they were slowly weaned throughout infancy. Some of these infants received phenobarbital for prolonged times.

Diazepam can also be used as an additional or adjuvant drug for infants withdrawing from opiates. This agent helps relieve irritability and improve infant comfort and should be used on a discretionary basis. Diazepam should not to be used as the sole medication for the treatment of withdrawal. The usual starting dose is 0.1 mg/kg, given as an oral dose for intermittent use in treating withdrawal signs (Anand and Arnold, 1994, Levy and Sino, 1993).

Adverse effects have been reported with the use of paregoric in preterm infants. Paregoric has been associated with acidosis, CNS depression, respiratory distress, hypotension, renal failure, seizures, and death (Anand and Arnold, 1994). Because of these significant limitations, this medication may have limited usefulness in patients with opiate withdrawal.

Although methadone has not been studied in neonates, and certainly not in premature infants, it has been used in the treatment of opiate withdrawal in older infants and children (Tobias, 2000; Tobias et al, 1990). Methadone has a long duration of action and can be administered by either the oral or the parenteral route. The initial methadone dose recommended for older infants and children is 0.05 to 0.1 mg/kg given every 6 to 12 hours, with increases of 0.05 mg/kg until symptoms are controlled. Tobias and colleagues (1990) showed that methadone could be given every 12 to 24 hours because of its longer half-life.

Once medications have been titrated to a level that controls the severity of opiate withdrawal, a judicious tapering of the dosage should be begun. A common method is to decrease the opiate dose by 10%, with continued surveillance of the infant for tolerance of this decrease. It is not unusual to note increased signs of opiate withdrawal during the medication tapering. The goal of tapering is to allow the infant to acclimate to a new and lower dose of medication while ensuring that he or she is comfortable and consolable, and is able to sleep, eat, and gain weight appropriately. Objective measurements using established withdrawal scoring systems should be used to determine the rate and efficacy of medication tapering.

#### *Sudden Infant Death Syndrome and Opiates*

Numerous small studies and reports have suggested a link between maternal opiate use during pregnancy and an increased risk for sudden infant death syndrome (SIDS). A large 10-year study from New York showed, after data were controlled for known associated high-risk factors, that the risk ratio for SIDS was two to four times greater among opiate-exposed infants than among infants not exposed to any perinatal drugs (Kandall et al, 1993). Others, in a case-control study of SIDS in California, found that after adjustment of data for maternal smoking during pregnancy, there was no apparent association between maternal drug use and the occurrence of SIDS (Klonoff-Cohen et al, 2001; Ostrea et al, 1997). Using a meta-analysis of neonatal mortality rates in relation to opiate exposure, Hulse and colleagues (1998) found no support for a higher mortality rate among heroin- or methadone-exposed infants.

Interestingly, investigators have shown an increase in the rate of infant death (1 to 2 years after birth) in low-birth-weight infants (<2501 g) who had been exposed in utero to cocaine or cocaine plus opiates (Ostrea et al, 1997). It is unclear from this report how many of these infants represented cases of SIDS and how many were immature rather than growth-retarded at birth. To date, it is unclear whether there is an additional risk for SIDS for preterm infants who were exposed to opiates during gestation. A number of confounding maternal risk factors may be associated with both opiate use and SIDS. Reports point to the stronger association between maternal smoking and SIDS (Taylor and Sanderson, 1995).

### Prognosis

Because the typical opiate drug abuser uses multiple drugs, including cigarettes, alcohol, cocaine, PCP, and amphetamines, it is impossible to ascribe all adverse developmental effects in the infant of an opiate abuser to opiates alone. A woman's socioeconomic status has significant effects on her children's performances on intelligence measures and social adaptive behaviors. Because of multiple confounding factors in neurodevelopmental studies of opiate-exposed infants, controversy remains regarding the long-term effects of opiates on normal child development.

A number of studies suggests that exposure to exogenous opiates during fetal development may influence lifelong alterations in the developing brain. Infants who have been exposed to opiates in utero have a higher risk for fetal growth retardation and smaller head circumference than those who have not (Bauer, 1999). Also, significant developmental and learning deficits have been described in both methadone-exposed and heroin-exposed children (Soepatmi, 1994; van Baar and de Graaf, 1994; van Baar et al, 1994). Bunikowski and associates (1998) have reported a higher incidence of abnormalities in intellectual performance, developmental retardation, and neurologic abnormalities in a group of opiate-exposed infants compared with a control group of infants. However, the treated infants in the study had an unusually high incidence of seizures during withdrawal treatment (with phenobarbital alone) as well as a higher incidence of prematurity than the control infants. These important considerations temper the findings of the study.

Other investigators have shown normal development for opiate-exposed infants during the first 2 years of life after data have been controlled for socioeconomic status and birth weight (Bauer, 1999). Using regression analysis, researchers have shown that the amount of prenatal care obtained by the mother and the postnatal home environment were more predictive of the infant's future intellectual performance. Conversely, the amount of maternal opiate use during pregnancy was not found to be predictive. Others have pointed to the adverse environmental effects of poverty and poor learning environment on the development of methadone-exposed children. A multifactorial model has been proposed that encompasses both prenatal and postnatal influences on childhood development in drug-exposed infants (Zuckerman and Bresnahan, 1991). Ornoy and colleagues (2001) have shown that children exposed to heroin but adopted at an early age performed better on intelligence testing than opiate-exposed infants who were raised in their biologic homes. The same investigators found a higher rate of attention deficit disorders in children exposed to opiates regardless of home environment, with the highest incidence in children who were raised in their biological homes. Thus, numerous studies point to the importance of the home environment in optimizing child development.

## COCAINE

Cocaine is a highly psychoactive stimulant with a long history of abuse. A naturally occurring anesthetic of the tropane family of alkaloids, cocaine is obtained from the *Erythroxylon coca* plant, which is indigenous to the mountain slopes of Central and South America. The coca leaf has been chewed or made into a stimulant tea for centuries by the natives of these areas to decrease fatigue and hunger. Introduced to Europe in the 16th century, cocaine was isolated in 1860. Cocaine's euphoria-producing effect was exploited extensively in the United States in the late 19th and early 20th centuries, when the agent was an active ingredient in a number of widely used over-the-counter elixirs and tonics. Easy access became a major medical problem. Cocaine use markedly decreased after the Harrison Narcotic Act of 1914, which regulated the distribution of narcotics and cocaine, and the supervening Comprehensive Drug Abuse Prevention and Control Act of 1970, which classified cocaine as a Schedule II drug (i.e., one of "high abuse potential with restricted medical use," similar to opiates, barbiturates, and amphetamines). Until the mid-1980s, cocaine held the status of an expensive and exotic drug used primarily by the affluent as well as a performance enhancer by people in sports and entertainment. Its reputation as a glamour drug, the widely held misconception that cocaine is nonaddicting, and the development and marketing of crack, a cheap version of cocaine, were major factors in the resurgence of drug use. Cocaine and other stimulants have become the drugs of choice for women in the United States (Berger et al, 1990), with estimates that up to 13% of women 18 to 25 years old use cocaine regularly. Studies based on urine toxicology screening report a prevalence ranging from 5% of parturients in New York City, to 1.1% of those in a geographic sample in California, and to less than 0.5% of those in private hospitals in Denver, Colorado (Burke and Roth, 1993). Prevalence increases to 18% when both self-report and urine testing are used, and the highest prevalence rates are reported from studies using meconium testing. In these studies, up to 31% of women delivering in a high-risk urban setting and 3.4% of women randomly tested in more representative urban samples tested positive for cocaine use (Ostrea et al, 1992a, 1992b).

The pharmacologic actions of cocaine include inhibition of postsynaptic re-uptake of norepinephrine, dopamine, and serotonin neurotransmitters by sympathetic nerve terminals. Cocaine allows higher concentrations of neurotransmitters to interact with receptors. Higher levels of epinephrine and norepinephrine produce vasoconstriction, hypertension, and tachycardia. In adults, cocaine binds strongly to neuronal dopamine re-uptake transporters, thereby increasing postsynaptic dopamine at the mesolimbic and mesocortical levels and producing the addictive cycle of euphoria and dysphoria (Malanga and Kosofsky, 1999). Tryptophan uptake is similarly inhibited, altering serotonin pathways with resultant effects on sleep. Sodium ion permeability is blocked, producing the anesthetic effect of cocaine. The metabolites of cocaine are pharmacologically active and may produce neurotoxicity in the pregnant woman or her fetus. Two forms of cocaine are commonly used, cocaine hydrochloride and cocaine base (either extracted by organic solvents or precipitated as "crack" through the use of ammonia and baking soda). Cocaine hydrochloride is a water-soluble white powder that is used orally, intranasally ("snorting"), or intravenously ("running"). Intravenous users are more likely to have a history of heroin abuse and often use the drug in combination with heroin ("speedballing"). Cocaine hydrochloride decomposes on heating and is, therefore, cocaine converted to the free base for inhalation. "Freebasing" involves extraction of cocaine from aqueous solution into an organic solvent such as ether. "Crack," the most widely available form of free-base, is almost pure cocaine, and when it is smoked, it readily enters the blood stream to produce levels similar to those occurring with intravenous use. Crack cocaine is popular in urban minority communities, where it may be smoked in combination with PCP ("spacebasing"). Crack smoking appears to be particularly reinforcing and is associated with compulsive use, binges, and acceleration of the addictive process.

Many adverse perinatal outcomes associated with cocaine use are due to the effects of cocaine on uterine blood supply (Woods et al, 1987). An increase in maternal mean arterial blood pressure, a decrease in uterine blood flow, and a transient rise in fetal systemic blood pressure after an intravenous cocaine infusion have been described in fetal sheep (Moore et al, 1986). Animal studies demonstrated significant fetal hypoxemia associated with changes in uterine blood flow after cocaine infusion (Woods et al, 1987). Maternal hypertension and intermittent fetal hypoxia contribute to the higher risks for abruptio placentae and IUGR seen in cocaine-exposed infants.

Cocaine and some of its metabolites readily cross the placenta and achieve pharmacologic levels in the fetus (Schenker et al, 1993). Amniotic fluid may serve as a reservoir for cocaine and its metabolites and prolong exposure to vasoactive compounds. The extent to which cocaine or its metabolites are responsible for aberrant fetal growth, neurodevelopmental sequelae in exposed infants, and the range of congenital malformations reported in the literature may be less than suggested by uncontrolled case reports early in the cocaine-epidemic era. The confounding effects of increased use of multiple drugs, tobacco, or alcohol, nutritional deficits, and decreased use of prenatal care among cocaine-using women make interpretation of the causal relationships between gestational cocaine exposure and intrauterine growth and subsequent neurobehavioral development difficult (Chiriboga, 1993). These identified confounders may explain much or all of the reported effects attributed to cocaine in clinical series (Dempsey et al, 1996).

## Maternal Effects of Cocaine

Cocaine use leads to a sense of well-being, increased energy, increased sexual achievement, and an intense euphoria, or "high." The sympathomimetic action can have potentially devastating physiologic effects on the cardiovascular system. In adults, cocaine has been associated with cerebral hemorrhage, cardiac arrest, cardiac arrhythmias, myocardial infarction, intestinal ischemia, and seizures. Chronic use is associated with anorexia, nutritional problems, and paranoid psychosis. Chronic use of cocaine ultimately results in neurotransmitter depletion and a "crash," characterized by lethargy, depression, anxiety, severe insomnia, hyperphagia, and cocaine craving.

Women who use cocaine during pregnancy are at higher risk for stillbirths, spontaneous abortions, abruptio placentae, intrauterine growth restriction (IUGR), anemia and malnutrition, and maternal death from intracerebral hemorrhage (Table 12–6). Cocaine directly stimulates uterine contractions because of its alpha-adrenergic, prostaglandin, or dopaminergic effects, with resulting greater risks for fetal distress and premature deliveries. Abruptio placentae appears to be related to cocaine only when the drug is used shortly before delivery (Ostrea et al, 1992b). Other problems are evidence of fetal distress associated with abnormal fetal heart rate tracing and meconium staining (but not aspiration syndrome). Such women are at high risk for premature labor, low-birth-weight infants, premature rupture of the membranes, and perinatal infections. The higher prevalence of sexually transmitted disease in cocaine-using women has been associated with the trading of sex for drugs. In a high-risk, inner city population of New York City, Greenberg and colleagues (1991) found fourfold higher odds of cocaine exposure among infants with congenital syphilis. Both intravenous injection and noninjection use of cocaine increase the risks for acquisition of HIV, with a 3.5-fold higher risk among women who trade sex for crack cocaine (Lindsay et al, 1992).

**TABLE 12–6**

**Associated Clinical Features in the Mother and Infant with Cocaine Use During Pregnancy**

| | |
|---|---|
| Pregnancy | Spontaneous abortions<br>Abruptio placentae<br>Stillbirths<br>Premature delivery |
| Growth | Low birth weight<br>Intrauterine growth restriction<br>Small head |
| Infections | Perinatal human immunodeficiency virus<br>Congenital syphilis |
| Malformations | Urogenital<br>Brain<br>Midline defects (agenesis of the corpus callosum, septo-optic dysplasia)<br>Skull defects, encephaloceles<br>Ocular<br>Vascular disruption (limb reduction, intestinal atresia)<br>Cardiac |
| Neurodevelopmental findings | Neonates<br>Impaired organizational state<br>Hypertonia, tremor<br>Strokes, porencephaly<br>Seizures<br>Brainstem conduction delays<br>Sudden infant death syndrome<br>Infants and children<br>Hypertonia in infancy<br>Abnormal behaviors(?) |

Adapted with permission from Chiriboga CA: Cocaine and the fetus: Methodological issues and neurologic correlates. In Konkol RJ, Olsen GD: Prenatal Cocaine Exposure. Copyright CRC Press, Boca-Raton, FL, 1996.

## Fetal Growth

Multiple studies early in the cocaine epidemic documented diminished intrauterine growth as the most common fetal effect of gestational cocaine exposure, with weight, height, and head circumference affected at birth (Table 12–7). Investigators have demonstrated asymmetric IUGR (head circumference affected) among newborns exposed to high levels of exposure, but not in infants with low levels or no exposure to cocaine (Bateman and Chiriboga, 2000). Zuckerman and colleagues (1989) reported that abstinence after the first trimester reduces the intrauterine growth–retarding process but may not prevent diminished head growth or neurobehavioral abnormalities. Their large prospective study suggested direct cocaine effects on intrauterine growth as well as indirect effects of cocaine-associated undernutrition. The effects of suboptimal intrauterine growth on subsequent neurodevelopmental outcome abnormalities have not been distinguished from those of cocaine or its metabolites.

### Congenital Malformations

Cocaine has been reported to be associated with a variety of congenital anomalies in animals. A fourfold rise in genitourinary anomalies has been reported (Martin et al, 1992). Some of the malformations reported in cocaine-exposed

**TABLE 12-7**

**Neonatal Neurobehavioral Symptoms After Fetal Drug Exposure**

| Drug | Onset (days) | Peak (days) | Duration | Relative Severity |
|---|---|---|---|---|
| Alcohol | 0-1 | 1-2 | 1-2 days | Mild |
| Cocaine | 0-3 | 1-4 | ? mos | Mild–moderate |
| Amphetamine | 0-3 | | 2-8 wks | Mild–moderate |
| Phencyclidine | 0-2 | 5-7 | 2-6 mos | Moderate–severe |
| Heroin | 0-3 | 3-7 | 2-4 wks | Mild–moderate |
| Methadone | 3-7 | 10-21 | 2-6 wks | Mild–severe |

infants may be explained by effects of norepinephrine-mediated vasoconstriction (e.g., limb reduction deformities, intestinal atresia or infarction, and other vascular disruption sequences) during organogenesis (Mahalik and Hitner, 1994). CNS ischemic and hemorrhagic lesions have been inconsistently reported (Dusick et al, 1993; Konkol et al, 1994) in both term and premature infants. Cardiac malformations, including cardiomegaly, atrial septal defects, and ventricular septal defects, have also been reported (Lipschultz et al, 1991). Ocular abnormalities in infants that have been attributed to cocaine exposure include retinopathy, persistent hyperplastic vitreous, dilated and tortuous iris blood vessels, delayed visual maturation, palpebral edema, and structural anomalies of the eye (Dominguez et al, 1991). To date, no well-defined cocaine-associated syndrome has been identified, and the teratogenic potential of cocaine remains controversial. The association between fetal cocaine exposure and malformations may be confounded by higher rates of maternal tobacco, marijuana, or alcohol use among the cocaine-exposed groups. Overall, the preponderance of data from multiple studies fails to demonstrate higher rates of other congenital anomalies among cocaine-exposed infants (Behnke et al, 2001).

### Cocaine and Premature Delivery

Of all the problems attributed to cocaine use in the pregnant woman, the most common problem is premature delivery (Bateman et al, 1993). Infants born to women who use cocaine may experience sequelae of prematurity, including cerebral palsy, developmental delay, diminished intellectual capacity, and behavioral impairment. Most studies with sample sizes large enough to assess independent effects of cocaine on prematurity demonstrated this association (Gillogley et al, 1990; Handler et al, 1991). One study showed no such association in woman receiving prenatal care, suggesting that in the absence of prenatal care, cocaine may bear an independent association with prematurity (Zuckerman et al, 1989). A number of studies shows that prematurity and IUGR due to cocaine appear to be closely related to maternal lifestyle. In populations studied in which the mother receives good prenatal care in association with drug treatment, the incidence of prematurity and IUGR is low (Shiono et al, 1995). In the presence of poor prenatal care and no documented drug treatment, the rates of premature birth and IUGR are high. These findings have obvious implications for the development of effective treatment strategies to minimize adverse perinatal outcome in substance-abusing women, as has been suggested by cohort studies demonstrating lower rates of prematurity in women with adequate prenatal care. Overall, because of the higher risks of premature delivery, the frequency of respiratory distress syndrome is greater in cocaine-exposed infants. Cocaine-exposed infants less frequently require surfactant administration and intubation for respiratory distress syndrome; however, the risks of bronchopulmonary dysplasia are similar in infants who have and those who have not been exposed to cocaine during gestation (Hand et al, 2001).

### Neurobehavioral Abnormalities

Cocaine-exposed infants manifest a range of neurobehavioral abnormalities that were initially described as drug withdrawal but are more likely due to acute intoxication (Dempsey et al, 1996). Signs are present at birth or a few days thereafter and wane as cocaine and the metabolite, benzoylecgonine, are cleared from plasma. The infants are hypertonic, irritable, and tremulous (Chiriboga, 1993) and may have abnormal crying, sleep, and feeding patterns, although controlled, blinded studies have demonstrated cocaine withdrawal signs in a lower proportion of cocaine-exposed infants than in unblinded studies. Tachycardia, tachypnea, and apnea have been noted in two blinded, controlled studies, with significant elevations in cardiac output, stroke volume, mean arterial blood pressure, and cerebral artery flow velocity resolving by day 2, consistent with an intoxicant effect of cocaine (van de Bor et al, 1990a, 1990b). Other early and late patterns of neurobehavioral abnormalities are a depressed state occurring immediately after birth and lasting 3 to 4 days (resembling the adult cocaine crash) and a later hyperirritable phase with onset from 3 to 30 days (Mott et al, 1994). Cocaine-exposed infants may have abnormal electroencephalograms or clinical seizures, perhaps the result of toxicity from the metabolite, benzoylecgonine (Konkol et al, 1994). Although up to 50% of exposed infants in one series had seizures (Doberczak et al, 1989), this finding was not confirmed by another study (Legido et al, 1992), and in our experience, neonatal seizures stemming directly from maternal use of cocaine are rare. Seizures may occur because of complications associated with maternal cocaine use. Prospective studies have demonstrated increased rates of hypertonia, peaking at 6 months after birth and resolving in most children over the next 2 to 3 years (Chiriboga et al, 1995; Hurt et al, 1995).

Persisting behavioral, neurologic, and rearing problems are reported in children exposed to cocaine (Chasnoff et al, 1989a, 1992). Significant impairment of orientation, motor, and state regulation among infants with documented cocaine exposure during only the first trimester has been reported (Chasnoff et al, 1989a). In contrast, Chasnoff and colleagues (1992) noted no significant differences in mean developmental scores between a group of children exposed to cocaine plus polydrugs and a group without drug exposure. Other investigators report no differences between infants who have and those who have not been exposed to cocaine in mean cognitive, psychomotor, or language quotients at age 36 months (Kilbride et al, 2000). Compromised motor performance in late infancy has been reported in exposed infants in a controlled longitudinal study (Fetters and Tronick, 1996). These motor abnormalities did not persist at 15 months, and both the exposed infants and the control group had motor scores significantly below norms for age. Variable outcomes of these studies may depend on amounts and style of drug use, which vary with geographic area, or on other covariates, such as nutritional status, poverty, and parental educational level.

The neurodevelopmental problems among children exposed to cocaine may occur either from a direct encephalopathic drug effect during gestation or from the effects of the social environment in which the developing infant is reared. Singer and colleagues (2002) reported that cocaine-exposed infants are twice as likely to have significant cognitive but not motor delays at 2 years of age and raised the concern that exposed infants demonstrate a downward trend in mean developmental scores by age 2 consistent with a deleterious effect of the environment, parental stimulation, socioeconomic status, or possibly other, indirect effects of drugs on the developing CNS. Other studies have not consistently demonstrated this association (Frank et al, 2001). To date, little is known about subsequent effects on adult behavior and learning.

### Postnatal Growth

Growth-retarded infants exposed to cocaine generally exhibit catch-up growth. Their height at 18 months does not differ from that of control subjects not exposed to cocaine. By 2 years, the mean height of cocaine-exposed infants does not differ significantly from that of alcohol-exposed or marijuana-exposed infants. At all ages, infants exposed to drugs (cocaine, ethanol, or marijuana) have lower mean head circumferences than unexposed infants. Some studies, however, have questioned the belief that growth aberrations result from gestational cocaine exposure (Shankaran et al, 1998).

## AMPHETAMINES

Amphetamine (methylphenethylamine) was synthesized in 1887 and introduced in the United States in 1931, being marketed as Benzedrine. A number of other isomers soon followed, the D-isomer dextroamphetamine (marketed as Dexedrine) having four times greater CNS effects than the L-isomer. The *N*-methylated form, methamphetamine ("crystal"), is increasingly abused because it readily dissolves in water for injection and it "sublimes" (goes directly from a solid to gas) when smoked. The amphetamine isomers have similar clinical effects and can be distinguished only in the laboratory. Amphetamines were initially marketed for the treatment of obesity and narcolepsy and continue to be used for treatment of attention deficit disorders in children. Amphetamines are classified as Schedule II drugs, like cocaine and narcotics.

The clinical effects of amphetamines resemble those of cocaine. Like cocaine, amphetamines are sympathomimetics, and they potentiate the actions of norepinephrine, dopamine, and serotonin. In contrast to cocaine, amphetamines appear to exert their CNS effects primarily by enhancing the release of neurotransmitters from presynaptic neurons. Amphetamines may block re-uptake of released neurotransmitters. They may also exert a weaker direct stimulatory action on postsynaptic catecholamine receptors.

Amphetamines are taken orally, inhaled, or injected. The clinical effects and toxicity of these agents are often indistinguishable from those of cocaine. The primary difference is in the duration of action. The psychotropic effects of cocaine are of short duration, 5 to 45 minutes. The effects of amphetamines may last from 2 to 12 hours. Amphetamines have usurped cocaine as the primary illicit drugs used by pregnant women in many areas of California and other states. Methamphetamine ("crystal") has been the primary form abused. The appearance of a new smokable form of methamphetamine, ("ice"), has made methamphetamine the principal abused drug in several parts of the United States, especially Hawaii and California. Both crystal and ice can be produced locally and fairly cheaply. Greater restrictions on the importation of cocaine has also contributed to a resurgence in amphetamine use. Amphetamines have always been popular among adolescents, especially females, and accordingly, women of child-bearing age are at high risk for perinatal abuse. A California study of drug-exposed infants in the social welfare system documented a higher prevalence of amphetamine use among white pregnant women than in women of other ethnicities (Sagatun-Edwards et al, 1995).

The medical and obstetric complications of amphetamine use are similar to those described for cocaine use. Amphetamine toxicity has been described as more intense and prolonged than cocaine toxicity. Visual, auditory, and tactile hallucinations are common, and microvascular damage has been seen in the brains of chronic users. Amphetamine withdrawal is characterized by prolonged periods of hypersomnia, depression, and intense, often violent paranoid psychosis. Obstetric complications include a higher incidence of stillbirth. Like the pregnancies of cocaine-using women, the pregnancies of amphetamine users are characterized by poor prenatal care, sexually transmitted diseases, and cardiovascular problems including abruptio placentae and postpartum hemorrhage. The risk of cerebrovascular accidents is lower in pregnant amphetamine users than in pregnant cocaine users, but the mechanism for this difference is not understood.

Neonatal problems associated with amphetamine use during pregnancy include prematurity and IUGR. Fetal growth restriction, leading to smaller head circumference and lower birth weight, may result from the vasoconstrictive effects of norepinephrine or other vasoactive amines, or from diminished maternal nutrient delivery as a consequence of the anorectic effect of amphetamine. Systemic effects from altered norepinephrine metabolism explain the transient bradycardia and tachycardia reported in exposed infants. Studies have failed to show consistent patterns of malformations in amphetamine-exposed infants, although several studies report cleft lip and palate in association with amphetamine and methamphetamine exposure during early gestation (Plessinger, 1998). Neurodevelopmental abnormalities have been described during the neonatal period and appear to persist, as documented by follow-up studies, as late as 14 years (Cernerud et al, 1996). Intellectual capacity does not appear to be diminished among exposed infants. These children are described as exhibiting disturbed behavior, including hyperactivity, aggressiveness, and sleep disturbances. Eriksson and colleagues (2000) report that neurobehavioral abnormalities appear to be associated with the extent and the duration of fetal exposure and with the severity of head growth restriction. In this study, children with the most severe problems were those born to mothers who abused amphetamines throughout pregnancy and were reared in homes with an addicted parent. Alterations in growth have been reported after prenatal exposure, with striking gender differences (Cernerud et al, 1996). Drug-exposed boys in Sweden were taller and heavier, and girls smaller and lighter, than national standards. This finding suggests that fetal amphetamine exposure accelerates onset of puberty in boys and delays it in girls. There may be an added mechanism by which amphetamines interfere with neurodevelopment of the adenohypophysis. Children of amphetamine abusers appear to be at high risk for social problems, including abandonment, abuse, and neglect. In two Swedish studies, only 22% of 10-year-old children who had been exposed to amphetamine in utero remained in the care of their biologic mothers, whereas 70% were in foster care (Cernerud et al, 1996; Eriksson and Zetterstrom, 1994).

Substitution of aryloxy groups on the benzene ring of amphetamines produces "designer drugs," which are chemically similar to mescaline, the active ingredient in peyote cactus. These drugs have potent psychostimulant effects in addition to the serotonergic effects demonstrated in animals. Methylenedioxymethamphetamine (MDMA, "Ecstasy") and methylenedioxyethamphetamine (MDEA, "Eve") are increasingly used as recreational drugs. Their use during pregnancy has been reported in association with an overall higher incidence of a wide variety of congenital defects, including limb anomalies and cardiac septal defects (McElhatton et al, 1999), although the data from the case series are insufficient to establish a causal relationship between MDMA (in the absence of other drug use) and any specific anomaly. Other investigators have not found a consistent association between MDMA use during pregnancy and congenital anomalies (van Tonningen-van Driel et al, 1999). Because MDMA is often used in conjunction with other drugs, vigorous exercise, and poor diets, it is not clear whether reported fetal effects of its use during pregnancy are due to MDMA alone or to confounding factors.

## PHENCYCLIDINE

Phencyclidine hydrochloride (1-phenyl cyclohexyl piperidine) is an arylcyclohexamine developed in 1956 and marketed for the first time in 1963 as an anesthetic (Sernyl) and in the early 1970s as a veterinary drug (Sernylan). PCP was withdrawn from the market after reports of delirium and hallucinations and the recognition of its potential for abuse. No longer legally manufactured, PCP is still included in the Comprehensive Drug Abuse Prevention and Control Act of 1970. The first reports of the illicit use of PCP came in 1967 from the Haight-Ashbury district of San Francisco. Epidemic use of PCP began in the mid-1970s and peaked in 1983, when it was the most frequently used hallucinogen among young adults in the United States. Since it developed a reputation as a dangerous drug, its popularity has been episodic and often geographically and demographically concentrated. Use of PCP is common among polysubstance users, particularly in combination with marijuana, heroin, and alcohol, but not in combination with cocaine (Mvula et al, 1999).

PCP, also known as "angel dust," is a white crystalline powder that is soluble in water and alcohol. It can be inhaled, taken orally, or injected intravenously. Its popularity among young adults, especially women, however, relates to its low cost and the fact that it can be smoked. PCP is usually smoked by being sprinkled (dusted) on cigarettes ("lovely") or marijuana ("sherm"). PCP increases epinephrine release, but its exact mechanism of action is not clearly understood. PCP receptors have been identified in the brain, but their physiologic function and how they interact with PCP are unclear. The effects of the drug are dose-related and differ according to the duration of exposure. Low doses primarily cause euphoria associated with disturbances in body image. Moderate doses result in confusion, disorientation, and impaired sensory perception (analgesic and anesthetic effects). High doses are followed by hypertension, seizures, hyperpyrexia, an acute toxic paranoid psychosis, coma, and death. Chronic, continuing use of PCP results in violent behaviors, depressive anxiety, an organic brain syndrome, and, rarely, schizophrenia-like reactions. The toxic psychosis is treated with sensory isolation and diazepam, whereas the prolonged PCP psychosis requires antipsychotic medications.

PCP readily crosses the placenta to the fetus and is secreted in breast milk. Although animal studies demonstrate alterations in septohippocampal cholinergic innervations with later behavioral consequences (Yanai et al, 1992), data on the effects of PCP on pregnancy and the newborn are limited. From 1981 to 1984, PCP was the primary drug of abuse among parturients in some urban areas of the United States. In 1985, crack cocaine replaced PCP as the drug of choice for substance-abusing women. Subsequently, use of PCP has decreased in this country. Its use was more prevalent among pregnant Latinas in one study in California (Sagatun-Edwards et al, 1995).

The effects of PCP on the outcome of pregnancy appear to be dose related. In low doses, PCP has few side effects, although the anesthetic nature of the drug increases the frequency of precipitous deliveries at home, in ambulances, and in emergency departments. Although some studies have shown that up to 40% of PCP-exposed infants are small for gestational age, PCP is not necessarily associated with higher risk of prematurity or low birth weight (Mvula et al, 1999). Other obstetric complications are not known, but associated polydrug use, syphilis, and diabetes mellitus increase perinatal risks among infants exposed to phencyclidine (Mvula et al, 1999).

A severe syndrome associated with PCP exposure in utero has been reported, with onset shortly after birth (Rahbar et al, 1993). The timing and severity of the symptoms, often present at birth, raise the question whether the neurologic findings represent drug intoxication rather than drug withdrawal effects, because PCP persists in the body, and especially in the fetal brain, for prolonged periods (Ahmad et al, 1987). The neurologic findings in PCP-exposed infants include severe hypertonicity and hyperreflexia, often associated with spontaneous clonus and persisting for several weeks. Sudden episodes of agitation and fluctuating levels of consciousness have been described. Gastrointestinal symptoms, including abdominal distension, vomiting, and diarrhea, are also present in about 20% of the infants. The morbidity of significant PCP withdrawal can be attributed to gastrointestinal complications and the prolonged duration of symptoms. The mean duration of hospitalization in the authors' population was 14 days (range 10 to 21 days) (Ahmad et al, 1987). The withdrawal syndrome seen in infants exposed to PCP in combination with other drugs appears to be less intense, most likely in relation to a lower dose exposure or to inadvertent or erratic exposure when other drugs, such as cocaine, are "cut" with PCP.

Congenital anomalies have been inconsistently reported in association with PCP use during pregnancy. A clear causal association with PCP has not been verified. The reported somatic growth of PCP-exposed infants appears similar to that of polydrug-exposed infants. Isolated microcephaly, usually less severe than that seen in cocaine-exposed infants, has also been described and may be dose related (Rahbar et al, 1993).

Early alterations in state lability and consolability more severe than in all other drug-exposed groups have been documented in infants exposed in utero to PCP but do not appear to persist later in infancy. Neurobehavioral abnormalities, temperament problems, sleep disturbances, and aberrant attachment have been reported in infants with gestational exposure to PCP. Some long-term outcome studies of chronically PCP-exposed infants show a higher prevalence of severe developmental and behavioral problems.

## ALCOHOL

First described in Europe in 1968 and subsequently in the United States, fetal alcohol syndrome (FAS) is an extensively documented teratogenic syndrome. The incidence of FAS in the United States has been estimated to vary from 1.95 to 5 cases per 1000 live births (Abel, 1995; American Academy of Pediatrics [AAP], 2000; Sampson et al, 1997; Surveillance, 1997). Fetal alcohol syndrome is recognized more frequently in the United States than in other countries and is most common (4.3%) among women who report "heavy" drinking (Abel, 1995). Accurate incidence and prevalence rates of FAS are difficult to obtain because of wide variations in methodologies used for estimation of rates and because the clinical diagnosis is often missed in the neonatal period. In fact, most cases (up to 89%) are not diagnosed until after a child is 6 years old (Surveillance, 1997).

It is unclear how much alcohol exposure is necessary to cause fetal teratogenicity, and even high consumption levels do not always result in the birth of a child with FAS (Abel and Hannigan, 1995). However, a woman with a previous affected child is at increased risk for having a child with FAS if she consumes alcohol during a subsequent pregnancy. The adverse effects of alcohol on the fetus are related to gestational age at exposure, the amount of alcohol consumed and the pattern of consumption (binge drinking), maternal peak blood alcohol concentrations, maternal alcohol metabolism, and the individual susceptibility of the fetus. Studies show that maternal peak blood alcohol levels are affected by maternal nutrition, age, body size, and genetic disposition (Eckardt et al, 1998; Maier and West, 2001). Additionally, various risk factors increase susceptibility to FAS, including advanced maternal age and confounding factors such as nonwhite race, poverty, and socioeconomic status (Abel, 1995; Bagheri et al, 1998; May and Gossage, 2001). In the United States, the incidence of FAS is ten times higher for African-Americans living in poverty than for white middle class people (Abel, 1995). Indeed, despite the differences in incidence of FAS worldwide, reports consistently point to poverty (or socioeconomic status) as a major determinant of FAS (Abel 1995; May et al, 2000).

Accurate data quantifying fetal exposure are difficult to amass because of unreliable maternal history, the numerous methods of estimating alcohol exposure, and the lack of an objective measurement tool. Women with higher rates of alcohol intake are at the highest risk for fetal effects, but whether there is a dose-dependent response to fetal alcohol exposure or a threshold for fetal effects is unclear (Abel, 1999; Jones and Chambers, 1999). Our understanding of the effects of alcohol on the developing fetus, the importance of timing of exposure, and the effects of other agents (nutrition, smoking) in raising the incidence of FAS is incomplete (Abel, 1995). Because of these limitations, there is no absolutely safe level of alcohol ingestion during pregnancy (AAP, 2000).

The three major components of FAS are prenatal and postnatal growth deficiencies, characteristic facial features, and microcephaly associated with mental retardation (AAP, 2000; Jones and Smith, 1973; Stratton et al, 1996). The facial features consist of short palpebral fissures, midface hypoplasia, broad flat nasal bridge, a broad and indistinct philtrum, and thin upper vermilion. Other facial abnormalities have also been described, including ptosis, strabismus, and low-set or dysplastic ears. The CNS is the organ system most affected by fetal alcohol exposure. Microcephaly is the most serious finding with FAS. Investigators have also reported dysgenesis of the corpus callosum as well as hypoplasia of the basal ganglia and cerebellum in children with FAS (Archibald et al, 2001; Riley et al, 1995; Roebuck et al, 1998). A finding of FAS associated with facial dysmorphology is a hearing deficit with neurosensory hearing loss (AAP, 2000; Hannigan and

Armant, 2000). Children with FAS have poor coordination, hypotonia, and feeding impairment as infants. Attention deficit–hyperactivity disorder and speech and behavioral problems contribute to learning disabilities characteristic of these children (AAP, 2000). IUGR is one of the most consistent findings of prenatal exposure to alcohol (Hannigan and Armant, 2000). Growth deficit begins in utero and continues throughout childhood (AAP, 2000). The facial features and the growth restriction become less noticeable during adolescence and puberty (Streissguth, 1991, 1993). Skeletal anomalies, abnormal hand creases, and renal and cardiac anomalies have been described in children with FAS.

Children do not always exhibit the full FAS, but may have "partial FAS," manifesting a few malformations or neurodevelopmental disabilities believed to be secondary to fetal alcohol exposure (AAP, 2000; Stratton et al, 1996). Other terms developed to describe the spectrum of fetal alcohol effects include alcohol-related neurodevelopmental disorder (ARND) and alcohol-related birth defects (ARBDs). Children with a history of significant fetal alcohol exposure and subsequent behavioral, cognitive, or developmental disabilities are classified as having ARND; children with alcohol exposure and malformations are classified as having ARBDs. These clinical conditions have been reproduced in animal models and represent plausible consequences of fetal alcohol exposure (Abel and Hannigan, 1995). Although these terms are used to describe incomplete FAS, the clinical manifestations can be quite severe and disabling and should not be regarded as "mild" consequences of alcohol exposure (Abel, 1999). Indeed, children with heavy alcohol exposure during pregnancy but without the physical stigmata of FAS have been shown to have lower IQ scores, significant cognitive impairment, and abnormalities on testing of verbal learning and memory skills (Mattson et al, 1997, 1998).

Fetal alcohol syndrome is diagnosed from the history and physical findings. No laboratory tests are available for clinical use to quantify the extent of alcohol exposure during fetal life. There also are no clinical methods for validating maternal self-reporting of alcohol use, quantifying the level of fetal exposure, or predicting future disability after fetal exposure (Jones and Chambers, 1999). Koren and associates (2002) have proposed meconium fatty acid ethyl ester levels as a potential biologic marker for fetal alcohol exposure. Whether this finding is shown to correlate with childhood outcomes remains to be seen. The development of a screening tool for recognition of fetal alcohol exposure may help diagnose children at an earlier age than is currently seen. Investigators have shown that pediatricians fail to recognize FAS in the newborn and do not always inquire about alcohol exposure during pregnancy (Stoler and Holmes, 1999).

FAS is not a problem just for pediatricians. Patients with FAS continue to have serious disabilities into adulthood (Streissguth, 1991, 1993). Although the facial features and growth restriction are no longer as distinctive as during childhood, mental retardation continues to have a significant effect. Adults with FAS have behavior, socialization, and communication dysfunction, and on average, they function at the second or third grade level. A significant number of patients does not achieve fully independent living. Earlier recognition and intervention for children with FAS (and its variants) may help minimize eventual adulthood disabilities and help prepare adolescents and young adults with the disorder for independent living.

The approach to a newborn with suspected FAS is to establish the diagnosis by ruling out other causes of malformations, determining the extent of malformation, and establishing long-term care for both the mother and her infant. A reasonable postnatal assessment consists of head, renal, and cardiac ultrasonography as well as consultations with genetics, neurology, ophthalmology, and social services professionals.

## CIGARETTES AND NICOTINE

Cigarettes and nicotine are the drugs most often used during pregnancy. Although smoking in the United States has decreased over the last 2 decades, 26% of reproductive-aged women smoke, and 15% to 20% of women smoke during their pregnancies (Andres and Day, 2000). Cigarette smoking has been associated with numerous perinatal complications, often in a dose-dependent fashion. Smoking has been shown to raise the risk of spontaneous abortion, stillbirth, fetal growth retardation, prematurity, perinatal mortality, and SIDS (Andres and Day, 2000; Kallen, 2001; Lambers and Clark, 1996; Tuthill et al, 1999). Cigarette smoking represents the most influential and most common factor adversely affecting perinatal outcomes.

Nicotine crosses the placenta and concentrates in fetal blood, amniotic fluid, and breast milk (Haustein, 1999). Nicotine can be detected in the fetal circulation and in amniotic fluid at levels that significantly exceed maternal concentrations. The serum concentration of cotinine, the primary metabolite of nicotine, is used to quantitate the level of smoking and fetal exposure. Cotinine has a half-life of 15 to 20 hours, and because its serum levels are 10-fold higher than those of nicotine, this substance may represent a better marker for exposure (Lambers and Clark, 1996).

Although the exact mechanism of the adverse effect on pregnancy is unknown, cigarettes contain numerous potentially toxic compounds that presumably affect fetal health in a number of ways. In animal models, nicotine has been shown to raise maternal blood pressure and to be associated with a decrease in uterine blood flow. Additionally, with cigarette smoking, increased levels of carbon monoxide cross the placenta and form carboxyhemoglobin in the fetus (Lambers and Clark, 1996). Erythropoietin levels are also higher in smoking exposed infants at delivery, a finding presumed to reflect fetal hypoxia (Beratis et al, 1999; Jazayeri et al, 1998). Investigators have shown an association between the number of cigarettes a woman smokes and umbilical cord plasma erythropoietin levels (Jazayeri et al, 1998). Most theories of the adverse effects of smoking on fetal health involve the induction of fetal hypoxia from carbon monoxide production, nicotine-induced vasospasm, or both. A direct cytotoxic effect is also possible. Investigators have shown decreased levels of amino acids in umbilical cord blood samples for infants exposed to maternal smoking during pregnancy, suggesting a disturbance of protein metabolism during gestation (Jauniaux et al, 2001).

The effect of smoking on fetal growth is significant. Smoking affects fetal growth in a dose-dependent manner (Kyrklund-Blomberg and Cnattingius, 1998; Nordentoft et al, 1996). Investigators report that lower birth weights are associated with levels of exposure as measured by cotinine levels (Eskenazi et al, 1995; Perkins et al, 1997; Savitz et al, 2001). A 1-g reduction in birth weight has been observed for every μg/mL increase in maternal serum cotinine level (Eskenazi et al, 1995; Perkins et al, 1997). IUGR is also related to the number of cigarettes smoked. Investigators have shown a dose-dependent relationship between amount of smoking and extent of fetal growth restriction and birth weight reduction (Horta et al, 1997; Jaakkola et al, 2001; Savitz et al, 2001; Sprauve et al, 1999). The risk ratio for fetal growth restriction in heavy smokers (>20 cigarettes/day) was reported as 2.4 (95% confidence intervals, 1.4, 4.0) (Savitz et al, 2001). Smoking has also been show to affect the length of gestation in a dose-dependent manner, a higher risk of preterm delivery being associated with higher maternal cotinine levels (Jaakkola et al, 2001; Savitz et al, 2001). Investigators also report a twofold increase in the incidence of placental abruption in women who smoke (Ananth et al, 1996). Perinatal mortality is increased in pregnant smokers, likely reflecting the increases in rates of prematurity, growth retardation, placental abruption, and placenta previa in women who smoke. Mothers who smoke during pregnancy commonly continue to smoke during their infants' childhood. Asthma as well as recurrent otitis media are more common in infants exposed to passive smoking (Ey et al, 1995; Martinez et al, 1995).

Potential mechanisms for the effects of smoking on fetal growth have included direct effects of nicotine on placental vasoconstriction, decreased uterine blood flow, increased levels of fetal carboxyhemoglobin, fetal hypoxia, adverse maternal nutritional intake, and altered maternal and placental metabolism (Andres and Day, 2000; Pastrakuljic et al, 1999).

Both reducing and ceasing cigarette smoking during pregnancy have been shown to be beneficial and to improve fetal growth. Lieberman and colleagues (1994) have shown that if women stop smoking during the third trimester, their infants' weights are indistinguishable from those of a nonsmoking population. Other investigators report even a reduction in smoking is associated with improved fetal growth (Li et al, 1993; Walsh et al, 2001).

### Sudden Infant Death Syndrome (SIDS) and Cigarette Smoking

Numerous reports have shown a strong association between smoking and SIDS (Mitchell et al, 1997; Taylor and Sanderson, 1995; Tuthill et al, 1999). Among the numerous risk factors associated with the syndrome, maternal smoking was found to be independently associated with SIDS (Taylor and Sanderson, 1995). Prenatal, postnatal, and passive smoking exposures have all been shown to be associated with increased risk for SIDS (Blair et al, 1996; Mitchell et al, 1993; Schoendorf et al, 1992). Additionally, a dose-response relationship has been reported, consisting of an increased incidence of SIDS in association with a higher amount of maternal smoking (MacDorman et al, 1997; Mitchell et al, 1993). Investigators have found cotinine levels in pericardial fluid to be significantly higher in infants dying from SIDS than in infants with infectious causes of death (Milerad et al, 1998). Researchers in Germany have shown that in a population of heavy smokers during pregnancy, IUGR (lower birth weight, lower body mass index) was more common in infants dying from SIDS than in a population of surviving infants born to heavy smokers. The growth restriction effects were even more pronounced in preterm infants exposed to heavy smoking during pregnancy (Schellscheidt et al, 1998). This study suggests that preterm infants who are born to heavy smokers and have IUGR are at a high risk for crib death.

The direct physiologic link between smoking and SIDS has not been identified. Theories are proposed that cigarette smoking may alter lung function or may alter CNS control of respiration, arousal, or both (Andres and Day, 2000). Slotkin and colleagues (1995), documenting loss of neonatal hypoxia tolerance after prenatal nicotine exposure, suggest this finding as a causative factor in the increased risk of SIDS among offspring of mothers who smoke.

## MARIJUANA

Marijuana is probably the illegal drug most frequently used during pregnancy. It is derived from the hemp plant *Cannabis*, and its most active ingredient being delta-9-tetrahydrocannabinol. Use of marijuana during pregnancy is associated with growth retardation. Neurologic abnormalities similar to a mild withdrawal syndrome, consisting of hypertonicity, irritability, and jitteriness, have been seen in the newborn but without documented evidence of long-term sequelae. Marijuana is often used in combination with other drugs and may potentiate risks for prematurity, low birth weight, or the teratogenic effects of other drugs (Cornelius et al, 1995).

## CAFFEINE

Fetal exposure to caffeine may occur in 75% of pregnancies in the United States (Eskenazi, 1993). Caffeine is contained in coffee, tea, colas, and chocolate (100 mg/cup of coffee). Most studies detect an increased risk of IUGR with caffeine intake in excess of 300 mg/day—that is to say, a detectable and significant increase of growth retardation occurs (relative risk about 1.5). Many studies also report a higher risk of spontaneous abortion with higher amount of caffeine exposure (e.g., risk of abortion increases by 1.017 for each cup of coffee per day in the first trimester [Armstrong et al, 1992]). Most studies of caffeine, like those of other licit and illicit drugs, share problems of ascertainment, dose, duration, response, and confounding factors. For example, genetic differences may affect susceptibility to caffeine. Caffeine may have fetotoxic additive effects when combined with smoking, and drinks such as coffee may contain ingredients with effects on pregnancy that are independent of the effects of caffeine. Granted these considerations, and to a greater degree than with other drugs discussed in this chapter, it is usually not possible to attribute growth retardation or spontaneous abortion in a specific case to caffeine. It is prudent to advise women to limit maximum caffeine intake to less than 100 mg/day both when pregnant and when anticipating pregnancy (Infante-Rinard et al, 1993).

## MANAGEMENT OF GESTATIONAL SUBSTANCE USE

### Intrapartum Management

The pregnant woman with suspected or admitted gestational or intrapartum substance use should undergo urine toxicology screening after informed consent; clinicians should recognize, however, that both self-report and urine screening are neither sensitive nor specific tools for identifying intrapartum complications, neonatal morbidity, long-term outcome, or families at risk of child neglect or abuse. Identification of gestational substance use offers the potential benefits of screening for sexually transmitted diseases, closer obstetric monitoring of maternal and fetal well-being, drug counseling, support and referrals for rehabilitation, and social service needs assessment. Use of prenatal care should be encouraged on the basis of the benefits to the mother and fetus rather than enforced by incarceration or prosecution. Obstetric care should be given in a nonjudgmental manner, and the givers of such care should avoid being codependent or punitive. Recommendations for intrapartum medications in substance users do not differ from those for drug-free women; however, drug-using women may require treatment for hypertension, agitation, or low tolerance of pain.

We recommend using standardized criteria for perinatal toxicology screening to avoid the risks of differential screening and reporting. Routine prenatal laboratory tests, including third-trimester (or intrapartum) syphilis serology, should be performed. We also strongly encourage HIV antibody testing for drug-using women, in keeping with current obstetric recommendations for routine perinatal care. Postpartum education should stress general health, routine postpartum teaching, breast-feeding risks, neonatal care, parenting skills, and the need for obstetric and neonatal follow-up. Referrals for drug treatment and counseling should be facilitated before discharge, with the recognition that resources available to substance-using women with children are scarce. Follow-up by a public health nurse is recommended.

### Neonatal Care

Although at higher risk for medical complications, the majority of infants of drug-using women do not require intensive neonatal care. Symptomatic infants often need more nursing care. Admission physical examination should document a maturational age assessment, birth weight, head circumference, and length. Infants should be examined for any evidence of malformations or complications of prematurity. Hypertonic, tremulous infants usually respond to swaddling, being held, decreases in ambient environmental stimuli (light and noise), pacifiers, and more frequent feedings. Studies such as electroencephalography, brain imaging, and renal ultrasonography may add diagnostic or prognostic information when physical or neurologic abnormalities are noted, but these procedures are not indicated for all drug-exposed infants. Neurologic or ophthalmologic evaluation may document tone and ocular abnormalities in some infants, but it is not clear that all drug-exposed infants should be referred for such examination. Feedings in premature infants with cocaine exposure should be started with diluted formula in lower than usual volume increments, because premature infants exposed to cocaine have been found to be at increased risk for both early-onset and late-onset necrotizing enterocolitis. Maternal cocaine use exposes infants to a higher than expected risk of problems with postasphyxial syndrome, and organ malfunction from this cause should be sought and treated.

Toxicology testing should be performed on neonatal urine (or meconium, as a potential substitute method) as soon as possible. Infants should undergo screening for anemia, polycythemia, hypoglycemia, congenital syphilis, and perinatal HIV exposure. Discharge planning should identify a continuity provider as well as support services for the mother and infant (e.g., nutritional, social/familial, parenting) and a plan for neurodevelopmental follow-up.

### Mother-Infant Care

Breast-feeding has the benefits of improved bonding, but the risks of HIV and continued drug exposure may outweigh these benefits. Women who wish to breast-feed despite these potential risks should undergo drug monitoring of breast milk and sequential HIV antibody testing. Close observation of mother-infant interaction should be documented in the infant's chart. Parenting and child-care skills should be stressed as part of the discharge education for the mother. All physician interactions with the family should be documented in detail.

## BREAST-FEEDING AND DRUG EXPOSURE

Psychotropic drugs, which are of low molecular weight and lipophilic, are readily excreted in breast milk. Breast-feeding by women using methadone is not recommended by the American Academy of Pediatrics (American Academy of Pediatrics Committee on Drugs, 1994). Methadone is excreted in small quantities in breast milk regardless of the daily maternal methadone dose and is probably safe for infants (Geraghty et al, 1997; McCarthy and Posey, 2000). Seizures and symptoms of overdose have been reported in an infant whose mother used cocaine. Amphetamines appear in large quantities in breast milk. PCP has also been found to cross into breast milk readily. Because of the risk of toxicity, breast-feeding should be discouraged for known abusers of these drugs. An exception is made for mothers enrolled in drug treatment programs in which the methadone use is monitored closely. Judicious evaluation of other safety considerations must be made on a case-by-base basis before allowing the infant to breast-feed, although we recommend caution if the mother is using a high methadone dose, and we actively discourage breast-feeding when mothers are not compliant with their maintenance programs or are infected with or at high risk for HIV. Alcohol use while breast-feeding is not listed as a contraindication by the

American Academy of Pediatrics, but excessive maternal alcohol intake during breast-feeding may be deleterious for the infant and should be avoided (see Chapter 33). Smoking in the postnatal period as well as during breast-feeding also has deleterious effects on the newborn. Smoking is associated with measurable levels of nicotine and cotinine in maternal breast milk.

## SUDDEN INFANT DEATH SYNROME IN DRUG-EXPOSED INFANTS

The incidence of SIDS is greater in drug-exposed infants, although the increase appears less significant for cocaine-exposed infants (Chasnoff et al, 1989b; Kandall et al, 1993) than for methadone-exposed or heroin-exposed infants (Bauchner and Zuckerman, 1990). A meta-analysis of 10 studies demonstrated a 4.1 odds ratio for SIDS among cocaine-exposed infants (Fares et al, 1997) in comparison with infants not exposed to perinatal drugs. However, after data were controlled for concurrent use of other drugs, the increased risk for SIDS could not be attributed to intrauterine cocaine alone, but was believed to be due to exposure to illicit drugs in general. Additionally, a higher risk for SIDS in infants exposed to maternal smoking appears to be present whether the exposure is antenatal or postnatal (Blair et al, 1996; Mitchell et al, 1993; Schoendorf and Kiely, 1992). Despite the increased risks of SIDS among drug-exposed infants, neither polysomnography nor home apnea monitoring are indicated in the absence of other risk factors for SIDS.

## HUMAN IMMUNODEFICIENCY VIRUS INFECTION

Nationwide, intravenous drug abusers are the second largest risk group for HIV infection. Drug abusers also may be the primary source of infection for non-using heterosexuals as well as for children (Chamberland and Dondero, 1987). Nationwide, 75% of cases of acquired immunodeficiency syndrome in children are perinatally acquired. The seropositivity rate varies across the country; the rate among female intravenous drug users in New York City and northern New Jersey is estimated at 50% to 70%, compared with 5% to 20% in California. Heroin and cocaine addicts often resort to prostitution to support their habits. Amphetamine and methamphetamine users often inject drugs several times daily. Alcohol decreases sexual inhibition, impairs judgment, and increases the incidence of unsafe sexual activity. Every infant born to a substance abuser should be evaluated for HIV infection, and universal precautions should be observed.

## DISPOSITION OF COCAINE-EXPOSED INFANTS

Many states include maternal substance abuse among reasons for mandated reporting of an infant to child protective services for evaluation of potential foster care placement. Cocaine exposure increases the risk for foster care placement from a general background rate of 1% to 2% among nonexposed infants to 26% to 58% in exposed infants (U.S. General Accounting Office, 1990). Cocaine use has become the dominant characteristic of child welfare caseloads in 22 states and the District of Columbia (Besharov, 1989). Variations in screening and reporting protocols lead to inconsistent reporting practices. In a Florida study, for example, referrals to child protective services were more frequent for black women using crack cocaine (Chasnoff et al, 1990). In California, cases involving maternal cocaine use are more apt to reach court adjudication for foster care placement than are cases involving maternal use of amphetamines (Chasnoff et al, 1990; Sagatun-Edwards et al, 1995).

The number of children in foster care rose by 81% in the first 4 years of the crack cocaine epidemic (County Welfare Directors Association of California, 1990). This increase was attributed to the cocaine epidemic and was associated with a decrease in the average age of children in foster care and with rapidly increased numbers of out-of-home placements (Halfon et al, 1990). Maltreatment of infants of cocaine-using women has been described in a controlled cohort study (Wasserman and Leventhal, 1993). However, the neurobehavioral abnormalities seen in foster children suggest that the separation of mother and infant should occur only in high-risk cases.

Costs of care for cocaine-exposed infants are significantly higher than for nonexposed infants and outweigh the costs of providing prenatal care (Joyce et al, 1995). The added costs of gestational cocaine exposure include those of perinatal care for the substance-using woman, of neonatal intensive care, and of boarding infants awaiting release to foster care, in addition to the costs of later specialized services to infants with the anatomic or neurodevelopmental sequelae of cocaine exposure.

## IDENTIFICATION AND GOALS OF INTERVENTION

The abuse of a variety of drugs during pregnancy has adverse consequences for the mother, fetus, and newborn. Clearly, it is important to ascertain and distinguish the causes of fetal and neonatal consequences of IUGR, vascular problems, and acute neurobehavioral symptoms. It is often less clear why one should identify infants who have been exposed to drugs in utero if they are asymptomatic. Reasons offered are that a positive toxicology screen result (sometimes backed by the potential loss of her newborn to foster care) may break through the mother's denial of drug abuse and enable her to accept treatment. In addition, courts are more apt to accept hard evidence such as a positive toxicology test result than historical data of drug abuse that may be denied by the mother.

History of drug and alcohol use should be routinely included in the initial contact with every pregnant patient. To be effective, the history-taking must be nonjudgmental and must occur in the context of other lifestyle questions. When a positive history of use is obtained, intervention should begin immediately. The person taking the history should be prepared to offer preliminary counseling on risk reduction and concrete referrals for treatment programs, although access to drug programs is often restricted, inadequate, or delayed.

A more controversial method of identification is using drug screening of mothers and infants in cases in which drug abuse is suspected. Rapid reliable drug testing using urine or blood is readily available in most clinical laboratories. Drug screening has proved reliable in both high-prevalence urban and in low-prevalence rural settings (O'Connor et al, 1997). Drug screening should be combined with a history and should be a part of a well-delineated protocol that clearly defines which infants and mothers should be screened. Screening protocols should be based on well-defined, high-risk behavior documented to be associated with perinatal drug abuse. High-risk behavior during the prenatal period consists of a history of drug abuse, physical evidence of drug use (track marks or altered mental status), noncompliance with medical treatment and appointments, history of child abuse or removal of children from the home, and history of a partner who uses drugs or excessive alcohol. Homelessness, prostitution, and recent incarceration are also risk factors. A large percentage of drug abusers has no prenatal care or inadequate prenatal care (beginning in the last trimester or consisting of only a few visits), and this group has a high rate of complicated deliveries. In addition, screening may include patients being admitted to the hospital with the complications associated with drug abuse, such as hemorrhage, untreated sexually transmitted diseases, and premature labor. Infants born to mothers who received no prenatal care and those born precipitously or prematurely should also be included in a toxicology screening protocol. Screening should always be done in a manner to ensure as much as possible the right of privacy of the mother while allowing physicians to provide optimal medical care to both mother and infant. Also, the infant should never be screened unless the mother is informed of the testing and the reasons for it.

In the absence of intervention, infants discharged to mothers who abuse alcohol or illegal drugs are at high risk for subsequent physical abuse and neglect, but the extent of risk is unknown. Most states require some form of reporting of such cases to a child protective service agency. States differ in the aggressiveness with which they deal with this issue. In some states, the child's drug exposure may be considered prima facie evidence of abuse. In general, however, the mother's addiction is evaluated in the context of its effect on her ability to care for her child. The primary focus of physicians caring for the mother and infant should be to ensure that all interventions are therapeutic and designed to foster the health of both patients.

## REFERENCES


Abel E: An update on incidence of FAS: FAS is not an equal opportunity birth defect. Neurotoxicol Teratol 17:437, 1995.

Abel E: What really causes FAS? Teratology 59:4, 1999.

Abel E, Hannigan J: Maternal risk factors in fetal alcohol syndrome: Provocative and permissive influences. Neurotoxicol Teratol 17: 445, 1995.

Agarwal P, Rajadurai V, Bhavani S, Tan KW: Perinatal drug abuse in KK Women's and Children's Hospital. Ann Acad Med Singapore 28:795, 1999.

Ahmad G, Halsall LC, Bondy SC: Persistence of phencyclidine in fetal brain. Brain Res 415:194, 1987.

American Academy of Pediatrics Committee on Drugs: The transfer of drugs and other chemicals into human milk. Pediatrics 93:137, 1994.

American Academy of Pediatrics Committee on Substance Abuse and Committee on Children with Disabilities: Fetal alcohol syndrome and alcohol-related neurodevelopmental disorders. Pediatrics 106:358, 2000.

Anand K, Arnold J: Opioid tolerance and dependence in infants and children. Crit Care Med 22:334, 1994.

Ananth C, Savitz D, Luther E: Maternal cigarette smoking as a risk factor for placental abruption, placenta previa, and uterine bleeding in pregnancy: Am J Epidemiol 144:881, 1996.

Andres R, Day M: Perinatal complications associated with maternal tobacco use. Semin Neonatol 5:231, 2000.

Annas G: Testing poor pregnant women for cocaine: Physicians as police investigators. N Engl J Med 344:1729, 2001.

Archibald S, Fennema-Notestine C, Gamst A, et al: Brain dysmorphology in individuals with severe prenatal alcohol exposure. Dev Med Child Neurol 43:148, 2001.

Armstrong BG, McDonald AD, Sloan M: Cigarettes, alcohol and coffee consumption and spontaneous abortion. Am J Public Health 82:85, 1992.

Bagheri M, Burd L, Martsolf J, Klug M: Fetal alcohol syndrome: Maternal and neonatal characteristics. J Perinat Med 26:263, 1998.

Barr G, Jones K: Opiate withdrawal in the infant. Neurotoxicol Teratol 16:219, 1994.

Bateman DA, Chiriboga CA: Dose-response effect of cocaine on newborn head circumference. Pediatrics 106:E33, 2000.

Bateman DA, Ng SK, Hansen CA, Heagarty MC: The effects of intrauterine cocaine exposure in newborns. Am J Public Health 83:190, 1993.

Bauchner H, Zuckerman BS: Cocaine, sudden infant death syndrome, and home monitoring. J Pediatr 117:904, 1990.

Bauer C: Perinatal effects of prenatal drug exposure. Clin Perinatol 26:87, 1999.

Behnke M, Eyler F: The consequences of prenatal substance use for the developing fetus, newborn and young child. Int J Addict 28:1341, 1993.

Behnke M, Eyler FD, Garvan CW, Wobie K: The search for congenital malformations in newborns with fetal cocaine exposure. Pediatrics 107:E74, 2001.

Beratis N, Varvarigou A, Christophidou M, et al: Cord blood α-fetoprotein concentrations in term newborns of smoking mothers. Eur J Pediatr 158:583, 1999.

Berger CS, Sorenson L, Gendler B, Fitzsimmons J: Cocaine and pregnancy: A challenge for health care providers. Health Soc Work 15:310, 1990.

Besharov D: The children of crack: Will we protect them? Public Welfare 47:6, 1989.

Blair P, Fleming P, Bensley D, et al: Smoking and the sudden infant death syndrome: Results from 1993-5 case-control study for confidential inquiry into stillbirths and deaths in infancy. BMJ 313:195, 1996.

Boer K, Smit B, van Huis A, Hogerzeil H: Substance use in pregnancy: Do we care? Acta Paediatr 404(Suppl):65, 1994.

Brown H, Britton K, Mahaffey D, et al: Methadone maintenance in pregnancy: A reappraisal. Am J Obstet Gynecol 179: 459, 1998.

Bunikowski R, Grimmer I, Heiser A, et al: Neurodevelopmental outcome after prenatal exposure to opiates. Eur J Pediatr 157:724, 1998.

Burke MS, Roth D: Anonymous cocaine screening in a private obstetric population. Obstet Gynecol 81:354, 1993.

Cernerud L, Eriksson M, Jonsson B: Amphetamine addiction during pregnancy: 14-year follow-up of growth and school performance. Acta Paediatr 85:204, 1996.

Chamberland ME, Dondero TJ: Heterosexually acquired infection with human immunodeficiency virus (HIV): A view from the III International Conference on AIDS. Ann Intern Med 107:763, 1987.

Chang G, Carroll K, Behr H, Kosten T: Improving treatment outcome in pregnant opiate-dependent women. J Subst Abuse Treat 9:327, 1992.

Chasnoff IJ, Griffith DR, MacGregor S: Temporal patterns of cocaine use in pregnancy: Perinatal outcome. JAMA 261:1741, 1989a.

Chasnoff IJ, Hunt CE, Kletter R, Kaplan D: Prenatal cocaine exposure is associated with respiratory pattern abnormalities. Am J Dis Child 143:583, 1989b.

Chasnoff IJ, Landress HJ, Barrett ME: The prevalence of illicit-drug or alcohol use during pregnancy and discrepancies in mandatory reporting in Pinellas County, Florida. N Engl J Med 332:1202, 1990.

Chasnoff IJ, Griffith DR, Freier C, Murray J: Cocaine/polydrug use in pregnancy: Two-year follow-up. Pediatrics 89:284, 1992.

Chiriboga CA: Neurologic complications of drug and alcohol abuse: Fetal effects. Neurol Clin 11:707, 1993.

Chiriboga CA, Vibbert M, Malouf R: Neurological correlates of fetal cocaine exposure: Transient hypertonia of infancy and early childhood. Pediatrics 96:1070, 1995.

Cornelius MD, Taylor PM, Geva D, Day N: Prenatal tobacco and marijuana use among adolescents: Effects on offspring gestational age, growth and morphology. Pediatrics 95:738, 1995.

Coyle M, Ferfuson A, Lagasse L, et al: Diluted tincture of opium (DTO) and phenobarbital versus DTO alone for neonatal opiate withdrawal in term infants. J Pediatr 140:561, 2002.

Dashe J, Jackson G, Olscher D, et al: Opioid detoxification in pregnancy. Obstet Gynecol 92:854, 1998.

Dempsey DA, Ferriero DM, Jacobson SN: Critical review of evidence for neonatal cocaine intoxication and withdrawal. In Konkol R, Olsen G (eds): Effects of Cocaine Exposure: Mechanisms and Outcome. Boca Raton, FL, CRC Press, 1996.

Doberczak TM, Shanzer S, Senie RT, Kandall SR: Neonatal neurologic and electroencephalographic effects of intrauterine cocaine exposure. J Pediatr 113:354, 1989.

Doberczak TM, Kandall S, Friedmann P: Relationships between maternal methadone dosage, maternal-neonatal methadone levels and neonatal withdrawal. Obstet Gynecol 81:936, 1993.

Dominguez R, Aguirre V, Coro A: Brain and ocular abnormalities in infants with in utero exposure to cocaine and other street drugs. Am J Dis Child 145:688, 1991.

Dusick A, Covert R, Schreiber M: Risk of intracranial hemorrhage and other adverse outcomes after cocaine exposure in a cohort of 323 very low birth weight infants. J Pediatr 122:438, 1993.

Eckardt M, File S, Gessa G, et al: Effects of moderate alcohol consumption on the central nervous system. Alcohol Clin Exp Res 22:998, 1998.

Eriksson M, Zetterstrom R: Amphetamine addiction during pregnancy: 10-year follow-up. Acta Paediatr 404(Suppl):27, 1994.

Eriksson M, Jonsson B, Zetterstrom R: Children of mothers abusing amphetamine: Head circumference during infancy and psychosocial development until 14 years of age. Acta Paediatr 89:1474, 2000.

Eskenazi B: Caffeine during pregnancy: Grounds for concern? JAMA 270:2973, 1993.

Eskenazi B, Prehn AW, Christianson RE: Passive and active maternal smoking as measured by serum cotinine: The effect on birthweight. Am J Public Health 85:395, 1995.

Ey JL, Holberg CJ, Aldous MB: Passive smoke exposure and otitis media in the first year of life. Pediatrics 95:670, 1995.

Fares I, McCulloch KM, Raju TN: Intrauterine cocaine exposure and the risk for sudden infant death syndrome: A meta-analysis. J Perinatal 17:1790, 1997.

Fetters L, Tronick EZ: Neuromotor development of cocaine-exposed and control infants from birth through 15 months: Poor and poorer performance. Pediatrics 98:938, 1996.

Finnegan L: Perinatal substance abuse: Comments and perspectives. Semin Perinatol 15:331, 1991.

Finnegan L, Connaughton J, Kron R: Neonatal abstinence syndrome: Assessment and management. Addict Dis 2:141, 1975.

Franck L, Vilardi J: Assessment and management of opioid withdrawal in ill neonates. Neonatal Network 14:39, 1995.

Frank D, Augustyn M, Grant-Knight W, et al: Growth, development, and behavior in early childhood following prenatal cocaine exposure: A systematic review. JAMA 285:1613, 2001.

Geraghty B, Graham E, Logan B, Weiss E: Methadone levels in breast milk. J Hum Lact 13:227, 1997.

Gillogley K, Evans A, Hansen R: The perinatal impact of cocaine, amphetamine and opiate use detected by universal intrapartum screening. Am J Obstet Gynecol 163:1535, 1990.

Green M, Suffet F: The Neonatal Narcotic Withdrawal Index: A device for the improvement of care in the abstinence syndrome. Am J Drug Alcohol Abuse 8:203, 1981.

Greenberg MS, Singh T, Htoo M, Schultz S: The association between congenital syphilis and cocaine/crack in New York City: A case control study. Am J Public Health 81:1316, 1991.

Hagopian G, Wolfe H, Sokol R, et al: Neonatal outcome following methadone exposure in utero. J Matern Fetal Med 5:348, 1996.

Halfon N, Berkowitz G, Klee L: Health and mental health utilization by children in foster care in California: Policy seminar brief. Berkeley, California, University of California, 1990.

Hand I, Noble L, McVeigh T, et al: The effects of intrauterine cocaine exposure on the respiratory status of the very low birth weight infant. J Perinatol 21:372, 2001.

Handler A, Kistin N, Davis F, Ferre C: Cocaine use during pregnancy: Perinatal outcome. Am J Epidemiol 133:818, 1991.

Hannigan J, Armant D: Alcohol in pregnancy and neonatal outcome. Semin Neonatol 5:243, 2000.

Harper R, Solish G, Feingold E: Maternal ingested methadone, body fluid methadone, and the neonatal withdrawal syndrome. Am J Obstet Gynecol 129:417, 1977.

Hartnoll R: Opiates: Prevalence and demographic factors. Addiction 89:1377, 1994.

Haustein K: Cigarette smoking, nicotine, and pregnancy. Int J Clin Pharmacol Ther 37:417, 1999.

HHS/Substance Abuse and Mental Health Services Administration: Summary of findings from the 2000 National Household Survey on Drug Abuse. Office of Applied Studies. (NHSDAH 13, DHHS publication No. [SMA] U 3549.) Substance Abuse and Mental Health Services Administration. Rockville, MD, 2001.

Horta B, Victora C, Menezes A, et al: Low birthweight, preterm births and intrauterine growth retardation in relation to maternal smoking. Paediatr Perinat Epidemiol 11: 140, 1997

Hulse G, O'Neill G: Methadone and the pregnant use: A matter for careful clinical consideration. Aust N Z J Obstet Gynaecol 41:329, 2001.

Hulse G, Milne E, English D, Holman C: The relationship between maternal use of heroin and methadone and infant birth weight. Addiction 92:1571, 1997.

Hulse G, Milne E, English D, Holman C: Assessing the relationship between maternal opiate use and neonatal mortality. Addiction 93:1033, 1998.

Human Resources Division. U. S. General Accounting Office: Drug Exposed Infants: A Generation at Risk. (USGAO publication No. 238209. GAO/HRD-90.138), Washington, DC, 1990.

Hurt H, Brodsky NL, Betancourt L: Cocaine-exposed children: Follow-up through 30 months. J Dev Behav Pediatr 16:29, 1995.

Infante-Rinard C, Fernandez A, Gauthier R: Fetal loss associated with caffeine intake before and during pregnancy. JAMA 270:2940, 1993.

Jaakkola J, Jaakkola N, Zahlsen K: Fetal growth and length of gestation in relation to prenatal exposure to environmental tobacco smoke assessed by hair nicotine concentrations. Environ Health Perspect 109:557, 2001.

Jauniaux E, Biernaux V, Gerlo E, Gulbis B: Chronic maternal smoking and cord blood amino acid and enzyme levels at term. Obstet Gynecol 97:57, 2001.

Jazayeri A, Isibris J, Spellacy W: Umbilical cord plasma erythropoietin levels in pregnancies complicated by maternal smoking. Am J Obstet Gynecol 178:433, 1998.

Jones H: Shorter dosing interval of opiate solution shortens hospital stay for methadone babies. Fam Med 31:327, 1999.

Jones K, Chambers C: What really causes FAS? A different perspective. Teratology 60:249, 1999.

Jones K, Smith D: Recognition of the fetal alcohol syndrome in early infancy. Lancet 3:999, 1973.

Joyce T, Racine AD, McCalla S, Wehbeh H: The impact of prenatal exposure to cocaine on newborn costs and length of stay. Health Serv Res 30:341, 1995.

Kallen K: The impact of maternal smoking during pregnancy on delivery outcome. Am J Public Health 11:329, 2001.

Kandall S, Doberczak T: The methadone-maintained pregnancy. Clin Perinatol 26:173, 1999.

Kandall S, Doberczak T, Mauer K, et al: Opiate vs CNS depressant therapy in neonatal drug abstinence syndrome. Am J Dis Child 137:378, 1983.

Kandall S, Gaines J, Habel L, et al: Relationship of maternal substance abuse to subsequent sudden infant death syndrome in offspring. J Pediatr 123:120, 1993.

Kilbride H, Castor C, Hoffman E, Fuger KL: Thirty-six month outcome of prenatal cocaine exposure for term or near-term infants: impact of early management. J Develop Behav Pediatr 21:19, 2000.

Klonoff-Cohen H, Lam-Kruglick P: Maternal and paternal recreational drug use and sudden infant death syndrome. Arch Pediatr Adolesc Med 155:765, 2001.

Konkol RJ, Murphey L, Ferriero DM, et al: Cocaine metabolites in the neonate: Potential for toxicity. J Child Neurol 9:242, 1994.

Koren G, Chan D, Klein J, Karaskov T: Estimation of fetal exposure to drugs of abuse, environmental tobacco smoke, and ethanol. Ther Drug Monit 24:23, 2002.

Kyrklund-Blomberg N, Cnattingius S: Preterm birth and maternal smoking: Risk related to gestational age and onset of delivery. Am J Obstet Gynecol 179:1051, 1998.

Lam S, To W, Duthie S, Ma H: Narcotic addiction in pregnancy with adverse maternal and perinatal outcome. Aust N Z J Obstet Gynaecol 32:216, 1992.

Lambers D, Clark K: The maternal and fetal physiologic effects of nicotine. Semin Perinatol 20:115, 1996.

Legido A, Clancy RR, Spitzer AR, Finnegan LP: Electroencephalographic and behavioral-state studies in infants of cocaine-addicted mothers. Am J Dis Child 146:748, 1992.

Lester B, ElSohly M, Wright L, et al: The maternal lifestyle study: Drug use by meconium toxicology and maternal self-report. Pediatrics 107:309, 2001.

Levy M, Sino M: Neonatal withdrawal syndrome: Associated drugs and pharmacologic management. Pharmacotherapy 13:202, 1993.

Li C, Windsor R, Perkins L, et al: The impact on infant birth weight and gestational age of cotinine-validated smoking reduction during pregnancy. JAMA 269:1519, 1993.

Lieberman E, Gremy F, Lang JM, Cohen AP: Low birthweight at term and the timing of fetal exposure to maternal smoking. Am J Public Health 84:1127, 1994.

Lindsay MK, Peterson HB, Boring J: Crack/cocaine: A risk factor for human immunodeficiency virus infection type I among inner-city parturients. Obstet Gynecol 80:981, 1992.

Lipshultz SE, Frassica JJ, Orav EJ: Cardiovascular abnormalities in infants prenatally exposed to cocaine. J Pediatr 118:44, 1991.

Little B, Snell L, Klein V, et al: Maternal and fetal effects of heroin addiction during pregnancy. J Reprod Med 35:159, 1990.

Maas U, Kattner E, Weingart-Jesse B, et al: Infrequent neonatal opiate withdrawal following maternal methadone detoxification during pregnancy. J Perinat Med 18:111, 1990.

MacDorman M, Cnattingius S, Hoffman H, et al: Sudden infant death syndrome and smoking in the United States and Sweden. Am J Epidemiol 146:249, 1997.

Mack G, Giles W, Thomas D, Buchanan N: Methadone levels and neonatal withdrawal. J Paediatr Child Health 27:96, 1991.

Madden J, Chappel J, Zuspan F, et al: Observation and treatment of neonatal narcotic withdrawal. Am J Obstet Gynecol 127:199, 1977.

Mahalik M, Hitner H: Antagonism of cocaine-induced fetal anomalies by prazosin and diltiazem in mice. Reprod Technol 6:161, 1994.

Maier S, West J: Drinking patterns and alcohol-related birth defects. Alcohol Res Health 25:168, 2001.

Malanga C, Kosofsky B: Mechanisms of action of drugs of abuse on the developing fetal brain. Clin Perinatol 26:17, 1999.

Malpas T, Darlow B, Lennox R, Horwood L: Maternal methadone dosage and neonatal withdrawal. Aust N Z J Obstet Gynaecol 35:175, 1995.

Martin ML, Khoury MJ, Cordero JF, Waters GD: Trends in rates of multiple vascular disruption defects, Atlanta 1968-1989: Is there evidence of a cocaine teratogenic epidemic? Teratology 45:647, 1992.

Martinez FD, Wright AL, Taussig LM, et al: Asthma and wheezing in the first six years of life. N Engl J Med 332:133, 1995.

Mattson S, Riley E, Gramling L, et al: Heavy prenatal alcohol exposure with or without physical features of fetal alcohol syndrome leads to IQ deficits. J Pediatr 131:718,1997.

Mattson S, Riley E, Gramling L, et al: Neuropsychological comparison of alcohol-exposed children with or without physical features of fetal alcohol syndrome. Neuropsychology 12:146,1998.

Mauri A, Piccione E, Deiana P, Volpe A: Obstetric and perinatal outcome in human immunodeficiency virus-infected pregnant women with and without opiate addiction. Eur J Obstet Gynecol Reprod Biol 58:135, 1995.

May P, Gossage J: Estimating the prevalence of fetal alcohol syndrome: A summary. Alcohol Res Health 25:159, 2001.

May P, Brooke L, Gossage P, et al: Epidemiology of fetal alcohol syndrome in a South African community in the Western Cape Province. Am J Public Health 90:1905, 2000.

McCarthy J, Posey B: Methadone levels in human milk. J Hum Lac 16:115, 2000.

McCarthy J, Siney C, Shaw N, Ruben S: Outcome predictors in pregnant opiate and polydrug users. Eur J Pediatr 158:748, 1999.

McElhatton PR, Bateman DN, Evans C, et al: Congenital anomalies after prenatal ecstasy exposure Lancet 354:1441, 1999.

Milerad J, Vege A, Opdal S, Rognum T: Objective measurement of nicotine exposure in victims of sudden infant death syndrome and in other unexpected child deaths. J Pediatr 133:232, 1998.

Mitchell E, Ford R, Steward A, et al: Smoking and sudden infant death syndrome. Pediatrics 91:893, 1993.

Mitchell E, Tuohy P, Brunt J, et al: Risk factors for sudden infant death syndrome following the prevention campaign in New Zealand: A prospective study. Pediatrics 100:835, 1997.

Moore TR, Sorg J, Thomas CK, et al: Hemodynamic effects of intravenous cocaine on the pregnant ewe and fetus. Am J Obstet Gynecol 155:883, 1986.

Mott SH, Packer RJ, Soldin SJ: Neurological manifestations of cocaine exposure in childhood. Pediatrics 93:557, 1994.

Mvula MM, Miller JM Jr, Ragan FA: Relationship of phencyclidine and pregnancy outcome. J Reprod Med 44:1021, 1999.

Nair P, Othblum S, Hebel R: Neonatal outcome in infants with evidence of fetal exposure to opiates, cocaine, and cannabinoids. Clin Pediatr 33:280, 1994.

Neonatal drug withdrawal: American Academy of Pediatrics Committee on Drugs. Pediatrics 101:1079, 1998.

Nordentoft M, Lou H, Hansen D, et al: Intrauterine growth retardation and premature delivery: The influence of maternal smoking and psychosocial factors. Am J Public Health 86:347, 1996.

O'Connor TA, Bondurant HH, Siddiqui J: Targeted perinatal drug screening in a rural population. J Matern Fetal Med 6:108, 1997.

Ornoy A, Segal J, Bar-Humburger R, Greenbaum C: Developmental outcome of school-age children born to mothers with heroin dependency: Importance of environmental factors. Dev Med Child Neurol 43:668, 2001.

Ostrea E, Brady M, Parks P, et al: Drug screening of meconium in infants of drug-dependent mothers: An alternative to urine testing. J Pediatr 115:474, 1992a.

Ostrea EM Jr, Brady MJ, Gause S, et al: Drug screening of newborns by meconium analysis: A large-scale, prospective, epidemiological study. Pediatrics 89:107, 1992b.

Ostrea E, Ostrea A, Simpson P: Mortality within the first 2 years in infants exposed to cocaine, opiate, or cannabinoid during gestation. Pediatrics 1997; 100:79, 1997.

Pastrakuljic A, Derewlany LO, Koren G: Maternal cocaine use and cigarette smoking in pregnancy in relation to amino acid transport and fetal growth. Placenta 20:499, 1999.

Perkins S, Belcher J, Livesey J: A Canadian tertiary care center study of maternal and umbilical cord cotinine levels as markers of smoking during pregnancy: Relationship to neonatal effects. Can J Public Health 88:232, 1997.

Plessinger M: Prenatal exposure to amphetamines. Obstet Gynecol Clin North Am 25:119, 1998.

Rahbar F, Fomufod A, White D, Westney LS: Impact of intrauterine exposure to phencyclidine (PCP) and cocaine on neonates. J Natl Med Assoc 85:349, 1993.

Riley E, Mattson S, Sowell E, et al: Abnormalities of the corpus callosum in children prenatally exposed to alcohol. Alcohol Clin Exp Res 19:1198, 1995.

Roebuck T, Mattson S, Riley E: A review of the neuroanatomical findings in children with fetal alcohol syndrome or prenatal exposure to alcohol. Alcohol Clin Exp Res 22:339, 1998.

Rosen T, Pippenger C: Pharmacologic observations on the neonatal withdrawal syndrome. J Pediatr 88:1044, 1976.

Sagatun-Edwards IJ, Saylor C, Shifflett B: Drug exposed infants in the social welfare system and juvenile court. Child Abuse Neglect 19:83, 1995.

Sampson P, Streissguth A, Bookstein F, et al: Incidence of fetal alcohol syndrome and prevalence of alcohol-related neurodevelopmental disorder. Teratology 56:317, 1997.

Savitz D, Dole N, Terry J, et al: Smoking and pregnancy outcome among African-American and white women in Central North Carolina. Epidemiology 12:636, 2001.

Schellscheidt J, Jorch G, Menke J: Effects of heavy maternal smoking on intrauterine growth patterns in sudden infant death victims and surviving infants. Eur J Pediatr 157:246, 1998.

Schenker S, Yang Y, Johnson RF: The transfer of cocaine and its metabolites across the term human placenta. Clin Pharmacol Ther 53:329, 1993.

Schoendorf K, Kiely J: Relationship of sudden infant death syndrome to maternal smoking during and after pregnancy. Pediatrics 90:905, 1992.

Shankaran S, Bauer CR, Bada HS: Effects of cocaine-opiate exposure during pregnancy on outcome at 1 year: A multicenter prospective, group-matched study. Pediatr Res 43:195A, 1998.

Shiono PH, Klebanoff MA, Nugent RP: The impact of cocaine and marijuana use on low birth weight and preterm birth: A multicenter study. Am J Obstet Gynecol 172:19, 1995.

Singer LT, Arendt R, Minnes S, et al: Cognitive and motor outcomes of cocaine-exposed infants. JAMA 287:1952, 2002.

Slotkin TA, Lappi SE, McCook EC, et al: Loss of neonatal hypoxia tolerance after prenatal nicotine exposure: Implications for sudden infant death syndrome. Brain Res Bull 38:69, 1995.

Soepatmi S: Developmental outcomes of children of mothers dependent on heroin or heroin/methadone during pregnancy. Act Paediatr 404(Suppl):36, 1994.

Spittal P, Craib K, Wood E, et al: Risk factors for elevated HIV incidence rates among female injection drug users in Vancouver. CMAJ 166:894, 2002.

Sprauve M, Lindsay M, Drews-Botsch C, Graves W: Racial patterns in the effects of tobacco use on fetal growth. Am J Obstet Gynecol 181:S22, 1999.

Stoler J, Holmes L: Under-recognition of prenatal alcohol effects in infants of known alcohol abusing women. J Pediatr 135:430, 1999.

Stratton K, Howe C, Battaglia F: Fetal Alcohol Syndrome: Diagnosis, Epidemiology, Prevention, and Treatment. Committee to Study Fetal Alcohol Syndrome, Division of Biobehavioral Sciences and Mental Disorders, Institute of Medicine. Washington, DC, National Academy Press, 1996, pp 4-21.

Streissguth A: Fetal alcohol syndrome in adolescents and adults. JAMA 265:1961, 1991.

Streissguth A: Fetal alcohol syndrome in older patients. Alcohol Alcohol Suppl 2: 209, 1993.

Suresh S, Anand K: Opioid tolerance in neonates: A state-of-the-art review. Pediatr Anaesth 11:511, 2001.

Surveillance for fetal alcohol syndrome using multiple sources: Atlanta, Georgia, 1981-1989. Morb Mortal Wkly Rep MMWR 46:1118, 1997.

Taeusch HW Jr, Carson S, Wang NS, et al: Heroin induction of lung maturation and growth retardation in fetal rabbits. J Pediatr 82:869, 1973.

Taylor J, Sanderson M. A reexamination of the risk factors for the sudden infant death syndrome. J Pediatr 126:887, 1995.

Tobias J: Tolerance, withdrawal, and physical dependency after long-term sedation and analgesia of children in the pediatric intensive care unit. Crit Care Med 28: 2122, 2000.

Tobias J, Schleien C, Haun S: Methadone as treatment for iatrogenic narcotic dependency in pediatric intensive care unit patients. Crit Care Med 18:1292, 1990.

Tuthill D, Steward J, Coles E, et al: Maternal cigarette smoking and pregnancy outcome. Paediatr Perinatal Epidemiol 13:245, 1999.

Vaccarino A, Kastin A: Endogenous opiates: 1999. Peptides 21:1975, 2000.

van Baar A, de Graaff B: Cognitive development at preschool-age of infants of drug-dependent mothers. Dev Med Child Neurol 36:1063, 1994.

van Baar A, Soepatmi S, Gunning W, Akkerhuis G: Development after prenatal exposure to cocaine, heroin and methadone. Acta Paediatr 404(Suppl):40, 1994.

van de Bor M, Walther FJ, Ebrahimi M: Decreased cardiac output in infants of mothers who abused cocaine. Pediatrics 85:30, 1990a.

van de Bor M, Walther F, Sims M: Increased cerebral blood flow velocity in infants of mothers who abuse cocaine. Pediatrics 85:733, 1990b.

van Tonningen-van Driel M, Garbis-Berkvens J, Reuvers-Lodewijks W: [Pregnancy outcome after Ecstasy use: 43 cases followed by the Teratology Information Service of the National Institute for Public Health and Environment]. Med Tijdschr Geneeskd 143:237, 1999.

Vega W, Kolody B, Hwang J, Noble A: Prevalence and magnitude of prenatal substance exposures in California. N Engl J Med 329:850, 1993.

Walsh R, Lowe J, Hopkins P: Quitting smoking in pregnancy. Med J Aust 175:320, 2001.

Ward J, Hall W, Mattick R: Role of maintenance treatment in Opioid dependence. Lancet 353:221, 1999.

Wasserman D, Leventhal J: Maltreatment of children born to cocaine-dependent mothers. Am J Dis Child 147:1324, 1993.

Woods J Jr, Plessinger M, Clark K: Effects of cocaine on uterine blood flow. JAMA. 257:957, 1987.

Yanai J, Avraham Y, Levy S: Alterations in septohippocampal cholinergic innervations and related behaviors after early exposure to heroin and phencyclidine. Brain Res 69:207, 1992.

Yawn B, Thompson L, Lupo V, et al: Prenatal drug use in Minneapolis, St. Paul, Minnesota: A 4 year trend. Arch Fam Med 3:520, 1994.

Zuckerman B, Bresnahan K: Developmental and behavioral consequences of prenatal drug and alcohol exposure. Pediatr Clin North Am 38:1387, 1991.

Zuckerman B, Frank DA, Hingson R: Effects of maternal marijuana and cocaine on fetal growth. N Engl J Med 320:762, 1989.

# ISSUES IN LABOR AND DELIVERY

Editor: ROBERTA A. BALLARD

PART IV

CHAPTER 13

# Antepartum Fetal Assessment

Andrew D. Hull and Thomas R. Moore

Fetal death in utero is a tragedy that patients and obstetricians wish to avoid. Figure 13–1A is a graph showing the incidence of fetal death in utero from 1959 through 1996. In the 1950s, approximately 1 in every 50 pregnancies ended in fetal death before delivery. Among women of African heritage, the rate was almost double that figure. Thanks to changes in obstetric practice and the institution of progressively more widely applied antepartum tests of fetal well-being beginning in the 1970s, the current risk of fetal death is approximately 1 in 150 pregnancies. However, as can be seen in Fig. 13–1A, substantial progress is needed, because no change has been noted in the rates for white or African-American women in the last decade.

In an ideal world, astute clinicians would be able to correct any inadequacies of the intrauterine environment so as to optimize fetal growth, development, and well-being. With such corrections, fetal outcome would be uniformly excellent. Because this is, as yet, an unattainable goal, clinicians must carefully observe fetal status and effect delivery when extrauterine life seems safer or more desirable than continuing the pregnancy. To that end, obstetricians have developed a set of tests that can assist in determining the timing of delivery so as to minimize unexpected fetal morbidity (American College of Obstetricians and Gynecologists [ACOG], 1999).

Although the primary aim of antenatal fetal surveillance is the prevention of stillbirth, a secondary, although no less important, aim is minimizing fetal and neonatal morbidity. A comparison of the efficacy of various surveillance methods reveals that reduction in fetal mortality is a convenient outcome measure. The best tests, however, result in the birth of healthier newborns. The various current methods of assessing fetal status are listed in Table 13–1, and the details of each are discussed subsequently.

## GENERAL PRINCIPLES OF FETAL BIOPHYSICAL ASSESSMENT

The ideal test of fetal well-being would be simple, cheap, and accurate and would generate clear, reproducible results not subject to variable interpretation. Equally, the test would be easy to apply to an entire patient population and thus to identify all patients at significant risk of poor fetal outcome. Unfortunately, such a test does not yet exist. Given the problems with designing the perfect test, clinicians have, over time, begun testing more and more pregnancies in order to minimize poor fetal outcome.

Platt and colleagues (1987) studied the impact of the increasing use of antepartum fetal testing in the period from 1971 through 1986. The results are shown in Table 13–2. Clearly, although the outcomes for the small tested population improved, the largest number of fetal deaths occurred in the larger untested population, in spite of a marked rise in the percentage of patients undergoing expensive antepartum testing.

The financial impact of this trend can be roughly calculated. Using estimated charges of approximately $125 per test, one can calculate that the cost of fetal testing in a cohort of 1000 pregnant patients would be $37,500, discounting the expense to the patient associated with child care or absence from a job to visit the testing center. If, as Platt and colleagues (1987) showed, such testing reduces fetal mortality rate by 2 per 1000 births, the cost per fetal life saved equals $18,750.

In reviewing the data, Platt and colleagues (1987) suggested that better means of identifying the at-risk fetus should be devised so that antepartum testing could be applied to the population most likely to experience benefit. On the basis of the accumulated experience with traditional biophysical testing, further increasing the indications for nonstress or biophysical profile testing is not likely to be economical or effective in reducing the fetal mortality rate.

### Indications for Fetal Testing

As noted previously, 30% or more of stillbirths occur in patients without identifiable risk factors (Hovatta et al, 1983). Thus, simply screening or testing high-risk patients is not enough. Nevertheless, conditions in which fetal surveillance is traditionally considered mandatory are listed in Table 13–3. This list can almost be expanded indefinitely. Optimally, fetal testing should involve use of an inexpensive, widely applied test, with further specific testing limited to those pregnancies identified as being at risk.

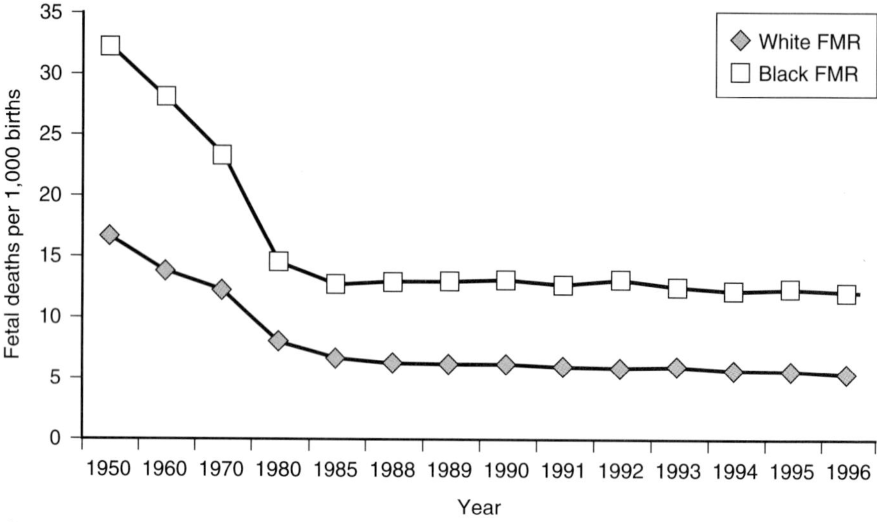


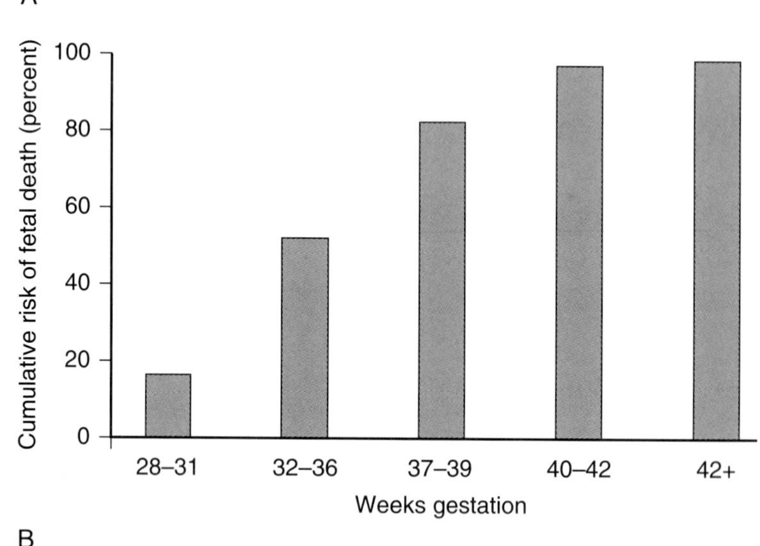


**FIGURE 13–1.** **A,** The incidence of fetal death in utero in the United States from 1959 to 1996. **B,** Cumulative likelihood of fetal death versus gestational age. *(**A** adapted from National Vital Statistics Reports, vol 49, no 8. Hyattsville, MD, National Center for Health Statistics, 2001; **B** adapted from McIlwaine, GM, Dunn FH, Howat RC, et al: A routine system for monitoring perinatal deaths in Scotland. Br J Obstet Gynaecol 92: 9-13, 1985.)*

## When to Begin Fetal Testing

Given that testing is indicated in an individual pregnancy, the next question is when to begin testing. Because there is little to be gained in identifying a fetus in distress before viability, testing typically begins after 24 to 26 weeks. As shown in Fig. 13–1B, the incidence of fetal death during pregnancy rises somewhat linearly in the third trimester. More than half of fetal deaths occur before 37 weeks. If performance of fetal testing is restricted to the estimated delivery date and beyond, the testing regimen will fail to detect more than 90% of fetuses at risk of death. Thus, the best test regimen includes all pregnancies after 32 weeks (83% sensitivity). Gestational age at entry into a surveillance program for specific diagnostic groups is most commonly based on risk assessment. For example, in insulin dependent diabetic women, routine testing is typically begun at 32 to 34 weeks of gestation, because the risk of stillbirth rises at that time. For women otherwise without complications, in whom the cost of universal testing could be substantial, testing is initiated after 41.5 weeks of gestation, when the risk of fetal death is fivefold higher than before the estimated delivery date.

**TABLE 13–1**

**Fetal Biophysical Assessment Modalities**

| | |
|---|---|
| Maternal assessment of fetal movement | Biophysical profile |
| Cardiotocography | Doppler flow studies |
| Nonstress testing | Amniocentesis |
| Contraction stress testing | Cordocentesis |
| Assessment of amniotic fluid volume | |

## Frequency of Fetal Testing

Fetal assessment clearly lends itself to the use of algorithms both for selecting patients and for designing a cascade of testing methods. Such a sequential approach is commonly used (Devoe et al, 1990) and potentially nullifies some of the subjective shortcomings of fetal testing.

Clearly, if clinicians are willing to use methods of fetal surveillance, they must be willing to act on the results.

**TABLE 13–2**

**Antepartum Fetal Deaths in Tested and Untested Pregnancies over 15 Years**

| | 1971-1975 | 1976-1980 | 1981-1985 |
|---|---|---|---|
| No. pregnancies tested | 1233 | 4163 | 11,263 |
| Death rate (per 1000) | 10.5 | 6.3 | 4.4 |
| Percentage of all deaths | 1.9 | 3.4 | 6.7 |
| No. pregnancies untested | 51,254 | 61,963 | 69,677 |
| Death rate (per 1000) | 13.3 | 11.9 | 10.0 |
| Percentage of all deaths | 98 | 96 | 93 |

Adapted from Platt LD, Paul RH, Phelan J, et al: Fifteen years of experience with antepartum fetal testing. Am J Obstet Gynecol 156:1509, 1987.

**TABLE 13–3**

**Indications for Fetal Surveillance**

| | |
|---|---|
| Threatened preterm delivery | Chronic maternal illness: |
| Post-term pregnancy | Diabetes |
| Hypertensive disorders | Anemia |
| Intrauterine growth restriction | Hemoglobinopathies |
| Previous stillbirth | Cyanotic heart disease |
| Decreased fetal movement | Collagen vascular disease |
| Multiple gestation | Renal impairment |

Given that for the most part the action required is delivery, it is imperative that the testing method chosen yields few false-positive results and even fewer false-negative results. This topic is addressed after the descriptions of each testing modality.

## ULTRASONOGRAPHY

Ultrasonography has become an increasingly important tool in the evaluation of high-risk obstetric patients. In many obstetric practices, all pregnant women are offered an ultrasonographic evaluation of the fetus at some point in pregnancy. Although this practice is controversial, there are several well-recognized indications for ultrasonography.

### Determination of Gestational Age

Accurate determination of pregnancy duration is a central goal of prenatal care. Although precise dating is valuable in even uncomplicated pregnancies, this information is critical in situations of marginal fetal viability and salvageability. A typical scenario involves the problem of performing or avoiding cesarean delivery in a pregnancy with fetal distress at 23 (<5% survival) to 26 (50% survival) weeks of gestation. Typical dating criteria and their accuracy are listed in Table 13–4. Although a crown-rump length measurement obtained between 7 and 10 weeks of gestation provides the smallest error (±3 days), a single ultrasonographic study performed between 16 and 22 weeks affords acceptable dating accuracy (±10 days) while allowing visualization of most of the fetal organs.

### Diagnosis of Fetal Anomalies

A major additional benefit of routine ultrasonographic scanning of pregnancies is the diagnosis of unexpected fetal anomalies. The following secondary benefits are associated with antenatal identification of the anomalous fetus:

1. Selection of appropriate level of obstetric and neonatal care. *Antenatal counseling by pediatric and neonatal specialists provides a smoother transition for both parents and the newborn.* Typical anomalies in which antenatal counseling improves postnatal care are congenital diaphragmatic hernia and cyanotic heart disease.
2. *Identification of lethal anomalies, avoiding unnecessary cesarean delivery and futile neonatal intervention.* Examples are anencephaly, holoprosencephaly, thanatophoric dwarfism, and bilateral renal agenesis, all of which have a

**TABLE 13–4**

**Accuracy of Gestational Age Estimation**

| Parameter | Accuracy | Comment |
|---|---|---|
| **Clinical** | | |
| Last menstrual period | ±2 wks | Depends on cycle length and maternal recollection |
| First-trimester uterine size | ±2 wks | Depends on operator skill |
| Auscultation of fetal heart tones | ±2 wks | Typically at 20 wks (fetoscope); 12 wks with Doppler scope |
| Fundal height measurements | ±3 wks | Varies with maternal body habitus |
| **Ultrasonographic** | | |
| Gestational sac diameter | ±5 days | Variable shape distorts measurements. Performed from 4.5 to 5.5 wks |
| Embryonic crown-rump length | ±3 days | Performed from 6.0 to 12 wks |
| Biparietal diameter, femur length, cerebellar transverse diameter | ±10 days; ±14-20 days | If performed from 15 to 22 wks; if performed after 22 wks |

high incidence of distress during labor that often leads to emergency cesarean delivery. Antenatal recognition of these lethal conditions permits families to make rational choices about the route of delivery.

3. Identification of chromosome anomalies *in otherwise low-risk women*. Most major chromosome anomalies have typical ultrasonographic features, which may suggest further diagnostic procedures, such as amniocentesis and umbilical cord blood sampling. Up to 50% to 60% of chromosome anomalies may be identified from the presence of structural abnormalities evident on midtrimester ultrasonogram.
4. Identification of nonlethal but significantly debilitating fetal anomalies *before viability permits the option of pregnancy termination or in utero fetal therapy*. Examples are large meningomyelocele, multiple amputations associated with the amniotic band syndrome, and fetal hydrops arising from perinatal viral infections such as cytomegalovirus. Conditions that may be amenable to in utero therapy include congenital hydrothorax and posterior urethral valves.

Factors that may adversely affect the accuracy and sensitivity of ultrasonographic screening for fetal anomalies include fetal position, maternal obesity, and decreased amniotic fluid volume. Further, accurate evaluation of fetal anatomy requires a skilled team of experienced ultrasonographers and perinatologists using equipment with optimal image resolution. Counseling of the affected family and formulation of the management plan should involve neonatologists, pediatric subspecialists, and geneticists. Even with optimal equipment and personnel, up to 25% of significant structural defects may be missed.

## ASSESSMENT OF FETAL MOVEMENT

The use of maternally perceived fetal activity to identify fetuses at risk for distress or death has been proposed because of its relatively low cost, convenience, and applicability to a large population. The optimal technique, frequency, and duration of fetal movement monitoring have not been clarified. Factors such as fetal waking and quiet cycles, maternal attention span, compliance, and motivation must be considered. The roles of maternal body habitus, placental position, and amniotic fluid volume may also be important. An understanding of the biology of fetal movement may provide important clues that will be helpful to the development of an effective program of fetal testing.

### Maturational and Circadian Influences

Patrick and colleagues (1982) monitored fetal body movements in third-trimester human pregnancy from 30 to 40 weeks of gestation using continuous 24-hour ultrasonographic observation. The results of their study are shown in Table 13–5. They observed no statistically significant change in the number of movements per hour as gestational age advanced. This finding was confirmed by three other studies (Manning et al, 1979; Rayburn, 1982; Valentin and Marsal, 1986). Valentin and Marsal (1986) documented a mean of 85 fetal movements in a 45-minute period, with a 95% confidence interval of 14 to 232 movements.

**TABLE 13-5**

**Frequency of Fetal Body Movements (FBMs) in the Human Fetus**

| | 30-31 Wks Gestation | 34-35 Wks Gestation | 38-39 Wks Gestation |
|---|---|---|---|
| No FBMs per hour* | 33 ± 2 | 28 ± 2 | 32 ± 2 |
| Percentage of time spent in FBMs* | 9.3 ± 0.9 | 98 ± 0.7 | 11.2 ± 0.9 |

*Expressed as mean ± SD.

Adapted from Patrick J, Campbell K, Carmichael L, et al: Patterns of gross fetal body movements over 24 hour observation intervals during the last 10 weeks of pregnancy. Am J Obstet Gynecol 142:363, 1982.

### Effect of Fetal Oxygenation on Body Movements

The thesis that fetal movements decrease with hypoxia is central to understanding of the nonstress test (NST) and biophysical profile. Bekedam and Visser (1985) monitored fetal body movements in growth-retarded fetuses before, during, and after uterine contractions. During contractions associated with late decelerations, the frequency of fetal body movements was 85% lower than the frequency before such contractions. In contractions associated with normal fetal heart rate, no change in fetal body movements occurred. The exquisite sensitivity of fetal movement frequency to reductions in oxygenation is similar to that reported by Natale and associates (1981).

Valentin and Marsal (1986) found that the 97.5th percentile for absence of fetal activity was 28 minutes, suggesting an ideal observation interval of approximately 1 hour. Moore and Piacquadio (1989) reported that the mean time to perceive 10 fetal movements was 18 ± 12 (standard deviation) minutes. A 1-hour observation period lacking 10 movements represented 3.5 standard deviations (99th percentile).

On the basis of these observations, various methods of "kick counting" have been proposed. Perhaps the simplest of proven worth is that of Moore and Piacquadio (1989), in which the patient records the time taken for 10 fetal movements to occur between 7 and 11 PM (the period of peak fetal activity). If the requisite 10 movements are not obtained after 1 hour of recording, further fetal evaluation is performed. An example of the card used for patient recording of fetal movement times is shown in Figure 13–2.

Other investigators have confirmed the utility of fetal movement counting in normal and high-risk patients (Neldham, 1980). The results of general population screenings are mixed, ranging from no benefit in a British multicenter randomized trial (Grant et al, 1989) to a significant reduction in stillbirth rate in a case-control study of patients in a military population (Moore and Piacquadio, 1989). Despite the varied results, it is difficult to formulate a good argument against maternal kick counting, and thus this method should probably be widely used as an initial screen from 28 weeks of gestation onward.

Fetal movement assessment thus is a simple screening test that enables the pregnant patient to participate in her

**FETAL MOVEMENT RECORD**

Name:________________________

Due Date:________________________

| Start Date | Number of weeks pregnant |
|---|---|
| | |

INSTRUCTIONS

1. Count the baby's movements EVERY NIGHT.
2. A movement may be a kick, swish or roll. Do not count hiccups or small flutters.
3. You can start counting any time in the evening when the baby is active. BUT: COUNT EVERY NIGHT.
4. Count baby's movements while lying down, preferably on your left side.
5. Mark down the time you feel the baby move for the first time.
6. Mark down the time you feel the 10th fetal movement.
7. You should feel at least 10 fetal movements within one hour. Call Labor and Delivery (543-6600) Immediately if
   a) you do not feel 10 movements within 1 hour .
   b) it takes longer and longer for your baby to move 10 times.
   c) you have not felt the baby move all day.

DO NOT WAIT UNTIL TOMORROW.

| Date | Time First Movement Felt | Time 10th Movement Felt | Total Time |
|---|---|---|---|
| EXAMPLE 11/4/91 | 6:50 p.m. | 7:28 p.m. | 38 minutes |
| | | | |
| | | | |
| | | | |
| | | | |
| | | | |
| | | | |
| | | | |
| | | | |
| | | | |
| | | | |
| | | | |
| | | | |
| | | | |
| | | | |
| | | | |
| | | | |
| | | | |
| | | | |
| | | | |
| | | | |
| | | | |
| | | | |

**FIGURE 13–2.** Sample card for patient recording of fetal movements. The patient records the starting time and the time at which she feels the 10th fetal movement. If 10 movements cannot be appreciated in less than 60 minutes, the patient is instructed to contact her physician.

pregnancy care in a useful way. Although the method is subjective and shows poor correlation with objective assessments of fetal movement, maternal reporting of fetal movement is an important first step in monitoring fetal well-being.

## CARDIOTOCOGRAPHY (CONTRACTION STRESS TEST, NONSTRESS TEST)

The most widely used method of assessing fetal well-being combines electronic monitoring of both fetal heart rate and uterine contractions. Antenatal fetal heart rate monitoring arose from the finding that certain intrapartum fetal heart rate patterns were associated with poor fetal outcomes, hypoxia, acidemia, and asphyxia.

### Contraction Stress Test

The earliest fetal wellness test involving fetal heart rate monitoring was the contraction stress test (CST). This test assesses the response of the fetal heart rate to uterine contractions produced by administration of exogenous oxytocin or by nipple stimulation (Evertson et al, 1979). In an oxygen-compromised fetus, contractions typically lead to

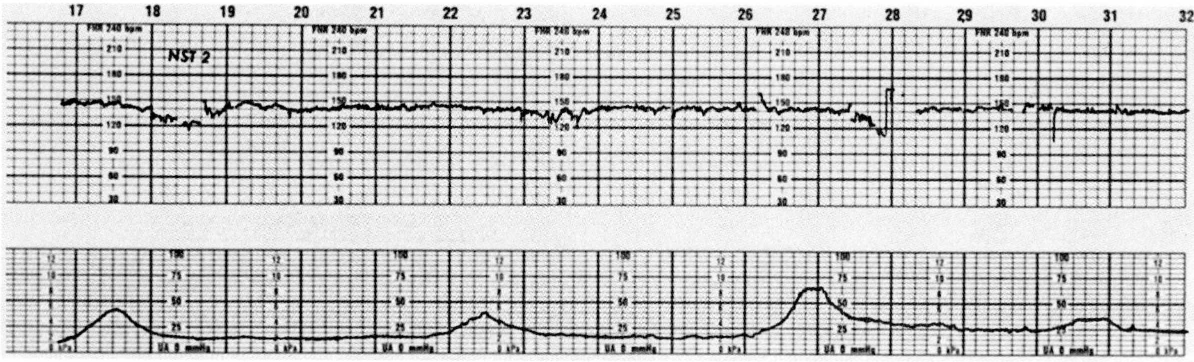


**FIGURE 13–3.** A contraction stress test. The fetal heart rate (FHR) is plotted above the uterine contraction signal. Note the late deceleration after a contraction. NST, nonstress test.

late decelerations in the fetal heart rate; such a test result is shown in Figure 13–3. Although the CST remains a useful test, its disadvantages include significant time investment (45 to 60 minutes), the high frequency of uterine contraction hyperstimulation, and the need for close supervision. Furthermore, the CST is contraindicated in the following high-risk groups:

- Threatened preterm delivery
- Premature ruptured membranes
- Previous classic cesarean section
- Placenta previa

The criteria for a satisfactory result are a minimum of three contractions in 10 minutes and a continuous fetal heart rate signal. Test results are categorized as negative (reassuring), equivocal, positive, and unsatisfactory. A negative CST result requires the absence of late decelerations after all contractions. The diagnostic categories of the CST are summarized in Table 13–6. If more than three contractions occur in 10 minutes and late decelerations are noted, the CST result is classified as hyperstimulatory or unsatisfactory, requiring further testing. In a woman with a reassuring CST result, testing can be repeated weekly. The risk of fetal death with a negative CST result is less than 1 per 1000 (Freeman et al, 1982).

**TABLE 13–6**

**Diagnostic Categories of the Contraction Stress Test Result**

| Result | Criteria | Comment |
|---|---|---|
| Negative (reassuring) | No late FHR decelerations after a minimum of 3 contractions in 10 min | Retest weekly |
| Positive | Late FHR decelerations after >50% of contractions | Further testing or delivery indicated |
| Equivocal | Late FHR decelerations noted, but after <50% of contractions | Retest in <24 hrs |
| Unsatisfactory | Hyperstimulation noted (>3 contractions/10 min with FHR decelerations or inadequate FHR tracing) | Retest immediately |

FHR, fetal heart rate.

## Nonstress Test

Several observers noted that CST results were rarely abnormal when fetal heart rate accelerations were present in association with movement. This clinical observation led to omission of the contractions, with simple monitoring for fetal heart rate accelerations (Lee et al, 1976; Rochard et al, 1976). Because of its ease of use, universal applicability, and lack of contraindications, the NST has replaced the CST as a first-line surveillance tool.

The NST is carried out with the patient supine with a lateral tilt. The fetal heart rate and uterine activity are recorded with an external transducer for up to 40 minutes. Usually, uterine activity is monitored simultaneously, and the patient records perceived fetal movement with an event marker. A normal (reactive) NST result is shown in Figure 13–4.

Criteria for a reassuring NST result are as follows:

- Observation period of 20 minutes
- Baseline fetal heart rate between 110 and 160 beats/min
- Short-term variability of <5 beats/min
- Two or more fetal heart rate accelerations of at least 15 beats/min lasting at least 15 seconds
- No nonreassuring features (decelerations, tachycardia, bradycardia)

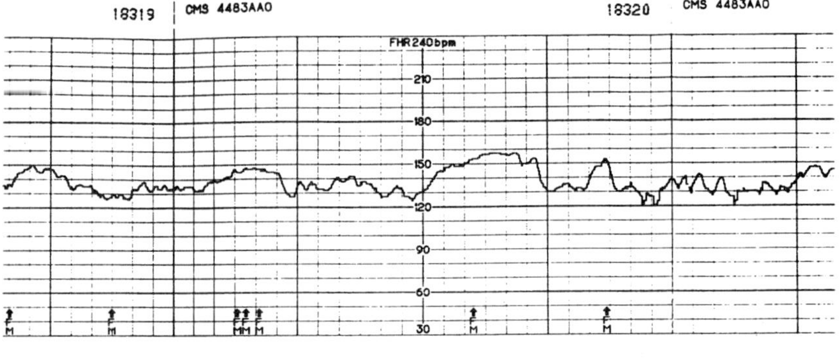


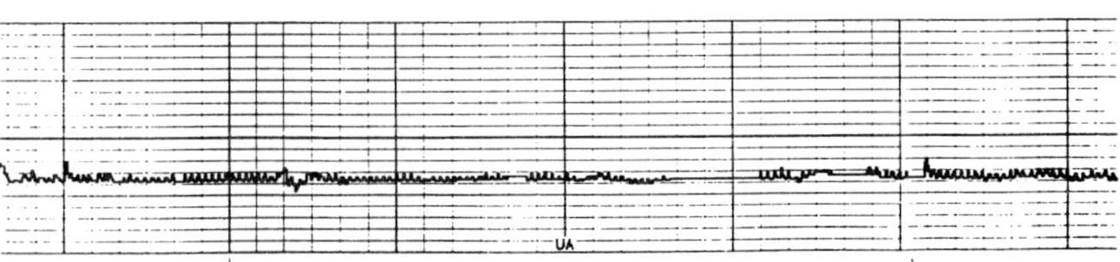


**FIGURE 13–4.** A reassuring nonstress test. Note two fetal heart rate (FHR) accelerations exceeding 15 beats/min and lasting at least 15 seconds during the monitoring period.

Although the risk of fetal death with a nonreactive NST result is approximately 40/1000, a reactive result has a risk of 1 to 5 per 1000.

### Factors Influencing the Nonstress Test Result

Fetal heart rate is modified by autonomic activity and may show reduction or absence of reactivity in the presence of hypoxia, neurologic depression, maternal drug ingestion, or acidosis. Fetal behavioral state influences the cardiac reactivity. The human fetus commonly exhibits periods of lowered activity referred to as "sleep cycles." These periods may produce a decrease or absence of reactivity on an NST. The sleep cycles rarely last more than 20 minutes and may be discounted by observing the fetus for up to 40 minutes.

Adjustments must be made for monitoring of the fetus remote from term (Lagrew, 1987). Between 24 and 32 weeks, the fetus may show accelerations of lesser amplitude that are of shorter duration, reduced reactivity (Druzin et al, 1985; Lavin et al, 1984), and spontaneous low-amplitude decelerations with movement (Sorokin et al, 1982), which do not carry the same ominous portent as in later gestations.

### Indications for and Frequency of Nonstress Testing

The typical indications for the NST are as follows:

- Multiple gestation
- Post-term pregnancy
- Intrauterine growth restriction (IUGR)
- History of previous stillbirth
- Maternal chronic illness (e.g., hypertension, renal or cardiac disease)
- Decreased fetal movement
- Maternal collagen vascular disorders
- Maternal diabetes mellitus

Although NSTs were originally performed weekly, studies suggest that the fetal death rate with weekly testing is excessive, especially compared with the CST (Freeman et al, 1982). Twice-weekly NST, often coupled with simultaneous measurement of amniotic fluid volume, is the mainstay of fetal monitoring for most complicated pregnancies today (Boehm et al, 1986).

It has been suggested that diabetes mellitus and post-term pregnancy increase the risk of fetal mortality and morbidity and thus are ideally suited to the application of fetal monitoring (Slavensen et al, 1993). Several studies have convincingly shown that waiting for spontaneous labor to occur as late as 42 weeks of gestation in women for whom fetal testing results are reassuring leads to healthy newborns and lower cesarean section rates than when a more aggressive labor induction policy is followed. Nonetheless, the growing risk to the fetus with pregnancy extending beyond 42 completed weeks leads many obstetricians to terminate pregnancy arbitrarily by induction at that point.

Sequential NSTs performed in fetuses with IUGR provide an ideal way of following fetal well-being and aid significantly in timing delivery for optimal outcome, especially when combined with assessment of amniotic fluid volume.

## ASSESSMENT OF AMNIOTIC FLUID VOLUME

Abnormalities of amniotic fluid volume are associated with suboptimal pregnancy outcome. *Oligohydramnios* (inadequate fluid volume) is associated with increased frequency of fetal urinary obstruction, placental insufficiency, umbilical cord compression, fetal distress, meconium passage, and fetal asphyxia (Hill et al, 1984). Prolonged oligohydramnios interferes with normal lung growth, resulting in potentially lethal pulmonary hypoplasia (Nimrod et al, 1984). *Hydramnios* (excessive amniotic fluid volume) is associated with maternal diabetes, fetal esophageal obstruction, and duodenal atresia. Pregnancies complicated by hydramnios have higher rates of abnormal fetal lie, cesarean delivery, and abruptio placentae (Hill et al, 1987). The major diagnostic entities associated with abnormal amniotic fluid volume are listed in Tables 13–7 through 13–9.

### Normal Amniotic Fluid Volume

Twelve studies devoted to the direct quantitation of human amniotic fluid volume have been published since 1965. Brace and Wolf (1989) summarized the changes in amniotic fluid volume during gestation derived from 705 observational studies of normal pregnancies as follows:

- Amniotic fluid volume rises progressively during gestation until approximately 32 weeks.
- From 22 to 39 weeks, the mean volume remains relatively constant, ranging from 630 to 817 mL.
- After 40 weeks, amniotic fluid volume declines at a rate of 8% per week, averaging only 400 mL at 42 weeks. Although amniotic fluid volume varies significantly during pregnancy, the lower 5th percentile in the third trimester (oligohydramnios) is approximately 300 mL. Hydramnios (>95th percentile) is greater than approximately 2000 mL.

### Ultrasonographic Assessment of Amniotic Fluid Volume

Although the increase in perinatal complications associated with abnormal amniotic fluid volume has been recognized for many decades, only the availability of ultra-

**TABLE 13–7**

**Diagnostic Categories of the Amniotic Fluid Index (AFI)**

| Amniotic Fluid Volume | % Patients | AFI Value (cm) |
|---|---|---|
| Very low | 8 | 5 |
| Low | 20 | 5.1-80 |
| Normal | 66 | 8.1-18.0 |
| High | 6 | >18 |

Adapted from Phelan JP, Smith CV, Broussard P, Small M: Amniotic fluid volume assessment using the four-quadrant technique in the pregnancy between 36 and 42 weeks' gestation. J Reprod Med 32:540, 1987.

**TABLE 13–8**

**Principal Diagnoses Associated with Oligohydramnios**

Occult or overt premature rupture of membranes
Placental insufficiency:
- Maternal hypertensive disease
- Autoimmune condition
- Chronic abruption
- Placental crowding in multiple-fetus pregnancy

Urinary tract anomaly:
- Renal agenesis
- Ureteral obstruction
- Urethral obstruction
- Polycystic or multicystic dysplastic kidneys

**TABLE 13–9**

**Principal Diagnoses Associated with Polyhydramnios**

| **Gastrointestinal obstruction** | **Other** |
|---|---|
| Esophageal atresia | Fetal anemia |
| Thoracic mass, pleural effusion | Fetomaternal hemorrhage |
| Duodenal atresia | Blood group isoimmunization |
| **Central nervous system abnormalities** | Parvovirus infection |
| Structural | Twin-twin transfusion syndrome |
| Chromosomal | Maternal diabetes |
| | Constitutional macrosomia |

sonography has enabled the estimation of amniotic fluid volume. Because of the complex shape of the fetus within the uterus, however, direct calculation of the volume of amniotic fluid surrounding the fetus is not currently feasible. Current techniques to estimate with ultrasonography the relative amount of fluid include subjective estimates (Moore et al, 1989), measurement of the largest pocket of amniotic fluid (Chamberlain et al, 1984), and sampling of pocket depths in several areas of the uterus (Rutherford et al, 1987). The amniotic fluid index (AFI) appears to offer better reproducibility and predictive value.

Measuring the AFI involves imaging the amniotic fluid pockets in each of four uterine quadrants and adding the deepest measurements (in mm). Longitudinal measurements of the AFI in normal pregnancies have shown that the AFI varies significantly during gestation (Moore and Cayle, 1990). The normal and boundary values for the AFI are depicted in Figure 13–5.

Although the percentile lines of Figure 13–5 define the limits of normal AFI, the values of AFI that constitute *action* points are less clear. Currently accepted values are shown in Table 13–7, although they have not necessarily been rigorously established. Typically, AFIs greater than 70 mm are regarded as normal, values between 50 and 70 mm require further evaluation, and values less than 50 mm mandate further, more complex testing or delivery.

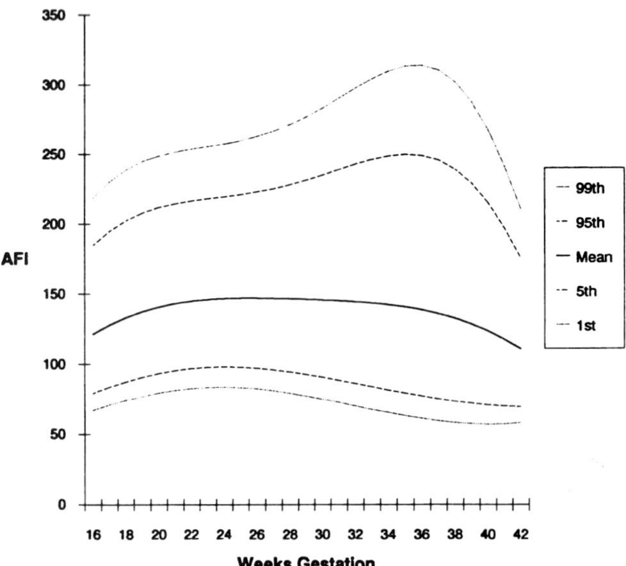


**FIGURE 13–5.** Amniotic fluid index (AFI; in mm) plotted against gestational age. The *darker line* represents the 50th percentile, and the *thinner lines* represent the 10th and 90th percentiles.

## BIOPHYSICAL PROFILE

Theoretically, identification of the compromised fetus could be improved by assessing several biophysical variables by means of real-time ultrasonography rather than simple monitoring of the fetal heart rate, as is done in cardiotocography. Manning and associates (1980) recognized the limitations of existing means of fetal heart rate monitoring and developed the biophysical profile (BPP), which encompasses observations of fetal behavioral activity on ultrasonography in addition to fetal heart rate reactivity. Prospective clinical studies have demonstrated generally good but varying predictive accuracies for each variable, but a combination of these measures improves the predictive accuracy substantially (Manning et al, 1987). The components of this BPP are listed in Table 13–10.

**TABLE 13–10**

**Elements of the Biophysical Profile Score**

| Parameter | Criterion Earning 2 Points* |
|---|---|
| Nonstress test | Reactive test |
| Fetal breathing movements | At least one episode of fetal breathing of 60 sec duration |
| Gross fetal body movements | At least three discrete episodes of fetal movement |
| Fetal tone | At least one episode of extension and return to flexion of extremities or spine or hand open/close |
| Amniotic fluid volume | At least one pocket of amniotic fluid ≥1 cm in depth |

*Total of 10 points available.

A positive finding in each of the BPP parameters is awarded a value of 2 to give a total BPP score of 10. Outcomes in the initial study were collected prospectively, and scores of 8 to 10 were found to correlate with good outcome. Scores of 2 and 4 are associated with high perinatal mortality and warrant intervention. A summary of possible scores and recommended actions is given in Table 13–11. The risk of fetal death with a BPP score of 8 is less than 1 per 1000.

Although a number of studies have demonstrated the efficacy of the BPP, its performance is time-consuming and expensive in resources. Many centers now use the so-called *modified BPP*, in which the NST provides the estimate of short-term fetal acid-base status and the AFI assesses comparatively longer-term alterations in placental function and fetal well-being (Clark et al, 1989; Vintzileos and Knuppel, 1994). Adding AFI measurements to the NST reduces the risk of fetal death from approximately 2 per 1000 to less than 1 per 1000.

## DOPPLER FLOW STUDIES

Reports of the use of Doppler ultrasonography for the evaluation of maternal and fetal conditions have increased in frequency in the obstetric literature. Despite the increasing number of publications reporting a variety of applications of Doppler ultrasonography in obstetrics, however, there is still considerable question as to the reliability of and the indications for its use.

It is possible to study flow in many fetal vessels using Doppler ultrasonography. The umbilical artery has been widely studied, but considerable interest has been generated by studies of cerebral blood flow and other regional circulations. Despite the enthusiasm of the proponents of Doppler ultrasonography, it remains an investigational tool only and is never required in any given situation, although it may aid decision-making.

### Physiology of Doppler Velocimetry

In fetal hypoxia or other forms of stress, abnormalities of the fetal velocity waveforms develop. Although the systolic component reflects the vigor of fetal cardiac function, the *diastolic component* of the fetal velocity waveforms is of greatest value in assessing fetal status because it reflects the amount of peripheral resistance that the downstream vascular bed presents to the heart. As peripheral resistance increases, blood flow velocity decreases during cardiac diastole. Therefore, the fetus with an infarcted placenta and associated increase in intraplacental resistance demonstrates rising systolic-to-diastolic ratios over time. If resistance rises high enough, flow in diastole may cease completely. In extreme cases, reversed diastolic flow may be seen. The association of absence of end-diastolic velocities (AEDV) in the umbilical artery with IUGR, meconium aspiration, intrauterine fetal death, and birth asphyxia has been reported by many investigators.

**TABLE 13–11**

**Interpretation and Management of Biophysical Profile (BPP) Score**

| Score (of 10) | Comment | Perinatal Mortality Within 1 Wk Without Intervention (per 1000) | Management |
|---|---|---|---|
| 10 | Risk of fetal asphyxia extremely rare | <1 | Intervention only for obstetric and maternal factors |
| 8: Normal fluid | No indication for intervention for fetal disease | — | — |
| Nonstress test (NST) not performed | Equivalent to BPP score of 10 with NST | — | — |
| Abnormal fluid | Probable chronic fetal compromise | 89 | Determine whether there is functioning renal tissue and membranes are intact; if so, deliver for fetal indications |
| 6: Normal fluid | Equivocal test, possible asphyxia | Variable | If the fetus is mature, deliver<br>In the immature fetus, repeat test within 24 hrs; if BPP score is <6, deliver |
| Abnormal fluid | Probable fetal asphyxia | 89 | Deliver for fetal indications |
| 4 | High probability of fetal asphyxia | 91 | Deliver for fetal indications |
| 2 | Fetal asphyxia almost certain | 125 | Deliver for fetal indications |
| 0 | Fetal asphyxia certain | 600 | Deliver for fetal indications |

Adapted from Manning FA, Morrison I, Harman CR, et al: Fetal assessment based on fetal biophysical profile scoring: Experience in 19,221 referred high-risk pregnancies. Am J Obstet Gynecol 157:880, 1987.

In pregnancies complicated by IUGR, between two thirds and three quarters of fetuses exhibit an excessively high index of placental resistance (systolic-to-diastolic ratio or resistance index) (Trudinger et al, 1991). Fetuses with abnormal flow-velocity waveforms have a higher incidence of neonatal morbidity than those with normal study findings.

Histologically, the high placental resistance evidenced by the abnormal umbilical Doppler flow velocity waveform is associated with reduced numbers of small (diameter $<90$ μm) arteries in the tertiary villi of the placenta (the resistance vessels) (Giles et al, 1985) and obliterative changes in the remaining vessels.

Abnormalities of blood flow velocity may occur in other vascular beds in the fetus experiencing hypoxemia. As the oxygen level in the umbilical venous blood drops, the cerebral circulation compensates by increasing flow in the carotid arteries. Accordingly, with progressive hypoxia, intracerebral vascular resistance typically falls, and diastolic velocity increases. Flow velocity in the descending aorta, supplying the majority of the fetus's visceral organs, may be adversely affected. The level of intrauterine hypoxemia at any given time may be best expressed as the sum of effects on umbilical, cerebral, and aortic circulations.

Because the relationship of the fetal heart to the placental, cerebral, and visceral circulations is in a dynamic state of flux during pregnancy, the fetal velocity waveform indices must be corrected for gestational age. *Normative tables* for the pulsatility index and systolic-to-diastolic ratio have been published by Schulman and coworkers (1984).

Abnormalities in the fetal velocity waveform (particularly the diastolic changes) generally become evident 1 to 3 weeks before the onset of abnormalities in other clinical parameters, such as fetal heart rate, amniotic fluid volume, and fetal BPP. During pregnancy, uterine blood flow is markedly increased with minimal resistance secondary to the effects of estrogen on the uterine circulation. From reasonably early in gestation, the fetal velocity waveforms of the uteroplacental circulation can be documented, and in certain maternal diseases, such as chronic hypertension and pregnancy-induced hypertension, abnormalities in the uteroplacental fetal velocity waveforms can be documented. In fact, Campbell and associates (1986) noted abnormalities in uteroplacental circulation from approximately 20 weeks onward in pregnancies in which either severe IUGR or pregnancy-induced hypertension developed.

## Applications of Doppler Waveform Analysis in Fetal Management

### Rule Out Chronic Fetal Hypoxia

Despite the flurry of papers concerning the use of Doppler ultrasonography throughout pregnancy, its most common indication is as an advisory adjunct in the evaluation of fetal status. As an example, in pregnancies remote from term with no evidence of IUGR, decreased amniotic fluid volume, or abnormal fetal heart rate changes, it is unlikely that one would deliver the fetus on the basis of a grossly abnormal Doppler blood flow unless the BPP score also was less than 4. The controversy surrounding use of Doppler ultrasonography in fetal testing has been well characterized by Low (1991).

Later investigators have used pulsed Doppler ultrasonography to examine blood flow in the carotid artery or descending aorta. They have found that under normal conditions, diastolic blood flow in the carotid arteries is decreased. With the development of IUGR or hypoxia, there is a dilation of the cerebral blood flow during diastole. These findings are consistent with the known increase in cerebral blood flow with hypoxia in laboratory animals.

Overall, the decision to intervene in a pregnancy at risk for IUGR is strengthened by knowing the trend in Doppler flow velocity ratios. Most experts believe that Doppler velocimetric findings alone are not adequate evidence of urgent fetal compromise unless diastolic flow is actually reversed. Doppler velocimetry should be used to guide the use of more traditional biophysical tests (e.g., NST, CST).

However, two findings (AEDV and reversed end-diastolic velocity [REDV)) should be viewed with concern. These two entities, marked by absence or reverse of umbilical artery flow during cardiac diastole, are associated with significantly increased placental resistance and fetal cardiac failure. The incidence of meconium staining, admission to a neonatal intensive care unit, and fetal growth restriction is several times higher with AEDV than if some diastolic flow is present. If fetal blood flow to the placenta reverses during the resting part of the cardiac cycle, cardiac pump function and placental resistance are at end stage; more than 60% of fetuses die within 48 hours of this finding.

### Investigate Discordant Growth in Twins

In a twin gestation, finding one large, possibly hydramniotic twin and the other twin smaller by 4 to 6 weeks of gestation in a sac with markedly diminished amniotic fluid can present a difficult diagnostic challenge, especially if the genders are concordant. The entity of severe growth discordance can be due to twin-twin transfusion syndrome (TTS) or associated with placental discordance and IUGR. Use of serial Doppler velocimetry measurements can help differentiate TTS from IUGR: in TTS, the systolic-to-diastolic ratio in umbilical fetal velocity waveforms of the small twin is usually normal or decreased, whereas the Doppler studies in a growth-restricted twin with small or infarcted placenta displays absence of diastolic velocity. Following such pregnancies with Doppler velocimetry studies can help identify the starting point for biophysical testing (when systolic-to-diastolic ratios rise or end-diastolic velocity disappears) and may provide an early signal of the need for urgent delivery.

Doppler ultrasonography is a helpful tool in the evaluation of fetal status. In some cases, the results can be predictive of abnormal future fetal or maternal outcomes, but the method is neither sensitive nor specific enough at this time to be completely reliable unless extremes of flow velocity are present.

## AMNIOCENTESIS

Examination of amniotic fluid in late pregnancy for biochemical evidence of lung maturity may precede elective delivery or aid in timing of delivery in a compromised pregnancy. The following tests are available:

- Lecithin-sphingomyelin ratio
- Phosphatidyl glycerol
- TDx-FLM (TDx–fetal lung maturity) fluorescence polarization assay

In certain cases of apparent fetal compromise, it may be necessary to exclude potentially lethal chromosome anomalies before intervention and delivery. Amniocentesis for karyotyping or the more rapid fluorescent in situ hybridization for identification of trisomies 13, 18, and 21 may thus be indicated.

## CORDOCENTESIS

Access to fetal blood provides the ultimate means of assessing fetal status—although not without significant procedural risk, carrying a fetal loss rate of 1%. Acid-base status and blood gas levels may be determined (Soothill et al, 1992), although critical values for intervention have not been firmly established (Sonek and Nicolaides, 1994).

## SUMMARY

Clearly, fetal surveillance encompasses a wide range of modalities, each with advantages and disadvantages. A suggested cascade of complexity is shown in Figure 13–6. There is no agreement among authorities as to the ideal tests for fetal well-being. Because there are no large randomized, prospective studies comparing the various methods available, none may be considered superior to others. The key is to identify the fetus potentially at risk and then to ensure that a reassuring test result is obtained at each scheduled encounter. Avoidable mortality occurs most often when the practitioner does not act on concerning test results.

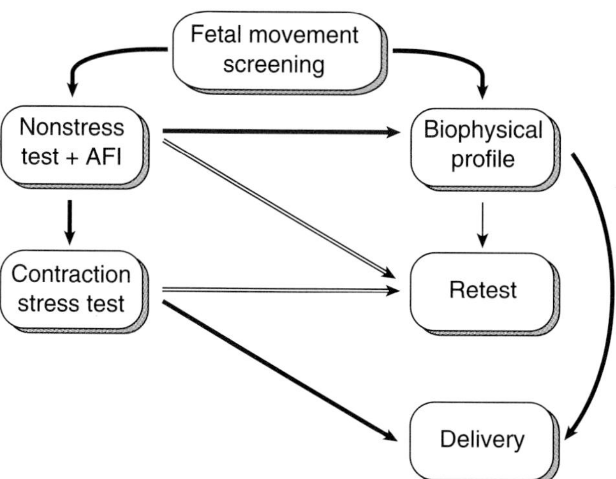


**FIGURE 13–6.** Fetal testing cascade. *Filled lines* indicate abnormal, or nonreassuring, test result. *Open lines* indicate normal, or reassuring, test result. AFI, amniotic fluid index.

## REFERENCES


American College of Obstetricians and Gynecologists: Clinical Management Guidelines For Obstetrician-Gynecologists: Antepartum Surveillance. Number 9, October 1999.

Bekedam MD, Visser GHA: Effects of hypoxemic events on breathing, body movements, and heart rate variation: A study in growth-retarded human fetuses. Am J Obstet Gynecol 153:52, 1985.

Boehm FH, Salyer S, Shah DM, Vaughn WK: Improved outcome of twice weekly nonstress testing. Obstet Gynecol 67:566, 1986.

Brace RA, Wolf EJ: Normal amniotic fluid volume changes throughout pregnancy. Am J Obstet Gynecol 161:382, 1989.

Campbell S, Pearch JMF, Hackett G, et al: Qualitative assessment of uteroplacental bloodflow: Early screening test for high-risk pregnancies. Obstet Gynecol 68:649, 1986.

Chamberlain MB, Manning GA, Morrison I, et al: Ultrasound evaluation of amniotic fluid. I: The relationship of marginal and decreased amniotic fluid volume to perinatal outcome. Am J Obstet Gynecol 150:245, 1984.

Clark SL, Sabey P, Jolley K: Nonstress testing with acoustic stimulation and amniotic fluid volume assessment: 5973 tests without unexpected fetal death. Am J Obstet Gynecol 160:694, 1989.

Devoe LD, Gardner P, Dear C, et al: The diagnostic values of concurrent nonstress testing, amniotic fluid measurement, and Doppler velocimetry in screening a general high-risk population. Am J Obstet Gynecol 163:1040, 1990.

Druzin ML, Fox A, Kogut E, et al: The relationship of the nonstress test to gestational age. Am J Obstet Gynecol 153:386, 1985.

Evertson LR, Gauthier RJ, Schifrin BS, et al: Antepartum fetal heart rate testing. I: Evolution of the nonstress test. Am J Obstet Gynecol 133:29, 1979.

Freeman RK, Anderson G, Dorchester W: A prospective multi-institutional study of antepartum fetal heart rate monitoring. II: Contraction stress test versus nonstress test for primary surveillance. Am J Obstet Gynecol 143:778, 1982.

Giles WB, Trudinger BJ, Baird P: Fetal umbilical artery flow velocity waveforms and placental resistance: Pathological correlation. Br J Obstet Gynaecol 92:31, 1985.

Grant A, Valentin L, Elbourne D, Alexander S: Routine formal fetal movement counting and risk of antepartum late death in normally formed singletons. Lancet 2:345, 1989.

Hill LM, Breckle R, Wolfgram KR, O'Brien PC: Oligohydramnios: Ultrasonically detected incidence and subsequent fetal outcome. Am J Obstet Gynecol 147:407, 1984.

Hill LM, Breckle R, Thomas ML, et al: Polyhydramnios: Ultrasonically detected prevalence and neonatal outcome. Obstet Gynecol 69:21, 1987.

Hovatta O, Lipasti A, Rapola J, et al: Causes of stillbirth: A clinicopathological study of 243 patients. Br J Obstet Gynaecol 90:691, 1983.

Lagrew DC: Fetal evaluation in early gestational ages. Clin Obstet Gynecol 30:992, 1987.

Lagrew DC, Pircon RA, Nageotte M, et al: How frequently should the amniotic fluid index be repeated? Am J Obstet Gynecol 167:1129, 1992.

Lavin JP, Miodovnik M, Barden TP: Relationship of nonstress reactivity and gestational age. Obstet Gynecol 63:338, 1984.

Lee CY, DiLoreto PC, Logrand B: Fetal activity acceleration determination for the evaluation of fetal reserve. Obstet Gynecol 48:19, 1976.

Low JA: The current status of maternal and fetal blood flow velocimetry. Am J Obstet Gynecol 164:1049, 1991.

Manning FA, Platt LD, Sipos L: Fetal movements in human pregnancies in the third trimester. Obstet Gynecol 6:699, 1979.

Manning FA, Platt LD, Sipos L: Antepartum fetal evaluation: Development of a fetal biophysical profile. Am J Obstet Gynecol 136:787, 1980.

Manning FA, Morrison I, Harman CR, et al: Fetal assessment based on fetal biophysical profile scoring: Experience in 19,221 referred high-risk pregnancies. Am J Obstet Gynecol 157:880, 1987.

Moore TR, Cayle JE: The amniotic fluid index in normal human pregnancy. Am J Obstet Gynecol 162:1168, 1990.

Moore TR, Piacquadio K: A prospective evaluation of fetal movement screening to reduce the incidence of antepartum fetal death. Am J Obstet Gynecol 162:1168, 1989.

Moore TR, Longo J, Leopold G, et al: The reliability and predictive value of an amniotic fluid scoring system in severe second trimester oligohydramnios. Obstet Gynecol 73:739, 1989.

Natale R, Clelow F, Dawes GS: Measurement of fetal forelimb movements in lambs in utero. Am J Obstet Gynecol 140:545, 1981.

Neldham S: Fetal movements as an indicator of fetal well-being. Lancet 1:1222, 1980.

Nimrod C, Varela-Gittings F, Machin G, et al: The effect of very prolonged membrane rupture on fetal development. Am J Obstet Gynecol 148:540, 1984.

Patrick J, Campbell K, Carmichael L, et al: Patterns of gross fetal body movements over 24 hour observation intervals during the last 10 weeks of pregnancy. Am J Obstet Gynecol 142:363, 1982.

Platt LD, Paul RH, Phelan J, et al: Fifteen years of experience with antepartum fetal testing. Am J Obstet Gynecol 156:1509, 1987.

Rayburn WF: Clinical applications of monitoring fetal activity. Am J Obstet Gynecol 144:967, 1982.

Rochard F, Schifin BS, Goupil F, et al: Nonstressed fetal heart rate monitoring in the antepartum period. Am J Obstet Gynecol 126:699, 1976.

Rutherford SE, Phelan JP, Smith CV, Jacobs N: The four-quadrant assessment of amniotic fluid volume: An adjunct to antepartum fetal heart rate testing. Obstet Gynecol 70:353, 1987.

Schulman H, Fleischer A, Sterm W, et al: Umbilical velocity wave ratios in human pregnancy. Am J Obstet Gynecol 148:986, 1984.

Slavesen DR, Freeman J, Brudenell JM, et al: Prediction of fetal acidemia in pregnancies complicated by maternal diabetes mellitus by biophysical profile scoring and fetal heart rate monitoring. Br J Obstet Gynaecol 100:227, 1993.

Sonek J, Nicolaides K: The role of cordocentesis in the diagnosis of fetal well being. Clin Perinatol 21:743, 1994.

Soothill PW, Ajayi RA, Campbell EM, et al: Relationship between fetal acidemia at cordocentesis and subsequent neurodevelopment. Ultrasound Obstet Gynecol 2:80, 1992.

Sorokin Y, Dierker LJ, Pillay SK, et al: The association between fetal heart rate patterns and fetal movements in pregnancies between 20 and 30 weeks gestation. Am J Obstet Gynecol 143:243, 1982.

Trudinger BJ, Cook CM, Giles WB, et al: Fetal umbilical artery velocity waveforms and subsequent neonatal outcome. Br J Obstet Gynaecol 98:378, 1991.

Valentin L, Marsal K: Fetal movement in the third trimester of normal pregnancy. Early Hum Dev 14:295, 1986.

Vintzileos AM, Knuppel RA: Multiple parameter biophysical testing in the prediction of fetal acid-base status. Clin Perinatol 21:823, 1994.

CHAPTER 14

# Prematurity: Causes and Prevention

George A. Macones

## TRENDS IN RATES OF PRETERM BIRTH

Preterm birth continues to be one of the major challenges in perinatal medicine. Despite years of research, the rate of preterm birth has remained constant over the past 20 years (Goldenberg and Rouse, 1998). If anything, the incidence of preterm birth may be rising somewhat, due in part to the increasing rates of multiple gestations resulting from advanced reproductive technologies. Fortunately, advances in neonatal medicine have led to drastic improvements in survival as well as reductions in morbidity among infants born preterm. These advances are well-described in other sections of this book.

In this chapter, we focus on the etiology, prediction, and prevention of preterm birth. We describe a current approach to prevention of preterm birth from the perspective of the obstetrician.

### Etiology of Preterm Birth

A *preterm birth*, defined as one occurring before 37 completed weeks of gestation, can occur for a variety of reasons. This diversity of etiologies is one reason why the prevention of preterm birth has been so problematic. In general, preterm births are categorized as either spontaneous or indicated (Meis et al, 1995). *Spontaneous* preterm births occur secondary to either preterm labor or preterm premature rupture of the amniotic membranes (PPROM). *Indicated* preterm births are those that occur because of a medical or obstetric problem that places either the mother or the fetus at risk; delivery is undertaken to preserve or improve the maternal or fetal status. Notably, spontaneous preterm births account for more than two thirds of all preterm births in the United States, and indicated preterm births account for the remaining third (Goldenberg and Rouse, 1998).

There are a variety of reasons for an indicated preterm birth, and they may be divided into maternal and fetal indications (Meis et al, 1995). The maternal indications for preterm delivery are as follows:

- Preeclampsia
- Placental abruption
- Placenta previa
- Any maternal medical condition requiring delivery (e.g., cancer)

Fetal indications for preterm delivery are:

- Severe fetal growth retardation
- Nonreassuring fetal status

As one can see from the preceding lists, the etiology of indicated preterm births is very heterogeneous, and it should not be surprising that spontaneous and indicated preterm births differ in epidemiology. For this reason, most preventive strategies for reducing preterm birth are focused on spontaneous, rather than indicated, preterm births. The remainder of the chapter focuses on spontaneous preterm births.

## RISK FACTORS FOR SPONTANEOUS PRETERM BIRTHS

Spontaneous preterm births occur because the labor process begins early (without any other identifiable maternal or fetal conditions). Preterm births resulting from preterm labor or PPROM account for a majority of preterm deliveries in the United States (Goldenberg and Rouse, 1998). There is considerable but not complete overlap in the risk factors for these two conditions. *Spontaneous preterm labor* is defined as the onset of uterine contractions with cervical change before 37 weeks of gestation. PPROM is rupture of the amniotic membranes before 37 weeks of gestation. The variety of risk factors for these spontaneous preterm deliveries is described in this discussion.

### Multiple Gestation

Multiple gestation is one of the strongest risk factors for either a spontaneous or indicated preterm birth. With advances in the treatment of infertility by means of ovulation induction and in vitro fertilization, the rate of multiple gestations both in the United States and in other developed countries is rising. It is generally believed that the risk of preterm labor and PPROM is increased with multiple gestation because of excessive uterine distension (because the same higher risk is observed with polyhydramnios). In addition, the more fetuses present, the higher the rate of preterm birth. The mean gestational age at delivery is approximately 37 weeks for twins, approximately 33 weeks for triplets, and approximately 28 weeks for quadruplets. Rates of preterm birth are higher for monochorionic than for dichorionic multiple gestations.

Because of the concerns with high-order multiple gestations (triplets or higher), patients are often offered fetal reduction. Fetal reductions are performed in the late first trimester. Under ultrasonographic guidance, potassium chloride is injected into the thorax of one or more of the fetuses. This procedure carries a small procedure-related loss rate, approximately 4%. Patients whose multiple gestations are reduced to twins seem to have perinatal outcomes similar to those of women with nonreduced twin gestations. The only exception to this is that there may be a higher rate of growth retardation in pregnancies that have been reduced to twins. Most physicians are comfortable with offering a fetal reduction to a patient with triplet or greater gestations, although there is controversy about the role of fetal reduction in triplet pregnancies (Macones et al, 1993; Melgar et al, 1991; Porreco et al, 1991; Yaron et al, 1999).

## Maternal Uterine Abnormalities

Maternal uterine abnormalities are also associated with spontaneous preterm birth, accounting for approximately 5% of all preterm births. Such anomalies include bicornuate uterus, uterus didelphys, and unicornuate uterus. The usual obstetric history of someone with a uterine abnormality would be the occurrence of multiple preterm births, with advancing gestational ages in subsequent pregnancies. At the University of Pennsylvania, any patient with a spontaneous preterm birth is counseled to undergo a postpartum evaluation for uterine abnormalities. This evaluation can be done via either hysterography or a hysterosalpingogram. Such an evaluation is essential, because some abnormalities are amenable to surgical correction, which in theory could lessen the chances of a subsequent preterm delivery.

## Fetal Abnormalities

Some fetal abnormalities also raise the risk of a spontaneous preterm birth. They include anomalies that might increase the volume of amniotic fluid, which through overdistension of the uterus can lead to preterm delivery—such as bowel obstruction and tracheoesophageal fistula. Because of the relationship between fetal abnormalities and preterm birth, it is essential to review findings of prior scans or to perform a targeted ultrasonogram for any woman presenting with preterm labor.

## Maternal Infection

Maternal infections are risk factors for preterm birth as well. Infections such as pneumonia and pyelonephritis have been linked to preterm birth. Genital tract infections, including *Chlamydia* and gonorrhea, have also been related to preterm birth. Attention has now turned to the relationship between maternal bacterial vaginosis and preterm birth. A number of observational studies both in the United States and around the world link bacterial vaginosis to spontaneous preterm birth (Hillier et al, 1995; Kurki et al, 1992; Riduan et al, 1995). The mechanism of this association is unclear, though some researchers have theorized that the bacterial vaginosis–associated organisms can ascend and cause a subclinical infection in the decidua. In theory, this smoldering infection could lead to activation of the inflammatory cascade, which in turn could lead to the activation of proteases and matrix metalloproteinases, weakening the amniotic membranes and causing preterm birth. Interestingly, the association between infection and preterm birth is strongest at earlier gestational ages.

## Maternal Cervical Abnormalities

Maternal cervical abnormalities can be associated with preterm birth. Traditionally, obstetricians have believed that cervical abnormalities lead to an incompetent cervix. Incompetent cervix has been associated with midtrimester cervical dilation and delivery. Substantial research has now been conducted on the relationship between the length of the cervix and preterm birth. On the basis of this work, it is now believed that the shorter the cervix, the higher the rate of preterm birth. Thus, the traditional teaching of an incompetent versus a competent cervix is being reconsidered (Iams et al, 1995, 1996).

## History of Spontaneous Preterm Birth

A history of a spontaneous preterm birth is among the strongest risk factors for a subsequent preterm birth. For example, in the United States, the baseline rate of preterm birth is approximately 8%. In women who had experienced a previous preterm birth, the rate rises to almost 16%. Table 14–1 demonstrates results from a landmark study describing rates of preterm birth based on pregnancy history. If an individual has a single preterm birth, the rate in the subsequent pregnancy rises to 17.2%. With two consecutive preterm births, the rate rises to more than 28% in the next pregnancy (Bakketeig and Hoffman, 1981).

## Ethnicity

Ethnicity is also a risk factor for preterm delivery. Specifically, rates of preterm birth in those of African-American descent are nearly twice as high as those in whites (Meis et al, 2000; Mercer et al, 1996). There are probably many reasons, but one commonly cited is the association between African-American race and bacterial vaginosis (Meis et al, 2000).

## Genetic Susceptibility

There is a great deal of ongoing work on whether or not there is a genetic susceptibility to preterm birth. The following lines of evidence support such a susceptibility:

- A history of a prior preterm birth is a strong risk factor for its subsequent occurrence (Bakketeig and Hoffman, 1981; Goldenberg et al, 1998).
- There appears to be an intergenerational risk of preterm birth (Klebanoff et al, 1989).
- Twin studies support a higher concordance of preterm birth in monozygotic twins than in dizygotic twins (Treolar et al, 2000).

Because of this work as well as the advances in genetic research, many investigators are looking for candidate genes

**TABLE 14-1**

**Risk of Preterm Birth in Subsequent Births**

| First Birth | Second Birth | Subsequent Preterm Birth (%) |
|---|---|---|
| Not preterm | | 4.4 |
| Preterm | | 17.2 |
| Not preterm | Not preterm | 2.6 |
| Preterm | Not preterm | 5.7 |
| Not preterm | Preterm | 11.1 |
| Preterm | Preterm | 28.4 |

From Bakketeig LS, Hoffman HJ: Epidemiology of preterm birth: Results from longitudinal study of births in Norway. In Elder MG, Hendricks CH (eds): Preterm Labor. London, Butterworths, 1981, p 17.

that might increase or decrease the risk of preterm birth. Interestingly, consideration is being given to both maternal and fetal candidates. Much of this current work is focused on polymorphisms that relate to the host inflammatory response to infection.

## SCREENING FOR PRETERM BIRTH

Conditions for screening for a given condition have been well described. Following are some of the tenets for a successful screening program:

- The screening test must be acceptable.
- The disease must be prevalent.
- The disease must have serious consequences.
- The screening test must have acceptable discriminatory ability (i.e., high sensitivity and specificity).
- There must be interventions to reduce disease burden in those with positive screening results.

Preterm birth meets many, though not all, of these requirements. Certainly, from an individual and societal perspective, a screening strategy that could reduce preterm births would be welcome. However, screening for preterm birth is limited because of the lack of interventions that could reduce preterm birth in women with positive results. Thus, most screening tests currently available have little, if any, clinical application. Rather, they are often used in research studies of new interventions. Despite these limitations, there are three methods of screening for preterm birth.

First, there are well-described *risk scoring indices* for preterm birth (Creasy et al, 1980; Mercer et al, 1996). Several of these indices have been published, and they are based on large epidemiologic studies of risk factors for preterm birth. The sensitivity of these indices approximates 50%, suggesting that at least half of preterm births would be missed by evaluations based on these clinical grounds alone.

Second, *biochemical markers* have been assessed as screening tests for preterm birth. Fetal fibronectin has undergone an extensive evaluation in this setting (Bartnicki et al, 1996; Goldenberg et al, 1996, 1997; Jones and Poston, 1998; Leitich et al, 1999; Lockwood et al, 1991). Fibronectin is a glycoprotein that is released when the extracellular matrix degrades. It is believed that fibronectin may be released when subclinical infections develop. These subclinical infections (such as bacterial vaginosis) can lead to activation of the cytokine cascade, which in turn leads to release of proteases and collagenases. The action of these enzymes on the extracellular matrix can then lead to the release of fetal fibronectin. Fetal fibronectin is measured in the cervix and vagina, and rapid tests are available (and have been approved by the U.S. Food and Drug Administration). The presence of fetal fibronectin at 16 to 22 weeks of gestation has been associated with a higher risk of spontaneous preterm birth (Goldenberg et al, 2000). Unfortunately, no interventions are available to reduce the risk of preterm birth in women with positive results. In fact, one large, multicenter study (Andrews et al, 2003) tested whether administration of antibiotics to women who test positive for fetal fibronectin could reduce preterm birth. Unfortunately, this study did not demonstrate any benefit in women who were treated with antibiotics compared with those who received placebo. For this reason, screening for risk of preterm birth using fibronectin is rarely performed in clinical practice.

Lastly, there are *physical screening tests* for preterm birth. They are digital and transvaginal ultrasonographic assessments of the cervix (Iams et al, 1995, 1996). Although a short cervix, as detected either digitally or ultrasonographically, is associated with preterm birth, as is testing positive for fibronectin, no interventions have been demonstrated to improve perinatal outcomes.

## CURRENT TREATMENTS TO REDUCE PRETERM BIRTHS

Although screening strategies have been disappointing, mainly because of the lack of efficacy of interventions, a number of treatments are commonly employed in those at risk of preterm birth.

### Screening for Bacterial Vaginosis

As has been mentioned earlier, maternal bacterial vaginosis has been associated with spontaneous preterm birth (Hillier et al, 1995; Kurki et al, 1992; Riduan et al, 1995). Given this association, it was hoped that screening and treating bacterial vaginosis in pregnancy could reduce the occurrence of preterm birth. Results of studies in women with a history of a prior preterm birth were conflicting, with some suggesting that screening and treatment could reduce the occurrence of preterm birth in high risk subjects, and others showing no benefit (Hauth et al, 1995; Morales et al, 1994). Still, these studies led to optimism that screening and treating all pregnant women could reduce the burden of preterm births in the United States. A large clinical trial performed within the Maternal-Fetal Medicine Units Network of screening and treating bacterial vaginosis in low-risk women did not demonstrate any benefit of treatment (Carey et al, 2000). Thus, screening for bacterial vaginosis in low-risk women is not currently recommended. On the basis of results of small clinical trials, some authorities still advocate screening and treating bacterial vaginosis in women with a previous spontaneous preterm birth.

### Avoidance of High-Order Multiple Gestations

The occurrence of preterm birth has been well documented to increase with increasing fetal number. Thus, limiting high-order multiple gestations that are achieved with advanced reproductive technologies is paramount. In addition, women with high-order multiple gestations should be counseled about the option of fetal reduction.

### Tocolysis for Preterm Labor

Neonatologists are very familiar with the treatment of an acute episode of preterm labor. *Preterm labor* is defined as the occurrence of regular uterine contractions accompanied by a change in the cervix (dilation or effacement). Depending on the gestational age, the arrest of preterm labor with various medications can be attempted. The oldest class of medications used for tocolysis are the beta-agonists, such as ritodrine and terbutaline. Ritodrine, in fact, is the only drug approved by the U.S. Food and Drug Administration for tocolysis (though no one manufactures it in the United States). Although these medications seem to be effective for a short-term delay in delivery (i.e., 48 hours), they do not reduce the rate of preterm birth (Barden et al, 1980; Downey and Martin, 1983; Larsen et al, 1986; Leveno et al, 1986). Nevertheless, a 48-hour delay allows for the administration of steroids, which can reduce the rate of various neonatal complications. The use of beta-agonists is limited by the occurrence of maternal side effects. Beta-agonist infusion has been associated with the following maternal complications (Alper and Cohen, 1983; Armson et al, 1992; Ferguson et al, 1989; Goyert et al, 1987; Ron-El et al, 1983):

- Hyperglycemia (and diabetic ketoacidosis in women with diabetes mellitus)
- Tachycardia
- Pulmonary edema
- Anxiety and restlessness
- Myocardial ischemia

Because of these complications, most centers in the United States do not use beta-agonists as a first line treatment for preterm labor.

Magnesium sulfate is commonly used for the arrest of preterm labor (Chau et al, 1992; Elliott, 1983; Macones et al, 1997; Madden et al, 1990; Miller et al, 1982; Smith et al, 1992; Tchilinguirian et al, 1984; Wilkins et al, 1988). Magnesium sulfate is usually administered intravenously—first as a loading dose and then as a constant infusion. The mechanism of action of magnesium sulfate is largely unknown, although it is believed to be related to calcium influx or efflux in smooth muscle. Magnesium sulfate is believed to be safe to use in pregnancy, although it has maternal side effects, such as lethargy, anxiety, chest heaviness, and pulmonary edema. Importantly, at very high levels of magnesium sulfate, maternal respiratory depression or cardiac arrest can occur.

There has been some concern about the fetal or neonatal safety of magnesium sulfate when used for preterm labor (Mittendorf et al, 1997). The MagNet Study was designed to evaluate whether the administration of magnesium sulfate to women at high risk of preterm delivery could reduce the occurrence of cerebral palsy. This clinical trial was stopped early because of an excess of pediatric deaths in the group receiving magnesium sulfate. However, many of the pediatric deaths reported in this study would be difficult, if not impossible, to ascribe to magnesium sulfate (e.g., accidents, congenital abnormalities). Thus, many maternal-fetal medicine specialists are skeptical of these findings. A large multicenter clinical trial is currently underway to assess whether the administration of magnesium sulfate to women at risk of preterm birth (e.g., those in preterm labor or with ruptured amniotic membranes) reduces the risk of cerebral palsy and neurodevelopmental disability.

Prostaglandin synthetase inhibitors, such as indomethacin, have also been tested and used to arrest an acute episode of preterm labor (Blake et al, 1980; Carlan et al, 1992; Keirse, 1995; Morales et al, 1989; Nieby et al, 1980; Zuckerman et al, 1974, 1984). These medications can be administered either orally or as vaginal or rectal suppositories. Although these agents are believed to have few serious maternal side effects, there has been concern about their safety for the fetus and neonate. Specifically, indomethacin freely crosses the placenta and has an extremely long half-life in preterm fetuses. Indomethacin has the following actions on the fetus:

- Reduction of renal blood flow
- Alteration of regional gastrointestinal blood flow
- Interference with platelet aggregation
- Closure of the ductus arterious

Because of these well-described physiologic changes associated with indomethacin, a number of observational studies have assessed the occurrence of necrotizing enterocolitis and intraventricular hemorrhage in infants who received antenatal indomethacin and in those who did not (Dudley and Hardie, 1985; Eronen et al, 1994; Goldenberg et al, 1989; Major et al, 1994; Norton et al, 1993). These studies have had conflicting results, with some showing higher rates of both disorders in infants who were exposed to indomethacin, and others demonstrating no relationship between indomethacin and adverse neonatal outcome (Gardner et al, 1996). Thus, at this point it is unclear whether the benefits of delaying delivery with indomethacin are outweighed by the neonatal or fetal risks of therapy (Macones and Robinson, 1997; Macones et al, 2001; Merrill et al, 1994). Most authorities agree that if indomethacin is to be used, it should be for a short course only (48 hours or less) and that this agent not be used beyond 34 weeks of gestation (when the fetal ductus arteriosus is more responsive to closure with indomethacin).

## Conservative Management of Preterm Premature Rupture of the Amniotic Membranes

Conservative management has become the standard method of managing PPROM at most centers around the country. Basically, when PPROM is confirmed at a gestational age of 30 weeks or less, the patient is admitted to the hospital and observed for signs of infection (chorioamnionitis) and for signs of labor. During this period, the following therapies are undertaken and the following procedures performed:

- Administration of corticosteroids
- Administration of antibiotics
- Fetal assessment via nonstress testing or biophysical profile
- Monitoring of maternal vital signs

The role of antenatal steroids in the setting of PPROM has been a topic of debate for many years. The concern had been that the administration of steroids in this setting could increase the rate of both maternal and fetal infections. However, a National Institute of Child Health and Human Development (NICHD) consensus panel has advocated the use of steroids in PPROM at less than 30 to 32 weeks of gestation. Beyond that gestational age, the risk-to-benefit ratio is less clear.

Administration of maternal antibiotics, irrespective of group B beta-hemolytic streptococci status, has been demonstrated to have benefits for the neonate (Mercer and Arheart, 1995; Mercer et al, 1997). Mercer and Arheart performed a meta-analysis to assess the role of maternal administration of antibiotics in patients with PPROM. This meta-analysis demonstrated that antibiotics improved outcomes as follows:

- Reduced occurrence of chorioamnionitis and postpartum maternal infection
- Reduced risk of neonatal sepsis (Table 14–2)
- Reduced risk of neonatal pneumonia
- Greater proportion of women undelivered after 7 days (Table 14–3)

**TABLE 14–2**

**Neonatal Sepsis and Antimicrobial Therapy in PPROM**

| | Cases of Sepsis in Treated Patients | | Cases of Sepsis in Control Group | | |
|---|---|---|---|---|---|
| **Study** | **No.** | **Percentage** | **No.** | **Percentage** | **Odds Ratios** |
| Amon | 23/43 | 53.5 | 28/39 | 71.8 | 0.45 |
| Johnston | 22/40 | 55.0 | 37/45 | 82.2 | 0.26 |
| McGregor | 14/28 | 50.0 | 18/27 | 66.7 | 0.50 |
| Mercer | 77/106 | 72.6 | 94/114 | 82.5 | 0.57 |
| Christmas | 28/48 | 58.3 | 39/46 | 84.8 | 0.25 |
| Blanco | 95/154 | 61.7 | 100/152 | 65.8 | 0.84 |
| Lockwood | 22/38 | 57.9 | 33/37 | 89.2 | 0.17 |
| Total all trials* | 281/457 | 61.5 | 349/460 | 75.9 | 0.51† |
| Total placebo-controlled trials‡ | 230/366 | 62.8 | 282/375 | 75.2 | 0.56§ |

*Breslow Day: 11.7; $P = .07$.

†95% confidence interval [CI], 0.38-0.68.

‡Breslow Day: 9.2; $P = .06$.

§95% CI, 0.41-0.76.

Adapted from Mercer B, Arheart K: Antimicrobial therapy in expectant management of preterm premature rupture of the membranes. Lancet 346:1271-1279, 1995.

**TABLE 14–3**

**Proportion of Women Undelivered After 7 Days and Antimicrobial Therapy in PPROM**

| | Undelivered Women in Treated Group | | Undelivered Women in Control Group | | |
|---|---|---|---|---|---|
| **Study** | **No.** | **Percentage** | **No.** | **Percentage** | **Odds Ratios** |
| Dunlop | 5/24 | 20.8 | 1/24 | 4.2 | 6.06 |
| Amon | 1/42 | 2.4 | 6/36 | 16.7 | 0.12 |
| Morales | 4/81 | 4.9 | 8/87 | 9.5 | 0.49 |
| Johnston | 3/40 | 7.5 | 11/45 | 24.4 | 0.25 |
| Mercer | 14/108 | 13.0 | 15/111 | 13.5 | 0.95 |
| Christmas | 2/48 | 4.2 | 0/45 | 0.0 | — |
| Kurki | 0/57 | 0.0 | 1/58 | 1.7 | — |
| Blanco | 0/153 | 0.0 | 5/150 | 3.3 | — |
| Lockwood | 2/37 | 5.4 | 3/36 | 8.3 | 0.63 |
| Owen | 2/59 | 3.4 | 6/56 | 10.3 | 0.30 |
| Total all trials* | 33/649 | 5.1 | 56/647 | 8.7 | 0.57† |
| Total placebo-controlled trials‡ | 19/395 | 4.8 | 35/400 | 8.8 | 0.53§ |

*Breslow Day: 18.9; $P = .03$.

†95% confidence interval [CI], 0.36-0.88.

‡Breslow Day: 6.8; $P = .15$.

§95% CI, 0.30-0.93.

Adapted from Mercer B, Arheart K: Antimicrobial therapy in expectant management of preterm premature rupture of the membranes. Lancet 346:1271-1279, 1995.

There are some unanswered questions regarding the use of antibiotics in the setting of PPROM. Specifically, a variety of antibiotics appears to be effective, but it is unclear which regimen, including duration of treatment, is most effective (Cox and Leveno, 1995). Another controversy in the management of PPROM is at what gestational age elective delivery should be considered. This decision should be made jointly by the neonatal group and obstetric group. At the Hospital of the University of Pennsylvania, we generally deliver patients electively with PPROM at 34 weeks of gestation.

## SUMMARY

Preterm birth remains one of the great challenges in perinatal medicine. Currently, there is active research on developing additional screening tests for preterm birth. More importantly, interventional studies on those who screen positive are ongoing.

## REFERENCES


Alper M, Cohen W: Pulmonary edema associated with ritodrine and dexamethasone treatment of threatened premature labor: A case report. J Reprod Med 28:349-352, 1983.

Andrews W, Sibai B, Thom E, et al: Randomized clinical trial of metronidazole plus erythromycin to prevent spontaneous preterm delivery in fetal fibronectin positive women. Obstet Gynecol 101:847-855, 2003.

Armson B, Samuels P, et al: Evaluation of maternal fluid dynamics during tocolytic therapy with ritodrine hydrochloride and magnesium sulfate. Am J Obstet Gynecol 167:758-765, 1992.

Bakketeig L, Hoffman H: Epidemiology of preterm birth: Results from a longitudinal study in Norway. In Elder MG, Hendricks CH (eds): Preterm Labor. London, Butterworths, 1981, p 17.

Barden T, Peter J, et al: Ritodrine hydrochloride: A betamimetic agent for use in preterm labor. Obstet Gynecol 56:1-6, 1980.

Bartnicki J, et al: Fetal fibronectin in vaginal specimens predicts preterm delivery and very-low-birthweight infants. Am J Obstet Gynecol 174:971-974, 1996.

Blake D, Niebyl J, et al: Treatment of premature labor with indomethacin. Adv Prostaglandin Thrombox Res 8:1465-1467, 1980.

Carey J, Klebanoff M, et al: Metronidazole to prevent preterm delivery in pregnant women with asymptomatic bacterial vaginosis. N Engl J Med 342:534-540, 2000.

Carlan S, O'Brien W, et al: Randomized comparative trial of indomethacin and sulindac for the treatment of refractory preterm labor. Obstet Gynecol 79:223-228, 1992.

Chau A, Gabert H, et al: A prospective comparison of terbutaline and magnesium for tocolysis. Obstet Gynecol 80:847-851, 1992.

Cox S, Leveno K: Intentional delivery versus expectant management with preterm ruptured membranes at 30-34 weeks' gestation. Obstet Gynecol 86:875-879, 1995.

Creasy R, Gremmer B, et al: System for predicting preterm birth. Obstet Gynecol 55:692-695, 1980.

Downey L, Martin A: Ritodrine in the treatment of preterm labour: A study of 213 patients. Br J Obstet Gynaecol 90: 1046-1053, 1983.

Dudley D, Hardie M: Fetal and neonatal effects of indomethacin used a tocolytic agent. Am J Obstet Gynecol 151:181-184, 1985.

Elliott J. Magnesium sulfate as a tocolytic agent. Am J Obstet Gynecol 147:277-284, 1983.

Eronen M, Pesonen E, et al: Increased incidence of bronchopulmonary dysplasia after antenatal administration of indomethacin to prevent preterm labor. J Pediatr 124:782-788, 1994.

Ferguson J, Dyson D, et al: Cardiovascular and metabolic effects associated with nifedipine and ritodrine tocolysis. Am J Obstet Gynecol 161:788-795. 1989.

Gardner M, Owen J, et al: Preterm delivery after indomethacin: A risk factor for neonatal complications? J Reprod Med 41: 903-906, 1996.

Goldenberg R, Rouse D: Prevention of preterm birth. N Engl J Med 339:313-320, 1998.

Goldenberg R, Davis R, et al: Indomethacin-induced oligohydramnios. Am J Obstet Gynecol 160:1196-1197, 1989.

Goldenberg R, Mercer B, et al: The preterm prediction study: Fetal fibronectin testing and spontaneous preterm birth. Obstet Gynecol 87:643-648, 1996.

Goldenberg R, Mercer B, et al: The preterm prediction study: Patterns of cervicovaginal fetal fibronectin as predictors of spontaneous preterm delivery. Am J Obstet Gynecol 177:8-12, 1997.

Goldenberg R, Iams J, et al: The preterm prediction study: The value of new vs standard risk factors in predicting early and all spontaneous preterm births. Am J Public Health 88:233-238, 1998.

Goldenberg R, Klebanoff M, et al: Vaginal fetal fibronectin measurements from 8 to 22 weeks' gestation and subsequent spontaneous preterm birth. Am J Obstet Gynecol 183:469-475, 2000.

Goyert G, Bhatia R, et al: Does intravenous ritodrine therapy cause capillary endothelial damage? Am J Perinatol 4:331-333, 1987.

Hauth J, Goldenberg R, et al: Reduced incidence of preterm delivery with metronidazole and erythromycin in women with bacterial vaginosis. N Engl J Med 333:1732-1736, 1995.

Hillier S, Nugent R, et al: Association between bacterial vaginosis and preterm delivery of a low birth weight infant. N Engl J Med 333:1737-1741, 1995.

Iams J, Johnson F, et al: Cervical competence as a continuum: A study of ultrasonographic cervical length and obstetric performance. Am J Obstet Gynecol 172:1097-1106, 1995.

Iams J, Goldenberg R, et al: The length of the cervix and the risk of spontaneous premature delivery. N Engl J Med 334: 567-572, 1996.

Jones G, Poston L: The diagnostic accuracy of cervico-vaginal fetal fibronectin in predicting preterm delivery: An overview. Br J Obstet Gynaecol 105:244-245, 1998.

Keirse M: Indomethacin tocolysis in preterm labour. London, BMJ Publishing Group, 1995.

Klebanoff M, Meirick O, et al: Second-generation consequences of small for dates birth. Pediatrics 84:343-347, 1989.

Kurki T, Sivonen A, et al: Bacterial vaginosis in early pregnancy and pregnancy outcome. Obstet Gynecol 80:173-177, 1992.

Larsen J, Eldon K, et al: Ritodrine in the treatment of preterm labor: Second Danish multicenter study. Obstet Gynecol 67:607-613, 1986.

Leitich H, Egarter C, et al: Cervicovaginal fetal fibronectin as a marker for preterm delivery: A meta-analysis. Am J Obstet Gynecol 180:1169-1176, 1999.

Leveno K, Guzick D, et al: Single-centre randomised trial of ritodrine hydrochloride for preterm labour. Lancet 1(8493): 1293-1295, 1986.

Lockwood C, Senyel A, et al: Fetal fibronectin in cervical and vaginal secretions as a predictor of preterm delivery. N Engl J Med 325:669-674, 1991.

Macones G, Schemmer G, et al: Multifetal reduction of triplets to twins improves perinatal outcome [see comments]. Am J Obstet Gynecol 169:982-986, 1993.

Macones G, Robinson C: Is there justification for using indomethacin in preterm labor? An analysis of risks and benefits. Am J Obstet Gynecol 177:819-824, 1997a.

Macones G, Sehdev H, et al: Evidence for magnesium sulfate as a tocolytic agent. Obstet Gynecol Surv 52:652-658, 1997b.

Macones G, Marder S, et al: The controversy surrounding indomethacin for tocolysis. Am J Obstet Gynecol 184:264-272, 2001.

Madden C, Owen J, et al: Magnesium tocolysis: Serum levels versus success. Am J Obstet Gynecol 162:177-180, 1990.

Major C, Lewis D, et al: Tocolysis with indomethacin increases the incidence of necrotizing enterocolitis in the low birth weight neonate. Am J Obstet Gynecol 170:102-106, 1994.

Meis P, Michielutte R, et al: Factors associated with preterm birth in Cardiff, Wales. II: Indicated and spontaneous preterm births. Am J Obstet Gynecol 173:597-602, 1995.

Meis P, Goldenberg R, et al: Preterm prediction study: Is socioeconomic status a risk factor for bacterial vaginosis in black or in white women. Am J Perinatol 17:41-45, 2000.

Melgar C, Rosenfeld D, et al: Perinatal outcome after multifetal reduction to twins compared with nonreduced multiple gestations. Obstet Gynecol 78:763-767, 1991.

Mercer B, Arheart K: Antimicrobial therapy in expectant management of preterm premature rupture of the membranes. Lancet 346:1271-1279, 1995.

Mercer B, Goldenberg R, et al: The preterm prediction study: A clinical risk assessment system. Am J Obstet Gynecol 174: 1885-1895, 1996.

Mercer B, Miodvnik M, et al: Antibiotic therapy for reduction of infant morbidity after preterm premature rupture of the membranes. JAMA 278:989-995, 1997.

Merrill J, Clyman R, et al: Indomethacin as a tocolytic agent: The controversy continues. J Pediatr 124:734-736, 1994.

Miller J, Keane M, et al: A comparison of magnesium sulfate and terbutaline for the arrest of premature labor. J Reprod Med 27:348-351, 1982.

Mittendorf R, Covert R, et al: Is tocolytic magnesium sulfate associated with increased total paediatric mortality? Lancet 350:1517-1518, 1997.

Morales W, Smith S, et al: Efficacy and safety of indomethacin versus ritodrine in the management of preterm labor: A randomized study. Obstet Gynecol 74:567-572, 1989.

Morales W, Schorr S, et al: Effect of metronidazole in patients with preterm birth in preceding pregnancy and bacterial vaginosis: A placebo-controlled, double-blind study. Am J Obstet Gynecol 171:345-348, 1994.

Niebyl J, Blake D, et al: The inhibition of premature labor with indomethacin. Am J Obstet Gynecol 136:1014-1019, 1980.

Norton M, Merrill J, et al: Neonatal complications after the administration on indomethacin for preterm labor. N Engl J Med 25:1603-1067, 1993.

Porreco R, Burke S, et al: Multifetal reduction of triplets and pregnancy outcome. Obstet Gynecol 78:335-339, 1991.

Riduan J, Hillier S, et al: Bacterial vaginosis and prematurity in Indonesia: Association in early and late pregnancy. Am J Obstet Gynecol 169:175-178, 1995.

Ron-El R, Caspi E, et al: Unexpected cardiac pathology in pregnant women treated with beta-adrenergic agents (ritodrine). Obstet Gynecol 61:10S-12S, 1983.

Smith L, Burns P, et al: Calcium homeostasis in pregnant women receiving long-term magnesium sulfate therapy for preterm labor. Am J Obstet Gynecol 167:45-51, 1992.

Tchilinguirian N, Najem R, et al: The use of ritodrine and magnesium sulfate in the arrest of preterm labor. Int J Gynecol Obstet 22:117-123, 1984.

Treolar S, Macones G, et al: Genetic influences on premature parturition in an Australian twin sample. Twin Research 3:80-82, 2000.

Wilkins I, Lynch L, et al: Efficacy and side effects of magnesium sulfate and ritodrine as tocolytics. Am J Obstet Gynecol 159:685-689, 1988.

Yaron Y, Bryant-Greenwood P, et al: Multifetal pregnancy reduction of triplets to twins: Comparison with nonreduced triplets and twins. Am J Obstet Gynecol 180:1268-1271, 1999.

Zuckerman H, Reiss U, et al: Inhibition of human premature labor by indomethacin. Obstet Gynecol 44:787-792, 1974.

Zuckerman H, Shalev E, et al: Further study of the inhibition of premature labor by indomethacin. Part II double-blind study. J Perinat Med 12:25-28, 1984.

CHAPTER 15

# Complicated Deliveries: Overview

**Sameer Gopalani and Thomas J. Benedetti**

In the past, childbirth was often regarded as a perilous undertaking. However, over the last century in the United States, perinatal and maternal mortality rates have dramatically fallen with advances in modern obstetric care, such as the widespread use of antibiotics, easy access to expedient cesarean delivery, and a better understanding of the proper use of instruments such as forceps and vacuum extraction (National Vital Statistics System, 2001). Indeed, adverse outcomes are in general uncommon in modern obstetrics, and unlike in the past, labor and delivery sessions conclude in most cases with a healthy mother and neonate. Nevertheless, complicated deliveries still occur, and knowledge of their conduct and sequelae are still required for the administration of proper maternal and infant care.

In this chapter we first address the complicated vaginal delivery, with particular attention to neonatal outcomes. We then discuss cesarean delivery and vaginal birth after a prior cesarean delivery (VBAC), and what neonatal implications they may have. However, prior to discussing complicated labor and its neonatal impact, we briefly consider the conduct of normal labor and delivery. A comprehensive discussion of labor and delivery is beyond the scope of this chapter; the interested reader is directed to any standard obstetric textbook chapter on normal labor (Fig. 15–1).

The *first stage of labor* begins with the onset of regular uterine contractions with concomitant cervical dilation and effacement, and ends with complete cervical dilation. The first stage is further subdivided into a *latent phase*, the length of which is quite variable and can last for several hours. The second part of the first stage of labor is the *active phase*, which usually begins when the cervix has dilated to 3 to 4 cm; this phase is marked by further rapid, progressive cervical dilation and effacement. Often the diagnosis of the transition from latent phase to active phase labor is retrospective, because the time of onset of active labor varies from patient to patient. The *second stage of labor* begins with complete cervical dilation and terminates with the expulsion of the fetus from the birth canal. The *third stage of labor* concludes with the delivery of the placenta.

Disorders of the conduct of labor are either of *protraction*, in which cervical dilation or fetal descent occurs but at a rate much less than expected, or *arrest*. Both disorders, if unresponsive to active medical management, are addressed by operative delivery. This delivery can be performed abdominally through cesarean section or vaginally with obstetric forceps or vacuum extraction if the cervix is fully dilated and specific criteria are fulfilled (see later). All these modalities can have neonatal and maternal effects, and the choice of instrument or mode of delivery must always take these potential morbidities into account.

## CESAREAN SECTION

Neonatal mortality within 7 days of birth was 20.5 per 1000 live births in 1950; this figure has fallen to 4.5 per 1000 (National Vital Statistics System, 2003). Certainly much of the improvement in neonatal survival stems from advances in neonatal intensive care and resuscitative techniques. Along with improved technology available to the pediatricians, however, is the fact that the last 50 years have also seen a dramatic increase in the universal access to safe cesarean section, which affords quick and timely fetal delivery. The National Center for Health Statistics (NCHS) records that in 1999, 20.8% of all infants born were delivered by cesarean section; in the 1950s and 1960s, the operative delivery rate was closer to 5% (NCHS, on line).

Cesarean section is usually performed through either a Pfannenstiel or vertical skin incision. The uterine incision is often made transversely in the lower uterine segment, as this approach minimizes intraoperative blood loss and future rupture risk during subsequent labor compared with a vertical or *classic* incision. The rupture risk in future labor is thought to be 0.5% to 1% for a low transverse incision, compared with 4% to 9% for a classic incision (American College of Obstetricians and Gynecologists [ACOG], 1999).

The accepted obstetric indications for operative delivery are as follows:

- Fetal malpresentation (e.g., shoulder or breech)
- Placenta previa
- Prior classic uterine incision
- Nonreassuring fetal status, remote from vaginal delivery
- Higher-order multiple gestation (triplets or more fetuses)
- Fetal contraindications to labor (alloimmune thrombocytopenia, neural tube defect)
- Maternal contraindication to labor (e.g., history of rectal or perineal fistulas from inflammatory bowel disease; large lower-uterine segment or cervical leiomyoma preventing vaginal delivery)

Cesarean section is also performed for disorders of protraction or arrest in the first stage of labor when conservative measures, such as oxytocin and amniotomy, fail to augment delivery or in the second stage, when assisted or operative vaginal delivery is deemed to be not feasible or not safe.

## THE COMPLICATED VAGINAL DELIVERY: OBSTETRIC FORCEPS AND VACUUM EXTRACTION

### Obstetric Forceps

Obstetric forceps have been employed for thousands of years to terminate difficult labors. However, many of these instruments were furnished with hooks and other accessories of destruction, being intended to save the mother but certainly not the fetus. It is only over the last

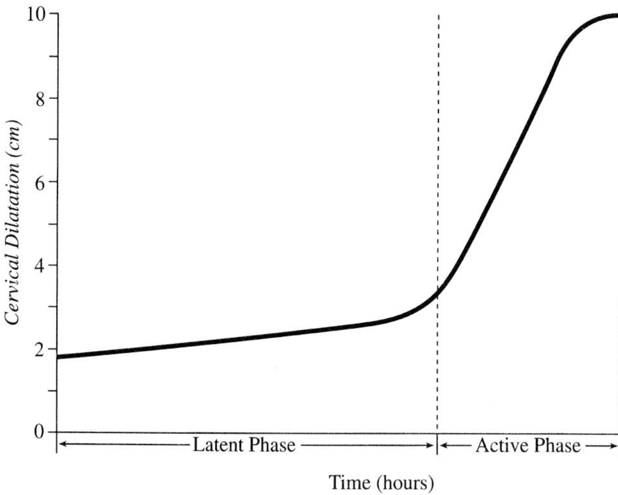


**FIGURE 15–1.** A graphic representation of normal labor, showing the variable time of onset to the active phase (3 to 4 cm), with a subsequent increase in the slope of cervical dilation.

400 years that ancestors of the modern instruments employed today came into existence, with the hope of delivering an intact, living baby.

Current obstetric forceps were first devised for practical use in the 17th and 18th centuries. They have been perfected over the past 200 years into the models that we currently use. There are many variations on the standard blueprint, depending on the indication for its use, but all obstetric forceps have a similar anatomy.

Forceps are devised of stainless steel and all have a *handle*, whereby the instrument is grasped by the obstetrician. There are long *shanks*, which are either parallel, divergent, or convergent, depending on the type of instrument, and a *lock*, which allows the two separate halves of the forceps to articulate. The two most common types of lock are the *sliding lock*, which can articulate anywhere along the shanks of the blade, and the *English lock*, which is fixed. The part of the forceps which grasps the fetal head is the *blade*. The blade can either be fenestrated, meaning that the body of the blade is hollow, or solid. Obstetric forceps also possess a rounded *cephalic curve*, which accommodates the fetal vertex, and a *pelvic curve*, which mirrors the curve of the mother's pelvis (Fig. 15–2).

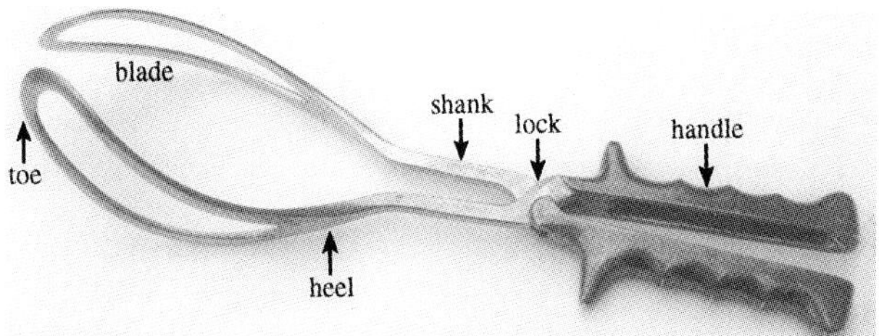


**FIGURE 15–2.** Simpson forceps: a standard obstetric forceps with features common to all such instruments.

More than 60 different types of obstetric forceps have been described in the literature, but most of these are not employed in current practice. The forceps most commonly used today are described in Table 15–1, along with the variations in anatomy that distinguish one from the other and their indications for use.

### Indications for and Use of the Obstetric Forceps

To an individual without obstetric training, the employment of forceps seems a dangerous and difficult undertaking, fraught with potential trauma for both the mother and fetus. It is certainly true that this instrument, if not handled carefully or appropriately, can have serious consequences. Nevertheless, in properly trained hands and with a proper appreciation of its use, forceps can be life-saving for both mother and fetus.

The criteria for safe application of obstetric forceps are as follows:

1. The cervix must be fully dilated.
2. The position of the fetal vertex must be known. *Forceps should not be applied when the fetal presentation is in doubt.*
3. The fetal vertex must be engaged. Often in difficult or challenging labors, significant edema of the fetal scalp can lead to the false impression that fetal station is lower than it actually is. For this reason, the obstetrician must be confident that the actual biparietal diameter has passed the pelvic inlet and that the leading part of the fetal skull is beyond the level of the ischial spines. In addition, when the presentation is occiput

**TABLE 15–1**

**Types of Obstetric Forceps in Most Common Use**

| Obstetric Forceps Type | Anatomic Modification | General Use |
|---|---|---|
| Simpson | Parallel shanks | Molded vertex or significant caput |
| Elliot | Convergent shanks | Nonmolded vertex |
| Tucker-McClane | Solid blade | Nonmolded vertex |
| Laufe | Pseudofenestrated blade; divergent shanks | For infants who are preterm or with estimated fetal weight <2500 g |
| Kielland | English lock; no pelvic curve | For rotation of fetal vertex >45 degrees |

posterior, the leading point of the fetal skull may appear to be lower in the pelvis even though the biparietal diameter has not yet passed through the pelvic inlet; this situation can also lead to an erroneous conclusion about fetal station.

4. When the forceps are properly applied, the sagittal suture must be exactly midway between the blades, and the lambdoidal sutures should be equidistant (usually a fingerbreadth) from the edge of the blade.

If the preceding conditions are not met, application of the forceps should be reconsidered. Furthermore, in 1988, the ACOG revised its classification of the type of forceps delivery according to the station of the fetal vertex before forceps application, as follows (ACOG, 2000b):

- *Outlet forceps*: The fetal vertex is visible at the labia without manually separating them, and the fetal skull has reached the pelvic floor.
- *Low forceps*: The leading point of the fetal skull is more than 2 cm beyond the ischial spines.
- *Mid-forceps*: The fetal head is engaged and is beyond the level of the ischial spines; *the forceps should be applied only if (1) cesarean delivery cannot be performed quickly or imminently and the fetus is in distress or (2) there is a high likelihood that the forceps operation will be successful*.
- *High forceps*: The vertex is not engaged (i.e., not at the level of the ischial spines or beyond); *under these circumstances, the forceps must never be applied*.

Obstetric forcep deliveries are further divided according to whether they are *rotational* (sagittal suture is more than 45 degrees from the midline) or *nonrotational* (sagittal suture less than 45 degrees from the midline).

The indications for use of the obstetric forceps are as follows:

- Maternal exhaustion or inability to push (endotracheal intubation with sedation or paralysis; neuromuscular disease)
- Nonreassuring fetal heart tracing or "fetal distress"
- Maternal contraindications to pushing (cardiopulmonary disease, cerebrovascular aneurysm)
- Aftercoming head in a vaginal breech delivery
- Facilitation of difficult extraction of the fetal vertex during cesarean delivery

### Forceps and Potential Neonatal Morbidity

As stated previously, forceps were employed for hundreds of years without thought for fetal survival, being needed primarily to terminate difficult labors for maternal benefit. Today with the widespread availability of cesarean delivery, considerations turn to providing the best neonatal outcome possible. Thus, the difficult forceps deliveries of the past have been abandoned. Nevertheless, forceps still play a crucial role in modern obstetrics and, if judiciously used, can provide a safer alternative to cesarean delivery for both mother and baby.

The difficulty in interpreting the obstetric literature with regard to neonatal morbidity incurred by forceps use is that the classification for type of forceps was revised by ACOG in 1988, and thus, studies performed before then did not use the same clinical criteria employed today in modern practice to select appropriate candidates for the use of forceps. Furthermore, residency training in operative vaginal delivery has dramatically decreased over the past 30 years, potentially increasing fetal risk (Hankins and Rowe, 1996). Consequently, for proper interpretation of adverse outcomes, one must look to studies performed after the ACOG revised its classification.

The prevalence of forceps use varies widely by region and accounts for approximately 5% to 10% of all vaginal deliveries (Duchon et al, 1988). National statistics show that of the 3,063,870 deliveries in 1999, 3.2% were forceps-assisted and 6.2% were vacuum-assisted, for a total national operative vaginal delivery rate of 9.4% (NCHS, on line). Unfortunately, the national prevalence of low forceps, outlet forceps, and mid-forceps deliveries is not known, nor is the rate of use of rotational and nonrotational forceps. Neonatal outcome according to type of forceps application is also not generally known, and collection of data on this issue is hindered by the fact that even with the universal ACOG classification scheme, the determination of fetal station and type of forceps can be quite subjective as well as dependent on the experience and examining skill of the obstetrician. Moreover, the indication for forceps use varies widely by clinical situation, and the neonatal morbidity that can result from a "difficult pull" in a patient with a transverse arrest and marked fetal asynclitism may well be different from the quick delivery of a 2600-g fetus whose mother is unable to push, even if both are low-forceps deliveries.

Nevertheless, what large studies exist show that long-term or even short-term neonatal morbidity from outlet or low forceps delivery is uncommon. Towner and colleagues (1999) analyzed 583,340 live-born singleton infants of nulliparous women born between 1992 and 1994 and weighing between 2500 and 4000 g for neonatal intracranial injury according to mode of delivery. These investigators found that risks of subdural and intraventricular hemorrhage as well as nerve injury are higher with operative than with spontaneous vaginal delivery; however, the rates of morbidity from operative vaginal delivery were not different from those for cesarean delivery with labor (Towner et al, 1999). The rate of birth injury was lowest in patients with nonlabored cesarean delivery, a finding that illuminates an important fact that has heretofore not been clearly evaluated: It is the process of labor itself, and not necessarily the operative delivery, that can lead to adverse neonatal outcome. This provocative conclusion bears further investigation. Furthermore, the overall risk of intracranial injury was very low for all modalities, as listed in Table 15–2.

Few randomized prospective trials have specifically addressed the issue of neonatal morbidity arising from forceps operations, yet those that have been published suggest no significantly higher risk from operative vaginal delivery than from spontaneous birth. Yancey and colleagues (1991) randomly assigned 364 women giving birth at term whose deliveries were at +2 station to either elective outlet forceps delivery or unassisted birth. Women with suspected fetal macrosomia or chorioamnionitis were excluded from the study. Neonates were examined at birth and at 72 hours of age, and cranial ultrasonography was performed by neonatologists 24 to 72 hours after

**TABLE 15-2**

**Risk of Intracranial Injury According to Type of Delivery**

| Mode of Delivery | Incidence of Intracranial Injury |
|---|---|
| Vacuum | 1/860 |
| Forceps | 1/664 |
| Combined vacuum-forceps | 1/256 |
| Cesarean | |
| In labor | 1/907 |
| Without labor | 1/2750 |
| Spontaneous vaginal delivery | 1/1900 |

Adapted from Towner D, Castro MA, Eby-Wilkens E, Gilbert WM: Effect of mode of delivery in nulliparous women on intracranial injury. N Engl J Med 341: 1709-1714, 1999.

birth. The spontaneous and forceps-assisted births showed no statistically significant differences in the incidence of scalp abrasions, facial bruising, cephalhematoma, subconjunctival hemorrhage, or abnormal cranial ultrasonograms (Yancey et al, 1991).

Carmona and associates (1995) conducted a prospective, randomized, controlled trial to evaluate neonatal morbidity arising from low forceps procedures. They selected nulliparous women giving birth at 38 to 42 weeks gestation, excluding pregnancies with suspected fetal macrosomia or growth restriction, and randomly assigned them at 0 to +1 station to either a low forceps-assisted delivery or spontaneous birth once the fetal vertex had reached +2 station. These investigators found no clinically significant differences in Apgar scores, rates of admission to neonatal intensive care units (NICU), or umbilical artery pH between the groups (Carmona et al, 1995).

Several retrospective, population-based studies have further examined the issue of potential adverse neonatal sequelae arising from forceps procedures. Robertson and coworkers (1990) reclassified forceps operations in accordance with the 1988 revised ACOG guidelines and examined neonatal outcomes according to type of forceps operation, matching them to cesarean sections with a second stage of at least 30 minutes from a similar station. These researchers found that mid-forceps operations resulted in greater neonatal resuscitation requirements, lower umbilical artery pH, greater/higher "birth trauma," defined as nerve injuries or fractures, than cesarean section from comparable station. There was no greater risk of trauma from low forceps procedures compared with cesarean section, although the prevalence of arterial cord pH less than 7.10 was increased with forceps deliveries (Robertson et al, 1990). It must be remembered, however, that this study was not randomized as to treatment and that women undergoing abdominal delivery do not necessarily make an appropriate control group for operative vaginal delivery. Nevertheless, this large population-based study (from a database of 20,831) emphasizes the relative safety of outlet and low forceps procedures, casting some doubt on the safety of mid-forceps operations.

The role of mid-forceps delivery in modern obstetrics, specifically with regard to rotation greater than 45 degrees, has incited much controversy. The difficulty lies in the fact that no randomized trials comparing mid-forceps operations with other modes of delivery have been performed, and it is unlikely that any will be done in the near future because training in this type of delivery has declined among obstetric residents in the United States (Hale and Dennen, 2002; Laufe, 1992). Our evaluation of the potential neonatal morbidity arising from these procedures is mainly from retrospective, population-based studies, and we must interpret them with an appreciation for their inherent biases.

Hankins and associates (1999) reported a case-controlled study of 113 rotational forceps deliveries with rotation of 90 degrees or more matched to 167 controls with rotation of 45 degrees or less. They found no significant differences in major injuries, defined as skull fracture, brachial plexus, facial or sixth nerve palsy, and subdural hemorrhage. There were also no differences in the prevalence of cephalhematoma, clavicular fracture, or superficial laceration. All deliveries were performed with Kielland forceps by resident staff, with supervision by attending physicians as required. The prevalence of nerve injury in these forceps operations ranged from 2% to 3%; there were no skull fractures.

A retrospective study comparing 104 rotational deliveries with 163 low or outlet forceps deliveries found similar results, although a higher rate of NICU admissions (9.3% vs. 2.5%, respectively; $P = .015$) was seen in the rotation group (Feldman et al, 1999). Another study comparing 55 deliveries involving Kielland forceps rotations with 213 nonrotational forceps deliveries found no significant differences in neonatal morbidity between the groups, save for a 1-minute Apgar score in the Kielland focus group of less than 6 (Krivak et al, 1999).

In conclusion, the available literature supports the fact that neonatal morbidity from outlet or low forceps delivery is exceedingly low and is comparable with that of spontaneous vaginal delivery. This conclusion comes from both prospective data and large population-based investigations. The evidence concerning neonatal safety from more advanced forceps operations (mid-forceps and rotations) shows that morbidity is slightly increased with these procedures, although whether the increase arises from the operative vaginal delivery itself or from difficult labor is at present impossible to discern (Bashore et al, 1989; Dierker et al, 1985). The benefit of appropriately selected candidates for mid-forceps or rotational forceps delivery in well-trained hands, may be justifiable, although the numbers of residents in the United States who are adept at these procedures are steadily declining.

## Vacuum Delivery

Operative vaginal delivery for the indications listed previously can also be alternatively performed with the vacuum extractor. The situations that call for the use of this device and the requirements that must be fulfilled for its correct use are identical to those for obstetric forceps. The vacuum extractor usually has a metal or plastic cup (flexible or semirigid) that is applied to the fetal vertex. Care is taken in its application to ensure that an adequate seal has been created and that no maternal soft tissue is trapped between the suction device and the fetus. Traction is then applied to the fetal head in the line of the birth canal, in an effort to assist delivery. Also, rocking movements and torque should not be applied to the cup. Prematurity of the fetus is a relative contraindication to vacuum application. It is also generally advised that no more than two "pop-offs" (unintended release of the vacuum from the fetal head) occur before attempts at vacuum extraction are abandoned, although this recommendation stems from an era in which the metal cup, and not the softer polymeric silicone (Silastic) cups currently employed, were more widely used (Hankins et al, 1999).

In a laboratory experiment, Duchon and colleagues (1988) compared the maximum force at suggested vacuum pressures (550 to 600 mm Hg) prior with "pop-offs" for different types of vacuum devices. They found that the average force of traction exerted before "pop-offs" ranged from 18 to 20 kg. This finding is of interest when one considers the older report by Wylie (1935), who estimated the average tractive force required for delivery of 15.95 kg for a primigravida and 11.33 kg for a multiparous woman (Fig. 15–3).

The vacuum extractor is widely used in the United States but can still be associated with neonatal injury. In addition to superficial scalp lacerations or abrasions, which usually heal without incident, and local soft tissue swelling or bruising, use of the vacuum extractor has been associated with cephalhematoma and subgaleal hemorrhages.

*Cephalhematoma* results when the force created by the vacuum results in ruptures of *diploic or emissary vessels* between the periosteum and outer table of the skull. The potential space between the two fills with blood. Luckily, although cephalhematomas are often cosmetically alarming, they are limited to traveling along one cranial bone, because the firm periosteal attachments limit further extravasation of blood across suture lines. Thus, large amounts of blood cannot usually collect in this space, and serious neonatal compromise from this bleeding is rare. Bofill and associates (1997), in a randomized trial of continuous or intermittent vacuum application, examined factors associated with raising the risk of cephalhematoma. They found that only asynclitism and traction time were independently related to this complication. There was a clear relationship between longer time of vacuum application (up to 6 minutes) and cephalhematoma. Interestingly, these researchers did not find a significant independent association of neonatal injury with continuous or intermittent vacuum, nor with decreasing gestational age or increasing birth weight. Furthermore, the number of "pop-offs" was not correlated with cephalhematoma. These results were corroborated by Teng and Sayre (1997), who conducted a prospective observational study of 134 vacuum extractions and found that only increasing total duration of vacuum application was associated with neonatal injury (Fig. 15–4).

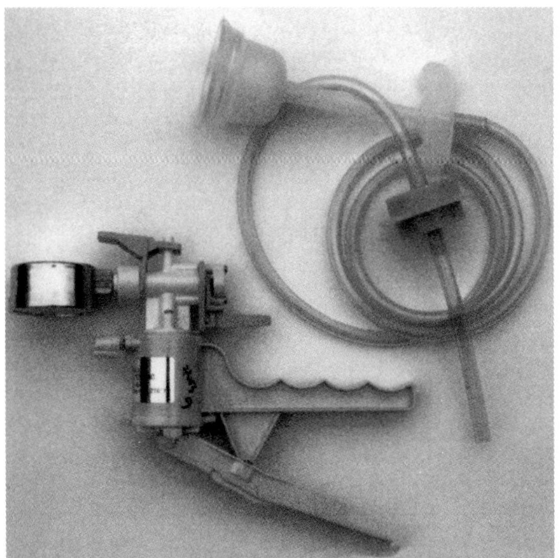

**FIGURE 15–3.** A soft-cup polymeric silicone (Silastic) vacuum extractor (MityVac device), along with a device used to generate negative pressure.

*Subgaleal hemorrhage* poses much more of a potential risk for the neonate. It occurs when emissary veins above the skull and periosteum rupture, and blood dissects through the loose tissue underlying the cranial aponeurosis, unimpeded by suture lines. A tremendous amount of blood, potentially the entire neonatal blood volume (approximately 250 mL), can fill this space; thus, this complication can significantly compromise the neonate (Plauche, 1980). Much of the literature about this unusual complication of vacuum extraction was published in the 1970s and early 1980s, with few later studies to detail associated risk factors. Plauche (1979), in his classic paper on vacuum extraction–related neonatal injury, identified only 18 cases of subgaleal hematomas among 14,276 cases of vacuum-assisted births, in contrast to a mean incidence of cephalhematoma of 6%. These morbidity estimates are derived from data that is nearly 30 to 40 years old; nevertheless, in a later investigation, Teng and colleagues (1997) noted an incidence of 8% for cephalhematoma and 0.7% for subgaleal hemorrhage, which agree well with Plauche's estimates.

Australian investigators evaluated 37 cases of subgaleal hemorrhage at a single tertiary care center accrued over a period of 23 years, with an estimated prevalence of 1.54 per 10,000 total births. They found that this complication occurred most often in primigravidas and that a large proportion of the cases (89.1% compared with 9.8% in the general control population) was associated with attempted vacuum extraction (Chadwick et al, 1996) (Fig. 15–5).

It must be kept in mind that the overall neonatal morbidity of the vacuum extractor is low, as ascertained from the large population-based study by Towner and coworkers (1999), which showed that the risk of intracranial injury is only 1 in 664. Yet as outlined previously, there are definite neonatal risks associated with the use of vacuum extraction. In 1998, the U.S. Food and Drug Administration (FDA) issued a statement warning obstetric care providers to use the vacuum device with caution and only for definite indications. This recommendation was made in response to the fact that from 1994 to 1998, there were 12 neonatal deaths and 9 serious injuries attributable to the vacuum, a five-fold increase in comparison with previous years. One must remember that during this period, the overall number of vacuum extractions in the United States nearly doubled, a development that could potentially account for the increase in adverse outcomes (NCHS, on line).

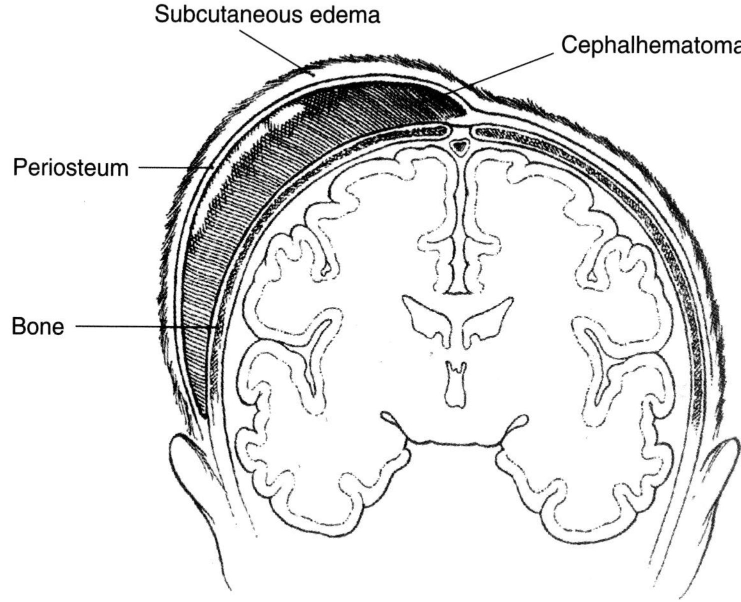


**FIGURE 15–4.** A cephalhematoma is a hemorrhage that occurs under the periosteum of the skull and is thus confined to a defined space with limited capacity for expansion. *(Adapted from Gilstrap LC, Cunningham FG, Hankins GDV, et al: Operative Obstetrics, 2nd ed. Appleton & Lange Publishers, 2002.)*

The FDA further suggested that infants delivered with the vacuum undergo close monitoring for subgaleal or subaponeurotic hematoma and that a high index of suspicion be maintained for this rare complication.

We emphasize here that the overall risk of adverse events attributable to the vacuum is extremely low, in that the FDA estimated only 5 serious complications per year of use during a time when 228,354 vacuum deliveries were performed. However, there is a definite possibility that sequelae related to vacuum extraction are often underreported.

The choice of instrument, forceps or vacuum, is usually determined by the skill level and experience of the obstetric care provider with the two methods. Several randomized trials have explored this issue (Bofill et al, 1996; Broekhuizen et al, 1987; Johanson, 1997; Williams et al, 1991). The Cochrane Library has pooled the results from 10 randomized trials comparing these two devices in terms of neonatal morbidity and successful vaginal delivery (Johanson and Menon, 2001). This analysis found that the vacuum was more likely to fail than the forceps (odds ratio [OR] 1.69; 95% confidence interval [CI] 1.31 to 2.19) and was associated with a greater likelihood of Apgar scores less than 7 at 5 minutes (OR 1.67; 95% CI .99 to 2.81), cephalhematoma (OR 2.38; 95% CI 1.68 to 3.37), and retinal hemorrhage (OR 1.99; 95% CI 1.35 to 2.98). However, the overall rate of serious complications was low, and there was no difference in long-term morbidity between the two devices.

The largest danger in the use of either vacuum or forceps comes from the combined use of the two instruments together. Towner and colleagues (1999) showed that the

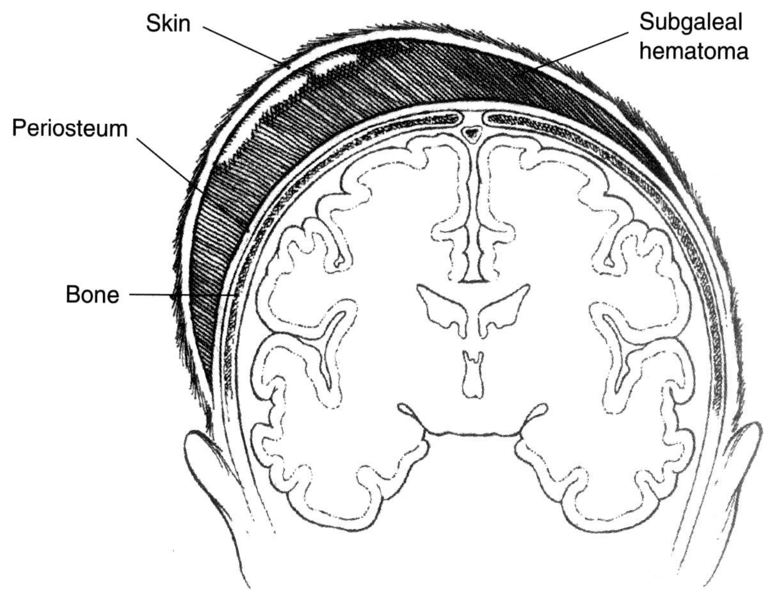


**FIGURE 15–5.** A subgaleal hematoma spreads along subcutaneous soft tissue planes and has no immediate barrier to expansion, creating the potential for significant neonatal hemodynamic compromise. *(Adapted from Gilstrap LC, Cunningham FG, Hankins GDV, et al: Operative Obstetrics, 2nd ed. Appleton & Lange Publishers, 2002.)*

use of one instrument after the other had failed carries a 1 in 256 risk of neonatal intracranial injury, significantly greater than that for either modality alone. This finding was further supported by the work of Gardella and associates (2001), who matched 11,223 women—one third of whom underwent combined forceps and vacuum instrumentation, one third vacuum alone, and one third forceps alone) to an equivalent number of women having spontaneous vaginal deliveries. These investigators found no statistically significant difference in risk of intracranial hemorrhage between use of either single instrument and vaginal delivery; however, use of both instruments markedly increased the risk not only of intracranial hemorrhage but also of seizures and low 5-minute Apgar scores (Gardella et al, 2001). The overall risk of nerve injury and scalp injury was greater for single-instrument delivery than for spontaneous delivery, but the overall incidence of each complication is rare.

Thus, the vacuum extractor is an acceptable instrument if used judiciously and in the proper circumstances, carrying an overall minimal risk of serious neonatal complications. Its safety is comparable with that of the obstetric forceps, although the vacuum extractor is associated with a higher incidence of cephalhematoma and a lower potential for facial nerve injury. The chance of failure is greater with the vacuum, which could then potentially tempt the care provider to employ the forceps. *The use of forceps or vacuum extractor after the other instrument has failed carries a higher risk of adverse outcomes and should be undertaken only with an understanding of this higher likelihood of neonatal morbidity.*

## SHOULDER DYSTOCIA

Shoulder dystocia is arguably the most dreaded complication in obstetrics. The problem it poses is that although much anticipated, shoulder dystocia is quite unpredictable and can appear despite the most cautious measures taken to prevent its occurrence. *Shoulder dystocia* is defined as the delivery of the fetal head with an impaction of the fetal shoulder girdle or trunk against the pubic symphysis, making subsequent delivery of the body either difficult or impossible without the performance of auxiliary delivery maneuvers.

Once shoulder dystocia occurs, a series of maneuvers (which, because of the sporadic and unpredictable nature of this complication, has never been tested in a prospective fashion) is employed to resolve it. The first step is the *McRoberts maneuver*, which consists of hyperflexing the maternal thighs onto the abdomen in hopes of increasing the anteroposterior dimensions of the pelvis to facilitate delivery. If unsuccessful, this step is usually followed by *suprapubic pressure* to disimpact the anterior shoulder from behind the pubic symphysis. The *Woods screw maneuver* or the Rubin rotational maneuver may also be used to attempt to rotate the infant's shoulders and thereby relieve the impaction of the shoulder against the pubic bone. If these measures fail, *delivery of the posterior arm* can be attempted: The operator inserts a hand in the vagina, grasps the posterior fetal arm, and extracts the arm across the fetal chest and through the vaginal introitus. It is often necessary to perform an episiotomy to have sufficient room in the vagina to accomplish this maneuver. If the dystocia continues, the *Zavanelli maneuver* or *cephalic replacement* is performed. After the fetal head is rotated from occiput transverse to occiput anterior, it is flexed and pushed back in the birth canal, and the child is delivered by emergency cesarean section. The McRoberts maneuver or suprapubic pressure will relieve more than 50% of shoulder dystocias. Cephalic replacement should be necessary in less than 5% of cases.

The prevalence of shoulder dystocia varies according to the population studied and to the presence of various risk factors known to predispose women to this obstetric emergency. Estimates range from 0.2% to 1% in a low-risk population to 20% in higher-risk groups (ACOG, 1997, 2000b; Gross et al, 1987; Lipscomb et al, 1995; Nesbitt et al, 1998). Maternal obesity, fetal macrosomia, history of shoulder dystocia in previous birth, and maternal diabetes mellitus are the most common associated variables, but they are not of sufficient prognostic power to be clinically useful in predicting shoulder dystocia (ACOG, 1997, 2000b; Nesbitt et al, 1998).

Because shoulder dystocia has the potential to cause significant neonatal morbidity and mortality, efforts have been made to predict its occurrence; unfortunately, no clinical guidelines have been clinically tested or proven. Ultrasonography is commonly used in patients with suspected fetal macrosomia or maternal diabetes mellitus to detect high-birth-weight infants who might be more likely to experience shoulder dystocia. Third-trimester ultrasonographic examination has an accuracy of 10% to 15% in the prediction of fetal weight and is thus not completely reliable (Delpapa and Mueller-Huebach, 1991; Gross et al, 1987; Rouse et al, 1996). In addition, even if ultrasonography was completely reliable, what fetal weight cutoff would prompt an elective cesarean section in an effort to avoid shoulder dystocia? These questions have been the subject of much debate in the obstetric literature.

Lipscomb and associates (1995), evaluating the deliveries of 227 mother-infant pairs at their institution with birth weights greater than 4500 g, found a shoulder dystocia rate of 18.5%; thus, the majority of women delivering vaginally did so without any adverse event. Of the infants who experienced shoulder dystocia, 51.7% suffered a neurologic injury, but at 2 months, all of the affected infants had normal neurologic findings. Thus, even the occurrence of shoulder dystocia does not necessarily guarantee permanent neurologic morbidity.

This conclusion has been reinforced by several other studies. Gherman and coworkers (1998) reviewed 285 cases of shoulder dystocia. They found that 77 of the infants (24.9%) suffered fetal injury, most commonly brachial plexus injury (16.8%) or fracture of the clavicula (9.5%) or humerus (4.2%). Nearly half of the shoulder dystocias resolved with the McRoberts maneuver alone; the rest required the Woods maneuver, posterior arm extraction, or the Zavanelli maneuver. The requirement of additional fetal manipulative procedures raised the risk of humeral fracture only and not of clavicular fracture or brachial plexus injury. As with previous studies, the incidence of permanent musculoskeletal injury was only 1.4% (Gherman et al, 1998).

A prospective investigation evaluated the natural history of recovery after a birth-related brachial plexus injury in infants referred to a tertiary care multidisciplinary neurologic center. Enrollment required identification of injury in the newborn period, initial evaluation at the center between 1 and 2 months of age, and persistence of lack of antigravity movement in the shoulder or elbow until 2 weeks of age. Even in this group of children subject to ascertainment bias (because injuries that resolved before 2 weeks of age would not have been included in the results), complete neurologic recovery was documented in 66%, and only 14% had persistent, severe weakness (Noetzel et al, 2001).

Rouse and colleagues (1996) performed a decision analysis showing that if one chose to perform an elective cesarean section for all nondiabetic women with ultrasonographically predicted macrosomia (estimated fetal weight >4000 g), 2345 cesarean sections would have to be performed to prevent one permanent brachial plexus injury. Even in the diabetic mother, if one chose a cutoff of 4500 g, 443 cesareans would be needed to prevent one permanent injury. The conclusions from this decision analysis have been borne out by several other investigators, who have established that the risk of nerve injury certainly increases with rising birth weight but that the large number of macrosomic infants who undergo normal, spontaneous vaginal delivery without sequelae does not justify a policy of elective cesarean delivery for macrosomia alone, especially in a nondiabetic population (Ecker et al, 1997; Gilbert et al, 1999; Gordon et al, 1973; Gregory et al, 1998; McFarland et al, 1986; Ouzounian et al, 1998; Roberts et al, 1995).

Therefore there is at present no universally accepted method to prevent shoulder dystocia. Studies have shown that operative vaginal delivery of a fetus suspected to have macrosomia on either clinical or ultrasonographic grounds could increase the risk of shoulder dystocia (Benedetti et al, 1978). It seems wise to avoid difficult forceps or vacuum delivery in a patient who is thought to have an infant larger than 4000 g, especially if she has diabetes or a history of shoulder dystocia. In addition, the ACOG (ACOG Bulletin, Shoulder Dystocia, 1997; ACOG Bulletin, Fetal Macrosomia, 2000a) states that "for pregnant women with diabetes who are suspected of carrying macrosomic fetuses, a planned cesarean delivery may be a reasonable course of action, depending on the incidence of shoulder dystocia, the accuracy of predicting macrosomia, and the cesarean delivery rate within a specific population."

## VAGINAL BREECH DELIVERY

Three percent to 4% of all full-term infants are in breech presentation at the time of delivery. There are three main types of breech presentations. In the *footling breech*, either one (single footling) or both (double footling) lower extremities are presenting. In the *frank breech*, both thighs are flexed but the legs are extended. An infant in *complete breech* has both thighs and legs flexed. Because the vaginal delivery of a singleton footling breech carries attendant risks of cord prolapse and head entrapment, the consensus among obstetricians is that the infant with this presentation should be delivered operatively (unless the fetus is a second twin, as discussed later). The baby in frank breech with buttocks presenting has a lower risk of these adverse events and thus could potentially be delivered vaginally. The complete breech presentation converts to frank or footling breech during labor, and the appropriate management scheme for delivery depends on which leading fetal part descends.

The feasibility of vaginal breech delivery and its safety have been the subject of much debate throughout the past half-century. With the advent of safe, expedient cesarean delivery in the United States, many obstetricians have favored the operative approach as the method of choice for management of the breech presentation at term. The literature to support this point of view has produced conflicting conclusions, and its interpretation is consequently quite difficult. The delivery of the vaginal breech is also an emotional issue; physicians trained in the art of the vaginal breech delivery maintain that for an appropriately selected candidate, vaginal breech delivery has acceptable neonatal risk as well as the advantage of sparing the mother significant operative morbidity. Proponents of cesarean delivery further state that the level of resident training in the art of the singleton vaginal breech delivery has markedly diminished, with most graduating senior residents having performed only a few such deliveries.

There has been an extensive body of literature over the previous half-century examining this issue. Unfortunately, only two randomized trials have explored the question of which delivery route is best for the term singleton frank breech fetus, but there are several large retrospective series describing neonatal outcomes with the vaginal approach, most of which suggest that vaginal delivery in carefully selected patients carries a low risk of long-term neonatal morbidity and mortality. Diro and colleagues (1999) evaluated 1021 term singleton breech deliveries occurring at their institution over a 4-year period. Women with clinically adequate pelvic dimensions and frank breech presentation whose infants weighed less than 3750 g were allowed a trial of labor. These researchers found an overall cesarean delivery rate of 85.6%; however, for women allowed to deliver vaginally, the "success" rate, defined as vaginal delivery, was 50% (19/38 patients) for nulliparous women and 75.8% (116/153 patients) for multiparous women. The need for admission to the NICU was higher for the group delivered vaginally (17.4% vs. 12.1%; $P = .036$), but major morbidities between operative and vaginal deliveries were not significantly different. Long-term outcome was not evaluated. It is notable that evaluation of the pelvic dimensions of the women in this cohort was clinical rather than radiographic or by computed tomography (CT) pelvimetry, as has been done in other studies.

Norwegian investigators examined their similar policy of vaginal breech delivery and evaluated maternal and neonatal outcomes in a large cohort of women (Albrechtsen et al, 1997). Patients were allowed a trial of vaginal delivery if radiographic pelvimetry showed adequate pelvic dimensions and were excluded for an estimated fetal weight greater than 4500 g or a footling presentation. Each vaginal breech birth was matched to a term vaginal vertex birth; each cesarean birth was matched to the appropriate vertex control. The researchers evaluated 1212 breech deliveries, 639 (52.7%) of which were vaginal, 172 (11.4%) intrapartum cesarean section, and 138 (11.4%) planned cesarean section. Once major or lethal anomalies and fetal disorders not related to delivery were excluded from the data, no perinatal deaths were attributable to mode of delivery. When births planned vaginally were compared with operative deliveries, there was a higher risk of 1-minute Apgar score of less than 7 and "traumatic morbidity" in the vaginal group but no significant differences in the rates of NICU admissions, 5-minute Apgar scores, or "uneventful course." The researchers concluded that short-term morbidity was worse in the group delivered vaginally but long-term outcomes were similar in the groups. It must be remembered, however, that this study was not randomized, and the infants selected for vaginal delivery or cesarean section were intrinsically different. Also, all deliveries occurred in a tertiary care institution.

The truly interesting point raised by these investigators is that aside from the issue of cesarean delivery versus a trial of labor, singleton breech infants regardless of mode of delivery have a higher risk of morbidity than their vertex counterparts. Breech infants had higher incidences of NICU admissions, "eventful courses," hip dislocation, and traumatic morbidity (soft tissue trauma, fracture, facial nerve paralysis, and brachial plexus palsy). Thus, both the obstetrician and the pediatrician must be aware of these potential factors at the birth of a breech infant.

Christian and associates (1990) evaluated their policy of offering a trial of vaginal breech delivery to women in whom estimated fetal weight was between 2000 and 4000 g and CT pelvimetry documented adequate pelvic dimensions. Of 122 women evaluated, 85 were judged appropriate by these standards for vaginal delivery, of whom 81.2% had a successful vaginal delivery. The only indices of neonatal outcome evaluated were the Apgar score, which was not different between groups; and neonatal cord pH, which was lower in a statistically but not clinically significant manner in the vaginal delivery group.

The greatest difficulty in interpreting the large number of retrospective studies examining the issue of vaginal breech delivery in the obstetric literature is that even the best-designed reports have relatively small numbers of patients, and the possibility of a type II or beta error is quite high; in addition, the groups being compared (those undergoing planned cesarean section and vaginal deliveries) are different because the patients are not randomly assigned to the two treatments (Christian et al, 1990; Westgren et al, 1985). Often the women chosen to undergo cesarean section tend to have factors that would place their neonates at higher risk than those of women allowed a trial of labor. A meta-analysis evaluating seven cohort studies and two randomized trials compared 1825 patients given trials of labor with 1231 patients undergoing elective cesarean section and found a statistically significant (but clinically questionable) higher risk with vaginal breech delivery of 1.10% (Gifford et al, 1995).

This controversy has been clarified by a large, multicentered, multinational trial that randomly assigned 2088 women at 121 centers in 26 countries to either planned vaginal birth or planned elective cesarean section (Hannah et al, 2000). Criteria for enrollment were frank or complete term singleton breech with no evidence of fetal macrosomia. The investigation was halted when preliminary results showed that there was significantly higher neonatal mortality and severe morbidity in the vaginal breech arm than in the cesarean arm of the study (5.0% vs. 1.6%, respectively). This conclusion was not altered by experience of the delivering obstetrician or maternal demographic factors such as parity and race. Maternal morbidities of the two groups were comparable. The difference in outcome for vaginal breech versus cesarean section was even more striking in countries with low national perinatal mortality rates, such as the United States (5.7% vs. 0.4%).

Criticisms of this study include the fact that patients enrolled did not undergo CT pelvimetry, which in some institutions is standard practice before a vaginal breech delivery is considered. Furthermore, intermittent fetal auscultation every 15 minutes was performed rather than continuous fetal monitoring. In addition, the capabilities of various centers to perform emergency cesarean section differ markedly, with potential effects on neonatal morbidity and mortality rates. Nevertheless, it is unlikely that another large study will ever be performed to examine this issue, and the ultimate results are difficult to dispute given the excellent study design and adequate sample size. Indeed, the ACOG (2001) has issued a statement that "planned vaginal delivery of a term singleton breech may no longer be appropriate . . . . Patients with a persistent breech presentation at term in a singleton gestation should undergo a planned cesarean delivery." As is discussed further, this statement does not apply to the vaginal delivery of a nonvertex second twin.

## MULTIPLE-FETUS DELIVERY

With the advent of in vitro fertilization (IVF) and the sophisticated assisted reproductive technologies and techniques (ARTs), the incidence of multiple-fetus pregnancies is steadily rising, in particular higher-order multiples. The mode of delivery for twins is well delineated by several studies, and the issues surrounding the choice of vaginal birth versus cesarean is outlined here.

### Twin Delivery

#### Vertex-Vertex Twins

It is almost universally accepted that the appropriate method of delivery if both twins are vertex is vaginal. The first infant is delivered like a singleton infant. The second infant is delivered in a similar fashion, but care must be taken not to rupture membranes before the head is well engaged, so as not to increase the risk of cord accident. It is notable that the delivery of the second twin does not necessarily occur immediately after the first.

#### Vertex-Nonvertex Twins

The first twin of a vertex-nonvertex pair is usually delivered vaginally. The options for delivery of the second twin are cesarean section, breech extraction, or attempts at external cephalic version and, if they are successful, vertex delivery. The optimal delivery choice for the second twin has been a subject of much controversy. Many obstetricians claim that cesarean section is the safest approach to the nonvertex twin, whereas others claim that vaginal delivery affords equivalent neonatal outcome while sparing the mother an unnecessary surgical procedure. Fortunately, there is a large body of evidence in the literature addressing these issues.

If the vaginal approach is chosen for the second, nonvertex twin, the obstetrician inserts a hand into the uterine cavity and, under ultrasonographic guidance if necessary, finds the feet of the second twin. Once the feet are firmly grasped, they are brought down into the vagina, and the membranes are ruptured. Traction is applied to the fetus along the pelvic curve; once the body has been delivered through the introitus, delivery of the arms, shoulders, and aftercoming head proceeds in a fashion similar to that of a singleton breech delivery (see earlier discussion).

Several large cohort studies have examined the issue of the feasibility and safety of total breech extraction of the nonvertex second twin. These have almost unanimously come to the conclusion that the neonatal outcome for nonvertex second twins delivered vaginally not only is similar to that for the vertex first twin but also is not statistically different from that of second twins delivered by cesarean section, regardless of birth weight or gestational age (Adam et al, 1991; Berglund and Axelsson, 1989; Chervenak et al, 1985; Davison et al, 1992; Fishman et al, 1989; Gocke et al, 1989; Winn et al, 2001).

Although several retrospective studies have evaluated the outcomes of vaginally born nonvertex second twins, there is only one randomized trial. Rabinovici and colleagues (1987) allocated 60 women with vertex-nonvertex twins to either operative or vaginal delivery. Maternal morbidity and hospital stay were higher in the surgical group, but there were no differences in neonatal outcome.

Thus, the available body of evidence supports attempts at vaginal delivery of the nonvertex second twin. Of course, the responsible obstetrician must choose a management plan most compatible with his or her experience and training, and for an obstetricians not versed in techniques of successful vaginal breech extraction, cesarean delivery might be a more prudent plan.

The third option for a nonvertex twin is *external cephalic version* (attempting to turn a nonvertex fetus to vertex by abdominal manipulation). Studies have shown that this option is associated with a higher failure rate for vaginal delivery and with other complications (such as cord accidents and malpresentations unamenable to vaginal delivery) compared with primary breech extraction and cesarean section (Chauhan et al, 1995; Gocke et al, 1989).

### Nonvertex-Nonvertex Twins

Due to the theoretic risk of "interlocking twins" as well as data showing greater morbidity for the singleton vaginal breech (see preceding discussion), cesarean section is the recommended choice for delivery of this presentation.

### Monochorionic, Monoamniotic Twins

Monochorionic, monoamniotic twins share a single intra-amniotic space and thus have a higher risk of cord and extremity entanglement during the course of delivery. It is thus commonly accepted that the optimal mode of delivery is a planned cesarean section before labor ensues.

### Higher-Order Multiple Gestations

Most perinatologists suggest cesarean section for triplets and higher-order multiple gestations (ACOG, 1998). Although this is a common practice, data mandating operative delivery are far from conclusive. At present, quadruplets and higher-order multiples are usually delivered by cesarean section.

## VAGINAL BIRTH AFTER CESAREAN: NEONATAL ISSUES

Cesarean section accounts nationally for one quarter of all deliveries (NCHS, on line). Surgery, of course, carries maternal risks for increased blood loss, prolonged hospital stay, and longer recovery period compared with vaginal delivery. Thus, in the 1980s and 1990s, efforts were made to encourage women to attempt vaginal birth after a previous cesarean (VBAC), success rates for which vary from 60% to 80%, depending on the indications for the previous cesarean (ACOG, 1999). Unfortunately, VBAC can result in uterine dehiscence, in which the scar from the cesarean separates asymptomatically, or, more seriously, uterine rupture. A full discussion of VBAC, studies supporting its safety, and controversies surrounding its feasibility are beyond the scope of this chapter; the interested reader is urged to consult an obstetric textbook for further details. We instead focus on neonatal risks of VBAC, particularly from its most dreaded complication, uterine rupture.

Studies have uniformly shown a risk of uterine rupture with VBAC on the order of 0.5% to 1% (ACOG, 1999; Lydon-Rochelle et al, 2001). In a large, retrospective study, Lydon-Rochelle and colleagues (2001) evaluated 20,095 women with a history of previous cesarean section and found that rupture risk was 0.16% if the woman elected a second operative delivery; 0.52% if VBAC occurred as a result of spontaneous labor, 0.77% if labor was induced without prostaglandins, and 2.5% if labor was induced with prostaglandins. Thus, VBAC carries the lowest risk if labor is spontaneous and non-augmented.

There are few large, well-designed studies specifically evaluating neonatal rather than maternal outcomes in VBAC. Socol and Peaceman (1999) compared 1677 successful with 920 unsuccessful VBACs, and further compared these neonatal outcomes with those in 22,863 spontaneous vaginal births without a history of prior cesarean section as well as in 2432 patients undergoing primary cesarean section during labor. These researchers found that neonates born of successful VBAC had a higher likelihood of a 5-minute Apgar score of less than 7 (but not less than 4), and an umbilical artery pH of less than 7.10 (but not less than 7.00) compared with those from spontaneous vaginal births. However, long-term outcome was not evaluated in this study, and the generally good outcome of all infants with a cord blood pH higher than 7.00 does not necessarily support a clinically significant greater neonatal risk with VBAC (Socol and Peaceman, 1999).

Yap and associates (2001) retrospectively evaluated 38,027 deliveries occurring at a single tertiary care institution and found 21 cases of uterine rupture; 17 had occurred in women with prior cesarean deliveries. Two neonatal deaths occurred, one the result of prematurity (23-week fetus) and the other of multiple congenital anomalies; all live-born infants were discharged from the hospital without neurologic sequelae. Thus, the ultimate neonatal outcome despite uterine rupture was favorable. However, all deliveries occurred in a tertiary care institution with rapidly available obstetric anesthesiologists, neonatologists, and obstetricians. Most deliveries after diagnosis of rupture occurred within 26 minutes.

A second group of investigators retrospectively identified 99 cases of uterine rupture occurring during a period in which 159,456 births occurred (Leung et al, 1993). Thirteen of the ruptures occurred before the onset of labor. There were six neonatal deaths, but four of them occurred in women who presented at admission with uterine rupture (and thus were never given a "trial of labor"). There were five cases of perinatal asphyxia; however, the study does not mention whether they occurred in women allowed a trial of labor or in women with uterine rupture on presentation to the hospital. Moreover, many of these women had an undocumented prior scar, which in some institutions would warrant an elective repeat cesarean section. The study by Lydon-Rochelle and colleagues (2001) evaluating 20,095 women with previous cesarean delivery and the subsequent risk of rupture found a neonatal mortality of 5.5%. However, this population-based study did not specify whether these deliveries occurred in tertiary care institutions with the capability of performing emergency operative rescue procedures in the event of uterine rupture. Thus, the true neonatal risk of VBAC, especially in the event of uterine rupture, cannot be precisely estimated at present. There are no studies adequately evaluating long-term outcomes of infants surviving after uterine rupture.

In conclusion, it appears that the risk of uterine rupture after a previous cesarean is low but rises when labor is augmented with oxytocin or prostaglandins. It is appropriate to offer women VBAC but they must carefully be counseled about the potential risk of uterine rupture. Moreover, VBAC should ideally occur in a tertiary care institution or in facilities capable of rapidly performing an emergency cesarean section, to improve the likelihood of minimizing adverse neonatal sequelae.

## CORD ACCIDENTS

*Cord accident* usually refers to adverse events affecting the fetus that occur as a result of some problem with the umbilical cord. This heterogeneous term encompasses umbilical cord prolapse, in which the cord delivers through the cervix and compression of the cord by a fetal part results in a significantly higher risk of asphyxia. It also includes such entities as cord entanglements and "true knots," which can lead to fetal compromise as well.

The incidence of such an event is not clearly known, as the diagnosis is often one of exclusion. One large population-based study compared 709 cases of cord prolapse occurring in 313,000 deliveries with matched controls and found that low birth weight, male sex, multiple gestation, breech presentation, and congenital anomalies all increased the risk of umbilical cord prolapse (Critchlow et al, 1994). Not surprisingly, cord prolapse was associated with a high mortality rate (10%), which was reduced if cesarean rather than vaginal delivery was performed.

The standard of care in cases of cord prolapse is to proceed immediately with cesarean section while an assistant elevates the presenting fetal part with a hand in the vagina to prevent compression of the umbilical cord. It is also of paramount importance to have appropriate pediatric support available at the time of delivery, because the newborn is likely to be depressed and to require resuscitation.

Cord accident or in utero compromise secondary to entanglement of the umbilical cord as a clinical entity is difficult to understand. Often in cases of in utero fetal demise (IUFD), a diagnosis or cause of fetal death is never found. It is tempting to attribute the demise to the occurrence of some event that compromises umbilical blood flow to the developing pregnancy. The literature on this subject is quite scarce. Hershkovitz and colleagues (2001) identified 841 cases of true knots from a population of 69,139 deliveries (for a prevalence of 1.2%) and, in a case-controlled study, found that grand multiparity (>10 deliveries), maternal chronic hypertension, history of genetic amniocentesis, male gender of the fetus, and umbilical cord prolapse were all independently associated with true knots of the umbilical cord. The presence of a true knot was associated with both IUFD and greater likelihood of cesarean delivery (Hershkovitz et al, 2001) (Fig. 15–6).

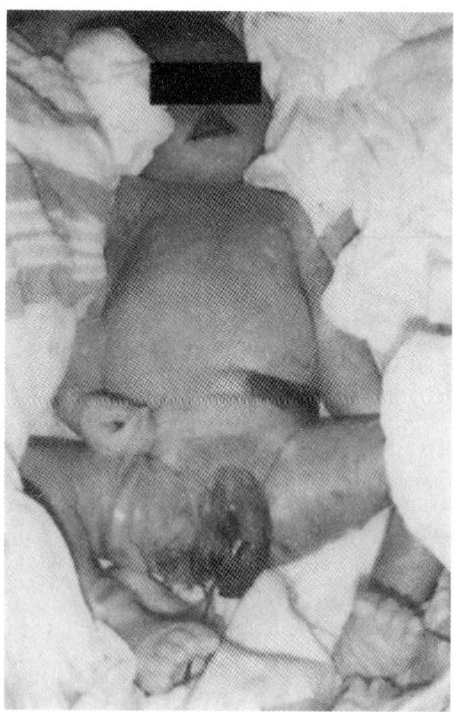

**FIGURE 15–6.** (See also Color Plate 15–6.) A 28-year-old woman presented to the labor and delivery department with an intrauterine demise. Examination of the fetus shows the cord wrapped tightly around the torso, leg, and ankle, suggesting cord accident as a cause of death. No other pathologic abnormalities were found on autopsy. *(Photo courtesy of Thomas R. Easterling, MD.)*

## REFERENCES


American College of Obstetricians and Gynecologists: Shoulder Dystocia. (ACOG Practice Patterns No. 7.) Washington, DC, ACOG, October 1997.

American College of Obstetricians and Gynecologists: Special Problems of Multiple Gestation. (ACOG Educational Bulletin # 253.) Washington, ACOG, November 1998.

American College of Obstetricians and Gynecologists: Vaginal Birth After Previous Cesarean Delivery. (ACOG Practice Bulletin No. 5.) Washington, DC, ACOG, July 1999.

American College of Obstetricians and Gynecologists: Operative Vaginal Delivery. (ACOG Practice Bulletin No. 17.) Washington, DC, ACOG, June 2000a.

American College of Obstetricians and Gynecologists: Fetal Macrosomia. (ACOG Practice Bulletin No. 22.) Washington, DC, ACOG, November 2000b.

American College of Obstetricians and Gynecologists: Mode of Term Singleton Breech Delivery. (ACOG Committee Opinion # 265.) Washington, DC, ACOG, December 2001.

Adam C, Allen AC, Baskett TF: Twin delivery: Influence of the presentation and method of delivery on the second twin. Am J Obstet Gynecol 165:23-27, 1991.

Albrechtsen S, Rasmussen S, Reigstad H, et al: Evaluation of a protocol for selecting fetuses in breech presentation for vaginal delivery or cesarean section. Am J Obstet Gynecol 177:586-592, 1997.

Bashore RA, Phillips WH, Brinkman CH: A comparison of the morbidity of midforceps and cesarean delivery. Am J Obstet Gynecol 162:1428-1433, 1989.

Benedetti TJ, Gabbe SG: Shoulder dystocia: A complication of fetal macrosomia and prolonged second stage of labor with midpelvic delivery. Obstet Gynecol 52:526, 1978.

Berglund L, Axelsson O: Breech extraction versus cesarean section for the remaining second twin. Acta Obstet Gynecol Scand 68:435-438, 1989.

Bofill JA, Rust OA, Devidas M, et al: Neonatal cephalohematoma from vacuum extraction. J Reprod Med 42:565-569, 1997.

Bofill JA, Rust OA, Schorr SJ, et al: A randomized trial of the obstetric forceps versus the M-cup vacuum extractor. Am J Obstet Gynecol 175:1325-1330, 1996.

Broekhuizen FF, Washington JM, Johnson F, Hamilton PR: Vacuum extraction versus forceps delivery: Indications and complications, 1979 to 1984. Obstet Gynecol 69:338-342, 1987.

Carmona F, Martinez-Roman S, Manau D, et al: Immediate maternal and neonatal effects of low-forceps delivery according to the new criteria of the American College of Obstetricians and Gynecologists compared with spontaneous vaginal delivery in term pregnancies. Am J Obstet Gynecol 173:55-59, 1995.

Chadwick LM, Pemberton PJ, Kurinczuk JJ: Neonatal subgaleal haematoma: Associated risk factors, complications and outcome. J Paediatr Child Health 32:228-232, 1996.

Chauhan SP, Roberts WE, McLaren RA, et al: Delivery of the nonvertex second twin: Breech extraction versus external cephalic version. Am J Obstet Gynecol 173:1015-1020, 1995.

Chervenak FA, Johnson RE, Youcha S, et al: Intrapartum management of twin gestation. Obstet Gynecol 65:119-124, 1985.

Christian SS, Brady K, Read JA, Kopelman JN: Vaginal breech delivery: A five-year prospective evaluation of a protocol using computed tomographic pelvimetry. Am J Obstet Gynecol 163:848-855, 1990.

Collea JV, Chien C, Quilligan EJ: The randomized management of term frank breech presentation: A study of 208 cases. Am J Obstet Gynecol 137:235-244, 1980.

Critchlow CW, Leet TL, Benedetti TJ, Daling JR: Risk factors and infant outcomes associated with umbilical cord prolapse: A population-based case-control study among births in Washington State. Am J Obstet Gynecol 170:613-618, 1994.

Davison L, Easterling TR, Jackson JC, Benedetti JC: Breech extraction of low-birth-weight second twins: Can cesarean section be justified? Am J Obstet Gynecol 166:497-502, 1992.

Delpapa EH, Mueller-Huebach E: Pregnancy outcome following ultrasound diagnosis of macrosomia. Obstet Gynecol 78:340-343, 1991.

Dierker LJ, Rosen MG, Thompson K, et al: The midforceps: Maternal and neonatal outcomes. Am J Obstet Gynecol 152:176-183, 1985.

Diro M, Puangsricharen A, Royer L, et al: Singleton term breech deliveries in nulliparous and multiparous women: A 5-year experience at the University of Miami/Jackson Memorial Hospital. Am J Obstet Gynecol 181:247-252, 1999.

Dommergues M, Mahieu-Caputo D, Madelbrot L, et al: Delivery of uncomplicated triplet pregnancies: Is the vaginal route safer? A case-control study. Am J Obstet Gynecol 172:513-517, 1995.

Duchon MA, DeMund MA, Brown RH: Laboratory comparison of modern vacuum extractors. Obstet Gynecol 71:155-158, 1988.

Ecker JL, Greenberg JA, Norwitz ER, et al: Birth weight as a predictor of brachial plexus injury. Obstet Gynecol 89:643-647, 1997.

Feldman DM, Borgida AF, Sauer F, Rodis J: Rotational versus nonrotational forceps: Maternal and neonatal outcomes. Am J Obstet Gynecol 181:1185-1187, 1999.

Fishman A, Grubb DK, Kovacs BW: Vaginal delivery of the nonvertex second twin. Am J Obstet Gynecol 161:861-864, 1989.

Gardella C, Taylor M, Benedetti T, et al: The effect of sequential use of vacuum and forceps for assisted vaginal delivery on neonatal and maternal outcomes. Am J Obstet Gynecol 185:896-902, 2001.

Gherman RB, Ousounian JG, Goodwin TM: Obstetric maneuvers for shoulder dystocia and associated fetal morbidity. Am J Obstet Gynecol 178:1126-1130, 1998.

Gifford DS, Morton SC, Fiske M, Kahn K: A meta-analysis of infant outcomes after breech delivery. Obstet Gynecol 85:1047-1054, 1995.

Gilbert WM, Nesbitt TS, Danielson B: Associated factors in 1611 cases of brachial plexus injury. Obstet Gynecol 93:536-540, 1999.

Gocke SE, Nageotte MP, Garite T, et al: Management of the nonvertex second twin: Primary cesarean section, external version, or primary breech extraction. Am J Obstet Gynecol 161:111-114, 1989.

Gordon M, Rich H, Deutschberger J, Green M: The immediate and long-term outcome of obstetric birth trauma. I: Brachial plexus paralysis. Am J Obstet Gynecol 117:51-56, 1973.

Gregory KD, Henry OA, Ramicone E, et al: Maternal and infant complications in high and normal weight infants by method of delivery. Obstet Gynecol 92:507-513, 1998.

Grobman WA, Peaceman AM, Haney EI, et al: Neonatal outcomes in triplet gestations after a trial of labor. Am J Obstet Gynecol 179:942-945, 1998.

Gross SJ, Shime J, Farine D: Shoulder dystocia: Predictors and outcome, a five-year review. Am J Obstet Gynecol 156:334-336, 1987.

Hale RW, Dennen EH: Dennen's Forceps Deliveries. 4th ed. American College of Obstetrics & Gynecology, 2002.

Hankins GDV, Rowe TF: Operative vaginal delivery—year 2000. Am J Obstet Gynecol 175:275-282, 1996.

Hankins GDV, Leicht T, Van Hook J, Uckan EM: The role of forceps rotation in maternal and neonatal injury. Am J Obstet Gynecol 180:231-234, 1999.

Hannah ME, Hannah WJ, Hewson SA, et al: Planned cesarean section versus planned vaginal birth for breech presentation at term: A randomized multicentre trial. Lancet 356:1375-1383, 2000.

Hershkovitz R, Silberstein T, Sheiner E, et al: Risk factors associated with true knots of the umbilical cord. Eur J Obstet Gynecol 98:36-39, 2001.

Johanson R: Choice of instrument for vaginal delivery. Curr Opin Obstet Gynecol 9:361-365, 1997.

Johanson RB, Menon BKV: Vacuum extraction versus forceps for assisted vaginal delivery (Cochrane Review). In: The Cochrane Library, Issue 4, 2001. Oxford, Update Software.

Krivak TC, Drewes P, Horowitz GM: Kielland v nonrotational forceps for the second stage of labor. J Reprod Med 44:511-517, 1999.

Laufe LE, Berkus MD: Assisted Vaginal Delivery: Obstetric Forceps and Vacuum Extraction Techniques. McGraw-Hill, 1992.

Leung AS, Leung EK, Paul RH: Uterine rupture after previous cesarean delivery: Maternal and fetal consequences. Am J Obstet Gynecol 169:945-950, 1993.

Lipscomb KR, Gregory K, Shaw K: The outcome of macrosomic infants weighing at least 4500 grams: Los Angeles county + University of Southern California Experience. Obstet Gynecol 85:558-564, 1995.

Lydon-Rochelle M, Holt VL, Easterling TR, Martin DP: Risk of uterine rupture during labor among women with a prior cesarean delivery. N Engl J Med 345:3-8, 2001.

McFarland LV, Raskin M, Daling JR, Benedetti TJ: Erb/Duchenne's palsy: A consequence of fetal macrosomia and method of delivery. Obstet Gynecol 68:784-788, 1986.

National Center for Health Statistics: Births—Method of Delivery, at www.cdc.gov/nchs

National Center for Health Statistics: Total and primary cesarean rates and vaginal births after previous cesarean delivery, 1989-1997. National Vital Statistics Report Supplements.

National Vital Statistics System: Infant mortality rates, fetal mortality rates, and perinatal mortality rates by Race: United States 1950-1998.

Nesbitt TS, Gilbert WM, Herrchen B: Shoulder dystocia and associated risk factors with macrosomic infants born in California. Am J Obstet Gynecol 179:476-480, 1998.

Noetzel MJ, Park TS, Robinson S, Kaufman B: Prospective study of recovery following neonatal brachial plexus injury. J Child Neurol 16:488-492, 2001.

Ouzounian JG, Korst LM, Phelan JP: Permanent Erb's palsy: A lack of a relationship with obstetrical risk factors. Am J Perinatol 15:221-223, 1998.

Plauche WC: Fetal cranial injuries related to delivery with the Malmstrom vacuum extractor. Obstet Gynecol 53:750-757, 1979.

Plauche WC: Subgaleal hematoma: A complication of instrumental delivery. JAMA 244:1597-1598, 1980.

Rabinovici J, Barkai G, Reichman B, et al: Randomized management of the second nonvertex twin: Vaginal delivery or cesarean section. Am J Obstet Gynecol 156:52-56, 1987.

Roberts SW, Hernandez C, Maberry MC, et al: Obstetric clavicular fracture: The enigma of normal birth. Obstet Gynecol 86:978-981, 1995.

Robertson PA, Laros RK, Zhao R: Neonatal and maternal outcome in low-pelvic and midpelvic operative deliveries. Am J Obstet Gynecol 162:1436-1444, 1990.

Rouse DJ, Owen J, Goldenberg RL, Cliver SP: The effectiveness and costs of elective cesarean delivery for fetal macrosomia diagnosed by ultrasound. JAMA 276:1480-1486, 1996.

Socol ML, Peaceman AM: Vaginal birth after cesarean: An appraisal of fetal risk. Obstet Gynecol 93:674-679, 1999.

Teng FY, Sayre JW: Vacuum extraction: Does duration predict scalp injury? Obstet Gynecol 89:281-285, 1997.

Towner D, Castro MA, Eby-Wilkens E, Gilbert WM: Effect of mode of delivery in nulliparous women on neonatal intracranial injury. N Engl J Med 341:1709-1714, 1999.

U.S. Food and Drug Administration, Center for Devices and Radiological Health. FDA Public Health Advisory: Need for Caution when Using Vacuum Assisted Delivery Devices. May 21, 1998. Available online at www.fda.gov

Westgren LMR, Songster G, Paul RH: Preterm breech delivery: Another retrospective study. Obstet Gynecol 66:481-484, 1985.

Wildschut HIJ, Roosmalen JV, Van Leeuwen E, Keirse MJNC: Planned abdominal compared with planned vaginal birth in triplet pregnancies. Br J Obstet Gynecol 102:292-296, 1995.

Williams MC, Knuppel RA, O'Brien W, et al: A randomized comparison of assisted vaginal delivery by obstetric forceps and polyethylene vacuum cup. Obstet Gynecol 78:789-794, 1991.

Winn HN, Cimino J, Powers J, et al: Intrapartum management of nonvertex second-born twins: A critical analysis. Am J Obstet Gynecol 185:1204-1208, 2001.

Wylie B: Traction in forceps deliveries. Am J Obstet Gynecol 29:425, 1935.

Yancey MK, Helpolsheimer A, Jordan GD, et al: Maternal and neonatal effects of outlet forceps delivery compared with spontaneous vaginal delivery in term pregnancies. Obstet Gynecol 78:646-650, 1991.

Yap OWS, Kim ES, Laros RK: Maternal and neonatal outcomes after uterine rupture in labor. Am J Obstet Gynecol 184:1576-1581, 2001.

CHAPTER 16

# Maternal and Fetal Anesthesia and Analgesia

Mark A. Rosen and Samuel C. Hughes

Modern obstetric anesthesia was born in Scotland on January 19, 1847, when James Young Simpson used diethyl ether to anesthetize a woman with a contracted pelvis. Morton's historic demonstration of the anesthetic properties of ether at the Massachusetts General Hospital in Boston had occurred only 3 months earlier. Fanny Longfellow, wife of Henry Wadsworth Longfellow, was the first American woman to receive anesthesia for childbirth, publicly proclaiming in 1847, "This is certainly the greatest blessing of this age."

Although anesthesia for surgery was immediately accepted, Simpson's contemporaries in obstetrics in the United States, France, and England were opposed to the use of anesthesia in obstetrics, presenting both medical and religious arguments—for example, that the Bible (Genesis 3:16) states, " . . . in sorrow, thou shalt bring forth children." However, this reading was likely based on a poor translation of the ancient Hebrew word meaning "labor." Certainly, the public outcry in 1853 was vehement; the reaction from Thomas Wolsley, editor of *The Lancet*, after John Snow administered ether for Queen Victoria's eighth child, Leopold, was so strong that court physicians denied that anesthesia had been used. The great debate was largely settled when Victoria delivered her ninth and last child, Beatrice, 4 years later and the use of a royal anesthetic was acknowledged.

Patients' demand for pain relief had won the argument as Simpson had predicted. Still, it was not until 1957 that Pope Pius XII felt the need for a special encyclical about the spiritual value of childbirth pain, in which it was explained that there was no prohibition of the use of labor analgesia in the tradition of the Catholic Church. The church had finally caught up with the public's opinion.

During the second half of the 20th century, anesthesiologists made significant advances in techniques and advances in the safety of delivering analgesia. The continuous caudal catheter developed by Hingson and Edwards (1943) was followed by the epidural catheter. Virginia Apgar (1953) proposed a simple scoring system for neonatal evaluation as a guide for neonatal resuscitation. Other early pioneers in the emerging specialty of obstetric anesthesia were Gertie Marx (Marx and Orkin, 1958), John Bonica (1967), and Sol Shnider (1963). They helped characterize the normal changes in maternal physiology related to pregnancy, confirm the safety and efficacy of obstetric analgesia, determine the effects of these techniques on uterine blood flow as well as the placental transfer of anesthetic agents, and evaluate the effects of these techniques and agents on newborn well-being.

The purposes of this chapter are to introduce the neonatal practitioner to the scientific background and clinical techniques of modern obstetric anesthesia and to discuss the consequences of these techniques for the fetus and neonate. Obstetric analgesia may benefit the parturient in painful labor, facilitate safe and painless use of forceps or vacuum devices for vaginal delivery, and facilitate safe vaginal delivery of twins or a fetus in a breech presentation, and is certainly required to permit delivery by cesarean section. Although the effects of modern obstetric anesthesia on the fetus and newborn are ordinarily benign, they can rarely have an adverse effect that the neonatal practitioner should learn to recognize, comprehend, and manage. Simpson observed that the umbilical cords of babies born to mothers given ether smelled of the agent.

## ANATOMY OF LABOR PAIN

Pain during labor and delivery is caused by uterine contractions, dilatation of the cervix, and distention of the perineum. Somatic and visceral afferent sensory fibers from the uterus and cervix travel with sympathetic nerve fibers to the spinal cord (Fig. 16–1). These fibers pass through the paracervical tissue, with the uterine artery, and then through the inferior, middle, and superior hypogastric plexuses to the sympathetic chain. Nerve impulses from the uterus and cervix enter the spinal cord through the 10th, 11th, and 12th thoracic nerves (T10 to T12) and the 1st lumbar nerve (L1). Somatic perineal pain impulses travel to the 2nd, 3rd, and 4th sacral nerves primarily via the pudendal nerve (S2 to S4). Pain in the perineum, caused by distention of the vagina, perineum, and pelvic floor muscles, is associated with descent of the fetus into the pelvis during the second stage of labor, and with delivery.

Somatic pain and visceral pain are very different types of pain sensation. *Somatic pain* (e.g., incision pain, second-stage labor pain) is well localized and typically described as "sharp." *Visceral pain* (e.g., uterine contractions in the first stage of labor) is poorly localized and usually described as "dull but intense aching." Along with the subjective sensation of pain, nerve impulses of labor pain lead to stimulation of the autonomic nervous system and create reflex cardiovascular, respiratory, endocrine, and musculoskeletal effects, such as maternal tachycardia, hypertension, hypotension, elevation in catecholamines, and reduced uterine blood flow.

## CHANGES IN MATERNAL PHYSIOLOGY AND THE IMPLICATIONS FOR ANESTHESIA

During pregnancy, labor, and delivery, women undergo fundamental changes in anatomy and physiology due to altered hormonal activity, biochemical changes associated with increasing metabolic demands of a growing fetus, placenta, and uterus, and mechanical displacement by an enlarging uterus (Cheek and Gutsche, 2002; Parer et al, 2002).

Hypotension may occur when a pregnant woman assumes the supine position, because of aortocaval compression by the gravid uterus: Significant aortoiliac artery

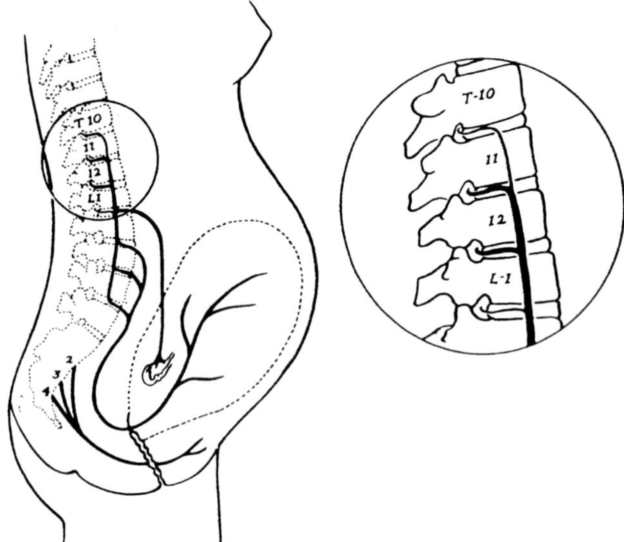


**FIGURE 16–1.** Parturition pain pathways. Nerves that accompany sympathetic fibers and enter the neuraxis at the T10, T11, T12, and L1 spinal levels carry afferent pain impulses from the cervix and uterus. Pain pathways from the perineum travel to S2, S3, and S4 via the pudendal nerve. *(From Bonica JJ: The nature of pain of parturition. Clin Obstet Gynaecol 2:511, 1975.)*

compression occurs in 15% to 20% of parturients and vena caval compression in all. Vena caval compression may contribute to lower extremity venous stasis, resulting in ankle edema and varices.

Physiologic (dilution) anemia of pregnancy occurs as a result of a greater increase in plasma volume than in red blood cell (RBC) mass. Average blood loss at delivery—300 to 500 mL for vaginal delivery and 600 to 1000 mL for cesarean section—is well tolerated because of this expanded blood volume.

Venous compression by the gravid uterus diverts some blood returning from the lower extremities through the internal vertebral venous plexus, the azygos and epidural veins, increasing the likelihood of epidural venous puncture with epidural or spinal techniques of anesthesia. Supine positioning is avoided in pregnant women during anesthetic administration in the second and third trimesters. Anesthetic techniques that interfere with increased sympathetic tone will further compromise compensatory mechanisms for vena caval compression induced by supine positioning, potentially causing profound hypotension.

The stomach is displaced cephalad and anterior, and the pylorus cephalad and posterior, by the gravid uterus. Gastric pressure is increased by the gravid uterus and by the lithotomy position. Plasma gastrin levels rise, probably by placental production of the hormone, increasing gastric acidity. Higher progesterone and estrogen levels reduce esophageal sphincter tone, and progesterone inhibits plasma motilin. Gastric reflux is common during gestation. Labor or opioids considerably slow gut motility and gastric emptying.

Beyond mid-gestation, women are at increased risk for pulmonary aspiration of acidic gastric contents because of decreased competence of the lower esophageal sphincter as well as delayed gastric emptying with onset of labor or administration of opioids. This risk has important consequences for both the method of induction of general anesthesia and airway management by the anesthesiologist.

### Uterine Blood Flow

Uterine weight rises, and blood flow increases to about 700 mL/min (about 10% of cardiac output) at term, with about 80% of the uterine blood flow perfusing the intervillous space (placenta) and 20% going to the myometrium. Uterine vasculature is not autoregulated, and remains (essentially) maximally dilated under normal conditions during pregnancy. Although the uterus is capable of marked vasoconstriction in response to α-adrenergic agents, pregnancy is associated with reduced uterine artery response and sensitivity to vasoconstrictors.

Uterine blood flow (UBF) decreases because of decreased uterine arterial blood pressure, which results from systemic hypotension (shock or general, epidural, or spinal anesthesia). UBF also decreases with aortocaval compression or increased uterine venous pressure, which results from vena caval compression (e.g., supine position) or uterine contractions (particularly uterine hyperstimulation, for instance by oxytocin hyperstimulation, or placental abruption).

## ANALGESIC TECHNIQUES FOR LABOR AND VAGINAL DELIVERY

The pain of labor is highly variable, described by many women as severe. Analgesia for labor and childbirth reduces the psychological or subjective component of pain. Factors that may influence a woman's perception of labor pain include duration of labor, maternal pelvic anatomy in relation to fetal size, use of oxytocin, parity, participation in childbirth preparation classes, fear and anxiety about childbirth, attitudes about and experience of pain, and coping mechanisms. Labor analgesia may prevent reflex effects that can be deleterious for certain high-risk patients or their fetuses (e.g., patients with severe preeclampsia, valvular heart disease, myasthenia gravis). However, a maternal request for pain relief is sufficient justification for administration of analgesics during labor. According to the 4th edition of the *Guidelines for Perinatal Care*, published by the American Academy of Pediatrics and the American College of Obstetricians and Gynecologists, "Of the various pharmacologic methods used for pain relief during labor and delivery, lumbar epidural block is the most flexible, effective, and least depressing to the central nervous system, allowing for an alert, participating mother" (Guidelines, 1997).

The choice of analgesic technique resides primarily with the parturient. The medical condition of the parturient, stage of labor, condition of the fetus, and availability of qualified personnel also are factors. Many different techniques are used to alleviate labor and delivery pain. *Analgesia* refers to pain relief without loss of consciousness; *regional analgesia* denotes partial sensory blockade in a specific area of the body, with or without partial motor blockade. *Regional anesthesia* is the loss of all sensation, motor function, and reflex activity in a specific area of the body. *General anesthesia* results in the loss of consciousness; goals for providing general anesthesia typically include hypnosis, amnesia, analgesia, and skeletal muscle relaxation. (It is of interest that agents that produce general anesthesia are not necessarily analgesic when administered in low concentrations.)

Techniques for labor analgesia must be safe for mother and fetus and individualized to satisfy the analgesic requirement and desires of the parturient; they also must accommodate the changing nature of labor pain as well as the evolving, varied course of labor and delivery (e.g., spontaneous vaginal delivery, instrumental vaginal delivery, and cesarean delivery). The current approaches to pain relief are outlined in Table 16–1.

## Nonpharmacologic Analgesia: Psychological and Alternative Techniques

Psychological and alternative techniques of obstetric analgesia include hypnosis, "natural childbirth" as described by Dick-Read, the breathing techniques described by Lamaze, acupuncture, acupressure, the LeBoyer technique (LeBoyer, 1975), transcutaneous nerve stimulation, hydrotherapy, and biofeedback. Psychoanalgesic techniques require a high level of personal concentration and are not entirely reliable or applicable to all deliveries.

## Systemic Medications

Systemic medications for labor and delivery are widely utilized but are administered in limited doses because they readily cross the placenta and can depress the fetus in a dose-dependent fashion. The use of sedative-hypnotics (barbiturates, phenothiazine derivatives and hydroxyzine, benzodiazepines), and dissociative agents (ketamine, scopolamine) is uncommon, but the use of opioid analgesics is very widespread. Opioids are the most effective systemic medications for relief of pain. However, excessive maternal sedation, maternal respiratory depression, loss of maternal protective airway reflexes, and the risk of neonatal depression limit the amount that can be administered for labor analgesia. The most commonly utilized opioid analgesics in obstetrics are the opiate morphine and the synthetic opioids fentanyl, butorphanol, nalbuphine, and meperidine.

Systemic administration of opioids at doses safe for mother and newborn provides some analgesia but cannot substitute for the analgesia provided by regional anesthetic techniques. Systemic opioids are recommended for administration in the smallest doses possible with minimization of repeated dosing to reduce the accumulation of drug and metabolites in the fetus. Opioids are most useful in primiparas in early labor, as adjuncts to major regional anesthetics, and in multiparas who have relatively short, predictable labors with minimal pain.

**TABLE 16–1**

**Techniques for Labor Analgesia**

| |
|---|
| Nonpharmacologic analgesia |
| Psychological techniques |
| Alternative techniques |
| Systemic medications |
| Sedatives and tranquilizers |
| Dissociative analgesia |
| Opioid analgesics |
| Inhalation analgesia |
| Regional analgesia |
| Spinal |
| Epidural |
| Combined spinal-epidural |
| Paracervical block |
| Lumbar sympathetic block |
| Pudendal block |

### Sedatives and Tranquilizers

Sedatives and tranquilizers are administered to parturients to diminish the adverse motivational-affective component of labor pain. Examples of such drugs are barbiturates, phenothiazines, and benzodiazepines.

Secobarbital and pentobarbital have been used in obstetrics. Due to the prolonged effects of these agents, their use is confined principally to facilitate maternal sleep in the early latent stage of labor, when delivery is not likely to occur for 12 to 24 hours. Barbiturates have been described as having an "antianalgesic effect" and may convert a minimally uncomfortable, controlled patient into a hyperventilating, confused, and unmanageable one. For this reason, they are used rarely today.

Promethazine and propiomazine are phenothiazines. Hydroxyzine, although not a phenothiazine, has similar properties. These drugs are useful for relieving anxiety, modifying the response to painful stimulation, and potentiating the actions of opioid analgesics. In addition, they are useful in controlling nausea and vomiting, which may be severe enough to produce maternal dehydration during labor. In recommended dosages, these drugs appear to have minimal depressant effects on both mother and fetus, although they rapidly cross the placenta and have been noted to cause a decrease in fetal beat-to-beat heart rate variability (Powe et al, 1962).

Diazepam and midazolam are used as anxiolytic agents in obstetrics. They rapidly cross the placenta, yielding approximately equal maternal and fetal blood levels within minutes of intravenous (IV) administration (Cree et al, 1973). In addition, the neonate has a limited ability to excrete diazepam, so the drug and its active metabolite may persist in significant amounts in the neonate for a week (Scher and Hailey, 1972). The use of benzodiazepines remains somewhat controversial, but these agents can reduce maternal anxiety, can decrease opioid dosage, and are useful for treatment of convulsions associated with local anesthetic toxicity or eclampsia. Benzodiazepines may produce hypotonia, lethargy, and hypothermia when used in large maternal doses (30 mg) (Cohen et al, 1993); however, when it is used in small doses (2.5 to 10 mg IV), minimal sedation and hypotonia have been observed (McAllister, 1980).

### Dissociative Analgesia

The intramuscular or IV administration of low-dose ketamine (0.25 mg/kg) produces a state called *dissociative analgesia*, which is characterized by good analgesia and amnesia without loss of consciousness or protective airway reflexes (Galloon, 1976). This state is accompanied by a dreaming phenomenon, which may be unpleasant but can be minimized by co-administration of benzodiazepines. Used in divided doses totaling less than 1 mg/kg, ketamine can provide adequate analgesia for vaginal delivery and episiotomy repair. As the dose administered increases, however, airway protection cannot be guaranteed, so aspiration may occur. This agent is best reserved for use as a supplement (in low doses) to other techniques or for situations in which (1) more reliable and safer agents or techniques are contraindicated or (2) rapid control is required because the mother's pain is compromising the fetus (e.g., mother thrashing in pain, unable to push cooperatively with contractions, while the fetal head is crowning with a prolonged deceleration of the fetal heart rate).

### Opioid Analgesics

The opioid analgesics act by stimulating opiate receptors found in many locations throughout the central nervous system (CNS). The majority of opiate receptors in the brain and spinal cord that produce analgesia are the $\mu$ receptors (Yaksh, 1981). These receptors are also responsible for respiratory depression and may affect thermoregulation. Binding of opiate agonist agents, probably at synaptic junctions, alters neural transmission. Another class of opioid drugs binds to the receptor with high affinity but does not produce analgesia. These drugs are capable of displacing the agonist drugs from the receptor and reversing their effects; they are known as *opioid antagonists* (e.g., naloxone, naltrexone). A third class of agents interacts with the receptors and results in both agonist and antagonist activity. Unlike the pure antagonists, these drugs, with high receptor affinity, are capable of having some analgesic effect (e.g., levallorphan, pentazocine, nalbuphine, and butorphanol). It is possible that the receptor specificity is the explanation for the peculiar actions of the agonist-antagonist agents (Bullingham et al, 1983).

In general, all opioids, at equipotent doses, have similar effects on the fetus and newborn, crossing the placental barrier through passive diffusion. Although systemic opioids can alleviate labor pain, large doses would be necessary, risking excessive maternal sedation, maternal respiratory depression, loss of protective airway reflexes, newborn respiratory depression, impairment of early breastfeeding and neurobehavior. In clinical use, large doses of opioids are avoided, and the doses used to relieve labor pain should not have adverse effects on either the mother or baby. All opioids readily cross the placental barrier and exert neonatal effects in normal doses, including decreased fetal heat rate variability. Normal doses also have maternal side effects, including nausea, vomiting, pruritus, and decreased motility of the gastrointestinal system (with delayed gastric emptying).

Intramuscular administration of opioids is technically easy but leads to uneven analgesia, the possibility of late respiratory depression, and profound neonatal effects if not properly timed (Shnider and Moya, 1960). For many parturients, opioids do not provide adequate analgesia during labor and delivery (Olofsson et al, 1996; Bricker and Lavender, 2002). For these reasons, many centers have abandoned this method of analgesia (Douglas and Levinson, 2002).

Intravenous administration is the most widely used technique to give opioids to a woman in labor, with effects that are more predictable and doses more easily timed. However, achievement of a steady blood level of opiate sufficient to provide analgesia is difficult, with the parturient frequently suffering underdosage (rarely overdosage). Continuous IV infusion of short-acting opiates (e.g., alfentanil, remifentanil) or self-administration of IV opiates may overcome this limitation.

Patient-controlled analgesia (PCA) is becoming a popular method of IV administration of these drugs, because the patient usually titrates her dose to the minimum required for analgesia with the lowest blood levels of opiates and, hence, considerably less placental transfer (McIntosh and Rayburn, 1991). With the introduction of remifentanil, which is rapidly metabolized by nonspecific serum esterases, it is possible that PCA with remifentanil will prove an effective method for continuous intravenous opiate analgesia, presuming that the drug does not accumulate in the fetus. It has been demonstrated that remifentanil rapidly crosses the placenta but appears to be rapidly metabolized and redistributed (Kan et al, 1998). PCA with remifentanil has been successful but it appears difficult to achieve satisfactory analgesia without the real potential of maternal respiratory depression (Olufolabi et al, 2000; Thurlow and Waterhouse, 2000; Volikas and Male, 2001).

Overall, the epidural injection of opiates alone has proven to be of limited utility for labor analgesia. Intraspinal opiates were demonstrated in 1979 to be capable of producing profound analgesia in humans (Behar et al, 1979; Wang et al, 1979). Shortly thereafter, several researchers attempted to apply this technique for the relief of labor pain. In one study, high doses of epidural morphine (7.5 mg) provided satisfactory but not excellent analgesia for 6 hours in the first stage of labor, whereas 2 mg or 5 mg produced barely satisfactory analgesia in less than half the patients (Hughes et al, 1984). Besides the inadequate analgesia, and the long time of onset (about 1 hour), the side effect of pruritus was significant. When rapidly acting, lipid-soluble opioids are administered alone into the epidural space, analgesia achieved is equivalent to that of systemic administration (Camann et al, 1992), inferior to that of dilute concentrations of local anesthetics, and less effective for somatic pain associated with the second stage of labor.

Subarachnoid (i.e., spinal) injections of fentanyl, meperidine, and sufentanil have been more promising, having analgesic effects that are more potent than that with epidural or systemic administration but are of short duration (2 hours) and less effective than dilute solutions of local anesthetics for analgesia in the second stage (Honet et al, 1989). This method is commonly performed with a combined spinal-epidural (CSE) technique. Reports of fetal heart rate changes after intrathecal administration of fentanyl or sufentanil (Cohen et al, 1993) may be due to rapid onset of analgesia and rapid decrease in circulating catecholamines, epinephrine faster than norepinephrine, resulting in unopposed oxytocic effect on the uterus, which increases uterine tone and decreases uterine blood flow. This mechanism is speculative but is suggested by observed cases and case reports (Friedlander et al, 1997). However, prospective, randomized studies have suggested no difference in incidence of fetal bradycardia between epidural administration of local anesthetics and intrathecal opioids administered with the CSE technique (Fogel et al, 1999; Nageotte et al, 1997).

When administered into the epidural or intrathecal spaces, these agents can be useful primarily in the first stage of labor but do not provide adequate analgesia for the second stage of labor or for obstetric surgical procedures. They have been most useful when co-administered into the epidural (or intrathecal) space with local anesthetics.

After maternal administration, the lipid-soluble, poorly ionized opioid analgesics rapidly enter the fetal circulation, where they cause a dose-related respiratory depression, as evidenced by a rightward shift in the carbon dioxide response curve. The severity of depression is a function of the amount of drug administered, the timing, and the route of administration. Intramuscular administration is associated with a high incidence of neonatal depression 2 to 4 hours after injection. Intravenous or epidural injection produces peak neonatal depression at 30 to 60 minutes. In addition, some opioids, most notably meperidine, have active metabolites that prolong their fetal effects far longer than the action of the parent drug.

### Inhalation Analgesia

Some birthing centers use nitrous oxide, which is usually administered by a device that delivers 50% oxygen and 50% nitrous oxide, a concentration that alone (without co-administration of opioids, etc.) is insufficient to cause unconsciousness or loss of protective airway reflexes. Appropriate equipment and fully trained personnel are essential to ensure safety (limiting the nitrous oxide concentration, avoiding administration of a hypoxic mixture, avoiding co-administration of other agents, minimizing risk of maternal loss of protective airway reflexes).

Nitrous oxide can provide satisfactory pain relief for some parturients and can be utilized during the first, second, or third stage of labor and either alone or to supplement a block or local infiltration. Use of 50% nitrous oxide in a supervised fashion is safe and rapid acting, causes minimal maternal cardiovascular or respiratory depression, and does not affect uterine contractility; its effects are rapidly reversed, and it does not cause neonatal depression regardless of duration of administration (Rosen, 2002). However, 50% nitrous oxide is a weak analgesic.

## REGIONAL ANALGESIA

Regional analgesia, including epidural, spinal, and CSE techniques, has become the most widely used regional block for labor analgesia. Lumbar sympathetic blocks and paracervical blocks are rarely performed for labor analgesia, but pudendal blocks are utilized for delivery. Regional blocks usually involve local anesthetic administration, and some include co-administration of opioid analgesics; the future will see administration of other agents that modulate interneuronal communication (Bouaziz et al, 1995; Eisenach et al, 1996).

### Local Anesthetics

The clinically useful compounds consist of amine moieties linked by an intermediate chain containing an ester or amides. Local anesthetics reversibly block impulse conduction in sensory and motor nerves; their chemical structures are of secondary or tertiary amines, which are weak bases, marketed as the hydrochloride salts to achieve aqueous solubility.

The ester-linked local anesthetics (procaine, chloroprocaine, tetracaine) are rapidly metabolized by plasma cholinesterase, limiting the risk of maternal toxicity and placental drug transfer (O'Brien et al, 1979). The amide-linked local anesthetics (lidocaine, bupivacaine, ropivacaine, levobupivacaine) are slowly degraded by the liver and bind to plasma protein. Ropivacaine and levobupivacaine, the newest local anesthetics, are *S*-enantiomers, amino amide–type local anesthetic agents with a chemical formula similar to that of bupivacaine. The significant difference from the other two congener local anesthetic agents is that ropivacaine is an *S*-isomer rather than a racemic mixture. Vascular absorption of local anesthetics limits the safe dose that can be administered; toxic plasma concentrations produce neurologic toxicity (seizures) or cardiovascular toxicity (myocardial depression, ventricular arrhythmia). Accidental intravascular injection of bupivacaine has resulted in maternal death.

Effects of mild overdoses of local anesthetic are exhibited by the neonate as decreases in neuromuscular tone similar to those seen with magnesium. If a direct intravascular or intrafetal injection of local anesthetics occurs, significant depression can develop, signified by bradycardia, ventricular arrhythmia, and severe cardiac depression with acidosis.

### Epidural Analgesia and Combined Spinal-Epidural Analgesia

In many centers, epidural analgesia for labor and delivery is the technique of choice. The parturient remains awake and alert without sedative side effects, maternal catecholamine concentrations are reduced (Shnider et al, 1983), hyperventilation is avoided (Levinson et al, 1974), cooperation and capacity to participate actively during labor are facilitated, and excellent, predictable analgesia can be achieved, superior to the analgesia provided by all other techniques.

The technique involves insertion of a specialized needle between vertebral spinous processes in the back, through the ligamentum flavum, and into the (potential) epidural space (but not through the dura, which forms the perimeter of the intrathecal or subarachnoid space) using a tactile technique of "loss of resistance" with an air- or saline-filled syringe (Fig. 16–2). Once the needle is properly placed, a catheter is inserted through the needle and left in place, and the needle removed. The catheter is secured in place (with

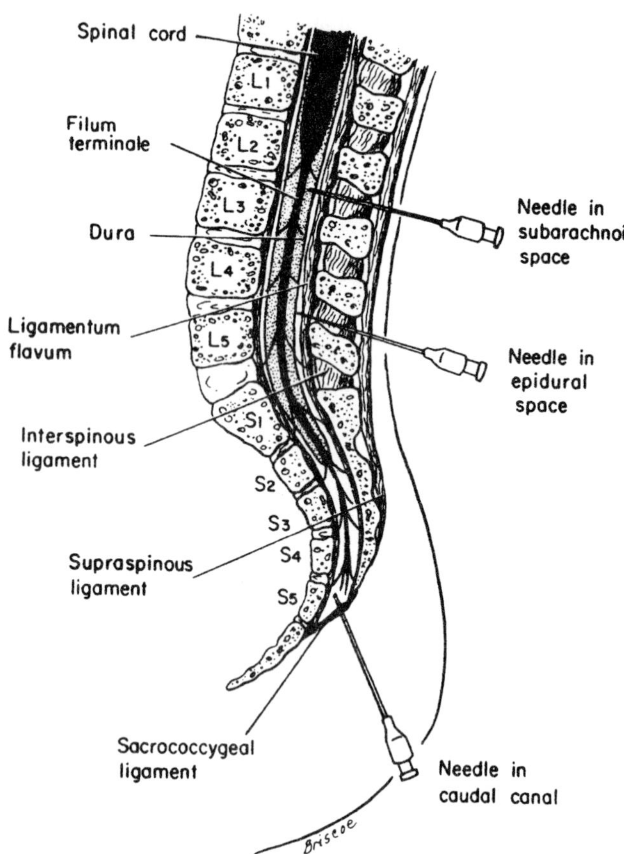


**FIGURE 16–2.** Schematic diagram of lumbosacral anatomy showing needle placement for subarachnoid, lumbar epidural, and caudal blocks. *(From Rosen MA, Hughes SC, Levinson G: Regional anesthesia for labor and delivery. In Hughes SC, Levinson G, Rosen MA [eds]: Shnider and Levinson's Anesthesia for Obstetrics, 4th ed. Baltimore, Lippincott Williams & Wilkins, 2002, p 125.)*

tape and adhesives) for intermittent or continuous injections. Most commonly, the needle is inserted at the lumbar epidural level (L1-L2, L2-L3, or L3-L4); caudal anesthesia is a similar technique, with placement of needle, catheter, and medication in the caudal epidural space rather than the lumbar epidural space.

Careful monitoring of the fetus and uterus is important after administration of regional analgesia. Fetal bradycardia from uterine hyperactivity causing decreased uteroplacental perfusion can occur, although rarely, most likely from the rapid decrease in maternal catecholamines after administration of analgesia (Friedlander et al, 1997). When resolution does not occur spontaneously and promptly, administration of nitroglycerin is an effective method to achieve fast onset and brief duration of uterine relaxation (Segal et al, 1998).

Epidural block can be performed early in labor, as soon as satisfactory progress of labor is established and the patient requests analgesia (i.e., usually 3 to 4 cm of cervical dilation in nulliparas, less in multiparas). During early labor, many anesthesiologists strive to provide a segmental block, to provide analgesia for the pain of uterine contractions and cervical dilation (T10 to L1). Later, a larger volume can be administered to provide perineal analgesia for spontaneous vaginal delivery, if necessary or desired, or for an instrumental vaginal delivery. Once the catheter is placed, analgesia may be attained and continued throughout the active stage of labor and delivery or for operative anesthesia (cesarean delivery) as well as postoperative analgesia, when necessary.

Local anesthetics are typically infused continuously after incremental bolus doses, to produce reliable pain relief with similar or lower blood levels of local anesthetics than repetitive, intermittent boluses of these drugs (Hicks et al, 1988; Rosenblatt et al, 1983). Most important, the possibility of disastrous complications of total spinal anesthesia or massive intravascular injections with cardiovascular collapse secondary to large doses of local anesthetics is decreased. If an epidural catheter enters an epidural vein during continuous infusion, the analgesia merely ceases without producing neurologic or cardiovascular toxicity (Dathis et al, 1988). If the catheter enters the subarachnoid space instead, the level of sensory and motor blockade increases slowly without the sudden onset of complete subarachnoid blockade that may occur with bolus techniques (Li et al, 1985).

The choice of drug for continuous epidural infusion includes dilute solutions of lidocaine, bupivacaine, ropivacaine or chloroprocaine (Lee et al, 2002). The concentration and volume of the loading dose, which is administered before initiation of the continuous infusion, and the volume and concentration of the infusion are quite variable. With higher concentrations of local anesthetics, the density of the motor blockade increases. With larger volumes, a greater dermatomal spread of analgesia is achieved. Most practitioners routinely use reduced concentrations of local anesthetics and co-administer an opioid with both the bolus and the infusion. Dilute solutions of local anesthetics minimize the motor blockade and preserve the perception of pelvic pressure with descent of the fetus. The administration of both agents, local anesthetics and opioids, results in an additive (perhaps synergistic) effect (Chestnut et al, 1988). Some practitioners use extremely dilute concentrations of local anesthetics combined with an opioid and allow the parturient to ambulate (after careful neurologic testing) (Rosen et al, 2002).

One variation of the lumbar epidural technique is CSE. After placement of the epidural needle but before insertion of the epidural catheter, a long spinal needle is passed through the indwelling epidural needle to puncture the dura, and a small dose of either local anesthetic or opioid or both is administered. If opioid alone is administered and the epidural catheter is not activated, analgesia without motor blockade or sympathectomy is achieved. This method allows the parturient to ambulate safely. The side effects pruritus, nausea, and vomiting are usually not substantial with lipid-soluble opioids such as fentanyl or sufentanil, but the analgesia is limited (about 2 hours in the early active stage) and is rarely effective for the second stage of labor.

If small doses of local anesthetics are administered through the spinal needle, a segmental analgesia results more rapidly than with epidural administration of local anesthetics. The epidural placement of the catheter allows continuation of the segmental analgesia initiated by the spinal technique. Although some practitioners use this technique routinely and allow the patient to walk after careful evaluation, most use the more straightforward epidural technique.

## Contraindications to and Complications of Regional Anesthesia

Certain conditions contraindicate regional anesthesia, such as patient refusal, infection at the needle insertion site, coagulopathy, and hypovolemic shock. Human immunodeficiency virus (HIV) infection is not a contraindication to regional technique in the parturient (Hughes et al, 1995).

Infrequent but occasionally life-threatening complications can result from administration of regional anesthesia. The most serious complications are from accidental intravenous or intrathecal injections of local anesthetics. After careful test dosing, administration of the therapeutic dose as incremental fractionation of doses is an important method of ensuring safety.

Hypotension secondary to sympathetic blockade is the most common complication of major regional block for parturition (Rosenblatt et al, 1983). Prophylactic measures include adequate hydration, avoidance of the supine position, and displacement of the uterus off the abdominal great vessels. Treatment consists of further uterine displacement, IV fluids, and vasopressor administration (e.g., ephedrine, 10 to 20 mg, which has primarily β-adrenergic effects, restoring uterine blood flow to normal values as well as correcting hypotension, unlike primarily α-adrenergic drugs, which increase uterine vascular tone, resulting in restoration of maternal pressure but not uterine blood flow). If treated promptly, maternal hypotension does not lead to fetal depression or neonatal morbidity. Other relatively common complications of epidural analgesia include headache from cerebrospinal fluid leak after accidental dural puncture. Resuscitation and support of the mother will reestablish uterine blood flow and allow adequate fetal oxygenation and excretion of local anesthetic (Morishima and Adamsons, 1967). Unless the mother cannot be resuscitated, delivery of the fetus should be delayed, because the neonate has an extremely limited ability to excrete local anesthetics and may have prolonged convulsions (Ralston and Shnider, 1978). Measures that minimize the likelihood of accidental intravascular injection include careful aspiration before injection, test dosing, and incremental administration of therapeutic doses.

An excessive level of neural blockade (high or total spinal) may develop during initiation of a spinal, epidural, or caudal block or during an infusion, leading to blockade of the motor nerves to the respiratory muscles (Yentis, 2001). Treatment consists of endotracheal intubation, ventilation with oxygen, and avoidance of aortocaval obstruction. Maternal circulation must be supported by avoidance of aortocaval compression and administration of additional fluids and vasopressors (e.g., ephedrine), if needed. If these measures are not promptly effective, epinephrine (0.5 to 1.0 mg) should be administered.

In any situation of maternal cardiac arrest with unsuccessful resuscitation, consideration must be given to urgent delivery of the fetus. If the fetus is delivered within 5 minutes of the arrest, the chances for survival are maximized, and evacuation of the uterus relieves aortocaval compression, improving the chances of maternal resuscitation (American Heart Association, 1997; Lee et al, 1986).

A rise in core maternal body temperature has been associated with epidural analgesic infusions during labor and may be influenced by several factors, including duration, ambient temperature, administration of systemic opioids, and, possibly most important, the presence of shivering. During the first 5 hours of epidural analgesia, there is no significant rise in body temperature (Mercier and Benhamou, 1997). If labor is prolonged, temperature increases at about 0.10 degrees C/hour, and may reach 38° C in as many as 15% of cases by 12 hours (Lieberman et al, 1997). Lieberman and colleagues (1997) suggested a significant increase in newborn sepsis work-up (SWU) rate with epidural analgesia, but 67.3% of the SWUs were ordered in infants born to mothers without fever. Kaul and associates (2001) found no association between epidural analgesia and SWU. However, patients who received epidural analgesia and their neonates had an increased body temperature at delivery and about 6% of women had temperatures equal to or exceeding 38° C. Although maternal temperature had no predictive value for SWU, Kaul and colleagues found other risk factors associated with SWU, including low birth weight, gestational age, meconium or respiratory distress requiring intubation at birth, hypothermia at birth, group-B β-hemolytic streptococcus colonization, and maternal preeclampsia or hypertension. Although the etiology of the maternal temperature rise remains uncertain, it need not affect neonatal SWU. Labor epidural analgesia does not increase the incidence of neonatal sepsis. Although some suggest that the fever may be associated with noninfectious inflammatory activation or altered thermoregulation, it is not associated with a change in white blood cell (WBC) count or with an infectious process, and treatment is not necessary.

## Spinal Analgesia

When utilized, spinal anesthesia is administered immediately before delivery. A small dose of a local anesthetic dissolved in a hypertonic dextrose solution is injected into the subarachnoid space, typically with the patient in the sitting position. Injection produces immediate analgesia of the lumbosacral nerve roots and provides excellent anesthesia for episiotomy, forceps application, and delivery.

### Paracervical and Lumbar Sympathetic Blocks

Paracervical block is occasionally used by obstetricians to provide pain relief in the first stage of labor. The technique consists of submucosal administration of local anesthetics immediately lateral and posterior to the uterocervical junction, which blocks transmission of pain impulses at the paracervical ganglion. Analgesia is not as profound as with epidural or spinal regional block, and the duration of analgesia is short (45 to 60 minutes), but the complications and side effects of epidural analgesia, such as hypotension, hypoventilation, and motor blockade, are avoided. Convulsions, however, may occur as a result of systemic absorption of local anesthetic.

The obstetrician performing a paracervical block should closely monitor the fetus, should inject just beneath the vaginal mucosa after aspiration for blood in the needle is negative, and should allow a 5-minute interval between injections on the two sides. 2-Chloroprocaine is often used for this block because it undergoes rapid intravascular hydrolysis and has a very short intravascular half-life if accidentally injected intravascularly or into the fetus. Lidocaine is also used, but bupivacaine is contraindicated.

Paracervical block is associated with a relatively high incidence of fetal bradycardia. The mechanism of this phenomenon is unclear but probably involves decreased uterine blood flow secondary to the vasoconstrictor properties of local anesthetics. The bradycardia is usually limited to less than 15 minutes, and treatment is supportive, consisting of lateral positioning and administration of oxygen. Because the fetal bradycardia is associated with increased neonatal morbidity and mortality, this block is rarely performed and should be avoided in patients with evidence of uteroplacental insufficiency or nonreassuring fetal heart rate patterns (Thiery and Vroman, 1972).

### Pudendal Block

The obstetrician performs a pudendal block with a transvaginal technique, guiding a sheathed needle to the vaginal mucosa and sacrospinous ligament just medial and posterior to the ischial spine. Although the technique provides analgesia for vaginal delivery or uncomplicated instrumental vaginal delivery, the rate of failure is high, and the block achieved is often inadequate for mid-forceps application, examination of the cervix and upper vagina, or manual exploration of the uterus after delivery. In many centers, this technique is used when epidural or spinal blocks are unavailable. Complications in addition to failure include vaginal lacerations, systemic local anesthetic toxicity, ischiorectal or vaginal hematoma, and, rarely, fetal injection of local anesthetic.

### Perineal Infiltration

Infiltration of the perineum is commonly performed by obstetricians to provide anesthesia for episiotomy and its repair. Care is taken to avoid both injection into the fetal scalp and excessive (total) doses of local anesthetic agents. This is a common and useful technique when used either alone or in conjunction with other regional blocks.

### Anesthesia For Cesarean Delivery

Although the majority of cesarean deliveries are performed with regional anesthesia, the use of general anesthesia is sometimes required by the severity of the fetal condition (e.g., severe fetal heart rate deceleration) or when regional anesthesia is contraindicated. Regardless, in preparation for cesarean delivery, all women should receive an oral antacid (nonparticulate, such as sodium citrate) to reduce gastric content pH; some anesthesiologists routinely co-administer an agent to accelerate gastric emptying—metoclopramide, an histamine$_2$ receptor antagonist (e.g., ranitidine) or both—to reduce production of gastric acid.

### Epidural Anesthesia

Epidural anesthesia is an excellent choice for surgical anesthesia when an indwelling, functioning epidural catheter had been placed for labor analgesia. It is also ideal for patients who cannot tolerate the sudden onset of a sympathectomy, such as some patients with cardiac disease. The volume and concentration of local anesthetic agents used for surgical anesthesia are larger than those used for labor analgesia; however, the technique of catheter placement, test dosing, and potential complications are similar. Typically, the anesthesiologist attempts to provide a dense block from the T4 level to the sacrum. This technique may not always alleviate the visceral pain associated with peritoneal manipulation, and adjuvant drugs may be necessary.

### Spinal Anesthesia

For the patient without an epidural catheter (e.g., a patient undergoing elective cesarean delivery or a laboring patient who has not been given an epidural block), spinal anesthesia is the most common regional anesthetic technique used for cesarean delivery. The block is technically easier than epidural blockade, more rapid in onset, and more reliable in providing surgical anesthesia from the mid-thoracic level to the sacrum (Riley et al, 1995). The incidence of post–dural puncture headache has fallen with the introduction of noncutting, "pencil point" spinal needles. However, the risk of hypotension is much higher and the hypotension more profound with spinal anesthesia than with epidural anesthesia, because the onset of the sympathectomy is more rapid. Prehydration, avoidance of aortocaval compression, and aggressive use of ephedrine (even as a prophylactic) results in very favorable conditions and outcome. Data also suggest that spinal anesthesia can be safely used for patients with preeclampsia (Wallace et al, 1995; Hood and Curry, 1999).

### Local Anesthesia

Although cesarean delivery can be performed with local infiltration, it is accompanied with considerable discomfort to the woman and risks the possibility of local anesthetic overdose; also, most obstetricians have not been trained to perform the technique. However, in rare circumstances, such as acute fetal distress, inadequacy of a regional block, and in patients for whom induction of general anesthesia is considered dangerous (e.g., morbid obesity), local infiltration can be helpful to at least deliver the baby. Then general anesthesia can be induced after the patient's airway has been secured while she is awake (using fiberoptic or other techniques).

## GENERAL ANESTHESIA

General anesthesia is used in obstetric practice for cesarean section typically when regional anesthesia is contraindicated (e.g., coagulopathy, certain cardiac lesions, hemorrhage) or for emergencies because of its rapid and predictable action (e.g., placental abruption, uterine rupture, fetal bradycardia, prolapsed umbilical cord). General anesthesia should be administered after placement of a cuffed endotracheal tube, due to the risks of pulmonary aspiration of acidic gastric contents as previously described.

After induction of anesthesia by "rapid sequence," anesthesia is maintained by administration of a combination of inhaled nitrous oxide, an inhaled potent halogenated agent (e.g., isoflurane), sedative-hypnotics, and opioid analgesics, and intravenous skeletal muscle relaxants are administered to decrease muscle tone and facilitate surgery.

## Induction Agents

A number of different agents are used by anesthesiologists to rapidly induce unconsciousness. Among the most common are thiopental, ketamine, and, to a lesser extent, etomidate and propofol. Each agent represents a different biochemical class, and each has specific advantages and cardiovascular effects.

Sodium thiopental is a highly lipid-soluble, protein-bound barbiturate that rapidly crosses the placenta and produces a dose-related global depression in the neonate. It is the most commonly used agent for induction of general anesthesia in obstetrics. Intravenous administration of an appropriate dose (4 to 6 mg/kg) renders the patient unconscious within 30 seconds and has no significant clinical effect on neonatal well-being. Although the drug undergoes hepatic oxidation to inactive, water-soluble metabolites, patients awaken within 15 minutes of initial administration because of rapid redistribution of the drug from vessel-rich organs (including the brain) to muscle and fat. Neonatal depression is found with higher dosages of barbiturates, however, which must be treated by cardiorespiratory supportive techniques until the neonate can excrete the drug; this process may take up to 2 days (Fox et al, 1979).

Ketamine, a structural analogue to phencyclidine, is more lipid soluble and less protein bound than thiopental. These characteristics lead to rapid brain uptake and subsequent redistribution, with awakening due to redistribution to peripheral tissue rather than metabolism. Ketamine is biotransformed in the liver to active metabolites, such as norketamine. In contrast to thiopental, ketamine increases arterial pressure, heart rate, and cardiac output through central stimulation of the sympathetic nervous system. Doses above those appropriate for induction of unconsciousness can increase uterine tone, reducing uterine arterial perfusion. In low doses (0.25 mg/kg), ketamine has profound analgesic effects, unlike barbiturates, but has been associated with undesirable psychotomimetic side effects (e.g., illusions, bad dreams), which can be lessened by co-administration of benzodiazepines. Many authorities consider this agent a more appropriate choice for the parturient who is actively hemorrhaging, for whom blood volume is uncertain and there is risk of profound hypotension in response to intravenous thiopental.

Etomidate contains a carboxylated imidazole ring, which provides water solubility in acidic solutions and lipid solubility at physiologic pH. Like thiopental, etomidate has a rapid onset of action because of its high lipid solubility, and redistribution results in a relatively short duration of action. Unlike thiopental and ketamine, etomidate has minimal effects on the cardiovascular system, but it is painful on injection and induces extrapyramidal motor activity and so is rarely used in obstetrics.

Propofol is a diisopropylphenol, available as a 1% aqueous solution in an oil-in-water emulsion containing soybean oil, glycerol, and egg lecithin. Because this preparation is preservative free, it does not lend itself to use in many labor and delivery units, where it is crucial to have syringes of induction agents ready to administer for rapid response to urgent situations requiring induction of general anesthesia (e.g., fetal distress). For an elective cesarean section, this highly lipid-soluble drug results in a rapid onset of action (about that of thiopental) and a very short initial distribution half-life, with less "hangover" effect than thiopental. However, propofol has not been demonstrated to be superior to thiopental in maternal or neonatal outcome. Further, it has been associated with maternal bradycardia when administered with succinylcholine for induction of general anesthesia for cesarean section.

## Nitrous Oxide

See previous discussion of this agent under "Inhalation Analgesia."

## Halogenated Hydrocarbons

Halothane, enflurane, isoflurane, sevoflurane, and desflurane are all halogenated hydrocarbons that differ in chemical composition, physical properties, biotransformation, potencies, and rates of uptake and elimination. In clinical use, specialized vaporizers deliver these volatile liquid agents, so the inhaled concentrations can be carefully titrated by anesthesiologists due to their relatively profound cardiovascular effects and potential for uterine muscle relaxation. These agents are important components of general anesthesia for cesarean section but readily cross the placenta. Without use of these agents, the incidence of maternal recall of intraoperative events is unacceptably high (Schultetus et al, 1986; Tunstall, 1979).

Placental transfer of inhalation agents is rapid because these are non-ionized, highly lipid-soluble substances of low molecular weight. The concentrations of these agents in the fetus depend directly on the concentration and duration of anesthetic in the mother. If excessive concentrations of anesthetic are given for inordinately long times, neonatal anesthesia, evidenced by flaccidity, cardiorespiratory depression, and decreased tone, can be anticipated (Moya, 1966). It cannot be overemphasized that if the neonatal depression is due to transfer of anesthetic drugs, the infant is merely lightly anesthetized and should respond easily to simple treatment measures. Treatment should include effective ventilation; cardiopulmonary resuscitation is rarely necessary. Ventilation will allow excretion of the inhalation anesthetic by the infant's lungs. Rapid improvement of the infant should be expected; if not, a search for other causes of depression is imperative.

Clinicians often confuse the use of general anesthesia, "fetal distress," and the depressed neonate. A "depressed" fetus will likely become a depressed neonate, and general anesthesia may be employed because it is the most rapidly acting anesthetic to allow cesarean delivery. However, for a healthy fetus, the use of general anesthesia is not contraindicated; the induction–delivery interval is not as important in neonatal outcome as the uterine incision–delivery interval, during which uterine blood flow may be compromised and fetal asphyxia may occur. A long induction–delivery time may result in a neonate who is lightly anesthetized but not asphyxiated.

The opioid analgesics have already been described. During typical general anesthesia for cesarean delivery, opioids are administered after the baby is delivered, to avoid placental transfer of these agents to the neonate.

### Neuromuscular Blocking Agents

Succinylcholine remains the skeletal muscle relaxant of choice for obstetric anesthesia because of its rapid onset and short duration of action. This depolarizing neuromuscular blocking agent is normally hydrolyzed in maternal blood by the enzyme pseudocholinesterase and usually does not interfere with fetal neuromuscular activity. If the hydrolytic enzyme is present either in low concentrations (Shnider, 1965) or in a genetically determined atypical form (Brada et al, 1975), prolonged maternal or neonatal respiratory depression secondary to muscular paralysis can occur.

Nondepolarizing neuromuscular blocking agents are titrated to the response shown by neuromuscular stimulation monitoring for continued neuromuscular blockade. Under normal circumstances, the poorly lipid-soluble, highly ionized, nondepolarizing neuromuscular blockers (e.g., D-tubocurarine, pancuronium, atracurium, vecuronium) do not cross the placenta in amounts significant enough to cause neonatal muscle weakness (Kivalo and Saaroski, 1972). This placental impermeability is only relative, however, and when large doses are given over long periods, as in the treatment of maternal tetanus or status epilepticus, neonatal neuromuscular blockade can occur (Older and Harris, 1968).

The diagnosis of neonatal depression secondary to neuromuscular blockade may be made on the basis of the maternal history (e.g., prolonged administration of neuromuscular blockers, history of atypical pseudocholinesterase), the response of the mother to neuromuscular blocking drugs, and the physical examination of the newborn. The paralyzed neonate has normal cardiovascular function and good color but lacks spontaneous ventilatory movements, has muscle flaccidity, and shows no reflex responses. The anesthesiologist can place a nerve stimulator on the neonate and demonstrate the classic signs of neuromuscular blockade (Ali and Savarese, 1976). Treatment consists of respiratory support until the neonate excretes the drug, up to 48 hours. Reversal of nondepolarizing relaxants with cholinesterase inhibitors may be attempted (e.g., neostigmine, 0.06 mg/kg), but adequate respiratory support is the mainstay of treatment.

### Adjuvant Medications

In addition to opioids, anesthesiologists may administer benzodiazepines, antiemetic agents, and other agents, but they typically do so only after the baby is delivered and the cord has been clamped. These drugs are rarely administered before delivery in doses large enough that placental transfer has a clinically important neonatal effect.

## SUMMARY

Maternal anesthetics may affect the fetus and neonate through diffusion from the maternal circulation to the fetal circulation, causing direct drug effects. However, these drugs are the same as those used for neonatal surgery in which they are directly administered to the neonate. Properly managed, these drugs are not toxic to the neonate. Serial dilutions, protein-tissue binding, and maternal administration of restricted doses usually protect the fetus from the effects of anesthetic drugs administered to the mother.

An anesthetic drug or technique may affect the fetus indirectly, producing the signs and symptoms of fetal distress and asphyxia; treatment is based on restoring placental exchange, perfusion, and gas exchange. Any technique that results in maternal hypotension, hypoxia, or both will decrease maternal-fetal oxygen exchange and produce fetal distress. Examples are overdose with opioid or inhalation analgesia, total spinal anesthesia, and maternal aspiration of gastric contents.

Uteroplacental blood flow depends on an adequate maternal cardiac output and perfusion pressure. Anesthetic techniques that interfere with maternal cardiovascular integrity can produce fetal depression by (1) increasing uterine arterial tone (e.g., use of drugs with primarily α-adrenergic activity), (2) decreasing cardiac output (e.g., decreased venous return caused by vena caval compression by the gravid uterus; venodilation and bradycardia secondary to the sympathectomy accompanying spinal or epidural block; myocardial depression due to overdose of potent inhalation anesthetic or local anesthetic drug) or (3) decreasing systemic blood pressure (e.g., sympathectomy due to high spinal or epidural anesthesia).

An increase in uterine muscular tone can reduce uteroplacental perfusion by impeding venous outflow from the intervillous space (Vasicka and Kretchmer, 1961). High levels of local anesthetics (e.g., after intravascular injection) or of α-adrenergic vasopressors may produce increased myometrial tone and fetal distress, particularly when combined with oxytocin stimulation.

In general, modern techniques of obstetric analgesia for labor and anesthesia for instrumental vaginal delivery or cesarean delivery are safe and effective for the mother and safe for the fetus and neonate. The analgesics and anesthetics, however, must be administered by skilled clinicians who observe appropriate precautions and understand the physiologic changes in pregnancy. Skillful labor analgesia coupled with emotional support for the parturient may not only reduce maternal stress but decrease intrapartum stress for the fetus as well (Jouppila et al, 1978; Morishima et al, 1978).

## REFERENCES

Ali HH, Savarese JJ: Monitoring of neuromuscular function. Anesthesiology 45:216, 1976.

American Heart Association: Advanced Cardiac Life Support: Special Resuscitation Situations. 11-8, 11-9, 1997.

Apgar V: A proposal for a new method of evaluation of the newborn infant. Curr Res Anesth Analg 32:260, 1953.

Behar M, Magora F, Olshwang D, Davidson JT: Epidural morphine in treatment of pain. Lancet 1:527, 1979.

Bonica JJ: Principles and Practice of Obstetric Analgesia and Anesthesia. Philadelphia, F.A. Davis Co, 1967.

Bouaziz H, Tong C, Eisenach JC: Postoperative analgesia from intrathecal neostigmine in sheep. Anesth Analg 80:1140, 1995.

Brada A, Haroun S, Bassili M, et al: Response of the newborn to succinylcholine injection in homozygotic atypical mothers. Anesthesiology 43:115, 1975.

Bricker L, Lavender T: Parenteral opioids for labor pain relief: A systematic review. Am J Obstet Gynecol 186(5 Suppl Nature): S49, 2002.

Bullingham RE, McQuay HJ, Moore RA: Clinical pharmacokinetics of narcotic agonist-antagonist drugs. Clin Pharmacokinet 8:139, 1983.

Camann WR, Denney RA, Holby ED, Datta S: A comparison of intrathecal, epidural, and intravenous sufentanil for labor analgesia. Anesthesiology 77:884, 1992.

Cheek TG, Gutsche BB: Maternal physiologic alterations during pregnancy. In Hughes SC, Levinson G, Rosen MA (eds): Shnider and Levinson's Anesthesia for Obstetrics. Baltimore, Lippincott Williams & Wilkins, 2002.

Chestnut DH, Owen CL, Bates JN, et al: Continuous infusion epidural analgesia during labor: A randomized double-blind comparison of 0.0625% bupivacaine/0.0002% fentanyl versus 0.125% bupivacaine. Anesthesiology 68:754, 1988.

Cohen SE, Cherry CM, Holbrook RH, et al: Intrathecal sufentanil for labor analgesia—sensory changes, side effects, and fetal heart rate changes. Anesth Analg 77:1155, 1993.

Cree IE, Meyer J, Hailey DM: Diazepam in labour. Br Med J 4:251, 1973.

Dathis F, Macheboeuf M, Thomas H, et al: Epidural analgesia with a bupivacaine-fentanyl mixture in obstetrics: Comparison of repeated injections and continuous infusion. Can J Anaesth 35:116, 1988.

Douglas MJ, Levinson G: Systemic medications for labor and delivery. In Hughes SC, Levinson G, Rosen MA (eds): Shnider and Levinson's Anesthesia for Obstetrics. Baltimore, Lippincott Williams & Wilkins, 2002.

Eisenach JC, De Kock M, Klimscha W: Alpha-adrenergic agonists for regional anesthesia. Anesthesiology 85:655, 1996.

Fogel ST, Daftary AR, Norris MC, et al: The incidence of clinically important fetal heart rate abnormalities: Combined spinal/epidural vs epidural anesthesia for labor. Reg Anesth Pain Med 24:A75, 1999.

Fox FS, Smith JB, Namba Y, et al: Anesthesia for cesarean section. Am J Obstet Gynecol 133:15, 1979.

Friedlander JD, Fox HE, Cain CF, et al: Fetal bradycardia and uterine hyperactivity following subarachnoid administration of fentanyl during labor. Reg Anesth 22:378, 1997.

Galloon S: Ketamine for obstetric delivery. Anesthesiology 44:522, 1976.

Guidelines for Perinatal Care, 5th ed. Elk Grove, IL, American Academy of Pediatricians; Washington, DC, American College of Obstetricians and Gynecologists, 2002.

Hicks JA, Jenkins JG, Newton MC, et al: Continuous epidural infusion of 0.075% bupivacaine for pain relief in labour: A comparison with intermittent top-ups of 0.5% bupivacaine. Anaesthesia 43:289, 1988.

Hingson RA, Edwards WB: Continuous caudal anesthesia: An analysis of the first ten thousand confinements thus managed with the report of the authors' first thousand cases. JAMA 123:538, 1943.

Honet JE, Arkoosh VA, Norris MC, et al: Comparison among intrathecal fentanyl, meperidine, and sufentanil for labor analgesia. Anesth Analg 69:122, 1989.

Hood DD, Curry R: Spinal versus epidural anesthesia for cesarean section in severely preeclamptic patients—a retrospective survey. Anesthesiology 90:1276, 1999.

Hughes SC, Rosen MA, Shnider SM, et al: Maternal and neonatal effects of epidural morphine for labor and delivery. Anesth Analg 63:319, 1984.

Hughes SC, Dailey PA, Landers D, et al: Parturients infected with human immunodeficiency virus and regional anesthesia: Clinical and immunologic response. Anesthesiology 82:32, 1995.

Jouppila R, Jouppila P, Hollmen A: Effect of segmental extradural analgesia on placental blood flow during normal labour. Br J Anaesth 50:563, 1978.

Kan, R, Hughes S, Rosen M, et al: Intravenous remifentanil, placental transfer, maternal and neonatal effects. Anesthesiology 88:1476, 1998.

Kaul B, Vallejo M, Ramanathan S, Mandell G: Epidural labor analgesia and neonatal sepsis evaluation rate: A quality improvement study. Anesth Analg 93:986, 2001.

Kivalo I, Saaroski S: Placental transmission and foetal uptake of C-dimethyltubocurarine. Br J Anaesth 44:557, 1972.

LeBoyer F: Birth without Violence. London, Wildwood House, 1975.

Lee BB, Ngan Kee WD, Lau WM, Wong AS: Epidural infusions for labor analgesia: A comparison of 0.2% ropivacaine, 0.1% ropivacaine, and 0.1% ropivacaine with fentanyl. Reg Anesth Pain Med 27:31, 2002.

Lee RV, Rodgers BD, White LM, Harvey RC: Cardiopulmonary resuscitation of pregnant women. Am J Med 81:311, 1986.

Levinson G, Shnider SM, DdeLorimier AA, et al: Effect of maternal hyperventilation on uterine blood flow and fetal oxygenation and acid-base status. Anesthesiology 40:340, 1974.

Li DF, Rees GA, Rosen M: Continuous extradural infusion of 0.0625% or 0.125% bupivacaine for pain relief in primigravid labour. Br J Anaesth 57:264, 1985.

Lieberman E, Lang JM, Frigoletto F, et al: Epidural analgesia, intrapartum fever, and neonatal sepsis evaluation. Pediatrics 99:415, 1997.

Marx GF, Orkin LR: Physiological changes during pregnancy. JAMA 19:258, 1958.

McAllister CB: Placental transfer and neonatal effects of diazepam when administered to women just before delivery. Br J Anaesth 52:423, 1980.

McIntosh DG, Rayburn WF: Patient-controlled analgesia in obstetrics and gynecology. Obstet Gynecol 78:1129, 1991.

Mercier FJ, Benhamou D: Hyperthermia related to epidural analgesia during labor. Int J Obstet Anesth 7:19, 1997.

Morishima HO, Adamsons K: Placental clearance of mepivacaine following administration to the guinea pig fetus. Anesthesiology 28:343, 1967.

Morishima HO, Pederson H, Finster M: The influence of maternal psychological stress on the fetus. Am J Obstet Gynecol 131:286, 1978.

Moya F: Volatile inhalation agents and muscle relaxants in obstetrics. Acta Anesthesiol Scand Suppl 25:368, 1966.

Nageotte MP, Larson D, Rumney PJ, et al: Epidural analgesia as compared with combined spinal epidural analgesia during labor in nulliparous women. N Engl J Med 337:1715, 1997.

O'Brien JE, Abbey V, Hinsvark O, et al: Metabolism and measurement of 2-chloroprocaine, an ester-type local anesthetic. J Pharm Sci 68:75, 1979.

Older PO, Harris JM: Placental transfer of tubocurarine. Br J Anaesth 40:459, 1968.

Olofsson C, Ekblom A, Ekman-Ordeberg G, et al: Lack of analgesic effect of systemically administered morphine or pethidine on labour pain. Br J Obstet Gynaecol 103:968, 1996.

Olufolabi AJ, Booth JV, Wakeling HG, et al: A preliminary investigation of remifentanil as a labor analgesic. Anesth Analg 91:606, 2000.

Parer JT, Rosen MA, Levinson G: Uteroplacental circulation and respiratory gas exchange. In Hughes SC, Levinson G, Rosen MA (eds): Shnider and Levinson's Anesthesia for Obstetrics, 4th ed. Baltimore, Lippincott Williams & Wilkins, 2002.

Powe CE, Kiem IM, Fromhagen C, et al: Propiomazine hydrochloride in obstetrical analgesia. JAMA 181:290, 1962.

Ralston DH, Shnider SM: The fetal and neonatal effects of regional anesthesia in obstetrics. Anesthesiology 48:34, 1978.

Riley ET, Cohen SE, Macario A, et al: Spinal versus epidural anesthesia for cesarean section: A comparison of time efficiency, costs, charges, and complications. Anesth Analg 80:709, 1995.

Rosen MA: Nitrous oxide for relief of labor pain: A systematic review. Am J Obstet Gynecol 186(5 Suppl Nature):S127, 2002.

Rosen MA, Hughes SC, Levinson G: Regional anesthesia for labor and delivery. In Hughes SC, Levinson G, Rosen MA (eds): Shnider and Levinson's Anesthesia for Obstetrics, 4th ed. Baltimore, Lippincott Williams & Wilkins, 2002.

Rosenblatt R, Wright R, Denson D, et al: Continuous epidural infusions for obstetric analgesia. Reg Anaesth 8:10, 1983.

Scher J, Hailey DM: The effects of diazepam on the fetus. J Obstet Gynaecol Br Commonw 79:635, 1972.

Schultetus RR, Hill CR, Dharamay CM, et al: Wakefulness during cesarean section after anesthetic induction with ketamine, thiopental, or ketamine and thiopental combined. Anesth Analg 65:723, 1986.

Segal S, Csavoy AN, Datta S: Placental tissue enhances uterine relaxation by nitroglycerin. Anesth Analg 86:304, 1998.

Shnider SM: Clinical and biochemical studies of cyclopropane analgesia in obstetrics. Anesthesiology 24:11, 1963.

Shnider SM: Serum cholinesterase activity during pregnancy, labor and puerperium. Anesthesiology 26:355, 1965.

Shnider SM, Moya F: Effects of meperidine on the newborn infant. Am J Obstet Gynecol 89:1009, 1960.

Shnider SM, Abboud TK, Artal R, et al: Maternal catecholamines decrease during labor after lumbar epidural anesthesia. Am J Obstet Gynecol 147:13, 1983.

Thiery M, Vroman S: Paracervical block analgesia during labour. Am J Obstet Gynecol 113:988, 1972.

Thurlow JA, Waterhouse P: Patient-controlled analgesia in labour using remifentanil in two parturients with platelet abnormalities. Br J Anaesth 84:411, 2000.

Tunstall ME: The reduction of amnesic wakefulness during caesarean section. Anaesthesia 34:316, 1979.

Vasicka A, Kretchmer H: Effect of conduction and inhalation anesthesia on uterine contractions. Am J Obstet Gynecol 82:600, 1961.

Volikas I, Male D: A comparison of pethidine and remifentanil patient-controlled analgesia in labor. Int J Obstet Anesth10:1, 2001.

Wallace DH, Leveno KJ, Cunningham FG, et al: Randomized comparison of general and regional anesthesia for cesarean delivery in pregnancies complicated by severe preeclampsia. Obstet Gynecol 86:193, 1995.

Wang JK, Nauss LA, Thomas JE: Pain relief by intrathecally applied morphine in man. Anesthesiology 50:149, 1979.

Yaksh TL: Spinal opiate analgesia: Characteristics and principles of action. Pain 11:293, 1981.

Yentis S: High regional block—the failed intubation of the new millenium? Int J Obstet Anesth 10:159, 2001.

PART V

# GENETICS

Editor: H. WILLIAM TAEUSCH

CHAPTER 17

## Impact of the Human Genome Project on Neonatal Care

DeWayne M. Pursley and Gary A. Silverman

### OVERVIEW AND HISTORY OF THE INTERNATIONAL HUMAN GENOME PROJECT

Since the 1970s, nearly all avenues of biomedical research have led to the gene, for genes contain the basic information about how the human body carries out its duties from conception until birth.

*Francis S. Collins, 1999*

Almost 50 years after Watson and Crick (1953) described the crystal structure of DNA, the International Human Genome Project (IHGP) completed sequencing the human genome. Inaugurated in October of 1990, this herculean task was achieved ahead of schedule (2 years shy of the 15-year goal) and under budget (0.3 billion dollars less than the 3 billion dollars allocated) and will radically change our understanding of human development, the pathogenesis of disease, and the diagnosis and treatment of constitutional and somatically acquired disorders. Although the impact of this new knowledge on clinical decision-making may be subtle at first, there is no doubt that the paradigms for clinical education and practice have been transformed.

The next major challenge for physicians and scientists is to unravel the complex links between genes and physiology (Duyk, 2003). Consider, for example, the complexity of a Boeing 747 jet. Imagine how difficult it might be to provide routine maintenance of this aircraft with only a rudimentary understanding of the location of its assembled parts, such as the engines, wings, and fuselage, and a limited knowledge of how these parts work together to achieve flight. In contrast, maintenance practices would be dramatically enhanced if a complete list of the aircraft's 6 million parts and an exact blueprint of how they are assembled were provided. Historically, physicians have cared for patients with a limited knowledge of their parts (gross anatomy) and how they function (physiology). Although the last 50 years have provided significant insight into the genetic basis of human development, anatomy, physiology, and disease, only a fraction of the molecular components that compose our body mass has been catalogued. Decoding the approximately 3 billion nucleotides that constitute our genome is a sentinel event in our quest to understand the complexity of human life. In essence, the IHGP has provided medicine with a "parts list" for creating a human. The daunting challenge ahead will be to synthesize the "blueprint" by determining how, when, and where the parts fit together during the human journey from conception to death.

The first concepts of a genome project were formulated at the Alta, Utah, conference in 1984 and the Santa Cruz, California, conference in 1985 (Watson, 1990). The concept was promulgated further by the U.S. Department of Energy (DOE). The DOE's interest stemmed from its Congressional mandate to track the heritable effects of radiation-induced DNA mutations. After vigorous scientific debate on the merits and costs of undertaking such a monumental task, a subcommittee of the National Research Council (NRC) in 1988 proposed that the United States, in collaboration with the international scientific community, undertake the task of sequencing the human genome. However, the subcommittee urged that the first 5 years of the project be focused on the generation of molecular and genetic maps as well as on improving the technology for mapping, DNA sequencing, and data handling (the birth of bio-informatics). Moreover, there was considerable interest in performing DNA mapping and sequencing projects for organisms that were the mainstays of biologic experimentation. As a consequence, the IGHP also included the analysis of model organisms such as bacteria (*Escherichia coli*), yeast (*Saccharomyces cerevisiae*), the roundworm (*Caenorhabditis elegans*), the fruit fly (*Drosophila melanogaster*), and the laboratory mouse (*Mus musculus*).

The inclusion of model organisms in the analysis was critical to the overall success of the program, for several reasons. First, by analyzing smaller genomes before more complex genomes (Table 17–1), scientists were able to develop more sophisticated sequencing, automation, and data management technologies. This "ramp-up" in technology was essential before an assault on the mega-sized, highly repetitive human sequence could even be considered. Second, by providing the sequence of model organisms, sequencing centers became integrated into the mainstream of experimental biology. Much as the 5′ end of RNA is processed while the 3′ end is still being synthesized,

**TABLE 17-1**

**Comparison of Genome Sizes**

| Organism | Haploid Genome Size (kilobases) | Approximate Number of Genes |
|---|---|---|
| Small DNA virus (SV40) | 5 | 6 |
| Bacteria (*Escherichia coli* K-12) | 4600 | 4400 |
| Yeast (*Saccharomyces cerevisiae*) | 12,000 | 6000 |
| Roundworm (*Caenorhabditis elegans*) | 100,000 | 19,000 |
| Fruit fly (*Drosophila melanogaster*) | 160,000 | 13,700 |
| Mouse (*Mus musculus*) | 3,000,000 | 30,000-40,000 |
| Human (*Homo sapiens*) | 3,000,000 | 30,000-40,000 |

biologists were analyzing data well before the complete sequences were available. As the genomes of prokaryotes, single-cell eukaryotes, and more complex multicellular organisms were unraveled (Table 17–2), the landscape for conducting science was shifting rapidly to a more global perspective in terms of how genes function within cellular systems and how they have been modified throughout evolution. Instead of thinking about single genes or molecules, scientists began to contemplate systems that were orders of magnitude more complex than could have been appreciated before complete genomic DNA sequences from multiple organisms were available. Third, the sequence of model organisms, with their increasing complexity, provided a reference point from which to compare the human sequence. Comparative genomic analysis is a powerful tool used to identify elements conserved throughout

**TABLE 17-2**

**International Human Genome Project (IHGP) Timeline**

| Year | Event |
|---|---|
| 1953 | Watson and Crick report on structure of DNA |
| 1996 | Genetic code revealed by Nirenberg, Khorana, and Holley |
| 1972 | Cohen and Boyer develop recombinant DNA technology |
| 1977 | DNA sequencing described by Sanger, Gilbert, and Maxam |
| 1982 | GenBank established |
| 1983 | First disease-related gene mapped (Huntington disease) |
| 1985 | Polymerase chain reaction (PCR) developed by Mullis |
| 1986 | First disease-related gene cloned by position (dystrophin) |
| 1987 | U.S. Department of Energy (DOE) recommends that the nation commit to a large, multidisciplinary, scientific, and technologic undertaking to map and sequence the human genome |
| 1988 | National Research Council (NRC) and U.S. Office of Technology Assessment (OTA) recommend that the United States map and sequence the human genome with National Institutes of Health (NIH) and DOE support |
| 1989 | Cystic fibrosis transmembrane conductance regulator (CFTR) cloned |
| 1988 | DOE establishes three genome centers |
| 1989 | NIH Director James Wyngaarden establishes National Center for Human Genome Research, with James Watson as director; Francis Collins becomes director in 1993, and Center becomes an Institute (NHGRI) in 1997 |
| 1990 | IHGP begins at an estimated cost of $200 million/year × 15 years ($3 billion) |
| 1991 | First NIH-funded genome centers established |
| 1995 | *Haemophilus influenzae* genome completed (first prokaryotic genome sequenced) |
| 1996 | *Saccharomyces cerevisiae* (yeast) genome completed (first unicellular eukaryotic genome sequenced |
| 1997 | *Escherichia coli* genome completed |
| 1998 | *Caenorhabditis elegans* (roundworm) genome completed (first multicellular eukaryote sequenced) |
| 1999 | Large-scale sequencing of the human genome begins |
| 1999 | Human chromosome 22 completed |
| 2000 | Human genome draft sequence completed |
| 2000 | *Drosophila melanogaster* (fruit fly) genome completed |
| 2000 | *Arabidopsis thaliana* (plant) genome completed |
| 2001 | Human genome draft published |
| 2002 | Mouse genome draft published |
| 2002 | Rat genome draft completed |
| 2003 | Human genome completed |

Adapted from Collins FS, Green ED, Guttmacher AE, Guyer MS: A vision for the future of genomics research. Nature 422:835-847, 2003.

evolution or those unique to individual lines of descent. In general, the conservation of genes between humans and other organisms provides insight into human gene function by facilitating the study of their homologues (related by local duplication events) or orthologues (related by direct descent) in more tractable experimental systems. These model systems (see later) have been crucial in elucidating fundamental biologic and disease-related processes (Table 17–3).

The DOE in 1987 and the National Institutes of Health (NIH) in 1988 began to allocate funds for genomic research. With a more substantial fiscal appropriation in 1989, the NIH Office of Genome Research became the National Center for Human Genome Research. A joint NIH-DOE subcommittee further defined the program's first 5-year goals, and the IHGP began officially on October 1, 1990 (Collins, 1999). The United Kingdom, Canada, France, Germany, Italy, Australia, Japan, and China also joined the effort. The first draft sequence of the human genome was reported in 2001 (Lander et al, 2001; Venter et al, 2001). Although obtaining the complete human genomic DNA sequence (99%) with 99.99% accuracy (and no gaps) was the primary goal of the project, the program also yielded a series of accomplishments and technologic advances, which are outlined in Table 17–2. In addition, the project provided scientists with a treasure trove of cloned resources (genomic DNA clones and complementary DNA [cDNA]) that could be used for functional and diagnostic studies.

A rough scorecard shows that the human genome contains between 30,000 and 40,000 genes. This number does not, however, take into account all of the genes encoding nontranslated RNAs—for example, transfer RNAs (tRNAs), ribosomal RNAs (rRNAs), rRNA-processing small nucleolar RNAs (snoRNAs), splicing-associated small nuclear RNAs (snRNAs), telomerase RNA, signal recognition particle 7SL RNA, and Xist RNA. Many of these RNAs are likely to mediate important regulatory roles and possibly epigenetic alterations of the genome in a cell-specific fashion. Only 2% of the genome encodes for proteins, whereas more than 50% of the genome contains various types of repetitive elements (e.g., short interspersed elements [SINEs], long interspersed elements [LINEs]). Of the protein-coding genes, approximately 60% are alternatively spliced. Alternative splicing combined with a myriad of post-translational modifications (e.g., glycosylation, prenylation, phosphorylation) add to the diversity of protein function.

**TABLE 17–3**

**Fundamental Biologic Processes Studied in Model Organisms**

| Organism | Process |
|---|---|
| Bacteria | Gene regulation |
| Yeast | Cell cycle control, mitosis, proteosome function |
| Nematodes | Apoptosis, aging, stress response, chemoreception, neural development, axonal guidance, ion channels, receptor tyrosine kinase signaling |
| Fruit flies | Innate immunity, development |
| Zebrafish | Hematopoiesis and cardiac, retinal, and vertebrate development |
| Mice and rats | Models for many human diseases including hypertension and cancer, genomic imprinting |

A more important set of instruction books will never be found by human beings.

*James Watson (1990)*

## IMPACT ON CLINICAL PRACTICE

### Identification and Molecular Diagnosis of Disease-Related Genes

#### Individual Gene Assessments and Antecedents to Adult Disease

Diseases primarily attributable to single genes are termed *monogenic* or *mendelian disorders*, because their heritability follows the heritability of the classic autosomal dominant, autosomal recessive, and sex-linked modes of inheritance (Guttmacher and Collins, 2002). Mutations in regulatory regions of genes may have profound effects on the rates of RNA synthesis, splicing, and stability. All of these factors can result in an abnormal phenotype through a quantitative effect on gene activity. Mutations in coding regions may be due to single-nucleotide changes or to small insertions and deletions (*indels*). Single-nucleotide changes may result in silent (no change in the amino acid encoded), missense (conservative or nonconservative amino acid change), or nonsense (stop codon) mutations. Although most silent mutations appear to be benign, single-nucleotide variants may effect codon usage or activate cryptic splice sites, leading to alternative splicing or *frame-shifts*. Similar events can occur with indels, even if they appear within introns. Other modes of monogenic inheritance associated with disease are mitochondrial inheritance, tri-nucleotide repeat expansion with successive generations (anticipation), genomic imprinting, and uniparental disomy.

The target genes have now been identified for well over 100 monogenic disorders. Many of these disorders manifest in the newborn period (Table 17–4). Although the locations of some of these genes were pinpointed at the breakpoints of chromosomal aberrations—for example, the cloning of dystrophin was facilitated by the identification of rare females with Duchenne muscular dystrophy and constitutional translocations involving Xp21 (Ray et al, 1985)—most were isolated by positional cloning. *Positional cloning* is a multiple-step technique whereby a disease-related gene is identified from its location in the genome and without any prior knowledge of its function (Collins, 1992). For example, a disease phenotype is segregating within an extended family (*pedigree*) with an apparent autosomal recessive mode of inheritance. DNA is collected from both affected and unaffected family members and scored for the presence of highly polymorphic genetic markers that map to precise locations throughout the genome. Linkage analysis is used

**TABLE 17-4**

**Monogenic Disorders Presenting in Newborns**

| Disorder | Gene | Location | OMIM Number |
|---|---|---|---|
| α1-Antitrypsin deficiency | *SERPINA1* | 14q32.1 | 107400 |
| Achondroplasia | *FGFR3* | 4p16.3 | 134934, #100800 |
| Adrenoleukodystrophy | *ABCD2* | 12q11 | 601081, #300100 |
| Alport syndrome | *COL4A5* | Xq22.3 | 303630 |
| Angelman syndrome | *UBE3A* | 15q11.2 | 601623, #105830 |
| Cockayne syndrome | *CKN1* | 5q12 | 216400, |
| | *ERCC6* | 10q11 | 133540 |
| Congenital adrenal hyperplasia | *CYP21* (most common cause) | 6p21.3 | 201910 |
| Cystic fibrosis | CFTR | 7q31 | 602421, #219700 |
| Diastrophic dysplasia | *SLC26A2* | 5q32 | 606718 |
| Fragile X syndrome | *FMR1* | Xq27.3 | 309550 |
| Gaucher disease | *GBA* | 1q22 | 606463 |
| Hereditary hemochromatosis | *HFE* | 6p21.3 | 235200 |
| Lesch-Nyhan syndrome | *HPRT1* | Xq26 | 308000 |
| Long QT syndrome-1 | *KCNQ1* | 11p15.5 | 607542 |
| Maple syrup urine disease | *BCKDH* | 19q13.1 | 248600 |
| Marfan syndrome | *FBN1* | 15q21.1 | 134797, #154700 |
| Menkes disease | *ATP7A* | Xq12 | 300011 |
| Myotonic dystrophy | *DMPK* | 19q13.2 | 605377 |
| Neurofibromatosis | *NF1* | 17q11.2 | 162200 |
| | NF2 | 22q12.2 | 101000 |
| Pendred syndrome | *SLC26A4* | 7q31 | 605646 |
| Phenylketonuria | *PAH* | 12q24.1 | 261600 |
| Refsum disease | *PHYH* | 10p11.2 | 602026 |
| Retinoblastoma | *RB1* | 13q14.1-q14.2 | 180200 |
| Rett syndrome | *MECP2* | Xq28 | 300005 |
| Severe combined immunodeficiency | *ADA* | 20q13.11 | 102700 |
| | *JAK3* | 19p13.1 | 600173 |
| | *IL2RG* | Xq13 | 308380 |
| | *LCK* | 1p35 | 153390 |
| Spinal muscular atrophy | *SMN1* | 5q12.2 | 600354 |
| Tay-Sachs disease | *HEXA* | 15q23 | 606869 |
| Tuberous sclerosis | *TSC1* | 9q34 | 605284 |
| | *TSC2* | 16p13.3 | 191092 |
| Von Hippel–Lindau syndrome | *VHL* | 3p26-p25 | 193300 |
| Waardenburg syndrome type 1 | *PAX3* | 2q35 | 606597, #193500 |
| Werner syndrome | *RECQL2* | 8p12 | 604611 |
| Williams syndrome | *ELN* | 7q11.2 | 130160, #194050 |
| | *LIMK1* | 7q11.2 | 601329 |
| Wilson disease | *ATP7B* | 13q14.3 | 606882 |
| Zellweger syndrome | *PXR1* | 12p13.3 | *600414 |

OMIM, Online database of Mendelian Inheritance in Man.

*Modified from Genes and Disease. Available online at www.ncbi.nlm.nih.gov/books/bv.fcgi?call = bv.View..ShowSection&rid = gnd

to determine which allelic variant is most closely linked (*segregating*) with the disease phenotype. Because the position of the linked marker is known, the area surrounding this locus is analyzed for the presence of genes. In turn, these genes are screened for mutations in individuals with the disease phenotype and compared with those of unaffected family members. Depending on the genomic region to be searched, investigators might have to identify and then sift through tens or hundreds of genes for mutations. This arduous, labor-intensive task commonly required tens to hundreds of personnel years to identify the correct gene. However, by having the complete genomic DNA sequence and list of genes for a region, investigators can make intelligent decisions about which genes to analyze before conducting a single mutation screen. This candidate gene approach has significantly shortened the time (months) and person power (a few workers) needed to successfully isolate a disease-related gene.

Unlike for monogenic disorders, the identification of genes associated with complex traits, such as cancer, Alzheimer's disease, cardiovascular disease, and diabetes, is more difficult (Nabel, 2003; Nussbaum and Ellis, 2003; Wooster and Weber, 2003). In part, this difficulty is due to the limited contribution of many or at least several genes to a disease process as well as to the profound effects of environmental, behavioral, and epigenetic factors on disease prevalence. Moreover, the effects of variable penetrance and expressivity of individual genes and the presence of heterogeneous disease phenotypes limit the use of simple pedigree analysis to analyze these disorders. Although any two individuals are 99.9% identical at the nucleotide level, the 0.1% difference translates to single-nucleotide polymorphisms (SNPs) occurring about once every thousand base-pairs. This inherent variability within the human genome provides an opportunity to combine SNP analysis with population studies to pinpoint *haplotypes* (clusters of SNPs that are inherited together on the same chromosomal segment and tend to be passed from generation to generation owing to their tight linkage) associated with disease phenotypes (Gibbs et al, 2003; Goldstein et al, 2003). By identifying common haplotypes associated with different individuals who have similar disease phenotypes (*linkage dysequilibrium*), investigators can begin to identify regions of the genome (due to their common haplotypes) containing genes that contribute to the disease process or increase the risk of development of an abnormal phenotype.

### Newborn Screening

The expansion of newborn screening programs to detect amino acidemias, organic acidemias, and disorders of fatty acid oxidation has been facilitated by the use of tandem mass spectrometry (Wilcken et al, 2003). The use of mass spectrometry along with DNA sequence–based techniques to detect disease-related genes and their mutations, genotype-phenotype correlations are providing greater insight into the molecular basis and developmental import of these genetic disorders. See Chapter 27 for a more detailed discussion of this topic.

### Molecular Cytogenetics

Classic karyotyping using Giemsa-banded chromosomes has been a diagnostic stalwart for aneuploidy syndromes (trisomies and monosomies) and for segmental chromosomal deletions and translocations for decades. The advent of fluorescence in situ hybridization (FISH) and spectral karyotyping (SKY) permits the diagnosis of many of these disorders more precisely and rapidly with the use of interphase nuclei or standard metaphase spreads (Tonnies, 2002). These techniques have also proved invaluable for pre-conception testing of polar bodies, chorionic villus cells, and amniocytes for trisomies 13, 18, and 21 and aneuploidies of the sex chromosomes (Lim et al, 2002). Also, FISH has been useful in identifying subsegmental deletions associated with, for example, the DiGeorge and Miller-Dieker syndromes and single-gene defects (Table 17–5). Subtelomeric fluorescent probes have been used in detecting submicroscopic deletions (<4 megabases [Mb]) in a subset of children with mental retardation (Clarkson et al, 2002). The availability of bacterial artificial chromosomes (BACs) and other types of clones spanning the entire human genome provide a complete array of probe material for identifying additional disorders associated with subtle chromosomal aberrations.

**TABLE 17–5**

**Disorders Detected by Fluorescence In Situ Hybridization or Spectral Karyotyping**

| Disorder | Locus | Gene(s) |
|---|---|---|
| Wolf-Hirschhorn syndrome (4p- syndrome, del[4p] syndrome, monosomy 4p) | 4p16.3 | *WHCR* |
| Cri du chat syndrome (5p-syndrome) | 5p15.2 | |
| Sotos syndrome (cerebral gigantism) | 5q35 | *NSD1* |
| Williams syndrome | 7q11.2 | *WBSCR* |
| Prader-Willi syndrome | 15q11.2-q13 | (*PWCR*) |
| Angelman syndrome | 15q11.2-q13 | Ubiquitin-protein ligase E3A (*UBE3A*) |
| Rubinstein-Taybi syndrome (broad thumbs-hallux syndrome) | 16p13.3 | CREB-binding protein (*CREBBP*) |
| 17-linked lissencephaly (17-linked subcortical band heterotopia, isolated 17-linked lissencephaly, Miller-Dieker syndrome) | 17p13.3 | Platelet-activating factor acetylhydrolase IB alpha subunit (*PAFAH1B1*) |
| Hereditary neuropathy with liability to pressure palsies | 17p11.2 | Peripheral myelin protein 22 (*PMP22*) |
| Smith-Magenis syndrome (del[17][p11.2]) | 17p11.2 | Retinoid-acid induced protein 1 (*RAI1*) |
| 22q11.2 deletion syndrome (Cayler cardiofacial syndrome, conotruncal anomaly face syndrome, DiGeorge syndrome, Opitz G/BBB, Sedlackova syndrome, Shprintzen syndrome, velocardiofacial syndrome) | 22q11.2 | *DGCR* |
| Chromosome 22q13.3 deletion syndrome | 22q13.3 | Arylsulfatase A (*ARSA*) |
| Ichthyosis, X-linked (steroid sulfatase deficiency) | Xp22.32 | Steryl-sulfatase (*STS*) |
| Kallmann syndrome, X-linked (hypogonadotropic hypogonadism/anosmia) | Xp22.3 | Anosmin 1 (*KAL1*) |
| Aneuploidy for chromosomes 21, 18, 13, X, and Y | — | — |
| Subtelomeric regions | — | — |

## Molecular Therapeutics

### Gene Replacement

The realization that genes are an underlying component of all human disease led to the anticipation that once the human genome was deciphered, clinicians would set about manipulating the genes for therapeutic purposes. For example, monogenic disorders (e.g., sickle cell disease, galactosemia, and cystic fibrosis) might be cured by providing endogenous cells with functional copies of wild-type genes, and tumor cells could be killed by giving them genes that make them more susceptible to inducible cell death signals. Although multiple gene therapy trials are under way and there have been some limited successes (as well as some well-publicized failures), this discipline is in its infancy (Balicki and Beutler, 2002).

The treatment of a monogenic disorder such as cystic fibrosis underscores the current difficulties in translating genomic science into effective gene therapy (West and Rodman, 2001). Cystic fibrosis is an autosomal recessive disorder associated with a variety of mutations involving the cystic fibrosis transmembrane conductance regulator (CFTR). The disease is characterized by multi-organ dysfunction due to decreased (or null) CFTR-mediated chloride channel activity. In the lung, a mutant CFTR is associated with thickened secretions, bacterial overgrowth, inflammation, and tissue destruction. Attempts to cure or ameliorate this disorder via gene replacement techniques illustrates many of the barriers that must be overcome before gene therapies become a mainstay of clinical practice. Initial studies using a recombinant adenoviral vector containing the CFTR cDNA showed a low transfection efficiency, transient expression, and a limited effect on overall chloride transport. Immune reactivity to the adenovirus precluded subsequent dosing using the same vector. Several trials using liposomes to deliver the CFTR cDNA to respiratory epithelium achieved greater transfection efficiency and higher levels of CFTR activity, but in general, the response waned over time.

The reasons for these suboptimal effects are multifactorial. Regardless of the mechanism of gene delivery in vivo, the transgene must traverse several physical barriers and access the correct cell types. The barriers include secretions, blood components, phagocytes, innate or acquired immune system molecules, extracellular matrix proteins such as sticky proteoglycans, proteases, and nucleases, and cell membranes (Balicki and Beutler, 2002). Upon entering the cell, the transgene must evade destruction in the endosomal compartment and gain access to the nucleus. In the nucleus, the transgene may remain episomal or may integrate into the host genome. If the host cell is capable of proliferating and the transgene remains episomal and does not replicate autonomously, it will eventually be lost with successive cell divisions. Integration of the transgene may lead to activation or disruption of other genes. These integration events could have profound effects, including transformation to a malignant state. For example, several children with the X-linked severe combined immunodeficiency type XI (SCID-XI) syndrome underwent immunologic correction, in which hematopoietic stem cells were transduced with a retrovirus containing $\gamma_c$ chain cytokine receptor (Hacein-Bey-Abina et al, 2003). Subsequently, a few patients demonstrated a leukemia-like disorder driven by activation of the *LMO2* oncogene. Integration of the retroviral vector near *LMO2* appeared to be the inciting event. Expression of the transgene in the nucleus is also subject to silencing mechanisms such as DNA methylation. Finally, if the transgene is transcribed, it is unlikely to contain the correct *cis*-acting elements to ensure that it will be properly regulated. Unregulated expression of certain proteins could lead to the accumulation of toxic aggregates or polymers that injure or kill cells.

The delivery mechanisms for gene replacement strategies include simple transformation using naked DNA, cationic complexes of DNA with lipids or peptides, and an array of viral vectors (Balicki and Beutler, 2002) (Table 17–6). Although each method has a unique set of advantages and disadvantages, none currently possesses all of the features that allow precise cellular targeting of the appropriate stem cell or long-lived cell population at high efficiency and with the capacity to sustain appropriate levels of expression (Thomas and Klibanov, 2003; Thomas et al, 2003). Viral vectors themselves, viral and transgene proteins, and transduced or transformed cells may also prove to be immunogenic and thereby limit the effectiveness of any protocol. Also, these immune responses can lead to untoward systemic reactions, as occurred in the fatal episode of shock and multi-organ dysfunction during an ornithine transcarbamylase (OTC) deficiency gene therapy trial using an adenovirus vector.

### Gene Repair

A major problem associated with gene replacement strategies is that the defective gene remains within the host genome and the inserted transgene is unlikely to contain enough surrounding control elements to ensure proper regulation. In some situations, the mutations of the endogenous alleles can lead to the production of a mutant gene product with dominant negative effects. In Marfan syndrome, an abnormal fibrillin-1 gene can yield an aberrant protein that interferes with normal microfibrillar assembly. Thus, gene replacement would be ineffective unless the mutant allele were silenced.

Targeted genetic repair offers an attractive alternative to simply infusing a cell with multiple copies of a wild-type allele. The advantages of gene repair strategies include elimination of the mutant gene product, use of the endogenous regulatory elements, and, owing to the site-specific nature of the repair process, minimization of random genome integration events (Sullenger, 2003). Gene repair strategies are also in their infancy but are currently focused on targeting either the pre–messenger RNA (Garcia-Blanco, 2003; Long et al, 2003; Sazani and Kole, 2003) or the gene itself (Gruenert et al, 2003; Kmiec, 2003; Seidman and Glazer, 2003). RNA repair strategies either pre-empt (*trans*-splicing ribozymes) or utilize the normal splicing process (*trans*-splicing or the use of antisense oligonucleotides to stimulate alternative splicing) (see Table 17–6). DNA repair strategies employ oligonucleotides or short DNA fragments to stimulate nucleotide excision or repair, homologous recombination, or gene conversion events (see Table 17–6).

**TABLE 17-6**

**Genetic Therapy of Mutant Gene Products or Alleles**

| Gene Therapy | Method | Mechanism | Advantages | Disadvantages |
|---|---|---|---|---|
| Gene replacements | Naked DNA | Direct transformation | No vectors needed | Small size<br>Not all cells transformed<br>Can elicit innate immunity |
| | Nonviral: Cationic liposomes (lipoplexes)<br>Cationic polymers (polyplexes) | Endosomal uptake | No vectors | Targeting difficult<br>Transformation efficiency<br>Complex stability |
| | Viral (capacity):<br>Adenovirus (8-30 kb)<br>Adeno-associated (AAV) (5 kb)<br>Retrovirus (8 kb)<br>Lentivirus (8 kb)<br>Herpes simplex virus-1 (HSV-1) (40-150 kb) | Infection or transduction | Some target specificity (HSV for neurons, transductional targeting by modifying vector capsids or by pseudotyping) Some vectors do not need dividing cells to integrate (lentivirus), whereas others do (retrovirus) | Some viruses induce potent immune response<br>Gene silencing<br>Possible integration of vector into genome, causing gene inactivation or activation (retroviruses and lentiviruses)<br>Repeated dosing in most cases may be necessary but difficult if immune reaction (adenovirus) |
| RNA repair | *Trans*-splicing using ribosomes | Group I or II introns (ribozymes) used to introduce new exon | No change in transcriptional regulation of gene<br>Control specificity | Route of delivery<br>Must get to nucleus<br>Need continuous source of construct |
| | *Trans*-splicing using spliceosome | Spliceosome-mediated RNA trans-splicing (SMaRT) used to introduce new exon | Control specificity | Route of delivery<br>Must get to nucleus<br>Need continuous source of construct |
| | Alternative splicing using oligonucleotides | Binding of oligonucleotide to splice sites suppresses splicing | Can control specificity | May get antisense (RNase H) effect and loss of message<br>Route of delivery<br>Must get to nucleus<br>Need to provide continuous source of oligonucleotide |
| DNA repair | Triplex-forming oligonucleotides | Triplex formation can induce nucleotide excision repair mechanism and recombination and/or gene conversion | Can be used for site specific DNA mutagenesis/ repair if triplex-forming oligonucleotide is bound to a short DNA segment, with the desired base change that is homologous to the target site<br>Can be used systemically, but oligonucleotides cannot cross blood-brain barrier | Targets limited to poly purine/polypyrimidine tracts<br>Limited access to nucleus<br>Inhibited by nucleosomes<br>Unique chemistries needed to synthesize oligonucleotides with good binding kinetics and stability |
| | Chimeric RNA-DNA oligonucleotides | Nucleotide exchange, mismatch repair | Specificity<br>Changes in situ<br>One-time fix | Delivery of oligonucleotides to cell<br>Poor uptake<br>Low frequency of correction |
| | Small single-stranded or double-stranded DNA fragments | Small fragment homologous replacement | Functions in vivo and in vitro<br>Transcription of target gene not necessary | |

The use of gene repair processes in vivo requires targeting the correct cells and is likely to suffer the same hurdles associated with the delivery of transgenes by viral and nonviral methods. One attractive use of gene repair, especially in the newborn period, involves ex vivo stem cell repair. In this scenario, a population of stem cells from an affected fetus or newborn is harvested from cord blood. The cells are cultured and transfected with a repair construct. Clones are analyzed molecularly for evidence of DNA repair and protein expression. The repaired clones are expanded and infused into the patient. Greater understanding of the identity, plasticity and function as well as the purification and culturing conditions for various stem cell and progenitor pools make this approach a realistic possibility within the next decade.

## RNA Interference

Most gene therapy strategies attempt to achieve a gain of gene function. However, under certain conditions, a loss of gene function (*gene silencing*) may be desirable. Gene silencing can occur at the transcriptional, post-transcriptional, or post-translational steps. Post-transcriptional strategies such as the use of antisense oligonucleotide technologies have been available for at least 25 years (Pirollo et al, 2003). However, their clinical use has been limited by delivery systems and their unpredictable mechanisms of action.

Another type of post-transcriptional gene silencing can occur when cells are exposed to double-stranded RNA (dsRNA) molecules (Paddison and Hannon, 2002). Although the mechanism has not been fully elucidated, dsRNA molecules are cleaved into shorter, 21- to 25-nucleotide fragments (small interfering RNAs [siRNAs]) by the RNAse III endonuclease Dicer (Shi, 2003). In turn, these siRNAs (presumably the antisense strand) bind to their target RNAs and guide their destruction by an RNA-induced silencing complex (RISC). This process, termed *RNA interference* (RNAi), is conserved among all eukaryotes and appears to be a natural defense against viruses and their dsRNA genomes or replication intermediates. RNAi-like processes also play a regulatory role in development. Initially, RNAi was thought to be impaired in higher eukaryotes, because the presence of dsRNA molecules more than 30 nucleotides in length induce a potent interferon response. This latter activity can result in a complete termination of protein synthesis and eventual cell death. However, if dsRNAs or short RNA "hairpins" (<30 nucleotides in length) are introduced into mammalian cells, RNAi can function (Brummelkamp et al, 2002). Under as yet undefined conditions, a modified or attenuated interferon response can still occur in the presence of small dsRNAs, but this response does not appear to disrupt the RNAi pathway (Sledz et al, 2003). RNAi is exquisitely sequence specific, and single-nucleotide mismatches may disrupt the process.

The clinical applications of RNAi require the delivery into cells of small dsRNA sequences or of vectors (plasmids or viral) expressing a small hairpin RNA construct driven by an RNA polymerase III promoter. Although this technology suffers from the delivery system limitations associated with all gene therapy strategies, RNAi will eventually be applied to the treatment of human disease. RNAi could be used to disrupt viral infection within the cell or to inactivate oncogenes within tumors. In the newborn period, RNAi might prove effective in quelling a vigorous immune response or repair processes associated with chronic lung disease or interfering with prostaglandin synthesis in a patent ductus arteriosus. Other applications are suppressing the production of misfolded (mutated) proteins, whose accumulation over time is toxic to cells (e.g., mutant $\alpha_1$-antitrypsin).

## DNA Vaccines

For many infectious agents, it has been difficult to develop vaccines using intact organisms or purified subcellular components. Also, many vaccination strategies preferentially stimulate humoral (antibody) responses and not cytolytic T ($CD8^+$) cell responses (Srivastava and Liu, 2003). Cytolytic T cells are important effectors in limiting the propagation of obligate intracellular pathogens, such as viruses and certain parasites and bacteria. The skewing of this immune response is due, in part, to the mechanism of protein handling by antigen-presenting cells (APCs). Exogenous proteins taken up by APCs are processed through the endosomal compartment, where the digested peptides combine with class II major histocompatibility (MHC) molecules. Class II MHC molecules loaded with peptides are transported to the surface, where they are presented to $CD4^+$ helper T cells. In turn, these activated, helper T cells can stimulate B cells to differentiate into antibody-producing plasma cells. In contrast, foreign proteins that gain access to the cytoplasm of APCs (e.g., by a viral infection) can be degraded and shuttled into the endoplasmic reticulum–Golgi pathway, where they encounter class I MHC molecules. After peptide loading, these MHC molecules are transported to the surface, where they can stimulate a $CD8^+$ cytolytic T cell response.

Because it is possible to construct bacterial plasmids or viral vectors to express either foreign or endogenous proteins in human cells, transgenes can be used to direct the synthesis and disposition (cytosolic or secreted) of any potential antigen (Garmory et al, 2003). DNA vaccines have been used to protect mice, guinea pigs, ferrets, and non-human primates against viral infections (e.g., influenza, herpes simplex virus [HSV], human immunodeficiency virus [HIV], hepatitis B virus [HBV]) and parasitic infections. However, phase 1 clinical trials in humans using genes from influenza, HIV, HBV, and *Plasmodium falciparum* have failed to generate significant protection. Vector modifications and combinations with more conventional vaccines or adjuvants are being used to augment the response to DNA vaccines. The results are too preliminary to allow one to determine whether these modalities will lead to a more effective use of DNA vaccines in humans.

## Pharmacogenomics

The individual response to a drug is governed by a multitude of factors, including age, environment, body mass, gender, intercurrent illness, and the presence of other medications (Johnson, 2003). Variations in absorption, volume of distribution, transporters, metabolism, and excretion (traditional pharmacokinetic variables) as well as the reactivity of intended and unintended targets also influence overall drug effect and toxicity (Weinshilboum, 2003). Genes associated with a number of these latter factors have already been determined (Table 17–7).

As the drug-associated effects of different genes and their variants are revealed, comprehensive genotyping or haplotyping at birth, possibly on a sequencing microchip, will provide physicians with a patient's comprehensive drug response profile. The goal is to use this profile to predict whether a particular patient is capable of responding to a drug to achieve a beneficial therapeutic index with minimal risks for toxicity and idiosyncratic reactions. Although current technology and knowledge of gene function preclude the ascertainment of individual drug response profiles at this time, genetic analysis already precedes treatment in some patients. For example, individuals with the Leiden variant (R506Q) of factor V are at increased risk for thrombotic events (Weinshilboum, 2003). This risk is even higher in women who are using birth control pills. Thus, prior knowledge of the presence of this variant in a woman would deter a physician from prescribing birth control pills for her. Mercaptopurine and azathioprine are purine antimetabolites used to treat acute lymphoblastic leukemia and autoimmune disorders. These drugs are metabolized by *S*-methylation via thiopurine *S*-methyltransferase (TPMT). Individuals with homozygous mutations of TMTP who are receiving standard doses of thiopurines are at risk for development of fatal bone-marrow suppression through the buildup of active 6-thioguanine nucleotides. Thus, in many candidates for thiopurine therapy, TMPT activity is commonly analyzed to determine whether the dosing regimen should be adjusted.

## Host-Pathogen Interactions

### Vaccine Development

Killed, live attenuated, and subunit conjugate vaccines have proved to be extremely effective in inducing protective immunity. In certain cases, however, traditional approaches fail to yield vaccines that are immunogenic or protective against different strains of the same species. One of the best examples is that of *Neisseria meningitidis* serotype B. The main capsular polysaccharide of this meningococcus is identical to a carbohydrate moiety (polysialic acid) in humans. Attempts to produce a vaccine against major surface proteins failed because of the antigenic variability between strains. To circumvent these problems, Pizza and colleagues (2000) used the genomic DNA sequence of *N. meningitidis* serotype B to search for genes encoding for novel surface-exposed or secreted proteins. Of 650 candidates, about half were amenable to expression and purification using standard *E. coli* expression systems. Thirty-five of these recombinant proteins, when injected into mice, yielded bactericidal antisera. Comparative genomic sequence analyses from 34 heterologous *N. meningitidis* serotype B clinical isolates showed that 5 of the protein antigens were highly conserved among these strains. These antigens are now being tested in phase 1 clinical trials.

### Microbial Genomics and Virulence Factors

To date, more than 140 bacterial (and ~1600 viral) genomes have been sequenced. Many of these organisms are significant human pathogens, including *Chlamydia trachomatis* and *Chlamydia pneumoniae*, *E. coli*, *Haemophilus influenzae*, *Listeria monocytogenes*, *Pseudomonas aeruginosa*, *Staphylococcus aureus*, *Streptococcus agalactiae* (group B

**TABLE 17–7**

**Examples of Types of Variant Genes That Effect Drug Responses**

| Phase I Drug-Metabolizing Enzymes | Phase II Drug-Metabolizing Enzymes | Drug Transporters | Drug Targets | Unintended Drug Targets |
|---|---|---|---|---|
| Cytochrome P-450 (CYP) enzymes | Thiopurine *S*-methyltransferase | ATP-binding cassette membrane transporters (e.g., *MDR1*) | $\beta_2$-adrenergic receptors | Factor V Leiden |
| CYP3A5 | *N*-Acetyltransferase 2 | | Angiotensin-converting enzyme (ACE) | Apolipoprotein E (ApoE) |
| CYP3A4 | Uridine diphosphate-glucuronosyltransferase 1A1 | | Arachidonate-5-lipoxygenase | Ion channels |
| CYP2D6 | | | Dopamine receptors | Prothrombin |
| CYPD2C9 | | | Serotonin transporters | Cholesterol ester transfer protein (CETP) |
| CYP2C19 | | | | |
| Butyrylcholinesterase | | | | |

Modified from Evans WE, McLeod HL: Pharmacogenomics: Drug disposition, drug targets, and side effects. N Engl J Med 348:538-549, 2003; and Weinshilboum R: Inheritance and drug response. N Engl J Med 348:529-537, 2003.

streptococcus), *Streptococcus pneumoniae*, and *Streptococcus viridans* (see The Institute for Genomic Research Web site, the Internet address of which is listed in Table 17–8). These bacterial genomes range in size from 580 kilobases (kb) (*Mycoplasma genitalium*) to 6300 kb (*P. aeruginosa*), with an average gene density of 1 per kilobase. Unlike DNA in the human genome, of which only about 2% contains coding sequence, 90% of DNA in bacterial genomes contains coding sequence (Chan, 2003; Fraser et al, 2000).

One of the most astonishing features of bacterial genome analysis is the significant variability among organisms. Depending on the species, 7% to 30% of the identified genes are unique to that species. Moreover, the variability between members of the same species can be significant. For example, the genome of the *E. coli* K-12 strain is 4600 kb in size and encodes for about 4300 genes, whereas the genome of the pathogenic *E. coli* O157:H7 strain is 5500 kb and encodes for about 5400 genes (Perna et al, 2001). Thus, the pathogenic strain contains about 1000 more genes, 25% of which are unique to that organism. On the basis of the percentage of similarity between the coding regions, these two *E. coli* strains appear to be more diverse evolutionarily than mice and humans.

Although some of this genomic diversity between strains may be due to local genomic duplications (e.g., O157:H7 strain) or deletions (e.g., K-12 strain), horizontal gene transfer appears to account for many of the differences between related bacterial genomes. *Horizontal gene transfer* is the acquisition of foreign DNA by various means such as simple transformation, phage infection, and conjugation (Chan, 2003). This type of genomic material frequently occurs in clusters or islands within the host genome and may encode for virulence factors (pathogenicity

**TABLE 17–8**

**Genomic and Genetic Web Resources**

| Site | Internet Address | Description |
|---|---|---|
| National Center for Biotechnology Information (NCBI) | www.ncbi.nlm.nih.gov/ | National resource for molecular biology information, biomedical information, public databases, and software tools for analyzing genome data |
| Ensembl | www.ensembl.org/ | Joint project between European Molecular Biology Laboratory-European Bioinformatics Institute (EMBL–EBI) and the Sanger Institute to develop a software system that produces and maintains automatic annotation on eukaryotic genomes |
| University of California, Santa Cruz (UCSC) Genome Bioinformatics Site | genome.cse.ucsc.edu/ | Human genome browser gateway |
| Human genome resources | www.ncbi.nlm.nih.gov/genome/guide/human/ | NCBI site for human genomic data |
| Gene expression atlas | expression.gnf.org/ | Expression data for many genes |
| Online database of Mendelian Inheritance in Man (OMIM) | www.ncbi.nlm.nih.gov/omim/ | Database describes correlations between genes and disease phenotypes |
| Human Gene Mutation Database (HGMD) | www.hgmd.org | Database of mutations associated with disease-related genes |
| The Institute for Genomic Research | www.tigr.org/ | Keeps track of microbial genome sequences |
| GeneTests/GeneClinics | www.geneclinics.com/ | Resource for finding laboratories that perform different types of genetic testing; locations of genetics clinics; and reviews on genetic diseases |
| The Transgenic/Targeted Mutation Database | tbase.jax.org/ | Database and lists of phenotypes for transgenic and knockout mice |
| Mouse Genome Database Project (MGD) | www.informatics.jax.org/ | Central repository for mouse genomic and genetic data |
| Mouse knockout and mutation database | research.bmn.com/mkmd | Biomednet's comprehensive database of phenotypic and genotypic information on mouse knockouts and classic mutations |
| The Journal of Gene Medicine Clinical Trial site | www.wiley.co.uk/genmed/clinical/ | Comprehensive source of information on gene therapy clinical trials |
| Silicon Genetics | www.silicongenetics.com/cgi/SiG.cgi/index.smf | Source for software for analyzing, interpreting, and managing microarray data |
| Whitehead Institute for Genomic Research | www.broad.mit.edu/cancer/software/software.html | Source for microarray data analysis software |

islands). Because these pathogenicity islands commonly distinguish virulent from nonvirulent strains, an understanding of their function will help identify potential therapeutic targets. The DNA sequence of these islands also may serve as unique diagnostic markers. For example, comparative genomic analyses of several pathogenic gram-negative organisms revealed the presence of a secretion system (type III) capable of using a syringe-like structure to inject bacterial toxins into eukaryotic cells (Blocker et al, 2003; Cornelis and Van Gijsegem, 2000). Because the activity of this secretion system can injure host cells, the development of drugs capable of interfering with bacterial secretory function should have clinical import. In the future, it should be possible to use genomic analysis to rapidly identify all types of bacteria as well as their virulence factors and their susceptibilities to antimicrobial agents.

Another important advantage of using genomic data is to obtain a comprehensive understanding of the interplay between pathogen and host (Rappuoli, 2000). Indeed, many host responses are far more damaging to the organism than the pathogen itself. Exposing mammalian cells in vitro to whole bacteria or bacterial products (cellular microbiology) and assaying their RNA profiles with microarrays (see later) enables one to discern how these organisms respond to each other at a molecular level. Extension of these studies to in vivo models of infection should make it possible to reconstruct the host response to a variety of infectious agents and determine how these responses can be modified to eliminate the infectious organism while minimizing collateral damage to the host and normal flora.

## DNA Microarry Analysis

Nearly 30 years ago, Southern (1975) published his seminal article describing the analysis of DNA by restriction endonuclease digestion, agarose gel electrophoresis, blotting to nitrocellulose, and hybridization with a radiolabeled probe (*Southern blot*). The simplicity and specificity of this technique are based on a fundamental aspect of nucleic acid chemistry: Complementary DNA strands anneal by Watson-Crick base-pairing.

Nucleic acid hybridization is also the basis for DNA microarray analysis. Instead of using nucleic acids to probe DNA blotted to nitrocellulose, microarrays contain thousands of nucleic acid probes attached to a solid support, such as a glass slide. The probes contain short oligonucleotides (≈25 bp), long oligonucleotides (50 to 120 bp) or PCR products (typically, 100- to 3000-bp cDNA fragments) (Stears et al, 2003). Individual oligonucleotides are synthesized on the chip, whereas PCR products are spotted on the chip using photolithography or ink jet–like printing technology. Fluorescently or chemically modified targets can be derived from a complex mixture of RNA (e.g., labeled first-strand cDNAs or labeled cRNAs synthesized from linear amplification reactions) prepared from selected populations of cells or tissues (e.g., leukemia cells, bronchiolar lavage cells, peripheral blood leukocytes) or genomic DNA (e.g., PCR products of different alleles for sequencing or SNP analysis). Labeled targets are applied to the array under conditions that permit high-stringency hybridization.

Target-probe annealing is detected with the use of a scanning confocal laser device and captured digitally with a charge-coupled device. Transformed and normalized data are displayed with one of several computer algorithms. Computer programs are also used, for example, to show hierarchical clustering or to create self-organizing maps, which can illustrate the relationships among the expression patterns of thousands of genes (Leung and Cavalieri, 2003). Much of this software is freely available and can be utilized effectively by the uninitiated (see Table 17–8). The major advantages of microarray analysis are the requirement of small sample volumes and the detection and analysis of highly specific binding in a format that lends itself to automation and high throughput.

### Disease Phenotyping by Expression Profiling

DNA microarray analysis is a rapidly evolving technology that permits a semiquantitative assessment of the transcriptional activity of thousands of genes in parallel (Staudt, 2003). These types of analyses can be ascertained by comparing the hybridization patterns of RNA-derived targets from different tissues (or cells), from diseased or nondiseased tissue, from the same tissues over time, or from the same tissues before and after exposure to a drug or toxin. For example, a subset of very low-birth-weight infants with surfactant deficiency experience severe chronic lung disease, whereas other surfactant-deficient infants have a more benign neonatal course. What accounts for this difference? Can it be explained by genetic or environmental factors? One means to differentiate among these possible explanations is to assay the expression profiles of the two cohorts of patients over time. Cells in bronchiolar alveolar lavage fluid or tracheal aspirates might serve as sources of RNA. Identification of differentially expressed genes could provide critical insights into why these patient populations differ (e.g., an increase in levels of cytokines or inflammatory mediators in the patients who experience chronic lung disease might suggest that infection alters the course of postnatal lung development).

The development of microarrays using proteins, peptides, and other organic molecules (e.g., carbohydrates) as features or probes is improving steadily. These arrays should be useful in determining protein-protein interactions, the detection of ligand or toxins, the measurement of post-translational protein modifications, protein-based diagnostics, and transcriptional factor DNA–chromatin binding.

## Analyses of Constitutional and Somatically Acquired Human Diseases by Comparative Genomic Analysis

The complete genomic DNA sequences of humans and other organisms provide a more expeditious means of selecting tractable biologic platforms (model organisms) to help decipher the functions of human genes and biochemical pathways (see Table 17–3) (Hariharan and Haber, 2003). The study of human genes in simpler biologic systems during the pre-genomic era entailed the tedious process of screening multiple cDNA or genomic libraries from multiple species. Library screening could take several months or years. If a clone was identified, the DNA sequence was obtained, and its homology confirmed. However, even if a similar gene was obtained, there was no guarantee that it was a true orthologue rather than a more distantly related family member.

With the advent of comparative genomic analysis, the amino acid or nucleotide sequence of a human gene is used to probe sequence databases with a simple search algorithm such as BLAST (basic local alignment search tool) (Altschul et al, 1990). With the touch of a keystroke, an entire list of closely related genes from different species can be displayed. The presence of other family members can be ascertained and, depending on the question being asked, a model system selected. Frequently, the cDNA and genomic clones can be obtained from ordered arrays of clones in public or private repositories. In turn, these reagents could be used to synthesize recombinant proteins or to prepare wild-type or mutant vectors capable of probing gene function in cells or intact organisms.

Approximately 20% of human disease–related genes show amino acid sequence similarity to those of the relatively simpler unicellular organism *S. cerevisiae*. Experimental genetics in yeast are very powerful because of their high degree of genomic annotation (i.e., the functions of many open reading frames have been identified), the ability to score phenotypes easily, the precision by which their genetic background can be modified by DNA transformation and high fidelity homologous recombination, the presence of haploid and diploid forms that facilitate the detection of lethal mutations, and the use of synthetic screens to detect the combined effects of multiple mutations. For example, *S. cerevisiae* has proved useful in defining the iron-binding function and mitochondrial localization of frataxin, the gene mutated in Friedreich ataxia (Walberg, 2000).

A search of the *C. elegans* genome for similarities to 100 human genes associated with inborn errors of metabolism as the query sequences revealed a worm orthologue for about 70% of the human genes (Culetto and Sattelle, 2000; Kuwabara and O'Neil, 2001; O'Kane, 2003). These findings suggest that many metabolic pathways are well conserved throughout evolution. Although the human pathways are likely to be more complex, the worm can be used to identify other proteins in the biochemical pathway, evaluate the effects of pathologic mutations on gene function, and test the effects of drugs in ameliorating the defect. Owing to the ease of creating transgenic worms (by micro-injection of naked DNA into the gonad), human diseases can be partially recapitulated in this simpler organism. For example, transgenic worms expressing human β-amyloid peptide or mutant huntingtin show peptide deposits or neuronal cell injury, respectively (Culetto and Sattelle, 2000). This model system will prove useful in identifying factors that contribute to deposit formation and cellular injury. Moreover, suppressor screens conducted on these animals may identify other genes that contribute to the disease phenotype. In worms, this screen is achieved by treating the mutant animals with a chemical mutagen and screening for progeny in which the mutant phenotype is suppressed.

Approximately 60% of human disease–associated genes have orthologues in *D. melanogaster* (Bernards and Hariharan, 2001). These genes are implicated in a multitude of disorders, including cancer, neurodegeneration, metabolic derangements, renal disease, and malformation syndromes. Conversely, genes isolated in *Drosophila* have provided insight into human gene function. For example, *sonic hedgehog* (*SHH*), which is critical for brain development and is associated with one form of holoprosencephaly in humans, was characterized initially in *Drosophila*. Transgenic approaches combined with enhancer-suppressor screens are also useful in delineating pathologic pathways in *Drosophila*. A model system for spinocerebellar ataxia type 1 (SCA1) was generated through expression of a wild-type and mutant form (containing a polyglutamine expansion) of ataxin-1 in flies (Fernandez-Funez et al, 2000). Genes capable of modifying the degenerative effect were identified, including ubiquitin conjugases, glutathione-S-transferases, and a nucleoporin. In turn, these genes may serve as therapeutic targets that can be tested subsequently in mouse models and eventually in humans. The ability to identify such a diverse array of modifier genes is simply not possible in human systems at this time, underscoring the utility of model organisms in gleaning important insights into human disease processes.

The use of mutagenesis screens in zebrafish is providing unparalleled insights into human developmental disorders and malformations. Although mutagenesis screens and natural mutations in mice yield similar types of disease phenotypes, the ease of cultivation, the ability to generate transgenic animals inexpensively, and the accessibility of developing embryos make zebrafish a preferred platform for the study of vertebrate morphogenesis (Dooley and Zon, 2000). With the use of positional cloning techniques, multiple genes associated with hematopoiesis have been cloned and characterized. Orthologues of some of these genes are associated with human diseases, such as sideroblastic anemia (D-aminolevulinate synthase) and a type of porphyria (uroporphyrinogen decarboxylase). This work in zebrafish has provided valuable insights into the genesis of developmental defects of the heart (coarctation of the aorta, rhythm disturbances, cardiomyopathy), kidney (polycystic kidney disease), and brain (holoprosencephaly).

For the study of specific mammalian developmental disorders and diseases, the laboratory mouse continues to serve as an irreplaceable resource. More than 3000 genes have been characterized by targeted deletions (knockouts) or by natural mutations. Information on many of these strains can be obtained through the Internet (see Table 17–8). With the advent of chromosomal engineering techniques, the mouse can also be used to study contiguous gene deletion disorders, such as those associated with DiGeorge syndrome, or aneuplodies (complete or partial) such as trisomy 21 (Baldini, 2002).

## Molecular Imaging in Vivo

Intermolecular interactions and biochemical pathways associated with normal or pathologic processes can be assayed in vitro with the use of isotope- or fluorescent-labeled probes by direct (e.g., a ligand to a receptor) or indirect (e.g., an enzyme substrate or a marker of channel permeability) techniques. The concentration or spectral emissions of the probes change upon association of the probes with targets in the pathway under investigation. These types of markers can also be detected in real time in vivo with positron emission tomography (PET), magnetic resonance imaging (MRI), and charge-coupled device (CCD) cameras to measure isotope-, radiowave- and light- (fluorescent or near-infrared) emitting probes, respectively (Herschman, 2003).

The opportunity to follow the fates of these probes over time allows for a longitudinal and in situ evaluation of multiple biologic processes, such as disease progression, growth and development of organs, response to drug therapy, activation of specific biochemical pathways under different experimental conditions, and the correct targeting and activity of gene therapy vectors. For example, a recombinant reporter construct containing a luciferase (reporter) gene flanked by caspase-cleavable silencing domains can be transfected into cells (Laxman et al, 2002). Upon activation of apoptosis, caspase-3 cleaves the silencer domains, allowing the recombinant enzyme to oxidize luciferin with the release of a photon. Bioluminescence imaging is used to detect the cells undergoing programmed cell death within these animals. The use of genomics and proteomics to identify and to expand upon biochemical pathways will aid in the identification of specific probes that could be used, for example, to help pinpoint the location and extent of gastrointestinal injury in the presence of a systemic inflammatory response associated with necrotizing enterocolitis.

### Resources

Nearly all of the species-specific genomic databases are freely available. Many of these repositories are accompanied by useful programs that permit a novice to explore the world of genomic biology. In addition, numerous Web sites offer a variety of software tools that facilitate the manipulation of nucleic acid and protein sequences as well as links to databases that help explore their clinical relevance. A selected set of sites is listed in Table 17–8.

## ETHICAL, LEGAL, AND SOCIAL IMPLICATIONS

Together with the research efforts focusing on the characterization of the human genome and its related technology development, the identification and analysis of the ethical, legal, and social implications of this field are integral and essential goals of the IHGP (Collins et al, 1998). Although the benefits of determining the human genome sequence and understanding the implications of genetic variation among individuals and groups are clear, several concerns have been raised (Table 17–9). They include the ethically sound (as well as scientifically sound) conduct of genetic research, the interpretation and use of genetic information, the integration of genetic information into clinical medicine, and the effect of this information in nonclinical and research settings.

These research issues will be of particular importance among communities of people who traditionally have not been the focus of genetic research. The exclusion of certain groups from research studies has contributed to well-documented disparities in health and available diagnostic and treatment options. There is equal, if not greater, concern among those communities that have been adversely affected by genetic research in the past. The potential for stigmatization and discrimination in employment, health care, and insurance as well as more broadly in society is of great concern. These issues will be particularly important as data on the interactions among genotype, diseases, or traits, and traditional concepts of race, ethnicity, and culture emerge. The great strides that have been made to ensure that research is safe for human subjects will have to be matched by efforts to ensure that the research is also fair (Greely, 1998).

The concerns that genetic information might be used in ways that will harm people have been reflected in recent policy development, particularly as it relates to privacy and the fair use of genetic information in health insurance, employment, and medical research. The passage of the Health Insurance Portability and Accountability Act (HIPAA), in which Congress specifically banned certain uses of genetic information in determining insurance eligibility, is one example of this focus (Collins, 1999). The issues are complex, because the tools of genomic medicine may reveal information about health risks faced by family members as well as the patient. One could argue effectively that physicians should inform their patients about the risks faced by family members, but whether the physicians are permitted or obligated to contact the relatives themselves has been a topic of debate and litigation (Clayton, 2003).

Our approach to population screening is likely to undergo tremendous change. Currently, population screening involving genetics has greatly focused on the perinatal field, including the identification of babies with certain mendelian disorders before the appearance of symptoms (e.g., phenylketonuria), the testing of selected populations for carrier status (e.g., sickle cell trait), and the use of prenatal diagnosis to reduce the frequency of disease in subsequent generations (e.g., Tay-Sachs). In the future, genetic information will increasingly be used in screening pediatric and adult populations to determine individual susceptibility to common disorders, such as heart disease, diabetes, and cancer. The responses to these findings will be more complex and will require efforts in primary prevention (e.g., diet and exercise) or secondary prevention (early detection or pharmacologic intervention). The American Academy of Pediatrics (AAP) has recommended that persons younger than 18 years be tested only if (1) testing offers immediate medical benefits or (2) another family member benefits and there is no anticipated harm to the person being tested. The AAP further currently recommends against predictive testing for adult-onset disorders in persons younger than 18 years. Informed consent processes with specific information on the clinical validity and value of genetic testing will be developed, much like the specific language in drug labeling requirements, over the coming years. Legislation to prevent discrimination on the basis of genetic information and substantive regulatory and professional oversight of genetic testing will necessarily evolve (Khoury et al, 2003).

It has been stated that the study, scope, and funding of the ethical, legal, and social implications of the Human Genome Project have made it the world's largest bioethics

**TABLE 17-9**

**Societal Concerns Arising from the IGHP**

| Concerns | Considerations |
|---|---|
| Fairness in the use of genetic information by insurers, employers, courts, schools, adoption agencies, and the military, among others | Who should have access to personal genetic information, and how will it be used? |
| Privacy and confidentiality of genetic information | Who owns and controls genetic information? |
| Psychological effect and stigmatization due to an individual's genetic differences | How does personal genetic information affect an individual's self-perception and society's perceptions of the individual?<br>How does genomic information affect members of minority communities? |
| Reproductive issues, including adequate informed consent for complex and potentially controversial procedures, use of genetic information in reproductive decision-making, and reproductive rights | Do health care personnel properly counsel parents about the risks and limitations of genetic technology?<br>How reliable and useful is fetal genetic testing?<br>What larger societal issues are raised by new reproductive technologies? |
| Clinical issues, including the education of doctors and other health service providers, patients, and the general public in the capabilities, scientific limitations, and social risks of genetic testing and the implementation of standards and quality-control measures in testing procedures | How will genetic tests be evaluated and regulated for accuracy, reliability, and utility?<br>How do we prepare health care professionals for the new genetics?<br>How do we prepare the public to make informed choices?<br>How do we as a society balance current scientific limitations and social risks with long-term benefits? |
| Uncertainties associated with gene tests for susceptibilities and complex conditions linked to multiple genes and gene-environment interactions | Should testing be performed when no treatment is available?<br>Should parents have the right to have their minor children tested for adult-onset diseases?<br>Are genetic tests reliable and interpretable by the medical community? |
| Conceptual and philosophical implications regarding human responsibility, free will versus genetic determinism, and concepts of health and disease | Do people's genes make them behave in a particular way?<br>Can people always control their behavior?<br>What is considered acceptable diversity?<br>Where is the line between medical treatment and enhancement? |
| Health and environmental issues concerning genetically modified foods and microbes | Are genetically modified foods and other products safe to humans and the environment?<br>How will these technologies affect developing nations' dependence on the West? |
| Commercialization of products, including property rights (patents, copyrights, and trade secrets) and accessibility of data and materials | Who owns genes and other pieces of DNA?<br>Will patenting DNA sequences limit their accessibility and their development into useful products? |

program. This development is clearly fortunate, given the great complexities of these issues and the potential effects on individuals, families, communities, and society.

## REFERENCES


Altschul SF, Gish W, Miller W, et al: Basic local alignment search tool. J Mol Biol 215:403-410, 1990.

Baldini A: DiGeorge syndrome: The use of model organisms to dissect complex genetics. Hum Mol Genet 11:2363-2369, 2002.

Balicki D, Beutler E: Gene therapy of human disease. Medicine (Baltimore) 81:69-86, 2002.

Bernards A, Hariharan IK: Of flies and men: Studying human disease in *Drosophila*. Curr Opin Genet Dev 11:274-278, 2001.

Blocker A, Komoriya K, Aizawa S: Type III secretion systems and bacterial flagella: Insights into their function from structural similarities. Proc Natl Acad Sci U S A 100:3027-3030, 2003.

Brummelkamp TR, Bernards R, Agami R: A system for stable expression of short interfering RNAs in mammalian cells. Science 296:550-553, 2002.

Chan VL: Bacterial genomes and infectious diseases. Pediatr Res 54:1-7, 2003.

Clarkson B, Pavenski K, Dupuis L, et al: Detecting rearrangements in children using subtelomeric FISH and SKY. Am J Med Genet 107:267-274, 2002.

Clayton EW: Ethical, legal, and social implications of genomic medicine. N Engl J Med 349:562-569, 2003.

Collins FS: Positional cloning: Let's not call it reverse anymore. Nat Genet 1:3-6, 1992.

Collins FS: Shattuck lecture: Medical and societal consequences of the Human Genome Project. N Engl J Med 341:28-37, 1999.

Collins FS, Patrinos A, Jordan E, et al: New goals for the U.S. Human Genome Project: 1998-2003. Science 282:682-689, 1998.

Cornelis GR, Van Gijsegem F: Assembly and function of type III secretory systems. Annu Rev Microbiol 54:735-774, 2000.

Culetto E, Sattelle DB: A role for *Caenorhabditis elegans* in understanding the function and interactions of human disease genes. Hum Mol Genet 9:869-877, 2000.

Dooley K, Zon LI: Zebrafish: A model system for the study of human disease. Curr Opin Genet Dev 10:252-256, 2000.

Duyk G: Attrition and translation. Science 302:603-605, 2003.

Fernandez-Funez P, Nino-Rosales ML, de Gouyon B, et al: Identification of genes that modify ataxin-1-induced neurodegeneration. Nature 408:101-106, 2000.

Fraser CM, Eisen JA, Salzberg SL: Microbial genome sequencing. Nature 406:799-803. 2000.

Garcia-Blanco MA: Messenger RNA reprogramming by spliceosome-mediated RNA trans-splicing. J Clin Invest 112:474-480, 2003.

Garmory HS, Brown KA, Titball RW: DNA vaccines: Improving expression of antigens. Genet Vaccines Ther 1:2-6, 2003.

Gibbs RA, Belmont JW, Hardenbol P, et al: The International HapMap Project. Nature 426:789-796, 2003.

Goldstein DB, Ahmadi KR, Weale ME, Wood NW: Genome scans and candidate gene approaches in the study of common diseases and variable drug responses. Trends Genet 19:615-622, 2003.

Greely HT: Genomics research and human subjects. Science 282:625, 1998.

Gruenert DC, Bruscia E, Novelli G, et al: Sequence-specific modification of genomic DNA by small DNA fragments. J Clin Invest 112:637-641, 2003.

Guttmacher AE, Collins FS: Genomic medicine: A primer. N Engl J Med 347:1512-1520, 2002.

Hacein-Bey-Abina S, von Kalle C, Schmidt M, et al: A serious adverse event after successful gene therapy for X-linked severe combined immunodeficiency. N Engl J Med 348:255-256, 2003.

Hariharan IK, Haber DA: Yeast, flies, worms, and fish in the study of human disease. N Engl J Med 348:2457-2463, 2003.

Herschman HR: Molecular imaging: Looking at problems, seeing solutions. Science 302:605-608, 2003.

Johnson JA: Pharmacogenetics: Potential for individualized drug therapy through genetics. Trends Genet 19:660-666, 2003.

Khoury MJ, McCabe LL, McCabe ER: Population screening in the age of genomic medicine. N Engl J Med 348:50-58, 2003.

Kmiec EB: Targeted gene repair—in the arena. J Clin Invest 112:632-636, 2003.

Kuwabara PE, O'Neil N: The use of functional genomics in *C. elegans* for studying human development and disease. J Inherit Metab Dis 24:127-138, 2001.

Lander ES, Linton LM. Birren B, et al: Initial sequencing and analysis of the human genome. Nature 409:860-921, 2001.

Laxman B, Hall DE, Bhojani MS, et al: Noninvasive real-time imaging of apoptosis. Proc Natl Acad Sci U S A 99:16551-16555, 2002.

Leung YF, Cavalieri D: Fundamentals of cDNA microarray data analysis. Trends Genet 19:649-659, 2003.

Lim HJ, Kim YJ, Yang JH, et al: Amniotic fluid interphase fluorescence in situ hybridization (FISH) for detection of aneuploidy: Experiences in 130 prenatal cases. J Korean Med Sci 17:589-592, 2002.

Long MB, Jones JP 3rd, Sullenger BA, Byun J: Ribozyme-mediated revision of RNA and DNA. J Clin Invest 112:312-318, 2003.

Nabel EG: Cardiovascular disease. N Engl J Med 349:60-72, 2003.

Nussbaum RL, Ellis CE: Alzheimer's disease and Parkinson's disease. N Engl J Med 348:1356-1364, 2003.

O'Kane CJ: Modeling human diseases in *Drosophila* and *Caenorhabditis*. Semin Cell Dev Biol 14:3-10, 2003.

Paddison PJ, Hannon GJ: RNA interference: The new somatic cell genetics? Cancer Cell 2:17-23, 2002.

Perna NT, Plunkett G 3rd, Burland V, et al: Genome sequence of enterohaemorrhagic *Escherichia coli* O157:H7. Nature 409: 529-533, 2001.

Pirollo KF, Rait A, Sleer LS, Chang EH: Antisense therapeutics: From theory to clinical practice. Pharmacol Ther 99:55-77, 2003.

Pizza M, Scarlato V, Masignani V, et al: Identification of vaccine candidates against serogroup B meningococcus by whole-genome sequencing. Science 287:1816-1820, 2000.

Rappuoli R: Pushing the limits of cellular microbiology: Microarrays to study bacteria-host cell intimate contacts. Proc Natl Acad Sci U S A 97:13467-13469, 2000.

Ray PN, Belfall B, Duff C, et al: Cloning of the breakpoint of an X;21 translocation associated with Duchenne muscular dystrophy. Nature 318:672-675, 1985.

Sazani P, Kole R: Therapeutic potential of antisense oligonucleotides as modulators of alternative splicing. J Clin Invest 112:481-486, 2003.

Seidman MM, Glazer PM: The potential for gene repair via triple helix formation. J Clin Invest 112:487-494, 2003.

Shi Y: Mammalian RNAi for the masses. Trends Genet 19:9-12, 2003.

Sledz CA, Holko M, de Veer MJ, et al: Activation of the interferon system by short-interfering RNAs. Nat Cell Biol 5:834-839, 2003.

Southern EM: Detection of specific sequences among DNA fragments separated by gel electrophoresis. J Mol Biol 98: 503-517, 1975.

Srivastava IK, Liu MA: Gene vaccines. Ann Intern Med 138:550-559, 2003.

Staudt LM: Molecular diagnosis of the hematologic cancers. N Engl J Med 348:1777-1785, 2003.

Stears RL, Martinsky T, Schena M: Trends in microarray analysis. Nat Med 9:140-145, 2003.

Sullenger BA: Targeted genetic repair: An emerging approach to genetic therapy. J Clin Invest 112:310-311, 2003.

Thomas M, Klibanov AM: Non-viral gene therapy: Polycation-mediated DNA delivery. Appl Microbiol Biotechnol 62:27-34, 2003.

Thomas CE, Ehrhardt A, Kay MA: Progress and problems with the use of viral vectors for gene therapy. Nat Rev Genet 4: 346-358, 2003.

Tonnies H: Modern molecular cytogenetic techniques in genetic diagnostics. Trends Mol Med 8:246-250, 2002.

Venter JC, Adams MD, Myers EW, et al: The sequence of the human genome. Science 291:1304-1351, 2001.

Walberg MW: Applicability of yeast genetics to neurologic disease. Arch Neurol 57:1129-1134, 2000.

Watson JD: The human genome project: Past, present, and future. Science 248:44-49, 1990.

Watson JD, Crick FH: Molecular structure of nucleic acids: A structure for deoxyribose nucleic acid. Nature 171:737-738, 1953.

Weinshilboum R: Inheritance and drug response. N Engl J Med 348:529-537, 2003.

West J, Rodman DM: Gene therapy for pulmonary diseases. Chest 119:613-617, 2001.

Wilcken B, Wiley V, Hammond J, Carpenter K: Screening newborns for inborn errors of metabolism by tandem mass spectrometry. N Engl J Med 348:2304-2312, 2003.

Wooster R, Weber BL: Breast and ovarian cancer. N Engl J Med 348:2339-2347, 2003.

CHAPTER

# 18

# Prenatal Genetic Diagnosis

Diana W. Bianchi

As a result of the ever-expanding number of prenatal diagnostic tests that are performed on pregnant women, clinicians know a lot about their patients long before they even touch them. This chapter discusses the common methods of prenatal genetic diagnosis, the information they convey, and the implications for the newborn.

## NONINVASIVE TECHNIQUES

### Maternal Serum Screening

Maternal serum screening has been incorporated into routine obstetric care. It is used to identify a high-risk pregnancy in a low-risk population of pregnant women. Currently, maternal serum screening consists of measurement of alpha-fetoprotein (AFP), human chorionic gonadotropin (hCG), unconjugated estriol (uE$_3$), and inhibin A, proteins that are made by the fetus or placenta. More than 20 years of clinical experience has accrued with the assay of AFP.

AFP is one of the major proteins in fetal serum. Its precise physiologic role is unknown. It can be detected as early as 4 weeks of gestation, when it is synthesized by the yolk sac (Bergstrand, 1986). Subsequently, it is produced in the fetal liver and peaks in the fetal serum between 10 and 13 weeks of gestation. AFP is then excreted into the fetal urine or leaks into the amniotic fluid through the skin before keratinization at 20 weeks of gestation. It is also present in cerebrospinal fluid. AFP in maternal serum is exclusively fetal in origin (Crandall, 1981). Maternal serum AFP peaks at 32 weeks of gestation owing to greater placental permeability for the protein (Ferguson-Smith, 1983). Most clinical assays of AFP are performed at 16 weeks of gestation. Accurate gestational dating as well as race, weight, and presence or absence of diabetes in the mother are critical to the interpretation of results.

In 1972, Brock and Sutcliffe observed that there were markedly increased levels of AFP in the amniotic fluid of fetuses with anencephaly and open neural tube defects. Subsequently, it was shown that elevated amniotic fluid AFP levels were associated with increased maternal serum AFP (Ferguson-Smith, 1983). The possibility of a screening test for open neural tube defects became apparent. In the initial collaborative efforts aimed at studying maternal serum AFP, results were expressed as multiples of the median (MoM) to allow comparisons between laboratories. It has become a convention to describe results greater than 2.5 MoM as abnormally high and less than 0.6 MoM as abnormally low. Both findings require further investigation.

If the AFP is elevated, the patient is offered an ultrasonographic examination to verify gestational age, determine fetal viability, and diagnose many of the structural abnormalities that can be associated with an elevated AFP. Although the AFP test was developed to screen for neural tube defects, abnormally high results are not specific for this condition (Table 18–1). If the ultrasonographic examination is unrevealing, the patient undergoes amniocentesis to assay the amniotic fluid for the presence of AFP and acetylcholinesterase, which are elevated in open spina bifida (Crandall et al, 1983). Even though an elevated AFP is compatible with a normal diagnosis, a study of 277 infants with elevations of maternal serum AFP and normal levels of amniotic fluid AFP revealed a higher incidence of intrauterine growth restriction and non–neural tube anomalies (Burton and Dillard, 1986).

Maternal serum AFP screening has also been used to detect chromosomally abnormal fetuses since the observation was made that a low AFP value was more likely in a fetus with trisomy 18 or 21 than in a normal fetus (Merkatz et al, 1984). Several prospective studies have demonstrated that, expressing risk for Down syndrome as a combined function of maternal age and AFP value and offering amniocentesis to all women with a risk of 1 in 270 or greater (the equivalent risk in a 35-year-old woman based on age alone) makes it possible to detect approximately one third of otherwise unexpected cases of Down syndrome in fetuses (Dimaio et al, 1987; Palomaki and Haddow, 1987). Low AFP values are probably caused by decreased hepatic production in the affected fetus. Although it would make sense to ascribe this phenomenon to the small size of the liver, one study found no association between fetal weight and low AFP values in chromosomally abnormal fetuses (Librach et al, 1988). The differential diagnosis of a decreased AFP level is shown in Table 18–2. Because a low AFP value detects only one third of fetuses with Down syndrome, a normal AFP value does not rule out trisomy 21.

Experience with using low maternal AFP levels as a screen for fetal chromosome abnormalities has led to the evaluation of many other proteins produced by both the fetus and placenta. Three of these, uE$_3$, hCG, and inhibin A, have been incorporated into maternal serum screening panels (Wenstrom et al, 1999). Measurements of all four can be combined to improve the sensitivity and specificity of Down syndrome detection. AFP, uE$_3$, and hCG are only weakly correlated with one another, and their values are all independent of maternal age (Norton, 1994). Elevations of hCG are the most specific markers for fetal trisomy 21 (Bogart et al, 1987; Rose and Mennuti, 1993), whereas estriol levels are approximately 25% less than normal. Pregnancies affected by fetal trisomy 18 also have reduced levels of uE$_3$ and hCG. Each measurement is compared with population-specific normal values (MoM), which are then converted to a likelihood ratio, which is expressed as a numeric risk for Down syndrome. Women whose serum screen results indicate a fetal Down syndrome risk of greater than 1 in 270 are offered amniocentesis. Approximately 5% of all serum screen values are calculated to be false-positive results in order to achieve a sensitivity of detection of at least 70% for cases of Down syndrome.

**TABLE 18-1**

**Differential Diagnosis of Abnormally High Maternal Serum Alpha-Fetoprotein Levels**

| |
|---|
| Incorrect gestational dating |
| Multiple pregnancies |
| Threatened pregnancy loss |
| Fetomaternal hemorrhage |
| Anencephaly |
| Open spina bifida |
| Anterior abdominal wall defects |
| Congenital nephrosis |
| Acardia |
| Lesions of the placenta and umbilical cord |
| Turner syndrome |
| Cystic hygroma |
| Renal agenesis |
| Polycystic kidney disease |
| Epidermolysis bullosa |
| Hereditary persistence (autosomal dominant trait) |

**TABLE 18-2**

**Differential Diagnosis of Abnormally Low Maternal Serum Alpha-Fetoprotein Levels**

| | |
|---|---|
| Incorrect gestational dating | Trisomy 18 |
| Trisomy 21 | Intrauterine growth restriction |

Future trends in maternal serum screening include measurements during the first trimester of pregnancy. Particularly promising are pregnancy-associated plasma protein A (PAPP-A) and the free β subunit of hCG (β-hCG) (Brambati et al, 1994), both of which are abnormal in cases of fetal trisomy 21. Initial studies indicate that sensitivity and specificity of fetal Down syndrome detection using PAPP-A and free β-hCG are the same in the first trimester as in second trimester (Haddow et al, 1998).

## Ultrasonographic Examination of the Fetus

Recommendations regarding the routine use of ultrasound imaging for all pregnant women have been controversial in the United States (Bakketeig et al, 1984; Eik-Neis et al, 1984; Ewigman et al, 1993). Nevertheless, it remains the best noninvasive method for gestational dating, definition of fetal anatomy, serial measurements of fetal growth, and evaluation of dynamic parameters such as cardiac contractility, fetal urine production, and fetal movement. Additionally, it has been suggested that antenatal visualization of the fetus promotes maternal-infant bonding (Fletcher and Evans, 1983). Despite controversies, 40% of obstetric patients are estimated to undergo at least one ultrasonographic examination during pregnancy (Hill et al, 1983). The advent of antenatal ultrasonography has had a large impact on the types of patients who present to the neonatal intensive care unit.

### Structural Assessment

Within the context of prenatal genetic diagnosis, ultrasonography may be used to detect congenital anomalies. In 2% to 3% of live births, a malformation is present (Nelson and Holmes, 1989). This risk is doubled in twins. Fetal structures that are normally filled with fluid are especially well visualized by ultrasonography. In approximately 10% of infants with anomalies, the central nervous system is involved (Hill et al, 1983). Ultrasonography is particularly useful in the diagnosis of anencephaly, microcephaly, encephalocele, and hydrocephalus. By 20 weeks of gestation, the fetal facial structures may be examined with this method for cyclopia, cleft lip, and micrognathia. Nuchal membrane thickening is suggestive of Down syndrome, familial pterygium coli, and other chromosome abnormalities (Benacerraf et al, 1987; Chervenak et al, 1983). Fetal cardiovascular structures may be reliably examined at 20 weeks of gestation. The presence or absence of four cardiac chambers, the dynamic relationships between the cardiac valves, and the locations of the vessels allow such diagnoses as hypoplastic left heart, double-outlet right ventricle, tricuspid atresia, tetralogy of Fallot, and Ebstein anomaly to be made. Pericardial effusion and arrhythmias may be similarly observed.

Gastrointestinal anomalies occur in approximately 0.6% of live births, and one third of them are associated with chromosome abnormalities (Barss et al, 1985). The decrease in fetal swallowing seen in some cases of bowel obstruction (from atresia, stenosis, annular pancreas, or diaphragmatic hernia) may lead to polyhydramnios that results in a uterine size greater than expected for gestational dates. Although gastroschisis and omphalocele are readily diagnosed on ultrasonography, they may be confused with each other, and their differing prognoses may cause considerable parental anxiety (Griffiths and Gough, 1985). Gastroschisis usually occurs as an isolated anomaly; infants generally do well after surgical repair. The kidneys are identifiable by 14 weeks of gestation, but the presence of perirenal fat and large adrenal glands may obscure the diagnosis of renal agenesis (Hill et al, 1983). Renal cysts, hydronephrosis, and obstructive uropathy are easily visualized. Oligohydramnios is indicative of poor renal function.

Multiple standard curves have been developed for fetal anthropometric measurements (Elejalde and Elejalde, 1986; Saul et al, 1988). These instruments are particularly helpful in the diagnosis of skeletal dysplasias and the evaluation of growth retardation. Fetal genitalia may be reliably determined by 24 weeks of gestation (Birnholz, 1983). Additionally, ultrasonographic examination is of benefit in the diagnosis and management of multiple pregnancies.

Although there have been no documented adverse outcomes related to ultrasound exposure during human pregnancy, the reported experimental biologic effects—altered immune response, cell death, change in cell membrane functions, formation of free radicals, and reduced cell reproductive potential—necessitate judicious use of this technology. Another concern is the appropriate pediatric follow-up for prenatally observed conditions with unclear clinical significance, such as minimal hydronephrosis and echogenic bowel.

The accuracy of ultrasonographic diagnosis has been addressed in several papers. In one study of 1737 referrals,

244 malformations were correctly diagnosed; six results were falsely called abnormal (0.3%), and 16 were incorrectly called normal (0.9%) (Campbell and Pearce, 1983). Of 596 women referred for ultrasonography, fetal anomalies were diagnosed in 81, with a falsely abnormal rate of 0.6% and a falsely normal rate of 0.5% (Sabbagha et al, 1985). The limitations of ultrasonography were delineated in a study correlating anatomic pathologic findings at autopsy with prenatal diagnosis (Rutledge et al, 1986). Fifty-two malformations in 45 fetuses were correctly diagnosed antenatally, but 90 additional malformations were missed.

The RADIUS (Routine Antenatal Diagnostic Imaging with Ultrasound) trial was a randomized study involving 15,151 pregnant women to determine whether the routine use of ultrasonographic screening decreased the occurrence of adverse perinatal outcomes (Ewigman et al, 1993). This study, which received considerable attention, did not show that ultrasonographic screening improved rates of preterm delivery or birth weight. Approximately 35% of the fetuses with anomalies were detected by antenatal ultrasonography in the screened population versus only 11% in the control group (Crane et al, 1994). Despite this difference, neither clinical management nor outcome of the pregnancy was significantly improved in the screened population.

Continuous ultrasonographic fetal imaging is important to improvement of the safety and efficacy of the more invasive diagnostic procedures, such as amniocentesis, chorionic villus sampling (CVS), and cordocentesis, which are discussed later.

### Nuchal Translucency Measurement or Absence of Nasal Bone

Ultrasonographic visualization and quantification of the fluid-filled space at the back of the fetal neck is known as the *nuchal translucency measurement*. This particular fluid-filled space is especially well seen in the first-trimester fetus (10 to 14 weeks of gestation) (Fig. 18–1). In normal fetuses, the maximal thickness of the subcutaneous translucency between the skin and soft tissue overlying the fetal spine increases as a function of crown-rump length. Normal standards have been established for each gestational week. An increased nuchal translucency (NT) thickness is associated with a higher risk of fetal trisomy 21 (Snijders et al, 1998), cardiac defects in chromosomally normal fetuses (Hyett et al, 1996), and other genetic syndromes and chromosome abnormalities. In a study of 96,127 pregnant women in the United Kingdom, Snijders and associates (1998) developed likelihood ratios for the extent of deviation of NT thickness from normal. Using a combination of maternal age and fetal NT thickness, these investigators detected 82.2% of the cases of trisomy 21 at a false-positive rate of 8.3%. Assessment of the risk of fetal chromosomal abnormalities in the first trimester allows pregnant women the option of earlier (invasive) diagnostic testing. The disadvantage of this approach is that earlier diagnosis of aneuploidy may preferentially identify fetuses already destined for miscarriage.

First-trimester ultrasonographic examination of the fetus, which is routinely performed in the United Kingdom and Europe, has identified other new markers for the noninvasive prenatal diagnosis of trisomy 21. In one study, absence of the nasal bone in the fetal facial profile was noted in 43 of 59 (73%) of fetuses with trisomy 21 and 3 of 603 (0.5%) of chromosomally normal fetuses (Cicero et al, 2001). Absence of the nasal bone is independent of NT thickness. Combination of the two ultrasonographic markers increases the sensitivity and specificity of detection of fetal Down syndrome.

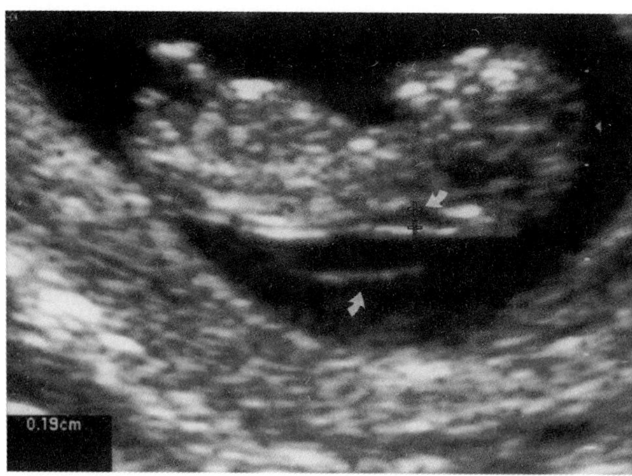


**FIGURE 18–1.** Sagittal ultrasonographic image of a first trimester fetus. The nuchal translucency measurement is the distance between the two crosses. A measurement larger than normal standards for gestational age indicates that the fetus is at high risk for Down syndrome, congenital heart disease, or both. *(Image courtesy of Dr. Fergal Malone.)*

## AMNIOCENTESIS

*Amniocentesis* refers to the removal of up to 20 mL of amniotic fluid from the pregnant uterus. Contained within this fluid are cellular components (desquamated fetal epithelial and bladder cells) that serve as sources of chromosomes, DNA, or enzymes. Most of the cellular elements are nonviable. Hence, amniocytes generally require tissue culture under specific conditions to provide enough material for diagnosis (Gosden, 1983). Herein lies one of the major disadvantages of the procedure, in that results are received late in the second trimester after fetal movement has been perceived by the pregnant woman. In contrast, the amniotic fluid itself may be assayed biochemically right after being removed for the presence of AFP, acetylcholinesterase, bilirubin, lecithin, sphingomyelin, or phosphatidylcholine.

The indications for genetic amniocentesis are (1) maternal age 35 years or older at the time of delivery, because there is an increased risk for fetal chromosome abnormalities, (2) a previous pregnancy that resulted in a fetus or an infant with chromosome abnormalities, (3) one parent with a balanced chromosome translocation, (4) an abnormal maternal serum screen value, (5) a family history of a child with a neural tube defect, (6) a family history of a metabolic disorder for which the enzyme defect is known, (7) maternal history of an X-linked disorder, and (8) a family history of a disorder for which DNA diagnosis is available.

Extensive clinical experience with amniocentesis has accrued since the results of the first large-scale randomized trials were published in the 1970s (Simpson et al, 1976; U.S. National Institutes of Health [NIH], 1976). Most institutions in the United States currently quote a 1% to 2% incidence of minor complications, such as amniotic fluid leakage, uterine cramping, and vaginal spotting after the procedure; the incidence of more serious complications, such as chorioamnionitis and miscarriage, is 0.25% to 0.5% (Chorionic villus sampling, 1995). There is a significant inverse relationship between the operator's experience with the procedure and the risk of miscarriage (Verjaal and Leschot, 1981).

In a series of 3000 amniocenteses performed at a single institution over 8 years, the diagnostic accuracy rate exceeded 99%. Chromosome abnormalities were detected in 2.4% of 2404 women with advanced maternal age, in 1.2% of 240 women who had previously had an infant with trisomy 21, and in 9.1% of 55 women with other cytogenetic indications for the procedure (Golbus et al, 1979).

Because results of amniocentesis are received relatively late in the pregnancy, research efforts have focused on evaluation of the procedure if performed between 12 and 15 weeks of gestation. Unfortunately, the Canadian Early and Mid-Trimester Amniocentesis Trial (CEMAT) showed both a higher fetal loss rate and a 1.3% risk of fetal clubfoot when amniocentesis was performed between 11 and 13 weeks of gestation (Randomised trial, 1998). The rate of clubfoot in the early amniocentesis group was 10 times the risk in the general population. The cause of clubfoot is thought to be a disruption of normal foot development secondary to transient oligohydramnios (Farrell et al, 1999). For these reasons, early amniocentesis is not generally recommended.

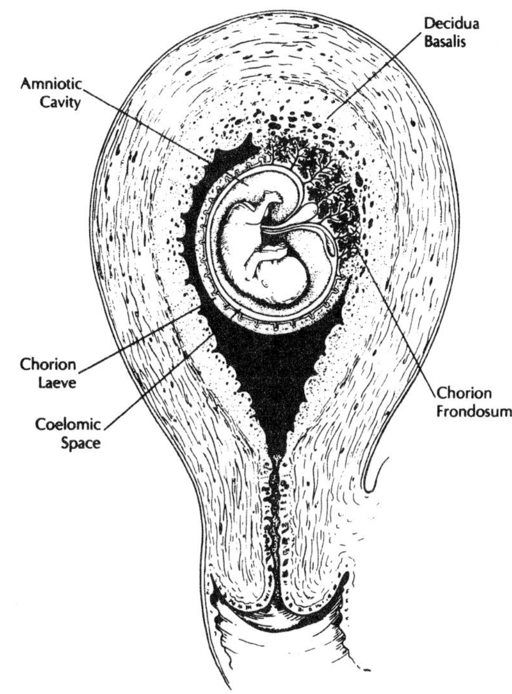


**FIGURE 18–2.** A pregnant uterus containing a fetus at about 9 weeks of gestation. The chorion frondosum, if sampled for biopsy, can provide fetal cells for chromosome, enzyme, or DNA analysis. *(From Jackson LG: First trimester diagnosis of fetal genetic disorders. Hosp Pract [Off Ed] 20:40 1985.)*

## CHORIONIC VILLUS SAMPLING

Despite the wealth of experience with amniocentesis, its usefulness has been somewhat limited by the late timing of the procedure. Since the publication of the first English language report on sampling of the chorion (Kazy et al, 1982), medical and scientific interest in first-trimester prenatal diagnosis has been significant.

*Chorionic villus sampling* involves the aspiration of the chorion frondosum between 10 and 11 weeks of gestation (Fig. 18–2). The fact that the procedure is performed early is advantageous, because most women at this point do not have external manifestations of pregnancy and have not yet perceived fetal movement. The chorionic villi are composed of syncytiotrophoblast and mesenchymal core cells that are actively growing and dividing. In contrast to the dying epithelial cells shed into the amniotic fluid, chorionic villus cells do not require prolonged culture to provide enough mitoses for a cytogenetic diagnosis. Karyotype results are generally available within 1 week of the procedure. Initially, direct preparations derived from syncytiotrophoblast were used for analysis, but the number of apparently mosaic abnormal results proved unacceptable. Cultured preparations derived from the cell of the mesenchymal core are more closely related in embryonic origin to the actual fetus (Bianchi et al, 1993). It is currently recommended that both direct and cultured preparations be used for cytogenetic analysis. *Mosaicism*, defined as the presence of two or more cell lines carrying different chromosomal constitutions, is a true biologic (not technical) problem in CVS. In several large studies, 0.8% to 1.7% of 1000 cases demonstrated a chromosome abnormality that was present in the villus but not in the fetus (Hogge et al, 1986; Ledbetter et al, 1992). This finding has led to the observation that postzygotic nondisjunction is more common than was previously suspected.

The indications for CVS are the same as those for amniocentesis, with two exceptions. First, neural tube defects cannot be diagnosed by this procedure, and AFP or other serum screening is not routinely offered at this early point in gestation. Second, evidence shows that the fetomaternal hemorrhage associated with placental biopsy results in elevated maternal serum AFP immediately after the procedure (Brambati et al, 1988).

CVS is performed transcervically or transabdominally. With the transcervical technique, the inherent risks of fetal and maternal infection appear to be greater because it is impossible to sterilize the cervix. Under ultrasonic guidance, a flexible catheter is passed through the endocervix and placed into the chorion frondosum. A small segment of placenta is then aspirated into sterile tissue culture medium, and the catheter is withdrawn (Jackson, 1985). In contrast, the transabdominal technique uses a needle to obtain villus material; sterilization of the skin surface is straightforward (Brambati et al, 1988). With either method, approximately 10 to 50 mg of tissue are obtained.

Subsequently, the villi are dissected from maternal decidua and processed for tissue culture or DNA extraction.

The safety and accuracy of these techniques have been extensively monitored. A randomized NIH clinical trial compared amniocentesis with CVS (Rhoads et al, 1989). The Centers for Disease Control and Prevention and the NIH held a consensus conference to summarize worldwide experience. After adjustment for confounding factors such as gestational age, the risk of miscarriage after CVS was found to be on the order of 0.5% to 1.0% (Chorionic villus sampling, 1995).

The advantages and disadvantages of CVS are summarized in Table 18–3. For patients at high risk for single-gene disorders amenable to DNA diagnosis (e.g., cystic fibrosis, sickle cell anemia, Duchenne muscular dystrophy), CVS is probably the preferred prenatal diagnostic method. On the other hand, for patients with relatively low risk (e.g., a 35-year-old woman being tested for chromosome abnormalities), an amniocentesis may be more appropriate. There have been a few reports of serious maternal sepsis and transient bacteremia in association with transcervical CVS (Barela et al, 1986; Blakemore et al, 1985; Silverman et al, 1994).

The 1% incidence of mosaicism in villus samples may necessitate a further invasive technique, such as amniocentesis or cordocentesis, to confirm or refute diagnoses. However, the detection of mosaicism in a CVS sample may identify a fetus at risk for uniparental disomy (UPD). *Uniparental disomy* refers to the inheritance of both copies of a chromosome pair from a single parent. This occurs when a trisomic fetus undergoes "rescue" and loses the extra copy of the chromosome. One third of the time, the fetus will be left with two chromosomes that originated in a single parent. UPD is an important mechanism in conditions such as Prader-Willi syndrome.

The biggest concern regarding CVS is the risk of limb deficiencies in infants whose mothers underwent the procedure. The risk of limb malformations was initially suggested by a number of studies describing an increased incidence of transverse limb anomalies and the hypoglossia-hypodactyly syndrome in infants whose mothers had undergone CVS (Burton et al, 1992; Firth et al, 1991, 1994; Hsieh et al, 1995). The overall rate of non–syndrome-related transverse limb deficiency from 65 centers performing CVS is 7.4 per 10,000 procedures (Chorionic villus sampling, 1995). This number is reasonably similar to that in population-based registries that monitor infants with all limb deficiencies, which give a rate of 5 to 6 per 10,000 live births (Chorionic villus sampling, 1995). Of concern, however, are studies in which cases of limb malformation were classified to match the phenotype of CVS-exposed infants with limb deficiencies. In these studies, a background rate of 1.5 to 2.3 per 10,000 live births was found, suggesting that CVS does raise the risk for limb malformations (Chorionic villus sampling, 1995). Factors likely to influence the rate of limb malformations include gestational age (risk of limb deficiencies being greatest at or before 9 weeks of gestation and decreased at or after 10 weeks of gestation), type of catheter used, and operator experience. The overall risk of limb deficiency appears to be on the order of 1 per 3000 procedures (Chorionic villus sampling, 1995). Furthermore, a higher incidence of hemangioma has been suggested in infants born after CVS (Burton et al, 1995).

**TABLE 18–3**

**Advantages and Disadvantages of Chorionic Villus Sampling (CVS)**

| |
|---|
| **Advantages of CVS** |
| Performed in first trimester; results available quickly |
| Cells obtained are mitotically active |
| Amount of tissue obtained is preferable for DNA analysis |
| Placental mosaicism is detected |
| **Disadvantages of CVS** |
| Miscarriage rate slightly higher |
| Increased fetomaternal hemorrhage after procedure |
| Risk of serious maternal infection |
| Risk of fetal limb and jaw malformations |

## CORDOCENTESIS

Percutaneous umbilical blood sampling (PUBS), or cordocentesis, was first described as a means of obtaining fetal immunoglobulin M (IgM) measurements in the prenatal diagnosis of congenital toxoplasmosis (Daffos et al, 1985). Under continuous ultrasonographic imaging, the insertion site of the umbilical cord into the placenta is identified. The umbilical vein is punctured with a 20-gauge needle, the sample is withdrawn, and the umbilical cord is observed for signs of hemorrhage. The technique has been used diagnostically in many clinical settings (Forestier et al, 1988) (Table 18–4). With regard to genetic diagnosis, the lymphocytes are a source of cells for a rapid karyotype. This is helpful in two situations: (1) when anomalies have been noted on ultrasonographic examination but it is too late in gestation to perform an amniocentesis (antenatal diagnosis of trisomy 13 or 18 influences delivery room management) and (2) for confirmation of a fetal karyotype when amniocentesis or CVS has shown mosaicism (Gosden et al, 1988).

## PREIMPLANTATION GENETIC DIAGNOSIS

The desire to avoid termination of pregnancy for fetuses affected with genetic disease has led to the development of techniques of preimplantation genetic diagnosis (PGD)

**TABLE 18–4**

**Indications for Fetal Blood Sampling**

| | |
|---|---|
| Thrombocytopenia | Acid-base abnormalities |
| Rapid third-trimester diagnosis of chromosome abnormalities* | Metabolic disorders* |
| Immunodeficiency | Fetal blood type incompatibility* |
| Congenital infection | Hemoglobinopathy* |

*Diagnosis can also be made by a DNA-based test performed on any nucleated fetal material, such as amniocytes.

(Handyside et al, 1992). In a limited number of laboratories, it is possible to analyze the DNA or chromosomal constitution from the polar body of the oocyte, a blastomere, or a blastocyst. The underlying rationale is that if disease-causing genes are identified in the embryo, the embryo will not be transferred into the uterus for implantation. Various forms of assisted reproductive technology are needed for the performance of PGD. In a worldwide survey, only approximately 15% of couples with normal fertility who underwent PGD procedures have ended with a "take home" baby (Harper, 1996). Furthermore, misdiagnoses have been reported (Harper and Wells, 1999).

More than half of the PGD cycles carried out to date worldwide have been performed for age-related aneuploidy (Harper and Wells, 1999). Other indications for PGD are the couple in which one partner carries a balanced translocation and couples at risk for a single-gene disorder such as cystic fibrosis. PGD is technically challenging, in that analysis is carried out on DNA or chromosomes from the nucleus of only a single cell. It is likely that new developments in DNA analysis, such as comparative genomic hybridization and microarrays, will be applied to the preimplantation embryo to improve pregnancy success rate.

## THE FUTURE

### Fetal Cells in Maternal Blood

All nucleated fetal cells from the same individual contain identical genetic information. As a result, research efforts are currently focused on noninvasive methods of fetal genetic diagnosis. An attractive potential population are the rare fetal cells that cross the placenta and circulate within the mother. The fetal cell types currently being studied include the trophoblast (Johansen et al, 1995) and nucleated erythrocyte (Bianchi et al, 1990). Genetic diagnoses that have already been made successfully in fetal cells isolated from maternal blood include trisomies 18 and 21, triploidy, Klinefelter syndrome (47,XXY), exclusion of beta globin mutations, inheritance of HLA-DR and DQ alpha types, and Rhesus D genotype (Bianchi, 1995; Simpson and Elias, 1993). On the basis of these encouraging preliminary results, the National Institutes of Child Health and Human Development sponsored a multicenter clinical evaluation designed to evaluate cytogenetic accuracy of fetal cells in maternal blood in comparison with that of amniocentesis and CVS (de la Cruz et al, 1995). Results of this trial have shown a 78% detection rate for at least one aneuploid cell in maternal blood when the fetus has aneuploidy (Bianchi et al, 2002). The major limitation in the clinical use of this technique appears to be the very small number of fetal cells present in most maternal blood samples.

### Cell-Free Fetal DNA in Maternal Plasma and Serum

In 1997, Lo and associates first described the circulation of large amounts of cell-free fetal DNA in maternal plasma and serum samples. A multitude of potential clinical applications for the noninvasive diagnosis of the complications of pregnancy from this DNA has been reported (Pertl and Bianchi, 2001). These applications have largely focused on the *quantitation* of male fetal DNA in maternal plasma or serum samples and its associated increase in conditions such as fetal trisomy 21, maternal hyperemesis gravidarum, preeclampsia, invasive placenta, and preterm labor. In addition, *qualitative* detection of uniquely fetal DNA sequences in maternal plasma or serum has facilitated the noninvasive prenatal diagnosis of Rhesus D genotype, myotonic dystrophy, and achondroplasia. It is likely that in the near future, noninvasive diagnosis of fetal Rhesus D genotype will be performed exclusively through the analysis of fetal DNA in maternal plasma or serum. The presence of amplified Rh D product in a sample from an Rh D–negative woman can come only from an Rh D–positive fetus.

## REFERENCES


Bakketeig LS, Eik-Neis SH, Jacobsen G, et al: Randomised controlled trial of ultrasonographic screening in pregnancy. Lancet 2:207, 1984.

Barela AL, Kleinman GE, Golditch IM, et al: Septic shock with renal failure after chorionic villus sampling. Am J Obstet Gynecol 154:1100, 1986.

Barss VA, Benacerraf BR, Frigoletto FD: Antenatal sonographic diagnosis of fetal gastrointestinal malformations. Pediatrics 76: 445, 1985.

Benacerraf BR, Gelman R, Frigoletto FD: Sonographic identification of second trimester fetuses with Down's syndrome. N Engl J Med 317:1371, 1987.

Bergstrand CG: Alpha-fetoprotein in paediatrics. Acta Paediatr Scand 75:1, 1986.

Bianchi DW: Prenatal diagnosis by analysis of fetal cells in maternal blood. J Pediatr 127:847, 1995.

Bianchi DW, Flint AF, Pizzimenti MF, et al: Isolation of fetal DNA from nucleated erythrocytes in maternal blood. Proc Natl Acad Sci U S A 87:3279, 1990.

Bianchi DW, Wilkins-Haug LE, Enders AC, Hay ED: Origin of extraembryonic mesoderm: Relevance to chorionic villus sampling. Am J Med Genet 46:542, 1993.

Bianchi DW, Simpson JL, Jackson LG, et al: Fetal gender and aneuploidy detection using fetal cells in maternal blood: Analysis of NIFTY I data. National Institute of Child Health and Development Fetal Cell Isolation Study. Prenat Diagn 22:609, 2002

Birnholz JC: Determination of fetal sex. N Engl J Med 309:942, 1983.

Blakemore KJ, Mahoney MJ, Hobbins JC: Infection and chorionic villus sampling. Lancet 2:338, 1985.

Bogart MH, Pandian MR, Hobbins JC: Abnormal maternal serum chorionic gonadotropin levels in pregnancies with fetal chromosome abnormalities. Prenat Diagn 7:623, 1987.

Brambati B, Lanzani A, Oldrini A: Transabdominal chorionic villus sampling: Clinical experience of 1,159 cases. Prenat Diagn 8:609, 1988.

Brambati B, Tului L, Shrimanker K, et al: Serum PAPP-A and free β-hCG are first-trimester screening markers for Down syndrome. Prenat Diagn 14:1043, 1994.

Brock DJH, Sutcliffe RG: Alpha fetoprotein in the antenatal diagnosis of anencephaly and spina bifida. Lancet 2:197, 1972.

Burton BK, Dillard RG: Outcome in infants born to mothers with unexplained elevations of maternal serum alpha fetoprotein. Pediatrics 77:582, 1986.

Burton BK, Schulz CJ, Burd LI: Limb anomalies associated with chorionic villus sampling. Obstet Gynecol 79:726, 1992.

Burton BK, Schulz CJ, Angle B, et al: An increased incidence of haemangiomas in infants born following chorionic villus sampling (CVS). Prenat Diagn 15:209, 1995.

Campbell S, Pearce JM: Ultrasound visualization of congenital malformations. Br Med Bull 39:322, 1983.

Chervenak FA, Isaacson G, Blakemore KJ: Fetal cystic hygroma: Cause and natural history. N Engl J Med 309:822, 1983.

Chorionic villus sampling and amniocentesis: Recommendations for prenatal counseling. Centers for Disease Control and Prevention. MMWR Recomm Rep 44RR-9):1, 1995.

Cicero S, Curcio P, Papgeorghiou A, et al: Absence of nasal bone in fetuses with trisomy 21 at 11-14 weeks of gestation: An observational study. Lancet 358:1658, 2001

Crandall BF: Alpha-fetoprotein: The diagnosis of neural tube defects. Pediatr Ann 10:38, 1981.

Crandall BF, Robertson RD, Lebherz TB: Maternal serum alpha-fetoprotein screening for the detection of neural tube defects. West J Med 138:524, 1983.

Crane JP, LeFevre ML, Winborn RC: A randomized trial of prenatal ultrasonographic screening: Impact on the detection, management, and outcome of anomalous fetuses. Am J Obstet Gynecol 171:392, 1994.

Daffos F, Capella-Pavlovsky M, Forestier F: Fetal blood sampling during pregnancy with use of a needle guided by ultrasound: A study of 606 consecutive cases. Am J Obstet Gynecol 153:655, 1985.

de la Cruz F, Shifrin H, Elias S, et al: Prenatal diagnosis by use of fetal cells isolated from maternal blood. Am J Obstet Gynecol 173:1354, 1995.

Dimaio MS, Baumgarten A, Greenstein RM, et al: Screening for fetal Down's syndrome in pregnancy by measuring maternal serum alpha fetoprotein levels. N Engl J Med 317:342, 1987.

Eik-Neis SH, Okland O, Aure JC, et al: Ultrasound screening in pregnancy: A randomised controlled trial. Lancet 1:1347, 1984.

Elejalde BR, Elejalde MM: The prenatal growth of the human body determined by the measurement of bones and organs by ultrasonography. Am J Med Genet 24:575, 1986.

Ewigman BG, Crane JP, Frigoletto FD, et al: Effect of prenatal ultrasound screening on perinatal outcome. RADIUS Study Group. N Engl J Med 329:821, 1993.

Farrell SA, Summers AM, Dallaire L, et al: Club foot, an adverse outcome of early amniocentesis: Disruption or deformation? CEMAT. Canadian Early and Mid-Trimester Amniocentesis Trial. J Med Genet 36:843, 1999.

Ferguson-Smith MA: The reduction of anencephalic and spina bifida births by maternal serum alpha-fetoprotein screening. Br Med Bull 39:365, 1983.

Firth HV, Boyd PA, Chamberlain PF, et al: Limb abnormalities and chorionic villus sampling. Lancet 338:51, 1991.

Firth HV, Chamberlain PF, MacKenzie IZ, et al: Analyses of limb reduction defects in babies exposed to chorionic villus sampling. Lancet 343:1069, 1994.

Fletcher JC, Evans MI: Maternal bonding in early fetal ultrasound examinations. N Engl J Med 308:392, 1983.

Forestier F, Cox WJ, Daffos F, et al: The assessment of fetal blood samples. Am J Obstet Gynecol 158:1184, 1988.

Golbus MS, Longman WD, Epstein CJ, et al: Prenatal genetic diagnosis in 3,000 amniocenteses. N Engl J Med 300:157, 1979.

Gosden C, Nicolaides KH, Rodeck CH: Fetal blood sampling in investigation of chromosome mosaicism in amniotic fluid cell culture. Lancet 1:613, 1988.

Gosden CM: Amniotic fluid cell types and culture. Br Med Bull 39:348, 1983.

Griffiths DM, Gough MH: Dilemmas after ultrasonographic diagnosis of fetal abnormality. Lancet 1:623, 1985.

Haddow JE, Palomaki GE, Knight GJ, et al: Screening of maternal serum for fetal Down's syndrome in the first trimester. N Engl J Med 338:955, 1998.

Handyside AH, Lesko JG, Tarín JJ, et al: Birth of a normal girl after in vitro fertilization and preimplantation diagnostic testing for cystic fibrosis. N Engl J Med 327:905, 1992.

Harper J: Preimplantation diagnosis of inherited disease by embryo biopsy: An update of the world figures. J Assist Reprod Genet 13:90, 1996.

Harper J, Wells D: Recent advances and further developments in PGD. Prenat Diagn 19:1193, 1999.

Hill LM, Breckle R, Gehrking WC: The prenatal detection of congenital malformations by ultrasonography. Mayo Clin Proc 58:805, 1983.

Hogge WA, Schonberg SA, Golbus MS: Chorionic villus sampling: Experience of the first 1,000 cases. Am J Obstet Gynecol 154:1249, 1986.

Hsieh F-J, Shyu M-K, Sheu B-C, et al: Limb defects after chorionic villus sampling. Obstet Gynecol 85:84, 1995.

Hyett J, Moscoso G, Papanagiotou G, et al: Abnormalities of the heart and great arteries in chromosomally normal fetuses with increased nuchal translucency thickness at 11-13 weeks of gestation. Ultrasound Obstet Gynecol 7:245, 1996.

Jackson LG: First trimester diagnosis of fetal genetic disorders. Hosp Pract (Off Ed) 20:39, 1985.

Johansen M, Knight M, Maher EJ, et al: An investigation of methods for enriching trophoblast from maternal blood. Prenat Diagn 15:921, 1995.

Kazy Z, Rozovsky IS, Bakharev VA: Chorion biopsy in early pregnancy: A method of early prenatal diagnosis for inherited disorders. Prenat Diagn 2:39, 1982.

Ledbetter DH, Zachary JM, Simpson JL, et al: Cytogenetic results from the U. S. Collaborative Study on CVS. Prenat Diagn 12:317-345, 1992.

Librach CL, Hogdall CK, Doran TA: Weights of fetuses with autosomal trisomies at termination of pregnancy: An investigation of the etiologic factors of low serum alpha-fetoprotein values. Am J Obstet Gynecol 158:290, 1988.

Lo YMD, Corbetta N, Chamberlain PF, et al: Presence of fetal DNA in maternal plasma and serum. Lancet 350:485, 1997.

Merkatz IR, Nitowsky HM, Macri JN, et al: An association between low maternal serum alpha-fetoprotein and fetal chromosome abnormalities. Am J Obstet Gynecol 148:886, 1984.

Nelson K, Holmes LB: Malformations due to presumed spontaneous mutations in newborn infants. N Engl J Med 320:19, 1989.

Norton ME: Biochemical and ultrasound screening for chromosomal abnormalities. Semin Perinat 18:256, 1994.

Palomaki GE, Haddow JE: Maternal serum alpha-fetoprotein, age, and Down syndrome risk. Am J Obstet Gynecol 156:460, 1987.

Pertl B, Bianchi DW: Fetal DNA in maternal plasma: Emerging clinical applications. Obstet Gynecol 98:483, 2001.

Randomised trial to assess safety and fetal outcome of early and midtrimester amniocentesis. Canadian Early and Mid-Trimester Amniocentesis Trial (CEMAT) Group. Lancet 351:242, 1998.

Rhoads G, Jackson L, Schlesselman S, et al: The safety and efficacy of chorionic villus sampling for early prenatal diagnosis of cytogenetic abnormalities. N Engl J Med 320:609, 1989.

Rose NC, Mennuti MT: Maternal serum screening for neural tube defects and fetal chromosome abnormalities. West J Med 159:312, 1993.

Rutledge JC, Weinberg AG, Friedman JM: Anatomic correlates of ultrasonographic prenatal diagnosis. Prenat Diagn 6:51, 1986.

Sabbagha RE, Sheikh Z, Tamura R, et al: Predictive value, sensitivity, and specificity of ultrasonic targeted imaging for fetal anomalies in gravid women at high risk for birth defects. Am J Obstet Gynecol 152:822, 1985.

Saul RA, Stevenson RE, Rogers RC, et al: Growth references from conception to adulthood. Proceedings of the Greenwood Genetics Center, Greenwood, SC, (Suppl 1): pp 1-214, 1988.

Silverman NS, Sullivan MW, Jungkind DL, et al: Incidence of bacteremia associated with chorionic villus sampling. Obstet Gynecol 84:1021, 1994.

Simpson JL, Elias S: Isolating fetal cells from maternal blood: Advances in prenatal diagnosis through molecular technology. JAMA 270:2357, 1993.

Simpson NE, Dallaire L, Miller JR, et al: Prenatal diagnosis of genetic disease in Canada: Report of a collaborative study. Can Med Assoc J 115:739, 1976.

Snijders RJ, Noble P, Sebire N, et al: UK multicentre project on assessment of risk of trisomy 21 by maternal age and fetal nuchal-translucency thickness at 10-14 weeks of gestation. Fetal Medicine Foundation First Trimester Screening Group. Lancet 351:343, 1998.

U.S. National Institutes of Health. National Institute of Child Health and Human Development (NICHHD) National Registry for Amniocentisis Study Group: Midtrimester amniocentesis for prenatal diagnosis: Safety and accuracy. JAMA 236:1471, 1976.

Verjaal M, Leschot NJ: Risk of amniocentesis and laboratory findings in a series of 1,500 prenatal diagnoses. Prenat Diagn 1:173, 1981.

Wenstrom KD, Owen J, Chu DC, Boots L: Prospective evaluation of free β subunit of human chorionic gonadotropin and dimeric inhibin A for aneuploidy detection. Am J Obstet Gynecol 181:887, 1999.

CHAPTER 19

# Evaluation of the Dysmorphic Infant

**Sulagna C. Saitta and Elaine H. Zackai**

Genetic disorders have a major impact on public health, as indicated by several large epidemiologic studies (Cassidy et al, 2000; Hall et al, 1978; Scriver et al, 1973; Table 19–1). The latest data indicate that genetic factors contribute to approximately two thirds of the conditions prompting admission to a children's hospital (Cassidy et al, 2000). Early identification of the genetic nature of a given condition may then help to appropriately focus resources for providing better care to these individuals. It is therefore critical to implement a systematic approach to evaluating a dysmorphic, or malformed, infant. This chapter outlines such a general approach.

The clinical geneticist incorporates the following five essential tools in the evaluation of a child suspected of having a primary genetic disorder:

1. History: prenatal, birth, and medical
2. A pedigree analysis or family history
3. A specialized clinical evaluation that includes a detailed dysmorphology examination
4. A comprehensive literature search
5. Focused special cytogenetic and molecular genetic laboratory analyses

## HISTORY

### Prenatal History

A complete gestational history should be generated, including results of prenatal testing such as serum triple-screen test, ultrasonography, chorionic villus sampling (CVS), and amniocentesis (Table 19–2). The maternal age at conception should be documented, because the risk of chromosomal anomalies such as improper separation and nondisjunction rises with maternal age. It is important to identify prenatal exposures to infection and medications, maternal habits such as alcohol and drug use, maternal chronic illnesses, and pregnancy-related complications.

It is also important to identify exposure to environmental agents that might act as teratogens. *Teratogens* are environmental agents that may cause structural and functional diseases in an exposed fetus. Each teratogen may have a characteristic expression pattern, with a specific range of associated structural anomalies and dysmorphic features. Effects and the extent of effect depend on the time of exposure, duration, and dosage as well as interactions with maternal and genetic susceptibility factors. In general, more severe effects are typically correlated with exposure early in the pregnancy and with more extensive (higher-dose) exposure. The list of well-documented human teratogens is short, and if history of an exposure is documented, an effort should be made to identify the developmental time and level of exposure. This information is critical, because the counseling and calculation of recurrence risk for a given malformation are vastly different if environmental exposures are involved.

### Birth History

Another important component of the gestational history is obtaining information on fetal activity, size, and position. Often, the mother's subjective impressions can be further confirmed by examining obstetric records of the perinatal period. A history of hypotonia may be further supplemented by reports of poor fetal movements and breech presentation. Perinatal information including gestational age, fetal position at delivery, the length of labor and type of delivery, and any evidence of fetal distress, such as passage of meconium, are all relevant data (Table 19–3). Apgar scores, the need for resuscitation, birth parameters, any malformations noted at birth, and all abnormal test results should be noted.

### Medical History

A full review of the medical issues of the child should include the baby's general health, results of tests, identification of any chronic medical issues, and need for hospitalization. Evaluation of growth, review of systems, developmental assessment, and notation of unusual behaviors can also provide important clues to a diagnosis.

## PEDIGREE ANALYSIS AND FAMILY HISTORY

A critical part of any genetic evaluation is to obtain the family history (Table 19–4). This is best accomplished by creating a three-generation *pedigree*, or schematic diagram depicting familial relationships using standard accepted symbols (Fig. 19–1). This formal record can also be used to summarize positive responses elicited during the interview. Special attention should be paid to ethnic origins of both sides of the family, consanguinity, and any first-degree relatives with similar malformations to those of the patient being evaluated, also known as the index case, *proband*, or *propositus*. An extended family history should be used to identify relatives with congenital anomalies, developmental abnormalities, or physical differences. Often photographs can provide clear objective evidence of a descriptive history.

Reproductive histories, especially of the parents, should be elicited. Specifically, questions should be asked about infertility, miscarriages, and stillbirths. The occurrence of more than two first-trimester miscarriages increases the probability of finding a balanced translocation in one parent (Campana et al, 1986; Castle and Bernstein, 1988). A *balanced translocation* is a rearrangement of genetic material such that two chromosomes have an equal exchange without loss or gain of material. There are

**TABLE 19-1**

**Genetic Disorders in Pediatric Hospital Admissions**

| Genetic disorders (%) | Montreal (1973) | Seattle (1978) | Cleveland (2000) |
|---|---|---|---|
| Chromosome/single gene | 7.3 | 4.5 | 8.5 |
| Polygenic | 29 | 49 | 55 |
| Nongenetic disorders (%) | 64 | 47 | 35 |
| Total number of admissions | 12,801 | 4115 | 4200 |

Data from Scriver et al (1973), Hall et al (1978), and Cassidy et al (2000).

**TABLE 19-2**

**Elements of Prenatal History for the Dysmorphic Infant**

| | |
|---|---|
| Maternal health | Age<br>Disease: diabetes, hypertension, seizure disorder |
| Exposures | Medications<br>Alcohol<br>Environmental agents<br>Infections (gestational age at exposure) |
| Prenatal testing | Ultrasonography (gestational age performed)<br>Triple screen<br>Chorionic villus sampling/amniocentesis and indications |

**TABLE 19-3**

**Elements of Perinatal/Birth History for the Dysmorphic Infant**

Fetal activity
Delivery:
- Type (indication for cesarean section, etc.)
- Gestational age
- Fetal presentation
- Apgar scores; history of distress/resuscitation
- Growth parameters
- Malformations noted

typically no associated clinical features with such a rearrangement. However, when chromosomes align to recombine for meiosis in the sperm or egg, this exchange produces a risk of unequal distribution and an unbalanced translocation in the resulting fetus. In this case, there would be aneuploidy for part of a chromosome. It has been estimated that 25% of stillbirths exhibit single or multiple malformations, and in at least half of these cases

**TABLE 19-4**

**Elements of Pedigree Analysis and Family History for the Dysmorphic Infant**

Identification of relatives with:
- Congenital anomalies (especially those similar to proband's)
- Mental retardation

Photographs (objective evidence)
Parental reproductive history:
- Pregnancy losses (gestational ages)
- Infertility

Medical histories of primary relatives
Ethnic origin(s)
Consanguinity

there is a genetic etiology for the malformations. Couples with two or more pregnancy losses should undergo routine chromosome analysis or karyotyping, and when possible, such analysis should be performed on the stillborn fetus or on products of conception.

Obtaining a formal family history is helpful in bringing out information that is often critical to making a diagnosis. Positive responses may help discern the mendelian pattern of inheritance of a given genetic disorder. For example, a disease affecting every generation, with both males and females involved, such as Marfan syndrome, would most likely be autosomal dominant. A pattern of X-linked recessive disease, such as hemophilia, would show affected males related through unaffected or minimally affected females; transmission in this pattern should not occur from father to son.

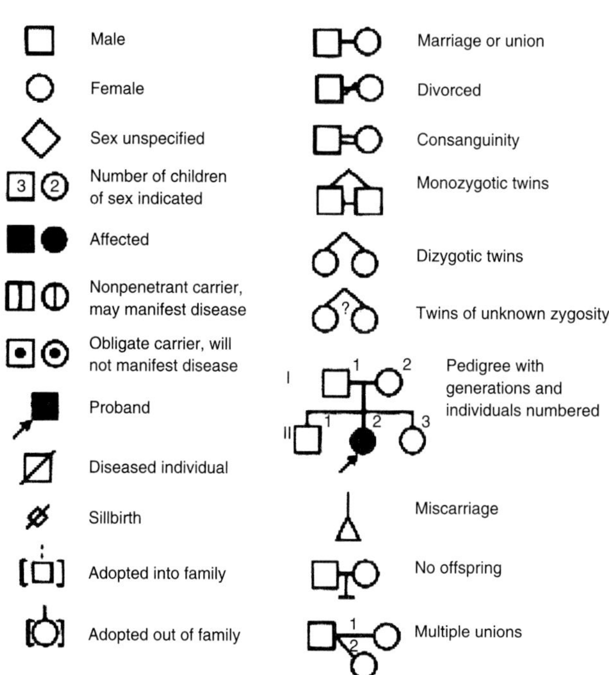


**FIGURE 19-1.** Symbols commonly used for pedigree notation. *(From Nussbaum RL, McInnes RR, Willard HF [eds]: Thompson and Thompson's Genetics in Medicine, 6th ed. Philadelphia, WB Saunders, 2001.)*

## PHYSICAL EXAMINATION FOR DYSMORPHOLOGY

A congenital *malformation* can be described as a "morphologic defect of an organ, part of an organ, or larger region of the body resulting from an intrinsically abnormal developmental process" (Jones, 1997). *Dysmorphology* was introduced by Dr. David Smith in the 1960s to describe the study of human congenital malformations. This study of "abnormal form" emphasizes a focus on structural errors in development with an attempt to identify the underlying genetic etiology and pathogenesis of the disorder.

In a landmark study, Feingold and Bossert (1974) examined more than 2000 children to define normal values for a number of physical features. These standards were devised as screening tools to objectively identify children with differences possibly attributable to a genetic disorder. Important measurements that are further discussed here include head circumference, inner and outer canthal distances, interpupillary distances, ear length and ear placement, internipple distances, chest circumference, and hand and foot lengths. Other graphs and measurements using age-appropriate standards can be found in compendia such as the *Handbook of Normal Physical Measurements* (Hall et al, 1989).

The assessment should begin with newborn growth parameters that can reflect the degree of any prenatal insult. Measurements such as height, weight (usually reflecting nutrition), and head circumference should be plotted on newborn graphs. Gestational age–appropriate graphs should be used for premature infants. It is often helpful to express values that are outside the normal range as 50th percentile for a different gestational age. For example, a full-term baby with microcephaly may have a head circumference of less than the 5th percentile for 38 weeks. This can be expressed as a measurement at the 50th percentile for 33 weeks, which imparts the degree of microcephaly more clearly.

A complete physical examination should include assessment of patient anatomy for features varying from usual or normal standards. This assessment can often provide clues to embryologic mechanisms. The data obtained should then be interpreted with respect to normal standards using comprehensive standard tables that are available for these purposes. Special attention to familial variants should be given.

The shape and size of the *head* and fontanels should be noted as well as the cranial sutures, with assessment for evidence of craniosynostosis or an underlying brain malformation. Any scalp defects should also be noted. The shape of the forehead, appearance of eyebrows (noting synophrys, or "mono-brow"), and the texture and distribution of hair should be noted. The spacing of the *eyes*, or canthal measurements (Fig. 19–2), the interpupillary distances (Fig. 19–3; see also Fig. 19–2), palpebral fissure lengths (Fig. 19–4), presence or absence of colobomata and epicanthal folds, and noting whether the palpebral fissures are turned upward or downward are components of the dysmorphology examination. Examination of the *ears* should include a search for preauricular and postauricular pits, or ear tags, and assessment of the placement (Fig. 19–5), length (Fig. 19–6), and folding of the ear is important. Ear development occurs in a temporal frame similar to that of the kidneys, and often, external ear anomalies are associated with renal anomalies. Evaluation of the *nose* should cover the shape of nasal tip, the alae nasi, presence of anteverted nares, the length of the columella, and patency of the choanae. The *mouth* and throat are examined for the presence of a cleft lip or palate; the shape of the palate and uvula are noted, and the presence of unusual features, such as tongue deformities, lip pits, frenula, and natal teeth, are recorded. A small retrognathic or receding chin, which can be a part of several syndromes or an isolated finding, should be noted. The neck is inspected for excess nuchal folds or skin and evidence of webbing. Any bony abnormalities in the neck should prompt an evaluation of the cervical vertebrae to confirm cervical and airway stability.

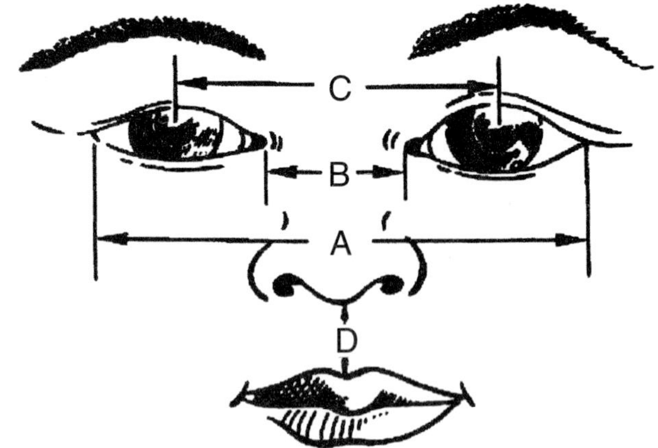


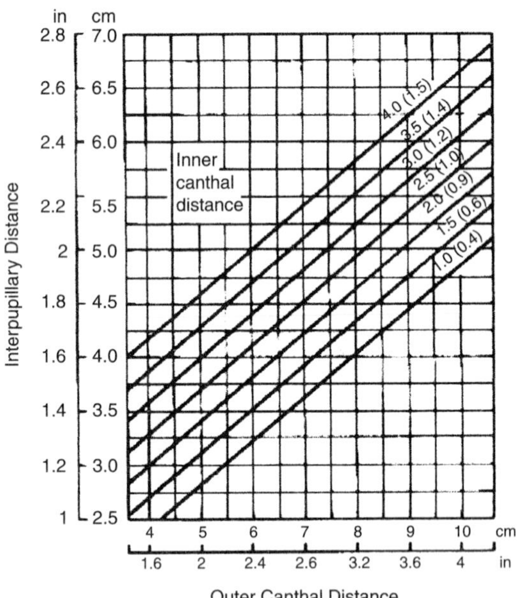


**FIGURE 19–2. Top,** Various eye measurements are depicted. A indicates the outer canthal distance, B the inner canthal distance, and C the interpupillary distance (IPD), which is difficult to measure directly. The IPD can be determined using the graph at the **bottom** or with the Pryor formula: IPD = (A − B) 2 + B. *(From Feingold M, Bossert WH: Normal values for selected physical parameters: An aid to syndrome delineation. Birth Defects 10:1-16, 1974).*

Evaluation of the *chest* and thorax involves lung auscultation and cardiac examination. Abnormal findings should

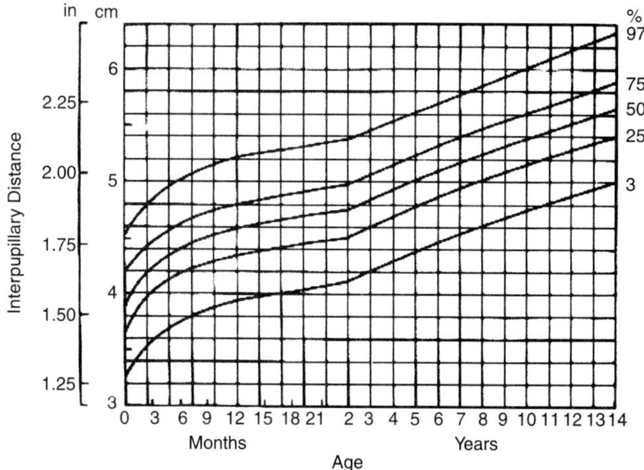


**FIGURE 19–3.** A nomogram for interpupillary distance (IPD) at different ages for both sexes *(From Feingold M, Bossert WH: Normal values for selected physical parameters: An aid to syndrome delineation. Birth Defects 10:1-16, 1974.)*

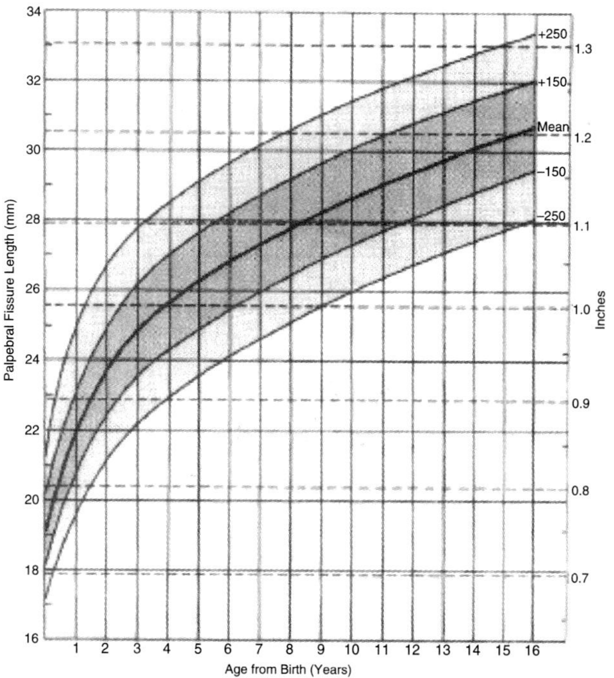


**FIGURE 19–4.** A graph of palpebral fissure length from birth to age 16 years for both sexes. *(From Hall JG, Froster-Iskenius UG, Allanson JE: Handbook of Normal Physical Measurements. Oxford, UK, Oxford University Press, 1989.)*

prompt consultation with a cardiologist and appropriate echocardiographic or invasive studies as needed. External measurements include determining the internipple distance and its ratio with respect to the chest circumference (Fig. 19–7). The *abdominal* examination is focused on determining whether organomegaly is present, a finding typically associated with an inborn error of metabolism. The umbilicus should also be examined, with any hernias as well the number of vessels present in the newborn cord noted. A two-vessel cord, in which only a single artery is present, can be associated with renal anomalies. The *genitourinary* examination concentrates on determining whether anomalies such as hypospadias, chordee, cryptorchidism, microphallus, and ambiguous genitalia are present. These external anomalies may be associated with internal anomalies involving the upper urinary tract as well. The anus is examined for evidence of tags, its placement, and its patency.

The *back* should be assessed especially for the shape of the *spine* and any associated defects, such as myelomeningocele. These defects prompt further radiologic evaluation to assess for potential functional limitations. Additionally, a sacral dimple or hair tuft at the base of the spine should be noted because either could signify developmental abnormalities in the underlying neural tissue.

Minor anomalies are often manifested in the extremities. Gross differences in the hands and feet include polydactyly (more than five digits; whether the extra digits are located in a pre-axial or post-axial position should be noted, syndactyly (fusion of the digits), clinodactyly (incurving of the digits), and extremity length, which should be expressed as

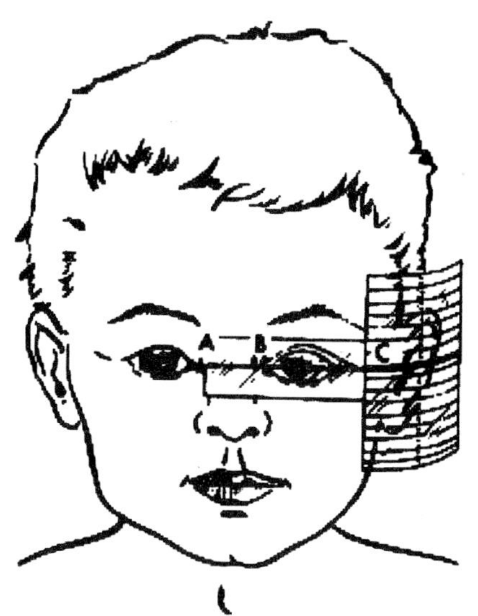


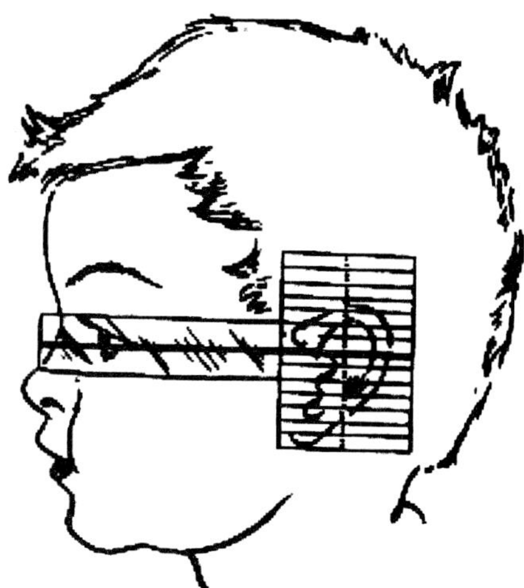

**FIGURE 19–5.** Ear placement. Using the medial canthi (A and B) as landmarks, one draws a central horizontal line and extends it to a point (C) on the side of the face. Ears placed below this line are considered low set.

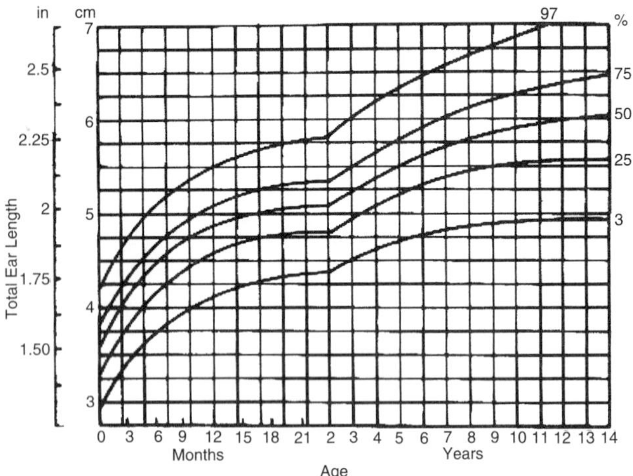


**FIGURE 19–6.** Graph showing various percentiles for ear length plotted against age. *(From Feingold M, Bossert WH: Normal values for selected physical parameters: An aid to syndrome delineation. Birth Defects 10:1-16, 1974.)*

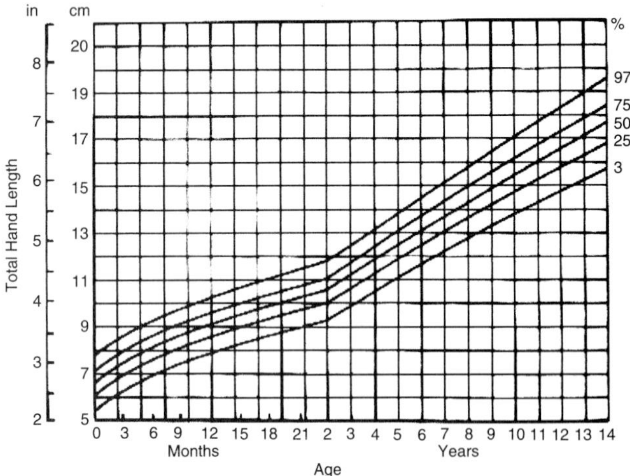


**FIGURE 19–8.** The total hand length plotted against age for both sexes. *(From Feingold M, Bossert WH: Normal values for selected physical parameters: An aid to syndrome delineation. Birth Defects 10:1-16, 1974.)*

a percentile measured on age-appropriate graphs (Figs. 19–8 and 19–9). Often these data can provide important clues to a unifying syndrome.

Dermal ridge patterns, or *dermatoglyphics*, are formed on the palms and soles early in embryonic life, and vary considerably among individuals. This variation can be inherited and can be influenced by disturbances to the development of the peripheral limb buds. Environmental exposures and chromosomal aberrations can greatly affect the formation of these structures and are reflected by the dermatoglyphic pattern of an individual. Each of the distal phalanges has one of three basic dermal ridge patterns: arches, whorls, or loops (Fig. 19–10). The predominance of a single pattern can be an associated feature of a genetic disorder; for example, the occurrence of arches on eight or more digits is a very rare event but is frequently encountered in children with trisomy 18 (Table 19–5).

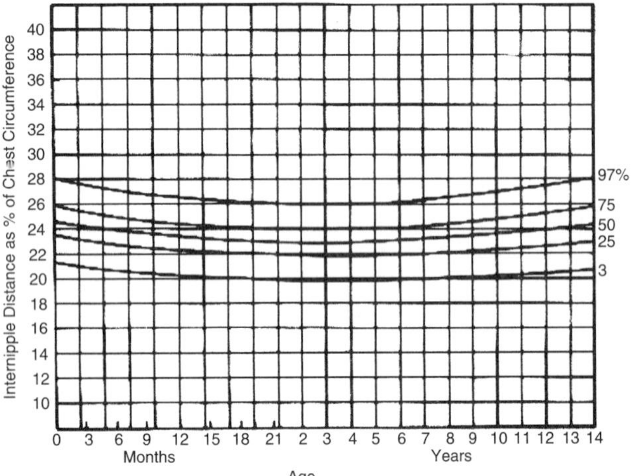


**FIGURE 19–7.** The internipple distance as a percentage of the chest circumference plotted against age for both sexes. *(From Feingold M, Bossert WH: Normal values for selected physical parameters: An aid to syndrome delineation. Birth Defects 10:1-16, 1974.)*

Deltas, or *triradii*, form at the convergence of three sets of ridges on the palm. This junction is where the hypothenar, thenar, and distal palmar patterns converge. There are typically no triradii in the hypothenar area of the palm, but when patterning is present or is large, a distal triradius arises, which is found in only 4% of normal white persons but in 85% of patients with trisomy 21 (Down syndrome). A single transverse (simian) crease is found in 4% of controls, but in more than half of patients with trisomy 21 (Fig. 19–11) and in even greater proportions in patients with other trisomies. The hallucal area of the foot, located at the base of the big toe, also has a dermal ridge pattern, usually a loop or whorl. A simple pattern or *open field* in this region is found in less than 1% of controls but in more than 50% of patients with Down syndrome (Fig. 19–12). This unusual dermal pattern is also associated with hypoplasia of the hallucal pad and a wide space between the great and second toes in these patients.

An examination of the *skin* is also important, to look for *phakomatoses* or skin manifestations that herald the presence of an underlying disorder. Examples are café-au-lait spots (associated with neurofibromatosis type 1) and ash leaf spots (associated with tuberous sclerosis and detected with the use of a Wood's lamp). Hemangiomas, irregular pigmentation, and skin diseases are noteworthy.

Finally, a careful neurologic examination with input from a specialist is often warranted in the child with multiple anomalies, because the neurologic status is often the most reliable prognostic indicator. Evaluation of tone, feeding, unusual movements, and the presence of seizure activity are critical pieces of diagnostic information.

## Adjunct Studies

An exhaustive physical examination often reveals differences that require further evaluation for diagnostic, prognostic, and treatment purposes (Table 19–6). Poor feeding

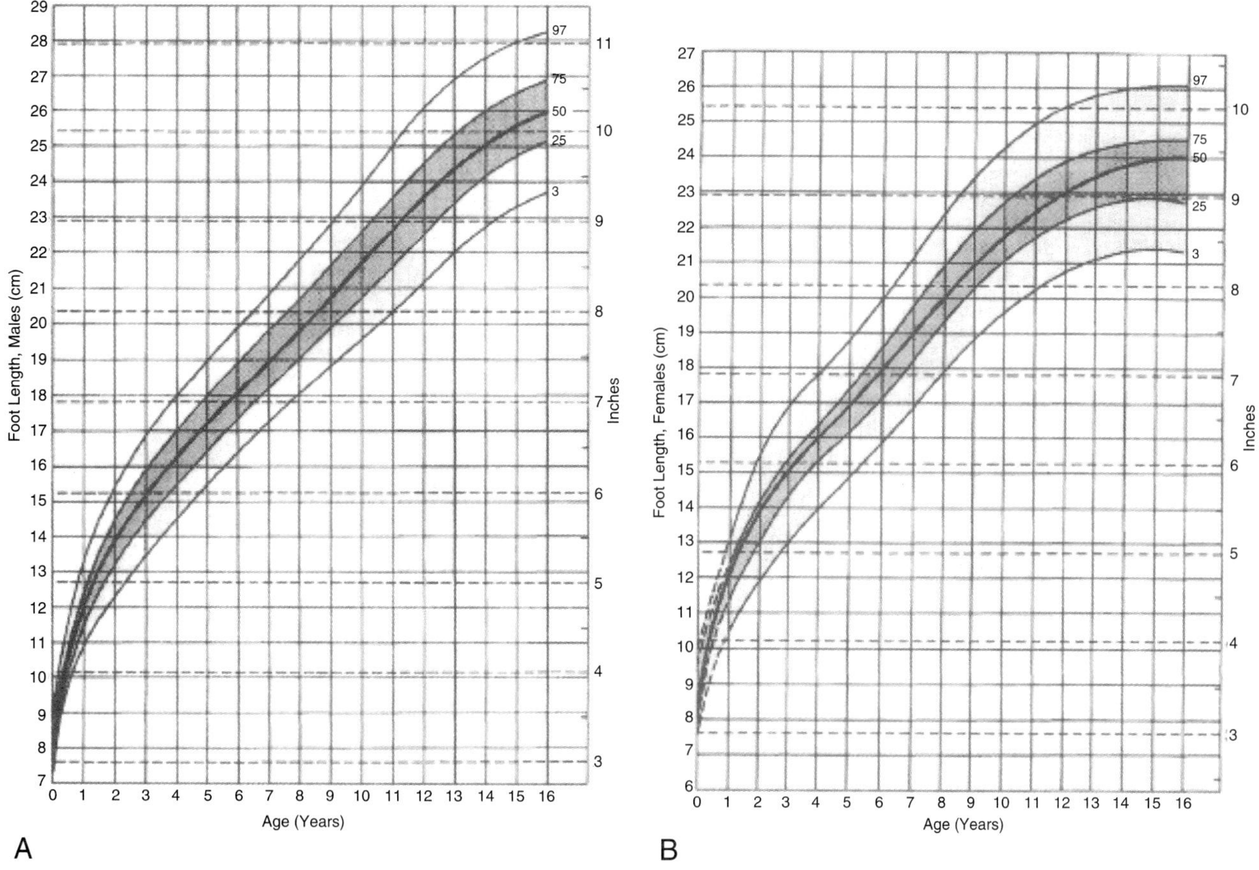


**FIGURE 19–9.** Total foot lengths plotted against age for boys (**A**) and girls (**B**). *(From Hall JC, Froster-Iskenius UG, Allanson JE: Handbook of Normal Physical Measurements. Oxford, UK, Oxford University Press, 1989.)*

or cyanosis may lead to detection of internal organ malformations on echocardiogram or abdominal ultrasonography. Differences in head shape suggest the need for skull films, three-dimensional computed tomography (CT), or magnetic resonance imaging (MRI) of the brain. A disproportion of the limbs prompts a skeletal survey and bone age measurement.

It is prudent, in children with anomalies involving multiple systems, to obtain the input of relevant specialists. This step is often essential to medical decision-making and the planning of interventions. Abnormal neurologic findings consultation from a trained specialist and interpretation of studies such as head ultrasonography, brain MRI, brainstem auditory evoked responses, and electroencephalogram (EEG) for seizure activity. Muscle dysfunction might result in the ordering of electromyography (EMG) or nerve conduction studies. Visual involvement requires a funduscopic examination by an experienced pediatric ophthalmologist, and sometimes, studies of visual evoked responses or electroretinograms are needed to predict visual prognosis. Often, there are well-characterized genetic disorders that have a specific pattern of abnormal findings on these highly specialized studies. Even when a unifying diagnosis is reached, there is often variation in the clinical phenotype, and determining the patient's prognosis on a system-by-system basis is typically the most appropriate and accurate way to proceed.

## LITERATURE REVIEW

The occurrence of malformations can fit into one of several categories (Table 19–7). The next step toward reaching a diagnosis is to analyze the data generated from the evaluation and attempt to categorize the findings. A *syndrome* is a "collection of anomalies involving more than one developmental region or organ system." The word itself means a "running together" or "pattern of multiple anomalies thought to be pathogenetically related." Thus, a given congenital anomaly may be an isolated defect in an otherwise normal person or part of a multiple malformation syndrome. Further, the primary malformation itself can determine additional defects through an interrelated cascade of physical and functional processes; if ensuing malformations are related to one primary defect, factor, or event, a pathogenetic *sequence* has occurred. A classic example is the Pierre-Robin sequence or constellation, consisting of a small recessed jaw, midline U-shaped cleft palate, and relatively large and protruding tongue. The primary anomaly is the small jaw, which does not allow adequate room for the tongue and displaces it superiorly. The displaced tongue prevents closure of the palatine shelves, causing the cleft palate. The recurrence risk with this isolated occurrence is negligible. However, one should also remember that such sequences can also be part of a larger constellation of findings that does fit into a

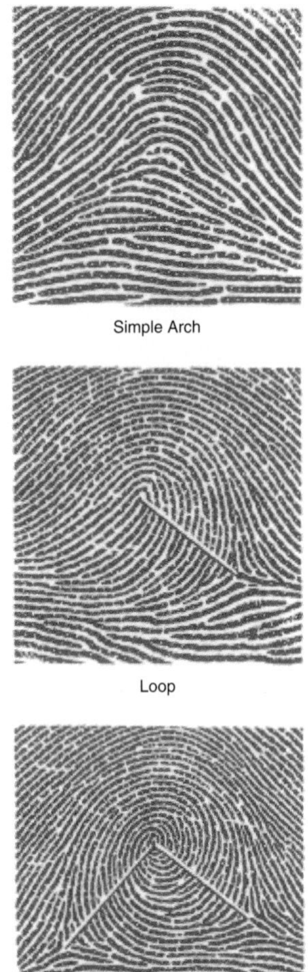


**FIGURE 19–10.** Basic fingerprint patterns (dermatoglyphics). *(From Holt SB: The Genetics of Dermal Ridges. Springfield, IL, Charles C Thomas, 1968.).*

syndrome, as Pierre-Robin sequence can when it is part of velocardiofacial syndrome (caused by a deletion of chromosome 22q11) or Stickler syndrome (associated with mutations in the type II collagen gene). The recurrence risk for an affected individual passing on these syndromes to their children is 50%.

**TABLE 19–5**

**Dermatoglyphic Patterns Associated with Specific Dysmorphic Disorders**

| Dermatoglyphic Pattern | Associated Disorder(s) |
|---|---|
| Excess arches | Trisomy 13, trisomy 18, Kline felter syndrome(47,XXY)<br>Deletion chr 5p (cri du chat), fetal phenytoin exposure |
| Excess ulnar loops | Trisomy 21 |
| Excess whorls | Smith-Lemli-Opitz syndrome<br>Turner syndrome (45,X0) |

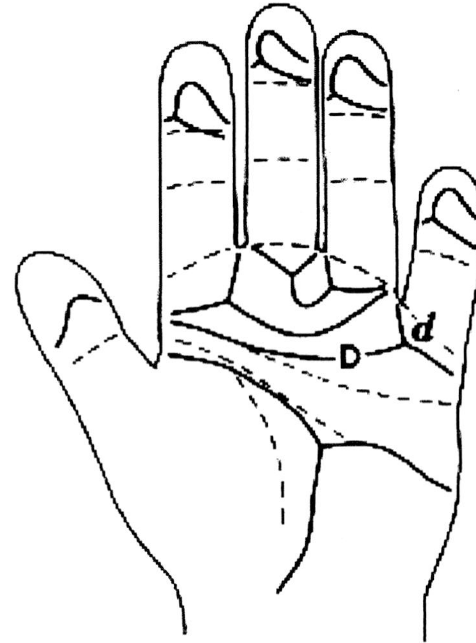


**FIGURE 19–11.** The patterns on the hand of a patient with trisomy 21 (Down syndrome) depicting the palmar crease (D). *(From Holt SB: The Genetics of Dermal Ridges. Springfield, IL, Charles C Thomas, 1968.)*

Additionally, a cluster of several malformations that are not developmentally related can occur in a nonrandom fashion called an *association* that may appear without characteristic dysmorphic features. The CHARGE association (coloboma, heart disease, atresia choanae, retarded growth and development, genital anomalies, and ear anomalies/deafness) is an example. It should be noted that not all features need to be present and that the extent of involvement of each system is widely variable. Another such statistically nonrandom association of defects consists of vertebral defects, imperforate anus, tracheoesophageal fistula, and radial or renal dysplasia (VATERR). Cardiac defects can also be a feature of the VATERR spectrum.

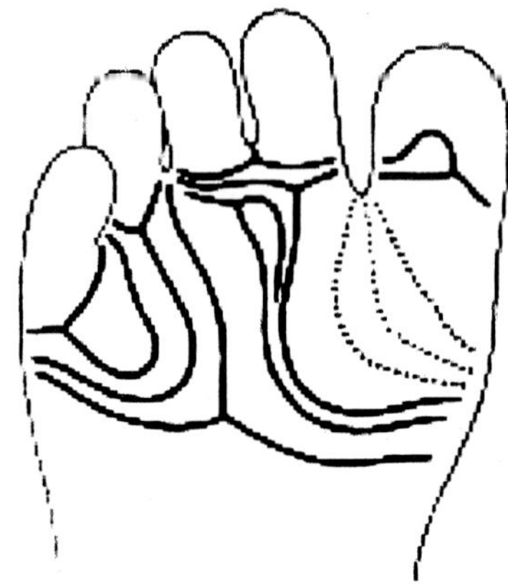

**FIGURE 19–12.** The distal sole of the foot of a patient with trisomy 21, depicting the characteristic "open field" pattern. *(From Holt SB: The Genetics of Dermal Ridges. Springfield, IL, Charles C Thomas, 1968.)*

**TABLE 19–6**

**Adjunct Studies in the Evaluation of the Dysmorphic Infant**

| | |
|---|---|
| Investigation of internal malformation | Ultrasonography<br>Magnetic resonance imaging |
| Assessment of neurologic function | Brain imaging<br>Electroencephalography as indicated<br>Electromyography as indicated |
| Identification of organ systems involved | Prognosis<br>Treatment and intervention |

These associations often manifest as sporadic rather than familial occurrences. Because they are not clearly related by a common etiology or pathogenesis, they are not considered syndromes and do not technically constitute a diagnosis. Instead, they are a recognition of a statistically significant association of features. It is important to remember that many of these same anomalies can occur as features of chromosomal aneuploidy or other syndromes. Syndromic malformations tend to occur in more than one developmental field. A *field defect* or complex is a set of primary malformations in a developmental field that originates from a single or primary abnormality in embryonic development (see Table 19–7).

When generating a differential diagnosis of malformations that might occur together, the evaluator must also consider structures that may look "abnormally formed" but in fact are structures that underwent normal development and then received some insult that distorted their true form (Table 19–8). For example, a *deformation* describes the abnormal form, shape, or position of a part of the body that was caused by mechanical forces. Examples are clubfoot, a hip dislocation, and craniofacial asymmetry. They can result from intrinsic (embryonic) or extrinsic (intrauterine) mechanical forces that alter the shape or position of an organ or part that had already undergone *normal* differentiation. Deformations are estimated to occur in 2% of births, and such factors as fetal crowding from the presence of multiple fetuses and uterine malformations, as well as oligohydramnios and a face presentation during delivery can cause them.

**TABLE 19–7**

**Underlying Mechanisms of Malformation**

| | |
|---|---|
| Syndrome | Pathogenetically related pattern of anomalies |
| Sequence | Pattern of anomalies derived from a presumed or known prior anomaly or mechanical disturbance |
| Association | Nonrandom occurrence of multiple anomalies |
| Field defect | Disturbance of a developmental field leading to a pattern of anomalies |

**TABLE 19–8**

**Processes Leading to Altered Form or Structure**

| | |
|---|---|
| Deformation | Abnormal form resulting from mechanical forces |
| Disruption | Morphologic defect caused by interference with a previously *normal* developmental process |
| Dysplasia | Altered morphology due to abnormal organization of cells into a given tissue |

Along similar lines, a *disruption* describes a "morphologic defect of an organ, part of an organ, or larger region of the body resulting from the extrinsic breakdown of, or an interference with, an originally normal developmental process." The classic example of a disruption is entanglement of the fetus in amniotic bands. Amniotic bands are ribbons of amnion that have ruptured in utero and cause disruptions of normal developmental processes in the fetus, either through physical blockage or interruption of the blood supply or by entangling and tearing of developing structures. This effect is most often seen with digits and limbs, and remnants of the bands, or constriction marks, can frequently be seen at birth. If the fetus should swallow a band, a cleft palate might result; the etiology is a very different etiology from that of cleft palate occurring as a primary malformation. Counseling of the parent would be very different in these two scenarios.

*Dysplasias* occur when there is "an abnormal organization of cells into tissue(s) and its morphologic results." Dysplasia tends to be tissue specific rather than organ specific (e.g., skeletal dysplasia) and can be localized or generalized.

In summary, structural or morphologic changes identified at birth can occur during intrauterine development as a result of malformations, deformations, disruptions, or dysplasia. However, approximately 90% of deformations undergo spontaneous correction. Malformations and disruptions often require surgical intervention, when possible. Dysplasias are typically not correctable, and the affected individual experiences the clinical effects of the underlying cell or tissue abnormality for life (see Table 19–8). Examples of these entities are listed in Table 19–9.

After the history and physical evaluation are complete, a cross-reference of two or more anomalies is useful to generate a differential diagnosis. When the rest of the baby's physical and history findings are added, the possibilities can often be narrowed down to a few entities that

**TABLE 19–9**

**Examples of Morphologic Differences**

| | |
|---|---|
| Malformation | Cardiac septal defects, cleft lip |
| Deformation | Club foot |
| Disruption | Amniotic bands |
| Dysplasia | Localized: hemangioma<br>Generalized (skeletal): achondroplasia |

may be amenable to diagnostic testing. If multiple anomalies are present, it is usually best to start with the least common. As Aase (1992) has stated, "The best clues are the rarest. The physical features that will be the most helpful on differential diagnosis are those infrequently seen either in isolation or as part of syndromes. Quite often, these are not the most obvious anomalies or even the ones that have the greatest significance for the patient's health." Cross-referencing is usually best accomplished by using published compendia of malformation syndromes. These compendia have been supplemented by databases that are accessible on line (GeneTests, on line; OMIM, on line; PubMed, on line). The availability of such tools allows the cross-referenced features to be easily compared with those of other described syndromes that may include similar malformations. This systematic review produces a differential diagnosis for the constellation of features described and identifies references to pertinent literature.

Thus, the recognition of patterns of genetic entities involves the comparison of the proband with the examiner's personal experience of known cases and a search of the literature. Multiple anomalies may be causally related, may occur together in a statistically associated basis, or may occur together merely by chance. Diagnosis of a genetic disorder relies heavily on the ability of the clinician to suspect, detect, and correctly interpret physical and developmental findings and to recognize specific patterns. Accurate diagnosis of a syndrome in a child is important to the identification of major complications and their treatment if possible. It is also crucial for long-term management of patients and for parental counseling about recurrence in future offspring.

## SPECIALIZED LABORATORY TESTS

In sorting through the array of possibilities listed, the geneticist utilizes one other important tool: the availability of highly specialized cytogenetic and molecular genetic testing, including:

- Karyotype
- Fluorescence in situ hybridization (FISH)
- Subtelomeric FISH
- Molecular analysis

The standard *karyotype*, or analysis of stretched and stained chromosome preparations usually taken from a peripheral blood sample, can often confirm a suspected diagnosis or explain a set of major malformations not classically encountered together. Further description of specific chromosomal abnormalities is addressed in Chapter 20; it is sufficient to note here that multiple malformation syndromes can result from large visible chromosome rearrangements that lead to deletion or addition of material (aneuploidy). These rearrangements can involve an entire arm of a chromosome or can be submicroscopic, requiring further special testing. Such small deletions can often be detected by *fluorescence in situ hybridization* (FISH) analysis, which is performed using a probe specific for the deleted region. FISH analysis utilizing probes from the tips of all chromosomes (*subtelomeric FISH*) has uncovered previously undetectable rearrangements that could explain the patient's clinical findings.

It has become the standard of care in several centers to offer such testing as an adjunct to karyotype analysis for newborns with multiple malformations that do not clearly fit into a recognizable syndrome. Additionally, as more information is becoming available about the role of mutations in specific individual genes, testing for these mutations is also becoming clinically available as an important confirmatory test. It can be useful to check with a geneticist or genetics counselor for the availability of gene mutation testing that may be performed on a research or diagnostic basis. GeneTests (on line) is one Web-based database of laboratories worldwide that provides such services. A more extensive discussion of single-gene disorders that can manifest in newborns is provided in Chapter 17.

## DIAGNOSIS

There are, however, cases in which, even after a detailed examination, exhaustive literature search, and genetic testing, no unifying diagnosis is evident. Aase (1992), a dysmorphologist, advises, "Don't panic! The absence of a diagnosis may be distressing to the diagnostician and the family, but it is much less dangerous than the possibility of assigning the wrong diagnosis with the risk of erroneous genetic and prognostic counseling and possibly hazardous treatment." Thus, in cases in which there is no clear diagnosis, prognosis and treatment should be determined according to the organ systems involved and the extent of their impairment. Additionally, when the infant has a severe untreatable impairment or the patient's condition is critical, it may be prudent to offer and obtain consent for a full postmortem examination by an experienced pathologist. A blood or skin sample should also be taken for establishing a cell line or for extracting DNA for future testing. Information gained from such investigations may often become relevant for family members, including the parents, allowing one to provide accurate recurrence risk counseling and perhaps offer prenatal testing of a new pregnancy. Such information can often help provide closure for the family as well.

When should a genetics evaluation be considered? The following clinical situations prompt a further genetic evaluation and counseling by a specialist:

- Multiple anatomic anomalies
- History of maternal exposure to teratogens
- Familial disorders
- Increased carrier frequency or ethnic risk
- Multiple pregnancy losses

As described previously, if a birth defect is identified in the presenting patient or *proband*, especially if the defect is associated with other anatomic anomalies, short stature, or developmental delays, the features of a specific genetic syndrome may be present. A known history of maternal exposure to a potential teratogen would also be an indication for consultation. Conditions appearing to be familial, or a family history of hereditary disorders involving malformation of a major organ, or major physical differences such as unusual body proportions, short stature, or irregular skin pigmentation, would warrant genetic investigation. Mental retardation, blindness, hearing loss, or neurologic deterioration in multiple family members suggests a genetic etiology. Likewise, a strong family history of cancer or a defined ethnic risk such as Ashkenazi Jewish heritage and its association with a higher carrier frequency for Tay-Sachs disease would be an indication for genetic evaluation. The occurrence of multiple pregnancy losses would also raise the suspicion of a genetically influenced cause and indicate the need for further investigation and counseling.

## CONCLUSION

Diseases with underlying genetic bases have significant effects on health care and its delivery. An appreciation of these entities, coupled with an organized, systematic evaluation, can help define the nature of a given disorder and aid in development of the optimal plan of treatment and care for the patient.

## SELECTED READINGS

Gehlerter TD, Collins FS, Ginsburg D (eds): Principles of Medical Genetics, 2nd ed, Baltimore, Williams & Wilkins, 1998.

Gorlin RJ, Cohen MM Jr, Hennecam RCM: Syndromes of the Head and Neck. New York, Oxford University Press, 2001.

Rimoin DL, Connor JM, Pyeritz RE (eds): Emery and Rimoin's Principles and Practice of Medical Genetics, 3rd ed. New York, Churchill Livingstone, 1996.

Schinzel A: Catalogue of Unbalanced Chromosome Aberrations in Man. Berlin, Walter de Gruyter, 1984.

Spranger J, Benirschke K, Hall JG, et al: Errors of morphogenesis: Concepts and terms. J Pediatr 100:160-165, 1982.

Stevenson RE, Hall JG, Goodman RM: Human Malformations and Related Anomalies, vol 2. New York, Oxford University Press, 1993.

## REFERENCES

Aase JM: Diagnostic Dysmorphology. New York, Plenum, 1992.

Campana M, Serra A, Neri G: Role of chromosome aberrations in recurrent abortion: A study of 269 balanced translocations. Am J Med Genet 24:341-356, 1986.

Cassidy SB, Brunger JW, Moussavand S, et al: Now more than ever: The burden of genetic disease in over 4,000 consecutive pediatric hospital admissions. Am J Hum Genet 67:32, 2000.

Castle D, Bernstein R: Cytogenetic analysis of 688 couples experiencing multiple spontaneous abortions. Am J Med Genet 29:549-556, 1988.

Feingold M, Bossert WH: Normal values for selected physical parameters: An aid to syndrome delineation. Birth Defects 10:1-16, 1974.

GeneTests. Available on line at www.genetests.org/

Hall JG, Powers EK, McIlvane RT, et al: The frequency and financial burden of genetic disease in a pediatric hospital. Am J Med Genet 1:417-436, 1978.

Hall JG, Froster-Iskenius UG, Allanson JE: Handbook of Normal Physical Measurements. Oxford, UK, Oxford University Press, 1989.

Holt SB: The Genetics of Dermal Ridges. Springfield, IL, Charles C Thomas, 1968.

Jones KL: Smith's Recognizable Patterns of Human Malformation, 5th ed. Philadelphia, WB Saunders, 1997.

Nussbaum RL, McInnes RR, Willard HF (eds): Thompson and Thompson's Genetics in Medicine, 6th ed. Philadelphia, WB Saunders, 2001.

OMIM: Available on line at www.ncbi.nlm.nih.gov:80/entrez/query.fcgi?db = OMIM/

PubMed: Available on line at www.ncbi.nlm.nih.gov/entrez/query.fcgi?db = PubMed/

Scriver CR, Neal JL, Saginur R, et al: The frequency of genetic disease and congenital malformation among patients in a pediatric hospital. Can Med Assoc J 108:1111-1115, 1973.

CHAPTER

# 20

# Specific Chromosome Disorders in Newborns

Sulagna C. Saitta and Elaine H. Zackai

It has been estimated that 3% of newborns have a major structural anomaly that will affect their quality of life. Although most of these patients have a single malformation, 0.7% of infants have multiple major malformations. In an additional 2%, a major anomaly is discovered by age 5 years. Early identification of the genetic nature of a given condition can aid in treatment and help to identify resources for providing better health care to these individuals. Here we focus on genetic disorders and syndromes with underlying chromosomal abnormalities that typically manifest in the newborn period (see OMIM for a detailed online database).

## HUMAN KARYOTYPE

Chromosomes consist of tightly compacted DNA whose structure is maintained by association with histones and other proteins. When treated and stretched, chromosomes from dividing cells can be visualized under the light microscope as linear structures with two *arms* joined by a *centromere*. The short arm is designated *p* (petit) and the long arm is designated *q*. The ends of the p and q arms are known as *telomeres*. Human chromosomes were first visualized in 1956 (Lejeune and Turpin et al), and each pair shows a distinctive size, centromeric position, and staining or banding pattern after treatment with special dyes, allowing it to be identified and classified. Each chromosome is identified by a number, in general from largest to smallest, in standard international cytogenetic nomenclature. This presentation, or *karyotype* (Fig. 20–1), normally consists of 46 chromosomes, with 22 pairs of autosomes and one set of sex chromosomes—two X chromosomes for females (46,XX), and an X and Y for males (46,XY).

Karyotype analysis is performed in cells undergoing *mitosis*, or cell division, in which the chromosomes condense and can be stained and visualized. Thus, cells that can be stimulated to divide and grow in culture, such as peripheral blood lymphocytes, skin fibroblasts, and amniocytes, are typically used. Alternatively, cells normally undergoing rapid cell division, such as bone marrow and chorionic villus, can also be used successfully. Historically, several different staining methods have been described, however, G-banding (Giemsa staining) is the standard cytogenetic method used. This technique permits a resolution of at least 400 bands among all of the chromosomes and can be adapted to allow for high-resolution analysis of up to 800 bands to analyze subtle differences.

Gamete formation, either spermatogenesis or oogenesis, is accomplished by a process known as *meiosis*. In the first part of meiosis (*meiosis I*), homologous chromosomes line up as pairs and cross over, exchanging genetic material, also known as *recombination*. In the next stage, *meiosis II* or reduction division, the recombined pairs separate, and the typical *diploid* content (46 chromosomes) of the cell is reduced by half to a *haploid* complement of 23 chromosomes. The full diploid state of the cell will be restored at the time of fertilization.

An imbalance of genetic material, or *aneuploidy*, can occur from a net loss or gain of genetic material during sperm or egg formation or, less commonly, during the initial divisions of the embryo. This missing or extra genetic material can be small pieces or parts of chromosomes or an entire chromosome itself. The classic recognizable aneuploidy syndromes involve *trisomy* (three copies of a given chromosome) such as those of chromosomes 13, 18, 21, or *monosomy* (only a single copy) of a complete chromosome, such as X. Trisomies, especially, can occur from *non-disjunction*, a failure of normal chromosome separation. In such cases, a pair of homologues does not separate in meiosis; one daughter cell receives both homologues of that pair, and the other cell receives none. This can occur in either part of gamete division, meiosis I or meiosis II. Most human meiotic non-disjunctions occur in oocyte formation, specifically in maternal meiosis I. This is especially pronounced in trisomies of the acrocentric chromosomes (13, 14, 15, 21, and 22) and in XXX trisomy (MacDonald et al, 1994; Zaragoza et al, 1994). The occurrence of meiotic non-disjunction increases significantly with maternal age. Thus, prenatal karyotyping from amniocentesis or chorionic villus sampling (CVS) is offered to women ages 35 years and older (Hook and Cross, 1982).

Non-disjunction can also occur in mitosis, with uneven division of genetic material during early embryonic cell division. This can result in two cell lines, one *trisomic* lineage that is potentially viable and another *monosomic* line. If this event occurs after the first postzygotic division, cells with a normal chromosome complement may also exist with cells containing an aneuploid complement as a *mosaic* chromosome constitution.

Partial aneuploidies can occur through several mechanisms, such as rearrangements of material between nonhomologous chromosomes that can occur in the gametes of a balanced translocation carrier. The carrier parent who has no net loss or gain of genetic material is usually phenotypically normal; however the offspring are at increased risk for an unbalanced rearrangement and its phenotypic consequences. Attention has also been focused on deletion syndromes caused by the loss of genetic material from several chromosomes (e.g., 1p-, 4p-, 5p-), with a resulting, often recognizable phenotype. Other microdeletions have been associated with segmental duplications, or large blocks of DNA that contain chromosome-specific repetitive sequences. It is thought that the repeats can mediate misalignment between two homologues and have been shown to be present in regions of the genome prone to instability, such as the pericentromeric regions of

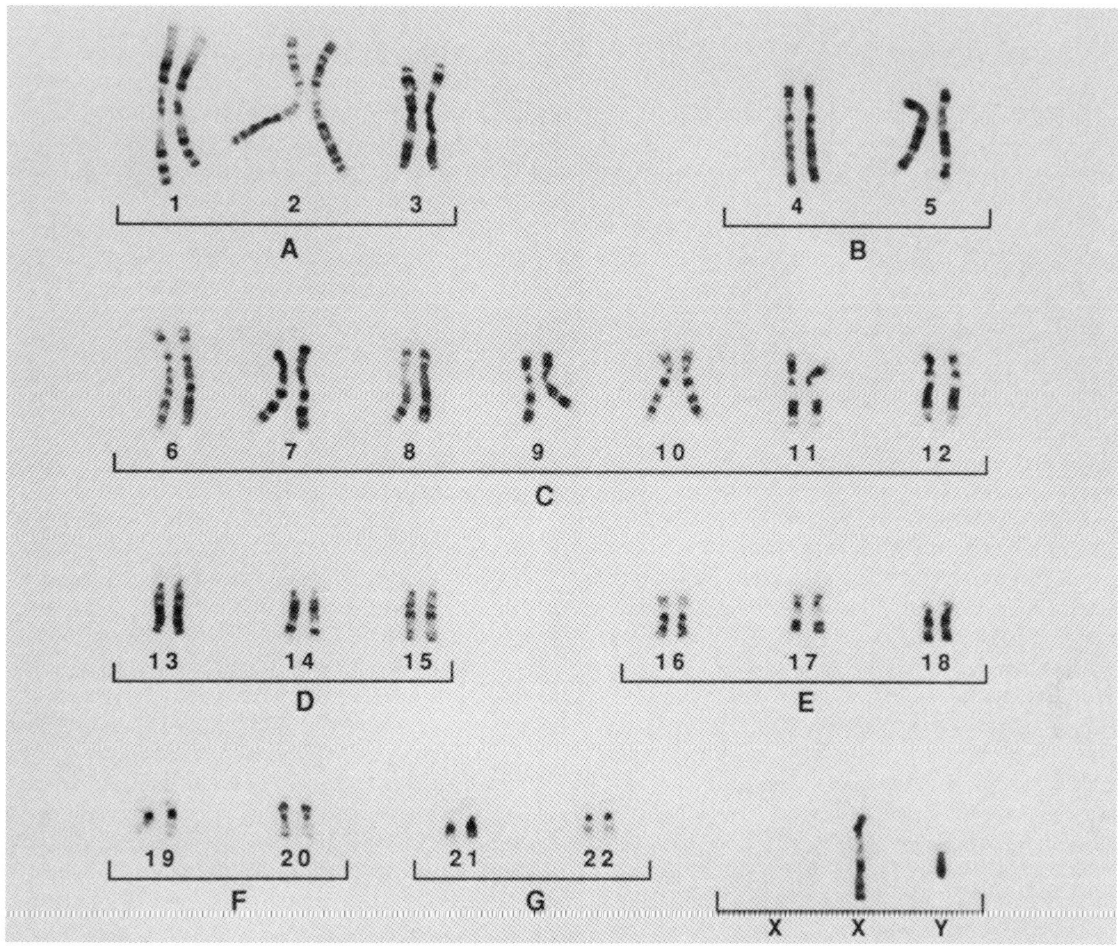


**FIGURE 20–1.** G-banded human male karyotype. The 46 chromosomes are arranged into 23 pairs, each with a specific banding pattern.

chromosomes 7q11, 15q11, 17q11, and 22q11, leading to the phenotypes seen in Williams-Beuren syndrome, Prader-Willi or Angelman syndrome, Charcot-Marie-Tooth disease or hereditary neuropathy with liability to pressure palsies (HNPP), and DiGeorge or velocardiofacial syndrome, respectively (Emanuel and Shaikh, 2001; Lupski, 2002). The advent and application of highly specific *fluorescent in situ hybridization* (FISH) probes to assess for these submicroscopic deletions as well as of chromosome-specific subtelomeric FISH (see later) has allowed the identification of smaller chromosomal rearrangements that were largely unrecognized only a decade ago.

## TRISOMIES

### Trisomy 21 (Down Syndrome)

In 1959, Lejeune and coworkers demonstrated that trisomy of human chromosome 21 caused the constellation of findings recognized as Down syndrome (Fig. 20–2). This was the first described chromosome disorder and is the most common viable autosomal trisomy, occurring in about 1 in 700 to 800 live births (Hook, 1992). The vast majority (>90%) occurs secondary to meiotic non-disjunction, and a pronounced maternal age effect is encountered. Approximately 3% to 5% of cases are due to a translocation, passed

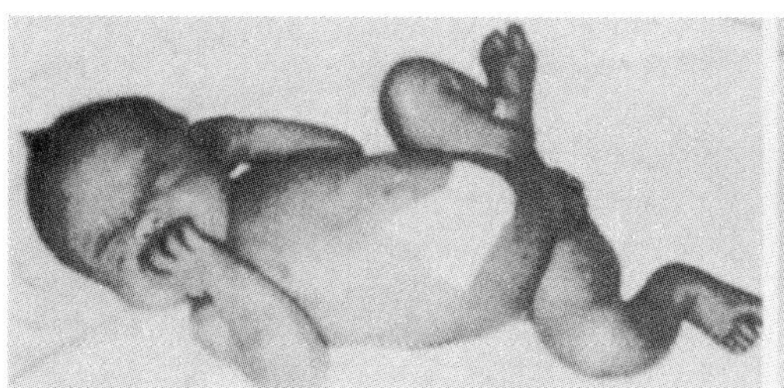

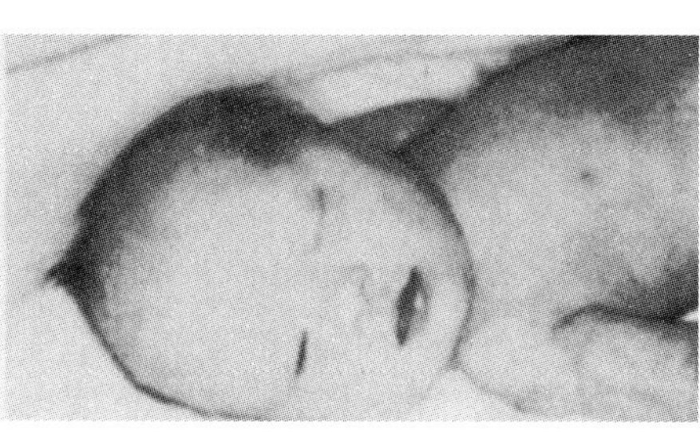

**FIGURE 20–2.** Newborn with Down syndrome (trisomy 21) illustrating some of the characteristic facial features, including upslanting palpebral fissures and a flat facial profile.

from a balanced translocation-carrier parent, that becomes unbalanced and trisomic in the baby. Typically, the translocated chromosome 21 rearranges with another acrocentric chromosome (often chromosome 14), resulting in a robertsonian translocation. Mitotic non-disjunction, or mosaic Down syndrome, has been demonstrated in approximately 3% of cases as well, with variable features ranging from normal to a typical Down syndrome phenotype.

## Clinical Features

It is the more common occurrence of Down syndrome in the babies of older mothers that has led to the use of prenatal karyotyping for advanced maternal age (>35 years) at the time of conception, with samples typically obtained by amniocentesis after 15 weeks of gestation, or CVS at 10 to 12 weeks. Maternal serum analyte (triple- or quad-screen) testing is for prenatal screening purposes. Associated ultrasonographic findings for trisomy 21, including a cardiac defect, shortened long bones, nuchal translucency or thickening, echogenic small bowel, and duodenal atresia (double-bubble sign), may be seen in 50% to 60% of fetuses with trisomy 21. Most patients with Down syndrome, if not diagnosed prenatally, are usually recognized at birth because of the typical phenotypic features, which then prompt karyotype analysis.

The constellation of physical findings associated with trisomy 21 consists of brachycephaly, presence of a third fontanelle, upslanted palpebral fissures, epicanthal folds, Brushfield spots in the irises, flattened nasal root, small posteriorly rotated ears, prominent tongue, short neck with excess nuchal skin, single palmar creases, brachydactyly, fifth-finger clinodactyly, exaggerated gap between first and second toe, open field hallucal pattern, and hypotonia (see Fig. 20–2). Often the physical features conform to an easily distinguishable phenotype, but in some cases, prematurity or ethnic variations may make a clinical diagnosis difficult. In any case, an immediate karyotype is indicated to confirm the diagnosis and as preparation for counseling of the family.

Malformations involving many organ systems have been described in trisomy 21, and whether the diagnosis is known prenatally or determined in the newborn period, several clinical investigations are warranted when this diagnosis is suspected. The most common malformation is congenital heart disease (up to 60%; Epstein, 2001), which typically requires surgical intervention. Atrioventricular canal defects are often encountered (mean of 40%), although ventricular septal defects (VSDs), atrial septal defects (ASDs), tetralogy of Fallot, and patent ductus arteriosus (PDA) are all described in the disorder. Thus, an echocardiogram is indicated in all cases, and medical and surgical intervention of cardiac lesions is routine. Gastrointestinal malformations, especially duodenal atresia (2% to 5%), and Hirschsprung disease as well as less frequently encountered conditions, such as esophageal atresias, fistulas, and webs throughout the tract, have been described. It is critical to carefully monitor the baby's feeding and bowel function before considering discharge.

Although growth parameters can be in the range of 10% to 25% at birth, significantly decreased postnatal growth velocity is encountered in these patients (Clementi et al, 1990). Separate growth curves have been devised for patients with trisomy 21 (Fernandes et al, 2001), because growth retardation involving height, weight, and head circumference has been well documented. An initial ophthalmologic evaluation is also indicated in the first few months of life and then annually, because strabismus, cataracts, myopia, and glaucoma have been shown to be more common in children with trisomy 21. Additionally, hearing loss of heterogenous origin is present in approximately half of patients, with middle ear disease contributing to this problem.

Spinal cord compression due to atlantoaxial subluxation and subsequent neurologic sequelae can be a complication of the disorder, and physicians should be vigilant in evaluating the cervical spine especially before administration of anesthesia as well as before an older child's participation in sports. The instability is thought to be due to ligamentous laxity in the region. Other associated disorders that merit screening are hypothyroidism, described in approximately 5% of patients with trisomy 21, often with the presence of thyroid autoantibodies. Additionally, bone marrow dyscrasias, such as neonatal thrombocytopenia, and transient self-resolving myeloproliferative disorders, such as leukemoid reaction, have been observed in the first year of life. An elevated rate of leukemia with a relative risk of 10 to 18 times normal up to age 16 years has been described. Acute nonlymphoblastic leukemia (ANLL) is seen at higher rates in congenital or newborn cases, but the distribution becomes similar to that of non–trisomy 21 patients after age 3 years. Survival of patients with Down syndrome is shorter after a diagnosis of acute lymphoblastic leukemia (ALL) than in diploid patients (Epstein, 2001).

Patients with trisomy 21 demonstrate a wide range of developmental abilities, with highly variable personalities and behavioral phenotypes as well (Pueschel et al, 1991). Central hypotonia with concomitant motor delay is most pronounced in the first 3 years of life, as are language delays. Thus, immediate and intensive early intervention and developmental therapy are critical for maximizing the developmental outcome. A wide IQ range has been described, with conflicting data on genetic and environmental modifiers of outcome (Epstein, 2001). Seizure disorders occur in 5% to 10% of patients, often manifesting in infancy.

The most common causes of death in patients with trisomy 21 are related to the congenital heart disease, to infection that is thought to be associated with defects in T-cell maturation and function, and to malignancy (Fong and Brodeur, 1987). Once medical and surgical interventions for correction of associated congenital malformations are complete and successful, the long-term survival rate is good. However, less than half of patients survive to 60 years, and less than 15% past 68 years. Neurodegenerative disease with features of Alzheimer disease is encountered in most patients with trisomy 21 who are older than 40 years, although frank dementia is not typical. Men with trisomy 21 are almost always infertile, while small numbers of affected women have reproduced (Epstein, 2001).

In counseling the family of a newborn diagnosed with trisomy 21 or Down syndrome, it is important to include the organ systems affected in their baby and the severity of each malformation when defining a prognosis. Above all, the wide variability of the phenotype should be emphasized, with a care plan tailored to the needs of the individual patient.

### Genetic Counseling

If a complete (full chromosome) or mosaic trisomy 21 is found, parental karyotypes are generally not analyzed, because in virtually all cases, the karyotypes are normal. After having one child with trisomy 21, a mother's recurrence risk for another affected child is approximately 1% higher than her age-specific risk (Hook, 1992). This fact is especially significant in younger mothers, whose age-specific risks are low. If a de novo translocation resulting in trisomy 21 is found, the recurrence risk is less than 1%. If the mother is found to carry a constitutional balanced robertsonian translocation, the risk for another translocation Down syndrome fetus is about 15% at the gestational age when amniocentesis is offered, and 10% at birth. However, if the father is the translocation carrier, the recurrence risk is significantly smaller, approximately 1% to 2% (Epstein, 2001).

## Trisomy 18 (Edwards Syndrome)

Trisomy 18 is encountered in 1 in 6000 live births and is associated with a high rate of intrauterine demise. It is estimated that only 5% of conceptuses with trisomy 18 survive to birth and that 30% of fetuses diagnosed by second-trimester amniocentesis die before the end of the pregnancy (Hook, 1992). Findings on prenatal ultrasonography can raise suspicion for the disorder—growth retardation, oligohydramnios or polyhydramnios, heart defects, myelomeningocele, clenched fists, excess of arches on dermatoglyphic examination, and limb anomalies. Maternal serum analyte or triple screening can show low values for alpha-fetoprotein, estradiol, and total human chorionic gonadotropin, indicating subsequent karyotype analysis and fetal ultrasonographic monitoring.

### Clinical Features

Phenotypic features present at birth consist of intrauterine growth restriction (1500 to 2500 g at term), small narrow cranium with prominent occiput, open metopic suture, low-set posteriorly rotated ears, micrognathia with small mouth, clenched hands with overlapping digits, hypoplastic nails, and "rocker-bottom" feet or prominent heels with convex soles (Fig. 20–3). Additional malformations encountered in this syndrome are congenital heart disease (ASD, VSD, PDA, pulmonic stenosis, aortic coarctation), cleft palate, clubfoot deformity, renal malformations, brain anomalies, choanal atresia, eye malformations, vertebral anomalies, hypospadias, cryptorchidism, and limb defects, especially of the radial rays.

The prognosis in this disorder is extremely poor, with more than 90% of babies succumbing in the first 6 months of life and only 5% alive at 1 year. Death is due to central apnea, infection, and congestive heart failure. The newborn period is characterized by poor feeding and growth, typically requiring tube feedings. A few patients have been described who have survived into childhood and beyond. Universal poor growth and profound mental retardation with developmental progress not beyond that of a 6-month-old infant (Baty et al, 1994) have been documented. Malignant tumors such as hepatoblastoma, and Wilms tumor, have been described in some of the survivors. In the few patients in whom cardiac surgery was performed, outcome was not shown to be improved.

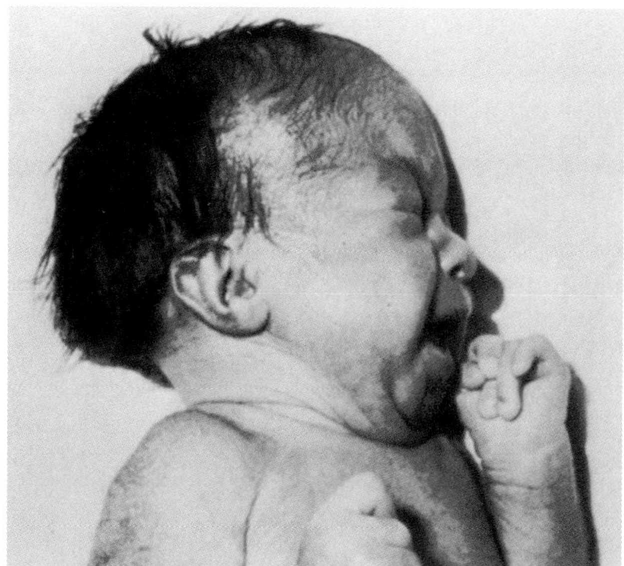

**FIGURE 20–3.** Newborn with trisomy 18, showing prominent occiput, characteristic facial appearance, and clenched hands.

### Genetic Counseling

The typical estimate of a recurrence risk for trisomy 18 in a future pregnancy is a 1% risk over the maternal age–specific risk for *any* viable autosomal trisomy (Hook, 1992). Trisomy occurring from a structural rearrangement such as a translocation warrants parental karyotype analysis before the recurrence risk can be assessed.

## Trisomy 13 (Patau Syndrome)

It has been estimated that only about 2% to 3% of fetuses with trisomy 13 survive to birth, with a frequency of 1 in 12,500 to 21,000 live births (Hook, 1992). As with other trisomies, amniocentesis performed for advanced maternal age or indicated by fetal ultrasonographic findings may lead to a prenatal diagnosis of trisomy 13.

### Clinical Features

Trisomy 13–associated malformations include congenital heart disease, cleft palate, holoprosencephaly, renal anomalies, and postaxial polydactyly (Fig. 20–4). Additionally, microcephaly, eye anomalies, and scalp defects can suggest the diagnosis. Brain malformations such as

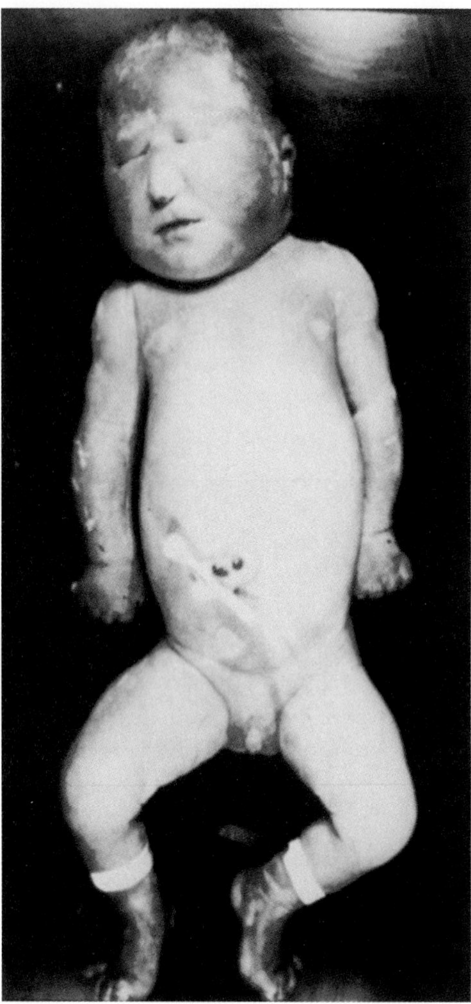

**FIGURE 20–4.** Stillborn with trisomy 13. The facial appearance is that of cebocephaly, which is associated with holoprosencephaly. There is an extra digit on the ulnar border of the right hand.

holoprosencephaly are found in more than half the patients, with concomitant seizure disorders. Microcephaly, split sutures, and open fontanelles are encountered. A scalp defect (cutis aplasia) that can sometimes be mistakenly attributed to a fetal scalp monitor is quite specific to the disorder, being found in 50% of cases. Eye malformations, including iris colobomas and hamartomatous cartilage "islands," can be found on funduscopic examination.

Congenital heart disease is present in about 80% of patients, usually VSD, ASD, PDA, or dextrocardia. Limb anomalies, such as postaxial polydactyly, single palmar creases, and hyperconvex narrow fingernails, are also seen. The fingers can be flexed and overlapped, and can show camptodactyly as well. An increased frequency of nuclear projections in neutrophils, giving a "drumstick" appearance similar to that of Barr bodies, can also be found. This finding would be especially striking in males, in whom Barr bodies would not be expected.

As with trisomy 18, prognosis for the fetus with trisomy 13 is extremely poor, with 80% mortality in the neonatal period, and less than 5% of patients surviving to age 6 months. Mental retardation is profound, and many patients are blind and deaf as well. Feeding difficulties are typical.

### Genetic Counseling

Recurrence risk data suggest that as with trisomy 18, the chance that a woman will have a child with any trisomy after a pregnancy affected by trisomy 13 is rare. The estimated risk is 1% higher than the maternal age–related risk for the recurrence of any viable autosomal trisomy in a subsequent pregnancy.

## Turner Syndrome (45,XO)

In early embryogenesis, two active X chromosomes are required for normal development. Turner syndrome, a phenotype associated with loss of all or part of one copy of the X chromosome in a female conceptus, occurs in approximately 1 in 2500 female newborns. The 45,XO karyotype or loss of one entire X chromosome accounts for roughly half the cases. A variety of X chromosome anomalies, including deletions, isochromosomes, and translocations, account for the remainder of the causes. It is important to note that only about 0.1% of fetuses with a 45,XO complement survive to term, the vast majority (>99%) being spontaneously aborted; this fact underscores the requirement for both X chromosomes during embryonic development. Further studies indicate that in approximately 80% of cases, it is the paternally derived X chromosome that is lost (Willard, 2001).

### Clinical Features

There is wide phenotypic variability in patients with Turner syndrome. Features present at birth include short stature, webbed neck, craniofacial differences (epicanthal folds and high arched palate), hearing loss, shield chest, renal anomalies, lymphedema of the hands and feet with nail hypoplasia, and congenital heart disease. Typical cardiac defects are bicuspid aortic valve, coarctation of the aorta, valvular aortic stenosis, and mitral valve prolapse.

Growth issues, especially short stature, are the predominant concern in childhood and adolescence; the mean adult height of patients with Turner syndrome is 135 to 150 cm without treatment. Growth hormone therapy, which is routinely offered starting around age 4 to 5 years, can lead to an average gain of 6 cm or more in final adult height (Willard, 2001). Primary ovarian failure due to gonadal dysplasia (streak gonads) can result in delay of secondary sexual characteristics and primary amenorrhea. Cyclic hormonal therapy is initiated at the age of puberty to aid the development of secondary sex characteristics and menses as well as to help bone mass. Infertility, related to gonadal dysplasia, is typical and has been successfully treated with assisted reproduction techniques and donor oocytes. It is important to evaluate for structural cardiovascular defects in the patient before pregnancy.

In terms of intellectual development, specific difficulties with spatial and perceptual thinking lead to a lower performance IQ; however, this syndrome is not characterized by mental retardation.

### Triploidy (69,XXX or 69,XXY)

As its name implies, *triploidy* is a karyotype containing three copies of each chromosome. Mechanisms that can lead to this state include fertilization of the egg by two different sperm, (dispermy) and complete failure of normal chromosome separation in maternal meiosis. The vast majority of triploid fetuses are spontaneously aborted, accounting for up to 15% of chromosomally abnormal pregnancy losses. Live births of affected fetuses are rare, and reports of survival beyond infancy are only anecdotal. Mosaicism with combinations of diploid and triploid cells (*mixoploid*) has also been documented. Malformations, including hydrocephalus, neural tube defects, ocular and auricular malformations, cardiac defects, and 3-4 syndactyly of the fingers, are associated findings. Additionally, the placenta is often abnormal, typically large and cystic.

## DELETION SYNDROMES

In addition to the aneuploid conditions described previously, monosomy or partial monosomy of a chromosome can lead to a recognizable pattern of malformation as well. Two classic syndromes are described that are associated with the deletion or loss of genetic material from the *p* arms of chromosomes 4 and 5. A newer constellation of findings consistent with loss of material from chromosome 1p has also been reported (Shaffer et al, 2001). All of these syndromes are associated with deletions that involve the loss of many genes located in a specific region.

### Cri du Chat Syndrome (5p-)

Partial monosomy of chromosome 5p is seen in approximately 1 in 50,000 live births and is associated with a multiple congenital anomaly syndrome named for the unusual cry of the affected babies, which sounds like a cat's. The constellation of features associated with this disorder includes low birth weight, microcephaly, round face, hypertelorism or telecanthus, down-slanting palpebral fissures, epicanthi, and broad nasal bridge. Hypotonia and cardiac defects are also seen, including ASD, VSD, and tetralogy of Fallot. Early issues include failure to thrive and pronounced developmental delay. The cat's cry usually resolves during infancy, and survival into adulthood is possible but often with severe mental retardation. Intensive therapy appears to provide some benefit, and more sensitive measures of cognition demonstrate clearly better language receptive skills than expressive language ability. Thus, children may understand more complex verbal language than their expressive skills might demonstrate (Cornish et al, 1999).

It is estimated that nearly 100 genes are lost when the putative critical region from 5p15.2 to p15.3 is deleted (Shaffer et al, 2001). Close to 90% of 5p deletions arise de novo in the affected child, incurring a minimal risk of recurrence(<1%). The remainder arise from malsegregation of a balanced translocation in a carrier parent, which would be associated with a 10% to 15% risk of recurrence of an unbalanced karyotype in a future liveborn. Parental karyotype analysis is indicated for proper recurrence risk counseling.

### Wolf-Hirschhorn Syndrome (4p-)

Distal deletions of the short arm of chromosome 4 are associated with a recognizable pattern of malformation. This syndrome is estimated to occur in 1 in 50,000 births and has features such as intrauterine growth restriction, microcephaly, midline structural defects such as cleft lip and cleft palate, cardiac septal defects, and hypospadias. The characteristic facial features are described as the "Greek helmet" facies, as evidenced by hypertelorism with epicanthi, a high forehead with a prominent glabella, and a beaked nose. Prominent, low-set ears are also seen. Hypotonia, failure to thrive, and developmental delay are the rule, with one third of infants dying in the first year of life. Many patients have lived well into childhood and even into adulthood, although profound growth and mental retardation, often accompanied by seizures, is typical.

Although most deletions are cytogenetically visible on karyotype analysis, small submicroscopic deletions have also been described. In cases in which the clinical features are suggestive but the karyotype is not revealing, further cytogenetic analysis using specific probes from the 4p region for FISH analysis is indicated. More than 80% of 4p deletions arise de novo in the patient, with minimal risk of recurrence. In the 10% to 15% of cases resulting from a translocation, obtaining parental karyotypes is clinically indicated for appropriate recurrence risk counseling.

### Chromosome 1p Deletion Syndrome (1p-)

Monosomy for the distal short arm of chromosome 1, or deletion of 1p36, has been associated with a constellation of clinical findings. A characteristic facies, consisting of frontal bossing, large anterior fontanelle, flattened midface with deep set eyes and developmental delay, has been described (Fig. 20–5). Orofacial clefting, hypotonia, seizures, deafness, and cardiomyopathy are also noted.

This deletion syndrome is estimated to occur in approximately 1 in 10,000 live births, a figure that is most probably an underestimate; the availability of a specific FISH test and greater recognition of the phenotype will likely lead to improved diagnosis of this condition. The vast majority of deletions arise de novo in the patient, with about 3% attributable to malsegregation of a balanced parental translocation. The size of the deletion varies, from submicroscopic (<5 Mb) to 32 cm. There appears to be a correlation between the size of the deletion and the severity of clinical features.

Diagnosis has been made with karyotype analysis, but 50% of patients do not have a cytogenetically visible deletion. FISH studies targeted to this region in cases with suggestive clinical features have uncovered most of the other cases. The use of subtelomeric FISH to screen for deletions in any chromosome, as an adjunct to routine karyotyping, has led to the diagnosis in a number of patients.

### Subtelomeric FISH

The subtelomeric regions of human chromosomes have been difficult to evaluate with standard cytogenetic means (karyotype), small rearrangements being undetectable at

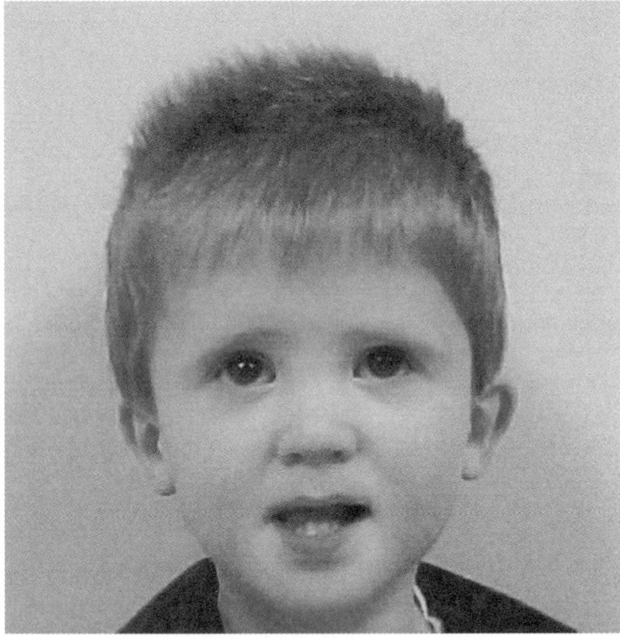

A

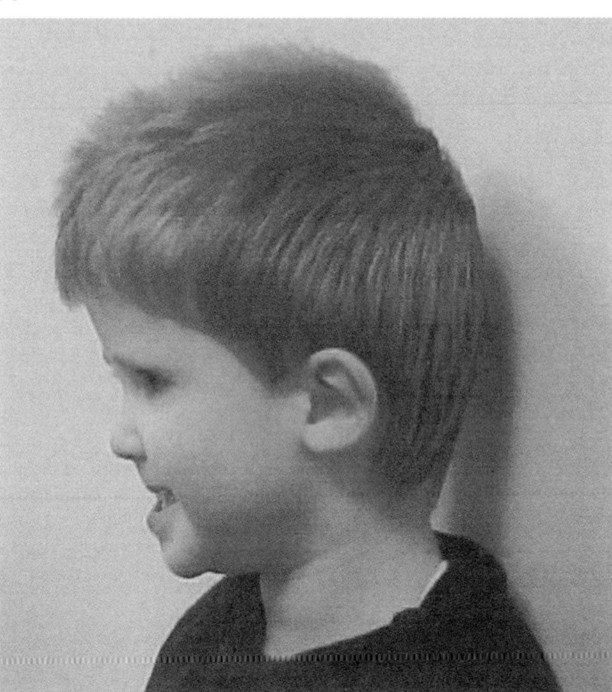

B

**FIGURE 20–5.** Child with deletion of chromosome 1p.

the current threshold of resolution. The development of commercially available chromosome-specific probes for use in subtelomeric FISH has emerged as the newest breakthrough in the identification of many submicroscopic rearrangements in these genomic regions. Use of subtelomeric repeat sequences that are distinctive for each chromosome for FISH analysis allows one to scan an entire karyotype for small rearrangements that were previously undetectable by high-resolution banding. Subtelomeric FISH has rapidly become part of routine genetic evaluations as an important adjunct to the standard or high-resolution karyotype for many situations.

Clinical indications for subtelomeric FISH include the evaluation of a newborn with multiple congenital anomalies that do not clearly fit into a recognizable pattern of malformation associated with a known chromosomal abnormality. As more subtelomeric rearrangements are characterized at the cytogenetic level, a greater recognition of their associated phenotypic features will emerge, ultimately leading to earlier diagnosis and better care for affected infants.

## SEGMENTAL DUPLICATIONS AND MICRODELETION SYNDROMES

A greater appreciation of the complexity of the human genome and an initial glimpse at its structure has now been afforded with the completion of the human genome sequence (see Chapter 17). This work has focused attention on regions of the genome that are prone to rearrangement. The presence of such "unstable" regions appears to play a significant role in the etiology of several genetic disorders (Emanuel and Shaikh, 2001). These disorders result from inappropriate dosage of crucial genes in a given genomic segment via either structural mechanisms (deletion or duplication) or functional mechanisms (imprinting, uniparental disomy). It has also been demonstrated that many of these regions of genomic instability have a common element: the presence of large, chromosome-specific low copy repeats that most likely mediate misalignment and unequal cross-over during recombination, leading to rearrangements such as a deletion and duplication (Fig. 20–6). Many of these large repeat structures are localized to a single chromosome or within a single chromosomal band. Examples of such "genomic" disorders are hemophilia A (inversion of Xq28), Charcot-Marie-Tooth disease (interstitial duplication on 17p12), the deletion of this same region of 17p12 leading to hereditary neuropathy with liability to pressure palsies (HNPP), and a small percentage of patients with neurofibromatosis type I (deletion involving 17q11.2).

In this section, we focus on several deletion syndromes that occur on chromosomes whose underlying genomic structure contains such segmental duplications: Williams-Beuren syndrome (involving chromosome 7q11.2), Prader Willi syndrome or Angelman syndrome (involving an imprinted region of chromosome 15q11 through 15q13) and DiGeorge or velocardiofacial syndrome (DGS/VCFS), the most commonly occurring microdeletion syndrome in humans, involving chromosome 22q11.2.

### Williams-Beuren Syndrome (7q11 Deletion)

The estimated incidence of Williams-Beuren syndrome is 1 in 20,000 to 50,000 live births. The phenotype has a variable spectrum but usually consists of distinctive facies, growth and developmental retardation, cardiovascular anomalies, and, occasionally, infantile hypercalcemia (see Fig. 24–8). Babies with Williams-Beuren syndrome usually show some degree of intrauterine growth restriction with mild microcephaly. Facial features are epicanthal folds

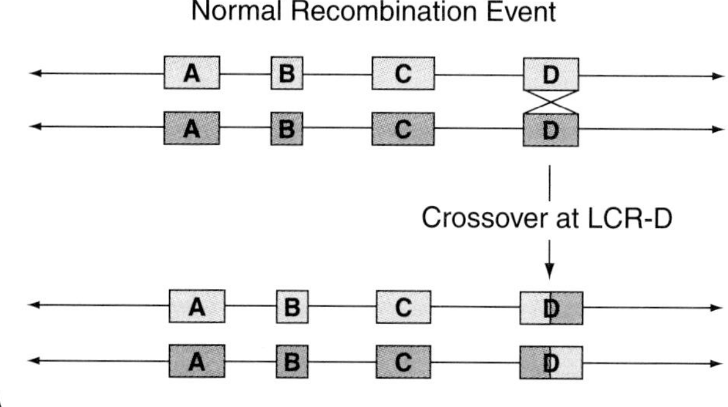


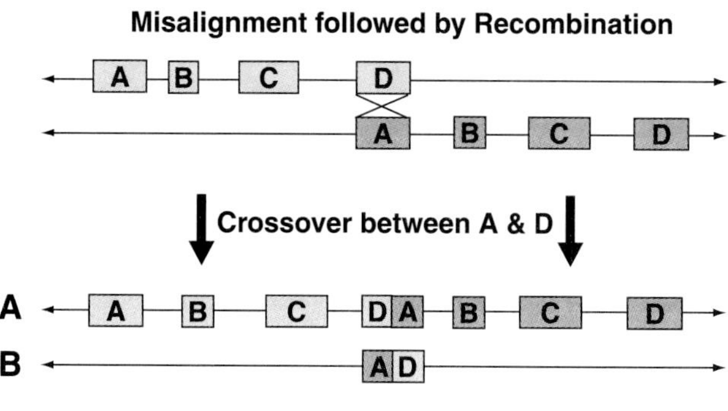


**FIGURE 20–6.** **A**, Alignment of low copy repeats (LCRs) before exchange. **B**, Misalignment of LCRs before exchange can result in rearrangement.

with periorbital fullness of subcutaneous tissues, flat midface, anteverted nostrils, long philtrum, thick lips, large open mouth, and stellate irises that may not be discernible at birth. Most infants have a cardiovascular abnormality; supravalvular aortic stenosis (SVAS) is the most commonly associated defect, seen in over 50% of cases. Pulmonary artery stenosis is also often encountered. It is interesting to note that isolated SVAS can also exist as a separate autosomal dominant trait and has been shown to occur from mutations of the elastin gene that is located within the region on 7q11 that is deleted in patients with Williams-Beuren syndrome. Patients with Williams-Beuren syndrome are typically missing one copy of the elastin gene as well (Shaffer et al, 2001).

Hypercalcemia, which is manifested in about 10% of patients with this disorder, is severe and persists through infancy. Umbilical and inguinal hernias are also associated features. Issues in infancy include feeding and growth problems, with pronounced irritability and "colicky" behavior. Hoarse voice, strabismus, hypertension, and joint mobility restrictions may develop later in childhood. In terms of development, the typical mild to moderate mental retardation can be masked by advanced language skills, although gross motor and visual-motor integration skills are especially affected. Attention deficit disorders are common, and a characteristic outgoing personality is often described in affected children.

Many of the classic features of Williams-Beuren syndrome are not clearly discernible in the newborn period, but the diagnosis should be suspected in any child with SVAS, hypercalcemia, and facial features consistent with the disorder. The diagnosis can be quickly confirmed by performing FISH using probes specific for the deleted region of chromosome 7q11. Because the condition is typically sporadic and most deletions arise de novo, the risk of recurrence in subsequent pregnancies is minimal. An affected adult, however, would pass on the condition in an autosomal dominant manner, with a 50% risk of the disorder in his or her child.

## The 22q11 Deletion Syndrome

A deletion of chromosome 22q11.2 has been identified in the majority of patients with the DiGeorge syndrome, VCFS, and conotruncal anomaly face syndrome (CAFS), leading to the realization that these clinical entities all reflect features of the same genomic disorder (McDonald-McGinn et al, 1997). The list of findings associated with the 22q11.2 deletion is extensive and varies from patient to patient. Estimates indicate that the 22q11 deletion occurs in approximately 1 in 3000 live births (Burn and Goodship, 1996). This disorder is the most common microdeletion syndrome occurring in humans and is a significant health concern in the general population.

The phenotype is characterized by a conotruncal cardiac anomaly and, often, aplasia or hypoplasia of the thymus and parathyroid glands. The majority of patients diagnosed with a deletion can present as newborns or infants with significant cardiovascular malformations, including interrupted aortic arch (IAA) type B, truncus arteriosus (TA), or tetralogy of Fallot, along with functional T-cell abnormalities and hypocalcemia. In addition, facial dysmorphia (Fig. 20–7), including hooded eyelids, hypertelorism, overfolded ears, bulbous nasal tip, a small mouth, and micrognathia, may be present. Since the initial report by DiGeorge in 1965, the spectrum of associated clinical features has been expanded to include anomalies such as vascular rings, cleft palate, renal agenesis, neural tube defects, and hypospadias (McDonald-McGinn et al, 1997). Before advances in the medical and surgical management of children with complex congenital cardiac disease and immune deficiencies, this disorder was associated with significant morbidity and mortality.

Developmental delays or learning disabilities have been reported in 90% to 100% of patients with the 22q11.2 deletion, and a wide range of developmental and behavioral findings have been observed in young children (Emanuel and Shaikh, 2001). In the preschool years, children with a 22q11.2 deletion were most commonly found to be hypotonic and developmentally delayed with language and speech difficulties. Severe or profound retardation was not seen, and a few patients functioned within the average range.

The vast majority of patients (80% to 90%) has the *same* large deletion, approximately 3 million base pairs (3 Mb), that is detected by FISH (Fig. 20–8). The deletion remains unchanged when inherited from an affected parent. However, the phenotype can be widely variable, even

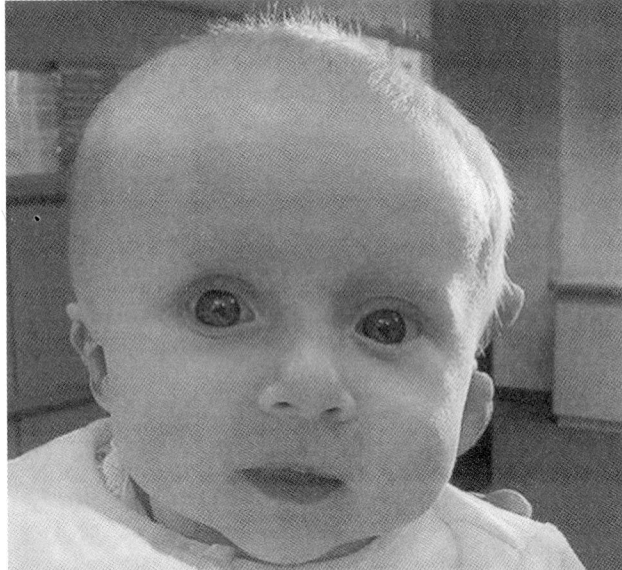

A

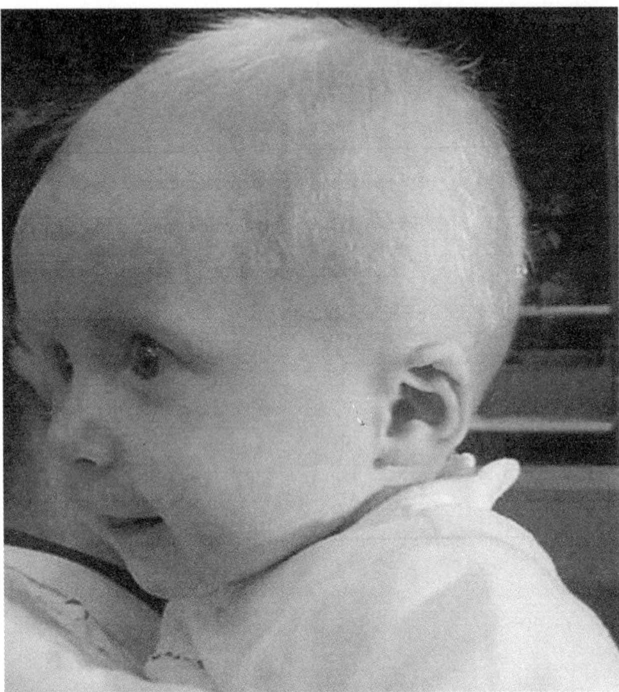

B

**FIGURE 20–7.** Facial differences associated with the 22q deletion.

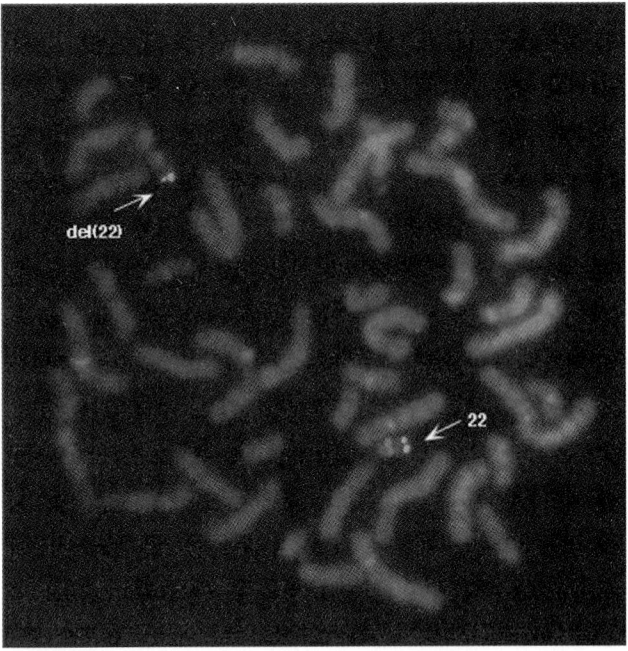


**FIGURE 20–8.** (See also Color Plate 20–8.) FISH study of a 22q deletion. *(Photograph courtesy of Dr. Beverly S. Emanuel.)*

within a family. Although smaller recurrent deletions that are half the size of the common deletion occur (1.5 Mb), a smaller size does not indicate milder symptoms, making genotype-phenotype correlations difficult. To date, no explanation for the great phenotypic variability has been forthcoming, and it is currently an area of active investigation (Emanuel and Shaikh, 2001).

Most 22q11 deletions occur as de novo lesions, less than 10% of them being inherited from an affected parent. The prevalence of these de novo 22q11.2 deletions indicates an extremely high mutation or rearrangement rate within this genomic region that is probably related to the presence of "recombination-permissive" duplicated DNA sequences or low copy chromosome 22–specific repeats in 22q11 (Emanuel and Shaikh, 2001).

## DISORDERS OF IMPRINTED CHROMOSOMES

A growing recognition of mechanisms regulating gene expression has emerged in the last decade. Two of the most exciting concepts with important clinical correlates are imprinting and uniparental disomy. *Genomic imprinting* implies that a whole region of a chromosome or a group of genes in a given region are subject to a difference in their expression that depends on whether they reside on the maternally inherited or paternally inherited chromosome. In these cases, a genetic disorder might manifest according to which parent the genomic region was inherited from. The genes in an imprinted region are not necessarily mutated, but they are marked such that the cell can distinguish between the maternal and paternal copies and coordinate expression on the basis of that distinction. At the molecular level, it appears that differences in the methlyation of the DNA, and its replication and regulation at the transcriptional level, appear to be involved in this mechanism.

### Prader-Willi Syndrome

It has been demonstrated that occasionally, instead of inheriting one copy of each chromosome from each parent, both copies of a given chromosome can come from the same parent. This phenomenon, known as *uniparental disomy* (UPD), is associated with advanced maternal age. It becomes a significant issue when the involved chromosome is imprinted or has regions on it that are imprinted.

Prader-Willi syndrome (PWS) involves the loss of activity from the *paternally* derived proximal long arm of chromosome 15 (15q11). This loss can occur through deletion or disruption of this region or through maternal uniparental disomy such that no paternal chromosome 15 is present at all (Nicholls et al, 1989). Newborns have pronounced central hypotonia and weak cry. Hyporeflexia is often encountered as well. The poor tone manifests as sucking and swallowing difficulties that can lead to failure to thrive and the need for feeding tubes in infancy. Facial differences that have been described include bifrontal narrowing, "almond-shaped" eyes, and a small, downturned mouth. Genitalia are often hypoplastic, with cryptorchidism quite common in boys with the syndrome. The commonly reported small hands and feet are not usually demonstrated in the newborn. Strabismus and hypopigmentation relative to the family are also common.

A history of poor fetal activity during the pregnancy can often be elicited, especially if the mother has had prior pregnancies. Consistent with the hypotonia, breech presentation and perinatal insults are found more frequently than usual. The extreme hypotonia begins to improve in the first year of life, as does motor development, although developmental delay is the rule, especially for gross motor skills and speech. The feeding improves in the first few years of life and gives way to often uncontrollable hyperphagia and obesity. This issue and other behavioral problems, including severe temper tantrums, are encountered throughout life. The majority of patients manifests mild to moderate mental retardation. Early diagnosis and preemptive implementation of behavioral therapy are essential components of the optimal management of these issues.

Deletions of the region critical in Prader-Willi syndrome have been demonstrated in up to 70% of patients. The deletion can be detected by FISH analysis using a probe specific for this region of chromosome 15. A small number of patients has a disruption of this area as the result of a rearrangement such as a translocation. To date, no single gene in this region has been implicated as the cause, but expression of the genes in this region is under intense investigation. It has been noted, however, that patients who have Prader-Willi syndrome as a result of a deletion of the region are more likely to be hypopigmented. This feature has been attributed to deletion of a gene involved in pigmentation, the so-called P gene (Rinchik et al, 1993). Recurrence risks are negligible in cases in which de novo deletions are found, and sporadic occurrence is usually encountered.

Approximately 20% to 25% of patients with Prader-Willi syndrome show maternal UPD that can be detected by means of a molecular assay designed to assess specific methylation differences between maternal and paternal alleles. A maternal age effect has been demonstrated in UPD cases, and recurrence risks in families without deletions are estimated at 1 in 1000. Additionally, this region of the genome is subject to regulation by imprinting. Large chromosome-specific segmental duplications are found in 15q11 and have been implicated in mediating the recurrent deletion of this genomic region (Emanuel and Shaikh, 2001).

## Angelman Syndrome

Loss of genetic material from the 15q11 region from the *maternal* copy of chromosome 15 is associated with Angelman syndrome. Clinical features are not evident in the newborn period and infancy but include significant mental retardation, seizures, ataxic gait, tongue thrusting, inappropriate bursts of laughter, and facial differences including protruding jaw, wide mouth, thin upper lip, and widely spaced teeth. The mental retardation and hypopigmentation overlap with features of Prader-Willi syndrome, but Angelman syndrome is a distinct entity.

Seventy percent to 75% of patients have a deletion of 15q11 that is detectable by FISH analysis. A small percentage (3% to 5%) have evidence of *paternal* isodisomy (two paternal copies) of the entire chromosome 15, with no apparent maternal chromosome. Unlike in Prader-Willi syndrome, Angelman syndrome has been associated with mutations in a single gene, UBE3A, an enzyme involved in the ubiquitin pathway of protein degradation, detected in up to 10% of patients. Additionally, mutations of an imprinting center locus on chromosome 15 are thought to be associated with 1% to 2% of Angelman phenotypes (Shaffer et al, 2001). Thus, the vast majority of cases result from a sporadic event, and risk of recurrence can be best evaluated once the genetic mechanism has been determined for a given patient.

## Beckwith-Wiedemann Syndrome

Beckwith-Wiedemann syndrome affects about 1 in 14,000 newborns and manifests as an overgrowth syndrome in the neonatal period. The characteristic findings are macrosomia, abdominal wall defect, and macroglossia (Fig. 20–9). Affected babies are large for gestational age with proportionate length and weight. Infants of diabetic mothers also manifest with macrosomia, but are more likely to have a weight disproportionately greater than length. Advanced bone age is also noted in Beckwith-Wiedemann syndrome. Hemihypertrophy due to asymmetric growth is common, as is visceromegaly of various organs, including the spleen, kidneys, liver, pancreas, and adrenal glands.

Other characteristic features of the syndrome are macroglossia, linear creases of the earlobe with indentations on the posterior helix, and severe hypoglycemia. Although the hypoglycemia responds quickly to therapy, it can be present for several months; thus, recognition of the condition and immediate therapeutic intervention are critical in these cases. The hypoglycemia resolves spontaneously with age, and the physical diagnostic features also become less prominent with age, making the diagnosis more difficult to ascertain.

Equally important is the establishment of routine ultrasonographic surveillance at regular intervals, because children with Beckwith-Wiedemann syndrome are at increased risk of malignant tumors, especially Wilms tumor. The estimated risk is 5% for patients with hemihypertrophy. Many centers currently perform ultrasonography at 3-month intervals until the school-age years and at least annually through adolescence. Monitoring of serum alpha-fetoprotein levels at the same intervals

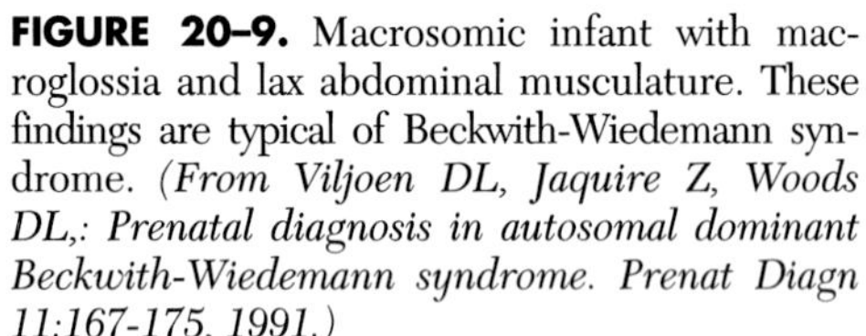

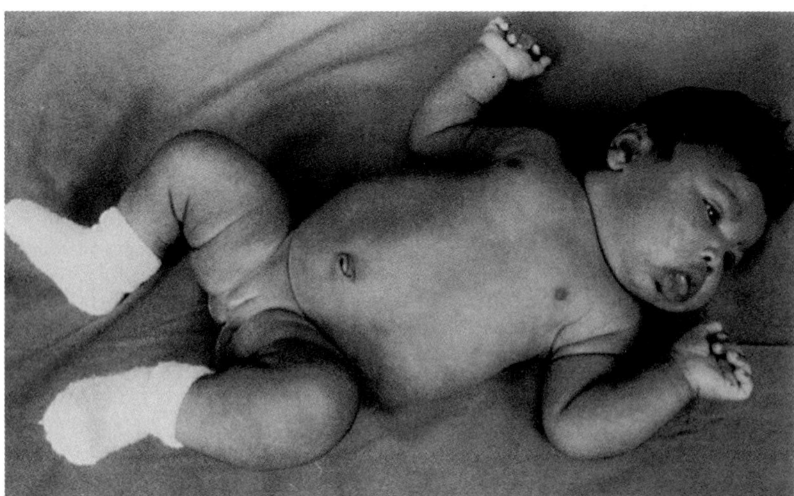

**FIGURE 20–9.** Macrosomic infant with macroglossia and lax abdominal musculature. These findings are typical of Beckwith-Wiedemann syndrome. *(From Viljoen DL, Jaquire Z, Woods DL,: Prenatal diagnosis in autosomal dominant Beckwith-Wiedemann syndrome. Prenat Diagn 11:167-175, 1991.)*

has proved valuable, as several cases of hepatoblastoma have also been reported and detected with this adjunct study.

Although most cases of Beckwith-Wiedemann appear to arise de novo, up to 15% may be familial. In familial cases, autosomal dominant transmission but with variable phenotype seems to be the mode of inheritance. Additionally, this region of the genome (11p15) appears to be imprinted such that the maternal allele is not usually expressed. The insulin-like growth factor type 2 (IGF2) gene is located in this region and encodes an important factor involved in fetal growth. Mutations causing overexpression of the paternal allele or underexpression of the maternal allele can result in an imbalance of expression leading to the overgrowth and tumor formation encountered in these patients. Paternal UPD has proved to be a mechanism involved in up to 20% of sporadic cases of Beckwith-Wiedemann syndrome.

## CONCLUSION

We have summarized the rapidly expanding field of chromosomal or genomic disorders, concentrating on those that commonly manifest in the newborn. The widespread development and clinical implementation of molecular cytogenetic techniques such as FISH and subtelomeric FISH have allowed the identification of subtle rearrangements that were previously undetectable. These advances now enable the discernment of "new" syndromes in which the chromosomal anomaly may be defined before a characteristic phenotype is recognized. Additionally, a greater understanding of the role of segmental duplications and their effects on human genetic disorders as well as of the influence of mechanisms that regulate gene expression, such as imprinting, is emerging. The tremendous advances in genomics lead by the completion of the Human Genome Sequencing Project and the development of new molecular diagnostic tools present new challenges for clinicians to better diagnose, understand, and care for patients with genetic disorders and their families.

## REFERENCES


Baty BJ, Blackburn BL, Carey JC: Natural history of trisomy 18 and trisomy 13. I: Growth, physical assessment, medical histories, survival, and recurrence risk. Am J Med Genet 49:175-188, 1994.

Burn J, Goodship J: Developmental genetics of the heart. Curr Opin Genet Dev 6:322-325, 1996.

Cornish KM, Bramble D, Munir F, Pigram J: Cognitive functioning in children with typical cri du chat (5p-) syndrome. Dev Med Child Neurol 41:263-266, 1999.

Emanuel BS, Shaikh TH: Segmental duplications: An "expanding" role in genomic instability and disease. Nat Rev Genet 2:791-800, 2001.

Emanuel BS, McDonald-McGinn D, Saitta SC, Zackai EH: The 22q11.2 deletion syndrome. Adv Pediatr 48:39-73, 2001.

Epstein CJ: Down syndrome (trisomy 21). In Scriver CR, Beaudet al, Sly WS, Valle D (eds): The Metabolic and Molecular Bases of Inherited Disease, 8th ed. New York, McGraw-Hill, 2001, pp 1223-1256.

Fernandes A, Mourato AP, Xavier MJ, et al: Characterisation of the somatic evolution of Portuguese children with Trisomy 21—preliminary results. Downs Syndr Res Pract 6:134-138, 2001.

Fong CT, Brodeur GM: Down's syndrome and leukemia: Epidemiology, genetics, cytogenetics and mechanisms of leukemogenesis. Cancer Genet Cytogenet 28:55-76, 1987.

Hook EB: Ultrasound and fetal chromosome abnormalities. Lancet 340:1109-1113, 1992.

Hook EB, Cross PK: Paternal age and Down's syndrome genotypes diagnosed prenatally: No association in New York state data. Hum Genet 62:167-174, 1982.

Jones KL: Smith's Recognizable Patterns of Human Malformation, 5th ed. Philadelphia, WB Saunders, 1997.

Lejeune J, Turpin R: Human chromosomal aberrations. C R Seances Soc Biol Fil 1960:54, 1956-1960.

Lupski JR: 2002 Curt Stern Award Address: Genomic disorders: Recombination-based disease resulting from genomic architecture. Am J Hum Genet 72:246-252, 2003.

MacDonald M, Hassold T, Harvey J, et al: The origin of 47,XXY and 47,XXX aneuploidy: Heterogeneous mechanisms and role of aberrant recombination. Hum Mol Genet 3:1365-1371, 1994.

McDonald-McGinn DM, LaRossa D, Goldmuntz E, et al: The 22q11.2 deletion: Screening, diagnostic workup, and outcome of results: Report on 181 patients. Genet Test 1:99-108, 1997.

McPherson JD, Marra M, Hillier L, et al: A physical map of the human genome. Nature 409:934-941, 2001.

Mitelman F (ed): An International System for Human Cytogenetic Nomenclature (ISCN) 1995: Recommendations of the International Standing Committee on Human Cytogenetic Nomenclature. Basel, S Karger, 1995.

Nicholls RD, Knoll JH, Butler MG, et al: Genetic imprinting suggested by maternal heterodisomy in nondeletion Prader-Willi syndrome. Nature 342:281-285, 1989.

Nussbaum RL, McInnes RR, Willard HF (eds): Thompson and Thompson's Genetics in Medicine, 6th ed. Philadelphia, WB Saunders, 2001.

OMIM. Available online at http://www3.ncbi.nlm.nih.gov/entrez/query.fcgi?db=omim

Pueschel SM, Bernier JC, Pezzullo JC: Behavioural observations in children with Down's syndrome. J Ment Defic Res 35: 502-511, 1991.

Rimoin DL, Connor JM, Pyeritz RE (eds): Emery and Rimoin's Principles and Practice of Medical Genetics, 3rd ed. New York, Churchill Livingstone, 1996.

Rinchik EM, Bultman SJ, Horsthemke B, et al: A gene for the mouse pink-eyed dilution locus and for human type II oculocutaneous albinism. Nature 361:72-76, 1993.

Schinzel A: Catalogue of Unbalanced Chromosome Aberrations in Man, 2nd ed. Berlin, Walter de Gruyter, 2001.

Shaffer LG, Ledbetter DH, Lupski JR: Molecular cytogenetics of contiguous gene syndromes: Mechanisms and consequences of gene dosage imbalance. In Scriver CR, Beaudet AL, Sly WS, Valle D (eds): The Metabolic and Molecular Bases of Inherited Disease, 8th ed. New York, McGraw-Hill, 2001, pp 1291-1324.

Willard HF: The sex chromosomes and X chromosome inactivation. In Scriver CR, Beaudet AL, Sly WS, Valle D (eds): The Metabolic and Molecular Bases of Inherited Disease, 8th ed. New York, McGraw-Hill, 2001, pp 1191-1211.

Zaragoza MV, Jacobs PA, James RS, et al: Nondisjunction of human acrocentric chromosomes: Studies of 432 trisomic fetuses and liveborns. Hum Genet 94:411-417, 1994.

# PART VI

# CONGENITAL METABOLIC PROBLEMS

Editors: **ROBERTA A. BALLARD** and **GERARD T. BERRY**

CHAPTER 21

## Introduction to the Metabolic and Biochemical Genetic Diseases

Gerard T. Berry

For the sake of simplicity, genetic diseases may be divided into the chromosome disorders, the contiguous gene deletion syndromes, nucleotide repeat disorders, imprinting/methylation silencing disorders, the single-gene defects, the polygenic disorder, and mitochondrial DNA diseases. Biochemical genetic disease is almost always the consequence of a single-gene defect, and most inborn errors of metabolism are inherited as autosomal recessive traits. However, not all biochemical genetic disorders are usually thought of as metabolic diseases. The clinician caring for sick newborns tends to consider metabolic diseases in terms of certain well-recognized clinical presentations—the catastrophically ill, comatose newborn infant; the baby with failure to thrive, recurrent feeding problems and emesis, hypotonia, or seizures; and the infant with physical stigmata such as hepatosplenomegaly, characteristic of the storage diseases. Acidosis, ketosis, hypoglycemia, or hyperammonemia frequently alerts the pediatrician or neonatologist to initiate evaluation for a metabolic disorder in the infant with life-threatening disease. In contrast, cystic fibrosis, a biochemical genetic disorder, has little in common with these kinds of inborn errors, except perhaps autosomal recessive transmission. The examples of the inborn errors described in Chapters 22 through 24 help clarify this clinical nosologic concept. A list of general references or reviews that emphasize the genetic metabolic diseases is provided at the end of this chapter.

The purpose of this section on Congenital Metabolic Problems is to review the biochemical genetic diseases and, specifically, the metabolic diseases that manifest in the extended newborn period, considering the appropriate laboratory testing for diagnosis and the therapeutic modalities for treatment of these disorders. With the exception of some rare contiguous gene deletion syndromes, the non–single-gene defects, such as the chromosome and polygenic genetic disorders, are not causes of metabolic disease. Yet as discussed in the context of biochemical genetic diseases producing dysmorphism, the distinction between what constitutes classic clinical genetics and metabolic diseases is becoming blurred. Although a few metabolic disorders are inherited as X-linked traits, autosomal dominant inheritance is not considered common, particularly in the group of inborn errors that can be readily detected by measuring the levels of chemicals such as amino and organic acids in body fluids. The biochemical genetic defects due to expansion of trinucleotide repeats, such as the fragile X syndrome, and disorders due to mitochondrial DNA mutations rarely manifest during the newborn period. Defects in the imprinting of a single parental gene of maternal or paternal origin, such as in the Prader-Willi, Angelman, and Beckwith-Wiedemann syndromes, are covered in other chapters.

In general, metabolic diseases in the newborn are the consequence of the malfunctioning of both the maternally and paternally inherited alleles at one specific gene locus. Some biochemical genetic diseases transmitted in such an autosomal recessive manner are not covered here because of the unique involvement of one organ or physiologic system, which places that disease within a particular subspecialty. Examples are cystic fibrosis, disorders of hemostasis and coagulation, methemoglobinemias, and immunodeficiencies. Other metabolic disorders, such as familial hyperinsulinism, congenital adrenal hyperplasia, and Crigler-Najjar syndrome, are thoroughly discussed in other chapters.

Of the 10,000 genetic diseases or polymorphic traits that follow a mendelian inheritance pattern, more than 500 are considered biochemical genetic diseases and have been defined at the protein or gene level. As discussed earlier, not all manifest during the newborn period. Almost 50 inborn errors of amino acid, organic acid, or ammonia metabolism can be recognized in the first weeks or months of life (Table 21–1). The primary lactic acidoses are rare, as are the storage, peroxisomal, and connective tissue diseases, which individually number few. Aside from hyperinsulinism, galactosemia is the most common of the defects in carbohydrate metabolism. Because of the number and rarity of these metabolic diseases, a practical general approach to patients with a potential metabolic disease is essential. For the clinician, it is helpful to focus not on the individual diseases, except when characteristic syndromes are readily recognizable, but rather on the different general modes of presentation and the classes or types of inborn errors that fit a particular mode of presentation.

In general, the metabolic diseases affecting the newborn can be divided into those involving complex molecules, such as the storage diseases, and those concerning the intermediary metabolism of small molecules, such as glucose,

**TABLE 21–1**

**Inborn Errors of Metabolism with Newborn Presentation**

| |
|---|
| Amino acid disorders |
| Organic acid disorders |
| Disorders of ammonia metabolism |
| Disorders of carbohydrate metabolism |
| Disorders of gluconeogenesis/hypoglycemia |
| Disorders of fatty acid oxidation |
| Primary lactic acidoses |
| Disorders of vitamin/metal metabolism |
| Storage diseases |
| Peroxisomal disorders |
| Disorders of sterol metabolism |
| Congenital defects in glycosylation |
| Connective tissue diseases |

pyruvate, lactate, amino acids, organic acids, ammonia, and mitochondrial respiration and oxidative phosphorylation. Overwhelming, acute, life-threatening illness is the outstanding feature of the group of metabolic diseases involving metabolism of small molecules. Acute encephalopathy may be due to the buildup of metabolic poisons such as ammonia and organic acids (Table 21–2), to hypoglycemia (Table 21–3), or to the failure to convert glucose to $CO_2$ and $H_2O$ associated with diminished mitochondrial adenosine triphosphate formation and lactate buildup (see Table 21–2).

**TABLE 21–2**

**Metabolic Diseases with Newborn Coma Secondary to Toxic Metabolite Accumulation or Mitochondrial Failure**

| |
|---|
| Galactosemia |
| Inborn errors of ammonia metabolism |
| Ornithine transcarbamylase deficiency |
| Argininosuccinic aciduria |
| Citrullinemia |
| Carbamylphosphate synthetase deficiency |
| Maple syrup urine disease |
| Nonketotic hyperglycinemia |
| Methylmalonic acidemia ± homocystinuria |
| Propionic acidemia |
| Isovaleric acidemia |
| Multiple carboxylase deficiency |
| Glutaric aciduria type 2 |
| Fatty acid oxidation defects |
| Short-chain acyl-CoA dehydrogenase deficiency |
| Medium-chain acyl-CoA dehydrogenase deficiency* |
| Very-long-chain acyl-CoA dehydrogenase deficiency |
| Long-chain 3-hydroxy acyl-CoA dehydrogenase deficiency |
| Carnitine transporter deficiency |
| Carnitine translocase deficiency |
| Carnitine palmitoyltransferase I and II deficiencies |
| Primary lactic acidosis |
| Pyruvate dehydrogenase deficiency |
| Pyruvate carboxylase deficiency |
| Mitochondrial respiratory chain or electron transport chain defects |

*Rare cause of sudden infant death syndrome.

**TABLE 21–3**

**Metabolic Diseases with Newborn Coma Secondary to Hypoglycemia**

| |
|---|
| Hyperinsulinism |
| 3-Hydroxy-3-methylglutaryl-CoA lyase deficiency |
| Fructose-1,6-diphosphatase deficiency |
| Hereditary fructose intolerance |
| Glycogen storage disease type I |

As is well known to neonatologists and pediatricians, the newborn or young infant has a limited array of responses to acute, severe illness with encephalopathy. The signs are nonspecific and include poor feeding, spitting up, lethargy, skin color changes, hypothermia, and poor weight gain. In fact, few newborn infants in whom a metabolic disease is suspected should have escaped evaluation for sepsis. In many of these diseases, respiratory distress is also a presenting feature because of the presence of an acid-base disturbance. Metabolic acidosis and hyperammonemia both produce hyperventilation. During the progression of metabolic coma, cerebral edema or other complications such as intracranial hemorrhages may develop in the patient, making it more difficult to establish the diagnosis.

Because a specific metabolic disorder may be associated with different amounts of residual enzyme activity—as the exact gene mutations often vary from patient to patient—or because different rates of protein ingestion lead to a variable accumulation of amino or organic acids, there may be different modes of presentation even for the same metabolic disorder. Examples of the different modes of presentation are shown in Table 21–4. A characteristic odor may provide the clue to the presence of phenylketonuria (musty), maple syrup urine disease (maple syrup), isovaleric aciduria (sweaty socks), and glutaric aciduria type 2 (sweaty socks). Often the physical findings are not specifically helpful in metabolic diseases involving small molecules. Conversely, the diseases involving cellular processing of complex molecules such as the storage diseases are usually associated with characteristic or unique physical findings (Table 21–5).

Although there are exceptions to both of these rules, this approach represents an easy and diagnostically helpful way to think about these rare disorders of metabolism. The characteristic unique or physical findings that

**TABLE 21–4**

**Modes of Presentation of Metabolic Diseases**

| |
|---|
| Acute life-threatening illness with coma |
| Seizures |
| Respiratory distress |
| Feeding problems and poor growth |
| Developmental delay or failure with hypotonia |
| Unique or characteristic findings on physical examination |
| Dysmorphic features or multiple malformations |
| Hydrops fetalis or neonatal ascites |
| Persistent diarrhea |

**TABLE 21–5**

**Metabolic Diseases in Which Physical Examination is Usually Helpful in Diagnosis**

| |
|---|
| Storage diseases |
| Peroxisomal diseases |
| Connective tissue diseases |
| Disorders of sterol metabolism |
| Congenital defects in glycosylation |

underscore the complex molecule diseases, as well as those that may be detected in the diverse group of small molecule disorders, are summarized in Table 21–6. With regard to Table 21–4, one should note that feeding problems and poor growth as well as developmental delay may be seen in both categories of metabolic disease. Characteristic or unique laboratory or diagnostic testing findings seen in some of these illnesses are shown in Table 21–7. Measurements such as blood pH, total $CO_2$

*Text continues on page 224*

**TABLE 21–6**

**Unique or Characteristic Physical Findings in Inborn Errors***

| | |
|---|---|
| Hepatomegaly | Hereditary galactosemia |
| | Glycogen storage diseases |
| | Hereditary fructose intolerance |
| | Fructose-1,6-bisphosphatase deficiency |
| | Methylmalonic acidemia |
| | Propionic acidemia |
| | Glutaric acidemia type 2 |
| | Very-long-chain acyl-CoA dehydrogenase deficiency |
| | Medium-chain acyl-CoA dehydrogenase deficiency |
| | Short-chain acyl-CoA dehydrogenase deficiency |
| | Long-chain 3-hydroxy acyl-CoA dehydrogenase deficiency |
| | Carnitine transporter defect |
| | Carnitine palmitoyltransferase type I deficiency |
| | Carnitine palmitoyltransferase type II deficiency |
| | Acyl carnitine translocase deficiency |
| | 3-Hydroxy-3-methylglutaryl CoA lyase deficiency |
| | Phosphoenolpyruvate carboxykinase deficiency |
| | Mitochondrial respiratory/electron transport chain defects |
| | Hereditary tyrosinemia type 1 |
| | Argininosuccinicaciduria |
| | $\alpha_1$-antitrypsin deficiency |
| | Smith-Lemli-Opitz syndrome |
| | Zellweger disease |
| | Neonatal adrenoleukodystrophy |
| | Niemann-Pick type C disease |
| | Congenital defects in glycosylation |
| Hepatosplenomegaly | $G_{M1}$ gangliosidosis |
| | I-cell disease |
| | Gaucher disease type 2 |
| | Niemann-Pick disease type A |
| | Niemann-Pick disease type C |
| | Galactosialidosis |
| | Sialidosis |
| | Mucopolysaccharidosis type VII |
| | Wolman disease |
| | Ceramidase deficiency |
| Macrocephaly | Glutaric acidemia type 1 |
| | Canavan disease |
| Microcephaly | Short-chain acyl-CoA dehydrogenase deficiency |
| | Mitochondrial respiratory/electron transport chain defects |
| | Leigh disease |
| | Methylmalonic acidemia with homocystinuria |
| Coarse facial features | $G_{M1}$ gangliosidosis |
| | I-cell disease |
| | Mucopolysaccharidosis type VII |
| | Sialidosis |
| | Galactosialidosis |

*Continued*

**TABLE 21-6**

**Unique or Characteristic Physical Findings in Inborn Errors*—Cont'd**

| | |
|---|---|
| Macroglossia | Pompe disease<br>$G_{M1}$ gangliosidosis |
| Dystonia or extrapyramidal signs | Gaucher disease type 2<br>Glutaric acidemia type 1<br>Krabbe disease<br>Crigler-Najjar syndrome<br>Phenylketonuria due to a biopterin defect |
| Macular "cherry red spot" | $G_{M1}$ gangliosidosis<br>Galactosialidosis<br>Niemann-Pick disease type A<br>Tay-Sachs disease ($G_{M2}$ gangliosidosis) |
| Retinitis pigmentosa | Mitochondrial respiratory/electron transport chain defects<br>Methylmalonic acidemia/homocystinuria<br>Sjögren-Larsson syndrome<br>Zellweger disease<br>Neonatal adrenoleukodystrophy<br>Infantile Refsum disease<br>Abetalipoproteinemia<br>Long-chain 3-hydroxy acyl-CoA dehydrogenase deficiency |
| Otic atrophy or hypoplasia | Pyruvate dehydrogenase complex deficiency<br>Leigh disease<br>Zellweger disease |
| Corneal clouding or opacities | I-cell disease<br>Steroid sulfatase deficiency |
| Cataracts | Hereditary galactosemia<br>Lowe syndrome<br>Mitochondrial respiratory/electron transport chain defects<br>Zellweger disease<br>Rhizomelic chondrodysplasia punctata<br>Mevalonic aciduria<br>Carbohydrate-deficient glycoprotein syndrome<br>Congenital defects in glycosylation |
| Dislocated lens | Methionine synthetase deficiency<br>Sulfite oxidase deficiency |
| Bone or limb deformities/contractures | Storage, peroxisomal, or connective tissue disorders<br>Inborn errors of cholesterol biosynthesis<br>Hypophosphatasia |
| Thick skin | I-cell disease<br>$G_{M2}$ gangliosidosis<br>Mucopolysaccharidosis type VII<br>Sialidosis<br>Galactosialidosis |
| Skin nodules | Ceramidase deficiency |
| Desquamating, eczematous, or vesiculobullous skin lesions | Acrodermatitis enteropathica<br>Multiple carboxylase deficiency<br>Methylmalonic acidemia<br>Propionic acidemia<br>Hepatoerythropoietic porphyria<br>Congenital erythropoietic porphyria |
| Ichthyosis | Gaucher disease type 2<br>Sjögren-Larsson syndrome<br>Steroid sulfatase deficiency |
| Alopecia | Multiple carboxylase deficiency |
| Steely or kinky hair | Menkes disease |
| Persistent diarrhea | Glucose galactose malabsorption<br>Congenital lactase deficiency<br>Congenital chloride diarrhea<br>Sucrase isomaltase deficiency<br>Acrodermatitis enteropathica<br>Congenital folate malabsorption<br>Wolman disease<br>Hereditary galactosemia |

*For discussion of specific disorders, see Chapters 22 through 24.

**TABLE 21–7**

**Characteristic or Unique Laboratory or Diagnostic Testing Outcomes in Inborn Errors**

| | |
|---|---|
| Metabolic acidosis ± increased anion gap | Methylmalonic acidemia<br>Propionic acidemia<br>Isovaleric acidemia<br>Multiple carboxylase deficiency<br>Maple syrup urine disease<br>Glutaric acidemia type 1<br>Glutaric acidemia type 2<br>Short-chain acyl-CoA dehydrogenase deficiency<br>Long-chain 3-hydroxy acyl-CoA dehydrogenase deficiency<br>Ketothiolase deficiency<br>Acetoacetate-CoA ligase deficiency<br>3-Hydroxy-3-methylglutaryl-CoA lyase deficiency<br>Pyruvate dehydrogenase complex deficiency<br>Pyruvate carboxylase deficiency<br>Phosphoenolpyruvate carboxykinase deficiency<br>Mitochondrial respiratory/electron transport chain defects<br>Leigh disease<br>Hereditary galactosemia<br>Glycogen storage disease type 1<br>Hereditary fructose intolerance<br>Fructose-1,6-diphosphatase deficiency<br>Hereditary tyrosinemia type 1 |
| Respiratory alkalosis | Ornithine transcarbamylase deficiency<br>Carbamylphosphate synthetase deficiency<br>Argininosuccinic aciduria<br>Citrullinemia |
| Hyperammonemia | Ornithine transcarbamylase deficiency<br>Carbamylphosphate synthetase deficiency<br>Argininosuccinic aciduria<br>Citrullinemia<br>Methylmalonic acidemia<br>Propionic acidemia<br>Isovaleric acidemia<br>Multiple carboxylase deficiency<br>Glutaric acidemia type 2<br>Very-long-chain acyl-CoA dehydrogenase deficiency<br>Medium-chain acyl-CoA dehydrogenase deficiency<br>Short-chain acyl-CoA dehydrogenase deficiency<br>Acylcarnitine translocase deficiency |
| Ketosis | Methylmalonic acidemia<br>Propionic acidemia<br>Isovaleric acidemia<br>Multiple carboxylase deficiency<br>Maple syrup urine disease<br>Glutaric acidemia type 2<br>Short-chain acyl-CoA dehydrogenase deficiency<br>Ketothiolase deficiency<br>Acetoacetate-CoA ligase deficiency<br>Pyruvate carboxylase deficiency<br>Glycogen storage disease type 1<br>Fructose-1,6-diphosphatase deficiency |
| Lactic acidosis | Methylmalonic acidemia<br>Propionic acidemia<br>Isovaleric acidemia<br>Multiple carboxylase deficiency<br>Glutaric acidemia type 2<br>Short-chain acyl-CoA dehydrogenase deficiency<br>Long-chain 3-hydroxy acyl-CoA dehydrogenase deficiency<br>Ketothiolase deficiency<br>Acetoacetate-CoA ligase deficiency |

*Continued*

**TABLE 21-7**

**Characteristic or Unique Laboratory or Diagnostic Testing Outcomes in Inborn Errors—Cont'd**

| | |
|---|---|
| | 3-Hydroxy-3-methylglutaryl-CoA lyase deficiency<br>Pyruvate dehydrogenase complex deficiency<br>Pyruvate carboxylase deficiency<br>Phosphoenolpyruvate carboxykinase deficiency<br>Mitochondrial respiratory/electron transport chain defects<br>Leigh disease<br>Glycogen storage disease type 1<br>Hereditary fructose intolerance<br>Fructose-1,6-diphosphatase deficiency |
| Hypoglycemia | Hyperinsulinism<br>Glycogen storage disease type 1<br>Hereditary fructose intolerance<br>Fructose-1,6-diphosphatase deficiency<br>Glutaric acidemia type 1<br>Glutaric acidemia type 2<br>Very-long-chain acyl-CoA dehydrogenase deficiency<br>Medium-chain acyl-CoA dehydrogenase deficiency<br>Short-chain acyl-CoA dehydrogenase deficiency<br>Long-chain 3-hydroxy acyl-CoA dehydrogenase deficiency<br>Carnitine transporter defect<br>Carnitine palmitoyltransferase type I deficiency<br>Carnitine palmitoyltransferase type II deficiency<br>Acyl carnitine translocase deficiency<br>Ketothiolase deficiency<br>Acetoacetate-CoA ligase deficiency<br>3-Hydroxy-3-methylglutaryl-CoA lyase deficiency<br>Hereditary galactosemia<br>Neonatal hemochromatosis<br>Mitochondrial respiratory/electron transport chain defects |
| Lipemia | Glycogen storage disease type 1 |
| Positive urinary-reducing substances | Hereditary galactosemia<br>Hereditary fructose intolerance<br>Essential fructosuria<br>Lowe syndrome |
| Discolored urine | Congenital erythropoietic porphyria<br>Alkaptonuria<br>Tryptophan malabsorption |
| Leukopenia | Methylmalonic acidemia<br>Propionic acidemia<br>Isovaleric acidemia<br>Multiple carboxylase deficiency<br>Glycogen storage disease type 1B<br>Mevalonic aciduria<br>Barth syndrome<br>Pearson syndrome |
| Thrombocytopenia | Methylmalonic acidemia<br>Propionic acidemia<br>Isovaleric acidemia<br>Multiple carboxylase deficiency<br>Pearson syndrome<br>Mevalonic aciduria |
| Anemia | $\alpha_1$-antitrypsin deficiency<br>Methylmalonic acidemia/homocystinuria/vitamin $B_{12}$ defects<br>Propionic acidemia<br>Isovaleric acidemia<br>Multiple carboxylase deficiency<br>Wolman disease<br>Pearson syndrome<br>Neonatal hemochromatosis<br>Abetalipoproteinemia |

**TABLE 21-7**

**Characteristic or Unique Laboratory or Diagnostic Testing Outcomes in Inborn Errors—Cont'd**

| | |
|---|---|
| | Mevalonic aciduria<br>Hereditary galactosemia |
| Prolonged prothrombin and partial thromboplastin times | Hereditary galactosemia<br>Hereditary fructose intolerance<br>$\alpha_1$-antitrypsin deficiency<br>Neonatal hemochromatosis<br>Hereditary tyrosinemia type 1 |
| Vacuolated lymphocytes or neutrophils | Storage diseases |
| Acanthocytosis | Abetalipoproteinemia<br>Wolman disease |
| Cardiomegaly | Pompe disease<br>Barth syndrome<br>Carnitine palmitoyltransferase type II deficiency<br>Carbohydrate-deficient glycoprotein syndrome |
| Electrocardiographic abnormalities | Pompe disease (short PR interval, large QRS)<br>Acyl carnitine translocase deficiency<br>Very-long-chain acyl-CoA dehydrogenase deficiency<br>Long-chain 3-hydroxy acyl-CoA dehydrogenase deficiency<br>Carnitine palmitoyltransferase type II deficiency |
| Ventricular hypertrophy | Pompe disease<br>Propionic acidemia<br>Isovaleric acidemia<br>Multiple carboxylase deficiency<br>Glutaric acidemia type 2<br>Very-long-chain acyl-CoA dehydrogenase deficiency<br>Long-chain 3-hydroxy acyl-CoA dehydrogenase deficiency<br>Carnitine transporter defect<br>Carnitine palmitoyltransferase type II deficiency<br>Acyl carnitine translocase deficiency<br>Ketothiolase deficiency<br>Mitochondrial respiratory/electron transport chain defects<br>Leigh disease |
| Dysostosis multiplex | $G_{M1}$ gangliosidosis<br>Mucopolysaccharidosis type VII<br>I-cell disease<br>Sialidosis<br>Galactosialidosis |
| Stippled calcifications of patellae | Zellweger disease |
| Adrenal calcifications | Wolman disease |
| Rhizomelism | Rhizomelic chondrodysplasia punctata |
| Pili torti | Menkes disease |
| Trichorrhexis nodosa | Argininosuccinicaciduria |
| Basal ganglia lesions on MRI | Methylmalonic acidemia<br>Propionic acidemia<br>Pyruvate dehydrogenase complex deficiency<br>Mitochondrial respiratory/electron transport chain defects<br>Leigh disease<br>Krabbe disease |
| Cerebellar atrophy or hypoplasia | Pyruvate dehydrogenase complex deficiency<br>Mitochondrial respiratory/electron transport chain defects<br>Leigh disease<br>Carbohydrate-deficient glycoprotein syndrome |
| Agenesis of corpus callosum | Pyruvate dehydrogenase complex deficiency<br>Pyruvate carboxylase deficiency<br>Mitochondrial respiratory/electron transport chain defects |

content, glucose, ammonia, and amino acids are not particularly helpful in the evaluation of these infants with abnormalities in the metabolism of complex molecules whose evaluation must be dictated by the history and important findings on physical examination. The enigmatic picture of hydrops fetalis, although uncommon as a mode of presentation, is exclusively associated with the storage diseases. Neurologic signs including seizures may also be seen in the storage diseases. Congenital chloride malabsorption, glucose-galactose malabsorption, and acrodermatitis enteropathica may manifest as congenital or persistent diarrhea.

Severe liver disease with jaundice or elevated serum transaminase determinations is characteristic of a few metabolic diseases; they are listed in Table 21–8. Of these disorders, only $\alpha_1$-antitrypsin deficiency, the peroxisomal disorders such as Zellweger disease and neonatal adrenoleukodystrophy, and Niemann-Pick type C disease are secondary to impaired disposition of complex molecules. Mild or transient liver function test abnormalities may also be seen in the glycogen storage diseases, fructose-1,6-bisphosphatase deficiency, and hyperammonemic conditions, but bridging fibrosis is not usually detected. A renal tubulopathy may also be detected in galactosemia, hereditary fructose intolerance, tyrosinemia type 1, and the mitochondrial respiratory chain or electron transport chain deficiencies. Hyperchloremic metabolic acidosis, therefore, may be an important clue to their presence.

Significantly, it is now recognized that some patients with multiple malformations may have a metabolic disease. The best example is Smith-Lemli-Opitz syndrome. Congenital craniofacial dysmorphic features, microcephaly, limb malformations, and progressive liver disease are secondary to a deficiency of the enzyme 7-dehydrocholesterol reductase. Another example of an autosomal recessive disorder resulting in malformations is Zellweger disease. In the classic form, the cellular organelle, the peroxisome, is not formed, resulting in multiple enzyme deficiencies such as those involved in very-long-chain fatty acid oxidation and plasmalogen biosynthesis. As a consequence, the brain, cranium, face, long bones, and kidney fail to develop normally. A list of the different metabolic diseases that can, but do not always, produce congenital dysmorphism or malformations is shown in Table 21–9. It is important, when confronted with an infant with these types of findings, that the physician not assume that a chromosome disorder is the cause or that congenital disease excludes a single-gene defect. In Chapter 18 the state of newborn screening, including metabolic diseases, is reviewed.

The next three chapters discuss various inborn errors of metabolism, including key clinical and laboratory findings, sophisticated biochemical and molecular diagnostic testing, therapy, and newborn screening. It is impractical to cover all known biochemical genetic diseases exhaustively and still provide useful and readily accessible information for the clinician. For this reason, the succeeding chapters focus on the major categories of disease as discussed earlier.

In Chapter 22, the metabolic defects involving small and simple molecules such as glucose, galactose, amino and organic acids, ammonia, and lactate are reviewed. These include the inborn errors that can produce acute, life-threatening disease with coma in the newborn infant. In Chapter 23, the storage diseases that manifest in the extended neonatal period are reviewed. This includes the disorders that involve handling of complex molecules. The lysosomal enzyme deficiencies are the most notable members of the group. They include the storage diseases that may manifest as nonimmune hydrops fetalis. Because physical examination is the key to the diagnosis of complex molecule diseases, the defects in peroxisomal metabolism such as Zellweger disease and Smith-Lemli-Opitz syndrome are also included in the chapter on storage diseases. In Chapter 24, the connective tissue diseases that involve metabolism of the complex molecules, collagen, fibrillin, and elastin and the osteochondrodystrophies that present in the newborn period are reviewed. Most metabolic diseases discussed in Chapters 22 through

**TABLE 21-8**

**Newborn Metabolic Disorders with Severe Hepatocellular Disease Potentially Leading to Cirrhosis**

Hereditary galactosemia
Hereditary fructose intolerance
Tyrosinemia type 1
Newborn iron storage disease
$\alpha_1$-antitrypsin deficiency
Long-chain acyl-CoA dehydrogenase deficiency
Long-chain 3-hydroxy acyl-CoA dehydrogenase deficiency
Mitochondrial respiratory/electron transport chain defects
Smith-Lemli-Opitz syndrome
Zellweger disease
Neonatal adrenoleukodystrophy
Niemann-Pick type C disease

**TABLE 21-9**

**Metabolic Diseases with Congenital Malformation(s) or Dysmorphic Features**

Smith-Lemli-Opitz syndrome
Zellweger disease
Neonatal adrenoleukodystrophy
Rhizomelic chondrodysplasia punctata
Glutaric aciduria type 2
Glutaric aciduria type 1
Primary lactic acidoses
- Pyruvate dehydrogenase deficiency
- Pyruvate carboxylase deficiency
- Mitochondrial respiratory/electron transport chain defects

Congenital defects in glycosylation
Mevalonic aciduria
I-cell disease
Galactosialidosis
Neuraminidase deficiency
Sialic acid storage disease
Menkes disease
Nonketotic hyperglycinemia
Lowe syndrome

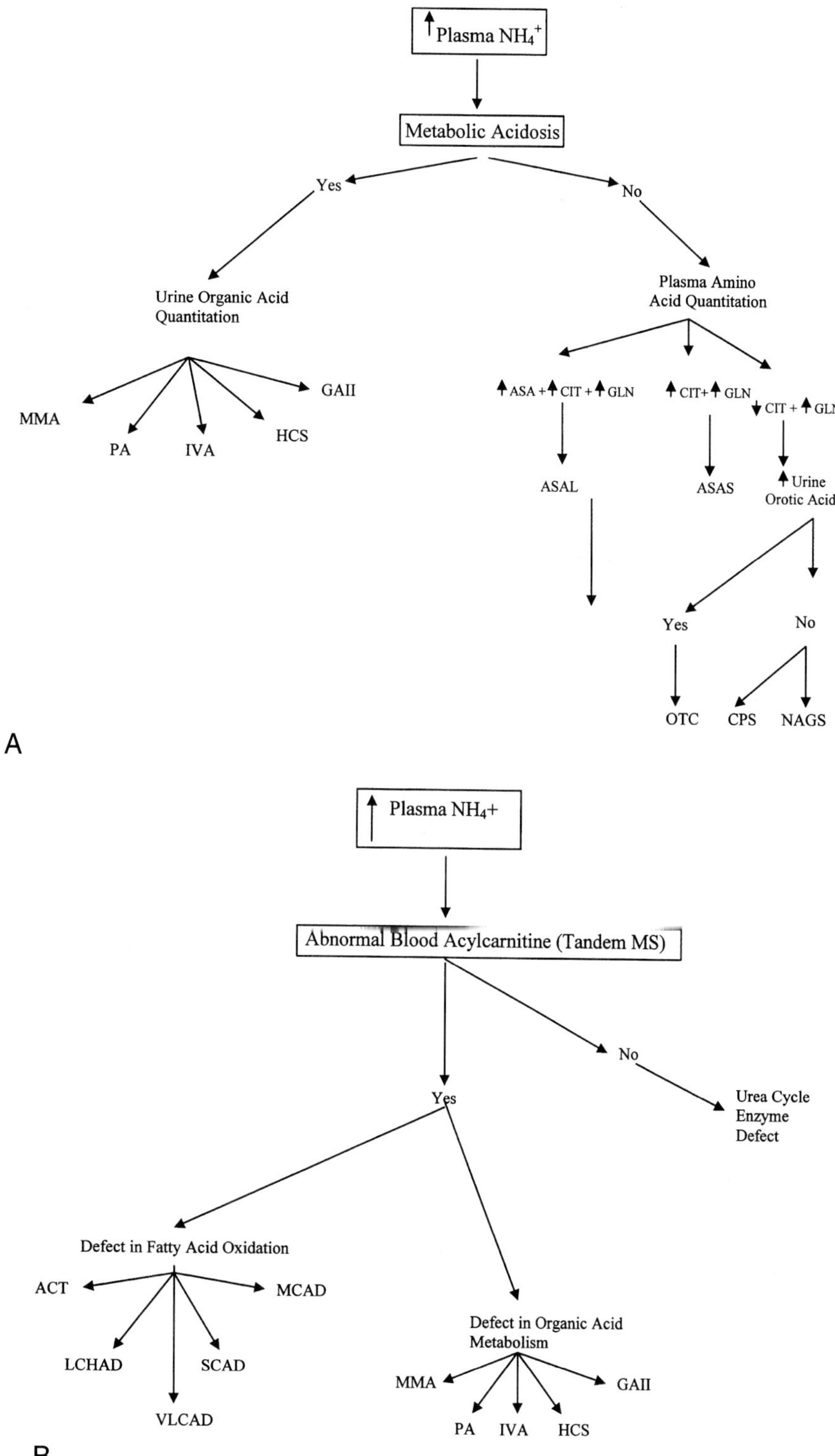


**FIGURE 21–1.** Algorithm for the metabolic work-up of a comatose infant with hyperammonemia. **A,** The presence of a metabolic acidosis is a key factor in the identification of the underlying disorder. Most infants with urea cycle defects present with a primary respiratory alkalosis. Please note that some infants with defects in organic acid metabolism and usually fatty acid oxidation display no acidosis. **B,** Defects in organic and fatty acid can be detected by the analysis of acyl carnitines by tandem mass spectrometry (MS-MS), as well as by the use of gas chromatography–MS for analysis of organ acids in urine. ACT, acyl carnitine translocase deficiency; ASA, argininosuccinic acid; ASAL, argininosuccinic acid lyase deficiency; ASAS, argininosuccinic acid synthetase deficiency; CIT, citrulline; CPS, carbamyl phosphate synthetase deficiency; GAII, glutaric aciduria type 2; GLN, glutamine; HCS, holocarboxylase synthetase deficiency; IVA, isovaleric acidemia; LCHAD, 3-hydroxy long-chain acyl CoA dehydrogenase deficiency; MCAD, medium-chain acyl CoA dehydrogenase deficiency; MMA, methylmalonic acidemia; NAGS, *N*-acetyl glutamate synthetase deficiency; OTC, ornithine transcarbamylase deficiency; PA, propionic acidemia; SCAD, short-chain acyl CoA dehydrogenase deficiency; VLCAD, very-long-chain acyl CoA dehydrogenase deficiency.

24 are not detected in the newborn screening programs currently in place. Accordingly, another purpose of this section is to help the clinician develop a conceptual framework to fashion a useful and practical approach to diagnostic testing.

To illustrate the effective use of the metabolic laboratory, an algorithm for the work-up of a comatose infant with hyperammonemia described in the following case study is shown in Fig. 21–1.

**CASE STUDY 1**

A full-term infant was breast-fed from birth. During the first 2 weeks of life, she failed to regain her birth weight and had decreased interest in feeding, with vomiting and progressive lethargy. By 3 weeks of age, the baby exhibited obtundation, tachypnea, hypothermia, hypotonia, and an ileus.

Laboratory studies performed on her admission to the neonatal intensive care unit (NICU) showed respiratory alkalosis, neutropenia, thrombocytopenia, and slight increase in urinary ketones. In addition, there were elevated plasma values for ammonium (900 μmol/L), glycine (1485 μmol/L) and lactate (3.0 mmol/L). Urine organic acid analysis by gas chromatography–mass spectrometry revealed the presence of 3-hydroxypropionate, methylcitrate, propionylglycine, and tiglyglycine, consistent with propionyl–coenzyme A carboxylase deficiency. Acyl carnitine analysis of a plasma sample by tandem mass spectrometry (MS-MS) showed elevated propionylcarnitine content.

Hemodialysis was utilized primarily for the management of hyperammonemia. Plasma ammonium levels were less than 100 μmol/L after 24 hours of treatment. A modified parenteral nutritional therapy with insulin was employed. Intravenous L-carnitine and metronidazole were added on the second day of hospitalization. Finally, a low-protein diet was initiated, and after a period of convalescence in the NICU, the patient was discharged. At 4 years of age, the patient has hypotonia, developmental delay, and anorexia requiring gastrointestinal tube feeding.

This case shows how an infant with a life-threatening hyperammonemic syndrome due to a defect in organic acid metabolism may not have a severe metabolic acidosis. In this instance, newborn screening with plasma acyl carnitine analysis by MS-MS led to the diagnosis of propionic acidemia because of the diagnostic elevation in plasma propionylcarnitine.

## REFERENCES

Berry GT, Yudkoff M: Metabolism. In Polin RA, Ditmer MF (eds): Pediatric Secrets, 3rd ed. Philadelphia, Hanley & Belfus, 2001.

Cohn RM, Roth KS: Metabolic Disease: A Guide to Early Recognition. Philadelphia, WB Saunders, 1983.

Fernandes J, Saudubray J-M, van den Berghe G (eds): Inborn Metabolic Diseases: Diagnosis and Treatment, 2nd ed. Berlin, Springer-Verlag, 1995.

Jones KL: Smith's Recognizable Patterns of Human Malformation, 5th ed. Philadelphia, WB Saunders, 1997.

Lyon G, Adams RD, Kolodny EH (eds): Neurology of Hereditary Metabolic Diseases of Children, 2nd ed. New York, McGraw-Hill, 1996.

Nyhan WL, Sakati NO: Diagnostic Recognition of Genetic Disease. Philadelphia, Lea & Febiger, 1987.

Online Mendelian Inheritance in Man (OMIM) Available on line at www.ncbi.nln. nih.gov/Omim/

Saudubray J-M, Charpentier C: Clinical phenotypes: Diagnosis/algorithms. In Scriver CR, Beaud et al, Sly WS, et al (eds): The Metabolic and Molecular Bases of Inherited Disease, 7th ed, vol 1. New York, McGraw-Hill 1995, pp 327-400.

Saudubray J-M, Ogier de Baulny H, Charpentier C: Clinical approach to inherited metabolic disorders. In Fernandes J, Saudubray J-M, van den Berghe G (eds): Inborn Metabolic Diseases: Diagnosis and Treatment, 2nd ed. Berlin, Springer-Verlag, 1995, pp 3-39.

Scriver CR, Beaud et al, Sly WS, et al (eds): The Metabolic and Molecular Bases of Inherited Disease, 7th ed. New York, McGraw-Hill, 1995.

CHAPTER 22

# Inborn Errors of Carbohydrate, Ammonia, Amino Acid, and Organic Acid Metabolism

Gerard T. Berry

The inborn errors of carbohydrate, ammonia, amino acid, and organic acid metabolism have one factor in common: All may be associated with acute, life-threatening disease during the newborn period. The most notable exception in this broad group of small-molecule disorders is phenylketonuria (PKU). There are often few signs secondary to classic PKU in the first 6 months of life, underscoring the importance of newborn screening in establishing the diagnosis of this disease. As discussed in Chapter 21, a single biochemical genetic defect may be associated with more than one mode of presentation. This chapter presents the most common phenotype for each disorder. The disorders that constitute each group are listed in Tables 22–1 to 22–4. The interrelationships among the major metabolites, biochemical cycles, and organelle pathways in the most critical facets of intermediary metabolism are simplified and depicted in Fig. 22–1. The primary lactic acidosis and mitochondrial respiratory chain disorders, as well as the defects in fatty acid oxidation, are included in the section on inborn errors of organic acid metabolism.

## INBORN ERRORS OF CARBOHYDRATE METABOLISM

### Hereditary Galactosemia

#### Galactose-1-Phosphate-Uridyltransferase (GALT) Deficiency

Galactose-1-Phosphate + UDP glucose $\xrightarrow{\text{GALT}}$ UDPgalactose + Glucose-1-Phosphate

- Enzyme: homodimer
- Gene location: chromosome 9p13
- Frequency: 1 in 35,000 to 60,000

**CASE STUDY 1**

A gravida 3, para 2 mother delivered a 10 lb, 3 oz male infant. On discharge from the nursery, the mother continued breast-feeding. The baby was noted to be jaundiced, with a total serum bilirubin of 28 mg/dL on day 4. He was readmitted to the local hospital, intravenous fluids were administered, and phototherapy was instituted. A sepsis work-up was performed, and the infant was treated with ampicillin. A second serum total bilirubin value was 24 mg/dL with a direct bilirubin value of 1 mg/dL, and 3+ reducing substances were detected in a urine specimen. Because galactosemia was suspected, the baby was switched to Nutramigen formula. The serum aspartate transaminase (AST) value was 232, and the γ-glutamyl-transferase (GGT) value was 132. On day 7, a trial of breast-feeding was resumed, and the urinary reducing substances value again became positive. On day 8, a bleeding diathesis was noted, and the prothrombin time (PT) and partial thromboplastin time (PTT) were longer than 30 and 150 minutes, respectively. Only a urine culture revealed the growth of *Escherichia coli*. The breast-feeding was again discontinued, and ProSobee formula was started. A Beutler fluorescent spot test performed on a filter paper specimen showed no fluorescence compatible with a diagnosis of hereditary galactosemia secondary to galactose-1-phosphate-uridyltransferase (GALT) deficiency. The infant's jaundice and laboratory abnormalities disappeared with the soy-based, lactose-free formula regimen.

After discharge, another blood specimen was obtained for confirmation of the enzyme deficiency. However, instead of a quantitation of erythrocyte GALT activity, an erythrocyte galactokinase (GALK) analysis was performed by a commercial laboratory that, not unexpectedly, demonstrated normal activity. Although the parents were reassured by the testing result that the diagnosis of galactosemia was incorrect, they continued to administer the lactose-free formula. Over the next year of life, the infant demonstrated normal growth and development.

Subsequently, the mother became pregnant and delivered a female infant, who was started on breast-feeding because the parents believed that galactosemia had been dismissed in the older infant. The newborn female infant began to have jaundice with vomiting. Despite the use of broad-spectrum antibiotics, she died of *E. coli* sepsis on day 13. A Beutler fluorescent spot test revealed no GALT activity compatible with classic galactosemia. Quantitation of erythrocyte GALT activity in the male confirmed the severe reduction in enzyme activity, and a GALT molecular analysis on DNA extracted from blood showed that the two siblings were homoallelic for the most common GALT gene defect, the Q188R mutation.

The three enzymes of the galactose metabolic pathway that are responsible for the rapid hepatic conversion of galactose to glucose after ingestion of dietary lactose are GALK, GALT, and uridine diphosphate (UDP) galactose-4-epimerase (Fig. 22–2). All three enzymes have been associated with inborn errors of galactose metabolism (Segal and Berry, 1996). However, when one refers to the disease galactosemia or hereditary galactosemia in clinical medicine, the reference is usually to GALT deficiency. The most common of these disorders, GALT deficiency is probably the most common of the inborn errors of carbohydrate metabolism that come to clinical attention in the newborn period. The clinical syndrome of transferase-deficiency galactosemia has changed since the advent of newborn screening for galactosemia. In the past, a severe multiorgan toxicity syndrome was a much more common occurrence, associated with weeks of unlimited intake of lactose in the proprietary formula or breast milk. However, as Case Study 1 illustrates, the disease can be devastating even in the first 1 or 2 weeks of life because of *E. coli* sepsis.

The most common initial clinical sign of GALT deficiency is poor growth; vomiting and poor feeding also occur in most patients. Jaundice may be present in the

**TABLE 22-1**

**Inborn Errors of Carbohydrate Metabolism**

| |
|---|
| Hereditary galactosemia |
| Glycogen storage diseases |
| Hereditary fructose intolerance |
| Fructose-1,6-bisphosphatase deficiency |

first few weeks of life and may persist. Initially the jaundice may be due to indirect hyperbilirubinemia, and only later associated with an elevation of direct bilirubin as well. While consuming lactose, many infants with galactosemia manifest in the first 2 to 3 weeks with only poor feeding and growth, jaundice, and mild irritability or lethargy. With continual ingestion, multiorgan toxicity syndrome ensues, associated with liver disease that may progress to cirrhosis with portal hypertension, splenomegaly, ascites, renal tubular dysfunction, sometimes the full-blown renal Fanconi syndrome, with anemia primarily due to decreased red blood cell (RBC) survival, lethargy, and brain edema associated with a bulging fontanelle. Two clinical phenomena deserve further mention, cataracts and *E. coli* sepsis. Cataracts may be evident in the first few weeks of life, but often, they are detected after 2 weeks of age. However, some infants are born with congenital cataracts that are associated with abnormalities of the embryonal lens; they are central in nature and require slit-lamp examination for documentation. *E. coli* sepsis is the most devastating complication in the newborn period, the mortality rate exceeding 50%. The reason that *E. coli* or gram-negative bacteria are uniquely present in newborns with GALT deficiency remains unknown.

After initiation of a lactose-free diet in the newborn period, the problems related to liver and kidney disease, anemia, and brain edema usually disappear, unless there has been severe organ damage such as hepatic cirrhosis. Most infants begin to grow and develop at a normal rate. However, we know now that even prospectively treated patients may manifest long-term complications related to speech defects, delays in language acquisition, learning problems in school, and hypergonadotropic hypogonadism in most of the females. The cause of these so-called dietary-independent complications is unknown. Patients with galactosemia must continue with a lactose-restricted diet for their entire lives. When an infant is initially diagnosed,

**TABLE 22-2**

**Inborn Errors of Ammonia Metabolism**

| |
|---|
| Ornithine transcarbamylase deficiency |
| Argininosuccinicaciduria |
| Citrullinemia |
| Carbamylphosphate synthetase deficiency |
| Transient hyperammonemia of the newborn |

**TABLE 22-3**

**Inborn Errors of Amino Acid Metabolism**

| |
|---|
| Maple syrup urine disease |
| Hereditary tyrosinemia type 1 |
| Nonketotic hyperglycinemia |
| Methionine synthetase deficiency |
| Phenylketonuria |

either through the newborn screening program or because of the recognition of clinical signs, blood galactose levels may be as high as 5 to 20 mM, and the RBC galactose-1-phosphate level is significantly elevated, as are urine galactitol levels. During this phase of severe hypergalactosemia, positive reducing substances are present in the urine.

One of the first abnormalities to be detected—albuminuria—reflects a poorly understood renal glomerular component. This develops within 24 to 48 hours of ingestion of lactose and disappears as quickly after elimination of lactose from the diet. In addition to hyperbilirubinemia, there may be mild to severe elevations of serum alanine transferase (ALT) and AST levels and various abnormalities related to renal tubular dysfunction, such as hyperchloremic metabolic acidosis, hypophosphatemia, glucosuria, and generalized aminoaciduria. Vitreous hemorrhages are newly recognized complications in the

**TABLE 22-4**

**Inborn Errors of Organic Acid Metabolism**

| |
|---|
| Methylmalonic acidemia |
| Propionic acidemia |
| Isovaleric acidemia |
| Multiple carboxylase deficiency |
| Glutaric acidemia type 1 |
| Fatty acid oxidation disorders |
|   Glutaric acidemia type 2 |
|   Very-long-chain acyl-CoA dehydrogenase deficiency |
|   Medium-chain acyl-CoA dehydrogenase deficiency |
|   Short-chain acyl-CoA dehydrogenase deficiency |
|   Long-chain 3-hydroxy acyl-CoA dehydrogenase deficiency |
|   Carnitine transporter defect |
|   Carnitine palmitoyltransferase type I deficiency |
|   Carnitine palmitoyltransferase type II deficiency |
|   Acylcarnitine translocase deficiency |
| Defects in ketone metabolism |
|   Ketothiolase deficiency |
|   Succinyl-CoA: 3-ketoacid-CoA transferase deficiency |
|   3-Hydroxy-3-methylglutaryl-CoA lyase deficiency |
| Primary lactic acidoses |
|   Pyruvate dehydrogenase complex deficiency |
|   Pyruvate carboxylase deficiency |
|   Phosphoenolpyruvate carboxykinase deficiency |
|   Mitochondrial respiratory/electron transport chain defects |
|     Barth syndrome |
|     Pearson syndrome |
|     Leigh disease |

CoA, coenzyme A.

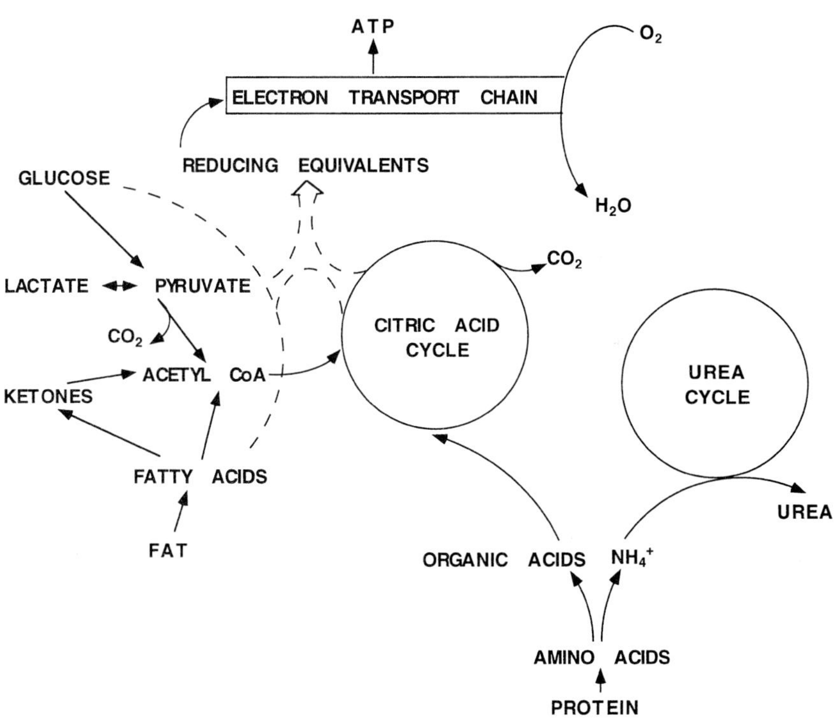


**FIGURE 22–1.** Intermediary metabolism interactions among the glycolytic, citric acid, mitochondrial respiratory–electron transport chain (ETC), amino acid, organic acid, and urea cycle pathways. Defects in these primarily catabolic pathways are the chief source of inborn errors of metabolism that involve the small, simple—not the large—complex molecules. ATP, adenosine triphosphate. *(Adapted from Cowett RM [ed]: Principles of Perinatal-Neonatal Metabolism, 2nd ed. New York, Springer-Verlag, 1998, p 800.)*

newborn period. After the patient is started on a lactose-free diet, the RBC galactose-1-phosphate levels in patients with classic galactosemia fall, but they never return to the normal range, remaining mildly elevated for the lifetime of the patient. This is also true for the urinary metabolite galactitol and may be related to endogenous galactose production (Berry et al, 1995).

The deficiency of the enzyme GALT may be detected in RBCs in patients with most common forms of galactosemia. The newborn screening programs in various states use an enzymatic method, a metabolite method, or both. When metabolites are assayed, either galactose-1-phosphate or total galactose and galactose-1-phosphate in RBCs are usually measured. Most of the gene defects that

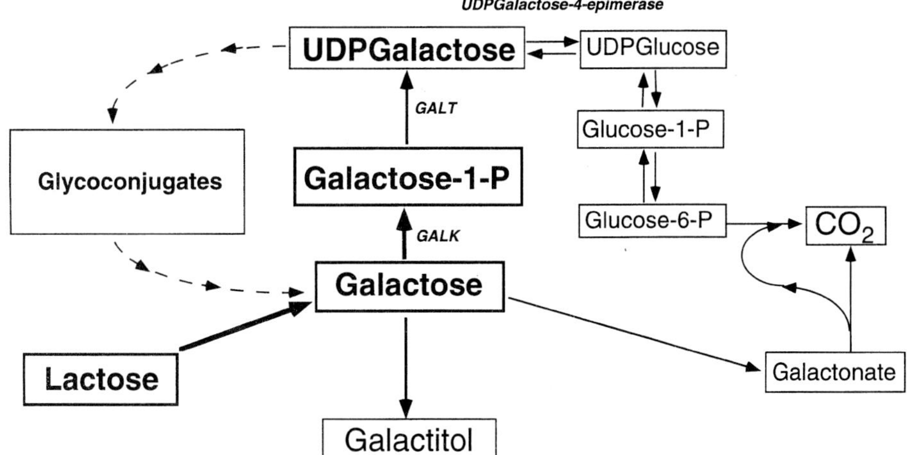


**FIGURE 22–2.** The important reactions in the galactose metabolic pathway are shown in relation to exogenous, via lactose primarily, and endogenous de novo synthesis of galactose. The reactions catalyzed by enzymes that have not been well delineated or are purported to exist are shown by *broken* or *dotted lines*. Carbon skeletons exit the galactose pool via galactokinase (GALK)–mediated conversion to galactose-1-phosphate (galactose-1-P), aldose reductase–mediated conversion to galactitol, and as galactonate. In patients with severe galactose-1-P-uridyltransferase (GALT) deficiency, there is little or no conversion of galactose-1-P to uridine diphosphate galactose (UDPgalactose). The epimerization of UDPglucose to UDPgalactose by UDPgalactose-4-epimerase, the utilization of UDPgalactose in the synthesis of glycoconjugates such as glycoproteins, and their subsequent degradation may constitute the pathways of de novo synthesis of galactose. *(Adapted from Berry GT, Nissim I, Gibson JB, et al: Quantitative assessment of whole body galactose metabolism in galactosemic patients. Eur J Pediatr 156:S44, 1997.)*

produce galactosemia are now known; therefore, some patients or siblings may be screened for the disease or for being carriers via genotype analyses. Liver disease of any cause and congenital hepatic vascular shunts may lead to impaired galactose tolerance and a positive newborn screening test result for galactosemia (Gitzelmann et al, 1992; Matsumoto et al, 1993).

## Glycogen Storage Diseases

The glycogen storage diseases (GSDs) may be divided into those types that primarily affect the liver and those that affect striated muscle (Chen and Burchell, 1995; Cornblath and Schwartz, 1991; Fernandes, 1988; Hirschhorn, 1995). With some forms, such as GSD type 3, or debrancher deficiency, both striated muscle and the liver may be affected. According to European prevalence data, the overall frequency of GSD is 1 in 20,000 to 25,000 (Chen and Burchell, 1995). With the exception of GSD type 2, or Pompe disease (a lysosomal defect), most of the patients with glycogenosis do not come to clinical attention in the newborn period. As Case Study 2, of a child with GSD type 1a illustrates, however, there are exceptions. Patients with the three most common forms of GSD—types 1, 3, 6—have a phenotype that mimics a small-molecule disorder because glucose homeostasis is affected.

### Glucose-6-Phosphatase Deficiency

Glucose-6-Phosphate + $H_2O \rightarrow$ Glucose + Phosphate

- Enzyme: heterodimer (catalytic and regulatory subunit)
- Catalytic subunit gene location: chromosome 17
- Frequency: 1 in 100,000

**CASE STUDY 2**

A 6 lb, 11 oz boy was born to consanguineous Lebanese parents. Despite hypoglycemia, for which he received intravenous glucose in the first 48 hours of life, the baby was discharged from the newborn nursery on day 2. He was fed Carnation Good Start formula. At 10 weeks of age, he demonstrated gastroenteritis and was treated with Pedialyte at home. He was subsequently admitted to a local hospital because of respiratory distress associated with fever and lethargy. Laboratory studies revealed a blood glucose value of 5 mg/dL, serum total $CO_2$ value of 5 mEq/L, an increased anion gap, and 3+ ketonuria. A chest radiograph was normal. The baby was intubated, started on ventilatory support, and given intravenous fluids with glucose, sodium bicarbonate, and antibiotics. He was subsequently transferred to the neonatal intensive care unit (NICU) at Children's Hospital of Philadelphia. Physical examination showed the patient to be lethargic with generalized hypotonia and enlarged liver. The liver edge was full, rounded, and palpated 7 cm below the right costal margin with a span of more than 10 cm. A liver ultrasonogram showed hepatomegaly with a coarsened echogenic texture. On the day of admission, a seizure was detected, in association with focal leg and jaw twitching and an increase in blood pressure. There was no recurrence of seizures after phenobarbital administration, which was later discontinued. Urine organic acid quantitation showed increased excretion of 3-hydroxybutyrate, acetoacetate, and lactate. A plasma amino acid quantitation showed alanine to be elevated, at 769 μM (normal is 88 to 440 μM).

After correction of the acid-base imbalance and hypoglycemia, the patient appeared to stabilize while receiving intravenous fluids with glucose. He was subsequently restarted on a proprietary formula, the Carnation Good Start formula. Results of a sepsis work-up were negative, and antibiotics were discontinued. Findings of a head magnetic resonance imaging (MRI) scan were normal. Subsequently, a blood glucose reagent strip test (Dextrosix) reading was 46 mg/dL 4 hours after a feeding. The blood lactate level was slightly increased at 2.2 mM (normal <2.0 mM). The liver remained enlarged, and a liver biopsy was performed. The histologic examination showed microsteatosis. The periodic acid–Schiff (PAS) stain response was positive but sensitive to diastase. Electron microscopy demonstrated increased glycogen. The glycogen content in the liver was high, at 6.8% (control, 2.3%). Glucose-6-phosphatase activity was measured in frozen liver homogenate and found to be markedly decreased (0.4 units; control value is 3.8 units), a finding compatible with glucose-6-phosphatase deficiency, specifically glycogen storage disease type 1a. A fasting study showed that the infant had a blood glucose level in the range of 40 mg/dL or lower 4 hours after a bottle feeding. This finding was associated with an increase in blood lactate levels. The serum uric acid and triglyceride levels were also elevated.

The baby was stabilized on ProSobee formula, given every 2 hours during the day, and a continuous glucose infusion administered at night via nasogastric tube. The baby was discharged with this regimen. The parents were instructed on home glucose monitoring. At discharge, the liver remained palpable to the level of the umbilicus, but the spleen was not enlarged. There were no further episodes of symptomatic hypoglycemia. By 4 months of age, the boy's weight was at the 95th percentile, and his length at the 90th percentile.

GSD type 1 is due to a decreased activity of glucose-6-phosphatase, the enzyme that is perched at the terminus of both glycogenolysis and gluconeogenesis. Several different biochemical abnormalities can result in this phenotype, now classified as GSD types 1a, 1b, and 1c. The enzyme that resides on the anticytoplasmic side of internal membrane spaces of the hepatocyte catalyzes the hydrolysis of glucose-6-phosphate to glucose and phosphate. Impairments in the transport of either glucose-6-phosphate or phosphate may result in decreased function of this enzyme. The major clinical findings are poor growth and enlarged abdominal girth, hepatomegaly, and any of the signs that may be related to hypoglycemia. The major laboratory findings are fasting hypoglycemia, ketosis, lactic acidosis, hyperlipidemia (specifically, hypertriglyceridemia), and hyperuricemia. In patients with type 1b disease due to a defect in the microsomal transporter of glucose-6-phosphate, there may be a history of recurrent infections due to neutropenia and defective neutrophil function. Diagnosis is based on hepatic enzyme analyses or, in some instances, molecular diagnostic testing (Burchell and Waddell, 1993; Chen and Burchell, 1995). The most important aspect of therapy is to prevent brain damage from hypoglycemia and growth failure. The mainstay of therapy is frequent feedings and restriction of lactose and sucrose (Chen and Burchell, 1995; Fernandes, 1988). The use of continuous nasogastric feedings or uncooked cornstarch, particularly during the night, has significantly improved the care of affected children, and although it does not correct all the biochemical perturbations, it does improve growth and can prevent hypoglycemic spells.

### Lysosomal α-Glucosidase Deficiency

$$\text{Glycogen}_{(n)} + H_2O \rightarrow \text{Glycogen}_{(n-1)} + \text{Glucose}$$

- Enzyme: α-1,4-glucosidase monomer
- Gene location: chromosome 17q23
- Frequency: 1 in 100,000

GSD type 2, or Pompe disease, is a deficiency of the lysosomal enzyme α-glucosidase. In the newborn period, the main clinical finding relates to heart disease. There is usually marked cardiomegaly and a typical abnormal electrocardiogram, with biventricular hypertrophy and a short PR interval. Decreased cardiac output may lead to heart failure and passive congestion. Infants may also have generalized hypotonia, not just because of heart failure but also because of skeletal myopathy. There is increased deposition of glycogen within striated muscle. Except in the instance of passive congestion, the liver is not usually enlarged. Diagnosis is based on muscle enzyme analysis (Hirschhorn, 1995). Cardiac transplantation has been performed to prevent death in infancy.

## Hereditary Fructose Intolerance

### Fructose-1,6-Bisphosphate Aldolase B Deficiency

$$\text{Fructose-1-Phosphate} + H_2O \rightarrow \text{Dihydroxyacetone Phosphate} + \text{Glyceraldehyde}$$

- Enzyme: homotetramer
- Gene location: chromosome 9q13-q32
- Frequency: very rare, except approximately 1 in 20,000 in Swiss persons

Hereditary fructose intolerance is secondary to a deficiency of the enzyme fructose-1,6-bisphosphate aldolase (Cornblath and Schwartz, 1991; Gitzelmann et al, 1995). There are different isoforms of aldolases in human tissues. The enzyme deficiency in this disease results in an impairment in the conversion of fructose-1-phosphate to glyceraldehyde and dihydroxyacetone phosphate and, to a much lesser degree, in the conversion of fructose-1,6-bisphosphate to glyceraldehyde-3-phosphate and dihydroxyacetone phosphate. The disorder is inherited as an autosomal recessive trait. Manifestations of clinical disease depend on sucrose or fructose ingestion. Thus, it usually does not come to clinical attention in the newborn period unless fruits are started early in the diet or the patients are started on a formula that contains sucrose or fructose.

The major clinical findings are poor feeding, vomiting, loose stools, poor growth, hepatomegaly, and any sign that could be related to hypoglycemia. Classically, the infants become ill soon after ingesting fructose. The acute signs may include pallor and lethargy, an altered state of central nervous system (CNS) function due to hypoglycemia. The major laboratory findings consist of hypoglycemia; hypophosphatemia; elevations of serum ALT and AST, including any of the findings that may be associated with hepatocellular disease per se; and the presence of reducing substances in the urine. The liver disease may be severe. Patients may be jaundiced with hyperbilirubinemia. There may be a bleeding diathesis. In addition to liver disease, renal tubular dysfunction may lead to full-blown renal Fanconi syndrome. Thus, one may detect metabolic acidosis due to a renal tubular acidosis, hypophosphatemia, impaired urate handling, spillage of glucose as well as fructose into the urine, and generalized amino aciduria. It is believed that the severity of the clinical findings is related to the amount of fructose ingested. Infants, however, probably because of decreased intake, may manifest only the signs of poor growth and may have few findings related to liver disease, except perhaps intermittent hypertransaminasemia. The suspicion of the physician is crucial in establishing the diagnosis. An intravenous fructose test may be performed under controlled circumstances, such as in the NICU or clinical research center, to determine whether, after 15 to 30 minutes of fructose administration, serum phosphate and glucose levels decrease and serum AST and ALT values rise. In the past, diagnosis depended on enzyme analysis, but molecular diagnostic testing is more available now. The treatment consists of elimination of dietary fructose and sucrose.

## Fructose-1,6-Bisphosphatase Deficiency

$$\text{Fructose-1,6-Bisphosphate} + H_2O \rightarrow \text{Fructose-6-Phosphate} + \text{Phosphate}$$

- Enzyme: homotetramer
- Gene location: unknown
- Frequency: very rare

The deficiency of the enzyme fructose-1,6-bisphosphatase results in an inability to hydrolyze fructose-1,6-bisphosphate to fructose-6-phosphate (Baker and Winegrad, 1970; Gitzelmann et al, 1995). This enzyme is key in gluconeogenesis. The main clinical features of the disease are hypoglycemia and the signs related to glucose deprivation in the CNS. The disease is primarily brought on by fasting, not by fructose ingestion, although fructose may exacerbate the abnormalities induced by fasting adaptation. Enlargement of the liver due to diffuse steatosis may be present only during periods of fasting and enhanced gluconeogenesis. The laboratory findings consist of hypoglycemia, ketosis, and lactic acidosis. The acidosis due to accumulation of lactic, 3-hydroxybutyric, and acetoacetic acids may be severe in this disease. Diagnosis depends on enzymatic analysis. The therapy consists primarily of avoidance of fasting.

# INBORN ERRORS OF AMMONIA METABOLISM

## Ornithine Transcarbamylase (OTC) Deficiency

$$\text{Ornithine} + \text{Carbamylphosphate} \xrightarrow{\text{OTC}} \text{Citrulline}$$

- Enzyme: homotrimer
- Gene location: chromosome X p21.1
- Frequency: 1 in 70,000 to 100,000

### Argininosuccinate Lyase (ASAL) Deficiency

$$\text{Argininosuccinate} \xrightarrow{\text{ASAL}} \text{Arginine} + \text{Fumarate}$$

- Enzyme: homotetramer
- Gene location: chromosome 7 cen-p21
- Frequency: 1 in 70,000 to 100,000

### Argininosuccinate Synthetase (ASAS) Deficiency

$$\text{Citrulline} + \text{Aspartate} \xrightarrow{\text{ASAS}} \text{Argininosuccinate}$$

- Enzyme: homotetramer
- Gene location: chromosome 9q34
- Frequency: 1 in 70,000 to 100,000

### Carbamylphosphate Synthetase I (CPSI) Deficiency

$$NH_3 + \text{Adenosine triphosphate (ATP)} + HCO_3 \xrightarrow{\text{CPSI}} \text{Carbamylphosphate}$$

- Enzyme: homodimer
- Gene location: chromosome 2p
- Frequency: 1 in 70,000 to 100,000

**CASE STUDY 3**

A male infant born at term after an uncomplicated pregnancy, labor, and delivery was noted to be lethargic with poor feeding at 2 days of age. Laboratory studies showed his plasma ammonium level to be more than 1500 μM. A plasma amino acid quantitation revealed massive elevations of glutamine (2640 μM; normal is 422 to 849 μM) and alanine (2540 μM; normal is 120 to 449 μM) and an undetectable level of citrulline. The most likely diagnosis was the X-linked disease ornithine transcarbamylase (OTC) deficiency in a male infant. Because of hyperammonemic coma, arrangements were immediately made for hemodialysis. Before catheter placements, the infant was given an intravenous bolus of sodium benzoate and sodium phenylacetate, both at 250 mg/kg per 24 hours. Intravenous arginine hydrochloride at 400 mg/kg per 24 hours was administered as a continuous infusion. In addition, the infant was given 10% glucose intravenously to suppress catabolism. The medications were continued during hemodialysis. After several hours of hemodialysis, the plasma ammonium level had fallen to the 200-μM range, and peritoneal dialysis was instituted. Normalization of the plasma alanine and glutamine levels occurred more gradually. After 3 days of peritoneal dialysis therapy, the plasma ammonium levels were within the normal range, and the severe encephalopathy resolved.

The patient was discharged at $2^1/_2$ weeks of age on a very-low-protein diet (0.7 g/kg per day) with supplementation of essential amino acids (0.7 g/kg per day), oral sodium benzoate (250 mg/kg per day), sodium phenylacetate (250 mg/kg per day) and arginine (174 mg/kg per day). He suffered no further episodes of hyperammonemia during the first year of life, and at 15 months of age, he underwent a liver transplantation. The OTC activity in the liver that was removed was undetectable. An analysis of genomic DNA revealed a CGA to CAA mutation in codon 141 of exon 5 of the OTC gene, thus producing an arginine to glutamine substitution (R141Q), which is a severe mutation involving the active site of the OTC enzyme. After transplantation, the therapy was discontinued, and although the patient has been on a regular-protein diet, plasma ammonium levels have completely normalized. Plasma citrulline levels remained undetectable.

Genetic diseases involving each of the five enzymes of the hepatic mitochondrial urea cycle have been described (Brusilow and Horwich, 1995). In the urea cycle, carbamylphosphate, which carries the nitrogen atom from ammonia, condenses with ornithine to form citrulline in a reaction catalyzed by the enzyme OTC. The most common defect among the inborn errors of the urea cycle is OTC deficiency. Citrulline subsequently interacts with aspartate to form argininosuccinate (ASA), and in the process, another waste nitrogen atom is shuttled into the urea cycle substrate. Arginine is formed from ASA, and the terminal enzyme in this cycle, arginase, converts arginine to urea for urinary excretion while regenerating ornithine to complete the cycle (Fig. 22–3). The first step in this cycle involves the synthesis of carbamylphosphate, and this reaction, catalyzed by carbamylphosphate synthetase type I (CPS-I), requires an activator, *N*-acetylglutamate, which is synthesized from acetyl coenzyme A (CoA) and glutamate via the enzyme *N*-acetylglutamate synthetase (NAGS). Rare patients may have reduced activity of NAGS.

With the exception of arginase deficiency, each of these enzyme deficiencies has been associated with disease in the newborn period. Clinical presentation in the newborn period is similar for all these defects (Batshaw, 1984). Almost all the infants are well in the first 12 to 24 hours of life when they begin to manifest poor feeding, vomiting, hyperventilation, lethargy, and coma, usually with seizures. When these diseases are untreated, they are almost always fatal. The treatment requires specific therapy to lower the waste nitrogen burden, including the toxic substance ammonia. An additional clinical finding is increased intracranial pressure. As with maple syrup urine disease (MSUD), the severe encephalopathic and life-threatening features may be related to brain edema. Chronic hepatomegaly has been reported in patients with argininosuccinic aciduria, whereas in the other urea cycle disorders, hepatomegaly is evident only during hyperammonemic episodes. Histologic examination of the liver shows modest fatty infiltration and fibrosis. Children with argininosuccinic aciduria may also manifest a specific abnormality of the hair, *trichorrhexis nodosa*.

The main laboratory finding in the urea cycle enzyme defects (UCEDs) is a plasma ammonium elevation. Plasma ammonium values may vary in different laboratories. In general, however, with automated chemistry testing for ammonia, the normal plasma values in older infants, children, and adults range between 10 and 35 μmol/L. However, in the Clinical Chemistry Laboratory at the Children's Hospital of Philadelphia, the normal plasma ammonium value in newborns may be as high as 110 μmol/L. In patients with newborn-onset UCEDs who are acutely ill, the plasma ammonium levels are often higher than 1000 or 2000 μmol/L. Patients with UCEDs usually do not have metabolic acidosis unless they are in a terminal state with vascular collapse or respiratory failure. Instead, the characteristic acid-base abnormality associated with hyperammonemia is respiratory alkalosis due to the effect of ammonia on the respiratory control centers in the brainstem.

The various UCEDs can usually be distinguished on the basis of the pattern and levels of plasma amino acids. Because citrulline is the product of the CPS-I and OTC reactions and the substrate for argininosuccinate synthetase

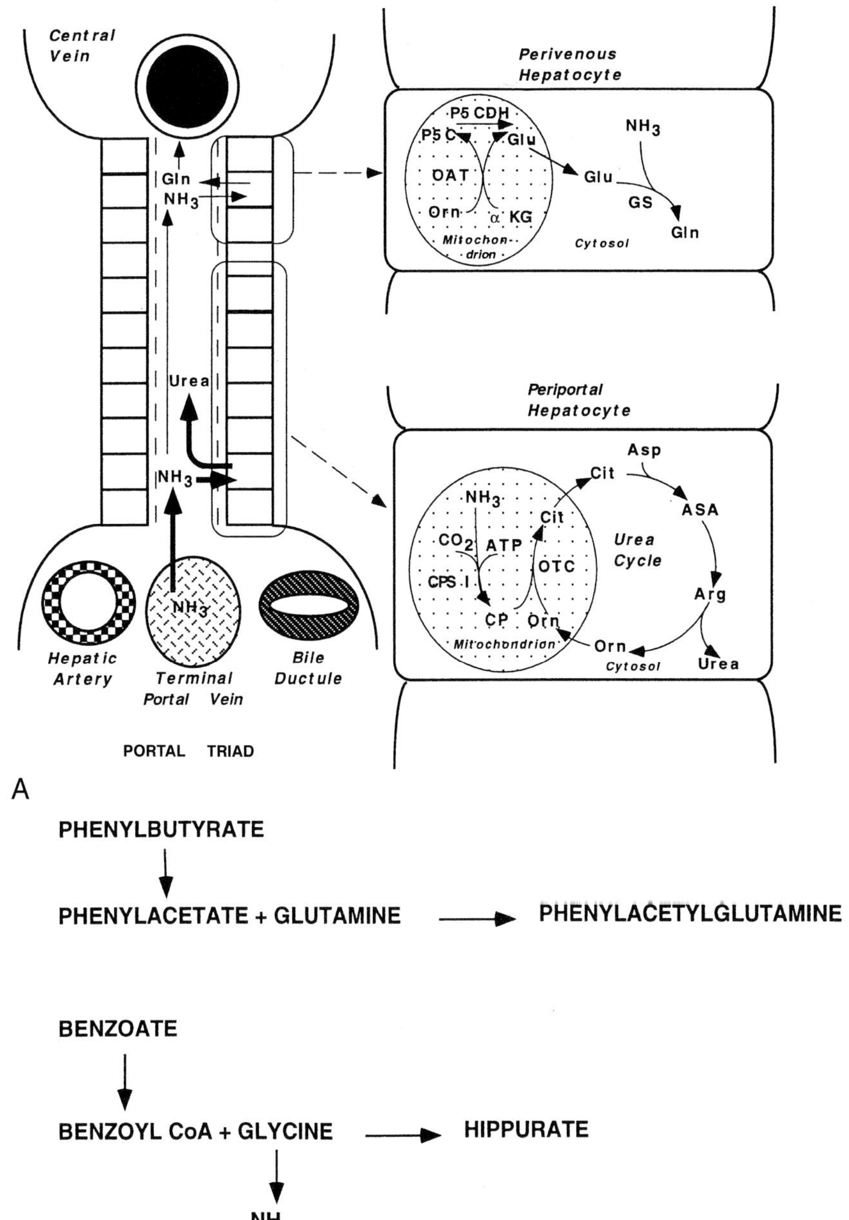


**FIGURE 22-3.** **A,** Depicted is the nonhomogeneous distribution of enzymes involved in ammonia metabolism in the hepatocytes of an acinar sinusoid as they are linearly distributed from the portal triad to the region of the central vein or terminal hepatic venule. The specific enzymatic reactions are shown for an individual periportal and perivenous hepatocyte. The glutamine synthetase (GS) and ornithine aminotransferase (OAT) enzyme activities are expressed exclusively in the one to three cell layers surrounding the central vein, that is, the region of zone 3 of the liver lobule, whereas the urea cycle enzymes are concentrated within the periportal hepatocytes. However, the urea cycle enzyme activities are higher in zone 1 immediately surrounding the portal triad than in the middle zone 2. The hepatocytes are shown as *squares*, the hepatic mitochondria as *shaded circles*, and the lining of the space of Disse as the *interrupted lines* on either side of the linear array of hepatocytes. Arg, arginine; ASA, argininosuccinate; Asp, aspartate; ATP, adenosine triphosphate; Cit, citrulline; CP, carbamylphosphate; CPS-I, carbamylphosphate synthetase type 1; Gln, glutamine; Glu, glutamate; α-KG, α-ketoglutarate; $NH_3$, ammonia; $CO_2$, $CO_2$ or bicarbonate; Orn, ornithine; P5C, pyrroline 5-carboxylate; P5CDH, pyrroline-5-carboxylate dehydrogenase. **B,** The medications sodium phenylacetate and phenylbutyrate and sodium benzoate promote alternative waste nitrogen disposal by participating in these two mitochondrial reactions. *(Adapted from Tuchman M, Lichenstein GR, Rajagopal BS, et al: Hepatic glutamine synthetase deficiency in fatal hyperammonemia after lung transplantation. Ann Intern Med 127:447, 1997.)*

(ASAS), its value is critical. In newborn-onset CPS-I and OTC deficiencies, plasma citrulline concentrations are zero to trace. With *OTC deficiency*, there is increased urinary orotate excretion secondary to carbamylphosphate accumulation and pyrimidine synthesis. With *CPS-I deficiency*, carbamylphosphate production is decreased or absent, and orotate excretion is decreased. Theoretically, a defect in the production of the activator of CPS-I, namely NAG, resembles a partial CPS-I deficiency. In citrullinemia, the plasma citrulline concentrations are markedly elevated. With argininosuccinic aciduria, plasma citrulline concentration is moderately elevated, in the range of 100 to 300 μmol/L, and can be readily detected during an analysis of plasma by amino acid column chromatography.

Because the ability of infants with these disorders to excrete waste nitrogen as urea is impaired, therapy initially centered around on the reduction of nitrogen intake by decreasing dietary protein and providing essential amino acids or the ketoacid analogues. This approach theoretically permits adequate growth without an excess nitrogen load. Excessive protein leads to hyperammonemia. However, too great a restriction of protein during long-term therapy leads to poor growth. Actually, this approach fails when the patient is in negative nitrogen balance, as occurs in the catastrophically ill infant presenting in the first week of life with massive hyperammonemia. For such an infant with hyperammonemia and coma, the mainstay of therapy is dialysis treatment. Hemodialysis is the most effective way of reducing plasma ammonium levels because it affords the greatest clearance of ammonia (Rutledge et al, 1990). Next in efficacy is continuous arteriovenous hemofiltration (CAVH) (Thompson et al, 1991). Although the clearance rate is not as great as with hemodialysis, the method has the added benefit of not being administered intermittently; with steady administration, there is less likelihood of major swings in intravascular volume that may exacerbate an already catabolic state. Ammonia clearance with peritoneal dialysis is only approximately one tenth that of CAVH and is not recommended for specific UCED therapy in the newborn period.

While the intensive care personnel are waiting for dialysis therapy to be instituted, alternative waste nitrogen therapy using intravenous sodium benzoate, sodium phenylacetate, and, for patients with ASAS and ASAL deficiencies, arginine hydrochloride should be initiated (Brusilow, 1991; Brusilow and Batshaw, 1979; Brusilow et al, 1979). (The medications as well as the proper dose for a bolus and 24-hour sustaining infusion are available from Ucyclyd Pharma, Inc., Scottsdale, AZ.) Patients with OTC and CPS-I deficiencies should also receive intravenous arginine hydrochloride, because body arginine pools can begin to deplete as arginine becomes an essential amino acid with a complete block in cycle function (Brusilow, 1984). The plasma arginine levels are usually low in all sick newborns with UCED. Unless corrected, arginine deficiency accentuates the hyperammonemia by promoting negative nitrogen balance and, theoretically, by failing to provide its usual stimulation of NAGS. A second role of arginine is to stimulate alternative pathways of waste nitrogen excretion. It does so by promoting synthesis and excretion of citrulline and ASA in citrullinemia and argininosuccinic aciduria, respectively. Argininosuccinate contains both waste nitrogen atoms destined for excretion as urea. It has a renal clearance rate equal to the glomerular filtration rate, provided that it is continuously synthesized and excreted. Accordingly, ASA should serve as an effective substitute for urea as a waste nitrogen product.

Like ASA, citrulline can be a means to excrete waste nitrogen, but it contains only the one nitrogen atom derived from ammonium, lacking the second nitrogen derived from aspartate. Citrulline also has a more limited urinary excretory capacity than ASA. Thus, therapy with arginine is less effective for citrullinemia. With citrullinemia and the other urea cycle disorders, arginine therapy is combined with sodium benzoate and sodium phenylacetate, both of which promote excretion of waste nitrogen. Sodium benzoate is conjugated with glycine to form hippurate, which is cleared by the kidney at five times the glomerular filtration rate (see Fig. 22–3). Theoretically, 1 mole of waste nitrogen is synthesized and excreted as hippurate for each mole of benzoate ingested. The hippurate synthetic mechanism resides primarily in the hepatic mitochondria and depends on an intact mitochondrial energy system for adenosine triphosphate (ATP) synthesis. The glycine consumed in this reaction can be replaced by either serine or the glycine cleavage pathway. Sodium phenylacetate, as well as sodium phenylbutyrate, which is used for long-term therapy in the absence of sodium benzoate, conjugates with glutamine to form phenylacetylglutamine, which is excreted by the kidney (see Fig. 22–3). Sodium phenylbutyrate is converted to phenylacetate in the liver. Glutamine contains two nitrogen atoms, whereas glycine contains one. Two moles of waste nitrogen are removed for each mole of phenylacetate administered. This acetylation reaction occurs in the kidney and the liver.

The outcome for patients with severe newborn-onset CPS-I and OTC deficiencies is poor. Sometimes, even dialysis therapy cannot rescue severely affected boys with X-linked OTC deficiency in the first few days of life. Prospectively administered alternative pathway therapy in conjunction with administration of high-calorie fluids usually prevents death and severe hyperammonemia in these patients. Even after institution of successful therapy, the morbidity and mortality rates are high in such patients. At present, liver transplantation is recommended for patients with CPS and OTC deficiencies who present in the newborn period and have almost no residual enzyme activity. Alternative pathway therapy has led to a 92% 1-year survival rate in newborns who recover from hyperammonemic coma, but most of the survivors are mentally retarded (Msall et al, 1984). There is a significant correlation between the duration of newborn hyperammonemic coma and the developmental quotient (DQ) score at 12 months of age (Msall et al, 1984). Four of five reported children in whom duration of coma was 2 days or less had normal IQ scores, whereas all seven children in whom coma lasted 5 days or longer were severely mentally retarded. This fact points to the devastating effects of prolonged newborn hyperammonemic coma and the importance of early diagnosis and treatment. Mutational analysis of DNA is available for most of these disorders (Brusilow and Horwich, 1995). If the lesion in a particular family is known, prenatal diagnosis by means of direct DNA analysis is also feasible. With the exception of OTC deficiency, all the UCEDs are inherited as autosomal recessive traits.

## Transient Hyperammonemia of the Newborn

Transient hyperammonemia of the newborn (THAN) is a distinct clinical syndrome that was first identified by Ballard and colleagues in 1978. The disease usually develops in premature infants during the course of treatment for respiratory distress syndrome. The plasma ammonium level may be enormously elevated, as high as that found in any of the patients with the most severe type of UCED. Its onset is usually in the first 24 hours after birth, when the infant is undergoing mechanical ventilatory support. Affected babies can manifest all the signs associated with hyperammonemic coma. The diagnosis may be difficult to determine, however, because many of these same infants are receiving sedatives and muscle relaxants to optimize therapy of their life-threatening pulmonary disease. Important clues are the absence of deep tendon reflexes, the absence of the normal newborn reflexes, and decrease or absence of response to painful stimuli. As with hyperammonemic coma in the UCED, this medical emergency requires dialysis therapy.

The cause of this disease is unknown. The plasma amino acid levels are similar to those found in CPS-I or OTC deficiency. Investigators have hypothesized that the disorder may be caused by impairment of hepatic mitochondrial energy production or shunting of portal blood away from the liver, such as in patent ductus venosus. However, patients with congenital portal shunting defects have been described with disturbances in liver function such as impaired galactose metabolism, but they are not premature and do not have life-threatening hyperammonemia (Gitzelmann et al, 1992; Matsumoto et al, 1993). The mortality rate in THAN is high. A patient who can be treated early and aggressively may survive the episode. There is no evidence that any of the survivors has suffered any further episodes of hyperammonemia, nor has there been any further evidence of impaired ammonia metabolism.

## INBORN ERRORS OF AMINO ACID METABOLISM

### Maple Syrup Urine Disease

#### Branched-Chain 2-Keto Dehydrogenase (BCKAD) Complex Deficiency

$$\text{Leucine} \longleftrightarrow \text{2-Ketoisocaproate} \xrightarrow{\text{BCKAD}} \text{Isovaleryl-CoA}$$

$$\text{Isoleucine} \longleftrightarrow \text{2-Keto-3-Methylvalerate} \xrightarrow{\text{BCKAD}} \text{2-Methylbutyryl-CoA}$$

$$\text{Valine} \longleftrightarrow \text{2-Ketoisovalerate} \xrightarrow{\text{BCKAD}} \text{Isobutyryl-CoA}$$

- Enzyme: 6 subunits:
  - BCKA decarboxylase subunits ($E_1$), 2α and 2β
  - 1 dihydrolipoyl transacylase ($E_2$) subunit
  - 1 dihydrolipoyl dehydrogenase ($E_3$) subunit
  - 1 BCKAD kinase subunit
  - 1 BCKAD phosphatase subunit
- Gene locations:
  - $E_1\alpha$ on chromosome 1q13.1-q13.2
  - $E_1\beta$ on chromosome 6p21-p22
  - $E_2$ on chromosome 2p31
  - $E_3$ on chromosome 7q31-q32
- Frequency: for MSUD, 1 in 200,000; except for Pennsylvania Mennonites, in whom frequency is 1 in 358.

MSUD is a rare inborn error of amino acid metabolism (Chuang and Shih, 1995; Menkes et al, 1954). It is inherited as an autosomal recessive trait and is secondary to a deficiency of the enzyme branched-chain 2-keto dehydrogenase (BCKAD) complex. This enzyme catalyzes the conversion of each of the 3-ketoacid derivatives of the branched-chain amino acids (BCAAs) into their decarboxylated coenzyme metabolites within the mitochondria (Fig. 22–4). The disease occurs in 1 in 200,000 newborn infants around the world, but in the Mennonite communities of the United States, the frequency is 1 in 358 because of a founder effect for a point mutation in the $E_1\alpha$ gene. In most of the patients around the world, as well as in the Mennonite community, the classic form of the disease occurs. It is associated with severe and catastrophic illness in the newborn period and usually results

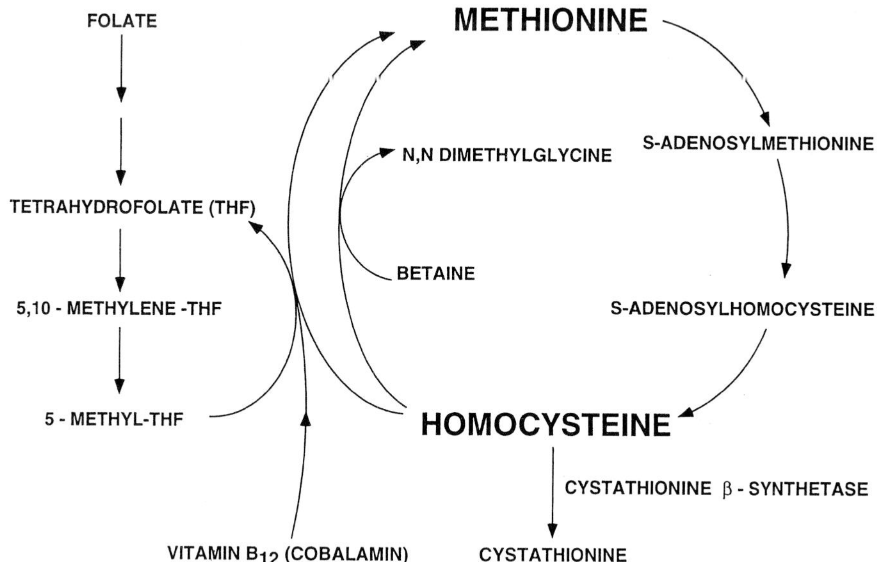


**FIGURE 22–4.** The pathways, metabolites, and vitamin cofactors important in the interconversion of methionine and homocysteine are shown in this abbreviated scheme of the trans-sulfuration pathway. In a methyl-transfer reaction, homocysteine is converted to methionine; the reaction is catalyzed by a cobalamin-containing enzyme, 5-methyl-tetrahydrofolate-homocysteine methyltransferase or methionine synthase. An alternate reaction involves betaine-homocysteine methyltransferase. Thus, vitamin $B_{12}$ and folate are important vitamins in homocysteine and methionine metabolism. The 5,10-methylene tetrahydrofolate (THF) derived from dietary folate is converted to 5-methyl THF by the enzyme 5,10-methylene THF reductase. In classic homocystinuria, the deficient enzyme is the cystathionine β-synthetase, which catalyzes the conversion of homocysteine to cystathionase, a precursor of cysteine. This pathway is readily operative in the adult so that cysteine is a nonessential amino acid. In newborn infants, however, synthesis of cysteine does not occur at the same rate as in adults. Adenosylmethionine-dependent methyl transfer may be extremely important in the central nervous system. Most of the patients who come to clinical attention in the newborn period have defects in the remethylation of homocysteine to methionine, and thus, these patients may have a severe deficiency of adenosylmethionine in the brain and spinal cord.

in death without specific medical intervention. Typically, the infants are well at birth; only after 2 or 3 days of ingestion of breast milk or formula do they begin to manifest poor feeding and spitting up. Lethargy becomes evident; the cry may be shrill and high pitched. There may be hypotonia alternating with hypertonia and opisthotonic posturing. The odor of maple syrup may be detected in the saliva, on the breath, in the urine and feces, and in cerumen obtained from the ear. The babies become more and more obtunded and eventually lapse into a deep coma. The anterior fontanelle may be bulging. Seizures may develop. The life-threatening encephalopathic features may simply be related to brain edema (Lungarotti et al, 1982; Riviello et al, 1991).

Laboratory findings consist of metabolic acidosis. The anion gap may be raised but not necessarily so. There is almost always ketonuria. The plasma ammonium values are not usually elevated. The complete blood count (CBC) is not usually abnormal. The levels of the plasma BCAAs leucine, isoleucine, and valine are elevated, with striking elevation in leucine. The normal ranges for plasma leucine, isoleucine, and valine in the newborn period are 29 to 152 μmol/L (or 0.4 to 2.0 mg/dL), 11 to 87 μmol/L (0.1 to 1.1 mg/dL), and 71 to 236 μmol/L (0.8 to 2.8 mg/dL), respectively. In these patients who are critically ill, the leucine levels may range between 1.9 and 6.9 mM (or 25 and 90 mg/dL). In the past, almost every newborn infant who was recognized to have MSUD and was in a severely decompensated state received peritoneal dialysis in a tertiary care center. The treatment was successful in most instances, but it did not allow for as rapid a rate of reduction in plasma BCAA levels as did hemodialysis or CAVH (Rutledge et al, 1990; Thompson et al, 1991).

It is now clear that a nutritional approach works just as well as peritoneal dialysis in newborns with MSUD (Berry et al, 1991; Parini et al, 1993; Shih et al, 1975; Townsend and Kerr, 1982). The approach consists of the use of a BCAA–free modified parenteral nutrition therapy for infants as well as older children with acute metabolic decompensation (Berry et al, 1991). Usually, insulin therapy is also necessary to curtail the effects of catabolic stress (Berry et al, 1991; Wendel et al, 1982). On the basis of the rate of plasma leucine decline, my colleagues and I have found that this nutritional therapy is comparable to peritoneal dialysis when the plasma leucine levels are as high as 25 to 40 mg/dL. It is unclear, however, whether CAVH or hemodialysis is more beneficial in achieving a greater rate of reduction of the plasma BCAAs and their corresponding branched-chain ketoacids (BCKAs) when the levels of leucine are in the range of 60 to 90 mg/dL. Most patients who are successfully treated by 7 days of age do not have mental retardation. Patients whose diagnosis and therapy are delayed, however, and perhaps even in those whose disorder is diagnosed in the first week of life but who have suffered such severe damage because of increased intracranial pressure often have substantial decreases in DQ or IQ, as well as signs compatible with spastic diplegia or quadriplegia.

The mainstay of long-term therapy for patients with MSUD who survive the newborn period is a special formula devoid of the BCAAs. The amount of BCAAs necessary to sustain growth but maintain the plasma, leucine, isoleucine, and valine levels in the normal range is supplied with a regular proprietary formula in limited amounts. In the first week of life, this is about 100 mg of leucine per kilogram of body weight daily and 50 mg/kg daily of both isoleucine and valine. The BCAA requirements and thus the rates of utilization of the BCAAs for protein accretion drop rapidly in the first year of life in conjunction with the decline in growth velocity in young infants. As with PKU, it is imperative that the administration of the special amino acid formula be carefully monitored by means of frequent plasma amino acid quantitations. One of the most common errors made in the treatment of MSUD is the failure to administer adequate amounts of supplemental isoleucine and valine solutions to maintain the normal plasma levels, because proprietary formulas alone do not always meet the needs of each growing baby (i.e., adequate amounts of each BCAA are not supplied by a formula alone). Deficiency of BCAAs may result in a severe exfoliative rash and anemia. The rash may mimic that of severe acrodermatitis enteropathica (Diliberti et al, 1973; Giacoia and Berry, 1993).

As with many of the inborn errors of amino acid, organic acid, and ammonia metabolism, protein administration in the infant whose disease is under previous good control and in metabolic balance with diet therapy must be discontinued during periods of intercurrent infections because catabolism, possibly driven by counter-regulatory hormones or cytokines, triggers metabolic decompensation through release of BCKA from skeletal muscle. Metabolic decompensation is further exacerbated by poor nutritional intake. It is imperative that during these times, adequate calories and fluids be given to prevent the crisis from escalating into a medical emergency.

In selected instances, a molecular diagnosis of MSUD may be undertaken; such a diagnosis is especially useful in targeted populations such as the Mennonites. Rarely, patients may have a defect in the $E_2$ component (Danner et al, 1985) or, as discussed in the Primary Lactic Acidosis section, in the $E_3$ component.

## Hereditary Tyrosinemia Type 1

### Fumarylacetoacetate Hydrolase (FAH) Deficiency

Fumarylacetoacetate $\xrightarrow{\text{FAH}}$ Fumarate + Acetoacetate

- Enzyme: homodimer
- Gene location: chromosome 15q23-q25
- Frequency: very rare, except in French-Canadians in Quebec

Tyrosinemia type 1 is due to a deficiency of the enzyme fumarylacetoacetate hydrolase (FAH) (Lindblad et al, 1977; Mitchell et al, 1995). This enzymatic reaction is distal in the phenylalanine and tyrosine pathway, and the disorder is actually an inborn error of organic acid metabolism, with hypertyrosinemia being a secondary and variable biochemical effect. Tyrosinemia type 1 is a rare disease inherited in an autosomal recessive manner. The highest incidence is found in those of French-Canadian ancestry as a result of a founder effect (De Bracketeer and Larochelle, 1990).

Two clinical phenotypes may be detected. The first occurs in early infancy and is a severe, usually fatal disease in which liver disease dominates the clinical picture. The second is a more chronic phenotype, and patients present with hypophosphatemic rickets related to renal Fanconi syndrome. These patients usually also have evidence of liver disease, albeit milder. Most of the patients with the severe liver disease phenotype do not come to clinical attention in the newborn period. Careful search, however, may reveal the laboratory findings compatible with this disease even in newborn infants (Hostetter et al, 1983). When the disease does manifest in the newborn period, the abnormalities are related to liver disease. Like hereditary fructose intolerance and hereditary galactosemia, tyrosinemia type 1 is one of the inborn errors of metabolism in which hepatocellular disease is also associated with renal Fanconi syndrome. In the phenotype seen in early infancy, the clinical findings are hepatomegaly, bleeding from coagulation defects, and jaundice. Ascites is not uncommon. The laboratory findings consist of abnormal liver function tests with increases in serum AST, ALT, and direct and indirect bilirubin; prolongations of PT and PTT; and the findings related to renal Fanconi syndrome, such as glycosuria, hypophosphatemia, hypouricemia, proteinuria due to $\beta_2$-microglobulin hyperexcretion, and generalized amino aciduria and organic aciduria.

More specific laboratory abnormalities consist of an increase in serum alpha-fetoprotein levels. In fact, levels of this protein may be elevated even in cord blood (Hostetter et al, 1983). There may be an elevation of plasma tyrosine. However, the hypertyrosinemia is due to a secondary impairment in the function of the liver enzyme, *p*-hydroxyphenylpyruvic acid oxidase, and is not seen in all patients at all times. This statement also is true for the hypermethioninemia. Some patients may have only hypertyrosinemia or only hypermethioninemia. The most important metabolites are those related to the substrate, fumarylacetylacetic acid, the handling of which is defective. Increased levels of the diagnostic metabolite succinylacetone can be detected on urine organic acid quantitation by gas chromatography–mass spectrometry (GC-MS) and in RBCs by the δ-aminolevulinic acid dehydratase inhibition assay. One must be careful about the interpretation of these test results. We have encountered patients who, because of the severity of their illness and poor dietary intake or because they were receiving intravenous fluids, had elevations of neither methionine nor tyrosine in plasma and only minute amounts of succinylacetone detectable in urine or RBCs. In any infant with severe liver disease and renal Fanconi syndrome that is not obviously due to other causes, I suggest that succinylacetone, FAH activity, or both be measured in RBCs, even if the urinary succinylacetone metabolites cannot be detected by GS-MS.

In the past, most of the infants with the hepatic form of tyrosinemia type 1 died in early to late infancy. It is now recommended that patients with this disease receive a liver transplantation. However, a medical therapy has been developed that uses the agent 2-(2-nitro-4-trifluoromethylbenzoyl)-1,3-cyclohexanedione (NTBC), which inhibits *p*-hydroxyphenylpyruvate dioxygenase (Lindstedt et al, 1992), thus blocking the conversion of *p*-hydroxyphenylpyruvate, the transamination product of tyrosine, to fumarylacetoacetate and thereby retarding the synthesis and accumulation of succinylacetate and succinylacetone. This therapy has been used successfully to improve liver and renal function as well as to normalize or improve the various laboratory abnormalities. It is unclear, however, whether NTBC therapy will eliminate the need for liver transplantation.

One of the most devastating complications for older infants with tyrosinemia type 1 who have become stabilized is the development of hepatocellular carcinoma. This complication is quite prevalent in tyrosinemia, and most patients who survive infancy or who have a chronic phenotype succumb to the liver disease. Unfortunately, several older infants who underwent successful liver transplantation had pulmonary metastases from liver cancer at the time of the transplant and did not survive. It is recommended that NTBC therapy be started in infants who are acutely ill while they are waiting for a liver transplantation. Tyrosinemia type 1 has no effect on the CNS in this disease other than as a secondary complication of the severe liver disease. So far, most of the liver transplantations have been successful, and the patients have done well on immunosuppressive therapy with only minimal persistent evidence of renal tubular dysfunction while eating a normal diet.

This entity is not to be confused with *transient tyrosinemia of the newborn*, which is prevalent in premature infants and is probably the most common disturbance of amino acid metabolism in humans, secondary to a delayed maturation of *p*-hydroxyphenylpyruvate dioxygenase activity (Levine et al, 1939; Mitchell et al, 1995) or with the *hypertyrosinemia* secondary to liver disease, per se (David et al, 1970).

## Nonketotic Hyperglycinemia

### Glycine Cleavage Complex (GCC) Deficiency

$$\text{Glycine} + \text{Tetrahydrofolate} \xrightarrow{\text{GCC}} CO_2 + NH_3 + \text{Methylenetetrahydrofolate}$$

- Enzyme complex: 4 subunits:
  - 1 pyridoxal-phosphate–dependent glycine decarboxylase P protein
  - 1 lipoate-containing hydrogen carrier H protein
  - 1 tetrahydrofolate-dependent T protein
  - 1 lipoamide dehydrogenase L protein
- P protein gene location: chromosome 9p13
- Frequency: 1 in 250,000; except 1 in 12,000 for P protein gene mutation in Finns

Nonketotic hyperglycinemia (NKH) is a rare defect of glycine metabolism (Gerritsen et al, 1965; Hamosh et al, 1995; Tada and Hayasaka, 1987). Inherited as an autosomal recessive trait, the disorder is due to deficient activity of the glycine cleavage enzyme complex (GCC). Its frequency is fewer than 1 in 200,000 newborn infants. Although several variant forms exist, most infants who come to clinical attention in the newborn period—presumably most patients with this disease—have a severe, catastrophic type of disease that mimics the most acute forms of ammonia, amino acids, or organic acid metabolism. The infants are usually well at birth but begin to manifest hypotonia and seizures after 12 to 36 hours. They quickly become comatose, and there is a loss of all the newborn reflexes as well as the deep tendon reflexes.

The clinical findings relate predominantly to those associated with CNS intoxication. The electroencephalogram (EEG) usually shows a characteristic pattern of spike and slow waves. The babies may manifest hiccups due to diaphragmatic spasms. The main laboratory finding is a massive elevation of plasma glycine. The urine glycine is usually also elevated. The cerebrospinal fluid (CSF) glycine value is elevated and out of proportion to the elevation in blood. A fraction of patients with an atypical biochemical form of NKH have elevated levels of glycine only in CSF. The amino acid serine, which is also a product of the defective enzyme reaction, is depressed in plasma, and there is a corresponding increase in the glycine-to-serine ratio in body fluids. Prenatal CNS lesions have been reported (Dobyns, 1989).

The pathophysiology of this brain disease is not well understood; it is believed that glycine may interfere with the activity of specific chloride channels, thus perturbing the membrane potential and depolarization of neurons. There also appears to be an impairment in alpha-motor neuron outflow tract activity, producing a clinical state that mimics Werdnig-Hoffmann disease. Uncommonly, the plasma ammonium value may be elevated. However, no acidosis or ketosis is seen in this disease—thus the name, *nonketotic hyperglycinemia*. Many of the disorders of organic acid metabolism, such as methylmalonic acidemia and propionic acidemia, are also associated with elevations of plasma glycine, presumably due to a secondary impairment in the GCC, and have been referred to in the past as the *ketotic hyperglycinemia syndromes*.

Although many therapies have been tried in this disease, such as protein restriction, benzoate to trap glycine as the byproduct hippurate, strychnine to affect the lower motor neuron function, and dextromethorphan to block *N*-methyl-D-aspartate (NMDA) receptors, there is no effective therapy. Most affected babies die in the newborn period despite medical support with assisted ventilation. A transient form of NKH has also been reported in newborns (Luder et al, 1989; Schiffman et al, 1989). Valproate may result in hyperglycinemia due to secondary inhibition of the GCC, as is postulated to explain secondary hyperglycinemia in the disorders of organic acid metabolism, such as propionic acidemia.

## Methionine Synthetase Deficiency

In humans, the essential amino acid methionine is converted to homocysteine, and in the process, a methyl group is transferred to an acceptor molecule from *S*-adenosylmethionine that serves as a donor for methyl groups in many different reactions (see Fig. 22–4) (Mudd et al, 1995). Subsequently, the homocysteine may either be completely metabolized through the cysteine pathway to sulfate or it may be remethylated back to methionine. Defective methionine remethylation or a deficiency in methionine synthetase leads to an uncommon remethylation form of homocystinuria. Patients with classic homocystinuria, due to a deficiency of the cystathionine beta-synthase enzyme, rarely manifest signs in early infancy (Mudd et al, 1995). In contrast, patients with methionine synthetase deficiency or methionine remethylation defect may come to clinical attention in the newborn period (Fenton and Rosenberg, 1995b). The patients may have either an abnormality in vitamin $B_{12}$ metabolism, which may also produce methylmalonic acidemia as well as homocystinuria, or an isolated defect in folate metabolism or the methionine synthetase enzyme (Rosenblatt, 1995). In this reaction, the methyl group from 5-methyltetrahydrofolate, which is derived from 5,10-methylene tetrahydrofolate, is transferred to methylcobalamin and subsequently to homocysteine.

The clinical findings associated with methionine synthetase deficiency are poor growth and development. There may be severe cortical atrophy and possible brain lesions due to thromboses of the arteries or veins, as in classic homocystinuria. The laboratory findings consist of an elevation in plasma homocysteine values and a normal or decreased methionine value. Often the homocysteine values are not as elevated as in classic cystathionine β-synthetase deficiency. If there is a defect in folate or vitamin $B_{12}$ metabolism that produces secondary impairment in methionine and synthetase activity, there may also be megaloblastic anemia.

Some patients with a defect in cobalamin metabolism may show response to megadose therapy with hydroxycobalamin. The treatment of the methionine synthetase deficiency is methionine supplementation to restore methionine levels in plasma to normal and to restore CNS pools of methionine, which may be critical in one carbon transfer reaction within the CNS. One can also retard homocysteine accumulation as well as restore methionine levels by administering betaine, which can enhance remethylation of homocysteine to methionine through the alternate betaine methyltransferase pathway. Some investigators have also used pharmacologic doses of cobalamin, folate, and pyridoxine to stimulate flux either through the methionine synthetase or the classic homocysteine pathway. Unfortunately, if infants with this type of disorder are not treated early, there is usually a permanent and devastating effect on cognitive and motor function.

## Phenylketonuria

### Phenylalanine Hydroxylase (PAH) Deficiency

$$\text{Phenylalanine} + O_2 + \text{Tetrahydrobiopterin} \xrightarrow{\text{PAH}} \text{Tyrosine} + \text{Biopterin} + H_2O$$

- Enzyme: multimer; identical subunits
- Gene location: chromosome 12q22-q24.1
- Frequency: 1 in 10,000

**CASE STUDY 4**

The patient was an 8 lb, 1 oz boy born after a full-term, uncomplicated gestation. Apgar scores were 8 at both 1 minute and 5 minutes. The newborn period passed without difficulty. He demonstrated bronchiolitis at 5 months of age. During the hospitalization for this event, no neurologic abnormalities were detected on physical examination. His parents reported that he walked at $1^1/_2$ years of age.

At 4 years of age, the patient was referred for neurologic evaluation because of lack of speech development. A behavioral problem was evident: He was noted to be hyperactive. In addition, he was not toilet trained, was unable to feed or undress himself, related poorly to other people, and occasionally engaged in rocking and head banging. Physical examination found a plantar extension response in the right toe. An EEG showed discharges consistent with seizure activity, and he was started on phenytoin.

At 6 years of age, because this blonde, blue-eyed boy with eczema of the palms had a chronic, nonprogressive encephalopathy manifested as severe mental retardation and idiopathic seizure disorder, a plasma sample was submitted for amino acid column chromatography analysis. The plasma phenylalanine level was 23 mg/dL (normal is 0.4 to 1.6 mg/mL). Result of a urinary ferric chloride test was positive for phenylketonuric derivatives despite the absence of a musty or mousy odor. Further research into the neonatal history showed that the original newborn filter-paper screen for PKU had been omitted.

---

PKU is the most common inborn error of amino acid metabolism that can result in mental retardation (Scriver et al, 1995). It is due to a defect in the activity of the enzyme phenylalanine hydroxylase (PAH), which converts phenylalanine to tyrosine, a reaction that resides primarily in the liver. Thus, in PKU, it is the deficiency of this liver enzyme that results in brain disease. Because of the paucity of findings in the newborn period or even early infancy, PKU usually went undiagnosed before newborn screening was instituted. As discussed in Chapter 27, newborn screening has enabled us to routinely prevent mental retardation from PKU. It is important for physicians caring for newborns to be aware of the pitfalls of screening that are summarized in Chapter 27. This disease, inherited as an autosomal recessive trait, has an overall frequency of about 1 in 12,000 newborns. It exemplifies the interaction of a gene and the manipulatable environment (i.e., diet) in the expression of a disease (Scriver and Clow, 1980a, 1980b).

The preceding case study illustrates that patients may easily escape detection even during childhood. After birth, the baby with PKU who is ingesting adequate amounts of breast milk or a proprietary formula will experience a gradual and persistent increase in plasma phenylalanine levels. The cutoff value for newborn screening results in most states is 4 mg/dL, with the upper range of normal being approximately 2 mg/dL. In the first 24 hours after birth, the plasma phenylalanine value in most infants with PKU readily exceeds the 4 mg/dL cutoff, but by the end of the first week of life, it is usually between 20 and 40 mg/dL. At that time, the derivatives of phenylalanine, the so-called phenylketonuric compounds, are excreted in urine in excess, and the greater excretion of phenylpyruvic acid gives rise to the positive ferric chloride test result, in which the urine turns green. The odor in PKU is due to increased production of the derivative phenylacetic acid, which has a musty or mousy odor. This odor may be detected when the levels of phenylalanine exceed 10 to 15 mg/dL, but it is not detected in every patient.

In the first 6 months of life, the affected babies may have difficulties with feeding and vomiting. In some instances, the persistent vomiting has been associated with the diagnosis of pyloric stenosis, for which corrective surgery has been performed, perhaps inappropriately. Developmental delay is usually evident in the second 6 months of life. Patients may have seizures, sometimes infantile spasms in early infancy associated with a hypsarrhythmic EEG pattern. Persistent elevation of plasma phenylalanine levels above 10 mg/dL is sufficient to result in mental retardation.

The mechanism of brain disease in PKU is still unknown. It may be related to the effect of high phenylalanine levels on transport of amino acids across the blood-brain barrier and then into brain neurons or glial elements. The plasma levels of tyrosine may be decreased, especially in those patients not receiving tyrosine supplementation in the special amino acid powder used as a daily nutrient. For many years investigators have speculated that hypotyrosinemia may also play a role in the CNS deficits because tyrosine (only a liver enzyme) cannot be synthesized within the CNS by PAH. Older infants often exhibit long tract findings, such as spastic quadriparesis and spastic quadriplegia. The untreated infant demonstrates postnatally acquired microcephaly and may also have severe behavioral problems. Average findings consist of elevated serum plasma phenylalanine levels, normal or subnormal plasma tyrosine levels, and increased urinary excretion of phenylpyruvic acid, phenyllactic acid, and phenylacetic acid.

The mainstay of therapy is a low-protein diet and the use of a special amino acid-containing formula that does not include phenylalanine. The patients must receive an adequate amount of phenylalanine from the protein in proprietary formulas and later from table foods, which is tracked by means of a phenylalanine exchange system, to allow for the normal daily utilization of phenylalanine for protein synthesis while maintaining plasma phenylalanine levels in a range as close as possible to normal. Deviations from normal plasma levels are believed to be associated with chronic, perhaps even acute, effects on CNS function and testing performance. Thus, the diet should be one for life. The phenylalanine hydroxylase gene has been cloned and sequenced, and the mutations that are responsible for most abnormalities in humans are known. DNA sequencing and mutational analysis may be used to identify carriers in families and to provide a scientific rationale during family counseling.

Some rare patients with hyperphenylalaninemia have a most severe disease not because of the deficiency of the phenylalanine hydroxylase apoenzyme but rather because of deficiency of the active cofactor of this enzyme, tetrahydrobiopterin. Several defects in the metabolism of biopterin can produce this type of hyperphenylalaninemia. Patients with these uncommon types of PKU usually come to attention in the newborn period because of severe seizure activity. Patients with the biopterin deficiency can have evidence of severe brain damage despite treatment with a low-phenylalanine diet. This may be related to deficiencies of other neurotransmitters whose synthesis also depends on adequate levels of tetrahydrobiopterin. These various other defects, such as the dihydropteridine reductase, 6-pyruvoyl tetrahydropterin synthetase, and the guanosine triphosphate cyclohydrolase deficiencies, can be ascertained by urinary measurements of neopterin and biopterin in urine.

## INBORN ERRORS OF ORGANIC ACID METABOLISM

Defects in the catabolism of the BCAAs are responsible for most of the disorders of organic acid metabolism (Fig. 22–5). Typical examples are methylmalonic, propionic,

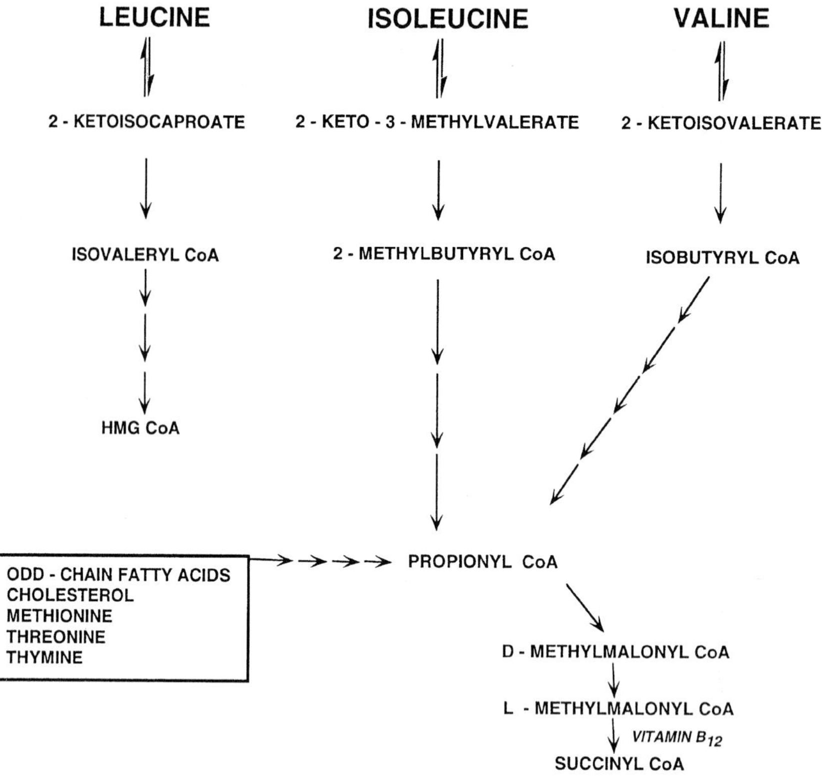


**FIGURE 22–5.** The branched-chain amino acids leucine, isoleucine, and valine are reversibly transaminated to their corresponding 2-keto analogues, which are the substrates for the single decarboxylase (branched-chain 2-keto dehydrogenase) ([BCKAD]) enzyme deficient in maple syrup urine disease. Reduced activity of isovaleryl coenzyme A (CoA) dehydrogenase, the next enzyme in the leucine degradative pathway, is the cause of isovaleric acidemia. The immediate precursor of ketones, 3-hydroxy-3-methylglutaryl CoA (HMG-CoA), is the final product of the leucine catabolic pathway. However, its production more strongly depends on oxidation of fatty acids as in ketogenesis and in cholesterol biosynthesis. Propionyl CoA, which accumulates in both propionic and methylmalonic acidemia, may be synthesized from isoleucine, valine, odd-chain fatty acids, cholesterol, methionine, threonine, and thymine. The adenosyl form of vitamin $B_{12}$ is the important cofactor in the L-methylmalonyl CoA mutase–catalyzed conversion of L-methylmalonyl CoA to the citric acid cycle intermediate, succinyl CoA.

and isovaleric acidemias. An organic acid is any organic compound that contains a carboxy functional group but no α-amino group as in an amino acid. In this section, we consider the disorders of fatty acid oxidation, ketone body metabolism, and lactic acid metabolism as well as the more classic inherited defects in organic acid metabolism. What is true for all these disorders is that the ability to establish a diagnosis depends primarily on the suspicion of the clinician caring for the sick infant. Most of the disorders also require sophisticated testing such as GC-MS to identify the specific organic compound responsible for the toxic syndrome. As discussed earlier, acidosis and encephalopathy are usually the hallmarks of these syndromes when they manifest in the newborn period.

## Methylmalonic Acidemia

### L-Methylmalonyl-CoA Mutase (MCM) Deficiency

$$\text{L-Methylmalonyl CoA} \xrightarrow[\text{adenosylcobalamin}]{\text{MCM}} \text{Succinyl-CoA}$$

- Enzyme: homodimer
- Gene location: chromosome 6p12-p21.2
- Frequency: 1 in 20,000

**CASE STUDY 5**

A 2954-g boy was the product of an uncomplicated pregnancy and delivery. He was breast-feeding at discharge, but on day 4 he began to feed less and sleep more. On day 5, the parents noted him to be unarousable at times and to be breathing fast. He was brought to the local hospital, where he was found to be obtunded and severely tachypneic. A sepsis work-up was performed, and antibiotics were administered. A serum total $CO_2$ value was 6 mEq/L. The urine ketone test result was strongly positive. The arterial blood pH was 7.15, the $P_{CO_2}$ 40 mm Hg, and the $P_{O_2}$ 62 mm Hg. Because of impending respiratory failure, the patient was intubated and started on mechanical ventilation.

Despite the use of intravenous fluids with glucose and sodium bicarbonate, he remained comatose. By day 8, his pupils were not reactive to light and he was unresponsive to painful stimuli. A plasma $NH_4^+$ level was 2059 μM. By this time, the results of the newborn screen performed on day 2 using the technology of tandem mass spectrometry on filter paper cards revealed elevated levels of propionylcarnitine in blood. Subsequently, GC-MS analysis of urine revealed a massive increase in methylmalonic acid along with the other metabolites such as 3-hydroxypropionate, propionylglycine, and methylcitrate, confirming the diagnosis of methylmalonic acidemia. Because of the terminal neurologic condition, dialysis therapy was not instituted and life support was withdrawn; the baby died on day 9.

Methylmalonic acidemia, along with propionic acidemia, is the most common of the disorders of organic acid metabolism (Fenton and Rosenberg, 1995a, 1995b). Although more than one enzyme defect may result in methylmalonic acidemia, all are inherited as autosomal recessive traits. The enzyme that is most often deficient is L-methylmalonyl-CoA mutase (see Fig. 22–5). This enzyme is present in mitochondria, and it depends on adenosyl-cobalamin for activity. Impaired function may result from either a mutation of the L-methylmalonyl-CoA mutase apoenzyme or deficient availability of the adenosyl form of vitamin $B_{12}$. The latter may result from impaired cellular metabolism of vitamin $B_{12}$, including defective activity of the enzyme adenosylcobalamin synthetase.

Some patients, but not usually newborn infants with methylmalonic acidemia, are responsive to pharmacologic therapy with vitamin $B_{12}$. Methylmalonic acidemia, therefore, is one of the important disorders that can be considered a vitamin-responsive inborn error of metabolism. Because of the deficient activity of L-methylmalonyl-CoA mutase, the substrate L-methylmalonyl CoA accumulates in mitochondria and is subsequently hydrolyzed to methylmalonic acid. Methylmalonic acid is capable of diffusing out of cells in which it is being produced, so it may be detected in excess in the blood, CSF, and urine of patients with these various forms of the disease. The precursors of L-methylmalonyl CoA are the BCAAs isoleucine and valine, as well as methionine, threonine, thymine, and odd-chain fatty acids (see Fig. 22–5).

There are many different phenotypes of methylmalonic acidemia. They range from severe, catastrophic newborn-onset disease in the first week of life to an almost benign form that has been detected in adults with partial L-methylmalonyl-CoA mutase deficiency. The phenotypes are the newborn-onset type, the intermediate variety with onset in early and late infancy, the intermittent form with onset usually in late infancy and childhood, and an adult or benign phenotype.

Most patients who present in the newborn period have a severe phenotype. In some of the patients who present in the first week of life with catastrophic illness, even dialysis therapy is not effective, possibly because of a delay in diagnosis and treatment. The most striking presentation is in the second or third day of life. The baby is usually well at birth, as in the UCEDs, but then gradually begins to manifest problems with feeding, vomiting, lethargy, and perhaps seizures. There may be respiratory distress as a manifestation of metabolic acidosis. The liver may be enlarged as a consequence of diffuse steatosis. The important laboratory findings include a metabolic acidosis usually associated with an increased anion gap, ketosis, and hyperammonemia. The elevation of plasma ammonium may be as high as in the severe newborn-onset hyperammonemic syndromes. Because ketonuria is relatively uncommon in newborn infants, even in stressed infants with hypoglycemia due to poor feeding, and because diabetes mellitus is so uncommon in the newborn period, the physician caring for newborn infants must always consider an inborn error of organic acid metabolism when confronted with an acutely ill baby with ketosis. Other laboratory findings are thrombocytopenia, leukopenia, and anemia due to effects of the metabolite on the hematopoietic elements in bone marrow. Older patients with methylmalonic acidemia during crisis have suffered acute pancreatitis as well as devastating lesions to the basal ganglia. Plasma amino acid analysis may reveal elevations of several amino acids such as glycine and alanine. Secondary carnitine deficiency with elevations of carnitine esters is expected (Chalmers et al, 1984). Methylmalonic acid may be detected in urine with GC-MS.

The diagnosis can be confirmed with an assay of the activity of L-methylmalonyl-CoA mutase enzyme in cultured skin fibroblasts. In addition, the various other disturbances in vitamin $B_{12}$ metabolism can also be studied by analyzing skin fibroblasts in culture. The treatment of acute disease consists of protein restriction, empirical therapy with vitamin $B_{12}$ (1 mg IM per day), intravenous fluids with 10% glucose and sodium bicarbonate to correct dehydration, electrolyte imbalance and acidosis, high-calorie feeds via a nasogastric tube, and, often, dialysis. The use of carnitine, 25 to 200 mg/kg/day intravenously or orally, is controversial. The treatment of the chronic state centers on the judicious use of a low-protein diet and administration of alkali to eliminate any acid-base imbalance.

## Propionic Acidemia

### Propionyl CoA Carboxylase (PCC) Deficiency

$$\text{Propionyl CoA} + \text{ATP} + \text{HCO}_3 \xrightarrow[\text{biotin}]{\text{PCC}} \text{D-Methylmalonyl CoA} + \text{AMP} + \text{Pyrophosphate}$$

- Enzyme: 6 $\alpha$ subunits and 6 $\beta$ subunits
- Gene locations: $\alpha$ subunits, chromosome 13q32; $\beta$ subunits, chromosome 3q13.3-q22
- Frequency: rare

Propionic acidemia was the first classic defect in organic acid metabolism to be described in humans (Fenton and Rosenberg, 1995a). The first patient, described by Childs and colleagues in 1961, was sick on the first day of life with severe metabolic acidosis and ketosis. He responded to massive alkali therapy and survived the newborn period. He subsequently suffered multiple episodes of recurrent attacks of metabolic decompensation with ketoacidosis usually precipitated by infections or protein ingestion; he also had developmental delay, a seizure disorder, and episodic neutropenia and thrombocytopenia. He died at age 7. His sister also demonstrated ketosis and metabolic acidosis in the first week of life, but because of better control of her disease, there were few severe episodes of decompensation in the first and second decades of life.

Propionic acidemia, due to a selective deficiency of propionyl-CoA carboxylase, is inherited as an autosomal recessive trait. This disorder was originally called *ketotic hyperglycinemia* because of the elevations of plasma glycine in conjunction with ketosis. The precursors of propionyl CoA include the amino acids isoleucine, and valine plus methionine, threonine, the pyrimidine compound, thymine, and odd-chain fatty acids (see Fig. 22–5). Of the several hundred patients described with this disease, most present in the newborn period with poor feeding, vomiting, lethargy, and hypotonia. Not uncommonly, the patients manifest seizures and hepatomegaly due to steatosis. The metabolic acidosis may be severe with or without an increase in the anion gap. Ketosis is usually but not always present. Please refer to the case report in Chapter 21. Patients who survive may often manifest choreoathetosis because of persistent damage to the basal ganglia. Usually, episodes of metabolic decompensation characterized by acidosis and ketosis can be precipitated by excessive protein intake or infection. Such episodes may result in permanent neurologic damage. Subsequent findings therefore include developmental delay, seizures, cerebral atrophy, and EEG abnormalities. During the acute attacks, leukopenia, thrombocytopenia, and, less rarely, anemia, probably due to suppression of maturation of bone marrow hematopoietic precursors, may occur.

The diagnosis may be confirmed by GC-MS analysis of urine in an organic acid quantitation. The urine has excess concentrations of various propionate metabolites, such as methylcitrate, propionylglycine, 2-methyl-3-hydroxybutyrate, 2-methylacetoacetate, as well as several other, rarer compounds. The plasma glycine value may be elevated, and during acute attacks, the plasma ammonium value is frequently increased. The enzyme activity of propionyl-CoA carboxylase may be assayed in white blood cells (WBCs) or extracts of cultured skin fibroblasts for definitive diagnosis. Several mutations have been identified in the genes that encode the two nonidentical subunits ($\alpha$ and $\beta$) of the propionyl-CoA carboxylase enzyme.

Therapy consists of a low-protein diet and adequate calories. As in L-methylmalonyl, there is secondary carnitine deficiency with elevations of propionylcarnitine. The use of L-carnitine to relieve a deficiency of free carnitine and promote greater urinary excretion of propionylcarnitine to lower mitochondrial propionyl CoA levels is controversial. This therapy has never been shown to result unequivocally in an improvement in the clinical state. Because gut bacteria can also contribute to propionate production, antimicrobial therapy with metronidazole has been used during an acute attack. In the acutely ill newborn, the immediate treatment consists of elimination of protein administration or total parenteral nutrition; administration of an adequate amount of calories (10% glucose intravenously and/or administration of a nonprotein formula, such as Mead-Johnson 80056 or Ross Prophree products, via nasogastric tube infusion); administration of alkali to eliminate metabolic acidosis; and platelet transfusion if warranted by thrombocytopenia. Often, because of the severe acidosis and coma, patients may need dialysis therapy. It is unclear whether administration of sodium benzoate and sodium phenylacetate, as in the treatment of hyperammonemia associated with UCEDs, is of benefit to the patient with secondary hyperammonemia. Several patients with propionic acidemia have undergone liver transplantation, with mixed success. Most of the patients with severe newborn-onset disease do not survive the first decade of life.

## Isovaleric Acidemia

### Isovaleryl-CoA Dehydrogenase (IVCD) Deficiency

$$\text{Isovaleryl CoA} \xrightarrow{\text{IVCD}} \text{3-Methylcrotonyl CoA}$$

- Enzyme: homotetramer
- Gene location: chromosome 15q14-q15
- Frequency: very rare

Isovaleric acidemia is caused by a selective deficiency of the enzyme isovaleryl-CoA dehydrogenase (Budd et al, 1967; Sweetman and Williams, 1995; Tanaka et al, 1966). It is inherited as an autosomal recessive trait. There are two major phenotypes; an acute form manifests as catastrophic disease in the newborn period, and the late-onset type is characterized by chronic, intermittent episodes of metabolic decompensation. In the acute form, the infants become extremely sick in the first week of life. There is usually a history of poor feeding, vomiting, lethargy, and, often, seizures. The characteristic sweaty feet or rancid cheese odor due to isovaleric acid (IVA) is noted. Metabolic acidosis, usually with an elevated anion gap and ketosis, is present. There may be secondary hyperammonemia, thrombocytopenia, neutropenia, and sometimes anemia, resulting in pancytopenia. The babies usually lapse into a coma. Dialysis therapy may be necessary. As with other organic acid disorders for which an amino acid determines organic acid production (see Fig. 22–5), treatment also consists of protein or total parenteral nutrition restriction, intravenous fluids with glucose and perhaps sodium bicarbonate, protein-free formula with calories via nasogastric tube, and glycine, 250 mg/kg/day (Cohn et al, 1978). Intravenous L-carnitine may be beneficial.

In the chronic, intermittent form of isovaleric acidemia, the patients have repeated episodes of metabolic decompensation precipitated by infections or protein intake. Some of these episodes may mimic Reye syndrome. The same principles are applied to therapy for acute metabolic decompensation beyond the newborn period; they are no protein content, sufficient calories, and administration of alkali to correct acidosis, glycine (Krieger and Tanaka, 1976; Naglak et al, 1988; Velazquez and Prieto, 1980), and L-carnitine (De Sousa et al, 1986; Roe et al, 1984). The mainstay of long-term therapy is a low-protein diet. Patients may benefit from the long-term administration of glycine (Berry et al, 1988), which enhances the production of the nontoxic compound isovalerylglycine and serves to reduce the free levels of IVA in body fluids (Krieger and Tanaka, 1976; Yudkoff et al, 1978). In addition, carnitine administration may augment the excretion of isovalerylcarnitine (Berry et al, 1988; Mayatepek et al, 1991); the benefit of carnitine treatment in the chronic state, however, remains unknown.

Most patients with the late-onset type of isovaleric acidemia are mentally retarded. In contrast, most of the patients with the acute phenotype are not severely retarded, but most have not survived the newborn period, attesting to the severely toxic nature of this organic acid disorder in the newborn period. The diagnosis may be made from measurement of marked elevations of isovalerylglycine in urine. There is usually also increased excretion of 3-hydroxyisovaleric acid. The enzyme isovaleryl-CoA dehydrogenase can be assayed in extracts of cultured skin fibroblasts. The gene has been identified and assigned to human chromosome 15. Various mutations have been described.

## Multiple Carboxylase Deficiency

There are two specific forms of multiple carboxylase deficiency, holocarboxylase synthetase deficiency and biotinidase deficiency (Wolf, 1995). All the carboxylase enzymes, such as propionyl-CoA carboxylase, pyruvate carboxylase, 3-methylcrotonyl-CoA carboxylase, and acetyl-CoA carboxylase, require covalent linkage with biotin for normal activity. In form, holocarboxylase synthetase deficiency, the enzyme that accomplishes the addition of biotin to these various carboxylases is deficient. In the second form of the disorder, the absence of the enzyme biotinidase does not allow for biotin recycling after a carboxylase enzyme is degraded and hydrolyzed. The biotinidase deficiency does not usually manifest in the newborn period.

Patients with the holocarboxylase synthetase deficiency, however, have a severe disease and characteristically are catastrophically ill in the newborn period. Few cases have been reported (Michalski et al, 1989). Patients have severe metabolic acidosis with lactic acidosis and are in coma. As with the biotinidase deficiency, administration of biotin is life-saving. Holocarboxylase synthetase deficiency is one of the few disorders of organic acid metabolism for which the administration of a vitamin in megadoses produces a dramatic turnabout in the clinical and laboratory findings. Diagnosis depends on GC-MS analysis of urine and the demonstration of markedly increased levels of lactate, 3-methylcrotonylglycine, and propionate metabolites. In most patients the affinity of the holocarboxylase synthetase enzyme for biotin is diminished, and for the biochemical disturbances to normalize or improve, patients need between 10 and 60 mg of biotin daily. The enzyme deficiency may be confirmed in cultured skin fibroblasts. The disorder is inherited as an autosomal recessive trait. There are also rare cases of isolated 3-methylcrotonyl-CoA carboxylase deficiency; these patients usually do not come to clinical attention until after early infancy. Of great interest, however, is our new understanding that previously asymptomatic women have demonstrated "acute fatty liver of pregnancy" syndrome. Recurrent episodes of this potentially lethal syndrome have now also been reported in heterozygous mothers who were carrying infants with fatty acid oxidation defects (Schoeman et al, 1991).

## Glutaric Acidemia Type 1

### Glutaryl-CoA Dehydrogenase (GCDH) Deficiency

$$\text{Glutaryl-CoA} + \text{Flavin adenine dinucleotide (FAD)} \xrightarrow{\text{GDCH}} \text{Crotonyl CoA} + CO_2 + FADH_2$$

- Enzyme: homotetramer
- Gene location: chromosome 19p13.2
- Frequency: very rare, except in Saulteaux-Ojibway Canadian Indians and Pennsylvania Old-Order Amish

An isolated deficiency of glutaryl-CoA dehydrogenase (GCDH) causes glutaric acidemia type 1 (GA-1) (Goodman and Frerman, 1995; Goodman et al, 1975). Multiple phenotypes are known. In the most dramatic presentation, which accounts for less than half of the known patients with GA-1, the illness develops acutely in the first year of life, usually after an infection. Acute encephalopathy is followed by the development of what appears to be a severe form of extrapyramidal cerebral palsy (Hoffmann et al, 1991). In essence, the affected infants have incurred bilateral damage to the caudate and putamen in the basal ganglia, resulting in an incapacitating dystonic syndrome. Some patients have a slowly progressive course with developmental delay, hypotonia, dystonia, and dyskinesia in the first couple years of life. Other patients are relatively asymptomatic.

In general, GA-1 is not a disorder that is associated with acute disease in the newborn period. However, macrocephaly at birth is common (Iafolla and Kahler, 1989). The etiology of any of the CNS lesions is unknown. Magnetic resonance imaging (MRI) of the head typically shows bilateral widening of the sylvian fissures associated with hypo-opercularization, resulting in the "bat-wing" appearance. Sometimes the fluid accumulation mimics subdural hygromas, and a few patients have actually been noted to have subdural hematomas. The congenital nature of these findings suggests that GA-1 has its onset in utero and affects CNS development. Usually infants do not demonstrate bilateral damage to the basal ganglia in the newborn period. Diagnosis depends on the demonstration of glutaric acid and 3-hydroxyglutaric acid in urine and is confirmed by the demonstration of deficiency of GCDH activity or protein levels on Western analysis in cultured fibroblasts.

A rare disorder, GA-1 is especially common in the Saulteaux-Ojibway Indians in Canada (Greenberg et al, 1993) and in the Old-Order Amish of Lancaster County, Pennsylvania (Morton et al, 1991). A low-protein diet may help in the treatment of these patients; acute illnesses, usually viral in nature, should be treated vigorously with fluids containing glucose and adequate amounts of calories to prevent catabolism. Bicarbonate may be necessary to correct acid-base imbalance. Carnitine has also been used to reduce mitochondrial glutaryl-CoA levels.

## Fatty Acid Oxidation Disorders

### Glutaric Acidemia Type 2

Glutaric acidemia type 2 (GA-2) is due to multiple acyl-CoA dehydrogenase deficiency (Frerman and Goodman, 1995; Przyrembel et al, 1976). The mitochondrial acyl-CoA dehydrogenases are the very-long-chain acyl-CoA dehydrogenase, the medium-chain acyl-CoA dehydrogenase, the short-chain acyl-CoA dehydrogenase (all of which are involved in fatty acid oxidation), isovaleryl-CoA dehydrogenase and 2-methylbutaryl-CoA dehydrogenase (important in BCAA catabolism), glutaryl-CoA dehydrogenase (important in lysine, hydroxylysine, and tryptophan metabolism), and the dimethylglycine and sarcosine dehydrogenases (important in choline degradation). All of these dehydrogenase proteins have in common the binding of a protein called *electron transfer flavoprotein* (ETF). This protein is responsible for accepting the electrons in any of these oxidative dehydrogenation reactions; a deficiency of either ETF or the ETF dehydrogenase enzyme, which is responsible for further transferring the electrons from ETF to coenzyme $Q_{10}$ within the mitochondria, causes GA-2. The three phenotypes of GA-2 are (1) a newborn-onset type with congenital anomalies, (2) a newborn-onset type without anomalies, and (3) a milder or later-onset type, sometimes called *mild acyl-CoA dehydrogenase deficiency* or *ethylmalonic adipic aciduria*.

Patients with GA-2 who have multiple malformations are often premature; severe disease is usually evident in the first week of life (Lehnert et al, 1982). The patients demonstrate hypotonia, encephalopathy, hepatomegaly, hypoglycemia, and metabolic acidosis; often the odor of IVA is present, because these patients also have a defect in metabolism of isovaleryl CoA as in isolated IVA. There may be facial dysmorphism consisting of a high forehead, low-set ears, hypertelorism, and a hypoplastic mid-face. The kidneys may be palpably enlarged associated with large renal cysts (Böhm et al, 1982), rocker-bottom feet, muscular defects of the inferior abdominal wall, and anomalies of the external genitalia, including hypospadias and chordee. Most of the patients with GA-2 and multiple malformations do not survive the first weeks of life. In some, the malformations are not so noticeable, and only renal cysts are identified at autopsy. Infants without the congenital abnormalities usually present in the first 24 to 48 hours of life with hypotonia, tachypnea due to a metabolic acidosis, liver enlargement, hypoglycemia, and the sweaty feet odor. Some of these patients have cardiomyopathy. In contrast, some of these infants can survive the newborn period.

The phenotype in the third form of GA-2 is quite variable. Some patients are relatively disease free and have intermittent episodes of vomiting, dehydration, hypoglycemia, and acidosis during childhood or adult life. In some, there may be hepatomegaly and muscle disease.

Laboratory studies in patients with the newborn-onset type usually show severe metabolic acidosis with lactic acidosis and increased anion gap, mild to moderate hyperammonemia, and hypoglycemia without a moderate or large ketonuria. The liver function values may be abnormal, with increases in the serum transaminases and prolongations of PT and PTT. A chest radiograph may show heart enlargement due to hypertrophic cardiomyopathy. Abdominal ultrasonography or computed tomography (CT) may reveal the renal cysts. The diagnosis is made from the characteristic pattern of organic acid metabolites on urine GC-MS analysis. It consists of glutarate, ethylmalonate, 3-hydroxyisovalerate, 2-hydroxyglutarate, 5-hydroxyhexanoate, adipic, subaric, sebacic, and dodecanedioic acids, isovalerylglycine, isobutyrylglycine, and 2-methylbutyrylglycine. The ketones, acetoacetic acid, and 3-hydroxybutyric acid are usually not present or are only minimally elevated if present, being inappropriate for the degree of fatty acid metabolites that indicate free fatty acid mobilization and the potential for enhanced ketogenesis. The renal cystic disease may also be associated with evidence of impaired renal tubular function. Generalized aminoaciduria may be present. The amino-containing compound sarcosine may be elevated in serum as well as in urine. There may be secondary carnitine deficiency, and abnormal carnitine esters such as isovalerylcarnitine and butyrylcarnitine can be detected in blood. The ETF and ETF dehydrogenase deficiency may be detected through the use of specific antibodies on Western analysis of cultured skin fibroblasts or of functional assays in skin cells.

Prenatal diagnosis can be achieved by demonstration of glutarate in amniotic fluid or from results of dehydrogenase assays in cultured amniocytes. The ETF and the α and β subunits of the ETF dehydrogenase genes have been cloned and sequenced. Several mutations of the α subunit of the ETF dehydrogenase have been described. In the future, in certain families, mutational analysis of DNA from the probands, as well as other family members, may be performed to establish the diagnosis or to perform prenatal testing using chorionic villus samples or cultured amniotic cells. A complete deficiency of the ETF dehydrogenase is often associated with the newborn type of GA-2 with congenital anomalies.

Although treatment with intravenous glucose, riboflavin, carnitine, and diets low in protein and fat generally have not been successful for catastrophically ill newborns, there has been some success in patients with milder or later-onset disease. Riboflavin is suggested to be administered to the newborn with severe disease, but riboflavin at a dosage of 100 to 300 mg/day has been effective in only a few older patients (Gregersen et al, 1982; Harpey et al, 1983). The rationale behind this therapy is that riboflavin, being a precursor of flavin adenine dinucleotide (FAD), may increase the concentrations of FAD and allow for better interaction with mutated and defective ETF or ETF dehydrogenase proteins. Finally, some artificial electron acceptors such as methylene blue have been used in the newborn period without success.

## Very-Long-Chain Acyl-CoA Dehydrogenase, Medium-Chain Acyl-CoA Dehydrogenase, and Short-Chain Acyl-CoA Dehydrogenase Deficiencies

In general, the defects in fatty acid oxidation have been associated with coma, hypoglycemia, liver disease, cardiomyopathy, and skeletal myopathy (Roe and Coates, 1995; Saudubray et al, 1997; Stanley, 1987). All of these defects involve abnormalities in the enzymes that participate in or facilitate the mitochondrial beta oxidation of fatty acids. In general, the pathophysiology associated with these disorders has the potential to put the patient in a life-threatening condition in which there is a state of catabolism and enhanced liberation of free fatty acids by adipose stores.

### *Medium-Chain Acyl-CoA Dehydrogenase Deficiency*

#### Medium-Chain Acyl-CoA Dehydrogenase (MCAD) Deficiency

$$\text{R-CH}_2-\text{CH}_2\text{-}\overset{\overset{\text{O}}{\|}}{\text{C}}\text{-S CoA} + \text{FAD} \xrightarrow{\text{MCAD}} \text{R-CH} = \text{CH-}\overset{\overset{\text{O}}{\|}}{\text{C}}\text{-S CoA} + \text{FADH}_2$$

- Enzyme: homotetramer
- Gene location: chromosome 1p31
- Frequency: approximately 1 in 20,000

The most common of these disorders is the medium-chain acyl-CoA dehydrogenase (MCAD) deficiency (Roe and Coates, 1995). More than 200 patients with this disorder have been described. Most patients do not present until late infancy. The typical patient is an older infant who, after an infection, experiences anorexia, vomiting, dehydration, lethargy, and hypoglycemia that may be associated with seizures. Similarly, older patients have features that mimic those of Reye syndrome and can die because of brain edema. Onset of symptoms in the newborn period is rare. However, some patients in the extended newborn period or in the first 6 months of life were originally believed to have sudden infant death syndrome (Ding et al, 1991; Mowat et al, 1984) but in retrospect turned out to have nonketotic hypoglycemia with coma after the development of fasting associated with an infection.

In MCAD deficiency, the initial episode is associated with a high mortality rate. The laboratory studies usually show hypoglycemia and an absence of moderate to large ketones in urine that would be expected to accompany hypoglycemia. The plasma ammonium values may be mildly elevated, the liver may be enlarged, and the serum ALT and AST levels may be slightly increased. During an acute episode, urine GC-MS analysis of organic acids characteristically shows increased levels of adipic, subaric, and sebacic acids as well as the unsaturated analogues of these medium-chain dicarboxylic acids. Greater urinary excretion of dicarboxylic acids is common in many of the defects of carnitine or fatty acid metabolism. However, this is not pathognomonic of a disorder of fat metabolism, because infants fed medium-chain triglyceride–enriched formulas also manifest dicarboxylic aciduria (Whyte et al, 1986). Fatty acid analysis of plasma from patients with MCAD deficiency demonstrates increased levels of octanoic and 4-decenedioic acids. Urine also contains glycine conjugates such as suberylglycine and hexanoylglycine. A secondary carnitine deficiency can be present, and the acylcarnitines analyzed by tandem MS have higher concentrations of 4-, 5-, 6-, 8-, and 10-carbon monounsaturated acylcarnitine species. The MCAD enzyme may be assayed in cultured skin fibroblasts.

The MCAD gene has been cloned and sequenced, and several mutations have been identified. The most conspicuous one is the *R329E*, a highly prevalent mutation in people of Northern European ancestry. The major treatment is the avoidance of fasting; if an episode occurs with hypoglycemia or encephalopathy, intravenous administration of glucose and calorie support should be instituted quickly. Because of the possibility of the development of brain edema, patients may have to be aggressively treated if obtunded to relieve increased intracranial pressure. Avoidance of free fatty acid mobilization during relative insulin deficiency and catabolic stress and prevention of hypoglycemia are the cornerstones of therapy.

### *Very-Long-Chain Acyl-CoA Dehydrogenase Deficiency*

Most of the patients who were previously diagnosed as having long-chain acyl-CoA dehydrogenase (LCAD) deficiency (Hale et al, 1985; Roe and Coates, 1995) actually had very-long-chain acyl-CoA dehydrogenase (VLCAD) deficiency (Yamaguchi et al, 1993). Patients with this disease may be ill in the newborn period because of liver disease with hypoglycemia, cardiomyopathy, and skeletal myopathy (Treem et al, 1991). The membrane-bound VLCAD, as opposed to the soluble LCAD, whose specific metabolic role is unknown, is the main enzyme for initiating the oxidation of free fatty acids that are derived from adipose stores, such as palmitic, stearic, and oleic acids. The fasting state may include coma. Even in its absence, however, the patients may exhibit hypotonia, hepatomegaly, and cardiomegaly. With an acute metabolic decompensation, urine organic acid analysis may demonstrate dicarboxylic aciduria. However, acylglycine excretion is not usually present. There may be a secondary carnitine deficiency with increased concentrations of the long-chain fatty acids (LCFAs) bound to carnitine.

VLCAD deficiency may be fatal; sudden death in early infancy has been reported. Therapy is directed toward replenishment of glucose, calorie administration, and treatment of any potential brain edema. The myopathy and cardiomyopathy, however, may proceed even in the absence of fasting. Most investigators suggest a reduction in dietary fat intake or supplementation in medium-chain triglyceride. However, it is important not to provoke an essential fatty acid deficiency by too severe dietary fat restriction. Diagnosis can be made through enzyme assay in cultured skin fibroblasts.

### Short-Chain Acyl-CoA Dehydrogenase Deficiency

The short-chain acyl-CoA dehydrogenase (SCAD) deficiency is a rare disorder (Amendt et al, 1987; Roe and Coates, 1995). Only a few patients have been reported. One patient manifested severe newborn-onset disease with feeding problems and vomiting, lethargy, and hypotonia in the first week of life. Laboratory findings indicated metabolic acidosis, hypoglycemia, and moderate hyperammonemia. The organic acid analysis of urine showed increased levels of lactate, ketone bodies, butyrate, ethylmalonate, and adipic acid. The patient died at 6 days of age. Postmortem examination showed brain edema, hepatosplenomegaly with steatosis, cholestasis, and focal hepatocellular necrosis. Other cases, however, suggest a disease associated with neurologic abnormalities with later onset as well as neuromuscular disease in adults. Diagnosis can be made by assaying the SCAD enzyme in cultured skin fibroblasts. The human gene has been cloned and sequenced, and mutations have been described; this development should enable a more rapid genetic diagnosis as well as make prenatal diagnosis feasible.

### Long-Chain 3-Hydroxy Acyl-CoA Dehydrogenase Deficiency

The long-chain 3-hydroxy acyl-CoA dehydrogenase (LCHAD) deficiency is associated with acute illness, fasting-induced hypoketosis, hypoglycemia, cardiomegaly, and muscle weakness (Bertini et al, 1992; Duran et al, 1991; Roe and Coates, 1995). As with LCFA oxidative abnormalities, some older patients may have episodes of illness associated with elevated serum creatine phosphokinase levels and myoglobinuria. A few patients have had sensory motor neuropathy and pigmentary retinopathy (Bertini et al, 1992). Half of the patients have not survived. Some patients may have severe liver disease with fibrosis in addition to necrosis and steatosis. Women who are carriers for this disease may also have acute fatty liver of pregnancy syndrome.

The diagnosis may be suggested by the demonstration of 3-hydroxydicarboxylic acids on urine organic acid analysis. However, some patients with liver disease per se may also manifest 3-hydroxydicarboxylic aciduria. The demonstration of an enzyme deficiency in fibroblasts may be difficult in some patients. The specific LCHAD defect was demonstrated in cultured skin fibroblasts through the use of an antibody directed against its analogous activity associated with the short-chain 3-hydroxy acyl-CoA dehydrogenase. Treatment of this disorder has involved frequent high-carbohydrate feedings, dietary fat restriction, and supplementation with uncooked cornstarch. Administration of medium-chain triglycerides may be helpful. Carnitine and riboflavin have also been tried without benefit. As in the other defects of fatty acid oxidation, the treatment of the acute episode is associated with hypoglycemia and potential brain swelling. Liver and neurologic disease may progress despite any intervention.

### Carnitine Transporter Defect and Deficiencies of Carnitine Palmitoyltransferase I and II and Acylcarnitine Translocase

Carnitine is essential for fatty acid oxidation because transport of LCFAs into mitochondria depends on an adequate amount of carnitine and the presence of two enzymes that covalently link carnitine to the fatty acid or remove the linkage and one transporter that carries it across the inner mitochondrial membrane (Roe and Coates, 1995; Stanley, 1987). These enzymes are carnitine palmitoyltransferase I and II and a carnitine translocase. Cellular levels of carnitine in turn depend on a sodium-dependent carnitine transporter.

Primary carnitine deficiency appears to be primarily associated with the carnitine transporter defect (Treem et al, 1988). Since the first report of the carnitine transporter defect in 1988, more than 25 cases have been reported. However, many other patients previously reported as having cardiomyopathy or Reye syndrome may have had the transporter defect (Waber et al, 1982). Patients with the transporter defect may present in infancy or in childhood. Earliest reports concern the extended newborn period or early infancy. The disease is characterized by hypoketotic hypoglycemia, hyperammonemia, elevations of transaminases, cardiomyopathy, and skeletal muscle weakness. In some of the older patients, cardiomyopathy may be the presenting sign. The characteristic laboratory finding in this disease is extremely low plasma carnitine levels. The total carnitine levels are usually less than 10 μM in plasma. A dicarboxylic aciduria is not usually evident on urine organic acid analysis. This is probably the only disorder in which pharmacologic administration of carnitine has dramatic effects on the clinical and laboratory abnormalities. The treatment is 100 to 400 mg of L-carnitine/kg/day. (Please note that investigators have used doses as high as 400 mg/kg/day, but because of limited GI absorption the clinical benefit of the higher doses remains unclear).

#### *Carnitine Palmitoyltransferase Type I Deficiency*

Carnitine palmitoyltransferase I (CPT-I) is responsible for covalently linking LCFAs such as palmitate to carnitine. Although one patient with deficiency of CPT-I presented in the newborn period, most come to attention in early to late infancy (Roe and Coates, 1995). The clinical findings are hypoketotic hypoglycemia, encephalopathy, and hepatomegaly; there is usually no evidence of cardiomyopathy or skeletal myopathy in CPT-I deficiency. Renal tubular acidosis, which is due to impaired distal hydrogen ion secretion, has been reported in two patients. Characteristic laboratory findings are the absence of dicarboxylic aciduria and high plasma levels of total carnitine and free carnitine; however, the plasma acylcarnitine profile is not abnormal. The definitive diagnosis rests on measuring CPT-I enzyme activity in cultured skin fibroblasts. Frequent feeding, reduction of dietary fat, supplementation with medium-chain triglyceride oils, and avoidance of fasting all have been beneficial in the long-term management of patients with CPT-I deficiency.

#### *Acylcarnitine Translocase Deficiency*

Acylcarnitine translocase deficiency is an exceedingly rare defect. It was initially reported in a male infant who suffered a cardiac arrest at 36 hours of age in association with fasting stress and ventricular dysrhythmias (Stanley et al, 1992). Because of the failure to transport long-chain acylcarnitines across the intermitochondrial membrane after the synthesis by CPT-I, the patient had very low total plasma levels of carnitine, most of which was long-chain esterified carnitine; he also had recurrent episodes of hypoglycemia, vomiting, gastroesophageal reflux, and mild chronic hyperammonemia as well as severe skeletal myopathy and mild hypertrophic cardiomyopathy. The continuous nasogastric feeding of a low-fat, high-carbohydrate formula failed to normalize the clinical abnormalities, and the patient died at 3 years of age. At that time, liver failure had also developed. Pathophysiology in this patient suggests that accumulation of long-chain acylcarnitine species may be toxic for several organs, including the heart, liver, and skeletal muscle. In addition, the acute development of ventricular dysrhythmias may be related to the accumulation of such species in cardiac tissue.

#### *Carnitine Palmitoyltransferase Type II Deficiency*

There are two phenotypes of carnitine palmitoyltransferase type II (CPT-II ) deficiency (Roe and Coates, 1995). The enzyme is responsible for the hydrolysis of the LCFA bound to carnitine after transport across the intermitochondrial membrane. Most of the patients reported with CPT-II deficiency have a mild deficiency of the enzyme and present in adulthood with episodes of muscle weakness and myoglobinuria brought on by prolonged exercise. The other phenotype is caused by a more serious enzyme defect and manifests in early infancy. The first detailed report was of a 3-month-old boy with hypoketotic hypoglycemia, coma, seizures, hepatomegaly, cardiomegaly, cardiac arrhythmias associated with an increase in long-chain acylcarnitine levels in tissues, and the absence of urinary dicarboxylic aciduria (Demaugre et al, 1991). The enzyme is also expressed in renal tissue as well as in skeletal muscle. Renal dysgenesis has been noted in three patients

(Zinn et al, 1991). Reports of onset in the newborn period (Hug et al, 1991) and in later infancy have been recorded. The gene for the human CPT-II is on chromosome 1. Several mutations have been described. Decreased activity of the CPT-II enzyme may be demonstrated in cultured skin fibroblasts.

## Defects in Ketone Metabolism

After LCFAs are broken down to medium-chain fatty acids and finally to short-chain fatty acids such as acetoacetyl CoA, they must be converted in the liver to 3-hydroxy-3-methylglutaryl CoA (HMG-CoA) before hydrolysis to acetoacetate. Depending on the mitochondrial redox potential—that is, the ratio of the reduced form of nicotinamide adenine dinucleotide (NAD) to its oxidized form ($NADH/NAD^+$)—some of the acetoacetate is converted to 3-hydroxybutyrate, and both ketone bodies are transported out of liver mitochondria and hepatocytes into blood, where they may be used by other tissues, especially brain. Acetoacetyl CoA derived from the last turn of the beta oxidation spiral together with acetyl CoA forms HMG-CoA in a reaction catalyzed by HMG-CoA synthetase. Normally, acetoacetyl CoA can also be hydrolyzed to acetyl CoA by the mitochondrial acetoacetyl-CoA thiolase. Patients with a deficiency of this thiolase have not a defect in ketone body synthesis but, rather, metabolic acidosis associated with excess ketosis (Cornblath et al, 1971; Daum et al, 1971; Sweetman and Williams, 1995).

The clinical features of the thiolase deficiency are variable. Severe acute metabolic decompensation has been reported in infants, but there are also asymptomatic adults with the disorder. The episodes are heralded by fasting or increased protein intake, because isoleucine is a precursor of 2-methylacetoacetyl CoA, which is also a substrate for the mitochondrial acetoacetyl-CoA thiolase enzyme. Thus, this block leads to a defect in the distal catabolism of isoleucine and in the processing of the precursor of ketone body formation, namely, acetoacetyl CoA. Cardiomyopathy has been identified in rare patients. The characteristic urinary metabolite pattern detected on urine organic acid quantitation centers on the presence of the isoleucine metabolites, such as 2-methylacetoacetate, 2-methyl-3-hydroxybutyrate, and tiglylglycine. During acute decompensation, lactate as well as the traditional ketone bodies are detected in excess amounts in the urine. Some older children have been mistakenly identified as having ketotic hypoglycemia. The amino acid glycine may be elevated in plasma. Deficiency in the mitochondrial acetoacetyl-CoA thiolase can be demonstrated in cultured skin fibroblasts. The gene has been cloned and sequenced. Several mutations have been identified. Treatment of the acute episodes consists of intravenous glucose and administration of alkali to correct metabolic acidosis, which may be severe. Long-term therapy involves protein restriction and avoidance of fasting.

The synthesis of acetoacetate from HMG-CoA depends on the HMG-CoA lyase enzyme. A deficiency of this enzyme represents the most profound defect in ketone body synthesis (Gibson et al, 1988; Sweetman and Williams, 1995). About one third of the patients with this disease present in the first week of life. The onset is dramatic and the disease is catastrophic, being characterized by vomiting, lethargy, coma, seizures, hepatomegaly, hypoglycemia, little or no ketones in the urine, and hyperammonemia. Most of the complications are related to the severe effects of hypoglycemia on the CNS in addition to the acidemia, which may be profound. The characteristic urine metabolites detected by GC-MS analysis are 3-hydroxy-3-methylglutaric acid, 3-methylglutaconic acid, and 3-hydroxyisovaleric acid. Only small, inappropriate amounts of acetoacetic acid and 3-hydroxybutyric acid may be detected. Lactate values may be elevated during the acute metabolic decompensation. Inherited as an autosomal recessive trait, the HMG-CoA lyase deficiency can be demonstrated in cultured skin fibroblasts. Treatment of the acute episode consists of administration of intravenous glucose and alkali to correct the metabolic acidosis. Most long-term therapy consists of a high-carbohydrate diet. Some patients are put on protein-restricted diets, but the most important element in long-term care is the avoidance of fasting.

The last defect to be discussed in the area of disturbances in ketone body metabolism is the succinyl-CoA: 3-ketoacid-CoA transferase deficiency (Cornblath et al, 1971; Middleton et al, 1987; Sweetman and Williams, 1995). In this disease, the ketone bodies, acetoacetic acid, and 3-hydroxybutyric acid are synthesized adequately in the liver, but they cannot be metabolized in the extrahepatic tissues because of the failure of activation of acetoacetate to acetoacetyl CoA by the transferase enzyme. Conversion to a CoA derivative is required for hydrolysis to acetyl CoA for final metabolism in the Krebs citric acid cycle. This is a rare disorder, and most of the affected patients who have presented in the newborn period have not survived. Such patients usually exhibit severe ketolactic acidosis. The hallmark of the disease is that ketosis never disappears, even after correction of the overt metabolic acidosis and the institution of frequent feedings with the avoidance of fasting. Plasma values of acetoacetate and 3-hydroxybutyrate are always mild to moderately elevated, resulting in intermittent ketonuria. The most important aspect of therapy is the avoidance of fasting, during which time acidosis and ketosis can be overwhelming. The gene that encodes this enzyme has been cloned, and several mutations have been detected.

## Primary Lactic Acidosis

The term *primary lactic acidosis* (PLA) refers to a group of diseases in which impaired lactate metabolism is due to a defect in the mitochondrial respiratory or electron transport chain (ETC), the tricarboxylic acid (TCA) (Krebs) cycle, or the accessory components that support mitochondrial function and shuttling of reducing equivalents, or in which there is a primary defect in pyruvate metabolism that secondarily leads to impaired lactate handling (see Fig. 22–1) (Robinson, 1995; Shoffner and Wallace, 1995). However, there are a limited number of reports on inborn errors of the TCA cycle (Blass et al, 1972). Most of the information on PLA focuses on mitochondrial ETC, pyruvate dehydrogenase (PDH) complex, and pyruvate carboxylase (PC) defects, all of which have been masterfully reviewed by Shoffner and Wallace (1995) and Robinson (1995). The approach taken in this section has been influenced by their reviews, as well as by the pioneering work of DeVivo and colleagues (1977, 1979), DiMauro and associates (1973, 1980, 1983, 1987), Blass and coworkers (1972), and Brown and colleagues (1987, 1988), to which the reader is directed for details beyond the scope of this chapter.

Some patients present with overwhelming lactic acidosis (Robinson, 1989). In others, lactate may be elevated only in CSF, a "cerebral" lactic acidosis syndrome (Brown et al, 1988). Depending on the nature of the enzyme deficiency, lactate and pyruvate as well as alanine can be elevated in blood. The ratio of blood lactate to pyruvate (L/P ratio) can be helpful in distinguishing the different types of inborn errors. For example, the L/P ratio is often normal (10 to 20) in the PDH and PC deficiencies but elevated in an ETC defect.

## Pyruvate Dehydrogenase Deficiency

### *Pyruvate Dehydrogenase (PDH) Complex Deficiency*

$$\text{Pyruvate} + \text{CoA} \xrightarrow{\text{PDH}} \text{Acetyl CoA} + CO_2$$

- Enzyme: 12 subunits per functional component
  - 4 pyruvate decarboxylase ($E_1$) subunits, 2 $E_1\alpha$ and 2 $E_1\beta$
  - 1 dihydrolipoyl transacylase ($E_2$) subunit
  - 1 X-lipoate component
  - 2 dihydrolipoyl dehydrogenase ($E_3$) subunits
  - 2 PDH kinase subunits
  - 2 PDH phosphatase subunits
- Gene locations:
  - $E_1\alpha$ on Chromosome X p22.1-22.2
  - $E_1\beta$ on Chromosome 3 p13-q23
  - $E_3$ on Chromosome 7 q31-32
- Frequency: <1 in 250,000

**CASE STUDY 6**

A boy, the product of a 36-week gestation, was delivered by cesarean section because of breech presentation. He required assistance with ventilation at birth. The Apgar scores were 5 at 1 minute and 9 at 5 minutes. At 1 hour of life, the infant had generalized seizures. An arterial blood pH was 7.38, and the $P_{CO_2}$ was 13 mm HG. Serum total $CO_2$ was 5 mmol/L, and glucose was 76 mg/dL. Blood lactate and pyruvate values were 9.93 mmol/L (normal ≤2.0 mmol/L) and 0.53 mmol/L (normal ≤0.20 mmol/L), respectively; the L/P ratio was 18.8 (normal ≤20).

Physical examination showed the infant to be lethargic and hypotonic. His weight (1770 g) and length (42 cm) were below the third percentile, and his head circumference (31 cm) was below the 10th percentile. Several minor craniofacial abnormalities, including hypertelorism, micrognathia, and low-set, posteriorly rotated ears, were detected. He also had a pectus excavatum, first-degree hypospadias, and rocker-bottom feet. There were few spontaneous movements, but he showed withdrawal in response to tactile stimulation. Neurologic findings included bilateral ptosis, bifacial palsy, and weak bulbar function.

The metabolic acidosis persisted, necessitating large amounts of intravenous sodium bicarbonate, and on day 2, the infant needed mechanical ventilation. By the third day of life, the baby was completely unresponsive. An EEG showed a burst suppression pattern, and a head CT demonstrated bilateral grade II intraventricular hemorrhages, a subarachnoid hemorrhage, and agenesis of the corpus callosum. Phenobarbital was started. The infant had received only intravenous glucose since his initial resuscitation. Before initiation of total parenteral nutrition with triglycerides at 1 week of age, the neonatal reflexes, doll's eye, and pupillary light reflexes were absent.

Over the next few days, the infant's level of consciousness improved, he was weaned off the ventilator, and the metabolic acidosis resolved. The phenobarbital was eventually discontinued. Analysis of organic acids in urine by gas chromotography showed increased lactate excretion. Before discharge at 1 month of age with a proprietary formula, he had had several episodes of bradycardia and was still hypotonic.

Over the next several months, the patient failed to grow despite adequate caloric intake. The metabolic acidosis had returned and was associated with elevated blood lactate levels. He required more than 4 mEq of sodium bicarbonate per kilogram per day for partial correction. He was given a high-fat diet and megadoses of thiamine hydrochloride. Despite normalization of blood lactate levels, there was no clinical improvement. At age 7 months, his length, weight, and head circumference were less than the fifth percentile.

The patient remained extremely hypotonic, did not appear to have vision, and had normal reflexes in the upper limbs but none in the lower extremities. He was resuscitated from a respiratory arrest at 7 months, but at 8 months, he died of a nocturnal primary respiratory arrest.

In cultured skin fibroblasts, there was 20% residual activity of the PDH complex. Western blot analysis revealed trace amounts of both $E_1a$ and $E_1ß$ subunits, but only the $E_1a$ peptide had abnormal electrophoretic mobility.

The most common cause of a primary defect in pyruvate metabolism is PDH complex deficiency (Robinson, 1995). This complex, located in the mitochondria, has several components, the $E_1\alpha$ and $E_1\beta$ subunits, the $E_2$ subunit, the $E_3$ subunit, the X-lipoate subunit, and the PDH phosphatase and kinase subunits. Most mutations have been reported in the $E_1$ subunit (Robinson et al, 1987). Unlike the other components, the $E_1\alpha$ subunit is encoded on the X chromosome. Because of the key importance of the PDH complex in energy metabolism, even partial defects of the complex may be associated with severe CNS disease. In addition, even though the $E_1\alpha$ subunit defect is an X-linked disease, many females are also affected, so it can be considered a dominant mutation. All the other defects are inherited as autosomal recessive disorders.

There are several different phenotypes of PDH complex deficiency based on the severity of the enzyme deficiency. Most of the patients with less than 20% residual enzyme activity in cultured skin fibroblasts present in the newborn period with overwhelming lactic acidosis (Farrel et al, 1975; Federico et al, 1990; Robinson et al, 1987; Stromme et al, 1976). Some patients, but perhaps those without life-threatening acidosis, even have congenital lesions associated with cystic lesions in the cerebral hemisphere; cerebral atrophy; cystic lesions in the basal ganglia; and facial dysmorphism, including features that resemble those of fetal alcohol syndrome, such as a narrowed head, frontal bossing, wide nasal bridge with upturned nose, a long poorly developed philtrum, and flared nostrils. In addition, there may be partial or complete agenesis of the corpus callosum and impaired migration of neurons within the cerebral hemispheres, identified as heterotopic dysplasia on neuropathologic examination of brain tissue. Patients with less severe defects manifest progressive psychomotor retardation (Miyabayashi et al, 1985), including the entity termed *Leigh disease*, or *subacute necrotizing encephalomyelopathy* (SNE) (DeVivo et al, 1979), as discussed later, and older male patients with variant lesions may manifest only intermittent ataxia during childhood (Blass et al, 1970) with a mild or intermittent lactic acidosis. Secondary hyperammonemia has been detected (Brown et al, 1987).

The $E_1\alpha$ subunit gene on the X chromosome has been cloned and sequenced, and multiple mutations have been identified. The $E_2$ and protein X-lipoate defects are rare and usually result in chronic psychomotor retardation syndrome in late infancy and childhood (Robinson et al, 1990). The $E_3$ subunit defect is a unique syndrome (Taylor et al, 1978), because the subunit is important not only in the PDH complex but also in the BCKAD complex and the α-ketoglutarate dehydrogenase (KGDH) complex. Thus, these patients have multiple deficiencies involving the BCAA as in MSUD, as well as Krebs cycle metabolites indicative of a block in the TCA cycle (Munnich et al, 1982). Most of the patients present later than the newborn period and have severe progressive neurodegenerative disease. The key laboratory findings are elevations of lactic acid in blood, BCAAs in plasma, and detection of α-ketoglutarate in urine by urine organic acid analysis. PDH phosphatase deficiency is a rare cause of congenital lactic acidosis (Robinson and Sherwood, 1975).

There is no effective treatment for any of the defects in PDH complex metabolism that manifest in the newborn period. A response to thiamine megatherapy has been reported in a few patients. Metabolic imbalance in the patient with PDH deficiency, as well as in other PLA defects, may be further compromised by high- or selective-carbohydrate feedings. There has been some success in reducing lactate accumulation with the use of a ketogenic diet. Dichloracetate, an inhibitor of the PDH kinase, is being studied as a treatment for several PLAs (Kuroda et al, 1986; McCormick et al, 1985; Stacpoole et al, 1983).

## Pyruvate Carboxylase Deficiency

### *Pyruvate Carboxylase (PC) Deficiency*

$$\text{Pyruvate} + \text{ATP} + \text{HCO}_3 \xrightarrow{\text{PC}} \text{Oxaloacetate} + \text{AMP} + \text{PP}_1$$

- Enzyme: homotetramer
- Gene location: chromosome 11q13
- Frequency: 1 in 250,000

There are three types of PC deficiency (Robinson, 1995; Robinson et al, 1984). Type A is characterized by lactic acidosis in the newborn period and delayed development (DeVivo et al, 1977). However, the disease is of a chronic nature. In type B, the catastrophic form of the disorder, the infant is acutely ill, usually in the first week of life, with encephalopathy, severe metabolic acidosis with lactic acidosis, and hyperammonemia (Saudubray et al, 1976). The mortality rate in this form is high. In one case, referred to as type C, the patient presented with mild episodic metabolic acidosis and lactic acidosis, but with no evidence of CNS dysfunction (Van Coster et al, 1991).

As discussed earlier, PC is a biotin-containing enzyme. Most of the patients presenting with a type B form of PC deficiency have been of French or English origin. Unlike patients with a type A defect, in whom the blood L/P ratio is normal because both lactate and pyruvate are comparably elevated, patients with the type B defect often have an elevated L/P ratio. Because of the importance of the PC product oxaloacetate in providing adequate cellular levels of aspartate, citrulline metabolism in the urea cycle is defective, leading to elevations of plasma citrulline as well as plasma ammonium concentrations. Although PC is also an important enzyme in gluconeogenesis, hypoglycemia has not been commonly reported. The liver may be enlarged. There is no effective treatment for PC deficiency when it is associated with progressive neurodegeneration. The gene that encodes the PC subunits, of which four combine to make an active enzyme, has been cloned and sequenced. Several mutations have been identified. PC deficiency may be detected in cultured skin fibroblasts or in liver biopsy samples.

## Phosphoenolpyruvate Carboxykinase Deficiency

Phosphoenolpyruvate carboxykinase (PEPCK) enzyme also functions in gluconeogenesis, and there are two forms in liver, one in the cytosol, and the other in the mitochondrial compartment. Only three cases of PEPCK deficiency have been documented (Fiser et al, 1974; Robinson, 1995). In each, the activity of PEPCK was found to be deficient in liver tissue. Patients do not usually come to attention until childhood with hypotonia, failure to thrive, hepatomegaly, lactic acidosis, and hypoglycemia. One patient had a more severe phenotype associated with severe liver disease and died at 6 months of age (Clayton et al, 1986). The accuracy of the diagnosis of PEPCK in some other patients is in question. Although there is no adequate experience to draw from in identifying the optimal therapy for these patients, it is reasonable to assume that frequent feedings and avoiding of fasting are important in avoiding severe metabolic imbalance.

## Mitochondrial Respiratory Chain or Electron Transport Chain Defects

Oxidative phosphorylation is the key process performed by the mitochondria of cells. Any inborn error of metabolism that involves the tightly coupled and regulated process of mitochondrial energy metabolism may have profound effects on health and disease, because oxidative phosphorylation is the process by which we convert food into energy. The various derivatives of foodstuffs such as pyruvate and fatty acids are converted to $CO_2$ in mitochondria. The energy derived from such controlled chemical combustion is harnessed by allowing the reducing equivalences (in the form of NADH or the reduced form of flavin adenine dinucleotide [$FADH_2$], which are derived from such metabolism) to combine with oxygen to form $H_2O$, and in the process, the synthesis of ATP is coupled to the orderly flow of electrons down the respiratory chain components.

The important components in the mitochondrial respiratory chain are complex 1 (NADH dehydrogenase), complex 2 (ETF dehydrogenase); complex 3 (cytochromes $b$, $c_1$) and the terminal complex in this chain; and complex 4, which is cytochrome $c$ oxidase (COX) (Shoffner and Wallace, 1995). In addition, there is a complex 5, or ATP synthetase, and an adenine nucleotide translocase, which permits transport of adenosine diphosphate (ADP) into and ATP out of the mitochondria. Complex 2 is involved primarily in fatty acid oxidation and oxidation of succinate derived from the Krebs cycle, because the reducing equivalents extracted from fatty acids, glutaric acid, and succinate flow from ETF into complex 2. The polypeptides that compose these various complexes are derived from both the nuclear genes and the genes on mitochondrial DNA (mtDNA). Except for complex 2, mtDNA is important in production of the subunits of all the respiratory chain complexes. PLA involving the ETC components has been associated with both nuclear and mtDNA mutations.

On the basis of molecular diagnostic testing, the oxidative phosphorylation diseases can be divided into the following four genetic groups (Shoffner and Wallace, 1995):

- Group 1: nuclear DNA mutations
- Group 2: mtDNA point mutations
- Group 3: mtDNA deletions and duplications
- Group 4: unidentified genetic defects

The relationship between phenotype and mtDNA mutations is not straightforward, probably because of the phenomenon of heteroplasmy. Mitochondria with their unique mtDNA are inherited solely from the mother (Hutchinson et al, 1974). Random segregation of mitochondria having mtDNA mutations leads to heteroplasmy and, ultimately, a variable concentration of defective mitochondria within cells and among tissues (Shoffner and Wallace, 1995). Most of our understanding of the detailed molecular mechanisms that contribute to or produce the ETC gene disturbances concern the mtDNA mutations. However, with the exception of the neurogenic muscle weakness, ataxia, retinitis pigmentosa (NARP) mutation, few of the primary mtDNA defects actually manifest in the newborn period. Examples are the MELAS (mitochondrial encephalopathy, lactic acidosis, and stroke-like episodes) (Ciafaloni et al, 1992; Goto et al, 1990), MERRF (myoclonic epilepsy with ragged-red fiber) (Noer et al, 1991), Leber hereditary optic neuropathy (Wallace et al, 1988), and sporadic deletion syndromes (Holt et al, 1988),. The diseases that affect young infants are benign infantile mitochondrial myopathy, cardiomyopathy, or both; lethal infantile mitochondrial disease; lethal infantile cardiomyopathy; SNE or Leigh disease; Pearson syndrome; Alpers disease; lethal infantile cardiomyopathy; and the most dramatic form, with presentation often in the first few days of life, during which an acid-base disturbance dominates the clinical picture.

### Benign Infantile Mitochondrial Myopathy, Cardiomyopathy, or Both

Benign infantile mitochondrial myopathy is associated with congenital hypotonia and weakness at birth, feeding difficulties, respiratory difficulties, and lactic acidosis. In this poorly understood, developmental-like disorder, only skeletal muscle appears to be affected, and histochemical analyses show a COX deficiency that returns to normal levels after 1 to 3 years of age (DiMauro et al, 1983; Jerusalem et al, 1973; Roodhooft et al, 1986; Tritschler et al, 1991; Zeviani et al, 1987). A nuclear DNA mutation in a gene important in a fetal isoform of an ETC polypeptide specific for muscle oxidative phosphorylation is believed to be the cause of this problem, and a developmental switch from the defective fetal gene to the adult form may be responsible for the gradual improvement. This disorder may be inherited in an autosomal recessive or autosomal dominant fashion. It is the only example of a developmental defect in oxidative phosphorylation that is probably nuclear encoded and in which the treatment is only support during the early newborn period to prevent death from respiratory disease.

The form also associated with cardiomyopathy may just be a variant of the benign isolated myopathy and involves striated muscle in both skeletal and cardiac muscle. It manifests in the newborn period with lactic acidosis and a cardiomyopathy that improves during the first year of life. The exact gene defect is unknown. More attention must be paid to these two disease entities, because with early optimal medical care, affected infants may have excellent prognoses.

### Lethal Infantile Mitochondrial Disease

Infants with lethal infantile mitochondrial disease are severely ill in the first few weeks of life or in the extended newborn period (DiMauro et al, 1980; Zeviani et al, 1986). They present with hypotonia, muscle weakness, failure to thrive, and severe lactic acidosis. Death occurs by 6 months of age and almost always is associated with overwhelming lactic acidosis. Skeletal muscle shows lipid and glycogen accumulation and abnormally shaped mitochondria on electron microscopic examination. Hepatic dysfunction may be a prominent finding in these patients. Generalized proximal renal tubular dysfunction may occur, leading to full-blown renal Fanconi syndrome (DiMauro et al, 1980; Heiman et al, 1982; Zeviani et al, 1986). The ETC defects reported in these patients include defects in complexes 1, 3, and 4, (Birch-Machin et al, 1989; Moreadith et al, 1984; Robinson et al, 1985; Sengers et al, 1984; Shoffner and Wallace, 1995; Zheng et al, 1989). Original reports concerned infants with a phenotype resembling severe Wernig-Hoffman disease with COX deficiency and renal Fanconi syndrome (DiMauro et al 1980; Heiman et al, 1982).

This entity is probably more than one disease. Some studies have suggested that the cause is tissue-specific depletions of mtDNA (Boustany et al, 1983). The cause of the depletion is believed to be a nuclear-encoded gene, perhaps inherited as an autosomal recessive trait. There are molecular precedents for this mechanism, in that mutations in the genes thymidine kinase and deoxyguanosine kinase have been shown to cause "myopathic" and "hepatocerebral" forms of mitochondrial DNA depletion syndromes (Mandel et al, 2001; Saada et al, 2001). In addition, some patients may have selective COX deficiency due to a defective nuclear-encoded complex 4 gene.

### Lethal Infantile Cardiomyopathy

Defects of the mitochondrial respiratory chain have varied neonatal presentations and are commonly due to isolated COX deficiency (DeVivo et al, 2002). Clinical features of COX deficiency reflect involvement of one or more tissues and include encephalopathy, myopathy, cardiopathy, liver disease, and nephropathy (Munnich et al, 2001). The heterogeneous clinical features are due, in part, to the dual genetic control of COX: the three catalytic subunits—COX I, COX II, COX III—are encoded by mtDNA, whereas the remaining subunits (COX IV to COX VIII) are encoded by nuclear DNA (nDNA). In addition, proper assembly of COX requires several nDNA-encoded proteins. The various syndromes due to COX deficiency are only partially understood at the genetic level. Most infants with isolated complex IV deficiency are likely to have nDNA gene defects in COX assembly genes, including *SURF1* (Zhu et al, 1998), *SCO2* (Papadopoulou et al, 1999), *SCO1* (Valnat et al, 2000a), *COX10* (Valnat et al, 2000b), and COX15 (Antonicka et al, 2003).

**CASE STUDY 7**

A boy was born to non-consanguineous, healthy parents after a full-term gestation. Biventricular hypertrophy with a predominant right-sided component had been observed on a fetal ultrasonography at 24 weeks of gestation. He was delivered by cesarean section due to variable decelerations, and he emerged without meconium staining or passage. Respiratory distress developed shortly after birth. An echocardiogram showed concentric right ventricular hypertrophy with elevated right ventricular pressure (70 mm Hg). Initial laboratory studies showed acute metabolic acidosis (blood lactate >18 mmol/L, arterial pH 6.91).

His weight was 2.36 kg (10th percentile), his length 46 cm (5th percentile), and his head circumference 31 cm (5th percentile). He had a right ventricular heave and an intermittent fourth heart sound. There was no liver enlargement. Muscle bulk was normal, and deep tendon reflexes were intact. Metabolic investigations showed persistent arterial lactic acidemia (range 3 to 11 mM) with increased pyruvate (range 0.02 to 0.44 mM). The L/P ratio ranged from 25 to 290. The activities of the respiratory chain complexes II, III, and IV were normal in cultured skin fibroblasts. A left quadriceps muscle biopsy was used for histochemical analysis and to prepare a 10% extract for respiratory chain studies. Histochemistry showed no ragged-red fibers with the modified Gomori trichrome stain but a diffusely weak response to staining for cytochrome *c* oxidase (COX, ETC complex 4); biochemistry showed markedly reduced COX activity, contrasting with normal activities of other complexes. Direct sequencing of the three COXs and all 22 transfer RNA genes of mtDNA, all the COX-assembly nuclear genes known to harbor pathogenic mutations (*SURF1, SC01, SC02, COX10*, and *COX15*), and the two other nuclear ancillary genes (*COX11* and *COX17*) showed no mutations. Southern blot analysis showed no deletions but results were inconclusive regarding mtDNA depletion. However, sequencing of the two genes known to be associated with the "myopathic" (Saada et al, 2001) and the and the "hepatocerebral" (Mandel et al, 2001) mtDNA depletion syndromes (*TK2* and *dGK*) did not show any mutations.

A series of echocardiograms documented biventricular, hypertrophic, nonobstructive cardiomyopathy. The patient expired on the seventh hospital day after a sudden episode of hemoglobin desaturation. An autopsy was performed 4 hours after death. The right ventricle was found to be thickened and enlarged, with relative sparing of the left side. The pulmonary vasculature of the lungs showed hypertrophy that extended to the most distal vessels. Routine microscopic findings in skeletal muscle were normal, and the CNS was without microscopic or macroscopic abnormalities.

This baby had a fatal syndrome defined clinically by prenatal cardiomyopathy and severe pulmonary hypertension in the newborn period. The syndrome was due to isolated ETC complex 4 deficiency. The pathophysiology centered on the heart and lungs. How much disease was due to the involvement of other organs remains unclear. As discussed later, this is an example of a mitochondrial metabolic disorder but without a specific molecular genetic cause.

### Barth Syndrome

Barth syndrome is an X-linked disorder associated with cardiomyopathy, skeletal muscle disease, and neutropenia (Barth et al, 1983; Neustein et al, 1979). Skeletal muscle shows abnormal mitochondrial morphology. Important laboratory findings include decreased plasma free carnitine, increased urinary excretion of 3-methylglutaconate on GC-MS analysis of urine organic acids, and decreased levels of serum cholesterol in early infancy (Kelley et al, 1991). Positional cloning identified a gene for this disorder on Xq28 that encodes for a phospholipid remodeling enzyme, cardiolipin acyl transferase. Several mutations have been identified. It was hypothesized that the organic acid, 3-methylglutaconate, accumulates because of defective mitochondrial transport. Patients must be supported from birth to early infancy. Investigators speculate that if severe cholesterol deficiency can be avoided, affected infants may survive and may be relatively free of cardiomyopathy during childhood. Of diagnostic importance, not all patients with 3-methylglutaconic aciduria have Barth syndrome. A few have isolated leucine-dependent 3-methylglutaconyl-CoA hydratase deficiency or Costeff syndrome, but most suffer from ill-defined mitochondropathies (Gibson et al, 1993).

### Subacute Necrotizing Encephalomyelopathy or Leigh Disease

Probably because of a failure to recognize the clinical signs, infants with SNE or Leigh disease usually come to clinical attention after the newborn period. This disease is best characterized as a progressive neurodegenerative disorder with severe hypotonia, seizures, extrapyramidal movement disorders, optic atrophy, and defects in automatic ventilation or respiratory control (Pincus, 1972). It is clear that there are many causes of SNE. As discussed earlier, PDH complex deficiency may lead to Leigh disease. Patients with defects in the ETC have also been reported to have findings compatible with SNE. Many neuropathologists believe that the diagnosis of SNE depends on an analysis of CNS tissue at autopsy. However, MRI characteristically shows bilateral symmetrical lesions of the basal ganglia.

There is no effective treatment for this disease. It is possible that most of the patients with Leigh disease have disturbances in nuclear-encoded genes. Although, as discussed later, the NARP lesion due to a group 2 mtDNA mutation is one important cause in early infancy. Clearly, this is not one disease entity, because the specific neuropathologic findings for SNE have also been reported in a patient with Menke disease, in which there exists a secondary ETC complex 4 deficiency because copper is an important metal cofactor of cytochrome *c* oxidase.

The following clinical findings have been noted in infants with SNE: optic atrophy, ophthalmoplegia, nystagmus, respiratory abnormalities, ataxia, hypotonia, spasticity, seizures, developmental delay, psychomotor retardation, myopathy, and renal tubular dysfunction. Some patients may manifest hypertrophic cardiomyopathy, liver dysfunction, and microcephaly. The neuropathologic lesions include demyelination, gliosis, necrosis, relative neuronal sparing, and capillary proliferation in specific brain lesions. There are lesions of the basal ganglia, which are bilaterally symmetrical, as well as of the brainstem, cerebellum, and, to a much lesser degree, the cerebral cortex. Commonly, the elevation in blood lactate is only slight to moderate, as well as intermittent, in this diverse group of patients. In some instances, lactate values may be elevated only in the CSF. The most commonly reported biochemical abnormalities are deficiencies in COX or complex 4 (DiMauro et al, 1987; Hoganson et al, 1984; Miranda et al, 1989; Willems et al, 1977), NADH dehydrogenase or complex 1 (Hoppel et al, 1987), and PDH. In a few rare patients, the abnormality in oxidative phosphorylation has been reported to be secondary to the NARP mutation. This involves a T→C transition at base pair 8993 of the adenosine triphosphatase (ATPase) 6 gene, changing a leucine to a proline at position 156 in the ATPase 6 polypeptide. Investigators have speculated that defects such as those in COX and the NADH dehydrogenase, when associated with the neuropathology of Leigh disease, are due to nuclear gene mutations (Miranda et al, 1989) and not to mtDNA gene defects such as the NARP point mutation in the ATPase 6 gene (Santorelli et al, 1993; Shoffner et al, 1992; Tatuch et al, 1992).

The diseases in group 3 (see earlier), exemplified by the Kearns-Sayre and chronic progressive external ophthalmoplegia syndromes (Shoffner and Wallace, 1995), are not familial and are due to mtDNA deletions (Morales et al, 1989) or duplications (Poulton et al, 1989) that are spontaneous mutations. These disorders do not usually come to clinical attention in infancy. The only example of such a mutation manifesting in early infancy is the Pearson syndrome (Cormier et al, 1991; Rotig et al, 1989). This is a systemic disorder that primarily affects the hematopoietic system and pancreas function. The characteristics are severe macrocytic anemia with varying degrees of neutropenia and thrombocytopenia. Bone marrow examination shows normal cellularity but extensive vacuolization of erythroid and myeloid precursors, hemosiderosis, and ringed sideroblasts. This disease of the bone marrow may lead to death in infancy. However, patients who are able to recover or who benefit from aggressive therapy may demonstrate other signs of this systemic disorder in late infancy or childhood, such as poor growth, pancreas dysfunction, mitochondrial myopathy, lactic acidosis, and progressive neurologic damage (Majander et al, 1991; Nelson et al, 1992).

### *Unidentified Genetic Defects*

A number of diseases are believed to be caused by mitochondrial respiratory chain problems, but the specific mutations remain unknown. These constitute the group 4 mutations, or the disorders of unknown inheritance (Shoffner and Wallace, 1995). Alpers disease is one such example. It has also been called *progressive infantile poliodystrophy*. Infants and children with this progressive disease experience progressive cerebral cortical damage, sometimes also involving the cerebellum, basal ganglia, and brainstem; in some, liver disease may progress to cirrhosis. The neuropathologic lesions consist of spongiform or microcystic cerebral degeneration, gliosis, necrosis, and capillary proliferation (Sandbank and Lerman, 1972). Seizures are prominent, including myoclonus. Laboratory abnormalities include abnormal NADH oxidation or complex 1 defects, impaired pyruvate handling, and PDH complex deficiency, TCA cycle malfunction, and decreased mitochondrial cytochrome $a + a_3$ content (Prick et al, 1983). The diversity of these findings suggests that this may be more than one disease. Finally, some patients in this "wastebasket" category have manifested lethal infantile cardiomyopathy, as described in Case Study 7, in association with cardiac failure and cardiac dysrhythmias, including Wolff-Parkinson-White syndrome. The pathologic abnormalities have included a reduced number of myofibrils, cardiac fibers with high lipid and glycogen content, and abnormal number of mitochondria. Both cytochrome $b$ and cytochrome $c + c_1$ deficiencies have been reported. The exact gene defects remain unknown.

### *Early Lethal Lactic Acidosis*

In an unknown fraction of patients with primary disturbances in mitochondrial oxidative phosphorylation or ETC defects, massive lactic acidosis develops within 24 to 72 hours after birth. Not uncommonly, the condition is untreatable, because it is relentless and unresponsive to alkali therapy. Dialysis is a remedy but not a cure. Often, affected infants have no obvious organ damage early in the course or evidence of malformations. This statement is also true for infants with the PDH complex deficiency, which is probably a more common cause of overwhelming acidosis in the first week of life. In addition, acidemia per se can easily explain the coma or impaired cardiac contractility that may be encountered. Some infants have survived with aggressive therapy. Anecdotal reports also suggest the existence of a transient disease process.

The care of babies with these different forms of severe lactic acidosis almost always brings an ethical and moral dilemma to the forefront for the physicians and nurses of the NICU as well as for the babies' families. To further complicate the issues, enzymatic and molecular analyses usually are not immediately available. The disease in most patients probably remains idiopathic, and no DNA mutation, nuclear or mitochondrial, can be identified. A rigid approach to care is impractical and unwise. Decisions regarding management must be individualized because the mitochondrial dysfunction and resultant pathophysiology may vary among infants.

## REFERENCES


Amendt BA, Green C, Sweetman L, et al: Short-chain acyl-coenzyme A dehydrogenase deficiency: Clinical and biochemical studies in two patients. J Clin Invest 79:1303, 1987.

Antonicka H, Mattman A, Carlson CG, et al: Mutation in COX15 produces a defect in the mitochondrial heme biosynthetic pathway, causing early-onset fatal hypertrophic cardiomyopathy. Am J Hum Genet 72:101, 2003.

Baker L, Winegrad AI: Fasting hypoglycaemia and metabolic acidosis associated with deficiency of hepatic fructose-1, 6-diphosphatase activity. Lancet 2:13, 1970.

Ballard RA, Vinocur B, Reynolds JW, et al: Transient hyperammonemia of the preterm infant. N Engl J Med 299:920, 1978.

Barth PG, Scholte HR, Berden JA, et al: An X-linked mitochondrial disease affecting cardiac muscle, skeletal muscle, and neutrophil leucocytes. J Neurol Sci 62:327, 1983.

Batshaw ML: Hyperammonemia. Curr Prob Pediatr 14:1, 1984.

Berry GT, Yudkoff M, Segal S: Isovaleric acidemia: Medical and neurodevelopmental effects of long-term therapy. J Pediatr 113:58, 1988.

Berry GT, Heidenreich R, Kaplan P, et al: Branched-chain amino acid–free parenteral nutrition in the treatment of acute metabolic decompensation in patients with maple syrup urine disease. N Engl J Med 324:175, 1991.

Berry GT, Nissim I, Zhiping L, et al: Endogenous synthesis of galactose in normal man and patients with hereditary galactosemia. Lancet 346:1073, 1995.

Bertini E, Dionisi-Vici C, Garavaglia B, et al: Peripheral sensory-motor polyneuropathy, pigmentary retinopathy, and fatal cardiomyopathy in long-chain 3-hydroxyacyl-CoA dehydrogenase deficiency. Eur J Pediatr 151:121, 1992.

Birch-Machin MA, Shepherd IM, Watmough NJ, et al: Fatal lactic acidosis in infancy with a defect of complex III of the respiratory chain. Pediatr Res 25:553, 1989.

Blass JP, Avigan J, Uhlendorf BW: A defect of pyruvate decarboxylase in a child with an intermittent movement disorder. J Clin Invest 49:423, 1970.

Blass JP, Schulman JD, Young DS, et al: An inherited defect affecting the tricarboxylic acid cycle in a patient with congenital lactic acidosis. J Clin Invest 51:1845, 1972.

Böhm N, Uy J, Kiessling M, et al: Multiple acyl-CoA dehydrogenation deficiency (glutaric aciduria type II), congenital polycystic kidneys, and symmetric warty degeneration of the cerebral cortex in two newborn brothers. II: Morphology and pathogenesis. Eur J Pediatr 139:60, 1982.

Boustany RN, Aprille JR, Halperin J, et al: Mitochondrial cytochrome deficiency presenting as a myopathy with hypotonia, external ophthalmoplegia, and lactic acidosis in an infant and as fatal hepatopathy in a second cousin. Ann Neurol 14:462, 1983.

Brown GK, Scholem RD, Hunt SM, et al: Hyperammonemia and lactic acidosis in a patient with pyruvate dehydrogenase deficiency. J Inherit Metab Dis 10:359, 1987.

Brown GK, Haan EA, Kirby DM, et al: "Cerebral" lactic acidosis: Defects in pyruvate metabolism with profound brain damage and minimal systemic acidosis. Eur J Pediatr 147:10, 1988.

Brusilow SW: Arginine, an indispensable amino acid for patients with inborn errors of urea synthesis. J Clin Invest 74:2144, 1984.

Brusilow SW: Treatment of urea cycle disorders. In Desnick RJ (ed): Treatment of Genetic Disease. New York, Churchill Livingstone, 1991, p 79.

Brusilow SW, Batashaw ML: Arginine therapy of argininosuccinase deficiency. Lancet 1:124, 1979.

Brusilow SW, Horwich AL: Urea cycle enzymes. In Scriver CR, Beaudet AL, Sly WS, et al (eds): The Metabolic and Molecular Bases of Inherited Disease, 7th ed. New York, McGraw-Hill, 1995, p 1187.

Brusilow SW, Valle DL, Batshaw ML: New pathways of nitrogen excretion in inborn errors of urea synthesis. Lancet 2:452, 1979.

Budd MA, Tanaka K, Holmes LB, et al: Isovaleric acidemia: Clinical features of a new genetic defect of leucine metabolism. N Engl J Med 277:321, 1967.

Burchell A, Waddell ID: The molecular basis of the genetic deficiencies of five of the components of the glucose-6-phosphatase system: Improved diagnosis. Eur J Pediatr 152(Suppl 1):S18, 1993.

Chalmers RA, Roe CR, Stacey TE, et al: Urinary excretion of L-carnitine and acylcarnitines by patients with disorders of organic acid metabolism: Evidence for secondary insufficiency of L-carnitine. Pediatr Res 18:1325, 1984.

Chen Y-T, Burchell A: Glycogen storage diseases. In Scriver CR, Beaudet AL, Sly WS, et al (eds): The Metabolic and Molecular Bases of Inherited Disease, 7th ed. New York, McGraw-Hill, 1995, p 935.

Childs B, Nyhan WL, Borden M, et al: Idiopathic hyperglycinemia and hyperglycinuria: A new disorder of amino acid metabolism. Pediatrics 27:522, 1961.

Chuang DT, Shih VE: Disorders of branched-chain amino acid and keto acid metabolism. In Scriver CR, Beaudet AL, Sly WS, et al (eds): The Metabolic and Molecular Bases of Inherited Disease, 7th ed. New York, McGraw-Hill, 1995, p 1239.

Ciafaloni E, Ricci E, Shanske S, et al: MELAS: Clinical features, biochemistry, and molecular genetics. Ann Neurol 31:391, 1992.

Clayton PT, Hyland K, Brand M, et al: Mitochondrial phosphoenolypyruvate carboxykinase deficiency. Eur J Pediatr 145:46, 1986.

Cohn RM, Yudkoff M, Rothman R, et al: Isovaleric acidemia: Use of glycine therapy in neonates. N Engl J Med 299:996, 1978.

Cormier V, Rotig A, Bonnefont JP, et al: Pearson's syndrome. Pancytopenia with exocrine pancreatic insufficiency: New mitochondrial disease in the first year of childhood. Arch Fr Pediatr 48:171, 1991.

Cornblath M, Schwartz R: Disorders of glycogen metabolism. In Disorders of Carbohydrate Metabolism in Infancy, 3rd ed. Boston, Blackwell Scientific, 1991, p 247.

Cornblath M, Gingell RL, Fleming GA, et al: A new syndrome of ketoacidosis in infancy. J Pediatr 79:413, 1971.

Danner DJ, Armstrong N, Heffelfinger SC, et al: Absence of branched-chain acyltransferase as a cause of maple syrup urine disease. J Clin Invest 75:858, 1985.

Daum RS, Lamm PH, Mamer OA, et al: A "new" disorder of isoleucine metabolism. Lancet 2:1289, 1971.

David M, Michel M, Collombel C, et al: Transient hypertyrosinemia secondary to hepatic involvement: Two cases of different etiologies (galactosemia, hepatitis). Pediatrie 25:459, 1970.

De Bracketeer M, Larochelle J: Genetic epidemiology of hereditary tyrosinemia in Quebec and in Saguenay-Lac St-Jean. Am J Hum Genet 47:302, 1990.

Demaugre F, Bonnefont J-P, Colonna M, et al: Infantile form of carnitine palmitoyltransferase II deficiency with hepatomuscular symptoms and sudden death: Physiopathological approach to carnitine palmitoyltransferase II deficiencies. J Clin Invest 87:859, 1991.

De Sousa C, Chalmers RA, Stacey TE, et al: The response to L-carnitine and glycine therapy in isovaleric acidaemia. Eur J Pediatr 144:451, 1986.

DeVivo D, Haymond MW, Leckie MP, et al: Clinical and biochemical implications of pyruvate carboxylase deficiency. J Clin Endocrinol Metab 45:1281, 1977.

DeVivo DC, Haymond MW, Obert KA, et al: Defective activation of the pyruvate dehydrogenase complex in subacute necrotizing encephalomyelopathy (Leigh disease). Ann Neurol 6:483, 1979.

Diliberti JH, DiGeorge AM, Auerbach VH: Abnormal leucine/isoleucine ratio and the etiology of acrodermatitis enteropathica–like rash in maple syrup urine (MSUD). Pediatr Res 7:154, 1973.

DiMauro S, DiMauro PMM: Muscle carnitine palmityltransferase deficiency and myoglobinuria. Science 182:929, 1973.

DiMauro S, Mendell JR, Sahenk Z, et al: Fatal infantile mitochondrial myopathy and renal dysfunction due to cytochrome-C-oxidase deficiency. Neurology 30:795, 1980.

DiMauro S, Nicholson JF, Hays AP, et al: Benign infantile mitochondrial myopathy due to reversible cytochrome C oxidase deficiency. Ann Neurol 14:226, 1983.

DiMauro S, Lombes A, Nakase H, et al: Cytochrome C oxidase deficiency in Leigh syndrome. Ann Neurol 22:498, 1987.

Ding J-H, Roe CR, Iafolla AK, et al: Medium-chain acyl-coenzyme A dehydrogenase deficiency and sudden infant death. N Engl J Med 325:61, 1991.

Dobyns WB: Agenesis of the corpus callosum and gyral malformations are frequent manifestations of nonketotic hyperglycinemia. Neurology 39:817, 1989.

Duran M, Wanders RJA, de Jager JP, et al: 3-Hydroxydicarboxylic aciduria due to long-chain 3-hydroxyacyl-coenzyme A dehydrogenase deficiency associated with sudden neonatal death: Protective effect of medium-chain triglyceride treatment. Eur J Pediatr 150:190, 1991.

Farrel DF, Clark AF, Scott CR, et al: Absence of pyruvate decarboxylase activity in man: A cause of congenital lactic acidosis. Science 187:1082, 1975.

Federico A, Doti MT, Fabrizi GM, et al: Congenital lactic acidosis due to a defect of pyruvate dehydrogenase complex (E1). Eur Neurol 30:123, 1990.

Fenton WA, Rosenberg LE: Disorders of propionate and methylmalonate metabolism. In Scriver CR, Beaudet AL, Sly WS, et al (eds): The Metabolic and Molecular Bases of Inherited Disease, 7th ed. New York, McGraw-Hill, 1995a, p 1423.

Fenton WA, Rosenberg LE: Inherited disorders of cobalamin transport and metabolism. In Scriver CR, Beaudet AL, Sly WS, et al (eds): The Metabolic and Molecular Bases of Inherited Disease, 7th ed. 1995b, p 3129.

Fernandes J, Chen Y-T: Glycogen storage diseases. In Fernandes J, Saudubray J-M, van den Berghe G (eds): Inborn Metabolic Diseases: Diagnosis and Treatment, 2nd ed. Berlin, Springer-Verlag, 1995, p 71.

Fernandes J, Leonard JV, Moses SW, et al: Glycogen storage disease: Recommendations for treatment. Eur J Pediatr 147:226, 1988.

Fiser RHJR, Melsher HL, Fisher DA: Hepatic phosphoenolpyruvate carboxylase (PEPCK) deficiency: A new cause of hypoglycemia in childhood. Pediatr Res 10:60, 1974.

Frerman FE, Goodman SI: Nuclear-encoded defects of the mitochondrial respiratory chain, including glutaric acidemia type II. In Scriver CR, Beaudet AL, Sly WS, et al (eds): The Metabolic and Molecular Bases of Inherited Disease, 7th ed. New York, McGraw-Hill, 1995, p 1611.

Gerritsen T, Kaveggia E, Waisman HA: A new type of idiopathic hyperglycinemia with hypooxaluria. Pediatrics 36:882, 1965.

Giacoia GP, Berry GT: Acrodermatitis enteropathica–like syndrome secondary to isoleucine deficiency during treatment of maple syrup urine disease. Am J Dis Child 147:954, 1993.

Gibson KM, Breuer J, Nyhan WL: 3-Hydroxy-3-methylglutaryl-coenzyme A lyase deficiency: Review of 18 reported patients. Eur J Pediatr 148:180, 1988.

Gibson KM, Elpeleg ON, Jakobs C, et al: Multiple syndromes of 3-methylglutaconic aciduria. Pediatr Neurol 9:120, 1993.

Gitzelmann R, Arbenz UV, Willi UV: Hypergalactosaemia and portosystemic encephalopathy due to persistence of ductus venosus Arantii. Eur J Pediatr 151:564, 1992.

Gitzelmann R, Steinmann B, Van den Berghe G: Disorders of fructose metabolism. In Scriver CR, Beaudet AL, Sly WS, et al (eds): The Metabolic and Molecular Bases of Inherited Disease, 7th edition. New York, McGraw-Hill, 1995, p 905.

Goodman SI, Frerman FE: Organic acidemias due to defects in lysine oxidation: 2-Ketoadipic acidemia and glutaric acidemia. In Scriver CR, Beaudet AL, Sly WS, et al (eds): The Metabolic and Molecular Bases of Inherited Disease, 7th ed. New York, McGraw-Hill, 1995, p 1451.

Goodman SI, Markey SP, Moe PG, et al: Glutaric aciduria: A "new" disorder of amino acid metabolism. Biochem Med 12:12, 1975.

Goto Y, Nonaka I, Horai S: A mutation in the tRNA (Leu) (UUR) gene associated with the MELAS subgroup of mitochondrial encephalomyopathies. Nature 348:651, 1990.

Gregersen G, Wintzensen H, Kolvraa S, et al: C6-C10-Dicarboxylic aciduria: Investigations of a patient with riboflavin-responsive multiple acyl-CoA dehydrogenation defects. Pediatr Res 16:861, 1982.

Hale DE, Batshaw ML, Coates PM, et al: Long-chain acyl-coenzyme A dehydrogenase deficiency: An inherited cause of nonketotic hypoglycemia. Pediatr Res 19:666, 1985.

Hamosh A, Johnston MV, Valle D: Nonketotic hyperglycinemia. In Scriver CR, Beaudet AL, Sly WS, et al (eds): The Metabolic and Molecular Bases of Inherited Disease, 7th ed. New York, McGraw-Hill, 1995, p 1337.

Harpey JP, Charpentier C, Goodman SI, et al: Multiple acyl-CoA dehydrogenase deficiency occurring in pregnancy and caused by a defect in riboflavin metabolism in the mother. J Pediatr 103:394, 1983.

Heiman PTD, Bonilla E, DiMauro S, et al: Cytochrome-C-oxidase deficiency in a floppy infant. Neurology 328:898, 1982.

Hirschhorn R: Glycogen storage disease type II: Acid a-glucosidase (acid maltase) deficiency. In Scriver CR, Beaudet AL, Sly WS, et al (eds): The Metabolic and Molecular Bases of Inherited Disease, 7th ed. New York, McGraw-Hill, 1995, p 2443.

Hoffmann GF, Trefz FK, Barth PG, et al: Glutaryl-CoA dehydrogenase deficiency: A distinct encephalopathy. Pediatrics 88:1194, 1991.

Hoganson GE, Paulson DJ, Chun R, et al: Deficiency of muscle cytochrome C oxidase in Leigh's disease. Pediatr Res 18:222, 1984.

Holt IJ, Harding AE, Morgan-Hughes JA: Deletions of muscle mitochondrial DNA in patients with mitochondrial myopathies. Nature 331:717, 1988.

Hommes FA, Bendien K, Elema JD, et al: Two cases of phosphoenolpyruvate carboxykinase deficiency. Acta Paediatr Scand 65:233, 1976.

Hoppel CL, Kerr DS, Dahms B, et al: Deficiency of the reduced nicotinamide adenine dinucleotide dehydrogenase component of complex I of mitochondrial electron transport: Fatal infantile lactic acidosis and hypermetabolism with skeletal-cardiac myopathy and encephalopathy. J Clin Invest 80:71, 1987.

Hostetter MK, Levy HL, Winter HS, et al: Evidence for liver disease preceding amino acid abnormalities in hereditary tyrosinemia. N Engl J Med 308:1265, 1983.

Hug G, Bove KE, Soukup S: Lethal neonatal multiorgan deficiency of carnitine palmitoyltransferase II. N Engl J Med 325:1862, 1991.

Hutchinson CAI, Newbold JA, Potter SS, et al: Maternal inheritance of mammalian mitochondrial DNA. Nature 251:536, 1974.

Iafolla AK, Kahler SG: Megaloencephaly in the neonatal period as the initial manifestation of glutaric aciduria type I. J Pediatr 114:1004, 1989.

Jerusalem F, Angelini C, Engel A, et al: Mitochondria-lipid-glycogen (MLG) disease of muscle: A morphologically regressive congenital myopathy. Arch Neurol 29:162, 1973.

Kelley RI, Cheatham JP, Clark BJ, et al: X-linked dilated cardiomyopathy with neutropenia, growth retardation, and 3-methylglutaconic aciduria. J Pediatr 119:738, 1991.

Krieger I, Tanaka K: Therapeutic effects of glycine in isovaleric acidemia. Pediatr Res 10:25, 1976.

Kuroda Y, Ito M, Toshima K, et al: Treatment of chronic congenital lactic acidosis by oral administration of dichloroacetate. J Inherit Metab Dis 9:244, 1986.

Lehnert W, Wendel U, Lindenmaier S, et al: Multiple acyl-CoA dehydrogenation deficiency (glutaric aciduria type II), congenital polycystic kidneys, and symmetric warty dysplasia of the cerebral cortex in two brothers. I: Clinical, metabolical, and biochemical findings. Eur J Pediatr 139:56, 1982.

Levine SZ, Marples E, Gordon HH: A defect in the metabolism of aromatic amino acids in premature infants: The role of vitamin C. Science 90:620, 1939.

Lindblad B, Lindstedt S, Steen G: On the enzyme defects in hereditary tyrosinemia. Proc Natl Acad Sci U S A 74:4641, 1977.

Lindstedt S, Holme E, Lock EA, et al: Treatment of hereditary tyrosinaemia type I by inhibition of 4-hydroxyphenylpyruvate dioxygenase. Lancet 340:813, 1992.

Luder AS, Davidson A, Goodman SI, et al: Transient nonketotic hyperglycinemia in neonates. J Pediatr 114:1013, 1989.

Lungarotti MS, Calabro A, Signorini E, et al: Cerebral edema in maple syrup urine disease. Am J Dis Child 136:648, 1982.

Majander A, Suomalainen A, Vettenranta K, et al: Congenital hypoplastic anemia, diabetes, and severe renal tubular dysfunction associated with a mitochondrial DNA deletion. Pediatr Res 30:327, 1991.

Mandel H, Szargel R, Labay V, et al: The deoxyguanosine kinase gene is mutated in individuals with depleted hepatocerebral mitochondrial DNA. Nature Genet. 29:337, 2001.

Matsumoto T, Ikano R, Sakura N, et al: Hypergalactosaemia in a patient with portal-hepatic venous and hepatic arteriovenous shunts detected by neonatal screening. Eur J Pediatr 152:990, 1993.

Mayatepek E, Kurczynski TW, Hoppel CL: Long-term L-carnitine treatment in isovaleric acidemia. Pediatr Neurol 7:137, 1991.

McCormick K, Viscardi RM, Robinson BH, et al: Partial pyruvate decarboxylase deficiency with profound lactic acidosis and hyperammonemia: Responses to dichloroacetate and benzoate. Am J Med Genet 22:291, 1985.

Menkes JH, Hurst PL, Craig JM: A new syndrome: Progressive familial infantile cerebral dysfunction associated with an unusual urinary substance. Pediatrics 14:462, 1954.

Michalski AJ, Berry GT, Segal S: Holocarboxylase synthetase deficiency: Nine-year follow-up of a case and a review of the literature. J Inherit Metab Dis 12:312, 1989.

Middleton B, Day R, Lombes A, et al: Infantile ketoacidosis associated with decreased activity of succinyl-CoA: 3-ketoacid CoA-transferase. J Inherit Metab Dis 10(Suppl 2):273, 1987.

Miranda DF, Ishii S, DiMauro S, et al: Cytochrome C oxidase (COX) deficiency in Leigh's syndrome: Genetic evidence for a nuclear DNA-encoded mutation. Neurology 39:697, 1989.

Mitchell GA, Lambert M, Tanguay RM: Hypertyrosinemia. In Scriver CR, Beaudet AL, Sly WS, et al (eds): The Metabolic and Molecular Bases of Inherited Disease, 7th ed. New York, McGraw-Hill, 1995, p 1077.

Miyabayashi S, Ito T, Narisawa K, et al: Biochemical study in 28 children with lactic acidosis in relation to Leigh's encephalomyelopathy. Eur J Pediatr 143:278, 1985.

Morales CT, DiMauro S, Zeviani M, et al: Mitochondrial DNA deletions in progressive external ophthalmoplegia and Kearns-Sayre syndrome. N Engl J Med 320:1293, 1989.

Moreadith RW, Batshaw ML, Ohnishi T, et al: Deficiency of the iron-sulfur clusters of mitochondrial-reduced nicotinamide-adenine dinucleotide-ubiquinone oxidoreductase (complex I) in an infant with congenital lactic acidosis. J Clin Invest 74:685, 1984.

Morton DH, Bennett MJ, Seargeant LE, et al: Glutaric aciduria type I: A cause of episodic encephalopathy and spastic paralysis in the Amish of Lancaster County, Pennsylvania. Am J Med Genet 41:89, 1991.

Mowat AJ, Bennett MJ, Variend S, et al: Deficiency of medium chain fatty acyl coenzyme A dehydrogenase presenting as the sudden infant death syndrome. Br Med J 288:976, 1984.

Msall M, Batshaw ML, Suss R, et al: Neurologic outcome in children with inborn errors of urea synthesis. N Engl J Med 310:1500, 1984.

Mudd SH, Levy HL, Skovby F: Disorders of trans-sulfuration. In Scriver CR, Beaudet AL, Sly WS, et al (eds): The Metabolic and Molecular Bases of Inherited Disease, 7th ed. New York, McGraw-Hill, 1995, p 1279.

Munnich A, Saudubray JM, Taylor J, et al: Congenital lactic acidosis, alpha-ketoglutaric aciduria and variant form of maple syrup urine disease due to a single enzyme defect: Dihydrolipoyl dehydrogenase deficiency. Acta Paediatr Scand 71:161, 1982.

Munnich A, Rotig A, Cormier-Daire V, Rustin P: Clinical presentation of respiratory chain deficiency. In Scriver CR, Beaudet AI, Sly WS, Valle D, Childs B, Kinzler KW, Vogelstein B (eds): The Molecular and Metabolic Bases of Inherited Disease. New York, McGraw-Hill, 2001, pp 2261-2275.

Naglak M, Salvo R, Madsen K, et al: The treatment of isovaleric acidemia with glycine supplement. Pediatr Res 24:9, 1988.

Nelson I, Bonne G, Degoul F, et al: Kearns-Sayre syndrome with sideroblastic anemia: Molecular investigations. Neuropediatrics 23:199, 1992.

Neustein HB, Lurie PR, Dahms B, et al: An X-linked cardiomyopathy with abnormal mitochondrial. Pediatrics 64:24, 1979.

Noer AS, Sudoyo H, Lertrit P, et al: A tRNA (Lys) mutation in the mtDNA is the causal genetic lesion underlying myoclonic epilepsy and ragged-red fiber (MERRF) syndrome. Am J Hum Genet 49:715, 1991.

Papadopoulou LC, Sue CM, Davidson MM, et al: Fatal infantile cardioencephalomypathy with COX deficiency and mutations in SCO2, a COX assembly gene. Nature Genet. 23:333, 1999.

Parini R, Sereni LP, Bagozzi DC, et al: Nasogastric drip feeding as the only treatment of neonatal maple syrup urine disease. Pediatrics 92:280, 1993.

Pincus JH: Subacute necrotizing encephalomyelopathy (Leigh's disease): A consideration of clinical features and etiology. Dev Med Child Neurol 14:87, 1972.

Poulton J, Deadman ME, Gardiner RM: Duplications of mitochondrial DNA in mitochondrial myopathy. Lancet 1:236, 1989.

Prick MJJ, Gabreels FJM, Trijbels JMF, et al: Progressive poliodystrophy (Alpers disease) with a defect in cytochrome aa3 in muscle: A report of two unrelated patients. Clin Neurol Neurosurg 85:57, 1983.

Przyrembel H, Wendel U, Becker K, et al: Glutaric aciduria type II: Report on a previously undescribed metabolic disorder. Clin Chim Acta 66:227, 1976.

Riviello JJ Jr, Rezvani I, diGeorge AM, et al: Cerebral edema causing death in children with maple syrup urine disease. J Pediatr 119:42, 1991.

Robinson BH: Lactic acidemia: Biochemical, clinical and genetic considerations. Adv Hum Genet 18:151, 1989.

Robinson BH: Lactic acidemia (disorders of pyruvate carboxylase, pyruvate dehydrogenase). In Scriver CR, Beaudet AL, Sly WS, et al (eds): The Metabolic and Molecular Bases of Inherited Disease, 7th ed. New York, McGraw-Hill, 1995, p 1479.

Robinson BH, Sherwood WG: Pyruvate dehydrogenase phosphatase deficiency: A cause of chronic congenital lactic acidosis in infancy. Pediatr Res 9:935, 1975.

Robinson BH, Oei J, Sherwood WG, et al: The molecular basis for the two different clinical presentations of classical pyruvate carboxylase deficiency. Am J Hum Genet 36:283, 1984.

Robinson BH, McKay N, Goodyer P, et al: Defective intramitochondrial NADH oxidation in skin fibroblasts from an infant with fatal neonatal lacticacidemia. Am J Hum Genet 37:938, 1985.

Robinson BH, MacMillan H, Petrova-Benedict R, et al: Variable clinical presentation in patients with deficiency of the pyruvate dehydrogenase complex: A review of 30 cases with a defect in the E1 component of the complex. J Pediatr 111:525, 1987.

Robinson BH, MacKay N, Petrova-Benedict R, et al: Defects in the E2 lipoyl transacetylase and the X-lipoyl containing component of the pyruvate dehydrogenase complex in patients with lactic acidemia. J Clin Invest 85:1821, 1990.

Roe CR, Coates PM: Mitochondrial fatty acid oxidation disorders. In Scriver CR, Beaudet AL, Sly WS, et al (eds): The Metabolic and Molecular Bases of Inherited Disease, 7th ed. New York, McGraw-Hill, 1995, p 1501.

Roe CR, Millington DS, Maltby DA, et al: L-Carnitine therapy in isovaleric acidemia. J Clin Invest 74:2290, 1984.

Roodhooft AM, Van AKJ, Martin JJ, et al: Benign mitochondrial myopathy with deficiency of NADH-CoQ reductase and cytochrome C oxidase. Neuropediatrics 17:221, 1986.

Rosenblatt DS: Inherited disorders of folate transport and metabolism. In Scriver CR, Beaudet AL, Sly WS, et al (eds): The Metabolic and Molecular Bases of Inherited Disease, 7th ed. New York, McGraw-Hill, 1995, p 3111.

Rotig A, Colonna M, Blanche S, et al: Mitochondrial DNA deletions in Pearson's marrow/pancreas syndrome. Lancet 1:902, 1989.

Rutledge SL, Havens PL, Haymond MW, et al: Neonatal hemodialysis: Effective therapy for the encephalopathy of inborn errors of metabolism. J Pediatr 116:125, 1990.

Saada A, Shaag A, Mandel H, et al: Mutant mitochondrial thymidine kinase in mitochondrial DNA depletion myopathy. Nature Genet. 29:342, 2001.

Sandbank U, Lerman P: Progressive cerebral poliodystrophy: Alpers disease—disorganized giant neuronal mitochondria on electron microscopy. J Neurol Neurosurg Psychiatry 35:749, 1972.

Santorelli FM, Shanske S, Jain KD, et al: A new mtDNA mutation in the ATPase 6 gene in a child with Leigh syndrome. Neurology 43:A171, 1993.

Saudubray JM, Marsac C, Charpentier C, et al: Neonatal congenital lactic acidosis with pyruvate carboxylase deficiency in two siblings. Acta Paediatr Scand 65:717, 1976.

Saudubray J-M, Martin D, Poggi-Travert F, et al: Clinical presentations of inherited mitochondrial fatty acid oxidation disorders: An update. Int Pediatr 12:34, 1997.

Schiffman R, Kaye EM, Willis JK III, et al: Transient neonatal hyperglycinemia. Ann Neurol 25:201, 1989.

Schoeman MN, Batey RG, Wilcken B: Recurrent acute fatty liver of pregnancy associated with a fatty acid oxidation defect in the offspring. Gastroenterology 100:544, 1991.

Scriver CR, Clow CL: Phenylketonuria: Epitome of human biochemical genetics (first of two parts). N Engl J Med 303:1336, 1980a.

Scriver CR, Clow CL: Phenylketonuria: Epitome of human biochemical genetics (second of two parts). N Engl J Med 303:1394, 1980b.

Scriver CR, Kaufman S, Eisensmith RC, et al: The hyperphenylalaninemias. In Scriver CR, Beaudet AL, Sly WS, et al (eds): The Metabolic and Molecular Bases of Inherited Disease, 7th ed. New York, McGraw-Hill, 1995, p 1015.

Segal S, Berry GT: Disorders of galactose metabolism. In Scriver CR, Beaudet AL, Sly WS, et al (eds): The Metabolic and Molecular Bases of Inherited Disease, 7th ed. New York, McGraw-Hill, 1996, p 967.

Sengers RCX, Trijbels JMF, Bakkeren JAJM, et al: Deficiency of cytochromes b and aa3 in muscle from a floppy infant with cytochrome C oxidase deficiency. Eur J Pediatr 141:178, 1984.

Shih VE, Herrin JT, Erickson AM: Hyperalimentation and peritoneal dialysis during acute metabolic decompensation in maple syrup urine disease. Pediatr Res 9:355, 1975.

Shoffner JM, Fernhoff PM, Krawiecki NS, et al: Subacute necrotizing encephalopathy: Oxidative phosphorylation defects and the ATPase 6 point mutation. Neurology 42:2168, 1992.

Shoffner JM, Wallace DC: Oxidative phosphorylation diseases. In Scriver CR, Beaudet AL, Sly WS, et al (eds): The Metabolic and Molecular Bases of Inherited Disease, 7th ed. New York, McGraw-Hill, 1995, p 1535.

Stacpoole PW, Harman EM, Curry SH, et al: Treatment of lactic acidosis with dichloroacetate. N Engl J Med 309:390, 1983.

Stanley CA: New genetic defects in mitochondrial fatty acid oxidation and carnitine deficiency. Adv Pediatr 34:59, 1987.

Stanley CA, Hale DE, Berry GT, et al: A deficiency of carnitine-acylcarnitine translocase in the inner mitochondrial membrane. N Engl J Med 327:19, 1992.

Stromme JH, Borud O, Moe PJ: Fatal lactic acidosis in a newborn attributable to a congenital defect of pyruvate dehydrogenase. Pediatr Res 10:60, 1976.

Sweetman L, Williams JC: Branched-chain organic acidurias. In Scriver CR, Beaudet Al, Sly WS, et al (eds): The Metabolic and Molecular Bases of Inherited Disease, 7th ed. New York, McGraw-Hill, 1995, p 1387.

Tada K, Hayasaka K: Nonketotic hyperglycinaemia: Clinical and biochemical aspects. Eur J Pediatr 146:221, 1987.

Tanaka K, Budd MA, Efron ML, et al: Isovaleric acidemia: A new genetic defect of leucine metabolism. Proc Natl Acad Sci U S A 56:236, 1966.

Tatuch Y, Chrisrodoulou J, Feigenbaum A, et al: Heteroplasmic mitochondrial DNA mutation (T to G) at 8993 can cause Leigh disease when the percentage of abnormal mtDNA is high. Am J Hum Genet 50:852, 1992.

Taylor J, Robinson BH, Sherwood WG: A defect in branched-chain amino acid metabolism in a patient with congenital lactic acidosis due to dihydrolipoyl dehydrogenase deficiency. Pediatr Res 12:60, 1978.

Thompson GN, Butt WW, Shann FA, et al: Continuous venovenous hemofiltration in the management of acute decompensation in inborn errors of metabolism. J Pediatr 118:879, 1991.

Townsend I, Kerr DS: Total parenteral nutrition therapy of toxic maple syrup urine disease. Am J Clin Nutr 36:359, 1982.

Treem WR, Stanley CA, Finegold DN, et al: Primary carnitine deficiency due to a failure of carnitine transport in kidney, muscle, and fibroblasts. N Engl J Med 319:1331, 1988.

Treem WR, Stanley CA, Hale DE, et al: Hypoglycemia, hypotonia, and cardiomyopathy: The evolving clinical picture of long-chain acyl-CoA dehydrogenase deficiency. Pediatrics 87:328, 1991.

Tritschler HJ, Bonilla E, Lombes A, et al: Differential diagnosis of fatal and benign cytochrome C oxidase–deficient myopathies of infancy: An immunohistochemical approach. Neurology 41:300, 1991.

Valnot I, Osmond S, Gigarel N, et al: Mutations of the SCO1 gene in mitochondrial cytochrome C oxidase deficiency with neonatal-onset hepatic failure and encephalopathy. Am J Hum Genet. 67:1104, 2000a.

Valnot I, von Kleist-Retzow J-C, et al: A mutation in the human heme-A:farnesyltransferase gene (COX 10) causes cytochrome c oxidase deficiency. Hum Mol Genet 9:1245, 2000b.

Van Coster RN, Fernhoff PM, DeVivo DC: Pyruvate carboxylase deficiency: A benign variant with normal development. Pediatr Res 30:1, 1991.

Velazquez A, Prieto EC: Glycine in acute management of isovaleric acidemia. Lancet 1:313, 1980.

Waber LJ, Valle D, Neill C, et al: Carnitine deficiency presenting as familial cardiomyopathy: A treatable defect in carnitine transport. J Pediatr 101:700, 1982.

Wallace DC, Singh G, Lott MT, et al: Mitochondrial DNA mutation associated with Leber's hereditary optic neuropathy. Science 242:1427, 1988.

Wendel U, Langenbeck U, Lombeck I, et al: Maple syrup urine disease: Therapeutic use of insulin in catabolic states. Eur J Pediatr 139:172, 1982.

Whyte RK, Whelan D, Hill R, et al: Excretion of dicarboxylic and ω-1 hydroxy fatty acids by low-birth-weight infants fed with medium-chain triglycerides. Pediatr Res 20:122, 1986.

Willems JL, Monnens LAH, Trijbels LMF, et al: Leigh's encephalomyelopathy in a patient with cytochrome C oxidase deficiency in muscle tissue. Pediatrics 60:850, 1977.

Wolf B: Disorders of biotin metabolism. In Scriver CR, Beaudet A, Sly WS, et al (eds): The Metabolic and Molecular Bases of Inherited Disease, 7th ed. New York, McGraw-Hill, 1995, p 3151.

Yamaguchi S, Indo Y, Coates PM, et al: Identification of very-long-chain acyl-CoA dehydrogenase deficiency in three patients previously diagnosed with long-chain acyl-CoA dehydrogenase deficiency. Pediatr Res 34:111, 1993.

Yudkoff M, Cohn RM, Pushak R, et al: Glycine therapy in isovaleric acidemia. J Pediatr 92:813, 1978.

Zeviani M, Van Dyke DH, Servidei S, et al: Myopathy and fatal cardiopathy due to cytochrome C oxidase deficiency. Arch Neurol 43:1198, 1986.

Zeviani M, Peterson P, Servidei S, et al: Benign reversible muscle cytochrome C oxidase deficiency: A second case. Neurology 37:64, 1987.

Zheng X, Shoffner JM, Lott MT, et al: Evidence in a lethal infantile mitochondrial disease for a nuclear mutation affecting respiratory complexes I and IV. Neurology 39:1203, 1989.

Zhu Z, Yao J, Johns T, et al: SURF1, encoding a factor involved in the biogenesis of cytochrome C oxidase, is mutated in Leigh syndrome. Nature Genet 20:337, 1998.

Zinn AB, Zurcher VL, Kraus F, et al: Carnitine palmitoyltransferase B (CPT B) deficiency: A heritable cause of neonatal cardiomyopathy and dysgenesis of the kidney. Pediatr Res 29:73A, 1991.

CHAPTER 23

# Lysosomal Storage, Peroxisomal, and Glycosylation Disorders and Smith-Lemli-Opitz Syndrome Presenting in the Neonate

**Janet A. Thomas, Carol L. Greene, and Robert M. Cohn**

Lysosomal storage diseases, peroxisomal disorders, congenital disorders of glycosylation (CDGs), and Smith-Lemli-Opitz syndrome (SLO syndrome) are single-gene disorders, most of which demonstrate autosomal recessive inheritance. The incidence of peroxisomal disorders is estimated to be approximately 1 in 25,000 to 50,000. No collective estimate of frequency for the many disorders of lysosomal dysfunction exists, but most individual diseases affect less than 1 in 100,000 births in the general population. The most current estimate for SLO syndrome is 1 in 20,000. A similar frequency of 1 in 20,000 is estimated for congenital disorders of glycosylation.

These four categories of metabolic diseases involve molecules important in cell membranes and share overlapping clinical presentations. Clinical presentations are heterogeneous, with a broad range of age of presentation and severity of symptoms. All are chronic and progressive. Age of onset varies from prenatal to adulthood, and severity may range from severe disability and early death to nearly normal lifestyle and life span. For each condition, interfamilial variability is greater than intrafamilial variability. The genetic and clinical characteristics of conditions in these categories that may manifest in the neonatal period (except Pompe disease, which is addressed in Chapter 22) are also summarized in the tables.

Important presentations that should lead the neonatologist to consider these disorders in the differential diagnosis are as follows:

1. "In utero infection:" hepatosplenomegaly and hepatopathy, possibly with extramedullary hematopoiesis.
2. Nonimmune hydrops fetalis and/or ichthyotic or collodion skin.
3. Neurologic only: early and often difficult to control seizures, hypertonia or hypotonia, with or without altered head size, and with or without eye findings.
4. Coarse features with bone changes, dysostosis multiplex, or osteoporosis.
5. Dysmorphic facial features with or without major malformations.
6. Rarely, known family history or positive prenatal diagnosis.

Only for the last three presentations are these conditions likely to be considered early in the differential diagnosis. Most babies with these conditions are born to healthy, nonconsanguineous couples with normal family histories, and these disorders are usually considered late, if at all, as in Case Study 1.

### CASE STUDY 1

CJ was a 2200-g girl, born to a 24-year-old mother (third pregnancy, second viable child) after a 32-week gestation, by cesarean section performed for fetal distress. Pregnancy was complicated by the finding on ultrasonography of fetal hydrops and ascites and possible hepatosplenomegaly at 24 weeks of gestation. Fetal blood sampling showed a hematocrit of 31% and elevations of γ-glutamyl-transferase (GGT) and aspartate transaminase (AST) values. Results of viral studies were negative, and chromosomes were normal. At delivery, the infant was limp and blue with a heart rate of 60 beats/min. Physical examination and chest radiograph showed marked abdominal distention, hepatosplenomegaly, multiple petechiae and bruises, a bell-shaped thorax, generalized hypotonia, talipes equinovarus, contractures at the knees, a large heart, and hazy lung fields with low volumes. Disseminated intravascular coagulopathy and evidence of liver disease, with elevated AST, GGT, and increasing hyperbilirubinemia, rapidly developed. The patient was maintained on a ventilator and treated with antibiotics for suspected sepsis.

Results of evaluations for bacterial and viral agents were negative. Metabolic studies, including ammonia, lactate, very-long-chain fatty acids (VLCFAs), and urine amino and organic acids, yielded unremarkable measurements. The white blood cells were noted to have marked toxic granularity consistent with overwhelming bacterial sepsis or metabolic storage disease.

The patient experienced continued cardiorespiratory deterioration, had bilateral pneumothoraces and pneumopericardium, and died on the third day of life. Consent for autopsy was obtained from the family. A standard autopsy was performed and showed the presence of large, membrane-bound vacuoles within hepatocytes, endothelial cells, pericytes, and bone marrow stromal cells, typical of a metabolic storage disorder. Similar cells were also found within the placenta. There was no evidence of an infectious cause. Unfortunately, because a lysosomal storage disorder was not considered as a possible etiology at the time of death, no frozen tissue or cultured fibroblasts were available to pursue the diagnosis. As a result of efforts by a research laboratory and the recurrence of disease in the couple's subsequent pregnancy, a diagnosis of β-glucuronidase deficiency, or mucopolysaccharidosis type VII, was confirmed.

### CASE STUDY 2

ME was born by normal spontaneous vaginal delivery, at full term according to dates based on early ultrasonography, with weight 2.2 kg, length 45 cm, and head circumference 31.5 cm. On the basis of physical examination, gestational age was assessed as 36 weeks. A heart murmur was noted, and investigation showed presence of a small ventricular septal defect with no hemodynamic significance. Submucous cleft palate was noted. Examination for dysmorphic features showed simple, posteriorly rotated ears, mild epicanthic folds, micrognathia, and unilateral simian crease. Tone was moderately decreased. Irritability and severe feeding problems were noted, and gavage feeding was required; growth was poor despite adequate calories. Karyotype was normal, and results of studies for velocardiofacial syndrome were negative. Vomiting developed, and further evaluation showed no acidosis, hypoglycemia, or hyperammonemia; liver-associated values and cholesterol level were normal, as were results of studies of amino acids, organic acids, and acylcarnitine profile. Vomiting became more severe and did not respond to elemental formula, and pyloric stenosis was detected. Feeding problems persisted after successful surgical correction. Delivery of more than 140 kcal/kg by gavage was poorly tolerated but did result in weight gain; however, length and head growth remained very poor.

Smith-Lemli-Opitz syndrome was suspected despite the normal cholesterol value obtained on analysis in the hospital laboratory. Studies performed in a specialized laboratory showed the 7- and 8-dehydrocholesterol values to be elevated and the cholesterol value decreased. Cholesterol supplementation led to some improvement in behavior and feeding. Decrease to 110 kcal/kg/day was tolerated without worsening of growth, and weight for height gradually returned to normal. Review of records confirmed that the pregnancy had been accurately dated by ultrasonography at 10 weeks of gestation, confirming that ME was small for gestational age and microcephalic at birth with subsequent growth typical for SLO syndrome. The incorrect assessment of gestational age as 36 weeks on examination was found to result from failure to appreciate the effect of hypotonia on the findings for gestational age. The family was counseled about autosomal recessive inheritance, including the availability of prenatal diagnosis.

**CASE STUDY 3**

HK was born at term to healthy parents by cesarean section performed for breech presentation after an otherwise uncomplicated pregnancy. Hypotonia and dysmorphic features were noted in the delivery room, including inner epicanthic folds, flat occiput, large fontanelles, shallow orbital ridges and low nasal bridge, micrognathia and redundant skin folds at the neck, and unilateral simian crease. Brushfield spots were present. Investigation of a heart murmur revealed patent ductus arteriosus and a small atrial septal defect. There was mild hepatomegaly but normal liver function, no acidosis, and no hypoglycemia. Suck was poor, and gavage feeding was required.

Karyotype was normal and there was no evidence of trisomy 21 in blood in 50 interphase cells examined; the option of skin biopsy to search further for evidence of mosaicism for trisomy 21 was considered. Thyroid function values were normal. Urine amino and organic acid values were normal, as was the acylcarnitine profile. Plasma VLFCA analysis showed elevation consistent with a diagnosis of Zellweger syndrome, along with a typical increase in pipecolic acid value and impaired capacity for fibroblast synthesis of plasmalogens. The baby died at 3 months, and autopsy showed polymicrogyria and small hepatic and renal cysts. The family was counseled about autosomal recessive inheritance, including availability of the prenatal diagnosis.

**CASE STUDY 4**

MJ presented with hypotonia at birth after an uncomplicated pregnancy. Minor dysmorphic features were noted, including high nasal bridge, large ears, and inverted nipples. Feeding difficulties were significant, and growth was poor. Findings of head ultrasonography were unremarkable, as were those of head magnetic resonance imaging, although the radiologist questioned whether the cerebellum might be slightly small. Karyotype was normal. Hypothyroidism, discovered on newborn screening, was promptly treated and closely monitored. There was no acidosis or hypoglycemia, and liver enzyme values were normal; results of amino and organic acid analyses and acylcarnitine profile were all normal.

The baby was discharged on 130 kcal/kg/day. On follow-up, growth remained poor, and development was severely delayed. At age 6 month, she was admitted to the hospital for an episode of acutely altered mental status and low blood pressure. Mild acidosis, borderline elevations of lactate and ammonia, and significant elevation of liver enzymes all resolved over the course of the hospital stay. Cardiac ultrasonography showed mild ventricular dysfunction, which also resolved. Amino and organic acid values were normal, as was the acylcarnitine profile. Urine oligosaccharide levels showed an unusual pattern, and urine mucopolysaccharide values were normal.

At 2 years of age, developmental delay remained marked, and hypotonia persisted with reflexes now absent. The creatinine phosphokinase level was normal, but liver function values were again abnormal. Because mitochondrial disease was suspected, the patient was scheduled for liver biopsy, but clotting values were abnormal. A congenital disorder of glycosylation was suspected, and a transferrin assay confirmed the diagnosis. Review of neonatal records revealed a comment from a neurology consultant about the unusual distribution of fat on the buttocks and thighs of MJ as a neonate. The family was counseled about autosomal recessive inheritance, including availability of prenatal diagnosis.

## LYSOSOMAL STORAGE DISORDERS

In this section, we first consider lysosomes in general, then the neonatal clinical presentation of individual diseases. We finish with a discussion of diagnosis and treatment.

*Lysosomes* are single–membrane-bound intracellular organelles that contain enzymes called *hydrolases*. These lysosomal enzymes are responsible for splitting large molecules into simple, low-molecular-weight compounds, which can be recycled. The material digested by lysosomes is either exogenous material taken up by endocytosis or endogenous material separated from other intracellular materials by autophagy. The common element of all compounds digested by lysosomal enzymes is that they contain a carbohydrate portion attached to a protein or lipid. These glycoconjugates include glycoproteins, glycosaminoglycans, and glycolipids.

*Glycolipids* are large molecules with carbohydrates attached to a lipid moiety. Sphingolipids, globosides, gangliosides, cerebrosides, and lipid sulfates all are glycolipids. The different classes of glycolipids are distinguished from one another primarily by different polar groups at C1. *Sphingolipids* are complex membrane lipids composed of one molecule each of the amino alcohol sphingosine, a long-chain fatty acid, and various polar head groups attached by a β-glycosidic linkage. Sphingolipids occur in the blood and nearly all tissues of the body, the highest concentration being found in the white matter of the CNS (CNS).

Additionally, various sphingolipids are components of the plasma membrane of practically all cells. The core structure of the natural sphingolipids is ceramide, a long-chain fatty acid amide derivative of sphingosine. Free ceramide, an intermediate in the biosynthesis and catabolism of glycosphingolipids and sphingomyelin, makes up 16% to 20% of the normal lipid content of the stratum corneum of the skin. Sphingomyelin, a ceramide phosphocholine, is one of the principal structural lipids of the membranes of nervous tissue.

*Cerebrosides* are a group of ceramide monohexosides with a single sugar, either glucose or galactose, and an additional sulfate group on galactose. The two most common cerebrosides are galactocerebroside and glucocerebroside. The largest concentration of galactocerebroside is found in the brain. Glucocerebroside is an intermediate in the synthesis and degradation of more complex glycosphingolipids.

*Gangliosides*, the most complex class of glycolipids, contain several sugar units and one or more sialic acid residues. Gangliosides are normal components of cell membranes and are found in high concentrations in the ganglion cells of the CNS, particularly in the nerve endings and dendrites. $G_{MI}$ is the major ganglioside in the brain of vertebrates. Gangliosides function as receptors for toxic agents, hormones, and certain viruses, are involved in cell differentiation, and may also play a role in cell-cell interaction by providing specific recognition determinants on the surface of the cells.

Ceramide oligosaccharides, *globosides*, are a family of cerebrosides that contain two or more sugar residues, usually galactose, glucose, or *N*-acetylgalactosamine. Glycosaminoglycans and oligosaccharides are essential constituents of connective tissue, parenchymal organs, cartilage, and the nervous system.

*Glycosaminoglycans*, also called *mucopolysaccharides*, are complex heterosaccharides consisting of long sugar chains rich in sulfate groups. The polymeric chains are bound to specific proteins (core proteins). *Glycoproteins* contain oligosaccharide chains (long sugar molecules) attached covalently to a peptide core. Glycosylation occurs in the endoplasmic reticulum and the Golgi apparatus. Most glycoproteins are secreted from cells and include transport proteins, glycoprotein hormones, complement factors, enzymes, and enzyme inhibitors. There is extensive diversity in the composition and structure of the oligosaccharides.

The degradation of glycolipids, glycosaminoglycans, and glycoproteins takes place especially within the lysosomes of phagocytic cells, related to histiocytes and macrophages, in any tissue or organ. A series of hydrolytic enzymes cleaves specific bonds, resulting in the sequential, stepwise removal of constituents such as sugars and sulfate, degrading the complex glycoconjugates to the level of their basic building blocks. Lysosomal storage diseases most commonly result when an inherited defect causes significantly decreased activity in one of these hydrolases. Other causes are failure of transport of an enzyme, substrate, or product. Whatever the specific etiology, incompletely metabolized molecules accumulate, especially within the tissue responsible for the catabolism of the glycoconjugate. Additional excess storage material may be excreted in the urine.

Lysosomal storage diseases are classified according to the stored compound. Clinical phenotype depends partially on the type and amount of storage substance. The disorders selected for discussion in this chapter all have known presentation in the neonatal period.

## Clinical Presentations

Table 23–1 summarizes the clinical characteristics of the neonatal presentations of the lysosomal storage disorders.

### Niemann-Pick A Disease (Acute, Sphingomyelinase Deficient)

#### Etiology

Niemann-Pick A disease is caused by a deficiency of sphingomyelinase. Sphingomyelinase catalyzes the breakdown of sphingomyelin to ceramide and phosphocholine, and its deficiency results in sphingomyelin storage within lysosomes. Cholesterol is also stored, suggesting that its metabolism is tied to that of sphingomyelin. Sphingomyelin normally makes up 5% to 20% of phospholipid in the liver, spleen, and brain. In these disorders, it may make up to 70% of the phospholipids. Patients with Niemann-Pick A disease usually have less than 5% of normal enzyme activity.

#### Clinical Features

Clinical features of this disorder may appear in utero or up to 1 year of age. Affected infants usually present with massive hepatosplenomegaly (hepatomegaly greater than splenomegaly), constipation, feeding difficulties, and vomiting with consequent failure to thrive. Patients eventually appear strikingly emaciated with a protuberant abdomen and thin extremities. Neurologic disease is evident by 6 months of age, with hypotonia, decrease or absence of deep tendon reflexes, and weakness. Later, loss of motor skills, spasticity and rigidity, and loss of vision and hearing occur. Seizures are rare. A retinal cherry-red spot is present in about half of cases, and the electroretinograhic findings are abnormal. Respiratory infections are common. The skin may have an ochre or brownish yellow color, and xanthomas have been observed. Radiographic findings consist of widening of the medullary cavities, cortical thinning of the long bones, and osteoporosis. In the brain and spinal cord, neuronal storage is widespread, leading to cytoplasmic swelling together with atrophy of the cerebellum. Bone marrow and tissue biopsies may show foam cells or sea-blue histiocytes, which represent lipid-laden cells of the monocyte-macrophage system. Similarly, vacuolated lymphocytes or monocytes may be present in the peripheral blood. Tissue cholesterol levels may be three to ten times normal, and patients may have a microcytic anemia and thrombocytopenia. Death occurs by 2 to 3 years of age.

### Niemann-Pick C Disease

#### Etiology

Niemann-Pick C disease is due to an error in the intracellular transport of exogenous low-density lipoprotein (LDL)–derived cholesterol, which leads to impaired esterification

*Text continues on page 266*

**TABLE 23–1**

**Lysosomal Storage Disorders Presenting in the Newborn Period: Genetic and Clinical Characteristics of Neonatal Presentation**

| Disorder | Onset | Facies | Neurologic Findings | Distinctive Features | Eye Findings | Cardiovascular Findings | Dysostosis Multiplex | Hepatomegaly/ Splenomegaly | Defect | Gene Location and Molecular Findings | Ethnic Predilection |
|---|---|---|---|---|---|---|---|---|---|---|---|
| Niemann-Pick disease Type A | Early infancy | Frontal bossing | Difficulty feeding, apathy, deafness, blindness, hypotonia | Brownish-yellow skin, xanthomas | Cherry-red spot (50%) | – | – | ++/+ | Sphingo-myelinase deficiency | *ASM* gene at 11p15.1-p15.4 3 of 18 mutations account for ≈92% of mutant alleles in the Ashkenazi population | 1/40,000 in Ashkenazi Jews with carrier frequency of 1/60 |
| Type C | Birth–3 mo | Normal | Develop-mental delay, vertical gaze paralysis, hypotonia, later spasticity | – | – | – | – | +/++ | Abnormal cholesterol esterifica-tion | *NPC1* gene at 18q11 accounts for >95% of cases; *HE1* gene mutations may account for remaining cases | Increased in French Canadians of Nova Scotia and Spanish Americans in the southwest United States |

*Continued*

**TABLE 23-1**

**Lysosomal Storage Disorders Presenting in the Newborn Period: Genetic and Clinical Characteristics of Neonatal Presentation—Cont'd**

| Disorder | Onset | Facies | Neurologic Findings | Distinctive Features | Eye Findings | Cardiovascular Findings | Dysostosis Multiplex | Hepatomegaly/Splenomegaly | Defect | Gene Location and Molecular Findings | Ethnic Predilection |
|---|---|---|---|---|---|---|---|---|---|---|---|
| Gaucher disease type 2 | In utero–6 mo | Normal | Poor suck and swallow, weak cry, squint, trismus, strabismus, opsoclonus, hypertonic, later flaccidity | Congenital ichthyosis, collodion skin | – | – | – | +/++ | Gluco-cerebro-sidase deficiency | 1q21; large number of mutations known; 5 mutations account for ≈97% of mutant alleles in the Ashkenazi population, but only ≈ 75% in the non-Jewish population | Panethnic |
| Krabbe disease | 3-6 mo | Normal | Irritability: tonic spasms with light or noise stimulation, seizures, hypertonia, later flaccidity | Increased CSF protein | Optic atrophy | – | – | –/– | Galacto-cerbro-sidase deficiency | 14q 24.3-q32.1; >60 mutations with some common mutations in specific populations | Increased in Scandi-navian countries and in a large Druze kindred in Israel |
| $G_{M1}$ ganglio-sidosis | Birth | Coarse | Poor suck, weak cry, lethargy, exaggerated startle, blindness, hypotonia, later spasticity | Gingival hypertrophy, edema, rashes | Cherry-red spot (50%) | – | + | +/+ | β-galacto-sidase deficiency | 3 pter-3p21; hetero-geneous mutations; common mutations in specific populations | Panethnic |

| | | | | | | | | | | | |
|---|---|---|---|---|---|---|---|---|---|---|---|
| Farber disease Type I | 2 wk-4 mo | Normal | Progressive psychomotor impairment, seizures, decreased reflexes, hypotonia | Joint swelling with nodules, hoarseness, lung disease, contractures, fever, granulomas, dysphagia, vomiting, increased CSF protein | Grayish opacification surrounding retina in some patients, subtle cherry-red spot | Occasional | – | Hepatomegaly in 50%, splenomegaly less common | Lysosomal acid ceramidase | 8p21.3-22; 9 disease-causing mutations identified | Panethnic |
| Types II and III | Birth–9 mo (≤20 mo) | Normal | | Joint swelling with nodules, hoarseness | Normal macula, ±corneal opacities | – | – | HSM less common than in type I | | 8p21.3-p22 | Panethnic |
| Type IV (neonatal) | Birth | Normal | Nodules not consistent findings | Corneal opacities (1/3) | – | – | | ++/++ | | Unknown | Panethnic |
| Congenital sialidosis | In utero–birth | Coarse, edema | Mental retardation, hypotonia | Neonatal ascites, inguinal hernias, renal disease | Corneal clouding | – | + | +/+ | Neuraminidase deficiency | *NEU 1* gene (sialidase) at 6p21 | Panethnic |
| Galactosialidosis | In utero–birth | Coarse | Mental retardation, occasional deafness, hypotonia | Ascites, edema, inguinal hernias, renal disease, telangiectasias | Cherry-red spot, corneal clouding | Cardiomegaly progressing to failure | + | +/+ | Absence of a protective protein that safeguards neuraminidase and beta-galactosidase from premature degradation | 20q13.1 | Panethnic |
| Wolman disease | First weeks of life | Normal | Mental deterioration | Vomiting, diarrhea, steatorrhea, abdominal distention, failure to thrive, anemia, adrenal calcifications | – | – | – | +/+ | Lysosomal acid lipase deficiency | 10q23.2-q23.3; variety of mutations identified | Increased in Iranian Jews and in non-Jewish and Arab populations of Galilee |

Continued

**TABLE 23–1**

**Lysosomal Storage Disorders Presenting in the Newborn Period: Genetic and Clinical Characteristics of Neonatal Presentation—Cont'd**

| Disorder | Onset | Facies | Neurologic Findings | Distinctive Features | Eye Findings | Cardiovascular Findings | Dysostosis Multiplex | Hepatomegaly/ Splenomegaly | Defect | Gene Location and Molecular Findings | Ethnic Predilection |
|---|---|---|---|---|---|---|---|---|---|---|---|
| Infantile sialic acid storage disease | In utero–birth | Coarse, dysmorphic | Mental retardation, hypotonia | Ascites, anemia, diarrhea, failure to thrive | – | Congestive heart failure | + | +/+ | Defective transport of sialic acid out of the lysosome | SLC17A5 gene at 6q | Panethnic |
| I-cell disease | In utero–birth | Coarse | Mental retardation, ±deafness | Gingival hyperplasia, restricted joint mobility, hernias | Corneal clouding | Valvular disease, congestive heart failure, cor pulmonale | ++ | +++/+++ | Lysosomal enzymes lack mannose-6-$PO_4$ recognition marker and fail to enter the lysosome (phosphotransferase deficiency, 3-subunit complex [$\alpha_2\beta_2\gamma_2$]) | Enzyme encoded by 2 genes; α and β subunits encoded by gene at 12p; γ subunit encoded by gene at 16p | Panethnic |

| | | | | | | | | | | | |
|---|---|---|---|---|---|---|---|---|---|---|---|
| Mucolipidosis type IV | Birth–3 mo | Normal | Mental retardation, hypotonia | – | Severe corneal clouding, retinal degeneration, blindness | – | – | –/– | Unknown; some patients with partial deficiency of ganglioside sialidase | *MCOLN1* gene at 19p13.2-13.3 encoding mucolipin; 2 founder mutations accounting for 95% of mutant alleles in Ashkenazi population | Increased in Ashkenazi Jews |
| Mucopolysaccharidosis type VII | In utero–childhood | Variable coarseness | Mild–severe mental retardation | Hernias | Variable corneal clouding | Variable | ++ | Variable | β-Glucuronidase deficiency | *GUSB* gene at 7q21.2-q22; heterogeneous mutations | Panethnic |

CSF, cerebrospinal fluid; HSM, hepatosplenomegaly; –, not seen; +, typically present, usually not severe; ++, usually present, and moderately severe; +++, always present, usually severe.

of cholesterol and trapping of unesterified cholesterol in lysosomes. Cell lines from patients can be divided into two complementation groups, NPC1 and NPC2, corresponding to different genes (Millat et al, 2001). In each group, the primary defect is abnormal cholesterol esterification, but the enzyme responsible for cholesterol esterification, acyl–coenzyme A (CoA):cholesterol acyltransferase (ACAT), is not deficient. The storage of sphingomyelin is secondary. It has been suggested that the defect is in the transport of cholesterol out of the lysosome, making cholesterol unavailable to ACAT (Natowicz et al, 1995). Sphingomyelinase activity appears normal or elevated in most tissues but partially deficient (60% to 70%) in fibroblasts from most patients with this disorder. Storage of sphingomyelin in tissues is much less than in Niemann-Pick A or B disease and is accompanied by additional storage of unesterified cholesterol, phospholipids, and glycolipids in the liver and spleen. Only glycolipids are increased in the brain.

### Clinical Features

The age of onset, clinical features, and natural history of Niemann-Pick C disease are highly variable. Onset may occur from birth to 18 years of age. Fifty percent of children with onset in the neonatal period have conjugated hyperbilirubinemia, which usually resolves spontaneously but is followed by neurologic symptoms later in childhood. In the severe infantile form, hepatosplenomegaly is common, accompanied by hypotonia and delayed motor development. Further mental regression is usually evident by the age of 1 to 1.5 years, in association with behavior problems, vertical supranuclear ophthalmoplegia, progressive ataxia, dystonia, spasticity, dementia, drooling, dysphagia, and dysarthria. Seizures are rare. Foam cells and sea-blue histiocytes may be found in many tissues. Neuronal storage with cytoplasmic ballooning, inclusions, meganeurites, and axonal spheroids are also seen. Death may occur in infancy or as late as the third decade. Niemann-Pick C disease may also manifest as fatal neonatal liver disease, often misdiagnosed as fetal hepatitis. Patients with mutations in the *NPC2* gene (*HE1*) may have remarkable features consisting of pronounced pulmonary involvement leading to early death due to respiratory failure (Millat et al, 2001).

## Gaucher Disease Type 2 (Acute Neuropathic)

### Etiology

Three types of Gaucher disease have been defined. Type 1, the nonneuropathic form, is the most common type and is distinguished from types 2 and 3 by the lack of CNS involvement. Type 1 disease most commonly manifests in early childhood but may do so in adulthood. Type 2 disease, the acute neuropathic form, is characterized by infantile onset of severe CNS involvement. Type 3 disease, the subacute neuropathic form, is also late in onset with slow neurologic progression. Almost all types of Gaucher disease are caused by a deficiency of lysosomal glucocerebrosidase and result in the storage of glucocerebroside in visceral organs; the brain is affected in types 2 and 3. Although there is significant variability in clinical presentation among individuals with the same mutations, there is a clear correlation between certain mutations and clinical symptoms involving the CNS (Beutler and Grabowski, 2001). The enzyme splits glucose from cerebroside, yielding ceramide and glucose. A few patients with Gaucher disease type 2 have a deficiency of saposin C, a cohydrolase required by glucocerebrosidase.

### Clinical Features

Typically, the age of onset of Gaucher disease type 2 is approximately 3 months, consisting of hepatosplenomegaly (splenomegaly predominates) with subsequent neurologic deterioration. Hydrops fetalis, congenital ichthyosis, and collodion skin, however, are well-described presentations (Fujimoto et al, 1995; Ince et al, 1995; Lipson et al, 1991; Liu et al, 1988; Sherer et al, 1993; Sidransky et al, 1992). In a review of 18 cases of Gaucher disease manifesting in the newborn period, Sidransky and associates (1992) found 8 of the patients to have associated dermatologic findings and 6 patients to have presented with hydrops. The etiology of the association of such findings and Gaucher disease is unclear, although the enzyme deficiency appears to be directly responsible (Sidransky et al, 1992). Ceramides have been shown to be major components of the intracellular bilayers in epidermal stratum corneum and play an important role in skin homeostasis (Fujimoto et al, 1995). Thus, Gaucher disease should be considered in the differential diagnosis for infants presenting with hydrops fetalis and congenital ichthyosis. For the subset of patients presenting prenatally or at birth, death frequently occurs within hours to days, or at least within 2 to 3 months.

## Krabbe Disease (Globoid Cell Leukodystrophy)

### Etiology

The non-eponymic synonym for Krabbe disease, globoid cell leukodystrophy, is derived from the finding of large numbers of multinuclear macrophages in the cerebral white matter that contain undigested galactocerebroside. Disease is caused by a deficiency of lysosomal galactocerebroside β-galactosidase, which normally degrades galactocerebroside to ceramide and galactose. Deficiency of the enzyme results in storage of galactocerebroside. Galactocerebroside is present almost exclusively in myelin sheaths. Accumulation of a toxic metabolite, psychosine, also a substrate for the enzyme, has been postulated to lead to early destruction of the oligodendroglia. Impaired catabolism of galactosylceramide is also important in the pathogenesis of the disease.

### Clinical Features

Age of onset ranges from the first weeks of life to adulthood. The typical age of onset of infantile Krabbe disease is between 3 and 6 months, but there are cases of very early onset in which neurologic symptoms are evident within weeks after birth. Symptoms and signs are confined to the nervous system; no visceral involvement is present. The clinical course has been divided into three stages. In stage I, patients who appeared relatively normal after birth present with hyperirritability, vomiting, episodic fevers, hyperesthesia, tonic spasms with light or noise stimulation, stiffness, and seizures. Peripheral neuropathy is present, but reflexes are increased. Stage II is marked by CNS deterioration and hypertonia that progresses to hypotonia and flaccidity. Deep tendon reflexes are eventually lost. Patients with stage III disease are decerebrate, deaf, and blind with hyperpyrexia, hypersalivation, and frequent seizures. Routine laboratory findings are unremarkable with the exception of an elevation of cerebrospinal fluid protein. Cerebral atrophy and demyelination become evident in the CNS, and segmental demyelination, axonal degeneration, fibrosis, and macrophage infiltration are common in the peripheral nervous system. The segmental demyelination of peripheral nerves is demonstrated by the finding of decreased motor nerve conduction. The white matter is severely depleted of all lipids, especially glycolipids, and nerve and brain biopsies show globoid cells. Death from hyperpyrexia, respiratory complications, or aspiration occurs at a median age of 13 months.

## $G_{M1}$ Gangliosidosis

### Etiology

Infantile $G_{M1}$ gangliosidosis is caused by deficiency of lysosomal β-galactosidase. The enzyme cleaves the terminal galactose in a β linkage from oligosaccharides, keratan sulfate, and $G_{M1}$ ganglioside. Deficiency of the enzyme results in storage of $G_{M1}$ ganglioside and oligosaccharides. Clinical severity correlates with the extent of substrate storage and residual enzyme activity. The same enzyme is deficient in Morquio disease type B.

### Clinical Features

Age of onset ranges from prenatal to adult life. Infantile or type 1 $G_{M1}$ gangliosidosis may be evident at birth as coarse and thick skin, hirsutism on the forehead and neck, and coarse facial features consisting of a puffy face, frontal bossing, depressed nasal bridge, maxillary hyperplasia, large and low-set ears, wide upper lip, moderate macroglossia, and gingival hypertrophy. These dysmorphic features, however, are not always obvious in the neonate. A retinal cherry-red spot is seen in 50% of patients, and corneal clouding is often observed. Shortly after birth, or by 3 to 6 months of age, failure to thrive and hepatosplenomegaly become evident, as does neurologic involvement with poor development, hyperreflexia, hypotonia, and seizures. Cranial imaging shows diffuse atrophy of the brain, enlargement of the ventricular system, and evidence of myelin loss in the white matter.

The neurologic deterioration is progressive, resulting in generalized rigidity and spasticity and sensorimotor and psychointellectual dysfunction. By 6 months of age, skeletal features are present, including kyphoscoliosis and stiff joints with generalized contractures, and striking bone changes are seen—vertebral beaking in the thoracolumbar region, broadening of the shafts of the long bones with distal and proximal tapering, and widening of the metacarpal shafts with proximal pinching of the four lateral metacarpals. Tissue biopsies demonstrate neurons filled with membranous cytoplasmic bodies and various types of inclusions as well as foam cells in the bone marrow. Death generally occurs before 2 years of age. A severe neonatal-onset type of $G_{M1}$ gangliosidosis with cardiomyopathy has also been described (Kohlschütter et al, 1982).

## Farber Lipogranulomatosis

### Etiology

Farber lipogranulomatosis results from a deficiency of lysosomal acid ceramidase. Ceramidase catalyzes the degradation of ceramide to its long-chain base, sphingosine, and a fatty acid. Clinical disease is a consequence of storage of ceramide in various organs and body fluids.

### Clinical Features

Four types of Farber lipogranulomatosis may manifest in the neonatal period. Type I, classic disease, is a unique disorder with onset from approximately 2 weeks to 4 months of age. Patients present with hoarseness progressing to aphonia, feeding and respiratory difficulties, poor weight gain, and intermittent fever due to granuloma formation and swelling of the epiglottis and larynx. Palpable nodules appear over joints and pressure points, and joints become painful and swollen. Later, joint contractures and pulmonary disease appear. Liver and cardiac involvement may occur, and patients may have a subtle retinal cherry-red spot. Severe and progressive psychomotor impairment may occur, as may seizures, decreased deep tendon reflexes, hypotonia, and muscle atrophy. Affected patients die in early infancy, usually from pulmonary disease.

Type 2, or intermediate, Farber lipogranulomatosis manifests from birth to 9 months of age as joint and laryngeal involvement and nodules. Death occurs in early childhood. Type 3 , or mild, disease, manifests slightly later, from approximately 2 months to 20 months of age, with survival into the third decade. Clinically, types 2 and 3 are both dominated by subcutaneous nodules, joint deformity, and laryngeal involvement. Liver and pulmonary involvement may be absent. Two thirds of patients have a normal intelligence quotient. Type 4, or neonatal visceral, Farber lipogranulomatosis manifests at birth as hepatosplenomegaly due to massive histiocyte infiltration of the liver and spleen, with infiltration also in the lungs, thymus, and lymphocytes. Subcutaneous nodules and laryngeal involvement may be subtle. Death occurs by 6 months of age.

In all types of Farber lipogranulomatosis, tissue biopsies show granulomatous infiltration, foam cells, and lysosomes with comma-shaped, curvilinear tubular structures called *Farber bodies*. Cerebrospinal fluid protein may be elevated in patients with type I disease.

## Sialidosis

### Etiology

Sialidosis is caused by a deficiency of neuraminidase, which is responsible for the cleavage of terminal sialyl linkages of several oligosaccharides and glycopeptides. The defect results in the multisystem lysosomal accumulation of sugars rich in sialic acid.

### Clinical Features

Type I sialidosis is characterized by retinal cherry-red spots and generalized myoclonus with onset generally in the second decade of life. Type II is distinguished from type I by the early onset of a progressive, severe phenotype with somatic features. Type II is often subdivided into juvenile, infantile, and congenital forms. Congenital sialidosis begins in utero and manifests at birth as coarse features, facial edema, hepatosplenomegaly, ascites, hernias, and hypotonia, and, occasionally, frank hydrops fetalis. Radiographs demonstrate dysostosis multiplex and epiphyseal stippling. Delayed mental development is quickly apparent. The patient may have recurrent infections. Severely dilated coronary arteries, excessive retinal vascular tortuosity, and an erythematous macular rash may also be features of this disease (Buchholz et al, 2001). Most patients are stillborn or die before 1 year of age. Age of onset for the infantile form of sialidosis ranges from birth to 12 months. Clinical features are coarse features, organomegaly, dysostosis multiplex, retinal cherry-red spot, and mental retardation. Death occurs by the second or third decade. In both types of sialidosis, vacuolated cells can be seen in almost all tissues, and bone marrow foam cells are present.

## Galactosialidosis

### Etiology

Galactosialidosis results from a deficiency of two lysosomal enzymes, neuraminidase and β-galactosidase. The primary defect in galactosialidosis has been found to be a defect in protective protein–cathepsin A (PPCA), an intralysosomal protein that protects the two enzymes from premature proteolytic processing. The protective protein has catalytic as well as protective functions, and the two functions appear to be distinct. Deficiency of the enzymes results in the accumulation of sialyloligosaccharides in tissue lysosomes and in excreted body fluids.

### Clinical Features

Galactosialidosis has been divided into three phenotypic subtypes on the basis of age of onset and severity of clinical manifestations. Most patients present in adolescence and adulthood, but early infantile and late infantile presentations occur. Patients with early infantile galactosialidosis present between birth and 3 months of age with ascites, edema, coarse facial features, inguinal hernias, proteinuria, hypotonia, and telangiectasias, and, occasionally, frank hydrops fetalis. Patients subsequently demonstrate organomegaly, including cardiomegaly progressing to cardiac failure, psychomotor delay, and skeletal changes, particularly in the spine. Ocular abnormalities, including corneal clouding and retinal cherry-red spots, may occur. Death occurs at an average age of 8 months, usually from cardiac and renal failure. Galactosialidosis may be a cause of recurrent fetal loss or recurrent hydrops fetalis.

Late infantile galactosialidosis manifests in the first months of life as coarse facial features, hepatosplenomegaly, and skeletal changes consistent with dysostosis multiplex. Cherry-red spots and corneal clouding may also be present. Neurologic involvement may be absent or mild. Valvular heart disease is a common feature, as is growth retardation, partially because of spinal involvement and often in association with muscular atrophy. Early death is not a feature of the late infantile form. In all forms of galactosialidosis, vacuolated cells in blood smears and foam cells in bone marrow are present.

## Wolman Disease

### Etiology

Wolman disease is caused by deficiency of lysosomal acid lipase, an enzyme involved in cellular cholesterol homeostasis and responsible for the hydrolysis of cholesterol esters and triglycerides. The result of the enzyme deficiency is the defective release of free cholesterol from lysosomes, which leads to up-regulation of the LDL receptors and 3-hydroxy-3-methylglutaryl-CoA reductase activity. De novo synthesis of cholesterol and activation of receptor-mediated endocytosis of LDL then occur, leading to further deposition of lipid in the lysosomes. The result is the accumulation of cholesterol esters and triglycerides in most tissues of the body, including the liver, spleen, lymph nodes, heart, blood vessels, and brain. An extreme level of lipid storage occurs in the cells of the small intestine, particularly in the mucosa. Additionally, the neurons of the myenteric plexus demonstrate a high level of storage, with evidence of neuronal cell death, which may account for the prominence of gastrointestinal symptoms (Wolman, 1995).

### Clinical Features

Patients with Wolman disease present within weeks of birth with evidence of malnutrition and malabsorption, including symptoms of vomiting, diarrhea, steatorrhea, failure to thrive, abdominal distention, and hepatosplenomegaly. Adrenal calcifications may be seen on radiographs, and adrenal insufficiency appears. The presence of adrenal calcifications in association with hepatosplenomegaly and gastrointestinal symptoms is strongly suggestive of Wolman disease. Later, mental deterioration becomes apparent. Laboratory findings include anemia secondary to foam cell infiltration of the bone marrow and evidence of adrenal insufficiency. The serum cholesterol level is normal. Death usually occurs before 1 year of age.

## Infantile Sialic Acid Storage Disease

### Etiology

A defective lysosomal sialic acid transporter that is responsible for the efflux of sialic acid and other acidic monosaccharides from the lysosomal compartment is the cause of infantile sialic acid storage disease. The defective transporter results in greater storage of free sialic acid and glucuronic acid within the lysosomes and increased sialic acid excretion.

### Clinical Features

Infantile sialic acid storage disease often manifests at birth as mildly coarse features, hepatosplenomegaly, ascites, hypopigmentation, and generalized hypotonia. Mild dysostosis multiplex may be seen on radiographs. Failure to thrive and severe mental and motor retardation soon appear. Cardiomegaly may be present. Corneas are clear, but albinoid fundi have been reported (Lemyre et al, 1999). Vacuolated cells are seen on tissue biopsy, and electron microscopy demonstrates swollen lysosomes filled with finely granular material. CNS changes include myelin loss, axonal spheroids, gliosis, and neuronal storage. Death occurs in early childhood. Infantile sialic acid storage disease may also manifest as fetal ascites, nonimmune fetal hydrops, or infantile nephrotic syndrome (Lemyre et al, 1999).

### I-Cell Disease (Mucolipidosis Type II)

#### Etiology

In normal cells, targeting of the enzymes to the lysosomes is mediated by receptors that bind a mannose-6-phosphate recognition marker on the enzyme. The recognition marker is synthesized in a two-step reaction in the Golgi complex, and it is the enzyme that catalyzes the first step of this process, uridine diphosphate–*N*-acetylglucosamine: lysosomal enzyme *N*-acetylglucosaminyl-1-phosphotransferase, that is defective in I-cell disease. As a result, the enzymes lack the mannose-6-phosphate recognition signal, and the newly synthesized lysosomal enzymes are secreted into the extracellular matrix instead of being targeted to the lysosome. Consequently, multiple lysosomal enzymes are found in the plasma in 10 to 20 times their normal concentrations. Affected cells, especially fibroblasts, show dense inclusions of storage material that probably consists of oligosaccharides, glycosaminoglycans, and lipids. These are the "inclusion bodies" from which the disease name is derived.

#### Clinical Features

I-cell disease may manifest at birth as coarse features, corneal clouding, organomegaly, hypotonia, and gingival hyperplasia. Birth weight and length are often below normal. Kyphoscoliosis, lumbar gibbus, and restricted joint movement are often present, and there may be hip dislocation, fractures, hernias, or bilateral talipes equinovarus. Dysostosis multiplex may be seen on radiographs. Severe psychomotor retardation, evident by 6 months of age, and progressive failure to thrive occur. The facial features become progressively more coarse with a high forehead, puffy eyelids, epicanthal folds, flat nasal bridge, anteverted nares, and macroglossia. Linear growth slows during the first year of life and halts completely thereafter. The skeletal involvement is also progressive, with the development of increasing joint immobility and claw-hand deformities. Respiratory infections, otitis media, and cardiac involvement are common complications. Death usually occurs in the first decade of life due to cardiorespiratory complications.

### Mucolipidosis Type IV

#### Etiology

Although mucolipidosis type IV is associated with a partial deficiency of the lysosomal enzyme, ganglioside sialidase, it is not certain that the deficiency is the root cause of the disorder. Nevertheless, deficiency of this enzyme causes lysosomal storage of gangliosides and glycosaminoglycans. Mutations in a novel transient receptor potential cation channel gene have been found in patients with mucolipidosis type IV (Sun et al, 2000). The gene, *MCOLN1*, encodes a protein, mucolipin 1, which is a member of a new protein family of unknown function (Bach, 2001).

#### Clinical Features

The age of onset for mucolipidosis type IV ranges from infancy to 5 years. Presenting features are corneal clouding, retinal degeneration, blindness, hypotonia, and mental retardation. Survival of affected patients into the fourth decade has been reported (Chitayat et al, 1991). Cytoplasmic inclusions are noted in the conjunctiva, fibroblasts, liver, and spleen.

### Mucopolysaccharidosis Type VII (Sly Disease)

#### Etiology

Sly disease is a member of a group of lysosomal storage disorders that are caused by a deficiency of enzymes catalyzing the stepwise degradation of glycosaminoglycans. Skeletal and neurologic involvement is variable. There is a wide spectrum of clinical severity among the mucopolysaccharidoses and even within a single enzyme deficiency. Most of these disorders manifest in childhood, but type VII is included in this chapter because of its well-recognized neonatal and infantile presentations. Sly disease is caused by β-glucuronidase deficiency and results in lysosomal accumulation of glycosaminoglycans, including dermatan sulfate, heparan sulfate, and chondroitin sulfate, causing cell, tissue, and organ dysfunction.

#### Clinical Features

Sly disease may manifest as a wide spectrum of severity. Patients with the early-onset or neonatal form may present with coarse features, hepatosplenomegaly, moderate dysostosis multiplex, hernias, and nonprogressive mental retardation. Corneal clouding is variably present. Frequent episodes of pneumonia during the first year of life are common. Short stature becomes evident. Granulocytes have coarse metachromic granules. A severe neonatal form associated with hydrops fetalis, and, frequently, early death has been recognized. Milder forms of the disease with later onset are also known.

## Diagnosis, Management, and Prognosis

Growing recognition of lysosomal storage disorders in the neonate has led to expansion of the spectrum of possible clinical presentation in the newborn period. Diagnostic tools and options for treatment also continue to advance, and any textbook is likely to be out of date, especially with respect to therapeutic options, immediately upon publication. For example, efforts are currently under way to develop newborn screening for mucopolysaccharidoses (Whitley et al, 2002), with the goal to offer treatment with enzyme infusion or bone marrow transplantation (BMT) to affected babies (Vogler et al, 1999). The neonatologist is urged to work closely with appropriate experts to explore diagnostic and treatment protocols on an individual basis.

Recognition of lysosomal storage disorders in the newborn period can be difficult because they often mimic more common causes of illness in newborns, such as respiratory distress, nonimmune hydrops fetalis, liver disease, and sepsis. The initial step in the diagnosis of these disorders is, therefore, to consider them in the differential diagnosis for a sick or unusual-appearing newborn. At times, the phenotype may suggest a specific diagnosis, such as respiratory distress and painful, swollen joints in Farber lipogranulomatosis or gastrointestinal symptoms, hepatosplenomegaly, and adrenal calcifications in Wolman disease. Subtle dysmorphic features, coarsening of features, and radiographic evidence of dysostosis multiplex are also strong indications that lysosomal storage disorders should be considered. Routine laboratory findings are often normal or nonspecific. Affected infants do not have episodes of acute metabolic decompensation. Anemia and thrombocytopenia may be seen due to bone marrow involvement. Vacuolated cells may be found in peripheral blood, but absence of this finding does not rule out lysosomal storage disease. Elevated cerebrospinal fluid protein is seen in Krabbe disease and Farber lipogranulomatosis type I.

Directed analysis of urine is helpful for those conditions in which characteristic metabolites are excreted in urine. One- or two-dimensional electrophoresis or thin-layer chromatography can detect excess excretion of urine glycosaminoglycans, oligosaccharides, or free sialic acid, but all urinary tests for the diagnosis of lysosomal storage disorders can have false-negative results. Examination of the bone marrow or other tissues may demonstrate storage macrophages in Gaucher disease and in Niemann-Pick A and C diseases. Small skin or conjunctival biopsy specimens may demonstrate storage within lysosomes in most of these disorders.

Definitive diagnosis for all lysosomal storage disorders, with the exception of Niemann-Pick C disease, is confirmed by enzymatic assays in serum, leukocytes, fibroblasts, or a combination of these. The diagnosis of Niemann-Pick C disease requires measurement of cellular cholesterol esterification and documentation of a characteristic pattern of filipin-cholesterol staining in cultured fibroblasts during LDL uptake. Analysis of DNA mutations may be helpful for the diagnosis of Gaucher disease and some other conditions. Additionally, prenatal diagnosis is available for most lysosomal storage disorders through the use of enzyme assays performed on amniocytes or chorionic villus cells or measurements of levels of stored substrate in cultured cells or amniotic fluid.

These conditions must also be considered in the dying infant, and the neonatologist must be prepared to request the appropriate samples for diagnosis at the time of death. In the surviving patients, treatment and management must be considered. All of the lysosomal storage disorders are chronic and progressive conditions for which there is no curative treatment. Gene transfer therapy holds promise but is not currently available for lysosomal storage disorders. With few exceptions, current standard medical management is supportive and palliative. Patients must be continually reassessed for evidence of disease progression and associated complications. These complications, which may include hydrocephalus, valvular heart disease, joint limitation, and obstructive airway disease, manifest at variable ages.

For several disorders, particularly neonatal Gaucher disease and Niemann-Pick C disease, splenectomy may be indicated to improve severe anemia and thrombocytopenia. This procedure enhances the risk of serious infections, however, and may accelerate the progression of the disease at other sites. Patients with Krabbe disease may suffer from significant pain from radiculopathy and spasms, and alleviation of that pain is important for the comfort of the patient. The administration of the glutamic acid transaminase inhibitor vigabatrin has been used in a small number of patients with Krabbe disease, because part of the pathology may involve a secondary deficiency of γ-aminobutyric acid (Barth, 1995). Low-dose morphine has also been reported to improve the irritability associated with this disorder (Stewart et al, 2001).

Enzyme replacement therapy is available for Gaucher disease. Alglucerase (Ceredase), replacement enzyme purified from placentas, and imiglucerase (Cerezyme), recombinant enzyme, are available for use in affected patients. Although enzyme replacement therapy has successfully reversed many of the systemic manifestations of the disease, it has been suggested that enzyme replacement therapy should not be given to patients with Gaucher disease type 2 who already have severe neurologic signs, because no substantial improvement has been demonstrated to occur in the neurologic symptoms of patients treated (Erikson et al, 1993; Gaucher disease, 1996).

Bone marrow transplantation has been tried for a variety of lysosomal storage disorders. The rationale for the procedure is that circulating blood cells derived from the transplanted marrow become a source of the missing enzyme. Results of bone marrow transplantation in disorders of glycosaminoglycans show that after successful engraftment, leukocyte and liver tissue enzyme activity normalizes, organomegaly decreases, and joint mobility increases. Skeletal abnormalities stabilize but do not improve. Whether brain function can be improved in patients with CNS disease remains questionable. Some patients maintained their learning capability or intelligence quotient, but others continued to deteriorate. Clinical experience and studies in animal models indicate that BMT before the onset of neurologic symptoms can prevent or delay the occurrence of symptoms, whereas there is no clear benefit if transplantation is performed when symptoms are already present (Hoogerbrugge et al, 1995). BMT in patients with nonneuropathic Gaucher disease may result in complete disappearance of all symptoms. The procedure is associated with significant risks, however (Hoogerbrugge et al, 1995), which must be balanced against lifelong enzyme replacement therapy. Currently, it is unclear to what extent patients with the neuropathic types of Gaucher disease (types 2 and 3) would benefit from transplantation.

BMT has also been attempted in a small number of patients with infantile Krabbe disease, Farber lipogranulomatosis, and Niemann-Pick A disease. The outcome after transplantation for these few patients has been poor, with continued disease progression and death. Krivit and associates (2000) reported successful long-term bone marrow engraftment in a patient with Wolman disease that resulted in normalization of peripheral leukocyte lysosomal acid lipase enzyme activity; the patient's diarrhea resolved, cholesterol, triglyceride and liver function values normalized, and the patient was gaining developmental milestones. Lysosomal storage diseases are not all equally amenable to BMT, and the use of BMT as a treatment modality for most lysosomal storage disorders remains uncertain. In a small number of cases, BMT has been performed in utero after prenatal diagnosis showing an affected infant, and experimental protocols are available for families who wish to pursue this option.

The goal of therapy for a dietary protocol proposed for the treatment of Wolman disease is lessened accumulation of storage material in the intestine and phagocytes. The diet, which should be started as soon as the diagnosis of Wolman disease is suspected, consists of (1) discontinuing breast-feeding or feeding with a formula containing triglycerides and cholesterol esters and (2) keeping the infant on a fatty ester–free diet (Wolman, 1995). The diet should include all the necessary vitamins, including the fat-soluble vitamins. In addition, daily smearing of the skin of a different extremity with a small amount (10 to 50 μL) of sunflower or safflower oil or preferably soy, canola, flax, cod liver, or algal oil is required for the prevention of essential fatty acid deficiency, which complicates the restricted diet (Wolman, 1995). The absorption of fatty acids through the skin spares the gastrointestinal tract from accumulation and is associated with the formation of phospholipids and triglycerides (Wolman, 1995). Preliminary results of this approach suggest that treatment appears to halt disease progression.

## CONGENITAL DISORDERS OF GLYCOSYLATION

### Etiology

Congenital disorders of glycosylation, previously called "carbohydrate deficient glycoprotein syndromes," are a group of disorders similar to the lysosomal storage diseases. In these conditions, there may be liver disease characterized by fibrosis, and electron microscopy shows myelin-like and granular lysosomal inclusions as well as abnormalities of the endoplasmic reticulum in hepatocytes. These disorders are due to the partial deficiency of carbohydrates on many glycoproteins with evidence of a defect in the addition of *N*-linked carbohydrates. Abnormalities of all classes of glycoproteins have been identified in CDG. These disorders are due to defective post-translational *N*-glycosylation of numerous proteins. Glycosylation occurs frequently and serves a number of functions, such as aiding in correct folding of the nascent protein, participating in cell adhesion phenomena, protecting against premature proteolytic destruction, and modifying biologic function. Given the ubiquitous occurrence of glycoproteins, it is not surprising that CDGs display diverse clinical manifestations. The description and classification of this group of disorders continue to expand (Jaeken et al, 2001).

Two main classes of congenital disorders of glycosylation are distinguished, and eleven subcategories of CDG type I (CDG-I) have been identified (types Ia through Ik), with Ia remaining the "classic" as well as the most common presentation. The basic defect in CDG-Ia has been shown to be a deficiency of the enzyme, phosphomannomutase, an enzyme required for the early steps of protein glycosylation (Jaeken et al, 2001; van Schaftingen and Jaeken, 1995). Type I CDG appear to be caused by defects in the biosynthesis of the dolichol-linked precursor oligosaccharides and their transfer to proteins (Westphal et al, 2000). This results in an insufficient amount of precursor oligosaccharide for glycosylation or an oligosaccharide that is poorly transferred to the protein. Type II disorders, of which four forms have been described (IIa through IId), appear to result from defects in oligosaccharide processing, the addition of other kinds of sugar chains to the proteins, or both (Westphal et al, 2000).

A number of patients with features of CDG defy disease classification, as no specific biochemical defect has been identified. The number of patients described with CGS-II and unclassified CDG-x remains small. Because there are more than 40 enzyme and transport steps in the *N*-glycosylation pathway, one can anticipate that additional defects will be identified. Table 23–2 summarizes the current clinical and biochemical information on CDG. Autosomal recessive inheritance is most likely for all forms of CDG.

### Clinical Features

The clinical spectrum of CDG continues to expand as greater understanding of its biochemistry permits recognition of additional conditions and clinical variability (Grunewald and Matthijs, 2000). Patients with CDG-Ia present at birth with dysmorphic features, consisting of high nasal bridge, prominent jaw, large ears, and inverted nipples, feeding difficulties and subsequent growth failure, hypotonia, lipocutaneous abnormalities (including prominent fat pads on the buttocks), and mild to moderate hepatomegaly. The clinical progression of this disorder is divided into four stages. In stage I, the infantile, multisystem stage, patients show evidence of multisystem involvement, including variable stroke-like episodes, thrombotic disease, liver dysfunction, pericardial effusions and cardiomyopathy, proteinuria, and retinal degeneration. The coagulopathy likely stems from the number of clotting and anti-clotting proteins that are *N*-linked glycoproteins. Mental retardation, peripheral neuropathy, and decreased nerve conduction velocities are observed. Strabismus and alternating esotropia are present in nearly all patients, and retinitis pigmentosa and abnormalities of the electroretinogram in most. Cranial imaging shows varying degrees of cerebral, cerebellar, and brainstem hypoplasia. Electroencephalogram results are usually normal. Liver biopsies typically show steatosis and fibrosis, and multicystic changes in the kidneys have been noted.

Stage II, the childhood stage, is characterized by ataxia and mental retardation. Skeletal abnormalities may become more prominent, consisting of contractures, kyphoscoliosis, pectus carinatum, and short stature. Stage III, generally occurring in the teenage years, is characterized primarily by lower extremity atrophy. Adulthood, or stage IV, is characterized by hypogonadism. In general, patients have an extroverted disposition and happy appearance. About 20% of patients die during the first year of life due to severe infection, liver failure, or cardiac insufficiency.

Patients with CDG-Ib are unique among patients with these disorders. They may present with vomiting and diarrhea as well as hypoglycemia and liver disease (coagulopathy, hepatomegaly, hepatic fibrosis). In addition, they often have a protein-losing enteropathy. Development is normal. The remaining forms of CDG are similar in presentation

**TABLE 23–2**

## Common Congenital Disorders of Glycoprotein (CDGs)

| Finding(s) | Types of CDG | | | | | | | |
|---|---|---|---|---|---|---|---|---|
| | Ia | Ib | Ic | Id | Ie | IIa | IIb | x |
| Enzyme defect | Phosphomannomutase | Phosphomannose isomerase | α1,3-Glucosyltransferase | α1,3-Mannosyl transferase | Dol-P-Man synthase | GlcNAc transferase 2 | Glucosidase I | Unknown |
| Dysmorphic features | + | +/– | +/– | +/– | + | + | + | + |
| Psychomotor retardation | + | – | + | + | + | + | + | + |
| Hypotonia | + | +/– | + | + | + | + | + | + |
| Cerebellar hypoplasia | + | – | +/– | – | +/– | – | – | – |
| Seizures | +/– | +/– | +/– | + | + | + | + | – |
| Eye findings | Strabismus, esotopia | – | Strabismus | Optic atrophy | Cortical blindness | – | – | – |
| Liver disease | + | + | – | – | + | + | + | – |
| Coagulopathy | + | + | + | – | + | + | + | – |
| Other | Multiorgan involvement, peripheral neuropathy, subcutaneous fat distribution, inverted nipples, stroke-like episodes, cardiomyopathy, ataxia, microcephaly, hypothyroidism | Protein-losing enteropathy, cyclic vomiting, diarrhea, hypoglycemia | Microcephaly, feeding difficulties, ataxia | Microcephaly, reduced responsiveness, adducted thumbs | Microcephaly, delayed myelination | Stereotype behavior, frequent infections, ventricular septal defect, widely spaced nipples, delayed myelination | Early death, generalized edema, hypoventilation, apnea, demyelinating polyneuropathy | Leukocyte adhesion deficiency syndrome type II (guanosine diphosphate–fucose transporter); phenotype: elevated peripheral leukocytes, absence of CD 15, Bombay blood group phenotype, failure to thrive, recurrent infections, short arms and legs, simian crease |

Adapted from Westphal V, Srikrishna G, Freeze H: Congenital disorders of glycosylation: Have you encountered them? Genet Med 2:329-337, 2000.

+, present; –, absent; +/–, occasionally present.

to type Ia. Additional features include seizures, normal cerebellar development, delayed myelination, optic atrophy, blindness, frequent infections, hypoventilation and apnea, and further dysmorphic features, such as adducted thumbs, high-arched palate, coarse facies, widely spaced nipples, and low-set ears.

The presence of carbohydrate-deficient transferrin in serum and cerebrospinal fluid is a distinctive biochemical feature of CDG. Normal serum transferrin is composed mainly of tetrasialotransferrin. When a protein is underglycosylated, it bears fewer negatively charged sialic acid residues, altering its migration on isoelectric focusing. Patients have prominent increases in asialotransferrin and disialotransferrin, and a pronounced decrease of tetrasialotransferrins, pentasialotransferrins, and hexasialotransferrins. Additionally, low serum levels of thyroxine-binding globulin, haptoglobin, transcortin, apolipoprotein B, cholesterol, coagulation factors, and various peptide and glycopeptide hormones are common.

### Diagnosis

CDG should be considered in newborns presenting with several of the following features:

- Neurologic signs, including hypotonia, hyporeflexia, or seizures
- Ophthalmic signs, including esotropia
- Abnormal eye movements or retinitis pigmentosa
- Hepatic and gastrointestinal signs, such as ascites or hydrops, hepatomegaly, diarrhea, and protein-losing enteropathy
- Endocrinologic signs, including hyperinsulinemic hypoglycemia and hypothyroidism
- Signs of renal or cardiac disease

Diagnosis of a CDG requires isoelectric focusing to analyze transferrin and quantitation of carbohydrate-deficient transferrin. Similar transferrin changes are also found in people with chronic alcoholism and galactosemia. Confirmatory testing via enzyme assay is now available for many forms of CDG. Patients with CDG can often be identified through neonatal screening for congenital hypo-thyroidism, because of an associated thyroid-binding globulin deficiency and an increased thyroid-stimulating hormone level. Prenatal diagnosis may be available with chorionic villus sampling (CVS) or cultured amniocytes. Prenatal diagnosis by transferrin isoelectric focusing is not reliable.

### Treatment and Management

The treatment and management for most types of CDG are primarily supportive and palliative. There is no curative or corrective treatment. In infancy, evidence of multisystem involvement and the resulting complications must be treated promptly. The exception is the treatment of CDG-Ib with oral mannose therapy. In this disorder, oral mannose effectively bypasses the impaired pathway and allows glycosylation to continue (Freeze, 1998). Therapy improves the protein-losing enteropathy and liver disease.

## PEROXISOMAL DISORDERS

In this section we first consider peroxisomes in general, then the clinical presentation of individual disorders of peroxisome biogenesis and disorders of peroxisomal β-oxidation. Diagnosis and treatment are discussed at the end of the section.

### Disorders of Peroxisome Biogenesis

Peroxisomes are single–membrane-bound cellular organelles that contain no internal structure or DNA and are characterized by an electron-dense core and a homogeneous matrix. Peroxisomes are found in all cells and tissues except mature erythrocytes and are in highest concentration in the liver and kidneys. They are formed by growth and division of preexisting peroxisomes and are randomly destroyed by autophagy. Their half-life is 1.5 to 2 days. Peroxisomal proteins are encoded by nuclear genes, synthesized in the cytosol, and imported post-translationally into the peroxisome. The import of the proteins into the peroxisome is mediated by receptors and requires adenosine triphosphate hydrolysis.

Peroxisomes contain enzymes that use oxygen to oxidize a variety of substrates, thereby forming peroxide. The peroxide is decomposed within the organelle by the enzyme catalase to water and oxygen. This process protects the cell against peroxide damage through compartmentalization of peroxide metabolism within the organelle. Peroxisomes may also function to dispose of excess reducing equivalents and may contribute to thermogenesis, producing heat from cellular respiration (Gould et al, 2001).

More than 50 enzymes have been found within peroxisomes (Gould et al, 2001). The proteins have multiple functions, both synthetic and degradative (Wanders et al, 2001). The primary synthetic functions are plasmalogen synthesis and bile acid formation. Plasmalogens constitute 5% to 20% of the phospholipids in cell membranes and 80% to 90% of the phospholipids in myelin. They are involved in platelet activation and may also protect cells against oxidative stress. Degradative functions include (1) β-oxidation of VLCFA (≥C23), fatty acids (down to C8 to C6), long-chain dicarboxylic acids, prostaglandins, and polyunsaturated fatty acids; oxidation of bile acid intermediates, pipecolic acid and glutaric acid (intermediates in lysine catabolism), and phytanic acid, (2) deamination of D- and L-amino acids, (3) metabolism of glycolate to glyoxylate, (4) polyamine degradation (spermine and spermidine), and (5) ethanol clearance. At least 16 conditions due to single peroxisomal enzyme deficiencies have been confirmed so far (Wanders et al, 2001).

Peroxisomal disorders constitute a clinically and biochemically heterogeneous group of inherited diseases that result from the absence or dysfunction of one or more peroxisomal enzymes. Conditions in which multiple peroxisomal enzymes are affected may result from disturbance of biogenesis or the organelle. Pathophysiology apparently involves either deficiency of necessary products of peroxisomal metabolism or excess of unmetabolized substrates. Disorders with similar biochemical defects may have markedly different clinical features, and disorders with similar clinical features may be associated with different biochemical findings. General features of peroxisomal disorders, each of which may manifest or may be evident in the newborn period, are as follows:

- Dysmorphic craniofacial features
- Neurologic dysfunction, primarily consisting of severe hypotonia, possibly associated with hypertonia of the extremities and seizures
- Hepatodigestive dysfunction, including hepatomegaly, cholestasis, and prolonged hyperbilirubinemia

Rhizomelic shortening of the limbs, stippled calcifications of epiphyses, renal cysts, and abnormalities in neuronal migration may also be seen.

Peroxisomal biogenesis disorders are composed of at least 12 complementation groups. All involve defects in the import of proteins into the organelle. Peroxins, which are encoded by PEX genes, are proteins necessary for the importation of targeted proteins into the peroxisome. The PEX genes responsible for 11 of the 12 complementation groups are known. Approximately 65% of patients with peroxisomal biogenesis disorders have mutations in *PEX1*.

We discuss here the peroxisomal disorders that may manifest in the newborn period. Zellweger syndrome is the prototype of neonatal peroxisomal disease. It is a disorder of peroxisome biogenesis due to failure to import newly synthesized peroxisomal proteins into the peroxisome. The proteins remain in the cytosol, where they are rapidly degraded. In this condition, peroxisomes are absent from liver hepatocytes or exist as "ghosts." Neonatal adrenoleukodystrophy and infantile Refsum disease are also disorders of peroxisome biogenesis in which, as in Zellweger syndrome, disruption of function of more than one peroxisomal enzyme is demonstrable. A few residual peroxisomes, however, may be seen in the liver. These disorders represent a continuum of clinical severity. Rhizomelic chondrodysplasia punctata is caused by a defect in a subset of peroxisomal enzymes; in this disorder, liver peroxisomes are demonstrable and normal in number, but their distribution and structure are abnormal.

There is circumstantial evidence that in utero elevations of VLCFAs may be key to the congenital CNS abnormalities. Powers and Moser (1998) proposed that the VLCFAs and phytanic acid that accumulate in these peroxisomal disorders are incorporated into myelin and cell membranes and that alteration of the normal constituents of the membrane adversely affects membrane function. Specifically, these investigators suggest that the abnormal constituents accelerate cell death and impede neuronal migration, accounting for the conspicuous CNS abnormalities in disorders of peroxisomal biogenesis.

To date, four disorders of peroxisomal fatty acid β-oxidation have been defined: acyl-CoA oxidase deficiency, D-bifunctional protein deficiency, peroxisomal thiolase deficiency, and 2-methylacyl-CoA racemase deficiency (Wanders et al, 2001). The clinical presentation of the first three disorders resembles that of the biogenesis disorders. Individuals with the fourth disorder, 2-methylacyl-CoA racemase deficiency, do not present early in life but, rather, have a late-onset neuropathy.

## Clinical Presentations

Table 23–3 summarizes the clinical features of the congenital disorders of peroxisome biogenesis.

### *Zellweger Syndrome*

Zellweger syndrome is most often evident at birth, affected babies having dysmorphic facial features, including large fontanels, high forehead, flat occiput, epicanthus, hypertelorism, up-slanting palpebral fissures, hypoplastic supraorbital ridges, abnormal ears, severe weakness and hypotonia, hepatomegaly, multicystic kidneys, and congenital heart disease. Seizures, feeding difficulties, and postnatal growth failure soon manifest. Ophthalmologic examination may detect cataracts, corneal clouding, glaucoma, optic atrophy, retinitis pigmentosa, and Brushfield spots. Somatic sensory evoked responses and electroretinograms are abnormal. Hearing assessment often shows an abnormal brainstem auditory evoked response consistent with sensorineural hearing loss. Skeletal radiographs demonstrate epiphyseal stippling, and cranial imaging shows leukodystrophy and neuronal migration abnormalities. Later, hepatic cirrhosis and severe psychomotor retardation occur. Laboratory analysis may demonstrate abnormal liver function values, hyperbilirubinemia, or hypoprothrombinemia. Death usually occurs within the first year of life, the average life span being 12.5 weeks.

### *Neonatal Adrenoleukodystrophy*

Clinically, neonatal adrenoleukodystrophy is similar to, but less severe than, Zellweger syndrome. Differences include less dysmorphology, absence of chondrodysplasia punctata and renal cysts, and fewer neuronal and gray matter changes. Patients with neonatal adrenoleukodystrophy may have striking white matter disease, however, and often show degenerative changes in the adrenal glands. They also have slow psychomotor development followed by neurodegeneration that usually begins before the end of the first year of life. Disease progression is slower than that observed in Zellweger syndrome, and longer survival is usual, to an average of approximately 15 months of age.

### *Infantile Refsum Disease*

Patients with infantile Refsum disease also present at birth with relatively mild dysmorphic features, such as epicanthic folds, midface hypoplasia with low-set ears, and mild hypotonia. Early neurodevelopment is normal, possibly up to 6 months of age, but then slow deterioration begins. Later, sensorineural hearing loss (100%), anosmia, retinitis pigmentosa, hepatomegaly with impaired function, and severe mental retardation are evident. Patients learn to walk, although their gait may be ataxic and broad-based. Diarrhea and failure to thrive may also be seen. Chondrodysplasia punctata and renal cysts are absent. Neuronal migration defects are minor, and adrenal hypoplasia occurs. The life span of patients with infantile Refsum disease ranges from 3 to 11 years.

**TABLE 23–3**

**Disorders of Peroxisomal Biogenesis Presenting in the Newborn Period**

| Feature | Zellweger Syndrome | Neonatal Adrenoleukodystrophy | Infantile Refsum Disease | Rhizomelic Chondrodysplasia Punctata |
|---|---|---|---|---|
| Onset | Birth | Birth–3 mo | Birth–6 mo | Birth |
| Facies | High forehead, large fontanelles, upslanting palpebral fissures, hypoplastic supraorbital ridges, epicanthic folds, micrognathia, abnormal ears | Milder features of Zellweger syndrome | Epicanthic folds, midface hypoplasia, low-set ears | Depressed nasal bridge, hypertelorism, microcephaly |
| Neurologic findings | Weakness, hypotonia, seizures, psychomotor retardation, sensorineural hearing loss | Hypotonia, seizures, slow psychomotor development and neurodegeneration | Mild hypotonia, normal early development followed by degeneration, ataxia, sensorineural hearing loss | Severe psychomotor retardation |
| Ophthalmologic findings | Cataracts, glaucoma, corneal clouding, retinitis pigmentosa, optic nerve dysplasia, Brushfield spots | Retinopathy | Retinitis pigmentosa | Cataracts |
| Other findings | Hepatomegaly, multicystic kidneys, congenital heart disease, growth failure, chondrodysplasia punctata | Impaired adrenal function | Hepatomegaly, anosmia, diarrhea | Severe shortening of proximal limbs, joint contractures, ichthyosis |
| Diagnosis | ↑ plasma VLCFA, phytanic acid, pipecolic acid, and bile acid intermediates, ↓ plasmalogens | Same as for Zellweger syndrome | Same as for Zellweger syndrome | ↑ phytanic and pipecolic acids, ↓ plasmalogens, normal VLCFA and bile acid intermediates |

VLCFA, very-long-chain fatty acid.

### *Rhizomelic Chondrodysplasia Punctata*

Patients with rhizomelic chondrodysplasia punctata present at birth with facial dysmorphia, microcephaly, cataracts, rhizomelic shortening of the extremities with prominent stippling, and coronal clefting of vertebral bodies. The chondrodysplasia punctata is more widespread than in Zellweger syndrome and may involve extraskeletal tissues. Infants with this disorder have severe psychomotor retardation from birth onward and severe failure to thrive. Additionally, patients may have joint contractures, and 25% experience ichthyosis. Neuronal migration is normal. Life span is usually less than 1 year.

## Disorders of Peroxisomal β-Oxidation

More than 40 patients have now been described with D-bifunctional protein deficiency. In general, children present with severe CNS involvement, consisting of profound hypotonia, uncontrolled seizures, and failure to acquire any significant developmental milestones. Children are usually born full term without evidence of intrauterine growth restriction. Dysmorphic features, similar to those seen in Zellweger syndrome, are notable in most children. Also, in most cases, neuronal migration is disturbed with areas of polymicrogyria and heterotopic neurons in the cerebrum and cerebellum. Death generally occurs before 1 year of age, but survival to at least 3 years of age is possible.

Eight patients from six families have been described with acyl-CoA oxidase deficiency. Patients present with global hypotonia, deafness, and delayed milestones with or without facial dysmorphic features. Patients may demonstrate early developmental gains, but then show regression of skills. Retinopathy with extinguished electroretinograms, failure to thrive, hepatomegaly, areflexia, and seizures have also been reported.

One patient with peroxisomal thiolase deficiency has been described (Goldfischer et al, 1986). The child presented with marked facial dysmorphia, muscle weakness, and hypotonia. She demonstrated no psychomotor development during her 11 months of life. Autopsy showed renal cysts, atrophic adrenal glands, minimal liver fibrosis, hypomyelination in the cerebral white matter, foci of neuronal heterotopia, and a sudanophilic leukodystrophy (Goldfischer et al, 1986).

## Diagnosis, Management, and Prognosis of Peroxisomal Disorders

The key to the diagnosis of peroxisomal disease is a high index of suspicion. Peroxisomal disorders should be considered in newborns with dysmorphic facial features, skeletal abnormalities, shortened proximal limbs, neurologic abnormalities (including hypotonia or hypertonia), ocular abnormalities, and hepatic abnormalities. Babies with abnormal visual, hearing, or somatosensory evoked potentials should also be considered for these diagnoses.

Peroxisomal disorders are not associated with acute metabolic derangements or abnormal routine laboratory tests. Measurements of VLCFAs, phytanic acid, pipecolic acid, bile acid intermediates, and plasmalogens are required for diagnosis. Zellweger syndrome is associated with elevations of VLCFAs, phytanic acid, pipecolic acid, and bile acid intermediates, and a decrease in plasmalogen synthesis. Neonatal adrenoleukodystrophy and infantile Refsum disease have similar biochemical findings; however, the defect in plasmalogen synthesis and the degree of VLCFA accumulation are less severe. Laboratory findings in rhizomelic chondrodysplasia punctata are elevations of phytanic and pipecolic acids, a decrease in plasmalogen, and normal levels of VLCFAs and bile acid intermediates. Thus, screening that uses only levels of VLCFA fails to detect rhizomelic chondrodysplasia punctata. D-bifunctional protein deficiency is associated with deficient oxidation of C23:0 and pristanic acid, leading to elevations of pristanic acid and, to a lesser extent, phytanic acid. This results in an elevated pristanic acid-to-phytanic acid ratio (this ratio is generally not elevated in peroxisomal biogenesis disorders). Abnormal VLCFA and elevation of varanic acid (an intermediate metabolite in β-oxidation) are also seen. Accumulation of bile acid intermediates is a variable finding. Abnormalities in phytanic acid and plasmalogens are age dependent. The elevation of phytanic acid may not be demonstrable in young infants, and the reduction in red blood cell plasmalogen levels may not be evident in children older than 20 weeks (Lazarow and Moser, 1995). A liver biopsy, to assess for the presence or absence and structure of peroxisomes, may be a useful adjunct diagnostic tool. Definitive diagnoses for all types of peroxisomal disease require cultured skin fibroblasts for measurement of VLCFA levels and their β-oxidation, and, as needed, assay of the peroxisomal steps of plasmalogen synthesis, phytanic acid oxidation, the subcellular localization of catalase, enzyme assays, and immunocytochemistry studies. Prenatal diagnosis with a variety of methods is available.

Treatment for all peroxisomal disorders presenting in the newborn period remains supportive. These disorders are chronic, progressive diseases with no currently available curative therapy. Setchell and associates (1992) described the effects of the administration of primary bile acids on the liver function in a 6-month-old infant with Zellweger syndrome. The effects included normalization of serum bilirubin and liver enzyme levels and a decrease in hepatic inflammation, bile duct proliferation, and canalicular plugs; the patient also showed an improvement in growth and neurologic function (Setchell et al, 1992).

Martinez (1992) reported the use of docosahexaenoic acid ethyl ester (DHA-EE) in two patients with neonatal adrenoleukodystrophy. Both patients had an increase in erythrocyte omega fatty acid levels and plasmalogens accompanied by significant improvement in clinical parameters, including alertness, motor performance, vocabulary, and visual evoked responses. Martinez and colleagues (2000) also reported on the effects of DHA supplementation in 13 patients with generalized peroxisomal disorders; the effects were normalization of blood DHA levels, increased plasmalogen concentrations, decreased plasma VLCFA, and improvement to near normal of liver enzymes. Although the patients with the severe neonatal Zellweger syndrome presentation did not benefit, patients with milder peroxisomal biogenesis disorders—in which clinical course is more variable—did experience improvement in vision, liver function, muscle tone, and social contact. Three patients showed normalization of brain myelin, and in three others, myelination improved (Martinez et al, 2000).

Further studies are underway to explore the question of the relationship between the DHA supplementation and clinical course. In addition, a "triple" dietary approach has been proposed that consists of the oral administration of ether lipids, decreased phytanic acid intake, and the oral administration of glyceryl trioleate and glyceryl trierucate (Lorenzo's oil) (Lazarow and Moser, 1995). This approach is now being tested in patients with mild forms of disordered peroxisomal biogenesis. Hence, future treatment protocols may be available for infants affected with peroxisomal disease, but long-term outcome remains unknown.

## SMITH-LEMLI-OPITZ SYNDROME

### Etiology

SLO syndrome is a well-recognized autosomal recessive malformation syndrome, with an estimated incidence ranging from 1 in 10,000 to 100,000 in various populations (Kelley and Hennekam, 2000). Because of the identification of an underlying biochemical defect, SLO syndrome has now been "reclassified" as an inborn error of metabolism. In 1993, it was discovered that SLO syndrome is caused by a defect in cholesterol biosynthesis that results in low levels of cholesterol and elevated levels of 7-dehydrocholesterol (7DHC) and its isomer, 8-dehydrocholesterol (8DHC). Patients have markedly reduced activity of the enzyme 7DHC reductase, the enzyme responsible for the conversion of 7DHC to cholesterol (Salen et al, 1995), which is located on chromosome 11 (Kelley and Hennekam, 2000). Patients are also noted to be deficient in bile acids, a problem that can interfere with absorption of dietary lipids (Natowicz and Evans, 1994).

The pivotal connection between cholesterol and SLO syndrome involves development and differentiation of the vertebrate body plan, although additional metabolic effects have not been ruled out. Among those proteins exerting decisive influence on patterning during embryogenesis are the Hedgehog proteins. One variant, Sonic hedgehog (Shh), becomes covalently linked to cholesterol at the protein's amino-terminal signaling domain. This linkage is needed to restrict the locus of action of the Shh to the region of the plasma membrane. Although it was originally suggested that failure to so modify Shh could account for the multiplicity of structural abnormalities in patients with SLO syndrome (Farese and Herz, 1998), the process is now thought to be more complex and to involve other signaling proteins (Farese and Herz, 1998; Kelley and Hennekam, 2000).

### Clinical Features

Recognition of the biochemical defect in SLO syndrome provided the diagnostic test required to recognize the most mild and most severe cases, substantially expanding the clinical spectrum of the condition. Classic SLO syndrome is often evident at birth; affected patients have microcephaly and facial dysmorphism, including bitemporal narrowing, ptosis, epicanthic folds, anteverted nares, broad nasal tip, prominent lateral palatine ridges, micrognathia, and low-set ears. Other features are 2- to 3-syndactyly of the toes, small proximally placed thumbs, and occasionally postaxial polydactyly and cataracts. Males usually have hypospadias, cryptorchidism, and a hypoplastic scrotum. Pyloric stenosis, cleft palate, pancreatic anomalies, and lung segmentation defects have also been reported (Baraitser and Winter, 1996). Hypotonia progressing to hypertonia and moderate to severe mental deficiencies are also present. Feeding difficulties and vomiting are common problems in infancy. Irritable behavior and shrill screaming may also pose problems during infancy. Cranial imaging studies show (and autopsy confirms) defects in brain morphogenesis, including hypoplasia of the frontal lobes, cerebellum, and brainstem, dilated ventricles, irregular gyral patterns, and irregular neuronal organization.

Historically, approximately 20% of patients die within the first year of life, although others may survive for more than 30 years. Life expectancy appears to correlate inversely with the number and severity of organ defects and with the kinds and numbers of limb, facial, and genital abnormalities (Kelley and Hennekam, 2000; Tint et al, 1995). Developmental outcomes are also highly variable, ranging from severe mental retardation to normal intelligence. Development of treatment protocols for SLO syndrome may contribute to improvements in prognosis, but improved recognition of more mildly affected patients may explain the increasing reports of SLO syndrome in patients with mild mental retardation or normal intelligence.

Some patients have a severe lethal form of SLO, type II. In this form, the external genitalia of male infants may be ambiguous or female. Postaxial polydactyly of the hands, valgus deformities of the feet with syndactyly of several toes, cleft palate, and hypoplasia of the anterior portion of the tongue are common. Other findings are unilobar lungs, hypoplastic kidneys, agenesis of the gallbladder, cerebellar hypoplasia, cardiac defects, and enlarged pancreatic islets with giant cells.

### Diagnosis

The diagnosis of SLO syndrome types I and II is based on the findings of elevated levels of 7DHC and 8DHC. Plasma cholesterol levels are usually but not always low; as many of 10% of patients at all ages have normal cholesterol levels (Kelley and Hennekam, 2000). In addition, the standard method for analysis of cholesterol in most hospital laboratories identifies 7DHC and 8DHC as cholesterol. Therefore, most laboratories report normal cholesterol levels in patients who have low cholesterol but elevations of 7DHC and 8DHC sufficient to bring the total level into the "normal" range (Kelley and Hennekam, 2000). The biochemical defect and findings are the same for both types. The difference between type I and type II appears to be one of degree: the enzyme defect is more severe and the block is more complete in patients with type II disease (Kelley and Hennekam, 2000; Tint et al, 1995). Prenatal diagnosis is possible. A mother carrying an affected fetus may have an abnormally low unconjugated estriol value. Ultrasonography detects many but not all affected fetuses, and biochemical analysis of amniotic fluid and of chorionic villus samples is accurate and umambiguous in most cases (Kelley and Hennekam). When molecular mutations are known, analysis may be useful.

### Treatment

The goal of therapy for SLO syndrome is twofold, (1) to increase the level of cholesterol in plasma and other body fluids and (2) to lower the level of 7DHC. Treatment consists of providing exogenous cholesterol, in the form of either dietary cholesterol or cholesterol suspension, to replenish body stores of cholesterol and to down-regulate the patient's endogenous cholesterol synthesis, thus decreasing the amount of 7DHC produced. A goal of cholesterol supplementation of 20 to 60 mg/kg per day was initially advocated, but doses higher than 300 mg/kg per day have been used without adverse outcome (Irons et al, 1995; Kelley and Hennekam, 2000). Provision of bile acids to facilitate adequate absorption of the dietary cholesterol is controversial, especially because fat malabsorption is unusual and certain bile acids may decrease tissue uptake of cholesterol (Kelley and Hennekam, 2000). Use of 3-hydroxy-3-methyl-CoA (HMG-CoA) lyase inhibitors such as lovastatin has also been suggested as a mechanism to decrease levels of 7DHC. However, because animal studies suggest that down-regulation of cholesterol synthesis may not decrease 7DHC, and because of concern about decrease in synthesis of other essential isoprenoid compounds, HMG-CoA reductase inhibitors are not routinely used in therapy (Kelley and Hennekam, 2000). In infants with SLO syndrome, the use of breast milk should be encouraged, because it supplies approximately 133 mg/L of cholesterol (Irons et al, 1995).

Although many questions remain about optimal therapy and outcomes, therapeutic interventions do appear to increase plasma cholesterol levels, decrease 7DHC levels, and improve irritability, behavior, and growth (Elias et al, 1997; Irons et al, 1995; Kelley and Hennekam, 2000). Parents report children to be more alert, active, and happier during therapy. Gain in developmental skills may be noted, and improvement in hypotonia may occur. Therapy appears to be well tolerated.

For maximal benefit, it has been suggested that treatment should begin prenatally, because SLO syndrome has many features consistent with in utero involvement of the disease process. Antenatal supplementation by fetal intravenous and intraperitoneal transfusions of fresh frozen plasma were shown in one patient to increase fetal cholesterol (Irons et al, 1999). Treatment should otherwise begin as soon as possible after birth or as soon as the diagnosis is confirmed. Patients with severe SLO syndrome may need gavage or gastrostomy feeding for management of reflux and gastrointestinal dysmotility, and many have protein allergies and require elemental formulas. Growth is often a problem, but the temptation to overfeed must be avoided because overfeeding would contribute to feeding problems and could not rescue the intrauterine growth restriction in severe SLO syndrome (Kelley and Hennekam, 2000).

## REFERENCES


Bach G: Mucolipidosis type IV. Mol Genet Metab 73:197-203, 2001.

Baraitser M, Winter RM: Color Atlas of Congenital Malformation Syndromes. London, Mosby-Wolfe, 1996, p 61.

Barth PG: Sphingolipids. In Fernandes J, Saudubray J-M, van den Berghe G (eds): Inborn Metabolic Diseases: Diagnosis and Treatment, 2nd ed. Berlin, Springer-Verlag, 1995, pp 375-382.

Beutler E, Grabowski GA: Gaucher Disease. In Scriver CR, Beaudet AL, Sly WS, Valle D, et al (eds): The Metabolic and Molecular Bases of Inherited Disease, 8th ed. New York, McGraw-Hill, 2001, pp 3635-3668.

Buchholz T, Molitor G, Lukong KE, et al: Clinical presentation of congenital sialidosis in a patient with a neuraminidase gene frameshift mutation. Eur J Pediatr 160:23-30, 2001.

Chitayat D, Meunier CM, Hodgkinson KA, et al: Mucolipidosis type IV: Clinical manifestations and natural history. Am J Med Genet 41:313-318, 1991.

Elias ER, Irons MB, Hurley AD, et al: Clinical effects of cholesterol supplementation in six patients with the Smith-Lemli-Opitz syndrome (SLOS). Am J Med Genet 683:305-310, 1997.

Erikson A, Johansson K, Mansson J-E, et al: Enzyme replacement therapy of infantile Gaucher disease. Neuropediatrics 24:237-238, 1993.

Farese RV, Herz J: Cholesterol metabolism and embryogenesis. Topics in Genetics 14:115-120, 1998.

Freeze H: Disorders in protein glycosylation and potential therapy: Tip of an iceberg? J Pediatr 133:593-600, 1998.

Fujimoto A, Tayebi N, Sidransky E: Congenital ichthyosis preceding neurologic symptoms in two sibs with type 2 Gaucher disease. Am J Med Genet 59:356-358, 1995.

Gaucher disease: Current issues in diagnosis and treatment. NIH Technology Assessment Panel on Gaucher Disease, JAMA 275:548-553, 1996.

Goldfischer S, Collins J, Rapin I, et al: Pseudo-Zellweger syndrome: Deficiencies in several peroxisomal oxidative activities. J Pediatr 108:25-32, 1986.

Gould S, Raymond G, Valle D: The peroxisome biogenesis disorders. In Scriver CR, Beaudet AL, Sly WS, Valle D, et al (eds): The Metabolic and Molecular Bases of Inherited Disease, 8th ed. New York, McGraw-Hill, 2001, pp 3181-3217.

Grunewald S, Matthijs G: Congenital disorders of glycosylation (CDG): A rapidly expanding group of neurometabolic disorders. Neuropediatrics 31:57-59, 2000.

Hoogerbrugge PM, Brouwer OF, Bordigoni P, et al: Allogenic bone marrow transplantation for lysosomal storage diseases. Lancet 345:1398-1402, 1995.

Ince Z, Coban A, Peker O, et al: Gaucher disease associated with congenital ichthyosis in the neonate. Eur J Pediatr 154:418, 1995.

Irons M, Elias ER, Abuelo D, et al: Clinical features of the Smith-Lemli-Opitz syndrome and treatment of the cholesterol metabolic defect. Int Pediatr 10:28-32, 1995.

Irons MD, Nores J, Steward TL, et al: Antenatal therapy of Smith-Lemli-Opitz syndrome. Fetal Diagn Ther 14:133-137, 1999.

Jaeken J, Matthijs G, Carchon H, VanSchaftingen E: Defects of *N*-glycan synthesis. In Scriver CR, Beaudet AL, Sly WS, Valle D, et al (eds): The Metabolic and Molecular Bases of Inherited Disease, 8th ed. New York, McGraw-Hill, 2001, pp 1601-1622.

Kelley RI, Hennekam RCM: The Smith-Lemli-Opitz syndrome. J Med Genet 37:21-335, 2000.

Kohlschütter A, Sieg K, Schulte FJ, et al: Infantile cardiomyopathy and neuromyopathy with beta-galactosidase deficiency. Eur J Pediatr 139:75-81, 1982.

Krivit W, Peters C, Dusenbery K, et al: Wolman disease successfully treated by bone marrow transplantation. Bone Marrow Transplant 23:567-570, 2000.

Lemyre E, Russo P, Melancon SB, et al: Clinical spectrum of infantile free sialic acid storage disease. Am J Med Genet 82:385-391, 1999.

Lipson AH, Rogers M, Berry A: Collodion babies with Gaucher's disease: A further case. Arch Dis Child 66:667, 1991.

Liu K, Commens C, Choong R, et al: Collodion babies with Gaucher's disease. Arch Dis Child 63:854-856, 1988.

Martinez M: Treatment with docosahexaenoic acid favorably modifies the fatty acid composition or erythrocytes in peroxisomal patients. In Coates PM, Tanaka K (eds): New Developments in Fatty Acid Oxidation. New York, Wiley-Liss, 1992, pp 389-397.

Martinez M, Vazquez E, Garcia-Silva MT, et al: Therapeutic effects of docosahexaenoic acid ethyl ester in patients with generalized peroxisomal disorders. Am J Clin Nutr 71(Suppl): 376S-385S, 2000.

Millat G, Chikh K, Naureckiene S, et al: Niemann-Pick disease type C: Spectrum of HE1 mutations and genotype/phenotype correlations in the NPC2 group. Am J Hum Genet 69: 1013-1021, 2001.

Natowicz MR, Evans JE: Abnormal bile acids in the Smith-Lemli-Opitz syndrome. Am J Med Genet 50:364-367, 1994.

Natowicz MR, Stoler JM, Prence EM, et al: Marked heterogeneity in Niemann-Pick disease, type C: Clinical and ultrastructural findings. Clin Pediatr 34:190-197, 1995.

Powers J, Moser H: Peroxisomal disorders: Genotype, phenotype, major neuropathologic lesions, and pathogenesis. Brain Pathol 8:101-120, 1998.

Salen G, Shefer S, Batta AK, et al: Biochemical abnormalities in the Smith-Lemli-Opitz syndrome. Int Pediatr 10:33-36, 1995.

Setchell KDR, Bragetti P, Zimmer-Nechemias L, et al: Oral bile acid treatment and the patient with Zellweger syndrome. Hepatology 15:198-207, 1992.

Sherer DM, Metlay LA, Sinkin RA, et al: Congenital ichthyosis with restrictive dermopathy and Gaucher disease: A new syndrome with associated prenatal diagnostic and pathology findings. Obstet Gynecol 81:842-844, 1993.

Sidransky E, Sherer DM, Ginns EI: Gaucher disease in the neonate: A distinct Gaucher phenotype is analogous to a mouse model created by targeted disruption of the glucocerebrosidase gene. Pediatr Res 32:494-498, 1992.

Stewart WA, Gordon KE, Camfield PR, et al: Irritability in Krabbe's disease: Dramatic response to low-dose morphine. Pediatr Neurol 25:344-345, 2001.

Sun M, Goldin E, Stahl S, et al: Mucolipidosis type IV is caused by mutations in a gene encoding a novel transient receptor potential channel. Hum Mol Genet 9:2471-2478, 2000.

Tint GS, Salen G, Batta AK, et al: Correlation of severity and outcome with plasma sterol levels in variants of the Smith-Lemli-Opitz syndrome. J Pediatr 127:82-87, 1995.

van Schaftingen E, Jaeken J: Phosphomannomutase deficiency as a cause of carbohydrate-deficient glycoprotein syndrome type I. FEBS Letters 377:318-320, 1995.

Vogler C, Levy B, Galvin NJ, et al: Enzyme replacement in murine mucopolysaccharidosis type VII: Neuronal and glial response to β-glucuronidase requires early initiation of enzyme replacement therapy. Pediatr Res 45:838-844, 1999.

Wanders R, Barth P, Heymans H: Single peroxisomal enzyme deficiencies. In Scriver CR, Beaudet AL, Sly WS, Valle D, et al (eds): The Metabolic and Molecular Bases of Inherited Disease, 8th ed. New York, McGraw-Hill, 2001, pp 3219-3256.

Westphal V, Srikrishna G, Freeze H: Congenital disorders of glycosylation: Have you encountered them? Genet Med 2: 329-337, 2000.

Whitley CG, Spielmann RC, Herro G, Teragawa SS: Urinary glycosaminoglycan excretion quantified by an automated semimicro method in specimens conveniently transported from around the globe. Mol Genet Metab 75:56-64, 2002.

Wolman M: Wolman disease and its treatment. Clin Pediatr 34:207-212, 1995.

CHAPTER 24

# Skeletal Dysplasias and Connective Tissue Disorders

**Paige Kaplan**

The *skeletal dysplasias*, or osteochondrodysplasias, are disorders of the development and growth of cartilage and bone. The *connective tissues* disorders involve abnormalities of the cell's supporting and connecting structures in the matrix. With the growing use and accuracy of ultrasonography for prenatal care, a greater number of osteochondrodysplasias and connective tissue disorders are diagnosed in the second trimester (Gordienko et al, 1996; Rasmussen et al, 1996). In one series of 126,316 deliveries monitored over 15 years, the incidence of skeletal dysplasias was 2.14 in 10,000 (Rasmussen et al, 1996).

This chapter focuses on several of the more common dysplasias and connective tissue disorders that manifest prenatally or perinatally (Gordienko et al, 1996; Rasmussen et al, 1996), but the discussion is not exhaustive (Table 24–1). The osteochondrodysplasias are reviewed extensively by Cohen (2002), Rimoin and Lachman (1997), Spranger and Maroteaux (1990), and Superti-Furga and associates (2001).

There are a large number of different *connective tissue* molecules, including collagen (at least 16 types), elastin, fibrillin (2 types), and microfibril-associated glycoproteins. These are components of tissues such as bone, cartilage, vascular media, tendon, skin, basement membranes in the renal glomeruli and other organs, and the suspensory ligament of the lens. The heritable disorders of connective tissue are varied, may be very dissimilar clinically, and may manifest in utero or at any age postnatally. Most are rare, but some of the more common conditions that manifest at birth are discussed here.

## CLASSIFICATION

The *skeletal dysplasias* have been classified into 24 groups on the basis of radiologic criteria (Beighton et al, 1992). Other classifications vary according to etiologic, clinical, pathologic, and radiologic criteria and may be confusing; for example, osteogenesis imperfecta (OI) can be classified as either a skeletal dysplasia or a connective tissue disorder.

*Connective tissue disorders* that may manifest at birth include Marfan syndrome, congenital contractural arachnodactyly (Beals syndrome), cutis laxa, and Ehlers-Danlos and Williams syndromes.

### Molecular Basis

With advances in molecular knowledge, several different dysplasias have been recognized to have mutations in the same genes. In some of these disorders, clinical similarities had been noted previously. An example is achondroplasia, hypochondroplasia, severe achondroplasia with developmental delay and acanthosis nigricans (SADDAN), and thanatophoric dysplasia, all of which are due to mutations in the fibroblast growth factor receptor 3 (*FGFR3*) gene (Francomano et al, 1994; Le Merrer et al, 1994; Rousseau et al, 1995; Tavormina et al, 1995). Another group of disorders with mutations in the same gene comprises, from mildest to most severe, Kniest dysplasia, spondyloepiphyseal dysplasias, spondyloepimetaphyseal dysplasia, Stickler syndrome, hypochondrogenesis, and achondrogenesis type II. They are caused by mutations in the gene for collagen type II, *COL2A1* (Rousseau et al, 1995; Spranger et al, 1994; Wilkin et al, 1994; Winterpacht et al, 1993), encoded on chromosome 12q13.11 to q13.2. In other groups of disorders, the common cause is not as obvious clinically: Diastrophic dysplasia (the mildest), atelosteogenesis type II, and achondrogenesis type 1B (the most severe) are caused by mutations in the diastrophic dysplasia sulfate transporter (*DTDST*) gene, on chromosome 5q31 to q34 (Hastbacka et al, 1994, 1996; Kaitila et al, 1989; Rousseau et al, 1995; Superti-Furga et al, 1996). This affects the transport of sulfate to proteoglycans (mucopolysaccharides), especially chondroitin sulfate B–containing proteoglycans, which is prevalent in cartilage.

## APPROACH TO DIAGNOSIS

Early and precise diagnoses are important for prognosis, optimal immediate and long-term management, and genetic counseling about other possible affected family members. An example is the group of disorders with punctate calcifications ("stippling") in epiphyses, called chondrodysplasia punctata; there are at least three types, each of which has a different cause and mode of inheritance—autosomal recessive , X-linked recessive, and X-linked dominant (Table 24–2). Multiple factors must be considered—complete physical examination, family history, radiologic studies, and histochemical and/or molecular tests.

Most skeletal dysplasias cause *short stature*, which may be proportionate or disproportionate. In considering a diagnosis, one must know whether the skull, vertebrae (trunk), ribs, or limbs are affected. If the limbs are disproportionately shortened compared with the trunk, there may be segmental (disproportionate) or proportionate involvement of one of the three parts of the limbs: upper arms and thighs (rhizomelic), forearms and legs (mesomelic), and hands and feet (acromelic). Most skeletal dysplasias that manifest at birth involve short limbs. Accurate measurements of length on a rigid board, arm span, and head and chest circumferences must be plotted on standard growth curves.

*Other characteristics* may give important clues for specific disorders:

- Children with achondroplasia and thanatophoric dysplasia have very large heads. Cloverleaf skull deformity is present in thanatophoric and, occasionally, diastrophic dysplasias.

**TABLE 24-1**

**Most Common Types of Osteochondrodysplasias Detected Prenatally and Perinatally**

| Diagnosis | No. Cases (%) Gordienko et al (1996) | Rasmussen et al (1996) |
|---|---|---|
| Thanatophoric | 3 (8) | 5 (20) |
| Osteogenesis imperfecta | | |
| Type II | 10 (26) | 3 (12) |
| Type III | | 2 (7) |
| Achondroplasia | 5 (13) | 3 (11) |
| Spondyloepiphyseal dysplasia congenita | | 3 (11) |
| Campomelic | 2 (5) | 2 (7) |
| Short-rib polydactyly | | |
| Type I | 2 (5) | 1 (4) |
| Type II | 2 (5) | 1 (4) |
| Other diagnoses | 15 (38) | 3 (11) |
| No diagnosis | — | 4 (13) |
| Total no. cases | 39 | 27 |

- A relatively long chest is seen in asphyxiating thoracic dystrophy.
- The hand in achondroplasia is short and the fingers are trident; in diastrophic dysplasia, there are distinctive "hitchhiker" thumbs.
- Deformations of feet ("clubfeet") occur in diastrophic dysplasia, Kniest syndrome, spondyloepiphyseal dysplasias, and OI type II.
- Multiple joint dislocations manifest at birth in Larsen and Ehlers-Danlos type VII syndromes as well as atelosteogenesis.

The presence of other abnormalities can be valuable clues to diagnosis, as follows:

- Cleft palate or uvula can occur in campomelic, Kniest, spondyloepiphyseal, short-rib polydactyly (Majewski), atelosteogenesis types I and II, hypochondrogenesis, and diastrophic dysplasias.
- Congenital cataracts occur in chondrodysplasia punctata.
- Congenital cardiac defects occur in short-rib polydactyly dysplasias (conotruncal malformations in type I and transposition of the great arteries in type II).

**TABLE 24-2**

**Skeletal Dysplasias Manifesting Prenatally or Perinatally**

| Dysplasia | Skeletal Features | Nonskeletal Features | Radiographic Features | Inheritance, Gene, Chromosome | Comment(s) |
|---|---|---|---|---|---|
| Lethal | | | | | |
| Thanatophoric | Large cranium, "proptosis," flat nose bridge, narrow chest, very short limbs (all segments) | Polyhydramnios, hydrocephalus, brain anomalies, congenital cardiac abnormalities | Large calvarium, short base, small magnum foramen, cloverleaf skull; short, splayed, cupped ribs; small, flat, U-shaped vertebrae; short, small, flat pelvis; short, bowed limbs, metaphyseal flare with spike | AD; most are new mutations<br>*FGFR3*<br>4p16.3 | Same gene as for achondroplasia, hypochondroplasia |
| Campomelic | Large cranium; small face with flat nose bridge, small chin, (cleft soft palate); small, narrow chest; bowed thighs and legs, with dimple on leg | Polyhydramnios, congenital cardiac abnormalities, female external genitalia in XY males | Large dolichocephalic calvarium with shallow orbits; short and wavy ribs, often 11 pairs; small, flat vertebrae; tall, narrow pelvis; relatively long, thin limbs with bowed femurs, short tibias | AD; most are new mutations<br>*SOX9*<br>17q24.1-q25.1 | |
| Achondrogenesis type IB | Soft cranium; round face; short, round chest; very short limbs | Polyhydramnios | Poorly ossified calvarium; ribs short with fractures (beading); nonossified vertebrae; small pelvis; short broad femurs with metaphyseal spikes, short broad tibias and fibulas | AR<br>DTDST<br>5q32-q33 | Same gene as diastrophic dysplasia (milder disease) and atelosteogenesis II |

*Text continues on page 283*

**TABLE 24–2**

**Skeletal Dysplasias Manifesting Prenatally or Perinatally—Cont'd**

| Dysplasia | Skeletal Features | Nonskeletal Features | Radiographic Features | Inheritance, Gene, Chromosome | Comment(s) |
|---|---|---|---|---|---|
| Short-rib polydactyly | | | | | |
| Types I and III | Hydropic appearance; round flat face; micrognathia; extremely narrow chest; very short limbs; postaxial polydactyly | Cardiac, renal, anal malformations | Normal calvarium; very short, horizontal ribs; flat wide intervertebral disc spaces; small pelvis; short limbs with lateral and medial metaphyseal spurs | AR | |
| Types II and IV | Hydropic; short face, flat nose, cleft lip±palate, low-set ears; narrow chest, protuberant abdomen; moderately short limbs | Cardiac, renal (dysplastic kidneys), respiratory malformations | Very short, horizontal ribs; normal pelvis and vertebrae; short limbs with round metaphyses; premature epiphyseal ossification; polydactyly | AR | |
| Asphyxiating thoracic dystrophy | Normal face; narrow, long chest; variable limb shortening | Lethal pulmonary insufficiency | Normal calvarium and vertebrae; very short ribs with anterior cupping; short limbs with wide proximal femoral metaphyses; premature ossification of proximal femoral epiphysis | AR | Patients who survive newborn period have renal disease (proteinuria, hypertension). Possibly, a variant of short-rib polydactyly III |
| Atelosteogenesis | | | | | |
| Type I (Fig. 24–9) | Flat face with cleft palate, micrognathia; very narrow chest; very short limbs (rhizomelic) with equinovalgus deformities; joint dislocations | Prematurity; stillbirth | Flat vertebrae with coronal and sagittal clefts; scoliosis; short ribs (11 pairs); small pelvis with enlarged sacrosciatic notch; short limbs, "drumstick" humeri and femurs; absence of fibulas; short metacarpals, triangular first metacarpals, dysharmonic ossification of hand bones; dislocated knees | AD | Similar to boomerang dysplasia; also known as spondylo-humero-femoral dysplasia |
| Type II | Cleft palate; narrow chest; short limbs with dislocations; equinovarus deformities; gap between first and second digits | Laryngeal stenosis; patent foramen ovale | Occasional coronal and sagittal vertebral clefts; short ribs; normal sacrosciatic notch; short "dumbbell" humeri and femurs, small fibulas; large second and third metacarpals; small round midphalanges | AR *DTDST* 5q32-q33.1 | Same gene as for diastrophic dysplasia (milder disease) and achondrogenesis type IB (more severe disease), and multiple epiphyseal dysplasia (MED) |

*Continued*

**TABLE 24–2**

**Skeletal Dysplasias Manifesting Prenatally or Perinatally—Cont'd**

| Dysplasia | Skeletal Features | Nonskeletal Features | Radiographic Features | Inheritance, Gene, Chromosome | Comment(s) |
|---|---|---|---|---|---|
| Dyssegmental (Silverman-Handmaker) | Flat midface, flat orbits, cleft palate, micrognathia; short neck; narrow chest; extremely small limbs | Encephalocele; patent ductus arteriosus | Midface hypoplasia; vertebrae variable sizes with coronal and sagittal clefts; very short, flared ribs; round scapulae with abnormal shape; very short, broad, bowed long bones; small first metacarpals; small, round pelvis | AR<br>*PERLECAN*<br>1p36.1 | Resembles dyssegmental dysplasia of Roland-Desbuquois (less severe) and Kniest syndrome |
| Chondrodysplasia punctata, rhizomelic type 1 (RCDP1) (Fig. 24-10) | Face flat; very flat nose bridge and tip; proximal shortening of limbs | Cataracts; joint contractures; skin: ichthyosiform erythroderma | Wide coronal vertebral clefts; short humeri and femurs; stippled epiphyses of long bones and pelvis and periarticular areas; pelvis: trapezoid ilia | AR<br>*PEX7*<br>6q22-q24 | Patients who survive newborn period can live a few years; severe growth and mental retardation. Biochemical abnormalities: decreased rbc plasmalogens and increased phytanic acid |
| **Nonlethal** | | | | | |
| Chondrodysplasia punctata X-linked recessive | Hypoplasia of the distal phalanges; severe hypoplasia of nose; short stature; congenital icthyosis | | | *ARSE* XR<br>Xp22.3 | Milder than X-linked dominant form, CDPX2. Variable clinical severity; neonatal death to longevity and diagnosis in adulthood. Males usually milder than females. (Brunetti-Pierri et al, 1999) |
| Chondrodysplasia punctata X-linked dominant (Conradi Hunermann Happle syndrome) | Asymmetric rhizomesomelia | Congenital cataracts; icthyosis; patchy alopecia | | *ESP*<br>3β hydroxy Δ8-Δ7 sterol isomerase<br>Xp11.23-11.22 | Severe form of disease; usually lethal in males; females vary from stillborn to mild (diagnosis in adulthood); intrafamilial variability |
| Achondroplasia | Large cranium; bossed forehead, flat nose bridge, prominent chin, short neck; slightly narrow chest; proximal limb shortening, short trident hands; short proximal and middle phalanges; later genu varum; thoracolumbar kyphosis; lumbar lordosis | Hypotonia: delayed motor milestones; spinal stenosis causes spinal compression; small foramen magnum can cause hydrocephalus; short mean adult height: males 131 cm, females 124 cm | Large calvarium, small foramen magnum, short base; diminished lumbosacral interpedicular space, short pedicles; short ribs with anterior cupping; short humeri and femurs; relatively long fibulas; metaphyseal flare; small iliac wings | AD; most cases are new mutations, associated with advanced paternal age<br>*FGFR3*<br>4p16.3 | Same gene as for hypochondroplasia (milder) SADDAN, and thanatophoric dysplasia (very severe) Hypochondroplasia is usually not apparent until 1-2 yrs |

TABLE 24–2

**Skeletal Dysplasias Manifesting Prenatally or Perinatally—Cont'd**

| Dysplasia | Skeletal Features | Nonskeletal Features | Radiographic Features | Inheritance, Gene, Chromosome | Comment(s) |
|---|---|---|---|---|---|
| Diastrophic dysplasia (Fig. 24–11) | Normal cranium; cleft palate, micrognathia; normal chest at birth; very short limbs; thumbs proximally placed and adducted ("hitchhiker thumb"); severe equinovarus of feet; limited movement of many joints | Cystic masses in external ears ("cauliflower ears") during infancy; deafness due to lack or fusion of ossicles; narrow external canal; scoliosis in childhood | Premature ossification of rib cartilage; narrow L1-L5 interpedicular spaces; scoliosis; short limbs; disproportionately short ulna and fibula (mesomelic); broad flared metaphyses; ovoid first metacarpals; variable symphalangism of proximal interphalangeal joints; irregular delayed epiphyseal ossification except accel-erated carpals | AR<br>*DTDST*<br>5q32-q33 | Intrafamilial variability; normal life span if scoliosis does not impair respiratory function; normal intelligence |
| Kniest syndrome | Large cranium; flat face with "large" eyes, flat nasal bridge, cleft palate; short limbs with proximal shortening (more severe in lower limbs), enlarged joints, flexion contractures | Infancy: tracheomalacia; childhood: myopia and retinal detachment; hearing loss; delayed motor development; normal intelligence | Frontal and maxillary hypoplasia with shallow orbits; slightly short ribs; flat vertebrae with coronal clefts; anisospondyly (different sizes); small pelvis with irregular acetabular roof; short limbs with broad and flared metaphyses ("dumbbell"), lateral bowing of femurs and upper tibias; slightly short and broad/normal tubular bones of hands and feet; epiphyses at knees not ossified | AD<br>*COL2A1*<br>12q13.1-13.2 | Same gene as for some spondylo-epiphyseal dysplasias, spondyloepi-metaphyseal dys-plasia, Stickler syndrome, hypo-chondrogenesis, achondrogenesis type II (more severe) |

- Postaxial polydactyly occurs in short-rib polydactyly and thoracic asphyxiating and chondroectodermal dysplasias; occasionally, preaxial polydactyly also occurs in the short-rib dysplasias.

## TESTS

*Radiographs* of the entire skeleton, including the hands and feet, are essential for accurate diagnosis. If the infant or fetus dies, specimens of cartilage and skin fibroblasts should be obtained for histochemical tests and molecular-gene mutation analysis; if photographs and skeletal radiographs were not obtained premortem, they should be obtained postmortem. Detailed family history and measurements of family members may be helpful; more mildly affected members might have gone undiagnosed.

*Tissue samples* are also needed. Lymphocytes and fibroblasts (from cultured skin) should be obtained in all cases for enzyme and molecular diagnoses. These can be used to make or confirm diagnoses and permit accurate prenatal diagnosis. Even if the molecular or enzymatic basis is not understood at the time, the tissue may be useful in the future.

## OSTEOGENESIS IMPERFECTA TYPES II AND III

OI is characterized by increased bone fragility. As mentioned, it can be classified as either a connective tissue disorder or a skeletal dysplasia. There are four clinical types: Types II and III are the most severe, manifesting prenatally and perinatally. OI type I rarely causes prenatal or perinatal fractures.

### Etiology

OI is caused by abnormalities in type I collagen, which is composed of three polypeptide chains, two α-1 (I) and one α-2 (I) fibrils, coiled in a triple helix (Byers, 1993; Byers et al, 1988, 1991). Two genes, *COL1A1* and *COLIA2*, on chromosomes 17q21 and 7q22.1, respectively, encode the chains. Mutations in either of the genes result in abnormal collagen. In OI type I, there is secretion of normal collagen but only half as much as usual, with a milder phenotype. In the other types, the altered procollagen chains are incorporated into the helix, causing 50% to 75% of collagen fibers to be abnormal, resulting in more severe phenotypes (Byers, 1993). Most, if not all, cases of OI are inherited as autosomal dominant traits.

### Presentation

*OI type II (perinatal lethal type)* is estimated to affect 1 in 20,000 to 60,000 infants. Affected infants may be born prematurely, with low birth weight and disproportionately short stature. The limbs are short and bowed with extra, circular skin creases; the hips are abducted and flexed. The head is soft and boggy, and minimal calvarial bone can be felt. The sclerae are dark blue, the nose may be prominent, and the chest is narrow. The infant cries with handling because there are many fractures at different stages of healing. Sixty percent of affected babies are stillborn or die during the first day of life, and 80% die by 1 month (Byers et al, 1988). With the growing use of ultrasonography, affected fetuses may be detected in the early second trimester because of short and bowed or angulated limbs and narrow thoraces (Fig. 24–1A).

Radiographs show the femurs in OI type II to be short, broad, and "telescoped" or "crumpled"; the tibias are short and bowed, and the fibulas may be thin (see Fig. 24–1B). There is minimal or no calvarial mineralization, with occasional wormian bones (small islands of bone in the suture spaces). The vertebrae are very flat (platyspondyly). The ribs are short, wavy, and thin or broad, with "beading" from callus formation.

Prenatal histochemical or molecular diagnosis is possible through analysis of chorionic villi or amniocytes, if a previously affected sibling's mutation is known. The bone deformations in OI type II may be detectable with ultrasonography in the second trimester but may not be 100% accurate.

*OI type III (progressive deforming type)* may manifest prenatally and perinatally as well as in the first 2 years of life (Byers, 1993). Prenatal and perinatal clinical features resemble those in OI type II but are less severe (Fig. 24–2A). Perinatal death is common. If not present at birth, fractures and deformations of the limbs develop in the first and second years. The highest prevalence of fractures in OI, up to 200, occur in type III. Extremely short stature, with adult heights of 92 to 108 cm, may result from microfractures in the growth plates. The head may be large because the calvarium is soft with a large anterior fontanelle. The sclerae may be blue initially but are white by puberty. The head assumes a triangular shape, with bossed, broad forehead and tapered, pointed chin. Later in childhood, dentinogenesis imperfecta and hearing loss may develop. Severe kyphoscoliosis may occur, leading to cardiopulmonary compromise, the major cause of early death. On radiographs, the femurs are short and deformed but not crumpled as in OI type II (see Fig. 24–2B and C). The other long bones are thinner than usual with healing fractures incurred in utero, bowing, and deformations. The calvarium is undermineralized with a large

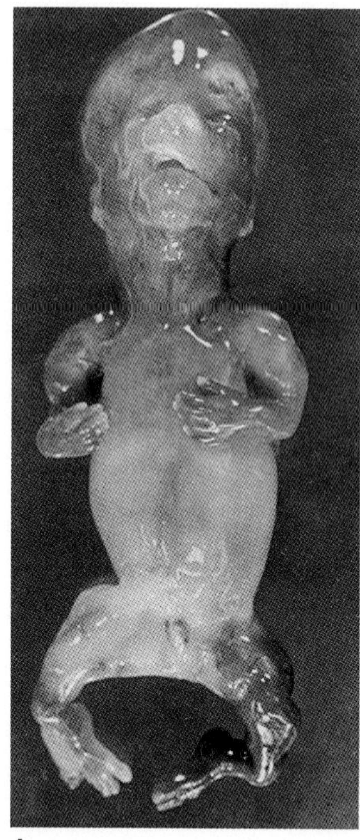
A

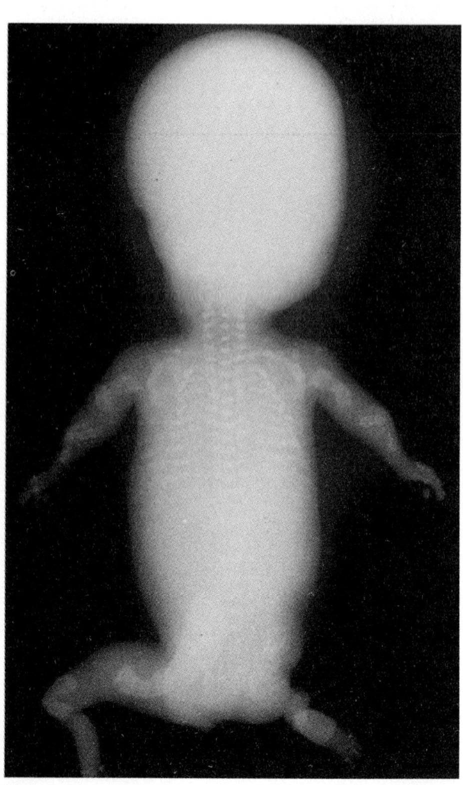
B

**FIGURE 24–1.** Osteogenesis imperfecta type II. **A,** 14-week fetus. The calvarium is deformed; limbs are angulated and deformed from multiple fractures. **B,** Radiograph of fetus (14 weeks) showing absence of ossification in calvarium, short telescoped or crumpled humeri and femurs, short and wavy ribs.

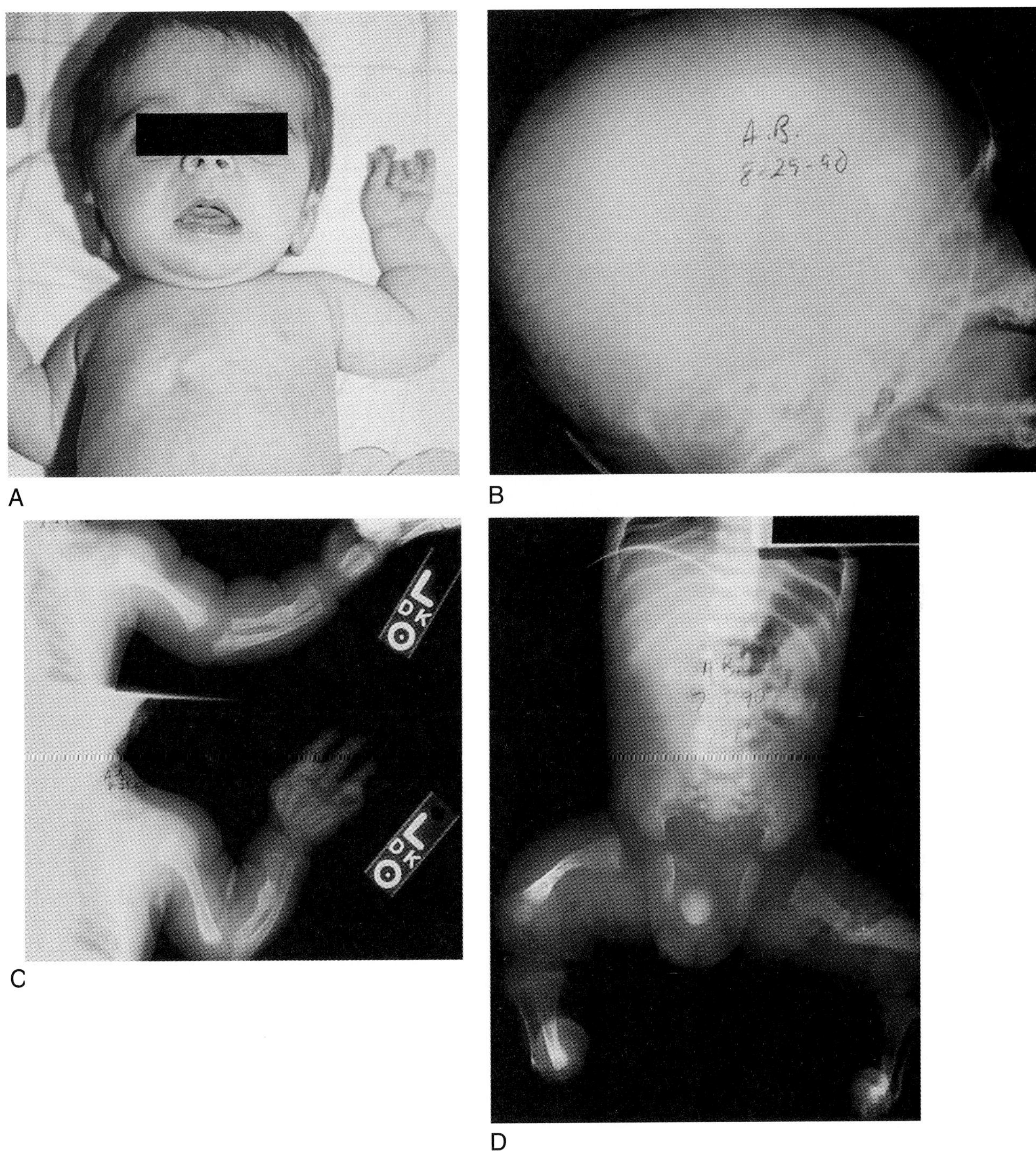


**FIGURE 24–2.** Osteogenesis imperfecta type III. **A,** Neonate with normal face, short neck, slightly short limbs. **B,** Radiograph shows that the calvarium is undermineralized with wormian bones. **C,** Radiograph shows the upper limbs, which have bowed humeri and callus in the ulnae. **D,** Radiograph shows lower limbs with moderately short, thick femora and angulated tibias and fibulas.

anterior fontanelle, and there are many wormian bones (see Fig. 24–2D). The ribs are thin and gracile.

The diagnosis can be confirmed with collagen studies performed on cultured fibroblasts from a skin biopsy. It is difficult to differentiate OI types III and IV histochemically.

### Differential Diagnosis

The four lethal skeletal dysplasias below have similar abnormalities to those in OI and can be diagnosed in the first half of pregnancy by means of ultrasonography. It may be difficult to differentiate the dysplasias; therefore, experienced ultrasonographers are required for accurate diagnoses. These four dysplasias have similar abnormal features in utero on ultrasound examination:

1. Thanatophoric dysplasia (Fig. 24–3; see also subsequent discussion).
2. Campomelic dysplasia (Fig. 24–4; see also subsequent discussion).

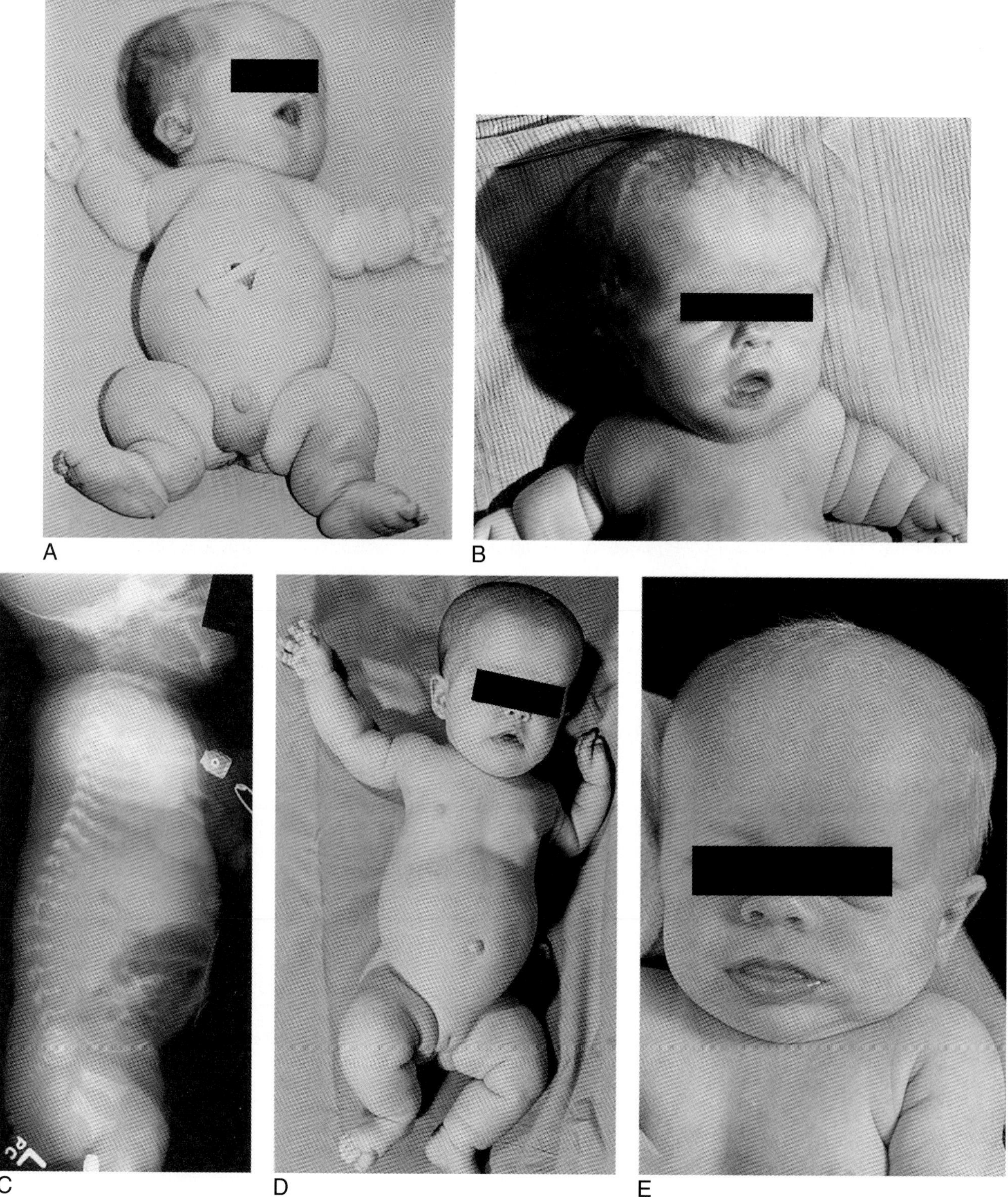


**FIGURE 24–3.** Thanatophoric dysplasia (**A** to **C**) and achondroplasia (**D** and **E**). **A,** Neonate with thanatophoric dysplasia has a large head, narrow chest, very short limbs and extra creases on the limbs, short hands with trident fingers, and angulated abducted thighs. **B,** Neonate with thanatophoric dysplasia has a face with bossed forehead, flat nose bridge, short neck, very short limbs with extra creases, and trident fingers. **C,** Radiograph of an infant with thanatophoric dysplasia demonstrates a large calvarium, short ribs with anterior splaying, and short bowed femurs with medial metaphyseal spike. **D,** Infant with achondroplasia has a bossed forehead and proximal limb shortening. **E,** Infant with achondroplasia has a bossed forehead and flat nasal bridge. (*__A__ and __B__, courtesy Montreal Children's Hospital, Montreal, Quebec, Canada; __D__ and __E__, courtesy Charles I. Scott, MD, AI DuPont Institute, Wilmington, DE.*)

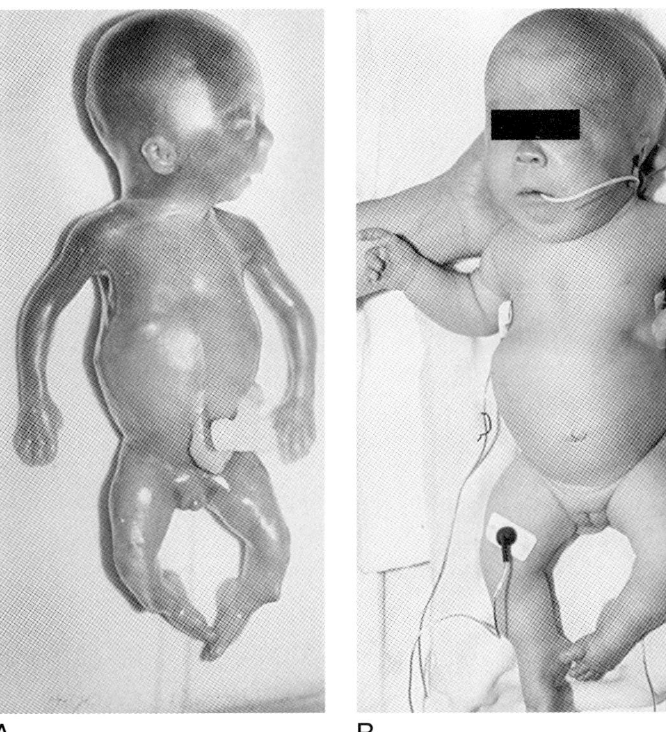

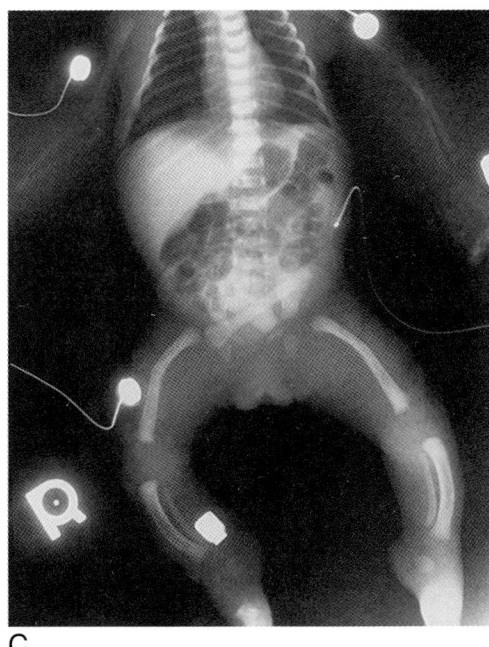

A B C

**FIGURE 24–4.** Campomelic dysplasia. **A,** 46,XY "female" 22-week-old fetus with normal head, long philtrum, micrognathia, low-set ears, mild narrowing of chest, proximally placed thumbs, and bowed or angulated lower limbs resembling those of osteogenesis imperfecta type II but less shortened; the external genitalia are female. **B,** Neonate with the long-limb form of the disorder has a relatively large head, micrognathia, narrow chest, and bowing of lower limbs with characteristic dimpling of lower leg. **C,** Radiograph shows the narrow chest; relatively long, thin limb bones with bowing of the femurs and tibias, and a long, narrow pelvis.

3. Achondrogenesis type IA (Fig. 24–5; see also subsequent discussion).
4. Perinatal hypophosphatasia (see subsequent discussion).

### Inheritance

A fetus or infant with OI type II or III is usually a sporadic occurrence in a family, but there is a risk of recurrence of approximately 6% in subsequent siblings because the gene mutation might be present in some of a parent's somatic cells or germline (parental mosaicism) (Byers et al, 1988). The parent is usually asymptomatic but may have minimal manifestations, such as short stature. *Prenatal diagnosis* is possible with ultrasonography and gene mutation analysis.

### Treatment

If the diagnosis of OI is made prenatally, delivery by cesarean section is recommended to avoid more fractures and intracranial bleeding that could occur with vaginal delivery. The neonate needs careful handling to minimize pain and prevent further fractures. Analgesia alleviates pain. In OI type III, consideration can be given to treatment with bisphosphonates (using intravenous pamidronate), which increase bone density, reduce the frequency of fractures and pain, possibly prevent short stature and deformations, and permit ambulation (Rauch et al, 2002). It is unknown whether the resultant marked decrease in cancellous bone remodeling and the increase in the amount of residual calcified cartilage within secondary spongiosa have sequelae or whether treatment with these agents has other potential adverse effects. It is prudent to treat only severely affected children in whom the clinical benefits outweigh potential long-term effects.

### Handling an Infant with OI

When changing the diapers of an infant with OI, one should place a hand behind the buttocks with the forearm supporting the legs; similarly, when the infant is lifted, the buttocks and head and neck must be supported. The infant can be laid on a pillow to be carried. To transport the infant, an infant seat that reclines as much as possible and allows easy placement or removal should be used. The seat can be padded with egg crating or 1-inch foam. A layer of foam can be placed between the seat's harnesses and the child for extra protection. The car seat must always be placed in the back seat. Sling carriers and "umbrella" strollers should not be used for infants with OI because they do not give sufficient leg or head and neck support.

## PERINATAL HYPOPHOSPHATASIA

Perinatal hypophosphatasia is a lethal condition characterized by short deformed limbs, a soft skull, and undermineralization of the entire skeleton, so that many bones

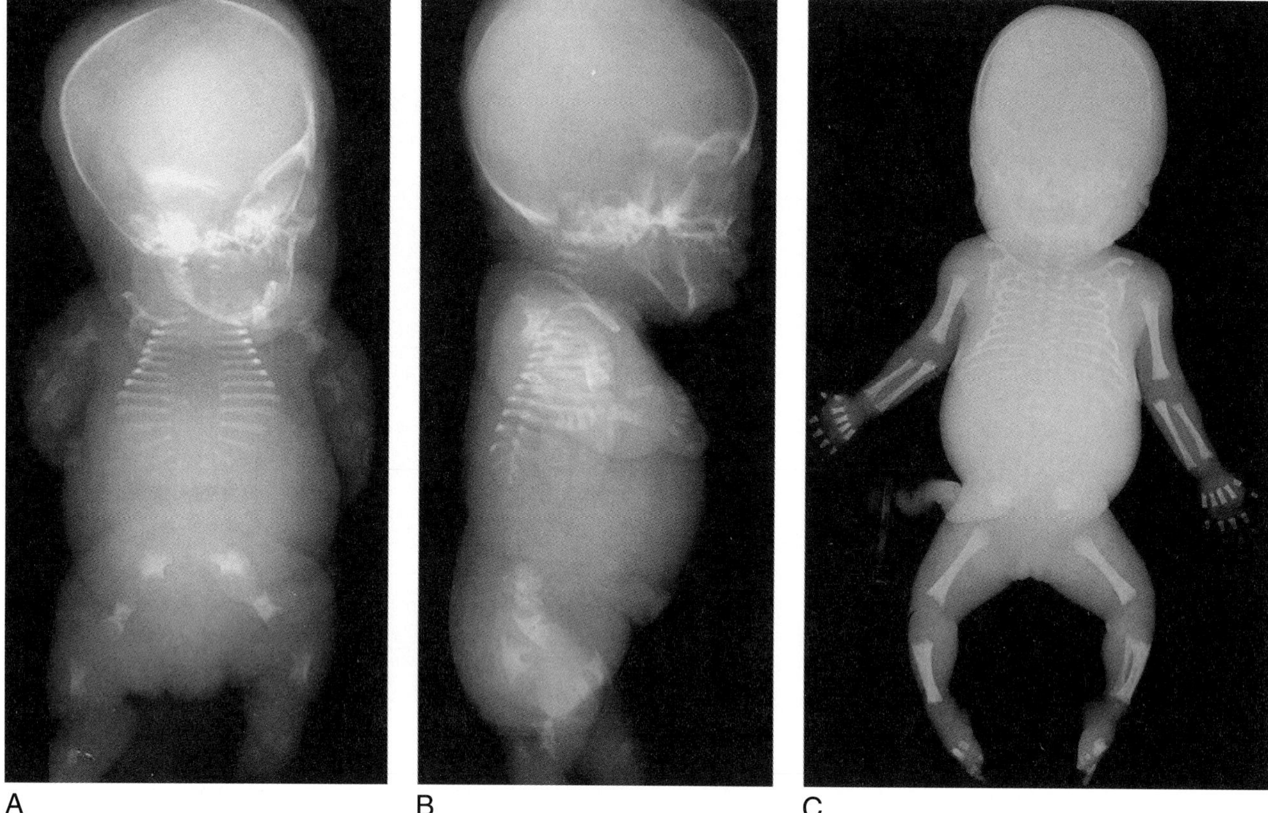


**FIGURE 24–5.** **A** and **B,** Radiographs showing characteristics of achondrogenesis type I: Cervical, thoracic, and lumbar vertebral bodies are not ossified, the sacrum is unossified, the ribs are short, and the limbs are extremely short with medial femoral metaphyseal spikes. **C,** Radiograph showing hypochondrogenesis in a midgestation fetus with underossified calvarium and vertebral bodies (although better ossified than in achondrogenesis), unossified pubis, longer limb bones but irregular metaphyses, short ribs, and a narrow thorax. *(Courtesy Elaine Zackai, MD, Children's Hospital of Philadelphia.)*

cannot be visualized and may seem on radiography to be absent. In the skull, only the base may be visualized radiologically. There may be rachitic changes and fractures. Seizures that are responsive to pyridoxine may occur. During pregnancy, there is polyhydramnios, and in utero death can occur. The disorder affects approximately 1 in 100,000 live births; neonatal death is usual (Whyte, 1995).

### Etiology

Deficiency of tissue-nonspecific isoenzyme of alkaline phosphatase (TNSALP) causes perinatal hypophosphatasia. The gene for TNSALP is mutant and is located on chromosome 1p34 to p36.1. Many mutations have been linked to severe perinatal hypophosphatasia (Orimo et al, 2001). The serum alkaline phosphatase (ALP) value is very low. Serum values of phosphoethanolamine, inorganic pyrophosphate, and pyridoxal 5′-phosphate, putative natural substrates for TNSALP, may be elevated.

TNSALP acts on multiple substrates: the essential function of TNSALP is in osteoblastic bone matrix mineralization. TNSALP hydrolyzes inorganic pyrophosphate to phosphate, thought to be critical in promoting osteoblastic mineralization. If TNSALP is deficient, there is extracellular accumulation of inorganic pyrophosphate, which inhibits hydroxyapatite crystal formation and mineralization of the skeleton. TNSALP is also needed for delivery of pyridoxal-5-phosphate into cells where it is a cofactor (vitamin $B_6$).

### Treatment

Treatment of perinatal hypophosphatasia with enzyme replacement has been unsuccessful.

### Inheritance

Perinatal hypophosphatasia is inherited as an autosomal recessive trait; each of a couple's subsequent children has a 25% risk for the disease. Prenatal diagnosis is optimized through the use of ultrasonography, assay of TNSALP activity in amniocytes, DNA mutation analysis if the previously affected child's mutation was known, or a combination of these methods.

## CAMPOMELIC DYSPLASIA

Campomelic dysplasia is characterized by short stature (birth length 35 to 49 cm), large dolichocephalic skull, large anterior fontanelle, high forehead, flat face, widely spaced eyes with short palpebral fissures, low-set ears, cleft soft palate, micrognathia, relatively long, slender thighs and upper arms, short bowed legs with dimples in the midshaft (in most cases), narrow chest, and kyphoscoliosis. Sex reversal or ambiguous genitalia affects 75% of the chromosomal males; there may be internal and external genital abnormalities (from mild anomalies to complete sex reversal) in XY males (Houston et al, 1983) (see Fig. 24–4A and B). Absence of the olfactory bulbs and tracts as well as heart and renal malformations occur. Death, usually in infancy, results from respiratory compromise. Survivors are usually retarded. A few more mildly affected people without bowed limbs have been reported.

### Radiology

In the second trimester, on ultrasonography, the limbs of a fetus with campomelic dysplasia may appear short, bowed, and angulated, and the disease may be mistaken for OI (see Fig. 24–4C). However, the two disorders are distinguishable because the calvarium in campomelic dysplasia is better ossified, the palate may be cleft, and the chin is small. Specific postnatal abnormalities are very small, bladeless scapulas and hypoplastic pedicles of thoracic vertebrae. Other features are as follows:

- Hypoplastic, undermineralized cervical vertebrae and thoracic pedicles
- Small iliac wings and relatively wide pelvic outlet
- Dislocated hips
- Short phalanges of the hands and feet; talipes equinovarus; anterior bowing of tibia; short fibula; mildly bowed femur
- Absence of ossification of proximal tibial and distal femoral epiphyses
- Ribs may be thin and wavy, with only 11 pairs

### Differential Diagnosis

See osteogenesis types II and III.

### Etiology

The mutant gene, *SOX9* (a transcription factor gene), is located at chromosome 17q24.1 to 25.1 (Tommerup, 1993). *SOX9*, with homology to the *SRY*- gene, is involved in both bone formation and control of testis development.

### Inheritance

Campomelic dysplasia is an autosomal dominant trait. Most cases are new sporadic occurrences in a family. Siblings may be affected if there is gonadal mosaicism.

### Management

Chromosome studies to determine gender and ultrasonography to examine internal genitalia should be performed in survivors. Cleft palate may need repair.

## ACHONDROGENESIS TYPES IA AND IB

Achondrogenesis types IA and IB are characterized by short stature, extremely short limbs (with "flipper" hands in type IA), relatively large head with round face, short nose, small mouth, soft skull, and very short neck (Borochowitz et al, 1988). Polyhydramnios during pregnancy, premature delivery, and hydrops are common. The affected infant is stillborn or dies within hours of birth.

### Radiology

The long bones are extremely short, with square, globular, or triangular shapes and medial spikes in the metaphyses of the femurs (see Fig. 24–5A and B). The calvarium is poorly ossified, the vertebrae are either unossified (type IA) or poorly ossified (type IB), and the ribs are short (with multiple fractures and callus [beading] in type IA).

### Inheritance and Cause

Achondrogenesis type 1B is caused by mutations in the *DTDST* gene, which also cause another lethal disorder, atelosteogenesis type 2 (AO2), and two nonlethal disorders, diastrophic dysplasia (DTD) and recessive multiple epiphyseal dysplasia (rMED). The gene product is a sulfate-chloride exchanger of the cell membrane (Superti-Furga et al, 1996).

### Differential Diagnosis

Achondrogenesis type II and hypochondrogenesis are the same condition, caused by different mutations in the same gene for type II collagen but with variable phenotypic expression. The short stature and the limb, calvarial, and vertebral abnormalities are somewhat less severe than in achondrogenesis type I, but there is also hydrops, with stillbirth, or death within hours after birth. Cleft palate may occur in hypochondrogenesis (see Fig. 24–5C).

### Inheritance

The inheritance pattern of achondrogenesis types IA and IB is autosomal dominant, usually a new sporadic mutation.

## ACHONDROPLASIA

Achondroplasia is the most common of the nonlethal chondrodysplasias; it affects 1 in 15,000 live births. It is characterized at birth by short limbs, particularly rhizomelic (proximal) and acromelic (hands) with trident fingers, large head with frontal prominence, flat nose bridge, flat midface, long narrow trunk, and thoracolumbar gibbus deformity (see Fig. 24–3D and E). The lateral cerebral ventricles may be large, but hydrocephalus is not common in affected children, although it is more prevalent than in the general population. The child with achondroplasia is hypotonic; together with the large head, the hypotonia leads to delayed motor milestones.

Most achondroplastic children have normal intelligence. However, development can be impaired if there is hydrocephalus, which can result from perinatal bleeds associated with vaginal deliveries, or impaired respiratory function (Hecht et al, 1991). The foramen magnum and the lumbar spinal canal may be narrow, causing compression of the spinal cord. Compression of the lower brainstem and cervical spinal cord can lead to hypotonia, retardation, quadriparesis, obstructive or central apnea, and sudden death (Pauli et al, 1984). Perinatal or infantile death is unusual (3%); most children die between 2 and 5 months, often during the day, and death may be precipitated by sleeping upright without support for the head.

In the achondroplastic infant who dies suddenly, the head circumference is usually not larger than average for achondroplasia, the neurologic state is not abnormal, and development is average.

Radiologic imaging of the skull and brain is recommended for monitoring; surgical decompression of foramen magnum or lumbar stenosis may prevent neurologic damage. In older persons with achondroplasia, untreated spinal stenosis can cause paresthesias, numbness, bladder and bowel incontinence, and impotence. Standard growth curves for achondroplasia should be used routinely (Horton et al, 1978); deviation from the expected should alert the physician to a possible new complication, such as hydrocephalus. Average adult height in this disorder is 118 to 145 cm (men) and 112 to 136 cm (women) and is diminished because of lumbar lordosis and mild thoracolumbar kyphosis. A controversial surgical technique to lengthen limbs, the Ilizarov method (Ilizarov, 1988), can add as much as 25 cm. It is used in adolescents. Pins are inserted into the limbs on either side of the epiphyses or fractured bone with callus formation, and the areas are stretched by millimeters daily.

### Radiology

The proximal long bones, the humeri and femurs, are short, especially the femoral neck. Fibulas are longer than tibias. There is metaphyseal flaring. The hand is short and trident with short proximal and midphalanges. The calvarium is large with a small foramen magnum and a short base. Vertebrae are small and cuboid with short pedicles and anterior beaking of the first or second lumbar vertebrae; there is progressive narrowing of interpedicular distance in the lumbar vertebrae. The pelvis has small, round iliac wings, a narrow greater sciatic notch, and flat acetabular roofs.

### Inheritance

The inheritance pattern in achondroplasia is autosomal dominant. Approximately 90% of cases are sporadic occurrences in a family, representing new mutations. Many cases are associated with advanced paternal age, with molecular confirmation that the new mutations are of paternal origin. Affected individuals are fertile, and achondroplasia is transmitted as a fully penetrant autosomal dominant trait, meaning that each person who inherits the mutant gene will show the condition.

### Etiology

The cause of achondroplasia is a mutation of the gene for *FGFR3* (fibroblast growth factor receptor 3), a membrane-spanning tyrosine kinase receptor. *FGFR3* is encoded on chromosome 4p16.3. More than 97% of persons with achondroplasia have a mutation in the transmembrane domain of the *FGFR3* gene, in which glycine is substituted by arginine, Gly380Arg (Shiang et al, 1994). The same gene is mutated, at different sites, in hypochondroplasia, thanatophoric dysplasia, SADDAN, Muenke craniosynostosis, and Crouzon craniosynostosis syndrome with acanthosis nigricans (Vajo et al, 2000). Histopathologic examination demonstrates a defect in the maturation of the cartilage growth plates of long bones.

### Differential Diagnosis

The differential diagnosis for achondroplasia includes the following disorders:

1. SADDAN (Vajo et al, 2000). Affected infants have seizures and hydrocephalus. This disorder represents the part of the spectrum between lethal thanatophoric dysplasia ( see later) and achondroplasia, with survival past infancy into young adulthood without prolonged ventilatory assistance. Some infants with SADDAN have the same Lys650Met mutation as some infants with thanatophoric dysplasia type I yet have skeletal abnormalities different from both thanatophoric dysplasia types I and II. These include absence of craniosynostosis or cloverleaf skull anomaly and only moderate bowing of the femurs with reverse bowing of the tibia and fibula.
2. Hypochondroplasia (usually not apparent at birth, as the face is normal). Although limbs are usually short, there is no rhizomelia, mesomelia, or acromelia, and final height is greater than in achondroplasia. There may be mild metaphyseal flaring, brachydactyly, and mild limitation of elbow extension. Hypochondroplasia may be genetically heterogeneous, because not all affected people have *FGFR3* mutations; those who do often have an Asn540Lys mutation.

### Management in the Newborn Period

Development of thoracolumbar kyphosis in a patient with achondroplasia is associated with unsupported sitting before trunk muscle strength is adequate. Infants should not be carried in flexed positions (including soft sling-carriers, "swingomatics," "jolly jumpers," and "umbrella" strollers), which may increase the risk for gibbus. Unsupported sitting should be avoided. Car safety seats should always be used.

Hydrocephalus may develop during the first 2 years, so the head circumference should be carefully measured monthly during the first year and plotted on achondroplasia growth charts. A disproportionate increase may indicate development of hydrocephalus.

Parents should be counseled about the clinical and hereditary aspects of the disorder and given a copy of the guidelines for health supervision of children with achondroplasia issued by the American Academy of Pediatrics (Health supervision, 1995).

## THANATOPHORIC DYSPLASIA

Thanatophoric dysplasia is one of the most common lethal dysplasias (Rimoin and Lachman, 1996; Spranger and Maroteaux, 1990), occurring in 1 in 35,000 births. It is characterized by extremely short limbs, long narrow trunk, large head with bulging forehead, prominent eyes, flat nose bridge, wide fontanelle, and, occasionally, cloverleaf skull deformity (see Fig. 24–3A). It is differentiated into types I and II on the basis of radiologic features. Death occurs in the neonatal period from respiratory insufficiency. Polyhydramnios is common during pregnancy.

Radiography shows that the femurs are short, flared at the metaphyses, with a medial spike, bowed (type I) or straight (type II); other long bones are also short and bowed (see Fig. 24–3B and C and Table 24–2). The calvarium is large with a short base and small foramen magnum; cloverleaf skull is sometimes present in type I thanatophoric dysplasia and is severe in type II. Vertebrae are flat with notching of superior and inferior aspects on lateral views; lumbar vertebrae have an inverted-U appearance on anteroposterior views. Ribs are short, cupped, and splayed anteriorly (Tavormina et al, 1995). A subtype of thanatophoric dysplasia type I is the platyspondylic San Diego type, in which there are metaphyseal spikes, better-preserved growth plates, and large inclusion bodies in the rough endoplasmic reticulum.

### Differential Diagnosis

The differential diagnosis for thanatophoric dysplasia consists of the following disorders:

1. OI types II and III
2. Achondroplasia (see earlier discussion)
3. Achondrogenesis and hypochondrogenesis

### Etiology

Thanatophoric dysplasia types I and II are caused by distinct mutations in the gene for *FGFR3*. In thanatophoric dysplasia type I, most mutations have been in the extracellular domain, with single amino acid substitutions by cysteine (Rousseau et al, 1995; Tavormina et al, 1995; Wilcox et al, 1998). In most European, North American, and Japanese studies, the most common mutation has been Arg248Cys. In all studied cases of thanatophoric dysplasia type II, the lysine at amino acid 650 has been substituted by glutamate (Lys650Glu) (Tavormina et al, 1995; Wilcox et al, 1998). More than 98% of studied cases of achondroplasia have substitution of the same amino acid, glycine, by arginine (Gly380Arg) (Shiang et al, 1994). In several patients with hypochondroplasia, mutations have been found at one specific nucleotide coding for asparagine, which has been substituted by lysine (Asp540Lys) (Bellus et al, 1995a and 1995b).

### Inheritance

Most cases of thanatophoric dysplasia, as with achondroplasia and hypochondroplasia, occur sporadically, resulting from new autosomal dominant mutations. Nevertheless, there is a small risk of recurrence in siblings of the patient with a sporadic case, because of possible parental mosaicism.

## CONGENITAL (NEONATAL, INFANTILE) MARFAN SYNDROME

Congenital Marfan syndrome (cMFS), the most severe form of Marfan syndrome, is caused by mutations in the same gene associated with classic Marfan syndrome (Dietz et al, 1991). The affected neonate has a long, thin body with an aged appearance because of a lack of subcutaneous tissue and wrinkled, sagging skin (cutis laxa) (Morse et al, 1990) (Fig. 24–6A). The characteristic facies has dolichocephaly, deep-set eyes with large or small corneas (and occasionally cataracts), high nose bridge, high palate, small pointed chin with a horizontal skin crease, and large simple or crumpled ears (see Fig. 24–6B and C). The fingers and toes are long and thin (arachnodactyly). Some joints are hyperextensible, and others have flexion contractures, causing equinovarus or equinovalgus, dislocated hips, or adducted thumbs. The infant tends to be hypotonic, with low muscle mass. Occasional features are diaphragmatic or inguinal hernias and retinal detachment. Lenses are usually not subluxated at birth. The most important cause of morbidity and mortality is severe cardiovascular disease, which affects almost every neonate with cMFS, namely, mitral and tricuspid valve prolapse and insufficiency and aortic root dilation. The ascending aorta may be dilated and tortuous. Congestive cardiac failure associated with mitral and tricuspid regurgitation develops; most infants die in the first year. Survivors have continuing hypotonia and contractures, are unable to walk, and require many surgical procedures.

### Inheritance

Marfan syndrome is an autosomal dominant disorder. Most neonates with cMFS are sporadic occurrences in a family (Dietz et al, 1991; Godfrey et al, 1995; Morse et al, 1990). However, there is one well-documented neonate with cMFS whose father had classic Marfan syndrome except for average height (Lopes et al, 1995). Routine ultrasonography at 34 weeks of gestation showed oligohydramnios and cardiomegaly. Fetal echocardiography demonstrated the typical severe features and pleural effusion.

### Etiology

Congenital MFS is caused by abnormalities of a connective tissue, fibrillin, which is encoded by the gene fibrillin 1 (*FBN1*) on the long arm of chromosome 15 (15q21.1) (Dietz et al, 1991; Godfrey et al, 1995). Fibrillin, together with other proteins (microfibril-associated glycoproteins), is a component of microfibrils, which form linear bundles in the matrices of many tissues, such as aorta, periosteum, perichondrium, cartilage, tendons, muscle, pleura, and meninges. Microfibrils have the following functions: (1) as scaffolding onto which elastin is deposited, for example, in the tunica media of the aorta, (2) as scaffolding for nonelastic tissues, for example, the ciliary zonule of the eye, periodontal ligament, and mesangium of renal glomeruli, and (3) as connections between elastin and other matrix components, for example, in the skin between elastin bundles and the dermoid-epidermoid junction.

There is a region of two "hot spots" in *FBN1* in which mutations causing congenital Marfan syndrome occur. These are missense mutations (mainly), small deletions or insertions and one exon skipping mutation in exons 24 to 27, and exon skipping mutations affecting exons 31 and 32 (Booms et al, 1999). It is possible that exon skipping mutations could cause very severe disruption of microfibril assembly by interfering with the exact lateral alignment of fibrillin monomers that must be incorporated into polymeric microfibrils.

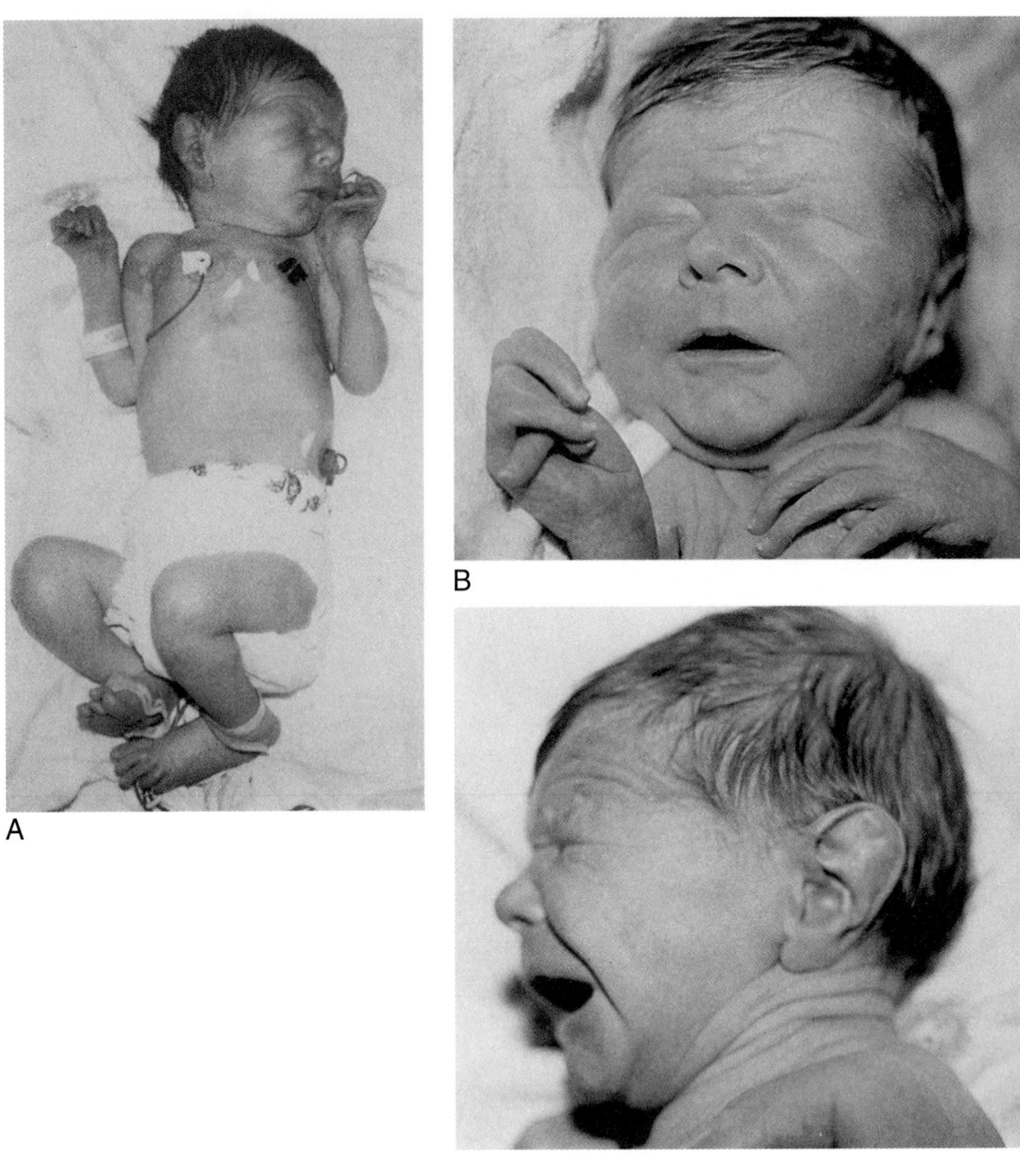


**FIGURE 24–6.** Congenital Marfan syndrome. **A,** Neonate with long thin trunk and limbs (particularly the feet), lack of adipose tissue, and multiple skin creases giving an aged appearance. The ears are large and simple, and the chin is small with a horizontal crease. There are flexion contractures at the joints. **B,** Neonate's face shows laxity of skin, typical horizontal chin crease, and pointed chin. The fingers are long with adduction contractures of the thumbs, which extend past the edge of the palm, and floppy wrists. **C,** Lateral view of the neonate's head showing simple "large" ears and redundant skin on the neck.

### Tests

Blood and skin should be obtained for gene mutation studies in lymphocytes and skin fibroblasts, although it has not been possible to detect the mutation in each case.

### Prenatal Diagnosis

Recurrences of congenital Marfan syndrome are not usual, but, if parents want assurance, prenatal diagnosis by chorionic villous biopsy and amniocentesis is feasible if the gene mutation is known. Prenatal detection by ultrasonography is possible in the second half of pregnancy. It is not known whether the cardiovascular and joint abnormalities are detectable before 20 weeks of gestation.

### Differential Diagnosis

The differential diagnosis for cMFS includes the following disorders.

1. Beals syndrome, or congenital contractural arachnodactyly (CCA), is characterized by a similar thin, wasted appearance with minimal muscle and fat mass and contractures of the large and small joints (Fig. 24–7A). Cardiovascular involvement is usually limited to mitral valve prolapse, contractures improve to some degree with time, and life span is normal. CCA is an autosomal dominant condition caused by mutations in the fibrillin 2 (*FBN2*) gene on chromosome 5 (5q23-31).

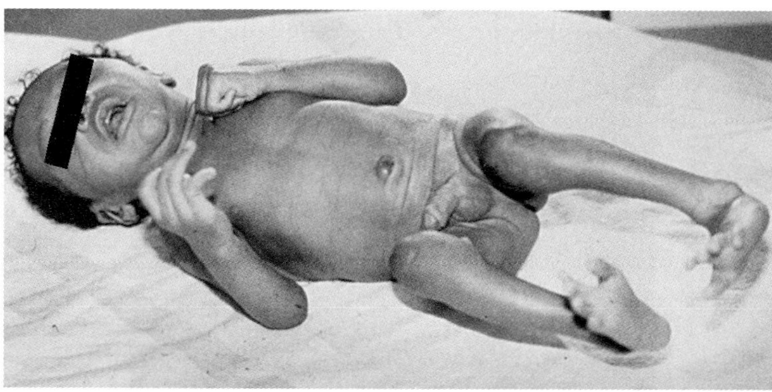

A

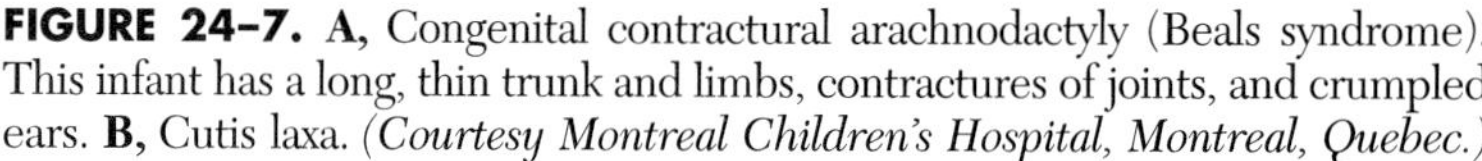

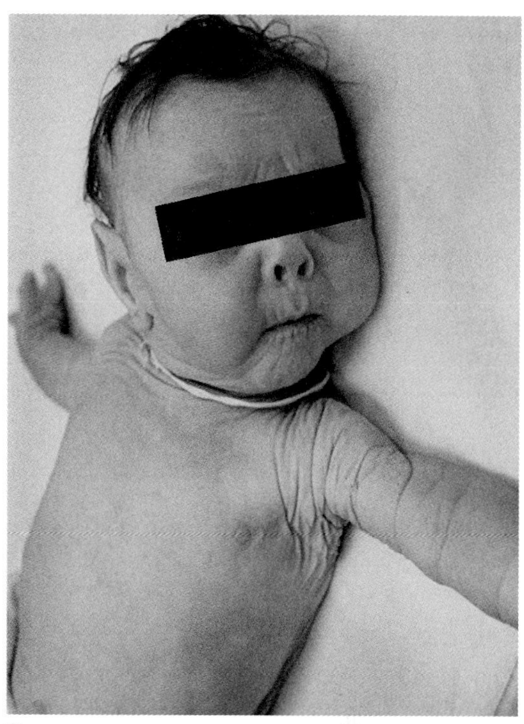

B

**FIGURE 24–7.** **A,** Congenital contractural arachnodactyly (Beals syndrome). This infant has a long, thin trunk and limbs, contractures of joints, and crumpled ears. **B,** Cutis laxa. *(Courtesy Montreal Children's Hospital, Montreal, Quebec.)*

2. The autosomal recessive form of cutis laxa syndrome is severe and can manifest at birth with loose, sagging skin, pulmonary emphysema, and gastrointestinal and urinary tract diverticula (Fig. 24–7B). The cardiovascular abnormality seen in Marfan syndrome does not occur in cutis laxa.

## WILLIAMS SYNDROME

Williams syndrome is difficult to diagnose in the newborn period, but the astute clinician notes an irritable infant with a coarse "swollen" face with periorbital fullness and thick lips who may have a cardiac murmur (Morris et al, 1988) (Fig. 24–8A and B). Supravalvar aortic stenosis and peripheral pulmonic stenosis may manifest in the newborn period, with occasional atrial or ventricular septal defects and, rarely, coarctation of the aorta. The presence of such an unusual vascular lesion, supravalvar aortic stenosis, should bring to mind the possibility of either isolated autosomal dominant supravalvar aortic stenosis or Williams syndrome. Supravalvar aortic stenosis affects more than 50% of children with Williams syndrome. Gestational age is usually approximately 42 weeks, with birth weight and length in the lower half of or below the normal growth curves. The facies in infancy may be coarse or fine, with periorbital fullness, medial flare of the eyebrows, common blue irises with a stellate pattern, epicanthic folds, flat nose bridge with full nasal tip and anteverted nares, long or undefined philtrum, chubby "low-set" cheeks, small chin, and large ears (see Fig. 24–8C and D). The lips may be thick at birth or may thicken later; the "Cupid's bow" is diminished or absent. The head may be dolichocephalic (increased anteroposterior diameter), and the hair curly.

Clinodactyly (incurving) of the fifth fingers is common. The skin is very soft, with fine creases on the palms, and ages prematurely. There is occasional inability to pronate and supinate the forearm. The limbs are short compared with the trunk but this characteristic may not be obvious in the newborn period. Mild hypotonia is common. Frequent vomiting starts soon after birth, and it is not unusual for the infant to scream most of the day and to refuse feedings. This behavior may be due to gastroesophageal reflux, causing esophagitis, or to hypercalcemia. The irritability can persist for most of the first year.

Moderate global developmental delay with a specific pattern of strengths and weaknesses is usual; rare individuals have normal IQ or severe retardation. Strengths include good expressive language, recognition of faces, friendliness (which may be inappropriate), and, sometimes, short-term memory. These qualities can hide or mask for the casual observer the patient's difficulties with visuomotor abilities such as writing and drawing figures, mathematical reasoning, understanding money, and subtle social interactions. The voice is deep and hoarse. Hyperactivity is common and can be controlled with methylphenidate and similar drugs, thereby improving learning and performance (Power et al, 1997).

In addition to supravalvar aortic and peripheral pulmonic artery stenoses, narrowing (stenosis or coarctation) of other vessels, including the aortic, renal, and cerebral

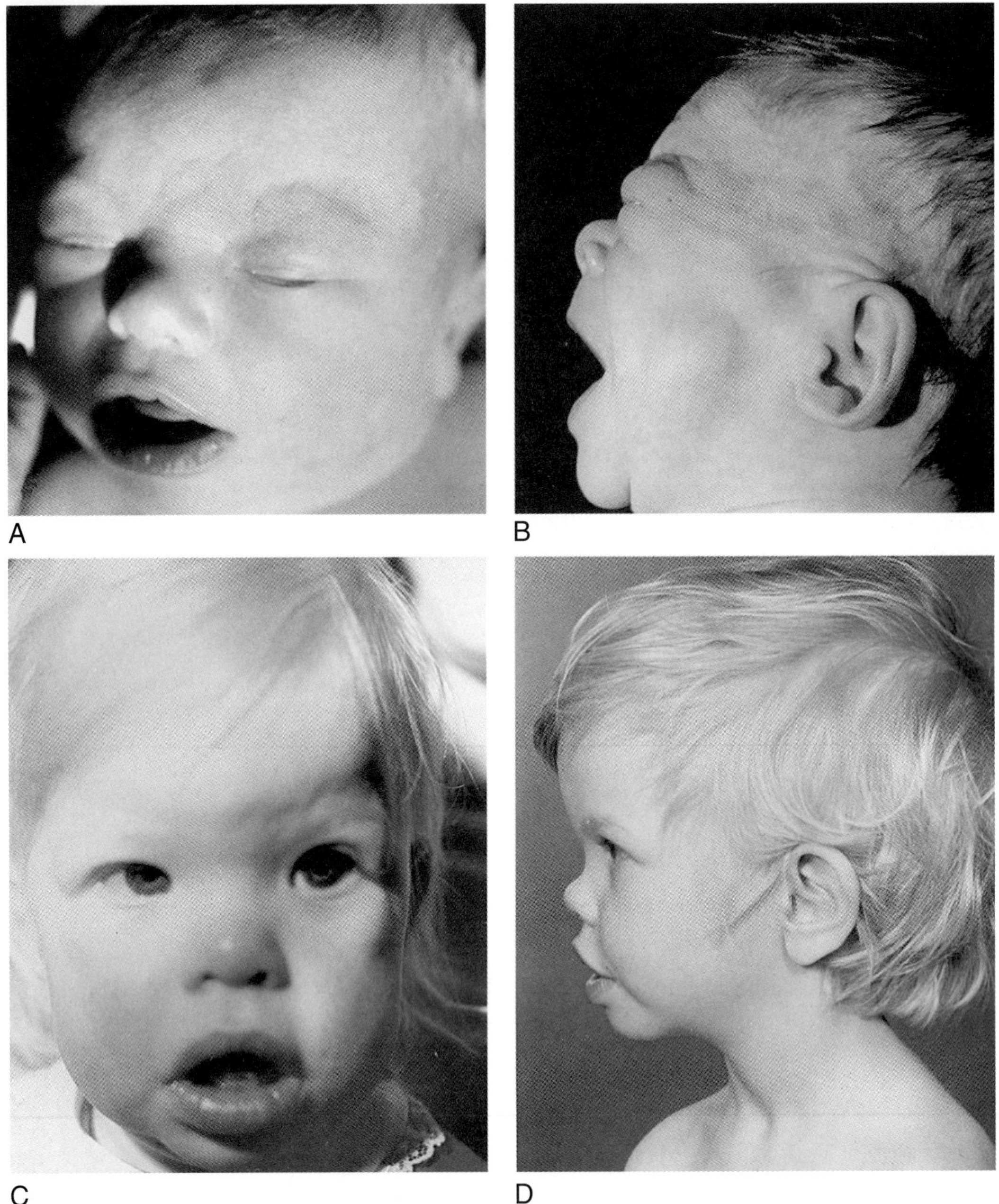


**FIGURE 24–8.** Williams syndrome. **A,** Neonate with a coarse face, periorbital fullness, wide mouth, and thick lips with decreased Cupid's bow. **B,** Neonate profile showing periorbital fullness, flat nasal bridge with full tip, and prominent cheeks. **C,** This infant has periorbital fullness, flat nasal bridge, thick lips with decreased Cupid's bow, pouty lower lip, and "low-set" full cheeks. **D,** Infant profile showing dolichocephaly (increased anteroposterior diameter of head), higher nasal bridge than in neonate, full nasal tip, pouty lower lip, long neck, sloping shoulders, and part of pectus excavatum.

arteries, may occur (Kaplan et al, 1995). Hypertension may develop because of arterial stenosis or renal disease. Life span may be shortened by cardiac or renal failure. Cardiac failure is less common than a decade ago because of earlier diagnosis and cardiac intervention with medications or surgery. Diverticulosis of the bowel (associated with chronic constipation) and bladder (associated with chronic dys-synergia of bladder emptying) may develop in adolescence or adulthood (Schulman et al, 1996). Contractures can impair daily function (Kaplan et al, 1989). Rarely, renal failure develops (Pober et al, 1993).

### Etiology

Williams syndrome is a contiguous gene deletion syndrome resulting from a deletion at 7q11.23 on one chromosome 7 only (Ewart et al, 1993). Many genes have been deleted, including elastin (Ewart et al, 1993) and replication factor C subunit 2 (Peoples et al, 1996), and LIM-kinase 1 (Frangiskakis et al, 1996).The function of all the deleted genes has not yet been elucidated. The lack of elastin accounts for many features, such as arterial narrowing, diverticula, skin and joint problems, some facial characteristics, and deep voice. The replication factor may be important for cell growth. The LIM-kinase has been linked to the visuomotor dysfunction in one series (Frangiskakis et al, 1996), but this finding is not substantiated in other series. The frequency of deletion in chromosomes of maternal and paternal origins is the same. The deletion can be demonstrated with fluorescent in situ hybridization (FISH) with use of a probe that includes the elastin gene and extends beyond the 3′ and 5′ borders.

### Inheritance

Most cases of Williams syndrome are sporadic occurrences in a family. There are reports of several sibling pairs with Williams syndrome with neither parent affected (Kara-Mostefa et al, 1999; CI Scott Jr, personal communication, 1997). This occurrence could be due to germline mosaicism in one parent; the risk for recurrence in a sibling of a sporadic case is approximately 5%, on the basis of experience in other disorders (Byers et al, 1988). Each child of a person with Williams syndrome has a 50% chance of inheriting the chromosome 7 with the deletion and manifesting the disorder (Morris et al, 1993); there are known families in which a parent and a child have Williams syndrome.

### Prenatal Diagnosis

Prenatal diagnosis of Williams syndrome is established with FISH of chorionic villus cells and amniocytes.

### Differential Diagnosis

The differential diagnosis of Williams syndrome in a newborn consists of the following disorders:

1. Lysosomal storage disease, particularly $G_{M1}$ gangliosidosis or mucolipidosis type II (I-cell disease), may cause coarse facial features and joint contractures in the newborn period. There may be cardiomyopathy but not arterial narrowing and other features.
2. Noonan syndrome may cause coarse features and valvar pulmonic stenosis but not usually peripheral pulmonic stenosis.
3. Autosomal dominant supravalvar aortic stenosis is not associated with all the other features of Williams syndrome. Often there are other affected family members.

### Management

A multispecialty team approach is needed for the life of a person with Williams syndrome. However, in the newborn period, the most immediate problems are the feeding difficulty, hypotonia, and narrowing of the great vessels (Kaplan, et al, 2001). The infant may be irritable, crying constantly, and refusing to feed. Recognition and treatment of contributory factors, as follow, will help:

- Sucking may be weak because of hypotonia; breastfeeding may not be feasible.
- Swallowing may be incoordinated.
- Gastroesophageal reflux causes profuse vomiting and pain from esophagitis.
- Idiopathic hypercalcemia adds to the vomiting and irritability and causes constipation; the ionized calcium value should be measured, and a low-calcium formula may be needed.
- Stenoses of the great vessels impair energy; an echocardiogram should be performed.

## EHLERS-DANLOS SYNDROMES

There are at least eight types of Ehlers-Danlos syndrome, which are characterized by varying degrees and extents of joint and skin hypermobility, excessive bruising, thin wide scars, and fragility of tissues (Steinmann et al, 1993). Ehlers-Danlos syndrome types I and VII are the most likely to manifest in the newborn period. Type I is characterized by premature delivery of a fetus with Ehlers-Danlos syndrome as a result of rupture of the amniotic membranes. The infant may be floppy and in breech position. There may be joint laxity and instability. In type VII, the major involvement is in the ligaments and joint capsules. Large and small joints are hypermobile and dislocatable; severe congenital dislocation of hips occurs. Dislocations are recurrent.

In type IV Ehlers-Danlos syndrome, the greatest danger is to the pregnant affected woman, for whom there is a high risk of uterine rupture. Although there is a 50% risk that the fetus will be affected, the problems of blood loss and prematurity are more important in the newborn period than the disorder itself.

### Etiology

Collagen type V has been implicated in causing (some) cases of Ehlers-Danlos syndrome types I and II (Burrows et al, 1996; De Paepe et al, 1997). Type IV of the syndrome is caused by mutations in collagen type III. Type VII is caused by a deleted exon 6 in the α-1 (COL1A1) or α-2 chain (COL1A2) of type I collagen.

### Inheritance

The types of Ehlers-Danlos syndrome discussed here are inherited as autosomal dominant traits. Each child of an affected person has a 50% chance of inheriting and manifesting the disorder.

### Prenatal Diagnosis

If the molecular defect has been characterized, chorionic villus sampling or amniocentesis is feasible. This had been difficult for type I, because the connective tissue was not known. However, amniocentesis in a fetus affected with Ehlers-Danlos syndrome type I may cause amniotic tears and fluid leaking.

## OTHER SKELETAL DYSPLASIAS

For information on atelosteogenesis (Fig. 24–9), chondrodysplasia (Fig. 24–10), and diastrophic dysplasia (Fig. 24–11), see Table 24–2.

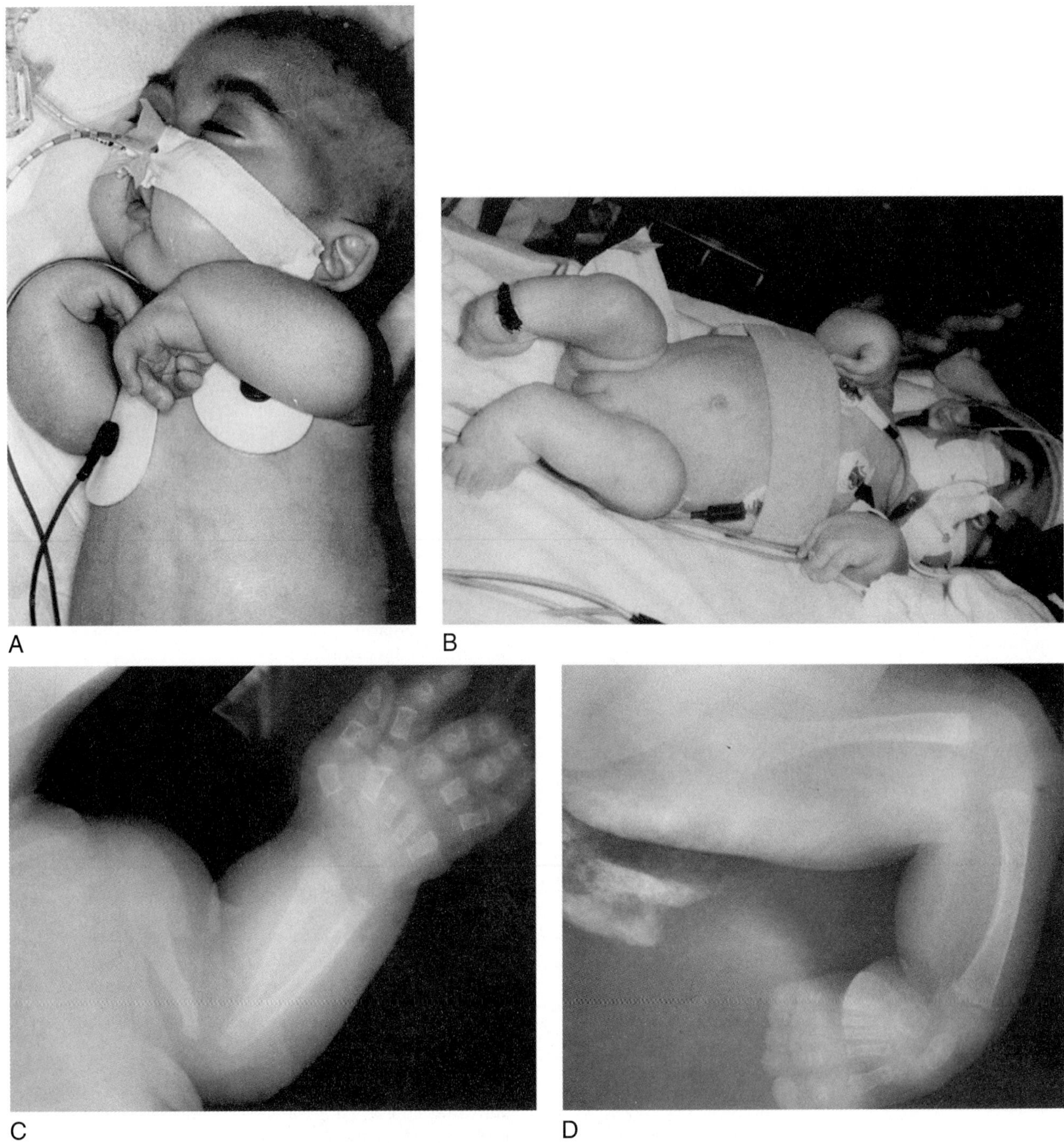


**FIGURE 24–9.** Atelosteogenesis (see Table 24–2). **A** and **B,** Infant with proximal limb shortening and equinovalgus deformities of the hands and feet. **C,** Radiograph of the upper limb showing distal tapering of humerus; metacarpals and phalanges are short and broad or irregular. **D,** Radiograph of the lower limb showing "clubbing" of foot; fibula is not visualized and may be hypoplastic or absent. *(Courtesy Charles I. Scott, MD, AI DuPont Institute, Wilmington, DE.)*

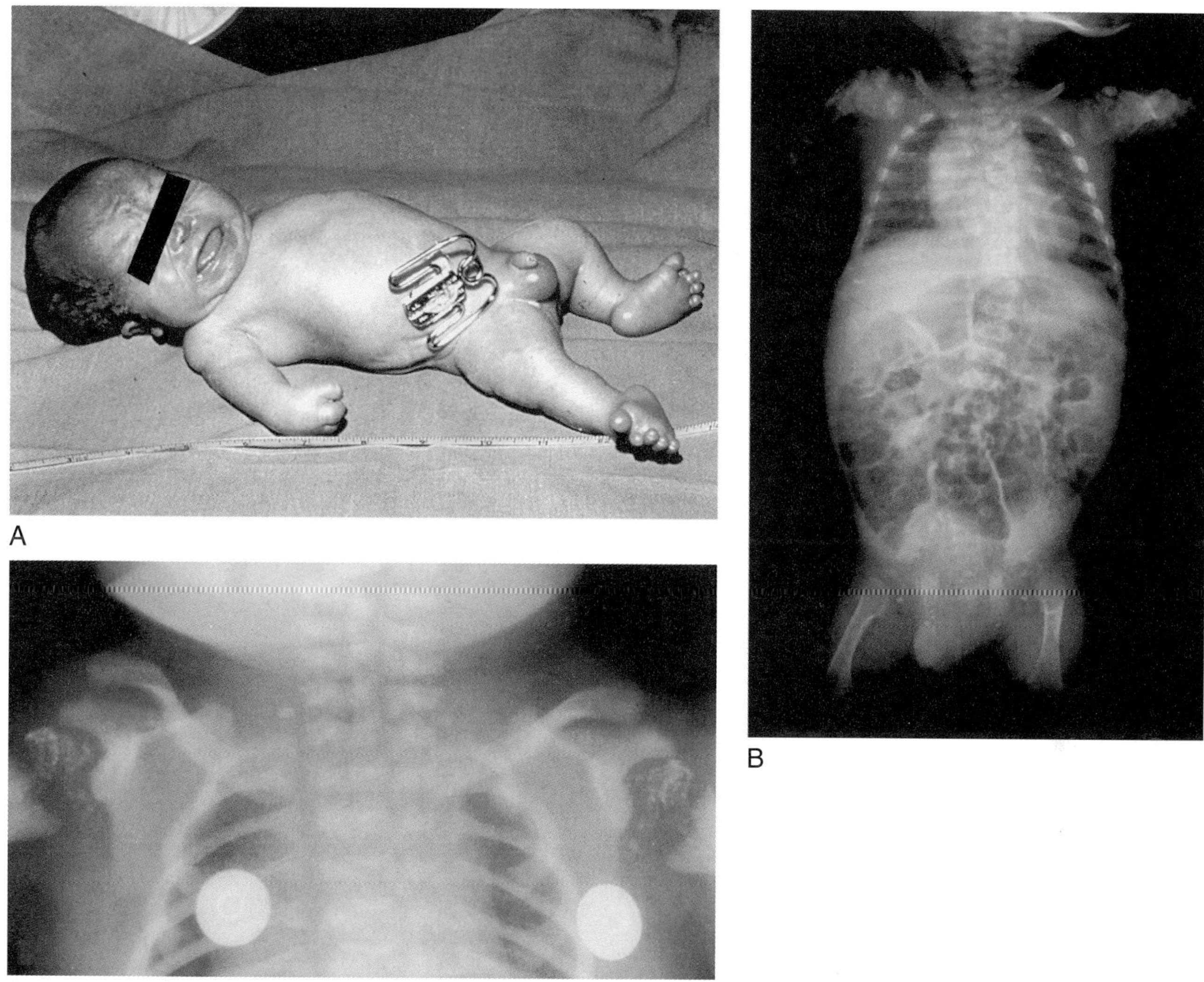


**FIGURE 24–10.** Chondrodysplasia punctata, rhizomelic type (see Table 24–2). **A,** Neonate with a flat face, very flat nasal bridge, marked shortening of limbs (especially proximally), and joint contractures. **B,** Radiograph shows shortening of the humeri and femora, and stippled epiphyses. **C,** Radiograph shows stippling of the shoulder joints. *(Courtesy Charles I. Scott, MD, AI DuPont Institute, Wilmington, DE.)*

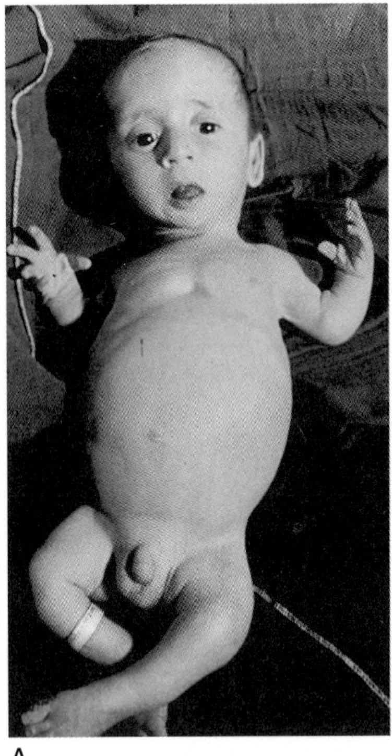
A

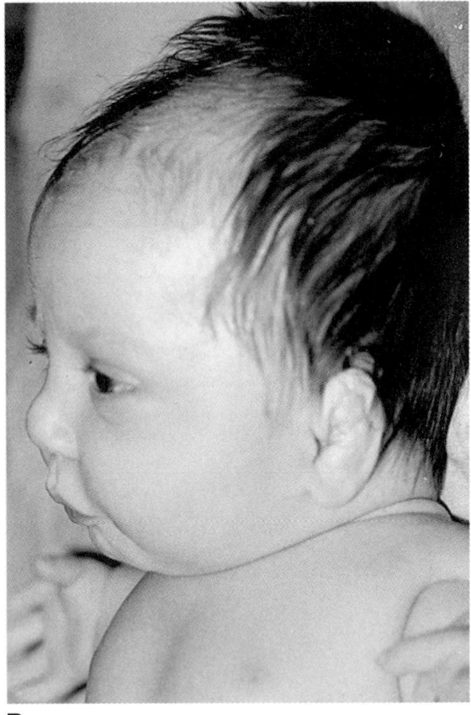
B

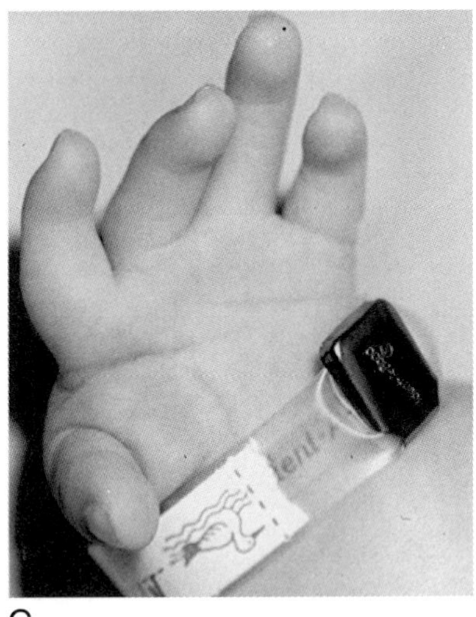
C

**FIGURE 24–11.** Diastrophic dysplasia (see Table 24–2). **A,** Infant has prominent eyes, small chin, slightly narrow chest, proximally placed angulated thumbs, and short limbs. **B,** Neonate profile showing small chin, swollen ears, and short neck. Note the proximally placed, angulated thumb. **C,** View of the neonate's hand shows the proximally placed angulated thumb and mild syndactyly.

## REFERENCES


American Academy of Pediatrics: Health supervision for children with achondroplasia (RE9514). Pediatrics 95:443, 1995.

Banerjee I, Shortland GJ, Evans WD, Gregory JW: Osteogenesis imperfecta and intravenous pamidronate. Arch Dis Child 87:562, 2002.

Beighton P, Giedion A, Gorlin R, et al: International classification of osteochondrodysplasias. Am J Med Genet 44:223, 1992.

Bellus GA, McIntosh I, Smith EA, et al: A recurrent mutation in the tyrosine kinase domain of fibroblast growth factor receptor 3 causes hypochondroplasia. Nat Genet 10:357, 1995a.

Bellus GA, Szabo JK, McIntosh I, et al: Hypochondroplasia: A second recurrent mutation of fibroblast growth factor receptor 3 (FGFR3) at nucleotide 1620. Am J Hum Genet 57:47, 1995b.

Booms P, Cisler J, Mathews KR, et al: Novel exon skipping mutation in the fibrillin-1 gene: Two "hot spots" for the neonatal Marfan syndrome Clin Genet 55:110, 1999.

Borochowitz Z, Lachman R, Adomian GE, et al: Achondrogenesis type I: Delineation of further heterogeneity and identification of two distinct subgroups. J Pediatr 112:23, 1988.

Brunetti-Pierri N, Andreucci MV, et al: X-linked recessive chondrodysplasia punctata: Spectrum of arylsulfatase E gene mutations and expanded clinical variability. Am J Med Genet 22:164, 1999.

Burrows NP, Nicholls AC, Yates JRC, et al: The gene encoding collagen alpha 1(V) (COL5A1) is linked to mixed Ehlers-Danlos syndrome type I/II. J Invest Dermatol 106:1273, 1996.

Byers PH: Osteogenesis imperfecta. In Royce PM, Steinmann B (eds): Connective Tissue and Its Heritable Disorders: Medical and Genetic Aspects. New York, Wiley-Liss, 1993, pp 317-350.

Byers PH, Tsipouras P, Bonadio JF, et al: Perinatal lethal osteogenesis imperfecta (OI type II): A biochemically heterogeneous disorder usually due to new mutations in the genes for type I collagen. Am J Hum Genet 42:37, 1988.

Byers PH, Wallis GA, Willing MC: Osteogenesis imperfecta: Translation of mutation to phenotype. J Med Genet 28:433, 1991.

Cohen MM Jr: Some chondrodysplasias with short limbs: Molecular perspectives. Am J Med Genet 112:304, 2002.

De Paepe A, Nuytinck L, Hausser I, et al: Mutations in the COL5A1 gene are causal in the Ehlers-Danlos syndromes I and II. Am J Hum Genet 60:547, 1997.

Dietz HC, Cutting GR, Pyeritz RE, et al: Marfan syndrome caused by a recurrent de novo missense mutation in the fibrillin gene. Nature 352:337, 1991.

Ewart AE, Morris CA, Atkinson D, et al: Hemizygosity at the elastin locus in a developmental disorder: Williams syndrome. Nat Genet 5:11, 1993.

Francomano CA, Ortiz de Luna RI, Hefferon TW, et al: Localization of the achondroplasia gene to the distal 2.5 Mb of human chromosome 4p. Hum Mol Genet 3:787, 1994.

Frangiskakis JM, Ewart AK, Morris CA, et al: LIM-kinase 1 hemizygosity implicated in impaired visuospatial constructive cognition. Cell 86:1, 1996.

Godfrey M, Raghunath M, Cisler J, et al: Abnormal morphology of fibrillin microfibrils in fibroblast cultures from patients with neonatal Marfan syndrome. Am J Pathol 146:1414, 1995.

Gordienko IY, Grechanina EY, Sopko NI, et al: Prenatal diagnosis of osteochondrodysplasias in high risk pregnancy. Am J Med Genet 63:90, 1996.

Hastbacka J, de la Chapelle A, Mahtani MM, et al: The diastrophic dysplasia gene encodes a novel sulfate transporter: Positional cloning by fine-structure linkage dysequilibrium mapping. Cell 78:1078, 1994.

Hastbacka J, Superti-Furga A, Wilcox W, et al: Atelosteogenesis type II is caused by mutations of the diastrophic dysplasia sulfate transporter gene (DTDST): Evidence for a phenotypic series involving three chondrodysplasias. Am J Hum Genet 58:255, 1996.

Hecht JT, Thompson NM, Weir T, et al: Cognitive and motor skills in achondroplastic infants: Neurologic and respiratory correlates. Am J Hum Genet 41:208, 1991.

Horton WA, Rotter JI, Rimoin DL, et al: Standard curves for achondroplasia. J Pediatr 93:435, 1978.

Houston CS, Opitz JM, Spranger JW, et al: The campomelic syndrome: Review, report of 17 cases and follow-up of the currently 17-year old boy first reported by Maroteaux et al in 1971. Am J Med Genet 15:3, 1983.

Ilizarov GA: The possibilities offered by our method for lengthening various segments in upper and lower limbs. In Nicoletti B, Kopits SE, Ascani E, McKusick VA (eds): Human Achondroplasia: A Multidisciplinary Approach. New York, Plenum Press, 1988, pp 323-324.

Kaitila I, Marttinnen E, Merikanto J, et al: Clinical expression and course of diastrophic dysplasia. Am J Med Genet 34:141, 1989.

Kaplan P, Kirschner M, Watters G, et al: Contractures in patients with Williams syndrome. Pediatrics 84:895, 1989.

Kaplan P, Levinson M, Kaplan BS: Cerebral artery stenoses in Williams syndrome cause strokes in childhood. J Pediatr 126:943, 1995.

Kaplan P, Wang PP, Franke U: Williams (Williams-Beuren) syndrome: A distinct neurobehavioral disorder. J Child Neurol. 16:177, 2001.

Kara-Mostefa A, Raoul O, Lyonnet S, et al: Recurrent Williams-Beuren syndrome in a sibship suggestive of maternal germ-line mosaicism. Am J Hum Genet 64:1475, 1999.

Le Merrer M, Rousseau F, Legeai-Mallet L, et al: A gene for achondroplasia-hypochondroplasia maps to chromosome 4p. Nat Genet 6:314, 1994.

Lopes LM, Cha SC, De Moraes EA, Zugaib M: Echocardiographic diagnosis of fetal Marfan syndrome at 34 weeks gestation. Prenat Diagn 15:183, 1995.

Morris C, Thomas IT, Greenberg F: Williams syndrome: Autosomal dominant inheritance. Am J Med Genet 47:478, 1993.

Morris CA, Demsey SA, Leonard CO, et al: Natural history of Williams syndrome: Physical characteristics. J Pediatr 113:318, 1988.

Morse RP, Rockenmacher S, Pyeritz RE, et al: Diagnosis and management of infantile Marfan syndrome. Pediatrics 86:888, 1990.

Orimo H, Girschick HJ, Goseki-Sone M, et al: Mutational analysis and functional correlation with phenotype in German patients with childhood-type hypophosphatasia. J Bone Miner Res 16:2313, 2001.

Pauli RM, Scott CI, Wassman ER Jr, et al: Apnea and sudden unexpected death in infants with achondroplasia. J Pediatr 104:342, 1984.

Peoples R, Perez Jurado LA, Wang Y-K, et al: The gene for replication factor C subunit 2 (RFC2) is within the 7q11.23 Williams syndrome deletion. Am J Hum Genet 58:1370, 1996.

Perez Juardo LA, Peoples R, Kaplan P, et al: Molecular definition of the chromosome 7 deletion in Williams syndrome and parent-of-origin effects on growth. Am J Hum Genet 59:781, 1996.

Pober BR, Lacro RU, Rice C, et al: Renal findings in 40 individuals with Williams syndrome. Am J Med Genet 46:271, 1993.

Power TJ, Blum NJ, Jones S, et al: Brief report: Response to methylphenidate in two children with Williams syndrome. J Autism Dev Disord 27:79, 1997.

Rasmussen SA, Bieber FR, Benacerraf BR, et al: Epidemiology of osteochondrodysplasias: Changing trends due to advances in prenatal diagnosis. Am J Med Genet 61:49, 1996.

Rauch F, Travers R, Plotkin, Glorieux FH: The effects of intravenous pamidronate on the bone tissue of children and adolescents with osteogenesis imperfecta. J Clin Invest 110:1293, 2002.

Rimoin DL, Lachman RS: Chondrodysplasias. In Rimoin DL, Pyeritz R (eds): Emery & Rimoin's Principles and Practice of Medical Genetics, 3rd ed. New York, Churchill Livingstone, 1997, p 2779.

Rousseau F, Saugier P, Le Merrer M, et al: Stop codon FGFR3 mutations in thanatophoric dysplasia type I. Nat Genet 10:11, 1995.

Schulman SL, Zderic S, Kaplan P: Increased prevalence of urinary symptoms and voiding dysfunction in Williams syndrome. J Pediatr 129:466, 1996.

Shiang R, Thompson LM, Zhu Y-Z, et al: Mutations in the transmembrane domain of FGFR3 cause the most common genetic form of dwarfism, achondroplasia. Cell 78:335, 1994.

Spranger J, Maroteaux P: The lethal osteochondrodysplasias. Adv Hum Genet 19:1, 1990.

Spranger J, Winterpacht A, Zabel R: The type II collagenopathies: A spectrum of chondrodysplasias. Eur J Pediatr 153:56, 1994.

Steinmann B, Royce PM, Superti-Furga A: The Ehlers Danlos syndrome. In Royce PM, Steinmann B (eds): Connective Tissue and Its Heritable Disorders: Medical and Genetic Aspects. New York, Wiley-Liss, 1993, pp 351-407.

Superti-Furga A, Hastbacka A, Wilcox W, et al: Achondrogenesis type IB is caused by mutations in the diastrophic dysplasia sulfate transporter gene. Nat Genet 12:100, 1996.

Superti-Furga A, Bonafe L, Rimoin DL: Molecular-pathogenetic classification of genetic disorders of the skeleton. Am J Med Genet 106:282, 2001.

Tavormina P, Shiang R, Thompson L, et al: Thanatophoric dysplasia (types I and II) caused by distinct mutations in the fibroblast growth factor receptor 3. Nat Genet 9:321, 1995.

Tommerup N: Assignment of an autosomal sex reversal locus (SRA1) and campomelic dysplasia (CMPD1) to 17q24.3-q25.1. Nat Genet 4:170, 1993.

Vajo Z, Francomano CA, Wilkin DJ: The molecular and genetic basis of fibroblast growth factor receptor 3 disorders: The achondroplasia family of skeletal dysplasias, Muenke craniosynostosis, and Crouzon syndrome with acanthosis nigricans. Endocrine Rev 21:23, 2000.

Whyte MP: Hypophosphatasia. In Scriver CR, Beaudet al, Sly WS, Valle D (eds): The Metabolic and Molecular Bases of Inherited Disease, 7th ed, vol III. New York, McGraw-Hill, 1995, pp 4095-4111.

Wilcox WR, Tavormina PL, Krakow D, et al: Molecular, radiologic, and histopathologic correlations in thanatophoric dysplasia. Am J Med Genet 78:274, 1998.

Wilkin DJ, Rogaert R, Lachman RS, et al: A single amino acid substitution (G103D) in the type II collagen triple helix produces Kniest dysplasia. Hum Mol Genet 3:1999, 1994.

Winterpacht A, Hilbert M, Schwarze U, et al: Kniest and Stickler dysplasia phenotypes caused by collagen type II gene (COL2A1) defect. Nat Genet 3:323, 1993.

# PART VII

# EVALUATION AND CARE OF THE NORMAL NEWBORN

Editor: H. WILLIAM TAEUSCH

CHAPTER 25

## Initial Evaluation: History and Physical Examination of the Newborn

Susan Sniderman and H. William Taeusch

Most newborn infants are normal, that is, free from disease and birth defects. Most are able to adapt easily to extrauterine life. Most parents, although having some degree of ambivalence, are excited by their newborn child and are able to care for the infant. When this scenario pertains, physicians must offer parents support and information about the major issues, risks, and achievements that they can expect for their infant over the next few months.

When an infant is born prematurely or is found to have anomalies or illnesses, the history and physical examination may have to be performed at the same time as the parents are informed of the infant's problems and likely course.

Specifics of the examination of various systems are given throughout this book. Therefore, the points relevant to newborns, particularly sick and anomalous infants, are emphasized in this chapter.

### EMERGENCY ASSESSMENT

Assessment of the newborn ranges from routine evaluation of a healthy full-term infant nearing the time of discharge to the emergency assessment of a gray, evidently lifeless, 500-g newborn in the delivery room. The impressions gained in the first seconds to minutes often dictate the speed with which further assessment and treatment must occur. A rapid assessment, including both a brief history and physical examination, is warranted whenever an infant has an acute change in status. The evaluation should not impede attention to the infant's immediate needs. It is a novice's mistake to suspect overwhelming sepsis, then to take several hours to obtain the history and perform the physical examination and a leisurely lumbar puncture before ensuring that antibiotics have been given to the infant. Another mistake is to wait for a chest radiograph to be obtained for an infant with hypotension and a clinically evident tension pneumothorax. A third mistake is to allow an infant to suffer thermal and oxygen insufficiency while hidden under sterile drapes during a protracted insertion of an umbilical artery catheter. A list of perinatal and postnatal conditions necessitating emergency assessment is given in Table 25–1. Delivery room assessment and resuscitation are discussed in Chapter 28.

### HISTORY

The first interview with the parents should occur, if possible, before birth. With rapidly expanding genetic diagnostic capabilities and identification of high-risk fetuses with prenatal ultrasonography, the need for pediatricians to meet with the parents before birth is increasingly common.

The first evaluation of the newborn infant is often said to be the most important routine examination that a person receives in his or her lifetime. If the infant is sick or has anomalies, this statement is particularly pertinent. However, for well infants, remarkably few studies have examined which elements of the initial history and physical examination are most important and which professional personnel should conduct them. If the infant is born at term with no complications, the parents are delighted with the good news. If the infant needs intensive care (approximately 3% of live births), the tendency to focus on ventilators, monitors, laboratory tests, radiographs, and ultrasonography makes it difficult for the parents to focus on the more mundane but possibly very important and pertinent medical history.

Frequently, infants enter the neonatal intensive care unit (NICU) without the parents having been able to anticipate this occurrence. When the parents first visit the NICU, they confront a strange environment in which the life of their infant is entrusted to nurses and doctors not known to them. Both parents may be exhausted and anxious in the hours after the delivery, at the time they become aware that the infant is seriously ill. Some parents are fatalistic and accept opinions about diagnosis and prognosis less out of trust than from a belief that they have little effect on events. Others attempt to exert control over the caregivers in the belief that their infant's plight can be fixed only if they (the parents) determine the correct decisions and treatments to be made.

Therefore, the style with which the initial interview is conducted must be adapted to the parents' as well as the infant's needs. The interview serves several purposes. First, it allows the collection of information that affects the management of the infant. Second, a therapeutic bond may be

**TABLE 25–1**

**Neonatal Conditions Requiring Emergency Assessment**

| | |
|---|---|
| Probably lethal conditions | Anencephaly, hydranencephaly, severe hydrops with hypoplastic lungs, extremely low birth weight (previability), nonresponsiveness to resuscitation |
| Respiratory conditions | |
| Airway obstruction | Mucus, meconium, kinked endotracheal tube, webs, cysts, large tongue, stenosis, tumors, vascular rings |
| Space-occupying lesions | Pneumothorax, pleural effusions, tracheoesophageal fistula, diaphragmatic hernia, adenomatoid malformation, tumors |
| Insufficient respiratory drive | Immaturity, asphyxia, maternal drugs, central nervous system depression, neuromuscular disease |
| Parenchymal disease | Respiratory distress syndrome, meconium aspiration pneumonia, infectious pneumonitis, hypoplastic lungs |
| Cardiovascular conditions | Hypovolemia, hypotension, bradycardia or other arrhythmia, hydrops, congestive heart failure, decreased pulmonary blood flow due to structural cyanotic congenital heart disease or persistent pulmonary hypertension, anemia, hyperviscosity |

formed with the parents, the first stage in enlisting them as allies rather than adversaries in the days, weeks, and possibly months ahead while the infant is in the NICU. Third, the clinician can make an initial assessment of the adequacy of the home and the parents with regard to the care of the infant. Fourth, the interview gives the parents an opportunity to receive an initial report on the status of the infant.

If the infant is being transferred to another hospital, giving the mother a "belonging" of the infant (e.g., a bracelet or Polaroid picture) can help her contend with the birth and immediate separation (to the NICU) from her infant. Realistically allaying the parents' anxiety about their infant's condition is often not possible at the first interview, but the manner and conduct of the history-taking can help the parents feel that their infant will receive competent care. Frightening though the illness or anomaly may be, the parents' concept of their infant's problem may be even more frightening; thus, some reassurance can be offered in most cases, especially after the parents have seen the infant. Novice caregivers, as a symptom of their own insecurity, may emphasize data in these discussions. This tactic, particularly at the first meeting, usually does more harm than good. The error of the opposite approach is to patronize the parents in an abbreviated interview. The worst mistake is to minimize contact with the parents altogether.

Usually, parents are justly intolerant of the professional who waits until after all history-taking, examinations, and laboratory data are in hand before giving them any notion of the problems. It may be wise to start an interview with an overview and follow with the history-taking. At the conclusion of the interview, the clinician should outline the next steps (diagnostic and therapeutic), describe real and potential problems, seek questions from the parents, and close with plans for the next contact.

The initial history and physical examination are screening tools. All systems and areas of the body are evaluated in a feed-forward mode; that is, if the initial screening result is positive (e.g., a problem with the heart or lungs), then that system immediately receives a more thorough evaluation, not only through the physical examination but also through expansion of the history and laboratory examinations. The equally weighted and relentlessly thorough history and physical examination performed by the compulsive novice are rightfully replaced by a balanced examination suitable for the individual circumstances of the infant.

The examiner, throughout the history and physical examination, seeks answers to a series of questions, the first and most important of which is whether the infant is acutely ill. Next, the examiner seeks whether there are problems with regard to the following aspects of the infant:

- Any specific organ system
- Infection
- Inadequate oxygen or nutrients (acute or chronic)
- Abnormal in utero environment
- Growth
- Anomalies or genetic disease
- Trauma
- Maturity
- Transition from in utero existence
- Home environment

The history, physical examination, and laboratory evaluations are never complete for sick infants in an intensive care setting. Information is constantly being compiled from diagnostic studies, physicians, nurses, respiratory therapists, family members, and so forth. Integration of these data with clear and appropriate communication in interviews with parents is one of the hardest tasks to learn. One of the best techniques is the use of careful, succinct, system- or problem-oriented, dated, and timed notes in the infant's hospital chart, including information about what has been told to the parents as well as their particular concerns.

## MATERNAL HISTORY

The history of the newborn is principally the history of the mother's pregnancy, general health, and previous pregnancies. Table 25–2 outlines the array of maternal conditions that can affect the newborn. Maternal influences on the fetus are thoroughly reviewed by Creasy and Resnik (2004).

The major problem of newborns throughout the world is low birth weight with prematurity. The complex and interrelated risk factors for low birth weight are summarized in Table 25–3. Each of these factors is important. If any of these factors is present in the maternal history, their relative weights must be individualized, because none of the items listed is necessarily associated with preterm delivery.

**TABLE 25–2**

**Maternal History**

| |
|---|
| **Social, educational, and economic factors** |
| Age, rage, primary language, work stress, education, religion, reasons for becoming pregnant, preparation for infant care, home support, health care access, history of child abuse |
| **Behavioral factors and habits** |
| Smoking, drugs, alcohol, exercise (duration and amount) |
| **Exposure to toxins or teratogens** |
| Radiation, radiochemicals, hormones (including diethylstilbestrol), thyroid suppressants, aminopterin, anticancer agents, mercury, chlorobiphenyls and other organic substances, hydantoins, anticoagulants, isotretinoin |
| **Nutrition** |
| Diet, vitamin and mineral supplements, weight gain |
| **Genetic/familial disorders** |
| See Table 25–4 |
| **Chronic medical problems predating pregnancy, and outcome(s) of prior pregnancy(ies)** |
| Fetal death, twins, prematurity, blood group incompatibilities, birth weight or gestational age of previous child(ren) |
| **Prenatal care** |
| Number of visits, trimester of first visit, ultrasonography |
| **Problems of current pregnancy*** |
| Central nervous system or psychiatric |
| Endocrine: diabetes, thyroid status, thyroid medication |
| Metabolic: cholestasis |
| Cardiopulmonary: mitral insufficiency or asthma |
| Hypertensive disorder, preeclampsia |
| Hematologic: anemia, Rh incompatibility, idiopathic or alloimmune thrombocytopenia |
| Third-trimester bleeding: placenta previa, abruptio placentae, ruptured uterus |
| Immunologic: systemic lupus erythematosus |
| Surgery or trauma |
| Infectious |
| Medications: tocolytics, glucocorticoids, antibiotics, antihypertensives |
| Renal |
| Neoplastic |
| Reproductive: incompetent cervix, hydramnios, oligohydramnios, in vitro fertilization |
| **Special tests during pregnancy** |
| Ultrasonographic examinations, karyotyping, alpha-fetoprotein testing, chorionic villus biopsy, percutaneous umbilical blood sampling of the fetus, stress and nonstress testing, amniotic fluid testing for bilirubin, fetal maturity assessment, biophysical profile |
| **Infection screening** |
| Rubella, syphilis, acquired immunodeficiency syndrome, toxoplasmosis, herpes, hepatitis B and C, cytomegalovirus, tuberculosis, gonorrhea (for close contacts as well as the mother) |
| **Onset and events of labor** |
| Fetal heart rate monitoring, fetal scalp pH, meconium, rupture of membranes, amnioinfusion, fever, maternal oxygen, vena caval compression, blood pressure, ventilation, analgesia or anesthesia, other medications, duration of stages of labor,† mode of delivery |

*Pregnancy-associated diseases and fetal exposure to tobacco, marijuana, alcohol, or illicit drugs are included on the U.S. Standard Certificates of Live Birth and Fetal Death (Freedman MA, Gay GA, Brookert JE, et al: The 1989 revisions of the U.S. Standard Certificates of Live Birth and Death and the U.S. Standard Report of Fetal Death. Am J Public Health 78:168, 1988.)

†Stage 1 = onset to full cervical dilation; stage 2 = dilation to delivery of fetus; stage 3 = delivery of fetus to delivery of placenta.

## Prenatal Care

The reasons that only some women receive prenatal care are of vital interest. Even though birth weight–specific mortality in the United States is among the world's lowest, the high neonatal mortality rate is directly related to a high rate of low-birth-weight deliveries. Deficiency or absence of prenatal care is associated with an increased risk of prematurity. All people who care for mothers and infants share a responsibility for disseminating these facts and uncovering and correcting the causes of lateness or absence of prenatal care.

## Duration of Pregnancy

Estimates of the length of gestation should be obtained from (1) the date of the mother's last menstrual period, (2) the date of quickening, that is, when the mother first

**TABLE 25-3**

**Principal Maternal Risk Factors for Low Birth Weight Infants**

| | |
|---|---|
| Demographic risks | Age (<18 or >35 yrs)<br>Ethnicity<br>Low socioeconomic status<br>Unmarried<br>Low level of education |
| Medical risks predating pregnancy | Parity (0 or >4)<br>Low weight for height<br>Genitourinary problems, renal insufficiency, or uterine surgery<br>Selected diseases, e.g., diabetes and hypertension<br>Poor obstetric history, including previous low-birth-weight baby or multiple abortions<br>Genetic factors, e.g., the mother herself was a low-birth-weight infant |
| Medical risks in current pregnancy | Multiple pregnancy<br>Poor weight gain<br>Short interpregnancy interval<br>Hypotension<br>Hypertension, preeclampsia, or toxemia<br>Infections, e.g., rubella, symptomatic bacteriuria, or cytomegalovirus infection<br>First- or second-trimester bleeding<br>Placental problems, e.g., placenta previa, abruptio placentae<br>Hyperemesis<br>Oligohydramnios or polyhydramnios<br>Anemia or abnormal hemoglobin level<br>Isoimmunization<br>Fetal anomalies<br>Incompetent cervix<br>Spontaneous premature rupture of membranes |
| Behavioral and environmental risks | Smoking<br>Poor nutritional status<br>Alcohol and other substance abuse, particularly cocaine<br>Diethylstilbestrol exposure and exposure to other toxins<br>High altitude |
| Health care risks | Insufficient prenatal care<br>Iatrogenic prematurity |
| Other possible correlates of premature labor | Physical and psychosocial stress or abuse<br>Uterine irritability<br>Cervical changes before labor<br>Infections, e.g, with *Mycoplasma* and *Chlamydia*<br>Immune interactions between the mother and fetus |

Adapted from the Institute of Medicine Committee to Study the Prevention of Low Birthweight: Preventing Low Birthweight. Washington, DC, National Academy Press, 1985.

feels the fetus move (16 to 18 weeks), (3) the first occurrence of fetal heart sounds (14 to 16 weeks with a fetoscope), and (4) ultrasonographic measurements. Nägele's rule is used to estimate the time of term delivery; with this rule, 3 calendar months are subtracted from the first day of the last menstrual period, and 7 days are added to the result. The uterine fundus is usually at the umbilicus by the fifth month after the last menstrual period.

## Genetic and Familial Factors

A history of genetic and familial disorders is becoming increasingly important as the diagnosis of genetic disease of the fetus during pregnancy becomes more widely available (see Part V of this text). Table 25–4 contains a list of maternal genetic screening questions adapted from the one recommended by the American College of Obstetricians and Gynecologists.

## Complications of Pregnancy

Complications of pregnancy (e.g., gestational diabetes mellitus, preeclampsia) may put the fetus at risk for specific abnormalities after birth, such as hypoglycemia and intrauterine growth restriction. Medications used to treat other complications may be important because they may have certain effects on the fetus (e.g., hydantoin causes dysmorphic features; diuretics may cause fetal thrombocytopenia). Even though they may be subclinical in the mother, infectious illnesses may lead to the birth of an infant with evidence of chronic in utero infection.

**TABLE 25-4**

**Maternal Prenatal Genetic Screening Questions**

1. Are you more than 34 years of age?
2. Has anyone in your family or the father's family had: Down syndrome ("mongolism"), chromosome problems or abnormalities, back (midline) defects at birth or later in life (spina bifida), prolonged or excessive bleeding (hemophilia), muscle weakness problems (muscular dystrophy), or childhood lung problems (cystic fibrosis)?
3. Do you or does the baby's father have a birth defect? Do any members of your or the father's family have birth defects of any kind?
4. Have any members of your family or the father's family, or any of your prior infants, had problems that were inherited or "passed down" through family members to their children?
5. Do you or the baby's father have any close relatives with mental retardation or learning disabilities in school?
6. Have you or the baby's father ever been tested for these genetic problems (relevant to specific ethnic group): Tay-Sachs disease, sickle cell trait or disease, β-thalassemia?
7. Have you lost any early pregnancies (had any miscarriages)?

Adapted from the American College of Obstetricians and Gynecologists: Antenatal Diagnosis of Genetic Disorders. ACOG Technical Bulletin No. 108. Washington, DC, ACOG, 1987, p 3.

## General Health of Mother

In the same way, chronic diseases in the mother may have important consequences for her infant. A mother with systemic lupus erythematosus may have certain antibodies that may cause heart block in the fetus, or a mother with long-standing renal disease may have a growth-retarded infant. Maternal diabetes mellitus with elevated glucose levels in the first trimester is associated with at least a fivefold increase in serious congenital anomalies including congenital heart disease, caudal regression syndrome, and left microcolon. Even diseases that have resolved in the mother (e.g., Graves disease and idiopathic thrombocytopenic purpura) may continue to affect the fetus because of the presence of serum factors that persist and cross the placenta, causing problems in the fetus and newborn infant.

## Onset and Events of Labor

The timing of the onset of labor and the events that occur around it are important. Examples are an automobile accident, premature rupture of membranes, and sharp, near-continuous low back pain with vaginal bleeding. Indications for risk of acute infections in the fetus should be sought. Has the mother had a recent infection? Did she have a fever around the time of delivery? The diagnosis of maternal chorioamnionitis has been associated with a high risk of neonatal encephalopathy and cerebral palsy. Has the mother received antibiotics? How long did labor last, and how long were the membranes ruptured before delivery?

The fetal heart rate in conjunction with uterine contractions is the best signal during labor of the condition of the fetus (see Chapter 13). Adjuncts include the use of fetal scalp pH monitoring.

The presentation of the fetus in the birth canal and the route of delivery are of obvious importance. Breech position occurs in 8% of women in labor. In approximately 25% of breech deliveries, conditions such as placenta previa, malformations of the fetus or uterus, twinning, and premature labor may coexist. Risks of vaginal delivery for the fetus in the breech position include prolapse of the cord, trapping of the head at the level of the cervix, asphyxia, trauma, and congenital hip dysplasia.

## Amniotic Fluid

The infant at term is immersed in about 1 L of amniotic fluid. Sources of this fluid are fetal urine, lung secretions, and transudate from surrounding membranes. Before birth, ultrasonographic assessment of amniotic fluid volume is part of the biophysical profile. Although standards vary, normal volumes are associated with the presence of one or more pockets of fluid with a total vertical diameter greater than 4 cm. Oligohydramnios is indicated by less than 500 mL of fluid. Polyhydramnios indicates more than 2 L of fluid at birth. Near term, the fetus drinks approximately 125 mL/kg body weight of amniotic fluid per day (equivalent to the volume of postnatal milk intake). The fluid has a pH of 7.2 and is alkaline with respect to vaginal fluid. Therefore leakage of amniotic fluid from the vagina can be tested for by checking the pH of the vaginal fluid.

Oligohydramnios or polyhydramnios is most common when fetal swallowing or micturition is increased or decreased. Either condition can be a matter of degree and is best assessed with fetal ultrasonography. Phelan and colleagues (1987) have described the simplest method, in which the largest pockets of fluid visualized on ultrasonography in each of four uterine quadrants are summed. If the sum is less than 6 cm, oligohydramnios is diagnosed. Causes of oligohydramnios include conditions in which there is decreased urination (e.g., bilateral cystic dysplastic kidneys, posterior urethral valves, maternal use of indomethacin), severe placental insufficiency, and chronic leaking of amniotic fluid resulting from premature membrane rupture. The consequences of oligohydramnios are joint contractures and limb deformities, lung hypoplasia, and Potter facies. Conditions listed in Table 25–5 are associated with polyhydramnios. High intestinal obstruction and anencephaly (presumably caused by decreased clearance of amniotic fluid by swallowing) are the most common.

## Timing of Umbilical Cord Clamping

Many events affect the relative volumes of blood left in the newborn and the placenta after birth. Prenatal asphyxia shifts blood from the placenta to the fetus, and, in these cases, because of the need to suction meconium and resuscitate the infant, no delay in cord clamping appears to be useful. If the cord of a normal infant is clamped within 5 seconds of delivery, before a contraction compresses the placenta, and if the infant is held well above the mother's introitus before cord clamping, the infant may be hypovolemic. In contrast, if the obstetrician zealously "strips" the cord toward the infant and delays clamping it, the resulting shift of blood volume from the placenta to the newborn may result in polycythemia, delayed absorption of lung fluid, and hyperbilirubinemia.

**TABLE 25–5**

**Conditions Associated with Polyhydramnios**

| |
|---|
| Agnathia |
| Anencephaly and other central nervous system defects |
| Beckwith-Wiedemann syndrome |
| Chylothorax |
| Conjoined twins |
| Cystic adenomatoid malformation of the lung |
| Diaphragmatic hernia |
| Fetal akinesis |
| Fetal death |
| Hydrops |
| Gastroschisis |
| Hemangioma |
| Maternal diabetes |
| Teratoma |
| Trisomies |
| Tumors of the lungs, placenta, or ovaries |
| Umbilical cord compression |
| Upper gastrointestinal obstruction (e.g., duodenal atresia) |
| Werdnig-Hoffmann disease |

Despite years of research, there is little consensus on the optimal timing of cord clamping. In the absence of asphyxia and isoimmunization, 30 to 45 seconds is a reasonable period to allow to lapse while the infant is held at the level of the introitus. This interval usually allows for an inspiratory gasp on the part of the newborn and a uterine contraction on the part of the mother. Both occurrences favor transfer of blood from the placenta to the newborn (Table 25–6). The obstetrician can suction the nares and oropharynx during this time. Few pediatricians and obstetricians note the timing and nature of the separation of the newborn infant from the placenta, although such information would be helpful in infants with anemia or polycythemia.

Blood volumes are between 85 and 100 mL/kg of body weight in term infants and up to 110 mL/kg in preterm infants. Values can be 35% higher with large shifts of blood volume from the placenta. At term, 75 to 100 mL (20 to 35 mL/kg) of blood is available to the newborn from the placenta.

## PLACENTA AND UMBILICAL CORD

The problems of the placenta are discussed in Chapter 4. The placenta at term (cord and membranes excised 2 cm from the insertion) weighs between 400 and 500 g, with approximately 50% of the weight representing maternal blood and approximately 15% composed of fetal blood. A fetal-placental weight ratio at birth greater than 10 implies that nutrient delivery and gas exchange may have been suboptimal. The cord may demonstrate one umbilical artery (0.7% of live births), true knots, evidence of vascular rupture, compression, hematoma, or edema. In some infants with intrauterine growth restriction, the cord and chorionic plate may be stained greenish brown, the cord may be long and thin, and diminished Wharton jelly may be present. The insertion of the cord may be central or marginal, or it may be incorporated into the membranes (velamentous), sometimes with vasa previa (splitting of the vessels in the membranes before insertion into the placenta). The umbilical cord is usually longer than 40 cm at term, and a shorter cord may indicate relative fetal akinesia from a variety of causes, the inference being that fetal activity contributes to lengthening of the cord. Amniotic membranes may show evidence of banding or thickening, often in association with amniotic fluid infection. In twins, there may be no membrane between cord insertions (monochorionic monoamniotic), a thin transparent membrane (monochorionic diamniotic), or a thick but separable opaque membrane (dichorionic diamniotic). About 20% of all monochorionic diamniotic twin pregnancies have placental vascular anastomoses with the risk of twin-twin transfusion syndrome (see also Chapter 4).

**TABLE 25-6**

**Factors Determining Neonatal and Placental Blood Volumes**

Prenatal drugs (e.g., ergot derivatives)
Maternal vascular disease (preeclampsia or diabetes)
Placental and fetal sizes
Maternal hypotension
Fetal asphyxia or placental insufficiency
Rate of umbilical artery constriction
Position of fetus relative to placenta
Uterine contractions (frequency, amplitude, duration, and baseline)
Time of cord clamping
Neonatal cardiac output
Fetal blood volume (hydrops)
Time of placental separation
Route of delivery
Cord compression
Timing of first breaths relative to cord clamping

## PHYSICAL EXAMINATION

The examiner always faces the dilemma of needing to be thorough while needing to be gentle and quick so as not to destabilize the smallest and sickest infants. The physical examination of newborn infants is tailored to fit both the gestational age and the postnatal age of an infant. The evaluation in the delivery room of a gasping 25-week premature infant is different from the routine examination at 12 hours of age of a full-term infant in the well baby nursery. (Compare Figures 25–1, 25–2, and 25–3 with the full-term infants in subsequent figures; then look at Figure 25–4.)

Ideally, the neonatal examination should take place with the infant under a radiant warmer. The clinician needs patience to be able to return frequently to resume performing parts of the examination, so as to stay within the limits of an infant's tolerance. It is fruitless to examine the abdomen of an infant who is crying and risky to do so in one who has just had a full feeding. At the same time, it is embarrassing to miss an imperforate anus or extra digits in an infant whose respiratory problems have captivated the examiner's initial interest. Table 25–7 outlines the elements of a complete history and physical examination for a newborn infant.

### Nosocomial Infection

Before one touches an infant for any purpose, he or she should perform hand-washing after removing rings and watches. The hand-washing should be done immediately before and immediately after the examination. A "low level of mysophobia" is prevalent among nursery personnel, no doubt contributing to the nosocomial infection rate approaching 50% for small sick infants who have spent more than several months in a NICU. If the prevalence of hand-washing is suboptimal in most nurseries, the use of insufficiently cleaned stethoscopes and other equipment is ever present. With concern provoked by the prevalence of acquired immunodeficiency syndrome (AIDS), many nurseries use universal precautions, meaning that a fresh gown and gloves are used for each direct contact with each patient, whether or not bodily fluids are directly handled. Reason dictates that patients should receive at least the same protection against common nosocomial bacteria as caregivers afford themselves against the much smaller risk of AIDS.

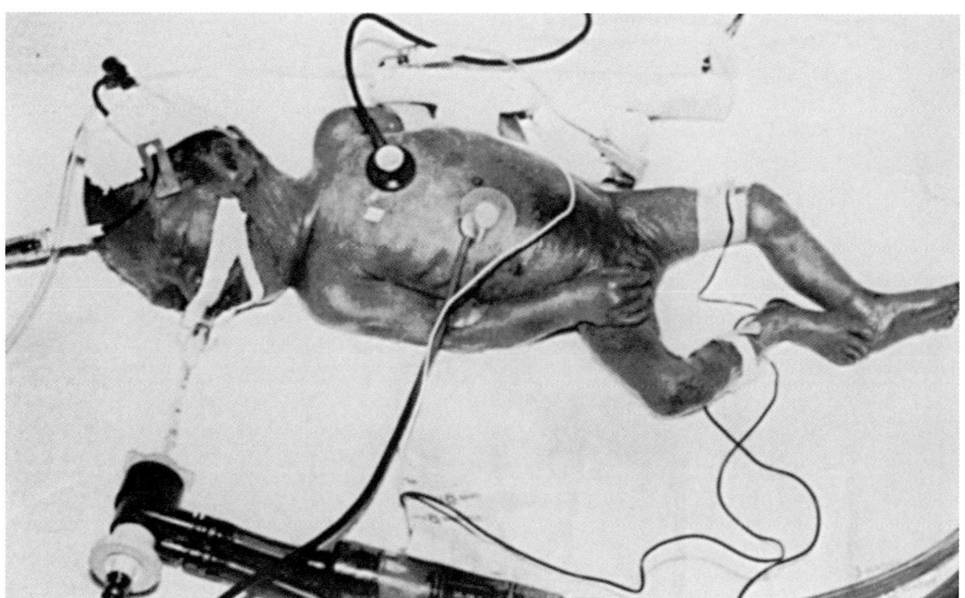

**FIGURE 25–1.** The problems of physical examination are illustrated by comparing this 25-week, 710-g infant, A.W., with respiratory distress syndrome with the full-term newborn shown in Figure 25–5. The story of this premature infant is the subject of a book entitled *Born Early*. *(From Avery ME, Litwack G: Born Early: The Story of a Premature Baby. Copyright © 1983 by Mary Ellen Avery, MD, and Georgia Litwack. By permission of Little, Brown and Company.)*

## Vital Signs

Vital signs are usually assigned the first place in write-ups of the physical examination. For small sick newborns, single measurements are less important than trends, which can be recorded as such. For example, "Axillary temperature was 34° C at 20:05 on arrival in the NICU and was 36.8° C after 2 hours in the servo-controlled overhead warmer supplemented with heat lamps." Without a good indication of the times of the measurements, vital sign

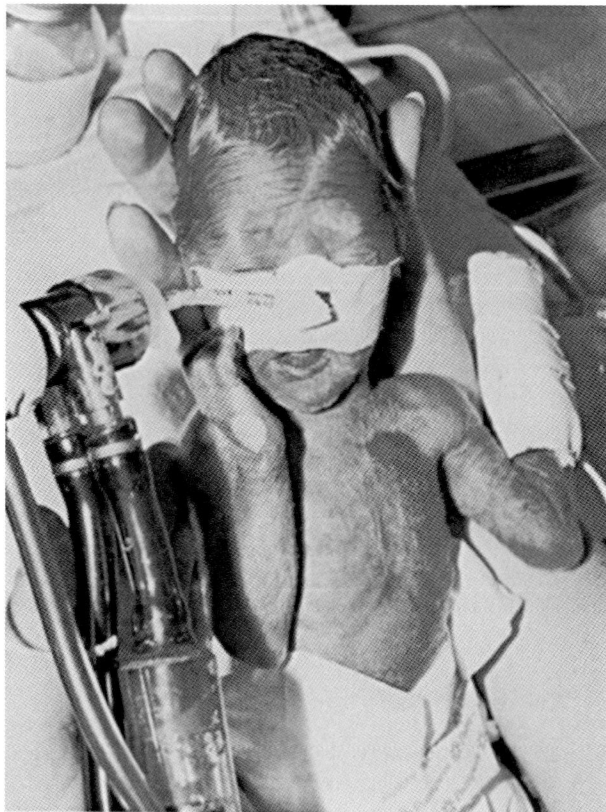

**FIGURE 25–2.** The infant A.W. is shown after the first week of life. Note the size of the skull relative to the adult hand supporting the head. Abundant lanugo is evident. *(Courtesy of G. Litwack.)*

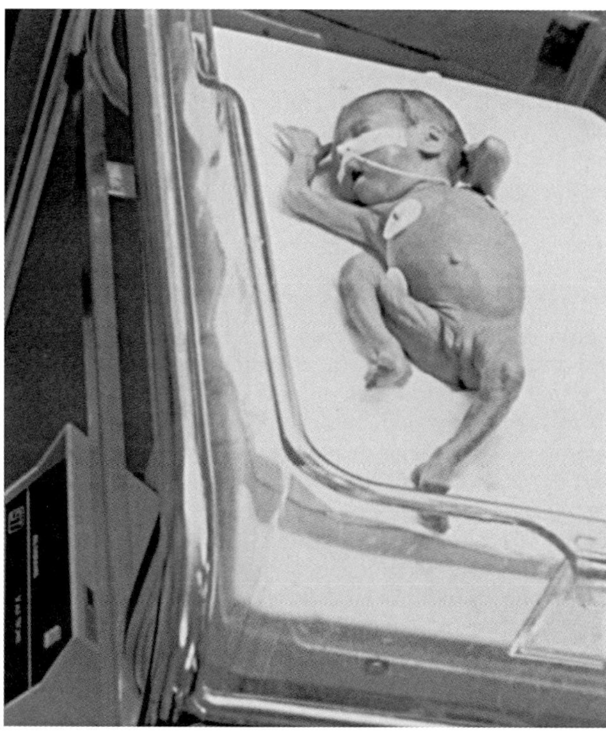

**FIGURE 25–3.** The infant A.W. at 6 weeks of age and 850 g. She required 33 days of ventilator support and underwent surgical ligation of a patent ductus arteriosus. With the head to the right, the infant manifests a strong spontaneous tonic neck reflex posture. She needed an incubator for temperature control but is shown here during a weight measurement. *(Courtesy of G. Litwack.)*

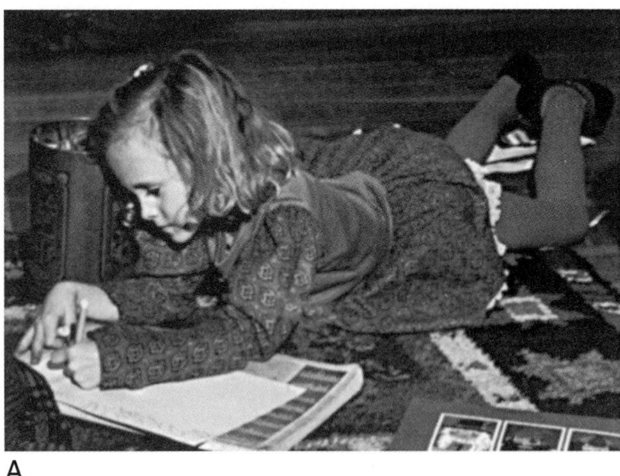


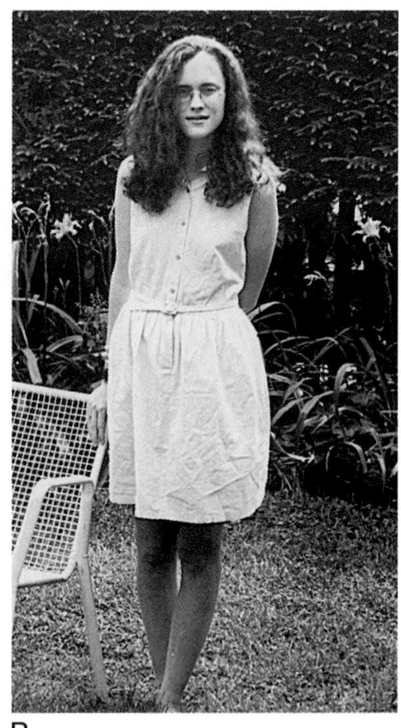


**FIGURE 25–4.** **A,** A.W., at 5 years of age, is thriving. **B,** A.W. at 15 years of age. She excels in academic studies and in athletics. *(Courtesy of G. Litwack.)*

data for newborns have little meaning. Temperature for the most part is measured in the axilla with electronic thermometers with disposable tips (see Chapter 29). Rectal temperatures, because of the greater risk of trauma or perforation associated with obtaining them, are useful only when core temperature may be in question. When the infant's temperature is more than 37.5° C, it is important to assess whether this elevation is a fever associated with infection or is related to an overly warm environment or excessive bundling. If the core temperature is elevated but the extremities are cool, sepsis is likely. When the extremities are warm, the cause is likely to be environmental or, rarely, "warm shock."

For all spontaneously breathing infants, term and premature, respiratory rates normally fall within a range of 40 to 60 breaths/min by 1 hour of age. Rarely, a term infant has a persisting respiratory rate of 100 breaths/min on the second day of life with no evident clinical, radiographic, or laboratory abnormality. In these cases, the respiratory rate becomes normal by the end of the first week. Persistent bradypnea is rare, seen only in extremely premature infants who are ill, infants whose respiratory drive is depressed from maternal narcotic administration, and infants with persisting central hypoventilation (Ondine's curse). Apneic episodes and periodic breathing should be described. In recorded observations, description rather than opinion is preferable; for example, "The infant had about six respiratory pauses of 4 to 7 seconds each without bradycardia or evident desaturation during a 5-minute period while lying undisturbed in apparent REM sleep."

Blood pressure is not usually measured routinely in well infants, and the cost-to-benefit ratio of this procedure for normal infants is unknown. For sick infants, blood pressure is assessed, for example, by direct intra-arterial measurement, oscillometry, auscultation, and Doppler flow. Intra-arterial catheters permit continuous blood pressure monitoring as a matter of routine. In infants being evaluated for a heart problem, blood pressure should be measured in all four extremities, primarily to check for problems of juxtaductal coarctation and left ventricular and outflow tract hypoplasia. Blood pressure correlates directly with gestational age and birth weight. In general, hypotension must be considered when mean blood pressure is less than gestational age. In the smallest, sickest newborns, blood pressures are usually measured intra-arterially with transducers that often receive suboptimal calibration. The transducer must be at the level of the ventricles, and with lower blood pressures, errors of leveling may cause large errors in blood pressure readings. Trends in blood pressure, skin perfusion, recent clinical events, urine output, and arterial pH are essential data for the diagnosis of clinically significant hypotension. Hypertension is a consideration with mean pressures of more than 50 to 70 mm Hg in preterm or term infants.

## Weight, Length, and Head Circumference

Weight should be measured in grams for greatest accuracy. For infants with birth weights between 500 and 800 g, differences of only 100 g are associated with differences in mortality of 50%. Length is more easily measured with an inflexible meter rule laid beside the baby rather than with a flexible measuring tape. Measurements of length carried out by one person using a measuring tape on a

**TABLE 25-7**

**Outline of History and Physical Examination for a Newborn Infant**

Time and date of history
Address and telephone numbers for day and night contact
Maternal history (see Table 25–2)
Neonatal course
- Delivery room events, resuscitation, Apgar scores, cord blood gases, evident anomalies, maternal condition after birth, weight and gross appearance of placenta, results of initial laboratory tests, and other events before the physical examination

Newborn physical examination
- Date and time of examination
- Vital signs
- Overall appearance, symmetry, and general proportions
- Assessment of gestational age
- Height, weight, head circumference, and growth percentile
- Skin: rash, birthmarks, tumors, angiomas
- Head: size, shape, sutures, fontanelles
- Ears: tags, anatomy of folds, placement on skull
- Eyes: size, spacing, colobomas, cataracts
- Mouth: filtrum, size, clefts
- Neck: fistulas, swellings
- Lungs and chest: malformations, air entry
- Heart and vascular: pulses, rhythm, murmurs, point of maximal intensity
- Abdomen: cord, vessels, masses, distention, scaphoid, bowel sounds, musculature, organ size
- Extremities: extra digits, bands, duplications, fusions
- Spine: scoliosis, sinus, masses
- Genitourinary and anus
- Musculoskeletal: range of motion, movement, pain
- Neurologic: movement, responses, tone, sensorium, cranial nerves, reflexes

Impressions, problems
Common laboratory results
- Initial neonatal blood gas levels, oxygen saturation, $FiO_2$
- Complete blood count and hematocrit
- Blood sugar (reagent strip)
- Cultures taken: blood or cerebrospinal fluid
- Screenings: syphilis, rubella, human immunodeficiency virus, hepatis, tuberculosis, genetic and metabolic diseases, illicit drugs

Initial radiography and imaging results
Plan
Signature and title

squirming infant are commonly inaccurate by several centimeters. The tonic neck reflex can occasionally help in straightening the leg during the measurement. The ponderal index (multiply the weight in grams by 100, then divide by the length in centimeters) may be useful in identifying the occasional baby who is underweight for length and therefore small for gestational age, who nonetheless is not so identified by standard weight, gestation, and length norms. Head circumference is determined by placing a soft tape measure just above the eyebrows and finding the largest circumference over the occiput (Fig. 25–5).

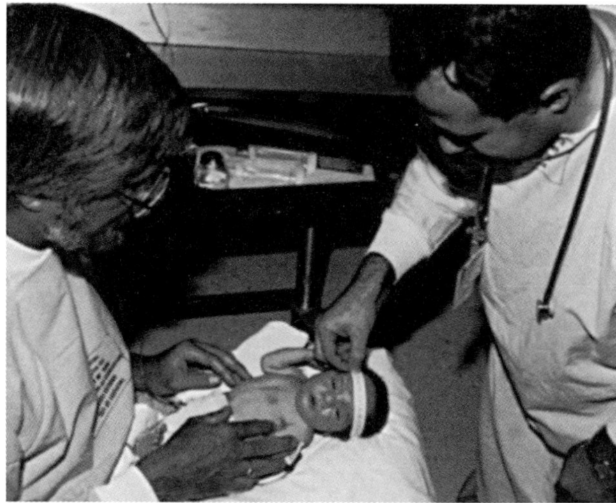

**FIGURE 25-5.** Positioning of tape for head circumference measurement.

## Gestational Age Assessment

Gestational age assessment is best achieved by recording all the available data, that is, by recording duration of gestation based on last menstrual period, prenatal ultrasonographic estimates, and, after birth, the gestational age that matches the 50th percentile for the child's head circumference, length, and weight, and the estimate of gestational age based on physical characteristics. These indicators can be combined to give "obstetric" duration and "pediatric" estimates of gestation that can be combined into a "clinical" estimate. We believe that the physical assessments of gestational age have been overemphasized because the skin and the central nervous system, which contribute the most to the score, can be affected by factors other than the duration of gestation, such as respiratory distress, asphyxia, and antenatal steroid therapy. The scoring examination by Ballard and associates (1991) is one of the simplest and should be consulted for detailed assessments. In terms of weight, as a rule of thumb, 24-week infants are about 600 g (the usual limit of viability), 28-week infants are 1200 g (600 × 2), and 33-week infants are 1800 g (600 × 3).

## Overall Appearance

Observing the infant is the most important aspect of the physical examination. It is best performed with the infant quiet and nude. Occasionally, these two states are incompatible, in which case the infant can usually be quieted by being rocked to and fro while the examiner makes faces and babbles. This time-honored method usually catches the surprised attention of the infant (and other personnel who happen by). The state of alertness, the muscle tone, the activity, obvious anomalies or injuries, respiratory pattern, and the skin are assessed during inspection. The infant may appear sick or well, responsive or lethargic. The muscle tone in a term infant should be sufficient for the hips, knees, and elbows to be flexed while the infant is lying supine or prone. Some spontaneous movements should be evident, and the well infant should appear alert at some point during the examination, unless the examiner is an extraordinarily boring person. The color should be pink rather than sallow or pale or blue. Cyanosis may be generalized or may be limited to the distal extremities or to the lower part of the body, as is seen occasionally with massive right-to-left shunting through a still patent ductus arteriosus. When only the hands and feet are blue, the infant may be cold with resulting peripheral vasoconstriction; this appearance is called acrocyanosis.

The appearance of the small premature infant after stabilization is different from the preceding description. The 900-g infant with respiratory distress syndrome may be intubated or ventilated and may have an arterial line or peripheral intravenous lines in place. Usually, a thermistor for temperature regulation and leads for cardiac and respiratory monitoring are also attached. Such an infant may also be sedated or paralyzed by muscle relaxants. Regardless, the infant is usually flaccid and minimally responsive. The infant may be covered in various ways to minimize heat loss and restrained to maintain the vascular lines. Stimulation during the examination may cause arterial desaturation, silent crying attempts around the endotracheal tube, decreased blood pressure, tachycardia or bradycardia, and decreased skin perfusion. In these cases, continual information on gas exchange, blood pressure, temperature, ventilation, and heart rate is gained at the price of access to the infant, which in any case can be harmful, especially if the examination is lengthy, inept, or both. Nonetheless, a careful head-to-foot examination can be gently and quickly carried out by one or two (not four or five) examiners. The cardiac and pulmonary examinations are often difficult because of ventilator noise (water accumulation in the inspiratory tube) and because of difficulties obtaining a good seal on the chest of premature babies with stethoscope bells designed for larger babies. The examination of the abdomen with a single index finger is often easier than the examination of full-term infants because of the thinness and diminished tone of the anterior abdominal wall.

Anomalies and birth injuries are often apparent on inspection. When observing the infant, one must look carefully at the facial features and the shape of the ears and head for any obviously dysmorphic or malformed features. Are there any obvious anomalies? Is the infant well proportioned or are the limbs short or long compared with the trunk? If any anomaly or dysmorphic feature is noted, a search should begin for other major or minor abnormalities that may help lead to diagnosis of isolated malformations, a malformation sequence or syndrome, or a deformation or disruption caused by external environmental factors. Malformations, deformations, and chromosome problems are discussed in Part V of this text. The most common anomalies are listed in Table 25–8. Birth injuries are often signified by lack of motion or asymmetries of movement of the limbs or face. There may be obvious pain when an extremity or clavicle is palpated, and bruising may be apparent after a few hours of life. Birth injuries occur with greater frequency in breech deliveries and other abnormal presentations. The most common birth injuries are listed in Table 25–9.

The chest should be inspected for symmetry. A prominent left chest may indicate cardiac hypertrophy from an obstructive lesion. A visible cardiac impulse may indicate a patent ductus arteriosus with left-to-right shunt. A small chest in an infant manifesting respiratory distress or failure may indicate pulmonary hypoplasia or, in a more severe form, asphyxiating thoracic dystrophy.

Much information is obtained by watching the infant breathe. Regular respiratory movements of less than 60 breaths/min without suprasternal, intercostal, or subcostal retractions make pulmonary disease unlikely. Apneic spells and periodic breathing can also be observed.

**TABLE 25–8**

**Most Common Anomalies Noted on the Initial Examination of a Newborn**

| Anomaly | Frequency (per 1000 live births) |
|---|---|
| Skin tags | 10-15 |
| Polydactyly | 10-15 |
| Cleft lip or palate | 1-4 |
| Congenital heart defects | 1-4 |
| Congenital hip dislocation | 1-4 |
| Down syndrome | 1-4* |
| Talipes equinovarus | 1-4 |
| Spina bifidas, anencephaly, or encephalocele | 1-4/10,000 live births |

*Frequency increases with maternal age greater than 33 years.

## Inspection by System

After gaining a general impression of the infant's status and being convinced that emergency intervention (intubation, relief of pneumothorax, or transfusion) is unnecessary, the clinician may continue observation of the infant by system, usually starting at the head and working caudad. Then the examination is repeated with palpation, auscultation, reflex testing, the shining of lights into various orifices, and, finally,

**TABLE 25–9**

**Most Common Birth Injuries and Insults**

Decreased gas exchange: placental insufficiency, prolapsed cord, premature placental separation*
Broken clavicle
Facial palsy
Brachial plexus injuries (especially Erb palsy)
Fractures of the humerus or skull
Ruptured internal organs
Testicular trauma
Fat necrosis
Lacerations or scalpel injury
Cephalhematoma and subgaleal hematoma
Scalp lesions from fetal scalp electrode or forceps
Umbilical cord accidents

*Acute prepartum asphyxia of sufficient duration and severity to be associated with hypoxic-ischemic encephalopathy. The incidence for each of these conditions is roughly 1-3 per 1000 live births.

range of motion. Auscultation and abdominal examination require a quiet if not cooperative infant. The hip examination and the Moro reflex testing should be the finale, because these assessments frequently leave the infant displeased with the whole concept of being examined.

## The Cry

As the clinician performs various parts of the newborn examination, he or she should listen for the infant's cry. Is it husky, loud, and sustained or is it shrill and high-pitched, indicating a possible central nervous system abnormality? The cry may be low pitched and husky in hypothyroidism, or hoarse with vocal cord injury or recurrent laryngeal nerve palsy. A weak whimper may indicate overwhelming sepsis or neuromuscular disease. Inspiratory stridor from airway obstruction may be heard only when the infant is crying. Complete aphonia usually indicates bilateral vocal cord injury or paralysis.

## Skin

Vernix usually covers the skin, especially in the skinfolds of the axillas, neck, and groin at birth. Post-term infants characteristically have little vernix, and their skin is dry, cracked, and wrinkled. The texture of the skin is evaluated with regard to scaliness, elasticity, thickness, and local or generalized edema. Hemangiomas, nevi, and urticarial, pustular, vesicular, or nodular rashes are sought. Particularly in infants with vascular catheters, evidence of partial or complete arterial or venous obstruction should be sought at regular intervals. Dermal sinuses occur in the midline of the back from occiput to coccyx and near the ears and in the neck. Dimples, sinuses, hirsute areas, or cystic swellings suggest the presence of cranial or vertebral sinuses or underlying defects. Preterm infants may have fine downy hair (lanugo) over the shoulders, back, thighs, forehead, and ears. The lanugo regresses as they mature over weeks.

Ecchymoses or petechiae may relate to birth trauma and may herald a higher than normal hyperbilirubinemia as the blood products break down and are absorbed over 24 to 36 hours. Generalized and recurring petechiae, especially those not on the head and necklace region, may signify serious infectious or hematologic problems.

Common findings include milia, white papules less than 1 mm in diameter that are scattered across the forehead. These and white vesicles with a red base (erythema toxicum) are transient and benign. In black infants, a similar but more dramatic benign condition is transient neonatal pustular melanosis. These conditions at times are impossible to differentiate on inspection from infectious pustules. Jaundice in the third day of life or later is common, but jaundice that is evident on the first day of life is unusual and needs laboratory investigation.

## Head

The most common findings after birth are caput succedaneum and cephalohematoma. Caput succedaneum is edema of the scalp skin and crosses suture lines. Cephalohematomas are subperiosteal and therefore do not cross suture lines. Frequently, the clinician gains the impression of a depressed skull fracture while palpating the rim of a cephalohematoma. This (false) perception is so common that we do not routinely obtain skull radiographs of an infant with a cephalohematoma unless other worrisome signs are present as well. Rarely, subgaleal hemorrhage may occur, especially after a birth assisted with vacuum extraction. The hemorrhage is under the aponeurosis of the scalp but above the periosteum. The swelling crosses suture lines and can be differentiated from a caput succedaneum on the basis of its firmness and other signs of loss of blood from the intravascular space.

On the first day of life, molding of the head from descent through the birth canal may be present, and the skull plates are overriding. After a few days, the clinician can better estimate the size of the fontanelles, their flatness, fullness, or tenseness, and the width of suture lines (Faix, 1982; Popich and Smith, 1972). Fontanelles may tense normally with vigorous crying. A bulging or tense fontanelle has a feel on palpation nearly equivalent to that of bone. In contrast, a full fontanelle may be normal and is easily distinguished from bone on palpation. The clinician may note the fusion of the sagittal, metopic, or coronal sutures as either total, partial, or unilateral. Large fontanelles and split sutures are most often a normal variant, but they can be associated with increased intracranial pressure or conditions that impair bone growth. Likewise, small fontanelles and overriding sutures are generally of little significance but may be associated with conditions in which brain growth has been retarded (Table 25-10). A small (third) fontanelle anterior to the posterior fontanelle is occasionally found and is associated with Down syndrome and hypothyroidism. Unusual whorls or other hair patterns and asymmetries of the skull may indicate problems in global or regional brain development.

## Skull Defects

Craniotabes is a demineralized area or softening of the skull. The skull bone can be indented with gentle pressure like a table tennis ball. When this finding is appreciated to a mild degree near the suture lines in newborn

**TABLE 25-10**

**Disorders Sometimes Associated with Abnormal Fontanelles**

| | |
|---|---|
| Fontanelles too large | Skeletal disorders (e.g., hypophosphatasia, osteogenesis imperfecta)<br>Chromosome abnormalities<br>Hypothyroidism<br>Increased intracranial pressure, hydrocephalus |
| Fontanelles too small | Hyperthyroidism<br>Craniosynostosis<br>Microcephaly |
| Third fontanelle | Down syndrome<br>Hypothyroidism |

infants, it is commonly a normal variant. When present over most of the skull, craniotabes may be associated with conditions in which calcification has been deficient (e.g., syphilis, osteogenesis imperfecta). By contrast, craniosynostosis is a condition wherein sutures are fused, thereby constraining brain growth.

Transillumination is useful for detecting severe hydrocephaly and hydranencephaly before obtaining an ultrasonographic evaluation. The heads of premature infants normally have a greater degree of transillumination than the heads of term infants.

## Eyes

Eyes are difficult to examine in the newborn, especially when instillation of silver nitrate has occurred. The use of this substance, which is currently not preferred over other antibacterials, is associated with swelling and conjunctivitis during the first 36 hours of life. Often, an infant soothed with to-and-fro rocking, during which the head is elevated, spontaneously opens the eyes, allowing their inspection and as well as assessment of visual tracking of the examiner's face or a bright object as it moves from side to side (Fig. 25–6).

Gross vision can also be assessed by observing whether the infant turns to light. Pupils should be equal in size, reactive to light, and symmetrical. The corneas should be clear. The pupil can be inspected with a light, and the pink retina (red reflex) discerned to rule out lenticular, anterior, and posterior chamber opacities. (With the ophthalmoscope about 6 inches from the infant, the clinician uses the +10 diopter lens.) Fixed strabismus should be absent, and the eye movements for the most part should be coordinated. The examiner can assess eye movements by checking for oculovestibular nystagmus, which consists of holding the infant under the axillas facing the examiner while the examiner turns in a circle. The infant's eyes should slowly deviate in the direction of spin with quick movements in the opposite direction. If other disease is present or a more complete examination is indicated, the pupils should be dilated for a complete retinal examination.

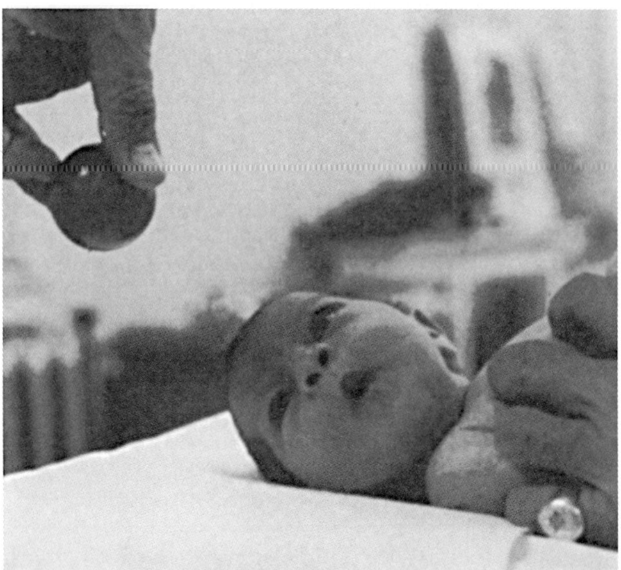

**FIGURE 25–6.** Head turning to follow a ball. *(Courtesy of Dr. B. Brazelton.)*

## Ears

The ears are examined for placement and deformation. Low-set or posteriorly rotated ears may be associated with other more major anomalies. Usually, the tips of the ears are cephalad to an imaginary circumferential line drawn around the skull through the inner and outer canthi of both eyes. Gross hearing is often inaccurately assessed by observing whether the infant blinks in response to a loud noise. More formal hearing screening for all newborns has now been recommended (see "Laboratory Screening"). In the immediate newborn period, the ear canals are usually occluded by vernix and are not routinely examined.

## Mouth and Lower Face

The lips may be good indicators of whether the infant is cyanotic. Retention cysts on the alveolar ridge may look like teeth; natal teeth occur rarely and are usually shed in a few days. Retention cysts, also called Epstein pearls, disappear in a few weeks. The frenulum, which in years past was occasionally cut to prevent "tongue-tie," can usually be ignored. The palate is examined for cleft, the tongue for size, and the sublingual area for masses. The two corners of the mouth should move symmetrically when the infant cries or grimaces; asymmetry is most usually caused by a seventh cranial nerve palsy. A long philtrum, thin upper lip, cleft lip, cleft palate, and small jaw are other significant findings associated with abnormal fetal development sometimes caused by chromosome abnormalities, alcohol, or other fetal toxins.

## Nose

Patency of each naris can be checked by holding a wisp of cotton at the orifice while occluding the other naris with the mouth closed. Newborn infants breathe preferentially through the nose, so bilateral choanal atresia may cause severe respiratory distress. Flaring of the nostrils occurs whenever respiratory effort is increased regardless of cause.

Almost half of all infants have nonfunctional nasolacrimal ducts for 1 to 5 days. Swelling is common at the inner canthal region, but infection (dacryocystitis) is rare. In more than 80% of cases, the ducts open spontaneously by age 3 months.

## Neck

The neck of the newborn always seems short. A very short, webbed neck may be associated with Klippel-Feil or Turner syndrome. The neck is palpated for cysts or masses. A thyroglossal duct cyst is usually palpable in the midline and retracts with tongue protrusion. The infant may have congenital muscular torticollis with or without a fibrous mass in the sternocleidomastoid muscle, associated with head tilt. A cystic hygroma is a spongy mass that may increase with increased intrathoracic pressure and may transilluminate. Hemangiomas are similar to hygromas to palpation but are commonly associated with skin discoloration. Branchial cleft cysts may have associated fistulas. They are palpable anterior to the sternocleidomastoid and may retract with swallowing. Thyroid masses are usually visible and are easily palpable with the head extended.

## Chest and Lungs

The circumference of the chest of the newborn is roughly equivalent to that of the head. Continued inspection of the chest may show a protruding xiphisternum (pectus carinatum), which is usually a normal variant. In contrast, a pectus excavatum deformity may be present at birth or may be associated with prolonged low-compliance respiration. While the infant is breathing, nasal flaring may be present along with retractions and "grunting," which is partial glottic closure during the first part of expiration. Suprasternal retractions and gasping, as opposed to substernal retractions, may indicate upper airway obstruction; in an infant with this finding, laryngoscopy should be performed rapidly. Almost any cardiopulmonary disease in the newborn period reduces lung compliance and is associated with subcostal retractions. The appearance of flaring, grunting, tachypnea, and retractions is called respiratory distress. Respiratory distress may be associated with pneumonia, delayed resorption of lung fluid, respiratory distress syndrome, or any number of cardiorespiratory problems.

Asymmetry of the chest may indicate fetal obstructive cardiac anomalies, a tension pneumothorax, or other forms of air trapping or mass lesions.

The nipples and underlying breast tissue are usually 1 cm in diameter in term infants, both boys and girls, and may be asymmetric. Under maternal hormonal influence, the breast bud may become as large as 3 to 4 cm in diameter and may excrete a watery whitish fluid for a few days or weeks ("witch's" milk). The enlargement occurs in both sexes and is usually symmetric. Redness or asymmetry indicates probable infection, which requires the administration of antibiotics. Widely spaced nipples and accessory nipples should be noted.

Single-finger percussion can be useful for detection of consolidated pneumonias or pleural effusions. Suspicion of clinically significant pneumothorax should lead to instant confirmatory checks of blood pressure, transillumination, and chest radiographs. Transillumination is carried out with high-energy fiberoptic transillumination devices in a darkened room. Some practice is necessary before the examiner can clearly distinguish the normal from excessive coronas of pink transillumination around the closely applied light source.

Auscultation of the lungs is best carried out with a cleaned and warmed stethoscope bell. Rhonchi can be inspiratory or expiratory. Inspiratory stridor implies large-airway obstruction, and expiratory prolongation indicates small-airway obstruction. Rales are moist crackling sounds emulated by licking a thumb and forefinger and separating them close to one's ear. The burst of fine crackles on separation of the thumb and forefinger is of the same quality and intensity as rales in the newborn. Gurgling and bubbling sounds come from secretions in large airways and often indicate the need for tracheal suctioning. Harsher bubbling sounds may be from water accumulating in the tubing of a ventilator. Listening alternately in the right and left axillas may indicate diminished breath sounds on one side. These asymmetries may indicate unilateral pneumothorax or that an endotracheal tube has inadvertently advanced into the right main bronchus. Rarely, bowel sounds may be heard high in the chest in the absence of breath sounds. If so, diaphragmatic hernia is possible, and emergency radiologic examination and surgical consultation are necessary. Meanwhile, a nasogastric tube should be inserted to prevent distention of the stomach and bowel within the chest cavity.

## Heart and Vascular System

The most common cardiac conditions in the newborn period are perinatal adaptations involving the ductus arteriosus (see Chapter 56), with right-to-left shunting through the ductus arteriosus of term infants with persistent pulmonary hypertension and left-to-right shunting through the ductus arteriosus of premature infants. Significant structural heart anomalies are diagnosed in the first week of life in about 1% of live-born children. The most common serious anomalies recognized in the first week of life are ventricular septal defects, patent ductus arteriosus, transpositions, hypoplastic left heart syndromes, tetralogy of Fallot, and coarctations.

The most common findings for an infant with heart disease in the newborn period are tachypnea, cyanosis, or both with an increased $O_2$ requirement. These findings are observed in the most common pathophysiologic conditions associated with congenital heart disease—low cardiac output, congestive heart failure from left-to-right shunts, obstruction to outflow, and insufficient pulmonary blood flow. The general appearance can often signal a cardiac problem, for example, the shocky underperfused infant on the third day of life with a hypoplastic left ventricle versus the contented cyanotic infant in no distress with transposition of the great vessels. Other aspects of heart disease detectable on general inspection are markedly increased precordial activity, hypertrophy of the left chest, and, rarely, venous engorgement (e.g., in an infant with thrombosis of a central venous line leading to a vena cava syndrome).

### *Auscultation*

The clinician should listen for cardiovascular problems first in "noncardiac" areas, such as the axilla (peripheral pulmonic stenosis), the neck (aortic obstruction), and the head and liver (arteriovenous malformations). Timing of the onset of murmurs is important. Frequently, murmurs that depend on pulmonary vascular tone (e.g., left-to-right shunt through a patent ductus arteriosus) may not be heard until pulmonary vascular resistance has decreased in the second to third day of life in an infant with respiratory distress syndrome or within 12 hours of birth in a normal full-term infant. The murmur of tricuspid insufficiency associated with a dilated heart after severe perinatal asphyxia may be present only in the first hours of life. Obstructive murmurs characteristically are heard from birth unless low cardiac output is present. Other characteristics that are important to note are the site where the murmur is heard best, the timing of the murmur with regard to systole and diastole, the quality, and the loudness. The murmurs that are of low intensity, that occur near the sternum or only in noncardiac areas, and that occur early in systole are often innocent.

A detailed history and physical examination, including four-extremity blood pressures, a chest radiograph, blood gas analysis, pre- and post-ductal oxygen saturation, and electrocardiogram, and ultrasonography, are usually sufficient to clarify whether congenital heart disease is present. Neonatologists and pediatricians who commonly care for newborns should be able to evaluate the heart using chest radiography, electrocardiography, and auscultation.

Irregularities in heart rhythm may also be auscultated. Sinus arrhythmia sounds like a periodic slowing and then speeding up of the heart rate, whereas premature atrial and ventricular contractions make the heart rhythm sound very irregular.

**CASE STUDY 1**

Baby B was transferred to the NICU at 6 hours of age because of tachypnea. The history of pregnancy and delivery was unremarkable. Physical examination showed the patient to be a well-formed, full-term infant breathing at a rate of 78 breaths/min. Lungs had occasional rales. The heart rate was 180 beats/min. A gallop rhythm was heard, but no murmurs. The liver was palpable 4 cm below the costal margin and was thought to be enlarged. The physical findings suggested heart failure, which was confirmed by a chest radiograph that showed an enlarged heart and pulmonary congestion. Arterial blood gas analysis on a specimen collected while the baby was receiving 30% oxygen showed a $PaO_2$ of 68, a $PCO_2$ of 48, and a pH of 7.2 with a base deficit. An electrocardiogram indicated a modest reduction of voltage in all leads. Ultrasonography of the heart showed that the organ was large with poor contractility. A number of diagnoses were considered including various cardiomyopathies, pericardial effusion, and anomalous pulmonary venous drainage with obstruction. The infant underwent cardiac catheterization, by which a large and inoperable arteriovenous malformation of the brain was diagnosed after injection of dye for cardiac angiography. After the infant returned to the unit, a large bruit was easily heard with the stethoscope applied to the anterior fontanelle or to the skull lateral to the eyes.

This case serves as a reminder that heart failure may occur from arteriovenous fistulas anywhere in the body.

## Abdomen

The abdomen is assessed by inspection and palpation for organomegaly, masses, inflammation, and distention. Unusual flatness or a scaphoid shape to the abdomen may be associated with congenital diaphragmatic hernia. Examination by inspection, palpation, auscultation, transillumination, and ultrasonography can usually discriminate between air within or outside the gastrointestinal tract and enlarged viscus or viscera, and a cystic or solid tumor. Normally, the examiner palpates a 1- to 2-cm liver edge below the right costal margin, a spleen tip overlying the stomach, and the lower pole of the left kidney in the pelvic gutter (Fig. 25–7). The examiner also looks for dilated veins on the abdominal wall indicating venous distention. Visible gastric or bowel patterns may be considered a certain sign of ileus or other obstruction. The umbilical stump should be examined for bleeding, abnormal vessels, increased or decreased Wharton jelly, meconium staining, polyps, granuloma, exudative discharge, or other evidence of inflammation (redness, tenderness, edema of abdominal wall, induration) or abnormal communication with intra-abdominal viscera. Omphaloceles and gastroschisis are readily apparent, but small umbilical hernias and diastasis recti abdominis may be less so.

Abdominal masses occur in approximately 1 of 1000 live births (Table 25–11). Evaluation is carried out by history, physical examination, ultrasonography, and radiography. Some masses are transitory and of little significance (e.g., intraluminal stool, gaseous dilation of the stomach or colon, distended bladder, or large but normal kidneys) (Table 25–12).

## Genital System

Maturation of the genitalia is apparent over the last 3 months of gestation, and the changes serve as one index on the scoring of physical attributes for gestational age

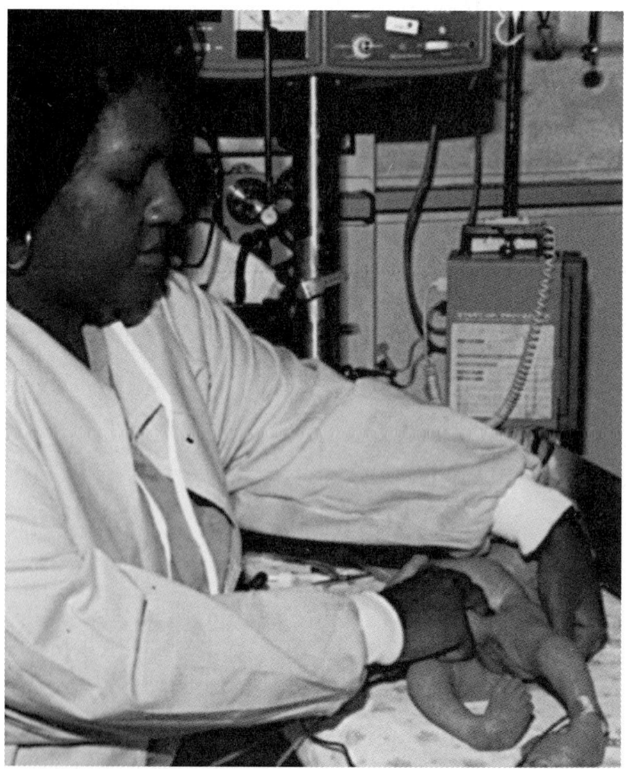

**FIGURE 25–7.** Abdominal palpation is carried out using counter-pressure in the flank with one hand. The lower pole of each kidney is usually palpable with this technique in the first days of life, before abdominal muscle tone increases. Note the bilateral clubfoot.

TABLE 25-11

**Most Common Congenital Abdominal Masses**

| | |
|---|---|
| Renal (55% of total abdominal masses) | Hydronephrosis<br>Multicystic or polycystic kidneys<br>Renal malformations<br>Renal vein thrombosis<br>Renal neoplasms |
| Genital (15%) | Hydrometrocolpos<br>Ovarian cyst |
| Gastrointestinal (15%) | Obstructions<br>Cysts or tumors<br>Duplications |
| Liver and biliary (5%) | Cysts<br>Tumors |
| Retroperitoneal (5%) | Solid tumors<br>Anterior meningomyelocele |
| Adrenal (5%) | Hemorrhage<br>Neuroblastoma |

Data from Griscom NT: The roentgenology of neonatal abdominal masses. AJR AM J Roentgenol 93:447, 1965, and Kirks D, Marten DE, Grossman H, Bowie JD: Diagnostic imaging of pediatric abdominal masses: An overview. Radiol Clin North Am 19:527, 1981.

TABLE 25-12

**Common Findings in the Neonate that are of Little Clinical Significance***

| | |
|---|---|
| Head | Caput succedaneum, cephalohematoma, asymmetries, bony protrusions, molding |
| Ears | Skin tags |
| Eyes | Position (close-set), conjunctival hemorrhage |
| Nose | Asymmetric nares |
| Mouth | Ranula, sucking calluses, epulis, frenulum, natal teeth, Epstein pearls |
| Face | Unusual features not consistent with known syndromes |
| Skin | Sparse petechiae on the head, erythema toxicum, mongolian spot, nevus flammeus, telangiectasia, nevi, inclusion cysts, bruises, prominent lanugo or vernix, milia, miliaria, dark pigmentation over genital skin, mild jaundice after 2nd day, peeling of skin, skin tags, sacrococcygeal dimple |
| Neck | Relative absence |
| Chest | Nipple spacing, extra nipples, breast hypertrophy, witch's milk |
| Umbilicus | Erythema or umbilicus cutis |
| Abdomen | Evanescent masses |
| Heart | Evanescent murmurs and adventitious sounds |
| Genitalia | Mild hypospadias, prominent labia, mucous secretion, transient vaginal blood, phimosis |
| Extremities | Extra digits, syndactyly, hips tight to abduction, neck in extension after breech delivery |
| Neurologic system | Transient tone asymmetries or abnormality, jitters, sudden jerky movements |

*Some of the items on this list may be associated with significant disease (e.g., jitteriness may be associated with metabolic problems or drug withdrawal). However, when findings on this list are mild and transient, they are most commonly not associated with significant disease. If the significance of a finding is in doubt, it is prudent to ask for another opinion and to follow up.

assignment. The spectrum of differences that nonetheless fall within the normal range are surprising. For a discussion of ambiguous genitalia, see Chapter 91.

Penile length and clitoral size are assessed. A clear white mucus is often present in the vagina of term infants for the first few days as a result of estrogens from the mother. The location of the urethral meatus and the presence or absence of palpable gonads are noted, and inguinal hernias are sought. Most "congenital" hernias are apparent only after a month or two, and these are most common in premature infants. The anus should be checked for patency and distance from the genitalia. The perineum should be checked for palpable masses. Rarely, with variants of imperforate anus with fistula, stool exudes from the vagina.

### Musculoskeletal System

The musculoskeletal system is assessed by observation and palpation for obvious trauma, inflammation, and malformation. The most common alterations in the musculoskeletal system are deformations caused by adverse mechanical forces in utero. Oligohydramnios that limits fetal movement and neuromuscular problems of the fetus can both be associated with multiple contractures known as *arthrogryposis*. Most positional deformities are mild and resolve with time. The hips deserve special attention because the physical examination is the only method of detecting hip problems before permanent damage has occurred by 1 year of age or so. Examination of the hips should be undertaken repeatedly in the first year of life, because a dislocation may not be demonstrable for several months after birth (Place et al, 1978).

Developmental dysplasia of the hip (DDH) occurs in about 1 of 800 live births, more commonly in white infants and girls. During pregnancy, circulating maternal hormones may contribute to joint capsule laxity, particularly in the female fetus. The condition represents a spectrum of conditions from the dislocatable hip found in approximately 5 of 100 live births to the fixed dislocation that may occur in the second trimester in association with some forms of arthrogryposis. It is found more commonly in infants delivered in breech position and in those with a positive family history for DDH. In utero conditions that limit hip movement as well as specific syndromes and chromosome disorders may be associated with hip dislocation. Such dislocation is often unilateral, occurring more commonly in the left hip for reasons that are unclear.

There are two major tests (with a number of variations) for determining whether the femoral head is fixed in the acetabulum (Fig. 25–8). The Barlow test determines whether the femoral head can be dislocated posteriorly. As the knees are brought together (adducted) or held in midabduction, the examiner pushes laterally on the upper inner thigh (lesser trochanter). A click or clunk indicates that the femoral head in slipping over the lateral ridge of the acetabulum during this maneuver. With the fingers on the greater trochanter, the examiner can alternately push the hip into and out of the acetabulum by alternating pressure with the thumb and the fingers. The Ortolani test is carried out by abducting the flexed hips while pushing upward on the posterior proximal femur. The hips are

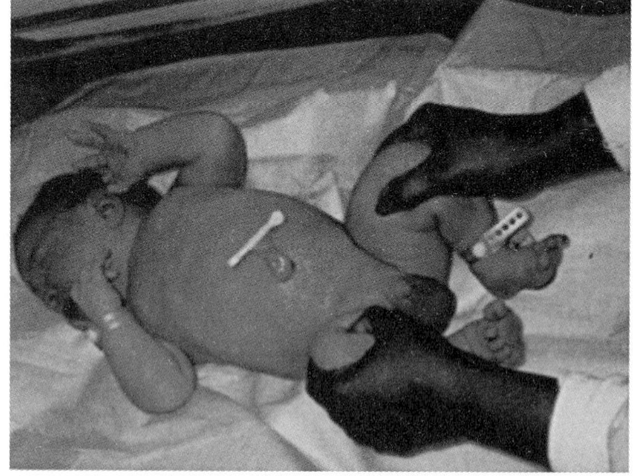
A

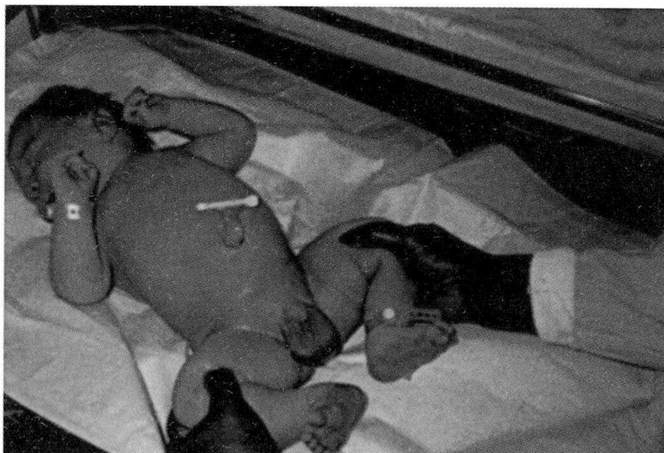
B

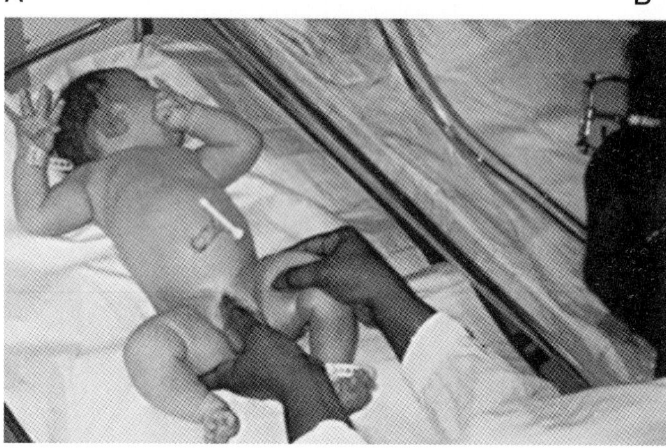
C

**FIGURE 25–8.** **A,** The hips are checked with the Ortolani maneuver. The examiner's second and third fingers press up against the heads of the femurs, and the hands press the shafts of the femurs toward the mattress while simultaneously abducting the hips. A palpable clunk during this maneuver indicates that the femoral head has slipped over the lip of the acetabulum and is dislocatable. **B,** Full abduction. **C,** For the Barlow maneuver, the examiner stabilizes the pelvis with the left hand and attempts to move the shaft of the femur upward and downward without flexing the hip. This maneuver checks whether the femoral head can be displaced posteriorly out of the acetabulum; instability of the femoral head is palpable during this maneuver in infants with congenitally dislocated hips (see Chapter 94).

adducted and flexed to 90 degrees; downward pressure is exerted on the knee while the hips are simultaneously abducted. A positive result consists of a click or clunk as the laterally dislocated femoral head is pushed over the acetabular ridge into the acetabulum. A modification of the Barlow test is to move the thigh anteriorly and posteriorly while holding the midthigh firmly with one hand and stabilizing the pelvis with the other. With this maneuver, the femoral head can alternately be dislocated and relocated, and in our experience, this test has been successful when the Ortolani maneuver has not (see Fig. 25–8).

Fixed dislocations that occurred early in fetal life often cannot be detected by the tests described because the femoral head is locked outside of the acetabulum as a result of joint capsule contractures. The diagnosis is made from palpation of the femoral head in a posterior location and by detecting limitation of hip mobility, in association with other problems, such as spina bifida and arthrogryposis. The sine qua non for diagnosis of DDH is real-time ultrasonography (Aronsson, 1994). (For a fuller discussion of DDH, including a discussion of Galeazzi and Klisic signs, see Morrissy, 1990.)

The four extremities should be checked for fractures, and the joints for hypermobility and hypomobility. A hypotonic arm or wrist drop implies brachial palsy on the affected side. The digits should be examined for polydactylism, syndactylism, edema, unusual skin ridge whorls and creases, nail growth, and unusual digit placement or contractures. Amputations or other evidence of amniotic bands may be present.

A variety of malformations of the lower extremities is common. Genu recurvatum is characterized by abnormal hyperextensibility of the knee joint. This condition affects females significantly more commonly than males. Genu recurvatum is associated with the breech position. The disorder may also be a feature of a number of disorders, such as the Ehlers-Danlos, Marfan, Klinefelter, and Turner syndromes, but it usually occurs as an in utero deformation not associated with other conditions. The extended leg or legs describe a concave arc when hyperextended at the knee. Hyperextensibility is mild or severe; that is, the arc is shallow or deep. In severe cases, there may be actual posterior dislocation of the knee. Nothing need be done for cases of mild or moderate severity. Posterior splinting or, rarely, casting for 2 to 4 weeks is indicated for the most severe forms.

Pes calcaneovalgus is the absolutely flat and sometimes slightly convex foot that often lies at rest dorsiflexed at an acute angle to the foreleg. When gentle pressure is applied to the sole of the foot, dorsiflexion increases easily until its dorsal surface lies in contact with the shin. Such feet should be casted in the equinovarus position for 4 to 6 weeks, and this therapy should be repeated several times if necessary. Continued treatment may be needed for several years.

In pes metatarsovarus, the heel and posterior half of the foot appear normal, but the forefoot angulates sharply inward. Thus, the outer border of the foot is convex, whereas its inner border is concave. If the foot can be straightened by gentle traction, with the examiner's thumb held firmly over the apex of the convexity, no immediate treatment is needed. If, however, the angulation is difficult or impossible to overcome, casting is probably indicated. Later use of corrective shoes may or may not be necessary.

Pes equinovarus is the classic clubfoot with sharp and tight hyperextension and in-curving of the entire foot. It is often a solitary defect, but not infrequently, it is associated with congenital dislocation of the hip, myelomeningocele, arthrogryposis, or other defects. It requires immediate and long-term orthopedic care. Most cases can be corrected by casting and subsequent shoe corrections. A few cases require open operation.

## Neurologic System

The neurologic examination is discussed in detail in Chapter 61. For most infants, the aim is to find whether a neurologic problem exists (Table 25–13); if so, the examination can be expanded to fully describe the findings. For a paralyzed 800-g infant undergoing mechanical ventilation, a complete neurologic examination is impossible. Nonetheless, neurologic assessment should not be deferred altogether. For example, attention to head size, shape, and possible abnormality, fontanelle size and pressure, pupil size and equality, lability of blood gases and blood pressure, variability of heart rate, and limb muscle mass are all available information about an infant's central nervous system status.

The quality and quantity of spontaneous movements are the best indicators of neuromuscular function and are assessed by inspection. Decreased tone may be one of the first detectable abnormalities in a full-term infant with sepsis. Tone is gestation and illness dependent, with smaller and sick infants having decreased tones. Tone may also vary in different muscle groups. The examiner checks the range of passive rotation of the neck by turning the infants' head to the left and right. He or she assesses flexor tone in the neck and arms by pulling the infant to a sitting position (Fig. 25–9), and extensor tone in the neck by holding the infant prone. Shoulder tone is assessed by an examiner either holding the infant in a vertical sling, that is, under the axillas, or performing the scarf maneuver (Fig. 25–10). Tone in the lower extremities is checked by the hip examination and with the heel-to-ear maneuver.

An array of primitive reflexes is present in the term newborn infant, but its expression is highly dependent on state—the most optimal being an awake alert state. Premature infants have diminished responses with decreasing gestational age, although this belief may be confounded by the growing frequency of illness with decreasing gestation and by the fact that sick infants respond poorly to elicitation of these reflexes. The Moro and tonic neck reflexes disappear by 6 months of age, but others (e.g., the parachute and Landau reflexes) make their appearance as these wane.

The most obvious primitive reflex of the newborn is the Moro. The infant can be supported behind the upper back by the examiner's hand, then dropped back 1 cm or so to the mattress. The arms are flung open followed by a flexion and an adduction (i.e., an "embrace"). The eyes open, as if in surprise, and the baby commonly emits a lusty cry, making this reflex a good stopping point for the examination. The examiner can elicit the grasp reflex in both hands and feet by placing a thumb on the infant's palm. With palmar pressure, the infant may open the mouth and yawn (palmar-mental reflex). When the examiner stimulates the dorsum of the foot, the infant lifts the stimulated foot and places it on a surface (placing). When the examiner allows the plantar surface of the other foot to contact a table top, the infant makes crude sequential walking movements (stepping). To obtain the tonic neck reflex, the examiner rotates the infant's head to the right or left while keeping the supine infant's shoulders flat.

**TABLE 25–13**

**Outline of Neurologic Screening Examination**

Appearance
Behavior, state, cry, abnormal movements
Visual responses
Hearing responses
Head size and shape
Active and passive tone of major muscle groups:
- Neck shoulders and upper extremities (pull to sit–traction response, vertical sling)
- Trunk (horizontal suspension)
- Lower extremities

Cranial nerves
Primitive neonatal reflexes (grasp, root, suck, Moro, withdrawal, tonic neck)
Deep tendon reflexes

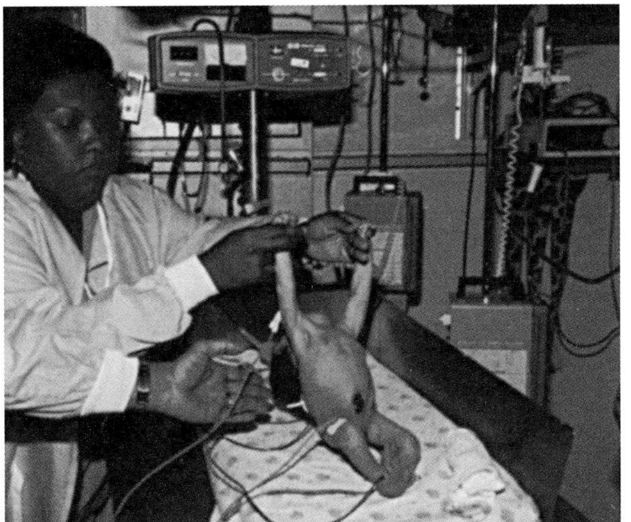

**FIGURE 25–9.** Tone of the neck flexors is assessed by pulling the infant off the mattress by both hands. In this infant, marked head lag is present.

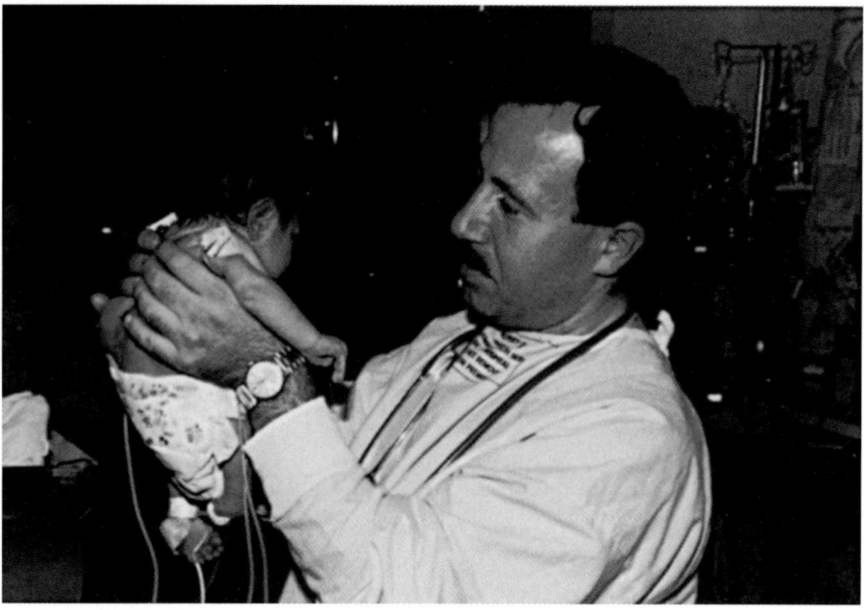

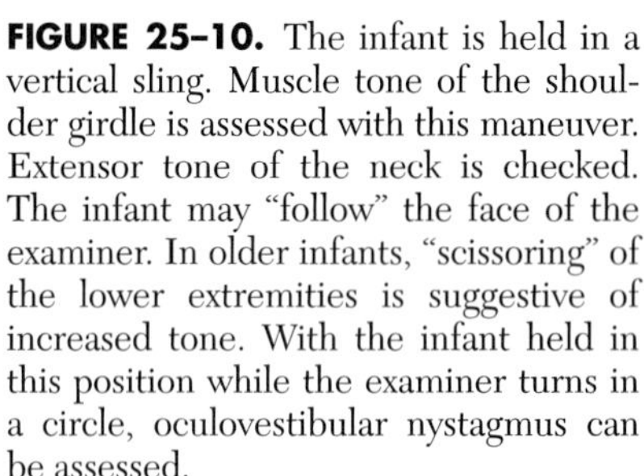

**FIGURE 25–10.** The infant is held in a vertical sling. Muscle tone of the shoulder girdle is assessed with this maneuver. Extensor tone of the neck is checked. The infant may "follow" the face of the examiner. In older infants, "scissoring" of the lower extremities is suggestive of increased tone. With the infant held in this position while the examiner turns in a circle, oculovestibular nystagmus can be assessed.

The arm and leg to the side of the occiput flex, and the other arm and leg extend (fencer's stance). When the infant is supported prone by the examiner's hand, tickling the area of the lateral spine causes the buttocks to swing to the side of stimulation (trunk incurvation reflex). Holding the infant in the same position and running a finger from the base of the spine toward the neck elicits spinal extension and, with a full bladder, micturition. Light pressure applied with the examiner's fingers to the soles of the feet causes the legs to extend (magnet reflex). Extending one of the infant's legs while the infant is supine and stimulating the plantar surface of the same foot causes the contralateral leg to flex, adduct, and extend (crossed extension reflex).

The examiner can best assess the infant's deep tendon reflexes by tapping with an index finger.

Other physical findings of clinical significance are listed in Table 25–14. Table 25–15 summarizes the various evaluations and issues for a "typical" high-risk premature infant during hospitalization.

**TABLE 25–14**

**Common Physical Findings that are of Clinical Significance in the Neonate**

| |
|---|
| Apnea |
| Tachypnea |
| Grunting |
| Bradycardia |
| Cyanosis |
| Hypotonia |
| Decreased breath sounds |
| Heart murmurs |
| Organomegaly |
| Evident anomalies other than of ears and digits |
| Jaundice |
| Plethora or pallor |
| Diffuse petechiae |

## ULTRASONOGRAPHY

Whenever a problem is defined that consists of anomalies or involves the head, heart, abdomen, or kidneys, the physician should conduct a screening ultrasonographic examination. Although the physician of newborns may not be an expert in imaging techniques, he or she should be capable of performing a screening examination in the same way that one carries out auscultation of the heart even if one is not a cardiologist. Obstetricians subspecializing in perinatology have surpassed neonatologists in their proficiency with ultrasonography screening. Using a 5-MHz sector scanner, the examiner can gain useful information by manipulating only gain and depth controls (Walther and Leighton, 1996).

### Head

The head is examined in the coronal and parasagittal planes through the anterior fontanelle. Ventricular size and the presence or absence of paraventricular and intraventricular blood are noted. Severe ventricular enlargement can be appreciated even by the relatively untrained examiner.

### Heart

The examiner should be able to identify all four chambers of the heart by aiming the probe, held in a transverse plane, cephalad from the substernal area. The atria are smaller than the ventricles and are symmetrical. At birth, the ventricles appear to be of equal size. Good contractility can be appreciated. Pericardial fluid may be signified by the presence of an echo-free area around

**TABLE 25-15**

**Changing Issues During Hospitalization of a "Typical" High-Risk Premature Infant**

| Evaluation | Pertinent Issues |
|---|---|
| Initial | Major malformations<br>Severe cardiopulmonary conditions<br>Viability<br>Postasphyxial complications<br>Hypotension<br>Intrauterine growth and length of gestation<br>Meeting with parents |
| Midweek | Patent ductus arteriosus<br>Intraventricular hemorrhage<br>Pneumothoraces and air leaks<br>Jaundice<br>Culture reports<br>Meeting with parents |
| First week | Metabolic<br>Renal<br>Gastrointestinal (necrotizing enterocolitis)<br>Intraventricular hemorrhage<br>Meeting with parents |
| First month | Chronic lung disease<br>Cystic periventricular lesions or ventricular enlargement<br>Retinopathy<br>Nutritional status<br>Nosocomial infection<br>Meeting with parents |
| Second and third months | Parental issues<br>Anemia<br>Feeding<br>Hydrocephalus<br>Growth<br>Chronic central nervous system disability<br>Apnea |
| Before discharge | Meeting with parents<br>Special (e.g., home oxygen)<br>Primary care vs. special medical follow-up planning<br>Other support services<br>Review of hospital course and global follow-up plans |

the heart that is surrounded by the echo-dense pericardium.

### Renal System

The paravertebral areas and the locale of the bladder are examined. Size, shape, and presence of large cysts or dilated collection systems are noted. The bladder can be visualized if filled with urine.

## LABORATORY SCREENING

At the time of the initial history and physical examination, the infant should be screened for a number of conditions, the precise nature of which depend on the characteristics of the population being served. For example, in an inner-city population, we tend to screen particularly for the conditions described in the following sections.

**Hematocrit, Rh, Blood Type, and Direct Antiglobulin Test (DAT, Direct Coombs' Test).** We collect heelstick blood specimens from all live-born infants. In our inner-city population, in which there is a greater risk of poor placentation and less than optimal use of prenatal care, we find about a 4% risk of clinical polycythemia (one venous hematocrit value >65% in an infant with symptoms or >70% in an infant without symptoms).

**Hearing Screening.** Only 50% of infants with significant hearing loss have identifiable risk factors. Fifty percent of hearing loss in newborns is genetic, with over half of cases being autosomal recessive traits. Nongenetic causes of hearing loss include fetal infection, teratogens, maternal disease, and perinatal events such as asphyxia, hyperbilirubinemia, and meningitis. Behavioral testing of hearing is crude in the newborn. Therefore, we follow the American Academy of Pediatrics (AAP) recommendation to screen all newborns with automated auditory brainstem response (ABR), a technique using three scalp electrodes that record brain waves and wave-form responses to auditory stimulation, thereby providing information on pathways from the outer ear to the cortex. Sensitivity is 100%, and specificity is 96%. Depending on the cause and extent of hearing loss, language acquisition may be improved by fitting a newborn with a hearing aid as early as 1 to 3 months. (Eilers and Oller, 1994; Joint Committee on Infant Hearing, 1995; Kuhl, 1993; J Stewart, Codirector, Newborn Hearing Screening Program, Beth Israel Deaconess Medical Center, Boston: Personal communication, 1997).

**Syphilis.** Standard immunologic tests for syphilis are a routine part of prenatal care in the United States. Because it is possible for exposure to *Treponema pallidum* to occur between the first trimester and delivery, mothers or infants in high-risk populations should be screened at delivery as well.

**Human Immunodeficiency Virus.** We offer testing for the human immunodeficiency virus (HIV) antibody to the newborn of any mother who has not been tested for HIV during pregnancy. Risk varies widely in different geographic areas.

**Hepatitis B.** We screen all mothers for hepatitis B, giving greater attention to those at special risk—for example, women who are involved in prostitution, who are from high-risk areas (Asia, Africa, Pacific islands, and inner cities of the United States), who have occupational exposure to blood products, who have been rejected for blood donation, who have received multiple frequent blood transfusions, who use intravenous drugs, who have had no prenatal care, and who have a history of liver disease or live with family members who have liver disease or are undergoing dialysis. Current risk estimates for infants born in Los Angeles are approximately 3 per 1000 live births (hepatitis data courtesy of L. Mascola, Los Angeles Department of Health Services). We administer hepatitis vaccine to all newborns according to current AAP recommendations. If the mother is hepatitis B positive, then hepatitis immune globulin is administered in addition to the vaccine.

**Drug Abuse.** Toxicology screening tests are performed on the urine of newborns whose mothers have a history of illicit drug use or who received little prenatal care, and (for our inner-city population) all infants admitted to the NICU. The screen used in our hospital identifies metabolites of amphetamines, phencyclidine (angel dust), opiates, and cocaine. It does not identify alcohol or cannabis. Approximately 12% of inner-city infants admitted to NICUs test positive for illicit drugs (see Chapter 12).

**Tuberculosis.** Mothers in groups at high risk for tuberculosis should undergo skin testing near delivery, and those who have positive results should be followed up with a chest radiograph and a careful history to look for active tuberculosis which requires treatment.

**Metabolic Diseases.** All states screen newborns for phenylketonuria and hypothyroidism (although different screening tools are used for hypothyroidism). Most states screen for galactosemia and hemoglobinopathies (such as sickle cell disease). Less than half the states screen for branched-chain amino acidemia, biotinidase deficiency, congenital adrenal hyperplasia, and homocystinuria. Only a few states currently screen for cystic fibrosis and toxoplasmosis (Stoddard and Farrell, 1997).

## WELL-BABY CARE

The principles of routine care for normal infants are screening for disease, prophylaxis for common problems (eye care and vitamin $K_1$ oxide), parent education when needed about infant care, and anticipatory guidance. These are discussed in the next chapter. The initial and discharge histories and examinations are truncated versions of complete procedures.

A welcome current trend "demedicalizes" routine delivery and postpartum care. This concept means delivery in a "homey" rather than operating room setting. More choices are offered to the parents concerning issues of childbirth, such as anesthesia and route and timing of delivery. The infant and mother are kept together as much as possible after birth. Fathers are often present during delivery, and liberal visiting policies that allow children to see their mother and new sibling are encouraged. Both before and after birth, nonmedically oriented classes are offered for discussing problems of both the mother and the infant. Forces in favor of these trends come from parents and (with regard to shorter hospital stays) financial considerations. Forces against these trends stem from administrative difficulties in handling the desires of parents and concerns about cross-infection.

How long should a mother and newborn stay in the hospital after delivery? Nobody knows. Since the last edition of this book, managed care has, to a growing extent, replaced fee for service as a medical reimbursement scheme in the United States. This change has provided a new impetus to find ways of reducing medical costs. Discharging mothers and newborn infants sooner after delivery is believed to be one way of achieving this goal. In California, the current norm is a hospital stay of 48 hours for a mother and infant after a vaginal delivery, and 4 days after a cesarean section. Although the benefit for cost savings in the short term appears obvious, it is not known whether this practice carries significant increased risk, especially for inner-city women and their infants (Braveman et al, 1995). Lee and associates (1995) found that readmission rates for infants nearly doubled after the duration of hospital stay after delivery was halved. Readmissions were largely for jaundice and poor milk intake.

Table 25–16 lists questions for which answers are needed before discharge of the mother and infant. The length of the list illustrates the difficulties presented by discharge of the mother within 24 hours of delivery.

In the delivery rooms of most U.S. hospitals, every newborn's eyes are instilled with erythromycin or 1% silver nitrate drops from single-use containers for prophylaxis of gonococcal eye infection. Vitamin $K_1$, 0.5 to 1.0 mg, is given intramuscularly to prevent hemorrhagic disease of the newborn. The infant is then bathed with a nonmedicated mild soap. No antiseptic is routinely applied to the umbilical cord stump.

**TABLE 25–16**

**Pre-Discharge Screening Questions for Newborns**

1. Is the infant at least 35 weeks of gestation at time of discharge?
2. Is the infant feeding well? If the mother is breast-feeding, does she know how to get support or where to call if she is having problems?
3. Has the infant been voiding and stooling appropriately?
4. Has the infant been able to maintain normal body temperature in a regular crib?
5. Does the infant have any significant anomalies or medical problems that need further investigation and/or follow-up and have the appropriate visits been scheduled?
6. Is the infant at risk for hyperbilirubinemia and has appropriate follow-up been arranged?
7. Has it been at least 5 days since the last episode of apnea that required stimulation?
8. Do parents want the infant to be circumcised prior to discharge?
9. Do the parents have a medical home for the baby?
10. Does the family have health insurance for the infant or does it need help with this issue?
11. Has the mother recovered from her childbirth experience well enough to adequately care for her infant? Does she have help or support at home?
12. Is the family able to contend with minor problems that may arise soon after discharge?
13. Is the family aware of the customary newborn prophylaxis and screening that their infant has received (e.g., eye prophylaxis, Vitamin K, state screening for metabolic errors, hearing screening, hepatitis B immunization)?
14. Have the parents received anticipatory guidance and instruction with regard to feeding problems, jaundice, signs of infection, use of infant car seats, immunizations, well-baby visits, sleeping position on the back to reduce sudden infant death syndrome (SIDS)?
15. Is the initial maternal-infant interaction appropriate?
16. Have the parents had an opportunity to discuss questions and concerns with hospital caregivers?

## DISCHARGE PLANNING

Discharge of a premature infant from the intermediate care unit can take place when the parents have made adequate preparations (actual and psychological) for the care of the infant. Meeting this need may take weeks of preparation on the part of the staff and may include arranging in-home support and equipment, teaching feeding and medication techniques, and providing anticipatory guidance. Other criteria for discharge are adequate feeding and weight gain and physiologic stability (e.g., absence of apnea and steady body temperature).

Detailed recording of the major events of the infant's stay—diagnoses, results of meetings with parents and case conferences, most recent evaluations, medications, and future needs—all should be summarized, and the information disseminated appropriately. Most importantly, the primary physician should know the parents and the infant well by the time of discharge, so that trust and confidence exist on both sides.

### Discharge Summary

An array of computerized data collection systems is available that should soon permit vastly improved transfer of information, freeing physicians from the tyranny of the handwritten medical record. We currently use a custom-programmed computerized database for data entry and retrieval, which deals with daily hospital notes for a hospital delivery service of 1700 inner-city births per year, including well babies, intermediate care babies, and babies requiring intensive care.

## FOLLOW-UP CARE

A variety of support groups is available for parents of infants with special problems. Pediatric follow-up care for normal infants is detailed in the *Guidelines for Health Supervision* published by the American Academy of Pediatrics and available in standard pediatric texts (Avery and First, 1989). California has also published detailed infant and child health assessment guidelines (Children's Medical Services, 1997). Follow-up care of high-risk infants is described in detail by Ballard (1988) and by Taeusch and Yogman (1987). Current changes in immunization recommendations can be ascertained through the Centers for Disease Control and the latest Academy of Pediatrics listing.

## SELECTED READINGS

Avery G: Neonatology: Pathophysiology and Management of the Newborn, 3rd ed. Philadelphia, JB Lippincott, 1987.

Avery M, First L: Pediatric Medicine. Baltimore, Williams & Wilkins, 1989.

Ballard R: Pediatric Care of the ICN Graduate. Philadelphia, WB Saunders, 1988.

Balsan MJ, Holyman IR: Slide Atlas of Pediatric Physical Diagnosis. 2: Neonatology. New York, Gower Medical, 1992.

Barness L: Manual of Pediatric Physical Diagnosis, 4th ed. Chicago, Year Book Medical, 1976.

Bates B: A Guide to Physical Diagnosis and History Taking, 4th ed. Philadelphia, JB Lippincott, 1987.

Cloherty J, Stark A: Manual of Neonatal Care, 2nd ed. Boston, Little, Brown, 1985.

Coen R, Koffler H: Primary Care of the Newborn. Boston, Little, Brown, 1987.

Crelin E: Anatomy of the Newborn—An Atlas. Philadelphia, Lea & Febiger, 1969.

Duncan R: Cedars Sinai Teaching Files: Detailed Newborn Exam. http://www.neonatology.org.

Dunn P, Evans T, Thearle M, et al: Congenital dislocation of the hip: Early and late diagnosis and management compared. Arch Dis Child 60:407, 1985.

Eden R, Boehm F: Assessment and Care of the Fetus. Norwalk, CT, Appleton & Lange, 1990.

Fanaroff A, Martin R: Neonatal-Perinatal Medicine, 7th ed. St. Louis, CV Mosby, 2002.

Fenichel G: Neurological exam of the newborn. Int Pediatr 9:77, 1994.

Fletcher MA: Physical Diagnosis in Neonatology. Philadelphia, Lippincott-Raven, 1998.

Gottfried A, Garter J: Infant Stress Under Intensive Care: Environmental Neonatology. Baltimore, University Park Press, 1985.

Graham J: Smith's Recognizable Patterns of Human Deformation. Philadelphia, WB Saunders, 1988.

Hoeckelman R: The physical examination of infants and children. In Bates B (ed): A Guide to Physical Exam and History Taking, 4th ed. Philadelphia, JB Lippincott, 1987, pp 525-598.

Hoeckelman R: The physical examination of infants and children. In Bates B (ed): A Guide to Physical Exam and History Taking, 4th ed. Philadelphia, JB Lippincott, 1987, pp 525-598.

Illingworth R: The Development of the Infant and Young Child, 2nd ed. Baltimore, Williams & Wilkins, 1963.

Illingworth R: The Development of the Infant and Young Child, 2nd ed. Baltimore, Williams & Wilkins, 1963.

Jones, KL: Smith's Recognizable Patterns of Human Malformation. 5th ed. Philadelphia, WB Saunders, 1997.

Larson E: A causal link between hand washing and risk of infection? Examination of the evidence. Infect Control 9:28, 1988.

Morrissy RT: Lovell and Winter's Pediatric Orthopedics, 3rd ed. Philadelphia, JB Lippincott, 1990.

Oski F, DeAngelis C, Feigin R, et al: Principles and Practice of Pediatrics. Philadelphia, JB Lippincott, 1990.

Roberton N: Textbook of Neonatology. Edinburgh, Churchill Livingstone, 1987.

Scanlon J: A System of Newborn Physical Exam. Baltimore, University Park Press, 1979.

Vulliamy D, Johnston : The Newborn Child, 6th ed. Edinburgh, Churchill Livingstone, 1987.

Yu V, Wood C: Prematurity. Edinburgh, Churchill Livingstone, 1987.

Ziai M, Clarke T, Merritt A: Assessment of the Newborn—A Guide for the Practitioner. Boston, Little, Brown, 1984.

Zitelli BJ, Davis HW: Slide Atlas of Pediatric Physical Diagnosis. St. Louis, CV Mosby, 1992.

## REFERENCES

Academy of Pediatrics, Task Force on Newborn and Infant Hearing. Newborn and Infant Hearing Loss: Detection and Intervention. Pediatrics 103:527, 1999.

American Academy of Pediatrics: Report of the Committee on Infectious Diseases: Red Book, 25th ed. Elk Grove, IL, American Academy of Pediatrics, 2003. http://www.cispimmunize.org.

Aronsson DD, Goldberg MJ, Kling TF, Roy DR: Developmental dysplasia of the hip. Pediatrics 94:201-208, 1994.

Ballard JL, Khoury JC, Wedig K, et al: New Ballard score expanded to include extremely premature infants. J Pediatr 119:417, 1991.

Braveman P, Egerter S, Pearl M, et al: Problems associated with early discharge of newborn infants. Pediatrics 96:716, 1995.

Children's Medical Services: Health Assessment Guidelines of the Child Health and Disability Prevention Program. Sacramento, CA, Department of Health Services, 1997.

Creasy R, Resnik R: Maternal-Fetal Medicine: Principles and Practice, 5th ed. Philadelphia, WB Saunders, 2004.

Eilers RE, Oller DK: Infant vocalizations and the early diagnosis of severe hearing impairment. J Pediatr 582:248, 1994.

Faix R: Fontanel size in black and white infants. J Pediatr 100:304, 1982.

Kuhl PK: Development of speech perception. Ann N Y Acad Sci 582:248, 1993.

Lee KS, Perlman M, Ballantyne M, et al: Association between duration of neonatal hospital stay and readmission rate. J Pediatr 127:758, 1995.

Phelan J, Smith C, Broussard P, et al: Amniotic fluid volume assessment using the four quadrant technique in the pregnancy between 36 and 42 weeks' gestation. J Reprod Med 32:540, 1987.

Place M, Parkin PM, Fitton M: Effectiveness of neonatal screening for congenital dislocation of the hip. Lancet 2:249, 1978.

Popich G, Smith D: Fontanels: Range of normal size. J Pediatr 80:749, 1972.

Stoddard JJ, Farrell PM: State-to-state variations in newborn screening policies. Arch Pediatr Adolesc Med 151:561, 1997.

Taeusch HW, Yogman Y: Follow-up Management of the High-Risk Infant. Boston, Little, Brown, 1987.

Walther FJ, Leighton JO: Diagnostic ultrasound screening of infants. In Pediatric and Neonatal Tests and Procedures. Philadelphia, WB Saunders, 1996, pp 387-405.

CHAPTER 26

# Routine Newborn Care

Carol A. Miller and Thomas B. Newman

The normal newborn nursery has a unique position within the hospital. It is probably the only inpatient unit focused on the care of the relatively well patient. It is also a unit where care of the patient is intimately connected to care of the mother. The mother-newborn dyad should be treated as an integral unit, promoting bonding and developing the mother's expertise as her infant's caregiver. With this goal in mind, many units are designed for the rooming-in of mother and infant and encourage physicians and nurses to give routine care to newborns in those locations rather in the nursery, as was previously practiced (Kennell and Klaus, 1998; Klaus, 1998; Prodromidis et al, 1995). The mother then becomes an important observer of her infant's behavior and a relevant member of the infant's care team. Some practitioners may find practicing this way a challenge and a bit awkward but with time may come to prefer the chance to include the mother in their assessment and care of her baby.

The shortening of the length of hospital stay for both mothers and newborns was an additional change that raised concern regarding the ability to adequately follow the newborn's successful transition to the outside world (Boodman, 1995). Current average stays for the healthy newborn range from about 24 to 48 hours after a vaginal delivery and from 72 to 96 hours after cesarean section (National Center for Health Statistics, 1999). Reliable assessment tools that can help identify which infants might eventually require intervention for problems such as breast-feeding or hyperbilirubinemia and reasonable strategies for prevention are obvious areas for future research. Fortunately, despite these challenges, most healthy infants born at term or close to term proceed through transition smoothly, are stable at discharge, and continue to be so at home (Escobar et al, 2001).

Nevertheless, care of the normal newborn within the hospital setting remains an important aspect of pediatric care and requires expertise and training. Routine procedures should be re-evaluated continually for efficacy and efficiency. Uncomfortable interventions should be minimized, as should practices that disrupt the mother's close contact with her baby. Pediatricians and other care providers should keep abreast of new technologies that might enhance the ability to deliver high-quality care in the least intrusive manner possible.

This chapter focuses on current routine newborn care practices. The physical examination assessment as well as the delivery room care are covered in detail in Chapters 25 and 27. In areas of controversy, we attempt to explore all sides of the issues and present national consensus when available. The reader is encouraged to view this material as we do—as a work in progress subject to change because of new research and experience.

## ROUTINE ASSESSMENT AND SCREENING TESTS

### Initial Assessment, Vital Signs, and Monitoring

A major goal of the initial care of the newborn is to identify potentially serious problems at an early stage while taking pains to minimize any maneuvers that cause discomfort to the infant or require separation from the mother. The initial assessment is made in the delivery room (see Chapter 25), including review of the mother's history with particular attention to risk factors for infection (see Chapter 39), a cursory examination of the infant, and assignment of Apgar scores. The purpose of this first assessment is to determine whether there is any reason to take the infant to the nursery for medical attention rather than placing him or her "skin to skin" on the mother's chest, the preferred place for infants to begin life after birth (Kennell and Klaus, 1998; Sinusas and Gagliardi, 2001). Most infants with good Apgar scores should be able to stay skin-to-skin with their mothers for at least the first hour or so, and given the opportunity to find their way to the breast and begin nursing (Righard and Alade, 1990). This important time should not be disturbed without sound medical justification, because the early contact facilitates bonding between mother and infant. Randomized trials have shown that this initial close contact enhances the relationship between mother and infant (Anisfeld and Lipper, 1983) and may increase the likelihood of successful breast-feeding (Renfrew et al, 2000; Sinusas and Gagliardi, 2001). For thess reasons, the routine procedures discussed here (e.g., eye prophylaxis, vitamin K administration) should be deferred until the baby has spent at least the first hour with the mother.

Although the infant should spend much of the first few hours with the mother, he or she should be assessed frequently. Many infants with significant illnesses have good Apgar scores and appear fine initially, only to deteriorate over the first 12 to 24 hours after birth. For this reason, the newborn's vital signs, tone, color, perfusion, and level of activity and consciousness should be monitored and recorded at least every 30 minutes until stable for 2 hours (American Academy of Pediatrics [AAP], 1997), and at least every 6 hours thereafter for the first 24 hours. Many normal infants have some initial respiratory distress soon after birth, which improves rapidly over the first 4 hours. Frequent assessments are necessary to determine whether the infant's status is deteriorating rather than showing the expected improvement.

The highest priority of the complete physical examination of the newborn infant is to identify abnormalities likely to have significant health consequences, particularly those for which early treatment has been demonstrated to improve outcome. However, another important reason for the physical examination is to anticipate and answer parents' questions. Performing the physical examination with the parents present facilitates this process. Many findings that do not require intervention but may be unfamiliar to parents, such as subconjunctival hemorrhages, the Moro reflex, and Mongolian spots, can be demonstrated and named; see Chapter 25.

## Routine Laboratory Testing

### Glucose and Hematocrit

The performance of routine laboratory tests in the first several hours after birth is controversial. A spun hematocrit and a glucose measurement using a chemical strip on a heelstick blood specimen are routinely done at 2 to 4 hours of age in some hospitals. The rationale for screening is that both hypoglycemia and polycythemia can be asymptomatic, both are associated with increased risk of adverse neurologic outcome, and both can be treated—the former with supplemental glucose and the latter by partial-exchange transfusion, in which aliquots of the infant's blood are withdrawn and replaced with saline solution.

However, the Committee on the Fetus and Newborn of the AAP does not recommend routine screening of infants for these entities, because there is no evidence that identifying and treating asymptomatic infants with polycythemia or hypoglycemia improves their outcome (Committee on Fetus and Newborn, 1995). That is, although low plasma glucose levels can be raised with supplemental glucose and high blood counts can reduced by partial-exchange transfusion, and although it makes sense that this approach might benefit the infant, there are no randomized trials showing that this is the case. Proponents of screening argue that our understanding of the body is sufficient to project that screening and intervention will be beneficial; opponents favor obtaining evidence of benefit before screening and intervention in asymptomatic people. One dilemma proponents of screening have is that in the absence of randomized trials, it is hard to know the level of asymptomatic laboratory abnormality at which treatment should be initiated. Thus different nurseries not only have different protocols for screening, they have different ranges for what constitutes the lower limit of normal and different protocols for treatment (Bonacruz et al, 1996; Koh and Vong, 1996). Given the lack of data on these tests, a wide range of clinical practices is acceptable, and parental preferences for more or less screening and intervention should be respected.

### Routine Metabolic Screens

Newborn metabolic screening for rare diseases like hypothyroidism and PKU is discussed in Chapter 27. Requirements for screening vary from state to state and over time. In general, there has been a trend toward screening for more diseases as new tests have become available. Unfortunately, in many cases the ability to diagnose metabolic diseases has preceded studies demonstrating the benefits of early intervention. Because of the low prevalence of the diseases being screened for, even with very specific tests most positive results will turn out to be falsely positive. Nonetheless, the incremental cost of testing for additional diseases is low and early results with a new technique called tandem mass spectrometry are promising, suggesting the ability to diagnose a wide range of metabolic disorders, with a retest rate of only about 1 in 1000 and a positive predictive value of about 10% (Wiley et al, 1999; Zytkovicz et al, 2001).

In order to avoid unnecessarily alarming families with these falsely positive results, it may be helpful to explain to families at the time the test is being drawn that the testing is for very rare diseases, that there are occasional false-alarms and inadequate specimens, and that therefore they should not panic if they are asked to bring the infant back for a repeat test.

### Hearing Screening

The rationale for newborn hearing screening comes from evidence that early detection and intervention in hearing-impaired children lead to improved language development (Moeller, 2000; Yoshinaga-Itano et al, 1998) and that in the absence of screening many children with hearing loss are not identified until 2 or 3 years of age. Although the data relating early intervention to improved outcome are from observational studies, rather than experiments, the strength and consistency of the association, the biologic plausibility, and the lack of another equally plausible explanation suggest that the relationship is causal.

The development of objective physiologic measures of hearing in newborns has made universal newborn hearing screening possible. Two technologies commonly used are measurements of otoacoustic emissions (OAE) and auditory brainstem responses (ABR). OAEs are *sounds* generated by the outer hair cells of the cochlea that can be measured by sensitive microphones. OAEs are not necessary for hearing, but are an indirect measure of the integrity of the cochlea (Folsom and Diefendorf, 1999). Measurements of OAEs will be abnormal in the face of conductive hearing loss due to obstruction of the external auditory canal or due to middle ear disease. Conversely, because OAEs only measure cochlear function, they will be normal in infants with neural but not sensory hearing loss (Joint Committee on Infant Hearing, 2000). Measurement of ABRs involves averaging electroencephalographic responses to multiple clicks. By subtracting baseline brain wave activity from the signal just after the clicks, brainwaves related to hearing can be separated and displayed, including the cochlea, auditory nerve, and auditory brainstem pathways. Because the clicks used include mainly mid- to high frequencies (2000 to 8000 Hz), low frequency hearing loss and steeply downsloping high frequency hearing loss (i.e., severe hearing loss at 8000 Hz with normal hearing at 2000 Hz) can be missed.

Although there are likely to be benefits from early identification of infants with hearing loss, they do not come without costs. Because the prevalence of hearing loss in newborns is low—only about 1 per 1000—(Fortnum et al, 2001) and the tests have imperfect specificity, most infants that fail the hearing screens will subsequently be found to have normal hearing. If the referral rate is 4% (the upper limit of what is recommended) (Joint Committee on Infant Hearing, 2000), this means that only about 1 in 40 referred infants (2.5%) will actually have hearing loss. Opponents of universal hearing screening suggest that we need data that the benefits of early detection of hearing loss in the true positives exceed the potential but largely unstudied adverse effects on the much more numerous false positives. These include expense (which may not be covered by third-party payers), parental anxiety, and possible adverse effects on the parent child relationship related to additional testing (Paradise, 1999).

Clinicians caring for newborns should take steps to minimize adverse effects in infants failing newborn hearing screening tests. The easiest step is simply repeating the test before discharge. Clemens and Davis (2001) reported that this reduced the number of referrals by 80%. For those still testing positive, the most important step is to provide accurate information to the parents. If the "refer" rate for the screening test used on the infant is known, a ball-park estimate for parents of the chance that their child truly has hearing loss is simply the prevalence of the disease (in this instance, 1 per 1000) divided by that referral rate. For example, a referral rate of 2% = 20 per 1000 means that the chance that a positive screen is truly positive is about 1 in 20.

Infants still failing the screen on retesting should receive confirmatory audiologic testing and medical evaluations before 3 months of age. Because the goal of screening is not only early identification but early treatment of affected infants, it is important that resources be available for further diagnosis and treatment of infants testing positive. If resources and expertise to provide these services at an affordable cost to families are not available, screening could do more harm than good.

## ROUTINE AND COMMON MEDICAL TREATMENTS

For any therapy given routinely to all infants, there must be compelling evidence that the benefits exceed the risks. Parents who question the need for these therapies should be supported for their interest in protecting their infant from unnecessary medical intervention, and treated with respect, not condescension or antagonism. Certainly the history of medicine provides ample justification for a skeptical attitude about conventionally accepted medical interventions. A collaborative approach to helping parents make informed decisions is likely to be more helpful than one that is overly directive or dogmatic. Such an approach requires clinicians caring for newborns to be familiar with the risks and benefits of common therapies, in order to help interested parents make informed decisions about providing or withholding them.

### Prevention of Ophthalmia Neonatorum and Conjunctivitis

Severe conjunctivitis in the newborn ("Ophthalmia neonatorum") was a major cause of blindness until the prophylactic instillation of antibiotic eye drops or ointment to newborns became routine. It is now required by law in most states. The most severe cases leading to risk of blindness are due to Neisseria gonorrhea, but other organisms, including Chlamydia trachomatis, Hemophilus influenzae and Streptococcus pneumoniae also cause conjunctivitis in the first few months after birth (Krohn et al, 1993). Among patients with good prenatal care that has included cervical cultures for gonorrhea, the risk of gonococcal conjunctivitis is low. For this reason, some of these patients may question the need for prophylaxis, because of concerns about causing chemical conjunctivitis. However, Bell and colleagues (Bell et al, 1993) in a randomized trial of such low-risk infants, found that either 1% silver nitrate drops or 0.5% erythromycin ointment reduced the total risk of conjunctivitis (both infectious and noninfectious) compared with no treatment. Most of the cases in all 3 groups were mild, and all of the benefit was in the first two weeks. The rates of conjunctivitis were 15% with no treatment, 8% with silver nitrate (P = .03), and 9% with erythromycin (P = .05), for a risk difference favoring treatment of 6%-7% and the number needed to treat to prevent one case of conjunctivitis, about 15.

Isenberg et al (1995) performed a randomized trial in Kenya, comparing 2.5% povidone-iodine solution with 1% silver nitrate solution and 0.5% erythromycin ointment. They reported that povidone-iodine was less expensive and slightly more effective at preventing both infectious (risk difference 2%-4%) and noninfectious (risk difference about 4%) conjunctivitis in newborns. However, 2.5% povidone-iodine ophthalmic solution has not been approved by the U.S. Food and Drug Administration for this indication.

### Vitamin K

Vitamin K is routinely administered to newborns to prevent vitamin K deficiency bleeding (VKDB; Chapter 76). Vitamin K deficiency beyond the newborn period is usually associated with fat malabsorption, because intake is generally adequate from the diet and from synthesis of vitamin K by intestinal flora. Newborns are at risk of vitamin K deficiency, and hence of prolonged clotting times and hemorrhage, because vitamin K is poorly transferred across the placenta, is present only at low levels in breast milk, and because their intestines have not yet been sufficiently colonized to make vitamin K.

Vitamin K deficiency bleeding is divided into three categories: early (first 24 hours), classic (1 to 7 days), and late (>7 days). Early VKDB is most often associated with maternal use of anticoagulants or other drugs that interfere with vitamin K metabolism, and is not prevented by prophylactic vitamin K administration. Classic VKDB, most often from the skin, gastrointestinal tract, or circumcision site, was reported to occur in about 1% of unsupplemented infants (Lane et al, 1985) and can be prevented by either oral or parenteral Vitamin K (Zipursky, 1999). Late VKDB is much less common, occurring in only about 5-10 per 100,000 untreated infants (McNinch and Tripp, 1991; Schubiger et al, 1999), but is much more serious, with about half the cases presenting with CNS bleeding, leading to death or serious neurologic sequelae (Bor et al, 2000; Brousson, 1996).

Late VKDB is more effectively prevented by intramuscular (1 mg, about 95% effective) than by oral vitamin K (e.g., 1 mg per week; about 80% effective) (Cornellissen et al, 1997), partly because compliance with oral vitamin K is incomplete and because some children with undiagnosed liver disease will fail adequately to absorb the oral vitamin K (Schubiger, 1999). Thus, the excess risk of late VKDB after oral vitamin K, compared with parenteral vitamin K is about 1-2/100,000.

A clear advantage of oral compared with intramuscular vitamin K is that it is not painful for the infant. A more controversial advantage is that it has not been associated with an increased risk of childhood cancer (particularly leukemia), as has intramuscular vitamin K. This association was initially suggested from two studies in Bristol, England, mostly of children born in the 1970s, which found the risk of childhood cancer was more than doubled among those that had received intramuscular vitamin K (Golding et al, 1992). Many subsequent studies in other populations have failed to confirm the association (Ekelund et al, 1993; Klebanoff et al, 1993; McKinney et al, 1998; von Kries et al, 1996), and childhood leukemia incidence did not increase in the years following intramuscular vitamin K (Miller, 1992; Olsen et al, 1994). Thus, an association of anywhere near the magnitude suggested by the initial studies from Bristol has been effectively ruled out. However, the issue has not entirely been put to rest because point estimates for the relative risk of leukemia in several studies, although not statistically significant, have been in the range of 1.2 to 1.3 (Ansell et al, 1996; McKinney et al, 1998; Parker et al, 1998; Passmore et al, 1998) and even a 10% increase in leukemia risk would be clinically relevant because leukemia is more than ten times as common than severe VKDB (Golding et al, 1992; Hey, 1999; von Kries, 1998). Because current studies have not had the power or consistency of results to rule out a small increase in risk of cancer following IM Vitamin K, vitamin K is given orally, rather than parenterally in some European countries. Unfortunately, there is currently (2001) no oral vitamin K preparation approved by the U.S. Food and Drug Administration for prophylactic use in newborns. When parents decline intramuscular vitamin K, the parenteral preparation (Aquamephyton) can be given orally. However, gagging and vomiting due to its bad taste are common, and it is not clear that oral use of the parenteral preparation is as effective as the oral preparations that have been studied in Europe. The American Academy of Pediatrics has recommended continuing to give vitamin K intramuscularly, while encouraging the licensing of an oral vitamin K preparation in the United States (American Academy of Pediatrics Ad Hoc Task Force, 1993).

## Circumcision

Few medical treatments generate as much heated debate as circumcision of newborn boys. Many parents will have already made a decision about circumcision by the time their son is born, and they may not wish to discuss the risks and benefits. Others, however, will request medical information on the medical risks and benefits, in order to make an informed decision. Unfortunately, misinformation abounds, particularly on the Internet, and the biases of authors color what looks to parents like objective information. The authors of this chapter are neither strong proponents nor opponents of circumcision, but like the American Academy of Pediatrics (1999) and the American College of Obstetrics and Gynecology (2001) we strongly oppose circumcision without anesthesia and we believe parents should be informed of the risks and benefits so that they can make the decision based upon accurate information (Learman, 1999).

The principal risks of circumcision include bleeding, infection, pain, and an unsatisfactory cosmetic result. The risks are probably operator dependent and also depend on the method used. The three most commonly used methods are the Mogen and Gomco clamps and the Plastibell device. Studies of circumcision complications have been case reports or retrospective series, likely underestimating minor complications. The Mogen clamp is the fastest method, but carries a low but poorly quantified (perhaps 1 in 5,000-10,000) risk of partial amputation of the glans (Strimling, 1996). The Plastibell device leads to ischemic necrosis and eventual sloughing of the foreskin. Plastibell circumcision has been associated with a slightly higher risk of infection than Gomco circumcision (.72% vs .14% in one series) (Gee and Ansell, 1976) and necrotizing fasciitis has been reported only with Plastibell circumcision (Bliss et al, 1997; Woodside, 1980). The risk of bleeding with either the Gomco or Plastibell devices is about 1%; this usually responds to local measures (Amir et al, 2000; Gee and Ansell, 1976). "Degloving" injuries that required skin grafting have been reported following Gomco circumcision (Patel et al, 2001). Infections related to neonatal circumcisions occur rarely. A recent study of over 130,000 circumcised neonates reported only 2 infections (Christakis et al, 2000). The risk of pain from circumcision can be minimized with anesthesia. A ring block or dorsal penile nerve block is easy to learn and more effective than topical anesthesia at reducing crying and physiologic pain responses (Butler-O'Hara et al, 1998; Lander et al, 1997). In addition, a few drops of a concentrated (~35%) sucrose solution on a pacifier help reduce apparent pain (Blass and Hoffmeyer, 1991; Herschel et al, 1998). The pain from circumcision with inadequate anesthesia may have consequences beyond the neonatal period. Taddio and colleagues have shown that boys circumcised without anesthesia cried longer following routine vaccinations at 4 and 6 months than uncircumcised boys or those circumcised with anesthesia (Taddio et al, 1997).

Data on satisfaction with the cosmetic result are sparse, of questionable generalizability, and probably subject to publication bias, as authors might be less eager to report on a high prevalence of dissatisfied patients. In one study of Gomco circumcisions, 99.7% of parents were satisfied with the result (Amir et al, 2000). Parents of uncircumcised infants in another study were more likely to be dissatisfied with their decision than were parents of circumcised infants (27% vs. 14%) (Adler et al, 2001). This is not an argument in favor of circumcision, however, because dissatisfaction with circumcision (i.e., wishing it had not been done) is less easily remedied than dissatisfaction with lack of circumcision, which presumably can be remedied (albeit expensively) with later circumcision. It does, however, suggest that information about circumcision and care of the intact foreskin should be provided to all families, not just those requesting circumcision.

The benefits of circumcision include reduced risk of foreskin problems, including infections and irritations, phimosis and paraphimosis; reduced risk of human immunodeficiency virus (HIV) and other sexually transmitted diseases, reduced risk of penile cancer, and reduced risk of urinary tract infections. The reduced risk of HIV infection was particularly compelling in a recent study of couples in sub-Saharan Africa discordant for HIV infection (Quinn et al, 2000). Over a follow-up period of about 2 years, seroconversions occurred among 40 of 137 uncircumcised men (29%) and none of 50 circumcised men ($P < 0.001$). Opponents of circumcision argue that most uncircumcised males will not have any of these problems, that they could be prevented by good hygiene and safer sexual practices, and that men wishing the benefits of reduced risk of sexually transmitted diseases or penile cancer may undergo elective circumcision at a later age, when they are old enough to provide their own consent. Unlike the other benefits, the approximately 10-fold reduction in risk of urinary tract infections (from 1%-2% to 0.1%-0.2%) (Schoen & Fischell, 1991) is mainly a benefit from circumcision in the neonatal period. Although most urinary tract infections have a benign course, even in infancy bacteremia accompanies UTI in about 10% of cases under 3 months, thus not surprisingly meningitis and death from UTI in infancy have been reported (Bergstrom et al, 1972; Wiswell and Geschke, 1989).

A recent task force of the American Academy of Pediatrics (1999) concluded that there were both risks and "potential medical benefits" of circumcision. This unfortunate phrasing has been widely misinterpreted. The medical benefits of circumcision are established beyond any reasonable doubt. They are "potential" only in that the most uncircumcised males will not develop conditions circumcision would have prevented, just as most infants immunized against meningitis would not have developed meningitis anyway. Routine immunization to prevent meningitis is recommended while circumcision is not, because the risks, irreversible changes, and nonmedical significance of circumcision are much greater than those associated with immunization (Newman, 2001).

## ONGOING CARE

### Infant Security Systems

Sentinel events, such as the switching of babies in the hospital, kidnappings from newborn nurseries, and liberal rooming-in policies heightened awareness that hospital systems were needed to accurately identify newborns throughout their hospital stay and to prevent unauthorized persons from gaining access. Accreditation agencies are encouraging that newborn security systems be put in place beyond those set up for the general hospital. Infant identification systems include immediate banding of newborns and their mothers before they leave the delivery room with the infant's name and medical record number along with the mother's name and medical record number. Every time a newborn is separated and subsequently reunited with the mother, banding checks should be made to confirm the correct match-up of mother and baby. Generally one other person, specified by the mother is also banded, allowing that person independent access to the newborn (Appelbaum, 2000-2001; Rabun et al, 1992).

The newborn's band is generally attached to a sensor that will alert unit staff and hospital security personnel when passage near or through exits occurs. These alerts are tied to immediate response procedures (i.e., "Code Pink") designed to prohibit the infant's unauthorized removal from the hospital. There are several such systems available with many of the newer ones attached to computer programs that will identify the exact location of the infant at the time the alert is sounded (Secure Care Systems of Virginia, *www.securecaresystemsofva.com*).

Infant security systems, while well-intentioned are not yet perfect and are troubled by false alarms, often because someone mistakenly takes the infant down the wrong corridor and passes a sensor. Sometimes there are mechanical problems, temporarily disabling the system. Additionally, as the newborn normally loses weight after birth, bands become loose and frequently fall off the legs or arms. Data assessing the effectiveness of electronically tracking newborns are currently unavailable and it will probably take some time before measurable change can be documented as these are uncommon though frightening events. Until the perfect electronic system is developed, mothers should be instructed regarding precautions they can take to safeguard their babies.

### Temperature and Bathing

Monitoring the newborn's ability to thermoregulate and maintain body temperature within normal range should be as simple as taking the temperature and comparing the reading with a norm. However, there are many questions that can complicate such a seemingly simple procedure, such as how and at what body site to take the temperature and, more importantly, what the normal temperature for a newborn is? Generally, comparing and noting trends of repeated measurements on the same baby gives much more valuable information than a single value at a single point in time.

Temperatures taken either axillary or rectally are common practices. The time required to obtain a stabilized reading using a digital thermometer is about 30-45 seconds at either site. Placement of the thermometer for axillary temperatures should be with the tip at the apex of the axilla midway between the anterior and posterior axillary borders. For rectal (not deep rectal) temperatures insert the thermometer gently to about 1 cm (May and Mahlmeister, 1994). Comparison studies show that temperatures taken rectally range between 0.1-0.3° C higher than those taken axillary. Results from both sites are about 0.2-0.5° C lower than core rectal temperatures. The advantage of using the axillary site is its' relative safety. Taking temperatures rectally has been associated with rectal perforation (Frank and Brown, 1978; Young, 1979).

There is no consensus as to what should be considered the normal temperature of a term healthy newborn. Studies of newborn thermoregulation most often focus on the newborn's response to extreme ambient conditions and seldom attempt to define what the normal range should be for clinical use. Mayfield and colleagues (1984) recommended core (deep rectal) temperatures between 36.5° C and 37.5° C as normal. The American Academy of Pediatrics Policy Statement of 1995 has set 36.1° C-37.0° C taken axillary as a discharge criteria (American Academy of

Pediatrics Committee on the Fetus and Newborn, 1995). Maternal fever (Takayama et al, 2000), birth weight (Takayama et al, 2000), bundling (Strothers et al, 1977), environmental temperature (CDC, 1988), and sleep state can alter (sometimes only temporarily) newborn temperature (Nako et al, 2000). For clinical use, interpreting trends over several hours rather than a single value in asymptomatic healthy newborns before instituting aggressive interventions such as septic work-ups seems prudent.

Bathing newborns within the first 24 hours of life continues to be common practice while daily bathing routines have been eliminated. Bathing to remove the blood and maternal body fluids is in keeping with universal precautions against blood borne pathogens such as hepatitis C and HIV (CDC, 1988). Proponents of no bathing cite preserving vernix for as long as possible because of reported infection protection properties, avoiding the disruption of mother-infant contact (which might adversely affect bonding and breast-feeding), and risk of hypothermia as their reasons. Bathing using a mild ph neutral soap or cleanser after the infant's temperature has reached 36.5°-36.8° C, followed by drying with a warm towel, results in very little change in temperatures (Nako et al, 2000). Babies do not need to be placed under radiant warmers routinely after their baths (Anderson et al, 1995). Having the mother give the first bath under supervision is an opportunity to teach this skill as well as encourage intimate touching by the mother and enhancing her attachment to her infant (Karl, 1999).

## Cord Care

Care of the umbilical cord is aimed at preventing or lowering the risk of omphalitis and sepsis. Cord care routines include simple cleaning, applying antiseptics, or antibiotics. The 1999 Cochrane review of randomized or quasi-randomized trials found no reported infections or deaths regardless of the method used (Zupan and Garner, 1999). The length of time to cord separation did vary. With cleaning only, the time to cord separation was about 8 days compared with 10 days after alcohol and 12 days with antibiotics (Zupan and Garner, 1999). One study found significantly higher maternal satisfaction with alcohol versus no care. Antibiotic use does lower the bacterial count significantly more and may be preferable to use under conditions when bacterial contamination of the cord might be higher such as out-of-hospital births (Zupan and Garner, 1999). Practitioners who choose to recommend no cleaning (Dore et al, 1998) at all should remember to advise the mother of the expected odor and unsightliness.

## Feeding

Breast-feeding is highly recommended for newborns. Few would dispute the Academy of Pediatrics statement in 1997 that "human milk is the preferred feeding for all infants, including premature and sick newborns with rare exceptions" (American Academy of Pediatrics, 1997). The benefits ascribed to breast milk include nutritional (Fomon, 1993), enhancement of bonding associated with early contact (Klaus, 1998), infection protection (Lawrence, 1994), diminished risk of serious atopic disease (Saarinen and Kajosaari, 1995), and economic (Weimer, 2001). Enhanced cognitive development has been suggested by some including a recent Norwegian study (Angelsen et al, 2001) finding of higher MDI scores at 13 months and higher WPPSI-R scores at 5 years of age with breast-feeding duration of 6 months compared with three months, despite correcting for signficant confounders such as maternal age, intelligence, and smoking. Lowered risk of chronic bowel disease may also be a benefit (Corrao et al, 1998). Regarding childhood cancer, a weak association with reduced risk was found by the UK Childhood Cancer Study Investigators which was a consistent trend in other smaller studies reviewed by the same group (Beral et al, 2001).

The protective effect of breast-feeding against sudden infant death syndrome (SIDS) is not as clear as was once thought from earlier studies. Sullivan's review of SIDS risk factors includes an analysis of several large studies from several countries. Although the two- to threefold decreased risk was a consistent finding among the studies, the magnitude of difference compared with bottle feeding lowers considerably when strong confounding factors such as maternal smoking, maternal age, and socio-economic levels were removed (Sullivan and Barlow, 2001). Nevertheless, even after rigorous analysis and care to remove the confounders, the association of breast-feeding with lowered risk for SIDS remains. Because breast-feeding moms tend to be nonsmoking, older age (i.e., non-adolescent), and of higher socio-economic level, breast-feeding may be a marker of lifestyle practices protective against SIDS. By promoting breast-feeding, practitioners potentially could introduce other healthy practices such as smoking cessation while encouraging more mothers to adopt "breast is best."

Earlier reports of decreased risk of insulin dependent diabetes mellitus (Gerstein, 1994; Mayer et al, 1998) have not been supported by more recent reports (Dahlquist and Mustonen, 2000; Jones et al, 1998; Norris et al, 1996). Jones and associates reported data from the Oxford Record Linkage Study of 311 diabetic children and found no association (Norris et al, 1996). The DAISY study in Colorado (Jones et al, 1998) as well as The Swedish Childhood Diabetes Study Group (Dahlquist and Mustonen, 2000) failed to find an association between breast-feeding and risk of developing diabetes.

Benefits of breast-feeding are not limited to the infant but extend to mothers by improving postpartum recovery, partial birth control, reduction in postmenopausal hip fractures, and reduced risk of ovarian and breast cancers. For these reasons and others, breast-feeding through the first six months of life and continuing at least until twelve months of life continues to be strongly recommended (American Academy of Pediatrics, 1997).

If such an ambitious recommendation is to be successfully accomplished, breast-feeding should be encouraged and supported prenatally, perinatally, and postnatally. The message should be consistent from physicians, nurses, dieticians, other health care providers, family, friends, the community, and the media. Current rates of both initiation of breast-feeding as well as continuation among mothers in the United States are disappointingly low. Ryan reported 1995 newborn breast-feeding rates (both exclusive as well as in combination with formula) of about 59%. By six months only 21.6% of mothers were still breast-feeding and many were supplementing feeds with formula (Ryan, 1997). By 2001 there has been only slight improvement with 64% of mothers initiating breast-feeding and 29% still breast-feeding at 6 months (Weimer, 2001).

The international community's interest in promoting breast-feeding worldwide comes as no surprise when the challenges of access to good nutritional sources, poverty, adequate sanitation, clean water sources, and infection control are prevalent and especially life-threatening to infants in developing countries. However, tangible benefits to developed countries, including the tremendous cost savings, justifies worldwide attention. Focusing on the United States, the U.S. Department of Agriculture issued its 2001 report analyzing the economic benefits if the Surgeon General's goal of early postpartum breast-feeding rates of 75% and 29% continuing at six months were achieved. This analysis only considered the reduction in incidence, medical care, and lost parental wages associated with three infectious diseases: otitis media, gastroenteritis, and premature deaths associated with necrotizing enterocolitis (Weimer, 2001). By the investigators' estimation, an impressive $3.6 billion per year would be saved. By inference, if the same analysis was applied to all the recognized benefits of breast-feeding the dollar amount would be staggering.

Recognizing the important role of newborn care providers and hospitals in the initiation of breast-feeding and that many hospital practices actually presented barriers to successful breast-feeding, the Baby-Friendly Hospital Initiative as an international approach was put forth. Presented in the 1989 joint statement by the World Health Organization (WHO) and United Nations Children's Fund (UNICEF), ten steps to successful breast-feeding were delineated (Joint WHO/UNICEF Statement, 1989). World recognition as a designated Baby-Friendly Hospital is given to those hospitals successfully completing the ten steps (Table 26–1). Accomplishing these ten steps requires cooperation between physicians, nurses, lactation specialists, hospital administration, and other key hospital departments.

**TABLE 26–1**

**Ten Steps to Successful Breast-feeding**

1. Have a written breast-feeding policy that is routinely communicated to all health-care staff.
2. Train all health-care staff in the skills necessary to implement the breast-feeding policy.
3. Inform all pregnant women about the benefits and management of breast-feeding.
4. Help mothers initiate breast-feeding soon after birth.
5. Show mothers how to breast-feed and how to maintain lactation even if they are separated from their babies.
6. Give newborn infants no food or drink other than breast milk, unless medically indicated.
7. Practice rooming-in, allowing mothers and infants to remain together 24 hours a day.
8. Encourage breast-feeding on demand.
9. Give no artificial teats or dummies to breast-feeding infants.
10. Foster the establishment of breast-feeding support groups and refer mothers to them on discharge from the hospital or clinic.

## Obstacles to Breast-Feeding

Obstacles to the establishment of breast-feeding include inadequate prenatal education and promotion, physician under-education and lack of support, cultural views, promotion of commercial formula, hospital practices, and lack of timely post-discharge follow-up (Weimer, 2001). Numerous studies have documented the lack of physician knowledge about breast-feeding. Two recent representative studies are those of Schanler and colleagues (1999) and Lee and associates (2000). Both studies involved surveying factual knowledge using a questionnaire which included clinical scenarios where physicians would be asked their advice regarding breast-feeding. Schanler in Texas found that whereas 65% of physicians recommended breast-feeding exclusively in the first month of life, only 37% followed the AAP guideline, recommending breast-feeding for the first twelve months. Many advised against breast-feeding for medical conditions known to be compatible with breast-feeding. Most were unaware of the Baby-Friendly Hospital Initiative. Nursing staff's lack of support for breast-feeding has been identified as influential in mothers' decision not to breast-feed. One study found a correlation between nurse attitude and behavior with their level of knowledge and personal experience. Those with more lactation knowledge and who had breastfed themselves were more likely to promote breast-feeding to their patients (Patton et al, 1996).

Cultural attitudes reflective of ethnicity, maternal age (adolescents), socio-economic level, and family have been identified as obstacles to successful breast-feeding. Forste and colleagues (2001) reported a strong relationship between race and the decision to breast-feed. In their analysis of data on 1088 women from the National Survey of Family Growth, they found that after correcting for confounders, African-American mothers were still 60% less likely to breast-feed as were non–African-American mothers. They went on to suggest that the gap in breast-feeding largely explains the higher rates of infant mortality and low birth weight among African-Americans. The reason given by these women for choosing not to breast-feed most often was "preferred to bottle-feed" without further elaboration. Adolescents' decision to breast-feed closely aligns that of peer and family influences and breast-feeding knowledge. Lizarraga and associates (1992) found a positive correlation between teens who had been breastfed themselves and their intent to breast-feed. A study comparing Japanese students in Japan with those in Michigan found that significantly more Japanese students perceived their mothers to have positive attitudes about breast-feeding as did the students themselves compared with the Michigan girls (Yeo et al, 1994). A study of African-American and Latina teen women by Hannon and colleagues (2000) identified fear of pain, embarrassment with public exposure, and unease with the act of breast-feeding, as well as concern for excessive attachment between mother and baby as reasons to not breast-feed.

Differences in socio-economic levels continue to be associated with differing rates of breast-feeding independent of race. Review of data presented in the Healthy People

2000 Final Review (National Center for Health Statistics, 2001) clearly illustrates the disparity between low-income women and those in higher income brackets despite targeted efforts to increase breast-feeding over the past ten years. Target goals for all women were 75% breast-feeding in the early postpartum period and 50% still breast-feeding by 6 months. Actual figures in 1999 showed 67% of mothers initiated breast-feeding and 31% were breast-feeding at 6 months. For low-income women, while progress was made, the comparable rates were 49% in the early postpartum period and 20% at 6 months. Possible reasons are suggested in two studies (Guttman and Zimmerman, 2000; Humphreys et al, 1998) and include lack of social support from peer groups, interference with working, breast-feeding experience, and perceived public disapproval.

Additional barriers to breast-feeding include parental educational level and knowledge about breast-feeding (Susin et al, 1999), partner's attitude (Arora et al, 2000), maternal employment (Gielen et al, 1991), commercial formula promotion (Henderson et al, 2000; Howard et al, 2000), and hospital practices (Perez-Escamilla et al, 1994; Snell et al, 1992; Zimmerman and Bernstein, 1996). Identifying obstacles to breast-feeding has resulted in multi-targeted approaches to the promotion of breast-feeding. Examples include the Baby-Friendly Hospital Initiative and its associated ten steps as discussed above. Studies have shown that even accomplishing some of the recommended changes results in demonstrable increases in breast-feeding rates in both the initiation and duration (Cattaneo and Buzzetti, 2001; DiGirolamo et al, 2001; Phillipp et al, 2001). Powers and colleagues (1994) reviewed 16 hospital practice changes friendly to the establishment and support of breast-feeding. These included educating and training of staff, allowing a close companion continuous access to the laboring mother, putting the baby to breast as soon after birth as possible (i.e., in the delivery room), rooming-in, encouraging frequent feedings, minimizing procedures that disrupt mother-infant closeness, discontinuing the dispensing of commercial gift packs containing formula, trained staff readily available to monitor progress and offer helpful instruction, and arranging for early post-discharge visits.

### Contraindications to Breast-Feeding

There are few conditions under which breast feeding would not be advisable because of the adverse effects on the infant. These include illegal drugs of abuse, maternal HIV infections, untreated maternal tuberculosis, and galactosemia (American Academy of Pediatrics, 1997; American Academy of Pediatrics, 2001; Mbori-Ngacha et al, 2001). Use of some medications may require temporary cessation of breast-feeding. In these situations, extra education and support should be given to the mother to reduce any anxiety regarding returning to breast-feeding when safety has been restored. These medications include cancer chemotherapy, radioactive isotopes, and antimetabolites. When maternal medications have been prescribed and there is not enough information to determine clearly the effects on the newborn, parents should be given the best available information to aid in their decision-making regarding breast-feeding. Smoking, while not a contraindication to breast-feeding should be discouraged. Around the time of the birth of a new baby, mothers who smoke may be receptive to smoking cessation interventions. It is appropriate to offer these interventions to women and to encourage the use of local resources to aid in stopping or at least decreasing cigarette use.

### Hepatitis C and Breast-Feeding

The current data are inconclusive regarding the clinical risk to the breast-feeding infant whose mother is infected with hepatitis C virus. Studies have recovered virus in samples of breast milk, however, no documented transmission has been reported. At this time the AAP recommends informing mothers of available information regarding the risk and support their decision to breast-feed or not (American Academy of Pediatrics, 1998; European Pediatric Hepatitis C Virus Network, 2001). Regardless of the breast-feeding decision, some pediatric hepatologists (for example, Rosenthal) advise PCR testing for hepatitis C virus be done shortly after birth and again between 9-12 months of life to assess the infant's infection status. PCR is recommended rather than antibody (ELISA) testing to avoid misinterpretation due to the presence of passively transferred maternal antibody.

The anatomy, physiology, and biochemistry relevant to lactation are well described in a textbook by Ruth A. Lawrence and will not be reviewed in this chapter (Lawrence, 1994).

### Bottle Feeding

For those infants whose mothers choose formula feeding, the standard 20 calorie per ounce, iron-fortified cow's milk based formulas are recommended (American Academy of Pediatrics, 1998). Feedings are usually begun within the first 4-6 hours of life after an initial sterile water feeding is given to test the integrity of the sucking and swallowing competency of the infant and to reduce the likelihood of formula aspiration into the lungs should a defect such as tracheo-esophageal fistula exist. The intake of term newborns on the first day of life, feeding and libitum, averages about 10-30 cc/kg/day and about twice this amount on day 2 (Dollberg et al, 2001). As the volume is considerably larger than the intake of breastfed newborns during the first 2 days, the percentage of weight loss of formula fed newborns is lower and may not reach the 7%-9% decrease from birth weight common with exclusive breast-feeding.

## Sleep Position

The importance of sleep position and the prevention of SIDS has clearly been demonstrated. Following the AAP's 1992 statement (American Academy of Pediatrics, 2000) strongly recommending supine sleeping position for infants, along with the "Back to Sleep" campaign, a greater than 40% reduction in the incidence of SIDS in the United States between 1992 and 1998 was achieved (American Academy of Pediatrics, 2000) Anticipatory guidance to educate parents and increase the likelihood of acceptance of this practice as routine should begin prenatally and continue throughout the postpartum hospital stay. Talking to parents, giving them appropriate informational material to read, as well as directing them to other informational sources such as the Newborn Channel (a 24-hour closed-circuit television channel on newborn care) are all helpful strategies (U.S. Public Health Service, 1994; Newborn Channel, *www.newborn.com/about.html*). Especially powerful is modeling behavior. Hospitals should examine their own sleep position practices and change to that of supine positioning (Braveman et al, 1995).

Parents should be instructed to avoid placing soft objects, pillows, or loose bedding under or in the infant's crib. If blankets are to be used, safe ways to wrap the infant to avoid obstructing the nose and mouth should be demonstrated. Education of staff may be needed to ensure consistency of complying with hospital policy. Special efforts to educate and address myths common in cultural groups with longstanding prone positioning practices may be necessary. African-Americans have been identified as one group where the acceptance of supine sleep positioning has lagged behind. SIDS rates for African-Americans, while lowered over the past ten years, remain disproportionately higher than for Caucasians (American Academy of Pediatrics, 2000). Special efforts to educate and encourage change in practice are clearly needed to reduce this continuing disparity.

## Anticipatory Guidance

The postpartum period presents an opportune time to begin anticipatory guidance. To avoid overloading the mother with information at a time when she is mentally and physically recovering from labor and delivery, trying to establish breast-feeding, and trying to connect with her new infant, staff and physicians should consider carefully and prioritize the information delivered. One approach might be to consider what the mother is most likely to encounter during the first 2-4 weeks (2 weeks if she appears especially inexperienced) at home with her infant. Easily readable handouts in the mother's primary language are helpful aids. Topics related to benign newborn skin findings, common behaviors such as snorting noises, sneezing hiccups, spitting-up, brief jerks while sleeping and facial grimaces, urate crystals, breast enlargement, pseudomenses, and crying responses are some examples. General care guidance should include bathing, appropriate clothing and how much, diapering, skin care, optimal environmental temperature, crib and bassinet use, care of circumcision site, and expected feeding, stooling, and voiding patterns. Family adjustment concerns should be addressed as well, especially sibling acceptance and housepets as well as postpartum depression or the "blues." Safety items might include proper sleeping surfaces, the pros and cons of co-bedding, passive exposure to smoking, safe carry-alls, and car seats. Warning signs of illness and how to respond should be reviewed (Table 26–2). Phone numbers and names of available resources should be provided.

## Discharge and Follow-up

The optimal length of hospital stay has not been determined (Braveman et al, 1995). Over the past two decades the average length of stay has decreased, initially driven by parents seeking to de-medicalize the birthing experience and finding the hospital's highly technical environment inconsistent with an experience that could include family members, individual comforting practices to be used during labor, and close contact with their infants. As labor, delivery, postpartum, and nursery practices responded to these requests, discharge timing became less driven by patient preferences and more driven by third party payor reimbursement policies. The medical backlash to early newborn discharge included reports of sentinel events such as kernicterus from extreme hyperbilirubinemia (Sola, 1995), inadequately established feedings resulting in readmission for severe dehydration and hypernatremia (Cooper et al, 1995), missed congenital heart defects (Kuehl et al, 1999), and general dissatisfaction by both the patients and doctors because of the interruption of the time honored practice of physician-directed timing of discharge. Federal and state legislation was passed modulating this behavior, requiring that minimal lengths of stays of 48 hours and 96 hours for uncomplicated vaginal and cesaerean section deliveries of healthy term infants be financially covered. The AAP policy statement issued in 1995 emphasized the need to time discharge according to the stability of the mother and infant. The statement details minimal medical and psychosocial criteria which should be met before consideration for discharge. The importance of specifying an identified and timely follow-up plan before discharge is emphasized (American Academy of Pediatrics, 1995). Table 26–3 summarizes these criteria.

**TABLE 26–2**

**Newborn Warning Signs of Illness for Parents**

- Refusal of feedings two or more times in a row. Breast-fed newborns generally feed every 2-3 hours and formula fed newborns feed every 3-4 hours
- Fewer than six wet diapers per day
- Fewer than two stools per day
- Difficulty waking baby for feedings (lethargy)
- Persistent difficulties with breast-feeding technique, such as inadequate latch, no let-down, inadequate suck/swallow pattern, and persistent pain with feedings
- Yellow coloring (jaundice) of the eyes or skin, especially if it extends to or beyond the belly button (umbilicus)
- Blue color or pale skin
- Repeated projectile vomiting
- Distended, tight abdomen
- Redness, swelling, or discharge from the eyes or umbilicus

## Car Seats

Promoting the safe and proper use of car seats can be appropriately addressed as a part of discharge teaching. Hospital policy might also include having trained hospital personnel observe and assist the parents in positioning the infant in the car seat and securing it properly in the vehicle prior to discharge. Infants are most safe if placed in a rear-facing seat installed in the back seat of the vehicle (American Academy of Pediatrics, 2002). Some hospitals support programs providing car seat purchasing and/or rental programs

**TABLE 26-3**

**Criteria for Newborn Discharge**

- Uncomplicated antepartum, intrapartum, and postpartum courses
- Vaginal delivery
- Singleton birth at term gestation and appropriate for gestational age
- Vital signs within normal ranges and stable for 12 hours before discharge
- Spontaneous voiding and stooling at least once
- Completion of two successful feedings
- Physical findings within normal ranges
- Circumcision site free of excessive bleeding for 2 hours
- Jaundice appropriately evaluated
- Mother demonstrating competency in providing adequate care for her baby
- Adequate support readily available to mother after discharge
- Laboratory data reviewed and screening tests performed
- Hepatitis B vaccine administered appropriate to the newborn's risk status
- Completion of hearing screening
- Identification of post-discharge continuing medical care
- Family, environmental, and social risk factors assessed
- Follow-up within 48 hours of discharge possible

for families who are unprepared at the time of discharge. The AAP recommends that parents purchase a car seat that meets federal safety standards, is the right size for the child, fits the vehicle's seats and seat belt systems, and is easy to use (American Academy of Pediatrics, 2002).

## COMMON PROBLEMS DURING NURSERY STAY

### Hyperthermia and Hypothermia

Elevated temperature in newborns can be the result of maternal fever present prior to delivery, excessive swaddling, environmental, hypermetabolic states such as drug withdrawal, dehydration, or true fever associated with infection. In an otherwise healthy infant, less than 3 days old, the first three of the previously mentioned causes are much more common than infection. Therefore, if the newborn is without other abnormal signs and symptoms, causes other than sepsis should be ruled out first.

Mild to moderate hypothermia is not uncommon during the first day or two after birth. Infants experiencing excessive heat loss feed poorly, act somewhat sluggish and may become hypoglycemic and develop metabolic acidosis. Causes of hypothermia include environmental, as well as sepsis or hypovolemia. The infant's internal response to cold stress depletes lipid substrates necessary to generate heat. Lack of feeding secondary to hypothermia then becomes a secondary cause of continuing hypothermia creating a cyclical pattern of cause and effect. The approach to hypothermia starts by determining the underlying cause, addressing the identified cause(s), followed by measures to rewarm the infant. Rewarming the otherwise healthy newborn can be effectively and easily accomplished by placing the infant skin-to-skin next to the mother and covering both with warm blankets. This method has the additional advantage of not disrupting mother-infant contact and encouraging feeding. Occasionally, placing the infant in a heated enclosed incubator unit or under a radiant warmer may be temporarily necessary.

Preventive measures aimed at reducing the thermal gradient known to promote heat loss from the infant to the environment are commonly incorporated into general hospital practices. Starting in the delivery room, newborns should be delivered into a dry warm towel and immediately wiped of surface fluids. Special attention should be directed to drying the head and face which together represent a large surface area from which evaporative heat loss can be significant. The initial drying can be followed by skin-to-skin swaddling against the mother or complete swaddling in dry warm blankets. Placing a cap on the head gives additional protection against excessive heat loss. Warming the room a few degrees is helpful, however the mother's comfort needs to be considered as well.

### Maternal Conditions Affecting the Baby

Maternal conditions such as chorioamnionitis, prenatal infections (HIV, GBS colonization), substance abuse, and diabetes, and other chronic immunologic diseases are examples of conditions that may affect the newborn. Maternal health should be reviewed as part of obtaining the medical history of the newborn. The approach to the infant varies with the specific condition, details of which can be found through this textbook. For the asymptomatic, healthy newborn, a determination should be made as to whether the condition is likely to be transferable to the infant and whether measures can be taken to prevent or lessen the likelihood of transmission as in the case of group B streptoccocus or HIV. Some conditions such as maternal substance abuse or diabetes have direct effects that may require treatment during the first few days of life.

### Abnormal Prenatal Ultrasounds

Prenatal ultrasonography has improved remarkably over the past decade, resulting in the detection of many findings at variance from normal. The dilemma for physicians is sorting out which findings are of clinical significance to the health of the newborn and requre intervention. Examples of sonographic findings associated with variable clinical outcomes include isolated abnormal or absent corpus callosum, small intracranial cysts, nonspecific dilation of the renal pelvices, isolated choroid plexus cysts, and echogenic cardiac foci (Maizels et al, 2002). The decision to obtain postnatal reimaging and other investigative studies depends on the presence of other sonographic abnormalities and/or abnormal postnatal physical examination. Subspecialty consultation may be helpful in determining further work-up.

### Breast-Feeding Problems

Common early problems are generally associated with the initiation of breast-feeding such as sleepy baby (disinterest), poor latch, sore nipples, pain with latching on, maternal anxiety regarding breast milk production and supply, and maternal breast engorgement. Much of the time, with proper management of the breast-feeding couple, many of these problems can be minimized or avoided altogether.

Creating a supportive environment is key to the successful establishment of breast-feeding. This would include allowing the mother ready access to her infant in the delivery room and facilitating breast-feeding at that time, should the infant show interest in nursing. Rooming-in should be encouraged so that the mother can readily respond to her infant's feeding cues. Nursing staff from all areas of the perinatal unit—labor and delivery, postpartum, and nursery—should be trained and experienced in the management of breast-feeding. The advice should be consistent and free from personal bias. Physicians as well should be knowledgeable regarding the science of breast-feeding, able to recognize problems, and understand the appropriate intervention approaches.

While a detailed discussion of the management of specific problems is beyond the scope of this chapter, there are important points that should be mentioned. The diagnosis of breast-feeding problems begins with an assessment of risk factors such as previous breast surgery, prolonged or difficult labor, cesarean section delivery, excessive maternal blood loss, or need for newborn resuscitation. Examination of the mother's breasts includes assessing the presence of engorgement, flat, inverted, or cracked nipples. Note mother's position for feeding. Is she sitting or reclining comfortably? Is the infant being held in a comfortable, supportive position with ready access and alignment to the breast? Direct observation of the latch, position of the infant's tongue, and quality of the suck and the pattern of suckling and swallowing are keys to proper diagnosis and intervention decisions. Lactation specialists can be especially helpful in developing a reasonable and appropriate management plan (Lawrence, 1994) While all newborns normally lose weight during the first few days of life, breastfed infants are at risk for excessive weight loss. By 72 hours after birth most breastfed newborns have generally lost about 7%-8% of their birthweight. Any newborn whose weight loss reaches 10% risks becoming dehydrated and should be carefully evaluated and monitored. In these instances short term supplementation many be required while continuing to work on establishing breast-feeding.

## Respiratory Problems

The normal respiratory rate of the fullterm newborn after transition is 35 to 60 breaths per minute. Tachypnea, one of the more common problems encountered in the newborn nursery may occur as an isolated finding or in combination with other signs of respiratory distress including nasal flaring, grunting, retractions, or cyanosis. The possible causes of tachypnea in the newborn range from benign conditions such as transient tachypnea of the newborn (TTNB) to more serious conditions such as primary pulmonary disease, sepsis, cardiac disease, metabolic problems, hypovolemia, anemia, polycythemia, and neurologic abnormalities. Identifying those infants needing aggressive intervention and transfer to a neonatal intensive care unit quickly requires using a reasoned approach combining assessment of maternal risk factors (e.g., GBS status, substance abuse), the labor and delivery experience (meconium, cesarean section, ashyxia, trauma, excessive blood loss), presence of additional findings on physical exam (e.g., respiratory distress, cardiovascular dysfunction, dysmorphic features), and a few key tests (blood gas, complete blood count, glucose, chest x-ray).

TTNB, thought to result primarily from retained fetal lung fluid, occurs in near-term and fullterm newborns following vaginal and cesarean section deliveries. The disorder, as described in 1966 by Avery and associates, presents typically shortly after birth (Avery et al, 1966). Tachypnea is often the only finding, however some infants may become more symptomatic with retractions, grunting respirations, and mild cyanosis. Chest radiographs characteristically show hyperaeration, pleural fluid, and prominent pulmonary vascular markings. The condition resolves by the third or fourth day. Management for many infants is limited to close observation. These babies generally are able to continue oral feedings. More symptomatic infants respond readily to oxygen supplementation and may require intravenous fluids to avoid hypoglycemia if the tachypnea prevents oral feedings.

## Cardiovascular Issues

Distinguishing the otherwise healthy newborn who is progressing normally through cardiovascular transition with an associated benign, transient murmur from the occasional newborn whose murmur is associated with a serious heart defect presents a common challenge for practitioners in the normal newborn nursery. The situation is further complicated if the mother is ready for discharge after a shortened hospital stay prior to completion of the major components of physiologic transition from fetal to neonatal circulation, which generally occurs over 2-3 days but may take as long as 7 days.

Further cardiac investigation is indicated if a murmur is found in association with other abnormal findings. The evaluation of newborns with murmurs includes taking note of maternal medications or drugs taken just before or during pregnancy. Infants whose family history is positive for first-degree relatives with congenital heart defects have a higher risk of also having congenital heart disease compared with those infants without a positive family history. The physical examination should focus on determining the presence of other anomalies and evidence of cardiac dysfunction such as tachypnea, tachycardia, cyanosis or pallor, absence of peripheral pulses, or poor perfusion. The reader is referred to Chapter 57 for a detailed discussion on the evaluation and management of cardiac disease.

## Voiding and Stooling

Delayed voiding or stooling is a common complaint during, however, the first void or stool is often missed and unrecorded because it may have happened shortly after birth in the delivery room, or a diaper may have been inadvertently discarded without being documented in the chart.

Ninety-five percent of newborns regardless of gestational age will spontaneously void for the first time by 24 hours of age (Clark, 1997). If a newborn has not voided by 48 hours, diagnostic investigation should be considered. Clues from the physical examination include palpable enlarged kidneys or enlarged bladder. The genitalia and lower back should be inspected for abnormalities as well as a carefully performed neurologic examination of the lower extremities, noting the anal "wink." Dysfunctional voiding may be a sign of a tethered spinal cord.

The first stool passed by newborns may be later than the first void, however most newborns will pass a meconium stool within the first 48 hours of life and certainly by 72 hours (Clark, 1997). Infants who have not spontaneously stooled by 72 hours should be assessed for any of the numerous obstructive causes. Retrieval of stool by artificial stimulation methods such as rectal insertion of a thermometer or suppository is discouraged as these maneuvers may delay the diagnosis of a serious condition.

## Jaundice

The important issues are to be aware of risk factors that may increase the likelihood of nonphysiologic hyperbilirubinemia. Those risk factors include siblings who required treatment for hyperbilirubinemia, maternal blood group type O, Rh negative or positive antibody screen, maternal diabetes, male gender, Asian race, preterm gestation, jaundice presenting in the first 24 hours of life, cephalohematoma or excessive bruising, and breast-feeding infants, especially those with excessive weight loss.

Reports of kernicterus associated with early hospital discharge and delay of recognition of significant jaundice (American Academy of Pediatrics Subcommittee on Neonatal Hyperbilirubinemia, 2001) have led to the development of predictive models based on the timing of an initial bilirubin prior to discharge (Bhutari et al, 1999). These models are intended to help the practitioner determine which infants should have repeated bilirubin determinations made or even a delay in discharge in order to avoid the development of extreme untreated hyperbilirubinemia. If a jaundiced infant has been cleared for discharge, follow-up within 24-48 hours should be arranged for further assessment and a possible redraw of bilirubin levels. Treatment guidelines are suggested by the AAP Task Force on Hyperbilirubinemia published in 1994 (American Academy of Pediatrics Provisional Committee for Quality Improvement and Subcommittee on Hyperbilirubinemia Practice Parameter, 1994).

## Family and Social Issues

Hospital policies should encourage the involvement of family and important support persons. This includes such practices as attendance during labor and delivery by the father or other support person and unrestricted postpartum visiting by family and friends. The provision of a professional support person such as a doula during labor, delivery, and immediately postpartum has been associated with fewer obstetric complications, greater breast-feeding success, and faster postpartum recovery. Allowances for sibling visitation have also become popular in many institutions. Guidelines addressing visitation by children are institution specific and generally focus on infection control as well as proper supervision of young siblings. Siblings should be free of contagious illnesses. Some guidelines require a brief screening by nursing. Visits should occur in the mother's room, limiting contact with non-sibling neonates. Siblings should be adequately supervised throughout their visits by a responsible adult other than the neonate's mother. The adult should be someone familiar to the visiting child and who can reliably monitor behavior, the child's handling of the neonate, and attend to the child's needs.

While the primary concern of hospital providers is caring for the mother and newborn in a supportive and medically safe hospital environment, the post-discharge environment should not be neglected. Determination of the adequacy of the home should address space, supplies and equipment, availability of support from family or friends, heating, telephone access, and other basic needs. Single, first-time mothers, and teenage mothers living on their own are especially vulnerable to inadequate support following hospital discharge. Lack of a supportive home environment is associated with mothers who are less likely to sustain successful breast-feeding and are at higher risk for postpartum depression and child abuse. The presence or likelihood of domestic violence should also be determined prior to discharge. When social challenges are identified, enlisting the help from the unit's social worker before discharge is recommended.

## REFERENCES


AAP Subcommittee on Neonatal Hyperbilirubinemia: Commentary: Neonatal jaundice and kernicterus. Pediatrics 108: 763-765, 2001.

Adler R, Ottaway MS, Gould S: Circumcision: We have heard from the experts; now let's hear from the parents. Pediatrics 107:E20, 2001.

American Academy of Pediatrics Committee on Fetus and Newborn: Routine evaluation of blood pressure, hematocrit, and glucose in newborns. Pediatrics 92:474-476, 1993.

American Academy of Pediatrics Vitamin K Ad Hoc Task Force: Controversies concerning vitamin K and the newborn. Pediatrics 91:1001-1003, 1993.

American Academy of Pediatrics, American College of Gynecologists and Obstetricians: Guidelines for Perinatal Care, 4th Edition: Elk Grove Village, IL, American Academy of Pediatrics, 1997.

American Academy of Pediatrics. Committee on Drugs: The transfer of drugs and other chemicals into human milk. Pediatrics 108:776-789, 2001.

American Academy of Pediatrics. Committee on Nutrition: Soy protein-based formulas: Recommendations for use in infant feeding. Pediatrics 101:148-153, 1998.

American College of Obstetricians and Gynecologists. Committee on Obstetric Practice: ACOG Committee Opinion. Circumcision. Number 260, October 2001. Obstet Gynecol 98:707-708, 2001.

Amir M, Raja MH, Niaz WA: Neonatal circumcision with Gomco clamp—a hospital-based retrospective study of 1000 cases. J Pak Med Assoc 50:224-227, 2000.

Anderson GC, et al: Axillary temperature in transitional newborn infants before and after tub bath. Appl Nurs Res 8: 123-128, 1995.
Angelsen NK, et al: Breastfeeding and cognitive development at age 1 and 5 years. Arch Dis Child 85:183-188, 2001.
Anisfeld E, Lipper E: Early contact, social support, and mother-infant bonding. Pediatrics 72:79-83, 1983.
Ansell P, Bull D, Roman E: Childhood leukaemia and intramuscular vitamin K: Findings from a case-control study. Br Med J 313:204-205, 1996.
Appelbaum A: Infant kidnapping: A tragic incident provokes a new HCFA response. J Healthc Prot Manage 17:80-88, 2000-01.
Arora S, et al: Major factors influencing breastfeeding rates: Mother's perception of father's attitudes and milk supply. Pediatrics 106:E67, 2000.
Avery ME, et al: Transient tachypnea of newborn: Possible delayed reabsorption of fluid at birth. Am J Dis Child 111:380, 1966.
Bell TA, et al: Randomized trial of silver nitrate, erythromycin, and no eye prophylaxis for the prevention of conjunctivitis among newborns not at risk for gonococcal ophthalmitis. Eye Prophylaxis Study Group. Pediatrics 92:755-760, 1993.
Beral V, et al: Breastfeeding and childhood cancer. Br J Cancer 85:1685-1694, 2001.
Bergstrom T, et al: Studies of urinary tract infections in infancy and childhood. XII: Eighty consecutive patients with neonatal infection. J Pediatr 80:858-866, 1972.
Bhutani VK, et al: Predictive ability of a predischarge hour-specific serum bilirubin for subsequent significant hyperbilirubinemia in healthy term and near-term newborns. Pediatrics 103:6-14, 1999.
Blass EM, Hoffmeyer LB: Sucrose as an analgesic for newborn infants. Pediatrics 87:215-218, 1991.
Bliss DP Jr, Healey PJ, Waldhausen JH: Necrotizing fasciitis after Plastibell circumcision. J Pediatr 131:459-462, 1997.
Bonacruz GL, et al: Survey of the definition and screening of neonatal hypoglycaemia in Australia. J Paediatr Child Health 32:299-301, 1996.
Boodman AG: Discharged too soon? Washington Post Health June 27, 1995.
Bor O, et al: Late hemorrhagic disease of the newborn. Pediatr Int 42:64-66, 2000.
Braveman P, et al: Early discharge of newborns and mothers: A critical review of the literature. Pediatrics 96:716-726, 1995.
Breastfeeding and the use of human milk. American Academy of Pediatrics. Work Group on Breastfeeding. Pediatrics 100: 1035-1039, 1997.
Brousson MA, Klein MC: Controversies surrounding the administration of vitamin K to newborns: A review. CMAJ 154: 307-315, 1996.
Butler-O'Hara M, LeMoine C, Guillet R: Analgesia for neonatal circumcision: A randomized controlled trial of EMLA cream versus dorsal penile nerve block. Pediatrics 101:E5, 1998.
Cattaneo A, Buzzetti R: Effect on rates of breastfeeding of training for the Baby Friendly Hospital Initiative. BMJ 323: 1358-1362, 2001.
Changing concepts of sudden infant death syndrome: Implications for infant sleeping environment and sleep position. American Academy of Pediatrics. Task Force on Infant Sleep Position and Sudden Infant Death Syndrome. Pediatrics 105:650-656, 2000.
Christakis DA, et al: A trade-off analysis of routine newborn circumcision. Pediatrics 105:246-249, 2000.
Circumcision policy statement. American Academy of Pediatrics. Task Force on Circumcision. Pediatrics 103:686-693, 1999.
Clark DA: Times of first void and first stool in 500 newborns. Pediatrics 60:457-459, 1977.
Clemens CJ, Davis SA: Minimizing false-positives in universal newborn hearing screening: A simple solution. Pediatrics 107:E29, 2001.
Committee on Fetus and Newborn. Hospital stay for healthy term newborns. American Academy of Pediatrics. Pediatrics 96:788-790, 1995.
Committee on Injury and Poison Prevention; American Academy of Pediatrics: Selecting and using the most appropriate car safety seats for growing children: Guidelines for counseling parents. Pediatrics 109:550-553, 2002.
Cooper WO, et al: Increased incidence of severe breastfeeding malnutrition and hypernatremia in a metropolitan area. Pediatrics 96:957-960, 1995.
Cornelissen M, et al: Prevention of vitamin K deficiency bleeding: Efficacy of different multiple oral dose schedules of vitamin K. Eur J Pediatr 156:126-130, 1997.
Corrao G, et al: Risk of inflammatory bowel disease attributable to smoking, oral contraception and breastfeeding in Italy: A nationwide case-control study. Cooperative Investigators of the Italian Group for the Study of the Colon and the Rectum (GISC). Int J Epidemiol 27:397-404, 1998.
Dahlquist G, Mustonen L: Analysis of 20 years of prospective registration of childhood onset diabetes time trends and birth cohort effects. Swedish Childhood Diabetes Study Group. Acta Paediatr 89:1231-1237, 2000.
DiGirolamo AM, et al: Maternity care practices: Implications for breastfeeding. Birth 28:94-100, 2001.
Dollberg S, et al: A comparison of intakes of breast-fed and bottle-fed during the first two days of life. J Am Coll Nutr 20:209-211, 2001.
Dore S, et al: Alcohol versus natural drying for newborn cord care. J Obstet Gynecol Neonatal Nurs 27:621-627, 1998.
Ekelund H, et al: Administration of vitamin K to newborn infants and childhood cancer. Br Med J 307:89-91, 1993.
Escobar GJ, et al: A randomized comparison of home visits and hospital-based group follow-up visits after early postpartum discharge. Pediatrics 108:719-724, 2001.
European Paediatric Hepatitis C Virus Network: Effects of mode of delivery and infant feeding on the risk of mother-to-child transmission of hepatitis C virus. BJOG 108:371-377, 2001.
Folsom RC, Diefendorf AO: Physiologic and behavioral approaches to pediatric hearing assessment. Pediatr Clin North Am 46:107-120, 1999.
Fomon SJ: Human milk and breastfeeding. In Fomon SJ: Nutrition of Normal Infants. St. Louis, Mosby-Year Book, 1993, pp 409-423.
Forste R, et al: The decision to breastfeed in the United States: Does race matter? Pediatrics 108:291-296, 2001.
Fortnum HM, et al: Prevalence of permanent childhood hearing impairment in the United Kingdom and implications for universal neonatal hearing screening: questionnaire based ascertainment study. Br Med J 323:536-540, 2001.
Frank JD, Brown S: Thermometers and rectal perforations in the neonate. Arch Dis Child 53:824-825, 1978.
Gee WF, Ansell JS: Neonatal circumcision: A ten-year overview, with comparison of the Gomco clamp and the Plastibell device. Pediatrics 58:824-827, 1976.
Gerstein HC: Cow's milk exposure and type I diabetes mellitus. Diabetes Care 17:13-19, 1994.
Gielen AC, et al: Maternal employment during the early postpartum period: Effects on initiation and continuation of breastfeeding. Pediatrics 87:298-305, 1991.
Golding J, et al: Childhood cancer, intramuscular vitamin K, and pethidine given during labour. Br Med J 305:341-346, 1992.
Guttman N, Zimmerman DR: Low-income mothers' views on breastfeeding. Soc Sci Med 50:1457-1473, 2000.
Hannon PR, et al: African-American and Latina adolescent mothers' infant feeding decisions and breastfeeding practices: A qualitative study. J Adolesc Heal 26:399-407, 2000.

Henderson L, et al: Representing infant feeding: Content analysis of British media portrayals of bottle feeding and breastfeeding. Br Med J 321:1196-1198, 2000.

Hepatitis C virus infection. American Academy of Pediatrics. Committee on Infectious Diseases. Pediatrics 101:481-485, 1998.

Herschel M, et al: Neonatal circumcision: Randomized trial of a sucrose pacifier for pain control. Arch Pediatr Adolesc Med 152:279-284, 1998.

Hey E: Prevention of vitamin K deficiency in newborns. Br J Haematol 106:255-256, 1999.

Howard C, et al: Office prenatal formula advertising and its effect on breastfeeding patterns. Obstet Gynecol 95:296-303, 2000.

Humphreys AS, et al: Intention to breastfeed in low-income pregnant women: The role of social support and previous experience. Birth 25:169-174, 1998.

Isenberg SJ, Apt L, Wood M: A controlled trial of povidone-iodine as prophylaxis against ophthalmia neonatorum. N Engl J Med 332:562-566, 1995.

Joint Committee on Infant Hearing, American Academy of Audiology, American Academy of Pediatrics, American Speech-Language-Hearing Association, and Directors of Speech and Hearing Programs in State Health and Welfare Agencies: Year 2000 position statement: principles and guidelines for early hearing detection and intervention programs. Pediatrics 106:798-817, 2000.

Jones ME, et al: Pre-natal and early life risk factors for childhood onset diabetes mellitus: A record linkage study. Int J Epidemiol 27:444-449, 1998.

Karl DJ: The interactive newborn bath. MCN Am J Matern Chil Nurs 24:280-286, 1999.

Kennell JH, Klaus MH: Bonding: recent observations that alter perinatal care. Pediatr Rev 19:4-12, 1998.

Klaus M: Mother and infant: Early emotional ties. Pediatrics 102:S1244-S1246, 1998.

Klebanoff MA, et al: The risk of childhood cancer after neonatal exposure to vitamin K. N Engl J Med 329:905-908, 1993.

Koh TH, Vong SK: Definition of neonatal hypoglycaemia: Is there a change? J Paediatr Child Health 32:302-305, 1996.

Kotagal UR, et al: Safety of early discharge for Medicaid newborns. JAMA 283:1150-1156, 1999.

Krohn MA, et al: The bacterial etiology of conjunctivitis in early infancy. Eye Prophylaxis Study Group. Am J Epidemiol 138:326-332, 1993.

Kuehl KS, et al: Failure to diagnose congenital heart disease in infancy. Pediatrics 103:743-747, 1999.

Lander J, et al: Comparison of ring block, dorsal penile nerve block, and topical anesthesia for neonatal circumcision: A randomized controlled trial. JAMA 278:2157-2162, 1997.

Lane PA, Hathaway WE: Vitamin K in infancy. J Pediatr 106:351-359, 1985.

Lawrence RA: Host-resistance factors and immunologic significance of human milk. In Breastfeeding: A Guide for the Medical Profession, 4th ed. St. Louis, Mosby-Year Book, 1994, pp 149-180, 215-273.

Learman LA: Neonatal circumcision: A dispassionate analysis. Clin Obstet Gynecol 42:849-859, 1999.

Lee A, et al: Choice of breastfeeding and physicians' advice: A cohort study to women receiving propylthiouracil. Pediatrics 106:27-30, 2000.

Lizarrage JL, et al: Psychosocial and economic factors associated with infant feeding intentions of adolescent mothers. J Adolesc Health 13:676-681, 1992.

Maizels M, et al: Fetal Anomalies: Ultrasound diagnosis and Postnatal Management. New York, Wiley-Liss, 2002.

May KA, Mahlmeister LR: Assessment of the neonate. In Maternal and Neonatal Nursing: Family-Centered Care. Philadelphia, JB Lippincott, 1994.

Mayer EJ, et al: Reduced risk of IDDM among breast-fed children. Diabetes 37:1625-1632, 1998.

Mayfield SR, et al: Temperature measurement in term and preterm neonates. J Pediatr 104:271-275, 1984.

Mbori-Ngacha D, et al: Morbidity and mortality in breastfed and formula-fed infants of HIV-1-infected women: A randomized clinical trial. JAMA 286:2413-2420, 2001.

McKinney PA, et al: Case-control study of childhood leukaemia and cancer in Scotland: Findings for neonatal intramuscular vitamin K. Br Med J 316:173-177, 1998.

McNinch AW, Tripp JH: Haemorrhagic disease of the newborn in the British Isles: Two year prospective study. Br Med J 303:1105-1109, 1991.

Miller RW: Vitamin K and childhood cancer. Br Med J 305:1016, 1992.

Moeller MP: Early intervention and language development in children who are deaf and hard of hearing. Pediatrics 106:E43, 2000.

Nako Y, et al: Effects of bathing immediately after birth on early neonatal adaptation and morbidity: A prospective randomized comparative study. Pediatr Int 42:517-534, 2000.

National Center for Health Statistics: Healthy People 2000 Final Review. Hyattsville, MD, Public Health Service, 2001, pp 211-212.

Newborn Channel. http://www.newborn.com/About.html.

Newman T, et al: Urine testing and urinary tract infections in febrile infants seen in office settings: The Pediatric Research in Office Settings Febrile Infant Study. Arch Pediatr Adolesc Med 156:44-54, 2002.

Newman TB. Circumcisions: Again. Pediatrics 108:522-524, 2001.

Norris JM, et al: Lack of association between early exposure to cow's milk protein and beta-cell autoimmunity. Diabetes Autoimmunity Study in the Young (DAISY). JAMA 276: 609-614, 1996.

Olsen JH, et al: Vitamin K regimens and incidence of childhood cancer in Denmark. Br Med J 308:895-896, 1994.

Paradise JL: Universal newborn hearing screening: Should we leap before we look? Pediatrics 103:670-672, 1999.

Parker L, et al: Neonatal vitamin K administration and childhood cancer in the north of England: Retrospective case-control study. Br Med J 316:189-193, 1998.

Passmore SJ, et al: Case-control studies of relation between childhood cancer and neonatal vitamin K administration. Br Med J 316:178-184, 1998.

Patel HI, et al: Genitourinary injuries in the newborn. J Pediatr Surg 36:235-239, 2001.

Patton CB, et al: Nurses' attitudes and behaviors that promote breastfeeding. J Hum Lact 12:111-115, 1996.

Perez-Escamilla R, et al: Infant feeding policies in maternity wards and their effect on breast-feeding success: An analytical overview. Am J Public Health 84:89-97, 1994.

Phillipp BL, et al: Baby-Friendly Hospital Initiative improves breastfeeding initiation rates in a US hospital setting. Pediatrics 108:677-681, 2001.

Popovic JR: 1999 National Hospital Discharge Survey: Annual summary with detailed diagnosis and procedure data. Vital Health Stat 13:44-49, 2001.

Powers NG, et al: Hospital policies: Crucial to breastfeeding success. Semin Perinatol 18:517-524, 1994.

Practice Parameter: Management of hyperbilirubinemia in the healthy term newborn. American Academy of Pediatrics, Provisional Committee for Quality Improvement and Subcommittee on Hyperbilirubinemia. Pediatrics 94:558-565, 1994.

Prodromidis M, et al: Mothers touching newborns: A comparison of rooming-in versus minimal contact. Birth 22:196-200, 1995.

Protecting, Promoting and Supporting Breast-Feeding: The Special Role of Maternity Services. Joint WHO/UNICEF Statement. Geneva, World Health Organization, 1989.

Quinn TC, et al: Viral load and heterosexual transmission of human immunodeficiency virus type 1. Rakai Project Study Group. N Engl J Med 342:921-929, 2000.

Rabun JB Jr, et al: Guidelines on preventing abduction of infants from the hospital. National Center for Missing and Exploited Children. J Healthc Prot Manage 8:36-49, 1992.

Renfrew MJ, Lang S, Woolridge MW: Early versus delayed initiation of breastfeeding. Cochrane Database Syst Rev (2): CD000043, 2000.

Righard L, Alade MO: Effect of delivery room routines on success of first breast-feed. Lancet 336:1105-1107, 1990.

Ryan AS: The resurgence of breastfeeding in the United States. Pediatrics 99:E12, 1997.

Saarinen UM, Kajosaari M: Breastfeeding as prophylaxis against atopic disease: Prospective follow-up study until 17 years old. Lancet 346:1065-1069, 1995.

Schanler RJ, et al: Pediatricians' practices and attitudes regarding breastfeeding promotion. Pediatrics 103:E35, 1999.

Schoen EJ, Fischell AA: Pain in neonatal circumcision. Clin Pediatr (Phila) 30:429-432, 1991.

Schubiger G, et al: Oral vitamin K1 prophylaxis for newborns with a new mixed-micellar preparation of phylloquinone: 3 years experience in Switzerland. Eur J Pediatr 158:599-602, 1999.

Secure Care Systems of Virginia: Kinderguard nursery security. Available on line at www.securecaresystemsofva.com/

Sinusas K, Gagliardi A: Initial management of breastfeeding. Am Fam Physician 64:981-988, 2001.

Snell BJ, et al: The association of formula samples given at hospital discharge with the early duration of breastfeeding. J Hum Lact 8:67-72, 1992.

Sola A: Changes in clinical practice and bilirubin encephalopathy in "healthy term newborns." Pediatr Res 37:145A, 1995.

Strimling BS: Partial amputation of glans penis during Mogen clamp circumcision. Pediatrics 97:906-907, 1996.

Strothers JK, et al: Thermal balance and sleep states in the newborn infant in a cool environment. J Physiol (Lond) 273:57, 1977.

Sullivan FM, Barlow SM: Review of risk factors for sudden infant death syndrome. Paediatr Perinat Epidemiol 15:144-200, 2001.

Susin LRO, et al: Does parental breastfeeding knowledge increase breastfeeding rates?. Birth 26:149-156, 1999.

Taddio A, et al: Effect of neonatal circumcision on pain response during subsequent routine vaccination. Lancet 349:599-603, 1997.

Takayama JL, et al: Body temperature of newborns: What is normal? Clin Pediatr (Phila) 39:503-510, 2000.

U.S. Public Health Service, American Academy of Pediatrics, SIDS Alliance, and Association of SIDS and Infant Mortality Programs: Back to Sleep (Parent Pamphlet). Washington, DC, 1994.

Update: Universal precautions for prevention of transmission of human immunodeficiency virus, hepatitis B virus, and other bloodborne pathogens in health-care settings. MMWR Morbid Mortal Wkly Rep 37:377-388, 1988.

von Kries R, et al: Vitamin K and childhood cancer: A population based case-control study in Lower Saxony, Germany. Br Med J 313:199-203, 1996.

von Kries R: Neonatal vitamin K prophylaxis: The Gordian knot still awaits untying. Br Med J 316:161-162, 1998.

Weimer J: The economic benefits of breastfeeding: A review and analysis. U. S. Department of Agriculture. Economic Research Service. ERS Food Assistance and Nutrition Research Report 13:1-20, 2001.

Wiley V, Carpenter K, Wilcken B: Newborn screening with tandem mass spectrometry: 12 months' experience in NSW Australia. Acta Paediatr Suppl 88:48-51, 1999.

Wiswell TE, Geschke DW: Risks from circumcision during the first month of life compared with those for uncircumcised boys. Pediatrics 83:1011-1015, 1989.

Woodside JR: Necrotizing fasciitis after neonatal circumcision. Am J Dis Child 134:301-302, 1980.

Yeo S, et al: Cultural views of breastfeeding among high-school female students in Japan and the United States: A survey. J Hum Lact 10:25-30, 1994.

Yoshinaga-Itano C, et al: Language of early- and later-identified children with hearing loss. Pediatrics 102:1161-1171, 1998.

Young DG: Thermometers and rectal perforations in the neonate. Arch Dis Child 54(3):242, 1979.

Zimmerman DR, Bernstein WR: Standing feeding orders in a well-baby nursery: "Water, water everywhere" J Hum Lact 12:189-192, 1996.

Zipursky A: Prevention of vitamin K deficiency bleeding in newborns. Br J Haematol 104:430-437, 1999.

Zupan J, Garner P: Topical umbilical cord care at birth (Cochrane Review). The Cochrane Library 1999, issue 2. Oxford: Update Software, 1999.

Zytkovicz TH, et al: Tandem mass spectrometric analysis for amino, organic, and fatty acid disorders in newborn dried blood spots: A two-year summary from the New England Newborn Screening Program. Clin Chem 47:1945-1955, 2001.

CHAPTER

# 27

# Newborn Screening

**Simone Albers and Harvey L. Levy**

Newborn screening is directed primarily at disorders in which the clinical complications develop postnatally. In metabolic diseases, these complications result from biochemical abnormalities that appear after birth, when the infant is no longer protected by fetal-maternal exchange. The infant with phenylketonuria (PKU), for instance, has a normal blood phenylalanine level at birth but within a few hours demonstrates hyperphenylalaninemia. If this and other biochemical abnormalities of PKU are not corrected or at least controlled by dietary treatment, the infant begins to show signs of developmental delay and, subsequently, becomes mentally retarded. If dietary therapy begins during the first weeks of life and the blood phenylalanine level is controlled, mental retardation is prevented (Levy and Cornier, 1994).

PKU was the first metabolic disorder known to benefit from dietary therapy. This fact was established by the mid-1950s. By the late 1950s, it was evident that the diet could prevent mental retardation if initiated in the neonatal period. Detecting PKU in all affected infants at that early age, before irreversible brain damage occurred, then became the challenge. This meant neonatal screening for a biochemical marker of the disease. In 1962, Guthrie developed a simple bacterial assay for phenylalanine that required only a small amount of whole blood soaked into filter paper (Guthrie and Susi, 1963). Thus, infants in newborn nurseries could be routinely tested for PKU in blood specimens obtained by lancing the heel and blotting the drops of blood onto a filter paper card. This filter paper blood specimen (Guthrie specimen) could be mailed to a central laboratory for PKU testing. An increased concentration of phenylalanine in the specimen indicated PKU in the infant.

By the mid-1960s, many states had established routine newborn screening programs for PKU using the Guthrie method. Infants with PKU were identified in larger numbers than anticipated and were showing normal development while receiving treatment (O'Flynn, 1992). The success of PKU screening led to the addition of tests for other metabolic diseases, including galactosemia, maple syrup disease (MSUD), and homocystinuria. These additional tests could be applied to the same blood specimen obtained for PKU screening. Later, a test for an endocrine disorder, congenital hypothyroidism, was added, followed by screening tests for sickle cell disease, congenital adrenal hyperplasia (CAH), biotinidase deficiency, cystic fibrosis, and others. Furthermore, urine soaked into filter paper was used to screen for neuroblastoma.

In 1990, tandem mass spectrometry (MS/MS) was first applied to the Guthrie specimen, opening a new era in newborn screening (Levy, 1998; Millington et al, 1990). The technology allows for the detection of more than 20 biochemical genetic disorders with a single assay of high specificity and an extremely low rate of false-positive results (Chace and Naylor, 1999) (Table 27–1). By the early 1990s, Naylor in Pittsburgh (Chace and Naylor, 1999) and Rashed and collaborators (1995) in Saudi Arabia were routinely screening neonates with this technology. Today, more and more state programs in the United States and screening programs in Europe and elsewhere have integrated MS/MS into newborn screening, thereby greatly expanding their possibilities for early detection of metabolic diseases in the newborn period (Levy and Albers, 2000). This single method is replacing the multiple procedures traditionally used by programs in screening for metabolic disorders.

Molecular testing (DNA) analysis has been another addition to newborn screening. As secondary or "second-tier" testing for diseases such as cystic fibrosis or medium-chain acyl–coenzyme A (CoA) dehydrogenase deficiency (MCADD), molecular testing substantially improves the positive predictive value of a primary screening result that is based on metabolite testing only (Ranieri et al, 1994; Wilcken et al, 1995; Ziadeh et al, 1995). The use of molecular testing for second-tier testing will most likely further expand with advances in DNA technology.

## SCREENING PROCEDURE

### Specimen

The blood specimen is obtained from the heel of the infant. This simple sampling method, conceived and introduced by Guthrie, has had an enormous effect on newborn screening. The specimen is not only easily obtained but also easily and inexpensively sent by mail to a central testing facility. There are no complications in obtaining the specimen from the newborn, contrary to early fears that its collection would lead to infection or result in excessive bleeding.

### Specimen Collection Procedure

The blood specimen should be obtained from the lateral or the medial side of the heel (Fig. 27–1). Blood should be applied to only one side of the filter paper card but should saturate each circle on the card. Contamination of the filter paper specimen with iodine, alcohol, petroleum jelly, stool, urine, milk, or a substance such as oil from the fingers can adversely affect the results of the screening tests. Also, exposure to heat and humidity can inactivate enzymes and produce false results. The specimen should be dried in air at room temperature for at least 3 hours before being placed in an envelope.

Specimens are sometimes collected in capillary tubes, by venipuncture of a dorsal vein or from a central line, and then spotted on filter paper. There is little or no substantial difference in analyte levels between blood collected

**TABLE 27-1**

**The Most Likely Disorders Identifiable in Expanded Newborn Screening**

| | |
|---|---|
| Amino acid disorders | Phenylketonuria (PKU) |
| | Homocystinuria and other hypermethioninemias |
| | Maple syrup urine disease (MSUD) |
| | Tyrosinemia |
| | Citrullinemia |
| | Argininosuccinic acidemia (ASA) |
| | Argininemia (arginase deficiency) |
| Organic acid disorders | Propionic acidemia (PPA) |
| | Methylmalonic acidemia (MMA) |
| | Isovaleric acidemia (IVA) |
| | Glutaric acidemia type I (GA I) |
| | β-Ketothiolase deficiency |
| | 3-Methylcrotonyl–coenzyme A (CoA) carboxylase (3-MCC) deficiency |
| | 3-Hydroxy-3-methylglutaryl (HMG)–CoA lyase deficiency |
| Fatty acid oxidation disorders | Medium-chain acyl-CoA dehydrogenase deficiency (MCADD) |
| | Short-chain acyl-CoA dehydrogenase deficiency (SCADD) |
| | Very-long-chain acyl-CoA dehydrogenase deficiency (VLCADD) |
| | Long-chain hydroxyacyl-CoA dehydrogenase deficiency (LCHADD) |
| | Carnitine deficiency |
| | Carnitine palmitoyltransferase II (CPT II) deficiency |
| | Glutaric acidemia type II (GA II) |

directly from the heel and that collected by any of these other methods (Lorey and Cunningham, 1994). However, there is the danger of introducing amino acids from total parental nutrition (TPN) solutions given through a central line into blood collected from this line, resulting in a false-positive increase in amino acids in the Guthrie specimen. In general, it is preferable that blood for screening be spotted on filter paper directly from the heel.

## Timing of the Collection

The specimen should be obtained from every newborn infant before nursery discharge or by the third day of life (whichever is first). With the practice of early nursery discharge, often during the first day of life, there is concern that some infants with metabolic disorders will not have ingested sufficient protein for an amino acid elevation to occur and, therefore, may not be identified. Lack of amino acid elevation is unlikely for severe forms of PKU but could occur in mild PKU and in disorders such as homocystinuria. In addition, because of maternally transferred thyroxine,

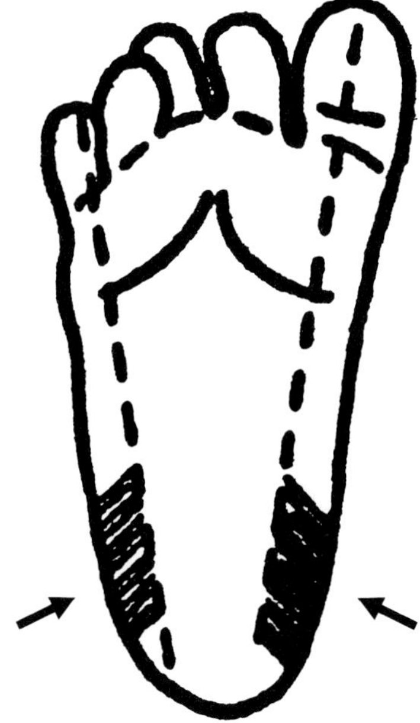

**FIGURE 27-1.** *Hatched areas* at medial and lateral sides of the heel in this drawing of the sole indicate the proper sites for heel-stick in the newborn.

testing of an early specimen could result in missing an infant with congenital hypothyroidism in programs that use a low thyroxine ($T_4$) level as the indicator of this disorder. Consequently, to be certain that an infant with a disorder is not missed, a second blood specimen should be obtained no later than 7 days of age from infants whose initial specimen was obtained within the first 24 hours of life.

Since the introduction of MS/MS, the reliability of newborn screening has considerably improved, even in very early specimens (Chace and Naylor, 1999). With MS/MS, PKU can be detected within the first 24 hours of life (Chace et al, 1998). Lowering the cutoff level for methionine in screening for homocystinuria, which MS/MS readily accommodates, is likely to enhance the reliability of early detection of this disorder (Peterschmitt et al, 1999).

Special circumstances require specific attention to newborn blood specimen collection. For *premature* or *very low birth weight* infants as well as infants who are sick, especially those in neonatal intensive care units (NICUs), additional specimens should be collected and submitted for rescreening for all disorders at 2 weeks of age or at discharge, whichever is earlier. Moreover, additional thyroid testing should be performed for these infants at 6 and 10 weeks of age or until they reach a 1500-g body weight.

In a newborn who is to receive *a blood transfusion*, a screening specimen should be collected before transfusion and a second specimen collected 2 days after the transfusion. In addition, a third screening specimen should be obtained 2 months after the transfusion, when most of the donor red blood cells (RBCs) have been replaced. This practice ensures reliable testing for analytes present in RBCs, if a pretransfusion specimen has not been obtained.

A blood specimen should be collected before transfer from any infant who is being *transferred* to a different hospital or to a NICU, regardless of age, and a second specimen collected at the receiving hospital by 4 days of age. This dual collection policy covers the infant from whom a newborn specimen might not have been obtained in the turmoil that frequently accompanies the transfer of neonates.

## Screening Laboratory

Newborn screening tests are usually performed in a centralized state, provincial, or regional laboratory. In a regional program, the specimens may be received by the state program and then delivered to the regional state or private laboratory, or they may be sent directly to the regional laboratory. In either case, the individual state programs serve as the state data and follow-up centers.

## Screening Tests

The testing procedure begins with the punching of small discs (each usually 3 mm in diameter) from the Guthrie specimen. In the bacterial assays for PKU and several other inborn errors of metabolism (galactosemia, homocystinuria, and MSUD), the discs are placed on agar or silica gels that contain bacteria, growth media, and other necessary factors. The constituents of each bacterial plate are specified for response to a particular metabolite, and the amount of bacterial growth around the disc is proportional to the concentration of the metabolite in the blood. In many newborn screening programs, the bacterial assays have been replaced by MS/MS, which allows for coverage of many inborn errors of metabolism (see Table 27–1) and offers many advantages over alternative methods of analysis.

Immunoassays, including radioimmunoassay (RIA), fluoroimmunoassay (FIA), and enzyme-linked immunosorbent assays (ELISA), are used to test for endocrinopathies such as congenital hypothyroidism and CAH, for infectious diseases such as congenital toxoplasmosis and human immunodeficiency virus (HIV) seropositivity, and for cystic fibrosis. Hemoglobin electrophoresis of blood eluted from the filter paper disc is employed for sickle cell disease screening. An enzyme assay is often used to screen for galactosemia and always used to screen for biotinidase deficiency.

## Secondary Tests

An abnormal finding on a newborn screening test is not diagnostic of a disorder. Abnormalities in the newborn specimen can be transient or artifactual. Accordingly, when an abnormality is identified, additional tests may be performed by the screening laboratory to substantiate the original finding. Also, the original specimen is retested for the analyte that was abnormal.

In screening for congenital hypothyroidism, the original newborn blood specimen in which a low $T_4$ level was found is further tested by immunoassay for an increased level of thyroid-stimulating hormone (TSH), which would indicate congenital hypothyroidism. A normal TSH level would suggest transient low $T_4$, a common finding in premature infants, or thyroxine-binding globulin (TBG) deficiency. Confirmation of PKU, galactosemia, or other inborn errors of metabolism requires additional specimens. Consequently, a second blood specimen (filter paper or plasma) and, on occasion, a urine specimen are necessary for specific testing when the newborn blood specimen suggests a disorder. Urine may also be valuable in confirmatory testing (e.g., organic acid and fatty acid oxidation disorders).

DNA analysis is now commonly used for the confirmation of disorders identified by newborn screening. The combination of gene amplification by the polymerase chain reaction (PCR) and either hybridization with specific oligonucleotide probes ("dot blotting") or analysis using restriction enzymes and band staining allows for the application of DNA analysis to the Guthrie specimen. DNA analysis is the second tier in cystic fibrosis screening (Wilcken et al, 1995). This two-tiered immunoreactive trypsinogen/DNA approach can identify up to 95% of patients with cystic fibrosis with a greatly increased specificity (Wilcken, 1993). Molecular testing for the prevalent A985G mutation in MCADD and the predominant E474Q mutation in long-chain 3-hydroxyacyl-CoA dehydrogenase deficiency (LCHADD), major metabolic causes of sudden infant death (SIDS), is performed as second-tier screening of specimens identified by MS/MS (Dobrowolski et al, 1999). Table 27–2 lists the disorders for which molecular testing is conducted and the corresponding second-tier mutations. It is likely that the use of molecular testing for second-tier screening will expand with advances in DNA technology.

**TABLE 27–2**

**Molecular Testing Performed as Second-Tier Newborn Screening**

| Disorder | Primary Analyte | Mutation(s) |
|---|---|---|
| Cystic fibrosis | Immunoreactive trypsinogen (IRT) | ΔF508, others |
| Medium-chain acyl-CoA dehydrogenase deficiency | Fatty acylcarnitine (C8) | A985G |
| Long-chain hydroxyacyl-CoA dehydrogenase deficiency | Fatty acylcarnitine (C16-OH) | E474Q |
| Galactosemia | Galactose, galactose-1-phosphate uridyltransferase (GALT) | Q188R, N314D |

### Physician Contact for Abnormal Results

Table 27–3 indicates disorders or other reasons for abnormal screening results and the initial evaluation required when the primary care physician (medical home) is contacted. For instance, a low $T_4$ level together with an elevated TSH concentration indicates congenital hypothyroidism. A specific markedly elevated level of phenylalanine, galactose, methionine, or leucine indicates, respectively, the probability of PKU, galactosemia, homocystinuria, or MSUD. A marked elevation of 17-hydroxyprogesterone (17-OHP) indicates the likelihood of CAH. An elevation of an acylcarnitine could point to an organic acid or fatty acid oxidation disorder.

Any infant for whom such a screening result is reported should be seen as soon as possible and evaluated with a careful history and physical examination. If the infant is ill or if the likely disorder requires immediate attention (see Table 27–3), a metabolic physician should be contacted; also, the baby should be admitted to a special care nursery, preferably in a center that has a pediatric metabolic unit with experience in the diagnosis and treatment of inborn errors of metabolism, where further evaluation and therapy for the illness can be initiated without delay. If the infant is active and alert with good feeding and shows no abnormal signs on initial evaluation, and the suspected disorder does not require immediate attention, a second filter paper blood specimen can be obtained and sent to the screening laboratory for repeat testing. If the second test confirms a disorder, the infant should be referred to a pediatric metabolic center.

Less striking abnormalities found by newborn screening are followed up with a letter sent to the physician from the screening program requesting another specimen. The physician should be notified of these results as soon as possible.

Most infants with a positive screening result, particularly when this result is only mildly or moderately abnormal, do not have a disorder (see later discussion of false-positive results). Transient or nonspecific abnormalities are quite common. Although all infants with an abnormal screening result must undergo repeat testing, the families should be informed that an initial positive result may have no medical implications. This approach can alleviate excessive anxiety and prevent unnecessary diagnostic procedures and treatment.

The physician should contact the screening laboratory when an infant has symptoms that suggest a metabolic disorder. The screening laboratory can check the results in the infant's newborn specimen. If the testing has been completed and the newborn specimens retained in storage, the laboratory may wish to recover the specimen and repeat the tests. The physician should also contact the screening laboratory for the results of repeat tests and inform the family of the results as soon as possible. If the second result is normal, the duration of family anxiety is thereby shortened.

## DISORDERS MOST COMMONLY SCREENED FOR

Following are brief summaries of the disorders most commonly screened for and detected by newborn screening. There is no attempt to describe any of the disorders in detail nor their very rare variants.

### Phenylketonuria

PKU is the paradigm for the disorders screened in the newborn. The cardinal screening feature is an increased level of phenylalanine. PKU should always be identified by newborn screening. If untreated, patients with PKU experience severe mental retardation and other neurologic abnormalities. The average incidence of the disorder is approximately 1 in 12,000 live births. With screening by MS/MS, PKU can reliably be identified as early as on the first day of life (Chace et al, 1998).

Not all infants with an elevation of phenylalanine have PKU. Mild elevations can indicate benign mild hyperphenylalaninemia. Liver disease, such as that associated with galactosemia or tyrosinemia I, can also produce increased phenylalanine. Therefore, treatment for PKU should never be given on the basis of a positive screening test result alone. The dietary therapy is complicated and can be hazardous to an infant who does not have PKU. If the screening test reveals a marked elevation of phenylalanine (≥6 mg/dl), the infant should be referred directly to a metabolic center for confirmatory testing and prompt consideration of dietary treatment. If the screening level of phenylalanine is only slightly increased (<6 mg/dl), a second specimen should be tested.

### Congenital Hypothyroidism

Congenital hypothyroidism is the most common disorder identified by routine newborn screening. It is found in 1 in 3000 to 5000 screened infants (Dussault, 1993). The major clinical features of untreated congenital hypothyroidism are growth retardation and delayed cognitive development leading to mental deficiency. If treatment with pharmacologic doses of thyroxine is initiated early, growth and mental development are normal.

Two screening approaches are used. One is primary screening for low $T_4$ with secondary screening for high TSH. The other is primary screening for high TSH. Either procedure reliably identifies congenital hypothyroidism. Nevertheless, in either approach, affected infants can be missed. This situation may be due to lack of the identifying marker. Specifically, the $T_4$ level during the first 24 hours of life in an affected infant might not yet be sufficiently decreased for identification due to persistence of maternally transmitted $T_4$. Moreover, in the premature infant with congenital hypothyroidism, it might take 2 weeks or more for a TSH elevation to develop.

The rate of false-positive results of screening for congenital hypothyroidism is approximately 0.04% to 0.5% (Table 27–4). Infants with false-positive results have transiently low $T_4$ or elevated TSH. Many of those with low $T_4$ are premature infants with a normal TSH concentration or infants with perinatal stress and elevated TSH. To avoid missing congenital hypothyroidism, screening programs require a second blood specimen from each of these infants. In addition to false-positive results, a low $T_4$ level with a normal TSH value can result from benign TBG deficiency (Dussault, 1993; Mandel et al, 1993) or hypothyroidism secondary to pituitary deficiency.

Infants with a positive screening test result should not be labeled as having congenital hypothyroidism or treated

**TABLE 27-3**

**Abnormal Newborn Screening Results: Possible Implications and Initial Evaluation Required**

| Newborn Screening Finding* | Differential Diagnosis | Initial Evaluation Required |
|---|---|---|
| **Medical emergency; immediate action required (admission to neonatal intensive care unit if infant is critically ill)** | | |
| ↑ Leucine | Maple syrup urine disease | Clinical evaluation, urinary ketone measurement, acid-base status determination, blood amino acid and urine organic acid measurements |
| ↑ 17-hydroxyprogesterone | Congenital adrenal hyperplasia, prematurity, low birth weight, stress in neonatal period, early specimen | Clinical evaluation including examination of genitals, serum electrolyte determination |
| ↑ Galactose (galactose-1-phosphate) | Galactosemia, liver disease, portosystemic shunt, transferase deficiency variant | Clinical evaluation, analysis of urine for reducing substances |
| ↑ Citrulline | Citrullinemia, argininosuccinic acid lyase deficiency | Clinical evaluation, blood ammonia and amino acid measurements, acid-base status determination |
| ↑ Arginine | Arginase deficiency | Clinical evaluation, blood ammonia and amino acid measurements, acid-base status determination |
| ↑ C3 (propionylcarnitine) | Propionic acidemia, methylmalonic acidemia | Clinical evaluation, urine organic acid and blood amino acid analysis, urinary ketone measurements, acid-base status determination |
| ↑ C5 (isovalerylcarnitine) | Isovaleric acidemia, antibiotic treatment of mother during delivery | Clinical evaluation, urine organic acid and ketone measurements, acid-base status determination |
| **Medical urgency; rapid but not immediate action required** | | |
| ↑ Phenylalanine | Phenylketonuria (PKU), non-PKU hyperphenylalaninemia, pterin defect | Second blood specimen for screening; if result is positive, send infant to metabolic center for urine pterins and dietary treatment |
| ↓ Thyroxine ($T_4$), ↑ thyroid-stimulating hormone (TSH) | Congenital hypothyroidism, iodine exposure | Second blood specimen for screening; if result is positive, send infant to endocrinologist for thyroxine treatment |
| ↑ C4 (butyrylcarnitine) | Short-chain acyl-CoA dehydrogenase deficiency (SCADD) | Second blood specimen for screening; avoid fasting >4 hr until diagnosis ruled out |
| ↑ C8 (octanoylcarnitine) | Medium-chain acyl-CoA dehydrogenase deficiency (MCADD) | Second blood specimen for screening and DNA analysis; avoid fasting >4 hr until diagnosis ruled out |
| ↑ C14:1 (tetradecanoylcarnitine) | Very-long-chain acyl-CoA dehydrogenase deficiency (VLCADD) | Second blood specimen for screening; avoid fasting >4 hr until diagnosis ruled out |
| ↑ C16OH (hydroxydecanoylcarnitine) | Long-chain hydroxyacyl-CoA dehydrogenase deficiency (LCHADD) | Second blood specimen for screening; avoid fasting >4 hr until diagnosis ruled out DNA analysis |
| ↑ C16 (palmitoylcarnitine), ↑ C18:1 (octadecanoylcarnitine) | Carnitine palmitoyltransferase (CPT) II deficiency | Second blood specimen for screening |
| ↑ C5OH (3-hydroxyisovalerylcarnitine) | Hydroxymethylglutaryl (HMG)-CoA lyase, β-ketothiolase, or 3-methylcrotonyl-CoA carboxylase deficiency | Second blood specimen for screening |
| ↑ Ornithine | Hyperammonemia-hyperornithinemia-homocitrullinemia (HHH) syndrome | Second blood specimen for screening |

**TABLE 27–3**

**Abnormal Newborn Screening Results: Possible Implications and Initial Evaluation Required—Cont'd**

| Newborn Screening Finding* | Differential Diagnosis | Initial Evaluation Required |
|---|---|---|
| Medical necessity; action required without urgency | | |
| ↑ Methionine | Homocystinuria, isolated hypermethioninemia, liver dysfunction, tyrosinemia type I | Second blood specimen for screening |
| ↑ Tyrosine | Tyrosinemia type I, II, or III, liver disease | Second blood specimen for screening |
| ↑ Trypsinogen | Cystic fibrosis, intestinal abnormalities, perinatal stress, trisomy 13 or 18, renal failure | Second blood specimen for repeat screening and DNA analysis; sweat test may be needed |
| ↓ Biotinidase | Biotinidase deficiency | Serum biotinidase assay |
| ↑ C5 (glutarylcarnitine) | Glutaric acidemia (GA) type I or II | Second blood specimen for screening |
| Presence of S-hemoglobin | Sickle cell disease, sickle cell trait | Hemoglobin electrophoresis |

*Every finding could also be transient or a false-positive result, especially if it is mild.

until testing of a second specimen confirms the disorder. This is especially true if the TSH concentration reported by the screening program is normal. If congenital hypothyroidism is confirmed, however, administration of thyroxine should be started without delay to prevent irreversible brain damage.

## Galactosemia

Galactosemia typically manifests in the neonatal period as failure to thrive, vomiting, and liver disease. Death from bacterial sepsis, usually due to *Escherichia coli*, occurs in a high percentage of untreated neonates (Levy et al, 1977). The average incidence of the disorder is 1 in 62,000.

Some screening programs use a metabolite assay for total galactose (galactose and galactose-1-phosphate) to detect galactosemia. Other programs screen the newborn specimen with a specific enzyme assay for activity of galactose-1-phosphate uridyltransferase (GALT), which is undetectable in severe galactosemia. The enzyme assay identifies only galactosemia, however, whereas the metabolite assay also identifies other galactose metabolic disorders, such as deficiencies of galactokinase and epimerase. Severe neonatal liver disease and portosystemic shunting due to anomalies in the portal system can also increase the galactose level.

**TABLE 27–4**

**Approximate Rates of False-Positive Results in Newborn Screening**

| Abnormal Analyte or Result | Disorder for Which Screening is Conducted | Rate of False-Positive Results (%) |
|---|---|---|
| 17-Hydroxyprogesterone | Congenital adrenal hyperplasia | 0.2-0.5 |
| Thyroxine/thyroid-stimulating hormone | Congenital hypothyroidism | 0.04-0.5 |
| Galactose or galactose-1-phosphate uridyltransferase | Galactosemia | 0.05-0.7 |
| Tyrosine | Tyrosinemia | 0.03 |
| Phenylalanine | Phenylketonuria | 0.03-0.1 |
| Leucine | Maple syrup urine disease | 0.05 |
| Methionine | Homocystinuria | 0.01-0.06 |
| Hemoglobins | Hemoglobinopathies | 0.03 |
| Biotinidase | Biotinidase deficiency | 0.05 |
| Immunoreactive trypsinogen/DNA analysis | Cystic fibrosis | 0.09 |
| C8 (octanoylcarnitine) | Medium-chain acyl-CoA dehydrogenase deficiency | 0.02 |

The most rapid confirmatory test for a positive result in galactosemia screening is urine testing for reducing substance. In almost all cases of severe galactosemia, this test produces a strongly positive reaction. Galactosemia with residual GALT activity, however, may be accompanied by a negative or only slightly positive result for urine reducing substance. If the urine contains reducing substance and the infant has clinical signs of galactosemia (e.g., poor feeding, jaundice, hepatomegaly), a blood specimen for confirmatory testing should be collected, and milk feeding (breast or formula) should be discontinued with substitution of a non-lactose formula such as soy or elemental. The infant should then be referred immediately to a pediatric metabolic center, where confirmatory testing should include the measurement of RBC galactose-1-phosphate and an enzyme assay for RBC GALT activity (Levy and Hammersen, 1978). Molecular testing for GALT mutations should also be performed (see Table 27–2). About 70% of the patients with galactosemia carry the Q188R mutation (Elsas and Lai, 1998). Variant galactosemia is produced by mutations such as S135L. The N314D mutation produces the benign Duarte variant.

If the urine test is negative for reducing substance, the newborn screening result is most likely to be false-positive or to indicate a benign GALT enzyme variant (e.g., Duarte variant). Nevertheless, urine reducing substance may be absent in infants with clinically significant variants of galactosemia. Consequently, screening should be repeated for all infants with an initial positive galactosemia screening result.

## Homocystinuria

Individuals with homocystinuria are clinically normal at birth but, if untreated, experience ectopia lentis (dislocation of the lens), thromboembolism, osteoporosis, mental retardation, or a combination of these problems. The worldwide frequency of all forms of homocystinuria has been estimated at about 1 in 344,000.

The newborn blood screening marker for detection of homocystinuria is an increased level of methionine. Infants with homocystinuria are missed, however, if the screening program does not include methionine in its list of measured analytes or because the blood methionine concentration was not elevated at the time the newborn specimen was collected (Whiteman et al, 1979). Reducing the cutoff value for methionine can substantially increase the frequency of identified infants (Peterschmitt et al, 1999). The introduction of MS/MS to newborn screening will most likely further improve the detection rates because it has a greater sensitivity for methionine than the bacterial assay. Moreover, because MS/MS measures methionine along with other amino acids (e.g., phenylalanine) without requiring a separate assay, many programs that formerly have not screened for homocystinuria will include the disorder (Chace et al, 1996).

A high methionine level by itself is not diagnostic of homocystinuria. Liver disease can produce a strikingly high methionine level, as can isolated hypermethioninemia (methionine-S-adenosyltransferase [MAT] I/III deficiency), a metabolic disorder that may be benign. Tyrosinemia type I (hereditary tyrosinemia) is usually associated with a high methionine level, most likely due to the liver disease. Furthermore, transient hypermethioninemia may occur in newborn infants. The initial action required when a methionine elevation is detected on newborn screening is submission of a second screening blood specimen. If the methionine level is increased in that specimen, the infant should be seen at a pediatric metabolic center, where quantitative amino acid analyses of plasma and urine should be performed. In the infant with homocystinuria, homocystine is usually detectable in plasma and urine, plasma total homocysteine is increased as is methionine, and cystine is reduced. In isolated hypermethioninemia, methionine is markedly increased in plasma, but there is no detectable homocystine in plasma or urine, and the plasma cystine concentration is normal. Hypermethioninemia secondary to liver disease or tyrosinemia type I is usually accompanied by increased tyrosine.

## Maple Syrup Urine Disease

The marker for MSUD is an increase in leucine in the newborn blood specimen. Newborns with classic MSUD almost always have at least a fourfold elevation of leucine. Transient increases in the blood leucine concentration are uncommon and are usually no more than twice the normal concentration. The average incidence of classic MSUD is 1 in 185,000.

MSUD can be a fulminant disease associated with severe ketoacidosis, vomiting, and lethargy and may rapidly progress to coma and death. Consequently, the finding of a substantially increased leucine level in the newborn blood specimen should prompt an immediate phone call from the screening program to the attending physician. If the infant is ill, he or she should be immediately transported to a NICU at a medical center with a metabolic specialist. Confirmatory plasma and urine specimens should be obtained, and emergency therapy initiated. Plasma amino acid analysis in the infant with MSUD will show marked increases in leucine, isoleucine, and valine (the branched-chain amino acids). The urine specimen will test strongly positive for ketones and will contain large quantities of the branched-chain ketoacids and amino acids. The characteristic odor reminiscent of maple syrup, which appears earliest in cerumen and only later in urine, will probably be detected on a cotton-tipped swab inserted in the infant's ear.

Milder variants of MSUD can be missed by newborn screening. The newborn with the *intermediate* variant may not have a blood leucine elevation or the increase may be so mild as to be below the cutoff value. In the *intermittent* variant, the blood leucine concentration is normal in the newborn period, becoming elevated only in later infancy or childhood during acute metabolic episodes precipitated by febrile illness or surgery.

## Congenital Adrenal Hyperplasia

A decidedly increased level of 17-OHP suggests CAH due to 21-hydroxylase deficiency. Infants with the salt-losing form of CAH can rapidly become hyperkalemic and die precipitously, often without a specific diagnosis. The clinical diagnosis may be suspected in the newborn girl because of ambiguous genitalia. However, the diagnosis is usually unsuspected in boys and in girls with atypical forms of CAH in which ambiguous genitalia may not occur. Even infant girls with ambiguous genitalia may be unrecognized as having CAH if the ambiguity is not obvious, or may be misassigned as boys, if the ambiguity is advanced. Because accurate gender assignment and initiation of hormone therapy as soon as possible are critical to a favorable prognosis in CAH, newborn screening is important in leading to early diagnosis and prompt therapy with pharmacologic doses of hydrocortisone. Consequently, testing for CAH has been incorporated into routine newborn screening in a number of programs in North America, Europe, and Asia (Pang and Clark, 1993).

Unfortunately, false-positive results in newborn screening for CAH are relatively common, the rate often as high as 0.5% (see Table 27–4). The finding may be truly increased 17-OHP such as in perinatal stress and early specimen collection (within the first 24 hours of life), or due to cross-reacting steroids, such as in prematurity and low birth weight (al Saedi et al, 1996). Cross-reacting steroids are produced by residual fetal adrenal cortex or result from decreased metabolic clearance by an immature liver.

A second blood specimen is required from any infant found on screening to have increased 17-OHP. If the infant shows signs of illness or has ambiguous genitalia, serum electrolytes should be measured. If these results indicate hyponatremia and hyperkalemia, the infant should be hospitalized without delay, and the electrolyte imbalance should be corrected immediately. Pediatric endocrinology consultation should also be sought.

### Biotinidase Deficiency

Biotin recycling is necessary for the maintenance of sufficient intracellular biotin to activate carboxylase enzymes. Biotinidase is a key enzyme in biotin recycling. Lack of biotinidase activity results in reduced carboxylase activities and an organic acid disorder known as multiple carboxylase deficiency (Wolf and Heard, 1991). The clinical features of the disorder are developmental delay, seizures, hearing loss, alopecia, and dermatitis. The developmental delay and seizures usually manifest at 3 to 4 months of age. Death during infancy has also been reported.

The initiation of biotin therapy in early infancy, when the disorder is presymptomatic, prevents all of the features of biotinidase deficiency. For this reason, a screening test has been developed and added to newborn screening in a number of newborn screening programs throughout the world (Hart et al, 1992). The frequency of identified newborns in these programs has a wide range, from 1 in 30,000 to 235,000. The average frequency is about 1 in 70,000. Almost all identified infants have been asymptomatic and have remained normal with biotin treatment.

### Sickle Cell Disease

In most newborn screening programs in the United States, the blood specimen is routinely tested for hemoglobin abnormalities. The major goal of this testing is to identify infants with sickle cell disease so that they can be given penicillin prophylaxis to prevent pneumococcal septicemia. Additional benefits of early detection are early referral to a comprehensive sickle cell program and early education and genetic counseling for parents (Smith and Kinney, 1993). Unfortunately, the long-term complications are not yet preventable.

Sickle cell screening is usually performed by means of hemoglobin electrophoresis of blood eluted from a disc of the Guthrie specimen. This procedure identifies not only sickle cell disease but also sickle cell trait and several other abnormal hemoglobins. Other than sickle cell disease, most of these abnormalities are benign. The finding of a hemoglobin abnormality on screening must be followed by confirmatory testing. This is especially critical in differentiating the common and benign sickle cell trait from the much rarer sickle cell disease (homozygosity for S hemoglobin). For instance, sickle cell disease affects approximately 1 in 600 African-American persons, whereas sickle cell trait (carrier status for S hemoglobin) is present in 1 in 12. Infants with sickle cell trait do not have complications and should not be stigmatized as having sickle cell disease.

When sickle cell disease is confirmed, penicillin prophylaxis should be initiated as soon as possible, and the infant referred to a sickle cell disease center or hematologist. The combination of screening and careful follow-up has been very effective in preventing pneumococcal sepsis in infants with sickle cell disease.

## OTHER DISORDERS DETECTED BY NEWBORN SCREENING

### Amino Acid Disorders

In addition to the amino acid disorders traditionally detected in newborn screening (PKU, MSUD, and homocystinuria), three disorders of the urea cycle as well as the tyrosinemias can be identified by expanded screening using MS/MS technology. These disorders are listed in Table 27–1.

The urea cycle disorders manifest as episodes of hyperammonemia, often in the neonatal period, producing poor feeding, tachypnea, lethargy, and vomiting. Respiratory alkalosis is characteristic. The clinical picture of presentation after the newborn period is very like that of Reye syndrome. Severe hyperammonemia in the newborn is a medical emergency and should trigger prompt consultation with a metabolic specialist or referral to a NICU at a metabolic center. Discontinuation of protein and provision of intravenous fluids with very high caloric content are the first steps to take. Administration of L-arginine or L-citrulline, sodium phenylbutyrate, and sodium benzoate, as well as hemodialysis, are required to control the neurotoxic hyperammonemia, which can lead to irreversible brain damage, coma, and death. It is hoped that with early identification through newborn screening, patients with urea cycle disorders will be protected through presymptomatic therapy in the neonatal period.

Tyrosinemia type I is an amino acid disorder that may be diagnosed through an elevation of tyrosine on the MS/MS profile. This disorder leads to liver and renal tubular disease and can later result in hepatocellular carcinoma. It is treated with administration of NTBC (2-nitro-4-trifluoro-methylbenzoyl-1,3-cyclohexanedione) and a diet low in phenylalanine and tyrosine. Unfortunately, moderate elevations of tyrosine that are transient occur frequently in neonates, especially those who have low birth weights and are sick, necessitating a cutoff value for tyrosine that is higher than the level in many neonates with tyrosinemia type I. Consequently, the newborn detection of tyrosinemia type I by a tyrosine marker is problematic. Tyrosinemia type II, which can result in mental retardation, painful hyperkeratoses, and keratoconjunctivitis, and tyrosinemia type III, which possibly causes cognitive loss, may also be detected by expanded newborn screening.

## Medium-Chain Acyl-CoA Dehydrogenase Deficiency and Other Fatty Acid Oxidation Disorders

The fatty acid oxidation disorders can be identified in programs that have adopted MS/MS technology. These disorders include those in which the long-chain fatty acids cannot traverse the mitochondrial membranes to be oxidized within the mitochondrial matrix and those that constitute defects in fatty acid oxidation per se. In either category, the problem is the inability to fully oxidize fatty acids. Fatty acid oxidation is essential to supply energy as adenosine triphosphate (ATP) via the Krebs cycle and as ketones in the presence of a low supply of glucose. The disorders involving defective *transport* concern carnitine, where those with defective *oxidation* are named according to the enzyme that is deficient (see Table 27–1). The clinical consequence of these disorders is fasting intolerance resulting in hypoketotic hypoglycemia, lethargy, hyperammonemia, metabolic acidosis, hepatomegaly and, not uncommonly, sudden death. Cardiomyopathy and developmental delay are additional features of very-long-chain acyl-CoA dehydrogenase deficiency (VLCADD) and LCHADD. Each fatty acid disorder is associated with a specific or almost specific acylcarnitine pattern on MS/MS analysis.

The most common fatty acid oxidation disorder is MCADD. Tragically, this disorder has often been diagnosed only retrospectively after a sudden unexplained death, usually when postmortem examination disclosed a fatty liver. This devastating outcome and a frequency of 1 in 15,000 to 20,000 (Zytkovicz et al, 2001), comparable with that of PKU, has made MCADD the primary reason for the addition of MS/MS technology to newborn screening. To reduce the rate of false-positive results in screening for MCADD, some programs have added molecular testing of the A985G MCADD mutation as second-tier screening. Because this mutation occurs in as many as 90% of persons with MCADD, this additional analysis of a newborn blood specimen with an elevation of the octanoylcarnitine (C8) marker for MCADD substantially improves the predictive value of the screening abnormality (Zytkovicz et al, 2001).

The most important treatment for fatty acid oxidation disorders in general is avoidance of fasting with frequent high-carbohydrate, low-fat feedings. Some centers also include carnitine supplements. Any infant diagnosed with a fatty acid oxidation disorder should be evaluated at a metabolic center. Most of these disorders are treatable, but even when early treatment may not be effective, such as in neonatal carnitine palmitoyltransferase II (CPT II) deficiency, screening enables early diagnosis and genetic counseling of the family (Albers et al, 2001a).

## Organic Acid Disorders

Organic acid disorders are a heterogenous group of disorders with a combined frequency of approximately 1 in 50,000 (Zytkovicz et al, 2001). Many of them can now be identified through MS/MS screening (see Table 27–1). The marker for this disease group, as for the fatty acid oxidation disorders, is an abnormal acylcarnitine pattern (see Table 27–3). If a screening result suggests an organic acidemia, a metabolic specialist should be consulted immediately.

Any of the organic acidemias can manifest in the neonatal period as a life-threatening, sepsis-like picture of feeding difficulties, lethargy, vomiting, and seizures. Metabolic acidosis virtually always accompanies this presentation, and hyperammonemia is common. In this situation, protein administration should be discontinued and replaced by administration of intravenous fluids with very high caloric content and carnitine. The hyperammonemia rarely requires specific treatment.

The effects of early diagnosis and treatment on the clinical and neurologic development of individuals affected by an organic acid disorder are currently under investigation (Albers et al, 2001b).

## Cystic Fibrosis

The frequency (1 in 2000 to 3000) and severity of cystic fibrosis explain its inclusion in routine newborn screening. As with sickle cell disease, therapy that can prevent the ultimate complications of cystic fibrosis is not yet available. However, early and usually presymptomatic diagnosis through screening leads to early nutritional therapy, pancreatic enzyme replacement, and antibiotic prophylaxis for pulmonary infection. Data from newborn screening suggests better growth in children identified by screening (Farrell et al, 2001). Other benefits of newborn screening are identifying the parents' genetic potential for producing additional children with cystic fibrosis and, through presymptomatic identification, allowing the family to avoid months or years of delay in the correct diagnosis of a child with chronic respiratory problems or poor growth (Farrell and Mischler, 1992; Wilcken, 1993).

The analyte marker in newborn screening for cystic fibrosis is increased immunoreactive trypsinogen (IRT). Transient increases in IRT are common in normal newborns as a result of perinatal stress or for unknown reasons. Consequently, the rate of false-positive results in cystic fibrosis screening is relatively high (see Table 27–4). To reduce this rate, screening programs have adopted a second-tier DNA analysis for one or more of the cystic fibrosis mutations when the specimen has increased IRT (Ferec et al, 1995). Despite this expanded approach to screening detection, a substantial number of infants who do not have cystic fibrosis must undergo a sweat test before the diagnosis can be eliminated. The high false-positive rate and the need for this somewhat complicated follow-up test have inhibited most programs from adopting screening for cystic fibrosis.

Gene therapy for cystic fibrosis has been intensively investigated. If gene therapy becomes available, advocacy for cystic fibrosis screening would greatly increase, because screening would then enable potentially curative treatment before the onset of irreversible pulmonary damage.

### Neuroblastoma

Neuroblastoma is the most common solid tumor of childhood, accounting for a significant number of deaths in preschool children. It is characterized by the excretion of increased vanillylmandelic acid (VMA) and homovanillic acid (HVA). In Japan and in some European programs, screening for neuroblastoma is conducted on filter paper urine specimens collected when infants are 6 months old. VMA and HVA are measured by high-performance liquid chromatography on urine eluted from the paper (Sawada, 1992). In a large, externally controlled study conducted in Quebec, filter paper urine specimens collected at 3 weeks and again at 6 months of age were screened for VMA and HVA by thin-layer chromatography with confirmatory follow-up by gas chromatography–mass spectrometry. The results indicated that screening does not reduce mortality from neuroblastoma. Notably, in almost all of the affected children with poor-prognosis neuroblastoma, screening results were falsely negative, the children being subsequently diagnosed clinically; in contrast, most of the infants identified by screening as having the disease had good-prognosis neuroblastoma, which either spontaneously regresses or can be effectively treated after clinical detection (Woods et al, 2003). Consequently, screening for neuroblastoma seems to be unnecessary and counterproductive, causing inappropriate anxiety and intervention.

## SPECIFIC ISSUES IN NEWBORN SCREENING

### False-Positive Results

The majority of positive results in newborn screening are not due to metabolic or any other disease. Table 27–4 lists the approximate rates of false-positive results for the most important inborn errors of metabolism. The rates are highest when the indicator is an abnormal metabolite level, such as thyroxine in congenital hypothyroidism, 17-OHP in CAH, or galactose in galactosemia. False-positivity rates are also high when the indicator is low activity of an enzyme, such as GALT in galactosemia. When the gene product can be directly examined, as for the hemoglobinopathies, the rate of false-positive results is low.

False-positive results are more common in preterm and low-birth-weight infants than in full-term babies. For example, up to 85% of preterm babies have transiently low thyroxine levels (Paul et al, 1998). Transient increases in 17-OHP are another common abnormality in infants who are preterm or have low birth weights or have experienced perinatal stress (Pang and Shook, 1997). Finally, transient tyrosinemia is commonly observed in preterm and low-birth-weight babies, although it can also occur in full-term infants (Levy et al, 1969).

Artifacts produced in the collection or transport of the Guthrie specimen account for some false-positive results. As mentioned in the discussion of the specimen collection procedure, collection of the specimen from a central line can result in mixing with amino acids in TPN solution and a false increase of amino acids in the specimen. Contamination with milk (or coffee containing milk) can result in a false elevation in the bacterial assay result for galactose and the mistaken suspicion of galactosemia. Prolonged exposure to heat can reduce the activity of GALT in the specimen and also produce a false impression of galactosemia when the Beutler spot enzyme assay is used to screen for this disorder; this error is common during the summer, especially when the specimens remain in a mailbox for a period of time.

With the expansion of molecular testing as second-tier screening, which is now commonly performed for cystic fibrosis and galactosemia, and the substitution of MS/MS for the traditional bacterial or specific assays, such as those for PKU and MSUD, the number of false-positive results will most likely be significantly reduced (Chace and Naylor, 1999). Nevertheless, false-positive results cannot be entirely eliminated, in particular among high-risk infants in NICUs. Therefore, it is important to reassure the parents that not every abnormal result of newborn screening inevitably implies a disorder.

### Missed Cases

Infants with PKU, congenital hypothyroidism, and other screened disorders have been missed in newborn screening. Laboratory or program error is the usual cause of these missed cases (Holtzman et al, 1974). In some instances, a specimen was never collected, particularly for an infant who was transferred to another hospital. In other instances, mistakes occurred because the laboratory was not properly supervised. Thus, physicians must exercise clinical judgment and not fall into the trap of excluding a diagnosis because an infant has presumably been screened. Specific testing for metabolic and endocrine disorders should be performed in any infant or child with symptoms that suggest the presence of such a disorder, regardless of the assumed or actual newborn screening result.

## REFERENCES

al Saedi S, Dean H, Dent W, et al: Screening for congenital adrenal hyperplasia: The Delfia Screening Test overestimates serum 17-hydroxyprogesterone in preterm infants. Pediatrics 97:100-102, 1996

Albers S, Marsden D, Quackenbush E, et al: Detection of neonatal carnitine palmitoyltransferase II deficiency by expanded newborn screening with tandem mass spectrometry. Pediatrics 107:E103, 2001a.

Albers S, Waisbren SE, Ampola MG, et al: New England Consortium: A model for medical evaluation of expanded newborn screening with tandem mass spectrometry. J Inherit Metab Dis 24:303-304, 2001b.

Chace D, Naylor E: Expansion of newborn screening programs using automated tandem mass spectrometry. Ment Retard Dev Disabil Res Rev 5:150-154, 1999.

Chace DH, Millington DS, Terada N, et al: Rapid diagnosis of phenylketonuria by quantitative analysis for phenylalanine and tyrosine in neonatal blood spots by tandem mass spectrometry. Clin Chem 39:66-71, 1993.

Chace DH, Hillman SL, Millington DS, et al: Rapid diagnosis of homocystinuria and other hypermethioninemias from newborns' blood spots by tandem mass spectrometry. Clin Chem 42:349-355, 1996.

Chace DH, Sherwin JE, Hillman SL, et al: Use of phenylalanine-to-tyrosine ratio determined by tandem mass spectrometry to improve newborn screening for phenylketonuria of early discharge specimens collected in the first 24 hours. Clin Chem 44:2405-2409, 1998.

Dobrowolski SF, Banas RA, Naylor EW, et al: DNA microarray technology for neonatal screening. Acta Paediatr Suppl 88:61-64, 1999.

Dussault JH: Neonatal screening for congenital hypothyroidism. Clin Lab Med 13:645-652, 1993.

Elsas LJ, Lai K: The molecular biology of galactosemia. Genet Med 1:40-48, 1998.

Farrell PM, Mischler EH: Newborn screening for cystic fibrosis. The Cystic Fibrosis Neonatal Screening Study Group. Adv Pediatr 39:35-70, 1992.

Farrell PM, Kosorok MR, Rock MJ, et al: Early diagnosis of cystic fibrosis through neonatal screening prevents severe malnutrition and improves long-term growth. Wisconsin Cystic Fibrosis Neonatal Screening Study Group. Pediatrics 107:1-13, 2001.

Ferec C, Verlingue C, Parent P, et al: Neonatal screening for cystic fibrosis: Result of a pilot study using both immunoreactive trypsinogen and cystic fibrosis gene mutation analyses. Hum Genet 96:542-548, 1995.

Guthrie R, Susi A: A simple phenylalanine method for detecting phenylketonuria in large populations of newborn infants. Pediatrics 32:338-343, 1963.

Hart PS, Barnstein BO, Secor McVoy JR, et al: Comparison of profound biotinidase deficiency in children ascertained clinically and by newborn screening using a simple method of accurately determining residual biotinidase activity. Biochem Med Metab Biol 48:41-55, 1992.

Holtzman NA, Mellits ED, Kallman CH: Neonatal screening for phenylketonuria. II: Age dependence of initial phenylalanine in infants with PKU. Pediatrics 53:353-357, 1974.

Levy HL: Newborn screening by tandem mass spectrometry: A new era. Clin Chem 44:2401-2402, 1998.

Levy H, Albers S: Genetic screening of newborns. Ann Rev Genomics Hum Genet 1:139-177, 2000.

Levy HL, Cornier AS: Current approaches to genetic metabolic screening in newborns. Curr Opin Pediatr 6:707-711, 1994.

Levy HL, Hammersen G: Newborn screening for galactosemia and other galactose metabolic defects. J Pediatr 92:871-877, 1978.

Levy HL, Shih VE, Madigan PM, MacCready RA: Transient tyrosinemia in full-term infants. JAMA 209:249-250, 1969.

Levy HL, Sepe SJ, Shih VE, et al: Sepsis due to Escherichia coli in neonates with galactosemia. N Engl J Med 297:823-825. 1977.

Lorey FW, Cunningham GC: Effect of specimen collection method on newborn screening for PKU. Screening 3:57-65, 1994.

Mandel S, Hanna C, Boston B, et al: Thyroxine-binding globulin deficiency detected by newborn screening. J Pediatr 122: 227-230, 1993.

Millington DS, Kodo N, Norwood DL, Roe CR: Tandem mass spectrometry: A new method for acylcarnitine profiling with potential for neonatal screening for inborn errors of metabolism. J Inherit Metab Dis 13:321-324, 1990.

O'Flynn ME: Newborn screening for phenylketonuria: Thirty years of progress. Curr Probl Pediatr 22:159-165, 1992.

Pang S, Clark A: Congenital adrenal hyperplasia due to 21-hydroxylase deficiency: Newborn screening and its relationship to the diagnosis and treatment of the disorder. Screening 2:105-139, 1993.

Pang S, Shook MK: Current status of neonatal screening for congenital adrenal hyperplasia [see comments]. Curr Opin Pediatr 9:419-423, 1997.

Paul DA, Leef KH, Stefano JL, Bartoshesky L: Low serum thyroxine on initial newborn screening is associated with intraventricular hemorrhage and death in very low birth weight infants. Pediatrics 101:903-907, 1998.

Peterschmitt MJ, Simmons JR, Levy HL: Reduction of false negative results in screening of newborns for homocystinuria. N Engl J Med 341:1572-1576, 1999.

Ranieri E, Lewis BD, Gerace RL, et al: Neonatal screening for cystic fibrosis using immunoreactive trypsinogen and direct gene analysis: Four years' experience. BMJ 308:1469-1472, 1994.

Rashed MS, Ozand PT, Bucknall MP, Little D: Diagnosis of inborn errors of metabolism from blood spots by acylcarnitines and amino acids profiling using automated electrospray tandem mass spectrometry. Pediatr Res 38:324-331, 1995.

Sawada T: Screening infants for neuroblastoma in Japan. Screening 1:253-272, 1993.

Smith J, Kinney T: Clinical practice guidelines, quick reference guide for clinician: Sickle cell disease: Screening and management in newborns and infants. Am Fam Physician 48:95-102, 1993.

Whiteman PD, Clayton BE, Ersser RS, et al: Changing incidence of neonatal hypermethioninaemia: Implications for the detection of homocystinuria. Arch Dis Child 54:593-598, 1979.

Wilcken B: Newborn screening for cystic fibrosis: Its evolution and a review of the current situation. Screening 2:43-62, 1993.

Wilcken B, Wiley V, Sherry G, Bayliss U: Neonatal screening for cystic fibrosis: A comparison of two strategies for case detection in 1.2 million babies. J Pediatr 127:965-970, 1995.

Wolf B, Heard GS: Biotinidase deficiency. Adv Pediatr 38:1-21, 1991.

Woods WG, Gao RN, Shuster JJ, et al: The effect of screening on population based mortality in neuroblastoma: A report from the Quebec Neuroblastoma Screening Project. N Engl J Med 346:1041-1046, 2003.

Ziadeh R, Hoffman EP, Finegold DN, et al: Medium chain acyl-CoA dehydrogenase deficiency in Pennsylvania: Neonatal screening shows high incidence and unexpected mutation frequencies. Pediatr Res 37:675-678, 1995.

Zytkovicz TH, Fitzgerald EF, Marsden D, et al: Tandem mass spectrometric analysis for amino, organic, and fatty acid disorders in newborn dried blood spots: A two-year summary from the New England Newborn Screening Program. Clin Chem 47:1945-1955, 2001.

# CARE OF THE HIGH-RISK INFANT

Editor: ROBERTA A. BALLARD

PART VIII

CHAPTER 28

# Resuscitation in the Delivery Room

Jeffrey D. Merrill and Roberta A. Ballard

## PHYSIOLOGY OF BIRTH

During normal gestation, labor, and delivery, powerful biochemical and mechanical forces act on the fetus to prepare it to adapt to extrauterine life. However, a myriad of adverse circumstances—genetic, maternal, and fetal—that vary in duration, degree, and implication for outcome can occur during the antepartum and intrapartum periods and impair the infant's ability to make this adaptation successfully. Hence, there is a need for resuscitative efforts to assist in this process. The approach to the resuscitation of any infant depends on a keen appreciation of the historical factors behind the need, an understanding of the physiologic mechanisms of adaptation, and sensitivity to the individual infant's responses as well as skill in resuscitative techniques. Thus, successful resuscitation depends on much more than the "mechanical" application of practiced routines; it requires a clear understanding of basic physiologic principles and excellent assessment skills as well as the essential equipment and practiced teamwork.

### "Stress" of Birth

As Lagercrantz and Slotkin (1986) point out, "At first thought, being born would seem to be a terrible and dangerous ordeal. The human fetus is squeezed through the birth canal for several hours, during which the head sustains considerable pressure, and the infant is intermittently deprived of oxygen. . . . then delivered from a warm, dark, sheltered environment into a cold, bright hospital room. . . . (In response) the fetus produces unusually high levels of the "stress" hormones, adrenalin and noradrenalin, . . . typically used to prepare the body to fight or flee from a perceived threat to survival." Surely, the process of labor and delivery is the time of greatest jeopardy that occurs during life, but would avoidance of this stress and the consequent elevation of catecholamine levels lead to better outcomes? Catecholamines clearly contribute to the regulation of many processes important to the infant's adaptation at birth, including resorption of lung liquid, release of surfactant into the alveoli, mobilization of readily usable fuel for nutrition, defense against cold stress, and modulation of cardiac output to ensure the preferential flow of blood to vital organs, such as the heart and brain. Perhaps, as some researchers have suggested, elevations of catecholamines even promote attachment between mother and child by increasing the appearance of alertness of the infant (Fig. 28–1).

The normal preterm infant has lower catecholamine levels at birth than the normal term infant, a feature that contributes to the disadvantages of preterm infants in establishing ventilation and maintaining temperature. In both term and preterm infants, catecholamine levels are higher with delivery after labor and also higher in girls than in boys. Levels are proportionately very much higher in each of these groups when there is asphyxia (Greenough et al, 1987; Newnham et al, 1984). The endogenous opiate peptides (enkephalins and endorphins) also probably modulate the cardiovascular response to stress and play a role in the infant's adaptation at birth (Martinez et al, 1988). It is hoped that greater understanding of the interaction of these and other agents will eventually allow optimal preparation of the fetus for labor. This understanding may also provide insight as to which interventions should be used during labor and at birth to ensure an optimal outcome.

### Transition from Fetal to Neonatal Circulation

Before birth, the placenta serves as the gas-exchange organ for the fetus and provides a low-resistance "shunt" compared with the high resistance of the fetus's peripheral circulation. As a result, the fetus normally has two large right-to-left shunts, one from the right atrium to the left atrium through the foramen ovale, and the other from the pulmonary artery to the aorta across the ductus arteriosus (Fig. 28–2). In utero, as a result of constricted pulmonary arterioles that produce high pulmonary vascular resistance, only a small percentage of the fetal cardiac output flows through the lungs. The fetus accommodates well to a normal $PO_2$ of 20 to 25 mm Hg in its best-oxygenated blood, which comes through the umbilical vein from the placenta. As a result of the right-to-left shunts through the foramen ovale and the ductus arteriosus, the best-oxygenated blood streams from the umbilical vein to the inferior vena cava, through the foramen ovale into the left atrium and ventricle, and then out the aorta, thus

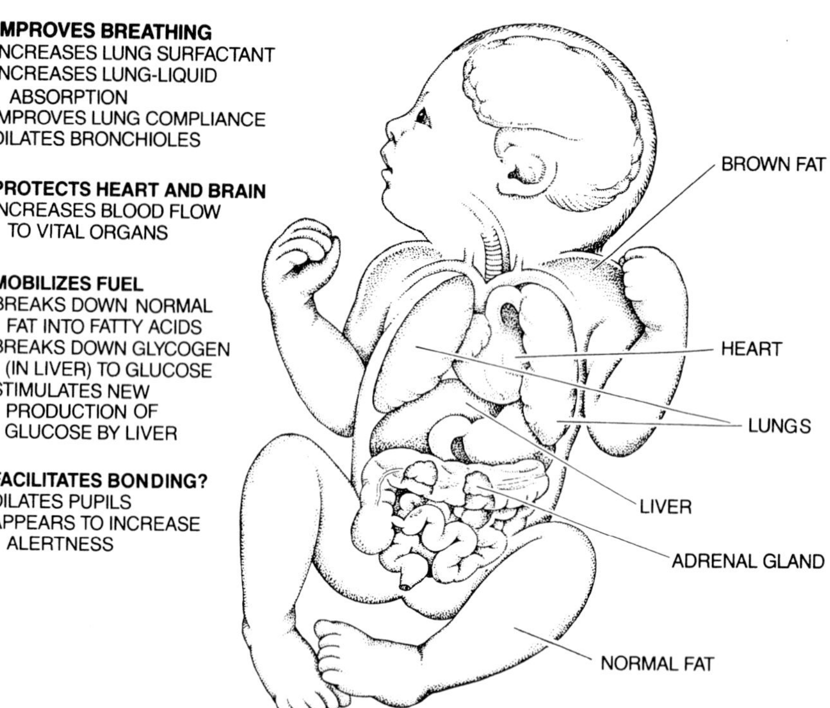


**FIGURE 28–1.** Adaptational effects of a catecholamine surge during delivery include promotion of normal breathing, alteration of blood flow to protect the heart and brain against potential asphyxia, immediate mobilization of fuel for energy and, possibly, enhancement of maternal-infant attachment. *(From Lagercrantz H, Slotkin TA: The "stress" of being born. Sci Am 254:100, 1986. Copyright 1986 by Scientific American, Inc. All rights reserved.)*

supplying best-oxygenated blood to the brain and myocardium of the fetus (see Fig. 28–2).

At delivery, two major changes occur in this system. First, the umbilical cord is clamped, eliminating the placenta as a gas-exchange organ and low-resistance "shunt." Second, respiration is initiated by the fetus. Expansion of the lungs results in a marked decrease in pulmonary vascular resistance that is furthered by the higher level of oxygenation that occurs as the infant begins to breathe (Fig. 28–3). With these changes, the flow of blood to the left atrium via the pulmonary veins increases, so that left atrial pressure exceeds right atrial pressure and functionally closes the foramen ovale. When pulmonary vascular resistance decreases to a level lower than the systemic vascular pressure, the ductus arteriosus is functionally closed.

At birth, the lungs normally are partially filled with fluid. Therefore, the initial breaths taken by the infant must inflate the lungs and effect a change in vascular pressures so that lung water is absorbed into the pulmonary arterial system and cleared from the lung. At the same time, inflation is a powerful mechanism for the release of pulmonary surface–active material, which increases compliance of the lung and enables stabilization of functional residual capacity (Massaro and Massaro, 1983; Taeusch et al, 1974).

### Fetal Reserve

Because the fetus is normally relatively hypoxemic ($PO_2$ of 20 to 24 mm Hg) and during labor is subjected to stresses associated with both increased oxygen consumption and interrupted gas exchange, the fetus is at particular risk for asphyxia at the time of birth. However, the fetus has several compensatory mechanisms that help protect it. Fetal hemoglobin has greater oxygen affinity than adult hemoglobin, fetal tissues have an increased ability to extract oxygen, and the fetus has greater tissue resistance to acidosis than the adult. In addition, the fetus has mechanisms that compensate for asphyxia. These include bradycardia and the "diving reflex" (similar to that found in diving mammals), which allows a preferential distribution of blood flow to the brain, adrenal glands, and heart and away from the lungs, gut, liver, spleen, kidney, and carcass. The fetus is also capable of reducing oxygen consumption and switching to anaerobic glycolysis, as long as liver glycogen stores are adequate.

## ASPHYXIA

### Physiology

*Asphyxia* is defined as a combination of *hypoxemia*, *hypercapnia*, and *metabolic acidemia* (Strang, 1977). If lung expansion does not occur in the minutes after birth and the infant is unable to establish ventilation and pulmonary perfusion, a progressive cycle of worsening hypoxemia, hypercapnia, and metabolic acidemia evolves. Pulmonary vascular resistance remains high, the ductus arteriosus remains widely patent (Fig. 28–4), and right-to-left shunting through the foramen ovale also persists. Once this process begins, it tends to be self-perpetuating and may result in serious tissue hypoxia, ischemia, and acidosis, which ultimately may lead to irreversible organ damage. Asphyxia may be caused by maternal, placental, or fetal factors that reduce the fetal reserve (Table 28–1). The duration of asphyxia is critical to the outcome of the infant, so it is important to evaluate rapidly all of the factors contributing to the asphyxia and to interrupt the process as soon as possible.

Figure 28–5 demonstrates the classic cardiopulmonary changes seen in the animal model of asphyxia, as described

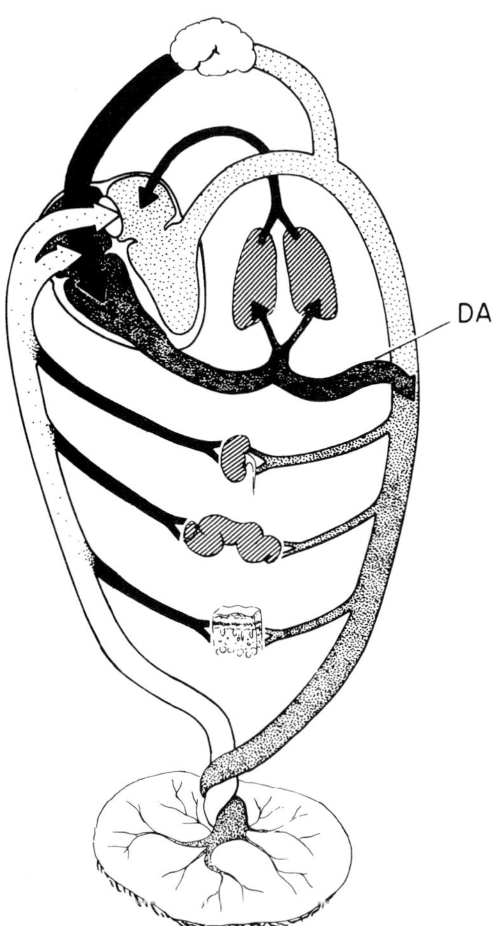


**FIGURE 28–2.** The fetal circulation. Oxygenated blood leaves the placenta by way of the umbilical vein (vessel without stippling). It flows into the portal sinus in the liver (not shown), and a variable portion of it perfuses the liver. The remainder passes from the portal sinus through the ductus venosus into the inferior vena cava, where it joins blood from the viscera (represented by the kidney, gut, and skin). About half of the inferior vena cava flow passes through the foramen ovale to the left atrium, where it mixes with a small amount of pulmonary venous blood. This relatively well-oxygenated blood (light stippling) supplies the heart and brain by way of the ascending aorta. The other half of the inferior vena cava stream mixes with superior vena cava blood and enters the right ventricle (blood in the right atrium and ventricle has little oxygen, which is denoted by heavy stippling). Because the pulmonary arterioles are constricted, most of the blood in the main pulmonary artery flows through the ductus arteriosus (DA) so that the descending aorta's blood has less oxygen (heavy stippling) than blood in the ascending aorta (light stippling). *(From Avery GN: Neonatology. Philadelphia, JB Lippincott, 1987.)*

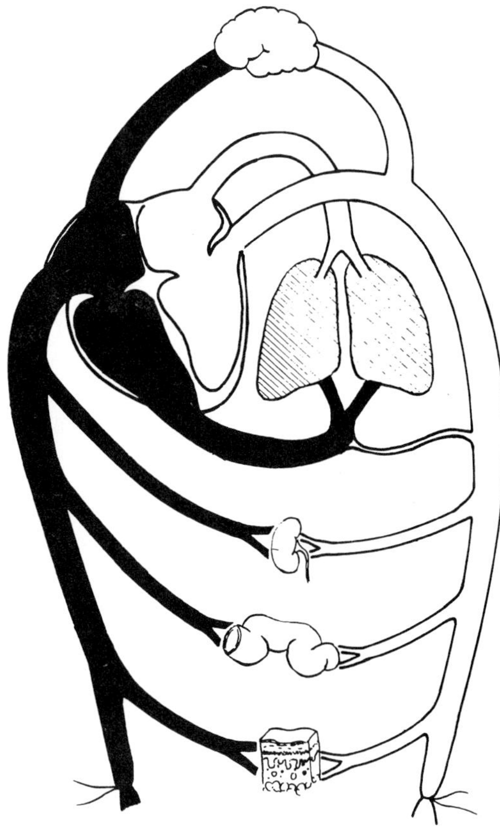

**FIGURE 28–3.** The circulation in the normal newborn. After expansion of the lungs and ligation of the umbilical cord, pulmonary blood flow increases and left atrial and systemic arterial pressures increase while pulmonary arterial and right heart pressures decrease. When the left atrial pressure exceeds right atrial pressure, the foramen ovale closes so that all of the inferior and superior vena cava blood leaves the right atrium, enters the right ventricle, and is pumped through the pulmonary artery toward the lung. With the increase in systemic arterial pressure and decrease in pulmonary arterial pressure, flow through the ductus arteriosus becomes left to right, and the ductus constricts and closes. The course of the circulation is the same as in the adult. *(From Avery GN: Neonatology. Philadelphia, JB Lippincott, 1987.)*

by Dawes (1968). The initial phase of asphyxia is marked by increased respiratory effort (*primary hyperpnea*). This is followed by *primary apnea*, which lasts approximately 1 minute. Rhythmic gasping then begins and is maintained at a rate of 8 to 10 gasps per minute for several minutes, after which the gasps become weaker and slower until they cease, which is called *secondary apnea*. Some variation occurs in the period of gasping as a result of prior maternal and fetal medications or conditions that may have affected the infant's level of asphyxia at the moment of birth.

## Universal Prerequisites for Resuscitation

### Skilled Personnel

In the United States, 4 million babies per year are born in 5000 hospitals with delivery services (Martin et al, 2002). Ninety percent of these hospitals are small, level 1 services; 5% are level 2; and another 5% are level 3 (Bloom and Cropley, 1987). Thus, most infants are born in hospitals that do not have sophisticated perinatal programs. Yet 10% of newborns require some assistance at birth, and 1% require a more extensive resuscitation (Wu and Carlo, 2002).

The Neonatal Resuscitation Program (NRP), a combined effort of the American Heart Association (AHA) and the American Academy of Pediatrics (AAP), began in the 1980s as a means to ensure that all personnel in hospital delivery rooms have the knowledge and skills to provide optimal care to newborns immediately after birth. Implementation of the

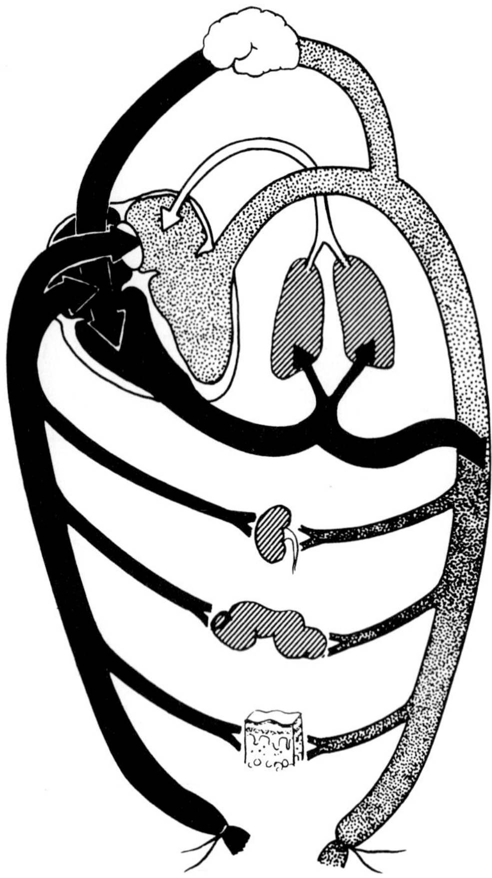

**FIGURE 28–4.** The circulation in an asphyxiated newborn with incomplete expansion of the lungs. Pulmonary vascular resistance is high, pulmonary blood flow is low (normal number of pulmonary veins), and flow through the ductus arteriosus is high. With little pulmonary arterial flow, left atrial pressure decreases below right atrial pressure, the foramen ovale opens, and vena cava blood flows through the foramen into the left atrium. Partially venous blood goes to the brain via the ascending aorta. The blood of the descending aorta that goes to the viscera has less oxygen than that of the ascending aorta (heavy stippling) because of the reverse flow through the ductus arteriosus. Thus, the circulation is the same as in the fetus except that there is less well-oxygenated blood in the inferior vena cava and umbilical vein. *(From Avery GN: Neonatology. Philadelphia, JB Lippincott, 1987.)*

**TABLE 28–1**

**Conditions Affecting Fetal Reserve**

| Determinants | Common Disorders |
|---|---|
| **Maternal** | |
| Infection | Amnionitis |
| Lungs | Pneumonia, asthma, adult respiratory distress syndrome |
| Heart | Arrhythmia, structural defect, failure |
| Blood | Anemia, hemoglobinopathy |
| Blood vessels | Systemic lupus erythematosus, diabetes, hypertension, hypotension |
| Uterus | Hypertonus, malformation, rupture |
| Other | Genetic, drugs, deformities, preterm labor, multiple gestation, abnormal fetal presentation |
| **Placental** | |
| Age | Postmaturity |
| Size, morphology | Abruptio placentae, placenta previa |
| **Fetal** | |
| Umbilical cord | Knot, entanglement, prolapse, compression, thrombosis |
| Blood | Anemia |
| Metabolic | Inborn error, aneuploidy |
| Other | Infection, hydrops, malformations, multiple gestation |

Data from Jacobs M, Phibbs R: Prevention, recognition, and treatment of perinatal asphyxia. Clin Perinatol 16:785, 1989.

NRP has been associated with improvement in Apgar scores (Patel et al, 2001). The NRP emphasizes the basic principle that effective resuscitation must begin with the awareness that *well-trained personnel must be immediately available in any setting where an infant is likely to be delivered.* (The American College of Obstetrics and Gynecology [ACOG], the American Society of Anesthesiology, the American Academy of Family Physicians, and the Canadian Pediatric Society have also stated their support for this principle.) Identification and training of staff are, therefore, the first steps in preparation for neonatal resuscitation. The second step is close communication between obstetricians and pediatricians to identify women with high-risk fetuses before labor if possible, to prevent abnormal labors, and to focus planning for the resuscitation of infants thus identified. Understanding the special needs of different kinds of infants enables caregivers to anticipate and prepare for various types of resuscitation appropriately.

## Equipment

Resuscitation of the newborn is best performed in the delivery room or immediately adjacent to it, to minimize the time lapse between delivery and initiation of resuscitation. The equipment that should be available for neonatal resuscitation is listed in Table 28–2 ; it is divided into (1) items needed in every institution for resuscitation of low-risk term infants with unexpected problems and (2) additional equipment required for resuscitation of high-risk or known preterm infants.

# MANAGEMENT AT DELIVERY

## Initial Assessment

The NRP algorithm for resuscitation in the delivery room begins with an initial evaluation of the newborn (Fig. 28–6). Abnormalities in breathing, tone, and color as well as the presence of meconium or evidence of prematurity are indicative of the need for further resuscitation. One begins by placing the infant under a radiant heater, positioning the infant's head to open the airway, clearing upper

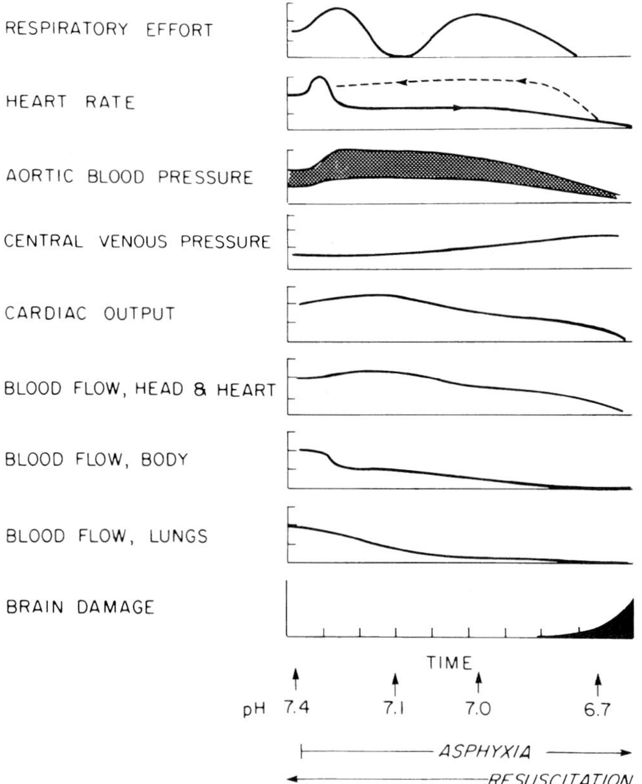


**FIGURE 28–5.** The sequence of cardiopulmonary changes with asphyxia and resuscitation. Time is on the horizontal axis. Asphyxia progresses from left to right; resuscitation proceeds from right to left. Units of time are not given. If there is complete interruption of respiratory gas exchange, the entire process of asphyxia from extreme left to right could occur in about 10 minutes. It could take much longer with an asphyxiating process that only partly interrupts gas exchange or does so completely, but only for repeated brief periods. With resuscitation, the process reverses, beginning at the point to which asphyxia has proceeded. *(Adapted from Dawes G: Foetal and Neonatal Physiology. Chicago, Year Book, 1968, and Avery GN: Neonatology. Philadelphia, JB Lippincott, 1987.)*

airway secretions, and drying and stimulating the infant. A brief delivery of oxygen, blown over the face, may be given as necessary for cyanosis. It is important to remember that at birth, the newborn infant's lungs are normally full of fluid which is cleared by resorption into the pulmonary vascular system (Walters, 1978). Excessive suctioning of clear fluid from the nasopharynx is not helpful and may contribute to atelectasis. The infant is next quickly assessed for respiration, heart rate, and color. The presence of apnea or a heart rate of less than 100 beats/min indicates the need for positive-pressure ventilation.

## Assisted Ventilation

*Effective ventilation* of the lung is the single most important step in the resuscitation of the compromised newborn. Previous studies demonstrate that reversal of hypoxia, bradycardia, and acidosis depends on adequate inflation (Wu and Carlo, 2002). The airway must be cleared before attempts to expand the lung are made. Initial inflation of a gasless fluid-filled lung may require relatively high inflation pressures (sufficient to move the chest, usually 25 to 40 cm $H_2O$) using a relatively long inspiratory time (0.5 to 1 second). The objective is to inflate the lung as well as to trap some gas during exhalation, thereby creating a functional residual capacity. This process occurs over a series of breaths. The term infant with a strong chest wall and large terminal airways is better able to generate the necessary forces to achieve lung inflation than the premature infant, who may need to be assisted. Lung inflation also stimulates surfactant secretion in mature lungs, and this response is enhanced by large-volume inflation. Once lung expansion is achieved, subsequent inflation pressure should be reduced to that necessary to sufficiently move the chest.

Concerns have been raised about the value of resuscitation with 100% oxygen versus room air. Traditionally, 100% oxygen has been used for rapid reversal of hypoxia (Rootwelt et al, 1992). Saugstad (1990, 1996) and others (Ramji et al, 1993) have raised concerns about the possibility that oxygen radicals produced in excess during the post-hypoxic reoxygenation period may cause tissue damage, particularly to the brain. One study has shown that asphyxiated infants resuscitated with room air exhibit shorter time to spontaneous respirations and first cry, with no differences in mortality or neurologic morbidity, than those resuscitated with 100% oxygen; in addition, biochemical markers of oxidative stress were reduced in the room air resuscitation group (Vento et al, 2001). Present data, however, are insufficient to change the current recommendation that 100% oxygen be used if assisted ventilation is required. If oxygen is not available, resuscitation should be initiated with room air.

Assisted ventilation should continue until the heart exceeds 100 beats/min and the infant begins spontaneous respiratory effort. For newborns requiring bag-and-mask ventilation for longer than several minutes, an orogastric tube should be inserted and left in place. If the need for positive-pressure ventilation lasts beyond several minutes, one should consider intubation of the trachea to improve efficiency of ventilation. Figure 28–7 shows landmarks of the larynx that should be visualized for successful intubation of the newborn. No attempt at intubation should last longer than 30 to 45 seconds before a return to bag-and-mask ventilation to support the neonate. If severe respiratory decompensation persists despite restoration of normal heart rate and color, and the mother has been given narcotics within 4 hours of delivery, one may consider naloxone administration. Naloxone should not be given to infants of mothers with a history of narcotic abuse during pregnancy. Once naloxone is administered, the infant should be observed for recurrence of respiratory depression, because of the shorter duration of effect of naloxone in comparison with opiates.

## Chest Compressions

Most infants respond to assisted ventilation alone during neonatal resuscitation. In a study by Perlman and Risser (1995), only 0.12% of infants required chest compressions,

**TABLE 28–2**

**Equipment for Neonatal Resuscitation**

| | |
|---|---|
| Low-risk and term infants | Radiant warmer to maintain temperature control<br>Stethoscope<br>Source of warm, humidified oxygen with flowmeter<br>Bulb syringe<br>Suction source<br>Suction catheter and meconium aspirator<br>Nasogastric tube and syringe<br>Oral airway<br>Apparatus for bag-and-mask ventilation of infant, either an anesthesia bag, or A bag with masks for different-sized infants<br>Laryngoscope with straight blades Nos. 0 and 1<br>Endotracheal tubes—sizes 2.5, 3.0, 3.5, 4.0—and stylet<br>Gloves, gowns, masks, hats for sterile procedures<br>Tape<br>Scissors<br>Fluids (10% dextrose in water, normal saline)<br>Medications (naloxone hydrochloride [Narcan], sodium bicarbonate [4.2%], calcium gluconate, epinephrine)<br>Clock or stopwatch<br>Volume expander (normal saline preferred) and/or blood available on emergency basis<br>Tubes for obtaining blood gas or other samples<br>Equipment for placing umbilical catheter<br>Equipment for microtechnique of measuring blood gases<br>Portable radiographic equipment |
| High-risk and preterm infants | All of the equipment listed for low-risk and term infants, plus:<br>Spotlight<br>Manometer for gauging pressure being used in ventilation<br>Blender for delivering oxygen in concentrations ranging from room air to 100%, with heated nebulizer<br>Oxygen analyzer<br>Electrocardiographic electrodes<br>Heart rate monitoring equipment<br>Blood pressure monitoring equipment<br>Hemoglobin saturation monitor<br>Blood gas syringes, heparinized and ready to use<br>Blood gas laboratory immediately available (10-minute processing time)<br>Umbilical artery and vein catheters set up and ready to insert, with vascular pressure monitor<br>Gowns, masks, hats, for sterile procedures<br>Emergency medications with estimated dosages calculated |

epinephrine, or both during resuscitation. In approximately two thirds of these infants, ineffective initial ventilatory support was the presumed mechanism for continued neonatal depression. Because chest compressions interfere with ventilation, they should not be initiated until adequate ventilation is established.

If, after 30 seconds of *effective* ventilation, the heart rate remains less than 60 beats/min, chest compressions should be initiated. The two-thumb technique is preferred over the two-finger technique for chest compressions, because it is more controlled and may offer some advantage in generating higher peak perfusion pressure (Menegazzi et al, 1993). NRP guidelines recommend a compression depth of one third to one half of the anteroposterior diameter of the chest to generate a pulse, at a ratio of three compressions to one breath.

## Epinephrine

If the infant's heart rate remains less than 60 beats/min despite at least 30 seconds of *effective* ventilation and 30 seconds of cardiac compression, epinephrine should be administered either endotracheally or, preferably, intravenously (McCrirrick and Kestin, 1992; Perlman and Risse, 1995). Standard dosage is 0.01 mg/kg of epinephrine using a 1:10,000 standard dilution. Higher doses of epinephrine have been suggested for adults and older children if there is no response to the lower dose, on the base of animal and human studies demonstrating better output and better coronary perfusion (Gonzalez et al, 1989; Paradis et al, 1991). However, such an enhancement of coronary blood flow may not be beneficial in neonates, because the usual terminal rhythm is a bradyarrhythmia from hypoxia, despite

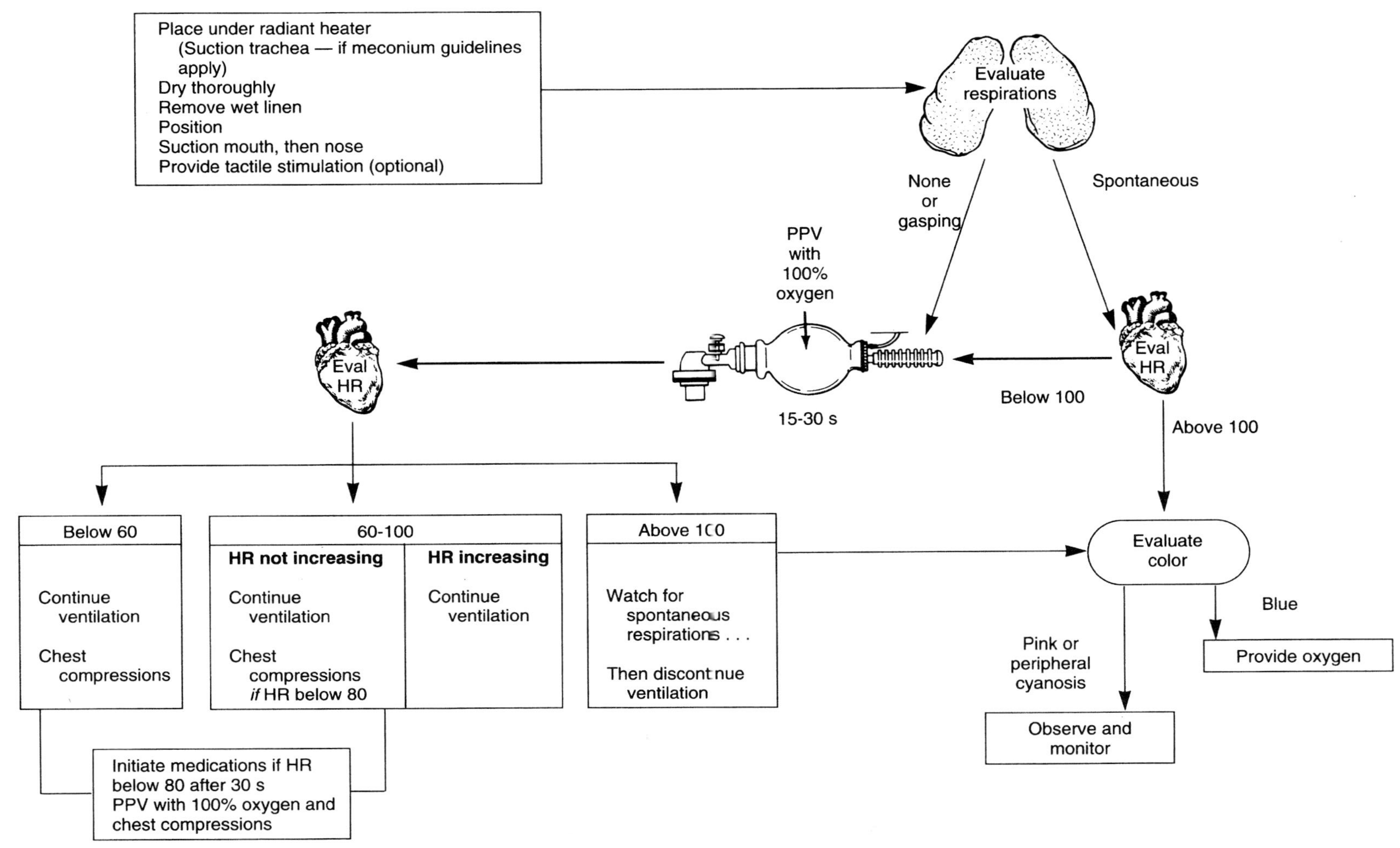


**FIGURE 28–6.** Overview of resuscitation in the delivery room. *(From Bloom RS, Cropley C: American Heart Association—American Academy of Pediatrics Textbook of Neonatal Resuscitation. Dallas, American Heart Association National Center, 1994. Copyright American Heart Association.)*

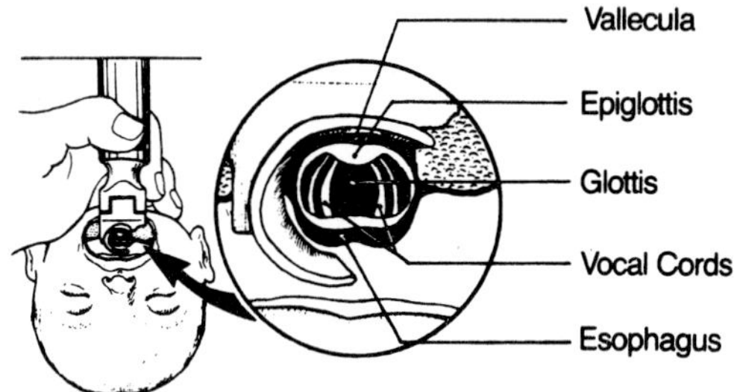


**FIGURE 28-7.** Landmarks of the larynx that should be visualized for intubation of the newborn. *(From Bloom RS, Cropley C: American Heart Association–American Academy of Pediatrics Textbook of Neonatal Resuscitation. Dallas, American Heart Association National Center, 1994. Reproduced with permission. Copyright American Heart Association.)*

an initial transient rise in cardiac and myocardial ischemia, as seen in adults (Burchfield, 1999). In addition, higher-dose epinephrine administration is associated with significant hypertension after recovery, with a greater risk of intracranial hemorrhage (Pasternak et al, 1983; Reynolds et al, 1979).

Although use of the standard dose via the endotracheal route results in lower serum concentrations than intravenous administration, efficacy of the routine endotracheal dose has been demonstrated (Lindemann, 1984). In addition, use of higher doses of epinephrine via the endotracheal route produces a prolongation of post-resuscitation hypertension that is seen with the intravascular route (Ralston et al, 1985). Therefore, the standard dose is recommended regardless of route of administration.

## Support of the Cardiovascular System

Most infants are not hypovolemic in the delivery room; however, infants are occasionally compromised secondary to acute hemorrhage. It is often a challenge to assess the infant's circulatory status to determine whether hypovolemia is the cause of hypotension or whether the infant is suffering cardiovascular depression because of some other problem. Physiologic variables to be remembered are as follows:

1. Falsely high arterial blood pressure readings have been associated with acidosis (which may respond to administration of sodium bicarbonate).
2. Hypocapnia may be associated with hypotension, so that infants who are being overventilated may have falsely low arterial blood pressure readings.
3. An infant with normal blood pressure who has poor perfusion may be maximally vasoconstricted; therefore, significant hypotension may be masked.
4. An infant who is distressed and in pain may have a falsely elevated blood pressure level.
5. The normal range of blood pressure for very small premature infants may be low. The physician should assume that the blood pressure is normal in an infant with good oxygenation and good peripheral perfusion and no signs of circulatory collapse, particularly if the infant passes urine. In the infant who is not voiding, use of low-dose dopamine (2 to 5 μg/kg/min) may improve renal perfusion.
6. Monitoring an infant's hematocrit levels over time can be enormously helpful. A decrease in hematocrit value during the first 2 hours after birth may indicate hypovolemia, because infants have the ability to mobilize fluid rapidly.
7. Preterm newborn infants ordinarily do not exhibit tachycardia as a sign of shock; therefore, a rapid heart rate generally is not useful as an indicator of volume status.

Volume expansion may be accomplished with the use of normal saline or lactated Ringer's solution. Albumin infusion is no longer recommended (Wu and Carlo, 2002). It may be appropriate to administer small (10 mL/kg) transfusions of packed red blood cells in cases of hypovolemic shock and severe anemia. It is of the utmost importance that volume replacement be given slowly, because some vascular beds (particularly those of the brain) may already be maximally dilated in response to systemic hypotension, and excessive pressure may be transmitted to the fragile capillaries, leading to intracranial hemorrhage.

In infants who have had prolonged or severe asphyxia, myocardial failure resulting from poor contractility may occur, evidenced by hypotension that persists after initial resuscitation. Such infants may show response to dopamine at a starting dose of 5 μg/kg/min which may be increased as needed up to 20 μg/kg/min to produce an adequate response. Rarely, dobutamine may be added, at 5 μg/kg/min (up to 15 μg/kg/min). It may be useful in these infants to pass a second umbilical catheter through the umbilical vein, via the ductus venosus, and into the right atrium to monitor central venous pressure in addition to arterial pressure.

## Sodium Bicarbonate

If an infant requires substantial resuscitation, samples for infant blood gas determination should be obtained whenever possible. Administration of sodium bicarbonate in neonatal resuscitation is controversial, and routine use of bicarbonate is discouraged. One may consider sodium bicarbonate use in cases of documented severe metabolic acidosis, but only after establishment of *adequate* ventilation and oxygenation.

The most severely asphyxiated infants are those with an arterial pH of 7.0 or less and a calculated base deficit of 25 mEq/L or greater in the presence of a marked elevation of $Pa_{CO_2}$. By means of artificial ventilation alone, this calculated deficit can be reduced by approximately 10 mEq/L if the infant's circulation is normal and oxygenation is achieved. This effect results from a significant bicarbonate shift that occurs when $Pa_{CO_2}$ exceeds 70 mm Hg and therefore must be taken into consideration in calculations for correcting base deficit. Some additional correction occurs with ventilation at pH levels above 7.0; therefore, the dose of bicarbonate administered should always be no more than one fourth of the initially calculated value. Blood gas studies should be repeated before further increments of bicarbonate are given. The equation for calculation of base replacement is

$$\frac{\text{mEq}}{\text{Base}} = \frac{0.3 \times \text{weight in kg} \times \text{base deficit in mEq/L}}{4}$$

Given the hyperosmolarity and $CO_2$-generating properties of sodium bicarbonate, this substance should be diluted to a strength of 4.2% with sterile water and administered slowly. Arterial blood pressure should be measured both before and after bicarbonate is given, because the administration of sodium bicarbonate may unmask hypovolemia that has not been apparent because of peripheral vasoconstriction. Table 28–3 provides the recommended drug dosages for neonatal resuscitation.

If an infant remains compromised despite adequate ventilation, chest compressions, and resuscitative medications, one should consider other causes, including pneumothorax, congenital airway malformations such as congenital diaphragmatic hernia, and complex congenital heart disease.

### Umbilical Vessel Catheterization

In the high-risk or significantly asphyxiated infant, it is important to place an umbilical catheter, preferably in the umbilical artery (although commonly a venous catheter can be placed more rapidly), to obtain samples for arterial blood gas and other determinations as well as to monitor arterial pressure. Changes in arterial pulse pressure and mean pressure can thus be followed up during the resuscitation, providing important indicators of cardiovascular responsiveness. In addition, appropriate medications can be administered easily through the catheter, although one should avoid administration of hypertonic medications, calcium, and blood products through an umbilical venous catheter, the tip of which is below the level of the diaphragm and therefore near the portal circulation.

### Continuation of Support after Resuscitation

The Apgar score was initially introduced to help quantitate the initial evaluation of newborn infants (Table 28–4). Apgar scores should be assigned at 1, 5, and 10 minutes, and, if the infant still requires resuscitation, at 15 and 20 minutes as well. The score is an indicator of responsiveness to therapy as well as a way of identifying infants who are at high risk for further difficulty. The score at 5 minutes and later is more predictive of survival and neurologic status than the 1-minute score, because the ability to interrupt and reverse the process of asphyxia indicates not only successful intervention but also that the process was not established for a long period in utero.

One of the factors essential to successful resuscitation is the ability to identify the infant who has continuing difficulties after resuscitation and, thus, to facilitate prevention of a relapse. This applies particularly to the premature infant with respiratory distress syndrome (RDS) who initially responds favorably to treatment with ventilation and sodium bicarbonate but then requires continued cardiorespiratory support to prevent respiratory distress from becoming severe and causing another cycle of hypoxia and acidosis. Another example is in the infant born after undergoing an episode of fetal distress, who may have reactive pulmonary vasculature. If such an infant is allowed to become hypoxic, pulmonary vasoconstriction may occur (or worsen) and may progress to persistent pulmonary hypertension of the newborn.

## THINGS TO AVOID IN RESUSCITATION

Successful resuscitation of a newborn infant involves not only interrupting the cycle of hypoxia and acidemia and bringing the infant back toward the physiologic norm but also avoiding iatrogenic damage. The following are, therefore, some important "rules" of resuscitation:

1. *Do not panic if an endotracheal tube cannot be placed immediately*. Concentrate on bag-and-mask ventilation and call for help. Do not assume that medication is a substitute for ventilation.
2. *Do not perform excessive suctioning of clear fluid from the infant's nasopharynx*. Fluid is normally absorbed into the lungs.
3. *Do not use excessive oxygen concentrations to resuscitate the premature infant unless the infant clearly requires it*.
4. *Do not use too much ventilatory pressure to expand the infant's lungs*. The required initial pressure for expanding the lung may be briefly higher right after birth than it is within just 15 to 30 minutes after birth. Use good clinical judgment. Watch the infant's chest and listen to breath sounds. Try reducing ventilation with hand ventilation to ensure that the lowest pressure necessary is being used. Excessive pressure on lungs that are normalizing may decrease venous return to the heart and decrease cardiac output and cause injury to lung tissue.
5. *Avoid hypocapnia*. There is evidence that even brief overdistention of the lung may raise the risk of bronchopulmonary dysplasia (BPD) (Garland et al, 1995).
6. *Do not give volume replacement or sodium bicarbonate automatically*. Each of these agents has been associated with production of intracranial hemorrhage in animal models.
7. *Do not focus or rely too heavily on cardiac resuscitation*, because, the most likely problem by far in neonatal resuscitation is the need for ventilatory support.
8. *Maintain normoxia in the term or post-term infant with meconium aspiration or asphyxia*, because such an infant may have reactive pulmonary blood vessels, and pulmonary vasoconstriction may develop if hypoxia persists.

## SPECIAL CONDITIONS REQUIRING ATTENTION DURING RESUSCITATION

### Extremely Premature Infant (<1000 g)

Resuscitation of very premature infants begins in utero; therefore, whenever possible, such infants should be born in a perinatal center with skilled staff from the obstetric, anesthetic, and neonatal teams in attendance. The fragility of these infants requires gentleness in handling and a high level of skill in the staff performing the resuscitation. Because of the relatively large surface area of extremely premature infants, attention to immediate drying and

**TABLE 28–3**

**Medications for Neonatal Resuscitation**

| Medication | Concentration to Administer | Preparation | Dosage and Route | Total Dose/Infant | | | Rate and Precautions |
|---|---|---|---|---|---|---|---|
| Epinephrine | 1:10,000 | 1 mL | 0.1-0.3 mL/kg IV or ET | **Weight (kg)** | **Total mL** | | Give rapidly<br>May dilute with normal saline to 1-2 mL if giving ET |
| | | | | 1 | 0.1-0.3 | | |
| | | | | 2 | 0.2-0.6 | | |
| | | | | 3 | 0.3-0.9 | | |
| | | | | 4 | 0.4-1.2 | | |
| Volume expanders | Saline<br>Normal saline | | 10 mL/kg IV | **Weight (kg)** | **Total mL** | | Give over 5-10 minutes |
| | | | | 1 | 10 | | |
| | | | | 2 | 20 | | |
| | | | | 3 | 30 | | |
| | | | | 4 | 40 | | |
| Sodium bicarbonate | 0.5 mEq/mL (4.2% solution) | 10-mL prefilled syringes | 2 mEq/kg IV | **Weight (kg)** | **Total Dose (mEq)** | **Total mL** | Give slowly, over at least 2 minutes<br>Give only if infant is being effectively ventilated |
| | | | | 1 | 2 | 4 | |
| | | | | 2 | 4 | 8 | |
| | | | | 3 | 6 | 12 | |
| | | | | 4 | 8 | 16 | |
| Naloxone hydrochloride | 0.4 mg/mL | 1 mL | 0.1 mg/kg (0.25 mL/kg) IV, ET, IM, SC | **Weight (kg)** | **Total Dose (mg)** | **Total mL** | Give rapidly IV, ET preferred; IM, SC acceptable |
| | | | | 1 | 0.1 | 0.25 | |
| | | | | 2 | 0.2 | 0.50 | |
| | | | | 3 | 0.3 | 0.75 | |
| | | | | 4 | 0.4 | 1.00 | |
| | 1.0 mg/mL | 1 mL | 0.1 mL/kg (0.1 mL/kg) IV, ET, IM, SC | 1 | 0.1 | 0.1 | |
| | | | | 2 | 0.2 | 0.2 | |
| | | | | 3 | 0.3 | 0.3 | |
| | | | | 4 | 0.4 | 0.4 | |
| Dopamine | | | Begin at 5 µg/kg/min (may increase to 20 µg/kg/min if necessary)* | **Weight (kg)** | **Total µg/min** | | Give as a continuous infusion using an infusion pump<br>Monitor heart rate and blood pressure closely<br>Seek consultation |
| | | | | 1 | 5-20 | | |
| | | | | 2 | 10-40 | | |
| | | | | 3 | 15-60 | | |
| | | | | 4 | 20-80 | | |

*There is evidence that 2-3 µg/kg/min may be adequate in many infants (Seri, 1995).

ET, endotracheal; IM, intramuscular; IV, intravenous; SC, subcutaneous.

Data from Bloom RS, Cropley CS: American Heart Association–American Academy of Pediatrics Textbook of Neonatal Resuscitation. Dallas, American Heart Association National Center, 1994.

TABLE 28-4

**Apgar Scoring System**

| Feature Evaluated | 0 Points | 1 Point | 2 Points |
|---|---|---|---|
| Heart rate (beats/min) | 0 | <100 | >100 |
| Respiratory effort | Apnea | Irregular, shallow, or gasping respirations | Vigorous and crying |
| Color | Pale, blue | Pale or blue extremities | Pink |
| Muscle tone | Absent | Weak, passive tone | Active movement |
| Reflex irritability | Absent | Grimace | Active avoidance |

temperature control is of even greater importance for them than for the normal newborn. When possible, these infants should be moved to a small warm room adjacent to the delivery room, carefully dried, and placed under a radiant warmer for resuscitation. It is essential that the gas used for very small infants, even for resuscitation, be warmed and humidified.

Many extremely premature infants are at risk for respiratory distress syndrome and may benefit from surfactant therapy. Although clinical trials have demonstrated that both synthetic and natural surfactant preparations are effective, several trials documented the benefit of natural surfactant products over synthetic surfactant, including a reduction in pneumothorax and mortality (Soll and Blanco, 2001). The timing of the first dose of surfactant is controversial. Previous studies of extremely immature human infants demonstrated a benefit of surfactant given prophylactically—that is, within minutes after birth—over rescue surfactant therapy given later as symptoms develop (Soll and Morley, 2001). However, later attention has focused on variations in incidence of bronchopulmonary dysplasia among various neonatal intensive care units, and the association of intubation and prolonged ventilation with the development of this disorder (Van Marter et al, 2000). Therefore, many nurseries have instituted early and aggressive use of continuous distending pressure given via nasal prongs (nasal continuous positive airway pressure [CPAP]) in the delivery room, in an attempt to decrease barotrauma and the subsequent development of bronchopulmonary dysplasia. Because surfactant given prophylactically is more effective than late rescue therapy for respiratory distress syndrome, earlier delivery of surfactant, followed by rapid extubation to nasal CPAP, may benefit those extremely premature infants likely to progress to respiratory failure (Verder et al, 1999).

If an infant is intubated, it is critical to avoid overdistention of the lungs—which may lead to volutrauma, interstitial emphysema, and pneumothorax and may interfere with cardiac output—as well as hyperventilation and hypocarbia. Rapid changes in carbon dioxide, or prolonged hypocarbia, may alter cerebral blood flow and produce hypertension and have been associated with higher risk of periventricular leukomalacia (Wiswell et al, 1996). During resuscitation of very small infants, it is also important to avoid hyperoxia; therefore, the oxygen blender should be set at an $F_IO_2$ of 0.40 when resuscitation is begun, then turned down as rapidly as possible, and thereafter increased only if the infant has clinical signs of cyanosis.

Most of these tiny infants also benefit from placement of an umbilical artery catheter so that the initial monitoring of their blood gas values does not require painful procedures for obtaining blood or for the administration of fluid, drugs, or volume replacement. At many centers, umbilical venous lines are also placed. Arterial blood pressure monitoring is important in this group of infants as an adjunct to assessing adequacy of circulating blood volume. The range of mean blood pressure for the tiny infant is wide and initially may be as low as 24 to 30 mm Hg. In an infant who is well oxygenated at low inspired oxygen concentrations and who has good peripheral perfusion, low blood pressure alone should never be used as the basis for volume administration. One may consider initial blood pressure support with low-dose dopamine (2 to 5 μg/kg per minute) to augment diminished urinary output (Seri, 1995). Careful administration and monitoring of blood glucose concentrations are also critical.

Finally, it is important to move these infants from the resuscitation area to the nursery with as little disruption of their support systems as possible. Therefore, a resuscitation bed that is fully equipped to be moved from the delivery area to the nursery is essential to maintain stabilization. Such a bed also enables continuous observation of these fragile infants, whose courses may change rapidly during the first few hours after birth.

## Meconium Aspiration

Approximately 11% of all pregnancies are complicated by passage of meconium, and 2% of infants have some degree of aspiration syndrome, ranging from some minor initial tachypnea to very severe meconium aspiration pneumonia with pulmonary hypertension. Skilled personnel must be present at the delivery of an infant born through meconium. All infants born through meconium should undergo immediate suctioning of the oropharynx, preferably while still at the perineum and before initiation of respiration (Gregory et al, 1974).

If the infant is born through meconium and has depression of respiratory drive, decreased tone, and a heart rate of less than 100 beats/min, direct suctioning of the trachea soon after delivery is indicated. Vigorous infants may not benefit from tracheal suctioning. One study found no differences in respiratory outcomes of vigorous infants randomly assigned either to immediate tracheal suctioning or to expectant management alone (Wiswell et al, 2000). The passage of meconium indicates that an infant has been in trouble at some point during gestation. Such infants are more susceptible to having reactive pulmonary vessels, which may reconstrict with hypoxia. They need careful initial evaluation and close observation to ensure that oxygenation is adequate and to prevent the gradual development of hypoxia and consequent pulmonary vasoconstriction, which would set off the cycle that ultimately may result in persistent pulmonary hypertension of the newborn.

### Hydrops

The evaluation and resuscitation of the infant with hydrops, as of the very small premature infant, begins with interdisciplinary management by the perinatal team to assess the fetus and to arrive at decisions as to the optimal time of delivery. Ultrasonographic evaluation is recommended to determine whether the infant would benefit from removal of excessive fluid from either the abdominal or the thoracic cavity before delivery. In preparing for resuscitation of a hydropic infant, it is critical that equipment be set up and a member of the team assigned to perform paracentesis, thoracentesis, or both immediately after the birth, if the amount of fluid interferes with the ability to ventilate the infant. In addition, packed red cells must be available at the resuscitation site if the cause of the hydrops is related to anemia.

The hydropic infant has extremely stiff lungs and may require high ventilatory pressures, including high end-expiratory pressure, for initial stabilization until the infant begins to mobilize and clear fluid. It is always appropriate to catheterize both the umbilical vein and the umbilical artery so that central venous pressure, as well as systemic pressures, can be measured for evaluation of volume status. In addition, for severely anemic infants, the hematocrit value can be augmented by immediate, isovolemic exchange transfusion through the two catheters. Staff should be aware that skin electrodes and saturation monitors commonly do not function accurately when used for infants with hydrops.

### Infants with Severe Malformations

Sometimes the resuscitation team is faced with an infant who has severe malformations. Resuscitation should proceed in a normal fashion unless (1) the staff present at the delivery has enough experience and skill to recognize that the malformations are associated with conditions incompatible with life and (2) there has been some foreknowledge of the possibility of malformations and the family has requested that there be no resuscitation of a severely malformed infant. Otherwise, it is appropriate to proceed with the resuscitation and stabilize the infant so that an accurate diagnosis can be made and the family can see the baby and participate in further decision-making about the child.

### Resuscitation of the Previable Infant

Survival remains extremely low for infants born at less than 23 weeks of postmenstrual age or with birth weights of less than 400 g (El-Metwally et al, 2000). If dating appears accurate, one should discuss the poor survival and the option of comfort care without resuscitation with the parents before the delivery.

### Duration of Resuscitation

Resuscitation should rarely be pursued beyond 15 minutes in an infant who continues to have no pulse and who does not respond rapidly to adequate ventilation, appropriate cardiac compression, and resuscitative medications. In infants showing response after 15 minutes of resuscitation, the incidence of death or very severe, irreversible neurologic damage is unacceptably high (Casalaz et al, 1998; Davis, 1993; Jain et al, 1991).

## LONG-TERM OUTCOME

The two central questions to be considered in thinking about the outcome of an infant after perinatal asphyxia are as follows:

- What is the contribution of perinatal asphyxia to mental retardation and cerebral palsy in the population?
- How often does documented perinatal asphyxia result in cerebral palsy and mental retardation?

The etiology of severe mental retardation without cerebral palsy is usually not related to perinatal events; rather, it is primarily of genetic, infectious, or developmental origin (Blair and Stanley, 1988; Nelson, 1988; Perlman, 1997). Studies suggest that at least 70% of cases of cerebral palsy are antepartum in origin. Therefore, the number of cases of cerebral palsy related to perinatal asphyxia are few, approximately 20%. Only cases of cerebral palsy associated with severe mental retardation may have a peripartum cause (ACOG/AAP statement, 2003).

The attempt to delineate which cases of perinatal asphyxia lead to cerebral palsy began in 1862, when Little noted the association of suboptimal perinatal events with subsequent poor neurologic outcome. A number of studies since that time have attempted to relate outcome to Apgar score, to the interval between birth and spontaneous respiration, and to various biochemical and biophysical markers of oxygen deprivation. The Collaborative Perinatal Project, conducted from 1959 to 1966, reported on the outcomes of 49,000 infants as correlated with Apgar scores (Nelson and Ellenberg, 1981; Niswander et al, 1975) (Table 28–5). The conclusions of this study were that low Apgar scores are risk factors for cerebral palsy; other findings, however, are as follows:

- 55% of children with cerebral palsy had Apgar scores of 7 to 10 at 1 minute.
- 73% of children with cerebral palsy had Apgar scores of 7 to 10 at 5 minutes.
- Of 99 children who had Apgar scores of 0 to 3 at 10, 15, or 20 minutes, only 12 (12%) had cerebral palsy; however, the mortality rate in the last group was more than 50% in infants weighing more than 2500 g and more than 90% in infants weighing less than 2500 g.
- 11 of the 12 infants with cerebral palsy were mentally retarded.

TABLE 28–5

**Prevalence Rates of Cerebral Palsy by Apgar Score and Birth Weight**

| | Infants < 2500 g | | | Infants > 2500 g | | |
|---|---|---|---|---|---|---|
| **Apgar Score** | **Mortality in 1st Year (%)** | **Survivors with Cerebral Palsy (%)** | **No. of Cases of Cerebral Palsy** | **Mortality in 1st Year (%)** | **Survivors with Cerebral Palsy (%)** | **No. of Cases of Cerebral Palsy** |
| 7-10 @ 1 minute | 3.8 | 0.6 | 13 | <1 | 0.2 | 53 |
| 0-3 @ 1 minute | 50 | 2.9 | 9 | 6 | 1.5 | 22 |
| 0-3 @ 5 minutes | 75 | 6.7 | 5 | 15 | 4.7 | 13 |
| 0-3 @ 10 minutes | 85 | 3.7 | 1 | 34 | 16.7 | 11 |
| 0-3 @ 15 minutes | 92 | 0 | 0 | 52 | 36.0 | 9 |
| 0-3 @ 20 minutes | 96 | 0 | 0 | 59 | 36.0 | 8 |

Data from Nelson KB, Ellenberg JH: Apgar scores as prediction of chronic neurologic disability. Pediatrics 68:36, 1981. Reproduced by permission of Pediatrics.

## Hypoxic-Ischemic Encephalopathy

Sarnat and Sarnat (1975) developed a clinical staging system for evaluating hypoxic-ischemic encephalopathy (HIE) (Table 28–6), and Robertson and Finer (1985) reported on the follow-up of infants after HIE (Table 28–7). The latter investigators found that 100% of infants with severe HIE either died or had significant handicaps. Among those with moderate HIE, 26% died or were handicapped; among those with mild HIE, none died subsequently or were handicapped (Robertson and Finer, 1985). Robertson and associates (1989) also noted no differences in school performance (at 8 years of age) between neurologically unimpaired children who suffered mild or moderate HIE and a matched peer group.

Holden and colleagues (1982) noted that the incidence of seizures was associated with a 17-fold increase in the likelihood of cerebral palsy over that in the absence of seizures. Some investigators have attempted to use injuries to other organs as indicators to help predict eventual outcome. Perlman and Tack (1988) found that oliguria in the perinatal period was significantly associated with signs of HIE, including seizures, death, and long-term neurologic deficits. In general, it can be assumed that an infant who has experienced an asphyxial event severe enough to produce permanent brain damage will show evidence of

TABLE 28–6

**Clinical Staging of Posthypoxia Encephalopathy**

| **Factor** | **Stage I** | **Stage II** | **Stage III** |
|---|---|---|---|
| Level of consciousness | Alert | Lethargic | Comatose |
| Muscle tone | Normal | Hypotonic | Flaccid |
| Tendon reflexes | Increased | Present | Depressed or absent |
| Myoclonus | Present | Present | Absent |
| Complex reflexes | | | |
| Sucking | Active | Weak | Absent |
| Moro response | Exaggerated | Incomplete | Absent |
| Grasping | Normal to exaggerated | Exaggerated | Absent |
| Oculocephalic response (doll's eyes) | Normal | Overreactive | Reduced or absent |
| Autonomic function | | | |
| Pupils | Dilated | Constricted | Variable or fixed |
| Respiration | Regular | Variations in rate and depth, periodic | Ataxic, apneic |
| Heart rate | Normal or tachycardia | Bradycardia | Bradycardia |
| Seizures | None | Common | Uncommon |
| Electroencephalogram | Normal | Low voltage, periodic and/or paroxysmal | Periodic or isoelectric |

Data from Sarnat HB, Sarnat MS: Neonatal encephalopathy following fetal distress. Arch Neurol 33:696, 1975.

**TABLE 28-7**

**Outcome 3 to 5 Years after Hypoxic-Ischemic Encephalopathy (HIE)**

| Severity of HIE | Total No. of Infants | No. of Infants for whom Information was Available at 3-5 Yrs | Number of Deaths | Outcome at 3–5 Years | |
|---|---|---|---|---|---|
| | | | | Normal | Handicapped |
| Mild | 79 | 69 | 0 | 69 | 0 |
| Moderate | 119 | 103 | 6* | 75 | 22 |
| Severe† | 28 | 28 | 21 | 0 | 7 |
| Total | | | | | |
| Number | 226 | 200 | 27 | 144 | 29 |
| Percentage | 100 | 88.5 | 13.5‡ | 83.2§ | 16.8§ |

*One death was due to an unrelated accident.

†All infants died or became handicapped.

‡Percentage of the 200 infants for whom information was available.

§Percentage of the 173 survivors for whom information was available.

Classification data from Sarnat HB, Sarnat MS: Neonatal encephalopathy following fetal distress. Arch Neurol 33: 696, 1975; data from Robertson C, Finer H: Term infants with hypoxic-ischemic encephalopathy: Outcome at 3-5 years. Dev Med Child Neurol 27:473, 1985.

significant damage to other organs within hours to days after birth.

Sunshine (1989) concluded that infants with perinatal asphyxia should be evaluated for structural abnormalities with current imaging techniques and that if such abnormalities are identified, an attempt should be made to determine whether the abnormalities can be explained by intrapartum asphyxia or are developmental aberrations or abnormalities that occurred before labor. In addition, Sunshine pointed out that infants who are small for gestational age compose a significant percentage of the total number of patients who experience neonatal asphyxia, HIE, and seizures as well as cerebral palsy. Therefore, attempts to improve outcome should focus on recognition of infants who are small for gestational age and on possible types of intervention in pregnancies complicated by intrauterine growth restriction. Other investigations have been directed at the prevention of intracellular calcium accumulation, free radical formation, or excitatory amino acid release—all of which are associated with hypoxic ischemic injury (Perlman, 1997).

The most accurate prediction of neurologic outcome comes from a full knowledge of perinatal and neonatal events, combined with biochemical and imaging studies and careful clinical evaluations performed throughout the first years of life.

## REFERENCES

American Academy of Pediatrics Committee on Drugs: Emergency drug doses for infants and children. Pediatrics 81:462, 1988.

American Academy of Pediatrics, American Heart Association: Textbook of Neonatal Resuscitation, 4th ed. Elk Grove Village, IL, American Academy of Pediatrics, American Heart Association, 2000.

American College of Obstetricians and Gynecologists (ACOG) Task Force on Neonatal Encephalopathy and Cerebral Palsy: Neonatal Encephalopathy and Cerebral Palsy: Defining the Pathogenesis and Pathophysiology. Washington, DC, American College of Obstetricians and Gynecologists, 2003.

Amiel-Tison C: Neurologic disorders in neonates associated with abnormalities of pregnancy and birth. Curr Probl Pediatr 3:1, 1973.

Apgar V: A proposal for new method for evaluation of the newborn infant. Anesth Analg 32:260, 1953.

Blair E, Stanley J: Intrapartum asphyxia: A rare cause of cerebral palsy. J Pediatr 112:515, 1988.

Bloom RS, Cropley CS: American Heart Association–American Academy of Pediatrics Textbook of Neonatal Resuscitation. Dallas, American Heart Association National Center, 1994.

Burchfield DJ: Medication use in neonatal resuscitation. Clin Perinatol 26:683, 1999.

Carson BS, Lasey BW, Bowes WA, et al: Combined obstetric and pediatric approach to prevent meconium aspiration syndrome. Am J Obstet Gynecol 126:712, 1976.

Casalaz DM, Marlow N, Spiedel BD: Outcome of resuscitation following unexpected apparent stillbirth. Arch Dis Child Fetal Neonatal Ed 78:112, 1998.

Davis DJ: How aggressive should delivery room cardiopulmonary resuscitation be for extremely low-birth-weight neonates? Pediatrics 92:447, 1993.

Dawes G: Foetal and Neonatal Physiology. Chicago, Year Book, 1968.

El-Metwally D, Vohr B, Tucker RB: Survival and neonatal morbidity at the limits of viability in the mid-1990s: 22 to 25 weeks. J Pediatr 137:616, 2000.

Garland JS, Buck RK, Allred EN, Leviton A: Hypocarbia before surfactant therapy appears to increase bronchopulmonary dysplasia risk in infants with respiratory distress syndrome. Arch Pediatr Adolesc Med 149:617, 1995.

Gonzalez ER, Ornato JP, Garnett AR, et al: Dose dependent vasopressor response to epinephrine during CPR in human beings. Ann Emerg Med 18:920, 1989.

Greenough H, Lagercrantz H, Pool J, et al: Plasma catecholamine levels in preterm infants: Effect of birth asphyxia and Apgar score. Acta Paediatr Scand 76:54, 1987.

Gregory GA, Gooding CA, Phibbs RH, et al: Meconium aspiration in infants: A prospective study. J Pediatr 85:807, 1974.

Holden KR, Mellits ED, Freeman JM: Neonatal seizures. I. Correlation of prenatal and perinatal events with outcomes. Pediatrics 70:165, 1982.

Jain L, Ferre C, Vidyasagar D, et al: Cardiopulmonary resuscitation of apparently stillborn infants: Survival and long term outcome. J Pediatr 118:778, 1991.

Lagercrantz H, Slotkin TA: The "stress" of being born. Sci Am 254:100, 1986.

Lindemann R: Resuscitation of the newborn with endotracheal administration of epinephrine. Acta Paediatr Scand 73:210, 1984.

Little WJ: On the influence of abnormal parturition, difficult labours, premature birth, and asphyxia neonatorum on the mental and physical condition of the child, especially in relation to deformities. Trans Obstet Soc (London) 3:293, 1861-1862.

Martin JA, Hamilton BE, Ventura SJ, et al: Births: Final data for 2001. Nat Vital Stat Rep 51:1, 2002.

Martinez A, Padbury J, Shames L, et al: Naloxone potentiates epinephrine release during hypoxia in fetal sheep: Dose response and cardiovascular effects. Pediatr Res 23:343, 1988.

Massaro GD, Massaro D: Morphologic evidence that large inflations of the lung stimulate secretion of surfactant. Ann Rev Respir Dis 127:235, 1983.

McCrirrick A, Kestin I: Haemodynamic effects of tracheal compared with intravenous adrenaline. Lancet 340:868, 1992.

Menegazzi JJ, Auble TE, Nicklas KA, et al: Two-thumb versus two-finger chest compression during CPR in a swine infant model of cardiac arrest. Ann Emerg Med 22:240, 1993.

Nelson KB: What proportion of cerebral palsy is related to birth asphyxia? J Pediatr 112:572, 1988.

Nelson KB, Ellenberg JH: Apgar scores as prediction of chronic neurologic disability. Pediatrics 68:36, 1981.

Newnham JP, Marshall CL, Padbury JF, et al: Fetal catecholamine release with preterm delivery. Am J Obstet Gynecol 149:888, 1984.

Niswander KR, Gordon M, Drage JS: The effect of intrauterine hypoxia on the child surviving to 4 years. Am J Obstet Gynecol 121:892, 1975.

Paradis NA, Martin GB, Rosenberg J, et al: The effect of standard- and high-dose epinephrine on coronary perfusion pressure during prolonged cardiopulmonary resuscitation. JAMA 265:1139, 1991.

Pasternak JF, Grootthuis DR, Fischer JM, et al: Regional cerebral blood flow in the beagle puppy model of neonatal intraventricular hemorrhage: Studies during systemic hypertension. Neurology 33:559, 1983.

Patel D, Piotrowski ZH, Nelson MR, et al: Effect of a statewide neonatal training program on Apgar scores among high-risk neonates in Illinois. Pediatrics 107:648, 2001.

Perlman JM: Intrapartum hypoxic-ischemic cerebral injury and subsequent cerebral palsy: Medicolegal issues. Pediatrics 99:851, 1997.

Perlman JM, Risser R: Cardiopulmonary resuscitation in the delivery room. Arch Pediatr Adolesc Med 149:2025, 1995.

Perlman JM, Tack ED: Renal injury in the asphyxiated newborn infant: Relationship to neurologic outcome. J Pediatr 113:875, 1988.

Ralston SH, Tacker WA, Showen L, et al: Endotracheal versus intravenous epinephrine during electromechanical dissociation with CPR in dogs. Ann Emerg Med 14:1044, 1985.

Ramji S, Ahuja S, Thirupuram S, et al: Resuscitation of asphyxic newborn infants with room air or 100% oxygen. Pediatr Res 34:809, 1993.

Reynolds ML, Evans CA, Reynolds EO, et al: Intracranial hemorrhage in the preterm sheep fetus. Early Hum Develop 3:163, 1979.

Robertson C, Finer N: Term infants with hypoxic-ischemic encephalopathy: Outcome at 3.5 years. Dev Med Child Neurol 27:473, 1985.

Robertson CMT, Finer NN, Grace MGA: School performance of survivors of neonatal encephalopathy associated with birth asphyxia at term. J Pediatr 114:753, 1989.

Rootwelt T, Loberg EM, Moen A, Saugstad OS: Hypoxemia and reoxygenation with 21% or 100% oxygen in newborn pigs: Changes in blood pressure, base deficit and hypoxanthine and brain morphology. Pediatr Res 32:107, 1992.

Sarnat HB, Sarnat MS: Neonatal encephalopathy following fetal distress. Arch Neurol 33:696, 1975.

Saugstad OD: Oxygen toxicity in the neonatal period. Acta Paediatr Scand 79:881, 1990.

Saugstad OD: Resuscitation of newborn infants: Do we need new guidelines? Prenatal Neonatal Med 1:26, 1996.

Seri I: Cardiovascular, renal, and endocrine actions of dopamine in neonates and children: Medical progress. J Pediatr 126:333, 1995.

Soll RF, Blanco F: Natural surfactant extract versus synthetic surfactant for neonatal respiratory distress syndrome. Cochrane Database Syst Rev CD000144, 2001.

Soll RF, Morley CJ: Prophylactic versus selective use of surfactant in preventing morbidity and mortality in preterm infants. Cochrane Database Syst Rev CD000510, 2001.

Strang LB: Neonatal Respiration: Physiological and Clinical Studies. Oxford, Blackwell Scientific, 1977.

Sunshine P: Epidemiology of perinatal asphyxia. In Stevenson DK, Sunshine P (eds): Fetal and Neonatal Brain Injury. Philadelphia, BC Decker, 1989.

Taeusch HW, Wyszogrodski I, Wang NS, et al: Pulmonary pressure-volume relationships in premature fetal and newborn rabbits. J Appl Physiol 37:809, 1974.

Van Marter LJ, Allred EN, Pagano M, et al: Do clinical markers of barotrauma and oxygen toxicity explain interhospital variation in the rate of chronic lung disease? The neonatal committee for the developmental network. Pediatrics 105: 1194, 2000.

Vento M, Asensi M, Sastre J, et al: Resuscitation with room air instead of 100% oxygen prevents oxidative stress in moderately asphyxiated term neonates. Pediatrics 107:642, 2001.

Verder H, Albertsen P, Ebbsen F, et al: Nasal continuous positive airway pressure and early surfactant therapy for respiratory distress syndrome in newborns of less than 30 weeks' gestation. Pediatrics 103:E24, 1999.

Walters DV, Olver RE: The role of catecholamines in lung liquid absorption at birth. Pediatr Res 12:239, 1978.

Wiswell TE, Graziani LJ, Kornhauser MS, et al: Effects of hypocarbia on the development of cystic periventricular leukomalacia in premature infants with high frequency jet ventilation. Pediatrics 98:918, 1996.

Wiswell TE, Gannon CM, Jacob J, et al: Delivery room management of the apparently vigorous meconium-stained neonate: Results of a multicenter, international collaborative trial. Pediatrics 105:1, 2000.

Wu T-J, Carlo WA: Neonatal resuscitation guidelines 2000: Framework for practice. J Matern Fetal Neonatal Med 11:4, 2002.

CHAPTER

# 29

# Temperature Regulation of the Premature Infant

Sudhish Chandra and Stephen Baumgart

The human neonate is a homeothermic mammal. Even the smallest premature infants respond adaptively to changes in their environment. Response, however, may be insufficient to maintain core body temperature and render preterm babies functionally poikilothermic, even in moderately temperate environments. Morbidity (e.g., poor brain and somatic growth) and mortality rates increase when core body temperature is permitted to decline much below 36° C (96.8° F).

## THE PROBLEM OF COLD STRESS

Evaporative heat loss is widely regarded as the most stressful cooling event on any infant's delivery at birth. Severe nonevaporative heat loss is also problematic, however, for several reasons. First, the baby's exposed surface area is much larger than the adult's relative to metabolically active body mass (Table 29–1). Especially for the extremely low-birth-weight (ELBW) infant, the heat-dissipating area is proportionately five to six times greater than that of the adult. Second, the tiny baby's small size presents a much smaller heat sink to store thermal reserve. Finally, the radius of curvature of the body is less in the infant than in the adult, resulting in a thinner protective boundary layer of warm, still air.

Aside from these geometric considerations, characteristics of the premature infant's skin contribute to the problem of excessive heat loss. The skin and subcutaneous fascia provide little insulation against the flow of heat from the core to the surface. Moreover, the lack of a keratinized epidermal barrier exposes infants to vastly greater evaporative heat loss.

Finally, premature infants may not induce effective thermogenesis in response to cold stress. They lack shivering, and nonshivering thermogenesis may be compromised by low stores of brown fat. Furthermore, the presence of hypoxia (common with preterm birth) seriously reduces nonshivering thermogenesis by reducing mitochondrial oxidative capacity.

## PHYSICAL ROUTES OF HEAT LOSS

### Convection

Convective heat loss in newborns occurs when ambient air temperature is less than the infant's skin temperature. Convective heat loss occurs through (1) natural convection, or passage of heat from the skin to the ambient still air, and (2) forced convection, in which mass movement of air over the infant conveys heat away from the skin. The quantity of heat lost is proportional to the difference between air and skin temperatures and to air speed. The effect of forced convection in disrupting the microenvironment of warm, humid air layered near an infant's skin is usually not appreciated in the nursery, where drafts, air turbulence, and, consequently, heat loss may occur even within the relatively protective environment of an incubator (Okken, 1982).

### Evaporation

Passive transcutaneous evaporation of water from a newborn's skin (insensible water loss) results in the dissipation of 0.58 kcal/mL latent heat. As shown in Figure 29–1, transcutaneous water loss increases exponentially with decreasing body size and gestation. The tiniest premature baby, least able to tolerate cold stress, may incur evaporative heat loss in excess of 4 kcal/kg/hour ($\approx$7 mL water/kg/hour). Evaporation is enhanced by low vapor pressure (high temperature and low relative humidity) and air turbulence. The highest evaporative losses occur on the first day of life. During the first week of life in infants of 25 to 27 weeks of gestation, evaporative heat losses may be higher than radiant losses (Hammarlund et al, 1986).

### Radiation

Radiant heat loss constitutes the transfer of heat from an infant's warm skin via infrared electromagnetic waves to the cooler surrounding walls that absorb this heat. Radiant heat loss is proportional to the temperature gradient between the skin and surrounding walls. An infant's posture may affect radiant heat loss by increasing or reducing the exposed radiating surface area. In a humid environment (relative humidity $\approx$50%), babies experience an ambient temperature (termed *operant temperature*) determined 60% by wall temperature and 40% by air temperature.

### Conduction

Conductive heat loss to cooler surfaces in contact with an infant's skin depends on the conductivity of the surface material as well as its temperature. Usually, babies are nursed on insulating mattresses and blankets that minimize conductive heat loss.

## PHYSIOLOGY OF COLD RESPONSE

### Afferents

Homeothermic response to a cold environment begins with the sensation of temperature. Traditional physiology identifies two temperature-sensitive sites, the hypothalamus and the skin. Sensing of cold by the neonatal skin triggers a cold-adaptive response long before core sensors in the hypothalamus become chilled. Some investigators conjecture that neonatal cold reception resides primarily

**TABLE 29–1**

**Body Surface Area to Body Mass Ratio**

| | Body Weight (kg) | Surface Area ($m^2$) | Ratio ($cm^2/kg$) |
|---|---|---|---|
| Adult | 70 | 1.73 | 250 |
| Very premature infant | 1.5 | 0.13 | 870 |
| Extremely premature infant | 0.5 | 0.07 | 1400 |

in the skin, whereas warm reception resides in the hypothalamus. Both sensors are probably integrated, however, because cold sensory response is inhibited by core sensor hyperthermia, and vice versa. Peripheral skin cold sensation is teleologically important, because early detection of heat loss from the skin aids in the infant's timely response for maintaining core temperature.

### Central Regulation

Integration of multiple skin temperature inputs probably occurs in the hypothalamus. No single control temperature seems to exist, however. Under different environmental conditions, temperature of the skin may fluctuate by 8° C to 10° C, and temperature of the hypothalamus may vary by 0.5° C. There are also diurnal temperature fluctuations, variations with general sympathetic tone, and blunted regulation with asphyxia, hypoxemia, and other central nervous system defects. Because important thermoregulatory processes are triggered by changes as little as 0.5° C, deviation at any temperature-sensitive site is important (Mayfield, 1984).

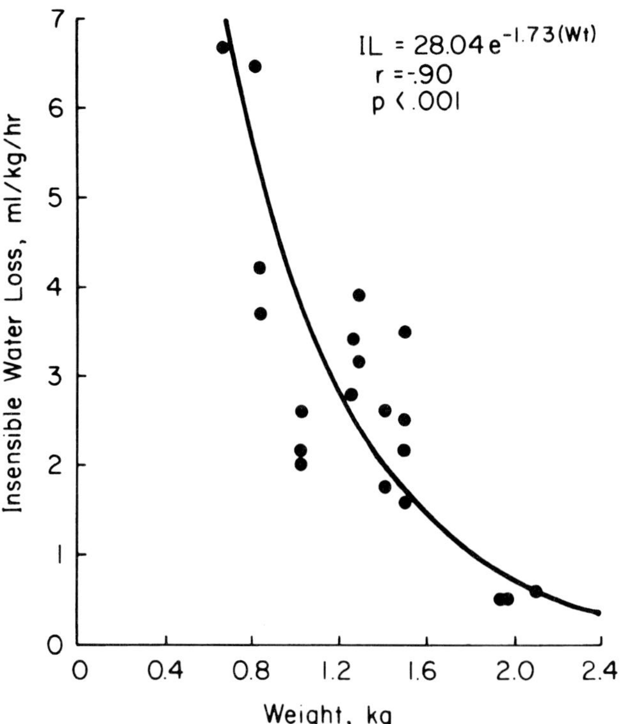


**FIGURE 29–1.** Exponential rise in evaporative water loss from the skin of very low-birth-weight infants nurtured under radiant warmers. *(Adapted with permission from Baumgart S, Langman CB, Sosulski R, et al: Fluid, electrolyte and glucose maintenance in the very low birth weight infant. Clin Pediatr 21:199–206, 1982.)*

### Efferents

The effector limb of the neonatal thermal response is mediated primarily by the sympathetic nervous system, although infant behavior may also be involved. The earliest maturing response is vasoconstriction in deep dermal arterioles, resulting in reduced flow of warm blood from the infant's core into the exposed periphery. Additionally, reduction of blood flow effectively places a layer of insulating fat between the core and the exposed skin in the term infant. Reduced fat content in LBW babies, however, diminishes this effective insulating property. Vasoconstriction nevertheless remains the newborn's first line of defense, and the response is present even in the most premature infant.

Brown fat constitutes a second sympathetic effector organ that provides a metabolic source of nonshivering thermogenesis (babies do not shiver like adults do to generate heat). Brown fat located in axillary, mediastinal, perinephric, and other regions of the newborn is especially innervated and equipped with an abundance of mitochondria to hydrolyze and re-esterify triglycerides and to oxidize free fatty acids. In the term infant, these reactions are exothermic and may increase metabolic rate twofold or more. Preterm babies, however, have little brown fat and may not be capable of more than a 25% increase in metabolic rate despite the most severe cold stress (Hull, 1966).

Finally, evidence suggests that control of voluntary muscle tone, posture, and increased motor activity with agitation may serve to augment heat production in skeletal muscle via glycogenolysis and glucose oxidation. Clinical observations of infant posture, behavior, and skin perfusion, and measurements of skin and core temperature gradients may ultimately provide the most useful guidelines for assessing infant comfort during incubation.

## MODERN INCUBATION: INCUBATORS AND RADIANT WARMERS

The lifesaving requirement of an appropriate thermal environment was demonstrated conclusively by Day and colleagues (1964) and further defined by Silverman and associates (1966). Minor changes in heat balance exact oxygen and energy costs, inducing an increase in metabolic rate that can be met only by an increase in ventilation or inspired oxygen and appropriate cardiovascular response.

### Thermal Neutral Zone

The thermal neutral zone is a narrow range of environmental temperatures within which an infant's metabolic rate is at a minimum and normal body temperature is maintained. When thermally neutral, infants regulate temperature through vasomotor tone alone without regulatory changes in metabolic heat production. A range of "critical" environmental temperatures relevant to modern incubators was clearly articulated by Hey and Katz (1970) (Fig. 29–2; Table 29–2). Below this range, these researchers observed an increase in the infant's minimal metabolic rate. The thermal neutral temperature range, therefore, was defined as the optimal incubator operating (operant) temperature. Several important considerations in regulating incubator temperature were included in these studies; (1) incubator wall temperature was maintained identical to air temperature, (2) relative humidity was controlled near 50%, and (3) the environment was kept in a steady state, uninterrupted by turbulence or invasion of the incubator's enclosed perimeter.

Rigid application of older air temperature recommendations should be modified. Many modern incubators now incorporate a double-walled design that results in lower radiant heat loss to cold incubator walls than is encountered in single-walled designs. Therefore, slightly cooler air temperature may be required (Bell and Rios, 1983a; Marks, 1981). Also, many nurseries do not humidify incubators artificially, fearing the occurrence of condensation ("rain-out") resulting in bacterial colonization, particularly around door openings. Finally, it is important to recognize that the incubator's steady-state temperature control is frequently interrupted for nursing and medical procedures that require opening doors to care for the infant. More than an hour may be required to recover previous steady-state conditions after such procedures. Therefore, the thermal neutral zone must be redefined in practical terms.

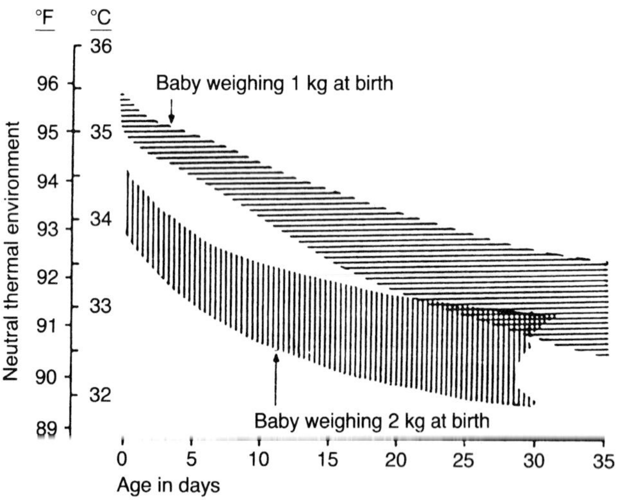


**FIGURE 29–2.** The range of temperature needed to provide neutral environmental conditions for a baby lying naked on a warm mattress in draft-free surroundings of moderate humidity (50% saturation) when mean radiant temperature is the same as air temperature. The *hatched areas* indicate the average neutral temperature range for a healthy baby weighing 1 kg or 2 kg at birth. Optimum temperature probably approximates the lower limit of neutral range as defined here. Approximately 1° C should be added to these operative temperatures to derive the appropriate neutral air temperature for a single-walled incubator when room temperature is less than 27° C (80° F), and more should be added if room temperature is very much less. *(From Hey EN, Katz G: The optimum thermal environment for naked babies. Arch Dis Child 45:328,1970, with permission BMJ Publishing Group.)*

**TABLE 29–2**

**Mean Temperature Needed to Provide Thermal Neutrality for a Healthy Baby Nursed Naked in Draft-Free Surroundings of Uniform Temperature and Moderate Humidity after Birth**

| Birth Weight (kg) | Operative Environmental Temperature* | | | |
|---|---|---|---|---|
| | **35° C** | **34° C** | **33° C** | **32° C** |
| 1.0 | For 10 days | After 10 days | After 3 weeks | After 5 weeks |
| 1.5 | — | For 10 days | After 10 days | After 4 weeks |
| 2.0 | — | For 2 days | After 2 days | After 3 weeks |
| >2.5 | — | | For 2 days | After 2 days |

*To estimate operative temperature in a single-walled incubator, subtract 1° C from incubator air temperature for every 7° C by which this temperature exceeds room temperature.

Data from Hey E: Thermal neutrality. Br Med Bull 31:69-74, 1975.

Silverman and colleagues (1966) used a modified concept of the thermal neutral zone to simplify clinical application. Reasoning that infants sense environmental temperature first on the skin, electronic negative-feedback (servo-controlled) regulation of the incubator heater in response to skin temperature was used. These investigators demonstrated minimal metabolic expenditure near 36.5° C (97.7° F) abdominal skin temperature measured by a shielded thermistor in a less rigidly defined incubator environment. The importance of frequently checking core temperatures (axillary or rectal) must be emphasized, however, before the infant's environment can be delegated to such thermostatic control (Bell and Rios, 1983b). In addition, Chessex and associates (1988) have demonstrated that incubator temperature may vary by more than 2° C when skin temperature is servo-controlled rather than air temperature control is used.

Finally, with the modern use of open radiant warmer beds (improving access to the critically ill premature infant without interrupting heat delivery), skin temperature servo-control is the only practical method for approximating the thermal neutral zone (Malin and Baumgart, 1987). These variations in incubator design and technique, and the extension of infant warming to include extremely LBW (ELBW), critically ill premature babies, have generated new problems for determining a universally accepted optimal environment.

## Partitioning Infant Heat Losses and Heat Gains

Wheldon and Rutter (1982) demonstrated the special problems encountered in incubating very LBW (VLBW) infants in a convection-warmed, closed-hood incubator environment. The top graph of Figure 29–3A, reproduced from their study, demonstrates the thermal balance achieved by a series of 12 infants (mean weight 1.58 kg). Heat losses to radiation (R), convection (C), and evaporation (E) are modest, and their sum (S) is balanced by the infant's metabolic heat production (M). Used in this fashion, the incubator reduces physical heat losses such that the infant's minimal metabolism (larger than any single avenue of heat loss) delicately balances minimal physical heat losses within the controlled thermal environment.

In contrast, a VLBW subject (1.08 kg) is evaluated in Figure 29–3B. As the incubator servo-control increases warming power (to accommodate massive evaporative heat loss), convective "loss" becomes a net "gain" (negative histogram bar). Radiant loss is diminished by warm walls inside the incubator. These conditions differ strikingly from those discussed previously in the following ways: (1) the incubator truly warms the infant rather than modestly attenuating convective heat loss and (2) evaporative heat loss vastly exceeds the infant's metabolism. The very small infant's body temperature is balanced, therefore, between opposing physical parameters of evaporative and convective heat transfer, and metabolism plays a secondary role.

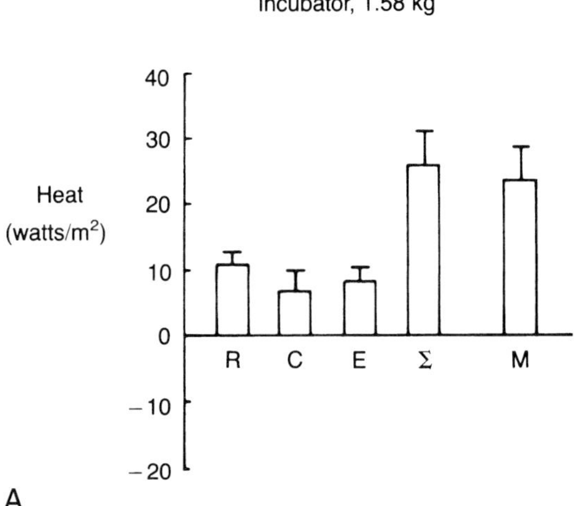


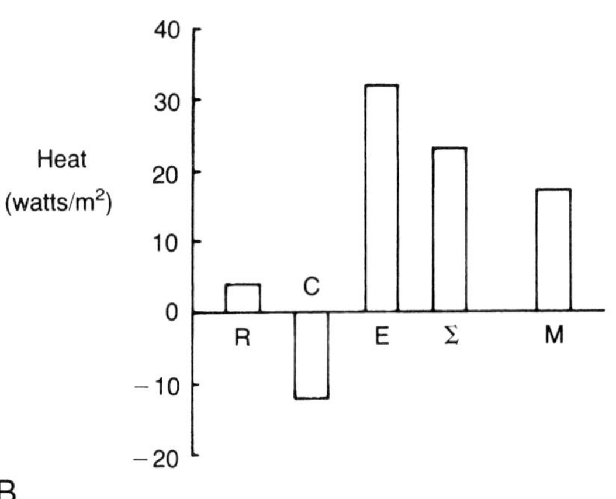


**FIGURE 29–3.** **A,** Partition of heat losses and gains in 12 premature infants nursed in incubators. **B,** Partition in a 1.08 kg low birth weight newborn. See text for detailed discussion. *(From Wheldon AE, Rutter N: The heat balance of small babies nursed in incubators and under radiant warmers. Early Hum Dev 6:131–143, 1982.)*

The modern use of radiant warmers that are servo-controlled to maintain infant abdominal skin temperature between 36.5° C and 37° C (97.7° F to 98.6° F) also demonstrates the opposition of physical forces described earlier. Figure 29–4 demonstrates the heat balance partition for 10 critically ill premature infants (mean weight 1.39 kg) nursed on open radiant warmer beds (Baumgart, 1985, 1990). Because ambient room air temperature is 5° C to 10° C cooler than air inside an incubator, convective heat loss is nearly double the infant's metabolic heat production. Evaporation adds to the net physical heat loss. Also, small amounts of heat are lost to conduction and radiation (to cooler room walls). The infant's metabolism provides only one third of the energy required to maintain body temperature, with the majority of heat supplied by the servo-controlled radiant heat source. In this instance, radiant warming (not convection, as in the incubator discussed earlier) delicately balances the infant's physical temperature environment. Wheldon and Rutter (1982) demonstrated similar results in their studies.

## LESS CONVENTIONAL TECHNIQUES

### Plastic Hoods

Plastic hoods are rigid body shields sometimes used as miniature incubator hoods placed over infants on open radiant beds. Hoods are usually made of 1- to 3-mm thick plastic and, when placed between an infant and the radiant warming element, may obstruct the delivery of radiant heat to the baby's skin. The plastic may form a heat sink, warming to 42° C to 44° C, but disrupts the radiant warmer's servo-control mechanism; in our opinion, use of such hoods is a poor strategy. In addition, such devices may not diminish insensible water loss, especially when used without humidity (Bell and Weinstein et al, 1980). Their use with humidity (a technique never validated) encourages bacterial colonization with waterborne pathogens.

A new development in commercial convection-warmed incubator and radiant warming technology is a hybrid design, combining the two separate warming modes into one device. In the incubator mode, movable plastic walls enclose the tiny premature infant, providing servo-controlled air warming, and the overhead radiant warmer is turned off. In the radiant warmer mode, the plastic walls are retracted to the sides, and the radiant warmer rapidly heats up to maintain servo-controlled skin temperature during procedures. The infant is not moved during the transition, and no plastic barrier is interposed between the infant and the radiant heater when it is on. The servo-control algorithms and the integrity of the plastic enclosure in incubator mode are critical to the performance of such devices, and the utility of these products is yet to be proven.

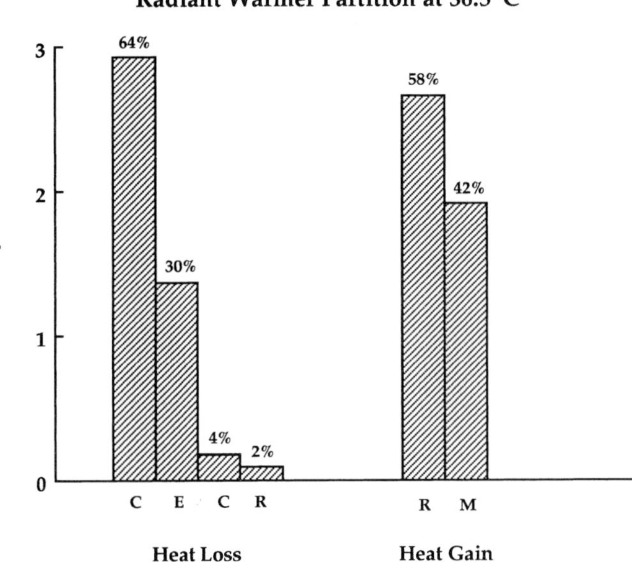


**FIGURE 29-4.** Partitional calorimetry in ten critically ill, low-birth-weight, premature newborns nursed under open radiant warmers. *(From Baumgart S: Radiant heat loss vs. radiant heat gain in premature neonates under radiant warmers. Biol Neonate 57:10-20, 1990; reproduced with permission of S. Karger AG, Basel.)*

## Plastic Blankets

As an alternative, a thin, flexible saran or polyethelene plastic "blanket" was introduced for covering premature infants under radiant warmers (Baumgart, 1984; Baumgart et al, 1982a, 1982b). This blanket prevents convective heat loss and is thin enough to transmit radiant heat from the warmer almost completely. The flexible plastic molds closely around the infant's body (with care taken to avoid skin adhesion), conserves evaporation, and forms a microenvironment near the baby's body. The plastic is enough of a mechanical barrier to prevent convective turbulence from disrupting this microenvironment. A two-thirds reduction in insensible water (and evaporative heat) loss under radiant warmers is achieved, so that less servo-controlled radiant heat delivery is required to maintain body temperature in even the smallest infants. Through moderation of heat losses, oxygen consumption is reduced by about 10%. Risks of plastic blankets include sticking to immature skin (causing skin breakdown) and accidental airway obstruction in non-intubated patients. In rare cases, partial detachment of the skin thermistor may result in life-threatening hyperthermia. Diligence is required to avoid these complications. The risk of abnormal bacterial colonization with the use of plastic blankets has not been evaluated.

Vohra and colleagues (1999) evaluated the capacity of a polyethylene plastic bag to promote temperature maintenance during resuscitation performed at delivery (under radiant warmers) and the transport of infants to the neonatal intensive care unit (NICU). Significantly higher admission rectal temperatures and subsequent survival rates were reported for infants younger than 28 weeks of gestation with use of the bag. A larger, randomized trial of this technique is underway.

## Semipermeable Polyurethane "Skin"

A semipermeable, semi-occlusive polyurethane dressing (Tegaderm or Op-Site) can be applied like an artificial skin to shield VLBW premature infants. These "breathing" polyurethane plastics do not cause skin breakdown and are often used to dress central venous catheter sites. Because such dressings adhere to the skin, the temperature probe is less likely to become detached. These dressings can be tailored to avoid airway obstruction. Insensible water loss may be reduced more than 30% with these dressings, and after their careful removal, the skin's naturally developing keratin moisture barrier may be preserved (Knauth et al, 1988). Porot and associates (1993) demonstrated that an adherent polyurethane layer over the torso and extremities of VLBW infants not only improved fluid and electrolyte balance but also reduced the occurrences of PDA and IVH and improved survival rates. Further studies are required to demonstrate the safety of this technique.

## Petroleum Ointments

Another occlusive dressing for the skin of LBW preterm infants during the first week of life is the application of Aquaphor™. Early results were encouraging for preservation of skin integrity and perhaps control of excessive dehydration in incubators (Nopper et al, 1996). However, the findings of a multicenter randomized trial have not yet been published, and some anecdotal reports suggest that bacterial infections may actually be more common with the use of this technique (Edwards, 2001; Oski, 2001). Until the results of the multicenter trial are conclusive, clinicians should exercise critical judgment about adopting this practice.

## Kangaroo Care

*Kangaroo care* is the warming of the infant through skin-to-skin contact with the mother or father; the parent holds the naked premature infant against her or his skin between the axilla or the breasts, mimicking a kangaroo's pouch. First implemented in Bogota, Columbia, this method was popularized for non-intubated premature infants in Scandinavian and European countries in the 1980s. Early studies suggested a significant reduction in early mortality and morbidity in premature infants weighing less than 1.5 kg who were nursed by kangaroo care. Furthermore, randomized clinical trials demonstrated enhanced mother-infant attachment, greater maternal self-esteem, prolonged and enhanced lactation, increased infant alertness, and better weight gain with earlier hospital discharge. Behavioral studies found more stable sleep patterns, less irritability at 6 months of age, and more eye contact with caregivers in infants nursed with kangaroo care. Kangaroo care has been shown to promote a thermal neutral metabolic response and temperature stability in stable growing premature babies. Moreover, during kangaroo nursing, infants with bronchopulmonary dysplasia have better oxygenation, and other infants show less periodic breathing and reduced apnea. In the modern nursery, kangaroo care may be initiated even during mechanical ventilation for patients without other complications. The infant should be put between the breasts with maximum skin contact and then should be covered with a blanket to avoid outward convective and evaporative heat losses. After initial sessions of 30 minutes to 1 hour with careful intermittent temperature monitoring, kangaroo care can be practiced for up to 4 hours. Kangaroo care integrates the family into the neonatal intensive care team. To our knowledge, no adverse reports about the approach have been published, and its use in many nurseries is on the rise.

## SPECIAL CASE MANAGEMENT

**CASE STUDY 1**

A 510-g baby boy was born at 23 weeks and 4 days of gestation; he was limp and cyanotic, with no respiratory effort and a heart rate higher than 100 beats/min. The baby was resuscitated under a radiant warmer and dried, and a stocking cap was placed over his head. The warmer's temperature probe was recording a low skin temperature because it did not attach well to the skin. The radiant warmer was on full power to compensate for this low probe reading. After resuscitation, the baby was transported to the NICU in an incubator preheated to a temperature of 35° C.

On arrival in the NICU, the baby was weighed quickly and put onto a preheated radiant warmer bed. Skin probe (servo-control) temperature registered as 33° C, rectal temperature as 35° C, and axillary temperature as 34° C. The radiant warmer set point was targeted at 37° C, and temperatures were monitored every 15 minutes. A saran blanket was used to minimize heat loss. Heated and 100%-humidified air from a respiratory pack was run underneath the saran blanket. Then the baby's skin was prepared with iodine solution and he was draped completely for umbilical catheterization (a 30-minute procedure). Over the first 2 hours of life, rectal temperature increased to only 34.5° C. The baby was transferred into a preheated and humidified incubator regulated by a skin probe set at 37° C. Two 250-watt light bulbs were positioned over the incubator hood for supplemental heat and for warming during any procedure that required opening of the incubator (e.g., serial weight determinations). Over the next 12 hours, the baby had difficulty maintaining his temperature even though the incubator air temperature was running near the set temperature of 37° C and sometimes above at 38.5° C.

Temperature maintenance of an extremely premature infant should be part of resuscitation from the time of delivery. Despite radiant warming in the delivery room and convective incubation during transport, this baby was nevertheless hypothermic on admission to the NICU. Low admission temperature correlates with increased mortality rates in these infants. They are born wet and prone to excessive transepidermal evaporative and convective heat losses. In addition, suboptimal radiant heating, blowing noncontrolled warm, humidified air under plastic blankets (probably not as effective as the still air envelope conserved by the blanket), and the pressure for performing procedures with surgical drapes blocking radiant heat delivery may worsen heat loss.

Quickly drying such babies, properly placing them directly under a radiant heater at birth, and covering the head are small but important steps in temperature resuscitation. Other techniques described in this chapter might be considered from birth, such as the use of a plastic bag described by (Vohra and colleagues, 1999) or of a saran blanket or polyurethane drape during umbilical catheterization. Finally, transferring such an infant into an incubator before adequately rewarming him or her under a radiant warmer may prolong thermal recovery in a hypoxic subject incapable of generating enough metabolic heat to do so. The use of light bulbs to provide supplemental radiant heat in incubators attests to the incubator's intrinsic operating power deficiency (seeking to reduce heat loss rather than to rewarm a cold baby). Moreover, such supplemental radiant heat sources are not controlled, produce more radiation in the visible light range, and are inefficient if not potentially dangerous, as they promote burns if placed too close to the infant.

There are no data describing the best rate of rewarming. Cold-stressed babies should probably be nursed under a servo-controlled radiant heat source, and heat losses minimized. During rewarming, they should be closely monitored and the heat delivery should be servo-controlled. A rate of about +1° C to +2° C per hour seems reasonable but may not be achievable. Alternatively, a preheated and humidified incubator may also be used for rewarming infants, although the rate may be slower. The incubator air or skin servo-control temperature can be set 1° C higher than the baby's temperature and gradually increased until a normal core temperature is achieved. Hybrid incubators that can also be used as radiant warmer beds are now available and may be helpful in rewarming scenarios.

## NEONATAL FEVER—A PROBLEM OF TEMPERATURE ELEVATION

There is no universally accepted definition of neonatal fever. Craig (1963) defined *neonatal pyrexia* as a rectal (core body) temperature higher than 37.4° C; however, other investigators accept normal temperatures up to 37.8° C. Between 1% and 2.5% of all newborns admitted to the normal nursery have fever as judged from rectal or axillary temperatures and depending on the limits chosen. Fever is an inconsistent and uncommon sign of sepsis (fewer than 10% of febrile neonates have culture-proven sepsis), and temperature elevation may be seen with several other clinical entities.

### Mechanisms Producing Neonatal Fever

The mechanisms producing neonatal fever are incompletely understood. They result from disturbances in the complex interactions between heat conservation and heat dissipation mechanisms. Fever may occur when immunogenic pyrogens (commonly, prostaglandin $E_2$) lead to upward displacement of the normal thermal set point in the hypothalamus, leading to activation of heat conservation and heat generation physiologic responses. Generally, heat conservation starts with peripheral vasoconstriction and is followed by thermogenesis (usually the nonshivering type in neonates) while the new set point is achieved. It is important to note that newborn infants of different animal species react in peculiar ways to different known pyrogens. Thus, human newborns may suffer severe documented bacterial infections without increased body temperature.

Phenomena besides pyogenic mechanisms of febrile response in newborns may lead to the elevation of body temperature. In fact, newborn infants have poor heat dissipation mechanisms (absence of sweating), so exposure to excess heat or insulation (too much swaddling) can quickly raise the core temperature. Such overheating commonly occurs when term babies are nursed in uncontrolled incubators or under radiant warmers. Temperature elevation may also occur with increased infant metabolic rate, such as that seen with skeletal muscle rigidity and status epilepticus.

Temperature elevation is occasionally observed in well, breast-feeding newborn infants on the third to fourth day of life; it is believed to result from dehydration due to insufficient milk production. Finally, a higher incidence of neonatal fever has been reported in infants of mothers receiving epidural analgesia. The mechanisms for temperature elevation in these latter two cases (see later) are unknown.

## Determining the Cause of Fever

Sepsis is an uncommon cause of fever; paradoxically, septic neonates more commonly present with hypothermia. However, sepsis is probably the most treatable life-threatening illness occurring in febrile newborn infants, especially those with temperature elevations exceeding 38° C to 39° C, who are more likely to have bacteremia, purulent meningitis, and pneumonia. Most neonatal febrile episodes are noted in the first day of life (54% in one series); however, any fever occurring on the third day of life and fever above 39° C have both been correlated with a significantly higher chance of bacterial disease. Severe temperature elevation is also associated with viral disease, particularly herpes simplex encephalitis, so septic evaluations in these infants should include a lumbar puncture.

Hyperthermia has been reported in tiny premature infants as a complication of the improper use of shielding devices either in convection-warmed incubators or under radiant warmers. When incubated, babies should always have a strictly monitored and controlled source of heat. Fever secondary to overheating (particularly in association with incubators) is more common in equatorial and tropical countries.

Dehydration is an uncommonly recognized cause of fever in the newborn period. Dehydration occurring in healthy term infants between the third and fourth days of life as noted previously, is probably due to an inadequate intake of milk. Dehydration fever is commonly seen in large breast-fed babies whose milk intake is poor and who may be exposed to high environmental temperatures in the summer or in the tropics. Temperature may be anywhere between 37.8° C and 40° C. Rehydration leads to resolution of fever and is key to the diagnosis of this entity.

Two studies have found fever is much more common in neonates whose mothers received epidural analgesia during labor than in those whose mothers did not (7.5% vs 2.5% and 14.5% vs 1%) (Lieberman et al, 1997; Pleasure and Stahl, 1990). One of these reports observed more common sepsis evaluations and use of antibiotics in the offspring of women receiving epidural analgesia. With the growing use of epidural analgesia during labor, the recognition of epidural neonatal fever is an important consideration in the evaluation of the febrile neonate.

Unusual and uncommon causes of neonatal fever include neonatal typhoid fever and congenital malaria, which should be considered in immigrant populations or in third world countries. An increase in unexplained neonatal fevers was associated with the introduction of routine hepatitis B vaccination (compared with historical controls). In addition, temperature elevations may be seen with hypothalamic or other central nervous system malformations or masses. Subarachnoid or other intracranial hemorrhages may also be associated with temperature elevation. On rare occasions, neonatal spinal neurenteric cysts can manifest as long-lasting neonatal fever and should be considered in the differential diagnosis of acute myelopathy with persistent fever in infancy (>3 weeks in duration). The presence of myelopathy helps establish this diagnosis.

## Management

The clinical problem is that fever may be the only indication of severe bacterial disease. The relevant perinatal history should be evaluated for risk factors so as to mitigate a laboratory evaluation or presumptive treatment for infection. Furthermore, signs suggestive of sepsis (diminished activity, irritability, seizures) should be considered. All neonates with fever should be evaluated for hydration, weight loss, and foci of infection (cellulitis, septic arthritis or osteomyelitis, omphalitis, and presence of colonized foreign bodies; e.g., in a central venous line).

However, febrile neonates without clinical histories or any signs of infection present a challenge, and there are insufficient data in our literature about appropriate management. An infant's environment should be examined for overheating, and in breast-feeding infants with fever at 3 to 4 days of life and excessive weight loss, dehydration fever should be considered and treated to establish this diagnosis. Mothers receiving epidural analgesia often manifest shivering with their temperature rise, and they experience a rapid defervescence after discontinuation of the epidural infusion; recognition of this pattern may avoid unnecessary sepsis evaluations in neonates with early fever.

## CONCLUSION

The LBW premature newborn is extremely vulnerable to harsh fluctuations in physical environment. These infants require frequent assessments of skin, core, and air temperatures and relative humidity so that an optimal strategy may be designed for thermal regulation. In the care of smaller babies, heat replacement is often required, and refinement of techniques to accomplish heat replacement without inducing hyperthermia is needed.

## SUGGESTED READINGS

Bruck K: Heat production and temperature regulation. In Stave U (ed): Perinatal Physiology. New York, Plenum, 1978, pp 455-498.

Dawkins MJR, Hull D: The production of heat by fat. Sci Am 213:62, 1965.

Scopes JW: Thermoregulation in the newborn. In Avery CB (ed): Neonatology, Pathophysiology and Management of the Newborn, 2nd ed. Philadelphia, JB Lippincott, 1981, pp 171-181.

## REFERENCES

Baumgart S: Reduction of oxygen consumption, insensible water loss and radiant heat demand with use of a plastic blanket for low-birth-weight infants under radiant warmers. Pediatrics 74:1022-1028, 1984.

Baumgart S: Partitioning of heat losses and gains in premature newborn infants under radiant warmers. Pediatrics 75:89-99, 1985.

Baumgart S: Radiant heat loss vs. radiant heat gain in premature neonates under radiant warmers. Biol Neonate 57:10-20, 1990.

Baumgart S, Fox WW, Polin RA: Physiologic implications of two different heat shields for infants under radiant warmers. J Pediatr 100:787-790, 1982a.

Baumgart S, Langman CB, Sosulski R, et al: Fluid, electrolyte and glucose maintenance in the very low birthweight infant. Clin Pediatr 21:199-206, 1982b.

Bell EF, Rios GR: A double-walled incubator alters the partition of body heat loss of premature infants. Pediatr Res 17:135B140, 1983a.

Bell EF, Rios GR: Air versus skin temperature servo control of infant incubators. J Pediatr 103:954-959, 1983b.

Bell EF, Weinstein MR, Oh W: Heat balance in premature infants: Comparative effects of convectively heated incubator and radiant warmer, with and without plastic heat shield. J Pediatr 96:460-465, 1980.

Chessex P, Blouet S, Vaucher J: Environmental temperature control in very low birth weight infants (<1000 gms) cared for in double-walled incubators. J Pediatr 113:373-380, 1988.

Craig WS: The early detection of pyrexia in the newborn. Arch Dis Child 41:448-450, 1963.

Day RL, Caliguiri L, Kamenski C, et al: Body temperature and survival of premature infants. Pediatrics 34:171-181, 1964.

Edwards WH, Conner JM, Soll RF, for the Vermont Oxford Network: The effect of Aquaphor™ original emollient ointment on nosocomial sepsis rates and skin integrity in infants of birth weight 501-1000 grams. Pediatr Res 49:388A, 2001.

Hammarlund K, Strömberg B, Sedin G: Heat loss from the skin of preterm and full-term newborn infants during the first weeks after birth. Biol Neonate 50:1-10, 1986.

Hey EN, Katz G: The optimum thermal environment for naked babies. Arch Dis Child 45:328-334, 1970.

Hull D: The structure and function of brown adipose tissue. Br Med Bull 22:92-96, 1966.

Knauth A, Gordin P, McNelis W, Baumgart S: A semipermeable polyurethane membrane as an artificial skin for the premature neonate. Pediatrics 83:945, 1988.

Lieberman E, Lan JM, Frigoletto F Jr, et al: Epidural analgesia, intrapartum fever, and neonatal sepsis evaluation. Pediatrics 99:415-419.

Malin S, Baumgart S: Optimal thermal management for low birth weight infants nursed under high-power radiant warmers. Pediatrics 79:47-54, 1987.

Marks KH, Lee CA, Bolan CD, Maisels MJ: Oxygen consumption and temperature control of premature infants in a double-wall incubator. Pediatrics 68:93-98, 1981.

Mayfield SR, Bhatia J, Nakamura KT, et al: Temperature measurement in term and preterm neonates. J Pediatr 104:271-275, 1984.

Nopper AJ, Horii KA, Sookdeo-Drost S, et al: Topical ointment therapy benefits premature infants. J Pediatr 128:660, 1996.

Okken A, Blijham C, Franz W, Bohn E: Effects of forced convection of heated air on insensible water loss and heat loss in preterm infants in incubators. J Pediatr 101:108-112, 1982.

Oski K, Pappagallo M, Lerer T, Hussain N: Does use of Aquaphor™ (Aq) in extremely low birth weight infants (ELBW) increase the risk for nosocomial sepsis? Pediatr Res 49:227A, 2001.

Pleasure JR, Stahl GE: Do epidural anesthesia-related maternal fevers alter neonatal care? Pediatr Res 27:221A, 1990.

Porat R, Brodsky N: Effect of Tegederm use on outcome of extremely low birth weight (ELBW) infants. Pediatr Res 33:231(A), 1993.

Silverman WA, Sinclair JC, Agate FJ: The oxygen cost of minor changes in heat balance of small newborn infants. Acta Paediatr Scand 55:294-300, 1966.

Vohra S, Frent G, Campbell V, et al: Effect of polyethylene occlusive skin wrapping on heat loss in very low birth weight infants at delivery: A randomized trial. J Pediatr 134:547-551, 1999.

Wheldon AE, Rutter N: The heat balance of small babies nursed in incubators and under radiant warmers. Early Hum Dev 6:131-143, 1982.

CHAPTER 30

# Acid-Base, Fluid, and Electrolyte Management

Istvan Seri, Rangasamy Ramanathan, and Jacquelyn R. Evans

## FLUID AND ELECTROLYTE BALANCE

Maintenance of fluid and electrolyte balance is essential for normal cell and organ function both during intrauterine development and throughout extrauterine life. Pathologic conditions in the newborn often lead to disruption of the complex regulatory mechanisms of fluid and electrolyte homeostasis and may result in irreversible cell damage. Thus, a thorough understanding of the physiologic changes in neonatal fluid and electrolyte homeostasis and the provision of appropriate fluid and electrolyte therapy based on the principles of developmental fluid and electrolyte physiology are among the cornerstones of modern neonatal intensive care.

### Developmental Changes in Body Composition, Fluid Compartments, and Organ Function Affecting Prenatal, Perinatal, and Postnatal Fluid and Electrolyte Balance

Protection of the intracellular milieu implies that the organism must be able to monitor and correct changes in the composition and volume of the extracellular (ECF) compartment resulting from its interaction with the ever-changing environment. Recognition of this basic physiologic requirement along with the advances in our understanding of the developmental changes in body composition, fluid compartments, and organ functions regulating fluid and electrolyte balance have resulted in the emergence of the modern principles of neonatal fluid and electrolyte therapy.

#### Developmental Changes in Body Composition and Fluid Compartments

Dynamic changes occur in body composition and fluid distribution during intrauterine life, labor and delivery, and the early postnatal period. Thereafter, the rate of change in body composition and fluid distribution gradually decreases, with more subtle changes taking place especially after the first year of life (Friis-Hansen, 1961).

##### *Changes During Intrauterine Development*

In early gestation, body composition is characterized by a high proportion of TBW (TBW) and a large extracellular compartment (Brans, 1986; Friis-Hansen, 1983). There also appears to be a prolactin-mediated increase in the water-binding capacity of fetal cells and perhaps the interstitium, contributing to the maintenance of increased total fetal body water content (Coulter, 1983). As gestation advances, however, the rapid cellular growth, accretion of body solids, and fat deposition result in gradual reductions in TBW content and extracellular water volume while the intracellular fluid compartment increases (Friis-Hansen, 1983). In the 16-week fetus, TBW represents approximately 94% of total body weight, and roughly two thirds of the TBW are distributed in the extracellular and one third in the intracellular compartment. In the term neonate, TBW are only about 75% of body weight, and almost half is located in the intracellular space (Fig. 30–1). Thus, infants born prematurely are in a state of TBW excess and extracellular volume expansion compared with their term counterparts, with the majority of the expanded extracellular volume being distributed in the interstitium (Brace, 1992).

During intrauterine development, the placenta provides an ample supply of nutrients and electrolytes for the fetus. To maintain normal weight gain, especially during the third trimester when an acceleration of fetal mass accumulation occurs, the fetus must be in a positive electrolyte balance.

##### *Changes During Labor and Delivery*

Additional and more acute changes in TBW and its distribution take place during labor and delivery. Arterial blood pressure rises a few days before delivery in response to increases in catecholamine, vasopressin, and cortisol plasma concentrations and translocation of blood from the placenta into the fetus. The rise in arterial blood pressure and the changes in the fetal hormonal milieu, along with the borderline intrapartum hypoxia-induced increase in capillary permeability, result in a shift of fluid from the intravascular to the interstitial compartment. This fluid shift results in an approximately 25% reduction in circulating plasma volume in the human fetus during labor and delivery (Brace, 1992). Because the expanded interstitial fluid is not immediately accessible for filtration and excretion by the kidneys, it may serve as a source of volume supply until maternal milk production becomes adequate. Thus, the translocation of fluid from the intravascular to the interstitial compartment during labor and delivery is a part of the physiologic adaptation for the transition to extrauterine life. The postnatal increase in oxygenation and changes in vasoactive hormone production then restore capillary membrane integrity and favor absorption of interstitial fluid into the intravascular compartment. The ensuing gradual movement of fluid from the expanded interstitial space into the vessels aids in maintaining intravascular volume during the first 24 to 48 hours, when oral fluid intake may be limited. However, prematurity, pathologic conditions, or both may disrupt this delicate process and interfere with the physiologic contraction of the ECF compartment in the immediate period.

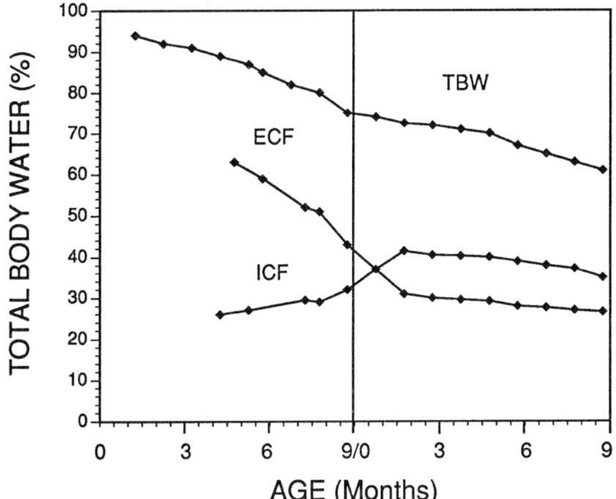


**FIGURE 30–1.** Total body water (TBW) content and its distribution between the extracellular fluid (ECF) and intracellular fluid (ICF) compartments in the human fetus, newborn, and infant from conception until 9 months of age. The data represent average values from Friis-Hansen (1961).

In the fetus, body composition and fluid balance depend on the electrolyte and water exchange among mother, fetus, and amniotic space (Brace, 1986). Therefore, several antenatal events influencing this exchange may have significant effects on the postnatal fluid balance. Maternal indomethacin treatment or excessive administration of intravenous fluids during labor may result in neonatal hyponatremia with expanded extracellular water content (Heijden et al, 1988; Rojas et al, 1984). Hydrops fetalis is the ultimate example of extreme fetal extracellular volume expansion. On the other hand, placental insufficiency or maternal diuretic therapy may impair fetal hydration, leading to decreases in extracellular volume, urine output, and amniotic fluid volume (Van Otterlo et al, 1977). Infants born under such conditions have an attenuated postnatal diuresis and weight loss and initially require greater fluid intake to correct the state of prenatal dehydration. Finally, there is no evidence that the mode of delivery influences neonatal extracellular water content (Cheek et al, 1982).

The timing of cord clamping after delivery is another important factor significantly affecting total circulating blood volume and extracellular volume in the neonate. Immediate clamping of the cord results in an average hematocrit of 48% to 51%, and there is little change in the neonate's hematocrit value over the next days (Linderkamp, 1982; Yao and Lind, 1974). However, if the cord is clamped only 3 to 4 minutes after delivery with the newborn positioned at or below the level of the placenta, up to 25 to 50 mL/kg of blood is transfused into the neonate, representing an approximately 25% to 50% increase in the total blood volume (Linderkamp, 1982; Yao and Lind, 1974). Because in these cases the higher transcapillary hydrostatic pressure forces an additional 25 to 30 mL/kg of intravascular fluid into the interstitium, the hematocrit may gradually increase to 60% to 65% or higher over the first 3 to 4 hours of life (Brace, 1992; Linderkamp, 1982; Yao and Lind, 1974). Thus, if the neonate is suspected to have received a prolonged placental transfusion and the initial hematocrit value is between 60% and 65%, the hematocrit should be checked again 4 to 6 hours later. The effects of the timing of cord clamping on intravascular and extracellular volumes are modified by the presence of asphyxia and neonatal breathing.

### *Changes in the Postnatal Period*

In the first few days and weeks after birth, the most important effects on the pace of further changes in body composition, TBW content, and its distribution are exerted by gestational and postnatal ages, the presence or absence of pathologic conditions, the immediate environment, and the type of nutrition.

During the early transitional period, the healthy newborn loses weight. It is generally accepted that this postnatal weight loss is primarily due to the contraction of the expanded ECF compartment (Cheek et al, 1961) and that it approximates the total body fluid loss (Shaffer et al, 1986). However, water loss from the intracellular space may also contribute to the physiologic weight loss (Coulter, 1983; MacLaurin, 1966), especially if there are rapid changes in serum osmolality. Such changes in serum osmolality may be seen in extremely low-birth-weight (LBW) infants with increased transepidermal water losses (Costarino and Baumgart, 1991, Sedin, 1995).

Although the exact mechanisms of the ECF contraction are unknown, several studies have suggested that atrial natriuretic peptide plays a role in this process (Kojima et al, 1987; Ronconi et al, 1995; Rozycki and Baumgart, 1991; Tulassay et al, 1987). The postnatal increase in capillary membrane integrity favors absorption of the interstitial fluid into the intravascular compartment. The ensuing rise in circulating blood volume stimulates release of atrial natriuretic peptide from the heart, which in turn enhances renal sodium and water excretion (Sagnella and MacGregor, 1984). The concomitant diminution in the release of vasoconstrictive and antidiuretic hormones further enhances the diuretic action of atrial natriuretic peptide.

The TBW excess and extracellular volume expansion of the preterm infants imply that their negative water and sodium balance during the first 5 to 10 postnatal days (Fig. 30–2) (Shaffer and Meade, 1989) represent an appropriate adaptation to extrauterine life and should not be compensated for by increased fluid administration and sodium supplementation. If this principle is not followed and a positive fluid balance (i.e., weight gain) is achieved during the transitional period, preterm infants are at higher risk of a more severe course of respiratory distress syndrome (Shaffer and Weismann, 1992) as well as a higher incidence of patent ductus arteriosus (Bell et al, 1980), congestive heart failure (Bell et al, 1980), pulmonary edema (Shaffer and Weismann, 1992), necrotizing enterocolitis (Bell et al, 1979), and bronchopulmonary dysplasia (Van Marter et al, 1990). Only the thorough understanding of the principles of developmental fluid and electrolyte physiology will enable the clinician to adjust fluid and caloric requirements appropriately during the transitional period in the sick term and preterm neonate and, thus, minimize the impact of abnormalities in postnatal fluid and electrolyte homeostasis on different short- and long-term outcome measures (see section on fluid and electrolyte management).

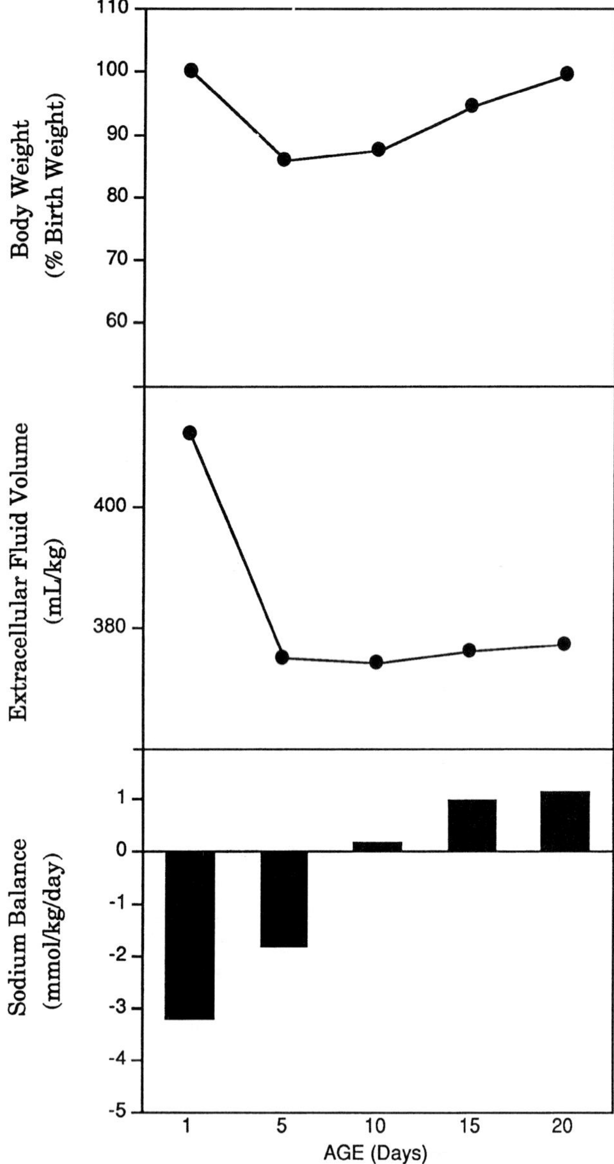


**FIGURE 30–2.** Postnatal changes in body weight (expressed in percent of birth weight), extracellular fluid volume (estimated by the bromide dilution method), and sodium balance (defined as the difference between sodium intake and urinary sodium excretion). *(From Shaffer SG, Weismann DN: Fluid requirements in the preterm infant. Clin Perinatol 19:233-250, 1992).*

Healthy term newborns lose an average of 5% to 10% of their body weight during the first 4 to 7 days of life (Brace, 1992). Thereafter they establish a pattern of steady weight gain. Because preterm infants have an increased TBW content and extracellular volume, they lose on average 15% of their body weight during transition (Shaffer et al, 1987) and, depending on the degree of prematurity and associated pathologic conditions, these neonates regain their birth weight only at 10 to 20 days after birth. However, because TBW content at birth is also influenced by factors other than maturity, as discussed earlier, weight loss may differ significantly among patients of the same gestational age, and there is no established optimal rate or extent of weight loss in infants born prematurely (Lorenz et al, 1982).

The healthy term infant is born after having developed adequate macromineral stores. After the extracellular volume contraction, these infants maintain an appropriate positive macromineral balance and steadily gain weight. On the other hand, preterm infants, especially those born before the third trimester, have missed the period of intrauterine life when the highest rate of macromineral retention takes place. To achieve and maintain normal growth, these neonates must be in a positive macromineral balance after their transitional period. However, certain pathologic conditions and the long-term administration of diuretics may hinder their ability to achieve a positive macromineral balance and, thus, appropriate growth rate.

## Physiology of the Regulation of Body Composition and Fluid Compartments

Although human cells have the ability to adjust their intracellular composition, ultimate regulation of the intracellular volume and osmolality relies on the control of the extracellular compartment. Therefore, the human body must be able to monitor the volume and osmolality of the extracellular compartment and to correct the changes resulting from its interaction with the environment.

### *Regulation of the Intracellular Solute and Water Compartment*

The major intracellular solutes are the cellular proteins necessary for cell function, the organic phosphates associated with cellular energy production and storage, and the equivalent cations balancing the phosphate and protein anions (MacKnight and Leaf, 1977). As a result of the activity of the cell membrane-bound sodium-potassium adenosine triphosphatase, potassium is the major intracellular cation and sodium is the major extracellular cation. The energy derived from the concentration differences for sodium and potassium between the intracellular and extracellular compartments is used for cellular work.

Because changes in osmolality of the extracellular compartment are reflected as net movements of water in or out of the cell, regulation of ECF concentration ultimately controls the osmolality and size of the intracellular compartment (MacKnight and Leaf, 1977). This physiologic principle must be kept in mind by the neonatologist managing sick term and preterm neonates with disturbances of sodium homeostasis. Rapid changes in serum sodium concentration and thus in extracellular osmolality directly affect the osmolality and size of the intracellular compartment and may lead to irreversible cell damage, especially in the central nervous system (see later).

### *Regulation of the Intracellular-Extracellular Interface: The Interstitial Compartment*

There are small but important differences in the composition of the interstitial and intravascular fluid compartments that allow the movement of water, solute, and nutrients from the blood into the interstitium and the transport of cellular waste products into the circulation for final elimination. The tightly regulated differences in the composition of the interstitium and the intravascular fluid space result from the interaction of the intravascular and interstitial hydrostatic and oncotic pressures (Starling, 1896). According to this principle, water movement across the capillary wall can be described by the equation

$$J_V = K_F\,[(P_C - P_T) - \delta\,(\pi_P - \pi_T)]$$

where $J_V$ = the net flow across the capillary, $K_F$ = filtration coefficient, $P_C$ = capillary hydrostatic pressure, $P_T$ = interstitial hydrostatic pressure, $\delta$ = protein reflection coefficient, $\pi_P$ = plasma oncotic pressure, and $\pi_T$ = interstitial oncotic pressure. Thus, the movement of fluid out of the capillary is determined by the product of the water permeability characteristics of the capillary wall ($K_F$) and the net driving pressure $[(P_C - P_T) - \delta\,(\pi_P - \pi_T)]$ that forces fluid out from the capillary. The net driving pressure is the difference between the hydrostatic ($P_C - P_T$) and oncotic ($\pi_P - \pi_T$) pressures on either side of the capillary wall (Fig. 30–3).

Under physiologic conditions, a small amount of fluid leaves the plasma at the arterial end of the capillary circulation as a result of the balance of these forces. As capillary hydrostatic pressure falls and plasma oncotic pressure increases along the capillary bed, filtration ceases and much of the filtered fluid reenters at the venous end of the capillary circulation. The difference between the filtered fluid and the reabsorbed fluid is cleared from the interstitium by the lymphatic system (Taylor, 1981). The reflection coefficient ($\delta$) describes the protein permeability characteristics of the capillary wall, which is tissue specific. In tissues with capillaries that are virtually impermeable to proteins (brain, skin: $\delta$ = 0.8), the oncotic pressure difference plays an important role in counterbalancing the tendency of the hydrostatic forces to move fluid out from the capillaries. In tissues with high capillary permeability to protein (liver, spleen: $\delta$ = 0.2), the lymphatic circulation plays a more important role in regulating the volume of the interstitial fluid compartment.

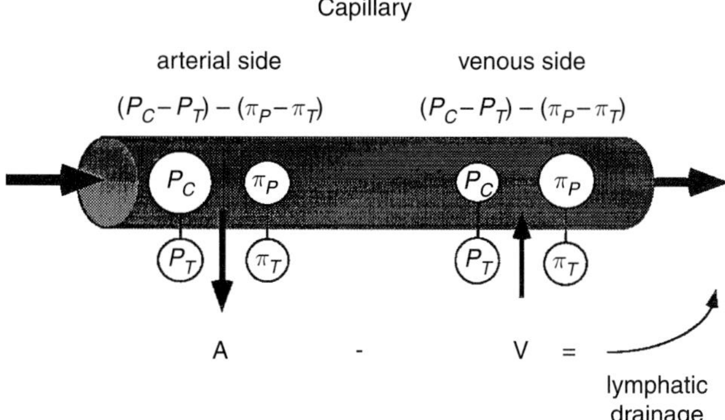


**FIGURE 30–3.** Filtration and reabsorption of fluid along the capillary under physiologic conditions. Movement of fluid across the capillary is determined by the direction of the net driving pressure $[(P_C - P_T) - (\pi_P - \pi_T)]$ and the water and protein permeability characteristics of the capillary wall. At the arterial end of the capillary, intracapillary hydrostatic pressure ($P_C$) is high, and plasma oncotic pressure ($\pi_P$) is relatively low, resulting in a net movement of fluid out of the capillary. As filtration of relatively protein-poor fluid continues along the capillary, plasma oncotic pressure rises and intracapillary hydrostatic pressure drops. Therefore, on the venous side, fluid moves from the interstitium into the capillary, so that much of the filtered fluid is reabsorbed at the end of the capillary bed. The fluid remaining in the interstitium (arterial-venous side of the capillary) is drained by the lymphatic system. Interstitial hydrostatic ($P_T$) and oncotic ($\pi_T$) pressures remain virtually unchanged along the capillary bed. See text for details.

In the healthy term neonate, hydrostatic and oncotic pressures are well balanced, being roughly half of those in the adult (Sola and Gregory, 1981). However, pathologic conditions readily disturb the delicate balance between the hydrostatic and oncotic forces, leading to an expansion of the interstitial compartment at the expense of the intravascular volume. The increased interstitial fluid volume (edema) then further affects tissue perfusion by altering the normal function of the extracellular-intracellular interface. Table 30–1 summarizes the conditions resulting in increased edema formation in the neonate.

There also are some important developmentally regulated differences between the newborn and the adult relating to the pathomechanisms of edema formation. Capillary permeability to proteins is increased during the early stages of development; this increase is reflected by a lower tissue-specific protein reflection coefficient ($\delta$) in the fetus and newborn than in the adult (Brace, 1992; Gold and Brace, 1988). Because, under pathologic conditions, neonatal capillary permeability is further increased (see Table 30–1), protein concentration in the interstitial compartment may approach that of the intravascular space, favoring further intravascular volume depletion and interstitial volume expansion. When neonates with such conditions are treated with frequent albumin boluses, much of the infused albumin leaks into the interstitium, creating a vicious cycle of intravascular volume depletion and edema formation. If the cycle is not interrupted, the result may be the formation of anasarca with an extremely poor prognosis. As mentioned previously, when the permeability of the capillary endothelium to protein is increased, the final balance between fluid filtration and reabsorption is more dependent on an effective lymphatic drainage (Taylor, 1981). However, because lymph flow in the neonate is readily disrupted by even a small elevation in venous pressure (Brace, 1992), pathologic conditions and therapeutic maneuvers that increase venous pressure are commonly associated with decreased lymphatic clearance and thus edema formation in the sick infant.

In summary, the sick neonate has a limited capacity to maintain appropriate intravascular volume and to regulate the volume and composition of the interstitium. The ensuing intravascular hypovolemia and edema formation result in vasoconstriction and disturbances in tissue perfusion and cellular function with further impairments in the regulation of extracellular volume distribution.

### *Regulation of the Extracellular Solute and Water Compartment*

The regulation of the volume and osmolality of the extracellular compartment ensures the integrity of the circulation and maintains the osmolality of the extracellular compartment within 2% of the osmolar set point between 275 and

**TABLE 30-1**

**Mechanisms Promoting Fluid Accumulation in the Interstitial Compartment**

**Conditions favoring fluid accumulation in the interstitial space by causing a dysequilibrium between filtration and reabsorption of fluid by the capillaries**

- Increased hydrostatic pressure
  - Elevated capillary hydrostatic pressure
    - Increased cardiac output
    - Venous obstruction
  - Decreased tissue hydrostatic pressure
    - Conditions associated with changes in the properties of the interstitial gel (edematous states, effects of hormones including prolactin)
- Decreased oncotic pressure gradient
  - Decreased capillary oncotic pressure
    - Prematurity, hyaline membrane disease
    - Malnutrition, liver dysfunction
    - Nephrotic syndrome
  - Increased interstitial oncotic pressure is usually the result of increased capillary permeability (see later)
- Elevation of the filtration coefficient
  - Increased capillary permeability
    - Organs with large-pore capillary endothelium (liver, spleen)
    - State of maturity (preterm infants > term newborns > adults)
    - Production of pro-inflammatory cytokines (sepsis, anaphylaxis, hypoxic tissue injury, tissue ischemia, ischemia-reperfusion, soft tissue trauma, extracorporeal membrane oxygenation)
  - Increased capillary surface area
    - Vasodilation

**Conditions associated with decreased lymphatic drainage**

- Decreased muscle movement
  - Neuromuscular blockade and/or heavy sedation
  - Central and/or peripheral nervous system disease
- Obstruction of lymphatic flow
  - Increased central venous pressure
  - Scar tissue formation (bronchopulmonary dysplasia)
  - Mechanical obstruction (dressings, high mean airway pressure in mechanically ventilated newborns)

Modified from Costarino AT, Baumgard S: Neonatal water metabolism. In Cowett RM (ed): Principles of Perinatal/Neonatal Metabolism. New York, Springer Verlag, 1991, pp 623-649.

290 mOsm (Robertson and Berl, 1986). Blood pressure and serum sodium concentration (i.e., osmolality) are monitored by baroreceptors and osmoreceptors, respectively. The effector limb of the regulatory system consists of the heart, the vascular bed, the kidneys, and the gastrointestinal intake of fluid in response to thirst. The latter part of the effector system is inactive in the critically ill term and preterm neonates whose fluid intake is completely controlled by the caregivers. By regulating the function of the effector organs, several hormones play a role in the control of the extracellular compartment, including the renin-angiotensin-aldosterone system, vasopressin, atrial natriuretic peptide, bradykinin, prostaglandins, and catecholamines.

Because volume changes in the extracellular compartment must be reflected by similar changes in the intravascular volume for effective operation of the regulatory mechanisms, regulation of the extracellular compartment relies on intact cardiovascular function as well as on the integrity of the capillary endothelium (Robertson and Berl, 1986). For instance, under physiologic conditions, an increase in the extracellular volume is reflected by an increase in the circulating plasma volume, leading to rises in blood pressure and renal blood flow. The ensuing increase in glomerular filtration and urine output returns the extracellular volume to normal.

In critically ill neonates, however, the capillary leak and reduced myocardial responsiveness resulting from immaturity and the underlying pathologic condition limit the increase in the circulating blood volume when extracellular volume expands. Thus, especially in sick preterm infants, blood pressure may rise only transiently, and renal blood flow and glomerular filtration rate remain low after volume boluses as fluid rapidly leaks out into the interstitium. By causing peripheral vasodilation, inappropriate central regulation of vascular tone further decreases effective circulating blood volume. With the concomitant release of catecholamines, vasopressin, and renin-angiotensin-aldosterone, renal tubular sodium and water reabsorption continue to be favored in order to increase diminished intravascular volume. However, this compensatory mechanism fails as the retained fluid continues to leak from the intravascular space into the interstitium, further compromising tissue perfusion. This leads to impaired gas exchange in the lungs, resulting in hypoxia with further increases in capillary leak. Thus, unless interrupted by appropriate therapeutic measures (see later), a vicious cycle with further deterioration rather than an effective extracellular volume regulation occurs in the sick preterm and term neonate.

### Maturation of Organs Regulating Body Composition and Fluid Compartments

The heart, the kidneys, the skin, and the endocrine system play the most important roles in the regulation of extracellular (and thus intracellular) fluid and electrolyte balance in the neonate. Immaturity of these organ systems, especially in very LBW infants, results in a compromised regulatory capacity, which one must remember when estimating daily fluid and electrolyte requirements in these patients. Other organs, including the gastrointestinal tract, are also involved in the physiologic regulation of fluid and electrolyte homeostasis. However, the impact of the maturational state of these organs is less significant for the fluid and electrolyte management in the critically ill newborn.

#### *Maturation of the Cardiovascular System*

There is a direct relationship between gestational maturity and the ability of the neonatal heart to respond to acute volume loading (Baylen et al, 1986). The blunted Starling response of the immature myocardium results from its lower content of contractile elements and incomplete sympathetic innervation (Mahony, 1995). Because central vasoregulation and endothelial integrity are also developmentally regulated (Brace, 1992; Gold and Brace, 1988), an appropriate effective intravascular volume is seldom maintained in a critically ill preterm infant. Since regulation of the extracellular volume requires the maintenance of an adequate effective circulating blood volume, the immaturity of the cardiovascular system contributes to the limited capacity of sick preterm infants to effectively regulate the total volume of their extracellular compartment.

#### *Maturation of Renal Function*

The kidney plays a crucial role in the physiologic control of fluid and electrolyte balance. It regulates extracellular volume and osmolality through the selective reabsorption of sodium and water, respectively. In the fetus, nephrogenesis is incomplete until 34 to 36 weeks of gestation (Robillard et al, 1990; see also Chapter 80). Thus, in addition to immaturity of tubular functions, preterm infants have a decreased number of glomeruli and the postnatal increase in their renal blood flow and glomerular filtration rate is attenuated compared with that of the term neonate (Arant, 1978). Tubular immaturity in preterm infants is reflected by their increased sodium, bicarbonate, and free water excretion and decreased renal concentrating capacity (Jones and Chesney, 1992; see also Chapter 80).

Some aspects of developmental renal physiology significantly influence the clinical management of the sick neonate. Because prenatal steroid administration accelerates maturation of renal function (van den Anker et al, 1994), preterm infants treated with steroids in utero have a better capacity to regulate their postnatal ECF contractions, which may facilitate their pulmonary recovery. Immaturity of their renal function renders preterm infants susceptible to both excessive sodium losses and sodium as well as volume overloading (El-Dahr and Chevalier, 1990). Sodium losses occur in spite of the low glomerular filtration rate and are mainly due to the immaturity of the tubular membrane transport processes and their hormonal regulation (Spitzer, 1982, Sulyok et al, 1985, Tulassay et al, 1986). The high urinary sodium excretion may be of clinical benefit during the period of transition because it promotes contraction of the expanded extracellular volume. Sodium retention is necessary for normal growth, however, so a negative sodium balance beyond the first 1 to 2 weeks of postnatal life may hinder appropriate weight gain (Sulyok et al, 1985). The inability of the preterm infant to respond promptly to a sodium or volume load results in a tendency of extracellular volume expansion with edema formation. This is a consequence primarily of the limited glomerular filtration rate, and it occurs despite the preterm infant's ability to produce a dilute urine (El-Dahr and Chevalier, 1990).

#### *Maturation of the Skin*

Although term infants have a well-developed cornified layer of the epidermis, extremely immature neonates have only two to three cell layers in the epidermis (Cartlidge-Patrick and Rutter, 1992). Because of the lack of an effective barrier to diffusion of water through the immature skin, transepidermal free water losses in the immature infant may be extremely high during the first few days of life. Gestational age, postnatal age, the pattern of intrauterine growth, and environmental factors play crucial roles in the magnitude of transepidermal free water losses (Fig. 30–4). Although skin cornification rapidly increases even in the extremely immature (23 to 26 weeks of gestational age) infant during the first few days of life, full maturation of the epidermis does not occur for more than 28 days after birth (Sedin, 1995). Chronic intrauterine stress (Hammarlund et al, 1983) and prenatal steroid treatment (Aszterbaum et al, 1993) also enhance maturation of the skin.

Because regulation of ECF volume and osmolality ultimately controls the intracellular compartment, increases in free water losses through the immature skin in the very LBW infant may result in early postnatal hypertonic dehydration with rapid changes in intracellular volume and osmolality. In many organs, especially the brain, the abrupt changes in intracellular volume and osmolality may lead to cellular dysfunction and ultimately to cell death (see later).

#### *Maturation of End-Organ Responsiveness To Hormones Involved in the Regulation of Fluid and Electrolyte Balance*

Several hormones, including but not limited to the renin-angiotensin-aldosterone system, vasopressin, atrial natriuretic peptide, dopamine and noradrenaline, directly

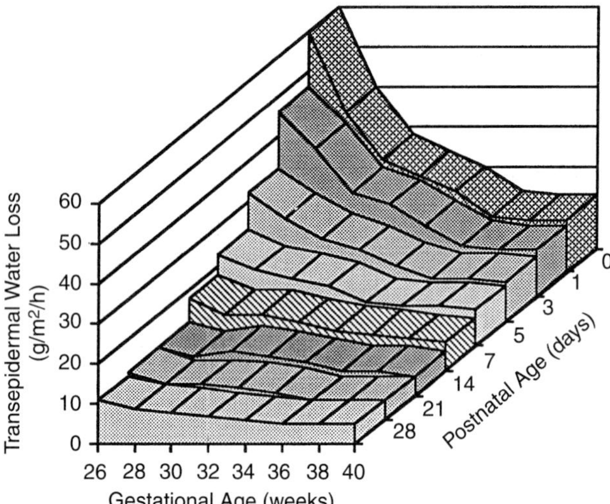


**FIGURE 30–4.** Transepidermal water loss in relation to gestational age during the first 28 postnatal days in appropriate-for-gestational-age infants. There is an exponential relationship between transepidermal water loss and gestational age, the water loss being higher in preterm infants than in term infants. Transepidermal water loss is also significantly affected by postnatal age, especially in the immature preterm infant. The measurements were performed at an ambient air humidity of 50% and with the infants calm and quiet. *(From Hammarlund K, Sedin G, Stromberg B: Transepidermal water loss in newborn infants. VIII: Relation to gestational age and postnatal age in appropriate and small for gestational age infants. Acta Paediatr Scand 72:721-728, 1983.)*

regulate the volume or composition of the extracellular compartment. These hormones exert their effects mainly by altering renal sodium and water excretion and by inducing changes in systemic vascular resistance and myocardial contractility. Other hormones, including the prostaglandins, bradykinin, and prolactin, modulate the actions of many of the regulatory hormones.

***Renin-Angiotensin-Aldosterone System.*** Decreases in renal capillary blood flow and tubular sodium delivery to the juxtaglomerular apparatus stimulate renin secretion, which in turn initiates the production of angiotensin. Angiotensin induces vasoconstriction, increases in tubular sodium and water reabsorption, and release of aldosterone (Riordan, 1995). Aldosterone increases potassium secretion and further enhances sodium reabsorption in the distal tubule. Thus, the primary function of this system is to protect the volume of the extracellular compartment and maintain adequate tissue perfusion (Bailie, 1992). However, its effectiveness in the neonate is somewhat limited by the decreased responsiveness of the immature kidney to the sodium- and water-retaining effects of these hormones (Sulyok et al, 1985). This is also one of the reasons why this system remains activated for several weeks to months after birth especially in the more immature or critically ill neonate (Godard et al, 1979; Sulyok et al, 1979).

Vasodilatory and natriuretic prostaglandins generated in the kidney (Gleason, 1987) are the main counter-regulatory hormones balancing the renal actions of the renin-angiotensin-aldosterone system. Therefore, when prostaglandin production is inhibited by indomethacin, the unopposed vasoconstrictive and sodium-retentive actions of the activated renin-angiotensin-aldosterone system contribute to the development of the drug-induced renal failure in the preterm infant (Gleason, 1987; Seri, 1995; Seri et al, 2002).

***Vasopressin (Antidiuretic Hormone).*** The rise in serum osmolality is a much more potent stimulus for vasopressin secretion than the decrease in systemic blood pressure (Dunn et al, 1973). This indicates that vasopressin is more important for maintaining the osmolality of the extracellular compartment than it is for regulating total extracellular volume and effective circulating blood volume. By midgestation, the fetus is able to respond to both osmotic and baroreceptor stimulation as well as to hypoxia with increased vasopressin release (Kelly et al, 1983, Leake, 1992; Weitzman et al, 1978). The primary renal action of vasopressin is to selectively raise free water reabsorption via the insertion of water channels into the luminal membrane of the distal tubular and collecting duct epithelium (Elliott et al, 1996). This free water retention is counterbalanced by locally generated prostaglandins (Bonvalet et al, 1987). Administration of indomethacin abolishes this regulatory effect, and the unopposed vasopressin-induced free water reabsorption contributes to the development of the drug-induced renal side effects (Gleason, 1987; Seri, 1995; Seri et al, 2002).

The primary cardiovascular action of vasopressin is peripheral vasoconstriction resulting in blood pressure elevation and redistribution of blood flow (Leake, 1992). Plasma levels of vasopressin are markedly elevated in the neonate, especially after vaginal delivery, and its cardiovascular actions facilitate neonatal adaptation (Pohjavouri and Raivio, 1985). The high vasopressin levels are in part also responsible for the diminished urine output of the healthy term neonate during the first day of life.

Under certain pathologic conditions, the dysregulated release of, or the end-organ unresponsiveness to, vasopressin significantly affects renal and cardiovascular functions in the sick preterm and term infant. In the syndrome of inappropriate secretion of antidiuretic hormone (SIADH), an uncontrolled release of vasopressin occurs in sick preterm and term infants. SIADH may be associated with birth asphyxia, intracerebral hemorrhage, respiratory distress syndrome, pneumothorax, and the use of continuous positive-pressure ventilation (El-Dahr and Chevalier, 1990; Leake, 1992). The syndrome is characterized by renal-free water retention, with decreased serum sodium values and serum osmolality, as well as by oliguria, increased urine concentration, and weight gain with edema formation. However, because the urinary concentrating capacity of the newborn is limited, a less than maximally diluted urine satisfies the diagnosis of SIADH in the presence of the other symptoms. The treatment is based on fluid and sodium restriction despite the oliguria and hyponatremia as well as on appropriate circulatory and ventilatory support. The clinician must remember that total body sodium is normal but TBW is elevated in such an infant, and that it is particularly dangerous to treat the hyponatremia caused by free water retention with large amounts of sodium. Owing to their more immature renal functions, extremely LBW infants during the first few weeks of life usually do not present with the full-blown syndrome in spite of their sometimes excessively high plasma vasopressin levels (Aperia et al, 1983).

Diminished vasopressin secretion or complete unresponsiveness of the renal tubules results in polyuria, diluted urine production, and increased serum osmolality (Leake, 1992). The treatment of these neonates consists of allowing for adequate free water intake. During the first few weeks of life, hemodynamically stable but extremely immature infants produce a dilute urine and may become polyuric despite appropriate vasopressin production, because of their renal tubular immaturity. As tubular functions mature, their concentrating capacity gradually improves from the second to fourth week of life. However, it takes years for the developing kidney to reach the concentrating capacity of the adult kidney. Finally, diminished vasopressin release may contribute to the development of vasopressor-resistant vasodilatory shock in critically ill preterm and term neonates (see Chapter 31).

***Atrial Natriuretic Peptide.*** Via its direct vasodilatory and renal natriuretic actions, atrial natriuretic peptide regulates the volume of the extracellular compartment in the fetus and neonate in a fashion opposite to that of the renin-angiotensin-aldosterone system (Iwamoto, 1992; Needleman and Greenwald, 1986; Seymour, 1985,). This opposing action is further reflected by its direct inhibitory effect on renin production and aldosterone release (Christensen, 1993). The stretch of the atrial wall caused by an increase in the circulating blood volume is the most potent stimulus for the release of this hormone. During early development, atrial natriuretic peptide is produced by all the chambers of the heart, and plasma levels of the hormone are high in the fetus (Claycomb, 1988).

There are a few specific conditions in which the actions of atrial natriuretic peptide are directly relevant for the neonatologist. For instance, the hormone is involved in the regulation of both the fluid shifts during labor (Brace, 1992) and the extracellular volume contraction during postnatal transition (Kojima et al, 1987; Ronconi et al, 1995; Rozycki and Baumgart, 1991; Tulassay et al, 1987). Furthermore, the oliguric effects of positive end-expiratory pressure ventilation are due in part to a decrease in atrial natriuretic peptide secretion (Christensen, 1993) along with the enhanced release of vasopressin (El-Dahr and Chevalier, 1990).

***Dopamine, Noradrenaline, and Adrenaline.*** Dopamine produced in the renal proximal tubule cells and the dopaminergic nerve endings of the kidneys and mesenterium regulates total ECF volume by enhancing sodium excretion and selectively increasing blood flow to the kidney and the intestine (Seri, 1995). In general, adrenaline and locally produced noradrenaline exert opposite renal vascular and tubular effects in the fetus and neonate (Robillard et al, 1990). Both the dopaminergic and α-adrenergic systems appear to be functionally mature even in the preterm neonate, as evidenced by the cardiovascular and renal response to dopamine treatment (Seri, 1995; Seri et al, 1998a, 2002).

***Prostaglandins.*** Prostaglandins play a well-documented counter-regulatory role for the renal vascular and tubular effects of renin-angiotensin-aldosterone and vasopressin (Bonvalet et al, 1987). The inhibition of these actions of prostaglandins by indomethacin results in clinically important and sometimes detrimental renal vascular and tubular effects in the preterm infant (see later). The actions of prostaglandins modulating the effects of the other regulatory hormones of the neonatal fluid and electrolyte homeostasis are less well studied.

***Kallikrein-Kinin System.*** The renal cortical enzyme kallikrein catalyzes the formation of the vasodilator and natriuretic hormone bradykinin. The kallikrein-kinin system is activated at birth and stimulates renal prostaglandin production. Bradykinin also antagonizes the renal actions of vasopressin, renin, and angiotensin (Siegel, 1982).

***Prolactin.*** Prolactin plays a permissive role in the regulation of fetal and neonatal water homeostasis (Coulter, 1983; Pullano et al, 1989). High fetal plasma prolactin levels contribute to the increased tissue water content of the fetus. Interestingly, postnatal prolactin levels remain high in the preterm neonate until around the 40th postconceptional week (Perlman et al, 1978). Dopamine inhibits prolactin secretion in the preterm and term neonate (de Zegher et al, 1993; Seri et al, 1985), potentially resulting in a decrease in water-binding capacity of the tissues (Coulter, 1983). However, the clinical significance of this hypolactotropic effect in the dopamine-treated edematous preterm infant remains to be demonstrated. Finally, it is important to note that prolactin also modulates certain immune and inflammatory responses and T-cell proliferation (Yu-Lee, 2002). Whether the hypolactotropic effects of dopamine would negatively affect neonatal immune function is unknown.

## Fluid And Electrolyte Management in Preterm and Term Neonates

### Patient Evaluation

Maternal conditions during pregnancy, drugs and fluids administered to the mother during labor and delivery, and specific fetal and neonatal conditions all affect the fluid and electrolyte balance of the newborn and should be taken into consideration by the clinician prescribing the infant's initial daily fluid intake.

Clinical evaluation of the newborn's fluid and electrolyte status should be based on clinical signs of dehydration or edema formation and on accurate serial measurements of body weight. Laboratory studies aiding in daily fluid and electrolyte management are serial measurements of serum electrolytes, blood urea nitrogen, serum creatinine, serum albumin, and serum osmolality. The frequency of monitoring depends on the extent of immaturity as well as the severity of the fluid and electrolyte disturbance and of the underlying pathologic condition.

### General Principles of Fluid and Electrolyte Management

The most important principle of fluid and electrolyte management of the sick preterm or term infant is to prevent, or at least to decrease the likelihood of, significant pulmonary and extrapulmonary edema formation. The measures to achieve this goal are (1) provision of a negative fluid and electrolyte balance during the first few postnatal days through restriction of fluid and salt administration, (2) avoidance of excessive fluid intake during the rest of the first months of life, (3) early closure of the ductus arteriosus, (4) the use of blood transfusions rather than that of colloid or crystalloid boluses for volume support if appropriate, and (5) the provision of sufficient nutrition. Because peripheral vasodilation due to disturbed regulation of vascular tone almost always contributes to the development of hypotension in the sick neonate, early administration of low to moderate doses of dopamine may further reduce the need for volume boluses, and via its renal and hormonal effects, dopamine may facilitate the process of extracellular volume contraction (Seri, 1995).

Water and electrolyte requirements depend on the daily losses and the state of metabolic activity. Water requirement should be estimated on the basis of the volume status and the sensible and insensible losses in the given infant. Because abrupt alterations in serum sodium concentration are associated with similar changes in serum osmolality, they may have severe central nervous system sequelae and should be avoided.

## Abnormalities of Sodium Homeostasis

### *Hyponatremia*

Hyponatremia (serum sodium <130 mEq/L) represents a deficit of sodium in relation to body water content and may be due to either total body sodium deficit or free water excess. When hyponatremia is caused by total body sodium deficit, free water may be decreased (hyponatremia with volume contraction), normal, or increased (hyponatremia with volume expansion). Similarly, when hyponatremia is caused by free water excess, total body sodium may be low, normal, or high. Depending on the osmolality of the serum, hyponatremia may be hypotonic, isotonic, or hypertonic. The most common manifestation of hyponatremia in the neonate is hypotonic hyponatremia due to excessive administration or retention of free water.

***Hypotonic Hyponatremia.*** Serum osmolality is reduced in hypotonic hyponatremia (<280 mOsm/L). In cases of *hypotonic hyponatremia with volume contraction*, there is a disproportionally greater loss of sodium than of water. In the preterm or term neonate, volume contraction with hypotonic hyponatremia may occur secondary to excessive renal losses of sodium due to renal immaturity, use of diuretics, and adrenal insufficiency as well as in cerebral salt wasting and during recovery from an acute renal insult (asphyxia, shock). Although cerebral salt wasting is uncommon in newborn infants (Ganong and Kappy, 1993), this condition must be differentiated from SIADH. In contrast to patients with SIADH, patients with cerebral salt wasting have decreases in plasma volume as well as plasma aldosterone and vasopressin levels and a normal plasma uric acid concentration. Treatment of hypotonic hyponatremia with volume contraction consists of replacement of both the free water and the sodium deficit.

*Hypotonic hyponatremia with volume expansion* results from positive water balance, and the diagnosis is based on the clinical signs of edema and weight gain as well as the history of increased free water administration or medical conditions associated with enhanced vasopressin production (central nervous system injury, congestive heart failure). Total body sodium is usually normal or somewhat elevated. Thus, appropriate restriction of free water intake, not administration of sodium, is the treatment of choice for this disorder.

***Isotonic Pseudohyponatremia.*** Hyponatremia in the presence of normal serum osmolality (285 to 295 mOsm/L) is referred to as *pseudohyponatremia*. Under physiologic conditions, 93% of the total plasma volume is an aqueous phase that contains the electrolytes, and the remaining 7% is a solid phase composed primarily of lipids and proteins. In hyperlipidemia or hyperproteinemia, the solid phase increases at the expense of the aqueous phase, and serum sodium concentration measured in the total plasma compartment decreases. Thus, in patients with pseudohyponatremia, total body sodium, TBW content, and sodium concentration in the aqueous phase are all within normal limits, but sodium concentration measured in the total plasma compartment is reduced. In these patients, the laboratory test results indicate hyponatremia, but serum osmolality is normal, and additional tests reveal the presence of hyperproteinemia or hyperlipidemia.

***Hypertonic Hyponatremia.*** In patients with hypertonic hyponatremia, the hyponatremia is associated with increased serum osmolality (>295 mOsm/L). This condition occurs because of the presence of an osmotically active substance in the plasma, such as glucose, which results in hypertonicity. Hypertonicity, in turn, causes water to shift from the intracellular space into the interstitium and the intravascular compartment, leading to a decrease in the plasma sodium concentration. With a serum glucose concentration in excess of 100 mg/dL, every 100-mg/dL rise in plasma glucose results in a 1.6-mEq/L decrease in the serum sodium concentration. This diagnosis should be suspected if hyponatremia is detected along with a serum osmolality of greater than 295 mOsm/L or if the measured serum osmolality is 20 mOsm/L higher than the calculated serum osmolality.

***Treatment of Hyponatremia.*** If serum sodium concentration is less than 120 mEq/L, correction of hyponatremia is recommended with 3% saline solution (513 mEq of sodium per liter) up to 120 mEq/L of serum sodium concentration over 4 to 6 hours depending on the severity of hyponatremia (Avner, 1995). Although rapid intravenous bolus administration of 4 to 6 mL/kg of 3% saline solution has been effective in children with seizures or coma (Sarnaik et al, 1991), one must keep in mind that rapid and complete correction of low serum sodium concentration in adults with chronic hyponatremia has been shown to be associated with pontine and extrapontine myelinolysis. Therefore, once the risk of central nervous system symptoms has been minimized and serum sodium concentration has reached 120 mEq/L, complete correction of hyponatremia should be performed more slowly, over 24 to 48 hours. In patients with asymptomatic hyponatremia whose serum sodium concentration exceeds 120 mEq/L, hypertonic infusions are not indicated. The use of 5% dextrose in water with 0.45% to 0.9% saline is reasonable. Figure 30–5 summarizes the clinical evaluation and therapy of neonates with hyponatremia.

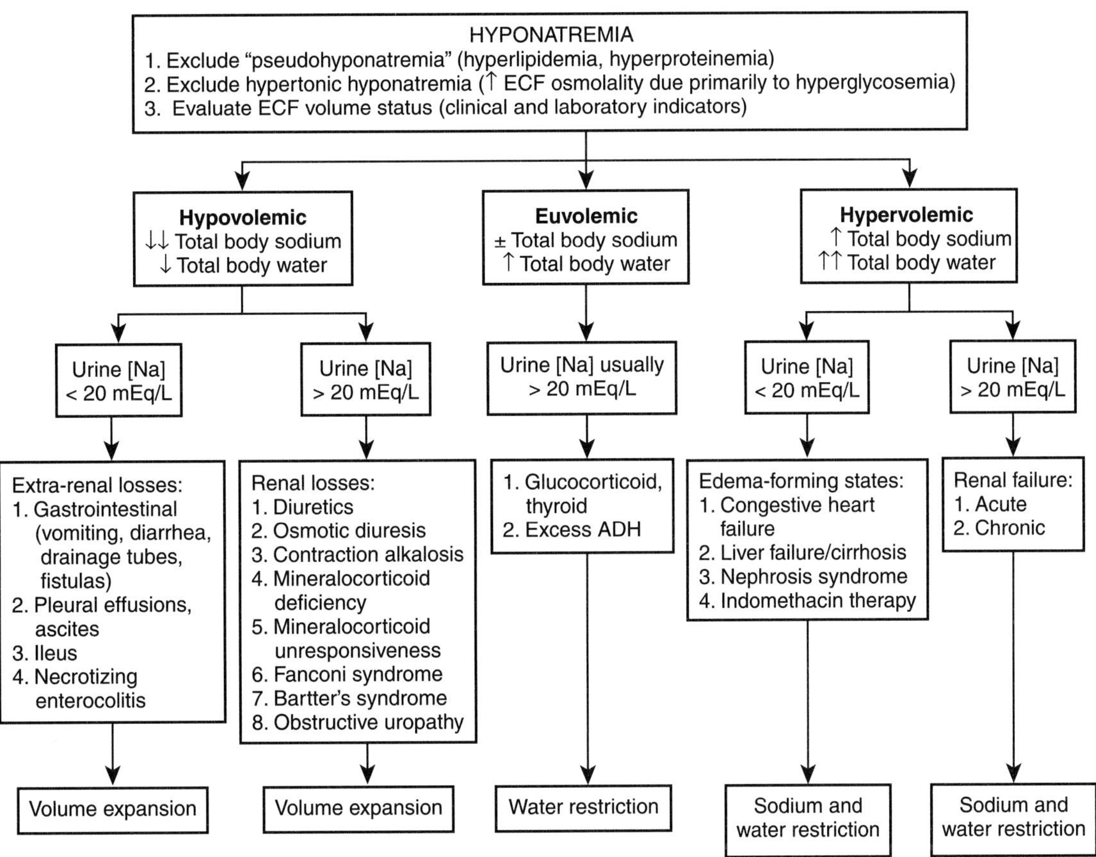


**FIGURE 30–5.** Flow diagram for the clinical evaluation and therapy of neonates with hyponatremia. ECF, extracellular fluid. *(Modified from Avner ED: Clinical disorders of water metabolism: Hyponatremia and hypernatremia. Pediatr Ann 24:23-30, 1995).*

### *Hypernatremia*

Hypernatremia (serum sodium >150 mEq/L) reflects the deficiency of water relative to total body sodium and is most often a disorder of water rather than sodium homeostasis. Hypernatremia does not indicate total body sodium content, which can be high, normal, or low depending on the etiology of the condition. If the primary cause is a disorder of water homeostasis, hypernatremia can result from pure water loss, from water loss coupled with a lesser degree of sodium deficit, or from sodium gain, and it can be associated with hypovolemia, normovolemia, or hypervolemia (Table 30–2). If hypernatremia is primarily due to changes in sodium balance, it can result from pure sodium gain or, more commonly, sodium gain coupled with a lesser degree of water accumulation or, rarely, sodium gain coupled with water loss. The hypernatremia-induced hypertonicity causes water to shift from the intracellular to the extracellular compartment, resulting in intracellular dehydration and the relative preservation of the extracellular compartment. This is the main reason that neonates with chronic and severe hypernatremic dehydration do not demonstrate overt clinical signs of dehydration until late in the course of the condition.

Compared with the other organs, the central nervous system has a unique adaptive capacity to respond to the

**TABLE 30–2**

**Conditions Causing Hypernatremia**

**Hypovolemic hypernatremia:**
- Inadequate breast milk intake
- Diarrhea
- Radiant warmers
- Excessive sweating
- Renal dysplasia
- Osmotic diuresis

**Euvolemic hypernatremia:**

*Decreased production of antidiuretic hormone:*
- Central diabetes insipidus, head trauma, central nervous system tumors (craniopharyngioma), meningitis, or encephalitis

*Decrease or absence of renal responsiveness:*
- Nephrogenic diabetes insipidus, extreme immaturity, renal insult and medications such as amphotericin, hydantoin, aminoglycosides

**Hypervolemic hypernatremia:**
- Improperly mixed formula
- $NaHCO_3$ administration
- NaCl administration
- Primary hyperaldosteronism

hypernatremia-induced hypertonicity, leading to a relative preservation of neuronal cell volume. The shrinkage of the brain stimulates the uptake of electrolytes such as sodium, potassium, and chloride (immediate effect) as well as the synthesis of osmoprotective amino acids and organic solutes (more delayed response). Osmoprotective amino acids include glutamate, glutamine, phosphocreatine and taurine; organic solutes, known as idiogenic osmols, include myo-inositol, glycerophosphoryl-choline, and betaine. The idiogenic osmols aid in maintaining normal brain-cell volume and protect intracellular proteins during longer periods of hyperosmolar stress (Trachtman, 1991). As long as hypernatremia develops rapidly (within hours), as in accidental sodium loading, a relatively rapid correction of the condition improves the prognosis without raising the risk of edema formation. This occurs because the accumulated electrolytes (sodium, potassium, and chloride) are rapidly extruded from the brain cells and effective idiogenic osmol synthesis has not yet taken place. In these cases, reducing serum sodium concentration by 1 mEq/L per hour (24 mEq/L per day) is appropriate (Adrogue and Madias, 2000).

However, because of the slow dissipation of idiogenic osmols over a period of several days (Adrogue and Madias, 2000), in cases of chronic hypernatremia, such as that in the breast-fed neonate with hypernatremic dehydration, the hypernatremia should be corrected more slowly, at a maximal rate of 0.5 mEq/L per hour (12 mEq/L per day). If correction is performed more rapidly in cases of chronic hypernatremia, the abrupt fall in the extracellular tonicity results in the movement of water into the brain cells, which have a relatively fixed hypertonicity because of the presence of the osmoprotective molecules. The result is the development of brain edema with deleterious consequences (Adrogue and Madias, 2000; Molteni, 1994).

In the *exclusively breast-fed neonate*, hypernatremia is usually due to high sodium levels in maternal breast milk as well as poor overall intake and dehydration. Reduction in breast-feeding frequency has been shown to be associated with a marked rise in the sodium concentration of breast milk (Neville et al, 1991). A vicious cycle can ensue in which the infant sucks poorly, breast milk production drops and sodium concentration rises, and the infant becomes increasingly dehydrated, hypernatremic, and lethargic. Hypernatremia associated with breast-feeding usually manifests at the end of the first to the third week after birth and may be delayed because these infants may appear quiet and content early on. The combination of inadequate fluid intake and hyperosmolarity can be devastating, with complications such as seizures, diffuse intravascular coagulation, and permanent neurologic and vascular injury.

In the *extremely immature neonate*, hypernatremia most commonly occurs from excessive transepidermal free water losses. The condition usually develops rapidly, within 24 to 48 hours after birth; it has become less common probably because of the more frequent use of antenatal steroids and humidified incubators. The diagnosis is based on the attendant decrease in body weight and clinical signs of extracellular volume contraction. Prevention of this condition by frequent monitoring of serum electrolyte levels, appropriate adjustments of free water intake, and the use of humidified incubators has been successful in the majority of immature neonates.

In the *breast-fed term neonate*, hypernatremia most commonly develops because of dehydration due to inadequate breast milk intake (Molteni, 1994). Because this is a more chronic process, usually occurring over 7 to 14 days, signs of extracellular volume contraction are less prominent until the development of the full clinical presentation consisting of lethargy, irritability, abnormal muscle tone with or without seizures, and cardiovascular collapse with renal failure. This presentation can be associated with especially significant central nervous system morbidity from both the hypertonicity (saggital or other venous sinus thrombosis, subdural capillary hemorrhage, white matter injury) and inappropriately rapid rehydration therapy (brain edema, myelinolysis).

*The central and nephrogenic forms of diabetes insipidus* are much less commonly encountered and result in hypernatremia due to the lack of production of and renal responsiveness to ADH, respectively. Because ADH is the primary neuroendocrine mechanism protecting against the rapid development of hypernatremia, central nervous system and renal immaturity make the sick preterm infant especially vulnerable to the rapid development of hypernatremia due to excessive free water losses. Finally, hypernatremia may also develop in response to excessive sodium supplementation, mainly in the sick neonate receiving repeated volume boluses for cardiovascular support. In these cases, clinical signs of edema, increased body weight, and the history of volume boluses help establish the diagnosis.

In the critically ill infant, the etiology of the serum sodium abnormality may be multifactorial, and the treatment less straightforward. However, thorough analysis of the medical history and the changes in clinical signs, laboratory findings, and body weight usually aid in determining the major etiologic factor and thus the treatment of the more complex cases of serum sodium abnormalities. Because sodium does not freely cross the cell membrane, serum sodium concentration is the major determinant of serum tonicity and, as mentioned previously, correction of its abnormalities should be carried out in a stepwise manner.

The following calculations may be used to govern the fluid and electrolyte replacement therapy in neonates with abnormal fluid and electrolyte status. Sodium deficit (or excess) may be calculated using the formula

$$\text{Na}^+ \text{ deficit (or excess)} = (0.75 \times \text{BW}) \times ([\text{Na}^+]_{\text{desired}} - [\text{Na}^+]_{\text{actual}}).$$

In this formula, sodium deficit (or excess) and body weight (BW) are expressed in mEq/L and kg, respectively, and (0.75 × BW) is the estimation of TBW.

Similarly, free water deficit (or excess) may be calculated as

$$\frac{\text{H}_2\text{O deficit}}{\text{(or excess)}} = (0.75 \times \text{BW}) \times \frac{[\text{Na}^+]_{\text{desired}}}{[\text{Na}^+]_{\text{actual}} - 1}$$

In this formula, $H_2O$ deficit (or excess) and body weight are given in L and kg, respectively, and (0.75 × BW) is the estimation of TBW.

Serum osmolality may be calculated by the formula

$$\text{serum osmolality} = 2[Na^+_{plasma}] + \frac{BUN}{2.8} + \frac{\text{blood glucose}}{18}$$

Serum osmolality, $[Na^+_{plasma}]$, BUN (blood urea nitrogen), and blood glucose should be expressed in mOsm/L, mEq/L, mg/dL, and mg/dL, respectively.

Total free water deficit is calculated as follows

$$\text{free water deficit} = 0.75 \times BW \times \frac{[1 - (\text{current Na concentration})}{145}$$

In this formula, free water deficit, body weight (BW), and sodium concentrations are given in L, kg, and mEq/L, respectively. The amount of free water required to decrease serum sodium by 12 mEq/L over a 24-hour period if serum sodium is ≥195 mEq/L is calculated as

$$\text{free water required} = \text{current weight (kg)} \times 3\ \text{mL/kg} \times 12\ \text{mEq/L}$$
$$\text{or current weight (kg)} \times 36\ \text{mL/kg/day}$$

3 mL/kg is used here because it is approximately the amount of free water required to decrease serum sodium concentration by 1 mEq/L when the serum sodium concentration is 195 mEq/L (Molteni, 1994).

***Treatment Guidelines for Cases of Severe, Chronic Hypernatremia.*** The patient with severe, chronic hypernatremia is usually an exclusively breast-fed neonate with inadequate milk supply. The amount of free water required to decrease serum sodium concentration by 1 mEq/L is 4 mL/kg under physiologic circumstances. However, as described previously, when the serum sodium concentration is 195 mEq/L, ≤3 mL/kg of free water is needed to achieve the same effect. Therefore, the maximum total amount of free water for *deficit replacement* over a 24-hour period should be around 36 mL/kg. *Maintenance fluid* calculations must take into consideration the usually significantly decreased urine output. Therefore, free water maintenance fluid administration should be based only on calculated insensible losses (30 to 40 mL/kg/day), and urine output should initially be replaced volume for volume every 4 to 6 hours with a solution tailored to the urinary sodium and free water losses (usually 0.45% sodium chloride saline and 50 to 75 mEq of sodium bicarbonate per L). To calculate the replacement and maintenance free water requirements, one must also know the free water content of the intravenous fluids used (Table 30–3).

The major goals of fluid therapy in the treatment of severe and chronic hypernatremic dehydration are (1) establishment and maintenance of appropriate intravascular volume, (2) replacement of water and electrolyte deficits, (3) replacement of ongoing urine and stool water and electrolyte losses as well as insensible water losses, and (4) establishment of a rate of decline in serum sodium concentration that does not exceed 12 mEq/L/day. Boluses used for stabilization of the intravascular volume should be given through the use of intravenous fluids with a sodium concentration *either equal to the serum sodium concentration or at most 10 mEq/L less than that concentration.* This practice limits free water delivery and avoids sudden drops in serum sodium concentration and thus in tonicity. One should then calculate the amount of free water required to decrease the serum sodium concentration by 12 mEq/L during the first 24 hours (see preceding calculation), subtract the free water content (if any) of the initial fluid boluses, add the insensible losses and remaining free water deficit-replacement volumes, and provide the resulting volume as 0.2% saline in 5% or 10% dextrose in water. Finally, ongoing urine losses should be replaced volume for volume with the use of a solution adjusted to the urinary electrolyte losses.

Serum electrolyte, blood urea nitrogen, and serum creatinine values should be monitored every 2 to 4 hours until an appropriate rate of decline in serum sodium concentration has been established. At this point, the frequency of the laboratory measurements can be relaxed to every 4 to 6 hours (and later to 8 to 12 hours), until the serum sodium concentration is less than 145 mEq/L. This approach provides

**TABLE 30–3**

**Free Water Content as Volume % of Common Intravenous Solutions at Normal and High Serum Sodium Concentrations***

| | Serum Sodium Concentration | | | |
|---|---|---|---|---|
| | 145 mEq/L | | 195 mEq/L | |
| **Intravenous Fluid** | **Isotonic (%)** | **Water (%)** | **Isotonic (%)** | **Water (%)** |
| D5W | 0 | 100 | 0 | 100 |
| 0.2% saline | 22 | 78 | 17 | 83 |
| 0.45% saline | 50 | 50 | 39 | 61 |
| 0.9% saline | 100 | 0 | 79 | 21 |
| Lactated Ringer's solution | 86 | 14 | 68 | 32 |

*Note that isotonic saline provides 21% free water when given to a patient with a serum sodium concentration of 195 mEq/L and therefore will induce undesirable decreases in serum sodium concentration when used for volume resuscitation in the severely dehydrated hypernatremic neonate. See text for details.

Modified from Molteni KH: Initial management of hypernatremic dehydration in the breastfed infant. Clin Pediatr 33:731-740, 1994.

a reasonable chance to gradually decrease serum sodium concentration to the normal range over 5 to 7 days depending on the initial sodium values.

Once serum sodium concentration, urine output, and renal function are normal, the patient should receive standard maintenance fluids, either intravenously or orally, depending on his or her condition. At this time, electrolyte status must still be monitored for an additional 24 hours to ensure that complete recovery has occurred. Hyperglycemia and hypocalcemia commonly accompany hypernatremia. Treatment of hyperglycemia with insulin is not recommended because it may increase brain idiogenic osmol content. Hypocalcemia should be corrected with appropriate calcium supplementation.

Although magnetic resonance imaging of the brain before discharge provides information on potential insults associated with the condition and its treatment, long-term neurodevelopmental follow-up should be arranged for every neonate who has experienced severe hypernatremic dehydration.

## Water Requirements

To appropriately estimate the daily free water requirements of the sick neonate, all sources of water losses must be taken into account—the insensible, sensible, and surgical water losses. Free water losses occurring through the skin and the respiratory tract are considered insensible losses, whereas the sensible water losses are composed of the amounts lost through urine and feces.

### *Insensible Losses*

As described in the earlier discussion of the maturation of the skin, gestational age, postnatal age and environmental factors determine the amount of daily insensible water losses through the skin (see Fig. 30–4). During the first few postnatal days, transepidermal water losses may be 15 times higher in extremely premature infants born at 24 to 26 weeks of gestation than in term neonates (Sedin, 1995). Although the skin rapidly matures shortly after birth even in extremely immature infants, the insensible water losses in such patients are still somewhat higher at the end of the first months than those of their term counterparts.

Among the environmental factors, ambient humidity has the greatest impact on transepidermal water loss. In extremely immature neonates, a rise in the ambient humidity of the incubator from 20% to 80% decreases the transepidermal water loss by approximately 75% (Sedin, 1995). The difference in daily free water losses between 20% and 80% ambient humidity values is around 150 mL/kg. On the other hand, the use of an open radiant warmer more than doubles transepidermal water losses. However, if a plastic heat shield is applied while the infant is under the warmer, transepidermal water loss may be decreased by 30% to 50% (Costarino and Baumgart, 1991). At low ambient humidity, phototherapy increases transepidermal water losses by approximately 30%. However, in infants older than 28 weeks gestation, phototherapy does not increase the transepidermal water loss if the ambient humidity is 50% in the incubator (Sedin, 1995). Other factors, including activity, airflow, and prenatal steroid treatment, also influence the magnitude of transepidermal free water losses (Aszterbaum et al, 1993; Sedin, 1995).

Insensible water losses from the respiratory tract depend mainly on the temperature and humidity of the inspired gas mixture and on the respiratory rate, tidal volume, and dead space ventilation. In a healthy term newborn, the water loss through the respiratory tract is approximately half of the total insensible water loss if the ambient air temperature is 32.5° C and the humidity is 50% (Sedin, 1995). However, the respiratory water loss in critically ill preterm and term infants undergoing mechanical ventilation is zero if the gas mixture is saturated with water at body temperature.

### *Sensible Losses*

Free water loss in the urine is the most important form of sensible water loss. Smaller preterm infants without systemic hypotension or prerenal renal failure usually lose 30 to 40 mL/kg/day water in the urine on the first postnatal day and around 120 mL/kg/day on the third day after birth. In stable, more mature preterm infants born after the 28th week of gestation, urinary water loss is around 90 mL/kg/day on the first postnatal day and 150 mL/kg/day on the third day (Coulthard and Hey, 1985). Owing to their renal immaturity, preterm neonates have a tendency to produce dilute urine, thereby increasing their obligatory free water losses.

Water losses in the stool are less significant, amounting to approximately 10 mL/kg/day in term infants and 7 mL/kg/day in preterm infants during the first week of life (Sedin, 1995). Water losses in the stool increase thereafter and are influenced by the type of feeding and the frequency of stooling.

### *Surgical Losses*

The most commonly encountered surgical water losses occur when a nasogastric tube is placed under continuous suction to provide relief for the gastrointestinal tract in conditions such as necrotizing enterocolitis and postoperative management after abdominal surgery. Because these losses may be substantial, their replacement every 8 to 12 hours is necessary to maintain appropriate water and electrolyte balance. However, free water retention often develops after surgery, so full replacement of the nasogastric free water loss is not usually recommended. The composition of the replacement solution depends on the electrolyte concentration of the fluid loss. Gastric fluid usually contains 50 to 60 mEq/L of sodium chloride, and the sodium loss should also be replaced.

## Electrolyte Requirements

Because sodium, potassium, chloride, and bicarbonate have the most profound effects on TBW volume and fluid balance, only the requirements for these electrolytes are considered here.

### *Sodium and its Anions*

In the preterm infant, sodium chloride supplementation should be started only after completion of the postnatal extracellular volume contraction. In general, as long as the infant's fluid balance is stable, daily sodium requirement does not exceed 3 to 4 mEq/kg/day, and provision of this amount usually ensures the positive sodium balance necessary for adequate growth. Extreme prematurity and pathologic conditions associated with delayed transition or disturbance of fluid and electrolyte balance may significantly reduce or increase the infant's daily sodium requirement. Neonates recovering from an acute renal insult and preterm infants with immature proximal tubule functions who are in a state of extracellular volume expansion (Ramiro-Tolentino et al, 1996) may need daily sodium bicarbonate supplementation to compensate for their greater renal bicarbonate losses.

### *Potassium*

In the early postnatal period, neonates, especially immature preterm infants, have higher serum potassium concentrations than older persons. The etiology of the relative hyperkalemia of the newborn is multifactorial and involves developmentally regulated differences in renal function, $Na^+$,$K^+$-ATPase activity (Vasarhelyi et al, 2000), and hormonal milieu. In general, potassium chloride supplementation should be started only after urine output has been well established, usually during the second day of life. In the majority of cases, potassium requirement is 2 to 3 mEq/kg/day. However, after the completion of the postnatal volume contraction, preterm infants may need more potassium because of their increased plasma aldosterone concentrations, prostaglandin excretion, and disproportionately high urine flow rates as well as the use of diuretics.

## Clinical Conditions Associated with Fluid and Electrolyte Disturbances

### Extreme Prematurity

Infants born between 23 and 27 weeks of gestation are at particular risks for acute abnormalities of the fluid and electrolyte status in the immediate postnatal period. Their transepidermal water loss is much higher than that in more mature preterm neonates (see Fig. 30–4), and it is difficult to maintain their water balance unless the excessive losses are prevented. It should be kept in mind that such an infant, when cared for in an open warmer without the use of a plastic heat shield, may lose 150 to 300 mL/kg/day of free water through the skin during the first 3 to 5 days of life. Although the insensible water loss primarily affects the extracellular volume, the intracellular compartment ultimately shares the loss of free water as osmotic pressure in the extracellular compartment rises. As water leaves the cells, intracellular osmolality rises and cell volume diminishes. In the central nervous system, as described earlier, these changes stimulate the generation of idiogenic osmols, resulting in selective increases in intracellular osmolality and a tendency toward normalization of neuronal cell volumes. This protective mechanism has significant clinical implications for the rate at which hypernatremia should be corrected, and the decrease in serum sodium concentration should not exceed 12 mEq/L/24 hours, especially in the infant in whom the hypernatremia has been chronic (>12 hours).

Because serum sodium concentration is a reliable clinical indicator of extracellular tonicity, monitoring of this parameter every 6 to 8 hours during the first 2 to 3 postnatal days coupled with daily measurements of body weight provide valuable information and appropriate guidance for the fluid and electrolyte management of the extremely immature preterm neonate, especially in the absence of prenatal steroid exposure and if the infant is not cared for in a humidified incubator. Serum osmolality should be directly measured in patients in whom calculated serum osmolality is more than 300 to 320 mOsm/L.

Because immature neonates cared for in an incubator with an ambient air humidity of 50% to 80% require significantly less free water as well as less frequent measurements of serum electrolyte and osmolality (Sedin, 1995), open radiant warmers should be used only for critically ill, extremely labile preterm infants requiring frequent hands-on medical management. In these cases, the use of a protective plastic heat shield decreases excessive evaporative losses, and total daily fluid intake may be started at 80 to 100 mL/kg/day with 5% dextrose in water. Daily fluid intake is then increased by 10 to 30 mL/kg/day every 6 to 8 hours if the serum sodium concentration rises from the baseline, the goal being to keep serum sodium concentration below 150 mEq/L. As skin integrity improves during the course of the second to third days, serum sodium concentration starts to fall. At this time, a significant stepwise limitation of total fluid intake is obligatory to allow a complete contraction of the extracellular volume to occur and to minimize the possibility of free water overload with its attendant risks for the development of ductal patency, pulmonary edema, and worsening lung disease.

Potassium chloride supplementation may be started as soon as urine output has been established and the serum potassium concentration is below 5 mEq/L. Extremely premature infants are at risk for the development of both oliguric and nonoliguric hyperkalemia, so the serum potassium concentration should be monitored closely, and supplementation discontinued if warranted by changes in serum potassium values or in renal function. Critically ill, extremely immature neonates often receive excess sodium with volume boluses, medications, and the maintenance infusion of their arterial lines. Therefore, extra sodium supplementation usually should not be started during the first few postnatal days so as to prevent a rise in total body sodium concentration and thus in extracellular volume.

Many critically ill preterm infants, however, retain their originally high extracellular volumes even when sodium and water intakes are restricted, and such neonates also tend to lose more bicarbonate in the urine. Interestingly, proximal tubular bicarbonate reabsorption may be appropriate even in the very LBW infant despite the immaturity of their renal functions, as long as extracellular volume contraction takes place (Ramiro-Tolentino et al, 1996). Therefore, the presence of the extracellular volume expansion appears to be an important factor in the renal bicarbonate wasting in these infants. The diagnosis of functional proximal tubular acidosis in such cases should not rely solely on the finding of an alkaline urine pH, because the distal tubular function is usually mature enough to acidify the urine once serum bicarbonate has decreased to its new threshold. Provided that liver function is normal, daily supplementation of bicarbonate in the form of sodium acetate, potassium acetate, or both normalizes blood pH and serum bicarbonate in these infants and also increases urine pH, aiding in the diagnosis. Once extracellular volume contraction occurs, these neonates generally achieve a positive bicarbonate balance (Ramiro-Tolentino et al, 1996), and supplementation becomes unnecessary.

Other general guidelines in the fluid and electrolyte management of the immature preterm infant during the first week of life are (1) daily calculation of fluid balance and estimation of sodium balance, (2) testing of all urine samples for glucose, albumin, and hemoglobin as well as osmolality or specific gravity, and (3) the daily measurements of serum electrolytes and creatinine, plasma glucose, and blood urea nitrogen. The frequency of testing and the addition of other tests, including the measurement of serum albumin concentration and osmolality, depend on the clinical status, severity of underlying disease, and fluid and electrolyte disturbance of the given patient.

## Respiratory Distress Syndrome

There is a well-established relationship between fluid and electrolyte balance and respiratory distress syndrome. Surfactant deficiency results in pulmonary atelectasis, elevated pulmonary vascular resistance, poor lung compliance, and decreased lymphatic drainage. In addition, preterm infants have low plasma oncotic and critical pulmonary capillary pressures and suffer pulmonary capillary endothelial injury from mechanical ventilation, oxygen administration, and perinatal hypoxia (Dudek and Garcia, 2001; Sola and Gregory, 1981). These abnormalities alter the balance of the Starling forces in the pulmonary microcirculation, leading to interstitial edema formation with further impairment in pulmonary functions.

In the pre-surfactant era, an improvement in pulmonary function occurred only during the third to fourth postnatal day. This improvement was usually preceded by a period of brisk diuresis characterized by small increases in glomerular filtration rate and sodium clearance and a larger rise in free water clearance (Costarino and Baumgart, 1991). Although the exact mechanism of the diuresis is not known, it is likely that improving endogenous surfactant production and capillary integrity promoted the recovery of the pulmonary capillary endothelium and lymphatic drainage. The ensuing changes in Starling forces then favored reabsorption of the hypotonic interstitial lung fluid into the circulation, and a delayed "physiologic diuresis" took place.

Currently, with the routine use of surfactant and the more common use of prenatal steroids, the pulmonary compromise and its consequences are less severe. However, because significant improvements in lung function take place only after the majority of the excess free water is excreted (Costarino and Baumgart, 1991), daily fluid intake should still be restricted to allow for the extracellular volume contraction to take place. If this principle is not followed and a positive fluid balance occurs, preterm infants with hyaline membrane disease are at higher risk for a more severe course of acute lung disease and for presenting with a higher incidence of patent ductus arteriosus, congestive heart failure, and necrotizing enterocolitis as well as a higher incidence and greater severity of the ensuing chronic lung disease.

Antenatal administration of steroids and postnatal use of surfactants have clearly altered the course and clinical presentation of hyaline membrane disease (Ballard and Ballard, 1995; Ishisaka, 1996; Kari et al, 1994). Antenatal steroid administration accelerates maturation of organs including those involved in the regulation of fluid and electrolyte balance (Ballard and Ballard, 1995), while the use of exogenous surfactant decreases pulmonary capillary leak and edema formation (Carlton et al, 1995). Furthermore, surfactant administration does not alter the rate and timing of ductal closure (Reller et al, 1993) although it may affect the pattern of shunting through the ductus arteriosus in the acute period (Kaapa et al, 1993; Kluckow and Evans, 2000). Thus, these interventions generally enhance extracellular volume contraction and aid in the stabilization of fluid and electrolyte homeostasis in preterm neonates with hyaline membrane disease. However, maintenance of a negative water and sodium balance during the first few days of life remains the cornerstone of fluid and electrolyte management in these infants (Tammela, 1995; Van Marter et al, 1990).

On the basis of the events in the pathophysiology of pulmonary edema formation in infants with hyaline membrane disease previously described, the use of furosemide has long been suggested to promote a negative fluid balance and directly inhibit pulmonary epithelial transport processes involved in edema formation in the lungs (Green et al, 1988; Yeh et al, 1984). However, furosemide induces only short-term improvements in pulmonary function in these patients, and no beneficial effects on long-term morbidity or mortality has been documented. Moreover, prophylactic use of the drug during the first postnatal days may lead to intravascular volume depletion with hypotension, tachycardia, and decreased peripheral perfusion as well as to acute and chronic disturbances in serum electrolytes and, thus, osmolality (Green et al, 1988; Shaffer and Weismann, 1992; Yeh et al, 1984). Furthermore, its chronic administration may be associated with an increased incidence of patent ductus arteriosus (Green et al, 1983). Therefore, the use of furosemide during this period should be restricted to patients with oliguria of renal origin whose intravascular volume appears to be adequate.

## Chronic Lung Disease

Low gestational age and birth weight, lack of antenatal steroid administration, severe hyaline membrane disease with oxygen toxicity, volu- and barotrauma, air leak, inflammation, patent ductus arteriosus, and insufficient nutrition are among the known etiologic factors for the development of bronchopulmonary dysplasia. In addition, a high fluid and salt intake during the first weeks of life have been shown to increase the incidence and severity of chronic lung disease. Therefore, careful fluid and electrolyte management during the first weeks of life is of great importance in decreasing the incidence and severity of this condition (see Chapter 49).

## Shock and Edema

In the uncompensated phase of shock, blood pressure is low, cardiac output may be low, normal, or high, effective circulating blood volume is usually decreased, transcapillary hydrostatic pressure is elevated, and capillary integrity and lymphatic drainage are impaired, resulting in edema formation and increased interstitial compliance. The latter condition further enhances fluid accumulation in the interstitium. The changes in the effective circulating blood volume also trigger the release of antidiuretic hormones, including the catecholamines, renin-angiotensin-aldosterone, and vasopressin, resulting in retention of sodium and free water. The specific cause of shock (infection, asphyxia, myocardial insufficiency, hypovolemia, etc.) may independently contribute to this chain of events, further compromising fluid and electrolyte balance. In affected infants, treatment is directed at normalizing tissue perfusion and oxygen delivery by restoring effective intravascular volume, cardiac output, and renal function with the use of vasopressor and inotropic support, as well as with the judicious use of volume expanders while monitoring blood pressure, cardiac output, and changes in organ blood flow (see Chapter 31). In shock refractory to this management, early initiation of low-dose glucocorticoid and mineralocorticoid replacement may help break the vicious cycle by improving capillary integrity and thus effective circulating blood volume, and by potentiating the cardiovascular response to vasopressors and inotropic agents (Seri et al, 2000).

## Patent Ductus Arteriosus

A patent ductus arteriosus significantly increases morbidity and mortality, especially in the very LBW preterm infant. Several conditions, including severe hypoxemia, unstable cardiovascular status, acute deterioration, metabolic acidosis, and increases in extracellular volume and ductal prostaglandin synthesis, have been recognized to promote the patency of the ductus arteriosus (Hammerman, 1995; see also Chapter 56). Accordingly, clinical management aimed at preventing the occurrence of ductal patency involves interventions that keep the cardiovascular status and oxygenation stable, restrict fluid intake, and maintain low levels of local prostaglandin synthesis by the administration of indomethacin (Clyman, 1996). Pharmacologic ductal closure with indomethacin is indicated only during the first two postnatal weeks, because ductal sensitivity to prostaglandins rapidly diminishes thereafter (Clyman, 1996; Van Overmeire et al, 2000).

In the sick preterm infant, indomethacin administration almost always has clinically significant, although mostly transient, renal side effects. Ibuprofen may cause less severe renal dysfunction (Van Overmeire et al, 2000) and cerebral vasoconstriction (Patel et al, 2000). However, further trials are necessary before ibuprofen can be used in this setting, especially since ibuprofen displaces bilirubin from albumin. If not recognized and treated promptly, the untoward renal actions of the inhibition of prostaglandin synthesis may alter the infant's fluid and electrolyte balance and could potentially reduce the effectiveness of the therapy. Under physiologic circumstances in the immediate postnatal period, renal prostaglandin production is increased to counterbalance the renal actions of vasoconstrictor and sodium- and water-retaining hormones released during labor and delivery (Bonvalet et al, 1987; Gleason, 1987). Thus, compared with the renal function of the adult kidney in euvolemia, the neonatal kidney is more dependent on the increased production of vasodilatory and natriuretic prostaglandins, rendering it more sensitive to the vasoconstrictive and sodium- and water-retaining actions of cyclooxygenase inhibition.

In the indomethacin-treated neonate, the unopposed renal vasoconstriction and sodium and water reabsorption lead to decreases in renal blood flow and glomerular filtration rate and to increases in sodium and free water reabsorption. These side effects occur despite the diminishing left-to-right shunt through the closing ductus. Characteristic clinical findings include a rise in serum creatinine level, oliguria, and hyponatremia (Cifuentes et al, 1979). Hyponatremia occurs because the free water retention caused by the unopposed renal actions of high plasma vasopressin levels is out of proportion to the sodium retention induced by angiotensin and noradrenaline. This pattern of renal response can most likely be explained by the fact that in a preterm infant, function of the distal tubule is more mature than that of the proximal tubule (Lumbers et al, 1988), leading to an expanded but somewhat hypotonic extracellular space. Therefore, treatment must focus on maintaining an appropriately restricted fluid intake and avoiding extra sodium supplementation. As the prostaglandin inhibitory effects of indomethacin diminish after the last dose, renal prostaglandin production returns to normal, and the retained sodium and excess free water are rapidly excreted, especially with the improvement in the cardiovascular status as the ductus closes. Similar but somewhat milder changes in renal function have been observed with the use of ibuprofen (Van Overmeire et al, 2000).

Because furosemide increases prostaglandin production, the drug may be used to attenuate the renal side effects of indomethacin if the intravascular volume is judged to be adequate (Yeh et al, 1982). However, furosemide administration may increase the incidence of ductal patency (Green et al, 1983), so routine use of the drug may not be prudent in preterm infants treated with indomethacin, because of the theoretical risk of reopening the ductus arteriosus (Seri, 1995). In cases of hemodynamic instability or to avoid the potential effect of furosemide on ductal closure, dopamine infusion may be used to support the cardiovascular status and attenuate the indomethacin-induced oliguria (Cochran et al, 1989; Seri et al, 1984, 1993). However, there is controversy regarding the efficacy and clinical significance of these interventions (Baenziger et al, 1999; Fajardo et al, 1992; Seri, 1995).

### Growing Premature Infant with Negative Sodium Balance

The 2- to 6-week-old growing preterm neonate who is without significant chronic lung disease and is not undergoing diuretic treatment may present with hyponatremia (serum sodium concentration 125 to 129 mEq/L) due to a relative sodium deficiency (Sulyok et al, 1979, 1985). Despite the low total body sodium and high activity of sodium retaining hormones, such an infant continues to lose sodium in the urine mainly because of the immaturity of the renal function. Although the infant is usually in a positive sodium balance, it is insufficient to keep up with the increased sodium demand of their growth. The treatment of this condition is to provide extra sodium supplementation in the form of sodium chloride (usually 2 to 4 mEq/kg/day) to keep serum sodium values higher than 130 mEq/L.

### Surgical Conditions

Surgery has a major effect on metabolism and fluid and electrolyte balance in the newborn. Preterm infants with acute or chronic lung disease are especially sensitive and respond to the procedure with significant catabolic responses, increases in capillary permeability with the attendant shift of fluid into the interstitial space, and retention of sodium and free water (John et al, 1989). The retention of sodium and free water is secondary to the decrease in effective circulating blood volume and to the increased plasma levels of sodium- and water-retaining hormones, including catecholamines, renin-angiotensin-aldosterone, and vasopressin.

Preoperative management has a significant effect on outcome and should be aimed at maintaining adequate effective circulating blood volume as well as cardiovascular and renal functions. In preterm infants who have evidence of absolute or relative adrenal insufficiency (Watterberg, 2002), the provision of stress doses of steroids may be necessary. In the postoperative period, maintenance of the integrity of the cardiovascular system through the judicious use of volume expanders and pressor support, prompt correction of any acute acid-base disorder, meticulous replacement of ongoing surgical and nonsurgical fluid and electrolyte losses, close monitoring, and intense and effective communication between the neonatal and surgical teams are essential to ensure a successful outcome. As capillary integrity improves, reabsorption and excretion of the expanded interstitial fluid volume takes place, with normalization in the secretion of hormones regulating fluid and electrolyte balance. At this time, the provision of maximized nutritional support becomes essential to restore the anabolic state and growth of the infant.

## ACID-BASE BALANCE

### Physiology of Acid-Base Balance Regulation

Like adults, newborns must maintain their extracellular pH, or hydrogen ion concentration, within a narrow range. A normal pH is essential for intact functioning of all enzymatic processes and, therefore, the intact functioning of all organ systems of the body. Newborns are subjected to many stresses that may affect their acid-base balance. In addition, infants, especially if they are premature, have a limited ability to compensate for acid-base alterations. Therefore, acid-base disturbances are common in the neonatal period. An understanding of the principles of acid-base regulation is essential for proper diagnosis and treatment of these disturbances.

In the healthy human, the normal range of ECF hydrogen ion concentration is 35 to 45 mEq/L. As pH is defined as the negative logarithm of hydrogen ion concentration ($pH = -\log [H^+]$), these values of hydrogen ion concentration correspond to a pH range of 7.35 to 7.45. Acidosis is a shift downward in pH to less than 7.35, and alkalosis is a shift upward in pH to more than 7.45. Alterations in normal pH are resisted by complex physiologic regulatory mechanisms. The main systems that maintain pH are the body's buffer systems, the respiratory system, and the kidneys. Some of these systems respond immediately to sudden alterations in hydrogen ion concentration, whereas others respond more slowly to changes but maintain the overall balance between acid and base production, intake, metabolism, and excretion over the long term.

The systems that respond immediately in the physiologic regulation of acid-base balance include the various intracellular and extracellular buffers as well as the lungs. A buffer is a substance that can minimize changes in pH when acid or base is added to the system. The extracellular buffers, which include the bicarbonate-carbonic acid system, phosphates, and plasma proteins, act rapidly to return the extracellular pH toward normal. The intracellular buffers, which include hemoglobin, organic phosphates, and bone apatite, act more slowly, taking several hours to reach maximum capacity.

The most important extracellular buffer is the plasma bicarbonate–carbonic acid buffer system, in which the acid component (carbonic acid [$H_2CO_3$]) is regulated by the lungs, and the base component (bicarbonate [$HCO_3^-$]) is regulated by the kidneys. The buffer equation is

$$H^+ + HCO_3^- \leftrightarrow H_2CO_3 \leftrightarrow H_2O + (CO_2)_d$$

At equilibrium, the amount of dissolved carbon dioxide [$(CO_2)d$] exceeds that of $H_2CO_3$ by a factor of 800:1; thus, for practical purposes, $(CO_2)_d$ and $H_2CO_3$ can be treated interchangeably. The fact that $CO_2$ excretion can be controlled by the respiratory system markedly improves the efficiency of this buffer system at physiologic pH. The enzyme carbonic anhydrase allows rapid interconversion of $H_2CO_3$ to $H_2O$ and $CO_2$. If the hydrogen ion ($H^+$) concentration increases for any reason, hydrogen combines with $HCO_3^-$, driving the buffer reaction toward greater production of $H_2CO_3$ and $CO_2$. Carbon dioxide crosses the blood-brain barrier and stimulates central nervous system chemoreceptors, leading to increased alveolar ventilation and decreased concentration of extracellular $CO_2$. This respiratory compensation begins within minutes after a pH change and is complete within 12 to 24 hours. A similar compensation occurs in response to a decrease in $H^+$ concentration, with a decreased $HCO_3^-$ concentration leading to decreased alveolar ventilation and a resultant increase in extracellular $CO_2$.

The relationship of the two components of the bicarbonate–carbonic acid buffer system to pH is expressed by the Henderson-Hasselbalch equation

$$pH = pK + \log \frac{[HCO_3^-]}{[H_2CO_3]}$$

Because $H_2CO_3$ is in equilibrium with the dissolved $CO_2$ in the plasma, and because the amount of *dissolved* $CO_2$ depends on the *partial pressure* of $CO_2$, the equation can be modified as

$$pH = pK + \log \frac{[HCO_3^-]}{0.03} \times P_aCO_2$$

Both the original equation and the modified equation are clinically difficult to use. Therefore, the modified Henderson-Hasselbalch equation can be rewritten as the Henderson equation, without logarithms for an easier clinical use

$$[H^+] = 24 \times \frac{P_aCO_2}{[HCO_3^-]}$$

This last equation clearly points out the clinically most important aspect of acid-base regulation by the bicarbonate-carbonic acid buffer system, that the change in the *ratio* of $P_aCO_2$ to $HCO_3^-$ concentration, and not in their absolute values, determines the direction of change in $H^+$ concentration and thus in pH. The status of the plasma bicarbonate–carbonic acid buffer system can be easily monitored by serial blood gas measurements, making understanding of this buffer system important in clinical care.

The system that responds more slowly in the physiologic regulation of acid-base balance is the renal system. There must be a long-term balance between net acid increase due to intake and production and net acid decrease due to excretion and metabolism. Although formula and protein-containing intravenous fluids have small amounts of preformed acid, most of the daily acid load results from metabolism. A large amount of the acid produced is in the form of the *volatile* $H_2CO_3$ that can be excreted in the lungs. *Nonvolatile* or *fixed* acids are also produced, which must be excreted through the kidneys. Nonvolatile acids normally are sulfuric acid produced in the metabolism of the amino acids methionine and cysteine as well as smaller contributions from phosphoric acid, lactic acid, hydrochloric acid, and incompletely oxidized organic acids. In addition to excretion of nonvolatile acids, however, the kidneys play a role in long-term acid-base regulation by controlling renal $HCO_3^-$ excretion.

Two regions of the kidney act to achieve urinary acidification, the proximal tubule and the collecting tubule. The proximal tubule acidifies the urine by two mechanisms. The first mechanism is the reabsorption of any $HCO_3^-$ already present in the blood that is being constantly filtered through the glomeruli. The proximal tubule reabsorbs 60% to 80% of all filtered $HCO_3^-$ and performs this role through an exchange of $Na^+$ for $H^+$ across the luminal membrane of the proximal tubular cells via the $Na^+/H^+$ exchanger. The excreted $H^+$ combines with filtered $HCO_3^-$, producing $H_2CO_3$ through the activity of carbonic anhydrase in the cellular brush border. The $H_2CO_3$ is then quickly converted to $CO_2$, which crosses into the tubular cell, where $HCO_3^-$ is regenerated and reabsorbed back into the blood stream, probably in exchange for chloride ($Cl^-$). The regenerated $H^+$ ion reenters the cycle at the $Na^+/H^+$exchanger.

The second mechanism by which the proximal tubule acidifies urine is by the production of ammonia ($NH_3$). Inside the tubular cell, $NH_3$ is produced by the deamination of glutamine. The $NH_3$ is secreted into the tubular lumen, where it combines with and "traps" free $H^+$ to form ammonium ($NH_4^+$).

The remaining urinary acidification occurs mostly in the collecting tubule. $H^+$ secretion in this region of the kidney is sufficient to combine with or *titrate* any remaining filtered $HCO_3^-$ or any filtered anions, such as phosphate and sulfate. Hydrogenated phosphate and sulfate anions produce the *titratable acid* of the urine. The collecting tubule also takes up $NH_3$ from the medullary interstitium and secretes it into the urine, where again it can combine with and trap $H^+$ as $NH_4^+$. This urinary $NH_4^+$ can act as a cation and be excreted with urinary anions such as $Cl^-$, $PO_4^-$, and $SO_4^-$, thereby preventing loss of cations such as $Na^+$, $Ca^{++}$, and $K^+$. Total acid secretion in the kidney can be represented by

$$\text{titratable acid} + NH_4^+ - HCO_3^-$$

and under normal conditions should equal the net production of acid from diet and metabolism that is not excreted in the form of $CO_2$ through the lungs.

In adults, the steady state for renal compensation for respiratory alkalosis is reached within 1 to 2 days and for respiratory acidosis within 3 to 5 days. Newborns are able to compensate for acidemia through the previously described renal mechanisms, although the renal response to acid loads is limited, especially in premature infants born before 34 weeks of gestation. Reabsorption of $HCO_3^-$ in the proximal tubule and distal tubular acidification are also decreased, with a fairly rapid gestational age-dependent maturation of these functions after birth (Jones and Chesney, 1992).

To accomplish the tight regulation of pH necessary for survival, $H^+$ ions generated in the form of the volatile acid $H_2CO_3$ are excreted by the lungs as $CO_2$. $H^+$ ions generated in the form of nonvolatile acids are buffered rapidly by extracellular $HCO_3^-$ and more slowly by intracellular buffers. $HCO_3^-$ is then replenished by the kidneys via the reabsorption of much of the filtered $HCO_3^-$ and by the excretion of $H^+$ in the urine as $NH_4^+$ and titratable acids.

## Disturbances of Acid-Base Balance in the Newborn

### General Principles

The plasma bicarbonate–carbonic acid buffer system is the reference base for acid-base equilibrium, and the status of this system can be monitored with blood gas measurements. Therefore, the blood gas measurement should be the starting point for the evaluation of any acid-base disorder. In the blood gas measurement, the pH and $PaCO_2$ levels are directly measured, and from these the $HCO_3^-$ level is calculated.

The whole blood buffer base, defined as the conjugate sum of the $HCO_3^-$ and non- $HCO_3^-$ buffer systems, is the

**TABLE 30–4**

**Expected Compensatory Mechanisms Operating in Primary Acid-Base Disorders**

| Acid-Base Disorder | Primary Event | Compensation | Rate of Compensation |
|---|---|---|---|
| Metabolic acidosis | | | |
| Normal anion gap | ↓ $[HCO_3^-]$ | ↓ $PCO_2$ | For 1 mEq/L ↓ $[HCO_3^-]$, $PCO_2$ ↓ by 1-1.5 mm Hg |
| Increased anion gap | ↑ acid production<br>↑ acid intake | ↓ $PCO_2$ | For 1 mEq/L ↓ $[HCO_3^-]$, $PCO_2$ ↓ by 1-1.5 mm Hg |
| Metabolic alkalosis | ↑ $[HCO_3^-]$ | ↑ $PCO_2$ | For 1 mEq/L ↑ $[HCO_3^-]$, $PCO_2$ ↑ by 0.5-1 mm Hg |
| Respiratory acidosis<br>Acute (<12-24 hr) | ↑ $PCO_2$ | ↑ $[HCO_3^-]$ | For 10 mm Hg ↑ $PCO_2$, $[HCO_3^-]$ ↑ by 1 mEq/L |
| Chronic (3-5 days) | ↑ $PCO_2$ | ↑ $[HCO_3^-]$ | For 10 mm Hg ↑ $PCO_2$, $[HCO_3^-]$ ↑ by 4 mEq/L |
| Respiratory alkalosis<br>Acute (<12 hr) | ↓ $PCO_2$ | ↓ $[HCO_3^-]$ | For 10 mm Hg ↑ $PCO_2$, $[HCO_3^-]$ ↑ by 1-3 mEq/L |
| Chronic (1-2 days) | ↓ $PCO_2$ | ↓ $[HCO_3^-]$ | For 10 mm Hg ↓ $PCO_2$, $[HCO_3^-]$ ↓ by 2-5 mEq/L |

Modified from Brewer ED: Disorders of acid-base balance. Pediatr Clin North Am 37:430-447, 1990.

other important blood gas value used in evaluating acid-base disturbances. The difference between the observed whole blood buffer base of any blood gas sample and the expected normal buffer base of that sample is called the *base excess* or *base deficit*. The base excess and base deficit give an accurate measure of the amount of strong base and acid, respectively, that have been added to the ECF. For example, a base excess of 10 mEq/L indicates the addition of 10 mEq of base per liter (or loss of 10 mEq of $H^+$ per liter). A base deficit of 10 mEq/L indicates the addition of a similar amount of strong acid (or loss of base).

Acid-base disorders are classified according to their cause as being either *metabolic* or *respiratory*. *Metabolic acidosis* occurs as a result of the accumulation of increased amounts of nonvolatile acid or decreased amounts of $HCO_3^-$ in the ECF. *Metabolic alkalosis* occurs as a result of increased amounts of $HCO_3^-$ in the ECF. *Respiratory acidosis* is due to hypoventilation and decreased excretion of volatile acid ($CO_2$), whereas *respiratory alkalosis* is due to hyperventilation and increased excretion of volatile acid ($CO_2$).

Acid-base disorders are also classified according to the number of conditions causing the disorder. When only one primary acid-base abnormality and its compensatory mechanisms occur, the disorder is classified as a *simple acid-base disorder*. When a combination of simple acid-base disturbances occurs, the patient has a *mixed* (*or complex*) *acid-base disorder*. Because secondary physiologic regulatory mechanisms often compensate for the alteration in pH caused by primary disturbances, it sometimes is difficult to differentiate simple from mixed disorders or even a simple disorder from its resulting compensation. One important principle that allows determination of primary acid-base disturbance is that the compensatory regulatory mechanisms do not completely normalize the pH.

Nomograms, such as the one shown in Fig. 30–6, can help in the diagnosis of the primary disturbance. The nomogram describes the 95% confidence limits of the expected compensatory response to a primary abnormality in either $PaCO_2$ or $HCO_3^-$. Table 30–4 summarizes the expected respiratory and metabolic compensatory mechanisms for primary acid-base disorders (Brewer, 1990). If the compensation in a given patient differs from that predicted in Fig. 30–6 or Table 30–4, the patient either has not had enough time to compensate for a simple acid-base disturbance or has a mixed acid-base disorder. Furthermore, the complete correction of an acid-base disturbance occurs only when the

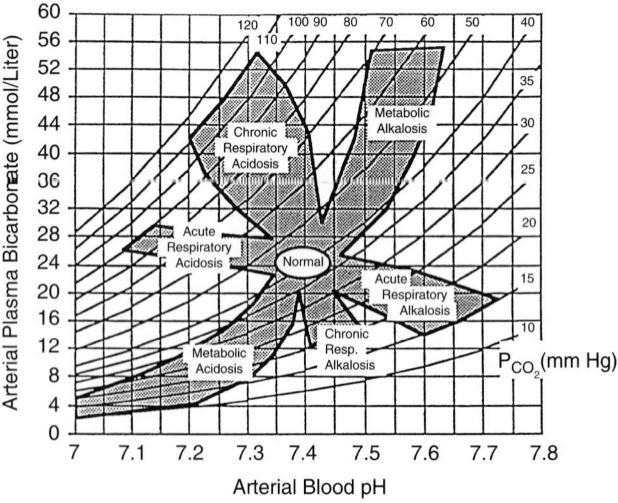


**FIGURE 30–6.** Acid-base nomogram illustrating the 95% confidence limits for compensatory responses to primary acid-base disorders. *(From Cogan MG, Rector FC Jr: Acid-base disorders, In Brenner BM, Rector FC Jr [eds]: The Kidney. Philadelphia, WB Saunders, 1986.)*

underlying process responsible for the abnormality has been effectively treated.

For identification of the primary disturbance, the analysis of blood gas values must be considered in light of the patient's history and physical findings and with an understanding of expected compensatory responses. Further laboratory evaluation is indicated if the problem is not immediately obvious or if the response to therapy is not as expected. The evaluation of the acid-base disturbance should always involve efforts to determine the underlying cause of the disturbance, because adequate treatment requires correction of the underlying disorder, if possible.

### Metabolic Acidosis

Metabolic acidosis is a common problem, particularly in the critically ill newborn. Metabolic acidosis occurs when the drop in pH is caused by the accumulation of acid other than $H_2CO_3$ by the ECF, resulting in loss of available $HCO_3^-$, or by the direct loss of $HCO_3^-$ from body fluids. Cases of metabolic acidosis are divided into those with an *elevated anion gap* and those with a *normal anion gap*.

The anion gap reflects the unaccounted-for acidic anions and certain cations in the ECF. The unmeasured anions normally include the serum proteins, phosphates, sulfates, and organic acids, whereas the unaccounted-for cations are the serum potassium, calcium, and magnesium. Thus, in clinical practice, the anion gap is estimated using the formula

$$\text{anion gap} = [Na^+]_{serum} - ([Cl^-]_{serum} + [HCO_3^-]_{serum})$$

The normal range of the serum anion gap in newborns is 8 to 16 mEq/L, with slightly higher values in very premature newborns. Accumulation of strong acids due to increased intake or production or to decreased excretion results in an increased anion gap acidosis, whereas loss of $HCO_3^-$ or accumulation of $H^+$ results in a normal anion gap acidosis. A decrease in serum potassium, calcium, and magnesium concentrations, an increase in serum protein concentration, or a falsely elevated serum sodium concentration may also result in an increased anion gap in the absence of metabolic acidosis. In clinical practice, although a serum anion gap value greater than 16 mEq/L is highly predictive of lactic acidosis and a value less than 8 mEq/L is highly predictive of the *absence* of lactic acidosis, an anion gap value between 8 and 16 mEq/L cannot be used to differentiate between lactic and nonlactic acidosis in the critically ill newborn (Lorenz et al, 1999). Therefore, the measurement of serum lactate is indicated when one suspects lactic acidosis and the anion gap is in the normal range.

An increased anion gap metabolic acidosis in the newborn is most commonly due to lactic acidosis secondary to tissue hypoxia, as seen in asphyxia, hypothermia, severe respiratory distress, sepsis, and other severe neonatal illnesses. Other important, but much less common causes of an increased anion gap metabolic acidosis in the neonatal period are inborn errors of metabolism, renal failure, and intake of toxins (Table 30–5). Table 30–6 lists inborn errors of metabolism that can manifest as increased anion gap metabolic acidosis in the newborn period.

**TABLE 30–5**

**Common Causes of Metabolic Acidosis**

| Increased Anion Gap | Normal Anion Gap |
|---|---|
| Lactic acidosis due to tissue hypoxia | Renal bicarbonate loss |
| + Asphyxia, hypothermia, shock | + Bicarbonate wasting due to immaturity |
| + Sepsis, respiratory distress syndrome | + Renal tubular acidosis |
| Inborn errors of metabolism | + Carbonic anhydrase inhibitors |
| + Congenital lactic acidosis | Gastrointestinal bicarbonate loss |
| + Organic acidosis | + Small bowel drainage: ileostomy, fistula |
| Renal failure | + Diarrhea |
| Late metabolic acidosis | Extracellular volume expansion with bicarbonate dilution |
| Toxins (e.g., benzyl alcohol) | Aldosterone deficiency |
| | Excessive chloride in intravenous fluids |

In the syndrome of late metabolic acidosis of prematurity, first described in the 1960s, otherwise healthy premature infants at several weeks of age demonstrated mild to moderate increased anion gap acidosis and decreased growth. All the infants were receiving high-protein cow's milk formula, and they demonstrated higher net acid excretion compared with controls. This type of late metabolic acidosis is now rarely seen, probably because of the use of special premature infant formulas and changes in regular formulas with decreased casein-to-whey ratios and lower fixed acid loads.

A normal anion gap metabolic acidosis most commonly occurs in the newborn as a result of $HCO_3^-$ loss from the extracellular space through the kidneys or the gastrointestinal tract. Hyperchloremia develops with the $HCO_3^-$ loss because a proportionate rise in serum chloride concentration must occur to maintain the ionic balance or to correct the volume depletion in the extracellular compartment. The most common cause of normal anion gap metabolic acidosis in the preterm newborn is a mild, developmentally regulated, proximal renal tubular acidosis with renal

**TABLE 30–6**

**Inborn Errors of Metabolism Associated with Metabolic Acidosis**

- Primary lactic acidosis
- Organic acidemias
- Pyruvate carboxylase deficiency
- Pyruvate hydroxylase deficiency
- Galactosemia
- Hereditary fructose intolerance
- Type I glycogen storage disease

$HCO_3^-$ wasting. In infants with this disorder, the serum $HCO_3^-$ usually stabilizes at 14 to 18 mEq/L in the early postnatal period. The urinary pH is normal once the serum $HCO_3^-$ falls to this level, because the impairment in proximal tubular $HCO_3^-$ reabsorption is not associated with an impaired distal tubular acidification of similar magnitude (Jones and Chesney, 1992). The diagnosis of this temporary cause of acidosis can be established by the recurrence of a urinary alkaline pH when serum $HCO_3^-$ is raised above the threshold after $HCO_3^-$ or acetate supplementation. Even term newborns have a lower renal threshold for $HCO_3^-$, with normal plasma $HCO_3^-$ levels in the range of 17 to 21 mEq/L. In most infants, plasma $HCO_3^-$ increases to adult levels over the first year as the proximal tubule matures. Other common causes of normal anion gap metabolic acidosis seen in neonatal intensive care units are gastrointestinal $HCO_3^-$ losses often due to increased ileostomy drainage, diuretic treatment with carbonic anhydrase inhibitors, and dilutional acidosis with rapid expansion of the extracellular space through the use of non-$HCO_3^-$ solutions in the hypovolemic newborn.

The presence of metabolic acidosis in the newborn should be suspected from the clinical presentation and the history of predisposing conditions, including perinatal depression, respiratory distress, blood or volume loss, sepsis, and congenital heart disease associated with poor systemic perfusion or cyanosis. Metabolic acidosis is confirmed by blood gas measurements. The cause of metabolic acidosis is often readily discernible from the history and physical examination; specific laboratory evaluation of electrolytes, renal function, lactate, and serum and urine amino acids may be undertaken, depending on the diagnosis that is suspected clinically. Fig. 30–7 shows a simple flow diagram outlining an approach to diagnosis of metabolic acidosis in the newborn.

The morbidity and mortality of metabolic acidosis depend on the severity of the acidosis and the responsiveness of the underlying pathologic process to clinical management. Because experimental data suggest that even a very low pH is compatible with neurologically intact survival (von Planta et al, 1993), and because a clear benefit of buffer therapy in the management of metabolic acidosis has not been demonstrated (Basir et al, 1996; Brewer, 1990; Nudel et al, 1993), indications for the use of buffers in newborns remain uncertain. At present, the judicious use of temporizing buffer therapy aimed at increasing the arterial pH to 7.25 to 7.30 in cases of severe acidosis is recommended and practiced by most neonatologists to avoid the complications of acidosis per se (Brewer, 1990; von Planta et al, 1993). These complications include arteriolar vasoconstriction followed by dilation, depression of cardiac contractility, systemic hypotension, pulmonary hypertension, pulmonary edema, and arrhythmias. This practice is supported by findings on the cardiovascular effects of sodium bicarbonate in preterm newborns with an arterial pH of less than 7.25 and term newborns with an arterial pH of less than 7.30 (Fanconi et al, 1993). The use of sodium bicarbonate in this study induced an increase in myocardial contractility and a reduction in afterload.

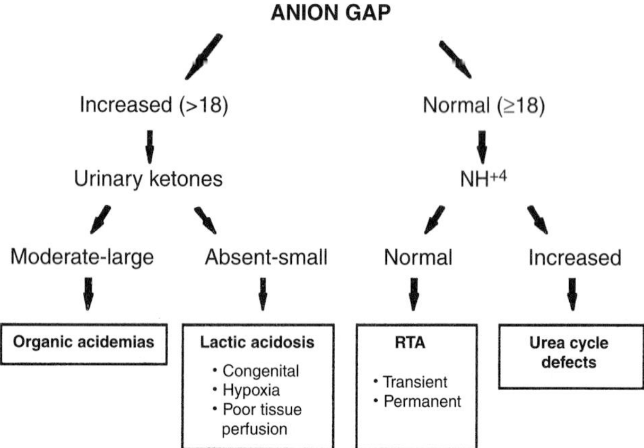


**FIGURE 30–7.** Flow diagram summarizing a diagnostic approach in cases of increased anion gap and normal anion gap metabolic acidosis in the newborn. TRA, renal tubular acidosis.

Sodium bicarbonate is the most widely used buffer in the treatment of metabolic acidosis in the neonatal period. Bicarbonate should not be given if ventilation is inadequate, because its administration results in an increase in $P_aCO_2$ with no improvement in pH and an increase in intracellular acidosis. Therefore, sodium bicarbonate should be administered slowly and in its diluted form only to newborns with documented metabolic acidosis and adequate alveolar ventilation. Once a blood gas measurement has been obtained, the dose of sodium bicarbonate required to correct the pH can be estimated with the use of the formula

$$\text{dose of NaHCO}_3\text{ (mEq)} = \text{base deficit (mEq/L)} \times \text{body weight (kg)} \times 0.3$$

Sodium bicarbonate is confined mostly to the ECF compartment, and the 0.3 value in the formula represents its volume of distribution. Most clinicians would use half of the calculated total correction dose for initial therapy to avoid overcorrection of metabolic acidosis. Subsequent doses of sodium bicarbonate are then based on the results of further blood gas measurements.

In certain clinical situations, tromethamine (Tham) may be used as an alternative buffer to sodium bicarbonate. The theoretical advantages of tromethamine over sodium bicarbonate in the treatment of metabolic acidosis of the newborn include its more rapid intracellular buffering capability, its ability to lower $P_aCO_2$ levels directly, and the lack of an increase in the sodium load (Schneiderman et al, 1993). Tromethamine lowers $P_aCO_2$ by covalently binding $H^+$ and thus shifting the equilibrium of the reaction

$$H^+ + HCO_3^- \leftrightarrow H_2CO_3 \leftrightarrow H_2O + CO_2$$

to the left resulting in a decrease in $CO_2$ and an increase in $HCO_3^-$. Because the end-product (chelated tromethamine) is a cation that is excreted by the kidneys, oliguria is a relative contraindication to the repeated use of this buffer. Tromethamine administration also has been associated with the development of acute respiratory depression, most likely secondary to an abrupt decrease in $PaCO_2$ levels as well as from rapid intracellular correction of acidosis in the cells of the respiratory center (Robertson, 1970). Furthermore, because hypocapnia is associated with decreases in brain blood flow and a higher incidence of white matter damage, especially in the immature preterm neonate, close monitoring of $P_aCO_2$ is of paramount importance when tromethamine is being used. Finally, when large doses of tromethamine are administered, hyponatremia (Seri et al, 1998b), hypoglycemia, hyperkalemia, an increase in hemoglobin oxygen affinity, and diuresis followed by oliguria may occur. Because the solution is hyperosmolal, and because rapid infusion of tromethamine may also lower blood pressure and intracranial pressure (Duthie et al, 1994), slow infusion is recommended.

Despite these disadvantages, tromethamine has a major advantage over sodium bicarbonate in that it acts to increase pH by also lowering $P_aCO_2$. Therefore, *tromethamine is the recommended buffer therapy in life-threatening situations of combined metabolic and respiratory acidosis.* Some centers also use tromethamine as initial therapy for neonatal resuscitation until adequate ventilation is documented by blood gas measurements. The suggested initial dose is 1 to 2 mEq/kg or 3.5 to 6 mL/kg given intravenously using the 0.3 M solution, with the rate of administration not exceeding 1 mL/kg/min. Once a blood gas measurement has been obtained, the dose of tromethamine required to raise the pH can be estimated using the formula

$$\text{dose of tromethamine in mL} = \text{base deficit (mEq/L)} \times \text{body weight (kg)}$$

A third buffer, dichloroacetate, has been successfully used in critically ill adults as an alternative to sodium bicarbonate and tromethamine. Dichloroacetate enhances cardiac output and increases oxidation of pyruvate and lactate through the stimulation of pyruvate dehydrogenase activity (Brewer, 1990). Because only limited experimental information regarding its effectiveness in the newborn period is available, however, its use cannot be recommended at this time (Nudel et al, 1993).

Regardless of the buffer used, care should be taken to avoid overtreatment, to minimize adverse effects of the buffer itself and of rapid swings in pH, and to direct therapy toward the underlying problem. In most conditions, correcting the pH to 7.25 to 7.30 is adequate. In addition, the recommendations for buffer treatment in metabolic acidosis, although widely practiced, are largely empiric without the backing of substantial experimental evidence.

Finally, during the correction of metabolic acidosis, particular attention should be paid to ensure an appropriate potassium balance. Because potassium moves from the intracellular space to the extracellular space in exchange for $H^+$ when acidosis occurs, the presence of a total body potassium deficit may not be appreciated during metabolic acidosis. Hypokalemia may become evident only as the pH increases and potassium returns to the intracellular space. Furthermore, intracellular acidosis cannot be completely corrected until the potassium stores are restored. Therefore, close monitoring of serum electrolytes and, if necessary, potassium supplementation are important during the correction of metabolic acidosis in the sick newborn.

## Respiratory Acidosis

Respiratory acidosis occurs when a primary increase in $P_aCO_2$ develops secondary to impairments in alveolar ventilation that result in an arterial pH of less than 7.35. Primary respiratory acidosis is a common problem in the newborn, and causes include hyaline membrane disease, pneumonia due to infection or aspiration, patent ductus arteriosus with pulmonary edema, chronic lung disease, pleural effusion, pneumothorax, and pulmonary hypoplasia. The initial increase in $P_aCO_2$ is buffered by the non-$HCO_3^-$ intracellular buffers without noticeable renal compensation for at least 12 to 24 hours (see Table 30–4). Renal metabolic compensation reaches its maximum levels within 3 to 5 days, and its effectiveness in the newborn is influenced mainly by the functional maturity of proximal tubular $HCO_3^-$ transport.

Management of respiratory acidosis is directed toward improving alveolar ventilation and treating the underlying disorder. In the sick newborn, adequate ventilation must often be provided by mechanical ventilation. In severe respiratory acidosis, tromethamine, because it lowers $CO_2$, may be used to raise pH. Tromethamine, however, produces only a transient decrease in $P_aCO_2$, and toxic doses would quickly be reached if it were used to buffer all the $CO_2$ produced by metabolism over a sustained period. Therefore, tromethamine should be used only as a temporizing measure in severe respiratory acidosis until alveolar ventilation can be improved.

## Metabolic Alkalosis

Metabolic alkalosis is characterized by a primary increase in the extracellular $HCO_3^-$ concentration sufficient to raise the arterial pH above 7.45. In the newborn, metabolic alkalosis occurs when there is a loss of $H^+$, a gain of $HCO_3^-$, or a depletion of the extracellular volume with the loss of more chloride than $HCO_3^-$. It is important to understand that metabolic alkalosis generated by any of these mechanisms can be maintained only when factors limiting the renal excretion of $HCO_3^-$ are also present.

Metabolic alkalosis can result from a *loss of* $H^+$ from the body, from either the gastrointestinal tract or the kidneys, that induces an equivalent rise in the extracellular $HCO_3^-$ concentration. The most common causes of this type of metabolic alkalosis in the newborn period are continuous nasogastric aspiration, persistent vomiting, and diuretic treatment. Less common causes of $H^+$ losses are congenital chloride-wasting diarrhea, certain forms of congenital adrenal hyperplasia, hyperaldosteronism, posthypercapnia, and Bartter syndrome.

Metabolic alkalosis can also result from a *gain of* $HCO_3^-$, such as occurs during the administration of buffer solutions to the newborn. In the past, a metabolic alkalosis was intentionally created when sodium bicarbonate or tromethamine was used to maintain an alkaline pH to decrease pulmonary vasoreactivity in infants with persistent pulmonary hypertension, a practice not recommended anymore. Currently, however, iatrogenically produced metabolic alkalosis is primarily unintentional and due to chronic excessive administration of $HCO_3^-$, lactate, citrate, or acetate in intravenous fluids and blood products. Because excretion of $HCO_3^-$ is normally not limited in the newborn, metabolic alkalosis resulting from $HCO_3^-$ gain alone should rapidly resolve after administration of $HCO_3^-$ is discontinued. However, if the alkalosis is severe and urine output is limited, inhibition of the carbonic anhydrase enzyme by the administration of acetazolamide may enhance elimination of $HCO_3^-$.

Metabolic alkalosis can also result from a *loss of ECF* containing disproportionally more chloride than $HCO_3^-$, so-called contraction alkalosis. During the diuretic phase of normal postnatal adaptation, preterm and term newborns retain relatively more $HCO_3^-$ than chloride (Ramiro-Tolentino et al, 1996). The obvious clinical benefits of allowing this physiologic extracellular volume contraction to occur, especially in the critically ill newborn, clearly outweigh the clinical importance of a mild contraction alkalosis that develops after recovery. No specific treatment is needed in such cases, because with the stabilization of the extracellular volume and renal function after recovery, acid-base balance rapidly returns to normal. Contraction alkalosis due to other causes, however, may need treatment as discussed subsequently.

For metabolic alkalosis to persist, *factors limiting the renal excretion of* $HCO_3^-$ must be present. The kidneys are usually effective in excreting excess $HCO_3^-$, but this ability can be limited under certain conditions, such as decreased glomerular filtration rate, increased aldosterone production, and the more common clinical situation of volume contraction–triggered metabolic alkalosis with potassium deficiency. In the last-mentioned condition, there is a direct stimulation of $Na^+$ reabsorption coupled with $H^+$ loss in the proximal tubule, and an indirect stimulation of $H^+$ loss in the distal nephron by the increased activity of the renin-angiotensin-aldosterone system. Contraction alkalosis responds to administration of saline to replete the intravascular volume and potassium supplementation. In the other disorders, however, the primary problem of reduced glomerular filtration rate or elevated aldosterone must be treated for the alkalosis to resolve.

One of the most commonly encountered clinical scenarios of chronic metabolic alkalosis actually occurs most often in the form of a mixed acid-base disorder in a preterm infant with chronic lung disease on long-term diuretic treatment. Such a newborn initially has a chronic respiratory acidosis that is partially compensated by renal $HCO_3^-$ retention. Prolonged or aggressive use of diuretics can lead to total-body potassium depletion and contraction of the extracellular volume, thus exacerbating the metabolic alkalosis. By stimulating proximal tubular $Na^+$ reabsorption and thus $H^+$ loss, distal tubular $H^+$ secretion, and renal ammonium production, the diuretic induced hypokalemia contributes to the severity and maintenance of the metabolic alkalosis in such a patient. Furthermore, metabolic alkalosis per se worsens hypokalemia, because potassium moves intracellularly to replace hydrogen as the latter shifts into the extracellular space. Although the serum potassium concentration may be decreased, the serum levels in the newborn do not accurately reflect the extent of total-body potassium deficit because potassium is primarily an intracellular ion, with around 98% of the total body potassium being in the intracellular compartment. In addition, the condition is often accompanied by marked hypochloremia and hyponatremia. Hyponatremia occurs in part because sodium shifts into the intracellular space to compensate for the depleted intracellular potassium. If the alkalosis is severe, alkalemia ($pH > 7.45$) can supervene and result in hypoventilation. In this situation, potassium chloride, and not sodium chloride supplementation, reverses hyponatremia and hypochloremia, corrects hypokalemia and metabolic alkalosis, and increases the effectiveness of diuretic therapy. Because chloride deficiency is the predominant cause of the increased pH, ammonium chloride or arginine chloride also corrects the alkalosis. These agents do not affect the other electrolyte imbalances such as the hypokalemia, so they should not be the only therapy given.

It is important to keep ahead of the potassium losses in infants receiving long-term diuretic therapy, rather than to attempt to replace potassium after intracellular depletion has occurred. Because the rate of potassium repletion is limited by the rate at which potassium moves intracellularly, correction of total body potassium deficits can take days to weeks. In addition, there is also a risk of acute hyperkalemia if serum potassium levels are driven too high during repletion, particularly in newborns in whom an acute respiratory deterioration may occur, with worsened respiratory acidosis and the subsequent movement of potassium from the intracellular to the extracellular space. The routine use of potassium chloride supplementation and close monitoring of serum sodium, chloride, and potassium levels are therefore recommended during long-term diuretic therapy to prevent these common iatrogenic problems.

### Respiratory Alkalosis

When a primary decrease in $P_aCO_2$ results in an increase in the arterial pH beyond 7.45, respiratory alkalosis develops. The initial hypocapnia is acutely titrated by the intracellular buffers, and metabolic compensation by the kidneys returns pH toward normal within 1 to 2 days (see Table 30–4). Interestingly, this is the only simple acid-base disorder in which, at least in the adult, the pH may completely be normalized by the compensatory mechanisms (Brewer, 1990). The cause of respiratory alkalosis is hyperventilation, which in the spontaneously breathing newborn is most often caused by fever, sepsis, retained fetal lung fluid, mild aspiration pneumonia, or central nervous system disorders. In the neonatal intensive care unit, the most common cause of respiratory alkalosis is iatrogenic secondary to hyperventilation of the intubated newborn. Because findings suggest an association between hypocapnia and the development of periventricular leukomalacia (Okumura et al, 2001; Wiswell et al, 1996) and chronic lung disease (Garland et al, 1995) in ventilated preterm infants, avoidance of hyperventilation during resuscitation and mechanical ventilation is of utmost importance in the management of the sick preterm newborn. The treatment of neonatal respiratory alkalosis consists of the specific management of the underlying process causing hyperventilation.

## REFERENCES

Adrogue HJ, Madias NE: Hypernatremia. N Engl J Med 342:1493-1499, 2000.

Aperia A, Broberger O, Herin P, et al: Postnatal control of water and electrolyte homeostasis in preterm and fullterm infants. Acta Paediatr Scand 305:61-65, 1983.

Arant BS Jr: Developmental patterns of renal functional maturation compared in the human neonate. J Pediatr 92:705-712, 1978.

Aszterbaum M, Feingold KR, Menon GK, Williams ML: Glucocorticoids accelerate fetal maturation of the epidermal permeability barrier in the rat. J Clin Invest 91:2703-2708, 1993.

Avner ED: Clinical disorders of water metabolism: Hyponatremia and hypernatremia. Pediatr Ann 24:23-30, 1995.

Baenziger O, Waldvogel K, Ghelfi D: Can dopamine prevent the renal side effects of indomethacin? A prospective randomized clinical study. Klin Paediatr 211:438-484, 1999.

Bailie MD: Development of the endocrine function of the kidney. Clin Perinatol 19:59-68, 1992.

Ballard PL, Ballard RA: Scientific basis and therapeutic regimens for use of antenatal glucocorticoids. Am J Obstet Gynecol 173:254-262, 1995.

Basir MA, Bhatia J, Brudno DS, Kleinman LI: Effects of Carbicarb and sodium bicarbonate on hypoxic lactic acidosis in newborn pigs. J Invest Med 44:70-74, 1996.

Baylen BG, Ogata H, Ikegami M, et al: Left ventricular performance and contractility before and after volume infusion: A comparative study in preterm and fullterm newborns. Circulation 73:1042-1049, 1986.

Bell EF, Warburton D, Stonestreet, BS, Oh W: High-volume fluid intake predisposes premature infants to necrotizing enterocolitis. Lancet 2:90, 1979.

Bell EF, Warburton D, Stonestreet BS, Oh W: Effect of fluid administration on the development of symptomatic patent ductus arteriosus and congestive heart failure in premature infants. N Engl J Med 302:598-604, 1980.

Bonvalet JP, Pradelles P, Farman N: Segmental synthesis and actions of prostaglandins along the nephron. Am J Physiol 253: F377-F387, 1987.

Brace RA: Amniotic fluid volume and its relationship to fetal fluid balance: Review of experimental data. Semin Perinatol 10:103-112, 1986.

Brace RA: Fluid distribution in the fetus and neonate. In Polin RA and Fox WW (eds): Fetal and Neonatal Physiology. Philadelphia, WB Saunders, 1992, pp 1288-1298.

Brans YW: Body fluid compartments in neonates weighing 1000 grams or less. Clin Perinatol 13:403-417, 1986.

Brewer ED: Disorders of acid-base balance. Pediatr Clin North Am 37:430-447, 1990.

Carlton DP, Cho SC, Davis P, et al: Surfactant treatment at birth reduces lung vascular injury and edema in preterm lambs. Pediatr Res 1995 37:265-270, 1995.

Cartridge-Patrick HT, Rutter N: Skin barrier function. In Polin RA and Fox WW (eds): Fetal and Neonatal Physiology. Philadelphia, WB Saunders, 1992, pp 569-585.

Cheek DB, Madison TG, Malinek M, Coldbeck JH: Further observation on the corrected bromide space of the neonate and investigation of water and electrolyte status in infants born of diabetic mothers. Pediatrics 28:861-869, 1961.

Cheek DB, Wishart J, MacLennan AH, et al: Hydration in the first 24 hours of postnatal life in normal infants born vaginally or by caesarean section. Early Hum Dev 7:323-330, 1982.

Christensen G: Cardiovascular and renal effects of atrial natriuretic factor. Scand J Clin Lab Invest 53:203-209, 1993.

Cifuentes RF, Olley PM, Balfe JW, et al: Indomethacin and renal function in premature infants with persistent patent ductus arteriosus. J Pediatr 95:583-587, 1979.

Claycomb WC: Atrial natriuretic factor mRNA is developmentally regulated in heart ventricles and actively expressed in cultured ventricular cardiac muscle cells of the rat and human. Biochem J 255:617-620, 1988.

Clyman RI: Recommendations for the postnatal use of indomethacin: An analysis of four separate treatment strategies. J Pediatr 128:601-607, 1996.

Cochran J, Reddy R, Devaskar U: Effect of indomethacin vs indomethacin + dopamine on serum BUN and creatinine, urinary output and the closure of patent ductus arteriosus in preterm neonates with hyaline membrane disease. Pediatr Res 25:211A, 1989.

Costarino AT, Baumgart S: Neonatal water metabolism. In Cowett RM (ed): Principles of Perinatal/Neonatal Metabolism. New York, Springer Verlag, 1991, pp 623-649.

Coulter MD: Prolactin: A hormonal regulator of the neonatal tissue water reservoir. Pediatr Res 17:665-668, 1983.

Coulthard MG, Hey EN: Effect of varying water intake on renal function in healthy preterm babies. Arch Dis Child 60:614-620, 1985.

de Zegher F, Van den Berghe G, Devlieger H, et al: Dopamine inhibits growth hormone and prolactin secretion in the human newborn. Pediatr Res 34:642-645,1993.

Dudek SM, Garcia JG: Cytoskeletal regulation of pulmonary vascular permeability. J Appl Physiol 91:1487-1500, 2001.

Dunn FL, Brennan TJ, Nelson AE, Robertson GL: The role of blood osmolality and volume in regulating vasopressin secretion in the rat. J Clin Invest 52:3212-3219, 1973.

Duthie SE, Goulin GD, Zornow MH, et al: Effects of THAM and sodium bicarbonate on intracranial pressure and mean arterial pressure in an animal model of focal cerebral injury. J Neurosurg Anesthesiol 6:201-208, 1994.

El-Dahr SS, Chevalier RL: Special needs of the newborn infant in fluid therapy. Pediatr Clin North Am 37:323-336, 1990.

Elliot S, Goldsmith P, Knepper M, et al: Urinary excretion of aquaporin-2 in humans: A potential marker of collecting duct responsiveness to vasopressin. J Am Soc Nephrol 7:403-409, 1996.

Fajardo CA, Whyte RK, Steele BT: Effect of dopamine on failure of indomethacin to close the patent ductus arteriosus. J Pediatr 121:771-775, 1992.

Fanconi S, Burger R, Ghelfi D, et al: Hemodynamic effects of sodium bicarbonate in critically ill neonates. Intensive Care Med 19:65-69, 1993.

Friis-Hansen B: Body water compartments in children: Changes during growth and related changes in body composition. Pediatrics 28:169-181, 1961.

Friis-Hansen B: Water distribution in the foetus and newborn infant. Acta Paediatr Scand 305(Suppl):7-11, 1983.

Ganong CA, Kappy MS: Cerebral salt wasting in children. Am J Dis Child 147:167-169, 1993.

Garland JS, Buck RK, Allred EN, Leviton A: Hypocarbia before surfactant therapy appears to increase bronchopulmonary dysplasia risk in infants with respiratory distress syndrome. Arch Pediatr Adolesc Med 149:617-622, 1995.

Gleason CA: Prostaglandins and the developing kidney. Semin Perinatol 11:12-21, 1987.

Godard C, Geering JM, Geering K, Vallotton MB: Plasma renin activity related to sodium balance, renal function and urinary vasopressin in the newborn infant. Pediatr Res 13:742-745, 1979.

Gold PS, Brace RA: Fetal whole-body permeability-surface area product and reflection coefficient for plasma proteins. Microvasc Res 36:262-274, 1988.

Green TP, Thompson TR, Johnson D, Lock JE: Furosemide promotes patent ductus arteriosus in premature infants with the respiratory distress syndrome. N Engl J Med 308:743-748, 1983.

Green TP, Johnson DE, Bass JL, et al: Prophylactic furosemide in severe respiratory distress syndrome: Blinded prospective study. J Pediatr 112:605-612, 1988.

Hammarlund K, Sedin G, Strömberg B: Transepidermal water loss in newborn infants. VIII: Relation to gestational age and post-natal age in appropriate and small for gestational age infants. Acta Paediatr Scand 72:721-728, 1983.

Hammerman C: Patent ductus arteriosus: Clinical relevance of prostaglandins and prostaglandin inhibitors in PDA pathophysiology and treatment. Clin Perinatol 22:457-479, 1995.

Heijden AJ, Provoost AP, Nauta J, et al: Renal functional impairment in preterm neonates related to intrauterine indomethacin exposure. Pediatr Res 24:644-648, 1988.

Ishisaka DY: Exogenous surfactant use in neonates. Ann Pharmacother 30:389-398, 1996.

Iwamoto HS: Endocrine regulation of the fetal circulation. In Polin RA and Fox WW (eds): Fetal and Neonatal Physiology. Philadelphia, WB Saunders, 1992, pp 646-655.

John E, Klavdianou M, Vidyasagar D: Electrolyte problems in neonatal surgical patients. Clin Perinatol 16:219-232, 1989.

Jones DP, Chesney RW: Development of tubular function. Clin Perinatol 19:33-57, 1992.

Kaapa P, Seppanen M, Kero P, Saraste M: Pulmonary hemodynamics after synthetic surfactant replacement in neonatal respiratory distress syndrome. J Pediatr 123:115-119, 1993.

Kari MA, Hallman M, Eronen M, et al: Prenatal dexamethasone treatment in conjunction with rescue therapy of human surfactant: A randomized placebo-controlled multicenter study. Pediatrics 93:730-736, 1994.

Kelly RT, Rose JC, Meis PJ, et al: Vasopressin is important for restoring cardiovascular homeostasis in fetal lambs subjected to hemorrhage. Am J Obstet Gynecol 146:807-812, 1983.

Kluckow M, Evans N: Ductal shunting, high pulmonary blood flow, and pulmonary hemorrhage. J Pediatr 13:768-772, 2000.

Kojima T, Hirata Y, Fukuda Y, et al: Spare plasma atrial natriuretic peptide and spontaneous diuresis in sick neonates. Arch Dis Child 62:667-670, 1987.

Leake RD: Fetal and neonatal neurohypophyseal hormones. In Polin RA and Fox WW (eds): Fetal and Neonatal Physiology. Philadelphia, WB Saunders, 1992, pp 1815-1819.

Linderkamp O: Placental transfusion: Determinants and effects. Clin Perinatol 9:559-592, 1982.

Lorenz JM, Kleinman LI, Kotagal UR: Water balance in very low-birth-weight infants: Relationship to water and sodium intake and effect on outcome. J Pediatr 101:423-432, 1982.

Lorenz JM, Kleinman LI, Markarian K, et al: Serum anion gap in the differential diagnosis of metabolic acidosis in critically ill newborns. J Pediatr 135:751-755, 1999.

Lumbers ER, Hill KJ, Bennett VJ: Proximal and distal tubular activity in chronically catheterized fetal sheep compared with the adult. Can J Physiol Pharmacol 66:697-702, 1988.

MacKnight ADC, Leaf A: Regulation of cellular volume. Physiol Rev 57:510-573, 1977.

MacLaurin JC: Changes in body water distribution during the first two weeks of life. Arch Dis Child 41:286-291, 1966.

Mahony L: Development of myocardial structure and function. In Emmanouilides GC, Riemenschneider TA, Allen HD, Gutgesell HP (eds): Heart Disease in Infants, Children, and Adolescents Including the Fetus and the Young Adult. Baltimore, Williams & Wilkins, 1995, pp 17-28.

Molteni KH: Initial management of hypernatremic dehydration in the breastfed infant. Clin Pediatr 33:731-740, 1994.

Needleman P, Greenwald JE: Atriopeptin: A cardiac hormone intimately involved in fluid, electrolyte, and blood pressure regulation. N Engl J Med 314:828-834, 1986.

Neville MC, Allen JC, Archer PC, et al: Studies in human lactation: Milk volume and nutrient composition during weaning and lactogenesis. Am J Clin Nutr 54:81-92, 1991.

Nudel DB, Camara A, Levine M: Comparative effects of bicarbonate, *tris*-(hydroxymethyl)aminomethane and dichloroacetate in newborn swine with normoxic lactic acidosis. Dev Pharmacol Ther 20:20-25, 1993,

Okumura A, Hayakawa F, Kato T, et al: Hypocarbia in preterm infants with periventricular leukomalacia: The relation between hypocarbia and mechanical ventilation. Pediatrics 107:469-475, 2001.

Patel J, Roberts I, Azzopardi R, et al: Randomized double-blind controlled trial comparing the effects of ibuprofen with indomethacin on cerebral hemodynamics in preterm infants with patent ductus arteriosus. Pediatr Res 47:36-42, 2000.

Perlman M, Schenker J, Glassman M, Ben-David M: Prolonged hyperprolactinemia in preterm infants. J Clin Endocrinol Metab 47:894-897,1978.

Pohjavuori M, Raivio KO: The effects of acute and chronic perinatal stress on plasma vasopressin concentrations and renin activity at birth. Biol Neonate 47:259-264, 1985.

Pullano JG, Cohen-Addad N, Apuzzio JJ, et al: Water and salt conservation in the human fetus and newborn. I: Evidence for a role of fetal prolactin. J Clin Endocrinol Metab 69:1180-1186, 1989.

Ramiro-Tolentino SB, Markarian K, Kleinman LI: Renal bicarbonate excretion in extremely low birth weight infants. Pediatrics 98:256-261, 1996.

Reller MD, Rice MJ, McDonald RW: Review of studies evaluating ductal patency in the premature infant. J Pediatr 122:S59-S62, 1993.

Riordan JF: Angiotensin II: Biosynthesis, molecular recognition, and signal transduction. Cell Mol Neurobiol 15:637-651, 1995.

Robertson GL, Berl T: Water metabolism. In Brenner BM, Rector FC (eds): The Kidney. Philadelphia, WB Saunders, 1986, pp 385-431.

Robertson NR: Apnea after THAM administration in the newborn. Arch Dis Child 45:306-214, 1970.

Robillard JE, Smith FG, Nakamura KT, et al: Neural control of renal hemodynamics and function during development. Pediatr Nephrol 4:436-441, 1990.

Rojas J, Mohan P, Davidson KK: Increased extracellular water volume associated with hyponatremia at birth in premature infants. J Pediatr 105:158-161, 1984.

Ronconi M, Fortunato A, Soffiati G, et al: Vasopressin, atrial natriuretic factor and renal water homeostasis in premature newborn infants with respiratory distress syndrome. J Perinat Med 23: 307-314, 1995.

Rozycki HJ, Baumgart S: Atrial natriuretic factor and postnatal diuresis in respiratory distress syndrome. Arch Dis Child 662:43-47, 1991.

Sagnella GA, MacGregor GA: Cardiac peptides and the control of sodium excretion. Nature 309:666-667, 1984.

Sarnaik AP, Meert K, Hackbarth R, et al: Management of hyponatremic seizures in children with hypertonic saline: A safe and effective therapy. Crit Care Med 19: 758-762, 1991.

Schneiderman R, Rosenkrantz TS, Knox I, et al: Effects of a continuous infusion of *tris* (hydroxymethyl)aminomethane on acidosis, oxygen affinity, and serum osmolality. Biol Neonate 64: 287-294, 1993.

Sedin G: Fluid management in the extremely preterm infant. In Hansen TN, McIntosh N (eds): Current Topics in Neonatology. London, WB Saunders, 1995, pp 50-66.

Seri I: Cardiovascular, renal, and endocrine actions of dopamine in neonates and children. J Pediatr 126:333-344, 1995.

Seri I, Tulassay T, Kiszel J, Csömör S: The use of dopamine for the prevention of the renal side effects of indomethacin in premature infants with patent ductus arteriosus. Int J Pediatr Nephrol 5:209-214, 1984.

Seri I, Tulassay T, Kiszel J, et al: Effect of low-dose dopamine infusion on prolactin and thyrotropin secretion in preterm infants with hyaline membrane disease. Biol Neonate 47: 317-322, 1985.

Seri I, Rudas G, Bors ZS, et al: Effects of low-dose dopamine on cardiovascular and renal functions, cerebral blood flow, and plasma catecholamine levels in sick preterm neonates. Pediatr Res 34:742-749, 1993.

Seri I, Abbassi S, Wood DC, et al: Effect of dopamine on regional blood flows in sick preterm infants. J Pediatr 133:728-734, 1998a.
Seri I, Jew RK, Drott HR, et al: Administration of large doses of thromethamine (THAM) causes pseudohyponatremia in addition to dilutional hyponatremia in critically ill preterm and term neonates. Pediatr Res 43:194A, 1998b.
Seri I, Tan R, Evans J: The effect of hydrocortisone on blood pressure in preterm neonates with pressor-resistant hypotension. Pediatrics 107:1070, 2000.
Seri I, Abbasi S, Wood DC, et al: Regional hemodynamic effects of dopamine in the indomethacin-treated preterm infant. J Perinatol 22:300-305, 2002.
Seymour AA: Renal and systemic effects of atrial natriuretic factor. Clin Exp Hypertens 5:887-906, 1985.
Shaffer SG, Meade VM: Sodium balance and extracellular volume regulation in very low birth weight infants. J Pediatr 115: 285-290, 1989.
Shaffer SG, Weismann DN: Fluid requirements in the preterm infant. Clin Perinatol 19:233-250, 1992.
Shaffer SG, Bradt SK, Hall RT: Postnatal changes in TBW and extracellular volume in the preterm infant with repiratory distress syndrome. J Pediatr 109:509-514, 1986.
Shaffer SG, Quimiro CL, Anderson JV, Hall RT: Postnatal weight changes in low birth weight infants. Pediatrics 79:702-705, 1987.
Siegel SR: Hormonal and renal interaction in body fluid regulation in the newborn infant. Clin Perinatol 9:535-557, 1982.
Sola A, Gregory GA: Colloid osmotic pressure of normal newborns and premature infants. Crit Care Med 9:568-572, 1981.
Spitzer A: The role of the kidney in sodium homeostasis during maturation. Kidney Int 21:539-545, 1982.
Starling EH: On the absorption of fluid from the connective tissue spaces. J Physiol (London) 19:312-326, 1896.
Sulyok E, Nemeth M, Tenyi I, et al: Relationship between maturity, electrolyte balance and the function of the renin-angiotensin-aldosterone system in newborn infants. Biol Neonate 35:60-65, 1979.
Sulyok E, Kovacs L, Lichardus B, et al: Late hyponatremia in premature infants: Role of aldosterone and arginine vasopressin. J Pediatr 106:990-994, 1985.
Tammela OK: Appropriate fluid regimens to prevent bronchopulmonary dysplasia. Eur J Pediatr 154:S15-18, 1995.
Taylor AE: Capillary fluid filtration. Circ Res 49:557-575, 1981.
Trachtman H: Cell volume regulation: A review of cerebral adaptive mechanisms and implications for clinical treatment of osmolal disturbances. Pediatr Nephrol 5:743-750, 1991.
Tulassay T, Rascher W, Seyberth HW, et al: Role of atrial natriuretic peptide in sodium homeostasis in premature infants. J Pediatr 109:1023-1027, 1986.
Tulassay T, Seri I, Rascher W: The role of atrial natriuretic peptide in extracellular volume contraction after birth. Acta Paediatr Scand 76:144-146, 1987.
van den Anker JN, Hop WCJ, de Groot R, et al: Effects of prenatal exposure to betamethasone and indomethacin on the glomerular filtration rate in the preterm infant. Pediatr Res 36:578-581, 1994.
Van Marter LJ, Leviton A, Allred EN, et al: Hydration during the first days of life and the risk of bronchopulmonary dysplasia in low birth weight infants. J Pediatr 116:942-949, 1990.
Van Otterlo LC, Wladimiroff JW, Wallenburg HCS: Relationship between fetal urine production and amniotic volume in normal pregnancy and pregnancy complicated by diabetes. Br J Obstet Gynecol 84:205-209, 1977.
Van Overmeire B, Smets K, Lecoutere D, et al: A comparison of ibuprofen and indomethacin for closure of patent ductus arteriosus. N Engl J Med 343:674-681, 2000.
Vasarhelyi B, Tulassay T, Ver A, et al: Developmental changes in erythrocyte $Na^+$,$K^+$-ATPase isoform expression and function in the preterm and term neonate. Arch Dis Child 83:F135-138, 2000.
von Planta M, Bar-Joseph G, Wiklund L, et al: Pathophysiologic and therapeutic implications of acid-base changes during CPR. Ann Emerg Med 22:404-410, 1993.
Watterberg KL: Adrenal insufficiency and cardiac dysfunction in the preterm infant. Pediatr Res 51:422-424, 2002.
Weitzman RE, Fisher DA, Robillard J, et al: Arginine vasopressin response to an osmotic stimulus in the fetal sheep. Pediatr Res 12:35-38, 1978.
Wiswell TE, Graziani LJ, Kornhauser MS, et al: Effects of hypocarbia on the development of cystic periventricular leukomalacia in premature infants treated with high-frequency jet ventilation. Pediatrics 98:918-924, 1996.
Yao AC, Lind J: Placental transfusion. Am J Dis Child 127: 128-141, 1974.
Yeh TF, Shibli A, Leu ST, et al: Early furosemide therapy in premature infants (less than or equal to 2000 gm) with respiratory distress syndrome: A randomized controlled trial. J Pediatr 105:603-609, 1984.
Yeh TF, Wilks A, Singh J, et al: Furosemide prevents the renal side effects of indomethacin therapy in premature infants with patent ductus arteriosus. J Pediatr 101:433-437, 1982.
Yu-Lee LY: Prolactin modulation of immune and inflammatory responses. Recent Prog Horm Res 57:435-455, 2002.

CHAPTER 31

# Cardiovascular Compromise in the Newborn Infant

Nick Evans and Istvan Seri

When oxygen delivery is inadequate to meet oxygen demand, the organs fail, and if the situation is not corrected, irreversible damage and, ultimately, death result. Oxygen delivery to the organs depends on many factors but, most fundamentally, on the oxygen content of the blood and the volume of blood flowing to those organs. Because *oxygen content* is determined primarily by the hemoglobin concentration and oxygen saturation with less contribution from the dissolved oxygen ($O_2$ content = [Hgb × 1.39 × $O_2$ saturation] + [$PaO_2$ × 0.0031]), it is relatively easily evaluated and monitored in the newborn intensive care unit. However, reliably measuring *organ blood flow* (tissue perfusion) at the bedside is difficult because it depends on cardiac output and end-organ vascular resistance.

In clinical practice, tissue perfusion is routinely assessed by monitoring heart rate, blood pressure, capillary refilling time, acid-base status, and urine output. However, Doppler ultrasound and near infrared spectroscopy data have shown that these parameters are relatively poor indicators of acute changes in organ blood flow in preterm neonates immediately after birth (Kluckow and Evans, 1996 and 2000b; Lopez et al, 1997; Pladys et al, 1999; Tyszczuk et al, 1998). This observation may herald the need for a shift in thinking about the pathophysiology, diagnosis, and treatment of neonatal circulatory compromise especially *in the preterm neonate during the period of immediate postnatal adaptation*, and should lead us to incorporate blood flow and its relationship to systemic blood pressure.

## PATHOPHYSIOLOGY AND PATHOGENESIS OF NEONATAL SHOCK

### Cardiac Output and Its Determinants

Cardiac output is the product of stroke volume and heart rate and is determined by the amount of blood returning to the heart *(preload)*, the strength of myocardial contractility, and the resistance against which the heart must pump *(afterload)*. If myocardial function is intact, cardiac output depends solely on preload and afterload according the relationships described by the Starling curve.

*Low cardiac output and thus low systemic blood flow* can result from various combinations of the following three factors: low cardiac preload, poor myocardial contractility, and high cardiac afterload. Decreases in preload lead to diminution in stroke volume and cardiac output. Low circulating blood volume is the main cause of the decreases in preload. It can be due to loss of circulating blood volume after hemorrhage (absolute hypovolemia), or the circulating volume may be inadequate for the vascular space, as in vasodilatory shock (relative hypovolemia). Because preload is also augmented by the negative intrathoracic pressure generated at each spontaneous inspiration, the positive intrathoracic pressure associated with excessive positive-pressure mechanical ventilation may reduce venous return and, hence, preload and cardiac output.

The strength of myocardial contractility depends on the filling volume and pressure as well as on the maturity and integrity of the myocardium. Thus, decreases in preload (hypovolemia, cardiac arrhythmia) as well as prematurity (especially extreme immaturity), hypoxic insults, and infectious (viral or bacterial) agents all negatively affect the ability of the myocardium to contract, leading to decreases in cardiac output.

If cardiac afterload (i.e., systemic vascular resistance) is too high, the ability of the myocardium to pump against the increased resistance may become compromised, and cardiac output will fall (Osborn et al, 2002; Roze et al, 1993). Such increases in afterload may be associated with the enhanced endogenous catecholamine release during the period of immediate postnatal adaptation. High afterload can also be a problem in hypovolemia, hypothermia, and when inappropriately high doses of vasopressor inotropic agents are being administered to a patient with intact cardiovascular adrenoreceptor responsiveness. High afterload can affect either ventricle, and if the output of one of the ventricles is reduced, the function of the other ventricle is also affected. For instance, if the right ventricular output is low owing to high pulmonary vascular resistance, the amount of blood getting through the lungs to the left ventricle is reduced, leading to low systemic blood flow with blood pooling in the systemic venous system.

Finally, during transition to extrauterine life, shunts through a persistently patent ductus arteriosus, foramen ovale, or both may compromise circulation (Kluckow and Evans, 2000b). Particularly in the preterm infant, normal postnatal closure of these fetal channels can fail. As the right-sided pressures fall, blood shunts left to right, from the systemic circulation back into the pulmonary circulation. This situation may occur soon after birth, especially when surfactant is administered. It may have greater impact on the circulatory status than has been traditionally appreciated (Evans and Iyer, 1994; Kluckow and Evans, 2000a) and is thought to contribute to the occurrence of pulmonary hemorrhage after administration of surfactant.

### Systemic Blood Pressure

Systemic blood pressure is the product of systemic blood flow and systemic vascular resistance. Although there may be an association between low blood pressure and central nervous system injury in the preterm neonate, blood pressure only weakly correlates with blood flow in this patient population during the period of immediate postnatal adaptation (Kluckow and Evans, 2000b). Thus, in preterm infants during the first postnatal day, blood pressure may be low because resistance is low in the presence of normal or even high blood flow, or blood pressure may be normal or high because resistance is high in the presence of normal or low blood flow.

## Organ Blood Flow Autoregulation

Even very immature preterm neonates appear to be capable of autoregulation of cerebral blood flow (Seri et al, 1998; Tyszczuk et al, 1998). However, organ blood flow autoregulation is impaired in a subset of preterm neonates in whom changes in blood pressure are mirrored by changes in cerebral blood flow, and these babies are at higher risk for cerebral injury (Tsuji et al, 2000). Factors that impair organ blood flow autoregulation include birth asphyxia, acidosis, infection, tissue hypoxia and ischemia, and sudden alterations in arterial carbon dioxide tension. Whether the impairment of autoregulation in the preterm neonate immediately after birth is the cause of the cerebral injury or a consequence of a preceding ischemic insult remains to be clarified.

## Pathogenesis of Neonatal Shock

### Conditions Affecting All Babies

#### *Hypovolemia*

Hypovolemia is probably overdiagnosed in neonatology; it is a relatively uncommon primary cause of circulatory compromise, especially during the first postnatal days. Among preterm newborns, there is no evidence that hypotensive babies as a group are hypovolemic (Wright and Goodhall, 1994). However, when hypovolemia occurs, it can be difficult to detect clinically.

Hypovolemia in the newborn can be due to several conditions. *Intrapartum fetal blood loss* is usually caused by an open bleed from the fetal side of the placenta and therefore is likely to be detected. More difficult to diagnose is the closed bleeding of an acute fetomaternal hemorrhage or an acute fetoplacental hemorrhage. The latter can occur in delivery situations in which the umbilical cord comes under some pressure (breech presentation or nuchal cord). Because the umbilical vein is occluded before the artery, blood continues to be pumped into the placenta, and if the cord is clamped early, this blood remains trapped in the placenta. This scenario probably happens to some degree in all babies with tight nuchal cords who, as a group, have lower hemoglobin levels. A tight nuchal cord may also cause severe circulatory compromise. *Postnatal hemorrhage* may occur from any site and is frequently associated with endothelial damage induced by perinatal infection or severe asphyxia and the ensuing disseminated intravascular coagulation. Finally, *acute abdominal surgical problems and conditions associated with the nonspecific inflammatory response syndrome* and subsequent increased capillary leak with loss of fluid into the interstitium can lead to significant decreases in the circulation blood volume.

#### *Sepsis*

Although clinical evidence of circulatory compromise is a feature of many infectious processes in the newborn, the hemodynamics in neonatal septic shock have not been systematically studied. In older subjects, two distinct hemodynamic patterns occur. "Warm shock" is characterized by loss of vascular tone, increased systemic blood flow and low blood pressure, and "cold shock" by increased vascular tone, low systemic blood flow, and, eventually, falling blood pressure. Cold shock has been well described in the newborn (Meadow and Rudinsky, 1995), but the warm shock phase is more difficult to recognize clinically unless the blood pressure is being closely monitored. The mediators of neonatal warm septic shock remain unclear; in adult sepsis, however, in addition to dysregulated cytokine release, nitric oxide and deficiency of vasopressin seem to play a role. The significance of this observation to newborn sepsis remains unclear but it may have relevance to the late inotrope unresponsive hypotension seen in preterm babies (Ng et al, 2001; Seri et al, 2001).

#### *Severe Respiratory Distress and Pulmonary Hypertension*

Term babies with severe respiratory failure have a high incidence of low ventricular output (Evans et al, 1998). The low output state is most common in the early course of the disease, resolving spontaneously with time, clinical improvement, or both. The causes of such circulatory compromise are probably multifactorial but include postnatal cardiovascular adaptation, the negative effects of excessive positive-pressure ventilation, and the systemic effect of raised pulmonary vascular resistance as previously described.

#### *Heart Disease*

Circulatory compromise can result from primary heart disease, either congenital or acquired. Structural heart defects that produce a ductus-dependent systemic circulation, such as the hypoplastic left heart syndrome, critical coarctation, and critical aortic stenosis, classically manifest as acute circulatory compromise with pallor, tachypnea, impalpable pulses, and hepatomegaly as the duct starts closing. The presentation is often initially misdiagnosed as sepsis.

Acquired heart diseases that can manifest as circulatory compromise include primary cardiomyopathies and post-asphyxial myocardial dysfunction. Studies have shown a high incidence of ischemic changes on electrocardiography (ECG), raised blood cardiac enzyme levels, and low cardiac output in babies after intrapartum asphyxia (Tapia-Rombo et al, 2000). There is more detail on structural heart disease and cardiomyopathies in the chapters on congenital heart disease.

## Circulatory Compromise in the Extremely Preterm Infant

### *Transitional Circulatory Compromise*

The transitional circulatory changes in the first 12 to 24 hours after birth are a period of unique circulatory vulnerability for the extremely preterm infant. During normal postnatal adaptation, pulmonary vascular resistance falls, systemic vascular resistance rises when the placenta is removed from the circulation, the ductus arteriosus closes, and the foramen ovale is closed by the reversal of the atrial pressure gradient. As these changes occur, the left ventricle has to double its output. Given that very preterm infants' cardiovascular systems are adapted to the low-resistance intrauterine environment and that their myocardium is immature, it is not surprising that these babies often have difficulties during this critical period. However, because blood pressure is not an accurate reflection of systemic and organ blood flow in this patient population during the immediate postnatal period, it is important to recognize that successful treatment of hypotension may not necessarily ensure normalization of organ blood flow. Furthermore, blood pressure in the low-normal to normal range does not necessarily translate into normal organ blood flow and tissue perfusion in these patients. Indeed, it is only when mean blood pressure is higher than 40 mm Hg during the first postnatal day in the preterm neonate born before 30 weeks of gestation that the systemic blood flow can definitely be assumed to be normal (Osborn et al, 2004).

Another special characteristic of the process of cardiovascular adaptation in this patient population is that early shunts through the preterm ductus arteriosus and foramen ovale are not balanced and, thus, can produce left-to-right shunts of significant clinical importance. The immediate postnatal physical constriction of the ductus is characterized by great variation, but if constriction fails, very large shunts can occur within a few hours of birth, leading to high, not low, pulmonary blood flow as previously thought. These abnormal hemodynamic changes may be further augmented by the administration of surfactant.

In the transitional circulation of the preterm infant, neither ventricular output will consistently reflect systemic blood flow because of the shunts across the ductus arteriosus and foramen ovale. Consequently, measurement of either ventricular output can overestimate systemic blood flow by more than 100% in some cases (Evans and Kluckow, 1996). Superior vena cava (SVC) flow can be used as a marker of total systemic blood flow, and serial measurement of SVC flow has been used to describe the natural history of systemic blood flow changes in preterm neonates in the early postnatal period (Fig. 31–1). These studies have found that at least one third of preterm neonates born before 30 weeks of gestation have a period of low systemic blood flow, mostly during the first 12 hours of life (Kluckow and Evans, 2000b). Gestational age is the predominant predicator of the low-flow state; 70% of babies born before 26 weeks of gestation having a period of low systemic flow, compared with about 10% of those born at 29 weeks. A larger-diameter ductus arteriosus (Evans and Iyer, 1994) and the need for a higher mean airway pressure have also been shown to be associated with low SVC flow. As mentioned earlier, the correlation between SVC flow and blood pressure is statistically significant but weak, in that some babies have low flow and normal blood pressure and others have low pressure and normal flow. The low-flow state can persist for up to 24 hours but usually improves after thereafter. There is a strong relationship between recovery from the low-flow state and subsequent intraventricular hemorrhage (IVH) (Kluckow and Evans, 2000b; Osborn, 2003). The finding that IVH occurs after systemic blood flow has improved indicates the involvement of a hypoperfusion-reperfusion cycle in the pathogenesis of this injury. Follow-up for up to 3 years of 96 of the 126 patients enrolled in the first phase of these studies identified the low-flow state as a significant risk factor for poor neurodevelopmental outcome (Hunt et al, 2002).

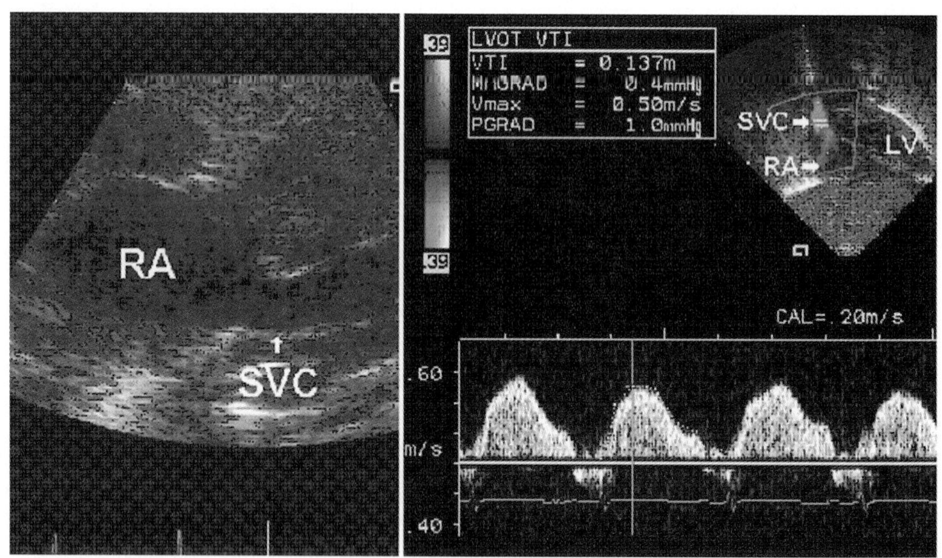


**FIGURE 31–1.** Assessment of superior vena cava (SVC) flow with measurement of the diameter from the low parasternal saggital view *(left)* and measurement of the velocity time (VTI) integral (area under the Doppler envelope) *(right)*. LV, left ventricle; RA, right atrium. *(From Kluckow M, Evans N: Superior vena cava flow in newborn infants: A novel marker of systemic blood flow. Arch Dis Child Fetal Neonatal Ed 82:F182-F187, 2000.)*

As for the pathogenesis of the abnormal circulatory adaptation of the very premature neonate, there is indirect evidence that the sudden increase in the systemic vascular resistance after separation from the placenta combined with myocardial immaturity plays an important role in the development of the low-flow state afflicting primarily the more immature patient population. Because the preterm myocardium is adapted to a low-resistance intrauterine environment and is characterized by reduced contractile elements and a limited ability to respond to an increase in afterload (Hawkins et al, 1989; Takahashi et al, 1997), it struggles to cope with the sudden increase in vascular resistance immediately after birth. The situation is compounded by both shunts out of the systemic circulation through the fetal channels and the negative circulatory effects of positive-pressure ventilation. In some babies, the result is a critically low systemic circulation. Then, as treatment and endocrine, neuroendocrine, and other compensatory responses to stress are initiated, the cardiovascular system adapts, and systemic blood flow improves. However, if the low-flow state is severe, a reperfusion injury may occur during the period of cardiovascular stabilization, especially in the extremely vulnerable immature central nervous system.

### Persistent Hypotension in Preterm Infants

Although the above-described transitional problems may or may not manifest as low blood pressure, there are a group of preterm babies in whom a persistent hypotension develops that is resistant to conventional inotropic support (Ng et al, 2001; Seri et al, 2001). Although this condition is well recognized, the underlying systemic hemodynamic changes are not well defined. Affected babies are more likely to be extremely preterm (<27 weeks in gestational age), have been critically ill or suffered a degree of perinatal asphyxia, or both. The problem may be apparent on the first postnatal day but typically persists beyond that time and may represent a state of vasodilatory shock with normal to high systemic blood flow and possibly supranormal cardiac output (Fig. 31–2) (Lopez et al, 1997). There are striking analogies between this presentation in preterm neonates with the vasodilatory shock as described in adults, particularly the lack of responsiveness to vasopressor inotropic agents (Landry and Oliver, 2001). Potential mechanisms of the uncontrolled vasodilation include dysregulated cytokine release, excess nitric oxide synthesis, vasopressin deficiency, overactivation of the potassium–adenosine triphosphate ($K_{ATP}$) channels in the vascular smooth muscle cell membrane in response to tissue

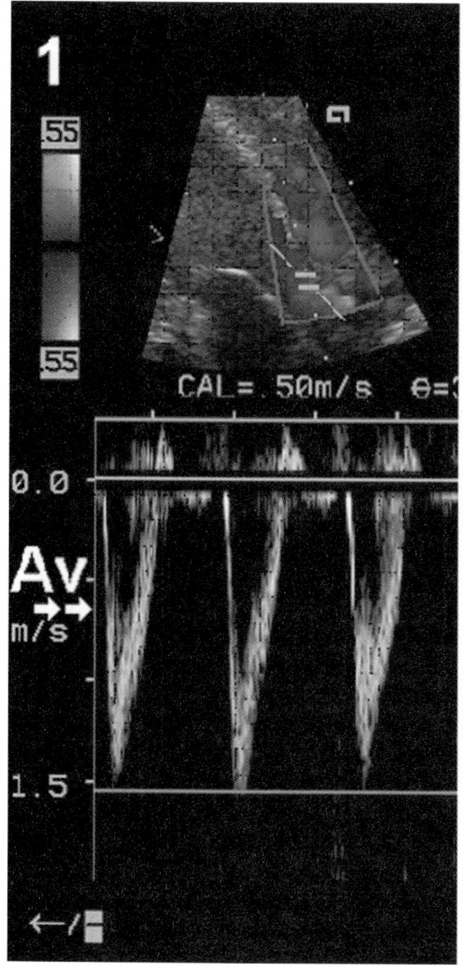


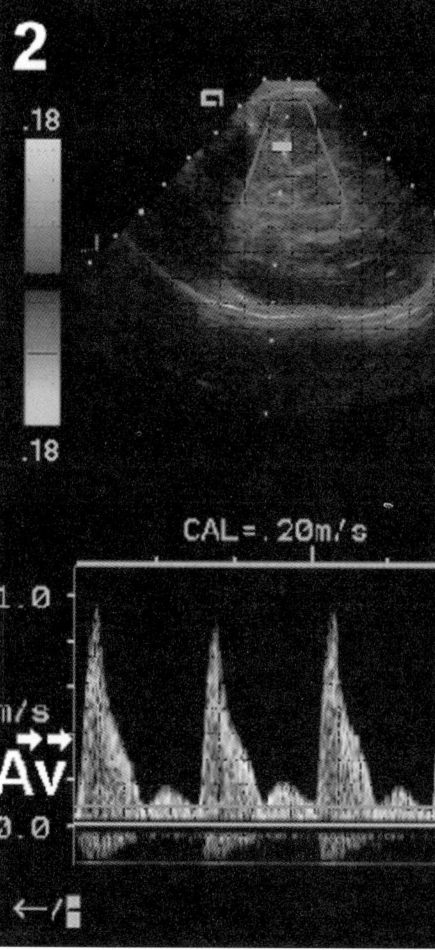


**FIGURE 31–2.** Doppler velocity in the ascending aorta (**1**) and middle cerebral artery (**2**) in a preterm infant, born at 27 weeks of gestation, with septic shock due to *Pseudomonas* cepticemia. The baby had a mean blood pressure of 20 mm Hg despite vasopressor and inotropic support. The high flow velocity can be seen from the normal average maximum velocity marked by the arrows (*Av*). The calculated left ventricular output was about 600 mL/kg/min (normal 150 to 300 mL/kg/min).

hypoxia, and down-regulation of the cardiovascular adrenergic receptors (Seri et al, 2001).

### *Summary*

The circulation of the very preterm infant exists in a state of precarious balance. The peripheral circulation is balanced between overconstriction, which may compromise systemic blood flow, and overdilation, which may result in vasodilatory shock. Data now suggest that the former situation dominates in the first 24 hours and the latter becomes increasingly important after that time. This suggestion creates a difficult therapeutic dilemma, because the correct approach for a circulatory compromise due to vasoconstriction is counterproductive if the underlying abnormality is vasodilation, and vice versa. Therefore, accurate diagnosis of the type of the circulatory failure is imperative.

## DIAGNOSIS OF CIRCULATORY COMPROMISE

What the "gold standard" for the diagnosis of circulatory compromise should be is far from clear. Conventionally, blood pressure has been and still is used as that standard. As mentioned earlier, data now suggest that this approach may not be appropriate and that sole reliance on blood pressure will lead to inaccurate and sometimes significantly delayed diagnosis of circulatory compromise, especially in the very preterm infant immediately after birth. On the other hand, many clinicians believe that over-reliance on blood pressure measurement will lead to overdiagnosis of shock. The other commonly used clinical signs of circulatory compromise, such as increased heart rate, slow skin capillary refill time, increased core-peripheral temperature difference, low urine output, and acidosis, have limited value in aiding the diagnosis of circulatory compromise in the preterm or term infant (Osborn et al, 2004).

### Heart Rate and Blood Pressure

Heart rate is accurately and routinely monitored in neonates requiring admission to the newborn infant care unit. Because many factors other than those regulating the cardiovascular system affect heart rate, it has a limited yet widely utilized role in the diagnosis of circulatory compromise.

In babies with invasive intra-arterial access, continuous and accurate measurement of blood pressure is possible. The accuracy of the noninvasive oscillometric method is less certain. Normal ranges for blood pressure in babies of different gestations have been defined in the literature, and it is clear that gestation and postnatal age are the dominant influences on blood pressure (Lee et al, 1999; Nuntnarumit et al, 1999). The nomogram in Figure 31–3, constructed from data of Nuntnarumit and colleagues (1999), shows the 10th percentile for mean blood pressure for babies of different gestations at different postnatal ages. A simple rule of thumb is that the number of the mean blood pressure in mm Hg should be higher than the number of weeks of the baby's gestation at the time of birth (Lee et al, 1999).

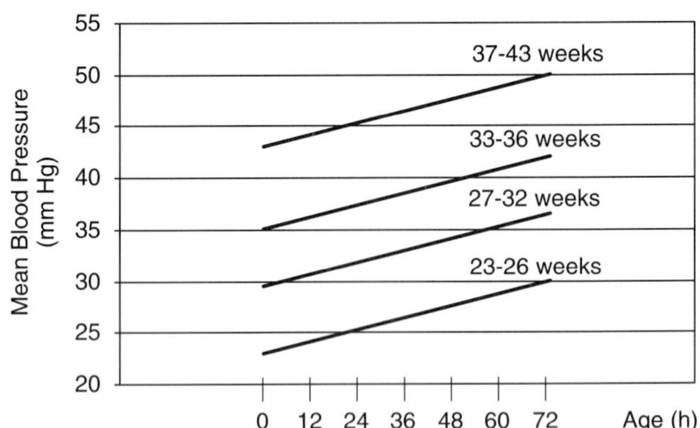


**FIGURE 31–3.** Gestational age– and postnatal age–dependent normogram for mean blood pressure values in neonates during the first 3 days of life. The normogram is derived from continuous arterial blood pressure measurements obtained from 103 neonates with gestational ages between 23 and 43 weeks. Each line represents the lower limit of 80% confidence interval of mean blood pressure for each gestational age group. Thus, 90% of infants for each gestational age group are expected to have a mean blood pressure equal to or greater than the value indicated by the corresponding line (the lower limit of confidence interval). *(From Nuntnarumit P, Yang W, Bada-Ellzey HS: Blood pressure measurements in the newborn. Clin Perinatol 26:981-996, 1999.)*

How accurately blood pressure defines the state of the systemic circulation in preterm neonates, however, is less clear. As mentioned earlier, there is only a weak relationship between mean blood pressure and measures of systemic blood flow in preterm neonates immediately after birth (Fig. 31–4). Thus, if blood pressure alone is

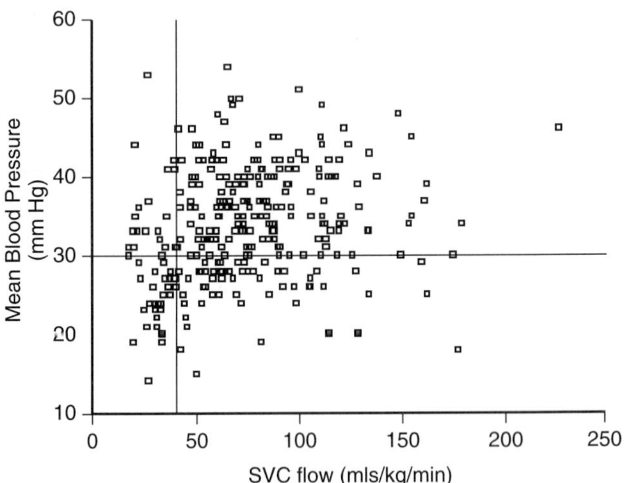


**FIGURE 31–4.** The relationship between superior vena cava (SVC) flow and mean blood pressure (MBP) during the first 24 hours in a cohort of 126 babies born before 30 weeks of gestation. Normal values are marked by the *line*. The 30–mm Hg value is chosen arbitrarily for MBP because the change in normal MBP with gestation cannot be marked. Although there is a relationship between the two measures ($r = 0.21$; $P = .023$), it is not strong, with some babies having normal pressure and low flow and others having low pressure and normal flow. *(From Kluckow M, Evans N: Low superior vena cava flow and intraventricular hemorrhage in preterm infants. Arch Dis Child Fetal Neonatal Ed 82:F188-F194, 2000.)*

used to guide treatment, some of these babies may not be treated appropriately. Available data indicate that only when mean blood pressures in very preterm babies are ≤20 mm Hg and ≥40 mm Hg does blood pressure become a more accurate indicator of abnormal and normal systemic blood flow, respectively. Thus, in the extremely preterm neonate with mean blood pressures between 20 and 40 mm Hg in the immediate postnatal period, the state of systemic blood flow is unclear, and the situation can be clarified only with Doppler flow measurements (Osborn et al, 2004).

## Capillary Refill Time

Although capillary refill time is a widely used clinical sign, there is little validation of its accuracy. A capillary refill time of less than 3 seconds is traditionally accepted as normal. In older infants in a pediatric intensive care setting, there is little relationship between capillary refill time and measures of systemic blood flow (Tibby et al, 1999). A similar lack of tight relationship has been found in preterm neonates born before 30 weeks of gestation; only when capillary refill time exceeds 5 seconds does it have any degree of specificity (Osborn et al, 2004).

## Core-Peripheral Temperature Difference

As with capillary refill, there is little data to support the accuracy of core-peripheral temperature difference in older babies (Tibby et al, 1999). In preterm neonates born before 30 weeks of gestation, no relationship has been found between this measure and systemic blood flow in the immediate postnatal period (Osborn et al, 2004).

## Low Urine Output and Hyperkalemia

A strong relationship has been documented in very preterm babies between low systemic blood flow and subsequent low urine output and hyperkalemia (Kluckow and Evans, 2001). However, there is a time delay between the development of the circulatory compromise and the recognition of oliguria or hyperkalemia, making these signs somewhat less valuable for the early diagnosis of shock.

## Lactic Acid, pH, and Base Excess

In a large series, pH and base excess was found to have little relationship with low systemic blood flow in preterm babies immediately after birth. This finding is likely explained by the lack of a strong relationship among pH, base excess, and lactic acid levels (Deshpande and Platt, 1997). Although the lactic acid concentration has been proposed as a measure of circulatory compromise, there is little evidence to support its accuracy. One study found that there also was no relationship between lactic acid level and SVC flow measured at two different time points during the first postnatal day (Kluckow and Evans, 1999). At both times, lactic acid level had a stronger relationship with the events of the preceding hours than with what was going on at the time of its measurement. Thus, as with urine output and hyperkalemia, by the time lactic acidosis develops and is detected, the initiating event may not be present anymore. In support of this assumption is the finding that a rising lactate level is more predictive of adverse outcome than a high early level that then falls (Deshpande and Platt, 1997).

## Organ Blood Flow

Much of the attention in the newborn has focused on measuring blood flow to the brain. Several methodologies have been studied, including Doppler velocity measurements, xenon clearance, and near-infrared spectroscopy (Tsuji et al, 2000; Tyszczuk et al, 1998). Because peripheral arteries tend to be too small for size measurement, Doppler studies in such vessels tend to be limited to parameters of velocity, from which it is not possible to derive blood flow. Consequently, peripheral artery Doppler ultrasonography tends to be more useful for assessing changes over time frames in which it is unlikely that vessel size will have changed (Seri et al, 1998). Xenon clearance is not practical outside a research setting. Near-infrared spectroscopy, which uses changes in oxygenation over time, or the difference between oxygenated and deoxygenated hemoglobin, to assess flow, has been very useful as a research tool (Tsuji et al, 2000; Tyszczuk et al, 1998). Whether it can be implemented in the clinical arena remains unclear.

## Echocardiographic Systemic Blood Flow Measures

In the mature circulation, systemic blood flow is the cardiac output. Although the outputs of the two ventricles are the same, cardiac output is traditionally measured from the left ventricular output. In the clinical practice, Doppler ultrasonography offers a noninvasive method to measure cardiac output. Measuring blood flows directly in the pulmonary artery and ascending aorta enables us to evaluate outputs from the right and left ventricles, respectively (Alverson et al, 1982; Evans and Kluckow, 1996; Walther et al, 1985). Unfortunately, in the transitional circulation of the newborn infant, neither ventricular output will consistently reflect systemic blood flow because of the shunts across the fetal channels. Because SVC flow measures blood flow returning from the upper body and brain, which must be the same as the blood flow going out to this area of the body, and because SVC lends itself well to Doppler flow studies in the early postnatal period, SVC flow has been introduced to evaluate systemic blood flow in preterm babies in the early postnatal period (see Fig. 31–1) (Kluckow and Evans, 2000).

Measurement of ventricular output is exceedingly difficult in the preterm infant because of atelectasis and multiple shunts. In addition, Doppler flow measures rely on a level of ultrasonographic technology and echocardiographic skill that are often not available 24 hours a day in many neonatal intensive care units. However, this may change in the future as increasing numbers of neonatologists are developing these skills (Evans, 2000).

### Summary

The mainstay of the diagnosis of neonatal circulatory compromise has been a combination of blood pressure measurement and evaluation of the previously described clinical parameters. However, none of these parameters has sufficient accuracy to be used on its own to evaluate systemic blood flow and tissue perfusion. Therefore, the addition of echocardiographic hemodynamic assessment to blood pressure monitoring and thorough continuous clinical evaluation of the patient are necessary to better understand changes in organ blood flow and tissue perfusion, especially in preterm neonates during the vulnerable period of immediate transition to extrauterine life. The goal should be to maintain normal systemic blood flow in the presence of an acceptable blood pressure, with use of the normal range for blood pressure that controls for gestation and postnatal age. If there is no immediate access to echocardiography, the clinician must rely on blood pressure monitoring while keeping in mind the limitations of this approach.

## TREATMENT

Selection of the most appropriate treatment strategy for neonatal shock requires identification of its pathogenesis (Seri, 2001). As described previously, the most common etiologic factors of neonatal cardiovascular compromise are (1) inappropriate peripheral vasoregulation resulting in vasodilation or vasoconstriction and (2) the dysfunction of the immature myocardium (Gill and Weindling, 1993; Osborn et al, 2002; Seri, 1995). Absolute hypovolemia is a much less frequent primary cause of neonatal hypotension, especially in preterm infants in the immediate postnatal period.

### Volume Administration

The findings that hypotensive neonates as a group are not hypovolemic, that low blood pressure is frequently associated with normal or even high ventricular output and low index of resistance (Pladys et al, 1999) and that dopamine is more effective than volume administration in normalizing blood pressure (Lundstrom et al, 2000) provide evidence that absolute hypovolemia is an uncommon primary cause of neonatal hypotension. Therefore, particularly in the preterm infant in the immediate postnatal period, fluid resuscitation should be minimized. Furthermore, because myocardial dysfunction frequently contributes to the development of neonatal hypotension (Gill and Weindling, 1993) and because aggressive volume administration in this patient population is associated with higher pulmonary, cardiovascular, gastrointestinal and central nervous system morbidity and mortality (Kavvadia et al, 2000; Lundstrom et al, 2000; Van Marter et al, 1990), judicious use of fluid administration is indeed of utmost importance.

Concerning the type of fluid administration, isotonic saline has been shown to be as effective as 5% albumin in raising the blood pressure (Oca et al, 2003; So et al, 1997). In addition, albumin may cause an impairment of gas exchange, may induce a fluid shift from the intracellular compartment (Ernest et al, 1999), and may be associated with increased mortality (Nadel et al, 1998). Therefore, unless evidence of serum or blood loss or hypoalbuminemia is present, volume support in hypotensive preterm infants should be provided in the form of 10 to 20 mL/kg of isotonic saline (Seri, 2001). However, it is important to mention that, owing to the unbalanced nature of normal saline, its administration in large amounts over a short time may worsen the metabolic acidosis. If the limited volume administration is ineffective, pharmacologic cardiovascular support with dopamine, dobutamine, or both should be initiated (Seri, 1995 and 2001; Osborn et al, 2002).

If there is an identifiable volume loss, the kind of fluid lost should be replaced. In cases of blood loss, transfusion with packed red blood cells after the initial bolus of crystalloid or colloid or with packed red blood cells suspended in fresh frozen plasma with a hematocrit around 55% may be used. In cases of greater transepidermal water losses, administration of larger amounts of free water without an increase in sodium supplementation is indicated.

### Dopamine And Dobutamine

Dopamine and dobutamine were introduced into the management of neonatal hypotension in the early and middle 1980s, respectively, without appropriately designed randomized and blinded clinical trials of their effectiveness. Thus, we have only indirect evidence that the use of these sympathomimetic amines improves neonatal mortality or morbidity. A few studies have extended their focus beyond the dopamine- and dobutamine-induced heart rate and blood pressure changes by examining the drugs' effects on neonatal myocardial contractility and organ blood flow (Lundstrom et al, 2000; Osborn et al, 2002; Roze et al, 1993; Seri et al, 1998, 2002; Zhang et al, 1999). However, there is still only limited information available about the effects of dopamine and dobutamine on tissue oxygen delivery and consumption (Wardle et al, 1999) and systemic blood flow in the newborn (Osborn et al, 2002).

#### Hemodynamic Effects

Dopamine, an endogenous catecholamine, is the sympathomimetic amine most commonly used in the treatment of hypotension in preterm infants (Seri, 1995; Noori et al, 2003). It exerts its cardiovascular actions via the dose-dependent stimulation of the cardiovascular dopaminergic, α- and β-adrenergic and serotonin receptors. In addition, by stimulating epithelial and peripheral neuronal dopaminergic and adrenergic receptors, the drug exerts significant renal and endocrine effects independent of its cardiovascular actions. Although dopamine affects all three major determinants of cardiovascular function (preload, myocardial contractility, and afterload), the drug-induced increases in myocardial contractility (Lundstrom et al, 2000; Zhang et al, 1999) and peripheral vascular resistance (afterload) (Lundstrom et al, 2000; Roze et al, 1993; Zhang et al, 1999) are the most important factors in raising systemic blood pressure and improving the cardiovascular status.

The original dose range recommendation for dopamine, 2 to 20 μg/kg/min, was based on pharmacodynamic data obtained in healthy adults. However, changes in cardiovascular adrenergic receptor expression by critical illness (Hausdorff et al, 1990) as well as the dysregulated production of local vasodilators during severe illness decrease the sensitivity of the cardiovascular system to dopamine, resulting in the emergence of hypotension resistant to "conventional" doses of the drug (Ng et al, 2001). Thus, with the advancement of the disease process, larger doses of dopamine and other sympathomimetic amines may be needed to generate the same magnitude of cardiovascular response. Dopamine administration should therefore be tailored to the drug's pharmacodynamic effects in the given patient at the bedside, rather than driven by the conventional dose recommendations based on data obtained in healthy adults. Indeed, although many neonatologists do not increase the dose of dopamine beyond 20 μg/kg/min, there is no evidence that, when required to normalize blood pressure, higher-dose dopamine treatment with or without additional administration of epinephrine has detrimental vasoconstrictive effects. However, there are no data available on changes in cardiac output and organ blood flow in response to high-dose catecholamine treatment in vasopressor-resistant neonatal shock, so close attention should be paid to signs of inappropriate vasoconstriction when this therapy is applied.

Unlike dopamine, dobutamine is a relatively cardioselective sympathomimetic amine with significant α- and β-adrenoreceptor–mediated direct inotropic effects and limited chronotropic actions (Ruffolo, 1987). Dobutamine administration is usually also associated with a variable drop in total peripheral vascular resistance and, at least in adults, with improvements in coronary blood flow and myocardial oxygen delivery. Furthermore, unlike dopamine, dobutamine increases myocardial contractility exclusively through the direct stimulation of the myocardial adrenergic receptors. Because myocardial norepinephrine stores are immature and rapidly depleted in the newborn, and because dobutamine may decrease afterload, newborns with primary myocardial dysfunction and elevated peripheral vascular resistance are most likely to benefit from dobutamine treatment (Martinez et al, 1992; Osborn et al, 2002; Noori et al, 2004). Interestingly, though addition of dobutamine to dopamine in preterm infants with RDS was effective in increasing blood pressure, it was associated with supranormal cardiac output states and low systemic vascular resistance (Lopez et al, 1997). Whether the benefits of supranormal cardiac output, through provision of adequate tissue oxygen delivery throughout the body, outweigh the risks of sustained hypercontractility, which potentially results in myocardial injury, remains to be investigated.

Some randomized studies have demonstrated that dopamine is more effective than dobutamine in raising blood pressure in the preterm infant. A meta-analysis of the findings confirmed that dopamine was more successful than dobutamine in treating hypotension and found that fewer infants in the dopamine-treated groups experienced treatment failure (Subdehar and Shaw, 2000). However, there was no difference in incidence of short-term adverse neurologic outcome between the two groups, and in the absence of long-term outcome data, no firm recommendations could be made regarding the first choice of drug to treat hypotension in preterm infants in the immediate postnatal period.

Because of the weak relationship between blood pressure and systemic blood flow *in very preterm neonates during the immediate postnatal period*, an increase in blood pressure does not necessarily guarantee that tissue perfusion has improved along with the blood pressure. Indeed, a randomized trial comparing the effects of dopamine and dobutamine on blood pressure and SVC blood flow found that, although dopamine is more effective in improving blood pressure, it is less effective in improving systemic blood flow in the very low-birth-weight neonate on the first postnatal day (Osborn et al, 2002). These findings may be explained by the difficulties extremely low-birth-weight neonates face during the immediate postnatal adaptation, when their immature myocardium struggles to maintain appropriate systemic blood flow against the suddenly increased peripheral vascular resistance. Under these circumstances, high doses of dopamine may further increase afterload without effectively improving myocardial function, and systemic blood flow may not improve or may worsen. Therefore, if there is evidence of peripheral vasoconstriction, especially in very low-birth-weight neonates during the first postnatal day, high-dose dopamine treatment should be attempted only if systemic blood flow can be monitored, because this treatment approach may result in further impairment in systemic blood flow despite improvements in blood pressure. At present, the neonatologist must rely on monitoring blood pressure and the indirect measures of cardiovascular function and must accept lower-end blood pressure values for gestational and postnatal age if evidence of vasoconstriction is present with higher doses of dopamine, while decreasing the dose of the drug below 10 μg/kg/min, at which significant α-adrenoreceptor stimulation is less likely (Seri, 1995; Noori et al, 2003). A combination of dobutamine and low- to medium-dose dopamine may achieve the most important goals of treatment by maintaining blood pressure and systemic blood flow in acceptable ranges, if monitoring of both cardiovascular parameters is possible. In summary, since both hypotension and low systemic blood flow may be associated with impairment of neurodevelopmental outcome, the primary goal of management of the hypotensive, very preterm neonate should be the correction of both measures of cardiovascular function.

The vasodilatory dopamine receptors are expressed primarily in the renal, mesenteric, and coronary circulation (Seri, 1995). Dopamine has been shown to selectively reduce renal vascular resistance (Seri et al, 1998, 2002) and raise glomerular filtration rate (Seri et al, 1993) in preterm infants as early as the 23rd week of gestation. However, dopamine decreases mesenteric vascular resistance in preterm infants only after the first postnatal day (Hentschel et al, 1995; Seri et al, 1998, 2000), and the effect may be variable (Zhang et al, 1999). Similarly, there are some differences in the reported magnitude of the drug-induced increases in ventricular function, cardiac output, and systemic vascular resistance (Clark et al, 2002; Lundstrom et al, 2000; Roze et al, 1993; Zhang et al, 1999). These differences may be best explained by variations in the intravascular volume status, the postnatal age, the developmentally regulated expression of cardiovascular adrenergic and dopaminergic receptors, and the severity of adrenoreceptor down-regulation among the different populations of critically ill preterm infants studied. It is important to note that none of the studies found evidence for a direct effect of dopamine on cerebral blood flow (Lundstrom et al, 2000; Seri et al, 1998, 2000; Zhang et al, 1999). Thus, dopamine administration appears to be devoid of potentially harmful selective hemodynamic effects in the brain. Finally, in addition to increasing afterload, dopamine may increase pulmonary vascular resistance in some preterm neonates (Liet et al, 2002). However, because the drug-induced increases in systemic blood pressure are not associated with impaired oxygenation in the majority of the preterm infants (Wardle et al, 1999), there is no evidence for consistent increases in extrapulmonary right-to-left shunting during dopamine treatment, especially in term neonates with persistent pulmonary hypertension.

There are no data available on the direct renal, cerebral, or pulmonary hemodynamic effects of dobutamine in the newborn (Noori et al, 2004). However, one nonrandomized study comparing the effects of dopamine and dobutamine on blood pressure and mesenteric blood flow in preterm infants found that the two drugs increased blood pressure and were equally effective in decreasing mesenteric vascular resistance (Hentschel et al, 1995). Dobutamine does not stimulate the dopaminergic receptors, so a β-adrenoreceptor–induced selective vasodilation may be responsible for the observed mesenteric vasodilation in the dobutamine-treated patients.

### Epithelial and Neuroendocrine Effects

Independent of the cardiovascular effects already described, dopamine exerts direct renal and endocrine (Seri, 1993 and 1995) actions in the newborn. Via its direct effects on sodium, phosphorus, and water transport processes and $Na^+,K^+$-ATPase activity in the renal tubules, dopamine increases excretion of sodium, phosphorous, and free water and may raise the hypoxic threshold of renal tubular cells during episodes of hypoperfusion and hypoxemia. Via its renal vascular and epithelial actions, dopamine also potentiates the diuretic effects of furosemide (Tulassay and Seri, 1986) and theophylline (Bell et al, 1998). Although dopamine has the theoretical potential to attenuate the renal side effects of indomethacin, published data for this issue are contradictory. Differences in the level of maturity, disease severity, ductal shunting, intravascular volume status, and indomethacin dose may be responsible for the conflicting results.

Among its endocrine actions, the dopamine-induced decreases in plasma prolactin and thyrotropin levels may be of clinical importance. The decrease in plasma prolactin may attenuate the preterm infant's propensity to edema formation. The inhibition of thyrotropin release, on the other hand, necessitates the postponement of routine neonatal thyroid screening until after dopamine administration has been discontinued. The potential effects on long-term neurodevelopmental outcome and immunologic function of the drug-induced alterations in the neuroendocrine function have not been investigated in the preterm or term neonate. Because dobutamine does not directly stimulate the dopaminergic receptors, its administration is devoid of neuroendocrine effects.

### Other Sympathomimetic Amines and Hormones

Despite the lack of peer-reviewed publications of controlled studies in the neonatal patient population, both epinephrine (Campbell and Byrne, 1998; Seri and Evans, 1998) and norepinephrine (Derleth, 1997) have been used in the treatment of hypotension in preterm infants. It is not known whether there is a difference in the cardiovascular response or side effects between the combined use of epinephrine and dopamine and the use of increasing doses of dopamine beyond 20 μg/kg/min with or without dobutamine. No detrimental vasoconstrictive effects have been reported for either high doses of epinephrine with or without dopamine or norepinephrine in these preliminary publications; this finding is best explained by the decreased cardiovascular sensitivity of these critically ill preterm infants to catecholamines, necessitating the high sympathomimetic support in the first place. In addition to sympathomimetic amines, arginine-vasopressin has been reported to improve cardiovascular function in a small number of newborns with vasodilatory shock after cardiac surgery (Rosenzweig et al, 1999).

## Corticosteroids

There is some limited evidence that brief corticosteroid treatment may stabilize the cardiovascular status and decrease the need for pressor support in the critically ill newborn with vasopressor-resistant hypotension. During the course of critical illness, down-regulation of adrenergic receptors may lead to gradual desensitization of the cardiovascular system to catecholamines, resulting in the need for escalation of vasopressor support. The finding that glucocorticoids regulate the expression of cardiovascular adrenergic receptors and some components of the second messenger systems (Hausdorff et al, 1990) explains the effectiveness of brief steroid treatment in stabilizing the cardiovascular status and reversing vasopressor resistance. In addition to regulating cardiovascular adrenergic receptor expression via their "genomic" effects, steroids exert certain "non-genomic" actions (Wehling, 1997), such as the inhibition of catecholamine metabolism and the production of vasoactive factors, including nitric oxide. Moreover, physiologic doses of mineralocorticoids and pharmacologic doses of glucocorticoids have been shown to instantly improve intracellular availability of calcium (Wehling, 1997), resulting in enhanced myocardial and vascular smooth muscle cell responsiveness to catecholamines. Indeed, some data suggest that hydrocortisone treatment in preterm infants with vasopressor-resistant hypotension is associated with significant increases in blood pressure within 2 hours of its administration (non-genomic effects) and that decreases in vasopressor requirement occur only after 8 to 12 hours of the first dose of the drug (genomic effects) (Fig. 31–5; Seri

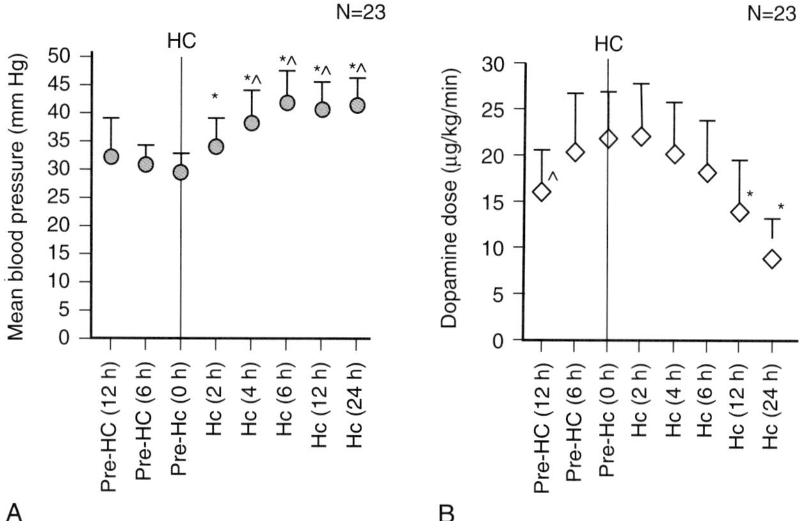


**FIGURE 31–5.** Effect of hydrocortisone (HC) on mean blood pressure (mean ± SD; **A**) and the dose of dopamine (mean ± SD; **B**) during the first 24 hours of hydrocortisone treatment in 23 preterm neonates with pressor-resistant shock. The mean blood pressure and dopamine requirement during 12 hours before and the first 24 hours after the first dose of hydrocortisone are shown. Before hydrocortisone administration, blood pressure remained low, despite significantly increased dopamine doses (**B**; ^, $P < .05$ vs. baseline [0 h]). However, mean blood pressure increased significantly by 2 hours after the first dose of hydrocortisone (**A**; °, $P < .05$ vs. baseline [0 h]) and continued to rise until 6 hours of hydrocortisone therapy, remaining stable thereafter (**A**; °, $P < .05$ vs. baseline [0 h]; ^, $P < .05$ vs. HC [2 h]). The dose of dopamine significantly decreased at 12 and 24 hours of hydrocortisone therapy (**B**; °, $P < .05$ vs. baseline [0 h]). *(From Seri I, Tan R, Evans J: Cardiovascular effects of hydrocortisone in preterm neonates with pressor-resistant hypotension. Pediatrics 107:1070-1074, 2001.)*

et al, 2001). However, there is growing concern about the potential short-term and long-term side effects of systemic steroid administration.

### Supportive Measures

Maintenance of a normal arterial pH and serum ionized calcium concentrations is necessary for the optimum cardiovascular response to catecholamines. Because some clinicians believe that a metabolic acidosis in which pH is less than 7.25 may compromise myocardial function in the preterm infant (Fanconi et al, 1993), it has been recommended that the arterial pH be maintained above this range in cases of acidosis with a significant metabolic component.

## SUMMARY

Sustained stabilization of the cardiovascular status with provision of appropriate blood pressure, cardiac output, tissue perfusion, and oxygenation remains a difficult task in most critically ill hypotensive newborns. Treatment of these patients requires the ability to monitor the most important measures of cardiovascular function (blood pressure and systemic blood flow) as well as a thorough understanding of the pathogenesis and pathophysiology of neonatal shock and the mechanisms of actions, pharmacodynamics, and potential side effects of the sympathomimetic amines and other medications used in the management of neonatal shock.

## REFERENCES


Alverson DC, Elridge M, Dillon T, et al: Noninvasive pulsed Doppler determination of cardiac output in neonates and children. J Pediatr 101:46-50, 1982.

Bell M, Jackson E, Mi Z, et al: Low-dose theophylline increases urine output in diuretic-dependent critically ill children. Intensive Care Med 24:1099-1105, 1998.

Campbell ME, Byrne PJ: Outcome after intravenous epinephrine infusion in infants <750 g birthweight. Pediatr Res 43:209A, 1998.

Clark SJ, Yoxall CW, Subhedar NV: Right ventricular performance in hypotensive preterm neonates treated with dopamine. Pediatr Cardiol 23:167-170, 2002.

Derleth DP: Clinical experience with norepinephrine infusions in critically ill newborns. Pediatr Res 145A, 1997.

Deshpande SA, Platt MP: Association between blood lactate and acid-base status and mortality in ventilated babies. Arch Dis Child Fetal Neonatal Ed 76:F15-F20, 1997.

Di Sessa TG, Leitner M, Ti CC, et al: The cardiovascular effects of dopamine in the severely asphyxiated neonate. J Pediatr 99:772-776, 1981.

Ernest D, Belzberg AS, Dodek PM: Distribution of normal saline and 5% albumin infusions in septic patients. Crit Care Med 27:46-50, 1999.

Evans N: Echocardiography on neonatal intensive care units in Australia and New Zealand. J Paediatr Child Health 36:169-171, 2000.

Evans N, Iyer P: Assessment of ductus arteriosus shunt in preterm infants supported by mechanical ventilation: Effects of interatrial shunting. J Pediatr 125:778-785, 1994.

Evans N, Kluckow M: Early determinants of right and left ventricular output in ventilated preterm infants. Arch Dis Child Fetal Neonatal Ed 74:F88-F94, 1996.

Evans N, Kluckow M, Currie A: Range of echocardiographic findings in term neonates with high oxygen requirements. Arch Dis Child Fetal Neonatal Ed 78:F105-F111, 1998.

Fanconi S, Burger R, Ghelfi D, et al: Hemodynamic effects of sodium bicarbonate in critically ill neonates. Intensive Care Med 19:65-69, 1993.

Gill AB, Weindling AM: Echocardiographic assessment of cardiac function in shocked very low birthweight infants. Arch Dis Child 68:17-21, 1993.

Hausdorff WP, Caron MG, Lefkowitz RJ: Turning off the signal: Desensitization of beta-adrenergic receptors. FASEB J 4: 2881-28889, 1990.

Hawkins J, Van Hare GF, Schmidt KG, et al: Effects of increasing afterload on left ventricular output in fetal lambs. Pediatr Cardiol 65:127-134, 1989.

Hentschel R, Hensel D, Brune T, et al: Impact on blood pressure and intestinal perfusion of dobutamine or dopamine in hypotensive preterm infants. Biol Neonate 68:318-324, 1995.

Hunt R, Kluckow M, Reiger I, Evans N: Low superior vena cava flow and neurodevelopmental outcome at 3 years in very preterm babies. Pediatr Res 49:336A, 2001.

Kavvadia V, Greenough A, Dimitrioe G, et al: Randomized trial of fluid restriction in ventilated very low birth weight infants. Arch Dis Child Fetal Neonatal Ed 83:F91-F96, 2000.

Kluckow M, Evans N: Relationship between blood pressure and cardiac output in preterm infants requiring mechanical ventilation. J Pediatr 129:506-512, 1996.

Kluckow M, Evans N: Ductal shunting, high pulmonary blood flow, and pulmonary hemorrhage. J Pediatr 137:68-72, 2000a.

Kluckow M, Evans N: Low superior vena flow and intraventricular haemorrhage in preterm infants. Arch Dis Child Fetal Neonatal Ed 82:F188-F194, 2000b.

Kluckow M, Evans N: Superior vena flow in preterm infants: A novel marker of systemic blood flow. Arch Dis Child Fetal Neonatal Ed 82:F182-F187, 2000c.

Kluckow M, Evans N: Low systemic blood flow and hyperkalemia in preterm infants. J Pediatr 139:227-232, 2001.

Landry DW, Oliver JA: The pathogenesis of vasodilatory shock. N Engl J Med 345:588-595, 2001.

Lee J, Rajadurai VS, Tan KW: Blood pressure standards for very low birthweight infants during the first day of life. Arch Dis Child Fetal Neonatal Ed 81:F168-F170, 1999.

Liet JM, Boscher C, Gras-Leguen C, et al: Dopamine effects on pulmonary artery pressure in hypotensive preterm infants with patent ductus arteriosus. J Pediatr 140:373-537, 2002.

Lopez SL, Leighton JO, Walther FJ: Supranormal cardiac output in dopamine and dobutamine dependent preterm infants. Pediatric Cardiol 18:292-296, 1997.

Lundstrom K, Pryds O, Greisen G: The hemodynamic effects of dopamine and volume expansion in sick preterm infants. Early Hum Dev 57:157-163, 2000.

Martinez AM, Padbury JF, Thio S: Dobutamine pharmacokinetics and cardiovascular responses in critically ill neonates. Pediatrics 89:47-51, 1992.

Meadow W, Rudinsky B: Inflammatory mediators and neonatal sepsis. Rarely has so little been known by so many about so much. Clin Perinatol 22:519-536, 1995.

Nadel S, De Munter C, Britto J, et al: Albumin: Saint or sinner? Arch Dis Child 79:384-385, 1998.

Ng PC, Lam CW, Fok TF, et al: Refractory hypotension in preterm infants with adrenocortical insufficiency. Arch Dis Child Fetal Neonatal Ed 84:F122-F124, 2001.

Noori S, Friedlich P, Seri I: Developmentally regulated cardiovascular, renal, and neuroendocrine effects of dopamine. NeoReviews 4:E283-E288, 2003.

Noori S, Friedlich P, Seri I: Cardiovascular and renal effects of dobutamine in the neonate. NeoReviews 5:E22-E26, 2004.

Nuntarumit P, Yang W, Bada-Ellzey HS: Blood pressure measurements in the newborn. Clin Perinatol 26:981-996, 1999.

Oca MJ, Nelson M, Donn SM: Randomized trial of normal saline versus 5% albumin for the treatment of neonatal hypotension. J Perinatol 23:473-476, 2003.

Osborn D, Evans N, Kluckow M: Randomised trial of dopamine and dobutamine in preterm infants with low systemic blood flow. J Pediatr 140:183-191, 2002.

Osborn DA, Evans N, Kluckow M: Hemodynamic and antecedent risk factors of early and late periventricular/intraventricular hemorrhage in premature infants. Pediatrics 112: 33-39, 2003.

Osborn DA, Kluckow M, Evans N: Blood pressure, capillary refill, and central-peripheral temperature difference. Clinical detection of low upper body blood flow in very premature infants. Arch Dis Child Fetal Neonatal Ed (in press), 2004.

Pladys P, Wodey E, Beuchee A, et al: Left ventricle output and mean arterial blood pressure in preterm infants during the 1st day of life. Eur J Pediatr 15:817-824, 1999.

Rosenzweig EB, Starc TJ, Chen JM, et al: Intravenous arginine-vasopressin in children with vasodilatory shock after cardiac surgery. Circulation 100:II182-II186, 1999.

Roze JC, Tohier C, Maingureneau C, et al: Response to dopamine and dobutamine in hypotensive very preterm infants. Arch Dis Child 69:59-63, 1993.

Ruffolo RR: The pharmacology of dobutamine. Am J Med Sci 294:244-248, 1987.

Seri I: Cardiovascular, renal, and endocrine actions of dopamine in neonates and children. J Pediatr 126:333-344, 1995.

Seri I: Circulatory support of the sick preterm infant. Semin Neonatol 6:85-95, 2001.

Seri I, Abbassi S, Wood DC, et al: Effect of dopamine on regional blood flows in sick preterm infants. J Pediatr 133: 728-734, 1998.

Seri I, Evans J: Addition of epinephrine to dopamine increases blood pressure and urine output in critically ill extremely low birth weight neonates with uncompensated shock. Pediatr Res 43:194A, 1998.

Seri I, Rudas G, Bors ZS, et al: Effects of low-dose dopamine on cardiovascular and renal functions, cerebral blood flow, and plasma catecholamine levels in sick preterm neonates. Pediatr Res 34:742-749, 1993.

Seri I, Tan R, Evans J: Cardiovascular effects of hydrocortisone in preterm neonates with pressor resistant hypotension. Pediatrics 107:1070-1074, 2001.

Seri I, Abbasi S, Wood DC, et al: Regional hemodynamic effects of dopamine in the indomethacin-treated preterm infant. J Perinatol 22:300-305, 2002.

So KW, Fok TF, Ng PC, et al: Randomized controlled trial of colloid or crystalloid in hypotensive preterm infants. Arch Dis Child Fetal Neonatal Ed 76:F43-F46, 1997.

Subhedar, NV Shaw NJ: Dopamine versus dobutamine for hypotensive preterm infants. Cochrane Database Syst Rev (2):CD001242, 2000.

Takahashi Y, Harada K, Kishkurno S, et al: Postnatal left ventricular contractility in very preterm infants. Pediatr Cardiol 18:112-117, 1997.

Tapia-Rombo CA, Carpio-Hernandez JC, Salazar-Acuan AH, et al: Detection of transitory myocardial ischaemia secondary to perinatal asphyxia. Arch Med Res 31:377-383, 2000.

Tibby SM, Hatherill M, Murdoch IA: Capillary refill and core-peripheral temperature gap as indicators of haemodynamic status in paediatric intensive care patients. Arch Dis Child 80:163-166, 1999.

Tsuji M, Saul JP, du Plessis A, et al: Cerebral intravascular oxygenation correlates with mean arterial pressure in critically ill premature infants. Pediatrics 106:625-632, 2000.

Tulassay T, Seri I: Interaction of dopamine and furosemide in acute oliguria of preterm infants with hyaline membrane disease. Acta Paediatr Scand 75:420-424, 1986.

Tyszczuk L, Meek J, Elwell C, et al: Cerebral blood flow is independent of mean arterial blood pressure in preterm infants undergoing intensive care. Pediatrics 102:337-341, 1998.

Van Marter LJ, Leviton A, Allred EN, et al: Hydration during the first days of life and the risk of bronchopulmonary dysplasia in low birth weight infants. J Pediatr 116:942-949, 1990.

Walther FJ, Siassi B, Ramadan NA, et al: Pulsed Doppler determinations of cardiac output in neonates: normal standards for clinical use. Pediatrics 76:829-833, 1985.

Wardle SP, Yoxall CW, Weindling AM: Peripheral oxygenation in hypotensive preterm babies. Pediatr Res 45:343-349, 1999.

Wehling M: Specific, nongenomic actions of steroid hormones. Annu Rev Physiol 59:365-393, 1997.

Wright IMR, Goodhall SR: Blood pressure and blood volume in preterm infants. Arch Dis Child Fetal Neonatal Ed 70: F230-F232, 1994.

Zhang J, Penny DJ, Kim NS, et al: Mechanisms of blood pressure increase induced by dopamine in hypotensive preterm neonates. Arch Dis Child Fetal Neonatal Ed 81:F99-F104, 1999.

CHAPTER 32

# Care of the Extremely Low-Birth-Weight Infant

**Eric C. Eichenwald**

Few medical specialties have experienced the amount of progress in medical care and impact on overall patient survival than neonatology over the past two decades. Improvements in technology, greater use of prenatal glucocorticoids and surfactant replacement therapy, better regionalization of perinatal and high-risk neonatal care, and a more comprehensive understanding of the physiology of the immature infant have all contributed to dramatic increases in survival of very preterm infants. Care of premature infants with birth weights between 1000 and 1500 g has become almost routine in most newborn intensive care units (NICUs) in the United States.

The newest frontier in neonatology is the care of extremely low-birth-weight infants (ELBW) (birth weight <1000 g), sometimes referred colloquially as "micropremies." These infants present one of the greatest medical and ethical challenges to the field. Although they represent a small percentage of overall births and NICU admissions, ELBW infants are often the most critically ill and at the highest risk for mortality and long-term morbidity of any NICU patient. They also contribute disproportionately to overall hospital days and consume a large percentage of NICU personnel time, effort, and costs of care. Care of these infants is in constant evolution, owing to new discoveries in both basic and clinical research as well as to growing clinical experience. In this chapter, I review some of the special challenges in and practical aspects of the management of the ELBW infant. The reader is referred to specific chapters throughout the text for a more comprehensive review of specific problems and conditions.

## EPIDEMIOLOGY

The percentage of babies born preterm in the United States has risen slowly over the past two decades (Martin et al, 2002). In the year 2000, preterm (<37 weeks of gestation) births accounted for 11.6% of all births, and births of infants before 28 weeks of gestation for just below 1%. There is a significant racial disparity in the incidence of extreme preterm birth, the African-American ELBW birth rate being nearly double that of the Hispanic and non-Hispanic white populations. Associated with this increase in frequency of preterm births is the greater availability of assisted reproductive technologies. These technologies result in a higher incidence of LBW infants, due in part to the higher frequency of multiple gestations (Schieve et al, 2002). Twins, triplets, and higher-order multiple gestations currently represent almost a quarter all LBW deliveries in the United States (Martin et al, 2002), and contribute to the ELBW population. Multiple gestations add to the potential morbidity of extremely premature birth because of a higher frequency of intrauterine growth restriction (IUGR) and other medical complications of pregnancy.

Several studies have shown increased survival in the smallest and most premature infants over the past decade (Figs. 32–1 through 32–3) (Horbar et al, 2002; Lemons et al, 2000). See also Chapter 1 for a complete discussion of these changes.)

Improved survival has been accompanied by a change in the incidence of several major morbidities among survivors (Figs. 32–4 and 32–5). Little change in the frequency of severe intracranial hemorrhage or necrotizing enterocolitis was observed in the National Institute of Child Health and Development (NICHD) cohort of infants born in institutions participating in the Neonatal Research Network between 1991 and 1996 (Lemons et al, 2001). In contrast, the Vermont-Oxford NICUs reported a reduction in the incidence of severe intracranial hemorrhage in the early part of the 1990s, which has remained static into the late 1990s (Horbar et al, 2002). The incidence of chronic lung disease (defined as oxygen requirement at 36 weeks of postmenstrual age) rose slightly from 1991 to 1996 in the NICHD cohort, likely related to the greater survival of infants in the lowest weight group. With the current trends in survival and in hospital morbidity, the absolute number of extremely premature infants who survive to NICU discharge and are diagnosed with a major morbidity in the neonatal period has increased (Fig. 32–6). A significant percentage of these infants continue to suffer from neurodevelopmental and neurosensory disability into childhood (Wood et al, 2000).

## PERINATAL MANAGEMENT

Short-term outcomes of extremely premature infants are improved if they are delivered in a high-risk center rather than being transported after birth (Arad et al, 1999; Chien et al, 2001; Cifuentes et al, 2002; Towers et al, 2000). Therefore, if clinically feasible, the pregnant woman who seems likely to deliver an extremely premature infant should be transferred to a high-risk perinatal center for the expertise in obstetrical and neonatology management. Upon arrival, she should be evaluated for factors that may have predisposed to preterm labor and assessed for the status of the fetal membranes and the presence or absence of chorioamnionitis. In addition, best obstetrical estimate of gestational age (by date of last menstrual period and early ultrasonographic dating, if available), ultrasonographic assessment of fetal size and position, and the presence of other medical or obstetrical complications (preeclampsia, placenta previa, abruptio placentae) should be documented. Specimens for rectovaginal cultures to detect the presence of group B streptococcus should also be obtained on admission (Schrag et al, 2002), and treatment with penicillin (or vancomycin for the penicillin-allergic patient) initiated until culture results

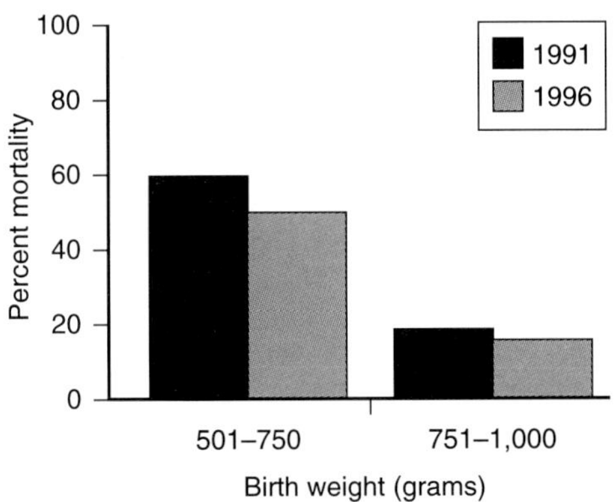


**FIGURE 32–1.** Mortality in extremely low-birth-weight infants cared for in the National Institute of Child Health and Human Development Neonatal Research Network Centers in 1991 to 1996. *(Adapted from Lemons J, Bauer C, Oh W, et al: Very low birth weight outcomes of the National Institute of Child Health and Human Development Neonatal Research Network, January 1995 through December 1996. Pediatrics 197:1-8, 2001.)*

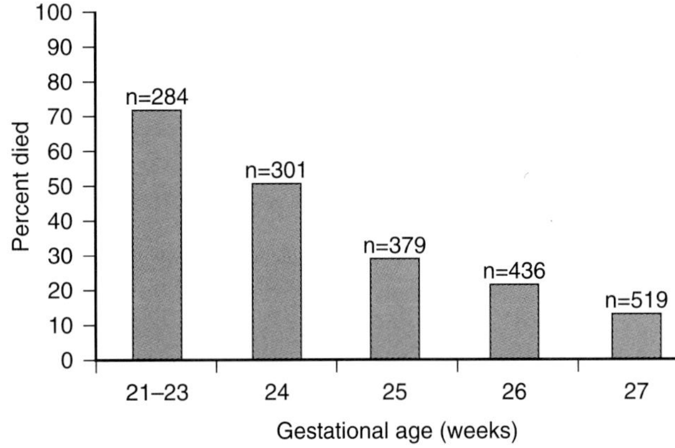


**FIGURE 32–3.** Mortality before discharge, by gestational age as estimated by best obstetrical estimate, among infants born at 21 to 27 weeks of gestation in National Institute of Child Health and Human Development Neonatal Research Network Centers between January 1, 1995, and December 31, 1996. *(Adapted from Lemons et al, 2001).*

are available. There is widespread agreement that prenatal glucocorticoids should be offered to any woman in whom delivery at 24 to 34 weeks of gestation threatens; treatment at earlier gestational ages is controversial and of unclear benefit. Although unlikely to arrest labor for an extended period, tocolytic agents (ritodrine, terbutaline, magnesium sulfate) should be considered for women with preterm uterine contractions without evidence of chorioamnionitis.

Premature rupture of the fetal membranes (PROM) occurs in 30% to 40% of women who deliver prematurely (Mazor et al, 1998). If PROM is diagnosed without evidence of chorioamnionitis, consideration should be given to use of prophylactic antibiotic therapy (ampicillin or erythromycin) for the mother. Several studies have shown that such therapy prolongs the latency period, reduces the incidence of chorioamnionitis and endometritis, and improves neonatal outcome (Gibbs and Eschenbach, 1997; Mazor et al, 1998; Mercer et al, 1997). Tocolytic and antibiotic therapy in the setting of PROM may prolong latency by 48 to 72 hours in many extremely preterm pregnancies in which delivery threatens, allowing administration of a complete course of glucocorticoids to the mother. (See also Chapters 42 and 47.)

## PRENATAL CONSULTATION

If possible, all parents who are at risk for delivery of an extremely premature infant should meet in consultation with a neonatologist before the infant's birth, preferably jointly with a perinatologist caring for the mother (Finer and Barrington, 1998). There are several goals of this consultation. First, the neonatologist and perinatologist should inform the parents about the proposed management of the pregnancy and delivery of the infant, including

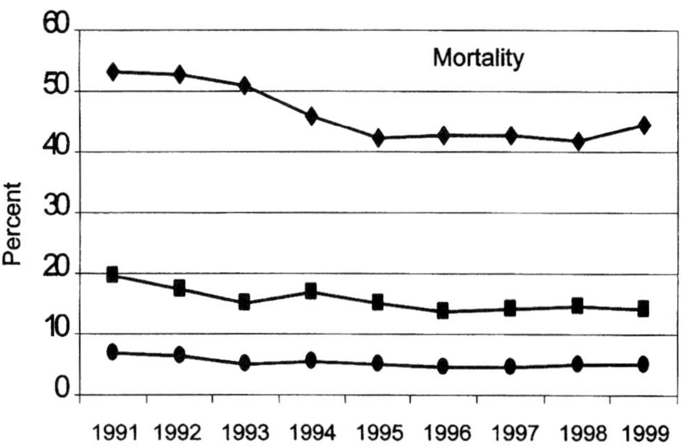


**FIGURE 32–2.** Mortality for infants 501 to 1500 g, 1991 to 1999, by birth weight category from 362 Vermont-Oxford Network centers. *Diamonds* indicate 501 to 750 g birth weight; *squares*, 750 to 1000 g; and *circles*, 1000 to 1500 g. *(From Horbar J, Badger G, Carpenter J, et al: Trends in mortality and morbidity for very low birth weight infants, 1991-1999. Pediatrics 110:143-151, 2002.)*

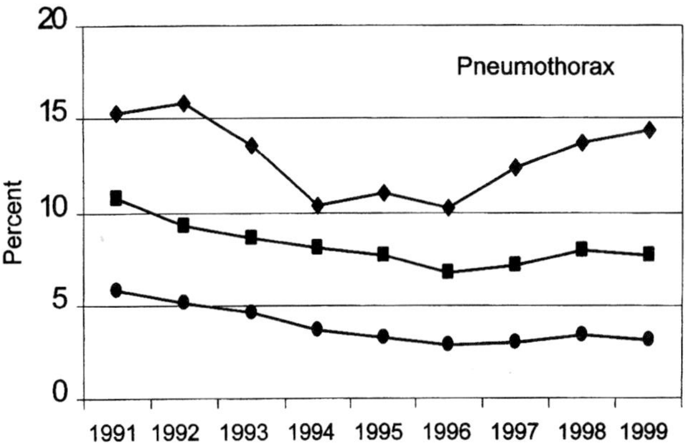


**FIGURE 32–4.** Incidence of pneumothorax for infants 501 to 1500 g by birth weight category from 362 Vermont-Oxford Network centers, 1991 to 1999. *Diamonds* indicate 501 to 750 g birth weight; *squares*, 750 to 1000 g; and *circles*, 1000 to 1500 g. *(From Horbar J, Badger G, Carpenter J, et al: Trends in mortality and morbidity for very low birth weight infants, 1991-1999. Pediatrics 110:143-151, 2002.)*

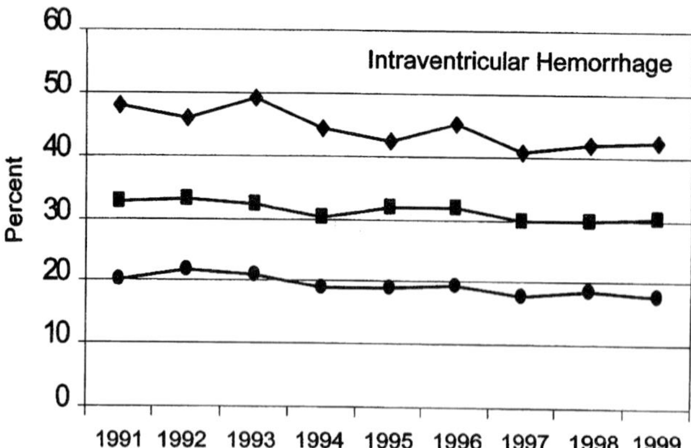


**FIGURE 32–5.** Incidence of intraventricular hemorrhage for infants 501 to 1500 g by birth weight category from 362 Vermont-Oxford Network centers, 1991 to 1999. *Diamonds* indicate 501 to 750 g birth weight; *squares*, 750 to 1000 g; and *circles*, 1000 to 1500 g. *(From Horbar J, Badger G, Carpenter J, et al: Trends in mortality and morbidity for very low birth weight infants, 1991-1999. Pediatrics 110:143-151, 2002.)*

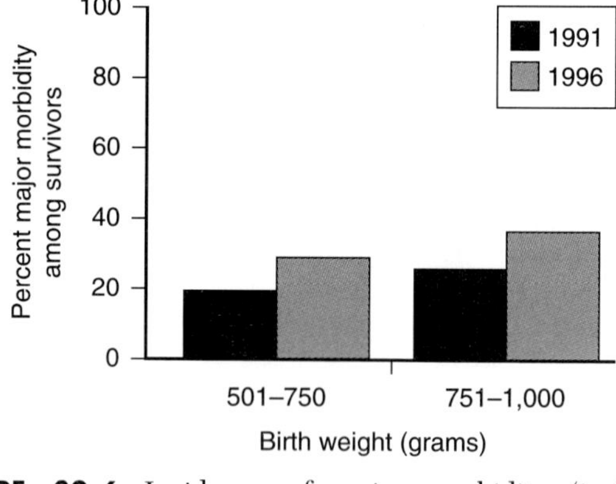


**FIGURE 32–6.** Incidence of major morbidity (including severe intracranial hemorrhage, chronic lung disease, and proven necrotizing enterocolitis) among surviving extremely low-birth-weight infants cared for in National Institute of Child Health and Human Development Neonatal Network Research Centers in 1991 to 1996. *(Adapted from Lemons et al, 2001.)*

a discussion of the advantages of administration of glucocorticoids to the mother, the possible need for cesarean delivery, and delivery room care and resuscitation of the baby. Second, the parents should be informed about the potential risks of both the extent of prematurity and the proposed therapeutic interventions (Tables 32–1 and 32–2). Third, the neonatologist should investigate the parents' beliefs and attitudes about delivery of an extremely premature infant and the potential for long-term morbidity. This outline for prenatal consultation is especially impor-

**TABLE 32–1**

**Major Problems of Extremely Low-Birth-Weight Infants**

| | Short-Term Problems | Long-Term Problems |
|---|---|---|
| Respiratory | Respiratory distress syndrome<br>Air leaks<br>Bronchopulmonary dysplasia<br>Apnea of prematurity | Chronic lung disease<br>Reactive airway disease |
| Gastrointestinal/nutritional | Feeding intolerance<br>Necrotizing enterocolitis<br>Growth failure | Growth failure<br>Failure to thrive<br>Inguinal hernias |
| Immunologic/infection | Immune deficiency<br>Perinatal infection<br>Nosocomial infection | Respiratory syncytial virus |
| Central nervous system | Intraventricular hemorrhage<br>Periventricular white matter disease | Cerebral palsy<br>Neurodevelopmental delay<br>Hearing loss |
| Ophthalmologic | Retinopathy of prematurity | Blindness, retinal detachment<br>Myopia<br>Strabismus |
| Cardiovascular | Hypotension<br>Patent ductus arteriosus | |
| Renal | Water/electrolyte imbalance<br>Acid-base disturbances | |
| Hematologic | Iatrogenic anemia<br>Frequent transfusions<br>Anemia of prematurity | |
| Endocrine | Transient hypothyroxinemia<br>?Cortisol deficiency | |

TABLE 32-2

**Incidence of Specific Interventions and Outcomes of Extremely Low-Birth-Weight Infants (<1000 g) in the Canadian NICU Network**

| | Birth Weight Category | |
|---|---|---|
| | <750 g (n = 744) | 750 to 999 g (n = 874) |
| Survival (%) | 62 | 86 |
| Respiratory morbidity | | |
| Chronic lung disease (%) | 54 | 33 |
| Postnatal steroids (% received) | 44 | 39 |
| Median days on oxygen | 28 | 16 |
| Median days on ventilation | 42 | 25 |
| Retinopathy of prematurity | | |
| Eye examination performed | 54 | 70 |
| None (%) | 30 | 47 |
| Stages 1-2 disease(%) | 41 | 41 |
| ≥Stage 3 disease (%) | 29 | 12 |
| Laser/cryotherapy (% treated) | 9 | 4 |
| Intraventricular hemorrhage (IVH) | | |
| Cranial ultrasound examination | 74 | 88 |
| No IVH (%) | 54 | 63 |
| Grade 1-2 (%) | 27 | 25 |
| ≥Grade 3 (%) | 19 | 12 |
| Ventriculoperitoneal shunt (%) | 1 | 2 |
| Patent ductus arteriosus (%) | | |
| Indomethacin treatment only (%) | 30 | 30 |
| Surgical ligation only (%) | 7 | 3 |
| Combination (indomethacin/surgical ligation) (%) | 10 | 8 |
| Nosocomial infection (%) | 29 | 29 |
| Necrotizing enterocolitis | | |
| Medical treatment (%) | 6 | 6 |
| Surgical treatment (%) | 5 | 3 |
| Survival without major morbidity (%) | 37 | 56 |

Data from Lee S, McMillan D, Ohlsson A, et al: Variations in practice and outcomes in the Canadian NICU network: 1996-1997. Pediatrics 106:1070-1079, 2000.

tant if delivery is expected at the borderline of viability (23 to 24 weeks of gestation).

Data are sparse about the process and results of prenatal consultation with parents of an extremely preterm infant. Some studies suggest that significant incongruity exists among the attitudes of obstetricians, nurses, neonatologists, and parents about active delivery room resuscitation and treatment of extremely premature infants (Streiner et al, 2001; Zupancic et al, 2002). Reuss and Gordon (1995) have shown that the obstetrical judgment of fetal viability was associated with an 18-fold increase in survival for infants with a birth weight less than 750 g, indicating that obstetrical attitudes and decisions influence outcome. Obstetricians and nurses tend to overestimate, and parents tend to underestimate, mortality and morbidity in premature infants (Doron et al, 1998; Haywood et al, 1994). Parents report being more in favor of intervening irrespective of gestational age or condition at birth compared with health care professionals (Streiner et al, 2001). In a survey by Ballard and colleagues (2002), the majority of neonatologists responded that they would respect parents' wishes about resuscitation of a borderline viable infant. In practice, when parental preferences about active resuscitation are known before delivery of an extremely preterm infant, neonatologists report that they would alter their management of the infant in the delivery room accordingly (Doron et al, 1998), indicating the important role for prenatal consultation. However, parental attitudes likely are strongly influenced by physician recommendations about aggressive resuscitation conveyed during the prenatal consultation.

The earliest gestational age at which resuscitation should be initiated remains controversial among neonatologists (Finer et al, 1999), making firm recommendations for the actual content of prenatal consultation difficult. Most studies that describe the outcome of premature infants are based on birth weight rather than gestational age and thus confound the effects of extremely preterm birth with those of intrauterine growth restriction. However, both parents and physicians are usually faced with making decisions based on the anticipated gestational age at delivery. Data from several studies suggest that in terms of survival and potential for long-term disability, encouragement of active management is appropriate for pregnancies expected to deliver at 25 weeks of gestation or later (Piecuch et al, 1997; Wood et al, 2000). The risk of death and severe morbidity is significantly higher before 25 weeks of gestation (El-Metwally et al, 2000). Mortality approaches 80% for infants delivered at 23 completed weeks of gestation, with the majority of survivors suffering from neurodevelopmental sequelae (Vohr et al, 2000; Wood et al, 2000). These data should be shared with parents during prenatal consultation, and appropriate guidance given for decision-making about the pregnancy, delivery, and resuscitation of the infant.

## GENERAL PRINCIPLES OF CARE SPECIFIC TO THE EXTREMELY LOW-BIRTH-WEIGHT INFANT

### The First Hours

The first few hours after admission to the NICU are critical for the ELBW infant, although there are significant variations in practice among hospitals and practitioners. Careful adherence to details in the delivery room and during the first few hours after birth is essential to help avoid some of the immediate and long-term complications of the ELBW infant. All NICUs should have a consistent approach to the initial care of these fragile infants in the delivery room and upon admission to the NICU. A suggested treatment guideline for the first few hours after birth is presented in Table 32–3, and screening guidelines for common complications are shown in Table 32–4.

### Delivery Room

At delivery, strict attention to maintenance of body temperature by means of rapid, gentle drying of the infant and the use of adequate heat sources is paramount to avoid cold stress. Use of a polyethylene occlusive skin wrap immediately after delivery may also help prevent initial evaporative heat losses (Vohra et al, 1999). Many ELBW infants need some form of assisted ventilation immediately after birth. If positive-pressure ventilation is required, it should be provided with low inspiratory pressure to prevent overdistention of the lungs, which can result in air leak and other lung injury, and adequate positive end-expiratory pressure (PEEP) to maintain lung

**TABLE 32–3**

**Treatment Guidelines for Initial Management of Extremely Low-Birth-Weight Infants**

| | |
|---|---|
| Delivery room | Ensure good thermoregulation<br>“Gentle” ventilation as required<br>Avoid hyperventilation and hyperoxia<br>Administer surfactant (if prophylaxis approach) |
| NICU admission | Obtain weight<br>Administer surfactant within first hour (if rescue approach)<br>Establish vascular access:<br>Peripheral intravenous catheter<br>Umbilical arterial catheter<br>Umbilical venous catheter (central, double-lumen)<br>Start intravenous fluids as soon as possible with dextrose solution<br>Limit evaporative water losses (humidified incubator)<br>Minimize stimulation<br>Avoid hyperventilation and hyperoxia<br>Obtain specimens for complete blood count with differential, blood culture, blood glucose measurement<br>Give antibiotics as indicated<br>Give parents information about their child |
| First 24 to 48 hours | |
| Cardiovascular | Monitor blood pressure; give vasopressors as required<br>Maintain vigilance for presence of patent ductus arteriosus<br>Obtain echocardiogram as indicated |
| Respiratory | Give additional surfactant doses as indicated<br>Maintain low tidal volume ventilation<br>Avoid hyperventilation and hyperoxia<br>Extubate infant and start on continuous positive airway pressure when possible |
| Fluid Management | Obtain weight every 12 to 24 hours<br>Monitor serum electrolyte, blood glucose, and calcium concentrations every 4 to 8 hours<br>Limit evaporative water losses<br>Administer skin care |
| Hematologic | Obtain second blood count<br>Administer transfusion support as indicated<br>Monitor bilirubin; give phototherapy as indicated |
| Infection | Consider discontinuing antibiotics if blood culture results negative at 48 hours |
| Nutrition | Start amino acid solution/parenteral nutrition |
| Neurologic | Minimize stimulation<br>Perform screening head ultrasonography |
| Social | Arrange to meet with family |

**TABLE 32-4**

**Recommended Screening for Common Complications of Extremely Low-Birth-Weight Infants**

| | |
|---|---|
| Intraventricular hemorrhage (IVH): | Head ultrasonography (HUS) on day 1-3; repeat on day 7-10 |
| Germinal matrix hemorrhage | Repeat HUS weekly until findings normal |
| Intraventricular hemorrhage | Repeat HUS every 3 to 7 days until stable/resolved |
| IVH with ventricular dilation or intraparenchymal bleeding | Repeat HUS every 3 to 7 days until stable/resolved<br>Consider measurement of resistive indices for progressive ventricular dilatation |
| Periventricular white matter disease | HUS at day 30; repeat at 36 weeks of postmenstrual age or at discharge<br>Consider magnetic resonance imaging if HUS findings equivocal |
| Retinopathy of prematurity (ROP): | Perform ophthalmologic examination (OE) exam at 4 to 6 weeks of postnatal age<br>Repeat every 2 weeks if no ROP<br>Repeat weekly if ROP present<br>Repeat twice weekly for pre-threshold disease or rapidly progressive ROP |
| Absence of ROP | Repeat OE every 2 weeks |
| Presence of ROP | Repeat OE weekly |
| Presence of prethreshold disease or rapidly progressive ROP | Repeat OE twice weekly |
| Audiology screening | Hearing screen no earlier than 34 weeks of postmenstrual age but prior to discharge home |

volume. Hyperventilation and hyperoxia also should be avoided. The use of room air for resuscitation of these infants has been proposed to protect them from hyperoxia and damage to the lungs by oxygen free radicals. This issue is under active investigation (Lefkowitz, 2002), but most centers continue to use either 100% or blended oxygen for initial resuscitation. (See also Chapter 28.)

Some centers routinely intubate all ELBW infants in the delivery room for respiratory support, and prophylactic surfactant administration (Egberts et al, 1997; Kendig et al, 1998). Soll and Morley (2001) have reported on their meta-analysis of eight randomized trials of the use of natural surfactant as prophylaxis versus as a rescue strategy for established respiratory distress syndrome (RDS) in the ELBW infant. Administration of exogenous surfactant before 15 minutes of age resulted in a reduction in rates of neonatal mortality, air leak, and the combined outcome of bronchopulmonary dysplasia (BPD) or death compared with a selective rescue approach. However, no trials comparing prophylactic administration with very early rescue administration of exogenous surfactant (within the first 30 to 60 minutes) have been performed (see Chapter 46). In some centers, ELBW infants are observed briefly after birth, and if respiratory distress develops, they are intubated and hand-ventilated for transfer to the NICU. Exogenous surfactant is given within 1 hour of birth, after endotracheal tube position and the presence of RDS are confirmed on chest radiograph This strategy assures uniform distribution of surfactant to both lungs and allows initial stabilization and more intensive monitoring of the infant during its administration. Other centers report success with intubation and immediate administration of surfactant during resuscitation, and still others try to avoid mechanical ventilation in ELBW infants by applying continuous positive airway pressure (CPAP) immediately in the delivery room (Lindner et al, 1999).

If intubation is required, both oral and nasal routes for endotracheal tube placement are equally effective and have similar complication rates (Spence and Barr, 2002). Preference is usually institution specific, although successful placement of a nasal endotracheal tube takes longer.

## Admission to the Neonatal Intensive Care Unit

All infants should be weighed upon admission; frequent determination of subsequent weights is an invaluable tool in managing fluid intake. In many centers, ELBW infants are initially placed in a radiant warmer for easier access (i.e., for surfactant administration and catheter placement). Because of the very high transepidermal fluid losses in these infants, intravenous fluids with a 5% to 10% dextrose solution should be started immediately after admission, and efforts made to ameliorate evaporative water losses by increasing the relative humidity surrounding the infant. A plastic heat shield used in concert with the radiant warmer may decrease transepidermal water losses; alternatively, a polyethylene "tent" with an infusion of warmed humidified air may be used. Several studies suggest that fluid management is improved by utilization of a humidified incubator instead of a radiant warmer, because of smaller water losses (Gaylord et al, 2001; Meyer et al, 2001). Exposure to high humidity may raise the rate of skin colonization with gram-negative organisms, although no increase in the rate of nosocomial infections was observed in several randomized trials comparing incubators with radiant warmers (Flenady and Woodgate, 2002). However, temperature regulation for the smallest infants in the first few days may be more difficult in an incubator than in a servo-controlled radiant warmer because of rapid drops in air temperature as the incubator doors are opened to care for the infant (Meyer et al, 2001). (See also Chapter 29.)

## Vascular Access

Close monitoring of blood pressure, arterial blood gases, and serum chemistries during the first few days after birth is required in most sick ELBW infants, so it is advantageous to insert an umbilical arterial catheter for reliable access in infants who require assisted ventilation. Infusion of half-normal saline with 0.5 units of heparin per milliliter at a low rate (0.8 to 1 mL/hr) is usually enough to maintain catheter patency. Although using a saline solution rather than a dextrose-water solution in the umbilical arterial line may complicate fluid and electrolyte management, this disadvantage is offset by the advantage of reliable measurement of blood glucose levels, which are frequently required, without disturbing the infant. Placement of a central umbilical venous catheter (tip at the inferior vena cava–right atrial junction) at the same time the umbilical arterial catheter is placed also provides the clinician with reliable venous access for infusion of fluids, medications, and blood products. Use of a double-lumen umbilical venous catheter often obviates insertion of a peripheral intravenous line over the first few days after birth and helps preserve intravenous sites and skin integrity.

The length of time that umbilical catheters are left in place varies by hospital. In most centers, umbilical lines are generally discontinued after 7 to 10 days because of the potential for catheter-related infection and vascular complications, although it is unusual for arterial access to be needed beyond a few days after birth. Before the umbilical venous catheter is removed, insertion of a percutaneous central venous catheter with its tip at the junction of the superior or inferior vena cava and the right atrium, dedicated to infusion of parenteral nutrition (see later), is advisable. Such a catheter helps maintain intravenous access for nutritional purposes without raising the risk of catheter-related infections and reduces the need to establish and maintain peripheral intravenous lines (Janes et al, 2000; Parellada et al, 1999). The incidence of complications of percutaneous central catheters, including catheter-related infections, is lower if a limited number of NICU personnel insert and maintain the lines.

## Skin Care

The skin of an infant born at 23 to 26 weeks of gestation is extremely immature and is ineffective as an epidermal barrier. Poor epidermal barrier function in the extremely preterm infant leads to disturbances in temperature regulation and water balance as well as breakdown in skin integrity that may increase the risk of infection. The stratum corneum, which is responsible for epidermal barrier function, does not become functionally mature in the fetus until about 32 weeks of gestation (Rutter, 2000). However, acceleration of the maturation process occurs after birth, so most extremely premature infants have a mature epidermal barrier by about 2 weeks of postnatal age. Until that time, full-thickness skin injury can occur in the ELBW infant from seemingly innocuous causes, such as local pressure from body positioning, removal of adhesives, and prolonged exposure to products containing alcohol or iodine. Such injury can lead to larger transepidermal water losses, an even greater risk of nosocomial infection, and significant scarring.

Because of these risks, preservation of skin integrity should be incorporated into the care of the extremely preterm infant (Table 32–5). Limited use of adhesives and extreme care upon their removal, frequent repositioning of the infant to avoid pressure points on the skin, and use of soft bedding or a water mattress are the minimum requirements. Hydrocolloids (e.g., DuoDerm) applied to

**TABLE 32–5**

**Practical Guidelines for Skin Care of Extremely Low-Birth-Weight infants**

| Interventions | Guidelines |
|---|---|
| Adhesive application | Increase adhesive tack by applying to dry, clean skin surface<br>Avoid alcohol for skin cleansing<br>Use smallest amount of tape possible<br>Use a hydrocolloid or pectin-based layer on the skin, before application of heavy adhesive<br>Avoid using adhesive over areas of skin breakdown<br>Avoid adhesive bonding agents (e.g., benzoin)<br>Use hydrophilic gel or pectin-based adhesives preferentially |
| Adhesive removal | Avoid adhesive removers and solvents<br>Use warm, wet cotton ball to periodically saturate hydrogel adhesives (avoid over-drying and over-saturation)<br>Facilitate removal of adhesive with mineral oil, petrolatum, and emollients if reapplication is not necessary |
| Emollient application | Infants born at <27 weeks may benefit from emollient use<br>Avoid multidose containers (e.g., large jars)<br>Use non-perfumed, non-irritating hydrophilic emollients<br>Recognize potential for emollients to interfere with adhesive and conductive properties of monitoring devices |
| Emollient removal | Wipe off gently with a soft cloth/gauze if site is contaminated<br>Avoid repeated attempts to thoroughly cleanse the skin (undesired friction effect)<br>Remove emollients before attaching thermistors or other monitoring devices |

Data from Hoath S, Narendran V: Adhesives and emollients in the preterm infant. Semin Neonataol 5:289-296, 2000.

the baby in areas where adhesive tape may come in prolonged contact with the skin (i.e., umbilical catheter or endotracheal tube fixation) to prevent direct application of tape to the baby may be useful because it is more easily removed than standard adhesive tape. Polyurethane adhesive dressings (Tegaderm) or hydrogels (Vigilon) may also be used to protect areas of skin friction and superficial wounds.

Prophylactic application of preservative-free emollient ointments (Aquaphor) to protect the skin of the ELBW infant has been studied (Lane and Drost, 1993; Nopper et al, 1996). Several small studies demonstrated smaller transepidermal water losses, improved skin condition, and lower risk of suspected or proven nosocomial infection with prophylactic application of emollient ointments. However, one report documented an increase in rate of systemic yeast infections in a single NICU coincident with a change to use of prophylactic emollients in ELBW infants; they returned to baseline after such use was discontinued (Campbell et al, 2000). Data are insufficient to recommend routine use of prophylactic emollients; however, their selective use in ELBW infants at risk for significant skin breakdown may be effective as an adjunct to other types of local skin care already described.

## Mechanical Ventilation

A high percentage of ELBW infants require some level of assisted ventilation to survive. Data from animal models of RDS indicate that positive-pressure ventilation with large tidal volumes damages pulmonary capillary endothelium, alveolar and airway epithelium, and basement membranes. This mechanical damage results in leakage of fluid, protein, and blood into the airways, alveoli, and interstitial spaces, leading to inhibition of surfactant activity and further damage to the lungs. These data suggest that a ventilator strategy that avoids large changes in tidal volume may reduce ventilator-induced lung injury in ELBW infants. The optimal mode, timing, and application of ventilatory support used in the initial management of the ELBW infant to meet this goal remain controversial. However, the objectives of all strategies of assisted ventilation in the ELBW infant should be similar—(1) to provide the lowest level of ventilatory support possible that will both support adequate oxygenation and ventilation and prevent atelectasis and (2) to try to reduce acute and chronic lung injury secondary to barotrauma, volutrauma, and oxygen toxicity (Clark et al, 2000).

## Conventional Mechanical Ventilation

Most NICUs continue to use pressure-limited time-cycled conventional ventilators for the initial respiratory management of the ELBW infant. Synchronized intermittent mandatory ventilation (SIMV) is the preferred mode of conventional ventilation for the ELBW infant. In the premature infant, SIMV, in which the inspiratory cycle is synchronized with the patient's own effort, is better in terms of oxygenation, ventilation, work of breathing, and blood pressure variability than conventional IMV (Cleary et al, 1995; Hummler et al, 1996; Jarreau et al, 1996). Technologic limitations in the ability of some ventilators to synchronize breaths with very weak inspiratory efforts may prevent use of SIMV in the smallest infants. With further advances in ventilator design, other modes of patient-triggered ventilation, including volume-guarantee, assist-control, and pressure support, have become available to the clinician. These designs are under investigation but have not been proven to produce better pulmonary outcomes than SIMV in the ELBW infant (Donn and Sinha, 1998; Herrera et al, 2002).

Currently accepted conventional ventilatory strategies in the ELBW infant stress avoidance of excessive tidal volumes by limiting peak inspiratory pressures and provision of adequate PEEP to maintain lung volume (Thome et al, 1998). This strategy helps prevent repeated cycles of atelectasis and lung overdistention, a risk factor for ventilator-induced lung injury (Dreyfuss and Saumon, 1998). Hyperventilation ($Pa\text{CO}_2 < 35$ mm Hg) has been associated with a higher risk for the development of BPD (Garland et al, 1995; Van Marter et al, 2000) as well as neurodevelopmental sequelae in ELBW infants (Wiswell et al, 1996).

In response to this suggestion of worse pulmonary outcome in hyperventilated infants, a strategy of "minimal ventilation," or permissive hypercapnia, has been proposed for conventional ventilation in ELBW infants. In the largest study to date of this ventilatory strategy, Carlo and associates (2002) randomly assigned 220 infants with birth weights between 501 and 1000 g to receive either minimal ventilation (target $Pa\text{CO}_2 > 52$ mm Hg) or routine ventilation (target $Pa\text{CO}_2 < 48$ mm Hg). No difference in the rate of BPD, death, or other major short-term morbidities was seen between the two groups. Potential risks of a high $Pa\text{CO}_2$ include increases in both cerebral perfusion and pulmonary vascular resistance and lower pH. Without clear data to support the benefit and safety of permissive hypercapnia, most centers target their conventional ventilatory strategy to maintain $Pa\text{CO}_2$ between 45 and 55 mm Hg in the first several days of mechanical ventilation in the ELBW infant.

In infants whose lung disease prevents extubation in the first several days after birth, changes in lung dynamics over the first 1 to 2 weeks often necessitate a change in ventilatory strategy. In the early stages of chronic lung disease, increased airway resistance and decreased lung compliance may require higher values for mean airway pressure, peak inspiratory pressure, PEEP, and inspiratory time than are usually used in initial ventilatory management. Once the need for more prolonged mechanical ventilation is established, many centers tolerate higher target $Pa\text{CO}_2$ values in the attempt to limit further ventilator-induced lung injury.

## High-Frequency Ventilation

Considerable interest has been generated over the past 15 years in the application of high-frequency ventilation (HFV) in newborns who have respiratory failure because this technique allows ventilation with very small tidal volumes. Results of studies using HFV in animal models of RDS have been promising in the prevention of lung injury, but those of clinical studies of this ventilatory technique have not. Despite many clinical trials, controversy continues to surround the indications for HFV in ELBW infants, whether HFV is more effective than other modes of ventilation for RDS, whether HFV reduces adverse outcomes (specifically BPD), and whether HFV is more likely to have significant long-term complications than conventional mechanical ventilation.

Early trials of HFV before surfactant replacement therapy demonstrated no pulmonary advantage of HFV over conventional mechanical ventilation and suggested an increase in rates of air leak and intracranial abnormalities in the HFV-treated infants (HIFI Study Group, 1989). Later trials in ELBW infants who were treated with surfactant also failed to demonstrate any reduction in the incidence of BPD in the HF- treated infants (Johnson et al, 2002; Rettitz-Volk et al, 1998; Thome et al, 1999).

A rigorously controlled trial of HFV as the primary mode of assisted ventilation compared with conventional mechanical ventilation was the first to suggest a small advantage to the early use of HFV in reduction of BPD or death without an increase in the incidence of short-term complications in ELBW infants. Courtney and associates (2002) compared high-frequency oscillatory ventilation (HFOV) with synchronized IMV in a randomized trial that enrolled 500 ELBW infants. These investigators found a small but significant decrease in the incidence of BPD in survivors, requirement of fewer doses of exogenous surfactant, and shorter time to successful extubation in the HFOV-treated group. No differences in other complications of prematurity were observed between the two groups.

These results suggest that when used in experienced hands according to strict protocol, HFV may confer some protection from lung injury in ELBW infants. Whether this same advantage is gained when HFV is used under usual clinical circumstances in less experienced centers and whether the incidence of other complications may be affected by mode of ventilation remain unclear. Some NICUs with the most experience with HFV use it routinely as the initial mode of ventilation for ELBW infants. Most centers continue to use conventional ventilation with low tidal volumes and reasonable ventilation goals as the initial mode of ventilation for ELBW infants, reserving HFV for infants in whom conventional ventilation and surfactant fail. This latter practice seems advisable, given the potential risks of HFV, including inadvertent lung overdistention, impaired cardiac output, and increased central venous pressure that may lead to intracranial hemorrhage.

## Continuous Positive Airway Pressure

In a classic study comparing the incidence of BPD between NICUs, Avery and colleagues (1987) reported that the NICU with the lowest incidence used CPAP more frequently and more aggressively than the other units. Van Marter and associates (2000) confirmed these observations.

Theoretically, early CPAP may protect the very immature lung from injury due to positive pressure tidal breaths, by preserving surfactant function, increasing alveolar volume and functional residual capacity, enhancing alveolar stability, and improving ventilation-perfusion matching. It also may stimulate the growth of the immature lung. In some NICUs, CPAP, delivered via nasal prongs or nasopharyngeal tube at 5 to 7 cm $H_2O$, is used as the initial mode of assisted ventilation for ELBW infants, starting almost immediately in the delivery room (Lindner and Vobeck, 1999). CPAP used this way has been reported in retrospective studies to decrease the need for mechanical ventilation (Gittermann et al, 1997; Poets and Sens, 1996), the need for surfactant treatment, and the incidence of BPD (Aly, 2001; de Klerk and de Klerk, 2001; Lindner and Vobeck, 1999). Alternatively, CPAP may be used after prophylactic or rescue surfactant therapy is given during a brief period of intubation and positive-pressure ventilation (Verder et al, 1999). Although results of these observational studies are promising, it is important to note that early CPAP has not been compared with mechanical ventilation with surfactant administration as the initial mode of assisted ventilation for the ELBW infant in a randomized fashion, nor have long-term follow-up data been reported.

### Post-Extubation CPAP for Respiratory Distress Syndrome and Apnea

CPAP is commonly used in the ELBW infant after extubation to stabilize functional residual capacity and reduce the frequency of apneic spells after the lung disease has improved. All ELBW infants should be extubated as soon as they have recovered from acute RDS and should be given a trial of CPAP to protect them from further barotrauma. When used in combination with methylxanthine therapy, CPAP decreases the need for re-intubation due to progressive respiratory distress or apnea (Davis and Henderson-Smart, 2003). Methylxanthine (aminophylline or caffeine) treatment before extubation has also been shown to lower the incidence of apnea and the need for re-intubation in premature infants. Although almost universally used in ELBW infants as a treatment for apnea of prematurity, methylxanthines have not been rigorously studied in this population, and their use may need to be reassessed as follow-up data become available (Schmidt, 1999). Many ELBW infants benefit from prolonged use of CPAP by nasal prongs after extubation, especially those with frequent or severe episodes of apnea and bradycardia resistant to methylxanthines, and some centers are now providing assisted ventilation through nasal prongs in order to avoid intubation (Khalaf et al, 2001). However, the smallest and least mature infants may need prolonged mechanical ventilation because of frequent, severe apneic spells unresponsive to other therapies.

## Adjunctive Therapies to Prevent Bronchopulmonary Dysplasia

### Vitamin A Supplementation

ELBW infants have low stores of vitamin A. Because of the role of vitamin A in promoting lung healing, its deficiency has been linked to a higher risk for development of BPD. In a large multicenter trial, vitamin A supplementation (5000 IU given intramuscularly 3 times a week for 4 weeks) reduced biochemical evidence of vitamin A deficiency and decreased the incidence of BPD by 12% without adverse effects in ELBW infants who required mechanical ventilation or supplemental oxygen at 24 hours of age (Tyson et al, 1999). Given these efficacy data and apparent safety, vitamin A supplementation as described should be administered to all ELBW infants starting at 24 hours after birth.

### Superoxide Dismutase

One of the proposed contributory mechanisms in the development of BPD in ELBW infants is lung damage from oxygen free radicals. Preterm infants have inadequate antioxidant defenses and may not be able to induce antioxidant enzymes in response to oxidative stress (Davis, 1998). Exogenously administered superoxide dismutase (SOD), an important intracellular enzyme that dismutates the superoxide radical into hydrogen peroxide, has been studied as a potential therapy to prevent oxygen toxicity in the ELBW infant. No difference in the incidence of BPD was seen in a small randomized, masked study of recombinant human SOD administered intratracheally in ELBW infants who were treated with surfactant for RDS (Davis et al, 1997); no acute toxicity of the therapy was observed. Although SOD is apparently safe, available data do not support its use for the prevention of BPD in the ELBW infant outside clinical trials.

### Systemic Corticosteroids

Inflammation also plays an important role in the pathogenesis of BPD; therefore, pharmacologic doses of systemic corticosteroids have been widely used for prevention and treatment of BPD in ELBW infants. Several studies have examined early (<96 hours of age) administration of corticosteroids, usually dexamethasone, to prevent the development of BPD in infants at risk (Garland et al, 1999; Rastogi et al, 1996; Stark et al, 2001). A meta-analysis of studies in which corticosteroids were used to prevent rather than treat established BPD suggested that early corticosteroid treatment in ELBW infants results in more rapid extubation and a lower incidence of BPD (Halliday and Ehrenkranz, 2001), although no effect on mortality was observed. However, a higher incidence of short-term complications, including hyperglycemia, hypertension, poor growth, and intestinal perforations and bleeding, was observed in the corticosteroid-treated infants (Garland et al, 1999; Stark et al, 2001). More importantly, long-term follow-up data suggest that exposure to corticosteroid for prevention or treatment of BPD raises the risk of neurological sequelae in treated infants, including poor head growth, cerebral palsy, and developmental impairment (American Academy of Pediatrics, 2002).

The apparent higher risk of long-term sequelae without an effect on overall mortality has tempered enthusiasm for systemic corticosteroid treatment to prevent or treat BPD in ELBW infants. Studies are currently under way to examine the effect of lower doses of dexamethasone, the use of alternative corticosteroids that may have a different side effect profile (Andre et al, 2000), and replacement hydrocortisone (Watterberg et al, 1999) on the development of BPD as well as long-term outcome. Until further data become available, it seems prudent to avoid routine use of systemic corticosteroids in ELBW infants. An American Academy of Pediatrics (2002) statement on postnatal corticosteroids to treat or prevent chronic lung disease in preterm infants summarizes current recommendations as follows: "Outside of the context of a randomized, controlled trial, the use of corticosteroids should be limited to exceptional clinical circumstances (e.g., an infant on maximal ventilatory and oxygen support). In those circumstances, parents should be fully informed about the known short- and long-term risks and agree to treatment."

## Nutritional Management

Provision of adequate nutrition is central to effective care of ELBW infants (see Chapters 68 and 69). These infants are born with limited nutrient reserves, immature pathways for nutrient absorption and metabolism, and higher nutrient demands. In addition, medical conditions associated with extreme prematurity both alter requirements for and complicate the adequate delivery of nutrients. The goals of nutritional management of the ELBW infant are preservation of endogenous body stores, achievement of postnatal growth similar to intrauterine weight accretion and body composition, and maintenance of normal physiologic and metabolic processes concomitant with minimizing complications and side effects. However, few ELBW infants are able to meet these goals despite the use of central parenteral nutrition and caloric supplementation of enteral feedings, so significant growth failure is commonplace (Fig. 32–7) (Berry et al, 1997; Ehrenkranz et al, 1999).

Medical problems of ELBW infants often preclude initiation of enteral feedings for several days to weeks. The experience of the NICHD Neonatal Network centers is likely representative of the problems in nutritional management of these infants (Ehrenkranz et al, 1999).

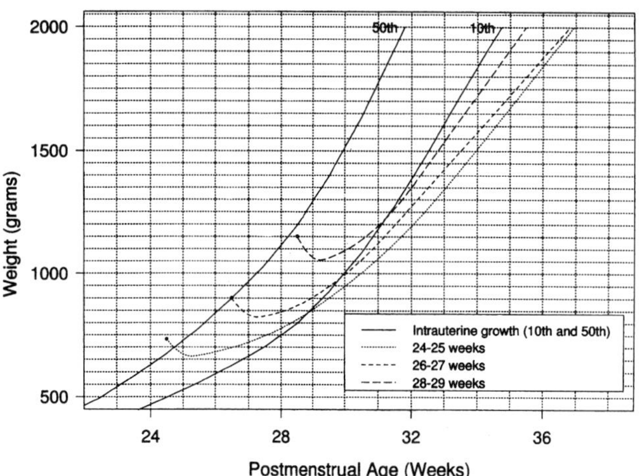


**FIGURE 32–7.** Average body weight versus postmenstrual age in weeks for 1660 very low-birth-weight infants plotted against the 50th and 10th percentiles for intrauterine growth. *(From Ehrenkranz R, Younes N, Lemons J, et al: Longitudinal growth of hospitalized very low birth weight infants. Pediatrics 104: 280-289, 1999.)*

In these centers, the mean age to first enteral feeding in the 500- to 1000-g weight group ranged from 6 to 9 days; mean age at which full enteral feedings were reached ranged from 21 to 34 days. Not surprisingly, the smallest and least mature infants were introduced to feedings and reached full enteral feedings later than larger, maturer infants did. Even after recommended enteral dietary intakes are reached, ELBW infants continue to have a cumulative energy and protein deficit, which in part explains their later growth failure (Embleton et al, 2001).

### Early Parenteral Nutrition

Protein losses in ELBW infants receiving a glucose infusion alone begin immediately after birth and can approach 1.5 g/kg/day in the first 24 to 72 hours. Fortunately, these losses can be offset by early administration of an amino acid solution, even at low caloric intakes. Several studies have demonstrated the safety of early administration (within 24 hours after birth) of an amino acid solution, with no abnormal elevations of ammonia or blood urea nitrogen even in the most immature infants (Rivera et al, 1993; Van Goudoever et al, 1995). To prevent early protein deficit, ELBW infants should be given a source of parenteral protein as soon as possible after birth. (See also Chapter 69.)

In most centers, parenteral nutrition is used exclusively during the first few days after birth and then gradually reduced as enteral feedings are introduced. Longer duration of parenteral nutrition is associated with the development of a number of complications, including cholestasis, osteopenia, and sepsis. For example, the risk of an episode of late-onset sepsis in premature infants is 22-fold higher if parenteral nutrition is continued for more than 3 weeks compared with is use for 1 week or less (Stoll et al, 2002b).

### Early Enteral Feedings

The structural and functional integrity of the gastrointestinal tract depends on the provision of enteral feedings. Withholding enteral feedings at birth imposes risks for all the complications of luminal starvation, including mucosal thinning, flattening of the villi, and bacterial translocation. Early initiation (within the first few days after birth) of low volumes of milk (trophic feedings, or “gut priming”) has been studied in several small trials in premature infants (McClure and Newell, 2000; Schanler et al, 1999a). Trophic feedings are not meant to give the infant significant nutrition but rather to promote continued functional maturation of the gastrointestinal tract. Documented benefits of trophic feedings include higher plasma concentrations of gastrointestinal hormones, a more mature gut motility pattern, lower incidence of cholestasis, increased calcium and phosphorus absorption, and better as well as sooner tolerance of enteral feedings. Trophic feedings have not been associated with a higher risk of necrotizing enterocolitis or other adverse outcomes; therefore, there is no clinical advantage to delaying initiation of feedings in the medically stable ELBW infant. (See also Chapter 68.)

Feeding intolerance, indicated by gastric residuals that exceed 25% to 50% of the volume fed, abdominal distention, or microscopic blood in the stool, is very common in ELBW infants and may be difficult to differentiate from early stages of necrotizing enterocolitis. Feeding intolerance may preclude the advance of enteral nutrition for days to weeks, complicating nutritional management and prolonging the need for parenteral nutrition. Numerous feeding strategies to avoid episodes of feeding intolerance have been employed in the ELBW infant, including very slow increase in enteral volume (<10 mL/kg/day), use of dilute rather than full-strength milk, continuous versus bolus tube-feeding, and use of prokinetic agents. None of these feeding strategies has been found to be clearly superior, although bolus feedings may decrease episodes of gastric residuals compared with continuous tube feedings and may allow a more rapid advance to full enteral volumes as well as promote better growth.

Episodes of feeding intolerance also are reduced in ELBW infants fed human milk rather than premature formulas (Schanler et al, 1999b). Other benefits of giving human milk in ELBW infants are a more rapid advance to full enteral volumes and the immunologic effects, with a reduction in the risk of necrotizing enterocolitis and late-onset sepsis. Human milk must be fortified with calcium, phosphorus, sodium, protein, and other minerals to provide adequate nutrition in the ELBW infant. In addition to commercially available human milk fortifiers, which increase the caloric density to approximately 24 calories per ounce, human milk may be fortified further to higher caloric densities with medium chain triglycerides, glucose polymers, and added protein.

Premature infants who are fed fortified human milk may grow more slowly than infants fed premature formulas (Schanler et al, 1999b), perhaps because of the variability in fat and caloric content of pumped breast milk or changes in the nutrient composition of human milk with fortification that affect fat absorption. Despite the potential for slower growth in infants fed human milk, its use should be strongly encouraged in ELBW infants because of the immunologic and other nutritional benefits. Further research on how best to fortify human milk is necessary to promote the best rate of growth in ELBW infants. (See also Chapter 68.)

## Management and Prevention of Infection

Bacterial and fungal infections are an important cause of illness and death among ELBW infants. In addition to the immediate morbidity and mortality, local and systemic inflammation caused by infections may increase the risk for development of other complications of prematurity, including BPD and brain injury. ELBW infants are frequently exposed to perinatal and delivery complications that raise their risk of early-onset (<7 days) infections. The need for prolonged intravenous access, exposure to parenteral nutrition, and mechanical ventilation also subject the ELBW infant to a high risk of late-onset (>7 days) nosocomial infections. The frequent infections seen in the ELBW population are related to immaturity of both humoral and cellular immunity (see Chapter 35). In addition to the judicious use of antimicrobial therapy, environmental controls, nursery surveillance, and modulation of the immature immune response have been proposed as possible interventions to prevent infections in extremely premature infants.

### Early-Onset Infections

The incidence of early-onset bacterial infections in very LBW (VLBW) infants is approximately 1% to 2%, with a mortality of approximately 40% to 50% (Stoll et al, 2002a; see also Chapter 39). The major risk factor for the development of perinatally acquired bacterial infections is PROM with chorioamnionitis, which frequently complicates premature deliveries. However, a significant percentage of extremely premature births may be associated with intrauterine infection before membrane rupture (Goldenberg et al, 2000); in one study, 41% of premature infants with early-onset sepsis were born less than 6 hours after membrane rupture (Stoll et al, 2002a).

Because the clinical signs of perinatally acquired infection are nonspecific, the index of suspicion and the concern about the possibility of intrauterine infection should always be high in the presence of premature birth. All ELBW infants should be evaluated for infection at birth by means of a complete blood count with differential and blood culture, and empiric antibiotic therapy with ampicillin and an aminoglycoside should be initiated. A white blood cell count less than 5000 cells/μL, a ratio of immature to total neutrophils ratio greater than 0.2 to 0.3, and neutropenia (absolute neutrophil count less than 1000 cells/μL) are all suggestive of infection but may also be seen in infants with other conditions, including maternal preeclampsia and hypertension. The duration of initial antibiotic therapy depends on the results of the blood culture, blood counts, the clinical course, and the perinatal history. If the blood culture is negative for bacterial growth at 48 to 72 hours and the infant has improved clinically, consideration should be given to discontinuation of antibiotics. Prolonged exposure to antibiotic therapy increases the likelihood of colonization with multiple antibiotic–resistant organisms and the development of fungemia, so should be reserved for those infants with documented infection or a very high index of suspicion of infection based on clinical or historical factors.

The distribution of pathogens causing early-onset sepsis in VLBW infants has changed, likely because of a greater use of intrapartum antibiotics for prevention of group B streptococcal infections and treatment of preterm PROM. As the rate of infections from group B streptococci has diminished with intrapartum antibiotic prophylaxis, the rate of documented infections from gram-negative organisms has risen (Table 32–6) (Stoll et al, 2002a). In a further change of the epidemiology of early-onset infections in premature infants, possibly related to greater use of intrapartum antibiotics, the frequency of infections due to ampicillin-resistant *Escherichia coli* strains has increased (Joseph et al, 1998; Stoll et al, 2002a). Current recommendations for empiric antibiotic therapy of the ELBW infant at risk of early-onset sepsis have not changed, but continued surveillance of the epidemiology and antibiotic resistance patterns of isolates within individual units is warranted. In infants with severe illness that may be caused by sepsis, broadening initial antibiotic coverage to include a third-generation cephalosporin should be considered.

**TABLE 32-6**

**Distribution of Pathogens among 84 Cases of Early-Onset Sepsis***

| Organism | No. | % |
|---|---|---|
| Gram-negative organism: | 51 | 60.7 |
| *Escherichia coli* | 37 | 44.0 |
| *Haemophilus influenzae* | 7 | 8.3 |
| *Citrobacter* | 2 | 2.4 |
| Other | 5 | 6.0 |
| Gram-positive organisms: | 31 | 36.9 |
| Group B streptococci | 9 | 10.7 |
| Viridans streptococcus | 3 | 3.6 |
| Other streptococci | 4 | 4.8 |
| *Listeria monocytogenes* | 2 | 2.4 |
| Coagulase-negative staphylococci | 9 | 10.7 |
| Other | 4 | 4.8 |
| Fungi: | 2 | 2.4 |
| *Candida albicans* | 2 | 2.4 |
| **Total** | 84 | 100 |

*Occurring in 5447 infants born between September 1, 1998, and August 31, 2000.

Data from Stoll B, Hansen N, Fanaroff A, et al: Changes in pathogens causing early onset sepsis in very low birth weight infants. N Engl J Med 347:240-247, 2002.

### Late-Onset Infections

Nosocomial infection is a common complication of intensive care of the ELBW infant. The incidence of late-onset sepsis in ELBW infants who survive beyond 3 days of age is 25% to 50%, depending on gestational age and birth weight, with the median age at onset of the first episode approximately 2 weeks (Fanaroff et al, 1998; Stoll et al, 2002b). The overall mortality rate is approximately 20% but may be as high as 80%, depending on the organism causing sepsis. Risk factors for the development of late-onset sepsis include prolonged hyperalimentation and lipid use, the presence of a central venous catheter, longer duration of mechanical ventilation, and delay in initiation of enteral feedings (Stoll et al, 2002b). These practices and procedures are common events that may be unavoidable in the care of ELBW infants. However, large variations have been observed among NICUs in the rate of late-onset infections in premature infants (Brodie et al, 2000; Stoll et al, 2002b), suggesting that individual NICU practices may affect the incidence of nosocomial infections.

The most common cause of late-onset infections in ELBW infants is coagulase-negative *Staphylococcus* (CoNS). The most significant risk factor for the development of CoNS infection is the use of a fat emulsion (e.g., Intralipid) infusion (Freeman et al, 1990). Infection with CoNS is almost never fatal but is associated with significant morbidity, such as more days of ventilator use and prolonged hospital stay (Gray et al, 1995). Other organisms that cause late-onset infections in ELBW infants are associated with a much higher morbidity and mortality. The distribution of pathogens associated with the first episode of late-onset sepsis among 1313 infants

**TABLE 32-7**

**Distribution of Pathogens Associated with the First Episode of Late-Onset Sepsis***

| Organism | No. | % |
|---|---|---|
| Gram-positive organisms: | 922 | 70.2 |
| Coagulase-negative staphylococci | 629 | 47.9 |
| *Staphylococcus aureus* | 103 | 7.8 |
| *Enterococcus* spp. | 43 | 3.3 |
| Group B streptococci | 30 | 2.3 |
| Other | 117 | 8.9 |
| Gram-negative organisms: | 231 | 17.6 |
| *Escherichia coli* | 64 | 4.9 |
| *Klebsiella* | 52 | 4.0 |
| *Pseudomonas* | 35 | 27 |
| *Enterobacter* | 33 | 2.5 |
| *Serratia* | 29 | 2.2 |
| Other | 18 | 1.4 |
| Fungi: | 160 | 12.2 |
| *Candida albicans* | 76 | 5.8 |
| *Candida parapsilosis* | 54 | 4.1 |
| Other | 30 | 2.3 |
| **Total** | 1313 | 100 |

*In National Institute of Child Health and Development Neonatal Research Network institutions, September 1, 1998, through August 31, 2000.

Data from Stoll B, Hansen N, Fanaroff A, et al: Late-onset sepsis in very low birth weight neonates: Experience of the NICDH Neonatal Research Network. Pediatrics 110:285-291, 2002.

in a cohort of VLBW babies over a 2-year period is shown in Table 32–7.

Presenting features of late-onset sepsis include increased apnea, feeding intolerance, abdominal distention or guaiac-positive stools, increased respiratory support, and lethargy and hypotonia (Fanarroff et al, 1998). Because these symptoms are nonspecific, ELBW infants are frequently evaluated for infection and treated with empiric antibiotic therapy. In one study, both use of vancomycin and antifungal therapy were inversely related to birth weight; approximately three-quarters of infants with a birth weight less than 750 g were treated with vancomycin during their hospital stay, and approximately one-third treated with antifungals (Stoll et al, 2002b). Central catheters should be removed immediately to ensure adequate treatment of infants in whom sepsis is diagnosed, except for that due to CoNS (Benjamin et al, 2001).

Endotracheal tube colonization with multiple organisms is common in infants who require prolonged mechanical ventilation. In general, such colonization should not be treated with antibiotics unless there is evidence of pneumonia or significant inflammation indicative of tracheitis. Prospective surveillance of common isolates and antimicrobial resistance patterns within individual NICUs can help guide empiric antibiotic therapy in the ELBW infant being evaluated and treated for presumed sepsis. However, indiscriminate use of broad-spectrum antibiotics in the absence of true infection can alter antimicrobial resistance patterns (Goldmann et al, 1996), raising the risk of late-onset infections and complicating therapy.

### Prevention of Nosocomial Infection

Because of the frequency and potential severity of late-onset sepsis in ELBW infants, several strategies to prevent infection have been proposed. Using these practices as a guideline, Horbar and colleagues (2001) observed a decrease in the CoNS infection rate from 22% to 16.6% over a 2-year period in VLBW infants in six study NICUs. Some NICUs routinely screen ELBW infants by stool or respiratory secretion cultures for the presence of multiple antibiotic–resistant organisms and isolate infants found to be colonized. Clusters of infections with unusual organisms should prompt surveillance cultures of infants, potential NICU environmental sources, and NICU staff (Foca et al, 2000). Restriction of broad-spectrum antibiotic use by hospital policy or treatment guidelines may limit local spread of resistant organisms (Goldmann et al, 1996). Strict adherence to hand-washing before and after every patient contact and avoidance of overcrowding within NICUs also help decrease the incidence of infection. Use of alcohol-based hand gels at the bedside may improve compliance with hand hygiene (Harbarth et al, 2002).

In addition to practice and environmental controls, prophylactic use of antibiotics and modulation of the immune response of ELBW infants have been studied as methods to reduce the incidence of late-onset sepsis. Low-dose vancomycin given continuously via hyperalimentation solutions (Baier et al, 1998; Spafford et al, 1994), or intermittently via peripheral vein (Cooke et al, 1997), has been shown to reduce the incidence of CoNS in premature infants at risk. Concern about emergence of vancomycin-resistant organisms and the low mortality associated with CoNS infections has prevented widespread use of this approach. In another study, prophylactic intravenous fluconazole given for 6 weeks lowered the incidence of fungal colonization and invasive disease in ELBW infants without associated complications or the emergence of resistant organisms (Kaufman et al, 2001). Such an approach might be advisable for NICUs with a high incidence of fungal infections in their ELBW population but needs considerably more study. Approaches that have been used with success in adult immunocompromised patients, such as antibiotic lock technique for central catheters and antiseptic-impregnated central catheters, are promising but have not yet been adequately studied in premature infants.

Prophylactic intravenous administration of polyclonal immunoglobulin (IVIG) to prevent late-onset sepsis has been extensively studied in premature infants. Several trials have shown a decrease in the incidence of documented sepsis by a small but significant amount in premature infants treated with prophylactic IVIG and no effect on mortality or other complications of prematurity (Lacy and Ohlsson, 1995). The costs associated with this therapy to achieve the small decrease in infection rates, as well as the increased exposure to blood products, have limited its use; whether selective prophylactic IVIG treatment of ELBW infants at highest risk for sepsis is warranted is unclear. However, IVIG therapy in addition to antibiotic therapy may be of benefit in reducing mortality in infants with established sepsis (Jenson and Pollock, 1997). Development of more targeted polyclonal or monoclonal $\gamma$-globulin preparations for specific organisms that cause sepsis in premature newborns may alter the use of IVIG in the future (Lamari et al, 2000).

Another promising strategy under investigation for modulation of the immature immune response to help prevent infections in premature infants is treatment with hemopoietic colony stimulating factors, including granulocyte colony-stimulating factor (G-CSF) and granulocyte-macrophage colony-stimulating factor (GM-CSF) (Modi and Carr, 2000). Most studies of these factors have been conducted in neutropenic, small-for-gestational-age infants or infants delivered to women with preeclampsia. Treatment with G-CSF in neutropenic infants resulted in an increase in neutrophil counts and reduced the incidence of sepsis (Kocherlakota and La Gamma, 1998). Prophylactic treatment with GM-CSF in premature infants with normal neutrophil counts prevented the development of neutropenia in episodes of sepsis, but whether this type of therapy to address cellular immune deficiency in ELBW infants will reduce the incidence of infection without additional complications remains unclear (Miura et al, 2001; Modi and Carr, 2000).

## Developmental and Parental Care

ELBW infants are particularly vulnerable to the potentially noxious stimuli of the NICU environment, including light, noise, frequent disturbances, and painful procedures. The ELBW infant reacts to the noisy and well-lit environment of many NICUs with greater variability of blood pressure, ventilatory requirements, and oxygen saturation as well as behavioral disorganization, which may have both short-term and long-term effects on outcome (Jacobs et al, 2002). Modification of the NICU environment to limit exposure of ELBW infants to such stresses—by lowering ambient light and reducing noise, clustering caregiving periods and procedures to allow periods of uninterrupted sleep, and using positioning aids to promote containment—is an intuitive part of their care. Whether individualized, developmentally supportive care or other developmental interventions started in the NICU improve long-term outcome in ELBW infants remains unclear (Feldman and Eidelman, 1998).

In addition to environmental modifications, NICUs should promote parental involvement with their infants, even when they are critically ill. Open visitation rules and encouragement of parental caregiving when appropriate may help parents bond with their baby. Skin-to-skin (kangaroo) care, in which the infant is placed unclothed on the mother or father's bare chest, was originally developed in nonindustrialized countries to maintain temperature regulation in premature infants. It is now used in many NICUs to promote parental attachment. Kangaroo care may have a positive effect on infant state organization and respiratory patterns, increase the rate of infant weight gain, improve maternal milk production, and have long-term benefits in infant development and parents' perceptions of their babies (Feldman et al, 2002). Kangaroo care can be initiated in ELBW infants within the first 2 weeks after birth, when they are more medically stable.

## FUTURE DIRECTIONS

In this chapter I present just some of the special needs of the ELBW infant. The medical care of the ELBW infant is a complex combination of knowledge of developmental physiology, evidenced-based interventions, and clinical experience. Wide variability in approach to care of these infants exists among practitioners and NICUs, as does variability in outcomes. Nevertheless, NICUs involved in treating ELBW infants should develop a coherent approach to the medical as well as ethical aspects of their care. Future research should focus on identification of best practices to narrow the variability in approach to care and with the goal to prevent long-term disability. As more of these tiny infants survive, it is the responsibility of neonatologists to stay abreast of clinical improvements and the short-term and long-term consequences of established and newly proposed medical interventions so as to provide the best care for these vulnerable infants and to keep parents informed and involved.

## REFERENCES


Aly H: Nasal prongs continuous positive airway pressure: a simple yet powerful tool. Pediatrics 108:759-760, 2001.

American Academy of Pediatrics, Committee on Fetus and Newborn: Postnatal corticosteroids to treat or prevent chronic lung disease in preterm infants. Pediatrics 109:330-338, 2002.

Andre P, Thebaud B, Odievre MH, et al: Methylprednisolone, an alternative to dexamethasone in very premature infants at risk of chronic lung disease. Intensive Care Med 26:1496-500, 2000.

Arad I, Gofin R, Baras M, et al: Neonatal outcome of inborn and transported very-low-birth-weight infants: relevance of perinatal factors. Eur J Obstet Gynecol Reprod Biol 83:151-157, 1999.

Avery ME, Tooley WH, Keller JB, et al: Is chronic lung disease in low birth weight infants preventable? A survey of eight centers. Pediatrics 79:26-30, 1987.

Baier RJ, Bocchini JA, Brown EG: Selective use of vancomycin to prevent coagulase-negative staphylococcal nosocomial bacteremia in high risk very low birth weight infants. Pediatr Infect Dis J 17:179-183, 1998.

Ballard DW, Yuelin, L, Evans J, et al: Fear of litigation may increase resuscitation of infants born near the limits of viability. J Pediatr 140:713-718, 2002.

Benjamin D, Miller W, Garges H, et al: Bacteremia, central catheters, and neonates: when to pull the line. Pediatrics 107:1272-1276, 2001.

Berry M, Abrahamowicz M, Usher R: Factors associated with growth of extremely premature infants during initial hospitalization. Pediatrics 100:640-646, 1997.

Brodie SB, Sands KE, Gray JE, et al: Occurrence of nosocomial bloodstream infections in six neonatal intensive care units. Pediatr Infect Dis J 19:56-65, 2000.

Campbell JR, Zaccaria E, Baker CJ: Systemic candidiasis in extremely low birth weight infants receiving topical petrolatum ointment for skin care: A case control study. Pediatrics 105:1041-1045, 2000.

Carlo WA, Stark AR, Wright LL, et al: Minimal ventilation to prevent bronchopulmonary dysplasia in extremely low birth weight infants. J Pediatr 141:370-374, 2002.

Chien LY, Whyte R, Aziz K, et al: Improved outcome of preterm infants when delivered in tertiary care centers. Obstet Gynecol 98:247-252, 2001.

Cifuentes J, Bronstein J, Phibbs C, et al: Mortality in low birth weight infants according to level of neonatal care at hospital of birth. Pediatrics 109:745-751, 2002.

Clark RH, Slutsky AS, Gerstmann DR: Lung protective strategies of ventilation in the neonate: What are they? Pediatrics 105:112-114, 2000.

Cleary JP, Bernstein G, Mannino FL, et al: Improved oxygenation during synchronized intermittent mandatory ventilation in neonates with respiratory distress syndrome: A randomized, crossover study. J Pediatr 126:407-411, 1995.

Cooke RWI, Nycyk JA, Okuonghuae H, et al: Low dose vancomycin prophylaxis reduces coagulase negative staphylococcal bacteraemia in very low birth weight infants. J Hosp Infect 37:297-303, 1997.

Courtney SE, Surand DJ, Asselin JM, et al: High-frequency oscillatory ventilation versus conventional mechanical ventilation for very low birth weight infants. N Engl J Med 347:643-652, 2002.

Davis JM: Superoxide dismutase: A role in the prevention of chronic lung disease. Biol Neonate 74(Suppl 1):29-34, 1998.

Davis JM, Rosenfeld WN, Richter SE, et al: Safety and pharmacokinetics of multiple doses of recombinant human CuZn superoxide dismutase administered intratracheally to premature neonates with respiratory distress syndrome. Pediatrics 100:24-30, 1997.

Davis PG, Henderson-Smart DJ: Nasal continuous positive airways pressure immediately after extubation for preventing morbidity in preterm infants. Cochrane Database Syst Rev (3):CD000143, 2003.

De Klerk, A, de Klerk R: Use of continuous positive airway pressure in preterm infants: Comments and experience from New Zealand. Pediatrics 108:761-762, 2001.

Donn SM, Sinha SK: Controversies in patient-triggered ventilation. Clin Perinatol 25:49-61, 1998.

Doron M, Veness-Meehan K, Margolis L, et al: Delivery room resuscitation decisions for extremely premature infants. Pediatrics 102:574-645, 1998.

Dreyfuss D, Saumon G: Ventilator-induced lung injury: Lessons from experimental studies. Am J Respir Crit Care Med 157:294-323,1998.

Egberts J, Brand R, Walti H, et al: Mortality, severe respiratory distress syndrome, and chronic lung disease of the newborn are reduced more after prophylactic than after therapeutic administration of the surfactant Curosurf. Pediatrics 100:E4, 1997.

Ehrenkranz R, Younes N, Lemons J, et al: Longitudinal growth of hospitalized very low birth weight infants. Pediatrics 104: 280-289, 1999.

El-Metwally D, Vohr B, Tucker, R: Survival and neonatal morbidity at the limits of viability in the mid 1990s: 22 to 25 weeks. J Pediatr 13:616-622, 2002.

Embleton N, Pang N, Cooke R: Postnatal malnutrition and growth retardation: An inevitable consequence of current recommendations in preterm infants? Pediatrics 107:270-273, 2001.

Fanaroff AA, Korones SB, Wright LL, et al: Incidence, presenting features, risk factors and significance of late onset septicemia in very low birth weight infants. The National Institute of Child Health and Human Development Neonatal Research Network. Pediatr Infect Dis J 17:593-598, 1998.

Feldman R, Eidelman A: Intervention programs for premature infants. How and do they affect development? Clin Perinatol 25:613-626, 1998.

Feldman R, Eidelman A, Sirota L, et al: Comparison of skin-to-skin (kangaroo) and traditional care: Parenting outcomes and preterm infant development. Pediatrics 110:16-26, 2002.

Finer N, Barrington K: Decision-making in delivery room resuscitation: A team sport. Pediatrics 100:644-645, 1998.

Finer N, Tarin T, Vaucher Y, et al: Intact survival in extremely low birth weight infants after delivery room resuscitation. Pediatrics 104:1-4, 1999.

Flenady VJ, Woodgate PG: Radiant warmers versus incubators for regulating body temperature in newborn infants. Cochrane Database Syst Rev (2):CD000435, 2002.

Foca M, Jakob K, Whittier S, et al: Endemic *Pseudomonas aeruginosa* infection in a neonatal intensive care unit. N Engl J Med 343:695-700, 2000.

Freeman J, Goldmann DA, Smith NE, et al: Association of intravenous lipid emulsion and coagulase-negative staphylococcal bacteremia in neonatal intensive care units. N Engl J Med 323:301-308, 1990.

Garland J, Colleen A, Pauly T, et al: A three-day course of dexamethasone therapy to prevent chronic lung disease in ventilated neonates: A randomized trial. Pediatrics 104:91-99, 1999.

Garland JS, Buck RK, Allred EN, et al: Hypocarbia before surfactant therapy appears to increase bronchopulmonary dysplasia risk in infants with respiratory distress syndrome. Arch Pediatr Adolesc Med 149:617-622, 1995.

Gaylord MS, Wright K, Lorch K, et al: Improved fluid management utilizing humidified incubators in extremely low birth weight infants. J Perinatol 21:438-443, 2001.

Gibbs RS, Eschenbach DA: Use of antibiotics to prevent preterm birth. Am J Obstet Gynecol 177:375-380, 1997.

Gittermann MK, Fusch C, Gittermann AR, et al: Early nasal continuous positive airway pressure treatment reduces the need for intubation in very low birth weight infants. Eur J Pediatr 156:384-388, 1997.

Goldenberg RL, Hauth JC, Andrews WW: Intrauterine infection and preterm delivery. N Engl J Med 342:1500-1507, 2000.

Goldmann DA, Weinstein RA, Wenzel RP, et al: Strategies to prevent and control the emergence and spread of antimicrobial-resistant microorganisms in hospitals: A challenge to hospital leadership. JAMA 275:234-240, 1996.

Gray JE, Richardson DK, McCormick MC, et al: Coagulase-negative staphylococcal bacteremia among very low birth weight infants: Relation to admission illness severity, resource use, and outcome. Pediatrics 95:225-230, 1995.

Halliday HL, Ehrenkranz RA, Doyle LW: Early postnatal (<96 hours) corticosteroids for preventing chronic lung disease in preterm infants. Cochrane Database Syst Rev (1): CD001146, 2002.

Harbarth S, Pittet D, Grady L, et al: Interventional study to evaluate the impact of an alcohol-based hand gel in improving hand hygiene compliance. Pediatr Infect Dis J 21:498-495, 2002.

Haywood JL, Goldenberg RL, Bronstein J, et al: Comparison of perceived and actual rates of survival and freedom from handicap in premature infants. Am J Obstet Gynecol 171:432-439, 1994.

Herrera CM, Gerhardt T, Claure N, et al: Effects of volume guaranteed synchronized intermittent mandatory ventilation in preterm infants recovering from respiratory failure. Pediatrics 110:529-533, 2002.

High frequency oscillatory ventilation compared with conventional mechanical ventilation in the treatment of respiratory failure in preterm infants. The HIFI Study Group. N Engl J Med 320:88-93, 1989.

Horbar J, Badger G, Carpenter J, et al: Trends in mortality and morbidity for very low birth weight infants, 1991-1999. Pediatrics 110:143-151, 2002.

Horbar J, Rogowski J, Plsek P, et al: Collaborative quality improvement for neonatal intensive care. Pediatrics 107:14-22, 2001.

Hummler H, Gerhardt T, Gonzalez A, et al: Influence of different methods of synchronized mechanical ventilation on ventilation, gas exchange, patient effort, and blood pressure fluctuations in premature neonates. Pediatr Pulmonol 22:305-313, 1996.

Jacobs S, Sokol J, Oklsson A: The newborn individualized developmental care and assessment program is not supported by meta-analyses of the data. J Pediatr 140:699-706, 2002.

Janes M, Kalyn A, Pinelli J, et al: A randomized trial comparing peripherally inserted central venous catheters and peripheral intravenous catheters in infants with very low birth weight. J Pedi Surg 35:1040-1044, 2000.

Jarreau PH, Moriette G, Mussat P, et al: Patient triggered ventilation decreases the work of breathing in neonates. Am J Respir Crit Care Med 153:1176-1181, 1996.

Jenson H, Pollock B: Meta-analyses of the effectiveness of intravenous immune globulin for prevention and treatment of neonatal sepsis. Pediatrics 99:1-11, 1997.

Johnson, AH, Peacock JL, Greenough A, et al: High-frequency oscillatory ventilation for the prevention of chronic lung disease of prematurity. N Engl J Med 347:633-642, 2002.
Joseph TA, Pyati SP, Jacobs N: Neonatal early onset *Escherichia coli* disease: The effect of intrapartum ampicillin. Arch Pediatr Adolesc Med 152:35-40, 1998.
Kaufman D, Boyle R, Hazen K, et al: Fluconazole prophylaxis against fungal colonization and infection in preterm infants. N Engl J Med 345:1660-1666, 2001.
Kendig JW, Ryan RM, Sinkin RA, et al: Comparison of two strategies for surfactant prophylaxis in very premature infants: A multicenter randomized trial. Pediatrics 101:1006-1012, 1998.
Khalaf MN, Brodsky N, Hurley J, et al: A prospective randomized, controlled trial comparing synchronized nasal intermittent positive pressure ventilation versus nasal continuous positive airway pressure as modes of extubation. Pediatrics 108:13-17, 2001.
Kocherlakota P, La Gamma E: Preliminary report: rhG-CSF may reduce the incidence of neonatal sepsis in prolonged preeclampsia-associated neutropenia. Pediatrics 102:1107-1111, 1998.
Lacy JB, Ohlsson A: Administration of intravenous immunoglobulins for prophylaxis or treatment of infection in preterm infants: Meta-analyses. Arch Dis Child Fetal Neonatal Ed. 72:F151-F155, 1995.
Lamari F, Anastassiou ED, Stamokosta E, et al: Determination of slime-producing *S. epidermidis* specific antibodies in human immunoglobulin preparations and blood sera by an enzyme immunoassay: Correlation of antibody titers with opsonic activity and application to preterm neonates. J Pharm Biomed Anal 23:363-374, 2000.
Lane AT, Drost SS: Effects of repeated application of emollient cream to premature neonates' skin. Pediatrics 92:415-419, 1993.
Lefkowitz W: Oxygen and resuscitation: Beyond the myth. Pediatrics 109:517-519, 2002.
Lemons J, Bauer C, Oh W, et al: Very low birth weight outcomes of the National Institute of Child Health and Human Development Neonatal Research Network, January 1995 through December 1996. Pediatrics 107:1-8, 211, 2001.
Lindner W, Vobeck S, Hummler H, et al: Delivery room management of extremely low birth weight infants: Spontaneous breathing or intubation? Pediatrics 103:961-967, 1999.
Martin JA, Hamilton BE, Ventura SJ, et al: Births: Final data for 2000. Nat Vital Stat Rep 50:1-101, 2002.
Mazor M, Chaim W, Maymon E, et al: The role of antibiotic therapy in the prevention of prematurity. Clin Perinatol 25: 659-685, 1998.
McClure RJ, Newell SJ: Randomised controlled study of clinical outcome following trophic feeding. Arch Dis Child Fetal Neonatal Ed 82:F29-F33, 2000.
Mercer BM, Miodovnik M, Thurnau GR, et al: Antibiotic therapy for reduction of infant morbidity after preterm premature rupture of the membranes. JAMA 278:989-995, 1997.
Meyer M, Payton M, Salmon A, et al: A clinical comparison of radiant warmer and incubator care for preterm infants from birth to 1800 grams. Pediatrics 108:395-401, 2001.
Miura E, Procianoy R, Bittar C, et al: A randomized, double-masked, placebo-controlled trial of recombinant granulocyte colony-stimulating factor administration to preterm infants with the clinical diagnosis of early-onset sepsis. Pediatrics 10:30-55, 2001.
Modi N, Carr R: Promising stratagems for reducing the burden of neonatal sepsis. Arch Dis Child Fetal Neonatal Ed 83: F150-F153, 2000.
Nopper AJ, Horii KA, Sookdeo-Drost S, et al: Topical ointment therapy benefits premature infants. J Pediatr 128:660-669, 1996.
Parellada JA, Moise AA, Hegemier S, et al: Percutaneous central catheters and peripheral intravenous catheters have similar infection rates in very low birth weight infants. J Perinatol 19:251-254, 1999.
Piecuch R, Leonard C, Cooper B, et al: Outcome of extremely low birth weight infants (500 to 999 grams) over a 12-year period. Pediatrics 100:633-639, 1997.
Poets CF, Sens B: Changes in intubation rates and outcome of very low birth weight infants: A population-based study. Pediatrics 98:24-27, 1996.
Rastogi A, Akintorin SM, Bez ML, et al: A controlled trial of dexamethasone to prevent bronchopulmonary dysplasia in surfactant-treated infants. Pediatrics 98:204-210, 1996.
Rettitz-Volk W, Veldman A, Roth B, et al: A prospective, randomized, multicenter trail of high-frequency oscillatory ventilation compared with conventional ventilation in preterm infants with respiratory distress syndrome receiving surfactant. J Pediatr 132:249-254, 1998.
Reuss ML, Gordon HR: Obstetrical judgments of viability and perinatal survival of extremely low birthweight infants. Am J Public Health 85:362-366, 1995.
Rivera A Jr, Bell EF, Bier DM: Effect of intravenous amino acids on protein metabolism of preterm infants during the first three days of life. Pediatr Res 33:106-111, 1993.
Rutter N: Clinical consequences of an immature barrier. Semin Neonatol 5:281-287, 2000.
Schanler R, Shulman R, Lau C, et al: Feeding strategies for premature infants: Randomized trial of gastrointestinal priming and tube-feeding method. Pediatrics 103:434-439, 1999a.
Schanler R, Shulman R, Lau C: Feeding strategies for premature infants: Beneficial outcomes of feeding fortified human milk versus preterm formula. Pediatrics 103:1150-1157, 1999b.
Schieve LA, Meikle SF, Ferre C, et al: Low and very low birth weight in infants conceived with use of assisted reproductive technology. N Engl J Med 346:731-737, 2002.
Schmidt B: Methylxanthine therapy in premature infants: Sound practice, disaster, or fruitless byway? J Pediatr 135:526-528, 1999.
Schrag S, Gorwitz R, Bultz-Butts K, et al: Prevention of perinatal group B streptococcal disease. MMWR Morbid Mortal Wkly Rep 51(RR-11):1-26, 2002.
Soll RF, Morley CJ: Prophylactic versus selective use of surfactant in preventing morbidity and mortality in preterm infants. Cochrane Database Syst Rev (2):CD001454, 2001.
Spafford PS, Sinkin RA, Cox C, et al: Prevention of central venous catheter related coagulase negative staphylococcal sepsis in neonates. J Pediatr 125:259-63, 1994.
Spence K, Barr P: Nasal versus oral intubation for mechanical ventilation of newborn infants. Cochrane Database Syst Rev (2):CD000948, 2002.
Stark A, Carlo W, Tyson J, et al: Adverse effects of early dexamethasone treatment in extremely low birth weight infants. N Engl J Med 344:95-101, 2001.
Stoll B, Hansen N, Fanaroff A, et al: Changes in pathogens causing early onset sepsis in very low birth weight infants. N Engl J Med 347:240-247, 2002a.
Stoll B, Hansen N, Fanaroff A, et al: Late-onset sepsis in very low birth weight neonates: Experience of the NICHD Neonatal Research Network. Pediatrics 110:285-291, 2002b.
Streiner D, Saigal S, Burrows E, et al: Attitudes of parents and health care professionals toward active treatment of extremely premature infants. Pediatrics 108:152-157, 2001.
Thome U, Topfer A, Schaller P, et al: The effect of positive end expiratory pressure, peak inspiratory pressure, and inspiratory time on functional residual capacity in mechanically ventilated preterm infants. Eur J Pediatr 157:831-837, 1998.
Thome U, Kossel H, Lipowsky G, et al: Randomized comparison of high-frequency ventilation with high-rate intermittent positive pressure ventilation in preterm infants with respiratory failure. J Pediatr 135:39-46, 1999.

Towers CV, Bonebrake R, Padilla G, et al: The effect of transport on the rate of severe intraventricular hemorrhage in very low birth weight infants. Obstet Gynecol 95:291-295, 2000.

Tyson J, Wright L, Oh W: Vitamin A supplementation for extremely low birth weight infants. N Engl J Med 340: 1962-1968, 1999.

Van Goudoever JB, Wattimena JL, Huijmans JG, et al: Immediate commencement of amino acid supplementation in preterm infants: Effect on serum amino acid concentrations and protein kinetics on the first day of life. J Pediatr 127:458-465, 1995.

Van Marter LJ, Allred EN, Pagano M, et al: Do clinical markers of barotrauma and oxygen toxicity explain interhospital variation in rates of chronic lung disease? The Neonatology Committee for the Developmental Network. Pediatrics 105:1194-1201, 2000.

Verder H, Albertsen P, Ebbesen F, et al: Nasal continuous positive airway pressure and early surfactant therapy for respiratory distress syndrome in newborns of less than 30 weeks' gestation. Pediatrics 103:1-6, 1999.

Vohr B, Wright L, Dusick A, et al: Neurodevelopmental and functional outcomes of extremely low birth weight infants in the National Institute of Child Health and Human Development Neonatal Research Network, 1993-1994. Pediatrics 105: 1216-1226, 2000.

Vohra S, Frent G, Campbell V, et al: Effect of polyethylene occlusive skin wrapping on heat loss in very low birth weight infants at delivery: A randomized trial. J Pediatr 134:547-551, 1999.

Watterberg K, Gerdes J, Gifford K, et al: Prophylaxis against early adrenal insufficiency to prevent chronic lung disease in premature infants. Pediatrics 104:1258-1263, 1999.

Wiswell TE, Graziani LJ, Kornhauser MS, et al: Effects of hypocarbia on the development of cystic periventricular leukomalacia in premature infants treated with high-frequency jet ventilation. Pediatrics 98:918-924, 1996.

Wood N, Marlow N, Costeloe K, et al: Neurologic and developmental disability after extremely preterm birth. N Engl J Med 343:378-384, 2000.

Zupancic JA, Kirpalani H, Barrett J, et al: Characterising doctor-parent communication in counseling for impending preterm delivery. Arch Dis Child Fetal Neonatal Ed. 87:F113-F117, 2002.

CHAPTER

# 33

# Pharmacologic Principles and Practicalities

Robert M. Ward and Ralph A. Lugo

The rapid application of new drug therapy in the neonatal intensive care unit (NICU) has made pharmacology in the newborn increasingly complex. Accompanying that complexity is the realization that even though drug treatment of newborns may be curative, it may also induce significant problems. Potential morbidity and mortality associated with drug treatment of newborns must be recognized and weighed against the expected benefits.

Drug therapy of newborns follows basic principles of pharmacology superimposed on dynamic, developmental changes during the newborn period. Patients cared for in the NICU are exposed to a wide variety of drugs, many of which are incompletely studied in newborns. Therapeutic drug monitoring is often an integral part of this drug exposure in the NICU. The effective use of drug concentration measurements requires a working knowledge of pharmacokinetics and thoughtful consideration of when such measurements are appropriate and helpful.

## PERINATAL DRUG EXPOSURE

Repeated warnings about fetal drug exposure were issued to physicians and the public after recognition of the teratogenic effects of thalidomide in the 1960s. Despite these warnings, drug exposure of the human fetus and newborn increased during subsequent decades and remains extensive today. The average number of drugs ingested during pregnancy rose from 3 in the 1950s to 11 in the 1970s (Ward and Green, 1988). Virtually all drugs administered to the pregnant woman reach the fetus, but careful interpretation of the significance of this exposure is needed because fetal drug concentrations and effects vary widely, from insignificant to life-threatening (Ward and Green, 1988; Ward et al, 1980).

For hospitalized newborns, a similar pattern of increasing drug exposure is evident. Serial observations from the same NICU reveal almost a doubling of the average number of drugs administered to newborns in less than a decade, from 3.4 per patient during 1974 and 1975 (Aranda et al, 1976) to 6.2 per patient during 1977 through 1981 (Aranda et al, 1982a). Unfortunately, drug exposure among NICU patients is disproportionately greater in the most susceptible (and least studied) patients—the most immature newborns and newborns with multiple organ dysfunction (Aranda, 1983).

## DRUG-INDUCED ILLNESS

The extensive exposure of newborns to drugs in the NICU is not benign. During their NICU hospitalization, 30% of newborns sustain one or more adverse drug reactions, of which 14.7% are fatal or life threatening (Aranda et al, 1982b). The causes of this NICU "epidemic" of drug-related morbidity and mortality are complex. Pharmacologic studies in pediatric patients are difficult because of a variety of problems from ethics to study design (Ward and Green, 1988). The difficulty of studying therapeutics in the newborn has created a situation in which a plethora of drugs is administered with a paucity of pharmacologic data. For the smaller and more immature newborns who are now surviving, there are no gestational age–appropriate pharmacologic data about efficacy, dose-response, and kinetics for most drugs they receive.

Furthermore, drug-induced illness is seldom considered in newborns. Failure to recognize drug-induced illness in the newborn often leads to further pharmacologic treatment as the first approach to correct unrecognized drug-induced problems. This fact may reflect an expectation that drug therapy is usually effective and safe. The observations of Aranda and colleagues suggest the opposite. Prudent management of newborns must recognize and weigh the potential benefits of unstudied drug therapy against potential drug-induced morbidity and mortality. Some examples from the history of drug-induced mortality and morbidity in newborns should serve as a reminder of how more harm than good may accrue from uncontrolled or unstudied drug therapy in the NICU.

### Lessons from Chloramphenicol

Chloramphenicol was released for use in the 1940s, and reports of its efficacy for treatment of *Salmonella* infections included pediatric patients. The manufacturer recommended dosages of 50 to 100 mg/kg per day for patients ≤15 kg. In 1959, when Sutherland reported three cases of sudden death in newborns treated with high dosages of chloramphenicol (up to 230 mg/kg per day), the drug was considered "well tolerated and nontoxic." Later the same year, Burns and colleagues (1959) reported the disturbing results of a controlled trial of the following four prophylactic treatment regimens for newborn sepsis: (1) no treatment, (2) chloramphenicol alone, (3) penicillin and streptomycin, and (4) penicillin, streptomycin, and chloramphenicol. The groups that received chloramphenicol (100 to 165 mg/kg per day), in regimens 2 and 4, had overall mortality rates of 60% and 68%, respectively, whereas groups receiving regimens 1 and 3 had mortality rates of 19% and 18%, respectively. The deaths of these newborns demonstrated the stereotyped sequence of symptoms and signs caused by chloramphenicol, designated the *gray syndrome*, which consisted of abdominal distention with or without emesis, poor peripheral perfusion and cyanosis, vasomotor collapse, irregular respirations, and death within hours of the onset of these symptoms. Weiss and coworkers (1960) attributed the gray syndrome in newborns to high concentrations of chloramphenicol secondary to its prolonged half-life in newborns who received dosages of more than 100 mg/kg per day, which are usually used in older children. They recommended maximum dosages of 50 mg/kg per day in term infants younger than 1 month, half that dose for premature infants, and careful monitoring of chloramphenicol blood concentrations.

The discovery and explanation of chloramphenicol toxicity in newborns illustrate several important aspects of neonatal pharmacology. Because chloramphenicol was considered well tolerated in older children and adults, it was regarded as nontoxic for newborns. Chloramphenicol was so effective in newborns that higher dosages were used without pharmacokinetic study. Higher doses were administered to newborns despite recognition that its clearance required glucuronide conjugation, which was known to be immature in newborns. The unexpected finding that chloramphenicol in doses of 100 to 165 mg/kg per day could be lethal to newborns was demonstrated because the study conducted by Burns and colleagues (1959) included appropriate control groups. In fact, because the mortality rate from the most effective antibiotic treatment regimen was equivalent to that of no antibiotic treatment, these investigators discontinued prophylactic use of antibiotics in the nursery.

Similar pharmacologic comparisons are needed for other drugs used in newborns. Even more, thoughtful consideration should be given to clinicians' response to therapeutic failure. Fewer drugs and lower dosages may be safer and more effective than additional drugs in higher dosages.

## REDUCTION AND PREVENTION OF MEDICATION ERRORS IN NEWBORN CARE

Drug treatment is one of the most common approaches used in the care of sick newborns. At Primary Children's Medical Center 35-bed NICU in Salt Lake City, Utah, with an average of 785 patient-days per month, patients receive an average of 8700 (range 6990 to 11,290) doses of medications, pharmacy-formulated intravenous solutions, and aerosols each month (unpublished observations, 1994). These are usually prepared by pharmacists and administered by nurses, respiratory therapists, and (rarely) physicians. In such a large and complex system that produces so many drug treatments per month, errors are virtually inevitable despite several levels of prospective and redundant reviews by nurses, pharmacists, and NICU unit secretaries involved in the drug treatment process. At Primary Children's NICU, the medication error rate averages 0.04% for nurses and pharmacists and 0.07% for physicians (unpublished observations, 1994). Many errors are inconsequential, whereas others have serious adverse effects. Medication errors incur significant costs, ranging from the obvious ones such as direct patient injury, prolonged hospital stays, and additional corrective treatments to the more subtle costs associated with monitoring and regulation of medication use within hospitals (ASHP, 1995).

In a study of 393 malpractice claims reported to the Physician Insurers Association of America, the second most common cause of malpractice claims was drug errors (Physician Insurers Association of America [PIAA], 1993). Among 16 medical specialties with two or more claims, pediatric practice ranked sixth in the number of claims, yet it had the third highest average cost per indemnity. The medications most frequently involved in all claims were antibiotics, glucocorticoids, narcotic or non-narcotic analgesics, and narcotic antagonists. In pediatric practice, the medications most frequently involved were vaccines (diphtheria-pertussis-tetanus) and bronchodilators (theophylline). In the PIAA review (1993), the five most common causes of drug errors were as follows:

- Incorrect doses
- Medications that were inappropriate for the medical condition
- Failure to monitor for drug side effects
- Failure of communication between physician and patient
- Failure to monitor drug levels

The primary opportunity for prevention of these five most common errors rests with the prescribing physician. Additional information as well as additional time for communication and documentation may be needed.

Prescriptions and drug orders are a means of communicating, yet clinicians often devote too little attention to making them legible, clear, and unambiguous (ASHP guidelines, 1993). Physicians should keep the following recommendations in mind to ensure that their medication orders communicate more effectively:

- Write out instructions rather than use abbreviations.
- Avoid vague instructions (e.g., "take as directed").
- Specify exact dosage strengths.
- Avoid abbreviations of drug names (e.g., MS could mean morphine sulfate or magnesium sulfate).
- Avoid trailing zeroes; use leading zeroes.
- Ensure that prescriptions and signatures are legible, even if it means printing the prescriber's name that corresponds to the signature.

The process for ordering, preparing, dispensing, and administering medications in an ICU with acutely ill patients is often complicated and may contribute directly to errors. The frequency of those errors, however, may be reduced in almost every NICU. Although complex and expensive computerized systems may help reduce medication errors, caregivers can take steps that are completely within their control to reduce medication errors without waiting for changes in the entire pharmacy process within the hospital (ASHP guidelines, 1993).

## PRINCIPLES OF NEONATAL THERAPEUTICS

A thorough understanding of factors that affect drug concentrations helps in the planning of accurate therapy and the identification of the causes of therapeutic failure. Many of these factors are not chosen consciously in a therapeutic plan but have tremendous impact on its effectiveness. Pharmacokinetics and pharmacodynamics in newborns follow the same general principles that govern drug actions in patients of any age: diagnosis, drug selection and administration, absorption, distribution, metabolism, and excretion. When applied to the newborn, these principles must accommodate several unique physiologic and pharmacologic features of the newborn, as outlined in Table 33–1 and discussed in detail here.

## Diagnosis

Effective treatment begins with an accurate diagnosis and accurate assessment of symptoms. Although this principle applies to all areas of therapeutics, treatment in newborns presents special diagnostic challenges because the small size and fragility of such patients may preclude useful, but inordinately invasive, diagnostic procedures. For example, many small immature newborns with chronic lung disease are given treatment for "bronchospasm" after decreased air entry associated with desaturation and abnormal breath sounds is observed. Relief of these symptoms with aerosolized bronchodilators may be interpreted as confirmation of the diagnosis. Although this interpretation may be correct, increased humidity, chest physiotherapy, or movement of the endotracheal tube bevel away from a pliable tracheal wall during an aerosol treatment may also account for the improvement. Evaluation of ineffective therapy should include reconsideration of the diagnosis.

**TABLE 33–1**

**Pharmacologic Principles and Pitfalls in Management of the Very-Low-Birth-Weight Infant**

I. Diagnosis:
  A. Limited diagnostic procedures
II. Absorption:
  A. Intravenous:
    1. Drug injection away from patient
    2. Uneven mixing of drugs and intravenous fluids
    3. Delayed administration due to very low flow
    4. Part of the dose discarded with tubing changes
  B. Intramuscular:
    1. Poor perfusion limits absorption
    2. Danger of sclerosis or abscess formation
    3. Depot effect
  C. Oral:
    1. Poorly studied
    2. Affected by delayed gastric emptying
    3. Potentially affected by reflux
    4. Passive venous congestion may occur with chronic lung disease, decreasing absorption
III. Distribution (affected by):
  A. Higher (85%) total body water (versus 65% in adults)
  B. Lower body fat, i.e., about 1% body weight (versus 15% in term infants)
  C. Low protein concentration
  D. Decreased protein affinity for drugs
IV. Metabolism:
  A. Half-life prolonged and unpredictable
  B. Total body clearance decreased
  C. Affected by nutrition, illness, and drug interaction
  D. Affected by maturational changes
V. Excretion:
  A. Decreased renal function, both glomerular filtration rate and tubular secretion

## Absorption

Although most types of drug therapy for acute problems involve *intravenous administration* to ensure drug delivery to the site of action, this route may *not* be reliable in newborns (Roberts, 1984). Drugs are often injected away from newborns, "up the IV line" through a Y-site injection port, with the expectation that the preset flow rate will deliver the drug over an appropriate infusion time. Inntravenous infusion rates for very-low-birth-weight (VLBW) infants may be less than 2 mL/hour, sometimes divided between two infusion sites. Consequently, a drug injected away from the infant may infuse so slowly that it does not reach the circulation for several hours and then enters over a prolonged period. Gould and Roberts (1979) estimated that as much as 36% of the total daily dose may be discarded when the intravenous solution tubing is changed. Infusion solution filters may also prevent drug delivery by direct adsorption of the drug or by allowing a heavier drug to settle in the filtration chamber and mix slowly with the infusion solution. For drug therapy in which the driving force for tissue entry is a concentration gradient between the circulation and the tissue (e.g., in meningitis), sustained low drug concentrations may provide suboptimal therapy.

*Intramuscular administration* of drugs to newborns is suboptimal and is generally used when there is difficulty maintaining intravenous access. Absorption of drugs from an intramuscular injection site is directly related to muscle perfusion. Patients with hypothermia or shock are unlikely to absorb intramuscular doses effectively. Intramuscular administration of drugs may sclerose tissue or create large intramuscular collections of the drugs, which are absorbed slowly, producing a "depot effect" in which serum concentrations rise slowly over a prolonged period. Intramuscular administration of drugs to newborns, especially for multiple doses, should be avoided because it may not deliver effective drug concentrations to the site of action and may cause disfiguring sterile abscesses in the limited muscle mass of small newborns.

Even though *oral administration* of drugs is preferred for treatment of chronic illnesses in newborns, this route is not well studied. In adults, less drug is usually absorbed from the stomach than from the intestinal tract because of the smaller surface area. Delayed gastric emptying postpones achievement of peak serum drug concentrations and prolongs the absorption phase while elimination continues. Many newborns experience gastroesophageal reflux associated with delayed gastric emptying, which may alter drug bioavailability. Passive venous congestion of the intestinal tract from elevated right atrial pressures decreases drug absorption in adults and may do so in premature infants with severe bronchopulmonary dysplasia complicated by cor pulmonale (Peterson et al, 1980). The administration of medications to newborns in small volumes of formula or during continuous gastric feedings may also alter drug absorption.

The possible effects of feeding patterns on drug absorption and action must be considered when enteral drug therapy fails.

### Distribution

In pharmacokinetics, *distribution* is the partitioning of drugs among various body fluids, organs, and tissues. The distribution of a drug within the body is determined by several factors, including organ blood flow, pH and composition of body fluids and tissues, physical and chemical properties of the drug (e.g., lipid solubility, molecular weight, and ionization constant), and the extent of drug binding to plasma proteins and other macromolecules (Ward et al, 1980).

Important differences among premature infants, children, and adults affect the distribution of drugs. Total body water varies from 85% in premature newborns to 75% in term newborns to 65% in adults (Boreus, 1982). Conversely, body fat content varies from 1% or less in premature infants to 15% in term newborns (Mirkin, 1978). These differences change the distribution of many drugs, especially polar, water-soluble drugs such as the aminoglycosides. Protein binding of drugs in the circulation is decreased in the premature newborn because of a smaller total amount of circulating protein and lower binding affinity of the protein itself. With rare exceptions, only the free (not bound to protein) drug molecules "are active," that is, cross membranes, exert pharmacologic actions, and undergo metabolism and excretion. Clinical measurements of serum or plasma drug concentrations usually reflect total circulating drug concentrations, which consist of both free and protein-bound drug. Thus, total circulating drug concentrations in the newborn, which are low by adult standards, may represent free drug concentrations that are equivalent to those of the adult because of the decreased protein binding in the newborn.

### Metabolism

Many drugs require metabolic conversion before elimination from the body. *Biotransformation* of a drug usually produces a more polar, less lipid-soluble molecule that can then be eliminated rapidly by renal, biliary, or other routes of excretion. Drug biotransformation is classified into two broad categories, (1) nonsynthetic (phase I) reactions, which include oxidation, reduction, and hydrolysis, and (2) synthetic or conjugation (phase II) reactions, which include glucuronidation, sulfation, and acetylation. Although the liver is considered the major organ responsible for drug biotransformation, many other organs carry out drug metabolism.

For most drugs in the newborn, the half-life is prolonged and total body clearance is decreased. Important variations occur, however, among drug classes and among individuals. Glucuronide conjugation of bilirubin is usually low at birth unless this enzyme has been induced in utero through maternal exposure to drugs, cigarette smoke, or other inducing agents (Ward et al, 1980). In contrast, conjugation through sulfation is usually active at birth. Various factors after birth, such as nutrition, illness, and drug interactions, may hasten or retard the maturation of enzymes and organs responsible for drug metabolism in the newborn. Maturational changes in hepatic blood flow, drug transport into hepatocytes, synthesis of serum proteins, protein binding of drugs, and biliary secretion—alone and in combination—confound accurate predictions about drug metabolism after birth, leading to empiric dose adjustments (Morselli et al, 1980). These factors must be studied again in the very immature, very-low-birth-weight infant.

### Excretion

Another major pathway for drug elimination from the body is renal excretion of metabolized and unchanged drug. Neonatal renal function is diminished both in absolute terms and when normalized to body weight or surface area. The neonatal glomerular filtration rate averages about 30% of the adult rate per unit surface area. Glomerular function rises steadily after birth, whereas tubular function matures more slowly, causing a glomerular and tubular imbalance (Aperia et al, 1981). The postnatal increase in glomerular function reflects greater cardiac output, reduced renal vascular resistance, redistribution of intrarenal blood flow, and changes in intrinsic glomerular basement membrane permeability (Morselli et al, 1980). The dynamics of neonatal renal function markedly influence drug excretion. The rate of change of renal function and its susceptibility to hypoxemia, nephrotoxic drugs, and underperfusion confound predictions of drug elimination rates in newborns, which must be measured empirically.

## PHARMACOKINETIC PRINCIPLES

*Pharmacokinetics* describes the time course of changes in drug concentrations within the body. Although rates of change are often described with differential equations, concepts useful at the bedside are emphasized here. More detailed mathematical discussions of pharmacokinetics can be found elsewhere (Gibaldi and Perrier, 1982; Greenblatt and Koch-Weser, 1975a, 1975b; Notari, 1980).

### Compartment

In pharmacokinetics, *compartment* refers to fluid and tissue spaces into which drugs penetrate. These compartments may or may not be equivalent to anatomic or physiologic fluid volumes. In the simplest case, the compartment may correspond to the vascular space and equal the volume of a real body fluid, blood. Large or quite polar molecules may be confined to this central compartment until they are eliminated by excretion or metabolism. Many drugs, however, diffuse reversibly out of the central compartment into tissues or other fluid spaces, referred to generically as peripheral or tissue compartments. Such compartments are seldom sampled directly, but their involvement in kinetic processes may be recognized from the graphic or mathematical description of the kinetics of a drug.

## Apparent Volume of Distribution

The apparent volume of distribution might be better termed "volume of dilution," because it is a mathematical description of the volume (L or L/kg) required for dilution of a dose (mg or mg/kg) to produce the observed circulating drug concentration (mg/L or μg/mL). (To simplify cancellation of units, concentrations are expressed here as mg/L, which is the same as μg/mL, the more conventional unit for drug concentrations.)

$$\text{Concentration (mg/L)} = \frac{\text{Dose (mg/kg)}}{\text{Apparent volume of distribution (L/kg)}}$$

For many drugs, the volume of distribution does not correspond to a specific physiologic body fluid or tissue—hence the term "apparent." In fact, the volume of distribution for drugs that are bound extensively in tissues may exceed 1.0 L/kg, a physiologic impossibility that emphasizes the arithmetic, nonphysiologic nature of the apparent volume of distribution. The calculation of distribution volume is described later.

## First-Order Kinetics

Removal of most drugs from the body can be described by first-order (exponential or proportional) kinetics, in which a constant proportion or percentage of a drug is removed over time, rather than a constant amount over time. For drugs exhibiting first-order kinetics, the higher the concentration, the greater the amount removed. The following equations describe the concentration (C) of a drug whose first-order kinetics have a rate constant, k ($\text{minute}^{-1}$), at time (t) and an initial concentration of $C_0$.

In differential form, the change in C with time is

$$\frac{dC}{dt} = -kC$$

In exponential form, C at time t is

$$C_t = C_0 e^{-kt}$$

If integrated, C at time t is expressed as the natural logarithm (ln)

$$\ln C_t = \ln C_0 - kt$$

The last equation fits the equation of a straight line, so that a graph that plots ln $C_t$ versus t has an intercept of ln $C_0$ at t = 0 and a slope of –k, the rate constant for the change in concentration, which can be used to calculate the half-life and dosages. Multiple rate constants in more complex equations are distinguished with the letter k and numbered subscripts or with Greek letters.

## Half-Life

The drug half-life ($t_{1/2}$) is the time required for a drug concentration to decrease by 50%. Half-life is a first-order kinetic process because the same proportion, 50%, of the drug is removed during equal periods. Half-life can be determined mathematically from the elimination rate constant, k, as

$$t_{1/2} = \frac{\text{natural logarithm 2}}{k} = \frac{0.693}{k}$$

Figure 33–1 illustrates a graphic method for determination of half-life. Drug concentrations measured serially are graphed on semilogarithmic axes, and the best-fit line is determined either visually or by linear regression analysis. In this illustration of first-order kinetics, the concentration decreases 50% (from 800 to 400) during the first hour and decreases another 50% (from 400 to 200) during the second hour. Thus, the half-life is 1 hour. More drug is removed during one half-life at higher concentrations, although the proportion removed remains constant. The exponential equation for this graph is

$$C = 800e^{-0.0116t}$$

where k = 0.0116/minute and $C_0$ = 800, allowing a mathematical calculation of half-life using the equation previously described:

$$t_{1/2} = \frac{0.693}{k(\text{minute}^{-1})} = \frac{0.693}{0.0116/\text{minute}} = 60 \text{ minutes}$$

## Multicompartment, First-Order Kinetics

The rate of removal of many drugs from the circulation is biphasic. The initial rapid decrease in concentration is the distribution (α) phase, often lasting 15 to 45 minutes, which is followed by a sustained slower rate of removal, the elimination (β) phase. Such biphasic processes are best visualized from semilogarithmic graphs of concentration versus time. When such semilogarithmic graphs show kinetics that best fit two straight lines, the kinetics are described as *biexponential*, or *two-compartment, and* first-order (Fig. 33–2). Two exponential terms are needed to describe such changes in concentration, as

$$C = Ae^{-\alpha t} + Be^{-\beta t}$$

In this equation, the rate constant for distribution is designated α to discriminate it from the rate constant for terminal elimination (β), where *A* and *B* are the time = 0

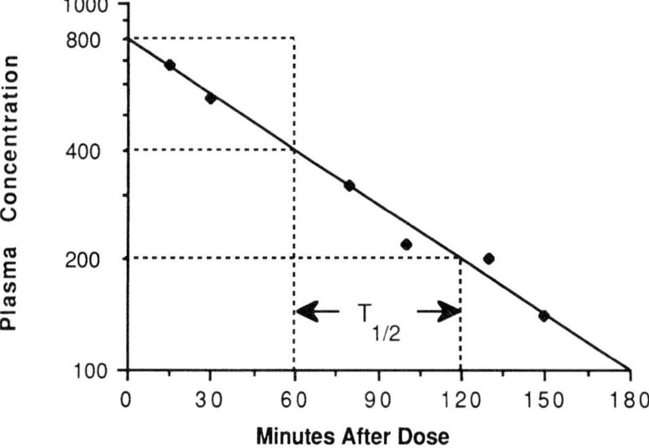


**FIGURE 33–1.** Apparent single-compartment, first-order plasma drug disappearance curve illustrating graphic determination of half-life from best-fit line of serial plasma concentrations.

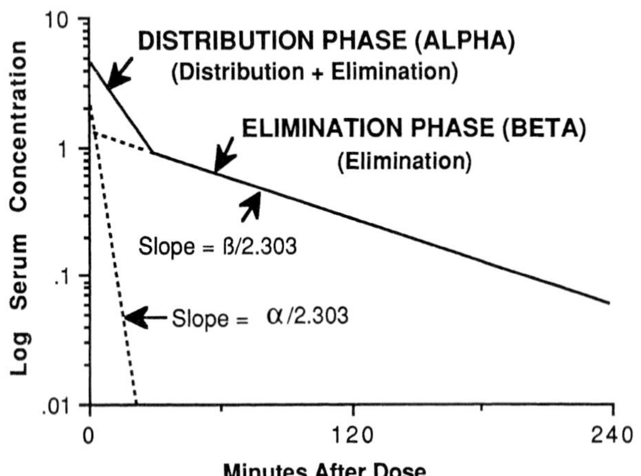


**FIGURE 33–2.** Multicompartment serum drug disappearance curve.

intercepts for the lines describing distribution and elimination, respectively. Division by 2.303 converts logarithms to natural logarithms.

After an intravenous dose, drug loss from the vascular space during the distribution phase occurs through both distribution and elimination (see Fig. 33–2). The rate constant of distribution (α) can be determined by plotting the difference between the total amount of drug lost initially and the amount of drug lost through elimination (Greenblatt et al, 1975a). This produces the line with the steeper slope (equal to α/2.303) below the serum concentration graph in Fig. 33–2. The single slope of the distribution phase and of the terminal elimination phase does not imply that distribution or elimination occurs through a single process. The observed rates usually represent the summation of several simultaneous processes, each with differing rates, occurring in various tissues.

When the time course of drug elimination is observed for prolonged periods, a third rate of elimination, or γ phase, may be observed that is usually attributed to elimination of drug that has reequilibrated from deep tissue compartments back into the plasma. Such kinetics are designated *three-compartment* and *first-order*. The kinetics of a drug are expressed with the smallest number of compartments that accurately describes its concentration changes over time.

## Apparent Single-Compartment, First-Order Kinetics

When a semilogarithmic graph of concentration versus time reveals a single slope with no distribution phase, the kinetics are characterized as *apparent single-compartment, first-order* (see Fig. 33–1). This may occur when a drug remains entirely within the vascular space or central compartment or when a drug passes very rapidly back and forth between the circulation and peripheral sites until it is metabolized or excreted by first-order kinetics. The adjective *apparent* is used because careful study often shows that distribution does occur even though the kinetic curve has only a single slope. Single-compartment kinetics implies that the drug rapidly and completely distributes homogeneously throughout the body, which rarely occurs clinically.

In many pharmacokinetic studies in newborns, blood samples are not obtained early enough to allow calculation of the distribution phase, and the kinetics are described as single-compartment. If sampling begins after the distribution phase, the concentration time points may fit a single-compartment, first-order model, which determines the elimination rate constant (β). The kinetics cannot be assumed, however, to fit a single-compartment model from such a limited study. The most accurate approach to kinetic analysis, *noncompartmental analysis*, makes no assumptions about the number of compartments (Gibaldi and Perrier, 1982; Notari, 1980).

## Zero-Order Kinetics

Some drugs demonstrate *zero-order kinetics*, in which a constant amount of drug, rather than a constant proportion or percentage, is removed over time, rather than a constant proportion or percentage. This relationship can be expressed as

$$\frac{dC}{dt} = -k$$

It is important to understand when zero-order kinetics occurs, how to recognize it, and how it affects drug concentrations. Zero-order kinetics is sometimes referred to as "saturation kinetics" because it may occur when excess amounts of drug completely saturate enzymes or transport systems so that they metabolize or transport only a *constant amount* of drug over time. Zero-order processes produce a curvilinear shape in a semilogarithmic graph of concentrations versus time (Fig. 33–3). When drug concentrations are high from inappropriate dosing or a drug overdose, kinetics may be zero-order, followed by first-order kinetics at lower concentrations. For drugs exhibiting zero-order kinetics, small increments in dose may cause disproportionately large increments in serum concentration. Certain drugs administered to newborns exhibit zero-order kinetics at therapeutic doses and concentrations and must be recognized for their potential accumulation (Table 33–2).

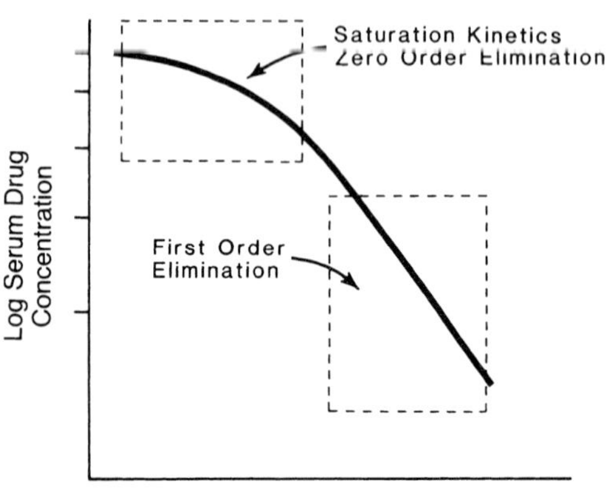


**FIGURE 33–3.** Representation of saturation, or zero-order (serum concentration–dependent), and first-order (serum concentration–independent) pharmacokinetics.

**TABLE 33-2**

**Drugs that Demonstrate Saturation Kinetics with Therapeutic Doses in Newborns**

| |
|---|
| Caffeine |
| Chloramphenicol |
| Diazepam |
| Furosemide |
| Indomethacin |
| Phenytoin |

## Target Drug Concentration Strategy

Drug treatment of newborns commonly uses the *target drug concentration strategy* (Table 33–3), in which drug therapy corrects a specific problem by producing an effective concentration of free drug at a specific site of action (Sheiner et al, 1978). The target site of drug action is usually inaccessible for monitoring of concentrations.

The requirements for effective and accurate application of the target drug concentration treatment in adults have been discussed by Spector and colleagues (1988). When applied to newborns, these requirements highlight the special problems of drug therapy in these patients and the special circumstances in which clinical drug concentration monitoring is appropriate. Some of these requirements are as follows:

- An available analytic procedure for accurate measurement of drug concentrations in small volumes of blood
- A wide variation in pharmacokinetics among individuals with the knowledge that population-based kinetics do not accurately predict individual kinetics
- Drug effects are proportional to plasma drug concentrations
- A narrow concentration range between efficacy and toxicity (narrow therapeutic index)
- Constant pharmacologic effect over time, in which tolerance does not develop
- Clinical studies that have determined the therapeutic and toxic drug concentration ranges

## Therapeutic Drug Monitoring

Table 33–3 illustrates the basic assumptions of therapeutic drug monitoring, that total plasma drug concentrations correlate with dose as well as with circulating unbound drug concentrations and unbound drug concentration at the site of action. Clinical measurements of drug concentrations usually include both bound and unbound drug, and the active portion is that portion that is unbound (see discussion of distribution). The two broad indications for monitoring drug concentrations are (1) attainment of effective concentrations and (2) avoidance of toxic concentrations. As Kauffman (1981) has pointed out, drug concentration ranges are not absolute reflections of effective therapy. Patient response, not a specific drug concentration range, is the endpoint of therapy.

Although concentrations of aminoglycoside antibiotics, such as gentamicin, are monitored frequently in newborns, toxicity is rare in newborns compared with its occurrence in adults (McCracken, 1986). Because of the limited evidence of toxicity in newborns, it is more important to measure aminoglycoside concentrations to achieve effective concentrations for treatment of culture-proven infections than to avoid toxicity. In newborns with serious therapeutic problems, measurement of serum drug concentrations should be used to achieve effective concentrations as well as to avoid toxicity. When the desired concentration range and kinetic parameters are known, doses may be estimated to reach that concentration with single bolus doses or bolus doses followed by continuous infusions.

## Kinetic Dosing

The following equations can be used both to guide dosing and to derive kinetic parameters for individual patients.

Where C = concentration and Vd = volume of distribution:

$$\underset{(mg/kg)}{\text{Dose}} = \underset{(mg/L)\,(L/kg)}{\Delta C \cdot Vd} = \underset{(mg/L)}{[C_{desired} - C_{initial}]} \cdot \underset{(L/kg)}{Vd}$$

This equation may be used to estimate dosage changes needed to increase or decrease concentration. For the first dose, the starting concentration is zero; for doses after the first, the calculation of distribution volume should use the change (Δ) in concentration from the preceding trough to the peak associated with that dose. To reach a desired concentration rapidly, a loading dose can be administered followed by a sustaining infusion. The equation for calculation of infusion doses to maintain a constant concentration is shown below.

Where C = concentration, Vd = volume of distribution, and k = rate constant of elimination,

$$\underset{(mg/kg)(min^{-1})}{\text{infusion rate}} = \underset{(min^{-1})}{k} \cdot \underset{(L/kg)}{Vd} \cdot \underset{(mg/L)}{C}$$

**TABLE 33-3**

**Target Drug Concentration Strategy**

| Drug dose | ↔ | Plasma total drug concentration | ↔ | Plasma unbound drug concentration | ↔ | Target site unbound drug concentration | ↔ | Desired pharmacologic effect |
|---|---|---|---|---|---|---|---|---|

Data from Shenier LB, Tozer TN: Clinical pharmacokinetics: The use of plasma concentrations of durgs. In Melmon KL, Morrelli HF (Eds): Clinical Pharmacology: Basic Principles in Therapeutics, 2nd ed. New York, Macmillan, 1978, p 71.

Steady state is reached when tissue concentrations are in equilibrium and the amount of drug removed equals the amount of drug infused. The time needed to reach a steady state depends on the elimination half-life and is *not* shortened by the administration of a loading dose.

## Repetitive Dosing and the "Plateau Principle"

During the typical course of drug therapy, drug doses are administered before complete elimination of previous doses, and the kinetics are more complex (Greenblatt et al, 1975b). During repeated administration, the peak and trough levels after each dose increase for a time. *Steady-state*, or *plateau*, concentrations are reached when the amount of drug eliminated equals the amount of drug administered during each dosing interval. During repetitive dosing, the steady-state concentrations achieved are related to the half-life, dose, and dosing interval relative to the half-life (Greenblatt et al, 1975b).

Fig. 33–4 illustrates a hypothetical concentration-time curve for a drug with a half-life of 4 hours administered orally every 4 hours, so the dosing interval corresponds to one half-life. Several important principles of pharmacokinetics are illustrated in this figure, with the mathematics described in detail elsewhere (Greenblatt et al, 1975b). Drug concentrations rise and fall with drug administration (absorption) and elimination. For dosing intervals of one half-life, accumulation is 88% complete after the third dose, 94% complete after the fourth dose, and 97% complete after the fifth dose. At steady state, the peak and trough concentrations between doses are the same after each dose. If a drug is administered with a dosing interval equal to one half-life, the steady-state peak and trough concentrations are two times those reached after the first dose. If the dosing interval is shortened to half of a half-life, the concentration decreases less before the next dose, more total drug is administered per day, and the steady-state peak and trough concentrations are considerably higher (3.4 times the peak and trough concentrations after the first dose). Thus, the shorter the dosing interval–to–half-life ratio, the higher the drug accumulation. As noted during infusions, the *length of time* required to reach steady-state concentrations depends primarily on the elimination half-life, not the dosing interval.

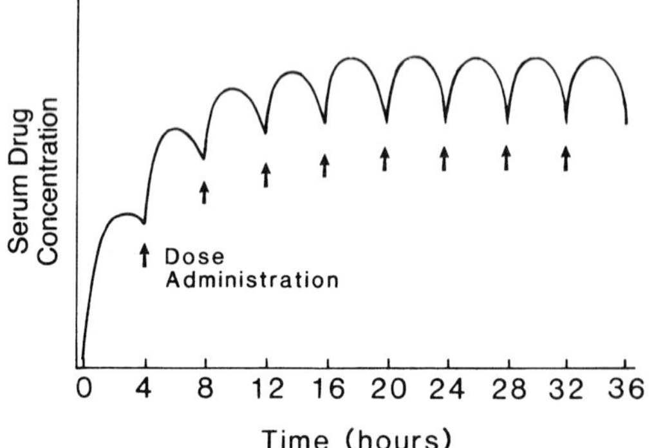


**FIGURE 33–4.** Representation of multiple dosing with accumulation of serum drug levels to steady-state concentration.

## Clearance

*Clearance* of drugs, as for creatinine, describes the volume of blood from which all the drug is removed per unit of time. Clearance is proportional to organ blood flow and the intrinsic capacity of organs to metabolize or remove drug from the circulation. In its simplest form, clearance is proportional to the flow to a single organ (Q) and to the arterial-venous difference in drug concentrations compared with the amount of drug in the circulation, expressed as

$$CL = Q \cdot \frac{C_{arterial} - C_{venous}}{C_{arterial}}$$

Total body clearance usually reflects the combined clearance of multiple organs with different enzyme activities and different rates of blood flow. Clearance can be measured by the rate of appearance of drug outside the body (such as urinary creatinine clearance) or by the rate of disappearance of drug from the circulation compared with the circulating concentration. For calculations, *clearance* (CL) is defined as the dose divided by the area under the plasma-concentration versus time curve (AUC) and by the rate of drug input per Css average, where rate of input is the dose/dosing interval ($\tau$) and Css is the steady-state concentration. For a drug administered by continuous infusion, this is simply the infusion rate (mg/kg)hr$^{-1}$ divided by Css as follows:

$$CL = \frac{\text{dose}}{\text{AUC}} = \frac{\text{dose}/\tau}{\text{Css}} = \frac{\text{infusion rate}}{\text{Css}}$$

Once clearance is known, this equation can be rearranged to solve for the dose necessary to achieve any desired steady state concentration, as

$$\begin{array}{ccccc} \text{Infusion rate} & = & \text{Css} & \cdot & \text{CL} \\ (\text{mg/kg})\text{hr}^{-1} & = & (\text{mg/L}) & & (\text{mL/kg})\text{hr}^{-1} \end{array}$$

Clearance changes significantly for some drugs during fetal and infant development because the activity of metabolic enzymes increases with advancing gestational and postnatal age. Values for clearance and volume of distribution at different stages of preterm development are available for a few drugs and can be used to estimate the dosages needed to achieve and maintain "therapeutic" concentrations associated with desired clinical responses.

Studies of the kinetics of fentanyl illustrate the developmental changes in its kinetics and how they may be used to calculate dosages to reach and maintain concentrations associated with effective analgesia. Analgesia has been associated with a serum fentanyl concentration of 1 to 2 ng/mL (Santeiro et al, 1997). If analgesic treatment is initiated with a continuous infusion of fentanyl, five half-lives are needed to reach a steady state. The fentanyl half-life ranges from 3 hours in term newborns to 12.7 hours in premature newborns (Koehntop et al, 1986; Santeiro et al, 1997). Because of this prolonged half-life, the patient may be inadequately treated for a long time, unless a loading dose is administered to reach an effective concentration more rapidly. In general, initiation of analgesic treatment and increases in infusion dosages of analgesics should begin with a loading dose based on the estimated volume of distribution in the central compartment (circulation) and desired concentration. Use of a loading dose shortens the time to reach higher effective analgesic concentrations but also increases the likelihood of toxicity, as has been reported with digoxin.

Limited data are available regarding the gestational age-related changes in fentanyl clearance, but two studies show that it increases with advancing gestational age (Koehntop et al, 1986; Santeiro et al, 1997) and with increasing age after birth (Gauntlett et al, 1988; Santeiro et al, 1997). The linear graph of clearance versus gestational age from 38 neonates who began treatment within 47 hours after birth was used to derive mean rates of clearance at different gestational ages as shown in Table 33–4.

Other investigators studied single-dose fentanyl kinetics during anesthesia and found an apparent central volume of distribution of fentanyl in neonates of 1.45 L/kg (Koehntop et al, 1986). Note that this distribution volume is smaller than the steady-state volume of distribution of 5.1 L/kg also calculated after a single dose of fentanyl (Koehntop et al, 1986). In turn, the apparent steady-state volume of distribution after a single bolus dose of a lipophilic drug is usually smaller than that associated with continuous drug infusions, during which tissues throughout the body become saturated with drug. The steady-state distribution volume for fentanyl during continuous infusions was calculated as 17 L/kg (Santeiro et al, 1997). It should be noted that because fentanyl is a lipid-soluble drug, it distributes rapidly from the central compartment into the peripheral tissue compartment. This much larger distribution volume likely reflects the period during the infusion when drug is leaving the circulation to penetrate peripheral tissues, such as fat. Because it may take 15 to 60 hours to achieve a steady-state concentration (5 half-lives) after a fentanyl infusion is begun or the infusion rate is increased, one may have to repeat the bolus dose in order to maintain effective plasma concentrations in the central compartment. The best approach is to repeat the calculated loading dose until the desired clinical effect is achieved. This also illustrates why, for sedation specifically, dosing should be adjusted to achieve the desired clinical effect. Clearance calculations, however, can guide the starting dosages to achieve effective sedation, as illustrated later.

The kinetic parameters for fentanyl in premature infants reported by Koehntop and associates (1986) can be used to calculate a loading and infusion dose to reach a fentanyl concentration of 2 ng/ml (Saarenmaa et al, 2000) in a premature at a gestational age of 33 weeks of (note that ng/ml is equivalent to μg/L) as

$$C\ (\mu g/L) = \frac{\text{load dose}\ (\mu g/kg)}{Vd_{central}\ (L/kg)}$$

$$\text{load dose}\ (\mu g/kg) = 2\ (\mu g/L) \cdot 1.45\ (L/kg)$$
$$= 2.9\ \mu g/kg$$

$$\text{infusion rate}\ (\mu g/kg \cdot hr) = C\ (\mu g/L) \cdot CL\ (mL/kg \cdot hr)$$
$$= 2\ \mu g/L \cdot 11.4\ mL/kg/min \cdot 1\ L/1000\ mL \cdot 60\ min/hr$$
$$= 1.4\ \mu g/kg \cdot hr$$

Two studies have observed rises in fentanyl clearance with increasing postnatal age (Gauntlett et al, 1988; Santeiro et al, 1997). This postnatal rise in clearance of fentanyl likely relates either to maturation of cytochrome P450 3A4 (the enzymes responsible for fentanyl metabolism) activity or to increased hepatic blood flow after birth, because fentanyl has a high hepatic extraction rate. For drugs, like fentanyl, with a high hepatic extraction ratio, the rate-limiting factor in clearance is the flow of blood to the liver (Saarenmaa et al, 2000). Some researchers have observed that increased intra-abdominal pressure reduces fentanyl clearance, a finding that is likely to be a consequence of reduced hepatic blood flow (Gauntlett et al, 1988; Koehntop et al, 1986). Clinical changes known to increase or decrease fentanyl clearance should be used to adjust starting dosages, but dosing should be adjusted primarily for the desired clinical effect.

**TABLE 33–4**

**Fentanyl Development Kinetics**

| Gestational Age (wk) | Clearance at 0-47 hours after birth (mL/[min · kg]) |
|---|---|
| 29 | 9.6 |
| 33 | 11.4 |
| 37 | 13.2 |
| 41 | 15.0 |

Data from Saarenmaa E, Neuvonen PJ, Fellman V: Gestational age and birth weight defects of plasma clearance of fentanyl in newborn infants. J Pediatr 136:67, 2000.

## PHARMACOKINETIC PRACTICALITIES

### Dose Adjustments

Gentamicin and phenobarbital can be used to illustrate the practical application of the principles of pharmacokinetics and therapeutic drug monitoring already discussed. The calculations may be carried out at the bedside with standard arithmetic calculators.

#### Gentamicin

Assume that optimal gentamicin concentrations are

$$\text{Peak} = 6\text{-}10\ \mu g/mL$$
$$\text{Trough} = 0.5\text{-}2\ \mu g/mL$$

Gentamicin peak concentration was 5.0 μg/mL; 18 hours later, the trough was 2.5 μg/mL after the fourth 2.5 mg/kg dose was administered intravenously to an edematous premature newborn. It is apparent that the distribution volume is greater than predicted because the peak concentration is lower than anticipated, and the half-life is longer than anticipated because the trough is higher than expected. The times of drug infusion and blood sampling were confirmed (an important step), so the half-life is 18 hours, because the concentration decreases 50% from 5.0 to 2.5 μg/mL in 18 hours. (This assumes that the kinetics are linear and first-order.)

$$\begin{aligned} \text{Vd (mL/kg)} &= \frac{\text{Dose (mg/kg)}}{\Delta\text{C } (\mu\text{g/mL}) \cdot 1 \text{ mg}/1000\ \mu\text{g}} \\ &= \frac{2.5 \text{ mg/kg} \cdot 1000\ \mu\text{g/mg}}{(5.0 - 2.5)\ (\mu\text{g/mL})} \\ &= 1000 \text{ mL/kg} \end{aligned}$$

To ensure a trough concentration of 2.0 μg/mL or less, doses are administered every two half-lives or every 36 hours. When two half-lives have passed after the fourth dose, the gentamicin concentration should be about 1.25 μg/mL (50% of 2.5 μg/mL). Increasing the concentration from the 1.25 μg/mL trough to >6 μg/mL requires a concentration difference of ≥4.75 μg/mL. With a distribution volume of 1000 mL/kg, a dose of 4.75 mg/kg should raise the concentration from a trough of 1.25 μg/mL to a peak of 6.00 μg/mL. In one half-life, this concentration will decrease to 3.0 μg/mL, and in two half-lives or 36 hours, to 1.5 μg/mL. Another 4.75-mg/kg dose will raise the peak concentration to 6.25 μg/mL, which will fall to 3.12 μg/mL in one half-life and to 1.6 μg/mL in two half-lives. The variation between the peak and trough concentrations after the last dose is within the measurement error for gentamicin and should achieve the optimum concentrations defined previously.

### Phenobarbital

Seizures that were hard to control developed in a 3.6-kg asphyxiated newborn. Seizures continued after two 20 mg/kg phenobarbital doses until an additional 10 mg/kg dose was administered. A maintenance dose of 7 mg/kg per day was started 24 hours after the loading doses were administered. At 10 days, this child was increasingly somnolent. The phenobarbital level measured in a blood specimen drawn 2 hours after administration of the oral maintenance dose was 50 μg/mL. Additional doses were withheld, and the phenobarbital concentration was checked daily; the results were as follows:

- 24 hours: 40 μg/mL
- 48 hours: 31 μg/mL
- 72 hours: 25 μg/mL
- 96 hours: 21 μg/mL

The maintenance dose (7 mg/kg) was resumed immediately after the 21 μg/mL concentration was measured and produced a concentration of 30 μg/mL. These concentrations and dosages can be used to calculate the volume of distribution and a dose to maintain the phenobarbital concentration between 20 and 30 μg/mL as

$$\begin{aligned} \text{Vd (L/kg)} &= \frac{\text{Dose (mg/kg)}}{\Delta\text{C } (\mu\text{g/mL} = \text{mg/L})} \\ &= \frac{7.0 \text{ (mg/kg)}}{(30 - 21) \text{ (mg/L)}} \\ &= \frac{7 \text{ (mg/kg)}}{9 \text{ (mg/L)}} \\ &= 0.78 \text{ L/kg} \end{aligned}$$

Half-life can be determined from inspection, because the concentration decreased from 50 to 25 μg/mL in 72 hours. Thus, it should take 72 hours for the concentration to decrease by one half-life from 30 to 15 μg/mL. The concentration will decrease approximately 5 μg/mL every 24 hours, or one third of a half-life. Dividing the half-life into fractions is an approximation because it estimates the change in concentration as linear rather than exponential. To be more accurate, the concentration decreases 59% in half of one half-life. Although this approximation violates certain principles of pharmacokinetics, it allows estimation of the change in concentration for each one third of a half-life as one third of the change during one half-life. Thus, the concentration decreases about 5 μg/mL in 24 hours. The following approach can be used to estimate the daily phenobarbital dose needed to return the concentration to 30 μg/mL, a change in concentration of 5 μg/mL:

$$\begin{aligned} \Delta\text{C (mg/L)} &= \frac{\text{Dose (mg/kg)}}{\text{Vd (L/kg)}} \\ 5 \text{ (mg/L)} &= \frac{\text{Dose (mg/kg)}}{(0.78) \text{ (L/kg)}} \\ 3.6 \text{ mg/kg} &= \text{Dose (mg/kg)} \end{aligned}$$

## DRUG EXCRETION IN BREAST MILK

The excretion of drugs in breast milk remains a source of confusion and concern for many physicians and families. Newer analytic techniques and more thorough pharmacokinetic studies have improved the available data in this area of neonatal pharmacology. The available data regarding drug exposure of the newborn through human milk have been organized, in decreasing levels of concern, from drugs that are associated with adverse effects on the infant during nursing to those that are of concern pharmacologically to those that have not been associated with problems during nursing. The list of drugs clearly contraindicated during nursing is surprisingly short (AAP, 2001).

## SUMMARY

The extensive drug exposure of the sick newborn in the NICU is dangerous because of the frequency of adverse, sometimes fatal, drug reactions. Unfortunately, in the rapidly changing fetus and newborn, drug therapy is often empiric owing to a lack of gestational age–appropriate kinetic data. Methods appropriate for the study of therapeutics in newborns present unique difficulties, but a review by Ward and Green (1988) may provide assistance for investigators. Drug therapy of newborns requires practical application of the principles of pharmacokinetics and pharmacodynamics—which describe the processes of drug absorption, distribution, metabolism, and excretion—to the estimation and individualization of dosages.

## REFERENCES

American Academy of Pediatrics, Committee on Drugs: The transfer of drugs and other chemicals into human breast milk. Pediatrics 108:776, 2001.

ASHP: Understanding and preventing drug misadventures. Proceedings of a conference. Chantilly, Virginia, October 21-23, 1994. Am J Health Syst Pharm 52:369, 1995.
ASHP guidelines on preventing medication errors in hospitals. Am J Hosp Pharm 50:305, 1993.
Aperia A, Broberger O, Elinder G, et al: Postnatal development of renal function in pre-term and full-term infants. Acta Paediatr Scand 70:183, 1981.
Aranda JV, Cohen S, Neims AH: Drug utilization in a newborn intensive care unit. J Pediatr 89:315, 1976.
Aranda JV, Collinge JM, Clarkson S: Epidemiologic aspects of drug utilization in a newborn intensive care unit. Semin Perinatol 6:148, 1982a.
Aranda JV, Portuguez-Malavasi A, Collinge JM, et al: Epidemiology of adverse drug reactions in the newborn. Dev Pharmacol Ther 5:173, 1982b.
Aranda JV: Factors associated with adverse drug reactions in the newborn. Pediatr Pharmacol 3:245, 1983.
Boreus LO: Principles of Pediatric Pharmacology. New York, Churchill Livingstone, 1982.
Burns LE, Hodgman JE, Cass AB: Fatal circulatory collapse in premature infants receiving chloramphenicol. N Engl J Med 261:1318, 1959.
Gauntlett IS, Fisher DM, Hertzka RE, et al: Pharmacokinetics of fentanyl in neonatal humans and lambs: Effects of age. Anesthesiology 69:683, 1988.
Gibaldi M, Perrier D: Pharmacokinetics, 2nd ed. New York, Marcel Dekker, 1982.
Gould T, Roberts RJ: Therapeutic problems arising from the use of the intravenous route for drug administration. J Pediatr 95:465, 1979.
Greenblatt DJ, Koch-Weser J: Clinical pharmacokinetics (First of two parts). N Engl J Med 293:702, 1975a.
Greenblatt DJ, Koch-Weser J: Clinical pharmacokinetics (Second of two parts). N Engl J Med 293:964, 1975b.
Kauffman RE: The clinical interpretation and application of drug concentration data. Pediatr Clin North Am 28:35, 1981.
Koehntop DE, Rodman JH, Brundage DM, et al: Pharmacokinetics of continuous infusion of fentanyl in neonates. Anesth Analg 65:227, 1986.
McCracken GH: Aminoglycoside toxicity in infants and children. Am J Med 80(Suppl 6B):172, 1986.
Mirkin BL: Pharmacodynamics and drug disposition in pregnant women, in neonates, and in children. In Melmon KL, Morrelli HF (eds): Clinical Pharmacology: Basic Principles in Therapeutics, 2nd ed. New York, Macmillan, 1978, p 127.
Morselli PL, Franco-Morselli R, Bossi L: Clinical pharmacokinetics in newborns and infants: Age-related differences and therapeutic implications. Clin Pharmacokinet 5:485, 1980.
Notari RE: Biopharmaceutics and Clinical Pharmacokinetics, 3rd ed. New York, Marcel Dekker, 1980.
Peterson RG, Simmons MA, Rumack BH, et al: Pharmacology of furosemide in the premature newborn infant. J Pediatr 97:139, 1980.
Physician Insurers Association of America: Medication Error Study. Washington, DC, June 1993.
Roberts RJ: Drug Therapy in Infants: Pharmacologic Principles and Clinical Experience. Philadelphia, WB Saunders, 1984, p 3.
Saarenmaa E, Neuvonen PJ, Fellman V: Gestational age and girth weight effects on plasma clearance of fentanyl in newborn infants. J Pediatr 136:67, 2000.
Santeiro ML, Christie J, Stromquist C, et al: Pharmacokinetics of continuous infusion of fentanyl in newborns. J Perinatol 17:135, 1997.
Sheiner LB, Tozer TN: Clinical pharmacokinetics: The use of plasma concentrations of drugs. In Melmon KL, Morrelli HF (eds): Clinical Pharmacology: Basic Principles in Therapeutics, 2nd ed. New York, Macmillan, 1978, p 71.
Spector R, Park GD, Johnson GF, et al: Therapeutic drug monitoring. Clin Pharmacol Ther 43:345, 1988.
Sutherland JM: Fatal cardiovascular collapse, of infants receiving large amounts of chloramphenicol. J Dis Child 13:761, 1959.
Ward RM, Singh S, Mirkin BL: Fetal clinical pharmacology. In Avery GS (Ed): Drug Treatment: Principles and Practice of Clinical Pharmacology and Therapeutics, 2nd ed. New York, Adis Press, 1980, p 76.
Ward RM, Green TP: Developmental pharmacology and toxicology: Principles of study design and problems of methodology. Pharmacol Ther 36:309, 1988.
Weiss CF, Glazko AJ, Weston JK: Chloramphenicol in the newborn infant: A physiologic explanation of its toxicity when given in excessive doses. N Engl J Med 262:787, 1960.

CHAPTER

# 34

# Neonatal Pain Management in the 21st Century

**Theresa J. Di Maggio and Mary Ann E. Gibbons**

In the last decade of the 20th century, the pool of resources and information available to support medical and surgical teams in neonatal pain management has expanded rapidly. Concurrently, the U.S. Department of Health and Human Services and the Joint Commission on Accreditation of Healthcare Organizations (JCAHO) have partnered with various professional organizations and mandated health care providers to look across the continuum of life at the complex nature of the pain experience so as to create new foundations for care. Organizations have commissioned interdisciplinary teams to incorporate regulatory directives and results of scientific investigation into institutional practice guidelines and standards for care. These guidelines include a patient's right to regular and systematic assessments of pain, interventions to relieve pain, evaluation of effectiveness of interventions, attention to long-term pain management needs, deleterious effects of unmanaged pain, and educational needs of families and staff who provide care (American Pain Society, 2001; Bell, 1994; Carrier and Walden, 2001; Joint Commission on Accreditation of Healthcare Organizations [JACHO], 2004).

Despite these initiatives, surveys of physicians and nurses continue to suggest that pain in the neonatal population is underassessed and undermanaged (Anand et al, 1996; Franck, 1987; Porter et al, 1997). Several investigations have substantiated the effectiveness of analgesia and comfort measures in attenuating acute pain responses and promoting long-term development; yet routine use of medications and comfort measures during performance of treatments remains inadequate in most NICUs (Anand et al, 1999; Fitzgerald et al, 1989; Guinsburg et al, 1998; Pokela, 1994). Concern about results of these studies is compounded by reports that infants born at 27 to 31 weeks of gestation may experience as many as 134 painful procedures in the first 2 weeks of life (Stevens et al, 1999a).

Finally, research and investigation have cautioned caregivers about the consequences of untreated and unmanaged pain. Several researchers have linked the stress induced by the pain response to the secondary development of adverse sequelae in multiple organ systems. Acute effects include elevations of cortisol, catecholamines, and lactate, hypertension, tachycardia, respiratory instability, glucose instability, and changes in cerebral blood flow. Chronic pain may affect growth, immune function, recovery, and discharge. In addition, a growing body of evidence has drawn attention to the potential deleterious effects of "growing up in a NICU environment," and the impact of repeated handling, stress, and pain on long-term memory, social and cognitive development, and neural plasticity (Anand, 1998; Anand et al, 1987, 1989; Evans, 2001; Fitzgerald et al, 1989; Pokela, 1994; Porter et al, 1999; Taddio et al, 1995a).

## COMPLEXITIES OF EFFECTIVE PAIN ASSESSMENT IN INFANTS

The broad spectrum of challenges to overcome the quest for effective pain management for the neonatal population cannot be underestimated. Despite efforts to dispel old myths about pain perception and safe, effective management strategies, remnants of conventional beliefs continue to interfere with progress in this area. To ensure that pain is managed reasonably and ethically, caregivers must be educated about infant pain physiology, neural development, and the differences in response patterns of term and preterm infants (Franck, 1997).

By 20 weeks of gestation, the fetus is served by a highly differentiated and fully functional sensory system. At this time, the pain experience is a dynamic process that links the nervous system to organ systems throughout the body, producing complex, measurable responses within those organ systems when stimulated. Pain perception may be more intense than in the adult, for several reasons. The large number of nociceptive nerve endings in the skin and mucous membranes of the fetus far exceed that in adults (Anand et al, 1987). Ascending pathways between the peripheral nervous system (PNS) and the spinal cord are rich in excitatory neurotransmitters, which potentiate pain transmission, but poor in mediating neurotransmitters, which blunt the pain response.

Although development of the complex structures of the central nervous system (CNS) parallels that in the PNS and a vast supply of neurons purveys the cortex itself, differentiation of structure and function in the cortex is a slower process and compromises preterm infants' ability to integrate and assimilate pain information (Anand et al, 1987, 1989). Their response patterns, both physiologic and behavioral, are less organized, less robust, less coordinated, and more difficult to interpret. They may become more easily disorganized with stress or may adapt to pain more readily. As many as 50% of premature infants do not exhibit crying behaviors during painful procedures (Evans et al, 1997; Johnston et al, 1993, 1995, 1999). Studies have also demonstrated that with repeated exposure to painful procedures, infants may lose the ability to distinguish between painful and nonpainful stimuli and maintain hypersensitive states for protracted periods of time. This hypersensitivity persists even if non-noxious stimuli are introduced (Evans, 2001; Fitzgerald et al, 1989). In addition, local tissue injury resulting from repeated heelsticks and invasive procedures trigger increased proliferation of nerve endings in surrounding tissues, particularly when this damage occurs early in gestation. As a result scars, old IV sites and surrounding tissues may remain hypersensitive well beyond the neonatal period (Fitzgerald et al, 1989; Reynolds and Fitzgerald, 1995). Pain assessment is most challenging in preterm infants who are exposed to the NICU environment for long periods (Johnston and Stevens, 1996).

## NEONATAL PAIN SCORING TOOLS

A review of current literature substantiates the importance of selecting a valid, reliable, and clinically useful pain scoring tool that is easily implemented at the bedside and allows for consistency in use and interpretation as part of clinical care. Caregivers are urged to keep in mind that the focus of these scoring tools is assessment of procedural pain, and their use may leave gaps in effective assessment for infants who are paralyzed, asphyxiated, or experiencing chronic pain. In addition, discriminating between pain and distress or agitation in the neonate is difficult, and a trial of therapies, both pharmacologic and nonpharmacologic, may occasionally be helpful. Assessments should be initiated on admission and then performed at regular intervals throughout the infant's hospitalization (JCAHO, 1999).

Scoring tools may use a unidimensional approach (e.g., The Neonatal Facial Coding System; Grunau et al, 1998), in which one specific behavior or group of related behaviors is evaluated, or a multidimensional approach (e.g., Neonatal Infant Pain Scale [*NIPS*]; Lawrence et al, 1993) in which complex behavioral and physiologic information is assessed simultaneously. With all gestational age groups, cry has been identified as the least reliable indicator of pain, and changes in facial expression, such as brow bulge, eye squeeze, nasolabial furrow, taut lips, and open mouth, as the most reliable (Grunau and Craig, 1987; Guinsburg et al, 1997; Stevens et al, 1993). Because of the complex nature of the pain experience, the infant's limited cognitive abilities, and the various ways that changes in physiologic parameters can be interpreted, the current recommendation has been to approach pain assessment with a multidimensional scoring tool. Such a tool adequately captures changes in both behavioral and physiologic domains (APS, 2001; Craig et al, 1993; Franck et al, 2000). A variety of pain scoring tools are available for use in the neonatal population. A few multidimensional tools that have been well studied and used extensively in the neonatal population are reviewed here.

The *CRIES* scoring system was established as a neonatal postoperative pain scoring tool and has been proven to be both clinically reliable and valid (Krechel and Bildner, 1995) (Table 34–1). CRIES is an acronym for an assessment approach that is comprised of five indicators, three behavioral and two physiologic. Each indicator is evaluated on a scale of 0 to 3. The total score ranges from 0 to 10, with a score of 4 or higher indicating pain. Although initially established as a tool to assess postoperative pain, CRIES has been useful in the broader range of neonates and is now widely used clinically.

The *Premature Infant Pain Scoring Tool* (*PIPP*) is a seven-indicator, multidimensional tool originally developed to assess acute pain in term and preterm infants (Stevens et al, 1996) (Table 34–2). Scoring with the PIPP is unique, in that special consideration is given to the infant's gestational age in addition to physiologic and behavioral indices. Each indicator is evaluated on a scale of 1 to 4, with a total score range of 21 for more premature infants and 18 for term and older infants. Given the complexities of pain appreciation and interpretation in premature infants, this tool may provide more accurate assessment and effective management for this group of patients. It is also the most tested neonatal pain scoring tool available. Because of its focus on acute pain experiences, additional study is needed with regard to its application to postoperative and more chronic pain situations.

The *Distress Scale for Ventilated Newborn Infants* (*DSVNI*) is another multidimensionsal, procedure-focused scoring tool that has been designed specifically for assessment of the ventilated infant (Sparshott, 1996). Although the CRIES and PIPP can be used in the ventilated population, their use does require the observer to make more subjective assessments about cry and changes in facial expression,

**TABLE 34–1**

**CRIES: Neonatal Postoperative Pain Assessment Score**

| | Scoring Criteria | | |
|---|---|---|---|
| **Indicator** | **0** | **1** | **2** |
| Crying | No cry, or cry not high pitched | High-pitched cry, but consolable | High-pitched cry, inconsolable |
| Requires oxygen for saturation >95% | No oxygen required from baseline | Oxygen requirement <30% from baseline | Oxygen requirement >30% from baseline |
| Increased vital signs[*] | Heart rate and blood pressure are both unchanged or at less than baseline | Heart rate or blood pressure is increased by <20% | Heart rate or blood pressure is increased by >20% |
| Expression[†] | None (no grimace) | Grimace only is present | Grimace and nonaudible grunt present |
| Sleeplessness[‡] | Continuously asleep | Awakens at frequent intervals | Awake constantly |

[*] Measure blood pressure last so as not to awaken infant.

[†] Grimace consists of lowered brow, eyes squeezed shut, deepening nasolabial furrow, and open lips and mouth.

[‡] Based on infant's state during preceding hour.

Adapted from Bildner J, Krechel S: Increasing staff nurse awareness of postoperative pain management in the NICU. Neonatal Netw 15:11-16, 1996. © S. Krechel, MD, and J. Bildner, RNC CHS. (Developed at University of Missouri–Columbia.)

TABLE 34–2

**Premature Infant Pain Profile (PIPP)**

| Process | Indicator | Description of Score 0 | 1 | 2 | 3 | Score |
|---|---|---|---|---|---|---|
| Chart | Gestational age | ≥36 wks | 32 wks-35 wks 6 days | 28 wks-31 wks 6 days | ≤28 wks | — |
| Score 15 seconds before event | Behavioral state | Active/ awake Eyes open Facial movements | Quite/ awake Eyes open No facial movements | Active/ sleep Eyes closed Facial movements | Quiet/ sleep Eyes closed No facial movements | — |
| Record baseline heart rate (—): Observe infant 30 seconds after event | Maximum heart rate | 0-4 beats/min increase | 5-14 beats/min increase | 15-24 beats/min increase | ≥25 beats/min increase | — |
| Record baseline oxygen saturation (—): | Minimum oxygen saturation | 0-2.4% decrease | 2.5%-4.9% decrease | 5%-7.4% decrease | ≥7.5% or decrease | — |
| Observe infant 30 seconds after event | Brow bulge | None (0-9% of time) | Minimum (10%-39% of time) | Moderate (40%-69% of time) | Maximum (≥70% of time) | — |
| Observe infant 30 seconds after event | Eye squeeze | None (0-9% of time) | Minimum (10%-39% of time) | Moderate (40%-69% of time) | Maximum (≥70% of time) | — |
| Observe infant 30 seconds after event | Nasolabial furrow | None (0-9% of time) | Minimum (10%-39% of time) | Moderate (40%-69% of time) | Maximum (≥70% of time) | — |
| **Total score** | | | | | | — |

*Scoring guidelines*:
1. Score the corrected gestational age before beginning.
2. Assess baseline heart rate and oxygen saturation:
   a. For procedural pain, assess before the event.
   b. If pain is already present, review the chart for earlier baseline.
3. Score behavioral state by observing the infant for 15 seconds immediately before the event.
4. Observe the infant for 30 seconds immediately after the event.

Adapted from Stevens B, Johnson C, Petryshen P, Taddio A: Premature infant pain profile: Development and initial evaluation. Clin J Pain 12:13-22, 1996.

because view of the infant may be obscured by an artificial airway. The DSVNI is more detailed and complex, but it may be more helpful in infants with special assessment needs.

## MANAGEMENT OF PAIN IN INFANTS

Effective pain management is a systematic approach that combines judicious use of pharmacologic and nonpharmacologic interventions. Because pain expression can be influenced by multiple contextual factors, management strategies should be comprehensive and should include the following aspects (Walden, 2001; Franck et al, 2001):

- Decrease in the number of painful interventions and noxious stimuli that infants are exposed to as part of bedside care
- Minimization of handling before invasive procedures
- Performance of procedures when the infant's state is most protective
- Timing of medication administration around necessary interventions
- Optimization of skill levels of staff performing procedures
- Use of an interdisciplinary team to evaluate the effectiveness of interventions
- Listening to family assessments and suggestions

### Nonpharmacologic Interventions

The complimentary effects of nonpharmacologic interventions have been well described in the literature. Additional information about various therapeutic modalities, including alternative therapies, massage, and music, are available on the selected reading list. A few of the more research-based interventions are discussed here.

#### Developmental Care

Als and colleagues (1994) reported the positive effects of an individualized, developmentally supportive approach to care of the preterm neonate. Review of current literature universally supports integration of this philosophy into pain management plans. This approach emphasizes the importance of assessing the individual strengths and limitations of an infant's development and then incorporating these cues into a caregiving approach that supports the infant at rest and protects the infant when handled. Highlights include protection from environmental stressors, promotion of self-regulatory behaviors, support during stressful interventions, and gentle, supportive handling. Suggested benefits include earlier time to extubation, earlier progression to oral feeds, better developmental outcomes, shorter time to discharge, and reduced hospital cost; however, these interventions have never been tested in a randomized, controlled fashion.

### Sucrose Pacifiers

Research-based evidence supports the use of single-dose sucrose as nonpharmacologic pain intervention in term and preterm infants (Stevens et al, 2000). Meta-analysis of four studies confirmed that a single dose of sucrose administered orally can reduce the time infants spend crying after completion of a painful procedure; this effect is thought to be mediated by the endogenous release of opioids stimulated by the sweet taste. Consensus has not been reached regarding dosage and method of administration. Beneficial effects have been documented in preterm infants after oral administration of 2 mL of 12% to 25% dextrose solution 2 minutes before painful procedures as well as with pacifiers dipped in 24% sucrose solutions and administered 2 and 5 minutes prior to painful procedures. Some concern has been raised about the potential for increased risk of necrotizing enterocolitis as a result of repeated administration of hyperosmolar dextrose solutions to the premature gut. Although no adverse effects were reported for use of the approaches in these studies, caregivers are urged to review the corresponding literature before incorporating this approach into guidelines for pain management practice.

### Positioning

Supportive positioning and containment have been effective in reducing procedural distress and promoting self-regulation (Porter et al, 1998). Facilitated tucking, a technique in which caregivers use their own hands to contain an infant's limbs close to the trunk, has also been shown to reduce pain responses in preterm infants (Corff et al, 1995) and can be used regularly throughout the course of bedside care.

## Pharmacologic Interventions

The severity of the pain, etiology, available administration routes, and consideration of potential side effects should all be evaluated for selection of an analgesic. Once medication administration has begun, careful monitoring for side effects can decrease potential adverse events related to administration of pain medications to infants. A key component of effective pain management is reassessment after a pain intervention. Evaluating the success or failure of a pain intervention and the need for modification of the pain regimen is essential.

### Nonopioid Analgesics

#### *Acetaminophen*

Acetaminophen is the most widely administered analgesic in patients of all ages. Acetaminophen inhibits the production of cyclooxygenase in the central nervous system and peripherally blocks pain impulse generation (Arana et al, 2001). Neonates are able to form the metabolite that results in hepatocellular damage (Arana et al, 2001); however, it is inappropriate to withhold acetaminophen in newborns because of concerns of liver toxicity. The immaturity of the newborn's cytochrome P-450 system may actually decrease the potential for toxicity by reducing production of toxic metabolites (Collins, 1981).

Current recommendations are for less frequent oral dosing, every 8 to 12 hours in preterm and term neonates, because of slower clearance times, and higher rectal dosing due to decreased absorption (Arana et al, 2001; van Lingen et al, 1999). Typical oral dosages for acetaminophen are 10 to 15 mg/kg/dose every 6 to 8 hours for neonates and 10 to 15 mg/kg/dose every 4 to 6 hours for infants. Administering 10 mg/kg may be inadequate for pain control as this dose is based on antipyretic dose-response studies. The maximum dose is 75 mg/kg/24 hours for infants, 60 mg/kg/24 hours for term and preterm neonates more than 32 weeks of postconceptual age, and 40 mg/kg/24 hours for preterm neonates 28 to 32 weeks of postconceptual age (Berde, 2002).

Rectally administered acetaminophen has a longer half-life, but absorption is highly variable because it depends on the individual infant and placement of the suppository. It should also be noted that the suppository may contain all of the drug in the tip and therefore should be divided lengthwise if a partial dose is desired. The analgesic effect of acetaminophen is additive when the agent is administered with opioids; this co-administration may enable a decrease in the opioid dose and therefore in corresponding opioid side effects.

#### *Nonsteroidal Anti-inflammatory Drugs*

Nonsteroidal anti-inflammatory drugs (NSAIDs) inhibit prostaglandin synthesis by inhibiting the action of cyclooxygenase. Cyclooxygenase enzymes are responsible for the breakdown of arachidonic acid to prostaglandins. NSAIDS have significant adverse effects, including decreased glomerular filtration rate and platelet dysfunction. These adverse effects are particularly worrisome for neonates and infants. NSAIDS are not generally recommended in neonates because of concerns about intestinal perfusion.

#### *Indomethacin*

Indomethacin has been widely used to promote closure of the patent ductus arteriosus (PDA) (Chapter 56) and also to prevent intraventricular hemorrhage (see also Chapter 64).

### Opioid Analgesics

Opioids provide the most effective treatment for moderate to severe pain in patients of all ages. There is a wide range of interpatient pharmacokinetic variability. Opioid dosing depends on the severity of the pain as well as the age and clinical condition of the infant. Opioids should be used in infants younger than 2 months only in a monitored setting such as an intensive or intermediate care unit (Yaster et al, 2003). Some clinicians propose a more conservative recommendation, restricting use of opioids to monitored settings for any infant younger than 6 months.

### *Morphine*

Morphine, the "gold standard" for pain management, is widely used in neonates. In older children and adults, morphine is metabolized in the liver and forms an active metabolite, morphine-6-glucuronide (M6G), and a second metabolite, morphine-3-glucuronide, that may be antianalgesic under some circumstances. However, little is known about the relative concentration of these metabolites in preterm infants. There is a potential for late respiratory depression due to a delayed release of morphine from less well perfused tissues and the sedating properties of the metabolite M6G (Anand et al, 2000).

Clearance or elimination of morphine and other opioids is prolonged in infants owing to the immaturity of the cytochrome P-450 system at birth. Hepatic function reaches adult levels at 1 or 2 months of age. The rate of elimination and clearance of morphine in infants 2 months and older is similar to that in adults. Chronologic age seems a better indicator than gestational age of how an infant metabolizes opioids (Scott et al, 1999; Yaster et al, 2003).

Infants are at greater risk of respiratory depression because of their immature responses to hypoxia and hypercarbia. There is an increase in unbound or free morphine available to reach the brain as a result of the reduced concentration of albumin and alpha$_1$ acid glycoproteins (Houck, 1998).

Hypotension, bradycardia, and flushing constitute the response to the histamine release and rapid intravenous administration of morphine. Histamine release may cause bronchospasm in infants with chronic lung disease, although this is not commonly seen (Anand et al, 2000).

There is a wide range of interpatient pharmacokinetic variability. For nonventilated infants, the initial opioid dose is approximately one fourth to one third the recommended dose for older children. For example, 0.03 mg/kg of morphine IV can be used as a starting dose (AHCPR, 1992). For ventilated infants, 0.05 to 0.1 mg/kg of morphine IV is an appropriate starting dose. Titration to the desired clinical effect is required in adjusting both the dose and the frequency of administration.

### *Fentanyl*

Fentanyl is 80 to 100 times more potent than morphine. Fentanyl causes less histamine release than morphine, making it a more appropriate choice for infants with hypovolemia, hemodynamic instability, or congenital heart disease. Another potential clinical advantage of fentanyl is its ability to reduce pulmonary vascular resistance, which can be of benefit for infants who have undergone cardiac surgery, have persistent pulmonary hypertension, or need extracorporeal membrane oxygenation (Anand et al, 2000). Fentanyl must be administered over a minimum of 3 to 5 minutes to avoid chest wall rigidity, a serious side effect observed after rapid infusion. Chest wall rigidity, which can result in difficulty or inability to ventilate, can be treated with naloxone or a muscle relaxant such as pancuronium or vecuronium.

Fentanyl is highly lipophilic. It has a quick onset and relative short duration of action. Owing to fentanyl's short duration of action, it is typically used as a continuous infusion for postoperative pain. In infants 3 to 12 months of age, total body clearance of fentanyl is greater than that of older children, and the elimination half-life is longer owing to its increased volume of distribution (Singleton et al, 1987). Fentanyl has been demonstrated to have a prolonged elimination half-life in infants with increased abdominal pressure (Gauntlett et al, 1988; Koehntop et al, 1986).

A rebound transient increase in plasma fentanyl levels is a phenomenon known to occur after discontinuation of therapy in neonates. It is a result of fentanyl's accumulation in fatty tissues, which may prolong its effects after continued use. Therefore, caution must be exercised in the use of repeated doses or a continuous infusion.

### Oral Opioids

Oral methadone can be used to wean infants from long-term opioid use. Methadone is widely used in neonates and children, although there are limited data on its efficacy and pharmacokinetics in this population (Chana and Anand, 2001; Suresh and Anand, 1998). The respiratory depressant effect of methadone is longer than its analgesic effect. Methadone is metabolized very slowly, and its half-life is very long.

Codeine is prescribed at 0.5 mg to 1 mg/kg orally every 4 hours as needed. Most pharmacies supply acetaminophen and codeine in a set formula, consisting of acetaminophen 120 mg and codeine phosphate 12 mg per 5 ml with alcohol 7%. The dose prescribed is limited by both the appropriate dose of codeine and the safe dose of acetaminophen.

Oxycodone dosing is 0.05 mg/kg to 0.15 mg/kg orally every 4 to 6 hours as needed. The liquid form is not universally available.

### Mixed Agonist-Antagonist Drug

Nalbuphine is a mixed agonist-antagonist drug; therefore its administration to infants of opioid-addicted mothers may precipitate withdrawal. This agent is equianalgesic with morphine. Nalbuphine has a ceiling effect for analgesia. Additional studies are needed on the safety and efficacy of nalbuphine use in infants.

### Sedatives-Benzodiazepines

Sedatives-benzodiazepines should not be used in place of an appropriate pain medication as this class of medication has no analgesic effect. Benzodiazepines are administered to decrease irritability and agitation in infants and to provide sedation for procedures. In ventilated infants, benzodiazepines can help avoid hypoxia and hypercarbia from breathing out of "sync" with the ventilator. For painful procedures, an analgesic must be used in conjunction with the benzodiazepine.

### Topical Anesthetics

#### *EMLA Cream*

For infants 37 weeks of gestation and older, EMLA (eutectic mixture of local anesthetics) cream to desired area and then cover with an occlusive dressing for 1 hour before the procedure. Longer application times provide deeper local anesthetic penetration but may potentially lead to toxicity. There is a slight risk of methemoglobinemia with use of EMLA cream in infants and G6PD-deficient patients. A rare occurrence, methemoglobinemia can occur when hemoglobin is oxidized by exposure to prilocaine. EMLA should not be used in patients with methemoglobinemia or infants younger than 12 months who are also receiving methemoglobinemia-inducing drugs, such as acetaminophen, sulfonamides, nitrates, phenytoin, and class I antiarrhythmics. (Refer to Table 34–3 recommended maximum doses of EMLA cream by age and weight) A study of 30 preterm infants found that a single 0.5-g dose of EMLA applied for 1 hour did not lead to a measurable change in methemoglobin levels (Taddio et al, 1995b).

## Procedural Pain

Some invasive procedures are obviously considered painful. Routine care performed in a neonatal unit, such as diaper changing and bathing, may not typically be thought of as painful but can be distressing to the neonate as indicated by changes in oxygen saturation and heart rate. Nonpharmacologic treatment should be routinely employed for stressful procedures, and pharmacologic treatment should be used for painful procedures. Infants are beginning to receive adequate pain management for postoperative pain, but unfortunately, little progress has been made in managing procedural pain for such patients.

## Circumcision

The Circumcision Policy Statement of the American Academy of Pediatrics (AAP) states that analgesia must be provided to infants undergoing circumcisions. EMLA cream, dorsal penile nerve block, and subcutaneous ring block are all possible options. AAP reports that subcutaneous ring block may provide the best analgesia (Circumcision, 1999).

Subcutaneous ring block has been found to be more effective than EMLA or dorsal penile nerve block in other studies (Lander et al, 1997). Dorsal penile nerve block has been found to be more effective than EMLA, but this method is not always available (Lee and Forrester, 1992).

EMLA has been established as superior to placebo for pain relief during circumcision (Bennini, 1993; Taddio, 1997). An effective method for applying EMLA in preparation for circumcision is to apply one third of the dose to the lower abdomen, extend the penis upward gently, pressing it against the abdomen, and then apply the remainder of the dose to an occlusive dressing placed over the penis. This dressing is then taped to the abdomen so the cream surrounds the penis. Another method is to apply the cream and then place plastic wrap (Saran Wrap) around the penis in a tubelike fashion to help direct the urine stream out and away from the cream.

Acetaminophen is ineffective for the management of severe pain associated with the circumcision procedure but does provide some analgesia in the postoperative period. Acetaminophen has been found to decrease pain 6 hours after circumcision (Howard et al, 1994).

## Blood Sampling and Monitoring

Heelsticks are routinely performed to obtain blood samples in neonates. The most appropriate method for relieving pain from a heelstick is yet to be determined. Heels should be warmed to aid blood sampling. EMLA does not relieve the pain of a heel lance (Stevens et al, 1999b; Taddio et al, 1998). Shah and colleagues (1997) demonstrated that neonates experiencing venipuncture had lower pain scores than those who underwent heelstick for blood sampling. In healthy neonates, venipuncture should be used preferentially over heelstick.

The pain of arterial puncture can be decreased by infiltrating around the site with 0.1 to 0.2 mL of 0.5 or 1% lidocaine using the smallest-gauge needle possible (Franck and Gregory, 1993). Buffering the lidocaine with sodium bicarbonate is recommended to decrease the burning caused by lidocaine. EMLA may reduce the pain of arterial puncture.

**TABLE 34–3**

**EMLA Cream: Recommended Maximum Dose by Age and Weight**

| Age and Body Weight | Maximum Total EMLA Dose | Maximum Application Area | Maximum Application Time |
|---|---|---|---|
| Birth–3 mo or <5 kg | 1 g | 10 $cm^2$ | 1 hr |
| 3-12 mo and >5 kg | 2 g | 20 $cm^2$ | 4 hr |

EMLA, eutectic mixture of local anesthetics.

Data Taketomo CK, Hodding JH, Kraus DM (eds): Pediatric Dosage Handbook, 2001-2002, p 595.

## Mechanical Ventilation

Because intubation can raise both blood pressure and intracranial pressure, a short-acting benzodiazepine such as midazolam can be beneficial. Midazolam can be used for infants with stable cardiovascular function; fentanyl can be used as an alternative for infants with compromised cardiovascular function (McClain and Anand, 1996). Any infant who is pharmacologically paralyzed during mechanical ventilation should receive adequate sedation. In addition, the infant should receive pain medication if pain is suspected from the infant's condition or because of the procedures being performed.

## Other Invasive Procedures

Placement of a central venous line requires topical anesthesia with EMLA or infiltration of the skin with lidocaine. Additionally, a parenteral opioid such as fentanyl is typically required.

The pain of a lumbar puncture is compounded by both the needle puncture and the distress caused by the body position required for the procedure. EMLA has been shown to decrease the pain of lumbar puncture in children (Halperin et al, 1989). Chest tube insertion requires an intravenous opioid, adequate local analgesia, or both.

## Antagonizing Pain Management

Small incremental doses of naloxone may make it possible to reverse respiratory depression without adversely affecting analgesia. Naloxone, 1 to 10 μg/kg given as an IV push (IVP) or subcutaneously (SC), is recommended for infants with mild somnolence. For apnea or respiratory arrest, an initial dose of 10 μg/kg IVP or SC followed by 1 μg/kg titrated to effect is recommended to avoid sudden hemodynamic effects. After the administration of naloxone, the infant must be observed, because the duration of naloxone is significantly shorter than the duration of an opioid. Naloxone can lead to seizures in opioid-dependent patients.

The use of flumazenil for reversal of benzodiazepines has not been investigated in infants.

## Physical Dependence, Tolerance, and Addiction

A clear distinction must be made between opioid or benzodiazepine dependence, tolerance, and addiction. Physical *dependence* is demonstrated by the need to continue the administration of the drug to prevent signs or symptoms of physical withdrawal. *Tolerance* is a reduction in the drug effects after repeated administration, or the need to increase the dose to achieve the same clinical effect. *Addiction* is compulsive drug-taking behavior (Gutstein and Akil, 2001). Infants are not capable of being addicted to a drug.

## Weaning Considerations

Baseline pain and weaning scores should be obtained prior to beginning the weaning process, and infants should be reassessed every 2 to 4 hours for signs of withdrawal. In addition, when an opioid dosage is being tapered, the infant must be assessed for the presence of pain a minimum of every 4 hours. If an infant is receiving both an opioid and a benzodiazepine, it is prudent to taper and stop only one class of medication at a time. Typically, a weaning schedule is 10% of the total initial dose per day, or 20% of the initial dose every other day. Many patients can tolerate a relatively large initial decrease in dose, but subsequent decreases may need to be smaller. Environmental stressors should be eliminated or reduced whenever possible. It should be noted that the potential onset of withdrawal symptoms varies according the half-life of the opioid or benzodiazepine and the half-life of active metabolites, which may be much longer than that of the parent compound (Tobias, 2000).

## SELECTED READINGS

Gibbins S, Stevens B: State of the art pain assessment and management in high risk infants. Newborn and Infant Nursing Reviews 1:85-96, 2001.
Harrison L: The use of comforting touch and massage to reduce stress for preterm infants in the neonatal intensive care unit. Newborn and Infant Nursing Reviews 1:235-241, 2001.
Jones J, Kassity N, Duncan K: Complimentary care: Alternatives for the neonatal intensive care unit. Newborn and Infant Nursing Reviews 1:207-210, 2001.
Ramsey T: An infant's first massage in the neonatal intensive care unit: A case report. Newborn and Infant Nursing Reviews 1:229-234, 2001.
Standley J: Music Therapy for the Neonate. Newborn and Infant Nursing Reviews 1:211-216.

## REFERENCES

AAP Circumcision Policy Statement. American Academy of Pediatrics. Task Force on Circumcision. Pediatrics 103: 686-693, 1999.
Acute Pain Management Guideline Panel: Acute Pain Management in Infants, Children, and Adolescents: Operative and Medical Procedures. Quick Reference Guide for Clinicians. (AHCPR Pub. No. 92-0020.) Washington, DC, Agency for Healthcare Policy and Research, Public Health Service, US Department of Health and Human Services, 1992, p12.
Als H, Lawhon G, Duffy FH, et al: Individualized developmental care for the very-low-birth-weight preterm infant. JAMA 272:853-858, 1994.
American Pain Society: Pain: The fifth vital sign. 1995. Available on line at www.ampainsoc.org.
Anand KJS.: Clinical importance of pain and stress in neonates. Biol Neonate 73:1-9, 1998.
Anand KJS, Phil D, Hickey P: Pain and its effects in the human neonate and fetus. N Engl J Med. 317:1321-1326, 1987.
Anand KJS, Phil D, Carr D: The neuroanatomy, neurophysiology, and neurochemistry of pain, stress, and analgesia in newborns and children. Pediatr Clin North Am 36:795-817, 1989.
Anand KJS, Selanikio JD, and the SOPAIN Study Group: Routine analgesic practices in 109 neonatal intensive care units. Pediatr Res 39:192a, 1996.
Anand KJS, McIntosh N, Lagercrantz H, et al: Analgesia and sedation in preterm neonates who require ventilatory support: Results from the NOPAIN Trial. Arch Pediatr Adolesc Med 153:331-338, 1999.

Anand KJS, Menon G, Narsinghani U, et al: Systemic analgesic therapy. In Anand KJS, Stevens BJ, McGrath PJ (eds): Pain in Neonates, 2nd ed. Amsterdam, Elsevier, 2000, pp 171-174.

Arana, A, Morton NS, Hansen TG: Treatment with paracetamol in infants. Acta Anaesthesiol Scand 45:20-29, 2001.

Bell S: The national pain management guideline: Implications for neonatal intensive care. Neonatal Netw 13:9-17, 1994.

Benini F, Johnston CC, Faucher D, Aranda JV: Topical anesthesia during circumcision in newborn infants. JAMA 270:850-853, 1993.

Berde CB, Sethna NF: Drug therapy: Analgesics for the treatment of pain in children. N Engl J Med. 347:1094-1103, 2002.

Carrier C, Walden M: Integrating research and standards to improve pain management practices for newborns and infants. Newborn Infant Nurs Rev 1:122-131, 2001.

Chana SK, Anand KJ: Can we use methadone for analgesia in neonates? Arch Dis Child Fetal Neonatal Ed 85:F79-F81, 2001.

Collins E: Maternal and fetal effects of acetaminophen and salicylates in pregnancy. Obstetrics and Gynecology 58:57S-62S.

Corff K, Seideman R, Venkataraman P, et al: Facilitated tucking: A nonpharmacologic comfort measure for pain in preterm infants. J Obstet Gynecol Neonatal Nurs 24:143-147, 1995.

Craig K, Whitfield M, Grunau R, et al: Pain in the preterm neonate: Behavioral and physiological indices. Pain 52:287-299, 1993.

Evans J: Physiology of acute pain in preterm infants. Newborn Infant Nurs Rev 1:75-85, 2001.

Evans J, Vogelpohl D, Bourguignon C, et al: Pain behaviors accompany some "nonpainful" procedures. Neo Network 16: 33-40, 1997.

Fitzgerald M, Millard C, McIntosh N: Cutaneous hypersensitivity following peripheral tissue damage in newborn infants and its reversal with topical anaesthesia. Pain 39:31-36, 1989.

Franck L: A national survey of the assessment and treatment of pain and agitation in the neonatal intensive care unit. J Obstet Gynecol Neonatal Nurs 16:387-393, 1987.

Franck L: The ethical imperative to treat pain in infants: Are we doing the best we can? Crit Care Nurse 17:80-87, 1997.

Franck LS, Gregory GA: Clinical evaluation and treatment of infant pain in the neonatal intensive care unit. In Schecter NL, Berde CB, Yaster M (eds): Pain in Infants, Children, and Adolescents. Baltimore, Williams & Wilkins, 1993, p 530.

Franck L, Greenberg C, Stevens B: Pain assessment in infants and children. Pediatr Clin North Am 47:487-511, 2000.

Franck L, Scurr K, Couture S: Parent views of infant pain and pain management in the neonatal intensive care unit. Newborn Infant Nurs Rev 1:106-113, 2001.

Gauntlett IS, Fisher DM, Hertzka RE, et al: Pharmacokinetics of fentanyl in neonatal humans and lambs: Effects of age. Anesthesiology 69:683-687, 1988.

Grunau R, Craig K: Pain expression in infants: Facial action and cry. Pain 28:395-410, 1987.

Grunau RE, Oberlander T, Holsti L, Whitfield MF: Bedside application of the Neonatal Facial Coding System in pain assessment of premature neonates. Pain 76:277-286, 1998.

Guinsburg R, Berenguel R, Xavier R, et al: Are behavioral scales suitable for preterm and term neonatal pain assessment? Proceedings of the 8th World Congress on Pain, Progress in Pain Research and Management. 8: ISAP Press, Seattle, 1997.

Guinsburg R, Kopelman B, Anand K, et al: Physiological, hormonal, and behavioral responses to a single fentanyl dose in intubated and ventilated preterm infants. J Pediatr 132:954-959, 1998.

Gutstein HB, Akil H: In Hardman JG, Limbird LE (eds): Goodman & Gilman's The Pharmacological Basis of Therapeutics, 10th ed. New York, McGraw-Hill, 2001, pp 586-587.

Halperin DL, Koren G, Attias D, et al: Topical skin anesthesia for venous, subcutaneous drug reservoir and lumbar punctures in children. Pediatrics 84:281-284, 1989.

Houck CS: In Ashburn MA, Rice LJ (eds): The Management of Pain. New York, Churchill Livingstone, 1998, pp 651-652.

Howard CR, Howard FM, Weitzman ML: Acetaminophen analgesia in neonatal circumcision: The effect on pain. Pediatrics 93:641-646, 1994.

Johnston C, Stevens B: Experience in a neonatal unit effects pain response. Pediatrics 98:925-930, 1996.

Johnston C, Stevens B, Craig K, et al: Developmental changes in pain expression in premature, full-term, two-, and four month old infants. Pain 52:201-208, 1993.

Johnston C, Stevens B, Yang F, et al: Differential response to pain by very premature neonates. Pain 61:471-479, 1995.

Johnston C, Stevens B, Franck L, et al: Factors explaining lack of response to heelstick in preterm newborns. J Obstet Gynecol Neonatal Nurs 28:87-594, 1999.

Joint Commission on Accreditation of Healthcare Organizations: Patient-Focused Functions. In 2004 Hospital Accreditation Standards. Oakbrook Terrace, Illinois, Joint Commission on Accreditation of Healcare Organizations, 2004, pp 113, 138, 140.

Koehntop DE, Rodman JH, Brundage DM, et al: Pharmacokinetics of fentanyl in neonates. Anesth Analg 65:227-232, 1986.

Krechel S, Bildner J: CRIES: A neonatal postoperative pain measurement score. Initial testing of validity and reliability. Pediatr Anaesth 5:53-61, 1995.

Lander J, Brady-Fryer, B, Metcalfe JB, et al: Comparison of ring block, dorsal penile nerve block, and topical anesthesia for neonatal circumcision. JAMA 278:2157-2162, 1997.

Lawrence J, Alcock D, McGrath P, et al: The development of a tool to assess neonatal pain. Neonatal Netw 12:59-66, 1993.

Lee JJ, Forrester P: EMLA for postoperative analgesia for day case circumcision in children: A comparison with dorsal nerve of penis block Anaesthesia 47:1081-1083, 1992.

McClain BS, Anand KJS: Neonatal pain management. In Deshpande JK, Tobias JD (eds): The Pediatric Pain Handbook, St. Louis, Mosby, 1996, pp 204-209.

Pokela M: Pain relief can reduce hypoxemia in distressed neonates during routine treatment procedures. Pediatrics 93:379-383, 1994.

Porter F, Wolf C, Gold J, et al: Pain and pain management in newborn infants: A survey of physicians and nurses. Pediatrics 100:626-632, 1997.

Porter F, Wolf C, Miller J: The effect of handling and immobilization on the response to acute pain in newborn infants. Pediatrics 102:1383-1389, 1998.

Porter F, Grunau R, Anand KJS: Long-term effects of pain in infants. Dev Behav Pediatr 20:253-261, 1999.

Reynolds M, Fitzgerald M: Long-term sensory hyperinnervation following neonatal skin wounds. J Comp Neurol 358:487-498, 1995.

Scott CS, Riggs KW, Ling EW, et al: Morphine pharmacokinetics and pain assessment in premature newborns. J Pediatr 135:423-429, 1999.

Shah VS, Taddio A, Bennett S, et al: Neonatal pain response to heel stick vs. venepuncture for routine blood sampling. Arch Dis Child Fetal Neonatal Ed 77:F143-F144, 1997.

Singleton MA, Rosen JI, Fisher DM: Plasma concentrations of fentanyl in infants, children, and adults. Can J Anesth 34: 152-155, 1987.

Sparshott M: The development of a clinical distress scale for ventilated newborn infants: Identification of pain and distress based on validated behavioural scores. J Neonatal Nurs 2:5-11, 1996.

Stevens B, Johnston C, Horton L: Multidimensional pain assessment in premature infants: A pilot study. J Obstet Gynecol Neonatal Nurs 22:531-541, 1993.

Stevens B, Johnston C, Petryshen P, et al: Premature Infant Pain Profile: Development and initial validation. Clin J Pain 12: 13-22, 1996.

Stevens B, Johnston C, Franck L, et al: The efficacy of developmentally sensitive behavioral interventions and sucrose for relieving procedural pain in very low birth weight neonate. Nurs Res 48:35-43, 1999a.

Stevens B, Johnston C, Taddio A, et al: Management of pain from heel lance with lidocaine-prilocaine (EMLA) cream: Is it safe and efficacious in preterm infants? J Dev Behav Pediatr 20:216-221, 1999b.

Stevens B, Gibbons S, Franck LS: Treatment of pain in the neonatal intensive care unit. Pediatr Clin North Am 47:633-650, 2000.

Suresh S, Anand KJ: Opioid tolerance in neonates: Mechanisms, diagnosis, assessment, and management. Semin Perinatol 22:425-433, 1998.

Taddio A, Goldbach M, Ipp M, et al: Effect of neonatal circumcision on pain responses during vaccination in boys. Lancet. 345:291-292, 1995a.

Taddio A, Shennan AT, Stevens B, et al: Safety of lidocaine-prilocaine cream in the treatment of preterm neonates. J Pediatr 127:1002-1005, 1995b.

Taddio A, Ohlsson A, Einarson TR, et al: A systematic review of lidocaine-prilocaine cream (EMLA) in the treatment of acute pain in neonates. Pediatrics 101:299, 1998.

Taddio A, Stevens B, Craig K, et al: Efficacy and safety of lidocaine-prilocaine cream for pain during circumcision. N Engl J Med 336:1197-1201, 1997.

Taketomo CK, Hodding JH, Kraus DM (eds). Pediatric Dosage Handbook. Lexi-Comp Inc. Hudson, Cleveland, 2001-2002, p 595.

Tobias JD: Tolerance, withdrawal, and physical dependency after long-term sedation and analgesia of children in the pediatric intensive care unit. Crit Care Med 28:2122-2132, 2000.

van Lingen RA, Deinum JT, Quak JM, et al: Pharmacokinetics and metabolism of rectally administered paracetamol in preterm neonates. Arch Dis Child Fetal Neonatal Ed 80: F59-F63, 1999.

Walden M: Pain assessment and management: Guideline for practice. (National Association of Neonatal Nurses Document 1222.) National Association of Neonatal Nurses. Glenview, Illinois, 2001.

Yaster M, Kost-Byerly S, Maxwell LG: Opioid agonists and antagonists. In Schecter NL, Berde CB, Yaster M (eds): Pain in Infants, Children, and Adolescent, 2nd ed. Baltimore, Lippincott Williams & Wilkins, 2003, pp193-194.

PART IX

# IMMUNOLOGY AND INFECTIONS

Editor: H. WILLIAM TAEUSCH

CHAPTER 35

# Immunology of the Fetus and Newborn

Calvin B. Williams and F. Sessions Cole

Understanding the contribution of the newborn infant's immunologic response to neonatal disease requires a review of the complex immunologic environment of pregnancy and the developmentally regulated changes in fetal and neonatal immunity. The contrasting functions of the fetal, neonatal, and maternal immunologic responses, that is, preservation of fetal well-being as an allogenic graft versus adequate immunologic protection in a nonsterile extrauterine environment, are regulated by a host of incompletely understood developmental and genetic mechanisms. The diversity and importance of these mechanisms are suggested by the heterogeneity and frequency of the infectious problems encountered in newborns. Differences in immunologic responsiveness between adults and newborns should not be considered defects or abnormalities. Just as the ductus arteriosus, a cardiopulmonary necessity in the intrauterine environment, closes at different rates in different infants, human fetal and newborn infant immunologic response mechanisms are developmentally and genetically programmed to change from graft preservation to identification and destruction of invading pathogens at different rates.

Fortunately, systemic antimicrobial chemotherapy can control microbial invasion and permit adaptation of the infected infant's immunologic system to an extrauterine existence exposed to multiple potential pathogens. However, antibiotics coupled with advances in support technology do not ensure survival of infected infants: Significant infectious morbidity and mortality persist in newborn infants (Polin and Harris, 2001; Shah et al, 1999).

## MATERNAL AND PLACENTAL IMMUNOLOGY

### Maternal Immunologic Response During Pregnancy

The survival of the fetal allogeneic graft in the uterus requires multiple adaptive immunologic mechanisms. Both tolerogenic and inflammatory mechanisms are at work during the different stages of reproduction (Mellor and Munn, 2000). Ovulation, copulation, and fertilization all induce changes in uterine physiology that alter immunologic responses and favor acceptance of the fetal allograft. For example, progesterone induced by ovulation can decrease the proliferation of T cells and inhibit the function of antigen-presenting cells (Ehring et al, 1998; Miyaura and Iwata, 2002). Prostaglandin (PE) $E_2$, which is present at high concentration in seminal fluid, has also been shown to inhibit lymphocyte activation and modify cytokine release in favor of interleukin (IL) 10 (Denison et al, 1999). IL-10 inhibits the production of IL-12, thereby favoring Th2 responses and tolerance. These and other data imply that a maternal shift from Th1-type immune responses to Th2-type responses may play a role in maternal tolerance to the fetal allograft (Mellor and Munn, 2000).

In contrast to $PGE_2$ and progesterone, which promote T-cell tolerance, other factors in seminal fluid, such as transforming growth factor-β1 (TGF-β1) have a pro-inflammatory effect (Tremellen et al, 1998). TGF-β1 stimulates production of granulocyte-macrophage colony stimulating factor (GM-CSF), which then acts by recruiting macrophages, dendritic cells, and neutrophils to the endometrial stroma. This pre-implantation inflammatory cascade may play a role in the tissue remodeling needed to prepare the endometrium for the fetal allograft (Norwitz et al, 2001). GM-CSF also has embryotrophic effects that promote fetal growth and viability. Knockout mice lacking GM-CSF have normal implantation rates but have 15% to 25% smaller litters (Robertson et al, 1999). In summary, the pregravid or gravid uterus is not ignored by the immune system, as suggested by the original notions of "immunologic privilege" (Billingham, 1964; Medawar, 1953; Simmons, 1969; Simmons and Russell, 1967). Instead, an orchestrated series of specific pro-inflammatory and tolerogenic mechanisms support implantation and fetal allograft survival.

Fetal antigenic maturity in eliciting a maternal immunologic response has been well documented (Beer and Billingham, 1976; Billington, 1987). Major histocompatibility complex (MHC) class I proteins are expressed at high levels on murine trophoblasts in early gestation (Chatterjee-Hasrouni and Lala, 1982; Philpott et al, 1988). The high frequency of alloreactive T cells in the maternal circulation (10% to 30%) makes it certain that maternal T cells will encounter fetal MHC class I alloantigens (Mellor and Munn, 2000). In the nonpregnant host, this high frequency of precursors results in potent T-cell responses to tissue allografts. The lack of such responses to fetal alloantigens has been studied in murine lineages genetically engineered to express a transgenic T-cell receptor restricted by MHC class I antigens (Jiang and Vacchio, 1998; Tafuri et al, 1995). These studies demonstrate that MHC class I expression on murine fetal trophoblasts results in the elimination of alloreactive class I–restricted maternal T cells and in induced unresponsiveness of the antigen-specific cells remaining.

Extrapolation of these data to humans is complicated by the fact that human trophoblasts do not express the conventional MHC class I molecules HLA-A or HLA-B. They do express HLA-C, but only during the first trimester (King et al, 1996a). Instead of these conventional MHC molecules, extravillous fetal cytotrophoblasts express HLA-G, a nonclassic MHC class I molecule (Kovats et al, 1990). HLA-G exhibits relatively little polymorphism (Klein et al, 1998), and the expression of this molecule is primarily limited to fetal tissue (Kovats et al, 1990; McMaster et al, 1995). On the cell surface, HLA-G is a trimolecular complex containing the HLA-G heavy chain in a complex with β-2 microglobulin and a short peptide in the antigen-binding grove. The peptides bound by HLA-G are similar to those bound by other class I molecules (Lee et al, 1995). In an ex vivo assay, investigators used a blocking monoclonal antibody to demonstrate that HLA-G was important in protecting the fetus from maternal natural killer (NK) cell–mediated cytolysis (Rouas-Freiss et al, 1997). Several receptors on human NK cells that bind HLA-G or a fragment of HLA-G bound to HLA-E (another nonclassic MHC molecule) have now been described (Llano et al, 1999; Ponte et al, 1999; Rajagopalan and Long, 1999; Soderstrom et al, 1997). Biochemical data suggest that ligand binding by certain receptors results in the inhibition of NK cell activity. In this regard, it is intriguing that virtually all human placental NK cells at term express the inhibitory receptor KIR2DL4, whereas circulating maternal NK cells do not (Ponte et al, 1999).

The lack of expression of MHC class II proteins by murine and human trophoblast cells contributes to maternal unresponsiveness to fetal antigens. MHC class II molecules are necessary for CD4$^+$ T cell responses, which contribute both effector and regulatory functions needed for graft rejection. MHC class II gene silencing in trophoblasts is partially the result of the transcriptional repression of class II transactivator (CIITA), a necessary transcription factor for class II gene expression (Morris et al, 1998; Murphy and Tomasi, 1998). Lack of CIITA may be the reason that attempts to force expression of MHC class II molecules in trophoblast cells in vivo have been largely unsuccessful (Mellor and Munn, 2000). Thus, it is an oversimplification to view the fetal tissues at the maternal-fetal interface as antigenically immature. Instead, tightly regulated expression of nonclassic MHC genes and silencing of several classic MHC genes help create an environment that favors survival of the fetal allograft.

Considerable evidence now supports the notion that the maternal-fetal interface is an immunologically active site, rather than an inert, impermeable barrier. Fetal cells enter the maternal circulation, where they may play a role in maternal T-cell tolerance. In mice, maternal splenic T cells show awareness of paternal alloantigens (Tafuri et al, 1995). In humans, fetal genetic microchimerism can be detected for years after parturition (Bianchi et al, 1996; Evans et al, 1999; Lo et al, 1996). Clearly, the placenta does not function as an impermeable barrier to cellular traffic (Medawar, 1953). However, several interesting features of the maternal-fetal interface document that this is a unique immunologic environment. Fas ligand (FasL) is expressed in both maternal and fetal components of the uteroplacental unit throughout gestation. Activated T cells express the Fas receptor, which delivers a death signal when bound by FasL. Implicit in these observations is the hypothesis that expression of FasL limits the reciprocal migration of activated fetal and maternal T cells. This idea is strengthened further by experiments examining the homozygous matings between *gld* mice, which make a nonfunctional FasL. Pregnant *gld* mice demonstrate leukocyte infiltration and necrosis at the decidual-placental interface, with many resorption sites and small litters (Hunt et al, 1997). In humans, the placenta restricts access of cytotoxic cells to the fetus (Beer et al, 1994; Sargent, 1993). However, evidence from infants with severe combined immunodeficiency (SCID) suggests that maternal T lymphocytes can cross the placenta and engraft in fetal bone marrow (Thompson et al, 1984). Whether aberrant regulation of maternal-fetal effector cell traffic plays a role in specific fetal or neonatal diseases, for example, intrauterine growth restriction, is poorly understood (Beer and Billingham, 1973; Beer et al, 1972).

In addition to FasL, placental products progesterone and prostaglandin $E_2$ both suppress Th1 responses (Abe et al, 1997; Piccinni et al, 1995). The Th1 cytokines interferon-γ (IFN-γ) and tumor necrosis factor-α (TNF-α) have been shown to inhibit the growth of trophoblasts as well as embryonic and fetal development (Haimovici et al, 1991). Th1 cytokines terminate normal pregnancy when injected into pregnant mice (Chaouat et al, 1990). When peripheral blood mononuclear cells from women with a history of recurrent spontaneous abortion were stimulated with trophoblast antigen extracts, the mononuclear cells produced high levels of factors that were toxic to mouse embryos. These factors, which included IFN-γ and TNF-α, were not seen in the control group, which produced IL-10 instead (Polgar and Anderson, 1995; Yamada et al, 1994). Finally, the local production of TGF-β and IL-10 provide additional lymphocyte immunosuppression. Although the placenta is not a physical barrier to immunologic recognition, it does seem reasonable to conclude that specific apoptotic mechanisms limit the trafficking of activated T cells, and the general cytokine milieu at the maternal-fetal interface favors the development of tolerogenic Th2 responses.

This body of evidence supports the hypothesis that tolerogenic mechanisms are important at the normal maternal-fetal interface. However, *scid* mice that lack an antigen-specific immune response are fertile even when bred with mice that carry the beige (*bg*) mutation that selectively impairs NK cell function (Croy, 1993; Croy and Chapeau, 1990; Roder and Duwe, 1979). Clark and associates (1994) reported that *scid/scid* mice bred with a different genetic background (CB-17) did not have a high rate of successful syngeneic pregnancies. The possibility of a TNF-α–induced vasculopathy triggered by an unidentified infectious agent was raised in these studies. These observations suggest that either multiple redundant systems contribute to successful pregnancy outcome or placental function does not require induction by immune recognition of lymphoid or cytokine functions (Croy, 1993; Ossa et al, 1994).

The placenta also regulates maternal-fetal and fetal-maternal transfer of immunologically important factors (Gitlin et al, 1964; Gurka and Rocklin, 1987; Hunziker and Wegmann, 1986; Jacoby et al, 1984). To accomplish these complex functions, the placenta has a wealth of cell populations that provide considerable regulatory diversity. The hemochorial placenta of the human is a chimeric organ. Fetal villi covered with invasive trophoblasts erode into layers of maternal epithelium, stroma, and vessel endothelium. In addition to the various cell types of the decidua, there are multiple immunologically competent cells in the placenta, as noted previously. The importance of these cell types has been emphasized by the immunotrophism model, which suggests that maternal immunologic recognition of fetal antigens induces production of cytokines that are necessary for placental growth, and by the important roles of IL-1, IL-6, TNF-α, and other immunoregulatory cytokines in the initiation of parturition (Guilbert et al, 1993; Romero et al, 1992, 1994; Tangri et al, 1994).

Besides local production of factors that regulate fetal and maternal well-being, the placenta can regulate passage of maternal immunologic effectors to the fetus (Tongio et al, 1975). For example, although maternal immunoglobulin (Ig) G is transported efficiently beginning at 20 weeks of gestation, maternal antibody can also be bound and degraded by the placenta (Swinburne, 1970; Wegmann et al, 1980). On the basis of observations in rabbits and mice, there is considerable antibody-binding capacity in the placenta: Radiolabeled maternal antibody is internalized and degraded by the placenta in 4 to 6 hours. Failure of this placental function may be due to elevated concentrations of maternal antibody that cannot be cleared by the placenta. Alternatively, specific antibodies may escape placental clearance and accumulate in the fetus because of a poorly understood lack of recognition of these antibodies. As understanding of the diverse immunologic functions of the placenta improves, more specific immunoregulatory clinical information will be derived from this important organ.

The fact that pregnant women are healthy and display all the appropriate immunologic defense mechanisms suggests strongly that pregnancy-induced systemic maternal immunosuppression is not necessary for successful pregnancy (Gill, 1992). The availability of genetically homogeneous murine lineages with altered immunologic responsiveness, the availability of reagents with which to evaluate regulation of expression of genes of the MHC, and greater understanding of the importance of cytokines have suggested that genetic and developmental mechanisms are responsible for successful human pregnancy (Beer and Billingham, 1976; Croy et al, 1993; Guilbert et al, 1993; Hunziker and Wegmann, 1986; Mellor and Munn, 2000; Tangri et al, 1994; Wegmann et al, 1991). Although not precisely understood, these mechanisms involve at a minimum antigen-specific T-cell tolerance, immune deviation (a propensity to develop Th2 responses), and the control of immunogenicity at the maternal-fetal interface as discussed above.

Abnormalities of maternal-fetal immunologic interaction can lead to spontaneous abortion or to morbidity or mortality for the fetus or newborn, as seen in pregnancies complicated by rhesus (Rh) isoimmunization. Approximately 75% of Rh-negative women with Rh-incompatible fetuses give birth to unaffected or mildly affected infants (Baskett et al, 1986; Berlin et al, 1985; Eklund and Nevanlinna, 1986; Mills and Napier, 1988). The regulation of the maternal immunologic response suggested by this heterogeneity is complex. Raum and colleagues (1984) studied the genetic immunoregulation of this response. These investigators demonstrated that a specific complotype of genetically determined allotypic variants of the second and fourth complement proteins of the classical complement pathway and factor B of the alternative complement pathway, all of which are encoded by genes within the MHC on the short arm of human chromosome 6, is tightly linked to a single extended haplotype, which is associated with fetal or neonatal morbidity and mortality. This observation suggests that genes that are closely linked to the MHC regulate maternal immunologic responsiveness to the Rh antigen. Preconceptual or antenatal determination of the complotype of Rh-negative women might supplement utilization of measurement of maternal anti-Rh titer to assess fetal risk. Genetic and developmental regulation of maternal immunologic response to polysaccharide antigens also plays a role in determining the risk of individual infants for systemic bacterial infection with polysaccharide-encapsulated organisms. Similar genetic markers may soon be available from studies of women in whose sequential infants group B streptococcal infection has developed within the first 3 months of life (Christensen and Christensen, 1988).

## Immunologically Mediated Fetal Loss Syndromes

Considerable experimental evidence derived from certain breeding combinations of mice shows that maternal immune responses can result in spontaneous fetal loss. The most extensively studied is the CBA/J × DBA/2 breeding combination, which results in a 20% to 30% rate of spontaneous fetal resorption (Bobe and Kiger, 1989; Bobe et al, 1986). This resorption rate is increased two- to three-fold when pregnant mice are treated with substances that induce IFN-γ, such as double-stranded RNA (dsRNA) and polyinosinic polycytidylic acid, a double stranded polymer, commonly used to mimic viral exposure (de Fougerolles and Baines, 1987; Kinsky et al, 1990). The IFN-γ effect can be partially reversed by antiserum that blocks NK cell activation. Immunohistochemical analysis of resorption sites showed infiltration with NK cells and macrophages and excessive production of nitric oxide and TNF-α (Duclos et al, 1994; Haddad et al, 1995, 1997). Pre-immunizing females with macrophages, pharmacologic inhibition of nitric oxide production, blocking of TNF-α, and administration of IL-10 all were found to reduce fetal loss (Gendron et al, 1990; Haddad et al, 1995). Collectively, these data argue that the inflammatory conditions at the maternal-fetal interface play a critical role in successful pregnancy.

Another series of murine investigations points to a clear-cut role for maternal T-cell alloresponses in mediating spontaneous fetal loss. When monocytes are induced to differentiate into macrophages in vitro using macrophage colony-stimulating factor, they become inhibitors of T-cell proliferation rather than activators. This inhibition was shown to be the result of selective degradation of tryptophan by the inducible enzyme indoleamine 2,3-dioxygenase (IDO). Serum tryptophan levels fall during pregnancy, possibly in response to IDO expression by syncytiotrophoblast cells, which make the enzyme as early as 7.5 days after coitus. Given the localization of IDO to the maternal-fetal interface and the immunosuppressive effects of tryptophan depletion, it seemed plausible to investigators that this pathway played a role in survival of the fetal allograft. This hypothesis was confirmed using either normal or recombinase-activating gene (RAG) knockout mice (which lack T and B cells) together with the IDO inhibitor 1-methyl-tryptophan. Normal mice carrying allogenic fetuses lost all their conceptuses by 11.5 days after coitus when they were treated with the inhibitor. In contrast, RAG-deficient mice treated with 1-methyl-tryptophan deliver healthy liters of normal size, demonstrating an immunologic basis for the observation (Munn et al, 1998, 1999). The fact that tryptophan levels fall during human pregnancy suggests that these data will have relevance to human fetal loss syndromes.

Other factors that may contribute to fetal loss syndromes are Th1 and Th2 cytokines. Data from mice demonstrate that Th2 cytokines such as IL-4 and IL-10 inhibit Th1-mediated graft rejection. These and other data have led to the hypothesis that Th2 cytokines produced at the maternal-fetal interface promote maternal tolerance. This broad concept is beyond the scope of this chapter. Several experiments, however, may elucidate mechanisms related to unexplained recurrent abortions. In murine models, leukemia inhibitory (LIF) factor is required for embryo implantation (Stewart, 1992). LIF-deficient mice are fertile, but their blastocysts fail to implant. LIF deficiency in women with unexplained recurrent abortions has been documented, and LIF production by maternal T cells from healthy pregnancies is positively associated with IL-4 production and inversely association with IFN-γ (Piccinni et al, 1998). These data suggest that the balance of Th1 and Th2 cytokines is important in both establishing and maintaining pregnancy and that LIF is a critical early regulator.

## DEVELOPMENTAL FETAL-NEONATAL IMMUNOLOGY

### Humoral Immunity

#### Complement

The complement system consists of approximately 40 plasma and cell surface proteins (Table 35–1) that interact dynamically to regulate multiple functions of this immunologic effector system (Frank, 2000). These functions include cytolysis of bacteria, nonspecific opsonization, release of anaphylotoxins, solubilization of immune complexes, and induction of B-cell proliferation and differentiation. Activation of the complement cascade can occur via the classical or alternative pathway. The activation steps in these pathways have been reviewed (Frank, 2000). Several characteristics of this cascade are important for the fetal-neonatal immunologic response. First, although the specificity of classical pathway activation results from interaction of antigens with antibodies of several isotypes, activation of the alternative pathway is antibody independent and may be initiated by structures such as endotoxin and polysaccharides that are frequently encountered among pathogenic organisms. For the fetus or infant who lacks type-specific IgG for immunologic recognition, the alternative pathway may be critical for triggering the effector functions of the complement cascade (Cole, 1987; Cole and Colten, 1984; Edwards, 1986; Stossel et al, 1973). Second, the enzymatic activation of the complement cascade permits prompt amplification of its functions: Deposition of a single immunoglobulin molecule or C3b fragment can generate enzymatic cleavage of thousands of later-acting components and, thus, multiple complement activities (Pangburn and Muller-Eberhard, 1984). In addition, the alternative pathway may be amplified via a positive feedback activation mechanism, because C3b, an activation product of the alternative pathway C3 convertase, is a component of this convertase (Volanakis, 1989). Because of the importance of antibody-independent recognition for the immunologic responsiveness of the fetus and infant, the positive amplification loop of the alternative pathway is critical for rapid generation of complement effector functions without specific immunologic recognition.

Complement activation via either pathway occurs in two distinct phases, proteolysis and assembly. First, early-acting components of the classical pathway (C1, C4, and C2) or alternative (factor B, factor D, and C3) pathway are activated by highly specific, limited proteolysis. Proteolytically activated components form specific enzymatic complexes composed of components of the classical (C2a and C4b) or alternative (C3bBb) pathway, which activate the third component of complement (C3). These two endopeptidases have identical substrate specificities: Each cleaves the single peptide bond $Arginine_{77}$-$Serine_{78}$ of the α chain of C3 (Volanakis, 1989). The rates of formation and dissociation of both C3 convertases are regulated by multiple soluble proteins (e.g., factor H, factor I, C4b-binding protein) and membrane-associated proteins (e.g., membrane cofactor protein, decay-accelerating factor [DAF]) (Schieren and Hansch, 1993). During activation of the early-acting classical components, small (8 to 10 kilodaltons [kd]) peptides are released by proteolytic cleavage from the second, third, and fourth components of complement. These fragments and an activation fragment of the fifth component of complement, C5a, have anaphylatoxin activities and modulate vascular permeability, smooth muscle reactivity, and chemotaxis of polymorphonuclear leukocytes and monocytes.

Upon activation of C3 by either convertase, the second phase of complement activation is initiated—assembly of the membrane attack complex by protein-protein interaction of terminal (C5 to C9) complement proteins (Muller-Eberhard, 1986). This complex alters membrane integrity

**TABLE 35-1**

**Summary of Recommendations for Immunization During Pregnancy**

| Immunization | Recommendation |
|---|---|
| **Live Virus Vaccines** | |
| Measles | Contraindicated |
| Mumps | Contraindicated |
| Poliomyelitis | Not routine; increased risk exposure; should be avoided |
| Rubella | Contraindicated |
| Yellow fever | Travel to high-risk areas only |
| Varicella | Contraindicated |
| **Inactivated Viral Vaccines** | |
| Influenza | Serious underlying diseases; >14 weeks of gestation |
| Rabies | Same as for nonpregnant woman |
| Hepatitis A | Safety not determined during pregnancy; individualized risk assessment |
| Hepatitis B | Pre- and post-exposure for at-risk women |
| **Inactivated Bacterial Vaccines** | |
| Cholera | To meet international travel requirements; individualized to reflect actual need |
| Meningococcus | Same as for nonpregnant woman |
| Plague | Selective vaccination of exposed persons |
| Typhoid | Travel to endemic areas; no data available for pregnant women |
| Pneumococcus | Same as for nonpregnant woman; safety during first trimester not evaluate |
| Bacille Calmette-Guérin (BCG) | Contraindicated |
| **Toxoids** | |
| Tetanus-diphtheria | Same as for nonpregnant woman |
| **Hyperimmune Globulin** | |
| Hepatitis B | Postexposure prophylaxis given along with hepatitis B vaccine initially, then vaccine alone at 1 and 6 months |
| Rabies | Postexposure prophylaxis |
| Tetanus | Postexposure prophylaxis |
| Varicella | Same as for nonpregnant woman |
| **Pooled Immune Serum Globulins** | |
| Hepatitis A | Postexposure prophylaxis |
| Measles | Postexposure prophylaxis |

Data from American College of Obstetricians and Gynecologists: Immunization During Pregnancy (Technical Bulletin No. 160). Washington, DC, ACOG, October 1991; and from Guidelines for vaccinating pregnant women, 1998. Available on line at www.cdc.gov/nip/publications/preg_guide.pdf.

via a transmembrane channel and thereby causes cytolysis of bacteria or cells.

Studies of fetal-neonatal complement have focused on quantification of serum concentrations of individual components, determining hepatic and extrahepatic synthesis rates, examining maternal-fetal transport of these proteins, and assessing specific effector functions of the classical and alternative pathways. In the human, Gitlin and Biasucci (1969) reported detectable concentrations of C3 (1% of adult levels) and C1 inhibitor (20% of adult levels) by immunochemical methods as early as 5 to 6 weeks of gestation. By 26 to 28 weeks of gestation, both C3 and C1 inhibitor concentration increased to 66% of adult levels (Gitlin and Biasucci, 1969). Since these studies, many investigators have demonstrated that functionally and immunochemically measured complement protein concentrations in cord blood increase with advancing gestational age and that they are only 50% to 75% of adult concentrations at full-term gestation (Davis et al, 1979, 1980; Fietta et al, 1987; Frank, 2000; Miyano et al, 1987; Shapiro et al, 1983; Sonntag et al, 1998; Strunk et al, 1979). The important roles of complement regulatory proteins, decay-accelerating factor, membrane cofactor protein (MCP), and CD59 prompted later examination of the ontogeny of these proteins in the human fetus (Simpson et al, 1993).

To examine the possible mechanisms of this developmental increase in serum concentrations of complement proteins, investigators have studied the hepatic synthesis rates of individual complement proteins in the human liver obtained at different gestational ages (Adinolfi and Colten, 1972; Gardner, 1967; Gitlin and Biasucci, 1969). They have shown that C2, C3, C4, C5, factor H, and C1 inhibitor are synthesized by the human fetal liver; C3 and C1 inhibitor synthesis can be demonstrated as early as 4 to 5 weeks of gestation. A marked increase in C4 synthesis by the fetal liver occurs at approximately 15 weeks of gestation, coincident with an increase in serum concentration.

The hepatic synthesis mechanisms that regulate this increase, either a change in the amount of C4 produced by individual hepatocytes or a change in the number of hepatocytes that produce C4, are not yet determined. Extrahepatic fetal synthesis of complement has been shown in the large and small intestines at 19 weeks of gestation (Colten et al, 1968) and in fetal monocytes obtained from cord blood (Sutton et al, 1986). An additional source of developmentally regulated complement proteins is the tissue fibroblast. Strunk and colleagues (1994) have demonstrated that regulation of endotoxin-induced synthesis of the third component of complement (C3) and factor B is pretranslationally regulated in the fetus, translationally regulated in the newborn, and transcriptionally regulated in the adult.

On the basis of studies of genetically determined, structurally distinct complement variants in maternal and cord serum, no transplacental passage from mother to fetus of C3, C4, factor B, or C6 has been observed (Colten et al, 1981; Propp and Alper, 1968). The presence of detectable amounts of C2 and C1 inhibitor in cord blood but not in the sera of mothers with genetic deficiencies of these proteins suggests that fetal-maternal transport of these components does not occur.

Regulation of complement effector functions in the fetus and newborn infant has not been as extensively examined. Opsonization of invading microorganisms without specific immunoglobulin recognition requires activation of the alternative pathway. For infants born prematurely or without organism-specific maternal IgG, alternative pathway activation provides a critical mechanism for triggering complement effector functions (Baker et al, 1986; Cole, 1987; Correa et al, 1994; Edwards, 1986). For example, Stossel and colleagues (1973) demonstrated opsonic deficiency in 6 of 40 cord sera specimens examined because of decreased factor B concentrations, despite normal C3 and IgG levels. The functional contribution of the classical pathway to neonatal effector functions has been assessed through the use of cord blood–mediated opsonophagocytosis by adult polymorphonuclear leukocytes of group B streptococci type Ia (Edwards et al, 1983). This serotype may be opsonized by classical pathway components in the absence of specific antibodies and thus permits evaluation of the function of classical pathway activation. In 8 of 20 neonatal sera examined, decreased bactericidal activity was detected and correlated with significantly lower functional activity of C1q and C4. These studies did not determine whether this decrease was mediated by an inhibitor of function or by an intrinsic change in functional activity of these components in neonatal sera. The importance of the terminal complement component C9 for cytolysis of multiple isolates of *Escherichia coli* was suggested by in vitro experiments in which killing of *E. coli* by neonatal serum samples was limited by C9 but not by other classical pathway components (Lassiter et al, 1992, 1994).

Even though lower serum concentrations of classical and alternative complement pathway proteins may contribute to enhanced susceptibility of infants to systemic infection, other complement functions important for fetal-neonatal well-being but not related to antimicrobial response may require decreased activation of the classical and alternative pathways. For example, reduced serum concentration of C4b-binding protein (8% to 35% of levels found in pooled adult plasma), a critical regulator of classical pathway C3 convertase activity, has been noted in fetal and neonatal sera (Fernandez et al, 1989; Malm et al, 1988; Melissari et al, 1988; Moalic et al, 1988). Lower C4b-binding protein concentration increases the functional anticoagulant activity of protein S with which it complexes and thereby contributes to reduced coagulation function of the fetus and newborn. Consideration of functions besides immunologic effector functions may be important to our understanding of the developmental regulation of complement component production.

Because of the low plasma concentrations of individual complement proteins, administration of purified, recombinant complement proteins has been considered as an adjunct to immunoglobulin replacement therapy and polymorphonuclear leukocyte transfusion in the treatment of neonatal systemic bacterial infection (Cairo et al, 1987; Hill et al, 1986; Kalli et al, 1994; Krause et al, 1989). Although a provocative idea, this approach must be studied thoroughly to ensure that effector functions of complement activation in resting and uninfected tissues are not triggered in an unregulated fashion. Peripheral administration of one or more complement proteins might result in the unregulated activation of complement at tissue sites that would compromise rather than enhance neonatal survival. Consequences of such unregulated activation have been suggested by the detection of the complement anaphylatoxin C5a in pulmonary effluent of infants with chronic pulmonary inflammation in whom bronchopulmonary dysplasia develops (Groneck et al, 1993, 1994). Concern has also been raised that unregulated complement activation may occur in some infants who undergo extracorporeal membrane oxygenation (Johnson, 1994).

Complement activation is the regulator of multiple effector functions of the host immunologic response. Further studies of the fetus and newborn infant will be aimed at understanding the developmental and genetic regulation of immunologic and nonimmunologic functions of this important group of plasma and cell surface proteins.

## Immunoglobulins

*Immunoglobulins* are a heterogeneous group of proteins detectable in plasma and body fluids and on the surface of B lymphocytes. Although these proteins have multiple, diverse functions, they are classified as a family of proteins because of their capacity to act as antibodies—that is, to recognize and bind specifically to antigens. The rapid advances in our understanding of molecular structure and regulation, genetic diversity, and differences in function of immunoglobulins have been reviewed (Colten and Gitlin, 1995). The functions of immunoglobulins relevant to fetal-neonatal immunity are summarized in Table 35–2.

The five known classes of immunoglobulins are IgG, IgM, IgA, IgE, and IgD. The prototype immunoglobulin molecule consists of a pair of identical heavy chains that

**TABLE 35–2**

**Proteins that Compose the Elements of the Complement System**

| Complement Protein | Molecular Weight (kd) | Serum Concentration (μg/mL) | Chromosomal Location |
|---|---|---|---|
| Regulatory Plasma Proteins | | | |
| C1 INH | 105 | 200 | 1q p11 |
| C4 binding protein | 540 | 200 | 1q 3.2 |
| H | 150 | 500 | 1q 3.2 |
| I | 88 | 34 | 4q 25 |
| S Protein | 80 | 400 | 17 |
| SP 40/40, Clusterin | 80 | 50 | 8q 21 |
| C3a/C5a INA | 305 | 35 | — |
| Membrane-Associated Receptors | | | |
| *Multiple types* | | | |
| C1q R | — | — | — |
| C1q Rp | 126 | — | — |
| C1q RO2 | — | — | — |
| C3a R | 100 | — | — |
| C5a R | 40 | — | 19q 13 |
| CR1 | 190-280 | — | 1q 3.2 |
| CR2 | 140 | — | 1q 3.2 |
| CR3 | | | |
| α chain | 165 | — | 16p 11 |
| β chain | 95 | — | 2q 22 |
| CR4 | | | |
| α chain | 140 | — | 16p 11 |
| β chain | 95 | — | 21p 22 |
| DAF | 700 | — | 1q 3.2 |
| MCP | 51-68 | — | 1q 3.2 |
| CD59 | 20 | — | 11p 13 |
| Plasma Proteins | | | |
| *Classic pathway proteins* | | | |
| C1q | 450 | 70 | 1p 34 |
| C1r | 85 | 34 | 12p 13 |
| C1s | 85 | 31 | 12p 13 |
| C4 | 206 | 600 | 6p 21 |
| C2 | 102 | 20 | 6p 21 |
| C3 | 190 | 1200 | 19p 21 |
| C5 | 190 | 85 | 9q 32 |
| C6 | 128 | 45 | 5q 13 |
| C7 | 120 | 55 | 5q 13 |
| C8 | | | |
| α, β chain | 150 | 80 | 1p 34 |
| λ chain | 20 | — | 9q 34 |
| C9 | 71 | 60 | 5p 13 |
| B | 90 | 225 | 6p 21 |
| D | 25 | 1 | — |
| Properdin | 53 | 25 | Xp11 |
| *Mannan-binding lectin pathway proteins* | | | |
| MBL | 96; trimer | — | 10q 21 |
| MASP1 | 83 | — | 3q 27 |
| MASP2 | ? Same | — | ? Same |

Data from Frank MM: Complement deficiencies. Pediatr Clin North Am 47:1339-1354, 2000.

determine the immunoglobulin class in combination with a pair of identical light chains. Disulfide bonds and electrostatic forces link the chains. Each immunoglobulin molecule contains two identical domains with antigen-binding activity (Fab) and a third fragment (Fc) devoid of antibody activity. The antigen-binding activity involves sites on both the heavy and light chains, whereas sequences in the Fc region of the heavy chain are involved in mediating immunoglobulin effector functions. Functions of individual immunoglobulin classes are different but overlapping.

### Immunoglobulin G

IgG is the most abundant immunoglobulin class in human serum, accounting for more than 75% of all antibody activity in this compartment. Its monomeric form circulates in plasma and has a molecular mass of approximately 155 kd; in adults, approximately 45% of total body IgG is in the extravascular compartment. The human conceptus is able to produce IgG by 11 weeks of gestation (Gitlin and Biasucci, 1969; Fudenberg, 1965) The importance of the contributions of IgG to immunologic function is illustrated by the clinical problems encountered in individuals who are genetically deficient in its production: These patients have recurrent infections if not treated with immunoglobulin replacement therapy (Sorensen and Polmar, 1987). The observations by several investigators that infants in whom group B streptococcal sepsis develops have low concentrations of type-specific IgG prompted attempts at acute or prophylactic treatment with immunoglobulin replacement therapy (Stiehm et al, 1987). Although successful in some trials, replacement therapy has not proved as efficacious in newborns as it has in individuals with genetically determined hypogammaglobulinemia (Noya and Baker, 1989). This difference may be due in part to the fact that fetal-neonatal IgG synthesis is regulated by both developmental and genetic mechanisms (Cates et al, 1988).

The kinetics of IgG placental transport suggest both passive and active transport mechanisms. Because IgG transport begins at approximately 20 weeks of gestation, preterm infants are born with lower IgG concentrations than term infants or their mothers. The full-term infant has a complete repertoire of maternal IgG antibodies. Thus, provided that relevant maternal IgG has been transported to the fetus, newborns are not susceptible to most viral and bacterial infections (e.g., measles, rubella, varicella, group B streptococci, and *E. coli*) until transplacentally acquired antibody titers decrease to biologically nonprotective concentrations at 3 to 6 months of age. The regulation of IgG production in preterm infants has been a topic of study for five decades (Ballow et al, 1986; Dancis et al, 1953). Although adults with antibody deficiency syndromes have a higher rate of infections when IgG concentrations fall below 300 mg/dL, the serum IgG concentrations of many preterm infants decrease to less than 100 mg/dL apparently without consequences. These observations suggest that preterm infants have additional immunologic protective mechanisms or that regulation of IgG function is not accurately assessed by serum IgG concentrations alone in preterm infants. Studies also suggest that low serum concentrations of IgG in the newborn may result from reduced ability of neonatal B cells to undergo immunoglobulin isotype switching because of decreased or ineffective expression of the ligand for the B cell surface protein CD40 on activated cord blood T cells (Brugnoni et al, 1994; Fuleihan et al, 1994).

IgG functions in host defenses in several ways. It can neutralize a variety of toxins in plasma by direct binding. After antigen binding, IgG can activate the complement cascade via interaction with the early-acting complement components. The Fc portion of IgG can interact with cell surface receptors on mononuclear phagocytes and polymorphonuclear leukocytes and thereby promote clearance of immune complexes and phagocytosis of particles or microorganisms. Finally, the presence of IgG on specific target cell antigens (e.g., tumors or allogeneic transplant tissues) can mediate antibody-dependent cellular cytotoxicity, a mechanism through which lymphocyte subpopulations recognize nonself antigens.

### Immunoglobulin M

IgM represents approximately 15% of normal adult immunoglobulin. IgM circulates in serum as a pentamer of disulfide-linked immunoglobulin molecules joined by a single cross-linking peptide. The size of IgM (molecular mass >900 kd) restricts its distribution to the vascular compartment. Although the antibody-binding affinity of monomeric IgM is low, the multivalent structure of the molecule provides high pentameric antibody avidity. IgM synthesis has been detected in the human conceptus at 10½ weeks of gestation (Rosen and Janeway, 1964). Because maternal-fetal transport of IgM does not occur, elevated concentrations of IgM in the fetus or newborn (>20 mg/dL) are suggestive of intrauterine infection or immunologic stimulation (Alford et al, 1969; Stiehm et al, 1966). However, because it is technically difficult to distinguish IgM molecules with specificity for individual organisms, diagnosis of infections through analysis for specific IgM antibody remains of limited usefulness.

IgM is important to fetal-neonatal host defenses for several reasons. First, the IgM molecule is the most efficient of any immunoglobulin isotype in activation of the classical complement pathway. It thus can trigger multiple effector functions of this cascade. Second, its pentameric structure provides conformational flexibility to accommodate multivalent ligand binding. Third, because of its localization in the vascular compartment and its high efficiency in complement activation, IgM plays a prominent role clearance of invading microorganisms from serum.

### Immunoglobulin A

Although IgA accounts for approximately 10% of serum immunoglobulins, it is detectable in abundance in all external secretions. In serum, IgA is present as a monomer (molecular weight, 160 kd), whereas in secretions, it exists as a dimer (molecular weight, 500 kd) attached to a J chain identical to that found in IgM. Besides the structural difference between serum and mucosal IgA, IgA found in secretions is attached to an additional protein called the secretory component (SC). This protein is a proteolytic cleavage fragment of the receptor involved in the secretion of polymeric IgA onto mucosal surfaces and into bile. Secretory IgA produced locally on mucosal surfaces by plasma cells is thus readily distinguishable from serum IgA. Although not rigorously quantified, the amount of IgA produced daily is estimated to exceed immunoglobulin production of all isotypes combined. Despite its relative abundance, and unlike IgM and IgG, IgA cannot activate the classical pathway of complement nor effectively opsonize particles or microorganisms for phagocytosis.

Although IgA is detectable on the surface of human fetal B cells at 12 weeks of gestation, adult concentrations of serum IgA and secretory IgA are not achieved until approximately 10 years of age. Because serum IgA is not transplacentally transferred in significant amounts, IgA is almost undetectable in cord blood. Colostrum-derived secretory IgA may provide a source of IgA found in both the gastrointestinal tract and other secretions of the newborn infant. Unlike other immunoglobulin isotypes, amino acid sequences of the hinge region of the IgA-2 subclass confer partial resistance to bacterial proteases. IgA is thus more resistant than other immunoglobulin isotypes to proteolytic effects of gastric acidity. Although considerable investigation suggests that passive immunization with IgA does occur with breast-feeding in humans, the overall importance of IgA in host defenses is currently not well characterized.

### Immunoglobulin E

The concentration of IgE in serum is undetectable by standard immunochemical techniques and accounts for approximately 1/10,000 of the immunoglobulin in adult serum. IgE circulates in the monomeric form (molecular weight, 190 kd). Structurally, IgE lacks a hinge region. It is produced by most lymphoid tissues in the body but in greatest amounts in the lung and gastrointestinal tract. It is not secreted, and the appearance of IgE in body fluids generally occurs only with induction of inflammation. IgE cannot activate complement nor act as an effective opsonin. Its primary function identified to date is to mediate immediate hypersensitivity reactions. Specifically, antigen-specific IgE triggers mast cell degranulation with resultant bronchoconstriction, tissue edema, and urticaria via interactions with IgE receptors on the mast cell surface. Because of the presence of IgE in lung secretions and its potential importance in mediating allergic pulmonary and gastrointestinal reactions, considerable interest has been focused on use of serum IgE concentrations to identify premature infants at risk for development of reactive airways disease or in the diagnosis of gastrointestinal hypersensitivity reactions (Bazaral et al, 1971; Jarrett, 1984).

### Immunoglobulin D

Although IgD is found in trace quantities in adult human serum and has neither complement-activating activity nor the capacity to opsonize particles or microorganisms, approximately 50% of cord blood lymphocytes exhibit IgD on their cell surface (Colten and Gitlin, 1995). These pre-B lymphocytes express surface IgM and IgD simultaneously. Because of its wide distribution on B cells, IgD may play an important role in primary antigen recognition for the fetus and newborn infant.

## Immunoglobulin Replacement Therapy

Klesius and coworkers (1973) suggested that lack of antibody to group B streptococci occurs in infants at risk for systemic infection with this organism. The maternal contribution to type-specific IgG was subsequently supported by the work of Hemming and associates (1976) and Baker and Kasper (1976). Animal and human studies have suggested that type-specific IgG can reduce mortality from systemic group B streptococcal infections. However, opsonization is not the sole mechanism of this protective effect (Fischer, 1988). Strain- and species-specific differences in protective effects of IgG have been noted. In addition, timing of administration and dosage of IgG can affect outcome. Prenatal administration has been attempted in only a small number of cases (Morell et al, 1986), but postnatal administration has been studied extensively. Although no major short-term adverse effects were noted, studies in the 1980s to test the efficacy of immunoglobulin replacement therapy to prevent or treat bacterial infection were generally inconclusive (Noya and Baker, 1989). Over the past 10 years, investigators have focused on assessment of intravenous immunoglobulin replacement to prevent nosocomial infections in preterm infants and to treat infection in infants.

Because of low serum immunoglobulin concentrations and a concurrent greater susceptibility to infection in preterm infants, several investigators have proposed prophylactic administration of immunoglobulin to prevent antibody deficiency and nosocomial infection in such patients (Baker et al, 1992; Clapp et al, 1989; Fanaroff et al, 1994; Kinney et al, 1991; Magny et al, 1991; Weisman et al, 1994). With one exception (Baker et al, 1992), these well-designed, placebo-controlled studies have failed to show consistent benefit of this strategy using different preparations of immunoglobulin, different treatment groups, and different dosage regimens.

In septic infants, the results of immunoglobulin replacement have been difficult to interpret because of the complexities in study design associated with enrolling acutely ill infants and the small numbers of enrolled infants. Sidiropoulos and colleagues (1986) and Haque and coworkers (1988) compared antibiotics alone with antibiotics plus intravenous immunoglobulin. Each study suggested therapeutic benefit, although neither was blinded nor placebo-controlled. A small, placebo-controlled pilot study of 22 patients reported by Christensen and associates (1991) demonstrated no difference between placebo-treated and immunoglobulin-treated groups with respect to survival but did show a marked rise in numbers of immature polymorphonuclear leukocytes in the immunoglobulin-treated group. In a study of prophylactic immunoglobulin therapy in infants who weighed 500 to 2000 g, Weisman and coworkers (1993a) randomly assigned 31 infants to receive either placebo or immunoglobulin treatment. Five of 17 placebo-treated infants died during the first 7 days after birth, but none of the 14 who received immunoglobulin died. Long-term survival rates were not significantly different in the two groups (Weisman et al, 1993a). Because group B streptococci are common causal organisms in neonatal bacterial sepsis, and because there are varying amounts of antibody against this organism in standard immunoglobulin preparations, Weisman and coworkers (1993a) have developed hyperimmune immunoglobulin for use in treatment of infected infants by immunizing plasma donors. Administration of this immunoglobulin preparation to 20 newborns significantly increased serum group B streptococci type–specific opsonic activity. Human monoclonal antibodies against group B streptococci, *E. coli* K1, and *Neisseria meningitides* have also been reported, but no large clinical trials have been reported as exploring the efficacy of these preparations (Hill, 1993a; Weisman et al, 1993b).

Cairo and colleagues (1992), comparing neutrophil transfusions with immunoglobulin replacement therapy in 35 newborns with sepsis, observed better survival in the neutrophil-treated group. Whitley (1994) has suggested the potential benefit of immunoglobulin therapy and concomitant administration of antiviral therapy for infants with herpes simplex encephalitis or disseminated infection. These studies suggest that intravenous immunoglobulin is more appropriate as a therapeutic agent for infants with established infection than as a preventive strategy, but further studies are required to document efficacy (Hill, 1993b; Weisman et al, 1993b).

Besides prophylactic or acute treatment of systemic infection, immunoglobulin replacement therapy has been used in other clinical situations. Oral immunoglobulin administration with a preparation that contains IgG and IgA has been proposed for prevention of necrotizing enterocolitis (Eibl et al, 1988). Necrotizing enterocolitis did not develop in any of 88 preterm infants who received 600 mg of an oral IgA-IgG preparation daily for 28 days, whereas the disorder did develop in 6 of 91 control infants studied concurrently. Confirmation was achieved with radiography (pneumatosis, pneumoperitoneum, or hepatic portal vein gas) or histopathologic examination of specimens obtained during surgery or autopsy. Similar results have been reported in an Italian study of 132 Italian infants with birth weight less than 1500 g (Rubaltelli et al, 1991). However, a multicenter, placebo-controlled trial of oral IgG to prevent necrotizing enterocolitis failed to demonstrate efficacy (Lawrence et al, 2001). Intravenous immunoglobulin has also been used with some success in small numbers of infants with neonatal isoimmune thrombocytopenia (Massey et al, 1987). Although immunoglobulin replacement therapy may be a promising intervention in selected clinical circumstances, its role in the newborn as acute treatment of or prophylaxis for systemic infections, prevention of necrotizing enterocolitis, or treatment of isoimmune thrombocytopenia warrants further study (Noya and Baker, 1989).

## Cellular Immunity

The newborn infant, especially the preterm infant, is at increased risk for development of infection by a considerable spectrum of opportunistic organisms, including *Candida* species, herpes simplex virus, and cytomegalovirus. Developmental and genetic differences between adults and infants in cell-mediated immunologic responsiveness account for this enhanced susceptibility. Considerable investigative interest has focused on the molecular, cellular, and functional definitions of these differences (Bellanti et al, 1994; Hogg et al, 1993; Krensky and Clayberger, 1994; Leung, 1994). This discussion focuses on those developmental aspects of cell-mediated immunity known to be important for fetal or neonatal responsiveness to opportunistic infections.

Lymphocytes play multiple critical roles in the cell-mediated immunologic response. The following three lymphocytic lineages have been identified from their cell surface and functional criteria: T, or thymus-dependent, lymphocytes; B, or bursa-derived, lymphocytes; and NK, or natural killer, lymphocytes (Abo et al, 1983; Baley and Schacter, 1985). All three types develop from $CD34^+$ $CD38^{dim}$ hematopoietic stem cells found in the fetal liver (Fig. 35–1). CD34 is also expressed on early committed progenitors, which differentially express other markers useful in lineage determination. Studies of a small subset of children with SCID have suggested, although not conclusively demonstrated, that defective development of all three cells occurs, implying the presence of a common lymphoid stem cell (Thompson et al, 1984).

### Lymphocytes

#### *T Lymphocytes*

T lymphocytes, or T cells, develop in the thymus (Fig. 35–2), which is formed from the third brachial cleft and the third or fourth brachial pouch. Thymic lobes are generated when tissue from these sites moves caudally to fuse in the midline. Each lobe can be divided into the following three regions on the basis of structure and function: the cortex, the corticomedullary junction, and the medulla. The thymic cortex is composed of specialized epithelial cells that express MHC class I and class II molecules and mediate the early stages of T-cell maturation.

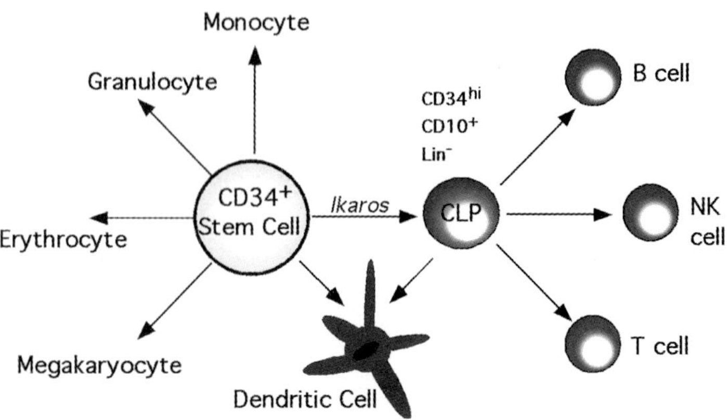


**FIGURE 35–1.** $CD34^+$ stem cells give rise to all cells in the hematopoietic lineage. This section focuses on the development of T, B, natural killer (NK), and dendritic cells, which develop from a common lymphoid precursor (CLP). Ikaros is a DNA binding protein involved in chromatin remodeling and is an essential regulator of lymphocyte development. $Lin^-$, lineage marker depleted. *(Data from Georgopoulos, 2002).*

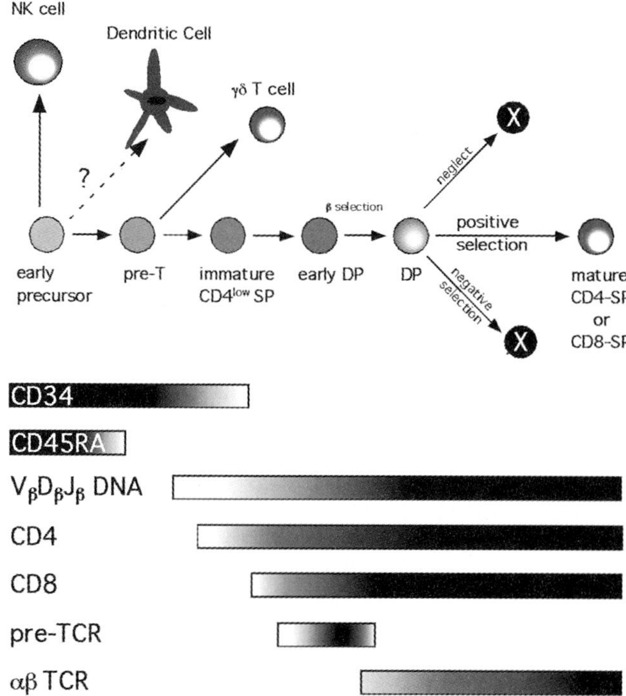


**FIGURE 35-2.** The stages of T-cell development that occur within the thymus. *Horizontal bar graphs* indicate the expression of lineage markers, important T-cell receptors/co-receptors, and complete *TCR*-β gene rearrangement. The gray scale approximates the level and timing of expression, with *black* indicating a higher level. DP, double positive ($CD4^+$ $CD8^+$); VDJ, variable, diversity and joining segment recombination. *(Data from Benoist and Mathis, 1999; Spits et al, 1998) (Adapted from Williams CB: Development of the immune system. In Rudolph C, Rudolph AM, Hostetter MK, et al [eds]: Rudolph's Pediatrics, 21st ed. New York, McGraw-Hill, 2002.)*

This complex developmental process begins when multipotent $CD1a^-$, $CD5^-$, $CD34^+$, $CD38^{low}$ stem cells enter the thymus at the corticomedullary junction and migrate into the outer cortex (Res et al, 1996). Maturation continues as cells migrate back through the cortex toward the corticomedullary junction. The first committed T cells express low levels of CD4 and show DNA rearrangement at the T-cell receptor (TCR) δ gene locus. These events are followed by low levels of CD8 expression and by rearrangement at the TCR β locus, which generates a pre-TCR on the cell surface (Spits et al, 1998). The pre-TCR is composed of several polypeptides, including a TCR β chain and the invariant pre-Tαchain. Expression of the pre-TCR serves as an important developmental checkpoint (βselection) (von Boehmer and Fehling, 1997). Cells that do not successfully rearrange their TCR β chain cannot express the pre-TCR and die by apoptosis (Falk et al, 2001). The remaining cells generate antigen-specific receptors when the TCR α chain replaces pre-Tα. These intermediate to late-stage progenitors also express both the CD4 and CD8 co-receptors and are called "double positives." The minor population of δγT cells follows a similar developmental pattern.

Small double-positive cells ($CD4^+$, $CD8^+$, $TCR^{low}$) constitute about three fourths of all thymocytes, reflecting the critical and rate-limiting developmental stage that follows. Further maturation requires that the unique TCR on each thymocyte interact with self-peptide–MHC complexes expressed on the surface of thymic epithelial cells. Several factors control the outcome of this interaction, including the strength and timing of the signal generated and the nature of the antigen-presenting cell (Bevan, 1997; Yun and Bevan, 2001). "Appropriate" interactions between thymocytes and thymic cortical epithelial cells stimulate sustained activation of the mitogen-activated signaling cascade (MAPK), resulting in continued development (positive selection). "Weak" interactions fail to generate a positive signal and result in T cell death by neglect. "Strong" interactions between T cells and bone marrow–derrived antigen-presenting cells cause transient activation of the MAPK pathway, which leads to activation-induced cell death (negative selection) (Gong et al, 2001). Negative selection in the thymus is the primary mechanism by which self-reactive T cells are eliminated. The precise mechanisms involved in positive and negative selection are not known.

Thymocytes in the medulla are mature, in that they express either CD4 or CD8 and a single TCR heterodimer. $CD4^+$ T cells recognize foreign antigenic peptide bound to HLA class II proteins, whereas those expressing CD8 are restricted to HLA class I molecules. In the human embryo, the first naïve, mature T cells appear at around 11 to 12 weeks of embryonic development. Thymopoieisis continues for many years thereafter. Naïve T cells express the adhesion molecule L-selectin (CD62L), which allows them to home to peripheral lymphoid organs. This process requires the interaction between L-selectin (CD62L) and GlyCAM-1, CD34 expressed on high endothelial venules, or both to promote adhesion. The first T-cell proliferative responses that occur are to mitogens and can be measured at about 12 weeks of gestational age. By 15 to 20 weeks, antigen-specific responses can be detected (Adkins, 1999; Garcia et al, 2001). Maturation of immune responses continues throughout the first year of life, a fact that affects vaccination schedules (Gans et al, 1998). Kennedy and associates (2001) have shown that thymopoiesis continues at some level into adulthood

The final component of T-cell development is independent of the thymus and involves peripheral (lymph nodes, spleen, and gut-associated lymphoid tissue) homeostatic mechanisms. These poorly understood events control the expansion of clones and the development of T-cell memory. Peripheral repertoire selection begins with activation of mature, naive T cells. T-cell activation requires a complex molecular cascade that results in reorganization of signaling molecules in the membrane into the "immunologic synapse" and in signal transduction (Bromley et al, 2001). Many of the important biochemical events in this process have been described. TCR engagement by an appropriate MHC-peptide ligand results in phosphorylation of components of the CD3 complex. The CD3 complex is composed of the αβTCR and γ, δ, ε and ζ chains. These later molecules all contain specific amino acid sequences called immune receptor tyrosine-based activation motifs (ITAMs), which serve as molecular targets for the tyrosine kinases fyn and lck. The ζ chain is thought to be the most critical component and is found as a homodimer. Each ζ chain contains three ITAMs, which will bind the tyrosine kinase Zap-70 when sequentially phosphorylated.

Appropriate phosporylation of ζ results in a downstream cascade involving the tyrosine phosphorylation of multiple cellular substrates, including phospholipase Cγ1, the guanine nucleotide exchange factor Vav, and the adaptor protein Shc. Ultimately the genetic program of the cells is altered, leading to the transcription of genes for cytokines, cytokine receptors, and transcription factors (Cantrell, 2002).

Initially after activation, all naïve T cells secrete IL-2. $CD4^+$ T cells will then differentiate into either Th1 or Th2 effectors. The mechanisms driving this differentiation continue to be the subject of considerable investigation. Th1 cells secrete IL-2, IFN-γ, lymphotoxin (LT), and TNF-β, and Th1 responses are generally pro-inflammatory. Th1 cytokines act synergistically to lyse virally infected cells, activate antigen-presenting cells as well as granulocytes. IFN-γ also promotes the development of the Th1 phenotype and inhibits the development of Th2 cells. Th2 cells secrete IL-4, IL-5, IL-10, and IL-13. IL-4 induces immunoglobulin heavy chain class switching to the IgE isotype and promotes the development of the Th2 phenotype. IL-5 is an eosinophil growth factor. Thus Th2 cells are thought to promote antibody production and the allergic response via multiple mechanisms (Ouyang et al, 2001).

Activation of naïve T cells requires a second signal, and the most potent co-stimulatory molecule is CD28. The ligands for CD28 are B7–1 and B7–2, which are present on the surface of antigen-presenting cells. Cytotoxic T-lymphocyte antigen (CTLA-4), a molecule expressed only on activated T cells, also binds B7–1 and B7–2 and functions as a negative regulator of T-cell activation. Experiments with knockout mice demonstrate that CD28 is the major co-stimulatory receptor and that signaling through CTLA-4 attenuates CD28-dependent responses (Alegre and Thompson, 2001; Wood et al, 2001).

Control of the clonal proliferation seen in a primary immune response involves Fas/FasL–mediated cell death. This mechanism resets the peripheral immune system, thereby maintaining adequate clonal diversity. A small number of activated T cells do survive, and they differentiate into memory cells. Memory cells are defined functionally (more rapid response) and by the expression of certain cell surface markers. Early memory T cells are L-selectin$^{low}$, CD45R0$^{high}$, and CD44$^{high}$. Late memory cells may become L-selectin$^{high}$, which is a surface marker seen in naïve T cells. The ultimate number of memory cells has been shown in mice to reflect the initial antigenic load and clonal burst size. Memory T cells allow the secondary response to be both more rapid and more potent, characteristics that form the basis for vaccinations. The memory phenotype is not seen early in life, but grows with age. The precise mechanisms that generate and maintain memory T cells have not been determined, although it is known that the persistence of $CD8^+$ memory T cells in mice does not depend on the persistence of specific antigen (Sprent, 2002; Williams and Brady, 2001).

Immunocompetent T cells capable of responding to foreign lymphocytes in the mixed lymphocyte reaction are found in the fetal liver at 5 weeks of gestation. Before 8 weeks of gestation, lymphocytes are not detectable in the fetal thymus. After 8 weeks, lymphoid follicles, T lymphocytes, and Hassall corpuscles can be identified. By 12 to 14 weeks, T lymphocytes can be found in the fetal spleen (Timens et al, 1987). By 15 to 20 weeks, the fetus has readily detectable numbers of peripheral T lymphocytes.

### *Natural Killer Cells*

NK cells are a component of the innate immune response and represent about 10% to 15% of all peripheral blood lymphocytes. NK cells are present in the spleen, lungs, and liver but rarely in lymph nodes and thoracic duct lymph (Cerwenka and Lanier, 2001). Interestingly, NK cells are the major type of lymphocyte found in the maternal decidual tissue, where they represent up to 95% of all lymphocytes (King et al, 1996b). NK cells are distinguished from other lymphocytes by their morphology, function, and expression of distinct surface molecules. Expression of the cell surface markers CD16 (FcγRIII) and CD56 (nerve cell adhesion molecule-1 [NCAM-1]) can be used to identify the NK population by analytical flow cytometry. Mature NK cells appear larger and more granular than T or B cells (Cooper et al, 2001). They are also distinguished by the presence of both activating and inhibitory receptors that are used to identify and kill selectively virally infected cells and tumors (Biassoni et al, 2001). NK receptors recognize MHC class I molecules on target cells, resulting in signals that suppress NK cell function. Target cells that are deficient or lacking in MHC class I activate NK cell function, leading to the release of lysosomal granules. These granules contain serine proteases, perforin, and TGF-β, which disrupt the target cell membrane and induce an inflammatory response. Studies show significant lower NK cell activity in the fetus and neonate compared to the adult (Georgeson et al, 2001; Kadowaki et al, 2001).

NK cells are derived from hematopoietic precursors, probably from a common T/NK progenitor, and first make their appearance in fetal liver as early as 6 weeks of gestation. Committed $CD34^+$, $CD56^-$ NK progenitors have been identified in the fetal thymus, bone marrow, and liver, although the thymus is probably not essential for NK cell development (Spits et al, 1998). Gene targeting experiments show that the transcription factors *Ets 1*, *IRF 1*, and *IRF 2* are required for NK cell development (Barton et al, 1998; Lohoff et al, 2000; Ogasawara et al, 1998). *Ets 1* is a 56 kd protein that contains a winged helix loop helix DNA-binding domain, capable of recognizing a purine-rich sequence containing the core consensus GGAA/T. Upon activation, *Ets 1* is phosphorylated, resulting in inhibition of DNA binding and rapid protein turnover. *Ets 1*–deficient mice lack both NK cells and NK cell activity (Barton et al, 1998). *IRF 1* appears to induce IL-15 expression, which promotes NK differentiation (Ogasawara et al, 1998). Initial studies also suggested the zinc finger transcription factor *Ikaros* was also essential. However, this interpretation was based on a knockout mouse that produced a dominant-negative form of *Ikaros* rather than a null allele (Guest et al, 1997). These later experiments do demonstrate that *Ikaros*-related proteins yet to be identified are essential for NK cell development. A lack of cell surface markers for NK precursors complicates these studies. In the human neonate, the NK population is immature:

Only half of all NK cells express CD56, and the NK cytolytic activity is lower (Dominguez et al, 1993). This functional reduction in NK activity has been proposed as a factor contributing to the severity of neonatal herpes simplex virus infections.

NK cell receptors are fundamentally different from the TCR and B-cell receptor. NK receptor gene expression does not require gene segment rearrangement, and the receptors are not clonally distributed. Instead, NK cells use an array of stimulatory and inhibitory receptors to regulate their cytolytic functions. A cluster of 10 or more genes encoding NK receptors, termed killer immunoglobulin–like receptors (KIRs), has been located on human chromosome 19q13.4 (Biassoni et al, 2001; Lanier, 1998). Each of these type I glycoproteins recognizes a different allelic group of HLA-A–, HLA-B–, HLA-C–, or HLA-G–encoded proteins, and each KIR is expressed by only a subset of NK cells. Another family of Ig-like receptor genes termed ILT is present near the KIR locus at 19q13.3. These receptors are not as restricted as the KIRs and bind multiple HLA class I molecules. A third inhibitory receptor gene locus has been identified on chromosome 12p12 to p13. These genes encode a C-type lectin inhibitory heterodimeric receptor called CD94/NKG2 that binds HLA-E. Importantly, those KIRs, ILT receptors, and CD94/NGK2s that have a long cytoplasmic tail with two immunoreceptor tyrosine-based inhibitory motifs (ITIMs) function as inhibitory receptors. Upon phosphorylation, the two ITIMs recruit and activate the Src homology domain 2 (SH2)-containing tyrosine phosphatases, which turn off the kinase-driven activation cascade (Ravetch and Lanier, 2000). The KIR family member KIR2DL4 is distinct from other KIRs in structure and distribution. KIR2DL4 binds HLA-G and has a single ITIM in its cytoplasmic tail and a lysine in the transmembrane region, which allow association with adaptor proteins. This inhibitory receptor was found on all NK cells in the placenta at term but not on circulating maternal NK cells, suggesting that expression of KIR2DL4 may be induced during pregnancy (Rajagopalan and Long, 1999). The colocalization of HLA-G on fetal trophoblasts and KIR2DL4-bearing NK cells certainly warrants further evaluation.

Other KIR or members of the C-type lectin superfamily serve as activating receptors (Moretta et al, 2001). These receptors lack the long cytoplasmic tail of the inhibitory receptors and therefore do not contain ITIMs. Instead, they have a charged amino acid in the transmembrane region that allows the receptor to associate with the adaptor molecule DAP12 (Lanier et al, 1998). This adaptor contains an immunoreceptor tyrosine–based activation motif (ITAM) that allows these receptors to activate NK cells. The physiologic role of these HLA class I–specific activating receptors remains unknown. Another group of NK cell–activating receptors has been identified, termed natural cytotoxicity receptors (NCRs) (Moretta et al, 2001). These proteins (NKp46, NKp30, NKp44) are Ig superfamily members with little similarity to one another or to other NK receptors. They are highly specific for NK cells, and they appear to interact with non-HLA molecules, although the precise ligands have yet to be identified.

### *B Lymphocytes*

B cells are lymphocytes that upon activation give rise to terminally differentiated, immunoglobulin-secreting plasma cells. Immunoglobulins form the humoral arm of the immune system and provide the main form of protection against many pathogens. B-cell development can be divided into embryonic and adult phases (Fig. 35–3). The embryonic phase begins in the fetal liver at the same gestational age as T-cell development, follows a similar time course, and utilizes similar developmental strategies. The adult phase occurs in the bone marrow and continues throughout life. In both phases, B-cell progenitors are selected at key developmental checkpoints for the presence of a functional BCR rearrangement and for the absence of BCR self-reactivity. The progenitors with self-reactive receptors either are eliminated or generate new antigen receptors by means of continued gene segment rearrangements that are not self-reactive. Both B-cell development and peripheral B-cell homeostasis require signal transduction through the BCR. Although the B-cell compartment is well formed before birth, diversification of the antibody repertoire and several important antibody responses are not developed until long after the neonatal period (Hardy and Hayakawa, 2001; Rohrer et al, 2000; Rolink et al, 2001; Yankee and Clark, 2000).

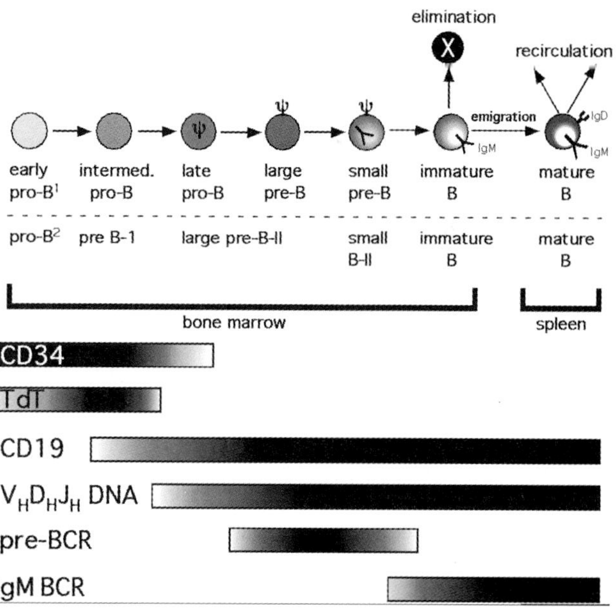


**FIGURE 35–3.** The stages of B-cell development in the bone marrow and spleen. Expression of the intracellular enzyme terminal deoxynucleotidyl transferase (TdT), the cell surface marker CD19, the pre-B cell receptor (pre-BCR) with the surrogate light chain (ψ), and complete heavy-chain gene segment rearrangement is shown. The gray scale estimates the timing and level of expression, with *black* indicating a higher level. VDJ, variable, diversity and joining segment recombination; IgM, immunoglobulin M. *(Kincade et al, 2000; Lassoued et al, 1883; Data from Melchers and Rolink, 1999; Rolink et al, 2001.) (Adapted from Williams CB: Development of the immune system. In Rudolph C, Rudolph AM, Hostetter MK, et al [eds]: Rudolph's Pediatrics, 21st ed. New York, McGraw-Hill, 2002.)*

B-cell development begins before 7 weeks of gestational age in the fetal liver, and by 8 weeks, pre-B cells in various stages of maturation are seen. By 8 to 10 weeks, $CD34^+$ hematopoietic stem cells are also found in the bone marrow, and B-cell development begins there as well. The early phase of B-cell development, as in T-cell development, is antigen independent. The first committed progenitors (pro/pre-B-I) express CD34, terminal deoxynucleotidyl transferase (TdT), recombinase-activating genes (RAGs), and CD19 (Li et al, 1993). They lack immunoglobulin gene rearrangement (Allman et al, 1999). The next lineage is marked by heavy chain (H) diversity to joining ($D_H$ to $J_H$) gene segment rearrangements, followed by variable to diversity/joining segment rearrangement. TdT is utilized during this process to insert nucleotides between the segments, creating additional diversity at a region that encodes the $V_H$ portion of antibody-binding sites. Late cells in this stage express an invariant surrogate light chain (SLC) (Kitamura et al, 1992). The normal light chain genes remain in germline configuration.

The first developmental checkpoint in B-cell development requires expression of SLC together with Igα and Igβ on the cell surface as the pre-BCR, marking the transition to the pre-B II stage. Expression of the pre-BCR is essential for positive selection of cells that have a functional μH chain rearrangement and for expansion of the pre-B cell lineage (Gong and Nussenzweig, 1996). Cells with a nonfunctional H chain rearrangement or with H chains that assemble poorly with SLC are unable to progress. $V_L$-to-$J_L$ rearrangement takes place next, and the newly expressed polymorphic L chain protein replaces the surrogate light chain. The completed BCR is antigen-specific and contains the mIgM molecule. A second selection developmental checkpoint occurs here, and those B cells with self-reactive receptors are eliminated or edited (Hartley et al, 1991). Only 10% to 20% of the immature B cells survive this negative selection and migrate to the spleen, which they enter through the terminal branches of the central arterioles. Once in the spleen, they rapidly differentiate into membrane $IgM^+$, membrane $IgD^+$, $B220^+$ mature B cells, which enter the recirculating pool of B lymphocytes (Hardy and Hayakawa, 2001).

When mature B cells contact antigen through the BCR, a signal is transduced that promotes further growth and differentiation into surface $Ig^+$ memory cells and plasma cells (Calamo, 2001). BCR signaling involves activation of the tyrosine kinases Syk and Btk, which are also involved in pre-BCR signal transduction. Certain mutations in Btk result in a failure of pre-BCR signaling, leading to X-linked agammaglobulinemia. Many B cell responses utilize the ability of B cells to capture antigen at vanishingly low concentrations, process the antigen into small peptide fragments, then present the antigen to Th cells in the context of MHC class II molecules. Antigen-specific T cells then form conjugates with antigen-presenting B cells. The T-cell membrane protein gp39 interacts with CD40 on B cells, triggering B clonal expansion, cytokine responsiveness, and isotype switching.

B lymphocytes with surface IgM are first found in the fetal liver at 9 weeks of gestation and in the fetal spleen at 11 weeks (Owen et al, 1977; Timens et al, 1987). Antigen-specific antibody production can be detected in the human fetus by 20 weeks of gestation. Fetal spleen cells can synthesize IgM and IgG in vitro by 11 and 13 weeks of gestation, respectively.

### *Functional Differences Between Fetal and Adult Lymphocytes*

Multiple studies have documented differences in the proportions of fetal-neonatal T-lymphocyte subpopulations and B cells at different gestational ages and in a variety of perinatal disease states (Baker et al, 1987; Lilja et al, 1984; Pittard et al, 1985). In addition, functional differences between cord blood and adult T cells and B cells have been identified (Andersson et al, 1983; Bussel et al, 1988; Hauser et al, 1985; Hayward and Mori, 1984; Hicks et al, 1983; Jacoby and Oldstone, 1983; Nelson et al, 1986; Olding and Oldstone, 1974; Oldstone et al, 1977; Papadogiannakis and Johnsen, 1988; Pittard et al, 1984, 1989). Because of the potential importance of both of these areas to future immunologic treatment of newborns, each is reviewed here.

Although multiple functional and cell surface characteristics have been used to identify and study T lymphocytes, less mitogen-induced proliferation, weaker ability to induce immunoglobulin synthesis by B cells, presence of different proportions of helper and regulatory cell surface markers, and smaller capacity to produce lymphokines have all been shown to differentiate fetal-neonatal T cells from adult T cells. Even though the in vivo significance of these differences has not been defined, the fetus and newborn infant can mount a cell-mediated immunologic response against certain antigens comparable to that of adults. Differences in the regulation of this responsiveness in the fetus and newborn are most likely the result of the necessity of preserving the fetus's immunologic role as a graft.

Availability of monoclonal antibodies directed at epitopes found on functionally distinct T-cell subsets has permitted identification of differences in T-cell regulation in certain common perinatal medical and infectious conditions (Ryhanen et al, 1984; Wilson et al, 1985). From a therapeutic perspective, the decreased production of lymphokines has considerable potential for clinical utilization. Specifically, it has been shown that neonatal T cells produce less IFN γ than adult T cells (Frenkel and Bryson, 1987; Wakasugi and Virelizier, 1985; Wilson et al, 1986; Winter et al, 1983). Other investigators have elucidated the molecular details of IFN-γ regulation in newborn T cells as follows: Methylation status of a specific nucleotide motif in the 5′ regulatory region of the IFN-γ gene correlates with transcription of the gene (Penix et al, 1993; Young et al, 1994).

These findings suggest that induction by IFN-γ may play a major role in developmental regulation of immunologic responsiveness and may thereby provide an important reagent with which to enhance the capacity of infected infants to respond to invading microbes. Systemic administration of IFN-γ to infants, as has been done in adults with chronic granulomatous disease, leprosy, and acquired immunodeficiency syndrome (AIDS) remains a possibility for further exploration. However, an alternative therapy in the neonatal period could be in vitro activation of autologous lymphocytes, which has been used in adults with malignancies. Such an approach might avoid the unanticipatable developmental regulatory problems of the systemic administration of a substance, such as IFN-γ, that has multiple, potentially deleterious effects. Similar approaches may be considered in specific infections with individual cytokines—for example, TNF-α and GM-CSF (Cairo et al, 1991; Wilson et al, 1993).

Considerable investigation has focused on the ontogeny of B lymphocytes (Bofill et al, 1985; Gathings et al, 1977; Pedersen et al, 1983; Pereira et al, 1982; Tedder et al, 1985a, 1985b). In the fetus, these cells are detectable during the first trimester, but their expression of immunoglobulins differs from that observed in adults. B-cell precursors (pre-B cells) are detectable in human fetal liver at 8 weeks of gestation and in the bone marrow at 12 weeks. By the 15th week of gestation, the proportions of fetal B cells that express different immunoglobulin heavy-chain isotypes are equivalent to those in adults. These cells exhibit intracytoplasmic heavy chains. They lack stable surface immunoglobulin molecules characteristic of mature B cells but are the precursors of $IgM^{+}$ B lymphocytes. The generation of immunoglobulin isotype diversity within the B-cell lineage occurs in the fetus without apparent stimulation by multiple foreign antigens. However, a fetal-neonatal characteristic of B lymphocytes is their concurrent expression of two or three immunoglobulin isotypes. The molecular events that regulate isotype switching and diversity are being investigated (Colten and Gitlin, 1995).

Although B cells of full-term and preterm infants can synthesize IgM, IgG, and IgA, the response of human infants to certain foreign antigens is qualitatively distinct from that of adults. For example, as noted in early studies of antibody responses to *Salmonella* organisms, infants can respond vigorously to protein H antigen but are incapable of responding to polysaccharide antigenic determinants (the O antigens of the cell wall). These differences appear to be due to both intrinsic differences in B-cell responsiveness and greater suppressor T-cell activity in the fetus and newborn. Further understanding of the mechanisms that regulate B-cell function may permit individualized immunologic manipulation of antibody responsiveness specific for the developmental stages of preterm and full-term infants. For example, systemic administration of pharmacologic agents, such as recombinant human cytokines, may permit enhanced B-cell or T-cell responsiveness to specific infectious agents. Alternatively, in vitro exposure of autologous T or B cells to these cytokines may also permit administration of focused immunoenhancing therapy.

## Polymorphonuclear Neutrophils

As observed for T and B lymphocytes, neonatal polymorphonuclear neutrophils (PMNs) are present at early stages of gestation, but thier functional capacities are different from those of adult PMNs. Progenitor cells that are committed to maturation along granulocyte or macrophage cell lineages (granulocyte-macrophage colony-forming units [CFU-GM]) are detectable in the human fetal liver between 6 and 12 weeks of gestation in proportions comparable to those observed in adult bone marrow (Christensen, 1989). Human fetal blood has detectable CFU-GM from the 12th week of gestation to term (Christensen, 1989; Liang et al, 1988;). Although these progenitor cells are detectable in the fetus and newborn infant, developmental differences between adult and neonatal mature PMNs have been demonstrated—in signal transduction, cell surface protein expression, cytoskeletal rigidity, microfilament contraction, oxygen metabolism, and intracellular antioxidant mechanisms (Hill, 1987; Ricevuti and Mazzone, 1987).

Besides intrinsic differences in PMN function, induction of specific functions as well as maturation of these cells are developmentally regulated by the availability in the microenvironment of specific inflammatory mediators and growth factors (Christensen, 1989; Vercellotti et al, 1987). For example, an activation product of the fifth component of complement, C5a, is a chemoattractant at sites of inflammation. Low concentrations of C5 in neonatal sera may not permit establishment of chemoattractant gradients at sites of inflammation in newborns comparable to those in adults. Differences between adult and fetal-neonatal PMN functions may thus reflect intrinsic cellular differences required for fetal well-being as well as differences in the availability or activity of substances that regulate PMN function.

The recognition that systemic bacterial infection in newborns is commonly accompanied by profound neutropenia prompted investigation of neutrophil kinetics in infected infants (Christensen et al, 1980, 1982; Santos et al, 1980). These studies have suggested diverse, developmentally specific regulatory mechanisms required for mobilization of the neutrophil response to infection. Lack of neutrophil precursors in bone marrow aspirates of infected infants and systemic neutropenia motivated several investigators to give neutrophil replacement therapy to neutropenic, infected infants (Christensen et al, 1980). Although this approach has been successful in some cases, the results have not been uniformly beneficial (Cairo, 1984, 1987; Menitove and Abrams, 1987; Stegagno et al, 1985;). Immunoglobulin replacement therapy treatment with recombinant cytokines has also been observed to have beneficial effects on mobilization of neutrophils during bacterial sepsis (Christensen et al, 1991). This heterogeneity emphasizes the importance of individualizing immunologic interventions for the developmental stage of the infant and the invading microorganism being treated. In vitro treatment of neutrophil precursors in peripheral neonatal blood with recombinant cytokines as well as adjunctive therapy with immunoregulatory proteins may provide future options for this therapy (Cairo, 1991; Gillan et al, 1994; Hill, 1993b; Hill et al, 1991).

## Monocytes and Macrophages

Cells committed to phagocyte maturation (granulocyte or monocyte-macrophage) are detectable in the human fetal liver by the 6th week of gestation and in peripheral fetal blood by the 15th week. Unlike granulocytes, whose tissue half-life is hours to days, macrophages migrate into tissues and reside for weeks to months. In a tissue-specific fashion, these cells regulate availability of multiple factors, including proteases, antiproteases, prostaglandins, growth factors, reactive oxygen intermediates, and a considerable repertoire of monokines.

The importance of macrophages in the neonatal response to infectious agents has been documented in multiple studies. For example, increased antibody response and protection from lethal doses of *Listeria monocytogenes* were induced in newborn mice by administration of adult macrophages (Lu et al, 1979). Functional differences in chemotaxis and phagocytosis between adult and neonatal cells have been observed and most likely result from both intrinsic fetal-neonatal monocyte-macrophage characteristics and nonmacrophage factors (e.g., decreased production of the lymphokine IFN-$\gamma$) (English et al, 1988; Stiehm et al, 1984; van Tol et al, 1984). Inducible expression of individual complement proteins by lipopolysaccharide (LPS), a constituent of gram-negative cell walls, has also been shown to differ in adult and neonatal monocyte-macrophages (Sutton et al, 1986, 1994). This difference suggests that even though signal transduction mediated by LPS, LPS-induced transcription, and accumulation of messenger RNAs (mRNAs), which direct the synthesis of the third component of complement and factor B, are comparable in adult and neonatal cells, a translational regulatory mechanism does not permit these important inflammatory proteins to be synthesized by LPS-induced neonatal cells. This observation emphasizes the fact that fetal-neonatal monocyte-macrophages may have functions developmentally distinct from those of adult cells. For example, in utero production of growth factors and removal of senescent cells during tissue remodeling may be critical to fetal development (Kannourakis et al, 1988). Concurrent induction of these functions and immunologic effector functions in fetal monocyte-macrophages would potentially elicit nonspecific inflammation in actively remodeling tissues.

Besides antibacterial functions, neonatal monocyte-macrophages contribute to tissue-specific regulation of the microenvironment in individual organs. For example, considerable attention has focused on the contributions of these cells to antioxidant defenses and to regulation of protease-antiprotease balance. Because of the importance of these functions in tissue injury and repair, tissue- and injury-specific treatment by appropriately targeted and primed monocyte-macrophages may provide therapeutic options for treatment of a spectrum of problems, from oxygen toxicity in the lung to hemorrhage in the brain.

## Specific Immunologic Deficiencies

The most common reason, besides prematurity, for the greater immunologic susceptibility to infection in neonates is administration of corticosteroids for treatment or prevention of bronchopulmonary dysplasia. Although pulmonary and neurodevelopmental benefits have been attributed to this therapy (Abman and Groothius, 1994; Cummings et al, 1989), caution has developed about the possible adverse effects of steroid administration (Bancalari, 2001; Barrington, 2002; Committee on the Fetus and Newborn, 2002). Even though the mechanisms that lead to steroid-induced amelioration of pulmonary disease have not been completely elucidated, pulmonary inflammatory response, as measured by concentrations of the anaphylatoxin C5a, leukotriene $B_4$, IL-1, elastase-$\alpha_1$-proteinase inhibitor, and a number of neutrophils, has been shown to be attenuated in steroid-treated infants (Groneck et al, 1993). Whereas shorter courses of steroids may reduce side effects, including immunosusceptibility, the availability of nebulized steroids may provide effective anti-inflammatory therapy with minimum toxicity (Cole et al, 1999).

Well over 100 primary immunodeficiency diseases are now recognized. The physician should attempt to differentiate infants with specific genetically regulated immunologic deficiencies from those with developmentally regulated, environmentally induced, or infection-related susceptibility to microbial invasion (Rosen, 1986; Rosen et al, 1984).

A careful family history during an antenatal visit may be helpful in identifying relatives removed by as many as two to four generations who have histories suggestive of genetic immunodeficiency. Because of the availability of antenatal diagnostic techniques for several of these diseases, initiation of treatment immediately after or possibly before birth can be considered (Flake et al, 1996; Harland et al, 1988; Holzgreve et al, 1984; Perignon et al, 1987; Puck et al, 1997).

### Severe Combined Immunodeficiency

SCID is a rare category of diseases affecting both B and T cells. The estimated frequency is 1 in 70,000 to 100,000 live births (Buckley et al, 1997; Stephan et al, 1993;). Before the identification of the genes involved in producing the SCID phenotype, investigators classified patients with the disorder by analyzing the number, cell surface proteins, and function of circulating lymphocytes. The most common subgroups are $T^-B^-$ SCID, $T^-B^+$ SCID, and adenosine deaminase deficiency.

$T^-B^+$ SCID accounts for more than half of all cases of SCID, and both X-linked and autosomal recessive forms exist (Fischer, 2000). About 80% of patients with $T^-B^+$ SCID are males with the X-linked form, which is the result of deleterious mutations in the "common" gamma chain ($\gamma_c$) shared by the IL-2, IL-4, IL-7, IL-9 and IL-15 cytokine receptors (Noguchi et al, 1993). Defects in the $\gamma_c$ protein abrogate development of T cells and NK cells and lead to B-cell dysfunction despite normal B-cell numbers. IL-7 receptor signaling is essential for T-cell development within the thymus, and the deficiency of this cytokine accounts for the absence of T cells (Cao et al, 1995; DiSanto et al, 1995; Peschon et al, 1994). IL-15 is implicated in NK-cell development, and reductions in IL-4 receptor signaling are thought to contribute to the poor B-cell function seen in $\gamma_c$-deficient patients (Mrozek et al, 1996). Nevertheless, the precise mechanisms involved in the NK-cell developmental defect and the B-cell functional defect are largely unknown.

The less common, autosomal recessive form of $T^-B^+$ SCID is primarily due to mutations in the Janus-associated tyrosine kinase JAK3 (Macchi et al, 1995; Russell et al,

1995). This kinase is expressed in cells of hematopoietic lineage and associates with $\gamma_c$ as part of the cytokine receptor–signaling cascade. The $T^-B^+NK^-$ immunophenotype of affected patients is identical to that seen in $\gamma_c$ deficiency. Rarely, patients with autosomal recessive $T^-B^+$ SCID have NK cells. In two such patients, a defect was found in the IL-7Rα chain (Puel et al, 1998). This finding was predicted by the phenotype of the IL7R knockout mouse, and the data imply that the IL-7 receptor is not essential for NK-cell development.

Clinically, the X-linked and autosomal recessive forms of $T^-B^+$ SCID are indistinguishable. Affected infants often appear normal at birth. In the neonatal period, a morbilliform rash, probably the result of attenuated graft-versus-host disease from transplacental passage of maternal lymphocytes, may be the only symptom of SCID (Rosen, 1986). Over the first several months of life, as the acquired maternal antibody levels drop, failure to thrive and undue susceptibility to infection become universal features. Intractable diarrhea, pneumonia, and persistent thrush, especially oral thrush, are the triad of findings most commonly seen in infants with this disease (Stephan et al, 1993).

Mutations in the gene encoding adenosine deaminase (ADA), an enzyme in the purine salvage pathway, account for about 20% of all cases of SCID. Mutations in another enzyme in the purine salvage pathway, purine nucleoside phosphorylase (PNP), are found in about 4% of patients with SCID (Fischer, 2000; Fischer et al, 1997). The ADA-deficient phenotype is variable, and neonatal onset, delayed onset, and partial forms have been described (Santisteban et al, 1993). In neonatal-onset ADA deficiency, patients have a profound T, B, and NK cell lymphopenia, with a clinical presentation similar to that of $T^-B^+$ SCID (Hirschhorn, 1990). Even though ADA is normally present in all mammalian cells, life-threatening disease in ADA deficiency is limited to the immune system. Less severe manifestations include flaring of the costochondral junction as seen on the lateral chest radiograph ("rachitic rosary") and pelvic dysplasia. Other findings associated with ADA deficiency are hepatic and renal dysfunction, deafness, and cognitive problems (Fischer, 2000; Rogers et al, 2001). Patients who lack ADA accumulate deoxy-adenosine triphosphate (dATP) in red blood cells and lymphocytes, and the concentration correlates with disease severity. The ADA substrates, adenosine and deoxyadenosine, are found at increased levels in the serum and urine. Studies in ADA-deficient mice suggest that developing thymocytes are particularly sensitive to these metabolic derangements and that the few T cells that do mature have signaling defects (Blackburn et al, 2001). The precise mechanism by which the accumulation of ADA substrates results in the immunologic disease seen in humans remains unclear (Yamashita et al, 1998).

The remaining 20% of patients with SCID lack mature T and B cells but have functional NK cells ($T^-B^-NK^+$). These patients exhibit an autosomal recessive pattern of inheritance and have defects in the V(D)J recombination machinery (Schwarz et al, 1996). Somatic recombination of variable, diversity, and joining DNA segments is a critical step in development of B and T cells. A rearranged IgM heavy chain and TCR β chain form components of the pre-B and pre-T receptors, which provide essential survival signals for developing lymphocytes. In the absence of recombination, these lymphocyte precursors do not receive a survival signal and so die, producing the $T^-B^-$ SCID phenotype. NK cells do not require somatic cell recombination and survive. In the recombination process, DNA cleavage is mediated by RAG1 and RAG2, the recombination-activating proteins, which recognize specific sequences flanking V, D, and J segments. The two proteins act in concert to introduce a double-stranded DNA break and leave hairpin-sealed coding ends. Recruitment of a DNA-dependent protein kinase, and other components of the general DNA repair machinery, completes the process.

Mutations in the genes encoding both RAG1 and RAG2 have been identified in patients with $T^-B^-NK^+$ SCID (Corneo et al, 2000). In some cases, the same RAG mutations have been found in patients with Omenn syndrome (Corneo et al, 2001). Omenn syndrome is clinically characterized by failure to thrive, diarrhea, erythroderma, alopecia, hepatosplenomegaly, and lymphadenopathy. This finding implies that factors other than RAG mutations also contribute to the Omenn phenotype. Finally, a small subset of patients with $T^-B^-NK^+$ SCID also have increased sensitivity to ionizing radiation, suggesting mutations affecting the DNA repair mechanism (Fischer, 2000). This supposition is strengthened by murine and equine SCID, in which specific defects in the DNA-dependent protein kinase involved in V(D)J recombination and DNA repair have been identified.

The diagnosis of SCID is often suggested by an opportunistic or unusually severe infection in the setting of profound lymphopenia (<1000 lymphocytes/mm$^3$)(Gennery and Cant, 2001). Only 10% of patients with SCID have lymphocyte counts in the normal range. T cells detectable in peripheral blood of affected infants shortly after birth may be either maternal T cells or circulating thymocytes. The thymus gland is not seen on chest radiographs. Histologically, the gland is composed of islands of endodermal cells that have not become lymphoid and contain no identifiable Hassall corpuscles. Lymphocyte subpopulation analysis using monoclonal antibodies to cell surface markers and analytical flow cytofluorometry (FACS) is the most important confirmatory test. As noted previously, each phenotypic pattern suggests a specific diagnosis and molecular defect. Other useful tests are measurements of ADA and PNP activity in red blood cells and of isohemagglutinins as a marker of specific IgM production. Quantitative immunoglobulin levels are not particularly helpful in the diagnosis of neonatal SCID, because most IgG is maternal in origin and IgA and IgM levels are often low in the neonatal period. Once the immunophenotype has been established, a precise molecular diagnosis should be obtained, and genetic counseling provided. Females carrying deleterious mutations in the *IL2RG* gene (X-linked SCID) can be identified by nonrandom inactivation of the X chromosome in lymphocytes. Prenatal diagnosis is available through gene identification from a chorionic villous biopsy.

When a fetus at risk for a genetic form of SCID is identified, treatment should begin in the delivery room and should be coordinated with antenatal diagnostic interventions.

Specifically, cord blood samples should be obtained for white blood cell count and differential, lymphocyte subset determinations, karyotype (if not performed antenatally), mitogen stimulation studies, and immunoglobulin measurements. Because the majority of children with genetic SCID do not become ill within the first week of life, care in an incubator should be provided, and staff should observe strict hand-washing technique.

SCID is a pediatric emergency and, if untreated, is invariably fatal. Most untreated patients die in the first year of life. Treatment of SCID begins with aggressive antibiotic and antiviral therapy for infections, intravenous immunoglobulin replacement, and prophylaxis for *Pneumocystis carinii* infection. Besides greater susceptibility to opportunistic infections, these infants are susceptible to development of graft-versus-host disease, either before birth, as a result of engraftment of maternal T lymphocytes, or after birth, as a result of the engraftment of T lymphocytes present in transfused blood products (Pollack et al, 1982; Thompson et al, 1984). Thus, infants in whom SCID is suspected should receive only irradiated blood products and should not be given live viral vaccines.

In 1968, Good and colleagues performed the first successful bone marrow transplantation (BMT) in a patient with SCID (Gatti et al, 1968). Allogeneic BMT, preferably from an HLA-matched sibling, is now the standard treatment for most types of SCID (Buckley, 2000). In these procedures, conditioning regimens are not required for engraftment. Recipients usually become chimeric, with T and NK cells only of donor origin. B-cell function is frequently deficient, and many patients continue to require monthly therapy with intravenous immune globulin. Survival rates for this type of BMT exceed 90%. When no HLA-identical donor is available, haploidentical transplants have been used successfully, although overall survival is lower with such transplants (Fischer, 2000). The rates of engraftment after haploidentical transplantation of patients with $T^-B^-NK^+$ SCID are low. This is likely due to host NK-cell function, and some form of preconditioning may be indicated in this subset of patients. In addition to BMT, ADA deficiency can be treated with enzyme replacement. This involves weekly injections of ADA coupled to polyethylene glycol. Response, consisting of decreasing deoxy-adenosine triphosphate levels and increasing T cell numbers, is seen in most patients within weeks. Finally, gene therapy of patients with ADA deficiency and γc SCID has been attempted. These protocols involve gene transfer into peripheral T cells or $CD34^+$ stem cells, which are then transfused into the patient. Results of some experiments have been encouraging (Kohn, 2001).

## Wiskott-Aldrich Syndrome

Wiskott-Aldrich syndrome (WAS), another form of immunodeficiency, is characterized by severe eczema, thrombocytopenia, higher risk of malignancy, and susceptibility to opportunistic infection. Other manifestations, which may be present in the newborn period, are petechiae and bruises, bloody diarrhea, and hemorrhage after procedures. WAS is inherited as a sex-linked recessive trait (Rosen, 1986). In untreated cases, children survive longer than infants with SCID (median survival, 5.7 years). T lymphocytes in affected patients are decreased in number and diminished in function. Reductions in platelet size and thrombopoiesis are also noted. Affected children can be treated with BMT, and the 5-year survival after HLA-identical sibling BMT is about 90% (Filipovich et al, 2001). Even though transplantation corrects the T-cell defects, thrombocytopenia persists. As for children with SCID, all blood products given to children with WAS should be irradiated before administration to avoid T-cell engraftment and graft-versus-host disease.

The gene responsible for the Wiskott-Aldrich syndrome was cloned in 1994 (Derry et al, 1994). It is composed of 12 exons and encodes a 502–aminoacid cytoplasmic protein (WASP) expressed in all hematopoietic cells. Other mamalian WASP family members include a more widely expressed N-WASP and three WAVE/Scar isoforms. These proteins have multiple domains and are important regulators of actin polymerization (Symons et al, 1996). They have a common carboxy-terminal region, through which they activate Arp2/3, an actin-nucleating complex involved in actin assembly and cytoskeletal structure. Their amino termini are distinct, allowing the proteins to couple Arp2/3 activation to a wide variety of different intracellular signals. More than 340 mutations in WASP have been described, which have profound effects on cell motility, signaling, and apoptosis (Rengan and Ochs, 2000).

## DiGeorge Syndrome

The embryologic anlage of the thymus gland and the parathyroid gland is the endodermal epithelium of the third and fourth pharyngeal pouches. When normal development of these structures is disturbed, thymic and parathyroid hypoplasia can occur (Rosen, 1986). Infants with this disorder, DiGeorge syndrome, may exhibit abnormalities of calcium homeostasis during the neonatal period (hypocalcemia and tetany) and variable T-cell deficits, which appear to depend on the presence and number of small, normal-looking ectopic thymic lobes. In addition, these infants have congenital conotruncal cardiac defects, low-set ears, midline facial clefts, hyomandibular abnormalities, and hypertelorism.

The availability of methodology for performing gene dosage studies and more refined cytogenetic techniques (fluorescence in situ hybridization [FISH]) has permitted description of a contiguous gene syndrome that includes DiGeorge phenotype (Hall, 1993). The DiGeorge syndrome is now known to result from various-sized deletions on chromosome 22q11 in more than 90% of patients (Markert et al, 1998). This deletion has been linked to several other diagnostic labels, including velocardiofacial (Shprintzen) syndrome, Cayler syndrome, and Opitz G/BBB syndrome. Collectively, these are now referred to as the *22q11 deletion syndromes*. The cardiac anomalies associated with the 22q11 deletion syndrome are variable but usually involve the outflow tract and the derivatives of the branchial arch arteries. These defects include interrupted aortic arch type B, truncus arteriosus, and tetralogy of Fallot.

Children with the 22q11 deletion syndrome also exhibit a higher incidence of receptive-expressive language difficulties, cognitive impairment, and behavioral problems including psychotic illness (Scambler, 2000). The cardiovascular defects have been shown to be the result of haploinsufficiency of TBX1 (Merscher et al, 2001). In the nursery, identification of infants with congenital conotruncal abnormalities should prompt consideration of this syndrome. Fetal thymic implants can correct the immunologic deficits (Reinherz et al, 1981).

## IMMUNIZATION

### Maternal Immunization

Immunization before pregnancy has been effective in preventing several specific neonatal infections, including diphtheria, pertussis, tetanus, hepatitis B, and rabies (American College of Obstetrician and Gynecologists, 1991; Hackley, 1999; Hepatitis B virus, 1991; Stevenson, 1999; Faix, 2002). For example, in developing countries, immunization during pregnancy with tetanus toxoid is a cost-effective method of preventing neonatal tetanus and of providing up to 10 years of protection for infants (Gill, Karasic et al, 1991; Schofield, 1986). The benefits for both mother and infant, from induction during pregnancy of maternal IgG antibody that can be transferred to the fetus and protect both the fetus and mother against postpartum morbidity and mortality, are substantial (Faix , 2002; Insel et al, 1994; Linder and Ohel 1994). However, immunization during pregnancy is biologically distinct from immunization of nonpregnant individuals. Vaccine epitopes may be shared with vital fetal or placental tissues, therefore, vaccination may lead to unanticipated maternal or fetal morbidity (Faix, 2002). Maternal immunization may induce an antibody response in the fetus, as has been demonstrated with tetanus toxoid (Gill et al, 1983), and thereby have potentially undesirable immunologic side effects (e.g., immunologic unresponsiveness or tolerance) in the infant.

Nevertheless, the increase in availability of potentially protective transplacentally transferred IgG through active maternal vaccination prompted the Institute of Medicine to recommend establishment of a program of active immunization to control early-onset and late-onset group B streptococcal disease in both infants and mothers (Institute of Medicine and National Academy of Sciences, 1985). Efforts to develop safe, effective vaccines for protection from group B streptococcal infections have encountered the same difficulties with immunogenicity and safety observed in the development of other vaccines that induce protection from polysaccharide-encapsulated organisms (Baker et al, 1988; Noya and Baker, 1992). The availability of conjugate vaccines, which include group B streptococcal polysaccharide antigens covalently linked either to tetanus toxoid or to a protein in the membrane of group B streptococci (beta C protein) (Madoff et al, 1994; Wessels et al, 1993) have shown considerable promise.

The indications for active vaccination during pregnancy rest on assessment of maternal risk of exposure, the maternal–fetal-neonatal risk of disease, and the risk from the immunizing agents (American College of Obstetricians and Gynecologists, 1991; Faix, 2002; Hackley, 1999; Stevenson, 1999). In general, immunization with live viral vaccines during pregnancy is not recommended. Preferably, immunizations with live viral vaccines are performed before pregnancy occurs. However, rare instances may occur in which live viral vaccine administration is indicated. For example, if a pregnant woman travels to an area of high risk for yellow fever, administration of that vaccine might be indicated because of the susceptibility of the mother and the fetus, the probability of exposure, and the risk to the mother and fetus from the disease. More common examples in the United States are influenza and polio virus vaccination. If a chronic maternal medical condition would be adversely affected by influenza, active immunization may be indicated during pregnancy. Similarly, if imminent exposure to live polio virus in an unprotected woman is anticipated, live oral polio virus vaccine may be used during pregnancy. If immunization can be completed before anticipated exposure, inactivated polio virus vaccine can be given. A summary of recommendations for immunizations during pregnancy is given in Table 35–3 and can be found at www.cdc.gov/nip/publications/preg_guide.pdf.

For the pediatrician, maternal immunization represents an important preventive intervention. Breast-feeding does not adversely affect immunization, and inactivated or killed vaccines pose no special risk for breast-feeding mothers or their infants (Atkinson et al, 2002; Recommended childhood immunization schedule, 2002b). Maternal immunizations with vaccines against polysaccharide-encapsulated organisms (e.g., *Haemophilus influenzae* type b and group B

**TABLE 35–3**

**Recommended Schedule of Hepatitis B Immunoprophylaxis to Prevent Perinatal Transmission**

| Vaccine Dose* and HBIG† | Age |
|---|---|
| Infant Born to Mother Known to be HBsAg-Positive | |
| First | Birth (within 12 hr) |
| HBIG | Birth (within 12 hr) |
| Second | 1-2 mo |
| Third | 6 mo |
| Infant Born to Mother Not Screened for HBsAg | |
| First‡ | Birth (within 12 hr) |
| HBIG | If mother is found to be HBsAg-positive, give 0.5 mL as soon as possible, i.e., not later than 1 wk after birth |
| Second | 1-2 mo |
| Third§ | 6-18 mo |

HBIG, hepatitis B immune globulin; HBsAg, hepatitis B surface antigen.

*Refer to www.cdc.gov/nip/recs/child-schedule.pdf for appropriate vaccine dose.

†HBIG (0.5 mL) given intramuscularly at a site different from that used for vaccine.

‡First dose is same as that for infant of HBsAg-positive mother. Subsequent doses and schedules are determined by maternal HBsAg status.

§Infants of HBsAg-positive mothers should be vaccinated at 6 mo.

Data from Peter G (ed): 1997 Red Book: Report of the Committee on Infectious Diseases, 24th ed. Elk Grove Village, IL, American Academy of Pediatrics, 1997, p 258.

streptococci) may decrease morbidity and mortality from these diseases during the first 3 to 6 months of the infant's life (Amstey et al, 1985; Baker et al, 1988; Faix, 2002; Walsh and Hutchins, 1989). The possibility of reducing the risks of development of hepatocellular carcinoma, cirrhosis, and chronic active hepatitis from perinatal transmission of hepatitis B through prenatal screening and active and passive immunization of the infant is substantial (Hepatitis B vaccination, 2002; Kao and Chen, 2002). The implications of maternal vaccination during pregnancy for preterm infants have not been studied.

The anthrax attacks of September 2001 have raised the possibility of the need for pre-exposure or post-exposure immunization programs that may include pregnant women. Currently available data suggest that the anthrax vaccine licensed since 1970 in the United States has no effect on pregnancy and does not increase adverse birth outcomes (Inglesby et al, 2002; Wiesen and Littell, 2002). A second infectious agent that might be used in a bioterrorist attack is variola virus (smallpox). Although eradicated in 1977, this virus remains a concern owing to its lethality, especially in pregnancy (Enserink, 2002; Suarez and Hankins, 2002). Pregnancy is a contraindication to smallpox immunization (Suarez and Hankins, 2002). However, if an intentional release of smallpox virus should occur, pregnant women should be immunized because of their high risk of mortality if unprotected (Suarez and Hankins, 2002).

## Infant Immunization

Advances in understanding of the developmental regulation of immunity have suggested that immunization during the neonatal period offers important advantages (Lawton, 1994). The recommendations of the American Academy of Pediatrics for immunization of infants are given in Table 35–3 (Committee on Infectious Diseases et al, 2002; Recommended childhood immunization schedule, 2002). Immunization against *H. influenzae* type b and pneumococci should be considered for infants who are discharged from intensive care nurseries at or after 2 months of age. For the preterm infant, although different clinical approaches are used by practitioners, including reducing the dosage of immunogen, postponing the first immunization until a corrected age of 2 months, and waiting for the infant to achieve an arbitrary body weight (e.g., 10 pounds), the American Academy of Pediatrics recommends administering full-dose diphtheria, tetanus, and pertussis (DTP) immunization beginning at 2 months of age (Atkinson et al, 2002). These recommendations, that no correction needs to be made for prematurity when routine immunization is initiated in preterm infants, have been supported by longitudinal evaluations of serum antibody response in preterm infants (Bernbaum et al, 1989; Conway et al, 1993; D'Angio, 1999; Siegrist, 2001).

The Committee on Infectious Diseases of the American Academy of Pediatrics and the Advisory Committee on Immunization Practices of the U.S. Public Health Service have recommended universal immunization of infants to reduce hepatitis B–associated morbidities (e.g., chronic hepatitis, hepatocellular carcinoma, cirrhosis) (Atkinson et al, 2002; Committee on Infectious Diseases et al, 2002). All infants born to women who test negative for hepatitis B surface antigen (HBsAg) should begin a hepatitis immunization schedule in the newborn period or within the first 2 months of life (Committee on Infectious Diseases et al, 2002). In 1999, the U.S. Agency for Toxic Substances and Disease Registry raised concern about the possibility that administration of thimerosal-containing vaccines, including the hepatitis B vaccines, might lead to mercury exposure that exceeded federal guidelines (Clark et al, 2001). This concern prompted the American Academy of Pediatrics and the U.S. Public Health Service to recommend jointly that hepatitis B immunization be postponed until 2 months of age in low-risk infants. By late 1999, the availability of thimerosal-free hepatitis vaccine was sufficient for the resumption of the immunization of all newborn infants in the United States.

All infants, regardless of gestational age at the time of birth, whose mothers test positive for HBsAg should receive passive immunization within 12 hours of birth and active immunization within 7 days of birth and then at 1 and 6 months of age. Special efforts should be made to complete the hepatitis B vaccination schedule within 6 to 9 months in populations of infants with high rates of childhood hepatitis B infection (Peter, 1994). For premature infants who weigh less than 2000 g at birth and are born to HBsAg-negative women, vaccination may be delayed until just before discharge or until 2 months of age, when other immunizations are given. These infants do not need routine serologic testing for anti-HBsAg after the third dose of vaccine. The infant whose mother tests negative for HBsAg but has received active or passive immunization during pregnancy because of exposure to hepatitis B should receive no treatment as long as the mother was HBsAg-negative at the time of birth.

Yeast-derived recombinant hepatitis B vaccines have excellent safety records, induce minimum adverse reactions, and are highly immunogenic (Greenberg, 1993). The recommended dose of hepatitis B vaccine for infants varies by manufacturer and the HBsAg status of the mother: For infants of HBsAg-negative mothers, 5.0 μg of Recombivax HB or 10.0 μg of Engerix-B are recommended; for infants of HBsAg-positive mothers, 5.0 μg of Recombivax HB or 10.0 μg of Engerix-B are recommended. The need for more than two booster doses and the feasibility of combining antigens in multivalent vaccines are currently under study. These guidelines for hepatitis immunization of infants have been developed for implementation for term and preterm infants. However, the extremely preterm infant whose mother is HBsAg-positive, a population seen with growing frequency owing to the coincidence of intravenous drug abuse and carriage of HBsAg, has not been studied.

Short-term and long-term neonatal immunologic protection after fetal exposure to maternally administered vaccines against anthrax or smallpox, the mass use of which might be prompted by a bioterrorist attack, has not been studied. Similarly, guidelines for neonatal immunization against these agents are not currently available. Before the eradication of smallpox, smallpox vaccine was routinely administered to older infants and children (Centers for Disease Control and Prevention, 2001). No data or experience are available on immunization of newborn infants with anthrax vaccine (Advisory Committee on Immunization Practices, 2000). For post-exposure prophylaxis in newborn infants, both chemotherapy (amoxicillin, ciprofloxacin, or doxycycline) and immunization should be considered (Atkinson et al, 2002). Clinicians faced with decisions concerning immunization strategies for newborn infants after a bioterrorist attack should consult the web site for the Centers of Disease Control and Prevention (www.cdc.gov).

## REFERENCES


Abe N, Katamura K, Shintaku N, et al: Prostaglandin E2 and IL-4 provide naive CD4+ T cells with distinct inhibitory signals for the priming of IFN-gamma production. Cell Immunol 181:86-92, 1997.

Abman SH, Groothius JR: Pathophysiology and treatment of bronchopulmonary dysplasia: Current issues. Pediatr Clin North Am 41:277-315, 1994.

Abo T Miller CA, Gartland GL, et al: Differentiation stages of human natural killer cells in lymphoid tissues from fetal to adult life. J Exp Med 157:273-284, 1983.

Adinolfi M, Gardner B: Synthesis of beta-1E and beta-1C components of complement in human foetuses. Acta Paediatr Scand 56:450-454, 1967.

Adkins B: T-cell function in newborn mice and humans [see comments]. Immunol Today 20:330-335, 1999.

Advisory Committee on Immunization Practices (ACIP): Use of anthrax vaccine in the United States. MMWR Morbid Mortal Wkly Rep 49(RR-15):1-20, 2000.

Alegre ML, Thompson CB: T-cell regulation by CD28 and CTLA-4. J Immunol 167:1036-1041, 2001.

Alford CA, Blankenship WJ, Straumfjord JB: The diagnostic significance of IgM globulin elevations in neonate infants with chronic intrauterine infections. Birth Defects 4:3, 1969.

Allman D, Li J, Hardy RR: Commitment to the B lymphoid lineage occurs before DH-JH recombination. J Exp Med 189:735-740, 1999.

American College of Obstetricians and Gynecologists: Immunization During Pregnancy (Technical bulletin No. 160). Washington, DC, ACOG, 1991.

Amstey MS, Insel R, Munoz J, et al: Fetal-neonatal passive immunization against *Hemophilus influenzae*, type b. Am J Obstet Gynecol 153:607-611, 1985.

Andersson U, Britton S, De Ley M, et al: Evidence for the ontogenic precedence of suppressor T cell functions in the human neonate. Eur J Immunol 13:6-13, 1983.

Atkinson WL, Pickering LK, Schwartz B, et al: Centers for Disease Control and Prevention. General recommendations on immunization. Recommendations of the Advisory Committee on Immunization Practices (ACIP) and American Academy of Family Physicians (AAFP). MMWR Morbid Mortal Wkly Rep 51(RR-2):1-36, 2002.

Baker CJ, Kasper DL: Correlation of maternal antibody deficiency with susceptibility to neonatal group B streptococcal infection. N Engl J Med 294:753-756, 1976.

Baker CJ, Webb BJ, Kasper DL, et al: The role of complement and antibody in opsonophagocytosis of type II group B streptococci. J Infect Dis 154:47-54, 1986.

Baker CJ, Rench MA, Edwards MS, et al: Immunization of pregnant women with a polysaccharide vaccine of group B streptococcus [see comments]. N Engl J Med 319:1180-1185, 1988.

Baker CJ, Melish ME, Hall RT, et al: Intravenous immune globulin for the prevention of nosocomial infection in low-birth-weight neonates. The Multicenter Group for the Study of Immune Globulin in Neonates [see comments]. N Engl J Med 327:213-219, 1992.

Baker DA, Hameed C, Tejani N, et al: Lymphocyte subsets in the neonates of preeclamptic mothers. American J Reproductive Immunology & Microbiology 14:107-109, 1987.

Baley JE, Schacter BZ: Mechanisms of diminished natural killer cell activity in pregnant women and neonates. J Immunol 134:3042-3048, 1985.

Ballow M, Cates KL, Rowe JC, et al: Development of the immune system in very low birth weight (less than 1500 g) premature infants: Concentrations of plasma immunoglobulins and patterns of infections. Pediatr Res 20:899-904, 1986.

Bancalari E: Changes in the pathogenesis and prevention of chronic lung disease of prematurity. Pediatrics 107:1425-1426, 2001.

Barrington KJ: Postnatal steroids and neurodevelopmental outcomes: A problem in the making. Pediatrics 109:330-338, 2002.

Barton K, Muthusamy N, Fischer C, et al: The Ets-1 transcription factor is required for the development of natural killer cells in mice. Immunity 9:555-563, 1998.

Baskett TF, Parsons ML, Peddle LJ: The experience and effectiveness of the Nova Scotia Rh program, 1964-84. CMAJ 134:1259-1261, 1986.

Bazaral M, Orgel HA, Hamburger RN: IgE levels in normal infants and mothers and an inheritance hypothesis. J Immunol 107:794-801, 1971.

Beer AE, Billingham RE: Maternally acquired runt disease. Science 179:240-243, 1973.

Beer AE, Billingham RE: The Immunobiology of Mammalian Reproduction. Englewood Cliffs, NJ, Prentice-Hall, 1976.

Beer AE, Billingham RE, Yang SL: Maternally induced transplantation immunity, tolerance, and runt disease in rats. J Exp Med 135:808-826, 1972.

Beer AE, Kwak JY, Ruiz JE: The biological basis of passage of fetal cellular material into the maternal circulation. Ann N Y Acad Sci 731:21-35, 1994.

Bellanti JA, Kadlec JV, Escobar-Gutierrez A: Cytokines and the immune response. Pediatr Clin North Am 41:597-621, 1994.

Benoist C, Mathis D: T-lymphocyte differentiation and biology. In Paul WE (ed): Fundamental Immunology, 4th ed. Philadelphia, Lippincott-Raven, 1999, pp 367-409.

Berlin G, Selbing A, Ryden G: Rhesus haemolytic disease treated with high-dose intravenous immunoglobulin. Lancet 1(8438):1153, 1985.

Bernbaum J, Daft A, Samuelson J, et al: Half-dose immunization for diphtheria, tetanus, pertussis: Response of preterm infants [see comments]. Pediatrics 83:471-476, 1989.

Bevan MJ: In thymic selection, peptide diversity gives and takes away. Immunity 7:175-178, 1997.

Bianchi DW, Zickwolf GK, Weil GJ, et al: Male fetal progenitor cells persist in maternal blood for as long as 27 years postpartum. Proc Natl Acad Sci U S A 93:705-708, 1996.

Biassoni R, Cantoni C, Pende D, et al: Human natural killer cell receptors and co-receptors. Immunol Rev 181:203-214, 2001.

Billingham RE: Transplantation immunity and the maternal-fetal relation. N Engl J Med 270:667-672, 1964.

Billington D: Evidence for trophoblast immunogenicity in the induction of maternal alloantibody formation in murine pregnancy: Reproductive immunology: Materno-fetal relationship. Colloque INSERM 154:17, 1987.

Blackburn MR, Kellems RE, Smith PT, et al: Adenosine deaminase deficiency increases thymic apoptosis and causes defective T cell receptor signaling. J Clin Invest 108:131-141, 2001.

Bobe P, Kiger N: Immunogenetic studies of spontaneous abortion in mice. III: Non-H-2 antigens and gestation. J Immunogenet 16:223-231, 1989.

Bobe P, Chaouat G, Stanislawski M, et al: Immunogenetic studies of spontaneous abortion in mice. II: Antiabortive effects are

independent of systemic regulatory mechanisms. Cell Immunol 98:477-485, 1986.
Bofill M, Janossy G, Janossa M, et al: Human B cell development. II: Subpopulations in the human fetus. J Immunol 134:1531-1538, 1985.
Bromley SK, Burack WR, Johnson KG, et al: The immunological synapse. Annu Rev Immunol 19:375-396, 2001.
Brugnoni D, Airo P, Graf D, et al: Ineffective expression of CD40 ligand on cord blood T cells may contribute to poor immunoglobulin production in the newborn. Eur J Immunol 24:1919-1924, 1994.
Buckley RH: Advances in the understanding and treatment of human severe combined immunodeficiency. Immunol Res 22:237-251, 2000.
Buckley RH, Schiff RI, Schiff SE, et al: Human severe combined immunodeficiency: Genetic, phenotypic, and functional diversity in one hundred eight infants. J Pediatr 130:378-387, 1997.
Bussel JB, Cunningham-Rundles S, LaGamma EF, et al: Analysis of lymphocyte proliferative response subpopulations in very low birth weight infants and during the first 8 weeks of life. Pediatr Res 23:457-462, 1988.
Cairo MS: Granulocyte transfusions in neonates with presumed sepsis. Pediatrics 80:738-740, 1987.
Cairo MS: Cytokines: A new immunotherapy. Clin Perinatol 18:343-359, 1991.
Cairo MS, Rucker R, Bennetts GA, et al: Improved survival of newborns receiving leukocyte transfusions for sepsis. Pediatrics 74:887-892, 1984.
Cairo MS, Worcester C, Rucker R, et al: Role of circulating complement and polymorphonuclear leukocyte transfusion in treatment and outcome in critically ill neonates with sepsis. J Pediatr 110:935-941, 1987.
Cairo MS, VandeVen C, Toy C, et al: GM-CSF primes and modulates neonatal PMN motility: Up-regulation of C3bi (Mo1) expression with alteration in PMN adherence and aggregation. Am J Pediatr Hematol Oncol 13:249-257, 1991.
Cairo MS, Worcester CC, Rucker RW, et al: Randomized trial of granulocyte transfusions versus intravenous immune globulin therapy for neonatal neutropenia and sepsis [see comments]. J Pediatr 120:281-285, 1992.
Calame KL: Plasma cells: finding new light at the end of B cell development. Nature Immunol 2:1103-1108, 2001.
Cantrell DA: T-cell antigen receptor signal transduction. Immunology 105:369-374, 2002.
Cao X, Shores EW, Hu-Li J, et al: Defective lymphoid development in mice lacking expression of the common cytokine receptor gamma chain. Immunity 2:223-238, 1995.
Cates KL, Goetz C, Rosenberg N, et al: Longitudinal development of specific and functional antibody in very low birth weight premature infants. Pediatr Res 23:14-22, 1988.
Centers for Disease Control and Prevention: Vaccinia (smallpox) vaccine recommendations of the Advisory Committee on Immunization Practices (ACIP), 2001. MMWR Morbid Mortal Wkly Rep 50(RR-10):1-25, 2001.
Cerwenka A, Lanier LL: Natural killer cells, viruses and cancer. Nature Rev Immunol 1:41-49, 2001.
Chaouat G, Menu E, Clark DA, et al: Control of fetal survival in CBA x DBA/2 mice by lymphokine therapy. J Reprod Fertil 89:447-458, 1990.
Chatterjee-Hasrouni S, Lala PK: Localization of paternal H-2K antigens on murine trophoblast cells in vivo. J Exp Med 155:1679-1689, 1982.
Christensen KK, Christensen P: IgG subclasses and neonatal infections with group B streptococci. Monogr Allergy 23:138-147, 1988.
Christensen RD: Hematopoiesis in the fetus and neonate. Pediatr Res 26:531-535, 1989.
Christensen RD, Shigeoka AO, Hill HR, et al: Circulating and storage neutrophil changes in experimental type II group B streptococcal sepsis. Pediatr Res 14:806-808, 1980.
Christensen RD, Anstall HB, Rothstein G: Use of whole blood exchange transfusion to supply neutrophils to septic, neutropenic neonates. Transfusion 22:504-506, 1982.
Christensen RD, Brown, MS, Hall, DC, et al: Effect on neutrophil kinetics and serum opsonic capacity of intravenous administration of immune globulin to neonates with clinical signs of early-onset sepsis [see comments]. J Pediatr 118:606-614, 1991.
Clapp DW, Kliegman RM, Baley JE, et al: Use of intravenously administered immune globulin to prevent nosocomial sepsis in low birth weight infants: report of a pilot study [see comments]. J Pediatrics 115:973-978, 1989.
Clark DA, Quarrington C, Banwatt D, et al: Spontaneous abortion in immunodeficient SCID mice. Am J Reprod Immunol (Copenh) 32:15-25, 1994.
Clark SJ, Cabana MD, Malik T, et al: Hepatitis B vaccination practices in hospital newborn nurseries before and after changes in vaccination recommendations. Arch Pediatr Adolesc Med 155:915-920, 2001.
Cole CH, Colton C, Shah BL, et al: Early inhaled glucocorticoid therapy to prevent bronchopulmonary dysplasia. N Engl J Med 340:1005-1010, 1999.
Cole FS: Complement function in the neonate. In Burgio GR, Hanson LA, Ugazio AG (eds): Immunology of the Neonate. Berlin, Springer Verlag, 1987, pp 76-82.
Cole FS, Colten HR: Complement. In Ogra PL (ed): Neonatal Infections, Nutritional and Immunologic Interactions. New York, Grune & Stratton, 1984, pp 37-49.
Colten HR: Ontogeny of the human complement system: In vitro biosynthesis of individual complement components by fetal tissues. J Clin Invest 51:725-730, 1972.
Colten HR, Gitlin JD: Immunoproteins. In Handin RI, Lux SE, Stossel TP (eds): Blood: Principles and Practice of Hematology. Philadelphia, JB Lippincott, 1995, pp 477-511.
Colten HR, Gordon JM, Borsos T, et al: Synthesis of the first component of human complement in vitro. J Exp Med 128:595-604, 1968.
Colten HR, Alper CA, Rosen FS: Genetics and biosynthesis of complement proteins. N Engl J Med 304:653-656, 1981.
Committee on Infectious Diseases, American Academy of Pediatrics, Advisory Committee on Immunization Practices of the Centers for Disease Control and Prevention, American Academy of Family Physicians: Recommended childhood immunization schedule—United States, 2002. Pediatrics 109:162, 2002.
Committee on the Fetus and Newborn: Postnatal corticosteroids to treat or prevent chronic lung disease in preterm infants. Pediatrics 109:330-338, 2002.
Conway S, James, J, Balfour, A, et al: Immunisation of the preterm baby. [see comments]. J Infection 27:143-150, 1993.
Cooper MA, Fehniger TA, Caligiuri MA: The biology of human natural killer-cell subsets. Trends Immunol 22:633-640, 2001.
Corneo B, Moshous D, Callebaut I, et al: Three-dimensional clustering of human RAG2 gene mutations in severe combined immune deficiency. J Biol Chem 275:12672-12675, 2000.
Corneo B, Moshous D, Gungor T, et al: Identical mutations in RAG1 or RAG2 genes leading to defective V(D)J recombinase activity can cause either T-B- severe combined immune deficiency or Omenn syndrome. Blood 97:2772-2776, 2001.
Correa AG, Baker CJ, Schutze GE, et al: Immunoglobulin G enhances C3 degradation on coagulase-negative staphylococci. Infect Immun 62:2362-2366, 1994.
Croy BA: The application of SCID mouse technology to questions in reproductive biology. Lab Animal Sci 43:123-126, 1993.

Croy BA, Chapeau C: Evaluation of the pregnancy immunotrophism hypothesis by assessment of the reproductive performance of young adult mice of genotype SCID/SCID.BG/BG. J Reprod Fertil 88:231-239, 1990.

Croy BA, Stewart CM, McBey BA, et al: An immunohistologic analysis of murine uterine T cells between birth and puberty. J Reprod Immunol 23:223-233, 1993.

Cummings JJ, D'Eugenio DB, Gross SJ: A controlled trial of dexamethasone in preterm infants at high risk for bronchopulmonary dysplasia. N Engl J Med 320:1505-1510, 1989.

Dancis J, Osborn JJ, Kunz HW: Studies of the immunology of the neonate infants. IV: Antibody formation in the premature infant. Pediatrics 12:151-157, 1953.

D'Angio CT: Immunization of the premature infant. Pediatr Infect Dis J 18:824-825, 1999.

Davis CA, Vallota EH, Forristal J: Serum complement levels in infancy: Age related changes. Pediatr Res 13:1043-1046, 1979.

Davis MM, Kim SK, Hood L: Immunoglobulin class switching: Developmentally regulated DNA rearrangements during differentiation. Cell 22:1-2, 1980.

de Fougerolles AR, Baines MG: Modulation of the natural killer cell activity in pregnant mice alters the spontaneous abortion rate. J Reprod Immunol 11:147-153, 1987.

Denison FC, Grant VE, Calder AA, et al: Seminal plasma components stimulate interleukin-8 and interleukin-10 release. Molec Hum Reprod 5:220-226, 1999.

Derry JM, Ochs HD, Francke U: Isolation of a novel gene mutated in Wiskott-Aldrich syndrome. Cell 78:635-644, 1994.

DiSanto JP, Muller W, Guy-Grand D, et al: Lymphoid development in mice with a targeted deletion of the interleukin 2 receptor gamma chain. Proc Natl Acad Sci U S A 92:377-381, 1995.

Dominguez M, Yacoub M, Dominguez E: Fetal natural killer cell function is suppressed. Immunology 70:110-121, 1993.

Duclos AJ, Pomerantz DK, Baines MG: Relationship between decidual leukocyte infiltration and spontaneous abortion in a murine model of early fetal resorption. Cell Immunol 159: 184-193, 1994.

Edwards MS: Complement in neonatal infections: An overview. Pediatr Infect Dis 5:S168-S170, 1986.

Edwards MS, Buffone GJ, Fuselier PA, et al: Deficient classical complement pathway activity in newborn sera. Pediatr Res 17:685-688, 1983.

Ehring GR, Kerschbaum HH, Eder C, et al: A nongenomic mechanism for progesterone-mediated immunosuppression: Inhibition of K+ channels, Ca2+ signaling, and gene expression in T lymphocytes. J Exp Med 188:1593-1602, 1998.

Eibl MM, Wolf HM, Furnkranz H, et al: Prevention of necrotizing enterocolitis in low-birth-weight infants by IgA-IgG feeding. N Engl J Med 319:1-7, 1988.

Eklund J, Nevanlinna HR: Perinatal mortality from Rh(D) hemolytic disease in Finland, 1975–1984. Acta Obstet Gynecol Scand 65:787-789, 1986.

English BK, Burchett SK, English JD, et al: Production of lymphotoxin and tumor necrosis factor by human neonatal mononuclear cells. Pediatr Res 24:717-722, 1988.

Enserink M: Bioterrorism: How devastating would a smallpox attack really be? Science 297:50-51, 2002.

Evans PC, Lambert N, Maloney S, et al: Long-term fetal microchimerism in peripheral blood mononuclear cell subsets in healthy women and women with scleroderma. Blood 93:2033-2037, 1999.

Faix RG: Immunization during pregnancy. Clin Obstet Gynecol 45:52-58, 2002.

Falk I, Nerz G, Haidl I, et al: Immature thymocytes that fail to express TCRbeta and/or TCRgamma delta proteins die by apoptotic cell death in the CD44(-)CD25(-) (DN4) subset. Eur J Immunol 31:3308-3317, 2001.

Fanaroff AA, Korones SB, Wright LL, et al: A controlled trial of intravenous immune globulin to reduce nosocomial infections in very-low-birth-weight infants. National Institute of Child Health and Human Development Neonatal Research Network [see comments]. N Engl J Med 330:1107-1113, 1994.

Fernandez JA, Estelles A, Gilabert J, et al: Functional and immunologic protein S in normal pregnant women and in full-term newborns. Thromb Haemost 61:474-478, 1989.

Fietta A, Sacchi F, Bersani C, et al: Complement-dependent bactericidal activity for *E. coli* K12 in serum of preterm newborn infants. Acta Paediatr Scand 76:37-41, 1987.

Filipovich AH, Stone JV, Tomany SC, et al: Impact of donor type on outcome of bone marrow transplantation for Wiskott-Aldrich Syndrome: Collaborative study of the International Bone Marrow Transplant Registry and the National Marrow Donor Program. Blood 97:1598-1603, 2001.

Fischer A: Severe combined immunodeficiencies (SCID). Clin Exp Immunol 122:143-149, 2000.

Fischer A, Cavazzana-Calvo M, De Saint Basile G, et al: Naturally occurring primary deficiencies of the immune system. Annu Rev Immunol 15:93-124, 1997.

Fischer GW: Immunoglobulin therapy of neonatal group B streptococcal infections: An overview. Pediatr Infect Dis J 7:S13-S16, 1988.

Flake AW, Roncarolo MG, Puck JM, et al: Treatment of X-linked severe combined immunodeficiency by in utero transplantation of paternal bone marrow. N Engl J Med 335:1806-1810, 1996.

Frank MM: Complement deficiencies. Pediatr Clin North Am 47:1339-1354, 2000.

Frenkel L, Bryson YJ: Ontogeny of phytohemagglutinin-induced gamma interferon by leukocytes of healthy infants and children: Evidence for decreased production in infants younger than 2 months of age. J Pediatr 111:97-100, 1987.

Fudenberg HH: $C_{III}$ genes and gamma globulin synthesis in the human fetus. J Immunol 94:514-520, 1965.

Fuleihan R, Ahern D, Geha RS: Decreased expression of the ligand for CD40 in newborn lymphocytes. Eur J Immunol 24:1925-1928, 1994.

Gans HA, Arvin AM, Galinus J, et al: Deficiency of the humoral immune response to measles vaccine in infants immunized at age 6 months. JAMA 280:527-532, 1998.

Garcia AM, Fadel SA, Cao S, et al: T cell immunity in neonates. Immunol Res 22:177-190, 2001.

Gathings WE, Lawton AR, Cooper MD: Immunofluorescent studies of the development of pre-B cells, B lymphocytes and immunoglobulin isotype diversity in humans. Eur J Immunol 7:804-810, 1977.

Gatti RA, Meuwissen HJ, Allen HD, et al: Immunological reconstitution of sex-linked lymphopenic immunological deficiency. Lancet 2(7583):1366-1369, 1968.

Gendron RL, Nestel FP, Lapp WS, et al: Lipopolysaccharide-induced fetal resorption in mice is associated with the intrauterine production of tumour necrosis factor-alpha. J Reprod Fertil 90:395-402, 1990.

Gennery AR, Cant AJ: Diagnosis of severe combined immunodeficiency. J Clin Pathol 54:191-195, 2001.

Georgeson GD, Szony BJ, Streitman K, et al: Natural killer cell cytotoxicity is deficient in newborns with sepsis and recurrent infections. Eur J Pediatr 160:478-482, 2001.

Georgopoulos K: Haematopoietic cell-fate decisions, chromatin regulation and Ikaros. Nature Rev Immunol 2:162-174, 2002.

Gill TJ 3rd: Reproductive immunology: A personal view. Am J Reprod Immunol (Copenh) 27:87-8, 1992.

Gill TJ 3rd, Repetti CF, Metlay LA, et al: Transplacental immunization of the human fetus to tetanus by immunization of the mother. J Clin Invest 72:987-996, 1983.

Gill TJ 3rd, Karasic RB, Antoncic J, et al: Long-term follow-up of children born to women immunized with tetanus toxoid during pregnancy. Am J Reprod Immunol (Copenh) 25:69-71, 1991.

Gillan ER, Christensen RD, Suen Y, et al: A randomized, placebo-controlled trial of recombinant human granulocyte colony-stimulating factor administration in newborn infants with presumed sepsis: Significant induction of peripheral and bone marrow neutrophilia. Blood 84:1427-1433, 1994.

Gitlin D, Kumate J, Urrusti J: The selectivity of the human placenta in the transfer of plasma proteins from mother to fetus. J Clin Invest 43:1938-1951, 1964.

Gitlin D, Biasucci A: Development of gamma G, gamma A, gamma M, beta IC-beta IA, C1 esterase inhibitor, ceruloplasmin, transferrin, hemopexin, haptoglobin, fibrinogen, plasminogen, alpha 1-antitrypsin, orosomucoid, beta-lipoprotein, alpha 2-macroglobulin, and prealbumin in the human conceptus. J Clin Invest 48:1433-1446, 1969.

Gong Q, Cheng AM, Akk AM, et al: Disruption of T cell signaling networks and development by Grb2 haploid insufficiency. Nature Immunol 2:29-36, 2001.

Gong S, Nussenzweig MC: Regulation of an early developmental checkpoint in the B cell pathway by Ig beta. Science 272:411-414, 1996.

Greenberg DP: Pediatr experience with recombinant hepatitis B vaccines and relevant safety and immunogenicity studies. Pediatr Infect Dis J 12:438-445, 1993.

Groneck P, Oppermann M, Speer CP: Levels of complement anaphylatoxin C5a in pulmonary effluent fluid of infants at risk for chronic lung disease and effects of dexamethasone treatment. Pediatr Res 34:586-590, 1993.

Groneck P, Gotze-Speer B, Oppermann M, et al: Association of pulmonary inflammation and increased microvascular permeability during the development of bronchopulmonary dysplasia: A sequential analysis of inflammatory mediators in respiratory fluids of high-risk preterm neonates [see comments]. Pediatrics 93:712-718, 1994.

Guest SS, Smale ST, Hahm K, et al: Lack of natural killer cell precursors in fetal liver of Ikaros knockout mutant mice. Cell 91:845-854, 1997.

Guilbert L, Robertson SA, Wegmann TG: The trophoblast as an integral component of a macrophage-cytokine network. Immunol Cell Biol 71:49-57, 1993.

Gurka G, Rocklin RE: Reproductive immunology. JAMA 258:2983-2987, 1987.

Hackley BK: Immunizations in pregnancy: A public health perspective. J Nurse-Midwifery 44:106-117, 1999.

Haddad EK, Duclos AJ, Baines MG: Early embryo loss is associated with local production of nitric oxide by decidual mononuclear cells. J Exp Med 182:1143-1151, 1995.

Haddad EK, Duclos AJ, Lapp WS, et al: Early embryo loss is associated with the prior expression of macrophage activation markers in the decidua. J Immunol 158:4886-4892, 1997.

Haimovici F, Hill JA, Anderson DJ: The effects of soluble products of activated lymphocytes and macrophages on blastocyst implantation events in vitro. Biol Reprod 44:69-75, 1991.

Hall JG: Catch 22. J Med Genet 30:801-802, 1993.

Haque KN, Zaidi MH, Bahakim H: IgM-enriched intravenous immunoglobulin therapy in neonatal sepsis. Am J Dis Child 142:1293-1296, 1988.

Hardy RR, Hayakawa K: B cell development pathways. Annu Rev Immunol 19:595-621, 2001.

Harland C, Shah T, Webster AD, et al: Dipeptidyl peptidase IV: Subcellular localization, activity and kinetics in lymphocytes from control subjects, immunodeficient patients and cord blood. Clinical Exp Immunol 74:201-205, 1988.

Hartley SB, Crosbie J, Brink R, et al: Elimination from peripheral lymphoid tissues of self-reactive B lymphocytes recognizing membrane-bound antigens. Nature 353:765-769, 1991.

Hauser GJ, Zakuth V, Rosenberg H, et al: Interleukin-2 production by cord blood lymphocytes stimulated with mitogen and in the mixed leukocyte culture. J Clin Lab Immunol 16:37-40, 1985.

Hayward AR, Mori M: Human newborn autologous mixed lymphocyte response: Frequency and phenotype of responders and xenoantigen specificity. J Immunol 133:719-723, 1984.

Hemming VG, Hall RT, Rhodes PG, et al: Assessment of group B streptococcal opsonins in human and rabbit serum by neutrophil chemiluminescence. J Clin Invest 58:1379-1387, 1976.

Hepatitis B vaccination—United States,1982–2002. MMWR Morbid Mortal Wkly Rep 51:549-563, 2002.

Hepatitis B virus: A comprehensive strategy for eliminating transmission in the United States through universal childhood vaccination. Recommendations of the Immunization Practices Advisory Committee (ACIP). MMWR Morbid Mortal Wkly Rep 40:1-25, 1991.

Hicks MJ, Jones JF, Thies AC, et al: Age-related changes in mitogen-induced lymphocyte function from birth to old age. Am J Clin Pathol 80:159-163, 1983.

Hill HR: Biochemical, structural, and functional abnormalities of polymorphonuclear leukocytes in the neonate. Pediatr Res 22:375-382, 1987.

Hill HR: Intravenous immunoglobulin use in the neonate: Role in prophylaxis and therapy of infection. Pediatr Infect Dis Journal 12:549-558, 1993a.

Hill HR: Modulation of host defenses with interferon-gamma in pediatrics. J Infect Dis 167(Suppl 1):S23-S28, 1993b.

Hill HR, Shigeoka AO, Pincus S, et al: Intravenous IgG in combination with other modalities in the treatment of neonatal infection. Pediatr Infect Dis 5:S180-S184, 1986.

Hill HR, Augustine NH, Jaffe HS: Human recombinant interferon gamma enhances neonatal polymorphonuclear leukocyte activation and movement, and increases free intracellular calcium. J Exp Med 173:767-770, 1991.

Hirschhorn R: Adenosine deaminase deficiency. Immunodefic Rev 2:175-198, 1990.

Hogg N, Harvey J, Cabanas C, et al: Control of leukocyte integrin activation. Am Rev Respir Dis 148:S55-S59, 1993.

Holzgreve B, Goldsmith PC, Holzgreve W, et al: A monoclonal antibody micromethod for studying fetal lymphocytes: Potential for prenatal diagnosis of inherited immunodeficiencies. J Reproductive Immunol 6:341-344, 1984.

Hunt JS, Vassmer D, Ferguson TA, et al: Fas ligand is positioned in mouse uterus and placenta to prevent trafficking of activated leukocytes between the mother and the conceptus. J Immunol 158:4122-4128, 1997.

Hunziker RD, Wegmann TG: Placental immunoregulation. Crit Rev Immunol 6:245-285, 1986.

Ingelsby TV, O'Toole T, Henderson DA, et al: Anthrax as a biological weapon, 2002: Updated recommendations for management. JAMA 287:2236-2252, 2002.

Insel RA, Amstey M, Woodin K, et al: Maternal immunization to prevent infectious diseases in the neonate or infant. Int J Technol Assess Health Care 10:143-153, 1994.

Institute of Medical and National Academy of Sciences: New vaccine development: Establishing priorities. Diseases of importance in the United States. Washington, DC, National Academy Press, 1985.

Jacoby DR, Oldstone MB: Delineation of suppressor and helper activity within the OKT4-defined T lymphocyte subset in human newborns. J Immunol 131:1765-1770, 1983.

Jacoby DR, Olding LB, Oldstone MB: Immunologic regulation of fetal-maternal balance. Adv Immunol 35:157-208, 1984.

Jarrett EE: Perinatal influences on IgE responses. Lancet 2:797-799, 1984.

Jiang SP, Vacchio MS: Multiple mechanisms of peripheral T cell tolerance to the fetal "allograft." J Immunol 160:3086-3090, 1998.

Johnson RJ: Complement activation during extracorporeal therapy: Biochemistry, cell biology and clinical relevance. Nephrol Dial Transplant 9(Suppl 2):36-45, 1994.
Kadowaki N, Antonenko S, Ho S, et al: Distinct cytokine profiles of neonatal natural killer T cells after expansion with subsets of dendritic cells. J Exp Med 193:1221-1226, 2001.
Kalli KR, Hsu P Fearon DT: Therapeutic uses of recombinant complement protein inhibitors. Springer Semin Immunopathol 15:417-431, 1994.
Kannourakis G, Begley CG, Johnson GR, et al: Evidence for interactions between monocytes and natural killer cells in the regulation of in vitro hemopoiesis. J Immunol 140:2489-2494, 1988.
Kao JH, Chen DS: Global control of hepatitis B virus infection. Lancet Infect Dis 2:395-403, 2002.
Kennedy B, Evans PA, Davies FE, et al: The human thymus during aging. Blood 98:29-35, 2001.
Kincade PW, Medina KL, Payne KJ, et al: Early B-lymphocyte precursors and their regulation by sex steroids. Immunol Rev 175:128-137, 2000.
King A, Boocock C, Sharkey AM, et al: Evidence for the expression of HLAA-C class I mRNA and protein by human first trimester trophoblast. J Immunol 156:2068-2076, 1996a.
King A, Burrows T, Loke YW: Human uterine natural killer cells. Nat Immun 15:41-52, 1996b.
Kinney J, Mundorf L, Gleason C, et al: Efficacy and pharmacokinetics of intravenous immune globulin administration to high-risk neonates. Am J Dis Child 145:1233-1238, 1991.
Kinsky R, Delage G, Rosin N, et al: A murine model of NK cell mediated resorption. Am J Reprod Immunol (Copenh) 23:73-77, 1990.
Kitamura D, KudoA, Schaal S, et al: A critical role of lambda 5 protein in B cell development. Cell 69:823-831, 1992.
Klein GL, Neibart SI, Hassman H, et al: Little evidence of HLA-G mRNA polymorphism in Caucasian or Afro Caribbean populations. Clin Pediatr 37:17-22, 1998.
Klesius PH, Zimmerman RA, Mathews JH, et al: Cellular and humoral immune response to group B streptococci. J Pediatr 83:926-932, 1973.
Kohn DB: Gene therapy for genetic haematological disorders and immunodeficiencies. J Intern Med 249:379-390, 2001.
Kovats S, Main EK, Librach C, et al: A class I antigen, HLA-G, expressed in human trophoblasts. Science 248:220-223, 1990.
Krause PJ, Herson VC, Eisenfeld L, et al: Enhancement of neutrophil function for treatment of neonatal infections. Pediatr Infect Dis J 8:382-389, 1989.
Krensky AM, Clayberger C: Transplantation immunology. Pediatr Clin North Am 41:819-839, 1994.
Lanier LL: NK cell receptors. Annu Rev Immunol 16:359-393, 1998.
Lanier LL, Corliss B, Wu J, et al: Association of DAP12 with activating CD94/NKG2C NK cell receptors. Immunity 8:693-701, 1998.
Lassiter HA, Watson SW, Seifring ML, et al: Complement factor 9 deficiency in serum of human neonates. J Infect Dis 166:53-57, 1992.
Lassiter HA, Wilson JL, Feldhoff RC, et al: Supplemental complement component C9 enhances the capacity of neonatal serum to kill multiple isolates of pathogenic *Escherichia coli*. Pediatr Res 35:389-396, 1994.
Lassoued K, Illges H, Benlagha K, Cooper MD: Fate of surrogate light chains in B lineage cells. J Exp Med 183:421, 1996.
Lawrence G, Tudehope D, Baumann K, et al: Enteral human Ig G for prevention of necrotizing enterocolitis: A placebo-controlled, randomised trial. Lancet 357:2090-2094, 2001.
Lawton AR: Immunization of the neonate. Int J Technol Assess Health Care 10:154-160, 1994.
Lee N, Malacko AR, Ishitani A, et al: The membrane-bound and soluble forms of HLA-G bind identical sets of endogenous peptides but differ with respect to TAP association. Immunity 3:591-600, 1995.
Leung DY: Mechanisms of the human allergic response: Clinical implications. Pediatr Clin North Am 41:727-743, 1994.
Li YS, Hayakawa K, Hardy RR: The regulated expression of B lineage associated genes during B cell differentiation in bone marrow and fetal liver. J Exp Med 178:951-960, 1993.
Liang DC, Ma SW, Lin-Chu M, et al: Granulocyte/macrophage colony-forming units from cord blood of premature and full-term neonates: Its role in ontogeny of human hemopoiesis. Pediatr Res 24:701-702, 1988.
Lilja G, Winbladh B, Vedin I, et al: Cord blood T lymphocyte subpopulations in premature and full-term infants. Int Arch Allergy Appl Immunol 75:273-275, 1984.
Linder N, Ohel G: In utero vaccination. Clin Perinatol 21:663-674, 1994.
Llano M, Bellon T, Colonna M, et al: How do NK cells sense the expression of HLA-G class Ib molecules? Eur J Immunol 29:277-283, 1999.
Lo YM, Lo ES, Watson N, et al: Two-way cell traffic between mother and fetus: Biologic and clinical implications. Blood 88:4390-4395, 1996.
Lohoff M, Duncan GS, Ferrick D, et al: Deficiency in the transcription factor interferon regulatory factor (IRF)-2 leads to severely compromised development of natural killer and T helper type 1 cells. J Exp Med 192:325-336, 2000.
Lu CY, Calamai EG, Unanue ER: A defect in the antigen-presenting function of macrophages from neonatal milk. Nature 282:327-329, 1979.
Macchi P, Villa, A, Giliani, S, et al: Mutations of Jak-3 gene in patients with autosomal severe combined immune deficiency (SCID). Nature 377:65-68, 1995.
Madoff LC, Paoletti LC, Tai JY, et al: Maternal immunization of mice with group B streptococcal type III polysaccharide beta C protein conjugate elicits protective antibody to multiple serotypes. J Clin Invest 94:286-292, 1994.
Magny JF, Bremard-Oury C, Brault D, et al: Intravenous immunoglobulin therapy for prevention of infection in high-risk premature infants: report of a multicenter, double-blind study [see comments]. Pediatrics 88:437-443, 1991.
Malm J, Bennhagen R, Holmberg L, et al: Plasma concentrations of C4b-binding protein and vitamin K-dependent protein S in term and preterm infants: Low levels of protein S-C4b-binding protein complexes. Br J Haematol 68:445-449, 1988.
Markert ML, Hummell DS, Rosenblatt HM, et al: Complete DiGeorge syndrome: Persistence of profound immunodeficiency. J Pediatr 132:15-21, 1998.
Massey GV, McWilliams NB, Mueller DG, et al: Intravenous immunoglobulin in treatment of neonatal isoimmune thrombocytopenia. J Pediatr 111:133-135, 1987.
McMaster MT, Librach CL, Zhou Y, et al: Human placental HLA-G expression is restricted to differentiated cytotrophoblasts. J Immunol 154:3771-3778, 1995.
Medawar PB: Some immunological and endocrinological problems raised by the evolution of viviparity in vertebrates. Symp Soc Exp Biol 7:320, 1953.
Melchers F, Rolink A: B-lymphocyte development and biology. In Paul WE (ed): Fundamental Immunology, 4th ed. Philadelphia, Lippincott-Raven, 1999, pp 183-224.
Melissari E, Nicolaides KH, Scully MF, et al: Protein S and C4b-binding protein in fetal and neonatal blood. Br J Haematol 70:199-203, 1988.
Mellor AL, Munn DH: Immunology at the maternal-fetal interface: Lessons for T cell tolerance and suppression. Annu Rev Immunol 18:367-391, 2000.
Menitove JE, Abrams RA: Granulocyte transfusions in neutropenic patients. Crit Rev Oncol Hematol 7:89-113, 1987.

Merscher S, Funke B, Epstein JA, et al: TBX1 is responsible for cardiovascular defects in velo-cardio-facial/DiGeorge syndrome. Cell 104:619-629, 2001.

Mills L, Napier JA: Massive feto-maternal haemorrhage: Effect of passively administered anti-D in the prevention of Rh sensitization and haemolytic disease of the newborn. Br J Obstet Gynaecol 95:1007-1012, 1988.

Miyano A, Nakayama M, Fujita T, et al: Complement activation in fetuses: Assessment by the levels of complement components and split products in cord blood. Diagn Clin Immunol 5:86-90, 1987.

Miyaura H, Iwata M: Direct and indirect inhibition of Th1 development by progesterone and glucocorticoids. J Immunol 168:1087-1094, 2002.

Moalic P, Gruel Y, Body G, et al: Levels and plasma distribution of free and C4b-BP-bound protein S in human fetuses and full-term newborns. Thromb Res 49:471-480, 1988.

Morell A, Sidiropoulos D, Herrmann U, et al: IgG subclasses and antibodies to group B streptococci in preterm neonates after intravenous infusion of immunoglobulin to the mothers. Pediatr Infect Dis 5:S195-S197, 1986.

Moretta A, Bottino C, Vitale M, et al: Activating receptors and coreceptors involved in human natural killer cell-mediated cytolysis. Ann Rev Immunol 19:197-223, 2001.

Morris AC, Riley JL, Fleming WH, et al: MHC class II gene silencing in trophoblast cells is caused by inhibition of CIITA expression. Am J Reprod Immunol 40:385-394, 1998.

Mrozek E, Anderson P, Caligiuri MA: Role of interleukin-15 in the development of human CD56+ natural killer cells from CD34+ hematopoietic progenitor cells. Blood 87:2632-2640, 1996.

Muller-Eberhard HJ: The membrane attack complex of complement. Annu Rev Immunol 4:503-528, 1986.

Munn DH, Shafizadeh E, Attwood JT, et al: Inhibition of T cell proliferation by macrophage tryptophan catabolism. J Exp Med 189:1363-1372, 1999.

Munn DH, Zhou M, Attwood JT, et al: Prevention of allogeneic fetal rejection by tryptophan catabolism. Science 281:1191-1193, 1998.

Murphy SP, Tomasi TB: Absence of MHC class II antigen expression in trophoblast cells results from a lack of class II transactivator (CIITA) gene expression. Mol Reprod Dev 51:1-12, 1998.

Nelson DL, Kurman CC, Fritz ME, et al: The production of soluble and cellular interleukin-2 receptors by cord blood mononuclear cells following in vitro activation. Pediatr Res 20:136-139, 1986.

Noguchi M, Yi H, Rosenblatt HM, et al: Interleukin-2 receptor gamma chain mutation results in X-linked severe combined immunodeficiency in humans. Cell 73:147-157, 1993.

Norwitz ER, Schust DJ, Fisher SJ: Implantation and the survival of early pregnancy. N Engl J Med 345:1400-1408, 2001.

Noya FJ, Baker CJ: Intravenously administered immune globulin for premature infants: A time to wait [letter; comment]. J Pediatr 115:969-971, 1989.

Noya FJ, Baker CJ: Prevention of group B streptococcal infection. Infect Dis Clin North Am 6:41-55, 1992.

Ogasawara N, Moszer I, Albertini AM, et al: Requirement for IRF-1 in the microenvironment supporting development of natural killer cells [erratum appears in Nature 1998 Apr 392:843, 1998]. Nature 390:249-256, 1998.

Olding LB, Oldstone MB: Lymphocytes from human newborns abrogate mitosis of their mother's lymphocytes. Nature 249:161-162, 1974.

Oldstone MB, Tishon A, Moretta L: Active thymus derived suppressor lymphocytes in human cord blood. Nature 269: 333-335, 1977.

Ossa JE, Cadavid AP, Maldonado JG: Is the immune system necessary for placental reproduction? A hypothesis on the mechanisms of alloimmunotherapy in recurrent spontaneous abortion. Med Hypotheses 42:193-197, 1994.

Ouyang W, Lohning M, Assenmacher M, et al: T helper subset development: Roles of instruction, selection, and transcription. J Exp Med 193:643-650, 2001.

Owen JJ, Wright DE, Habu S, et al: Studies on the generation of B lymphocytes in fetal liver and bone marrow. J Immunol 118:2067-2072, 1977.

Pangburn MK, Muller-Eberhard HJ: The alternative pathway of complement. Springer Semin Immunopathol 7:163-192, 1984.

Papadogiannakis N, Johnsen SA: Distinct mitogens reveal different mechanisms of suppressor activity in human cord blood. J Clin Lab Immunol 26:37-41, 1988.

Pedersen SA, Petersen J, Andersen V: Suppression of B lymphocytes in mature newborn infants. Acta Paediatr Scand 72: 441-447, 1983.

Penix L, Weaver WM, Pang Y, et al: Two essential regulatory elements in the human interferon gamma promoter confer activation specific expression in T cells. J Exp Med 178: 1483-1496, 1993.

Pereira S, Webster D, Platts-Mills T: Immature B cells in fetal development and immunodeficiency: Studies of IgM, IgG, IgA and IgD production in vitro using Epstein-Barr virus activation. Eur J Immunol 12:540-546, 1982.

Perignon JL, Durandy A, Peter MO, et al: Early prenatal diagnosis of inherited severe immunodeficiencies linked to enzyme deficiencies. J Pediatr 111:595-598, 1987.

Peschon JJ, Morrissey PJ, Grabstein KH, et al: Early lymphocyte expansion is severely impaired in interleukin 7 receptor-deficient mice. J Exp Med 180:1955-1960, 1994.

Peter G: Summary of major changes in the 1994 Red Book: American Academy of Pediatrics Report of the Committee on Infectious Disease. Pediatrics 93:1000-1002, 1994.

Philpott KL, Rastan S, Brown S, et al: Expression of H-2 class I genes in murine extra-embryonic tissues. Immunology 64: 479-485, 1988.

Piccinni MP, Giudizi MG, Biagiotti R, et al: Progesterone favors the development of human T helper cells producing Th2-type cytokines and promotes both IL-4 production and membrane CD30 expression in established Th1 cell clones. J Immunol 155:128-133, 1995.

Piccinni MP, Beloni L, Livi C, et al: Defective production of both leukemia inhibitory factor and type 2 T-helper cytokines by decidual T cells in unexplained recurrent abortions. Nature Med 4:1020-1024, 1998.

Pittard WB 3rd, Miller K, Sorensen RU: Normal lymphocyte responses to mitogens in term and premature neonates following normal and abnormal intrauterine growth. Clin Immunol Immunopathol 30:178-187, 1984.

Pittard WB 3rd, Miller KM, Sorensen RU: Perinatal influences on in vitro B lymphocyte differentiation in human neonates. Pediatr Res 19:655-658, 1985.

Pittard WB 3rd, Schleich DM, Geddes KM, et al: Newborn lymphocyte subpopulations: The influence of labor. Am J Obstet Gynecol 160:151-154, 1989.

Polgar K, Anderson DJ: Immune interferon gamma inhibits translational mobility of a plasma membrane protein in preimplantation stage mouse embryos: A T-helper 1 mechanism for immunologic reproductive failure. JAMA 273:1933-1936, 1995.

Polin RA, Harris MC: Neonatal bacterial meningitis. Semin Perinatol 6:157-172, 2001.

Pollack MS, Kirkpatrick D, Kapoor N, et al: Identification by HLA typing of intrauterine-derived maternal T cells in four patients with severe combined immunodeficiency. N Engl J Med 307:662-666, 1982.

Ponte M, Cantoni C, Biassoni R, et al: Inhibitory receptors sensing HLA-G molecules in pregnancy: Decidua-associated natural killer cells express LIR-1 and CD94/NKG2A and acquire

p49, an HLA-G1-specific receptor. Proc Natl Acad Sci U S A 96:5674-5679, 1999.
Propp RP, Alper CA: C′3 synthesis in the human fetus and lack of transplacental passage. Science 162:672-673, 1968.
Puck JM, Middelton L, Pepper AE: Carrier and prenatal diagnosis of X-linked severe combined immunodeficiency: Mutation detection methods and utilization. Human Genetics 99:628-633, 1997.
Puel A, Ziegler SF, Buckley RH, et al: Defective IL7R expression in T(-)B(+)NK(+) severe combined immunodeficiency. Nature Genet 20:394-397, 1998.
Rajagopalan S, Long EO: A human histocompatibility leukocyte antigen (HLA)-G-specific receptor expressed on all natural killer cells [erratum appears in J Exp Med 191:2027, 2000]. J Exp Med 189:1093-1100, 1999.
Raum DD, Awdeh ZL, Page PL, et al: MHC determinants of response to Rh immunization. J Immunol 132:157-159, 1984.
Ravetch JV, Lanier LL: Immune inhibitory receptors. Science 290:84-89, 2000.
Recommended childhood immunization schedule—United States, 2002. MMWR Morbid Mortal Wkly Rep 51:31-33, 2002b.
Reinherz EL, Cooper MD, Schlossman SF, et al: Abnormalities of T cell maturation and regulation in human beings with immunodeficiency disorders. J Clin Invest 68:699-705, 1981.
Rengan R, Ochs HD: Molecular biology of the Wiskott-Aldrich syndrome. Rev Immunogenet 2:243-255, 2000.
Res P, Martinez-Caceres E, Cristina Jaleco A, et al: CD34+ CD38dim cells in the human thymus can differentiate into T, natural killer, and dendritic cells but are distinct from pluripotent stem cells. Blood 87:5196-5206, 1996.
Ricevuti G, Mazzone A: Clinical aspects of neutrophil locomotion disorders. Biomed Pharmacother 41:355-367, 1987.
Robertson SA, Roberts CT, Farr KL, et al: Fertility impairment in granulocyte macrophage colony stimulating factor-deficient mice. Biol Reprod 60:251-261, 1999.
Roder J, Duwe A: The beige mutation in the mouse selectively impairs natural killer cell function. Nature 278:451-453, 1979.
Rogers MH, Lwin R, Fairbanks L, et al: Cognitive and behavioral abnormalities in adenosine deaminase deficient severe combined immunodeficiency. J Pediatr 139:44-50, 2001.
Rohrer J, Minegishi Y, Conley ME: Defects in early B-cell development: Comparing the consequences of abnormalities in pre-BCR signaling in the human and the mouse. Clin Rev Allergy Immunol 19:183-204, 2000.
Rolink AG, Schaniel C, Andersson J, et al: Selection events operating at various stages in B cell development. Curr Opin Immunol 13:202-207, 2001.
Romero R, Sepulveda W, Kenney JS, et al: Interleukin 6 determination in the detection of microbial invasion of the amniotic cavity. Ciba Found Symp 167:205-220; discussion 220-223, 1992.
Romero R, Mazor M, Munoz H, et al: The preterm labor syndrome. Ann N Y Acad Sci 734:414-429, 1994.
Rosen FS: Defects in cell-mediated immunity. Clin Immunol Immunopathol 41:1-7, 1986.
Rosen FS, Janeway CA: Immunologic competence of the newborn infant. Pediatrics 33:159-160, 1964.
Rosen FS, Cooper MD, Wedgwood RJ: The primary immunodeficiencies (2). N Engl J Med 311:300-310, 1984.
Rouas-Freiss N, Goncalves RM, Menier C, et al: Direct evidence to support the role of HLA-G in protecting the fetus from maternal uterine natural killer cytolysis. Proc Natl Acad Sci U S A 94:11520-11525, 1997.
Rubaltelli FF, Benini F, Sala M: Prevention of necrotizing enterocolitis in neonates at risk by oral administration of monomeric IgG. Dev Pharmacol Ther 17:138-143, 1991.
Russell SM, Tayebi N, Nakajima H, et al: Mutation of Jak3 in a patient with SCID: Essential role of Jak3 in lymphoid development. Science 270:797-800, 1995.
Ryhanen P, Jouppila R, Lanning M, et al: Effect of segmental epidural analgesia on changes in peripheral blood leucocyte counts, lymphocyte subpopulations, and in vitro transformation in healthy parturients and their newborns. Gynecol Obstet Invest 17:202-207, 1984.
Santisteban I, Arredondo-Vega FX, Kelly S, et al: Novel splicing, missense, and deletion mutations in seven adenosine deaminase-deficient patients with late/delayed onset of combined immunodeficiency disease: Contribution of genotype to phenotype. J Clin Invest 92:2291-2302, 1993.
Santos JI, Shigeoka AO, Hill HR: Functional leukocyte administration in protection against experimental neonatal infection. Pediatr Res 14:1408-1410, 1980.
Sargent IL: Maternal and fetal immune responses during pregnancy. Exp Clin Immunogenet 10:85-102, 1993.
Scambler PJ: The 22q11 deletion syndromes. Hum Molec Genet 9:2421-2426, 2000.
Schieren G, Hansch GM: Membrane-associated proteins regulating the complement system: Functions and deficiencies. Int Rev Immunol 10:87-101, 1993.
Schofield F: Selective primary health care: Strategies for control of disease in the developing world. XXII: Tetanus: A preventable problem. Rev Infect Dis 8:144-156, 1986.
Schwarz K, Gauss GH, Ludwig L, et al: RAG mutations in human B cell-negative SCID. Science 274:97-99, 1996.
Shah SS, Ehrenkranz RA, Gallagher PG: Increasing incidence of gram-negative rod bacteremia in a newborn intensive care unit. Pediatr Infect Dis J 18:591-595, 1999.
Shapiro R, Beatty DW, Woods DL, et al: Complement activity in the cord blood of term neonates with the amniotic fluid infection syndrome. S Afr Med J 63:86-87, 1983.
Sidiropoulos D, Boehme U, Von Muralt G, et al: Immunoglobulin supplementation in prevention or treatment of neonatal sepsis. Pediatr Infect Dis 5:S193-S194, 1986.
Siegrist CA: Neonatal and early life vacinology. Vaccine 19: 3331-3346, 2001.
Simmons RL: Histoincompatibility and the survival of the fetus: Current controversies. Transplant Proc 1:47-52, 1969.
Simmons RL, Russell PS: Immunologic interactions between the mother and fetus. Adv Obstet Gynecol 1:38, 1967.
Simpson KL, Houlihan JM, Holmes CH: Complement regulatory proteins in early human fetal life: CD59, membrane co-factor protein (MCP) and decay-accelerating factor (DAF) are differentially expressed in the developing liver. Immunology 80:183-190, 1993.
Soderstrom K, Corliss B, Lanier LL, et al: CD94/NKG2 is the predominant inhibitory receptor involved in recognition of HLA-G by decidual and peripheral blood NK cells. J Immunol 159:1072-1075, 1997.
Sonntag J, Brandenburg U, Pulzehl D, et al: Complement system in healthy term newborns: Reference values in umbilical cord blood. Pediatr Dev Pathol 1:131-135, 1998.
Sorensen RU, Polmar SH: Immunoglobulin replacement therapy. Ann Clin Res 19:293-304, 1987.
Spits H, Blom B, Jaleco AC, et al: Early stages in the development of human T, natural killer and thymic dendritic cells. Immunol Rev 165:75-86, 1998.
Sprent J: T cell memory. Microbes Infect 4:51-56, 2002.
Stegagno M, Pascone R, Colarizi P, et al: Immunologic follow-up of infants treated with granulocyte transfusion for neonatal sepsis. Pediatrics 76:508-511, 1985.
Stephan JL, Vlekova V, Le Deist F, et al: Severe combined immunodeficiency: A retrospective single-center study of clinical presentation and outcome in 117 patients. J Pediatr 123:564-572, 1993.
Stevenson AM: Immunizations for women and infants. J Obstet Gynecol Neonatal Nurs 28:534-544, 1999.
Stewart CL: Blastocyst implantation depends on maternal expression of leukaemia inhibitory factor. Nature 359:76-79, 1992.

Stiehm ER, Ammann AJ, Cherry JD: Elevated cord macroglobulins in the diagnosis of intrauterine infections. N Engl J Med 275:971-977, 1966.

Stiehm ER, Sztein MB, Steeg PS, et al: Deficient DR antigen expression on human cord blood monocytes: Reversal with lymphokines. Clin Immunol Immunopathol 30:430-436, 1984.

Stiehm ER, Ashida E, Kim KS, et al: Intravenous immunoglobulins as therapeutic agents [erratum appears in Ann Intern Med 107:946, 1987]. Ann Intern Med 107:367-382, 1987.

Stossel TP, Alper CA, Rosen FS: Opsonic activity in the newborn: Role of properdin. Pediatrics 52:134-137, 1973.

Strunk RC, Fenton LJ, Gaines JA: Alternative pathway of complement activation in full term and premature infants. Pediatr Res 13:641-643, 1979.

Strunk RC, Fleischer JA, Katz Y, et al: Developmentally regulated effects of lipopolysaccharide on biosynthesis of the third component of complement and factor B in human fibroblasts and monocytes. Immunology 82:314-320, 1994.

Suarez VR, Hankins GD: Smallpox and pregnancy: From eradicated disease to bioterrorist threat. Obstet Gynecol 100:87-93, 2002.

Sutton MB, Strunk RC, Cole FS: Regulation of the synthesis of the third component of complement and factor B in cord blood monocytes by lipopolysaccharide. J Immunol 136:1366-1372, 1986.

Swinburne LM: Leucocyte antigens and placental sponge. Lancet 2:592-594, 1970.

Symons M, Derry JM, Karlak B, et al: Wiskott-Aldrich syndrome protein, a novel effector for the GTPase CDC42Hs, is implicated in actin polymerization. Cell 84:723-734, 1996.

Tafuri A, Alferink J, Moller P, et al: T cell awareness of paternal alloantigens during pregnancy. Science 270:630-633, 1995.

Tangri S, Wegmann TG, Lin H, et al: Maternal anti-placental reactivity in natural, immunologically-mediated fetal resorptions. J Immunol 152:4903-4911, 1994.

Tedder TF, Clement LT, Cooper MD: Development and distribution of a human B cell subpopulation identified by the HB-4 monoclonal antibody. J Immunol 134:1539-1544, 1985a.

Tedder TF, Clement LT, Cooper MD: Human lymphocyte differentiation antigens HB-10 and HB-11. I: Ontogeny of antigen expression. J Immunol 134:2983-2988, 1985b.

Thompson LF, O'Connor RD, Bastian JF: Phenotype and function of engrafted maternal T cells in patients with severe combined immunodeficiency. J Immunol 133:2513-2517, 1984.

Timens W, Rozeboom T, Poppema S: Fetal and neonatal development of human spleen: An immunohistological study. Immunology 60:603-609, 1987.

Tongio MM, Mayer S, Lebec A: Transfer of HL-A antibodies from the mother to the child. Complement of information. Transplantation 20:163-166, 1975.

Tremellen KP, Seamark RF, Robertson SA: Seminal transforming growth factor beta-1 stimulates granulocyte-macrophage colony-stimulating factor production and inflammatory cell recruitment in the murine uterus. Biol Reprod 58:1217-1225, 1998.

van Tol MJ, Zijlstra J, Thomas CM, et al: Distinct role of neonatal and adult monocytes in the regulation of the in vitro antigen-induced plaque-forming cell response in man. J Immunol 133:1902-1908, 1984.

Vercellotti G, Stroncek D, Jacob HS: Granulocyte oxygen radicals as potential suppressors of hemopoiesis: Potentiating roles of lactoferrin and elastase; inhibitory role of oxygen radical scavengers. Blood Cells 13:199-206, 1987.

Volanakis JE: C3 convertases of complement. Year Immunol 4:218-230, 1989.

von Boehmer H, Fehling HJ: Structure and function of the pre-T cell receptor. Annu Rev Immunol 15:433-452, 1997.

Wakasugi N, Virelizier JL: Defective IFN-gamma production in the human neonate. I: Dysregulation rather than intrinsic abnormality. J Immunol 134:167-171, 1985.

Walsh JA, Hutchins S: Group B streptococcal disease: Its importance in the developing world and prospect for prevention with vaccines [see comments]. Pediatr Infect Dis J 8:271-277, 1989.

Wegmann TG, Barrington LJ, Carlson GA: Quantitation of the capacity of the mouse placenta to absorb monoclonal anti-fetal H-2k antibody. J Reprod Immunol 2:53, 1980.

Wegmann TG, Gill TJ, Nesbet-Brown E: Molecular and Cellular Immunobiology of the Maternal Fetal Interface. New York, Oxford University Press, 1991.

Weisman LE, Anthony BF, Hemming VG, et al: Comparison of group B streptococcal hyperimmune globulin and standard intravenously administered immune globulin in neonates. J Pediatr 122:929-937, 1993a.

Weisman LE, Cruess DF, Fischer GW: Standard versus hyperimmune intravenous immunoglobulin in preventing or treating neonatal bacterial infections. Clin Perinatol 20:211-224, 1993b.

Weisman LE, Stoll BJ, Kueser TJ, et al: Intravenous immune globulin prophylaxis of late-onset sepsis in premature neonates. J Pediatr 125:922-930, 1994.

Wessels MR, Paoletti LC, Rodewald AK, et al: Stimulation of protective antibodies against type Ia and Ib group B streptococci by a type Ia polysaccharide-tetanus toxoid conjugate vaccine. Infect Immun 61:4760-4766, 1993.

Whitley RJ: Neonatal herpes simplex virus infections: Is there a role for immunoglobulin in disease prevention and therapy? Pediatr Infect Dis J 13:432-439, 1994.

Wiesen AR, Littell CT: Relationship between prepregnancy anthrax vaccination and pregnancy and birth outcomes among U.S. Army women. JAMA 287:1556-1560, 2002.

Williams O, Brady HJ: The role of molecules that mediate apoptosis in T-cell selection. Trends Immunol 22:107-111, 2001.

Wilson CB, Westall J, Johnston L, et al: Decreased production of interferon-gamma by human neonatal cells: Intrinsic and regulatory deficiencies. J Clin Invest 77:860-867, 1986.

Wilson CB, Penix L, Melvin A, et al: Lymphokine regulation and the role of abnormal regulation in immunodeficiency. Clin Immunol Immunopathol 67:S25-S32, 1993.

Wilson M, Rosen FS, Schlossman SF, et al: Ontogeny of human T and B lymphocytes during stressed and normal gestation: Phenotypic analysis of umbilical cord lymphocytes from term and preterm infants. Clin Immunol Immunopathol 37:1-12, 1985.

Winter HS, Gard, SE, Fischer, TJ, et al: Deficient lymphokine production of newborn lymphocytes. Pediatr Res 17:573-578, 1983.

Wood CR, Chernova T, Chaudhary D, et al: The B7-CD28 superfamily. Nature Immunol 2:261-268, 2001.

Yamada H, Polgar K, Hill JA: Cell-mediated immunity to trophoblast antigens in women with recurrent spontaneous abortion. Am J Obstet Gynecol 170:1339-1344, 1994.

Yamashita Y, Thompson LF, Resta R: Insights into adenosine deaminase deficiency provided by murine fetal thymic organ culture with 2′-deoxycoformycin. Immunol Rev 161:95-109, 1998.

Yankee TM, Clark EA: Signaling through the B cell antigen receptor in developing B cells. Rev Immunogenet 2:185-203, 2000.

Young HA, Ghosh P, Ye J, et al: Differentiation of the T helper phenotypes by analysis of the methylation state of the IFN-gamma gene. J Immunol 153:3603-3610, 1994.

Yun TJ, Bevan MJ: The Goldilocks conditions applied to T cell development [letter; comment]. Nature Immunol 2:13-14, 2001.

CHAPTER 36

# Identification, Evaluation, and Care of the Human Immunodeficiency Virus–Exposed Neonate

Karen P. Beckerman

## EARLY HISTORY OF THE AIDS PANDEMIC

In the last months of 1980, previously healthy young men began to present for care with complaints of chronic illness without apparent etiology. Their complaints included fever, malaise, weight loss, lymphadenopathy, candidiasis, abdominal pain, headaches, and new-onset seizures. By late 1981, reports of an unprecedented clinical syndrome appeared in the U.S. Public Health Service's *Morbidity and Mortality Weekly Report* and several prominent medical journals. Two of these focused on nine young men who had been admitted to tertiary referral centers with *Pneumocystis carinii* pneumonia. At the time of publication, five of the nine men had died and the other four were severely and chronically ill. It quickly became clear that the fatality rate for this mysterious syndrome would approach 100%.

During these very early years of the epidemic, it appeared as if the syndrome could be defined by the groups who first presented for medical attention. Thus, "Gay Cancer" and "GRID" (gay-related immunodeficiency) were the names the world initially heard in connection with the human immunodeficiency (HIV). All too soon, however, the syndrome was identified in others, including intravenous drug users, transfusion recipients, and hemophiliacs. Inexplicably, Haitian immigrants started to present with identical symptoms and findings yet had no behavioral risks in common with other groups. Even so, the concepts of being either "at risk" or "not at risk" for the syndrome of opportunistic infections and immunodeficiency were universally adopted.

Dr. Peter Piot, Director of UNAIDS, has noted, "Denial has been a characteristic of this epidemic at all levels." In 1982, the first reports of infants with noncongenital (i.e., *acquired*) immunodeficiency were rejected, first by national meetings and then by prominent journals, with comments that these children certainly did not have "the homosexuals' disease" (Shilts, 2000). In 1983, Dr. Piot led a team cosponsored by the Centers for Disease Control and Prevention (CDC) and the National Institutes of Health (NIH) that studied an illness that was filling hospitals in Kinshasa, Zaire (now Congo), with equal numbers of previously healthy young men and women who were emaciated and dying. The team identified 36 cases of acquired immunodeficiency syndrome (AIDS). The report of their findings—that an identical immunodeficiency syndrome was heterosexually spread in Africa, and therefore that *everyone in the world* was at risk (Gellman, 2000)—was rejected for publication 12 times.

From our perspective two decades later, it is difficult to grasp the fear that accompanied the first scientific recognition of the spread of HIV type 1 (HIV-1) infection. In the United States and Europe, identification of at-risk groups helped investigators define transmission patterns, identify and isolate the etiologic agent, and develop diagnostic assays within several years of the first reports. However, the concept of "risk" also served to foster worldwide ignorance of what we now know to be a virtually universal risk of infection.

Recognition of this history is important precisely because most of society's attitudes and values that fostered the global spread of HIV/AIDS in the 1980s and 1990s persist today. Infected women are still routinely asked, by otherwise well-meaning caregivers, "Are you an intravenous drug user, a prostitute or both?" Questionnaires given to women entering prenatal care continue to inquire about HIV risk factors, even when we know that any pregnant woman has had unprotected exposure to semen and is at risk of infection. To this day, treatment, transmission prevention, and research among those "not at risk" (a euphemism for individuals who are not gay, do not have multiple sexual partners, are not hemophiliac, and do not use injection drugs) have been neglected. In parts of the developed world, where vertical (mother-to-child) transmission rates among treated pregnant women are less than 1% to 2%, infected infants continue to be born to "low-risk" mothers who were never tested during pregnancy. In the United States, hundreds of new cases of pediatric HIV/AIDS are reported annually. Tragically, many infected infants are often diagnosed only when they present with advanced AIDS. Even though some states mandate HIV screening for all infants before discharge from the newborn nursery, many do not. Determination of all infants' HIV exposure status will remain a major challenge in every newborn nursery for a long time to come. Excellent standard references on the management of pediatric HIV-1 infection are readily available, including comprehensive reviews (Khoury and Kovacs, 2001) and U.S. Public Health Service Guidelines, which are frequently updated and readily available on the Internet (Centers for Disease Control and Prevention [CDC], 2003).

## PATHOGENESIS OF HIV DISEASE

### Transmission of the Virus

Transmission of HIV requires the exchange of bodily fluids. Numerous studies have demonstrated that casual household or community contacts are not associated with transmission or acquisition of HIV/AIDS. The three general mechanisms by which the virus can be passed from one individual to another are sexual, parenteral, and perinatal.

Different types of exposure to infection are associated with different risks of infection (Royce et al, 1997). One sexual transmission occurs for every 100 to 1000 exposures.

Male-to-female transmission risk is about ten times greater than female-to-male transmission risk. Needlestick injury from an infected source carries a transmission risk between 0.5% and 1%, with the risk from needle sharing significantly greater. The risk of transmission through blood transfusion is greater than 90%. Without antiretroviral prophylaxis or maternal treatment, risk of mother-to-child transmission is about 25%.

### Sexual Transmission

Sexual transmission is the dominant mode of transmission of HIV worldwide. Increased rates of sexual transmission are associated with other sexually transmitted diseases, particularly those producing genital ulcers, such as genital herpes and syphilis. Inflammatory conditions of the male or female genital tract result in both higher HIV viral loads in genital secretions and decreased integrity of genital mucosal defenses. Chronic immune activation due to other infectious diseases, such as tuberculosis and intestinal parasitic diseases, may enhance susceptibility to infection by the virus and are also associated with greater HIV disease activity in persons already living with the virus.

Nonhuman primate studies of the closely related simian immunodeficiency virus (SIV) have revealed a dynamic picture of early events in HIV transmission. Spira and colleagues (1998) reported that vaginal inoculation of adult rhesus macaques was followed by infection of dendritic cells in the lamina propria of the cervicovaginal mucosa. Within 2 days, virus could be identified in draining internal iliac lymph nodes. By day 5, virus could be detected in the blood.

### Parenteral Transmission

Parenteral transmission is the dominant route of transmission in many regions. Eastern Europe and Central Asia have the world's fastest-growing epidemic, and 90% of 1.2 million infections have been officially attributed to injection drug use. The immediate site of viral replication after intravenous exposure is not well established, but it would stand to reason that after injection, the virus would have immediate access to tissues of the central immune compartment.

Transmission by injection drug use also fuels transmission by sexual and mother-to-child routes, because the virus spreads through populations of men and women of reproductive age.

### Mother-to-Child Transmission

Mother-to-child-transmission is incompletely understood. Transfer of virus from maternal to fetal or neonatal tissues is thought to occur during one of three discrete periods—antepartum (before the onset of labor), peripartum (during labor and delivery), and breast-feeding. Studies of early viral dynamics in infected neonates suggest that the peripartum period is the time of highest risk (Mofenson, 1997).

We do not know how the virus travels from mother to baby before delivery. Many investigators postulate that virus from maternal genital secretions access the fetus via mucosal routes. Others have studied transplacental routes of transmission. Regardless, no route of transmission except for blood transfusion is as successful as perinatal transmission (Royce et al, 1997).

After delivery, transmission through breast milk is responsible for up to 16% of transmissions to babies who were not perinatally infected (Nduati et al, 2000a). Neonatal primates that were inoculated orally required doses 10 times higher than those in vaginal and rectal inoculations to establish infection but, once infected, had demonstrable circulating virus within 1 week. Interestingly, breast milk from infected mothers contains HIV-specific cytolytic $CD8^+$ T cells, which may partially protect nursing infants from transmission of HIV through breast milk (Sabbaj et al, 2002).

## HIV and Immune Destruction

### Life Cycle

The life cycle of HIV-1 is summarized in Figure 36–1; details are also available on line in an animated format (HIV Life Cycle, 2002).Like these cartoons, most models of HIV-1 infection are based on experimental data derived from the infection of cell culture or animals with high titer free virus. We do not know whether transmission of HIV-1 can occur in vivo without critical cell-to-cell interactions. Regardless, whether cell-associated or free, HIV-1 depends on host cell surface receptor expression for cell entry. Once in a cell, the virus requires host cytoplasmic pathways for its journey to and from the host nucleus, where it utilizes the infected cell's transcriptional capacity for production of viral proteins. Immature viral particles bud out from the host cell, and the creation of infectious virions finally depends on the action of viral protease.

### Pathogenesis of Immune Destruction

HIV-1 infection appears to have three phases (Fig. 36–2). *Primary infection* is characterized by acute symptoms of viral illness and extremely high plasma viremia. With the onset of an antiviral immune response, signaled by the appearance of anti-HIV antibodies and cytotoxic T cells, plasma viremia falls by 2 or more logs, and a so-called *latent phase* begins; levels of virus and infected cells are detected in the peripheral circulation at an individual set point (Pantaleo et al, 1993b). Without antiretroviral therapy, plasma viremia slowly increases, and the latent phase ends after about 10 years with a rapid increase in circulating HIV-1 and a collapse of immune function (fully-expressed AIDS).

Our understanding of HIV disease was revolutionized in the early 1990s, when potent antiretrovirals, quantitative assays of viral replication based on the polymerase chain reaction (PCR), and in situ PCR techniques became available for study of HIV-1 cellular kinetics and viral dynamics in lymphoid tissues (Embretson et al, 1993; Pantaleo et al, 1993a). These techniques have demonstrated that HIV-1 infection is characterized by massive HIV-1 production and immune cell turnover during all phases of the disease, long before immunodeficiency sets in.

Many mechanisms of HIV-1–induced immunodeficiency have been described. Broadly speaking, they include

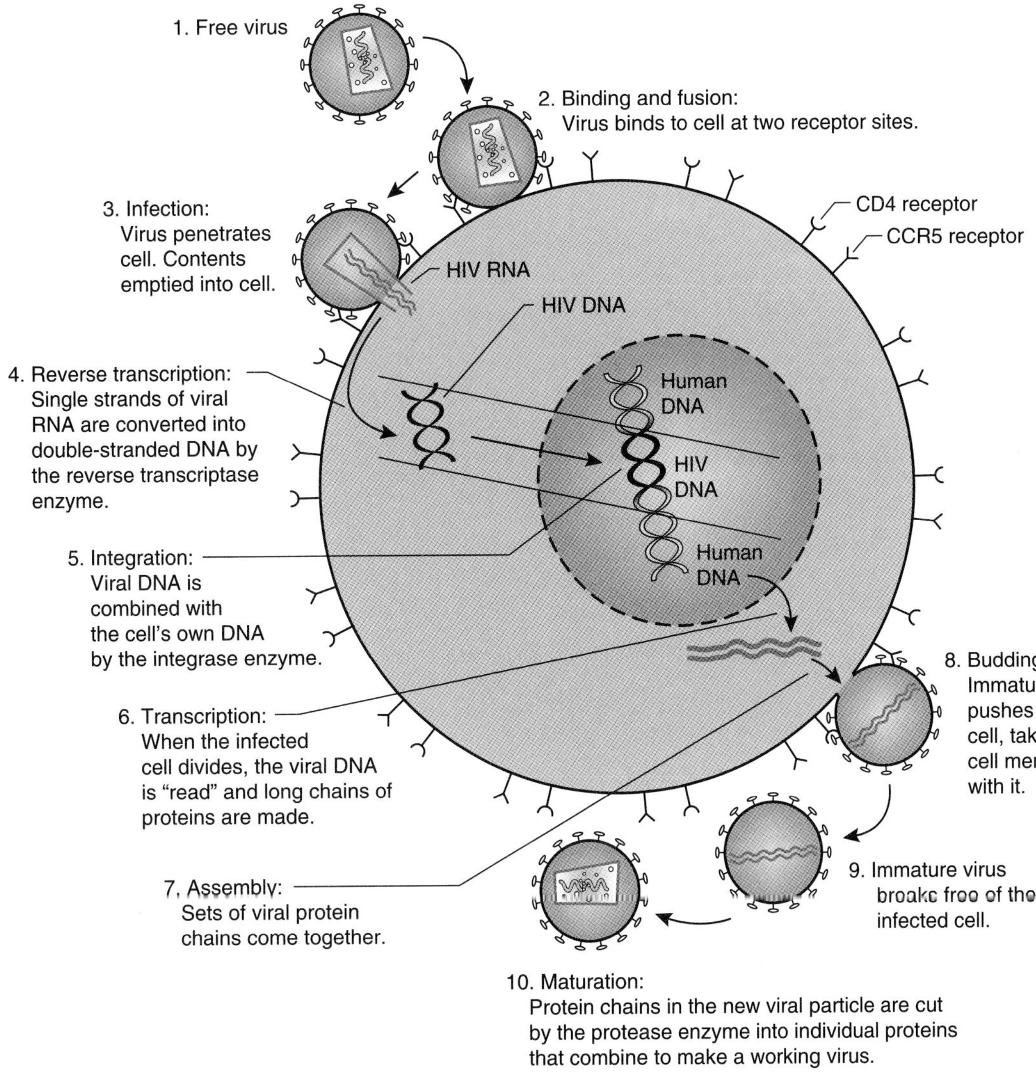

1. Free virus
2. Binding and fusion:
Virus binds to cell at two receptor sites.
CD4 receptor
CCR5 receptor
3. Infection:
Virus penetrates cell. Contents emptied into cell.
HIV RNA
HIV DNA
4. Reverse transcription:
Single strands of viral RNA are converted into double-stranded DNA by the reverse transcriptase enzyme.
Human DNA
HIV DNA
Human DNA
5. Integration:
Viral DNA is combined with the cell's own DNA by the integrase enzyme.
6. Transcription:
When the infected cell divides, the viral DNA is "read" and long chains of proteins are made.
7. Assembly:
Sets of viral protein chains come together.
8. Budding:
Immature virus pushes out of the cell, taking some cell membrane with it.
9. Immature virus breaks free of the infected cell.
10. Maturation:
Protein chains in the new viral particle are cut by the protease enzyme into individual proteins that combine to make a working virus.

**FIGURE 36–1.** Life cycle of the human immunodeficiency virus.

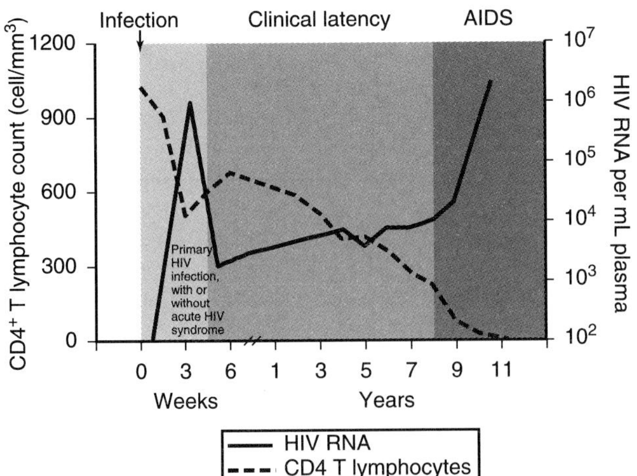


**FIGURE 36–2.** Three phases of HIV disease: Primary infection characterized by high viral load and normal but falling CD4 count. Clinical latency with stable viral load at an individual's set point and gradually falling CD4 count. AIDS or symptomatic HIV disease, with high viral load, low CD4 count and immunodeficiency.

direct killing of infected cells by the virus or the host, induction of programmed cell death *(apoptosis)*, induction of abnormal cytokine production by infected cells, disruption of the architecture of lymphoid tissues, disruption of hematopoiesis and lymphoid differentiation, and evolution or diversification of the virus during infection to variants with greater virulence (Coffin, 1995). Unifying all such theories is the observation that deterioration of immune function is driven by constantly repeated cycles of massive viral replication (more than $10^{10}$ virions/day) (Perelson et al, 1996) and immune cell turnover of more than $10^9$ cells/day.

## Immune Activation

Immune activation plays a key role in the pathogenesis of HIV-1 disease (Lawn et al, 2001). Commonly, immune activation due to co-infection (mycobacterial, parasitic, viral, or bacterial) renders infected individuals more infectious and may make the uninfected more susceptible to transmission. Although interactions between activation of the immune system and progression of HIV disease are complex, the inflammatory response clearly promotes cell-to-cell transmission of HIV-1. In fact, at least one clinical study has suggested that chorioamnionitis may be associated with higher rates of vertical transmission (Mofensen et al, 1999).

## MATERNAL-CHILD HEALTH AND HIV/AIDS

### The Global Pandemic

The HIV/AIDS pandemic has affected the health of women and children unlike any previous infectious scourge. Soon it will bypass the Black Death as the greatest cause of mortality in history. Typically, people are infected in their youth, during their prime productive and reproductive years. After acute infection, time to death ranges from 9 to 11 years (see Fig. 36–2). Those who die represent an irreplaceable loss to their families, communities, and society. They leave in their wake unfarmed land, untaught students, hospitals without doctors and nurses, depleted armies, civil services, and police forces, and, of course, orphans. The scope of the problem is difficult to grasp. Within the next few years, however, if the pandemic continues unchecked, 25% of children younger than 15 years in the most devastated regions will be orphans, numbering 44 million by the year 2010. By 2020, teenagers will outnumber adults in Sub-Saharan Africa.

The infection has been reported in all parts of the world (Fig. 36–3). Seventy percent of those living with HIV/AIDS occupy Sub-Saharan Africa. Eighty-one percent of infected women are African. More than 95% of infected children are African. No other region has reported the high seroprevalence seen in Africa; however, rapid and even explosive growth of the pandemic has been reported in Eastern Europe, the Baltic States, the Russian Federation, and several Central Asian Republics. China and India are experiencing serious localized epidemics affecting 5 million people. At current rates of spread, 45 million more people (in addition to the 42 million infected today) will have acquired the virus by 2010 (AIDS Epidemic Update, 2002).

### Women

HIV/AIDS spares no one, but it has become increasingly apparent that women are at special risk of infection. In 2002, 58% of people living with HIV in Southern Africa were women. Among residents of this region 15 to 19 years old, HIV seroprevalence is twice as high in young women as in young men. Women are likely to become infected at a significantly earlier age than men, for both biologic and demographic reasons—they become sexually active and marry at younger ages, and because of their position in many societies, they are more often unable to negotiate safer sex with their sexual partners. On a per exposure basis, women are ten times more likely than men to become infected (AIDS Epidemic Update, 2002).

### Children

HIV/AIDS threatens the health of children from multiple perspectives (see Fig. 36–3). The devastation of the epidemic undermines the health and safety of all members of a society, especially the most vulnerable. Older children are at great risk of becoming sexually infected. Indeed, given current trends, 50% of all Sub-Saharan 15-year-olds will someday themselves become infected with HIV. All babies of HIV-infected mothers face a 20% risk of dying before their second birthday, whether they themselves are infected or not (Nduati et al, 2000a). Less than half of the babies who are infected will survive to age 3 years.

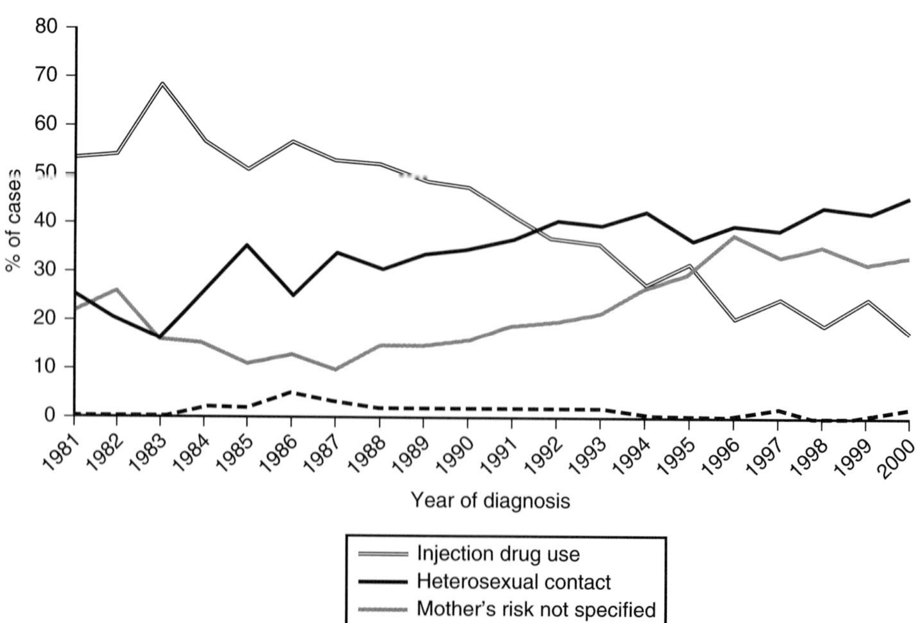


**FIGURE 36–3.** Centers for Disease Control and Prevention analysis of mother's exposure category, by year of diagnosis for perinatally acquired AIDS, 1981 to 2000, United States. Note that most women with "risk not specified" probably acquired HIV by heterosexual contact, raising that category to about 70% of total in 2000.

### Mothers

Our understanding of the impact of infectious disease on maternal health is incomplete. Before the introduction of antibiotics, pneumonia, tuberculosis, and influenza were associated with markedly higher mortality during pregnancy. Indeed, before the 1950s, active tuberculosis was considered a justifiable reason for abortion. Today, effective antibiotic therapies and supportive treatment have obscured any effects that these infections may have on maternal health as well as any effect that pregnancy and lactation may have on the course of infection.

A similar situation exists in our understanding of HIV disease and maternal health. Several comprehensive studies conducted both before and after the availability of effective antiretroviral therapies have shown that pregnancy does not alter the course of HIV disease in resource-rich settings. The same may not be true for resource-poor regions. Women in these latter areas lack access to not only effective antiretroviral treatment but also to prophylaxis and treatments for opportunistic infections and endemic scourges such as tuberculosis, parasitic disease diseases, and malaria, not to mention adequate sewage and clean water.

Two studies have appeared suggesting that in resource-poor settings, HIV-infected women are at markedly higher risk of death after the birth of a child. A multivariate analysis of 4000 pregnant Malawi women found that 3% of pregnant women infected with HIV died before their babies' first birthdays, vs. 0.3% of uninfected pregnant women (McDermott et al, 1996). Nduati and colleagues (2000b), at Kenyatta Hospital in Nairobi, noted that breast-feeding by HIV-infected breast-feeding women had an 11% risk of death by 2 years after delivery. Both studies noted markedly higher death rates among the infants of mothers who died, regardless of transmission status.

## HIV/AIDS in High-Income Countries

Only 1.6 million people, or 4% of the total global population infected with HIV, are living in high-income countries (AIDS Epidemic Update, 2002). In these resource-rich regions, routes of transmission were first identified among homosexuals and injection drug users. Rates of heterosexual transmission have risen every year (see Fig. 36–3), and the virus has spread disproportionately among marginalized populations over the last decade. In the United States, African-Americans and Latinos account for 62% of new infections yet make up only 20% of the population. This trend is even more marked among U.S. women: In 2001, 63% of newly diagnosed women were black, and 13% were Hispanic (CDC, 2001a). Forty percent of new AIDS diagnoses during 1999 occurred among residents of the poorest U.S. counties, with the Southeast disproportionately represented (Karon et al, 2001).

## Impact of Antiretroviral Agents

The introduction of potent antiretroviral therapies in the mid-1990s markedly reduced deaths due to AIDS in most regions of the developed world. Still, 23,000 HIV-related deaths were reported in these countries in 2002. In the United States, HIV/AIDS remains the leading cause of death for African-American men between the ages of 25 and 44 years and the third most common cause of death among Hispanic men of the same age.

Potent antiretroviral therapies not only have reversed AIDS mortality trends in the developed world (Fig. 36–4A); they have also completely altered patterns of transmission of HIV from mothers to children (Fig. 36–4B). Almost 10 years ago, the astonishing results of the Pediatric AIDS Clinical Trial Group (PACTG) Study 076 protocol were announced (Connor et al, 1994). This prospective, placebo-controlled, randomized trial demonstrated that zidovudine prophylaxis during pregnancy, delivery, and early infancy reduced the rate of vertical HIV transmission from 25% to 8%. It became evident that the efficacy of the strategy was even greater in the field, where experience in New York State and other areas soon showed that zidovudine prophylaxis was consistently associated with transmission risk of 5%. Less than 2 years later, additional antiretroviral agents became available for actual treatment of HIV, disease and it became possible to measure HIV disease activity via plasma HIV-1 RNA assays. Soon thereafter, clinicians observed that women who could achieve control of their disease did not transmit the virus to their offspring and that potent therapeutic combinations were associated with low transmission risk even when maternal HIV replication was not completely suppressed.

In contrast, antiretrovirals have not yet had a demonstrable effect on the incidence or mortality of HIV and AIDS in resource-poor regions. Sub-Saharan Africa, home to 29.4 million people living with HIV, lost 2.4 million citizens to death from HIV in the last year and will experience 3.5 million new infections in the coming year (AIDS Epidemic Update, 2003).

## Treatment of Maternal HIV-1 Infection

Nowhere in the epidemic has the impact of combination antiretroviral therapy and opportunistic infection prophylaxis been more far-reaching than in maternal-child health in resource-rich regions. Control of maternal HIV disease both improved maternal health and survival and virtually eliminated the problem of AIDS orphans in the West. Moreover, aggressive antiretroviral therapy during pregnancy appears to offer almost complete protection from perinatal HIV-1 infection to the fetus and neonate.

U.S. Public Health Service Guidelines for the management of HIV disease during pregnancy, antiretroviral therapy for adults and adolescents, and for opportunistic infection prophylaxis have been updated and are an excellent resource that all practitioners should consult. They are easily accessed as living documents on the CDC Web site (www.AIDSinfo.nih.gov/guidelines/).

### General Principles

General principles of HIV care during pregnancy have been articulated elsewhere and are summarized in Table 36–1.

Women diagnosed with HIV infection during pregnancy often present in crisis. As with any patient, the basics of safety, shelter, and nutrition must be attended to

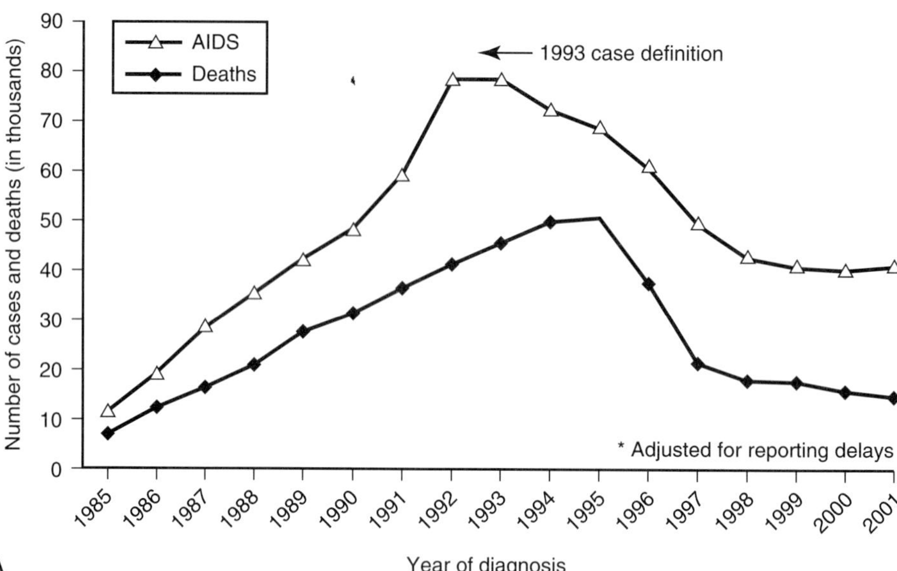


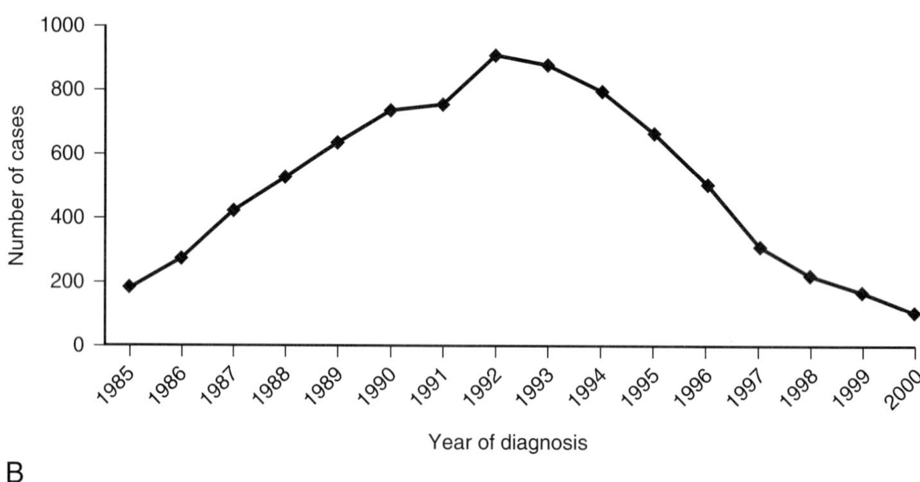


**FIGURE 36–4.** Centers for Disease Control and Prevention estimates of (**A**) Incidence of AIDS and deaths of adults and adolescents with AIDS (adjusted for reporting delays), 1985 to 2001, and (**B**) perinatally acquired AIDS cases, by year of diagnosis, 1985 to 2000.

**TABLE 36–1**

**Principles of Care of Human Immunodeficiency Virus (HIV) Disease During Pregnancy**

| |
|---|
| Self-determination of reproductive choice and HIV therapy |
| Nondirective, supportive education and counseling |
| Intensive monitoring of HIV disease activity, particularly as term approaches |
| Prophylaxis for opportunistic infections |
| Aggressive use of antiretrovirals to suppress maternal HIV replication |
| Protection of mothers from mono- and dual-drug therapies likely to induce antiretroviral resistance |
| Informed maternal choice regarding timing and route of delivery |

first. First assessment of a newly diagnosed woman must include definitive assessment of other family members, especially her other children. For those older than 12 to 18 months, HIV antibody testing may be enough. For those younger than 1 year, more involved virologic testing may be required (Table 36–2). The first few clinic visits should be directed at education and counseling, with clinical focus on assessment of the stage of maternal disease and, most important, prophylaxis or detection and treatment of opportunistic infection.

### *Prophylaxis Against Opportunistic Infection*

Opportunistic infection prophylaxis during pregnancy follows general adult guidelines. Individuals with CD4 T-cell

**TABLE 36–2**

**Diagnostic Testing Schedule for Infants Exposed to Human Immunodeficiency Virus Type 1**

| Laboratory Assay | Tube or Other Media Needed | Laboratory Instructions | Birth (1st 48 hrs of life) | Age 2 wks | Age 1 mo (4-6 wks) | Age 3 mos (12-14 wks) | Age 6 mos (24-28 wks) | Age 1 yr (50-54 wks) | Age $1^1/_2$ yrs (76-80 wks) | Until Sero-reversion |
|---|---|---|---|---|---|---|---|---|---|---|
| HIV-1 DNA PCR | Yellow-top (= acid citrate dextrose) | Room temperature | √ | May be considered for very-high-risk infants | √ | √ | √ | | | |
| HIV-1 RNA PCR | Lavender-top (= EDTA) | Send when repeating test because of positive DNA PCR result or when DNA PCR is not available See text and Table 36–1 | | | | | | | | |
| HIV Ab | | | | | | | | √ | √ | √ |
| HCV Ab (If mother tests positive) | | | | | | | | √ | | |
| CBC | Lavender-top (= EDTA) | | √ | | √ | √ | √ | √ | | |
| CD4 and CD8 counts | Run on same specimen as CBC | Call lab to confirm volume needed | | | √ | | √ | | | |
| AST/ALT | | | With nevirapine prophylaxis | | All | All | | | | |
| Bilirubin | | | When infant was exposed to indinavir | | | | | | | |
| Glucose | Reagent strip | | Test at 1 and 6 hrs after birth if infant was exposed to protease inhibitors | | | | | | | |

Ab, antibody; ALT, alanine transferase; AST, aspartate transaminase; CBC, complete blood count; EDTA, ethylenediaminetetraacetic acid; HCV, hepatitis C virus; HIV, human immunodeficiency virus; HIV-1, HIV type 1; PCR, polymerase chain reaction.

From Bay Area Perinatal AIDS Center, Departments of Obstetrics, Gynecology and Reproductive Sciences and Pediatrics, July 1, 2001.

counts lower than 200 cells/mm$^3$ should be started on *P. carinii* prophylaxis regardless of reproductive status. Trimethoprim-sulfamethoxazole (TMP-SMX) is the agent of choice. Theoretically, there is a risk of neonatal anemia when this agent is administered close to term, but the maternal benefits of prophylaxis far outweigh any theoretical fetal risk. Women with CD4 T-cell counts lower than 50 cells/mm$^3$ should receive *Mycobacterium avium* pneumonia prophylaxis with azithromycin; TMP-SMX also offers toxoplasmosis prophylaxis in this setting. Women who have had an opportunistic infection should receive appropriate prophylaxis regardless of CD4 count.

Many authorities now recommend that patients whose CD4 T-cell counts have been restored to more than 350 cells/mm$^3$ may be offered a trial of stopping opportunistic infection prophylaxis. Although some pregnant women with established HIV infection may be interested in this strategy, I have advised against stopping prophylaxis during pregnancy. There is ample time after pregnancy to consider such options.

### *Antiretrovrial Therapy*

Recommendations regarding the initiation of antiretroviral therapy for adults have changed significantly in the past few years (Guidelines, 2002). From earlier recommendations to "hit early, hit hard" in order to avoid immunodeficiency and other complications of HIV disease, guidelines have moved to stress the advantages of delaying therapy as long as possible in order to avoid, or at least postpone, the complications of antiretroviral therapy. These complications are summarized in Table 36–3. Of greatest concern are metabolic complications and the induction of antiretroviral resistance.

All individuals with symptomatic HIV infection should be counseled about the lifesaving nature of combination antiretroviral therapy. Therapy should be initiated when patients believe they are ready. Guidelines are less uniform for individuals with asymptomatic HIV infection. Generally, therapy should be started for anyone with a CD4 T-cell count less than 350 cells/mm$^3$ or a viral load

**TABLE 36–3**

**Antiretrovirals: Mechanisms of Action with Selected Toxic Effects and Complications**

| Agents | Mechanism of Action | Selected Toxic Effects/Complications |
|---|---|---|
| Nucleoside RT inhibitors (NRTIs):<br>Zidovudine<br>Lamivudine<br>Stavudine<br>Abacavir<br>Tenofovir | Phosphorylated intracellularly to the 5'-triphosphate metabolite that inhibits viral RT by competing with thymidine triphosphate for incorporation into viral DNA, then prematurely terminating DNA synthesis by preventing further 5′ to 3′ phosphodiester linkages | Bone marrow toxicity resulting in maternal and neonatal anemia<br>Most pronounced with zidovudine<br>Lactic acidosis and hepatomegaly/steatosis are most strongly associated with stavudine and stavudine/didanosine<br>Severe hypersensitivity in 3% of patients |
| Non-nucleoside RT inhibitors (NNRTIs):<br>Nevirapine<br>Delavirdine<br>Efavirenz | Specific noncompetitive inhibitors of viral RT<br>Bind directly to a hydrophobic cavity near the active site of RT and cause a conformational change in the enzyme | Cross-class drug resistance emerges rapidly and uniformly when administered as single agent<br>Rash is common and more frequent in women<br>Hepatotoxicity, hepatitis; may be severe or fatal, especially with nevirapine<br>Neural tube defects in non-human primates found in preclinical studies of efavirenz (see text)<br>CNS or psychiatric symptoms with efavirenz. |
| Protease inhibitors (PI):<br>Indinavir<br>Ritonavir<br>Nelfinavir<br>Lopinavir | Competitive inhibitors of HIV protease, an enzyme required for the formation of infectious virus<br>PIs block virus maturation and cause the formation of immature, noninfectious virions, limiting further infectious spread<br>Certain PIs given in combination with ritonavir exhibit markedly enhanced pharmacokinetics | Hyperbilirubinemia<br>Lipid abnormalities with increased triglycerides and LDL<br>Glucose intolerance, type 2 diabetes<br>Increase in gestational diabetes not reported<br>Body fat composition and distribution abnormalities† |
| Fusion inhibitors:<br>Enfuvirtide | Block HIV from entering human cells by blocking virus–cell membrane fusion | Requires subcutaneous injection†<br>Bacterial pneumonia, severe allergic reaction, injection site reaction, and infection |

CNS, central nervous system; HIV, human immunodeficiency virus; LDL, low-density lipoprotein; RT, reverse transcriptase (also known as viral RNA-dependent DNA polymerase)

†Also reported with non-PI regimens.

greater than 55,000 copies/mL. Considerable evidence exists to supporting a lower viral load cutoff for women, 35,000 copies/mL (Considerations, 2002).

International experience to date has consistently shown that the most powerful predictor of transmission risk is maternal viral load (Dorenbaum et al, 2002; Garcia et al, 1999) and that treatment with triple-antiretroviral combinations during pregnancy is associated with transmission risk of 1% to 2% or less (Ioannidis et al, 2000). HIV-infected pregnant women should be offered a combination of three or more antiretroviral agents regardless of the stage of their infection. For those with symptomatic infection or CD4 T cell counts less than 350 cells/mm$^3$, treatment should be initiated or continued as it would for anyone not pregnant, with the primary aim of achieving a durable suppression of maternal viral replication in order to preserve or restore maternal health. For women with asymptomatic infection, and CD4 T cell counts greater than 350 cells/mm$^3$, and viral loads less than 35,000 copies/mL, antiretrovirals are still indicated for the prevention of transmission of HIV to the fetus; therapy can safely be stopped after pregnancy is over as long as mother's health continues to be monitored.

## Antiretroviral Agents

### *Currently Available HIV Therapies*

Four classes of antiretroviral agents are now available for treating HIV infection (see Table 36–3). First-line combinations are made up of two nucleoside transcriptase inhibitors (NRTIs) and either a protease inhibitor (PI) or a non-nucleoside reverse transcriptase inhibitor (NNRTI). The fusion inhibitor enfurvidine is generally reserved for patients who are have received numerous antiretrovirals and have experienced virologic breakthrough using multiple different potent combinations.

All classes of antiretrovirals have serious side effects, advantages, and disadvantages. Determination of optimal combinations must factor in patient preference, other medications, stage of HIV disease, ease of administration, and reproductive plans. Protease inhibitors can now be taken either twice daily alone (as with nelfinavir) or along with small doses of ritonavir (as with indinavir and lopinavir), which markedly enhances pharmacokinetics. Efavirenz is a highly potent, once-daily NNRTI that has become very popular. Unfortunately, preclinical evaluation of efavirenz in nonhuman primates demonstrated serious neural tube defects in 2 of 20 exposed fetuses. A prospective registry of the use of antiretroviral agents in pregnancy has received no reports of neural tube defects in 84 cases reported with first-trimester efavirenz exposure. Still, the use of efavirenz during the first trimester remains of great concern.

### *Teratogenicity*

Teratogenicity of antiretrovirals has been of great concern since they first became available. Teratogenicity of these agents is being closely monitored by industry and the U.S. Food and Drug Administration (FDA). The Antiretroviral Pregnancy Registry has collected more than 4000 voluntary, prospective reports of antiretroviral exposure during pregnancy (Committee APRS, 2003). Overall, the prevalence of birth defects has been 2.5 per 100 live births. Among these exposures, 1242 occurred during the first trimester, and the prevalence of birth defects was 2.8 per 100 live births. These proportions compare favorably with the CDC's population-based birth defects surveillance system, in which total prevalence of birth defects identified among births from 1991 through 1995 was 3.1 per 100 live births (Table 36–4).

The registry now has sufficient enrollment to detect at least a twofold increase in risk of overall birth defects and of defects of cardiovascular and genitourinary systems for the commonly used antiretrovirals listed in Table 36–4. Retrospective reports are also collected by the Registry. No pattern of defects, isolated or syndromic, has been found in the evaluation of these reports.

**Efavirenz.** One NNRTI, efavirenz, has been of special concern ever since results of a developmental toxicity study of cynomolgus monkeys were released. Pregnant monkeys received efavirenz and achieved plasma levels equivalent to therapeutic human dosages. Three of 20 efavirenz-treated fetuses had birth defects (one with anencephaly and unilateral anophthalmia, another with microphthalmia, and a third with cleft palate). There were no birth defects in the 20 controls. The Registry has insufficient numbers of reports of infants exposed to efavirenz during organogenesis (i.e., before 12 weeks of gestation) to allow draw conclusions to be drawn regarding human teratogenicity of this agent. Of 118 first-trimester exposures, 4 infants (3.4%) had birth defects (polydactyly, hydronephrosis, bilateral hip dislocation, and urinary obstruction), but no prospective reports of neural tube defects have been received by the registry. Women anticipating pregnancy should be advised not to take efavirenz. When first-trimester exposure inadvertently occurs, women should be offered early ultrasonography and maternal serum screening for neural tube and other defects.

**TABLE 36–4**

**Summary of Birth Defect Rates Following First-Trimester Exposure to Frequently Used Antiretrovirals from the Antiretroviral Pregnancy Registry**

| Regimen | Rate (No. Defects/ No. Live Births) | Prevalence (95% Confidence Limits) |
|---|---|---|
| Lamivudine | 28/940 | 3.0% (2.0, 4.3) |
| Stavudine | 7/323 | 2.2% (0.9, 4.4) |
| Zidovudine | 25/886 | 2.8% (1.8, 4.1) |
| Nelfinavir | 10/343 | 2.9% (1.4, 5.3) |
| Nevirapine | 5/248 | 2.0% (0.7, 4.7) |
| | | 3.1% (3.1, 3.2) |

Committee APRS, 2003

### *Antiretrovirals and Neonatal Mitochondrial Dysfunction*

A study from France has described mitochondrial dysfunction in 8 (out of 1754) HIV-exposed, uninfected infants who were exposed to zidovudine or zidovudine-lamivudine in utero (Blanche et al, 1999). Two infants experienced progressive mitochondrial dysfunction and death; 6 others had various degrees of nonfatal illness, as diagnosed by screening for symptoms of mitochondrial dysfunction, such as seizures and other neurologic abnormalities, or laboratory evidence of mitochondrial dysfunction, such as persistent lactic acidosis, abnormal liver enzyme values, or abnormal nuclear magnetic resonance (NMR) findings.

Immediately after this report, U.S. investigators pooled all available data from the CDC and NIH. Of 23,000 children exposed in utero to zidovudine, lamivudine, or both, the investigators could identify no children with mitochondrial disease (MacIntosh, 1999).

### *Antiretrovirals and Prematurity*

In 1998, data appeared from three Swiss cohorts reporting preterm delivery in 10 of 30 infants exposed to protease inhibitors in utero (Lorenzi et al, 1998). Multiple reports from the United States do not show a link between the use of protease inhibitors and prematurity. In fact, many caregivers have the impression that optimization of maternal health using protease inhibitor–based and non–protease inhibitor–based regimens enhances pregnancy outcome and birth weight.

## Virologic Breakthrough During Pregnancy

Virologic breakthrough during pregnancy can occur both in antiretroviral-experienced women and in women who have just been diagnosed and started on therapy. Because plasma HIV-1 RNA levels are highly correlated with transmission risk, we measure viral loads at least monthly in most pregnant women. Transiently detectable viremia (or "blips") in those whose virus has been consistently undetectable is probably of limited consequence for both maternal and fetal health.

By far, the most common reasons for virologic breakthrough are difficulties with tolerance of and adherence to medication regimens. Patients should be counseled in detail, and practical, supportive advice should be given to improve adherence. Pill boxes and other aids are extremely helpful. Up to half of HIV-infected pregnant women have not disclosed their infection to their sexual partner. Some women are marginally housed. Support in connection with such issues of daily living may significantly help adherence.

Therapeutic recommendations in the setting of virologic breakthrough vary significantly. While caregivers are addressing adherence, they can obtain resistance testing and carefully consider switching a patient's medications. If a woman is experiencing virologic breakthrough near term with very high ($>10^4$ to $10^5$ copies/mL) viral loads, there may not be time to await resistance testing results, and it may be prudent to empirically (but thoughtfully) add or replace agents in order to achieve the maximum control possible around the time of delivery. Significantly, simply adding a single dose of the NNRTI nevirapine during labor to ongoing antiretroviral therapy did not decrease transmission rates and did induce NNRTI resistance among mothers with incomplete virologic control (Dorenbaum et al, 2002).

We do not know how virologic breakthrough in women receiving therapy may influence transmission rates. PACTG Study 367 has reported transmission rates of 1% among women on 3 or more medications at the time of delivery (Shapiro et al, 2000). The study has not yet included analysis of maternal plasma HIV-1 RNA among women on therapy. It may be that combination therapy is effective at preventing vertical transmission even when virologic control is not perfect. Generally, considerations of maternal health are the best guide to treatment decisions in this setting.

### *Antiretroviral Resistance and Maternal-Child Health*

**Viral Dynamics and the Development of Resistance.** From our earliest laboratory and clinical work with antiretroviral agents, it has been clear that HIV-1 is capable of rapidly evolving drug resistance to medications designed to block its replication. Two general phenomena contribute to the virus's extraordinary success at overcoming barriers to its production, high rates of viral replication and high rates of genomic mutation (Coffin, 1995). Several billion $CD4^+$ T cells are productively infected at any given time. More than a billion die and are replaced every day. Infected individuals produce on the order of $10^{10}$ particles of HIV-1 per day. Mutation rates are high, because (1) insertion and deletion mutations are common with two RNA copies per virion and (2) RNA strand breaks can force template switching. Furthermore, the two polymerases involved in HIV-1 production, HIV-1 reverse transcriptase and cellular RNA polymerase, both lack proofreading activity.

Early clinical success of antiretroviral therapy was significantly hindered by the lack of long-term effectiveness of single antiretroviral agents. The recognition in the mid-1990s that combination therapy could be given not only to enhance potency of single-drug therapy but also to forestall the development of antiretroviral resistance (both by creating multiple blocks to viral replication and decreasing mutation rates by suppressing replication rates) led to the ongoing success of HIV treatment and reversal of AIDS mortality trends in many parts of the developed world (see Fig. 36–4A).

Despite the dramatic reduction of HIV-related morbidity and mortality in the developed world, antiretroviral resistance has been a widespread problem that has limited the efficacy of treatment (Yerly et al, 1999). Little and associates (2002) have documented transmission of resistant HIV-1 variants among recently infected, antiretrovirally naïve, predominantly male groups, the rate of which has risen dramatically to as high as 23%. These investigators also found the rate of multiple-drug resistance to be more than 10%. Today, resistance poses a major threat to the management of antiretroviral therapy.

**Antiretroviral Resistance in Pregnant Women and Perinatally Infected Infants.** Data describing the prevalence of antiretroviral resistance among HIV-infected women of child-bearing age are limited, but it is reasonable to assume that women harbor resistant virus at rates similar to those for men.

Mother-to-child transmission of HIV-1 with high-level resistance to zidovudine was first reported in 1993 (Masquelier et al, 1993). Only low-level genotypic resistance was detected in samples from participants in the AIDS Clinical Trials Group Protocol 076 (ACTG 076) (all of whom had CD4 counts >200 cells/mm$^3$) and was not associated with transmission risk (Eastman et al, 1998). However, the Women and Infants Transmission Study Group found that 25% of maternal isolates had at least one zidovudine-associated resistance mutation and that the presence of resistance was independently associated with a fivefold greater risk of transmission (Welles et al, 2000). The high-level lamivudine resistance mutation, M184 V, has been reported in 4 of 5 pregnant women receiving zidovudine and lamivudine (Clarke et al, 1999).

We do not know how the rising rates of antiretroviral resistance will affect mother-to-child transmission rates. Virologic breakthrough—that is, increasing viral load in a woman receiving therapy—is commonly associated with development of antiretroviral resistance. Although high viral loads also are associated with increased rates of vertical transmission (Garcia et al, 1999), we do not know whether resistant virus can be transmitted to the fetus-neonate as efficiently as wild-type virus. Mathematical modeling using data from retrospective surveys of clinical data has suggested that sexual transmission of resistant HIV from patients receiving antiretroviral therapy is only 20% that of wild-type virus (Brown et al, 2003). The same could be true of perinatal transmission.

Regardless, optimal initial treatment for any infected individual provides the best chance of therapeutic success for the long term. Thus, prevention of the transmission of antiretroviral-resistant HIV to neonates requires potent therapy to suppress maternal replication of both wild-type and resistant viruses. Resistance testing for HIV-infected women can optimize initial treatment, prevent development of resistance, and lower fetal exposure to resistant as well as wild-type HIV-1 (Yerly et al, 1999).

## IDENTIFICATION OF THE HIV-EXPOSED NEONATE

### Prevalence of Perinatal HIV-1 Exposure and Infection

Even though many pediatricians and neonatologists are unlikely to encounter HIV-1 infection in their patients, the stark reality remains that all babies born today are at some risk, however large or small, of AIDS. Prevalence of HIV infection varies by a factor of more than 1000 in different parts of the world. Neonatal exposure and infection rates also vary greatly. In some areas of Sub-Saharan Africa, 30% of infants of the more than 30% of pregnant women who are HIV-infected, that is, 1 in 10 babies, are HIV-infected. In the developed world, fewer than 1 in 3000 newborns are exposed to HIV, and fewer than 2% of these (one in 150,000) are HIV-infected.

Perinatal HIV-1 exposure is diagnosed by demonstrating anti-HIV-1 antibodies in maternal, cord blood, or neonatal serum. Although anti-HIV-1 serologic results from these sources is diagnostic of maternal infection status, it does not reflect any infant's actual infection status, only the exposure status (Table 36–5).

### Prevention of Pediatric AIDS

Potent antiretroviral therapies and current highly sensitive and effective techniques of screening the blood supply have rendered pediatric AIDS a preventable disease. Pediatric AIDS can be prevented at two points. First, and by far the most effective, is the prevention of pediatric infection by ensuring a safe blood supply and by treating maternal HIV infection during pregnancy. Second, even if an infant does become infected, early recognition and treatment with potent combinations of antiretrovirals can forestall both destruction of the pediatric immune system and the development of AIDS (Krogstad et al, 1999; Luzariaga et al, 1997). It is therefore doubly critical that no infant leave the newborn nursery before his or her HIV-1 exposure is known. Transmission rates in the developed world should approach zero, and no HIV-1–infected infant should be allowed to progress to AIDS. Diagnosis of pediatric AIDS at the time of presentation with an opportunistic infection happens only when we have missed both the opportunity to prevent transmission *and* the opportunity to prevent immune deficiency after infection.

### Clinical Presentations

Perinatal HIV-1 exposure alone has no clinical manifestations. The only way to determine any infant's exposure status is to determine maternal infection status, usually through antibody screening of maternal or neonatal blood or secretions. Similarly, until immunodeficiency sets in, neonatal HIV-1 infection is diagnosed only by demonstration of viral genome in the infant (Tables 36–5 and 36–6).

Pediatric AIDS can have general, infectious, or organ-specific manifestations, which have been thoroughly reviewed elsewhere (Khoury and Kovacs, 2001). Failure to thrive, said to be universal among HIV-infected children (Pollack et al, 1997), is caused by multiple complications of HIV disease. Malignancy may be the presenting clinical problem, but recurrent and especially chronic bacterial or viral infections are often the first sign of HIV disease. Infections can be either minor (otitis, sinusitis, skin and soft tissue infections) or serious (bacteremia, pneumonia, bone and joint infections) and may be seen in the context of pronounced hepatosplenomegaly and lymphadenopathy. Dermatologic complications of HIV infection are common. They range from allergic reactions

**TABLE 36-5**

## A Neonatologist's Guide to Laboratory Evaluation of the HIV-exposed Infant*

| | Test | | | |
|---|---|---|---|---|
| | **HIV-1 Antibody Test** | **HIV-1 Culture** | **HIV-1 DNA PCR** | **Plasma HIV-1 RNA** |
| Common term used for test | "HIV test" | "Culture" | "PCR" | "Viral load" or "viral burden" |
| What it does | Detects the presence of antibody<br>Reflects infant's exposure status and maternal infection status but not infant infection status | Detects replicating HIV in infant PBMCs co-cultured with donor lymphocytes | Detects the presence of integrated, proviral DNA in the genome of infant's PBMCs by PCR | Also a PCR-based technique<br>Measures the amount of viral RNA in plasma of infant |
| What result means | Sero-reversion to negative at 12-18 months confirms negative PCR test finding that infant is uninfected<br>Remains the "gold standard," final determination of infant infection status | If result is positive, infant is infected | If result is positive, infant is infected<br>If negative at least twice, including once after 2 months of age, suggests strongly that infant is not infected | Quantitative result reflects HIV-1 disease activity<br>If unknown infection status, >3000 copies/mL, infant is likely infected. If below limits of detection at least twice, infant may be uninfected<br>Potential for false-positive results at <3000 copies/mL |
| Results reported | Qualitative: "positive" or "negative" | Qualitative: "positive" or "negative" | Qualitative: "positive" or "negative" | Quantitative: number of copies of HIV-1 RNA per mL plasma |
| Time required for results | 1-2 days | 30-40 days | 7-14 days | 3-10 days |
| Advantages | Sero-reversion (loss of detectable maternal HIV-1 antibody by 12-18 months of age) remains the gold standard for proof that an infant is uninfected | Very low false-positive rate<br>False-negative results reported | Low false-positive rate<br>False-negative results reported | Wider availability<br>Faster turnover |
| When indicated | If PCR results have all been negative, should be performed at 1 year of age and then every 6 months until result is negative | For diagnosis of infection when antibody status is not informative | For diagnosis of infection when antibody status is not informative | To assess HIV-1 disease activity in individuals known to be infected with HIV-1 |
| When performed? | Starting at 12 months of age, then every 6 months until result is negative | Has largely been replaced by PCR-based systems of HIV detection | First 48 hrs of life, then at 4-6 wks, 3 mos, and 6 mos of age | Used to quantify viral replication and disease activity in individuals known to be infected<br>May be used with caution during suspected primary HIV infection or in exposed infants |
| Disadvantages | May cause confusion regarding infant exposure and infection status when performed prior to 12 mo<br>Result will be negative during primary acute maternal HIV infection; see text | Long turnaround time | Send-out laboratory assay<br>False-positive results reported | Because of the possibility of false-positive reading of low copy numbers, not currently recommended for diagnosis of HIV-1 infection; this situation may change |

*Expert consultation is always recommended.

ELISA, enzyme linked immunosorbent assay; HIV-1, human immunodeficiency virus type 1; PBMC, peripheral blood mononuclear cell; PCR, polymerase chain reaction.

**TABLE 36-6**

**Commonly Used Terms Describing HIV Infection Status and Their Interpretation in Non–Breast-feeding Infants**

| Common-Usage Term | Usual meaning | Technical Meaning | Meaning in Infants Younger than 1 Yr | Source of Confusion |
|---|---|---|---|---|
| HIV-positive | Infected with HIV | Individual has anti-HIV antibodies in blood or other body fluids | Infant has been exposed to HIV during gestation and may or may not be infected with HIV | All infants of HI-infected mothers test "positive" for HIV antibodies until 12-18 months of age, regardless of whether they are infected or uninfected |
| HIV-negative | (1) not infected with HIV or (2) in acutely infected individual, seroconversion has not yet occurred | Individual does not have detectable HIV antibody | Infant is not infected with HIV: either was not exposed to HIV during gestation or was exposed to HIV and has already cleared maternal antibody | Even though viral tests give earlier, reliable assessment of infant's infection status, absence or loss of HIV antibody remains the "gold standard" for proof of uninfected status of perinatally exposed infants |
| HIV-DNA PCR–negative | Individual or infant older than 1 month is not infected with HIV | On highly sensitive testing for intracellular viral genome, no HIV DNA can be detected | If infant is older than 1 month, result suggests infant is not infected<br>A negative result at birth suggests that an exposed infant was not infected early, i.e., before the peripartum period. | Two thirds of infected infants are infected during the peripartum period and test DNA-PCR negative at birth Follow-up testing is required. |
| HIV-DNA PCR–positive | Individual is infected with HIV | HIV-DNA that has been integrated into the host's cellular DNA is detected | Detection before infant is 48 hours old suggests early transmission, before the peripartum period. With detection after this age, timing of transmission is indeterminate* | |
| HIV-RNA PCR undetectable | HIV viral replication is not detectable<br>Not usually used for diagnostic testing, but rather to monitor efficacy of treatment | | | |

*Identification of "late" i.e., breast milk, transmission of HIV, requires negative HIV-DNA PCR testing after 1 month of age followed by positive HIV DNA PCR result, or documentation of HIV antibody negativity followed by seroconversion.

to medications and noninfectious dermatoses to bacterial, viral, or fungal infections.

*P. carinii* pneumonia (PCP) is the most common AIDS-defining illness in children. It manifests in more than a third of infected infants, usually between 3 and 6 months of age (Simonds et al, 1993). It may be associated with other generalized signs of immunosuppression, such as failure to thrive and candidiasis. Short of demonstration of parasites in tissue or bronchiolar lavage specimens, PCP is difficult to diagnose. Tachypnea, hypoxia, and low-grade fever are common, but chest radiographs are often nondiagnostic, especially early in the illness (Simonds et al, 1993). Once infants require intubation, mortality approaches 90%, although it is considerably reduced with the use of antibiotics and corticosteroids (McGlaughlin et al, 1995). Even so, without antiretroviral therapy, median survival for infants who survive is only 19 months.

*Candida* esophagitis and oral candidiasis are common in pediatric AIDS. Other fungal infections are associated with profound immunodeficiency. Many AIDS-defining opportunistic infectious seen in adults are less common in children, although asymptomatic shedding of cytomegalovirus has been described (Kovacs et al, 1999).

Disorders of hematopoiesis are found in almost all pediatric AIDS patients. As disease progresses, the $CD4^+$ T-cell population decreases, followed by depletion of $CD8^+$ lymphocytes. Anemia, neutropenia, and thrombocytopenia occur regularly and result from both HIV and antiretroviral-induced bone marrow failure. Peripheral destruction of platelets may also contribute to thrombocytopenia.

Neurologic and developmental manifestations of pediatric AIDS are commonly seen by 2 years of age and are encountered in one of five perinatally infected children (Cooper et al, 1998). Progression of neurologic disease may be indolent or rapid and is generally thought to be secondary to viral replication and abnormal production of central nervous system cytokines rather than opportunistic infection.

Cardiac and pulmonary complications of HIV infection have been described. Cardiomyopathy with decreased cardiac output may be the result of myocardial infection by HIV or other organisms or the result of HIV-associated immune dysregulation (Shearer et al, 2000). Cardiac dysfunction caused by in utero antiretroviral exposure has not been demonstrated. Lymphoid interstitial pneumonitis affects young children, is associated with slow disease progression, and may result in chronic oxygen dependency.

Gastrointestinal, renal and malignant complications of HIV disease have been well described. Gastrointestinal illness can be due to enteric infections or to malabsorption syndromes. Hepatitis due to infection or medications is common and also contributes to growth failure (Khoury and Kovacs, 2001). In the pre-antiretroviral era, renal disease was found in 10% of infected children but was generally asymptomatic (Strauss et al, 1989). Cancer has become a very unusual presentation of pediatric HIV disease. By the late 1990s, national surveys reported less than 2% of infected children with AIDS-associated malignancy. Kaposi sarcoma, commonly seen in men with advanced HIV disease, has been reported only rarely in children (Granovsky et al, 1998).

### HIV Testing Beyond the Neonatal Period

Many caregivers are reluctant to consider AIDS in the differential diagnosis of ill children who are believed to be at low risk for HIV-1 infection. In the setting of recurrent pneumonia, nonspecific pulmonary problems, hepatosplenomegaly, or lymphadenopathy, to mention only a few manifestations of HIV disease in the neonatal period, AIDS must be ruled out. If the mother was screened during pregnancy, the possibility exists that she could have become infected after the test. Primary maternal infection is associated with negative serologic results during the so-called window period—placing the infant in double jeopardy: He or she will test negative on standard HIV-1 antibody screens and will be exposed to extremely high viral titers without the benefit of protection from antiretroviral drugs. In such cases, which have already been reported (Van Tine et al, 1999), diagnosis cannot be made without the assistance of PCR testing for viral genome (see Table 36–5).

## PREVENTION OF MOTHER-TO-CHILD TRANSMISSION

### Counseling and Care of HIV-Affected Families

HIV care services for women of reproductive age often neglect reproductive health. Reproductive choice and reproductive counseling must be nondirective, educational, and supportive. HIV-infected women must have access to the full range of reproductive health services, including family planning, contraception, abortion, and pregnancy care. Caregivers must inquire about a patient's long-term and short-term reproductive plans, provide access to reliable contraceptive and safer sex methods, and tailor antiretroviral therapy appropriately. For example, women who report that they might like to become pregnant should not be started on efavirenz, despite its convenience as a once-daily pill.

### Preconceptional and Prenatal Counseling by Pediatricians

Given the important implications for general family health, pediatricians may be asked to provide counseling to women or couples who are anticipating pregnancy or are already pregnant. Although there is no set formula for such counseling, it must be based on several fundamental issues. First, the right to found a family is a fundamental human right that has been articulated in international law. Second, with treatment, prospective HIV-infected parents in the developed world are likely to live out their natural lives and can expect to raise their children to adulthood. Third, with treatment, HIV-infected women are highly unlikely to transmit the virus to their babies. The odds that their baby will be born uninfected are greater than 98%.

By the same token, prospective parents need to know what they and their infants will experience because of their exposure to HIV. During pregnancy, women will be closely monitored and they will be offered aggressive treatment aimed at maximizing control of viral replication around the time of delivery. Concerns about the teratogenicity of antiretrovirals should be addressed (see earlier discussion). Parents should be aware that their perinatally exposed infant will receive antiretroviral prophylaxis as well as multiple venipuncture for blood sampling for the assessment of transmission status during the first year of life (see Table 36–2). They must also understand that the virus can be transmitted to the infant by breast milk and that formula feeding is therefore highly recommended. Finally, infected individuals must understand that although available therapies are effective, lifesaving, and improving, there is still no cure for the infection.

## Planning for Delivery and the Neonatal Period

### Maternal Adherence to Therapy

Maternal HIV plasma viremia is the most important predictor of perinatal transmission of HIV-1. Late pregnancy care is focused on maintaining control of maternal viremia or achieving the best control possible. Most data from the current era of highly active antiretroviral therapy suggest that use of antiretrovirals, and not necessarily route of delivery, is the most important determinant of HIV-1 perinatal transmission rates.

### Route of Delivery

Many factors determine the route of delivery in the setting of maternal HIV-1 infection. The first and most important is informed maternal choice. Women should be aware that elective cesarean section before rupture of membranes and before onset of labor has been shown in two retrospective (Mandelbrot et al, 1998; The mode of delivery, 1999) and one prospective study (Elective caesarean-section, 1999) to be associated with lower risk of transmission when mothers received either no antiretrovirals at all or zidovudine prophylaxis alone. Both CDC practice guidelines (CDC, 2003) and the American College of Obstetricians and Gynecologists state that scheduled cesarean section at 38 weeks of gestation should be recommended or offered to all HIV-infected women. Both groups acknowledge that data are insufficient to demonstrate benefit of elective abdominal delivery when maternal viral loads are lower than 1000 copies/mL or when rupture of membranes or labor has already occurred. These recommendations are based on studies performed before the current era of potent antiretroviral therapy; all participants of those studies received either no antiretrovirals or zidovudine alone during pregnancy.

In fact, lower transmission rates with elective cesarean section have not been demonstrated when mothers are taking potent combination antiretroviral therapy, regardless of maternal viral load. PACTG Study 316 reported on 1248 mother-baby pairs (Dorenbaum et al, 2002). Seventy-seven percent of them received combinations of two or more antiretrovirals, and 41% received protease inhibitor–based triple combinations; viral load at delivery was available for 95% of mothers. Only 34% delivered by elective cesarean section. The overall HIV transmission rate was 1.5%. Univariate analysis found that the risk for transmission was significantly higher for women with low CD4 T-cell counts and higher viral loads but did not differ significantly with route of delivery. Multivariate analysis revealed that the only significant predictor of transmission was maternal viral load at delivery. Significantly, 56% of the 18 infected infants had positive HIV DNA PCR results at birth, suggesting that the majority of transmissions occurred before the peripartum period and could not have been prevented by interventions at delivery such as elective cesarean section.

Several studies have shown a small but significant risk of respiratory complications among infants delivered electively by cesarean at term (Krantz et al, 1986), and any woman is at increased risk of bleeding and infection when delivered abdominally.

Our understanding of the mechanisms of the vertical transmission of HIV is incomplete. Elective abdominal delivery, performed according to a woman's choice, remains a reasonable alternative in the setting of HIV disease. An infected woman should be counseled, however, that if she is taking combination therapy, vaginal delivery may be as safe as cesarean section for her baby, particularly if her viral load is less than 10,000 copies/mL (Dorenbaum et al, 2002). Even at higher viral loads, the highest risk of transmission in PACTG Study 316 was 7%. Furthermore, elective cesarean delivery will not decrease the risk of transmission for babies infected before the peripartum period or if membranes rupture or labor occurs before the scheduled delivery date. Women must understand that combination therapy offers highly significant protection to the fetus throughout pregnancy, whenever and however it is born.

### Intrapartum Prophylaxis

Intrapartum prophylaxis, which has been standard for almost 10 years, is summarized in Table 36–7. Zidovudine should not be administered during labor if the patient is allergic to the medication. If a woman is doing well on a stavudine-based regimen, either she should not be given intravenous zidovudine or the stavudine should be stopped before the zidovudine infusion is initiated. Stavudine and zidovudine should not be administered together because they are mutually antagonistic (Havlir et al, 2000). In the setting of documented laboratory and clinical signs of high-level maternal resistance to zidovudine, many workers in the field find it pointless to initiate a maternal zidovudine infusion before delivery. Others believe that the infusion should still be given because the benefits of zidovudine are not completely understood. Expert consultation and patient education and choice, along with a plan clearly formulated before delivery, are extremely important.

### The Postpartum-Neonatal Period

Neonatal caregivers are in a key position to teach and reinforce the principle that in order to take care of their babies, women must also take care of themselves. The postpartum period is a time of challenges to adherence to therapy. Daily schedules are disrupted by irregular infant feeding and sleeping patterns. Many women shift their focus from their own therapy and health to their baby's health needs for general care, HIV prophylaxis, and testing. Attention to their own health, and especially to their own therapy, is likely to decrease substantially. These challenges can be met by prenatal planning for adequate support systems for both baby and mother. Coordination of infant prophylaxis and maternal dosing schedules by pediatric and maternal health care teams greatly facilitates adherence to both interventions and

**TABLE 36–7**

**Public Health Service Guidelines for Intrapartum, Neonatal Antiretroviral and Opportunistic Infection Prophylaxis for Perinatally HIV-1 Exposed Infants***

| Age | Dosage | Adjustment(s) |
|---|---|---|
| Intrapartum, given to mother (see text) | Zidovudine, 2 mg/kg intravenous loading dose, followed by zidovudine, 1 mg/kg continuous infusion | Discontinue when cord is clamped |
| 0-6 weeks, gestational age 35 weeks or greater at birth | Zidovudine, 2 mg/kg PO or IV q6 h | Per infant weight gain |
| 0-2 weeks, gestational age 30-35 weeks at birth | Zidovudine, 1.5 mg/kg IV q12 h or 2.0 mg/kg PO q12 h | Decrease dosing interval to q8 h at 2 weeks of age |
| 0-4 weeks, gestational age less than 30 weeks at birth | Zidovudine, 1.5 mg/kg IV q12 h or 2.0 mg/kg PO q12 h | Decrease dosing interval to q8 h at 2 weeks of age |
| 6 weeks to 1 year or until HIV infection is fully excluded | Trimethoprim-sulfamethoxazole, 150–750 mg/m²/day in 2 divided doses | Per infant's growth |

*Data from the Centers for Disease Control and Prevention (2003), and Khoury and Kovacs (2001).

should always be a part of obstetric-neonatal discharge planning.

### Neonatal Antiretroviral Prophylaxis

Antiretroviral and opportunistic infection prophylaxis guidelines for HIV-exposed neonates have been in place since 1994 (Connor et al, 1994), are summarized in Table 36–7, and are available as a living document on the Internet (CDC, 2003).

No guidelines exist for prophylaxis of infants in the setting of documented high-level clinical and laboratory maternal resistance to zidovudine, particularly that involving codon 215. Practice in this area is inconsistent and controversial. Planning for neonatal prophylaxis must begin during pregnancy and should be coordinated with those who will be caring for the baby. Consultation with pediatric virologists with experience in the use of non–zidovudine-containing regimens in infants is highly recommended. Parents must be counseled about the risks and benefits of alternative prophylaxis strategies for their infants and must be included in the decision-making process.

### Neonatal Prophylaxis Against Opportunistic Infection

Before the current era of antiretroviral prophylaxis, when 25% of HIV-exposed newborns were themselves infected, PCP was a common opportunistic infection during the first year of life and carried exceptionally high mortality (see earlier discussion). Even though perinatal HIV transmission has decreased markedly, recommendations for opportunistic infection prophylaxis in infants of indeterminate infection status remain in place (CDC, 2001b, 2003) Many parents question the necessity of opportunistic infection prophylaxis after they have been told their infants are not infected with HIV, and some authorities have suggested that prophylaxis may be terminated once HIV infection is fully excluded (CDC, 2003).

## Infant Feeding and HIV Transmission

Transmission of HIV-1 in breast milk has been well documented and occurs in 14% to 16% of exposed infants who were not infected perinatally. In resource-rich regions, feeding with breast milk substitutes has been a straightforward and acceptable method of eliminating such transmission. In the developing world, the risks and benefits of this intervention are very complex. In Thailand and certain sections of Nairobi, Kenya, where sanitary water supplies are available, breast milk substitutes have proved both safe and beneficial for mother and baby (Nduati et al, 2000a, 200b). Results of other studies have been less straightforward. Variables such as the extent of mixed feeding as well as availability of both clean water supplies and supplies of breast milk substitutes profoundly affect the risks and benefits of bottle-feeding HIV-exposed infants in the developing world.

Interestingly, viral load in breast milk is generally low (Sabbaj et al, 2002), and Aldrovandi (2003) reported viral load to be undetectable in the milk of five women who were taking potent combination therapy. The impact of combination therapy on breast milk transmission in the developing world is completely unknown. As with all other issues, planning for infant feeding and suppression of lactation are best dealt with long before the baby is born.

### Site-of-Care Issues for Mother and Baby

Every community has its own resources and limitations. Care can be provided for HIV-affected families in many different ways and by several different specialties and health care teams from different backgrounds. However, it is clear that pregnant women and women with children can attend only so many visits to so many clinics in the space of a week. It is also clear that women, even those with life-threatening illnesses, will neglect their own health in order to care for their children. For this reason, multidisciplinary clinics have been very successful in a variety of settings. A woman is far more likely to attend her own medical appointments when they occur in conjunction with care of her children. In some areas, the challenges to such "one-stop" family-centered programs may be insurmountable; in others, such programs can be put in place simply by manipulating caregivers' schedules.

The Bay Area Perinatal AIDS Center at San Francisco General Hospital has provided family-centered HIV care since 1989. Currently, care at the center is coordinated by a family nurse practitioner. This professional and an obstetrical/infectious disease specialist give prenatal and HIV care in consultation with primary HIV caregivers and neonatologists. Antepartum admission orders, postpartum orders, and nursery admission orders are all discussed and prepared in advance of the delivery admission. Neonatal, postpartum, and ongoing family care are given by the family nurse practitioner and family medicine faculty with a strong interest in HIV care.

## EVALUATION OF TRANSMISSION STATUS OF HIV-1–EXPOSED INFANTS

Careful follow-up and months of testing are required to evaluate the transmission of infants exposed to HIV (see Table 36–6). We generally accept that negative results of two viral tests, at least one of which has been performed after 1 month of age, are highly suggestive that an infant is not infected. Even so, authorities stress the importance of ongoing evaluation and care of exposed infants so that sero-reversion to "HIV-negative" status can be documented between 1 and 2 years of age. Parents should be counseled about the availability of national and international studies of children who have been HIV and referred to appropriate centers for participation.

Table 36–5 summarizes available HIV diagnostic tests and their meaning in the setting of perinatal exposure to HIV-1. Of greatest importance here is that HIV antibody status before a baby is 1 year old reflects the mother's infection status and the baby's own exposure status, but does not reflect the baby's infection status.

## CONCLUSION

Pediatric HIV infection has become a disease of the developing world, where more than 90% of HIV-exposed and more than 98% of HIV-infected children live (Fig. 36–5). Without therapy, morbidity and mortality are high for all infected individuals and are worse for children. Even exposed uninfected children face the virtual certainty of becoming orphans by their tenth birthdays and a 50% chance of some day becoming infected themselves. By 2010, the epidemic will have produced 44 million orphans.

Solutions to this crisis exist. HIV transmission, whether sexual, vertical, or parenteral, is virtually 100% preventable. Progression to AIDS and death is also preventable. The United States and rest of the developed world have not always been immune to devastation, and in the early 1990s, both a pediatric HIV epidemic and an AIDS orphan crisis loomed very large in a number of wealthy countries. Although the potential to arrest all HIV transmission remains a goal unfulfilled, potent antiretroviral combination therapy has not only reversed AIDS mortality trends (see Fig. 36–4A) but has virtually eliminated mother-to-child transmission of the virus in the United States (see Fig. 36–4B). The current challenge in this country is to miss no opportunity to treat disease and prevent transmission. Already, our tolerance for vertical transmission events has come close to zero.

Our attitudes must be no different regarding the epidemic in the developing world. Given global resources today, the death of a mother from AIDS is just as much a preventable tragedy in any other country as it is in our own. Similarly, the infection of a single baby represents our global failure to protect the world's children, whether that child was born in affluence to a U.S. woman who never suspected her own HIV infection or to a mother in the developing world with no access to testing or therapy.

Prevention of pediatric HIV infection is not easy but it is entirely possible. It requires universal screening, aggressive approaches to the management of maternal infection, and careful coordination of disparate services with a clear goal of family-centered care. With adequate newborn screening and follow-up, even the rarely infected neonate should never be allowed to progress to full blown AIDS.

Advocacy for those whose lives have been most devastated by the HIV/AIDS pandemic is not just a fundamental part of good global citizenship and humanitarian compassion. It is also a critical element of preserving the health of our own families and societies. We are now at the beginning of the third decade of HIV/AIDS, and we have long understood that the infection knows no social, economic, or geographic barriers. If global transmission remains unchecked and the global standard of treatment continues to consist of either no therapy or suboptimal therapy, the ensuing crisis in transmission and loss of antiretroviral efficacy will not stop at our collective door.

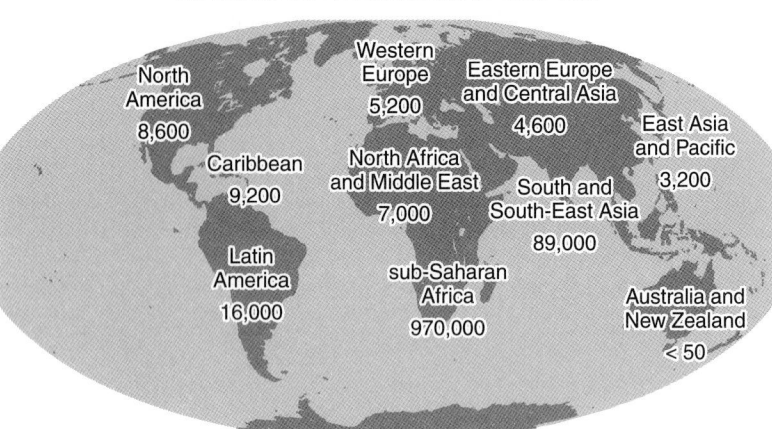

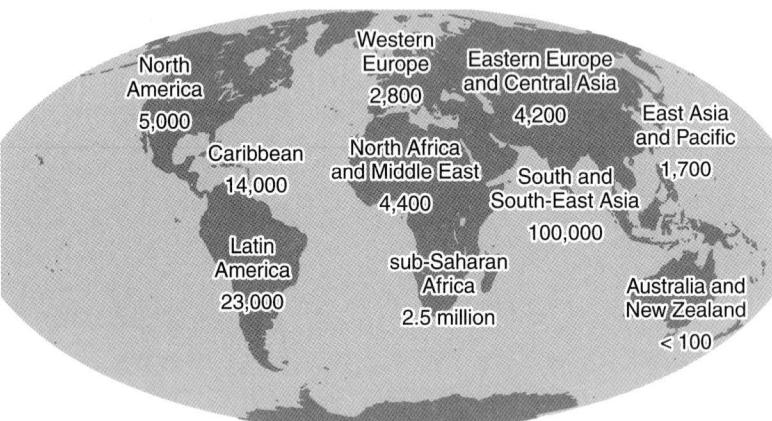


**FIGURE 36–5.** Global prevalence of pediatric HIV/AIDS. **A,** Children younger than 15 years estimated to be living with HIV/AIDS, 1997. **B,** Estimated child deaths due to HIV/AIDS from the beginning of the epidemic to the end of 1997.

## REFERENCES

AIDS Epidemic Update. UNAIDS and the World Health Organization; www.unaids.org, 2003, NY.

Aldrovandi G: 2003.

Beckerman KP: Principles of management of HIV disease during pregnancy. Topics in HIV Medicine, Vol 8, 2000.

Blanche S, Tardieu M, Rustin P, et al: Persistent mitochondrial dysfunction and perinatal exposure to antiretroviral nucleoside analogues. Lancet 354:1084-1989, 1999.

Brown AJL, Frost SDW, Mathews WC, et al: Transmission fitness of drug-resistant human immunodeficiency virus and the prevalence of resistance in the antiretroviral-treated population. J Infect Dis 187:683-686, 2003.

Centers for Disease Control and Prevention: HIV/AIDS Surveillance Report 13:1-44, 2001a.

Centers for Disease Control and Prevention: 2001 USPHS/IDSA Guidelines for the Prevention of Opportunistic Infections in Persons Infected with the Human Immunodeficiency Virus. Washington, DC, National Institutes of Health, 2001b.

Centers for Disease Control and Prevention: Public Health Service task force recommendations for the use of antiretroviral drugs in pregnant HIV–infected women for maternal health and interventions to reduce perinatal HIV-1 transmission in the United States. National Institutes of Health; 2003. Available on line at http://www.AIDSinfo.nih.gov/guidelines/perinatal/

Clarke JR, Braganza R, Mirza A, et al: Rapid development of genotypic resistance to lamivudine when combined with zidovudine in pregnancy. J Med Virol 59:364-368, 1999.

Coffin JM: HIV population dynamics in vivo: Implications for genetic variation, pathogenesis, and therapy. Science 267: 483-489, 1995.

Committee APRS: Antiretroviral Pregnancy Registry International Interim Report for 1 January 1989-31 January 2003. Washington, DC, PharmaResearch Corporation, 2003.

Connor EM, Sperling RS, Gelber R, et al: Reduction of maternal-infant transmission of human immunodeficiency virus type 1 with zidovudine treatment. New Engl J Med 331:1173-1180, 1994.

Considerations for Antiretroviral Therapy in Women. Washington, DC, United States Public Health Service, 2002.

Cooper ER, Hanson C, Diaz C, et al: Encephalopathy and progression of human immunodeficiency virus disease in a cohort of children with perinatally acquired human immunodeficiency virus infection. Women and Infants Transmission Study Group. J Pediatr 132:808-812, 1998.

Dorenbaum A, Cunningham CK, Gelber RD et al: Two-dose intrapartum/newborn nevirapine and standard antiretroviral therapy to reduce perinatal HIV transmission. JAMA 288:190-198. 2002.

Eastman PS, Shapiro DE, Coombs RW, et al: Maternal viral genotypic zidovudine resistance and infrequent failure of zidovudine therapy to prevent perinatal transmission of human immunodeficiency virus type 1 in Pediatric AIDS Clinical Trials Group Protocol 076. J Infect Dis 177:557-564, 1998.

Elective caesarean-section versus vaginal delivery in prevention of vertical HIV-1 transmission: A randomised clinical trial. European Mode of Delivery Collaboration. Lancet 353:1035-1039, 1999.

Embretson J, Zupancic M, Ribas J, et al: Massive covert infection of helper T lymphocytes and macrophages by HIV during the incubation period of AIDS. Nature 362:359-362, 1993.

Garcia PM, Kalish LA, Pitt J, et al: Maternal levels of plasma human immunodeficiency virus type 1 RNA and the risk of perinatal transmission. New Engl J Med 1999;341:394-402.

Granovsky MO, Mueller BU, Nicholson HS, et al: Cancer in human immunodeficiency virus-infected children: A case series from the Children's Cancer Group and the National Cancer Institute. J Clin Oncol 16:1729-1735, 1998.

Guidelines for the Use of Antiretroviral Agents in HIV-Infected Adults and adolescents. Washington, DC, United States Public Health Service, 2002.

Guidelines for the use of antiretroviral agents in pediatric HIV infection. Washington, DC, Centers for Disease Control and Prevention, 2003.

Havlir DV, Tierney C, Friedland GH, et al: In vivo antagonism with zidovudine plus stavudine combination therapy. J Infect Dis 182:321-325, 2000.

Ioannidis JP, Abrams EJ, Ammann A, et al: Perinatal transmission of human immunodeficiency virus type 1 by pregnant women with RNA virus loads <1000 copies/ml. J Infect Dis 183:539-545, 2000.

Karon JM, Fleming PL, Steketee RW, De Cock KM: HIV in the United States at the turn of the century: An epidemic in transition. Am J Public Health 91:1060-1068, 2001.

Khoury M, Kovacs A: Pediatric HIV infection. Clin Obstet Gynecol 44:243-275, 2001.

Kovacs A, Schluchter M, Easley K, et al: Cytomegalovirus infection and HIV-1 disease progression in infants born to HIV-1-infectedwomen. Pediatric Pulmonary and Cardiovascular Complications of Vertically Transmitted HIV Infection Study Group. New Engl J Med 341:77-84, 1999.

Krantz ME, Wennergren LG, Bengston LGW: Epidemiological analysis of the increased risk of disturbed neonatal respiratory adaptation after caesarean section. Acta Paediatr Scand 75: 832-839, 1986.

Krogstad P, Wiznia A, Luzariaga K, et al: Treatment of human immunodeficiency virus 1-infected infants and children with the protease inhibitor nelfinavir mesylate. Clin Infect Dis 28:1109-1118, 1999.

Lawn SD, Butera ST, Folks TM: Contribution of immune activation to the pathogenesis and transmission of human immunodeficiency virus type 1 infection. Clin Microbiol Rev 14:753-777, 2001

Little SJ, Holte S, Routy J-P, et al: Antiretroviral-drug resistance among patients recently infected with HIV. New Engl J Med 347:385-394, 2002.

Lorenzi P, Spicher VM, Laubereau B, et al: Antiretroviral therapies in pregnancy: Maternal, fetal and neonatal effects. AIDS 12:F241-F247, 1998.

Luzariaga K, Bryson YJ, Krogstad P, et al: Combination treatment with zidovudine, didanosine, and nevirapine in infants with human immunodeficiency virus type 1 infection. New Engl J Med.335:1343-1349, 1997

MacIntosh K: Mitochondrial toxicity of perinatally administered zidovudine. Presented at the 7th Conference on Retroviruses and Opportunistic Infections, San Francisco, 2000, p 21.

Mandelbrot L, Le Chenadec J, Berrebi A, et al: Perinatal HIV-1 transmission: Interaction between zidovudine prophylaxis and mode of delivery in the French Perinatal Cohort. JAMA 280:55-60, 1998.

Masquelier B, Lemoigne E, Pellegrin I, et al: Primary infection with zidovudine-resistant HIV. New Engl J Med 329:1123-1124, 1993.

McDermott JM, Slutsker L, Steketee RW, et al: Prospective assessment of mortality among a cohort of pregnant women in rural Malawi. Am J Trop Med Hyg 55:66-70, 1996.

McGlaughlin GE, Virdee SS, Schleien CL, et al: Effect of corticosteroids on survival of children with acquired immunodeficiency syndrome and *Pneumocystis carinii*-related respiratory failure. J Pediatr 126:821-824, 1995.

Mofenson LM: Mother-child HIV-1 transmission: Timing and determinants. Obstet Gynecol Clin North Am 24:759-784, 1997.

Mofenson LM, Lambert JS, Stiehm ER, et al: Risk factors for perinatal transmission of human immunodeficiency virus type 1 in women treated with zidovudine. New Engl J Med 341: 385-393, 1999.

Nduati R, John G, Mbori-Ngacha D, et al: Effect of breastfeeding and formula feeding on transmission of HIV-1: A randomized clinical trial. JAMA 283:1167-1174, 2000a.

Pantaleo G, Graziosi C, Demarest J, et al: HIV infection is active and progressive in lymphoid tissue during the clinically latent stage of the disease. Nature 362:355-358, 1993a.

Pantaleo G, Graziosi C, Fauci AS: New concepts in the immunopathogenesis of human immunodeficiency virus infection. New Engl J Med 328:327-335, 1993b.

Perelson AS, Neumann A, Markowitz M, et al: HIV-1 dynamics in vivo: Virion clearance rate, infected cell life-span, and viral generation time. Science 271:1582-1586, 1996.

Pollack H, Glasberg H, Lee E, et al: Impaired early growth of infants perinatally infected with human immunodeficiency virus: Correlation with viral load. J Pediatr.130:915-922, 1997.

Rousseau CM, Nduati RW, Richardson BA, et al: Longitudinal analysis of human immunodeficiency virus type 1 RNA in breast milk and of its relationship to infant infection and maternal disease. J Infect Dis 187:741-747, 2003.

Royce RA, Sena A, Cates W, Cohen MS: Sexual Transmission of HIV. New Engl J Med 336:1072-1078, 1977.

Sabbaj S, Edwards BH, Ghosh MK, et al: Human immunodeficiency virus-specific CD8+ T cells in human breast milk. J Virol 76:7365-7373, 2002.

Shapiro D, Tuomala R, Samelson R, et al: Antepartum antiretroviral therapy and pregnancy outcomes in 462 HIV-infected women in 1998-1999 (PACTG 367) [abstract 664]. Presented at the 7th Conference on Retroviruses and Opportunistic Infections. San Francisco, 2000.

Shearer WT, Lipshultz SE, Easley KA, et al: Alterations in cardiac and pulmonary function in pediatric rapid human immunodeficiency virus type 1 disease progressors. Pediatric Pulmonary and Cardiovascular Complications of Vertically Transmitted Human Immunodeficiency Virus Study Group. Pediatrics 105: e9, 2000.

Shilts R: And the Band Played On: Politics, People, and the AIDS Epidemic. St. Martin's Press, NY, 2000.

Simonds RJ, Oxtoby MJ, Caldwell MB, et al:. *Pneumocystis carinii* pneumonia among U.S. children with perinatally acquired HIV infection. JAMA 270:470-473, 1993.

Spira AI, Marx PA, Patterson BK, et al: Cellular targets of infection and route of viral dissemination following an intravaginal inoculation of SIV into rhesus macaques. AIDS Res Hum Retroviruses 14, 1998.

Strauss J, Abitbol C, Zilleruelo G, et al: Renal disease in children with the acquired immunodeficiency syndrome. New Engl J Med 321:625-630, 1989.

The mode of delivery and the risk of vertical transmission of human immunodeficiency virus type 1. International Perinatal HIV Group. New Engl J Med 340:977-986, 1999.

Van Tine BA, Shaw GM, Aldrovandi G: Mother-to-infant transmission of the human immunodeficiency virus during primary infection. New Engl J Med 341:1548-1557, 1999.

Welles SL, Pitt J, Colgrove R, et al: HIV-1 genotypic zidovudine drug resistance and the risk of maternal-infant transmission in the women and infants transmission study. AIDS 14:263-271, 2000.

Yerly S, Kaiser L, Race E, et al: Transmission of antiretroviral-drug-resistant HIV-1 variants. Lancet. 354:729-733, 1999.

CHAPTER 37

# Viral Infections of the Fetus and Newborn

**Erica S. Pan, F. Sessions Cole, and Peggy Sue Weintrub**

Many viral infections are acquired in utero, or congenitally. Alternatively, numerous infections may also occur perinatally or postnatally, although it is often difficult to ascertain the time of acquisition. The clinical manifestations and long-term effects differ according to when the infection was acquired.

*Congenital infection* is defined here as infection transmitted any time during gestation excluding the last 5 to 7 days. The most common infections acquired in utero are those due to cytomegalovirus (CMV), rubella virus, *Toxoplasma gondii, Treponema pallidum*, human immunodeficiency virus (HIV), and human parvovirus B19 (Kinney and Kumar, 1988; Stamos and Rowley, 1994). The somewhat misnamed TORCH group, an acronym first used in 1971, signifies toxoplasmosis, rubella, cytomegalovirus, and herpes simplex virus, with the O standing for "other infections" (Nahmias et al, 1971). The confusion generated by this acronym arises because "H," or herpes simplex, rarely belongs to the group and because syphilis and many other significant infections are omitted from it (Stamos and Rowley, 1994). For many years, numerous hospitals offered a panel of serologic tests for these four organisms, a practice that led to uncertainty about the significance of each test and an oversimplification of the approach to diagnosis. These congenital infections have clinical features in common, but they are distinguishable, and the differential diagnosis of congenital infection should not be limited to these four organisms alone (Cullen et al, 1998; Kinney and Kumar, 1988). HIV is covered in Chapter 36.

Clinical findings for congenital viral infections are listed in Table 37–1. The most common manifestations are hepatomegaly, splenomegaly, pneumonia, bone lesions, and cytopenias. The most significant congenital viral infections (excluding HIV) are CMV, rubella, parvovirus B19, and, less commonly, herpes simplex virus (HSV) and varicella.

Some viruses may rarely cause intrauterine infection but are more commonly transmitted just before or during delivery; this pattern is characteristic of herpes simplex virus, varicella, hepatitis B and C viruses, and others. Viruses such as enterovirus and hepatitis A can also be acquired in the perinatal period. Other viruses of importance that are more commonly transmitted postnatally, and sometimes nosocomially, are respiratory viruses, rotavirus, and, occasionally, hepatitis A. Figure 37–1 summarizes significant viruses and the relative distribution of intrauterine, perinatal, and postnatal infections.

## DIAGNOSTIC APPROACH

The incidence of congenital infection in the fetus and newborn infant is high (0.5% to 2.5%) (Alpert and Plotkin, 1986), and a significant number of congenitally infected infants are asymptomatic. Evaluation begins with a complete family and maternal history, including information on birth weights and medical problems of siblings, maternal illness during pregnancy, drug use, sexual orientation and medical history of sexual partners, and information about the mother's travels, country of origin, and blood transfusions.

Common clinical features associated with specific congenital infections in the neonate are listed in Table 37–2. Whether children born with a single finding—for example, birth weight less than the third percentile for gestational age without other signs—should be evaluated is unclear. Studies from Sweden and Canada suggest that isolated growth retardation is not associated with congenital infection (Andreasson et al, 1981; Primhak and Simpson, 1982). However, growth retardation has been described as the only manifestation of congenital infection with CMV, rubella, and toxoplasmosis (Alpert and Plotkin, 1986).

## CYTOMEGALOVIRUS

Cytomegalovirus (CMV) is a member of the herpes virus family and has the largest DNA genome of any known virus (Adler, 1986b). CMV infection at any age is usually asymptomatic. After a period of active replication, the virus usually becomes latent but retains the capability of reactivation under special circumstances. Such reactivation occurs commonly during pregnancy. A primary infection or reactivation during pregnancy can lead to congenital infection of the fetus. CMV is now the most common congenital viral infection in developed countries, overtaking rubella since the introduction of rubella immunizations (Demmler, 1991). Perinatal or postnatal infection is also common but rarely results in symptomatic infection.

### Incidence

In developed countries, CMV seroprevalence rates range widely from 50% to 90% among adult women (Mustakangas et al, 2000; Wong et al, 2000). Older age, lower socioeconomic and educational status, and non-white ethnicity are all associated with higher rates of detectable CMV antibody (Demmler, 1991; Mustakangas et al, 2000; Nelson and Demmler, 1997). The incidence of viral excretion in the cervix or urine appears to rise during pregnancy from approximately 3% in the first trimester to as much as 25% to 50% at term (Montgomery et al, 1972). Estimated seroconversion rates during pregnancy range from 0.7% to 4.1% (Stagno et al, 1984).

Approximately 40,000 infants are born with congenital CMV infection annually in the United States (Griffiths, 1993; Stagno and Whitley, 1985a). This infection rate

**TABLE 37–1**

**Clinical Features Commonly Associated with Congenital Viral Infections in Neonates**

Growth restriction
Hepatosplenomegaly
Jaundice (>20% direct-reacting bilirubin)
Hemolytic anemia
Petechiae and ecchymoses
Microcephaly and hydrocephaly
Intracranial calcification
Pneumonitis
Myocarditis
Cardiac abnormalities (especially peripheral pulmonic stenosis [rubella])
Chorioretinitis
Keratoconjunctivitis
Cataracts
Glaucoma
Nonimmune hydrops

Data from Kinney JS, Kumar ML: Should we expand the TORCH complex? A description of clinical and diagnostic aspects of selected old and new agents. Clin Perinatol 15:727-744, 1988.

**TABLE 37–2**

**Clinical Findings in Congenitally Infected Infants that Suggest a Specific Diagnosis**

| Congenital Infection | Findings |
|---|---|
| Rubella | Eye: cataracts, cloudy cornea, pigmented retina |
| | Skin: "blueberry muffin" syndrome |
| | Bone: vertical striation |
| | Heart: malformation (ductus, pulmonary artery stenosis) |
| Cytomegalovirus | Microcephaly with periventricular calcifications |
| | Petechiae with thrombocytopenia |
| | Jaundice |
| | Hearing loss |
| | Inguinal hernias in boys |
| Toxoplasmosis | Hydrocephalus with generalized calcifications |
| | Chorioretinitis |
| Syphilis | Osteochondritis and periostitis |
| | Eczematoid rash |
| | Mucocutaneous lesions (snuffles) |
| Herpes | Skin vesicles |
| | Keratoconjunctivitis |
| | Acute central nervous system findings |
| Varicella | Limb hypoplasia |
| | Dermatomal scarring |
| | Gastrointestinal tract atresia |
| Lymphocytic choriomeningitis virus | Hydrocephaly |
| | Chorioretinitis |
| | Intracranial calcifications |

Data from Stagno S, Pass RF, Alford CA: Perinatal infections and maldevelopment. In Bloom D, James LS (eds): The Fetus and the Newborn, vol 17, series 1. New York, Alan R. Liss, 1981.

(approximately 1%) is greater than rates observed in England, Denmark, and Sweden (approximately 0.3%) and comparable with the rate in Africa (1.4%) (Peckham, 1991; Starr et al, 1970). Similarly, worldwide estimates range from 0.4% to 2.3% of all live births (Stagno et al, 1982a). It has been estimated that approximately 40% of primary maternal infections transmit CMV to the fetus compared with only 1% to 2% of reactivated infections (Demmler, 1991). Most evidence has shown that a primary maternal CMV infection is more likely than a recurrent infection to cause congenital infection (Stagno et al, 1982b), but later data suggest that symptomatic congenital infection in children of women with non-primary CMV infection may occur more often than previously appreciated (Boppana et al, 1999). Estimated rates of CMV susceptibility and transmission in pregnancy are given in Figure 37–2.

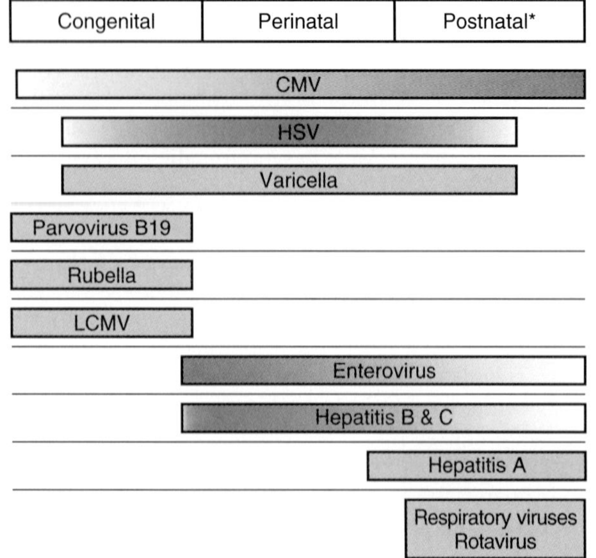


**FIGURE 37–1.** Routes of viral infections of the fetus and newborn. CMV, cytomegalovirus; HSV, herpes simplex virus; LCMV, lymphocytic choriomeningitis virus.

The incidence of *perinatal* (up to 1 month after birth) infection and *postnatal* (up to 12 months after birth) infection is still higher than that of intrauterine infection. Typically, the infant is exposed to virus shed from the cervix, excreted in breast milk, or, less commonly, shed from other infants infected with the virus. Approximately 50% of babies born to mothers excreting virus at term acquire infection in the first weeks of life (Reynolds et al, 1973). Many of these babies are infected through breast milk (Hayes et al, 1972). All infants, regardless of the route of infection, excrete virus for a prolonged period, usually for at least 1 year (Emanuel and Kenny, 1966). Although the incidence of perinatal and postnatal CMV infections is higher, these infants typically have asymptomatic or self-limited disease but do not have the neurologic sequelae seen in some congenitally infected infants (Demmler, 1991).

Nosocomial infant-to-infant transmission of CMV has been reported, but it occurs infrequently (Adler, 1986b; Spector, 1983; Yeager et al, 1972). Transfusion-related

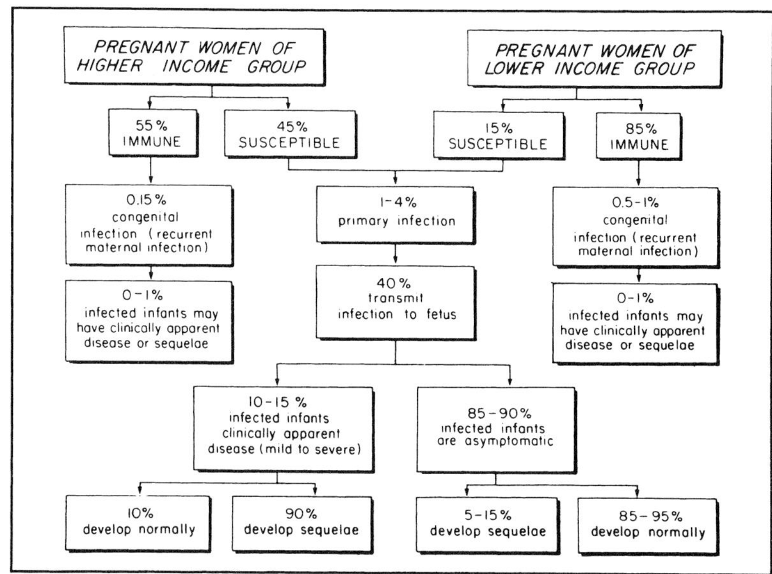


**FIGURE 37-2.** Characteristics of cytomegalovirus infection in pregnancy. *(From Stagno S, Whitley RT: Herpesvirus infections of pregnancy. Part I: Cytomegalovirus and Epstein-Barr virus infections. N Engl J Med 313:1270-1274, 1985.)*

infections were first reported in 1969, when infants in newborn intensive care units demonstrated a syndrome consisting of respiratory distress, hepatosplenomegaly, lymphocytosis, and a "septic appearance" (King-Lewis and Gardner, 1969; McCracken et al, 1969). In 1971, noting the connection between seropositive blood used for exchange transfusion and the acquisition of CMV by CMV-seronegative recipients, Luthardt and colleagues suggested that such infections could be prevented by selection of CMV-seronegative donors. Subsequent investigators observed that exclusive use of CMV-seronegative blood eliminated CMV infection in hospitalized seronegative infants (Adler, 1986a; Yeager et al, 1981). Between 3 and 12 CMV infections occur per 100 units of transfused blood, and in premature infants, seroconversion occurs in 10% of 30% of those transfused with CMV antibody–positive blood (Lamberson et al, 1988). Although the frequency of postnatal transfusion-acquired CMV has decreased with the use of leukodepletion and of CMV-seronegative donors, a high index of suspicion must be maintained when symptoms consistent with CMV infection occur in infants who have received multiple transfusions.

The prevalence of acquired CMV infection may be significantly increased in different populations by differences in prevalence of breast-feeding and child-rearing practices. In the United States, this effect may be greatest among infants born to women of higher socioeconomic status who send their children to daycare centers or are daycare center workers themselves (Stagno and Cloud, 1994). For CMV-seronegative women in the reproductive age range exposed to increasing numbers of CMV-seropositive children, the risk of primary infection rises.

### Maternal Exposures and History

Child care providers (including daycare workers, special education teachers, and therapists) appear to have a higher risk of occupational exposure to CMV from infants and young children, compared with other women of child-bearing age working with similar populations (CDC, 1985).

Health care workers using routine infection control practices are not at increased risk of CMV acquisition. Like most healthy individuals, more than 90% of pregnant women with primary CMV infections remain asymptomatic. When symptoms do occur, they are nonspecific and vague, often described as a "flu-like syndrome." Potential manifestations include fever, fatigue, headache, myalgia, lymphadenitis, and pharyngitis. Prenatal ultrasonography findings that would also raise concern for intrauterine CMV infection are oligohydramnios or polyhydramnios, nonimmune hydrops, fetal ascites, intrauterine growth restriction, microcephaly, cerebral ventriculomegaly or hydrocephalus, intracranial calcifications, pleural or pericardial effusion, hepatosplenomegaly, intrahepatic calcifications, echogenic bowel, and pseudomeconium ileus (Nelson and Demmler, 1997).

### Etiology and Pathogenesis

The fetus can be infected by either a primary maternal infection (Davis et al, 1971) or a reactivated maternal infection (Stagno et al, 1982b). A newborn infant without congenital infection can be infected perinatally by his or her mother at the time of delivery or postnatally through breast milk, by acquisition from the nursery or home environment, or by transfusion of blood from a donor.

CMV infection can occur throughout gestation, but there is a higher incidence of adverse fetal sequelae if primary maternal infection occurs during the first trimester. The virus is transmitted first to the placenta via infected leukocytes, then replicates within placental fibroblasts, syncytiotrophoblasts, and cytotrophoblast cells. From there the virus infects the fetus hematogenously via the umbilical cord (Trincado and Rawlinson, 2001). Once the fetus is infected, viral replication occurs primarily in the tubular epithelium of the kidneys (Scott et al, 1997). The virus is then excreted in fetal urine and subsequently in amniotic fluid. It is assumed that once infected amniotic fluid is ingested, the virus replicates further in the oropharynx, enters the fetal circulation, and hematogenously spreads to target organs (Lazzarotto et al, 1999b). The mechanism of hearing loss secondary to congenital CMV infection is not known.

Little is known about the effect of virulence factors in congenital CMV infections. Although all strains are serologically related, there appear to be some variations in antigenicity, and evidence is emerging that certain envelope glycoprotein B genotypes are predominant in congenital or perinatal infections (Bale et al, 2000; Lukacsi et al, 2001; Trincado et al, 2000). Newer evidence supports the theory that some women with pre-existing immunity who give birth to infants with symptomatic CMV infection may have a newly acquired strain rather than reactivated latent infection (Boppana et al, 2001).

### Clinical Spectrum

Prospective studies report that up to 90% of infants with congenital CMV infections are asymptomatic at birth and that milder manifestations of infections are more common than the classic syndrome.

In the classic form of congenital CMV infection, cytomegalic inclusion disease, newborn infants have acute progressive disseminated disease. They show petechiae and ecchymoses, and they are jaundiced at birth or jaundice appears within a few hours and becomes intense. The liver and spleen are enlarged and firm and may increase in size for a number of days. Fever, respiratory distress, or pallor may appear. Puncture wounds bleed for many minutes, and hemorrhage from internal organs may cause death. Infants infected with the virus are often born prematurely. Table 37–3 is a summary of the frequency of various clinical and laboratory findings in 285 infants in the National Congenital CMV Disease Registry (Istas et al, 1995). Petechiae, hepatosplenomegaly, and jaundice are the most common signs during the neonatal period. Although microcephaly was seen in only one third of the infants in the Registry at birth, a number of additional children may become microcephalic as they grow older. Nine percent (25 of 285) of infants in the Registry died of the CMV disease. Most fatalities occur before 3 months of age, primarily because of severe neurologic impairment.

Visual deficits, when present, are most commonly secondary to cortical visual impairment or sequelae of chorioretinitis such as optic atrophy or macular scars. One small prospective study of CMV-infected infants reported that approximately 20% of symptomatic patients had moderate to severe visual impairment, and approximately 30% had strabismus (Coats et al, 2000). Many other isolated defects have been reported in conjunction with congenital CMV infection, but because approximately 1% of all infants are infected, CMV may not always be the cause of abnormality.

A presumptive diagnosis may sometimes be made after the infant is several months of age if a virus is found and the clinical syndrome is classic. Other causes of congenital infection must be ruled out, because there is extensive overlap in the symptoms of several types of infections.

### Laboratory Evaluation

There is no universal standard regarding prenatal screening for CMV, and an optimal approach has not yet been delineated. Some countries administer routine prenatal screening for CMV, and various investigators are researching

**TABLE 37–3**

**Characteristics of the 285 Infants Enrolled in the National Congenital Cytomegalovirus Disease Registry (January 1, 1990, through December 31, 1993)**

| Characteristic | No. of Infants Affected | % of Infants Affected |
|---|---|---|
| Non-neurologic abnormalities: | | |
| Petechiae or purpura | 154 | 54 |
| Small for gestational age | 135 | 47 |
| Hepatosplenomegaly | 114 | 40 |
| Jaundice at birth | 108 | 38 |
| Pneumonia | 24 | 8 |
| Neurologic abnormalities: | | |
| One or more of the following abnormalities | 194 | 68 |
| Intracranial calcifications | 106 | 37 |
| Microcephaly | 104 | 36 |
| Unexplained abnormality | 78 | 27 |
| Hearing impairment | 70 | 25 |
| Chorioretinitis | 30 | 11 |
| Seizures | 30 | 11 |
| Neonatal death* | 25 | 9 |
| Laboratory findings: | | |
| Platelet count ≤75000/mm3 | 136 | 48 |
| Direct bilirubin level ≥3 mg/dL | 102 | 36 |
| Alanine aminotransferase level >100 U/L | 66 | 23 |
| Hemolytic anemia | 32 | 11 |

*Data not systematically collected.

Data from Istas AS, Demmler GH, Dobbins JG, Stewart JA: Surveillance for congenital cytomegalovirus disease: A report from the National Congenital Cytomegalovirus Disease Registry. Clin Infect Dis 20:665-670, 1995.

optimal protocols for testing and correlation with clinical outcomes. The use of immunoglobulin (Ig) M antibody testing in mothers and infants has been difficult to interpret, for several reasons. First, mothers with reactivation as well as primary infection may have positive CMV IgM. Second, IgM testing itself has wide variability in accuracy and reproducibility, although it has improved with enzyme immunoassay and immunoblot techniques (Trincado and Rawlinson, 2001). Third, it is estimated that only 10% of pregnant women in whom IgM is detected will transmit infection to their fetuses.

Some centers use the combination of anti-CMV IgM and IgG avidity results to screen pregnant women. Use of CMV-specific IgG avidity testing has proved to be helpful in discriminating between primary infection and recurrent infection. Typically, IgG avidity is greater than 80% in women with recurrent CMV infection, but low IgG avidity is demonstrated for 18 to 20 weeks after a primary infection (Grangeot-Keros et al, 1997; Lazzarotto et al, 1999a). These tests are not routinely available for clinical use. Some investigators have examined the potential correlation between maternal CMV antigenemia or viremia and neonatal outcomes, but study results are inconclusive (Lazzarotto et al, 1999b).

Prenatal diagnosis of congenital CMV can be established by isolation of the virus from amniotic fluid obtained by amniocentesis (Grose et al, 1992) or from fetal blood (Enders et al, 2001). A specific nucleic acid test (NAT) for CMV in amniotic fluid or chorionic villus sampling via polymerase chain reaction (PCR) has been studied, but these tests have not conclusively shown correlation with clinical symptoms (Dong et al, 1994; Jones et al, 2000; Liesnard et al, 2000; Revello et al, 1999). In Italy and the United States, researchers have found quantitative PCR in the amniotic fluid of women to be helpful in predicting symptomatic CMV infection of their fetus or newborn (Guerra et al, 2000; Lazzarotto et al, 2000; Lehman et al, 2001).

The laboratory diagnosis of congenital CMV infection in the infant can be made with certainty only through detection of the virus in organs or culture specimens at birth or within the first 2 to 3 weeks of life. The most sensitive detection system is growth of the virus from urine in tissue culture, and most neonatal culture results are positive within 3 to 7 days (Stagno and Whitley, 1985a; Kinney and Kumar, 1988). A more rapid method of viral isolation, called the shell vial assay, is available in many clinical viral laboratories. In this method centrifugation is performed to enhance viral attachment to cells; then, 16 to 72 hours after inoculation, the culture vials can be stained with fluorescein-conjugated monoclonal antibody to CMV antigen. This technique usually produces results within 24 hours (Rabella and Drew, 1990). It is impossible to determine whether CMV infection was acquired congenitally, perinatally, or postnatally in infants more than about 3 weeks old, because infection acquired during all three periods would result in positive culture results in such infants. Both symptomatic and asymptomatic congenitally infected infants shed virus in their urine for an average of 4 years and for as long as 10 years (Noyola et al, 2000).

Results of serologic testing of an infant at the time of delivery have often been difficult to interpret, because 50% to 75% of women have anti-CMV IgG, which is transplacentally transmitted to the infant, and serial antibody titers cannot absolutely differentiate between congenital infection and perinatally acquired infection. It is estimated that only 50% of congenitally infected infants produce IgM antibody (Nelson and Demmler, 1997).

The principal types of abnormalities found on other laboratory tests in infants with symptomatic CMV infection at birth are listed in Table 37–3. Elevations in liver transaminases and thrombocytopenia are common. Other cytopenias, such as anemia (usually hemolytic) and neutropenia, have also frequently been reported. The urine usually contains bile but no urobilin. Albumin is commonly present, as are some red and white blood cells. Sediment that has been dried, fixed, and stained with hematoxylin and eosin often demonstrates the characteristic inclusion bodies within desquamated renal epithelial cells, so-called owl's-eye cells.

Abnormal head computed tomography (CT) findings are noted in 70% to 80% of symptomatic infants, and 90% of those with abnormal CT findings demonstrate neurologic sequelae (Boppana et al, 1997; Noyola et al, 2001). Neuroradiographic findings include periventricular intracranial calcifications (which may also be seen on plain skull films), ventriculomegaly, cerebellar hypoplasia, and, less commonly, myelination delay consistent with migrational disorders such as lissencephaly, schizencephaly, and pachygyria (Barkovich and Lindan, 1994; Hayward et al, 1991).

Pathologic examination of aborted fetuses or autopsy of infants with symptomatic CMV infection shows characteristic multinuclear giant cells with both cytoplasmic and intranuclear inclusion bodies in many organs, including liver, lungs, brain, pancreas, and kidneys. Mononuclear cell infiltration and diffuse fibrosis may be intense. The brain contains areas of necrosis, often subependymal and periventricular, and glial overgrowth, containing heavy deposits of calcium. Petechiae and larger hemorrhages involve the skin and serous surfaces (Kasprzak et al, 2000; Ko et al, 2000).

### Treatment

The CMV virus differs from herpes simplex and varicella viruses in that it lacks the enzyme thymidine kinase. This feature renders it resistant to antiviral agents that depend on the enzyme for their action, such as acyclovir. Attempts to treat CMV infection with idoxuridine, cytosine arabinoside, adenine arabinoside, interferon inducers, interferon alpha, corticosteroids, cytotoxic agents, and CMV IgG have all failed. Transient reduction in the titer of virus excretion in the urine may be seen with such approaches, but no clinical benefit has been detected.

Anecdotal accounts and case series on the use of ganciclovir have reported variable results (Nigro et al, 1994). A phase II multicenter trial to test the safety and pharmacokinetics of using intravenous ganciclovir for 6 weeks in 47 severely symptomatic infants showed a transient decrease in viral urine titers, and at 2 years of follow-up, 24% of infants were developing normally. Side effects included neutropenia and thrombocytopenia, and 19% of subjects discontinued the drug due to toxicity (Whitley et al, 1997). This transient reduction in viral shedding is difficult to interpret, because other evidence suggests that duration of viral shedding does not correlate with clinical outcome

(Noyola et al, 2000). A phase III randomized, controlled study of 42 infants showed a higher proportion (68%) of infants in the placebo group with worsening of hearing based on BSER test results compared with 21% of infants treated with intravenous ganciclovir for 6 weeks. A significant proportion (63%) of treated infants also developed severe neutropenia during treatment compared with controls (21%) (Kimberlin et al, 2003). Thus, the risk to benefit ratio of administering this intravenous drug for 6 weeks with the frequent side effect of neutropenia makes its use controversial.

#### *Prognosis*

The fate of the congenitally infected infant who is normal at birth is still not clear. Two early series indicated variable risks of deafness and reduction of IQ scores (Hanshaw et al, 1976; Reynolds et al, 1974). In both instances, however, the case finding method was measurement of cord IgM level; an increase in this value might be found only in more severely affected infants (possibly reflecting primary infection in the mother). In another follow-up study, the children were found to be normal at 4 years, but audiometric screening was not performed (Kumar et al, 1973). A Swedish study monitored CMV-infected infants who remained asymptomatic (including no hearing loss) at 12 months of age, and no differences were noted in development or intelligence at 21 months and 7 years of age in these subjects compared with uninfected matched controls (Ivarsson et al, 1997). Thus, most early evidence suggested that infected infants who are asymptomatic at birth will have minimal to no sequelae other than potential hearing loss.

However, congenital CMV infection is currently the leading cause of sensorineural hearing loss in childhood in developed countries. It is now estimated that 7% to 15% of asymptomatic congenitally infected infants have sensorineural hearing loss (Fowler et al, 1997; Williamson et al, 1992). Severity of hearing loss ranges from mild to profound, and of those with hearing loss, approximately half have bilateral deficits, and half have progressive hearing loss. In one fifth of the infants with hearing loss, onset is delayed to 2 to 5 years of age (Fowler et al, 1997). Visual impairment in asymptomatic infants is rare (Coats et al, 2000).

For congenitally infected infants who are symptomatic at birth, mortality rates range from 4% to 30%, and at least 90% of symptomatic neonates have late complications (Griffiths, 1993; Stagno and Whitley, 1985a). Of those who survive, 60% to 75% have intellectual or developmental impairment (Berenberg and Nankervis, 1970), about one third have hearing loss, one third have neuromuscular disorders (spasticity or seizures), and a smaller proportion experience visual impairment due to reactivation or late-onset chorioretinitis. Of all the CMV-infected infants who eventually develop hearing loss, only one third are identifiable with newborn hearing screening at birth (Fowler et al, 1999); thus, these infants should have close audiologic follow-up for the first several years of life.

Neurologic outcomes in congenitally infected infants vary, but microcephaly (when adjusted for weight and gestational age) is the most specific predictor, and head CT scan abnormality the most sensitive prognostic factor, for poor cognitive outcome and motor disability (Noyola et al, 2001). Duration of viral shedding has no correlation with long-term outcomes (Noyola et al, 2000). Up to one third of infected infants are normal late in childhood, and those who demonstrated minimal abnormalities at birth have the greatest chance of being normal at long-term follow-up. Strabismus and amblyopia may develop, so these infants should have close ophthalmologic follow-up throughout their lives (Coats et al, 2000).

#### Prevention

There is currently no convincing evidence supporting the benefits of antiviral therapy for CMV infection during pregnancy. Preliminary research efforts to develop a vaccine are in progress. The most important means of prevention are basic hygiene and hand-washing for pregnant women, especially after contact with urine, diapers, oral secretions, and other body fluids.

## HERPES SIMPLEX VIRUS INFECTIONS

Herpes simplex viruses are classified into two types. HSV-1 causes approximately 98% of oral infections (gingivostomatitis and pharyngitis), 7% to 50% of primary genital herpes, and almost 100% of encephalitis after the newborn period. HSV-2 causes 90% of primary genital herpes, 99% of recurrent genital infections, and most cases of aseptic meningitis (Nahmias and Roizman, 1973; Freij and Sever, 1988). It is likely that most infections are acquired from the mother shortly before or at the time of delivery, though some are acquired from other sources. Considering the high frequency of oro-labial herpes in the adult population, however, acquisition of herpes simplex from such lesions must be extremely rare.

#### Incidence

Seroprevalence of HSV-2 ranges from 20% to 45% and varies with gender and ethnicity (Fleming et al, 1997). The incidence of genital herpes infections has risen steadily since the 1970s (Whitley, 1994), and the frequency of neonatal disease has concomitantly increased (Prober et al, 1988). Approximately 70% to 85% of neonatal herpes simplex infections are caused by HSV-2 (Kimberlin et al, 2001). Frequency of neonatal disease differs among populations according to socioeconomic status as well as incompletely understood immunologic factors (Nahmias and Roizman, 1973; Nahmias et al, 1971; Whitley, 1993). Estimated incidence of neonatal HSV infection is one in 3500-10,000 deliveries (Whitley, 1993). Primary genital herpes infection in a pregnant mother results in an attack rate of 33% to 50% for her infant, whereas recurrent maternal infection results in a 1% to 3% attack rate (Arvin, 1991; Brown et al, 1997; Prober et al, 1987).

#### Etiology and Pathogenesis

Some infants with HSV have been described with a syndrome more closely resembling congenital viral infection; they were probably infected in utero during the first or second trimester (Florman et al, 1973; Freij and Sever,

1988; South et al, 1969). These cases compose approximately 5% of neonatal HSV infections (Kimberlin, 2001). Primary genital HSV infections that occur during the first half of pregnancy are associated with a higher frequency of spontaneous abortions and stillbirths (Freij and Sever, 1988; Stagno and Whitley, 1985b).

Most HSV-infected infants (approximately 85%) acquire HSV from the maternal genital tract at the time of delivery, although only 15% to 30% of mothers who give birth to infants with neonatal HSV infection have a known history of genital HSV (Whitley, 1988). HSV lesions have been reported to develop at the site of intrapartum monitoring electrodes on the infant's scalp. A smaller number of infants are infected several days before delivery and are born with clinically evident disease. Cases proved to have been acquired from individuals other than the mother, or even from the mother at any time other than during delivery, are rare (Linnemann et al, 1978; Yeager et al, 1983). Postnatal infections are estimated to contribute approximately 10% of neonatal HSV infections. There are also anecdotal case reports of postnatally acquired HSV infection after procedures such as instrumentation during ophthalmologic examinations for premature infants and ritual circumcisions performed by Orthodox Jewish *mohelim* (Hutchinson et al, 2000; Rubin and Lanzkowsky, 2000).

The pathogenic mechanisms responsible for the newborn infant's susceptibility to herpes infection do not depend on a single key difference between adult and infant but are the results of a spectrum of immunologic deficiencies (Arvin, 1991; Burchett et al, 1992; Jenkins and Kohl, 1992). Among the currently identified cellular deficits are the inability of the neonatal macrophage and unstimulated neonatal lymphocyte to mediate early viral containment, and a profound defect in natural killer cell cytotoxicity (Kohl, 1985). The contribution of transplacentally acquired antibody is unresolved, but type-specific antibody is probably partially protective (Arvin, 1991; Arvin and Prober, 1993; Kohl, 1991). Antibody-dependent effector mechanisms, including antibody-dependent cellular cytotoxicity, which may rely on lymphocytes, macrophages, and polymorphonuclear leukocytes, may be responsible in different infants for the conflicting data concerning anti-HSV antibody titers and protection from infection. The genetic and developmental regulatory mechanisms of these varied immunologic defects suggest different immunoregulatory interventions that are individualized for specific infants.

Disseminated disease may infect and infiltrate several different organs. Macroscopic examination shows that many viscera, but chiefly the liver, lungs, and adrenal glands, are riddled with pale yellow, firm, necrotic nodules, measuring 1 to 6 mm in diameter. Under the microscope, massive coagulation necrosis can be seen to involve the parenchyma, stroma, and vessels in these areas. Necrotizing, calcifying lesions of the brain may also be found. Intranuclear eosinophilic inclusions as well as multinucleated giant cells, which represent the individual cell's response to viral infection, may be observed (Singer, 1981).

### Clinical Spectrum

Although most neonatal HSV infections occur perinatally, there are several case reports of infants born with congenital malformations more suggestive of in utero HSV infection. Clinical manifestations involve multiple systems, primarily the skin, central nervous system (CNS), and eyes. Reported findings include extensive dermatologic scarring or bullae, microencephaly or hydranencephaly, encephalitis, microphthalmia or chorioretinitis, and sometimes hepatosplenomegaly (Baldwin and Whitley, 1989; Hutto et al, 1987).

Most infants with perinatal or postnatal HSV infection are normal at birth, illness developing after 3 days of age. Approximately 40% to 50% of affected infants are less than 36 weeks in gestational age (Whitley, 1988). Overt herpetic disease in the maternal genital tract is evident in only about one third of patients (Overall, 1994). In the remaining two thirds, the virus likely originates from an asymptomatic maternal genital infection.

The clinical manifestations of disease have been classified into the following three groups: (1) localized skin, eye, and mouth (SEM) disease, (2) encephalitis or CNS disease, and (3) disseminated disease. SEM disease without overt CNS involvement represents approximately 20% of all cases of neonatal herpes. Localized CNS disease with or without skin, eye, or oral cavity involvement is seen in approximately 33% of infants with neonatal herpes. Approximately 50% of all cases of neonatal herpes manifest as disseminated disease (Whitley, 1993).

Less than half of infants with any form of HSV infection have fever, only 30% to 40% of patients have the classic vesicular skin lesions at presentation, and only two thirds of patients have skin lesions at any time during infection. On the neonatal skin, HSV produces the characteristic grouped vesicles seen in later life, although individual lesions may be large and even bullous, and late lesions are typically eroded, flat, irregular ulcers with an erythematous base.

Disseminated disease usually begins toward the end of the first week of life. Skin vesicles may be the first or a later sign, but they do not appear at all in almost half of patients. Systemic symptoms, although insidious in onset, progress rapidly. Poor feeding, lethargy, and fever may be accompanied by irritability or convulsions if the CNS is involved. These symptoms are followed rapidly by jaundice, hypotension, disseminated intravascular coagulation, apnea, and shock. This form of disease is indistinguishable at its onset from both neonatal enterovirus infection and bacterial sepsis. Thus, herpes infection should be considered in the differential diagnosis of infants who have fever during the first 2 weeks of life.

Localized disease may begin somewhat later, with most cases appearing in the second to third week of life. When the CNS is the primary site of infection, the skin or eyes may or may not be involved. The infants are lethargic, irritable, and tremulous, and seizures are common and difficult to control.

Other less common but potentially localized or disseminated findings are keratoconjunctivitis or chorioretinitis, which account for approximately 5% of HSV manifestations, and pneumonitis, which can begin as a focal infiltrate but may become generalized. Supraglottitis, intracranial hemorrhage, aseptic meningitis, and fulminant liver failure have also been described in association with neonatal HSV infection (Abzug and Johnson, 2000; Greenes et al, 1995; Kohl, 1994; Schlesinger and Storch, 1994).

### Laboratory Evaluation

Except when encephalitis is the only manifestation of disease, HSV is readily recovered from clinical samples. In the disseminated form, virus is present in blood, conjunctivae, respiratory secretions, urine, and, in approximately half of the patients, the central nervous system. In the localized form, the virus can usually be found at the site of disease. Definitive microbiologic diagnosis requires growth of the virus in tissue culture. Fortunately, HSV can be detected in culture because of its cytopathic effect in 24 to 48 hours in most instances. When herpes neonatorum is suspected, viral cultures of the throat, conjunctiva, blood, stool or rectum, and urine should all be obtained, as should scrapings of any suspicious skin lesions. Of these sites, skin and conjunctival HSV cultures have the highest yield (Kimberlin et al, 2001). The mother's genital tract should also be sampled if there is a high index of suspicion. Scrapings of skin vesicles may show giant, multinucleated cells when stained with Wright or Giemsa stain (the Tzanck smear), typical of either herpes or varicella virus infection, although this test has low sensitivity. Demonstration of viral antigens in cytologic smears by means of enzyme immunoassays is more sensitive than the Tzanck smear, and direct fluorescent antibody staining also provides rapid results (Alpert and Plotkin, 1986). Serologic assays are rarely helpful in neonatal infections.

CSF should be sent for cell count, protein, and glucose measurements, and HSV DNA PCR analysis. PCR of the CSF yields a much higher sensitivity for HSV than viral CSF culture. There is a wide variability of reliable PCR results, depending on individual laboratory expertise and experience. False-positive and false-negative results may occur early in the disease; thus, as with all tests, results should be interpreted cautiously and in conjunction with clinical evaluation. Usually if the CNS is involved, evaluation of the CSF reveals a lymphocytosis, often red blood cells, normal or high protein level, and low or normal glucose level. Some experts recommend obtaining a second CSF specimen for evaluation at the end of antiviral therapy, and it has been reported that persistence of HSV DNA may be a poor prognostic factor (Kimberlin et al, 1996b; Malm and Forsgren, 1999). Research is under way to investigate the utility of quantitative HSV PCR as well as PCR of serum and other respiratory, gastrointestinal, and urinary samples (Diamond et al, 1999; Revello et al, 1997).

In disseminated disease, liver transaminase elevations consistent with hepatocellular injury are usually found. Infants with CNS disease should also undergo neuroradiographic imaging with CT or magnetic resonance imaging (MRI). Imaging may demonstrate early, nonspecific lack of gray-white matter junction differentiation and general signs of encephalitis. Later findings include dilated ventricles, parenchymal echogenicity, cystic degeneration, and intracranial calcifications (O'Reilly et al, 1995). Newborn HSV encephalitis is not usually confined to the temporal lobes as is classically described in older patients. Electroenceephalography (EEG) should also be performed in infants with CNS or disseminated disease to evaluate for seizure activity; EEG findings will be abnormal in approximately 80% of such patients (Kimberlin et al, 2001).

### Treatment

After the appropriate specimens are collected and sent for viral culture and PCR analysis, the infant should receive acyclovir, 60 mg/kg/day intravenously divided into 3 doses given every 8 hours, for 14 days in SEM disease and 21 days in disseminated or CNS disease (American Academy of Pediatrics [AAP], 2003). This treatment has been shown to be effective in all forms of the disease, reducing mortality and, to a lesser extent, long-term sequelae. Shorter intervals between initiation of treatment and onset of symptoms have been shown to decrease mortality and morbidity (Whitley, 1991). Herpetic keratoconjunctivitis should receive topical ophthalmic antiviral therapy along with parenteral treatment. No persuasive human data currently exist supporting the use or efficacy of intravenous immunoglobulin or cytokines to treat HSV. Monoclonal antibodies have proved helpful in animal models and will likely be studied in humans within the next few years (Kimberlin, 2001).

The Collaborative Antiviral Study Group is currently conducting randomized controlled studies to evaluate long-term oral suppressive acyclovir therapy after neonatal HSV in the prevention of recurrent skin lesions and neurologic sequelae. Phase I and II trials demonstrated fewer cutaneous recurrences in the treatment group but did not have enough subjects to analyze the impact on neurologic outcomes (Kimberlin et al, 1996a). Neutropenia has been reported in 20% to 50% of neonates receiving long-term acyclovir therapy. The emergence of acyclovir-resistant HSV strains is also a concern (Kimberlin et al, 1996a; Oram et al, 2000).

### Prognosis

Overall mortality for neonatal HSV infection with treatment is approximately 20%. Infants with localized SEM disease typically have minimal mortality and lower morbidity. Despite a lack of detectable CNS disease upon presentation, neurologic abnormalities develop later in approximately 5% of this group. The survival results reported by the Collaborative Antiviral Study Group trials for infants with CNS or disseminated disease treated between 1981 and 1997 are shown in Figure 37–3 (Kimberlin et al, 2001).

The mortality rates in infants with localized CNS disease range from 4% to 14% with antiviral therapy, and most survivors have long-term neurologic sequelae. Risk factors for increased morbidity and mortality from CNS infection include prematurity and seizures upon initiation of therapy (Kimberlin et al, 2001; Kohl, 1999). Infants with disseminated disease have an even higher mortality without antiviral therapy; 80% die, and survivors have serious neurologic sequelae (Whitley, 1988). With antiviral therapy, 20% to 60% die, and 40% to 55% of survivors suffer neurologic sequelae (Freij and Sever, 1988). High-dose acyclovir has improved mortality rates but has had less impact on morbidity. Lethargy at initiation of therapy has been noted to be associated with a higher mortality rate in neonates with disseminated HSV infection (Kimberlin et al, 2001).

Even with antiviral treatment, the prognosis for survivors of disseminated HSV infection is poor. Microcephaly, spasticity, paralysis, seizures, deafness, blindness, or a combination of these conditions develops in more than half of infants with disseminated disease. Infants with skin

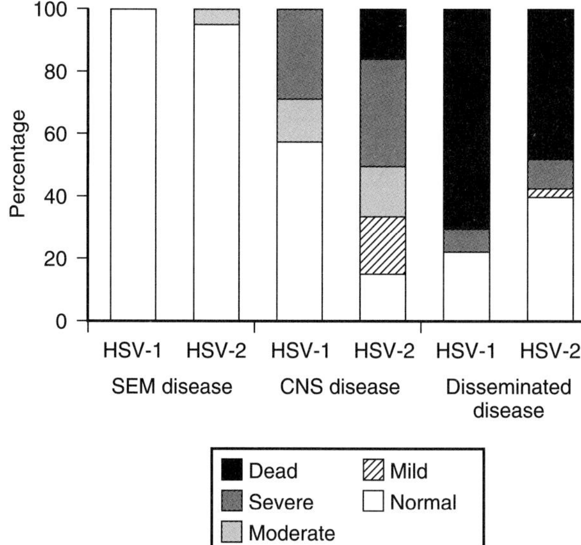


**FIGURE 37–3.** Morbidity and mortality among patients with herpes simplex virus (HSV) disease after 12 months of age by viral type, 1981 to 1997. CNS, CNS; SEM, localized skin, eye, and mouth. *(From Kimberlin DW, Lin CY, Jacobs DA, et al: Natural history of neonatal herpes simplex virus infections in the acyclovir era. Pediatrics 108:223, 2001.)*

involvement often have recurrent crops of skin vesicles for several years. More than three episodes of recurrent skin lesions within the first 6 months of life is a prognostic sign for poor neurologic outcome (Whitley, 1991).

### Prevention

If a mother has active genital herpes simplex infection at the time of delivery and if the membranes are either intact or have been ruptured for less than 4 hours, both the AAP and the American College of Obstetrics and Gynecology (ACOG) recommend delivery by cesarean section (AAP, 2003; ACOG practice bulletin, 2000). There is a 30% to 50% risk to the child inadvertently delivered vaginally during primary maternal infection; thus, most experts recommend surveillance HSV cultures of conjunctiva, oropharynx, and nares at 24 to 48 hours after birth. Some experts recommend empiric intravenous acyclovir treatment for 10 to 14 days of any infant born vaginally to a mother with known active primary HSV infection, whereas others advocate such a measure only if the infant is symptomatic or results of HSV cultures or other diagnostic tests are positive.

Because active recurrent maternal genital HSV infection at the time of delivery poses a less than 5% risk of infection to the infant, cesarean section is also strongly recommended in this situation, although the issue is more controversial. Many experts also recommend surveillance viral cultures of infants born to mothers with recurrent HSV infection. In all cases, infants should be observed closely for signs of infection, and parents should be educated about the signs and symptoms of neonatal HSV (AAP, 2003).

Infants in whom HSV infection is known or highly suspected should be put in isolation with contact precautions, and skin lesions should be covered. Any health care provider with active herpetic whitlow should not have direct patient care responsibilities for neonates (AAP, 2003).

Several clinical phase I, II, and III trials are ongoing to investigate the utility of various HSV vaccines to prevent genital infections (Stanberry, 1998).

## VARICELLA

Varicella zoster is a DNA virus in the herpes virus family. Primary varicella infection, commonly known as *chickenpox*, usually results in a fever and a characteristic vesicular exanthem beginning on the face or trunk. It is often accompanied by other systemic symptoms, such as headache and malaise. Secondary infection or reactivation, usually referred to as zoster or shingles, is characterized by a painful vesicular rash in a dermatomal distribution. Primary varicella infection during pregnancy can result in congenital malformations.

There is some confusion about the term *congenital varicella* that would probably be best resolved if the term were reserved for the rare cases transmitted to the fetus in the first or second trimester of pregnancy (Laforet and Lynch, 1947; Srabstein et al, 1974). Also often called "congenital varicella" but probably more appropriately termed *neonatal varicella* are those cases of perinatal varicella acquired late in the third trimester, which become apparent in the newborn on or before the tenth day of life.

### Incidence

Before the advent of routine varicella immunization in childhood in the United States, seroprevalence surveys estimated that approximately 95% of women were immune (Gershon, 1975). Primary varicella-zoster virus (VZV) infections occured during pregnancy with a frequency of 5 to 7 per 10,000 pregnancies in the United States (Balducci et al, 1992; Brunell, 1992). For pregnant women with primary varicella infection, the transmission rate to the fetus is estimated to be approximately 25%. Only 4% to 8% of infected fetuses have symptomatic disease, so congenital varicella syndrome (CVS) is rare (Enders et al, 1994; Liesnard et al, 1994).

At least 96 cases of CVS have been reported in the literature (Sauerbrei and Wutzler, 2000). The risk of symptomatic intrauterine VZV infection after maternal varicella during the first 20 weeks is approximately 1% to 2% (Enders et al, 1994; Paryani and Arvin, 1986; Pastuszak et al, 1994; Siegel, 1973). Unlike first-trimester mumps and rubella infection, first-trimester varicella infection does not commonly result in a detectable increase in fetal wastage (Brunell, 1992; Siegel and Fuerst, 1966). Paryani and Arvin (1986) reported that 1 of 11 infants born to women with varicella during the second trimester demonstrated herpes zoster during infancy; among 16 infants born to women with varicella during the third trimester, 2 had varicella at birth. Two thirds of symptomatic infected infants reported are female (Sauerbrei and Wutzler, 2000).

Neonatal varicella is much more common than congenital varicella. For infants whose mothers contract varicella 5 days or less before delivery or up to 2 days after delivery, the infant attack rate is 17% to 31% (Brunell, 1992; Feldman, 1986; Meyers, 1974). Neonatal varicella may develop despite the administration of varicella zoster immune globulin (VZIG) to the infant at birth.

Although primary maternal varicella infection has been associated with congenital infection and potential sequelae, transmission secondary to maternal reactivation with clinical zoster during pregnancy has not been reported. A prospective study of infants born to 366 mothers with a clinical history of zoster during pregnancy found no infants with congenital malformations consistent with intrauterine VZV infection (Enders et al, 1994). Of the few case reports of infants with malformations born to mothers with clinical zoster during pregnancy, none has had findings classically associated with CVS or laboratory evidence of intrauterine infection with VZV (Sauerbrei and Wutzler, 2000). See Figure 37–4 for an overview of perinatal varicella infection.

### Etiology and Pathogenesis

CVS is acquired from a maternal primary varicella infection that occurs during the first or second trimester. The virus is thought to be transmitted transplacentally during the viremia that precedes or accompanies the rash. Ascending infection from cervical infection has also been proposed as a potential mechanism of transmission (Sauerbrei and Wutzler, 2000). It has been suggested that some of the congenital malformations associated with maternal varicella infection may actually be the consequence of zoster reactivation of the fetus in utero rather than direct effects of the primary viral infection. This explanation is supported by the common clinical finding of a dermatomal distribution of skin lesions in the newborn. Immature fetal cell–mediated immune response may explain the short latency period as well as the inadequate protection from the consequences of reactivation infection (Higa et al, 1987; Kustermann et al, 1996). Pathology reports have noted destruction of neural tissue with residual dystrophic calcifications, chronic active inflammation in non-neural tissues surrounding viral inclusions, and chronic villitis of the placenta (Bruder et al, 2000; Petignat et al, 2001; Qureshi and Jacques, 1996).

Neonatal varicella is probably transplacentally acquired in most cases. Because the incubation period for varicella is between 10 and 21 days, cases beginning in the first 10 days of life are considered to have been acquired in utero. The prognosis, however, differs markedly between those cases in which maternal illness began 5 or more days before delivery and those in which maternal illness occurred from 5 days before to 2 days after delivery. In the first group, neonatal disease usually begins with the first 4 days of life, and the prognosis is good. Early case series reported survival in 27 of 27 infants (Gershon, 1975). Presumably, maternal immunity has appeared before delivery and has been transferred to the baby before birth. In the second group, neonatal disease begins between 5 and 10 days after delivery. Of 23 cases described, 7 infants (30%) died of overwhelming varicella, and 2 barely survived after severe disease (Brunell, 1966). Serious postnatal infection acquired from maternal varicella via breast-feeding has not been reported.

### Clinical Spectrum

As with many other congenital viral infections, there is likely a wide clinical range of VZV disease. In the only large prospective study, involving more than 1300 pregnant women with varicella infection, 7% to 12% of the infants had serologic evidence of disease postnatally but remained asymptomatic. At least 1% to 2% of congenitally infected infants may be asymptomatic at birth and demonstrate zoster in early infancy (Enders et al, 1994).

The rare cases of CVS are characterized by the presence of unusual cicatrices, often in a dermatomal distribution, asymmetric muscular atrophy with limb hypoplasia, low birth weight, neurologic abnormalities (cortical or spinal

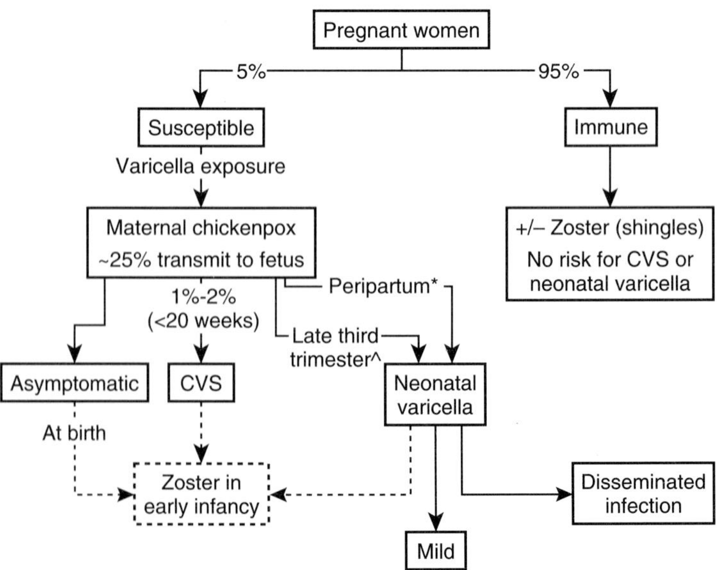


**FIGURE 37–4.** Overview of varicella infection during pregnancy. *Peripartum* is defined as between 5 days before and 2 days after delivery; *Late third trimester* is defined as between 2 weeks and 5 days before delivery. *Dotted lines* denote potential outcome. CVS, congenital varicella syndrome.

cord atrophy, seizures, microcephaly, encephalitis, Horner syndrome), and ophthalmologic abnormalities (chorioretinitis, microphthalmia, atrophy, and cataracts) (Brunell, 1992; Feldman, 1986; Sauerbrei and Wutzler, 2000). Gastrointestinal abnormalities are reported in 15% to 23% of cases; findings include duodenal stenosis, dilated jejunum, small left colon, intestinal atresia or bands, and hepatic calcifications (Alkalay et al, 1987; Jones et al, 1994). Table 37–4 summarizes the frequencies of clinical findings in 96 infant cases of CVS (Sauerbrei and Wutzler, 2000).

Neonatal varicella follows typical maternal varicella and thus can usually be anticipated. Disease that is evident at birth or that appears in the first 4 days of life is usually mild, with a few cutaneous lesions, presumably due to modification of the illness by maternal immunity. When the disease appears in the infant during the riskiest period (between 5 and 10 days of age), it closely resembles varicella in the immunodeficient or immunosuppressed host. Recurrent crops of skin vesicles develop over a prolonged period, reflecting the newborn infant's inability to control the infection. Typical presenting signs are fever, hemorrhagic rash, and visceral dissemination with involvement of the liver, lung, and brain. Secondary bacterial infection may occur.

### Laboratory Evaluation

Prenatal diagnosis, by means of quantification of varicella-specific IgM on fetal blood obtained by cordocentesis or through PCR analysis of chorionic villi, fetal blood, and amniotic fluid, has been attempted (Cuthbertson et al, 1987; Kustermann et al, 1996; Mouly et al, 1997). Although the yield of PCR on amniotic fluid or fetal blood is higher than that of serologic analysis of fetal IgM or viral cultures, large prospective studies of correlation of such findings with clinical outcomes have not been performed. Prenatal ultrasonographic findings include polyhydramnios, hydrops, progressive intrauterine growth restriction, microcephaly, limb hypoplasia, and liver hyperechogenicities (Pretorius et al, 1992). Abnormal ultrasonographic findings may not develop in a fetus for at least 5 weeks after maternal infection (Kerkering, 2001).

Serologic studies can be performed postnatally on infants (Paryani and Arvin, 1986). Suspected congenital infection with varicella may be confirmed by the finding of persistent VZV IgG beyond the presumed duration of passive transfer of maternal antibodies (at least 6 to 7 months). Detection of fetal IgM may also confirm infection, but it is less useful because only about one fourth of infants reported with classic CVS have positive VZV IgM titer values (Enders et al, 1994; Sauerbrei and Wutzler, 2000). Scrapings of skin lesions, as with herpes simplex infections, may show large multinucleated cells when stained with Wright or Giemsa stain (Tzanck smears), but this procedure is not commonly performed. The virus can be grown in tissue culture or detected by direct fluorescent antibody (DFA) staining of cells from skin and visceral lesions, but viral tests in infants with congenital infection are often extremely low yield compared with those infants with acquired varicella infections. Neuroradiographic

**TABLE 37–4**

**Main Symptoms of Infants with Congenital Varicella Syndrome Cited in the Literature (N = 96)***

| Symptom | No. of Infants Affected | % of Infants Affected |
|---|---|---|
| Skin lesions: cicatricial scars, skin loss | 70 | 76 |
| Neurologic defects or diseases: cortical atrophy, spinal cord atrophy, limb paresis, seizures, microcephaly, Horner syndrome, encephalitis, dysphagia | 55 | 60 |
| Eye diseases: microphthalmia, exophthalmia, chorioretinitis, cataracts, nystagmus, anisocoria, optic atrophy | 47 | 51 |
| Limb hypoplasia and other skeletal anomalies | 45 | 49 |
| Intrauterine growth retardation | 20 | 22 |
| Muscle hypoplasia | 19 | 21 |
| Gastrointestinal abnormalities | 14 | 15 |
| Developmental delay | 11 | 12 |
| Genitourinary abnormalities | 11 | 12 |
| Defects of the cardiovascular system | 7 | 8 |
| Defects of other organs | 6 | 7 |

*Symptoms of 4 children have not been described.

Data from Sauerbrei A, Wutzler P: The congenital varicella syndrome. J Perinatol 20:548-554, 2000.

demonstration of intracranial calcifications has been reported but is not common (Kerkering, 2001).

### Treatment

No controlled studies examining the effect of antiviral therapy to prevent or treat congenital varicella syndrome have been conducted. Treatment of the infected pregnant woman with acyclovir is unlikely to be effective in preventing fetal infection, because viremia with VZV typically takes place 1 to 2 days before the characteristic rash, and antiviral therapy shortens the duration of infection by only about 1 day. Anecdotal observations have noted a potential effect of acyclovir on the progression of eye disease in CVS (Sauerbrei and Wutzler, 2000). No recommendations can be made to use acyclovir for treatment or prevention of CVS.

If symptoms of neonatal varicella are severe, treatment with intravenous acyclovir, 60 mg/kg/day divided into doses every 8 hours, should be given.

### Prognosis

Prospective studies of the long-term outcomes of congenitally infected infants with VZV have not been performed, and there is probably a wide continuum of disease. Among the 96 congenitally infected infants reviewed by Sauerbrei and Wutzler (2000), 14 (15%) had clinical signs of zoster during early infancy. Some experts consider early zoster infection as one criterion for diagnosis of infection with VZV in utero. Mortality rates for CVS are estimated at 30%. Deaths generally occur within the first few months of life, usually secondary to severe pulmonary disease (Pastuszak et al, 1994; Sauerbrei and Wutzler, 2000). Before the use of VZIG and acyclovir, mortality rates for neonatal varicella were also approximately 30% (Isaacs, 2000).

### Prevention

If a susceptible pregnant woman has a significant exposure to varicella, administration of high-titered VZIG should be seriously considered. Infants of mothers in whom varicella develops from 5 days before to 2 days after delivery should receive VZIG as soon as possible (125 units) (AAP, 2003). Such preparations have been shown to prevent chickenpox in exposed older children (Brunell et al, 1969) but do not always prevent infection (Reynolds et al, 1999). Approximately 50% of exposed infants treated with VZIG may still have varicella infection, but the disease is often attenuated, and only approximately 10% have severe disease (Hanngren et al, 1985).

Follow-up of infants exposed to VZV and treated with VZIG may include consideration of serologic testing (enzyme immunoassay, latex agglutination, or indirect fluorescent antibody staining for IgG) to determine whether asymptomatic infection has elicited immune protection. Repeat exposure of infants in whom varicella did not develop more than 3 weeks after administration of VZIG should prompt administration of another dose of VZIG (AAP, 2003). If special globulin preparations are not available, standard intravenous immune globulin (IVIG) may be given. The infant should also be put in respiratory isolation for 28 days or until discharge, because administration of VZIG may prolong the incubation period.

In the event of a significant varicella exposure in a nursery situation, infants whose mothers have no history of chickenpox and who have undetectable anti-varicella antibody titers should be considered candidates for VZIG. All exposed infants less than 28 weeks of gestational age, regardless of maternal history, should receive VZIG (AAP, 2003). The recommended dosage is 125 units/10 kg. Little experience is available to guide treatment of extremely premature infants, but fractional doses are not recommended; currently, all infants should receive 125 units.

The best means of prevention is to follow current recommendations for universal varicella immunization of all children at 12 to 15 months of age as well as susceptible adolescents and adults at high risk of exposure to varicella. None of the 362 women followed in a pregnancy registry for inadvertent exposure to varicella vaccine during or within 3 months of pregnancy has given birth to an infant with congenital varicella syndrome (Shields et al, 2001). Nonetheless, it is recommended that adolescents and women of child-bearing age should avoid pregnancy for at least 1 month after immunization.

## HUMAN PARVOVIRUS B19

Parvovirus B19, a single-stranded, small DNA virus, is the only member of the parvovirus family that causes disease in humans. Infection with parvovirus B19 is more commonly known as *fifth disease* or *erythema infectiosum*; it is classically described as a childhood exanthem with a "slapped cheek" rash. Considerable interest in the role of human parvovirus B19 infection in neonatal hydrops fetalis (nonimmune) and fetal aplastic crisis has developed since cases of fetal deaths in humans associated with maternal parvovirus B19 infection were reported in the 1980s (Brown et al, 1984; Kinney et al, 1988).

### Incidence

Approximately 50% to 80% of adults in the United States are seropositive for human parvovirus B19 (Anderson, 1987). A significant proportion of child-bearing women is thus presumably susceptible to human parvovirus B19 infection. Although large studies are not available, the overall risk of maternal exposure or infection to the fetus appears low (Berry et al, 1992; Sheikh et al, 1992). It is estimated that one quarter to one third of maternal parvovirus infections are transmitted to the fetus (Alger, 1997; Gratacos et al, 1995). It is difficult to estimate risk of sequelae, but approximately 1% to 12% of pregnancies in which infection occurs before 20 weeks of gestational age have resulted in fetal loss, and up to 1% of those infected after 20 weeks may lead to fetal hydrops or death (Markenson and Yancey, 1998; Yaegashi et al, 1998). The risk of adverse sequelae appears to be highest during the second trimester. Thus, at most, the fetus of a pregnant woman with a significant exposure to parvovirus B19 has a 1% to 3% risk of hydrops or death.

Various estimates suggest that human parvovirus B19 infection contributes from 10% to 27% of cases of nonimmune hydrops fetalis (Essary et al, 1998; Markenson and Yancey, 1998; Yaegashi et al, 1994). Although there are case reports of neurologic and ophthalmologic anomalies associated with maternal parvovirus B19 infections, no prospective studies or characteristic anomalies have conclusively identified the virus as a human teratogen. Two studies undertaken to examine the association between human parvovirus B19 infection and congenital anomalies have failed to reveal any connection (Kinney et al, 1988; Mortimer et al, 1985). There have been at least three case reports of fetal encephalopathy associated with in utero infection with parvovirus B19 (Alger, 1997).

### Etiology and Pathogenesis

The most common route of transmission of parvovirus B19 is via respiratory droplets. Typically, once the virus establishes infection, viremia occurs along with systemic symptoms such as fever and malaise. It is important to note that viremia lasts only 1 to 3 days, and the characteristic immune-mediated rash develops 1 to 2 weeks later, when the host is no longer infectious.

Potential pathogenic mechanisms involve the recognized affinity of parvovirus B19 for progenitor erythroid cells of bone marrow. The blood group P antigen is a main cellular receptor for parvovirus B19, and it is found on red blood cells and on placental trophoblast cells (Jordan et al, 2001). Fetal infection most likely occurs hematogenously via the placenta during maternal viremia. Parvovirus B19 infection then causes a pronormoblast arrest, which leads to fetal anemia, nonimmune hydrops, and, sometimes, progressive congestive heart failure (Kinney et al, 1988). The fetus is especially susceptible to adverse consequences of red blood cell infection secondary to short erythrocyte life span and rapidly expanding blood volume, especially during the second trimester. It has been well established that antibody-mediated immune response is crucial to protection from acquired parvovirus B19 infection. Data also suggest that cell-mediated immune responses may contribute to the pathogenesis of congenital infection (Jordan et al, 2001).

Pathologic studies of human fetuses infected with parvovirus B19 have suggested that myocardial inflammation and subendocardial fibroelastosis may also contribute to fetal hydrops (Morey et al, 1992). It has also been postulated that parvovirus B19 infection leads to cytotoxicity and subsequent anemia by inducing apoptosis of infected red blood cells (Yaegashi et al, 1999). Neuropathologic findings in the infected hydropic fetus include perivascular calcifications, primarily in the cerebral white matter, as well as multinucleated giant cells. Viral DNA has been demonstrated in the brain and liver (Isumi et al, 1999).

### Clinical Spectrum

Parvovirus B19 infection causes erythema infectiosum, or fifth disease, in normal hosts, aplastic crisis in patients with hemolytic disorders, and chronic anemia in immunocompromised hosts. A substantial proportion of infected adult women may also have arthropathy in association with parvovirus B19 infection. Maternal symptoms have been present in up to two thirds of documented cases of nonimmune hydrops fetalis associated with parvovirus B19 infection (Yaegashi et al, 1998).

Little data are available regarding clinical outcomes of infected infant survivors, but two prospective studies in the United Kingdom of more than 300 congenitally exposed infants found the risk of major congenital or developmental abnormality to be less than 1% (Miller et al, 1998; Prospective study, 1990).

### Laboratory Evaluation

The diagnosis of human parvovirus B19 infection is most commonly made clinically. Serologic confirmation is necessary in high-risk situations, such as after a significant exposure of a pregnant woman. Both radioimmunoassays and enzyme-linked immunosorbent assays (ELISAs) are available for detection of human parvovirus B19–specific IgG and IgM (Kinney and Kumar, 1988). Presence of anti–parvovirus B19 IgM in fetal blood or amniotic fluid may confirm fetal infection but may be detected in only one fifth of infected fetuses (Torok et al, 1992). False-positive results of anti–parvovirus B19 IgM testing have also been reported, including cross-reactions with anti-rubella IgM (Dieck et al, 1999).

In the context of a human parvovirus B19 infection in a symptomatic, pregnant woman, elevated or rising weekly measurements of maternal serum alpha-fetoprotein may indicate that the fetus is infected. Elevated maternal alpha-fetoprotein concentration may also be a marker for an adverse outcome (Carrington et al, 1987). Serial fetal ultrasonographic evaluations of infected pregnant women are recommended to evaluate and follow for fetal hydrops or demise.

Other techniques to diagnose fetal parvovirus B19 infection have been studied and utilized, but most are not commonly available. Virus can be cultured from tissue in suspension cultures of bone marrow cells from persons with hemolytic anemias but it is difficult to isolate, so this is not a routinely feasible method of prenatal or postnatal diagnosis. Electron microscopy and histology have permitted visualization of parvovirus in fetal blood, ascitic fluid, tissue, and amniotic fluid, but the utility and sensitivity of these evaluations have not been well studied (Markenson and Yancey, 1998). Finally, molecular probes with DNA PCR can detect human parvovirus B19 DNA in tissues, maternal and fetal serum, amniotic fluid, and urine and may become the most useful and sensitive means of diagnosis once they are more widely available (Dieck et al, 1999; Kinney and Kumar, 1988).

### Treatment

Spontaneous resolution of fetal hydrops with normal neonatal outcome has been reported in approximately one third of cases (Humphrey et al, 1991; Rodis et al, 1998a; Sheikh et al, 1992). Because two thirds of fetuses do not recover without intervention, fetal transfusion is usually recommended to attempt to improve pregnancy outcome (Boley and Popek, 1993; Brown et al, 1994). The earlier fetal transfusion is attempted, the more likely it is to be successful. After appropriate serologic or molecular diagnosis, the clinician should care for each case individually because there are insufficient data to predict outcome with certainty. Treatment of the pregnant woman or the neonate with intravenous immune globulin (IVIG) has not been shown to improve fetal outcomes and so is not routinely recommended.

### Prognosis

Mortality rates for fetal hydrops due to all nonimmune causes have ranged from 50% to 98%, even in the 1990s with more aggressive therapies (Wy et al, 1999). Prognosis and survival do seem to vary with etiology, and hydrops secondary to parvovirus B19 seems to have a better outcome than that from other causes (Ismail et al, 2001). Although few long-term prospective studies of infants born to mothers with documented primary parvovirus B19 infection have been conducted, most reported infants appear to have normal development. One small case-control study, involving approximately 200 mother-infant pairs in each group, found no differences in frequency of developmental delay between infants born to women with confirmed primary parvovirus B19 infection during pregnancy and infants born to mothers with evidence of preconceptional immunity (Rodis et al, 1998b). Data on long-term neurodevelopmental outcomes for infants who received transfusions in utero because of hydrops secondary to parvovirus B19 infection are still insufficient, but most transfused hydropic fetuses with hemolytic disease appear to do well (Ismail et al, 2001).

### Prevention

If a pregnant woman has a significant exposure to an infectious case of parvovirus B19, she should be counseled regarding the potential risk of infection. Anti–parvovirus IgM and IgG serologic analyses should be performed, and if they show evidence of primary infection, serial fetal ultrasonographic evaluations should be performed. Postexposure passive immunization with immunoglobulin is not currently recommended, because the period of maternal viremia has passed by the time diagnosis with parvovirus B19 infection is made (Boley and Popek, 1993). Efforts are under way to research and develop vaccines to prevent parvovirus B19 infections (Franssila et al, 2001).

Pregnant health care providers should be counseled about the potential risks to the fetus from parvovirus B19 infections and should, at a minimum, wear masks when caring for immunocompromised patients with chronic parvovirus B19 infection or patients with parvovirus B19–induced aplastic crises. Some hospitals exclude pregnant health care providers from caring for these high-risk patients, but this issue remains controversial. Standard droplet precautions should be practiced for patients with transient aplastic crises during hospitalization to avoid transmission to health care providers (AAP, 2003).

## RUBELLA

Rubella virus is a single-stranded RNA virus belonging to the *Togaviridae* family. Humans are the only known natural hosts. Rubella infection, commonly known as *German measles*, usually results in a mild illness in adults and children but can have serious consequences when a fetus is infected. Physicians became aware of the teratogenicity of the rubella virus in 1941, when Gregg made the association of maternal rubella with cataracts in infants. Not until the global pandemic of 1964 to 1965, however, were the multiple manifestations of the congenital rubella syndrome (CRS) fully appreciated and the later consequences well delineated. The capacity to grow the virus in tissue culture led rapidly to the development of vaccines and a reduction in the incidence of congenital disease, at least in the United States and other developed countries. The United States has established the goal of elimination of indigenous rubella infections by the year 2010 (U.S. Department of Health and Human Services, 2000).

### Incidence

Since the availability of rubella vaccine in 1969, the incidence of rubella in the United States has significantly decreased. The annual incidence of rubella cases has dropped 99%, from 58 per 100,000 population in 1969 to less than 0.5 per 100,000 population in 1997 to 1999 (Danovaro-Holliday et al, 2001). Although the majority of cases in the past occurred in school-aged children, the proportion of cases has shifted since the mid- to late 1990s, with more than 80% occurring in adults. Three fourths of reported rubella infections since 1997 have been in Hispanic persons, and 80% of outbreak-related cases were in foreign-born persons (CDC, 2000).

The number of CRS cases in the United States has dramatically declined, and rubella in people emigrating from Latin America has now contributed a large portion of the cases (Control and prevention of rubella, 2001). From 1997 to 2000, 30 cases of CRS were reported, 23 of which (77%) were infants of mothers born in Latin America or the Caribbean (Danovaro-Holliday et al, 2001). In other parts of the world, where routine rubella immunization has not or has only lately been implemented, CRS continues to contribute significantly to pediatric morbidity and mortality. It is still the most common vaccine-preventable cause of birth anomalies in the world, as more than 100,000 cases of CRS are estimated to occur annually in developing countries (World Health Organization, 2000).

Maternal rubella infection that occurs in the period of time from 1 month before conception through the second trimester may be associated with disease in the infant. The classic findings of congenital rubella predominate with onset of maternal infection during the first 8 weeks of gestation (Miller et al, 1982). Both the risk and severity of fetal infection decline after the first trimester, and the risk of any congenital defects from infection is low after 17 weeks of gestation (Lee and Bowden, 2000). The incidence of congenital rubella defects after maternal rubella infection varies widely among reported series. A study of 1016 women with serologically confirmed rubella infection at different stages of pregnancy who were followed prospectively provides the most useful estimate of the risks of congenital rubella infection (Miller et al, 1982). The frequency of congenital infection after maternal rubella with a rash is 70% to 80% during the first 12 weeks of pregnancy, 30% to 54% at 13 to 14 weeks of gestation, and 10% to 25% at the end of the second trimester (Miller et al, 1982; South and Sever, 1985).

### Etiology and Pathogenesis

Rubella virus is transmitted from person to person via respiratory droplets. Once the oral or nasopharyngeal mucosa are infected, viral replication occurs in both the upper respiratory tract and nasopharyngeal lymphoid tissue. The virus then spreads contiguously to regional lymph nodes and hematogenously to distant sites. Fetal infection is presumed to occur during maternal viremia. The exact mechanism of teratogenesis is unknown, but theories include a virus-induced apoptosis of cells leading to a cytopathic effect and a virus-induced inhibition of cell division. Fetuses infected with rubella demonstrate cellular damage in multiple sites and a non-inflammatory necrosis in target organs, including eyes, heart, brain, and ears (Lee and Bowden, 2000).

Although positive rubella IgG titers should incur immunity, rare cases of documented maternal re-infection (typically subclinical) with rubella have been reported, and the estimated risk is approximately 8% (Morgan-Capner et al, 1991). Approximately 20 cases of CRS after maternal reinfection have been reported in the literature, and none has caused symptomatic CRS when the known re-infection occurred after 12 weeks of gestation (Bullens et al, 2000).

### Clinical Spectrum

Typical illness in adults and children with acquired rubella infection consists of an acute generalized maculopapular rash, fever, and arthralgias, arthritis, or lymphadenopathy. Conjunctivitis is also common. Often a mild prodrome of mild systemic symptoms precedes the rash by 1 to 5 days. The rash classically begins on the face and spreads caudally to the trunk and extremities. Symptoms generally last up to 3 days, and the incubation period ranges from 14 to 21 days.

Infants with congenital rubella are usually born at term but often are of low birth weight. The most common isolated sequela is hearing loss. The next most common findings are heart defects, cataracts, low birth weight, hepatosplenomegaly, and microcephaly. Table 37–5 summarizes the clinical findings for congenital rubella reported to the National Congenital Rubella Syndrome Registry (NCRSR). The triad of deafness, cataracts, and congenital heart disease constitutes the classic syndrome. Approximately one third of the infants in the NCRSR has only one or two defects, but more than 60% show at least three manifestations of the disease. In addition, systemic illness, characterized by purpura, hepatosplenomegaly, jaundice, pneumonia, and meningoencephalitis, can occur. A comparison of the frequency of clinical findings in prospective studies with those in past case series reports reveals a slightly different proportion of outcomes than previously noted. For instance, 45% to 70% of infants have cardiac lesions, including patent ductus arteriosus, peripheral pulmonic stenosis, and valve abnormalities (Reef et al, 2000; Schluter et al, 1998). A variety of other signs may be present. Additional ocular findings are pigmentary retinopathy, microphthalmia, and strabismus. The skin lesions have been described as resembling a "blueberry muffin," and represent extramedullary hematopoiesis within the skin (Brough et al, 1967).

Deafness, the most common manifestation, occurs, along with retinopathy as a consequence of both first and second trimester maternal infections (Miller et al, 1982; Ueda et al, 1979). In a prospective study following pregnant women with confirmed rubella infection by trimester, rubella-associated defects (primarily congenital heart disease and deafness) were observed in nine infants infected before the 11th week. Thirty-five percent of infants (9 of 26) infected between 13 and 16 weeks had deafness alone (Miller et al, 1982). Cataracts occur with maternal rubella before the 60th day after the 1st day of the last menstrual period; heart disease is found almost exclusively when maternal infection is before the 80th day (i.e., first trimester). Among the manifestations that may occur after the newborn period (late-onset disease) are a generalized rash with seborrheic features that may persist for weeks, interstitial pneumonia (either acute or chronic), abnormal hearing from involvement of the organ of Corti, central auditory imperception, and progressive rubella panencephalitis (Franklin and Kelley, 2001; Phelan and Campbell, 1969; Reef et al, 2000; Sever et al, 1985).

A higher than expected incidence of autoimmune diseases, such as thyroid disorders and diabetes mellitus, have also been reported years after the diagnosis of congenital rubella (McEvoy et al, 1988; Reef et al, 2000). Infants with late-onset disease sometimes have immunologic abnormalities, including dysgammaglobulinemia or hypogammaglobulinemia (Hancock et al, 1968; Hayes et al, 1967; Soothill et al, 1966). Others have also observed cellular immunity dysfunction (Fuccillo et al, 1974; South et al, 1975). The principal immunologic problem in late-onset disease may be defective cytotoxic effector cell function, which leads to defective elimination of virus and immune complex disease (Verder et al, 1986), but immunodeficiencies and autoimmune diseases in patients with congenital rubella are poorly understood.

**TABLE 37–5**

**Clinical Characteristics of Congenital Rubella Syndrome in Cases Reported to the National Congenital Rubella Syndrome Registry, United States, 1985 to 1996**

| Clinical Characteristics | No. of Cases | % of Cases |
|---|---|---|
| Heart disease (any congenital) | 86 | 70.5 |
| Patent ductus arteriosus | 62 | 50.8 |
| Pulmonary stenosis | 22 | 18.0 |
| Other congenital heart conditions | 36 | 29.5 |
| Hearing loss | 73 | 59.8 |
| Low birth weight | 70 | 57.4 |
| Very low birth weight (<1500 g) | 15 | 12.3 |
| Low birth weight (1500-2500 g) | 55 | 45.1 |
| Cataracts | 52 | 42.6 |
| Purpura | 45 | 36.9 |
| Hepatomegaly | 43 | 35.2 |
| Splenomegaly | 42 | 34.4 |
| Thrombocytopenia | 41 | 33.6 |
| Microcephaly | 28 | 23.0 |
| Radiolucent bone disease | 24 | 19.7 |
| Jaundice | 18 | 14.8 |
| Mental retardation | 15 | 12.3 |
| Pigmentary retinopathy | 10 | 8.2 |
| Meningoencephalitis | 9 | 7.4 |
| Glaucoma | 4 | 3.3 |

Data from Schluter WW, Reef SE, Redd SC, Dykewicz CA: Changing epidemiology of congenital rubella syndrome in the United States. J Infect Dis 178:636-641, 1998.

### Laboratory Evaluation

All pregnant women who are exposed to rubella should be screened for evidence of previous immunity, and if none is found, they should be tested for rubella IgG and IgM antibodies. A positive IgM titer or a rise in paired IgG titers is indicative of recent infection. Women with such findings should also be evaluated to try to determine the likely gestational age at time of infection in order to assess the potential risk to the fetus (CDC, 2001).

The laboratory diagnosis of congenital rubella can only be made definitively during the first year of life, unless the virus can be recovered later from an affected site, such as the lens. Diagnosis can be made with any one of the following four criteria: (1) positive anti-rubella IgM titer, preferably determined with enzyme immunoassays, but indirect assays are acceptable, (2) a significant rise in rubella IgG titer between acute and convalescent measurements 2 to 3 weeks apart, or persistence of high titers longer than expected from passive maternal antibody transfer; (3) isolation of rubella virus cultured from nasal, blood, throat, urine, or CSF specimens (throat swabs have the best yield), and (4) detection of virus by reverse transcriptase–PCR in specimens from throat swabs, CSF, or cataracts obtained from surgery (CDC, 2001).

The infected infant may excrete the virus for many months after birth despite the presence of neutralizing antibody and, thus, may pose a hazard to susceptible individuals in the environment. Only rarely can the virus be recovered after 1 year of age. An exception to this rule is the cataract, in which the virus may remain for as long as 3 years. In late-onset disease, the virus may also be found in affected skin and lung.

Other laboratory findings are thrombocytopenia, hyperbilirubinemia, and leukopenia. Radiographic findings include large anterior fontanelle, linear areas of radiolucency in the long bones ("celery stalking"), increased densities in the metaphyses, and irregular provisional zones of calcification. The radiographic changes seen in rubella are not pathognomonic of the disease but resemble those seen in other congenital infections, such as cytomegalic inclusion disease.

### Treatment

There is no specific therapy for congenital rubella. Initially, the infant may need general supportive care, such as administration of blood transfusion for anemia or active bleeding, seizure control, and phototherapy for hyperbilirubinemia. Long-term care requires a multidisciplinary approach consisting of occupational and physical therapy, close neurologic and audiologic monitoring, and surgical interventions as needed for cardiac malformations and cataracts.

### Prognosis

The consequences of fetal rubella infection may not be evident at birth. Infection in the first or second trimester may lead to deafness or persistent growth restriction (Miller et al, 1982). Although infection in the third trimester may also lead to intrauterine growth retardation, this growth problem does not persist, suggesting that the mechanism of growth restriction among infants infected in the first or second trimester may be different (Miller et al, 1982). In one study of 123 infants with documented congenital rubella, 85% were not diagnosed until after discharge from the nursery (Hardy, 1973). Communication disorders, hearing defects, some mental or motor retardation, and microcephaly by 1 to 3 years of age were among the major problems that were discovered after the newborn period. A predisposition to inguinal hernias was also noted.

Longitudinal studies of somatic growth show that most infants with congenital rubella remain smaller than average throughout infancy but grow at a normal rate. Stunting of growth was more common after rubella infection in the first 8 weeks of pregnancy than after later infection. Even in the absence of mental retardation, neuromuscular development is commonly abnormal. A study that followed up 29 children without mental retardation found that 25 had other abnormalities; hearing loss, difficulties with balance and gait, learning deficits, and behavioral disturbances were found in more than half of the affected children (Desmond et al, 1978).

### Prevention

There is no effective antiviral therapy against congenital rubella infection, so the most useful practice is to ensure that women who are considering pregnancy are immune to rubella. The Advisory Committee on Immunization Practices recommends screening of all pregnant women for rubella immunity and postpartum vaccination of those who are susceptible (CDC, 1998). Live attenuated rubella virus vaccine is safe and effective (Lepow et al, 1968), although the duration of immunity is uncertain. The vaccine is recommended for children at 12 to 15 months of age and at 4 to 5 years of age. It is also recommended for women of child-bearing age in whom results of both a hemagglutination inhibition antibody test and a pregnancy test are negative. Although no cases of symptomatic congenital rubella infection have been reported as a consequence of vaccination during pregnancy of the more than 500 cases monitored, vaccination is not recommended during pregnancy because of the theoretical hazard to the fetus (Control and prevention of rubella, 2001; Josefson, 2001; Tookey, 2001). A mild rubella-like illness is sometimes seen after immunization, with arthralgia occurring 10 days to 3 weeks after injection. Immunization in the postpartum period has infrequently led to polyarticular arthritis, neurologic symptoms, and chronic rubella viremia (Tingle et al, 1985).

The problem of management of the pregnant woman who is exposed to or who contracts the disease should be resolved after the known risks are weighed. If, at the time of exposure, serum antibody is detectable, the fetus is probably protected. Administration of immunoglobulin will not prevent rubella viremia or infection in the mother. Immunoglobulin may reduce the likelihood of fetal infection but will not eliminate the risk; thus, the CDC does not routinely recommend the use of immunoglobulin to a pregnant woman for postexposure prophylaxis unless she does not wish to terminate the pregnancy under any circumstances (CDC, 2001).

Decisions about the termination of pregnancy should be made only after maternal infection has been proven and should also take into account the risk of rubella-associated damage to the fetus, which is highest when maternal infection occurs during the first 8 weeks of pregnancy.

## LYMPHOCYTIC CHORIOMENINGITIS VIRUS

Lymphocytic choriomeningitis virus (LCMV) is a member of the Arenaviridae family, and rodents are the primary reservoir, primarily mice and hamsters. These rodents are infected asymptomatically in utero, can harbor chronic infection, and can excrete virus in urine, feces, saliva, nasal secretions, milk, and semen for life. Typically, mice remain asymptomatic but hamsters may demonstrate viremia and viruria with variable symptoms (Jahrling and Peters,

1992). Sequelae of human exposure to LCMV ranges from asymptomatic infection to nonspecific, flulike symptoms, and a proportion of infections have neurologic manifestations. LCMV was described as an etiology for congenital infection first in England in 1955, in a 12-day-old infant who died (Komrower et al, 1955) and later in the United States (Barton et al, 1993; Larsen et al, 1993). Because LCMV has only lately been recognized as a source of congenital infection, it is likely underdiagnosed.

### Incidence

Human seroprevalence ranges between less than 1% and 10% worldwide and varies extensively with geographic region (Ambrosio et al, 1994; Childs et al, 1991; Marrie and Saron, 1998; Stephensen et al, 1992). At least one small surveillance study noted a higher prevalence in women (Marrie and Saron, 1998). Lower socioeconomic status and older age are associated with higher seroprevalence. Studies conducted in the 1940s through the 1970s found that approximately 8% to 11% of cases of aseptic meningitis and encephalitis were associated with LCMV virus infection (Meyer et al, 1960; Park et al, 1997b). In temperate climates, human exposure may occur more often during the fall and winter seasons, when rodents move indoors. Several outbreaks have been reported in laboratory personnel working with hamsters and mice (Dykewicz et al, 1992; Hinman et al, 1975; Vanzee et al, 1975). Multiple outbreaks associated with pet hamsters have also been reported in the United States (Biggar et al, 1975; Maetz et al, 1976) and Europe (Brouqui et al, 1995; Deibel et al, 1975).

Congenital infection, however, is rarely reported. A total of 55 cases have been diagnosed worldwide since the first case in 1955, and 27 of those occurred in the United States (Barton and Mets, 2001; Greenhow and Weintrub, 2003). The true frequency of congenital LCMV infection, however, is unknown, because there are no surveillance studies of the disorder. As with other congenital infections, there may be a wide spectrum of disease, including asymptomatic and subclinical or nonspecific infections.

### Etiology and Pathogenesis

Humans acquire LCMV infection from aerosolized particles, bites, or fomite contact with virus excreted from rodents (Jahrling and Peters, 1992). Human-to-human horizontal transmission has not been documented. The pathogenesis of LCMV infection is poorly understood, although it likely involves both cell-mediated and antibody-mediated immunity. Like other arenaviruses, LCMV is not cytopathic. Both animal and in vitro models strongly suggest that disease is an immunopathologic process mediated by the host $CD8^+$ T-cell response (Craighead, 2000). It is also postulated that the high rate of spontaneous mutations allows both variability in pathogenicity and a mechanism of escape from humoral response during the initial phase of infection (Ciurea et al, 2001).

Like other arenaviruses, LCMV replicates either at the site of infection or in corresponding lymph nodes, and then produces a viremia. It is thought that during the viremic stage, the virus travels to parenchymal organs and potentially the CNS. Pathologic findings include lymphocytic infiltration and extramedullary hematopoiesis. In the two congenitally infected infants for whom neuropathology results were available, cerebromalacia, glial proliferation, and perivascular edema were reported (Barton et al, 1993). In adult mice inoculated intracranially with LCMV, subsequent viral proliferation in the ependyma, meninges, or both have been described (Peters, 1997). This viral infiltration, along with the host inflammatory response, may lead to aqueductal stenosis and subsequent hydrocephalus.

### Clinical Spectrum

It is estimated that asymptomatic or mild LCMV infections occur in approximately one third of patients infected. However, the classic presentation of LCMV infection is a nonspecific, "flulike" or "mononucleosis-like" illness that is often biphasic. Symptoms are fever, malaise, nausea, vomiting, myalgias, headache, photophobia, pharyngitis, cough, and adenopathy. After defervescence and resolution of these constitutional symptoms, a second phase of CNS disease may develop. Neurologic manifestations occur in approximately one fourth of infectious episodes and vary from aseptic meningitis to meningoencephalitis. Transverse myelitis, Guillain-Barré syndrome, and deafness have also been reported. Other manifestations are pneumonitis, arthritis, myocarditis, parotitis, and dermatitis. Recovery may take months but does usually occur without sequelae (Craighead, 2000; Peters, 1997).

When LCMV infection occurs during pregnancy, maternal symptoms, when present, typically appear during the first and second trimesters, but only 50% to 60% of mothers of infants diagnosed with LCMV congenital infection recall having symptoms (Wright et al, 1997). Known maternal exposure to rodents is reported in only about one fourth to one half of cases (Barton and Mets, 2001). Typically, exposed women are from rural settings or have substandard housing conditions.

The complete spectrum of disease secondary to congenital LCMV infection is still uncertain, because no prospective surveillance studies of outcome after infection have been performed. Of the cases reported, chorioretinitis is the most common manifestation, present in more than 90% of cases. Other ocular findings are chorioretinal scars, optic atrophy (usually bilateral), nystagmus, esotropia, exotropia, leukocoria, cataracts, and microphthalmia (Barton and Mets, 2001; Brezin et al, 2000; Enders et al, 1999). Some ophthalmologic findings resemble those seen in the lacunar retinopathy of Aicardi syndrome (Wright et al, 1997).

Most infants are born at term, and birth weights are generally appropriate or large for gestational age. Thirty-five percent to 40% of infants reported with congenital LCMV have had microcephaly or macrocephaly at birth (Barton and Mets, 2001). Systemic symptoms are rare, although hepatosplenomegaly and jaundice have been noted. Other individual case report findings are pes valgus, dermatologic findings consistent with staphylococcal scalded-skin syndrome (Wright et al, 1997), spontaneous abortion (Biggar et al, 1975), and intrauterine demise secondary to hydrops fetalis (Enders et al, 1999). It is important to note that because systemic symptoms are typically minimal at birth, diagnosis of LCMV infection often is not made until an affected infant is a few months of age, when microcephaly, macrocephaly, visual loss, or developmental delay may be noted.

### Laboratory Evaluation

Serology is the most reliable and feasible method to diagnose LCMV. In most reports, the diagnosis was established by testing of infant's serum, CSF, or both; in some, maternal serum testing was the key. Testing all three fluids provides the most information. Because of the low baseline population seroprevalence, positive titers for LCMV are much more useful for diagnosis than detection of antibodies to microbes such as CMV and toxoplasmosis. There is a commercially available immunofluorescent antibody (IFA) test that detects both IgM and IgG for LCMV. It has better sensitivity than the complement fixation and neutralizing antibody tests that also have been used (Lehmann-Grube et al, 1979; Lewis et al, 1975). Complement fixation titers generally do not rise until more than 10 days after onset of infection, but IFA results may be positive within the first few days of illness (Deibel et al, 1975). The CDC also has an enzyme-linked immunosorbent assay test for IgM and IgG; it may be more useful for diagnosis in an older child because it can detect increased IgG later than and persistent IgG for longer than the IFA test. Some studies have found antibody as late as 30 years after suspected exposure. Virus can be cultured in Vero cell lines or inoculated into newborn mice, but use of these methods is uncommon. Reverse transcriptase-PCR has been used in serum and CSF to diagnosis LCMV and as a surveillance tool; it may become more available in the future (Enders et al, 1999; Park et al, 1997a).

Information about routine laboratory data in patients diagnosed with congenital LCMV infection is minimal, but thrombocytopenia and hyperbilirubinemia have been reported. CSF findings are variable. Up to one half of cases demonstrate a mild increase in white blood cell count (up to 64 cells/μL in one case series of 18 infants), the serum protein concentration may be normal or mildly elevated, and the serum glucose concentration may be normal or mildly decreased (Wright et al, 1997). Among infants reported in whom neuroradiographic imaging was performed, 89% (17 of 19) had hydrocephalus or intracranial periventricular calcifications. "Flattened gyri" or lissencephaly, schizencephaly, and other findings consistent with a migrational disorder have also been reported (Barton and Mets, 2001).

### Treatment

Therapy for LCMV infection has never been attempted, but ribavirin has been used for management of other arenavirus infections and inhibits LCMV growth in vitro (Géssner and Lother, 1989). No current recommendations can be made regarding the use of antivirals in congenital LCMV infection.

### Prognosis

Because congenital LCMV infections have been recognized relatively recently and the existing data come from case reports, there may be a wider spectrum of disease than is currently appreciated. The proportion of asymptomatic infected infants is unknown. For the 25 infant cases reported, estimated mortality rates are 16% to 35% between birth and 21 months of age (Barton and Mets, 2001; Wright et al, 1997). Among infants who survived, 84% (32 of 38) have neurologic sequelae, including spastic quadriparesis, mental retardation, developmental delay, seizures, and visual loss (Barton and Mets, 2001). Sensorineural hearing loss is less common, and has only been reported in 2 infants (Barton and Mets, 2001; Wright et al, 1997).

Some ophthalmologists suggest that among patients with developmental delay and visual loss consistent with chorioretinitis, LCMV congenital infection may be underdiagnosed. A study in Chicago of prospectively diagnosed patients with chorioretinitis and patients in a home for severely mentally retarded children with chorioretinal scars found six children with elevated LCMV titers and normal toxoplasmosis, CMV, rubella, and HSV titers (Mets et al, 2000). Two children with chorioretinal scars and elevated LCMV titers have been reported in France (Brezin et al, 2000).

### Prevention

Public health officials and clinicians should be aware that (1) wild, laboratory, and pet rodent exposure can lead to intrauterine infection with LCMV virus and (2) congenital infection has been associated with potentially devastating ophthalmologic and neurologic sequelae. Pregnant women need to be educated about the potential risks of exposure to infected rodent excreta and instructed to avoid rodents and rodent droppings whenever possible.

## ENTEROVIRUSES

Enteroviruses are single-stranded RNA viruses belonging to the Picornaviridae family. The enteroviruses of humans include polioviruses 1, 2, and 3, coxsackieviruses A and B, and the echoviruses. Poliovirus infection of newborn infants has become extremely rare. According to early accounts, however, severe, often fatal diseases developed in infants infected in the perinatal period, with a high incidence of paralysis occurring in the survivors (Bates, 1955; Cherry, 1990). This review is limited to consideration of the neonatal diseases associated with coxsackieviruses and echoviruses most commonly seen today.

### Incidence

Enterovirus infections are seasonal, occurring most commonly during the summer and autumn in temperate climates. The incidence varies from year to year, with outbreaks sometimes caused by a single coxsackievirus or echovirus serotype, and sometimes by several (Sawyer et al, 1994). Disease in newborn infants is uncommon but reflects the frequency of infections in the population at large (Krajden and Middleton, 1983). Low socioeconomic status and bottle-feeding have been associated with increased risk of enteroviral infections in newborns (Jenista et al, 1984). Nursery outbreaks of both coxsackievirus B (Brightman et al, 1966; Rantakallio et al, 1970) and echovirus infections (Jankovic et al, 1999; Nagington et al, 1978) have been reported and associated with severe, and sometimes fatal, illnesses.

Enteroviral infections account for at least one third of neonatal febrile admissions for suspected sepsis overall, and for between half and two thirds of admissions during peak enteroviral season (Byington et al, 1999; Dagan, 1996). Neonatal aseptic meningitis is also frequently caused by enteroviral infections. In a review of neonatal meningitis seen over a 15-year period in Galveston, Texas, enterovirus was the most common cause of meningitis in newborn infants older than 7 days and accounted for 33% of all cases of neonatal (<28 days of age) meningitis (Shattuck and Chonmaitree, 1992). Enteroviruses, along with other viruses, have also been implicated as a potential cause of sudden infant death syndrome, possibly from myocarditis or pulmonary infection, but their role is still poorly delineated (Grangeot-Keros et al, 1996; Shimizu et al, 1995).

### Etiology and Pathogenesis

Infection may take place either in utero, intrapartum, or postnatally. Intrauterine infections likely occur transplacentally secondary to maternal viremia. Regardless of whether the mother, a family member, or some other caretaker is the source of the infection, severe disease results more often when the baby lacks antibody to the infecting strain (Jenista et al, 1984). Other potential factors determining severity of disease are the virus strain or serotype and the quantity of the inoculum. It is not clear why the newborn infant is so highly susceptible to overwhelming illness, but growing evidence suggests that lack of type-specific antibody is a crucial factor.

It appears that any of the non-polio enteroviruses can cause disease in the newborn infant. A retrospective chart review of 24 newborn infant enteroviral infections in Toronto found that 10 infants died, 12 had aseptic meningitis, and 5 had myocarditis (Krajden and Middleton, 1983). Of the 24 isolates, 7 were echovirus, 15 were coxsackievirus B, one was coxsackievirus A, and one was nontypable. Types of coxsackievirus B are associated primarily with myocarditis or aseptic meningitis or combinations of the two (Kibrick and Benirschke, 1958). Echoviruses, however, are seen more often with severe nonspecific febrile illnesses with disseminated intravascular coagulation (Nagington et al, 1978), aseptic meningitis (Cramblett et al, 1973), or hepatitis (Modlin, 1980). With both groups of viruses, nonspecific febrile illnesses, with or without a rash, are commonly seen.

Enterovirus infections primarily target the heart, CNS, liver, and adrenal glands. In coxsackievirus B infections, myocardial necrosis and inflammation may be seen that are patchy or diffuse, with extensive infiltration by lymphocytes, mononuclear cells, histiocytes, and some polymorphonuclear leukocytes. Similar infiltrates are seen in the meninges in both coxsackievirus and echovirus infections. When liver or adrenal glands are involved, there is usually extensive hemorrhage as well as inflammation and necrosis.

### Clinical Spectrum

As with many other viruses, most infections with enterovirus are asymptomatic. Well-recognized clinical syndromes associated with enteroviral infections in children include hand-foot-mouth disease, herpangina, aseptic meningitis, and acute hemorrhagic conjunctivitis. Enterovirus infection is also likely to cause a large proportion of nonspecific febrile illness, especially in young infants.

When neonatal disease is acquired vertically from the mother, the infant is characteristically well at birth, although premature delivery is more common in this group. The mother, however, may be febrile at this time or may have a history of recent high fevers and gastrointestinal symptoms. Fever, anorexia, and vomiting develop in the baby after an incubation period of 1 to 5 days. The onset of illness occurs in the first week of life in more than 50% of affected infants (Krajden and Middleton, 1983). At that point, the clinical evolution depends on the infecting virus and the extent of involvement.

In most instances, the disease is mild and self-limited. A rash may appear in some infants, and aseptic meningitis in others. A review of 29 infants with enteroviral infections younger than 2 weeks old reported that 5 of 29 infants had severe multisystem disease, and all survived (Abzug et al, 1993). In severe disseminated disease, disseminated intravascular coagulation (DIC), refractory hypotension, and death may follow quickly. If myocarditis is present, the liver rapidly enlarges, the heart dilates, and the heart sounds become muffled. However, in many infants, myocardial involvement is temporary, and recovery occurs over the course of several weeks.

The severity of CNS infection is also variable. Enteroviruses can produce overwhelming meningoencephalitis, sometimes with cranial nerve signs. It is more common, however, to see moderate or mild meningitis characterized by temporary irritability, lethargy, fever, and feeding difficulty.

Some infections, particularly those with echoviruses, are characterized by a rampant and overwhelming hepatitis (Modlin, 1980). Others exhibit primarily pulmonary disease or gastrointestinal involvement including diarrhea and necrotizing enterocolitis (Lake et al, 1976). Intracranial bleeding ranging from small, grade I to massive, severe hemorrhage has also been reported as a complication of neonatal enteroviral infection (Abzug, 2001; Abzug and Johnson, 2000; Swiatek, 1997). Other, rarely associated findings include disseminated vesicular rash, dermal hematopoiesis, and hemophagocytic syndrome (Barre et al, 1998; Bowden et al, 1989; Sauerbrei et al, 2000).

Acquired postnatal enteroviral disease in infants is characterized primarily by high fever, irritability, lethargy, or poor feeding. One fourth of infected infants presents with diarrhea or vomiting with or without an erythematous maculopapular rash. Mild conjunctivitis has also been observed. Respiratory tract symptoms are less common (Dagan, 1996). Unfortunately, there is significant overlap between enteroviral and bacterial neonatal infections, and the two syndromes are difficult to distinguish. Duration of illness varies from less than 24 hours to longer than 7 days but generally lasts 3 to 4 days.

### Laboratory Evaluation

Viral culture from stool or rectal swab, nasopharyngeal swab, blood, buffy coat, urine, or CSF remains a reliable diagnostic test. Stool or rectal swab and respiratory tract cultures have the highest yield. Cultures usually become positive within a few days and most often within 1 week (Dagan, 1996). The wider availability of PCR analysis provides greater sensitivity and more rapid results, especially when performed on CSF. PCR may also be performed on serum or mononuclear cell suspension (Prather et al, 1984). Serologic tests for enteroviruses have been reported but are less useful than culture and PCR (Swanink et al, 1993).

Infants with meningitis typically have moderate CSF pleocytosis. Thrombocytopenia, elevated transaminase values, hyperbilirubinemia, hyperammonemia, hematologic abnormalities consistent with disseminated intravascular coagulation, anemia, peripheral leukocytosis, and abnormal chest radiographs are among other potential laboratory findings. The echocardiogram and electrocardiogram may show diffuse myocardial inflammation. Liver biopsies have been performed in severe cases, and usually, viral cultures of the specimens are negative (Abzug, 2001).

### Treatment

The manifestations of myocarditis and heart failure must be treated with slow digitalization, diuretics, aggressive fluid management, and other supportive measures. Disseminated intravascular coagulation should be treated with vitamin K, fresh frozen plasma, platelets, and other supportive measures as indicated. Both plasma infusions (including maternal plasma transfusion) and exchange transfusions have been attempted in overwhelming enterovirus infections, with unclear beneficial effects (Jantausch et al, 1995). There is no evidence that steroids are of benefit.

IVIG has anecdotally been reported to treat neonatal enteroviral infections with various results (Kimura et al, 1999; Valduss et al, 1993). Only one randomized trial has systematically studied its use, in 16 neonates with severe enteroviral infection. Decreased viremia and viruria along with faster resolution of irritability, jaundice, and diarrhea was demonstrated in patients administered IVIG with high titers of neutralizing enteroviral-specific antibodies. However, there were no significant differences in other major clinical outcomes, such as duration of hospitalization, fever, and symptoms of acute illness between treatment and control groups (Abzug et al, 1995). Although further investigation with larger numbers of patients are needed, routine use of IVIG for neonatal enterovirus infections cannot be recommended at this time.

The antiviral drug pleconaril has been developed specifically to treat picornavirus infections (enteroviruses and rhinoviruses). Data in neonates are limited, but one center has reported that two of three treated infants with severe enteroviral hepatitis survived (Aradottir et al, 2001). The Pleconaril Treatment Registry Group reported that five of six neonates with severe enteroviral infection who were treated with pleconaril survived, with minimal or no sequelae (Rotbart and Webster, 2001). A multicenter study of pleconaril treatment for neonatal enteroviral meningitis sponsored by the National Institutes of Health showed disappointing results (Abzug et al, 2003). The drug is not currently licensed or used for the treatment of enteroviral infections.

### Prognosis

Prognostic factors for severe neonatal disease include peripartum maternal illness, earlier age of onset of neonatal disease, absence of serotype-specific antibody, and absence of fever and irritability (Abzug et al, 1993). All of these risk factors are most consistent with vertical intrauterine enteroviral infection rather than acquired infection.

By the time disseminated intravascular coagulation has developed, the prognosis is grave. Prothrombin time longer than 30 seconds was a risk factor for death in one retrospective case review (Abzug, 2001). Highest mortality rates are associated with the combination of severe hepatitis, coagulopathy, and myocarditis. Severe hepatitis due to enteroviral infection is associated with mortality rates ranging from 30% to 80% (Abzug, 2001; Modlin, 1986).

Few long-term follow-up studies have been published, but the available information suggests that infants who survive severe enteroviral neonatal disease have a complete recovery in most instances. Outcomes of 6 of 11 survivors with follow-up ranging from 9 to 48 months reported normal growth and no residual medical problems or liver dysfunction (Abzug, 2001).

The prognosis after CNS involvement is also unclear. Most patients do well. A number of early studies of infants younger than 3 months with aseptic meningitis suggested that there may be some impairment of intellectual development in comparison with carefully selected control groups (Farmer et al, 1975; Sells et al, 1975). However, in a series of nine children with enteroviral meningitis and nine matched controls evaluated for sequelae at approximately 4 years of age, no differences in mean IQ level, head circumference, detectable sensorineural hearing loss, or intellectual functioning were detected. Receptive language functioning of the meningitis group was significantly less than that in control subjects (Wilfert et al, 1981). A similar case-control follow-up study of 33 subjects, who were compared with siblings used as controls, reported no neurodevelopmental sequelae (Bergman et al, 1987).

### Prevention

Anecdotal reports of the use of IVIG in nursery outbreaks to prevent further horizontal transmission of enteroviral infection produce conflicting results (Carolane et al, 1985; Kinney et al, 1986; Nagington et al, 1983). Because there are multiple non-polio enteroviral serotypes that cause clinical disease, development of anti-enteroviral immunization is difficult. Standard contact precautions should be used for the treatment of hospitalized infants with known or suspected enteroviral infections (AAP, 2003).

## VIRAL HEPATITIS

There are now six distinct viruses known to cause viral hepatitis—hepatitis A, B, C, D (delta), E, and G viruses—although only B and C are of major importance in the newborn. The main features of each virus type are listed in Table 37–6 (Krugman, 1992). Hepatitis A virus (HAV) is passed by fecal-oral transmission and is a rare cause of neonatal disease, although it has been nosocomially transmitted in the setting of a neonatal intensive care unit. Hepatitis E virus (HEV) is similar to hepatitis A in its mode of transmission and clinical manifestations, except for an increased mortality in hepatitis E–infected pregnant women. There are no data regarding perinatal transmission of hepatitis E. Hepatitis D virus (HDV) may cause only co-infection or super-infection with hepatitis B virus. Its only clinical significance is that hepatitis B infection may become more severe when hepatitis D virus is present. Perinatal transmission is uncommon (AAP, 2003).

Hepatitis G virus (HGV), also known as GB virus type C (GBV-C), has been associated with acute and chronic hepatitis and usually is noted as a co-infection with hepatitis B or C. Perinatal transmission can occur in 60% to 80% of infants born to HGV-viremic mothers, but of infants studied for up to 2 years, none has demonstrated clinical hepatitis attributed to the HGV infection (Ohto et al, 2000; Wejstal et al, 1999; Zanetti et al, 1998; Zuin et al, 1999). The clinical

**TABLE 37–6**

**Viral Hepatitis Types A, B, C, D, E, and G: Comparison of Clinical, Epidemiologic, and Immunologic Features**

| Feature | Hepatitis A | Hepatitis B | Hepatitis C | Hepatitis D (delta) | Hepatitis E | Hepatitis G/GB Virus Type C |
|---|---|---|---|---|---|---|
| Virus | Hepatitis A virus (HAV) | Hepatitis B virus (HBV) | Hepatitis C virus (HCV) | Hepatitis D virus (HDV) | Hepatitis E virus (HEV) | Hepatitis G virus (HGC) (GB virus type C [GBV-C]) |
| Family | Picornavirus | Hepadnavirus | Flavivirus | Satellite | Calicivirus | Flavivirus |
| Genome | RNA | DNA | RNA | RNA | RNA | RNA |
| Incubation period | 15-40 days | 50-180 days | 1-5 mos | 2-8 wks | 2-9 wks | Unknown |
| Mode of transmission | | | | | | |
| Oral (fecal) | Usual | No | No | No | Usual | No |
| Parenteral | Rare | Usual | Usual | Usual | No | Usual |
| Perinatal | Rare | Yes | Yes | Only with HBV | Unknown | Yes |
| Other | Food- or water-borne | Sexual contact | Sexual contact less common | Sexual contact less common | Water-borne transmission in developing countries | Sexual contact; probably less common |
| Sequelae | | | | | | |
| Carrier state | No | Yes | Yes | Yes | No | Yes |
| Chronic disease | No cases reported | Yes | Yes | Yes | No cases reported | Yes; controversial |

Data from Krugman S: Viral hepatitis: A, B, C, D, and E—prevention. Pediatr Rev 13:245-247, 1992.

significance and impact of HGV infection are still poorly understood. Hepatitis B and C viruses are both transmitted vertically and are the primary focus of this discussion.

## Hepatitis B

The issues that are most important to neonatologists are the frequency with which hepatitis B virus (HBV) is transmitted to infants at the time of birth, the short-term and long-term consequences of these infections, the importance of greater surveillance for maternal carriage of HBV, and the availability of effective HBV immunoprophylaxis (Krugman, 1988).

### Incidence

In certain parts of the world and among certain ethnic groups, as many as 7% to 10% of all infants acquire hepatitis B infections at the time of birth, and almost all of these infections become chronic. In the United States, approximately 20,000 infants are born annually to mothers who are chronic HBV carriers (Mast et al, 1998). The frequency of transmission depends primarily on the prevalence of the hepatitis B carrier state among women of child-bearing age. The relationship of these infections to chronic liver failure and hepatic carcinoma in adult life has been noted (Balistreri, 1988; Beasley and Hwang, 1984).

The incidence of neonatal hepatitis B infection depends on a number of factors. Women with acute hepatitis B infection during the first or second trimester rarely transmit the virus to their infants (Krugman, 1988; Stevens, 1994). The carriage rate for hepatitis B surface antigen (HBsAg) varies from 0.1% in the United States and Europe to 15% in Taiwan and parts of Africa, with intermediate rates in Japan, South America, and Southeast Asia. Transmission rates among immigrant women in Western countries appear to parallel the rates in their countries of origin (Krugman, 1988).

Another factor is the potential of the infection to be transmitted from the mother at the time of delivery. The likelihood of transmission is great if symptomatic acute disease is present (60% to 70% transmission) (Gerety and Schweitzer, 1977). Infants of hepatitis B e antigen (HBeAg)–positive mothers have an 80% to 90% chance of becoming HBsAg carriers (Okada et al, 1976). Chronic neonatal infection occurs in less than 10% of infants of HBeAg antigen–negative mothers (Krugman, 1988). The serologic and biochemical courses of subclinical infection are outlined in Figure 37–5. Although HBsAg has been found in breast milk, breast-feeding does not appear to have any influence, either positive or negative, on the rate of transmission (Beasley et al, 1975).

### Etiology and Pathogenesis

HBV is a DNA virus that localizes primarily in hepatic parenchymal cells but circulates in the bloodstream, along with several subviral antigens, for periods ranging from a few days to many years. Transplacental leakage of HBeAg-positive maternal blood is a potential source of intrauterine infection (Lin et al, 1987). During either acute or persistent viremia in the mother, the virus itself or viral antigens may rarely cross the placenta and cause intrauterine infection, or more commonly, infection may occur perinatally during labor or delivery (Chisari and Ferrari, 1995; Xu et al, 2001). Most infants born to mothers

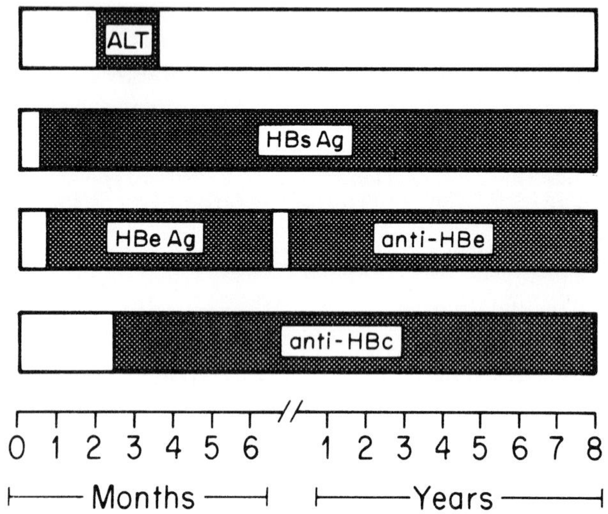


**FIGURE 37–5.** Serologic and biochemical courses of subclinical hepatitis B infection progressing to asymptomatic chronic carrier state. ALT, alanine aminotransaminase; anti-HBc, antibody to hepatitis B core antigen; anti-HBe, antibody to hepatitis B e antigen; HBeAg, hepatitis B e antigen; HBsAg, hepatitis B surface antigen. *(From Krugman S: Hepatitis B virus and the neonate. Ann N Y Acad Sci 549:129, 1988.)*

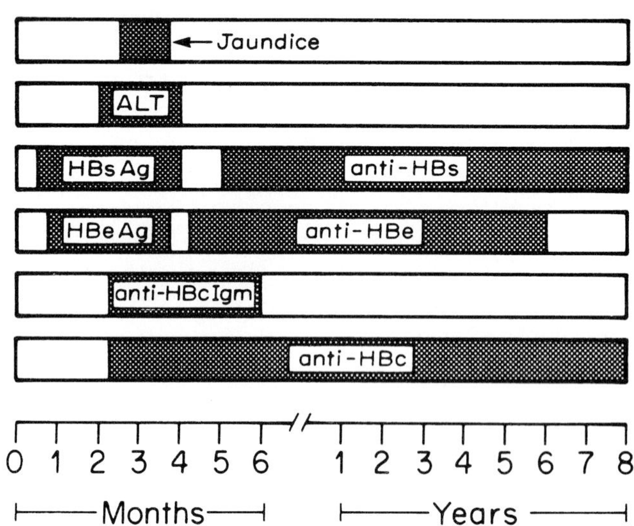


**FIGURE 37–6.** Chemical, serologic, and biochemical courses of acute hepatitis B infection followed by recovery. ALT, alanine aminotransaminase; anti-HBc, antibody to hepatitis B core antigen; anti-HBcIgm, immunoglobulin M antibody to hepatitis B core antigen; anti-HBe, antibody to hepatitis B e antigen; anti-HBs, antibody to hepatitis B surface antigen; HBeAg, hepatitis B e antigen; HBsAg, hepatitis B surface antigen. *(From Krugman S: Hepatitis B virus and the neonate. Ann N Y Acad Sci 549:129, 1988.)*

infected with HBV test negative for HBsAg at birth and, in the absence of prophylaxis, become HBsAg-positive during the first 3 months of life, suggesting that transmission is primarily peripartum (Krugman, 1988, 1992; Mulligan and Stiehm, 1994; Shapiro, 1993).

### Clinical Spectrum and Laboratory Evaluation

Infants with hepatitis B infection do not show clinical or chemical signs of disease at birth. Without immunoprophylaxis, the usual pattern is the development of chronic antigenemia with mild and often persistent enzyme elevations, beginning at 2 to 6 months of age (Mulligan and Stiehm, 1994). Less commonly, the infection becomes clinically manifest, with jaundice, fever, hepatomegaly, and anorexia, followed by either recovery or chronic active hepatitis. Rarely, fulminant hepatitis is seen and can be fatal (Delaplane et al, 1983).

Laboratory tests are essential in the diagnosis of hepatitis B infection. Evaluations of serum enzymes and of bilirubin reflect the extent of liver damage. Several helpful serologic tests identify the virus involved (Krugman, 1988) (Fig. 37–6 and Table 37–7). HBsAg appears early, usually before liver disease is found; it persists in those who become chronic carriers or disappears in the 5% of infants who resolve the infection. HBeAg and antibody against HBeAg (anti-HBe) testing can be employed to assess infectivity but are rarely used clinically.

### Prevention

For immunoprophylaxis to be successful, maternal screening is important (Cruz et al, 1987; Summers et al, 1987). The U.S. Public Health Service's Advisory Committee on Immunization Practices (ACIP) and the ACOG have recommended routine screening of all pregnant women (CDC, 1991; Guidelines for hepatitis B screening, 1993). In developing countries, such a strategy is neither feasible nor affordable. In areas where hepatitis B virus infection is hyperendemic, all newborn infants should be routinely immunized (Hsu et al, 2001).

In 1991, the ACIP recommended that universal childhood vaccination against hepatitis B virus begin in the neonatal period, with the intention of eliminating transmission of HBV in the United States (CDC, 1991). Hepatitis B vaccination is recommended for all infants, whether their mothers test HBsAg negative or positive. For infants born to HBsAg-negative mothers, the three-dose vaccination schedule should be initiated in the neonatal period or by 2 months of age (Table 37–8). The second dose is given 1 to 2 months after the first dose, and the third dose at 6 to 18 months of age (AAP, 2003). Vaccination may be delayed until just before hospital discharge in preterm (birth weight less than 2000 g) infants born to HBsAg-negative mothers.

All infants born to HBsAg-positive women should receive both active and passive immunization within 12 hours of birth. The dosage amounts of the two hepatitis B vaccines currently licensed in the United States are given in Table 37–9. If maternal HBsAg status is unknown, it should be checked immediately, and the infant should receive the first dose of HBV vaccine immediately. Infants of women who test positive should be given hepatitis B immune globulin (HBIG) as soon as possible and within 1 week after birth (AAP, 2003). The highest immunization failure rate (3 of 21 infants, or 14%) has been observed in infants of HBeAg-positive women and those infected in utero (Farmer et al, 1987; Tang et al, 1998). It is recommended that infants born to HbsAg-positive mothers undergo postimmunization testing for anti-HBS and HbsAg 3 to 9 months after completion of the series,

TABLE 37-7

**Diagnostic Tests for Hepatitis B Virus (HBV) Antigens and Antibodies**

| Factor to Be Tested | Hepatitis B Virus Antigen or Antibody | Use |
|---|---|---|
| HBsAg | Hepatitis B surface antigen | Detection of acutely or chronically infected persons<br>Antigen used in hepatitis B vaccine |
| Anti-HBs | Antibody to HBsAg | Identification of persons who have resolved infection with HBV<br>Determination of immunity after immunization |
| HBeAg | Hepatitis B e antigen | Identification of infected persons at increased risk for transmitting HBV |
| Anti-HBe | Antibody to HBeAg | Identification of infected persons with lower risk for transmitting HBV |
| Anti-HBc | Antibody to HBcAg* | Identification of persons with acute, resolved, or chronic HBV infection (not present after immunization) |
| Immunoglobulin M (IgM) anti-HBc | IgM antibody to HBcAg | Identification of acute or recent HBV infection (including those in HBsAg-negative persons during the "window" phase of infection) |

*No test is commercially available to measure hepatitis B core antigen (HBcAg).

Modified from and used with permission of the American Academy of Pediatrics: Hepatitis B. In Pickering JL, ed: *2003 Red Book: Report of the Committee on Infectious Diseases*. 26th ed. Elk Grove Village, IL: American Academy of Pediatrics, 2003, p 322.

for identification of breakthrough carriers and of infants who may benefit from revaccination (CDC, 1991).

### Treatment

There is no therapy for acute hepatitis B infection. Interferon (IFN-α) and antiretroviral drugs such as lamivudine, an antiretroviral drug that blocks HBV polymerase, have been approved for treatment of chronic hepatitis B in children, but success is widely variable. Based on small studies, lamivudine treatment results in clearance of HBeAg in 23%-37.5% of HBV-infected children followed for 6-12 months, but relapse and drug resistance remain important concerns (Hagmann, 2003; Jonas, 2002). Studies investigating the use and efficacy of adefovir dipivoxil for HBV treatment in pediatrics are currently under way (Rosenthal, 2003).

### Prognosis

Most long-term follow-up studies have shown that children vaccinated at birth have high levels of protection until at least 5 years of age. Approximately 5% to 10% of infants born to HbeAg-positive mothers become chronic HBV carriers despite combined active and passive immunoprophylaxis with HBIG and HBV vaccine (Kato et al, 1999). Failure of immunoprophylaxis may be associated with the level of maternal viremia and specific HBV genetic variants (Ngui et al, 1998). Infants who become infected with HBV perinatally have a 90% risk of chronic infection, and 15% to 25% of those with chronic infection die of HBV-related liver disease (primarily hepatocellular carcinoma) as adults (CDC, 1991).

## Hepatitis C

In 1989, hepatitis C virus (HCV) was found to be the main cause of non-A, non-B, parenterally transmitted hepatitis; subsequently, HCV has been found to account for a significant portion of the cases of sporadic acute and chronic hepatitis (Weiss and Persing, 1995). Vertically transmitted hepatitis C infection in infants is associated with a higher rate of chronic hepatitis but less liver injury compared with adult HCV infections (Tovo et al, 2000).

### Incidence

The seroprevalence for anti-HCV antibody in pregnant women ranges from 0.7% to 4.4% worldwide (Conte et al, 2000). In the United States, seroprevalence in pregnant women and the general population is estimated to be 1% to 2% (AAP, 2003). Forty percent to 50% of women with HCV have no identified known risk factors for infection (Bortolotti et al, 1998). The vertical transmission rate of HCV is approximately 5% to 11% from HIV-negative mothers and ranges from 10% to 20% from mothers co-infected with HIV (Hillemanns et al, 2000; Palomba et al, 1996; Polywka et al, 1997; Tajiri et al, 2001). One study has shown, in a multivariate analysis, that higher risk of vertical transmission is related more to maternal use of injection drugs than to HIV infection itself, although the mechanism for this finding is still unclear (Resti et al, 2002). The risk of HCV infection from transfused blood after the advent of HCV screening is estimated to be less than 1 in 1 million units transfused (AAP, 2003).

**TABLE 37-8**

**Recommended Schedule of Hepatitis B Immunoprophylaxis to Prevent Perinatal Transmission**

| Vaccine Dose* and HBIG | Age |
|---|---|
| Infant born to mother known to be HBsAg-positive | |
| First dose | Birth (within 12 hrs) |
| HBIG† | Birth (within 12 hrs) |
| Second dose | 1-2 mos |
| Third dose | 6 mos |
| Infant born to mother not screened for HBsAg | |
| First dose‡ | Birth (within 12 hrs) |
| HBIG† | If mother is found to be HBsAg-positive, give 0.5 mL as soon as possible, not later than 1 wk after birth |
| Second dose | 1-2 mos |
| Third dose | 6-18 mos§ |

*See Table 37–9 for appropriate vaccine dose.

†HBIG (0.5 mL) given intramuscularly at a site different from that used for vaccine.

‡First dose is same as that for infant of HBsAg-positive mother. Subsequent doses and schedules are determined by maternal HBsAg status.

§Infants of HBsAg positive mothers should be vaccinated at 6 mos.

HBIG, hepatitis B immune globulin; HBsAg, hepatitis B surface antigen.

Modified from and used with permission of the American Academy of Pediatrics: Hepatitis B. In Pickering JL, ed: *2003 Red Book: Report of the Committee on Infectious Diseases*. 26th ed. Elk Grove Village, IL: American Academy of Pediatrics, 2003, p 333.

## Etiology and Pathogenesis

HCV is less efficiently transmitted by sexual contact than HBV. Risk factors for HCV infection include transfusion, intravenous drug use, frequent occupational exposure to blood products, and household or sexual contact with an infected person (Weiss and Persing, 1995). Lots of IVIG contaminated with HCV were reported between April 1993 and February 1994, but since that time, routine screening for HCV with PCR and application of a viral inactivation process during manufacturing have been implemented to reduce the risk of transmission (AAP, 2003; Schiff, 1994).

Transmission of HCV from mother to child is thought to occur either in utero or at the time of delivery and rarely by breast-feeding. Viral genotypes and infection and replication in maternal peripheral blood monocytes may also affect the ability of the virus to infect the fetus or newborn (Azzari et al, 2000; Zuccotti et al, 1995). Data regarding the correlation of HCV RNA titer in the mother with the risk of vertical transmission are conflicting, although most studies have reported an association (Conte et al, 2000; Lynch-Salamon and Combs, 1992; Ohto et al, 1994; Resti et al, 1998; Tajiri et al, 2001). The effect of vaginal delivery versus cesarean section also remains controversial (Gibb et al, 2000; Paccagnini et al, 1995).

Transmission of HCV via breast milk has not been demonstrated conclusively, but HCV can be found in breast milk and colostrum (Gurakan et al, 1994; Zimmermann et al, 1995). Hepatitis C viral titers in the breast milk of infected women, when found, are typically much lower than in the serum, but variability of levels may correlate with maternal viremia (Kumar and Shahul, 1998; Lin et al, 1995). In a study following 65 HCV antibody–positive women and their exclusively breast-fed infants, 5 of the mothers became symptomatic with correlating higher HCV-RNA titers during or soon after delivery. The infants of all 5 of these women tested negative on HCV-RNA PCR at birth, but three became symptomatic and HCV-RNA positive by 3 months of age. The investigators of this study suggest that the higher viral load in the mothers may have raised the risk of transmission to the infants during breast-feeding (Kumar and Shahul, 1998). Other smaller studies have reported rare to no HCV transmission when infected mothers breast-feed their infants (Fischler et al, 1996; Polywka et al, 1999). Studies comparing breast-fed and bottle-fed infants born to HCV-infected mothers have not shown a statistically significant difference in vertical transmission, but both were small studies with sample sizes possibly insufficient for detection of a low level of transmission (Lin et al, 1995; Resti et al, 1998). No large, prospective studies have been performed to clarify whether breast-feeding is an independent mode of vertical transmission of HCV, so the topic remains controversial. Although HCV-RNA has also been described in saliva, cord blood, and amniotic fluid, the role of these fluids in vertical transmission is still uncertain (Delamare et al, 1999; Ogasawara et al, 1993).

## Clinical Spectrum and Laboratory Evaluation

Acquired HCV infection typically causes jaundice in one third of cases and significant increases in alanine aminotransferase (ALT) in almost all persons infected. Most neonates perinatally infected with HCV do not show clinical symptoms or at most have hepatomegaly. They may have elevated liver ALT either briefly or intermittently. The increases in ALT values, when tested, are most commonly noted between 3 and 6 months of age. HCV-RNA PCR results may be negative initially at birth or within the first few days of life but typically become positive by 1 to 2 weeks of age and remain so until at least 5 years of age. Highest sensitivity of PCR is reported to be after 1 month of age (Gibb et al, 2000; Thomas et al, 1997). Confirmatory serologic anti-HCV IgG antibody tests should be delayed until exposed infants are at least 15 to 18 months old, when at least 99% will have cleared maternal antibody (Dunn et al, 2001). Before 18 months of age, only a positive HCV PCR result can confirm diagnosis of neonatal infection; positive anti-HCV IgG results may still be due to passively acquired maternal antibody. IgM assays are not available or reliable for perinatal diagnosis of HCV. Liver ultrasonographic findings are usually normal or may consist of a mild diffuse increase in echogenicity. Liver biopsies, when performed, typically demonstrate mild to moderate chronic persistent hepatitis (Palomba et al, 1996; Tovo et al, 2000).

**TABLE 37–9**

**Recommended Dosages of Hepatitis Vaccines**

| | Vaccine and Dosage* | |
|---|---|---|
| | **Recombivax HB, μg (mL)†** | **Engerix-B, μg (mL)‡** |
| Infants of HBsAg-negative mothers, children and adolescents younger than 20 yrs | 5 (0.5) | 10 (0.5) |
| Infants of HBsAg-positive mothers (HBIG, 0.5 mL, also is recommended) | 5 (0.5) | 10 (0.5) |
| Adults (20 yrs or older) | 10 (1.0) | 20 (1.0) |
| Patients undergoing dialysis and other immunosuppressed adults | 40 (1.0)§ | 40 (2.0)¶ |

*Both vaccines are administered in a 3- or 4-dose schedule; 4 doses may be administered if a birth dose is given and a combination vaccine is used to complete the series. Only single-antigen hepatitis B vaccine can be used for the birth dose. Single-antigen or combination vaccine containing hepatitis B vaccine may be used to complete the series.

†Available from Merck & Co Inc, West Point, PA. A 2-dose schedule, administered at 0 mo and then 4 to 6 mo later, is available for adolescents 11 to 15 years of age using the adult dose of Recombivax HB (10 μg). In addition, a combination of hepatitis B (Recombivax, 5 μg) and *Haemophilus influenzae* type b (PRP-OMP) vaccine is licensed for use at 2, 4, and 12 to 15 months of age (Comvax).

‡Available from GlaxoSmithKline Biologicals, Rixensart, Belgium. The U.S. Food and Drug Administration has licensed this vaccine for use in an optional 4-dose schedule at 0, 1, 2, and 12 mo of age.

a) In addition, a combination of hepatitis B (Engerix-B, 20 μg) and hepatitis A (Havrix, 720 ELU) vaccine (Twinrix) is licensed for use in people 18 years of age and older in a 3-dose schedule administered at 0, 1, and 6 or more months later.
b) Also, a combination of diphtheria and tetanus toxoids and acellular pertussis (DTaP), inactivated poliovirus (IPV), and hepatitis B (Engerix-B, 10μg) is licensed for use in people from 6 weeks through 6 years of age in a 3-dose schedule administered preferably at 2, 4, and 6 months of age (Pediarix [GlaxoSmithKline Biologicals, Rixensart, Belgium]). For additional information, see Pertussis (p 479).

§Special formulation for patients undergoing dialysis.

¶Two 1.0-mL doses given in 1 site in a 4-dose schedule at birth and ages 1, 2, and 6-12 mos.

HBIG, hepatitis B immune globulin; HBsAg, hepatitis B surface antigen

Modified from and used with permission of the American Academy of Pediatrics: Hepatitis B. In Pickering JL, ed: *2003 Red Book: Report of the Committee on Infectious Diseases*. 26th ed. Elk Grove Village, IL: American Academy of Pediatrics, 2003, p 325.

### Treatment

Interferon and ribavirin are both approved by the U.S. Food and Drug Administration (FDA) to treat adults and children with chronic hepatitis C. Only 10% to 25% of adults treated with interferon have a sustained remission of disease (Bonkovsky and Woolley, 1999). Treatment with a combination of interferon and ribavirin achieves remission in closer to half of treated adults (Cornberg et al, 2002). Data on the use of these agents in infants and children are limited, and these therapies are not approved by the FDA for use in patients younger than 18 years. In Europe, Tovo and colleagues (2000) reported treating four pediatric patients with interferon for 1 year; viremia decreased to undetectable levels during treatment in all four patients, but two patients became viremic again once the treatment was stopped. Interferon therapy is still available only parenterally and is associated with significant side effects; thus, further research into its utility in pediatric HCV infection is needed.

Infants and children with persistent elevations in liver transaminases should be referred to a pediatric gastroenterologist for evaluation and management. The necessity for, as well as the frequency of, screening tests of liver function has not been established.

### Prognosis

In about one third of HCV-infected adults, chronic HCV infection leads to cirrhosis or liver failure within 20 years or hepatic cancer 20 to 30 years after infection (Iwarson et al, 1995). There are limited data regarding long-term follow-up in HCV-infected infants, but existing knowledge indicates that most children remain viremic until at least 5 to 6 years of age, and most develop chronic, persistent hepatitis. Studies monitoring infected children beyond 6 years of age have not been completed, but they are at risk for cirrhosis and, theoretically, hepatocellular carcinoma. Transient hepatitis C viremia with subsequent resolution has been reported (Padula et al, 1999; Ruiz-Extremera et al, 2000; Zanetti et al, 1995). All of the infants who have been followed up for an average of 3 to 4 years have been reported to have normal growth and development (Tovo et al, 2000). Concern has also emerged regarding the potential induction of autoimmune disorders by HCV.

### Prevention

There is currently no vaccine for hepatitis C, although research is under way. Like all other infants, infants with HCV should receive routine hepatitis B immunization. In addition, they should receive hepatitis A vaccination at 2 years of age. Parents should be advised to avoid unnecessary administration of medicines known to be hepatotoxic. Standard precautions are recommended for the hospitalized infant.

## RESPIRATORY VIRUSES

Any one of the large number of respiratory viruses can cause symptomatic respiratory disease in newborn infants. The association has been described for rhinoviruses, adenoviruses, parainfluenza viruses, influenza virus, and respiratory syncytial virus. Adenovirus, rhinovirus, and parainfluenza virus infections are generally characterized by mild rhinorrhea in neonates. All of these viruses, however, may at times cause clinical symptoms indistinguishable from those of bacterial infection, leading to increased diagnostic testing and unnecessary antibiotic treatment. Influenza virus infections are usually mild, but in the absence of maternally transmitted antibody, they can be life-threatening, with severe pneumonia, hypoxia, and a prolonged course.

The most extensive nursery outbreaks, however, have been caused by respiratory syncytial virus (RSV) (Hall et al, 1979; Wilson et al, 1989). Simultaneous outbreaks of RSV and parainfluenza virus type B have also been reported (Meissner et al, 1984).

### Respiratory Syncytial Virus

RSV is the major cause of viral pneumonia and bronchiolitis in infants and children. In temperate climates, it causes large annual epidemics during the cold months. Nosocomial infections are frequent during these times, and illness in the hospital staff is a major factor in its spread from infant to infant. Several nursery outbreaks have been described. In one of these outbreaks, cultures were obtained prospectively so that a full picture of the virus's pathogenicity and epidemiology could be drawn (Hall et al, 1979). Twenty-three of 66 infants hospitalized for 6 or more days were infected. Only 1 was asymptomatic. Clinical manifestations included pneumonia, upper respiratory infection, apneic spells, and nonspecific signs. Pneumonia and apnea were seen almost exclusively in infants older than 3 weeks, and nonspecific signs were most commonly observed in younger infants. Four (17%) infants died, 2 unexpectedly, during the course of infection. Infants in isolettes did not seem to be protected against acquisition of the infection. Eighteen of the 53 nursery personnel were infected during the outbreak; 83% of the infected nursery providers were symptomatic. RSV infection in preterm infants commonly appears to be associated with a new onset of apnea (Bruhn et al, 1977). After discharge from initial hospitalization, risk factors for infant rehospitalization secondary to RSV infection include premature gestational age, chronic lung disease, siblings in daycare or school, chronologic age of less than 3 months, and exposure to tobacco smoke (Carbonell-Estrany and Quero, 2001).

Diagnosis can be confirmed by direct fluorescent antibody (DFA) staining of nasopharyngeal or tracheal aspirate, nasopharyngeal swab, or other respiratory secretions. Culture of RSV may take 3 to 5 days and may be used if DFA staining is not available. The sensitivity of DFA staining for RSV varies from 80% to 90% (AAP, 2003).

Treatment and prevention of RSV infection in infants attracted considerable attention during the 1990s because of the clinical and economic impacts of these infections (Groothuis, 1994; Kinney et al, 1995; Levin, 1994; Meissner, 1994). Considerable debate has ensued concerning the efficacy, safety, and potential effect on health care workers of ribavirin therapy, so its use remains controversial (AAP, 2003; Wald and Dashefsky, 1994). Treatment consists of nebulization of ribavirin by a small-particle aerosol generator supplied by the manufacturer into an oxygen hood, tent, or mask from a solution containing 20 mg of ribavirin per mL of water. The aerosol has been administered on various schedules for 3 to 5 days (e.g., 12 to 20 hours/day). Use of ribavirin in controlled trials has not demonstrated a significant effect on duration of mechanical ventilation, intensive care unit, or hospitalization (Meissner, 2001). Corticosteroids are not effective in the treatment of RSV.

Prevention efforts have focused on passive and active immunization. Standard immune globulin has not been shown to be efficacious for prevention of RSV infection in high-risk infants (Meissner et al, 1993). The efficacy of monthly prophylactic administration of RSV-specific immune globulin (RSV-IG) (750 mg/kg or 150 mg/kg) in 249 infants with cardiac disease or bronchopulmonary dysplasia was examined in a multicenter trial (Groothuis, 1994). In the high-dose (750 mg/kg) group, there were fewer lower respiratory tract infections, hospitalizations, days in hospital, and days in the intensive care unit as well as less use of ribavirin. This therapy requires the placement of an intravenous line and 4 to 6 hours of infusion.

Subsequently, a mouse monoclonal antibody, palivizumab, was developed, which provides similar protection against RSV (Palivizumab,1998). Unlike anti-RSV immune globulin, which is a pooled human blood product, the monoclonal antibody does not confer the theoretical risk of acquiring blood-borne pathogens. Palivizumab is also substantially easier to administer because it is an intramuscular injection.

Recommendations by the American Academy of Pediatrics for the use of palivizumab and RSV-IGIV are as follows:

- Palivizumab or RSV-IGIV prophylaxis should be considered for infants and children younger than 2 years of age with chronic lung disease (CLD) who have required medical therapy (supplemental oxygen, bronchodilator, diuretic, or corticosteroid therapy) for CLD within 6 months before the start of the RSV season. Palivizumab is preferred for most high-risk children because of its ease of administration, safety, and effectiveness. Patients with more severe CLD may benefit from prophylaxis during a second RSV season if they continue to require medical therapy for respiratory or cardiac dysfunction.
- Recommendations for premature infants:
    - Infants born at 32 weeks of gestation or earlier may benefit from RSV prophylaxis, even if they do not have CLD. For these infants, major risk factors to consider include their gestational and chronologic ages at the start of the RSV season.
    - Infants born at 28 weeks of gestation or earlier may benefit from prophylaxis during their first RSV season, whenever that occurs during the first 12 months of life.
    - Infants born at 29 to 32 weeks of gestation may benefit most from prophylaxis up to 6 months of age.
- Most experts recommend that prophylaxis should be reserved for infants born between 32 and 35 weeks of

gestation who are younger than 6 months of age at the start of the RSV season AND two or more of the following risk factors:
    - Child care attendance, school-aged siblings, exposure to environmental air pollutants, congenital abnormalities of the airways, or severe neuromuscular disease.
- Prophylaxis against RSV should be initiated just before onset of the RSV season and terminated at the end of the RSV season. In most seasons and in most regions of the Northern Hemisphere, the first dose of palivizumab should be administered at the beginning of November and the last dose should be administered at the beginning of March, which will provide protection into April.
    - To understand the epidemiology of RSV in their area, physicians should consult with local health departments or diagnostic virology laboratories or the Centers for Disease Control and Prevention if such information is not available locally. Decisions about the specific duration of prophylaxis should be individualized according to the duration of the RSV season. Pediatricians may wish to use RSV rehospitalization data from their own region to assist in the decision-making process.
- Children who are 24 months of age or younger with hemodynamically significant cyanotic and acyanotic congenital heart disease will benefit from 5 monthly intramuscular injections of palivizumab (15 mg/kg).
    - Decisions regarding prophylaxis with palivizumab in children with congenital heart disease should be made on the basis of the degree of physiologic cardiovascular compromise. Infants younger than 12 months of age with congenital heart disease who are most likely to benefit from immunoprophylaxis include:
        - Infants who are receiving medication to control congestive heart failure
        - Infants with moderate to severe pulmonary hypertension
        - Infants with cyanotic heart disease
    - Because a mean decrease in palivizumab serum concentration of 58% was observed after surgical procedures that use cardiopulmonary bypass, for children who still require prophylaxis, a postoperative dose of palivizumab (15 mg/kg) should be considered as soon as the patient is medically stable.
    - The following groups of infants are not at increased risk from RSV and generally should not receive immunoprophylaxis:
        - Infants and children with hemodynamically insignificant heart disease (e.g., secundum atrial septal defect, small ventricular septal defect, pulmonic stenosis, uncomplicated aortic stenosis, mild coarctation of the aorta, and patent ductus arteriosus)
        - Infants with lesions adequately corrected by surgery unless they continue to require medication for congestive heart failure
        - Infants with mild cardiomyopathy who are not receiving medical therapy
    - Dates for initiation and termination of prophylaxis should be based on the same considerations as for high-risk preterm infants. Unlike palivizumab, RSV-IGIV is contraindicated in children with cyanotic congenital heart disease (AAP, 2003; Committee on Infectious Diseases and Committee on the Fetus and Newborn, 2003).

Additional preventive measures for high risk infants include eliminating or minimizing exposure to tobacco smoke, avoidance of crowds and situations in which exposure to infected individuals cannot be controlled, careful hand hygiene education of parents, vaccination against influenza beginning at 6 months of age, and restricted participation in child care during the RSV season whenever feasible.

The prospects for infant or maternal immunization with live attenuated and protein subunit vaccines are under active investigation and development (Piedra, 2000; Crowe, 2001).

Nosocomial spread of RSV and other respiratory viruses can be minimized by emphasis on hand washing by care providers between contacts with patients. Without additional special precautions, an attack rate of approximately 26% has been observed (Madge et al, 1992). Use of standard contact precautions, such as cohort nursing and the use of gowns and gloves for all contacts with RSV-infected children, can reduce the risk of nosocomial RSV infection to 9.5% (Madge et al, 1992).

## GASTROINTESTINAL VIRUSES

The best studied of the viruses that cause diarrhea are the rotaviruses. This important group of viruses, with at least four serotypes, is responsible for a large proportion of significant and sometimes severe diarrhea in infants 6 to 24 months of age (Cohen, 1991; Greenberg et al, 1994; Haffejee, 1991; Taylor and Echeverria, 1993). Nursery-acquired infections are common in parts of the world where they have been sought; surprisingly, such infections appear to be benign in most infants. Two studies performed in nurseries in Sydney, Australia, and in London found that 30% to 50% of 5-day-old babies excreted the virus (Chrystie et al, 1978; Murphy et al, 1977). However, more than 90% of the infected infants were asymptomatic. The remaining symptomatic infants had loose stools and vomiting, but this figure was only slightly higher than the proportion of uninfected infants with the same symptoms.

## REFERENCES


Abzug MJ: Prognosis for neonates with enterovirus hepatitis and coagulopathy. Pediatr Infect Dis J 20:758-763, 2001.

Abzug MJ, Johnson SM: Catastrophic intracranial hemorrhage complicating perinatal viral infections. Pediatr Infect Dis J 19:556-559, 2000.

Abzug MJ, Levin MJ, Rotbart HA: Profile of enterovirus disease in the first two weeks of life. Pediatr Infect Dis J 12: 820-824, 1993.

Abzug MJ, Cloud G, Bradley J, et al: National Institute of Allergy and Infectious Diseases Collaborative Antiviral Study Group. Double blind placebo-controlled trial of pleconaril in infants with enterovirus meningitis. Pediatr Infect Dis J 22:335-341, 2003.

Abzug MJ, Keyserling HL, Lee ML, et al: Neonatal enterovirus infection: virology, serology, and effects of intravenous immune globulin. Clin Infect Dis 20:1201-1206, 1995.

ACOG practice bulletin: Management of herpes in pregnancy. Number 8, October 1999: Clinical management guidelines for obstetrician-gynecologists. Int J Gynaecol Obstet 68:165-173, 2000.

Adler SP: Neonatal cytomegalovirus infections due to blood. Crit Rev Clin Lab Sci 23:1-14, 1986a.

Adler SP: Nosocomial transmission of cytomegalovirus. Pediatr Infect Dis 5:239-246, 1986b.

Alger LS: Toxoplasmosis and parvovirus B19. Infect Dis Clin North Am 11:55-75, 1997.

Alkalay AL, Pomerance JJ, Rimoin DL: Fetal varicella syndrome. J Pediatr 111:320-323, 1987.

Alpert G, Plotkin SA: A practical guide to the diagnosis of congenital infections in the newborn infant. Pediatr Clin North Am 33:465-479, 1986.

Ambrosio AM, Feuillade MR, Gamboa GS, Maiztegui JI: Prevalence of lymphocytic choriomeningitis virus infection in a human population of Argentina. Am J Trop Med Hyg 50:381-386, 1994.

American Academy of Pediatrics, Committee on Infectious Diseases: 2003 Red Book: Report of the Committee on Infectious Diseases, 26th ed. Elk Grove Village, IL, American Academy of Pediatrics, 2003.

Anderson LJ:. Role of parvovirus B19 in human disease. Pediatr Infect Dis J 6:711-718, 1987.

Andreasson B, Svenningsen NW, Nordenfelt E: Screening for viral infections in infants with poor intrauterine growth. Acta Paediatr Scand 70:673-676, 1981.

Aradottir E, Alonso EM, Shulman ST: Severe neonatal enteroviral hepatitis treated with pleconaril. Pediatr Infect Dis J 2):457-459, 2001.

Arvin AM: Relationships between maternal immunity to herpes simplex virus and the risk of neonatal herpesvirus infection. Rev Infect Dis 13(Suppl 11):S953-S596, 1991.

Arvin AM, Prober CG: Analysis of the epidemiology and pathogenesis of herpes simplex virus (HSV) infections in pregnant women and infants using the HSV-2 glycoprotein G antibody assay. Infect Agents Dis 2:375-382, 1993.

Azzari C, Resti M, Moriondo M, et al: Vertical transmission of HCV is related to maternal peripheral blood mononuclear cell infection. Blood 96:2045-2048, 2000.

Balducci J, Rodis JF, Rosengren S, et al: Pregnancy outcome following first-trimester varicella infection. Obstet Gynecol 79:5-6, 1992.

Baldwin S, Whitley RJ: Intrauterine herpes simplex virus infection. Teratology 39:1-10, 1989.

Bale JF Jr, Murph JR, Demmler GJ, et al: Intrauterine cytomegalovirus infection and glycoprotein B genotypes. J Infect Dis 182:933-936, 2000.

Balistreri WF: Viral hepatitis. Pediatr Clin North Am 35:637-669, 1988.

Barkovich AJ, Lindan CE: Congenital cytomegalovirus infection of the brain: Imaging analysis and embryologic considerations. AJNR Am J Neuroradiol 15:703-715, 1994.

Barre V, Marret S, Mendel I, et al: Enterovirus-associated haemophagocytic syndrome in a neonate. Acta Paediatr 87:469-471, 1998.

Barton LL, Mets MB: Congenital lymphocytic choriomeningitis virus infection: Decade of rediscovery. Clin Infect Dis 33: 370-374, 2001.

Barton LL, Budd SC, Morfitt WS, et al: Congenital lymphocytic choriomeningitis virus infection in twins. Pediatr Infect Dis J 12:942-946, 1993.

Bates T: Poliomyelitis in pregnancy, fetus and newborn. Am J Dis Child 90:189, 1955.

Beasley RP, Hwang LY: Hepatocellular carcinoma and hepatitis B virus. Semin Liver Dis 4:113-121, 1984.

Beasley RP, Stevens CE, Shiao IS, Meng HC: Evidence against breast-feeding as a mechanism for vertical transmission of hepatitis B. Lancet 2(7938):740-741, 1975.

Berenberg W, Nankervis G: Long-term follow-up of cytomegalic inclusion disease of infancy. Pediatrics 46:403-410, 1970.

Bergman I, Painter MJ, Wald ER, et al: Outcome in children with enteroviral meningitis during the first year of life. J Pediatr 110:705-709, 1987.

Berry PJ, Gray ES, Porter HJ, Burton PA: Parvovirus infection of the human fetus and newborn. Semin Diagn Pathol 9:4-12, 1992.

Biggar RJ, Woodall JP, Walter PD, Haughie GE: Lymphocytic choriomeningitis outbreak associated with pet hamsters: Fifty-seven cases from New York State. JAMA 232:494-500, 1975.

Boley TJ, Popek EJ: Parvovirus infection in pregnancy. Semin Perinatol 17:410-419, 1993.

Bonkovsky HL, Woolley JM: Reduction of health-related quality of life in chronic hepatitis C and improvement with interferon therapy. The Consensus Interferon Study Group. Hepatology 29:264-270, 1999.

Boppana SB, Fowler KB, Vaid Y, et al: Neuroradiographic findings in the newborn period and long-term outcome in children with symptomatic congenital cytomegalovirus infection. Pediatrics 99:409-414, 1997.

Boppana SB, Fowler KB, Britt WJ, et al: Symptomatic congenital cytomegalovirus infection in infants born to mothers with preexisting immunity to cytomegalovirus. Pediatrics 104:55-60, 1999.

Boppana SB, Rivera LB, Fowler KB, M. et al: Intrauterine transmission of cytomegalovirus to infants of women with preconceptional immunity. N Engl J Med 344:1366-1371, 2001.

Bortolotti F, Resti M, Giacchino R, et al: Changing epidemiologic pattern of chronic hepatitis C virus infection in Italian children. J Pediatr 133:378-381, 1998.

Bowden JB. Hebert AA, Rapini RP: Dermal hematopoiesis in neonates: Report of five cases. J Am Acad Dermatol 20:1104-1110, 1989.

Brezin AP, Thulliez P, Cisneros B, et al: Lymphocytic choriomeningitis virus chorioretinitis mimicking ocular toxoplasmosis in two otherwise normal children. Am J Ophthalmol 130:245-247, 2000.

Brightman VJ, Scott TF, Westphal M, Boggs TR: An outbreak of coxsackie B-5 virus infection in a newborn nursery. J Pediatr 69:179-192, 1966.

Brough AJ, Jones D, Page RH, Mizukami I: Dermal erythropoiesis in neonatal infants: A manifestation of intra-uterine viral disease. Pediatrics 404:627-635, 1967.

Brouqui P, Rousseau MC, Saron MF, Bourgeade A: Meningitis due to lymphocytic choriomeningitis virus: Four cases in France. Clin Infect Dis 20:1082-1083, 1995.

Brown KE, Green SW, Antunez de Mayolo J, et al: Congenital anaemia after transplacental B19 parvovirus infection. Lancet 343:895-896, 1994.

Brown T, Anand A, Ritchie LD, et al: Intrauterine parvovirus infection associated with hydrops fetalis. Lancet 2(8410):1033-1034, 1984.

Brown ZA, Selke S, Zeh J, et al: The acquisition of herpes simplex virus during pregnancy. N Engl J Med 337:509-515, 1997.

Bruder E, Ersch J, Hebisch G, et al: Fetal varicella syndrome: Disruption of neural development and persistent inflammation of non-neural tissues. Virchows Arch 437:440-444, 2000.

Bruhn FW, Mokrohisky ST, McIntosh K: Apnea associated with respiratory syncytial virus infection in young infants. J Pediatr 90:382-386, 1977.

Brunell PA: Placental transfer of varicella-zoster antibody. Pediatrics 38:1034-1038, 1966.

Brunell PA: Varicella in pregnancy, the fetus, and the newborn: Problems in management. J Infect Dis 166(Suppl 1):S42-S47, 1992.

Brunell PA, Ross A, Miller LH, Kuo B: Prevention of varicella by zoster immune globulin. N Engl J Med 280:1191-1194, 1969.

Bullens D, Smets K, Vanhaesebrouck P: Congenital rubella syndrome after maternal reinfection. Clin Pediatr (Phila) 39(2):113-116, 2000.

Burchett SK, Corey L, Mohan KM, et al: Diminished interferon-gamma and lymphocyte proliferation in neonatal and postpartum primary herpes simplex virus infection. J Infect Dis 165:813-818, 1992.

Byington CL, Taggart EW, Carroll KC, Hillyard DR: A polymerase chain reaction-based epidemiologic investigation of the incidence of nonpolio enteroviral infections in febrile and afebrile infants 90 days and younger. Pediatrics 103:e27, 1999.

Carbonell-Estrany X, Quero J: Hospitalization rates for respiratory syncytial virus infection in premature infants born during two consecutive seasons. Pediatr Infect Dis J 20:874-879, 2001.

Carolane DJ, Long AM, McKeever PA, et al: Prevention of spread of echovirus 6 in a special care baby unit. Arch Dis Child 60:674-676, 1985.

Carrington D, Gilmore DH, Whittle MJ, et al: Maternal serum alpha-fetoprotein—a marker of fetal aplastic crisis during intrauterine human parvovirus infection. Lancet 1(8530):433-435, 1987.

Centers for Disease Control and Prevention. Control and prevention of rubella: Evaluation and management of suspected outbreaks, rubella in pregnant women, and surveillance for congenital rubella syndrome. MMWR Morbid Mortal Wkly Rep 50(RR-12):1-23, 2001.

Centers for Disease Control and Prevention. Hepatitis B virus: A comprehensive strategy for eliminating transmission in the United States through universal childhood vaccination. Recommendations of the Immunization Practices Advisory Committee (ACIP). MMWR Morbid Mortal Wkly Rep 40(RR-13):1-25, 1991.

Centers for Disease Control and Prevention. Measles, rubella, and congenital rubella syndrome—United States and Mexico, 1997-1999. MMWR Morb Mortal Wkly Rep 49:1048-1050, 1059, 2000.

Cherry J: Enterovirus. In Remington J, Klein J (eds): Infectious Diseases of the Fetus and Newborn. Philadelphia, WB Saunders, 1990, pp 325-366.

Childs JE, Glass GE, Ksiazek TG, et al: Human-rodent contact and infection with lymphocytic choriomeningitis and Seoul viruses in an inner-city population. Am J Trop Med Hyg 44:117-121, 1991.

Chisari FV, Ferrari C: Hepatitis B virus immunopathogenesis. Annu Rev Immunol 13:29-60, 1995.

Chrystie IL, Totterdell BM, Banatvala JE: Asymptomatic endemic rotavirus infections in the newborn. Lancet 1(8075):1176-1178, 1978.

Ciurea A, Hunziker L, Zinkernagel RM, Hengartner H: Viral escape from the neutralizing antibody response: The lymphocytic choriomeningitis virus model. Immunogenetics 53:185-189, 2001.

Coats DK, Demmler GJ, Paysse EA, et al: Ophthalmologic findings in children with congenital cytomegalovirus infection. J AAPOS 4:110-116, 2000.

Cohen MB: Etiology and mechanisms of acute infectious diarrhea in infants in the United States. J Pediatr 118:S34-S39, 1991.

Committee on Infectious Diseases and Committee on Fetus and Newborn: Revised indications for the use of palivizumab and respiratory synctial virus immune globulin intravenous for the prevention of respiratory syncytial virus infections. Pediatrics 112:1442-1446, 2003.

Conte D, Fraquelli M, Prati M, et al: Prevalence and clinical course of chronic hepatitis C virus (HCV) infection and rate of HCV vertical transmission in a cohort of 15,250 pregnant women. Hepatology 31:751-755, 2000.

Cornberg M, Wedemeyer H, Manns MP: Treatment of chronic hepatitis C with PEGylated interferon and ribavirin. Curr Gastroenterol Rep 4:23-30, 2002.

Craighead JE: Lymphocytic Choriomeningitis Virus: Pathology and Pathogenesis of Human Viral Disease. San Diego, Academic Press, 2000, pp 427-429.

Cramblett HG, Haynes RE, Azimi PH, et al: Nosocomial infection with echovirus type II in handicapped and premature infants. Pediatrics 514:603-60, 1973.

Crowe JE Jr Respiratory syncytial virus vaccine development. Vaccine 20(Suppl 1):S32-S37, 2001.

Cruz AC, Frentzen BH, Behnke M: Hepatitis B: A case for prenatal screening of all patients. Am J Obstet Gynecol 156:1180-1183, 1987.

Cullen A, Brown S, Cafferkey M, et al: Current use of the TORCH screen in the diagnosis of congenital infection. J Infect 36:185-188, 1998.

Cuthbertson G, Weiner CP, Giller RH, Grose C: Prenatal diagnosis of second-trimester congenital varicella syndrome by virus-specific immunoglobulin M. J Pediatr 111:592-595, 1987.

Dagan R: Nonpolio enteroviruses and the febrile young infant: Epidemiologic, clinical and diagnostic aspects. Pediatr Infect Dis J 15:67-71, 1996.

Danovaro-Holliday MC, Zimmerman L, Reef SE: Preventing congenital rubella syndrome (CRS) through vaccination of susceptible women of childbearing age. J Womens Health Gend Based Med 10:617-619, 2001.

Davis LE, Tweed GV, Stewart JA, et al: Cytomegalovirus mononucleosis in a first trimester pregnant female with transmission to the fetus. Pediatrics 48:200-206, 1971.

Deibel R, Woodall JP, Decher WJ, Schryver GD: Lymphocytic choriomeningitis virus in man: Serologic evidence of association with pet hamsters. JAMA 232:501-504, 1975.

Delamare C, Carbonne B, Heim N, et al: Detection of hepatitis C virus RNA (HCV-RNA) in amniotic fluid: A prospective study. J Hepatol 31:416-420, 1999.

Delaplane D, Yogev R, Crussi F, Shulman ST: Fatal hepatitis B in early infancy: The importance of identifying HBsAg-positive pregnant women and providing immunoprophylaxis to their newborns. Pediatrics 72:176-180, 1983.

Demmler GJ: Infectious Diseases Society of America and Centers for Disease Control. Summary of a workshop on surveillance for congenital cytomegalovirus disease. Rev Infect Dis 13:315-329, 1991.

Desmond MM, Fisher ES, Vorderman AL, et al: The longitudinal course of congenital rubella encephalitis in nonretarded children. J Pediatr 93:584-591, 1978.

Diamond C, Mohan K, Hobson A, et al: Viremia in neonatal herpes simplex virus infections. Pediatr Infect Dis J 18:487-489, 1999.

Dieck D, Schild RL, Hansmann M, Eis-Hubinger AM: Prenatal diagnosis of congenital parvovirus B19 infection: Value of serological and PCR techniques in maternal and fetal serum. Prenat Diagn 19:1119-1123. 1999.

Dong ZW, Yan C, Yi W, Cui YQ: Detection of congenital cytomegalovirus infection by using chorionic villi of the early pregnancy and polymerase chain reaction. Int J Gynaecol Obstet 44:229-231, 1994.

Dunn DT, Gibb DM, Healy M, et al: Timing and interpretation of tests for diagnosing perinatally acquired hepatitis C virus infection. Pediatr Infect Dis J 20:715-716, 2001.

Dykewicz CA, Dato VM, Fisher-Hoch SP, et al: Lymphocytic choriomeningitis outbreak associated with nude mice in a research institute. JAMA 267:1349-1353, 1992.

Emanuel I, Kenny GE: Cytomegalic inclusion disease of infancy. Pediatrics 38:957-965, 1966.

Enders G, Miller E, Cradock-Watson J, et al: Consequences of varicella and herpes zoster in pregnancy: Prospective study of 1739 cases. Lancet 343:1548-1551, 1994.

Enders G, Varho-Gobel M, Lohler J, et al: Congenital lymphocytic choriomeningitis virus infection: An underdiagnosed disease. Pediatr Infect Dis J 18:652-655, 1999.

Enders G, Bader U, Lindemann L, et al: Prenatal diagnosis of congenital cytomegalovirus infection in 189 pregnancies with known outcome. Prenat Diagn 21:362-377, 2001.

Essary LR, Vnencak-Jones CL, Manning SS, et al: Frequency of parvovirus B19 infection in nonimmune hydrops fetalis and utility of three diagnostic methods. Hum Pathol 29:696-701, 1998.

Farmer K, MacArthur BA, Clay MM: A follow-up study of 15 cases of neonatal meningoencephalitis due to coxsackie virus B5. J Pediatr 87:568-571, 1975.

Farmer K, Gunn T, Woodfield DG: A combination of hepatitis B vaccine and immunoglobulin does not protect all infants born to hepatitis B e antigen positive mothers. N Z Med J 100:412-414, 1987.

Feldman S: Varicella zoster infections of the fetus, neonate, and immunocompromised child. Adv Pediatr Infect Dis 1:99-115, 1986.

Fischler B, Lindh G, Lindgren S, et al: Vertical transmission of hepatitis C virus infection. Scand J Infect Dis 28:353-356, 1996.

Fleming DT, McQuillan GM, Johnson RE, et al: Herpes simplex virus type 2 in the United States, 1976 to 1994. N Engl J Med 337:1105-1111, 1997.

Florman AL, Gershon AA, Blackett PR, Nahmias AJ: Intrauterine infection with herpes simplex virus: Resultant congenital malformations. JAMA 225:129-132, 1973.

Fowler KB, McCollister FP, Dahle AJ, et al: Progressive and fluctuating sensorineural hearing loss in children with asymptomatic congenital cytomegalovirus infection. J Pediatr 130:624-630, 1997.

Fowler KB, Dahle AJ, Boppana SB, Pass RF: Newborn hearing screening: Will children with hearing loss caused by congenital cytomegalovirus infection be missed? J Pediatr 135:60-64, 1999.

Franklin, SL, Kelley R: Congenital rubella and interstitial pneumonitis. Clin Pediatr (Phila) 40:101-103, 2001.

Franssila R, Hokynar K, Hedman K: T helper cell-mediated in vitro responses of recently and remotely infected subjects to a candidate recombinant vaccine for human parvovirus b19. J Infect Dis 183:805-809, 2001.

Freij BJ, Sever JL: Herpesvirus infections in pregnancy: Risks to embryo, fetus, and neonate. Clin Perinatol 15:203-231, 1988.

Fuccillo DA, Steele RW, Hensen SA, et al: Impaired cellular immunity to rubella virus in congenital rubella. Infect Immun 9:81-84, 1974.

Gerety RJ, Schweitzer IL: Viral hepatitis type B during pregnancy, the neonatal period, and infancy. J Pediatr 90:368-374, 1977.

Gershon AA: Varicella in mother and infant: Problems old and new. In Krugman S, Gershon AA (eds): Infections of the Fetus and the Newborn Infant. New York, Alan R Liss, 1975, pp 79-95.

Géssner A, Lother H: Homologous interference of lymphocytic choriomeningitis virus involves a ribavirin-susceptible block in virus replication. J Virol 63:1827-1832, 1989.

Gibb DM, Goodall RL, Dunn DT, et al: Mother-to-child transmission of hepatitis C virus: Evidence for preventable peripartum transmission. Lancet 356:904-907, 2000.

Grangeot-Keros L, Broyer M, Briand E, et al: Enterovirus in sudden unexpected deaths in infants. Pediatr Infect Dis J 15:123-128, 1996.

Grangeot-Keros L, Mayaux MJ, Lebon P, et al: Value of cytomegalovirus (CMV) IgG avidity index for the diagnosis of primary CMV infection in pregnant women. J Infect Dis 175:944-946m 1997.

Gratacos E, Torres PJ, Vidal J, et al: The incidence of human parvovirus B19 infection during pregnancy and its impact on perinatal outcome. J Infect Dis 171:1360-1363, 1995.

Greenberg HB, Clark HF, Offit PA: Rotavirus pathology and pathophysiology. Curr Top Microbiol Immunol 185:255-283, 1994.

Greenhow TL, Weintrub PS: Your diagnosis, please. Neonate with hydrocephalus. Pediatr Infect Dis J 22:1099, 1111-1112, 2003.

Greenes DS, Rowitch D, Thorne GM, et al: Neonatal herpes simplex virus infection presenting as fulminant liver failure. Pediatr Infect Dis J 14:242-244, 1995.

Griffiths PD: Current management of cytomegalovirus disease. J Med Virol Suppl 1:106-111, 1993.

Groothuis JR: Role of antibody and use of respiratory syncytial virus (RSV) immune globulin to prevent severe RSV disease in high-risk children. J Pediatr 124:S28-S32, 1994.

Grose C, Meehan T, Weiner CP: Prenatal diagnosis of congenital cytomegalovirus infection by virus isolation after amniocentesis. Pediatr Infect Dis J 11:605-607, 1992.

Guerra B, Lazzarotto T, Quarta S, et al: Prenatal diagnosis of symptomatic congenital cytomegalovirus infection. Am J Obstet Gynecol 183:476-482, 2000.

Guidelines for hepatitis B virus screening and vaccination during pregnancy. ACOG Committee Opinion: Committee on Obstetrics: Maternal and Fetal Medicine. Number 111–May 1992. Int J Gynaecol Obstet 40:172-174, 1993.

Gurakan B, Oran O, Yigit S: Vertical transmission of hepatitis C virus. N Engl J Med 331:399-400, 1994.

Haffejee IE: Neonatal rotavirus infections. Rev Infect Dis 13:957-962, 1991.

Hagmann S, Chung M, Rochford G, et al: Response to lamivudine treatment in children with chronic hepatitis B virus infection. Clin Infect Dis 37:1434-1440, 2003.

Hall CB, Kopelman AE, Douglas RG Jr, et al: Neonatal respiratory syncytial virus infection. N Engl J Med 300:393-396, 1979.

Hancock MP, Huntley CC, Sever JL: Congenital rubella syndrome with immunoglobulin disorder. J Pediatr 72:636-645, 1968.

Hanngren K, Grandien M, Granstrom G: Effect of zoster immunoglobulin for varicella prophylaxis in the newborn. Scand J Infect Dis 17:343-347, 1985.

Hanshaw JB, Scheiner AP, Moxley AW, et al: School failure and deafness after silent congenital cytomegalovirus infection. N Engl J Med 295:468-470, 1976.

Hardy JB: Clinical and developmental aspects of congenital rubella. Arch Otolaryngol 98:230-236, 1973.

Hayes K, Dudgeon JA, Soothill JF: Humoral immunity in congenital rubella. Clin Exp Immunol 2:653-657, 1967.

Hayes K, Danks DM, Gibas H, Jack I: Cytomegalovirus in human milk. N Engl J Med 287:177-178, 1972.

Hayward JC, Titelbaum DS, Clancy RR, Zimmerman RA: Lissencephaly-pachygyria associated with congenital cytomegalovirus infection. J Child Neurol 6:109-114, 1991.

Higa K, Dan K, Manabe H: Varicella-zoster virus infections during pregnancy: hypothesis concerning the mechanisms of congenital malformations. Obstet Gynecol 69:214-222, 1987.

Hillemanns P, Dannecker C, Kimmig R, Hasbargen U: Obstetric risks and vertical transmission of hepatitis C virus infection in pregnancy. Acta Obstet Gynecol Scand 79:543-547, 2000.

Hinman AR, Fraser DW, Douglas RG, et al: Outbreak of lymphocytic choriomeningitis virus infections in medical center personnel. Am J Epidemiol 101:103-110, 1975.

Hsu HM, Lee SC, Wang MC, et al: Efficacy of a mass hepatitis B immunization program after switching to recombinant hepatitis B vaccine: A population-based study in Taiwan. Vaccine 19:2825-2829, 2001.

Humphrey W, Magoon M, O'Shaughnessy R: Severe nonimmune hydrops secondary to parvovirus B-19 infection: Spontaneous reversal in utero and survival of a term infant. Obstet Gynecol 78:900-902, 1991.

Hutchinson AK, Coats DK, Langdale LM, et al: Disinfection of eyelid specula with chlorhexidine gluconate (Hibiclens) after examinations for retinopathy of prematurity. Arch Ophthalmol 118:786-789, 2000.

Hutto C, Arvin A, Jacobs R, et al: Intrauterine herpes simplex virus infections. J Pediatr 110:97-101, 1987.

Isaacs D: Neonatal chickenpox. J Paediatr Child Health 36:76-77, 2000.

Ismail KM, Martin WL, Ghosh S, et al: Etiology and outcome of hydrops fetalis. J Matern Fetal Med 10:175-181, 2001.

Istas AS, Demmler GJ, Dobbins JG, Stewart JA: Surveillance for congenital cytomegalovirus disease: A report from the National Congenital Cytomegalovirus Disease Registry. Clin Infect Dis 20:665-670, 1995.

Isumi H, Nunoue T, Nishida A, Takashima S: Fetal brain infection with human parvovirus B19. Pediatr Neurol 21:661-663, 1999.

Ivarsson SA, Lernmark B, Svanberg L: Ten-year clinical, developmental, and intellectual follow-up of children with congenital cytomegalovirus infection without neurologic symptoms at one year of age. Pediatrics 99:800-803, 1997.

Iwarson S, Norkrans G, Wejstal R: Hepatitis C: Natural history of a unique infection. Clin Infect Dis 20:1361-1370, 1995.

Jahrling PB, Peters CJ: Lymphocytic choriomeningitis virus: A neglected pathogen of man. Arch Pathol Lab Med 116:486-488, 1992.

Jankovic B, Pasic S, Kanjuh B, et al: Severe neonatal echovirus 17 infection during a nursery outbreak. Pediatr Infect Dis J 18:393-394, 1999.

Jantausch BA, Luban NL, Duffy L, Rodriguez WJ: Maternal plasma transfusion in the treatment of disseminated neonatal echovirus 11 infection. Pediatr Infect Dis J 14:154-155, 1995.

Jenista JA, Powell KR, Menegus MA: Epidemiology of neonatal enterovirus infection. J Pediatr 104:685-690, 1984.

Jenkins M, Kohl S: New aspects of neonatal herpes. Infect Dis Clin North Am 6:57-74, 1992.

Jonas Maureen M, Kelly, Deirdre A, Mizerski, Jacek, et al: The International Pediatric Lamivudine Investigator Group: Clinical trial of lamivudine in children with chronic hepatitis B. N Engl J Med 346:1706-1713, 2002.

Jones KL, Johnson KA, Chambers CD: Offspring of women infected with varicella during pregnancy: A prospective study. Teratology 49:29-32, 1994.

Jones RN, Neale ML, Beattie B, et al: Development and application of a PCR-based method including an internal control for diagnosis of congenital cytomegalovirus infection. J Clin Microbiol 38:1-6, 2000.

Jordan JA, Huff D, DeLoia JA: Placental cellular immune response in women infected with human parvovirus B19 during pregnancy. Clin Diagn Lab Immunol 8:288-292, 2001.

Josefson D: Rubella vaccine may be safe in early pregnancy. BMJ 322:695, 2001.

Kasprzak A, Zabel M, Wysocki J, et al: Detection of DNA, mRNA and early antigen of the human cytomegalovirus using the immunomax technique in autopsy material of children with intrauterine infection. Virchows Archiv 43:482-490, 2000.

Kato H, Nakata K, Hamasaki K, et al: Long-term efficacy of immunization against hepatitis B virus in infants at high-risk analyzed by polymerase chain reaction. Vaccine 18:581-587, 1999.

Kerkering KW: Abnormal cry and intracranial calcifications: Clues to the diagnosis of fetal varicella-zoster syndrome. J Perinatol 21:131-135, 2001.

Kibrick S, Benirschke K: Severe generalized disease (encephalohepatomyocarditis) occurring in the newborn period and due to infection with coxsackie virus, group B: Evidence of intrauterine infection with this agent. Pediatrics 22:857-875, 1958.

Kimberlin DW: Advances in the treatment of neonatal herpes simplex infections. Rev Med Virol 11:157-163, 2001.

Kimberlin D, Powell D, Gruber W, et al: Administration of oral acyclovir suppressive therapy after neonatal herpes simplex virus disease limited to the skin, eyes and mouth: results of a phase I/II trial. Pediatr Infect Dis J 15:247-254, 1996a.

Kimberlin DW, Lakeman FD, Arvin AM, et al: Application of the polymerase chain reaction to the diagnosis and management of neonatal herpes simplex virus disease. National Institute of Allergy and Infectious Diseases Collaborative Antiviral Study Group. J Infect Dis 174:1162-1167, 1996b.

Kimberlin DW, Lin CY, Jacobs RF, et al: Natural history of neonatal herpes simplex virus infections in the acyclovir era. Pediatrics 108:223-229, 2001.

Kimberlin DW, Lin CY, Sanchez PJ, et al: National Institute of Allergy and Infectious Diseases Collaborative Antiviral Study Group. Effect of ganciclovir therapy on hearing in symptomatic congenital cytomegalovirus disease involving the central nervous system: A randomized, controlled trial. J Pediatr 143:16-25, 2003.

Kimura H, Minakami M, Harigaya A, et al: Treatment of neonatal infection caused by coxsackievirus B3. J Perinatol 19:388-390, 1999.

King-Lewis PA, Gardner SD: Congenital cytomegalic inclusion disease following intrauterine transfusion. Br Med J 2(657): 603-605, 1969.

Kinney JS, Kumar ML: Should we expand the TORCH complex? A description of clinical and diagnostic aspects of selected old and new agents. Clin Perinatol 15:727-744, 1988.

Kinney JS, Onorato IM, Stewart JA, et al: Cytomegaloviral infection and disease. J Infect Dis 151:772-774, 1985.

Kinney JS, McCray E, Kaplan JE, et al: Risk factors associated with echovirus 11′ infection in a hospital nursery. Pediatr Infect Dis 5:192-197, 1986.

Kinney JS, Anderson LJ, Farrar J, et al: Risk of adverse outcomes of pregnancy after human parvovirus B19 infection. J Infect Dis 157:663-667, 1988.

Kinney JS, Robertsen CM, Johnson KM, et al: Seasonal respiratory viral infections: Impact on infants with chronic lung disease following discharge from the neonatal intensive care unit. Arch Pediatr Adolesc Med 149:81-85, 1995.

Ko HM, Kim KS, Park JW, et al: Congenital cytomegalovirus infection: Three autopsy case reports. J Korean Med Sci 15:337-342, 2000.

Kohl S: Herpes simplex virus immunology: Problems, progress, and promises. J Infect Dis 152:435-440, 1985.

Kohl S: Role of antibody-dependent cellular cytotoxicity in neonatal infection with herpes simplex virus. Rev Infect Dis 13(Suppl 11):S950-S952, 1991.

Kohl S: Herpes simplex virus infection—the neonate to the adolescent. Isr J Med Sci 30:392-398, 1994.

Kohl S: Herpes simplex infections in newborn infants. Semin Pediatr Infect Dis 10:154-160, 1999.

Komrower GM, Williams BL, Stones PB: Lymphocytic choriomeningitis in the newborn, probable transplacental infection. Lancet 1(6866):697-698, 1955.

Krajden S, Middleton PJ: Enterovirus infections in the neonate. Clin Pediatr (Phila) 22:87-92, 1983.

Krugman S: Hepatitis B virus and the neonate. Ann N Y Acad Sci 549:129-134,1988.

Krugman S: Viral hepatitis: A, B, C, D, and E—prevention. Pediatr Rev 13:245-247, 1992.

Kumar ML, Nankervis GA, Gold E: Inapparent congenital cytomegalovirus infection: A follow-up study. N Engl J Med 288:1370-1372, 1973.

Kumar RM, Shahul S: Role of breast-feeding in transmission of hepatitis C virus to infants of HCV-infected mothers. J Hepatol 29:191-197, 1998.

Kustermann A, Zoppini C, Tassis B, et al: Prenatal diagnosis of congenital varicella infection. Prenat Diagn 16:71-74, 1996.

Laforet E, Lynch C: Multiple congenital defects following maternal varicella. N Engl J Med 236:534, 1947.

Lake AM, Lauer BA, Clark JC, et al: Enterovirus infections in neonates. J Pediatr 89:787-791, 1976.

Lamberson HV Jr, McMillian JA, Weiner LB, et al: Prevention of transfusion-associated cytomegalovirus (CMV) infection in neonates by screening blood donors for IgM to CMV. J Infect Dis 157:820-823, 1988.

Larsen, PD, Chartrand SA, Tomashek KM, et al: Hydrocephalus complicating lymphocytic choriomeningitis virus infection. Pediatr Infect Dis J 12:528-531, 1993.

Lazzarotto T, Spezzacatena P, Varani S, et al: Anticytomegalovirus (anti-CMV) immunoglobulin G avidity in identification of pregnant women at risk of transmitting congenital CMV infection. Clin Diagn Lab Immunol 6:127-129, 1999a.

Lazzarotto T, Varani S, Gabrielli L, et al: New advances in the diagnosis of congenital cytomegalovirus infection. Intervirology 42:390-397, 1999b.

Lazzarotto T, Varani S, Guerra B, et al: Prenatal indicators of congenital cytomegalovirus infection [see comments]. J Pediatr 137:90-95, 2000.

Lee JY, Bowden DS: Rubella virus replication and links to teratogenicity. Clin Microbiol Rev 13:571-587, 2000.

Lehman D, Toyoda M, Jordan S, Silverman N: Prenatal diagnosis of congenital cytomegalovirus infection: Quantitative CMV PCR in amniotic fluid. Presented at the 39th Annual Meeting of the Infectious Diseases Society of America, San Francisco, Oct 25-28, 2001.

Lehmann-Grube F. Kallay M, Ibscher B, Schwartz R: Serologic diagnosis of human infections with lymphocytic choriomeningitis virus: Comparative evaluation of seven methods. J Med Virol 4:125-136, 1979.

Lepow ML, Veronelli JA, Hostetler DD, Robbins FC: A trial with live attenuated rubella vaccine. Am J Dis Child 115: 639-647, 1968.

Levin MJ: Treatment and prevention options for respiratory syncytial virus infections. J Pediatr 124:S22-S27, 1994.

Lewis VJ, Walter PD, Thacker WL, Winkler WG: Comparison of three tests for the serological diagnosis of lymphocytic choriomeningitis virus infection. J Clin Microbiol 2:193-197, 1975.

Liesnard C, Donner C, Brancart F, Rodesch F: Varicella in pregnancy. Lancet 344:950-951, 1994.

Liesnard C, Donner C, Brancart F, et al: Prenatal diagnosis of congenital cytomegalovirus infection: Prospective study of 237 pregnancies at risk. Obstet Gynecol 95:881-888, 2000.

Lin HH, Lee TY, Chen DS, et al: Transplacental leakage of HBeAg-positive maternal blood as the most likely route in causing intrauterine infection with hepatitis B virus. J Pediatr 111:877-881, 1987.

Lin HH, Kao JH, Hsu HY, et al: Absence of infection in breast-fed infants born to hepatitis C virus-infected mothers. J Pediatr 126:589-591, 1995.

Linnemann CC Jr, Buchman TG, Light IJ, Ballard JL: Transmission of herpes-simplex virus type 1 in a nursery for the newborn: Identification of viral isolates by DNA fingerprinting. Lancet 1(8071): 964-946, 1978.

Lukacsi A, Tarodi B, Endreffy E, et al: Human cytomegalovirus gB genotype 1 is dominant in congenital infections in South Hungary. J Med Virol 65:537-542, 2001.

Luthardt T, Siebert H, Losel I, et al: [Cytomegalo-virus infections in infants with blood exchange transfusions after birth]. Klin Wochenschr 49:81-86, 1971.

Lynch-Salamon DI, Combs CA: Hepatitis C in obstetrics and gynecology. Obstet Gynecol 79:621-629, 1992.

Madge P, Paton JY, McColl JH, Mackie PL: Prospective controlled study of four infection-control procedures to prevent nosocomial infection with respiratory syncytial virus. Lancet 340(8827):1079-1083, 1992.

Maetz H.M, Sellers CA, Bailey WC, Hardy GE Jr: Lymphocytic choriomeningitis from pet hamster exposure: A local public health experience. Am J Public Health 66:1082-1085, 1976.

Malm G, Forsgren M: Neonatal herpes simplex virus infections: HSV-DNA in cerebrospinal fluid and serum. Arch Dis Child Fetal Neonatal Ed 81:F24-F29, 1999.

Markenson GR, Yancey MK: Parvovirus B19 infections in pregnancy. Semin Perinatol 22:309-317, 1998.

Marrie TJ, Saron MF: Seroprevalence of lymphocytic choriomeningitis virus in Nova Scotia. Am J Trop Med Hyg 58:47-49, 1998.

Mast EE, Mahoney FJ, Alter MJ, Margolis HS: Progress toward elimination of hepatitis B virus transmission in the United States. Vaccine 16(Suppl):S48-S51, 1998.

McCracken GH Jr, Shinefield HM, Cobb K, et al: Congenital cytomegalic inclusion disease. A longitudinal study of 20 patients. Am J Dis Child 117:522-359, 1969.

McEvoy RC, Fedun B, Cooper LZ, et al: Children at high risk of diabetes mellitus: New York studies of families with diabetes and of children with congenital rubella syndrome. Adv Exp Med Biol 246:221-227, 1988.

Meissner HC: Economic impact of viral respiratory disease in children. J Pediatr 124:S17-S21, 1994.

Meissner HC: Uncertainty in the management of viral lower respiratory tract disease. Pediatrics 108:1000-1003, 2001.

Meissner HC, Murray SA, Kiernan MA, et al:. A simultaneous outbreak of respiratory syncytial virus and parainfluenza virus type 3 in a newborn nursery. J Pediatr 104:680-684, 1984.

Meissner HC, Fulton DR, Groothuis JR, et al: Controlled trial to evaluate protection of high-risk infants against respiratory syncytial virus disease by using standard intravenous immune globulin. Antimicrob Agents Chemother 37:1655-1658, 1993.

Mets MB, Barton LL, Khan AS, Ksiazek TS: Lymphocytic choriomeningitis virus: An underdiagnosed cause of congenital chorioretinitis. Am J Ophthalmol 130:209-215, 2000.

Meyer H, Johnson R, Crawford I, et al: CNS syndromes of viral etiology: A study of 713 cases. Am J Med 29:334-347, 1960.

Meyers JD: Congenital varicella in term infants: Risk reconsidered. J Infect Dis 129:215-217, 1974.

Miller E, Cradock-Watson JE, Pollock TM: Consequences of confirmed maternal rubella at successive stages of pregnancy. Lancet 2(8302):781-784, 1982.

Miller E, Fairley CK, Cohen BJ, Seng C: Immediate and long term outcome of human parvovirus B19 infection in pregnancy. Br J Obstet Gynaecol 105:174-178, 1998.

Modlin JF: Fatal echovirus 11 disease in premature neonates. Pediatrics 66:775-780, 1980.

Modlin JF: Perinatal echovirus infection: Insights from a literature review of 61 cases of serious infection and 16 outbreaks in nurseries. Rev Infect Dis 8:918-926, 1986.

Montgomery R, Youngblood L, Medearis DN Jr: Recovery of cytomegalovirus from the cervix in pregnancy. Pediatrics 49:524-531, 1972.

Morey AL, Keeling JW, Porter HJ, Fleming KA: Clinical and histopathological features of parvovirus B19 infection in the human fetus. Br J Obstet Gynaecol 99:566-574, 1992.

Morgan-Capner P, Miller E, Vurdien JE, Ramsay ME: Outcome of pregnancy after maternal reinfection with rubella. CDR (Lond Engl Rev) 1:R57-R59, 1991.

Mortimer PP, Cohen BJ, Buckley MM, et al: Human parvovirus and the fetus. Lancet 2(8462):1012, 1985.

Mouly F, Mirlesse V, Meritet JF, et al: Prenatal diagnosis of fetal varicella-zoster virus infection with polymerase chain reaction of amniotic fluid in 107 cases. Am J Obstet Gynecol 177:894-898, 1997.

Mulligan MJ, Stiehm ER: Neonatal hepatitis B infection: Clinical and immunologic considerations. J Perinatol 14:2-9, 1994.

Murphy AM, Albrey MB, Crewe EB: Rotavirus infections of neonates. Lancet 2(8049):1149-1150, 1977.

Mustakangas P, Sarna S, Ammälä P, et al: Human cytomegalovirus seroprevalence in three socioeconomically different urban areas during the first trimester: A population-based cohort study. Int J Epidemiol 29:587-591, 2000.

Nagington J, Wreghittt TG, Gandy G, et al: Fatal echovirus 11 infections in outbreak in special-care baby unit. Lancet 2(8092):725-728, 1978.

Nagington J, Gandy G, Walker J, Gray JJ: Use of normal immunoglobulin in an echovirus 11 outbreak in a special-care baby unit. Lancet 2(8347):443-446, 1983.

Nahmias AJ, Roizman B: Infection with herpes-simplex viruses 1 and 2. 1. N Engl J Med 289:667-674, 1973.

Nahmias AJ, Josey WE, Naib ZM, et al: Perinatal risk associated with maternal genital herpes simplex virus infection. Am J Obstet Gynecol 110:825-837, 1971.

Nelson CT, Demmler GT: Cytomegalovirus infection in the pregnant mother, fetus, and newborn infant. Clin Perinatol 24:151-160, 1997.

Ngui SL, Andrews NJ, Underhill GS, et al: Failed postnatal immunoprophylaxis for hepatitis B: Characteristics of maternal hepatitis B virus as risk factors. Clin Infect Dis 27:100-106, 1998.

Nigro G, Scholz H, Bartmann U: Ganciclovir therapy for symptomatic congenital cytomegalovirus infection in infants: A two-regimen experience. J Pediatr 124:318-322, 1994.

Noyola DE, Demmler GJ, Williamson WD, et al: Cytomegalovirus urinary excretion and long term outcome in children with congenital cytomegalovirus infection. Congenital CMV Longitudinal Study Group. Pediatr Infect Dis J 19:505-510, 2000.

Noyola DE, Demmler GJ, Nelson CT, et al: Early predictors of neurodevelopmental outcome in symptomatic congenital cytomegalovirus infection. J Pediatr 138:325-331, 2001.

Ogasawara S, Kage M, Kosai K, et al: Hepatitis C virus RNA in saliva and breastmilk of hepatitis C carrier mothers. Lancet 341(8844):561, 1993.

Ohto H, Terazawa S, Sasaki N, et al: Transmission of hepatitis C virus from mothers to infants. The Vertical Transmission of Hepatitis C Virus Collaborative Study Group. N Engl J Med 330:744-750, 1994.

Ohto H, Ujiie N, Sato A, et al: Mother-to-infant transmission of GB virus type C/HGV. Transfusion 40:725-730, 2000.

Okada K, Kamiyama I, Inomata M, et al: e antigen and anti-e in the serum of asymptomatic carrier mothers as indicators of positive and negative transmission of hepatitis B virus to their infants. N Engl J Med 294:746-749, 1976.

Oram RJ, Marcellino D, Strauss D, et al: Characterization of an acyclovir-resistant herpes simplex virus type 2 strain isolated from a premature neonate. J Infect Dis 181:1458-1461, 2000.

O'Reilly MA, O'Reilly PM, de Bruyn R: Neonatal herpes simplex type 2 encephalitis: Its appearances on ultrasound and CT. Pediatr Radiol 25:68-69, 1995.

Overall JC Jr: Herpes simplex virus infection of the fetus and newborn. Pediatr Ann 23:131-136, 1994.

Paccagnini S, Principi N, Massironi E, et al: Perinatal transmission and manifestation of hepatitis C virus infection in a high risk population. Pediatr Infect Dis J 14:195-199, 1995.

Padula D, Rodella A, Spandrio M, et al: Spontaneous recovery from perinatal infection due to hepatitis C virus. Clin Infect Dis 28:141-142, 1999.

Palivizumab, a humanized respiratory syncytial virus monoclonal antibody, reduces hospitalization from respiratory syncytial virus infection in high-risk infants. The IMpact-RSV Study Group. Pediatrics 102:531-537, 1998.

Palomba E, Manzini P, Fiammengo P, et al: Natural history of perinatal hepatitis C virus infection. Clin Infect Dis 23:47-50, 1996.

Park JY, Peters CY, Rollin PE, et al: Development of a reverse transcription-polymerase chain reaction assay for diagnosis of lymphocytic choriomeningitis virus infection and its use in a prospective surveillance study. J Med Virol 51:107-114, 1997a.

Park JY, Peters CJ, Rollin PE, et al: Age distribution of lymphocytic choriomeningitis virus serum antibody in Birmingham, Alabama: Evidence of a decreased risk of infection. Am J Trop Med Hyg 57:37-41, 1997b.

Paryani SG, Arvin AM: Intrauterine infection with varicella-zoster virus after maternal varicella. N Engl J Med 314:1542-1546, 1986.

Pastuszak AL, Levy M, Schick B, et al: Outcome after maternal varicella infection in the first 20 weeks of pregnancy. N Engl J Med 330:901-905, 1994.

Peckham CS: Cytomegalovirus infection: Congenital and neonatal disease. Scand J Infect Dis Suppl 80:82-87, 1991.

Peters CJ: Arenaviruses. In Richman DD, Whitley RJ, Hayden FG (eds): Clinical Virology. New York, Churchill Livingstone,1997, pp 973-996.

Petignat P, Vial Y, Laurini R, Hohlfeld P: Fetal varicella-herpes zoster syndrome in early pregnancy: Ultrasonographic and morphological correlation. Prenat Diagn 21:121-124, 2001.

Phelan P, Campbell P: Pulmonary complications of rubella embryopathy. J Pediatr 75:202-212, 1969.

Piedra PA: Respiratory syncytial virus vaccines: recent developments. Pediatr Infect Dis J 19:805-810, 2000.

Polywka S, Feucht H, Zollner B, Laufs R: Hepatitis C virus infection in pregnancy and the risk of mother-to-child transmission. Eur J Clin Microbiol Infect Dis 16:121-124, 1997.

Polywka S, Schroter M, Feucht HH, et al: Low risk of vertical transmission of hepatitis C virus by breast milk. Clin Infect Dis 29:1327-1329, 1999.

Prather S, Dagan R, Jenista JA, Menegus MA: The isolation of enteroviruses from blood: A comparison of four processing methods. J Med Virol 14:221-227, 1984.

Pretorius DH, Hayward I, Jones KL, Stamm E: Sonographic evaluation of pregnancies with maternal varicella infection. J Ultrasound Med 11:459-463, 1992.

Prevalence of cytomegalovirus excretion from children in five day-care centers—Alabama. MMWR Morb Mortal Wkly Rep 34:49-51, 1985.

Prevention of respiratory syncytial virus infections: Indications for the use of palivizumab and update on the use of RSV-IGIV. Committee on Infectious Diseases and Committee of Fetus and Newborn. Pediatrics 102:1211-1216, 1998.

Primhak RA, Simpson RM: Screening small for gestational age babies for congenital infection. Clin Pediatr (Phila) 21:417-420, 1982.

Prober CG, Sullender WM, Yasukawa LL, et al: Low risk of herpes simplex virus infections in neonates exposed to the virus at the time of vaginal delivery to mothers with recurrent genital herpes simplex virus infections. N Engl J Med 316:240-244, 1987.

Prober CG, Hensleigh PA, Boucher FD, et al: Use of routine viral cultures at delivery to identify neonates exposed to herpes simplex virus. N Engl J Med 318:887-891, 1988.

Prospective study of human parvovirus (B19) infection in pregnancy. Public Health Laboratory Service Working Party on Fifth Disease. BMJ 300:1166-1170, 1990.

Qureshi F, Jacques SM: Maternal varicella during pregnancy: Correlation of maternal history and fetal outcome with placental histopathology. Hum Pathol 27:191-195, 1996.

Rabella N, Drew WL: Comparison of conventional and shell vial cultures for detecting cytomegalovirus infection. J Clin Microbiol 28:806-807, 1990.

Rantakallio P, Lapinleimu K, Mantyjarvi R: Coxsackie B 5 outbreak in a newborn nursery with 17 cases of serous meningitis. Scand J Infect Dis 2:17-23, 1970.

Recommended childhood immunization schedule—United States, 1998. JAMA 279:495-496, 1998.

Reef SE, Plotkin S, Cordero JF, et al: Preparing for elimination of congenital rubella syndrome (CRS): Summary of a workshop on CRS elimination in the United States. Clin Infect Dis 31:85-95, 2000.

Resti M, Azzari C, Mannelli F, et al: Mother to child transmission of hepatitis C virus: Prospective study of risk factors and timing of infection in children born to women seronegative for HIV-1. Tuscany Study Group on Hepatitis C Virus Infection. BMJ 317:437-441, 1998.

Resti M, Azzari C, Galli L: Maternal drug use is a preeminent risk factor for mother-to-child hepatitis C virus transmission: Results from a multicenter study of 1372 mother-infant pairs. J Infect Dis 185:567-572, 2002.

Revello MG, Baldanti F, Sarasini A, et al: Quantitation of herpes simplex virus DNA in cerebrospinal fluid of patients with herpes simplex encephalitis by the polymerase chain reaction. Clin Diagn Virol 7:183-191, 1997.

Revello MG, Zavattoni M, Furione M, et al: Quantification of human cytomegalovirus DNA in amniotic fluid of mothers of congenitally infected fetuses. J Clin Microbiol 37:3350-3352, 1999.

Reynolds DW, Stagno S, Hosty TS, et al: Maternal cytomegalovirus excretion and perinatal infection. N Engl J Med 289:1-5, 1973.

Reynolds DW, Stagno S, Stubbs KG, et al: Inapparent congenital cytomegalovirus infection with elevated cord IgM levels: Casual relation with auditory and mental deficiency. N Engl J Med 290:291-296, 1974.

Reynolds L, Struik S, Nadel S: Neonatal varicella: Varicella zoster immunoglobulin (VZIG) does not prevent disease. Arch Dis Child Fetal Neonatal Ed 8:F69-F70, 1999.

Rodis JF, Borgida AF, Wilson M, et al: Management of parvovirus infection in pregnancy and outcomes of hydrops: A survey of members of the Society of Perinatal Obstetricians. Am J Obstet Gynecol 179:985-988, 1998a.

Rodis JF, Rodner C, Hansen AA, et al: Long-term outcome of children following maternal human parvovirus B19 infection. Obstet Gynecol 91:125-258, 1998b.

Rosenthal P: Recent studies of adefovir dipivoxil for hepatitis B. J Pediatr Gastroenterol Nutr 37:323-324, 2003.

Rotbart HA, Webster AD: Treatment of potentially life-threatening enterovirus infections with pleconaril. Clin Infect Dis 32:228-235, 2001.

Rubin LG, Lanzkowsky P: Cutaneous neonatal herpes simplex infection associated with ritual circumcision. Pediatr Infect Dis J 19:266-268, 2000.

Ruiz-Extremera A, Salmeron J, Torres C, et al: Follow-up of transmission of hepatitis C to babies of human immunodeficiency virus-negative women: The role of breast-feeding in transmission. Pediatr Infect Dis J 19:511-516, 2000.

Sauerbrei A, Wutzler P: The congenital varicella syndrome. J Perinatol 20:548-554, 2000.

Sauerbrei A, Gluck B, Jung K, et al: Congenital skin lesions caused by intrauterine infection with coxsackievirus B3. Infection 28:326-328, 2000.

Sawyer MH, Holland D, Aintablian N, et al: Diagnosis of enteroviral CNS infection by polymerase chain reaction during a large community outbreak. Pediatr Infect Dis J 13:177-182, 1994.

Schiff RI: Transmission of viral infections through intravenous immune globulin. N Engl J Med 331:1649-1650, 1994.

Schlesinger Y, Storch GA: Herpes simplex meningitis in infancy. Pediatr Infect Dis J 13:141-144, 1994.

Schluter WW, Reef SE, Redd SC, Dykewicz CA: Changing epidemiology of congenital rubella syndrome in the United States. J Infect Dis 178:636-641, 1998.

Scott LL, Hollier LM, Dias K: Perinatal herpesvirus infections. Herpes simplex, varicella, and cytomegalovirus. Infect Dis Clin North Am 11:27-53, 1997.

Sells CJ, Carpenter RL, Ray CG: Sequelae of central-nervous-system enterovirus infections. N Engl J Med 293:1-4, 1975.

Sever JL, South MA, Shaver KA: Delayed manifestations of congenital rubella. Rev Infect Dis 7(Suppl 1): S164-S169, 1985.

Shapiro CN: Epidemiology of hepatitis B. Pediatr Infect Dis J 12:433-437, 1993.

Shattuck KE, Chonmaitree T: The changing spectrum of neonatal meningitis over a fifteen-year period. Clin Pediatr (Phila) 31:130-136, 1992.

Sheikh AU, Ernest JM, O'Shea M: Long-term outcome in fetal hydrops from parvovirus B19 infection. Am J Obstet Gynecol 167:337-341, 1992.

Shields KE, Galil K, Seward J, et al: Varicella vaccine exposure during pregnancy: Data from the first 5 years of the pregnancy registry. Obstet Gynecol 98:14-19, 2001.

Shimizu C, Rambaud C, Cheron G, et al: Molecular identification of viruses in sudden infant death associated with myocarditis and pericarditis. Pediatr Infect Dis J 14:584-588, 1995.

Siegel M: Congenital malformations following chickenpox, measles, mumps, and hepatitis: Results of a cohort study. JAMA 226:1521-1524, 1973.

Siegel M, Fuerst HT: Low birth weight and maternal virus diseases: A prospective study of rubella, measles, mumps, chickenpox, and hepatitis. JAMA 197:680-684, 1966.

Singer DB: Pathology of neonatal herpes simplex virus infection. Perspect Pediatr Pathol 6:243-278, 1981.

Soothill JF, Hayes K, Dudgeon JA: The immunoglobulins in congenital rubella. Lancet 1(7452):1385-1388, 1966.

South MA, Sever JL: Teratogen update: The congenital rubella syndrome. Teratology 31:297-307, 1985.

South MA, Montgomery JR, Rawls WE: Immune deficiency in congenital rubella and other viral infections. Birth Defects Orig Artic Ser 11:234-238, 1975.

South MA, Tompkins WA, Morris CR, Rawls WE: Congenital malformation of the CNS associated with genital type (type 2) herpesvirus. J Pediatr 75:13-18, 1969.

Spector SA: Transmission of cytomegalovirus among infants in hospital documented by restriction-endonuclease-digestion analyses. Lancet 1(8321):378-381, 1983.

Srabstein JC, Morris N, Larke RP, et al: Is there a congenital varicella syndrome? J Pediatr 84:239-243, 1974.

Stagno S, Cloud GA: Working parents: The impact of day care and breast-feeding on cytomegalovirus infections in offspring. Proc Natl Acad Sci U S A 91:2384-2349, 1994.

Stagno S, Dworsky ME, Torres J, et al: Prevalence and importance of congenital cytomegalovirus infection in three different populations. J Pediatr 101:897-900, 1982a.

Stagno S, Pass RF, Dworsky ME, et al: Congenital cytomegalovirus infection: The relative importance of primary and recurrent maternal infection. N Engl J Med 306:945-949, 1982b.

Stagno S, Cloud G, Pass RF, et al: Factors associated with primary cytomegalovirus infection during pregnancy. J Med Virol 13:347-353, 1984.

Stagno S, Whitley RJ: Herpesvirus infections of pregnancy. Part I: Cytomegalovirus and Epstein-Barr virus infections. N Engl J Med 313:1270-1274, 1985a.

Stagno S, Whitley RJ: Herpesvirus infections of pregnancy. Part II: Herpes simplex virus and varicella-zoster virus infections. N Engl J Med 313:1327-1330, 1985b.

Stamos JK, Rowley AH: Timely diagnosis of congenital infections. Pediatr Clin North Am 41:1017-1033, 1994.

Stanberry LR: Herpes. Vaccines for HSV. Dermatol Clin 16:811-816, 1998.

Starr JG, Bart RD Jr, Gold E: Inapparent congenital cytomegalovirus infection: Clinical and epidemiologic characteristics in early infancy. N Engl J Med 282:1075-1078, 1970.

Stephensen CB, Blount SR, Lanford RE, et al: Prevalence of serum antibodies against lymphocytic choriomeningitis virus in selected populations from two U.S. cities. J Med Virol 38:27-31, 1992.

Stevens CE: In utero and perinatal transmission of hepatitis viruses. Pediatr Ann 23:152, 155-158, 1994.

Summers PR, Biswas MK, Pastorek JG 2nd, et al: The pregnant hepatitis B carrier: Evidence favoring comprehensive antepartum screening. Obstet Gynecol 69:701-704, 1987.

Swanink CM, Veenstra L, Poort YA, et al: Coxsackievirus B1-based antibody-capture enzyme-linked immunosorbent assay for detection of immunoglobulin G (IgG), IgM, and IgA with broad specificity for enteroviruses. J Clin Microbiol 31:3240-3246, 1993.

Swiatek B: Neonatal enterovirus infection. Neonatal Netw 16:85-88, 1997.

Tajiri H, Miyoshi Y, Funada S, et al: Prospective study of mother-to-infant transmission of hepatitis C virus. Pediatr Infect Dis J 20:10-14, 2001.

Tang JR, Hsu HY, Lin HH, et al: Hepatitis B surface antigenemia at birth: A long-term follow-up study. J Pediatr 133:374-377, 1998.

Taylor DN, Echeverria P: Diarrhoeal disease: Current concepts and future challenges: Molecular biological approaches to the epidemiology of diarrhoeal diseases in developing countries. Trans R Soc Trop Med Hyg 87(Suppl 3):3-5, 1993.

Thomas SL, Newell ML, Peckham CS, et al:. Use of polymerase chain reaction and antibody tests in the diagnosis of vertically transmitted hepatitis C virus infection. Eur J Clin Microbiol Infect Dis 16:711-719, 1997.

Tingle AJ, Chantler JK, Pot KH, et al: Postpartum rubella immunization: Association with development of prolonged arthritis, neurological sequelae, and chronic rubella viremia. J Infect Dis 152:606-612, 1985.

Tookey P: Pregnancy is contraindication for rubella vaccination still. BMJ 322:1489, 2001.

Torok TJ, Wang QY, Gary GW Jr, et al: Prenatal diagnosis of intrauterine infection with parvovirus B19 by the polymerase chain reaction technique. Clin Infect Dis 14:149-155, 1992.

Tovo PA, Pembrey LJ, Newell ML: Persistence rate and progression of vertically acquired hepatitis C infection. European Paediatric Hepatitis C Virus Infection. J Infect Dis 181:419-424, 2000.

Trincado DE, Rawlinson WD: Congenital and perinatal infections with cytomegalovirus. J Paediatr Child Health 37:187-192, 2001.

Trincado DE, Scott GM, et al: Human cytomegalovirus strains associated with congenital and perinatal infections. J Med Virol 61:481-487, 2000.

U.S. Department of Health and Human Services: Reduce or eliminate indigenous cases of vaccine-preventable diseases. In Healthy People 2010: Understanding and Improving Health. Washington, DC, U.S. Government Printing Office, 2000, p 1.

Ueda K, Nishida Y, Oshima K, Shepard TH: Congenital rubella syndrome: Correlation of gestational age at time of maternal rubella with type of defect. J Pediatr 94:763-765, 1979.

Valduss D, Murray DL, Karna P, et al: Use of intravenous immunoglobulin in twin neonates with disseminated coxsackie B1 infection. Clin Pediatr (Phila) 32:561-563, 1993.

Vanzee BE, Douglas RG, Betts RF, et al: Lymphocytic choriomeningitis in university hospital personnel: Clinical features. Am J Med 58:803-809, 1975.

Verder H, Dickmeiss E, Haahr S, et al: Late-onset rubella syndrome: Coexistence of immune complex disease and defective cytotoxic effector cell function. Clin Exp Immunol 63:367-375, 1986.

Wald ER, Dashefsky B: Ribavirin: Red Book Committee recommendations questioned. Pediatrics 93:672-673, 1994.

Weiss JB Jr, Persing DH: Hepatitis C: Advances in diagnosis. Mayo Clin Proc 70:296-297, 1995.

Wejstal R, Manson AS, Widell A, Norkrans G: Perinatal transmission of hepatitis G virus (GB virus type C) and hepatitis C virus infections—a comparison. Clin Infect Dis 28:816-821, 1999.

Whitley RJ: Natural history and pathogenesis of neonatal herpes simplex virus infections. Ann N Y Acad Sci 549:103-117, 1988.

Whitley RJ: Herpes simplex virus infections of the CNS: Encephalitis and neonatal herpes. Drugs 42:406-427, 1991.

Whitley RJ: Neonatal herpes simplex virus infections. J Med Virol Suppl 1:13-21, 1993.

Whitley RJ: Herpes simplex virus infections of women and their offspring: Implications for a developed society. Proc Natl Acad Sci U S A 91:2441-2447, 1994.

Whitley RJ, Cloud G, Gruber W, et al: Ganciclovir treatment of symptomatic congenital cytomegalovirus infection: results of a phase II study. National Institute of Allergy and Infectious Diseases Collaborative Antiviral Study Group. J Infect Dis 175:1080-1086, 1997.

Wilfert CM, Thompson RJ Jr, Sunder TR, et al: Longitudinal assessment of children with enteroviral meningitis during the first three months of life. Pediatrics 67:811-815, 1981.

Williamson WD, Demmler GJ, Percy AK, Catlin FI: Progressive hearing loss in infants with asymptomatic congenital cytomegalovirus infection. Pediatrics 90:862-866, 1992.

Wilson CW, Stevenson DK, Arvin AM: A concurrent epidemic of respiratory syncytial virus and echovirus 7 infections in an intensive care nursery. Pediatr Infect Dis J 8:24-29, 1989.

Wong A, Tan KH, Tee CS, Yeo GS: Seroprevalence of cytomegalovirus, Toxoplasma and parvovirus in pregnancy. Singapore Med J 41:151-155, 2000.

World Health Organization. Preventing congenital rubella syndrome. Wkly Epidemiol Rec 75:290-295, 2000.

Wright R, Johnson D, Neumann M, et al: Congenital lymphocytic choriomeningitis virus syndrome: A disease that mimics congenital toxoplasmosis or cytomegalovirus infection. Pediatrics 100:e9, 1997.

Wy CA, Sajous CH, Loberiza F, Weiss MG: Outcome of infants with a diagnosis of hydrops fetalis in the 1990s. Am J Perinatol 16:561-567, 1999.

Xu DZ, Yan YP, Zou S, et al: Role of placental tissues in the intrauterine transmission of hepatitis B virus. Am J Obstet Gynecol 185:981-987, 2001.

Yaegashi N, Okamura K, Yajima A, et al: The frequency of human parvovirus B19 infection in nonimmune hydrops fetalis. J Perinat Med 22:159-163, 1994.

Yaegashi N, Niinuma T, Chisaka H, et al: The incidence of, and factors leading to, parvovirus B19-related hydrops fetalis following maternal infection: Report of 10 cases and meta-analysis. J Infect 37:28-35, 1998.

Yaegashi N, Niinuma T, Chisaka H, et al: Parvovirus B19 infection induces apoptosis of erythroid cells in vitro and in vivo. J Infect 39:68-76, 1999.

Yeager AS, Jacobs H, Clark J: Nursery-acquired cytomegalovirus infection in two premature infants. J Pediatr 81:332-335, 1972.

Yeager AS, Grumet FC, Hafleigh EB, et al: Prevention of transfusion-acquired cytomegalovirus infections in newborn infants. J Pediatr 98:281-287, 1981.

Yeager AS, Ashley RL, Corey L: Transmission of herpes simplex virus from father to neonate. J Pediatr 103:905-907, 1983.

Zanetti AR, Tanzi E, Paccagnini S, et al: Mother-to-infant transmission of hepatitis C virus. Lombardy Study Group on Vertical HCV Transmission. Lancet 345(8945):289-291, 1995.

Zanetti AR, Tanzi E, Romano L, et al: Multicenter trial on mother-to-infant transmission of GBV-C virus. The Lombardy Study Group on Vertical/Perinatal Hepatitis Viruses Transmission. J Med Virol 54:107-112, 1998.

Zimmermann R, Perucchini D, Fauchere JC, et al: Hepatitis C virus in breast milk. Lancet 345(8954):928, 1995.

Zuccotti GV, Ribero ML, Giovannini M, et al: Effect of hepatitis C genotype on mother-to-infant transmission of virus. J Pediatr 127:278-280, 1995.

Zuin G, Saccani B, Di Giacomo S, et al: Outcome of mother to infant acquired GBV-C/HGV infection. Arch Dis Child Fetal Neonatal Ed 80:F72-F73, 1999.

CHAPTER 38

# Toxoplasmosis, Syphilis, Malaria, and Tuberculosis

**Pablo J. Sánchez and Amina Ahmed**

## TOXOPLASMOSIS

*Toxoplasmosis* refers to the disease state that results from infection with the obligate protozoan parasite, *Toxoplasma gondii. Toxoplasma* is a coccidian that is ubiquitous in nature, and the cat is the definitive host. The organism exists in the following three forms: (1) an oocyst in which sporozoites are formed within the intestinal tract of the cat and that is shed in feces, (2) a tachyzoite or endozoite that is the proliferative form and was formerly referred to as a trophozoite, and (3) a tissue cyst that has an intracystic form termed *cystozoite* or *bradyzoite*. Nonfeline mammals or birds ingest infective oocysts from contaminated soil. Tissue cysts then accumulate in the organs and skeletal muscle of these animals. The possible routes of transmission from animal to human are direct contact with cat feces, ingestion of undercooked meat containing infective cysts, and ingestion of fruits or vegetables that have been in contaminated soil. Congenital infection results from placental infection and subsequent hematogenous spread to the fetus.

### Epidemiology

Toxoplasmosis is a worldwide medical problem. High prevalence of infection has been documented in Europe, Central America, and parts of Africa. However, seroprevalence rates differ considerably from one country to another, from one region of a country to another, and even from one ethnic group to another in the same region. These widely disparate seroprevalence rates among different adult populations throughout the world have been explained by differences in eating and sanitation practices that contribute to acquisition of infection. Eating undercooked or raw meat or unwashed raw fruits and vegetables, large cat populations, and even certain climactic conditions have been associated with higher risks of infection.

Among women of child-bearing age in the United States, the prevalence of antibody to *T. gondii* varies from approximately 3% to 30%, depending on the region of the country (Boyer and McAuley, 1994, Remington et al, 2001). The lowest seroprevalence rates have been found in the Mountain and Pacific states, and the highest rates have been seen in the Northeastern and Southeastern United States. Seroprevalence rates for pregnant women seem to be decreasing, although regional and ethnic differences persist.

The prevalence of congenital infection in Massachusetts and New Hampshire has been documented to be 0.08 per 1000 births through immunoglobulin (Ig) M screening of newborn blood specimens collected on filter paper (Guerina et al, 1994). This finding compares with a rate of 3 to 10 per 1000 live births in Paris and Vienna, where maternal seroprevalence rates of about 70% and 40%, respectively, are observed. In Massachusetts, a case-control study involving 14 years of newborn screening for congenital toxoplasmosis found that the mother's birth outside the United States, particularly in Cambodia and Laos, as well as the mother's educational level and higher gravidity were strongly predictive of congenital infection (Jara et al, 2001).

### Natural History

Infection of the fetus occurs as a consequence of maternal primary infection during pregnancy or, rarely, just before conception (Villena et al, 1998b). Reactivation of latent *Toxoplasma* infection during pregnancy does not lead to fetal infection except among immunocompromised women such as those infected with the human immunodeficiency virus (HIV) (Dunn et al, 1997; Langer, 1983; Low incidence, 1996; Mitchell et al, 1990; O'Donohoe et al, 1991; Remington et al, 2001). Under these circumstances, however, the risk is low. In addition, maternal re-infection may result in congenital toxoplasmosis (Gavinet et al, 1997; Hennequin et al, 1997). Acute maternal infection which is usually acquired early in pregnancy may lead to fulminant fetal infection resulting in stillbirth, nonimmune fetal hydrops, preterm birth, and perinatal death (Wong and Remington, 1994). On the other hand, chronic *Toxoplasma* infection rarely has been associated with sporadic abortion (Remington et al, 1964).

Infection of the fetus occurs transplacentally during maternal parasitemia. Placental infection is an important intermediary step, and up to 16 weeks may elapse between placental infection and subsequent infection of the fetus. This time delay has been termed the *prenatal incubation period* (Remington et al, 2001). Congenital toxoplasmosis has occurred in twins and triplets (Couvreur et al, 1991; Sibalic et al, 1986; Wiswell et al, 1984). In monozygotic twins, the clinical manifestations are usually similar, whereas in dizygotic twins, discrepancies in clinical findings are common.

Approximately 40% of infants born to mothers who acquired toxoplasmosis during pregnancy are infected with *T. gondii*. The rate of vertical transmission varies according to the trimester in which the mother became infected, fetal infection rates increasing as pregnancy advances (Dunn et al, 1999; Remington et al, 2001; Wong and Remington, 1994). Specifically, when maternal infection occurs in the first trimester, 15% of infants are infected, whereas maternal infection in the second and third trimesters results in transmission rates of 30% and 60%, respectively. The severity of clinical manifestations is greatest, however, when maternal infection is acquired early in pregnancy. Maternal infection in the first trimester results in severe disease in as many as 40% of infected fetuses, and in stillbirth or perinatal death in an additional 35% of infants. Only about 15% of newborns have subclinical disease. However, maternal infection in the third trimester is rarely if ever associated with severe fetal disease or stillbirth, and about 90% of infants in such situations have subclinical infection.

Postnatally, transmission of *T. gondii* can occur from transfusion of blood or blood products or from transplantation of organ or bone marrow from a seropositive donor with latent infection. Although the organism has been detected in human milk, transmission by breast-feeding has not been documented.

The majority of newborns with congenital toxoplasmosis lack clinical signs of infection, although thorough evaluation may demonstrate eye or neurologic abnormalities in about 20% of cases. Clinically apparent disease is present in only about 10% to 25% of infected infants (Alford et al, 1969, 1974; Guerina et al, 1994). The clinical manifestations of toxoplasmosis are often indistinguishable from those seen with other congenital infections, such as cytomegalic inclusion disease and congenital syphilis. Approximately one third of infants has a generalized form of the disease that principally involves organs of the reticuloendothelial system. The abnormalities include temperature instability, hepatosplenomegaly, jaundice, pneumonitis, generalized lymphadenopathy, rash, chorioretinitis, anemia, thrombocytopenia, eosinophilia, and abnormal cerebrospinal fluid (CSF) indices (Table 38–1) (Boyer and McAuley, 1994; Eichenwald, 1960). The other two thirds of infected infants principally manifest neurologic disease.

**TABLE 38–1**

**Clinical Findings Among Infants with Congenital Toxoplasmosis**

| | Infants with Findings (%) | |
|---|---|---|
| **Finding** | **Neurologic Disease* (108 Cases)** | **Generalized Disease† (44 Cases)** |
| Chorioretinitis | 94 | 66 |
| Abnormal cerebrospinal fluid | 55 | 84 |
| Anemia | 51 | 77 |
| Convulsions | 50 | 18 |
| Intracranial calcification | 50 | 4 |
| Jaundice | 29 | 80 |
| Hydrocephalus | 28 | 0 |
| Fever | 25 | 77 |
| Splenomegaly | 21 | 90 |
| Lymphadenopathy | 17 | 68 |
| Hepatomegaly | 17 | 77 |
| Vomiting | 16 | 48 |
| Microcephaly | 13 | 0 |
| Diarrhea | 6 | 25 |
| Cataracts | 5 | 0 |
| Eosinophilia | 4 | 18 |
| Abnormal bleeding | 3 | 18 |
| Hypothermia | 2 | 20 |
| Glaucoma | 2 | 0 |
| Optic atrophy | 2 | 0 |
| Microphthalmia | 2 | 0 |
| Rash | 1 | 25 |
| Pneumonitis | 0 | 41 |

*Infants with otherwise undiagnosed central nervous system diseases in the first year of life.

†Infants with otherwise undiagnosed non-neurologic diseases during the first 2 months of life.

Adapted from Remington JS, McLeod R, Thulliez P, Desmonts G: Toxoplasmosis. In Remington JS Klein JO (eds): Infectious Diseases of the Fetus and Newborn Infant, 5th ed. Philadelphia, WB Saunders, 2001, p 246.

Central nervous system involvement is the hallmark of congenital *Toxoplasma* infection (Diebler et al, 1985; McAuley et al, 1994; Remington et al, 2001). Chorioretinitis, intracranial calcifications, and hydrocephalus are the most characteristic findings, occurring in approximately 86%, 37%, and 20% of symptomatic infants, respectively (see Table 38–1) (Boyer and McAuley, 1994; Eichenwald, 1960; Remington et al, 2001). This constellation of findings has been referred to as the "classic triad" of congenital toxoplasmosis; their presence should alert the clinician to the diagnosis. Intracranial calcifications may be single or multiple but typically are generalized and located in the caudate nucleus, choroid plexus, meninges, and subependyma (Müssbichler, 1968). They also may occur periventricularly as in cytomegalovirus infection. They are visualized best by computed tomography (CT) but are often detected on ultrasonography as well. Intracranial calcifications may resolve with appropriate antimicrobial therapy (McAuley et al, 1994). Hydrocephalus may be the only manifestation of disease. It results from the extensive periaqueductal and periventricular vasculitis with necrosis that causes obstruction of the ventricular system. Ventriculoperitoneal shunting is often required (Martinovic et al, 1982; McAuley et al, 1994). Abnormalities of the CSF are common; characteristically, they consist of lymphocytic pleocytosis and a markedly elevated protein content. Microcephaly, when present, indicates severe brain injury. Hypothermia as well as hyperthermia may occur secondary to hypothalamic involvement. *Toxoplasma* has been detected in the inner ear and mastoid, with the associated inflammation resulting in deafness. An ascending flaccid paralysis with myelitis has also been reported (Campbell et al, 2001).

Chorioretinitis secondary to congenital toxoplasmosis can manifest at any age. It usually manifests as strabismus in infants, and in older children, defects in visual acuity are more common. Typically, the eye lesion consists of a focal necrotizing retinitis that is often bilateral with involvement of the macula and even the optic nerve. Complications include blindness, iridocyclitis, and cataracts.

Other, less common manifestations of congenital toxoplasmosis are nonimmune hydrops fetalis, myocarditis, nephrotic syndrome, and immunoglobulin abnormalities with both hypergammaglobulinemia and hypogammaglobulinemia described. Bony abnormalities consisting of metaphyseal lucencies similar to those seen in congenital syphilis have also been reported (Milgram, 1974). A variety of endocrine abnormalities may occur, including hypothyroidism, diabetes insipidus (Oygur et al, 1998; Yamakawa et al, 1996), precocious puberty, and growth hormone deficiency.

### Diagnosis

Isolation of *T. gondii* from body fluids and tissues provides definitive evidence of infection. The organism can be isolated from placenta, amniotic fluid, fetal blood obtained by cordocentesis, umbilical cord blood, infant peripheral blood, and CSF by means of intraperitoneal and subcutaneous inoculation into laboratory mice (Foulon et al, 1999a; Remington et al, 2001; Wong and Remington, 1994). Mouse inoculation may require as long as 4 to 6 weeks for demonstration of the parasite. Although it is not a practical method, isolation of the organism should be attempted whenever possible. It is available at the *Toxoplasma* Serology Laboratory, Palo Alto Medical Foundation (860 Bryant St, Palo Alto, CA 94301; telephone: 415-326-8120). In addition, tissue culture has been used to isolate *T. gondii* from amniotic fluid.

Histopathologic examination of the placenta as well as tissues obtained at postmortem examination or by biopsy from stillborns or infants should be performed because the specimens may demonstrate the presence of tachyzoites. In addition, tachyzoites have been demonstrated in CSF, ventricular fluid, and aqueous humor by specialized staining techniques.

Polymerase chain reaction (PCR) analysis has been used successfully to detect *Toxoplasma* DNA in amniotic fluid, placenta, CSF, brain, urine, and fetal and infant blood (Foulon et al, 1999a; Fricker-Hidalgo et al, 1998; Grover et al, 1990; Guy et al, 1996; Hohlfield et al, 1994; Jenum et al, 1998; Romand et al, 2001). PCR performed on amniotic fluid obtained by amniocentesis has become the preferred method of confirming in utero infection. False-negative results have been reported, however, and interlaboratory variability in performance of PCR assays has been documented (Guy et al, 1996; Romand et al, 2001). PCR performed on neonatal CSF is recommended for the evaluation of possible central nervous system involvement.

Serologic assays for measurement of antibodies to *T. gondii* in serum and body fluids are the most widely used methods of diagnosing congenital toxoplasmosis (Boyer, 2001; Boyer and McAuley, 1994; Dannemann et al, 1990; Foudrinier et al, 1995; Guerina et al, 1994; Lappalainen et al, 1993; Naessens et al, 1999; Naot et al, 1991; Pinon et al, 2001; Remington et al, 1985; Robert-Gangneux, 2001; Robert-Gangneux et al, 1999a, 1999b; Villena et al, 1999; Wong and Remington, 1994). These tests are commercially available at the *Toxoplasma* Serology Laboratory. The more commonly used tests that detect *T. gondii*–specific IgG antibodies are the Sabin-Feldman dye test, which is considered the "gold standard" but requires live organisms, indirect immunofluorescent antibody (IFA) test, IgG enzyme-linked immunosorbent assay (ELISA), direct agglutination, and IgG avidity test.

In addition, a differential agglutination test has been developed as a confirmatory test to differentiate acute from chronic maternal infection. This test compares the IgG serologic titer obtained with the use of formalin-fixed tachyzoites (HS antigen) with those obtained with acetone- or methanol-fixed tachyzoites (AC antigen). The latter preparation contains stage-specific *Toxoplasma* antigens that are recognized by IgG antibodies only during early infection. An additional assay that may assist in ruling out maternal infection acquired in the first 3 months of pregnancy is the IgG avidity test performed by the ELISA technique. This test is based on the principle that although the antibody-binding avidity or affinity for an antigen is initially low after primary antigenic stimulation, IgG antibodies that are present from previous antigenic stimulation are usually of high avidity. Therefore, a high avidity result in the first trimester would exclude an infection acquired in the previous 12 weeks. Finally, an enzyme-linked immunofiltration assay (ELIFA) has been developed that allows discrimination between IgG antibodies of maternal origin and IgGs synthesized by the fetus as well as identification of antibody subtypes in infected neonates (Zufferey et al, 1999).

Tests that detect *T. gondii*–specific IgM are (1) the double-sandwich IgM ELISA, which has a sensitivity of 75% to 80% and a specificity of 100% (Guerina et al, 1994), (2) the IgM immunosorbent agglutination assay (ISAGA), which is the most sensitive test but should not be performed on umbilical cord blood, because even small quantities of maternal IgM antibodies contaminating the specimen will yield a false-positive result (Boyer and McAuley, 1994); and (3) the IgM immunofluorescent antibody test. The last test is not recommended because it has both a much lower sensitivity than either the IgM ELISA or IgM immunosorbent agglutination assay and poor specificity secondary to rheumatoid factors and antinuclear antibodies, contributing to false-positive results. Other tests that are still being investigated include a *T. gondii*–specific IgA ELISA and IgA immunofiltration assay; a *T. gondii*–specific IgE immunofiltration assay; and IgG, IgM, and IgA immunoblotting tests.

Because the majority of adults with acquired *Toxoplasma* infection are asymptomatic, evaluation of the pregnant woman and fetus is usually prompted by either seroconversion or an elevated maternal *Toxoplasma* IgG titer (Couvreur et al, 1988; Daffos et al, 1988). The latter may reflect chronic or past infection, so the acuity of the maternal infection is determined serologically with the HS-AC differential agglutination test. If recent maternal infection is documented by an acute pattern on the HS-AC test, seroconversion, or rising IgG antibody titers, the fetus should be evaluated by ultrasonography, and amniotic fluid should be tested for specific *Toxoplasma* DNA with PCR. The latter has supplanted the need for cordocentesis, and a positive result confirms fetal infection (Hohlfeld et al, 1994). Postnatally, serologic testing of paired maternal and infant sera should be performed at a reliable laboratory that will include assays for *Toxoplasma* IgG and IgM antibodies. Neonatal serum for *Toxoplasma* IgA determination by ELISA also should be considered because it may yield the only positive result in some infants.

Subinoculation of placental tissue, amniotic fluid, and umbilical cord blood into mice should be considered. If results of these tests suggest possible infection, the newborn should be evaluated fully with complete blood cell count and platelet determination, liver function tests, CSF evaluation (including tests for IgG and IgM antibodies and PCR) (Wallon et al, 1998), CT of the head, ophthalmologic examination, and hearing evaluation. The presence of neonatal IgM antibody in serum or CSF, or a positive PCR result for blood or CSF indicates congenital infection. In addition, at-risk infants should undergo serologic follow-up to detect rising serum IgG titers during the first year of life or persistence of IgG antibody beyond 12 to 15 months of age, when maternal IgG antibody has disappeared (Robert-Gangneux et al, 1999a, 1999b). Uninfected infants show a continuous decline in *Toxoplasma* IgG titer with no detectable IgM or IgA antibodies.

Low IgG titers and an HS-AC differential agglutination test that indicate remote maternal infection do not require further evaluation of the mother or infant unless the mother is infected with HIV. Because fetal infection has occurred during chronic *Toxoplasma* infection in HIV-infected pregnant women, their infants should be evaluated serologically at birth for evidence of congenital infection. It has been suggested that HIV-infected pregnant women who have low $CD4^+$ T lymphocyte counts and who are seropositive for *Toxoplasma* antibody receive prophylaxis to prevent fetal infection (Beaman et al, 1992; Wong and Remington, 1994). However, insufficient data currently are available to recommend that such therapy be given routinely for this indication. Nevertheless, if such women previously have had toxoplasmic encephalitis, prophylaxis with pyrimethamine, sulfadiazine, and leucovorin (folinic acid) should be considered (Masur et al, 2002).

### Therapy

It is currently recommended that fetuses and infants younger than 1 year who are infected with *T. gondii* receive specific therapy effective against this congenital pathogen, even if they have no clinical signs of disease (Couvreur et al, 1988; Daffos et al, 1988; Foulon et al, 1999; Friedman et al, 1999; Gilbert et al, 2001; Hohlfeld et al, 1989; Koppe et al, 1986; McAuley et al, 1994; McGee et al, 1992; Peyron and Wallon, 2001; Roizen et al, 1995; Vergani et al, 1998; Wallon et al, 1999; Wong and Remington, 1994). On the basis of comparison with untreated historic controls, outcome is improved substantially by maternal, fetal, and neonatal treatment. Spiramycin has been used in pregnant women with acute toxoplasmosis to reduce transplacental transmission of *T. gondii*. If fetal infection is confirmed after the 17th week of pregnancy, however, treatment with pyrimethamine, sulfadiazine, and folinic acid is recommended. Prenatal treatment of congenital toxoplasmosis reduces the clinical severity of infection in the newborn while shifting the disease to a more subclinical form. This effect in turn may ameliorate the long-term neurologic complications that are commonly seen among infants who have clinical manifestations in the neonatal period.

Neonatal treatment has also resulted in reductions in sensorineural hearing loss and neurodevelopmental and visual handicaps. Table 38–2 shows the recommended

**TABLE 38–2**

**Treatment Guidelines for Congenital Toxoplasmosis**

| | Therapy | Dosage (Oral Unless Specified) | Duration |
|---|---|---|---|
| In pregnant women with acute toxoplasmosis: | | | |
| For first 21 wks of gestation or until term if fetus not infected | Spiramycin* | 1 g q 8 hr without food | Until fetal infection documented or excluded at 21 wks; if fetal infection documented, replaced with pyrimethamine, leucovorin, and sulfadiazine (see below) |
| If fetal infection confirmed after 18th week of gestation or if infection acquired in last few weeks of gestation | Pyrimethamine *and* | Loading dose: 100 mg/day in 2 divided doses for 2 days followed by 50 mg/day | Until delivery |
| | Sulfadiazine* *and* | Loading dose: 75 mg/kg/day in 2 divided doses (maximum, 4 g/d) for 2 days; then 100 mg/kg/day in 2 divided doses (maximum, 4 g/day) | Until delivery |
| | Leucovorin† | 10-20 mg qd | Until delivery |
| Congenital *Toxoplasma* infection in infant | Pyrimethamine *and* | Loading dose: 2 mg/kg/day for 2 days; then 1 mg/kg/day for 2 or 6 months; then 1 mg/kg/day on Mon, Wed, and Fri each week | ≥1 yr |
| | Sulfadiazine* *and* | 100 mg/kg/day in 2 daily divided doses | ≥1 yr |
| | Leucovorin (folinic acid)† | 10 mg 3 times weekly | ≥1 yr |
| | Corticosteroids (prednisone)‡ | 1 mg/kg/daily in 2 daily divided doses | Until resolution of elevated (≥1 g/dL) CSF protein or active chorioretinitis that threatens vision |

*Available only on request from the U.S. Food and Drug Administration (301-827-2127; fax, 301-927-2475).

†Monitor blood and platelet counts weekly; adjust dosage for megaloblastic anemia, granulocytopenia, or thrombocytopenia.

‡When signs of inflammation or active chorioretinitis have subsided, dosage can be tapered and drug discontinued; use only in conjunction with pyrimethamine, sulfadiazine, and leucovorin.

Data from Boyer KM, McAuley B: Congenital toxoplasmosis. Semin Pediatr Dis 5:42, 1994; and Remington JS, McLeod R, Thulliez P, Desmonts G: Toxoplasmosis. In Remington JS, Klein JO (eds): Infectious Diseases of the Fetus and Newborn Infant. 5th ed. Philadelphia, WB Saunders, 2001, p 293.

guidelines for the treatment of congenital toxoplasmosis. In infants with congenital toxoplasmosis, the treatment consists of pyrimethamine, sulfadiazine, and folinic acids (Boyer and McAuley, 1994; McAuley et al, 1994; McLeod et al, 1992; Remington et al, 2001). The actual duration of therapy is not known, although prolonged courses, at least 1 year, are preferred. Currently, most experts recommend combined treatment until the patient is 1 year old (Remington et al, 2001; Villena et al, 1998a, 1998b).

Complete blood cell counts and platelet determination must be monitored closely while the patient is receiving therapy, because granulocytopenia, thrombocytopenia, and megaloblastic anemia may occur. These parameters usually improve once a higher dosage of folinic acid is administered or pyrimethamine and sulfadiazine are discontinued temporarily. The indications for adjunctive therapy with corticosteroids such as prednisone (0.5 mg/kg twice a day) are CSF protein concentration 1 g/dL or higher and chorioretinitis that threatens vision; corticosteroid treatment is continued until either condition resolves. Current therapies are not effective against encysted bradyzoites and therefore may not prevent reactivation of chorioretinitis and neurologic disease.

### Prognosis

Maternal toxoplasmosis acquired during the first and second trimesters has been associated with stillbirth and perinatal death secondary to severe fetal infection in approximately 35% and 7% of cases, respectively. Among infants born with congenital toxoplasmosis, the mortality rate has been reported to be as high as 12%. In addition, infants with congenital toxoplasmosis are at high risk for ophthalmologic, neurodevelopmental, and audiologic impairments, including mental retardation (87%), seizures (82%), spasticity and palsies (71%), and deafness (15%) (Eichenwald, 1960; Hohlfeld et al, 1989; Koppe et al, 1986; McAuley et al, 1994). Of neonates with subclinical infection, long-term follow-up reveals eye or neurologic disease in as many as 80% to 90% by the time they reach adulthood (Couvreur and Desmonts, 1962; Couvreur et al, 1984; McLeod et al, 2000; Saxon et al, 1973; Wilson et al, 1980). Data from the United States National Collaborative Treatment Trial show that treatment of neonates with congenital toxoplasmosis early and for 1 year resulted in more favorable outcomes than were reported for untreated infants or infants who were treated for only 1 month.

### Prevention

Pregnant women whose serologic status for *T. gondii* is negative or unknown, as well as women who are attempting to conceive, should be educated on the prevention of congenital toxoplasmosis through avoidance of at-risk behaviors that may expose them to cat feces or encysted bradyzoites in raw meat (Centers for Disease Control and Prevention [CDC], 2000; Eskild et al, 1996; Foulon et al, 2000; Jones et al, 2001; Wilson and Remington, 1980). Such women should be taught to wear gloves when changing cat litter boxes or gardening and to wash hands well after such activities. Daily changing of cat litter will also decrease the chance of infection, because oocysts are not infective during the first 1 to 2 days after passage. In addition, feeding cats commercially prepared foods rather than undercooked meats or wild rodents reduces the likelihood of their becoming infected and capable of transmitting the infection to a pregnant woman. Oral ingestion of *T. gondii* can be prevented by either cooking meat to well done, smoking it, or curing it in brine, and by washing kitchen surfaces that come into contact with raw meat. Vegetables and fruits should be washed, and hands and kitchen surfaces should be cleaned after handling fruits, vegetables, and raw meat. Flies and cockroaches may serve as transport hosts for *T. gondii*, so their access to food must be prevented.

Routine serologic screening of women during pregnancy has been an effective means of prevention in such countries as France and Austria, where the incidence of congenital toxoplasmosis is high. No such screening is currently recommended in the United States. However, high-risk women, including those who are immunocompromised, should be screened early in pregnancy. Neonatal screening for IgM antibody has also been advocated so that asymptomatic infants can be detected and treated before neurologic symptoms develop (Peterson and Eaton, 1999). This strategy, however, has been hampered by the lack of readily available and reliable IgM test kits. Moreover, such screening will not detect the approximately 25% of infected infants who lack anti-*Toxoplasma* IgM antibody. Further studies involving cost analyses are needed to define the best preventive strategy for congenital toxoplasmosis in specific populations, regions, and countries.

## SYPHILIS

Before 1945, a chapter on congenital syphilis in a textbook devoted to diseases of the newborn would have been the most important one in the infectious disease section because of the great number of newborns affected and the broad variety of clinical syndromes produced. If this chapter had been omitted in the 1950s and 1960s, it would have been scarcely missed. In many parts of the United States, a young pediatrician might have completed 3 years of residency in a large urban hospital without ever having encountered one case. The situation has changed, however, and a new syphilis epidemic developed during the late 1980s and 1990s (Berry and Dajani, 1992).

### Incidence

During the 1930s and 1940s, in the congenital syphilis clinic of the Harriet Lane Home in Baltimore, Maryland, 60 to 80 infants and children attended each week for arsenic therapy. Many more were lost to follow-up before completing their 2- to 3-year course of treatment. It was unusual if fewer than three or four new examples were discovered in the general outpatient department in the course of 1 week. Then, for several decades, the frequency of the disease declined. The curve of incidence has been rising since the 1970s, however (Fig. 38–1).

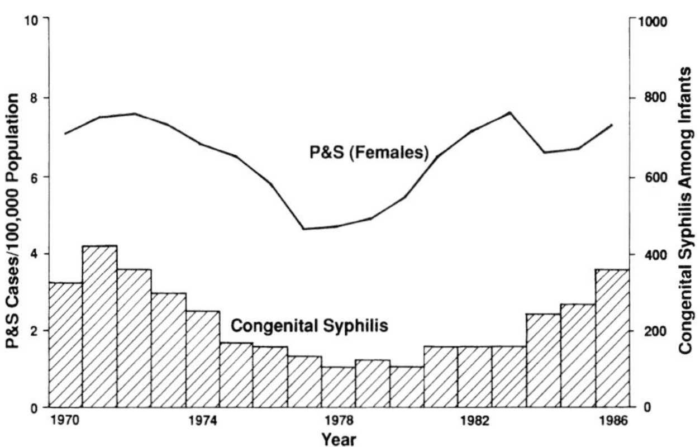


**FIGURE 38–1.** Case rates of primary and secondary (P&S) syphilis among females and congenital syphilis among infants less than 1 year of age in the United States, 1970 to 1986 showing the beginning of the epidemic in the United States. *(From Ingall D, Dobson SRM, Musher D: Syphilis. In Remington JS, Klein JO [eds]: Infectious Diseases of the Fetus and Newborn Infant. Philadelphia, WB Saunders, 1990, pp 367-394.)*

From 1980 to 1986, the number of cases of congenital syphilis rose from 111 cases to 365 cases per year in the United States. More than 600 cases were reported in 1989. In 48% of cases, there was inadequate or no prenatal care, and treatment failed in 19% of total cases and in 35% of women who had prenatal care (Congenital syphilis, 1986). During the 1990s, the epidemic has not been restricted to a single region of the country: The South (178%), the Midwest (244%), and the West (777%) have all experienced dramatic increases in incidence of congenital syphilis (Dunn et al, 1993). By 2001, the spike in number of cases has all but disappeared (www.cdc.gov/std/syphilis2001).

## Etiology and Pathogenesis

The organism responsible for syphilis is *Treponema pallidum*. This delicate, corkscrew-shaped, flagellated, highly motile spirochete is almost identical in appearance to *Treponema pertenue*, which causes yaws. These two diseases, like smallpox and cowpox, produce a cross-immunity for each other. This fact was established by Alexander Schaffer, the first editor of this textbook, when, after having spent 2 years on yaws-infested Fiji without encountering one case of syphilis, he was transferred to yaws-free India, where syphilis became one of his major medical preoccupations.

Syphilis can be acquired by introduction of *Treponema* through an abrasion in the skin or mucous membrane or by transplacental transmission. Whereas adults and some children become infected percutaneously, young infants almost invariably receive the organism from their mothers via the placenta and the umbilical vein. Transplacental transmission may take place at any time during gestation but ordinarily occurs during the second half of pregnancy. Fetuses infected early may die in utero or are at high risk for significant neurodevelopmental morbidity. The impact of the current epidemic on potentially preventable fetal deaths has not been evaluated. The usual outcome of a third-trimester infection is the birth of an apparently normal infant who becomes ill within the first few weeks of life. Whereas virtually all infants born to women with primary or secondary infection have congenital infection, only 50% are clinically symptomatic. Because of growing pressure from managed care organizations for early discharge of new mothers, which has occurred at the same time as the current epidemic, identification of congenitally infected, asymptomatic infants whose maternal infections occurred late in the third trimester and whose syphilis serologic test results are not yet positive at the time of delivery has presented an unusually difficult problem for tracking and treatment (Dorfman and Glaser, 1990). It is critical that all infants undergo serologic testing for syphilis at the time of delivery and have a source of primary health care capable of tracking both maternal and infant syphilis status (Chhabra et al, 1993; Zenker and Berman, 1991). Early latent infection results in a 40% infant infection rate, and late latent infection results in a 6% to 14% infant infection rate (Wendel, 1988).

## Pathology

Because *Treponema* enters the fetal bloodstream directly, the primary stage of infection is completely bypassed. There is no chancre and no local lymphadenopathy. Instead, the liver, the immediate target of the invasion, is flooded with organisms, which then penetrate all the other organs and tissues of the body to a lesser degree. Exactly where they take root and arouse local pathologic response, which in turn produces the presenting signs and symptoms, is unpredictable. Principal sites of predilection are the liver, skin, mucous membranes of the lips and anus, bones, and the central nervous system. If fetal invasion has taken place early, the lungs may be heavily involved in a characteristic *pneumonia alba*, but this condition is seldom compatible with life. *Treponema* may be found in almost any other organ or tissue of the body but seldom causes inflammatory and destructive changes in loci other than the ones named previously.

Under the microscope, the tissue alterations consist of nonspecific interstitial fibrosis with or without evidence of low-grade inflammatory response in the form of round cell inflammation. Necrosis follows fairly regularly in bone but only rarely in other tissues. Localization and gumma formation are not common in the neonate. Noteworthy is extensive extramedullary hematopoiesis in the liver, spleen, kidneys, and other organs.

## Diagnosis

The most common signs and symptoms of congenital infection in the neonatal period are listed in Table 38–3. Additional diagnoses associated with congenital syphilis are nonimmune hydrops, nephrosis, and myocarditis (Wendel, 1988). The earliest sign of congenital syphilis may be snuffles, in which the nose becomes obstructed and begins to discharge clear fluid at first, then purulent or even sanguineous material later.

Cutaneous lesions appear at any time from the second week on. They are sparse or numerous and are copper-colored and may be round, oval, or iris-shaped and circinate or desquamative. Even more characteristic than their appearance is their distribution, which most frequently

TABLE 38-3

**Clinical Features of Early Congenital Syphilis by Age**

| Feature | % of Patients with Finding: Age <4 Wks | Age >4 Wks |
|---|---|---|
| Hepatosplenomegaly | 91 | 87 |
| Joint swellings | 3 | 34 |
| Rash | 31 | 55 |
| Anemia | 64 | 89 |
| Jaundice | 49 | 7 |
| Snuffles | 12 | 50 |
| Metaphyseal dystrophy | 95 | 91 |
| Periostitis | 37 | 80 |
| Cerebrospinal fluid changes | 44 | 37 |

Modified from Hira SK, Bhad GJ, Patel JB, et al: Early congenital syphilis: Clinicoradiographic features in 202 patients. Sex Transm Dis 12:177, 1985.

includes the perioral, perinasal, and diaper regions. Palms and soles are also involved, but the rash is soon replaced there by diffuse reddening, thickening, and wrinkling. In heavily infected infants, the rash may become generalized. Mucocutaneous junctions become involved in typical fashion. The lips become thickened and roughened and tend to weep. Radial cracks appear that traverse the vermilion zone up to and a bit beyond the mucocutaneous margins of the lips. These are the beginnings of the radiating scars that may persist for many years as rhagades. Similar mucocutaneous lesions involve the anus and vulva, but in these locations, the white, flat, moist, raised plaques known as "condylomata" are also encountered, although less frequently.

Radiographs of the bones show characteristic osteochondritis and periostitis in 80% to 90% of infants with symptomatic congenital syphilis. In most cases, the bone lesions are asymptomatic, but in a few, they are severe enough to lead to subepiphyseal fracture and epiphyseal dislocation, an extremely painful pseudoparalysis of one or more extremities, may supervene. About 20% asymptomatic, congenitally infected infants have metaphyseal changes consistent with congenital syphilis. Radiographic alterations include an unusually dense band at the epiphyseal ends, below which is a band of translucency whose margins are at first sharp but that later become serrated, jagged, and irregular. The shafts become generally more opaque, but spotty areas of translucency throughout may give them a moth-eaten look. The periosteum of the long bones becomes more and more thickened. Epiphyses separate because the dense end plate breaks away from the shaft by fracture through the subepiphyseal zone of decalcification. This is exactly what happens in the pseudoparalysis of scurvy, although the reason for the weakening of the subepiphyseal bone is different. In syphilis, pseudoparalysis appears within the first 3 months of life; in scurvy, it seldom manifests before 5 months of life.

Signs of visceral involvement include hepatomegaly, splenomegaly, and general glandular enlargement. Palpable epitrochlear nodes are not pathognomonic but are highly suggestive of congenital syphilis. The liver may be greatly enlarged, firm, and nontender. Associated with this may be jaundice, which appears in the second or third week of life, is seldom intense, and does not persist for many days. Anemia, probably indicative of bone marrow infection and hematopoietic suppression, may become severe. Lesions in the gastrointestinal tract and pancreas may occur and may produce distention and delay in passage of meconium.

Clinical signs of central nervous system involvement seldom appear in the newborn infant, even though one third to one half of those infected suffer such involvement. The involvement is demonstrated by cerebrospinal fluid changes such as increased protein content, a mononuclear pleocytosis of up to 200 or 300 cells/mL, or by a positive result of the Venereal Disease Research Laboratories (VDRL) test (Table 38–4).

Diagnosis is confirmed by dark-field visualization of *Treponema* in scrapings from any lesion or from any body fluid, by visualization of characteristic bone changes on radiographs, and by positive serologic test results for syphilis. Serologic test results must be interpreted with caution, however. Because the IgG portion of reagin is transmitted across the placenta, its finding in the baby's serum means no more than that the mother has or has had syphilis. She may have been cured during pregnancy and yet still have quantities of reagin in her blood, or she may not have received treatment at all and still not have passed the disease on to her fetus. A

TABLE 38-4

**Severity of Disease and Cerebrospinal Fluid Findings in 108 Patients with High Risk for Congenital Syphilis**

| | Asymptomatic (normal) | Minimum Involvement | Intermediate Involvement | CNS Involvement |
|---|---|---|---|---|
| **% of infants affected:** | | | | |
| Age 91-180 days (n = 47) | 28 | 30 | 36 | 6 |
| Age 181-365 days (n = 31) | 45 | 32 | 20 | 3 |
| Age 366-731 days (n = 30) | 63 | 26 | 10 | 0 |
| **Cerebrospinal fluid findings:** | | | | |
| Cells/mL | 0-5 | 5-30 | 0-100 | 10-200 |
| Protein (mg/100 mL) | 15-30 | 30-75 | Moderate increase | 50-200 |
| VRDL titer result | Negative | Negative | Positive | Positive |

Modified from Moore JF: The Modern Treatment of Syphilis, 2nd ed. Springfield, IL, Charles C Thomas, 1943: and Platou RV: Adv Pediatr 4:35, 1949.

higher titer in the infant's blood than in the mother's is not evidence of fetal infection, nor is an elevated concentration of total IgM in the cord serum.

The most helpful specific test result is a positive finding in the newborn's blood of IgM antibody against *T. pallidum* on IgM-FTA-ABS (fluorescent treponemal antibody absorption) (Lewis, 1992; Stoll et al, 1993). This is fluorescent *Treponema* antibody from which antibodies from treponemes other than *T. pallidum* have been removed by absorption. This finding is usually an indicator of congenital syphilis, although in the presence of rheumatoid factor, false-positive results of this test are occasionally seen. However, the result is not always positive at first, even when infection is present in the infant, possibly because if the infection is acquired late in pregnancy, specific antibodies have not had time to form.

Thus, when an infant's blood VDRL test result is positive at birth, the diagnosis of congenital syphilis is not justified unless pathognomonic signs are also present. If they are not, serial determinations of reagin titer must be performed. If antibodies are passively acquired, the titer decreases to zero within 4 to 12 weeks; it increases if the disease is actually present. If the IgM-FTA-ABS result is also positive at birth, treatment may be initiated. If this result is negative, however, the test should be repeated several times at 3- or 4-week intervals.

### Treatment

Treatment is recommended for all pregnant women with syphilis regardless of the stage of pregnancy (Table 38–5). Recommendations from the CDC (2002) for treatment of symptomatic or asymptomatic infants are listed in Table 38–6. Long-term follow-up recommendations are outlined in Table 38–7.

Hardy and coworkers (1970) reported a rare case of a male infant who died of congenital syphilis. His mother had received penicillin G 10 days before delivery, and he was given massive doses for 17 days after birth. Even so, *T. pallidum* was recovered from the infant's eyes after his death.

## MALARIA

Malaria is a febrile disease caused by four species of *Plasmodium—P. falciparum, P. vivax, P. ovale*, and *P. malariae*. Humans acquire the infection from the bite of the female, nocturnally feeding *Anopheles* mosquito. Malaria remains the leading cause of death from parasitic infections in the world. An estimated 2 million deaths and 300 to 500 million cases of infection are attributed to malaria annually. Children have the highest mortality rate, followed by pregnant women (Alecrim et al, 2000). The greatest burden of disease and death is in Africa, where the rate *of P. falciparum* infection approaches 75% of the total population. In the United States, more than 1000 cases of malaria are reported annually to the CDC, and these occur almost exclusively in travelers and immigrants from endemic areas.

Congenital malaria, in contrast, remains rare, with only about 300 cases reported in the world literature (Balatbat et al, 1995). In the United States, an estimated 50 cases have been reported to the CDC in the last 50 years. A dramatic increase in the number of cases of congenital malaria that occurred in the United States from 1980 to 1981 was the result of a large influx of immigrants from endemic countries (Malviya and Shurin, 1984). With current

**TABLE 38-5**

**Recommended Treatment of Pregnant Patients with Syphilis**

| Stages of Syphilis | Drug (Penicillin) | Route | Dose (units) |
|---|---|---|---|
| Early (<1 yr duration) | Recommended | | |
| Primary, secondary, or early latent | | | |
| HIV antibody-negative | Benzathine | IM | 2.4 million single dose; possibly repeat in 1 wk |
| HIV antibody-positive* | Benzathine | IM | 2.4 million single dose; possibly repeat weekly × 2 |
| | *Alternative* | | |
| | Penicillin desensitization† | | |
| Latent (>1 yr duration)‡ | *Recommended* | | |
| | Benzathine | IM | 2.4 million weekly × 3 wk |
| | *Alternative* | | |
| | Penicillin desensitization | | |
| Neurosyphilis | *Recommended* | | |
| | Aqueous | IV | 3-4 million every 4 hr × 10-14 days |
| | *Alternative* | | |
| | Procaine§ | IM | 2.4 million daily × 10-14 days |

*With normal cerebrospinal fluid findings, if performed.

†For details, see MMWR Morb Mortal Wkly Rep 47:28, 1998.

‡Lumbar puncture to exclude neurosyphilis is recommended for HIV-antibody positive patients.

§Probenecid, 500 mg orally QID × 10-14 days, should also be prescribed.

HIV = human immunodeficiency virus; IM = intramuscular; IV = intravenous.

From Remington JS, Klein JO (eds): Infectious Diseases of the Fetus and Newborn Infant. 5th ed. Philadelphia, WB Saunders, 2001, p 666.

**TABLE 38-6**

**Recommended Treatment of the Newborn with Syphilis**

| Penicillin | Dose |
|---|---|
| Aqueous penicillin G | 50,000 u/kg/dose every 12 hours during first 7 days of life and every 8 hours thereafter for a total of 10-14 days |
| or | |
| Penicillin G, procaine | 50,000 u/kg per day, IM, in a single dose every day for 10 days |
| or | |
| (with low risk, no clinical signs, and uncertain follow-up) | |
| Penicillin G benzathine | 50,000 u/kg, IM, in a single dose |

From Remington JS, Klein JO (eds): Infectious Diseases of the Fetus and Newborn Infant. Philadelphia, WB Saunders, 5th ed. 2001, p 669, and Committee on Infectious Diseases: Red Book: 2003 Report of the Committee on Infectious Diseases. 26th ed. Elk Grove Village, IL: Academy of Pediatrics; 2003, p 602.

trends in immigration and foreign travel, congenital malaria not only will continue to be observed in the United States but also will probably increase in frequency in the years ahead. Because delay in diagnosis and treatment can result in significant morbidity and mortality, the differential diagnosis of fever in infants born to mothers who have lived or traveled in areas where malaria is endemic must include congenital malaria.

### Definition

*Congenital malaria* is defined as malaria acquired by the fetus or newborn directly from the mother, either in utero or during delivery (Moran and Couper, 1999). Application of the definition has not been consistent. Some investigators have based diagnosis of congenital malaria on detection of parasites in the newborn within 24 hours of birth (Larkin and Thuma, 1991) whereas others have used detection of the parasites within the first 7 days of age (Moran and Couper, 1999). These age-specific criteria are most applicable in endemic regions where, in older infants, it is difficult to distinguish congenital malaria from malaria acquired through mosquito transmission. Outside endemic areas, where postnatal transmission can be reasonably excluded, it is evident that clinical onset of disease in congenital malaria is usually delayed several weeks. These observations suggest that many cases of congenital malaria in endemic areas are likely misclassified as being postnatally acquired.

Congenital malaria also has been defined as umbilical cord blood parasitemia (Fischer, 1997), although the finding of parasites in cord blood is not uncommon in endemic areas and frequently clears without involving the peripheral circulation (Airede, 1991). Reinhardt (1978) found parasites in thick smears of cord blood in 22% of 198 infants born to women in the Ivory Coast, although the peripheral blood smears were negative for all of the infants. Similarly, 4% of 1009 infants born to Tanzanian women had parasites in umbilical cord blood, but in only 2 of 11 infants was evidence of parasitemia also detected on peripheral blood smear (McGregor, 1984). Parasitemia detected shortly after birth also may not evolve into clinically significant disease. In 10 of 35 congenitally infected newborns diagnosed at birth by Diallo (1983), parasites were no longer detectable in peripheral blood at 96 hours of age. In the remaining infants, blood smears for malaria

**TABLE 38-7**

**Follow-Up After Treatment or Prophylaxis for Congenital Syphilis**

| Patient Category | Follow-Up Procedures |
|---|---|
| Patients receiving diagnosis of congenital syphilis | 1. Reagin testing every 2-3 months for the first 15 months, then every 6 months until result is negative or stable at low titer.<br>2. Treponemal antibody test after 15 months of age.<br>3. Repeat cerebrospinal fluid evaluation 6 months after treatment if patient received treatment for or showed any signs of central nervous system disease.<br>4. Careful developmental evaluation, vision testing, and hearing testing before 3 years of age or at time of diagnosis. |
| Patients receiving treatment in utero or at birth because of maternal syphilis | 1. Reagin testing at birth and then every 3 months until test is negative.<br>2. Treponemal antibody test after 15 months of age. |
| Women receiving treatment for syphilis during pregnancy | 1. Reagin testing monthly until delivery, then every 6 months until test result is negative.<br>2. Retreatment any time there is a fourfold increase in reagin titer. |

Modified from Rathbun KC: Congenital syphilis: A proposal for improved surveillance, diagnosis and treatment. Sex Transm Dis 10:102, 1983.
From Remington JS, Klein JO (eds): Infectious Diseases of the Fetus and Newborn Infant. 5th ed. Philadelphia, WB Saunders, 2001, p 671.

were negative within 30 days of age. Larkin and Thuma (1991) found peripheral parasitemia within 24 hours of age in 19 (65%) of 65 newborns, but only 7 had clinical signs of disease. Because all 19 newborns received antimalarial therapy, it is not known how many of them would have shown clinical manifestations of malaria if left untreated.

### Epidemiology

The existence of congenital malaria was questioned in the early part of the 20th century. In 1950, Covell tabulated all reports of congenital malaria, defined as detection of the parasite in infants in the first 7 days after birth. Rates of placental parasitemia ranged from 5% to 74% and of maternal parasitemia from 1% to 68%. The prevalence of congenital malaria was estimated to be 0.3% (16 of 5324 births). The low frequency of vertical transmission was attributed to the effective barrier served by the placenta to the passage of the parasite as well as to the protective effect of transplacentally acquired maternal antibody in the fetus and newborn.

Covell's findings confirmed the existence of congenital malaria and have been cited repeatedly as evidence of the rarity of the disease in endemic areas. Bruce-Chwatt (1952) found a placental infection rate of 20% among 228 pregnancies in Nigeria, but only 1 (0.4%) of the 235 neonates had parasitemia. Similarly, McGregor (1984) found no peripheral parasitemia in blood samples collected within 24 hours of age from 147 infants born to mothers with placental malaria. In 1958, Cannon found that 26% of placentas were infected and, in 1970, Williams and McFarlane found 37% of placentas infected. Parasitemia, however, was not detected in any of the umbilical cord blood samples in either series.

Later studies have reported incidence rates for congenital malaria ranging from 4% to 15% (Nyirjesy et al, 1993). In Zambia during a season of heavy malaria transmission, Larkin and Thuma (1991) identified peripheral parasitemia in 19 (29%) of 65 newborns born to 63 women, although only 7 (37%) of the 19 infants had clinical signs of disease at the time of diagnosis. Peripheral blood smears from 700 peripartum mothers at seven sites in Sub-Saharan Africa revealed a 15% prevalence of maternal parasitemia (Fischer, 1997). Congenital malaria, defined as umbilical cord blood parasitemia, was found in 7% of newborns and ranged from 0% to 23% at the various centers. These researchers concluded that congenital malaria should no longer be considered rare in endemic areas.

A summary of studies from Africa reported from 1950 to the late 1980s divides the incidence of maternal and congenital malaria into low-frequency and high-frequency groups (MacLeod, 1988). In six studies of 2103 infants, the prevalence of congenital malaria ranged from 0% to 0.2%, whereas in another six studies of 1821 infants, the prevalence ranged from 4% to 44%. However, there was no consistent difference between the two groups to account for the discrepant findings. Even in the report by Covell (1950), the frequency of congenital malaria at various study sites ranged from 0% to 10%.

It is apparent from these observations that the true incidence of congenital malaria in endemic areas is unknown but highly variable among different populations. Underreporting of disease in endemic areas is likely, in part because of suboptimal data collection but also secondary to the difficulty in distinguishing congenital malaria from malaria acquired postnatally in young infants by mosquito transmission. Other confounding factors are location of the study, definition of congenital malaria, and selection of study participants, which varied from unselected mothers in labor to women with placental or peripheral parasitemia.

In contrast to the rarity of congenital malaria in indigenous populations, Covell (1950) found that the prevalence of congenital malaria among nonimmune populations (i.e., Europeans residing in or visiting endemic areas) to be approximately 7%. It is postulated that congenital malaria is more common in infants born to these women because their levels of immunity are lower than those of the native population. Congenital malaria also is more common among infants of women who emigrate from areas in which malaria is endemic to areas that are free of malaria, presumably as a result of waning immunity from lack of continued exposure.

In the United States, the occurrence of congenital malaria is well documented because the country has been free of indigenous disease since the 1950s. From 1950 to 1991, 49 cases of congenital malaria were reported (Hulbert, 1992), and at least five additional cases have been described subsequently (Balatbat et al, 1995; D'Avanzo et al, 2002; Gereige and Cimino, 1995; Starr and Wheeler, 1998; Viraraghavan and Jantausch, 2000). As expected, almost all of the cases were imported. Up to 1979, an average of one case per year was reported to the CDC (Hulbert, 1992; Malviya and Shurin, 1984). From 1980 to 1981, 16 cases were reported (Quinn et al, 1982). This abrupt increase followed a rise in the total number of cases of malaria in the United States that occurred as a result of a large influx of refugees and immigrants from Southeast Asia (Mertz et al, 1981). Fifteen of the 16 infants were born to mothers from that region. In contrast, in the past 20 years, mothers of infants with congenital malaria have come from Mexico, Central America, and Africa, reflecting changes in immigration patterns.

### Natural History

Congenital infection occurs with all four species of *Plasmodium*. Among the 107 cases tabulated by Covell (1950), mostly all from Africa, 64% were caused by *P. falciparum*, 32% by *P. vivax*, and 2% by *P. malariae*. In Hulbert's (1992) review of 49 cases in the United States since 1950, 82% of infections were due to *P. vivax*, reflecting immigration patterns in the United States. *P. falciparum* and *P. malariae* accounted for 6% and 10% of infections, respectively. Infection with more than one species also is possible. In one report, concurrent infection with *P. malariae* and *P. vivax* was documented in a 6-week-old infant (MacLeod et al, 1982).

In endemic regions, both the prevalence and density of malarial parasitemia are increased in pregnant versus nonpregnant women (Fisher, 1997; McGregor, 1984). Prevalence rates are highest in primigravid women and decline with rising parity (McGregor, 1984). The propensity of pregnant women to have malaria is hypothesized to be due to diminished immunity associated with pregnancy, which allows for reactivation of symptomatic or asymptomatic parasitemia. In addition, parasitemia in the placental tissue of women living in endemic areas is not an uncommon finding. In Africa, prevalence rates of placental malaria are 20% to 34%, although rates as high as 74% have been reported (McGregor, 1984).

Malaria in pregnancy may affect both the mother and fetus adversely. Several studies from areas where malaria is endemic have demonstrated an association between maternal peripheral or placental parasitemia and spontaneous abortion, premature delivery, and low birth weight (MacLeod, 1988; Nyirjesy et al, 1993; Subramanian et al, 1992). The best-documented sequela is low birth weight, secondary to either prematurity or intrauterine growth restriction. Bruce-Chwatt (1952) examined the placentas of 310 singleton deliveries in Lagos and found that 73 (24%) contained parasites. The average birth weight of infants born to mothers whose placentas were infected was 145 g less than that of those born with uninfected placentas. Similarly, Archibald (1956) and Jeliffe (1968) documented a decrease in birth weight of 170 g and 263 g, respectively, in infants born to mothers with placental parasitemia. With respect to peripheral parasitemia, Larkin and Thuma (1991) found a 469-g lower average birth weight without an increase in prematurity rate among 19 such infants compared with 46 infants without parasitemia. Additional supportive evidence of the effect of maternal malaria on birth weight is the rise in birth weight that is observed when pregnant women are given chemoprophylaxis (MacLeod, 1988; Nyierjesy et al, 1993).

The timing and mechanism of transmission of *Plasmodium sp.* from the mother to the fetus is not well understood. In utero transmission is supported by the finding of malarial parasites in fetal tissues at autopsy (Mertz et al, 1981), by umbilical cord blood parasitemia (McGregor, 1984), and by the onset of clinical signs of malaria within hours of birth (Brandenburg and Kenny, 1982; Covell, 1950; Gereige and Cimino, 1995). Alternatively, clinical findings in infants with congenital malaria may be delayed for several weeks after birth, suggesting infection at parturition (Hulbert, 1992). Transmission of malaria probably does not occur as a result of transplacental passage of the exoerythrocytic parasite. More likely, vertical transmission occurs by transfusion of parasitized maternal erythrocytes through a breach in the placental barrier that may occur either prematurely during pregnancy or during labor. Parasites in umbilical cord blood or fetal blood then may be cleared spontaneously, resulting in no disease manifestations, or may proliferate, with development of clinical signs of disease. Transmission of malaria by breast-feeding does not occur.

The clinical manifestations of congenital malaria, although occasionally seen within hours of birth (Brandenburg and Kenny, 1982; Gereige and Cimino, 1995), are typically delayed until an infant is several weeks of age. Among 49 infants with congenital malaria born in the United States, the mean age at onset of clinical signs was 5.5 weeks, with 96% of infants presenting between 2 and 8 weeks of age (Hulbert, 1992). The prolonged interval between birth and onset of clinical manifestations may be explained by transmission late in pregnancy or at delivery, so that multiple erythrocytic life cycles are required to produce clinically evident disease, or by the presence and amount of transplacentally acquired maternal antimalarial antibodies. When such antibodies are present in sufficient concentrations, as in infants born to immune mothers, parasitic replication may be prevented or attenuated, and clinical signs may be mild, delayed, or even absent. On the other hand, among infants born to mothers with low or nonexistent immunity, parasitic replication is uninhibited, and clinical signs of malaria supervene. Preterm infants, who do not benefit from passive immunity, may manifest clinical signs earlier than full-term infants. In a review of premature neonates with congenital malaria, 4 of 5 infants were diagnosed in the first week of life (Ahmed et al, 1998), although the prompt medical evaluation afforded these infants may have facilitated earlier detection.

The clinical features of congenital malaria are nonspecific and often resemble those due to sepsis or other congenital infections. Fever is almost uniformly present, but without the characteristic paroxysmal pattern. In Hulbert's review of congenital malaria (1992), fever occurred in all 44 infants for whom clinical information was available. Other clinical signs are anorexia, vomiting, and irritability (Brandenburg and Kenny, 1982). On physical examination, hepatosplenomegaly, suggestive of a transplacentally acquired infection, is found in the majority of infants (Hulbert, 1992). Anemia, often hemolytic, thrombocytopenia, and hyperbilirubinemia are the most commonly reported laboratory abnormalities. Additional physical and laboratory findings among 49 infants with congenital malaria reviewed by Hulbert (1992) are provided in Tables 38–8 and 38–9. Most abnormalities resolve within several days of initiation of treatment.

### Diagnosis

The diagnosis of congenital malaria is based on microscopic demonstration of parasites on thick and thin blood smears. For detection of organisms, a thick blood film is preferred because it concentrates the red blood cells. Identification of the *Plasmodium* species, however, requires a thin blood film. Specimens for smears should be obtained from both the infant and the mother, and quantification of the parasitemia is helpful to assess the response to therapy. Often, the diagnosis of congenital malaria is made incidentally. In all 4 cases of congenital malaria reported by Quinn and associates (1982), the diagnosis was established by a hematology technician who noted malarial parasites on routine blood smears.

**TABLE 38–8**

**Frequency of Physical Findings in 49 Infants with Congenital Malaria**

| Finding | Frequency* | % |
|---|---|---|
| Fever | 44/44 | 100 |
| Irritability | 11/13 | 85 |
| Jaundice | 11/14 | 79 |
| Hepatomegaly | 21/25 | 84 |
| Splenomegaly | 25/27 | 93 |

*Numerator = number of patients with finding; denominator = number of patients of the 49 for which data were available.

Adapted from Hulbert TV: Congenital malaria in the United States: Report of a case and review. Clin Infect Dis 14:922, 1992.

**TABLE 38-9**

**Frequency of Laboratory Findings in 49 Infants with Congenital Malaria**

| Finding | Mean (Range) | No. of Patients* |
|---|---|---|
| Hemoglobin (g/L) | 83 (40-165) | 22 |
| Reticulocyte count (%) | 7.5 (1.9-16) | 8 |
| Leukocyte count (cells/L) | $8.3 \times 10^9$ ($4.7\text{-}21 \times 10^9$) | 16 |
| Platelet count (cells/L) | $72 \times 10^9$ ($27\text{-}257 \times 10^9$)† | 10 |
| Total bilirubin (μmol/L) | 72 (7-154)‡ | 15 |

*Number of patients for whom data were available.

†Count in 90% of patients $<100 \times 10^9$ cells /L.

‡Value elevated in 71% of patients.

Adapted from Hulbert TV: Congenital malaria in the United States: Report of a case and review. Clin Infect Dis 14:922, 1992.

The diagnosis of congenital malaria is often delayed because of its nonspecific features and the lack of clinical suspicion. In Hulbert's review (1992) of 49 infants with congenital malaria, the diagnosis was established within 2 weeks of onset of clinical manifestations in 81% of cases. For the remaining 19%, diagnosis was delayed to between 3 and 24 weeks. Maternal history of recent travel to or emigration from an endemic area may suggest the diagnosis but is often obscured by the lack of clinical or laboratory findings in the mother. Depending on her immune status as well as the infecting species of *Plasmodium*, the mother may be completely asymptomatic or severely ill. In the review by Hulbert (1992), only 24 (69%) of 35 mothers reported having fever at some time during their pregnancies, and in only 42% of the mothers of 49 infants with malaria did blood smears show malarial parasites.

Further confounding the early recognition of congenital malaria is that the lapse between malaria exposure in the mother and in utero infection of the infant may be prolonged. *P. vivax* and *P. ovale* can remain dormant in the liver, especially if the infected individual did not receive therapy for the exoerythrocytic forms, and can cause a delayed relapse of malaria. *P. malariae* may persist for 20 to 40 years before demonstrable parasitemia or clinical symptoms appear (D'Avanzo et al, 2002). In the review by Hulbert (1992), among 35 mothers of infants with congenital malaria, 3 had resided in the United States for 36, 60, and 84 months, respectively. Sixty-one percent of the mothers had been in the United States for less than 10 months, and 91% for less than 18 months, before delivery. Congenital malaria due to *P. malariae* has been reported in an infant whose mother lived in the United States for 5 years before delivery and did not have any clinical signs or symptoms of malaria for more than 20 years (Harvey et al, 1969). In North Carolina, congenital *P. malariae* infection was reported in a 10-week-old infant who was born to a mother who had emigrated from the Democratic Republic of Congo 4 years before delivery (D'Avanzo et al, 2002).

## Therapy

The management of congenital malaria consists of supportive care and antimalarial therapy. Standard precautions are recommended. For all cases of congenital malaria, except those due to chloroquine-resistant *P. falciparum*, the recommended therapy is oral chloroquine sulfate (10 mg base/kg followed by 5 mg base/kg at 6, 24, and 48 hours later) (Quinn et al, 1982). Treatment with primaquine for *P. vivax* or *P. ovale* infection is not necessary because, as in transfusion-acquired malaria, congenital infection does not involve the transmission of exoerythrocytic parasites. If oral therapy is not possible, chloroquine may be administered by nasogastric tube (White et al, 1988). Parenteral administration of chloroquine has been associated with cardiovascular collapse and should be reserved for severe cases if oral administration is not possible (Quinn et al, 1982; White et al, 1988).

The treatment of congenital infection caused by chloroquine-resistant *P. falciparum* is not well defined. In older children, recommended regimens include quinine sulfate in combination with doxycycline or pyrimethamine-sulfadoxine and mefloquine (American Academy of Pediatrics [AAP], 2003a). The use of oral quinine sulfate (25 mg/kg/day divided in three doses for five days) and trimethoprim-sulfamethoxazole (8 mg/kg/day of trimethoprim in two divided doses for 5 days) is recommended by Quinn and associates (1982), who used this regimen to treat a 1-month-old infant. Ahmed and colleagues (1998) used a similar regimen for the treatment of an infant born at 28 weeks of gestation to a mother from Zaire. Other regimens used successfully in neonates are oral quinine sulfate and pyrimethamine-sulfadoxine (Gereige and Cimino, 1995) and intravenous quinine hydrochloride followed by oral quinine (Airede, 1991). Intravenous quinine hydrochloride is not available in the United States.

Parenterally administered quinidine gluconate may result in cardiac arrhythmias and should be reserved for severely ill infants, such as those with a higher than 5% parasitic load. These patients should be managed in the intensive care setting to allow for cardiac monitoring. Exchange transfusion may be considered when parasitemia exceeds 10% or if there is evidence of complications at lower parasite densities. With the rarity of *P. falciparum* congenital malaria in the United States, the growing pattern of resistance, and the potential toxicity associated with therapy, advice for the most current treatment recommendations should be sought from the CDC (telephone: 770-488-7788, www.cdc.gov).

The efficacy of antimalarial therapy should be monitored by means of sequential blood smears for percentage of parasitemia. Response to therapy with chloroquine for non–*P. falciparum* malaria is usually favorable (Brandenburg and Kenny, 1982; Dowell and Musher, 1991; Hindi and Azimi, 1980). The mother of an infant with congenital malaria should be screened for malaria. Even if the smear is negative, by definition she is harboring a *Plasmodium* infection and should be treated accordingly. Mothers may breast-feed while receiving antimalarial drugs. Only very small concentrations of antimalarial drugs are detected in breast milk; the amount is neither harmful to the infant nor protective against malaria.

### Prognosis

The incidence of infant mortality secondary to maternal or congenital malaria in endemic areas is unknown. On the basis of its association with low birth weight, malaria in pregnancy is likely to be an underappreciated risk factor for increased infant mortality. In a review of studies between 1985 and 2000, Steketee and colleagues (2001) determined population-attributable risks for maternal malaria of 8% to 14% for low birth weight and of 3% to 8% for infant mortality. They estimated that 75,000 to 200,000 infant deaths annually are associated with malaria infection in pregnancy.

Among the cases of congenital malaria reported outside malarious areas, short-term outcome generally has been favorable. Most cases respond rapidly to therapy, and no neonatal deaths were reported among the 49 cases described by Hulbert (1992). Five premature neonates with congenital malaria have been reported, two of whom were born outside indigenous areas, but prematurity could not be attributed solely to maternal malaria for these infants. All five infants were treated successfully. It remains unclear whether the outcome of infants reported in the literature is due to an overall favorable prognosis for congenital malaria or to reporting bias.

### Prevention

The prevention of congenital malaria is based on avoidance of exposure and use of chemoprophylaxis. The use of mosquito netting, mesh screens on windows, insecticides, and mosquito repellents can decrease potential exposure to malarial parasites. For pregnant women traveling to areas where there is no chloroquine-resistant *P. falciparum* malaria, prophylaxis with chloroquine is recommended. The safety of chloroquine used for chemosuppression of malaria in pregnant women is well established (MacLeod 1988). The World Health Organization (WHO) advises pregnant women against traveling to areas where there is transmission of chloroquine-resistant *P. falciparum*. If such travel is unavoidable, consultation with an infectious diseases or malaria expert is advised.

Currently, mefloquine is the prophylactic drug of choice, including during the first trimester, for pregnant women who may be exposed to chloroquine-resistant *P. falciparum* (AAP, 2003). Although the product labeling of mefloquine does not recommend its use during pregnancy, it has not been associated with adverse fetal or pregnancy outcomes. Doxycycline and atovaquone-proguanil should not be used during pregnancy to prevent malaria. For those who cannot take the recommended antimalarial drug, the CDC should be contacted for advice on alternative drugs. There is no commercially available vaccine against malaria.

Because of the high prevalence of malaria in pregnancy, the WHO also advocates chemoprophylaxis for pregnant women living in malaria-endemic areas (Steketee et al, 2001). Antimalarial chemoprophylaxis during pregnancy may reduce the risk of malaria infection in pregnant women and increase the birth weight of infants born to infected women. Nyirjesy and colleagues (1993) found that chloroquine prophylaxis, even in areas where chloroquine-resistant *P. falciparum* was endemic, protected against maternal and fetal malaria, low birth weight, and perinatal death. Other investigators have not found similar benefits, and the overall impact of prophylaxis on maternal and fetal outcome remains inconclusive. In practice, implementation of antenatal malaria prevention is limited by lack of access to medical care, poor compliance with therapy, and widespread presence of chloroquine-resistant organisms.

## TUBERCULOSIS

Tuberculosis remains the most extensive infectious epidemic in the world. Each year, an estimated 8 million new cases of tuberculosis occur worldwide, and approximately 3 million people die from the disease. Although 95% of cases occur in the developing world, there are approximately 18,000 new cases annually in the United States, and about 15 million people have latent tuberculosis. Given its impact on public health, the WHO has declared tuberculosis to be a global emergency.

Despite the prevalence of tuberculosis, congenital tuberculosis occurs rarely, with approximately 300 cases described in the world literature. Although the majority of cases was reported in the pre-chemotherapy era, a substantial number has been observed in the last few decades (Adhikari et al, 1997; Cantwell et al, 1994a; Mazade et al, 2001; Pejham et al, 2002). Given the propensity of tuberculosis to progress rapidly with immunodeficiency states, the current epidemic of HIV in countries with endemic tuberculosis is likely to result in active tuberculosis in many pregnant women with the potential for transmitting infection to their offspring (Adhikari et al, 1997). In addition, increased immigration from developing countries along with global mobility suggests that congenital tuberculosis will also be observed in developed nations. The clinician should maintain a high index of suspicion for tuberculosis in pregnant women and infants.

### Definition

Congenital tuberculosis is the result of in utero infection of the fetus with *Mycobacterium tuberculosis*. The fetus can acquire the infection transplacentally from a mother with hematogenous tuberculosis or by aspiration of amniotic fluid that has been infected from endometritis or the placenta. Infection of the newborn also can occur during delivery through aspiration of infected amniotic fluid or postnatally through contact with a tuberculous mother or ingestion of infected breast milk. Because of the difficulty in ascribing the precise mode of transmission, some researchers suggest that the term *perinatal tuberculosis* be used to describe the acquisition of tuberculosis before or shortly after birth (Lackmann, 1994). Historically, however, *congenital tuberculosis* has referred to tuberculous infection of infants that is acquired before birth, that is, either antenatally or intrapartum (Cantwell et al, 1994b).

In 1935, Beitzke proposed the following criteria to standardize the definition of congenital tuberculosis:

(1) tuberculosis must be established by isolation of *M. tuberculosis* from the infant, (2) a primary complex must be demonstrated in the liver as proof of dissemination of the tubercle bacilli from the umbilical vein, and (3) if the primary complex is not documented, either tuberculous lesions must be present in the neonate within a few days of age or postnatal infection must be excluded in the older infant with certainty—as for example, by immediate separation of the newborn from the infected mother. These criteria were developed before the introduction of chemotherapy, when infant mortality in congenital tuberculosis was high, thus allowing for demonstration of the primary liver complex at autopsy, and when prolonged separation of the mother and infant at birth was standard tuberculosis-control practice.

It is difficult and no longer practical to apply Bietzke's criteria for the diagnosis of congenital malaria. The higher survival rate makes the documentation of a primary complex impossible, and separation of the mother and infant at birth is unlikely because the disease in the mother is often unrecognized. Revised criteria were proposed that are more applicable to current practice and thus improve diagnostic sensitivity (Cantwell et al, 1994a). To meet these criteria, the infant must have proven tuberculous lesions and at least one of the following conditions must be present: (1) lesions in the infant in the first week of life, (2) a primary hepatic complex or caseating hepatic granulomas in the infant, the latter of which may be documented by percutaneous liver biopsy, (3) tuberculous infection of the placenta or maternal genital tract, and (4) exclusion of postnatal transmission by thorough investigation of contacts.

## Epidemiology

From 1953 through 1984, the incidence of tuberculosis in the United States declined an average of 5% per year, reaching a nadir of 9.4 cases per 100,000 population. From 1985 through 1992, there was a 20% increase in the total number of cases of tuberculosis in the United States. The resurgence of tuberculosis was attributed to (1) the co-epidemic of HIV infection, (2) the increase in immigration from countries with a high prevalence of tuberculosis, (3) increased tuberculosis transmission in congregate settings such as homeless shelters and prisons, and (4) a decline in public health funding for tuberculosis control. Since 1992, however, the number of cases in the United States has decreased each year, reaching a record low in 1998 with a case rate of 6.8 per 100,000. Despite the decrease in the total burden of disease, tuberculosis in the United States continues to disproportionately affect foreign-born individuals as well as the medically underserved—the urban poor and racial and ethnic minorities.

The current epidemiology of tuberculosis in pregnancy is not well delineated. With the resurgence of tuberculosis in the 1980s, the number of cases among women of child-bearing age rose by 40% (Cantwell et al, 1994a). In 1991, almost 40% of tuberculosis cases in minority women occurred in those between 15 and 35 years of age (Smith and Teele, 1995). In spite of the high incidence of tuberculosis in women of child-bearing age, congenital tuberculosis remains uncommon. Blackall (1969) reported only three cases among infants born to 100 mothers with tuberculosis, and Ratner and colleagues (1951) identified no cases among infants born to 260 mothers with the disease. In a study of 1369 infants separated at birth from their tuberculous mothers and placed in foster care, only 12 children became tuberculin-positive during the 4 years of observation, and in all 12 cases, there was a source of infection in the postnatal environment (Smith and Teele, 1995).

The majority of the 300 sporadically reported cases of congenital tuberculosis were described in the pre-chemotherapy era. In 1980, Hageman and associates reviewed 24 cases of congenital tuberculosis reported in the English literature since the introduction of isoniazid (INH) in 1952 as well as 2 additional cases from their own experience. In the subsequent 25 years, more than 30 additional cases have been cited (Abughali et al, 1994; Cantwell et al, 1994a; Mazade et al, 2001; Pejham et al, 2002) in the United States. As would be expected, the majority of infants with congenital tuberculosis were born to foreign-born mothers. The low incidence of congenital tuberculosis is in part attributed to the high likelihood of infertility in women who have endometrial tuberculosis (Balasubramanian et al, 1999). However, underreporting may be a contributing factor and the true incidence of congenital tuberculosis as the well as the rate of vertical transmission remain unknown.

## Natural History

The pathogenesis of tuberculosis in the pregnant woman is similar to that in nonpregnant adults. Tuberculous bacillemia can disseminate to the placenta, the endometrium, or the genital tract. Genital tuberculosis that occurred before pregnancy may be asymptomatic, although sterility in these cases frequently decreases the likelihood of congenital infection. Transmission to the fetus occurs by (1) hematogenous spread from the placenta via the umbilical vein, (2) aspiration in utero of infected amniotic fluid from either placental or endometrial infection, or (3) ingestion of infected amniotic fluid or secretions during delivery. The hematogenous route and in utero aspiration each probably account for approximately half of the cases of congenital tuberculosis. In addition, postnatal infection may occur from contact with a contagious mother or caregiver or ingestion of infected breast milk from a mother with tuberculous breast abscess. In the absence of a breast abscess, transmission of tuberculosis via breast milk has not been documented.

Tubercle bacilli have been demonstrated in the decidua, amnion, and chorionic villi of the placenta. It is unlikely that the fetus can be infected directly from the mother without the presence of a caseous lesion in the placenta, although even massive involvement of the placenta does not always result in congenital tuberculosis. When a tubercle ruptures into the fetal circulation, bacilli in the umbilical vein may infect the liver, forming a primary focus with involvement of periportal lymph nodes. The bacilli may also pass through the liver and right ventricle and into the lung, or may enter the left ventricle via the foramen ovale and pass into the systemic circulation. The organisms in the lung remain dormant until after birth, when oxygenation and circulation result in their multiplication and the subsequent development of a primary pulmonary focus. Alternatively, if the caseous lesion in the placenta ruptures directly into the uterine cavity and infects the amniotic fluid, the fetus may inhale or ingest the bacilli, leading to primary foci in the lung, intestine, or middle ear.

Pathologic examination of tuberculosis in the fetus and newborn usually demonstrates disseminated disease, with the liver and lungs being principally involved. In Siegel's study (1934) of 38 postmortem cases, the lungs were involved in 97%, the liver in 82%, and the spleen in 76% of the infants. Other sites described are the gastrointestinal tract, kidneys, adrenal glands, and skin (Agrawal and Rehman, 1995; Hageman, 1980; Sood, 2000). Central nervous system involvement occurs in fewer than 50% of cases (Starke, 1997). It is not always possible to determine whether sites represent multiple primary foci or are secondary to primary lesions in the lung or liver. The only lesion in the neonate that is unquestionably associated with congenital infection is a primary complex in the liver; all others may be acquired congenitally or postnatally.

The clinical manifestations of congenital tuberculosis are nonspecific and resemble those of bacterial sepsis and other congenital infections. The affected infant is commonly born prematurely (Davis et al, 1960), but clinical signs typically do not appear until he or she is 2 to 4 weeks of age. In a review of 29 cases of congenital tuberculosis, the median age at presentation was 24 days of life, with a range of 1 to 84 days (Cantwell et al, 1994a).

On the basis of findings from infants with congenital tuberculosis that have been reported in the post-INH era, respiratory distress, hepatomegaly with or without splenomegaly, and fever are the most common presenting manifestations of disease (Abughali et al, 1994; Cantwell et al, 1994a; Hageman, 1980). Such features as failure to thrive, meningitis, and jaundice, which were more prevalent in the pre-INH era, are present in only a minority of infants today. Additional features are listed in Table 38–10. Otitis media with aural discharge has been described as the first sign of congenital tuberculosis (Gordon-Nesbitt and Rajan, 1973; Ng et al, 1995). Skin manifestations also are infrequently reported. In the two cases reported by Hageman and colleagues (1980), the lesions were initially papular and later pustular with surrounding erythema; skin biopsy confirmed granulomatous inflammation. It is important to emphasize, however, that many infected infants lack clinical signs of infection and are identified only after a parent or caregiver is diagnosed with tuberculosis.

**TABLE 38–10**

**Clinical Signs of Congenital Tuberculosis in 58 Infants**

| Sign | No. of Patients | % of Patients |
|---|---|---|
| Respiratory distress | 44 | 76 |
| Hepatomegaly with/without splenomegaly | 38 | 65 |
| Fever | 33 | 57 |
| Lymphadenopathy | 19 | 33 |
| Poor feeding | 18 | 31 |
| Lethargy/irritability | 16 | 30 |
| Abdominal distention | 15 | 26 |
| Failure to thrive | 9 | 15 |
| Ear discharge | 9 | 15 |
| Rash | 5 | 9 |
| Abnormal fundoscopic findings | 4 | 7 |
| Jaundice | 4 | 7 |
| Seizure | 3 | 5 |
| Bloody diarrhea | 3 | 5 |
| Ascites | 3 | 5 |

Adapted from Abughali N, Van Der Kuyp F, Annable W, et al: Pediatr Infect Dis J 13:738-741, 1994.

## Diagnosis

Timely diagnosis of congenital tuberculosis requires a high index of suspicion. There are no typical clinical signs or radiographic findings. Diagnostic evaluation, consisting of a tuberculin skin test (TST), chest radiograph, lumbar puncture, and cultures of appropriate specimens (e.g., gastric aspirate, endotracheal aspirate, cerebrospinal fluid, and skin lesion), should be performed as soon as tuberculosis is suspected, and treatment should be initiated promptly.

Result of the Mantoux tuberculin skin test using 5 tuberculin units of purified protein derivative is usually "nonreactive" in neonates with tuberculosis. The lack of response, or anergy, is likely secondary to the poor cell-mediated immunity in young infants. Alternatively, it may be due to overwhelming tuberculous disease or even to the fact that specific tuberculosis hypersensitivity may be delayed for up to 12 weeks after infection. Hageman and colleagues (1980) reported that among 14 infants with congenital tuberculosis who underwent skin testing, only 2 had positive test results at presentation. Seven infants subsequently demonstrated positive tuberculin skin tests, the earliest at 6 weeks of age, almost 4 weeks after presentation with clinical signs. Similarly, results of tuberculin skin tests performed in 9 of 29 patients described by Cantwell and associates (1994a) were all negative, although results of tests performed later in 2 of the 9 infants were reactive.

Radiographic findings vary according to the route of infection and the cause of illness. In most infants with congenital tuberculosis, chest roentgenographic findings are abnormal at presentation. Typically, a nonspecific parenchymal infiltrate, adenopathy, or a miliary pattern is noted. Sixteen (62%) of 26 patients reviewed by Hageman and colleagues (1980) had abnormal radiographic findings on presentation, 7 with a miliary pattern and 9 with nonspecific changes. Radiographic abnormalities developed in 4 other infants later. Among 29 cases reviewed by Cantwell and associates (1994a), 23 (79%) infants had chest radiograph abnormalities, which consisted of nonspecific infiltrates in 18 (78%) of infants. Cavitation secondary to progressive pulmonary involvement is an uncommon feature of congenital tuberculosis (Cunningham et al, 1982).

Microbiologic confirmation of disease should be sought from multiple sites. Smear and culture of gastric aspirate for *M. tuberculosis* are the most expedient and reliable ways of establishing the diagnosis. Additional sources of culture are endotracheal aspirate, middle-ear discharge, and lymph node biopsy specimens. CSF should be evaluated and cultured, although the yield is low (Abughali et al, 1994; Cantwell et al, 1994a; Hageman et al, 1980). A biopsy of skin lesions is often helpful and definitive (Nemir and O'Hare, 1985). Hageman and colleagues (1980) found positive cultures of *M. tuberculosis* in 10 of 12 gastric aspirates, 3 of 3 liver biopsy specimens, 3 of 3 lymph node biopsy specimens, and 2 of 4 bone marrow biopsy specimens. In a later review by Cantwell and associates (1994a), biopsy and noninvasive procedures were useful for the diagnosis of 29 infants with congenital tuberculosis (Table 38–11).

Demonstration of a primary hepatic complex, which would require an open surgical procedure or autopsy, is not essential for diagnosis of congenital tuberculosis. In the appropriate clinical setting, a percutaneous liver biopsy specimen that demonstrates caseating granulomas is sufficient evidence for diagnosis (Cantwell et al, 1994a). PCR assays are available for testing of specimens such as gastric aspirates, respiratory secretions, and CSF, but they are not recommended for routine use because their sensitivity is similar to that of culture, and both false-positive and false-negative results occur.

The mother of a newborn in whom congenital tuberculosis is suspected should be evaluated for disease. Often, the mother is asymptomatic or has subclinical disease. Hageman and colleagues (1980) found that tuberculosis was diagnosed in only 10 (38%) of 26 mothers before the disease was discovered in their offspring. The majority of mothers (15, or 58%) were not diagnosed until after the disease became apparent in their infants. Similarly, Cantwell and associates (1994a) found that 50% of mothers of infants with congenital tuberculosis were not diagnosed with tuberculosis at the time their infants demonstrated clinical signs. It is evident that the lack of a maternal history of tuberculosis should not deter the clinician from thoroughly investigating its possibility in the infant. Examination of the mother should include a tuberculin skin test and chest radiograph. Histologic examination of the placenta, if available, is strongly recommended, and an endometrial biopsy may also help in confirming disease (Balasubramanian et al, 1999; Cooper et al, 1985; Niles, 1982). The mother with tuberculosis should also undergo serologic testing for HIV antibody, and, if she is seropositive, the infant should be evaluated for perinatally acquired HIV infection.

### Therapy

The successful management of congenital tuberculosis depends on early recognition and treatment of the disease. Empiric therapy is provided often to neonates and should not be delayed while awaiting culture results, epidemiologic investigation, and follow-up tuberculin skin testing. The optimal treatment regimen for congenital tuberculosis has not been established because the rarity of the disease precludes evaluation in clinical trials. It is assumed that the regimens used for the treatment of tuberculosis in older children and adults are safe and efficacious for congenital tuberculosis. Until susceptibility test results are known, all infants with suspected or proven congenital tuberculosis should receive the following four antituberculous drugs: INH (10 to 15 mg/kg/day PO); rifampin (10 to 20 mg/kg/day PO); pyrazinamide (20 to 40 mg/kg/day PO); and either streptomycin (20 to 40 mg/kg/day IM), kanamycin (15 to 30 mg/kg/day IM), amikacin (15 to 22.5 mg/kg/day IV or IM), or ethambutol (15 to 25 mg/kg/day PO) The adjunctive

**TABLE 38–11**

**Results of Diagnostic Procedures Performed on 29 Infants with Congenital Tuberculosis Reported from 1980 to 1994***

| Type of Specimen | Acid-Fast Smear | Mycobacterial Culture | Smear or Culture |
|---|---|---|---|
| Gastric aspirate | 8/9 | 8/9 | 9/11 |
| Endotracheal aspirate | 7/7 | 7/7 | 7/7 |
| Ear discharge | 2/2 | 1/1 | 2/2 |
| Cerebrospinal fluid | 1/2 | 1/2 | 1/2 |
| Urine | 0/2 | 0/2 | 0/2 |
| Peritoneal fluid | 1/1 | 1/1 | 1/1 |
| Bronchoscopic specimen | 1/1 | 1/1 | 1/1 |
| Biopsy specimen | 14/19 | 11/12 | 16/21 |
| Lymph node | 7/8 | 6/6 | 7/8† |
| Liver | 4/6 | 1/2 | 4/6† |
| Skin | 1/3 | 1/1 | 1/3 |
| Lung | 1/1 | 1/1 | 2/2 |
| Bone marrow | — | 1/1 | 1/1 |
| Ear | 1/1 | 1/1 | 1/1 |

*Results expressed as no. positive results/no. patients tested.

†All biopsy specimens of lymph node and liver that tested negative on smear and culture showed histopathologic changes consistent with tuberculosis (i.e., giant cell transformation of granulomas, with or without caseation).

Adapted from Cantwell MF, Shehab ZM, Costello AM, et al: Brief report: Congenital tuberculosis. N Engl J Med 330:1051, 1994.

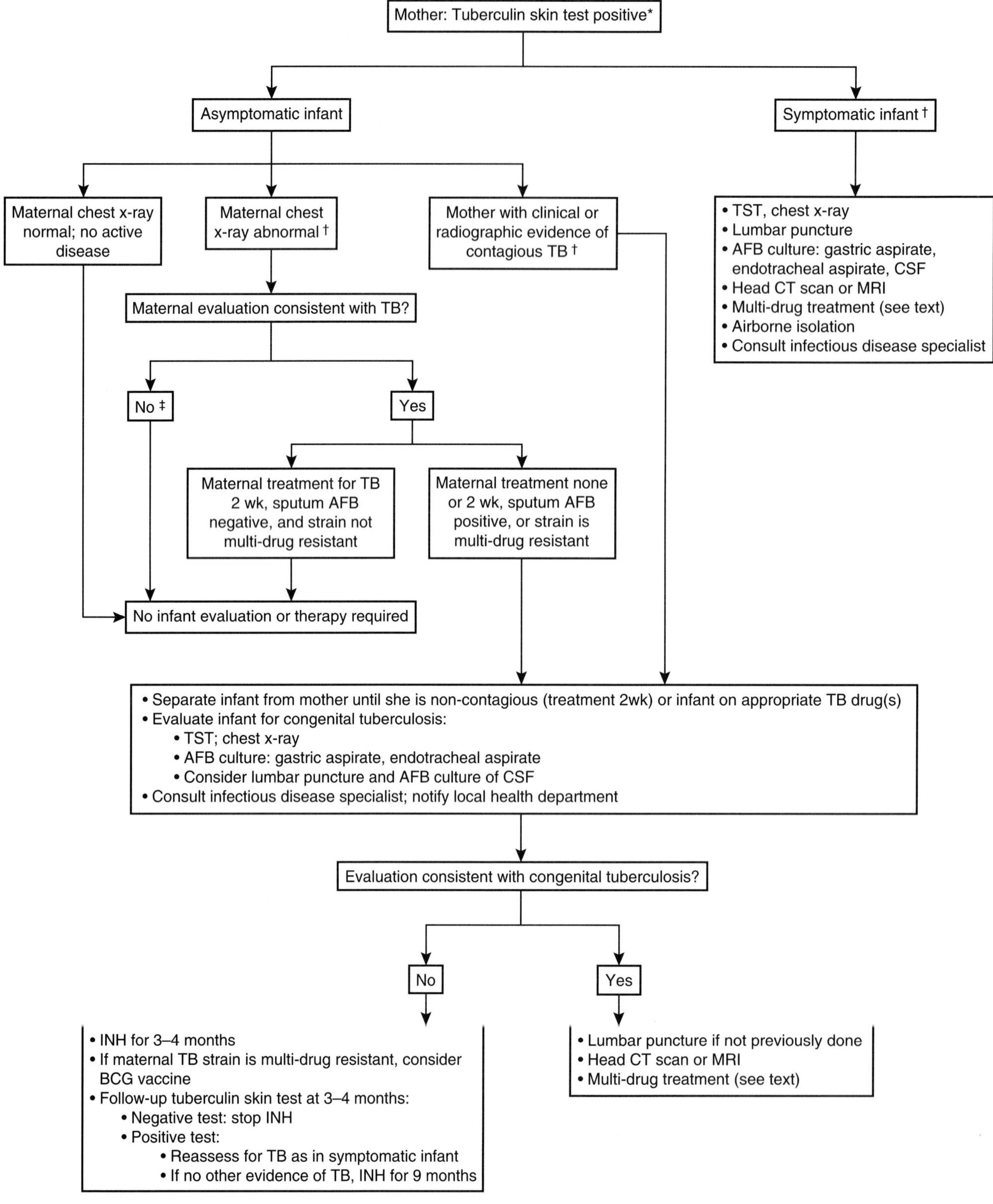


**FIGURE 38–2.** Management of infants born to mothers with a positive tuberculin skin test (TST) result.

*Household contacts should have a TST and further evaluation for contagious tuberculosis (TB). Consult local health department. The mother should receive treatment for latent tuberculosis infection. All persons with tuberculosis should be tested for human immunodeficiency virus (HIV) infection.

†Acid-fast bacillus (AFB) culture of amniotic fluid and placenta, if available; placenta for histopathologic examination.

‡Includes mother with chest radiographic findings consistent with old, healed tuberculosis.

BCG, bacille Calmette-Guérin; CSF, cerebrospinal fluid; CT, computed tomography; INH, isoniazid; MRI, magnetic resonance imaging. *(Adapted from American Academy of Pediatrics: Tuberculosis. In Pickering LK [ed]: 2003 Red Book: Report of the Committee on Infectious Diseases, 26th ed. Elk Grove Village, IL, American Academy of Pediatrics; 2003, p 642.)*

use of corticosteroids such as prednisone (1 to 2 mg/kg/day) is recommended for the treatment of meningitis, because it decreases mortality and improves long-term neurologic outcome (Girgis, 1991). Corticosteroids also may be considered for pleural and pericardial effusions, endobronchial disease, and severe miliary tuberculosis.

Although INH is safe in the neonate, data on the safety and pharmacokinetics of the other agents are limited. Monitoring for clinical signs of hepatotoxicity is recommended. Routine determination of serum transaminase concentrations is indicated for infants with severe (e.g., meningeal or miliary) tuberculosis or with concurrent or recent liver disease as well as those receiving other hepatotoxic drugs. The risks of optic neuritis with ethambutol and of auditory and vestibular toxicities with streptomycin and kanamycin should be considered when these agents are used, and hearing or vision should be periodically monitored.

If the isolate is found to be susceptible, the regimen can be narrowed to three drugs (INH, rifampin, and pyrazinamide) for the first 2 months of therapy, followed by INH and rifampin to complete therapy. Directly observed therapy (DOT) is recommended for treatment of tuberculosis in children to ensure adherence and successful treatment. The duration of therapy is not established. Most experts would treat for 9 to 12 months because of the relatively compromised immune system of the young infant and the high likelihood of disseminated disease. For drug-resistant tuberculosis, longer duration of therapy with daily administration of medications is recommended. Pyridoxine should be given to breast-fed infants receiving INH. Although antituberculous drugs are secreted in human milk, their concentrations are low, and breast-feeding should be encouraged.

Infants with suspected or proven congenital tuberculosis require airborne precautions. Most children with tuberculosis are not contagious, and isolation of the hospitalized pediatric patient is directed at adult contacts who may be source cases and potentially contagious. Visitation of the hospitalized pediatric patient should be restricted to adults in whom contagious tuberculosis has been excluded. (AAP, 2003b).

The management of infants born to mothers who have latent tuberculosis infection or disease is outlined in Figure 38–2. Recommendations are based on the categorization of infection in the mother and the potential risk of transmission of tuberculosis to the infant (AAP, 2003b). Infants born to mothers with potentially contagious tuberculosis should be evaluated for congenital tuberculosis. The mother with latent tuberculosis infection is not contagious. However, to prevent reactivation disease in the mother and to prevent subsequent exposure of the infant, the mother should receive treatment with INH. Additionally, latent tuberculosis infection in the mother may be a marker for contagious tuberculosis within the household, and it is recommended that all household members and close contacts of the mother be evaluated for tuberculosis.

### Prognosis

The prognosis for congenital tuberculosis was dismal in the pre-chemotherapy era, the diagnosis often being only made at autopsy. Although the survival rate has since improved, mortality remained about 50% secondary to delayed diagnosis. In the review by Hageman and colleagues (1980) of 26 cases of congenital tuberculosis reported between 1952 and 1980, 12 (46%) patients died, 9 of whom were untreated and were diagnosed at autopsy. In a subsequent review of 29 cases between 1980 and 1994, the mortality rate was 38% overall but decreased to 22% (5 of 23 infants) among infants who received antituberculous therapy (Cantwell et al, 1994a). Early diagnosis and initiation of antituberculous treatment are critical for a favorable outcome.

### Prevention

Prevention of congenital tuberculosis requires the control of the disease among women of child-bearing age. Collaboration between health care providers and the public health department is essential. Reporting of cases of tuberculosis to the local health department is mandatory for timely contact investigation, appropriate antituberculous therapy, and DOT services. In addition, tuberculin skin testing is recommended for pregnant women who are at increased risk of either acquiring tuberculosis or having latent infection. Risk factors include contact with a case of tuberculosis, recent family history of tuberculosis, positive TST result in a household member, immigration from or prolonged travel to countries with a high prevalence of tuberculosis, and frequent contact with people from such countries. Asymptomatic pregnant women with reactive TST results and normal chest radiographs should receive INH therapy along with pyridoxine after the first trimester of pregnancy.

Vaccination at birth with bacille Calmette-Guérin (BCG) vaccine, a live-virus vaccine prepared from attenuated strains of *M. bovis*, is recommended by the WHO for prevention of disseminated tuberculosis infection in infants and young children. Although the vaccine does not prevent infection with tuberculosis, it has a 50% to 80% protective efficacy against meningeal and miliary disease. In the United States, vaccination with BCG vaccines is not recommended except in rare circumstances in which continued exposure of the infant to individuals with untreated or ineffectively treated tuberculosis is completely unavoidable.

## REFERENCES

Abughali N, Van Der Kuyp F, Annable W, et al: Congenital tuberculosis. Pediatr Infect Dis J 13:738, 1994.

Adhikari M, Pillay T, Pillay DG: Tuberculosis in the newborn: An emerging disease. Pediatr Infect Dis J 16:1108, 1997.

Agrawal RL, Rehman H: Congenital miliary tuberculosis with intestinal perforations. Tuber Lung Dis 76:468, 1995.

Ahmed A, Cerilli LA, Sánchez PJ: Congenital malaria in a preterm neonate: Case report and review of the literature. Am J Perinatol 15:19, 1998.

Airede AI: Congenital malaria with chloroquine resistance. Ann Trop Paediatr 11:267-269, 1991.

Alecrim WD, Espinosa FEM, Alecrim MGC: *Plasmodium falciparum* infection in the pregnant patient. Infect Dis Clin North Am 14:83, 2000.

Alford CA Jr, Foft JW, Blanckenship WJ, et al: Subclinical central nervous system disease of neonates: A prospective study of infants born with increased levels of IgM. J Pediatr 75:1167, 1969.

Alford CA Jr, Stagno S, Reynolds DW: Congenital toxoplasmosis: Clinical, laboratory and therapeutic considerations, with special reference to subclinical disease. Bull N Y Acad Med 50:160, 1974.

American Academy of Pediatrics, Committee on Infectious Diseases: Drugs for parasitic infections. In Pickering LK (ed): 2003 Red Book: Report of the Committee on Infectious Diseases, 26th ed. Elk Grove Village, IL, American Academy of Pediatrics, 2003a, p 744.

American Academy of Pediatrics, Committee on Infectious Diseases: Tuberculosis. In Pickering LK (ed): 2003 Red Book: Report of the Committee on Infectious Diseases, 26th ed. Elk Grove Village, IL, American Academy of Pediatrics, 2003b, p 642.

Archibald HM: The influence of malarial infection of the placenta on the incidence of prematurity. Bull World Health Organ 15:842, 1956.

Balasubramanian S, Shivram R, Padmasani LN, et al: Congenital tuberculosis. Indian J Pediatr 66:148, 1999.

Balatbat ABN, Jordan GW, Halsted C: Congenital malaria in a nonidentical twin. West J Med 162:458, 1995.

Beaman MH, Luft BJ, Remington JS: Prophylaxis for toxoplasmosis in AIDS. Ann Intern Med 117:163, 1992.

Beitzke H: Ueber die angeborene tuberkuloese infektion. Ergeb Ges Tuberk Forsh 7:1, 1935.

Berry MC, Dajani AS: Resurgence of congenital syphilis. Infect Dis Clin North Am 6:19, 1992.

Blackall PB: Tuberculosis: Maternal infection of the newborn. Med J Austral 1:1055, 1969.

Boyer K: Diagnostic testing for congenital toxoplasmosis. Pediatr Infect Dis J 20:59, 2001.

Boyer KM, McAuley JB: Congenital toxoplasmosis. Semin Pediatr Infect Dis 5:42, 1994.

Brandenburg VR, Kenny JF: Neonatal malaria in an American born infant of an Asian immigrant. S D Med J 35:17, 1982.

Bruce-Chwatt LJ: Malaria in African infants and children in southern Nigeria. Ann Trop Med Parasitol 46:173, 1952.

Campbell AL, Sullivan JE, Marshall GS: Myelitis and ascending flaccid paralysis due to congenital toxoplasmosis. Clin Infect Dis 33:1778, 2001.

Cannon DSH: Malaria and prematurity in the western region of Nigeria. BMJ 2:877, 1958.

Cantwell MF, Shehab ZM, Costello AM, et al: Brief report: Congenital tuberculosis. N Engl J Med 330:1051, 1994a.

Cantwell MF, Valway SE, Onorato IM: Congenital tuberculosis [letter]. N Engl J Med 331:548, 1994b.

Centers for Disease Control and Prevention: CDC recommendations regarding selected conditions affecting women's health: Preventing congenital toxoplasmosis. MMWR Morb Mortal Wkly Rep 49(RR-2):57, 2000.

Centers for Disease Control and Prevention: Sexually transmitted diseases treatment guidelines—United States–2002. MMWR Recommend Rep 2002; 51(RR-6): 1-80.

Chhabra RS, Brion LP, Castro M, et al: Comparison of maternal sera, cord blood, and neonatal sera for detecting presumptive congenital syphilis: Relationship with maternal treatment. Pediatrics 91:88, 1993.

Congenital syphilis, United States, 1983-1985. MMWR Morb Mortal Wkly Rep Morb Mortal Wkly Rep 35:625, 1986.

Cooper AR, Heneghan W, Matthew D: Tuberculosis in a mother and her infant. Pediatr Infect Dis J 4:181, 1985.

Couvreur J, Desmonts G: Congenital and maternal toxoplasmosis: A review of 300 congenital cases. Dev Med Child Neurol 4:519, 1962.

Couvreur J, Desmonts G, Tournier G, et al: Study of a homogeneous series of 210 cases of congenital toxoplasmosis in infants aged 0 to 11 months detected prospectively. Ann Pediatr 31:815, 1984.

Couvreur J, Desmonts G, Thulliez P: Prophylaxis of congenital toxoplasmosis. Effect of spiramycin on placental infection. J Antimicrob Chemother 22:193, 1988.

Couvreur J, Thulliez P, Daffos F, et al: Six cases of toxoplasmosis in twins. Ann Pediatr (Paris) 38:63, 1991.

Covell S: Congenital malaria. Trop Dis Bull 47:1447, 1950.

Cunningham DG, McGraw TT, Griffin AJ, et al: Neonatal tuberculosis with pulmonary cavitation. Tuber Lung Dis 63:217, 1982.

D'Avanzo NJ, Morris VM, Carter TR, et al: Congenital malaria as a result of *Plasmodium malariae*—North Carolina 2000. MMWR Morb Mortal Wkly Rep 51:164, 2002.

Daffos F, Forestier F, Capella-Pavlovsky M, et al: Prenatal management of 746 pregnancies at risk for congenital toxoplasmosis. N Engl J Med 318:271, 1988.

Dannemann BR, Vaughan WC, Thurlliez P, et al: Differential agglutination test for diagnosis of recently acquired infection with *Toxoplasma gondii*. J Clin Microbiol 28:1928, 1990.

Davis SF, Finley SC, Hare WK: Congenital tuberculosis. J Pediatr 57:221, 1960.

Diallo S, Victorius A, N'Dir O, et al: Prévalence et évolution du paludisme congénital en zone urbaine: Cas de la ville de Thiès (Sénégal). Dakar Méd 28:133, 1983.

Diebler C, Dusser A, Dulac O: Congenital toxoplasmosis: Clinical and neuroradiologic evaluation of the cerebral lesions. Neuroradiology 27:125, 1985.

Dorfman DH, Glaser JH: Congenital syphilis presenting in infants after the newborn period. N Engl J Med 323:1299, 1990.

Dowell M, Musher DM: An unusual cause of fever in a newborn infant. Hosp Practice 26:40, 1991.

Dunn D, Newell M.L, Gilbert R: Low risk of congenital toxoplasmosis in children born to women infected with human immunodeficiency virus. Pediatr Infect Dis J 16:84, 1997.

Dunn D, Wallon M, Peyron F, et al: Mother-to-child transmission of toxoplasmosis: Risk estimates for clinical counselling. Lancet 353:1829, 1999.

Dunn RA, Webster LA, Nakashima AK, Sylvester GC: Surveillance for geographic and secular trends in congenital syphilis—United States, 1983-1991. MMWR Morb Mortal Wkly Rep Morb Mortal Wkly Rep 42:59, 1993.

Eichenwald HG: A study of congenital toxoplasmosis, with particular emphasis on clinical manifestations, sequelae, and therapy. In Siim JC (ed): Human Toxoplasmosis. Copenhagen, Munksgaard, 1960, p 41.

Eskild A, Oxman A, Magnus P, et al: Screening for toxoplasmosis in pregnancy: What is the evidence of reducing a health problem? J Med Screening 3:188, 1996.

Fischer PR: Congenital malaria: An African survey. Clin Pediatr 36:411, 1997.

Foudrinier F, Marx-Chemla C, Aubert D, et al: Value of specific immunoglobulin A detection by two immunocapture assays in the diagnosis of toxoplasmosis. Eur J Clin Microbiol Infect Dis 14:585, 1995.

Foulon W, Pinon JM, Stray-Pederson B, et al: Prenatal diagnosis of congenital toxoplasmosis: A multicenter evaluation of different diagnostic parameters. Am J Obstet Gynecol 181:843, 1999a.

Foulon W, Villena I, Stray-Pederson B, et al: Treatment of toxoplasmosis during pregnancy: A multicenter study of impact on fetal transmission and children's sequelae at age 1 year. Am J Obstet Gynecol 180:410, 1999b.

Foulon W, Naessens A, Ho-Yen D: Prevention of congenital toxoplasmosis. J Perinat Med 28:337, 2000.

Fricker-Hidalgo H, Pelloux H, Racinet C, et al: Detection of *Toxoplasma gondii* in 94 placentae from infected women by polymerase chain reaction, in vivo, and in vitro cultures. Placenta 19:545, 1998.

Friedman S, Ford-Jones LE, Toi A, et al: Congenital toxoplasmosis: Prenatal diagnosis, treatment and postnatal outcome. Prenat Diag 19:330, 1999.

Gavinet MF, Robert F, Firtion G, et al: Congenital toxoplasmosis due to maternal reinfection during pregnancy. J Clin Microbiol 35:1276, 1997.

Gereige RS, Cimino D: Congenitally acquired chloroquine resistant *P. falciparum* malaria in an infant born in the United States. Clin Pediatr 34:166, 1995.

Gilbert RE, Gras L, Wallon M, et al: Effect of prenatal treatment on mother to child transmission of *Toxoplasma gondii*: Retrospective cohort study of 554 mother-child pairs in Lyon, France. Int J Epidemiol 30:1303, 2001.

Girgis NI, Farid Z, Kilpatrick MG, et al: Dexamethasone adjunctive therapy for tuberculous meningitis. Pediatr Infect Dis J 10:179, 1991.

Gordon-Nesbitt DC, Rajan G: Congenital tuberculosis successfully treated. BMJ 27:233, 1973.

Gratzl R, Hayde M, Kohlhauser C, et al: Follow-up of infants with congenital toxoplasmosis detected by polymerase chain reaction analysis of amniotic fluid. Eur. J Clin Microbiol Infect Dis 17:853, 1998.

Grover CM, Thulliez P, Remington JS, et al: Rapid prenatal diagnosis of congenital *Toxoplasma* infection by using polymerase chain reaction and amniotic fluid. J Clin Microbiol 28:2297, 1990.

Guerina NG, Hsu H-W, Meissner HC, et al: Neonatal serologic screening and early treatment for congenital *Toxoplasma gondii* infection. N Engl J Med 330:1858, 1994.

Guy EC, Pelloux H, Lappalainen M, et al: Interlaboratory comparison of polymerase chain reaction for the detection of *Toxoplasma gondii* DNA added to samples of amniotic fluid. Eur J Clin Microbiol Infect Dis 15:836, 1996.

Hageman J, Shulman S, Schreiber M, et al: Congenital tuberculosis: Critical reappraisal of clinical findings and diagnostic procedures. Pediatrics 66:980, 1980.

Hardy JB, Hardy PH, et al: Failure of penicillin in a newborn with congenital syphilis. JAMA 212:1345, 1970.

Harvey B, Remington JS, Sulzer AJ: IgM malaria antibodies in a case of congenital malaria in the United States. Lancet 1:333, 1969.

Hennequin C, Dureau P, N'Guyen L, et al: Congenital toxoplasmosis acquired from an immune woman. Pediatr Infect Dis J 16:75, 1997.

Hindi RD, Azimi PH: Congenital malaria due to *Plasmodium falciparum*. Pediatr 66:977, 1980.

Hohlfeld P, Daffos F, Thurlliez P, et al: Fetal toxoplasmosis: Outcome of pregnancy and infant follow-up after in utero treatment. J Pediatr 115:765, 1989.

Hohlfeld P, Daffos F, Costa J-M, et al: Prenatal diagnosis of congenital toxoplasmosis with a polymerase-chain-reaction test on amniotic fluid. N Engl J Med 331:695, 1994.

Hulbert TV: Congenital malaria in the United States: Report of a case and review. Clin Infect Dis 14:922, 1992.

Jara M, Hsu HW, Eaton RB, Demaria A Jr: Epidemiology of congenital toxoplasmosis identified by population-based newborn screening in Massachusetts. Pediatr Infect Dis J 20:1132, 2001.

Jeliffe EFP: Low birthweight and malarial infection of the placenta. Bull World Health Organ 38:69, 1968.

Jenum PA, Holberg-Petersen M, Melby KK: Diagnosis of congenital *Toxoplasma gondii* infection by polymerase chain reaction (PCR) on amniotic fluid samples. The Norwegian experience. APMIS 106:680, 1998.

Jones JL, Lopez A, Wilson M, et al: Congenital toxoplasmosis: A review. Obstet Gynecol Surv 56:296, 2001.

Koppe JG, Loewer-Sieger DH, DeRoever-Bonnet H: Result of 20-year follow-up of congenital toxoplasmosis. Lancet 1:254, 1986.

Lackmann GM: Congenital tuberculosis. N Engl J Med 331:548, 1994.

Langer H: Repeated congenital infection with *Toxoplasma gondii*. Obstet Gynecol 21:318, 1983.

Lappalainen M, Koskela P, Koskiniemi M, et al: Toxoplasmosis acquired during pregnancy: Improved serodiagnosis based on avidity of IgG. J Infect Dis 167:691, 1993.

Larkin GL, Thuma PE: Congenital malaria in a hyperendemic area. Am J Trop Med Hyg 45:587, 1991.

Lewis LL: Congenital syphilis: Serologic diagnosis in the young infant. Infect Dis Clin North Am 6:31, 1992.

Low incidence of congenital toxoplasmosis in children born to women infected with human immunodeficiency virus. European Collaborative Study and Research Network on Congenital Toxoplasmosis. Eur J Obstet Gynecol Reprod Biol 68:93, 1996.

MacLeod CL, West R, Saloman WL, et al: Double malaria infection in a six week old infant. Am J Trop Med Hyg 31:893, 1982.

MacLeod CL: Malaria. In MacLeod CL (ed): Parasite Infections in Pregnancy and the Newborn. Oxford, Oxford University Press, 1988, p 8.

Malviya S, Shurin SB: Congenital malaria: Case report and review. Clin Pediatr 23:516, 1984.

Martinovic J, Sibalic D, Djordjevic M, et al: Frequency of toxoplasmosis in the appearance of congenital hydrocephalus. J Neurosurg 56:830, 1982.

Masur H, Kaplan JE, Holmes KK, et al: Guidelines for preventing opportunistic infections among HIV-infected persons: 2002 recommendations of the U. S. Public Health Service and the Infectious Diseases Society of America. MMWR Morb Mortal Wkly Rep 51(RR-8):5, 2002.

Mazade MA, Evans EM, Starke JR, Correa AG: Congenital tuberculosis presenting as sepsis syndrome: Case report and review of the literature. Pediatr Infect Dis J 20:439, 2001.

McAuley J, Boyer KM, Patel D, et al: Early and longitudinal evaluations of treated infants and children and untreated historical patients with congenital toxoplasmosis: The Chicago collaborative treatment trial. Clin Infect Dis 18:38, 1994.

McGee T, Wolters C, Stein L, et al: Absence of sensorineural hearing abnormalities in treated infants with congenital toxoplasmosis. Otolaryngol Head Neck Surg 106:75, 1992.

McGregor IA: Epidemiology, malaria and pregnancy. Am J Trop Med Hyg 33:517, 1984.

McLeod R, Mack D, Foss R, et al: Levels of pyrimethamine in sera and cerebrospinal and ventricular fluids from infants treated for congenital toxoplasmosis. The Toxoplasmosis Study Group. Antimicrob Agents Chemother 36:1040, 1992.

McLeod R, Boyer K, Roizen N, et al: The child with congenital toxoplasmosis. Curr Clin Topics Infect Dis 20:189, 2000.

Mertz GJ, Quinn TC, Jacobs R, et al: Congenital malaria in children of refugees—Washington, Massachusetts, Kentucky. MMWR Morb Mortal Wkly Rep 30:53, 1981.

Milgram JW: Osseous changes in congenital toxoplasmosis. Arch Pathol 97:150, 1974.

Mitchell CD, Erlich SS, Mastrucci MT, et al: Congenital toxoplasmosis occurring in infants perinatally infected with human immunodeficiency virus 1. Pediatr Infect Dis 9:512, 1990.

Moran NF, Couper ID: Congenital malaria in South Africa—A report of four cases. S Afr Med J 89:943, 1999.

Müssbichler H: Radiologic study of intracranial calcifications in congenital toxoplasmosis. Acta Radiol 7:369, 1968.

Naessens A, Jenum PA, Pollak A, et al: Diagnosis of congenital toxoplasmosis in the neonatal period: A multicenter evaluation. J Pediatr 135:714, 1999.

Naot Y, Desmonts G, Remington JS: IgM enzyme-linked immunosorbent assay test for the diagnosis of congenital *Toxoplasma* infection. J Pediatr 98:32, 1991.

Nemir RL, O'Hare D: Congenital tuberculosis: Review and diagnostic guidelines. Am J Dis Child 139:284, 1985.

Ng PC, Hiu J, Fok TF, et al: Isolated congenital tuberculosis otitis in a preterm infant. Acta Paediatr 84:955, 1995.

Niles RA: Puerperal tuberculosis with death of infant. Am J Obstet Gynecol 144:131, 1982.

Nyirjesy P, Kavasya T, Axelrod P, et al: Malaria during pregnancy: Neonatal morbidity and mortality and the efficacy of chloroquine chemoprophylaxis. Clin Infect Dis 16:127, 1993.

O'Donohoe JM, Brueton MJ, Holliman RE: Concurrent congenital human immunodeficiency virus infection and toxoplasmosis. Pediatr Infect Dis J 10:627, 1991.

Oygur N, Yilmaz G, Ozkaynak C, Guven AG: Central diabetes insipidus in a patient with congenital toxoplasmosis. Am. J Perinatol 15:191, 1998.

Pejham S, Altman R, Li KI, Munoz JL: Congenital tuberculosis with facial nerve palsy. Pediatr Infect Dis J 21:1085, 2002.

Peterson E, Eaton RB: Control of congenital infection with *Toxoplasma gondii* by neonatal screening based on detection of specific immunoglobulin M antibodies eluted from phenylketonuria filter-paper blood-spot samples. Acta Paediatr Suppl 88:36, 1999.

Peyron F, Wallon M: Options for the pharmacotherapy of toxoplasmosis during pregnancy. Expert Opin Pharmacother 2:1269, 2001.

Pinon JM, Dumon H, Chemla C, et al: Strategy for diagnosis of congenital toxoplasmosis: Evaluation of methods comparing mothers and newborns and standard methods for postnatal detection of immunoglobulin G, M, and A antibodies. J Clin Microbiol 39:2267, 2001.

Quinn TC, Jacobs RF, Mertz GJ, et al: Congenital malaria: A report of four cases and review. J Pediatr 101:229, 1982.

Ratner B, Rostler AE, Salgado PS: Care, feeding and fate of premature and full term infants born of tuberculous mothers. Am J Dis Child 81:471, 1951.

Reinhardt MC: Maternal anemia in Abidjan: Its influence on placenta and newborns. Helv Paediatr Acta 41:43, 1978.

Remington JS, Newell JW, Cavanaugh E: Spontaneous abortion and chronic toxoplasmosis: Report of a case, with isolation of the parasite. Obstet Gynecol 24:25, 1964.

Remington JS, Araujo FG, Desmonts G: Recognition of different *Toxoplasma* antigens by IgM and IgG antibodies in mothers and their congenitally infected newborns. J Infect Dis 152:1020, 1985.

Remington JS, McLeod R, Thulliez P, Desmonts G: Toxoplasmosis. In Remington JS, Klein JO (eds.): Infectious Diseases of the Fetus and Newborn Infant, 5th ed. Philadelphia, WB Saunders, 2001, p 205.

Robert-Gangneux F, Commerce V, Tourte-Schaefer C, Dupouy-Camet J: Performance of a Western blot assay to compare mother and newborn anti-*Toxoplasma* antibodies for the early neonatal diagnosis of congenital toxoplasmosis. Eur J Microbiol Infect Dis 18:648, 1999a.

Robert-Gangneux F, Gavinet MF, Ancelle T, et al: Value of prenatal diagnosis and early postnatal diagnosis of congenital toxoplasmosis: Retrospective study of 110 cases. J Clin Microbiol 37:2893, 1999b.

Robert Gangneux F: Contribution of new techniques for the diagnosis of congenital toxoplasmosis. Clin Lab 47:135, 2001.

Roizen N, Swisher CN, Stein MA, et al: Neurologic and developmental outcome in treated congenital toxoplasmosis. Pediatrics 95:11, 1995.

Romand S, Wallon M, Franck J, et al: Prenatal diagnosis using polymerase chain reaction on amniotic fluid for congenital toxoplasmosis. Obstet Gynecol 97:296, 2001.

Saxon SA, Knight N, Reynolds DW, et al: Intellectual deficits in children born with subclinical congenital toxoplasmosis: A preliminary report. J Pediatr 82:792, 1973.

Sibalic D, Djurkovic-Djakovic O, Nikolic R: Congenital toxoplasmosis in premature twins. Folia Parasitol (Praha) 33:1, 1986.

Siegel M: Pathological findings and pathogenesis of congenital tuberculosis. Am Rev Tuberc 29:297, 1934.

Smith MD, Teele DW: Tuberculosis. In Remington JS, Klein JO (eds): Infectious Diseases of the Fetus and Newborn Infant, 4th ed. Philadelphia, WB Saunders, 1995, p 1074.

Sood M, Trehan A, Arora S, et al: Congenital tuberculosis manifesting as cutaneous disease. Pediatr Infect Dis J 19:1109, 2000.

Starke JR: Tuberculosis: An old disease but a new threat to the mother, fetus, and neonate. Clin Perinatol 24:107, 1997.

Starr SR, Wheeler DS: Index of suspicion. Pediatr Rev 19:333, 1998.

Steketee RW, Nahlen BL, Parise ME, et al: The burden of malaria in pregnancy in malaria-endemic areas. Am J Trop Med Hyg 64:28, 2001.

Stoll BJ, Lee FK, Larsen S, et al: Clinical and serologic evaluation of neonates for congenital syphilis: A continuing diagnostic dilemma. J Infect Dis 167:1093, 1993.

Subramianian D, Moise KJ, White AC: Imported malaria in pregnancy: Report of four cases and review of management. Clin Infect Dis 15:408, 1992.

Vergani P, Ghidini A, Ceruti P, et al: Congenital toxoplasmosis: Efficacy of maternal treatment with spiramycin alone. Am J Reprod Immunol 39:335, 1998.

Villena I, Aubert D, Leroux B, et al: Pyrimethamine-sulfadoxine treatment of congenital toxoplasmosis: Follow-up of 78 cases between 1908 and 1997. Reims Toxoplasmosis Group. Scand J Infect Dis 30:295, 1998a.

Villena I, Chemla C, Quereux C, et al: Prenatal diagnosis of congenital toxoplasmosis transmitted by an immunocompetent woman infected before conception. Prenat Diag 18:1079, 1998b.

Villena I, Aubert D, Brodard V, et al: Detection of specific immunoglobulin E during maternal, fetal, and congenital toxoplasmosis. J Clin Microbiol 37:3487, 1999.

Viraraghavan R, Jantausch B: Congenital malaria: Diagnosis and therapy. Clin Pediatr 39:66, 2000.

Wallon M, Caudie C, Rubio S, et al: Value of cerebrospinal fluid cytochemical examination for the diagnosis of congenital toxoplasmosis at birth in France. Pediatr Infect Dis J 17:705, 1998.

Wallon M, Liou C, Garner P, Peyron F: Congenital toxoplasmosis: Systematic review of evidence of efficacy of treatment in pregnancy: BMJ 318:1511, 1999.

Wendel GD: Gestational and congenital syphilis. Clin Perinatol 15:287, 1988.

White NJ, Miller KD, Churchill FC, et al: Chloroquine treatment of severe malaria in children. N Engl J Med 319:1493, 1988.

Williams AIO, McFarlane H: Immunoglobulin levels, malarial antibody titres and placental parasitaemia in Nigerian mothers and neonates. Afr J Med Sci 1:369, 1970.

Wilson CB, Remington JS: What can be done to prevent congenital toxoplasmosis? Am J Obstet Gynecol 138:357, 1980.

Wilson CB, Remington JS, Stagno S, et al: Development of adverse sequelae in children born with subclinical congenital *Toxoplasma* infection. Pediatrics 66:767, 1980.

Wiswell TE, Fajardo JE, Bass JW, et al: Congenital toxoplasmosis in triplets. J Pediatr 105:59, 1984.

Wong S-Y, Remington JS: Toxoplasmosis in pregnancy. Clin Infect Dis 18:853, 1994.

Yamakawa R, YamashitaY, Yano A, et al: Congenital toxoplasmosis complicated by central diabetes insipidus in an infant with Down syndrome. Brain Dev 18:75, 1996.

Zenker PN, Berman SM: Congenital syphilis: Trends and recommendations for evaluation and management. Pediatr Infect Dis J 10:516, 1991.

Zufferey J, Hohlfeld P, Bille J, et al: Value of the comparative enzyme-linked immunofiltration assay for early neonatal diagnosis of congenital *Toxoplasma* infection. Pediatr Infect Dis J 18:971, 1999.

CHAPTER

# 39

# Bacterial Sepsis and Meningitis

Richard A. Polin, Elvira Parravicini, Joan A. Regan*, and H. William Taeusch

## NEONATAL BACTERIAL SEPSIS

The earliest description of infants with sepsis has been attributed to Ylppö, who first recognized sepsis as a cause of infant mortality in 1919 when he documented positive culture results from the heart in infants dying from a variety of pathologic conditions (Ylppö, 1919). It was his belief that the postmortem cultures were indicative of antemortem blood stream invasion. However, it was not until the 1930s that case reports began to appear in the pediatric literature in which the diagnosis of sepsis was confirmed before death occurred (Campbell, 1931). Subsequently, Dunham (1933) described 33 cases of neonatal sepsis at New Haven Hospital, most of which were diagnosed antemortem. In 60% of these cases, onset of sepsis was in the first week of life, but in only 10% were the infants symptomatic at birth. The most common pathogens responsible for neonatal sepsis during that time were hemolytic streptococci, staphylococci, and coliforms.

In her original report, Dunham (1928) noted the lack of specificity of the clinical manifestations of infections in the neonate and emphasized the difficulty in making the diagnosis. In 1949, Silverman and Homan described 25 infants with sepsis in whom blood stream infection appeared to be the major problem. Coliform organisms were responsible for the majority of cases of neonatal sepsis. In defining the syndrome, these researchers made the important observation that "the most rigorous definition of sepsis of the newborn confines itself to a group of infections which are presumably acquired at or shortly after birth." Although that definition ignored the large number of nosocomial infections, it did indicate the importance of perinatal events in the pathogenesis of neonatal sepsis.

Early-onset bacterial sepsis remains a major cause of neonatal morbidity and mortality. However, data indicate that the sepsis-associated death rate (per 100,000 live births) declined by 21% between 1979 and 1994 (Fig. 39–1) (Stoll et al, 1998). In contrast, the number of preterm births during that same period increased significantly. This finding suggests that the decline in sepsis deaths is probably due to changes in obstetric care resulting in a smaller number of sepsis cases, (e.g., intrapartum antibiotic therapy), to improvements in neonatal intensive care, or to earlier identification of infected infants, all of which have resulted in reduced case-fatality ratios. The basic treatment of infants with sepsis has not changed substantially over the last 50 years, (antibiotics with or without supportive care), so it is likely that further improvements in outcome will result from a greater understanding of the perinatal factors responsible for sepsis, interventions that address those factors, and better ways to identify the infected newborn.

### Pathogenesis and Pathways of Early-Onset Bacterial Infections

Early-onset bacterial sepsis can manifest as a fulminant disease with immediate onset of respiratory distress after delivery (with or without cardiovascular instability) or on day 1 to 3 of postnatal life after an asymptomatic period. The sequence of events responsible for both presentations begins with colonization of the maternal genital tract (Fig. 39–2). The flora colonizing the lower genital tract in pregnant women contains large numbers of bacteria and fungi. As pregnancy progresses, there is a gradual increase in the frequency of colonization with *Lactobacillus* spp. and a decrease in the colonization rate with *Escherichia coli* and anaerobes (Goldenberg et al, 2000). Organisms that inhabit the cervix, vagina, or rectum can spread upward into the amniotic cavity through intact or ruptured membranes and cause amnionitis. Initially, they spread into the choriodecidual space (Fig. 39–3), and in some instances, they cross intact chorioamnionic membranes. Intra-amniotic infection is usually polymicrobial in etiology (Gibbs et al, 1980). The organisms most commonly recovered are *Bacteroides* spp., group B streptococci, other aerobic streptococci, aerobic gram-negative bacteria, and genital mycoplasmas (Oshiro et al, 1993). Factors affecting colonization with group B streptococci (GBS) are discussed later. Among a cohort of 11,989 women followed throughout pregnancy, the recovery of *Gardnerella vaginalis*, a heavy growth of *Bacteroides* spp., or isolation of *Mycoplasma hominis* was associated with a greater likelihood of intra-amniotic infection (Krohn et al, 1995). The role of *Chlamydia trachomatis* as an intrauterine pathogen is uncertain (Pankuch et al, 1984).

Intra-amniotic infection can be subclinical or clinical, but both types of infection may result in serious neonatal morbidity (Barton et al, 1999). Subclinical chorioamnionitis may be a common cause of preterm labor and preterm premature rupture of membranes (pPROM) (Hillier et al, 1988). In some cases, intrauterine infection occurs quite early in pregnancy and is not detected for months (Cassell et al, 1983). Vaginal organisms associated with spontaneous preterm labor and pPROM are listed in Table 39–1. Microbial pathogens can be recovered from the amniotic cavity in 10% to 15% of cases of spontaneous preterm labor and in 32% to 35% of women with pPROM (Kenyon et al, 2001a, 2001b). Risk factors for clinical intra-amniotic infection include low parity, long labor, prolonged rupture of membranes, multiple vaginal examinations during labor, internal fetal monitoring, prolonged duration of monitoring, and bacterial vaginosis (Newton et al, 1989; Soper et al, 1989). Other variables that affect the incidence of amnionitis are the antibacterial properties of the amniotic fluid, the size of the bacterial

*Deceased.

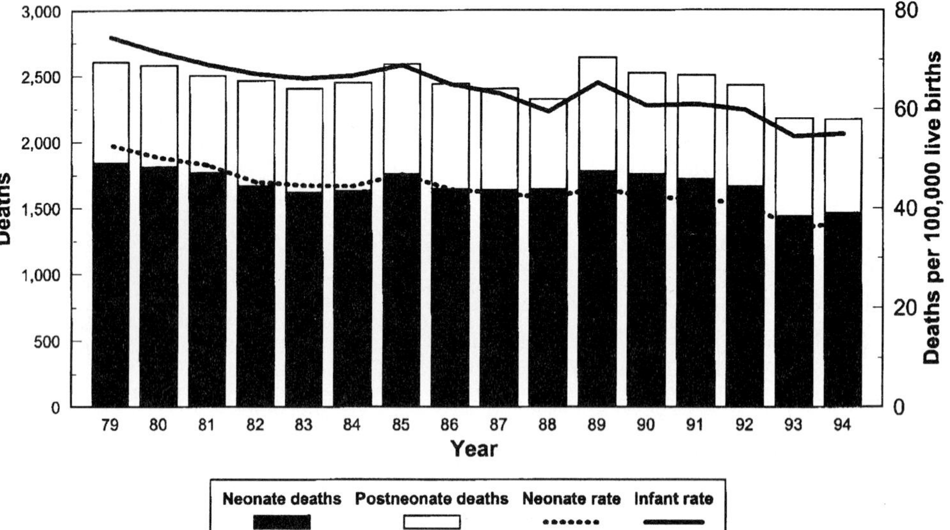


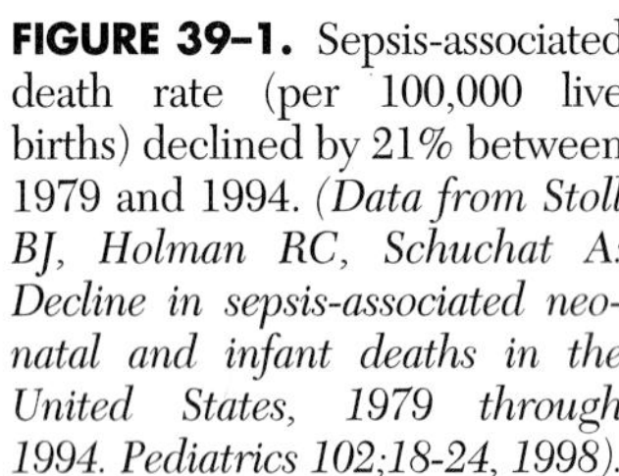

**FIGURE 39–1.** Sepsis-associated death rate (per 100,000 live births) declined by 21% between 1979 and 1994. *(Data from Stoll BJ, Holman RC, Schuchat A: Decline in sepsis-associated neonatal and infant deaths in the United States, 1979 through 1994. Pediatrics 102;18-24, 1998).*

inoculum, and the presence of urinary tract infection. Subclinical or clinical chorioamnionitis results in a vigorous inflammatory response (cytokines and inflammatory cells) within the amniotic cavity. The cytokines produced in response to infection have a key role in parturition and may contribute to brain and lung injuries in the newborn infant (Grether and Nelson, 1997; Van Marter et al, 2000).

In infants presenting with immediate onset of respiratory distress and sepsis, it is certain that the infection

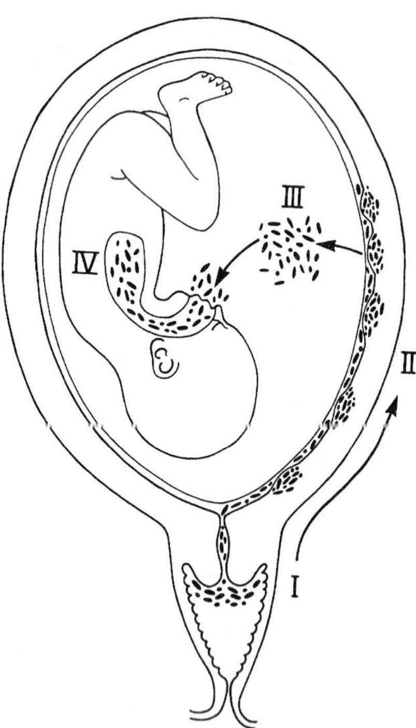


**FIGURE 39–2.** The sequence of events responsible for both early-onset and late-onset neonatal sepsis begins with colonization of the maternal genital tract. I, colonization of birth canal; II, upward spread of organisms leading to choriodeciduitis; III, development of chorioamnionitis; IV, inhalation and ingestion of contaminated amniotic fluid.

(bacteremia) must have begun antenatally (usually during labor and delivery). The fetus inhales the infected amniotic fluid, leading to pneumonia, blood stream invasion, and a systemic inflammatory response. Babies infected in this way exhibit the highest mortality rates. In babies who are initially asymptomatic, bacteremia can be somewhat delayed, although asymptomatic infants can be bacteremic (Escobar et al, 2000). Microorganisms acquired at the time of delivery colonize mucous membranes and proliferate locally before causing blood stream infection. Common sites of invasion are devitalized umbilical cord tissue and skin surfaces that have been compromised by monitoring or sampling (scalp monitoring, intravenous [IV] sites, etc.). The distinction between these two scenarios is important, because an early dose of antibiotics may effectively prevent overwhelming sepsis in an infant with the delayed presentation but will not do so in an infant whose sepsis began in utero. Transient bacteremia in the neonate is common, especially in babies undergoing procedures that bypass normal skin defense barriers (e.g., suctioning, intubation, or umbilical catheterization) (Storm, 1980). The bacteremia usually disappears within minutes. Persistent bacteremia occurs when the infant's local and systemic host defenses are overwhelmed.

The central cell in the cytokine response to bacterial sepsis is the activated macrophage (Fig. 39–4). Macrophages become activated when they come in contact with microbial cell wall products and toxins (e.g., endotoxin). Activated macrophages produce a variety of inflammatory substances (interleukins IL-1β, IL-6, and IL-8 and tumor necrosis factor-α [TNF-α]) that increase vascular permeability, alter vascular tone, depress myocardial function, increase pulmonary vascular resistance, activate clotting systems, and mobilize and activate other phagocytic cells (allowing them to move via chemotaxis to sites of inflammation and kill bacteria) (see Fig. 39–4). Regulated production of cytokines allows the host to recover from the infectious episode. Unregulated cytokine responses increase both morbidity and mortality. Furthermore, when bacteremia is persistent, organisms are likely to disseminate and lodge in organs at distant sites (lungs, bone, central nervous system, kidney, etc.).

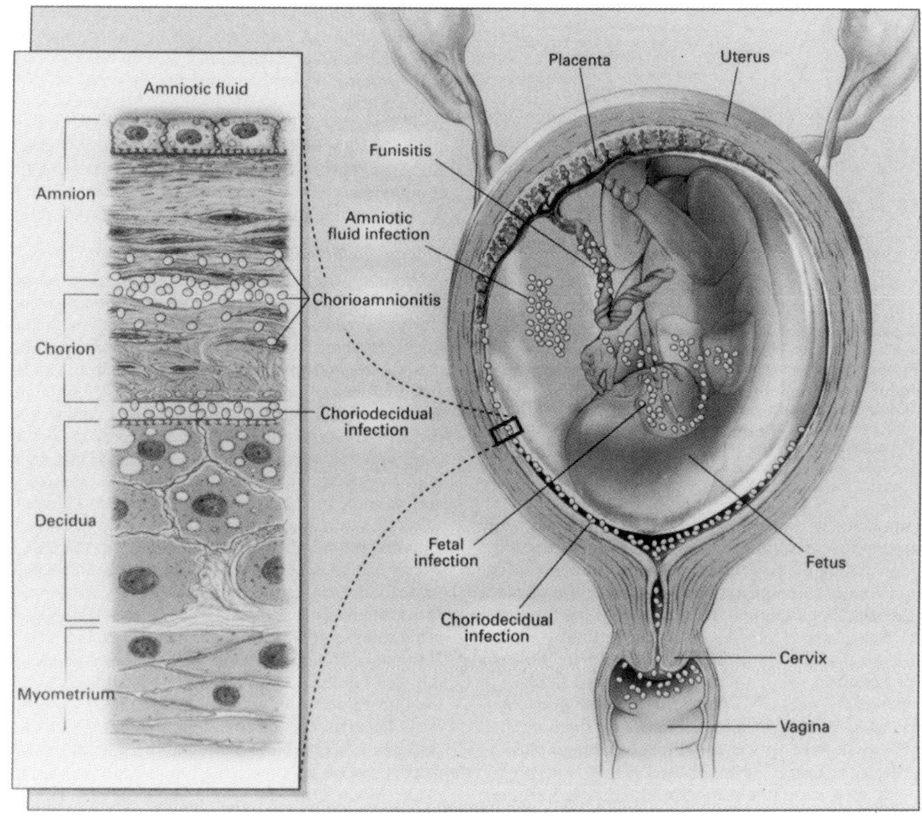


**FIGURE 39–3.** Organisms that inhabit the cervix, vagina, or rectum can spread upward into the amniotic cavity through intact or ruptured membranes and cause amnionitis. Initially, they spread into the choriodecidual space.

**TABLE 39–1**

**Vaginal Organisms and Conditions Associated with Spontaneous Preterm Labor and Preterm Premature Rupture of Membranes**

| Condition | Associated Organism or Condition |
|---|---|
| Premature preterm rupture of membranes | *Neisseria gonorrhoeae* |
| | *Chlamydia trachomatis* |
| | *Trichomonas vaginalis* |
| | *Prevotella* spp. |
| | *Bacteroides* spp. |
| | Bacterial vaginosis |
| Preterm labor | *Ureaplasma urealyticum* |
| | *Mycoplasma hominis* |
| | *Gardnerella vaginalis* |
| | *Peptostreptococcus* |
| | *Bacteroides* spp. |

## Epidemiology of Early-Onset Bacterial Infections

The incidence of early-onset bacterial infections ranges from 1 to 8 per 1000 live births (Klein, 2001). However, data now suggest that the incidence is declining as a result of intrapartum antibiotic therapy (Baltimore et al, 2001). In a surveillance study from Connecticut, in which the outcomes for 174,535 live births were recorded, the incidences of early-onset GBS sepsis and early-onset non-GBS sepsis were 0.23 and 0.67 per 1000 live births, respectively (Baltimore et al, 2001).

Infants who experience early-onset sepsis commonly have one or more identifiable risk factors. The risk factors can be divided into the following four categories: host immunity, socioeconomic factors, obstetric and nursery practices, and health and nutrition of mothers. Prematurity is the single greatest risk factor for early-onset bacterial infections. The strong association between preterm birth and infection is related both to the reasons for preterm birth (e.g., chorioamnionitis) and host defense impairments that exist in all newborn babies but are greatest in extremely low-birth-weight (ELBW) infants (see Chapter 32). In a study of more than 32,000 infants by Boyer and colleagues (1983a), the attack rate for early-onset GBS sepsis in infants of birth weight less than 1000 g was 26 times that in term newborn infants and accounted for the greatest number of deaths. Additional risk factors for early-onset sepsis are colonization with known pathogens (e.g., GBS), chorioamnionitis, higher number of vaginal examinations during labor, and rupture of membranes for 18 hours or longer.

In a recent multicenter case-control study involving seven regional medical centers, 49% of infants with GBS and 79% of other infants with sepsis had one or more of the three major maternal risk factors already noted (signs and symptoms of chorioamnionitis, prolonged [>18 hours] rupture of membranes, and colonization with GBS) (Schuchat et al, 2000). However, one must be cautious in using fever as the sole indicator of maternal infection, because fever is observed quite commonly in women who receive epidural anesthesia to alleviate pain during labor.

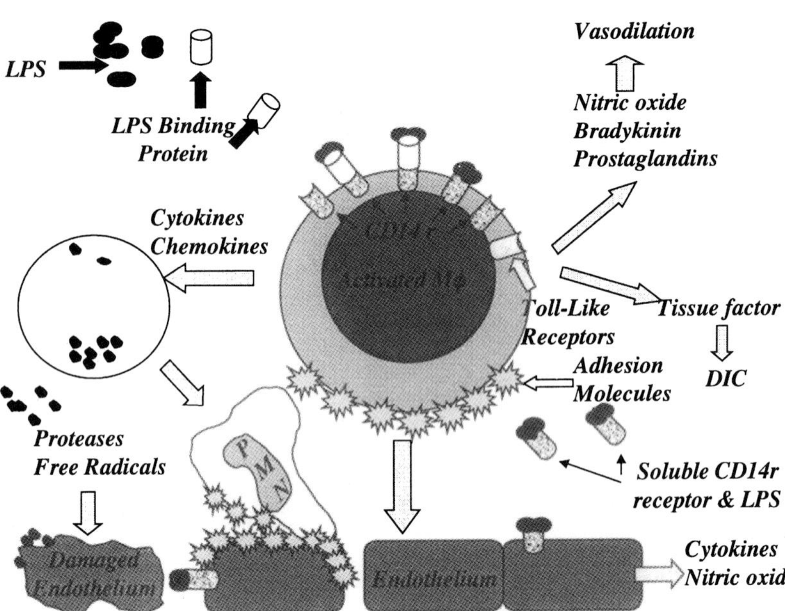


**FIGURE 39-4.** Macrophages become activated when they come in contact with microbial cell wall products and toxins (e.g., endotoxin). Activated macrophages produce a variety of inflammatory substances (interleukins IL-1β, IL-6, and IL-8; tumor necrosis factor-α [TNF-α]) that increase vascular permeability, alter vascular tone, depress myocardial function, increase pulmonary vascular resistance, activate clotting systems, and mobilize and activate other phagocytic cells (allowing them to move via chemotaxis to sites of inflammation and kill bacteria). CD14r, CD14 receptor; DIC, disseminated intravascular coagulation; LPS, lipopolysaccharide; PMN, polymorphonuclear (leukocyte).

In a prospective study, Lieberman and colleagues (1997) found that fever occurred in 14.5% of women who did receive epidural anesthesia and in 1.0% of women who did not. For labors lasting more than 18 hours, the incidence of fever was 36%. These investigators calculated that 96.2% of intrapartum fevers, 85.6% of sepsis evaluations, and 87.5% of neonatal antibiotic treatment in term infants were associated with use of epidural anesthesia. In the epidural group, fever accounted for the sepsis evaluations in about one third of cases. Even among afebrile women, the use of epidural anesthesia is associated with a higher incidence of major and minor risk factors for neonatal sepsis—fetal tachycardia, low-grade temperature elevation, and prolonged rupture of membranes (Goetzl et al, 2001). Commonly accepted criteria for diagnosis of chorioamnionitis are listed in Table 39–2.

A number of other risk factors for early-onset sepsis has been identified. In several studies, a low Apgar score and need for resuscitation were associated with a higher incidence of sepsis (Gluck et al, 1966). Because of the strong association with chorioamnionitis, pPROM is a well-established risk factor for sepsis (Romero et al, 1999). Fortunately, the incidence of sepsis after pPROM can be reduced by administering antibiotics as soon as the membranes rupture (Kenyon et al, 2001a). Race appears to be another important variable, and in several studies, black infants have exhibited higher rates of early-onset GBS sepsis than non-black infants (Schuchat et al, 1990). Data collected as part of the Collaborative Perinatal Research Study (n = 38,500 pregnancies) indicated that black women had higher rates of pPROM for longer than 24 hours, puerperal infection, and infants weighing less than 2500 g (Niswander and Gordon, 1972). The effect of race on the incidence of sepsis is complex and may relate to differences in nutrition, socioeconomic status, sexually transmitted diseases, or host immunity. Finally, in almost all studies, male infants have demonstrated a higher incidence of sepsis than female infants (Washburn et al, 1965). The immunologic basis for these differences is unknown.

**TABLE 39-2**

**Criteria for Diagnosis of Chorioamnionitis**

1. Fever (temperature >37.8° C) *plus* two or more of the following:
   a. Maternal tachycardia (>100 beats/min)
   b. Fetal tachycardia (>160 beats/min)
   c. Uterine tenderness
   d. Malodorous or cloudy amniotic fluid
   e. Maternal white blood cell count >15,000 cells/mm$^3$
2. No other site for infection

## Group B Streptococcal Infections

Among bacterial agents known to cause sepsis in the neonate during the first week of life, Group B streptococci are unique for two reasons. First, despite numerous studies of the pathophysiology and epidemiology of maternal colonization and infant disease, the reason for the emergence of this pathogen as the leading cause of serious, lethal sepsis in the newborn is not known (Baker and Edwards, 1995). Secondly, GBS are the only bacterial pathogens, which have been demonstrated to respond to maternal intrapartum antibiotic prophylaxis with a significant reduction in the incidence of disease. (Carey et al, 2000; Locksmith and Duff, 2001; Schuchat, 2001).

Lancefield (1933) designated *Streptococcus agalactiae* as group B streptococci after a pandemic of streptococcal disease during World War I. Although the organism had been known to be the leading cause of mastitis in cattle since the 1800s, it was not recognized as a human pathogen until 1938, when Fry recovered the organism from three patients with puerperal sepsis. Before the 1960s, GBS was infrequently recognized as a cause of human disease. However, GBS emerged in the late 1960s as the leading cause of neonatal sepsis in human newborn infants (Eickhoff et al, 1964).

Group B streptococci cause sepsis and other infections in newborns very early in life (early-onset sepsis) and also later in the newborn period and in infancy (late-onset sepsis). Early-onset disease was originally defined as that occurring during the first 5 days of life, and late-onset disease as that occurring at 10 days or later (Baker and Barrett, 1973). Subsequently, timing of the two forms of the disease has blurred (Baker and Edwards, 1995; Isaacs et al, 1996). All designations of timing have been empiric and independent of the epidemiology and clinical spectra of these two disease entities. Table 39–3 summarizes the features of early-onset and late-onset GBS sepsis.

Group B streptococci were first reported as the leading cause of neonatal sepsis in 1964 in a large Northeastern U.S. center by Eickhoff and colleagues. Subsequently, this same observation was made in many U.S. centers as well as in Great Britain, Scandinavia, and mainland Europe. The position of GBS as the leading cause of neonatal sepsis persisted until the implementation of prevention strategies in the late 1990s (see later). It has been suggested that shifts in the predominant subtypes of GBS causing disease in infants play a role in emergence of GBS as a major neonatal pathogen. However, this proposition has not been supported in seroepidemiologic studies (Lee et al, 2000; Lin et al, 1998).

### *Vertical Transmission from Mothers to Infants*

More than 98% of cases of early-onset GBS sepsis are the consequence of vertical transmission from the genital tract of the mother to the infant (Baker and Edwards, 1995). The mean rate of vertical transmission is about 50%. A very small number of cases are due to hematogenous transmission through the placenta. In these cases, the mother commonly displays signs and symptoms of chorioamnionitis—although hematogenous transmission does occur in the absence of symptoms. In cases of hematogenous transmission, results of maternal genital cultures are usually negative, as is the case for the very rare occurrences of transmission from a health care worker or from a nonhuman vector (Davis et al, 1978).

**TABLE 39–3**

**Characteristics of Early-Onset and Late-Onset Group B Streptococcal Sepsis**

| Characteristic | Early-Onset Sepsis | Late-Onset Sepsis |
|---|---|---|
| Age at onset | Birth through 5 day after birth | After day 7 |
| Symptoms | Respiratory distress<br>Apnea | Irritability<br>Fever<br>Poor feeding |
| Serotypes | All | All |
| Mode of transmission | Vertical | Nosocomial |
| Effect of intrapartum antibiotic prophylaxis recommended by the Centers for Disease Control and Prevention | Reduces incidence by 85%-90% | No effect |

Detection of maternal colonization presents an opportunity to identify infants at risk for early-onset GBS sepsis and offers an opportunity for intervention in the form of maternal treatment before delivery. Both antepartum and intrapartum types of antibiotic prophylaxis have been investigated; the U.S. Centers for Disease Control and Prevention (CDC) recommendations support an intrapartum regimen (see later). The following issues affect the accuracy of identifying women colonized with GBS: culturing methods, anatomic site of maternal culture specimens, and quantitation of cultures.

#### Culturing Methods

The majority of studies using selective broth media containing antibiotics (e.g., nalidixic acid, gentamicin, colistin) demonstrate at least a two-fold greater yield of positive results for genital and rectal cultures from adults in comparison with nonselective methods (Baker et al, 1976; Gray et al, 1979). This greater yield is made possible by the suppression of overgrowth by co-colonizing bacteria in selective methods. It is noteworthy that standard laboratory methods for isolation of GBS from the blood and cerebrospinal fluid (CSF) of mothers and infants are fully adequate. In addition, use of nonselective media (standard blood agar plates) increases the yield of positive results from surface cultures in newborns during the first 24 to 48 hours of life, because the antibiotics in selective media are slightly inhibitory to GBS and most GBS surface isolates grow as pure cultures in the first 2 days of life (San Giovanni et al, 1987).

#### Anatomic Site of Specimen Collection

Since 1977 there has been controversy in the literature regarding the best sampling site for identification of maternal colonization, genital or rectal (Badri et al, 1977; Anthony et al, 1981). The majority of studies reveals higher rates of rectal colonization (Baker and Edwards, 1995). However, Regan and colleagues (1987a), using culture methods that controlled for differences in behavior of lactobacilli at the two sites, found higher colonization rates at the genital site.

#### Quantitation of Culture Results

"Heavy" colonization was first suggested by Bobitt and Ledger in 1976 as a factor likely to enhance vertical transmission. However, quantitative cultures are difficult to perform, and interest in obtaining them never achieved popularity. In contrast, semiquantitative screening is more feasible for most laboratories, and women with heavy colonization (3+ to 4+) are more likely to pass the microorganism to their infants (Ancona et al, 1980; Schuchat et al, 1994). In the Vaginal Infections and Prematurity (VIP) multicenter trial, a significantly greater rate of vertical transmission as well as higher incidences of preterm delivery and low birth weight were observed among women with heavy colonization (Regan et al, 1991).

### *Maternal Colonization with Group B Streptococcal Infections*

In the United States, the prevalence of GBS in the genital or gastrointestinal tracts of pregnant women varies from 15% to 40% (Baker and Edwards, 1995). Carriage of GBS during pregnancy may be chronic, intermittent, or transient (Anthony et al, 1978). Therefore, a single culture of a specimen taken randomly during pregnancy may not be predictive of carriage at delivery. However, results of culture of specimens collected 1 to 5 weeks before delivery have a predictive value ranging from 60% to 100%, depending on site of culture (rectal, vaginal, or both) and interval between culture and delivery (Boyer et al, 1983b).

Although original studies reported no association between GBS colonization and risk factors for sepsis (Baker and Barrett, 1973), many subsequent reports have documented these associations (Bobitt et al, 1985; Regan et al, 1981; Stewardson-Krieger and Gotoff, 1978). Risk factors include preterm labor, preterm delivery, premature rupture of membranes, pPROM, prolonged rupture of membranes, and maternal fever. These risk factors form the basis of the CDC's consensus strategies for the intrapartum antibiotic prophylaxis risk factor-based strategy.

Other epidemiologic variables associated with an increased risk of maternal colonization are Hispanic race (both Mexican Americans and Caribbean Island Hispanics, especially patients of Dominican Republican Heritage) (Regan et al, 1987b), age less than 20 years, African-American ethnicity, and lower parity. In contrast, older age and lower parity, living with a partner (versus living alone), increased years of education, and smoking are associated with a reduced risk of colonization. Concurrent colonization with *Candida* species is associated with a higher risk of maternal colonization with GBS, but there is no relationship of GBS colonization with carriage of *C. trachomatis, Ureaplasma urealyticum, Trichomonas vaginalis*, or *M. hominis* (Regan et al, 1991).

### *Group B Streptococcal Sepsis in Neonates*

Only 1% to 2% of infants born to women who are colonized with GBS have early-onset sepsis. This incidence of infection rises with premature delivery (15%), prolonged (>18 hours) rupture of membranes (11%), presence of chorioamnionitis (6% to 20%), and twin pregnancy (35%). Other risk factors associated with early-onset sepsis are African-American race (Schuchat et al, 1990) and use of intrauterine monitoring (Davis et al, 1979).

Implementation of the CDC consensus strategies has lowered the incidence of sepsis in infants with these risk factors and changed the spectrum of risk factors describing early-onset sepsis (e.g., sepsis is more common among term than preterm infants) but has not yet altered GBS subtype distributions or prevalence in geographic locations.

Subtypes currently identified are Ia, II, III, IV, V, VI, VII, and VIII. Early studies of GBS disease in North America demonstrated a predominance of subtype III, which is thought also to be the most virulent subtype. It remains the most commonly isolated subtype causing meningitis in this country (Wilkinson, 1978). Since the 1970s, there has been a progressive change in predominance of subtypes, with Ia now the leading cause of early-onset infection (Lin et al, 1998).

During the last decade, several new subtypes have been identified. Subtype V, initially isolated from nonpregnant adults testing positive for human immunodeficiency virus (HIV) in the United States, has become a common colonizing subtype among healthy, pregnant patients. It is most prevalent in the Northeastern United States (Lin et al, 1998). Subtype V has been reported to cause sepsis in very premature infants (Eliott et al, 1998; Rench and Baker, 1993).

Subtype IV is more commonly isolated in Europe, whereas subtypes VI and VIII predominate in Asia (Lachenauer et al, 1999; Lee et al, 2000). From an immunologic and public health perspective, the recognition of multiple new subtypes has confounded the efforts of investigators to develop an effective multivalent vaccine to prevent the disease in newborns.

### Escherichia coli Infections

*E. coli* is one of the most common pathogens causing sepsis and meningitis in the neonate. Although the antigenic structure of *E. coli* is complex (145 different somatic "O" antigens, 50 flagellar "H" antigens, and 80 capsular "K" antigens), the antigenic diversity of strains that cause neonatal sepsis and meningitis is limited. Eighty percent of the strains causing meningitis and 40% of the strains causing sepsis possess the K1 antigen (Mulder et al, 1984). It is noteworthy that the K1 polysaccharide is identical to the capsule of group B meningococci. Furthermore, the outer capsules of K1 *E. coli* and group B streptococci contain sialic acid, which may prevent activation of the alternative complement pathway. Other possible explanations for the virulence of this organism are lower concentrations of the ninth component of complement and reduced recognition by neutrophils. Approximately 20% to 30% of newborn babies are colonized with *E. coli*, and that percentage increases over the first few weeks of life (Peter and Nelson, 1978). Fifty percent of women at the time of delivery are colonized with *E. coli* that are K1 positive, and vertical transmission occurs 70% of the time (Sarff et al, 1975). Disease occurs in 1 in 100 to 200 colonized babies.

### Listeria monocytogenes Infections

*Listeria monocytogenes* is commonly found throughout the environment. Higher rates of colonization have been found among farmers and veterinarians. Almost all cases in humans come from the ingestion of contaminated food (Fleming et al, 1985). There are no differences in carriage rates between pregnant and nonpregnant individuals. Fecal carriage ranges from 1% in hospitalized patients to 5% in household contacts (Schlech, 1991; Schlech et al, 1983). *Listeria* can be transmitted to the fetus through a hematogenous (transplacental route) or ascending infection. Infections with *Listeria* that occur early in gestation result in septic abortion. Later in pregnancy (after the fifth month), infection with this organism results in the premature delivery of a stillborn or infected newborn. Approximately 70% of *Listeria*-infected pregnant women deliver before 35 weeks. An influenza-like illness in the mother generally precedes delivery by 2 to 14 days and is demonstrable in about half of perinatal cases. During that time, the mother may be bacteremic. Treatment of *Listeria* sepsis during pregnancy can prevent infection in the fetus (Kalstone, 1991). *Listeria* tends to mimic GBS, with early-onset and late-onset presentations.

## Bacterial Pathogens

Since Dunham's original report in 1928, the bacteria responsible for early-onset neonatal sepsis have changed dramatically. However, the mechanisms responsible for the changes in incidence are not well understood. In the pre-antibiotic era, group A β-hemolytic streptococci accounted for the majority of perinatal infections. After the introduction of sulfonamides and then penicillin, gram-negative enteric organisms became the most common pathogens. In the 1950s, *Staphylococcus aureus* assumed a major dominance, followed once again by *E. coli* and gram-negative enterics in the 1960s. Beginning in the late 1960s, GBS (*S. agalactiae*) became the most common cause of neonatal sepsis in the United States. However, intrapartum antibiotic therapy has diminished the frequency of isolation of this pathogen.

Furthermore, there are regional differences in the kinds of organisms responsible for early-onset sepsis. These regional differences are important because they dictate the kinds of antibiotics used for empiric therapy. In the United States, the most common pathogens responsible for early-onset neonatal sepsis are *S. agalactiae* and *E. coli*. Other pathogens known to cause fulminant early-onset sepsis are *S. aureus, Haemophilus influenzae, Enterococcus* spp., *Streptococcus viridans, Klebsiella, Enterobacter* spp., *L. monocytogenes*, group A streptococci, and coagulase-negative staphylococci. There also, however, are dozens of bacteria known to be rare causes of early-onset neonatal sepsis.

## Clinical Manifestations

The clinical presentation of infants with early-onset bacterial sepsis is quite variable. The majority of infants present with respiratory distress and cardiovascular instability in the first 12 hours of life. In a subgroup of infected neonates, the signs appear after 12 hours of life. The delayed presentation in these infants suggests that the onset of bacteremia occurred at (or near) birth or during postnatal life. The signs of early-onset sepsis may be subtle (e.g., tachypnea) or overt (e.g., grunting, flaring, retractions). Almost any body system can be involved. Unfortunately, the signs of sepsis are nonspecific and common to many noninfectious disorders. Therefore, one must be cautious in ascribing an abnormal finding to a condition other than sepsis and must have a low threshold for initiating a sepsis evaluation. The common clinical signs of bacterial sepsis in the neonate are listed in Table 39–4.

Although the clinical manifestations of early-onset bacterial sepsis are nonspecific, a carefully performed physical examination is still the best way to identify infants with possible sepsis.

**TABLE 39–4**

**Clinical Signs of Neonatal Sepsis**

| Clinical Sign | % of Infants with Sign |
|---|---|
| Hyperthermia | 51 |
| Hypothermia | 15 |
| Respiratory distress | 33 |
| Apnea | 22 |
| Cyanosis | 24 |
| Jaundice | 35 |
| Hepatomegaly | 33 |
| Anorexia | 28 |
| Vomiting | 25 |
| Abdominal distention | 17 |
| Diarrhea | 11 |

Data from Klein JO: Current concepts of infectious diseases in the newborn infant. Curr Prob Pediatr 31:405, 1984.

## Laboratory Testing

### General Concepts

One must consider four characteristics of laboratory tests when evaluating an infant for possible sepsis—sensitivity, specificity, positive predictive accuracy, and negative predictive accuracy. The *sensitivity* of a laboratory test is defined as the proportion of infants with proven (or probable) sepsis in whom the result is abnormal; its *specificity* is the proportion of healthy (noninfected) infants in whom the result is normal. A sensitive test will rarely miss an infant with sepsis, and a specific test will rarely misclassify an infant who is healthy.

Although tests that have both high sensitivity *and* high specificity are desirable, one must make tradeoffs in the real world between these two properties. Sensitivity is a desirable characteristic when the condition is serious and treatable, as sepsis in infants certainly is. Specificity is an important characteristic when false-positive test results can lead to harm. For example, if the therapy used to treat a condition has serious side effects (e.g., chemotherapeutics for malignancy), one must choose a laboratory test with high specificity. Sepsis is generally treated with antimicrobial agents that have a low toxicity. Therefore, high specificity is not as important as high sensitivity in the choice of tests to rule out sepsis. The relationship between sensitivity and specificity can be expressed using a receiver operator characteristic (ROC) curve. ROC curves are constructed by plotting the rate of true-positive results (sensitivity) against the rate of false-positive results (specificity) (Fig. 39–5). Tests that discriminate well are localized to the upper left corner of the curve. The ROC curve can help determine the best cut-off value (i.e., the best combination of sensitivity and specificity).

Positive and negative predictive accuracies are variables that help clinicians interpret the laboratory test once a result is known. *Positive predictive accuracy* is the probability that an infant with an abnormal laboratory test result is infected; *negative predictive accuracy* is the probability that an infant with a normal result is healthy (free of infection). The more

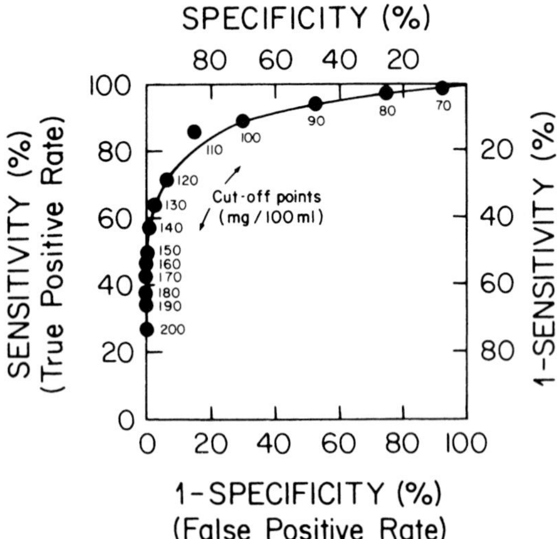


**FIGURE 39–5.** Receiver operator characteristic (ROC) curves are constructed by plotting the rate of true-positive results (sensitivity) against the rate of false-positive results (specificity).

sensitive a test, the greater its negative predictive value, and the more specific a test, the better its positive predictive value. Although we often order laboratory tests with the hope of identifying infants with sepsis, no single laboratory test or group of laboratory tests has a positive predictive value greater than 40%. In practice, the negative predictive value is a more important characteristic because it allows one to withhold or discontinue antibiotics when the probability of sepsis is low.

One other term deserves mention. The *likelihood ratio* is the likelihood that a given test result would be expected in an infant with sepsis compared with the likelihood that the same result would be expected in a healthy infant. Likelihood ratios focus on how likely a diagnostic test is to change our minds from what we thought before the test (pretest probability) to what we think afterward (post-test probability). A likelihood ratio greater than 1 (positive likelihood ratio) increases the probability that the infant has the disease in question (e.g., sepsis), and a likelihood ratio less than 1 (negative likelihood ratio) decreases the probability that the infant is infected. Likelihood ratios greater than 10 or less than 0.1 are considered large (conclusive) changes from pretest to post-test probability. Likelihood ratios between 5 and 10 and between 0.1 and 0.2 are considered moderate shifts in pretest to post-test probability. The relationships among sensitivity, specificity, positive predictive accuracy, negative predictive accuracy, and likelihood ratio are shown in Figure 39–6.

## Cultures

### *Surface Cultures and Analysis of Gastric Aspirates*

Cultures of superficial body sites (external auditory canal, gastric aspirate, nasopharynx, groin, axilla, and umbilicus), or surface cultures, have traditionally been used to identify pathogens in sick neonates when other culture results are negative. Although some centers still use surface culture specimens to make clinical decisions regarding discontinuation of antimicrobial therapy, most do not (Shenoy et al, 2000). Evans and colleagues (1988) analyzed data from 24,584 cultures obtained from 3371 infants and found that the sensitivity, specificity, and positive predictive accuracy of surface cultures were 56%, 82%, and 7.5%, respectively. They concluded that surface cultures were of limited value in predicting the etiology of sepsis in neonates. Similarly, the examination of gastric aspirates for polymorphonuclear leukocytes (PMNs) has been used as a screening procedure for neonatal sepsis (Leibovich et al, 1987; Mims et al, 1972; Scanlon, 1972; Yeung and Tam, 1972). The presence of increased numbers of white blood cells has been thought to represent amnionitis and a fetal inflammatory response. However, a careful analysis of the origin of the cells in gastric aspirate has indicated a maternal origin

| | | **Bacterial Infection Present** | | |
|---|---|---|---|---|
| | | **Yes** | **No** | |
| **Laboratory Test** | **Positive** | TRUE POSITIVES (a) | FALSE POSITIVES (b) | POSITIVE PREDICTIVE VALUE (a)/(a+b) |
| | **Negative** | FALSE NEGATIVES (c) | TRUE NEGATIVES (d) | NEGATIVE PREDICTIVE VALUE (d)/(c+d) |
| | | SENSITIVITY (a)/(a+c) | SPECIFICITY (d)/(b+d) | PREVALENCE (a+c)/(a+b+c+d) |
| | | LIKELIHOOD RATIO, POSITIVE sensitivity/1–specificity | LIKELIHOOD RATIO, NEGATIVE 1–sensitivity/specificity | |

**FIGURE 39–6.** Diagram of the relationships among sensitivity, specificity, positive predictive accuracy, negative predictive accuracy, and likelihood ratio.

(Vasan et al, 1977). Therefore, the presence of PMNs does not indicate fetal infection.

### *Blood Culture*

A positive blood culture result is the "gold standard" for detection of bacteremia in a neonate with suspected early-onset sepsis. However, the following variables affect the likelihood of recovering at least one colony-forming unit (CFU) in a blood culture specimen: (1) the number of CFUs in the blood at the time the culture specimen was obtained, (2) the culture techniques, (3) the volume of blood obtained, and (4) use of intrapartum antibiotics. Therefore, the blood culture is an imperfect reference standard. In one study, data obtained before the use of intrapartum therapy indicated that premortem blood culture results were positive in only 80% of infants in whom infection was proven by immediate postmortem cultures and autopsy (Squire et al, 1982). Furthermore, blood culture results are negative in up to 50% of neonates with a congenital bacterial pneumonia (positive tracheal aspirate culture result in the first 12 hours of life, and clinical signs) (Sherman et al, 1980). The use of intrapartum antibiotics has substantially reduced the number of positive blood culture results.

The number of CFUs is another important variable. In approximately 25% of infants with bacterial sepsis, the CFU count in the blood specimen is less than 5 CFU/mL (Dietzman et al, 1974). When the number of CFUs is that low, the volume of blood required to detect bacteremia is critical. In an in vitro study, Schelonka and associates (1996) demonstrated that when the CFU count in the blood specimen (original colony count) is 4 CFU/mL or less, a culture volume of 0.5 mL fails to detect at least one CFU 13% of the time. When the original colony count is 1 CFU/mL, the blood culture fails to detect bacteremia almost 60% of the time. Sending 1 mL of blood for culture will improve the recovery rates to 98% and 63% if the original colony counts are 4 CFU/mL and 1 CFU/mL, respectively. Unfortunately, the volume of neonatal blood sent for culture is frequently inadequate. In a study by Neal and colleagues (1986), 55% of neonatal blood specimens contained less than 0.5 mL of blood. Although 1 mL appears to be the ideal blood culture volume, it may be technically difficult to obtain in small, sick premature infants. In those circumstances, blood drawn through an indwelling arterial line appears to be an acceptable alternative (Cowett et al, 1976; Polin et al, 1981).

Another controversy is the time required for blood culture results to become positive. This is particularly relevant for the asymptomatic infant (or transiently symptomatic infant) who was started on antibiotic therapy because of risk factors for infection. In a study by Kumar and associates (2001), 97% of definite and "possible" bacterial pathogens were detected by 48 hours. The negative predictive value for isolation of definite bacterial pathogens was 99.8% at 48 hours. These data are similar to those reported by Garcia-Prats and coworkers (2000), who found that virtually all cultures growing clinically significant gram-positive and gram-negative organisms were positive by 36 hours (Garcia-Prats et al, 2000). In this study, there was no difference in time to positivity between cultures of specimens collected "pre-therapy" and "post-therapy." Therefore, in the term asymptomatic infant, it is reasonable to stop antibiotic therapy after 48 hours if culture results are negative *and* physical findings remain normal. In asymptomatic preterm infants started on antibiotic therapy because of risk factors for infection, a carefully performed physical examination is equally reassuring, but it is more difficult to do in these tiniest neonates. In such patients, the decision to continue or discontinue antibiotics is often based on results of other laboratory tests (see discussion of sepsis screens). Whenever the suspicion of sepsis is high (especially in a symptomatic infant), consideration should be given to continuing antibiotic therapy for a "complete course" despite a negative blood culture result (see later).

### *Urine Culture*

The rate of positive urine culture results in infants with early-onset sepsis is low. In the study by Visser and Hall (1979), the urine culture result was negative in eight of nine infants with early-onset sepsis in whom blood culture results were positive. In two other infants, the urine culture result was positive and the blood culture result was negative. Infants with late-onset sepsis had a higher rate of positive urine cultures. Similarly, DiGeronimo (1992) found only 1 infant with a positive urine culture result of 280 infants who were being evaluated for early-onset sepsis (16 of the infants had positive blood culture results), and no infants with negative blood culture results had bacteriuria.

Pyelonephritis in the neonate is thought to represent seeding of the kidney during an episode of bacteremia. Therefore, it makes intuitive sense that the blood culture result should be positive in any infant with a positive urine culture; however, this finding has not been substantiated in infants born to women who have received intrapartum antibiotic therapy. Given the low yield of positive urine culture results and costs of processing the specimens, urine culture should not be part of the traditional sepsis evaluation in the first 72 hours of life.

### Cerebrospinal Fluid

The controversies surrounding indications for lumbar puncture are discussed later. Lumbar puncture should be deferred in any infant with clinical instability or an uncorrected bleeding diathesis.

### White Blood Count and Neutrophil Indices

Total leukocyte counts are not very helpful in the diagnosis of neonatal sepsis (Schuchat et al, 1994). Normal counts range from 9000 to 30,000 cells/$mm^3$ at the time of birth, and differences in the site of sampling and the activity of the baby can affect this measurement. For example, in a study by Christensen and Rothstein (1979), venous blood leukocyte counts were 82% of simultaneously drawn capillary blood values, and arterial blood counts were 77% of capillary blood values. These investigators also reported that in samples collected after "violent crying," white blood counts increased to 146% of baseline values and a "shift to the left" occurred. Neutrophil indices—absolute neutrophil count (ANC), the absolute band count (immature neutrophil count), and the ratio of immature neutrophils to total neutrophils (I/T ratio)—have proved more useful than total leukocyte counts in the diagnosis of neonatal sepsis.

The reference ranges for each of these indices were established by Manroe and colleagues (Manroe, 1979). The lower limit or total neutrophil count is 1750 cells/mm$^3$ at birth and rises to 7200 cells/mm$^3$ by 12 hours of age. It then declines to approximately 1720 cells/mm$^3$ by 72 hours of age. The absolute band count undergoes similar changes postnatally. Peak values of 1400 cells/mm$^3$ occur at about 12 hours of life and then decline. In contrast, the I/T ratio is maximum at birth (0.16) and then declines to a value of 0.12 beyond age 72 hours. In this study, the mean gestational age of study infants was 38.9 weeks, and the mean weight was 2685 g. Mouzinho and coworkers (1994) published revised reference ranges for very low-birth-weight (VLBW) infants. They observed a wider reference range in total neutrophil counts for the VLBW population. The lower boundary ranged from 500 cells/mm$^3$ soon after birth to 2,200 cells/mm$^3$ by 18 to 20 hours of life. By day 5 of life, the lower boundary was 1,100 cells/mm$^3$. These researchers found no differences in the I/T ratio or absolute immature neutrophil counts in VLBW infants.

Although normal values for neutrophil indices have been fairly well established, the cutoff values indicative of sepsis remain controversial. Table 39–5 lists suggested cutoff values for the ANC, absolute band count, and I/T ratio. It is important to note, however, that there is considerable overlap of these indices between healthy and infected newborns. Schelonka and colleagues (1994) determined normal values for neutrophil indices in healthy term infants. As noted previously, the upper limits for absolute band count and I/T ratio overlap with the suggested cutoff values. Furthermore, the inter-reader variability in the identification of immature neutrophils renders the value of the I/T ratio and absolute band count open to question (Schelonka et al, 1995).

The total neutrophil count is abnormal in about two thirds of infants with sepsis. However, a variety of clinical conditions can affect total neutrophil counts (Table 39–6). Neutropenia is the best predictor of sepsis, and neutrophilia does not correlate very well. Counts obtained in specimens collected immediately after birth have an impaired sensitivity for identification of infected newborns (Rozycki et al, 1987). Therefore, collection of the initial laboratory screen specimen should be delayed for several hours or a second screen specimen should be obtained at about 12-24 hours of life. The absolute band count is an insensitive marker of sepsis but has a good positive predictive value and specificity. The I/T ratio has the best sensitivity of all the neutrophil indices (range 60% to 90%); however, a variety of perinatal conditions has been shown to affect this ratio (Manroe et al, 1979). The sensitivity, specificity, and positive and negative predictive values for the commonly used neutrophil indices are shown in Table 39–7.

**TABLE 39–5**

**Neutrophil Value Suggestive of Infection**

Neutropenia: neutrophil count <1750 cells/mm$^3$
Ratio of immature to total neutrophil count >0.2
Absolute band count >2000 cells/mm$^3$
Total white blood cell count <5000 cells/mm$^3$

### Platelet Counts

At the time of diagnosis of sepsis, about 25% of infants exhibit thrombocytopenia, and that percentage increases during the course of infection. The major mechanism responsible for thrombocytopenia in infected neonates is accelerated platelet destruction; a minority of infected infants has disseminated intravascular coagulation (DIC). In the absence of DIC, clinical bleeding abnormalities are rare.

### Acute Phase Reactants and Erythrocyte Sedimentation Rate

A wide variety of acute phase reactants has been used to identify infants with possible sepsis, including C-reactive protein (CRP), fibrinogen, ceruloplasmin, fibronectin, prealbumin, haptoglobin, and orosomucoid (Benitz et al, 1998; Gabay and Kushner, 1999; Sáez-Llorens and Lagrutta, 1993). Acute phase proteins are produced by hepatocytes in response to cytokine signals, principally IL-6. Gene expression for acute phase proteins is regulated mainly at the transcriptional level. Because the increase in acute phase proteins depends on an initial cytokine response, there is always some delay in the rise of these proteins. After an inflammatory stimulus (and after a delay of several hours) CRP and serum amyloid A are the first acute phase protein values to rise. The rise in the erythrocyte sedimentation rate (ESR) is slower and reflects elevated fibrinogen levels.

C-reactive protein is the most well studied acute phase protein in neonatal sepsis (Jaye and Waites, 1997). CRP was discovered in 1930 by Tillett and Francis in the sera of patients with pneumonia. It consists of five non–covalently bound identical subunits, each containing 187 amino acids, with one intrachain disulfide bond and no carbohydrate modifications. Monitoring of CRP levels has been widely promoted as a way to reduce the duration of antibiotic therapy in infants with suspected and proven sepsis (Bomela et al, 2000; Ehl et al, 1997; Philip and Mills, 2000). A CRP value of 10 mg/dL is generally accepted as the upper limit of normal, but some laboratories have used different cutoff values. The most widely used technique for measurement of CRP is laser nephelometry. Results can be available within 15 to 30 minutes and only 50 μL of serum is needed.

The largest prospective study evaluating CRP in the diagnosis of neonatal infection was performed by Benitz and colleagues (1998). In this study, CRP was measured in 1002 infants with suspected early-onset sepsis at the time of initial evaluation (CRP #1) and on each of the next

**TABLE 39-6**

**Frequency of Physical Findings in 49 Infants with Congenital Malaria**

| | Frequency in Neonates with Following Abnormal Values* | | | |
|---|---|---|---|---|
| **Complication** | **Decrease in Total Neutrophils** | **Increase in Total Neutrophils** | **Increase in Total Immature Neutrophil Forms** | **Increased Ratio of Immature Forms to Total Neutrophil Count** |
| Maternal hypertension | ++++ | 0 | + | + |
| Maternal fever, neonate healthy | 0 | ++ | +++ | ++++ |
| ≥6 hrs intrapartum oxytocin | 0 | ++ | ++ | ++++ |
| Asphyxia (5-min Apgar score ≤5) | + | ++ | ++ | +++ |
| Meconium aspiration syndrome | 0 | ++++ | +++ | ++ |
| Pneumothorax with uncomplicated hyaline membrane disease | 0 | ++++ | ++++ | ++++ |
| Seizures—no hypoglycemia, asphyxia, or central nervous system hemorrhage | 0 | +++ | +++ | ++++ |
| Prolonged (≥4 min) crying | 0 | ++++ | ++++ | ++++ |
| Asymptomatic blood glucose ≤30 mg/dL | 0 | ++ | +++ | +++ |
| Hemolytic disease | ++ | ++ | +++ | ++ |
| Surgery | 0 | ++++ | ++++ | +++ |
| High altitude | 0 | ++++ | ++++ | 0 |

*Frequency defined as follows: 0, not present; +, present in 0% to 25%; ++, present in 25% to 50%; +++, present in 50% to 75% ++++, present in 75% to 100%.

two mornings (CRP #2 and CRP #3). CRP #1 was found to have a poor sensitivity (35.0%) for proven sepsis; this finding is not surprising, given the delayed rise in CRP. In contrast, CRP #2 had a sensitivity of 78.9% for proven sepsis. The sensitivity of CRP #2 and CRP #3 (excluding CRP #1) for proven sepsis was 88.9%; the negative predictive value was 99.7% for proven or probable early-onset sepsis. Positive predictive values were low (<10%); however, marked elevations of CRP (>6 mg/dL) were associated with a higher (60%) probability of sepsis. Therefore, like most diagnostic tests for early-onset sepsis, the high negative predictive accuracy of serial CRP determinations (performed 8 to 12 hours after birth) was helpful in deciding which infants did not require antibiotic therapy and those in whom antibiotics could be discontinued after a brief course.

**TABLE 39-7**

**Performance of Hematologic Tests in the Diagnosis of Sepsis**

| Parameter | Neutropenia | I/T > 0.2 | Increased Band Count |
|---|---|---|---|
| Sensitivity (%) | 38-96 | 90-100 | 63-67 |
| Specificity (%) | 61-92 | 50-78 | 69-77 |
| PPV (%) | 20-77 | 11-51 | 17-46 |
| NPV (%) | 96-99 | 99-100 | 95 |

I/T, ratio of immature neutrophil forms to total neutrophil count; PPV, positive predictive value; NPV, negative predictive value.

Data from Gerdes JS: Clinicopathologic approach to the diagnosis of neonatal sepsis. Isr J Med Sci 30:435, 1994.

Determination of the erythrocyte sedimentation rate with the use of a micro-hematocrit tube was developed more than 50 years ago. During the first two weeks of life, an approximation of the upper limits of normal values for the ESR can be made by adding 2 or 3 to the age of the infant in days. The ESR is normal in most infants with noninfectious conditions, but significant elevations occur in infants with a Coombs-positive hemolytic anemia (Adler and Denton, 1975). The sensitivity of the ESR ranges from 30% to 70%. As for other measures of inflammation, there is a delay in the rise in ESR in infected neonates. Furthermore, once the ESR is elevated, the decline is very slow. However, the negative predictive accuracy of the micro-ESR is high (>95%), and in centers where CRP determinations are not available, it may be a suitable alternative.

## Cytokines

*Cytokines* are proteins, glycoproteins, and lipids that regulate the inflammatory response. A wide variety of cytokines has been identified in infants with sepsis, including IL-1, IL-6, IL-8, TNF-α, soluble IL-2 receptor, soluble intercellular adhesion molecule-1 (ICAM-1), soluble TNF-α receptor, E-selectin, IL-1 receptor antagonist, granulocyte-macrophage colony-stimulating factor (GM-CSF), and granulocyte CSF (G-CSF) (Mehr and Doyle, 2000).

The diagnostic value of IL-6 has been studied most extensively. Although the data are not definitive, the following generalizations about IL-6 and other cytokines in neonatal sepsis are possible:

1. There are marked variations in the assays used for cytokine determinations, which have resulted in variations in the cutoff values used to discriminate infected from noninfected infants.
2. The sensitivity of the IL-6 value is approximately 90%, and the negative predictive accuracy exceeds 95% (values for specificity have varied).
3. As the inflammatory response subsides, levels of IL-6 quickly return to a normal range (usually within 24 hours).
4. Persistent elevations of cytokines are associated with higher mortality.

A number of investigators has demonstrated that the combination of Il-6 and CRP determinations results in a higher sensitivity than either marker used alone (Doellner et al, 1998). IL-6 assays currently require hours to complete. Therefore, at present, cytokine determinations remain an unproven but promising diagnostic tool.

### Sepsis Screens

Because none of the diagnostic tests for sepsis is able to identify infants with proven sepsis with reasonable accuracy, investigators have used combinations of laboratory tests (neutrophil indices, measurements of acute phase proteins and ESR) to enhance the identification of infected neonates. Although these so-called sepsis screens do not have better positive predictive accuracy than individual laboratory tests, they have significantly better negative predictive accuracy and can provide greater reassurance that infection is not present. Philip and Hewitt (1980) utilized five tests—I/T ratio, absolute leukocyte count, CRP, micro-ESR, and haptoglobin—to screen infants admitted for suspected sepsis or meningitis. A positive sepsis screen result was defined as two or more abnormal test results. The sensitivity of the sepsis screen was 93%, and the positive predictive accuracy was 39%. When results of fewer than two tests were positive, the negative predictive accuracy was 99%.

Gerdes and Polin (1987) performed two sepsis screens 12 to 24 hours apart; the screens consisted of I/T ratio, white blood count, CRP, and micro-ESR. This method identified 100% of infected infants (n = 13) and had a negative predictive accuracy of 100%. With a hematologic scoring system employing seven variables, Rodwell and colleagues (1988, 1993) obtained similar results using a hematologic scoring system. Because of their high negative predictive accuracy, sepsis screens have been shown to result in a significant decrease in the use of antimicrobial agents. In addition, they permit discontinuation of antibiotic therapy at the earliest possible time with the greatest confidence.

## Diagnostic Approach to Neonates with Suspected Sepsis

### Symptomatic Infants

All symptomatic infants must be carefully evaluated for the possibility of sepsis, and most symptomatic infants are treated. Although the presence of risk factors should increase one's suspicion of sepsis, the absence of risk factors in a symptomatic infant is not totally reassuring. During the adjustment to postnatal life, some infants transiently exhibit abnormal signs (e.g., tachypnea) before becoming asymptomatic. Any infant who is still symptomatic at 6 hours of life should be treated as if infected. A suggested algorithm for the evaluation and treatment of symptomatic infants is shown in Figure 39–7. Antibiotic therapy can be stopped in a symptomatic infant when (1) the clinical suspicion of sepsis is low, (2) physical findings are normal at 48 hours of age, and (3) sepsis screen results remain negative.

### Asymptomatic Infants

The management of asymptomatic infants born to mothers with risk factors for infection is controversial. Unfortunately, there are almost no prospective data to guide decision-making. A carefully performed physical examination is the most important part of the diagnostic work-up. Our recommendations for the management of asymptomatic infants born to women with risk factors for infection are shown in Figures 39–8 and 39–9. Recommendations for infants born at 35 weeks of gestation or later and for those

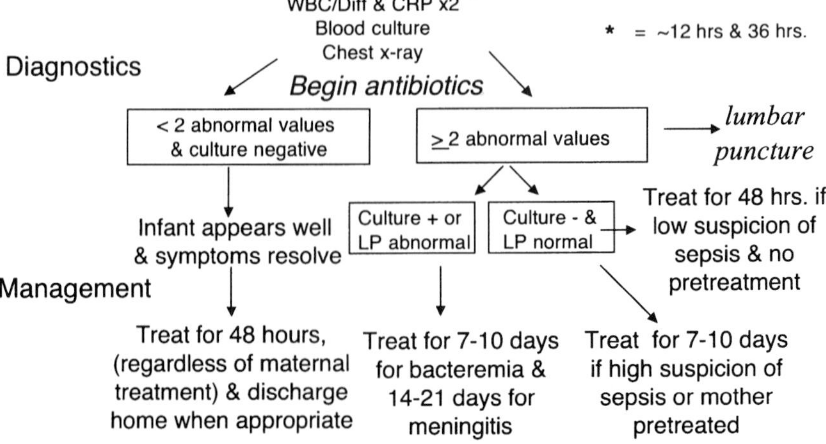


**FIGURE 39–7.** A suggested algorithm for the evaluation and treatment of symptomatic infants for neonatal sepsis. CRP, C-reactive protein value; LP, lumbar puncture (with examination of cerebrospinal fluid); Px, physical; WBC/Diff, white blood count with differential count.

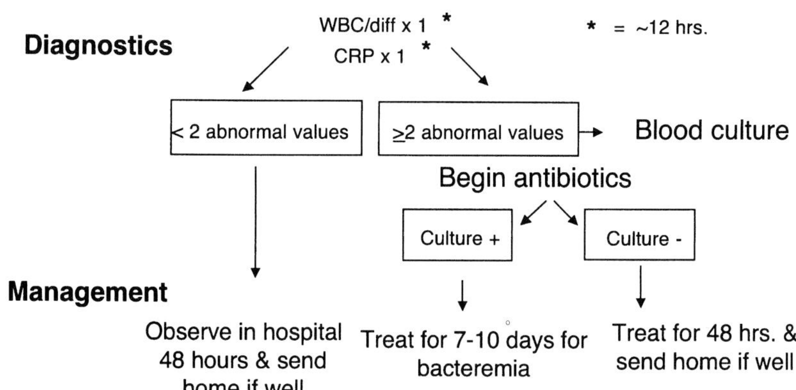


**FIGURE 39–8.** Recommendations for the management of asymptomatic infants born at 35 weeks of gestation or later to women with risk factors for infection. CRP, C-reactive protein value; WBC/Diff, white blood count with differential count.

born before 35 weeks of gestation are presented separately. As noted previously, the three main maternal risk factors for early-onset neonatal sepsis are colonization with GBS, signs and symptoms of chorioamnionitis, and prolonged (>18 hours) rupture of membranes. Intrapartum antibiotic therapy for women colonized with GBS is effective when administered more than 4 hours before delivery but does not guarantee that the infant will be well.

In asymptomatic infants born at or after 35 weeks of gestation to women with risk factors, there are two principal options, observation alone and observation plus diagnostic studies (see Fig. 39–8). The use of intrapartum antibiotics (more than 4 hours before delivery) is 90% effective when no other risk factors are present (Schrag et al, 2002). Therefore, observation alone is probably sufficient for asymptomatic infants born at or after 35 weeks of gestation to women who are colonized with GBS, have no other risk factors, and have received an appropriate antibiotic at least 4 hours before delivery. For any infant whose mother has other risk factors (PROM >18 hours or signs and symptoms of chorioamnionitis), we recommend that a sepsis screen be performed, due to the difficulty of observing infants closely enough for the early, subtle signs of sepsis. The sepsis screen specimen should be drawn at 12 hours of life rather than immediately after birth, because of the greater likelihood of a positive result in an infected infant with the passage of time. If the result is positive, our recommendation is to obtain a blood culture and give antibiotic therapy until culture results are confirmed negative (48 hours). A positive sepsis screen result places the risk of bacteremia at about 40% (Gerdes, 1994). Escobar and colleagues (2000) identified 1275 asymptomatic infants (>2000 g) who were evaluated for early-onset sepsis because of risk factors. In the study, asymptomatic status reduced the probability of proven sepsis (adjusted odds ratio 0.26 (95% confidence interval [CI], 0.11 to 0.63); however, 1% of asymptomatic infants born to untreated women were infected, and 0.9% of infants born to women receiving intrapartum antibiotics were infected. Both of these rates are still ten times the rate seen in the general population. Overall, intrapartum antibiotic therapy decreased the percentage of babies who

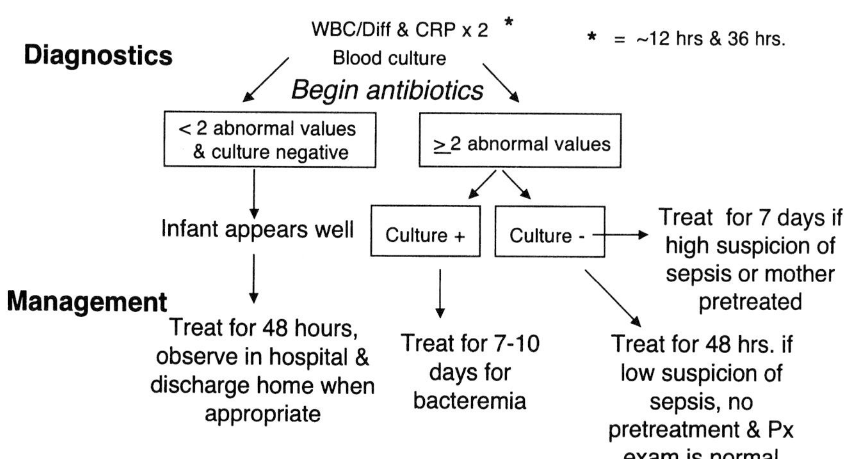


**FIGURE 39–9.** Recommendations for the management of asymptomatic infants born before 35 weeks of gestation and born to women with risk factors for infection. CRP, C-reactive protein value; Px, physical; WBC/Diff, white blood count with differential count.

were critically ill ($P$ = .001) and infected ($P$ = .066). These researchers suggest that screening, treatment, and observation protocols cannot be based on asymptomatic status alone.

Recommendations for asymptomatic infants born before 35 weeks of gestation are shown in Figure 39–9. With increasing degrees of prematurity, the physical findings become more difficult to assess. Therefore, in an asymptomatic infant born before 35 weeks of gestation to a woman with any risk factors for sepsis, we recommend that broad-spectrum antibiotic therapy be started after a blood culture specimen has been obtained. Sepsis screen specimens should be obtained at 12 and 36 hours of life. We believe that if the infant remains asymptomatic (and appears well) and the results of culture and sepsis screens are negative, antibiotic therapy can be discontinued, and the infant observed. In the asymptomatic infant with a positive sepsis screen result, the decision to continue antibiotic therapy should be individualized. If the mother has received intrapartum antibiotics, blood culture results are less reliable, and such an infant should probably be given a complete course of therapy. If the mother has not received intrapartum antibiotics and appears well, antibiotic therapy can be discontinued, and the infant observed. The decision whether to perform a lumbar puncture for CSF analysis is discussed later.

## Clinical Spectrum of Disease

### Streptococcus agalactiae (Group B Streptococcus)

The clinical picture of early-onset GBS sepsis is identical to that of early-onset sepsis due to other organisms. The case fatality rate is low in term infants, and morbid sequelae are rare. There are no characteristic physical findings. Furthermore, there are no distinguishing findings on complete blood count (CBC) or acute phase reactant determinations. Chest radiographs are indistinguishable from those seen in respiratory distress syndrome (RDS), transient tachypnea of the newborn, meconium aspiration syndrome, and pneumonia (Ablow, 1976).

### Staphylococcus aureus

As already mentioned, *S. aureus* was the most common cause of neonatal sepsis in the 1950s; it was replaced by gram-negative enteric organisms (*E. coli*) and GBS. Staphylococci are responsible for a wide variety of serious infections in newborn infants, including breast abscess, furunculosis, osteomyelitis, endocarditis, and septic arthritis. Furthermore, phage group II organisms are capable of producing an exotoxin that cleaves the skin at the granular cell layer, causing toxic epidermal necrolysis, bullous impetigo, and a scarlatiniform rash. Most strains of *S. aureus* are sensitive to semisynthetic penicillins (e.g., methicillin), but methicillin-resistant strains of *S. aureus* (MRSA) have assumed an increasing importance. There are many potential reservoirs for MRSA in the nursery environment. Risk factors for colonization are birth weight less than 1500 g, prolonged hospital stay, and the presence of central venous catheter, thoracostomy tubes, or shunts. MRSA generally cause nosocomial infections, and epidemics are not uncommon. Contact with the hands of colonized nursery personnel is usually how these organisms are spread. Coagulase-negative staphylococci can also cause early-onset bacterial sepsis; the clinical spectrum of disease is indistinguishable from that for other bacterial pathogens.

### Listeria monocytogenes

*L. monocytogenes* is responsible for early- and late-onset bacterial infections in a pattern similar to that seen with GBS. Infants with early-onset sepsis due to *Listeria* generally become symptomatic in the first day or two of life. There is often a history of an antecedent maternal illness (malaise, myalgia, and fever). Passage of meconium before birth is commonly noted. Infants infected with *Listeria* are generally indistinguishable from those infected with other pathogens; however a granulomatous rash has been described in critically ill infants with *L. monocytogenes* infection. Persistent pulmonary hypertension has also been observed in seriously ill infants. Laboratory features are nonspecific. The mortality rate with early-onset disease is 25%.

## Prevention

### Intrapartum Antibiotic Prophylaxis

#### *History*

In 1990, GBS infections caused an estimated 7600 serious illnesses and 310 deaths among U.S. infants 90 days or younger. Approximately 80% of these illnesses occurred in infants younger than 7 days—that is, those diagnosed with early-onset disease (Decreasing incidence, 1997). At that time and during the 2 years that followed, several well-designed studies demonstrated the efficacy of intrapartum antibiotic prophylaxis in reducing the incidence of early-onset GBS disease (Allen et al, 1993; Boyer and Gotoff, 1986). Professional and public demand encouraged the American Academy of Pediatrics (AAP) and the American College of Obstetricians and Gynecologists (ACOG) to publish guidelines for prevention of early-onset GBS sepsis (AAP, 1992; ACOG, 1992). The two organizations' recommendations differed in that one took a screening-based approach and the other a risk factor–based approach, leading to confusion.

In 1995, the CDC led representatives of the AAP and ACOG and other leaders in GBS research to develop a policy acceptable to all participants. In 1996, the CDC published consensus strategies recommending alternative strategies ("risk factor-based or culture-based") for prevention of early-onset streptococcal sepsis (Prevention, 1996). Assessment of the CDC consensus strategies and other studies of intrapartum antibiotic prophylaxis have been confounded by noncompliance issues. Nevertheless, the impact of implementation has been dramatic. Active population-based surveillance in eight states from 1993 to 1998 demonstrated a decrease in attack rate of early-onset GBS sepsis from 1.7 to 0.6 per 1000 live births. This drop was associated with a 75% reduction in the (excess) incidence of disease among African-American infants. Projecting the study findings to the entire United States, Schrag and colleagues (2000) estimated that 3900 cases of early-onset sepsis and 200 neonatal deaths were prevented by protocol-directed intrapartum antibiotic prophylaxis. In 2002, the CDC published new guidelines to take into account new information regarding the superiority of the culture-based strategy over the risk-based strategy (Prevention, 1996; Schrag et al, 2002).

### *Protocol—The "CDC Consensus Strategies"*

The CDC recommendations for intrapartum antibiotic prophylaxis to prevent early-onset group B streptococcal disease are summarized here (Schrag et al, 2002).

#### Antepartum Culture-Based Strategy

Originally, antepartum screening at 22 to 23 weeks and 35 to 37 weeks of gestation with the use of a combined vaginal-rectal swab specimen processed in selective media was advocated as the screening strategy. Later revisions of the screening strategy recommend screening only at 35 to 37 weeks of gestation. Antepartum treatment is recommended for women with the following characteristics:

- Previous infant with invasive disease
- GBS bacteriuria during pregnancy
- Positive GBS screening culture result during pregnancy (unless a planned cesarean delivery, in the absence of labor or amniotic membrane rupture, is performed)
- Unknown GBS status (culture not performed, culture incomplete, or results unknown) and any of the following features: delivery before 37 weeks of gestation, rupture of amniotic membranes for 18 hours or longer, and intrapartum temperature of 100.4° F (38° C) or higher.

#### Intrapartum Management of Parturients

Women who are able to receive penicillin should be given penicillin G, 5 million units as a loading IV dose followed by 2.5 million units q4h until delivery, *or* ampicillin, 2 g IV as a loading dose followed by 1 g q4h until delivery.

For any woman who is allergic to penicillin, the CDC recommends that during prenatal care, the history of penicillin allergy be assessed to determine whether the patient is at high risk for anaphylaxis (i.e., history of immediate hypersensitivity reactions). Women who *are not* at high risk for anaphylaxis should receive cefazolin, 2 g IV then 1 g IV q8h until delivery. Women who *are* at high risk for anaphylaxis should receive clindamycin, 900 mg IV q8h until delivery *or* erythromycin, 500 g IV q6h until delivery.

#### Postnatal Management of Infants Born to Mothers Treated with Intrapartum Antibiotics

The CDC guidelines recommend that all symptomatic infants undergo a full diagnostic evaluation, including CBC and differential, blood culture, and chest radiograph (if respiratory symptoms are present). If feasible, a lumbar puncture should be performed, and empiric therapy should be initiated with ampicillin and gentamicin. The duration of treatment might be as short as 48 to 72 hours, depending on the culture results and clinical course. The same recommendation (full diagnostic evaluation and treatment) is made for any infant born to a woman who has received antibiotics for suspected chorioamnionitis. For asymptomatic infants born before 35 weeks of gestation to women who are culture positive for GBS, a limited evaluation (CBC with differential and blood culture) is recommended. If sepsis is suspected in this population, a full diagnostic evaluation and empiric therapy are suggested.

Asymptomatic infants born at or after 35 weeks of gestation to mothers who have received 4 or more hours of intrapartum antibiotic prophylaxis require no additional evaluation or therapy; however, observation for a minimum of 48 hours is recommended. Asymptomatic infants of the same gestational age whose mothers received less than 4 hours of intrapartum antibiotic prophylaxis should undergo a limited evaluation, consisting of a CBC with differential and a blood culture, and should be observed for a minimum of 48 hours. In selected circumstances (fully compliant family and adequate therapy), such an infant may be discharged earlier.

#### Assessing the CDC Consensus Strategies—Noncompliance Issues, Cost-Versus-Benefit Analyses, Future Changes in Protocol

Despite the initiation of the standardized protocols recommended by the AAP, CDC, and ACOG, there have been many noncompliance issues. Chandran and associates (2001) presented an observational study in which clinician compliance with nationally recommended guidelines was evaluated. For the combined risk factor-based and culture-based algorithm, clinical compliance with intrapartum prophylaxis ranged from 75% to 84%. Twenty-two percent of women received antibiotics that were not indicated. Among the women for whom antenatal cultures were indicated, only 65% underwent the tests. More significantly, only 9% of culture specimens were obtained from the anogenital site. Fourteen percent to 75% of infants underwent the guideline-suggested evaluation, and 61% to 94% remained hospitalized for a minimum of 48 hours. The failure to process cultures with selective media is another common noncompliance issue, but it may be improving (Adoption, 1998).

#### Impact of Implementation of the CDC Consensus Strategies

The primary outcome of the implementation of the CDC consensus strategies for prevention of early-onset neonatal GBS sepsis has been a steady and dramatic decrease in the incidence of the disease, with rates currently at 40% to 60% of those in the pre-implementation era. With few exceptions, however, there has not been any reduction in the incidence of early-onset sepsis due to other organisms (Isaacs and Royle, 1999). The majority of published reports also shows that intrapartum prophylaxis is not 100% effective; 10% of infants with positive blood culture results are born to treated mothers.

Initial concerns about the risks of implementing these strategies have proved unwarranted. The principal risks were maternal anaphylaxis (Schuchat et al, 2000) and emergence of infections in mothers and infants due to resistant organisms (e.g., *E coli, Enterococcus* spp.) (Chen et al, 2001; Towers et al, 1998). A study by the Neonatal Network of the National Institute of Child Health and Human Development (NICHHD) demonstrated a change in the pathogens causing early-onset sepsis, with an increase in sepsis due to *E. coli* from 3.2 to 6.8 per 1000 live births. Most (85%) *E. coli* isolates were resistant to ampicillin (Stoll et al, 2002).

### *Preterm Premature Rupture of Membranes*

It is generally accepted that intrauterine infection plays a primary role in the pathogenesis of pPROM and preterm delivery. Furthermore, there are strong associations among pPROM, positive amniotic fluid culture results, clinical signs of chorioamnionitis, and histologically confirmed chorioamnionitis. The relationship between lower genital tract colonization and pPROM is not as conclusive; however, several studies have demonstrated an association between colonization with various microorganisms (GBS, *U. urealyticum, G. vaginalis, Bacteroides* spp., *C. trachomatis*, and *T. vaginalis*) and pPROM. Although there have been numerous controlled trials examining the benefits of antibiotics in women with pPROM, only two studies have had sufficient power to evaluate neonatal morbidity. In 1997, the Maternal Fetal Network at the NICHHD published the results of a multicenter trial (n = 614) in which women with pPROM (24 to 32 weeks of gestation) were randomly assigned to receive either antibiotic treatment (ampicillin or amoxicillin and erythromycin) for 1 week or placebo (Mercer et al, 1997). In the group receiving antibiotics, the incidence of clinical amnionitis was lower and gestation was significantly prolonged. Infants born to women treated with antibiotics exhibited lower incidences of respiratory distress syndrome and stage 2 or 3 necrotizing enterocolitis (NEC). Although the incidence of sepsis in infants younger than 72 hours was not reduced ($P = .26$), the overall incidence of sepsis was significantly lower ($P = .01$).

The ORACLE I study from the United Kingdom randomly assigned women with pPROM (n = 4286) to the following four treatment groups: amoxicillin–clavulanic acid, erythromycin, both antibiotics, or placebo (Kenyon et al, 2001a). Among 2260 singletons who were treated with erythromycin or placebo, the risk of death or major adverse outcome (chronic lung disease or major cerebral abnormality) was reduced. Use of erythromycin was associated with prolongation of pregnancy, reduced treatment with surfactant, and fewer positive blood culture results. There was no benefit to using amoxicillin–clavulanic acid with or without erythromycin; in fact, those combinations were associated with a higher risk of necrotizing enterocolitis. These studies suggest that administration of erythromycin for 7 to 10 days after pPROM offers substantial benefits to the preterm neonate and reduces the likelihood of sepsis.

### Intravenous Immune Globulin for Prevention of Early-Onset Sepsis

Reduced transplacental transfer of immunoglobulins (Ig) and decreased endogenous synthesis of IgG predispose premature infants to early-onset sepsis. This physiologic hypogammaglobulinemia provides a rationale for administering intravenous immune globulin (IVIG). However, few controlled studies of IVIG prophylaxis for early-onset sepsis have been undertaken.

Haque and colleagues (1986) studied VLBW (≤1500 g) infants who were given either IVIG shortly after delivery or nothing (control). The rates of infection (mean age of onset 8 to 76 hours) were 16% in the control group and 4% in the treated group ($P < .005$). Moreover, significantly higher serum Ig concentrations were found in the treated infants. Three randomized, placebo-controlled studies determined the overall incidence of both early-onset and late-onset infections in infants treated with IVIG since birth, in comparison with controls. Chirico and associates (1987) found a benefit of the treatment only in VLBW infants, whereas Conway and coworkers (1990) found no difference in sepsis incidence between treated and untreated infants when blood culture result was the diagnostic criterion. Sandberg and colleagues (2000) evaluated the effects of IVIG infusion in preterm infants with a plasma level of IgG less than 4 g/L at birth and were unable to demonstrate any benefit of the treatment.

### Recombinant Cytokines for Prevention of Early-Onset Sepsis

The recombinant forms of some hematopoietic cytokines have been cloned and purified and have been under clinical investigation for their possible role in modulating host defense in the prevention of neonatal sepsis. G-CSF has the ability to increase the number of circulating neutrophils and to augment the effectiveness of neutrophils and macrophages to kill infectious organisms.

Kocherlakota and La Gamma (1998) evaluated the ability of G-CSF to reverse neutropenia and reduce the incidence of early-onset sepsis in VLBW ventilator-dependent infants with preeclampsia-associated neutropenia. They found that the absolute neutrophil count (ANC) increased significantly in the treated infants in comparison with controls. Sepsis was observed in 2 of the 15 treated infants and in 7 of the 13 controls (13% and 54%, respectively; $P < .05$).

## Treatment

### Antimicrobial Therapy

The decision to treat a newborn infant for possible sepsis is based on clinical signs or risk factors with or without confirmatory laboratory data. The choice of antibiotics for an infant with suspected early-onset sepsis depends on the predominant pathogens and the antibiotic sensitivity patterns for the microorganisms causing early-onset sepsis in a given region. The algorithms presented in Figures 39–7, 39–8, and 39–9 are meant to serve as guidelines for the diagnosis and management of infants with suspected sepsis. Decisions to discontinue antimicrobial therapy should be based on the level of suspicion for sepsis at the time treatment was begun, culture results, laboratory test results, and the clinical course of the infant. Therefore, when sepsis is highly suspected, antibiotics should be given for a "full course" even if culture results are negative.

Empiric therapy for early-onset sepsis generally uses combinations of antibiotics effective against gram-positive and gram-negative pathogens. The two most commonly used combinations are ampicillin with an aminoglycoside (frequently gentamicin) and ampicillin with cefotaxime. Cefotaxime, a broad-spectrum third-generation cephalosporin, is used because of its reduced toxicity. However, the third-generation cephalosporins have been associated with rapid development of glycopeptide-resistant enterococci and with the selection of stably derepressed forms of β-lactamase–producing gram-negative bacteria (Bryan et al, 1985). Furthermore, none of the cephalosporins is effective against enterococci or *L. monocytogenes*.

After an organism has been isolated from culture, antibiotic therapy should be tailored according to its demonstrated sensitivities. *L. monocytogenes* is usually treated with ampicillin and an aminoglycoside until the blood culture result is negative. Enterococci are treated either with ampicillin and an aminoglycoside or with vancomycin, depending on sensitivity patterns. GBS can be safely treated with either ampicillin or penicillin. There are no data to suggest that the addition of an aminoglycoside improves morbidity or mortality in infants with bacteremia due to GBS. Most strains of *S. aureus* are resistant to ampicillin and penicillin because they produce β-lactamase. Therefore, infections with *S. aureus* are treated with penicillinase-resistant penicillins or cephalosporins. Methicillin-resistant *S. aureus* is sensitive to vancomycin. Gram-negative enteric organisms are generally sensitive to aminoglycosides. For gram-negative bacteria that are resistant to aminoglycosides, cefotaxime is a suitable alternative. Ceftriaxone is not commonly used because of the potential for displacement of bilirubin from albumin. *Pseudomonas aeruginosa* infections are commonly treated with ticarcillin or carbenicillin and an aminoglycoside, but most are also sensitive to ceftazidime.

Antibiotic therapy should be stopped as soon as the clinician believes the likelihood of infection is very low. Forty-eight hours are generally sufficient to determine that a blood culture result is truly negative. Infants with proven bacteremia (and without meningitis) are treated for 7 to 10 days. Dosing recommendations for commonly used antibiotics are presented in Appendix 1. Infants receiving potentially toxic antibiotics for more than 48 hours should undergo therapeutic drug monitoring.

## Adjunctive Immunologic Therapies for Treatment of Early-Onset Sepsis

In addition to conventional management (antibiotics and supportive care), adjunctive therapies, which attempt to modulate the immune status of the infant, have been investigated to reduce the mortality of neonatal sepsis. They include IVIG, granulocyte transfusions, and hematopoietic cytokines.

### *Intravenous Immune Globulin*

At the time of birth, the neonate has antibodies against any bacterial pathogens that the mother has been exposed to during her lifetime. These antibodies are actively transported across the placenta during the second half of gestation. There is very little endogenous production of antibody by the fetus unless infection occurs during fetal life (e.g., the TORCH [toxoplasmosis, other infections, rubella, cytomegalovirus, herpes simplex virus] infections). Furthermore, preterm birth limits the amount of antibody the fetus receives. The lack of protective levels of antibody against specific pathogens significantly increases the susceptibility to infection and impairs the ability to recover from an infectious episode. For example, the absence of type-specific antibody against the capsular polysaccharide antigen of GBS is a significant risk factor for early-onset GBS sepsis (Baker and Kasper, 1976). For these reasons, the efficacy of administering IVIG as an adjunct treatment for neonatal sepsis has been investigated.

In 1994, Acunas and colleagues (1994) randomly assigned 67 infants with possible sepsis to receive either fresh frozen plasma or IVIG. Before that time, there were anecdotal reports on the benefits of administering fresh frozen plasma to infants with bacterial sepsis (Shigeoka et al, 1978). After 24 hours, these researchers found the plasma concentrations of immunoglobulins and IgG subclasses to be increased only in infants treated with IVIG, confirming the rationale for treatment with immunoglobulin rather than plasma. Sidiropoulos and associates (1986) conducted a randomized study to evaluate the use of IVIG in term and preterm neonates with bacterial sepsis. Study infants either received antibiotics alone or antibiotics plus IVIG for 6 days. There was no difference in overall mortality between the two groups; however, IVIG was found to significantly decrease the mortality in the preterm subgroup.

In 1988, Haque and coworkers investigated the use of an IgM-enriched immunoglobulin preparation. Infants in their study were randomly assigned to receive either antibiotic alone (controls) or antibiotic in combination with intravenous IgM-enriched immunoglobulin. Mortality due to sepsis was 20% in the control group but 3.3% in the group treated with the IgM preparation. In a second trial, the same group randomly assigned 130 term and preterm infants with suspected sepsis to receive a standard IVIG preparation, an IgM-enriched immunoglobulin, or supportive care alone (controls) for 4 days (Haque et al, 1995). Mortality from infection was 6.8% in the group receiving IgM-enriched immunoglobulin, 14.2% in the group given standard IVIG, and 25.5% in the control group. Although the overall mortality from sepsis was lower in the two immunoglobulin-treated groups than the control group, no advantages were demonstrated for administration of IgM-enriched therapy over standard IVIG.

Shenoi and associates (1999) reported a multicenter, placebo-controlled trial in which 58 term and preterm neonates were randomly assigned to receive IVIG or placebo. Although the placebo group contained a significantly greater number of babies with positive blood culture results (principally gram-negative organisms), no difference was found in mortality. Ohlsson and Lacy (2002) analyzed data from 13 randomized clinical trials in which infants with suspected sepsis were treated with supportive care alone or IVIG plus supportive care. Some of the trials were placebo-controlled. Although the mortality was lower with IVIG treatment in six studies (n = 318) of infants in whom sepsis was suspected, there was no such reduction in mortality with IVIG in infants with subsequently proven infection (n = 262). The analysis of the published studies was complicated by differences in design, IVIG preparation and dose, severity of infection, and infecting organisms. Ohlsson and Lacy (2002) concluded that there were insufficient data to support the routine use of IVIG preparations to prevent death in suspected or proven infection in neonates.

Although data indicate that the use of IVIG in newborns appears safe, rare complications may occur. An outbreak of hepatitis C was reported in association with administration of IVIG (Flora et al, 1996), and dose-related immunosuppression with IVIG given at high doses (>2000 mg/kg) was detected in immunocompromised hosts (Cross et al, 1984). In addition, one report observed hemolysis in association with administration of IVIG to a neonate, secondary to an antigen-antibody reaction (Haque et al, 1988).

### Granulocyte Transfusion

The identification of functional and quantitative immaturity in neonatal phagocytic immunity has led investigators to postulate a role for granulocyte transfusions in the treatment of neonatal sepsis. In the early 1980s Laurenti and associates (1981) retrospectively analyzed data for infants who were given granulocyte transfusions as an adjuvant treatment for neonatal sepsis. A significant decrease in mortality (10% versus 72%) was observed, which was greatest in infants weighing less than 1500 g (10% versus 91%). A benefit of granulocyte transfusion was also demonstrated by Christensen and colleagues (1982), who performed a randomized controlled study on a population of neonates with overwhelming sepsis, neutropenia, and bone marrow neutrophil storage pool depletion. Survival was 100% in the seven treated neonates, and only 11% for the nine controls.

Both Baley and coworkers (1987) and Wheeler and associates (1987) evaluated the effects of stored buffy coat transfusion in neutropenic septic neonates. The total number of granulocytes transfused was approximately 50% less than in other studies. Neither of the studies was able to demonstrate effects on survival, and the researchers concluded that the efficacy of buffy coat transfusion remains questionable. Furthermore, in the study by Baley and coworkers, neutrophil storage pool depletion was rare among neutropenic infants.

In two studies published in 1984 and 1987, Cairo and associates demonstrated an increase in survival with granulocyte transfusions in infants with early-onset sepsis. These studies were unique, in that granulocytes were obtained by continuous-flow centrifugation and study patients received a total of five transfusions. In the first study, 23 septic and neutropenic infants (60% with positive blood culture results) were randomly assigned to receive either standard supportive care or granulocyte transfusions. Not one of the infants receiving granulocytes died, but mortality was 60% in the control group (Cairo et al, 1984). In 1992, the same group prospectively studied a population of neutropenic infants with early-onset sepsis in order to compare the effects of IVIG administration and granulocyte transfusion. Term and preterm infants, postnatal ages 3 to 8 days, were randomly selected to receive granulocyte transfusion or intravenous IVIG. Survival rate was 100% in the granulocyte-treated group and 64% in the IVIG-treated group (Cairo et al, 1992). A meta-analysis of 5 clinical studies designed to investigate the efficacy of granulocyte transfusion in treatment of neonatal sepsis concluded that granulocyte transfusion did not provide a statistically significant benefit to neonates with culture-proven infections. (Vamvakas and Pineda, 1996).

### Cytokines

The recombinant forms of some hematopoietic growth factors have been investigated for their possible role in modulating host defense in infants, especially during periods of increased demand, such as overwhelming sepsis complicated by a low neutrophil count. G-CSF has a powerful ability to induce proliferation of neutrophil precursors and to mobilize neutrophils from the bone marrow into the circulation (Lieschke and Burgess, 1992a, 1992b). GM-CSF can prime term and preterm neutrophils for enhanced chemotaxis and respiratory burst responses (Jawson et al, 1994). Studies in newborn rats with induced sepsis have demonstrated that both G-CSF (Cairo et al, 1990) and GM-CSF (Frenck et al, 1990) improve survival.

In a controlled trial, Schibler and colleagues (1998) randomly assigned 20 infants with neutropenia and presumed early-onset sepsis to receive either G-CSF for 3 days or placebo. No significant differences in mortality were observed. Kocherlakota and La Gamma (1997) studied whether recombinant human G-CSF (rhG-CSF) could reverse sepsis-associated neutropenia and improve survival in early- and late-onset sepsis. Administration of rhG-CSF led to higher ANCs than those seen in retrospectively selected, case-matched control patients with sepsis. In the early-onset sepsis group, 3 of the 5 neonates treated with antibiotics and supportive therapy died, but none of the neonates treated with rhG-CSF died. Miura and associates (2001) conducted a similar study in 44 preterm neonates with clinical diagnosis of early-onset sepsis. At 24 and 48 hours after treatment with G-CSF, the ANC significantly increased, but no effect on mortality was observed.

In a prospective controlled trial, 49 neutropenic infants with clinical signs of sepsis were randomly assigned to receive GM-CSF (for 7 consecutive days) or supportive care to determine whether G-CSF could reverse neutropenia and improve survival in early-onset sepsis (Bilgin et al, 2001). By day 7, the ANCs in the treated group were significantly higher than those in the control group. Furthermore, the mortality rate in the GM-CSF–treated group (10%) was significantly lower than in the control group (30%). In a small, randomized, placebo-controlled study of VLBW infants with neutropenia and clinical signs of sepsis, Bedford Russell and colleagues (2001) demonstrated that administration of rhG-CSF increased the ANC and lowered mortality. Bernstein and associates (2001) analyzed data from five randomized clinical trials in which infants with sepsis were treated with supportive care alone or a recombinant hematopoietic growth factor. Their analysis showed that the efficacy of G-CSF was unproven, even though there was a trend toward lower mortality. The lower-birth-weight neonates and neonates with neutropenia appeared most likely to benefit.

## NEONATAL BACTERIAL MENINGITIS*

Neonatal bacterial meningitis remains a dreaded disease because of its mortality and its morbidity (in general terms, 20% and 50%, respectively; see prognosis discussion). As with sepsis, the incidence of purulent meningitis of the newborn infant varies among institutions and is higher in inner city hospitals, where prenatal care for the poor is suboptimal, and in complicated pregnancies and deliveries, especially those resulting in premature births. Incidence rates for neonatal meningitis are approximately one fourth to one tenth those for bacterial sepsis. The same pathogens that cause sepsis cause meningitis, with GBS and *E. coli* strains accounting for approximately 70% of all cases, and *L. monocytogenes* for an additional 5% in the first week of life. The other more common pathogens are *H. influenzae* and pneumococcus. Among infants who are hospitalized for longer than one week in neonatal intensive care units, *S. epidermidis* is the most common isolate. Risk factors for meningitis are identical to those for sepsis because bacteremia, if not actual sepsis, precedes seeding of the meninges with bacteria. Why some infants with sepsis also experience meningitis but most do not is not clear.

GBS meningitis usually manifests after the first several days of life, and the principal organism encountered in these infants is serotype III. The mortality rate is 20% to 40%. Streptococcal disease that occurs in the first 48 hours after delivery commonly manifests as acute respiratory distress with or without shock. Although the organism is frequently isolated from postmortem CSF cultures taken from these infants, histologic evidence of meningeal inflammation may be lacking (Franciosi et al, 1973).

Approximately 80% of all types of *E. coli* that cause meningitis possess the K1 antigen. The O18 and O7 somatic types and H6 and H7 flagellar types are most commonly associated with K1 strains cultured from CSF (Sarff et al, 1975). The presence, concentration, and persistence of this capsular polysaccharide antigen in CSF and blood of infants with meningitis correlate directly with the outcome of the disease (Franco et al, 1992). The concentration and persistence of interleukin-1β and TNF-α, the principal mediators of meningeal inflammation, correlate with an adverse outcome (Dodge, 1994; McCracken et al, 1989; Mustafa et al, 1989; Velasco et al, 1991). The mortality rates for neonatal *E. coli* meningitis vary from 20% to 30% in some centers to 50% to 60% in others. These figures have been relatively constant despite improvements in overall perinatal mortality.

### Pathology

The pathologic findings in neonatal meningitis are similar regardless of the bacterial etiology. The most consistent findings at necropsy of babies who die of meningitis are purulent exudate of the meninges and of the ependymal surfaces of the ventricles associated with vascular inflammation. The inflammatory response of newborns is similar to that observed in adults with meningitis, except that babies have a paucity of plasma cells and lymphocytes during the subacute stage of meningeal reaction. Hydrocephalus and a noninfectious encephalopathy can be demonstrated in approximately 50% of infants who die of meningitis. Subdural effusions occur rarely in newborns; in contrast, this complication of meningitis is common in infants 3 to 12 months old. Varying degrees of phlebitis and arteritis of intracranial vessels can be found in all infants who die of meningitis. Thrombophlebitis with occlusion of veins may occur in the subependymal zones. K1 antigen has been demonstrated in the brain tissue of infants who die of *E. coli* K1 infection.

### Clinical Manifestations

The early signs and symptoms of neonatal meningitis are commonly indistinguishable from those of septicemia. Specific findings, such as stiff neck and Kernig and Brudzinski signs, are commonly absent (85% of the time) but should be sought because of their usefulness if present. Lethargy, feeding problems, and altered temperature are the most common presenting symptoms, and respiratory distress, anorexia, vomiting, apnea, jaundice, diarrhea, and abdominal distention are common findings. A bulging fontanelle may be a late sign of meningitis but can be confused with subgaleal hemorrhage, cephalohematoma, or caput succedaneum. Poor muscle tone (heel-to-head maneuver and vertical sling, for example) is extremely common for infants with either sepsis, meningitis, or both. Seizures are observed frequently and may be caused by direct central nervous system inflammation or may occur in association with hypoglycemia, hyponatremia, or hypocalcemia. Table 39–8 lists the differential diagnoses of infants presenting with the similar signs or symptoms of sepsis or meningitis.

### Diagnosis

Although analysis of the CSF is the gold standard for diagnosis of meningitis, it is imperfect for reasons similar to those previously discussed for blood cultures, and the interpretation of CSF cell counts in newborn infants may be difficult (Polk and Steele, 1988; Unhanand et al, 1993). Table 39–9 summarizes the characteristics of neonatal CSF for newborn infants as reviewed by Klein (2001). During the first week, the white cell count slowly diminishes in full-term infants but may remain high or may even increase in premature babies. Cell counts in the range of 0 to 10 cells/mm$^3$ are observed at 1 month of age. The percentage ratio of CSF glucose level to blood glucose level is 44% to more than 100% in both preterm and term infants. Although the CSF cell counts and protein and sugar concentrations from normal infants can overlap with those from infants with meningitis, less than 1% of babies with proven meningitis have totally normal results on a CSF analysis of a specimen from the initial lumbar puncture (Hristeva et al, 1993). Approximately 50% of all

*This portion of the chapter is revised from that of the prior edition by F. Sessions Cole. It includes contributions from previous authors: Drs. Alexander Schaffer, George H. McCracken, Jr., Jorge B. Howard, and Kenneth McIntosh.

**TABLE 39–8**

**Differential Diagnoses of Clinical Signs Associated with Neonatal Sepsis and Some Noninfectious Conditions**

| Clinical Sign | Differential Diagnoses |
|---|---|
| **Respiratory distress** (apnea, cyanosis, costal and sternal retraction, rales, grunting, diminished breath sounds, tachypnea) | Transient tachypnea of the newborn<br>Respiratory distress syndrome<br>Atelectasis<br>Aspiration pneumonia, including meconium aspiration<br>Pneumothorax<br>Pneumomediastinum<br>Central nervous system disease: hypoxia, hemorrhage<br>Congenital abnormalities, including tracheoesophageal fistula, choanal atresia, diaphragmatic hernia, hypoplastic lungs<br>Congenital heart disease<br>Cardiac arrhythmia<br>Hypothermia (neonatal cold injury)<br>Hypoglycemia<br>Neonatal drug withdrawal syndrome<br>Medication error with inhaled epinephrine |
| **Temperature abnormality** (hyperthermia or hypothermia) | Altered environmental temperature<br>Disturbance of central nervous system thermoregulatory mechanism, including anoxia, hemorrhage, kernicterus<br>Hyperthyroidism or hypothyroidism<br>Neonatal drug withdrawal syndrome<br>Dehydration<br>Congenital adrenal hyperplasia<br>Vaccine reaction |
| **Jaundice** | Breast milk jaundice<br>Blood group incompatibility<br>Red cell hemolysis, including blood group incompatibility, glucose-6-phosphate dehydrogenase (G6PD) deficiency<br>Resorption of blood from closed space hemorrhage<br>Gastrointestinal obstruction, including pyloric stenosis<br>Extrahepatic or intrahepatic biliary tract obstruction<br>Inborn errors of metabolism, including galactosemia, glycogen storage disease type IV, tyrosinemia, disorders of lipid metabolism, peroxisomal disorders, defective bile acid synthesis (trihydroxycoprostanic acidemia)<br>Hereditary diseases, including cystic fibrosis, α-antitrypsin deficiency, bile excretory defects (Dubin-Johnson, Rotor, Byler, Aagenaes syndromes)<br>Hypothyroidism<br>Prolonged parenteral hyperalimentation |
| **Hepatomegaly** | Red cell hemolysis, including blood group incompatibility, G6PD deficiency<br>Infant of a diabetic mother<br>Inborn errors of metabolism, including galactosemia, glycogen storage disease, organic acidemias, urea cycle disorders, hereditary fructose intolerance, peroxisomal disorders<br>Biliary atresia<br>Congestive heart failure<br>Benign liver tumors, including hemangioma, hamartoma<br>Malignant liver tumors, including hepatoblastoma, metastatic neuroblastoma, congenital leukemia |
| **Gastrointestinal abnormalities** (anorexia, regurgitation, vomiting, diarrhea, abdominal distention) | Gastrointestinal allergy<br>Overfeeding, aerophagia<br>Intestinal obstruction (intraluminal or extrinsic)<br>Necrotizing enterocolitis<br>Hypokalemia<br>Hypercalcemia or hypocalcemia<br>Hypoglycemia<br>Inborn errors of metabolism, including galactosemia, urea cycle disorders, organic acidemias<br>Ileus secondary to pneumonia<br>Congenital adrenal hyperplasia<br>Gastric perforation<br>Neonatal drug withdrawal syndrome |

TABLE 39-8

**Differential Diagnoses of Clinical Signs Associated with Neonatal Sepsis and Some Noninfectious Conditions—Cont'd**

| | |
|---|---|
| **Lethargy** | Central nervous system disease; including hemorrhage, hypoxia, or subdural effusion<br>Congenital heart disease<br>Neonatal drug withdrawal syndrome<br>Hypoglycemia<br>Hypercalcemia<br>Familial dysautonomia |
| **Seizure activity** (tremors, hyperactivity, muscular twitching) | Hypoxia<br>Intracranial hemorrhage or kernicterus<br>Congenital central nervous system malformations<br>Neonatal drug withdrawal syndrome<br>Hypoglycemia<br>Hypocalcemia<br>Hyponatremia, hypernatremia<br>Hypomagnesemia<br>Inborn errors of metabolism, including urea cycle disorders, organic acidemias, galactosemia, glycogen storage disease, peroxisomal disorders<br>Pyridoxine deficiency |
| **Petechiae and purpura** | Birth trauma<br>Blood group incompatibility<br>Neonatal isoimmune thrombocytopenia<br>Maternal idiopathic thrombocytopenic purpura<br>Maternal lupus erythematosus<br>Drugs administered to mother<br>Giant hemangioma (Kasabach-Merritt syndrome)<br>Thrombocytopenia with absent radii (TAR) syndrome<br>Disseminated intravascular coagulopathy<br>Coagulation factor deficiencies<br>Congenital leukemia<br>Child abuse |

Data from Klein JO: Bacterial sepsis and meningitis. In Remington JS, Klein JO (eds): Infectious Diseases of the Fetus and Newborn Infant, 5th ed. Philadelphia, WB Saunders, 2001, p. 966.

infants with positive results of CSF cultures for bacteria have negative blood culture results (Shattuck and Chonmaitree, 1992).

Stained smears of CSF must be examined carefully for every infant with suspected meningitis. Grossly clear fluid may contain few white blood cells and many bacteria. The stained smears from approximately 20% of newborns with proven meningitis are interpreted as showing no bacteria. As its name implies, *L. monocytogenes* commonly evokes a mononuclear cellular response in the CSF.

Difficult clinical choices must be made when (1) an infant is judged too unstable to undergo a lumbar puncture, (2) the puncture is traumatic or unproductive of fluid, or (3) the results of the CSF analysis are equivocal. Estimates of traumatic lumbar puncture, "dry tap," and inadequate volume of CSF together are as high as 25% depending on the experience and persistence of those performing the procedure. In my experience, bloody or dry lumbar punctures are minimized, and hypoxemia is reduced, when the infant is placed in the flexed sitting position. For infants receiving ventilator therapy, less extreme hip flexion in the lateral position may minimize stress (Gleason et al, 1983; Weisman et al, 1983). Both preoxygenation through an increase in fractional inspired oxygen ($FiO_2$) and local anesthesia have merit and are standard procedures among caring clinicians and nurses. For an infant who is too unstable to undergo a lumbar puncture or after a "dry tap," the clinician must rely on other features of the clinical picture and choose to treat for meningitis if those warrant it. Blood in the CSF does not necessarily indicate a traumatic puncture (meaning that a blood vessel has been nicked by the needle aiming for CSF). Depending on the ego of the clinician performing the procedure, other causes of blood in the CSF should be sought with more or less rigor.

## Therapy

It is the rare infant with meningitis who is not severely ill, and therefore, newborns with meningitis need multisystem, aggressive management in the setting of an intensive care unit. In addition to antibiotic therapy, these infants frequently require mechanical ventilation, compulsive fluid management to minimize the effects of cerebral edema and, inevitably, of capillary leak and inappropriate secretion of antidiuretic hormone (ADH), seizure control, vasopressor support, and cardiopulmonary monitoring. Selection of

**TABLE 39–9**

**Hematologic and Chemical Characteristics of Cerebrospinal Fluid in Normal Newborns: Results of Selected Studies**

| Newborns | | | | Red Blood Cells (per mm³), Mean (Range) | White Blood Cells (per mm³) | | | Protein (mg/dL), Mean (Range) | Glucose (mg/dL), Mean (Range) |
|---|---|---|---|---|---|---|---|---|---|
| Group | Reference No. | Age (days) | No. of Infants | | No. of Cells, Mean (Range) | No. of Polymorphonuclear Cells, Mean (Range) | No. of Mononuclear Cells, Mean (Range) | | |
| Premature | 1 | 1-3 | 22 | Not given | 2 (0-13) | | | 105 (50-180) | |
| | 2 | 0-7 | 21 | | 9 (4-18) | | | 100 (50-138) | |
| | 3 | 1-7 | 21 | (6-333) | 27 (4-112) | | | 150 (57-292) | |
| | 4 | <7-28* | 28 | | 9 (0-29) | 5 | 4 | 115 (65-150) | 50 (24-63) |
| | 5 | 8-14 | 15 | | 3 (4-44) | | | 128 (50-269) | 83† (66-106) |
| | 6 | 8-19 | 28 | | 20 (3-56) | | | 110 (74-189) | |
| | 7 | 15-28 | 30 | | 9 (1-31) | | | 75 (31-131) | 79‡ (64-106) |
| | 8 | 21-40 | 23 | | 17 (2-70) | | | 86 (55-166) | |
| Term | 9 | 1 | 135 | 9 (0-1070) | 5 (0-90) | 3 (0-70) | 2 (0-20) | 63 (32-240) | 51 (32-78) |
| | 10 | 0-13 | 22 | | 6 (0-15) | | | 67 (52-120) | |
| | 11 | 7 | 20 | 3 (0-48) | 3 (0-9) | 2 (0-5) | 1 (0-4) | 47 (27-65) | 55 (48-62) |
| | 12 | <7-10 | 87 | | 8 (0-32) | 5 | 3 | 90 (20-170) | 81 (44-248) |
| | 13 | 14-27 | 14 | | 5 (2-5) | | | 52 (26-88) | |
| | 14 | 28-55 | 16 | | 2 (1-8) | | | 48 (17-63) | |

*24 of 28 infants younger than 7 days.

†Three cases, 0-14 days.

‡Nine cases, 0-28 days.

Data from Klein JO: Bacterial sepsis and meningitis. In Remington JS, Klein JO: Infectious Diseases of the Fetus and Newborn Infant, 5th ed. Philadelphia, WB Saunders, 2001, p 973.

appropriate antibiotic therapy is based in part on the achievable CSF levels of these drugs in relation to the susceptibility of the organisms that cause the disease. The highest kanamycin and gentamicin concentrations in CSF are approximately 40% of the peak serum levels and are only equal to or slightly greater than the minimal inhibitory concentrations (MICs) for disease-causing coliform bacteria. In contrast, CSF penicillin and ampicillin concentrations may be only 10% of the corresponding peak serum levels, but these values are usually 10- to 100-fold higher than the greatest minimal inhibitory concentrations for group B streptococci and *L. monocytogenes*. The ability to attain CSF antimicrobial activity that is many times greater than is necessary to inhibit the pathogen may explain the rapid sterilization of CSF cultures from infants with gram-positive meningitis.

Delayed sterilization of CSF cultures from newborns with gram-negative meningitis may likewise be due to the low inhibitory and bactericidal CSF concentrations. Therefore, in some infants with coliform meningitis, one should alter the therapeutic regimens by adding a second antibiotic, selecting a different aminoglycoside, using one of the newer cephalosporin derivatives, or changing the route of administration. In addition, dosage and timing should be guided by renal, hepatic, and cardiopulmonary function. When possible, individualizing drug regimens on the basis of regular measurement of serum drug concentrations permits the attainment of therapeutic antibiotic effects and the avoidance of toxicity.

In the United States, ampicillin and either gentamicin or kanamycin are recommended as the initial therapy for neonatal meningitis. An alternative regimen of ampicillin and a cephalosporin (e.g., cefotaxime) can be used, but frequent use of such a regimen may lead to emergence of cephalosporin-resistant gram-negative bacterial isolates. Chloramphenicol, because of its capacity to diffuse readily into the CSF, has been used in neonatal meningitis and, with frequent measurement of blood levels.

It may be prudent to repeat a CSF examination and culture after initiation of therapy, especially if the clinical response is less than satisfactory. If organisms are seen on methylene blue-stained or gram-stained smears of the fluid, modification of the therapeutic regimen should be considered. In general, approximately 3 days are required for an antibiotic regimen to sterilize the CSF in infants with gram-negative meningitis. In infants with gram-positive meningitis, sterilization is usually seen within 36 to 48 hours. Neuroimaging should be considered to exclude parameningeal foci and abscess and to assist in the prognosis.

Some adjunctive therapies have been tried, and others appear promising, but none has widespread use at the present time. Neither intrathecal nor intraventricular administration of antibiotics significantly improves morbidity or mortality in infants with gram-negative meningitis. Although dexamethasone is clearly useful in experimental models of meningitis (Kim et al, 1995), it has not been proved useful in clinical trials for newborn infants (Daoud et al, 1999). New therapies that relate to inducible nitric oxide synthase or endothelin inhibition are being explored. These strategies aim at maintenance of adequate blood flow during inflammation and, thereby, minimization of ischemic injury, which is of major importance in the disease process (Leib et al, 1998; Pfister et al, 2000).

Once the pathogen has been identified and the susceptibility study results are available, the single drug or combination of drugs that is most effective should be used. In general, penicillin or ampicillin is preferred for GBS infection; ampicillin with or without kanamycin or gentamicin for infection with *L. monocytogenes* and *Enterococcus*; ampicillin plus gentamicin or kanamycin for infection with coliform bacteria; and carbenicillin plus gentamicin for *Pseudomonas* infections. There is no precise method for determining the duration of antimicrobial therapy. A useful guide is to continue therapy for approximately 2 weeks after sterilization of CSF cultures or for a minimum of 2 weeks for gram-positive meningitis and 3 weeks for gram-negative meningitis, whichever is longer.

## Prognosis

The mortality rate in neonatal meningitis is high. The overall mortality rate remains approximately 20% to 50%, depending on the pathogen, the time of onset of disease, the degree of maturity of the patient, and the timing and adequacy of treatment. Short-term and long-term sequelae of neonatal meningitis occur frequently (Dodge, 1994; Edwards et al, 1985; Franco et al, 1992; Unhanand et al, 1993). The complications include brain abscess, communicating or noncommunicating hydrocephalus, subdural effusions, ventriculitis, deafness, and blindness. The extent of damage in survivors is in general related to the severity of the disease that is evident in the neonatal period. The spectrum of outcomes is not dissimilar from those for infants with moderate to severe asphyxia, in part because of the central nervous system ischemia related to the meningitis. Like infants with moderate asphyxia, the infant who has experienced meningitis may appear relatively normal at the time of discharge, and only after prolonged and careful follow-up do perceptual difficulties, reading problems, or signs of minimal brain damage become apparent. Approximately 40% to 50% of survivors have some evidence of neurologic damage, with severe damage obvious in 11%. Infants who survive neonatal meningitis should have regular audiology, language, and neurologic evaluations until they enter school (Edwards et al, 1985; Stevens et al, 2003).

## REFERENCES

1993 sexually transmitted diseases treatment guidelines. Centers for Disease Control and Prevention. MMWR Recomm Rep 42(RR14):1-102, 1993.

Ablow RC: Comparison of early onset group B streptococcal infections and the respiratory distress syndrome of the newborn. N Engl J Med 294:96-107, 1976.

Acunas BA, Peakman M, Liossis G, et al: Effect of fresh frozen plasma and gammaglobulin on humoral immunity in neonatal sepsis. Arch Dis Child 70:F182-F187, 1994.

Adler SM, Denton RL: The erythrocyte sedimentation rate in the newborn period. J Pediatr 86:942-948, 1975.

Adoption of hospital policies for prevention of perinatal group B streptococcal disease—United States, 1977. MMWR Morb Mortal Wkly Rep 47:665-670, 1998.

Allen UD, Navas L, King SM: Effectiveness of intrapartum penicillin prophylaxis in preventing early-onset group B streptococcal infection: Results of a metaanalysis. Can Med Assoc J 149:1659-1665, 1993.

American Academy of Pediatrics Committee on Infectious Diseases and Committee on Fetus and Newborn: Guidelines for prevention of group B streptococcal (GBS) infection by chemoprophylaxis. Pediatrics 90:775-778, 1992.

American Academy of Pediatrics: 2003 Red Book: Report of the Committee on Infectious Diseases, 26th ed. Elk Grove Village, IL: American Academy of Pediatrics.

American College of Obstetricians and Gynecologists: Group B Streptococcal Infections in Pregnancy. (ACOG Technical Bulletin No. 170.) Washington, DC, American College of Obstetricians and Gynecologists, 1992.

Ancona RJ, Ferrieri P, Williams PP: Maternal factors that enhance the acquisition of group B streptococci by newborn infants. J Med Microbiol 13:273-280, 1980.

Anthony BF, Okada DM, Hobel C: Epidemiology of group B *Streptococcus*: Longitudinal observations during pregnancy. J Infect Dis 137:542-530, 1978.

Anthony BF, Eisenstadt R, Carter J, et al: Genital and intestinal carriage of group B streptococci during pregnancy. J Infect Dis 143:761-766, 1981.

Badri MS, Zawaneh S, Cruz AC, et al: Rectal colonization with group B streptococci: Relation to vaginal colonization of pregnant women. J Infect Dis 135:301-312, 1977.

Baker CJ, Barrett FF: Transmission of group B streptococci among parturient women and their neonates. J Pediatr 83:919-923, 1973.

Baker CJ, Edwards MS: Group B streptococcal infections. In Remington JS, Klein JO (eds): Infectious Diseases of the Fetus and Newborn Infant, 4th ed. Philadelphia, WB Saunders. 1995, pp 980-1054.

Baker CJ, Kasper DL: Correlation of maternal antibody with susceptibility to neonatal group B streptococcal infection. N Engl J Med 294:753-756, 1976.

Baker CJ, Goroff DK Alpert, SL, et al: Comparison of bacteriological methods for the isolation of group B streptococcus from vaginal cultures. J Clin Microbiol 4:40-48, 1976.

Baley JE, Stork EK, Warkentin PI, et al: Buffy coat transfusions in neutropenic neonates with presumed sepsis: A prospective, randomized trial. Pediatrics 80:712-720, 1987.

Baltimore RS, Huie SM, Meek JI, et al: Early-onset neonatal sepsis in the era of group B streptococcal prevention. Pediatrics 108:1094-1098, 2001.

Barton L, Hodgman JE, Pavlova Z: Causes of death in the extremely low birth weight infant. Pediatrics 103:446-451, 1999.

Bedford-Russell AR, Emmerson AJB, Wilkinson N, et al: A trial of recombinant human granulocyte colony stimulating factor for the treatment of very low birth weight infants with presumed sepsis and neutropenia. Arch Dis Child Fetal Neonatal Ed 84:F172-F176, 2001.

Benitz WE, Han MY, Madan A, Ramachandra P: Serial serum C-reactive protein levels in the diagnosis of neonatal infection. Pediatrics 102:1-10, 1998.

Bernstein HM, Pollok BH, Calhoun DA, et al: Administration of recombinant granulocyte colony-stimulating factor to neonates with septicemia: A meta-analysis. J Pediatr 138:917-920, 2001.

Bilgin K, Yaramis A, Haspolat K, et al: A randomized trial of granulocyte-macrophage colony-stimulating factor in neonates with sepsis and neutropenia. Pediatrics 107:36-41, 2001.

Bobitt JR, Ledger WJ: Obstetric observations in eleven cases of neonatal sepsis due to group B hemolytic streptococcus. Obstet Gynecol 47:439-445, 1976.

Bobitt JR, Damato JD, Sakakini J: Perinatal complications in streptococcal carriers: A longitudinal study of pregnant patients. Am J Obstet Gynecol 151:711-717, 1985.

Bomela HN, Ballot DE, Cory BJ, Cooper PA: Use of C-reactive protein to guide duration of empiric antibiotic therapy in suspected early neonatal sepsis. Pediatr Infect Dis J 19:531-535, 2000.

Boyer KM, Gotoff SP: Prevention of early-onset neonatal group B streptococcal disease. N Engl J Med 314:1665-1669, 1986.

Boyer KM, Gadzala CA, Burd LI, et al: Selective intrapartum chemoprophylaxis of neonatal group B streptococcal early-onset disease. I: Epidemiologic rationale. J Infect Dis 148:795-801, 1983a.

Boyer KM, Gadzala CA, Kelly PD, et al: Selective intrapartum chemoprophylaxis of neonatal group B streptococcal early onset disease. II: Predictive value of prenatal cultures. J Infect Dis 148:802-809, 1983b.

Bryan CS, John JF, Pai MS, et al: Gentamicin vs. cefotaxime for therapy of neonatal sepsis. Am J Dis Child 139:1086-1089, 1985.

Cairo MS, Rucker R, Bennetts GA, et al: Improved survival of newborns receiving leukocyte transfusions for sepsis. Pediatrics 74:887-892, 1984.

Cairo MS, Worcester C, Rucker R, et al: Role of circulating complement and polymorphonuclear leukocyte transfusion in treatment and outcome in critically ill neonates with sepsis. J Pediatr 110:935-941, 1987.

Cairo MS, Plunkett JM, Mauss D, et al: Seven-day administration of recombinant human granulocyte colony-stimulating factor to newborn rats: Modulation of neonatal neutrophilia, myelopoiesis and group B streptococcus sepsis. Blood 76:1788-1794, 1990.

Cairo MS, Worcester C, Rucker R, et al: Randomized trial of granulocyte transfusion versus intravenous immune globulin therapy for neonatal neutropenia and sepsis. J Pediatr 120:281-285, 1992.

Campbell GA: Septicaemia in children. Can Med Assoc J 24:674-675, 1931.

Carey C, Klebanoff MA, Hauth JC, et al: Metronidazole to prevent preterm delivery in pregnant women with asymptomatic bacterial vaginosis. N Engl J Med 342:534-540, 2000.

Cassell GH, Davis RO, Waites KB, et al: Isolation of *Mycoplasma hominis* and *Ureaplasma urealyticum* from amniotic fluid at 16-20 weeks of gestation: Potential effect on outcome of pregnancy. Sex Transm Dis 10:294-302, 1983.

Chandran L, Navaie-Waliser M, Zulqarni NJ, et al: Compliance with group B streptococcal disease prevention guidelines. MCN Am J Matern Child Nurs 26:313-319, 2001.

Chen KT, Tuomala RE, Cohen AP, et al: No increase in rates of early-onset neonatal sepsis by non-group B streptococcus or Ampicillin-resistant organisms. Am J Obstet Gynecol 4:854-858, 2001.

Chirico G, Rondini G, Plebani A, et al: Intravenous gammaglobulin therapy for prophylaxis of infection in high-risk neonates. J Pediatr 110:437-442, 1987.

Christensen RD, Rothstein G: Pitfalls in the interpretation of leukocyte counts of newborn infants. Am J Clin Pathol 72:608-611, 1979.

Christensen RD, Rothstein G, Anstall HB, et al: Granulocyte transfusions in neonates with bacterial infection, neutropenia and depletion of mature marrow neutrophils. Pediatrics 70:1-6, 1982.

Conway SP, Ng PC, Howel D, et al: Prophylactic intravenous immunoglobulin in pre-term infants: A controlled trial. Vox Sang 59:6-11, 1990.

Cowett RM, Peter G, Hakanson DO, et al: Reliability of bacterial culture of blood obtained from an umbilical artery catheter. J Pediatr 88:1035-1036, 1976.

Cross AS, Alving BM, Sadoff JC, et al: Intravenous immunoglobulin: A cautionary note [letter]. Lancet 1(8382):912, 1984.

Daoud AS, Baticha A, Al-Sheyyab M, et al: Lack of effectiveness of dexamethasone in neonatal bacterial meningitis. Eur J Pediatr 158:230-233, 1999.

Davis JP, Gutman LT, Higgins MV, et al: Nasal colonization with group B streptococcus associated with intrauterine pressure transducers. J Infect Dis 138:804-810, 1978.

Davis JP, Moggio MV, Klein D, et al: Vertical transmission of group B streptococcus: Relation to intrauterine fetal monitoring. JAMA 343:42-44, 1979.

Decreasing incidence of perinatal group B streptococcal disease—United States, 1993-1995. MMWR Morb Mortal Wkly Rep 46:473-477, 1997.

Dietzman DE, Fischer GW, Schoenknecht FD: Neonatal *Escherichia coli* septicemia: Bacterial counts in blood. J Pediatr 85:128-30, 1974.

DiGeronimo RJ: Lack of efficacy of the urine culture as part of the initial workup of suspected neonatal sepsis. Pediatr Infect Dis 11:764-766, 1992.

Dodge PR: Neurological sequelae of acute bacterial meningitis. Pediatr Ann 23:101, 1994.

Doellner H, Arntzen KJ, Haereid PE, et al: Interleukin-6 concentrations in neonates evaluated for sepsis. J Pediatr 132:295-299, 1998.

Dunham EC: Septicemia in newborn. Am J Dis Child 45:229-253, 1933.

Edwards MS, Rench MA, Haffar AAM, et al: Long-term sequelae of group B streptococcal meningitis in infants. J Pediatr 106:717-722, 1985.

Ehl S, Gering B, Bartmann P, et al: C-reactive protein is a useful marker for guiding duration of antibiotic therapy in suspected neonatal bacterial infection. Pediatrics 99:216-221, 1997.

Eickhoff TC, Klein JO, Daly AK, et al: Neonatal sepsis and other infections due to group B beta hemolytic streptococci. N Engl J Med 27:1221-1228, 1964.

Eliott JA, Farmer KD, Facklam RR: Sudden increase in isolation of group B streptococci serotype V is not due to emergence of a new pulsed field gel electrophoresis type. J Clin Microbiol 36:2115-2116, 1998.

Escobar GJ, Li DK, Armstrong MA, et al: Neonatal sepsis workups in infants ≥2000 grams at birth: A population-based study. Pediatrics 106:256-263, 2000.

Evans ME, Schaffner W, Federspiel CF, et al: Sensitivity, specificity, and predictive value of body surface cultures in a neonatal intensive care unit. JAMA 259:248-252, 1988.

Fleming DW, Cochi SL, MacDonald KL, et al.: Pasteurized milk as a vehicle of infection in an outbreak of listeriosis. N Engl J Med 312:404-407, 1985

Flora K, Schiele M, Benner K, et al: An outbreak of acute hepatitis C among recipients of intravenous immunoglobulin. Ann Allergy Asthma Immunol 76:160-162, 1996.

Franciosi RA, Knostman JD, Zimmerman RA: Group B streptococcal neonatal and infant infections. J Pediatr 83:707, 1973.

Franco SM, Cornelius VE, Andrews BF: Long-term outcome of neonatal meningitis. Am J Dis Child 146:567, 1992.

Frenck RW, Sarman G, Harper TE, et al: The ability of recombinant murine granulocyte-macrophage colony stimulating factor to protect neonatal rats from septic death due to *Staphylococcus aureus*. J Infect Dis 162:109-114, 1990.

Fry RM: Fatal infections by haemolytic streptococcus group B. Lancet 1:199-201, 1938.

Gabay C, Kushner I: Acute-phase proteins and other systemic responses to inflammation. N Engl J Med 340:448-454, 1999.

Garcia-Prats JA, Cooper RR, Schneider VF, et al: Rapid detection of microorganisms in blood cultures of newborn infants utilizing an automated blood culture system. Pediatrics 105:523-527, 2000.

Gerdes JS: Clinicopathologic approach to the diagnosis of neonatal sepsis. Isr J Med Sci 30:430-441, 1994.

Gerdes JS, Polin RA: Sepsis screen in neonates with evaluation of plasma fibronectin. Pediatr Infect Dis J 6:443-446, 1987.

Gibbs RS, Castillo MS, Rodgers PJ: Management of acute chorioamnionitis. Am J Obstet Gynecol 136:709-713, 1980.

Gleason CA, Martin FJ, Anderson JV, et al: Optimal position for a spinal tap in preterm infants. Pediatrics 71:31-35, 1983.

Gluck L, Wood HF, Fousek MD: Septicemia of the newborn. Pediatr Clin North Am 13:1131-1148, 1966.

Goetzl L, Cohen A, Frigoletto F, et al: Maternal epidural use and neonatal sepsis evaluation in afebrile mothers. Pediatrics 108:1099-1102, 2001.

Goldenberg RL, Hauth JC, Andrews WW: Intrauterine infection and preterm delivery. N Engl J Med.342:1500-1507, 2000.

Gray BM, Pass MA, Dillon HC: Laboratory and field evaluation of selective media for isolation of group B streptococci. J Clin Microbiol 9:466-470, 1979.

Grether JK, Nelson KB: Maternal infection and cerebral palsy in infants of normal birth weight. JAMA 278:207-211, 1997.

Haque KN, Zaidi MH, Haque SK, et al: Intravenous immunoglobulin for prevention of sepsis in preterm and low birth weight infants. Pediatr Infect Dis 5:622-625, 1986.

Haque KN, Zaidi MH, Bahakim H: IgM-enriched intravenous immunoglobulin therapy in neonatal sepsis. Am J Dis Child 142:1293-1296, 1988.

Haque KN, Remo C, Bahakim H: Comparison of two types of intravenous immunoglobulin in the treatment of neonatal sepsis. Clin Exp Immunol 101:328-333, 1995.

Hillier SL, Martius J, Krohn M, et al: A case-control study of chorioamnionic infection and histologic chorioamnionitis in prematurity. N Engl J Med 319:972-978, 1988.

Hristeva L, Bowler I, Booy R, et al: Value of cerebrospinal fluid examination in the diagnosis of meningitis in the newborn. Arch Dis Child 69:514-517, 1993.

Isaacs D, Royle JA: Intrapartum antibiotics and early onset neonatal sepsis caused by group B streptococcus and by other organisms in Australia. Australasian Study Group for Neonatal Infections. Pediatr Infect Dis J 6:524-528, 1999.

Isaacs D, Barfield C, Clothier T, et al: Late onset infections in neonatal units. J Paediatr Child Health 32:158-161, 1996.

Jaswon MS, Jones MH, Linch DC: The effects of recombinant human granulocyte-macrophage colony-stimulating factor on the neutrophil respiratory burst in the term and preterm infant when studied in whole blood. Pediatr Res 36:623-627, 1994.

Jaye DL, Waites KB: Clinical applications of C-reactive protein in pediatrics. Pediatr Infect Dis J 16:735-747, 1997.

Kalstone C: Successful antepartum treatment of listeriosis. Am J Obstet Gynecol 164:57-58, 1991.

Kenyon SL, Taylor DJ, Tarnow-Mordi W: Broad-spectrum antibiotics for preterm, prelabour rupture of fetal membranes: The ORACLE I randomised trial. Oracle Collaborative Group. Lancet 357:979-988, 2001a.

Kenyon SL, Taylor DJ, Tarnow-Mordi W: Broad-spectrum antibiotics for spontaneous preterm labour: The ORACLE II randomised trial. Oracle Collaborative Group. Lancet 357:989-994, 2001b.

Kim YS, Sheldon RA, Elliott BR, et al: Brain injury in experimental neonatal meningitis due to group B streptococci. J Neuropathol Exp Neurol 55:531-539, 1995.

Klein JO: Bacterial sepsis and meningitis In Remington JS, Klein JO (eds): Infectious Diseases of the Fetus and Newborn Infant, 5th ed. Philadelphia, WB Saunders. 2001, pp 943-998.

Kocherlakota P, La Gamma E: Human granulocyte colony-stimulating factor may improve outcome attributable to neonatal sepsis complicated by neutropenia. Pediatrics 100:1-6, 1997.

Kocherlakota P, La Gamma E: Preliminary report: rhG-CSF may reduce the incidence of neonatal sepsis in prolonged preeclampsia-associated neutropenia. Pediatrics 102:1107-1111, 1998.

Krohn MA, Hillier SL, Nugent RP, et al: The genital flora of women with intraamniotic infection. J Infect Dis 171:1474-1480, 1995.

Kumar Y, Qunibi M, Neal TJ, Yoxall CW: Time to positivity of neonatal blood cultures. Arch Dis Child Fetal Neonatal Ed 85: F182-F186, 2001.

Lachenauer CS, Kasper DI, Shimoda, J, et al: Serotypes VI and VIII predominate among group B streptococci isolated from pregnant Japanese women. J Infect Dis 1791030-1033, 1999.

Lancefield RC: Serological differentiation of human and other groups of hemolytic streptococci. J Exp Med 57:571-595, 1933.

Laurenti F, Ferro R, Isacchi G, et al: Polymorphonuclear leukocyte transfusion for the treatment of sepsis in the newborn infant. J Pediatr 98:118-123, 1981.

Lee K, Shin JW, Chang Y, et al: Trend in serotypes and antimicrobial susceptibility of group B streptococci isolated in Korea. J Infect Chemother 6:93-97, 2000.

Leib SL, Kim YS, Black SM, et al: Inducible nitric oxide synthase and the effect of aminoguanidine in experimental neonatal meningitis. J Infect Dis 177:692-700, 1998.

Leibovich M, Gale R, Slater PE: Usefulness of the gastric aspirate examination in the diagnosis of neonatal infection. Trop Geogr Med 39:15-17, 1987.

Lieberman E, Lang JM, Frigoletto F, et al: Epidural analgesia, intrapartum fever, and neonatal sepsis evaluation. Pediatrics 99:415-419, 1997.

Lieschke GJ, Burgess AW: Granulocyte colony stimulating factor and granulocyte macrophage colony stimulating factor (first of two parts): Review. N Engl J Med 327:28-35, 1992a.

Lieschke GJ, Burgess AW: Granulocyte colony stimulating factor and granulocyte macrophage colony stimulating factor (second of two parts): Review. N Engl J Med 327:99-106, 1992b.

Lin YF, Clemens JD, Azimi PH, et al: Capsular polysaccharide types of group B streptococcal isolates from neonates with early-onset systemic infection. J Infect Dis 177:790-792, 1998.

Locksmith G, Duff P: Infection, antibiotics and preterm delivery. Semin Perinatol 25:295-309, 2001.

Manroe BL, Weinberg AG, Rosenfeld CR, Browne R: The neonatal blood count in health and disease. I: Reference values for neutrophilic cells. Pediatrics 95:89-98, 1979.

McCracken GH, Mustafa MM, Ramilo O, et al: Cerebrospinal fluid interleukin 1-β and tumor necrosis factor concentrations and outcome from neonatal gram-negative enteric bacillary meningitis. Pediatr Infect Dis J 8:155-159, 1989.

Mehr S, Doyle LW: Cytokines as markers of bacterial sepsis in newborn infants: A review. Pediatr Infect Dis J 19:879-887, 2000.

Mercer BM, Miodovnik M, Thurnau GR, et al: Antibiotic therapy for reduction of infant morbidity after preterm premature rupture of the membranes: A randomized controlled trial. National Institute of Child Health and Human Development Maternal-Fetal Medicine Units Network. JAMA 278:989-955, 1997.

Mims LC, Medawar MS, Perkins JR, Grubb WR: Predicting neonatal infections by evaluation of the gastric aspirate: A study in two hundred and seven patients. Am J Obstet Gynecol 114:232-238, 1972.

Miura E, Procianoy RS, Bittar C, et al: A randomized, double-masked, placebo-controlled trial of recombinant granulocyte colony-stimulating factor administration to preterm infants with the clinical diagnosis of early-onset sepsis. Pediatrics 107:30-35, 2001.

Mouzinho A, Rosenfeld CR, Sanchez PJ, Risser R: Revised reference ranges for circulating neutrophils in very-low-birth-weight neonates. Pediatrics 94:76-82, 1994.

Mulder CJJ, van Alphen L, Zanen HC: Neonatal meningitis caused by *Escherichia coli* in the Netherlands. J Infect Dis 150:935-940, 1984.

Mustafa MM, Mertsola J, Ramko O, et al: Increased endotoxin and interleukin-1beta concentrations in cerebrospinal fluid of infants with coliform meningitis and ventriculitis associated with intraventricular gentamicin therapy. J Infect Dis 160:891-895, 1989.

Neal PR, Kleiman MB, Reynolds JK, et al: Volume of blood submitted for culture from neonates. J Clin Microbiol 24:353-356, 1986.

Newton ER, Prihoda TJ, Gibbs RS: Logistic regression analysis of risk factors for intra-amniotic infection. Obstet Gynecol 73:571-575, 1989.

Niswander KR, Gordon M: The women and their pregnancies. The Collaborative Perinatal Study of the National Institute of Neurological Diseases and Stroke. (U.S. Department of Health, Education and Welfare Publication No. [NIH] 73-379.) Washington, DC, USDHEW, 1972.

Ohlsson A, Lacy JB: Intravenous immunoglobulin for suspected or subsequently proven infection in neonates (Cochrane Review). Cochrane Library, Issue 1, 2002.

Oshiro BT, Monga M, Blanco D: Intra-amniotic Infections. Semin Perinatal 517:420-425, 1993.

Pankuch GA, Applebaum PC, Lorenz RP, et al. Placental microbiology and histology and the pathogenesis of chorioamnionitis. Obstet Gynecol 64:802-806, 1984.

Peter G, Nelson JS: Factors affecting neonatal *E. coli* K1 rectal colonization. J Pediatr 93:866-869 1978.

Pfister LA, Tureen JH, Shaw S, et al: Endothelin inhibition improves cerebral blood flow and is neuroprotective in pneumococcal meningitis. Ann Neurol 2000 47:329-335, 2000.

Philip AG, Hewitt JR: Early diagnosis of neonatal sepsis. Pediatrics 65:1036-1041, 1980.

Philip AG, Mills PC: Use of C-reactive protein in minimizing antibiotic exposure: experience with infants initially admitted to a well-baby nursery. Pediatrics 106:E4-E9, 2000.

Polin JI, Knox I, Baumgart S, et al: Use of umbilical cord blood cultures for detection of neonatal bacteremia. Obstet Gynecol 57:233-237, 1981.

Polk DB, Steele RW: Bacterial meningitis progressing with normal cerebrospinal fluid. Pediatr Infect Dis J 6:1040-1042, 1987.

Prevention of perinatal group B streptococcal disease: A public health perspective. Centers for Disease Control and Prevention. MMWR Morb Mortal Wkly Rep 45:1-24, 1996.

Regan JA, Chao S, James LS: Preterm delivery, premature rupture of membranes and maternal colonization with group B streptococci. Am J Obstet Gynecol 141:184-186, 1981.

Regan JA, Ruf C, Greenberg EM, et al: Increased risk of colonization with group B streptococci (GBS) among Hispanic Americans in New York City. Pediatr Res 21:402A-419A, 1987a.

Regan JA, Greenberg EM, Swamback S, et al: Is the primary site of group B streptococcal (GBS) colonization really the GI tract? Presented to ICAAC Proceedings, NYC, 1987b.

Regan JA, Klebanoff MA, Nugent RP: The epidemiology of group B streptococcal colonization in pregnancy. Obstet Gynecol 77:604-610, 1991.

Rench MA, Baker CJ: Neonatal sepsis caused by a new group B streptococcal serotype. J Pediatr 122:638-640, 1993.

Rodwell RL, Leslie AL, Tudehope DI: Early diagnosis of neonatal sepsis using a hematologic scoring system. J Pediatr 112:761-767, 1988.

Rodwell RL, Taylor K, Tudehope DI, Gray PH: Hematologic scoring system in early diagnosis of sepsis in neutropenic newborns. Pediatr Infect Dis J 12:372-376, 1993.

Romero R, Athayde N, Maymon E, et al: Premature rupture of the membranes. In Reece A, Hobbins J (eds): Medicine of the Fetus and Mother. Philadelphia, Lippincott-Raven, 1999, pp 1581-1625.

Rozycki HJ, Stahl GE, Baumgart S: Impaired sensitivity of a single early leukocyte count in screening for neonatal sepsis. Pediatr Infect Dis J 6:440-442, 1987.

Sáez-Llorens X, Lagrutta FS: The acute phase host reaction during bacterial infection and its clinical impact in children. Pediatr Infect Dis J 12:83-87, 1993.

San Giovanni T, Regan JA, Greenberg EM, et al: Selective media is not optimal for isolation of group B streptococci from surface cultures of newborns. Presented, ICAAC Proceedings, NYC, 1987.

Sandberg K, Fasth A, Berger A, et al: Preterm infants with low immunoglobulin G levels have increased risk of neonatal sepsis but do not benefit from prophylactic immunoglobulin G. J Pediatr 137:623-628, 2000.

Sarff LD, McCracken GH, Schiffer MS, et al: Epidemiology of *Escherichia coli* K1 in healthy and diseased newborns. Lancet 1(7916):1099-1104, 1975.

Scanlon J: Early recognition of neonatal sepsis. Clin Pediatr 11:258-260, 1972.

Schelonka RL, Chai MK, Yoder BA, et al: Volume of blood required to detect common neonatal pathogens. Pediatrics 129:275-278, 1996.

Schelonka RL, Yoder BA, desJardins SE, et al: Peripheral leukocyte count and leukocyte indexes in healthy newborn term infants. J Pediatr 125:603-606, 1994.

Schelonka RL, Yoder BA, Hall RB, et al: Differentiation of segmented and band neutrophils during the early newborn period. J Pediatr 127:298-300, 1995.

Schibler KR, Osborne KA, Leung LY, et al: A randomized, placebo-controlled trial of granulocyte colony-stimulating factor administration to newborn infants with neutropenia and clinical signs of early-onset sepsis. Pediatrics 102:6-13, 1998.

Schlech WF, Lavigne PM, Bortolussi R, et al. Epidemic listeriosis: Evidence for transmission by food. N Engl J Med 308:203-206, 1983.

Schlech WF: Listeriosis: Epidemiology, virulence and the significance of contaminated foodstuffs. J Hosp Infect 19:211-224, 1991.

Schrag SJ, Zywicki S, Farley MM, et al: Group B streptococcal disease in the era of intrapartum antibiotic prophylaxis. N Engl J Med 322:1367-1368, 2000.

Schrag S, Gorwitz R, Fultz-Butts K, Schuchat A: Prevention of perinatal group B streptococcal disease: Revised guidelines from CDC. MMWR Recomm Rep 51(RR-11):1-22, 2002.

Schuchat A: Group B streptococcal disease: From trial and tribulations to triumph and trepidation. Clin Infect Dis 133:751-756, 2001.

Schuchat A, Oxtoby M, Cochi S, et al: Population-based risk factors for neonatal group B streptococcal disease: Results of a cohort study in metropolitan Atlanta. J Infect Dis 162:672-677, 1990.

Schuchat A, Deaver-Robinson K, Plikaytis BD, et al: Multistate case-control study of maternal risk factors for neonatal group B streptococcal disease. Pediatr Infect Dis J 13:623-629, 1994.

Schuchat A, Zywicki SS, Dinsmoor MJ, et al: Risk factors and opportunities for prevention of early-onset neonatal sepsis: A multicenter case-control study. Pediatrics 105:21-26, 2000.

Shattuck KE, Chonmaitree T: The changing spectrum of neonatal meningitis over a fifteen-year period. Clin Pediatr 31:130, 1992.

Shenoi A, Nagesh NK, Maiya PP: Multicenter randomized placebo controlled trial of therapy with intravenous immunoglobulin in decreasing mortality due to sepsis. Indian Pediatr 36:1113-1118, 1999.

Shenoy S, Antony G, Shenoy UV: Value of superficial cultures in diagnosing neonatal sepsis. Indian J Pediatr 67:337-338, 2000.

Sherman MP, Goetzman BW, Ahlfors CE, Wennberg RP: Tracheal aspiration and its clinical correlates in the diagnosis of congenital pneumonia. Pediatrics 65:258-263, 1980,

Shigeoka AO, Hall RT, Hill HR: Blood-transfusion in group-B streptococcal sepsis. Lancet 1(9605):636-638, 1978.

Sidiropoulos D, Boehme U, von Muralt G, et al: Immunoglobulin supplementation in prevention or treatment of neonatal sepsis. Pediatr Infect Dis J 5(Suppl):S193-S194, 1986.

Silverman WA, Homan WE: Sepsis of obscure origin in the newborn. Pediatrics 3:157-176, 1949.

Soper DE, Mayhall CG, Dalton HP: Risk factors for intraamniotic infections: A prospective epidemiologic study. Am J Obstet Gynecol 161:562-566, 1989.

Squire EN, Reick HM, Merenstein GB, et al: Criteria for the discontinuation of antibiotic therapy during presumptive treatment of suspected neonatal infection. Pediatr Infect Dis 1:85-90, 1982.

Stevens JP, Eames M, Kent A, et al: Long term outcome of neonatal meningitis. Arch Dis Child Fetal Neonatal Ed. 88:F179-F184, 2003.

Stewardson-Krieger PB, Gotoff SP: Risk factors in early onset neonatal group B streptococcal colonization and disease. Infection 6:50-53, 1978.

Stoll BJ, Holman RC, Schuchat A: Decline in sepsis-associated neonatal and infant deaths in the United States, 1979 through 1994. Pediatrics 102:E18-E24, 1998.

Stoll BJ, Hansen N, Fanaroff AA, et al: Changes in pathogens causing early-onset sepsis in very-low-birth-weight infants. N Engl J Med 347:240-247, 2002.

Storm W: Transient bacteremia following endotracheal suctioning in ventilated newborns. Pediatrics 65:487-490, 1980.

Streptococci (GBS) among Hispanic Americans of Caribbean origin. Pediatr Res 21:402A-419A, 1987c.

Tillet WS, Francis T: Serological reactions in pneumonia with a non-protein somatic faction of pneumococcus. J Exp Med 52:561-571, 1930.

Towers CV, Carr MH, Padilla G, et al: Potential consequences of widespread antepartal use of ampicillin. Am J Obstet Gynecol 4:879-883, 1998.

Unhanand M, Mustafa MM, McCracken GH Jr, Nelson JD: Gram-negative enteric bacillary meningitis: A twenty-one–year experience. J Pediatr 122:15-21, 1993.

Vamvakas EC, Pineda AA: Meta-analysis of clinical studies of the efficacy of granulocyte transfusions in the treatment of bacterial sepsis. J Clin Apher 11:1-9, 1996.

Van Marter LJ, Allred EN, Pagano M, et al: Do clinical markers of barotrauma and oxygen toxicity explain interhospital variation in rates of chronic lung disease? Pediatrics 105:1194-1201, 2000.

Vasan U, Lim DM, Greenstein RM, Raye JR: Origin of gastric aspirate polymorphonuclear leukocytes in infants born after prolonged rupture of membranes. Pediatrics 91:69-72, 1977.

Velasco S, Tarlo M, Olsen K, et al: Temperature-dependent modulation of lipopolysaccharide-induced interleukin-1 beta and tumor necrosis factor alpha expression in cultured human astroglial cells by dexamethasone and indomethacin. J Clin Invest 87:1674-1680, 1991.

Visser VE., Hall RT: Urine culture in the evaluation of suspected neonatal sepsis. Pediatrics 94:635-638, 1979.

Washburn TC, Medearis DN, Childs B: Sex differences in susceptibility to infections. Pediatrics 35:57-64, 1965.

Weisman LE, Merenstein GB, Steenbarger JR: The effect of lumbar puncture position in sick neonates. Amer J Dis Child. 137: 1077, 1983.

Wheeler JG, Chauvenet AR, Johnson CA, et al: Buffy coat transfusions in neonates with sepsis and neutrophil storage pool depletion. Pediatrics 79:422-425, 1987.

Wilkinson HW: Analysis of group B streptococcal types associated with disease in human infants and adults. J Clin Microbiol 7:176-179, 1978 .

Yeung CY, Tam ASY: Gastric aspirate findings in neonatal pneumonia. Arch Dis Child 47:735-740, 1972.

Ylppö A: Pathologisch-anatomische Stüdien bei Frügeborenen. Ztschr f Kinderh 20:371, 1919.

CHAPTER 40

# Nosocomial Infections in the Nursery

**Ira Adams-Chapman and Barbara J. Stoll**

Nosocomial infections are a significant cause of morbidity and late mortality among neonates (Stoll et al, 1996). There are numerous risk factors for acquiring a nosocomial infection, but the most important are prematurity, interventions associated with intensive care, and prolonged length of hospital stay. The duration of hospital stay is inversely related to birth weight and gestational age and directly related to comorbidities, such as respiratory disease and nosocomial infection (Mahieu et al, 2001a; Pittet et al, 1994). In addition to the greater financial burden of nosocomial infections, there is growing concern that the deleterious effects of the inflammatory response to infection may adversely affect long-term outcomes, including bronchopulmonary dysplasia and neurodevelopmental impairment (Adams-Chapman and Stoll, 2001; Gonzalez et al, 1996; Jobe and Ikegami, 1998; Leviton et al, 1999; Rojas et al, 1995; Stoll et al, 2003).

The growing numbers of surviving very low-birth-weight (VLBW) infants magnifies the effect of this problem. Clinicians must be aware of and make efforts to minimize exposure of newborns to known risk factors for infection. Continuous surveillance and monitoring of endemic nosocomial infection rates and patterns of responsible pathogens are necessary to establish a reference point in each nursery and facilitate early identification of epidemics. This also provides the framework for the design of intervention strategies to reduce nosocomial infections in the nursery.

## DEFINITIONS

Infections that manifest early in the first week of life are typically related to perinatal risk factors and vertical transmission from the mother. Nosocomial infections are more often related to patient colonization and environmental risk factors. Unfortunately, there is no specific postnatal age that distinguishes maternally transmitted infections from hospital-acquired infections (Baltimore, 1998). Most sources define nosocomial infections as infections occurring after 3 days of age (Baltimore, 1998; Stoll et al, 2002a). The Centers for Disease Control and Prevention (CDC) defines nosocomial infection as any infection that occurs after admission to the neonatal intensive care unit (NICU) and that was not transplacentally acquired (Garner et al, 1988). Other authorities suggest that nosocomial infections be defined as infections occurring more than 5 to 7 days after birth (Baltimore, 1998).

The lack of uniform definitions for nosocomial infections makes surveillance and comparisons between hospitals difficult (Baltimore, 1998; Goldmann, 1989). The CDC has established uniform definitions for nosocomial infections in adult and neonatal patients, but these definitions are not universally accepted (Garner et al, 1988). Criteria for nosocomial infections common in the neonatal population are outlined in Table 40–1 (Garner et al, 1988). These definitions allow for comparisons between centers and serve as a tool to monitor quality improvement after instituting an intervention program. Of note, the diagnoses easiest to define and compare are blood culture–proven blood stream infections and necrotizing enterocolitis (NEC).

The majority of nosocomial infections in the neonatal population are blood stream infections associated with an intravascular device. Criteria for catheter-related blood stream infections (CRBSIs), as defined by the CDC, are (1) isolation of a recognized pathogen from one blood culture specimen or of a skin commensal from two blood culture specimens, (2) one or more clinical signs of infection, such as temperature instability, apnea, and bradycardia, and (3) presence of an intravascular device at the time the culture specimen is collected (Pearson, 1996).

## INCIDENCE

### Well Baby Nursery

Nosocomial infections are uncommon in the well baby nursery. Accurate rates of nosocomial infection in the well baby nursery are difficult to ascertain because there is no systematic reporting or surveillance network for this issue; however, the incidence appears to be exquisitely low. Some researchers estimate rates of less than 1 per 100 patients discharged (Baltimore, 1998). Typical risk factors for acquiring a nosocomial infection, such as an invasive procedure and presence of an intravascular device, are uncommon in the healthy newborn population. Discharge from the hospital within 48 hours of birth and rooming-in practices have helped further decrease the risk of exposure in modern mother-baby units. Early discharge may further limit surveillance efforts, because patients may be discharged home before they become symptomatic from hospital-acquired infections (Goldmann, 1989).

### Neonatal Intensive Care Unit

The majority of neonatal nosocomial infections occurs in term and preterm infants hospitalized in special care nurseries. It is difficult to determine and compare reports of endemic nosocomial infection rates in different NICU populations. Comparison of surveillance data between institutions is limited by differences in patient demographics (e.g., birth weight and gestational age distribution, underlying severity of disease, babies born in the hospital versus those born elswhere), back transport policies, and the use of different definitions for nosocomial infection.

Among a cohort of 6215 VLBW infants (<1500 g) who were monitored by the National Institute of Child Health and Human Development (NICHHD) Neonatal Research Network, 21% of those who survived beyond 3 days of age had at least one episode of late-onset sepsis (Stoll et al,

**TABLE 40–1**

**Definitions of Nosocomial Infections for Patients Younger than 12 Months, from the Centers for Disease Control and Prevention**

| | |
|---|---|
| Nosocomial blood stream infections | 1. Recognized pathogen isolated from blood culture and pathogen is not related to infection at another site.<br>2. Skin commensal isolated from two blood culture specimens on separate occasions or skin contaminant isolated from a patient with an intravascular device and clinical signs of infection (temperature instability, apnea, or bradycardia) and antimicrobial therapy is initiated.<br>3. Clinical sepsis, defined as clinical signs of infection (temperature instability, hypotension, apnea, or bradycardia) without a recognized cause and all of the following:<br>Blood culture specimen not collected or result negative<br>No apparent infection at another site<br>Therapy instituted for sepsis |
| Pneumonia | Chest radiograph with new or progressive infiltrate, cavitation, consolidation or pleural effusion and clinical evidence of increased respiratory secretions, purulent sputum or change in character of sputum<br>Isolation of pathogens from transtracheal aspirate, bronchial washing or biopsy specimen<br>Isolation of virus from secretions<br>Histopathologic evidence of pneumonia |
| Eye/ear/nose/throat infection | Superficial infections involving the eyes, external or middle ear, sinuses, or nares |
| Necrotizing enterocolitis | Two of the following symptoms with no other recognized cause:<br>Vomiting<br>Abdominal distention or pre-feeding residuals and persistent microscopic and gross evidence of blood in the stool<br>Radiographic findings consistent with pneumoperitoneum, pneumatosis intestinalis, or fixed bowel loops |

Modified from Garner JS, Jarvis WR, Emori TG, et al: CDC definitions for nosocomial infections, 1988. J Infect Control 16:128-140, 1988.

2002b). There was significant variability among the participating centers, with rates ranging from 10.6% to 31.7% at individual sites (Stoll et al, 2002b) Moreover, rates were inversely related to birth weight and gestational age, ranging from 43% for infants weighing 401 to 750 g at birth to 7% for infants weighing 1251 to 1500 g at birth. These data are similar to those reported by Brodie and colleagues (2000). In their study, 19% of 1354 infants weighing less than 1500 g at birth had nosocomial infections, and the rates were highest for infants at the lowest birth weights (39%, <750 g; 27%, 750-999 g; 10%, 1000-1499 g). A point prevalence survey conducted by the 29 level II to level IV nurseries participating in the Pediatric Prevention Network revealed a prevalence of 11.4% for nosocomial infection (Sohn, 2001).

Some investigators believe that reporting overall incidence rates may be misleading because of the wide variations in practice and patient populations in different units. Therefore, the National Nosocomial Infections Surveillance (NNIS) system monitors device-associated nosocomial infection rates by using an approach that accounts for variability in device utilization and length of hospital stay (Emori et al, 1991; Gaynes et al, 1996). These data are also stratified by birth weight categories and expressed as incidence density per 100 or 1000 patient-days. These two adjustments modify the relative risk on the basis of the severity of the illness and the duration of exposure to the risk factor. The small number of participating centers with high-risk nurseries confounds interpretation of NNIS data. However, these data are similar to institutional and collaborative epidemiologic data reported elsewhere. Rates of device-associated infections are presented in Table 40–2. These rates remained constant in the 1990s (Gaynes et al, 1996; National, 2000). The adverse effect of low birth

**TABLE 40–2**

**Rate of Device-Associated Nosocomial Infections**

| | Infections/1000 Device Days | | VAP/1000 Vent Days | |
|---|---|---|---|---|
| **Birth Weight (g)** | **Gaynes et al (1999)** | **Stover et al (2001)** | **Gaynes et al (1996)** | **Stover et al (2001)** |
| <1000 | 11.4 | 12.8 | 4.8 | 3.5 |
| 1001-1500 | 6.9 | 8.9 | 3.6 | 4.9 |
| 1501-2500 | 4.0 | 4.7 | 2.9 | 1.1 |
| >2500 | 3.8 | 4.4 | 2.6 | 0.9 |

VAP, ventilator-associated pneumonia.

weight on the rate of infection is evident for catheter-related blood stream infections. Of interest, the rates of ventilator-associated pneumonia are more consistent across weight groups.

## ANATOMIC SITES OF INFECTION

### Well Baby Nursery

Nosocomial infections in the well baby nursery are most commonly superficial, involving the skin, mouth, or eyes. These infections include omphalitis, pustules, abscesses, and bullous impetigo (Goldmann, 1989). Nursery epidemics of diarrhea caused by bacterial and viral enteropathogens have been reported, but they occur infrequently (Goldmann, 1989).

### Neonatal Intensive Care Unit

National and institutional surveillance data demonstrate that blood stream infections are responsible for the majority of nosocomial infections among NICU patients (Gaynes et al, 1996; National, 2000; Sohn et al, 2001). The remaining cases involve the respiratory tract, eye, ear, nose, and throat, or gastrointestinal tract (Fig. 40–1). Surveillance data for meningitis are limited. There are widespread differences in clinical practice regarding the inclusion of a lumbar puncture with cerebrospinal fluid analysis in the evaluation of an infant with suspected sepsis. Reports suggest that late-onset meningitis may be underdiagnosed in the high-risk population of VLBW infants (Stoll et al, 2002b).

## RISK FACTORS

Some risk factors for acquiring a nosocomial infection are reflections of the patient population and cannot be modified. Other risk factors are directly related to the level of supportive care associated with intensive care medicine. Risk factors for nosocomial infection are lower gestational age and low birth weight; invasive procedures; invasive devices, especially intravascular catheters and endotracheal tubes; parenteral nutrition and intravenous lipids; colonization of skin, gastrointestinal tract, and airway with invasive organisms; selected drugs administered to the neonate; and issues surrounding nursery staffing, nursery crowding, and hand washing (Table 40–3) (Gaynes et al, 1996; Kawogoe et al, 2001; Stoll et al, 1996, 2002a; Stover et al, 1996; Suara et al, 2000). Minimizing exposure to known risk factors for infection is important to attempts to reduce the rate of nosocomial infections in the nursery.

The risk for development of a nosocomial infection is inversely related to gestational age and birth weight (Gaynes et al, 1996, Kawogoe et al, 2001; National, 2000; Stoll et al, 1996, 2002a; Stover et al, 1996; Suara et al, 2000). Previous reports estimate that there is a 3% higher risk of acquiring a nosocomial infection with each 500-g increment in birth weight (Goldmann, 1989). Infants with birth weights less than 1000 g have twice the rate of nosocomial blood stream

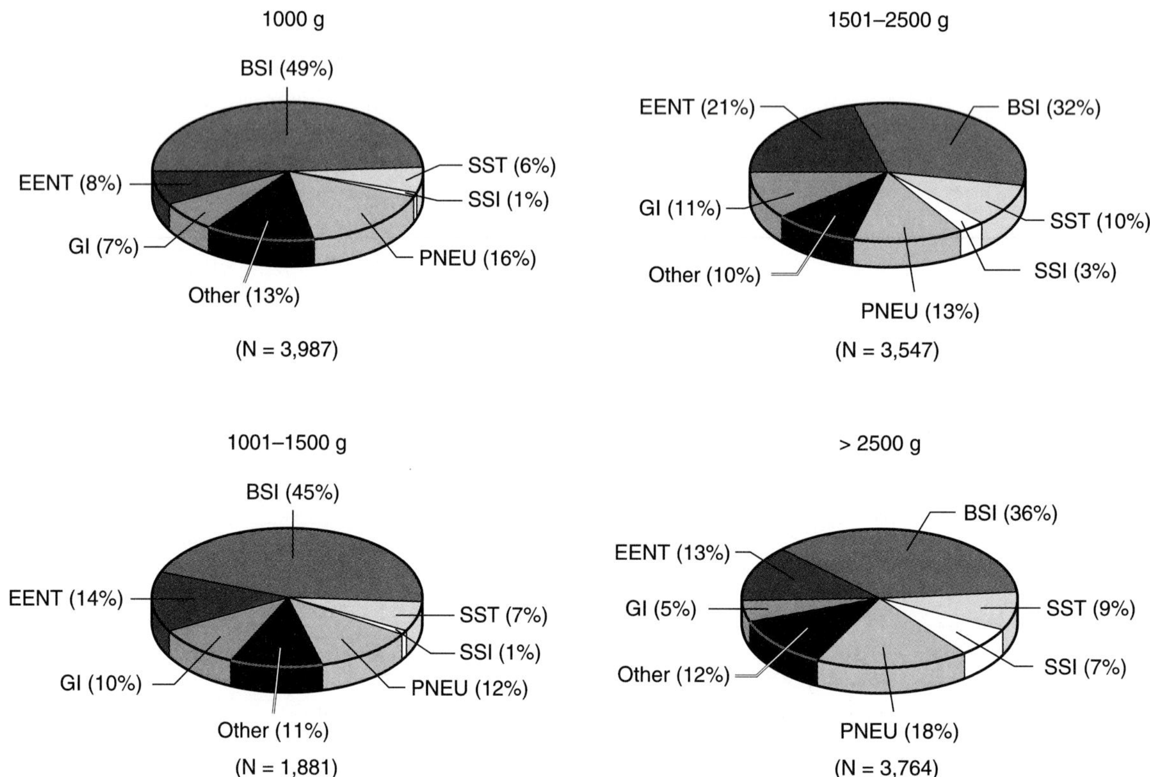


**FIGURE 40–1.** Distribution of nosocomial infections by site of infection. *(Data from Gaynes RP, Edwards JR, Jarvis WR, et al: Nosocomial infections among neonates in high-risk nurseries in the United States. Pediatrics 98:357-361, 1996.)*

**TABLE 40-3**

**Risk Factors for Acquiring Nosocomial Infection in the Neonatal Intensive Care Unit**

| |
|---|
| Prematurity |
| Low birth weight |
| Invasive device |
| Intravascular device (PIVC, umbilical catheter, PICC, CVC, PAL) |
| Mechanical ventilator |
| Urinary catheter |
| Ventriculoperitoneal shunt |
| Medications |
| Histamine$_2$-blocking agents |
| Steroids |
| Others |
| Prolonged administration of hyperalimentation |
| Intralipid administration |
| Delayed enteral feedings |
| Feeding with formula rather than human milk |
| Inadequate nursery staffing and overcrowding |
| Poor compliance with handwashing |

CVC, central versus catheter; PAL, percutaneous asterial line; PIVC, percutaneous intravenous catheter; PICC, peripherally inserted central catheter.

infections than infants with birth weights greater than 1000 g (Brodie et al, 2000; Gaynes et al, 1996; National, 2000; Stoll et al, 2002a; Stover et al, 1996). Severity of illness scores may be more predictive than birth weight alone, because they reflect physiologic stability and the cumulative need for intervention and invasive therapies (Goldmann, 1989; Gray et al, 1995).

The use of any type of invasive device increases the risk for infection. The most common invasive devices used in the nursery are intravascular catheters, mechanical ventilators, ventriculoperitoneal shunts, and urinary catheters. In general, the risk rises as the duration of exposure lengthens. Compared with adult patients, neonates are at higher risk for catheter-related blood stream infections and at lower risk for ventilator-associated and urinary tract infections. (Langley et al, 2001; National, 2000). These patterns correlate with the frequency with which these devices are used in the neonatal patient population.

Prolonged duration of mechanical ventilation is the primary risk factor for development of hospital-acquired pneumonia. Contamination of respiratory equipment—especially with gram-negative organisms that thrive in moist environments, such as *Acinetobacter, Pseudomonas*, and *Flavobacterium*—frequently lead to colonization of the respiratory tract. We speculate that aspiration of colonized gastric and oropharyngeal secretions around the uncuffed endotracheal tube may also occur. The various closed-system suctioning devices may decrease the risk of iatrogenic contamination during suctioning.

Intravascular devices commonly used in the neonatal population are peripheral intravenous catheters (PIVs), umbilical catheters, peripherally inserted central catheters (PICCs), surgically placed central venous catheters (CVCs) and percutaneous arterial catheters (PALs). Regardless of the type of device used, the rate of catheter-related blood stream infections is directly related to the number of days catheters are in place and inversely related to the gestational age and birth weight of the patients (Gaynes et al, 1996; Kawogoe et al, 2001; National, 2000; Stoll et al, 2000a; Suara et al, 2000). Coagulase-negative staphylococci (CONS) remain the primary pathogens associated with catheter-related blood stream infections.

PIVs are the most commonly used device for vascular access in the neonate. In adults, removal of such catheters after 72 hours is recommended. Data in neonates are insufficient to recommend elective removal of PIVs after 72 hours, because studies have not shown a clear correlation between the higher colonization rate noted after 72 hours and an increased rate of catheter-related blood stream infection (Oishi, 2001; Pearson, 1996). Additional studies are needed to answer this question.

At present, data comparing the infection rates of the various types of intravascular catheters are limited. Theoretically, the risk should be lower for tunneled catheters because the Dacron cuff proximal to the exit site of a surgically placed catheter may inhibit the migration of organisms into the catheter tract (Mermel et al, 2001). Adult data suggest that tunneled catheters have lower infection rates than nontunneled catheters. This issue needs further study in the neonatal population, especially because PICCs are being used with greater frequency for long-term vascular access in neonates (Stoll et al, 2002a). A retrospective cohort study comparing infection rates between infants with PICCs with those with PIVs found no difference in the rates of catheter-related blood stream infection (Parellada et al, 1999).

The use of intravenous lipid emulsions (e.g., Intralipid) increases the risk for infection (Freeman et al, 1990). Lipid emulsions decrease the flow rate through the intravenous catheter and potentiate the growth and proliferation of some microorganisms. Lipid emulsions may interfere with host defense mechanisms by impairing the function of neutrophils and reticuloendothelial macrophages (Freeman et al, 1990; Langevin et al, 1999; Nugent, 1984). Extrinsic contamination has been reported but rarely occurs in the United States (Hernandez-Ramos et al, 2000). Freeman and associates (1990) reported that the use of a lipid emulsion was positively and independently predictive for the development of CONS bacteremia. Infants who demonstrated CONS sepsis were 5.8 times more likely to have been exposed to lipid emulsions. Administration of such emulsions has also been linked to a higher risk for nosocomial infection with *Candida* and *Malassezia* spp. in neonates (Long and Keyserling, 1985; Redline et al, 1985; Saiman et al, 2000).

Histamine-blocking agents and postnatally administered corticosteroids are the medications most commonly associated with an increased risk of nosocomial infections among newborns. It is hypothesized that the reduced gastric pH associated with the use of histamine$_2$-blocking agents promotes bacterial overgrowth and invasion of pathogenic bacteria (Beck-Sague et al, 1994; Stoll et al, 1999). Others speculate that the use of these medications is a marker for infants with gastroesophageal reflux who may be at a higher risk for aspiration pneumonia (Stoll et al, 1999). Previously, dexamethasone was used in ventilator-dependent preterm infants to facilitate weaning from the ventilator and to minimize the risk of chronic lung disease. Current data support minimizing use of this drug in VLBW infants, secondary to concerns of spontaneous bowel perforation and an adverse effect on growth and neurodevelopmental outcome (O'Shea et al, 1999; Stark et al, 2001, Vohr et al, 2000). The use of dexamethasone has been associated with an increased risk of infection in VLBW infants (Stoll et al, 1999, Yeh et al, 1997).

Nursery design and staffing influence the risk of infection. Overcrowding and larger workloads decrease compliance with hand washing and raise the risk of nosocomial infection (Archibald et al, 1997, Fridkin et al, 1996; Harbarth et al, 1999; Robert et al, 2000; Vicca, 1999). Inadequate numbers of staff and the use of temporary or inexperienced staff both adversely affect the rate of infection. The adverse impact of inadequate staffing and overcrowding were nicely demonstrated by Haley and Bregman (1982), who showed a relationship between nurse-to-patient ratio and colonization of patients with methicillin-resistant *Staphylococcus aureus* (MRSA). Fridkin and colleagues (1996) found that patient-to-nurse ratio was an independent predictor of development of a catheter-related blood stream infection. Furthermore, strategic nursery design and improvement in nursing staffing correlate with a lower rate of nosocomial infections (Gladstone et al, 1990).

## DISTRIBUTION BY PATHOGEN

The predominant pathogens responsible for nosocomial blood stream infections have changed over time. Goldmann (1989) proposed that these trends are explained by changes in the neonatal intensive care patient population and advancing technology. *S. aureus* was the most common nosocomial pathogen in the 1950s and 1960s. In the 1960s and 1970s, gram-negative organisms emerged as the predominant pathogens; globally, these organisms remain the most important pathogens responsible for nosocomial infections in the nursery (Stoll, 2001). National surveillance data indicate that CONS are currently the most common nosocomial pathogens (Gaynes et al, 1996; National, 2000) (Table 40–4). In the United States, the distribution of pathogens has not changed significantly over the past decade (Gaynes et al, 1996; Stoll et al, 1996, 2002a) (Table 40–5). Among a cohort of infants of birth weights less than 1500 g with late-onset infections, the NICHHD Neonatal Research Network reported that gram-positive organisms were responsible for 70% of cases, gram-negative organisms for 18%, and fungi for 12% (Stoll et al, 2002a). These findings are similar to those of a 10-year retrospective analysis of pathogens in a single center, in which gram-positive organisms caused 57% of late-onset infections (Karlowicz et al, 2000). The distribution of infecting pathogens did not differ with birth weight or timing of infection (Stoll et al, 2002a).

For the clinician, understanding the specific colonization and resistance patterns in the individual NICU is perhaps more important than being aware of national trends. The emergence of nosocomial pathogens with antimicrobial resistance is a concern. In patients of all ages, reports estimate that 50% to 60% of nosocomial infections are caused by resistant organisms (Jones, 2001; Weinstein, 1998). Surveillance data indicate that the organisms showing patterns of increasing antibiotic resistance of importance to NICU patients are vancomycin-resistant enterococci (VRE), MRSA, and multidrug-resistant gram-negative organisms.

**TABLE 40–4**

**Distribution of Pathogens Responsible for Blood Stream Infections**

| Pathogen | No. | % |
|---|---|---|
| Coagulase-negative staphylococci | 3833 | 51.0 |
| *Staphylococcus aureus* | 563 | 7.5 |
| Group B streptococcus | 597 | 7.9 |
| *Enterococcus* spp. | 467 | 6.2 |
| *Candida* spp. | 518 | 6.9 |
| *Escherichia coli* | 326 | 4.3 |
| Other *Streptococcus* spp. | 205 | 2.7 |
| *Enterobacter* spp. | 219 | 2.9 |
| *Klebsiella pneumoniae* | 188 | 2.5 |

Data from Gaynes RP, Edwards JR, Jarvis WR, et al: Nosocomial infections among neonates in high-risk nurseries in the United States. Pediatrics 98:357-361, 1996.

### Gram-Positive Bacteria

CONS are the most common endemic nosocomial pathogens in neonates (Brodie et al, 2000; Gaynes et al, 1996; Gray et al, 1995; National, 2000; Stoll et al, 2002a). The majority of CONS infections are blood stream infections.

**TABLE 40–5**

**Common Pathogens Causing Nosocomial Infections**

| | |
|---|---|
| Gram-positive organisms | Coagulase-negative staphylococci<br>*Staphylococcus aureus*<br>*Enterococcus* spp.<br>Group B *Streptococcus* |
| Gram-negative organisms | *Escherichia coli*<br>*Klebsiella*<br>*Pseudomonas*<br>*Enterobacter* spp.<br>*Serratia*<br>*Haemophilus* spp.<br>*Acinetobacter*<br>*Salmonella* |
| Fungal organisms | *Candida albicans*<br>*Candida parapsilosis*<br>*Malassezia furfur* |
| Viral organisms | Respiratory syncytial virus<br>Influenza<br>Varicella zoster<br>Rotavirus<br>Enterovirus |

Data from Gaynes RP, Edwards JR, Jarvis WR, et al: Nosocomial infections among neonates in high-risk nurseries in the United States. Pediatrics 98:357-361, 1996; and Stoll BJ, Hansen N, Fanaroff AA, et al: Late-onset sepsis in very-low-birth-weight neonates: The experience of the HICHD Neonatal Research Network. Pediatrics 110:285-291, 2002.

Reported incidence ranges from 51% to 78% among VLBW infants (Gray et al, 1995; Isaacs et al, 1996; Stoll, 2002a; Stoll et al, 1996). Gray and colleagues (1995) reported a cumulative incidence of 17.5 episodes of CONS sepsis per 100 patient-days and an incidence density of 6.9 episodes of CONS sepsis per 1000 patient-days.

Known risk factors for CONS infection are low birth weight, lower gestational age, use of central venous catheters, prolonged administration of hyperalimentation, use of intravenous lipid emulsions, postnatal administration of corticosteroids, and prolonged hospital stay (Brodie et al, 2000; Freeman et al, 1990; Goldmann, 1989; Johnson-Robbins et al, 1996). CONS is the pathogen most commonly associated with catheter-related infections, partially because they produce capsular polysaccharide adhesin (poly-*N*-succinyl glucosamine), which enhances their ability to adhere to intravascular devices. Although preliminary studies suggest that prophylactic use of vancomycin reduces the risk of CONS catheter-related infections, this practice is not recommended because of the serious risk of encouraging antibiotic-resistant organisms, especially VRE and staphylococci.

Enterococci are responsible for both endemic and epidemic nosocomial infections in the NICU. Use of central venous catheters, prolonged hospital stay, and prior antibiotic use are recognized risk factors for colonization with these organisms. The gastrointestinal tract is often the primary source of infection; however, the pathogens are typically spread via the hands of health care workers or through environmental contamination. The widespread use of antibiotics has led to the emergence of VRE. There are published guidelines to prevent the spread of VRE, which include hand washing, isolation, barrier precautions, and cohorting of infected patients (Gross and Pujat, 2001; Recommendations, 1995). Educational programs to limit the indiscriminate use of antibiotics have been effective in decreasing the spread of VRE (Goldman et al, 1996; Isaacs, 2000).

*S. aureus* has caused epidemics in both the well baby nursery and the NICU. In the nursery, the major reservoir for staphylococci is colonized or infected infants. These infants transmit the organism to health care workers, who subsequently infect other infants. The skin, nares, and umbilicus are the most common sites of colonization. Unfortunately, routine surveillance cultures are not useful because colonization rates correlate poorly with infection rates. Studies in adult patients have shown that many patients who demonstrate *S. aureus* bacteremia were colonized with the identical strain at the time of admission to the hospital, suggesting that some of the infections with *S. aureus* are community acquired rather than hospital acquired (von Eiff et al, 2001). Similarly, health care workers may be colonized with a community-acquired strain of *S. aureus*, which they then transfer to vulnerable infants.

Group B streptococci (GBS) remain an important cause of late-onset infection in neonates. Intrapartum antibiotic treatment to prevent vertical transmission of GBS from a colonized mother to her infant has led to a dramatic decrease in early-onset GBS disease. In contrast, the incidence of late-onset GBS disease has remained unchanged, presumably because prophylaxis does not eradicate colonization of the genital tract or the environment.

## Gram-Negative Organisms

Gram-negative organisms are a particularly important cause of nosocomial blood stream infections, pneumonia, and meningitis because they generally cause severe disease. *Escherichia coli* is the most common gram-negative pathogen. Other gram-negative organisms responsible for nosocomial infections are *Klebsiella, Pseudomonas, Enterobacter, Acinetobacter, Serratia, Haemophilus* spp., and *Salmonella* spp. (see Table 40–5).

The attributable mortality is much higher for gram-negative infections than for gram-positive infections. Stoll and associates (2002a) report that infants with gram-negative infections had a 3.5-fold higher risk of death. Karlowicz and colleagues (2000) found that gram-negative infections were associated with fulminant death within 48 hours of a positive blood culture results in 69% of cases. *Pseudomonas* spp. appear to be particularly virulent, causing death in 42% to 75% of infected neonates (Karlowicz et al, 2000; Leigh et al, 1995; Stoll et al, 2002a).

## Fungal Organisms

Fungal infections are discussed in detail in Chapter 41.

Fungi are responsible for approximately 12% of nosocomial infections in the VLBW population (Makhoul et al, 2002; Stoll et al, 2002a). The reported incidence is 0.4 to 2 cases per 1000 live births (Benjamin et al, 2001; Makhoul et al, 2002). Rates and predominant fungal species vary among clinical centers. The smallest and most premature infants appear to be at the highest risk. Other identified risk factors are prolonged mechanical ventilation, use of broad-spectrum antibiotics, prolonged use of central venous catheters, and prior use of lipid emulsions (Benjamin et al, 2001; Long and Keyserling, 1985; Makhoul et al, 2002; Saiman et al, 2000).

## Viral Organisms

Viral organisms that cause nosocomial infection in the NICU are respiratory syncytial virus (RSV), influenza, varicella, rotavirus, and enterovirus. Isolated infections generally result from contact with infected caregivers or family members. Nursery epidemics may occur in addition to isolated individual cases.

### Respiratory Syncytial Virus

Careful hand washing is the most effective measure to prevent RSV infection.

Recommendations for prevention of RSV epidemics in the inpatient setting include cohorting of patients, barrier precautions, and careful hand washing (Goldmann, 2001; Hall, 2000; Karanfil et al, 1999; Mlinarvić-Galinović and Varda-Brkić, 2000; Snydman et al, 1988). Rapid testing to detect the virus in nasal washings facilitates efforts to cohort infected patients, which has been shown to be an effective control measure (Madge et al, 1992; Snydman et al, 1988). RSV is a fastidious organism capable of surviving on inanimate objects for prolonged periods; therefore, some authorities advocate the use of gowns and gloves because of the increased risk of contamination through casual contact between the patient and the environment (Goldmann, 2001; Hall, 2000; Karanfil et al, 1999; Mlinarić-Galinović and Varda-Brkić, 2000). Several case reports have described the use of palivizumab, an RSV monoclonal antibody, to control nosocomial outbreaks; however, the efficacy of administering monthly injections to hospitalized patients has not been critically or systematically evaluated (Cox et al, 2001; Maćartney et al, 2000). Preterm infants born before 32 weeks of gestation and those with chronic lung disease remain at high risk for RSV infection after hospital discharge; therefore, the American Academy of Pediatrics (AAP) recommends that all high-risk infants (<32 weeks in gestational age, chronic lung disease, or asymptomatic acyanotic congenital heart disease, such as a patent ductus arteriosus or ventricular septal defect) receive palivizumab throughout the RSV season (AAP Committee, 1998; Meissner et al, 1999). These guidelines were updated in 2003 to also include patients with cyanotic congenital heart disease.

### Influenza

Influenza is spread primarily via airborne transmission. Hand washing and immunization of health care workers are the primary tools to prevent nosocomial spread of this virus (Nichol and Hauge, 1997). Most infection control guidelines recommend that every health care worker wear a mask during contact with infected patients. Although several drugs are available for the prophylaxis and treatment of influenza, they have not been studied in newborns and cannot be recommended at this time (Meissner, 2001). At risk infants should receive the influenza vaccine during the winter months.

### Varicella

Potential exposures and epidemics of nosocomial varicella have been reported. After exposure, the rate of disease transmission is higher in pediatric units than in neonatal units. The index case is typically an asymptomatic infected health care worker or family member who has had contact with a susceptible infant before the onset of clinical disease in the health care worker/family member. The incubation period lasts 14 to 16 days, and infected persons are contagious 24 to 48 hours before the appearance of the rash. The relative risk of infection varies according to the intensity of the exposure and the presence of maternal antibody. The majority of transplacental antibody transfer occurs during the third trimester, therefore most extremely preterm infants are born before this process is complete. ELBW infants may be at risk even if their mothers have documented titer of varicella antibodies. The AAP recommends administration of varicella zoster immune globulin (VZIG) to any newborn whose mother shows signs of varicella infection within 5 days before delivery or within 2 days after delivery. An exposed preterm infant born before 28 weeks of gestation or at less than 1000 g should receive immunoprophylaxis regardless of the mother's varicella history or serologic status. An exposed preterm infant born after 28 weeks of gestation should receive VZIG only if the mother lacks clinical or serologic evidence of prior disease (AAP, 2000).

Airborne and contact precautions are recommended for all infants with active varicella disease for at least 5 days after vesicles appear and until all lesions have crusted. Airborne and contact precautions should be used for any exposed susceptible patient from 8 to 21 days after the exposure. Administration of VZIG potentially prolongs the incubation period; therefore, all exposed infants who receive this product should be isolated for up to 28 days after the exposure. An infant born to a mother with active varicella should be isolated for 21 days, or for 28 days if the infant received VZIG. The infants should also be isolated from the mother until all of her lesions have crusted.

### Rotavirus

Although rare, epidemics of rotavirus diarrhea may occur in the nursery (Jain and Glass, 2001; Lee et al, 2001; Widdowson et al, 2000). They are primarily due to inadequate hand washing and cross-contamination between patients. Standard and contact precautions should be adhered to throughout the duration of the illness. Some patients have prolonged fecal shedding of low concentrations of the virus; therefore, some infection control experts recommend contact precautions for the duration of the hospitalization of such patients. Rotavirus is an important cause of diarrhea in older infants and should be suspected with any apparent epidemic of diarrhea.

### Enterovirus

There are numerous serotypes of enteroviruses, including polioviruses, Coxsackie viruses A and B, and echovirus, as well as nonassigned subtypes (Chambon et al, 1999). Enterovirus infections have been described among neonates in the well baby nursery and the neonatal intensive care setting (Chambon et al, 1999; Isaacs et al, 1989; Sizun et al, 2000; Takami et al, 2000, Wreghitt et al, 1989). Both individual cases and epidemics can occur. The seasonal distribution of enterovirus infections in neonates mirrors what is seen in the community.

The clinical presentation associated with enteroviral infection is variable. Many patients are asymptomatic; however, several case reports describe overwhelming infection with multisystem organ dysfunction and death (Jankovic et al, 1999; Keyserling, 1997). Clinical manifestations of severe disease include meningoencephalitis, hepatic dysfunction, disseminated intravascular coagulation, myocarditis, pneumonitis, gastroenteritis, and muscle weakness (Abzug et al, 1993; Isaacs et al, 1989; Keyserling, 1997; Wreghitt et al, 1989). The severity of disease and the likelihood of death are often more pronounced in perinatally acquired cases than in nosocomially acquired cases, presumably related to the lack of maternal antibody present in the neonate (Isaacs et al, 1989; Modlin et al, 1981).

Infection control measures during an enteroviral epidemic include hand washing with alcohol-based preparations or antimicrobial soaps and cohorting of infected patients. Surveillance cultures of specimens from the throat and rectum may be helpful in identifying asymptomatic colonized infants. Blood and cerebrospinal fluid cultures should be obtained in any patient with clinical symptoms of disease. Polymerase chain reaction (PCR) analysis is helpful in making a rapid diagnosis (Nigrovic, 2001). No antiviral agents are currently available to treat enteroviral infections in newborns (Nigrovic, 2001). Although commercially available intravenous immunoglobulin preparations have high levels of neutralizing antibodies to common enterovirus serotypes, there is no clear evidence that administration of immunoglobulin alters the process or outcome of enteroviral infection (Abzug et al, 1993; Dagan et al, 1983; Keyserling, 1997). The use of these products remains controversial in patients with enteroviral infection.

**TABLE 40–6**

**Guidelines for Sibling Visitation in the Nursery**

- Siblings should not have been exposed to known communicable diseases (e.g., varicella).
- Siblings should not have fever or symptoms of acute illness (i.e., upper respiratory infection or gastroenteritis).
- Children should be supervised by their parents or a responsible adult during the entire visit.
- Children should be prepared in advance for the visit.

Adapted from the American Academy of Pediatrics Committee on the Fetus and Newborn. Postpartum (neonatal) sibling visitation. Pediatrics 76:650, 1985.

## EPIDEMICS

Numerous nursery epidemics have been reported. Common sources for infection are contaminated equipment (i.e., breast pump, thermometer, ventilator), environmental reservoirs, soaps, and lapses in hand hygiene practices (Focca et al, 2000; Hervas et al, 2001; Hoque et al, 2001; Jeong et al, 2001; Jones et al, 2000; McNeil et al, 2001; Reiss et al, 2000; van den Berg et al, 2000; Wisplinghoff et al, 2000; Yu et al, 2000). Clinicians must have a high index of suspicion to detect nursery outbreaks, especially when clusters of infections with unusual pathogens occur in a nursery. Continuous surveillance and monitoring of the endemic infection rate are crucial for determining when there has been a significant change in the baseline pattern of infection for a given nursery. Modern molecular technology facilitates identification and tracking of specific strains of bacteria to help determine the common source of infection (Chambon et al, 1999; Jeong et al, 2001; Jones et al, 2000; Takami et al, 2000).

Epidemics must be identified promptly, and immediate control measures instituted. Efforts should be made to identify the causal agent and the mode of transmission. Surveillance of staff may be necessary, even if they are asymptomatic. Reinforcement of hand-washing policies is of utmost importance. Cohorting of infected patients may be helpful in limiting the spread of organisms in the nursery. In an effort to minimize the risk of cross-contamination between patients, staff caring for colonized or infected infants should not care for infants who are not infected or colonized.

## INFECTION CONTROL

The CDC has developed a two-tier approach to infection control. Standard precautions should be used with all patient contact regardless of the underlying diagnosis or infectious status. These consist of universal precautions (designed to prevent blood and body fluid contamination) and body substance precautions (designed to prevent contamination with moist substances). Transmission-based precautions are necessary when a patient is infected with a known or suspected pathogen that is associated with a high risk of contamination via airborne or droplet transmission or contact with skin or contaminated surfaces (Garner, 1996).

The routine use of gowns is not an effective measure to decrease the endemic nosocomial infection rate in the nursery (Garner, 1996; Goldmann, 1989, 1991). Gowns should be used in specific circumstances in which the risk for contamination is high or the infant is being held. Gowns should be changed after each patient encounter.

Visitation policies are nonrestrictive in most modern nurseries. Various regulatory agencies have developed guidelines for sibling visitation (Table 40–6) (AAP, 1985). Infection and colonization rates have not risen with use of the current standards. Siblings should be screened for infection or recent exposures prior to visitation.

## PREVENTION OF NOSOCOMIAL INFECTIONS

There will always be a baseline rate of nosocomial infection in the NICU because of inherent risk factors associated with the patient population, such as low birth weight, prematurity, and the need for supportive and invasive care. However, the wide variability of endemic nosocomial infection rates among centers with similar patient populations suggests that some risk factors are modifiable. Effective prevention strategies focus on these "modifiable" risks, such as strategic nursery design, adequate staffing, hand-washing compliance, minimization of catheter days, and promotion of enteral nutrition, especially with human milk (Adams-Chapman and Stoll, 2002; Goldmann, 1989; Horbar et al, 2001). Programs that include education and frequent feedback from staff, and active participation by health care providers at all levels are more likely to achieve sustained improvement in compliance. Monitoring and surveillance of the nosocomial infection rates in the nursery are also critical components of any prevention program (Table 40–7).

### Hand Hygiene

#### Historic Perspective

Hand washing has clearly been shown to be the most effective and least expensive means of preventing the spread of nosocomial infection; however, even today, compliance with this simple practice is poor (Jarvis, 1994; Larson, 1999; Pittet, 2000; Pittet et al, 2000). Historically, the benefits of hand washing have been known since the early 19th century. Labarraque, a French pharmacist, was one of the first to demonstrate that cleansing the hands with solutions containing lime or soda could be used as disinfectants and antiseptics (Boyce et al, 2002). The issue was further elucidated by Ignaz Semmelwies, who noted that the mortality and puerperal infection rates were higher among women cared

**TABLE 40–7**

**Principles for the Prevention of Nosocomial Infection in the NICU**

- Observe recommendations for standard precautions with all patient contact
- Observe recommendations for transmission-based precautions as indicated:
  - Gowns
  - Gloves
  - Masks
  - Isolation
- Use good nursery design/engineering:
  - Appropriate nursing-to-patient ratio
  - Avoidance of overcrowding and excessive workload
  - Readily accessible sinks, antiseptic solutions, soaps, and paper towels
- Maintain hand-washing practices:
  - Improving hand-washing compliance
  - Washing of hands before and after each patient encounter
  - Appropriate use of soap, alcohol-based preparations, or antiseptic solutions
  - Alcohol-based antiseptic solution at each patients bedside
  - Emollients provided for nursery staff
  - Education and feedback for nursery staff
- Minimize risk of contamination of central verous catheters (CVCs):
  - Maximal sterile barrier precautions during CVC insertion
  - Local antisepsis with chlorhexidine gluconate
  - Minimal entries into the line for laboratory tests
  - Aseptic technique when entering the line
  - Minimal CVC days
  - Sterile preparation of all fluids to be administered via a CVC
- Provide meticulous skin care
- Encourage early and appropriate advancement of enteral feedings
- Provide education and feedback for nursery personnel
- Perform continuous monitoring and surveillance of nosocomial infection rates in the NICU

for by physicians than in those cared for by midwives. He postulated that the puerperal fever in these patients was caused by "cadaverous particles" transmitted from the autopsy suite on the hands of the students and physicians. After he instructed physicians to cleanse their hands with a chlorine solution between patients, the maternal infection and mortality rates dropped significantly (Boyce et al, 2002; Carter, 1983). This intervention represents the first clinical evidence suggesting that cleansing contaminated hands with an antiseptic agent was more effective than washing them with plain soap and water and that hand antisepsis could reduce the spread of contagious disease via the hands of health care workers (Boyce et al, 2002).

## Guidelines for Hand Hygiene Practices in the Neonatal Intensive Care Unit

### *Clinical Indications for Hand Hygiene*

Hand hygiene techniques are effective in decreasing the colonization rate of resident and transient flora and have been shown to reduce cross-contamination among patients. Several studies have shown that the hands of health care workers become contaminated during routine patient care activities, including "clean" procedures, such as lifting patients and checking vital signs, as well as during contact with intact skin (Casewell and Phillips, 1977; Pittet et al, 1999). Attempts have been made to stratify the type of activity with the likelihood of contamination, but they have not been validated by quantitative bacterial contamination analysis. Direct patient contact and respiratory tract care seem to be particularly associated with contamination (Pittet et al, 1999). Organisms such as RSV, *S. aureus*, and gram-negative bacilli are able to survive on inanimate objects, so changing diapers or holding an infant infected with one of these organisms, and even touching items in the infant's room, may result in contamination (Boyce et al, 2002; Goldmann, 1989; Hall, 2000).

Recommendations concerning indications for and the technique of hand washing are summarized in Table 40–8 (Boyce et al, 2002; Garner and Favero, 1986; Larson, 1995). Current recommendations strongly support the use of waterless alcohol-based preparations as the primary agents for hand hygiene except when the hands are soiled with organic material (Boyce et al, 2002).

### *Preparations for Hand Hygiene*

Washing the hands with soap causes suspension and mechanical removal of microorganisms and dirt from the hands. *Hand disinfection* refers to the same process but with the use of an antimicrobial product to kill or inhibit microorganisms. Table 40–9 compares properties of the various hand hygiene agents.

The cleansing activity of plain soap results from its detergent properties (Boyce et al, 2002). Hand washing with soap alone reduces bacterial colonization of the hands but has no significant antimicrobial activity and is ineffective at

**TABLE 40–8**

**Recommendations for Hand Hygiene Practices in the NICU***

| | |
|---|---|
| Indications for handwashing | ▪ Wash hands with a non-antimicrobial soap or an antimicrobial soap and water when hands are visibly soiled or contaminated with proteinaceous material.<br>▪ If the hands are not visibly soiled, alcohol-based waterless antiseptic agents are strongly preferred for routine decontamination of hands in all other clinical situations.<br>▪ Alcohol-based waterless antiseptic agents should be available at each patient area and other convenient locations, and in individual pocket-sized containers for health care providers.<br>▪ Antimicrobial soaps may be considered in settings with few time constraints and easy access to hand hygiene facilities.<br>▪ Decontaminate hands after contact with intact patient skin (i.e., checking pulse or lifting).<br>▪ Decontaminate hands after contact with body fluids or excretions, mucous membranes, non-intact skin, or wounds.<br>▪ Decontaminate hands before applying sterile gloves or inserting a central intravascular catheter.<br>▪ Decontaminate hands before inserting indwelling urinary catheters or other invasive devices not requiring surgical procedures.<br>▪ Decontaminate hands after removing gloves.<br>▪ Decontaminate hands before caring for patients with severe neutropenia or severe immunosuppression.<br>▪ Decontaminate hands after contact with inanimate objects in the immediate vicinity of the patient. |
| Recommended techniques for hand hygiene | ▪ When using a waterless antiseptic agent, apply enough of the product to cover all surfaces of the hands and fingers, and rub hands together until they are dry. Each manufacturer has guidelines for the volume to be used; in general, however, enough should be applied such that it takes 15 to 25 seconds to dry.<br>▪ When using a non-antimicrobial or antimicrobial soap, wet hands, apply 3 to 5 mL of solution to the hands, and rub for at least 15 seconds. Be sure to cover all surfaces of the hands and fingers. Rinse hands with warm water, and dry thoroughly. Foot pedals or towels should be used to turn off the water |

Adapted from Boyce, 2002.

removing pathogenic flora. Soaps containing antimicrobial agents are typically used in the NICU environment.

The antimicrobial activity of alcohol stems from its ability to denature proteins (Boyce et al, 2002). Because proteins are not readily denatured in the absence of water; solutions containing 50% to 80% alcohol are most effective (Boyce, 2000; Boyce et al, 2002). Alcohol has a rapid onset of action and reduces bacterial colonization but has no residual activity. The efficacy of alcohol-based products is influenced by the type of alcohol used, concentration, contact time, volume used, and whether the hands are wet when the product is applied (Boyce et al, 2002; Mackintosh and Hoffman, 1984). When used in adequate amounts, alcohol is usually more effective than other hand hygiene products (Boyce, 2000; Boyce et al, 2002).

Chlorhexidine gluconate is a cationic bis-biguanide whose antimicrobial activity is due to attachment and disruption of cytoplasmic membranes (Boyce et al, 2002). The onset of action is slower than the alcohol-based preparations; however its major benefit is the persistent antimicrobial activity, which may last up to 6 hours after application (Boyce et al, 2002; Larson, 1995). Varying percentages of this product have been added to other hand hygiene preparations, especially the alcohol-based preparations to confer greater residual activity.

Hexachlorophene is a bisphenol compound with bacteriostatic properties. Its activity is due to its ability to inactivate essential enzymes systems. It has good activity against *S. aureus* but weak activity against gram-negative bacteria, fungi, and *Mycobacterium tuberculosis*. Hexachlorophene also has residual activity. Hexachlorophene was used for routine bathing of newborn infants until 1972, when the U.S. Food and Drug Administration (FDA) warned against its use because infants bathed in the 3% solution were found to have cystic degeneration of the cerebral white matter (Shuman et al, 1975). This product should be used only on term infants during a severe outbreak of *S. aureus*. Most experts recommend diluting the material 1:4 with water to minimize the risk of systemic absorption.

Iodine and iodophors penetrate the cell walls of organisms, impairing protein synthesis and altering the cellular membranes (Boyce et al, 2002). The amount of iodine present determines the level of antimicrobial activity. Combining iodine with polymers (i.e., povidone or poloxamers) increases the solubility, promotes sustained release of iodine, and decreases skin irritation. The activity of this product is affected by pH, exposure time, temperature, presence of organic (blood or sputum) or inorganic material, and the concentration of iodine.

TABLE 40–9

**Antimicrobial Spectrum and Characteristics of Hand Hygiene Antiseptic Agents***

| Group | Gram-Positive Bacteria | Gram-Negative Bacteria | Mycobacteria | Fungi | Viruses | Speed of Action | Comments |
|---|---|---|---|---|---|---|---|
| Alcohols | +++ | +++ | +++ | +++ | +++ | Fast | Optimum concentration 60%-90%<br>No persistent activity |
| Chlorhexidine (2% and 4% aqueous) | +++ | +++ | + | + | +++ | Intermediate | Persistent activity<br>Rare allergic reactions |
| Iodine compounds | +++ | +++ | +++ | ++ | +++ | Intermediate | Causes skin burns<br>Usually too irritating for hand hygiene |
| Iodophors | +++ | +++ | + | ++ | ++ | Intermediate | Less irritating than iodine |
| Phenol derivatives | +++ | + | + | + | + | Intermediate | Activity neutralized by non-ionic surfactants |
| Triclosan | +++ | ++ | + | − | +++ | Intermediate | Acceptability varies |
| Quaternary ammonium compounds | + | ++ | − | − | + | Slow | Used only in combination with alcohols<br>Ecologic concerns |

+++, excellent; ++, good, but does not include the entire bacterial spectrum; +, fair; −, no activity or not sufficient.

*Note: Hexachlorophene is not included because it is no longer an accepted ingredient of hand disinfection.

Reprinted with permission from Boyce JM, Pittet D, 2002.

### Compliance

Despite the fact that the benefits of hand washing have been reported since the 19th century, compliance with hand-washing protocols remains unacceptably low. The overall compliance rate is approximately 40% (Pittet, 2000). Reported barriers to compliance with hand hygiene recommendations include skin irritation, poor accessibility of sinks or cleansing agents, greater priority for patient needs, insufficient time, heavy workload and understaffing, and lack of information (Table 40–10). A common misconception is that using gloves obviates adequate hand hygiene. Leakage and contamination of gloves have been reported (Boyce et al, 2002; Larson, 1995). Disposable single-use gloves should be removed after each patient encounter, and hands should be washed before and after their use.

Hand hygiene is extremely cost effective. The additional hospital charges associated with a single nosocomial infection almost equal the yearly hand hygiene budget. Pittet and colleagues (2000) estimated the cost of a hand hygiene intervention program to be less than $57,000 per year. Assuming that only 25% of the observed decrease in infections was attributable to improved hand hygiene practices, they estimated a savings of $2,100 for every infection averted.

## Prevention of Catheter-Related Blood Stream Infections

The care and maintenance of central venous catheters may affect the risk of catheter-related blood stream infection. Before insertion of an intravascular device, attempted sterilization of the skin insertion site is of utmost importance. The recommended technique for skin antisepsis is to use two consecutive 10-second applications or a single 30-second application of the selected antibacterial agent. Sterile water rather than alcohol should be used to remove antiseptics from the skin. Providone-iodine (10%) solution is commonly used for skin antisepsis; however, recent reports suggest that chlorhexidine gluconate is more effective at decreasing skin colonization and subsequent CRBSI in adults as well as colonization of peripheral intravenous catheters in neonates (Darmstadt and Dinulos, 2000; Garland et al, 1995).

Hub colonization and repeated entry into the line for administration of medications or collection of specimens

**TABLE 40-10**

**Factors Influencing Compliance with Hand Hygiene Practices**

| | |
|---|---|
| Observed risk factors for poor adherence to recommended practices | Physician status (rather than a nurse) |
| | Nursing assistant status (rather than a nurse) |
| | Working in an intensive care unit |
| | Working during the week compared with the weekend |
| | Wearing gowns and gloves |
| | Automated sink |
| | Activities with high risk of contamination |
| | High numbers of indications for hand hygiene per hour of patient care |
| Self-reported factors for poor adherence to recommended practices | Agents irritating or drying |
| | Inconvenient location of sinks and supplies |
| | Inadequate supply of soap, paper, etc. |
| | Too busy/patient needs take priority |
| | Perceived low risk of acquiring infection |
| | Gloves obviate the need for hand hygiene |
| | Lack of knowledge of guidelines and recommendations |
| | Disagreement with recommendations |

Data from Pittet D: Improving compliance with hand hygiene in hospitals. Infect Control Hosp Epidemiol 21: 381-386, 2000; and Boyce JM: Using alcohol for hand antiseptics: Dispelling old myths. Infect Control Hosp Epidemiol 21: 438-441, 2000.

for laboratory studies are both associated with an increased risk for infection. Salzman and coworkers (1993) conducted a prospective study in which surveillance cultures of catheter hubs were performed three times per week, and blood cultures and hub cultures were conducted for any suspected episode of sepsis. These investigators found that 54% of 28 episodes of CRBSI were preceded by or coincided with colonization of the catheter hub with the same pathogen. Mahieu and associates (2001b) reported that catheter manipulation for blood sampling and fluid or tubing changes raised the risk of colonization. Despite the lack of large randomized controlled trials, the available data suggest that the use of heparin is associated with a lower risk of bacterial colonization and thrombosis (Appelgren et al, 1996; Mahieu et al, 2001b). It is hypothesized that heparin prevents bacteria from adhering to the catheter and that the preservatives in heparin preparations have some limited antibacterial properties.

Various products have been designed to decrease the risk of catheter-related infection in adult patients. Although data on their use are promising, many of the currently available products are not specifically designed for the neonate, and their safety and efficacy have not been tested in this patient population. Antiseptic- or antibiotic-impregnated catheters have been shown to significantly decrease the risk of CRBSI in adults (Elliott, 2000; Marin et al, 2000; Pai et al, 2000; Tennenberg et al, 1997; Veenestra et al, 1999). Pierce and colleagues (2000) reported that pediatric patients randomly assigned to the use of a heparin-bonded device had a lower incidence of CRBSI than controls (4% versus 33%; $P < .005$). Studies are in progress to evaluate the efficacy of antibiotic lock therapy in neonates. Johnson and associates (1994) treated a small group of pediatric patients with CRBSIs with antibiotic lock therapy for 10 days. They reported that 10 out of 12 catheters were salvaged. There are very limited data describing the use of antibiotic lock therapy in neonates. Garland and coworkers (2002) randomly assigned 82 VLBW infants to saline control or vancomycin antibiotic lock therapy of catheters in an effort to prevent CRBSI. These researchers found a significantly lower incidence density of catheter-related infections, no evidence of toxicity, and no cases of VRE in the neonates receiving antibiotic lock therapy.

## Umbilical Cord Care

Umbilical cord infections remain a significant cause of neonatal mortality in developing nations, although not in the United States (Zupan and Garner, 2001). In clinical practice, there are numerous approaches to umbilical cord care in the healthy term infant because the available data are insufficient to recommend the use of a specific agent or regimen (Zupan and Garner, 2001). Most authorities agree that the umbilical cord should be separated from the placenta with the use of good aseptic technique. Subsequently, some experts recommend "natural drying," but others support the use of an antiseptic agent such as alcohol, silver sulfadiazine, chlorhexidine, triple dye, or gentian violet (Darmstadt et al, 2000; Hsu et al, 1999; Pezzati et al, 2002; Zupan and Garner, 2001). Hexachlorophene and iodine are used sparingly because of concerns about their systemic absorption and toxicity. Studies have shown that antiseptic products decrease umbilical cord colonization. Unfortunately, this decrease has not clearly resulted in a lower incidence of umbilical cord infections. In a meta-analysis that included "no intervention" as an alternative, Zupan and Garner (2001) were unable to determine which regimen was superior. In general, they found that time to cord separation is prolonged when antiseptics are used, but there were no significant differences in the incidence of infection or death with the use of a particular agent for cord care.

## Skin Care

The skin of VLBW preterm infants is immature and functions as an ineffective barrier to prevent transepidermal loss of water and invasion of bacteria. The stratum corneum (the outermost layer of skin) has both mechanical and chemical properties that decrease the risk of infection (Darmstadt and Dinulos, 2000). This layer of skin matures at approximately 32 weeks of gestation. In a prematurely born neonate, the maturation process is accelerated and is usually complete by 2 to 4 weeks after birth (Darmstadt and Dinulos, 2000).

Unfortunately, there is no consensus on the most effective skin care practices for VLBW infants (Baker et al, 1999; Munson et al, 1999). Neonatologists had hoped that the application of a topical emollient would be the "magic bullet" to protect the developing epidermal layer, reduce the risk of infection, and prevent transepidermal water loss. Several studies have documented that such a practice decreases water loss; however, there was no significant reduction in nosocomial infection in VLBW infants randomly assigned to receive routine application of one emollient product (Aquaphor) in a study performed by Edwards and colleagues (2001). Infants randomly assigned to emollient therapy had more nosocomial blood stream infections, particularly with CONS. This difference was most evident in infants with birth weights of 501 to 750 g.

The efficacy of other topical agents warrants further study. Efforts to prevent traumatic injury to the skin of VLBW infants include the use of transparent dressing over bony prominences, semipermeable barriers between the skin and adhesive tape, and water-activated electrodes and the avoidance of agents such as tincture of benzoin, mastisol, and adhesive removers (Adams-Chapman and Stoll, 2002; Darmstadt and Dinulos, 2000; Hoath and Narendran, 2000).

## MANAGEMENT OF NOSOCOMIAL INFECTIONS

### Catheter-Related Blood Stream Infections

Management of neonates with CRBSIs is problematic because of the limited intravenous access in most such patients as well as the lack of consensus among clinicians. Current recommendations for adults regarding catheter removal with associated CRBSI suggest the removal of nontunneled central venous catheters (umbilical venous catheters, PICCs) associated with bacteremia or fungemia, unless the pathogen is CONS (Mermel et al, 2001). A patient with a catheter-related infection due to CONS should undergo catheter removal if culture results are persistently positive or if the patient is unstable (Benjamin et al, 2001; Karlowicz et al, 2000).

Benjamin and colleagues (2001) retrospectively reviewed data on infants with CRBSIs and compared outcomes in patients in whom catheters were removed at the onset of infection with those in whom catheters remained in place. Forty-six percent (59 of 128) of infants in whom catheter sterilization was attempted had complications, compared with 8% (2 of 25) of those in whom catheters were removed. In particular, infants with gram-negative infections were more likely to have complications if their catheters remained in place. A study of infants with CRBSIs due to CONS found no difference in the complication or mortality rate in patients in whom removal of the catheter was delayed (Karlowicz et al, 2000). Such patients were more likely to have persistently positive culture results (43%, versus 13% for immediate catheter removal), and the attempt to retain the catheter was never successful if culture results remained positive for more than 4 days. Further prospective randomized trials are needed to validate these observational data.

### Antibiotic and Adjunctive Therapies

Antibiotic therapy effective against a culture-proven or suspected pathogen is the primary treatment for nosocomial infections. Awareness of the colonization patterns for a particular infant or a nursery influence the choice of antibiotics. One should consider coverage for *Pseudomonas* spp. or other resistant gram-negative organisms in patients with a rapid clinical deterioration (Karlowski et al, 2000; Stoll et al, 2002a).

Many high-risk neonates with late-onset infections have evidence of multisystem organ dysfunction. Supportive therapy (i.e., colloid infusions, ionotropic agents, mechanical ventilation) should be used as indicated by the clinical status of the patient.

A meta-analysis of the prophylactic use of intravenous immune globulin (IVIG) in preterm neonates found only a 3% reduction in nosocomial infection and no reduction in mortality (Modi and Carr, 2000; Ohlsson and Lacy, 2001a). The benefit in patients with culture-proven sepsis remains unclear, and IVIG is therefore not recommended for routine use in such patients (Modi and Carr, 2000). Some authorities speculate that the benefit of IVIG would be greater if products containing high concentrations of specific antibodies against pathogens frequently responsible for neonatal infections were developed (Hill, 2000; Ohlsson and Lacy, 2001b; Weisman et al, 1994). Hemopoietic colony-stimulating factors (G-CSF and GM-CSF) are effective in raising the neutrophil count but have not consistently decreased nosocomial infection rates or mortality (Modi and Carr, 2000; Modi et al, 2001). Studies are being conducted in adults to evaluate the efficacy of administering various cytokine preparations known to modulate the inflammatory response.

## CONCLUSION

Interventions to reduce nosocomial infection are urgently needed. Infants with nosocomial infections have significantly longer hospital stays (79 versus 60 days; $P < .001$) and higher hospital costs (Gray et al, 1995; Mahieu et al, 2001a; Pittet et al, 1994; Stoll et al, 2002a). The higher costs are primarily secondary to daily hospital charges and pharmaceutical fees (Mahieu et al, 2001a). The attributable cost of nosocomial infection has been estimated to be approximately $40,000 per adult case and $1200 per neonatal case (Mahieu et al, 2001a; Pittet et al, 1994). The magnitude of these costs is significant, especially when one considers the growing number of surviving VLBW infants, who are at the highest risk for acquiring a nosocomial infection. Moreover, infants who experience a nosocomial infection are significantly more likely to die than are those who remain uninfected (Stoll et al, 1996, 2002a).

A variety of new therapeutic alternatives are currently being investigated. Clinicians must continue to focus on developing effective prevention strategies, including strict hand-washing policies, minimal use of invasive devices, promotion of enteral nutrition surveillance of infection patterns, and education for the nursery staff.

## REFERENCES


Abzug MJ, Levin MJ, Rotbart HA: Profile of enterovirus disease in the first two weeks of life. Pediatr Infect Dis J 12:820-824, 1993.

Adams-Chapman I, Stoll BJ: Systemic inflammatory response syndrome. Semin Pediatr Infect Dis 12:5-16, 2001.

Adams-Chapman I, Stoll BJ: Prevention of nosocomial infections in the neonatal intensive care unit. Curr Opin Pediatr 14: 157-164, 2002.

American Academy of Pediatrics: Postpartum (neonatal) sibling visitation. Committee on the Fetus and Newborn. Pediatrics 76: 650, 1985.

American Academy of Pediatrics: Varicella zoster infections. In Pickering LK (ed): 2003 Red Book: Report of the Committee on Infectious Diseases, 25th ed. Elk Grove Village, IL, American Academy of Pediatrics, 2003, pp 672-686.

Appelgren R, Ransjo U, Bindsley L, et al: Surface heparinization of central venous catheters reduces microbial colonization in vitro and in vivo: Results from a prospective, randomized trial. Crit Care Med 24:1482-1489, 1996.

Archibald LK, Manning ML, Bell LM, et al: Patient density, nurse-to-patient ratio and nosocomial infection risk in a pediatric cardiac intensive care unit. Pediatr Infect Dis J 16:1045-1048, 1997.

Baker SF, Smith BJ, Donohue PK, et al: Skin care management practices for premature infants. J Perinatol 19:426-431, 1999.

Baltimore RS: Neonatal nosocomial infections. Semin Perinatol 22:25-32, 1998.

Beck-Sague CM, Azimi P, Fonseca SN, et al: Bloodstream infections in neonatal intensive care unit patients: Results of a multicenter study. Pediatr Infect Dis J 13:1110-1116, 1994.

Benjamin DK, Miller W, Harmony G, et al: Bacteremia, central catheters, and neonates: When to pull the line. Pediatrics 107:1272-1276, 2001.

Boyce JM: Using alcohol for hand antisepsis: Dispelling old myths. Infect Contr Hosp Epidemiol 21: 438-441,2000.

Boyce JM, Pittet D, et al: Guidelines for Hand Hygiene in Health-Care Settings: Recommendations of the Healthcare Infection Control Practices Advisory Committee and the HICPAC/SHEA/APIC/IDSA Hand Hygiene Task Force. Infect Control Hosp Epidemiol 23:(12 Suppl):33-40, 2002.

Brodie SB, Sands KE, Gray JE, et al: Occurrence of nosocomial bloodstream infections in six neonatal intensive care units. Pediatr Infect Dis J 19:56-62, 2000.

Carter KC: In Semmelweis, I: The Etiology, Concept and Prophylaxis of Childbed Fever. Translated and edited by KC Carter. Madison, WI, University of Wisconsin Press, 1983.

Casewell M, Phillips I: Hands as route of transmission for *Klebsiella* species. Br Med J 2:1315-1317, 1977.

Chambon M, Bailly JL, Beguet A, et al: An outbreak of echovirus type 30 in a neonatal unit in France in 1997: Usefulness of PCR diagnosis. J Hosp Infect 43:63-68, 1999.

Cox RA, Rao P, Brandon-Cox C: The use of palivizumab monoclonal antibody to control an outbreak of respiratory syncytial virus infection in a special care baby unit. J Hosp Infect 48:186-192, 2001.

Dagan R, Prather SL, Powell KR, et al: Neutralizing antibodies to non-polio enteroviruses in human immune serum globulin. Pediatr Infect Dis 2:454-456, 1983.

Darmstadt GL, Dinulos JG: Neonatal skin care. Pediatr Clin North Am 47:757-782, 2000.

Edwards WH, Conner JM, Soll RF: The effect of Aquaphor original emollient ointment on nosocomial sepsis rates and skin integrity in infants of birth weight 501 to 1000 grams. Vermont Oxford Neonatal Network. Pediatric Research 49(Suppl):338A, 2001.

Elliott T: Intravascular catheter-related sepsis-novel methods of prevention. Intensive Care Med 26(Suppl):45-50, 2000.

Emori TG, Culver DH, Horan TC, et al: National nosocomial infections surveillance system (NNIS): Description of surveillance methods. Am J Infect Control 19:19-35, 1991.

Focca M, Jakob K, Whittier S, et al: Endemic *Pseudomonas aeruginosa* infection in a neonatal intensive care unit. N Engl J Med 343:695-700, 2000.

Freeman J, Goldmann DA, Smith NE, et al: Association of intravenous lipid emulsion and coagulase-negative staphylococcal bacteremia in neonatal intensive care units. N Engl J Med 323:301-308, 1990.

Fridkin SK, Pear SM, Williamson TH, et al: The role of understaffing in central venous catheter-associated bloodstream infections. Infect Control Hosp Epidemiol 17:150-158, 1996.

Garland JS, Buck RK, Maloney P, et al: Comparison of 10% povidone-iodine and 0.5% chlorhexidine gluconate for the prevention of peripheral intravenous catheter colonization in neonates: A prospective trial. Pediatr Infect Dis J 14:510-516, 1995.

Garland J, Alex C, Henrickson K, et al: A randomized pilot trial of a vancomycin-heparin lock solution for prevention of catheter related bloodstream infection in neonates. Pediatr Res 51 (Suppl): 298A, 2002.

Garner JS: Guideline for isolation precautions in hospitals. Part I: Evolution of isolation practices. Infect Contr Hosp Epidemiol 17:54-80, 1996.

Garner JS, Favero MS: CDC guidelines for the prevention and control of nosocomial infections: Guideline for handwashing and hospital environmental control, 1985. Supersedes guideline for hospital environmental control published in 1981. Am J Infect Control 14:110-115, 1986.

Garner JS, Jarvis WR, Emori TG, et al: CDC definitions for nosocomial infections, 1988. J Infect Control 16:128-140, 1988.

Gaynes RP, Edwards JR, Jarvis WR, et al: Nosocomial infections among neonates in high-risk nurseries in the United States. Pediatrics 98:357-361, 1996.

Gladstone IM, Ehrenkrannz RA, Edberg SC, et al: A ten-year review of neonatal sepsis and comparison with the previous fifty-year experience. Pediatr Infect Dis J 9:819-825, 1990.

Goldmann DA: Prevention and management of neonatal infections. Infect Dis Clin North Am 3:779-813, 1989.

Goldmann DA: The role of barrier precautions in infection control. J Hosp Infect 18(Suppl A):515-523, 1991.

Goldmann DA: Epidemiology and prevention of pediatric viral respiratory infections in health-care institutions. Emerg Infect Dis 7:249-253, 2001.

Goldmann DA, Weinstein RA, Wenzel RP, et al: Strategies to prevent and control the emergence and spread of antimicrobial-resistant microorganisms in hospitals: A challenge to hospital leadership. JAMA 275:234-240, 1996.

Gonzalez A, Sosenko IR, Chandar J, et al: Influence of infection on patent ductus arteriosus and chronic lung disease in premature infants weighing 1000 grams or less. J Pediatr 128:470-478, 1996.

Gray JE, Richardson DK, McCormick MC, et al: Coagulase-negative staphylococcal bacteremia among very low birth weight infants: Relation to admission illness severity, resource use, and outcome. Pediatrics 95:225-230, 1995.

Gross PA, Pujat D: Implementing practice guidelines for appropriate antimicrobial usage. Med Care 39(Suppl II):55-69, 2001.

Hall CB: Nosocomial respiratory syncytial virus infections: The "cold war" has not ended. Clin Infect Dis 31:590-596, 2000.

Harbarth S, Sudre P, Dharan S, et al: Outbreak of *Enterobacter cloacae* related to understaffing, overcrowding and poor hygiene practices. Infect Control Hosp Epidemiol 20:598-603, 1999.

Hayley RP, Bregman DA: The role of understaffing and overcrowding in recurrent outbreaks of staphylococcal infection in a neonatal special-care unit. J Infect Dis 145:875-885, 1982.

Hernandez-Ramos I, Gaitan-Meza J, Garcia-Gaitan E, et al: Extrinsic contamination of intravenous infusates administered children in Mexico. Pediatr Infect Dis J 19:888-890, 2000.

Hervas JA, Ballesteros F, Alomar A, et al: Increase of *Enterobacter* in neonatal sepsis: A twenty-two-year study. Pediatr Infect Dis J 20:134-140, 2001.

Hill HR: Additional confirmation of the lack of effect of intravenous immunoglobulin in the prevention of neonatal infection. J Pediatr 137:595-597, 2000.

Hoath SB, Narendran V: Adhesives and emollients in the preterm infant. Semin Neonatol 5:289-296, 2000.

Hoque SN, Graham J, Kaufmann ME, et al: *Chryseobacterium (Flavobacterium) meningosepticum* outbreak associated with colonization of water taps in a neonatal intensive care unit. J Hosp Infect 47:188-192, 2001.

Horbar JD, Rogowski J, Plsek PE, et al: Collaborative quality improvement for neonatal intensive care. Pediatrics 107:14-22, 2001.

Hsu CF, Wang CC, Yuh YS, et al: The effectiveness of single and multiple applications of triple dye on umbilical cord separation time. Eur J Pediatr 158:144-146, 1999.

Isaacs D: Rationing antibiotic use in neonatal units. Arch Dis Child Fetal Neonatal Ed 82:F1-F2, 2000.

Isaacs D, Wilkinson AR, Eglin R, et al: Conservative management of an echovirus 11 outbreak in a neonatal unit. Lancet 1(8637):543-545, 1989.

Isaacs D, Barfield C, Clothier T, et al: Late-onset infections of infants in neonatal units. J Paediatr Child Health 32:158-161, 1996.

Jain VP, Glass RI: Epidemiology of rotavirus in India. Indian J Pediatr 68:855-862, 2001.

Jankovic B, Pasic S, Kanjuh B, et al: Severe neonatal echovirus 17 infection during a nursery outbreak. Ped Infect Dis J 18:393-394, 1999.

Jarvis WR: Handwashing—the Semmelweis lesson forgotten? Lancet 344:1311-1312, 1994.

Jeong SH, Kim WM, Chang CL, et al: Neonatal intensive care unit outbreak caused by a strain of *Klebsiella oxytoca* resistant to aztreonam due to overproduction of chromosomal β-lactamase. J Hops Infect 48:281-288, 2001.

Jobe AH, Ikegami M: Mechanisms initiating lung injury in the preterm. Early Hum Dev 53:81-94, 1996.

Johnson DC, Johnson FL, Goldman S: Preliminary results treating persistent central venous catheter infections with the antibiotic lock technique in pediatric patients. Ped Infect Dis J 13:930-931, 1994.

Johnson-Robbins LA, El-Mohandes AE, Simmens SJ, Keiser JF: *Staphylococcus epidermidis* sepsis in the intensive care nursery: A characterization of risk associations in infants $< 1{,}000$ g. Biol Neonate 69:249-256, 1996.

Jones BL, Gorman LJ, Simpson J: An outbreak of *Serratia marcescens* in two neonatal intensive care units. J Hosp Infect 46:314-319, 2000.

Jones RN: Resistance patterns among nosocomial pathogens: Trends over the past few years. Chest 119(Suppl):397S-404S, 2001.

Karanfil LV, Conlon M, Lykens K, et al: Reducing the rate of nosocomially transmitted respiratory syncytial virus. Am J Infect Control 27:91-96, 1999.

Karlowicz MG, Buescher S, Surka AE: Fulminant late-onset sepsis in a neonatal intensive care unit, 1988-1997, and the impact of avoiding empiric vancomycin therapy. Pediatrics 106:1387-1390, 2000.

Kawagoe JY, Segre CA, Pereira CR, et al: Risk factors for nosocomial infections in critically ill newborns: A 5-year prospective cohort study. Am J Infect Control 29:109-114, 2001.

Keyserling HL: Other viral agents of perinatal importance: Varicella, parvovirus, respiratory syncytial virus, and Enterovirus. Clin Perinatol 24:193-211, 1997.

Langevin PB, Gravenstein N, Doyle TJ, et al: Growth of *Staphylococcus aureus* in Diprivan and Intralipid: Implications on the pathogenesis of infections. Anesthesiology 9: 1394-1404, 1999.

Langley JM, Hanakawski M, Leblanc JC: Unique epidemiology of nosocomial urinary tract infection in children. Am J Infect Control 29:94-98, 2001.

Larson EL: APIC guideline for handwashing and hand antisepsis in health care setting. Am J Infect Control 23:251-269, 1995.

Larson E: Skin hygiene and infection prevention: More of the same or different approaches? Clin Infect Dis 29:1287-1294, 1999.

Lee CN, Lin CC, Kao CL, et al: Genetic characterization of the rotaviruses associated with a nursery outbreak. J Med Virol 63:311-320, 2001.

Leigh L, Stoll BJ, Rahman M, et al: *Pseudomonas aeruginosa* infection in very low birth weight infants: A case-control study. Pediatr Infect Dis J 14:367-371, 1995.

Leviton A, Paneth N, Reuss ML, et al: Maternal infection, fetal inflammatory response, and brain damage in very low birth weight infants. Developmental Epidemiology Network Investigators. Pediatr Res 46:566-575, 1999.

Long JG, Keyserling HL: Catheter-related infection in infants due to an unusual lipophilic yeast: *Malassezia furfur*. Pediatrics 76:896-900, 1985.

Macartney KK, Gorelick MH, Manning ML, et al: Nosocomial respiratory syncytial virus infections: The cost effectiveness and cost-benefit of infection control. Pediatrics 106:520-526, 2000.

Mackintosh CA, Hoffman PN: An extended model for transfer of microorganisms via the hands: Differences between organisms and the effect of alcohol disinfection. J Hyg (Lond) 92: 345-355, 1984.

Madge P, Paton JY, McColl JH, et al: Prospective controlled study of four infection-control procedures to prevent nosocomial infection with respiratory syncytial virus. Lancet 340: 1079-1083, 1992.

Mahieu LM, Buitenweg N, Beutels PH, et al: Additional hospital stay and charges due to hospital-acquired infections in a neonatal intensive care unit. J Hosp Infect 47:223-229, 2001a.

Mahieu LM, De Dooy JJ, Lenaerts AE, et al: Catheter manipulations and the risk of catheter-associated bloodstream infection in neonatal intensive care unit patients. J Hosp Infect 48:20-26, 2001b.

Makhoul IR, Kassis I, Smolkin T, et al: Review of 49 neonates with acquired fungal sepsis: Further characterization. Pediatrics 104:61-66, 2002.

Marin MG, Lee JC, Skurnick JH: Prevention of nosocomial bloodstream infections: Effectiveness of antimicrobial-impregnated and heparin-bonded central venous catheters. Crit Care Med 28:3332-3338, 2000.

McNeil SA, Foster CL, Hedderwick SA, et al: Effect of hand cleansing with antimicrobial soap or alcohol-based gel on microbial colonization of artificial fingernails worn by health care workers. Clin Infect Dis 32:367-372, 2001.

Meissner HC: Antiviral drugs for prophylaxis and treatment of influenza. Pediatr Infect Dis 20:1165-1167, 2001.

Meissner HC, Long SS: American Academy of Pediatrics Committee on Infectious Diseases and Committee on Fetus and Newborn. Revised indications for the use of palivizumab and respiratory syncytial virus immune globulin intravenous for the prevention of respiratory syncytial virus infections. Pediatrics 112:1447-1452, 2003.

Meissner HC, Welliver RC, Chartrand SA, et al: Immunoprophylaxis with palivizumab, a humanized respiratory syncytial virus monoclonal antibody, for prevention of respiratory syncytial virus infection in high risk infants: A consensus opinion. Pediatr Infect Dis J 18:223-231, 1999.

Mermel LA, Farr BM, Sheretz RJ, et al: Guidelines for the management of intravascular catheter-related infections. Clin Infect Dis 32:1249-1272, 2001.

Mlinarić-Galinović G, Varda-Brkić D: Nosocomial respiratory syncytial virus infections in children's wards. Diagn Microbiol Infect Dis 37:237-246, 2000.

Modi N, Carr R: Promising stratagems for reducing the burden of neonatal sepsis. Arch Dis Child Fetal Neonatal Ed 83:F150-F153, 2000.

Modi N, Carr R, Dore C: G-CSF and GM-CSF for treating or preventing neonatal infections. Cochrane Database Syst Rev (3), 2001.

Modlin JF, Polk BF, Horton P, et al: A perinatal echovirus infection: Risk of transmission during a community outbreak. N Engl J Med 305:368-371, 1981.

Munson KA, Bare DE, Hoath SB, et al: A survey of skin care practices for premature low birth weight infants. Neonat Netw 18:25-31, 1999.

National Nosocomial Infections Surveillance (NNIS) system report, data summary from January 1992-April 2000, issued June 2000. Am J Infect Control 28:429-448, 2000.

Nichol KL, Hauge M: Influenza vaccination of healthcare workers. Infect Control Hosp Epidemiol 18:189-194, 1997.

Nigrovic LE: What's new with enteroviral infections? Curr Opin Pediatr 13:89-91, 2001.

Nugent KM: Intralipid effect on reticuloendothelial function. J Leukoc Biol 36:123-132, 1984.

Ohlsson A, Lacy JB: Intravenous immunoglobulin for preventing infection in preterm and/or low-birthweight infants. Cochrane Database Syst Rev (2):CD0000361, 2001a.

Ohlsson A, Lacy JB: Intravenous immunoglobulin for suspected or subsequently proven infection in neonates. Cochrane Database Syst Rev (2):CD0001239, 2001b.

Oishi LA: The necessity of routinely replacing peripheral intravenous catheters in hospitalized children. J Intraven Nursing 24:174-179, 2001.

O'Shea TM, Kothadia JM, Klinepeter KL, et al: Randomized placebo-controlled trial of a 42 day tapering course of dexamethasone to reduce the duration of ventilator dependency in very low birthweight infants: Outcome of study participants at 1 year adjusted age. Pediatrics 104:15-21, 1999.

Pai MP, Pendland SL, Danziger LH: Antimicrobial-coated/bonded and impregnated intravascular catheters. Ann Pharmacother 35:1255-1263, 2000.

Parellada JA, Moise AA, Hegemier S, et al: Percutaneous central catheters and peripheral intravenous catheters have similar infection rates in very low birthweight infants. J Perinatol 19:251-254, 1999.

Pearson ML: Guideline for prevention of intravascular device-related infections. Part I: Intravascular device-related infections: An overview. The Hospital Infection Control Practices Advisory Committee. Am J Infect Control 24: 262-277, 1996.

Pezzati M, Biagioli EC, Martelli E, et al: Umbilical cord care: The effect of eight different cord-care regimens on cord separation time and other outcomes. Biol Neonate 81:38-44, 2002.

Pierce CM, Wade A, Mok Q: Heparin-bonded central venous lines reduce thrombotic and infective complications in critically ill children. Intensive Care Med 26:967-972, 2000.

Pittet D: Improving compliance with hand hygiene in hospitals. Infect Control Hosp Epidemiol 21:381-386, 2000.

Pittet D, Tarara D, Wenzel RP: Nosocomial bloodstream infection in critically ill patients: Excess length of stay, extra costs, and attributable mortality. JAMA 271:1598-1601, 1994.

Pittet D, Dharan S, Touveneau S, et al: Bacterial contamination of the hands of hospital staff during routine patient care. Arch Intern Med 159:821-826, 1999.

Pittet D, Hugonnet S, Harbarth S, et al: Effectiveness of a hospital-wide programme to improve compliance with hand hygiene. Infection Control Programme. Lancet 356(9238): 1307-1312, 2000.

Prevention of respiratory syncytial virus infections: Indications for the use of palivizumab and update on the use of RSV-IGIV. AAP Committee on Infectious Diseases and Committee of Fetus and Newborn. Pediatrics 102:1211-1216, 1998.

Recommendations for preventing the spread of vancomycin resistance. Hospital Infection Control Practices Advisory Committee (HICPAC). Infect Control Hosp Epidemiol 16:105-113, 1995.

Redline RW, Redline SS, Boxerbaum B, et al: Systemic *Malassezia furfur* infections in patients receiving Intralipid therapy. Hum Pathol 16:815-822, 1985.

Reiss I, Borkhardt A, Fussle R, et al: Disinfectant contaminated with *Klebsiella oxytoca* as a source of sepsis in babies. Lancet 356(9226):310, 2000.

Robert J, Fridkin SK, Blumberg HM, et al: The influence of the composition of the nursing staff on primary bloodstream infection rates in a surgical intensive care unit. Infect Control Hosp Epidemiol 21:7-12, 2000.

Rojas M, Gonzalez A, Bancalari E, et al: Changing trends in the epidemiology and pathogenesis of neonatal chronic lung disease. J Pediatr 126:506-510, 1995.

Saiman L, Ludington E, Pfaller M, et al: Risk factors for candidemia in neonatal intensive care unit patients. Pediatr Infect Dis J 19:319-324, 2000.

Salzman MB, Isenberg HD, Shapiro JF, et al: A prospective study of the catheter hub as the portal of entry for microorganisms causing catheter-related sepsis in neonates. J Infect Dis 167:487-490, 1993.

Shuman RM, Leech RW, Alvord EC: Neurotoxicity of hexachlorophene in humans. II: A clinicopathological study of 46 premature infants. Arch Neurol 32:320-325, 1975.

Sizun J, Yu MW, Talbot PJ: Survival of human coronaviruses 229 E and OC43 in suspension and after drying on surfaces: A possible source of hospital acquired infections. J Hosp Infect 46:55-60, 2000.

Snydman DR, Greer C, Meissner HC, et al: Prevention of nosocomial transmission of respiratory syncytial virus in a newborn nursery. Infect Control Hosp Epidemiol 9:105-108, 1988.

Sohn AH, Garrett DO, Sinkowitz-Cochran RL, et al: Prevalence of nosocomial infections in neonatal intensive care unit patients: Results from the first national point-prevalence survey. J Pediatr 139:821-827, 2001.

Stark AR, Carlo WA, Tyson JE, et al: Adverse effects of early dexamethasone in extremely low birth weight infants. Neonatal Institute of Child Health and Human Development Neonatal Research Network. N Engl J Med 344:95-101, 2001.

Stoll BJ: Neonatal infections: A global perspective. In Remington JS, Klein JO (eds): Infectious Diseases of the Fetus and Newborn Infant, 5th ed. Philadelphia, WB Saunders. 2001, pp 139-168.

Stoll BJ, Adams-Chapman I, et al: Abnormal neurodevelopmental outcome of ELBW infants with infection. Pediatr Res Suppl (Apr) vol. 53, No 4 Abstract, p 2212, 2003.

Stoll BJ, Gordon T, Korones SB, et al: Late-onset sepsis in very low birth weight neonates: A report from the National Institute of Child Health and Human Development Neonate. J Pediatr 129:63-71, 1996.

Stoll BJ, Temprosa M, Tyson JE, et al: Dexamethasone therapy increases infection in very low birthweight infants. Pediatrics 104:E63, 1999.

Stoll BJ, Hansen N, Fanaroff AA, et al: Late-onset sepsis in very-low-birth-weight neonates: The experience of the NICHHD Neonatal Research Network. Pediatrics 110:285-291, 2002a.

Stoll BJ, Hansen N, Wright LL, et al: High likelihood of meningitis without sepsis among VLBW infants. Pediatr Res 51(Suppl): 265A, 2002b.

Stover BH, Shulman ST, Bratcher DF, et al: Nosocomial infection rates in US children's hospitals' neonatal and pediatric intensive care units. Am J Infect Control 29:152-157, 2001.

Suara RO, Young M, Reeves I: Risk factors for nosocomial infection in a high-risk nursery. Infect Control Hosp Epidemiol 21:250-251, 2000.

Takami T, Sonodat S, Houjyo H, et al: Diagnosis of horizontal enterovirus infections in neonates by nested PCR and direct sequence analysis. J Hosp Infect 45:283-287, 2000.

Tennenberg S, Lieser M, McCurdy B, et al: A prospective randomized trial of an antibiotic- and antiseptic-coated central venous catheter in the prevention of catheter-related infections. Arch Surg 132:1348-1351, 1997.

van den Berg RW, Claahsen HL, Niessen M, et al: *Enterobacter cloacae* outbreak in the NICU related to disinfected thermometers. J Hosp Infect 45:29-34, 2000.

Veenstra DL, Saint S, Saha S, et al: Efficacy of antiseptic impregnated central venous catheters in preventing catheter-related bloodstream infection. JAMA 281:261-267, 1999.

Vicca AF: Nursing staff workload as a determinant of methicillin-resistant *Staphylococcus aureus* spread in an adult intensive therapy unit. J Hosp Infect 43:109-113, 1999.

Vohr BR, Wright LL, Dusick AM, et al: Neurodevelopmental and functional outcomes of extremely low birth weight (ELBW) infants in the NICHHD Neonatal Research Network. Pediatrics 105:1216-1226, 2000.

von Eiff C, Becker K, Machka K, et al: Nasal carriage as a source of *Staphylococcus aureus* bacteremia. Study Group. N Engl J Med 344:11-16, 2001.

Weinstein RA: Nosocomial infection update. Emerg Infect Dis 4:416-420, 1998.

Weisman LE, Stoll BJ, Kueser TJ, et al: Intravenous immune globulin prophylaxis of late-onset sepsis in premature neonates. J Pediatr 125:922-930, 1994.

Widdowson MA, van Doornum GJ, van der Poel WH, et al: Emerging group-A rotavirus and a nosocomial outbreak of diarrhoea. Lancet 356(9236):1161-1162, 2000.

Wisplinghoff H, Edmond MB, Pfaller MA, et al: Nosocomial bloodstream infections caused by *Acinetobacter* species in United States hospitals: Clinical features, molecular epidemiology, and antimicrobial susceptibility. Clin Infect Dis 31:690-697, 2000.

Wreghitt TG, Sutehall GM, King A, et al: Fatal echovirus 7 infection during an outbreak in a special care baby unit. J Infect 19:229-236, 1989.

Yeh TF, Yuh JL, Wu SH, et al: Early postnatal dexamethasone therapy for the prevention of chronic lung disease in preterm infants with respiratory distress syndrome: A multicenter clinical trial. Pediatrics 100:E3, 1997.

Yu WL, Cheng HS, Lin HC, et al: Outbreak investigation of nosocomial *Enterobacter cloacae* bacteraemia in a neonatal intensive care unit. Scand J Infect Dis 32:293-298, 2000.

Zupan J, Garner P: Topical umbilical cord care at birth. Cochrane Database Syst Rev (2), 2001.

CHAPTER

# 41

# Fungal Infections in the Neonatal Intensive Care Unit

Margaret K. Hostetter

## OVERVIEW OF FUNGAL INFECTION IN THE NEWBORN

Invasive fungal infection occurs in approximately 6% to 7% of all infants admitted to the neonatal intensive care unit (NICU) (Stoll et al, 1996), but the incidence is inversely correlated with birth weight: the lower the birth weight, the greater the risk of invasive fungal infection. For example, in a survey of 2847 infants from six different nurseries, the risk of candidemia in infants weighing less than 800 g was 8%; the risk fell to 3% for infants weighing 801 to 1000 g, to 1% for infants weighing 1101 to 1500 g, and to 0.31% for infants weighing more than 1500 g (Saiman et al, 2000). According to these data, the infant weighing 800 g or less has a 25-fold increased risk of invasive candidemia. This markedly increased risk correlates with a mortality rate exceeding 25% in most studies (Chapman and Faix, 2000; Saxen et al, 1995; Weese-Mayer et al, 1987).

Colonization with ubiquitous fungal species occurs in at least 25% of very low-birth-weight (VLBW) infants (Baley et al, 1986), and both the number of *Candida* organisms in the gastrointestinal tract (Pappu-Katikaneni et al, 1990) and colonization at sites such as endotracheal tubes (Rowen et al, 1994) have been correlated with increased risk of invasive disease due to *Candida* species. Prospective studies correlating colonization by other fungal genera (e.g., *Aspergillus, Malassezia*) with risk of invasive disease have not been done.

Host factors that contribute to the susceptibility of the NICU infant to fungal infection include birth weight of less than 1500 g, 5-minute Apgar scores of less than 5, disruption of cutaneous barriers by percutaneous catheters (Faix et al, 1989; Saiman et al, 2000; Stoll et al, 1996), and relative immunocompromise ascribable to reduced numbers of T cells, impaired neutrophil number and function, and reduced levels of complement (Rebuck et al, 1995; Zach and Hostetter, 1989). Concomitants of nursery care that are thought to increase the risk of fungal infections include prolonged use of antimicrobials (especially third-generation cephalosporins), indwelling central venous catheters, abdominal surgery, parenteral nutrition, parenteral lipid formulations, histamine $H_2$ receptor antagonists, endotracheal intubation, and length of stay more than 1 week (Saiman et al, 2000).

This combination of factors has made *Candida* the third most common cause of late-onset sepsis in the NICU. Other fungi encountered include the non-*albicans* species *Candida parapsilosis, Candida glabrata*, and *Candida lusitaneae; Aspergillus fumigatus* and *Aspergillus flavus*; and *Malassezia furfur* and *Malassezia pachydermatis*. All of these fungi have in common a ready ability to colonize the infant's gastrointestinal tract (*Candida albicans*), the skin of caregivers (*Candida parapsilosis, M. furfur* or *M. pachydermatis*), various parenteral nutrition formulations (*Candida* and *Malassezia* species), and sinks, drainage pipes, air ducts, or new construction (*Aspergillus* species). Of interest, the yeast *Cryptococcus neoformans* and the fungi *Histoplasma capsulatum, Blastomyces dermatitidis*, and *Coccidioides immitis* are virtually never seen in the NICU.

## INFECTIONS DUE TO *CANDIDA* SPECIES

### Risk Factors and Epidemiology

Approximately 7% of infants weighing less than 1500 g will develop evidence of invasive candidal disease such as candidemia or disseminated candidiasis. This relatively high incidence contrasts with the logarithmically smaller incidence (0.6%) of candidemia in infants weighing more than 2500 g; most of these infants acquire blood-borne candidal infection in association with congenital anomalies, especially those of the gastrointestinal tract (Rabalais et al, 1996).

A number of environmental factors other than birth weight and gestational age are thought to facilitate colonization with *Candida* species as stated above. Hand carriage of *C. albicans* was found in approximately 5% of health care workers; *C. parapsilosis* was present in 19%.

Of interest, a number of variables appear not to be associated with candidal colonization, including use of antibiotics in the mother, premature rupture of the membranes, the infant's gender, intubation, use of antimicrobial agents other than third-generation cephalosporins in the infant, surgical procedures, and frequency of intubation (Saiman et al, 2001). The role of some environmental factors is controversial. One study found that infants receiving intravenous hydrocortisone were approximately 7 times as likely as uninfected infants to develop disseminated candidal infection within the first 35 days of life (Botas et al, 1995). Use of topical petrolatum was associated with systemic candidal infection in a case-control study (Campbell et al, 2000). Table 41–1 shows the typical species involved in colonization versus candidemia.

### Congenital Candidiasis

Presenting within the first 24 hours of life in both full-term and premature infants, congenital candidiasis, a very rare entity, manifests as a deeply erythematous skin rash in the setting of pronounced neutrophilia, with white

TABLE 41-1

**Colonization and Disease Due to *Candida***

| Species | Percent of Cases | | |
|---|---|---|---|
| | Colonization (n = 486/2157) | Candidemia (n = 35/2847) | Disseminated Candidiasis (n = 19) |
| *Candida albicans* | 62% | 63% | 68% |
| *Candida parapsilosis* | 32% | 29% | 32% |
| Other *Candida* spp. | 6% | 8% | |

Data from Saiman 2001; Saiman 2000; Noyola, 2001.

blood cell (WBC) counts often rising to 50,000/mm$^3$ or more. In the full-term infant, the infection appears to be limited to the dermatologic involvement, and desquamation typically ensues within 2 to 3 days. Although the condition appears extremely painful and is reminiscent of staphylococcal scalded skin syndrome, full-term infants remain stable and continue to feed well.

In contrast, congenital candidiasis in the premature infant is a life-threatening condition (Dvorak and Gavaller, 1966; Johnson et al, 1981). Again, the clinical manifestations develop within the first 24 hours of life, but the rash is often accompanied by multiple pustules, as well as hazy infiltrates on chest radiograph. Results of blood cultures may be positive on occasion. The premature infant is thought to acquire the organism from inhalation of infected amniotic fluid; the accompanying pneumonitis is the most frequent cause of death, even in the face of rapid diagnosis and initiation of systemic antifungal therapy with amphotericin B.

Diagnosis in both premature and full-term infants requires the visualization of the organism on Gram stain of a skin swab or a smear from an opened pustule. On rare occasions, the placenta has yielded the diagnosis. In full-term infants, cultures of blood, urine, and cerebrospinal fluid (CSF) are negative, and chest radiographic findings are normal. In premature infants, chest radiographs show fluffy infiltrates that can be confused with hyaline membrane disease, and the child may have accompanying candidemia.

Treatment for the full term infant requires only the full-body application of antifungal creams containing either nystatin or azoles such as miconazole or clotrimazole. In the premature infant, systemic treatment with amphotericin B at a dose of 1 mg/kg is mandatory, but respiratory involvement all too frequently heralds death despite antifungal therapy.

## Local Infections with *Candida* Species

### *Wound Infections*

Local infections due to *Candida* species occur mainly at wound sites and in the urinary tract. Candidal peritonitis may be seen in the rare infant receiving chronic ambulatory peritoneal dialysis. This entity also can occur in patients with necrotizing enterocolitis as a consequence of intestinal perforation and contamination of the peritoneal cavity. In this context, candidal peritonitis typically presages death.

Because *Candida* species may colonize the skin of patients or caregivers, isolation of *Candida* from a skin swab should not necessarily be construed as evidence for a wound infection. Visualization of the organism in polymorphonuclear leukocytes on Gram stain is a more convincing finding.

### Candidal Infection of the Urinary Tract

The growth of *Candida* species from urinary samples collected by bag is not a reliable indicator of infection (Lundstrom and Sobel, 2001). Isolation of *Candida* species from a catheterized specimen or suprapubic aspiration is a reliable indicator of infection, although asymptomatic colonization of urinary catheters, stents, or nephrostomy tubes can be difficult to distinguish from true infection.

The presence of candiduria in the NICU infant is associated with renal candidiasis—the latter manifested by cortical abscesses or fungal mycelia in the collecting system ("fungus balls")—nearly half the time (Bryant et al, 1999). Thus, in contrast to older children or adults, the finding of candiduria in the NICU infant should prompt blood cultures and renal imaging at the very least. If blood cultures prove to be positive, a full evaluation for disseminated candidiasis should be undertaken (see below). It is important to remember that almost 50% of premature infants with candiduria will have upper tract disease that may progress to frank obstruction if fungal mycelia occlude the calyces (Bryant et al, 1999).

Diagnosis requires the isolation of *Candida* species from suprapubic aspiration or catheterized urine specimens. Because of the high prevalence of associated upper tract disease, imaging of the kidneys by ultrasonography should be performed on isolation of the organism from a sterile urine specimen. Only about half of patients who eventually develop upper tract manifestations will display them on the first ultrasound study (Bryant et al, 1999). Therefore, follow-up imaging is recommended both to ensure the clearance of fungal mycelia, if initially present, and to monitor for later development of this complication. Unfortunately, no standard interval for monitoring has been proposed. However, in the infant who remains persistently funguric or candiduric, a negative result on a single ultrasound examination should not be considered presumptive evidence of cure.

Removal of a colonized urinary catheter may suffice for management of a patient without pyuria or systemic symptoms. Disease confined to the lower tract is best treated with oral azoles (e.g., fluconazole, 4 to 6 mg/kg/day). Treatment of upper tract disease requires systemic amphotericin B. In adults, less than 10% of candiduric patients develop candidemia; in the premature infant, this number is thought to be considerably higher. Therefore, the growth of *Candida* species from a urine specimen collected under sterile conditions demands a thorough search for systemic foci.

## Candidal Peritonitis

*Candida* peritonitis typically develops as a consequence of bowel perforation or rarely as a complication of peritoneal dialysis. In the former situation, multiple organisms such as gram-negative rods and enterococci also may be involved, and the neonate is at risk for sepsis with any one of them (Johnson et al, 1980). Resected tissue from infants suffering from a newly reported entity called "invasive *Candida* enteritis of the newborn" shows penetrating candidal hyphae at the site of an intestinal perforation; this finding is thought by some investigators to be distinct from candidal peritonitis accompanying necrotizing enterocolitis (Bond et al, 2000). Peritonitis associated with a peritoneal dialysis catheter usually occurs as an isolated process, and the outcome is much better.

Diagnosis requires visualization of the organism on a Gram stain of peritoneal fluid obtained by sterile technique or culture of the organism from the same source. Isolation of *Candida* species from the peritoneal fluid should always prompt a search for bowel perforation, either by radiology or by surgical exploration, depending on the clinical circumstances.

Treatment of *Candida* peritonitis due to necrotizing enterocolitis or bowel perforation requires surgical evaluation, supportive therapy, and pharmacologic coverage for all contaminating microorganisms in the peritoneal fluid. The typical regimen may include ampicillin and an aminoglycoside for enterococci and gram-negative rods, clindamycin for anaerobes, and systemic antifungal therapy, most likely with amphotericin B. The isolation of *Candida* species from peritoneal dialysate can be treated with a short course (for 7 to 10 days) of parenteral amphotericin B therapy in a dose of 0.3 to 0.5 mg/kg/day after removal of the catheter. The catheter typically can be reinserted within 24 to 48 hours, once the Gram stain is free of yeast cells.

## Candidemia/Line Infections

The association between prematurity and blood-borne candidal infections has been recognized since the 1980s (Baley et al, 1984; Faix et al, 1989). From that time up to the present, the incidence of candidemia has escalated from 25 to 123 cases per 10,000 NICU admissions (Kossoff et al, 1998; Saiman et al, 2000). *Candida* species are the third most frequent cause of late-onset sepsis, accounting for approximately 9% of infections in this category (Stoll et al, 1996). The median time of onset is at approximately 30 days of age (Baley et al, 1984). In a large multicenter study, colonization of the gastrointestinal tract preceded candidemia in 43% of cases, a frequency suggesting that other sites of colonization, such as intravascular catheters or endotracheal tubes, may contribute to the risk of candidemia (Saiman et al, 2000).

A variety of nonspecific clinical symptoms may be associated with this presentation of candidal disease, including respiratory decompensation, feeding intolerance, temperature instability, and mild thrombocytopenia. It is unclear whether this last manifestation relates more to the use of heparin in central venous catheters or to the presence of *Candida* species in the blood stream.

Although *C. albicans* and *C. parapsilosis* account for almost 90% of candidemias (see Table 41–1), other species such as *C. krusei* are increasing in prevalence and may be resistant to azoles (Faix, 1992; Huang et al, 1999). Despite the emergence of less sensitive species, however, morbidity and mortality rates are highest with *C. albicans* infection (Bayley et al, 1984; Faix, 1992).

*Candida* species isolated from a blood culture should never be regarded as a contaminant but should prompt an immediate search for evidence of disseminated disease, which occurs in approximately 10% of premature newborns (Noyola et al, 2001; Patriquin et al, 1980). A thorough evaluation includes ophthalmologic examination and ultrasonography of the heart, venous system, and abdomen. When lumbar puncture is performed in the evaluation for disseminated candidiasis, as many as 50% of candidemic infants may be found to have associated meningitis (Faix, 1992). Moreover, even with the prompt removal of the central venous catheter and institution of appropriate doses of antifungal therapy, a substantial proportion of infants may exhibit prolonged candidemia lasting 1 to 3 weeks (Chapman and Faix, 2000).

Numerous studies have shown that central venous catheters should be removed within 24 hours after the diagnosis of candidemia (Karlowicz et al, 2000); in particular, removal of the central venous catheter within 3 days is associated with a significantly shorter median duration of candidemia (3 versus 6 days) and a reduced mortality rate (0% versus 39%). Many experts recommend routine echocardiograms for patients with central venous catheters to look for catheter-associated thrombi prior to removal of the catheter.

The rapid institution of parenteral amphotericin B to a maximum dose of 1 to 1.5 mg/kg/day is of paramount importance. The lower dose is favored for candidemia, but the higher dose may be necessary for accompanying meningitis or disseminated disease. No more than 24 hours should elapse before the infant is receiving a dose of 0.7 to 1 mg/kg/day. Accompanying meningitis, if documented, should prompt the addition of 5-fluorocytosine in doses of approximately 25 mg/kg/day. Levels of this drug should be monitored in the newborn and kept at 25-50 μg/mL to avert bone marrow suppression or hepatotoxicity.

A rise in creatinine occurs in more than 80% of older patients receiving amphotericin B (Bennett, 1974), but infants in the NICU appear in large part to be protected against this complication. However, infants demonstrating a twofold rise in creatinine, evidence of tubular compromise, or renal tubular acidosis may benefit from use of one of the liposomal amphotericin preparations. One such agent, AmBisome, has been used in neonates (Juster-Reicher et al, 2000; Weitkamp et al, 1998). The particles in at least one other liposomal preparation appear to be too large to penetrate the adult kidney (Hell et al, 1999), and this author has seen a premature newborn whose persistent candiduria failed to resolve until the liposomal preparation (Abelcet) was changed to amphotericin B desoxycholate. If the central venous catheter is promptly removed and there is no evidence of dissemination, the duration of therapy is typically 10 to 14 days after the blood culture becomes negative (Donowitz and Hendley, 1995).

A recent prospective study of 100 premature newborns weighing less than 1000 g at birth has shown that 6 weeks of prophylaxis with intravenous fluconazole in an escalating dosage regimen (3 mg/kg, divided, every third day for 2 weeks; then every other day for 2 weeks; then every day for 2 weeks) reduced both colonization and infection in the treatment group. The incidence of candidemia was approximately 20% in the placebo group and zero in the treatment group (Kaufman et al, 2001). Although resistance to fluconazole did not emerge during the 6 months of the study, at least one institution in a separate multisite, prospective study of candidemia reported three *C. albicans* isolates that were resistant to fluconazole (minimal inhibitory concentration [MIC] greater than 64 μg/mL) (Saiman et al, 2000).

Molecular genotyping must be employed in attempting to differentiate a temporally related cluster of candidal infections from a true outbreak caused by a common source. Any of several methods of sufficient sensitivity and specificity may be utilized, but genotyping that relies solely on restriction fragment patterns frequently gives rise to erroneous conclusions (Faix et al, 1995; Vazquez et al, 1997).

### Disseminated Candidiasis

Mortality rates approach 30% for disseminated candidiasis, a dreaded complication of candidal infection. Once again, *C. albicans* is the leading pathogen. Organ involvement is most common in the vascular tree at catheter sites (15.2%), followed by the kidneys (7.7%) (Noyola et al, 2001; Patriquin et al, 1980). Eye involvement occurs in approximately 6% of infants. Thrombi within the vascular bed may be particularly difficult to eradicate with antifungal therapy; infants with right atrial thrombi may benefit from atriotomy (Foker et al, 1984). Other sites rarely involved include the liver (Noyola et al, 2001), spleen (Kretschmer et al, 1968), and skeletal system (Adler et al, 1972; Brill et al, 1979; Dan, 1983; Diament et al, 1982; Ho et al, 1989; Pittard et al, 1976; Pope, 1982; Svirsky-Fein et al, 1979; Ward et al, 1983). In infection of the bones and joints in premature newborns, *Candida* species typically are the second most likely pathogen, preceded by *Staphylococcus aureus* (Ho et al, 1989).

Both prospective and retrospective studies have established that *C. albicans* carries higher morbidity and mortality rates than those associated with *C. parapsilosis* (Faix, 1992; Saxen et al, 1995). Premature newborns infected with *C. albicans* have a considerably higher risk of prolonged fungemia, in many cases lasting more than 7 days (Chapman and Faix, 2000). Reasons underlying this propensity to delayed clearance despite adequate systemic antifungal therapy are poorly understood but may involve an insufficient cytokine response or immaturities of reticuloendothelial clearance (Mehr and Doyle, 2000). In animal models, tumor necrosis factor-α (TNF-α) appears to be the cytokine best correlated with clearance (Choi et al, 2001), but levels in premature infants are highly variable (Ng et al, 1997).

## INFECTIONS ASCRIBABLE TO OTHER FUNGI

### Invasive Fungal Dermatitis

Invasive fungal dermatitis typically manifests in the infant weighing less than 1000 g, who displays macerated or bruise-like lesions that are contaminated with fungal species. In the initial report, *C. albicans* was identified in three of seven confirmed cases; *C. parapsilosis, C. tropicalis, Trichosporon beigelii, Curvularia*, or *A. niger* or *A. fumigatus* were cultured from the remainder (Rowen et al, 1995). Among cases considered "probable," seven of eight had *C. albicans*. Systemic complications including fungemia, meningitis, or infection of the urinary tract occurred in four of seven confirmed cases and in seven of eight probable cases. In more cases than controls, the patient had received postnatal steroids and had had prolonged hyperglycemia. Disseminated infection occurred in 69% of the cases, all ascribable to *Candida* species.

Diagnosis requires a skin biopsy demonstrating fungal invasion beyond the stratum corneum or a positive potassium hydroxide preparation of skin scrapings; growth of the identical organism from an otherwise sterile site (blood, CSF, or urine obtained via supra pubic aspiration) is confirmatory. Treatment requires systemic doses of amphotericin B in the range of 0.7 to 1.0 mg/kg/day; in those infants who do not develop systemic infection, oral therapy with fluconazole or topical antifungal creams may suffice. Parenteral therapy is advisable for pathogens like *Aspergillus*, and repeated skin biopsies may be necessary to define duration of therapy.

### Line Infections Due to Lipophilic Organisms

*M. furfur* and *M. pachydermatis* are lipophilic organisms commonly carried on the skin, even in patients without tinea versicolor (Marcon and Powell, 1992). Cutaneous colonization can infect hyperalimentation fluids or parenteral lipid formulations. Infants typically present with mild but nonspecific symptoms: respiratory decompensation, glucose intolerance, or thrombocytopenia (Dankner et al, 1987; Stuart and Lane, 1992). Diagnosis requires isolation of the organism from blood by growth on fungal medium overlaid with olive oil, because *Malassezia* species will not grow in the absence of lipids (Marcon et al, 1986). Removal of the central venous catheter usually suffices for therapy, although some experts recommend the addition of amphotericin B in doses of 0.5 mg/kg/day for 7 days.

## Miscellaneous Fungal Infections

### *Aspergillus Infections*

Most infections with *Aspergillus* occur in severely immunocompromised patients such as those with DiGeorge syndrome or myeloperoxidase deficiency (Chiang et al, 2000; Marcinkowski et al, 2000), but disseminated disease has occurred in premature newborns without additional immunologic abnormalities (Rowen et al, 1992). Rare cases of *Aspergillus* osteomyelitis or brain abscess also have been reported (Marcinkowski et al, 2000; Simpson et al, 1977). Diagnosis requires isolation of the fungus from a normally sterile tissue site or visualization by Gomori-methenamine silver stain on biopsy of infected tissue. Of note, a commercially available ELISA for diagnosis of aspergillosis on serum specimens had an 83% rate of false-positives in premature newborns (Siemann et al, 1998). Treatment requires systemic amphotericin B in doses of 1.0 to 1.5 mg/kg/day. Fungistatic agents such as the triazoles are not recommended for treatment of aspergillosis. There is no published experience with itraconazole or voriconazole in the premature newborn.

### *Trichosporon beigelii Infection*

In a cluster of five neonatal cases of infection caused by *T. beigelii*, a yeast found ubiquitously in soil, no common source was identified (Fisher et al, 1993). Two of three premature infants infected with this organism died. Resistance to achievable concentrations of amphotericin B complicates therapy.

## REFERENCES


Adler S, Randall J, Plotkin SA: Candidal osteomyelitis and arthritis in a neonate. Am J Dis Child 123:595-596, 1972.

Baley JE, Kliegman RM, Boxerbaum B, et al: Fungal colonization in the very low birth weight infant. Pediatrics 78:225-232, 1986.

Baley JE, Kliegman RM, Fanaroff AA: Disseminated fungal infections in very low-birth-weight infants: Clinical manifestations and epidemiology. Pediatrics 73:144-152, 1984.

Bennett JE: Chemotherapy of systemic mycoses (first of two parts). N Engl J Med 290:30-32, 1974.

Bond S, Stewart DL, Bendon RW: Invasive *Candida* enteritis of the newborn. J Pediatr Surg 35:1496-1498, 2000.

Botas CM, Kurlat I, Young SM, et al: Disseminated candidal infections and intravenous hydrocortisone in preterm infants. Pediatrics 95:883-887, 1995.

Brill PW, Winchester P, Krauss AN, et al: Osteomyelitis in a neonatal intensive care unit. Radiology 131:83-87, 1979.

Bryant K, Maxfield C, Rabalais G: Renal candidiasis in neonates with candiduria. Pediatr Infect Dis J 18:959-963, 1999.

Campbell JR, Zaccaria E, Baker CJ: Systemic candidiasis in extremely low birth weight infants receiving topical petrolatum ointment for skin care: A case-control study. Pediatrics 105:1041-1045, 2000.

Chapman RL, Faix RG: Persistently positive cultures and outcome in invasive neonatal candidiasis. Pediatr Infect Dis J 19:822-827, 2000.

Chiang AK, Chan GC, Ma SK, et al: Disseminated fungal infection associated with myeloperoxidase deficiency in a premature neonate. Pediatr Infect Dis J 19:1027-1029, 2000.

Choi JH, Ko HM, Kim JW, et al: Platelet-activating factor–induced early activation of NF-kappa B plays a crucial role for organ clearance of *Candida albicans*. J Immunol 166: 5139-5144, 2001.

Dan M: Neonatal septic arthritis. Isr J Med Sci 19:967-997, 1983.

Dankner WM, Spector SA, Fierer J, et al: *Malassezia fungemia* in neonates and adults: Complication of hyperalimentation. Rev Infect Dis 9:743-753. 1987.

Diament MJ, Weller M, Bernstein R: *Candida* infection in a premature infant presenting as discitis. Pediatr Radiol 12:96-98, 1982.

Donowitz LG, Hendley JO: Short-course amphotericin B therapy for candidemia in pediatric patients. Pediatrics 95:888-891, 1995.

Dvorak AM, Gavaller B: Congenital systemic candidiasis. Report of a case. N Engl J Med 274:540-543, 1966.

Faix RG: Invasive neonatal candidiasis: Comparison of *albicans* and *parapsilosis* infection. Pediatr Infect Dis J 11:88-93, 1992.

Faix RG, Finkel DJ, Andersen RD, et al: Genotypic analysis of a cluster of systemic *Candida albicans* infections in a neonatal intensive care unit. Pediatr Infect Dis J 14:1063-1068, 1995.

Faix RG, Kovarik SM, Shaw TR, et al: Mucocutaneous and invasive candidiasis among very low birth weight (less than 1,500 grams) infants in intensive care nurseries: A prospective study. Pediatrics 83:101-107, 1989.

Fisher DJ, Christy C, Spafford P, et al: Neonatal *Trichosporon beigelii* infection: Report of a cluster of cases in a neonatal intensive care unit. Pediatr Infect Dis J 12:149-155, 1993.

Foker JE, Bass JL, Thompson T, et al: Management of intracardiac fungal masses in premature infants. J Thorac Cardiovasc Surg 87:244-250, 1984.

Holl W, Korn T, Klouche M. Failure of a lipid amphotericin B preparation to eradicate candiduria: Preliminary findings based on three cases. Clin Infect Dis 29:686-687, 1999.

Ho NK, Low YP, See HF: Septic arthritis in the newborn—17 years' clinical experience. Singapore Med J 30:356-358, 1989.

Huang YC, Lin TY, Leu HS, et al: Outbreak of *Candida parapsilosis* fungemia in neonatal intensive care units: Clinical implications and genotyping analysis. Infection 27:97-102, 1999.

Johnson DE, Conroy MM, Foker JE, et al: *Candida* peritonitis in the newborn infants. J Pediatr 97:298-300, 1980.

Johnson DE, Thompson TR, Ferrieri P: Congenital candidiasis. Am J Dis Child 135:273-275, 1981.

Juster-Reicher A, Leibovitz E, Linder N, et al: Liposomal amphotericin B (AmBisome) in the treatment of neonatal candidiasis in very low birth weight infants. Infection 28:223-226, 2000.

Karlowicz MG, Hashimoto LN, Kelly RE Jr, et al: Should central venous catheters be removed as soon as candidemia is detected in neonates? Pediatrics 106:E63, 2000.

Kaufman D, Boyle R, Hazen KC, et al: Fluconazole prophylaxis against fungal colonization and infection in preterm infants. N Engl J Med 345:1660-1666, 2001.

Kossoff EH, Buescher ES, Karlowicz MG: Candidemia in a neonatal intensive care unit: Trends during fifteen years and clinical features of 111 cases. Pediatr Infect Dis J 17:504-508, 1998.

Kretschmer R, Say B, Brown D, et al: Congenital aplasia of the thymus gland (DiGeorge's syndrome). N Engl J Med 279:1295-1301, 1968.

Lundstrom T, Sobel J: Nosocomial candiduria: A review. Clin Infect Dis 32:1602-1607, 2001.

Marcinkowski M, Bauer K, Stoltenburg-Didinger G, et al: Fatal aspergillosis with brain abscesses in a neonate with DiGeorge syndrome. Pediatr Infect Dis J 19:1214-1216, 2000.

Marcon MJ, Powell DA: Human infections due to *Malassezia* spp. Clin Microbiol Rev 5:101-119, 1992.

Marcon MJ, Powell DA, Durrell DE: Methods for optimal recovery of *Malassezia furfur* from blood culture. J Clin Microbiol 24:696-700, 1986.

Mehr S, Doyle LW: Cytokines as markers of bacterial sepsis in newborn infants: A review. Pediatr Infect Dis J 19:879-887, 2000.

Ng PC, Cheng SH, Chui KM, et al: Diagnosis of late onset neonatal sepsis with cytokines, adhesion molecule, and C-reactive protein in preterm very low birthweight infants. Arch Dis Child Fetal Neonatal Ed 77:F221-F227, 1997.

Noyola DE, Fernandez M, Moylett EH, et al: Ophthalmologic, visceral, and cardiac involvement in neonates with candidemia. Clin Infect Dis 32:1018-1023, 2001.

Pappu-Katikaneni LD, Rao KP, Banister E: Gastrointestinal colonization with yeast species and *Candida* septicemia in very low birth weight infants. Mycoses 33:20-23, 1990.

Patriquin H, Lebowitz R, Perreault G, et al: Neonatal candidiasis: Renal and pulmonary manifestations. AJR Am J Roentgenol 135:1205-1210, 1980.

Pittard WB 3rd, Thullen JD, Fanaroff AA; Neonatal septic arthritis. J Pediatr 88:621-624, 1976.

Pope TL Jr: Pediatric *Candida albicans* arthritis: Case report of hip involvement with a review of the literature. Prog Pediatr Surg 15:271-283, 1982.

Rabalais GP, Samiec TD, Bryant KK, et al: Invasive candidiasis in infants weighing more than 2500 grams at birth admitted to a neonatal intensive care unit. Pediatr Infect Dis J 15:348-352, 1996.

Rebuck N, Gibson A, Finn A: Neutrophil adhesion molecules in term and premature infants: normal or enhanced leucocyte integrins but defective L-selectin expression and shedding. Clin Exp Immunol 101:183-189, 1995.

Rowen JL, Atkins JT, Levy ML, et al: Invasive fungal dermatitis in the ≤ 1000-gram neonate. Pediatrics 95:682-687, 1995.

Rowen JL, Correa AG, Sokol DM, et al: Invasive aspergillosis in neonates: Report of five cases and literature review. Pediatr Infect Dis J 11:576-582, 1992.

Rowen JL, Rench MA, Kozinetz CA, et al: Endotracheal colonization with *Candida* enhances risk of systemic candidiasis in very low birth weight neonates. J Pediatr 124:789794, 1994.

Saiman L, Ludington E, Dawson JD, et al: Risk factors for *Candida species* colonization of neonatal intensive care unit patients. Pediatr Infect Dis J 20:1119-1124, 2001.

Saiman L, Ludington E, Pfaller M, et al: Risk factors for candidemia in neonatal intensive care unit patients. The National Epidemiology of Mycosis Survey study group. Pediatr Infect Dis J 19:319-324, 2000.

Saxen H, Virtanen M, Carlson P, et al: Neonatal *Candida parapsilosis* outbreak with a high case fatality rate. Pediatr Infect Dis J 14:776-781, 1995.

Siemann M, Koch-Dorfler M, Gaude M: False-positive results in premature infants with the Platelia *Aspergillus* sandwich enzyme-linked immunosorbent assay. Mycoses 41:373-377, 1998.

Simpson MB Jr, Merz WG, Kurlinski JP, et al: Opportunistic mycotic osteomyelitis: Bone infections due to *Aspergillus* and *Candida* species. Medicine (Baltimore) 56:475-482, 1977.

Stoll BJ, Gordon T, Korones SB, et al: Late-onset sepsis in very low birth weight neonates: A report from the National Institute of Child Health and Human Development Neonatal Research Network. J Pediatr 129:63-71, 1996.

Stuart SM, Lane AT: *Candida* and *Malassezia* as nursery pathogens. Semin Dermatol 11:19-23, 1992.

Svirsky-Fein S, Langer L, Milbauer B, et al: Neonatal osteomyelitis caused by *Candida tropicalis*. Report of two cases and review of the literature. J Bone Joint Surg Am 61:455-459, 1979.

Vazquez JA, Boikov D, Boikov SG, et al: Use of electrophoretic karyotyping in the evaluation of *Candida* infections in a neonatal intensive-care unit. Infect Control Hosp Epidemiol 18:32-37, 1997.

Ward RM, Sattler FR, Dalton AS Jr: Assessment of antifungal therapy in an 800-gram infant with candidal arthritis and osteomyelitis. Pediatrics 72:234-238, 1983.

Weese-Mayer DE, Fondriest DW, Brouillette RT, et al: Risk factors associated with candidemia in the neonatal intensive care unit: A case-control study. Pediatr Infect Dis J 6:190-196, 1987.

Weitkamp JH, Poets CF, Sievers R, et al: *Candida* infection in very low birth-weight infants: Outcome and nephrotoxicity of treatment with liposomal amphotericin B (AmBisome). Infection 26:11-15, 1998.

Zach TL, Hostetter MK: Biochemical abnormalities of the third component of complement in neonates. Pediatr Res 26:116-120, 1989.

# PART X

# RESPIRATORY SYSTEM

Editor: ROBERTA A. BALLARD

CHAPTER 42

## Lung Development: Embryology, Growth, Maturation, and Developmental Biology

Susan Guttentag and Philip L. Ballard

The primary function of the lung is to accomplish exchange of oxygen and carbon dioxide, to accommodate the needs of aerobic cellular respiration. Oxygen consumption in the adult human ranges from 250 mL/minute at rest to 5500 mL/minute at peak exercise (reviewed in Warburton et al, 2000). To accommodate these needs, a large surface area, up to 70 $m^2$, and a thin alveolar-capillary membrane are required. Therefore, a primary component of lung organogenesis is to expand the lung surface area to meet these needs, a process known as *lung branching morphogenesis*. A second goal of lung organogenesis is to minimize the alveolar-capillary membrane, coordinating the development of an extensive capillary network with a thin, expansive alveolar epithelial surface. A third goal of lung development is production of a protective aqueous barrier overlying the delicate alveolar epithelium that is constantly exposed to air. This liquid layer, however, creates a surface tension sufficient to collapse alveoli in the course of air breathing. Hence, another goal of lung development is to produce a surface-active agent, or surfactant, to reduce surface tension, thereby preventing alveolar collapse, or atelectasis, at end-expiratory alveolar volumes. This allows for air to remain within the lung at end-expiration, the functional residual capacity, which significantly reduces the work required to generate the next breath.

The trachea, airways, and alveoli are in constant contact with the external environment. Consequently, with every inhalation these epithelial surfaces come into contact with large numbers of microorganisms and toxic particles. Another important goal of lung organogenesis is to develop mechanisms for clearance of microorganisms and allergens that may result in epithelial infection or injury (Crouch and Wright, 2001).

Finally, the lung needs to develop defenses against nonparticulate substances that are potentially harmful. Oxygen, so critical to cellular function, can be the source of harmful reactive oxygen species (Chabot et al, 1998). Inhaled pollutants also must be detoxified by the lung. The lung, like other organs, has multiple strategies for handling reactive oxygen species and toxic metabolites to minimize tissue damage.

Appropriate development and integration of these lung functions are critical to the health and survival of newborn infants. This chapter focuses on developmental aspects of each function that place the premature neonate at increased risk for lung injury and disease.

### DEVELOPMENT OF GAS EXCHANGE SURFACE

Lung formation begins early in human gestation (by day 25) and growth extends well into childhood, reaching completion by approximately 8 years of age (Davies and Reid, 1970). Lung development can be organized into five stages: embryonic, pseudoglandular, canalicular, terminal sac, and alveolar. The timing of these stages is somewhat imprecise, however, and considerable overlap may occur between stages (Hislop and Reid, 1981). Figure 42–1 shows a time line for fetal and postnatal lung development that incorporates salient events in the development of airway, alveolar, and vascular components as a reference for the discussion that follows. Because of the interrelatedness of these events, it is possible to examine how disruptions in the developmental program can have profound effects on lung morphogenesis. Disruption in the final common pathway of altered lung development often results in pulmonary hypoplasia. Table 42–1 lists genetic defects and disorders associated with pulmonary malformations, organized by mechanism of disease. Pulmonary hypoplasia can result from primary defects in lung morphogenesis as well as from neurologic diseases associated with decreased fetal breathing movements, derangements of the chest wall that restrict fetal breathing movements, renal disorders that compromise amniotic fluid volume and thereby restrict fetal breathing, or space-occupying masses that restrict lung growth. In each case, disorders that manifest early in fetal development have the most profound effects on lung development, resulting in the most severe pulmonary hypoplasia.

#### The Embryonic Phase

The lung bud develops initially as a laryngotracheal groove of the ventral foregut at 25 days of human gestation; within a few days, the groove closes in such a fashion that the only

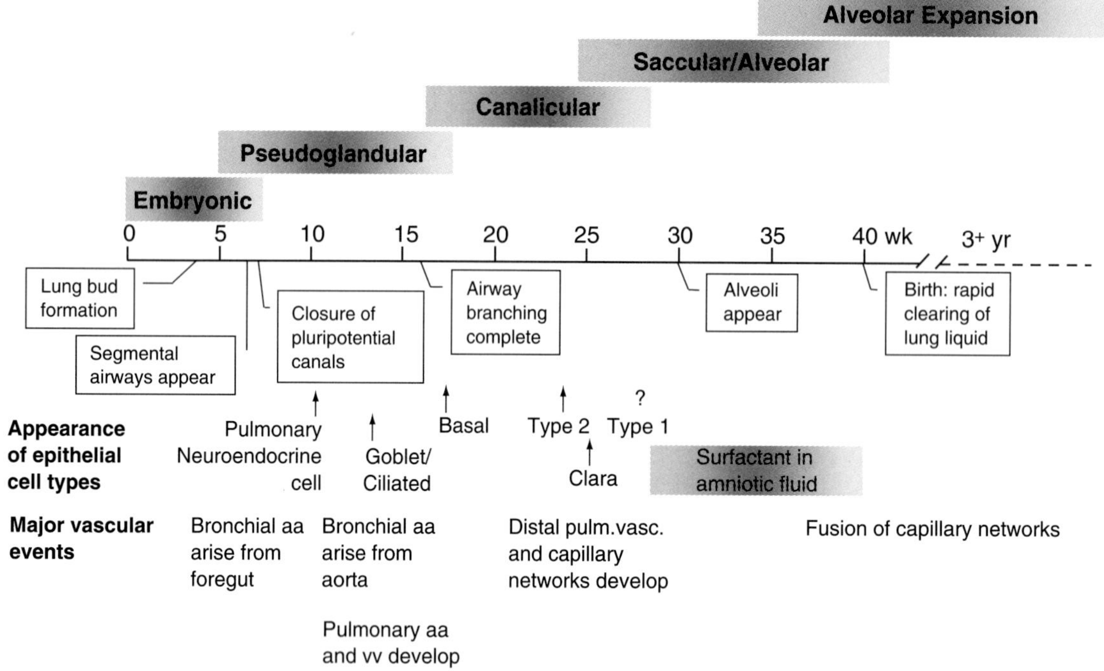


**FIGURE 42–1.** Timeline for fetal and postnatal lung development that incorporates salient events in the development of airway and alveolar and vascular components. aa,vv, arteries, veins.

remaining luminal attachment to the foregut is in the region of the developing hypopharynx and larynx. The lung bud, consisting of epithelium and surrounding mesenchyme, then begins the first of a series of dichotomous branchings that give rise to the conducting airways and five primordial lung lobes (two on the left and three on the right).

The process of branching morphogenesis requires extensive communication between the cells lining the tubular lung bud and those cells contained within the invested mesenchyme (reviewed in Kaplan, 2000; Warburton et al, 2000). Classic recombination experiments using mesenchyme dissected away from the epithelium of either the trachea or more distal bronchi indicate that the mesenchyme plays an important role in dictating the branching pattern and cell fate of the expanding epithelium (Shannon and Deterding, 1997). Branching involves growth arrest of the epithelial cells at branch points, with continued or accelerated growth of epithelial cells lateral to branch points (Hogan and Yingling, 1998). This is governed by the expression of transcription factors that in turn control the expression of growth factors and their receptors—for example, Sonic hedgehog, secreted from epithelial cells, and its receptor patched (Ptc) on adjacent mesenchyme cells—in a complex array of both positive and negative feedback loops. Activation of Ptc results in the release of an intracellular gene product smoothened (Smo), which activates the Gli family of transcription factors. Although the downstream targets for this signaling pathway are unclear, the net result is local proliferation of mesenchymal cells at the tips of the growing epithelial tubules. The Gli family of transcription factors also are necessary for dorsolateral patterning that separates the trachea from the esophagus. Left-right asymmetry of the lung, studied in mice, is governed by another family of transcription factors related to transforming growth factor-β (TGF-β), specifically, lefty 1 and 2, nodal, and gdf1 (Rankin et al, 2000).

Tracheoesophageal fistulas and tracheal atresia and stenosis result from errors in partitioning of the laryngotracheal groove. Transgenic mouse models have shown that targeted knockout of genes encoding Gli family members recapitulates these developmental errors and may contribute to these malformations (Rankin et al, 2000; Warburton et al, 2000). Failure of partitioning of the lung bud also can result in pulmonary agenesis, typically of the right lung.

## The Pseudoglandular and Canalicular Phases

Branching continues such that by 7 weeks, the trachea and the segmental and subsegmental bronchi are evident, marking the end of the embryonic phase. The pseudoglandular phase extends from 7 to 16 weeks of human gestation. By the end of 16 weeks, all bronchial divisions are complete, resulting in a total of 16 divisions responsible for gas conduction. The canalicular phase, extending from 16 to 28 weeks, is marked by the development of the rudimentary gas exchange units that are no longer invested with supportive cartilaginous structures. Furthermore, parallel development of vascular structures occurs to supply ever-increasing numbers of potential air spaces.

Successive branching of the lung bud is dependent on a number of growth factors and transcription factors (reviewed in Kaplan, 2000; Warburton et al, 2000). A critical component is the mesenchymal product fibroblast growth factor-10 (FGF-10) and its receptor fibroblast growth factor receptor-2 (FGFR-2) on epithelial cells. The

**TABLE 42–1**

**Genetic Disorders and Syndromes Associated with Pulmonary Abnormalities**

| Genetic Condition | Pulmonary Abnormality | Associated Finding(s) | OMIM Ref.* |
|---|---|---|---|
| **Syndromes Associated with Primary Defects in Lung Development** | | | |
| Trisomy 21 | Pulmonary hypoplasia, tracheoesophageal fistula, alveolar dysplasia | Chylothorax | |
| Trisomy 18 | Pulmonary malsegmentation to aplasia of right lung; tracheoesophageal fistula | | |
| Trisomy 13 | Situs inversus of lungs; calcified pulmonary arterioles; congenital diaphragmatic hernia | | |
| Pallister-Hall syndrome | Laryngeal cleft, dysplastic tracheal cartilage, absent lung, abnormal lung lobation | Hypoplasia/absent epiglottis | 146510 |
| Pfeiffer syndrome | Tracheal stenosis, laryngotracheomalacia | Broad short thumbs and big toes; FGFR-2 defects | 101600 |
| Smith-Lemli-Opitz syndrome type II | Unilobar lung | Postaxial polydactyly, cleft palate, cataracts, heart disease | 268670 |
| G syndrome, Opitz-Frias syndrome | Laryngotracheoesophageal cleft | Hypertelorism, hoarse cry; X-linked | 145410 |
| Hydrolethalus syndrome | Tracheal stenosis, abnormal lung lobation | | 236680 |
| Lung agenesis | May be bilateral; if unilateral, usually right is missing | | 601612 |
| Type 1 total anomalous pulmonary venous return | Unilateral pulmonary hypoplasia | Total anomalous pulmonary venous return | 106700 |
| Thymic aplasia with fetal death | Unilateral pulmonary agenesis, pulmonary hypoplasia | No parathyroid tissue, truncus arteriosis | 274210 |
| Matthew-Wood syndrome | Pulmonary hypoplasia | Anophthalmia, microphthalmia | 601186 |
| Familial pulmonary hypoplasia | Pulmonary hypoplasia | | 265430 |
| Larsen-like syndrome, lethal type | Pulmonary hypoplasia, tracheomalacia | Collagen fiber dysmaturity | 245650 |
| Aphalangy with hemivertebrae | Pulmonary hypoplasia | Aphalangy of hands, feet | 207620 |
| **Syndromes Associated with Hypotonia and Decreased Fetal Breathing** | | | |
| Pena-Shokeir syndrome type I | Pulmonary hypoplasia | Fetal akinesia sequence | 208150 |
| COFS syndrome (Pena-Shokeir syndrome type II) | Pulmonary hypoplasia | Hypotonia, large ears, arthrogryposis, camptodactyly | 214150 |
| Myasthenia gravis | Pulmonary hypoplasia | Similar to fetal akinesia sequence | 254200 |
| **Syndromes Associated with Restriction of Thoracic Volume** | | | |
| Pulmonary cystic lymphangiectasis | Pulmonary hypoplasia | Bilateral chylothoraces | 265300 |
| Lethal congenital contracture syndrome | Pulmonary hypoplasia | Contractures, short thorax, hydrops | 253310 |
| Tight skin contracture syndrome | Pulmonary hypoplasia | Contractures, tight thin skin | 275210 |
| Pterygium syndrome | Pulmonary hypoplasia | Arthrogryposis | 265000 |
| Spondylospinal thoracic dysostosis | Pulmonary hypoplasia | Arthrogryposis, micrognathia | 601809 |
| Jeune asphyxiating thoracic dystrophy | Pulmonary hypoplasia | Small narrow thorax, polydactyly, hepatic and renal abnormalities | 208500 |
| Neonatal osseous dysplasia I | Pulmonary hypoplasia, laryngeal stenosis, tracheobronchomalacia | Skeletal dysplasia | 256060 |
| Short rib–polydactyly syndrome types II and IV | Pulmonary hypoplasia | Hydrops, narrow chest | 269860<br>263520 |
| Osteosclerotic bone dysplasia, lethal | Pulmonary hypoplasia | Craniofacial defects, osteosclerosis | 259775 |

*Continued*

**TABLE 42-1**

**Genetic Disorders and Syndromes Associated with Pulmonary Abnormalities—Cont'd**

| Genetic Condition | Pulmonary Abnormality | Associated Finding(s) | OMIM Ref.* |
|---|---|---|---|
| Dyssegmental dysplasia, Silver-Handmaker type | Pulmonary hypoplasia | Short-limbed dwarfism, abnormal vertebral bodies; defect in perlecan | 224410 |
| Tetra-amelia | Pulmonary hypoplasia | Amelia, pulmonary vascular anomalies | 276695 |
| **Syndromes Associated with Decreased Amniotic Fluid** | | | |
| Renal tubular dysgenesis | Pulmonary hypoplasia | Potter phenotype | 267430 |
| Renal dysplasia–limb defects syndrome | Pulmonary hypoplasia | Potter phenotype | 266910 |
| Hereditary urogenital adysplasia | Pulmonary hypoplasia | Potter phenotype | 191830 |
| Nephronophthisis 2 | Pulmonary hypoplasia | Potter phenotype | 602088 |
| Diffuse cystic renal dysplasia | Pulmonary hypoplasia | Potter phenotype | 601331 |
| Diaphragmatic defects, limb deficiency, and ossification defects | Congenital diaphragmatic hernia, pulmonary hypoplasia | Potter phenotype | 601163 |
| Meckel syndrome (Meckel-Gruber syndrome) | Pulmonary hypoplasia | Potter phenotype, posterior encephalocele, polydactyly | 249000 |
| PKD1 | Pulmonary hypoplasia | Potter phenotype | 601313 |
| Autosomal recessive PKD | Pulmonary hypoplasia | Potter phenotype | 263200 |

COFS, cerebro-oculofacial-skeletal; FGFR, fibroblast growth factor receptor; OMIM, Online Mendelian Inheritance in Man; PKD, polycystic kidney disease.

*Numbers are those used in OMIM classification. Data available at http://www.ncbi.nlm.nih.gov:80/entrez/query.fcgi?db = OMIM

expression of FGFR-2 in key positions along the expanding tubule determines the location of primary, secondary, and tertiary branches. In another complex feedback network, FGF-10 signaling from the epithelium also induces the expression of bone morphogenetic protein-4 (BMP-4), another member of the TGF-β superfamily, by the mesenchyme, which inhibits epithelial proliferation, thus limiting tubule length. Other families of growth and transcription factors assist in the regulation of lung morphogenesis, including the epithelial growth factor (EGF)/EGF receptor family, insulin-like growth factors/receptors, platelet-derived growth factors and their receptors, and other members of the TGF-β superfamily. The complex interplay of these networks is reviewed elsewhere (Cardoso, 1995; Costa et al, 2001). Components of extracellular matrix are vital to branching morphogenesis and microvascular development by influencing cell adhesion, cell shape, and cytoskeletal organization, as well as providing a scaffold for cell-cell signaling (Dunsmore and Rannels, 1996). For example, interference in the assembly of fibronectin matrix, which is thought to provide positional information for cell migrations, inhibits branching in embryonic lungs.

Errors in the developmental program during the later embryonic and/or pseudoglandular stages may result in a form of pulmonary hypoplasia that is characterized by decreased numbers of bronchial segments that contain an appropriate number of alveoli per bronchiole as indicated by radial alveolar counting (Hislop and Reid, 1981). Congenital diaphragmatic hernia results from a developmental error in this period. Closure of the pleuriperitoneal canals occurs by 7 weeks of gestation, thereby separating the pleural from the peritoneal cavity. Failure of closure results in a diaphragmatic defect permitting continuity between these spaces. With this defect, at 10 weeks, when the midgut returns to the peritoneal cavity, abdominal contents are free to pass into the thoracic cavity and restrict the space into which the lung grows. The molecular mechanisms governing the development of the pleuroperitoneal folds and their closure, and the migration of myoblasts into these membranes to form the diaphragm, are poorly understood. Administration of nitrofen, a herbicide with structural similarity to thyroid hormone, early in rodent gestation induces unilateral or bilateral diaphragmatic defects. This line of evidence has been a valuable model of congenital diaphragmatic hernia.

As branching morphogenesis continues, maturation of more proximal epithelium follows. Some of the same growth factors modulating branching also influence cell fate of the once-undifferentiated epithelium. Thyroid transcription factor-1 (TTF-1), a product of the *Nkx2.1* gene, plays an important role in embryonic lung branching; transgenic mice null for *Nkx2.1* exhibit complete absence of lung branching (reviewed in Cardoso, 1995). However, *Nkx2.1* also plays a prominent role in establishing cell fate, specifically of alveolar type II cells. The physiologic role of endogenous corticosteroids, thyroid hormones, and potentially other circulating hormones is limited to modulation of the rate of differentiation of both mesenchymal and epithelial cells after completion of airway branching. This role is well illustrated for glucocorticoids by the arrest of lung cellular differentiation at about fetal day 16, after branching morphogenesis is complete, in transgenic mice with knockout of either corticotrophin-releasing hormone or glucocorticoid receptor (Muglia et al, 1995; Schmid et al, 1995).

## The Terminal Sac and Alveolar Phases

The *acinus* is the gas exchange unit of the lung and encompasses a respiratory bronchiole and all of its associated alveolar ducts and alveoli (West, 1990). A terminal bronchiole with all of its associated acinar structures constitutes a *lobule*. Ultimately, the zone of gas exchange will attain a surface area of 50 to 100 $m^2$, with a volume of 2.5 to 3.0 L in the adult human. Branching of the most distal air spaces continues on a more limited basis during the terminal sac and alveolar phases, finally achieving a total of 23 airway subdivisions by the end of the terminal sac phase, while evolution of the relationships between the air spaces, capillaries, and mesenchyme takes on more significance.

Lengthening and widening of the terminal sacs serve to expand the surface area available for gas exchange. Each saccule will give rise to two to three alveolar ducts, further expanding the available surface area. The expansion of surface area and luminal volume compresses the interstitium, bringing the capillary networks in close proximity to potential air spaces, thereby promoting alveolar development and later capillary bed fusion. At this stage, a complete capillary network is available for each acinus, effectively creating a double circulation between acini. Capillary networks investing separate acini will fuse as the interstitium separating alveoli thins toward birth, a process that is not complete until 18 months of postnatal age.

The basement membrane and interstitial extracellular matrix components appear to play important roles in alveologenesis as well as in the differentiation of types I and II epithelial cells (Dunsmore and Rannels, 1996; Wright et al, 1999). Production of elastic fibers, composed of elastin and microfibrillar proteins, begins at mid-gestation and extends through the neonatal period (reviewed in Dunsmore and Rannels, 1996; Mariani et al, 1997; Schuger, 1997). Elastin is a polymer of cross-linked tropoelastin precursor protein and constitutes approximately 90% of the mass of the fibers. A variety of glycoproteins makes up the microfibrils that serve as a scaffold for elastin deposition. Elastin, localized to the walls of alveoli and pulmonary vessels, allows for repetitive deformations in the shape and size of these structures. Excess elastin or diminished content of elastin in diseases such as pulmonary hypertension and fibrotic conditions can severely compromise the strength and formation of blood vessels and alveoli.

The alveolar basement membrane includes laminin, entactin, types IV and V collagen, chondroitin sulfate and chondroitin sulfate proteoglycan, heparan sulfate proteoglycans, and fibronectin. Basement membrane components are important in the regulation of epithelial differentiation into surfactant-producing type II cells and the thin type I cell that participates in gas exchange and alveolar fluid homeostasis. The local concentration of basement membrane components may regulate the location of type II cells (at the corners of alveoli) and the relative ratio of types I and II alveolar cells. There is evidence that the type II cell basement membrane is discontinuous, allowing maintenance of direct cell-cell interactions with cells of the interstitium, specifically fibroblasts (Adamson, 1992). In addition, in vitro studies have shown that extracellular matrix can have dramatic effects on maintenance of type II cell phenotype in isolated cell culture. The developmental program governing extracellular matrix composition during alveolar epithelial cell differentiation probably is recapitulated after epithelial damage by airborne or blood-borne toxic agents. Because type II cells are the source of type I cells after injury, alterations in extracellular matrix composition are essential to reconstitute a functional, differentiated alveolar lining. Moreover, aberrant signaling during the repair process may lead to abnormalities in extracellular matrix deposition and reconstitution of the alveolar lining, thereby contributing to the pathobiology of lung diseases such as bronchopulmonary dysplasia. The interplay of extracellular matrix (ECM) components and proteases involved in the remodeling of ECM reinforces the dynamic nature of ECM during lung development and injury repair (reviewed in Parks and Shapiro, 2001). For example, the aberrant alveologenesis that occurs in EGF receptor–knockout mice is associated with a dramatic reduction in matrix metalloproteinase-2 (MMP-2). The MMP-2–knockout mouse model phenocopies the alveolar defects of the EGF receptor knockout, indicating that the abnormal alveologenesis of the EGF receptor knockout is due in part to abnormal modulation of ECM components (Kheradmand et al, 2002).

The development of primary alveoli is followed by a further expansion of the gas exchange surface area through the formation of septa, or secondary crests. Primitive saccules develop low ridges that subdivide the saccule into an alveolar duct (primary septa) and outpouchings between the ridges (secondary septa) (Fig. 42–2). Regions destined for secondary septation exhibit increased elastin deposition (Mariani et al, 1997). Septa contain a connective tissue core separating two capillary membranes, suggesting that the septum is formed by the folding of the capillary on itself. This folding occurs in regions in which the double capillary network is preserved between acini or, alternatively, at pleural surfaces or adjacent to large blood vessels and conducting airways. Septation also leads to the development of the pores of Kohn, allowing gaseous continuity between acini.

There is controversy regarding the completion of alveolarization. Current estimates suggest that the formation of new alveoli is complete by approximately 2 to 3 years of postnatal life, achieving a total of between 200 million and 600 million alveoli (Davies and Reid, 1970). Lung growth is not complete at this stage, however. Between 4 years of age and adulthood, there is extensive linear growth, which includes expansion of the thoracic cavity. Increased intrathoracic volume increases the negative pressure generated by diaphragmatic excursions, thereby allowing three- dimensional stretch of alveoli, which increases alveolar volume. In total, lung volume increases 23-fold between birth and adulthood. The capillary bed expands at a greater pace, achieving a 34-fold expansion over the same period. Thus, compared with adult lung, the term

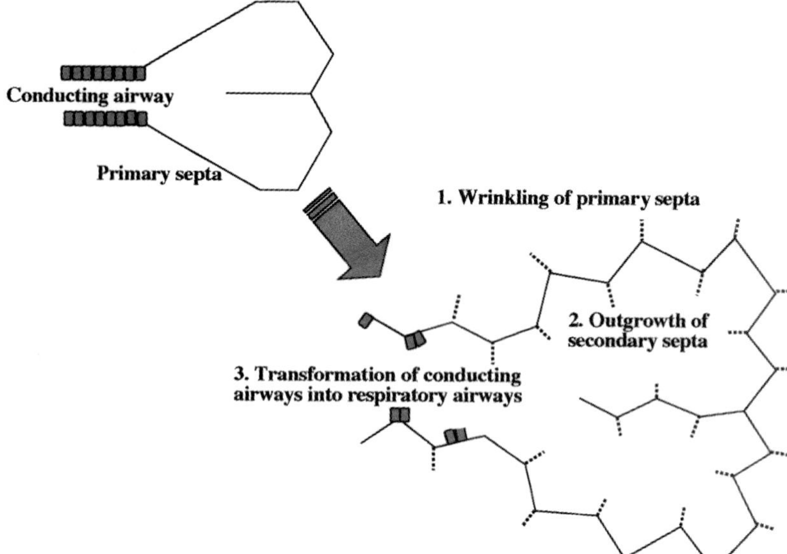


**FIGURE 42–2.** Primary and secondary septa.

newborn has relatively less lung volume per kilogram of body weight, increased interstitial components relative to air space, and a smaller capillary bed.

The physiologic factors regulating growth of the lung during postnatal life are not well understood. Treatment of animals with corticosteroids, can reduce lung weight through direct effects on cell replication (e.g., in newborn rats) and indirectly in the fetus by accelerating placental senescence and impairing function (Okajima et al, 2001; Tschanz et al, 1995). Postnatally, lung growth is stimulated after partial pneumonectomy but there is little information on mediating agents and mechanism of action (Holmes and Thurlbeck, 1979).

## PHYSICAL FACTORS INFLUENCING LUNG DEVELOPMENT

The role of physical factors in modulating lung size is well established. Normal growth requires adequate space in the chest cavity and appropriate tonic and cyclic distending forces. Genetic defects that compromise the thoracic skeleton are associated with pulmonary hypoplasia as a result of the restriction of intrathoracic space. In animal models, denervation of the diaphragm to eliminate fetal breathing movements also is associated with pulmonary hypoplasia. Finally, manipulation of fetal lung fluid volume can modulate lung growth in utero, although the mechanisms for this effect remain unclear.

### Fetal Lung Fluid

In fetal animals, lung growth is reduced by maneuvers such as cervical spinal cord transection (denervating the diaphragm); removing a portion of the rib cage, thereby reducing chest wall rigidity; chronic drainage of amniotic fluid; and tracheostomy that allows free efflux of lung fluid. The common thread is reduction of the tonic or cyclic stretch imposed on the developing lung (Dobbs and Gutierrez, 2001). In contrast, tracheal occlusion, which increases intraluminal pressure, increases lung dry weight. These and other experimental observations have led to the proposal that fetal breathing movements retard loss of lung liquid and maintain lung expansion in the face of decreased upper airway resistance, whereas during periods of nonbreathing there is tonic inflation secondary to laryngeal abduction (Harding, 1984; Harding et al, 1986). Both of these stretching events may stimulate production of growth-mediating factors such as insulin-like growth factor-II and platelet-derived growth factor B by lung fibroblasts. The mechanisms by which mechanical forces are transduced into epithelial cell proliferation and differentiation are largely unexplored.

Fetal lung fluid is a product of the epithelial lining of the developing lung (reviewed in Hooper and Harding, 1995). Its composition is distinct from that of both amniotic fluid and plasma, as illustrated in Table 42–2. The increased chloride content of fetal lung fluid as compared with serum is due to the ability of the tracheal and distal pulmonary epithelium to actively secrete chloride into the potential air spaces. The identity of the chloride pump remains unclear; however, its action can be inhibited by a variety of mediators, including beta-adrenergic agonists, arginine vasopressin, and prostaglandin $E_2$. Production of fetal lung fluid averages 4 to 6 mL/kg/hour. Because of the resistance imparted by laryngeal abduction, fluid accumulates to a total volume of 20 to 30 mL/kg during gestation, providing end-expiratory pressure of approximately 4 cm $H_2O$.

Despite the importance of fetal lung fluid to lung growth and development, the transition to an air-breathing environment must be coupled with the conversion from a secretory pulmonary epithelium to one that is absorptive. Enhanced sodium transport across the alveolar epithelium is in part responsible for this change. Much evidence suggests that induction of components of the epithelial sodium channels (ENaC) around the time of birth is a major factor in promoting sodium transport,

**TABLE 42-2**

**Composition of Human Fetal Lung Liquid Compared with Other Body Fluids**

| Component | Lung Liquid | Interstitial Fluid | Plasma | Amniotic Fluid |
|---|---|---|---|---|
| Sodium (mEq/L) | 150 | 147 | 150 | 113 |
| Potassium (mEq/L) | 6.3 | 4.8 | 4.8 | 7.6 |
| Chloride (mEq/L) | 157 | 107 | 107 | 87 |
| Bicarbonate (mEq/L) | 3 | 25 | 24 | 19 |
| pH | 6.27 | 7.31 | 7.34 | 7.02 |
| Protein (g/dL) | 0.03 | 3.27 | 4.09 | 0.10 |

with water passively following the movement of sodium (reviewed in Jain, 1999). Transgenic knockout animals devoid of the α subunit of ENaC die at birth due to failure to clear fetal lung fluid. The α-ENaC subunit is dramatically up-regulated just before birth, whereas the β and γ subunits are not up-regulated until shortly after birth. Induction of ENaC components occurs at a transcriptional level in response to changes in ECM components, glucocorticoids, aldosterone, and oxygen. By contrast, agents that increase intracellular cyclic adenosine monophosphate (cAMP) levels (i.e., beta agonists, phosphodiesterase inhibitors, and cAMP analogues), although not increasing the number of sodium channels, increase the probability of a channel being open to sodium transport as a result of phosphorylation of the subunits.

Water channels, consisting of aquaporins, also are induced during the late fetal period to facilitate fluid movement (Song et al, 2000). Aquaporin 5 is expressed by alveolar type I cells, whereas aquaporin 4 is expressed in airway epithelial cells and aquaporin 1 in pulmonary endothelial cells. In contrast with the α-ENaC −/− mice, newborn transgenic animals deficient in aquaporin 5 or both 5 and 1 survive despite reduced water permeabilities (reviewed in Verkman et al, 2000).

On delivery of the head and neck, continued uterine contractions on the fetal thorax promote expulsion of bulk fluid from the fetal lung. The absence of uterine contractions is associated with an increased incidence of retained fetal lung fluid in infants delivered by cesarean section without the benefit of labor. However, animal studies have shown that the magnitude of the benefit of thoracic compression during labor is modest (reviewed in Bland, 2001). The primary mechanism by which labor facilitates clearance of lung fluid, thereby reducing the incidence of transient tachypnea of the newborn, is through hormonal effects on fluid clearance, such as α-ENaC, especially through catecholamines. The onset of air breathing, associated with increased intrathoracic negative pressure, assists in the clearance of residual fetal lung fluid into the loose interstitial tissues surrounding alveoli. Fluid is then reabsorbed via lymphatics and pulmonary blood vessels.

### Fetal Breathing Movements

Fetal breathing is an essential stimulus for lung growth and for successful respiratory effort after birth (Blanco, 1994; Harding, 1997). Fetal breathing is readily detectable as early as 10 weeks of gestation in the human fetus. Fetal breathing occurs for 10% to 20% of the time at 24 to 28 weeks and for 30% to 40% of the time after 30 weeks of gestation. Originating from the diaphragm, fetal breathing is erratic in frequency and amplitude, and changes throughout gestation. The volume of fluid moved is small and insufficient to be cleared from the trachea. Respiratory rates ranging from 30 to 70 breaths/minute, in addition to periods of apnea of up to 2 hours, have been recorded. Sustained periods of fetal breathing increase in duration with advancing gestation. The frequency of fetal breathing varies with sleep state (inhibited during quiet sleep) and exhibits diurnal variation, with the lowest rates recorded early in the morning. Fetal breathing is hormonally responsive, and the inhibition of fetal breathing at the onset of labor is attributed to the action of increased circulating prostaglandins (Rigatto, 1996). Similarly, maternal medications can influence the frequency of fetal breathing movements. Central nervous system stimulants (e.g., caffeine, amphetamines) are associated with increased fetal breathing, whereas depressants (e.g., anesthetics, narcotics, ethanol) are associated with decreased fetal breathing. Maternal smoking is associated with reduced fetal breathing, largely as a result of the associated relative hypoxemia. Animal studies have clearly shown that permanent cessation of fetal breathing, regardless of the insult, is associated with impaired fetal lung growth. However, the impact of short-term alterations in frequency and amplitude of fetal breathing on fetal lung development is unknown.

After delivery, the breathing pattern changes from episodic and erratic to continuous and regular. There are several mechanisms by which postnatal breathing patterns are established (Jansen and Chernick, 1991). Animal studies suggest that delivery triggers the withdrawal of inhibitory signaling on the midbrain. Similarly, it has been suggested that withdrawal of a placental inhibitory factor is in part responsible for the initiation of continuous breathing, although no substance has been identified to date. Skin cooling and a concomitant reduction in core temperature are potent sensory stimuli for initiating and maintaining continuous breathing. The most detailed studies, however, have been related to the roles of oxygen and carbon dioxide in postnatal breathing. Central and peripheral chemoreceptors are reset with the onset of continuous breathing, allowing for increased sensitivity to $P_{CO_2}$ immediately after birth as a primary mechanism for continuous breathing. By contrast, hypoxemia does not appear to play a role in maintaining continuous breathing for several days postnatally.

## LUNG EPITHELIAL CELL DIFFERENTIATION

As branching morphogenesis proceeds, the epithelium lining the successive generations of airways and, ultimately, alveoli give rise to specialized cells that participate in gas exchange, mucociliary clearance, and host defense. Differentiation proceeds in a centrifugal fashion from proximal to distal air spaces, lagging behind branching. Temporal as well as contextual signals foster the regionalization of epithelial cell types.

### Proximal Airways

The airway epithelial cells are tall and columnar, decreasing to a more cuboidal appearance in the most distal segments (Jeffrey, 1998). The endodermal epithelial lining cells of the conducting airways differentiate into four cell types: ciliated, mucus-secreting goblet, indeterminate, and basal cells. A fifth cell, the pulmonary neuroendocrine cell, is not endodermal in origin but originates from neural crest cells migrating into the lung during development (reviewed in Warburton et al, 1998). Cartilaginous support of the tracheobronchial tree begins and proceeds in a centrifugal fashion, beginning in the primitive trachea at approximately 10 weeks and proceeding to the most distal terminal bronchioles by approximately 25 weeks.

### Distal Airways

The bronchiolar epithelium differs from the more proximal airway epithelium in the contribution of Clara cells to the epithelial cell population. The nonciliated, secretory Clara cell is found in increasing numbers and density down the conducting airways, such that the Clara cell is the most abundant cell of the terminal bronchiole (reviewed in Massaro et al, 1994; Plopper, 1997). Clara cells are critical to the host defense and detoxification functions of the lung. This specialized cell produces the highest levels of cytochrome P-450 and flavin mono-oxygenases of the 40 known lung cell types. These enzyme systems are important in detoxification but also participate in the bioactivation of procarcinogens, placing the Clara cell in a delicate balance between these two activities. Accordingly, Clara cells are one of the primary targets of toxic metabolites. Other important products of the Clara cell include Clara cell secretory protein (CCSP or CC10); surfactant proteins A, B, and D (SP-A, SP-B, SP-D); leukocyte protease inhibitor; and a trypsin-like protease. CC10, SP A, and SP D have important roles in regulating inflammatory responses within the lung, both from pathogens and allergens. Despite SP-B immunoreactivity, Clara cells are incapable of completing the proteolysis of SP-B to its mature, surface-active form, implying that the other products of SP-B processing have additional function in the airways. The secretion of antiproteases from Clara cells indicates that these cells play an important role in maintaining the protease-antiprotease balance in the lung. Clara cells are detected in proximal bronchi as early as 15 weeks of gestation, appearing in scattered bronchioles by 18 weeks. Between 23 and 34 weeks, there is a dramatic increase in Clara cell numbers as well as in CC10 expression in distal bronchioles. Although transcription factors known to be important in type II cell differentiation and in the expression of type II cell–specific genes also control the expression of Clara cell–specific genes (e.g., TTF-1, GATA6), little is known about the regulation of Clara cell differentiation. However, like type II cells, the Clara cell is responsive to injury, proliferating in response to epithelial injury and transdifferentiating into ciliated epithelial cells to repopulate the airway.

### Alveolar Epithelium

During months 4 to 6 of gestation, the epithelial cells lining the acini begin to differentiate further (Brody and Williams, 1992; Mallampalli et al, 1997). The cuboidal epithelial cells accumulate large glycogen stores and develop small vesicles containing loose lamellae. In cells destined to become type II cells, lamellar bodies become larger, more numerous, and more densely packed with surfactant phospholipids and proteins, whereas those cells destined to become type I cells, on losing their relationship to mesenchymal fibroblasts, lose the prelamellar vesicles and thin progressively, thereby adopting a phenotype more suitable for gas exchange. Type I and type II cells are readily identified early in the terminal sac stage of fetal lung development. Induction of the components of pulmonary surfactant results in the increased synthesis and storage of surfactant in the increasing numbers of lamellar bodies within type II cells (Fig. 42–3). From approximately 24 weeks of human gestation, the acini and the alveolar-capillary membrane are sufficiently developed to support gas exchange, but the limiting factor for successful air breathing is the maturation of the surfactant system.

Differentiation of precursor epithelial cells into type II cells, and subsequently into type I cells, is under both negative and positive regulation, and these effects occur primarily through altered gene expression. Type II cell differentiation in vitro is blocked by TGF-β, which acts in part by restricting the availability of transcription factors (e.g., TTF-1, hepatic nuclear factor-3) that are required for synthesis of type II cell–specific genes. It is likely that TGF and other growth-promoting factors inhibit the differentiation process in developing lung in vivo; in later gestation, a decline in level or activity of these factors promotes cell differentiation. Glucocorticoids and agents that stimulate production of cAMP antagonize TGF-β effects and stimulate cell differentiation through induction and repression of specific genes. In culture systems, these hormones cause precocious development of type II cells, inducing approximately 2% of genes that are expressed in lung epithelial cells. The spectrum of the hormonal response includes proteins of all categories of structural and functional activity in addition to type II cell—specific genes such as surfactant components. A number of transcription factors is induced, some with known function related to surfactant production (e.g., TTF-1, CAAT enhancer–binding protein), and these in turn control expression of target genes. Regulation of gene transcription involves many different proteins that often interact with each other and/or nucleic acid. Categories of these nuclear proteins include transcription factors, coactivators, corepressors, histones, enzymes that modify nuclear proteins, DNA or RNA, proteins of the transcriptional machinery (e.g., RNA polymerase), and receptors for ligands such as corticosteroids and retinoic

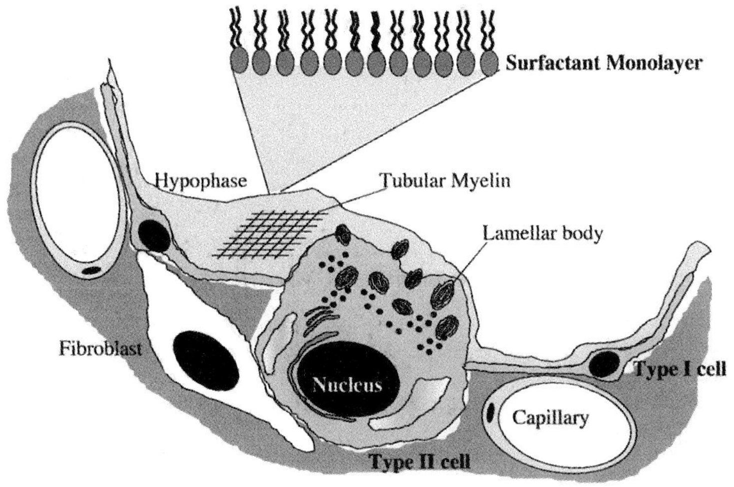


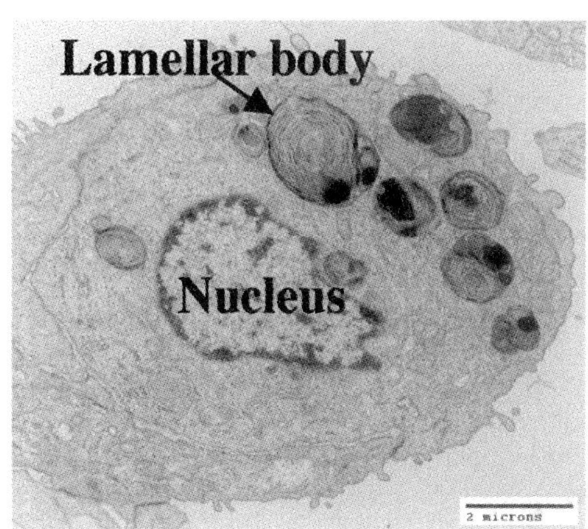


**FIGURE 42–3.** Lamellar bodies within type II cells.

acid. Clearly, regulation of epithelial cell differentiation is a complex molecular process that incorporates actions of a variety of signaling molecules and target genes.

## Surfactant

After bulk removal of fetal lung fluid at birth, a thin layer of lung liquid remains to protect the delicate alveolar epithelium. The surface tension generated by this aqueous layer opposes alveolar inflation and promotes alveolar collapse at the low alveolar volumes at end-expiration. The film of surfactant at the air-liquid interface lowers surface tension as alveolar surface area decreases, thereby preventing alveolar collapse, maintaining functional residual capacity, and lowering the force required for subsequent alveolar inflation.

Surfactant is a mixture of phospholipids, neutral lipids, and proteins that are synthesized, packaged, and secreted by alveolar type II cells (reviewed in Hawgood and Clements, 1990) (Table 42–3). Storage of surfactant occurs in a lysosome-derived, membrane-bound organelle, the lamellar body, which undergoes regulated secretion in response to a variety of stimuli, most of which result in increased intracellular calcium levels. In the alveolus, surfactant phospholipids undergo transition through an extracellular storage form, tubular myelin, in association with SP-A and SP-B. The hydrophobic SP-B and SP-C are necessary to liberate surfactant phospholipids from this structure and to order phospholipids in the monolayer at the air-liquid interface. Phospholipid and protein components are recycled out of the monolayer and back into the alveolar type II cell, where they can be repackaged into lamellar bodies. Alternatively, alveolar macrophages are able to phagocytize and degrade surfactant components (Wright, 1990).

**TABLE 42–3**

**Composition of Pulmonary Surfactant**

| Component | Percentage (by weight) |
|---|---|
| Lipid | 90 |
| Saturated phosphatidylcholine | 45 |
| Unsaturated phosphatidylcholine | 25 |
| Phosphatidylglycerol | 5 |
| Other phospholipids | 5 |
| Neutral lipids | 10 |
| Protein | 10 |
| Surfactant proteins | 5 |
| Serum proteins | 5 |

The predominant surfactant phospholipid is disaturated phosphatidylcholine (specifically, dipalmitoyl phosphatidylcholine [DPPC]), with the remaining phospholipids consisting of monounsaturated phosphatidylcholine and other phospholipids (Rooney, 1989). Disaturated phospholipids are compressible, allowing for packing of the surface film at end-expiration that reduces surface tension to nearly zero. The amounts of DPPC and phosphatidylglycerol in fetal lung increase with advancing gestation due to increased activity of enzymes responsible for phospholipid synthesis. The expression and activity of enzymes of the choline incorporation pathway, the predominant pathway for surfactant phospholipid synthesis, not only are developmentally regulated but are also induced by hormones, specifically glucocorticoids, thyroid hormone, and agents that increase intracellular cAMP.

Surfactant contains a group of specific proteins with functions relevant to many of the primary functions of the lung (Kuroki and Voelker, 1994). The four surfactant proteins—SP-A, SP-B, SP-C, and SP-D—are subdivided on the basis of their physical characteristics into hydrophobic (SP-B and SP-C) and hydrophilic (SP-A and SP-D) proteins. The hydrophobic surfactant proteins play a major role in the surface-active properties of surfactant, whereas the primary roles of the hydrophilic surfactant proteins are in host defense (see later on) and surfactant clearance and metabolism. SP-B is a secretory protein that exhibits strong association with membranes; SP-C contains a membrane-spanning domain that integrates the protein into phospholipid layers (reviewed in Weaver and Conkright, 2001). Both are synthesized as large precursor pro-proteins that undergo extensive post-translational processing through the secretory pathway, ultimately leading to the lamellar body. SP-B is essential for the process of lamellar body genesis, and the alveolar type II cells of infants with inherited deficiency of SP-B are devoid of lamellar bodies. Lamellar bodies are the site of final events in SP-C processing, and infants with inherited deficiency of SP-B are therefore deficient in mature SP-C, instead accumulating a larger precursor of SP-C. Thus, patients with inherited deficiency of SP-B, despite having relatively normal surfactant phospholipid profiles, make a pulmonary surfactant with very poor surface tension properties due to the combined defects in SP-B and SP-C synthesis. Together, the hydrophobic proteins facilitate the release of surfactant phospholipid from tubular myelin to the surface monolayer and promote spreading of lipids in the film and film stability at the end-expiration (Veldhuizen and Haagsman, 2000).

SP-B and SP-C exhibit developmental and hormonal regulation of expression (reviewed in Mendelson, 2000). In human fetuses, SP-C mRNA is detected as early as 12 weeks of gestation and SP-B mRNA by 14 weeks of gestation, yet the mature proteins are not detectable in fetal lung tissue until after 24 weeks of gestation. Furthermore, SP-B protein is not detectable in amniotic fluid until after 30 weeks of gestation (Fig. 42–4), increasing toward term (Pryhuber et al, 1991). This is due to developmental regulation of post-translational events in the proteolytic processing of pro-SP-B and pro-SP-C. Consequently, infants delivered prematurely have reduced levels of both surface-active components of surfactant, phospholipid, and hydrophobic surfactant proteins.

In the absence of adequate amounts of mature pulmonary surfactant, preterm infants develop progressive atelectasis and respiratory distress syndrome. The rate of type II cell differentiation and, secondarily, of surfactant production by the fetal lung, is modulated by levels of endogenous corticosteroids and is accelerated by administration of glucocorticoid (Mendelson, 2000). The response of the surfactant system to glucocorticoid involves all of the lipid and protein components and occurs primarily through increased gene expression, thus representing precocious maturation mimicking the normal developmental pattern and processes. Glucocorticoids probably also enhance maturation of other cell types, as well as the extracellular matrix, but these effects are less well characterized. Endogenous thyroid hormones, prostaglandins, and catecholamines also have stimulatory effects on type II cell maturation as well as clearance of lung fluid at birth. Certain cytokines (e.g., tumor necrosis factor-α [TNF-α], TGF-β) inhibit surfactant production in experimental systems and may down-regulate surfactant in conditions such as sepsis and inflammation. A partial list of hormones capable of inducing or inhibiting surfactant components is presented in Table 42–4.

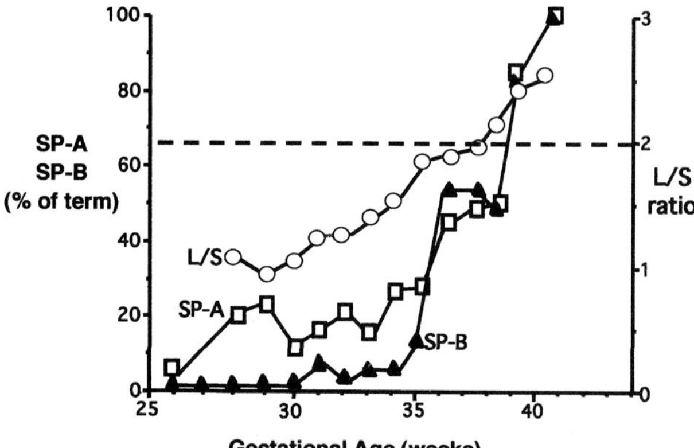


**FIGURE 42–4.** Levels of SP-A and SP-B proteins in amniotic fluid plotted against gestational age.

## Development of the Pulmonary Vasculature

The pulmonary vasculature consists of the vascular supply to the acini and the bronchial circulation (Burri, 1997). Branching of the pulmonary arteries follows branching of bronchi and bronchioli up to the acinar level, and for each airway branch, the pulmonary artery branches are 2 to 3 times more numerous. Pulmonary venous development occurs in the connective tissue septa between airway branches and parallel arterial divisions. The proximal pulmonary arteries and veins develop through the process of

**TABLE 42–4**

**Regulators of Alveolar Type II Cell Differentiation**

| Agent | Proposed Physiologic Role |
|---|---|
| **Inducers** | |
| Glucocorticoids (cortisol) | Major endogenous modulator of alveolar development and surfactant production |
| Beta-adrenergic agonists (epinephrine) | Increase surfactant production and secretion, especially during labor and delivery |
| Cyclic AMP | |
| Thyroid hormones ($T_3$, $T_4$) | Enhance glucocorticoid effects on lipid synthesis |
| Retinoic acid | May interact with glucocorticoids to regulate lipid and SP-B production |
| Bombesin-related peptides | May contribute to surfactant lipid synthesis |
| Parathyroid hormone–related protein (PTHrP) | |
| **Inhibitors** | |
| Protein kinase C activators (proinflammatory cytokines) | Inhibit surfactant protein gene transcription during infection, inflammation |
| TGF-β family | Inhibit type II cell maturation during early gestation and with inflammation |
| TNF-α | Inhibit SP-B and SP-C gene transcription during infection |
| Insulin | Inhibit surfactant protein gene transcription in infants of diabetic mothers with poorly controlled disease |
| Dihydrotestosterone | Delayed type II cell maturation in males |

SP-B, SP-C, surfactant proteins B, C; $T_3$, triiodothyronine; $T_4$, thyroxine; TGF, transforming growth factor; TNF, tumor necrosis factor.

angiogenesis, whereby new vascular structures arise from existing vessels; endothelial cells migrate out and organize to form a central lumen, thereby extending the length of the existing vessel. The second vascular supply to the lung, the bronchial circulation, arises first from the dorsal aorta in close proximity to the celiac axis (6 weeks) and is then replaced by definitive bronchial arteries arising from the aorta by 12 weeks. Persistence of rudimentary bronchial arteries is associated with developmental anomalies such as pulmonary sequestration.

The capillary network investing the acinus expands to match the increasing surface area of the developing acinar structures. Unlike the preacinar and resistance arteries that are present by 28 weeks of gestation, which arise through the process of *angiogenesis*, the more distal pulmonary vascular plexus arises de novo from the mesoderm surrounding the developing lung bud, a process known as *vasculogenesis* (reviewed in Baldwin, 1996). Angioblasts within the mesenchyme surrounding the acini differentiate into endothelial cells, proliferate, and organize into clusters that send out endothelial cells to establish a lumen. This network ultimately connects to the developing pulmonary arteries and veins. Alveolar-capillary dysplasia, an unusual and fatal cause of respiratory failure in the term neonate, is the result of developmental errors that prevent the appropriate interconnection of these vascular networks. Thinning of the interstitial mesenchyme surrounding the capillary network proceeds such that by 28 weeks, the alveolar-capillary membrane is similar in thickness to that in the adult (0.6 μm).

Muscularization of the preacinar and resistance arteries extends through the canalicular stage to term (reviewed in Stenmark and Mecham, 1997). The developing endothelial cells recruit smooth muscle cells and pericyte precursors, which are important in maintaining vascular integrity, through the action of growth factors such as angiopoietin-1. Muscularization normally occurs from pulmonary arteries to the level of the terminal bronchiole and is minimal in the vessels supplying respiratory bronchioles. Abnormal extension of smooth muscle along arterioles supplying acinar structures occurs in infants dying from persistent pulmonary hypertension of the newborn and in severe bronchopulmonary dysplasia.

## DEVELOPMENT OF PULMONARY HOST DEFENSE

The adult human lung takes in approximately 7 L/minute of air contaminated with a variety potential pathogens and particulates that can cause epithelial injury. An integrated system of host defense maintains the sterility and integrity of the gas exchange surface. The proximal and distal airway epithelia play a major role in clearance of potential pathogens. Components of mucociliary clearance appear at 11 to 13 weeks in human gestation with the differentiation of ciliated epithelial cells and the expression of mucus in mucus-secreting goblet cells within the epithelium as well as submucosal glands. The number of goblet cells peaks in mid-gestation (30% to 35% of total airway epithelial cells), decreasing toward term to levels lower than in adults and then increasing after birth. The postnatal increase in goblet cells occurs after preterm birth as well, resulting in greater numbers of goblet cells in preterm infants than in term infants. Therefore, premature infants are prone to more mucus production in smaller airways than term infants and have relatively fewer ciliated cells to assist in mobilization of secretions.

A number of microbial defense molecules are produced and secreted into the airways. They include lysozyme, C-reactive protein, lactoferrin (Wilmott et al, 2000), defensins (Weiss, 1994), cathelicidins (Lehrer and Ganz, 2002), and collectins. Collectins are molecules possessing collagen-like domains and a calcium-dependent lectin domain that recognizes and binds carbohydrates on proteins and lipids. The lung collectins, the hydrophilic SP-A and SP-D, are secreted by epithelial cells lining airways (Clara cells) and alveoli (type II cells) (reviewed in Crouch and Wright, 2001; McCormack and Whitsett, 2002). They interact with microorganisms, inflammatory cells, and leukocytes to facilitate clearance of microorganisms from the air space. They interact in similar ways with inhaled pollens and other antigens to facilitate clearance and to modulate allergic responses.

The basis for the interactions of the lung collectins with microbes and antigens centers on the binding of sugars by the lectin domain, or carbohydrate recognition domain (Hakansson and Reid, 2000). Differences in the structure of the carbohydrate recognition domain provide SP-A and SP-D with altered affinities for different sugar molecules, allowing complementary functions and improving the diversity of microbial interactions. Collectins enhance the uptake of microorganisms and antigens in part through aggregation of multiple organisms by the carbohydrate recognition domain. Each individual collectin trimerizes through interactions between the collagen-like domains. The trimers further associate into octadecamers (six groups of 3) in the case of SP-A, conferring an appearance similar to a bouquet of tulips, or dodecamers (four groups of 3) in the case of SP-D, which associate in the form of a cross. This arrangement of SP-D facilitates the aggregation of multiple organisms and inflammatory cell surface receptors. Studies of the role(s) of the lung collectins in pulmonary infections have been greatly aided by the availability of knockout mouse models. Interactions with gram-negative organisms frequently depend on the ability of SP-A and SP-D to bind lipopolysaccharide, whereas the mechanism of SP-A interactions with gram-positive organisms, including group B beta-hemolytic streptococci, are not as clear (Fig. 42–5). Both collectins bind a variety of fungi as well as *Pneumocystis carinii* and play an important role in inhibiting a variety of respiratory viruses, including influenza A virus and respiratory syncytial virus.

The lung collectins also modulate the functions of a variety of immune cells, including macrophages, neutrophils, eosinophils, and lymphocytes (Wright, 1997). In addition to opsonizing microorganisms, functions of the lung collectins include stimulating chemotaxis of macrophages and neutrophils, enhancing cytokine production by macrophages and eosinophils, attenuating lymphocyte responses, and modulating the production of reactive oxygen and nitrogen species used in killing microorganisms.

Two highly homologous SP-A genes (*SPA1* and *SPA2*) lie in close proximity to the SP-D gene on chromosome 10 in

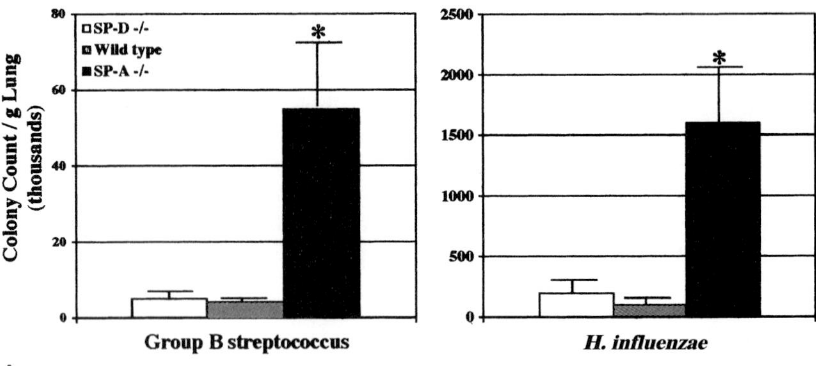


A

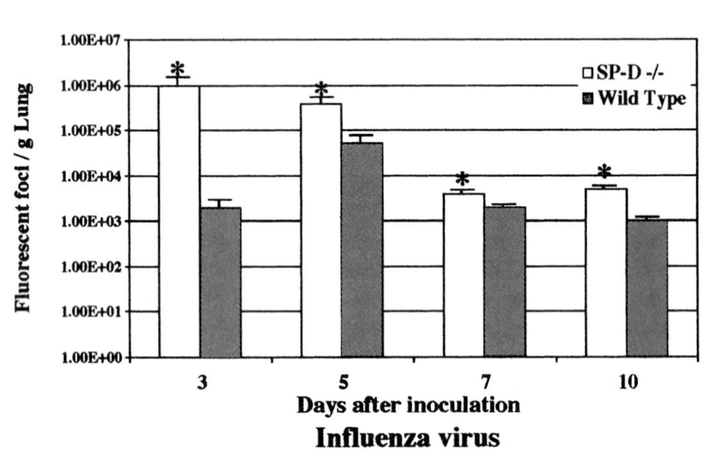


B

**FIGURE 42–5.** Presence of group B streptococci, *H. influenzae*, and influenza virus after inoculation into SP-A or SP-D knockout mice.

the human. Like the hydrophobic surfactant proteins, SP-A and SP-D exhibit both developmental and hormonal regulation of expression (reviewed in Mendelson, 2000). In human fetuses, SP-A mRNA is undetectable before 20 weeks of gestation, and SP-A protein is first detectable in amniotic fluid by 30 weeks (see Fig. 42–4), increasing toward term (Pryhuber et al, 1991). In humans, SP-A gene expression is induced by cAMP and glucocorticoids, although the response to glucocorticoids is biphasic, showing attenuation at higher doses. Retinoids, insulin, and growth factors such as TGF-β and TNF-α inhibit SP-A gene expression. SP-A is produced and secreted by both alveolar type II cells and bronchiolar Clara cells. SP-D is produced in tracheobronchial glands as well as by type II and Clara cells. Like SP-A, SP-D levels in human lung are quite low during the second trimester (Dulkerian et al, 1996), increase toward term, and are detectable in amniotic fluid (Miyamura et al, 1994). Levels of both SP-A and SP-D increase markedly in the first days after preterm birth.

## Development of Detoxification Systems

Although oxygen is essential to cellular processes, excessive oxygen is damaging through direct toxicity of oxygen free radicals or indirectly from altered physiologic processes (reviewed in Weinberger et al, 2002). The lung is particularly susceptible to the damaging effects of free radicals. Oxygen free radicals are byproducts of the electron transport reactions of mitochondria that generate adenosine triphosphate (ATP) from molecular oxygen. Superoxide, produced by reduction of molecular oxygen with the addition of a single electron, is formed by all cells and occurs in high concentrations in phagocytic cells to facilitate the killing of microorganisms. Hydrogen peroxide is generated from the transfer of a single electron to superoxide. Hydroxyl radicals are generated from the interaction of hydrogen peroxide with superoxide. The free electrons of each of these species of free radicals can interact with membrane lipids resulting in lipid peroxidation, with proteins to oxidize sulfhydryl groups, and with DNA causing direct damage. This leads to damage of airway and alveolar epithelial cells as well as capillary endothelial cells. Compromise of epithelial integrity leads to interstitial and air space edema, followed by infiltration of neutrophils. The damaged alveolar epithelium heals through proliferation of the alveolar type II cell and can be accompanied by various degrees of pulmonary fibrosis.

Hyperoxia is a potent regulator of a variety of processes. Prolonged exposure to oxygen results in influx of neutrophils into the lung. Oxygen regulates the activity of plasminogen activator inhibitor-1 and other proteases and antiproteases within the air spaces, thereby modulating the destructive effects of proteases elaborated from inflammatory cells. Oxygen can also regulate growth responses by inhibiting the secretion of growth factors and reducing DNA synthesis. Therefore, it is understandable that oxygen toxicity is a central component of bronchopulmonary dysplasia.

Multiple defenses exist to attenuate the effects of oxygen free radicals in the lung. Enzymes such as superoxide dismutase, glutathione peroxidase, and catalase catalyze the detoxification of superoxide and hydrogen peroxide. Vitamins, especially vitamin E, and other antioxidants such as beta-carotene, selenium, and taurine assist in the trapping of free radicals. The fetal lung is exposed to oxygen tensions of 20 to 25 mm Hg in utero, and the transition to air breathing is associated with a four- to sevenfold increase in oxygen tension, presenting a significant oxidant stress. Animal studies indicate that many of the antioxidant enzymes are induced before term delivery, and limited data suggest that the same is true for human fetuses (reviewed in Weinberger et al, 2002). Premature animals fail to up-regulate antioxidant enzymes in response to oxygen-induced lung injury (Frank and Sosenko, 1991). Thus, preterm infants are more significantly compromised in antioxidant defenses, and because of the need for oxygen in the treatment of respiratory distress syndrome, they are more susceptible to oxygen toxicity.

## SUMMARY

Lung branching morphogenesis is coordinated with both epithelial cell proliferation and pulmonary vascular development to provide a large surface area and thin alveolar-capillary membrane for gas exchange. Many of the syndromes listed in Table 42–1 illustrate how abnormalities of early fetal lung development compromise gas exchange as a result of pulmonary hypoplasia. Although the fetal lung developmental program requires an array of transcription factors, hormones, and growth factors promoting branching morphogenesis, lung growth is equally dependent on intact neural input to modulate fetal breathing, stability of an appropriate-size thorax, and the production of adequate lung and amniotic fluid. Although it occurs late in fetal lung development, maturation of the surfactant system also is crucial to the transition to air breathing. Furthermore, the maturation of the host defense and detoxification systems minimizes the effects of increased oxygen tension and exposure to potential pathogens accompanying the transition to air breathing. Premature birth affects all of these functions, as illustrated in Table 42–5. Bronchopulmonary dysplasia is the end result of multiple injuries to the underdeveloped lungs of premature newborns that further compromise postnatal growth and development and impair function. Thus, integrated approaches to therapy that reflect the interdependency of these lung functions, rather than single "therapeutic bullets," will have the most promise for minimizing the impact of premature birth on childhood and, ultimately, adult lung function.

**TABLE 42–5**

**Impact of Pregnancy Abnormalities, Prematurity, and Infant Lung Disease on Lung Development and Maturation**

| Event | Impact | Potential Consequence(s) |
|---|---|---|
| Development of conducting airways | *Branching*: no effect; completed to level of the respiratory bronchi by 24 weeks | None |
| | *Tone*: Increased secondary to lung disease in part reflecting developmental deficiency of nitric oxide and proliferation of smooth muscle cells | Increased airways resistance |
| Alveolization | Variable inhibition depending on timing of delivery and severity of lung disease; also may be compromised by excess glucocorticoids | Reduced lung growth and total lung surface area with increased alveolar size (hypoplasia with emphysemic changes); impaired pulmonary function |
| Development of alveolocapillary membrane | Approaches adult diameter by week 24; glucocorticoids induce precocious thinning | Underdevelopment impairs gas exchange and contributes to RDS |
| Type II cell differentiation | Variable immaturity and deficient surfactant production depending on timing of delivery; induced by antenatal glucocorticoids | Developmental deficiency of surfactant content and composition results in RDS |
| Hydrophobic surfactant proteins (SP-B, SP-C) | Variable deficiency depending on timing of delivery and infection; necessary for lamellar body formation and optimal surfactant function | High alvedar surface tension; RDS |
| Hydrophilic surfactant proteins (SP-A, SP-D) | Variable deficiency depending on timing of delivery; participate in lung host defense and immunomodulation | Compromised ability to clear microorganisms from airways/alveolar space; pneumonia<br>Unmodulated inflammatory response contributes to chronic lung disease |
| Type I cell differentiation | Variable deficiency depending on timing of delivery and type II cell hyperplasia secondary to lung disease; cells develop from type II cells | Thickened epithelium impairs gas exchange |
| Clara cell differentiation | Variable deficiency depending on timing of delivery; reduction in number of cells | Impaired antioxidant and antimicrobial defenses; may contribute to chronic lung disease and pneumonia |

*Continued*

**TABLE 42-5**

**Impact of Pregnancy Abnormalities, Prematurity, and Infant Lung Disease on Lung Development and Maturation—Cont'd**

| Event | Impact | Potential Consequence(s) |
|---|---|---|
| Induction of antioxidant systems | Low expression until just prior to term | Lung injury from oxidant stress exacerbated by need for increased oxygen |
| Mucociliary clearance | Goblet cells decrease in number toward term | Increased mucus production may obstruct small airways |
| Development of pulmonary capillary bed | Normally parallels alveolar development; thus, variable effects depending on timing of delivery and severity of lung disease | In the extreme, alveolar capillary dysplasia; probably associated with variable degrees of impaired gas exchange; pulmonary hypertension |
| Pulmonary arteries | Medial hypertrophy and increased muscularization of peripheral vessels with lung disease | Pulmonary hypertension associated with chronic lung disease |
| Fetal lung liquid | *Fluid loss*: variable effects depending on magnitude and duration of fluid loss as well as timing of delivery; reduced content occurs secondary to prolonged premature rupture of membranes or intrinsic defect in fluid secretion | Pulmonary hypoplasia |
| | *Fluid retention*: Hormone surges near term and labor promote reabsorption before delivery | Transient tachypnea of the newborn |
| Fetal breathing movements | Contribute to lung growth; reduced movements associated with severe neurologic impairment and asphyxia | Pulmonary hypoplasia |
| | Postnatal transition to regular respiratory pattern disrupted with premature delivery | Apnea of prematurity |
| Respiratory musculature | Underdeveloped and easily fatigued in premature newborn | Apnea of prematurity |

RDS, respiratory distress syndrome.

## KEY REFERENCES


Blanco CE: Maturation of fetal breathing activity. Biol Neonate 65:182-188, 1994.

Burri P: Structural aspects of prenatal and postnatal development and growth of the lung. In McDonald J (ed): Lung Growth and Development. New York, Marcel Dekker, 1997, pp 1-36.

Cardoso WV: Transcription factors and pattern formation in the developing lung. Am J Physiol Lung Cell Mol Physiol 269:L429-L42, 1995.

Chabot F, Mitchell JA, Gutteridge JM, et al: Reactive oxygen species in acute lung injury. Eur Respir J 11:745-757, 1998.

Crouch E, Wright, JR: Surfactant proteins A and D and pulmonary host defense. Annu Rev Physiol 63:521-554, 2001.

Dunsmore SE, Rannels DE: Extracellular matrix biology in the lung. Am J Physiol Lung Cell Mol Physiol 270:L3-L27, 1996.

Jain L: Alveolar fluid clearance in developing lungs and its role in neonatal transition. Clin Perinatol 26:585-599, 1999.

Jeffrey PK: The development of large and small airways. Am J Respir Crit Care Med 157:S174-S180, 1998.

Mallampalli RK, Acarregui MJ, Snyder JM: Differentiation of the alveolar epithelium in the fetal lung. In McDonald JA (ed): Lung Growth and Development. New York, Marcel Dekker, 1997, pp 119-162.

Shannon JM, Deterding RR: Epithelial-mesenchymal interactions in lung development. In McDonald JA (ed): Lung Growth and Development. New York, Marcel Dekker, 1997, pp 81-118.

Stenmark KR, Mecham RP: Cellular and molecular mechanisms of pulmonary vascular remodeling. Annu Rev Physiol 59: 89-144, 1997.

Warburton D, Schwarz M, Tefft D, et al: The molecular basis of lung morphogenesis. Mech Dev 92:55-81, 2000.

Weaver TE, Conkright JJ: Function of surfactant proteins B and C. Annu Rev Physiol 63:555-578, 2001.


## REFERENCES


Adamson IY: Relationship of mesenchymal changes to alveolar epithelial cell differentiation in fetal rat lung. Anat Embryol (Berl) 185:275-280, 1992.

Baldwin HS: Early embryonic vascular development. Cardiovasc Res 31 Spec: E34-E45, 1996.

Bland RD: Loss of liquid from the lung lumen in labor: More than a simple "squeeze." Am J Physiol Lung Cell Mol Physiol 280:L602-L605, 2001.

Brody JS, Williams MC: Pulmonary alveolar cell differentiation. Ann Rev Physiol 54:351-371, 1992.

Costa RH, Kalinichenko VV, Lim L: Transcription factors in mouse lung development and function. Am J Physiol Lung Cell Mol Physiol 280:L823-L838, 2001.

Davies P, Reid LM: Growth of the alveoli and pulmonary arteries in childhood. Thorax 25:669-681, 1970.

Dobbs LG, Gutierrez JA: Mechanical forces modulate alveolar epithelial phenotypic expression. Comp Biochem Physiol A Mol Integr Physiol 129:261-266, 2001.

Dulkerian SJ, Gonzales LW Ning, Y, et al: Regulation of surfactant protein D in human fetal lung. Am J Respir Cell Mol Biol 15:781-786, 1996.

Frank L, Sosenko IR: Failure of premature rabbits to increase antioxidant enzymes during hyperoxic exposure: Increased susceptibility to pulmonary oxygen toxicity compared with term rabbits. Pediatr Res 29:292-296, 1991.

Hakansson K, Reid KB: Collectin structure: A review. Protein Sci 9:1607-1617, 2000.

Harding R: Function of the larynx in the fetus and newborn. Annu Rev Physiol 46:645-659, 1984.

Harding R: Fetal pulmonary development: The role of respiratory movements. Equine Vet J Suppl:32-39, 1997.

Harding R, Bocking AD, Sigger JN: Influence of upper respiratory tract on liquid flow to and from fetal lungs. J Appl Physiol 61:68-74, 1986.

Hawgood S, Clements JA: Pulmonary surfactant and its apoproteins. J Clin Invest 86:1-6, 1990.

Hislop A, Reid L: Growth and development of the respiratory system: Anatomical development. In Davis JA, Dobbing J (eds): Scientific Foundations of Paediatrics. London, Heinemann Medical Publications, 1981, pp 390-431.

Hogan BL, Yingling JM: Epithelial/mesenchymal interactions and branching morphogenesis of the lung. Curr Opin Genet Dev 8:481-486, 1998.

Holmes C, Thurlbeck WM: Normal lung growth and response after pneumonectomy in rats at various ages. Am Rev Respir Dis 120:1125-1136, 1979.

Hooper SB, Harding R: Fetal lung liquid: A major determinant of the growth and functional development of the fetal lung. Clin Exp Pharmacol Physiol 22:235-247, 1995.

Jansen AH, Chernick V: Fetal breathing and development of control of breathing. J Appl Physiol 70:1431-1446, 1991.

Kaplan F: Molecular determinants of fetal lung organogenesis. Mol Genet Metab 71:321-341, 2000.

Kheradmand F, Rishi K, Werb Z: Signaling through the EGF receptor controls lung morphogenesis in part by regulating MT1-MMP-mediated activation of gelatinase A/MMP2. J Cell Sci 115:839-848, 2002.

Kuroki Y, Voelker DR: Pulmonary surfactant proteins. J Biol Chem 269:25943-25946, 1994.

Lehrer RI, Ganz T: Cathelicidins: A family of endogenous antimicrobial peptides. Curr Opin Hematol 9:18-22, 2002.

Mariani TJ, Sandefur S, Pierce RA: Elastin in lung development. Exp Lung Res 23:131-145, 1997.

Massaro GD, Singh G, Mason R, et al: Biology of the Clara cell. Am J Physiol Lung Cell Mol Physiol 266:L101-L106, 1994.

McCormack FX, Whitsett JA: The pulmonary collectins, SP-A and SP-D, orchestrate innate immunity in the lung. J Clin Invest 109:707-712, 2002.

Mendelson CR: Role of transcription factors in fetal lung development and surfactant protein gene expression. Annu Rev Physiol 62:875-915, 2000.

Miyamura K, Malhotra R, Hoppe HJ, et al: Surfactant proteins A (SP-A) and D (SP-D): Levels in human amniotic fluid and localization in the fetal membranes. Biochim Biophys Acta 1210:303-307, 1994.

Muglia L, Jacobson L, Dikkes P, et al: Corticotropin-releasing hormone deficiency reveals major fetal but not adult glucocorticoid need. Nature 373:427-432, 1995.

Okajima S, Matsuda T, Cho K, et al: Antenatal dexamethasone administration impairs normal postnatal lung growth in rats. Pediatr Res 49:777-781, 2001.

Parks WC, Shapiro SD: Matrix metalloproteinases in lung biology. Respir Res 2:10-19, 2001.

Plopper CG: Clara cells. In McDonald JA (ed): Lung Growth and Development. New York, Marcel Dekker, 1997, pp 181-210.

Pryhuber GS, Hull WM, Fink I, et al: Ontogeny of surfactant proteins a and b in human amniotic fluid as indices of fetal lung maturity. Pediatr Res 30:597-605, 1991.

Rankin CT, Bunton T, Lawler AM, et al: Regulation of left-right patterning in mice by growth/differentiation factor-1. Nat Genet 24:262-265, 2000.

Rigatto H: Regulation of fetal breathing. Reprod Fertil Dev 8:23-33, 1996.

Rooney SA: Fatty acid biosynthesis in developing fetal lung. Am J Physiol Lung Cell Mol Physiol 257:L195-L201, 1989.

Schmid W, Cole TJ, Blendy JA, et al: Molecular genetic analysis of glucocorticoid signalling in development. J Steroid Biochem Mol Biol 53:33-35, 1995.

Schuger L: Laminins in lung development. Exp Lung Res 23:119-129, 1997.

Song Y, Fukuda N, Bai C, et al: Role of aquaporins in alveolar fluid clearance in neonatal and adult lung, and in edema formation following acute lung injury: Studies in transgenic aquaporin null mice. J Physiol 525:771-779, 2000.

Tschanz SA, Damke BM, Burri PH: Influence of postnatally administered glucocorticoids on rat lung growth. Biol Neonate 68:229-245, 1995.

Veldhuizen EJ, Haagsman HP: Role of pulmonary surfactant components in surface film formation and dynamics. Biochim Biophys Acta 1467:255-270, 2000.

Verkman AS, Matthay MA, Song Y: Aquaporin water channels and lung physiology. Am J Physiol Lung Cell Mol Physiol 278:L867-L879, 2000.

Warburton D, Wuenschell C, Flores-Delgado G, et al: Commitment and differentiation of lung cell lineages. Biochem Cell Biol 76:971-995, 1998.

Weinberger B, Laskin DL, Heck DE, et al: Oxygen toxicity in premature infants. Toxicol Appl Pharmacol 181:60-67, 2002.

Weiss J: Leukocyte-derived antimicrobial proteins. Curr Opin Hematol 1:78-84, 1994.

West JB: Respiratory Physiology: The Essentials. Baltimore, Williams & Wilkins, 1990.

Wilmott RW, Khurana-Hershey G, Stark JM: Current concepts on pulmonary host defense mechanisms in children. Curr Opin Pediatr 12:187-193, 2000.

Wright C, Strauss S, Toole K, et al: Composition of the pulmonary interstitium during normal development of the human fetus. Pediatr Dev Pathol 2:424-431, 1999.

Wright JR: Clearance and recycling of pulmonary surfactant. Am J Physiol Lung Cell Mol Physiol 259:L1-L12, 1990.

Wright JR: Immunomodulatory functions of surfactant. Physiol Rev 77:931-962, 1997.

CHAPTER 43

# Control of Breathing

**Thomas N. Hansen and Anthony Corbet**

Rhythmic breathing is maintained by alternating discharges of inspiratory and expiratory neurons, located diffusely in the medulla oblongata, and is activated by nonspecific neuronal traffic in the brainstem. One concept is that expiratory neurons discharge continuously under the influence of the reticular activating system, but rhythmic breathing is produced by the central inspiratory activator, which intermittently discharges and temporarily inhibits expiratory neurons (Cohen, 1979). Some of the inspiratory neurons are organized into the nucleus paragigantocellularis lateralis, thought to be the central inspiratory activator, and located close to the central chemoreceptors on the ventral surface of the medulla (Von Euler, 1983).

In adults, inspiration is active, and expiration is passive. Expiration is divided into two phases. In the first phase, a group of inspiratory neurons apply postinspiratory "braking" to slow exhalation. In the second phase, exhalation continues passively, or it is accelerated by contraction of expiratory muscles. The main inspiratory muscles are the diaphragm, intercostals, and upper airway abductors. The main expiratory muscles are intercostal and abdominal groups, which accelerate expiration, and upper airway adductors, which retard expiration by narrowing the larynx.

Inspiration is controlled by an "off switch" (Fig. 43–1). During inspiration, the augmenting discharge of the central inspiratory activator to inspiratory motor neurons and specialized $R_b$ neurons suddenly causes the off switch neurons to discharge, transiently inhibiting the central inspiratory activator and allowing passive exhalation. The off switch also is controlled by the pulmonary volume sensors and the rostral pontine pneumotaxic center, which together decrease the depth and increase the rate of breathing (Kosch et al, 1986). The threshold of the off switch, and thus the depth and rate of breathing, are modulated up or down from a number of sources: peripheral chemoreceptors, central chemoreceptors, chest wall propriosensors, hypothalamus, and cerebral cortex (Von Euler, 1983).

The respiratory control mechanisms develop progressively throughout gestation and infancy, so the system does not attain maturity until late in the first year of life. During quiet sleep, modulation of breathing is metabolic, through central and peripheral chemoreceptors, which sense, respectively, $P_{CO_2}$ and $P_{O_2}$. During active sleep and wakefulness, there are additional behavioral controls such as crying, sucking, and gross body motions (Schulte, 1977; Thach et al, 1978).

## FETAL BREATHING

After many years of controversy, it is now established that the fetus breathes (Dawes, 1973). This breathing activity, which is essentially diaphragmatic, is present for 30% to 35% of the time in mothers examined with a real-time ultrasound scanner (Patrick et al, 1978). It is irregular in rate and amplitude; recorded rates in the human fetus range between 30 and 70 breaths/minute. The tidal volume of lung liquid is small, quite insufficient to clear the dead space. Owing to active lung liquid secretion, the net flow of liquid is out of the lung. Periods of apnea may last as long as 1 hour in the normal human fetus. In the lamb, breathing occurs during active sleep, associated with low-voltage electrocortical activity, and breathing is inhibited during quiet sleep, associated with high-voltage electrocortical activity. There appears to be a circadian rhythm, breathing activity being lowest in the early morning and rising during the afternoon to peak in the early evening (Dawes, 1974). Fetal breathing has been detected as early as 10 weeks of gestation. Fetal breathing is suppressed, however, during late pregnancy as labor approaches, probably due to a progressive rise of plasma prostaglandins (Kitterman et al, 1983), and remains suppressed during active labor (Boylan and Lewis, 1980).

Fetal breathing is increased by drugs that stimulate the central nervous system, such as caffeine, isoproterenol, serotonin, and substance P, and it is inhibited by anesthetics, narcotics, barbiturates, ethanol, and smoking (Manning, 1977). Fetal breathing also is inhibited by prostaglandins, endorphins, and adenosine. The inhibitory effect of maternal ethanol ingestion is mediated by prostaglandins (Smith et al, 1990). Hypoglycemia or maternal fasting is associated with decreased fetal breathing, whereas it is stimulated after maternal meals and by hyperglycemia.

Mild fetal hypoxemia severely depresses fetal breathing, by acting at a midbrain inhibitor, but more severe fetal hypoxemia induces primitive deep gasping by a direct action on the medulla. It is believed that the hypoxia-sensitive carotid body peripheral chemoreceptors are active in the fetus and provide a constant stimulus to breathing (Murai et al, 1985), but their effect on the central respiratory neurons is easily overridden by high-voltage electrocortical activity (quiet sleep) acting through the midbrain inhibitor or, under certain conditions, by endogenous depressants such as prostaglandins, endorphins, or adenosine, which may be present at high levels in the blood stream (Jansen and Chernick, 1988). Adenosine may be released under conditions of hypoxia, and adenosine antagonists such as theophylline have been found to decrease the depressant effect of hypoxia on ventilatory drive (Darnall, 1985; Runold et al, 1989). The hypoxic response with depression of fetal breathing may be blocked with dopamine antagonists (Lagercrantz, 1992), which suggests that a dopaminergic pathway may connect the midbrain inhibitor with the respiratory centers in the medulla.

Hypercarbia has a rapid stimulatory effect on fetal breathing, this effect being exerted by increased hydrogen ion concentration at central chemoreceptors on the surface

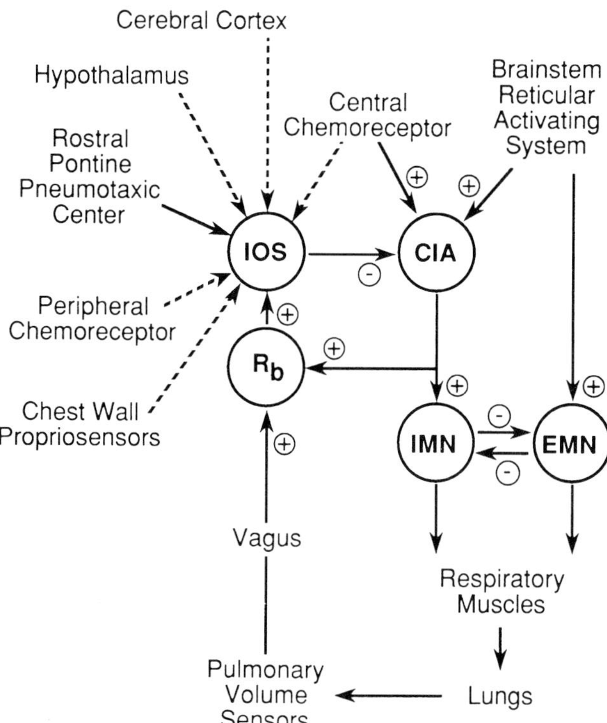


**FIGURE 43–1.** Possible functional organization of the central respiratory pattern generator. CIA, central inspiratory activator; IMN, inspiratory motor neurons; IOS, inspiratory "off switch"; $R_b$, respiratory neurones, which receive input from the pulmonary stretch receptors and the CIA; EMN, expiratory motor neurons. *Solid arrows* indicate direct effects. *Interrupted arrows* indicate modulatory effects. Effects are stimulatory (+) or inhibitory (−). *(Adapted from Von Euler C: On the central pattern generator for the basic breathing rhythmicity. J Appl Physiol 55:1647, 1983.)*

of the medulla; $CO_2$ diffuses rapidly into the cerebrospinal fluid surrounding these chemoreceptors. A similar stimulation occurs with the production of metabolic acidemia, but only after a latent interval to allow slow diffusion of organic acids into the cerebrospinal fluid (Harding, 1984). The pH-sensitive medullary cells are located at the midline on the ventromedial medulla; they are situated under the basilar artery with its penetrating arterial branches (Richerson et al, 2001). There are larger pH-sensitive cells that stimulate breathing, and there are smaller pH-sensitive cells that inhibit breathing; together they act as an accelerator and as a brake to modulate breathing. They are exquisitely sensitive to very tiny changes in local pH in the appropriate range, they are near arterial blood, they project to respiratory motor neurons, and the stimulatory cells contain neurotransmitters, such as serotonin, that are known to stimulate breathing. The firing rate of these cells is reduced during sleep. In the rat, the development of sensitivity in these cells corresponds with the development of respiratory control.

The purpose of fetal breathing appears to be at least twofold. To many physiologists, it is inconceivable that efficient postnatal breathing could be accomplished without prenatal practice. In addition, it appears that growth and development of the lungs (Wigglesworth and Desai, 1982), including the surfactant system (Higuchi et al, 1991), is highly dependent on the distensive forces produced by fetal breathing.

## Onset of Continuous Breathing at Birth

Before birth, fetal breathing is episodic and dependent on the low-voltage electrocortical state (active sleep), but after birth, breathing becomes continuous and independent of the electrocortical state. Experimentally in fetal lambs, breathing becomes continuous and independent of electrocortical state when the brainstem is sectioned just below the midbrain level (Dawes et al, 1983). Continuous breathing after birth may be due to suppression of this midbrain inhibitor. Brain sections in this region result in the abolition of the ventilatory depressive response to hypoxia and in the institution of continuous breathing in both fetal and newborn lambs (Gluckman and Johnston, 1987; Martin-Boddy and Johnston, 1988).

The somatic sensory stimulation associated with delivery can be a powerful stimulus to continuous breathing (Condorelli and Scarpelli, 1975). Similarly, cooling the skin without change in core temperature has been shown to stimulate continuous breathing in fetuses with normal blood gas levels (Gluckman et al, 1983). It is believed that these multiple stimuli, by increasing neuronal traffic in the brainstem, may suppress the midbrain inhibition of breathing during the high-voltage electrocortical state.

Before birth, mild fetal asphyxia with both hypoxemia and hypercarbia, produced by clamping the umbilical cord, always induces continuous fetal breathing, and it does this without cooling or somatic sensory stimulation (Adamson et al, 1987). Mild fetal hypoxemia by itself produces depression of fetal breathing, through the midbrain inhibitor, so breathing stimulated by mild fetal asphyxia is probably due not to hypoxia but rather to hypercarbia. After birth, the arterial $PO_2$ is much higher than before birth, increasing from 30 to 70 mm Hg within minutes, and the arterial $PCO_2$ decreases from 45 mm Hg in the fetus to 35 mm Hg in the newborn. On first examination, therefore, it would seem likely that neither hypoxemia nor hypercarbia could be responsible for continuous breathing after birth. Nevertheless, it is believed that continuous postnatal breathing must be associated with a resetting of the threshold for both peripheral and central chemoreceptors, so they are stimulated at the new levels for arterial $PO_2$ and $PCO_2$. Because the onset of breathing is not abolished by carotid body denervation (Jansen et al, 1981), it seems unlikely that hypoxemia is important in the onset of breathing. Furthermore, it is known that the peripheral chemoreceptors are inactive for several days after birth, both in the lamb (Blanco et al, 1984) and in the human (Hertzberg and Lagercrantz, 1987), presumably because the resetting to a higher-threshold $PO_2$ is delayed. On the other hand, although hypercarbia by itself, induced with $CO_2$ breathing by the mother, is a powerful stimulus to fetal breathing (Dawes et al, 1982), this is not true during the high-voltage electrocortical state (quiet sleep). If hypercarbia is given the prime responsibility for continuous breathing at birth, as seems most likely, there must still be a rapid downward adjustment in the central chemoreceptor threshold for

$CO_2$, about which little is known, and there must still be a reversal of the midbrain inhibition produced by the high-voltage electrocortical state, perhaps induced by increased brainstem neuronal traffic. In addition, clamping the umbilical cord at birth may cut off the supply of a placental inhibitor, possibly prostaglandin, endorphin, or adenosine, and this may facilitate the onset of breathing. It has been demonstrated in the fetal lamb in which breathing has been stimulated by a cord clamp, that when the cord is unclamped, breathing is soon inhibited (Adamson et al, 1987). Injection of a placental extract also produces inhibition of fetal breathing (Alvaro et al, 1993); the inhibitor may be a prostaglandin (Adamson et al, 1991), and recent evidence suggests that adenosine may be important (Herlenius et al, 2002). The conclusion must be that no single factor is responsible for the onset of continuous breathing at birth (Jansen and Chernick, 1988). In summary, hypoxemia does not play a role for several days after birth; hypercarbia probably is most important, but there must be a very rapid resetting of the central chemoreceptor threshold for $PCO_2$. In addition, the action of the midbrain inhibitor during the high-voltage electrocortical state must be abolished by increased neuronal traffic in the brainstem; and there must be removal of an unknown placental inhibitor.

## CONTROL OF BREATHING IN THE FULL-TERM NEWBORN INFANT

In adults, it is well known that mild hypoxia and hypercarbia stimulate breathing. The ventilatory response to hypercarbia in the full-term newborn is considered to be similar to that in the adult, but the response to hypoxia is more complex.

As discussed previously, before birth, mild hypoxia inhibits breathing, due to stimulation of the midbrain inhibitor. The term newborn infant responds to decreased oxygen by a transient weak hyperpnea, followed by a relative ventilatory depression of variable magnitude (Brady and Ceruti, 1966). This phenomenon suggests rapid exhaustion of the peripheral chemoreceptor in the face of moderate hypoxic respiratory center depression produced by the midbrain inhibitor. This biphasic response to hypoxia persists for a few days after birth in the full-term infant. In addition to the effect of the midbrain inhibitor, adenosine, released by hypoxia, also may be responsible for the depressed hypoxic ventilatory response (Koos and Matsuda, 1990).

If the term infant at age 2 to 6 hours is given 100% oxygen to breathe, no change in ventilation occurs, as would be expected in the normal adult; the absence of a transient depression suggests that the peripheral chemoreceptor is not functional and has not undergone upward resetting of the threshold from the low level operating in the fetus (Hertzberg and Lagercrantz, 1987). If the term infant older than a few days is given 100% oxygen to breathe, there is a transient depression of ventilation (Rigatto and Brady, 1972); this suggests that the normal expected activity of the peripheral chemoreceptor appears by 2 days of age in the full-term infant. The occurrence of mild apnea episodes is not uncommon in healthy term infants on the first day of life.

## CONTROL OF BREATHING IN THE PREMATURE INFANT

The sensitivity of the central chemoreceptor to $CO_2$ is reduced in premature infants and increases progressively with gestational age to adult levels by full term (Rigatto, 1977; Rigatto et al, 1975b). Higher oxygen concentrations increase sensitivity, and hypoxemia decreases sensitivity to $CO_2$ (Rigatto et al, 1975c). In small premature infants, adult levels of sensitivity are reached by 4 weeks of postnatal age (Fig. 43–2).

Although full-term infants have a biphasic response to hypoxia, in small preterm infants, there is no initial hyperpnea, only a sustained decrease in ventilatory activity (Alvaro et al, 1992). This finding indicates that peripheral chemoreceptor function is even worse in preterm infants.

In preterm infants given 100% oxygen, the peripheral chemoreceptor response initially is absent, but it improves

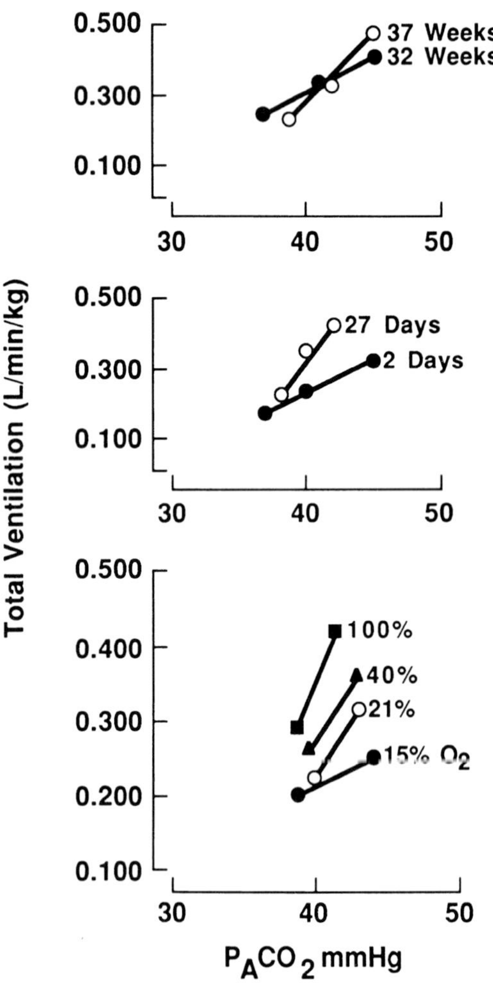


**FIGURE 43–2.** The relationship between ventilatory sensitivity to carbon dioxide and gestational age (**top panel**), postnatal age (**middle panel**), and the concentration of inspired oxygen (**bottom panel**). *(From Rigatto H, Brady J, Verduzco RT: Chemoreceptor reflexes in preterm infants: The effect of gestational and postnatal age on the ventilatory response to inhaled carbon dioxide. Pediatrics 55:614, 1975; and Rigatto H, Verduzco RT, Cates DB: Effects of $O_2$ on the ventilatory response to $CO_2$ in preterm infants. J Appl Physiol 39:896, 1975.)*

with time, and by 2 weeks of postnatal age the response is as good as that seen in term infants (Lagercrantz, 1992). Thus, the main problem in premature infants may be that the peripheral chemoreceptor function is relatively weak, at least in the first few weeks of life.

In larger premature infants, the central hypoxic depression of ventilation, mediated by the midbrain inhibitor, also disappears about 2 to 3 weeks after birth, when the mature response of sustained hypoxic stimulation of ventilation mediated by the peripheral chemoreceptor becomes dominant (Rigatto et al, 1975a). However, in very small premature infants, Martin and colleagues (1998) demonstrated that this insufficiency was persistent through 4 to 8 weeks of postnatal age and contributed to a prolonged vulnerability to depression of breathing.

## THE ROLE OF STRETCH RECEPTORS

Evidence for the presence of a Hering-Breuer reflex in newborn infants has been obtained, and the strength of the reflex increases with gestational age until term (Gerhardt and Bancalari, 1981), but declines after birth (Bodegard et al, 1969). The Hering-Breuer reflex is mediated by stretch and irritant receptors. The function of stretch receptors is to increase inspiratory flow and tidal volume without changing inspiration time (Haddad and Mellins, 1977). This means that stretch receptors increase the output of the respiratory center. The function of irritant receptors is to shorten inspiration and expiration times and to reduce tidal volume without changing inspiratory flow. The irritant receptors must operate the off switch neurons (see Fig. 43–1), but have no effect on respiratory center output. The combined activity of stretch and irritant receptors, the volume sensor, shortens both inspiration and expiration, reduces tidal volume, and increases the inspiratory flow. Thus, the increasing activity of the Hering-Breuer reflex throughout gestation is consistent with a maturational increase of respiratory drive induced by the stretch receptors, and may play a role in the reduced ventilatory drive seen in preterm infants.

## PERIODIC BREATHING

A periodic breathing pattern consists of breathing for 10 to 15 seconds followed by apnea for 5 to 10 seconds, without change of heart rate or skin color. The net effect may be hypoventilation (Rigatto and Brady, 1972). This pattern is common at high altitude and is abolished by supplemental oxygen (Graham et al, 1950) and by continuous positive airway pressure (CPAP). The more premature the infant, the more frequent its occurrence, but to a lesser extent it persists in term infants and during early infancy (Hoppenbrouwers et al, 1977). Periodic breathing does not occur during the first 2 days of life (Barrington and Finer, 1990) and is more frequent during active sleep. The prognosis is excellent, so no treatment is required. Although it initially was thought that periodic breathing was associated with a high risk for apnea of prematurity (Daily et al, 1969), this concept has been questioned by Barrington and Finer (1990), who found that periodic breathing does not immediately precede significant apnea spells in preterm infants.

Theoretical models suggest that periodic breathing is due to an imbalance between the peripheral and the central chemoreceptor effects on ventilatory drive (Khoo et al, 1982). Investigators have shown that periodic breathing in newborn guinea pigs can be induced by suppression of the central chemoreceptor, and then abolished by restoration of the balance with suppression of the peripheral chemoreceptor (Wennergren and Wennergren, 1983). In humans at high altitude, with spontaneous periodic breathing due to hypoxic stimulation of the peripheral chemoreceptor, stimulation of the central chemoreceptor with acetazolamide abolished periodic breathing, whereas further stimulation of the peripheral chemoreceptor with almitrine increased periodic breathing (Hackett et al, 1987). The hypothesis of Barrington and Finer (1990) is that periodic breathing in premature infants is often due to excessive stimulation by the peripheral chemoreceptor, promoting an imbalance; this concept is consistent with their observation that periodic breathing is not observed in the first 2 days of life, when the peripheral chemoreceptor is inactive, but is common thereafter, when the peripheral chemoreceptor is reset and again functional.

## APNEA OF PREMATURITY

During episodes of apnea, there is a cessation of respiratory activity—exchange of oxygen and carbon dioxide. This means that the term *apnea* is applied to the absence of both air flow and breathing effort (so-called central apnea) and also to the absence of air flow with breathing effort present (so-called obstructive apnea).

Apneic spells usually seen in infants are episodic and random (Daily et al, 1969). Episodes prolonged for 20 seconds or more or those accompanied by bradycardia or color change (desaturation) are considered significant. Perlman and Volpe (1985) have described the cerebral ischemia that accompanies severe bradycardia with a heart rate of less than 80 beats/minute. On neurodevelopmental follow-up evaluation, infants with significant apnea of prematurity do not perform as well as do similar premature infants without recurrent apneas (Cheung et al, 1999; Kitchen et al, 1987; Tudehope et al, 1986). The diagnosis of apnea of prematurity can be made only after the exclusion of all other causes of recurrent apnea.

The incidence of apneic spells is inversely related to gestational age (Henderson-Smart, 1981). Although commonly stated otherwise, apneic episodes frequently start on the first day of life (Barrington and Finer, 1991; Henderson-Smart, 1981). In many infants, only bradycardia is recognized by the hospital staff, but polygraphic recordings indicate that bradycardia is nearly always preceded by apnea (Dransfield et al, 1983). It is thought that 40% of the episodes are central or diaphragmatic, 10% are obstructive, and 50% are mixed, which may indicate either obstructive followed by central apnea (Martin et al, 1986) or central followed by obstructive apnea (Butcher-Puech et al, 1985). In an individual infant, one type tends to predominate. Central apneas tend to be shorter, whereas obstruction tends to prolong the episode and accelerate the onset of bradycardia. Obstructive apneas are particularly common on the first day of life in premature infants (Barrington and Finer, 1991).

Apnea of prematurity usually resolves by 38 weeks of postconceptional age, but sometimes resolution is delayed until 42 weeks; now that so many very small infants survive, it may be even more prolonged. In many infants there is a good correlation between the attainment of full nipple feeds and the cessation of apnea episodes (Darnall et al, 1997); but just as poor nipple feeding may be prolonged so may apnea be prolonged. In very small premature infants of 24 to 28 weeks of gestation, apnea of prematurity often is prolonged past full-term gestation (Eichenwald et al, 1997), especially if the infant has neurologic dysfunction (Cheung et al, 1999). In a recent study, infants who were still experiencing routine hospital monitor alarms at the time of possible hospital discharge were found to have lower oxygen saturation levels than those in similar infants who were not having routine hospital monitor alarms (Di Fiore et al, 2001); continuous pneumogram recordings showed that although occurrence rates for apneas were nearly the same, desaturation and bradycardia events were more likely in infants who had lower resting oxygen saturation levels (95%) in room air than in those who had normal resting oxygen saturation levels (99%). The investigators suggested that those with lower oxygen levels and more monitor alarms may have subtle residual lung disease or possibly increased neurologic dysfunction. In infants with prolonged apnea of prematurity, often sent home on apnea monitors, apnea, desaturation, and bradycardia events persist for up to 6 months or longer (Silvestri et al, 1994).

It was once thought that bradycardia was not related to hypoxemia (Hiatt et al, 1981), but rather had a central brainstem origin (Schulte, 1977) or was a reflex response to the cessation of lung inflation (Gabriel and Albani, 1976). Henderson-Smart and colleagues (1986) however, concluded that episodes of bradycardia were associated with oxygen desaturation, and Poets and associates (1993) confirmed this. In 80 premature infants, just before discharge from the hospital, 193 episodes of bradycardia were recorded; 83% were associated with apnea episodes, and 86% were associated with oxygen desaturation; when all three occurred together, the sequence of events was apnea followed by desaturation followed by bradycardia. The median interval between the onset of apnea and the onset of desaturation was 1 second, and between the onset of apnea and the onset of bradycardia the interval was 5 seconds. Although in such circumstances the bradycardia may be due to a direct effect on the heart, the short time interval suggests that the bradycardia is a peripheral chemoreceptor response to hypoxemia, as suggested by earlier workers (Storrs, 1977). There was no evidence that the onset of apnea and that of bradycardia were simultaneous, as would be expected in a lung or brainstem reflex.

### Pathogenesis

The cause of apnea of prematurity is unknown, but a number of theories have been considered for central, diaphragmatic, and obstructive apneas. The neurons of the central pattern generator are poorly myelinated and have a reduced number of dendrites and synaptic connections, thus impairing the capability for sustained ventilatory drive. Prolonged auditory conduction times have been demonstrated in infants with apnea, a problem assumed to reflect the function of the medulla in general (Henderson-Smart et al, 1983).

Along similar lines, because infants with apnea of prematurity have a deficiency of catecholamine excretion in the urine, other investigators have suggested a neurotransmitter deficiency (Kattwinkel et al, 1976b). Infants with apnea of prematurity have a decreased ventilatory response to $CO_2$ inhalation in comparison with premature infants of the same gestation without apnea of prematurity (Gerhardt and Bancalari, 1984a).

The chest wall of premature infants is highly compliant, so considerably more work is performed to generate adequate tidal ventilation. This results in substrate depletion and diaphragmatic failure from fatigue. Evidence for fatigue has been shown by examination of the diaphragmatic electromyogram (Muller et al, 1979).

There is some evidence that the diaphragm may activate before the upper airway abductors, which would predispose to upper airway closure during inspiration. The same problem may occur if abductor activation is insufficient (Mathew, 1985). Because airway obstruction imposes a load on the inspiratory muscles, the ability to load-compensate is important. It has been shown that load compensation is poor in small premature infants and increases as term is approached (Gerhardt and Bancalari, 1982). The poor load compensation is due to the high degree of compliance of the chest wall and the presence of an intercostal phrenic inhibitory reflex, which is activated by chest distortion and also shortens the duration of inspiration (Gerhardt and Bancalari, 1984b). This problem predisposes the infant to obstructive apnea, especially under conditions of excessive neck flexion, when the upper airway tends to narrow, and in the supine position, when the tongue falls backward.

### Relation to Sleep State

Most apneas occur during active sleep (Schulte, 1977) and are less common during states of quiet sleep or wakefulness. During active sleep, there is a low-voltage electrocortical state, as well as decreased arousal from sleep, decreased muscular tone, absence of upper airway adductor activity, decreased respiratory drive, irregular breathing, and inspiratory chest wall distortion. The loss of chest wall muscle tone and airway adductor activity causes a 30% reduction in lung volume and a decreased arterial $PO_2$ (Henderson-Smart and Read, 1979). Reduced ventilatory drive causes a slight elevation in arterial $PCO_2$. The ventilatory response to hypoxia is depressed during active sleep, much more than in quiet sleep. The ventilatory sensitivity to $CO_2$ also is thought to be more depressed in active sleep (Rigatto, 1982). The newborn and the premature infant are asleep 80% of the time, compared with the adult, who is asleep for 30% of the time. More than 50% of sleep is active in the small premature infant, and the mature amount of 20% is not reached until 6 months of age (Bryan and Bryan, 1986).

### Treatment

All infants at risk for apnea should have a heart rate monitor; monitoring should be continued until the infant is at least 34 weeks of postconceptional age, or after that time until the infant has been free of bradycardia for 1 week. Heart rate monitors are preferred because apnea without bradycardia is not significant apnea, obstructive apnea with bradycardia is detected reliably, and false alarms are infrequent. Most monitors in the neonatal intensive care unit also include an apnea monitor; the principal objections to the apnea monitor alone are that it misses obstructive apnea with the infant breathing, and it may confuse bradycardia with large stroke volumes for breathing. It has become common to monitor with pulse oximetry because of the importance of both oxygen desaturation and heart rate.

Because respiratory center output is dependent on general neuronal traffic, cutaneous stimulation is effective (Kattwinkel et al, 1975). The use of oscillation water beds has been helpful sometimes (Korner et al, 1975). It is reasonable to maintain the patient in the prone position (Kurlak et al, 1994) because in this position there is a significant reduction in the duration of episodes of desaturation and bradycardia. Even in larger premature infants nearing hospital discharge, there may be advantages to the prone position in the form of improved oxygenation and a better ventilatory response to hypercarbia (Martin et al, 1995). Because diaphragmatic fatigue has been implicated, it is essential to maintain the circulation and a general state of good nutrition; the infusion of amino acids may increase the ventilatory response to hypoxia and hypercarbia (Soliz et al, 1994).

If the patient is hypoxemic, oxygen supplementation is essential, but there is no evidence that significant apnea is reduced if the patient is hyperoxygenated, and harm to the immature retina may be inflicted with such a strategy. Upton and colleagues (1991), using pulse oximetry, found that if the baseline oxygen saturation was higher, the desaturation produced by apnea tended to be less severe, and it was less likely that bradycardia would result. In apneas without bradycardia, the median baseline oxygen saturation was 95% and the median reduction with apnea was 5%, whereas for those apneas with bradycardia, the median baseline oxygen saturation was 92% and the median reduction was 9%. Upton and colleagues concluded that it is important to keep the premature infant with recurrent apneas relatively well oxygenated. Pulse oximeters vary in their ability to detect hyperoxemia (arterial $PO_2$ greater than 90 mm Hg), but with one commonly used instrument, Adams and coworkers (1994) found that setting the upper limit at 95% detected nearly all instances of hyperoxemia. If the infant must be given occasional bag-mask ventilation, it is important to ensure that the oxygen concentration remains stable and is not increased.

Because an oxygen hood interferes with access to the infant, many centers prefer to use nasal cannulas to administer oxygen, usually at a flow of 1 to 2 L/minute, with use of blended oxygen to maintain the pulse oximeter reading in the range of 92% to 96% saturation. Some evidence suggests that nasal cannula therapy may lead to correction of chest wall distortion, with less asynchrony between chest and abdomen, resulting in a more efficient breathing strategy (Locke et al, 1993), perhaps by producing a small amount of continuous distending pressure in the nasopharynx; although this pressure may seem unregulated, pulmonary air leak complications have never been reported with this simple technique.

Most infants are treated with methylxanthines, which have been demonstrated to be effective in controlled trials (Murat et al, 1981). Because caffeine produces less tachycardia, has a more favorable therapeutic index, and produces less erratic blood level fluctuations, it may be preferred over theophylline (Aranda and Turmen, 1979). There is some evidence that theophylline, but not caffeine, decreases cerebral blood flow in premature infants (Pryds and Schneider, 1991; Saliba et al, 1989); high doses of caffeine may decrease cerebral and intestinal blood flow (Hoecker et al, 2002), perhaps related to antagonism of adenosine receptors. Theophylline may increase the metabolic rate (Walther et al, 1990), which may retard weight gain; increased oxygen consumption may be detrimental if organ blood flow is reduced at the same time. A significant fraction of theophylline is methylated to caffeine in premature infants (Aranda and Turmen, 1979). In a significant number of patients who do not respond to theophylline, a good response is obtained with caffeine (Davis et al, 1987). In a comparative trial, Larsen and colleagues (1995) found caffeine to be equally effective but associated with less tachycardia and less feeding intolerance than were found with theophylline. Either drug may be given for 2 weeks and then stopped to observe whether apnea has ceased, or it may be continued until 32 to 34 weeks of postconceptional age, by which time the problem of apnea has frequently resolved. Infants should not be discharged before caffeine or theophylline has been eliminated because there is evidence that theophylline is effective at quite low levels. Methylxanthines may increase $CO_2$ sensitivity, decrease diaphragmatic fatigue, and improve load compensation (Gerhardt et al, 1983). Methylxanthines reduce the ventilatory depression following hypoxia by blocking adenosine receptors (Lopes et al, 1994). Some investigators have suggested that theophylline increases the activity of the peripheral chemoreceptors in term infants (Cattarossi et al, 1993), which is consistent with experimental evidence in peripheral chemoreceptor–denervated lambs treated with caffeine (Blanchard et al, 1986).

The other mainstay of treatment is nasal CPAP (Kattwinkel et al, 1975). Although the effect of 5 cm $H_2O$ should be tried, frequently as much as 8 to 10 cm $H_2O$ is necessary for satisfactory control, perhaps because many of these infants have chest cage insufficiency and a low lung volume. Infants may be fed by continuous gastric infusion during this procedure. Care should be taken not to depress the circulation; the chest radiograph should be reviewed periodically to avoid overdistending the lungs. It has been postulated that CPAP provides increased ventilatory drive by directly stimulating the pulmonary stretch receptors (DiMarco et al, 1981; Speidel and Dunn, 1976), but this hypothesis could not be confirmed in premature infants by measurements of the rate of inspiratory flow (Krauss et al, 1986). Also, Krauss and colleagues could not find any improvement in the ventilatory response to inhaled $CO_2$. Other investigators consider that obstructive and mixed apneas are selectively relieved by CPAP (Miller et al, 1985), which suggests that CPAP may work by supporting the pharynx. Using fiberoptic laryngoscopy, it has been demonstrated that nasal CPAP produces dilation of the larynx in premature infants (Gaon et al, 1999). In addition, CPAP prevents chest wall distortion during inspiration (Locke et al, 1991), which may improve the efficiency of ventilation and suppress the intercostal phrenic inhibitory reflex; improved load compensation in small premature infants on CPAP has been demonstrated (Martin et al, 1977). Some centers use nasal cannula therapy with high flow (1.0 to 2.0 L/minute) as a simple form of nasal CPAP. In a controlled clinical trial, it has been shown that esophageal pressures generated with this technique are equivalent to levels generated with conventional nasal CPAP, and that the occurrence rate for apnea was similar (Sreenan et al, 2001b), indicating an improvement. Nasal humidification should be maintained with frequent nasal saline drops.

Another drug that has proved useful is doxapram (Barrington et al, 1987). At low doses, it stimulates the peripheral chemoreceptors, whereas at higher doses, it stimulates the respiratory center directly. In the United States, the preparation contains 0.9% benzyl alcohol as a preservative, but at a dose of 0.5 mg/kg/hour, the amount of benzyl alcohol administered is only 5.4 mg/kg/day, which is far below the levels associated with toxicity in premature infants (Barrington and Finer, 1986). Doxapram should be reserved for infants who fail to respond to optimal xanthine and CPAP therapy, in whom mechanical ventilation would be the next step; methylxanthine therapy should be continued during doxapram infusion (Eyal et al, 1985). In addition, doxapram should not be used in the first week of life or if the serum bilirubin is high, because an association with intraventricular hemorrhage and kernicterus has been reported (Jardine and Rogers, 1988). The drug may be started at 1.0 mg/kg/hour for a few hours as a loading dose, which may then be decreased to 0.5 mg/kg/hour. Higher doses may sometimes be associated with side effects, such as abdominal distention, increased gastric residuals, irritability, hyperglycemia, and mild hypertension (Hayakawa et al, 1986). Poets and colleagues (1999) treated small premature infants not responding to high levels of caffeine with intravenous (0.5 to 2.0 mg/kg/hour) or enteral (2 to 8 mg/kg every 2 hours) doxapram and described a significant reduction in the occurrence of apnea, desaturation, and bradycardia. Enteral administration was not tolerated in one third of the patients. Doxapram is quite widely used in Japan; a controlled trial in preterm infants who did not respond to xanthines showed an approximate 80% reduction in apnea with low-dose doxapram (0.2 to 1.0 mg/kg/hour) and only minimal side effects (Yamazaki et al, 2001). Doxapram may be associated with a moderate prolongation of the Q-Tc interval, and use of electrocardiographic monitoring has been suggested (Maillard et al, 2001). A recent case-control study suggested that isolated mental delay may occur in infants treated with longer courses of doxapram (Sreenan et al, 2001a), but a causal relationship was not proved.

It has been reported that inhalation of 0.5% to 1.5% carbon dioxide is effective at reducing the number of apnea spells in premature infants (Al-Aif et al, 2001). There was no change in transcutaneous $P_{CO_2}$ levels, presumably because minute ventilation was increased.

## Movement-Related Apnea Episodes

Mathew and associates (1991) observed a high incidence of apneas during squirming motions associated especially with arousal from sleep; they suggested that as many as one third of apneas in premature infants may be of this type. Using esophageal pressure measurements, Abu-Osba and coworkers (1982) showed that these motions were associated with increased abdominal expiratory muscle activity against a closed glottis (i.e., Valsalva maneuvers); they also observed some obstructed inspiratory breaths during squirming motions (i.e., Müller maneuvers). These episodes may be associated with greatly reduced minute ventilation and severe oxygen desaturation and bradycardia. These spells are unlikely to respond to methylxanthine therapy. A similar phenomenon without glottic closure may occur in infants on slow-rate mechanical ventilation.

## Cyanotic Spells without Apnea in Preterm Infants: "V/Q Spells"

In a study by Poets and colleagues (1993), about 15% of premature infants had episodes of bradycardia, which were associated with appropriate nasal air flow but significant oxygen desaturation. The rate at which oxygen desaturation developed was even more rapid with these spells than during apnea (Samuels et al, 1992). Poets and colleagues (1992) considered the likely causes of this phenomenon and concluded that there is sudden ventilation-perfusion (V/Q) mismatching secondary to peripheral airway dysfunction. The latter may respond to CPAP therapy or increased positive end-expiratory pressure (PEEP) if the infant is on a ventilator, but this has not been proved. Poets and colleagues (1995) also have described episodes of severe oxygen desaturation without bradycardia, without apnea, and without squirming motions, but they were not sure of the cause; they suggested that premature infants born at less than 32 weeks of gestation should be monitored with pulse oximeters until at least 36 weeks of postconceptional age. This recommendation is based on the frequency of these episodes and the inability of apnea and heart rate monitors to detect them reliably. Upton and coworkers (1991) also described many episodes of desaturation without bradycardia in premature infants and suggested that pulse oximetry may be the best way to monitor premature infants; it is more important to detect the effect of apnea on the heart rate and oxygen saturation than it is to detect the apnea itself.

Adams and colleagues (1997) analyzed similar episodes in premature infants using respiratory inductance plethysmography and concluded that many spells with air flow present were associated with reduced tidal breath volumes and hypopnea. Potential consequences could include small peripheral airway dysfunction, secondary V/Q mismatching, and oxygen desaturation.

Bolivar and coworkers (1995) described episodes of oxygen desaturation in premature infants on mechanical ventilation; these episodes were preceded by increased positive esophageal pressure resulting from active expiratory efforts, presumably produced during attempts at crying. The presence of an endotracheal tube prevented the larynx from closing and allowed the lung volume to decrease suddenly, causing a decrease in lung compliance and an increase in airway resistance; then continued mechanical ventilation or spontaneous breathing was relatively ineffective during a period of severe oxygen desaturation. These investigators suggested that increased positive end-expiratory pressure (PEEP) might be effective, that further sedation might prevent the attempts at crying, and that extubation would allow the larynx to function properly to maintain the lung volume and peripheral airway patency.

## SYMPTOMATIC RECURRENT APNEA EVENTS

Apnea events are a frequent manifestation of general problems in newborn and premature infants (Kattwinkel, 1977). The more common underlying disorders or conditions are (1) local infection such as a scalp abscess; (2) bacteremia or septicemia; (3) necrotizing enterocolitis; (4) hypoxic-ischemic encephalopathy; (5) intracranial hemorrhage, posthemorrhagic hydrocephalus, and periventricular leukomalacia; (6) patent ductus arteriosus with a large left-to-right shunt; (7) gastroesophageal reflux; (8) hypoglycemia; (9) hypocalcemia; (10) anemia; (11) drugs or anesthesia; (12) environmental overheating; (13) any condition causing hypoxemia or hypovolemia; and (14) causes of upper airway obstruction such as nasal stenosis, choanal atresia, or vocal cord paralysis. These should be excluded and appropriately treated before a diagnosis of apnea of prematurity is made.

### Apnea Associated with Infection

Small premature infants commonly have systemic infections, and the initial sign is often an increased frequency of apnea episodes. Such infections include *Staphylococcus epidermidis* bacteremia associated with venous catheters, *Candida* fungal sepsis associated with vaginal delivery and dexamethasone administration, and respiratory syncytial virus pneumonia associated with bronchopulmonary dysplasia and nosocomial spread. It is imperative that infection be definitively ruled out or diagnosed and treated in all cases of recurrent apnea events. This is an important part of clinical practice with premature infants. For suspected infection it is usual to take blood specimens for culture, examine the white cell count, and start antibiotics. The removal of indwelling catheters always becomes an important consideration.

### Apnea Associated with Gastroesophageal Reflux

It has been established that visible postfeeding regurgitation of formula into the pharynx or mouth is associated with an increased incidence of apnea in premature infants (Menon et al, 1985); the explanation for the reflux is considered to be an activation of the laryngeal chemoreflex by gastric fluids (Thach, 1997). This phenomenon has suggested that covert gastroesophageal reflux to the level of the mid-esophagus, which is common in small premature infants, may be associated with recurrent apnea; treatment with theophylline may exacerbate the reflux, making the situation worse. Several polygraphic studies in premature infants have failed to demonstrate a temporal relationship between episodes of apnea and episodes of acid reflux into the lower or mid-esophagus (Ajuriaguerra et al, 1991; Newell et al, 1989; Walsh et al, 1981). Examining older infants, Paton and colleagues (1990) concluded that although reflux and apnea may coexist in the same patient, acid events in the lower esophagus do not precede apnea events.

Newell and colleagues (1989) showed in a small subgroup of infants with xanthine-resistant apnea of prematurity that effective control of gastroesophageal reflux with use of a thickened formula and a more upright position was associated with a significant reduction in the number of apneic spells. Of importance, this reduction was not immediate but delayed by 1 to 2 days following treatment; also, the improvement was obtained without the use of cisapride or other drugs. It has been suggested that the decreased number of apneas was due to the resolution of esophagitis (Booth, 1992).

Barrington and colleagues (2002) found no relationship between acid reflux events and apnea events in premature infants just prior to discharge from the hospital. Arad-Cohen and associates (2000) also found in older infants that most apneas were not related to reflux, but when apnea and reflux occurred close together, the apnea event preceded the reflux event. It seems more logical that apnea and desaturation would lead to relaxation of the gastroesophageal junction, explaining why formula is often found in the pharynx of infants suctioned during an apnea event.

Other investigators have suggested that the pH probe method may not be sufficiently sensitive, as it does not detect non–acid reflux events (Wenzl et al, 2001); they have used the intraluminal impedance technique in larger infants to detect esophageal volume changes with reflux and claim this method to be more reliable. Using similar impedance methodology in premature infants, Peter and colleagues (2002) found no temporal relationship between apnea, desaturation, or bradycardia and lower esophageal reflux events.

It has become common practice in many centers to treat xanthine-resistant apnea of prematurity with metoclopramide, cisapride, and other antireflux agents, although no controlled trials have established the efficacy of these drugs in preventing apnea. Some evidence does suggest that cisapride is effective at reducing reflux in small premature infants (Ariagno et al, 2001), as in older infants. Kimball and Carlton (2001) performed a retrospective chart review in a large number of premature infants and found that the number of apneas in the 5 days after starting cisapride or metaclopramide was not less than the number of apneas during the 5 days before therapy. It is extremely doubtful if these drugs have an important role to play in the management of recurrent apnea events. Cisapride is currently restricted by the Food and Drug Administration (FDA) to only investigational use, related to an associated Q-T prolongation with possibly an increased risk for cardiac arrhythmias (Dubin et al, 2001).

### Apnea Associated with Anemia of Prematurity

Agreement is lacking on the problem of anemia of prematurity and its relationship to recurrent apnea. In many centers, blood transfusion is standard policy in premature infants with a hematocrit of less than 30%, and in any infant with signs of anemia, such as tachycardia, tachypnea, or episodes of apnea or bradycardia. Keyes and associates (1989) found no relationship between hematocrits of 19% to 64% and any of these signs, and found no consistent changes after transfusion. However, Joshi and colleagues (1987) found a significant reduction in the incidence of brief and intermediate apneas, and in the incidence of bradycardias, after transfusion. Other investigators have reported similar results (DeMaio et al, 1989). Ross and coworkers (1989) conducted a controlled trial of blood transfusion in a group of infants who all met the aforementioned criteria for transfusion. After transfusion there was a significant reduction in the heart rate, in the number of apnea and bradycardia episodes, and in the blood lactate levels in comparison with the group not transfused. Stute and coworkers (1995) found a significant reduction in the number of apneas and the number of bradycardias during the 3 days after transfusion in small premature infants.

### Apnea Associated with Anesthesia

Premature infants who undergo surgery with general anesthesia frequently have major recurrent apnea episodes for a few days after the procedure; the most common case is that of bilateral inguinal hernia repair (William et al, 2001). This susceptibility to apnea may persist until 50 to 60 weeks of postconceptional age, so older premature infants must be appropriately observed and treated for apnea following anesthesia (Scherer, 1991). Spinal anesthesia may be a better choice than general anesthesia when possible (Krane et al, 1995).

### Apnea Associated with Immunizations

An increased incidence of apneas is sometimes associated with routine vaccinations given at 2 months of postconceptional age (Stalker, 2000). Botham and colleagues (1997) described a group of preterm infants born at 24 to 31 weeks of gestation; only 1 infant had apnea before the diphtheria-tetanus-pertussis (DTP) injection, but 17 infants had apnea events afterward.

### Apnea Associated with Respiratory Syncytial Virus infection

Premature infants who have respiratory syncytial virus (RSV) infections frequently have recurrent apnea episodes accompanied by nasalitis and increased secretions in the pharynx. Lindgren and colleagues (1992) have described a hyperresponsive laryngeal chemoreflex in RSV-infected lambs with nasalitis and increased tracheal secretions.

## FEEDING HYPOXEMIA

Feeding hypoxemia (also called feeding apnea, feeding desaturation, and feeding bradycardia) is frequent in premature infants given nipple feeds too soon but sometimes occurs in term infants (Hanlon et al, 1997; Rosen et al, 1984). During sucking and swallowing, ventilation is severely impaired (Shivpuri et al, 1983). The rapid onset of bradycardia is thought to be reflex in origin, whereas the delayed onset of bradycardia is due to oxygen desaturation. Feeding hypoxemia resolves with maturation, usually by 44 weeks of postconceptional age but occasionally as late as 54 weeks. Infants are treated by frequent interruptions during a feed, by supplemental oxygen while feeding, and in extreme cases by gavage. Sometimes, atropine before feeds may be helpful for treating the rapid-onset reflex bradycardia (Kattwinkel et al, 1976a). These events are not sleep related and should be differentiated from events associated with apnea of prematurity. With a knowledgeable, trained mother, feeding events should not delay discharge from the hospital.

## CONGENITAL HYPOVENTILATION SYNDROME

Although congenital hypoventilation syndrome—an uncommon condition—is more frequently described in older infants (Brouillette et al, 1990), the severe form occurs in newborns and may need attention in the delivery room or the newborn nursery. These infants have significant hypoventilation with small tidal volumes and prolonged apneas while asleep, but tend to have more normal ventilation while awake. There is little evidence of a response to asphyxia, so severe oxygen desaturation and hypercarbia develop without signs of an increased effort to breathe. Because the arousal responses may be present but the ventilatory responses to hypoxia and hypercarbia are absent, it is thought that this condition is caused by a failure to integrate signals from the central and peripheral chemoreceptors into the respiratory centers (Marcus et al, 1991). Findings on sonography, computed tomography (CT), and magnetic resonance imaging (MRI) studies of the head usually are normal initially (Weese-Mayer et al, 1988); the auditory brainstem responses may be abnormal. No respiratory stimulant drugs have been found to be effective (Oren et al, 1986), at least in the severe newborn type of this syndrome, and most infants require prolonged home mechanical ventilation with a tracheostomy. Phrenic nerve pacemakers may be useful sometimes (Brouillette et al, 1983), but because the upper airway muscles are not activated by the phrenic nerve, a tracheostomy is still necessary. Initially the ventilator may be needed for much of the day, but some improvement may be noted at about the age of 6 months, after which the infant may need the ventilator only at night while sleeping (Oren et al, 1987). Some of these infants may have Hirschsprung disease (O'Dell et al, 1987), a dysautonomia syndrome, or a neuroblastoma (Lambert et al, 2000), suggesting a more widespread problem. Seizure disorder, mild cerebral atrophy, and developmental delay may occur, possibly as a result of multiple asphyxial episodes. Many families cope with management of these children surprisingly well, and some of the children may even go to school (Marcus et al, 1991).

Acquired forms of central hypoventilation syndrome may be associated with the Arnold-Chiari syndrome (Choi et al, 1999), hypoxic-ischemic encephalopathy, meningitis, brain tumor, and metabolic brain disease. Examples of the obesity-hypoventilation syndrome have not been reported in the newborn.

## APNEA OF INFANCY

Isolated apneas 5 to 15 seconds in duration, with or without periodic breathing, occur commonly in term infants during the first 6 months of life (Richards et al, 1984). There is no associated bradycardia or color change, and the episodes resolve spontaneously. Certain infants have significant apneas, usually more than 20 seconds in duration but sometimes shorter, and nearly always associated with bradycardia or skin color change. These too usually resolve spontaneously. The diagnosis of apnea of infancy is reserved for apneas with onset after 38 weeks of gestation, to distinguish them from apnea of prematurity persisting until 42 weeks of postconceptional age (Consensus Statement, 1987).

Usually after discharge from the nursery, some infants with apnea of infancy have an acute life-threatening event (ALTE), necessitating resuscitation by vigorous stimulation or positive pressure ventilation (Consensus Statement, 1987). Apnea of infancy is just one cause of an ALTE, perhaps representing 50% of the cases. Other causes include gastroesophageal reflux, pharyngeal incoordination, convulsions, infection, heart disease, breath-holding spells, central hypoventilation syndrome, central nervous system abnormality, and accidental or intentional smothering by the mother. Many infants with an ALTE, after appropriate investigation to exclude other causes, are considered to have *near-miss sudden infant death syndrome* (SIDS). Investigation of these infants, by a 24-hour recording of their breathing, reveals that they have an increased incidence of periodic breathing, brief apneas, and prolonged apneas, when compared with control infants (Guilleminault et al, 1979). It is not clear whether the infants had the same abnormalities before their ALTE, which were simply not recognized, but that scenario seems quite likely. A significant number of these infants later die suddenly; it seems reasonable to consider that they died of apnea of infancy with a fatal episode of ALTE.

## SUDDEN INFANT DEATH SYNDROME

SIDS describes the sudden unexpected death of an infant, which is unexplained by history, by a thorough death scene investigation, and by an adequate autopsy (Consensus Statement, 1987). Death occurs during sleep, most commonly at night. The incidence in the United States is 0.8 per 1000 live births (1995 data). It is a major cause of infant mortality, with a peak incidence between 2 and 4 months of age, and it is much less common after 6 months of age. Environmental risk factors include prone sleeping position, exposure to tobacco smoke, overheating, and upper respiratory infections. Other risk factors are soft bedding, bed sharing, and bottle feeding, although they may not be independent variables. A recent study found that parental bed sharing was not a factor if the infant was sleeping in the supine position (Gessner et al, 2001).

The occurrence rate for SIDS is 3 to 4 times higher in all premature infants, and 10 times higher in very low-birth-weight infants, but the increased risk is not related to apnea of prematurity (Hodgman, 1998). Subsequent siblings of infants who die of SIDS may be at increased risk for SIDS.

Considerations in the differential diagnosis include accidental suffocation, deliberate infanticide, congenital brain abnormalities, cardiac conduction defects, and rare metabolic disorders of fatty acid oxidation. It must be emphasized that the diagnosis of SIDS is one of exclusion. The autopsy evaluation is remarkable for subtle findings, pulmonary congestion, and multiple petechial hemorrhages on the surface of the lungs, thymus, and pericardium—signs of suffocation that suggest deep breaths against an obstructed airway.

### The Prolonged Q-T Syndrome Hypothesis

One hypothesis is that infants who die of SIDS have a prolonged corrected Q-T interval in the electrocardiogram (ECG) and die from a cardiac arrhythmia. Schwartz and colleagues (1998) examined the ECGs of 34,000 infants on day 4 of life. In 12 of 24 infants (50%) who subsequently died of SIDS, the Q-Tc was longer than 440 msecs. Of those who did not die of SIDS, only 2.5% had a Q-Tc longer than 440 msecs. Other investigators have examined this problem and not found similar results (Southall et al, 1986). Infants with the true long Q-T syndrome die with syncopal spells and ventricular tachycardia episodes. There is no evidence that infants with SIDS die with such cardiac arrhythmias; recordings at the time of death suggest severe sinus bradycardia from hypoxia (Meny et al, 1994). Death by cardiac arrhythmia would not explain the characteristic autopsy findings of SIDS. As a screening procedure for detecting high SIDS risk, analysis of the Q-T interval would not be efficient; the positive test predictive value would be only 1.5%. In view of the absence of any reliable preventive treatment for this problem, it does not seem prudent to subject millions of infants to routine ECG examinations (Hoffman and Lister, 1999). The long Q-T syndrome may be associated with sodium channel gene mutations; in a postmortem molecular analysis of 93 cases of SIDS, only 2 infants had such a gene mutation (Ackerman et al, 2001). Infants who die of a cardiac arrhythmia with the long Q-T syndrome should be considered in a separate category.

### Apnea of Infancy Hypothesis

A more widely accepted hypothesis has been that these infants die from obstructive apnea and that they have apnea of infancy before their demise. However, infants with apnea of infancy, diagnosed by pneumogram, who have not yet experienced an ALTE, have only a slightly increased risk for SIDS over that in the general population. If infants with apnea of infancy have a single ALTE, the risk for sudden death increases to 4%, and if they have several ALTE episodes the risk is enormous. Nevertheless, only 7% of infants diagnosed with SIDS have a preceding ALTE. In a study examining breathing patterns obtained with 24-hour recordings at the time of discharge from the birth hospital, nonselected infants destined to die of SIDS did not have a breathing pattern significantly different from that in closely matched infants who did not die of SIDS (Southall et al, 1982). Infants who die of SIDS seldom have a prior diagnosis of apnea of infancy or prolonged apnea of prematurity. It seems reasonable to conclude that the apnea of infancy hypothesis for SIDS remains unproved, and that SIDS and apnea of infancy should be considered separate problems. Thus, an infant who dies suddenly after episodes of apnea of infancy should be considered not to have died of SIDS but to have died of apnea of infancy with an ALTE.

### A Variation of the Apnea Hypothesis

Although the apnea of infancy hypothesis is widely discredited, a recent study in Belgium found that in pneumograms performed at ages 1 to 4 months, short obstructive and mixed sleep apneas were more common in infants destined to die of SIDS than in control infants (Kato et al, 2001). Such episodes are common in early infancy; they are mild and nonthreatening and do not warrant a diagnosis of apnea of infancy, in which the recorded events are more prolonged and severe. Consistent with this reported mild ventilatory instability, there is evidence that the medullary arcuate nucleus of infants who die of SIDS is hypoplastic and manifests reduced neuronal density (Matturri et al, 2000). The arcuate nucleus corresponds to the site of central chemoreceptor cells in experimental animals such as the rat. In addition, in the arcuate nucleus of infants who die of SIDS, there is reduced muscurinic receptor binding (Kinney et al, 1995) and reduced serotonergic receptor binding (Panigrahy et al, 2000). This finding is unique to this site in infants who die of SIDS. In other infants who die of chronic oxygen insufficiency not related to SIDS, the same defect often is found, but it occurs without specificity in many other sets of neurons; it does not occur in infants who die of other causes without chronic oxygen deprivation. Although not established, a defect in central chemoreception is a likely cause for SIDS.

### Prone Sleeping Position and Further Hypotheses About SIDS

The evidence that the prone sleeping position is associated with an increased incidence of SIDS is convincing. An American Academy of Pediatrics Task Force on sleeping position and SIDS recommended that infants should sleep in the supine or lateral position (Kattwinkel et al, 1992). The relative risk of SIDS associated with the prone sleeping position ranges from 3.5 to 9.3 in seven reported studies; no study has reported a relative risk of less than 1.0 (Guntheroth and Spiers, 1992). Critical review of reports from several countries has shown that previously observed large reductions in the SIDS rate with supine or lateral positioning were sustained over time; further reductions in the incidence of prone positioning were accompanied by further reductions in the incidence of SIDS (Centers for Disease Control and Prevention, 1996; Hunt, 1994). It was concluded that the supine position was not associated with an increase in complications such as upper airway obstruction or aspiration pneumonia, as had been believed previously (Hunt and Shannon, 1992; Malloy, 2002).

The decreased incidence of SIDS is more marked with supine than with lateral positioning (Fleming et al, 1996; Wigfield et al, 1992); while asleep, the infant placed in the side position may roll into the prone position. The lateral position is no longer recommended (AAP Task Force, 1996). It is emphasized that the American Academy of Pediatrics recommendations do not apply to small premature infants, to infants with significant gastroesophageal reflux, or to those with craniofacial abnormalities such as the Pierre Robin syndrome or laryngomalacia; such infants may do better sleeping in the prone position.

No consensus on the cause of the problem with prone positioning has been developed, but several suggestions have been published that constitute further related hypotheses for the cause of SIDS.

#### *The Face-Down Sleeping Hypothesis*

Chiodini and Thach (1993) showed that the prone position may be associated with rebreathing and hypoxia; this is especially true when the infant assumes a persistent face-down position, a not uncommon occurrence, and when the infant sleeps on soft bedding with pillows, rather than on a firm mattress. These authors could find little evidence for the development of any airway obstruction, but the development of hypoxia was significant. Associated with rebreathing, the reduction of inspired oxygen was significantly greater than the increased inspired carbon dioxide (Patel et al, 2001), and there was a related increase in minute ventilation. Waters and colleagues (1996) found a high incidence of face-down position among older infants, but noted that periodic arousals with head turning prevented serious hypercarbia in most cases. Constantin and associates (1999) noted that the face-down position was uncommon in older premature infants near the time of discharge; it may be that such infants are not prone to SIDS until they are old enough to move their head into the face-down position, at which time they become dependent on an adequate arousal response.

#### *The Decreased Arousability Hypothesis*

Kahn and coworkers (1993) demonstrated that the prone position was associated with significantly fewer and shorter arousals from sleep. During obstructive apneas, an arousal or deep sigh response is significantly more frequent in the supine position than in the prone position (Groswasser et al, 2001). Decreased arousability in the prone sleeping position is independent of quiet or active sleep (Goto et al, 1999; Horne et al, 2001). It seems possible that an insufficient arousal response to serious hypoxia, during sleep in the prone position, may be an important factor in SIDS. Nevertheless, the occurrence of airway obstruction in SIDS is poorly explained.

#### *The Laryngeal Chemoreflex Hypothesis*

Jeffery and colleagues (1999) showed in normal term infants that small pharyngeal infusions of water caused markedly slower swallowing and breathing rates in the prone position, but little change in the supine position. Larger infusions in piglets under similar conditions caused more severe apneas and sometimes death. These investigators hypothesized that any or all of three factors may be operating: (1) prone position, (2) active sleep, and (3) laryngeal chemoreflex activity. All three may dominate in early infancy, the time of peak occurrence for SIDS. Later in infancy, infants roll on their backs, sleep becomes predominantly quiet rather than active, and the chemoreflex is attenuated with maturation. In the supine position, the pyriform fossae on either side of the larynx are available to store pharyngeal fluid and may protect the upper airway. In the prone position, the esophagus is superior to the larynx, so fluid may flow easily over the laryngeal chemoreceptors, initiating apnea with bradycardia. Under these circumstances it is reasonable that the glottis or larynx may close, causing airway obstruction. It has been suggested that the airway obstruction is due to laryngospasm caused by reflux of acid gastric contents into the pharynx, a phenomenon that has been demonstrated repeatedly in newborn dogs (Duke et al, 2001).

Other environmental factors important in SIDS also may play parts: smoking, nasalitis, and overheating. Nicotine exposure in lambs is associated with reduced arousal responses and reduced ventilatory responses to hypoxemia (Hafstrom et al, 2000). Pooled secretions in upper respiratory infections may stimulate the laryngeal chemoreflex, and this may be accentuated by overheating (Jeffery et al, 1999), but diminished in the supine sleeping position (Lindgren, 1999).

In view of the strong evidence about the prone sleeping position, infants in the normal newborn nursery should be placed in the supine position. SIDS has been reported in the newborn infant in the hospital (Burchfield and Rawlings, 1993). Premature infants accustomed to sleeping prone should be encouraged into the supine position before being discharged; in the supine position, premature infants are more arousable (Goto et al, 1999). Mothers should be appropriately advised of the advantages of the supine position. The "Back to Sleep" campaign was initiated in 1994 by the National Institute of Child Health and Human Development to inform health care professionals and families of this important recommendation. There is evidence that health care professionals, families, and day care centers do not always follow this advice (Paris et al, 2001; Pollack et al, 2002), so there is considerable room for improvement.

## HOME APNEA MONITORING PROGRAMS

Controversy remains about whether some infants should have apnea monitoring at home. Infants may be candidates for home monitoring if they have unresolved apnea of prematurity or unresolved apnea of infancy or are considered to be at increased risk for SIDS. The hope of those who use home monitors is that the occurrence of ALTE or SIDS will be reduced by appropriate caretaker interventions. Parents must be skilled in the use of the monitor, in the interpretation of frequent false alarms, and in cardiopulmonary resuscitation. There is no evidence that home apnea monitoring reduces the number of deaths or the number of ALTE episodes in any of these conditions, and the incidence of SIDS remains unchanged related to the use of home monitors.

### Discharge Pneumogram for Premature Infants

The pneumogram performed in premature infants at the time of discharge appears to be of no help in deciding whom to monitor for SIDS and should not be used for this purpose (Consensus Statement, 1987). In one British study, 4% of 1157 premature infants discharged from the hospital had previously unrecognized prolonged apneas on the predischarge pneumogram. None of the infants with later SIDS had prolonged apneas at discharge, and none with prolonged apneas at discharge had SIDS (Southall et al, 1982). Some clinicians perform a predischarge pneumogram to assess the risk for an ALTE. Barrington and associates (1996) performed a pneumogram in small premature infants believed to be ready for discharge from intensive care. In a few with worrisome apneas, discharge was delayed until the recordings improved, but in the end, most infants had less worrisome apneas recorded just prior to discharge, and all infants were sent home without a home apnea monitor. During a 6-month follow-up period, only 3 of 176 infants had an ALTE, and the predischarge pneumogram could not distinguish these 3 infants from the others without an ALTE. Some authors justify the predischarge pneumogram because it may detect undiagnosed apneas (Razi et al, 1999); however, the significance of such apneas not detected clinically by the nursing staff is currently uncertain (Martin and Fanaroff, 1998). Some inconclusive evidence has been found in favor of the predischarge pneumogram under certain circumstances. Subhani and colleagues (2000) examined the predischarge event recordings of 106 infants, but all of the infants were still on caffeine for apnea of prematurity. These investigators found that 74 infants had normal recordings and none had complications at follow-up, whereas in 32 infants, the recordings were not considered normal and 3 infants had an ALTE after discharge. It was not claimed that those 3 infants with an ALTE could be differentiated from the 29 other infants with an abnormal pneumogram and no ALTE. Furthermore, criteria for indicating an abnormal pneumogram are not established at this time. Di Fiore and colleagues (2001) concluded that infants who continue to have clinical monitor alarms near the time of discharge have relatively short apnea events, but they are more prone to desaturation and bradycardia events because they have residual lung disease with lower oxygen saturation levels, or because they have subtle neurodevelopmental dysfunction.

Despite lack of conclusive evidence, some institutions still perform a pneumogram in most small premature infants before discharge, usually if there is a history of recurrent apnea events and even if the apneas appear to be resolved. If persistent apnea events are found, depending on the severity, infants may be kept in the hospital longer, they may be discharged home without a monitor, or they may be discharged home on a monitor with the apparent hope of preventing an ALTE. However, many institutions take a different approach: They keep premature infants in the hospital for 5 to 7 days after the last apnea event observed by the hospital staff and then discharge the infant without a home apnea monitor. Darnall and colleagues (1997) concluded that it is reasonable to wait for up to 8 days after an apnea event before discharging the premature infant without a monitor. In larger premature infants, Eichenwald and associates (2001) concluded that an interval of 5 to 6 days was appropriate before discharge without a home monitor. A national survey showed that home apnea monitoring is not the standard of care (Meadows et al, 1992), and that there is no evidence that the home apnea monitoring strategy prevents any deaths. Surprisingly, there is no evidence that use of the home monitor accelerates discharge and reduces the length of hospitalization (Sychowski et al, 2001); it takes additional time in the hospital to prepare the family for use of the monitor. However, despite lack of evidence, use of monitors is widely supported in the community, and in making decisions about their use, it may be unwise to alienate an anxious and insistent family. If an infant is sent home on caffeine, it seems reasonable to use a home monitor, especially as the drug should be discontinued a month or so after discharge.

### The CHIME Project

As mandated by Congress, a large multicenter study is being conducted by the Collaborative Home Infant Monitoring Evaluation (CHIME) group. The aim is to reach a better understanding of apnea events in early infancy and to explore the possible role of home monitoring in the prevention of SIDS. A new and improved monitor is used; it includes pulse oximetry and respiratory inductance plethysmography for evaluating both central and obstructive apneas (Weese-Mayer et al, 2000). Data from this group indicate that the median level of fractional oxygen saturation in healthy term infants in the first 6 months of life is 98%, with the lower limit at 95% (Hunt et al, 1999). Transient desaturations of more than 10% were common, found in 60% of the infants, and nearly always were associated with brief apneas. The desaturations decreased in frequency as the infants approached the age of 6 months. These data confirm the earlier studies by Poets and colleagues (1991), who found that desaturations to less than 80% associated with apneas were common in healthy infants.

The CHIME group has reported a comparison of four groups of infants: (1) healthy full-term infants, (2) discharged preterm infants, (3) siblings of infants who died of SIDS, and (4) infants who had a recent ALTE (Ramanathan et al, 2001). The latter three groups were considered to be at increased risk for SIDS. The authors adopted arbitrary definitions that can be approximated as follows: *conventional events* were apneas of 20 or more seconds or bradycardias with heart rates of less than 80 beats/minute for at least 15 seconds; *extreme events* were apneas of 30 or more seconds or bradycardias with heart rates of less than 60 beats/minute for at least 10 seconds. Conventional events occurred in 31% of all infants, and extreme events occurred in an additional 10% of infants. Conventional events were quite common, and occurrence rates were similar in all four groups of infants. Extreme events were common only in the preterm infant group and only up to 43 weeks of postconceptional age, well before the peak incidence of SIDS. There was a high frequency of obstructive apneas without bradycardias, which would not be detected by commercial home monitors using transthoracic impedance; about 50% of extreme events had no bradycardia even with oxygen desaturation. There are no data confirming that even the extreme events documented in this study, especially those without bradycardia, would have any deleterious effects or predictive values.

It is not known what effect parental interventions may have had on the data. However, based on about 700,000 hours of monitoring, events described as abnormal by many authorities were actually quite common even in healthy term infants during the first 6 months of life, as well as in premature infants. For commercial home monitors, if they are to be used without better evidence for their efficacy, it is clear that technical improvements must be made and that much broader limits for normal breathing behavior must be accepted. Jobe (2001), among others, has called for a radical reduction in the use of home apnea monitors for the purpose of preventing SIDS.

## REFERENCES


AAP Task Force on infant positioning and SIDS: Update. Pediatrics 98:1216, 1996.

Abu-Osba YK, Brouillette RE, Wilson SL, Thach BT: Breathing pattern and transcutaneous oxygen tension during motor activity in preterm infants. Am Rev Respir Dis 125:382, 1982.

Ackerman MJ, Siu BL, Sturner WQ, et al: Postmortem molecular analysis of SCN5A defects in sudden infant death syndrome. JAMA 286:2264, 2001.

Adams JA, Zabaleta IA, Sackner MA: Hypoxemic events in spontaneously breathing premature infants: Etiological basis. Pediatr Res 42:463, 1997.

Adams JM, Murfin K, Mort J, et al: Detection of hyperoxemia in neonates by a new pulse oximeter. Neonat Intensive Care 7:42, 1994.

Adamson SL, Kuipers IM, Olson DM: Umbilical cord occlusion stimulates breathing independent of blood gases and pH. J Appl Physiol 70:1796, 1991.

Adamson SL, Richardson BS, Homan J: Initiation of pulmonary gas exchange by fetal sheep in utero. J Appl Physiol 62:989, 1987.

Ajuriaguerra MD, Radvanyi-Bouvet MF, Huon C, Moriette G: Gastroesophageal reflux and apnea in prematurely born infants during wakefulness and sleep. Am J Dis Child 145:1132, 1991.

Al-Aif S, Alvaro R, Manfreda J, et al: Inhalation of low (0.5-1.5%) $CO_2$ as a potential treatment for apnea of prematurity. Semin Perinatol 25:100, 2001.

Alvaro R, de Almeida V, al-Alaiyan S, et al: A placental extract inhibits breathing induced by umbilical cord occlusion in fetal sheep. J Dev Physiol 19:23, 1993.

Alvaro R, Alvarez J, Kwiatkowski K, et al: Small preterm infants (<1500 g) have only a sustained decrease in ventilation in response to hypoxia. Pediatr Res 32:403, 1992.

Arad-Cohen N, Cohen A, Tirosh E: The relationship between gastroesophageal reflux and apnea in infants. J Pediatr 137:321, 2000.

Aranda JV, Turmen T: Methylxanthines in apnea of prematurity. Clin Perinatol 6:87, 1979.

Ariagno RL, Kikkert MA, Mirmiran M, et al: Cisapride decreases gastroesophageal reflux in preterm infants. Pediatrics 107:E58, 2001.

Barrington K, Finer N: The natural history of the appearance of apnea of prematurity. Pediatr Res 29:372, 1991.

Barrington KJ, Finer NN: Doxapram for apnea of prematurity [letter]. J Pediatr 109:563, 1986.

Barrington KJ, Finer NN: Periodic breathing and apnea in preterm infants. Pediatr Res 27:118, 1990.

Barrington KJ, Finer NN, Li D: Predischarge respiratory recordings in very-low-birth-weight newborn infants. J Pediatr 129:934, 1996.

Barrington KJ, Finer NN, Torok-Both G, et al: Dose-response relationship of doxapram in the therapy for refractory idiopathic apnea of prematurity. Pediatrics 80:22, 1987.

Barrington KJ, Tan K, Rich W: Apnea at discharge and gastroesophageal reflux in the preterm infant. J Perinatol 22:8, 2002.

Blanchard PW, Cote A, Hobbs S, et al: Abolition of ventilatory response to caffeine in chemodenervated lambs. J Physiol 61:133, 1986.

Blanco CE, Dawes GS, Hanson MA, et al: The response to hypoxia of arterial chemoreceptors in fetal sheep and newborn lambs. J Physiol (Lond) 351:25, 1984.

Bodegard G, Schweiler GH, Skoglund S, et al: Control of respiration in newborn babies: The development of the Hering-Breuer inflation reflex. Acta Paediatr Scand 58:567, 1969.

Bolivar JM, Gerhardt T, Gonzalez A, et al: Mechanisms for episodes of hypoxemia in preterm infants undergoing mechanical ventilation. J Pediatr 127:767, 1995.

Booth IW: Silent gastro-esophageal reflux: How much do we miss? Arch Dis Child 67:1325, 1992.

Botham SJ, Isaacs D, Henderson-Smart DJ: Incidence of apnea and bradycardia in preterm infants following DTPw and Hib immunizations: A prospective study. J Paediatr Child Health 33:418, 1997.

Boylan P, Lewis PJ: Fetal breathing in labor. Obstet Gynecol 56:35, 1980.

Brady JP, Ceruti E: Chemoreceptor reflexes in the newborn infant: Effects of varying degrees of hypoxia on heart rate and ventilation in a warm environment. J Physiol (Lond) 184:631, 1066.

Brouillette RT, Ilbawi MN, Hunt CE: Phrenic nerve pacing in infants and children: A review of experience and report on the usefulness of phrenic nerve stimulation studies. J Pediatr 102:32, 1983.

Brouillette RT, Weese-Mayer DE, Hunt CE: Breathing control disorders in infants and children. Hosp Pract 25:82, 1990.

Bryan AC, Bryan MH: Control of respiration in the newborn. In Thibeault DW, Gregory GA (eds): Neonatal Pulmonary Care. Norwalk, Conn, Appleton-Century-Crofts, 1986.

Burchfield DJ, Rawlings J: Sudden deaths and ALTE in hospitalized neonates presumed to be healthy. Neonatal Intensive Care May (12):46, 1993.

Butcher-Puech MC, Henderson-Smart DJ, Holley D, et al: Relation between apnea duration and type and neurological status of preterm infants. Arch Dis Child 60:953, 1985.

Cattarossi L, Rubini S, Macagno F: Aminophylline and increased activity of peripheral chemoreceptors in newborn infants. Arch Dis Child 69:52, 1993.

Centers for Disease Control and Prevention: Sudden infant death syndrome, United States, 1983-1994. MMWR 45:859, 1996.

Cheung PY, Barrington KJ, Finer NN, et al: Early childhood neurodevelopment in very low birth weight infants with predischarge apnea. Pediatr Pulmonol 27:14, 1999.

Chiodini BA, Thach BT: Impaired ventilation in infants sleeping facedown: Potential significance for sudden infant death syndrome. J Pediatr 123:686, 1993.

Choi SS, Tran LP, Zalzal GH: Airway abnormalities in patients with Arnold-Chiari malformation. Otolaryngol Head Neck Surg 121:720, 1999.

Cohen MI: Neurogenesis of respiratory rhythm in the mammal. Physiol Rev 59:1105, 1979.

Condorelli S, Scarpelli EM: Somatic-respiratory reflex and onset of regular breathing movements in the lamb fetus in utero. Pediatr Res 9:879, 1975.

Consensus Statement: National Institutes of Health Consensus Development Conference on Infantile Apnea and Home Monitoring. Pediatrics 79:292, 1987.

Constantin E, Waters KA, Morielli A, et al: Head turning and face down positioning in prone sleeping premature infants. J Pediatr 134:558, 1999.

Daily WJR, Klaus M, Meyer HB: Apnea in premature infants: Monitoring, incidence, heart rate changes and an effect of environmental temperature. Pediatrics 43:510, 1969.

Darnall RA: Aminophylline reduces hypoxic ventilatory depression: Possible role of adenosine. Pediatr Res 19:706, 1985.

Darnall RA, Kattwinkel J, Nattie C, Robinson M: Margin of safety for discharge after apnea in preterm infants. Pediatrics 100:795, 1997.

Davis JM, Spitzer AR, Stefano JL, et al: Use of caffeine in infants unresponsive to theophylline in apnea of prematurity. Pediatr Pulmonol 3:90, 1987.

Dawes GS: Breathing before birth in animals and man. N Engl J Med 290:557, 1974.

Dawes GS: Revolutions and cyclical rhythms in prenatal life: Fetal respiratory movements rediscovered. Pediatrics 51:965, 1973.

Dawes GS, Gardner WN, Johnston BM, et al: Breathing in fetal lambs: The effect of brainstem section. J Physiol (Lond) 335:535, 1983.

Dawes GS, Gardner WN, Johnston BM, et al: Effects of hypercapnia on tracheal pressure, diaphragm, and intercostal electromyograms in unanesthetized sheep. J Physiol (Lond) 326:461, 1982.

DeMaio JG, Harris MC, Deuber C, Spitzer AR: Effect of blood transfusion on apnea frequency in growing premature infants. J Pediatr 114:1039, 1989.

Di Fiore JM, Arko MK, Miller MJ, et al: Cardiorespiratory events in preterm infants referred for apnea monitoring studies. Pediatrics 108:1304, 2001.

DiMarco AF, Von Euler C, Romaniuk JR, Yamamoto Y: Positive feedback facilitation of external intercostal and phrenic inspiratory activity by pulmonary stretch receptors. Acta Physiol Scand 113:375, 1981.

Dransfield DA, Spitzer AR, Fox WW: Episodic airway obstruction in premature infants. Am J Dis Child 137:441, 1983.

Dubin A, Kikkert M, Mirmiran M, Ariagno R: Cisapride associated with QTc prolongation in very low birth weight infants. Pediatrics 107:1313, 2001.

Duke SG, Postma GN, McGuirt WF, et al: Laryngospasm and diaphragmatic arrest in immature dogs after laryngeal acid exposure: A possible model for sudden infant death syndrome. Ann Otol Rhinol Laryngol 110:729, 2001.

Eichenwald EC, Aina A, Stark A: Apnea frequently persists beyond term gestation in infants delivered at 24 to 28 weeks. Pediatrics 100:354, 1997.

Eichenwald EC, Blackwell M, Lloyd JS, et al: Inter-neonatal intensive care unit variation in discharge timing: influence of apnea and feeding management. Pediatrics 108:928, 2001.

Eyal F, Alpan G, Sagi E, et al: Aminophylline versus doxapram in idiopathic apnea of prematurity: A double blind controlled trial. Pediatrics 75:709, 1985.

Fleming PJ, Blair PS, Bacon C, et al: Environment of infants during sleep and risk of the sudden infant death syndrome: Results of 1993-1995 case control study for confidential inquiry into stillbirths and deaths in infancy. Br Med J 313:191, 1996.

Gabriel M, Albani M: Cardiac slowing and respiratory arrest in preterm infants. Eur J Pediatr 122:257, 1976.

Gaon P, Lee S, Hannan S, et al: Assessment of effect of nasal continuous positive pressure on laryngeal opening using fibre optic laryngoscopy. Arch Dis Child 80:F230, 1999.

Gerhardt T, Bancalari E: Maturational changes of reflexes influencing inspiratory timing in newborns. J Appl Physiol 50:1282, 1981.

Gerhardt T, Bancalari E: Components of effective elastance and their maturational changes in human newborns. J Appl Physiol 53:766, 1982.
Gerhardt T, Bancalari E: Apnea of prematurity: I. Lung function and regulation of breathing. Pediatrics 74:58, 1984a.
Gerhardt T, Bancalari E: Apnea of prematurity: II. Respiratory reflexes. Pediatrics 74:63, 1984b.
Gerhardt T, McCarthy J, Bancalari E: Effects of aminophylline on respiratory center and reflex activity in premature infants with apnea. Pediatr Res 17:188, 1983.
Gessner BD, Ives GC, Perham-Hester KA: Association between sudden infant death syndrome and prone sleeping position, bed sharing, and sleeping outside an infant crib in Alaska. Pediatrics 108:923, 2001.
Gluckman PD, Gunn TR, Johnston BM: The effect of cooling on breathing and shivering in unanesthetized fetal lambs in utero. J Physiol (Lond) 343:495, 1983.
Gluckman PD, Johnston BM: Lesions in the upper lateral pons abolish the hypoxic depression of breathing in unanesthetized fetal lambs in utero. J Physiol (Lond) 382:373, 1987.
Goto K, Mirmiran M, Adams MM, et al: More awakenings and heart rate variability during supine sleep in preterm infants. Pediatrics 103:603, 1999.
Graham BD, Reardon HS, Wilson JL, et al: Physiologic and chemical response of premature infants to oxygen enriched atmosphere. Pediatrics 6:55, 1950.
Groswasser J, Simon T, Scaillet S, et al: Reduced arousals following obstructive apneas in infants sleeping prone. Pediatr Res 49:402, 2001.
Guilleminault C, Ariagno R, Korobkin R, et al: Mixed and obstructive sleep apnea and near-miss for sudden infant death syndrome: 2. Comparison of near-miss and normal control infants by age. Pediatrics 64:882, 1979.
Guntheroth WG, Spiers PS: Sleeping prone and the risk of sudden infant death syndrome. JAMA 267:2359, 1992.
Hackett PH, Roach RC, Harrison GL, et al: Respiratory stimulants and sleep periodic breathing at high altitude: Almitrine versus acetazolamide. Am Rev Respir Dis 135:896, 1987.
Haddad GG, Mellins RB: The role of airway receptors in the control of respiration in infants: A review. J Pediatr 91:281, 1977.
Hafstrom O, Milerad J, Asokan N, et al: Nicotine delays arousal during hypoxemia in lambs. Pediatr Res 47:646, 2000.
Hanlon MB, Tripp JH, Ellis RE, et al: Deglutition apnea as indicator of maturation of suckle feeding in bottle fed preterm infants. Dev Med Child Neurol 39:534, 1997.
Harding R: Fetal breathing. In Beard RW, Nathanielsz PW (eds): Fetal Physiology and Medicine. New York, Marcel Dekker, 1984, p 255.
Hayakawa F, Hakamada S, Kuno K, et al: Doxapram in the treatment of idiopathic apnea of prematurity: Desirable dosage and serum concentrations. J Pediatr 109:138, 1986.
Henderson-Smart DJ: The effects of gestational age on the incidence and duration of recurrent apnea in newborn babies. Aust Pediatr J 17:273, 1981.
Henderson-Smart DJ, Butcher-Puech MC, Edwards DA: Incidence and mechanism of bradycardia during apnea in preterm infants. Arch Dis Child 61:227, 1986.
Henderson-Smart DJ, Pettigrew AG, Campbell DJ: Clinical apnea and brain-stem neural function in preterm infants. N Engl J Med 308:353, 1983.
Henderson-Smart DJ, Read DJC: Reduced lung volume during behavioral active sleep in the newborn. J Appl Physiol 46:1081, 1979.
Herlenius E, Aden U, Tang LQ, Lagercrantz H: Perinatal respiratory control and its modulation by adenosine and caffeine in the rat. Pediatr Res 51:4, 2002.
Hertzberg T, Lagercrantz H: Postnatal sensitivity of the peripheral chemoreceptors in newborn infants. Arch Dis Child 62:1238, 1987.
Hiatt IM, Hegyi T, Indyk L, et al: Continuous monitoring of $PO_2$ during apnea of prematurity. J Pediatr 98:288, 1981.
Higuchi M, Hirano H, Gotoh K, et al: Relationship of fetal breathing movement pattern to surfactant phospholipid levels in amniotic fluid and postnatal respiratory complications. Gynecol Obstet Invest 31:217, 1991.
Hodgman JE: Apnea of prematurity and risk for SIDS. Pediatrics 102:969, 1998.
Hoecker C, Nelle M, Poeschl J, et al: Caffeine impairs cerebral and intestinal blood flow velocity in preterm infants. Pediatrics 109:784, 2002.
Hoffman JIE, Lister G: The implications of a relationship between prolonged QT interval and the sudden infant death syndrome [letter]. Pediatrics 103:815, 1999.
Hoppenbrouwers T, Hodgman JE, Harper RM, et al: Polygraphic studies of normal infants during the first six months of life: III. Incidence of apnea and periodic breathing. Pediatrics 60:418, 1977.
Horne RS, Ferens D, Watts AM, et al: The prone sleeping position impairs arousability in term infants. J Pediatr 138:793, 2001.
Hunt CE: Infant sleep position and sudden infant death syndrome risk: A time for change. Pediatrics 94:105, 1994.
Hunt CE, Corwin MJ, Lister G, et al: Longitudinal assessment of hemoglobin oxygen saturation in healthy infants during the first 6 months of age. Collaborative Home Infant Monitoring Evaluation (CHIME) Study Group. J Pediatr 135:580, 1999.
Hunt CE, Shannon DC: Sudden infant death syndrome and sleeping position. Pediatrics 90:115, 1992.
Jansen AH, Chernick V: Onset of breathing and control of respiration. Semin Perinatol 12:104, 1988.
Jansen AH, Ioffe S, Russell BJ, et al: Effect of carotid chemoreceptor denervation on breathing in utero and after birth. J Appl Physiol 51:630, 1981.
Jardine DS, Rogers K: Relationship of benzyl alcohol to kernicterus, intraventricular hemorrhage, and mortality in premature infants. Pediatrics 83:721, 1988.
Jeffery HE, Megevand A, Page M: Why the prone position is a risk factor for sudden infant death syndrome. Pediatrics 104:263, 1999.
Jobe AH: What do home monitors contribute to the SIDS problem? JAMA 285:2244, 2001.
Joshi A, Gerhardt T, Shandloff P, Bancalari E: Blood transfusion effect on the respiratory pattern of preterm infants. Pediatrics 80:79, 1987.
Kahn A, Groswasser J, Sottiaux M, et al: Prone or supine position and sleep characteristics in infants. Pediatrics 91:1112, 1993.
Kato I, Groswasser J, Franco P, et al: Developmental characteristics of apnea in infants who succumb to sudden infant death syndrome. Am J Respir Crit Care Med 164:1464, 2001.
Kattwinkel J: Neonatal apnea: Pathogenesis and therapy. J Pediatr 90:342, 1977.
Kattwinkel J, Brooks J, Myerberg D: Positioning and SIDS: AAP task force on infant positioning and SIDS. Pediatrics 89:1120, 1992.
Kattwinkel J, Fanaroff AA, Klaus MH: Bradycardia in preterm infants: Indications and hazards of atropine therapy. Pediatrics 58:494, 1976a.
Kattwinkel J, Mars H, Fanaroff A, et al: Urinary biogenic amines in idiopathic apnea of prematurity. J Pediatr 88:1003, 1976b.
Kattwinkel J, Nearman HS, Fanaroff AA, et al: Apnea of prematurity: Comparative therapeutic effects of cutaneous stimulation and nasal continuous positive airway pressure. J Pediatr 86:588, 1975.

Keyes WG, Donohue PK, Spivak JL, et al: Assessing the need for transfusion of premature infants and role of hematocrit, clinical signs, and erythropoietin level. Pediatrics 84:412, 1989.

Khoo MCK, Kronauer RE, Srohl KP, Slutsky AS: Factors influencing periodic breathing in humans: A general model. J Appl Physiol 53:644, 1982.

Kimball AL, Carlton DP: Gastroesophageal reflux medications in the treatment of apnea in premature infants. J Pediatr 138:355, 2001.

Kinney HC, Filiano JJ, Sleeper LA, et al: Decreased muscarinic receptor binding in the arcuate nucleus in sudden infant death syndrome. Science 269:1446, 1995.

Kitchen WH, Doyle LW, Ford GW, et al: Cerebral palsy in very low birth weight infants surviving to 2 years with modern perinatal intensive care. Am J Perinatol 4:29, 1987.

Kitterman JA, Liggins GC, Fewell JE, et al: Inhibition of breathing movements in fetal sheep by prostaglandins. J Appl Physiol 54:687, 1983.

Koos BJ, Matsuda K: Fetal breathing, sleep state and cardiovascular responses to adenosine in sheep. J Appl Physiol 68:489, 1990.

Korner AF, Kraemer HC, Hoffner ME, et al: Effects of waterbed flotation on premature infants: A pilot study. Pediatrics 56:361, 1975.

Kosch PC, Davenport PW, Wozniak JA, et al: Reflex control of inspiratory duration in breathing. J Appl Physiol 60:2007, 1986.

Krane EJ, Haberkern CM, Jacobson LE: Postoperative apnea, bradycardia, and oxygen desaturation in formerly premature infants: Prospective comparison of spinal and general anesthesia. Anesth Analg 80:7, 1995.

Krauss AN, Goldstein RF, Alfero V, et al: Effect of endotracheal continuous positive airway pressure on sensitivity to carbon dioxide and on respiratory timing in preterm infants. Pediatr Pulmonol 2:103, 1986.

Kurlak LO, Ruggins NR, Stephenson TJ: Effect of nursing position on incidence, type, and duration of clinically significant apnoea in preterm infants. Arch Dis Child 71:F16, 1994.

Lagercrantz H: What does the preterm infant breathe for? Controversies on apnea of prematurity. Acta Paediatr 81:733, 1992.

Larsen PB, Brendstrup L, Skov L, Flachs H: Aminophylline versus caffeine citrate for apnea and bradycardia prophylaxis in premature infants. Acta Paediatr 84:360, 1995.

Lambert SR, Yang LL, Stone C: Tonic pupil associated with congenital neuroblastoma, Hirschprung's disease, and central hypoventilation syndrome. Am J Ophthalmol 130:238, 2000.

Lindgren C: Respiratory control during upper airway infection: Mechanism for prolonged reflex apnea and sudden infant death with special reference to infant sleep position. FEMS Immunol Med Microbiol 25:97, 1999.

Lindgren C, Jing L, Graham B, et al: Respiratory syncytial virus infection reinforces reflex apnea in young lambs. Pediatr Res 31:381, 1992.

Locke R, Greenspan JS, Shaffer TH, et al: Effect of nasal CPAP on thoraco-abdominal motion in neonates with respiratory insufficiency. Pediatr Pulmonol 11:259, 1991.

Locke RG, Wolfson MR, Shaffer TH, et al: Inadvertent administration of positive end distending pressure during nasal cannula flow. Pediatrics 91:135, 1993.

Lopes JM, Davis GM, Mullahoo K, Aranda JV: Role of adenosine in the hypoxic ventilatory response of the newborn piglet. Pediatr Pulmonol 17:50, 1994.

Maillard C, Boutroy MJ, Fresson J, et al: QT interval lengthening in premature infants treated with doxapram. Clin Pharmacol Ther 70:540, 2001.

Malloy MH: Trends in postneonatal aspiration deaths and reclassification of sudden infant death syndrome: impact of the back to sleep program. Pediatrics 109:661, 2002.

Manning FA: Fetal breathing movements as a reflection of fetal status. Postgrad Med 61:116, 1977.

Marcus CL, Bautista DB, Amihyia A, et al: Hypercapnic arousal responses in children with congenital central hypoventilation syndrome. Pediatrics 88:993, 1991.

Marcus CL, Jansen MT, Poulsen MK, et al: Medical and psychosocial outcome of children with congenital central hypoventilation syndrome. J Pediatr 119:888, 1991.

Martin RJ, DiFiore JM, Davis JL, et al: Persistence of the biphasic ventilatory response to hypoxia in preterm infants. J Pediatr 132:960, 1998.

Martin RJ, DiFiore JM, Korenke CB, et al: Vulnerability of respiratory control in healthy preterm infants placed supine. J Pediatr 127:609, 1995.

Martin RJ, Miller MJ, Carlo WA: Pathogenesis of apnea in preterm infants. J Pediatr 109:733, 1986.

Martin RJ, Nearman HS, Katona PG, et al: The effect of a low continuous positive airway pressure on the reflex control of respiration in the preterm infant. J Pediatr 90:976, 1977.

Martin RJ, Fanaroff AA: Neonatal apnea, bradycardia or desaturation: Does it matter? J Pediatr 132:758, 1998.

Martin-Boddy RL, Johnston BM: Central origin of the hypoxic depression of breathing in the newborn. Respir Physiol 71:25, 1988.

Mathew OP: Maintenance of upper airway patency. J Pediatr 106:863, 1985.

Mathew OP, Thoppil CK, Belan M: Motor activity and apnea in preterm infants. Am Rev Respir Dis 144:842, 1991.

Matturri L, Biondo B, Mercurio P, Rossi L: Severe hypoplasia of medullary arcuate nucleus: Quantitative analysis in sudden infant death syndrome. Acta Neuropathol 99:371, 2000.

Meadows W, Mendez D, Lantos J, et al: What is the legal standard of medical care when there is no standard of medical care? A survey of the use of home apnea monitoring for graduates of neonatal intensive care units. Neonat Intensive Care 5:43, 1992.

Menon AP, Schefft GL, Thach BT: Apnea associated with regurgitation in infants. J Pediatr 106:625, 1985.

Meny RG, Carroll JL, Carbone MT, Kelly DH: Cardiorespiratory recordings from infants dying suddenly and unexpectedly at home. Pediatrics 93:44, 1994.

Miller MJ, Carlo WA, Martin RJ: Continuous positive airway pressure selectively reduces obstructive apnea in preterm infants. J Pediatr 106:91, 1985.

Muller N, Volgyesi G, Eng P, et al: The consequences of diaphragmatic muscle fatigue in the newborn infant. J Pediatr 95:793, 1979.

Murai DT, Lee CH, Wallen LD, et al: Denervation of peripheral chemoreceptors decreases breathing movements in fetal sheep. J Appl Physiol 59:575, 1985.

Murat I, Morriette G, Blin MC, et al: The efficacy of caffeine in the treatment of recurrent idiopathic apnea in premature infants. J Pediatr 99:984, 1981.

Newell SJ, Booth IW, Morgan MEI, et al: Gastroesophageal reflux in preterm infants. Arch Dis Child 64:780, 1989.

O'Dell K, Staren E, Bassuk A: Total colonic aganglionosis (Zuelzer-Wilson syndrome) and congenital failure of autonomic control of ventilation (Ondine's curse). J Pediatr Surg 22:1019, 1987.

Oren J, Kelly DH, Shannon DC: Long term follow-up of children with congenital central hypoventilation syndrome. Pediatrics 80:375, 1987.

Oren J, Newth CJL, Hunt CE, et al: Ventilatory effects of almitrine bismesylate in congenital central hypoventilation syndrome. Am Rev Respir Dis 134:917, 1986.

Panigrahy A, Filiano J, Sleeper LA, et al: Decreased serotonergic receptor binding in rhombic lip derived regions of the medulla oblongata in the sudden infant death syndrome. J Neuropathol Exp Neurol 59:377, 2000.

Paris CA, Remler R, Daling JR: Risk factors for sudden infant death syndrome: Changes associated with sleep position recommendations. J Pediatr 139:771, 2001.

Patel AL, Harris K, Thach BT: Inspired $CO_2$ and $O_2$ in sleeping infants rebreathing from bedding: Relevance for sudden infant death syndrome. J Appl Physiol 91:2537, 2001.

Paton JY, Macfadyen U, Williams A, et al: Gastroesophageal reflux and apneic pauses during sleep in infancy: No direct relationship. Eur J Pediatr 149:680, 1990.

Patrick J, Fetherston W, Vick H, et al: Human fetal breathing movements at weeks 34 to 35 of gestation. Am J Obstet Gynecol 130:693, 1978.

Perlman JM, Volpe JJ: Episodes of apnea and bradycardia in the preterm newborn: Impact on cerebral circulation. Pediatrics 76:333, 1985.

Peter CS, Sprodowski N, Bohnhorst B, et al: Gastroesophageal reflux and apnea of prematurity: No temporal relationship. Pediatrics 109:8, 2002.

Poets CF, Darraj S, Bohnhorst B: Effect of doxapram on episodes of apnea, bradycardia and hypoxemia in preterm infants. Biol Neonate 76:207, 1999.

Poets CF, Samuels MP, Southall DP: Potential role of intrapulmonary shunting in the genesis of hypoxemic episodes in infants and young children. Pediatrics 90:385, 1992.

Poets CF, Stebbens VA, Richard D, Southall DP: Prolonged episodes of hypoxemia in preterm infants undetected by cardiorespiratory monitors. Pediatrics 95:860, 1995.

Poets CF, Stebbens VA, Samuels MP, Southall DP: The relationship between bradycardia, apnea, and hypoxemia in preterm infants. Pediatr Res 34:144, 1993.

Poets CF, Stebbens VA, Southall DP: Arterial oxygen saturation and breathing movements during the first year of life. J Dev Physiol 15:341, 1991.

Pollack HA, Frohna JG: Infant sleep placement after the Back to Sleep campaign. Pediatrics 109:608, 2002.

Pryds O, Schneider S: Aminophylline reduces cerebral blood flow in stable preterm infants without affecting the visual evoked potential. Eur J Pediatr 150:366, 1991.

Ramanathan R, Corwin MJ, Hunt CE, et al: Cardiorespiratory events recorded on home monitors: Comparison of healthy infants with those at increased risk for SIDS. JAMA 285:2244, 2001.

Razi NM, Humphreys J, Pandit PB, et al: Predischarge monitoring of preterm infants. Pediatr Pulmonol 27:113, 1999.

Richards JM, Alexander JR, Shinebourne EA, et al: Sequential 22-hour profiles of breathing patterns and heart rate in 110 full-term infants during their first 6 months of life. Pediatrics 74:763, 1984.

Richerson GB, Wang W, Tiwari J, Bradley SR: Chemosensitivity of serotonergic neurons in the rostral ventral medulla. Respir Physiol 129:175, 2001.

Rigatto H: Apnea. Pediatr Clin North Am 29:1105, 1982.

Rigatto H: Ventilatory response to hypercapnia. Semin Perinatol 1:363, 1977.

Rigatto H, Brady JP: Periodic breathing and apnea in preterm infants: Evidence for hypoventilation possibly due to central respiratory depression. Pediatrics 50:202, 1972.

Rigatto H, Brady JP, Verduzco RT: Chemoreceptor reflexes in preterm infants: The effect of gestational and postnatal age on the ventilatory response to inhalation of 100% and 15% oxygen. Pediatrics 55:604, 1975a.

Rigatto H, Brady J, Verduzco RT: Chemoreceptor reflexes in preterm infants: The effect of gestational and postnatal age on the ventilatory response to inhaled carbon dioxide. Pediatrics 55:614, 1975b.

Rigatto H, Verduzco RT, Cates DB: Effects of $O_2$ on the ventilatory response to $CO_2$ in preterm infants. J Appl Physiol 39:896, 1975c.

Rosen CL, Glaze DG, Frost JD: Hypoxemia associated with feeding in the preterm infant and full-term neonate. Am J Dis Child 138:623, 1984.

Ross MP, Christensen RD, Rothstein G, et al: A randomized trial to develop criteria for administering erythrocyte transfusions to anemic preterm infants 1-3 months of age. J Perinatol 9:246, 1989.

Runold M, Lagercrantz H, Prabhakar NR, et al: Role of adenosine in hypoxic ventilatory depression. J Appl Physiol 67:541, 1989.

Saliba E, Autret E, Gold F, et al: Effect of caffeine on cerebral blood flow velocity in preterm infants. Biol Neonate 56:198, 1989.

Samuels MP, Poets CF, Stebbens VA, et al: Oxygen saturation and breathing patterns in preterm infants with cyanotic episodes. Acta Paediatr 81:875, 1992.

Scherer LR: Surgical management. In Jones MD, Gleason CA, Lipstein SU (eds): Hospital Care of the Recovering NICU Infant. Baltimore, Williams & Wilkins, 1991.

Schulte FJ: Apnea. Clin Perinatol 4:65, 1977.

Schwartz PJ, Stramba-Badiale M, Segantini A, et al: Prolongation of the QT interval and the sudden infant death syndrome. N Engl J Med 338:1709, 1998.

Shivpuri CR, Martin RJ, Carlo WA, Fanaroff AA: Decreased ventilation in preterm infants during an oral feed. J Pediatr 103:285, 1983.

Silvestri JM, Weese-Mayer DE, Kenny AS, et al: Prolonged cardiorespiratory monitoring of children more than 12 months of age: Characterization of events and approach to discontinuation. J Pediatr 125:51, 1994.

Smith GN, Brien JF, Homan J, et al: Indomethacin reversal of ethanol-induced suppression of ovine fetal breathing movements and relationship to prostaglandin $E_2$. J Dev Physiol 14:29, 1990.

Soliz A, Suguihara C, Huang J, et al: Effect of amino acid infusion on the ventilatory response to hypoxia in protein-deprived neonatal piglets. Pediatr Res 35:316, 1994.

Southall DP, Richards JM, Rhoden KJ, et al: Prolonged apnea and cardiac arrhythmias in infants discharged from neonatal intensive care units: Failure to predict an increased risk for sudden infant death syndrome. Pediatrics 70:844, 1982.

Southall DP, Richards JM, Stebbens V, et al: Cardiorespiratory function in 16 full-term infants with sudden infant death syndrome. Pediatrics 78:787, 1986.

Speidel BD, Dunn PM: Use of nasal continuous positive airway pressure to treat severe recurrent apnea in very preterm infants. Lancet 2:658, 1976.

Sreenan C, Etches PC, Demianczuk N, et al: Isolated mental developmental delay in very low birth weight infants: Association with prolonged doxapram therapy for apnea. J Pediatr 139:832, 2001a.

Sreenan C, Lemke RP, Hudson-Mason A, et al: High flow nasal cannulae in the management of apnea of prematurity: A comparison with conventional nasal continuous positive airway pressure. Pediatrics 107:1081, 2001b.

Stalker DJ: Apnea following immunization in premature infants. Arch Dis Child 83:F74, 2000.

Storrs CN: Cardiovascular effects of apnea in preterm infants. Arch Dis Child 52:534, 1977.

Stute H, Greiner B, Linderkamp O: Effect of blood transfusion on cardiorespiratory abnormalities in preterm infants. Arch Dis Child 72:F194, 1995.

Subhani M, Katz S, DeCristofaro JD: Prediction of post discharge complications by predischarge event recordings in infants with apnea of prematurity. J Perinatol 20:92, 2000.

Sychowski SP, Dodd E, Thomas P, et al: Home apnea monitor use in preterm infants discharged from newborn intensive care units. J Pediatr 139:245, 2001.

Thach BT: Reflux associated apnea in infants: Evidence for a laryngeal chemoreflex. Am J Med 103:120S, 1997.

Thach BT, Frantz ID, Adler S, et al: Maturation of reflexes influencing inspiratory duration in human infants. J Appl Physiol 45:203, 1978.

Tudehope DI, Rogers YM, Burns YR, et al: Apnea in very low birth weight infants: Outcome at 2 years. Aust Paediatr J 22: 131, 1986.

Upton CJ, Milner AD, Stokes GM: Apnoea, bradycardia, and oxygen saturation in preterm infants. Arch Dis Child 66:381, 1991.

Von Euler C: On the central pattern generator for the basic breathing rhythmicity. J Appl Physiol 55:1647, 1983.

Walsh JK, Farrell MK, Keenan WJ, et al: Gastro-esophageal reflux in infants: Relation to apnea. J Pediatr 99:197, 1981.

Walther FJ, Erickson R, Sims ME: Cardiovascular effects of caffeine in preterm infants. Am J Dis Child 144:1164, 1990.

Waters KA, Gonzales A, Jean C, et al: Face straight down and face near straight down positions in healthy prone sleeping infants. J Pediatr 128:616, 1996.

Weese-Mayer DE, Brouillette RT, Naidich TP, et al: Magnetic resonance imaging and computerized tomography in central hypoventilation. Am Rev Respir Dis 137:393, 1988.

Weese-Mayer DE, Corwin MJ, Peucker MR, et al: Comparison of apnea identified by respiratory inductance plethysmography with that detected by end tidal $CO_2$ or thermistor. Am J Respir Crit Care Med 162:471, 2000.

Wennergren G, Wennergren M: Neonatal breathing control mediated by the central chemoreceptors. Acta Physiol Scand 119:139, 1983.

Wenzl TG, Schenke S, Peschgens T, et al: Association of apnea and non-acid gastroesophageal reflux in infants: Investigations with the intraluminal impedance technique. Pediatr Pulmonol 31:144, 2001.

Wigfield RE, Fleming PJ, Berry PJ, et al: Can the fall in Avon's sudden infant death rate be explained by changes in sleeping position? BMJ 304:282, 1992.

Wigglesworth JS, Desai R: Is fetal respiratory function a major determinant of perinatal survival? Lancet 1:264, 1982.

William JM, Stoddart PA, Williams SA, et al: Postoperative recovery after inguinal herniotomy in ex premature infants: Comparison between sevoflurane and spinal anaesthesia. Brit J Anaesth 86:366, 2001.

Yamazaki T, Kajiwara M, Itahashi K, et al: Low dose doxapram therapy for idiopathic apnea of prematurity. Pediatr Int 43:124, 2001.

CHAPTER

# 44

# Pulmonary Physiology of the Newborn

Thomas N. Hansen and Anthony Corbet

## LUNG MECHANICS AND LUNG VOLUMES

The lungs possess physical, or mechanical, properties that resist inflation, such as elastic recoil, resistance, and inertance. The dynamic interaction between these properties determines the effort that must be exerted during spontaneous breathing and the resting and extreme values for the volume of gas in the lung.

### Elastic Recoil

The lung contains elastic tissues that must be stretched for lung inflation to occur. Hooke's law requires that the pressure needed to inflate the lung must be proportional to the volume of inflation (Fig. 44–1). Conventionally, volume of inflation is plotted on the $y$-axis, and the distending pressure is plotted on the $x$-axis. In this way, the constant of proportionality is volume divided by pressure, or *lung compliance*. Throughout the range of tidal ventilation, the relationship between pressure and volume is linear. At higher lung volumes, as the lung reaches its elastic limit (*total lung capacity* [TLC]), this relationship plateaus.

The lungs and the chest wall function as a unit (the respiratory system) coupled with the interface between the parietal and the visceral pleura. The tendency for the lung to collapse at rest is balanced by the outward recoil of the chest wall, resulting in a negative (subatmospheric) intrapleural pressure. The volume at which this balance occurs is the functional residual capacity (FRC). Inflation of the respiratory system above FRC requires a positive distending pressure that, at higher lung volumes, must overcome the elastic recoil of both the lung and the chest wall. Deflation below FRC requires an active expiratory maneuver. Residual volume (RV) is defined as the volume of air that cannot be expired with a forced deflation.

As depicted in Figure 44–1, the relative compliance of the lung of the newborn is similar to that of the adult lung (Krieger, 1963); however, the infant's chest wall compliance (Table 44–1) is greater than the adult's (see Fig. 44–1), and the pleural pressure is only slightly subatmospheric. Measurements of lung and chest wall compliance suggest that the newborn should have a lower percent RV and a lower percent FRC than in the adult. In fact, the percent FRC in the newborn is equal to the adult's, and the infant's percent RV is slightly greater. This seeming paradox exists because FRC and RV are measured while the infant is breathing, and predictions from the pressure volume curves assume that there is no air movement and passive relaxation of all respiratory muscles (Bryan and England, 1984). Data suggest two mechanisms by which the newborn can maintain a normal FRC during spontaneous breathing: (1) by maintaining inspiratory muscle activity throughout expiration and splinting the chest wall or (2) by increasing expiratory resistance by glottic narrowing. The reason for the elevated RV is not entirely clear, but it could result from airway closure during an active expiration as part of a crying vital capacity maneuver.

### Resistance

Resistance to gas flow arises because of friction between gas molecules and the walls of airways (*airway resistance*) and because of friction between the tissues of the lung and the chest wall (*viscous tissue resistance*). Airway resistance represents approximately 80% of the total resistance of the respiratory system (Polgar and String, 1966). In the newborn, nasal resistance represents nearly half the total airway resistance; in the adult, it accounts for about 65% of the airway resistance (Polgar and Kong, 1965).

Gas flows only in response to a pressure gradient (Fig. 44–2). During laminar flow, the pressure difference needed to force gas through the airway is directly related to the flow rate times a constant—airway resistance. During turbulent flow, however, this pressure is directly proportional to a constant times the flow rate squared. Gas flow becomes turbulent at branch points in airways, at sites of obstruction, and with high flow rates. Turbulence occurs whenever flow increases to a point that Reynolds' number exceeds 2000. This dimensionless number is directly proportional to the volumetric flow rate and gas density, and it is inversely proportional to the radius of the tube and gas viscosity. Obviously, turbulent flow is most likely to occur in the central airways, where volumetric flow is high, rather than in lung periphery, where flow is distributed across a large number of airways. Both types of flow exist in the lung, so the net pressure drop is calculated as follows (Pedley et al, 1977):

$$\Delta P = (K_1 \times \dot{V}) + (K_2 \times \dot{V}^2) \qquad (1)$$

It is possible to take advantage of the differences between laminar and turbulent flows to determine the site of airway obstruction in the lung. If obstruction to gas flow is in the central airways, turbulent flow is affected the most. Because turbulent gas flow is density dependent, allowing the patient to breathe a less dense gas (such as helium mixed with oxygen) reduces the resistance to gas flow. If the site of obstruction is peripheral, the mixture of helium and oxygen does not appreciably affect resistance.

Inflation of the lung increases the length of airways and might therefore be expected to increase airway resistance. Lung inflation also increases airway diameter, however. Because airway resistance varies with the fourth to fifth power of the radius of the airway, the effects of changes in airway diameter dominate, and resistance is inversely proportional to lung volume (Rodarte and Rehder, 1986). Similarly, airway resistance is lower during inspiration than during

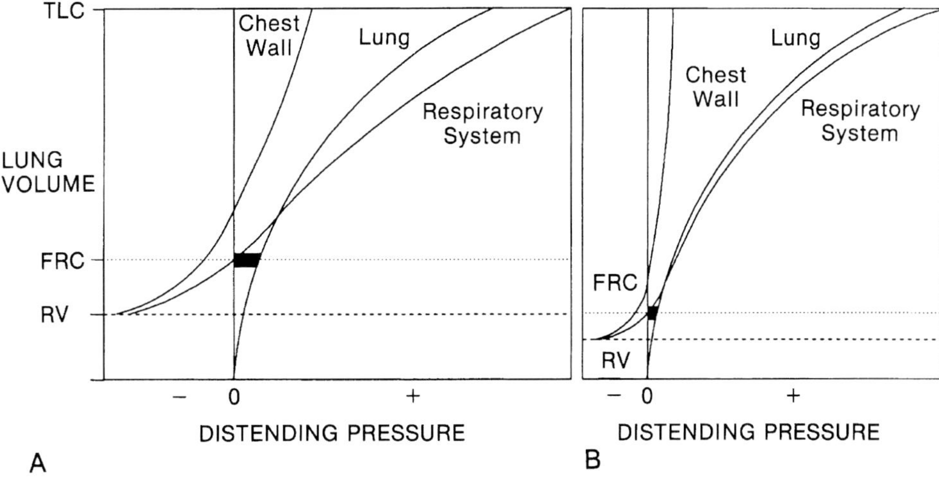


**FIGURE 44–1.** This is an idealized plot of volume as a function of distending pressure for the lung, chest wall, and respiratory system (lung plus chest wall) of an adult (**A**) and an infant (**B**). These curves are derived by instilling or removing a measured volume of gas from the lung and allowing the respiratory system to come to rest against a shuttered airway. At this point, only elastic forces are acting on the respiratory system, and airway pressure is equal to alveolar pressure. Intrapleural pressure can be measured using an esophageal balloon. Because airway pressure is equal to alveolar pressure, the distending pressure for the lung can be measured as *airway pressure – intrapleural pressure*. The distending pressure for the chest wall is *intrapleural pressure – atmospheric pressure*, and the distending pressure for the respiratory system is *airway pressure – atmospheric pressure*. Compliance is the change in volume divided by the change in distending pressure. The shaded area is the resting intrapleural pressure at functional residual capacity (FRC). Lung volumes depicted include residual volume (RV), functional residual capacity (FRC), and total lung capacity (TLC).

expiration because of the effects of changes in intrapleural pressure on airway diameter. During inspiration, pleural pressure becomes negative, and a distending pressure is applied across the lung. This distending pressure increases airway diameter as well as alveolar diameter and decreases the resistance to gas flow. During expiration, pleural pressure increases and airways are compressed. Collapse of airways is opposed by their cartilaginous support and by the pressure exerted by gas in their lumina. During passive expiration, these defenses are sufficient to prevent airway closure. When intrapleural pressure is high during active expiration, airways may collapse, and gas may be trapped in the lung. This problem may be accentuated in the small preterm infant with poorly supported central airways.

**TABLE 44–1**

**Lung Volumes and Mechanics in the Normal Newborn**

| **Lung Volumes** | **mL/kg** |
|---|---|
| Total lung capacity | 63 |
| Functional residual capacity | 30 |
| Residual volume | 23 |
| Tidal volume | 6 |
| **Compliance** | **mL/cm $H_2O$** |
| Total respiratory system | 3 |
| Chest wall | 20 |
| Lung | 4 |
| **Resistance** | **cm $H_2O$/mL/sec** |
| Total pulmonary resistance | 0.03-0.04 |

Data from Cook et al, 1957; Gerhardt and Bancalari, 1980; Polgar and Promadhat, 1971; Polgar and String, 1966; Reynolds and Etsten, 1966.

### Inertance

Gas and tissues in the respiratory system also resist accelerations in flow. Inertance is a property that is negligible during quiet breathing and physiologically significant only at rapid respiratory rates.

### Dynamic Interaction

Compliance, resistance, and inertance all interact during spontaneous breathing (Fig. 44–3). This interaction is described by the equation of motion for the respiratory system:

$$P(t) = (V[t] \times 1/C) + (\dot{V}[t] \times R) + (\ddot{V}[t] \times I) \quad (2)$$

where P(t) is the driving pressure at time t, V[t] is the lung volume above FRC, C is the respiratory system compliance, $\dot{V}$[t] is the rate of gas flow, R is the resistance of the respiratory system, $\ddot{V}$[t] is the rate of acceleration of gas in the airways, and I is the inertance of the respiratory system. If I is neglected, the equation simplifies to:

$$P(t) = (V[t] \times 1/C) + (\dot{V}[t] \times R) \quad (3)$$

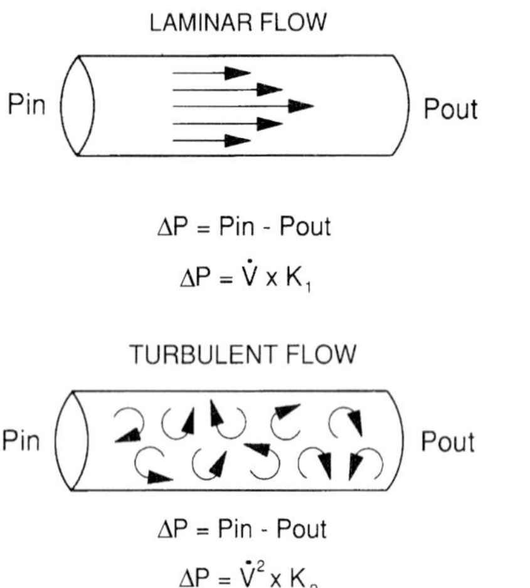


**FIGURE 44–2.** Gas flow ($\dot{V}$) through tubular structures occurs only in the presence of a pressure gradient (Pin > Pout). For laminar flow, P is directly proportional to

$$\Delta P = \dot{V} \times (8 \times L \times \mu)/(\pi \times r^4)$$

In this case, the constant of proportionality ($K_1$) is directly related to the length of the airway (L) and the viscosity of the gas ($\mu$) and indirectly proportional to the fourth power of the radius of the airway (r).

For turbulent flow, $\Delta P$ is proportional to $\dot{V}^2$. The constant of proportionality ($K_2$) is directly proportional to the length of the airway and the density of the gas and inversely proportional to the fifth power of the radius of the airway.

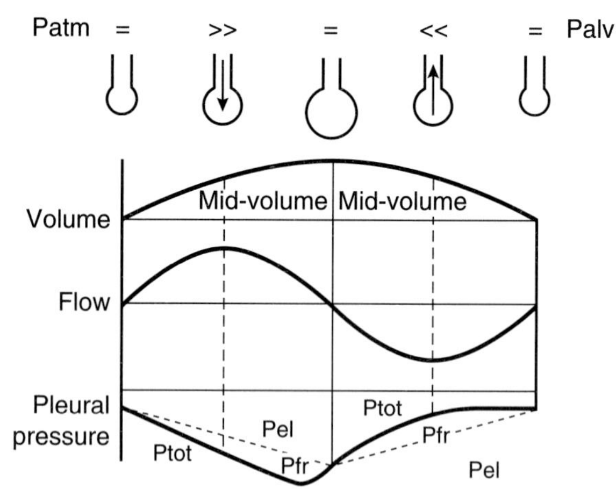


**FIGURE 44–3.** Gas flows from the atmosphere into the lung *only if atmospheric pressure* (Patm) *is greater than alveolar pressure* (Palv). At end-exhalation, when Patm equals Palv, there is no gas movement into or out of the lung. During a spontaneous inspiration, the diaphragm contracts, the chest wall expands, and the volume in the intrathoracic space increases. As a result, pleural pressure (Ppl) decreases relative to Patm, and a gradient is created between Ppl and Palv, distending the lung, increasing alveolar volume, and decreasing Palv. A gradient also is created between Patm and Palv, and gas flows from the atmosphere into the alveolar space. The rate of gas flow increases rapidly, reaches a maximum (peak flow), and then decreases as the alveolus fills with gas and Palv approaches Patm. At peak inspiration, Palv equals Patm, and lung volume is at its maximum, as is Ppl. The *curved solid line* connecting end-expiration to end-inspiration is the total driving pressure for inspiration (Ptot). The *dotted line* represents the pressure needed to overcome elastic forces alone (Pel). The difference between the two lines is the pressure dissipated overcoming flow-resistive forces (Pfr). During exhalation, this cycle is reversed.

At times of zero gas flow (end-expiration and end-inspiration), the equation further simplifies to:

$$P(t) = (V[t] \times 1/C) \text{ and } C = V(t)/P(t) \qquad (4)$$

This series of equations and Figure 44–3 demonstrate that at points of no gas flow (end-expiration and end-inspiration), only elastic forces are operating on the lung. During inflation or deflation of the lung, however, both elastic and resistive forces are important.

Although the solution to the equation of motion for the respiratory system is beyond the scope of this discussion, the behavior of the respiratory system during passive exhalation is a special situation for which a solution can be obtained relatively easily (Lesouëf et al, 1984; McIlroy et al, 1963). Before a passive exhalation maneuver, the infant is given a positive pressure breath, and the airway is occluded—invoking the Hering-Breuer reflex and a brief apnea. Airway pressure is measured, and the occlusion is released. Expired gas flow is measured using a pneumotachometer and integrated to volume; flow is then plotted as a function of volume (Fig. 44–4A). During a passive exhalation, there are no external forces acting on the respiratory system (P[t] = 0), so the equation of motion simplifies to:

$$(V[t] \times 1/C) + (\dot{V}[t] \times R) = 0$$

Rearranging gives

$$\dot{V}(t) = (-1/[RC]) \times V(t) \qquad (5)$$

This equation states that during passive exhalation, flow plotted against volume is a straight line with slope $-1/(RC)$.

The quantity RC has units of time and is termed the *respiratory time constant* (Trs). Trs defines the rate at which the lung deflates during a passive exhalation (see Fig. 44–4). Time constants affect the rate of lung inflation in the same manner in which they affect lung deflation (see Chapter 45).

## Measurements of Lung Mechanics

A true measurement of static lung compliance requires instilling a known volume of gas into the lung and then measuring airway pressure at equilibrium in the absence of respiratory muscle activity (see Fig. 44–1) (McCann et al, 1987). This technique is used to measure compliance during the passive exhalation maneuver described previously (see Fig. 44–4). Another technique for measuring compliance takes advantage of the fact that gas flow is transiently equal to zero at end-inspiration and end-expiration (see Fig. 44–3). Compliance is calculated by dividing the change in volume between these two points by the concomitant change in distending pressure. Because the measurement is made while the infant is breathing, it is termed *dynamic compliance*. In the normal infant, dynamic compliance should be equal to static compliance.

As was mentioned earlier, measurements of compliance are affected by lung size. For example, if a distending

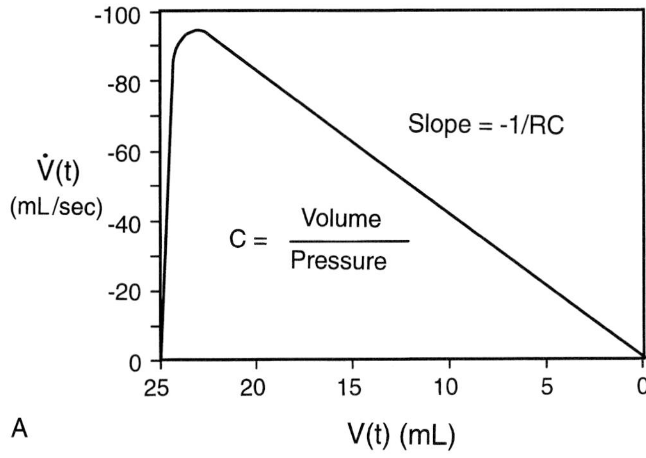


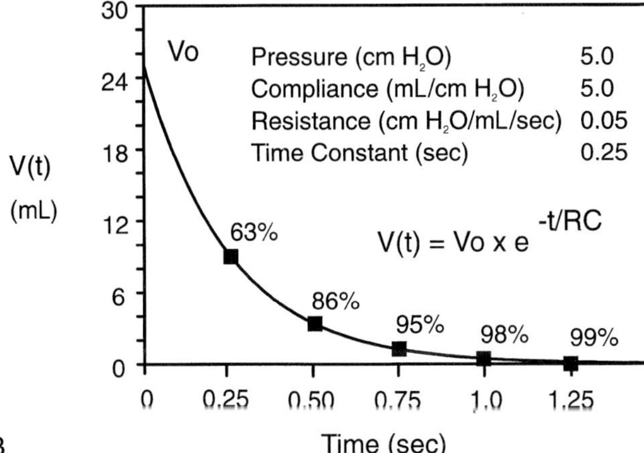


**FIGURE 44–4. A,** Plot of flow of gas out of the lung, $\dot{V}t$, versus volume of gas remaining in the lung, V(t), for a passive exhalation. Flow of gas out of the lung is negative by convention. After an initial sharp increase, flow decreases linearly as the lung empties. Static compliance of the respiratory system is obtained by dividing the exhaled volume by the airway pressure at the beginning of the passive exhalation. Resistance is calculated from the slope of the flow volume plot, −(1/RC), and the compliance. This technique has the advantages of not requiring measurements of pleural pressure and being relatively unaffected by chest wall distortion. **B,** V(t) is plotted as a function of time for a passive exhalation. The graph is an exponential with the equation

$$V(t) = V_0 \times e^{-t/(R \times C)}$$

$V_0$ is the starting volume, and *e* is a mathematical constant (roughly 2.72). For this example, the time constant of the respiratory system (Trs) is roughly 0.25 second. Calculations show that when exhalation persists for a time equal to one time constant (t = 0.25 sec = 1 × Trs), 63% of the gas in the lung is exhaled. For t = 2Trs, 86% of the gas is exhaled; for 3Trs, 95%; for 4Trs, 98%; and for 5Trs, 99%. If expiration is interrupted before a time t = 3Trs, gas is trapped in the lung.

pressure of 5 cm $H_2O$ results in a 25-mL increase in lung volume in a newborn, calculated lung compliance is 5 mL/cm $H_2O$. In an adult, the same distending pressure of 5 cm $H_2O$ increases the lung volume by roughly 500 mL, and calculated compliance is 100 mL/cm $H_2O$. Although the calculated lung compliances are different, the forces needed to carry out tidal ventilation are similar (i.e., lung function is normal in both circumstances). This example points out that if lung compliances are to be compared, they must be corrected for size. This is usually performed by dividing compliance by resting lung volume to get *specific compliance*. For the newborn, resting lung volume is roughly 100 mL, so specific compliance is 0.05 mL/cm $H_2O$/mL lung volume. For the adult, resting lung volume is nearly 2000 mL, so specific compliance is 0.05 mL/cm $H_2O$/mL lung volume—identical to that in the newborn.

Lung compliance changes with volume history, meaning that it decreases with fixed tidal volumes and increases after deep breaths that recruit air spaces that may have been poorly ventilated or atelectatic. The periodic sigh in spontaneous breathing is associated with an increase in lung compliance and in oxygenation.

Many respiratory disorders result in nonhomogeneous increases in small airway resistance in the lung. Therefore, if lung compliance remains relatively uniform, the product of resistance and compliance (Trs) varies throughout the lung. During lung inflation, units with normal resistance have the lowest Trs and fill rapidly. Units with high resistance have a longer Trs and fill more slowly. At rapid respiratory rates, when the duration of inspiration is short, only those lung units with a short Trs are ventilated. In effect, the ventilated lung becomes smaller. As discussed earlier, as the lung becomes smaller, its measured compliance decreases. Therefore, in infants with ventilation inhomogeneities, dynamic lung compliance decreases as respiratory rate increases. This decrease in lung compliance with increasing respiratory rate is termed *frequency dependence of compliance* and is suggestive of inhomogeneous small airway obstruction.

Resistance of the total respiratory system can be measured using the passive exhalation technique described previously (see Fig. 44–4), or it can be calculated from measurements of distending pressure, volume, and flow (see Fig. 44–3). Points of equal volume are chosen during inspiration and expiration. The gas flow and the distending pressure are measured at each point. The pressure needed to overcome elastic forces should be the same for inspiration and expiration; therefore, these pressures cancel out each other. Total resistance, consequently, is equal to distending pressure at the inspiratory point minus distending pressure at the expiratory point, divided by the sum of the respective inspiratory and expiratory point gas flows. Investigators have calculated compliance and resistance by measuring distending pressure, gas flow, and volume (see Fig. 44–3), then fitting these measurements to the equation of motion (see Equation 3) using multiple linear regression techniques, and solving for the coefficients 1/C and R (Bhutani et al, 1988).

FRC is measured by inert gas dilution techniques (helium dilution) or inert gas displacement (nitrogen washout) (Fig. 44–5). Both of these techniques measure gas that communicates with the airways. The total volume of gas in the thorax at end-expiration (thoracic gas volume [TGV]) can be measured using a body plethysmograph and applying Boyle's law. This technique measures all gas in the thorax—even trapped gas that is not in contact with the airways. Obviously, FRC measured by inert gas dilution is less than TGV if significant volumes of trapped gas are present.

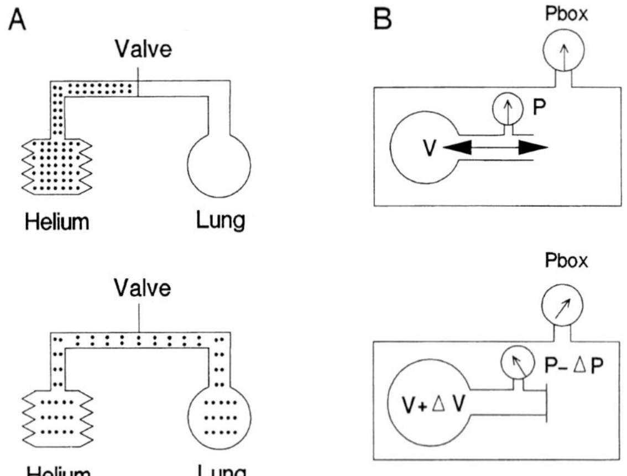


**FIGURE 44–5.** **A,** Measurement of functional residual capacity (FRC) by helium dilution. At end-exhalation, the infant breathes from a bag containing a known volume ($V_{bag}$) and (initial) concentration of helium ($He_i$) in oxygen. The gas in the infant's lungs dilutes the helium-oxygen mixture to a new concentration ($He_f$): FRC = Bag volume × ($He_i$ – $He_f$)/$He_f$. **B,** Measurement of thoracic gas volume (TGV) using a plethysmograph. The infant breathes spontaneously in a sealed body plethysmograph. At end-exhalation, the airway is closed with a shutter. As the infant attempts to inspire against the shutter, the volume of the thorax increases and airway pressure decreases. The increase in volume of the thorax can be measured from the change in the pressure inside the plethysmograph (Pbox). By Boyle's law: $P \times TGV = (P - \Delta P) \times (TGV + \Delta V)$, where P is atmospheric pressure, $(P - \Delta P)$ is airway pressure during occlusion, and $(TGV + \Delta V)$ is thoracic volume during occlusion. Therefore, $TGV = (P - \Delta P) \times \Delta V/\Delta P$. Because $\Delta P$ is small compared with P, this can be simplified to $TGV = P \times \Delta V/\Delta P$.

## ALVEOLAR VENTILATION

The tissues of the body continuously consume $O_2$ and produce $CO_2$ (Fig. 44–6). The primary function of the circulation is to pick up $O_2$ from the lungs and deliver it to the tissues, then to pick up $CO_2$ from the tissues and deliver it to the lungs. The exchange of $O_2$ and $CO_2$ with the blood occurs within the alveolar volume of the lungs. The alveolar volume acts as a "large sink" from which $O_2$ is continuously extracted by the blood and to which $CO_2$ is continuously added. This mechanism for acquiring $O_2$ from the atmosphere and excreting $CO_2$ into the atmosphere is the *alveolar ventilation* (Slonim and Hamilton, 1987).

The alveolar volume of the lung includes all lung units capable of exchanging gas with mixed venous blood: respiratory bronchioles, alveolar ducts, and alveoli. Because the conducting airways do not participate in gas exchange, they constitute the *anatomic dead space* (VD). At end exhalation, the FRC is the sum of the volume of gas in the alveolar volume and in the anatomic dead space. During normal breathing, the amount of gas entering and leaving the lung with each breath is the tidal volume (VT):

$$V_T \times \text{respiratory rate (RR)} = \text{minute ventilation } (\dot{V})$$

Part of each VT is wasted ventilation because it moves gas into and out of the VD. Therefore, alveolar ventilation ($\dot{V}_A$) can be expressed as:

$$\dot{V}_A = (V_T - V_D) \times RR \qquad (6)$$

Alveolar ventilation is an intermittent process, whereas gas exchange between the alveolar space and the blood occurs continuously. Because arterial $O_2$ and $CO_2$ tensions ($PaO_2$ and $PaCO_2$) are roughly equal to the $O_2$ and $CO_2$ tensions within the alveolar space, these fluctuations in breathing could result in intermittent hypoxemia and hypercarbia. Fortunately the lung has a large buffer—the FRC. The FRC is four to five times as large as the VT; therefore, only a fraction of the total gas in the lung is exchanged during normal breathing. This large buffer continues to supply $O_2$ to the blood during expiration and acts as a sump to accept $CO_2$ from the blood, so alveolar $O_2$ and $CO_2$ tensions ($P_AO_2$ and $P_ACO_2$) change little throughout the ventilatory cycle.

Alveolar ventilation is linked tightly to metabolism. When alveolar ventilation is uncoupled from the body's metabolic rate, hypoventilation or hyperventilation results. During hypoventilation, less $O_2$ is added to the alveolar space than is removed by the blood, and less $CO_2$ is removed from the alveolar space than is added by the blood. As a result, $P_AO_2$ decreases and $P_ACO_2$ increases. The net result of hypoventi-

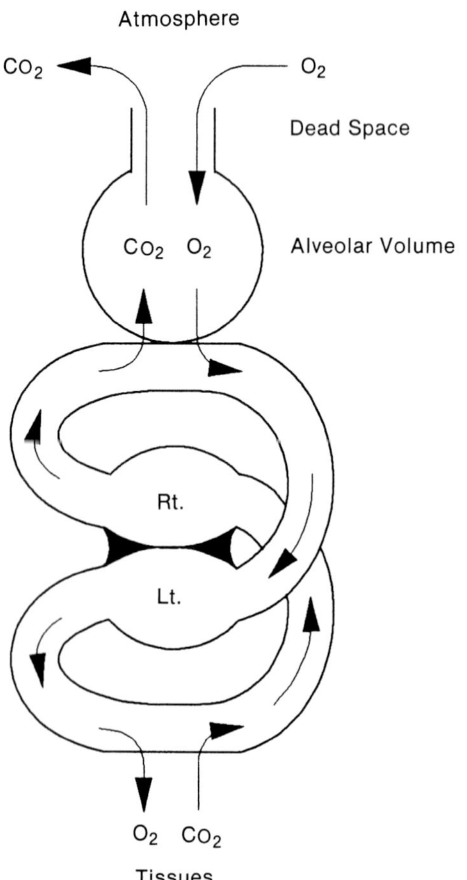


**FIGURE 44–6.** Schematic showing coupling of alveolar ventilation to tissue oxygen consumption.

lation is hypoxemia and hypercapnia. Administering supplemental $O_2$ increases the quantity of $O_2$ in each breath delivered to the alveolar space, and it may prevent arterial hypoxemia. For example, suppose a 1-kg male infant has a VT of 6 mL, an anatomic VD of 2 mL, and a respiratory rate of 40 breaths/minute. His alveolar ventilation is 160 mL/ minute ([6 mL − 2 mL] × 40/min). If he breathes room air (21% $O_2$), he delivers 33.6 mL of $O_2$ to the alveolar space every minute (160 mL/min × 0.21). If he maintains the same VT but breaths only 20 times per minute, his alveolar ventilation decreases to 80 mL/minute, only 16.8 mL of $O_2$ (80 mL/min × 0.21) is delivered to the alveolar space each minute, and his $PAO_2$ and $PaO_2$ decrease. If he is allowed to breathe 50% $O_2$, $O_2$ delivery to the alveolar space increases to 40 mL/minute (80 mL/min × 0.50), and both his $PAO_2$ and $PaO_2$ increase. Because $O_2$ administration has no effect on the accumulation of $CO_2$, it does not prevent hypercapnia.

Hyperventilation delivers more $O_2$ to the alveolar space than can be removed by the blood and removes more $CO_2$ than can be added by the blood. As a result, $PAO_2$ increases and $PACO_2$ decreases.

Measurements of alveolar ventilation and anatomic VD in the infant rely on the relationship between $CO_2$ production ($\dot{V}CO_2$), $\dot{V}A$, and $PACO_2$. The mathematical expression of this relationship states (Cook et al, 1955):

$$FACO_2 = \dot{V}CO_2/\dot{V}A \quad (7)$$

$FACO_2$ is the fraction of $CO_2$ in total alveolar gas, or

$$FACO_2 = PACO_2/(PB - 47) \quad (8)$$

PB is the barometric pressure, and 47 mm Hg is the vapor pressure of water at body temperature. Therefore,

$$\dot{V}A = [\dot{V}CO_2 \times (PB - 47)]/PACO_2 \quad (9)$$

If minute ventilation ($\dot{V}$) is measured, dead space ventilation ($\dot{V}D$) is calculated as:

$$\dot{V}D = \dot{V} - \dot{V}A \quad (10)$$

VD *volume* is calculated by dividing by the respiratory rate.

This method measures the anatomic VD in the lung. As seen in the next section, portions of some gas exchanging units in the lung can also function as VD; therefore, the total VD, or the physiologic VD, may be greater than the anatomic VD. Physiologic VD is calculated by substituting $PaCO_2$ into Equation 9 for $PACO_2$. When $PACO_2 = PaCO_2$, all the VD is anatomic VD, and the gas-exchanging units are all functioning normally. As physiologic VD increases, however, $PaCO_2$ increases relative to $PACO_2$. Therefore, the difference between $PaCO_2$ and $PACO_2$ (the $aA.DCO_2$) is a measure of efficiency of gas exchange in the lung.

For clinical purposes, $\dot{V}CO_2$ in Equation 9 is assumed to be a constant, so that $\dot{V}A$ is proportional to $1/PaCO_2$. Thus, increased $PaCO_2$ means that alveolar ventilation has decreased; decreased $PaCO_2$ means that alveolar ventilation has increased.

## VENTILATION-PERFUSION RELATIONSHIPS

Under ideal circumstances, ventilation and perfusion of the lung are evenly matched ($\dot{V}/\dot{Q} = 1$), both in the lung as a whole and in each individual air space. The air spaces receive $O_2$ from the inspired gas and $CO_2$ from the blood. $O_2$ is transported into the blood, while $CO_2$ is transported to the atmosphere. Even though $\dot{V}/\dot{Q}$ is 1, $CO_2$ and $O_2$ are exchanged in the lung at the same ratio at which they are exchanged in the tissues: A little less $CO_2$ is transported out than $O_2$ is transported in, so the respiratory exchange ratio R equals 0.8. If there is no diffusion defect, the gas composition of the air spaces and the blood comes into equilibrium. $N_2$ makes up the balance of dry gas. The sum of partial pressures of all gases in the air spaces must equal atmospheric pressure. The ideal alveolar gas composition is as follows: $PO_2 = 100$, $PCO_2 = 40$, $PN_2 = 573$, and $PH_2O = 47$, all in mm Hg, at an atmospheric pressure of 760 mm Hg. The ideal arterial blood composition is the same. Therefore, differences between alveolar and arterial gas compositions under ideal circumstances all are zero. Knowing the values for $PaCO_2$ and inspired gas, ideal alveolar gas composition can be calculated from the alveolar gas equations (Farhi, 1966):

$$PAO_2 = PIO_2 - PACO_2 \times [FIO_2 + (1 - FIO_2)/R] \quad (11)$$

where

$$PIO_2 = FIO_2 \times (PB - PH_2O) \quad (12)$$

$$PAN_2 = FIN_2 \times [PACO_2 \times (1 - R)/R + (PB - PH_2O)] \quad (13)$$

Under normal circumstances and certainly in the presence of lung disease, this ideal situation does not exist; some air spaces receive more ventilation than perfusion, and others receive more perfusion than ventilation. A reduction of ventilation may occur because of atelectasis, alveolar fluid, or airway narrowing. Reduced ventilation in one part of the lung may cause increased ventilation elsewhere. A reduction of perfusion may occur if air spaces are collapsed or overdistended or because of gravitational effects, and increased perfusion may occur in congenital heart disease. As with ventilation, reduced perfusion in one part of the lung may cause increased perfusion in other regions. If an air space is relatively overventilated (high $\dot{V}/\dot{Q}$), its gas composition tends toward that of inspired gas, which in the case of room air is $PO_2 = 150$ mm Hg and $PCO_2 = 0$ mm Hg. If an air space is relatively underventilated (low $\dot{V}/\dot{Q}$), its gas composition tends toward that of mixed venous blood, which is $PO_2 = 40$ mm Hg and $PCO_2 = 46$ mm Hg. What counts is the $\dot{V}/\dot{Q}$ ratio, not absolute values of $\dot{V}$ or $\dot{Q}$ (West, 1986).

To understand $\dot{V}/\dot{Q}$ imbalance, it is common to view the lung as a three-compartment model (Fig. 44–7), in which $\dot{V}/\dot{Q} = 0$ (see Fig. 44–7A), $\dot{V}/\dot{Q} = 1$ (see Fig. 44–7B), and $\dot{V}/\dot{Q}$ = infinity for the three compartments, respectively (see Fig. 44–7C). The $O_2$ saturation of blood in each compartment depends on the $PO_2$ and the $O_2$ dissociation curve. For illustrative purposes, in a badly diseased lung, 50% of ventilation goes to $\dot{V}/\dot{Q} = 1$ and 50% to $\dot{V}/\dot{Q}$ = infinity, whereas 50% of perfusion goes to $\dot{V}/\dot{Q} = 1$ and 50% to $\dot{V}/\dot{Q} = 0$. Perfusion of $\dot{V}/\dot{Q} = 0$ causes venous admixture, whereas ventilation of $\dot{V}/\dot{Q}$ = infinity causes alveolar VD. The mixed alveolar gas composition is easily calculated as the mean. For mixed arterial blood, the $PO_2$ must be read from the $O_2$ dissociation curve, but because the $CO_2$ dissociation curve is fairly linear, the values for $CO_2$ are easily calculated as the mean. The abnormalities in distribution of $\dot{V}$ and $\dot{Q}$ have created an $Aa.DO_2 = 70$, $aA.DCO_2 = 23$, and $aA.DN_2 = 32$ mm Hg (see Fig. 44–7). The $Aa.DO_2$

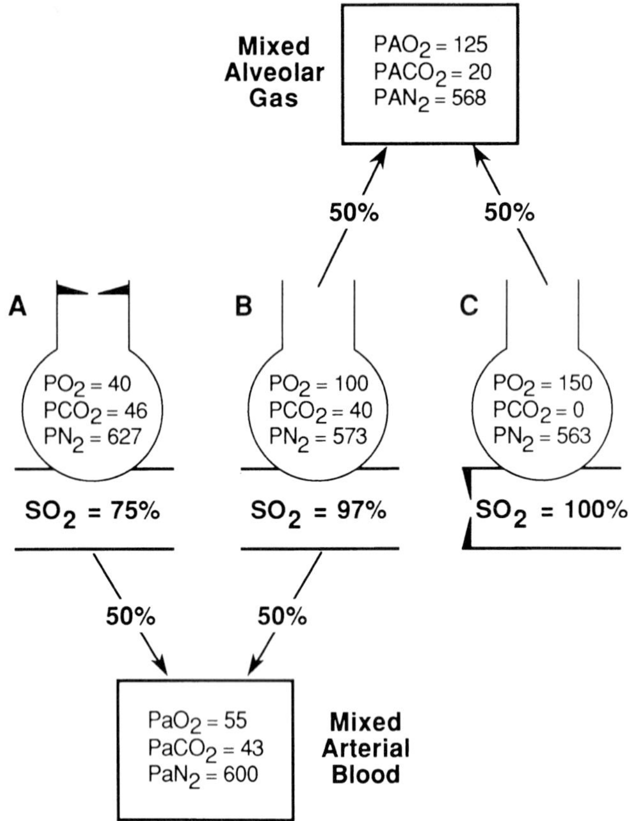


**FIGURE 44–7.** Three-compartment model of the lung with $\dot{V}/\dot{Q} = 0$ (**A**), $\dot{V}/\dot{Q} = 1$ (**B**), and $\dot{V}/\dot{Q}$ = infinity (**C**). The inspired gas is room air, and **B** is the ideal compartment. The sum of alveolar gas partial pressures is always 713 mm Hg. $SO_2$ is oxygen saturation in capillary blood. $PaO_2$ is read from the oxygen dissociation curve for a saturation of 86%. By calculated differences, $Aa.DO_2$ is 70 mm Hg, $aA.DCO_2$ is 23 mm Hg, and $aA.DN_2$ is 32 mm Hg.

is greater than the sum of the other two because the $O_2$ dissociation curve is not linear. Of course, the situation in most lungs is not as extreme as the one illustrated. From this case, however, it can be seen that

1. Open low $\dot{V}/\dot{Q}$ units produce increased $Aa.DO_2$, significant hypoxemia, and increased $aA.DN_2$, but because they are poorly ventilated and have a $PCO_2$ close to the ideal value, they do not change the $aA.DCO_2$ significantly.
2. High $\dot{V}/\dot{Q}$ units produce increased $Aa.DO_2$ without hypoxemia and increased $aA.DCO_2$, but because they are poorly perfused and have a $PN_2$ close to the ideal value, they do not change the $aA.DN_2$ significantly.

For the calculation of $Aa.DO_2$ and $aA.DN_2$, it is customary to calculate the ideal alveolar gas composition for $O_2$ and $N_2$ from the alveolar gas equations and use these values with those measured for arterial $PO_2$ and $PN_2$. This approach emphasizes that part of the $Aa.DO_2$ and $aA.DN_2$ responsible for hypoxemia. For $aA.DCO_2$, both arterial and mixed alveolar samples are required.

In the newborn, a fourth compartment in the model is important. A significant part of the venous return may be shunted from right to left at the foramen ovale, ductus arteriosus, pulmonary arteriovenous vessels, or lung mesenchyme without airway development, thus adding mixed venous to mixed arterial blood. This substantially increases the $Aa.DO_2$ but has little effect on $aA.DCO_2$ and no effect on $aA.DN_2$. The reason for the lack of effect on $aA.DN_2$ is that there is no significant exchange of $N_2$ in the body, so venous and arterial $PN_2$ are the same. The effect on $aA.DCO_2$ is small because venous $PCO_2$ is only slightly higher than arterial. From this analysis, it can be seen that hypoxemia is produced by a true right-to-left shunt and open low $\dot{V}/\dot{Q}$ units. Diffusional problems are not thought to be important in the newborn. Hypoxemia may be modeled as a venous admixture, the part of mixed venous blood expressed as a fraction of cardiac output, that when added to blood equilibrated with an ideal lung would produce the measured arterial oxygen saturation. It is calculated as follows:

$$\dot{Q}va/\dot{Q}t = (C\dot{c}O_2 - CaO_2)/(C\dot{c}O_2 - C\bar{v}O_2) \qquad (14)$$

where $\dot{Q}va/\dot{Q}t$ = venous admixture, $CO_2$ = oxygen content, $\dot{c}$ = pulmonary capillary, a = arterial, and $\bar{v}$ = mixed venous blood. For practical application, $CO_2$ is calculated from a constant $a\bar{V}.O_2$ difference, which does introduce an error.

If an infant breathes 100% $O_2$ for 15 minutes, most $N_2$ is washed out of the lung, and the $PO_2$ in open low $\dot{V}/\dot{Q}$ units becomes so high that associated blood is 100% saturated with $O_2$. The remaining venous admixture is attributed to true right-to-left shunt ($\dot{Q}s/\dot{Q}t$). If an infant has the total venous admixture $\dot{Q}va/\dot{Q}t$ measured while breathing room air and then the true shunt ($\dot{Q}s/\dot{Q}t$) measured while breathing 100% $O_2$, the venous admixture due to open low $\dot{V}/\dot{Q}$ units ($\dot{Q}o/\dot{Q}t$) can be calculated as the difference. The venous admixture due to open low $\dot{V}/\dot{Q}$ units also can be calculated from the $aA.DN_2$ (Markello et al, 1972):

$$\dot{Q}o/\dot{Q}t = (PaN_2 - PAN_2)/(PON_2 - PAN_2) \qquad (15)$$

where $PON_2$ is the $PN_2$ in the $\dot{V}/\dot{Q} - 0$ units (see Fig. 44–7), and $PaN_2$ is measured and $PAN_2$ is the ideal value calculated from the alveolar gas equation. In newborns with a significant value for true shunt, this value really represents venous admixture as a fraction of effective pulmonary blood flow ($\dot{Q}o/\dot{Q}\dot{c}$). A better estimate for $\dot{Q}o/\dot{Q}t$ can be obtained from simple arithmetic (Corbet et al, 1974):

$$\dot{Q}o/\dot{Q}t = (\dot{Q}o/\dot{Q}\dot{c}) \times (1 - \dot{Q}va/\dot{Q}t)/(1 - (\dot{Q}o/\dot{Q}\dot{c})) \qquad (16)$$

The true right-to-left shunt can then be estimated without 100% $O_2$ breathing, using the equation:

$$\dot{Q}s/\dot{Q}t = \dot{Q}va/\dot{Q}t - \dot{Q}o/\dot{Q}t \qquad (17)$$

The normal values for the various indices of ventilation-perfusion imbalance in normal newborn infants are shown in Table 44–2.

## HEART-LUNG INTERACTION

### Effects of the Lung on the Heart

There exists considerable potential for the lung to affect the heart. Because they share the thoracic cavity, changes in intrathoracic pressure accompanying lung inflation are

**TABLE 44–2**

**Indices of Ventilation-Perfusion Imbalance in the Normal Newborn Breathing Room Air**

| | Aa.$DO_2$ mm Hg | $\dot{Q}va/\dot{Q}t$ | aA.$DN_2$ mm Hg | $\dot{Q}o/\dot{Q}t$ | $\dot{Q}s/\dot{Q}t$ | aA.$DCO_2$ mm Hg |
|---|---|---|---|---|---|---|
| Newborn | 25 | 0.25 | 10 | 0.10 | 0.15 | 1 |
| Adult | 10 | 0.07 | 7 | 0.05 | 0.02 | 1 |

Data from Nelson NM: Respiration and circulation after birth. In Smith CA, Nelson NM (eds): The Physiology of the Newborn Infant. Springfield, Ill, Charles C Thomas, 1976.

transmitted directly to the heart. In addition, all of the blood leaving the right ventricle must traverse the pulmonary vascular bed, so changes in pulmonary vascular resistance may greatly affect right ventricular function.

## Effects of Changes in Intrathoracic Pressure on the Heart

### *Negative Intrathoracic Pressure*

During spontaneous inspiratory efforts, the chest wall and diaphragm move outward, intrathoracic volume increases, and intrathoracic pressure decreases (Fig. 44–8A). The heart also resides within the thoracic cavity and is subject to the same negative intrathoracic pressure during inspiration. With a decrease in intrathoracic pressure, the heart increases in volume, and the pressure within its chambers decreases relative to atmospheric pressure. Analogous to the lung, when the pressure within the heart decreases, blood is literally sucked back into the heart from systemic veins and arteries. On the right side of the heart, the phenomenon serves to increase the flow of blood from systemic veins into the right atrium, increasing right ventricular preload and ventricular output. On the left side of the heart, ventricular ejection is impaired. During systole, the left ventricle must overcome not only the load imposed by the systemic vascular resistance but also the additional load imposed by the negative intrathoracic pressure (McGregor, 1979).

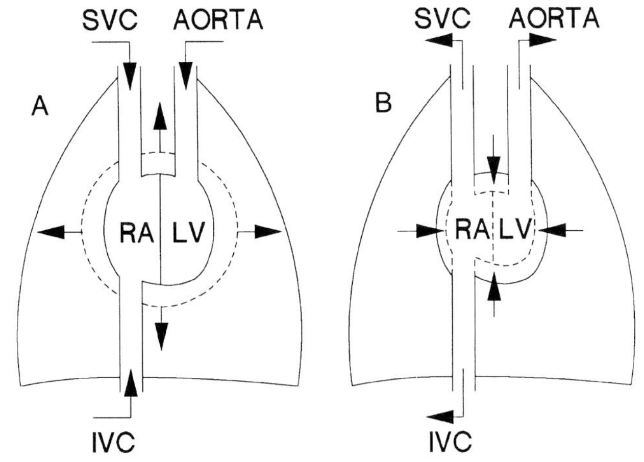

In infants with normal lungs, spontaneous respiratory efforts result in relatively small swings in pleural pressure (2 to 3 mm Hg) that have little effect on the pressure within the heart. With airway obstruction or parenchyma lung disease, however, swings in pleural pressure can be much greater (5 to 20 mm Hg), and systemic arterial pressure may fluctuate as much as 5 to 20 mm Hg, depending on where in the respiratory cycle ventricular systole occurs. In older children with asthma or some other form of airway obstruction, these fluctuations in blood pressure constitute pulsus paradoxus and are indicative of severe airway obstruction.

**FIGURE 44–8.** **A,** Negative intrathoracic pressure increases the volume of the heart and decreases the pressure within the chambers. This facilitates return of blood from the superior vena cava (SVC) and inferior vena cava (IVC) to the right atrium (RA) and impedes ejection of blood from the left ventricle (LV) into the extrathoracic aorta. **B,** Positive intrathoracic pressure decreases the volume of the heart and increases pressure within its chambers. This impedes blood return to the right atrium and augments ejection of blood from the left ventricle.

### *Positive Intrathoracic Pressure*

During positive pressure ventilation, the lung inflates and pushes the chest wall and diaphragm outward (see Fig. 44–8B). This outward push generates a pressure in the thoracic space that is greater than atmospheric pressure. The magnitude of the increase (relative transmission of airway pressure to the pleural space) is determined by the volume of lung inflation (which in turn is determined by the airway pressure and lung compliance) and by the compliance of the chest wall and diaphragm. If the lung is compliant and the chest wall rigid, little airway pressure is lost inflating the lung, but considerable pressure is generated in the thoracic cavity as the lung attempts to push the rigid chest wall outward. In this instance, intrathoracic pressure (intrapleural pressure) is much greater than atmospheric and in fact nearly equal to airway pressure. If the lung is poorly compliant and the chest wall highly compliant, most of the airway pressure is dissipated in efforts to inflate the lungs, and little is transmitted to the thoracic cavity.

The effects of positive intrathoracic pressure on the heart are opposite to those of negative intrathoracic pressure. The heart is compressed by the lungs and chest wall, and blood is squeezed out of the heart and the thoracic cavity. Return of blood from systemic veins is impaired, and right ventricular preload and output decrease. If the increase in intrathoracic pressure coincides with ventricular systole, the effect is to augment left ventricular ejection and reduce the load on the left ventricle.

In the infant undergoing positive pressure ventilation, the degree to which lung inflation compromises venous return is related to the relative compliances of the lung and chest wall. If the infant's lung is poorly compliant and the chest wall is compliant, as in hyaline membrane disease, there is little effect of lung inflation on venous return. If the infant's lung is normally compliant but tight abdominal distention prevents descent of the diaphragm, intrathoracic pressure increases dramatically during positive pressure ventilation, and venous return and cardiac output can be impaired. This mechanism may help explain the circulatory instability of infants after repair of gastroschisis or omphalocele. A similar situation may arise in the preterm infant with pulmonary interstitial emphysema and massive lung overinflation. In this case, the heart is tightly compressed between the hyperinflated lungs, the other structures of the mediastinum, and the diaphragm. Venous return may be severely limited and venous pressures so increased that massive peripheral edema often accompanies the reduction in cardiac output.

Although the effects of increased pleural pressure on the right atrium are detrimental, the effects on the left ventricle may be extremely beneficial (Niemann et al, 1980). During cardiopulmonary resuscitation, the chest wall is compressed against the lung, and intrathoracic pressure increases. Because the left ventricle is in the thorax, left ventricular pressure increases as well. A gradient is created favoring flow of blood out of the ventricle and thorax and into the extrathoracic systemic circulation. Between chest compressions, elastic recoil causes the chest wall to pull away from the lung and heart, decreasing pleural pressure and favoring return of venous blood and priming the heart for the next chest compression. A similar phenomenon may result in augmentation of systemic pressure when ventilator breaths coincide with ventricular systole.

### Effect of Lung Inflation on Pulmonary Vascular Resistance

The pulmonary interstitium comprises three different interconnected connective tissue compartments, each containing a different element of the pulmonary circulation (Fishman, 1986). The first—the perivascular cuffs—consists of a sheath of fibers that contain the preacinar pulmonary arteries, lymphatics, and bronchi. The second consists of the intersegmental and interlobular septa and contains pulmonary veins and additional lymphatics. The third connects these two within the alveolar septa and contains the majority of the pulmonary capillaries. The first and second compartments represent the extra-alveolar interstitium, whereas the third represents the alveolar interstitium. The perivascular cuffs are surrounded by alveoli and expand during lung inflation (Fig. 44–9A). As a result, pressure within each cuff decreases, distending extra-alveolar blood vessels and decreasing their resistance to blood flow. The alveolar interstitium lies between adjacent alveoli and contains the majority of gas-exchanging vessels in the lung. These vessels are exposed to alveolar pressure on both sides and during lung inflation (see Fig. 44–9B) are compressed so that their resistance to blood flow increases.

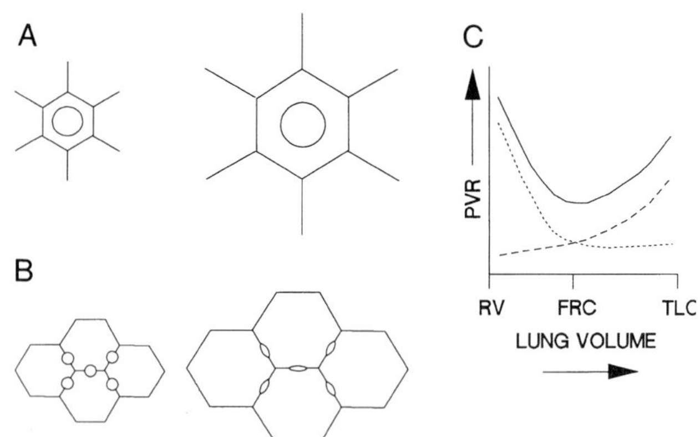


**FIGURE 44–9.** **A,** Effects of lung inflation on extra-alveolar vessels. **B,** Effects of lung inflation on alveolar vessels. **C,** Effect of lung volume on pulmonary vascular resistance (PVR) (*solid line*). Inflation is from residual volume (RV) to functional residual capacity (FRC) to total lung capacity (TLC). *Dashed line* represents alveolar vessels; *dotted line* represents extra-alveolar vessels.

Therefore, during lung inflation (see Fig. 44–9C), the resistance in extra-alveolar vessels (dotted line) decreases, while resistance in alveolar vessels (dashed line) increases. As a result, the overall pulmonary vascular resistance (solid line) decreases initially, with lung inflation reaching its nadir at FRC, and then increases with further inflation.

If transition from intrauterine life to extrauterine life is to be successful, after birth all of the right ventricular output must traverse the pulmonary vascular bed. To some extent, this adaptation is facilitated by a reduction in pulmonary vascular resistance that occurs with inflation of the lungs (see Fig. 44–9) to a stable FRC. Inflation of the lung beyond FRC increases pulmonary vascular resistance. If care is not taken during positive pressure ventilation, it is possible to inflate the lung to the point at which alveolar vessels close and blood flow through the lung is impaired. When this occurs, either cardiac output decreases or the blood bypasses the lung via the foramen ovale or ductus arteriosus. Clinically, this is manifested as circulatory insufficiency from impaired right ventricular output or hypoxemia from right-to-left shunting of blood, or both.

## Effects of the Heart on the Lung

### Pulmonary Edema

Pulmonary edema is the abnormal accumulation of water and solute in the interstitial and alveolar spaces of the lung (Bland and Hansen, 1985; Staub, 1974). In the lung, fluid is filtered from capillaries in the alveolar septa into the alveolar interstitium (Fig. 44–10A) and then siphoned into the lower pressure extra-alveolar interstitium. The extra-alveolar interstitium contains the pulmonary lymphatics, and under normal conditions, they remove fluid from the lung so that there is no net accumulation in the interstitium. Pulmonary edema results only when the rate of fluid filtration exceeds the rate of lymphatic removal. This can occur by one of only

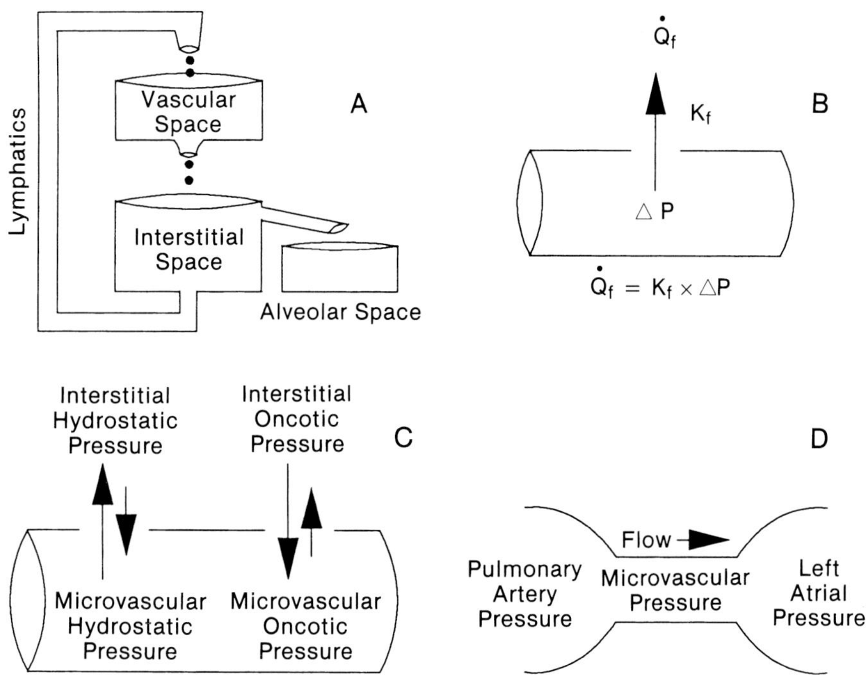


**FIGURE 44–10.** **A,** In the lung, fluid is continuously filtered out of vessels in the microcirculation into the interstitium and then returned to the intravascular compartment by the lymphatics. *Only when the rate of filtration exceeds the rate of lymphatic removal can fluid accumulate in the interstitium.* Spillover of fluid into the alveolar space occurs only when the interstitial space fills or when the alveolar membrane is damaged. **B,** Fluid flows out of vessels at a flow rate (f) that is equal to the driving pressure for fluid flow (ΔP) times the filtration coefficient ($K_f$): $\dot{Q}_f = K_f \times \Delta P$. $K_f$ can be thought of as the relative permeability of the vascular bed to fluid flux. $K_f$ in the normal lung is a small number, so that despite a driving pressure of roughly 5 mm Hg, the net rate of fluid filtration is approximately 1 to 2 mL/kg/hour. **C,** The driving pressure for fluid flow out of the microvascular bed represents a balance of two sets of pressures. Within the blood vessel, hydrostatic pressure tends to push fluid out of the vessel into the interstitium. This pressure is partially opposed by a smaller hydrostatic pressure within the interstitium pushing fluid back into the blood vessel. Within the blood vessel, there also exists a discrete oncotic pressure resulting predominantly from intravascular albumin, which tends to draw fluid from the interstitium back into the blood vessel. This pressure is partially opposed by an interstitial oncotic pressure tending to draw fluid from the blood vessel into the interstitium. **D,** The intravascular hydrostatic pressure must be less than pulmonary artery pressure (Ppa) for blood to flow into the microvascular bed and greater than left atrial pressure (Pla) for blood to flow out. Intravascular pressure within the microvascular bed is roughly equal to $0.4(Ppa - Pla) + Pla$. The interstitial hydrostatic pressure is roughly equal to alveolar pressure. The intravascular oncotic pressure can be calculated from the plasma albumin concentration. The interstitial oncotic pressure is roughly two thirds of the intravascular oncotic pressure. The balance of these pressures favors filtration out of the vessel (in the normal lamb, this pressure is roughly 5 mm Hg).

three mechanisms (see Fig. 44–10B): (1) the driving pressure for fluid filtration (filtration pressure) increases, (2) the permeability of the vascular bed (and hence the filtration coefficient $K_f$) increases, or (3) lymphatic drainage decreases.

### *Increased Driving Pressure*

Filtration pressure can be increased by increased intravascular hydrostatic pressure, decreased interstitial hydrostatic pressure, decreased intravascular oncotic pressure, or increased interstitial oncotic pressure (see Figs. 44–10C and D). By far the most common cause of increased filtration pressure is increased intravascular hydrostatic pressure (Table 44–3). In the newborn, intravascular hydrostatic pressure increases with increased left atrial pressure from volume overload or with any of a number of congenital and acquired heart defects. In the preterm and term newborn, evidence suggests that alterations in pulmonary blood flow that are independent of any change in left atrial pressure also may influence fluid filtration in the lung. Preterm infants with patent ductus arteriosus and left-to-right shunts exhibit signs of respiratory insufficiency before they develop any

**TABLE 44-3**

**Increased Intravascular Hydrostatic Pressure**

**Increased Left Atrial Pressure**
Intravascular volume overload
 Overzealous fluid administration
 Overtransfusion
 Renal insufficiency
Heart failure
 Left-sided obstructive lesions
 Left-to-right shunts
 Myocardiopathies

**Increased Pulmonary Blood Flow**
Normal pulmonary vascular bed
 Patent ductus arteriosus
 Increased cardiac output
Reduced pulmonary vascular bed
 Bronchopulmonary dysplasia
 Pulmonary hypoplasia

evidence of heart failure, and experiments performed in newborn lambs show that fluid filtration in the lung can be increased by increasing pulmonary blood flow without increasing left atrial pressure (Feltes and Hansen, 1986). In the newborn with a diminished pulmonary vascular bed, either from lung injury or from hypoplasia, cardiac output appropriate for body size may represent a relative overperfusion of the lung and can result in increased fluid filtration. This phenomenon has been invoked to explain the lung edema that often complicates the clinical course in the infant with bronchopulmonary dysplasia.

The exact cause of pulmonary edema that accompanies severe hypoxia or asphyxia in the newborn is still a controversial issue. Data suggest that it is the result of increased filtration pressure and not the result of any alteration in permeability. Heart failure accounts for some of the increased filtration pressure following severe asphyxia. In addition, there may be some element of pulmonary venous constriction. Finally, evidence indicates that hypoxia and acidosis may redistribute pulmonary blood flow to a smaller portion of the lung and result in relative overperfusion and edema, similar to that seen with anatomic loss of vascular bed (Hansen et al, 1984).

Several investigators have suggested that upper airway obstruction may cause pulmonary edema by decreasing interstitial hydrostatic pressure relative to intravascular hydrostatic pressure. Other workers suggest, however, that with airway obstruction vascular pressures decrease with intrapleural pressure in such a way that filtration pressure remains unchanged (Hansen et al, 1985).

Hypoproteinemia in infants results in a decrease in intravascular oncotic pressure. Its effects on filtration pressure, however, are blunted by the simultaneous decrease in protein concentration in the interstitial space of the lung. As a result, edema is unlikely to occur unless hydrostatic pressure also increases (Hazinski et al, 1986).

### *Increased Permeability*

Another possible mechanism for increased fluid filtration in the lung is a change in the permeability of the microvascular membrane to protein. In this form of edema, the sieving properties of the microvascular endothelium are altered so that $K_f$ increases, and patients may develop pulmonary edema despite relatively normal vascular pressures (Albertine, 1985). Furthermore, even small changes in vascular pressures can result in a dramatic worsening of pulmonary status. High-permeability pulmonary edema usually implies either direct or indirect injury to the capillary endothelium of the lung. Direct injuries result from local effects of an inhaled toxin such as oxygen. Indirect injuries imply that the initial insult occurs elsewhere in the body and that the lung injury occurs secondarily. An example of indirect lung injury is that due to sepsis: Neutrophils activated by bacterial toxins attack endothelial cells in the lung and increase permeability to water and protein (Brigham et al, 1974). Indirect injuries usually involve blood-borne mediators such as leukocytes, leukotrienes, histamine, or bradykinin. Alveolar overdistention can also cause high-permeability pulmonary edema, presumably by direct injury of the pulmonary vascular bed. This type of vascular injury probably accounts for some of the edema that accompanies diseases such as hyaline membrane disease and bronchopulmonary dysplasia, in which maldistribution of ventilation results in areas of alveolar overdistention (Carlton et al, 1990).

### *Decreased Lymphatic Drainage*

In the normal lung, the rate of lung lymph flow is equal to the net rate of fluid filtration, and as long as lymphatic function can keep up with the rate of fluid filtration, water does not accumulate in the lung. Although lymphatics can actively pump fluid against a pressure gradient, studies show that this ability is limited and that lung lymph flow varies inversely with the outflow pressure (pressure in the superior vena cava). Several groups of investigators have demonstrated that, in the presence of an increased rate of transvascular fluid filtration, the rate of fluid accumulation in the lung is substantially greater if systemic venous pressure is increased (Drake et al, 1985). Recent data suggest that the ability of the lymphatics to pump against an outflow pressure is impaired in the fetus and newborn. In fact, in fetal lambs, lymph flow ceases at an outflow pressure of roughly 15 mm Hg (Johnson et al, 1996). This explains why pulmonary edema often complicates the clinical course in infants with bronchopulmonary dysplasia and cor pulmonale and explains the particular problem of edema with pleural effusions complicating the postoperative course in patients following cavopulmonary shunt placement.

More recently, investigators have shown that the ability of the lymphatics to pump can be affected by other mediators, with pumping increased by alpha-adrenergics and certain leukotrienes and impaired by nitric oxide, beta-adrenergics (Von Der Weid, 2001), and products of hemolysis (Elias et al, 1990).

### Congenital Pulmonary Lymphangiectasis

Congenital pulmonary lymphangiectasis is a rare form of pulmonary lymphatic dysfunction that can be categorized as (1) that associated with congenital heart disease and (2) that not associated with congenital heart disease. The cardiac anomalies may include hypoplastic left heart syndrome, total anomalous pulmonary venous drainage, and pulmonary stenosis, including Noonan syndrome (France and Brown, 1971). The type that does not include associated cardiac anomalies may be of early or late onset and has a wide spectrum of severity. In some affected children, the lesion is asymptomatic, whereas in others, it can lead to severe respiratory failure, usually in the first hours after birth but sometimes during the first weeks or months of life. Most infants with this condition die early in the neonatal period. Pulmonary lymphangiectasis has been reported twice as often in males and has been seen in families (Scott Emaukpor et al, 1981).

Usually the radiologist is the first to suggest the diagnosis, after observing dilated lymphatic vessels and sometimes small accumulations of pleural fluid on the chest radiograph. The older infant may have no symptoms or mild to moderate tachypnea with varying degrees of hypoxemia. If pleural fluid has accumulated, examination of the fluid is important. If the infant has received milk feedings, pleural fluid is chylous; otherwise, there is an elevation in mononuclear cells and moderate protein of up to about 4%. These findings in the absence of fever or other signs of systemic illness are diagnostic of impaired lymphatic drainage.

Lung biopsy probably is not indicated and can be hazardous because once the distended lymphatic channels are severed, they can leak fluid for weeks. Only if the diagnosis is in doubt is open lung biopsy appropriate.

In non–cardiac lesion–associated diffuse lymphangiectasis, only supportive treatment is available. The long-term prognosis depends on the severity of the lesion, but this form of pulmonary lymphangiectasis is compatible with asymptomatic life as an adult (Wohl, 1989).

### Symptoms of Pulmonary Edema

As discussed previously, fluid filtered into the alveolar interstitium ordinarily moves rapidly along pressure gradients into the extra-alveolar interstitium, where it is removed by the lymphatics. A delay in this process at birth can result in clinical transient respiratory distress (see Chapter 47). The extra-alveolar interstitium has a large storage capacity. Fluid does not begin to spill over into the alveoli and airways until total lung water has increased by more than 50%, unless the alveolar membrane is damaged. Therefore, the first signs and symptoms of pulmonary edema are related to the presence of extra fluid in the interstitial cuffs of tissue that surround airways. As fluid builds up in these cuffs, airways are compressed, and signs of obstructive lung disease develop. The chest may appear hyperinflated, and auscultation reveals rales, rhonchi, and a prolonged expiration. Early in the course, chest radiographs reveal lung overinflation and an accumulation of fluid in the extra-alveolar interstitium—evident as linear densities of fluid that extend from the hilum to the periphery of the lung (the so called sunburst appearance) and fluid in the fissures. With more severe edema, fluffy densities appear throughout the lung as alveoli fill with fluid (Fig. 44–11). Heart size may be increased in infants with edema from increased intravascular pressure. Initially, infants present with increased $PaCO_2$ secondary to impaired ventilation. Later, $PaO_2$ decreases secondary to ventilation-perfusion mismatching and alveolar flooding. In adults, a ratio of protein concentration in tracheal aspirate to that in plasma greater than 0.5 may help to differentiate high-permeability pulmonary edema from high-pressure pulmonary edema (Fein et al, 1979).

### Treatment of Pulmonary Edema

Treatment of pulmonary edema is directed at relieving hypoxemia and lowering vascular pressures. Hypoxemia should be treated with the administration of oxygen and,

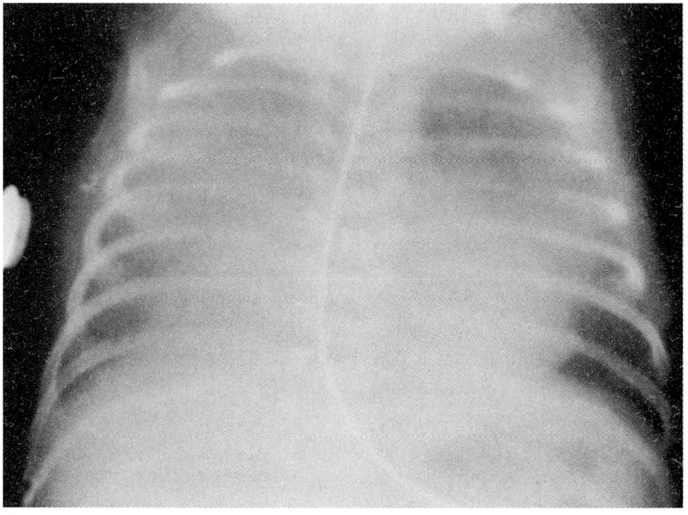


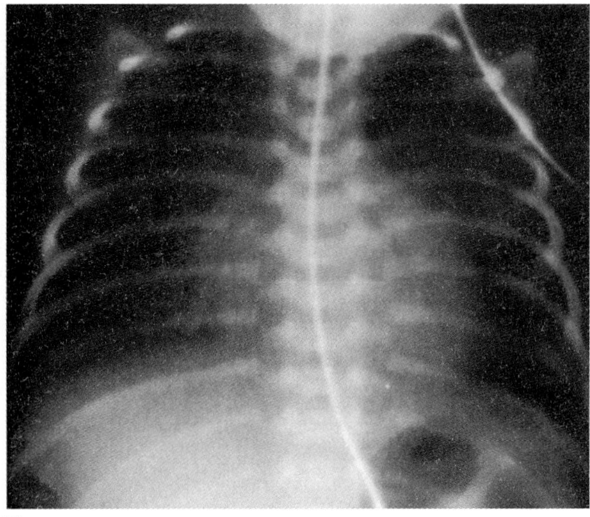


**FIGURE 44–11.** **A,** Preterm infant with a large patent ductus arteriosus and pulmonary edema. **B,** The same infant 24 hours after the patent ductus arteriosus was closed by administration of indomethacin.

if necessary, positive pressure ventilation. Positive end-expiratory pressure frequently improves oxygenation in persons with pulmonary edema by improving ventilation-perfusion matching within the lung. Available evidence suggests that positive pressure ventilation does *not* reduce the rate of transvascular fluid filtration in the lung (Woolverton et al, 1978). Optimal treatment of pulmonary edema requires correction of the underlying cause. In infants with patent ductus arteriosus (see Fig. 44–11) or other heart disease amenable to surgery, this is often easily accomplished. In cases of permeability edema or edema from nonsurgical heart defects, correction of the underlying cause may not be possible. In these instances, the only remaining option is to lower vascular pressures (even in permeability edema, lowering vascular pressures lowers the rate of fluid filtration and may also improve lymphatic function). This can be accomplished by lowering circulating blood volume by use of diuretics and fluid restriction, by improving myocardial function with the use of digitalis or other inotropic agents, or in severe cases by using a systemic vasodilator to reduce afterload and lower vascular pressures directly.

More recent data suggest that clearance of fluid from the alveolar space may be accelerated by beta-adrenergic agents (Frank et al, 2000) and by dopamine (Saldias et al, 1999). Whether these agents will have any clinical efficacy remains to be determined.

## *Pulmonary Hemorrhage*

Landing (1957) described pulmonary hemorrhage in 68% of lungs of 125 consecutive infants who died in the first week of life; massive pulmonary hemorrhage was found in 17.8% of neonatal autopsies at the Johns Hopkins Hospital (Rowe and Avery, 1966). Fedrick and Butler (1971) judged massive pulmonary hemorrhage to be the principal cause of death in about 9% of neonatal autopsies.

### Etiology and Pathogenesis

Pulmonary hemorrhage usually occurs between days 2 and 4 of life in infants who are receiving mechanical ventilation. It has been associated with a wide variety of predisposing factors, including prematurity, asphyxia, overwhelming sepsis, intrauterine growth restriction/retardation, massive aspiration, severe hypothermia, severe Rh hemolytic disease, congenital heart disease, and coagulopathies. It is often associated with central nervous system injury, such as asphyxia or intracranial hemorrhage. Cole and associates (1973) studied a group of infants with pulmonary hemorrhage to determine the clinical circumstances under which the illness occurred as well as the hematocrit and protein compositions of fluid obtained from lung effluent and arterial or venous blood. Their results indicated that the lung effluent was, in most cases, hemorrhagic edema fluid and not whole blood (i.e., as indicated by hematocrit values significantly lower than those of whole blood). In addition, they did not find that coagulation disorders initiated the condition but probably served to exacerbate it in some cases. They postulated that the important precipitating factor was acute left ventricular failure caused by asphyxia or other events that might increase the filtration pressure, thereby injuring the capillary endothelium of the lung. Thus, pulmonary hemorrhage may be considered to represent the extreme form of high-permeability pulmonary edema.

Pulmonary edema following central nervous system injury probably results from increased hydrostatic pressure and some increase in vascular permeability (Malik, 1985). With the massive sympathetic discharge that accompanies central nervous system injury, left atrial pressure increases, and pulmonary arteries and veins constrict. As a result, microvascular pressure increases dramatically, damaging the microvascular endothelium, increasing its permeability to proteins and red blood cells. In infants with overwhelming sepsis and endotoxin production, increased microvascular permeability is apparent in the pulmonary circulation as well, undoubtedly contributing to the massive pulmonary hemorrhage sometimes seen in this group of patients. Pulmonary hemorrhage also has been described occasionally in the presence of a large patent ductus arteriosus, with a left-to-right shunt that results in high flow and high pressure injurious to the vascular bed.

Pulmonary hemorrhage also is associated with surfactant replacement therapy. Presumably the hemorrhage results from the rapid increase in pulmonary blood flow that accompanies improved lung function after surfactant therapy. The contribution of the patent ductus arteriosus to this increased blood flow remains to be determined. A meta-analysis suggests that surfactant replacement may be associated with an increased risk of pulmonary hemorrhage. This risk, however, is still extremely small compared with the known benefits of surfactant replacement (Pappin et al, 1994; Raju and Langenberg, 1993).

### Diagnosis

Infants with any of the conditions mentioned previously should be observed carefully for possible pulmonary hemorrhage. Particular note should be made of any blood-stained fluid from endotracheal tube aspirates, especially if repeated suctioning shows an increase in the amount of hemorrhagic fluid. The infant's chest radiograph may show the fluffy appearance of pulmonary edema in addition to the underlying pathologic process, and the infant may have increased respiratory distress. Frank pulmonary hemorrhage, when it occurs, is an acute emergency, and the fluid has the appearance of fresh blood being pumped directly from the vascular system, although hematocrit values for the fluid are at least 15 to 20 points lower than the hematocrit of circulating blood, in keeping with hemorrhagic pulmonary edema.

### Treatment

Effective treatment of pulmonary hemorrhage requires (1) clearing the airway of blood to allow ventilation; (2) use of adequate mean airway pressure, particularly end-expiratory pressure; (3) resisting the temptation to administer large volumes of blood, because in most cases the infant has not had a large loss of volume, so that administration of excessive volume exacerbates the increase in left atrial pressure and hemorrhagic pulmonary edema; rather, red cell replacement should be done as a slow administration of packed cells after the infant's pulmonary status has been stabilized; and (4) evaluation of the possibility of coagulopathy and administration of vitamin K and platelets, if appropriate.

## REFERENCES


Albertine KH: Ultrastructural abnormalities in increased permeability pulmonary edema. Clin Chest Med 6:345, 1985.

Bhutani VK, Sivieri EM, Abbasi S, Shaffer TH: Evaluation of neonatal pulmonary mechanics and energetics: A two factor least mean square analysis. Pediatr Pulmonol 4:150, 1988.

Bland RD, Hansen TN: Neonatal lung edema. In Said SI (ed): The Pulmonary Circulation and Acute Lung Injury. Mount Kisco, NY, Futura Publishing, 1985, p 225.

Brigham KL, Woolverton W, Blake L, et al: Increased sheep lung vascular permeability caused by *Pseudomonas* bacteremia. J Clin Invest 54:792, 1974.

Bryan AC, England SJ: Maintenance of an elevated FRC in the newborn: Paradox of REM sleep. Am Rev Respir Dis 129:209, 1984.

Carlton DP, Cummings JJ, Scheerer RG, et al: Lung overexpansion increases pulmonary microvascular protein permeability in young lambs. J Appl Physiol 69:577, 1990.

Cole VA, Normand ICS, Reynolds EOR, et al: Pathogenesis of hemorrhagic pulmonary edema and massive pulmonary hemorrhage in the newborn. Pediatrics 51:175, 1973.

Cook CD, Cherry RB, O'Brien D, et al: Studies of respiratory physiology in the newborn infant: I. Observations on normal premature and full term infants. J Clin Invest 34:975, 1955.

Cook CD, Sutherland JM, Segal S, et al: Studies of respiratory physiology in the newborn infant: III. Measurements of mechanics of respiration. J Clin Invest 36:440, 1957.

Corbet AJS, Ross JA, Beaudry PH, et al: Ventilation-perfusion relationships as assessed by $aA.DN_2$ in hyaline membrane disease. J Appl Physiol 36:74, 1974.

Drake R, Giesler M, Laine G, et al: Effect of outflow pressure on lung lymph flow in unanesthetized sheep. J Appl Physiol 58:70, 1985.

Elias RM, Wandolo G, Ranadive NS, et al: Lymphatic pumping in response to changes in transmural pressure is modulated by erythrolysate/hemoglobin. Circ Res 67:1097, 1990.

Farhi LE: Ventilation-perfusion relationship and its role in alveolar gas exchange. In Caro CG (ed): Advances in Respiratory Physiology. Baltimore, Williams & Wilkins, 1966.

Fedrick J, Butler NR: Certain causes of neonatal death: IV. Massive pulmonary hemorrhage. Biol Neonate 18:243, 1971.

Fein A, Grossman RF, Jones JG, et al: The value of edema fluid protein measurement in patients with pulmonary edema. Am J Med 67:32, 1979.

Feltes TF, Hansen TN: Effects of a large aorticopulmonary shunt on lung fluid balance in newborn lambs. Pediatr Res 20:368A, 1986.

Fishman AP: Pulmonary circulation. In Fishman AP, Fisher AB, Geiger SR (eds): Handbook of Physiology. Bethesda, Md, American Physiological Society, 1986, p 131.

France NE, Brown RJK: Congenital pulmonary lymphangiectasis: Report of 11 examples with special reference to cardiovascular findings. Arch Dis Child 46:528, 1971.

Frank JA, Wang Y, Osorio O, Matthay MA: Beta-adrenergic agonist therapy accelerates the resolution of hydrostatic pulmonary edema in sheep and rats. J Appl Physiol. 89:1255, 2000.

Gerhardt T, Bancalari E: Chestwall compliance in full term and premature infants. Acta Paediatr Scand 69:359, 1980.

Hansen TN, Gest AL, Landers S: Inspiratory airway obstruction does not affect lung fluid balance in lambs. J Appl Physiol 58:1314, 1985.

Hansen TN, Hazinski TA, Bland R: Effects of asphyxia on lung fluid balance in baby lambs. J Clin Invest 741:370, 1984.

Hazinski TA, Bland RD, Hansen TN, et al: Effect of hypoproteinemia on lung fluid balance in awake newborn lambs. J Appl Physiol 61:1139, 1986.

Johnson SA, Vander Straten MC, Parellada JA, et al: Thoracic duct function in fetal, newborn, and adult sheep. Lymphology 29:50, 1996.

Krieger I: Studies on mechanics of respiration in infancy. Am J Dis Child 105:439, 1963.

Landing BH: Pulmonary lesions in newborn infants: A statistical study. Pediatrics 19:217, 1957.

Lesouef PN, England SJ, Bryan AC: Passive respiratory mechanics in newborns and children. Am Rev Respir Dis 129:552, 1984.

Malik AB: Mechanisms of neurogenic pulmonary edema. Circ Res 57:1, 1985.

Markello R, Winter P, Olszowka A: Assessment of ventilation-perfusion inequalities by arterial alveolar nitrogen differences in intensive care patients. Anesthesiology 37:4, 1972.

McCann EM, Goldman SL, Brady JP: Pulmonary function in the sick newborn infant. Pediatr Res 21:313, 1987.

McGregor M: Pulsus paradoxus. N Engl J Med 301:480, 1979.

McIlroy MB, Tierney DF, Nadel JA: A new method for measurement of compliance and resistance of lungs and thorax. J Appl Physiol 18:424, 1963.

Nelson NM: Respiration and circulation after birth. In Smith CA, Nelson NM (eds): The Physiology of the Newborn Infant. Springfield, Ill, Charles C Thomas, 1976.

Niemann JT, Rosborough J, Hausknect M, et al: Documentation of systemic perfusion in man and in an experimental model: A "window" to the mechanism of blood flow in external CPR. Crit Care Med 8:141, 1980.

Pappin A, Shenker N, Hack M, et al: Extensive intraalveolar pulmonary hemorrhage in infants dying after surfactant therapy. J Pediatr 124:621, 1994.

Pedley TJ, Sudlow MF, Schroter RC: Gas flow and mixing in the airways. In West JB (ed): Bioengineering Aspects of the Lung. New York, Marcel Dekker, 1977, p 163.

Polgar G, Kong GP: The nasal resistance of newborn infants. J Pediatr 67:557, 1965.

Polgar G, Promadhat V: Pulmonary Function Testing in Children: Techniques and Standards. Philadelphia, WB Saunders, 1971, p 273.

Polgar G, String ST: The viscous resistance of the lung tissues in newborn infants. J Pediatr 69:787, 1966.

Raju TNK, Langenberg P: Pulmonary hemorrhage and exogenous surfactant therapy: A meta-analysis. J Pediatr 123:603, 1993.

Reynolds RN, Etsten BE: Mechanics of respiration in apneic anesthetized infants. Anesthesiology 27:13, 1966.

Rodarte JR, Rehder K: Dynamics of respiration. In Fishman AP, Macklem PT, Mead J, Geiger SR (eds): Handbook of Physiology, Vol III. Bethesda, Md, American Physiological Society, 1986, p 131.

Rowe S, Avery ME: Massive pulmonary hemorrhage in the newborn: II. Clinical considerations. J Pediatr 69:12, 1966.

Saldias FJ, Lecuona E, Comellas AP, et al: Dopamine restores lung ability to clear edema in rats exposed to hyperoxia. Am J Respir Crit Care Med 159:626, 1999.

Scott Emaukpor AB, Warren ST, Kapur S, et al: Familial occurrence of congenital pulmonary lymphangiectasis: Genetic implications. Am J Dis Child 135:532, 1981.

Slonim NB, Hamilton LH: Respiratory Physiology, 5th ed. St. Louis, CV Mosby, 1987, p 52.

Staub NC: Pulmonary edema. Physiol Rev 54:678, 1974.

Von Der Weid, P-Y: Lymphatic vessel pumping and inflammation: The role of spontaneous constrictions and underlying electrical pacemaker potentials. Aliment Pharmacol Ther 15:1115, 2001.

West JB: Ventilation: Blood Flow and Gas Exchange, 4th ed. St. Louis, CV Mosby, 1986.

Wohl MEB: Case records of Massachusetts General Hospital. N Engl J Med 321:309, 1989.

Woolverton NC, Brigham KL, Staub NC: Effect of positive pressure breathing on lung lymph flow and water content in sheep. Circ Res 42:550, 1978.

CHAPTER

# 45

# Principles of Respiratory Monitoring and Therapy

Thomas N. Hansen, Anthony Corbet, Alfred L. Gest, and Alicia A. Moise

## OXYGEN THERAPY

In an emergency, high concentrations of oxygen may be administered by face mask, head hood, or endotracheal tube for the relief of cyanosis. If administration of oxygen must be continued beyond the emergency, it should be warmed, humidified, and delivered by a flow proportioner connected to compressed sources of air and oxygen. The concentration of oxygen should be analyzed continuously or at least every hour, using an oxygen analyzer that is calibrated with air and oxygen every 8 hours. The use of oxygen therapy beyond the emergency period should be monitored continuously by measuring oxygen saturation using a pulse oximeter or oxygen tension using a transcutaneous $PO_2$ electrode. When this is not possible, oxygen should be given in a concentration just sufficient to abolish central cyanosis; within a few hours, arrangements should be made for appropriate measurements. In older infants, it has become common to administer oxygen by nasal cannula, with adjustments to either the flow or the concentration, according to the results of pulse oximetry.

### Monitoring Oxygen Therapy

#### Indwelling Catheters

In infants with significant respiratory distress, it is common to monitor oxygen therapy during the first few days of life using an umbilical artery catheter. For most infants, the arterial oxygen pressure ($PaO_2$) should be maintained between 50 and 70 mm Hg, but in some patients with labile pulmonary hypertension, it may be necessary to keep the $PaO_2$ slightly higher. For infants requiring high ventilator pressures, however, levels between 30 and 40 mm Hg may be accepted, provided that the circulatory status is well maintained and metabolic acidosis does not occur.

The reported complications of umbilical artery catheters include perforation, vasospasm, thrombosis, embolism, and infection. The most obvious sign of vasospasm is ischemia of the ipsilateral leg, and if this persists after a brief period of warming the contralateral leg, the catheter should be removed. During a difficult insertion procedure, it is possible (although this rarely occurs) to perforate the umbilical artery and enter the peritoneum, with consequent hemoperitoneum and hemorrhagic shock. By far the most frequently feared complication is thrombosis, and small thrombi, as documented by contrast aortography, may develop around the catheter in up to 95% of infants (Neal et al, 1972). Minute emboli may explain transient episodes of ischemia that later result in bluish discoloration of the toes. Clinical evidence of obstruction to a mesenteric, renal, pelvic, or femoral artery or to the aorta itself is comparatively uncommon but has been found in 13% of autopsy cases (Cochran, 1976). Suggestive evidence was found serendipitously by Jackson and coworkers (1987) that aortic thrombosis, detected by ultrasound examination, is more common after 11 days than after 4 days of catheterization. Infants with thrombosis can usually be managed conservatively with removal of the catheter and supportive care. Renovascular hypertension may occur, necessitating antihypertensive therapy. The condition usually resolves in time (Caplan et al, 1989). Another significant complication of umbilical arterial catheterization is infection, with sepsis occurring in 5% of cases (Landers et al, 1991). The incidence, however, is clearly higher (13%) if the catheter remains in place more than 14 days. Although the umbilical artery catheter is the easiest and most reliable way to monitor oxygen therapy, the need for arterial access should always be weighed against the inherent risks of an indwelling line when a decision is made to leave a catheter in place for more than a few days.

As an alternative to the umbilical artery catheter, short catheters inserted percutaneously or by cut-down procedure into the radial, posterior tibial, or dorsalis pedis artery are now widely used. These catheters sometimes function only a few days to a week, but the rates of infection and other complications are quite low.

Unfortunately, these measurements of $PaO_2$ are intermittent and represent conditions at only a single point in time. Information derived from continuous estimates of arterial oxygenation using noninvasive devices has shown that arterial oxygenation can vary significantly over time. As a result, changes in oxygen therapy should be based on data from a continuous monitoring device as well as intermittent determinations of arterial oxygen tension ($PAO_2$).

#### Intermittent Punctures

Arterial samples can be obtained by percutaneous needle aspiration of brachial, radial, or temporal arteries. Unfortunately, unless the sample is obtained immediately on penetration, the infant will become agitated and the measurement will not reflect steady-state oxygenation.

"Arterialized" capillary blood samples also have been used to monitor oxygen therapy. These measurements require that the extremity be heated to 43° to 44° C and that blood be collected free-flowing and under anaerobic conditions. These conditions are extremely difficult to reproduce in clinical situations. In addition, this technique almost always disturbs the infant, causing actual arterial oxygenation to fall. As a result, estimates of $PaO_2$ from capillary samples are notoriously unreliable, and capillary sampling is not recommended.

## Noninvasive Monitors

### *Pulse Oximeter*

Pulse oximetry is now the standard noninvasive technique for monitoring oxygen therapy. In fact, pulse oximeters are now incorporated into most bedside monitors, and pulse oximeter estimates of arterial oxygen saturation ($SpO_2$) are considered by some authorities to be the "fifth vital sign." The pulse oximeter takes advantage of differences in light absorption between oxyhemoglobin and reduced hemoglobin in the red and infrared spectra (Fig. 45–1) (Pologe, 1987; Wukitsch, 1987). In the red region of the spectrum, reduced hemoglobin absorbs more light than oxyhemoglobin, whereas in the infrared region, oxyhemoglobin absorbs more light than reduced hemoglobin. Total light absorption (at any wavelength) is the sum of the independent absorptions. For whole blood, the ratio of absorption in the red region to that in the infrared region (see Fig. 45–1) decreases as oxygen saturation ($SaO_2$) increases.

Pulse oximeters are easy to calibrate and apply. They do not require heat, have a rapid response time, and are not affected by skin thickness. Although the pulse oximeter assumes that there are only two types of hemoglobin present in arterial blood, a consistent effect of fetal hemoglobin on the relationship between oxygen saturation measured by the pulse oximeter and arterial oxygen saturation has not been demonstrated (Jennis and Peabody, 1987; Ramanathan et al, 1987). In the presence of methemoglobin, the pulse oximeter will overestimate $SaO_2$, especially as actual $SaO_2$ decreases (Barker et al, 1989). Similarly, in the presence of carboxyhemoglobin, the $SpO_2$ will consistently overestimate actual $SaO_2$ (Barker and Tremper, 1987).

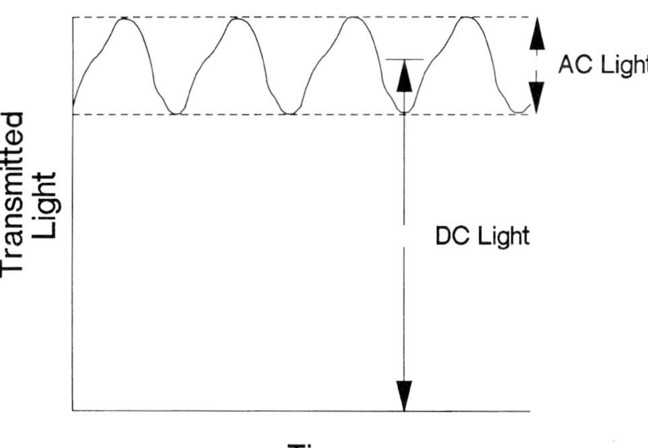


**FIGURE 45–1.** The pulse oximeter uses light-emitting diodes (LEDs) to send pulses of light of two different wavelengths through tissue containing a peripheral artery. A photodiode located opposite the LEDs measures the intensity of the transmitted light. At each wavelength, the light transmitted to the diode consists of two components: (1) an alternating current (AC) component, in which the intensity of transmitted light changes with the volume of blood (light absorber) in the artery, and (2) a direct current (DC) or constant component that results from light being transmitted through the tissues without being absorbed or scattered. The pulse oximeter measures the intensity of transmitted light as it illuminates one LED and then the other and then switches both off. With both LEDs off, the oximeter can measure and correct for the effects of external light incident on the photodiode. These cycles occur 480 times per second. The pulse oximeter focuses on the pulse-added component of the transmitted light by dividing the AC component by the DC component at each wavelength and creating the ratio $R = (AC_{Red}/DC_{Red})/(AC_{Ir}/DC_{Ir})$. (See text.) In this way, it ignores absorbances of venous blood, tissue, and pigmentation.

The alternating current (AC) signal detected by the pulse oximeter is small compared with the direct current (DC) background, so if changes in tissue perfusion reduce arterial pulsations, the pulse oximeter cannot function. In addition, motion artifacts can be confused with pulsatile flow resulting in $SpO_2$ values that are significantly different from the actual $SaO_2$. The magnitude of this error will be influenced by the magnitude of the movement, the degree of arterial pulsation, and venous oxygen saturation (Hay, 2000). Recently, signal-processing algorithms have been developed that have substantially reduced the number of "false hypoxemia" and "false bradycardia" episodes. The SET (signal extraction technology) algorithm validates measurements of $SpO_2$ using spectral data obtained before, during, and after movements to match measurements of $SpO_2$ to the frequency domain of the patient's heart rate. In one study, this algorithm reduced the number of episodes of false alarms by 86% (Hay et al, 2002).

Although $PaO_2$ can be roughly calculated from $SaO_2$, particularly at higher ranges of saturation, the range of $PaO_2$ values for any given confidence interval of saturations can be broad. A recent survey suggested that more than 70% of neonatal units were setting the upper alarm limit on the pulse oximeter at 96% or greater, and 32% were using 100% as the upper alarm limit (Vijayakumar et al, 1997). These upper limits will miss many, if not most, hyperoxic episodes. Poets and colleagues (1993) have shown that the upper alarm limit must be set at 95% to identify 95% of hyperoxic episodes while allowing the $PaO_2$ to be kept at greater than 60 mm Hg. Adams and coworkers (1994) found that an upper limit of 94% was necessary to detect 95% of hyperoxic episodes in their unit and that setting the limit at 95% allowed them to detect only 89% of hyperoxic episodes. Each center should generate acceptable ranges for $SaO_2$ for given clinical conditions. For example, if the goal is to keep $PaO_2$ between 50 and 80 mm Hg in a small preterm infant, ranges for $SaO_2$ must be developed that maintain the $PaO_2$ within this range.

### *Skin Surface Oxygen Monitoring*

The first noninvasive technique to gain widespread clinical acceptance was the skin surface oxygen ($PsO_2$) electrode (Huch et al, 1976; Landers and Hansen, 1994) (Fig. 45–2). The $PsO_2$ electrode does not measure $PaO_2$ directly; it simply measures the $PO_2$ on the surface of the skin. If certain conditions are met—an appropriate electrode temperature for a given skin thickness (Fig. 45–3) and normal circulation—the two measurements are highly correlated, and the $PsO_2$ provides a reasonable estimate of the $PaO_2$ for values between 15 and 150 mm Hg.

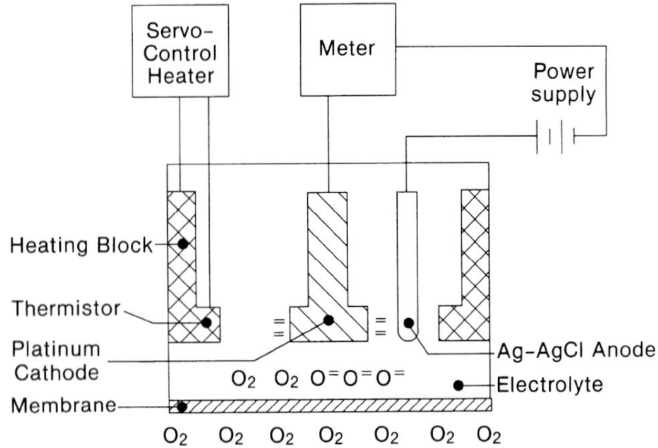


**FIGURE 45–2.** The $PsO_2$ electrode consists of a servo-controlled heater, a platinum cathode, and a silver–silver chloride anode that is immersed in an electrolyte solution and covered with semipermeable membrane. An external voltage maintains the cathode negative with respect to the anode. Oxygen diffuses across the membrane to the negatively charged cathode, and because it is extremely electrophilic, it readily accepts electrons from the cathode. The reduced oxygen species react with KCl in the electrolyte to form KOH, and liberated chloride ions are deposited on the anode. As electrons are removed from the cathode, electrons flow from the anode and generate an electrical current that can be measured in the external circuit. This current is proportional to the rate of diffusion of oxygen molecules across the membrane into the electrode. The rate of diffusion, in turn, is proportional to the $PsO_2$ and the permeability of the membrane to oxygen. Oxygen electrodes must be *zeroed* to compensate for the current produced by the external voltage, and a gain must be set to adjust the output for a given membrane permeability.

Problems arise when the $PsO_2$ differs from the $PaO_2$ (Table 45–1). Skin thickness, skin blood flow, oxygen consumption, and electrode temperature all affect the correlation (see Fig. 45–3). The $PsO_2$ electrode itself also may interfere with the correlation between $PsO_2$ and $PaO_2$. The electrode consumes oxygen at a rate limited by the membrane permeability. If membrane permeability increases, oxygen consumption by the electrode can lower the $PsO_2$. Because an infinite supply of oxygen exists at the time of calibration, the electrode calibrates normally.

### *Skin Surface Carbon Dioxide Monitoring*

The skin surface carbon dioxide ($PsCO_2$) electrode is a glass pH electrode modified so that it can be heated and mounted on the skin (Brunstler et al, 1982; Hansen and Tooley, 1979). $CO_2$ diffuses into the electrode, producing a change in pH. The $PsCO_2$ electrode measures the concentration of $CO_2$ on the surface of the skin and is little affected by skin thickness or membrane permeability. It is affected by blood flow to the skin and must be heated to 42° to 44° C to produce vasodilation. Heating increases

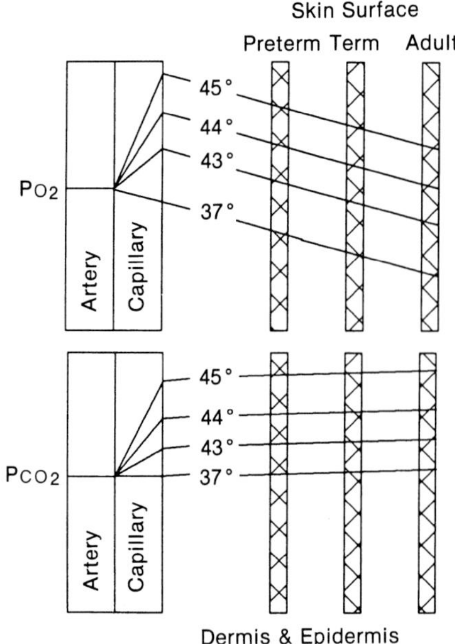


**FIGURE 45–3. Top,** In unheated skin, as oxygen diffuses from the capillary bed across the dermis and epidermis, $PO_2$ decreases relative to $PaO_2$ because of skin consumption of oxygen. As skin thickness increases (preterm infant versus term infant versus adult), this discrepancy increases. To counteract this effect, $PsO_2$ electrodes are heated. Heating increases capillary and tissue $PO_2$ by producing vasodilation, thereby increasing oxygen delivery to the skin, and by shifting the oxygen-hemoglobin dissociation curve to the right. The subsequent fall in $PO_2$ as oxygen diffuses to the skin surface counterbalances the effect of heating and lowers $PO_2$ at the skin surface to a value approaching $PaO_2$. Optimal correlation between $PaO_2$ and $PsO_2$ requires that electrode temperature be appropriate for skin thickness. **Bottom,** Because of local carbon dioxide production, the $PsCO_2$ of even unheated skin is greater than $PaCO_2$. Heating the electrode increases $PsCO_2$ further. The effect of electrode temperature on $PsCO_2$ is constant and predictable, so that correction factors can be built into the calibration procedure.

$PsCO_2$ relative to $PaCO_2$, and correction factors must be incorporated into the calibration procedure so that the digital or graphic readout of $PsCO_2$ equals $PaCO_2$ (see Fig. 45–3).

**TABLE 45–1**

**Factors Affecting Skin Surface $O_2$ and $CO_2$ Tensions**

| | |
|---|---|
| **Increase $PsO_2$** | **Increase $PsCO_2$** |
| Increased $PaO_2$ | Increased $PaCO_2$ |
| | Increased temperature |
| **Decrease $PsO_2$** | Increased skin $CO_2$ production |
| Decreased $PaO_2$ | Decreased perfusion |
| Decreased skin perfusion | |
| Increased skin thickness (age-related) | **Decrease $PsCO_2$** |
| Edema | Decreased $PaCO_2$ |
| Damaged membrane | Decreased temperature |

# MECHANICAL VENTILATION

## Continuous Positive Airway Pressure

### Treatment of Respiratory Distress Syndrome

Continuous positive airway pressure (CPAP) was developed as a technique to improve oxygenation in spontaneously breathing premature infants with hyaline membrane disease (Gregory et al, 1971). Positive pressure was applied through an endotracheal tube, endopharyngeal tube, nasal prongs, face mask, or head box, or by creating continuous negative pressure around the chest with the airway at atmospheric pressure.

The primary role of CPAP is to support small airways and prevent the generalized atelectasis of the surfactant-deficient lung. At the same time, CPAP improves oxygenation in infants with hyaline membrane disease by improving ventilation to open poorly ventilated air spaces, relieving local vasoconstriction and decreasing the right-to-left shunt and the alveolar-arterial oxygen tension difference ($Aa.DO_2$) (Corbet et al, 1975; Hansen et al, 1979). CPAP decreases tidal volume ($V_T$), minute ventilation, and the arterial-alveolar carbon dioxide tension difference ($aA.DCO_2$), suggesting that it improves alveolar ventilation (Bancalari et al, 1973; Hansen et al, 1979; Landers et al, 1986).

The infant flow driver is a relatively new device for delivering nasal CPAP that generates positive pressure at the airway, keeps the level of distending pressure constant throughout inspiration, and probably assists with inspiration (Moa and Nilsson, 1993). When compared with conventional modes for delivery of nasal CPAP, this device increases lung volume more for any change in distending pressure (Courtney et al, 2001) while increasing compliance and decreasing work of breathing (Pandit et al, 2001).

Between 1973 and 1976, four randomized controlled trials of CPAP to treat respiratory distress syndrome (RDS) were conducted (Belenky et al, 1976; Durbin et al, 1976; Fanaroff et al, 1973; Rhodes and Hall, 1973). A meta-analysis of the results of these trials (Bancalari and Sinclair, 1992) showed that CPAP reduced mortality from hyaline membrane disease, reduced the need for subsequent mechanical ventilation, and increased the risk of air leak. There was no detectable effect on the risk of bronchopulmonary dysplasia. Bancalari and Sinclair (1992) then analyzed results of five trials comparing early with late CPAP for the treatment of hyaline membrane disease (Allen et al, 1977; Gerard et al, 1975; Hegyi and Hiatt, 1981; Krouskop et al, 1975; Mockrin and Bancalari, 1975) and found that early application of CPAP reduced the need for subsequent mechanical ventilation without affecting mortality or the risk of air leak.

### Early Nasal Continous Positive Airway Pressure

Many clinicians believe that endotracheal CPAP alone is not likely to be successful in smaller infants (birth weight of less than 1500 g) and proceed directly to mechanical ventilation (Drew, 1982). This approach has come into question in recent years, however (Poets and Sens, 1996). A study comparing outcomes in different academic medical centers (Avery et al, 1987) noted that the institution reporting the best survival without chronic lung disease was also the one that used nasal CPAP early and extensively for stabilization of very low-birth-weight (VLBW) infants (Wung et al, 1975). Since that report, there has been a renewed interest in the use of very early nasal CPAP for the initial stabilization and management of VLBW infants. Several reports from Denmark suggested that more than half of infants weighing less than 1500 g could be managed exclusively with nasal CPAP and oxygen if high values for $PaCO_2$ were tolerated (Kamper and Ringsted, 1990; Kamper et al, 1993; Lundstrom and Greisen, 1993). Two trials compared outcomes in infants weighing less than 1500 g who were managed with early nasal CPAP with outcomes in historic controls. Early nasal CPAP was found to reduce the need for subsequent intubation and mechanical ventilation by roughly 50% without affecting overall mortality or the incidence of chronic lung disease (Gittermann et al, 1997; Jacobsen et al, 1993). Lindner and colleagues (1999) found that in infants weighing less than 1000 g, early nasal CPAP reduced the rate of intubation in the delivery room by 50% and that 25% of these infants could be managed by nasal CPAP alone. The infants who could be managed on nasal CPAP alone had a lower mortality rate and a reduced incidence of chronic lung disease and severe intracranial hemorrhage. DeKlerk and DeKlerk (2001) used historic controls to show that for infants weighing between 1000 and 1500 g, early nasal CPAP reduced the need for subsequent mechanical ventilation as well as a number of other problems including chronic lung disease, need for pressor support, and necrotizing enterocolitis. All of these studies suffer from the lack of a randomized group of control infants, and many of the outcomes may reflect other changes in practice or differences in underlying disease severity. However, their results are intriguing and call for randomized controlled trials to determine the safety and utility of early nasal CPAP.

Verder and colleagues (1994) studied the effects of routine surfactant administration in combination with early nasal CPAP in infants between 25 and 35 weeks of gestational age. They intubated the infants for surfactant administration, mechanically ventilated them briefly to allow the surfactant to distribute, and then extubated them and continued nasal CPAP. They found that surfactant administration significantly reduced the need for subsequent mechanical ventilation and, in a later study in infants born at less than 30 weeks of gestational age, found that this effect was magnified if surfactant was administered early (Verder et al, 1999).

### Techniques for Administration of Continuous Positive Airway Pressure for the Treatment of Respiratory Distress

Traditionally, endotracheal CPAP is used in larger infants (birth weight greater than 1500 g) with respiratory distress in the hope that mechanical ventilation will not be necessary; it should be started when the oxygen requirement reaches 50%. In these infants, the initial level of endotracheal CPAP used is 5 cm $H_2O$ at an oxygen requirement of 50%, and the pressure is increased in 1–cm $H_2O$ steps for each 10% increase in the oxygen requirement; the incidence of pulmonary air leak with this regimen is no higher than the spontaneous rate for RDS (Corbet and Adams, 1978). Infants who require an oxygen concentration of more than 80% with endotracheal CPAP of 8 to 10 cm $H_2O$ will usually need mechanical ventilation. However, with the advent of surfactant therapy, it is now common to omit the initial CPAP step, to start surfactant administration and mechanical ventilation when the oxygen requirement is 40% to 50%, or less, and to use CPAP only later when the infant is near clinical recovery and extubation. Another possible strategy in larger infants is the use of intubation and mechanical ventilation for surfactant administration and then endotracheal CPAP (Mandy et al, 1999).

In the past, nasal CPAP has usually been administered by a positive pressure ventilator set in the CPAP mode (ventilator CPAP), or by placing the expiratory limb of a constant-flow circuit into water at a depth sufficient to generate the required positive end-expiratory pressure (bubble CPAP) (Wung et al, 1975). In more recent years, nasal CPAP has been administered using the infant flow driver. When compared with ventilator CPAP, the infant flow driver produces a greater change in lung volume for any given change in pressure (Courtney et al, 2001), increases lung compliance, and decreases work of breathing (Pandit et al, 2001). The infant flow driver delivers slightly more oxygen than is provided by the other nasal CPAP devices (0.5% to 3%) (Ahluwalia et al, 1998; Kavvadia et al, 2000; Mazzella et al, 2001). A single controlled trial compared the infant flow driver with bubble CPAP in infants of less than 36 weeks of gestation eligible for CPAP and found that in infants managed with the infant flow driver, work of breathing was less, with lower respiratory rates and lower oxygen requirements. These studies all suggest that the infant flow driver probably assists with inspiration, improving overall gas exchange. Another controlled trial found that infants managed with bubble CPAP had lower minute ventilation and respiratory rates than in infants managed with ventilator CPAP, despite no differences in $SaO_2$ or $PsCO_2$ (Lee et al, 1998). This improvement in gas exchange may be the result of vibrations transmitted from the bubble chamber to the chest.

Typically, nasal CPAP is delivered using binasal prongs or an endotracheal tube shortened to fit 2 to 3 cm into the nose (mononasal prong) or left longer and placed in the pharynx (nasopharyngeal tube). Courtney and colleagues (2001) found that respiratory rate, thoracoabdominal asymmetry (a measure of inspiratory loading), and $FIO_2$ all were higher in infants receiving nasal CPAP through a mononasal prong than in infants receiving CPAP via binasal prongs. Davis and colleagues (2001) found that with ventilator CPAP, binasal prongs were more effective than mononasal prongs in preventing failure of extubation in infants weighing less than 1000 g. When binasal and mononasal prongs were compared using the infant flow driver, however, no differences in pressure transmitted to the nasopharynx were found (Pederson and Nielsen, 1994).

Of interest, two studies (Locke et al, 1993; Sreenan et al, 2001) have shown that the use of nasal cannulas to deliver oxygen may result in positive end-expiratory pressure. This seemed to occur only when the cannulas were 0.3 cm in outer diameter. Because the amount of end pressure delivered is difficult to assess in this instance, the use of nasal cannulas to deliver nasal CPAP should be discouraged.

Most authors suggest starting nasal CPAP at a pressure of 5 to 6 cm $H_2O$ and then increasing to a maximum of 8 to 10 cm $H_2O$ based on the clinical response and the oxygen requirement. Indications for subsequent intubation and mechanical ventilation include intractable apnea and persistent hypoxemia in 80% to 100% oxygen. Because CPAP may overdistend the lung, impairing the pulmonary circulation, attempts have been made to identify optimal levels. As CPAP is increased and approaches optimum, the $aA.DCO_2$ falls significantly; but as the optimal level is exceeded, both the $aA.DCO_2$ and the arterial $PCO_2$ rise significantly (Landers et al, 1986). Under clinical conditions, hypercarbia may indicate excessive CPAP, which should be recognized and corrected before oxygenation deteriorates.

## Intermittent Positive Pressure Ventilation

Advances in techniques for intermittent positive pressure ventilation have dramatically altered outcomes in infants with a variety of lung diseases. To use these techniques effectively, the clinician must have a thorough understanding of how the various components of intermittent positive-pressure ventilation affect the lung of the newborn.

### Positive Pressure Inflation of the Lung

During a positive pressure breath, gas flows into the lung because airway pressure is greater than alveolar pressure. The volume of gas entering the lung over time is a function of the peak inflation pressure (PIP), duration of inspiration (Ti), and respiratory system compliance (Crs) and resistance (Rrs) (Figs. 45–4 and 45–5). For purposes of this discussion, exhalation is considered to be passive.

Most ventilators that are currently in use in neonatal intensive care units (NICUs) are time cycled and pressure limited (Fig. 45–6). PIP, positive end-expiratory pressure (PEEP), Ti, and expiratory time (Te) are adjusted independently or linked by the Ti/Te ratio. The rate is altered by changing Ti or Te or both. Mean airway pressure (MAP) is the average pressure at the proximal airway over time. If the inspiratory pressure waveform resembles a square wave (see Fig. 45–6), then

$$MAP = (PIP - PEEP) \times (Ti/[Ti + Te]) + PEEP$$

### Effects of Positive Pressure Ventilation on Gas Exchange

#### *Determinants of Oxygenation*

In infants with parenchymal lung disease, hypoxemia is related to the presence of open but severely underventilated lung units (see Chapter 44). In these units, alveolar ventilation is not sufficient to maintain the alveolar oxygen tension ($PAO_2$) much above mixed venous $PO_2$. These lung units can cause arterial hypoxemia by two different mechanisms: (1) ventilation-perfusion mismatch and (2) right-to-left shunt.

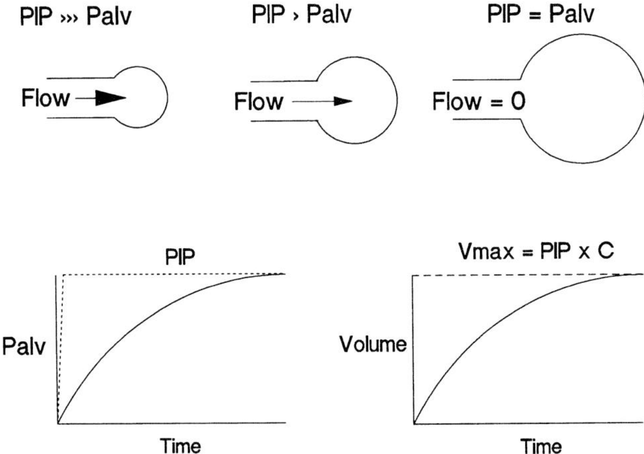


**FIGURE 45–4.** Positive pressure inflation of the lung. In this example, airway pressure increases rapidly to a plateau (peak inflation pressure [PIP]) (*dashed line*). Initially, alveolar pressure (Palv) is equal to atmospheric pressure and is much less than airway pressure (PIP >>> Palv). As a result of this large driving pressure, gas flows into the lung, and the volume of gas in the lung increases as a function of time. Obviously, because Palv is directly related to lung volume (Palv = volume/compliance), it also increases as a function of time. Therefore, the driving pressure for gas flow (PIP – Palv) and the rate of gas flow into the lung both decrease over time. Ultimately, Palv becomes equal to PIP, and flow ceases. Therefore, the maximal volume of gas that can enter the lung (Vmax) during any positive pressure breath is ultimately determined by PIP and compliance (C): Vmax = PIP × C.

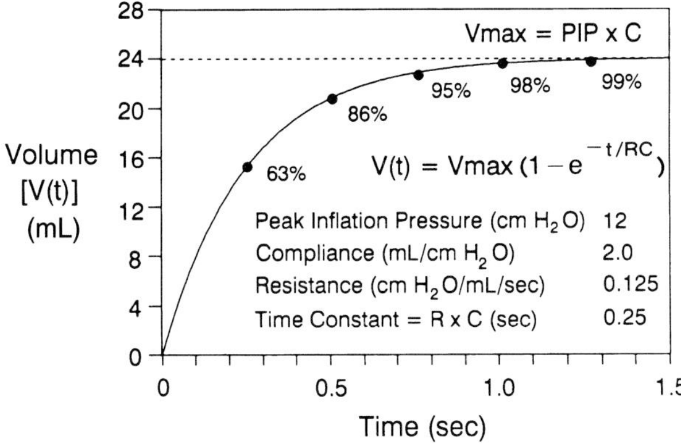


**FIGURE 45–5.** Lung inflation over time. As in Figure 45–4, airway pressure is rapidly increased to 25 cm $H_2O$ and then maintained at a plateau. The volume of gas in the lung, V(t), increases over time according to the relationship: $V(t) = Vmax \times (1 - e^{-t/RC})$, where R is the resistance of the respiratory system and C is the compliance. The maximal volume of gas that can flow into the lung (Vmax) is limited by the peak airway pressure (PIP) and C (i.e., Vmax = PIP × C). The rate of lung inflation, similar to the rate of deflation, is described by an exponential equation involving the respiratory time constant (Trs). As described in Chapter 44, Trs = R × C. For an inspiratory time equal to 1 time constant (Ti = 1 × Trs), the lung inflates to 63% of its maximal volume (Vmax). For Ti = 2 × Trs, it reaches 86% of Vmax; for 3 × Trs, 95%; for 4 × Trs, 98%; and for 5 × Trs, 99%. Therefore, the volume of gas entering the lung during a positive pressure breath is determined by the peak inflation pressure (PIP), the duration of inspiration (Ti), and respiratory system compliance (Crs) and resistance (Rrs).

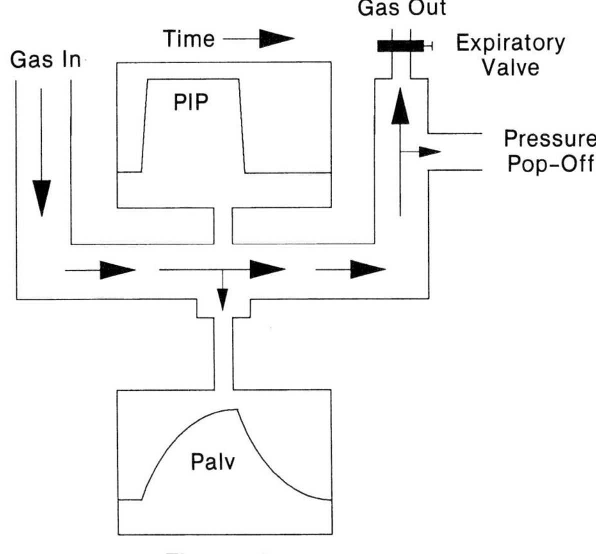


**FIGURE 45–6.** Time-cycled, pressure-limited ventilator. Gas flows continuously through the ventilator circuit while a flow resistor on the exhalation limb of the circuit provides positive end-expiratory pressure. During inspiration, the expiratory valve is closed, and pressure builds up in the circuit for a preset time (Ti). The rate of the pressure buildup is determined to a large extent by the system flow. In this example, flow is high, and the pressure waveform is a square wave. PIP is limited by venting excessive pressure to the atmosphere. Airway pressure increases rapidly and is held at a plateau. Alveolar pressure increases gradually as gas flows into the lung from the ventilator. The rate of gas flow to the patient is determined primarily by the driving pressure (PIP – Palv) and the resistance (R), so flow = (PIP – Palv)/R, not by the rate of gas flow through the ventilator circuit.

## Ventilation-Perfusion Mismatch

In term infants with meconium aspiration pneumonia or older infants with bronchopulmonary dysplasia, blood continues to flow past the poorly ventilated lung units and remains poorly oxygenated. When it mixes with the remainder of the pulmonary venous return, it decreases overall systemic oxygen saturation. The severity of the resultant hypoxemia is directly related to the severity of the hypoxia in the poorly ventilated lung units and to the quantity of blood flowing past them.

## Right-to-Left Shunt

In infants with RDS, the cause of hypoxemia is right-to-left shunt. In these infants, intense vasoconstriction occurs in blood vessels supplying severely underventilated lung units, causing blood to be directed away from these lung units through intrapulmonary and extrapulmonary shunts (Hansen et al, 1979). The magnitude of the right-to-left shunt—as well as, correspondingly, the severity of the arterial hypoxemia—is related to the severity of the hypoxia in the open, underventilated lung units and to the number of these units present in the lung. Therefore, regardless of the underlying parenchymal disease, the degree of arterial hypoxemia is determined by the $PAO_2$ in open but severely underventilated units of the lung; the only way to increase arterial $PO_2$ is to increase the $PAO_2$ in these lung units.

Several studies have shown that increasing the MAP increases $PaO_2$ in infants with lung disease, suggesting that increases in MAP must somehow increase the $PAO_2$ in poorly ventilated units of the lung (Herman and Reynolds, 1973; Stewart et al, 1981). As discussed previously, MAP is really a function of PIP, PEEP, and Ti. Increasing MAP by increasing PIP increases the driving pressure for gas flow into poorly ventilated lung units (Fig. 45–7). Increasing MAP by increasing Ti allows more time for gas to distribute to these units. Finally, increasing MAP by increasing PEEP splints small airways open, decreases airway resistance, decreases the time constant for inspiration, and allows more gas to enter the lung unit for any given PIP or Ti. All three techniques improve ventilation to the poorly ventilated lung units and increase their $PAO_2$. For a given increase in MAP, increasing PEEP or PIP results in a greater increase in $PaO_2$ than can be obtained by increasing Ti (Stewart et al, 1981). The reason for this discrepancy lies in the effects of mechanical ventilation on the normal parts of the lung.

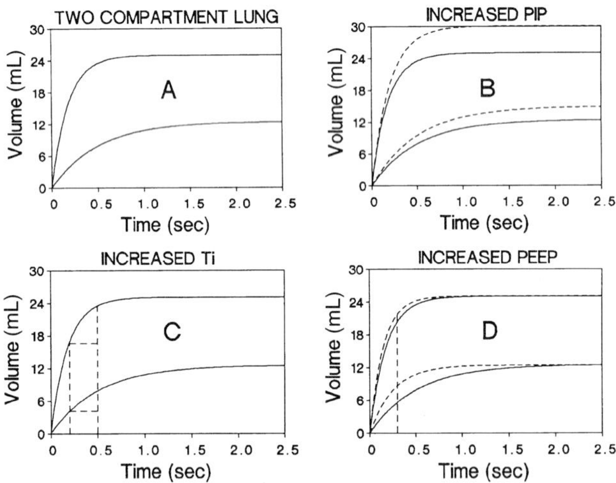


**FIGURE 45–7.** Effects of ventilatory manipulations on each compartment of a two-compartment lung. **A,** Plot of lung volume over time during a positive pressure inflation of the lung (PIP = 25 cm $H_2O$). The top curve represents normal lung units (compliance = 1 mL/cm $H_2O$, resistance = 0.150 cm $H_2O$/mL/second, and time constant = 0.15 second). These lung units inflate to a greater maximal volume (Vmax = PIP × C = 25 mL) and reach Vmax quickly (5 time constants = 0.75 second). The *lower curve* represents poorly ventilated lung units (compliance = 0.5 mL/cm $H_2O$, resistance = 1.0 cm $H_2O$/mL/second, and time constant = 0.5 second). Obviously, these units have a lower Vmax (12.5 mL) and take longer to reach Vmax (5 time constants = 2.5 seconds). As stated previously, the only ventilatory means of increasing the patient's $PaO_2$ is to increase the volume of gas entering poorly ventilated lung units. **B,** Increasing peak inflation pressure (*dashed curves*) increases the volume of gas entering each group of lung units. The increase is greater in normal lung units than in poorly ventilated lung units for any inspiratory time value (Ti). The net result is overdistention of normal parts of the lung incurred in an attempt to ventilate the poorly ventilated lung units. **C,** Increasing Ti from 0.2 to 0.5 seconds increases the volume of gas entering each group of lung units. As in **B,** the increase, as well as corresponding tendency for overdistention, is much more pronounced in the normal parts of the lung. **D,** Increasing positive end-expiratory pressure (PEEP) decreases the time constant in each group of lung units. The net effect is to allow more gas to enter each part of the lung for any given PIP or Ti. In this case, the effect is more pronounced in the poorly ventilated lung units. As a result, the likelihood of overdistention of normal lung units is less.

None of the parenchymal lung diseases, including RDS, is homogeneous (Richardson et al, 1992). Relatively normal lung units coexist with severely underventilated lung units. Because all are connected, however, all are exposed to the same airway pressures during mechanical ventilation. Relatively normal units may have a low airway resistance and high compliance and may be subject to overdistention with increases in MAP. The risk of overdistention is greatest when MAP is increased by increasing Ti, less with increases in PIP, and least with increases in PEEP (see Fig. 45–7). As discussed in Chapter 44, overdistended lung units compress intra-alveolar vessels and redirect blood flow past poorly ventilated lung units or through shunt pathways (Landers et al, 1986). This increase in ventilation-perfusion mismatching tends to offset any increase in $PaO_2$ that occurs because of increased oxygenation in poorly ventilated lung units. This phenomenon probably explains why $PaO_2$ increases less when MAP is increased by increasing Ti than when it is increased by increasing PEEP or PIP.

Besides its effects on oxygenation, alveolar overdistention carries the risk of alveolar rupture and pulmonary interstitial emphysema (PIE). The propensity for increases in Ti to result in alveolar overdistention is supported by its high correlation with pulmonary air leaks in one study that explored the antecedents of alveolar rupture (Primhak, 1983). It is also supported by the results of two controlled trials showing a higher incidence of pneumothorax in infants ventilated with a long Ti than in those ventilated with a short Ti (Heicher et al, 1981; Oxford Region Controlled Trial, 1991).

### *Determinants of Ventilation*

The other important function of mechanical ventilation is to ventilate adequately, to control $PaCO_2$. $PaCO_2$ is equal to the rate of $CO_2$ production divided by the alveolar ventilation ($\dot{V}A$). The latter is represented by the equation $\dot{V}A = (Vt - Vd) \times RR$, where VT is tidal volume, VD is dead space volume, and RR is respiratory rate. If VD and $CO_2$ production are relatively constant, $PaCO_2$ is proportional to 1/(RR × VT). $PaCO_2$ decreases if either RR or VT is increased, and $PaCO_2$ increases if RR or VT is decreased. On a pressure-limited respirator, at a constant inspiratory time, the VT is determined by the lung compliance and by PIP and PEEP (Fig. 45–8). If Ti is less than 3 time constants, increasing Ti will also increase VT but at the expense of overdistention of more normal lung units. $PaCO_2$ can be decreased by increasing RR, by increasing PIP, or by decreasing PEEP. Conversely, $PaCO_2$ can be increased by decreasing RR, by decreasing PIP, or by increasing PEEP.

Although it is attractive to try to lower the $PaCO_2$ by increasing the respirator rate, rather than by adjusting ventilatory pressures, data suggest that this approach may not be entirely without risk. As the respirator rate increases, the absolute time allotted for expiration decreases. If expiratory time decreases to less than 3 time constants for expiration, gas trapping (Simbruner, 1986) and alveolar overdistention may occur (Kano et al, 1993).

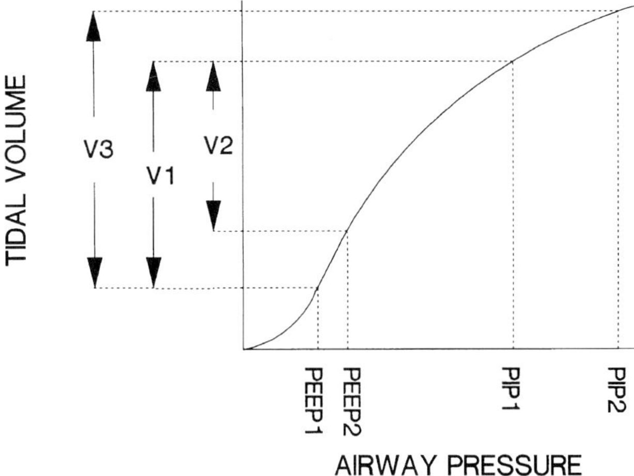


**FIGURE 45–8.** Determinants of tidal volume. Lung volume is plotted as a function of inflation pressure. As the ventilator cycles between positive end-expiratory pressure (PEEP1) and peak inflation pressure (PIP1), the lung volume changes, generating tidal volume (V1). Increasing PEEP to PEEP2 forces the ventilator to cycle between PEEP2 and PIP1 and results in a lower tidal volume (V2). Leaving PEEP at PEEP1 while increasing peak inflation pressure to PIP2 increases the tidal volume to V3.

### Implementation

Because tiny premature infants characteristically have structurally immature lungs and weak chest walls, many centers have a standard practice of providing some form of respiratory support (i.e., nasal CPAP or mechanical ventilation) for all infants who weigh between 1000 and 1250 g. For infants who weigh between 1250 and 1500 g and have RDS, respiratory support also may necessary. The use of early nasal CPAP in these circumstances has been discussed in detail previously.

#### *Intubation and Mechanical Ventilation*

Intubation and mechanical ventilation at birth still constitute routine practice in many centers for infants weighing between 1000 and 1250 g. In addition, infants in whom nasal CPAP is unsuccessful because of apnea or persistent hypoxemia will require intubation and mechanical ventilation. Infants usually are intubated orally with an endotracheal tube that allows an audible air leak to ensure that the tube is not too tight against the walls of the trachea. A 2.5-mm-internal-diameter (ID) tube is appropriate for infants weighing less than 1 kg, 3.0 mm for those weighing between 1 and 2 kg, and 3.5 mm for those weighing more than 2 kg. For standard use, orotracheal intubation is preferred over nasotracheal because nasotracheal intubation has been found to cause nasal deformities (McMillan et al, 1986).

During intubation, infants often require a fraction of inspired oxygen ($FIO_2$) that is 10% greater than they were receiving before the initiation of mechanical ventilation. It is always valuable to hand-ventilate an infant initially to determine the minimal PIP necessary to achieve good chest wall excursion and good bilateral breath sounds. A rate of 60 breaths/minute (which approximates the normal rate for a premature infant) and PEEP of 5 cm $H_2O$ are often used. In general, oxygenation can be improved by increasing MAP by increasing PEEP or PIP. Ti should rarely be prolonged, because of the risk of alveolar overdistention. An infant with poor pulmonary blood flow due to hypotension, hypovolemia, cardiac failure, or high pulmonary vascular resistance also may have a low $PaO_2$, and treatment should be directed to improving blood pressure and cardiac output.

Hypercarbia is treated by increasing PIP or respirator rate. To allow sufficient time for exhalation, the respirator rate should not ordinarily exceed 80 breaths/minute. The overall cardiopulmonary status of the infant must be kept in mind. Data have suggested that attempts to control $PaCO_2$ rigorously may result in worsened lung injury (Garland et al, 1995; Kraybill et al, 1989). Ventilation with large tidal volumes has been shown to damage the lung of immature animals (Carlton et al, 1990; Hernandez et al, 1989). Hypocapnia exacerbates lung injury following ischemia-reperfusion (Laffey et al, 2000) and may be a risk factor for periventricular leukomalacia (PVL) (Okumura et al, 2001) and cerebral palsy in preterm infants (Collins et al, 2001). Hypercapnia has been shown to protect the lungs of rabbits from ventilator-induced lung injury (Sinclair et al, 2002) and to protect the brains of neonatal rats from hypoxic-ischemic damage (Vannucci et al, 1995). Two published studies have compared *permissive hypercapnia* ($PaCO_2$ typically between 45 and 55 mm Hg) with normocapnia ($PaCO_2$ typically between 35 and 45 mm Hg) and have found no reduction in death or bronchopulmonary dysplasia (Carlo et al, 2002; Mariani et al, 1999). Comorbid conditions such as intraventricular hemorrhage (IVH) and PVL also were similar in frequency in both groups. Therefore, the data are not sufficient to recommend ventilator strategies that routinely target high arterial $CO_2$ tensions. However, many centers allow the $PaCO_2$ to increase to 50 to 60 mm Hg or above in infants with severe respiratory distress, in whom the risk of lung injury or air block is great.

If the infant's breathing is asynchronous, especially if the blood pressure is low, then it is common to find that the blood pressure wave fluctuates (Perlman and Thach, 1988). Asynchrony also is associated with an increased incidence of pneumothorax. Sometimes, an increase in the rate to 70 or 80 beats/minute may promote adequate synchrony (Greenough et al, 1987), or breathing can be suppressed with narcotics (Goldstein and Brazy, 1991). If narcotics are given, expiratory braking may be impaired, so it is again important to use generous levels of PEEP to promote the maintenance of lung volume (Miller et al, 1994).

The use of neuromuscular blockade to facilitate mechanical ventilation in the newborn remains controversial. Paralysis may result in decreased dynamic lung compliance and increased airway resistance and removes any contribution of the infant's own respiratory effort from tidal breathing (Bhutani et al, 1988). Therefore, it is often necessary to increase ventilator pressures after initiation of neuromuscular blockade. Venous return also is impaired by lack of movement and decreased muscle tone, and generalized edema may develop with this treatment.

Ventilator gas should be warmed to 34° to 36° C, and relative humidity should be greater than 90% to prevent excessive water loss from the respiratory tract and injury to the lung from exposure to cold dry air (Chatburn, 1989; Gomez and Hansen, 1999; Hanssler et al, 1992; Tarnow-Mordi et al, 1989). This warming is most easily accomplished by using a heated nebulizer with heated ventilator circuits to prevent condensation of water in the ventilator tubing. Tracheal suctioning and chest physiotherapy should be minimized in the infant with RDS in the first few days after birth because their secretions are scant, and there is little evidence that suctioning and chest physiotherapy are of benefit. Concern has been expressed that these interventions might increase the risk of intracranial hemorrhage (Greisen et al, 1985; Perlman and Volpe, 1983). Infants with secretions (e.g., meconium aspiration or pneumonia) and older infants with RDS may require suctioning of the trachea as often as every 2 to 4 hours. Even then, suctioning often is associated with acute side effects of hypoxia, hypertension, and bradycardia (Simbruner et al, 1981) and, with deep suctioning, the risk of airway injury (Miller et al, 1981). If hand ventilation accompanies suctioning, a manometer must be attached to the bag to prevent delivery of excessive PIP.

### *Weaning from Mechanical Ventilation*

#### Nasal CPAP to Facilitate Weaning from Mechanical Ventilation

For infants weighing less than 1500 g, when PIP is less than 20 cm $H_2O$ and $FIO_2$ is less than 0.30, it is possible to decrease gradually the respiratory rate to 15 to 20 breaths/minute and then to wean directly to nasal CPAP (Wung et al, 1975). For this group of infants, the resistance of the endotracheal tube is such that periods of endotracheal CPAP or ventilatory rates less than 15 breaths/minute cannot be tolerated (Lesouef et al, 1984). A more recent study has shown, in fact, that chest-abdomen asynchrony (a measure of inspiratory loading) is much less for infants breathing though nasal prongs than for those breathing through an endotracheal tube (Kiciman et al, 1998).

Seven randomized clinical trials comparing postextubation nasal CPAP with extubation to an oxygen hood (Annibale et al, 1994; Chan and Greenough, 1993b; Davis et al, 1998; Engelke et al, 1982; Higgins et al, 1991; So et al; 1995; Tapia et al, 1995) were recently summarized in a meta-analysis (Davis and Henderson-Smart, 1999). Nasal CPAP reduced extubation failure rates by roughly 62% but did not decrease the number of infants requiring oxygen support at 28 days. A subgroup analysis suggested that nasal CPAP greater than 5 cm $H_2O$ was necessary for efficacy. These findings were confirmed by a subsequent controlled trial and meta-analysis by Dimitriou and coworkers in 2000. Overall, these studies and the meta-analyses provide support for the use of nasal CPAP as a tool for weaning small premature infants from mechanical ventilation.

#### Nasal Ventilation to Facilitate Weaning from Mechanical Ventilation

Lin and colleagues (1998) compared nasal intermittent positive pressure ventilation (IPPV) with conventional nasal CPAP in a group of 34 infants between 590 and 1880 g and found that nasal IPPV was more effective in reducing apnea. More recently, Kiciman and colleagues (1998) noted that nasal synchronized intermittent ventilation (SIMV) (see later) was more effective in reducing chest-abdomen asynchrony than was endotracheal CPAP or nasal CPAP delivered by an infant flow driver, suggesting that nasal SIMV was particularly useful in unloading the respiratory system of the preterm infant. Three subsequent clinical trials (Barrington et al, 2001; Friedlich et al, 1999; Khalaf et al, 2001) all showed that nasal SIMV was more effective than nasal CPAP in weaning infants from mechanical ventilation. The single study that reported gastrointestinal outcomes noted no increase in distention, feeding intolerance, or perforation (Barrington et al, 2001). These trials are interesting and suggest that nasal SIMV requires additional study as a weaning tool from mechanical ventilation. However, nasal CPAP delivered by the infant flow driver was also effective in reducing chest-abdomen asynchrony when compared with conventional nasal CPAP (Kiciman et al, 1998) but slightly less than nasal SIMV. Additional trials should compare nasal SIMV and nasal CPAP delivered by the infant flow driver.

## Patient-Triggered Ventilation

The use of patient-triggered ventilation (PTV) is now relatively common in the NICU to achieve a greater degree of synchrony between the infant's breathing and the ventilator. Asynchronous breathing may impair oxygenation, increase ventilator requirements, necessitate heavy sedation or paralysis, or, more important, may result in blood pressure and cerebral blood flow fluctuations (Rennie et al, 1987), which have been linked to IVH (Perlman and Thach, 1988; Perlman et al, 1983).

PTV is used in four modes:

1. In *synchronized intermittent mandatory ventilation* (SIMV), a single triggered breath is given in equal windows of time, with the other patient-initiated breaths in each window not assisted; this means that the rate of supported breaths can be slowly reduced, with all assisted breaths well synchronized.
2. In *assist/control mode* (A/CV), all breaths are triggered, so the patient controls the ventilator rate, and weaning is accomplished by reducing the PIP; during apnea, controlled breaths are delivered at the preset rate.
3. In *pressure support ventilation* (PSV), a constant pressure is applied during inspiration and terminated when a decrease in air flow is sensed.
4. In *proportional assist ventilation* (PAV), the applied airway pressure is servo-controlled throughout each spontaneous breath. Pressure increases in proportion to the instantaneous tidal volume and inspiratory air flow generated by the patient.

These ventilators detect inspiratory activity (Bernstein, 1993) by measuring one of the following:

- flow of gas through the endotracheal tube using a hot-wire anemometer (Hird and Greenough, 1991a) or a variable-orifice pneumotachometer
- changes in airway pressure (Greenough et al, 1991) measured near the orifice of the endotracheal tube

- changes in chest wall impedance (Visveshwara et al, 1991) using a cardiorespiratory monitor
- diaphragm movements using a balloon-like pressure capsule (Graseby capsule) taped to the abdomen (Mehta et al, 1986)

The delay of a triggered breath from the beginning of a spontaneous respiration is the response time (in milliseconds) and includes both the "trigger" and "system" delay. In general, response times are less than 100 msec. As the response time increases, less of the spontaneous inspiratory effort is supported, and the likelihood increases that positive pressure support will interfere with expiration. Triggering mechanisms that are too sensitive or that are prone to artifacts can result in autocycling (inappropriate triggering of the ventilator due to artifact), and those that are not sensitive enough will cause the ventilator to miss spontaneous breaths. Several studies have investigated the performance of various trigger mechanisms. Although the results are somewhat inconsistent between the different trials, it appears that triggers that rely on measurements of air flow, pressure change, and diaphragm movement are roughly comparable and are faster and more reliable than those based on changes in impedance of the thorax (Bernstein et al, 1993; Dimitriou et al, 2001; Hummler et al, 1996; John et al, 1994). Of interest, differences in processing of the signal by the ventilator may contribute to greater differences than choice of triggering mechanism (Bernstein et al, 1993; Sanders et al, 2001). Finally, one study suggested that in infants with severe lung disease, changes in air flow and pressure at the airway may be damped, and measurements of diaphragm movement with the Graseby capsule may be superior (John et al, 1994).

Early trials comparing PTV (SIMV or A/CV) with conventional ventilation (CV) suggested that PTV resulted in greater synchrony between the ventilator and patient, improved oxygenation, improved weaning from mechanical ventilation (Bernstein et al, 1994; Cleary et al, 1995; Mizuno et al, 1994; Visveshwara et al, 1991), and reduced fluctuations in blood pressure (Hummler et al, 1996). Greenough and colleagues (2001) recently reported a meta-analysis of six trials comparing PTV (SIMV or A/CV) with CV (Baumer, 2000; Beresford et al, 2000; Bernstein et al 1996; Chan and Greenough, 1993c; Chen et al, 1997; Donn et al, 1994). They found that infants receiving PTV had a shorter duration of ventilation (roughly 32 hours) than that in infants receiving CV. There were no differences in the incidence of extubation failure, air leak, chronic lung disease, or severe IVH between the two groups. In this review, the authors also performed a meta-analysis of two studies comparing SIMV with A/CV (Chan and Greenough, 1994a; Dimitriou et al, 1995) and found no statistically significant difference in duration of weaning or frequency of weaning failure, extubation failure, or air leaks between the two techniques.

Although PSV would help overcome the resistance of the endotracheal tube and could facilitate weaning from mechanical ventilation in premature infants, no neonatal trials have been reported. Two trials have reported the use of PAV to reduce respiratory load in low-birth-weight infants. In one trial, PAV was compared with A/CV and CV in premature infants with acute respiratory distress. Arterial oxygenation was similar in all three groups, but the infants on PAV had lower airway and transpulmonary pressures and a lower oxygen index (Schulze et al, 1999). In another trial comparing PAV with CPAP in infants recovering from respiratory distress, PAV resulted in less chest wall distortion and thoracoabdominal asynchrony (Musante et al, 2001). There have been no controlled trials of the use of PAV for prolonged periods of time during acute respiratory distress or during weaning from respiratory support.

A more recent approach to PTV allows the user to set the volume to be delivered by the ventilator. Tidal volume is measured using the same hot-wire anemometer (HWA) that the ventilator uses to trigger breaths. In this mode, a maximum pressure can be set, but if the preset volume is reached before the ventilator reaches the maximum pressure, the breath is terminated. Volume guarantee (VG) can be used with SIMV or AC/V. Short clinical trials carried out in infants with acute respiratory distress or recovering from respiratory distress have found that PTV with VG results in less breath-to-breath variability in tidal volume and similar gas exchange at lower airway pressures when compared with standard PTV (Abubakar and Keszler, 2001; Cheema and Ahluwalia, 2001; Herrera et al, 2002; Mrozek et al, 2000). One trial in infants with acute respiratory distress found that when compared with PSV, PSV with VG resulted in a higher minute ventilation and mean airway pressure (Olsen et al, 2002). There are no randomized controlled trials of PTV with VG that have examined the effects on outcomes such as air leak or chronic lung disease. In addition, there is some concern about measurements of tidal volume in premature infants in the presence of leaks around the endotracheal tube.

## High-Frequency Ventilation

Respiratory rates on the ventilator between 60 and 80 breaths/minute represent conventional ventilation; high-frequency ventilation (HFV) refers to respirator rates between 150 and 3000 breaths/minute. Three modes of HFV have been used in the newborn (Slutsky, 1988): high-frequency jet ventilation (HFJV), high-frequency oscillatory ventilation (HFOV), and high-frequency flow-interrupted ventilation (HFIV) (Clark, 1994).

In HFJV, the ventilator delivers a high-pressure puff of gas through a small-bore cannula usually positioned in the airway at the proximal end of the endotracheal tube. The actual volume of gas delivered cannot be known because the volume delivered by the jet may be augmented by gas from the auxiliary circuit that is dragged along with the high-pressure puff. Exhalation is passive.

In HFOV, the ventilator uses a piston or moving diaphragm to pump gas into and out of the lung, making both inspiration and expiration active. The oscillator uses small tidal volumes (usually less than VD) and relies on a bias flow of gas to flush $CO_2$ out of the system and to maintain a supply of fresh gas at the proximal end of the endotracheal tube.

In HFIV, the ventilator uses a circuit similar to that of a conventional ventilator. Gas flow through the circuit is interrupted by a motorized rotating ball. Constant end-expiratory pressure is adjusted by a valve on the expiratory limb of the circuit. As for HFJV, exhalation is passive. A newer ventilator interrupts flow by a set of metered pneumatic valves. This ventilator also creates an active exhalation using a Venturi system and functions more like an HFOV ventilator than a classic flow interrupter.

## Mechanisms of Gas Exchange

The mechanism responsible for oxygenation with HFV is the same as for CV—it depends on increasing the $PAO_2$ in the poorly ventilated part of the lung (Froese and Bryan, 1987; Slutsky, 1988). As with CV, HFV accomplishes this by increasing MAP. Whether or not HFV results in comparable levels of oxygenation with lower MAPs is still controversial.

The difference between HFV and CV lies in the methods of removing $CO_2$. HFV seemingly defies conventional pulmonary physiology by removing $CO_2$ by rapid ventilation of the lung with tidal volumes less than the anatomic dead space. With HFV, removal of $CO_2$ may be accomplished by five mechanisms:

1. Some alveoli are located near enough to central airways that bulk convection of gas can play a role in $CO_2$ exchange.
2. Similar to CV, HFV relies on molecular diffusion for gas exchange within the terminal lung units.
3. At the high frequencies employed with HFV, gas exchange between lung units with uneven time constants (pendelluft) can set up circulating currents that enhance gas mixing in the lung and $CO_2$ exchange.
4. The velocity profile of gas in the airways is asymmetrical (i.e., in the center of the parabolic gas stream, forward transport is slightly greater than backward transport of gas, and at the edge of the stream, backward transport is greater than forward). At high frequencies, this results in a net forward flow of fresh gas down the center of the airway and a net backward flow of alveolar-airway gas up the airway.
5. At high frequencies, a form of facilitated diffusion occurs secondary to enhanced dispersion of both turbulent and laminar streams of gas flow (Taylor dispersion).

During HFV, these mechanisms combine so that the rate of $CO_2$ elimination is proportional to the respiratory frequency multiplied by the square of the tidal volume.

## Potential Problems

One of the major problems associated with HFV is related to humidification of inspired gas. This is a particular problem with HFJV, in which inadequate humidification combined with the high-pressure pulses of gas has resulted in cases of necrotizing tracheitis (Gomez and Hansen, 1999). It is much less of a problem with HFIV and HFOV, in which the bias flow can be adequately humidified. The other concern with the use of HFV is that of gas trapping. At high frequencies, expiration may be shortened to the point at which expiratory time is less than 3 time constants, and gas trapping may occur. This may be a particular problem when the inspiratory time–to–expiratory time ratio is increased from 1:2 to 1:1 (Gerstmann et al, 1990).

## Clinical Experience

### *High-Frequency Jet Ventilation*

Early studies in infants with hyaline membrane disease showed that HFJV could provide adequate oxygenation with low MAP and PIP over limited period of times (Carlo et al, 1984; Pagani et al, 1985). Three randomized controlled trials have compared HFJV with CV in premature infants with respiratory distress (Carlo et al, 1990; Keszler et al, 1997; Wiswell et al, 1996). Two of these studies (Carlo et al, 1990; Wiswell et al, 1996) used lower mean airway pressures (*low-volume strategy*) when switching from CV to HFJV, whereas the third (Keszler et al, 1997) used higher mean airway pressures (*high-volume strategy*). Surfactant was administered to infants in the two most recent trials (Keszler et al, 1997; Wiswell et al, 1996). There were no differences in mortality, pulmonary air leak, or IVH between the HFJV and CV groups in any of the studies. The study using the high-volume strategy (Keszler et al, 1997) noted a reduction in the incidence of chronic lung disease at 36 weeks of postmenstrual age in the HFJV group, as well as a reduction in the requirement for home oxygen. The other trials found no effect on chronic lung disease. The other more recent trial (Wiswell et al, 1996) found that the infants ventilated with HFJV were more likely to develop cystic PVL. Because a number of infants in the high-volume-strategy study (Keszler et al, 1997) was in fact ventilated using a low-volume strategy, the investigators were able to compare the two strategies within their trial. They noted that the incidence of PVL was increased only in those infants receiving HFJV with a low-volume strategy. A recent meta-analysis of these trials (Bhuta and Henderson-Smart, 2000) confirmed that HFJV was associated with a reduction in chronic lung disease in survivors at 36 weeks of postmenstrual age but cautioned against routine use of HFJV for premature infants with respiratory distress until issues regarding ideal strategies are resolved.

Descriptive reports suggest that HFJV may be useful in the management of newborn infants with severe respiratory failure who are on maximal ventilatory support and are being considered for treatment with extracorporeal membrane oxygenation (Baumgart et al, 1992; Davis et al, 1992) (see also Chapter 48). Trials in infants with persistent pulmonary hypertension of the neonate (PPHN) have shown that HFJV improves ventilation (Carlo et al, 1989) and oxygenation (Engle et al, 1997) at lower ventilatory pressures but has no effect on ultimate outcome. One study comparing HFJV with CV in an experimental model of meconium aspiration pneumonia found HFJV to be superior (Trindade et al, 1985), whereas another found CV to be superior (Mammel et al, 1983). (See Chapter 48, Respiratory Failure in the Term Infant.)

### *High-Frequency Flow-Interrupted Ventilation*

HFIV was used in a controlled trial in preterm infants with RDS; the results were not different from those with conventional mechanical ventilation (Pardou et al, 1993). In one nonrandomized trial, HFIV improved oxygenation in infants with PPHN without hypocarbia or alkalosis and appeared to reduce the duration of mechanical ventilation and the incidence of chronic lung disease (Jirapaet et al, 2001).

### *High-Frequency Oscillatory Ventilation for the Initial Management of Respiratory Distress Syndrome*

Nine randomized controlled trials compared HFOV with CV for primary management of premature infants with RDS (Clark et al, 1992; Gerstmann et al, 1996; HIFI Study Group, 1989; Johnson et al, 2002; Moriette et al, 2001; Ogawa et al, 1993; Plavka et al, 1999; Rettwitz-Volk et al, 1998; Thome et al, 1999). A recent review and meta-analysis have summarized the findings of the first eight of these trials (Henderson-Smart et al, 2001).

**Mortality.** There was no difference in mortality at 28 to 30 days or at 36 to 37 weeks of postmenstrual age in any of the individual trials or in the overall meta-analysis.

**Chronic Lung Disease.** In the four trials (Moriette et al, 2001; Ogawa et al, 1993; Plavka et al 1999; Thome et al, 1999) reporting need for oxygen at 28 days, there was no difference between the HFOV and CV groups in any of the individual trials or in the overall analysis. In another subgroup analysis, four trials defined chronic lung disease as the use of oxygen or mechanical ventilation plus an abnormal chest radiograph at 28 to 30 days (Clark et al, 1992; Gerstmann et al, 1996; HIFI Study Group, 1989; Ogawa et al, 1993). Two of these trials (Clark et al, 1992; Gerstmann et al, 1996) showed that HFOV reduced the incidence of chronic lung disease but the difference was not significant when all four trials were analyzed. However, if the meta-analysis was confined to three trials using a high-volume strategy, the incidence of chronic lung disease decreased significantly (Clark et al, 1992; Gerstmann et al, 1996; Ogawa et al, 1993). Chronic lung disease at 36 to 37 weeks of postmenstrual age was reported in six trials (Clark et al, 1992; Gerstmann et al, 1996; Johnson et al, 2002; Moriette et al, 2001; Plavka et al 1999; Rettwitz-Volk et al, 1998; Thome et al, 1999) and was decreased significantly in the HFOV group. Of interest, five of these six studies used a high-volume strategy.

**Air Leak.** The risk of air leak was increased by HFOV in the trial by Thome and coworkers (1999) and was increased in the overall analysis of six trials by meta-analysis (Henderson-Smart et al, 2001).

**Intraventricular Hemorrhage.** There was no difference in the rate of IVH between the two groups in the individual trials or in the overall analysis. Severe IVH (grade 3 or 4) was increased in the HFOV group in two individual trials (HIFI Study Group, 1989; Moriette et al, 2001) and in the meta-analysis of all eight trials.

**Periventricular Leukomalacia.** There was no significant increase in PVL in the seven studies reporting this outcome (Gerstmann et al, 1996; HIFI Study Group, 1989; Moriette et al, 2001; Ogawa et al, 1993; Plavka et al, 1999; Rettwitz-Volk et al, 1998; Thome et al, 1999). In a subgroup analysis of the two studies not using a high volume strategy (HIFI Study Group, 1989; Rettwitz-Volk et al, 1998), the incidence of PVL was increased significantly.

**Neurodevelopmental Outcome.** Follow-up evaluation at 16 to 24 months of age revealed more neurologic deficits in the HFOV group (HIFI Study Group, 1990), probably related to the increased incidence of severe IVH in this group. In the study by Gerstmann and colleagues (2001), neurodevelopmental outcome at age 6 years was normal and not different between the two groups. Frequency of significant retinopathy of prematurity was actually reduced in the HFOV group in a meta-analysis of two trials using a high-volume strategy (Gerstmann et al, 1996; Thome et al, 1999).

**Clinical Considerations**

The concern about high-frequency ventilation and severe IVH and PVL was addressed in a meta-analysis (Clark et al, 1996) that included four trials using HFOV for initial treatment of premature infants with respiratory distress (Clark et al, 1992; Gerstmann et al, 1996; HIFI Study Group, 1989; Ogawa et al, 1993), one trial of rescue therapy (HIFO Study Group, 1993), three trials of HFJV for the treatment of respiratory distress (Carlo et al, 1987, 1990; Wiswell et al, 1996), and one trial using HFJV for treatment of premature infants with PIE (Keszler et al, 1991). The investigators found no difference in the incidence of severe IVH between the HFV group and the CV group. However, they did find an increase in the rate of PVL in the HFV group. This difference disappeared if the HIFI study was excluded.

Two trials in 2002 compared HFOV with CV. Johnson and colleagues (2002) studied 797 patients. They found no differences between the two groups in mortality, survival with chronic lung disease, air leak, IVH, PVL, or retinopathy of prematurity. Courtney and colleagues (2002) compared HFOV with SIMV in 500 premature infants with respiratory distress. They found that the incidence of chronic lung disease was reduced in the HFOV group, and infants in this group were extubated 1 week earlier. The risk of pulmonary air leak was increased in the HFOV group. There were no differences in mortality, IVH, or PVL between the two groups.

Although it is possible that the use of HFOV for the initial therapy of premature infants with respiratory distress may reduce the incidence of bronchopulmonary dysplasia, the same studies suggest that it may increase the risk of pulmonary air leak and PVL. In addition, outcomes appear to be *very* dependent on the ventilator strategy employed. Until theses issues are resolved, HFOV cannot be recommended as the routine method of providing mechanical ventilation to premature infants with respiratory distress. Should CV and surfactant therapy fail, however, HFOV is a reasonable form of rescue therapy.

The usual recommendation for HFOV in the management of severe respiratory failure is to start at an MAP 2 to 3 cm $H_2O$ above the MAP being used for CV, at a rate of 10 Hz, at an inspiratory-expiratory ratio (I:E) of 1:2, and at a pressure difference that moves the chest visibly. Chan and

Greenough (1993a) recommended a rate of 10 Hz and an MAP of 5 cm $H_2O$ above the MAP used for CV. In general, oxygenation is controlled with MAP, and ventilation is controlled with amplitude and rate. Few changes are made in the rate, but if hypercarbia dictates a larger VT at the same Δ pressure, this can be accomplished by a reduction of the rate to 9 or 8 Hz. The reduction in rate allows a larger volume to be transmitted. If PIE dictates a smaller VT at the same Δ pressure, this can be accomplished by an increase in the rate as high as 15 Hz. The MAP may be increased to 25 cm $H_2O$ or higher, but depression of the circulation becomes an important factor, and volume support may be needed. When oxygenation is improved, it is usual to begin weaning from oxygen first and favor the continued use of high MAP. When the MAP has been decreased to 9 to 12 cm $H_2O$, it is usual to change the patient back to CV at a level of MAP 2 to 3 cm $H_2O$ lower.

### High-Frequency Ventilation in the Management of Air Leak Problems

In uncontrolled trials, HFIV (Frantz et al, 1983; Gaylord et al, 1987) and HFJV (Boros et al, 1985; Pokora et al, 1983) both appear to provide some benefit in the management of low-birth-weight infants with pulmonary interstitial emphysema (PIE). Keszler and colleagues (1991) reported the results of a large multicenter controlled trial in the management of premature infants with PIE, comparing HFJV with CV at rapid rates; the success criteria were prospectively defined, and provision was made for crossover as necessary. Overall, 61% of infants who started on HFJV and only 31% of those who started on CV were successfully managed—a significantly improved result with HFJV. More patients starting on CV had to be crossed over to HFJV. When patients were crossed over to HFJV, the success rate was much higher (45%) than when patients were crossed over to CV (9%). Radiographic improvement was clearly more rapid with HFJV. After excluding crossover, the mortality rate among infants who started on HFJV was 35%, compared with 53% among those who started on conventional ventilation. In this study of PIE, a low-volume strategy was pursued, with encouragement of the lung to derecruit; such a strategy can be followed with other forms of HFV in the management of PIE.

## Liquid Ventilation

For the past 30 years or so, investigations have been pursuing the possibility of treating ventilatory failure with liquid rather than gaseous ventilation (Shaffer et al, 1984; Wolfson et al, 1996). The discovery of a class of compounds known as fluorocarbons has led to significant advances because they are chemically and physiologically inert. Perfluorocarbon (PFC), the compound being used in both animal experimentation and human clinical studies, has a greater solubility for respiratory gases than the solubility of blood. It also has some of the properties of surfactant, with a low surface tension. When instilled into the lung, this radiopaque compound gradually recruits alveoli without barotrauma and, because of its low vapor pressure, is rapidly eliminated by vaporization.

The first human trials of liquid ventilation were conducted in "near-death" infants in 1989. The lungs were filled with the PFC liquid, and tidal volumes of liquid were cycled into and out of the lung using a gravity-assisted approach. The infants tolerated the procedure, and gas exchange and lung compliance improved. All three infants died after discontinuation of liquid ventilation (Greenspan et al, 1997). In 1996, Leach and colleagues reported on 10 preterm infants who received partial liquid ventilation (PLV) for up to 24 to 76 hours. For PLV, the lungs are filled with PFC to functional residual capacity (20 mL/kg) while gas ventilation is continued. They also noted dramatic improvements in gas exchange and lung compliance. Eight of the 10 infants in their study survived to 36 weeks of corrected gestational age. Although these findings are encouraging and suggest that PLV may be a feasible treatment for some infants with respiratory failure, animal studies have not been encouraging, and clearly, randomized controlled trials must be performed before more widespread use of this technology can be recommended.

## Complications of Respiratory Support

### Air Block

The most serious complication of mechanical ventilation is air block. PIE, pneumomediastinum, subcutaneous emphysema, pneumothorax, pneumopericardium, pneumoperitoneum, and intravascular air all are manifestations of the air block syndrome, and all begin with some degree of PIE (Kirkpatrick et al, 1974; Macklin and Macklin, 1944).

#### *Pulmonary Interstitial Emphysema*

**Pathophysiology**

PIE is the result of alveolar rupture from overdistention of alveoli abutting nonalveolar structures and marginal alveoli (Caldwell et al, 1970; Hansen and Gest, 1984) (Figs. 45–9 and 45–10). It occurs most commonly in preterm or term infants undergoing mechanical ventilation for some form of parenchymal lung disease. In these infants, distribution of inspired gas is nonuniform, with the bulk of each breath being distributed to the more normal lung units. As a result, these lung units may become overdistended and rupture. Gas trapping from an insufficient expiratory time also can result in alveolar overdistention and rupture. Once alveolar rupture occurs, air is forced from the alveoli into the loose connective tissue sheaths surrounding airways and pulmonary arterioles and into the interlobular septa containing pulmonary veins. The air follows a track along these sheaths to the hilum of the lung, producing the characteristic radiographic appearance of PIE (Fig. 45–11).

PIE increases the volume of gas within the lung parenchyma and splints the lung in full inflation, thereby decreasing lung compliance. Air trapped within the interstitial cuffs compresses airways and increases airway resistance. In addition, air in the interstitial space impairs lymphatic function, allowing fluid to accumulate in the interstitial cuffs and in alveoli (Leonidas et al, 1979). $Pa\text{CO}_2$

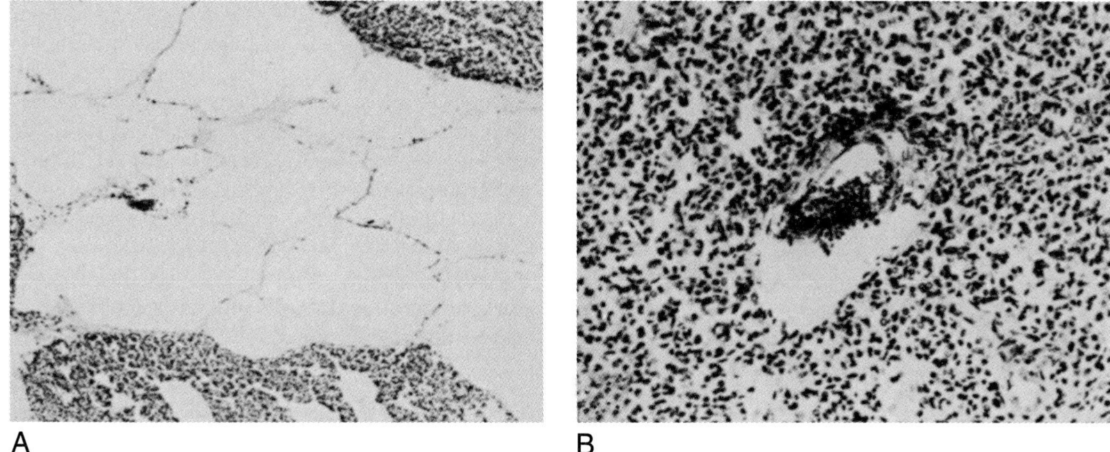


**FIGURE 45–9.** **A,** Photomicrograph of the lung of an infant who died of emphysema and bilateral pneumothorax. The alveoli in the center show much distention, their septa thinned. Some of the septa have ruptured. In the periphery, the lung is atelectatic. **B,** Higher-power view showing a blood vessel in cross section. The vessel is compressed by a surrounding collar of air that has filled and ballooned the perivascular space.

increases and $PaO_2$ decreases. The increase in $PaCO_2$ occurs early and is the result of increased respiratory dead space and reduced minute ventilation. The decrease in $PaO_2$ results in part from reduction in alveolar ventilation and in part from ventilation-perfusion mismatch secondary to mechanical obstruction of airways by interstitial air and edema fluid. It also results from compression of pulmonary arterioles by air in the perivascular cuffs with increased pulmonary vascular resistance (Brazy and Blackmon, 1977) and right-to-left shunting of blood.

Once interstitial air reaches the hilum of the lung, it coalesces to form large hilar blebs, or it tracks beneath the visceral pleura to form large subpleural pockets of air. In both instances, these accumulations of air can be large enough to compress normal lung and impair ventilation, or to cause circulatory embarrassment by encroaching on mediastinal structures (Plenat et al, 1978).

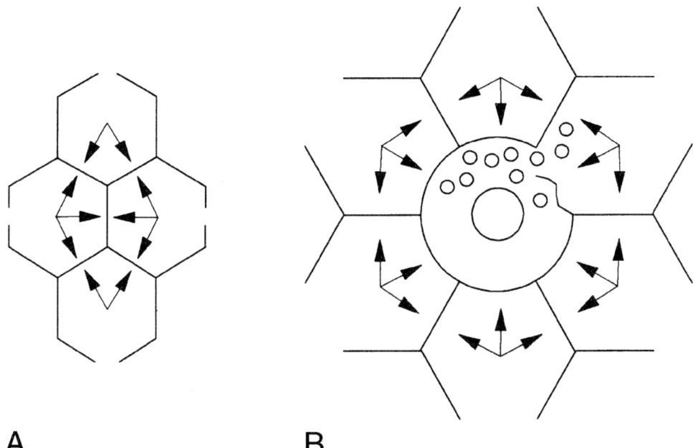


**FIGURE 45–10.** Mechanism of alveolar rupture. Partitional alveoli (**A**) have their bases lying against other alveoli, whereas marginal alveoli (**B**) abut bronchi, blood vessels, or pleura. During lung inflation, these two different types of alveoli behave quite differently. Partitional alveoli are free to expand equally in all directions, as they abut the equally distensible walls of adjacent alveoli. In addition, the pressure within each alveolus is balanced by an equal pressure inside surrounding alveoli, so no unbalanced forces occur across the alveolar wall. Marginal alveoli, especially those surrounding blood vessels, are tethered at the base to a less distensible structure and are not as free to expand in all directions. During lung inflation, the connective tissue sheaths surrounding pulmonary blood vessels attempt to expand with the alveoli, while the vessels themselves increase in size only slightly. As a result, unbalanced forces develop across the wall at the base of the alveolus, and air ruptures into the adjacent connective tissue sheath.

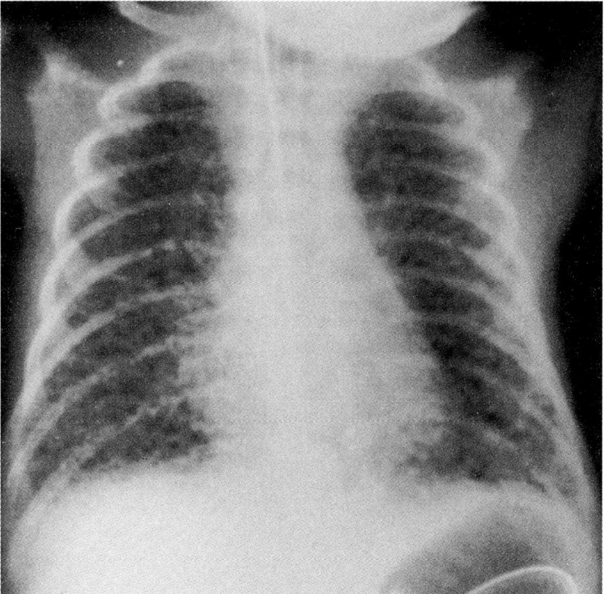

**FIGURE 45–11.** Pulmonary interstitial emphysema. The lung is grossly hyperinflated, with coarse radiolucencies extending from the pleura to the hilum. These radiolucencies represent bubbles of air in the perivascular and peribronchial interstitial cuffs.

### Prevention

The cause of PIE is alveolar overdistention and rupture. Therefore, ventilatory techniques that minimize alveolar overdistention would be expected to reduce the risk of PIE. Previous data have shown that increases in inspiratory time are associated with pulmonary air leaks (Primhak, 1983), and two controlled trials done prior to routine surfactant replacement showed that techniques for ventilation that rely on shorter inspiratory times decrease the incidence of PIE (Heicher et al, 1981; Oxford Region Controlled Trial, 1991).

### Treatment

Because the site of the air leak behaves like a check valve, gas trapping occurs, resulting in further alveolar overdistention and rupture. Therefore, the first step in treatment must be to interrupt this cycle by putting to rest the more severely involved areas in the lung. If PIE is unilateral, this can be done by positioning the infant with the involved side down (Swingle et al, 1984) or by selectively intubating the main bronchus on the uninvolved side (Brooks et al, 1977). If PIE is bilateral, the involved areas can be put to rest by taking advantage of regional differences in time constants in the lung. Areas with PIE have airway compression and long time constants for inspiration and expiration. Mechanical ventilation using short inspiratory times (0.1 second), low inflation pressures, and small tidal volumes is ineffective in inflating these areas of the lung and should not contribute to further gas trapping (Meadow and Cheromcha, 1985). Over time, these areas deflate and collapse. Unfortunately, it may be difficult to maintain oxygenation and ventilation while selectively underventilating the areas of the lung with PIE. If this happens, it may be necessary to increase the respirator rate to 80 to 100 breaths/minute. The advantage of rapid-rate ventilation is that it makes maximal use of the less severely involved lung units and may compensate for the respiratory deterioration associated with selective underventilation of areas with extensive PIE. A multicenter controlled trial in 1991 (Keszler et al, 1991) found that HFJV allowed the use of lower peak and mean airway pressures in the treatment of infants with PIE than did rapid-rate CV. Furthermore, HFJV led to more frequent and rapid improvement in PIE than did rapid-rate CV (see earlier section, "High-Frequency Ventilation").

### Prognosis

PIE is a serious complication of mechanical ventilation. Infants in whom PIE develops have a significantly increased risk of developing chronic lung disease, as well as higher mortality rates (Gaylord et al, 1985; Powers and Clemens, 1993). In fact, for infants in whom PIE develops on day 0 or 1 after birth, the gestational age–adjusted odds ratio for risk of dying is nearly 10 to 1 and for developing chronic lung disease is 3 to 1 (Powers and Clemens, 1993).

## *Pneumomediastinum and Pneumothorax*

### Epidemiology

The incidence of spontaneous pneumomediastinum and pneumothorax in term infants is 1% to 2%, presumably because high transpulmonary pressures exerted at birth, when coupled with some degree of ventilation inhomogeneity, result in alveolar overdistention and rupture (Chernick and Avery, 1963; Lubchenco, 1959). In the presence of underlying lung disease, the incidence of pneumothorax increases dramatically. Pneumothorax develops in 10% of infants with retained fetal lung fluid and in 5% to 10% of spontaneously breathing infants with hyaline membrane disease. CPAP increases the incidence of pneumothorax in infants with hyaline membrane disease only slightly, whereas positive pressure ventilation increases the risk dramatically. Treatment with surfactant, however, markedly lowers this risk.

### Natural History

Pneumomediastinum occurs when air that has tracked through the perivascular and peribronchial cuffs to the hilum ruptures into the mediastinum. From there, air can rupture through the mediastinum into the pleural space, producing tension pneumothorax. Available evidence suggests that air in the mediastinum seldom achieves enough tension to cause circulatory embarrassment, because as the tension increases, air can dissect into the soft tissues of the neck to produce subcutaneous emphysema or rupture into the intrapleural space. On the other hand, tension pneumothorax can result in very high pressures within the pleural space, collapsing the lung on the involved side and resulting in immediate hypoxia and hypercapnia. In addition, by compressing mediastinal structures and impeding venous return, pneumothorax may result in circulatory collapse.

### Diagnosis

Pneumomediastinum usually is asymptomatic or associated with mild tachypnea. In the spontaneously breathing infant, however, pneumothorax usually results in clinically significant tachypnea, grunting, irritability, pallor, and cyanosis. The cardiac point of maximum impulse may be shifted away from the pneumothorax, and often the affected hemithorax appears to bulge. Differential breath sounds are unreliable markers of pneumothorax in the infant. Arterial pressure tracings may reveal a reduction in pulse pressure. In the infant on a mechanical ventilator, signs may be more dramatic, with sudden onset of hypoxemia and cardiovascular collapse (Ogata et al, 1976). Transillumination of the chest is increased over the affected side. Pneumothorax should be confirmed by chest radiograph (Fig. 45–12), if at all possible. Needle aspiration of the chest to diagnose pneumothorax relieves acute distress but should be discouraged. If needle aspiration is necessary, it should ordinarily be followed by tube thoracostomy.

### Treatment

Asymptomatic or mildly symptomatic spontaneously breathing infants may simply be observed closely until spontaneous resolution occurs. Although having infants breathe 100% oxygen hastens reabsorption of intrapleural air (Chernick and Avery, 1963), the risk associated with prolonged hyperoxia limits usefulness of this therapy in preterm infants. Infants with moderate to severe symptoms and all infants receiving positive pressure ventilation

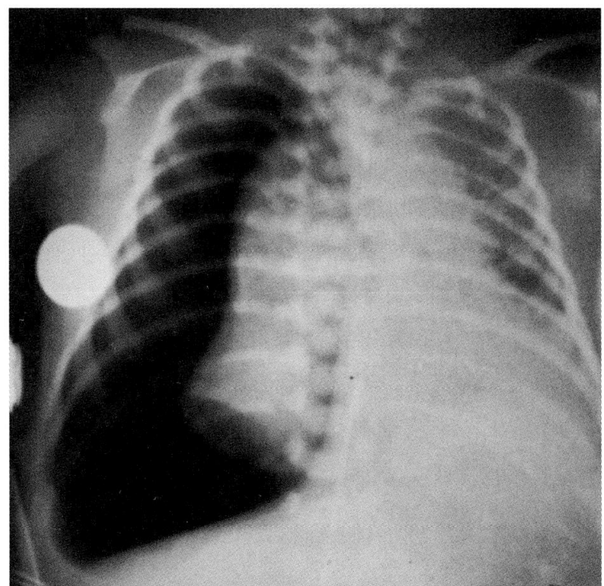

**FIGURE 45–12.** Tension pneumothorax. The lung on the involved side is collapsed, and the mediastinum is shifted to the opposite side. Pleura can be seen bulging into the intercostal spaces.

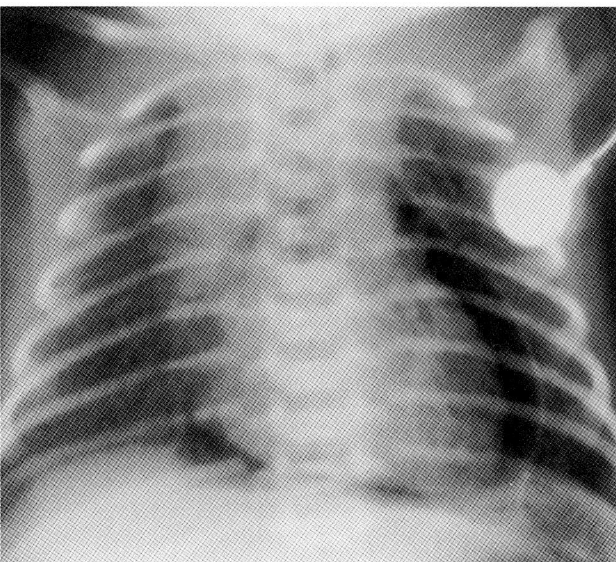

**FIGURE 45–13.** Pneumopericardium. A thin rim of pericardium is visible and clearly separated from the heart by air within the pericardial sac.

require tube thoracostomy. The tube may be inserted at the midaxillary line and directed anteriorly or placed in the second intercostal space in the midclavicular line and directed toward the diaphragm so that the tip lies between the lung and the anterior chest wall (Allen et al, 1981). When placing the tube, the operator must take care to avoid impaling the lung, especially if a trocar, rather than curved hemostats, is used to direct the tube. Care also must be taken to avoid placing the tube too far into the chest, compressing mediastinal structures (Gooding et al, 1981). It also is possible to drain pneumothoraces using pigtail catheters that are placed percutaneously into the pleural space. This technique involves less trauma but may not be effective in addressing large air leaks (Wood and Dubik, 1995). The thoracostomy tube or catheter usually is connected to a water seal with 10 to 20 cm $H_2O$ negative pressure and is left in place until it ceases to drain. The negative pressure should be discontinued, and the tube should be left under the water seal for 12 to 24 hours before removal. Infant chest tubes should never be clamped.

### *Pneumopericardium*

Pneumopericardium results from direct tracking of interstitial air along the great vessels into the pericardial sac (Varano and Maisels, 1974). Gas under tension in the pericardium impairs atrial and ventricular filling, decreases stroke volume, and ultimately decreases cardiac output and systemic blood pressure. Infants present with increasing cyanosis, muffled heart sounds, and decreased systemic blood pressure. The chest radiograph is diagnostic (Fig. 45–13). Needle aspiration alleviates the acute symptoms, but because recurrence rate is high (53%), continuous tube drainage is frequently necessary (Reppert et al, 1977). The mortality rate associated with pneumopericardium has been reported to be as high as 75%.

### *Pneumoperitoneum*

Pneumoperitoneum results from dissection of air from the mediastinum along the sheaths of the aorta and vena cava, with subsequent rupture into the peritoneal cavity. Infants with this condition present with abdominal distention of sudden onset and a typical abdominal radiograph. Occasionally, the pneumoperitoneum may be large enough to cause respiratory embarrassment by compromising descent of the diaphragm and may require drainage. A more common problem, however, is the difficulty in distinguishing this cause of peritoneal air from a primary gastrointestinal catastrophe, such as a perforated ulcer or necrotizing enterocolitis (Knight and Abdenour, 1981). Obtaining more than 0.5 mL of green or brown fluid on paracentesis is suggestive of primary bowel disease, especially if bacteria are present on Gram stain. Measurement of the $P_{O_2}$ of the gas aspirated from the abdomen also may be of some help, because it is likely to be very high if the gas is of pulmonary origin. Finally, a careful upper gastrointestinal series performed with water-soluble contrast may be of use in distinguishing the cause of intraperitoneal air (Cohen et al, 1982).

### *Intravascular Air*

The classic belief was that intravascular air resulted from pumping air directly into the pulmonary venous system when airway pressure was extremely high (70 cm $H_2O$). More recently, studies have found that the air is more commonly found in the systemic venous circulation, and it has been suggested that the air actually is pumped under high pressure through the pulmonary lymphatics into the systemic venous circulation (Booth et al, 1995). This theory is compatible with the observation of interstitial air in the loose connective tissue cuffs containing the pulmonary lymphatics. Intravascular air results in immediate cardiovascular collapse and is often diagnosed when air is seen in vessels on chest radiographs taken to determine the cause of cardiovascular collapse. Although intravascular air usually is fatal, placing the infant head down on the left side may favor displacement of cerebral emboli.

## Airway Complications

Prolonged orotracheal intubation may cause palatal grooving, potentially interfering with dentition (Duke et al, 1976; Moylan et al, 1980), whereas nasotracheal intubation may result in cosmetic deformities of the nose (Jung and Thomas, 1974) and even nasal obstruction. Subglottic stenosis, although rare, can be a disastrous complication of intubation. A too snug-fitting endotracheal tube, prolonged duration of intubation, and multiple reintubations all correlate with subsequent subglottic stenosis (Fan et al, 1983; Sherman et al, 1986). Some infants have required tracheostomy.

Necrotizing tracheobronchitis (Pietsch et al, 1985) is a necrotic inflammatory process involving the trachea and main bronchi that has been described in newborns requiring mechanical ventilation. Sloughing of the tracheal epithelium results in occlusion of the distal trachea. Infants present with acute respiratory deterioration with symptoms of airway obstruction, hyperexpansion on chest radiograph, and poor chest movement. Emergency bronchoscopy may be necessary to relieve airway obstruction. The lesion is thought to result from drying of the tracheal mucosa secondary to inadequate humidification in the presence of high rates of gas flow and high concentrations of oxygen.

Atelectasis occasionally occurs after extubation from mechanical ventilation, with the right upper lobe most commonly affected. In some instances, atelectasis may reflect injury to the bronchi from suction catheters. In small preterm infants, postextubation atelectasis may result from chest wall instability and may be prevented by weaning to nasal CPAP.

## REFERENCES


Abubakar KM, Keszler M: Patient-ventilator interactions in new modes of patient-triggered ventilation. Pediatr Pulmonol 32:71, 2001.

Adams JM, Murfin K, Mort J, et al: Detection of hyperoxemia in neonates by a new pulse oximeter. Neonat Intensive Care 7:42, 1994.

Ahluwalia JS, White DK, Morley CJ: Infant flow driver or single prong nasal continuous positive airway pressure: Short-term physiological effects. Acta Paediatr 87:325, 1998.

Allen LP, Reynolds EOR, Rivers RPA, et al: Controlled trial of continuous positive airway pressure given by face mask for hyaline membrane disease. Arch Dis Child 52:373, 1977.

Allen RW, Jung AL, Lester PD: Effectiveness of chest tube evacuation of pneumothorax in neonates. J Pediatr 99:629, 1981.

Annibale DJ, Hulsey TC, Engstrom PC, et al: Randomized, controlled trial of nasopharyngeal continuous positive airway pressure in the extubation of very low birth weight infants J Pediatr 124:455, 1994.

Avery ME, Tooley WH, Keller JB, et al: Is chronic lung disease in low birth weight infants preventable? A survey of eight centers. Pediatrics 79:26, 1987.

Bancalari E, Garcia OL, Jesse MJ: Effects of continuous negative pressure on lung mechanics in idiopathic respiratory distress syndrome. Pediatrics 51:485, 1973.

Bancalari E, Sinclair, JC: Mechanical ventilation. In Sinclair, JC and Bracken, MB (eds): Effective Care of the Newborn Infant. New York, Oxford University Press, 1992, p 200.

Barker SJ, Tremper KK, Hyatt J: Effects of methemoglobinemia on pulse oximetry and mixed venous oximetry. Anesthesiology 70:112, 1989.

Barker SJ, Tremper KK: The effect of carbon monoxide inhalation on pulse oximetry and transcutaneous $Po_2$. Anesthesiology 66:677, 1987.

Barrington KJ, Bull D, Finer NN: Randomized trial of nasal synchronized intermittent mandatory ventilation compared with continuous positive airway pressure after extubation of very low birth weight infants. Pediatrics 107:638, 2001.

Baumer JH: International randomised controlled trial of patient triggered ventilation in neonatal respiratory distress syndrome. Arch Dis Child Fetal Neonatal Ed 82:F5, 2000.

Baumgart S, Hirschl RB, Butler SZ, et al: Diagnosis-related criteria in the consideration of extracorporeal membrane oxygenation in neonates previously treated with high-frequency jet ventilation. Pediatrics 89:491, 1992.

Belenky DA, Orr RJ, Woodrum DE, et al: Is continuous transpulmonary pressure better than conventional respiratory management of hyaline membrane disease? A controlled study. Pediatrics 58:800, 1976.

Beresford MW, Shaw NJ, Manning D: Randomised controlled trial of patient triggered and conventional fast rate ventilation in neonatal respiratory distress syndrome. Arch Dis Child Fetal Neonatal Ed 82:F14, 2000.

Bernstein G, Cleary JP, Heldt GP, et al: Response time and reliability of three neonatal patient-triggered ventilators. Am Rev Respir Dis 148:358, 1993.

Bernstein G, Heldt GP, Mannino FL: Increased and more consistent tidal volumes during synchronized intermittent mandatory ventilation in newborn infants. Am J Respir Crit Care Med 150:1444, 1994.

Bernstein G, Mannino FL, Heldt GP, et al: Randomized multicenter trial comparing synchronized and conventional intermittent mandatory ventilation in neonates. J Pediatr 128:453, 1996.

Bhuta T, Henderson-Smart DJ: Elective high frequency jet ventilation versus conventional ventilation for respiratory distress syndrome in preterm infants. Cochrane Database Syst Rev CD000328, 2000.

Bhutani VK, Abbasi S, Sivieri EM: Continuous skeletal muscle paralysis: Effect on neonatal pulmonary mechanics. Pediatrics 81:419, 1988.

Booth TN, Allen BA, Royal SA: Lymphatic air embolism: A new hypothesis regarding the pathogenesis of neonatal systemic air embolism. Pediatr Radiol 25(Suppl 1):S220, 1995.

Boros SJ, Mammel MD, Coleman JM: Neonatal high-frequency jet ventilation: Four years' experience. Pediatrics 75:657, 1985.

Brazy JE, Blackmon LR: Hypotension and bradycardia associated with airblock in the neonate. J Pediatr 90:796, 1977.

Brooks JG, Bustamante SA, Koops BL, et al; Selective bronchial intubation for the treatment of severe localized pulmonary interstitial emphysema in newborn infants Pediatrics 91:648, 1977.

Brunstler I, Enders A, Versmold HT: Skin surface $Pco_2$ monitoring in newborn infants in shock: Effect of hypotension and electrode temperature. J Pediatr 100:454, 1982.

Caldwell EJ, Powell RD, Mullooly JP: Interstitial emphysema: A study of physiologic factors involved in experimental induction of the lesion. Am Rev Respir Dis 102:516, 1970.

Caplan MS, Cohn RA, Langman CB, et al: Favorable outcome of neonatal aortic thrombosis and renovascular hypertension. Pediatrics 115:291, 1989.

Carlo WA, Beoglos A, Chatburn RL, et al: High-frequency jet ventilation in neonatal pulmonary hypertension. Am J Dis Child 143:233, 1989.

Carlo WA, Chatburn RL, Martin RJ, et al: Decrease in airway pressure during high frequency jet ventilation in infants with respiratory distress syndrome. J Pediatr 104:11, 1984.

Carlo WA, Chatburn RL, Martin RJ; Randomized trial of high-frequency jet ventilation versus conventional ventilation in respiratory distress syndrome. J Pediatr 110:275, 1987.

Carlo WA, Siner B, Chatburn RL, et al: Early randomized intervention with high-frequency jet ventilation in respiratory distress syndrome. J Pediatr 117:765, 1990.

Carlo WA, Stark AR, Wright LL, et al: Minimal ventilation to prevent bronchopulmonary dysplasia in extremely-low-birth-weight infants. J Pediatr 141:370, 2002.

Carlton DP, Cummings JJ, Scheerer RG, et al: Lung overexpansion increases pulmonary microvascular protein permeability in young lambs. J Appl Physiol 69:577, 1990.

Chan V, Greenough A: Comparison of weaning by patient triggered ventilation or synchronous intermittent mandatory ventilation in preterm infants. Acta Paediatr 83:335, 1994a.

Chan V, Greenough A: Determinants of oxygenation during high frequency oscillation. Eur J Pediatr 152:350, 1993a.

Chan V, Greenough A: Randomised controlled trial of weaning by patient triggered ventilation or conventional ventilation. Eur J Pediatr 152:51, 1993b.

Chan V, Greenough A: Randomised trial of methods of extubation in acute and chronic respiratory distress. Arch Dis Child 68:570, 1993c.

Chatburn RL: Physiologic and methodologic issues regarding humidity therapy. J Pediatr 114:416, 1989.

Cheema IU, Ahluwalia JS: Feasibility of tidal volume-guided ventilation in newborn infants: A randomized, crossover trial using the volume guarantee modality. Pediatrics 107:1323, 2001.

Chen JY, Ling UP, Chen JH: Comparison of synchronized and conventional intermittent mandatory ventilation in neonates. Acta Paediatr Jpn 39:578, 1997.

Chernick V, Avery ME: Spontaneous alveolar rupture at birth. Pediatrics 32:816, 1963.

Clark RH: High frequency ventilation. J Pediatr 124:661, 1994.

Clark RH, Dykes FD, Bachman TE, et al: Intraventricular hemorrhage and high-frequency ventilation: A meta-analysis of prospective clinical trials. Pediatrics 98:1058, 1996.

Clark RH, Gerstmann DR, Null DM, et al: Prospective randomized comparison of high-frequency oscillatory and conventional ventilation in respiratory distress syndrome. Pediatr 89:5, 1992.

Cleary JP, Bernstein G, Mannino FL, et al: Improved oxygenation during synchronized intermittent mandatory ventilation in neonates with respiratory distress syndrome: A randomized, crossover study. J Pediatr 126:407, 1995.

Cochran WD: Umbilical artery catheterization. In Moore TD (ed): Iatrogenic Problems in Neonatal Intensive Care. Proceedings of the 69th Ross Conference on Pediatric Research. Columbus, Ohio, Ross Laboratories, 1976, p 28.

Cohen MD, Schreiner R, Lemons J: Neonatal pneumoperitoneum without significant adventitious pulmonary air: Use of metrizamide to rule out perforation of the bowel. Pediatrics 69:587, 1982.

Collins MP, Lorenz JM, Jetton JR, et al: Hypocapnia and other ventilation-related risk factors for cerebral palsy in low birth weight infants. Pediatr Res 50:712, 2001.

Corbet A, Adams J: Current therapy in hyaline membrane disease. Clin Perinatol 5:299, 1978.

Corbet AJS, Ross JA, Beaudry PH, et al: Effect of positive pressure breathing on aA.$DN_2$ in hyaline membrane disease. J Appl Physiol 38:33, 1975.

Courtney SE, Durand DJ, Asselin JM, et al: High-frequency oscillatory ventilation versus conventional mechanical ventilation for very-low-birth-weight infants. N Engl J Med 347:643, 2002.

Courtney SE, Pyon KH, Saslow JG, et al: Lung recruitment and breathing pattern during variable versus continuous flow nasal continuous positive airway pressure in premature infants: An evaluation of three devices. Pediatrics 107:304, 2001.

Davis JM, Richter SE, Kendig JW, et al: High-frequency jet ventilation and surfactant treatment of newborns with severe respiratory failure. Pediatr Pulmonol 13:108, 1992.

Davis P, Davies M, Faber B: A randomised controlled trial of two methods of delivering nasal continuous positive airway pressure after extubation to infants weighing less than 1000 g: Binasal (Hudson) versus single nasal prongs. Arch Dis Child Fetal Neonatal Ed 85:F82, 2001.

Davis P, Henderson-Smart D: Post-extubation prophylactic nasal continuous positive airway pressure in preterm infants: Systematic review and meta-analysis. J Paediatr Child Health 35:367, 1999.

Davis P, Jankov R, Doyle L, Henschke P: Randomised, controlled trial of nasal continuous positive airway pressure in the extubation of infants weighing 600 to 1250 g. Arch Dis Child Fetal Neonatal Ed 79:F54, 1998.

De Klerk AM, De Klerk RK: Nasal continuous positive airway pressure and outcomes of preterm infants. J Paediatr Child Health 37:161, 2001.

Dimitriou G, Greenough A, Cherian S: Comparison of airway pressure and airflow triggering systems using a single type of neonatal ventilator. Acta Paediatr 90:445, 2001.

Dimitriou G, Greenough A, Griffin F, et al: Synchronous intermittent mandatory ventilation modes compared with patient triggered ventilation during weaning. Arch Dis Child Fetal Neonatal Ed 72:F188, 1995.

Dimitriou G, Greenough A, Kavvadia V, et al: Elective use of nasal continuous positive airways pressure following extubation of preterm infants. Eur J Pediatr 159:434, 2000.

Donn SM, Nicks JJ, Becker MA: Flow synchronized ventilation of preterm infants with respiratory distress syndrome. J Perinatol 14:90, 1994.

Drew, JH: Immediate intubation at birth of the very low birth-weight infant. Am J Dis Child 136:207, 1982.

Duke PM, Coulson JD, Santos JI, et al: Cleft palate associated with prolonged orotracheal intubation in infancy. J Pediatr 89:990, 1976.

Durbin GM, Hunter NJ, McIntosh N, et al: Controlled trial of continuous inflating pressure for hyaline membrane disease. Arch Dis Child 51:163, 1976.

Engelke SC, Roloff DW, Kuhns LR: Postextubation nasal continuous positive airway pressure. A prospective controlled study. Am J Dis Child 136:359, 1982.

Engle WA, Yoder MC, Andreoli SP, et al: Controlled prospective randomized comparison of high-frequency jet ventilation and conventional ventilation in neonates with respiratory failure and persistent pulmonary hypertension. J Perinatol 17:3, 1997.

Fan LL, Flynn JW, Pathak DR: Risk factors predicting laryngeal injury in intubated neonates. Crit Care Med 11:431, 1983.

Fanaroff AA, Cha CC, Sosa R, et al: Controlled trial of continuous negative external pressure in the treatment of severe respiratory distress syndrome. J Pediatr 82:921, 1973.

Frantz ID, Werthammer J, Stark AR: High frequency ventilation in premature infants with lung disease: Adequate gas exchange at low tracheal pressure. Pediatrics 71:483, 1983.

Friedlich P, Lecart C, Posen R, et al: A randomized trial of nasopharyngeal-synchronized intermittent mandatory ventilation versus nasopharyngeal continuous positive airway pressure in very low birth weight infants after extubation. J Perinatol 19:413, 1999.

Froese AB, Bryan AD: High-frequency ventilation. Am Rev Respir Dis 135:1363, 1987.

Garland JS, Buck RK, Allred EN, et al: Hypocarbia before surfactant therapy appears to increase bronchopulmonary dysplasia risk in infants with respiratory distress syndrome. Arch Pediatr Adolesc Med 149:617, 1995.

Gaylord MS, Quissell B, Lair ME: High-frequency ventilation in the treatment of infants weighing less than 1,500 grams with pulmonary interstitial emphysema: A pilot study. Pediatrics 79:915, 1987.

Gaylord MS, Thieme RE, Woodall DL, et al: Predicting mortality in low-birth-weight infants with pulmonary interstitial emphysema. Pediatrics 76:219, 1985.

Gerard P, Fox WW, Outerbridge EW, Beaudry PH: Early versus late introduction of continuous negative pressure in the management of the idiopathic respiratory distress syndrome. J Pediatr 87:591, 1975.

Gerstmann DR, Fouke JM, Winter DC, et al: Proximal, tracheal, and alveolar pressures during high-frequency oscillatory ventilation in a normal rabbit model. Pediatr Res 28:367, 1990.

Gertsmann DR, Minton SD, Stoddard RA, et al. The Provo Multicenter Early High-Frequency Oscillatory Ventilation Trial: Improved pulmonary and clinical outcome in respiratory distress syndrome. Pediatrics 98:1044, 1996.

Gerstmann DR, Wood K, Miller A, et al: Childhood outcome after early high-frequency oscillatory ventilation for neonatal respiratory distress syndrome. Pediatrics 108:617, 2001.

Gittermann MK, Fusch C, Gittermann AR, et al: Early nasal continuous positive airway pressure treatment reduces the need for intubation in very low birth weight infants. Eur J Pediatr 156:384, 1997.

Goldstein RF, Brazy JE: Narcotic sedation stabilizes arterial blood pressure fluctuations in sick premature infants. J Perinatol 11:365, 1991.

Gomez MR, Hansen TN: Impact of respiratory care practices on the development of bronchopulmonary dysplasia. In Bland RD, Coalson J (eds): Chronic Lung Disease of Early Infancy. New York, Marcel Dekker, 1999, p 209.

Gooding CA, Kerlan RK, Brasch RC: Partial aortic obstruction produced by a thoracostomy tube. J Pediatr 98:471, 1981.

Greenough A, Greenall F, Gamsu H: Synchronous respiration: Which ventilator rate is best? Acta Paediatr Scand 76:713, 1987.

Greenough A, Hird MF, Chan V: Airway pressure triggered ventilation for preterm neonates. J Perinat Med 19:471, 1991.

Greenough A, Milner AD, Dimitriou G: Synchronized mechanical ventilation for respiratory support in newborn infants. Cochrane Database Syst Rev CD000456, 2001.

Greenspan JS, Fox WW, Rubenstein SD, et al: Partial liquid ventilation in critically ill infants receiving extracorporeal life support. Philadelphia Liquid Ventilation Consortium. Pediatrics 99:E2, 1997.

Gregory, GA, Kitterman, JA, Phibbs, RH, et al: Treatment of idiopathic respiratory distress syndrome with continuous positive airway pressure. N Engl J Med 284:1333, 1971.

Greisen G, Frederiksen PS, Hertel J, et al: Catecholamine response to chest physiotherapy and endotracheal suctioning in preterm infants. Acta Paediatr Scand 74:525, 1985.

Hansen TN, Corbet AJS, Kenny JD, et al. Effects of oxygen and constant positive pressure breathing on aA.$DCO_2$ in hyaline membrane disease. Pediatr Res 13:1167, 1979.

Hansen TN, Gest AL: Oxygen toxicity and other ventilatory complications of treatment of infants with persistent pulmonary hypertension. Clin Perinatol 11:653, 1984.

Hansen TN, Tooley WH: Skin surface carbon dioxide tension in sick infants. Pediatrics 64:942, 1979.

Hanssler L, Tennhoff W, Roll C: Membrane humidification—a new method for humidification of respiratory gases in ventilator treatment of neonates. Arch Dis Child 67:1182, 1992.

Hay WW Jr: Pulse oximetry: As good as it gets? J Perinatol 20:181, 2000.

Hay WW Jr, Rodden DJ, Collins SM, et al: Reliability of conventional and new pulse oximetry in neonatal patients. J Perinatol 22:360, 2002.

Hegyi T, Hiatt IM: The effect of continuous positive airway pressure on the course of respiratory distress syndrome: the benefits on early initiation. Crit Care Med 9:38, 1981.

Heicher DA, Kasting DS, Harrod JR: Prospective clinical comparison of two methods for mechanical ventilation of neonates: Rapid rate and short inspiratory time versus slow rate and long inspiratory time. J Pediatr 98:957, 1981.

Henderson-Smart DJ, Bhuta T, Cools F, et al: Elective high frequency oscillatory ventilation versus conventional ventilation for acute pulmonary dysfunction in preterm infants. Cochrane Database Syst Rev CD000104, 2001.

Herman S, Reynolds EOR: Methods for improving oxygenation in infants mechanically ventilated for severe hyaline membrane disease. Arch Dis Child 48:612, 1973.

Hernandez LA, Peevy KJ, Moise AA, et al: Chest wall restriction limits high airway pressure-induced lung injury in young rabbits. J Appl Physiol 66:2364, 1989.

Herrera CM, Gerhardt T, Claure N, et al: Effects of volume-guaranteed synchronized intermittent mandatory ventilation in preterm infants recovering from respiratory failure. Pediatrics 110:529, 2002.

HIFI Study Group: High-frequency oscillatory ventilation compared with conventional intermittent mechanical ventilation in the treatment of respiratory failure in preterm infants: Neurodevelopmental status at 16 to 24 months of postterm age. J Pediatr 117:939, 1990.

HIFI Study Group: High-frequency oscillatory ventilation compared with conventional mechanical ventilation in the treatment of respiratory failure in preterm infants. N Engl J Med 320:88, 1989.

HIFO Study Group: Randomized study of high-frequency oscillatory ventilation in infants with severe respiratory distress syndrome. J Pediatr 122:609, 1993.

Higgins RD, Richter SE, Davis JM: Nasal continuous positive airway pressure facilitates extubation of very low birth weight neonates. Pediatrics 88:999, 1991.

Hird MF, Greenough A: Patient triggered ventilation using a flow triggered system. Arch Dis Child 66:1140, 1991a.

Hird MF, Greenough A: Randomized trial of patient triggered ventilation versus high frequency positive ventilation in acute respiratory distress. J Perinat Med 19:379, 1991b.

Huch R, Huch A, Albani M, et al: Transcutaneous $PO_2$ monitoring in routine management of infants and children with cardiorespiratory problems. Pediatrics 57:681, 1976.

Hummler H, Gerhardt T, Gonzalez A, et al: Influence of different methods of synchronized mechanical ventilation on ventilation, gas exchange, patient effort, and blood pressure fluctuations in premature neonates. Pediatr Pulmonol 22:305, 1996.

Jackson JC, Truog WE, Watchko JF, et al: Efficacy of thromboresistant umbilical artery catheters in reducing aortic thrombosis and related complications. J Pediatr 110:102, 1987.

Jacobsen T, Gronvall J, Petersen S, et al: Minitouch treatment of very low birth weight infants. Acta Paediatr 82:934, 1993.

Jennis MS, Peabody JL: Pulse oximetry. An alternative method for the assessment of oxygenation in newborn infants. Pediatrics 79:524, 1987.

Jirapaet KS, Kiatchuskul P, Kolatat T, Srisuparb P: Comparison of high-frequency flow interruption ventilation and hyperventilation in persistent pulmonary hypertension of the newborn. Respir Care 46:586, 2001.

John J, Bjorklund LJ, Svenningsen NW, et al: Airway and body surface sensors for triggering in neonatal ventilation. Acta Paediatr 83:903, 1994.

Johnson AH, Peacock JL, Greenough A, et al: High-frequency oscillatory ventilation for the prevention of chronic lung disease of prematurity. N Engl J Med 347:633, 2002.

Jung AL, Thomas GK: Stricture of the nasal vestibule. A complication of nasotracheal intubation in newborn infants. J Pediatr 85:412, 1974.

Kamper J, Ringsted C: Early treatment of idiopathic respiratory distress syndrome using binasal continuous positive airway pressure. Acta Paediatr Scand 79:581, 1990.

Kamper J, Wulff K, Larsen C, et al: Early treatment with nasal continuous positive airway pressure in very low birth weight infants. Acta Paediatr 82:193, 1993.

Kano S, Lanteri CJ, Pemberton PJ, et al: Fast versus slow ventilation for neonates. Am Rev Respir Dis 148:578, 1993.

Kavvadia V, Greenough A, Dimitriou G: Effect on lung function of continuous positive airway pressure administered either by infant flow driver or a single nasal prong. Eur J Pediatr 159:289, 2000.

Keszler M, Donn SM, Bucciarelli RL, et al: Multicenter controlled trial comparing high frequency jet ventilation and conventional mechanical ventilation in newborn infants with pulmonary interstitial emphysema. J Pediatr 119:85, 1991.

Keszler M, Modanlou HD, Brudno DS, et al: Multicenter controlled clinical trial of high-frequency jet ventilation in preterm infants with uncomplicated respiratory distress syndrome. Pediatrics 100:593, 1997.

Khalaf MN, Brodsky N, Hurley J, et al: A prospective randomized, controlled trial comparing synchronized nasal intermittent positive pressure ventilation versus nasal continuous positive airway pressure as modes of extubation. Pediatrics 108:13, 2001.

Kiciman NM, Andreasson B, Bernstein G, et al: Thoracoabdominal motion in newborns during ventilation delivered by endotracheal tube or nasal prongs. Pediatr Pulmonol 25:175, 1998.

Kirkpatrick BV, Felman AH, et al: Complications of ventilator therapy in respiratory distress syndrome Am J Dis Child 128:496, 1974.

Knight PJ, Abdenour G: Pneumoperitoneum in the ventilated neonate: Respiratory or gastrointestinal origin? J Pediatr 98:972, 1981.

Kraybill EN, Runyan DK, Bose CL, et al: Risk factors for chronic lung disease in infants with birth weights 751 to 1000 grams. J Pediatr 115:115, 1989.

Krouskop RW, Brown EG, Sweet AY: The early use of continuous positive airway pressure in the treatment of idiopathic respiratory distress syndrome. J Pediatr 87:263, 1975.

Laffey JG, Engelberts D, Kavanagh BP: Injurious effects of hypocapnic alkalosis in the isolated lung. Am J Respir Crit Care Med 162:399, 2000.

Landers S, Hansen TN, Corbet AJS, et al: Optimal constant positive airway pressure assessed by aA.$D_{CO_2}$ in hyaline membrane disease. Pediatr Res 20:884, 1986.

Landers S, Hansen TN: Skin surface oxygen monitoring. Perinatol Neonatol 8:39, 1994.

Landers S, Moise AA, Fraley JK, et al: Factors associated with umbilical catheter-related sepsis in neonates. Am J Dis Child 145:675, 1991.

Leach CL, Greenspan JS, Rubenstein SD, et al: Partial liquid ventilation with perflubron in premature infants with severe respiratory distress syndrome. The LiquiVent Study Group. N Engl J Med 335:761, 1996.

Lee KS, Dunn MS, Fenwick M, et al: A comparison of underwater bubble continuous positive airway pressure with ventilator-derived continuous positive airway pressure in premature neonates ready for extubation. Biol Neonate 73:69, 1998.

Leonidas JC, Bhan I, McCauley GK: Persistent localized pulmonary interstitial emphysema and lymphangiectasia: A causal relationship? Pediatrics 64:165, 1979.

Lesouef PN, England SJ, Bryan AC: Total resistance of the respiratory system in preterm infants with and without an endotracheal tube. J Pediatr 104:108, 1984.

Lin CH, Wang ST, Lin YJ, et al: Efficacy of nasal intermittent positive pressure ventilation in treating apnea of prematurity. Pediatr Pulmonol 26:349, 1998.

Lindner W, Vossbeck S, Hummler H, et al: Delivery room management of extremely low birth weight infants: Spontaneous breathing or intubation? Pediatrics 103:961, 1999.

Locke RG, Wolfson MR, Shaffer TH, et al: Inadvertent administration of positive end-distending pressure during nasal cannula flow. Pediatrics 91:135, 1993.

Lubchenco LO: Recognition of spontaneous pneumothorax in premature infants. Pediatrics 24:996, 1959.

Lundstrom KE, Greisen G: Early treatment with nasal-CPAP. Acta Paediatr 82:856, 1993.

Macklin MT, Macklin CC: Malignant interstitial emphysema of the lungs and mediastinum as an important occult complication in many respiratory diseases and other conditions: An interpretation of the clinical literature in the light of laboratory experiment. Medicine 23:281, 1944.

Mammel MC, Gordon MJ, Connett JE, et al: Comparison of high-frequency jet ventilation and conventional mechanical ventilation in a meconium aspiration model. J Pediatr 103:630, 1983.

Mandy GT, Moise AA, Smith EO, et al: Endotracheal continuous positive airway pressure after rescue surfactant therapy. J Perinatol 18:444, 1999.

Mariani G, Cifuentes J, Carlo WA: Randomized trial of permissive hypercapnia in preterm infants. Pediatrics 104:1082, 1999.

Mazzella M, Bellini C, Calevo MG, et al: A randomised control study comparing the Infant Flow Driver with nasal continuous positive airway pressure in preterm infants. Arch Dis Child Fetal Neonatal Ed 85:F86, 2001.

McMillan DD, Rademaker AW, Buchan KA, et al: Benefits of orotracheal and nasotracheal intubation in neonates requiring ventilatory assistance. Pediatrics 77:39, 1986.

Meadow WL, Cheromcha D: Successful therapy of unilateral pulmonary emphysema: Mechanical ventilation with extremely short inspiratory time. Am J Perinatol 2:194, 1985.

Mehta A, Wright BM, Callan K, et al: Patient-triggered ventilation in the newborn. Lancet 5:17, 1986.

Miller J, Law AB, Parker RA, et al: Effects of morphine and pancuronium on lung volume and oxygenation in premature infants with hyaline membrane disease. J Pediatr 125:97, 1994.

Miller KE, Edwards DK, Hilton S, et al: Acquired lobar emphysema in premature infants with bronchopulmonary dysplasia: An iatrogenic disease? Pediatr Radiol 138:589, 1981.

Mizuno K, Takeuchi T, Itabashi K, et al: Efficacy of synchronized IMV on weaning neonates from the ventilator. Acta Paediatr Jpn 36:162, 1994.

Moa G, Nilsson K, Zetterstrom H, Jonsson LO: A new device for administration of nasal continuous positive airway pressure in the newborn: An experimental study. Crit Care Med 16:1238, 1988.

Mockrin LD, Bancalari EH: Early versus delayed initiation of continuous negative pressure in infants with hyaline membrane disease. J Pediatr 87:596, 1975.

Moriette G, Paris-Llado J, Walti H, et al: Prospective randomized multicenter comparison of high-frequency oscillatory ventilation and conventional ventilation in preterm infants of less than 30 weeks with respiratory distress syndrome. Pediatrics 107:363, 2001.

Moylan FMB, Seldin EB, Shannon DC, et al: Defective primary dentition in survivors of neonatal mechanical ventilation. J Pediatr 96:106, 1980.

Mrozek JD, Bendel-Stenzel EM, Meyers PA, et al: Randomized controlled trial of volume-targeted synchronized ventilation and conventional intermittent mandatory ventilation following initial exogenous surfactant therapy. Pediatr Pulmonol 29:11, 2000.

Musante G, Schulze A, Gerhardt T, et al: Proportional assist ventilation decreases thoracoabdominal asynchrony and chest wall distortion in preterm infants. Pediatr Res 49:175, 2001.

Neal WA, Reynolds JW, Jarvis CW, et al: Umbilical artery catheterization: Demonstration of arterial thrombosis by aortography. Pediatrics 50:6, 1972.

Ogata E, Gregory GA, Kitterman JA, et al: Pneumothorax in respiratory distress syndrome: Incidence and effect on vital signs, blood gases and pH. Pediatrics 58:177, 1976.

Ogawa Y, Miyasaka K, Kawano T, et al: A multicenter randomized trial of high frequency oscillatory ventilation as compared with conventional mechanical ventilation in preterm infants with respiratory failure. Early Hum Dev 32:1, 1993.

Okumura A, Hayakawa F, Kato T, et al: Hypocarbia in preterm infants with periventricular leukomalacia: The relation between hypocarbia and mechanical ventilation. Pediatrics 107:469, 2001.

Olsen SL, Thibeault DW, Truog WE: Crossover trial comparing pressure support with synchronized intermittent mandatory ventilation. J Perinatol 22:461, 2002.

Oxford Region Controlled Trial of Artificial Ventilation Study Group (OCTAVE): Multicentre randomised controlled trial of high against low frequency positive pressure ventilation. Arch Dis Child 66:770, 1991.

Pagani G, Rezzonico R, Marini A: Trials of high frequency jet ventilation in preterm infants with severe respiratory disease. Acta Paediatr Scand 74:681, 1985.

Pandit PB, Courtney SE, Pyon KH, et al: Work of breathing during constant- and variable-flow nasal continuous positive airway pressure in preterm neonates. Pediatrics 108:682, 2001.

Pardou A, Vermeylen D, Muller MF, et al: High frequency ventilation and conventional mechanical ventilation in newborn babies with respiratory distress syndrome: A prospective randomized trial. Intensive Care Med 19:406, 1993.

Pedersen JE, Nielsen K: Oropharyngeal and esophageal pressure during mono- and binasal CPAP in neonates. Acta Paediatr 83:143, 1994.

Perlman J, Thach BT: Respiratory origin of fluctuations in arterial blood pressure in premature infants with respiratory distress syndrome. Pediatrics 81:399, 1988.

Perlman JM, McMenamin JB, Volpe JJ: Fluctuating cerebral blood flow velocity in respiratory distress syndrome: Relation to the development of intraventricular hemorrhage. N Engl J Med 309:204, 1983.

Perlman JM, Volpe JJ: Suctioning in the preterm infant: Effects on cerebral blood flow velocity, intracranial pressure, and arterial blood pressure. Pediatrics 72:329, 1983.

Pietsch JG, Nagaraj HS, Groff DB, et al: Necrotizing tracheobronchitis: A new indication for emergency bronchoscopy in the neonate. J Pediatr Surg 20:391, 1985.

Plavka R, Kopecky P, Sebron V, et al: A prospective randomized comparison of conventional mechanical ventilation and very early high frequency oscillatory ventilation in extremely premature newborns with respiratory distress syndrome. Intensive Care Med 25:68, 1999.

Plenat F, Vert P, Didier F, et al: Pulmonary interstitial emphysema. Clin Perinatol 5:351, 1978.

Poets CF, Sens B: Changes in intubation rates and outcome of very low birth weight infants: A population-based study. Pediatrics 98:24, 1996.

Poets CF, Wilken M, Seidenberg J, et al: Reliability of a pulse oximeter in the detection of hyperoxemia. J Pediatr 122:87, 1993.

Pokora T, Bing D, Mammel M, et al: Neonatal high-frequency jet ventilation. Pediatr 72:27, 1983.

Pologe JA: Pulse oximetry: Technical aspects of machine design. Int Anesthesiol Clin 25:137, 1987.

Powers WF, Clemens JD: Prognostic implications of age at detection of air leak in very low birth weight infants requiring ventilatory support. J Pediatr 123:611, 1993.

Primhak RA: Factors associated with pulmonary air leak in premature infants receiving mechanical ventilation. J Pediatr 102:764, 1983.

Ramanathan R, Durand M, Larazabal C: Pulse oximetry in very low birthweight infants with acute and chronic lung disease. Pediatrics 79:612, 1987.

Rennie JM, South M, Morley CJ: Cerebral blood flow velocity variability in infants receiving assisted ventilation. Arch Dis Child 62:1247, 1987.

Reppert SM, Ment LR, Todres ID: The treatment of pneumopericardium in the newborn infant. J Pediatr 905:115, 1977.

Rettwitz-Volk W, Veldman A, Roth B, et al: A prospective, randomized, multicenter trial of high-frequency oscillatory ventilation compared with conventional ventilation in preterm infants with respiratory distress syndrome receiving surfactant. J Pediatr 132:249, 1998.

Rhodes PG, Hall RT: Continuous positive airway pressure delivered by face mask in infants with the idiopathic respiratory distress syndrome: A controlled study. Pediatrics 52:1, 1973.

Richardson P, Pace WR, Valdes E, et al: Time dependence of lung mechanics in preterm lambs. Pediatr Res 31:276, 1992.

Ryan CA, Finer NN, Peters KL: Nasal intermittent positive-pressure ventilation offers no advantages over nasal continuous positive airway pressure in apnea of prematurity. Am J Dis Child 143:1196, 1989.

Sanders RC Jr, Thurman TL, Holt SJ, et al: Work of breathing associated with pressure support ventilation in two different ventilators. Pediatr Pulmonol 32:62, 2001.

Schulze A, Gerhardt T, Musante G, et al: Proportional assist ventilation in low birth weight infants with acute respiratory disease: A comparison to assist/control and conventional mechanical ventilation. J Pediatr 135:339, 1999.

Shaffer TH, Lowe CA, Bhutani VK, Douglas PR: Liquid ventilation: Effects on pulmonary function in distressed meconium-stained lambs. Pediatr Res 18:47, 1984.

Sherman JM, Lowitt S, Stephenson C, et al: Factors influencing acquired subglottic stenosis in infants. J Pediatr 109:322, 1986.

Simbruner G, Coradello H, Fodor M, et al: Effect of tracheal suction on oxygenation, circulation, and lung mechanics in newborn infants. Arch Dis Child 56:326, 1981.

Simbruner G: Inadvertent positive end-expiratory pressure in mechanically ventilated newborn infants: Detection and effect on lung mechanics and gas exchange. J Pediatr 108:589, 1986.

Sinclair SE, Kregenow DA, Lamm WJ, et al: Hypercapnic acidosis is protective in an in vivo model of ventilator-induced lung injury. Am J Respir Crit Care Med 166:403, 2002.

Slutsky AS: Nonconventional methods of ventilation. Am Rev Respir Dis 138:175, 1988.

So BH, Tamura M, Mishina J, et al: Application of nasal continuous positive airway pressure to early extubation in very low birthweight infants. Arch Dis Child Fetal Neonatal Ed 72:F191, 1995.

Sreenan C, Lemke RP, Hudson-Mason A, et al: High-flow nasal cannulae in the management of apnea of prematurity: A comparison with conventional nasal continuous positive airway pressure. Pediatrics 107:1081, 2001.

Stewart AR, Finer NN, Peters KL: Effects of alteration of inspiratory and expiratory pressures and inspiratory/expiratory ratios on mean airway pressure, blood gases, and intracranial pressure. Pediatrics 67:474, 1981.

Swingle HM, Eggert LD, Bucciarelli RL: New approach to management of unilateral tension pulmonary interstitial emphysema in premature infants. Pediatrics 74:354, 1984.

Tapia JL, Bancalari A, Gonzalez A, et al: Does continuous positive airway pressure (CPAP) during weaning from intermittent mandatory ventilation in very low birth weight infants have risks or benefits? A controlled trial. Pediatr Pulmonol 19:269, 1995.

Tarnow-Mordi WO, Griffiths ERP, Wilkinson AR: Low inspired gas temperature and respiratory complications in very low birth weight infants. J Pediatr 114:438, 1989.

Thome U, Kossel H, Lipowsky G, et al: Randomized comparison of high-frequency ventilation with high-rate intermittent positive pressure ventilation in preterm infants with respiratory failure. J Pediatr 135:39, 1999.

Trindade W, Goldberg RN, Bancalari E, et al: Conventional versus high frequency jet ventilation in a piglet model of meconium aspiration: Comparison of pulmonary and hemodynamic effects. Pediatrics 107:115, 1985.

Vannucci RC, Towfighi J, Heitjan DF, et al: Carbon dioxide protects the perinatal brain from hypoxic-ischemic damage: An experimental study in the immature rat. Pediatrics 95:868, 1995.

Varano LA, Maisels MJ: Pneumopericardium in the newborn: Diagnosis and pathogenesis. Pediatrics 53:941, 1974.

Varughese M, Patole S, Shama A, et al: Permissive hypercapnia in neonates: The case of the good, the bad, and the ugly. Pediatr Pulmonol 33:56, 2002.

Verder H, Albertsen P, Ebbesen F, et al: Nasal continuous positive airway pressure and early surfactant therapy for respiratory distress syndrome in newborns of less than 30 weeks' gestation. Pediatrics 103:E24, 1999.

Verder H, Robertson B, Greisen G, et al: Surfactant therapy and nasal continuous positive airway pressure for newborns with respiratory distress syndrome. N Engl J Med 331:1051, 1994.

Vijayakumar E, Ward GJ, Bullock CE, et al: Pulse oximetry in infants of <1500 gm birth weight on supplemental oxygen: A national survey. J Perinatol 17:341, 1997.

Visveshwara N, Freeman B, Peck M, et al: Patient triggered synchronized assisted ventilation of newborns: Report of a preliminary study and 3 years experience. J Perinatol 11:347, 1991.

Wiswell TE, Graziani LJ, Kornhauser MS, et al: High frequency jet ventilation in the early management of respiratory distress syndrome is associated with a greater risk for adverse outcomes. Pediatrics 98:1035, 1996.

Wolfson MR, Greenspan JS, Shaffer TH: Pulmonary administration of vasoactive substances by perfluorochemical ventilation. Pediatrics 97:449, 1996.

Wood B, Dubik M: A new device for pleural drainage in newborn infants. Pediatrics 96:955, 1995.

Wukitsch MW: Pulse oximetry: Historical review and Ohmeda functional analysis. Int J Clin Monit Comput 4:161, 1987.

Wung JT, Driscoll JM, Epstein RA, et al: A new device for CPAP by nasal route. Crit Care Med 3:76, 1975.

CHAPTER 46

# Surfactant Treatment of Respiratory Disorders

H. William Taeusch, Daniela Ramierez-Schrempp, and Ian A. Laing

## HISTORIC OVERVIEW

The infant mortality rate in the United States has halved in the last 20 years or so, a drop explained largely by the use of replacement surfactant for premature babies and positioning infants on their backs for sleeping to reduce the occurrence of sudden infant death syndrome (SIDS). The increased survival due to the treatment of newborn infants with surfactant amounts to 3 lives per 10,000 births. If 10 million infants are born in developed countries each year, then an estimated 30,000 lives have been saved in the past 10 years with surfactant therapy. Morbidity is also reduced. Pneumothoraces and other forms of air leak have become a rarity for infants with respiratory distress syndrome (RDS) (Malloy and Freeman, 2000).

All current exogenous surfactants reduce the severity of RDS. Most also reduce the mortality rates associated with RDS by 40% to 60%, and they significantly reduce overall mortality among premature infants at risk for RDS.

The story of the development of surfactant therapy is now a well-told tale (Avery, 2000; Clements and Avery, 1998). In 1929, by comparing pressures after inflating lungs with air and with fluid, von Neergard first inferred that surface forces contribute in a major way to mechanical properties of the lung. Several investigators (e.g., Gruenwald, Macklin) suggested that the lung contains substances that result in low surface tension. Comparing foam from lungs with foams from other detergents, Pattle estimated that surface tension in the lung is near zero, a startling conclusion. Clements discovered that material in the aqueous layer lining alveolar spaces has the unique ability to change surface tension according to surface area (alveolar volume). Clements, among others, identified the major constituents of pulmonary surfactant as lipids and proteins. In 1959, Mary Ellen Avery working with Jere Mead established that insufficiency of surfactant was associated with RDS (Avery and Mead, 1959).

The 1960s and 1970s were marked by *successful* trials of surfactant in animals with surfactant deficiency and *unsuccessful* clinical studies of use of surfactant in human infants. In retrospect, lack of success in the early clinical trials was due to the use of inadequate formulations and delivery methods. Then Fujiwara and colleagues (1980) published a paper describing a series of 10 infants with severe RDS who were markedly improved after treatment with bovine surfactant compared with historic controls. Their success where others had failed was due to three essential factors: use of an animal-derived surfactant that was extensively tested in vitro; delivery as a liquid via the endotracheal tube; and the use of positive end-expiratory pressure, without which the effectiveness of surfactant therapy is limited. The work of these investigators was followed by a decade of clinical trials matched with basic science discoveries that led to the widespread use of surfactant throughout the developed world by around 1990. The review by Comroe (1977) illustrates the benefit of interactions among scientists and clinicians involved in surfactant research, and some of their contributions are listed in Table 46–1.

## COMPOSITION OF SURFACTANT

Human pulmonary surfactant consists of 90% lipids and 10% proteins. Phosphatidylcholines (lecithins), such as 1,2-dipalmitoyl-sn-phosphatidylcholine (DPPC) (36%), unsaturated phosphatidylcholine (32%), and phosphatidylglycerol (PG) (10%), constitute the bulk of the lipids (Fig. 46–1). In truth, because surfactant has multiple functions and is a mixture of several compounds, and because some of its constituents may be secreted into the alveoli from at least two cell types, it is impossible to say with exactitude what surfactant is. Operationally, surfactant is defined by its functions, by co-isolation of lipids and associated proteins from bronchoalveolar lavage fluid from normal humans and animals, and by measuring the secretions of alveolar type II cells. As the lung of the fetus matures in utero, lung fluid containing surfactant lipids and proteins enters the amniotic fluid, where it may be sampled, allowing estimation of lung maturity in cases of threatened premature delivery. In Table 46–2, the lipid constituents of human surfactant are compared with those of four exogenous surfactants used to treat surfactant deficiency in humans. Fig. 46–2 indicates the synthetic pathways by which the lipids are made. (see also relevant discussion in Chapter 42, Lung Development: Embryology, Growth, Maturation, and Developmental Biology.)

Four proteins are known to be associated with surfactant lipids (Table 46–3). They are known as surfactant proteins A to D: SP-A, SP-B, SP-C, and SP-D. SP-A is a hydrophilic, calcium-binding glycoprotein of 28 to 36 kDa synthesized by the alveolar type II cell and secreted as a large complex constructed from 18 polypeptide chains. SP-A consists of an N-terminal alpha-helical segment, a triple-helix coiled structure, an alpha helix, and a carbohydrate recognition domain. SP-B is a hydrophobic polypeptide of approximately 18 kDa with two identical polypeptide chains linked by a disulfide bridge. SP-C is very hydrophobic, and its main form is a 35-residue peptide chain containing two thioester-linked palmitoyl groups. SP-D is a hydrophilic glycoprotein. Like SP-A, SP-D has a collagen-like domain, a short linking region, and a C-lectin–like C-terminal domain. It is assembled as a multimer of 43-kDa subunits. SP-A and SP-D are members of a family of immunoprotective proteins termed collectins (collagen-lectins). SP-B and SP-C are stored in the lamellar bodies of the alveolar type II cell, whereas SP-A and SP-D are secreted separately both from alveolar

**TABLE 46–1**

**Historic Contributions to the Development of Surfactant Therapy**

| | |
|---|---|
| 1806 | Laplace describes the relationship *inflating pressure* = 2 × *surface tension/bubble radius*. |
| 1929 | Von Neergaard infers the importance of surface tension in the lungs. |
| 1950s | Macklin and Gruenwald suggest again the importance of surface forces; Pattle suggests that the lungs contain a surfactant that lowers surface tension. |
| 1957 | Clements infers that lung surfactant changes surface tension with changes in lung volume. |
| 1959 | Avery and Mead describe surfactant inadequacy in lungs of infants who died of RDS. |
| 1965 | Chu and others were unsuccessful in treating infants with aerosolized surfactant lipids. |
| 1973 | King and Clements characterize surfactant lipids and identify a surfactant-specific protein. |
| 1970s | Gluck, Clements, and coworkers find that amniotic fluid surfactant lipids predict RDS; Enhorning, Robertson, and coworkers show benefits of surfactant treatment of immature animals. |
| 1971 | Gregory demonstrates success of CPAP treatment for infants with RDS. |
| 1980 | Fujiwara successfully treats infants with a liquid preparation of bovine surfactant. |
| 1980s | Characterization of surfactant lipids and their synthesis and metabolism. |
| 1988 | TA surfactant approved for clinical use in Japan. Extensive clinical trials in Europe and the United States of a variety of surfactants. |
| 1990s | Approval of Exosurf and Survanta in the United States and Curosurf in Europe, leading to widespread use of surfactants. Cloning and regulation of surfactant proteins. Extensive clinical trials. Approval in the United States of Curosurf and Infasurf. |

CPAP, continuous positive airway pressure; RDS, respiratory distress syndrome; TA, tracheal aspirate.

type II cells and from other cells lining the entrance to the alveoli (McCormack and Whitsett, 2002) (see relevant discussion in Chapter 42). The proteins in natural mammalian surfactant are compared with the proteins contained in the modified surfactants that are available for therapy in Table 46–4. Fig. 46–3 shows current molecular models of the four surfactant-associated proteins.

Note that Exosurf contains no proteins. Due to extraction with organic solvents during the purification process, the other surfactants used clinically contain the hydrophobic proteins, SP-B and SP-C, but lack the more hydrophilic SP-A and SP-D.

## SURFACTANT PHENOMENA AND SURFACTANT FUNCTION

Surface tension results from intermolecular attractive forces of molecules (e.g., hydrogen bonds, electrostatic and van der Waals forces). Among fluids, the surface tension of water and

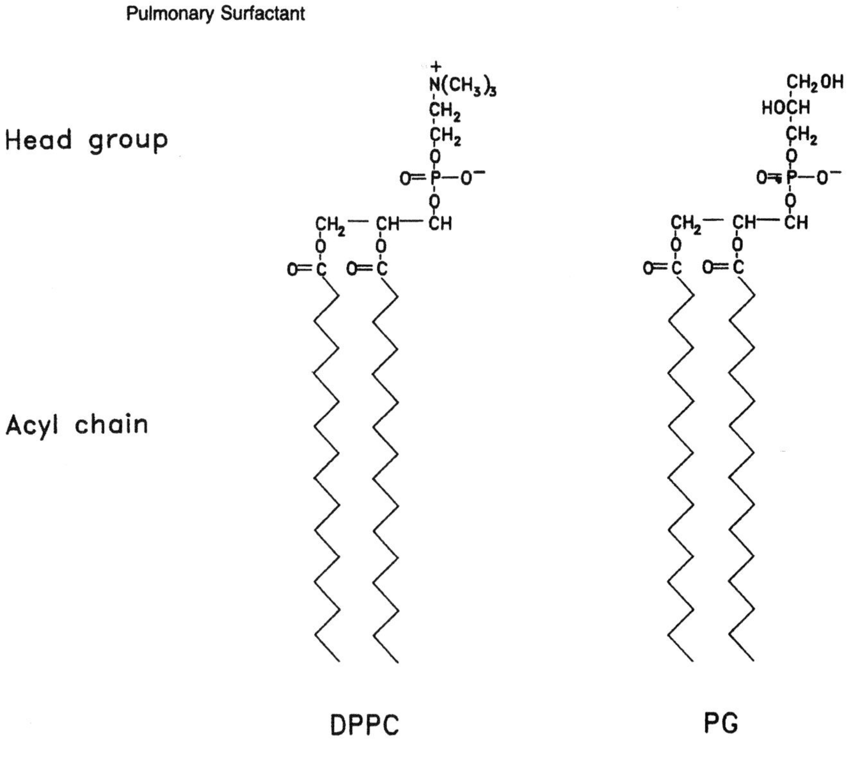

**FIGURE 46–1.** Molecular structures of dipalmitoyl phosphatidylcholine (DPPC) and phosphatidylglycerol (PG). Phospholipid molecules pack densely, forming membrane monolayers, bilayers, and vesicles and other aggregate forms. Strong molecular interactions occur between polar head groups. Distinct interactions occur between atoms composing the more hydrophobic acyl chains. *(From Polin RA, Fox WW: Fetal and Neonatal Physiology, 3rd ed. Philadelphia, Elsevier, 2003, p 944.)*

**TABLE 46–2**

**Lipid Composition of Surfactants***

| | Native Surfactant† | Curosurf‡ | Infasurf§ | Survanta‖ | Exosurf¶ |
|---|---|---|---|---|---|
| PC | 70-85 | 67-74 | 70-74 | 79-87 | 90 |
| DPPC (% PC) | 36-54 | 50-56 | 41-61 | 45-74 | 100 |
| LPC | 0.2 | 6.9 | — | 2.2 | 0 |
| Sphingomyelin | 2 | 8.1 | 2 | 4.8 | 0 |
| Cholesterol | 5 | 0 | 5 | 0 | 0 |
| PI | 4-7 | 3.3 | ca. 2 | 0.5 | 0 |
| PS | 5 | — | ca. 2 | ? | 0 |
| PE | 3 | 4.5 | 3 | 2.2 | 0 |
| PG | 7-10 | 1.2 | 6 | 3.2 | 0 |
| Unknown | — | — | 4.3 | — | — |
| Hexadecanol | 0 | 0 | 0 | 0 | 10 |
| Tyloxapol | 0 | 0 | 0 | 0 | 7 |

*%, g/g of total lipid.

†Data from Notter, 2000; Postle et al, 2001; Robertson and Taeusch, 1985.

‡Data from Bernhard and Mottaghian, 2000; Chiesi Farmaceutici; Robertson and Taeusch, 1985; Seeger et al, 1993.

§Data from Bloom et al, 1997; Kahn et al, 1995; ONY, 1998.

‖Data from Robertson and Taeusch, 1985; Ross, 1999; Seeger et al, 1993.

¶Data from Notter, 2000; Wellcome, 1996.

DPPC, dipalmitoyl phosphatidylcholine; LPC, lysophosphatidyl choline; PC, phosphatidylcholine; PE, phosphatidylethanolamine; PG, phosphatidylglycerol; PI, phosphatidylinositol; PS, phosphatidylserine.

salt solutions is relatively high, approximately 72 mN/m. The force of surface tension is measured in a number of ways—for example, by the size of a fluid drop in air hanging from a pipette, the downward pull on a plate hanging in a fluid surface, the pressure needed to inflate a bubble in fluid, the deformation characteristics of a bubble under increasing pressure in a fluid, or the lateral force needed to compress a surface film on an aqueous buffer (Fig. 46–4).

If the air spaces of the lung were lined with extracellular fluid alone (conferring a high surface tension), then the pressure needed to inflate the lungs would be high, lung compliance would be low, the work of breathing would be great, and the air spaces would tend to collapse at end-expiration, leaving a low functional residual capacity and limiting excretion of carbon dioxide and saturation of pulmonary venous blood with oxygen. In addition, the

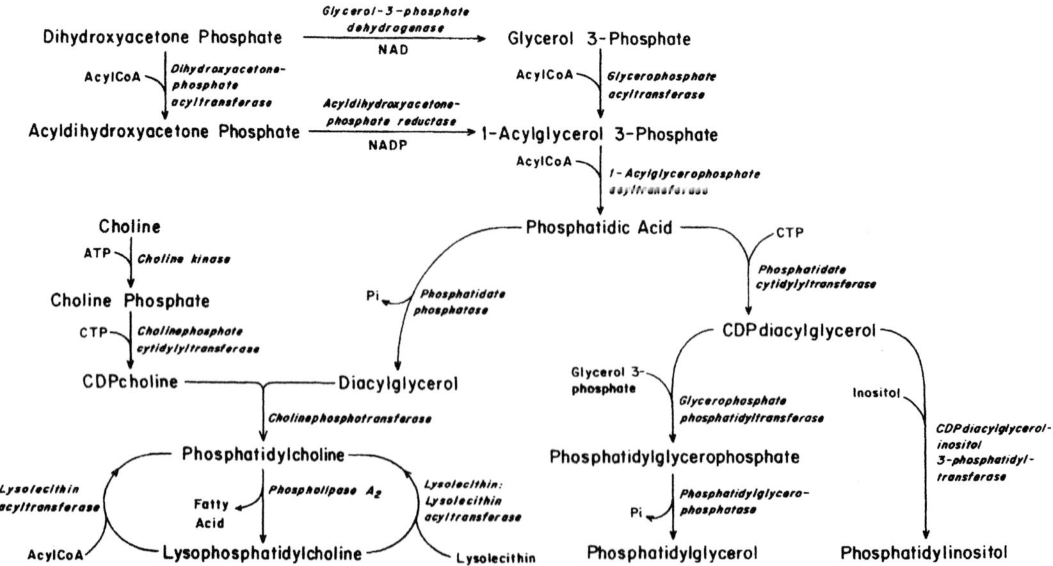


**FIGURE 46–2.** Pathways in the biosynthesis of phosphatidylcholine, phosphatidylglycerol, and phosphatidylinositol. *(From Polin RA, Fox WW: Fetal and Neonatal Physiology, 3rd ed. Philadelphia, Elsevier, 2003.)*

**TABLE 46–3**

**Characteristics of Surfactant Proteins**

**SP-A**
Most abundant surfactant-related protein
Enhances phospholipid aggregation and order
Immunoprotective
Reduces surfactant inactivation
Two genes located on chromosome 10
Hydrophilic
35-kDa monomer; mature form is an octadecamer of 630 kDa

**SP-B**
Essential for surfactant activity
Enhances rate of surface film creation
Creates "surfactant reservoirs"
Prevents surfactant inactivation
Anti-inflammatory
Affects intracellular processing of SP-C
Necessary for tubular myelin formation
Enhances phospholipid adsorption
Gene located on chromosome 2
Hydrophobic
79-amino-acid monomer; mature form is a homodimer of 18 kDa

**SP-C**
Decreases order and packing density in phospholipid bilayers
Enhances phospholipid adsorption
Increases respreading and contributes to film refining during cycling
Gene located on chromosome 8
Hydrophobic
35 aminoacids; mature form is a homodimer

**SP-D**
Immunoprotective
May have a role in controlling release of surfactant into alveoli
Gene located on chromosome 10
Hydrophilic
43-kDa monomer; four triplet monomers in cross-like form

law of Laplace ($P = 2ST/r$), if applied to air spaces that are in contiguity and are lined with liquid with invariant surface tension (ST), dictates that small alveoli (small radius, $r$) would tend to collapse into larger ones, driven by the tendency of their internal pressure ($P$) to increase. All of these phenomena are present to a variable degree in infants with RDS (and in children and adults with lung injuries and acute RDS).

Clements had the first insight that the unusual mixture of substances lining mammalian lungs—pulmonary surfactant—has the capability of changing its surface tension with changes in lung volume (i.e., in lung surface area). This feature stabilizes the lungs at low lung volumes (it allows partially inflated alveoli of unequal sizes to coexist) and allows increased recoil at higher lung volumes. If surface tension remains unequally distributed according to alveolar size, then the inflating pressure on the whole lung can maintain patency of large and small airways in parallel. This theory was directly proved by Schürch and colleagues (1976), who described the surface tension in the walls of air spaces of variable sizes by evaluating the spreading characteristics of microdroplets of fluorocarbons. How does pulmonary surfactant change surface tension with changing lung volume? Below the surface (air-liquid interface), a water molecule is attracted equally in all directions by neighboring molecules. Molecules beneath the surface attract molecules on the surface to a degree much greater than is true for molecules above the surface (in the gas phase). These forces make liquids with a high surface tension (mercury, water) bead on a solid surface.

A *surfactant*, or surface-active agent, is any molecule that localizes on aqueous surfaces. Surface tension reduces according to the number of surface-active molecules in a given surface area. An increase of surfactant molecules lowers surface tension, as the net attractive forces among surfactant molecules is less than those for water molecules. At very low surface tensions, an aqueous surface containing a surfactant can be viewed as a two-dimensional solid, excluding water, with surfactant molecules compacted contiguously.

Soaps and detergents are soluble surfactants and lower surface tension of water, but these compounds for the most part do not change surface tension as surface area changes. For that to occur, a relatively insoluble surfactant is necessary. An amphipathic molecule is one with both hydrophobic and hydrophilic regions, so that it concentrates at the surface, where the hydrophilic portion is in the water phase, while the hydrophobic part of the molecule extrudes in the air. Pulmonary surfactant contains (see Table 46–2) a specific amphipathic compound called dipalmitoyl phosphatidylcholine (DPPC) (formerly called dipalmitoyl lecithin). DPPC consists of a three-carbon glycerol backbone, with palmitate on the first and second carbons and with a phosphate linkage to choline on the third carbon.

**TABLE 46–4**

**Estimated Average Protein Content of Surfactants***

| | Native Surfactant | Curosurf | Infasurf | Survanta | Exosurf |
|---|---|---|---|---|---|
| SP-A | 300 | 0 | 0 | 0 | 0 |
| SP-D | 42 | 0 | 0 | 0 | 0 |
| SP-C | 22-34 | 5-11.6 | 8.1 | 1-20 | 0 |
| SP-B | 10-11 | 2-3.7 | 5.4 | 0-1.3 | 0 |

*μg of protein per μM of phospholipid.

Data from Bernhard and Mottaghian, 2000; Cheng, 2000 #1870; Chiesi Farmaceutici; Haagsman et al, 1997; ONY, 1998; Ramirez-Schrempp and Taeusch, 2002.

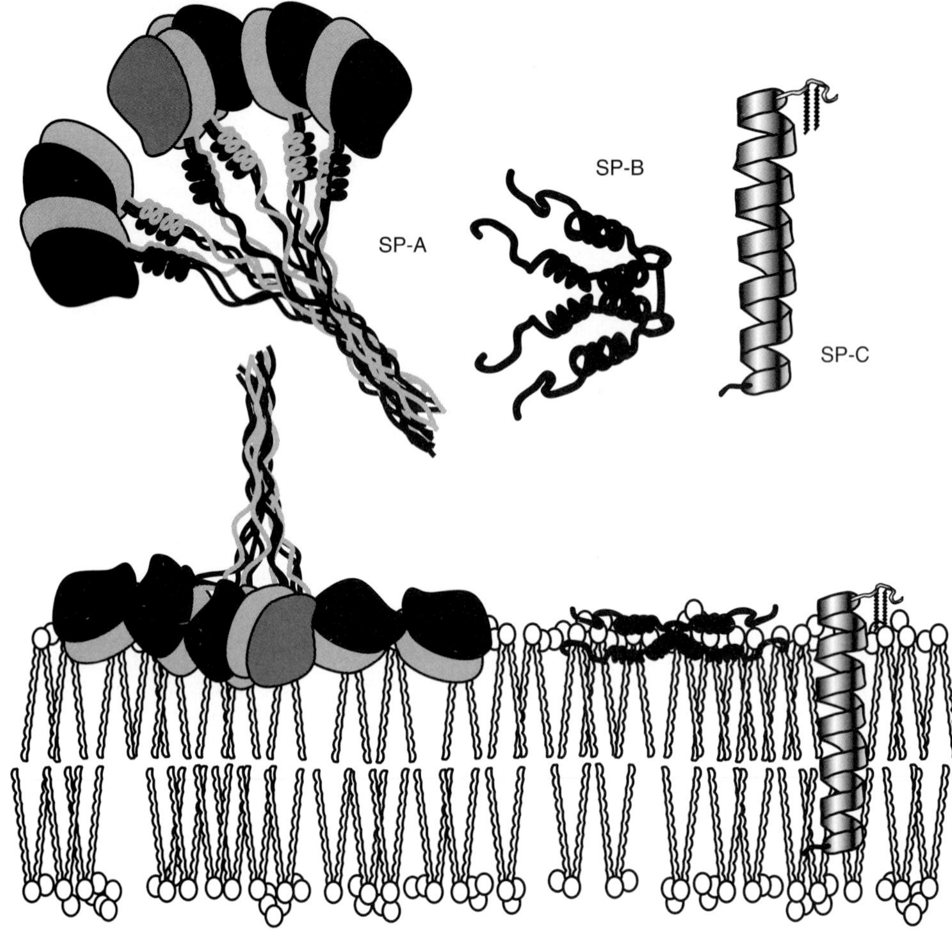


**FIGURE 46–3.** Current models on the structure and lipid-protein interaction of surfactant-associated apolipoproteins SP-A, SP-B, and SP-C. The drawings of the three proteins are not presented on the same scale. *(From Perez-Gil J: Molecular interactions in pulmonary surfactant films. Biol Neonate 81[suppl 1]: 6-15, 2002. © S. Karger AG, Basel.)*

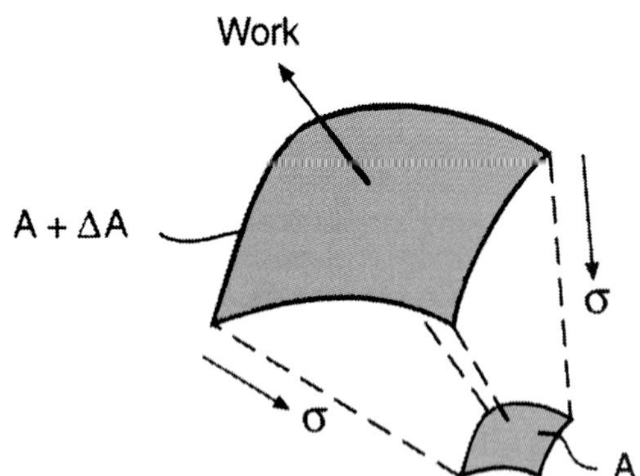


**FIGURE 46–4.** Surface tension is related to the work necessary to expand a surface. Surface tension has units of force per length or work or energy per area. Work must be done against surface tension in order to increase the surface area of a system. Surface tension is defined thermodynamically as a change in free energy per unit surface area. *(From Notter R: Lung Surfactants: Basic Science and Clinical Applications. New York, Marcel Dekker, 2000, p 11.)*

When DPPC is compressed on an aqueous surface, not only are attractive forces minimal among DPPC molecules, but net intermolecular forces become repulsive, leading to the concept of surface pressure—the tendency of such molecules to fly apart on the surface (Surface pressure is equal to the surface tension of clean water minus the surface tension of the surfactant film; therefore, the lower the surface tension, the higher the surface pressure.)

As the lung expands and contracts, the surfactant lining layer expands and contracts in an inhomogeneous manner. As lung volume reduces, the dispersed molecules of surfactant at the air water interface coalesce into islands of enriched DPPC surrounded by more fluid areas of other lipids and proteins. The DPPC islands join, and the surface becomes solid and homogeneous as lung volume reduces further. At lowest lung volumes, the surface is compacted, distorted, and pleated into multilayers. On reexpansion, the multilayers are reincorporated into the surface, and the process repeats. During lung injury, serum proteins and other substances that have leaked into alveoli can absorb into the expanded surface layer, preventing the reincorporation of the extruded surfactant back into the surface, an explanation for one mechanism of inactivation of surfactant (Warriner et al, 2002).

No clinical conditions have been described with genetic abnormalities specifically for surfactant lipids. Knockout mice with absent SP-A or SP-D have relatively normal surfactant activity and pulmonary mechanics in the newborn period. No humans with absence of either of these proteins have been described, although SP-A polymorphisms have been described that correlate with both increased and decreased risks of respiratory distress, for reasons that remain unclear (Hallman et al, 2001). Surfactant deficient in SP-A is more susceptible to inactivation in vitro and in vivo. In the presence of calcium, surfactant proteins act to aggregate lipids to form a specific protein-lipid structure in the alveoli called tubular myelin that represents a transition form of surfactant between the osmiophilic bodies secreted from alveolar type II cells and the surfactant surface film. The structure of tubular myelin may protect secreted surfactant from inactivating materials and may promote the rate of adsorption of surfactant lipids into a surface film.

About $20^8$ bacteria, in addition to particulate matter, viruses, fungi, and gaseous pollutants, are inhaled by adults breathing 12,000 liters of air per day. With a moist surface the size of a badminton court within the lungs, protective measures are necessary, and a major role for SP-A and SP-D is defense against infection (Fig. 46–5). SP-A and SP-D are large-molecular-weight, complement-like proteins that both have a collagen-like tail with a globular sugar-binding (lectin) head. Both help opsonize bacteria and prepare various particles for engulfment and destruction by alveolar macrophages. SP-A has been shown to bind and enhance the uptake of a number of microorganisms (McCormack and Whitsett, 2002). Mice in which the SP-A gene has been knocked out have increased susceptibility to infection with group B beta-hemolytic streptococci and *Pseudomonas aeruginosa*. SP-A similarly protects the lungs against *Escherichia coli*, *Klebsiella*, fungi, and respiratory syncytial virus (RSV). SP-D also has been shown to have a similar potential role in protection against *E. coli*, *Klebsiella*, and RSV.

Disruption of the gene encoding SP-B is lethal for newborn (knockout) mice, which die of RDS, and a similar rare lethal RDS has been described for human newborns (reviewed in Cole et al, 2001). Babies with SP-B deficiency present with severe respiratory distress in the neonatal period. Because the condition in some respects mimics severe RDS in premature infants, the deficiency is recognized most clearly in term infants. SP-B deficiency is not relieved by the administration of exogenous surfactant, and the condition is fatal (without lung transplantation). Therefore, SP-B is a single-gene product essential for life.

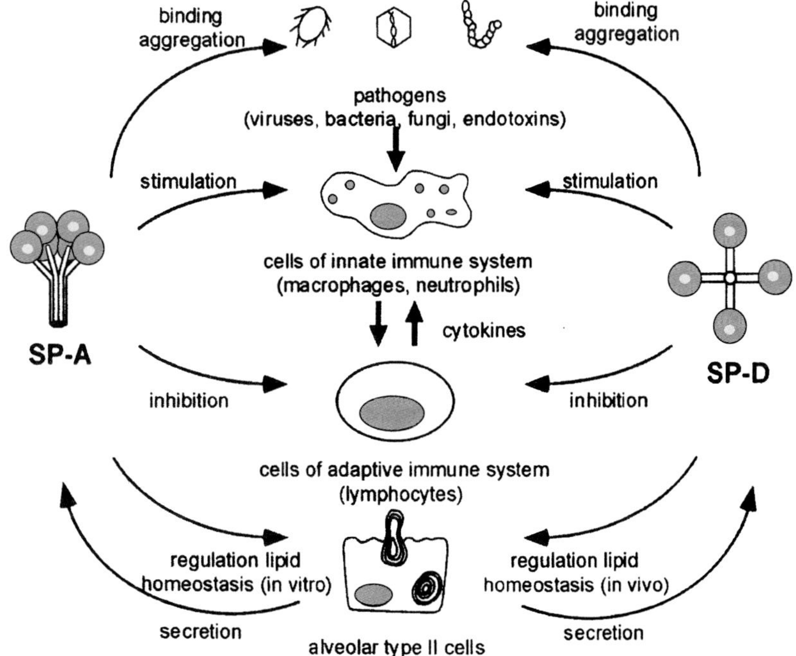


**FIGURE 46–5.** Mechanisms of SP-A– and SP-D–mediated host defenses in the lung. SP-A and SP-D are secreted by alveolar type II cells and Clara cells (not shown). SP-A and SP-D are large multimeric proteins and belong to a family of collagenous C-type lectins designated collectins. Besides a role in the homeostasis of lung surfactant (in the case of SP-A based on in vitro and in the case of SP-D based on in vivo studies), both lung collectins are believed to play a role in the innate immunity of the lung. SP-A and SP-D can bind to a broad spectrum of pathogens, including bacteria, viruses, fungi, and yeasts, but also lipopolysaccharides (LPSs, endotoxin) and allergens. Furthermore, SP-A and SP-D enhance the clearing of various pathogens by neutrophils and macrophages by aggregation of the pathogens or by direct interaction of the collectins with receptors on the phagocytic cells. Finally, the lung collectins are suggested to dampen an excessive inflammatory response by inhibiting the secretion of cytokines and the proliferation of lymphocytes. *(From Vaandrager A, Van Golde L: Lung surfactant proteins A and D in innate immune defense. Biol Neonate 77[suppl 1]:9-13, 2000. © S. Karger AG, Basel.)*

Absence of SP-C also has been described (Amin et al, 2001). This condition appears to cause interstitial lung disease manifesting in later childhood or even adulthood but does not cause neonatal RDS.

SP-B and SP-C facilitate the initial adsorption and the reincorporation of surfactant lipids into surface films and help prevent inactivation of surfactant, presumably by their ability to both order and disorder lipid membranes (Johansson and Curstedt, 1997; Kruger et al, 2002; Perez-Gil, 2002; Wang et al, 2002). Lung injuries of different causes can down-regulate surfactant proteins. A recent study, for example, finds that SP-A and SP-D are diminished in the lungs of children with gastroesophageal reflux (Griese et al, 2002).

An excellent and extensive review of pulmonary surfactant has recently been published (Notter, 2000).

**TABLE 46–5**

**Effects of Pulmonary Surfactant on the Lung**

| |
|---|
| Maintains a gas reservoir at the end of expiration (FRC) |
| Provides a protective yet gas-permeable barrier between air and tissue in the lungs; fosters clearance of foreign material from the lung |
| Maintains optimal compliance of the lung. (low at high lung volume and high at low lung volume) |
| Enhances liquid efflux from alveoli, thus reducing edema |
| Lowers work of breathing and hence oxygen consumption |
| Allows optimal ventilation-perfusion ratios (large and small alveoli coexist) |
| In part, self-regulates secretion and metabolism |
| FRC, forced residual capacity |

Data from Soll and Morley, 2001.

## PHYSIOLOGY AND PATHOPHYSIOLOGY

In the term infant, after clearance of alveolar fluid present during fetal life, with mature amounts of alveolar surfactant, the opening pressures (pressure at which air first enters the lung) are relatively low. Pulmonary compliance is normal, and the work of breathing is minimal. During expiration, a sizable functional residual capacity allows a reservoir of air between breaths. Low surface tension in alveoli helps increase egress of fluid from air spaces and keeps lungs edema-free. All of these attributes are reversed in premature infants with RDS or in older children or adults with acute RDS from lung injuries.

Why does surfactant deficiency matter in the lung? If surface tension in the lung is high, then air spaces tend to contract, lowering lung compliance and increasing the work of breathing. If the work of breathing is increased, then more respiratory drive from the brain is required to maintain normal alveolar ventilation and gas exchange. In premature infants with RDS, the increased work of breathing is manifested by intercostal and subcostal retractions as the infant generates higher negative pleural pressure to maintain alveolar ventilation. Alveolar ventilation is reduced, and the increased work of breathing generates high oxygen needs. Apneic spells may occur as respiratory drive becomes insufficient to inflate stiff (noncompliant) lungs. Smaller alveoli collapse into larger ones, creating the "Swiss cheese" or "ground-glass" appearance on chest radiographs; atelectasis and overinflated alveoli coexist, leading to ventilation-perfusion mismatching and right-to-left intrapulmonary shunting, resulting in hypoxemia. Hypercarbia may coexist with the hypoxemia. (see Chapter 47, Respiratory Distress in the Preterm Infant.)

The effects of pulmonary surfactant on the lung are summarized in Table 46–5.

Before the use of surfactant therapy, infants with RDS were treated with oxygen sufficient to overcome intrapulmonary shunting; constant distending airway pressure, that is, continuous positive airway pressure (CPAP); and ventilator support. CPAP is a mechanical partial substitute for surfactant, holding air spaces open at end-expiration. CPAP reduces *atelectrauma*, the damage done to lungs by repeatedly reopening collapsed air spaces. High levels of oxygen were required to maintain adequate $PaO_2$ in the face of widespread atelectasis, and this use "burned" the lung after several days (*oxytrauma*). High tidal volumes and inspiratory pressures were used on the ventilator to overcome low lung compliance (*volutrauma* and *barotrauma*). These therapeutic practices may combine to evoke inflammatory processes that could affect distant organs (*biotrauma*). Lung damage from ventilation and high levels of inspired oxygen also damage capillaries, so plasma (and in worst cases whole blood) leaks into air spaces, resulting in surfactant inactivation. Therefore, surfactant inactivation rapidly joins with surfactant insufficiency in RDS. Surfactant inactivation occurs not only in the preterm infant but also in association with lung injury states including meconium aspiration syndrome and pneumonia. Surfactant inactivation is a hallmark of acute (adult) RDS. Surfactant treatment acts to prevent or partially reverse all of these processes if given early in the course of the disease.

## SURFACTANT DEVELOPMENT, TURNOVER, SYNTHESIS, AND SECRETION

Lung surfactant is synthesized, processed, packed, secreted, and recycled by alveolar type II cells, which comprise 10% to 15% of the cells in the mature distal lung and are stem cells for alveolar epithelial (type I) cells. Type II cells produce, along with other cells, cytokines and growth factors that mediate lung growth, maturation, and repair. In the smooth endoplasmic reticulum, surfactant phospholipids and proteins are synthesized and exported in the Golgi system as osmiophilic lamellar bodies, where surfactant is stored and some of the final processing occurs. Lamellar bodies, which are storage sites for surfactant, are first observed at 22 weeks of gestation. From the lamellar bodies, surfactant is secreted by exocytosis into the liquid lining of the alveoli. Other cells in the distal lung also secrete surfactant proteins, and some assembly of lipid-protein complexes may occur after secretion. Surfactant secretion is stimulated by hyperventilation and mechanical stretch, catecholamines, ATP, protein kinases A and C, cyclic adenosine monophosphate (cAMP), phorbol esters, prostaglandins, and leukotrienes. Surfactant secretion is inhibited by SP-A and possibly by other surfactant lipids and proteins.

Pulmonary surfactant appears in the future air spaces at 23 to 24 weeks of gestation. Because of net efflux of pulmonary fluid from the fetal lung, surfactant lipids and proteins are seen in the amniotic fluid starting at about 24 weeks of gestation. These surfactant constituents can be sampled by amniocentesis, allowing assessment of biochemical maturity of the fetal lung by various methods including determination of lecithin-to-sphingomyelin (L/S) ratio, measurement of phosphatidylglycerol (PG), and tests of bubble stability. With the continuing development of thin-walled air spaces and sufficient production of surfactant, the incidence of RDS falls in linear fashion from 24 to 34 weeks of gestation. Mature levels of pulmonary surfactant usually are present after week 35 of gestation. (see Chapters 6 and 42).

The ontogeny, synthesis, and secretion of the constituents of pulmonary surfactant are elaborately regulated (Copland and Post, 2002; McCormack and Whitsett, 2002; Whitsett and Weaver, 2002) (Fig. 46–6 and Fig. 46–7). The clinical corollary is that some maternal diseases, conditions, and treatments may perturb the endocrine milieu of the fetus, thereby affecting rates of development of both the lung structure and pulmonary surfactant. To prevent RDS in the premature infant, prenatal glucocorticoids are now universally recommended for mothers at risk of giving birth before the infant's lungs are mature (see Chapters 6 and 42). Maternal diseases that stress the fetus and cause endogenous fetal secretion of catecholamines, hypothalamic hormones, thyroid hormones, and glucocorticoids may contribute to precocious surfactant production. Nevertheless, such diseases, including pregnancy-induced hypertension and chorioamnionitis, may involve poor placental function and may be associated with chronic and/or acute hypoxemia for the fetus, offsetting the benefit of the enhanced rate of appearance of surfactant. Maternal diabetes and male gender of the infant are associated with delay in lung maturation and in production of surfactant.

Catabolism of surfactant is slow. Most surfactant is taken up by endocytocis from the alveolar lumen. Approximately 5% of secreted surfactant is cleared from the lung every hour in newborn animals, compared with 25% to 50% every hour in adults. Approximately 95% of secreted phophatidylcholine is recycled. Endogenous phosphatidylcholine has a turnover rate of 13 hours in preterm lambs, and phosphatidylglycerol's estimated half-life is 30 hours. Recycling pathways for both endogenous and replacement surfactants are active in preterm human lungs. The effete surfactant is returned to the alveolar type II cell to provide the raw materials for recycling.

Clinical studies have shown that the incidence or severity of RDS is affected by many factors. Table 46–6 lists factors that may increase or decrease the amount of available surfactant. Humoral factors are important for control of surfactant synthesis, including glucocorticoids, catecholamines, thyroid hormones, and insulin. (see Chapters 6, 42, and 47).

Alveolar type II cells secrete osmiophilic bodies that contain most of the surfactant lipids and proteins. The catecholamine surge at birth serves two important lung functions: It stimulates the reversal of fluid production such that alveolar fluid is taken up rather than produced, and it stimulates the secretion of the stored intracellular osmiophilic bodies. In the extracellular fluid space in the

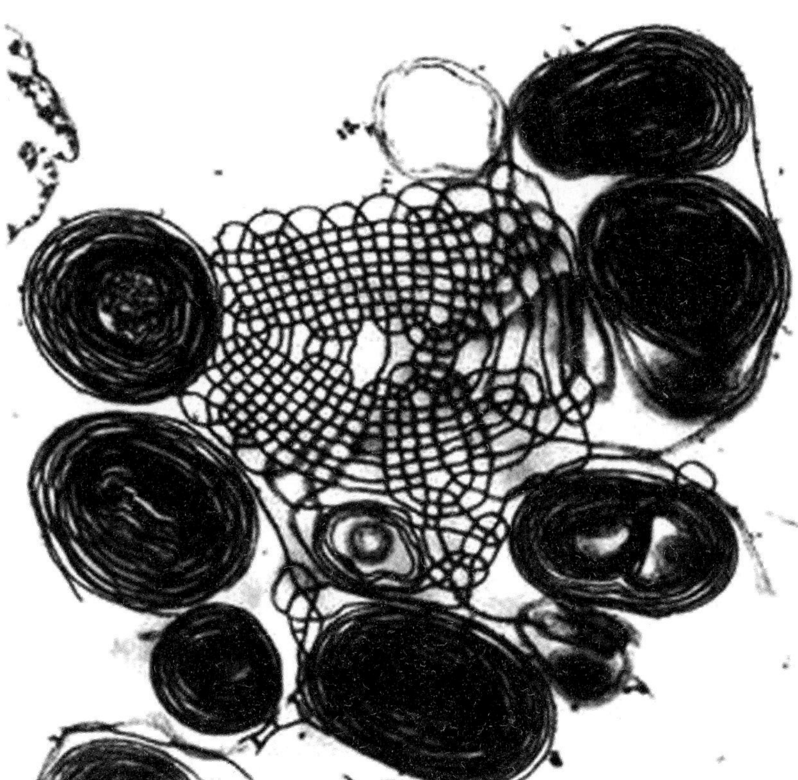

**FIGURE 46–6.** Transmission electron micrograph of lamellar bodies forming tubular myelin in the (fluid-filled) air space of a fetal rat. *(From Polin RA, Fox WW: Fetal and Neonatal Physiology, 3rd ed. Philadelphia, Elsevier, 2003, p 968.)*

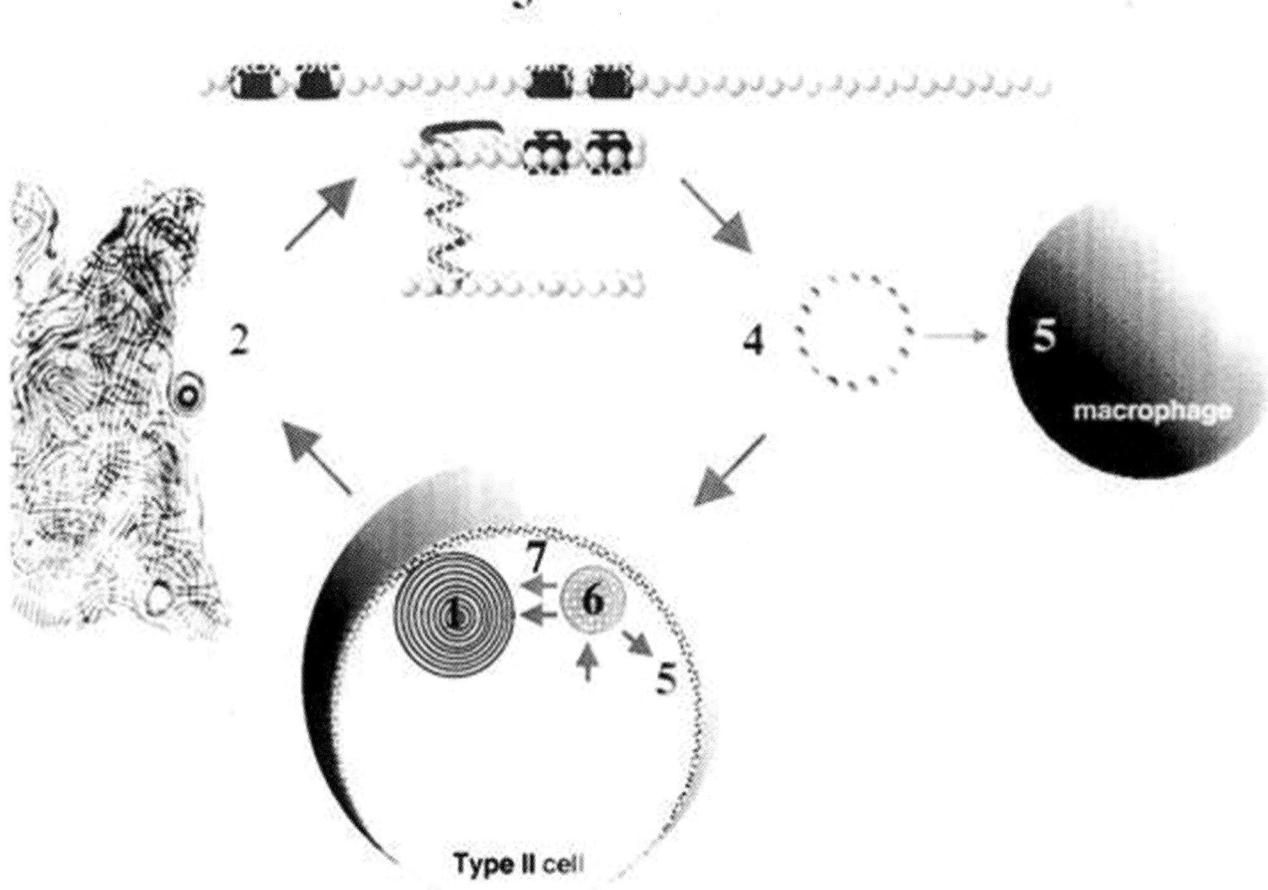


**FIGURE 46–7.** Surfactant homeostasis. 1, Lamellar body. 2, Large aggregate surfactant in alveolar hypophase. 3, Surface film. 4, Small aggregate surfactant. 5, Surfactant catabolic pathway. 6, Multivesicular body. 7, Recycling/biosynthetic pathway. Arrows represent anabolic pathways and catabolic pathways. Peptides are SP-B and SP-C. *(With permission from Weaver T, Conkright J: Functions of surfactant proteins B and C. Annu Rev Physiol 63:555-578, 2001.)*

alveoli, osmiophilic bodies transform into tubular myelin, which in turn form a monomolecular lipid surface film. In concert with the charged phospholipids, the three surfactant proteins—SP-A, SP-B, and SP-C—facilitate this process of adsorption of surfactant lipids to the surface.

**TABLE 46–6**

**Clinical Factors Affecting Fetal Lung Maturation and Presumably Surfactant Synthesis**

| Decrease | Increase |
|---|---|
| Prematurity | Maturity or postmaturity |
| Asphyxia | Maternal glucocorticoid therapy |
| Maternal diabetes | Opiate abuse |
| Elective cesarean section | Alcohol abuse |
| Family history | Black race |
| Maternal hypertension | Female gender |
| Second twin | |
| Erythroblastosis | |
| Male gender | |

From recurring expansion and contraction, the surface film desorbs into the alveolar liquid in the form of small vesicles that are not surface active. These vesicles are either engulfed by macrophages or pinocytosed into alveolar type II cells, where the lipid constituents are recycled. The uptake of used surfactant is under the control of granulocyte-macrophage colony-stimulating factor (GM-CSF), in the absence of which alveolar proteinosis occurs (Reed et al, 1999). The half-life for secreted surfactant in premature infants is over one day. Surfactant instilled in the trachea is thought to be catabolized by similar pathways.

## CLINICAL USES OF SURFACTANT

Today, replacement surfactant is used predominantly in the prophylaxis and treatment of respiratory distress syndrome in preterm infants. It is increasingly recognized, however, that exogenous surfactant has a role in conditions of surfactant inactivation in infants of any gestational age.

Clinical trials demonstrate that administration of surfactant, natural or synthetic, for treatment or prophylaxis is associated with decreased mortality rates and a decrease in the risk of pneumothorax. Suresh and Soll (2001) estimate from meta-analysis a reduction of 30% to 65% in the relative risk of pneumothorax, and up to 40% reduction in the relative risk of death. Surfactant administration reduces the severity of RDS but will not eliminate the mortality and morbidity associated with other complications of prematurity.

Before the use of therapeutic surfactants, RDS usually worsened for a few days after birth, followed by death or improvement. Now, if cost and availability are not problems, surfactant usually is administered in the delivery room to premature infants at significant risk for disease, thereby ameliorating the classic clinical and radiographic signs of RDS (Suresh and Soll, 2001).

### Indications and Timing of Treatment

If surfactant deficiency in the neonate could be confidently predicted antenatally, then early use of exogenous surfactant would be clearly beneficial. It is important to acknowledge, however, that gestational age is inversely related to the accuracy of the test results for fetal lung maturity. Screening tests such as the foam stability test, determination of optical density at 650 nm, and semiquantitative measurement of phosphatidylglycerol have a low positive predictive value and high sensitivity. Quantitative tests such as determination of L/S ratio and saturated phosphatidylcholine assay, on the other hand, have a high predictive value that tends to be associated with low sensitivity.

Prophylactic surfactant administration (defined as giving surfactant in the first minutes of life before overt signs of classic RDS have developed) improves clinical outcome over that obtained with surfactant treatment given later. Studies in preterm animals showed that surfactant treatment given before they breathe or receive positive pressure ventilation is associated with less epithelial damage (Jobe et al, 1993). If surfactant is given at the time of birth, there is a reduction in transvascular protein permeation and reduction in pulmonary edema (Carlton et al, 1995). Surfactant given within 15 minutes of birth produces better clinical outcomes in infants born at less than 31 weeks of gestation who require intubation (Egberts et al, 1997; Soll and Morley, 2001). If 100 such infants were administered prophylactic surfactant, there would be two fewer cases of pneumothorax and five fewer deaths than would occur with later treatment. Surfactant administered in the first 15 minutes of life is just as effective as surfactant given at or before the first breaths (Kendig et al, 1998).

Most infants born at a gestation of less than 27 weeks will be deficient in surfactant. The use of prophylactic surfactant for infants born at greater than 32 weeks of gestation would result in unnecessary treatment in a large number of infants, particularly those whose mothers had received a full course of antenatal corticosteroids. It is not yet clear where the cutoff should be to provide maximum benefit to infants with true surfactant deficiency, while protecting those more mature infants against unnecessary, costly, and possibly harmful administration of exogenous surfactant.

### Surfactant Delivery

In the delivery room, when surfactant is administered in the first minutes of life, the experienced clinician will have ensured that the endotracheal tube tip is truly in the trachea and not in the esophagus. It is equally important that the tube tip is not situated in the right main bronchus. Many endotracheal tubes are designed with a black tip, which, if still partly visible, testifies to the tube tip being in the larynx. When time is not critical, a chest radiograph should be carried out to ascertain that the tube tip position is optimal.

The initial recommendations for positioning during administration of surfactant in order to optimize distribution of surfactant throughout the lung are now often ignored. Survanta, Curosurf, or Infasurf are administered into the endotracheal tube as a liquid in aliquots. An endotracheal tube adaptor with a side hole for instillation obviates the need for disconnecting the infant from the ventilator during surfactant treatment and, in our experience, minimizes the oxygen desaturation sometimes seen with surfactant administration. Surprisingly, bolus administration probably gives better distribution than intratracheal infusions. In animal studies, slow infusions resulted in a non-homogenous distribution pattern (Suresh and Soll, 2001). Walther has found that cerebral blood flow may be altered during surfactant administration probably due to the desaturation episodes with reflex changes in blood pressure (van de Bor, 1991). The goal during administration should be to maintain homeostasis of the infant.

The dosage of surfactant is not well worked out, nor is it known what the dose-response relationships are for infants with RDS of varying degrees of severity. Particularly when surfactant is being instilled in the delivery room, the clinician may not yet know the weight of the infant. Dosages range from 2.5 to 5 mL/kg of body weight and from 50 to 200 mg/kg. Even with use of the smaller volumes, unknown quantities of surfactant may well up through or around the endotracheal tube. These effects can be minimized by two methods: First, while the bolus of surfactant is being instilled, gentle pressure on the cricoid will reduce the amount of surfactant returning around the endotracheal tube. Also, for some of the smallest infants who are unstable, we may give a half-dose, followed by another half-dose 30 minutes later.

Some authorities have suggested the use of surfactant given in the delivery room with immediate extubation, followed by continuous distending airway pressure (i.e., CPAP) administered by nasal prongs in an effort to reduce ventilator damage to the lungs. The decision must be made clinically. For an infant with good respiratory drive and an $FIO_2$ of less than 0.30 extubation after surfactant administration is likely to be successful. The early use of nasal CPAP is safe under these circumstances, but it is not yet known whether the combination of prophylactic surfactant and nasal CPAP will reduce the incidence of chronic lung disease (Thomson, 2002).

### Choice of Surfactant: Natural Versus Synthetic Surfactants

Although both synthetic, protein-free surfactants and natural (animal-derived) surfactants have both been shown to improve outcome, they vary in effectiveness. Natural surfactant has rapid action, and most natural surfactants contain both SP-B and SP-C. Meta-analysis of comparisons in clinical trials shows that natural surfactants are associated with fewer air leaks and improved survival compared with synthetic surfactants (Soll and Blanco, 2001). One study comparing the synthetic surfactant Pumactant with porcine surfactant Curosurf was stopped early because of the lower mortality rate for the infants receiving natural surfactant (Ainsworth et al, 2000). Despite the theoretical advantages of protein-free synthetic surfactants and their relative ease of manufacture with lesser costs, the improved clinical results with natural surfactants have resulted in their largely supplanting the protein-free synthetic surfactants.

### *Comparisons of Natural Surfactants*

Only a few large, well-controlled trials have compared modified natural surfactants. Bloom and colleagues (1997) carried out a prospective, randomized, double-blind, multicenter clinical trial that compared the relative safety and efficacy of Infasurf with Survanta. Thirteen neonatal intensive care units (NICUs) participated. A total of 608 infants with RDS were randomly assigned to receive Infasurf or Survanta in a dose of 100 mg/kg, with an initial dose of 4 mL/kg. Twenty-two percent of the infants who received Infasurf and 33% of those who received Survanta required a fourth dose. The interval between doses was significantly longer for Infasurf. The average fraction of inspired oxygen ($FIO_2$) was lower in the infants who received Infasurf during the first 24 hours, by about 5% to 10%. Differences were not apparent after 24 hours. These investigators also evaluated prophylaxis with Survanta versus Infasurf in 374 infants born at 29 weeks of gestation at birth weights of less than 1250 g. In this group of infants, those receiving Infasurf had longer interdose intervals after the second dose compared with those receiving Survanta, but equal numbers of doses of surfactant were administered to both groups of infants. No differences in inspired oxygen concentration or mean airway pressure were noted in the prevention group. The survival rate was higher in the Survanta treatment group by 6%, and the mortality rate for infants with weights of less than 600 g was extremely low (26%) in the Survanta treatment group, compared with 63% in the Infasurf treatment group. The investigators attributed the extremely low mortality rate to chance in the very low-birth-weight group of infants who received Survanta. Infants who received Survanta required more days of ventilation and oxygen support, primarily because of increased survival of those weighing only 600 g at birth. In both the treatment and prophylaxis groups, no significant differences were found for air leaks, complications associated with dosing, complications of prematurity, overall mortality, or survival without chronic lung disease.

A more recent retrospective review of 5169 records of neonates who received either Survanta or Infasurf concluded that there is no difference in mortality rates for infants receiving these two exogenous surfactants, in contrast with the study described before. There also was no difference found in the incidence of necrotizing enterocolitis or intraventricular hemorrhage or in length of hospital stay (Clark et al, 2001).

Speer and colleagues (1995) compared Survanta with Curosurf regimens in a randomized clinical trial. Seventy-five infants (birth weights 700 to 1500 g) with established RDS received an initial dose of Curosurf (200 mg/kg) or Survanta (100 mg/kg). Patients who remained ventilator dependent with an $FIO_2$ greater than 0.3 received up to two additional doses of Curosurf (each 100 mg/kg) or up to three additional doses of Survanta (each 100 mg/kg). Infants who received Curosurf had increased oxygenation and reduced ventilatory requirements compared with such requirements in infants who received Survanta, for up to 24 hours after initial treatment. The average total dose was 273 mg/kg in the Curosurf treatment group and 218 mg/kg in the Survanta treatment group. Differences in total duration of ventilation and total time of exposure to supplemental oxygen between the two groups were not significant. Although comparing Curosurf at twice the dose of Survanta, this study shows few differences that could be considered clinically significant; however, important differences could be masked by small numbers of enrolled infants.

A recently reported study comparing Curosurf with Survanta showed significantly less oxygen use over 6 days when Curosurf was administered (Ramanathan et al, 2002).

In summary, whereas large clinical differences were found in comparisons of natural with synthetic protein-free surfactants, relatively small differences are found in clinical trials that compare different natural surfactants. Whatever differences are evident may be due either to differences in the infants under study or the surfactants being compared or to the differing dosages. It remains unclear what the optimal concentrations and volumes for surfactant treatment should be. Based on animal experiments, it is probable that higher doses of surfactant will be necessary for lung injuries in which surfactant inactivation plays a role.

Although surfactant may be beneficial for lung diseases other than RDS (see later on), no comparative studies on the use of surfactants for these different diseases have been conducted.

## Interactions with Steroids

Corticosteroids given before preterm birth are effective in preventing RDS and neonatal mortality (see also Chapters 42 and 47). The efficacy of neonatal surfactant therapy is enhanced by antenatal exposure to corticosteroids (Jobe et al, 1993).

## Dosage of Exogenous Surfactant

Dosages between 50 and 200 mg/kg have been used successfully in animal and human studies, with retreatment occurring up to four times in the first 24 hours. These dosages form the basis for the manufacturers' recommendations for dosage and retreatment. (Repeated doses of surfactant are thought to be useful because they overcome inactivation that may result from soluble proteins and other factors present in the alveoli.) The meta-analysis of studies that compare single with multiple doses shows that repeated doses decrease the risk for pneumothoraces and death. No complications were reported with multiple doses (Suresh and Soll, 2001).

There is reason to follow the manufacturers' recommendations (maximum of four doses of Survanta, given every 6 hours; two of Curosurf, given every 12 hours; and three doses of Infasurf, also given every 12 hours). This phenomenon may be due to alveolar damage and inactivation occurring during the natural course of the disease. If an infant has responded to the first dose and has subsequently deteriorated, a second dose should be seriously considered, even if the recommended time gap has not yet elapsed, and even if the chest radiograph indicates relatively well-expanded lung fields. Usually the most remarkable responses are seen after the first dose. Rarely have we seen dramatic responses after a third or fourth dose.

### Clinical Responses

If extubation of the infant after instillation of exogenous surfactant is not clinically indicated, pediatricians should nevertheless be aware of the rapid improvements in pulmonary compliance that follow a dose of natural surfactant. Within minutes, the requirement for positive pressure and enriched oxygen are much diminished. To avoid damage to the alveoli from barotrauma, positive inspiratory pressures must be rapidly reduced, along with $FIO_2$. A not unusual scenario is the use of 80% $FIO_2$ and positive inspiratory pressure (PIP) of 22 cm $H_2O$ for respiratory support of the infant; then, after instillation of a dose of natural surfactant, the improved pulmonary compliance dictates reduction of PIP to 16 cm $H_2O$ and of $FIO_2$ to 25%. The data of Fujiwara (1990) and Charon (1989) and their colleagues indicate that about 65% of infants with RDS have a sustained improvement with exogenous surfactant; about 20% have a transient improvement, followed by a relapse requiring further surfactant treatment; and about 15% do not have a significant response (Fig. 46–8). Response to surfactant constitutes an indicator of survival (Hamvas et al, 1993; Kuint et al, 1994). In the case of Survanta, a poor response and the need for a fourth dose have been associated with the development of bronchopulmonary dysplasia.

Possible reasons for a poor response include:

- The patient may not have RDS, and particularly in the near-term infant, SP-B deficiency should be considered (see also Chapter 42).
- The patient may have RDS, but a severe complication in another organ may cause clinical deterioration—in particular, intraventricular hemorrhage.
- The patient may have RDS, but there may an additional problem in the lung, such as pneumonia, interstitial edema, or pulmonary edema due to patent ductus arteriosus or excessive fluid intake (Hallman et al, 1991). Poor responders, before treatment, may have a higher airway resistance than that in good responders (Wallenbrock et al, 1992). This may reflect the general level of injury and lung edema.
- The RDS may be so severe that the dose is insufficient.
- The ventilation settings may not be optimal.
- The surfactant preparation may not optimal.
- Surfactant activity may have been inhibited by plasma proteins and other serum or airway (meconium) substances.

Among infants with a clinical diagnosis of RDS, some may be found to have high levels of static respiratory compliance incompatible with a diagnosis of surfactant deficiency. A majority of such infants will respond poorly to treatment with exogenous surfactant (Stenson et al, 1994). Nevertheless, static respiratory compliance measurement has not lent itself to routine use in NICUs.

### Monitoring

During administration of the exogenous surfactant, heart rate, color, chest expansion, oximeter and endotracheal tube patency have to be monitored. If surfactant is being administered by infusion and the heart rate slows down or oxygen saturation falls more than 15%, dosing should be slowed down or stopped. The child should be carefully evaluated clinically to establish the cause of the deterioration. Pulmonary hemorrhage is a rare complication of surfactant administration. If chest expansion improves substantially after dosing, peak ventilator inspiratory pressures should be reduced immediately. Failure or delay to reduce pressures can result in lung overdistention and pulmonary air leak. The clinician must be in constant attendance of the child during the first 30 minutes, to compensate for the acute changes in compliance.

Although the incidence of patent ductus arteriosus may not increase after surfactant treatment, we have the strong clinical impression that the time of onset of left-to-right shunting may be affected—that is, the onset of manifestations of a clinically significant PDA may occur within 36 hours of birth, as pulmonary vascular resistance decreases sooner. In our experience, some infants have evidence of large left-to-right shunts at 12 to 18 hours of age after surfactant treatment, which may be a factor predisposing to intraventricular hemorrhage.

The most commonly experienced adverse effects of surfactant administration are cardiorespiratory or mechanical. In some infants, acute bradycardia or even cardiac arrest develops. Sometimes the endotracheal tube will become blocked with surfactant, and occasionally it is necessary to clear such a blockage urgently, or even to change the endotracheal tube. Intubation of the right main bronchus can result in delivery of the surfactant to the right side only, and this can cause overexpansion of the right lung and atelectasis of the left lung.

Surfactant instillation can cause transient suppression of the electroencephalogram (Lundstrom and Greisen, 1996). The cause of this suppression is not known, nor has it been linked to a long-term detrimental outcome.

No other significant toxicity has been documented. Concern has existed whether sensitivity to bovine surfactant and serum proteins would occur. No problems in this regard have been reported, and Chida and colleagues (1988) have indicated that surfactant treatment may actually suppress formation of autoantibody to surfactant proteins by reducing the alveolar-capillary leaks associated with lung damage incurred by the disease process and its treatment (e.g., barotrauma).

### Long-Term Outcome

Although surfactant has reduced significantly the mortality rate for preterm infants, there is no good evidence that the incidence of chronic lung disease has diminished significantly. The explanation for this lack of improvement in

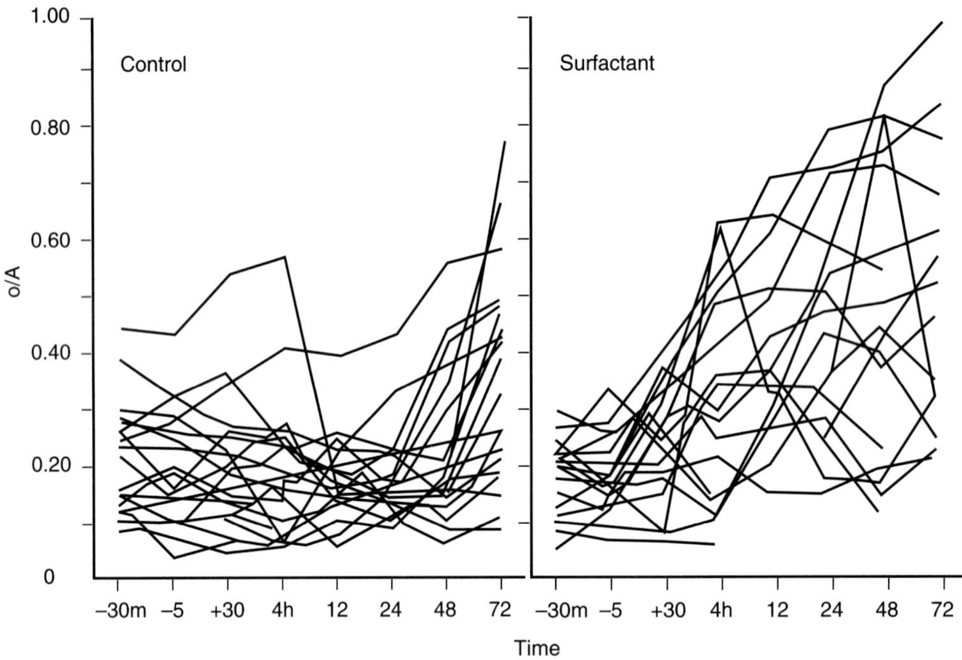


**FIGURE 46–8.** Sequential arterial-to-alveolar ratios are plotted against time for control infants or infants treated with surfactant. Variability is marked for both groups, but improvement from 4 to 48 hours after treatment is apparent in the group receiving surfactant. Arterial-alveolar ratios of more than 0.8 are expected for infants with normal lung function. The scale on the abscissa is nonlinear (−30 m, −5, +30 indicate minutes before and after treatment). *(Redrawn from Chida S, Phelps DS, et al: Surfactant-associated proteins in tracheal aspirates of infants with respiratory distress syndrome after exogenous surfactant therapy. Am Rev Resp Dis 137:943, 1988.)*

outcomes in these children may be due to the effect of surfactant itself. With exogenous surfactant therapy and prenatal steroids, smaller infants survive, and the pathogenesis of bronchopulmonary dysplasia may have changed from barotrauma and toxicity lesions to an inflammatory response due to prolonged ventilation and infection. However, the more severe cases have become less common (Bancalari and del Moral, 2001).

### Surfactant Use in Diseases Other than Respiratory Distress Syndrome

Many neonatal pulmonary conditions including RDS have an element of surfactant inactivation from leakage of plasma across damaged endothelial and epithelial membranes into alveoli (Landmann et al, 2002). The rationale for the use of surfactant for conditions other than RDS is that inactivation (usually by leakage of serum constituents into alveoli) may be reversed to some degree by surfactant treatment. Obviously, surfactant inactivation and surfactant insufficiency may be superimposed in some infants with RDS, such as those with severe birth asphyxia. Some clinical data suggest that surfactant is useful in infants with pneumonia, diaphragmatic hernia with lung hypoplasia, meconium aspiration, and ARDS and in some infants who require extracorporeal membrane oxygenation (ECMO) (Fig. 46–9). Infants and children with acute lung injuries, pulmonary hemorrhage, bronchiolitis, chronic bronchitis, asthma, and lung transplantation may eventually be candidates for therapy with newer surfactants.

If meconium constituents reach alveoli, surfactant can be inactivated. Meconium has a dose-dependent effect on surfactant that can be overcome by high doses of surfactant. Several reports have now shown that replacement surfactant has a role in the treatment of meconium aspiration syndrome, limiting disease severity and reducing the need for extracorporeal membrane oxygenation (Findlay et al, 1996; Halliday et al, 1996; Soll and Dargaville, 2002). It is not yet clear whether surfactant lavage provides any clinical benefit over surfactant instillation, although in preliminary work, Wiswell and colleagues (2002) found that lung lavage with fluid containing surfactant improves outcomes. Herting and colleagues (2000) conducted a study to evaluate surfactant effectiveness in neonates with respiratory failure and group B streptococcal (GBS) infection. They concluded that surfactant therapy improves gas exchange in a majority of patients with GBS pneumonia. The response is slower than in the treated patients with RDS, and repeated doses are often required. Surfactant therapy has a place in the management of respiratory failure in term infants even in the absence of known meconium aspiration syndrome or pneumonia (Lotze et al, 1998).

Other conditions suggested as indications for surfactant use include congenital diaphragmatic hernia, respiratory syncytial virus pneumonia, pulmonary hemorrhage, bronchopulmonary dysplasia, bronchiolitis, asthma, and adult (acute) RDS (Curley and Halliday, 2001; Wiswell, 2001).

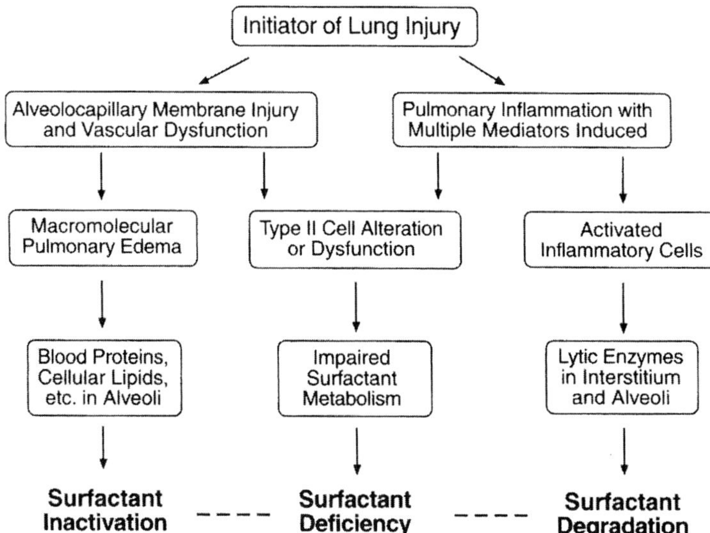


**FIGURE 46–9.** Schematic representation of surfactant-related events in acute respiratory distress syndrome (ARDS)-related lung injury. As part of the pathophysiology of acute lung injury (ALI) and ARDS, surfactant can be inactivated by biophysical interactions with inhibitory compounds present in the lungs through edema and inflammation. Active surfactant components also can be degraded or altered chemically, and surfactant can become deficient due to type II cell injury or alteration. Surfactant dysfunction/deficiency can also result from depletion or alteration of active large surfactant aggregate subtypes. Not shown are the multiple aspects of inflammatory lung injury unrelated to lung surfactant that also contribute to ARDS. *(From Notter R: Lung Surfactants: Basic Science and Clinical Applications. New York, Marcel Dekker, 2000, p 246.)*

## NEW APPROACHES

After all the clinical and laboratory-based evidence in favor of the use of surfactant, a reasonable question is whether this therapy is good enough. Because the most commonly used surfactants are derived from lung lavage or minced lung of animals, we remain in an era not dissimilar from the times when ground thyroid or animal-derived insulins were used for replacement therapy. Batch-to-batch variation, requirement for intratracheal administration, possible inclusion of unknown impurities, the remote possibility of transmission of infectious agents, the theoretical possibility of immunologic consequences, the susceptibility to inactivation, and, finally, cost per dose (about $400/vial, with 1 or 2 vials required per newborn) all are reasons to seek to improve what is already extraordinarily beneficial.

Theoretically, administration of surfactant by aerosolisation should be less of a physical challenge to the infant. Unfortunately, only small amounts of aerosolized surfactant are successfully delivered to the lung, and its use in combination with CPAP has shown no clear clinical benefits to surfactant administration via the trachea (Berggren et al, 2000).

Much current work is aimed at developing synthetic or partially synthetic surfactants using modified lipids or surfactant proteins that are synthesized or made by recombinant DNA technology—or by including organic polymers that mimic some of the activities of the surfactant proteins (Taeusch and Keough, 2001). Surfactants containing analogues of SP-C or SP-B show promise (Hafner et al, 1999; Palmblad et al, 2001; Walther, 2000).

## REFERENCES

Ainsworth S, Beresford M, Milligan D, et al: Pumactant and poractant alpha for treatment of respiratory distress syndrome in neonates born at 25-29 weeks' gestation. Lancet 355: 1387-1392, 2000.

Amin R, Wert S, Baughman R, et al: Surfactant protein deficiency in familial interstitial lung disease. J Pediatr 139:85-92, 2001.

Avery M: Surfactant deficiency in hyaline membrane disease. Am J Respir Crit Care Med 161:1074-1075, 2000.

Avery ME, Mead J: Surface properties in relation to atelectasis and hyaline membrane disease. Am J Dis Child 97:517, 1959.

Bancalari E, del Moral T: Bronchopulmonary dysplasia and surfactant. Biol Neonate 80(suppl 1):7-13, 2001.

Berggren E, Liljedahl M, Winbladh B, et al: Pilot study of nebulized surfactant therapy for neonatal respiratory distress syndrome. Acta Paediatr 89:460-464, 2000.

Bernhard W, Mottaghian J, Gebert A, et al: Commercial versus native surfactants. Am J Respir Crit Care Med 162:1524-1533, 2000.

Bloom B, Kattwinkel J, Hall R, et al: Comparison of Infasurf (calf lung surfactant extract) to Survanta (Beractant) in the treatment and prevention of respiratory distress syndrome. Pediatrics 100:31-38, 1997.

Carlton D, Cho S, Davis P, et al: Surfactant treatment at birth reduces lung vascular injury and edema in preterm lambs. Pediatr Res 37:265-270, 1995.

Charon A, Taeusch H, Fitzgibbon C, et al: Factors associated with surfactant treatment response in infants with severe respiratory distress syndrome. Pediatrics 83:348-354, 1989.

Chida S, Phelps DS, Soll RF, et al: Surfactant proteins and anti-surfactant antibodies in sera from infants with respiratory distress syndrome with and without surfactant treatment. Pediatrics 88:84-89, 1988.

Clark R, Auten R, Peabody J: A comparison of the outcome of the neonates treated with two different natural surfactants. J Pediatr 139:828-831, 2001.

Clements JA, Avery ME: Lung surfactant and neonatal respiratory distress syndrome. Am J Respir Crit Care Med 157:S59-S66, 1998.

Cole FS, Hamvas A, Nogee LM: Genetic disorders of neonatal respiratory function. Pediatr Res 50:157-162, 2001.

Comroe J Jr: Retrospectroscope: Insights into Medical Discovery. Menlo Park, Calif, Von Gehr Press, 1977.

Copland B, Post M: Understanding the mechanisms of infant respiratory distress and chronic lung disease. Am J Respir Cell Mol Biol 3:261-265, 2002.

Curley A, Halliday H: The present status of exogenous surfactant for the newborn. Early Hum Dev 61:67-83, 2001.

Curosurf package insert NDA 20-744: 1-7. Chiesi Farmaceutici, Parma, Italy.

Egberts J, Brand R, Walti H, et al: Mortality, severe respiratory distress syndrome and chronic lung disease of the newborn are reduced more after prophylactic than after therapeutic administration of the surfactant. Pediatrics 100:E4, 1997.

Findlay RD, Taeusch HW, et al: Surfactant replacement therapy for meconium aspiration syndrome. Pediatrics 97:48-52, 1996.

Fujiwara T, Konishi M, et al: Surfactant replacement therapy with a single, post-ventilatory dose of a reconstituted bovine surfactant in preterm neonates with respiratory distress syndrome: Final analysis of a multicenter, double-blind, randomized trial and comparison with similar trials. Pediatrics 86: 753-764, 1990.

Fujiwara T, Maeta H, et al: Artificial surfactant therapy in hyaline membrane disease. Lancet 1:55-59, 1980.

Griese M, Maderlechner N, et al: Surfactant proteins A and D in children with pulmonary disease due to gastroesophageal reflux. Am J Respir Crit Care Med 165:1546-1550, 2002.

Haagsman HP, Van Eijk M, et al: Protein composition and surface activity of commercial surfactant preparations. Am J Respir Crit Care Med 155:A213, 1997.

Hafner D, Germann P, et al: Effects of early treatment with rSP-C surfactant on oxygenation and histology in rats with acute lung injury. Pulmon Pharmacol Ther 12:193-201, 1999.

Halliday H, Speer C, Robertson B: Treatment of severe meconium aspiration syndrome with porcine surfactant. Eur J Pediatr 155:1047-1051, 1996.

Hallman M, Glumoff V, Ramet M: Surfactant in respiratory distress syndrome and lung injury. Comp Biochem Physiol 129:287-294, 2001.

Hallman M, Merritt T, Akino T, et al: Surfactant protein A, phosphatidylcholine, and surfactant inhibitors in epithelial lining fluid: Correlation with surface activity, severity of respiratory distress syndrome, and outcome in small premature infants. Am Rev Respir Dis 144:1376-1384, 1991.

Hamvas A, Devine T, Cole FS: Surfactant therapy failure identifies infants at risk for pulmonary mortality. Am J Dis Child 147:665-668, 1993.

Herting E, Gefeller O, Land M, et al: Surfactant treatment of neonates with respiratory failure and group B sreptococcal infection. Pediatrics 106:957-964, 2000.

Jobe AH, Mitchell BR, Gunkel JH: Beneficial effects of the combined use of prenatal corticosteroids and postnatal surfactant on preterm infants. Am J Obstet Gynecol 168:508-513, 1993.

Johansson J, Curstedt T: Molecular structures and interactions of pulmonary surfactant components. Eur J Biochem 244: 675-693, 1997.

Kahn M, Anderson G, Anyan WR, et al: Phosphatidylcholine molecular species of calf lung surfactant. Am J Physiol 13:L567-L573, 1995.

Kattwinkel J: Surfactant lavage for meconium aspiration: A word of caution. Pediatrics 109:1167-1168, 2002.

Kendig J, Ryan R, Sinkin RA, et al: Comparison of two strategies for surfactant prophylaxis in very premature infants: A multicenter randomized trial. Pediatrics 101:1006-1012, 1998.

Kruger P, Baatz J, Dhuly RA, et al: Effect of hydrophobic surfactant protein SP-C on binary phospholipid monolayers: Molecular machinery at the air/water interface. Biophys Chem 99:209-228, 2002.

Kuint J, Reichman B, Neumann L, et al: Prognostic value of the immediate response to surfactant. Arch Dis Child Fetal Neonat Ed 71:170-173, 1994.

Landmann E, Gortner L, Reiss L, et al: Protein content and biophysical properties of tracheal aspirates from neonates with respiratory failure. Klin Paediatr 214:1-7, 2002.

Lotze A, Mitchell B, Bulas DI, et al: Multicenter study of surfactant (Beractant) use in the treatment of term infants with respiratory failure. J Pediatr 132:40-47, 1998.

Lundstrom K, Greisen G: Changes in EEG: Systemic circulation and blood gas parameters following two or six aliquots of porcine surfactant. Acta Paediatr 85:708-712, 1996.

Malloy M, Freeman D: Respiratory distress syndrome mortality in the United States, 1987-1995. J Perinatol 20:414-420, 2000.

McCormack F, Whitsett J: The pulmonary collectins, SP-A and SP-D, orchestrate innate immunity in the lung. J Clin Invest 109:707-712, 2002.

Notter R: Lung Surfactants: Basic Science and Clinical Applications. New York, Marcel Dekker, 2000.

Palmblad M, Gustafsson M, Curstedt T, et al: Surface activity and film formation from the surface associated material of artificial surfactant preparations. Biochim Biophys Acta 1510:106-117, 2001.

Perez-Gil J: Molecular interactions in pulmonary surfactant films. Biol Neonate 81(suppl 1):6-15, 2002.

Postle A, Heeley E, Wilton DC: A comparison of the molecular species compositions of mamalian lung surfactant phospholipids. Comp Biochem Physiol 129:65-73, 2001.

Ramanathan R, Rasmussen M, Gertsmann D, et al: A randomized multicenter masked comparison trial of Curosurf and Survanta in the treatment of RDS in preterm infants [abstract]. Biol Neonate 81(suppl 1):36, 2002.

Reed J, Ikegami M, Cianciolo E, et al: Aerosolized GM-CSF ameliorates pulmonary alveolar proteinosis in GM-CSF–deficient mice. Am J Physiol 276: L556-L563, 1999.

Schürch S, Goerke J, Clements JA: Direct determination of surface tension in the lung. Proc Natl Acad Sci U S A 73:7720-7726, 1976.

Seeger W, Grube C, Gunther A, et al: Surfactant inhibition by plasma proteins: Differential sensitivity of various surfactant preparations. Eur Respir J 6:971-977, 1993.

Soll R, Blanco F: Natural surfactant extract versus synthetic surfactant for neonatal respiratory distress syndrome. Cochrane Database Syst Rev 2001.

Soll R, Dargaville P: Surfactant for meconium aspiration syndrome in full term infants. Cochrane Database Syst Rev CD002054, 2002.

Soll R, Morley C: Prophylactic versus selective use of surfactant in preventing morbidity and mortality in preterm infants. Cochrane Database Syst Rev CD000510, 2002.

Speer C, Gefeller O, Groneck P, et al: Randomised clinical trial of two treatment regimens of natural surfactant preparations in neonatal respiratory distress syndrome. Arch Dis Child 72: F8-F13, 1995.

Stenson B, Glover R, Parry GJ, et al: Static respiratory compliance in the newborn. III: Early changes after exogenous surfactant treatment. Arch Dis Child 70: F19-F24, 1994.

Suresh K, Soll R: Current surfactant use in premature infants. Clin Perinatol 28:671-690, 2001.

Taeusch HW, Keough KM: Inactivation of pulmonary surfactant and the treatment of acute lung injuries. Pediatr Pathol Mol Med 20:519-536, 2001.

Thomson M: Continuous positive airway pressure and surfactant: Combined data from animal experiments and clinical trials. Biol Neonate Suppl 1:16-19, 2002.

van de Bor M, Ma E, Walther F: Cerebral blood flow velocity after surfactant instillation in preterm infants. J Pediatr 118:285-287, 1991.

Wallenbrock M, Sekar K, Toubas P: Prediction of the acute response to surfactant therapy by pulmonary function testing. Pediatr Pulmonol 13:11-15, 1992.

Walther F, Gordon L, Zasadzinski J, et al: Surfactant protein B and C analogues. Mol Genet Metab 71:342-351, 2000.

Wang Z, Baatz J, Holm B, et al: Content-dependent activity of lung surfactant protein B in mixtures with lipids. Am J Physiol Lung Cell Mol Physiol 283:L897-L906, 2002.

Warriner H, Ding J, Waring A, et al: A concentration dependent mechanism by which serum albumin inactivates replacement lung surfactants. Biophys J 82:835-842, 2002.

Whitsett J, Weaver T: Hydrophobic surfactant proteins in lung function and disease. N Engl J Med 347:2141-2148, 2002.

Wiswell T: Expanded uses of surfactant therapy. Clin Perinatol 28:695-710, 2001.

Wiswell T, Knight G, Finer N, et al: A multicenter, randomized controlled trial comparing Surfaxin (lucinactant) lavage with standard care for treatment of meconium aspiration syndrome. Pediatrics 109:1081-1087, 2002.

CHAPTER

# 47

# Respiratory Distress in the Preterm Infant

**Stephen Welty, Thomas N. Hansen, and Anthony Corbet**

## RESPIRATORY DISTRESS SYNDROME

Respiratory distress syndrome (RDS), previously referred to as *hyaline membrane disease* (HMD), occurs after the onset of breathing in infants with insufficiency of the pulmonary surfactant system.

### Epidemiology

An estimated 40,000 cases of RDS occur annually in the United States (Farrell and Wood, 1976), affecting about 14% of all low-birth-weight infants (Farrell and Avery, 1975). The incidence is 60% at 29 weeks of gestation but declines with maturation to near zero by 39 weeks (Usher et al, 1971). The condition is more common in male than in female infants (Miller and Futrakul, 1968) and is more common in white than in nonwhite infants (Richardson and Torday, 1994); at each level of gestational age, RDS is less common in black infants, and this phenomenon is not explained by other factors that may influence lung maturity (Hulsey et al, 1993). At any given gestational age, the incidence is higher for infants born by cesarean section without labor than for those born by vaginal delivery (Fedrick and Butler, 1972); there is a significantly increased risk if elective cesarean section is performed before completion of 39 weeks of gestation (Morrison et al, 1995).

When the occurrence of RDS is corrected for the important effect of gestational age, the occurrence of RDS is significantly increased in gestational diabetes and in insulin-dependent mothers without vascular disease (Robert et al, 1976). Most such infants of diabetic mothers are large for gestational age, and similar overnourished infants in the absence of maternal diabetes also are at increased risk (Naeye et al, 1974). Evidence suggests that the incidence of RDS in infants of diabetic mothers is now much less, almost certainly because of improved medical control of diabetes (Kjos et al, 1990).

Early reports in comparatively large infants suggested that the risk is decreased in infants who are small for gestational age (Gluck and Kulovich, 1973). In the much less mature infants seen more recently, however, comparisons of appropriate (weight)-for-gestational-age (AGA) and small-for-gestational-age (SGA) infants, both weight-matched and gestation-matched, suggest that immature SGA infants do not have this advantage (Pena et al, 1988). In fact, there is some evidence that the risk of RDS at constant gestational age may be increased in SGA infants, that the mortality rate may be higher (Lemons et al, 2001; Thompson et al, 1992; Tyson et al, 1995), and that the development of bronchopulmonary dysplasia (BPD) is more likely. Maternal conditions that compromise fetal growth also may be associated with decreased risk, including pregnancy-induced hypertension (Yoon et al, 1980), chronic hypertension, subacute placental abruption, narcotic addiction (Glass et al, 1971), and maternal smoking. More recently, Tubman and colleagues (1991) found an increased risk for RDS in infants of hypertensive mothers; this was because of the high incidence of cesarean section delivery without benefit of labor. There is some evidence that the incidence of RDS may be reduced in infants of cocaine-addicted mothers (Zuckerman et al, 1991).

There has been controversy about whether prolonged rupture of membranes may protect against RDS (Jones et al, 1975). A more recent stepwise discriminant analysis suggested that when gestational age is carefully controlled, pulmonary maturation continues but is not accelerated after premature rupture of the membranes (PROM). In fact, there is a strong suggestion that PROM actually increases the risk of RDS at a given gestational age (Hallak and Bottoms, 1993). Suggestions that birth asphyxia predisposes infants to RDS (Table 47–1) are based on lower Apgar scores in human infants with RDS (James, 1975) and some experimental evidence in lambs (Orzalezi et al, 1965). In an examination of umbilical artery blood at birth, however, it was found that infants with RDS are not more acidemic at birth (Kenny et al, 1976), and that lower Apgar scores associated with RDS are better explained by relative immaturity and defective lung function. Other studies have confirmed that infants with RDS are not more acidemic at birth (Hibbard et al, 1991; Tejani and Verma, 1989). Furthermore, in a study of premature twins, although second-born twins had a higher incidence of RDS than first-born twins, as reported previously, and had much lower Apgar scores, there was no evidence for increased acidemia in cord blood samples of either all second-born twins or all second-born twins with RDS (Kenny et al, 1977).

### Pathology

The gross findings at autopsy include diffuse lung atelectasis, congestion, and edema; if the lungs are inflated at postmortem examination, distensibility is found to be greatly reduced, and the lungs collapse more readily with deflation (Gribetz et al, 1959). On histologic examination, the peripheral air spaces are collapsed, but more proximal respiratory bronchioles, lined with necrotic epithelium and hyaline membranes, have an overdistended appearance (Finlay-Jones et al, 1974) (Figs. 47–1 and 47–2). There is obvious pulmonary edema with congested capillaries, and the lymphatic and interstitial spaces are distended with fluid. The epithelial damage appears within 30 minutes of the onset of breathing; the hyaline membranes, composed of plasma exudation products and associated with damaged

**TABLE 47-1**

**Respiratory Distress Syndrome**

**Epidemiology**
Worldwide
Prematurity predisposes
Cesarean section without labor predisposes
Perinatal asphyxia predisposes
Male > female
White > black
Second-born twin at greater risk
PROM spares
IUGR spares
Maternal stress spares
Maternal diabetes predisposes if < 37 weeks
Maternal hemorrhage predisposes

**Clinical Signs**
Onset near the time of birth
Retractions and tachypnea
Expiratory grunt
Cyanosis
Systemic hypotension
Characteristic chest film
Course to death or improvement in 3 to 5 days
Fine inspiratory rales
Hypothermia
Peripheral edema
Pulmonary edema

**Pathophysiology**
Reduced lung compliance
Reduced FRC
Poor lung distensibility
Poor alveolar stability
Right-to-left shunts
Reduced effective pulmonary blood flow
If hypotensive and hypoxic, poor peripheral perfusion, poor renal perfusion, myocardial malfunction
Patent ductus arteriosus contributes

**Pathobiochemistry**
Respiratory acidosis
Decreased saturated phospholipids
Low AF L/S ratio
Low surfactant-associated proteins
Decreased total serum proteins
Decreased fibrinolysis
Low thyroxine levels

**Pathology**
Atelectasis
Injury to epithelial cells, edema
Membrane contains fibrin and cellular products
No tubular myelin
Osmiophilic lamellar bodies decreased early, increased later

**Etiology**
Surfactant deficiency during disease
Probable inadequate hormonal (corticoid) stimulus in utero
DPL synthesis impaired and/or destruction increased
Autonomic dysfunction

**Prevention**
Prenatal glucocorticoids for >24 hours
Surfactant replacement before 1–2 hours

AF, amniotic fluid; DPL, dipalmitoyl lecithin; FRC, functional residual capacity; IUGR, intrauterine growth retardation/restriction; L/S, lecithin/sphingomyelin; PROM, prolonged rupture of membranes (>16 hours).

capillaries, appear within 3 hours of birth (Gandy et al, 1970). In experimental animals, the bronchiolar lesions may be completely prevented (Nilsson et al, 1978), and the leakage of protein may be considerably reduced (Ikegami et al, 1992), by the administration of exogenous surfactant at birth. This finding indicates that the bronchiolar lesions are secondary to atelectasis in terminal air spaces and to disruptive overdistention of more proximal airways. Pulmonary edema is a common finding in infants with RDS and probably represents an acute inflammatory process. Studies in premature lambs demonstrate that there is a marked accumulation of neutrophils within the air spaces and capillaries within 2 hours of delivery and stabilization, which is associated with permeability pulmonary edema (Bland et al, 2000), and that neutrophil depletion totally abrogates the development of pulmonary edema. There is indirect evidence that neutrophils play a role in lung injury in infants with RDS. Circulating neutrophil counts are lower in infants with RDS than in infants without RDS, and the neutrophil count is inversely correlated with the severity of RDS (Brus et al, 1997). Circulating neutrophils from infants with RDS have more activation markers on their surface than are seen in neutrophils from infants without RDS (Nupponen et al, 2002), and neutrophil oxidation products are much higher in tracheal aspirates from infants with RDS than in those from infants without RDS (Buss et al, 2003). These findings indicate that neutrophil activation is a prominent feature in RDS, which then leads to vascular injury and subsequent pulmonary edema observed histologically.

### Pathophysiology

In RDS the respiratory rate is elevated, so despite a reduction in each tidal volume, the minute ventilation initially is increased. The functional residual capacity (FRC), analyzed by nitrogen washout, is reduced: the greater the

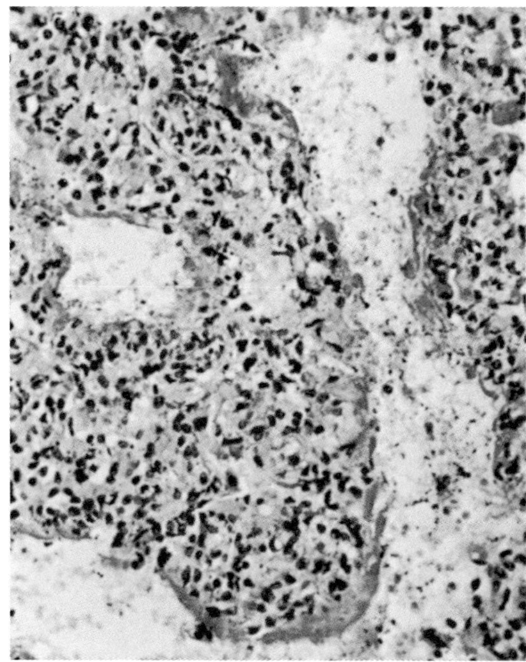

**FIGURE 47–1.** Photomicrograph of a section of lung of an infant born at 32 weeks of gestation and weighing 1640 g. He seemed well for 1 hour; then dyspnea appeared and gradually increased with deepening sternal and costal retractions. He died at 22 hours of age. Unexpanded lung, with dilated air spaces lined with thick, homogeneously staining membrane, can be seen.

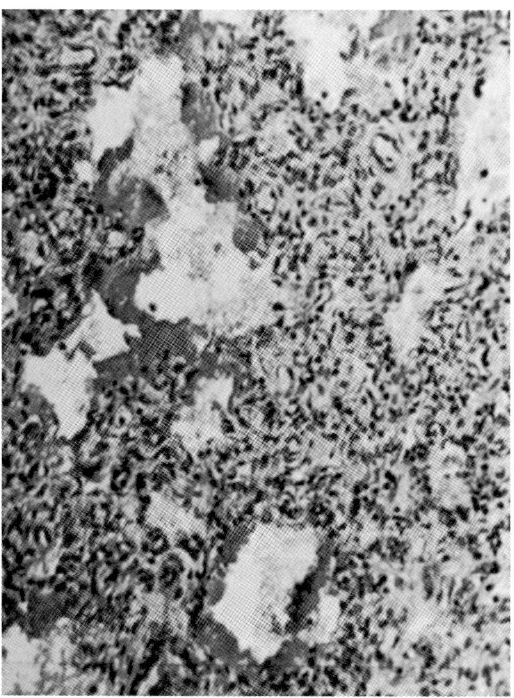

**FIGURE 47–2.** Photomicrograph of a section of lung of a premature infant weighing 2270 g at birth whose dyspnea was first noticed at 8 hours and who died after steadily increasing respiratory difficulty at 27 hours of age. The appearance of the section of lung is in all respects similar to that in Figure 47–1. The pattern of aeration and atelectasis has been described as Swiss cheese–like, in contrast with lace-like aeration.

need for oxygen, the smaller the measured value for FRC (Richardson et al, 1986). In keeping with the reduced static lung compliance found at autopsy (Gribetz et al, 1959), the static lung compliance measured by multiple airway occlusions during exhalation also is markedly reduced, the average value being only 0.5 mL/cm $H_2O$/kg (Dreizzen et al, 1988). As a result, the work of breathing is greatly increased. Measurements of airway resistance suggest values in the normal range, but there is a tendency toward an increase. In one study, the average value was 69 cm $H_2O$/L/second, compared with a reference value of 42 cm $H_2O$/L/second (Hjalmarson and Olsson, 1974). More recently, Edberg (1991) found decreased compliance, increased resistance, decreased lung volume, and reduced gas mixing efficiency in very low-birth-weight (VLBW) infants with RDS. From these data, it can be approximated that the overall time constant in RDS would be less than 0.05 seconds (see Chapter 44 on pulmonary physiology). Because the patency of small peripheral airways depends on proximal spread of surfactant (Macklem et al, 1970), in some regions of lung the local time constants may be more prolonged. The curvature of nitrogen washout traces is better represented by a two-space mathematical model than by a one-space assumption (Richardson and Jung, 1978). The postulated "slow" space may represent those parts of the lung with more prolonged time constants. Passive-exhalation flow-volume plots obtained in preterm lambs with HMD also exhibit curvature, suggesting the presence of both fast and slow spaces in the lung (Richardson et al, 1989). Mathematical modeling of these plots suggests that airway resistance in the slow space is significantly increased. Finally, clamping and unclamping of the airway of these lambs during passive exhalation reveal the presence of pendelluft, further suggesting that measurements of lung mechanics are time dependent and that a significant slow space exists (Richardson et al, 1992).

The alveolar-arterial oxygen tension difference ($Aa.DO_2$) and right-to-left shunt during breathing of 100% oxygen are greatly increased, many infants having values for shunt in the range of 50% to 90% of cardiac output (Strang and MacLeish, 1961). As there is no evidence for a diffusion limitation (Krauss et al, 1976), it is commonly stated that large shunts at the foramen ovale and ductus arteriosus and in atelectatic lung constitute the only cause of severe hypoxemia in HMD. If this were true and the shunt was 50%, it can be seen from Figure 47–3 that changing inspired oxygen would have little effect on arterial oxygen pressure, and oxygen therapy would be relatively ineffective. In fact, precipitous changes in arterial oxygen tension and calculated venous admixture occur if inspired oxygen is reduced. This effect indicates the presence of an open, poorly ventilated lung compartment with extremely low ventilation-perfusion ratio ($\dot{V}/\dot{Q}$), representing a significant proportion of the lung and producing variable hypoxic vasoconstriction and alterations in right-to-left shunt as the inspired oxygen changes (Corbet et al, 1974). Therefore, in infants with RDS the severity of arterial hypoxemia is directly related to the size of the open, poorly ventilated compartment. The relationship among $\dot{V}/\dot{Q}$, alveolar oxygen tension, and changing inspired oxygen (Fig. 47–4) indicates how oxygen concentration as high as 90% is required before the oxygen pressure in very low

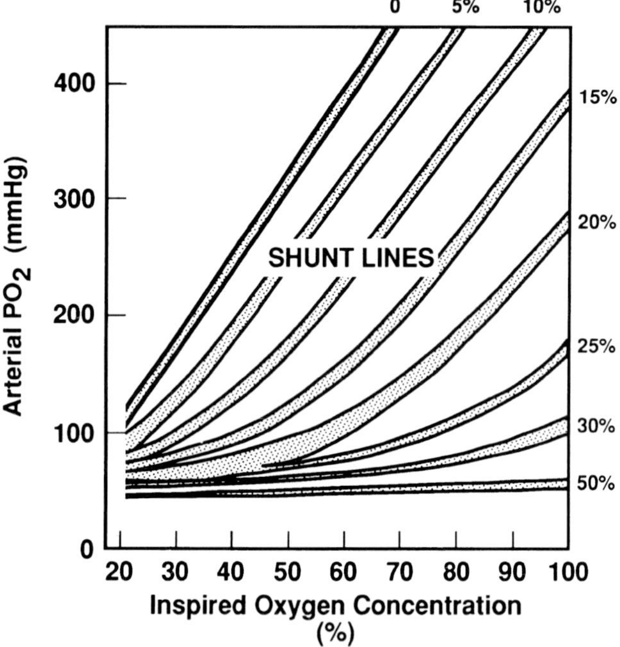


**FIGURE 47–3.** The relationship between inspired oxygen concentration and arterial oxygen tension as it is affected by true right to left shunting. The assumptions are a hemoglobin of 10 to 14 g/dL; arterial $P_{CO_2}$ of 25 to 40 mm Hg; and arterial–mixed venous oxygen tension difference ($a\bar{v}.D_{O_2}$) of 5 mL/100 cc. *(From Benatar SR, Hewlett AM, Nunn JF: The use of iso-shunt lines for control of oxygen therapy. Br J Anesthesiol 45:711, 1973.)*

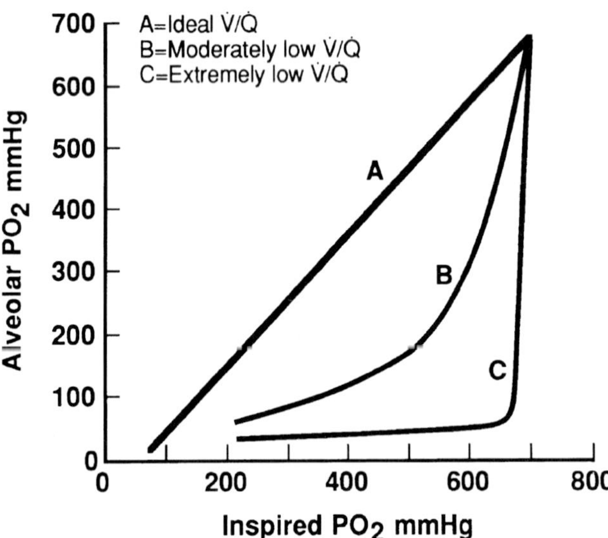


**FIGURE 47–4.** The relationship between inspired $P_{O_2}$ and alveolar $P_{O_2}$. In an open lung compartment with extremely low ventilation-perfusion ratio ($\dot{V}/\dot{Q}$), the alveolar $P_{O_2}$ rises very slowly until greater than 90% oxygen is reached, when it rises rapidly. This phenomenon accounts for the often dramatic changes in arterial $P_{O_2}$ with small changes in inspired $O_2$, especially reductions of inspired $O_2$, seen in patients with respiratory distress syndrome. *(From West JB: Ventilation-perfusion inequality and overall gas exchange in computer models of the lung. Respir Physiol 7:88, 1969.)*

$\dot{V}/\dot{Q}$ units will rise significantly (West, 1969). (See also Chapter 44.) Because perfusion of the open, extremely low $\dot{V}/\dot{Q}$ compartment is greatly reduced by hypoxic vasoconstriction, it makes only a small contribution to cardiac output, and measurements of arterial-alveolar partial pressure difference for nitrogen ($aA.D_{N_2}$) are not greatly increased in HMD (Corbet et al, 1974). It should not be overlooked that this lung compartment makes a significant contribution to the oxygenation defect in HMD.

Measurements of the arterial-alveolar tension difference for carbon dioxide ($aA.D_{CO_2}$) and alveolar dead space (VD) are markedly increased in HMD (Nelson et al, 1962). Although minute ventilation is increased, the alveolar ventilation is actually decreased, as reflected by the elevated values for arterial $CO_2$ tension. Because a large part of the lung is collapsed or poorly ventilated, most alveolar ventilation is diverted to a relatively small part of the lung, represented by the reduced FRC. Because this compartment is small, it is relatively overventilated, so the $\dot{V}/\dot{Q}$ and the measured $aA.D_{CO_2}$ are high (Hansen et al, 1979). Measurements of pulmonary blood flow, utilizing the disappearance of gases that enter ventilated parts of the lung, confirm that perfusion of ventilated lung is very low (Chu et al, 1967). Based on the foregoing considerations, an idealized model of the lung in RDS is shown in Figure 47–5, representing the three lung compartments: shunt, open low $\dot{V}/\dot{Q}$, and high $\dot{V}/\dot{Q}$. Under conditions of changed inspired oxygen and and changed levels of CPAP, there is a close correspondence between predicted and measured values for $aA.D_{CO_2}$, suggesting the validity of this model (Hansen et al, 1979; Landers et al, 1986).

In infants with RDS undergoing treatment in a neonatal intensive care unit (NICU), the pulmonary artery pressure declines more slowly after birth than in preterm infants without RDS (Seppanen et al, 1994). The systemic arterial pressure is maintained similar to that in controls and tends to rise slowly with time; by 24 hours the systemic

| | $\dot{V}/\dot{Q}>1$ | $\dot{V}/\dot{Q}<<1$ | $\dot{V}/\dot{Q}=0$ |
|---|---|---|---|
| **Ventilation** | 0.999 | 0.001 | 0.000 |
| **Perfusion** | 0.330 | 0.030 | 0.640 |
| | V/Q=3 | Qo/Qt | Qs/Qt |

**FIGURE 47–5.** Three-compartment model of hyaline membrane disease (high $\dot{V}/\dot{Q}$, open low $\dot{V}/\dot{Q}$, and shunt; the shunt includes shunt at the ductus, at the foramen, and at collapsed air spaces). The high $\dot{V}/\dot{Q}$ compartment receives nearly all the ventilation. From the measured value for arterial $P_{O_2}$, the calculated venous admixture is 0.67 of cardiac output. Thus, perfusion of the high $\dot{V}/\dot{Q}$ compartment is 0.33 of cardiac output, and the value for $\dot{V}/\dot{Q}$ is 3. From the latter value, a predicted value for the arterial-alveolar carbon dioxide tension difference ($aA.D_{CO_2}$) can be calculated and compared with the measured value. If a value of 0.03 is assumed for the fraction of blood flowing past "open" but very poorly ventilated lung units ($\dot{Q}_o/\dot{Q}_t$), then the calculated value for the shunt fraction ($\dot{Q}_s/\dot{Q}_t$) is 0.64. *(From Hansen TN, Corbet AJS, Kenny JD, et al: Effects of oxygen and constant positive pressure breathing on $aA.D_{CO_2}$ in hyaline membrane disease. Pediatr Res 13:1167, 1979.)*

arterial pressure is well above the pulmonary artery pressure. Extrapulmonary right-to-left shunting at the foramen ovale or the ductus arteriosus disappears by 24 hours (Seppanen et al, 1994), and left-to-right shunting at the ductus arteriosus is very common by age 24 hours (Dudell and Gersony, 1984). In experimental animals, it is not thought that this early left-to-right ductal shunt makes an important contribution to the overall lung dysfunction of RDS (Morrow et al, 1995), but as the pulmonary artery pressure continues to fall with time, the ductal shunt assumes a much greater importance. In preterm infants without RDS, the ductus arteriosus tends to close within 4 days of birth (Reller et al, 1988), whereas in those with RDS, the ductus tends to remain open (Reller et al, 1993), which may become a significant problem by 3 to 4 days of age (Corbet, 1996).

## Diagnosis

### *Clinical Diagnosis*

The infant with RDS untreated with surfactant replacement or end-expiratory pressure is almost always premature and is cyanotic in room air. Beginning at or immediately after birth, breathing is rapid or labored. Infants usually have a characteristic grunt during expiration, caused by closure of the glottis, the effect of which is to maintain lung volume and gas exchange during exhalation. Frequently, the unventilated infant requires 40% to 50% oxygen after birth for relief of central cyanosis but then develops an increasing oxygen requirement over 24 to 48 hours; this may reach as high as 100%. In other infants, the oxygen requirement transiently decreases as acidosis or hypothermia is corrected or fetal lung fluid is cleared; the oxygen requirement begins to increase only after 3 to 6 hours. More severely affected infants have an immediate high oxygen requirement that increases rapidly to 100%; without surfactant and mechanical ventilation, they may die within 24 hours. Another group of larger infants needs less oxygen initially and manifests a slowly progressive course of generalized atelectasis over 48 to 72 hours. The urine output is low for the first 24 to 48 hours, but soon thereafter, a diuresis ensues. If RDS is uncomplicated, recovery starts after 48 hours. The decline in oxygen requirement is relatively rapid after 72 hours, and usually oxygen can be discontinued after 1 week. The VLBW infant (less than 1500 g) usually will require mechanical ventilation and have a more prolonged course. A few infants with RDS also appear to have a contribution from pulmonary hypertension; they are easy to ventilate, especially after exogenous surfactant, but are difficult to oxygenate, and they have severe pulmonary hypertension as evaluated by echocardiographic criteria (Abman et al, 1993; Golan et al, 1995; Walther et al, 1985). Administration of exogenous surfactant has dramatically reduced the incidence and severity of RDS.

### *Laboratory Diagnosis*

Based on arterial blood gas values, infants with untreated RDS have a moderate to severe oxygenation defect, significant hypercarbia, and a mild metabolic acidosis with elevation of blood lactate (Sinclair, 1973). The lecithin-sphingomyelin (L/S) ratio and phosphatidylglycerol (PG) level remain low in serial tracheal aspirate samples for 48 hours and then increase with recovery; the saturated phosphatidylcholine (SP-C) levels remain low in RDS and reach normal levels after 4 to 7 days; the surfactant protein A (SP-A)–to–SPC ratio is low in RDS. (See Chapter 42 on lung development and Chapter 46 on surfactant.)

### *Radiographic Diagnosis*

Diffuse, fine granular densities that develop during the first 6 hours of life are seen on the chest radiograph (Fig. 47–6); occurrence of these densities is influenced by size of the infant, severity of disease, treatment with surfactant, and degree of ventilatory support. The densities may be more pronounced at the lung bases than at the apices. The lung volume may appear normal early, especially if the infant is strong enough to overdistend less affected regions, but ultimately the lung volume is decreased. Positive airway pressure frequently obliterates these diagnostic findings. Other conditions such as pneumonia or pulmonary edema may have very similar radiographic features.

## Etiology

RDS is primarily a developmental deficiency in the amount of surface-active material at the air-liquid interface of the lung, as demonstrated by pressure-volume curves with air and saline in infants who died from RDS (Avery and Fletcher, 1974). Saline extracts of minced lung from infants who died from RDS have higher surface tensions than those in lungs of controls (Avery and Mead, 1959); this finding is associated with lower levels of total tissue phospholipid (Brumley et al, 1967) and SP-C (Adams et al, 1970). Although on the basis of theoretical considerations of the amount required, a more than adequate amount of phospholipid evidently is present in total lung (Clements and Tooley, 1977), only a small proportion of lung phospholipid is surface-active material (Rieutort et al, 1986).

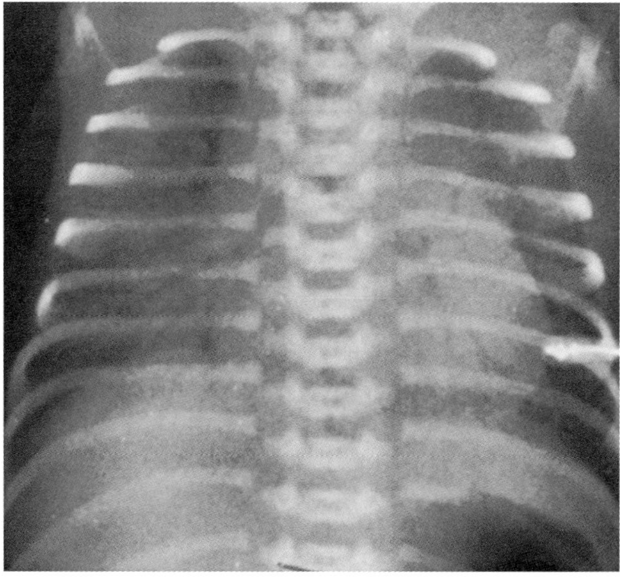

**FIGURE 47–6.** Typical chest radiograph of an infant with hyaline membrane disease.

Infants with RDS may synthesize adequate amounts of SP-C but cannot package and export it to the alveolar surface in a way that makes it function as surfactant. In infants who die, deMello and colleagues (1987) have demonstrated the complete absence of tubular myelin and a modest deficiency of lamellar bodies in type II cells, in comparison with controls. For further discussion of the role of surfactant proteins in RDS, see Chapter 42 on lung development and Chapter 46 on surfactant.

It has been suggested that surfactant function in infants with RDS is inhibited by plasma proteins (Ikegami et al, 1986), which leak into the respiratory bronchioles at the sites of overdistention and epithelial damage. In particular, a plasma protein of relative molecular weight 110,000 has been implicated. Fibrinogen, hemoglobin, and albumin are potent inhibitors of surfactant (Seeger et al, 1993). It is of critical importance for the lungs to have adequate surfactant at the gas-liquid interface from the earliest possible moment after birth; otherwise, acute lung injury and surfactant inhibition will supervene rapidly, contributing to a cycle of worsening disease (Nilsson et al, 1978). Thus, RDS is due to a developmental deficiency of surfactant at birth, but associated lung injury results in surfactant dysfunction as well.

Based on the results of animal experiments, it is estimated that the air spaces of the newborn infant at term contain about 75 mg/kg of SP-C; this compares with only 10 to 15 mg/kg in adults and only 1 to 10 mg/kg in premature infants with RDS (Ikegami et al, 1993). Aside from lower surfactant content, the surfactant from premature infants has decreased biophysical function and is more susceptible to inactivation than surfactant from adults, presumably because it contains lower amounts of surfactant proteins (Ueda et al, 1994). The pool size of alveolar surfactant in recovering premature infants has not been determined but has been measured in preterm monkeys recovering from RDS, in which the pool size increased to 100 mg/kg within 3 to 4 days of birth (Jackson et al, 1986). Dipalmitoyl phosphatidylcholine (DPPC) concentrations in tracheal aspirate samples increase in premature infants recovering from RDS (Hallman et al, 1976). These findings indicate that as premature infants recover from RDS, the alveolar pool size approaches that in the term infant. The evidence suggests that newborn infants need more surfactant than that required in adults for adequate function, which may mean that in the neonatal lung, more surfactant is present in an inactive or catabolic form and that more surfactant is inhibited by excessive fluid and protein. (See also Chapter 46 on surfactant.)

### Prevention

Because RDS is a problem of insufficient lung maturity, the best way to prevent it would be to prevent premature birth; for this purpose, the effective strategies are thought to be cervical cerclage, discovery and treatment of bacterial infections, and the liberal use of tocolytics (Joint Working Party, 1992). At present, however, the two major approaches to the problem are (1) prediction of the risk for RDS by antenatal testing of amniotic fluid samples and (2) antenatal treatment of women in preterm labor with glucocorticoid hormones to accelerate fetal lung maturation. In addition, the prophylactic administration of exogenous surfactant at birth is designed to prevent RDS, and this strategy has been successful, especially with the use of mammalian surfactants (see Chapter 46.)

#### *Prenatal Prediction*

In normal pregnancy, the L/S ratio displays a remarkably stable pattern, increasing slowly to a value of 1 at 32 weeks, rising more rapidly to 2 at 35 weeks, and accelerating very rapidly thereafter (Gluck and Kulovich, 1973) (Fig. 47–7). In an abnormal pregnancy, there is a much wider scatter of values, reflecting conditions that accelerate or decelerate lung maturation. The ratio may reach 2 as early as 28 weeks or remain at 1 until close to term. The incidence of RDS is only 0.5% for an L/S ratio of 2 or more but 100% for an L/S ratio below 1; between 1 and 2, the risk of RDS decreases progressively. The L/S ratio reflects the secretory activity of the lung, which is greatly accelerated at 35 weeks. Elective cesarean section delivery of infants who have an unrecognized low L/S ratio carries an unnecessary risk of RDS (Hack et al, 1976).

Phosphatidylinositol (PI) in amniotic fluid progressively increases until 36 weeks and then decreases (Hallman et al, 1976). At about this time, PG appears and increases until term (Fig. 47–8). The appearance time of PG may be accelerated or delayed in the same way as noted for the L/S ratio. Thin-layer chromatography is very sensitive, so values for PG of less than 1% of total phospholipid, by reflective

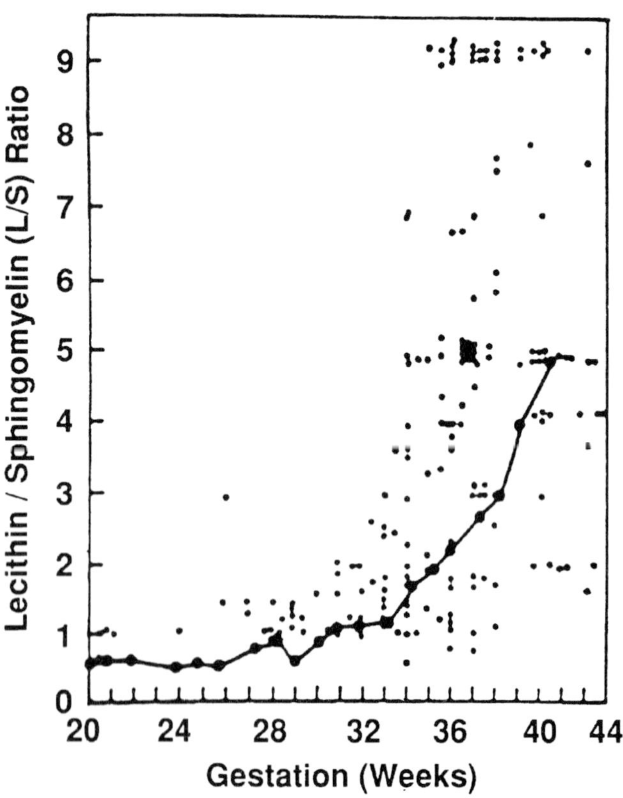


**FIGURE 47–7.** The lecithin-sphingomyelin (L/S) ratio in normal and abnormal pregnancies, indicating wide biologic scatter. *(From Gluck L, Kulovich MV: The evaluation of functional maturity in the human fetus. In Gluck L [ed]: Modern Perinatal Medicine. Chicago, Year Book Medical Publishers, 1974.)*

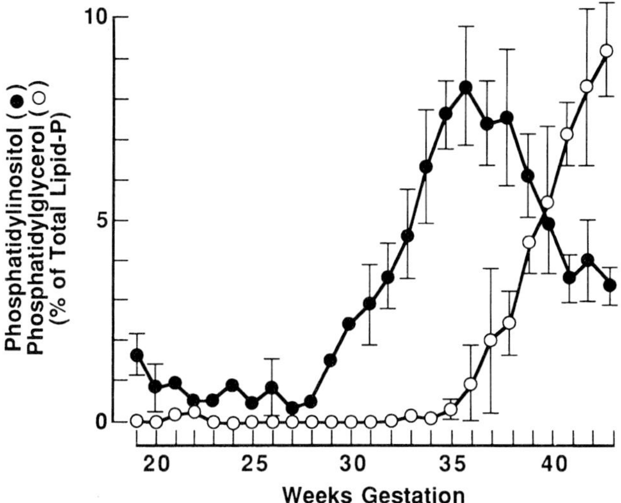


**FIGURE 47-8.** Phosphatidylglycerol and phosphatidylinositol content of amniotic fluid plotted against gestational age. *(From Hallman M, Kulovich MV, Kirkpatrick E, et al: Phosphatidylinositol and phosphatidylglycerol in amniotic fluid: Indices of lung maturity. Am J Obstet Gynecol 125:613, 1976.)*

densitometry on the chromatographic plate, should be considered negative; this correlates with the less sensitive but much faster immunologic detection methods for PG, such as the AmnioStat-FLM (Irvine Scientific, Santa Ana, CA) which has detection limits of 0.05 μg/mL (Towers and Garite, 1989). The presence of PG at 1% of total phospholipid indicates a remarkably low risk for RDS, less than 0.5%. If a patient has both an L/S ratio of less than 2 and a PG of less than 1%, the risk for RDS is greater than 80% (Hallman and Teramo, 1981). Besides an L/S ratio below 1, this combination is the best predictor of RDS available to the clinician. In certain pregnancies characterized by diabetes and Rh isoimmunization, the L/S ratio has proved less reliable, the risk of RDS at a value between 2 and 3 still being approximately 13% (Hallman and Teramo, 1981). However, in infants with both an L/S ratio above 2 and PG of 1% or more, the risk has been reduced to zero. Other factors must be considered in the interpretation of the L/S ratio: A low L/S ratio carries a much smaller risk at a more advanced gestation, and in black mothers, the risk of RDS in the infant is extremely low with an L/S ratio of more than 1.2 (Richardson and Torday, 1994).

The measurements of SP-A and SP-B by ELISA have been made in amniotic fluid samples for the purpose of predicting the occurrence of RDS (Dilger et al, 1994). Although SP-A and SP-B increased with advancing gestation, the excellent predictive values of L/S and PG were not improved by the additional measurement of surfactant proteins (Pryhuber et al, 1991).

A rapid test for the evaluation of amniotic fluid samples is the foam stability test, in which samples of variable dilution are shaken with 95% alcohol and the tubes examined for stable foam (Clements et al, 1972); it has not been found entirely satisfactory but may be used in conjunction with other tests. A modification of this "shake test" is the stable microbubble test, in which stable bubbles are counted under the microscope; fewer than 5 stable microbubbles/mm$^2$ are considered positive for RDS (Chida and Fujiwara, 1993; Chida et al, 1993). This test has been found to have a positive result predictive value of 95% to 100% and a negative result predictive value of 85% to 90%. This test is rapid and inexpensive and may be adapted for use with tracheal aspirate samples after birth.

Recently, amniotic fluid lamellar body counts have been studied to determine the predictive value of this method for the development of HMD and for comparison with traditional measurements of phospholipids in amniotic fluid samples (Dalence et al, 1995). In this method, amniotic fluid samples are analyzed by Coulter counter, and the lamellar bodies are read as platelets. Values of greater than 30,000/μL have a negative predictive value of 100%, and values less then 10,000/μL have a positive predictive value of 67%. This assessment is quick, cheap, and available and has advantages over many of the other tests of phospholipid concentrations.

### *Early Postnatal Prediction*

The L/S ratio may be used in tracheal aspirate samples to predict RDS, but the threshold level of 2.0 must be raised to 3.0 (Harker et al, 1992); the measurement of PG on tracheal aspirate samples also is very useful, and the combination of low L/S ratio and absent PG on tracheal aspirate samples gives a positive result predictive value of 89%. Skelton and Jeffery (1994) have obtained good results with the "click test," another modification of the shake test, in tracheal aspirate samples from preterm infants. After shaking a 0.2-mL sample of tracheal aspirate with an equal volume of 95% ethanol, the bubbles, suspended in airless water, are examined under the microscope; if the bubbles increase and decrease in size, this means an active surfactant and therefore a negative result. The positive result predictive accuracy was 100% and the negative result predictive accuracy was 93% for tracheal aspirate samples from preterm infants. Either this test or the stable microbubble test as described may be used in tracheal aspirate samples of small premature infants at birth for predicting the presence of RDS; in turn, the result may be used in deciding on the use of early surfactant therapy. The measurement of static lung compliance also is very useful for this purpose; with a value of less than 1.8 mL/cm $H_2O$/m of body length, the positive result predictive value is 100%; with a value of more than 1.8, the negative result predictive value is 92% (Wilkie et al, 1994). This test is complex and expensive, however.

### *Prophylaxis with Antenatal Glucocorticoid Hormones*

A vast literature on the effect of corticosteroid hormones on lung and surfactant maturation in animal and tissue culture models has accumulated (Ballard, 1986). Since 1972, when Liggins and Howie described decreased mortality, decreased incidence of RDS, and less severe RDS in a prospective blinded study done in New Zealand, more than 30 studies have been published worldwide. Unfortunately, not all of these studies have been of appropriate size, and not all have been of sufficient quality to exclude the problems of bias and error; these shortcomings have resulted in widespread misinterpretation of the results and a regrettable underutilization of glucocorticoid therapy (Ryan and Finer, 1995).

The National Perinatal Epidemiology Unit at Oxford University published the results of a meta-analysis of 12 randomized controlled trials (Crowley et al, 1990); to be included, the trials had to meet rigorous standards. The authors concluded that maternal steroid therapy significantly reduced the incidence of RDS, intraventricular hemorrhage (IVH), necrotizing enterocolitis (NEC), and neonatal death; in addition, they concluded that the duration and costs of hospital care for the newborn infant were greatly decreased. The benefits applied to all infants born at a gestational age of 24 to 34 weeks and were not affected by race or gender or by the presence of prelabor rupture of amniotic membranes (Crowley, 1992).

Recently, the National Institutes of Health reported the conclusions of a panel of experts; they commissioned an updated meta-analysis, a neonatal registry review, and a cost-benefit analysis and evaluated the scientific literature according to the rigorous standards of the U.S. Preventive Services Task Force (NIH Consensus Development Panel, 1995; NIH Consensus Development Conference Statement, 1995). The investigators concluded that the incidences of RDS, IVH, and neonatal death were significantly reduced (odds ratios of 0.5, 0.5, and 0.6, respectively), and they regarded the evidence as compelling. The benefits were not affected by race or gender or by the presence of PROM, and, most important, the benefits were still apparent in infants in whom exposure was less than 24 hours. In infants of 24 to 28 weeks, the evidence for a reduced incidence of RDS was less certain, but the severity of RDS and the incidence of severe IVH were significantly decreased.

There is no reasonable evidence that the incidence of infection is increased in either the mother or the infant. The results of long-term follow-up studies have shown no problems with general health or neurodevelopment that could be attributed to the use of hormone therapy (Ballard, 1986). The NIH panel estimated that if the use of prenatal steroids could be increased from the level of 15% in preterm infants at 24 to 34 weeks of gestation to a level of 60%, then the cost savings for initial hospital care alone would be $157 million each year in the United States.

The recommendations of the NIH panel are as follows: (1) all fetuses between 24 and 34 weeks of gestation are candidates for this therapy; (2) the decision should not be influenced by race, gender, PROM, or anticipated surfactant therapy; (3) all obstetric patients eligible for tocolytic therapy should receive steroids; (4) because therapy for less than 24 hours is effective, all patients should be treated unless immediate delivery is anticipated; (5) patients whose pregnancies have not reached 30 weeks of gestation should be treated because of the reduction in IVH; (6) treatment may be witheld in the presence of overt amnionitis; and (7) treatment consists of betamethasone, 12 mg every 24 hours for two doses, or dexamethasone, 6 mg every 12 hours for four doses. Liggins and Howie (1972) reported a high incidence of RDS in infants delivered more than 7 days after maternal steroid treatment, suggesting that the beneficial effect could be reversible. However, routine retreatment after 7 days is not recommended. Subsequent to the recommendations of the NIH consensus conference, use of repeat courses of antenatal steroids to mothers with threatened preterm labor became widespread. Animal studies of repeat antenatal steroid administrations were concerning because of evidence of deleterious effects on lung and somatic growth as well as on cerebral myelination and development (Jobe et al, 1998; Okajima et al, 2001; Uno et al, 1990). Data in humans are not well established, but possible decreases in somatic and brain growth, as well as increases in the incidence of chronic lung disease and neonatal sepsis and in the mortality rate, have been suggested (Banks et al, 1999; French et al, 1999). The revised recommendations reiterated those from the previous consensus conference and added: "Because of insufficient scientific data from randomized clinical trials regarding efficacy and safety, repeat courses of corticosteroids should not be used routinely. In general, repeat courses should be reserved for patients enrolled in randomized controlled trials. Several randomized trials are in progress" (National Institutes of Health Consensus Development Panel, 2001). Specific recommendations also were made directing clinical and basic scientific research efforts to characterize optimal treatment.

A number of recent studies has examined the use of antenatal steroids in mothers at risk for delivery of a very immature infant, a problem that has been of great concern to many obstetricians. To examine the question of treatment before 30 weeks of gestation, Kattner and colleagues (1992) carried out a meta-analysis with over 250 infants and found a significant reduction in the incidence of RDS with maternal steroid treatment. Then, in a prospective study, they enrolled 135 mothers in a trial of prenatal steroids and found a significant increase in survival in the infants whose mothers had received treatment. Garite and colleagues (1992) performed a small randomized controlled trial of prenatal corticosteroids in mothers without PROM at gestational age 24 to 28 weeks; they found no reduction in the incidence of RDS, but they found dramatic reductions in the incidences of severe IVH and the severity of RDS. The data obtained for the March of Dimes–sponsored Prematurity Prevention Program were analyzed for the effect of prenatal steroids; major reductions in the incidence of RDS, IVH, and death were found in infants between 26 and 31 weeks of gestation who had received prenatal steroids (Maher et al, 1994). The data for a controlled trial of indomethacin were examined for the effect of antenatal steroids; in infants between 600 and 1250 g birth weight, a large decrease in the incidence of IVH was found with antenatal steroid treatment (Ment et al, 1995).

Prenatal glucocorticoids appear to have several other beneficial effects in the small preterm infant (Ballard, 1986). Clyman and colleagues (1981) demonstrated a significant reduction in the incidence of clinically significant patent ductus arteriosus (PDA) with prenatal betamethasone therapy. Van Marter and associates (1990) reported data indicating that the incidence of BPD is reduced in preterm infants exposed to prenatal corticosteroids; this appears logical in view of the evidence relating RDS, especially severe RDS, to the occurrence of BPD. Other effects observed in animal models include decreased pulmonary protein leaks (Rider et al, 1989), induction of antioxidant enzymes in rat lung (Frank et al, 1985), and acceleration of renal function in the fetal lamb (Scholle and Braunlich, 1989; Stonestreet et al, 1983).

The results for prenatal steroid therapy can be further improved; the effects of prenatal steroid and exogenous surfactant therapy proved to be additive in several initial small trials (Jobe, 1993). The effect of prenatal steroids has been retrospectively analyzed in the large number of infants enrolled in the many large controlled trials of exogenous surfactant performed in the last 10 years or so. The beneficial effects of steroids are still clearly apparent (Wright et al, 1995), even in populations that also have benefited from the use of exogenous surfactant therapy.

Several other hormones, particularly thyroid hormone, are known to have a positive effect on lung development in tissue culture and animal models; because thyroid hormone does not cross the placenta, thyrotropin-releasing hormone (TRH) has been used instead. Early randomized controlled trials of prenatal TRH given in addition to corticosteroids have demonstrated further improvements in outcome, compared with controls treated with steroids alone; Ballard and colleagues (1992) noted a significant reduction in death and BPD at a postconceptional age of 36 weeks, and Knight and associates (1994) reported a New Zealand trial in which significant reductions in RDS incidence, RDS severity, frequency of BPD, and mortality rate were found. However, an Australian controlled trial of TRH, which used a smaller dose and a longer dosage interval, found an increased risk for severe RDS (ACTOBAT Study Group, 1995), and Pierce and colleagues (1992) found decreased survival rates in oxygen-exposed newborn rats given TRH prenatally. In a more recent large clinical trial, nearly 1000 mothers were randomized to either TRH or placebo antenatally in addition to steroids at less than 30 weeks of gestation. Of the 1134 infants delivered, 769 were born at less than 32 weeks of gestation. In these infants, at increased risk of RDS and chronic lung disease, there were no differences in the rate of RDS (66% for THRH versus 65% for placebo), death (11% versus 11%), or chronic lung disease (32% versus 34%) (Ballard et al, 1998). On the basis of the most recent studies, the addition of prenatal TRH to antenatal steroids given to mothers at risk for very preterm delivery cannot be recommended for clinical practice.

## Treatment

### *Resuscitation*

The mortality rate among all infants, including those with HMD, is increased by asphyxia. Therefore, the presence of a skilled resuscitation team at the delivery of high-risk infants can reduce the morbidity and mortality rates of the disease (see Chapter 28 on resuscitation).

### *Lung Expansion*

Because secretion of surfactant is impaired by inadequate expansion of the lungs at birth (Lawson et al, 1979), many experts believe that it is appropriate to intubate all infants weighing less than 1000 g at birth and to initiate mechanical ventilation with positive end-expiratory pressure (PEEP) in the delivery room. Another approach to obtaining lung expansion in this weight group is early utilization of nasal CPAP, without automatic intubation. These two approaches in this weight group have not been compared in a randomized study, but centers using the delivery room management approach of nasal CPAP have a low incidence of BPD, and these centers do not report differences in mortality rate or occurrence of IVH or other important morbidity (Van Marter et al, 2000). Intubation and mechanical ventilation may be used for larger premature infants if they have respiratory distress or are not vigorous in the delivery room. For infants with birth weights of less than 1000 g in whom intubation combined with mechanical ventilation is chosen, the administration of artificial replacement surfactant within the first 15 minutes of life is associated with lower mortality and less BPD than in infants who are given surfactant later in the course of RDS (see Chapter 46 on surfactant).

### *Thermal Neutrality*

Infants should be nursed in a warm environment so that oxygen consumption is maintained at minimal levels. This usually means servo-controlling the anterior abdominal skin temperature at 36.5° C, but in small premature infants, the skin temperature may need to be servo-controlled at 36.9° C in order to maintain the rectal temperature at 37° C. The measured energy expenditure is 55 calories/kg/day during the first 4 days (Samiec et al, 1994); unfortunately, the caloric intake is usually only 25 calories/kg/day, so it is very important to minimize overall caloric expenditure.

### *Blood Gas Monitoring*

Infants with RDS require monitoring of blood pressure, blood gases, electrolytes, calcium, and glucose. Blood samples may be obtained from an umbilical artery catheter.

### *Oxygen*

Oxygen therapy is beneficial despite the presence of large right-to-left shunts. Increased inspired oxygen produces (1) a rise of alveolar oxygen pressure in open low $\dot{V}/\dot{Q}$ units (see Fig. 47–4); (2) relief of regional hypoxic vasoconstriction in this compartment; (3) a reduction in true right-to-left shunt; and (4) an increase in arterial oxygen saturation (Hansen et al, 1979).

### *Fluid Restriction and Attention to Serum Electrolytes*

Because RDS is characterized by high-surface-tension pulmonary edema (Boughton et al, 1970), high-permeability pulmonary edema (Jefferies et al, 1984), and marked fluid retention, fluid restriction to 50 mL/kg/day is indicated for many infants with RDS for the first 48 hours or until the onset of diuresis. The complex hormonal responses to RDS result in high levels of arginine vasopressin and low concentrations of atrial natriuretic peptide, favoring a low urine output and fluid retention (Ronconi et al, 1995); subsequently, an increase in atrial natriuretic peptide concentration occurs with the onset of the diuretic phase observed in the course of RDS. A controlled trial of fluid restriction, compared with a modest increase in fluid intake, showed a significant reduction in the incidence of BPD at the age of 1 month and at a postconceptional age near term (Tammela et al, 1992). In addition, a meta-analysis in which fluid restriction was compared with a modest increase in daily fluid intakes found a reduction in the incidence of PDA, NEC, and death in the infants in whom fluid restriction was applied (Bell and Acarregui, 2001). Close attention should be paid to fluid intake, urine output, urine concentration, and serum electrolytes. Premature infants have an excess of extracellular fluid and are expected to lose at least 10% of body weight by the end of the first week of life. It is not necessary or beneficial to administer sodium in the first few days of life (Costarino et al, 1992), and potassium also should be restricted, as hyperkalemia may be troublesome (Stefano et al, 1993). In the infant who develops hyponatremia in the first few days of life in association with RDS, without an appropriate loss in weight, the hyponatremia does not represent a depletion in total body sodium but indicates excessive total body water, and consideration should be given to decreasing the rate of fluid administration further. In the very immature infant (24 to 26 weeks of gestation) with very permeable skin, evaporative losses may be excessive, and much higher amounts of fluid may be required. If the serum sodium rises sharply, especially if it approaches 150 mEq/L, it can be assumed that insensible water losses through the skin are excessive, and the fluid intake should be liberalized accordingly. To minimize insensible water losses, it is useful to manage the infant in a humidified incubator; or if the infant is on an open warmer, a transparent plastic cover can be placed across the infant and across the sides of the bassinet and then a gentle flow of heated mist directed into the infant's microenvironment. It should be noted that antenatal corticosteroid administration decreases permeability of the very preterm infant's skin. If fluids must be liberalized, the development of hyperglycemia is not uncommon; in this situation, a continuous enteric infusion of water may be useful to control the serum sodium (Gaylord et al, 1995).

### *Minimal Stimulation*

Manipulations such as heel sticks, tracheal suctioning, diaper changes, and even weighing should be kept to a minimum, as these procedures have been shown to reduce arterial oxygen tension (Lucey, 1981); they probably also increase oxygen consumption and may contribute to the genesis of cerebral hemorrhage by rapidly raising arterial blood pressure to excessive levels. It is not appropriate to give enteral feedings to infants with RDS, because this condition usually is accompanied by poor intestinal motility. Many centers now insert both an umbilical vein catheter and an umbilical artery catheter and use the venous catheter to infuse glucose and the arterial catheter to infuse saline. The major reason for use of the two catheters is that a source of glucose-free blood is needed to monitor glucose tolerance adequately without the use of heel sticks, which are painful to the infant and very disturbing.

### *Blood Pressure Support*

Premature infants with RDS frequently have a low arterial blood pressure in the first 12 hours of life, as defined by normative data (Versmold et al, 1981). Many extremely low-birth-weight (ELBW) infants with RDS probably have low blood pressure for many days after birth, which may predispose them to brain injury (Kopelman, 1990). A working party of the Royal College of Physicians has defined hypotension in small premature infants as a mean blood pressure of less than the gestational age in completed weeks (Joint Working Party, 1992). However, there is a tendency for the blood pressure to rise spontaneously in the first 12 hours of life (Moscoso et al, 1983).

Adequate oxygenation may be difficult in the presence of hypotension and reduced pulmonary blood flow. In infants with a low hematocrit, poor peripheral perfusion, and metabolic acidosis, the hypotension often is due to hypovolemia and will respond to a cautious infusion of 10 to 20 mL/kg of saline. Only a few infants have obvious signs of hypovolemia, however, and echocardiographic studies in small premature infants have shown that many have decreased cardiac contractility, which is reflected in a poor cardiac output and significant hypotension (Gill and Weindling, 1993a). If there are no signs of hypovolemia, the infusion of dopamine at 5 to 10 μg/kg/minute usually is effective at increasing the mean blood pressure. A randomized controlled trial of Plasmanate versus dopamine in hypotensive preterm infants showed that only 45% responded to Plasmanate, but 89% responded to dopamine (Gill and Weindling, 1993b). Some investigators have suggested that dopamine is superior to dobutamine for the correction of hypotension in small premature infants (Christophe Roze et al, 1993), and this was confirmed in a controlled trial (Klarr et al, 1994) in which dopamine was successful in elevating the mean blood pressure in 97% of infants and dobutamine was successful in 67% of infants. Serial echocardiographic data have shown dopamine dose–dependent increases in cardiac output and stroke volume, without significant changes in heart rate or systemic vascular resistance (Padbury et al, 1986).

Helbock and colleagues (1993) presented evidence that some small preterm infants with RDS have low cortisol levels and that their hypotension is corrected with hydrocortisone. Others have found that small premature infants with RDS needing inotrope support have lower cortisol levels than small premature infants with RDS not needing inotrope support (Scott and Watterberg, 1995). Other centers have found that dexamethasone often corrects the low blood pressure in these infants after an interval of 6 to 12 hours (Fauser et al, 1993). These investigators suggest that the mechanism involves protein induction of adrenergic receptors. Glucocorticoids given in the first 96 hours of life in premature infants, however, have been associated with an increased incidence of intestinal perforation and abnormal developmental outcomes, including cerebral palsy. The Committee on the Fetus and Newborn of the American Academy of Pediatrics (2002) has recommended that postnatal steroids not be given to premature infants unless the infant is on maximal support. (See also Chapter 49 on BPD.) One of the many benefits of prenatal corticosteroid therapy is that the mean blood pressure is higher in treated infants (Moise et al, 1995). In a study in which a single dose of dexamethasone was given within 2 hours of birth to infants born at less than 28 weeks of gestation, blood pressures were higher and ventilator pressures lower than in the infants receiving placebo (Kopelman et al, 1999); however, it is not clear that even this amount of exposure to dexamethasone is safe. Evans and Iyer (1993) found that the mean blood pressure increased after successful closure of the ductus arteriosus with indomethacin, but the effect was small. Adequate attention to the blood pressure is very important in the management of RDS.

### *Alkali Therapy*

Severe metabolic acidosis may increase pulmonary vascular resistance, impair surfactant synthesis, reduce cardiac output, and ultimately reduce ventilation. An early trial showed that continuous infusion of glucose-bicarbonate solutions reduced the mortality rate for RDS (Usher, 1963). With the introduction of better methods for oxygenating infants however, bicarbonate therapy no longer appears to have much benefit (Corbet et al, 1977), and it may be harmful in infants who are not being ventilated adequately and have a high arterial $P_{CO_2}$.

### *Closure of the Patent Ductus Arteriosus*

Especially in infants weighing less than 1000 g at birth, a PDA may contribute significantly to the overall problem during recovery from RDS and may predispose the infant to the development of BPD. If the ductus is demonstrated to be patent at the age of 3 to 4 days by two-dimensional echocardiography and pulsed Doppler ultrasonography, the evidence suggests that it is unlikely to close spontaneously within a reasonable time (Dudell and Gersony, 1984); therefore, it should be closed, either with indomethacin therapy or with surgery (see Chapter 56 on PDA).

### *Surfactant Replacement*

Infants with birth weights of less than 1000 g should receive prophylactic exogenous surfactant within 15 to 30 minutes of birth, but only after adequate stabilization; in larger infants, surfactant treatment should begin as early as possible, preferably before the age of 2 hours, and certainly before the age of 6 hours. A mammalian surfactant is currently preferred; the dose should be 100 mg/kg, the interval between doses should be between 6 and 12 hours, and two or three doses should be given. The drug should be given as rapidly as possible with a catheter passed into the endotracheal tube, followed by bag-tube ventilation to ensure even distribution, but it should not be given so rapidly as to obstruct the airways and promote hypercarbia. The number of aliquots for each dose does not matter, two aliquots being as good as four aliquots. After surfactant instillation, it is customary to maintain the patient on continuous mechanical ventilation (CMV), but Verder and colleagues (1994) have demonstrated that larger infants may be extubated to nasal CPAP and that the need for endotracheal intubation and CMV may be reduced. Trials of this approach in lower-birth-weight infants are underway.

### *Corticosteroids*

See Chapter 49 for a discussion of the potential role of glucocorticoids in the prevention and treatment of BPD.

### *Prognosis*

The chances of survival in RDS are directly related to birth weight and gestational age and are affected by prenatal treatment with glucocorticoids, by surfactant replacement therapy, and by the severity and complications of the disease.

## TRANSIENT TACHYPNEA OF THE NEWBORN

Transient tachypnea of the newborn (TTN) also is known as *delayed clearance of fetal lung fluid*. In 1966, Avery and coworkers reported on eight near-term infants with early onset of respiratory distress whose chest radiographs showed hyperaeration of the lungs, prominent pulmonary vascular markings, and mild cardiomegaly (Fig. 47–9). The respiratory symptoms were transient and relatively mild, and most infants improved within 2 to 5 days. The investigators named the disorder "transient tachypnea of the newborn" and speculated that it was the result of delayed clearance of fetal lung liquid.

### Pathophysiology

### *Fetal Lung Fluid*

Most authors agree with Avery and her coworkers that TTN represents a transient pulmonary edema resulting from delayed clearance of fetal lung liquid. The lung liquid that fills the potential air spaces of the lung (20 to 30 mL/kg of body weight) is quite distinct from amniotic fluid or plasma (Adams et al, 1963; Adamson et al, 1969; Humphreys et al, 1967) (Table 47–2). The possibility that the lung could contribute to amniotic fluid was first proposed by Jost and Policard (1948), when they demonstrated an increase in lung volume in the rabbit fetus after ligation of the trachea. Evidence for active secretion of lung liquid was provided by Strang (1967), who measured the ratios of cations and anions between lung liquid and plasma. Olver and Strang (1974) later demonstrated that lung liquid required active transport of chloride ions from plasma in excess of the bicarbonate movement in the opposite direction. This liquid contains large amounts of chloride, relatively small amounts of bicarbonate, and almost no protein. Its potassium concentration is similar to that of plasma until near term, when it increases in response to surfactant secretion. Fetal lung liquid is secreted by the lung at approximately 4 to 6 mL/kg/hour along an electrochemical gradient that is produced by the active pumping of chloride from the interstitium into the air space. Although the site of the chloride pump is unknown, it can be inhibited by a variety of mediators that include beta agonists, arginine vasopressin, and prostaglandin $E_2$ (Bland, 1988; Walters and Olver, 1978).

The potential airways of the fetus are in contact with amniotic fluid when the glottis is open. Rarely does amniotic fluid itself enter the developing lung, except in circumstances of fetal distress. When the fetus is stimulated to gasp, sufficient pressure is applied across the lung to allow entry of amniotic fluid and sometimes squamous debris and even meconium. The rapid, irregular respiratory movements described as fetal breathing do not, in effect, move much fluid, as fluid is approximately 100 times as viscous as air, and the rapid, small respiratory movements of the fetus are not associated with high transpulmonary pressures.

### *Clearance of the Fetal Lung Fluid*

In order for the fetus to complete the transition from intrauterine to extrauterine life, the lung must clear this liquid soon after birth. The process of clearing liquid from the lung actually begins 2 to 3 days prior to birth with a decrease in the rate of secretion of fetal lung liquid.

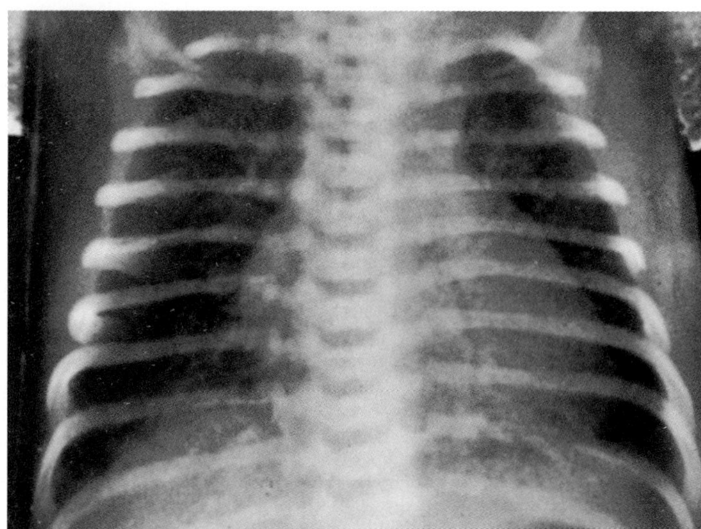


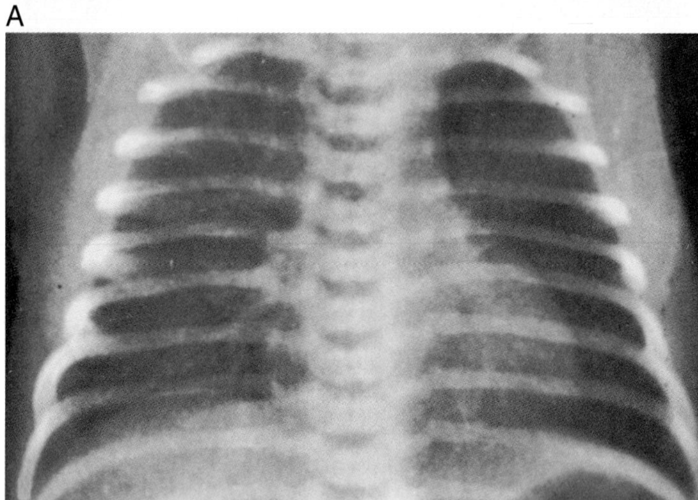


**FIGURE 47–9.** The large cardiovascular silhouette, air bronchogram, and streaky lung fields were seen at 2 hours of age (**A**) but had cleared by 24 hours of age (**B**), typical of transient tachypnea of the newborn or delayed clearance of lung liquid.

However, lung liquid begins to clear in earnest with the onset of labor. Data obtained from experiments using fetal lambs show that nearly two thirds of the total clearance of liquid that occurs during the transition from intrauterine to extrauterine life occurs during labor (Bland, 1983, 1988; Bland et al, 1982). With the onset of labor, the pulmonary epithelium changes from a chloride secreting membrane to a sodium-absorbing membrane, with reversal of the direction of flow of lung liquid. This change is an active metabolic process involving increased $Na^+$, $K^+$-ATPase activity in the epithelial cells and serves to drive liquid from the lung lumen into the interstitium. In addition, because lung liquid contains very little protein, oncotic pressure also favors the movement of water from the air space back into the interstitium, and from there into the vascular compartment (Berthiaume et al, 1987; Bland, 1988; Bland

**TABLE 47–2**

**Interstitial Fluid Estimated from Measurements in Lung Lymph**

| Component | Lung Liquid | Interstitial Fluid | Plasma | Amniotic Fluid |
|---|---|---|---|---|
| Sodium (mEq/L) | 150 | 147 | 150 | 113 |
| Potassium (mEq/L) | 6.3 | 4.8 | 4.8 | 7.6 |
| Chloride (mEq/L) | 157 | 107 | 107 | 87 |
| Bicarbonate (mEq/L) | 3 | 25 | 24 | 19 |
| pH | 6.27 | 7.31 | 7.34 | 7.02 |
| Protein (g/dL) | 0.03 | 3.27 | 4.09 | 0.10 |

Data from Adams et al, 1963; Adamson et al, 1969; Bland, 1983; and Humphreys et al, 1967.

and Nielson, 1992). In the past, physicians believed that some of the reduction in lung water at birth was caused by vaginal compression of the chest, which expelled liquid from the lung. However, although lung water content in fetal rabbits delivered vaginally with labor is less than the lung water of rabbits delivered by cesarean section without labor, the lung water content in fetal rabbits delivered by cesarean section during labor is not different (Bland et al, 1979). These data suggest that any mechanical effects on the clearance of fetal lung liquid are minimal.

### *Delayed Clearance of the Fetal Lung Fluid*

Infants born without labor do not have the opportunity for early lung liquid clearance and begin their extrauterine life with excess water in their lungs. In addition, the increase in $Na^+$, $K^+$-ATPase activity around the time of labor appears to be developmentally regulated, suggesting that preterm infants would not be able to use this pathway effectively to help clear fetal lung fluid. Infants with TTN often are hypoproteinemic, and decreased plasma oncotic pressure may delay the direct absorption of water into the blood vessels (Cummings et al, 1993). Finally, these infants can have elevated pulmonary vascular pressures and ventricular dysfunction (Halliday et al, 1981), which will increase central venous pressure and impair thoracic duct function and the removal of interstitial water by the lymphatics. This is especially true in infants who receive large transfusions of blood from the placenta as a result of delayed cord clamping or milking of the cord (Saigal et al, 1977).

### *Transient Pulmonary Edema*

The symptoms of TTN result from compression of the compliant airways by water that has accumulated in the perivascular cuffs of the extra-alveolar interstitium. This compression results in airway obstruction and hyperaeration of the lungs secondary to gas trapping. Hypoxia results from the continued perfusion of poorly ventilated lung units; hypercarbia results from mechanical interference with alveolar ventilation and from central nervous system depression. Lung function measurements in infants with TTN are compatible with airway obstruction and gas trapping. The FRC measured by gas dilution is normal or reduced, whereas measurements of thoracic gas volume by plethysmography are increased, suggesting that some of the gas in the lungs is not in communication with the airways (Krauss and Auld, 1971).

### Clinical Signs

It initially was thought that TTN was limited to term or larger preterm infants, but it is now clear that very small infants also may present with pulmonary edema from retained fetal lung liquid; this may complicate their surfactant deficiency, accounting for some of their need for supplemental oxygen and ventilation. There is often a history of heavy maternal sedation, maternal diabetes, or delivery by elective cesarean section. Affected infants may be mildly depressed at birth, which may mask many of their early symptoms. They are often very tachypneic, with respiratory rates ranging from 60 to 120 breaths/minute, and may have hyperinflation with grunting, chest wall retractions, and nasal flaring.

Arterial blood gas values often reveal a respiratory acidosis, which resolves within 8 to 24 hours, and mild to moderate hypoxemia. These infants seldom require more than 40% oxygen to maintain an adequate $PaO_2$ and usually are in room air by 24 hours of age. They have no evidence to indicate right-to-left shunting of blood at the ductus arteriosus or foramen ovale. They respond rapidly and well to nasal CPAP therapy.

Chest radiographs reveal hyperaeration, which often is accompanied by mild cardiomegaly (see Fig. 47–9). Water contained in the perivascular cuffs produces prominent vascular markings in a "sunburst pattern" emanating from the hilum. The interlobar fissures are widened, and pleural effusions may be present. Occasionally, coarse fluffy densities may be seen, indicating alveolar edema. The radiographic abnormalities resolve over the first 2 to 3 days after birth, or more rapidly with treatment with nasal CPAP.

### Clinical Course and Treatment

As its name implies, TTN is a benign, self-limited disease. The infant's need for supplemental oxygen usually is highest at the onset of the disease and then progressively decreases. Infants with uncomplicated disease usually recover rapidly, without any residual pulmonary disability. Although the symptoms of TTN relate to pulmonary edema, one controlled trial that assessed therapy with diuretics found no evidence for their efficacy (Wiswell et al, 1985). (See Chapter 46 for treatment with surfactant and Chapter 45 for a complete discussion of the principles of respiratory monitoring and therapy.)

## REFERENCES

Abman SH, Kinsella JP, Schaffer MS, et al: Inhaled nitric oxide in the management of a premature newborn with severe respiratory distress syndrome and pulmonary hypertension. Pediatrics 92:606, 1993.

ACTOBAT Study Group: Australian Collaborative Trial of Antenatal Thyrotropin Releasing Hormone (ACTOBAT) for prevention of neonatal respiratory disease. Lancet 345:877, 1995.

Adams FH, Fujiwara T, Emmanouilides GC, Raiha N: Lung phospholipids of human fetuses and infants with and without hyaline membrane disease. Pediatrics 77:833, 1970.

Adams FH, Fujiwara T, Rowshan G: The nature and origin of the fluid in the fetal lamb lung. J Pediatr 63:881, 1963.

Adamson TM, Boyd RDH, Platt HS, et al: Composition of alveolar liquid in the foetal lamb. J Physiol 204:159, 1969.

Avery ME, Fletcher BD: The Lung and Its Disorders in the Newborn Infant. Philadelphia, WB Saunders, 1974.

Avery ME, Gatewood OB, Brumley G: Transient tachypnea of newborn: Possible delayed resorption of fluid at birth. Am J Dis Child 111:380, 1966.

Avery ME, Mead J: Surface properties in relation to atelectasis and hyaline membrane disease. Am J Dis Child 97:517, 1959.

Ballard PL: Hormones and Lung Maturation. New York, Springer-Verlag, 1986.

Ballard RA, Ballard PL, Creasy R, et al: Respiratory disease in very low birth weight infants after prenatal thyrotropin releasing hormone and glucocorticoid. Lancet 339:510, 1992.

Ballard RA, Ballard PL, Cnann A, et al: Antenatal thyrotropin-releasing hormone to prevent lung disease in preterm infants. North American Thyrotropin-Releasing Hormone Study Group. N Engl J Med 338:493, 1998.

Banks BA, Cnann A, Morgan MA, et al: Multiple courses of antenatal corticosteroids and outcome of premature neonates. North American Thyrotropin-Releasing Hormone Study Group. Am J Obstet Gynecol 181:709, 1999.

Bell EF, Acarregui MJ: Restricted versus liberal water intake for preventing morbidity and mortality in preterm infants. Cochrane Database Syst Rev 3, 2001.

Benatar SR, Hewlett AM, Nunn JF: The use of iso-shunt lines for control of oxygen therapy. Br J Anaesthesiol 45:711, 1973.

Berthiaume Y, Staub NC, Matthay MA: Beta-adrenergic agonists increase lung liquid clearance in anesthetized sheep. J Clin Invest 79:335, 1987.

Bland RD, Albertine KH, Carlton DP, et al: Chronic lung injury in preterm lambs: Abnormalities of the pulmonary circulation and lung fluid balance. Pediatr Res 48:64, 2000.

Bland RD, Nielson DW: Developmental changes in lung epithelial ion transport and liquid movement. Annu Rev Physiol 54:373, 1992.

Bland RD, Bressack MA, McMillan DD: Labor decreases the lung water content of newborn rabbits. Am J Obstet Gynecol 35:364, 1979.

Bland RD: Dynamics of pulmonary water before and after birth. Acta Paediatr Scand 305(suppl):12, 1983.

Bland RD: Lung liquid clearance before and after birth. Semin Perinatol 12:124, 1988.

Bland RD, Hansen TN, Haberkern CM, et al: Lung fluid balance in lambs before and after birth. J Appl Physiol 53:992, 1982.

Boughton K, Gandy G, Gairdner D: Hyaline membrane disease II. Lung lecithin. Arch Dis Child 45:311, 1970.

Brumley GW, Hodson WA, Avery ME: Lung phospholipids and surface tension correlations in infants with and without hyaline membrane disease. Pediatrics 40:13, 1967.

Brus F, van Oeveren WV, Okken A, et al: Number and activation of circulating polymorphonuclear leukocyte and platelets are associated with neonatal respiratory distress syndrome severity. Pediatrics 99:672, 1997

Buss IH, Senthilmohan R, Darlow BA, et al: 3-Chlorotyrosine as a marker of protein damage by myeloperoxidase in tracheal aspirates from preterm infants: Association with adverse respiratory outcome. Pediatr Res 53:455, 2003.

Chida S, Fujiwara T: Stable microbubble test for predicting the risk of respiratory distress syndrome: comparisons with other predictors of fetal lung maturity in amniotic fluid. Eur J Pediatr 152:148, 1993.

Chida S, Fujiwara T, Konishi M, et al: Stable microbubble test for predicting the risk of respiratory distress syndrome: Prospective evaluation of the test on amniotic fluid and gastric aspirate. Eur J Pediatr 152:152, 1993.

Christopher Roze J, Tohier C, Maingueneau C, et al: Response to dobutamine and dopamine in the hypotensive very preterm infant. Arch Dis Child 69:59, 1993.

Chu J, Clements JA, Cotton EK, et al: Neonatal pulmonary ischemia: Clinical and physiological studies. Pediatrics 40:709, 1967.

Clements JA, Platzker ACG, Tierney DF, et al: Assessment of the risk of respiratory distress syndrome by a rapid test for surfactant in amniotic fluid. N Engl J Med 286:1077, 1972.

Clements JA, Tooley WH: Kinetics of surface active material in the fetal lung. In Hodson WA (ed): Development of the Lung. New York, Marcel Dekker, 1977.

Clyman RI, Ballard PL, Sniderman S, et al: Prenatal administration of betamethasone for prevention of patent ductus arteriosus. J Pediatr 98:123, 1981.

Committee on the Fetus and Newborn: Postnatal corticosteroids to treat or prevent chronic lung disease in preterm infants. Pediatrics 109:330, 2002.

Corbet A: Medical manipulation of the ductus arteriosus. In Garson A, Bricker JT, Fisher DJ, Neish SR (eds): The Science and Practice of Pediatric Cardiology. Philadelphia, Lea & Febiger, 1996.

Corbet AJS, Adams JM, Kenny JD, et al.: Controlled trial of bicarbonate therapy in high risk premature newborn infants. J Pediatr 91:771, 1977.

Corbet AJS, Ross JA, Beaudry PH, Stern L: Ventilation-perfusion relationships as assessed by aA.$DN_2$ in hyaline membrane disease. J Appl Physiol 36:74, 1974.

Costarino AT, Gruskay JA, Corcoran L, et al: Sodium restriction versus daily maintenance replacement in very low birth weight premature neonates: A randomized blind therapeutic trial. J Pediatr 120:99, 1992.

Crowley P, Chalmers I, Keirse MJNC: The effects of corticosteroid administration before preterm delivery: An overview of the evidence from controlled trials. Br J Obstet Gynecol 97:11, 1990.

Crowley P: Corticosteroids after preterm premature rupture of membranes. Obstet Gynecol Clin North Am 19:317, 1992.

Cummings JJ, Carlton DP, Poulain FR, et al: Hypoproteinemia slows lung liquid clearance in young lambs. J Appl Physiol 74:153, 1993.

Dalence CR, Bowie LJ, Dohnal JC, et al: Amniotic fluid lamellar body count: A rapid and reliable fetal lung maturity test. Obstet Gynecol 86:235, 1995.

deMello DE, Chi EY, Doo E, Lagunoff D: Absence of tubular myelin in lungs of infants dying with hyaline membrane disease. Am J Pathol 127:131, 1987.

Dilger I, Schwedler G, Dudenhausen JW: Determination of the pulmonary surfactant associated protein SP-B in amniotic fluid with a competition ELISA. Gynecol Obstet Invest 38:24, 1994.

Dreizzen E, Migdal M, Praud JP, et al.: Passive compliance of total respiratory system in preterm newborn infants with respiratory distress syndrome. J Pediatr 112:778, 1988.

Dudell GG, Gersony WM: Patent ductus arteriosus in neonates with severe respiratory disease. J Pediatr 104:915, 1984.

Edberg KE, Sandberg K, Silberberg A, et al: Lung volume, gas mixing, and mechanics of breathing in mechanically ventilated very low birth weight infants with idiopathic respiratory distress syndrome. Pediatr Res 30:496, 1991.

Evans N, Iyer P: Change in blood pressure after treatment of patent ductus arteriosus with indomethacin. Arch Dis Child 68:584, 1993.

Farrell PM, Avery ME: State of the art: Hyaline membrane disease. Am Rev Respir Dis 111:657, 1975.

Farrell PM, Wood RE: Epidemiology of hyaline membrane disease in the United States: Analysis of national mortality statistics. Pediatrics 58:167, 1976.

Fauser A, Pohlandt F, Bartmann P, Gortner L: Rapid increase of blood pressure in extremely low birth weight infants after a single dose of dexamethasone. Eur J Pediatr 152:354, 1993.

Fedrick J, Butler NR: Hyaline membrane disease. Lancet 2:768, 1972.

Finlay-Jones JM, Papadimitriou JM, Barter RA: Pulmonary hyaline membrane: Light and election microscopic study of the early stage. J Pathol 112:117, 1974.

Frank L, Lewis PL, Sosenko IRS: Dexamethasone-stimulated fetal rat lung antioxidant enzyme activity in parallel with surfactant stimulation. Pediatrics 75:569, 1985.

French NP, Hagan R, Evans SF, et al: Repeated antenatal corticosteroids: Size at birth and subsequent development. Am J Obstet Gynecol 180:114, 1999.

Gandy G, Jacobson W, Gairdner D: Hyaline membrane disease: Cellular changes. Arch Dis Child 45:289, 1970.

Garite TJ, Rumney PJ, Briggs GG, et al: A randomized placebo controlled trial of betamethasone for the prevention of respiratory distress syndrome at 24–28 weeks gestation. Am J Obstet Gynecol 166:646, 1992.

Gaylord MS, Lorch S, Lorch V, Wright P: The novel use of sterile water gastric drips for management of fluid and electrolyte abnormalities in extremely low birth weight infants. Neonat Intensive Care May:44, 1995.

Gill AB, Weindling AM: Echocardiographic assessment of cardiac function in shocked very low birth weight infants. Arch Dis Child 68:17, 1993a.

Gill AB, Weindling AM: Randomised controlled trial of plasma protein fraction versus dopamine in hypotensive very low birth weight infants. Arch Dis Child 69:284, 1993b.

Glass L, Rajegowda BK, Evans HE: Absence of respiratory distress syndrome in premature infants of heroin addicted mothers. Lancet 2:685, 1971.

Gluck L, Kulovich MV: The evaluation of functional maturity in the human fetus. In Gluck L (ed): Modern Perinatal Medicine. Chicago, Year Book Medical Publishers, 1974.

Gluck L, Kulovich MV: Lecithin-sphingomyelin ratios in amniotic fluid in normal and abnormal pregnancy. Am J Obstet Gynecol 115:539, 1973.

Golan A, Zalzstein E, Zmora E, et al: Pulmonary hypertension in respiratory distress syndrome. Pediatr Pulmonol 19:221, 1995.

Gribetz I, Frank NR, Avery ME: Static volume pressure relations of excised lungs of infants with hyaline membrane disease, newborn and stillborn infants. J Clin Invest 38:2168, 1959.

Hack M, Fanaroff A, Klaus M: Neonatal respiratory distress following elective delivery: A preventable disease? Am J Obstet Gynecol 126:43, 1976.

Hallak MB, Bottoms SF: Accelerated pulmonary maturation from preterm premature rupture of membranes: A myth. Am J Obstet Gynecol 169:1045, 1993

Halliday HL, McClure G, McCreid M: Transient tachypnoea of the newborn: Two distinct clinical entities? Arch Dis Child 56:322, 1981.

Hallman M, Kulovich MV, Kirkpatrick E, et al: Phosphatidylinositol and phosphatidylglycerol in amniotic fluid. Indices of lung maturity. Am J Obstet Gynecol 125:613, 1976.

Hallman M, Teramo K: Measurement of the lecithin-sphingomyelin ratio and phosphatidylglycerol in amniotic fluid: An accurate method for the assessment of fetal lung maturity. Br J Obstet Gynaecol 88:806, 1981.

Hansen TN, Corbet AJS, Kenny JD, et al: Effects of oxygen and constant positive pressure breathing on aA.D$CO_2$ in hyaline membrane disease. Pediatr Res 13:1167, 1979.

Harker LC, Merritt TA, Edwards DK: Improving the prediction of surfactant deficiency in very low birth weight infants with respiratory distress. J Perinatol 12:129, 1992.

Helbock HJ, Insoft RM, Conte FA: Glucocorticoid responsive hypotension in extremely low birth weight newborns. Pediatrics 92:715, 1993.

Hibbard JU, Hibbard MC, Whalen MP: Umbilical cord blood gases and mortality and morbidity in the very low birth weight infant. Obstet Gynecol 78:768, 1991.

Hjalmarson O, Olsson T: Mechanical and ventilatory parameters in healthy and diseased newborn infants. Acta Paediatr Scand (Suppl) 247:26, 1974.

Hulsey TC, Alexander GR, Robillard PY, et al: Hyaline membrane disease: The role of ethnicity and maternal risk factors. Am J Obstet Gynecol 168:572, 1993.

Humphreys PW, Normand ICS, Reynolds EOR, et al: Pulmonary lymph flow and the uptake of liquid from the lungs of the lamb at the start of breathing. J Physiol 193:1, 1967.

Ikegami M, Jobe AH, Berry D: A protein that inhibits surfactant in respiratory distress syndrome. Biol. Neonate 50:121, 1986.

Ikegami M, Jobe AH, Tabor BL, et al: Lung albumin recovery in surfactant treated preterm ventilated lambs. Am Rev Respir Dis 145:1005, 1992.

Ikegami M, Ueda T, Absolom D, et al: Changes in exogenous surfactant in ventilated preterm lamb lungs. Am Rev Respir Dis 148:837, 1993.

Jackson JC, Palmer S, Truog WE, et al: Surfactant quantity and composition during recovery from hyaline membrane disease. Pediatr Res 20:1243, 1986

James LS: Perinatal events and respiratory distress syndrome. N Engl J Med 292:1291, 1975.

Jefferies AL, Coates G, O'Brodovich H: Pulmonary epithelial permeability in hyaline membrane disease. N Engl J Med 311:1075, 1984.

Jobe AH: Pulmonary surfactant therapy. N Engl J Med 328:861, 1993.

Jobe AH, Wada N, Berry LM, et al: Single and repetitive maternal glucocorticoid exposures reduce fetal growth in sheep. Am J Obstet Gynecol 178:880, 1998

Joint Working Party of the Royal College of Physicians: Development of audit measures and guidelines for good practice in the management of neonatal respiratory distress syndrome. Arch Dis Child 67:1221, 1992.

Jones MD, Burd LI, Bowes WA, et al: Failure of association of premature rupture of membranes with respiratory distress syndrome. N Engl J Med 292:1253, 1975.

Jost A, Policard A: Contribution expérimentale a l'étude du développement du poumon chez le lapin. Arch Anat Microsc 37:323, 1948.

Kattner E, Metze B, Waib E, Obladen M: Accelerated lung maturation following maternal steroid treatment in infants born before 30 weeks gestation. J Perinatal Med 20:449, 1992.

Kenny JD, Adams, JM, Corbet AJS, Rudolph AJ: The role of acidosis at birth in the development of hyaline membrane disease. Pediatrics 58:184, 1976.

Kenny JD, Corbet AJS, Adams JM, Rudolph AJ: Hyaline membrane disease and acidosis at birth in twins. Obstet Gynecol 50:710, 1977.

Kjos SL, Walther FJ, Montoro M, et al: Prevalence and etiology of respiratory distress syndrome in infants of diabetic mothers: Predictive values of fetal lung maturation tests. Am J Obstet Gynecol 163:898, 1990.

Klarr JM, Faix RG, Pryce CJE, et al: Randomized blind trial of dopamine versus dobutamine in preterm infants with respiratory distress syndrome. J Pediatr 125:117, 1994.

Knight DB, Liggins GC, Wealthall SR: A randomized controlled trial of antepartum thyrotropin releasing hormone and betamethasone in the prevention of respiratory disease in preterm infants. Am J Obstet Gynecol 171:11, 1994.

Kopelman AE: Blood pressure and cerebral ischemia in very low birth weight infants. J Pediatr 116:1000, 1990.

Kopelman AE, Moise AA, Holbert D, et al: A single very early dexamethasone dose improves respiratory and cardiovascular adaptation in preterm infants. J Pediatr 135:345, 1999

Krauss AN, Auld PAM: Pulmonary gas trapping in premature infants. Pediatr Res 5:10, 1971.

Krauss AN, Klain DB, Auld PAM: Carbon monoxide diffusing capacity in newborn infants. Pediatr Res 10:771, 1976.

Landers S, Hansen TN, Corbet AJS, et al.: Optimal constant positive airway pressure assessed by arterial alveolar difference for $CO_2$ in hyaline membrane disease. Pediatr Res 20:884, 1986.

Lawson EE, Birdwell RL, Huang PS, Taeusch HW: Augmentation of pulmonary surfactant secretion by lung expansion at birth. Pediatr Res 13:611, 1979.

Lemons JA, Bauer CR, Oh W, et al: Very low birth weight outcomes of the National Institute of Child Health and Human Development Neonatal Research Network, January 1995 through December 1996. Pediatrics 107:E1, 2001

Liggins GC, Howie RN: A controlled trial of antepartum glucocorticoid treatment for prevention of the respiratory distress syndrome in premature infants. Pediatrics 50:515, 1972.

Lucey JF: Clinical uses of transcutaneous oxygen monitoring. Adv Pediatr 28:27, 1981.

Macklem PT, Proctor DF, Hogg JC: The stability of peripheral airways. Respir Physiol 8:191, 1970.

Ment LR, Oh W, Ehrenkranz RA, et al: Antenatal steroids, delivery mode, and intraventricular hemorrhage in preterm infants. Am J Obstet Gynecol 172:795, 1995.

Miller HC, Futrakul P: Birth weight, gestational age and sex as determining factors in the incidence of respiratory distress syndrome of prematurely born infants. J Pediatr 72:628, 1968.

Moise AA, Wearden ME, Kozinetz CA, et al: Antenatal steroids are associated with less need for blood pressure support in extremely premature infants. Pediatrics 95:845, 1995.

Morrison JJ, Rennie JM, Milton PJ: Neonatal respiratory morbidity and mode of delivery at term: Influence of timing of elective cesarian section. Br J Obstet Gynecol 102:101, 1995.

Morrow RW, Taylor AF, Kinsella JP, et al: Effect of ductal patency on organ blood flow and pulmonary function in the preterm baboon with hyaline membrane disease. Crit Care Med 23:179, 1995.

Moscoso P, Goldberg RN, Jamieson J, Bancalari E: Spontaneous elevation in arterial blood pressure during the first hours of life in the very low birth weight infant. J Pediatr 103:114, 1983.

Naeye RL, Freeman RK, Blanc WA: Nutrition, sex, and fetal lung maturation. Pediatr Res 8:200, 1974.

National Institutes of Health Consensus Development Panel: Antenatal corticosteroids revisited: Repeat courses—National Institutes of Health Consensus Development Conferences Statement, August 17–18, 2000. Obstet Gynecol 98:144, 2001.

Nelson NM, Prod'hom LS, Cherry RB, et al: Pulmonary function in the newborn infant. Perfusion, estimation by analysis of the arterial-alveolar carbon dioxide difference. Pediatrics 30:975, 1962.

NIH Consensus Development Conference Statement: Effect of corticosteroids for fetal maturation on perinatal outcomes, 1994. Am J Obstet Gynecol 173:246, 1995.

NIH Consensus Development Panel: Effect of corticosteroids for fetal maturation of perinatal outcomes. JAMA 273:413, 1995.

Nilsson R, Grossman G, Robertson B: Lung surfactant and the pathogenesis of neonatal bronchiolar lesions induced by artificial ventilation. Pediatr Res 12:249, 1978.

Nupponen I, Pesonen E, Andersson S, et al: Neutrophil activation in preterm infants who have respiratory distress syndrome. Pediatrics 110:36, 2002

Okajima S, Matsuda T, Cho K, et al: Antenatal dexamethasone administration impairs normal postnatal lung growth in rats. Pediatr Res 49:777, 2001

Olver RE, Strang LB: Ion fluxes across the pulmonary epithelium and secretion of lung liquid in the foetal lamb. J Physiol 241:327, 1974.

Orzalesi MM, Motoyama EK, Jacobson HN, et al: The development of the lungs of lambs. Pediatrics 35:373, 1965.

Padbury JF, Agata Y, Baylen BG, et al: Dopamine pharmacokinetics in critically ill newborn infants. J Pediatr 110:293, 1986.

Pena IC, Teberg AJ, Finella KM: The premature small for gestational age infant during the first year of life: Comparison by birth weight and gestational age. J Pediatr 113:1066, 1988.

Pierce MR, Sosenko IRS, Frank L: Prenatal thyroid releasing hormone and thyroid releasing hormone plus dexamethasone lessen the survival of newborn rats during prolonged high $O_2$ exposure. Pediatr Res 32:407, 1992.

Pryhuber GS, Hull WM, Fink I, et al: Ontogeny of surfactant proteins A and B in human amniotic fluid as indices of fetal lung maturation. Pediatr Res 30:597, 1991.

Reller MD, et al: Duration of ductal shunting in healthy preterm infants: An echocardiographic color flow Doppler study. J Pediatr 112:441, 1988.

Reller MD, Rice MJ, McDonald RW: Review of studies evaluating ductal patency in the premature infant. J Pediatr 122:S59, 1993.

Richardson CP, Jung AL: Effects of continuous positive airway pressure on pulmonary function and blood gases of infants with respiratory distress syndrome. Pediatr Res 12:771, 1978.

Richardson DK, Torday JS: Racial differences in predictive value of the lecithin/sphingomyelin ratio. Am J Obstet Gynecol 170:1273, 1994.

Richardson P, Bose CL, Carlstrom JR: The functional residual capacity of infants with respiratory distress syndrome. Acta Paediatr Scand 75:267, 1986.

Richardson P, Jarriel S, Hansen TN: Mechanics of the respiratory system during passive exhalation in preterm lambs. Pediatr Res 26:425, 1989.

Richardson P, Pace WR, Valdes E, et al: Time dependence of lung mechanics in preterm lambs. Pediatr Res 31:276, 1992.

Rider E, Jobe A, Ikegami M, et al: Effects of maternal corticosteroid dose on surfactant pool sizes, protein leaks and SPC precursor incorporation in preterm rabbits. Clin Res 37:207A, 1989.

Rieutort M, Farrell PM, Engle MJ, et al: Changes in surfactant phospholipids in fetal rat lungs from normal and diabetic pregnancies. Pediatr Res 20:650, 1986.

Robert MF, Neff RK, Hubbell JP, et al: Association between maternal diabetes and the respiratory distress syndrome in the newborn. N Engl J Med 294:357, 1976.

Ronconi M, Fortunato A, Soffiati G, et al: Vasopressin, atrial natriuretic factor and renal water homeostatis in premature newborn infants with respiratory distress syndrome. J Perinat Med 23:307-314, 1995

Ryan CA, Finer NN: Antenatal corticosteroid therapy to prevent respiratory distress syndrome. J Pediatr 126:317, 1995.

Saigal S, Wilson R, Usher R: Radiological findings in symptomatic neonatal plethora resulting from placental transfusion. Radiology 125:1851, 1977.

Samiec TD, Radmacher P, Hill T, Adamkin DH: Measured energy expenditure in mechanically ventilated very low birth weight infants. Am J Med Sci 307:182, 1994.

Scholle S, Braunlich H: Effects of prenatally administered thyroid hormones or glucocorticoids on maturation of kidney function in newborn rats. Dev Pharmacol Ther 112:162, 1989.

Scott SM, Watterberg KL: Effect of gestational age, postnatal age, and illness on plasma cortisol concentrations in premature infants. Pediatr Res 37:112, 1995.

Seeger W, Grube C, Gunther A, Schmidt R: Surfactant inhibition by plasma proteins: Differential sensitivity of various surfactant proteins. Eur Respir J 6:971, 1993.

Seppanen MP, Kaapa PO, Kiro PO, Saraste M: Doppler derived systolic pulmonary artery pressure in acute neonatal respiratory distress syndrome. Pediatrics 93:769, 1994.

Sinclair JC: Pathophysiology of hyaline membrane disease. In Winter RW (ed): The Body Fluids in Pediatrics. Boston, Little, Brown, 1973.

Skelton R, Jeffery H: Click test: Rapid diagnosis of the respiratory distress syndrome. Pediatr Pulmonol 17:383, 1994.

Stefano JL, Norman ME, Morales MC, et al: Decreased erythrocyte sodium-potassium-ATPase activity associated with cellular potassium loss in extremely low birth weight infants with non-oliguric hyperkalemia. J Pediatr 122:276, 1993.

Stonestreet BS, Hansen MB, Laptock AR, et al.: Glucocorticoids accelerate renal function maturation in fetal lambs. Early Hum Dev. 8:331, 1983.

Strang LB: Uptake of liquid from the lungs at the start of breathing. In DeReuch AVS, Porter R (eds): CIBA Foundation Symposium: Development of the Lung. London, J & A Churchill, 1967.

Strang LB, MacLeish MH: Ventilatory failure and right to left shunt in newborn infants with respiratory distress. Pediatrics 28:17, 1961.

Tammela KT, Lanning FP, Koivisto ME: The relationship of fluid restriction during the first month of life and the occurrence and severity of bronchopulmonary dysplasia in low birth weight infants: A 1 year radiological follow up. Eur J Pediatr 151:367, 1992.

Tejani N, Verma UL: Correlation of Apgar scores and umbilical artery acid base status to mortality and morbidity in the low birth weight infant. Obstet Gynecol 73:597, 1989.

Thompson PJ, Greenough A, Gamsu HR, Nicolaides KH: Ventilatory requirements for respiratory distresss syndrome in small for gestational age infants. Eur J Pediatr 151:528, 1992.

Towers CV, Garite TJ: Evaluation of the new AmnioStat-FLM test for the detection of phosphatidylglycerol in contaminated fluids. Am J Obstet Gynecol 160:298, 1989.

Tubman TRJ, Rollins MD, Patterson C, Halliday HL: Increased incidence of respiratory distress syndrome in babies of hypertensive mothers. Arch Dis Child 66:52, 1991.

Tyson JE, Kennedy K, Broyles S, Rosenfeld CA: The small for gestational age infant: Accelerated or delayed pulmonary maturation? Increased or decreased survival? Pediatrics 95:534, 1995.

Ueda T, Ikegami M, Jobe AH: Developmental changes of sheep surfactant: In vivo function and in vitro subtype conversion. J Appl Physiol 76:2701, 1994.

Uno H, Lohmiller L, Thieme C, et al: Brain damage induced by prenatal exposure to dexamethasone in fetal rhesus macaques. I. Hippocampus. Brain Res Dev Brain Res 53:157, 1990.

Usher R: Reduction in mortality from respiratory distress syndrome and prematurity with early administration of intravenous glucose and sodium bicarbonate. Pediatrics 32:966, 1963.

Usher RH, Allen AC, McLean FH: Risk of respiratory distress syndrome related to gestational age, route of delivery and maternal diabetes. Am J Obstet Gynecol 111:826, 1971.

Van Marter LJ, Allred EN, Pagano M, et al: Do clinical markers of barotrauma and oxygen toxicity explain interhospital variation in rates of chronic lung disease? The Neonatology Committee for the Developmental Network. Pediatrics 105:1194, 2000.

Van Marter LJ, Leviton A, Kuban KCK, et al: Maternal glucocorticoid therapy and reduced risk of bronchopulmonary dysplasia. Pediatrics 86:331, 1990.

Verder H, Robertson B, Greisen G, et al: Surfactant therapy and nasal continuous positive airway pressure for newborns with respiratory distress syndrome. N Engl J Med 331:1051, 1994.

Versmold HT, Kitterman JA, Phibbs RH, et al: Aortic blood pressure during the first 12 hours of life in infants with birthweight 610-4220 grams. Pediatrics 67:607, 1981.

Walters DV, Olver RW: The role of catecholamines in lung liquid absorption at birth. Pediatr Res 12:239, 1978.

Walther FJ, Siassi B, Ramadan NA, et al: Cardiac output in infants with transient myocardial dysfunction. J Pediatr 107:781, 1985.

West JB: Ventilation perfusion inequality and overall gas exchange in computer models of the lung. Respir Physiol 7:88, 1969.

Wilkie RA, Bryan MH, Tarnow-Mordi WO: Static respiratory compliance in the newborn. 2 Its potential for selection of infants for early surfactant treatment. Arch Dis Child 70:F16, 1994.

Wiswell TE, Rawlings JS, Smith FR, Goo ED: Effect of furosemide on the clinical course of transient tachypnea of the newborn. Pediatrics 75:908, 1985.

Wright LL, Horbar JD, Gunkel H, et al: Evidence from multicenter networks on the current use and effectiveness of antenatal corticosteroids in low birth weight infants. Am J Obstet Gynecol 173:263, 1995.

Yoon JJ, Kohl S, Harper RG: The relationship between maternal hypertensive disease of pregnancy and the incidence of idiopathic respiratory distress syndrome. Pediatrics 65:735, 1980.

Zuckerman B, Maynard EC, Cabral H: A preliminary report of prenatal cocaine exposure and respiratory distress syndrome in premature infants. Am J Dis Child 145:696, 1991.

CHAPTER 48

# Respiratory Failure in the Term Infant

Roberta A. Ballard, Thomas N. Hansen, and Anthony Corbet

The pathophysiology of respiratory failure in the term or near-term infant, although sharing some of the same developmental physiologic issues that affect the preterm infant, includes a number of etiologic disorders not commonly seen in the more immature infant. In particular, persistent pulmonary hypertension of the newborn (PPHN) and meconium aspiration syndrome tend to be seen most commonly in term or post-term infants. In addition, other entities such as perinatal-neonatal asphyxia or pneumonia, particularly those due to group B streptococcal infection, may cause profound respiratory failure in infants with otherwise normal mature lungs. Finally, a small but significant number of infants may have severe respiratory distress secondary to abnormalities or maldevelopment of the surfactant system or abnormal development of the alveoli or the pulmonary vascular system. Management of intractable pulmonary failure in these infants also includes therapies not available or established for the preterm infant, including use of inhaled nitric oxide (iNO) and extracorporeal membrane oxygenation (ECMO).

In the approach to the term infant with respiratory failure presented in this chapter, it is assumed that appropriate studies have ruled out the presence of anatomic anomalies of the airway (see Chapters 50 and 51). In the absence of such abnormalities, the evaluation should now be directed at (1) ruling out cyanotic congenital heart disease and (2) attempting to determine whether the primary underlying disorder is due to intrinsic parenchymal lung disease, such as meconium aspiration or pneumonia, or to entities causing inadequate pulmonary blood flow, such as shock, asphyxia, cardiomyopathy, or PPHN.

This chapter addresses the etiology, pathobiology, and therapy of disorders that commonly lead to respiratory failure in term infants, with the assumption that both airway anomalies and congenital heart disease have been ruled out.

## PERSISTENT PULMONARY HYPERTENSION OF THE NEWBORN

Gersony and coworkers (1969) described a group of term infants without structural heart disease who became cyanotic shortly after birth and had only mild respiratory distress. These infants all had suprasystemic pulmonary arterial pressures and evidence of right-to-left shunting of blood across persistent fetal pathways (the foramen ovale and ductus arteriosus). The nature of these shunts initially led to the name "persistence of the fetal circulation." Subsequently, the name was changed to *persistent pulmonary hypertension of the newborn* to describe the pathophysiology of the disorder more accurately.

### Pathogenesis

Successful transition from intrauterine to extrauterine life requires that the pulmonary vascular resistance decrease precipitously at birth. In infants with PPHN, this decrease either does not occur or the vascular resistance does not remain low. Pulmonary arterial pressure is elevated, and blood is shunted right to left across the ductus arteriosus and foramen ovale. In addition, the persistently high pulmonary vascular resistance increases right ventricular afterload and oxygen demand and impairs oxygen delivery to the right ventricle, the posterior wall of the left ventricle, and the subendocardial regions of the right ventricle. Increased right ventricular afterload often results in displacement of the septum into the left ventricle, impairing left ventricular filling and reducing cardiac output.

In some instances, pulmonary vascular resistance remains only transiently elevated at birth (Table 48–1) and decreases rapidly once the underlying condition is corrected. In a number of other conditions, however, the pulmonary vascular resistance remains persistently elevated, either because of active constriction of pulmonary vessels or because of some anatomic abnormality.

Active constriction of pulmonary vessels can complicate the course of bacterial sepsis or pneumonia in the newborn (Shankaran et al, 1982). Experiments in animals show that this increase in pulmonary vascular resistance is temporally related to increased plasma thromboxane concentrations (Hammerman et al, 1988) and can be blocked by the administration of inhibitors of prostaglandin synthesis (Rojas et al, 1983). Active constriction of pulmonary vessels can also complicate the course of meconium aspiration pneumonia. Some studies suggest that vasoactive substances present in meconium or amniotic fluid diffuse through the lung and either constrict pulmonary vessels directly or induce platelet aggregation in the microcirculation, with the subsequent release of thromboxane. Clinical data support this hypothesis and show an association among perinatal aspiration syndromes, transient thrombocytopenia, and PPHN. Moreover, pathologic data demonstrate platelet plugging in the microcirculation of the lung of infants dying of PPHN associated with meconium aspiration pneumonia (Levin et al, 1983). Alternatively, in utero hypoxia may lead both to changes in the pulmonary vessels and to passage of meconium, and some infants born through meconium *without* aspiration have PPHN (see later on).

Anatomic abnormalities of the pulmonary vascular bed fall into two general categories: those associated with underdevelopment of the lung and those that result from maldevelopment of the vessels. In the case of pulmonary hypoplasia, lung mass is reduced, yet cardiac output is appropriate for body size. As a result, the volume of blood

**TABLE 48–1**

**Causes of Persistent Pulmonary Hypertension**

| |
|---|
| **Transient Pulmonary Hypertension** |
| Hypoxia with or without acidosis |
| Hypothermia |
| Hypoglycemia |
| Polycythemia |
| **Persistent Pulmonary Hypertension** |
| Active vasoconstriction |
| Bacterial sepsis and/or pneumonia |
| Perinatal aspiration syndromes |
| Underdevelopment of the lung |
| Diaphragmatic hernia |
| Potter syndrome |
| Other causes of pulmonary hypoplasia |
| Maldevelopment of pulmonary vessels |
| Idiopathic |
| Chronic intrauterine asphyxia |
| Meconium aspiration pneumonitis |
| Premature closure of the fetal ductus arteriosus |

flowing through the existing pulmonary vessels is relatively high, pulmonary arterial pressures are high, and relative pulmonary vascular resistance is increased. In addition to this anatomic impediment to flow, infants with pulmonary hypoplasia are likely to have maldevelopment of the pulmonary vessels and an increased pulmonary vascular resistance from anatomic obstruction of existing vessels (Geggel et al, 1986; Naeye et al, 1976).

Maldevelopment of pulmonary vessels refers predominantly to abnormalities of vascular smooth muscle found in lungs of infants dying from PPHN (Murphy et al, 1981) (Fig. 48–1). In these infants, pulmonary arterial smooth muscle hypertrophies and extends from preacinar arteries into normally nonmuscular intra-acinar arteries, even to the level of the alveolus (Fig. 48–2). This thickened muscle encroaches on the vessel lumen, resulting in mechanical obstruction to blood flow. In extreme cases, vascular maldevelopment can cause a reduction in the number of arteries per unit of cross-sectional area of the lung. A review of the associated clinical entities and the available data from experiments in animals suggest that this vascular maldevelopment is the result of sustained pulmonary hypertension in utero. PPHN is strongly associated with low-grade chronic intrauterine hypoxia. In fact, it is likely that unrecognized asphyxia or ductal closure may account for a large proportion of cases labeled as "idiopathic." In chronically asphyxiated fetuses, pulmonary arterial pressure can be increased by active constriction of pulmonary arterioles secondary to hypoxia. Because the pulmonary circulation is parallel to the systemic circulation, it also can be increased secondary to asphyxia-induced increases in systemic arterial pressure. Experimental data from fetal rats and lambs support both of these hypotheses (Soifer et al, 1987); however, although systemic hypertension (even by itself) consistently results in vascular maldevelopment (Levin et al, 1978b), intrauterine hypoxia does not consistently result in vascular maldevelopment (Geggel et al, 1986).

Premature closure of the ductus arteriosus secondary to maternal ingestion of inhibitors of prostaglandin synthesis has been associated with PPHN. Experiments in animals show that premature closure of the ductus (Morin, 1989; Wild et al, 1989) results in maldevelopment of pulmonary vessels, presumably by forcing a greater portion of the combined ventricular output

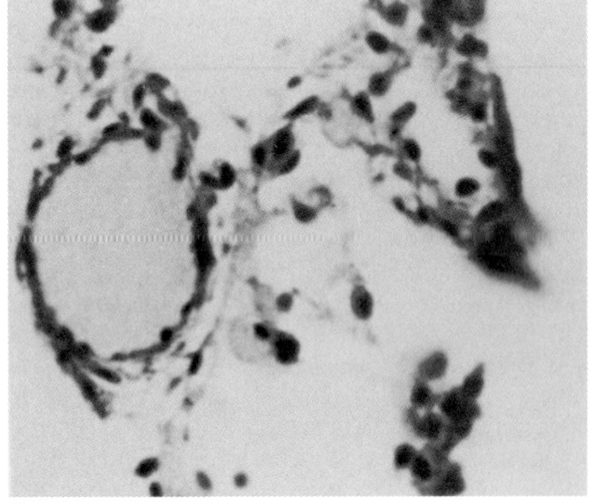
A

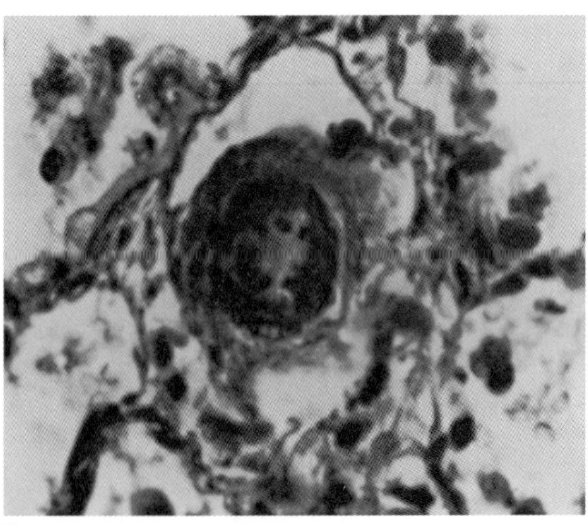
B

**FIGURE 48–1.** Photomicrographs of alveolar wall arteries distended with the barium gelatin suspension from a 3-day-old infant with normal lungs (**A**) and from a 3-day-old infant with persistent hypertension (**B**). The normal artery, seen in **A,** is nonmuscular, with a single-endothelial-cell lining surrounded by a thin layer of connective tissue. In **B,** the artery wall is composed of smooth muscle (darkly stained), two cell layers thick, surrounded by a thick connective tissue sheath enclosing a dilated lymphatic (located superiorly). (Elastin-van Gieson stain, × 250.) *(Courtesy of Dr. John Murphy.)*

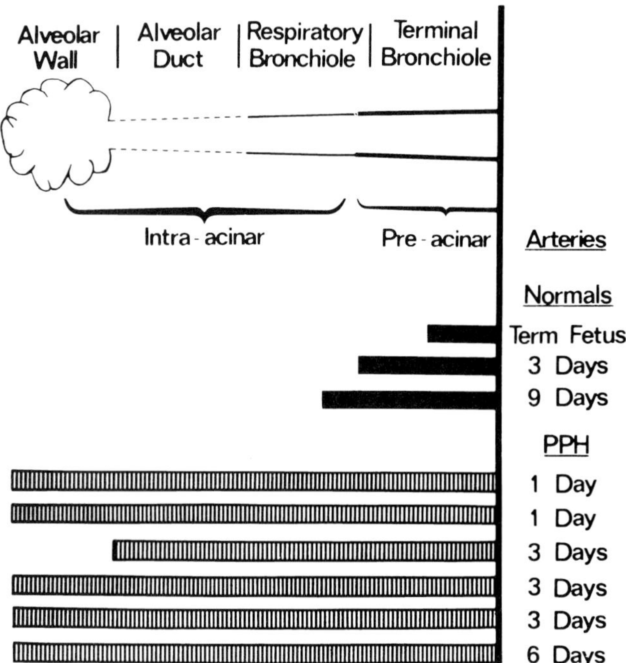


**FIGURE 48–2.** Vascular maldevelopment in persistent pulmonary hypertension of the newborn. In normal infants, no muscular arteries are found within the acinus. All patients with pulmonary hypertension had extension of muscle into intra-acinar arteries. *(From Murphy JD, Rabinovitch M, Goldstein JD, Reid LM: The structural basis of persistent pulmonary hypertension of the newborn infant. J Pediatr 98:962, 1981.)*

through the lungs at a significantly higher pressure (Levin et al, 1978a). The association between meconium aspiration pneumonia and vascular maldevelopment is interesting. Of 11 infants dying of meconium aspiration pneumonia, 10 were found to have significant vascular smooth muscle hypertrophy with extension of muscle into intra-acinar arteries (Murphy et al, 1984). This maldevelopment could be secondary to chronic intrauterine asphyxia, and recent work by Stenmark and Mecham (1997) suggests a complex interaction of epithelial and mesenchymal cells with growth factors in the developing lung and extracellular matrix protein changes that may be influenced by chronic hypoxia. Finally, because disorders associated with underdevelopment of the lung also result in intrauterine pulmonary hypertension, it is not too surprising that they also frequently are associated with maldevelopment of existing vessels. This is particularly true in infants with congenital diaphragmatic hernia, accounting for much of the respiratory instability of these infants (see Chapter 51).

It has become apparent that these anatomically abnormal vessels also exhibit certain functional abnormalities (Morin and Stenmark, 1995). One of the more important functions of the vascular endothelium is to produce the vasodilator NO. NO is produced in endothelial cells from L-arginine by the enzyme NO synthase. It diffuses rapidly into smooth muscle cells, where it stimulates production of cyclic guanosine monophosphate (cGMP) and smooth muscle relaxation. NO production by endothelial cells is responsible for the vasodilation that occurs in response to substances such as acetylcholine and bradykinin. Accordingly, these mediators are called *endothelial cell–dependent vasodilators*. Because NO is such a potent pulmonary vasodilator, it is tempting to speculate that impaired NO synthesis contributes to PPHN. In support of this speculation, investigators have shown that infants with PPHN have lower urinary nitrite and nitrate concentrations than those in infants without pulmonary disease, suggesting that their ability to produce NO may be impaired (Dollberg et al, 1995). Adults with pulmonary hypertension have reduced expression of NO synthase in their lungs (Giaid and Saleh, 1995), and chronic inhibition of NO production in the fetal lamb results in PPHN (Fineman et al, 1995). Data show that endothelial cell–dependent vasodilation is impaired in fetal lambs with pulmonary hypertension secondary to early closure of the ductus arteriosus (McQueston et al, 1995). How much of this impairment is at the level of NO synthase versus guanylate cyclase remains to be determined (Steinhorn et al, 1995).

In addition to production of the vasodilator NO, endothelial cells also produce many other factors including endothelin-1, which may act as a pulmonary vasoconstrictor in the newborn. Infants with PPHN have increased concentrations of endothelin-1 in arterial blood. These concentrations correlate with the severity of the pulmonary hypertension (Rosenberg et al, 1993). Many other factors including presence of oxygen free radicals (Sanderud, 1991) are associated with increased pulmonary vascular resistance. Table 48–2 (Kinsella and Abman, 1995) lists factors associated with either an increase or a decrease in pulmonary vascular resistance.

In their review of the cellular and molecular mechanisms of pulmonary vascular remodeling, Stenmark and Mecham (1997) discuss the vascular development in the lung and the cellular responses that occur in pulmonary hypertension. They review the evidence for endothelial cell replication in control of vasculogenesis with an interaction of epithelial cells and mesenchymal cells as well as the specific growth factors known to play a role in the developing lung. Smooth muscle cell replication in the pulmonary vasculature, which occurs at a very high rate in the embryo, decreases when the embryo becomes a fetus and decreases more than 2000-fold from embryonic to adult life. In addition, major changes in extracellular matrix protein occur during development that have an effect on the migration and differentiation of smooth muscle cells. These components include collagen, elastin, fibronectin, and tenascin-C (Cowan et al, 2000b). Cowan and colleagues provided further evidence that endothelial alterations may allow extravasation of a serum factor capable of stimulating smooth muscle cell production of a vascular serine-elastase. They found that tenascin-C amplifies the response of smooth muscle cells to growth factors that are liberated through matrix proteolysis. Reversal of fatal pulmonary hypertension in an animal model by a serine-elastase inhibitor also has been demonstrated (Cowan et al, 2000a).

TABLE 48–2

**Factors Known to Decrease or Increase Pulmonary Vascular Resistance**

| Decreases | Increases |
|---|---|
| **Mechanical Factors** | |
| Normal lung inflation | Overinflation or underinflation |
| Vascular cell structural changes | Excessive muscularization, vascular remodeling |
| Interstitial fluid and pressure changes | Altered mechanical properties of smooth muscle |
| Shear stress | Pulmonary hypoplasia |
| | Alveolar capillary dysplasia |
| | Pulmonary thromboemboli |
| | Main pulmonary artery distention |
| | Ventricular dysfunction, venous hypertension |
| **Endogenous Mediators and Mechanisms** | |
| Oxygen (but not hyperoxia) | Hypoxia |
| Nitric oxide | Oxygen-derived free radicals |
| Prostacyclin | Acidosis |
| Adenosine, ATP, magnesium | Endothelin-1 |
| Bradykinin | Leukotrienes |
| Atrial natriuretic factor | Thromboxanes |
| Alkalosis | Platelet-activating factor |
| $K^+$ channel activation | $Ca^{2+}$ channel activation |
| Histamine | α-adrenergic stimulation |
| Acetylcholine | Prostaglandin $F_{2\alpha}$ |
| β-adrenergic stimulation | |

Adapted from Kinsella and Abman, 1995.

### Clinical Manifestations

Affected infants usually are delivered at term or post-term and frequently are born through meconium-stained fluid. They often are thought to be normal after brief distress at birth. Then within the first 12 hours after birth, they are recognized as having cyanosis and tachypnea, without apnea and retractions or grunting. They frequently have a cardiac murmur that is compatible with tricuspid insufficiency, but systemic blood pressure is normal. Hypoglycemia frequently complicates many of the associated conditions, such as sepsis and meconium aspiration; hypocalcemia also frequently occurs. Arterial blood gas analysis reveals severe arterial oxygen desaturation, but $CO_2$ tensions may be relatively normal. In infants with significant ductal level right-to-left shunting, the oxygen saturation measured from the right brachial or radial artery is greater than that obtained from the umbilical artery. Chest radiographs may reveal cardiomegaly. For infants with idiopathic PPHN without parenchymal lung disease, the lung fields are clear and appear undervascularized (Fig. 48–3). For the remainder of the associated entities, chest radiographs reflect the underlying parenchymal disease. Electrocardiograms reveal ventricular hypertrophy appropriate for age; in more severe cases, they also reveal ST segment depression in the precordial leads, suggestive of ischemia. All infants suspected of having PPHN should undergo ultrasound examination of the heart to rule out cyanotic congenital heart disease, to document right-to-left shunting of blood at the foramen ovale and ductus arteriosus, and to measure systolic time intervals. Prolonged systolic time intervals support a diagnosis of pulmonary hypertension, but such findings are not definitive because the intervals also can be prolonged by right ventricular dysfunction. Please see Chapter 54 for further discussion of the evaluation of PPHN by echocardiography. At some point in the course of the disease, most infants with PPHN increase their $PaO_2$ above 100 mm Hg, at least transiently, in response to some therapeutic intervention. Infants who can never be oxygenated should be considered for additional echocardiographic studies or cardiac catheterization.

### Management

It is essential at each stage in the management of these infants to determine whether or not parenchymal lung disease is contributing to their respiratory failure. Initially, the most common contributing parenchymal diseases are aspiration of particulate meconium, severe overwhelming pneumonia, and cardiogenic pulmonary edema secondary to asphyxia. However, if the infant has no evidence of parenchymal lung disease, it is essential to avoid either excessive oxygen exposure or overventilation of the lungs. Oxygen toxicity as well as lung damage from stretch, along with decreased cardiac output secondary to decreased venous return due to excessive pressure applied to the respiratory system, contributes to worsening of the disease (Table 48–2) (Kinsella and Abman, 1995).

If adequate ventilation of the infant is possible (to achieve $PaCO_2$ in the normal range and good chest wall movement and good breath sounds), it is more likely that the hypoxic failure is secondary to decreased pulmonary blood flow and may be due to PPHN. Attention should

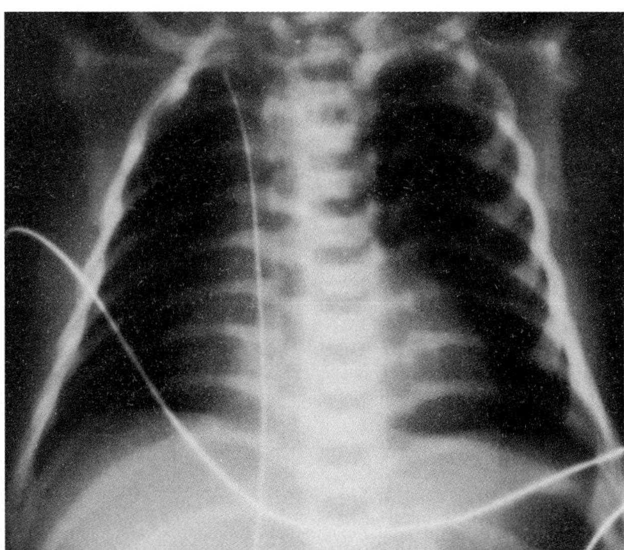

**FIGURE 48–3.** Chest radiograph from an infant with idiopathic persistent pulmonary hypertension of the newborn. Lung fields appear hyperlucent, with decreased vascularity.

first be paid to making sure that the infant is ventilated adequately, that blood pressure and cardiac output are supported, and that additional environmental stresses such as hypothermia, hyperthermia, excessive noise, or discomfort causing agitation in the infant have been minimized. All of these infants should be nursed in a neutral thermal environment. Cold stress raises the metabolic rate, increases oxygen consumption, and causes the infant to release norepinephrine, which is a pulmonary vasoconstrictor. Fluids should be restricted and hypoglycemia and hypocalcemia corrected. Systemic hypotension and acidosis should be corrected by judicious use of blood and alkali. Calcium, blood products, and hyperosmolar solutions are potentially vasoactive and should be infused with caution in this group of infants. Infusion of dopamine or, under some circumstances, dobutamine or epinephrine may increase cardiac output without affecting systemic or pulmonary vascular resistance. If the central hematocrit is greater than 60% to 65%, a partial exchange transfusion should be performed to lower the hematocrit and to reduce the effects of hyperviscosity on the pulmonary artery pressure.

Based on results from several centers suggesting that conservative medical management of infants with PPHN may reduce the need for extracorporeal membrane oxygenation and improve outcome (Dworetz et al, 1989; Wung et al, 1985), we have adopted an approach to therapy that seeks to reduce oxygen demand while maximizing oxygen delivery. A review by Walsh-Sukys and colleagues (1994) found, however, that use of gentler ventilation was slow to permeate standard management of PPHN. Subsequently, reporting for the NICHD Neonatal Network, Walsh-Sukys with other associates (2000) further noted that a wide range in clinical practice continued in the absence of controlled clinical trials.

In infants with PPHN, the pulmonary circulation seems to be exceptionally sensitive to changes in oxygen tension. Therefore, it is advisable to try to maintain the $Pa O_2$ between 70 and 100 mm Hg if possible. There is no evidence to suggest that maintaining $Pa O_2$ in excess of 100 mm Hg improves the outcome for the infant with PPHN, and prolonged exposure to excessively high $Pa O_2$ can injure other organs, such as the brain and the eye (Hansen and Gest, 1984). However, in patients with very severe PPHN, attempts to maintain $Pa O_2$ between 70 and 100 mm Hg may result in unacceptable complications of therapy. Therefore, many centers now tolerate much lower values for $Pa O_2$ (as low as 40 mm Hg) in infants with severe PPHN (Wung et al, 1985).

Oxygen should be given by nasal cannula or hood, in concentrations of up to 100% if necessary. If oxygen alone does not lower the pulmonary vascular resistance and improve arterial oxygen saturation, the next step is to induce alkalosis. Although several studies in animals have shown that both respiratory and metabolic alkalosis effectively lower pulmonary vascular resistance (Fike and Hansen, 1989; Schreiber et al, 1986), only respiratory alkalosis has been studied in infants (Drummond et al, 1981). Clearly, however, metabolic alkalization benefits these infants and many clinicians prefer metabolic alkalization over hyperventilation as the initial approach, as low $Pa CO_2$ levels are associated with poor neurodevelopmental outcome. The use of neuromuscular blockers such as pancuronium bromide in these infants is controversial and probably should be reserved for infants with parenchymal disease requiring extremely high inspiratory pressures. Because these infants are extremely sensitive to external stimuli, they should be sedated and handled as little as possible. To avoid alveolar overdistention, the inspiratory time is kept short (0.15 to 0.30 seconds). The lungs of infants with PPHN frequently have normal to prolonged expiratory time constants, so expiratory time must be kept relatively long to prevent gas trapping. Inspiratory pressure is adjusted to control the $Pa CO_2$. Positive end-expiratory pressure (PEEP) is useful only in patients with parenchymal lung disease. If the pulmonary hypertension is severe, however, the infant frequently develops surfactant deficiency and pulmonary edema over time and consequently may respond to end-expiratory pressure and/or surfactant replacement later in the course of the disease.

### *High-Frequency Ventilation*

For those infants with parenchymal lung disease underlying their PPHN, both high-frequency jet ventilation (HFJV) and high-frequency oscillatory ventilation (HFOV) are highly effective in controlling $Pa CO_2$. As a result, several groups have postulated that these ventilatory modalities may be effective in improving oxygenation in infants with PPHN associated with parenchymal disease. HFJV results in reductions in both $Pa CO_2$ and ventilator pressures in infants with PPHN but has no effect on ultimate outcome (Carlo et al, 1989).

Descriptive reports suggest that HFOV may be useful in the management of newborn infants with severe respiratory failure who are on maximal ventilatory support and are being considered for treatment with ECMO (Carter et al, 1990; Cornish et al, 1987). Clark and colleagues (1994) compared HFOV with conventional ventilation in

79 patients with PPHN in a randomized trial that allowed cross-over for treatment failures. There were no differences in mortality, treatment failures, or pulmonary outcomes between the two groups. Of interest, of the 24 patients in whom conventional ventilation failed, 15 (63%) responded to HFO, whereas only 4 (23%) of the 17 in whom HFO failed responded to conventional ventilation ($P$ = .03). A more recent trial (Kinsella et al, 1997) compared HFOV with conventional ventilation with iNO using a cross-over design that allocated patients in whom both therapies failed to a group for treatment with the combination of HFOV and iNO. Response to HFOV or iNO alone was similar between the two groups (23% and 28%, respectively), as was the response to the cross-over treatment (21% and 14%, respectively). Roughly one third of infants in whom both treatments failed, however, responded to the combination of HFOV and iNO. The response rates were best for infants with meconium aspiration syndrome or respiratory distress syndrome (RDS). Their results support the use of HFOV in combination with iNO, especially in infants in whom iNO alone fails. Both trials support the premise that HFOV for PPHN should be used only in hospitals that can also provide ECMO, because patients in whom HFOV therapy fails must be managed with conventional ventilation for the purpose of transportation.

### *Surfactant Replacement*

Data suggest that surfactant deficiency may play a role in several of the diseases associated with PPHN. Meconium aspiration pneumonia (Sun et al, 1993a, 1993b) and bacterial pneumonia both are associated with surfactant inactivation, and surfactant replacement therapy appears to improve gas exchange in infants with these conditions (Al-Mateen et al, 1994; Auten et al, 1991; Herting, 2000; Khammash et al, 1993). Although results with use of surfactant to treat severe respiratory failure in the term infant (Lotze et al, 1998) are promising, surfactant replacement therapy for infants with PPHN must still be considered experimental. For the infant in whom adequate ventilation with oxygen and appropriate cardiovascular support does not result in an acceptable $PaO_2$, the remaining alternative is to try to lower the pulmonary vascular resistance by pharmacologic means.

### *Inhaled Nitric Oxide Therapy*

It has long been postulated that vascular tone is an intrinsic property of the blood vessels. The observation that this was true only when the endothelium remained intact (Furchgott and Zawadzki, 1980) led to the suggestion that an endothelial cell–derived relaxing factor existed. In experiments done by Ignarro and colleagues (1987), it was shown that the endothelial cell–derived relaxing factor was identical with NO, a gas that could be delivered to the lung by inhalation. NO is produced in the endothelial cell by NO synthase, which catalyzes the conversion of arginine and oxygen to citrulline and NO (Palmer et al, 1988); the NO diffuses to the smooth muscle cell and activates guanyl cyclase, which converts guanosine triphosphate (GTP) into cGMP, producing smooth muscle relaxation.

Inhaled NO (iNO) initially was used in laboratory animal models to produce a specific decrease in pulmonary artery pressure (Frostell et al, 1991). No similar effect on the systemic circulation occurs because on entering the pulmonary bloodstream, NO is rapidly inactivated by combination with hemoglobin, forming first nitrosohemoglobin and then methemoglobin. Studies in the lamb and piglet models of PPHN (Etches et al, 1994; Kinsella et al, 1994; Roberts et al, 1993a; Zayek et al, 1993) demonstrate that iNO can reduce frequency of deaths and pulmonary artery pressure in a dose-related fashion from 0 to 80 parts per million (ppm).

#### Clinical Experience

These animal studies led to simultaneous reports by Roberts and colleagues (1992) and Kinsella and associates (1992b) showing that low-dose iNO (between 5 and 80 ppm) could produce a fall in pulmonary artery pressure, with improved systemic oxygenation, in newborn infants with severe respiratory failure due to PPHN. NO did this without decreasing systemic blood pressure or producing other toxic side effects.

This targeted delivery of dilator therapy by inhalation to the pulmonary vasculature with improved oxygenation had tremendous clinical appeal. Reports of improved oxygenation in PPHN (Kinsella et al, 1993), in congenital heart disease (Roberts et al, 1993b), in acquired RDS in children (Abman et al, 1994) and in adults (Zapol and Hurfor, 1993) rapidly followed the animal studies. Finer and coworkers (1994) found that most responding patients had a satisfactory response at NO levels of less than 20 ppm and that higher doses did not produce any improvement in the response. It is essential to remember that even though NO may improve pulmonary vascular resistance, it may have little effect if the lungs are not adequately recruited, if myocardial function is severely impaired, or if systemic circulatory insufficiency is present. On the other hand, infants with pure PPHN may respond to NO without much additional therapy. Gupta and colleagues (2002) reported their 5-year single-center experience with iNO combined with gentle ventilation (described in Wung et al, 1985): Their patients had 72% survival, and the need for ECMO was reduced compared with that in historical controls) from 23.9% to 12.8%.

#### Clinical Trials

Several large multicenter, multinational trials of iNO therapy have been conducted. Although there was considerable variation in the design of the trials with regard to entry criteria, prior treatments, randomization, blinding, placebo, dose ranges, and therapeutic outcomes, on the whole these trials represent a determined attempt to delineate the role of iNO therapy in the treatment of neonatal respiratory failure (Abman and Kinsella, 1995). Several controlled trials of iNO therapy have demonstrated clinically important outcome improvement. In the Neonatal Inhaled Nitric Oxide Study (NINOS) trial (1997), the mortality rates among 121 controls and 114 treated infants were the same, but the need for ECMO was reduced from 64% in control subjects to 46% in those

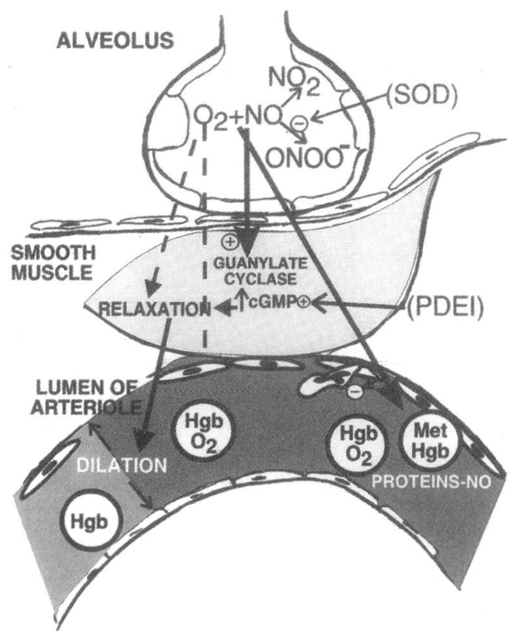


**FIGURE 48–4.** Nitric oxide (NO) synthesis. cGMP, cyclic guanosine monophosphate; Hgb, hemoglobin; Met Hgb, methemoglobin; PDEI, phosphodiesterase inhibitors; SOD, superoxide dismutase. *(From Davidson D: iNO for PPHN. Current evidence for safe and effective guidelines. Tufts University School of Medicine Reports in Neonatal Respiratory Disease 10[2], 2000.)*

given iNO treatment. Similarly, in a trial reported by Roberts and associates (1997), although mortality rate was unchanged, the need for ECMO was reduced from 71% in control subjects to 40% in treated infants. In three additional controlled trials, the need for ECMO was reduced (Clark et al, 2000; Cornfield et al, 1999; Davidson et al, 1998). It seems reasonable to conclude that iNO reduces the need for ECMO by about one third.

Promising new research into the biochemistry of iNO is ongoing that may lead over time to the use of lower doses of NO. It is possible that the vasodilatory effect of iNO may be enhanced by cGMP-specific phosphodiesterase inhibitors and that superoxide dismutase may enhance the response to iNO (see Fig. 48–4) (Davidson, 2000).

### Toxicity Of Nitric Oxide

With the exception of anesthesia, the use of inhaled gas therapy in medicine is rare. There continue to be concerns about the possible toxicity of NO. When exposed to oxygen, NO is slowly converted to $NO_2$. The Centers for Disease Control and Prevention recommendation is that $NO_2$ levels not exceed 5 ppm. The higher the oxygen concentration, the higher the rate of conversion of NO to $NO_2$; an NO concentration of 20 ppm exposed to 95% oxygen achieves an $NO_2$ level of 5 ppm after 5 minutes. In addition, when exposed to superoxide radicals in the lung lining liquid, NO is converted to peroxynitrite, which generates hydroxyl radicals, potentially producing significant injury to surfactant lipids and proteins (Haddad et al, 1993). There is no evidence, however, that NO treatment is associated with an increased incidence of BPD, and in fact, trials using iNO to prevent BPD are under way (see Chapter 49). Another concern has been that NO may inhibit platelet function or prolong bleeding time, promoting the occurrence of hemorrhagic complications (Edwards, 1995); however, bleeding has not been a problem in clinical trials.

### Clinical Safety

The inherent reactivity of NO and oxygen meant that new techniques needed to be developed to ensure safety. NO is fed into the inspiration line of the ventilator distal to the humidifier, so its exposure to oxygen is as short as possible before inhalation. Exhaled gas is collected at the PEEP valve and exhausted into the wall suction system of the hospital. The concentrations of NO and $NO_2$, sampled at the patient manifold, are measured constantly by electrochemical sensors. The level of methemoglobin in blood usually does not exceed 2%, and the level of $NO_2$ in the inspired gas usually does not exceed 2 ppm, but they both must be monitored. Because of the low inspired concentrations of NO, new delivery systems and new detection devices have been developed to provide safe, accurate methods of gas delivery. The inspired iNO concentration should be weaned to the minimal effective level once the oxygen concentration has been weaned (usually to less than 80%) and the infant is stable. The patient should be weaned from iNO over a period of 12 to 48 hours, as tolerated.

As a result of these trials, the Food and Drug Administration (FDA) has approved the use of iNO for treatment of pulmonary hypertension in the term and near-term newborn infant (Centers for Disease Control and Prevention recommendations, 1998). This is currently the only approved use of iNO, although a number of clinical trials are ongoing to examine use of iNO in the preterm infant to prevent BPD (see Chapter 49), as well as in the adult or older child with acute RDS.

### Outcome in Patients with Persistent Pulmonary Hypertension of the Newborn

In the past, mortality rates for infants with PPHN ranged from 20% to 40%, and the incidence of subsequent neurologic handicap ranged from 12% to 25% (Ballard and Leonard, 1984). Sell and coworkers (1985), however, found that only 40% of 40 infants with PPHN in their institution were developmentally normal at 1 to 4 years: 32% had abnormal or suspect findings on neurologic examination, and 20% had neurosensory hearing loss.

It should be noted, however, that most of the infants described before 1992 were managed with hyperventilation with significant hypocarbia (often with a $Pa\text{CO}_2$ of less than 20 to 25 mm Hg for hours to days), and the exposure to hypocarbia correlates with poor outcome. Marron and colleagues (1992) reported on 34 infants managed conservatively without induced alkalosis. All 34 survived. Of the 27 who returned for follow-up, 4 had severe neurologic deficits, 5 had minor abnormalities, and none had any evidence of sensorineural hearing loss. The outcome for infants with PPHN has been further improved with the careful use of iNO and of ECMO when appropriate (see later on).

### Outcome after Inhaled Nitric Oxide Therapy

Four reports have described the neurodevelopmental outcome for a group of newborns who received iNO for PPHN (Clark et al, 2003; Lipkin et al, 2002; Neonatal Inhaled Nitric Oxide Study Group, 2000; Rosenberg, 2002). Although all of these reports are follow-up studies showing an initial improved pulmonary outcome and decreased requirement for ECMO, this improvement has not translated into a reduced need for outpatient treatment of lung disease or reduced rehospitalization rates. On the other hand, there is no evidence that being treated with iNO and avoiding ECMO is associated with any increase in adverse pulmonary or neurologic effects. These follow-up studies, however, all are relatively short-term (including infants up to 1 year of age), and much longer follow-up will be necessary to determine that use of iNO has improved intact survival of critically ill term infants.

## MECONIUM ASPIRATION PNEUMONIA

Meconium, an odorless, thick, blackish green material, is first demonstrable in the fetal intestine during the third month of gestation. It is an accumulation of debris that consists of desquamated cells from the alimentary tract and skin, lanugo hairs, fatty material from the vernix caseosa, amniotic fluid, and various intestinal secretions. Meconium is biochemically composed of a mucopolysaccharide of high blood group specificity, a small amount of lipid, and a small amount of protein, which decreases throughout gestation. Its blackish green color is the result of bile pigments.

### Pathogenesis

Meconium staining of amniotic fluid (MSAF) occurs in roughly 10% to 26% of all deliveries (Nathan et al, 1994). The risk of MSAF is strongly correlated with gestational age. Before 37 weeks of gestation, the risk of MSAF is less than 2%, whereas the risk after 42 weeks of gestation is nearly 44%.

The cause of MSAF is controversial. At one time, the passage of meconium in utero was thought to be synonymous with ongoing fetal asphyxia. At present, however, the relationship between MSAF and fetal asphyxia is unclear. A number of studies have failed to show any consistent effects of MSAF on Apgar scores, fetal scalp pH, or incidence of fetal heart rate abnormalities (Abramovici et al, 1974; Baker et al, 1992; Miller et al, 1975). These studies led to speculation that asphyxial episodes too brief to decrease pH or Apgar scores may cause the passage of meconium in utero. These conclusions were supported by a study showing that there was no correlation between the consistency of meconium and markers of fetal asphyxia (Trimmer and Gilstrap, 1991). Several studies have suggested that the presence of meconium (Nathan et al, 1994), especially thick meconium (Berkus et al, 1994), increases the risk of fetal acidosis and an adverse neonatal outcome. Moreover, one study found that although MSAF correlated poorly with markers of acute intrauterine asphyxia (pH, lactate, and hypoxanthine concentrations), it correlated well with blood erythropoietin concentration (a marker of chronic intrauterine asphyxia). The strong correlation between MSAF and gestational age supports two additional theories: (1) It is possible that the passage of meconium in utero is the result of transient parasympathetic stimulation from cord compression in a neurologically mature fetus. (2) Passage of meconium in utero is a natural phenomenon that reflects the maturity of the gastrointestinal tract. Despite these theories, most authorities agree that MSAF in connection with fetal heart rate abnormalities is a marker for fetal distress and is associated with an increased perinatal morbidity.

Meconium may enter the trachea and airways in utero. In one study, meconium was recovered from the tracheas of 56% of meconium-stained infants in the delivery room (Gregory et al, 1970). Another study (Davis et al, 1985) described 12 infants who died with meconium aspiration pneumonia, even though their tracheas were suctioned vigorously in the delivery room. These findings suggest that in some instances, particularly with distressed fetuses who are gasping, considerable peripheral migration of meconium can occur before birth. Autopsy findings of meconium in the terminal airways of stillborn fetuses support this theory (Brown and Gleicher, 1981). It is highly unlikely, however, that significant intrauterine aspiration of meconium is the result of normal fetal breathing, because the rate of production of fetal lung fluid is such that the net movement of fluid is out of the lung. It is more likely that meconium is aspirated into the tracheobronchial tree when the fetus begins to gasp deeply in response to hypoxia and acidosis. Data showing that cord arterial pH is lower in meconium-stained infants with meconium in their tracheas at delivery support this hypothesis (Yeomans et al, 1989). It is unknown whether the reduced rate of production of fetal lung fluid that accompanies labor contributes to the movement of meconium into the trachea or to its migration peripherally.

If meconium is not removed from the trachea after delivery, with the onset of respiration it migrates from the central airways to the periphery of the lung. Initially, particles of meconium produce mechanical obstruction of the small airways that results in hyperinflation with patchy atelectasis. Later, small airway obstruction is the result of chemical pneumonitis and interstitial edema. During this later stage, hyperinflation persists, and areas of atelectasis become more extensive. In addition, there is infiltration of the alveolar septa by neutrophils, necrosis of alveolar and airway epithelia, and accumulation of proteinaceous debris within the alveolus.

Infants who die of meconium aspiration pneumonia complicated by pulmonary hypertension frequently have evidence of injury to the vascular bed of the lung. In these infants, vascular smooth muscle extends into the walls of normally nonmuscular intra-acinar arterioles, reducing their luminal diameter, which subsequently interferes with the normal postnatal drop in pulmonary vascular resistance. In addition, these infants may demonstrate plugs of platelets in their small vessels that reduce the overall cross-sectional area of the pulmonary vascular bed (Levin et al, 1983).

Airway resistance is increased in newborn infants and experimental animals with meconium aspiration pneumonia (Tran et al, 1980; Yeh et al, 1982). In addition, dynamic lung compliance is reduced while static lung compliance is unchanged, suggesting that airway obstruction is patchy and located in peripheral airways. Functional residual capacity is increased in animals with meconium aspiration pneumonia but not in humans. The effects of meconium on surfactant function have been studied in a number of animal models of meconium aspiration. Data suggest that meconium does inactivate surfactant (Davey et al, 1993; Moses et al, 1991; Sun et al, 1993a). Furthermore, several investigators have shown that surfactant replacement may improve gas exchange in animals with meconium aspiration pneumonia (Ohama et al, 1994; Paranka et al, 1992; Sun et al, 1993b). Gas exchange is inevitably altered in meconium aspiration pneumonia. In the absence of persistent pulmonary hypertension, hypoxia is the result of continued perfusion of poorly ventilated lung units, whereas hypercarbia is the result of a decrease in minute ventilation and increase in respiratory dead space. Some infants with meconium aspiration pneumonia have elevated pulmonary arterial pressures with shunting of blood right to left across the foramen ovale and ductus arteriosus (see discussion of pulmonary hypertension).

### Clinical Manifestations

Infants with meconium aspiration pneumonia are often postmature and have visible meconium staining of the nails, the skin, and the umbilical cord. Asphyxia is a finding in many cases, and much of the early distress may relate more to asphyxia and retained fetal lung fluid complicated by elevated pulmonary vascular resistance than to the presence of meconium in the airways. Infants with meconium aspiration pneumonia have clinical evidence of lung overinflation, with a barrel chest. Auscultation of the chest reveals diffuse rales and rhonchi. The chest radiograph shows patchy areas of atelectasis and areas of overinflation (Fig. 48–5). Pneumothorax and pneumomediastinum are common. The clinical symptoms progress over 12 to 24 hours as meconium migrates to the periphery of the lung. Because meconium must ultimately be removed by phagocytes, respiratory distress and requirements for supplemental oxygen may persist for days or even weeks after birth. Infants who present with a shorter course and with rapid resolution of symptoms are more likely to have had retained fetal lung fluid with some PPHN than meconium aspiration pneumonia.

### Therapy

Symptomatic infants with meconium suctioned from their tracheas should be given chest physiotherapy and warmed humidified oxygen to breathe. Lung lavage may result in deterioration of lung function. Because of the high incidence of air leaks, positive-pressure ventilation should be avoided, if possible. Judicious use of nasal or endotracheal continuous positive airway pressure (CPAP) (4 to 7 cm $H_2O$) may improve oxygenation in the patient who is unresponsive to oxygen administration alone. This improvement in oxygenation is achieved presumably by stabilizing the small airways and improving the ventilation of poorly ventilated lung units. However, many of these infants may also have some degree of delayed clearance of lung water as a result of perinatal asphyxia. High airway pressures may impair oxygenation by impeding blood flow to well-ventilated lung units. Mechanical ventilation should be reserved for infants with apnea from birth asphyxia or for those who cannot maintain their $PaO_2$ greater than 50 mm Hg in 100% oxygen, because infants with meconium aspiration pneumonia often are large and vigorous and tend to fight mechanical ventilation, and agitation increases the chances of air leak. If this occurs, the patient may require neuromuscular blockade. Because meconium aspiration pneumonia is an obstructive lung disease, the time constant for expiration is prolonged in severely involved areas of the lung. Careful attention must be paid to expiratory time (ventilatory rate) to prevent inadvertent PEEP, further gas trapping, and alveolar rupture.

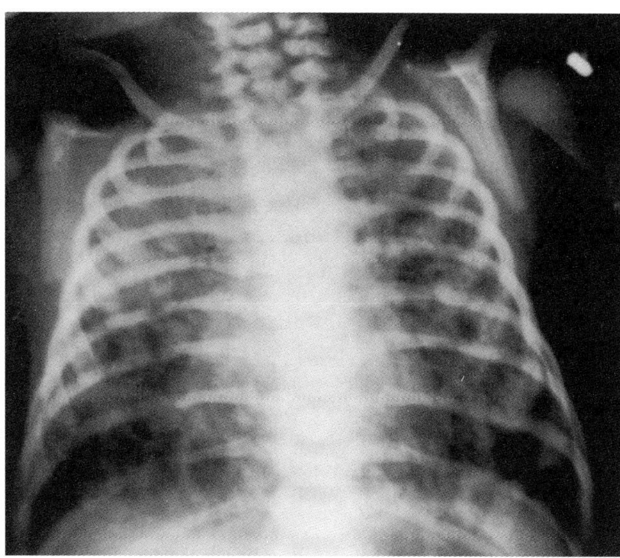

**FIGURE 48–5.** Chest radiograph from an infant with meconium aspiration pneumonia.

The role of antibiotics in the treatment of meconium aspiration pneumonia is controversial. Meconium enhances bacterial growth by reducing host resistance, and the risk of intra-amniotic infection is increased in the presence of MSAF (Romero et al, 1991; Wen et al, 1995). However, no studies have shown that infection plays a role in the pathogenesis of meconium aspiration pneumonia. Because of the difficulty in distinguishing this disorder from bacterial pneumonia, we routinely institute antibiotic therapy in infants with presumed meconium aspiration pneumonia, pending negative cultures.

The use of corticosteroids for treatment of meconium aspiration pneumonia is not recommended. The time to weaning to room air is prolonged by corticosteroids in infants with meconium aspiration pneumonia (Yeh et al, 1977), and the mortality rate for rabbits with experimental meconium aspiration pneumonia is increased by treatment with corticosteroids (Frantz et al, 1975).

As discussed earlier, there is some evidence that infants with meconium aspiration pneumonia have surfactant inactivation. A recent controlled trial studied the effects of surfactant replacement (up to 4 doses of 150 mg/kg of beractant every 6 hours) on infants who were being mechanically ventilated for meconium aspiration pneumonia (Findlay et al, 1996). The investigators found that surfactant replacement therapy, if started within 6 hours after birth, improved oxygenation and reduced the incidence of air leaks, severity of pulmonary morbidity, and duration of hospitalization. Other therapies for the infant with meconium aspiration pneumonia and PPHN, including the use of high-frequency ventilation, iNO, and ECMO, are covered elsewhere in this chapter.

#### Prevention of Meconium Aspiration Pneumonia

Several older studies have shown that by clearing the airway of meconium at the time of birth, meconium aspiration pneumonia can be virtually eliminated (Carson et al, 1976; Gregory et al, 1970; Ting and Brady, 1975). Based on these results, the American Heart Association and the American Academy of Pediatrics have recommended a combined obstetric and pediatric approach to the infant with MSAF (Bloom and Cropley, 2000). For infants born through thin watery meconium, no special management is necessary. For infants born through thick particulate or *pea soup* meconium, they recommend the following steps:

1. When the infant's head is delivered, the mouth, pharynx, and nose should be thoroughly suctioned by the obstetrician using a 10 F or larger suction catheter.
2. If the baby is vigorous, the mouth and nose are cleared of secretions, and oxygen is given as needed.
3. If the infant is not vigorous, the hypopharynx should be visualized and residual meconium removed by suctioning. Then the trachea should be intubated and meconium suctioned from the lower airway.

Tracheal suctioning should be performed using an appropriately sized endotracheal tube and a large-bore meconium aspirator. In the presence of severe asphyxia, it may not be possible to clear the trachea of all meconium, and clinical judgment must be used to determine the amount of suctioning. Studies have found that 7% to 10% of meconium-stained infants had meconium in their tracheas even when there was not any meconium visible at the vocal cords. A free flow of oxygen should be provided via oxygen tubing to minimize hypoxia during suctioning. After tracheal suctioning, the stomach should be emptied to prevent aspiration of swallowed meconium.

A number of investigators have tried to prevent meconium aspiration by infusing saline into the amniotic cavity of mothers with heavy meconium staining of the amniotic fluid. Several randomized trials have shown that amnioinfusion decreases the risk of meconium below the vocal cords, and a meta-analysis of five controlled trials found that amnioinfusion decreased the risk of meconium below the vocal cords and the risk of meconium aspiration pneumonia (Dye et al, 1994). One large retrospective study (Usta et al, 1995) and a randomized, controlled trial (Spong et al, 1994) found no benefit to a policy of routine amnioinfusion. Furthermore, in the controlled trial, the risk of endometritis-chorioamnionitis was increased in the amnioinfusion group. As a result, the role of amnioinfusion in the prevention of MAP is still controversial.

#### Outcome

The outcome for infants with meconium aspiration pneumonia has improved dramatically. In the past, meconium aspiration pneumonia carried a risk of pneumothorax and pneumomediastinum of between 10% and 20%. This risk increased to as high as 50% if the infant required mechanical ventilation. Now with improved approaches to the management of PPHN and the availability of extracorporeal membrane oxygenation, the mortality for meconium-stained infants is roughly 0.15% in the total population (Nathan et al, 1994). The mortality for severely affected infants with meconium aspiration pneumonia requiring extracorporeal membrane oxygenation is less than 7% in most centers and approaches zero in some units.

## OTHER CAUSES OF RESPIRATORY FAILURE IN THE TERM INFANT

### Postasphyxial Pulmonary Edema

Pulmonary edema in newborn lambs following asphyxia from umbilical cord occlusion was described by Adamson and colleagues (1970). The lambs showed transudation of fluid from the circulation into the lungs in the presence of elevated lung capillary pressures. Infants with this condition are often depressed in the delivery room and require mechanical ventilation immediately or soon after birth (Corbet, 1990). In other infants breathing unassisted, there may be severe respiratory distress because of pulmonary edema, transient cardiomegaly, and cerebral irritation; Strang (1977) called this condition *postasphyxial lung edema*. The radiologic appearance of the lungs is that of pulmonary congestion or pulmonary edema with diffuse coarse densities, and in some reports this may be called pneumonia. The heart may be enlarged on the chest radiograph with evidence of mitral or tricuspid valve insufficiency, hypotension, hepatomegaly, poor perfusion, and reduced urine output. On the echocardiogram, there may be evidence of poor myocardial contractability and low cardiac output. Some infants have ischemic changes on the electrocardiogram, and they may have elevated creatine kinase and liver transaminase levels in the blood.

Infants with postasphyxial pulmonary edema do not usually have physical evidence for prematurity as in the case of RDS, or tracheal evidence for meconium aspiration, or bacterial evidence for neonatal pneumonia; instead, they have evidence of asphyxia, heart failure, ventricular dysfunction, pulmonary edema, and often pulmonary hypertension. Some of these infants develop clinical pulmonary hemorrhage, which is now known to be hemorrhagic pulmonary edema, the most severe form of postasphyxial pulmonary edema. Treatment consists of oxygen supported with PEEP, mechanical ventilation, and circulation support, until spontaneous recovery occurs in a few days.

### Surfactant Protein Deficiencies

Several families have been described in which full-term infants developed prolonged and eventually fatal RDS; detailed tissue analysis suggested that they had what was originally called "congenital alveolar proteinosis" and is now known to be surfactant protein-B (SP-B) deficiency (deMello et al, 1994a). Other families have since been described. The condition is due to mutations in the SP-B gene; the most commonly described mutation (121 ins 2) involves a two-base-pair insertion at position 375 in codon 121 of the complementary DNA (Nogee et al, 1994); the additional two bases produce a frameshift signal for termination of translation after codon 214. There is no detectable messenger RNA (mRNA) for SP-B.

The chest radiograph shows the granular pattern characteristic of hyaline membrane disease (HMD) in preterm infants; hence, these infants initially may resemble other term infants with RDS. There is frequently evidence for severe pulmonary hypertension. The alveolar spaces are packed with a proteinaceous material rich in SP-A and SP-C but poor in SP-B or phospholipids, and surfactant function assessed by pulsating surfactometer is abnormal. The lamellar bodies in granular pneumocytes are poorly formed, and there may be basal rather than apical secretion, indicating defective transport protein signaling within the alveolar type II epithelial cells (deMello et al, 1994b).

Oxygen, mechanical ventilation, repeated administration of bovine surfactant containing relatively high levels of SP-B, and eventually ECMO have not been successful in changing the outcome. A few infants have survived for several months on mechanical ventilation (Ballard et al, 1995). More recently, several infants have undergone lung transplantation, with apparent success.

Prenatal amniotic fluid profiles have shown an L/S ratio of less than 2 and the absence of phosphatidylglycerol (PG) and SP-B at full-term gestation (Hamvas et al, 1994). To establish the diagnosis in newborn infants, tracheal aspirates or lung lavage aspirates should be examined for SP-B by either the enzyme-linked immunosorbent assay or by the Western blot procedure; the presence of even low levels of SP-B makes the diagnosis unlikely (Nogee, 1995). It may be possible to test the infant or the parents for the gene mutation in a DNA diagnostic laboratory. Biopsy or autopsy samples of the affected infant's lung may be examined for surfactant proteins by immunostaining.

Ballard and colleagues (1995) have described a term newborn infant with partial SP-B deficiency who needed ECMO and remained on mechanical ventilation until death at 9 months of age. The mother had the previously described point mutation in exon 4, and the father had a new point mutation at codon 236 in exon 7, which resulted in a single amino acid substitution. The infant's surfactant contained low levels of SP-B, more precursor than mature protein, and near-normal levels of mRNA for SP-B; these findings suggested a defect in translation or in post-translational processing. Other mutations have been reported, frequently occurring in conjunction with the 121 ins 2 mutation (Cole et al, 2001). Recently, infants with abnormalities of SPC also have been found to have significant respiratory distress (Amin et al, 2001; Nogee et al, 2001). (See also Chapter 42 on lung development and Chapter 46 on surfactant.)

## ALVEOLAR CAPILLARY DYSPLASIA

Alveolar capillary dysplasia is a rare cause of persistent pulmonary hypertension. This disorder is characterized by failure of formation and ingrowth of alveolar capillaries, medial muscle hypertrophy of pulmonary arteries, and anomalously located pulmonary veins running along with pulmonary arteries, instead of in their normal position in the interlobular septa. The patients sometimes present with symptoms similar to those of idiopathic PPHN and may be impossible to wean from ECMO. However, the early presentation may be mild (some cases have been discharged) (Boggs et al, 1994; Vassal et al, 1998). A familial occurrence has been reported. There is no gender predilection, but 50% of the patients have other anomalies (genitourinary, gastrointestinal, cardiovascular).

## EXTRACORPOREAL MEMBRANE OXYGENATION

In a group of infants with severe lung disease, progressive respiratory failure, and life-threatening hypoxemia who do not respond to maximal ventilatory support or iNO, ECMO may be considered as a treatment of last resort. This is a highly invasive procedure and should not be started without good reason. Physicians using ECMO should review their own experiences and determine appropriate criteria for selecting infants with at least an 80% risk of death from their condition. Most centers report that about 80% of such infants survive when treated with ECMO.

### Conduct of Extracorporeal Membrane Oxygenation

For venoarterial ECMO, the system consists of a venous pressure control module, a roller pump, a countercurrent membrane oxygenator, and a heat exchanger, connected in series and primed with heparinized buffered blood (Short and Pearson, 1986) (Fig. 48–6). A catheter (14 F) is inserted in the right internal jugular vein with its tip in the right atrium, and another catheter (8 to 12 F) is inserted in the right common carotid artery with its tip in the arch of the aorta. The infant is given a bolus dose of heparin and connected to the system, with venous blood drained by gravity from the right atrium and fully oxygenated blood infused at the aorta. The heart and lungs, to a variable extent, are bypassed. The venous control module regulates the operation of the pump, ensuring that the venous drainage from the patient and the pump output to the patient are balanced.

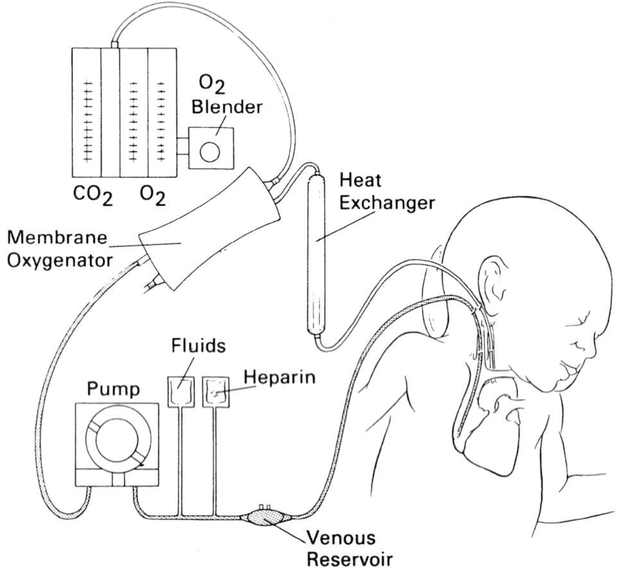


**FIGURE 48–6.** Extracorporeal membrane oxygenation (ECMO) system. *(From Short BL, Miller MK, Anderson KD: Extracorporeal membrane oxygenation in the management of respiratory failure in the newborn. Clin Perinatol 14:737, 1987.)*

Over 30 minutes, the flow is slowly increased to about 120 to 150 mL/kg/minute, after which the mechanical ventilator can be reduced to benign settings, 25% to 30% oxygen, 15 to 20 cm $H_2O$ peak pressure, 5 cm $H_2O$ PEEP, and a rate of 10 breaths/minute. The arterial oxygen pressure can be maintained between 50 and 70 mm Hg by adjusting the ECMO flow. The venous oxygen saturation may be used to assess the overall level of oxygenation; values below 70% suggest that the cardiac output may not be sufficient. Heparinization is continued by an adjustable infusion, to maintain the activated clotting time at 180 to 220 seconds, up to two times longer than normal. In addition, packed red blood cells are transfused to maintain the hematocrit above 40%, platelets are transfused to maintain the platelet count above 100,000/$mm^3$, and fresh frozen plasma is transfused to maintain the fibrinogen level above 200 mg/dL.

The ECMO flow can usually be decreased gradually to about 90 to 100 mL/kg/minute after the first day. An improvement in lung function may be recognized by increased lung compliance with the use of periodic bag-tube ventilation and increased pulse oximeter saturation. After 4 to 5 days, the ECMO flow is further reduced, and the ventilator settings are again increased to assume responsibility for gas exchange. Ideally, the settings should be comparatively benign, such as oxygen concentration 40% to 50%, rate 40 to 60 breaths/minute, PEEP 8 to 10 cm $H_2O$, and peak inflation pressure 20 to 25 cm $H_2O$. After a brief period at a low ECMO flow (30 mL/kg/minute), to ensure adequate pulmonary function, the infant can be decannulated and the vessels ligated; it is usual to place a Broviac central venous line in the right external jugular vein at this time for the purpose of continued parenteral nutrition.

### Patient Selection

Patients with meconium aspiration pneumonia, RDS, neonatal pneumonia, congenital diaphragmatic hernia, and PPHN are prime candidates for this therapy. Because of systemic heparinization, infants weighing less than 2000 g and less than 34 weeks of gestation at birth have a high incidence of cerebral hemorrhage (Cilley et al, 1986) and should be excluded, as should larger infants if they already have evidence for cerebral hemorrhage or cerebral infarction. All patients should undergo head ultrasound examination before initiation of ECMO. Those who are older than 7 to 14 days and have been exposed to prolonged mechanical ventilation with oxygen are not good candidates because their lung disease may not be reversible. Infants with severe malformations should be excluded. A thorough search for congenital heart disease should be made with echocardiography before ECMO (Palmisano et al, 1992), and occasionally an emergency chromosome analysis is necessary in patients with dysmorphic features.

The definition of life-threatening hypoxemia, sufficient to justify ECMO, is still somewhat controversial among neonatal centers. Many centers prefer to use the oxygenation index, the product of three factors: (1) the percent oxygen, (2) the mean airway pressure, and (3) the reciprocal of arterial $PO_2$ (Keszler et al, 1992). Failure to respond to iNO at 40 ppm for 2 to 3 hours is considered a reliable indication for ECMO. In our current practice, most patients who are placed on ECMO have an arterial $PO_2$ of less than 50 mm Hg. When the arterial oxygen tension is this low, despite intensive medical therapy, there is an increased risk that anaerobic metabolism may result in severe metabolic acidosis, which increases the likelihood of either death or significant morbidity. Patients with an arterial $PO_2$ of more than 50 mm Hg and a normal acid-base status, with no evidence of anaerobic metabolism, may survive without ECMO.

### Efficacy of Extracorporeal Membrane Oxygenation

The efficacy of ECMO was assessed in a randomized, controlled trial in adult patients and was found not to be superior to conventional therapy (Zapol et al, 1979). There have been two North American attempts to conduct a randomized, controlled trial of ECMO in newborn infants. In the first (Bartlett et al, 1985), an unusual trial design resulted in a small control group (only one patient), so the results in favor of ECMO were widely discounted. In the second controlled trial (O'Rourke et al, 1989), more appropriately randomized, 6 of 10 infants survived with conventional mechanical ventilation, and 9 of 9 infants survived with ECMO. Although this difference was not significant, further enrollment into the ECMO group suggested superior results with ECMO. Both of these trials reflected the bias of investigators in favor of ECMO. In the second trial, the mortality rate in controls was much lower than the 80% expected. It then became impossible to conduct a good randomized, controlled trial in North America, where ECMO has become universally accepted. A controlled trial in Great Britain demonstrated improved survival in infants with intractable respiratory failure with the use of ECMO (UK Collaborative ECMO Trial Group, 1996). Of 93 patients allocated randomly to ECMO, 3 improved and did not need ECMO, 5 were excluded (most for congenital heart disease), 7 died before ECMO could be started, and 78 were treated with ECMO. There were 30 deaths in these 93 patients (32% mortality rate), compared with 54 deaths among 92 control subjects who were not allocated to ECMO (59% mortality rate), a significantly better result. The improvement was most noticeable among those with idiopathic persistent pulmonary hypertension, but it was significant among those with meconium aspiration pneumonia, and even among those with congenital diaphragmatic hernia.

### Outcome with Extracorporeal Membrane Oxygenation

There has been much concern about the long-term outcome of infants who have received ECMO. Schumacher and colleagues (1988) reviewed multiple reports and found that at follow-up assessment, 81% of 643 patients were considered to be normal, 7% had borderline abnormalities, and 12% had serious disabilities. These results are considered to be as good as, and possibly better than, the results in infants with the same conditions treated without ECMO (Klein and Whittlesey, 1994). An evaluation of the effect of neonatal risk factors and treatment strategy on long-term outcome for ECMO survivors (Vaucher, 1996) found that compared with 52 infants who met criteria for use of ECMO but were successfully treated with conventional or high-frequency ventilation, the 138 ECMO survivors were more mature in spite of having earlier, more severe pulmonary disease. The ECMO survivors were also more likely to have had meconium aspiration. They had significantly fewer ventilator days (9 versus 11), hospital days (23 versus 29), and less chronic lung disease (12% versus 25%). At 12 to 30 months, the mean developmental scores of the ECMO survivors were similar to those of infants who survived without ECMO. Those infants who had chronic lung disease had significantly lower motor scores and were more likely to have cerebral palsy than were those without chronic lung disease (27% versus 6%). The investigators concluded that neonatal ECMO candidates who were treated with ECMO did as well as or better than neonates whose conditions were managed with alternate treatment strategies. It should be noted that these infants all were treated prior to the FDA approval of iNO as therapy for respiratory failure in term or near-term infants. The only follow-up from a randomized trial of neonatal ECMO is that reported by Bennett and colleagues (2001) for the UK Collaborative Trial. The 4-year follow-up demonstrated improved, intact survival in critically term neonates who received ECMO, compared with that in the control group.

### Problems with Extracorporeal Membrane Oxygenation

Because ECMO is an invasive procedure and because contact of blood with a plastic surface sets off a massive release of potent mediators, there are a large number of associated problems, for example:

1. The circuit must be constantly observed for large air bubbles and clots, which, if present on the arterial side of the circuit, may embolize into the patient's systemic circulation, with potentially disastrous results. Some centers use a trap on the patient's side of the circuit. In addition, an unnoticed disconnection anywhere in the circuit may rapidly cause hemorrhagic shock, so constant vigilance is necessary.
2. If the patient receives too much heparin, there may be hemorrhagic complications, such as bleeding at the operative site, bleeding into the brain, bleeding into the peritoneal or pleural space, or gastrointestinal bleeding. The use of cautery and fibrin glue at the surgical site or the use of systemic aminocaproic acid (Amicar) may help lessen the incidence of hemorrhage. In some cases, a consumptive coagulopathy (excessive consumption of coagulation factors) may develop, as the plastic surface of the circuit becomes coated with multiple fibrin thrombus layers; this condition may become so serious that decannulation or a change of the circuit may be necessary. The level of fibrin split products should remain less than 10 μg/mL during routine ECMO.
3. The patient may develop a low cardiac output, which does not increase when ECMO flow is reduced and which may prolong the length of time on ECMO; this condition is known as the *cardiac stun syndrome* (Hirschl et al, 1992). The reason for this problem may be twofold: that coronary perfusion is dependent on poorly oxygenated left ventricular blood (Kinsella et al, 1992a) and that retrograde flow from the aortic catheter may increase the afterload resistance to left ventricular ejection. This condition should not be confused with the universal reduction in cardiac output and myocardial contractility that occurs because the heart is unloaded in venoarterial ECMO (Kimball et al, 1991).
4. Within a few hours of initiation of ECMO, the lungs frequently develop a diffuse, dense opacification and further loss of compliance; this is thought to be caused by high-permeability pulmonary edema, possibly secondary to activated complement fragments and increased leukotriene production. This pulmonary edema lessens within a few days, especially if high PEEP levels (10 to 12 cm $H_2O$) are maintained (Keszler et al, 1992). Because surfactant may be inactivated by pulmonary edema fluid, exogenous surfactant therapy may be helpful (Lotze et al, 1993).
5. The urine output often decreases dramatically on ECMO, and the patient may become edematous. As in the case of the lungs, the edema is probably caused by capillary injury from activated complement fragments and increased leukotriene production. This injury cascade leads to hypotension, with the need for frequent infusions of colloid to raise the blood pressure; these infusions are in addition to those given to maintain the hematocrit, platelet, and fibrinogen levels. As the capillary injury resolves after a few days, the edema may be treated with loop diuretics, but sometimes hemofiltration becomes necessary, especially if pulmonary edema fails to resolve.

6. The use of the carotid artery for cannulation and its ligation at the time of decannulation have raised much concern about the circulation to the brain and the possibility of brain injury. Schumacher and colleagues (1988) reported an increased incidence of right-sided ischemic lesions of the brain. In some centers, the carotid artery is reconstructed at the time of decannulation (Taylor et al, 1992). Baumgart and colleagues (1994) found, using color-coded Doppler imaging, that the brain blood flow profile was improved with this procedure, but head computed tomography scans before discharge and neurodevelopmental status at age 1 year did not suggest any improvement in the outcome. Some centers use a second catheter placed in the cephalic segment of the internal jugular vein to improve the venous drainage of the brain; this measure improves the total ECMO flow but has not been shown to change the outcome.
7. Some patients develop systemic hypertension on ECMO; this effect may be related to circulation overload and may respond to diuresis or hemofiltration. Because the heart and lungs are bypassed, there may be a deficiency of epinephrine degradation; because renal blood flow is nonpulsatile, there may be high levels of plasma renin; and because the right atrium is decompressed, there may be high levels of arginine vasopressin. Hypertension may predispose the patient to cerebral hemorrhage, so treatment with hydralazine or enalapril may be necessary.
8. A few patients develop excessive hemolysis, related to high pressures in the circuit (greater than 300 mm Hg); this problem may be monitored by measurements of plasma free hemoglobin, which should remain below 40 mg/100 mL.
9. After ECMO, many patients have problems with feeding; the reason for this is not understood, but because the vascular catheters lie near the vagus nerve, there may be temporary injury causing esophageal dysfunction and gastroesophageal reflux. Some of these patients also may develop a superior vena cava syndrome (Zreik et al, 1995) or a chylothorax, and some may have transient vocal cord paralysis, again related to the catheters.

### Venovenous Extracorporeal Membrane Oxygenation

The initial development of ECMO was venoarterial, but there has been increasing use of venovenous ECMO, especially when a single dual-lumen catheter can be placed in the right atrium. The catheter must be carefully placed so that well-oxygenated blood is directed toward the tricuspid valve, to minimize recirculation into the venous drainage.

The major advantage of this technique is that the carotid artery does not have to be sacrificed. In addition, because the pulmonary and coronary circulations receive well-oxygenated blood, there may be significant improvements in pulmonary artery pressures and myocardial function. Because of the recirculation problem, the capacity to deliver oxygen is less than in venoarterial ECMO; the ECMO flow must usually be higher, frequently in the range of 120 to 140 mL/kg/minute, and lower levels of arterial $PO_2$, in the range of 40 to 60 mm Hg, must often be accepted. If the circulation and hemoglobin levels are well maintained and if the patient's acid-base status and blood lactate levels remain normal, it is unlikely that a state of oxygen deficiency exists. Also, because of the recirculation problem, the central venous oxygen saturation cannot be used as an assessment of overall oxygenation. Commonly a cephalic venous catheter is used to monitor cerebral venous oxygen saturation; values of less than 60% are considered evidence for oxygen deficiency.

Despite the use of pressors to maintain the circulation, venovenous ECMO must be changed to venoarterial ECMO in up to 10% of patients. Nevertheless, Cornish and associates (1993) found that most patients referred to an ECMO center could be managed effectively with venovenous ECMO; myocardial function usually improved, and pressors could be gradually withdrawn. The neurodevelopmental outcome of patients after venovenous ECMO is similar to that after venoarterial ECMO (van Meurs et al, 1994).

## LIQUID VENTILATION

During the past 25 years or so, investigators have been pursuing the possibility of treating ventilatory failure with liquid rather than gaseous ventilation (Shaffer et al, 1984; Wolfson et al, 1996). The discovery of a class of compounds known as fluorocarbons has led to significant advances because they are chemically and physiologically inert. Perfluorocarbon, the compound that has been used in both animal experimentation and human clinical studies, has a greater solubility for respiratory gases than that of blood. It has some of the properties of surfactant, with a low surface tension. When instilled into the lung, this radiopaque compound gradually recruits alveoli without barotrauma and, because of its low vapor pressure, is rapidly eliminated by vaporization. Although animal studies initially were encouraging, there are no successful controlled trials in humans at this time (Greenspan, 1990; Leach et al, 1993, 1995, 1996).

## REFERENCES


Abman SH, Griebel JL, Parker DK, et al: Acute effects of inhaled nitric oxide in children with severe hypoxemic respiratory failure. J Pediatr 124:881, 1994.

Abman SH, Kinsella JP, Schaffer MS, Wilkening RB: Inhaled NO in the management of a preterm newborn with severe respiratory distress and pulmonary hypertension. Pediatrics 92:606, 1993.

Abman SH, Kinsella JP: Inhaled NO for persistent pulmonary hypertension of the newborn: The physiology matters! Pediatrics 96:1153, 1995.

Abramovici J, Brandes JM, Fuchs K, Timor-Tritsch I: Meconium during delivery: A sign of compensated fetal distress. Am J Obstet Gynecol 118:251, 1974.

Adamson TM, Boyd RDH, Hill JR, et al: Effect of asphyxia due to umbilical cord occlusion in the foetal lamb on leakage of liquid from the circulation and on permeability of lung capillaries to albumin. J Physiol 207:493, 1970.

Al-Mateen KB, Dailey K, Grimes MM, et al: Improved oxygenation with exogenous surfactant administration in experimental meconium aspiration syndrome. Pediatr Pulmonol 17:75, 1994.

Amin RS, Wert SE, Baughman RP, et al: Surfactant protein deficiency in familial interstitial lung disease. J Pediatr 139:85, 2001.

Auten RL, Notter RH, Kendig JW, et al: Surfactant treatment of full-term newborns with respiratory failure. Pediatrics 87:101, 1991.

Baker PN, Kilby MD, Murray H: An assessment of the use of meconium alone as an indication for fetal blood sampling. Obstet Gynecol 80:792, 1992.

Ballard PL, Nogee LM, Beers MF, et al: Partial deficiency of surfactant protein B in an infant with chronic lung disease. Pediatrics 96:1046, 1995.

Ballard RA, Leonard CH: Development follow-up of infants with persistent pulmonary hypertension of the newborn. Clin Perinatol 11:737, 1984.

Bartlett RH, Roloff DW, Cornell RG, et al: Extracorporeal circulation in neonatal respiratory failure: A prospective randomized study. Pediatrics 76:479, 1985.

Baumgart S, Streletz LJ, Needleman L, et al: Right common carotid artery reconstruction after extracorporeal membrane oxygenation: Vascular imaging, cerebral circulation, electroencephalographic, and neurodevelopmental correlates to recovery. J Pediatr 125:295, 1994.

Bennett CC, Johnson A, Field DJ, et al: UK Collaborative randomized trial of neonatal ECMO: Follow-up to age 4 years. Lancet 357:1094, 2001.

Berkus MD, Langer O, Samueloff A, et al: Meconium-stained amniotic fluid: Increased risk for adverse neonatal outcome. Obstet Gynecol 84:115, 1994.

Bloom RS, Cropley C (eds): Lesson 2: Initial Steps in Resuscitation. Neonatal Resuscitation Textbook, 4th ed. Elk Grove Village, Ill, American Heart Association/Academy of Pediatrics, 2000, p 212.

Boggs S, Harris MC, Hoffman DJ, et al: Misalignment of pulmonary veins with alveolar capillary dysplasia: Affected siblings and variable phenotypic expression. J Pediatr 124:125, 1994.

Brown BL, Gleicher N: Intrauterine meconium aspiration. Obstet Gynecol 57:26, 1981.

Carlo WA, Beoglos A, Chatburn RL, et al: High-frequency jet ventilation in neonatal pulmonary hypertension. Am J Dis Child 143:233, 1989.

Carson BS, Losey RW, Bowes WA, Simmons MA: Combined obstetric and pediatric approach to prevent meconium aspiration syndrome. Am J Obstet Gynecol 126:712, 1976.

Carter JM, Gertsmann DR, Clark RH, et al: High frequency oscillatory ventilation and extracorporeal membrane oxygenation for the treatment of acute neonatal respiratory failure. Pediatrics 85:159, 1990.

Centers for Disease Control and Prevention recommendations for occupational safety and health standards. MMWR 37:21, 1998.

Cilley RE, Zwischenberger JB, Andrews AF, et al: Intracranial hemorrhage during extracorporeal membrane oxygenation in neonates. Pediatrics 78:699, 1986.

Clark RH, Yoder BA, Sell MS: Prospective, randomized comparison of high-frequency oscillation and conventional ventilation in candidates for extracorporeal membrane oxygenation. J Pediatr 124:447, 1994.

Clark RH, Keuser TJ, Walker MW, et al: Low dose nitric oxide therapy for persistent pulmonary hypertensino of the newborn. Clinical Inhaled Nitric Oxide Research Group. N Engl J Med 342:469, 2000.

Clark RH, Huckaby JL, Keuser TJ, et al: Low dose nitric oxide therapy for PPHN: 1 year follow-up. J Perinatol 23:300, 2003.

Cole FS, Hamvas A, Nogee LM: Genetic disorders of neonatal respiratory function. Pediatr Res 50:157, 2001.

Corbet A: Respiratory disorders in the newborn. In Chernick V, Kendig EL (eds): Disorders of the Respiratory Tract in Children. Philadelphia, WB Saunders, 1990, p 288.

Cornish JD, Gertsmann DR, Clark RH, et al: Extracorporeal membrane oxygenation and high-frequency oscillatory ventilation: Potential therapeutic relationships. Crit Care Med 15:831, 1987.

Cornish JD, Heiss KF, Clark RH, et al: Efficacy of venovenous extracorporeal membrane oxygenation for neonates with respiratory and circulatory compromise. J Pediatr 122:105, 1993.

Cowan KN, Heilbut A, Humpl T, et al: Complete reversal of fatal pulmonary hypertension in rats by a serine elastase inhibitor. Nat Med 6:698-702, 2000a.

Cowan KN, Jones PL, Rabinovitch M: Elastase and matrix metalloproteinase inhibitors induce regression, and tenascin-C antisense prevents progression of vascular disease. J Clin Invest 105:21, 2000b.

Davey AM, Becker JD, Davis JM: Meconium aspiration syndrome: Physiological and inflammatory changes in a newborn piglet model. Pediatr Pulmonol 16:101, 1993.

Davidson D, Barefield ES, Kattwinkel J, et al: Inhaled nitric oxide for the early treatment of persistent pulmonary hypertension of the term newborn: A randomized, double masked placebo-controlled dose-response, multicenter study. The INO/PPHN Study Group. Pediatrics 107:328, 1998.

Davidson D: iNO for PPHN: Current evidence for safe and effective guidelines. Tufts University School of Medicine Reports in Neonatal Respiratory Disease 10(2), 2000.

Davis RO, Philips JB, Harris BA, et al: Fetal meconium-aspiration syndrome occurring despite airway management considered appropriate. Am J Obstet Gynecol 151:731, 1985.

deMello DE, Heyman S, Phelps DS, et al: Ultrastructure of lung in surfactant protein B deficiency. Am J Respir Cell Mol Biol 11:230, 1994a.

deMello DE, Nogee LM, Heyman S, et al: Molecular and phenotypic variability in the congenital alveolar proteinosis syndrome associated with inherited surfactant protein B deficiency. J Pediatr 125:43, 1994b.

Dollberg S, Warner BW, Myatt L: Urinary nitrite and nitrate concentrations in patients with idiopathic persistent pulmonary hypertension of the newborn and effect of extracorporeal membrane oxygenation. Pediatr Res 37:31, 1995.

Drummond WH, Gregory GA, Heymann MA, Phibbs RH: The independent effects of hyperventilation, tolazoline and dopamine on infants with persistent pulmonary hypertension. J Pediatr 98:603, 1981.

Dworetz AR, Moya FR, Sabo B, et al: Survival of infants with persistent pulmonary hypertension without extracorporeal membrane oxygenation. Pediatrics 84:1, 1989.

Dye T, Aubry R, Gross S, et al: Amnioinfusion and the intrauterine prevention of meconium aspiration. Am J Obstet Gynecol 171:1601, 1994.

Edwards AD: The pharmacology of inhaled NO. Arch Dis Child 72:F127, 1995.

Etches PC, Finer NN, Barrington KJ, et al: NO reverses acute hypoxic pulmonary hypertension in the newborn piglet. Pediatr Res 35:15, 1994.

Fike C, Hansen TN: Effects of alkalosis on hypoxic pulmonary vasoconstriction in newborn rabbit lungs. Pediatr Res 25:383, 1989.

Findlay RD, Taeusch HW, Walther FJ: Surfactant replacement therapy for meconium-aspiration syndrome. Pediatrics 97:48, 1996.

Fineman JR, Wong J, Morin FCI, et al: Chronic nitric oxide inhibition in utero produces persistent pulmonary hypertension in newborn lambs. J Clin Invest 93:2675, 1995.

Finer NN, Etches PC, Kamstra BJ, et al: Inhaled nitric oxide in infants referred for extracorporeal membrane oxygenation: Dose response. J Pediatr 124:302, 1994.
Frantz ID, Wang NS, Thach BT: Experimental meconium aspiration: Effects of glucocorticord treatment. J Pediatr 86:438, 1975.
Frostell C, Fratacci MD, Wain J, et al: Inhaled NO: A selective pulmonary vasodilator reversing hypoxic pulmonary vasoconstriction. Circulation 83:2038, 1991.
Frostell CG, Zapol WM. Inhaled nitric oxide, clinical rationale and applications. Adv Pharmacol 34:439, 1995.
Furchgott RF, Zawadzki JV: The obligatory role of endothelial cells in the relaxation of arterial smooth muscle by acetylcholine. Nature 327:524, 1980.
Geggel RL, Aronovitz MJ, Reid LM: Effects of chronic in utero hypoxemia on rat neonatal pulmonary arterial structure. J Pediatr 108:756, 1986.
Gersony WM, Duc GV, Sinclair JC: "PFC" syndrome (persistence of the fetal circulation). Circulation 39(suppl):III87, 1969.
Giaid A, Saleh D: Reduced expression of endothelial nitric oxide synthase in the lungs of patients with pulmonary hypertension. N Engl J Med 333:214, 1995.
Greenspan JS, Wolfson MR, Rubenstein D, Shaffer TH: Liquid ventilation of human preterm neonates. J Pediatr 117:106, 1990.
Gregory GA, Gooding CA, Phibbs RH, Tooley WH: Meconium aspiration in infants—a prospective study. J Pediatr 85:848, 1970.
Gupta A, Rostogi S, Sahni R, et al: Inhaled NO and gentle ventilation in the treatment of pulmonary hypertension of the newborn—a single center 5-year experience. J Perinatol 22:435, 2002.
Haddad IY, Ischiropoulos H, Holm BA, et al: Mechanisms of peroxynitrite-induced injury to pulmonary surfactants. Am J Physiol 265:L555, 1993.
Hammerman C, Komar K, Abu-Khudair H: Hypoxic vs septic pulmonary hypertension. Am J Dis Child 142:319, 1988.
Hamvas A, Cole FS, deMello DE, et al: Surfactant protein B deficiency: Antenatal diagnosis and prospective treatment with surfactant replacement. J Pediatr 125:356, 1994.
Hansen TN, Gest AL: Oxygen toxicity and other ventilatory complications of treatment of infants with persistent pulmonary hypertension. Clin Perinatol 11:653, 1984.
Herting E, Gefeller O, Land M, et al, with Collaborative European Multicenter Study Group: Surfactant treatment of neonates with respiratory failure and GBS infection. Pediatrics 106:957, 2000.
Hirschl RB, Heiss KF, Bartlett RH: Severe myocardial dysfunction during extracorporeal membrane oxygenation. J Pediatr Surg 27:48, 1992.
Ignarro LJ, Buga GM, Wood KS, et al: Endothelial derived relaxing factor (EDRF): Produced and released from artery and vein. PNAS 84:9265, 1987.
Keszler M, Ryckman FC, McDonald JV, et al: A prospective multicenter randomized study of high versus low end expiratory pressure during extracorporeal membrane oxygenation. J Pediatr 120:107, 1992.
Khammash H, Perlman M, Wojtulewicz J, et al: Surfactant therapy in full-term neonates with severe respiratory failure. Pediatrics 92:135, 1993.
Kimball TR, Daniels SR, Weiss RG, et al: Changes in cardiac function during extracorporeal membrane oxygenation for persistent pulmonary hypertension in the newborn infant. J Pediatr 118:431, 1991.
Kinsella JP, Abman SH: Recent developments in the pathophysiology and treatment of persistent pulmonary hypertension of the newborn. J Pediatr 126:853, 1995.
Kinsella JP, Gerstmann DR, Rosenberg AA: The effect of extracorporeal membrane oxygenation on coronary perfusion and regional blood flow. Pediatr Res 31:80, 1992a.
Kinsella JP, Ivy DD, Abman SH: iNO improves gas exchange and lowers PVR in severe experimental HMD. Pediatr Res 36:402, 1994.
Kinsella JP, Neish SR, Ivy DD, et al: Clinical responses to prolonged treatment of persistent pulmonary hypertension of the newborn with low doses of inhaled NO. J Pediatr 123:103, 1993.
Kinsella JP, Neish SR, Shaffer E, Abman SH: Low dose inhalational NO in persistent pulmonary hypertension of the newborn. Lancet 340:818, 1992b.
Kinsella JP, Truog WE, Walsh WF, et al: Randomized, multicenter trial of inhaled nitric oxide and high-frequency oscillatory ventilation in severe, persistent pulmonary hypertension of the newborn. J Pediatr 131:55, 1997
Klein MD, Whittlesey GC: Extracorporeal membrane oxygenation. Pediatr Clin North Am 41:365, 1994.
Leach CL, Fuhrman BP, Morin FC III, Rath MG: Perfluorocarbon-associated gas exchange (partial liquid ventilation) in respiratory distress syndrome: A prospective, randomized, controlled study. Crit Care Med 21:1270, 1993.
Leach CL, Greenspan JS, Rubenstein SD, et al, for the LiquiVent Study Group: Partial liquid ventilation with perflubron in premature infants with severe respiratory distress syndrome. N Engl J Med 335:761, 1996.
Leach CL, Holm B, Morin FC III, et al: Partial liquid ventilation in preterm lambs and compatibility with exogenous surfactant. J Pediatr 126:412, 1995.
Levin DL, Fixler DE, Morriss FC, Tyson J: Morphologic analysis of the pulmonary vascular bed in infants exposed in utero to prostaglandin synthetase inhibitors. J Pediatr 92:478, 1978a.
Levin DL, Hyman AI, Heymann MA, Rudolph AM: Fetal hypertension and the development of increased pulmonary vascular smooth muscle: A possible mechanism for persistent pulmonary hypertension of the newborn infant. J Pediatr 92:265, 1978b.
Levin DL, Weinberg AG, Perkin RM: Pulmonary microthrombi syndrome in newborn infants with unresponsive persistent pulmonary hypertension. J Pediatr 102:299, 1983.
Linder N, Aranda JV, Tsur M, et al: Need for endotracheal intubation and suction in meconium-stained neonates. J Pediatr 112:613, 1988.
Lipkin P, Davidson D, Spivak I, et al: One-year neurodevelopmental and medical outcome of PPHN in term newborns treated with INO. J Pediatr 140:306, 2002.
Lotze A, Knight GR, Martin GR, et al: Improved pulmonary outcome after exogenous surfactant therapy for respiratory failure in term infants requiring extracorporeal membrane oxygenation. J Pediatr 122:261, 1993.
Lotze A, Mitchell BR, Bulas DI, et al: Multicenter study of surfactant (beractant) use in the treatment of term infants with severe respiratory failure. Survanta in Term Infants Study Group. J Pediatr 132:40, 1998.
Marron MJ, Crisafi MA, Driscoll JM Jr, et al: Hearing and neurodevelopmental outcome in survivors of persistent pulmonary hypertension of the newborn. Pediatrics 90:392, 1992.
McQueston JA, Kinsella JP, Ivy DD, et al: Chronic pulmonary hypertension in utero impairs endothelium-dependent vasodilatation. Am J Physiol 268:H288, 1995.
Miller FC, Sacks DA, Yeh SY, et al: Significance of meconium during labor. Am J Obstet Gynecol 122:573, 1975.
Morin FC III: Ligating the ductus arteriosus before birth causes persistent pulmonary hypertension in the newborn lamb. Pediatr Res 25:245, 1989.
Morin FC, Stenmark KR: Persistent pulmonary hypertension of the newborn. Am J Respir Crit Care Med 151:2010, 1995.

Moses D, Holm BA, Spitale P, et al: Inhibition of pulmonary surfactant function by meconium. Am J Obstet Gynecol 164:477, 1991.

Murphy JD, Rabinovitch M, Goldstein JD, Reid LM: The structural basis of persistent pulmonary hypertension of the newborn infant. J Pediatr 98:962, 1981.

Murphy JD, Vawter GF, Reid LM: Pulmonary vascular disease in fetal meconium aspiration. J Pediatr 104:758, 1984.

Naeye RL, Schochat SJ, Whitman V, Maisels MJ: Unsuspected pulmonary vascular abnormalities associated with diaphragmatic hernia. Pediatrics 58:902, 1976.

Nathan L, Leveno KJ, Carmody TJ III, et al: Meconium: A 1990s perspective on an old obstetric hazard. Obstet Gynecol 83:329, 1994.

Neonatal Inhaled Nitric Oxide Study Group: Inhaled NO in full-term and nearly full-term infants with hypoxic respiratory failure. N Engl J Med 336:597, 1997.

Neonatal Inhaled Oxide Study (NINOS) Group: INO in term and near-term infants: Neurodevelopmental follow-up of the NINOS. J Pediatr 136:611, 2000.

Nogee LM: Clinical significance of surfactant protein B deficiency. Neonatal Respir Dis 5:1, 1995.

Nogee LM, Dunbar AE III, Wert SE, et al: A mutation in the surfactant protein C gene associated with familial interstitial lung disease. N Engl J Med 344:573, 2001.

Nogee LM, Garnier G, Dietz HC, et al: A mutation in the surfactant protein B gene responsible for fatal neonatal respiratory disease in multiple kindreds. J Clin Invest 93:1860, 1994.

Ohama Y, Itakura Y, Koyama N, et al: Effect of surfactant lavage in a rabbit model of meconium aspiration syndrome. Acta Paediatr Jpn 36:236, 1994.

O'Rourke PP, Crone RK, Vacanti JP, et al: Extracorporeal membrane oxygenation and conventional medical therapy in neonates with persistent pulmonary hypertension of the newborn: A prospective randomized study. Pediatrics 84:957, 1989.

Palmer RM, Ashton DS, Moncada S: Vascular endothelial cells synthesize NO from L-arginine. Nature 333:664, 1988.

Palmisano JM, Moler FW, Custer JR, et al: Unsuspected congenital heart disease in neonates receiving extracorporeal life support: A review of 95 cases from the ELSO registry. J Pediatr 121:115, 1992.

Paranka MS, Walsh WF, Stancombe BB: Surfactant lavage in a piglet model of meconium-aspiration syndrome. Pediatr Res 31:625, 1992.

Roberts JD, Chen TY, Kawai N, et al: iNO reverses pulmonary vasoconstriction in the hypoxic and acidotic newborn lamb. Circ Res 72:246-254, 1993a.

Roberts JD, Fineman JR, Morin FC III, et al: Inhaled nitric oxide and persistent pulmonary hypertension of the newborn. N Engl J Med 336:605, 1997.

Roberts JD, Lang P, Bigatello LM, et al: Inhaled NO in congenital heart disease. Circulation 87:447, 1993b.

Roberts JD, Polaner DM, Lang P, et al: Inhaled NO in persistent pulmonary hypertension of the newborn. Lancet 340:818, 1992.

Rojas J, Larsson LE, Ogletree ML, et al: Effects of cyclooxygenase inhibition on the response to group B streptococcal toxin in sheep. Pediatr Res 17:107, 1983.

Romero R, Hanoaka S, Mazor M, et al: Meconium-stained amniotic fluid: A risk factor for microbial invasion of the amniotic cavity. Am J Obstet Gynecol 164:859, 1991.

Rosenberg AA, Kennaugh J, Koppenhafer SL, et al: Elevated immunoreactive endothelin-1 levels in newborn infants with persistent pulmonary hypertension. J Pediatr 123:109, 1993.

Rosenberg AA: Outcome in term infants treated with INO. J Pediatr 140:284, 2002.

Sanderud J, Norstein J, Saugstad J: Reactive oxygen metabolites produce pulmonary vasoconstriction in young pigs. Pediatr Res 29:543, 1991.

Schreiber ME, Heymann MA, Soifer SJ: Increased arterial pH, not decreased $PACO_2$, attenuates hypoxia-induced pulmonary vasoconstriction in newborn lambs. Pediatr Res 20:113, 1986.

Schumacher RE, Barks JDE, Johnston MV, et al: Right sided brain lesions in infants following extracorporeal membrane oxygenation. Pediatrics 92:155, 1988.

Sell EJ, Gaines JA, Gluckman C, Williams E: Persistent fetal circulation. Am J Dis Child 139:25, 1985.

Shaffer TH, Lowe CA, Bhutani VK, Douglas PR: Liquid ventilation: Effects on pulmonary function in distressed meconium-stained lambs. Pediatr Res 18:47, 1984.

Shankaran S, Farooki Q, Desai R: Beta-hemolytic streptococcal infection appearing as persistent fetal circulation. Am J Dis Child 136:725, 1982.

Short BL, Pearson GD: Neonatal extracorporeal membrane oxygenation: A review. J Intensive Care Med 1:47, 1986.

Soifer SJ, Kaslow D, Roman C, Heymann MA: Umbilical cord compression produces pulmonary hypertension in newborn lambs: A model to study the pathophysiology of persistent pulmonary hypertension in the newborn. J Dev Physiol 9:239, 1987.

Spong CY, Ogundipe OA, Ross MG: Prophylactic amnioinfusion for meconium-stained amniotic fluid. Am J Obstet Gynecol 171:931, 1994.

Steinhorn RH, Russell JA, Morin FCI: Disruption of cGMP production in pulmonary arteries isolated from fetal lambs with pulmonary hypertension. Am J Physiol 268:H1483, 1995.

Stenmark KR: New hope for the treatment of pulmonary hypertension: Novel approaches to a complex disease. Pediatr Res 48:421, 2000.

Stenmark KR, Mecham RP: Cellular and molecular mechanisms of pulmonary vascular remodeling. Ann Rev Physiol 59:89, 1997.

Sun B, Curstedt T, Robertson B: Surfactant inhibition in experimental meconium aspiration. Acta Paediatr Scand 82:182, 1993a.

Sun B, Curstedt T, Song GW, et al: Surfactant improves lung function and morphology in newborn rabbits with meconium aspiration. Biol Neonate 63:96, 1993b.

Taylor BJ, Seibert JJ, Glasier CM, et al: Evaluation of the reconstructed carotid artery following extracorporeal membrane oxygenation. Pediatrics 90:568, 1992.

Ting P, Brady JP: Tracheal suction in meconium aspiration. Am J Obstet Gynecol 122:767, 1975.

Tran N, Lowe C, Sivieri EM, Shaffer TH: Sequential effects of acute meconium obstruction on pulmonary function. Pediatr Res 14:34, 1980.

Trimmer KJ, Gilstrap LC: "Meconiumcrit" and birth asphyxia. Am J Obstet Gynecol 165:1010, 1991.

UK Collaborative ECMO Trial Group: UK collaborative randomised trial of neonatal extracorporeal membrane oxygenation. Lancet 348:75, 1996.

Usta IM, Mercer BM, Aswad NK, et al: The impact of a policy of amnioinfusion for meconium-stained amniotic fluid. Obstet Gynecol 85:237, 1995.

van Meurs KP, Nguyen HT, Rhine WD, et al: Intracranial abnormalities and neurodevelopmental status after venovenous extracorporeal membrane oxygenation. J Pediatr 125:304, 1994.

Vassal HB, Malone M, Petros AJ, et al: Familial PPHN resulting from misalignment of the pulmonary vessels (congenial alveolar capillary dysplasia) J Med Genet 35:58, 1998.

Walsh-Sukys MC, Cornell DJ, Houston LN, et al: Treatment of persistent pulmonary hypertension of the newborn without hyperventilation: An assessment of diffusion of innovation. Pediatrics 94:303, 1994.

Walsh-Sukys MC, Tyson JE, Wright LL, et al: Persistent pulmonary hypertension of the newborn in the era before nitric oxide: Practice variation and outcomes. Pediatrics 105:14, 2000.

Ward RM, Daniel CH, Kendig JW, Wood MA: Oliguria and tolazoline pharmacokinetics in the newborn. Pediatrics 77:307, 1986.

Wen TS, Eriksen NL, Blanco JD, et al: Association of clinical intra-amniotic infection and meconium. Am J Perinatol 10:438, 1995.

Wild LM, Nickerson PA, Morin FC III: Ligating the ductus arteriosus before birth remodels the pulmonary vasculature of the lamb. Pediatr Res 25:251, 1989.

Wolfson MR, Greenspan JS, Shaffer TH: Pulmonary administration of vasoactive substances by perfluorochemical ventilation. Pediatrics 97:449, 1996.

Wung J-T, James LS, Kichevsky E, James E: Management of infants with severe respiratory failure and persistence of the fetal circulation, without hyperventilation. Pediatrics 76:488, 1985.

Yeh TF, Lilien LD, Aiyanadar B, Pildes RS: Lung volume, dynamic lung compliance, and blood gases during the first 3 days of postnatal life in infants with meconium aspiration syndrome. Crit Care Med 10:588, 1982.

Yeh TF, Scrinivasan G, Harris V, Pildes RS: Hydrocortisone therapy in meconium aspiration syndrome: A controlled study. J Pediatr 90:140, 1977.

Yeomans ER, Gilstrap LC III, Leveno KJ, et al: Meconium in the amniotic fluid and fetal acid-base status. Obstet Gynecol 73:175, 1989.

Yoder BA: Meconium-stained amniotic fluid and respiratory complications: Impact of selective tracheal suction. Obstet Gynecol 83:77, 1994.

Zapol WM, Hurfor W: Inhaled NO in adult respiratory distress syndrome and other lung diseases. New Horizons 1:638, 1993.

Zapol WM, Snider MT, Hill DJ, et al: Extracorporeal membrane oxygenation in severe respiratory failure: A randomized prospective study. JAMA 242:2193, 1979.

Zayek M, Wild L, Roberts JD, et al: Effect of NO on the survival rate and incidence of lung injury in newborn lambs with PPHN. J Pediatr 123:947, 1993.

Zreik H, Bengur AR, Meliones JN, et al: Superior vena cava obstruction after extracorporeal membrane oxygenation. J Pediatr 127:314, 1995.

CHAPTER

# 49

# Bronchopulmonary Dysplasia

Beverly A. Banks-Randall
and Roberta A. Ballard

## HISTORICAL OVERVIEW

Bronchopulmonary dysplasia (BPD), which is referred to also as *chronic lung disease of prematurity*, is the most common chronic lung disease of childhood. BPD was first described by Northway and colleagues, in 1967, as a severe chronic lung injury in premature infants who survived hyaline membrane disease after treatment with mechanical ventilation and oxygen. Four distinct clinical and pathologic stages were described, progressing from typical respiratory distress syndrome (RDS), with alveolar interstitial edema as well as atelectasis, to massive fibrosis and consolidation of the lung with areas of cystic emphysema and overinflation.

BPD as originally described occurred predominantly in larger preterm infants born at 30 to 34 weeks of gestation with a history of severe respiratory distress necessitating high levels of ventilatory support and oxygen exposure for a prolonged period of time. These infants were born before the introduction of antenatal corticosteroids or postnatal surfactant replacement and at a time when ventilators were first being adapted for use in the newborn.

Since that time, much has been learned about BPD, and the disorder as originally described has virtually disappeared. The infants who are more commonly affected with BPD today are those of extremely low birth weight and born at less than 26 weeks of gestation. Following treatment with antenatal corticosteroids, combined with postnatal surfactant, these infants initially frequently do remarkably well, requiring only low concentrations of oxygen for treatment of RDS, which usually responds favorably to exogenous surfactant. They often then have several days during which there is minimal or no requirement for supplemental oxygen or ventilatory support. Although the initial definition of BPD was a requirement for oxygen at more than 28 days after birth, at present the definition has been revised to include oxygen *or* ventilatory support at 36 weeks of post-menstrual age. The definition of BPD was reviewed at a recent National Institutes of Health–sponsored workshop on BPD (Jobe and Bancalari, 2001). The new definition specifies diagnostic criteria including the need for oxygen, positive pressure ventilation, and/or continuous positive airway pressure (CPAP), along with postnatal age, to better characterize the severity of BPD (Table 49–1). The form of BPD seen in the tiny preterm infant who has had minimal initial respiratory distress is now being called the "new" BPD (Bancalari, 2001; Jobe, 1999).

## BRONCHOPULMONARY DYSPLASIA

### Epidemiology

BPD is now relatively rare in infants born beyond 32 to 34 weeks of gestation but may be increasing in infants born at less than 26 weeks of gestation at a weight of less than 1000 g. In the National Institute of Child Health and Development (NICHD) Neonate Network, the incidence of BPD at 36 weeks in all infants weighing 501 to 1500 g increased from 19% in 1990 to 23% in 1996 and remained at 22% in 2000. In addition, for those very low-birth-weight infants who require prolonged mechanical ventilation, approximately 60% are oxygen dependent at 28 days, and 30% are still oxygen dependent at 36 weeks post-menstrual age. For those weighing less than 1000 g, the incidence of BPD was 40% in the NICHD Neonatal Network; if the infant required mechanical ventilation, the incidence of BPD was as high as 77%, with an overall incidence for mild cases of 31%; for moderate cases, 28%; and for severe cases, 18% (Ehrenkranz et al, 2001).

Although there has been a marked decrease in BPD in larger infants, recent data from the NICHD Network as well as from the Vermont Oxford Database indicate that in the years since 1996, there has been no further decrease in the incidence of BPD (see Chapter 1). The odds of developing BPD increase by approximately two-to threefold for each lower week of gestational age (Palta et al, 1998).

### Pathobiology

BPD is fundamentally the result of abnormal reparative processes in response to injury and inflammation occurring in an immature lung of a genetically susceptible infant (Fig. 49–1). Thus, it is very clear that the pathogenesis of BPD begins with a very immature lung complicated by iatrogenic damage from therapy with oxygen and volume ventilation with superimposed infection and inflammation as well as pulmonary edema complicated by poor nutrition.

#### *Pathologic Stages of Disease*

The original description of BPD pathology by Northway divided the disease into four distinct clinicopathologic stages (Fig. 49–2). Stage 1 pathologic findings were consistent with hyaline membrane disease (now called "respiratory distress syndrome"). In stage 2 (age 4 to 10 days), atelectasis was more extensive, alternating with areas of emphysema, and the chest film again showed opaque lung fields with air bronchograms. It is worth noting that at the time of this description in the late 1960s, the usefulness of CPAP or positive end-expiratory pressure (PEEP) as we know it today had not yet been described. The ventilation of these infants was with zero PEEP, contributing to severe atelectasis. During stage 3, at 11 to 30 days of age, prominent features included extensive bronchial and

**TABLE 49-1**

**Diagnostic Criteria for Bronchopulmonary Dysplasia**

| | |
|---|---|
| Treatment with $FIO_2$ greater than 0.21 for at least 28 days | |
| PLUS | |
| Failure of room air challenge test at 36 weeks of post-menstrual age | |
| **Classification of Severity** | |
| Mild | Requires up to 0.30 effective $FIO_2$* |
| Moderate | Requires greater than 0.30 effective $FIO_2$* |
| Severe | Requires ventilatory support, usually with oxygen |

*Effective $FIO_2$ is based on infant's weight and the concentration and flow of oxygen through a nasal cannula or in a hood.

$FIO_2$, fraction of inspired oxygen.

Data from Jobe and Bancalari, 2001.

bronchiolar metaplasia and hyperplasia. On the chest film, the lung now began to show cystic areas. During stage 4, after 30 days of age, there was massive fibrosis of the lung with destruction of alveoli and airways. The radiographs revealed fibrosis and edema with areas of consolidation as well as areas of overinflation.

### *Pathologic Findings in the "New" Form of the Disease*

In the "new" BPD, the lungs are more uniformly inflated and actually have minimal airway injury or fibrosis. The major abnormality is a decrease in alveolar number, referred to as *alveolar hypoplasia* (Burri, 1997; Coalson et al, 1999; Husain et al, 1998). In the very preterm infants in whom

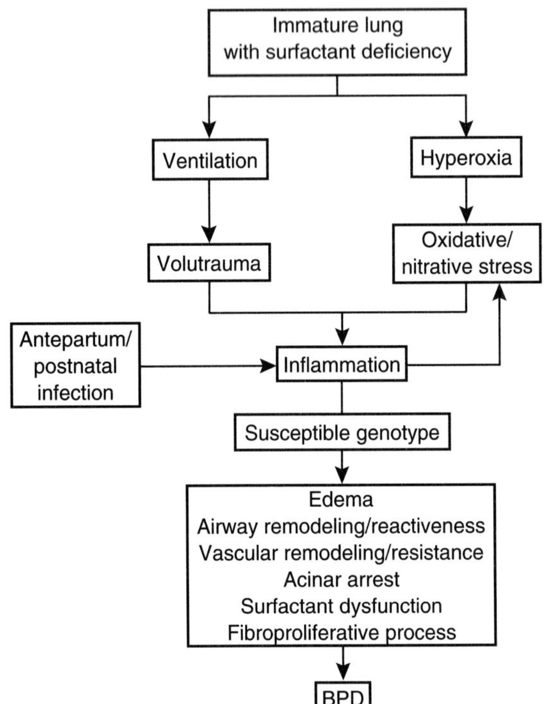


**FIGURE 49-1.** Immature lung with surfactant deficiency. BPD, bronchopulmonary dysplasia.

this "new" BPD is seen, the lung is just finishing the canalicular stage of development at the time of birth; consequently, a number of factors that interfere with the progress of alveolar development may contribute to the development of the "new" BPD.

## Etiologic Factors

Our current understanding of BPD indicates a multifactorial etiology incorporating many contributing factors.

### *Host Susceptibility and Genetic Predisposition*

By far the most important factor in the pathogenesis of BPD is prematurity. Intrauterine growth retardation/restriction also contributes to increased risk (Lal et al, 2003).

It has been known for some time that infants born to certain families are more likely to have RDS at any given gestational age than those in other families. In addition, it has been clear that a family history of asthma and reactive airway disease also puts an infant at additional disadvantage (Bertrand et al, 1985; Evans et al, 1998; Nickerson and Taussig, 1980). Little is known about the genetic contribution to the occurrence of BPD among premature infants. One small study demonstrated an association between BPD and human leukocyte antigen-A2 (HLA-A2). Infants with a family history of asthma are at greater risk for BPD. The availability of the human genome sequence, continuing characterization of single nucleotide polymorphisms (SNPs), and advances in genetic epidemiology give us the tools to identify polymorphisms that affect susceptibility to BPD.

Genetic polymorphisms may contribute to an infant's risk of developing BPD by influencing (1) degree of lung maturity, in particular the content or function of surfactant and the abundance of alveoli at the time of birth; (2) the intensity of the inflammatory response and the propensity to fibrosis; (3) the ability of antioxidant enzymes to protect the lung from free radical damage; and (4) the ability of the neonatal lung and vascular tissue to mature and form alveoli. Ideal candidate genes for genetic analysis would include those with clear biologic significance in pathogenesis of BPD, those with polymorphisms that affect protein level or function, and those with polymorphisms that are amenable to high throughput screening assays. The genes encoding surfactant proteins (SPs), transforming growth factor-$\beta_1$ (TGF-$\beta_1$), and vascular endothelial growth factor (VEGF) meet these criteria as ideal candidate genes. Nevertheless, it remains clear that immaturity of the lung is the single most important etiologic factor in BPD.

### *Inflammation*

A complex inflammatory response clearly plays a major role in the development of BPD (Yoon, 1999). This response may be triggered by a number of other factors thought to be a part of the pathobiology of BPD. These triggers include oxygen toxicity with oxidant damage, ventilation with volutrauma due to use of excessive tidal volumes, and infection prior to delivery, with increased concentrations of inflammatory cytokines in amniotic fluid, as well as cytokines produced as a result of neonatal infection.

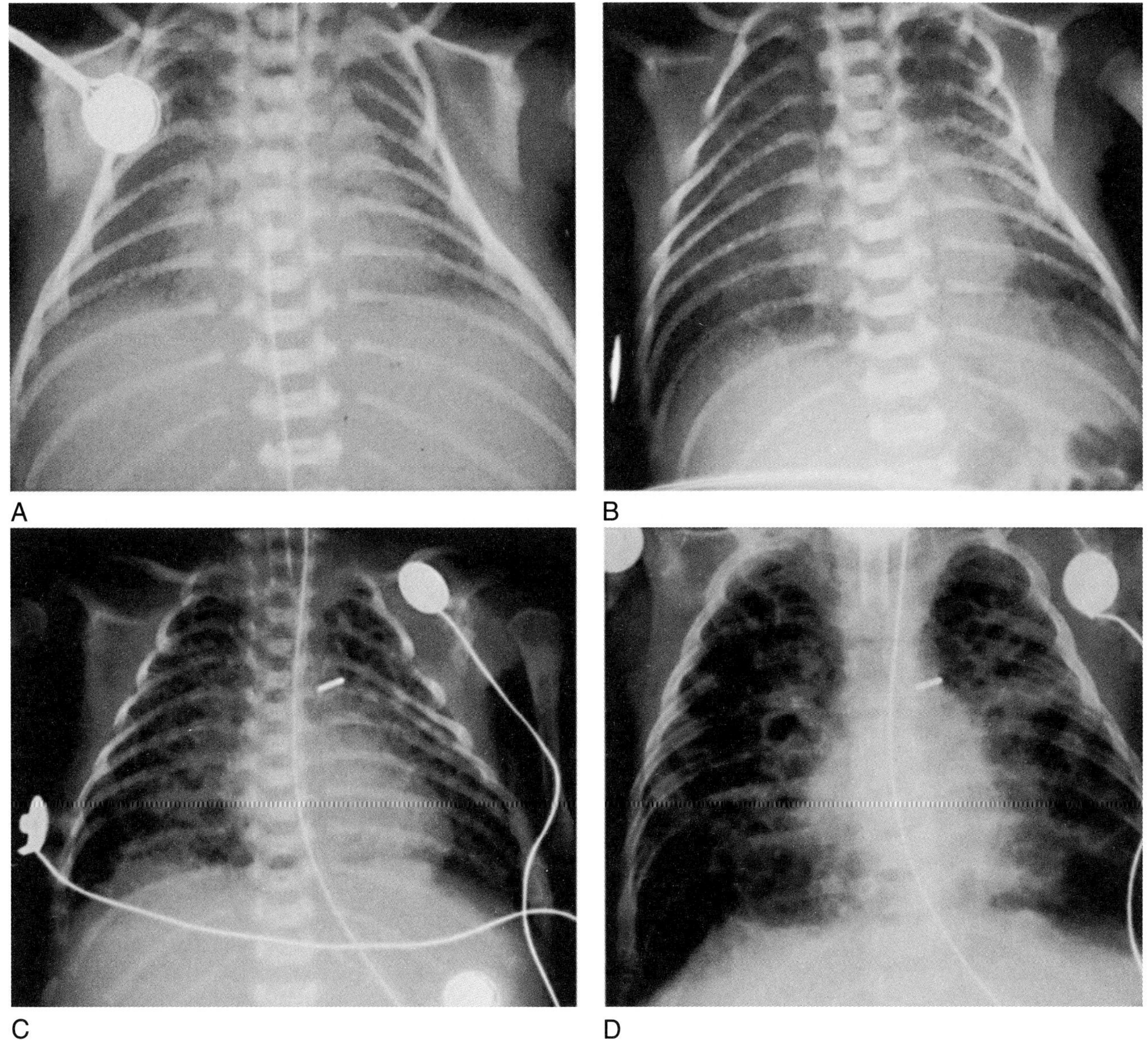


**FIGURE 49–2.** **A–D,** Radiographs illustrating the four stages of bronchopulmonary dysplasia.

The inflammatory response is reflected in increased numbers of neutrophils in tracheal aspirate samples as early as the second day of life (Arnon et al, 1993). Although alveolar macrophages are essential for recognition, ingestion, and elimination of lung pathogens, they also produce fibroblast, epithelial, and endothelial cell growth factors, leading to lung tissue repair. In addition, they can have deleterious effects through release of oxygen radicals and can release fibronectin, a large glycoprotein that is a growth factor for fibroblasts, as well as releasing the growth factor TGF-β, which stimulates the growth of mesenchymal cells and inhibits proliferation of epithelial cells. Among the markers of inflammation that have been found in high concentrations in tracheal aspirates of infants in whom BPD develops are interleukins IL-6, IL-8, IL-11; TNF-α and TGF-β; and elastase, type IV collagen, endothelin-1 (Groneck et al, 1996; Kotecha et al, 1995, 1996; Jonsson et al, 1997; Ohki et al, 2001; Niu et al, 1998; Ramsay et al, 1998), and soluble E-selectin and intercellular adhesion molecule-1 (ICAM-1). Table 49–2 lists the factors that have been found in tracheal aspirates and are associated with the development of BPD in the preterm infant.

### *Neonatal Infection*

Postnatal bacterial sepsis clearly increases the risk of BPD (Gonzalez et al, 1996; Romagnoli, 1998). Airway microbial colonization even without frank sepsis also may increase the risk of BPD. A study of tracheal aspirate samples from ventilated preterm infants revealed that those with positive bacterial, including *Ureaplasma urealyticum*, cultures in the first day of life had an increased airway inflammatory response (Groneck et al, 1996). Continued tracheal colonization with certain bacterial agents, including *Ureaplasma*, has also been associated with increased risk of BPD. If the concept of the new BPD in the tiny preterm infant is regarded

**TABLE 49-2**

**Inflammatory Markers in Tracheal Aspirate Associated with Bronchopulmonary Dysplasia**

| |
|---|
| Tumor necrosis factor-α |
| Interleukins IL-6, IL-8, IL-11 |
| Transforming growth factor-β |
| Elastase |
| Neutrophils |
| Interleukin-1β |
| Soluble E-selectin |
| Intracellular adhesion molecule-1 |
| Endothelin-1 |
| Type IV collagen |

as a syndrome of arrested lung development, then it may be that either infection or inflammatory cytokines may contribute to the arrest of normal alveolarization and development.

### *Oxygen Toxicity*

In the initial cases of BPD reported by Northway and colleagues (1967), it was clear that exposure to high oxygen concentration was a factor in development of the disease. Subsequent reports have continued to show an association between high levels of supplemental oxygen or prolonged oxygen exposure and lung damage in ventilated preterm infants. Recent evidence (STOP-ROP, 2000) suggests that even a slight increase in inhaled oxygen concentration over a prolonged time contributes to pulmonary pathology. In experimental animals, oxygen toxicity follows a course similar to that of BPD, and postmortem findings are similar (Chang et al, 2003; Coalson et al, 1995). The damage to the lung caused by oxygen toxicity appears to be mediated by reactive oxygen species that are produced during univalent reduction of molecular oxygen. These species include superoxide anion ($O_2^-$), hydrogen peroxide ($H_2O_2$), and hydroxyl radical ($OH^-$). Evidence suggests the presence of an oxidant-antioxidant imbalance in lungs that are at risk for BPD, and the higher concentrations of lipid peroxidation metabolites such as the $F_2$ isoprostanes found in preterm infants support this concept (Saugstad, 1996, 2001). The concept of oxidant-antioxidant imbalance is further supported by observations that preterm infants have lower levels of retinoic acid (Shenai et al, 2000), which has been shown to suppress both superoxide and hydrogen peroxide formation in stimulated neutrophils and macrophages. It is clear that reactive oxygen and nitrogen species, which are generated during pulmonary oxygen toxicity, are responsible for many of the pathologic features observed in the premature baboon model of BPD. There is some evidence (Chang et al, 2003) that treatment of the animals with a catalytic antioxidant metalloporphyrin can protect against some of the oxygen toxicity. The change in pattern in these animals, however, is similar to the original description of BPD in older preterm infants. It will be essential to observe whether or not blockage of oxidant damage with antioxidant therapy will have an effect on the known arrest of alveologenesis seen in the "new" BPD.

### *Ventilation with Volutrauma*

As is the case with exposure to high oxygen, the association between overdistention of the preterm lung and the development of BPD is well established. It is clear that overinflation produces stress fractures of the capillary endothelium, epithelium, and basement membrane. This mechanical injury causes leakage of fluid into the alveolar spaces, with additional inflammatory response and the release of additional proinflammatory cytokines. The relative contribution of high peak inspiratory pressures (*barotrauma*) versus overdistention of the lung (*volutrauma*) to lung injury previously was a source of some controversy. Hernandez and colleagues (1989) compared the respective roles of high tidal volume with high peak inspiratory pressure (PIP) in immature New Zealand white rabbits to look at the effect on microvascular permeability in animals that were treated with chest wall restriction with a full-body plaster cast. Preventing overdistention also prevented any significant increase in microvascular permeability, even when the manometer indicated pressures up to 45 cm $H_2O$. In contrast, when isolated excised lungs were ventilated with peak inspiratory pressures of only 15 cm $H_2O$ for 1 hour (with overdistention), there was an 850% increase in microvascular permeability. This finding suggests that preterm infants with relatively healthy lungs and highly compliant chest walls may experience significant lung injury even at apparently low ventilator pressures. In addition, in the preterm lamb model, manual ventilation with as few as 6 very large breaths at birth may compromise the therapeutic effect of subsequent surfactant administration, leading to significant lung damage (Bjorklund et al, 1997; Dreyfuss et al, 1998). Evidence that exposure to high tidal volumes in preterm human infants contributes to BPD comes from several sources. In particular, there is an association between hypocarbia and an increased incidence of BPD (Garland et al, 1995; Kraybill et al, 1989) as well as a known strong association between the occurrence of pneumothorax and pulmonary interstitial emphysema with lung overdistention.

Multiple attempts have been made to improve ventilatory strategies for the preterm infant that would result in a marked decrease in incidence of BPD. One such strategy is the use of high-frequency oscillatory ventilation (HFOV) (Courtney et al, 2002; Gerstmann et al, 1996; Johnson et al, 2002; Moriette et al, 2001). (See also Chapter 45 on the principles of respiratory care.) Although a statistically significant decrease in the incidence of BPD has been described, none of the studies using HFOV achieved large clinically relevant differences in outcome. On the other hand, attempts have been made to use a minimal ventilation strategy to prevent BPD (Carlo et al, 2002). Although the need for ventilatory support at 36 weeks of postmenstrual age was only 1% in the minimal ventilation group versus 16% in the routine conventional ventilation treatment group ($P < .01$), the major morbidities and long-term outcomes were comparable in the two treatment groups. Thus, this approach also requires additional study.

In 1987, Avery and associates published a descriptive review of treatment center differences in the incidence of BPD. At one neonatal center, use of nasal CPAP immediately after delivery was associated with a much lower incidence of BPD than that reported by the other centers.

Van Marter and colleagues (2000) compared the practices and outcomes for neonatal units in Boston and at Columbia University and again found that the incidence of BPD at Columbia overall was much lower, as were other care practices including use of mechanical ventilation, surfactant, indomethacin, and sedation. The use of nasal CPAP was higher and infants at Columbia were intubated less frequently than at the other centers. These investigators found that the best predictor of subsequent BPD was requirement for ventilation on the day of birth (odds ratio 13.4, with a 95% confidence interval [CI] of 5.9 to 30.7).

It must be remembered, however, that infants requiring initial ventilation are often the sickest infants, and even at Columbia, these infants usually die without intervention. Much work is now in progress to improve the delivery systems for nasal CPAP. Use of the recently developed variable-flow nasal CPAP systems, including those employing a nasal mask, appears to significantly decrease work of breathing associated with the use of other systems for applying nasal CPAP (DeKlerk and DeKlerk, 2001; Pandit et al, 2001) Unfortunately, to date, no large randomized trial of this technique has been done. However, multiple attempts are ongoing to study early application of nasal CPAP, thus avoiding intubation and mechanical ventilation. On the other hand, it is clear from review of the literature that nasal CPAP is effective in preventing failure of extubation in preterm infants following a period of endotracheal intubation and intermittent positive pressure ventilation (IPPV) (Ho et al, 2002).

It is clear that loss of functional residual capacity (FRC) with onset of generalized atelectasis also can be a major contributor to the development of BPD. In infants who are being ventilated below a normal FRC, repetitive opening and closing of lung units occur in the presence of maldistribution. This then leads to areas of significant overdistention. There is accumulating evidence from both animal and human newborns that the optimal use of PEEP is associated with a lower risk for BPD. Figure 49–3 demonstrates the appearance of static pressure-volume curves for infants with either normal lungs or with RDS and also depicts the potential areas of lung injury from either high-volume ventilation or low-volume ventilation with atelectasis. There is general agreement that the least injurious approach to supporting ventilation in the preterm infant would be to avoid intubation and stabilize FRC with CPAP. However, many preterm infants are too small or too sick to tolerate the use of nasal CPAP alone and therefore will require intubation and mechanical ventilation. At this time, the approach that would seem most likely to contribute to prevention of BPD is the use of an optimal PEEP to support a normal FRC combined with low-tidal-volume ventilation. Large trials are under way to examine this hypothesis.

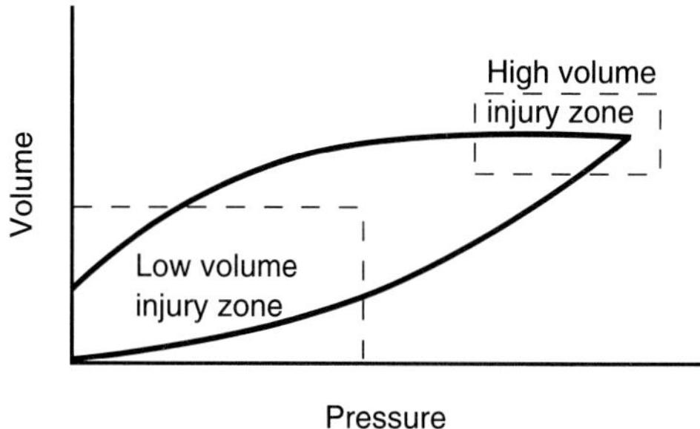


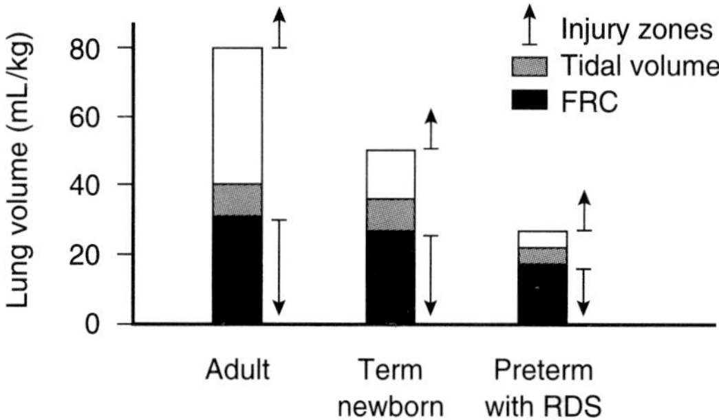


**FIGURE 49–3. Upper panel,** Static pressure-volume curve indicating areas of lung injury from either high-volume ventilation or low-volume ventilation with atelectasis. **Lower panel,** Lung volumes for a normal adult, a term newborn, and a preterm with RDS. The low and high volume injury zones are indicated by arrows. The preterm lung is susceptible to injury with ventilation because of the small volume/kg between the two injury zones. FRC, functional residual capacity; RDS, respiratory distress syndrome.

### *Pulmonary Edema and Patent Ductus Arteriosus*

It is clear from animal studies (Bland et al, 2000) that abnormalities of lung fluid balance contribute to BPD. In the human, several studies done before routine administration of antenatal steroids or postnatal surfactant became available suggested that pulmonary edema and patent ductus arteriosus (PDA) contributed to the pathogenesis of BPD (Brown et al, 1978; Van Marter et al, 1990a). Several investigators have also demonstrated that patency of the ductus arteriosus has a significant association with the incidence of BPD (Gonzalez et al, 1996). However, it is clear that excess flow through the ductus arteriosus can be controlled with appropriate levels of end-expiratory pressure and that the ductus itself can be closed pharmacologically with indomethacin. In addition, the more generalized use of antenatal steroids since the Consensus Conference in 1994 has reduced the incidence of PDA in the preterm infant.

### *Poor Nutrition*

All of the aforementioned etiologic factors are intensified by the inadequate nutritional status that is virtually always present in sick preterm infants. These infants have delayed feeding as well as difficulty receiving adequate parenteral nutrition because of the need to restrict fluid. Because of the increased work of breathing, they also are generally in a catabolic state. In addition, they have vitamin deficiencies, particularly of vitamin A; the latter condition that has been associated with disruption of epithelial cell integrity in the animal model. They also have diminished amounts of antioxidant agents including vitamin E, which probably leads to potentiation of oxygen free radical injury. Each of these factors leads to increased susceptibility to infection, which leads in turn to a further cycle of impaired defense against injury.

### Adrenal Insufficiency

It has been suggested (Watterberg and Scott, 1995; Watterberg et al, 1996) that preterm infants may have developmental immaturity of the hypothalamic-pituitary-adrenal axis and that the risk of BPD is increased secondary to inadequate response to inflammatory lung injury. Banks and colleagues (2001), reported, however, in a study of cortisol levels in 314 preterm infants, that even the earliest gestation infants (24 to 25 weeks) have an increase in cortisol after delivery and that levels were not associated with gestational age (Fig. 49–4). More important, there was only a weak association with severity of illness. Using the CRIB (Clinical Risk Index for Babies) score (International Neonatal Network, 1993) to adjust for clinical risk factors, low cortisol at 3 to 7 days of life contributed only very minimally to increasing the risk for BPD and there was no correlation at 14 to 28 days. It is possible that a high-risk subpopulation of preterm infants who have low cortisol levels or an inappropriate response to ACTH stimulation might benefit from low-dose hydrocortisone therapy; however, there is no evidence that adrenal insufficiency is a major contributor to BPD.

### *Inhibition of Normal Lung Development*

The insults contributing to BPD as described are occurring at a gestational age when alveolarization should be occurring. Development of alveoli can be delayed in a number of animal models by hypoxia, hyperoxia, glucocorticoids, and poor nutrition. In addition, cytokine overexpression also can interfere with normal septation (Albertine et al, 1999; Jobe, 1999; Massaro and Massaro, 2000).

Increasing evidence indicates that abnormal pulmonary vascular development is associated with all of these insults (Abman, 2001). Thus, with the arrest of alveolarization occurring in these infants, arrest of pulmonary vascular development also occurs (Bhatt et al, 2001).

### Preventive Factors

Jobe and Ikegami (2001) recently reviewed approaches to prevention of BPD. Among the practices they evaluated were antenatal maternal steroid administration, use of surfactant, nasal CPAP, and postnatal corticosteroids (PNCS).

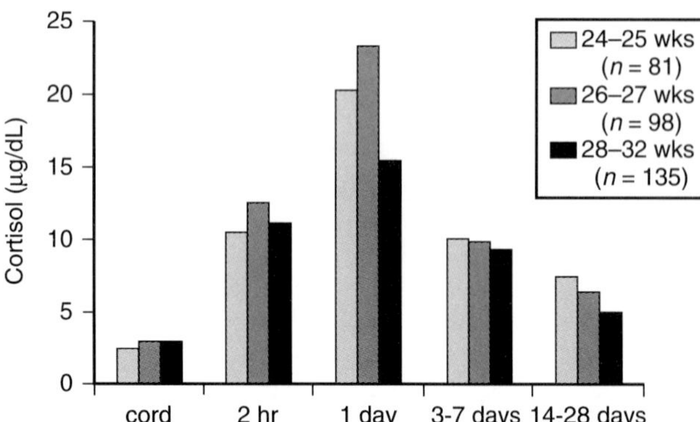


**FIGURE 49–4.** Plasma cortisol concentrations in premature infants during the first 4 weeks of life. Data are mean levels stratified by gestational age: 24 to 25 weeks ($n$ = 81), 26 to 27 weeks ($n$ = 98), and 28 to 32 weeks ($n$ = 135).

### *Antenatal Steroids*

Numerous clinical studies and several large meta-analyses have demonstrated that a single course of antenatal glucocorticoids administered to women at high risk for premature delivery results in a significant decrease in the mortality rate and in the morbidity associated with prematurity, including RDS, intraventricular hemorrhage (IVH), PDA, and necrotizing enterocolitis (NEC). However, the effect on the incidence of BPD among the survivors does not appear to be of substantial clinical importance (Van Marter et al, 1990b). This lack of clinical significance may be due to increased survival of more and smaller preterm infants (see also Chapter 47 on RDS).

### *Surfactant*

Although surfactant replacement therapy is clearly associated with decreased severity of RDS and with a lower associated mortality rate, there is no evidence overall that the survivors have a significantly decreased incidence of BPD. Again, this lack of correlation may be due to the improved survival of smaller, sicker infants.

### *Gentle Ventilation*

As described previously, there is evidence that volutrauma as well as atelectasis contribute directly to lung damage as well as releasing cytokines, which further the cycle of damage. Therefore, numerous trials of ventilatory modes including patient-triggered ventilation, high-frequency ventilation, and minimal ventilation (with the goal of keeping the $PaCO_2$ above 55 mm Hg), as well as trials with some newer modes of ventilation, have been attempted (Carlo et al, 2002; Stark, 2002). (See also Chapter 45 on the principles of respiratory care.) Thus far, none of these trials has resulted in a substantial clinical benefit supporting a given mode of ventilation for general use in care of the newborn.

### *Nasal Continuous Positive Airway Pressure*

Current attempts to accomplish randomized clinical trials of the "Columbia approach" are under way (Aly, 2001). This approach involves immediate administration of "bubble" CPAP in the delivery room to high-risk preterm infants and also involves an initial tolerance of quite high $PaCO_2$ values (in the range of 65 to 70 mm Hg) and subsequent tolerance of higher $PaCO_2$ (55 to 68 mm Hg) as well. These trials have raised the question of what the optimal level of $PaCO_2$ is in the preterm infant, as well as concern about the optimal oxygen saturation for these infants (Askie et al, 2003) (see later on).

### *Fluid Restriction*

Good evidence suggests that fluid overload contributes to an increased risk for BPD (Van Marter et al, 1990a), and some clinical trial data suggest that excessive fluid administration increases the risk of PDA, NEC, and death (Tammela, 1995). However, too-vigorous limitation of fluid administration contributes to the problem of undernutrition, thereby contributing to failure of development of alveoli.

### *Vitamin A*

Vitamin A is an essential nutrient for maintaining respiratory tract epithelial cells and also is stored in the septal cells of the alveoli involved in alveolar septation. Compelling animal data (Albertine et al, 1999) support the need for vitamin A as well (Fig. 49–5). Because vitamin A is accumulated predominantly in the third trimester, preterm infants have deficient liver stores of this vitamin (Zachman, 1989). These infants, who often are unable to tolerate enteral feedings, are at particular risk for vitamin A deficiency because vitamin A added to parenteral nutrition solutions is degraded by light and can adhere to the intravenous tubing, making it largely inaccessible. A number of clinical trials have investigated whether supplementation with vitamin A, typically by intramuscular injections, would result in a decrease in BPD. A large study by the NICHD Neonatal Network demonstrated a significant decrease in BPD (11%) with treatment with vitamin A (Tyson et al, 1999). A meta-analysis of clinical trials published in the Cochrane database in 1999 also revealed that vitamin A supplementation was associated with a reduction in BPD at 36 weeks (Darlow and Graham, 1999). Vitamin A is well tolerated, although it does involve intramuscular injections. It is also inexpensive and is to date the only intervention tested by randomized clinical trials demonstrated to produce a decrease in relative risk of death or BPD at 36 weeks of post-menstrual age. Although there has been a theoretical concern about potential skin or muscle complications from the injections, there was no evidence of damage at follow-up evaluation in the NICHD trial.

### *Postnatal Corticosteroids*

Preterm infants who were given PNCS demonstrate some decreased inflammatory markers and suppression of cytokine-mediated inflammatory reactions in their tracheal aspirates. Numerous theoretical reasons have been advanced regarding why postnatal administration of steroids might decrease the incidence of BPD, including the potential for increased surfactant synthesis, enhanced beta-adrenergic activity, increased antioxidant production, stabilization of cell and lysosomal membranes, and inhibition of prostaglandin and leukotriene synthesis (Watterberg et al, 1999). Although clinical trials have demonstrated increased dynamic compliance and decreased pulmonary resistance following treatment with PNCS, their overall impact on BPD and/or death are not compelling, and major concerns exist regarding both short- and long-term side effects.

A meta-analysis by Banks (2002) reviewed 40 clinical trials of dexamethasone and stratified outcome by time interval and duration of treatment, as shown in Figure 49–6. None of the regimens tried resulted in decreased mortality. Trials of 4-day or longer courses of dexamethasone in preterm infants less than 48 hours old, however, did demonstrate a decreased risk of death or BPD. Under these circumstances, one would need to treat approximately 9 infants with PNCS in order to prevent one adverse outcome of death or BPD.

On the other hand, significant adverse effects of dexamethasone are well known, including hypertension, hyperglycemia, adrenal suppression, and decreased growth. In addition, four large recently published trials (Garland et al, 1999, Sinkin et al, 2000; Stark et al, 2001; Vermont Oxford Network Steroid Study Group, 2001) have described an increased rate of early gastrointestinal perforation not associated with NEC in infants who received PNCS. Even more concerning, however, are results of follow-up in randomized trials involving large numbers of infants. It is now clear that administration of PNCS, particularly very early and/or prolonged administration, is associated with an increased incidence of cerebral palsy and adverse neurodevelopmental outcome (Finer et al,

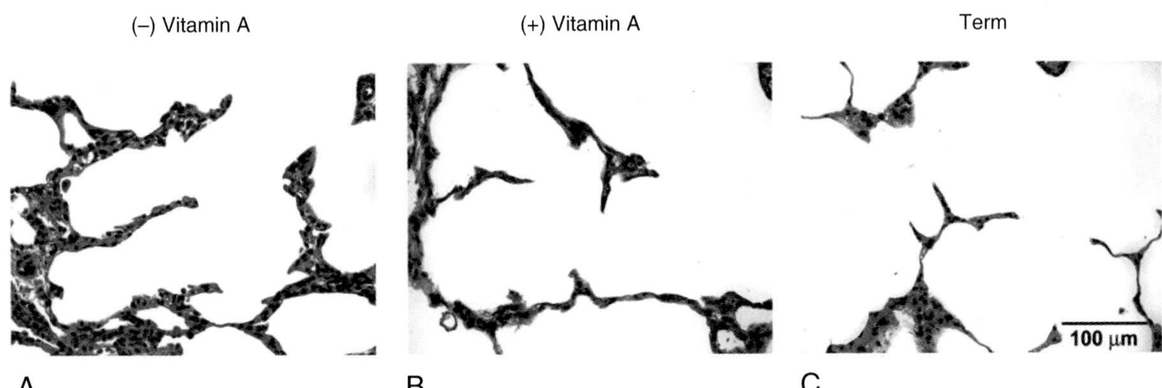


**FIGURE 49–5.** Histopathology of evolving chronic lung disease (CLD) of prematurity in lambs that were mechanically ventilated for 3 weeks at 20 breaths/minute (~15 mL/kg tidal volume). **A,** Preterm lamb ventilated for 3 weeks, treated daily with saline (the vehicle for vitamin A) given intramuscularly. **B,** Preterm lamb ventilated for 3 weeks, treated daily with vitamin A (5,000 U/day) given intramuscularly. **C,** Term lamb ventilated for 3 weeks (control). The most simplified distal air spaces and most thickened alveolar walls are in the lung tissue of the preterm lamb that was not treated with vitamin A (seen in **A**). Secondary septa also are least evident in the preterm lamb that was not treated with vitamin A. All panels are of the same magnification (scale bar = 100 µm).

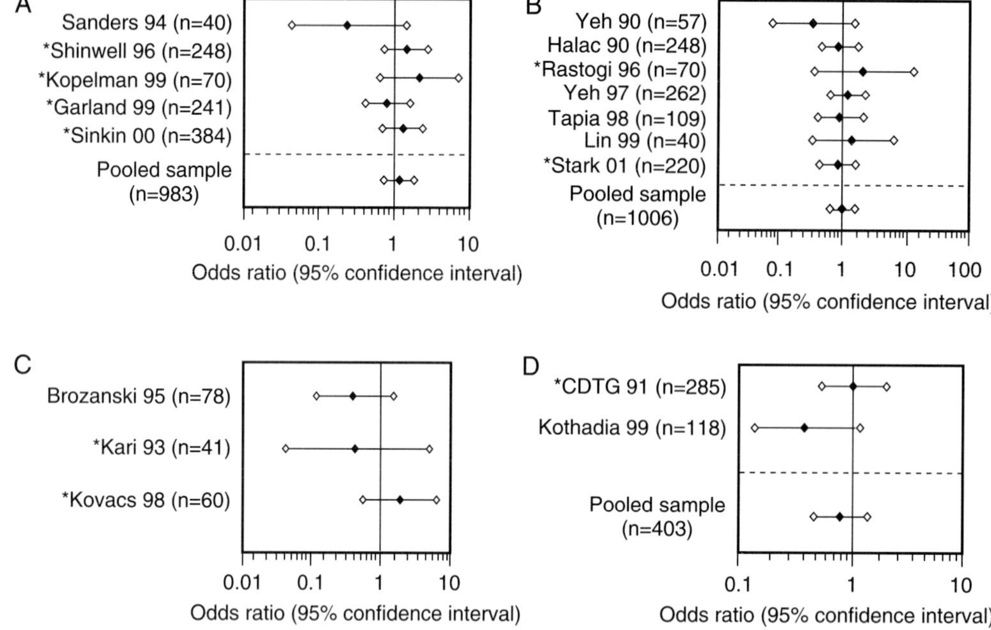


**FIGURE 49–6.** Odds ratios and 95% confidence intervals for the effect of dexamethasone therapy on mortality. Figures are stratified by age at initiation of treatment and duration of therapy. Studies that allowed the use of open-label steroids are indicated with an asterisk. The estimated odds ratio for each trial is shown with the *black diamond*, and the 95% confidence interval for the odds ratio is shown with *open diamonds*. Pooled odds ratios determined by the Mantel-Hanszel technique are shown in the *bottom bar*. No odds ratio is significantly different from 1. **A,** Effect of dexamethasone on mortality when treatment is begun at less than 48 hours and continued for 1 to 3 days. **B,** Effect of dexamethasone on mortality when treatment is begun at less than 48 hours and continued for 4 or more days. **C,** Effect of dexamethasone on mortality when treatment is begun at 7 to 14 days. Because of significant variability in the study design of these three trials, a pooled odds ratio is not calculated. **D,** Effect of dexamethasone on mortality when treatment is begun at more than 14 days.

2000; O'Shea et al, 1999; Shinwell et al, 2000; Yeh et al, 1997). Figure 49–7 shows the risk-benefit balances for treating preterm infants with PNCS.

The high risk of poor neurodevelopmental outcome has led the American Academy of Pediatrics (AAP) and the Canadian Pediatric Society along with the European Pediatric Society to strongly recommend that (1) postnatal steroids be used only within randomized controlled trials that have neurodevelopmental outcome as a part of their protocol; (2) if steroids are to be used, they be used only under exceptional clinical circumstances; and (3) there be documented full, informed consent of the family regarding the potential short- and long-term risks of steroids. In addition, the goal should be to give the minimum dose for the shortest possible period of time. At present, the optimal course with the least side effects would appear to be limiting treatment to infants with severe disease (requiring fraction of inspired oxygen [$FIO_2$] greater than 0.5 and mean airway pressure [MAP] greater than 12 to 14 cm of $H_2O$) who are older than 7 days of age, and to use brief bursts of a 3-day course of steroids beginning at a dose of less than 0.25 mg/kg.

Although other routes of steroid administration, including inhalation (Cole, 2002), as well as the possibility of using other types of glucocorticoids such as hydrocortisone, have been suggested, no data at this point suggest clinical improvement with either inhaled steroids or use of hydrocortisone. A trial of early administration of low-dose hydrocortisone for prevention of BPD was recently stopped due to an increased incidence of intestinal perforation in treated infants.

### *Antioxidant Therapy*

Some evidence in the baboon model of BPD indicates that a catalytic antioxidant metalloporphrin can protect against hyperoxia-induced lung injury (Chan et al, 2003; Tanswell and Jankov, 2003). Superoxide dismutase is a naturally occurring enzyme that protects against oxygen free radical injury. Preliminary trials in the human infant have suggested that administration of exogenous superoxide dismutase might be of benefit (Davis, 2002; Davis et al, 2000, 2003). Some investigators have raised caution concerning use of antioxidants as therapy in the newborn (Jankov et al, 2001). Further trials of this intervention are needed before it can be recommended as useful in preventing BPD.

### *Inhaled Nitric Oxide*

It has been hypothesized that inhaled nitric oxide (iNO) may potentially either prevent BPD or benefit infants with evolving BPD, as a result of several of its known effects. In fact, it may be that preterm infants with early BPD have a deficiency of endogenous NO, and that exogenous iNO, by causing pulmonary vasodilatation as

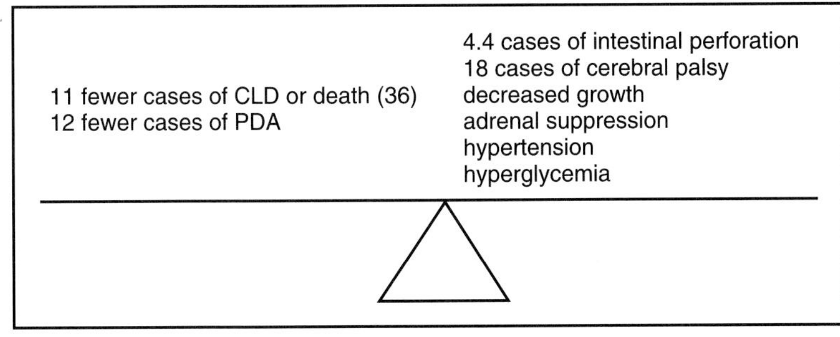


**FIGURE 49-7.** Balance of treatment of 100 ventilated preterm infants in the first 48 hours of life resulted in limited benefit and significant possibility for harm. CLD, chronic lung disease; PDA, patent ductus arteriosus.

well as bronchial dilatation (Martin et al, 2002), will reduce the need for oxygen and ventilatory support. Pilot data on iNO administration were obtained (Banks et al, 1999) in a group of preterm infants with severe BPD who were older than 28 days of age and still required mechanical ventilation with an MAP of greater than 10 cm $H_2O$ as well as inspired oxygen concentration of at least 45%, with a majority requiring greater than 75% oxygen. These infants were treated with iNO at 20 parts per million (ppm) and evaluated both within the first hour and after 72 hours. Approximately two thirds of the infants demonstrated marked improvement in oxygenation within 1 hour of beginning iNO therapy, and a similar number had significant decrease in oxygen requirement within 72 hours. Based on this pilot information as well as studies from Kinsella and colleagues (1999) confirming the safety of iNO, several randomized controlled trials of approaches preventing BPD with iNO are ongoing in North America. The hypothesis is that low-dose iNO administered to preterm infants with birth weights of 500 to 1250 g who require mechanical ventilation will increase survival without chronic lung disease at 36 weeks of post-menstrual age. In addition, it is hypothesized that the treatment will increase neither pulmonary inflammatory response nor level of oxidant stress and will have no adverse effect on either short- or long-term clinical outcome. Infants enrolled in these trials will be followed to at least 2 years of age to determine neurodevelopmental outcome as well.

### Clinical Course and Treatment

As mentioned earlier, the classic BPD described by Northway and colleagues is now extremely rare with the advent of antenatal steroids, postnatal surfactant, and ventilators and ventilator strategies better suited for newborn infants. Thus, here we address only the clinical course of the "new" BPD. As pointed out by Bancalari (2001) and others, a majority of infants who have BPD currently are extremely low-birth-weight (usually under 1000 g) infants who require prolonged ventilator support, often for management of apnea or poor respiratory effort. Following use of antenatal steroids and postnatal surfactant, these infants often initially require relatively low concentrations of oxygen and have fairly mild initial respiratory distress. They are extremely susceptible to infection, however, and often between 5 and 10 days of age they develop systemic sepsis and/or tracheitis and pneumonia. Infection contributes to the deterioration of respiratory status that occurs during this period in many of these infants. Although certainly high-level oxygen and ventilator support contribute to the developing BPD, a number of other factors are involved as well.

Barrington and Finer (1998) reviewed the treatment of BPD. Management of these infants should be directed at (1) minimizing ventilatory support and overdistention while (2) supporting and maintaining adequate FRC with end-expiratory pressure. These goals can best be achieved with the use of nasal CPAP with a variable-flow delivery system (Courtney et al, 2001; Pandit et al, 2001). Successful use of nasal CPAP requires tolerance of permissive hypercapnia both immediately after birth (the recommendation of the group at Columbia is to tolerate levels as high as 70 mm Hg) as well as subsequent tolerance of $PaCO_2$ values well into the 60s, along with avoidance of $PaCO_2$ values under 40. This recommendation has led to the need for further investigation of the appropriate level of $PCO_2$ in these preterm infants. There has been concern that elevated levels might be associated with IVH or other adverse neurodevelopmental effects. However, recent studies in the human rather suggest that both hypocapnia (not hypercapnia) and hyperoxia place infants at increased risk for disabling cerebral palsy (Collins et al, 2001). In addition, there is some evidence that high $PaCO_2$ levels may actually be neuroprotective (Vanucci et al, 1995, 1997). In fact, some data (Laffey et al, 2000) indicate that $PCO_2$ values up to 100 mm Hg actually protect the lung from reperfusion injury and that buffering the low pH that results from high $PCO_2$ negates the protective effect of the high $PCO_2$.

Another management issue that is crucial for maintaining infants on nasal CPAP is the expected level of oxygen saturation to be achieved. Again, there is enormous controversy regarding the appropriate oxygen status of these infants. It should be emphasized that in utero, the fetus is exposed to a $PaO_2$ of only 25 to 27 mm Hg and oxygen saturations below 80%. Yet, without any good data, keeping the preterm infant's oxygen saturation ($SaO_2$) in a range of 90% to 95% is commonplace. In some institutions, levels have routinely been kept above 95%. The data from a recent large clinical trial (STOP-ROP, 2000) did not demonstrate any major value for protection against retinopathy of prematurity with exposure to $SaO_2$ ranges that were greater than 96%, compared with 89% to 94%. However, the pulmonary outcomes for the infants in this trial exposed to higher oxygen indicated more evidence of damage. On the other hand, in a randomized trial involving 358 infants born at less than 30 weeks of gestation who remained dependent on supplemental $O_2$ at 32 weeks, there was no evidence that targeting the

$SaO_2$ ranges in the 91% to 94% rather than 95% to 98% range had any effect on growth or development. However, maintaining the higher $SaO_2$ range resulted in longer exposure to oxygen, higher rates of $O_2$ dependence at a postmenstrual age of 36 weeks, and higher frequency of home-based oxygen therapy (Askie et al, 2003). Trials are ongoing to evaluate whether keeping oxygen saturation at lower levels (even allowing $SaO_2$ to fall to under 80%) might result in improvement in both pulmonary and neurodevelopmental outcomes.

### *Ventilation*

In spite of the development of numerous sophisticated ventilators for the newborn, there is still no clear advantage to any one approach to ventilating the preterm infant (see also Chapter 47). The general approach should be one of preventing atelectasis, sustaining FRC, using a minimal tidal volume (usually 4 to 6 cc/kg) and allowing the infant to trigger his or her own ventilation as much as possible (Carlo et al, 2002). It is also clear that infants can be extubated more successfully if they are extubated directly to nasal CPAP.

### *Nutrition*

It is clear that maximizing both enteral and parenteral nutrition is essential to growth and recovery of preterm infants with BPD. Beginning parenteral nutrition within the first 2 or 3 days after birth, as well as the use of aggressive feeding regimens, is crucial to success in these infants. In addition, it is appropriate to treat such infants with vitamin A, as it is the only agent shown to decrease the incidence of BPD in clinical trials.

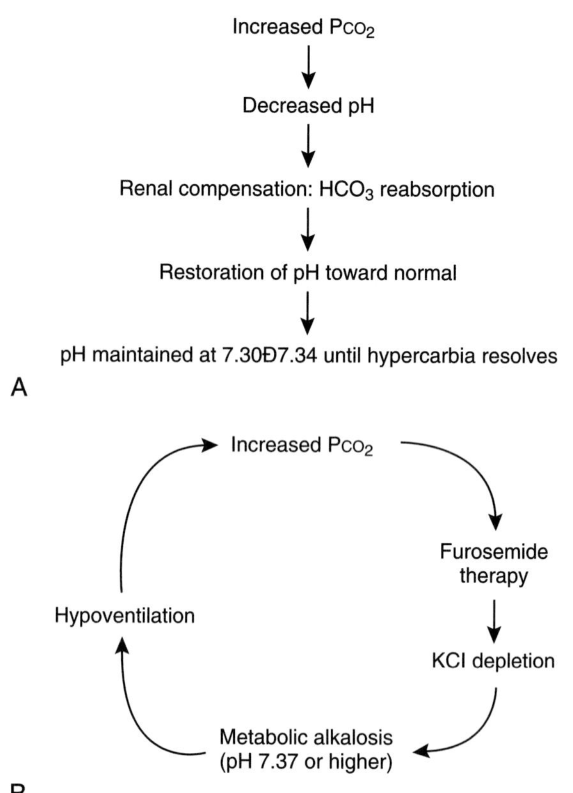


**FIGURE 49–8. A,** Compensated respiratory acidosis in BPD. **B,** Diuretic-induced metabolic alkalosis in BPD. (Data from Hazinski TA: Drug treatment for established BPD. In Bland RD, Coalson JJ [eds]: Chronic Lung Disease in Early Infancy. New York, Marcel Dekker, 2000, pp 257-283.)

### *Diuretics*

In infants with well-developed BPD, pulmonary edema is a major component of the illness. Diuretics, therefore, have been used for some time (Hazinski, 2000). There is clear evidence that either daily or alternate-day therapy with furosemide improves lung mechanics and gas exchange in infants with established BPD (Rush et al, 1990). Thiazide-type diuretics alone or in combination with spironolactone also have improved lung function in several studies. A major concern with diuretic usage, however, has been hypercalciuria along with metabolic alkalosis. There are no long-term trials of diuretic therapy; nevertheless, most centers use diuretics at some point in the management of infants with BPD. It is essential, if long-term diuretics are administered, that supplemental KCl also be administered to prevent the diuretic-induced metabolic alkalosis associated with hypochloremia as well as hypokalemia. The cycle that can be set up in these infants is demonstrated in Figure 49–8 (Hazinski, 2000). Diuretic-induced hypokalemia and alkalosis can be diagnosed by finding a blood pH (not the base deficit) that is inappropriate for the infant's clinical state. In chronic BPD, an infant who has become hypercarbic will, over time, have a compensated respiratory acidosis (pH of 7.3 to 7.35 in the presence of slightly elevated serum bicarbonate). However, if the infant is receiving diuretics and is not receiving adequate supplements of KCl, the infant's loss of potassium and chloride can lead to a primary metabolic alkalosis. The infant will hypoventilate to reduce blood pH, creating further inhibition of ventilation.

Another complication of concern for long-term diuretic therapy is hypercalciuria with potential calcium deposition in the renal interstitium with nephrocalcinosis.

### *Bronchodilator Therapy*

With established BPD, there is a significant increase in airway resistance, and there may also be persistent or intermittent wheezing. Several studies of either short-term, inhaled, or parenteral $beta_2$-adrenergic agonist therapy have demonstrated some improvement in ventilation with such therapy. Inhaled albuterol has been the most widely used agent. Systemic use of bronchodilators has been more restricted because of a high incidence of side effects and a very narrow therapeutic index (DeBoeck et al, 1998). Hazinski (2000) points out that there are two pitfalls to the use of $beta_2$ agonist drugs: (1) there can be beta agonist–induced vasodilatation, which may lead to hypoxia; and (2) beta agonist–induced augmentation of airway instability in an infant with both BPD and tracheomalacia may occur. Both of these pitfalls may lead to complex ventilation-perfusion ($\dot{V}/\dot{Q}$) relations. Discussions of these pitfalls as well as management are included in Hazinski's chapter in the textbook by Bland and Coalson (2000).

### *Postnatal Corticosteroids*

As discussed earlier, there has been a widespread effort to prevent chronic lung disease with the use of postnatal dexamethasone. Currently, recommendations of the American Academy of Pediatrics and the Canadian Pediatric Society are that use of postnatal steroids be restricted to randomized, controlled trials and, when these agents are given outside of such trials, that they be used only under exceptional circumstances of severity and after fully informing the parents of the potential problems with neurodevelopmental outcome.

### Outcome

The mortality rate among infants with the severest form of BPD with cor pulmonale can be as high as 40%. The mortality rate among infants who are discharged on therapy from the hospital is roughly 10%. In long-term follow-up assessments of preterm infants, BPD clearly is one of the major conditions associated with poor neurodevelopmental outcome (along with IVH and periventricular leukomalacia). Because there is a very powerful association of administration of postnatal steroids with increased cerebral palsy and poor outcome, however, it is unclear how much of the contribution to poor neurodevelopmental outcome in these infants is from the disease itself and how much is a result of treatment with postnatal steroids along with poor nutrition, impaired growth, and prolonged hospitalization. Long-term morbidity associated with BPD may include damage to supraglottic, glottic, subglottic, and tracheal tissues secondary to endotracheal intubation (Statement on the care of the child with chronic lung disease, 2003). Systemic hypertension has also been described in severe cases (Alagappan and Malloy, 1998).

## SUMMARY

BPD remains the most common form of chronic lung disease in children. It is estimated that there are between 10,000 and 12,000 infants with BPD at any one time in the United States. This disease remains very costly in terms of illness and long-term neurodevelopmental outcome, as well as the financial costs to families and society. The American Thoracic Society has recently published a well-referenced position paper on the care of the child with chronic lung disease of infancy and childhood that addresses many of the important ongoing issues in the care of these children (Statement on the care of the child with chronic lung disease, 2003).

It is hoped that combining treatment with vitamin A with new approaches to ventilation, including more vigorous use of nasal CPAP, along with the possibility of other interventions such as iNO, will lead to a significant decrease in the impact of this problem over the next 10 years.

## SUGGESTED READINGS

Bland RD, Coalson JJ (eds): Chronic Lung Disease in Early Infancy. New York, Marcel Dekker, 2000.

Statement on the care of the child with chronic lung disease of infancy and childhood. American Thoracic Society documents. Am J Respir Crit Care Med 168:356-396, 2003.

## REFERENCES

Abman SH: Bronchopulmonary dysplasia: A "vascular hypothesis." Am J Respir Crit Care Med 164:1955-1956, 2001.

Alagappan A, Malloy MH: Systemic hypertension in very low birth weight infants with bronchopulmonary dysplasia: Incidence and risk factors. Am J Perinatol 15:3-8, 1998.

Albertine KH, Jones GP, Starcher BC, et al: Chronic lung injury in preterm lambs: Disordered respiratory tract development. Am J Respir Crit Care Med 159:945-958, 1999.

Aly HZ: Nasal prongs CPAP: A simple yet powerful tool. Pediatrics 108:759-761, 2001.

Arnon S, Grigg J, Silverman M: Pulmonary inflammatory cells in ventilated preterm infants: Effect of surfactant treatment. Arch Dis Child 69:44, 1993.

Askie LM, Henderson-Smart DJ, Irwig L, et al: Oxygen-saturation targets and outcomes in extremely preterm infants. N Engl J Med 349:959-967, 2003.

Avery ME, Tooley WH, Keller JB, et al: Is chronic lung disease in low birth-weight infants preventable? A survey of eight centers. Pediatrics 79:26, 1987.

Bancalari E: Epidemiology and risk factors for the "new" BPD. Neo Reviews 1:e2-e5, 2001.

Banks BA, Seri I, Ischiropoulos H, et al: Changes in oxygenation with inhaled nitric oxide in severe bronchopulmonary dysplasia. Pediatrics 103:610-618, 1999.

Banks BA, Stouffer N, Cnaan A, et al: Association of plasma cortisol and chronic lung disease of preterm infants. Pediatrics 107:494-498, 2001.

Banks BA: Postnatal dexamethasone for bronchopulmonary dysplasia: A systematic review and meta-analysis of 20 years of clinical trials. NeoReviews 3:e24, 2002.

Barrington KJ, Finer NN: Treatment of bronchopulmonary dysplasia: A review. Clin Perinatol 25:177-202, 1998.

Bertrand JM, Riley SP, Popkin J, et al: The long-term pulmonary sequelae of prematurity: The role of familial airway hyperreactivity and the respiratory distress syndrome. N Engl J Med 312:742, 1985.

Bhatt AJ, Pryhuber GS, Huyck H, et al: Disrupted pulmonary vasculature and decreased vascular endothelial growth factor, FLT-1 and TIE-2 in human infants dying with bronchopulmonary dysplasia. Am J Respir Crit Care Med 164:1971-1980, 2001.

Bjorkund LJ, Imqimarsson J, Curstedt T, et al: Manual ventilation with a few large breaths at birth compromised the therapeutic effect of subsequent surfactant replacement in immature lambs. Pediatr Res 432:348-355, 1997.

Bland RD, Albertine KH, Carlton DP, et al: Chronic lung injury in preterm lambs: Abnormalities of the pulmonary circulation and lung fluid balance I. Pediatr Res 48:1-11, 2000a.

Bland RD, Albertine KH, Carlton DP, et al: Chronic lung injury in preterm lambs: Abnormalities of the pulmonary circulation and lung fluid balance II. Pediatr Res 48:64-74, 2000b.

Brown ER, Stark A, Sosenko I, et al: Bronchopulmonary dysplasia: Possible relationship to pulmonary edema. Pediatrics 92:982, 1978.

Brozanski BS, Jones JG, Gilmour CH, et al: Effect of pulse dexamethasone therapy on the incidence and severity of chronic lung disease in the very low birth weight infant. J Pediatr 126:769-776, 1995.

Burri PH. Structural aspects of prenatal and postnatal development and growth of the lung. In McDonald JA (ed): Lung Growth and Development. New York, Marcel Dekker, 1997.

Carlo WA, Stark AR, Wright LL, et al: Minimal ventilation to prevent BPD in extremely low birth weight infants. J Pediatr 141:370-375, 2002.

Chang LL, Subramanian M, Yoder BA, et al: A catalytic antioxidant attenuates alveolar structural remodeling in BPD. Am J Respir Crit Care Med 167:57-64, 2003.

Coalson JJ, Winter V, deLemos RA: Decreased alveolarization in baboon survivors with BPD. Am J Resp Crit Care Med 152:640-646, 1995.

Coalson JJ, Winter VT, Siler-Khodr T, et al: Neonatal CLD in extremely immature baboons. Am J Resp Crit Care Med 160:1333-1346, 1999.

Cole CH: Postnatal glucocorticoid therapy for prevention of bronchopulmonary dysplasia: Routes of administration compared. Semin Neonatol 6:343-350, 2001.

Collaborative Dexamethasone Trial Group: Dexamethasone therapy in neonatal chronic lung disease: An international placebo-controlled trial. Pediatrics 88:421-427, 1991.

Collins MP, Lorenz JM, Jettan JR, et al: Hypocapnea and other ventilation-related risk factors for cerebral palsy in low birth weight infants. Pediatr Res 50:712-719, 2001.

Courtney SE, Durand DJ, Asselin JM, et al: High-frequency OV vs. conventional ventilation for VLBW infants. N Engl J Med 347:643-652, 2002.

Courtney SE, Pyon KH, Saslow JG, et al: Lung recruitment and breathing pattern during variable vs continuous flow nasal CPAP in premature infants: An evaluation of 3 devices. Pediatrics 107:304-308, 2001.

Darlow BA, Graham PJ: Vitamin A supplementation for preventing morbidity and mortality in very low birthweight infants. Cochrane Database Syst Rev 2000. http://156.40.88/cochrane/Darlow/Darlow.htm

Davis JM, Parad RB, Michele T, et al: Pulmonary outcome at one year corrected age in premature infants treated at birth with recombinant human CuZn superoxide dismutase. Pediatrics 111:469-476, 2003.

Davis JM, Richter SE, Biswas S, et al: Long term follow-up of premature infants treated with prophylactic, intratracheal recombinant human CuZn superoxide dismutase. J Perinatol 4:213-216, 2000.

Davis JM: Role of oxidant injury in the pathogenesis of neonatal lung disease. Acta Paediatr Suppl 437:23-25, 2002.

DeBoeck K, Smith, VanLierde, et al: Response to bronchodilations in clinically stable 1-year-old patients with BPD. J Pediatr 157:75-79, 1998.

DeKlerk AM, DeKlerk RK: Use of CPAP in preterm infants: Comments and experience from New Zealand. Pediatrics 108:761-762, 2001.

Dreyfuss D, Saumon G: Ventilation-induced lung injury: Lessons from experimental studies. Amer J Respr Crit Care Med 157:294-323, 1998.

Ehrenkranz RA, Walsh-Sukys MC, Vohr BR, et al and The NICHD Neonatal Research Network: New consensus definition of bronchopulmonary dysplasia (BPD-DEF) predicts pulmonary and neurodevelopmental outcomes in early infancy. Pediatr Res 49:276A, 2001.

Evans M, Palta M, Sadek M, et al: Associations between family history of asthma, bronchopulmonary dysplasia, and childhood asthma in very low birth weight children. Am J Epidemiol 148:460-466, 1998.

Finer NN, Craft A, Vauchen YE, et al: Postnatal steroids: Short-term gain, long-term pain? J Pediatr 137:9-13, 2000.

Garland JS, Alex CP, Pauly TH, et al: A three-day course of dexamethasone therapy to prevent chronic lung disease in ventilated neonates: A randomized trial. Pediatrics 104:91-99, 1999.

Garland JS, Buck RK, Allred EN, et al: Hypocarbia before surfactant therapy appears to increase bronchopulmonary dysplasia risk in infants with respiratory distress syndrome. Arch Pediatr Adolesc Med 149:617-622, 1995.

Gerstmann DR, Minton SD, Stoddard RA, et al: The Provo multicenter early high-frequency oscillatory ventilation trial: Improved pulmonary and clinical outsome in RDS. Pediatrics 98:1044-1057, 1996.

Gonzalez A, Sosenko IRS, Chandar J, et al: Influence of infection on patent ductus arteriosus and chronic lung disease in premature infants weighting 1000 grams or less. J Pediatr 128:470-478, 1996.

Groneck P, Gotze-Speer B, Speer CP: Inflammatory bronchopulmonary response of preterm infants with microbial colonisation of the airway at birth. Arch Dis Child 74: F51-F55, 1996.

Halac E, Halac J, Begue EF, et al: Prenatal and postnatal corticosteroid therapy to prevent neonatal necrotizing enterocolitis: A controlled trial. J Pediatr 117:132-138, 1990.

Hazinski TA: Drug treatment for established BPD. In Bland RD, Coalson JJ (eds): Chronic Lung Disease in Early Infancy. New York, Marcel Dekker, 2000, pp 257-283.

Hernandez LA, Peevy KJ, Moise AA, et al: Chest wall restriction limits high airway pressure-induced lung injury in young rabbits. J Appl Physiol 66:2364, 1989.

Ho JJ, Subramaniam P, Henderson-Smart DJ, Davis PG: Continuous distending pressure for respiratory distress syndrome in preterm infants. The Cochrane Library, Issue 2, Oxford: Update Software Ltd, 2002.

Husain AN, Siddiqui NH, Stocker JT: Pathology of arrested acinar development in postsurfactant bronchopulmonary dysplasia. Hum Pathol 29:710-717, 1998.

International Neonatal Network: The CRIB (Clinical Risk Index for Babies) score: A tool for assessing initial neonatal risk and comparing performance of neonatal intensive care units. Lancet 342:193-198, 1993.

Jankov RP, Negus A, Tanswell AK: Antioxidants as therapy in the newborn: Some words of caution. Pediatr Res 50:681-687, 2001.

Jobe AJ: The new BPD: An arrest of lung development. Pediatr Res 46:641-643, 1999.

Jobe AH, Bancalari E: Bronchopulmonary dysplasia. Am J Respir Crit Care Med 163:1723-1729, 2001.

Jobe AH, Ikegami M: Lung development and function in preterm infants in the surfactant treatment era. Annu Rev Physiol 62:825-846, 2000.

Jobe AH, Ikegami M: Prevention of BPD. Curr Opin Pediatr 13:124-129, 2001.

Johnson AH, Peacock JL, Greenough A, et al: High frequency oscillatory ventilation for the prevention of CLD of prematurity. N Engl J Med 347:633-642, 2002.

Jonsson B, Tullus K, Brauner A, et al: Early increase of TNF-α and IL-6 in tracheobronchial aspirate fluid indicator of subsequent chronic lung disease in preterm infants. Arch Dis Child 77: F198-F201, 1997.

Kari MA, Heinonen K, Ikonen RS, et al: Dexamethasone treatment in preterm infants at risk for bronchopulmonary dysplasia. Arch Dis Child 68:566-569, 1993.

Kinsella JP, Walsh WF, Bose CL, et al: Inhaled nitric oxide in premature neonates with severe hypoxemic respiratory failure: A randomized controlled trial. Lancet 354:1061-1065, 1999.

Kopelman AE, Moise AA, Holbert D, Hegemier SE: A single very early dexamethasone dose improves respiratory and cardiovascular adaptation in preterm infants. J Pediatr 135:345-350, 1999.

Kotecha S, Chan B, Azam N, et al: Increase in Interleukin-8 and soluble intracellular adhesion molecule-1 in BAL fluid for premature infants who develop CLD. Arch Dis Child Fetal Neonatal Ed 72:F90-F96, 1995.

Kotecha S, Wangoo A, Silverman M, et al: Increase in the concentration of TGFβ in BAL fluid before development of CLD of prematurity. J Pediatr 128:464-469, 1996.

Kothadia JM, O'Shea TM, Roberts D, et al: Randomized placebo-controlled trial of a 42-day tapering course of dexamethasone to reduce the duration of ventilator dependency in very low birth weight infants. Pediatrics 104:22-27, 1999.

Kovacs L, Davis GM, Faucher D, Papageorgiou A: Efficacy of sequential early systemic and inhaled corticosteroid therapy in the prevention of chronic lung disease of prematurity. Acta Paediatr 87:792-798, 1998.

Kraybill EN, Runyan DK, Bose CL, et al: Risk factors for chronic lung disease in infants with birth weights of 751 to 1000 grams. J Pediatr 115:115, 1989.

Laffey JG, Engelberts D, Kavanagh BP: Buffering hypercapnic acidosis worsens acute lung injury. Am J Resp Crit Care Med 161:141-146, 2000.

Lal MK, Manktelow BN, Draper ES, et al: Chronic lung disease of prematurity and IUGR: A population-based study. Pediatrics 111:483-487, 2003.

Lin YJ, Yeh TF, Hsieh WS, et al: Prevention of chronic lung disease in preterm infants by early postnatal dexamethasone therapy. Pediatr Pulmonol 27:21-26, 1999.

Martin RJ, Mhanna MJ, Haxhiu MA: The role of endogenous and exogenous nitric oxide on airway function. Semin Perinatol 26:432-438, 2002.

Massaro DJ, Massaro GM: The regulation of the formation of pulmonary alveoli. In Bland RD, Coalson JJ (eds): Chronic Lung Disease in Early Infancy. New York, Marcel Dekker, 2000.

Moriette G, Paris-Llado J, Walti H, et al: Prospective randomized multicenter comparison of high-frequency oscillatory ventilation and conventional ventilation in preterm infants of less than 30 weeks with respiratory distress syndrome. Pediatrics 107:363-372, 2001.

Nickerson BG, Taussig LM: Family history of asthma in infants with bronchopulmonary dysplasia. Pediatrics 65:1140, 1980.

Niu JO, Munshi UK, Siddiq MM, Parton LA: Early increase in endothelin-1 in tracheal aspirates of preterm infants: Correlation with bronchopulmonary dysplasia. J Pediatr 132:965-970, 1998.

Northway WH, Rosan RC, Porter DY: Pulmonary disease following respiratory therapy of hyaline membrane disease. N Engl J Med 276:357-368, 1967

Ohki Y, Kato M, Kimura H, et al: Elevated type IV collagen in bronchoalveolar lavage fluid from infants with bronchopulmonary dysplasia. Biol Neonate 79:34-38, 2001.

O'Shea TM, Kothadia JM, Klinepeter KL, et al: Randomized placebo-controlled trial of a 42-day tapering course of dexamethasone to reduce the duration of ventilator dependency in very low birth weight infants: Outcome of study participants at 1-year adjusted age. Pediatrics 104:15-21, 1999.

Palta M, Sadek M, Barnet JH, et al: Evaluation of criteria for chronic lung disease in surviving very low birth weight infants. J Pediatr 132:57-63, 1998.

Pandit PB, Courtney SE, Pyon KH, et al: Work of breathing during constant- and variable-flow nasal CPAP in preterm neonates. Pediatrics 108:682-685, 2001.

Ramsay PL, Smith EO, Hegemier S, Welty SE: Early clinical markers for the development of bronchopulmonary dysplasia: Soluble E-Selectin and ICAM-1. Pediatrics 102:927-932, 1998.

Rastogi A, Akintorin SM, Bez ML, et al: A controlled trial of dexamethasone to prevent bronchopulmonary dysplasia in surfactant-treated infants. Pediatrics 98:204-210, 1996.

Romagnoli C, Zecca E, Tortorolo L, et al: A scoring system to predict the evolution of respiratory distress syndrome into chronic lung disease in preterm infants. Intensive Care Med 24:476-480, 1998.

Rush MG, Engelhardt B, Parker RA, Hazinski TA: Double-blind, placebo-controlled trial of alternate-day furosemide therapy in infants with chronic bronchopulmonary dysplasia. J Pediatr 117:112-118, 1990.

Sanders RJ, Cox C, Phelps DL, Sinkin RA: Two doses of early intravenous dexamethasone for the prevention of bronchopulmonary dysplasia in babies with respiratory distress syndrome. Pediatr Res 36:122-128, 1994.

Saugstad OD: Role of xanthine oxidase and its inhibitor in hypoxia: Reoxygenation injury. Pediatrics 98:103-107, 1996.

Saugstad OD: Mechanisms of tissue injury by oxygen radicals: Implications for neonatal disease. Acta Paediatr 85:1-4, 1996.

Saugstad OD: Chronic lung disease: The role of oxidative stress. Biol Neonate 74(suppl 1):21-28, 1998.

Saugstad OD: Is oxygen more toxic than currently believed? Pediatrics 108:1203-1205, 2001.

Shenai JP, Mellen BG, Chytil F: Vitamin A status and postnatal dexamethasone treatment in BPD. Pediatrics 106:547-553, 2000.

Shinwell ES, Karplus M, Zmora E: Failure of early postnatal dexamethasone to prevent chronic lung disease in infants with respiratory distress syndrome. Arch Dis Child Fetal Neonatal Ed 74:F33-F37, 1996.

Shinwell ES, Karplus M, Reich D, et al: Early postnatal dexamethasone treatment and increased incidence of cerebral palsy. Arch Dis Child Fetal Neonatal Ed 83: F177-F181, 2000.

Sinkin RA, Dweck HS, Horgan MJ, et al: Early dexamethasone—attempting to prevent chronic lung disease. Pediatrics 105:542-548, 2000.

Stark AR, Carlo W, Tyson JE, et al for the NICHD Neonatal Research Network: Adverse effects of early dexamethasone treatment in extremely-low-birth-weight infants. N Engl J Med 344:95-101, 2001.

Stark AR: HFOV to prevent BPD: Are we there yet? [editorial]. N Engl J Med 347:682-684:2002.

Statement on the care of the child with chronic lung disease of infancy and childhood. American Thoracic Society documents. Am J Respir Crit Care Med 168:356-396, 2003.

STOP-ROP (Supplemental Therapeutic Oxygen for Prethreshold Retinopathy of Prematurity): A randomized controlled trial. Pediatrics 105:295-310, 2000.

Tammela OKT. Appropriate fluid regimens to prevent bronchopulmonary dysplasia. Eur J Pediatr 154(Suppl 3):S15-S18, 1995.

Tanswell AK, Jankov RP: Bronchopulmonary dysplasia: One disease or two? [editorial]. Am J Respir Crit Care Med 167:1-6, 2003.

Tapia JL, Ramirez R, Cifuentes J, et al: The effect of early dexamethasone administration on bronchopulmonary dysplasia in preterm infants with respiratory distress syndrome. J Pediatr 132:48-52, 1998.

Tyson JE, Wright LL, Oh W, et al: Vitamin A supplementation for extremely low birth weight infants: NICHD Network. N Engl J Med 340:1962-1968, 1999.

Van Marter LJ, Allred EN, Pegano M, et al: Do clinical markers of barotrauma and oxygen toxicity explain interhospital variation in rates of CLD? Pediatrics 105:1194-1201, 2000.

Van Marter LJ, Leviton A, Allred EN, et al: Hydration during the first days of life and the risk of bronchopulmonary dysplasia in low birth weight infants. J Pediatr 116:942-949, 1990a.

Van Marter LJ, Leviton A, Kuban KCK, et al: Maternal glucocorticoid therapy and reduced risk of bronchopulmonary dysplasia. Pediatrics 86:331-336, 1990b.

Vannucci RC, Brucklacher RM, Vannucci SJ: Effect of carbon dioxide on cerebral metabolism during hypoxia-ischemia in the immature rat. Pediatr Res 42:24-29, 1997.

Vannucci RC, Towfighi J, Heitjan DF, et al: Carbon dioxide protects the perinatal brain from hypoxic-ischemic damage: an experimental study in the immature rat. Pediatrics 95:868-874, 1995.

Vermont Oxford Network Steroid Study Group: Early postnatal dexamethasone therapy for the prevention of chronic lung disease. Pediatrics 108:741-748, 2001.

Watterberg KL, Demers LM, Scott SM, Murphy S: Chorioamnionitis and early lung inflammation in infants in whom bronchopulmonary dysplasia develops. Pediatrics 97:210-215, 1996.

Watterberg KL, Gerdes JS, Gifford KL, Lin H: Prophylaxis against early adrenal insufficiency to prevent chronic lung disease in premature infants. Pediatrics 104:1258-1263, 1999.

Watterberg KL, Scott SM: Evidence of early adrenal insufficiency in babies who develop bronchopulmonary dysplasia. Pediatrics 95:120-125, 1995.

Yeh TF, Lin YJ, Hsieh WS, et al: Early postnatal dexamethasone therapy for the prevention of chronic lung disease in preterm infants with respiratory distress syndrome: A multicenter clinical trial. Pediatrics 100:e3, 1997.

Yeh TF, Lin YJ, Hsieh WS, et al: Early postnatal dexamethasone therapy for the prevention of chronic lung disease in preterm infants with respiratory distress syndrome: A multicenter clinical trial. Pediatrics 100:E3, 1997. http://www.pediatrics.org/cgi/content/full/100/4/e3

Yeh TF, Torre JA, Rastogi A, et al: Early postnatal dexamethasone therapy in premature infants with severe respiratory distress syndrome: A double-blind, controlled study. J Pediatr 117:273-282, 1990.

Yoon BH, Romero R, Kim KS, et al: A systemic fetal inflammatory response and the development of bronchopulmonary dysplasia. Am J Obstet Gynecol 181:773-779, 1999.

Zachman RD: Retinol (vitamin A) and the neonate: Special problems of the human premature infant. Am J Clin Nutr 50:413-424, 1989.

CHAPTER

# 50

# Anomalies of the Airways, Mediastinum, and Lung Parenchyma

Thomas N. Hansen and Anthony Corbet

## ANOMALIES OF THE AIRWAYS

### Nasal Obstructive Disorders

Because newborns are preferential nasal breathers for the first 2 to 3 weeks of life, nasal obstruction may be associated with chest retractions and severe cyanosis, particularly during feedings, with airway obstruction relieved only when the mouth is open to cry. Respiratory distress due to nasal obstruction may manifest as a serious, life-threatening event shortly after birth.

#### Congenital Nasal Stenosis

With birth trauma, the nasal septum may become buckled or, less commonly, dislocated. Most cases respond to decongestant and steroid nasal drops, but dislocations require surgical manipulation (Presscott, 1995).

Nasal congestion may be associated with congenital syphilis, viral infection, maternal reserpine ingestion, and maternal fluphenazine ingestion.

Nasal pyriform aperture stenosis is characterized by excessive bone formation in the nasal processes of the maxillary bone; manifestations include severe obstruction and difficulty in passing a catheter. Because the newborn is a preferential nasal breather, an oral airway may be necessary to relieve the breathing difficulty. The obstruction is best demonstrated by computed tomography (CT) scan (Truong and Oudjhane, 1994). In most cases, the problem is resolved with nasal drops, but in more severe cases, surgery to remove excessive bone and nasal stenting are required. The condition may be associated with a solitary maxillary central incisor tooth; in other cases there may be more serious problems, including midline defects such as pituitary hypoplasia with endocrine insufficiency (Beregszaszi et al, 1996), diabetes insipidus (Godil et al, 2000), other manifestations of holoprosencephaly, and craniosynostosis (Van den Abbeele et al, 2001).

Nasal hypoplasia has been associated with warfarin embryopathy. In some newborns a nasolacrimal duct cyst may cause nasal obstruction.

#### Congenital Choanal Atresia

##### Epidemiology

Congenital choanal atresia is caused by persistence of the bucconasal membrane, occurs in 1 per 10,000 births, and has a significant female preponderance. About half the cases are bilateral; these malformations necessarily constitute an immediate neonatal emergency at birth. Associated anomalies such as Treacher Collins syndrome are present in 50% of the cases (Hall, 1979). The most common collection of anomalies is called the *CHARGE association*, consisting of some combination of *c*olobomas of the eyes, *h*eart defects, *a*tresia of the choanae, *r*etardation of brain and body development, *g*enital hypoplasia, and *e*ar anomalies associated with deafness (Pagon et al, 1981).

##### Diagnosis

Because the newborn is a preferential nasal breather, there may be serious difficulties soon after birth. A catheter cannot be passed through the nose, and nasal instillation of radiopaque dye demonstrates obstruction. CT scan is the method of choice for making a definitive diagnosis (Crockett et al, 1987). Sometimes choanal stenosis rather than atresia may be present.

##### Treatment

Emergency prophylaxis consists of an oral anesthesia airway or even endotracheal intubation. Although 90% of cases involve bone rather than membrane, in some infants the bone is soft and easily penetrated. Surgery can be performed within a few days of birth. Correction can be accomplished using the transnasal approach with either Hegar dilators (Stahl and Jurkiewicz, 1985), or a carbon dioxide surgical laser (Healy et al, 1978). After the appropriate airway is created, polyvinyl tubes are sutured in place to prevent subsequent closure. The tubes are lavaged with saline and suctioned frequently, and after 6 weeks, they can be removed. The transnasal procedure with modern endoscopic biting and drilling instruments is often definitive (Josephson et al, 1998), or it can be followed by a transpalatal operation when the infant is much larger. If CT scan demonstrates a very thick bone component, transpalatal surgery during the newborn period is sometimes considered the best method of correction.

### Pharyngeal Deformities

#### Pierre Robin Syndrome

Pierre Robin syndrome has an incidence of 1 per 2000 births. The major feature is micrognathia with posterior displacement of the tongue into the pharynx, but 60% of the patients also have a cleft palate. Hereditary transmission may be through a dominant gene, with variable expressivity. Because the pharyngeal airway is narrowed by the tongue, obstructive respiratory distress and cyanosis are common during the newborn period; these episodes may progress to dangerous spells of apnea (Cozzi and Pierro, 1985). Obstruction is common when the infant is in the supine position, during feeding, and in active sleep, when pharyngeal muscle tone is absent. Excessive air swallowing, followed by gastric distention, vomiting, and tracheal aspiration, are frequent problems. The pharyngeal obstruction is maintained by the generation of large negative pressures in the lower pharynx during inspiration and swallowing (Fletcher et al, 1969). Chronic obstruction leads to carbon dioxide retention, failure to thrive, and development of pulmonary hypertension with right ventricular failure (Johnson and Todd, 1980).

In an emergency, tracheal intubation should be performed. For a less invasive procedure, it is now customary to pass a 3.5-mm tube through the nose and into the hypopharynx (Heaf et al, 1982; Stern et al, 1972). This prevents the generation of negative pressure and greatly relieves the respiratory difficulty. The nasopharyngeal tube may be left in place for weeks or even months with adequate lavage and suctioning. The infant should be placed in the prone position to prevent the tongue from falling backward. If a nasopharyngeal tube does not adequately relieve the obstruction, tracheostomy is indicated to prevent progression to cor pulmonale. Nutrition can be maintained with a hypercaloric formula fed by nasogastric tube or gastrostomy. With the passage of time, the problem becomes less threatening, especially after a few months, when the infant gains better control of the tongue (Mallory and Paradise, 1979). Oral feedings can be introduced, usually with a long lamb's nipple to help hold the tongue forward. With adequate nutrition and growth of the mandible, the problem usually resolves by 6 to 12 months of age.

### Glossoptosis-Apnea Syndrome

Pierre Robin syndrome is not the only condition characterized by the tongue obstructing the airway. Infants with Beckwith-Wiedemann syndrome may have considerable breathing and apnea difficulties with an enlarged tongue. Infants with a normal-sized tongue who also have conditions such as unilateral choanal atresia, choanal stenosis, or swelling of the nasal mucosa may generate large negative pressures in the pharynx; in the absence of adequate muscular control over the tongue, they may develop pharyngeal obstruction, with respiratory distress, cyanosis, and severe episodes of apnea (Cozzi and Pierro, 1985).

### Pharyngeal Incoordination

Pharyngeal incoordination causes choking and cyanosis with feedings and may be complicated by aspiration pneumonia (Avery and Fletcher, 1974). Affected infants have difficulties in swallowing their own secretions. The condition may be seen in infants with severe hypoxic-ischemic encephalopathy and pseudobulbar palsy, in those with Arnold-Chiari malformation, and in those with Möbius syndrome. Some improvement may be obtained with the use of atropinergic drugs, which decrease secretions. Although some infants may gradually improve, the long-term management includes tube feedings or even gastrostomy.

## Laryngeal Deformities

### Congenital Laryngeal Stridor (Laryngomalacia)

A relatively common condition, congenital laryngeal stridor is due to the prolapse of poorly supported supraglottic structures—the arytenoids, the aryepiglottic folds, and the epiglottis—into the airway during inspiration. Despite loud inspiratory stridor and significant chest retractions, usually from birth or the first month of life, the infant seldom has cyanosis, hypercarbia, notable feeding difficulty or growth failure, or an abnormal cry (Richardson and Cotton, 1984). Congenital stridor is worse in the supine position with the neck flexed and subsides in the prone position with the neck extended (Cotton and Richardson, 1981). Obstruction is worse during episodes of agitation and lessens when the infant is calmed. Radiographic demonstration of prolapse of the aryepiglottic folds supports the diagnosis; ultrafast cine CT scan is effective at demonstrating the abnormalities without disturbance to the airway structures (Galvin et al, 1994). Confirmation may be obtained at laryngoscopy (Friedman et al, 1990), but care must be taken not to fixate the supraglottic tissues with the instrument. Some practitioners prefer to pass a flexible fiberoptic bronchoscope through the nose (Berkowitz, 1998), which does not disturb the supraglottic tissues. In some cases, gastroesophageal reflux or episodes of obstructive apnea may be associated with this condition (Belmont and Grundfast, 1984). About 18% of infants with a congenital lesion of the airway have a second lesion of some kind. Thus, the evaluation of stridor must include the examination of the entire upper airway and upper digestive tract (Friedman et al, 1984). The treatment is conservative and consists of placing the infant in the prone position, tracheostomy rarely being required; the condition spontaneously improves over about 18 months (Smith and Catlin, 1984). A very few patients may have severe obstructive apneas, cor pulmonale, and failure to thrive. In these cases unilateral supraglottoplasty with a carbon dioxide laser has been effective (Kelly and Gray, 1995); if necessary, the other side may be operated on later.

### Vocal Cord Paralysis

Unilateral cord paralysis is usually left-sided; stridor and retractions are not marked, and the voice is weak and hoarse. The infant may cough and choke during feedings, as larygeal closure with swallowing is impaired. The condition is due to a lesion involving the recurrent laryngeal nerve, perhaps caused by excessive stretching of the neck during delivery. Another possible cause is trauma from ligation of a patent ductus arteriosus (Davis et al, 1988). Right-sided vocal cord paralysis has been reported as a complication of extracorporeal membrane oxygenation (ECMO) (Schumacher et al, 1989), presumably as a result of the surgical dissection for insertion of the catheters. Stridor may be less if the infant lies on the paralyzed side, when the affected cord can fall away from the midline (Cotton and Richardson, 1981). The condition often tends to improve over a period of several weeks or months.

Bilateral cord paralysis is a much more serious condition, accompanied by serious inspiratory stridor. Frequently, however, the cry is normal. The diagnosis may be suspected at laryngoscopy and then confirmed with flexible fiberoptic bronchoscopy in the neonatal intensive care unit (NICU), rigid bronchoscopy in the operating room, or ultrafast cine CT scan in the radiology department. Associated problems may include pharyngeal incoordination with swallowing difficulty and esophageal dysfunction, recurrent apnea episodes, and tracheal aspiration of mucous secretions and formula. Usually, severe central nervous system problems also are present, such as hypoxic-ischemic encephalopathy, cerebral hemorrhage, Arnold-Chiari malformation, hydrocephalus, or brainstem dysgenesis. The stridor may resolve slowly if brain swelling subsides after birth. Tracheostomy frequently is required (Smith and Catlin, 1984), and the prognosis usually is poor because of the underlying problems.

### Congenital Laryngeal Stenosis

The larynx may be partially obstructed by a web or cyst that causes inspiratory stridor from birth and a hoarse cry. The diagnosis of congenital laryngeal stenosis is made by laryngoscopy. Treatment consists of endoscopic lysis with microlaryngeal surgery or a carbon dioxide laser (Smith and Catlin, 1984). Usually, one application is sufficient to correct this difficulty, and the prognosis is excellent.

### Congenital Laryngeal Atresia

In laryngeal atresia, the larynx may be completely obstructed by a web, seen in the delivery room during attempts to intubate the cyanotic infant. An endotracheal tube sometimes can be forced beyond the obstruction into the trachea. Otherwise, a large-bore needle should be inserted percutaneously into the trachea to maintain marginal gas exchange while preparations for emergency tracheostomy are made. Most infants with laryngeal atresia have other lethal malformations (Smith and Catlin, 1984).

This diagnosis has been made on fetal ultrasound scan, which shows enlarged lungs with inverted hemidiaphragms and a dilated trachea (Hedrick et al, 1994). The mother may be investigated for ascites or hydrops fetalis due to impaired venous return to the heart. The amniotic fluid lecithin may be very low in such cases. Bui and colleagues (2000) managed one case by uterine incision, delivery of the head, fetal laryngoscopy to confirm the diagnosis, fetal tracheostomy, and then delivery of the infant. Alternatively, in the absence of other lethal malformations, the characteristic ultrasound diagnosis may permit preparations for emergency tracheostomy after delivery of the infant.

### Congenital Subglottic Stenosis

Congenital subglottic stenosis is secondary to malformation of the cricoid cartilage. In severe cases, stridor is present from birth, and respiratory distress is obvious. In milder cases, excessive *croup* in an older infant may indicate the presence of this malformation (Healy et al, 1988; McGill, 1984).

### Congenital Subglottic Hemangioma

Subglottic hemangioma, often occurring in association with cutaneous hemangioma, may cause inspiratory stridor and expiratory wheezing, which progress with slow enlargement of the tumor (Cotton and Richardson, 1981). The presence of a cutaneous hemangioma in the facial beard distribution is often associated with a subglottic hemangioma (Orlow et al, 1997). Although some practitioners have advocated high-dose corticosteroid therapy (Brown et al, 1972) and others have tried intralesional injections of steroids, in many cases intubation or tracheostomy is eventually required. Results with removal by carbon dioxide laser have been encouraging (Healy and McGill, 1984), enabling treatment without tracheostomy in many cases (Hughes et al, 1999).

### Acquired Subglottic Stenosis

Extubation after prolonged endotracheal intubation sometimes is followed by inspiratory stridor and expiratory wheezing, produced by subglottic edema and fibrosis. The risk is greatest in infants who have had tightly fitting endotracheal tubes, frequent intubations, and prolonged intubation and mechanical ventilation (Downing and Kilbride, 1995; Sherman et al, 1986). Couser and associates (1992) reported the results of a controlled trial in which three doses of dexamethasone were given, starting 4 hours before extubation, to premature infants at high risk for subglottic edema; the incidence of stridor in the treatment group was greatly reduced. The initial evaluation of these patients may be performed with a flexible bronchoscope after extubation in the NICU.

For management of this condition, adequate humidification of inspired gas, nebulization of racemic epinephrine, and systemic, nebulized, or topical dexamethasone have proved useful. It may be helpful to use nasal continuous positive airway pressure (CPAP) to dilate the upper airway until improvement is obtained with steroid medication. In cases with no response to these measures, reintubation with a smaller endotracheal tube for a short period, while growth occurs, may be helpful.

Difficult cases should be evaluated by rigid bronchoscopy and in some instances by ultrafast cine CT scan. In some infants, an anterior cricoid split procedure may be successful (Seid and Canty, 1985). In this operation, a vertical incision is made in the cricoid and the first two tracheal cartilages, after which the airway is stented open with a larger endotracheal tube, which prevents the cut ends of the cartilage from abutting. The tube is maintained in place for 7 to 14 days, with the help of heavy sedation, and then removed under cover of steroid treatment (Tavin et al, 1994). More severely affected infants may require tracheostomy, followed by a formal surgical procedure with rib grafts to reconstruct the subglottic space later in life (Rowe et al, 1991).

### Laryngotracheoesophageal Cleft (Congenital Laryngeal Cleft)

In laryngotracheoesophageal cleft, a longitudinal communication is present between the airway and the esophagus, stretching from the larynx into the upper trachea or sometimes as far as the carina. The condition is caused by failure of cephalic advancement of the tracheoesophageal septum. Affected infants have respiratory distress with inspiratory stridor and cyanosis, associated with tracheal aspiration of saliva and feedings. The chest radiograph may show evidence of aspiration pneumonia, and the cine esophagogram shows contrast material spilling into the trachea. The diagnosis can be established with direct laryngoscopy and bronchoscopy. Initially, the airway must be adequately secured with an endotracheal tube or tracheostomy (Richardson and Cotton, 1984). An esophagostomy can be fashioned to divert saliva from the trachea. These patients invariably have esophageal dysmotility and gastroesophageal reflux if fed with an orogastric tube; enteral feedings can be accomplished safely after gastric division and gastrostomy tube placement. Attempts at later operative repair through a lateral pharyngotomy with or without thoracotomy have been successful in a few infants (Burroughs and Leape, 1974; Cotton and Schreiber, 1981). Some practitioners prefer an anterior translaryngeal approach for laryngeal and esophageal repairs, with closure over an endotracheal tube (Evans et al, 1995).

## Tracheal Deformities and Other Tracheal Disorders

### Tracheal Agenesis Syndrome

In the rare condition of tracheal agenesis syndrome, the trachea is atretic just below the vocal cords, or it is absent all the way down to the carina (Altman et al, 1972). Clinical manifestations include severe distress, absence of vocal sounds, and severe cyanosis. Affected infants usually have a tracheoesophageal fistula as well as severe cardiac malformations, lung lobation defects, and sometimes renal and anal anomalies. Despite the presence of a larynx, intubation cannot be accomplished at delivery; however, if the tracheal tube is positioned in the esophagus and connected to a mechanical ventilator, reasonable gas exchange can be obtained through the tracheoesophageal fistula. When the tracheal atresia is high, a tracheostomy can be done. If survival seems possible, gastric division and a gastrostomy for feeding should be performed. Reconstructive surgery is not likely to be successful, however, and the prognosis is extremely poor, if not because of poor ventilation, then because of the underlying malformations.

### Congenital Tracheal Stenosis

In congenital tracheal stenosis, a segment of the trachea is narrowed, usually starting in the subglottic region. The affected segment may be short or long; occasionally, the entire trachea is hypoplastic, and the bronchi may be involved. The narrowing is caused by complete or nearly complete tracheal cartilage rings. The patient may have inspiratory stridor, expiratory wheezing, and often cyanotic episodes. Mild inflammation and small mucous plugs may cause life-threatening deterioration. In many cases, other congenital malformations are also present, such as vascular ring anomalies, congenital heart defects, tracheoesophageal fistula, especially the H type, and hemivertebrae (Benjamin et al, 1981); there also is an association with pulmonary agenesis (Voland et al, 1986). A series of cases without accompanying defects has been reported in premature infants, who presented with difficulties at tracheal intubation (Hauft et al, 1988).

Patients with this deformity usually can be intubated, but the endotracheal tube cannot be advanced and should not be forced; mechanical ventilation with generous levels of positive end-expiratory pressure (PEEP) may be helpful to stabilize the infant. Tracheostomy is not indicated and interferes with making the diagnosis (Nakayama et al, 1982). Sometimes the diagnosis can be made by chest radiographs, using air as the contrast medium, with inspiration and expiration films. Investigators have described a high-kilovoltage technique, the so-called lateral airways xeroradiogram (Benjamin, 1980). Fluoroscopy often is useful (Lobe et al, 1987). Either flexible fiberoptic bronchoscopy in the NICU or rigid bronchoscopy in the operating room is usually required. Because it is important to examine the lower limits of the stenosis, it may be necessary to proceed with tracheobronchography, but this may sometimes cause acute decompensation (Loeff et al, 1988). As an alternative, ultrafast cine CT scan has been developed as a useful diagnostic technique to define the lower limits of the stenosis (Galvin et al, 1994).

In most cases, the stenosis requires treatment of some kind in the operating room. Balloon dilation alone is not likely to be successful in the case of a complete tracheal cartilage ring, because cartilage cannot be stretched. For short-segment stenosis, the technique of balloon dilation with laser may be used; at rigid bronchoscopy the cartilage ring is split at the midline posterior aspect using the KTP laser, and the bronchoscope is advanced with the aid of serial balloon dilations (Otherson et al, 2000). For longer-segment stenosis Longaker and colleagues (1990) described segmental resection of the stenosis with end-to-end anastomosis, shortening the trachea, followed by serial balloon dilations through a rigid bronchoscope. Backer and colleagues (2000) described the successful use of free autografts of resected trachea for this type of tracheoplasty. However, for long-segment stenosis, a procedure called slide tracheoplasty is now commonly preferred (Lipshutz et al, 2000). The stenosis is transected in the middle; the upper segment is incised longitudinally along the anterior aspect; the lower segment is incised longitudinally at the posterior aspect; the incised segments are then slid over one another, shortening the trachea; and the edges are anastomosed.

The use of cardiopulmonary bypass has improved treatment, averting the need for complex anesthesiology techniques (Loeff et al, 1988). After midline sternotomy, tracheal resection, and tracheoplasty with shortening of the trachea, the patient may need fixation in a brace for at least 6 weeks to maintain neck flexion and prevent excessive stretching of the anastomosis (Nakayama et al, 1982).

For premature infants with congenital tracheal stenosis, patients who cannot undergo tracheal resection and tracheoplasty with cardiopulmonary bypass procedures, aggressive balloon dilations have been recommended, with splitting of the weaker posterior aspect of the tracheal rings (Messineo et al, 1992).

### Rupture of the Trachea

Tracheal rupture just below the cords is an uncommon lesion that may occur as a result of severe head traction with a difficult delivery; the infant presents with pneumomediastinum, pneumothorax, or subcutaneous emphysema, accompanied by other signs of birth trauma such as vocal cord or brachial or phrenic nerve palsy (Hogason et al, 1992). Tracheal intubation may be difficult because the trachea bends at the site of injury. At flexible fiberoptic bronchoscopy, the endotracheal tube can be positioned past the rupture and maintained in position using a total body brace for 10 to 14 days to ensure adequate healing. If tracheal stenosis occurs, this can later be resected with end-to-end anastomosis, making use of cardiopulmonary bypass if necessary.

### Acquired Tracheobronchial Stenosis

Lesions of the trachea and main bronchi are being increasingly recognized as acquired complications of prolonged intubation and mechanical ventilation of infants in the NICU. These lesions are thought to be inflammatory, related to movement of the endotracheal tube and suction catheter. To prevent these problems, the endotracheal tube should be adequately fixed in position, and it is recommended that in routine suctioning the catheter should not be pushed past the end of the endotracheal tube (Bailey et al, 1988). This lesion may be suspected in infants with recurrent lobar atelectasis, emphysema, or both, especially of the right lower lobe; with difficulties after extubation; or with a resistance noted during use of the suction catheter (Friedberg and Forte, 1987). Most of these stenoses are just above or below the carina. The usual time of diagnosis is at about 4 weeks of age.

The initial diagnostic approach may be with flexible fiberoptic bronchoscopy in the NICU (Cohn et al, 1988) or with rigid bronchoscopy in the operating room. These infants often are in poor condition; an alternative way to establish the length of the stenosis is by contrast tracheobronchography performed in the NICU. This procedure has been described by Betremieux and coworkers (1995). A fine catheter filled with water-soluble contrast material is positioned with its tip precisely at the end of the endotracheal tube; 0.2 mL of contrast material is injected rapidly, followed by 5 mL of air; then two plain films are taken with 30 seconds of bag tube ventilation in between; the contrast material is suctioned, and mechanical ventilation is resumed. In a significant number of infants, the findings suggest mucous plug obstruction, which responds to chest physical therapy, and further investigation can be avoided.

Mild inflammatory stenosis may respond to topical or inhaled steroids or racemic epinephrine, and systemic steroids may be used (Elkerbout et al, 1993). In some cases, granuloma tissue has been biopsy-excised through the rigid bronchoscope (Miller et al, 1987) or subjected to electroresection (Greenholz et al, 1987). In patients with a mature stenosis, balloon dilation may be undertaken with rigid bronchoscopy in the operating room; several operative sessions may be needed. The success rate is only 50%, however, and the mortality rate is as high as 33% (Betremieux et al, 1995). Alternatively, dilations may be accomplished with bougies through a rigid bronchoscope, which may allow a better "feel" for the operator (Albert, 1995). These infants are small and premature and have frequent complications, such as bronchopulmonary dysplasia and infection; a greatly feared risk is airway rupture by the dilation procedure, with pneumomediastinum or pneumothorax (Messineo et al, 1997). The use of alternative strategies, such as carbon dioxide laser ablation, operative stenting, and surgical resection with grafting, is limited by the small size and severe illness of these infants. If the stenosis is short, however, as is often the case, resection with end-to-end anastomosis can be accomplished with skilled anesthesiology techniques (Albert, 1995). As a last resort, cadaver tracheal transplantation or live donor heart-lung transplantation may be considered in larger and older infants who are candidates for cardiopulmonary bypass.

### Tracheobronchomalacia (Tracheomalacia)

This condition may be primary or associated with tracheoesophageal fistula, bronchopulmonary dysplasia, or extrinsic tracheal compression.

Rarely, development of tracheal cartilage support may be delayed, resulting in an excessively compliant trachea or tracheobronchomalacia, a condition characterized by expiratory wheezing and respiratory distress. Callahan (1998) has described infants with primary tracheomalacia and gastroesophageal reflux; they presented with cough, an unusual sign in the newborn, and with wheezing. In tracheomalacia the chest radiograph shows diffuse overinflation. The abnormalities of the trachea can be well demonstrated with ultrafast cine CT scan (Galvin et al, 1994; Kimura et al, 1990); in particular, a good idea of the peripheral extent of the lesion can be obtained. At bronchoscopy, the anterior and posterior walls of the trachea are approximated during expiration (Salzberg, 1983). The bronchoscope may support the walls of the trachea, so the respiratory distress may be alleviated by passage of the bronchoscope to the carina, but this may disguise the extent of the abnormalities.

Many affected infants with tracheomalacia improve by 6 to 12 months of age. Severe cases may benefit from tracheostomy and treatment with CPAP, which prevents the tracheal collapse; prolonged treatment for 1 to 2 years may be required (Wiseman et al, 1985). Prolonged tracheostomy alone without positive pressure may be useful, with the tube acting as a stent for the compliant trachea (Cogbill et al, 1983), but this is less useful when the bronchi also are involved. In some cases, use of a special long tracheostomy tube has been successful, even with bronchial involvement (Zinman, 1995), and in some patients the positive pressure could be discontinued.

A strong association with tracheoesophageal fistula has been reported (Benjamin et al, 1976), but tracheomalacia does not occur in patients with esophageal atresia without a fistulous connection to the trachea (Rideout et al, 1991). A diffuse insufficiency of tracheal cartilage in these patients has been described, and many of them have ectopic, stenotic, or absent bronchi (Usui et al, 1996). Filler and associates (1992) have reported a large series of infants in which the flaccid trachea was compressed between the aorta anteriorly and the dilated esophagus posteriorly; most of these patients responded to aortopexy, fixation of the aorta to the sternum, which has the effect of supporting the attached trachea. An alternative is tracheopexy, in which the trachea is fixed directly to the sternum (Benjamin et al, 1976).

Tracheomalacia has been seen in respirator-dependent infants with bronchopulmonary dysplasia (Sotomayor et al, 1986), who present with severe cyanotic episodes (bronchopulmonary dysplasia spells). Many of these patients also have gastroesophageal reflux (Jacobs et al, 1994). Penn and colleagues (1988) have described the effect of prolonged mechanical ventilation on lamb tracheas and demonstrated increased worsening of collapse and increased flow resistance correlated with deformation of the trachea. The trachea of premature infants is very compliant and may be excessively stretched and injured during mechanical ventilation; because the tracheal compliance decreases with maturity, it is the very immature infant who is prone to tracheomalacia. Some premature infants have greatly enlarged tracheas or tracheomegaly after mechanical ventilation (Bhutani et al, 1986). Downing and Kilbride (1995) found that the factors associated with the development of tracheomalacia were immaturity, higher mean airway pressure, and prolonged mechanical ventilation. Infants with bronchopulmonary dysplasia and tracheomalacia may have significant dynamic compression of the trachea; this is caused by reactive lower airway disease with forceful expiration compressing the trachea; such patients may show some improvement from bronchodilator therapy. However, increased smooth muscle tone may help support the trachea during expiration, so bronchodilator therapy may sometimes make the situation worse (McCubbin et al, 1989).

Flexible bronchoscopy in the NICU may be performed after hyperoxygenation with the patient extubated briefly. If the patient must remain intubated, then the ventilator can be turned off for a short time while the ultra thin flexible bronchoscope is passed through the endotracheal tube with the patient breathing spontaneously (Wood, 1985). In the case of rigid bronchoscopy in the operating room, there may be some difficulty in making the diagnosis; collapse of the trachea may be abolished by the positive pressure of the ventilator, and dynamic compression of the trachea during forced expiration may be abolished by general anesthesia (Jacobs et al, 1994). Ultrafast cine CT scan also has proved invaluable to help establish this diagnosis if the infant can be transported to the radiology department.

The usual treatment is continued tracheal intubation with high levels of CPAP or PEEP with mechanical ventilation, and empirical attempts to wean the infant from these modalities as he or she grows older (Jacobs et al, 1994). Many of these patients must have a tracheostomy to avoid laryngeal complications from intubation. McCoy and colleagues (1992) described a group of infants with bronchopulmonary dysplasia and severe cyanotic spells during episodes of agitation. These investigators observed tracheal collapse at flexible bronchoscopy, initiated by agitation and relieved by soothing the patient or by sedation; thus, adequate sedation is an important part of management in patients with bronchopulmonary dysplasia spells. Many of the most severely affected patients respond well to aortopexy (McCoy et al, 1992). Bullard and associates (1997) have described a limited operation using an approach through the mediastinum for aortopexy while avoiding a full thoracotomy.

### Malignant Lobar Hyperexpansion in Bronchopulmonary Dysplasia

Azizkhan and colleagues (1992) have described a complication they called *acquired lobar hyperinflation* in infants with bronchopulmonary dysplasia; this condition was due to bronchomalacia with diffuse involvement but more severe involvement in the affected lung lobe. These patients were evaluated by ultra thin flexible videobronchoscopy, performed during mechanical ventilation. Selective intubation of the less involved lung provided only transient benefit. These patients can sometimes be managed medically, but many benefit immediately from surgical lobectomy; a few infants are operated on under emergency circumstances involving malignant hyperexpansion of the affected lobe and compression of surrounding lung. In general, the results of surgery may be good, although some patients eventually die from underlying bronchopulmonary dysplasia and its complications.

### Tracheal Compression by Vascular Rings

The trachea may be compressed by (1) a double aortic arch, (2) a right aortic arch, (3) a left-sided origin of the (right) innominate artery, (4) a right-sided origin of the left common carotid artery, or (5) an anomalous origin of the left pulmonary artery from the right pulmonary artery (Hendren and Kim, 1978). With a right aortic arch, the trachea is compressed by the main pulmonary trunk, aortic arch, and ligamentum arteriosus. The anomalous innominate or common carotid arteries form a tight crotch, which impinges on the anterior trachea. The anomalous left pulmonary artery returns to the left by passing between the esophagus and the trachea, compressing the trachea between the right and the left pulmonary arteries. Infants with tracheal compression have inspiratory stridor and expiratory wheezing. The onset of symptoms is usually later in the neonatal period. These infants often lie with the head and neck hyperextended to stretch the trachea and make it less compressible. If the esophagus is compressed, feeding is associated with regurgitation. The chest radiograph may show mild overinflation, a right-sided aorta, and, with appropriate technique, evidence of tracheal narrowing. A barium swallow examination may show indentation of the esophagus. Magnetic resonance imaging (MRI) has proved to be accurate in defining most vascular malformations compressing the airway (Simoneaux et al, 1995). Bronchoscopy should reveal a pulsatile mass at the carina. Echocardiography may not be as accurate as the MRI scan in this situation (Rimell et al, 1997). After surgical relief, the respiratory distress may persist for weeks or longer because of localized tracheal deformity, either stenosis or tracheomalacia, and in some cases a second operation may be required to repair the trachea further.

### Tracheal Compression by Extrinsic Masses

The trachea may be compressed by a bronchogenic cyst, an enteric duplication cyst, a thoracic neurogenic tumor, or a mediastinal teratoma (Benjamin, 1980). These may be demonstrated by anteroposterior and lateral chest films and especially well by CT scan. They also may compress the esophagus and be demonstrated with a barium swallow.

### Bronchoscopy and Bronchography

Albert (1995) has described the advantages and disadvantages of the methods used in the diagnostic approach to tracheobronchial obstructions. The instillation of nonionic contrast material for tracheobronchography does not seem to cause serious bronchospasm and, despite the iodine, does not seem to affect thyroid function seriously in premature infants. The lower trachea and main bronchi beyond the stenosis are well demonstrated. The technique does not differentiate a soft stenosis with granulation tissue from a hard stenosis composed of fibrous tissue, and because it is two-dimensional, it does not identify a complete tracheal ring in congenital stenosis. An advantage is that it can be performed in the NICU (Betremieux et al, 1995).

Flexible fiberoptic bronchoscopy also can be performed in the NICU, usually after a period of hyperoxygenation to prevent oxygen desaturation. The instrument may be passed for short intervals through the endotracheal tube during mechanical ventilation (Dab et al, 1993). The smallest readily available flexible bronchoscope is 2.2 mm in outside diameter. It does not have a suction channel; however, it does have the capacity for distal angulation, and it can be passed through a 3.0-mm-internal-diameter endotracheal tube for brief periods. Flexible bronchoscopy can differentiate soft from hard stenoses, in contrast with tracheobronchography, and the instrument may sometimes penetrate easily beyond the stenosis; the images are of lower quality than those with a rigid bronchoscope, however, and continued ventilation is not always easily accomplished. Two other ultra thin flexible bronchoscopes also are available (with outside diameters of 1.8 mm and 2.3 mm), but they do not have a suction channel (Wood, 1985), although they have the capacity for modest distal angulation. These instruments can be passed through a small, 2.5-mm-internal-diameter endotracheal tube during mechanical ventilation to evaluate the lower trachea and the main bronchi in very small infants; they can be advanced and withdrawn repeatedly to assist in the maintenance of adequate ventilation. They may be most useful to evaluate obstruction from granulation tissue or tracheobronchomalacia in infants with bronchopulmonary dysplasia. A 2.7-mm-outside-diameter flexible bronchoscope with capacity for better distal angulation also is available (Wood, 1985); this scope can be passed through a 3.5-mm-internal-diameter endotracheal tube to examine the lower trachea, main bronchi, and segmental bronchi in larger infants, but there is no suction channel. The standard pediatric flexible bronchoscope is 3.5 mm in outside diameter, and it has a 1.2-mm suction channel for removal of mucous plugs. All flexible bronchoscopes can be used with reasonable-quality video recording, so that examinations can be reviewed later (Wood, 1985).

The rigid bronchoscope with a glass rod telescope requires transfer of the patient to the operating room, extubation, and general anesthesia with continued ventilation through the bronchoscope. It gives better images, anesthesia and ventilation are easily maintained through the bronchoscope, suction is available, biopsies can be performed, solutions can be injected, and it can be used for balloon or bougie dilation procedures. The smallest available rigid bronchoscope is 2.5 mm in outside diameter.

## DISORDERS OF THE MEDIASTINUM

In the posterior mediastinal space, thoracic neuroblastomas and neurenteric duplication cysts are most commonly encountered in the newborn. Bronchogenic cysts occur in the middle mediastinal space. An enlarged thymus and a mediastinal teratoma are the masses most often seen in the anterior mediastinum.

### Thymus

The thymus occupies the upper anterior mediastinum, and it is more prominent in the newborn period than at any other time of life. It may be so large as to reach the diaphragm or obscure both cardiac borders on radiographs. The normal thymus can be distinguished from an abnormal mass by the absence of tracheal deviation or compression. The thymus changes in position with respiration and is less prominent with deep inspiration. It also involutes with stress as well as with corticosteroid therapy. Absence of the thymic shadow in an infant should alert the clinician to the possibility of severe combined immune deficiency syndrome (SCIDS) or DiGeorge syndrome with hypocalcemia and cardiac anomalies.

The cardiothymic-to-thoracic ratio provides an index of thymic size. The shadow of the enlarged thymus is the most common radiopaque mass visualized in the anterior mediastinum of the newborn. The enlarged thymus causes little if any trouble in the neonatal period.

Fletcher and associates (1979), as well as Gewolb and colleagues (1979), noted that a large thymus is present on the first day of life in infants at risk for hyaline membrane disease, presumably because of less-than-normal levels of glucocorticoids before birth.

### Congenital Mediastinal Teratoma

Mediastinal teratomas rarely cause symptoms in the newborn infant. These teratomas are invariably not malignant, and surgical resection is sufficient treatment. When an anterior mediastinal mass is associated with respiratory distress in the newborn, the strong likelihood is that the lesion is a mediastinal teratoma. Mogilner and colleagues (1992) described a newborn with severe respiratory distress and tracheal compression who underwent emergency thoracotomy and mediastinal teratoma resection. Another infant had emergency resection for respiratory distress but died with poor cardiac function (Thambi Dorai et al, 1998); as in that case, the tumor may be large enough to cause underdevelopment of the heart with severe circulatory insufficiency. In other cases, the tumor has caused mild lung hypoplasia.

## Congenital Bronchogenic Cysts

In the newborn, bronchogenic cysts are encountered infrequently; most do not come to the attention of the practitioner until later in infancy or childhood. Bronchogenic cysts seldom attain a large size. They contain clear fluid, they are lined with columnar or cuboidal epithelium, and their walls generally contain smooth muscle and cartilage, the latter indicating their bronchial origin. These cysts lie near the carina in the middle mediastinal space. They produce lung overdistention or atelectasis, depending on whether airway obstruction is complete or partial, and this is accompanied by respiratory distress in the newborn infant. Opsahl and Berman (1962) reported a case that showed overinflation on the left followed by clearing and then similar overinflation on the right. Radiographic examination often shows a mass lesion at or just above the carina, and displacing the lower trachea forward (Fig. 50–1). Ultrasonography may help localize the lesion more accurately. The barium swallow examination may reveal indentation of the esophagus, the cyst pushing it backward at the level of the carina (see Fig. 50–1). Bronchoscopy reveals compression of the trachea and sometimes of one major bronchus, usually from the posterior aspect. Sometimes the bronchogenic cyst may communicate with the airway and contain air. In the immediate newborn period, there may be retention of fetal lung fluid in the lung compromised by the bronchogenic cyst; the fluid may take days to be cleared. This phenomenon produces a characteristic appearance on the chest radiograph (Fig. 50–2). Treatment for bronchogenic cyst consists of early surgical excision, with uniformly good results.

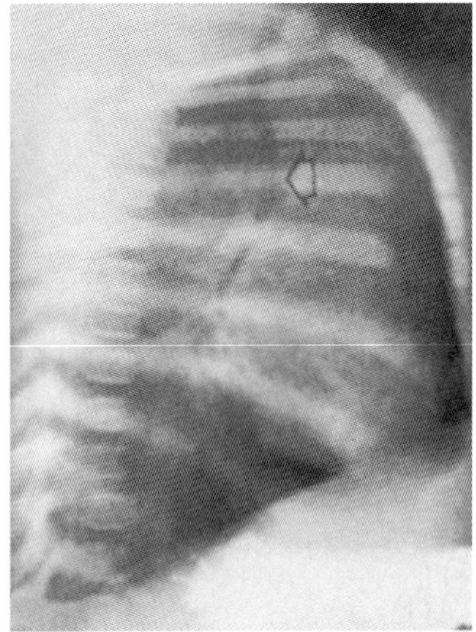


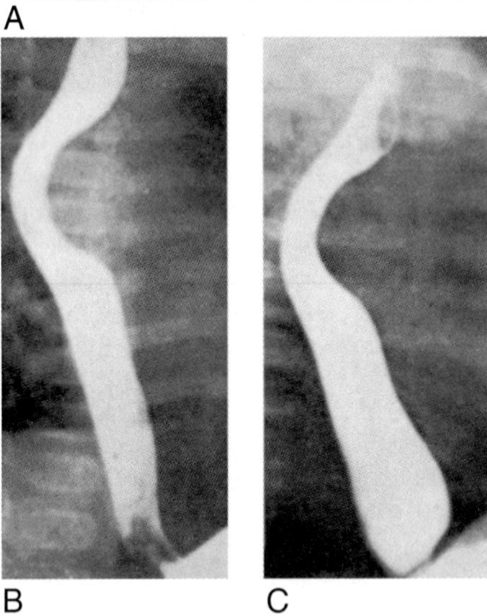


**FIGURE 50–1.** Bronchogenic cyst. **A,** The lateral film shows the trachea displaced anteriorly. **B,** The anteroposterior film shows the barium-filled esophagus displaced to the right. **C,** Another lateral film shows the barium-filled esophagus displaced posteriorly. *(From Hope JW, Koop CE: Differential diagnosis of mediastinal masses. Pediatr Clin North Am 3:379, 1959.)*

## Neurenteric Duplication Cysts

These mediastinal cysts may be derived from the esophagus, stomach, or small bowel, so they may also be called enterogenous cysts. Although they are not encountered frequently, they are far from uncommon in the newborn. They are duplicated segments of the foregut that have become partially or completely detached from the parent viscus. They lie in the posterior mediastinum but with increasing size may project far into one or the other hemithorax. Their walls are composed of a mucosal layer, characteristic of their site of origin, and one or more muscular layers. They contain secreted fluid that is the same as that of their parent viscus; the fluid in a gastrogenic cyst contains pepsin and hydrochloric acid in the same concentration as in gastric juice.

The foregut becomes duplicated in the course of embryonic development by failure of complete resorption of primitive occluding epithelium, resulting in the formation of a supernumerary wall and eventually a separate lumen and cyst. The high percentage of vertebral anomalies associated with neurenteric duplication cysts led Veeneklaas (1952) to suggest that the primary embryonic defect lies in abnormal persistence of the primitive foregut adherence to the notochord. When the foregut descends from its early position in the neck, this adhesion causes anomalies of the vertebral bodies derived from the notochord. This adhesion also breaks off the duplicated portion of the foregut and prevents its complete descent into the thorax and abdomen along with the mature foregut.

Clinical signs depend on the size and location of the duplication cyst. Because all of these cysts are posterior and lie close to the trachea, esophagus, and great vessels,

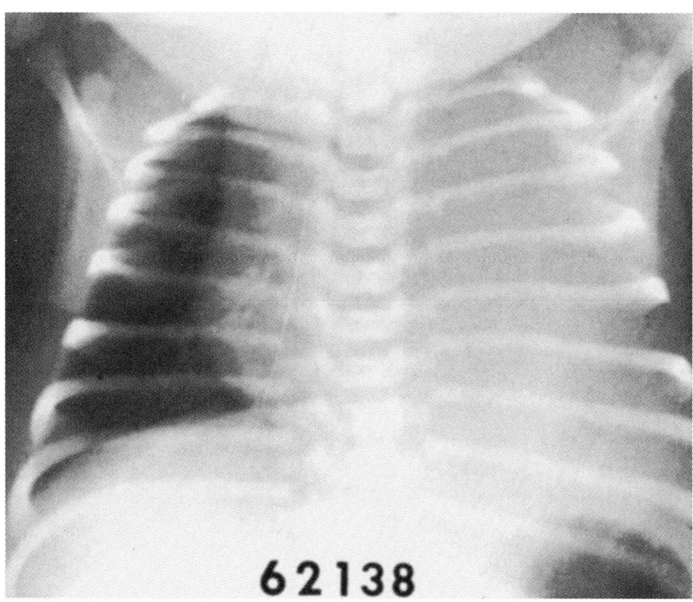


**FIGURE 50–2.** Bronchogenic cyst. The left lung shows delayed clearance of lung liquid, associated with bronchial obstruction by a bronchogenic cyst. *(From Griscom NT, Harris GBC, Wohl MEB, et al: Fluid filled lung due to airway obstruction in the newborn. Pediatrics 43:383, 1969.)*

they are seldom present without signs of abnormality. Cyanosis, tachypnea, and dyspnea often are present from birth. Swallowing difficulty and vomiting are less frequent. Recurrent lower respiratory tract infections are findings in a few older infants with such cysts. Frank hemorrhage from the lungs or stomach, or in the form of melena, is not at all uncommon. In most instances, hemorrhage indicates that the cyst is of gastrogenic origin, with peptic acid erosion into the trachea or esophagus. Technetium scans are useful for delineating cysts lined with gastric mucosa. Radiographs of the chest show abnormal densities that are often difficult to distinguish from unusual cardiac contours. The barium swallow examination commonly shows displacement of the esophagus, usually forward because the mass is in the posterior mediastinum. The cyst may partially or totally compress the bronchus, with consequent lung overdistention or atelectasis. Sometimes the symptoms are intermittent as the cyst enlarges or empties. Bronchoscopy may show compression of the trachea or bronchus from without, usually from the posterior aspect. Superina and colleagues (1984) reviewed 25 years of experience with neurenteric duplication cysts; they noted that a spinal component may accompany the mediastinal cyst in as much as 20% of the children. They recommended careful radiographic evaluation of the spinal canal with CT scan and then excision of the intraspinal cyst, if possible, before the onset of neurologic signs in later childhood. The MRI scan may give improved delineation of intraspinal cysts.

Operation is indicated as soon as the diagnosis of mediastinal mass is made. It is neither necessary nor wise to delay exploration until a specific diagnosis has been made.

## Congenital Thoracic Neuroblastoma

Neuroblastoma, the most common solid tumor in the mediastinum of infants, arises from sympathetic neural tissue along the vertebral column and is therefore located in the posterior mediastinum. It may extend into both lungs, causing respiratory distress, and it may extend into the spinal canal, later causing neurologic signs. The chest mass may be obvious on routine radiographs obtained for unrelated reasons in the newborn (Fig. 50–3), or on chest radiographs taken to evaluate significant respiratory distress (Li et al, 2001). In older infants the diagnosis may follow chest radiography for lower respiratory tract infection, or radiographs may be taken to investigate dyspnea with physical signs of a solid intrathoracic mass. In some cases the tumor mass shows calcification, well visualized with the CT scan. A thoracic neuroblastoma may sometimes be found on fetal ultrasound examination (Moppett et al, 1999).

Differentiation from other posterior mediastinal masses may be impossible before exploration; neuroblastoma is not likely to be so sharply demarcated as a neurenteric duplication cyst. Invasion of neighboring lung parenchyma strongly supports a diagnosis of neuroblastoma. The MRI scan is superior to the CT scan for discerning spread to lymph nodes, spinal canal, and chest wall (Slovis et al, 1997), and also for discerning liver metastases. Elevations of urinary vanillylmandelic acid and homovanillylic acid may be present, but this finding is less common in the newborn, and its absence does not rule out neuroblastoma. If the patient has systemic hypertension, plasma levels of epinephrine, norepinephrine, and dopamine may be elevated, but this has not been reported in a thoracic neuroblastoma. Also, results of assays for various clinical biologic markers may be positive; for example, serum ferritin and serum lactate dehydrogenase may be elevated, but this is not usual in the newborn. A bone marrow aspirate should be obtained for cytologic evaluation, and a nuclear bone scan should be performed to exclude the possible remote spread of metastases. A number of cytogenetic biologic markers may be detected in the excised tumor tissue (e.g., cellular DNA ditetraploidy, increased N-*myc* oncogene copy number); these usually indicate malignancy in older children

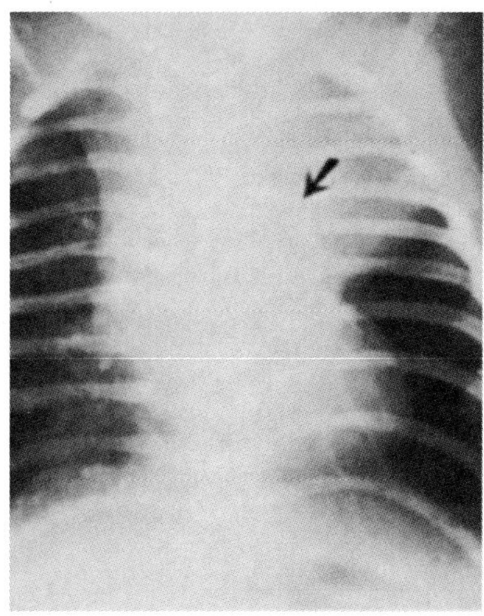
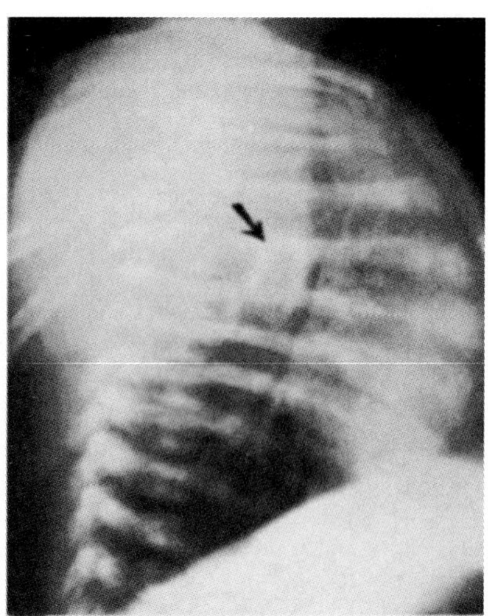

A B

**FIGURE 50–3.** Congenital thoracic neuroblastoma. The mass is in the left upper hemithorax (**A**) and in the posterior mediastinum (**B**). *(From Hope JW, Koop CE: Differential diagnosis of mediastinal masses. Pediatr Clin North Am 6:379, 1959.)*

(Ladenstein et al, 2001), but again, they are commonly negative in the newborn.

Surgical exploration is indicated for any intrathoracic mass. If the tumor proves to be a neuroblastoma, as much of it should be excised as is feasible. The tumor should be staged by histologic examination according to the system of Evans and colleagues (1971), and subsequent therapy should be dictated by the stage. In general, chemotherapy is not indicated unless distant metastases are present.

The outlook for neuroblastomas in extra-adrenal locations is better than that for their adrenal counterparts (Young et al, 1970). The outlook for neuroblastomas manifesting in the first year of life also is good. Many of these tumors are cystic in nature, and the histologic examination suggests that the neuroblasts are arranged in clumps rather than in sheets; this "neuroblastoma in situ" feature carries a high likelihood of spontaneous regression and therefore a good prognosis. Most neuroblastomas in the newborn are Evans stage A, with a good outlook. So-called stage D (S) also is quite common (Moppett et al, 1999); although there are metastases to the liver, marrow, or skin, the prognosis is still good because metastases to the bone are rare. The clinical markers are seldom elevated, and results of assays for the cytogenetic markers are seldom positive, all of which indicate a reasonable outlook. If the lesion can be completely removed and no bone metastases are found, then most infants survive. Some authors have suggested that the chance of spontaneous regression is so high in the newborn that even surgery may not be necessary (Li et al, 2001; Morgan, 1995). However, intraspinal spread may occur, in which case the later clinical course is more troublesome, with paraparesis and neurogenic bladder (Moppett et al, 1999); most authors consider surgery to be advisable.

## MALFORMATIONS OF THE LUNG PARENCHYMA

### Congenital Pulmonary Cysts

Congenital lung cysts are not common; they may be single or multiple but are always confined to one lobe of the lung; and other organs are not affected by cystic changes. Congenital cysts are persistent. All cysts have a communication with the peripheral airways, and for this reason they are filled with air except at birth, when they may be filled with fluid for several hours after birth.

#### Diagnosis

Newborns who develop signs of cystic disease of the lungs usually manifest the effects of rapid expansion of the cysts. The most common presentation is with air trapping, tension cyst, pneumothorax, and severe respiratory distress that necessitates lobectomy (Gwinn et al, 1970). Tachypnea or respiratory distress may begin at birth or any time thereafter and progress rapidly or slowly; the infant's condition may become critical within hours or remain static for weeks or months. In a few cases, older infants may present with recurrent episodes of pneumonia; it may then be difficult to decide whether the cyst is congenital or acquired (Fig. 50–4).

#### Radiographic Findings

Large balloon cysts filled with air under tension are often mistaken for a tension pneumothorax. One hemithorax is overfilled, the diaphragm is flattened or even concave, and the mediastinum and heart are pushed to the contralateral side. Points that may distinguish balloon cysts from a pneumothorax are (1) a delicate linear pattern within the translucent area denoting the cyst's fine trabeculation, which is not present in the case of a pneumothorax; (2) the presence of compressed lung at the apex and at the costophrenic and cardiohepatic angles, often demarcated from the cyst by a curving line visible in one or another projection; and (3) the absence of all hilar shadows. In pneumothorax, the collapsed lung often is visible as a dense shadow projecting from the hilar region or upward from the diaphragm. It may be difficult to distinguish between congenital pulmonary cyst and congenital lobar emphysema; a chest CT scan often demonstrates the cystic nature of the former lesion (Kravitz, 1994).

#### Treatment

The absolute indication for immediate surgical treatment is increasing air tension within the cyst. Repeated aspirations of air by needle and syringe or constant suction through a catheter introduced into the cyst may be neces-

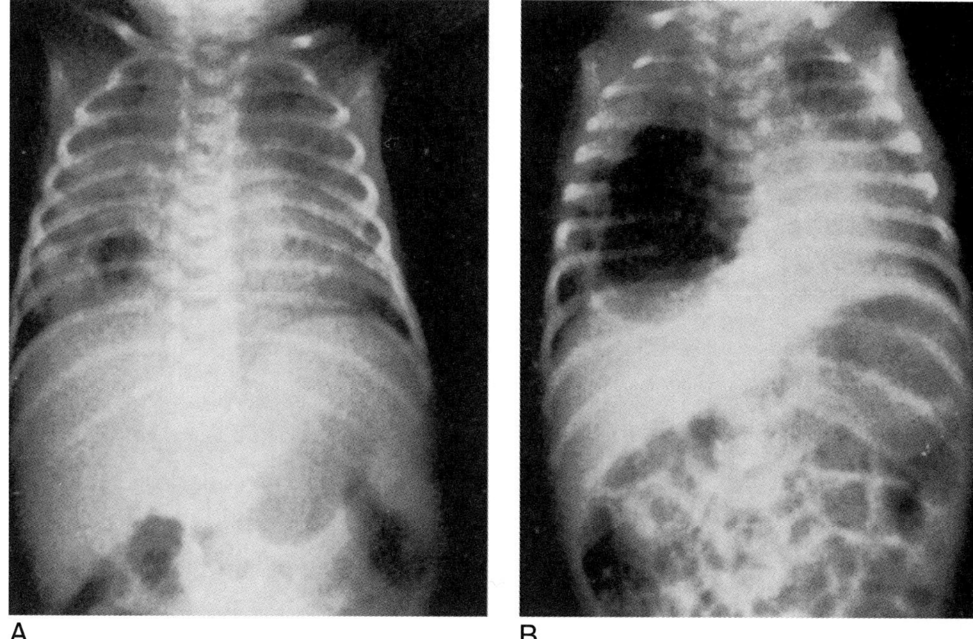


**FIGURE 50–4.** Congenital pulmonary cyst in right lower lung (**A**), with increase in size and displacement of the heart at age 30 days (**B**). *(From Swan H, Aragon GE: Surgical treatment of pulmonary cysts in infancy. Pediatrics 14:651, 1954.)*

sary in an emergency situation, but these maneuvers provide only temporary relief. Surgery should then consist of removal of as small a portion of the lung as possible, either a segment of a lobe or the entire lobe. If the older patient has recurrent bouts of infection, associated with a congenital cyst, lobectomy is again indicated.

### Prenatal Management

Large fluid-filled cysts, producing mass effects, polyhydramnios, and fetal hydrops, have been treated with thoracoamniotic catheters, with resolution of both the cyst and the hydrops condition (Revillon et al, 1993).

## Acquired Lung Cysts (Pneumatoceles)

Acquired lung cysts are not lung malformations, but they are much more common than congenital cysts. Most pulmonary cysts in the newborn are pneumatoceles acquired after an episode of pneumonia with necrosis of lung tissue, or they are acquired during the course of mechanical ventilation complicated by pulmonary interstitial emphysema or bronchopulmonary dysplasia. Unlike congenital cysts, acquired cysts tend to disappear with time, but like congenital cysts, they too may develop tension enlargement leading to compression of adjacent lung with severe embarrassment, they may rupture with the production of a pneumothorax, and they may ultimately require elective or emergency surgical lobectomy.

## Congenital Cystic Adenomatoid Malformation of the Lung

Congenital cystic adenomatoid malformation of the lung (CCAM) is due to an overgrowth of the terminal bronchioles with cysts of various sizes and no development of normal alveoli. This condition may affect any single lobe of the lung, causing a great increase in mass from multiple cystic proliferation (Merenstein, 1969), which may result in lung compression and significant pulmonary hypoplasia in adjacent lobes. The arterial blood supply and the venous drainage are connected with the pulmonary circulation. The lesion is a type of hamartoma with cystic structures, and on rare occasions there may be malignant change. Many of the affected infants are stillborn or premature or both. Associated malformations are present in about 20% of affected infants; there may be renal agenesis, jejunal atresia, diaphragmatic hernia, hydrocephalus, and skeletal anomalies. In the case of congenital heart disease, the lesion is frequently truncus arteriosus or tetralogy of Fallot (Morin et al, 1994). Due to its great mass, this malformation displaces the mediastinum and impedes venous return to the heart, accounting for a 50% incidence of hydrops fetalis. Another complication is polyhydramnios, which may be due to esophageal compression with impaired fetal swallowing (Revillon et al, 1993). In addition, polyhydramnios may occur because the cysts communicate with the airways and secrete fluid actively. After birth, because they are connected to the airways, the multiple cysts fill with air, producing further compression of the adjacent lung. If born alive, these infants have an early onset of respiratory distress, and the diagnosis is made by chest radiography (Fig. 50–5). This condition may be confused with congenital diaphragmatic hernia, but in cystic adenomatoid malformation, the abdominal gas pattern is normal, and a feeding catheter follows the normal path below the diaphragm.

### Natural Course

There are two major pathologic types of cystic adenomatoid malformation. In the macrocystic type, the cysts are

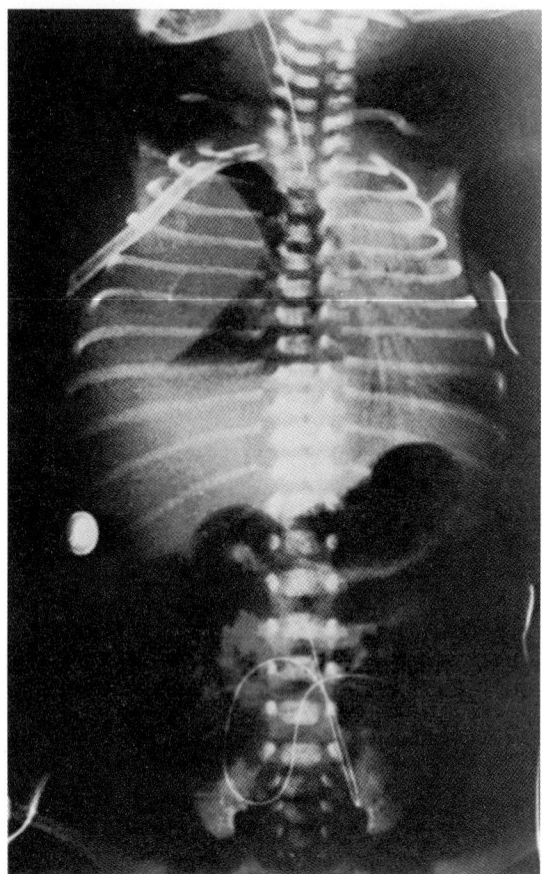

**FIGURE 50–5.** Cystic adenomatoid malformation of the lung with chest tube on the right side.

more than 5 mm in diameter and are visible and echolucent on fetal ultrasonography, and the prognosis is better. In the microcystic type, the cysts are less than 5 mm in diameter, the mass has a solid appearance on fetal ultrasound examination, and the prognosis is worse; a poor outcome is more commonly associated with large size, mediastinal shift, polyhydramnios, pulmonary hypoplasia, and hydrops fetalis. In a large series of these lesions diagnosed prenatally, Thorpe-Beeston and Nicolaides (1994) reported that 51% were on the left side, 35% were on the right, and 14% were bilateral. In this series, 59% of the cases were macrocystic and 41% were microcystic. In 33% of the cases, there was an elective termination of pregnancy; in 5%, there was intrauterine death; hydrops fetalis developed in 43%; the infant was liveborn in 62%; and in 26%, there was a neonatal death. It was considered that survival was better if the mass was macrocystic and if there was no hydrops or polyhydramnios. Spontaneous regression with near-normal lungs at birth has been described in several series; in one series, 13 out of 32 cases showed regression before birth (Revillon et al, 1993). Masses that disappear are usually the microcystic type, but this phenomenon does not occur in cases with hydrops fetalis (Morin et al, 1994). During the canalicular (acinar) phase of lung development it is thought that platelet growth factor is very active (Liechty et al, 1999); at term gestation, this growth factor activity was much less. These changes in growth factor activity may account for rapid proliferation in some masses and later regression in others. In addition to an increased proliferative index, there also may be decreased apoptosis in these lesions (Cass et al, 1998).

### Prenatal Diagnosis

In prenatal diagnosis with the ultrasound scan, there may be confusion with bronchopulmonary sequestration, in which case color flow Doppler studies should be used to distinguish the systemic blood supply of the bronchopulmonary sequestration (Morin et al, 1994). The MRI scan is very useful for distinguishing cystic adenomatoid malformation of the lung from diaphragmatic hernia (Hubbard et al, 1999). Chromosome analysis and fetal echocardiography should be performed, and the fetus should be followed for increasing mass size, mediastinal shift, and signs of hydrops fetalis.

### Prenatal Management

Those fetal patients at 32 weeks or more should have betamethasone prophylaxis against respiratory distress syndrome if necessary and then delivery as soon as possible. Those fetal patients at less than 32 weeks should be considered for fetal surgery if there are signs of hydrops fetalis. In the case of large cysts, it is possible to perform fetal thoracentesis, perhaps on a repeated basis, to drain the fluid from the mass, allowing the remaining lung to develop normally (Obwegeser et al, 1993). In another approach, a catheter may be placed from the cystic mass to the amniotic cavity, to provide a more prolonged decompression of the mass (Bernaschek et al, 1994). Adzick and colleagues (1993) reported three cases managed by placement of a thoracoamniotic shunt; two infants survived, but they had pulmonary hypoplasia and needed high-frequency oscillatory ventilation and ECMO. Dommergues and colleagues (1997) advocated thoracoamniotic shunting for cases with hydrops fetalis or severe polyhydramnios and expectant management for the other fetuses without hydrops.

As an alternative to shunting, surgeons have performed lobectomy in fetuses with large cystic adenomatoid malformations, particularly microcystic lesions, producing mass effects with mediastinal shift, lung hypoplasia, vena caval compression, and hydrops fetalis. Harrison and coworkers (1990) reported one fetus with early hydrops successfully operated on at 23 weeks of gestation. Adzick and colleagues (1993) reported a series of six cases with microcystic disease and hydrops; the first fetus died of premature delivery and pulmonary hypoplasia soon after operation, four fetuses survived with resolution of hydrops and good lung development, and the last was a fetal death occurring for unknown reasons in the postoperative phase. There are no established criteria for use of the radical lobectomy operation versus the more conservative thoracoamniotic shunt procedure.

Various authors have claimed that many cases improve spontaneously during the last trimester (Bagolan et al, 1999; Revillon et al, 1993; Roggin et al, 2000); however, in a large series the chance of this occurring was considered by the authors to be low (MacGillivray et al, 1993). Hydrops fetalis, the usual indication for surgery, is not known to resolve spontaneously and always signifies a poor outcome without surgery (Miller et al, 1996); however, if the lesion decreases in size with time, the outcome is usually good. Winters and colleagues (1997) reported a series of seven cases in which there was improvement or disappearance of the fetal lesion with time; on the postnatal radiograph, there were normal findings in one, subtle findings in four, and clearly abnormal findings in only two cases. Findings on the chest CT scan were abnormal in all seven infants, mostly air-filled cysts. It would appear that regression of these lesions is an important factor that must be considered in determinations about prenatal surgery, especially in the absence of hydrops fetalis.

#### Postnatal Management

Prenatal diagnosis may also allow plans to be made for resection of the tumor immediately after delivery (Adzick et al, 1985). If severe gas trapping is present, selective bronchial intubation and either needle or tube thoracostomy may give temporary relief, but the treatment of choice is lobectomy as soon as possible after delivery (Morin et al, 1994). In infants subjected to early lobectomy, pulmonary hypertension secondary to lung hypoplasia has been successfully managed with the use of ECMO (Njinimbam et al, 1999; Rescoria et al, 1990). Lobectomy is recommended for all lesions, even when there are no signs of illness.

## Bronchopulmonary Sequestration

More than 300 cases of bronchopulmonary sequestration (BPS) have been reported in the literature; these were reviewed by Carter in 1969 and by Landing in 1979. BPS has only rarely produced symptoms in newborn infants and usually has been detected on chest radiographs taken for other reasons; more commonly, a sequestered lobe manifests itself in children or young adults by repeated infections in a fluid-filled lung cyst. The lesion should be suspected in infants with cystic lesions, especially in the lower lobes. The malformation is slightly more common in males and is distinctly more likely on the left side; approximately two thirds of the cases involve the left lower lobe.

*Sequestration* is characterized by the presence of nonfunctioning lung tissue that does not communicate with the tracheobronchial tree and that derives its blood supply from the aorta. A single large anomalous vessel may be present, but sometimes multiple small anomalous arteries from above or below the diaphragm supply the sequestered lobe. The venous drainage may be pulmonary or systemic. In the latter case, drainage may be into the inferior vena cava, the azygous vein, or the portal vein; in the case of pulmonary venous return, there may be a large left-to-right shunt and possible congestive heart failure. In greater than 80% of the cases, a communication with the foregut can be demonstrated by contrast studies (Heithoff et al, 1976); the usual location is the lower esophagus or gastric fundus. The affected lung is highly abnormal, consisting of atelectatic areas interspersed with fluid-filled cysts. The incidence of associated malformations (e.g., diaphragmatic hernia, congenital heart disease, eventration of the diaphragm, duplication cysts, vertebral or rib anomalies) is increased.

Bronchopulmonary sequestration is thought to be caused by an accessory lung bud originating lower down in the primitive foregut. The lesion may be associated with abnormal expression of the homeobox gene product Hoxb-5, which is necessary for normal airway branching (Volpe et al, 2000). If the bud originates early, the normal and sequestered lungs have a common pleural covering, in which case the sequestration is considered to be intralobar; whereas if the supernumerary bud originates later, the sequestered lung has its own pleura and is considered to be extralobar; in some cases, an extralobar sequestration may be subdiaphragmatic in location. About 75% of cases are intralobar sequestrations, but in cases presenting in the newborn period, extralobar sequestrations are far more common. If the sequestered lobe is found to obtain its blood supply from the pulmonary system, rather than from the systemic system, it may be called an accessory lung lobe. Other malformations occur in 60% of extralobar sequestrations and in 10% of intralobar sequestrations.

#### Prenatal Diagnosis

The diagnosis of BPS may be made in the fetus, but in some cases solid chest masses have been known to resolve by the time of delivery (MacGillivray et al, 1993). A sequestration is a solid, highly echogenic chest mass, seen on the fetal ultrasound scan, and the systemic blood supply may be demonstrated by color-coded Doppler ultrasonography (Dolkart et al, 1992). The MRI scan is superior for confirming the diagnosis. In some cases, the lesions have been associated with mediastinal shift, polyhydramnios, and hydrops fetalis, in which case the prognosis is poor and stillbirth or early neonatal death is common. Unilateral or bilateral pleural effusions may be present; the pathomechanism is thought to be torsion of the lesion around a pedicle with obstruction of the venous or lymphatic drainage, leading to pleural effusion. According to Lopoo and colleagues (1999), the only reason for hydrops fetalis in BPS is the presence of a tension hydrothorax.

#### Postnatal Diagnosis

Most infants with BPS are not symptomatic in the neonatal period, but if the sequestration is sufficiently large, there may be persistent cyanosis and respiratory distress (Pearl, 1972), with or without lung hypoplasia. Some cases may manifest with a large unilateral hydrothorax, possibly secondary to lymphatic obstruction in the sequestration (Boyer et al, 1996; Hernanz-Schulman et al, 1991). Brus and colleagues (1993) described an infant with nonimmune hydrops fetalis, bilateral hydrothoraces, and severe pulmonary hypoplasia secondary to an extralobar pulmonary sequestration. Chan and associates (1996) reported a case in which a fetus with a pleural effusion was treated with a pleuroamniotic shunt; this infant did well after excision of the sequestration. Evans (1996) reported on three infants who did well after hydrops fetalis, mechanical ventilation, and surgical excision. Infants with a large left-to-right shunt through the sequestration may present with congestive heart failure in the newborn period, especially if born prematurely so that the pulmonary vascular resistance is low (Kolls et al, 1992; Spinella et al, 1998). Later in infancy, frequent bouts of pneumonia may occur. On the chest radiograph, the classic appearance consists of a triangular or oval-shaped basal lung mass on one side of the chest, usually the left side. Ultrasound examination confirms the presence of a thoracic mass (Schlesinger et al, 1994); the chest CT scan also is helpful (Boyer et al, 1996). The definitive diagnosis is made with angiography, which delineates the feeding vessels to the sequestration; the usual study is contrast aortography (Kravitz, 1994), but other less invasive techniques, such as magnetic resonance angiography (Doyle, 1992) and color-coded Doppler ultrasonography (Eisenberg et al, 1992; Smart and Hendry, 1991), have been used successfully. The barium swallow examination frequently demonstrates contrast material entering the sequestered lung from a communication originating in the foregut, either the esophagus or the gastric fundus.

#### Management

If a large hydrothorax is discovered before birth, this may be drained by insertion of a thoracoamniotic shunt to allow further lung development (Hernanz-Schulman et al, 1991). Depending on the degree of associated lung hypoplasia, the newborn infant may need no mechanical ventilation, only conventional ventilation, or high-frequency oscillatory ventilation and ECMO (Morin et al, 1994). Large pleural effusions present at birth should be treated with immediate tube thoracostomy drainage.

Further treatment consists of surgical resection of the involved lobe in all cases; resection is indicated even if there are no signs of respiratory distress, because repeated lung infections in the future are the rule. Resection of an extralobar lesion in the newborn infant causes no loss of functional lung tissue, unlike in the case of intralobar lesions in older infants who need a lobectomy. A preoperative angiographic study is helpful to alert the surgeon to the position of the anomalous vessels from the aorta and to the position of the venous drainage system. The arterial vessels may bleed postoperatively if not found and ligated, and the venous drainage may represent the sole venous drainage of the ipsilateral lung. There may be problems with management of pulmonary hypertension in the postoperative period.

If the lesion disappears before birth, the residual lesion should be sought with chest CT scans or chest MRI scans (Blau et al, 2002); if found, these lesions should be resected because of the risks for infection, hemorrhage, and malignant transformation. Although lung resection is recommended, resection of an intralobar sequestration may make the management of pulmonary hypoplasia more difficult; fortunately, most newborns have extralobar masses.

### Congenital Lobar Emphysema

Congenital lobar emphysema describes a pathologic condition characterized by respiratory distress caused by overinflation of one lobe of the lung, usually the left upper, right upper, or right middle lobe. There is no emphysematous destruction of lung tissue, as the name might imply. The onset may be at any time in the first 6 months of life, but 50% of cases manifest in the newborn period. The respiratory distress may be severe, but in many cases it is mild, without cyanosis in room air. The chest radiograph shows overdistention of one lobe, compression of the adjacent lung, herniation across the mediastinum, and diaphragmatic depression. The chest CT scan shows decreased vessels due to compression in the involved lung and increased vessels due to overperfusion on the opposite side. About 15% of the cases are associated with congenital heart disease, usually patent ductus arteriosus or ventricular septal defect, and other cases may be associated with rib anomalies and cystic renal lesions (Kravitz, 1994). Before this diagnosis is made, a mucous plug obstruction should be excluded by vigorous physical therapy or suction applied at rigid bronchoscopy in the operating room.

Some authors contend that most cases are caused by local bronchial cartilage deficiency, with airway collapse and gas trapping with exhalation (Campbell, 1969). Other causes have been suggested (e.g., redundant bronchial mucosal fold, stenosis of the bronchial wall, external compression by an anomalous pulmonary artery or a mediastinal mass). It is possible for a lobe to be rotated on its pedicle, with resultant obstruction (Hislop and Reid, 1971).

Sometimes the condition represents a polyalveolar lobe, in which, despite a normal number of airways, there is a fivefold increase in the number of alveoli in each acinus (Hislop and Reid, 1970). Infants with this condition tend to have prolonged retention of fetal lung liquid in the affected lobe after birth and to have early signs of respiratory distress on the first day of life (Cleveland and Weber, 1993).

Most cases can be evaluated with the chest radiograph, especially if films are taken on both inspiration and expiration. The chest CT scan is useful for defining a mediastinal mass or a vascular ring and in the evaluation of possible bronchial stenosis (Stigers et al, 1992). The ventilation-perfusion study is useful in assessing lung function, which may be surprisingly good in many cases. Some cases have been detected by increased echogenicity on the fetal ultrasound scan; continued observation suggests that the abnormalities tend to diminish with time; but postnatal assessment has confirmed the presence of congenital lobar emphysema (Olutoye et al, 2000).

In infants with congenital lobar emphysema and severe respiratory distress, the treatment is surgical lobectomy, the results of which have been excellent. In infants with mild tachypnea and no significant oxygen requirement, the treatment may be expectant (Shannon et al, 1977). The mild symptoms frequently subside by the age of 1 year. Stigers and coworkers (1992) managed five of their eight cases without surgery. Whether treated medically or surgically, at age 10 most such children have evidence of mild airway obstruction, suggesting a more generalized abnormality of the airways (McBride et al, 1980).

### Unilateral Pulmonary Agenesis

Unilateral pulmonary agenesis may be a unilateral lung agenesis without main bronchus development on one side, and therefore without a carina, or it may be a unilateral lung aplasia, with a carina and a rudimentary main bronchial pouch as evidence of arrested bronchial development. Left-sided lung agenesis is slightly more common and sometimes is associated with severe congenital heart disease, such as tetralogy of Fallot; however, cases have been described in asymptomatic adults. Right-sided lung agenesis may cause more problems from mediastinal shift, with obstruction of major vessels and airways, and is more frequently associated with congenital heart disease, such as obstructed anomalous pulmonary venous drainage (Finci et al, 1999), ventricular septal defect, and coarctation of the aorta. The contralateral lung may be enlarged and hypertrophied, it may be overdistended and overperfused with congestion, and it may herniate into the opposite hemithorax, usually through the anterior mediastinum. Thus, there may be no obvious evidence for asymmetry of the chest in the newborn, and asymmetry may develop only with further growth during later infancy. For this reason, breath sounds may be heard on the involved side, but not posteriorly.

Some patients with this condition may die in the delivery room. Others may have severe respiratory distress that does not respond to mechanical ventilation; the appearance may be that of total main bronchus obstruction from a mucous or meconium plug, which may lead to consideration for ECMO. Some patients may have only modest and transient respiratory distress at birth, or signs of illness may be absent in the newborn. The clinical presentation may be that of congenital heart disease, frequently with cyanosis. Signs of pulmonary hypertension may be present because the entire cardiac output must traverse only one lung; this may be the case especially if the ductus arteriosus closes early. In lung agenesis, the ipsilateral pulmonary artery is absent, so cyanosis cannot be attributed to perfusion of airless lung mesenchyme. There may be other anomalies, such as esophageal atresia and polycystic kidneys, and hemivertebrae are particularly common.

The chest radiograph shows homogeneous density in place of the lung in one hemithorax, the ribs may appear closer together on the involved side, and there is mediastinal shift with tracheal deviation. A chest CT scan may be necessary to confirm the absence of lung tissue on one side (Kravitz, 1994). Bronchoscopy shows the absence of the ipsilateral main bronchus, which may be confirmed by bronchography. The echocardiogram demonstrates the absence of the ipsilateral pulmonary artery, the contralateral pulmonary artery appears dilated, and there may be other signs associated with congenital heart disease. If there is confusion with dextrocardia, as in right lung agenesis, an electrocardiogram may be useful.

If affected infants survive beyond the neonatal period, recurrent pneumonia and reactive airways disease may develop, but the pathomechanism is not clear. One suggestion is that in the case of lung aplasia, the remnant bronchial pouch allows the accumulation of stagnant secretions and therefore predisposes to infection in the normal lung (Borja et al, 1970).

## Pulmonary Hypoplasia

Pulmonary hypoplasia is a pathologic condition in which the combined lung weight is less than 1.2% of body weight, the standardized autopsy lung volume is less than 60% of predicted lung volume, the lung DNA is less than 100 mg/kg of body weight, or the radial alveolar count is less than 4 (Langston and Thurlbeck, 1986). The incidence at autopsy is approximately 10% of newborns, and the overall incidence is thought to be approximately 2 per 1000 live births (Knox and Barson, 1986).

Infants with pulmonary hypoplasia present usually with respiratory distress and cyanosis in room air. On the chest radiograph, the lungs appear small, and they are clear unless another condition such as pneumonia is superimposed; the hemidiaphragms are elevated, and the thorax may appear bell-shaped. These infants have significant hypercarbia, which responds poorly to mechanical ventilation, and the risk of pneumothorax is high. They often have persistent pulmonary hypertension, as a result of a reduced vascular bed and secondary arterial muscle hypertrophy (Hislop et al, 1979). Conventional therapy may fail in these infants, who then become candidates for ECMO, in which case it will be necessary to make a clinical judgment concerning the permanent size of the lungs. In addition, the hypoplastic lung also may have an immature surfactant profile, so a significant number of infants also have respiratory distress syndrome (Nakamura et al, 1988; Wigglesworth et al, 1981), and require surfactant replacement therapy.

Normal lung growth depends on lung distention with stretch (Wigglesworth and Desai, 1982), which in turn depends on (1) lung expansion caused by lung liquid secretion and fetal breathing and (2) available space within the thorax. The fetal lung actively secretes lung liquid at a rate equivalent to about 10% of body weight per day (Kitterman, 1996). Escape of liquid from the lungs is resisted at the larynx. The resultant distending pressure maintains the fetal lung volume at levels very similar to those after birth. Experiments in which lung liquid is drained from the fetal lung showed that this causes severe lung hypoplasia (Alcorn et al, 1977). If fetal breathing is abolished by cervical spinal cord section above the phrenic nerve, the position of the diaphragm and therefore the lung volume are not changed; such experiments have shown the development of severe lung hypoplasia and indicate that fetal breathing also is necessary for lung development (Wigglesworth and Desai, 1979).

Conditions causing oligohydramnios and fetal thoracic compression are associated with pulmonary hypoplasia, due to increased loss of lung fluid into the amniotic cavity and reduced fetal lung volume. It is possible that in oligohydramnios the amniotic fluid pressure is low, so that when the larynx is opened periodically, excess lung fluid is expelled and fetal lung volume is reduced (Kitterman, 1984). It is also likely that increased anterior spinal flexion produced by oligohydramnios may elevate the fetal diaphragm, with resultant application of pressure to the lungs and consequent reduction in thoracic volume (Harding and Liggins, 1991). Clinical conditions associated with oligohydramnios include renal agenesis, renal dysplasia, obstructive uropathy (Thomas and Smith, 1974), and chronic amnion rupture (Thibeault et al, 1985).

Increased lung compression may be due to lesions within the thorax or outside the thorax; such problems include congenital diaphragmatic hernia, cystic lung disease, eventration of the diaphragm, ascites, and pleural effusion, all of which may cause reduced fetal lung volume and thus pulmonary hypoplasia. Patients with a giant omphalocele may have pulmonary hypoplasia because the lower chest cage is not adequately supported by abdominal contents and thoracic volume is reduced (Hershenson et al, 1985).

Effective fetal breathing may be impaired by brainstem malformations such as iniencephaly, by neuromuscular problems such as spinal muscular atrophy or congenital myotonic dystrophy, by skeletal chest cage insufficiency as in congenital thoracic dystrophy or short rib–polydactyly syndrome; these conditions would also result in reduced fetal lung volume and lung hypoplasia. In the fetal akinesia sequence there may be nemaline myopathy, multiple joint contractures, and pulmonary hypoplasia. Finally, in a significant number of infants, no cause for primary pulmonary hypoplasia can be found (Swischuk et al, 1979), although suppression of fetal breathing caused by maternal use of tobacco, barbiturates, or ethanol may be implicated (Collins et al, 1985; Inselman et al, 1985).

In many cases of lung hypoplasia, the number of bronchial generations is reduced, suggesting an insult occurring between 10 and 14 weeks of gestation during the glandular phase of lung development; this is a finding in diaphragmatic hernia or renal dysplasia. Although the total number of acini is reduced, along with the number of bronchi, the number of alveoli per acinus is relatively well preserved in these cases (Hislop et al, 1979). There may be a maturation arrest, especially in cases associated with oligohydramnios, with a wide blood-gas septal interface, immature epithelial cells, a lack of elastic tissue, and low surfactant phospholipid concentrations (Porter, 1999).

## Lung Hypoplasia Associated with Chronic Amnion Rupture

In chronic amnion rupture, Nimrod and colleagues (1984) concluded that serious lung hypoplasia was unlikely to occur if the membranes ruptured after 26 weeks of gestation, apparently because a sufficient number of acinar units with respiratory bronchioles and saccules may have developed by then. This is in agreement with the data of Moessinger and associates (1986), who found in a guinea pig model that hypoplasia was most likely if amnion rupture occurred in the canalicular (acinar) stage of lung development and was not significant if amnion rupture occurred in the saccular stage of lung development, with primitive alveoli (subsaccules) already present. McIntosh and Harrison (1994) found that the minimal duration of rupture for the development of lung hypoplasia was 2 weeks for survivors and 3 weeks for those who died. In addition, the median length of rupture for infants with compression deformities of the face and limbs was 28 days, and for those with pulmonary hypoplasia it was 31 days, indicating the close relationship of pulmonary hypoplasia with the fetal compression syndrome. In patients with membrane rupture before 25 weeks of gestation and with oligohydramnios lasting 14 days or more, the risk of death is more than 75% (Geary and Whitsett, 2002).

Although fetal breathing movements may disappear in oligohydramnios, thoracic compression and loss of lung liquid are the main causes of lung hypoplasia in chronic amnion rupture (Adzick et al, 1984). Blott and associates (1987), however, found that the presence of sustained fetal breathing movements may protect against the development of pulmonary hypoplasia.

In many cases of chronic amnion rupture, the onset is quite late, so the major effects are on elements that develop later, and the resultant lung hypoplasia is therefore less severe. The bronchial number is normal, the acinar number may be near normal, and only the number of alveoli per acinus is reduced, because the amnion rupture occurred during the saccular phase of lung development with primitive alveoli (subsaccules) already present.

In the Netherlands, Laudy and colleagues (2002) have assessed the obstetric prediction of lethal pulmonary hypoplasia before delivery; they were especially interested in cases in which the gestational age was less than 24 weeks, so that pregnancy termination might be an option for the mother. They found that amnion rupture before 20 weeks of gestation, associated with amniotic pockets less than 1 cm and presence of rupture for more than 8 weeks before delivery, was associated reliably with lethal lung hypoplasia, but this was not a common clinical finding. A reduced ratio of thoracic to abdominal circumference was helpful, as was a reduced Doppler flow velocity in the pulmonary artery, but neither of these alone or in combination could reliably predict lethal pulmonary hypoplasia.

The possibilities for treatment of lung hypoplasia are limited; the clinician can only manage the associated complications. A major objective of fetal surgery is the relief of fetal lung compression, such as that caused by diaphragmatic hernia, pleural effusion, lung cysts, and other problems. As these infants may have congenital pneumonia or respiratory distress syndrome, they usually are treated with antibiotics and surfactant replacement. They also may have persistent pulmonary hypertension and respond to inhaled nitric oxide therapy (Geary and Whitsett, 2002; Peliowski et al, 1995). Mechanical ventilation should be designed to avoid lung rupture and its complications. When all else fails, lobar lung transplantation for severe pulmonary hypoplasia may become possible in the future.

Kitterman (1993) has warned that many infants with severe respiratory distress syndrome, and born in clinical circumstances suggestive of pulmonary hypoplasia, in fact do not have any pulmonary hypoplasia and make a good recovery; he suggests that clinicians be skeptical of this diagnosis in infants who survive. McIntosh (1988) described three infants with prolonged amnion rupture, small lungs, and compression deformities who required high pressures with mechanical ventilation on the first day of life, but who markedly improved on the second day of life and recovered in room air.

## Pulmonary Hemangiomatosis

Pulmonary hemangiomatosis is a proliferation of small blood vessels that may be peribronchovascular, septal, or pleural in location. If the lesions also involve the airways, hemoptysis may occur.

### Natural History

Pulmonary hemangiomatosis may be a part of a disseminated hemangiomatosis that can involve the liver, gastrointestinal tract, central nervous system, and skin. Cutaneous lesions may be present at birth or develop within the first few weeks of life. In some instances, the hemangiomas may be confined to the lung and remain asymptomatic until childhood. Because the flow through the hemangiomas in the lung is right to left, venous admixture is significant, with associated clubbing of all digits. In some instances, clubbing may take place even in the absence of arterial desaturation. The major symptom is dyspnea, which is progressive. The most likely cause of death is bleeding or, in adults, pulmonary hypertension.

### Diagnosis

The diagnosis is suggested by appearance on the chest radiograph, which may resemble that of an interstitial infiltrate or thickened fissures. Pulmonary angiography and MRI are useful in diagnosis.

### Treatment

In at least one instance, a 12-year-old boy had a good response to treatment with interferon alfa-2a administered subcutaneously. He received daily interferon therapy for 14 months, during which his dyspnea remitted, his digital clubbing resolved, and results on pulmonary function tests were restored to normal. Abnormal vessels were still evident in the angiogram, but their density had been substantially reduced (White, 1990). This therapy seems to be less toxic than long-term corticosteroid and cyclophosphamide regimens, which have been used in the past.

### Prognosis

Experience with interferon is too recent to determine whether all visceral hemangiomas respond.

## Pulmonary Arteriovenous Malformations

A rare lesion, pulmonary arteriovenous fistula or angioma is characterized by persistent cyanosis in the newborn, but unless the fistula is large and compresses the surrounding lung, it does not cause respiratory distress (Hodgson et al, 1959). Lesions may be single or multiple and aneurysmal or microscopic in size. About 50% of the cases are associated with hereditary hemorrhagic telangiectasia (Rendu-Osler-Weber syndrome). The chest radiograph most commonly shows a small mass lesion, usually in the lower lobes; the electrocardiogram may suggest unusual left ventricular dominance. The diagnosis can be made at cardiac catheterization, in which a selective cine angiogram of the pulmonary artery shows the lesion in the lung (Mitchell and Austin, 1993). Alternatively, the diagnosis may be made with a radionuclide perfusion study or digital subtraction angiography. The best treatment is conservative surgical excision, with lobectomy or segmentectomy as necessary. For large lesions, embolotherapy may be useful. Multiple hemangiomas may respond to glucocorticoid therapy or newer inhibitors of angiogenesis. Mortality and morbidity rates in untreated cases are considerable (Dines et al, 1983). Most cases are diagnosed in adults; less than 10% are diagnosed in infancy.

## REFERENCES


Adzick NS, Harrison MR, Flake AW, et al: Fetal surgery for congenital cystic adenomatoid malformation of the lung. J Pediatr Surg 28:806, 1993.

Adzick NS, Harrison MR, Glick PC: Fetal cystic adenomatoid malformation: Prenatal diagnosis and natural history. J Pediatr Surg 20:483, 1985.

Adzick NS, Harrison MR, Glick PC, et al: Experimental pulmonary hypoplasia and oligohydramnios: Relative contributions of lung fluid and fetal breathing movements. J Pediatr Surg 19:658, 1984.

Albert D: Management of suspected tracheobronchial stenosis in ventilated neonates. Arch Dis Child 72:F1, 1995.

Alcorn D, Adamson TM, Lambert TF, et al: Morphological effects of chronic tracheal ligation and drainage in the fetal lamb lung. J Anat 123:649, 1977.

Altman RP, Randolph JG, Shearin RB: Tracheal agenesis: Recognition and management. J Pediatr Surg 7:112, 1972.

Avery ME, Fletcher BD: The Lung and Its Disorders in the Newborn Infant. Philadelphia, WB Saunders, 1974.

Azizkhan RG, Grimmer DL, Askin FB, et al: Acquired lobar emphysema (overinflation): Clinical and pathological evaluation of infants requiring lobectomy. J Pediatr Surg 27:1145, 1992.

Backer CL, Mavroudis C, Dunham ME, Holinger L: Intermediate term results of the free tracheal autograft for long segment congenital tracheal stenosis. J Pediatr Surg 35:813, 2000.

Bagolan P, Nahom A, Giorlandino C, et al: Cystic adenomatoid malformation of the lung. Clinical evolution and management. Eur J Pediatr 158:879, 1999.

Bailey C, Kattwinkel J, Teja K, Buckley T: Shallow versus deep endotracheal suctioning in young rabbits: Pathologic effects on the tracheobronchial wall. Pediatrics 82:746, 1988.

Belmont JR, Grundfast K: Congenital laryngeal stridor (laryngomalacia): Etiologic factors and associated disorders. Ann Otol Rhinol Laryngol 93:430, 1984.

Benjamin B: Endoscopy in congenital tracheal anomalies. J Pediatr Surg 15:164, 1980.

Benjamin B, Cohen D, Glasson M: Tracheomalacia in association with congenital tracheo-esophageal fistula. Surgery 79:504, 1976.

Benjamin B, Pitkin J, Cohen D: Congenital tracheal stenosis. Ann Otol Rhinol Laryngol 90:364, 1981.

Beregszaszi M, Leger J, Garel C, et al: Nasal pyriform aperture stenosis and absence of the anterior pituitary gland: Report of 2 cases. J Pediatr 128:858, 1996.

Berkowitz RG: Neonatal upper airway assessment by awake flexible laryngoscopy. Ann Otolaryngol 107:75, 1998.

Bernaschek G, Deutinger J, Hansmann M, et al: Feto-amniotic shunting: Report of the experience of four European centers. Prenat Diagn 14:821, 1994.

Betremieux P, Treguier C, Pladys P, et al: Tracheobronchography and balloon dilatation in acquired neonatal tracheal stenosis. Arch Dis Child 72:F3, 1995.

Bhutani VK, Ritchie WG, Shaffer TH: Acquired tracheomegaly in very preterm infants. Am J Dis Child 140:449, 1986.

Blau H, Barak A, Karmazyn B, et al: Postnatal management of resolving fetal lung lesions. Pediatrics 109:105, 2002.

Blott M, Greenough A, Nicolaides KH, et al: Fetal breathing movements as predictor of favorable pregnancy outcome after oligohydramnios due to membrane rupture in second trimester. Lancet 2:129, 1987.

Borja AR, Ransdell HT, Villa S: Congenital developmental arrest of the lung. Ann Thorac Surg 10:317, 1970.

Boyer J, Dozor A, Brudnicki A, et al: Extralobar pulmonary sequestration masquerading as a congenital pleural effusion. Pediatrics 97:115, 1996.

Brown SH, Neerhout RC, Fonkalsrud EW: Prednisone therapy in the management of large hemangiomas in infants and children. Surgery 71:168, 1972.

Brus F, Nikkels PGJ, Van Loon AJ, et al: Non-immune hydrops fetalis and bilateral pulmonary hypoplasia in a newborn infant with extralobar pulmonary sequestration. Acta Paediatr 82:416, 1993.

Bui TH, Grunewald C, Frenckner B, et al: Successful EXIT (ex utero intrapartum treatment) procedure in a fetus diagnosed prenatally with congenital high airway obstruction due to laryngeal atresia. Eur J Pediatr 10:328, 2000.

Bullard KM, Adzick NS, Harrison MR: A mediastinal window approach to aortopexy. J Pediatr Surg 32:680, 1997.

Burroughs N, Leape LL: Laryngotracheoesophageal cleft: Report of a case successfully treated and review of the literature. Pediatrics 53:516, 1974.

Callahan CW: Primary tracheomalacia and gastro-esophageal reflux in infants with cough. Clin Pediatr 37:725, 1998.

Campbell PE: Congenital lobar emphysema: Etiological studies. Aust Paediatr J 5:226, 1969.

Cass DL, Quinn TM, Yang EY, et al: Increased cell proliferation and decreased apoptosis characterize congenital cystic adenomatoid malformation of the lung. J Pediatr Surg 33:1043, 1998.

Carter R: Pulmonary sequestration: Collective review. Ann Thorac Surg 7:68, 1969.

Chan V, Greenough A, Nicolaides KN: Antenatal and postnatal treatment of pleural effusion and extralobar pulmonary sequestration. J Perinat Med 24:335, 1996.

Cleveland RH, Weber B: Retained fetal lung liquid in congenital lobar emphysema: A possible predictor of polyalveolar lobe. Pediatr Radiol 23:291, 1993.

Cogbill TH, Moore FA, Accurso FJ, et al: Primary tracheomalacia. Ann Thorac Surg 35:538, 1983.

Cohn RC, Kercsmar C, Dearborn D: Safety and flexibility of flexible endoscopy in children with bronchopulmonary dysplasia. Am J Dis Child 142:1225, 1988.

Collins MD, Moessinger AC, Kleinerman J, et al: Fetal lung hypoplasia associated with maternal smoking: A morphometric analysis. Pediatr Res 19:408, 1985.

Cotton RT, Richardson MA: Congenital laryngeal anomalies. Otolaryngol Clin North Am 14:203, 1981.

Cotton RT, Schreiber JH: Management of laryngotracheoesophageal cleft. Ann Otol 90:401, 1981.

Couser RJ, Ferrara TB, Falde B, et al: Effectiveness of dexamethasone in preventing extubation failure in preterm infants at increased risk for airway edema. J Pediatr 121:591, 1992.

Cozzi F, Pierro A: Glossoptosis-apnea syndrome in infancy. Pediatrics 75:836, 1985.

Crockett DM, Healy GB, McGill TJ, et al: Computed tomography in the evaluation of choanal atresia in infants and children. Laryngoscope 97:174, 1987.

Dab I, Malfroot A, Goosens A: Therapeutic bronchoscopy in ventilated neonates. Arch Dis Child 69:533, 1993.

Davis JT, Baciewicz FA, Suriyapa S, et al: Vocal cord paralysis in premature infants undergoing ductal closure. Ann Thorac Surg 46:214, 1988.

Dines DE, Seward JB, Bernatz PE, et al: Pulmonary arteriovenous fistulas. Mayo Clin Proc 58:176, 1983.

Dolkart LA, Reimers FT, Helmuth WV, et al: Antenatal diagnosis of pulmonary sequestration: A review. Obstet Gynecol Surv 47:515, 1992.

Dommergues M, Louis-Sylvestre C, Mandelbrot L, et al: Congenital adenomatoid malformation of the lung: When is active fetal therapy indicated? Am J Obstet Gynecol 177:953, 1997.

Downing GJ, Kilbride HW: Evaluation of airway complications in high risk preterm infants: Application of flexible fiberoptic airway endoscopy. Pediatrics 95:567, 1995.

Doyle AJ: Demonstration of blood supply to pulmonary sequestration by MR angiography. AJR Am J Roentgenol 158:989, 1992.

Eisenberg P, Cohen HL, Coren C: Color Doppler in pulmonary sequestration diagnosis. J Ultrasound Med 11:175, 1992.

Elkerbout SC, van Lingen RA, Gerritsen J, Roorda RJ: Endoscopic balloon dilatation of acquired airway stenosis in newborn infants: A promising treatment. Arch Dis Child 68:37, 1993.

Evans AE, D'Angio GJ, Randolph J: A proposed staging for children with neuroblastoma. Cancer 27:324, 1971.

Evans MG: Hydrops fetalis and pulmonary sequestration. J Pediatr Surg 31:761, 1996.

Evans KL, Courteney-Harris R, Bailey CM, et al: Management of posterior laryngeal and laryngotracheo-esophageal clefts. Arch Otolaryngol Head Neck Surg 121:1380, 1995.

Filler RM, Messineo A, Vinograd I: Severe tracheomalacia associated with esophageal atresia: Results of surgical treatment. J Pediatr Surg 27:1136, 1992.

Finci V, Beghetti M, Kalangos S, et al: Unilateral total and contralateral partial pulmonary agenesis with total anomalous pulmonary venous drainage. J Pediatr 134:510, 1999.

Fletcher BD, Masson M, Lisbona A, et al: Thymic response to endogenous and exogenous steroids in premature infants. J Pediatr 95:111, 1979.

Fletcher MM, Blum SL, Blanchard CL: Pierre-Robin syndrome: Pathophysiology of obstructive episodes. Laryngoscope 79:547, 1969.

Friedberg J, Forte V: Acquired bronchial injury in neonates. Int J Pediatr Otorhinolaryngol 14:223, 1987.

Friedman EM, Williams M, Healy GB, et al: Pediatric endoscopy: A review of 616 cases. Ann Otol 93:517, 1984.

Friedman EM, Vastola AD, McGill TJ, et al: Chronic pediatric stridor: Etiology and outcome. Laryngoscope 100:277, 1990.

Galvin JR, Gingrich RD, Hoffman E, et al: Ultrafast computed tomography of the chest. Radiol Clin North Am 32:775, 1994.

Geary C, Whitsett J: Inhaled nitric oxide for oligohydramnios induced pulmonary hypoplasia: A report of two cases and review of the literature. J Perinatol 22:82, 2002.

Gewolb IH, Lebowitz RL, Taeusch HW: Thymic size and its relationship to the respiratory distress syndrome. J Pediatr 95:108, 1979.

Godil MA, Galvin-Parton P, Monte D, et al: Congenital nasal pyriform aperture stenosis with central diabetes insipidus. J Pediatr 137:260, 2000.

Greenholz SK, Hall RJ, Lilly JR, Shikes RH: Surgical implications of bronchopulmonary dysplasia. J Pediatr Surg 22:1132, 1987.

Gwinn JL, Lee FA, Rao PS: Radiological case of the month. Am J Dis Child 119:341, 1970.

Hall BD: Choanal atresia and associated multiple anomalies. J Pediatr 95:395, 1979.

Harding R, Liggins GC: The influence of oligohydramnios on thoracic dimensions in fetal sheep. J Dev Physiol 16:355, 1991.

Harrison MR, Adzick NS, Jennings RW, et al: Antenatal intervention for congenital cystic adenomatoid malformation. Lancet 336:965, 1990.

Hauft SM, Perlman JM, Siegel MJ, et al: Tracheal stenosis in the sick premature infant: Clinical and radiologic features. Am J Dis Child 142:206, 1988.

Heaf DP, Helms PJ, Dimwiddie R, et al: Nasopharyngeal airways in Pierre Robin syndrome. J Pediatr 100:698, 1982.

Healy GB, McGill T: $CO_2$ laser in subglottic hemangioma—an update. Ann Otol Rhinol Laryngol 93:270, 1984.

Healy GB, McGill T, Jako GJ, et al: Management of choanal atresia with the carbon-dioxide laser. Ann Otol Rhinol Laryngol 87:658, 1978.

Healy GB, Schuster SR, Jonas RA, et al: Correction of segmental tracheal stenosis in children. Ann Otol Rhinol Laryngol 97:444, 1988.

Hedrick MH, Ferro MM, Filly RA, et al: Congenital high airway obstruction syndrome (CHAOS): A potential for perinatal intervention. J Pediatr Surg 29:271, 1994.

Heithoff KB, Sane SM, Williams HJ, et al: Bronchopulmonary foregut malformations: A unifying etiological concept. AJR Am J Roentgenol 126:46, 1976.

Hendren WH, Kim SH: Pediatric thoracic surgery. In Scarpelli EM, Auld PAM, Goldman HS (eds): Pulmonary Disease of the Fetus and Newborn and Child. Philadelphia, Lea & Febiger, 1978, p 166.

Hernanz-Schulman M, Stein SM, Neblett WW, et al: Pulmonary sequestration: Diagnosis with color Doppler sonography and a new theory of associated hydrothorax. Radiology 180:817, 1991.

Hershenson MB, Brouillette RT, Klemka L, et al: Respiratory insufficiency in newborns with abdominal wall defects. J Pediatr Surg 20:348, 1985.

Hislop A, Hey E, Reid L: The lungs in congenital bilateral renal agenesis and dysplasia. Arch Dis Child 54:32, 1979.

Hislop A, Reid L: New pathological findings in emphysema of childhood: Overinflation of a normal lobe. Thorax 26:190, 1971.

Hislop A, Reid L: New pathological findings in emphysema of childhood: Polyalveolar lobe with emphysema. Thorax 25:682, 1970.

Hodgson CH, Burchell HB, Good CA: Hereditary hemorrhagic telangiectasia and pulmonary arteriovenous fistula. N Engl J Med 261:625, 1959.

Hogason AKM, Boe G, Finne PH: Rupture of the trachea: An unusual complication of delivery. Acta Paediatr 81:911, 1992.

Hubbard AM, Adzick NS, Crombleholme TM, et al: Congenital chest lesions: Diagnosis and characterization with prenatal MR imaging. Radiology 212:43, 1999.

Hughes CA, Rezaee A, Ludemann JP, Holinger LD: Management of congenital subglottic hemangioma. J Otolaryngol 28:223, 1999.

Inselman LS, Fisher SE, Spencer H, et al: Effect of intra-uterine ethanol exposure on fetal lung growth. Pediatr Res 19:12, 1985.

Jacobs IN, Wetmore RF, Tom LWC, et al: Tracheobronchomalacia in children. Arch Otolaryngol Head Neck Surg 120:154, 1994.

Johnson GM, Todd DW: Cor pulmonale in severe Pierre Robin syndrome. Pediatrics 65:152, 1980.

Josephson GD, Vickery CL, Giles WC, Gross CW: Transnasal endoscopic repair of congenital choanal atresia: Long term results. Arch Otolaryngol Head Neck Surg 124:537, 1998.

Kelly SM, Gray SD: Unilateral endoscopic supraglottoplasty for severe laryngomalacia. Arch Otolaryngol Head Neck Surg 121:899, 1995.

Kimura K, Soper RT, Kao SCS, et al: Aortosternopexy for tracheomalacia following repair of esophageal atresia: Evaluation by cine CT and technical refinement. J Pediatr Surg 25:769, 1990.

Kitterman JA: The effects of mechanical forces on fetal lung growth. Clin Perinatol 23:727, 1996.

Kitterman JA: Fetal lung development. J Dev Physiol 6:67, 1984.

Kitterman JA: Transient severe respiratory distress mimicking pulmonary hypoplasia in preterm infants. J Pediatr 123:969, 1993.

Knox WF, Barson AJ: Pulmonary hypoplasia in a regional perinatal unit. Early Hum Dev 14:33, 1986.

Kolls JK, Kiernan MP, Ascuitto RJ, et al: Intralobar pulmonary sequestration presenting as congestive heart failure in a neonate. Chest 102:974, 1992.

Kravitz RM: Congenital malformations of the lung. Pediatr Clin North Am 41:453, 1994.

Ladenstein R, Ambros IM, Potschger U, et al: Prognostic significance of DNA di-tetraploidy in neuroblastoma. Med Pediatr Oncol 36:83, 2001.

Landing BH: Congenital malformations and genetic disorders of the respiratory tract (larynx, trachea, bronchi and lungs). Am Rev Respir Dis 120:151, 1979.

Langston C, Thurlbeck WM: Conditions altering normal lung growth and development. In Thibeault DW, Gregory GS (eds): Neonatal Pulmonary Care. Norwalk, Conn, Appleton-Century-Crofts, 1986.

Laudy JAM, Tibboel D, Robben SGF, et al: Prenatal prediction of pulmonary hypoplasia: Clinical, biometric, and Doppler velocity correlates. Pediatrics 109:250, 2002.

Li AM, Chang J, Kumar A: Neonatal neuroblastoma presenting with respiratory distress. J Paediatr Child Health 37:203, 2001.

Liechty KW, Crombleholme TM, Quinn TM, et al: Elevated platelet derived growth factor B in congenital cystic adenomatoid malformations requiring fetal resection. J Pediatr Surg 34:805, 1999.

Lipshutz GS, Jennings RW, Lopoo JB, et al: Slide tracheoplasty for congenital tracheal stenosis: A case report. J Pediatr Surg 35:259, 2000.

Lobe TE, Hayden CK, Nicolas D, et al: Successful management of congenital tracheal stenosis in infancy. J Pediatr Surg 22:1137, 1987.

Loeff DS, Filler RM, Vinograd I, et al: Congenital tracheal stenosis: A review of 22 patients from 1965 to 1987. J Pediatr Surg 23:744, 1988.

Longaker MT, Harrison MR, Adzick NS: Testing the limits of neonatal tracheal resection. J Pediatr Surg 25:790, 1990.

Lopoo JB, Goldstein RB, Lipshutz GS, et al: Fetal pulmonary sequestration: A favorable congenital lung lesion. Obstet Gynecol 94:567, 1999.

MacGillivray TE, Adzick NS, Harrison MR, et al: Disappearing fetal lung lesions. J Pediatr Surg 28:1321, 1993.

Mallory SF, Paradise JL: Glossoptosis revisited: On the development and resolution of airway obstruction in the Pierre Robin syndrome. Pediatrics 64:946, 1979.

McBride JT, Wohl MEB, Strieder DJ, et al: Lung growth and airway function after lobectomy in infancy for congenital lobar emphysema. J Clin Invest 66:962, 1980.

McCoy KS, Bagwell CE, Wagner M, et al: Spirometric and endoscopic evaluation of airway collapse in infants with bronchopulmonary dysplasia. Pediatr Pulmonol 14:23, 1992.

McCubbin M, Frey EE, Wagener JS, et al: Large airway collapse in bronchopulmonary dysplasia. J Pediatr 114:304, 1989.

McGill T: Congenital diseases of the larynx. Otolaryngol Clin North Am 17:57, 1984.

McIntosh N: Dry lung syndrome after oligohydramnios. Arch Dis Child 63:190, 1988.

McIntosh N, Harrison A: Prolonged premature rupture of membranes in the preterm infant: A seven year study. Eur J Obstet Gynecol Reprod Biol 57:1, 1994.

Merenstein GB: Congenital cystic adenomatoid malformation of the lung. Am J Dis Child 118:772, 1969.

Messineo A, Forte V, Joseph T, et al: The balloon posterior tracheal split: A technique for managing tracheal stenosis in premature infants. J Pediatr Surg 27:1142, 1992.

Messineo A, Narne S, Mognato G, et al: Endoscopic dilation of acquired tracheobronchial stenosis in infants. Pediatr Pulmonol 23:101, 1997.

Miller JA, Corteville JE, Langer JC: Congenital cystic adenomatoid malformation in the fetus: Natural history and predictors of outcome. J Pediatr Surg 31:805, 1996.

Miller RW, Woo P, Kellman RK, Slagle TS: Tracheobronchial abnormalities in infants with bronchopulmonary dysplasia. J Pediatr 111:779, 1987.

Mitchell RO, Austin EH: Pulmonary arteriovenous malformation in the neonate. J Pediatr Surg 28:1536, 1993.

Moessinger AC, Collins MH, Blanc WA, et al: Oligohydramnios-induced lung hypoplasia: The influence of timing and duration in gestation. Pediatr Res 20:951, 1986.

Mogilner JG, Fonseca J, Davies MR: Life threatening respiratory distrss caused by a mediastinal teratoma in a newborn. J Pediatr Surg 27:1519, 1992.

Moppett J, Haddadin I, Foot ABM, et al: Neonatal neuroblastoma. Arch Dis Child 81:F134, 1999.

Morgan E: Prenatal diagnosis of neuroblastoma: A non-invasive approach [letter]. Pediatrics 95:161, 1995.

Morin L, Crombleholme TM, D'Alton ME: Prenatal diagnosis and management of fetal thoracic lesions. Semin Perinatol 18:228, 1994.

Nakamura Y, Yamamoto I, Funatsu Y, et al: Decreased surfactant level in the lung with oligohydramnios: Amorphometric and biochemical study. J Pediatr 112:471, 1988.

Nakayama DK, Harrison MR, deLorimier AA, et al: Reconstructive surgery of obstructing lesions of the intrathoracic trachea in infants and small children. J Pediatr Surg 17:854, 1982.

Nimrod C, Varela-Gittings F, Machin G, et al: The effect of very prolonged membrane rupture on fetal development. Am J Obstet Gynecol 148:540, 1984.

Njinimbam CG, Hebra A, Kicklighter SD, et al: Persistent pulmonary hypertension in a neonate with cystic adenomatoid malformation of the lung following lobectomy: Survival with prolonged extracorporeal membrane oxygenation. J Perinatol 19:64, 1999.

Obwegeser R, Deutinger J, Bernaschek G: Fetal pulmonary cyst treated by repeated thoracentesis. Am J Obstet Gynecol 169:1622, 1993.

Olutoye OO, Coleman BG, Hubbard AM, Adzick NS: Prenatal management of congenital lobar emphysema. J Pediatr Surg 35:792, 2000.

Opsahl T, Berman EJ: Bronchogenic mediastinal cysts in infants: Case report and review of the literature. Pediatrics 30:372, 1962.

Orlow SJ, Isakoff MS, Blei F: Increased risk of symptomatic hemangiomas of the airway in association with cutaneous hemangiomas in a beard distribution. J Pediatr 131:514, 1997.

Otherson HB, Hebra A, Tagge EP: A new method of treatment for complete tracheal rings in an infant: Endoscopic laser division and balloon dilation. J Pediatr Surg 35:262, 2000.

Pagon RA, Graham JM, Zonana J, et al: Coloboma, congenital heart disease, and choanal atresia with multiple anomalies: CHARGE association. J Pediatr 99:223, 1981.

Pearl M: Sequestration of the lung. Am J Dis Child 124:706, 1972.

Peliowski A, Finer NN, Etches PC, et al: Inhaled nitric oxide for premature infants after prolonged rupture of membranes. J Pediatr 126:450, 1995.

Penn RB, Wolfson MR, Shaffer TH: Effect of ventilation on mechanical properties and pressure-flow relationships of immature airways. Pediatr Res 23:519, 1988.

Porter HJ: Pulmonary hypoplasia. Arch Dis Child 81:F81, 1999.

Presscott CAJ: Nasal obstruction in infancy. Arch Dis Child 72:287, 1995.

Rescoria FJ, West KW, Vane DW, et al: Pulmonary hypertension in neonatal cystic lung disease: Survival following lobectomy and extra corporeal membrane oxygenation in two cases. J Pediatr Surg 25:1054, 1990.

Revillon Y, Jan D, Plattner V, et al: Congenital cystic adenomatoid malformation of the lung: Prenatal management and prognosis. J Pediatr Surg 28:1009, 1993.

Richardson MA, Cotton RT: Anatomic abnormalities of the pediatric airway. Pediatr Clin North Am 31:821, 1984.

Rideout DT, Hayashi AH, Gillis DA, et al: The absence of clinically detected tracheomalacia in patients having esophageal atresia without tracheo-esophageal fistula. J Pediatr Surg 26:1303, 1991.

Rimell FL, Shapiro AM, Meza MP, et al: Magnetic resonance imaging of the pediatric airway. Arch Otolaryngol Head Neck Surg 123:999, 1997.

Roggin KK, Breuer CK, Carr SR, et al: The unpredictable character of congenital cystic lesions. J Pediatr Surg 35:801, 2000.

Rowe RW, Betts J, Free E: Peri-operative management of laryngotracheal reconstruction. Anesth Analg 73:483, 1991.

Saltzberg AM: Congenital malformations of the lower respiratory tract. In Kendig EL, Chernick V (eds): Disorders of the Respiratory Tract in Children. Philadelphia, WB Saunders, 1983, p 169.

Schlesinger AE, DiPietro MA, Statter MB, et al: Utility of sonography in the diagnosis of bronchopulmonary sequestration. J Pediatr Surg 29:52, 1994.

Schumacher RE, Weinfeld IJ, Bartlett RH: Neonatal vocal cord paralysis following extracorporeal membrane oxygenation. Pediatrics 84:793, 1989.

Seid AB, Canty TG: The anterior cricoid split procedure for the management of subglottic stenosis in infants and children. J Pediatr Surg 20:388, 1985.

Shannon DC, Todres ID, Moylan FMB: Infantile lobar hyperinflation: Expectant treatment. Pediatrics 59:1012, 1977.

Sherman JM, Lowitt S, Stephenson C, et al: Factors influencing acquired subglottic stenosis in infants. J Pediatr 109:322, 1986.

Simoneaux SF, Bank ER, Webber JB, Parks WJ: Magnetic resonance imaging of the pediatric airway. Radiographics 15:287, 1995.

Slovis TL, Meza MP, Cushing B, et al: Thoracic neuroblastoma: What is the best imaging modality for evaluating extent of disease? Pediatr Radiol 27:273, 1997.

Smart LM, Hendry GMA: Imaging of neonatal pulmonary sequestration including Doppler ultrasound. Br J Radiol 64:324, 1991.

Smith RJH, Catlin FI: Congenital anomalies of the larynx. Am J Dis Child 138:35, 1984.

Sotomayor JL, Godinez RI, Borden S, et al: Large airway collapse due to acquired tracheobronchomalacia in infancy. Am J Dis Child 140:367, 1986.

Spinella PC, Strieper MJ, Callahan CW: Congestive heart failure in a neonate secondary to bilateral intralobar and extralobar pulmonary sequestrations. Pediatrics 101:120, 1998.

Stahl RS, Jurkiewicz MJ: Congenital posterior choanal atresia. Pediatrics 76:429, 1985.

Stern LM, Fonkalsrud EW, Hassakis P, et al: Management of Pierre Robin syndrome in infancy by prolonged naso-esophageal intubation. Am J Dis Child 124:79, 1972.

Stigers KB, Woodring JH, Kanga JF: The clinical and imaging spectrum of findings in patients with congenital lobar emphysema. Pediatr Pulmonol 14:160, 1992.

Suporina RA, Ein SH, Humphreys R: Cystic duplications of the esophagus and neuro-enteric cysts. J Pediatr Surg 19:527, 1984.

Swischuk LE, Richardson CJ, Nichols NM, et al: Primary pulmonary hypoplasia in the neonate. J Pediatr 95:573, 1979.

Tavin E, Singer L, Bassila M: Problems in postoperative management after anterior cricoid split. Arch Otolaryngol Head Neck Surg 120:823, 1994.

Thambi Dorai CR, Muthu Alhagi V, Chee Eng N, et al: Mediastinal teratoma in a neonate. Pediatr Surg Int 14:84, 1998.

Thibeault DW, Beatty EC, Hall RT, et al: Neonatal pulmonary hypoplasia with premature rupture of fetal membranes and oligohydramnios. J Pediatr 107:273, 1985.

Thomas IT, Smith DW: Oligohydramnios, cause of the non-renal features of Potter's syndrome, including pulmonary hypoplasia. J Pediatr 84:811, 1974.

Thorpe-Beeston JG, Nicolaides KH: Cystic adenomatoid malformation of the lung: Prenatal diagnosis and outcome. Prenat Diagn 14:677, 1994.

Truong DT, Oudjhane K: Anterior nasal stenosis as a cause of neonatal nasal airway obstruction. Arch Pediatr Adolesc Med 148:279, 1994.

Usui N, Kamata S, Ishikawa S, et al: Anomalies of the tracheobronchial tree in patients with esophageal atresia. J Pediatr Surg 31:258, 1996.

Van den Abbeele T, Triglia JM, Francois M, Narcy P: Congenital nasal pyriform aperture stenosis: Diagnosis and management of 20 cases. Ann Otol Rhinol Laryngol 110:70, 2001.

Veeneklaas GMH: Pathogenesis of intrathoracic gastrogenic cysts. Am J Dis Child 83:500, 1952.

Voland JR, Benirschke K, Saunders B: Congenital tracheal stenosis with associated cardiopulmonary anomalies: Report of 2 cases with a review of the literature. Pediatr Pulmonol 2:247, 1986.

Volpe MV, Archavachotikul K, Bhan I, et al: Association of bronchopulmonary sequestration with expression of the homeobox protein Hoxb-5. J Pediatr Surg 35:1817, 2000.

White CW: Treatment of hemangiomatosis with recombinant interferon alfa. Semin Hematol 27:15, 1990.

Wigglesworth JS, Desai R: Effects on lung growth of cervical cord section in the rabbit fetus. Early Hum Dev 3:51, 1979.

Wigglesworth JS, Desai R: Is fetal respiratory function a major determinant of perinatal survival? Lancet 1:264, 1982.

Wigglesworth JS, Desai R, Guerrini P: Fetal lung hypoplasia: Biochemical and structural variations and their possible significance. Arch Dis Child 56:606, 1981.

Winters WD, Effmann EL, Nghiem HV, et al: Disappearing fetal lung masses: Importance of postnatal imaging studies. Pediatr Radiol 27:535, 1997.

Wiseman NE, Duncan PG, Cameron CB: Management of tracheobronchomalacia with continuous positive airway pressure. J Pediatr Surg 20:489, 1985.

Wood RE: Clinical applications of ultrathin flexible bronchoscopes. Pediatr Pulmonol 1:244, 1985.

Young LW, Rubin P, Hanson RE: The extra adrenal neuroblastoma: High radio-curability and diagnostic accuracy. AJR Am J Roentgenol 108:75, 1970.

Zinman R: Tracheal stenting improves airway mechanics in infants with tracheobronchomalacia. Pediatr Pulmonol 19:275, 1995.

CHAPTER

# 51

# Disorders of the Chest Wall, Pleural Cavity, and Diaphragm

**Thomas N. Hansen, Anthony Corbet, and Roberta A. Ballard**

## DISORDERS OF THE CHEST WALL

Abnormalities of the bone and muscle of the chest wall may be a mechanical hindrance to ventilation.

### Skeletal Disorders

Although abnormalities involving bone are rare, they may be recognized immediately and are sometimes amenable to operative correction.

#### Defects of Sternal Fusion

Defects in fusion of the sternum are uncommon. Complete separation of the two halves of the sternum allows protrusion of cardiovascular structures, a condition known as *ectopia cordis* (Maier and Bortone, 1949). Lethal malformations of the heart are commonly associated with this condition. Upper sternal clefts are more common. Early operation is advised to shield the underlying structures from injury, and because of the greater ease of approximating the separated parts in the first days of life compared with later (Sabiston, 1958). A lower sternal cleft and ectopia cordis with a congenital heart defect may be associated with congenital apertures in the upper abdominal wall, in the pericardium, and in the anterior diaphragm, with a Morgagni-type diaphragmatic hernia, the so-called pentalogy of Cantrell (Cantrell et al, 1958).

#### Pectus Excavatum

The most common of the sternal defects is pectus excavatum, sometimes associated with Pierre Robin syndrome or Marfan syndrome. Rarely is it a fixed or severe deformity until several months of postnatal age. A family history of some type of anterior thoracic deformity was found in 37% of patients, according to Welch (1980). The heart may be compressed between the sternum and the vertebral column and displaced to the left, impinging on the space of the left lung. There is usually no respiratory or cardiac distress. Only later in childhood may there be cosmetic and psychological distress sufficient to warrant intervention. The indications for operative correction are debatable. In our opinion, correction should not be undertaken until the child is several years of age and then only in those few children in whom the deformity appears to be progressing. Serial photographs are the best way to document changes in pectus excavatum. Periodic evaluation of cardiovascular status with ultrasonography and electrocardiography and assessment of pulmonary function are appropriate in the presence of progressive deformity. Results of operative correction are excellent in more than 80% of patients; surgery is almost always associated with functional improvement. Recurrences are possible during later active growth.

#### Poland Syndrome

Deficiency of pectoral muscles on one side, so-called Poland syndrome, may be associated with a deficiency of the second through the fifth ribs on the same side—the ribs of attachment for the pectoralis major muscle. There may be associated syndactyly, hemivertebrae and scoliosis, and later hypoplasia of breast development. Breathing may be paradoxical and the cardiac impulse easily observed through the soft tissues, but there usually is no distress. Later in childhood, and uncommonly, there may be increasing respiratory distress with scoliosis lung disease and heart failure. No operative intervention is required in infancy, although mammoplasty may be desirable later on in affected girls after puberty.

#### Thoracic Dystrophies

##### *Asphyxiating Thoracic Dystrophy*

A rare deformity of the thoracic cage, asphyxiating thoracic dystrophy is part of a serious generalized chondrodystrophy, with short-limbed dwarfism and often polydactyly (Fig. 51–1). It was first described by Jeune and coworkers (1954). The ribs are horizontal, hypoplastic, and short, with flared costochondral junctions. The thorax is small, bell-shaped, and rigid; this results in displacement of the liver and spleen well into the abdominal cavity. Some degree of lung hypoplasia may be present, often severe and lethal. The pelvis shows flaring of the iliac wings and acetabular abnormalities (Kohler et al, 1970). Prenatal diagnosis with ultrasonography is possible. Renal cystic dysplasia may be present, resulting in hypertension and renal failure. In the past, most patients with this condition did not survive the first month. Oberkaid and coworkers (1977) studied 10 cases and noted that only two patients were alive at the time of the report. One of the two was in excellent health at 15 years of age. The more severely affected infants had respiratory distress from birth. Three patients have been described in one family; as it is an autosomal recessive trait, the expectation would be for an occurrence in one of four siblings, so mutations must be common. No parent-child occurrence has been described. Recently, Davis and coworkers (2001) reported an operative technique for lateral thoracic expansion in 10 patients with chest wall deformities limiting thoracic capacity—including 8 patients

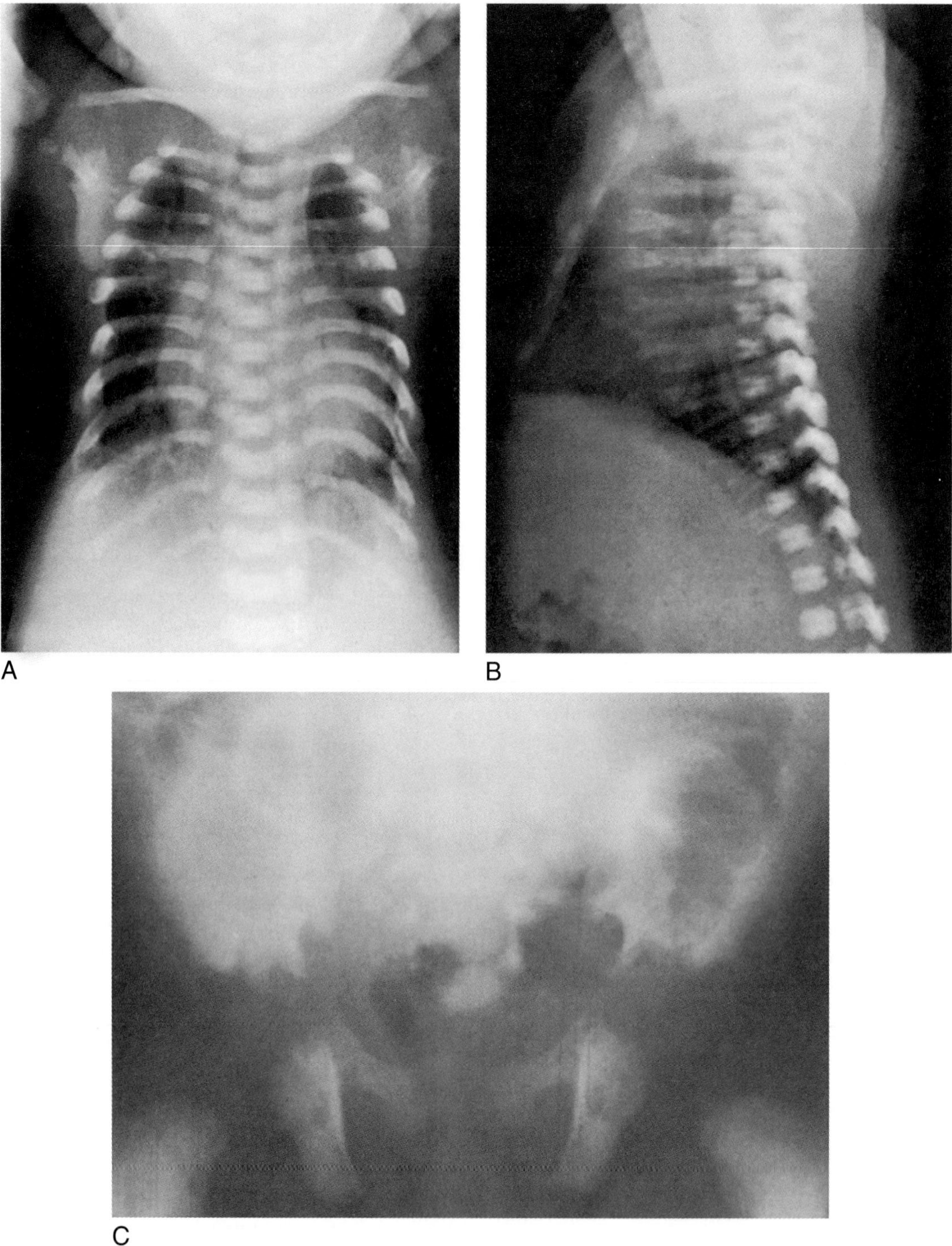


**FIGURE 51–1.** Radiographs from an infant with asphyxiating thoracic dystrophy. **A** and **B,** On anteroposterior and lateral views of the chest, the thoracic dimension is seen to be reduced in comparison with the abdominal dimension. **C,** Radiograph of the pelvis shows flaring of the iliac crests and bony protrusions of the acetabulae. (***A** and **B**, Courtesy of Dr John Kirkpatrick; **C**, from Avery ME, Fletcher BD, Williams RG: The Lung and Its Disorders in the Newborn Infant, 4th ed. Philadelphia, WB Saunders, 1981.*)

with classic Jeune syndrome. Three were younger than 1 year of age at the time of surgery, and 6 were ventilator dependent. All of the infants older than 1 year of age at the time of surgery improved, with measured lung volumes increasing in 2 of 3 studied, and thoracic volumes by computed tomography increasing in 4 of 5 studied. The only deaths were in 2 infants younger than 1 year of age at the time of surgery. These results suggest that lateral thoracic expansion is a safe and effective procedure for patients beyond the first year of age.

### *Other Thoracic Dystrophies*

Severe underdevelopment of the thoracic rib cage, accompanied usually by lethal pulmonary hypoplasia, may be seen in other conditions, such as the thanatophoric dwarfism syndrome, the short rib–polydactyly syndrome, and the camptomelic dwarfism syndrome. Affected infants do not survive for long after birth.

## Neuromuscular Disorders

Other causes of thoracic dysfunction are diseases of the nerves and muscles, including congenital myasthenia gravis, congenital spinal muscular atrophy (Werdnig-Hoffmann disease), congenital myotonic dystrophy, glycogen storage disease, and congenital spinal injury. Such conditions are usually recognized in the context of the associated systemic muscular weakness. Newborns with myasthenia gravis have episodes of muscle weakness, poor feeding, weak cry, hypoventilation, and apnea with a positive response to an anticholinesterase medication. In congenital spinal muscular atrophy, there is lung hypoplasia associated with absent fetal breathing, and as a result the thorax is small. Other features include severe hypotonia, muscle fasciculation, respiratory failure, and early death; the inheritance is autosomal recessive. In congenital myotonic dystrophy, there is lung hypoplasia from absent fetal breathing; affected infants have respiratory distress at birth, rapidly need mechanical ventilation, and are soon ventilator dependent. Mothers of these infants have myotonia, difficulty in relaxing muscle contractions; the inheritance is autosomal dominant.

# DISORDERS OF THE PLEURAL CAVITY

The pleural space exists between the parietal pleura of the chest wall and the visceral pleura of the lung. Each pleural surface is composed of a mesothelial layer that covers a layer of connective tissue containing lymphatics, blood vessels, and nerves. In the parietal pleura, lymphatic channels communicate with the pleural space to provide a direct pathway for fluid and protein reabsorption. It was initially believed that the blood supply to the parietal pleura emanated from the systemic circulation and that the blood supply to the visceral pleura emanated from the pulmonary circulation. The capillary hydrostatic pressure in the visceral pleura was believed to be correspondingly low, leading to the assumption that fluid was filtered out of the parietal pleura and reabsorbed by the visceral pleura. Data now show, however, that the blood supply to the visceral pleura emanates from the bronchial circulation. Both pleural surfaces filter fluid into the pleural space, and the lymphatics are responsible for most of the fluid reabsorption (Wiener-Kronish et al, 1985).

## Pathomechanisms of Pleural Effusion

Fluid accumulates in the pleural space only if the rate of filtration increases or if the rate of lymphatic clearance decreases or if both of these processes occur.

### *Increased Fluid Filtration*

The rate of fluid filtration can be increased by increasing the filtration pressure. The parietal pleura is drained by the systemic veins, and the visceral pleura is drained by the pulmonary veins. Therefore, filtration pressure is increased with increases in either systemic or pulmonary venous pressure (Mellins et al, 1970). Raised venous pressure is the most likely cause for pleural effusions that complicate heart failure, as well as for the effusions that occur with hydrops fetalis. It is not believed that hypoproteinemia plays a primary role in the accumulation of fluid (Moise et al, 1991), because low protein would be reflected in both the vascular and the interstitial spaces, with little change in the transvascular oncotic pressure. The rate of fluid filtration into the pleural space also is increased if the permeability of the pleura to water and protein is increased, as in the case of infections.

### *Decreased Fluid Clearance*

The rate of fluid clearance from the pleural space may be decreased by any impairment of lymphatic function caused by direct mechanical obstruction (Mellins et al, 1970). As the main lymphatic channels drain into the systemic venous system, elevated systemic venous pressure will also impair lymphatic clearance. The main thoracic duct on the left side drains into the angle of junction of the left subclavian and internal jugular veins; the right lymphatic duct drains into the angle of junction of the right subclavian and internal jugular veins. Small valves prevent the reflux of venous blood into the lymphatic ducts.

## Diagnosis of Effusion

Pleural effusions should be suspected in any infant with respiratory difficulty who is hydropic or who has been receiving intravenous nutrition. Infants who receive central venous alimentation should have the glucose content of the pleural fluid checked immediately to make sure that the catheter has not perforated into the pleural space. Differential breath sounds are valuable in localizing unilateral effusions. The chest radiograph is diagnostic (Fig. 51–2). Thoracentesis is useful to identify effusions secondary to infections and to distinguish chylothorax from other causes of pleural effusions.

## Congenital Chylothorax

Accumulations of chyle in the pleural space may be congenital or acquired. Congenital chylothorax occurs more commonly in males than in females (2:1), and it occurs more commonly on the right side. Chernick and Reed (1970) said that 53% of the cases were on the right side, 35% on the left side, and 12% were bilateral. In some classifications this condition may be called primary hydrothorax.

Congenital chylothorax is probably one part of the spectrum of anomalies that results from intrauterine obstruction of the thoracic duct (Chervenak et al, 1983; Smeltzer et al, 1986). It may occur alone or in combination with other lymphatic anomalies as part of the jugular lymphatic obstruction

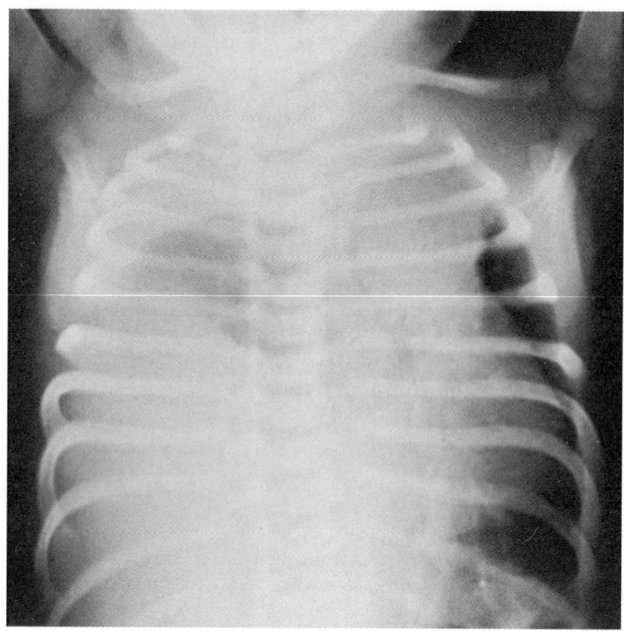

**FIGURE 51–2.** Chest radiograph from an infant with a right-sided chylothorax.

sequence. Infants may have cystic hygroma malformations or severe webbing of the neck, the residue of a fetal cystic hygroma that has resolved. Presumably, lymph flow obstruction results in the development of fistulas between the thoracic duct and the pleural space or in rupture of the thoracic duct. Dutheil et al (1998) described an infant with generalized lymphangiomatosis with skin lymphangiomas and congenital chylothorax. Njolstad and colleagues (1998) described several siblings with congenital pulmonary lymphangiectasia and nonimmune hydrops with congenital distal lymphedema. Chylothorax has been described as a complication of Down syndrome, in which there is presumably a significant maldevelopment of the lymphatic system (Yamamoto et al, 1996). Other patients may have Turner or Noonan syndrome.

Congenital chylothorax frequently is diagnosed in utero by ultrasonography (Devine and Malone, 2000). If the problem occurs early and is severe enough, the fetus may have significant pulmonary hypoplasia, and after birth the infant may have severe respiratory distress. If the chylothorax is large enough or bilateral, intrathoracic pressure may be sufficiently increased to cause esophageal dysfunction with polyhydramnios, and compression of central veins also may be sufficient to cause ascites or general hydrops, in which case the clinical picture may be very confusing. In some cases the chylothorax may resolve before birth, but this is unlikely if hydrops is present. Some fetuses have been treated by placement of a drainage tube from the pleural cavity into the amniotic fluid, a pleuroamniotic shunt (Rodeck et al, 1988; Schmidt et al, 1985). If the problem is present just before birth, it is better to drain the effusion after delivery, because drainage may cause hypovolemia, necessitating further treatment. Others have described ex utero treatment with intact placental circulation, by catheter aspiration of the effusions before cord clamping and tracheal intubation for mechanical ventilation (Prontera et al, 2002).

Bilateral chylothoraces should be considered in the differential diagnosis for any infant who cannot be ventilated in the delivery room. An emergency thoracentesis may be required and life-saving. In less severe cases, thoracentesis is still required for a definitive diagnosis. Chyle can be distinguished from a transudate by its high protein and lipid content; it can be distinguished from an exudate by its high lipid content, the characteristic preponderance of lymphocytes, and its slightly alkaline pH (Table 51–1). Differential count of the white cells reveals more than 80% lymphocytes. It should be remembered that the lipid characteristics depend on the infant's having been fed with a formula. Before feeding, it can be quite difficult to distinguish chylothorax from hydrothorax (Eddleman et al, 1991).

Treatment of chylothorax may require repeated thoracenteses or even thoracostomy tube drainage to prevent respiratory failure (Brodman, 1975). The clinician should be careful to replace plasma proteins lost in the pleural fluid. Once drainage is accomplished, these infants are placed on formulas containing medium-chain triglycerides (MCTs), rather than long-chain fatty acids, to reduce thoracic duct lymph flow. Oral intake of protein and water also stimulates thoracic duct lymph flow, so in resistant cases the infant is managed with nothing by mouth, with nutritional support provided through an indwelling intravenous catheter. Some researchers have claimed that total

**TABLE 51–1**

**Composition of Chyle**

| Measurement | Units | Mean | Range |
|---|---|---|---|
| Total protein | g/dL | 3.56 | 1.89-6.17 |
| Albumin | g/dL | 2.24 | 1.26-3.0 |
| Total lipids | mg/dL | 1180 | 56-3500 |
| Cholesterol | mg/dL | 81 | 48-200 |
| Triglycerides | mg/dL | 197 | 123-234 |
| White blood cells | /mm$^3$ | 15,200 | 0-29,000 |
| Lymphocytes | % | 90 | 70-100 |
| pH | — | 7.5 | 7.4-7.8 |
| Specific gravity | — | 1.013 | 1.008-1.027 |

Data from Brodman RF: Congenital chylothorax: Recommendation for treatment. NY State J Med 75:553, 1975.

parenteral nutrition (TPN) results in significantly earlier resolution of chylothorax than treatment with enteral MCT formula (Fernandez Alvarez et al, 1999).

A variety of approaches have been used with some success to treat the infant with persistent chylothorax, including direct attempts at repair, patching with fibrin glue (Stenzl et al, 1983), and obliteration of the pleural space with sclerosing agents. Congenital chylothorax also has been managed successfully using a pleuroperitoneal shunt (Azizkhan et al, 1983). Finally, some reports suggest that ligation of the thoracic duct below the area of leakage is highly effective (Stringel et al, 1984); this procedure appears to be surprisingly well tolerated without accumulations of fluid in the peripheral tissues or in the peritoneum.

The prognosis for infants with congenital chylothorax is good. In a review of 34 cases, two thirds of the infants with chylothorax responded to thoracentesis alone, without the need for indwelling drainage tubes, and only 5 infants died. The complications reported in this review included weight loss from malnutrition, hypoproteinemia, and lymphopenia (Brodman, 1975).

### Acquired Chylothorax

Acquired chylothorax results from damage to the thoracic duct. It has been reported as a surgical complication in the repair of diaphragmatic hernia, tracheoesophageal fistula, and a variety of congenital heart disorders. This complication may also occur following the use of extracorporeal membrane oxygenation (ECMO) catheters, following patent ductus arteriosus (PDA) ligation, and with insertion of chest tubes too far when such tubes are used for the treatment of pneumothorax. Acquired chylothorax usually is diagnosed by a chest radiograph obtained because of a change in respiratory status. The management is the same as for congenital chylothorax. It has been reported that a continuous infusion of somatostatin may be efficacious (Buettiker et al, 2001), presumably by reducing splanchnic blood flow and lymph production.

### Congenital Hydrothorax

Congenital hydrothorax may be unilateral or bilateral. It may be isolated but is more often associated with ascites or hydrops fetalis. Hydrothorax may manifest with difficulties in the delivery room and require immediate treatment by pleural drainage tube.

The following conditions should be considered in the differential diagnosis: (1) immune hydrops with fetal anemia and heart failure, usually due to Rh isoimmunization or a similar disorder; (2) nonimmune hydrops with fetal anemia and heart failure (e.g., with twin-to-twin transfusion syndrome, chronic fetal maternal transfusion syndrome, fetal parvoviral infection); (3) nonimmune hydrops without fetal anemia but with fetal heart failure (e.g., with fetal tachyarrhythmia, fetal bradyarrhythmia, arteriovenous malformations at various locations including the placenta and causing large systemic-to-venous shunts, cardiac malformations with ventricular hypoplasia and premature closure of the foramen ovale, fetal viral infections such as cytomegalovirus infection, probably with associated myocarditis); (4) large space-occupying lesions within the thorax that obstruct venous return to the heart (e.g., congenital cystic adenomatoid malformation, congenital mediastinal teratoma, congenital diaphragmatic hernia, large pleural effusions, enlarged fetal lungs associated with laryngeal atresia, large fetal chylothorax); and (5) chromosome abnormalities such as Turner syndrome and Down syndrome and other trisomies, which may be associated with more subtle lymphatic drainage malformations and hydrothoraces or chylothoraces. In some cases, but not all, once the underlying abnormality is corrected, the effusions may resolve without further need for drainage.

Thibeault and colleagues (1995) described two infants who had congenital hydrothoraces due to lymphatic hypoplasia, so that normal filtered fluid could not be drained from the pleural spaces. Small pleural effusions may be associated with "wet lung syndrome" or group B streptococcal pneumonia in the newborn. Pleural effusions also may be associated with bronchopulmonary sequestrations and with right-sided diaphragmatic hernias; in such cases the hydrothorax may be quite large.

### Acquired Hydrothorax

#### *Central Catheters*

Infants with central venous catheters for infusion of total parenteral nutrition solutions are at risk for the development of pleural effusions, sometimes associated with pericardial effusion and pericardial tamponade. The catheter tip may burrow directly through the pleura, or there may be localized damage from hypertonic solutions with diffusion of fluid into the pleural space. In an infant with severe clinical difficulties and a central catheter, this diagnosis must be considered immediately, especially if there is pericardial tamponade. The fluid aspirated from the pleural space or from the pericardial sac may look like TPN or lipid solution, but if there is doubt it should be checked for its high glucose or lipid content.

#### *Superior Vena Cava Syndrome*

In cases of superior vena cava obstruction with venous thrombosis, significant hydrothoraces may develop because of elevated central venous pressure (Dhande et al, 1983). Such hydrothoraces may be extremely troublesome and require repeated tube drainage or even a surgical shunt procedure. In some infants with superior vena cava thrombosis, chylothoraces rather than hydrothoraces may develop, presumably because lymphatic drainage into the venous system is impaired. Treatment of caval thrombosis may consist of long-acting heparin, tissue plasminogen activator, or a surgical procedure.

## DISORDERS OF THE DIAPHRAGM

### Congenital Diaphragmatic Hernia

Most infants with congenital diaphragmatic hernia (CDH) are mature, two thirds are male, and in 90% the hernia is left-sided. The incidence has been reported at between 1 in

2000 and 1 in 10,000 live births (Langham et al, 1996), with an overall estimate of 1 per 3500 live births. The incidence may be higher because some affected infants are not born alive; Morin and colleagues (1994) suggested an incidence of 1 per 2200 when all cases of fetal demise are included. In the newborn, nearly all hernias pass through the posterolateral foramen of Bochdalek. The pathophysiology of CDH has been reviewed by Glick and colleagues (1996).

### Pathogenesis

#### *Lung Hypoplasia and Arterial Muscle Hyperplasia*

The diaphragm develops anteriorly as a septum between the heart and liver and progresses backward to close last at the left Bochdalek foramen around 8 to 10 weeks of gestation. The bowel migrates from the yolk sac at about 10 weeks, and if it arrives in the abdominal cavity before the foramen has closed, a hernia into the left hemithorax may result. Lung compression from an early age is associated with pulmonary hypoplasia, most severe on the ipsilateral side but also present on the contralateral side if there is mediastinal shift to the right. There is a marked reduction in the number of bronchial generations, with a less marked reduction in the number of alveoli per acinus. In autopsy specimens from infants with CDH, expression of the mitogen insulin growth factor in macrophages and granular pneumocytes is increased, as demonstrated by in situ hybridization studies (Miyazaki et al, 1998), which may reflect a failure of the normal decrease with maturation of the lung. Expression of vascular endothelial growth factor is increased in infants with pulmonary hypertension (Shehata et al, 1999). In the rat nitrofen CDH model there is a marked reduction in mitogen-activated protein kinase activity levels associated with lung growth (Kling et al, 2001). In this same model, there may be alterations of fibroblast growth factors, which are important in branching morphogenesis of the airways (Jesudason et al, 2000).

The number of arterial generations is reduced proportionately to the reduction in airway numbers (Bohn et al, 1987), and there is a modest increase in the medial muscle of pulmonary arterioles, together with abnormal peripheral extension of muscle into arterioles at the acinar level (Geggel et al, 1985). In many cases, herniation occurs comparatively late in gestation, or the hernia is small, in which case the lung hypoplasia and developmental changes in the lung vessels are less marked (Adzick et al, 1985).

After birth, when the hernia fills with swallowed air, compression of the lungs is increased, thus superimposing atelectasis on pulmonary hypoplasia. The prognosis depends on the degree of pulmonary hypoplasia (Nguyen et al, 1983), with its associated reduction in alveolar and vascular surface area. There may be severe hypercarbia and hypoxemia with persistent pulmonary hypertension and large right-to-left shunts at the atrial and ductal levels. The pulmonary hypertension has a fixed element because of the vascular anatomic changes associated with lung hypoplasia, and a reactive vasoconstrictive element induced by mediators, which is more responsive to clinical conditions. Kobayashi and Puri (1994) have shown in this condition that pulmonary hypertension is accompanied by markedly elevated levels of endothelin in the plasma and markedly increased expression of endothelin immunoreactivity in lung endothelial cells. Pulmonary hypertension is markedly improved with selective endothelin receptor antagonists in the lamb CDH model (Kavanagh et al, 2001). Also, the pulmonary vascular resistance in CDH is very dependent on the concentrations of plasma thromboxane and other prostanoids during episodes of clinical deterioration (O'Toole et al, 1996a). Expression of vascular endothelial growth factor is enhanced, especially in pulmonary arterial smooth muscle cells, as demonstrated by immunohistochemical staining in autopsy specimens from infants with CDH (Shehata et al, 1999).

#### *Lung Immaturity and Surfactant Insufficiency*

The lungs are immature even at full-term gestation, appearing arrested in the saccular phase of development. The terminal saccules have fewer septa, the interstitium is thicker, and there are fewer capillaries. Granular pneumocytes are more numerous, but they contain more glycogen and fewer surfactant lamellar bodies. The saccular lining cells are more cuboidal, and thin membranous pneumocytes are less developed (George et al, 1987). In the lamb model of CDH, surfactant phospholipids and proteins are reduced in the lung lavage fluid and in the lung tissue residues, and the surfactant produced has impaired biophysical properties when compared with that from controls (Wilcox et al, 1996b). Such lungs are very susceptible to ventilator-induced injury. In the rat model it has been shown that CDH lungs have a reduced antioxidant response to oxygen breathing, suggesting they are also more prone to oxygen-induced injury. In the nitrofen rat model it has been shown that vitamin A reverses the effects on lung hypoplasia and surfactant depletion (Thebaud et al, 2001).

### Diagnosis

An increasing percentage of diaphragmatic hernias are now diagnosed antenatally by ultrasonography. Antenatal diagnosis allows evaluation of the fetus for possible additional anomalies, as well as counseling of the family about treatment approaches in a tertiary center and discussing with the family the likely short- and long-term prognoses. It is still unclear, however, what factors are the most accurate for predicting eventual outcome (Wilcox et al, 1996a). Among infants in whom CDH was not diagnosed in utero, the onset of symptoms is usually with respiratory distress in the first few hours or days of life. Patients with the most severe symptoms present in the delivery room with a difficult resuscitation and have a high incidence of pneumothorax in the more common left-sided hernias. Breath sounds are absent on the left side, the chest is barrel-shaped, the abdomen is scaphoid, and the heart beat is displaced to the right. The diagnosis is made easily with a chest radiograph, aided by a feeding tube placed in the stomach. The left hemithorax is filled with a mass, usually incorporating air-filled bowel loops, and the stomach tube enters the chest. The heart is displaced to the right, and the abdomen is remarkably devoid of gas patterns (Fig. 51–3).

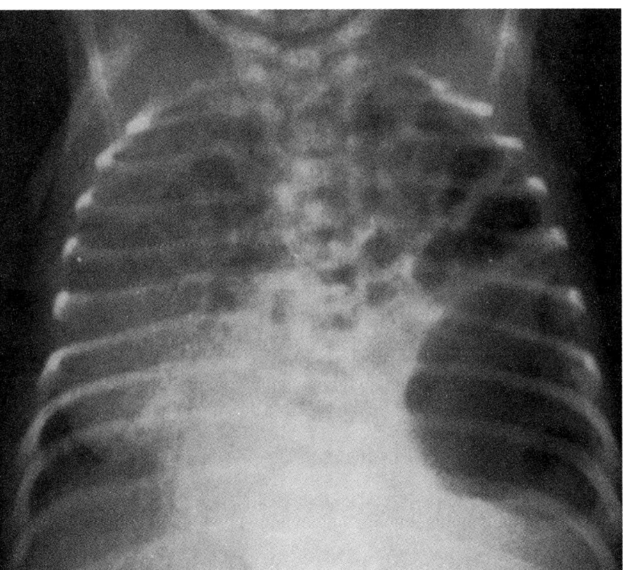

**FIGURE 51-3.** Left-sided congenital diaphragmatic hernia on day 2 of life. The chest is overexpanded and barrel-shaped. Translucencies of variable sizes fill the left hemithorax, reflecting herniated bowel. The heart is pushed into the right hemithorax.

### Associated Anomalies

Fauza and Wilson (1994) reviewed 166 cases of CDH and found that 39% had associated anomalies and 61% were isolated; many of the listed anomalies may not be clinically evident, but many have an adverse effect on the outcome. About two thirds of the anomalies were cardiac, including hypoplastic left heart syndrome, atrial septal defect, ventricular septal defect, coarctation of the aorta, and Ebstein anomaly. Other anomalies in this series included esophageal atresia, trisomy 18, hydronephrosis, hydrocephalus, and omphalocele. In the patients discussed by Langham and coauthors (1996), one third had a chromosomal defect or a multiple malformation syndrome involving the brain, heart, kidneys, bowel, or skeleton. Cases have been reported in association with Fryns syndrome, Beckwith-Wiedemann syndrome, Pierre Robin syndrome, and choanal atresia.

### The Cardiac Function Problem

In addition, there is evidence that cardiac function in these patients is not normal; it is important to assess these patients with echocardiography, but the study is often technically difficult because of the malposition of the heart (Ryan et al, 1994). This cardiac malposition is not corrected by surgical repair of the CDH (Baumgart et al, 1998). It has been reported that left ventricular mass is reduced in CDH and that this may adversely affect the outcome (Schwartz et al, 1994). The cause of the left side reduction in ventricular mass is not clear, but one suggestion is that during development the hernia presses on the left atrium and increases the vascular pressure; left-to-right shunting has been demonstrated in the fetus with diaphragmatic hernia. This reduces the venous return to the left atrium, resulting in underdevelopment of the left heart (Allan et al, 1996). Because there is increased flow in the right heart, pulmonary artery, and ductus arteriosus, these structures appear larger. In addition, the decreased lung size further reduces the venous return to the left atrium, contributing to the decreased left heart development. Experimentally, gene expression of growth factors in cardiac muscle of the rat diaphragmatic hernia model is reduced (Teramoto and Puri, 2001).

### Prediction of Outcome

In an early study, it was found that among infants diagnosed during the first 6 hours of life, the mortality rate was 68%, in those diagnosed at 6 to 24 hours of age the mortality rate was 59%, and in those diagnosed after 24 hours of age the mortality rate was 22% (Raphaely and Downes, 1973). In a more recent study, however, which may reflect improvements in care over time, it was found that in those needing treatment in the first 6 hours of life, the mortality rate was 44%, and in those needing treatment after 6 hours, the mortality rate was close to zero (Marshall and Sumner, 1982). These data imply that if the lungs are good enough to bridge the first 6 hours of life, the results of treatment are likely to be good.

Some investigators believe that the prognosis is best assessed by the arterial $P_{CO_2}$ and the intensity of conventional mechanical ventilation required, as a reflection of the degree of pulmonary hypoplasia. Bohn and coworkers (1987) assessed the mortality in terms of a critical arterial $P_{CO_2}$ of 40 mm Hg and a critical ventilation index of 1000 (where ventilation index is the product of mean airway pressure and ventilator rate). Their data were accumulated before the availability of ECMO. More recently they have used the product of peak inflation pressure and ventilator rate in a modified ventilation index; a value under 1250 with a $P_{CO_2}$ of less than 40 mm Hg indicates only a mild or modest degree of lung hypoplasia (Bohn et al, 1996). Wung and colleagues (1995), however, have reported excellent outcomes in infants who have been managed with gentle ventilation and permissive hypercarbia. This approach makes the predictive value of $Pa_{CO_2}$ much less important.

Wilson and colleagues (1991) and O'Rourke and colleagues (1988) have found that a postductal $Pa_{O_2}$ of greater than 100 mm Hg on at least one occasion during the first 24 hours of life was associated with much better survival (91%) than that in infants who never experienced this so-called honeymoon phenomenon (only 7% survival). Obviously, if this $Pa_{O_2}$ is associated with a normal $Pa_{CO_2}$ without vigorous ventilation, this combination is most promising.

Utilizing the 5-minute Apgar score, birth weight, ventilatory index, and arterial $P_{CO_2}$, Keshen and colleagues (1997) devised a complex regression equation for predicting survival.

Hasegawa and coworkers (1994) demonstrated the predictive value of the ratio of the left and right pulmonary artery dimensions, as measured at echocardiography. If the left artery was smaller than the right artery, severe pulmonary hypoplasia and severe pulmonary hypertension were more likely to be present. Suda and colleagues (2000) examined another echocardiographic index, the ratio of the dimensions for the combined left and right pulmonary arteries to the descending aorta, in assessing the likely outcome of CDH. They found that a value of less than 1.3 predicted death with considerable accuracy. With echocardiography, others have investigated an index of left ventricular mass and function as a tool for predicting survivability and have indicated that the results are promising (Springer et al, 2002).

### Initial Treatment

Mothers with infants known to have CDH should receive betamethasone prophylaxis for surfactant insufficiency, even at term gestation. In infants with a prenatal diagnosis, or as soon as the diagnosis is suspected after birth, a double-lumen orogastric tube should be passed and suctioned continuously to reduce the amount of air in the hernia and decrease compression of the lung. The infant should not be ventilated by bag and mask, but instead should be immediately intubated and ventilated using a low peak pressure (less than 30 cm $H_2O$) if possible and ventilator rates of 20 to 80 breaths/minute. Finer and colleagues (1998), in their protocol for the management of CDH, prefer to keep the peak inflation pressure less than 24 cm $H_2O$ to minimize lung injury. Because the danger of pneumothorax is high, with a substantial increase in risk of death (Hansen et al, 1984), paralysis with pancuronium and sedation with morphine, fentanyl, or sufentanyl are indicated; paralysis provides the additional benefit that swallowing air is abolished, which helps keep the hernia decompressed. Exogenous surfactant should be administered because there is accumulating evidence that the lungs in infants with severe diaphragmatic hernias are immature in addition to being hypoplastic (Bohn et al, 1996; Glick et al, 1992b; Wilcox et al, 1996b). This treatment should be performed very early if possible, because mechanical ventilation of the hypoplastic lung is likely to produce significant barotrauma, lung edema, and surfactant inactivation.

The infant should have an umbilical artery catheter inserted and, if possible, an umbilical vein catheter with its tip at the junction of the inferior vena cava and right atrium. In cases of CDH with the liver in the chest, the catheter does not go through the ductus venous, and it may be advisable not to leave it in place for long. In the absence of an umbilical vein catheter, venous access can be obtained with a Silastic catheter threaded into a central vein or with a larger Broviac catheter inserted by the surgeon. Right-to-left shunting can be followed by the use of pulse oximeters above and below the ductus. Blood pressure support should be given in the form of colloid or crystalloid and continuous dobutamine or dopamine infusion; the mean arterial blood pressure should be maintained at 50 mm Hg or greater to minimize any right-to-left shunt. It is prudent to restrict the volume of fluid administered because pulmonary edema may cause deterioration. Metabolic acidosis may be corrected by administration of sodium bicarbonate or tris(hydroxymethyl)aminomethane (Tham); Finer and colleagues (1998) suggested that the arterial pH should be maintained above 7.25 with the arterial $P_{CO_2}$ less than 60 mm Hg. To avoid excessive ventilation, they also suggested that oxygen saturation levels of 75% to 85% could be tolerated in the first 6 hours of life. An echocardiogram should be performed to assess pulmonary hypertension and left ventricular function. Chromosomal analysis should be undertaken as soon as possible, especially if other malformations are detected. Although the definitive treatment is surgical reduction of the hernia, there is no evidence that the condition constitutes an emergency, and time should be spent in adequately stabilizing the infant with mechanical ventilation (Bohn et al, 1996; Charlton et al, 1992; Goh et al, 1992). If possible, the preductal arterial oxygen saturation should be maintained close to 90%, but high peak pressures over 25 cm $H_2O$ should be avoided. A trial of high-frequency ventilation is often helpful. Inhaled nitric oxide may not be efficacious early in the course of this condition, but it may improve oxygenation modestly for a short time, assisting in the stabilization process. Finally, if all else fails, the infant should be managed using extracorporeal membrane oxygenation (ECMO).

### Advanced Treatment Approaches

#### *Hyperventilation and Alkalization Therapy*

Deliberate attempts to increase the arterial blood pH above 7.50 with the use of hyperventilation and alkali therapy may help to improve oxygenation in infants with pulmonary hypertension. In many centers this was once the only available approach. Using a newborn piglet model, Davis and colleagues (1989) showed that hyperventilation similar to that used in the clinical situation caused severe lung edema, marked lung inflammation and obvious cell necrosis by 48 hours. This therapy is now considered unwise, in view of the effects of hypocarbia on reduced cerebral circulation and neurodevelopmental outcome, and in view of the effects of high airway pressures and tidal volumes on hypoplastic lungs causing pulmonary air leaks and later bronchopulmonary dysplasia (Nobuhara et al, 1996).

#### *Surfactant Replacement Therapy*

There have been several isolated reports of low lecithin-sphingomyelin ratios in the amniotic fluid of mothers at term with a fetus having CDH. Lower levels of surfactant protein A and surfactant phospholipid have been demonstrated in amniotic fluid in the presence of a fetus with CDH (Moya et al, 1995). It has been shown that the alveolar lavage fluid of lambs with a surgically induced diaphragmatic hernia is deficient in surfactant phospholipids and that exogenous surfactant produces marked improvement in the blood gases and lung mechanics of these lambs (Wilcox et al, 1994). Also, in the rat model of CDH, insufficiency of surfactant development has been demonstrated, and lung surfactant maturation can be accelerated with antenatal betamethasone treatment or thyrotropin-releasing hormone (Suen et al, 1993, 1994a, 1994b). In this same rat model, immunostaining for surfactant protein A is reduced in the lungs of rats with a CDH (Mysore et al, 1998). Both in humans and in the lamb model, however, there is no systematic evidence that the lecithin-sphingomyelin ratio and phosphatidylglycerol profile in amniotic fluid samples accurately indicate lung surfactant immaturity (Sullivan et al, 1994; Wilcox et al, 1995b). It is possible that only the ipsilateral lung is immature (George et al, 1987), and this is hidden by the contribution of both lungs to the amniotic fluid samples. Administration of surfactant not only may treat surfactant deficiency and improve compliance but also may lower pulmonary vascular resistance and improve pulmonary blood flow (O'Toole et al, 1996b). Lotze and coworkers (1994) gave repeated doses of bovine surfactant to nine infants on ECMO and compared them with eight air-treated controls; they could find no advantage to surfactant treatment. Surfactant may need to be administered prophylactically to be effective, but not after prolonged periods of mechanical ventilation. Glick and colleagues (1992a) reported the outcomes in three infants, two of them premature, whose CDH was diagnosed prenatally and who were given a bovine surfactant in the delivery room. Although they all were high risk by ultrasound criteria, they all survived without ECMO, and despite there being no controls, the authors considered that exogenous surfactant had played an important part in the outcome. Many clinicians currently administer antenatal betamethasone in addition to prophylactic surfactant at birth.

### *High-Frequency Ventilation*

Tamura and colleagues (1988) reported on two infants with high-risk CDH treated successfully with high-frequency oscillatory ventilation (HFOV); the major advantage was improved control of the arterial $P_{CO_2}$. For infants with severe respiratory failure on maximal conventional mechanical ventilation and approaching ECMO inclusion criteria, the success rate for high-frequency jet ventilation (HFJV) in avoiding ECMO has been reported as 33% (Baumgart et al, 1992), and the success rate for HFOV in avoiding ECMO has been reported as 22% (Paranka et al, 1995). A trial of up to 6 hours of high-frequency ventilation is considered worthwhile, but most responsive patients improve within 1 hour, so the trial need not be prolonged and ECMO need not be unduly delayed. High-frequency ventilation also may be used in patients with less severe pulmonary hypoplasia. Although there is no evidence that high-frequency ventilation is superior to conventional ventilation, it may be a good choice if the patient develops a pneumothorax on conventional ventilation. Cacciari and associates (2001) reported greatly improved survival in infants managed with HFOV, but the comparison was made with historical controls.

### *Inhaled Nitric Oxide*

Inhaled nitric oxide has been used successfully in the treatment of persistent pulmonary hypertension of the newborn (see Chapter 48), and several investigators have tried this therapy in infants with persistent pulmonary hypertension of the newborn complicating the course of CDH (Bohn et al, 1996; Dillon et al, 1995; Finer et al, 1992; Henneberg et al, 1995). However, a multicenter randomized controlled trial of nitric oxide in CDH failed to show any reduction in the need for ECMO or any reduction in the number of deaths (Neonatal Inhaled Nitric Oxide Group, 1997). Karamanoukian and associates (1994) treated CDH infants with nitric oxide and found that before ECMO there was little response, but about 1 week later, after ECMO, the same patients responded to nitric oxide treatment with sustained improvements in oxygenation. In the lamb model of CDH, there was a good response to nitric oxide but only after the animals had received exogenous surfactant treatment (Karamanoukian et al, 1995). It is not yet clear whether this is true for the human infant.

### *Liquid Ventilation*

Observations on the use of perfluorocarbon to distend the lung and provide gas exchange (see Chapter 48) have led to current trials of partial liquid ventilation in infants with CDH, both before and during treatment with ECMO (Pranikoff et al, 1996). Animal studies have been promising (Wilcox et al, 1995a). The results of clinical trials have not been as encouraging as promised, so at this time liquid ventilation has not been approved by the Food and Drug Administration (FDA) for use in humans.

### *Extracorporeal Membrane Oxygenation*

No randomized controlled trials have specifically examined the efficacy of ECMO in the management of CDH. Many centers using ECMO have not seen an improvement in the survival of patients with CDH, but this may be because of a change in the referral pattern to these centers, with more severe cases being sent for treatment. Atkinson and coworkers (1991) analyzed data for infants with an oxygenation index of 40 or more; before the availability of ECMO, the mortality rate was 95%, and after the introduction of ECMO, the mortality rate was 31%. Infants who presented with respiratory distress in the first 6 hours of life were analyzed before and after the introduction of ECMO in the Netherlands (vanden Staak et al, 1995). Patients without exclusion criteria, who were suitable candidates for ECMO, were classified according to whether or not they met ECMO inclusion criteria. Before the availability of ECMO, in those who met ECMO inclusion criteria, the mortality rate was 100%, whereas after the introduction of ECMO, in those who met ECMO inclusion criteria, the mortality rate was 39%, a highly significant improvement.

Although most patients receive venoarterial ECMO, patients receiving venovenous ECMO survive at the same rate (Dimmitt et al, 2001). At present, the standard criteria for ECMO are used in CDH patients, but in general the results with ECMO have not been as good as in other conditions, such as meconium aspiration pneumonia. Attempts have been made to decrease the number of infants subjected to ECMO and to improve the results with ECMO treatment of CDH by changing the inclusion criteria. Some centers require that the patient show evidence of the so-called honeymoon period, in which the postductal arterial $P_{O_2}$ should be at least 100 mm Hg on at least one occasion (O'Rourke et al, 1988; Stolar et al, 1988); otherwise, the patient is considered to have severe pulmonary hypoplasia and not be a candidate for ECMO. Steimle and associates (1994) considered a honeymoon period to be represented by any arterial $P_{O_2}$ greater than 50 mm Hg. When they included infants who never had a honeymoon period, the results with ECMO overall were worse; they found that survival of the additional patients without a honeymoon period was only 27%. They considered lack of a honeymoon period, as they defined it, to be a relative contraindication to ECMO. This approach is associated with improved results only for those subjected to ECMO treatment, not for all cases of CDH.

Other investigators have wanted to use ECMO in more cases (Newman et al, 1990). Clinicians have argued that the overall results for survival in CDH patients might be improved if infants with CDH were started on ECMO earlier, at a higher level of arterial $Po_2$, to take into account that the arterial $Pco_2$ often is elevated in CDH (vanden Staak et al, 1993). No confirmation of this idea has appeared. Evidence suggests that in ECMO-treated patients, compared with similar patients not treated with ECMO, a favorable remodeling of the pulmonary arteries, especially a reduction in thickening of the arterial adventitia, occurs (Shehata et al, 1999; Shehata et al, 2000); this would favor the early use of ECMO.

In the final analysis, the degree of lung hypoplasia, along with the severity of pulmonary vascular disease, determines the outcome with ECMO. The aim of ECMO is to have the patient survive long enough for the reactive component of pulmonary hypertension to resolve, which may take up to 2 to 3 weeks. If there is severe lung hypoplasia with fixed pulmonary hypertension, however, death becomes inevitable. Antunes and coworkers (1995) evaluated the prognosis with preoperative measurements of lung volume by the helium dilution method; there were clear differences among those who survived without ECMO (16 mL/kg), those who survived with ECMO (12 mL/kg), and those who died despite ECMO (5 mL/kg). A lung volume of less than 9 mL/kg delineated infants with such severe lung hypoplasia that they were unlikely to survive, even after prolonged ECMO for up to 4 weeks.

Thibeault and Haney (1998) assessed the lung development of infants with CDH at autopsy, comparing these data with clinical and echocardiographic findings. All infants needing ECMO had pulmonary-to-systemic pressure ratios of near 1.0, and in nearly all such infants these values were reduced to less than 0.5 after 7 to 14 days of ECMO. Even with successful reduction of pulmonary-to-systemic pressure ratios, many of the infants still died, because lung hypoplasia was too severe. These authors considered that infants with lung volume, lung weight, and lung DNA values less than 45% of predicted normal values had lung hypoplasia too severe for survival following ECMO. More recently, and from a clinical point of view, it has been suggested that infants who never achieve a preductal oxygen saturation of at least 85% for at least an hour have lethal pulmonary hypoplasia and are not suitable candidates for ECMO (Boloker et al, 2002). Infants in whom the arterial $Pco_2$ cannot be reduced below 60 mm Hg are also poor candidates for ECMO.

The presence of congenital heart disease is a relative contraindication to ECMO, but only if the lesion is known to be untreatable (Ryan et al, 1994), as in the case in hypoplastic left heart syndrome. Overall, the mortality rate is doubled by the presence of congenital heart disease (Cunnif et al, 1990). When other system anomalies are present, it is important to assess the chromosome status as rapidly as possible to avoid using ECMO in infants with severe genetic problems. This may be difficult in an emergency situation, in which case the clinician may have to start ECMO and withdraw it later.

### *Surgery*

For many years, it was considered imperative to reduce the hernia surgically as soon as possible after birth (Langer et al, 1988). Cartlidge and associates (1986) reported a markedly improved survival when surgery, instead of being done immediately, was delayed for a period of 4 to 16 hours of stabilization; they recommended that surgery not be performed until the pH was at least 7.20. To explore why early surgery may be harmful, Sakai and colleagues (1987) measured the static respiratory system compliance before and after surgery in infants who presented with CDH in the first 6 hours of life and were operated on immediately. The surgical technique included, when considered necessary, the use of abdominal muscle flaps for diaphragm repair and nonclosure of abdominal muscle to avoid overfilling the abdominal cavity. These clinicians found no improvement in compliance after surgery, and most patients had major reductions in compliance, suggesting that surgery had made matters worse. The reduced compliance was thought to be due mostly to tension in the chest wall generated by the repaired diaphragm, and to tension generated by the abdominal wall after closure of the muscle layers, rather than to changes in the lung itself.

In a prospective controlled trial, Nakayama and coworkers (1991) compared a group of infants who had early emergency repair at about 11 hours of age with a group who had delayed repair, many of them after a period of ECMO, at about 5 to 6 days of age. These investigators confirmed that respiratory system compliance was not improved after surgery and was usually decreased, and this was true whether or not the infants had early or delayed surgery. Before surgery, the delayed surgery group demonstrated a significant improvement in respiratory system compliance, which may ultimately have been helpful. The mortality rate in the early surgery group was 54%, whereas in the delayed surgery group it was only 11%. Although the delayed surgery group was thought to have more severe disease initially, the results for delayed surgery looked better; however, results of this study, similar to others before it, may have been misleading because it was not properly randomized.

Nio and colleagues (1994) have reported the results of a randomized, controlled trial of early versus delayed surgical repair of CDH in 32 infants who presented with respiratory distress within 12 hours of birth. All patients were treated with ECMO according to standard criteria. The early surgery group had surgery at about 10 hours of age, and the delayed surgery group had surgery at about the age of 1 week. There was no difference in the need for ECMO or in the mortality rate between the two groups. The authors concluded that if the patient could be adequately stabilized with mechanical ventilation, early surgery was suitable, but if the patient could not be stabilized, preoperative ECMO with delayed surgery was a more reasonable course. The delay in surgery also helps to select patients with a higher likelihood of survival.

## Surgical Management

Some surgeons recommend placement of a thoracostomy tube to protect against the catastrophic development of tension pneumothorax, but the underwater seal should be at atmospheric pressure and not placed to suction. The latter may increase the transpulmonary pressure and overdistend the ipsilateral lung. Others believe that no chest tube should be placed and that air in the pleural cavity should not be removed, to prevent mediastinal displacement and discourage overdistention of the contralateral lung (Cloutier et al, 1983). They believe that overdistention may be sufficient to compress pulmonary capillaries and reduce pulmonary blood flow; Ramenofsky (1979) used a dog model of CDH to show that suction to the ipsilateral pleural space caused overdistention and deterioration of gas exchange, which could be reversed by instillation of air back into the ipsilateral pleural space. No matter what is done concerning the chest tube, every attempt should be made to keep the mediastinum in the midline and not to overdistend the contralateral lung. Such volutrauma may cause high-permeability pulmonary edema with surfactant inactivation. Wung and colleagues (1995) have reported excellent results emphasizing delayed surgery, avoidance of lung overdistention, and no chest tube.

The diaphragmatic defect may be repaired with sutures alone, but because increased tension may compromise total thoracic compliance, a synthetic patch or an abdominal muscle flap procedure may be used (Michalevicz and Chaimoff, 1989). Because abdominal cavity development may be reduced, closure of the abdominal wall may increase tension and cause problems. Surgeons have closed abdominal skin only, with a later repair of the ventral hernia, or they have used patch or silo procedures (Newman et al, 1985; Schnitzer et al, 1995).

### Postoperative Care

Postoperatively, patients often require quite large volumes of colloid to overcome the effects of third-space fluid losses on systemic perfusion. All too commonly, the course is complicated by the development of pulmonary hypertension. If the systemic arterial pressure is not well maintained with inotropics, there may be increased right-to-left shunting at the ductus arteriosus and foramen ovale. There is no evidence that hyperventilation is helpful in these infants; moreover, Wung and colleagues (1995) have been successful using permissive hypercarbia. Attempts to increase pulmonary blood flow with tolazoline, nitroprusside, magnesium sulfate, and other drugs have only occasionally been successful, and if they reduce systemic arterial pressure they may instead be harmful.

The left lung may take only a few days to expand and fully occupy the hemithorax, which means that atelectasis predominated over hypoplasia preoperatively. Otherwise the space initially filled with air becomes filled with fluid. The lung may slowly increase in size over the next few weeks, but in the most severe cases, growth may take several months. Histologically, growth in the number of alveoli and a reduction in the muscle mass of pulmonary arteries are seen, but these improvements are more marked on the contralateral side (Beals et al, 1992), and the time course is such that it is at least a week before improvement occurs.

### Surgery on or off Extracorporeal Membrane Oxygenation

Although delayed surgery has become common, some centers have performed surgery while the patient is still on ECMO (Breaux et al, 1991), and some centers wait until the patient can be taken off ECMO (Adolph et al, 1995). The technique of surgery on ECMO calls for the use of topical thrombin powder or fibrin glue, the use of less heparin with acceptance of shorter activated clotting times (180 to 200 seconds, instead of 200 to 220 seconds), and the use of antifibrinolytic agents (Wilson et al, 1994a). In the experience of many, the incidence of hemorrhagic complications is greater; surgical site hemorrhage requiring transfusion occurred in 38%, 18%, and 6% of cases of CDH repaired on, before, and after ECMO, respectively (Vasquez and Cheu, 1994). It is possible that these complications may contribute to a worse outcome (Lally et al, 1992).

The major reason for performing surgical repair on ECMO is the fear of rebound pulmonary hypertension after decannulation. In a large Canadian experience, however, Sigalet and colleagues (1995) have not found rebound pulmonary hypertension to be a problem in following their strategy of initial stabilization, ECMO if necessary, and delayed surgical repair after decannulation. Although it seems reasonable to temporarily maintain the catheters with concentrated heparin infusions, this approach has not proved practical while maintaining coagulation during surgery, and has been associated with an unacceptable incidence of thrombosis. Some centers find it useful to monitor the patient with serial echocardiography and to decannulate only after the pulmonary artery pressure reaches 30 to 50 mm Hg or a left-to-right shunt appears (Haugen et al, 1991). Some centers may decannulate for surgery and then offer a second course of ECMO if necessary; this approach may be quite useful in the case of CDH (Lally and Breaux, 1995). Surgical reinsertion of the catheters usually has been possible.

### Lobar Lung Transplantation

In infants who come off ECMO, perhaps after a second course, and then have respiratory failure on the ventilator, a few centers now consider lobar lung transplantation as a last resort (Adzick et al, 1985; Adzick, 1992; Van Meurs et al, 1994), but at the present time there are too many difficulties with this approach for it to be widely considered.

## Mortality

In the review by Langham and colleagues (1996), which involved 2024 patients with CDH, the overall mortality rate was 40%, lower in those with isolated lesions and much higher in those with significant other malformations. Nobuhara and associates (1996) reported that the mortality rate among infants without associated malformations was only 16%.

For those presenting in the first 6 hours of life, Adzick and colleagues (1985) found no difference in mortality rate for left-sided versus right-sided hernias, but all infants with bilateral hernias died. The mortality rate for infants with associated polyhydramnios was 89%, compared with 45% for those without associated polyhydramnios; presumably, the polyhydramnios reflects a larger hernia. Prematurity was associated with a higher mortality rate, as expected. The mode of delivery, whether vaginal or abdominal, and immediate surgery after birth made no difference to the outcome. Infants with a prenatal diagnosis and planned delivery have better resuscitation at birth, as reflected in the 5-minute Apgar score, but there is no evidence that this has improved the survival rate.

### Complications Following Treatment of Congenital Diaphragmatic Hernia

Failure to thrive is a common problem following treatment of CDH, even with optimization of caloric intake, possibly due to chronic respiratory distress and increased work of breathing (Nobuhara et al, 1996). Many patients remain below the 25th percentile for weight and have severe oral aversion (Muratore et al, 2001). It is common for infants with CDH to have evidence of esophageal dilation, esophageal dysfunction, and gastroesophageal reflux (Stolar et al, 1990), and some of these infants require a Nissen fundoplication and gastrostomy tube placement in the predischarge phase (Kieffer et al, 1995; Koot et al, 1993; Nagaya et al, 1994; Sigalet et al, 1994). Esophageal dilation and dysfunction are more common in infants who had polyhydramnios before birth, suggesting that the problem is caused by increased mediastinal pressure. There is often a minimal or absent left diaphragmatic crus, with insufficiency of the gastroesophageal junction, and it may be necessary to refashion this at the time of the hernia repair (Sigalet et al, 1994). It is also possible that a tight primary repair of the diaphragm may apply excessive tension at the gastroesophageal junction and that a synthetic patch should be used more often (Kieffer et al, 1995).

Some infants may develop intestinal obstruction related to volvulus and adhesions and require a laparotomy and "adhesionlysis." In a few instances of CDH repaired with a synthetic patch, a recurrent diaphragmatic hernia has developed, sometimes within a few months but often at about the age of 18 months, and the diaphragmatic patch may need to be repaired (Atkinson and Poon, 1992). Other infants have complications associated with chronic bronchitis (with cough), chronic aspiration pneumonitis, and the development of bronchopulmonary dysplasia. Of course, these infants may have the usual complications related to the use of ECMO, other invasive procedures, and indwelling venous catheters; the most notable have been extra-axial fluid collections in the brain, pleural effusions due to chylothorax, and superior vena cava syndrome with acquired hydrothorax.

### Outcome in Survivors

Van Meurs and colleagues (1993) found that neurodevelopmental outcome was the same in ECMO-treated infants with CDH and in ECMO-treated infants with other conditions. This finding may suggest that the outcome is determined by the treatment, not the condition of CDH itself.

D'Agostino and coworkers (1995) provided data for the first year of life in 16 surviving patients who were treated with ECMO during the years 1990 to 1992. Before discharge from the hospital, 13 infants had gastroesophageal reflux; 11 infants were poor oral feeders and needed tube feedings; and 10 infants had bronchopulmonary dysplasia, some of mild severity. At the age of 1 year, 11 infants had symmetrical hypotonia. In addition, three infants still needed ventilatory support for bronchopulmonary dysplasia. On the Bayley Scales of Infant Development, the mean mental score was 87, which was considered to be average, and the mean psychomotor score was 75, indicating a significant level of motor impairment in some infants. The scores were worse in infants who needed a synthetic patch for repair of the diaphragm and were better in those who did not need a patch (an indicator of severity). The authors considered that seven infants had normal cognitive and motor function. Only one out of 14 infants had a significant hearing loss.

Lund and colleagues (1994) followed 33 patients with CDH for a period of 2 to 3 years; 20 of these patients were treated with ECMO. They found deafness needing amplification in seven infants, seizure disorder that resolved by 12 months of age in four infants, developmental delays without evidence of cerebral palsy in 15 infants, and evidence of growth failure in many infants. Findings on head computed tomography scans were abnormal in 10 infants, usually including bifrontal brain atrophy or ventriculomegaly, both of uncertain significance. Six infants needed surgery for bowel obstruction, and six infants needed fundoplication for gastroesophageal reflux. Chest wall deformities were seen in one third of infants, usually pectus excavatum, presumably the result of chronic respiratory distress, and scoliosis developed in four infants, possibly the result of tight diaphragmatic repairs with more tension on one side than the other side. In other series of older children, although the chest radiograph may appear normal, lung volumes are slightly reduced, and there is persistent evidence of a reduced vascular bed in the left lung (Reid and Hutcherson, 1976; Wohl et al, 1977).

### Approaches to Congenital Diaphragmatic Hernia Before Birth

#### *Prenatal Diagnosis*

The pregnant woman whose fetus has CDH may have a low serum alpha-fetoprotein level on the routine screen, or she may present with polyhydramnios. With routine fetal ultrasound examination, most cases of CDH can be found. Findings commonly include polyhydramnios, absence of the abdominal stomach bubble, presence of a thoracic stomach bubble, mediastinal shift to the right, and fetal hydrops caused by obstructed venous return. Associated malformations should be sought. Amniocentesis for cell culture and chromosomal analysis may be helpful. The most likely abnormalities are trisomies 13 and 18, 3 p microdeletion, and 12 p tetrasomy. Associated problems greatly reduce the likelihood of a good outcome. With adequate prenatal diagnosis, the mother may be delivered in a tertiary care center and adequate preparation made for delivery of the infant.

#### *Assessment of the Risk before Birth*

It is important to know the mortality with conventional therapy when assessing the suitability of other therapies such as fetal surgery. There has been controversy over how to assess the results of therapy for CDH, especially whether the denominator should be all fetuses with the condition or all those infants referred for surgical treatment.

Harrison (1994) and Adzick (1985, 1989) and their colleagues at the University of California, San Francisco, have produced evidence that CDH is associated with large hidden mortality that is not reflected in the results reported from ECMO referral centers. A significant number of infants have associated lethal malformations, some are stillborn, some either are electively not resuscitated in the delivery room or cannot be resuscitated despite the best efforts of clinicians, and some are not transported to an appropriate center for surgery and ECMO. These authors concluded that when the diagnosis is made before birth, the true mortality rate is about 60% for those without lethal malformations and about 80% for the total population; this contrasts with the results from ECMO referral centers, which report mortality rates of 20% to 40%, depending on the patients included.

Two other groups of investigators, however, have failed to find relevant differences in mortality rates for those diagnosed before birth versus those diagnosed after birth (Sharland et al, 1992; Wilson et al, 1994b). Most of the difference was explained by a higher incidence of lethal malformations in those with a prenatal diagnosis. It is doubtful that prenatal diagnosis alone indicates an increased risk of death, but it may be that prenatal diagnosis is precipitated by an event such as polyhydramnios that may be associated with a poor prognosis.

It is a logically appealing notion that the earlier in gestation the hernia occurs and the larger the hernia, the more severe the degree of pulmonary hypoplasia and the worse the outcome. To improve the results, Harrison and coworkers (1993a, 1993b) suggested surgical reduction of the hernia before 30 weeks of gestation, and for this to be a viable alternative form of therapy, they needed to identify the fetus at greatest risk. In a group of infants who all had antenatal diagnosis, Adzick and colleagues (1989) found evidence that diagnosis before 24 weeks of gestation and the development of polyhydramnios, usually after 24 weeks, were poor prognostic signs. This finding has not been absolutely confirmed. After exclusion of malformations, Sharland and associates (1992) reported a 72% mortality rate for those diagnosed before 25 weeks of gestation and a 52% mortality rate for those diagnosed later in gestation. Wilson and colleagues (1994b) indicated a similar trend in their subpopulation of infants with prenatal diagnosis.

Harrison and coworkers (1994) found in a homogeneous group of infants, all of whom had prenatal diagnosis before 24 weeks of gestation, that the true mortality rate, after excluding malformations, was 58%, compared with a 37% mortality rate if only infants reaching an ECMO center were considered. Thus, in those with a prenatal diagnosis and without associated malformations, the evidence suggests that diagnosis before 24 weeks of gestation may be associated with a worse outcome; this may justify consideration for fetal surgery. Other data have suggested that the presence of polyhydramnios (Adzick et al, 1985), the presence of the liver in the left hemithorax (Albanese et al, 1998), the presence of stomach in the thoracic hernia (Burge et al, 1989; Hatch et al, 1992), a reduced lung-thorax area ratio (Kamata et al, 1992), a reduced right lung–to–head ratio (Lipschutz et al, 1997; Mychaliska et al, 1996), or a reduced left ventricular mass (Crawford et al, 1989; Sharland et al, 1992), all possibly reflections of a large hernia, also may predict a bad outcome and may be useful in selecting suitable candidates for fetal surgery. Recently, it has been shown that the prenatal magnetic resonance image also may be used to assess the fetal lung volume; in CDH, the median value for the observed-to-expected lung volume is markedly reduced and is much lower in patients who die than in those who survive (Mahieu-Caputo et al, 2001).

### *Fetal Surgical Repair of the Hernia*

The group at the University of California, San Francisco, performed fetal surgical repair of CDH before 30 weeks of gestation in highly selected cases (Harrison et al, 1990). One of the many difficulties of fetal surgery is in removal of the liver from the chest without kinking the umbilical vein and compromising the umbilical circulation (Harrison et al, 1993b). In their first summary, Harrison and colleagues reported that they operated on six infants chosen from a total of 45; three died intraoperatively, one died at birth, and two died in the late neonatal period. In their second summary, these investigators (1993a) reported that they operated on 14 new infants chosen from a total of 61 additional infants; five died during operation, three died within 48 hours after operation (these were considered fetal deaths), two died of prematurity, and four were survivors, none of whom needed ECMO. In a situation in which the investigators expected 40% survival, they obtained only a 30% survival. Furthermore, not all clinicians agree with the criteria used for selection; the prenatal identification of patients with the most severe lung hypoplasia, those most likely to fail after ECMO, remains a significant problem (Weinstein and Stolar, 1993). In addition, postsurgical premature labor with premature birth is a constant threat to the success of fetal surgery (Longaker et al, 1991). The National Institutes of Health sponsored a randomized trial of fetal surgical repair of CDH, excluding those cases with the liver included in the hernia (Harrison et al, 1997). It was concluded that there was no improvement in survival with fetal surgery over that obtained with the conventional approach, and there was no reduction in the requirement for ventilator or ECMO support. This approach has now been abandoned.

### *Tracheal Plug Operations on the Fetus with Congenital Diaphragmatic Hernia*

Several other approaches to fetal surgery have been suggested. DiFiore and coworkers (1994) and Hedrick and colleagues (1994) found that tracheal ligation in the lamb CDH model caused the lungs to enlarge with lung fluid, resulting in reduction of the hernia and excellent lung growth. As lung distention with saline does not have the same effect, it is clear that growth factors are important. Bealer and colleagues (1995) have used translaryngeal insertion of a hydrophilic plug to obstruct the trachea of fetal lambs; the plug can be removed at birth. On tissue examination, there is increased DNA content with a normal DNA-protein ratio, indicating substantial cell proliferation. The morphology appears more mature, with thin alveolar septal walls. The vascular development is greatly improved with abnormal muscular hypertrophy reduced (Bratu et al, 2001; Kanai et al, 2001; Sylvester et al, 1998); the resistance to blood flow is improved, and a more normal response to oxygen is restored in the pulmonary circulation. Despite these promising results, tracheal ligation had an adverse effect on the surfactant system, and granular pneumocytes were severely injured (O'Toole et al, 1997; Piedboeuf et al, 1997). Ongoing clinical trials of this technique have not produced definitive results (Mychaliska et al, 1996). Initially, a foam plug was inserted in the fetal trachea using an endoscopic technique, but tracheal injury resulted; a tracheal clip or a small balloon has since been used. Harrison and colleagues (1996) reported a series of eight human fetuses operated on at late second trimester, and there was only one survivor. They (1998) reported a further series of 34 cases, but the total survival in fetuses treated with tracheal occlusion was the same as in infants treated after birth. Several other single cases have been reported, but the results are not encouraging. Porter (1999) indicated after review that fetal tracheal occlusion offers no improvement over the standard clinical approach to CDH. Some centers continue to offer this approach in the most severe cases of isolated CDH: those with gestation of less than 26 weeks, with liver herniation present and a small lung-to-head ratio (Kitano et al, 1999). The use of lung growth factors in the future may offer a better approach to this problem.

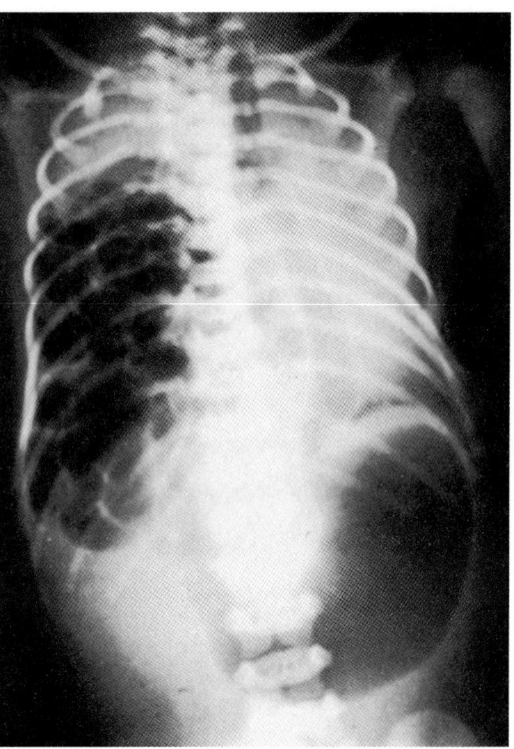

**FIGURE 51–4.** Right-sided congenital diaphragmatic hernia with herniated bowel in the right hemithorax and heart displaced further into the left hemithorax.

### Unilateral Agenesis of the Diaphragm

Among 31 newborns with CDH presenting in the first 6 hours of life, Muraskas and coworkers (1993) reported eight cases of unilateral diaphragmatic agenesis, in which no remnant of skeletal muscle could be found at the subcostal margin. A prenatal diagnosis was more common in agenesis of the diaphragm. Other investigators have found lower Apgar scores and a longer period of preoperative stabilization in this condition (Tsang et al, 1995). The affected infants have more severe gas exchange problems and more severe bilateral pulmonary hypoplasia than even in fatal cases of CDH. Despite repair with a synthetic patch and despite the use of ECMO, the outcome is frequently fatal, and the long-term survival rate is reported as less than 30%. Various muscle flap procedures have been described for the surgical construction of the hemidiaphragm (Samarakkody et al, 2001). Diaphragmatic agenesis has been observed more often in recent years, presumably because of antenatal diagnosis and the improved ability to resuscitate infants and transport them to referral centers. This group of infants should be considered separately in assessing the results for CDH.

### Right-Sided Diaphragmatic Hernia of Delayed Onset

This condition should not be confused with a right-sided hernia that is present at birth, as discussed earlier. Because the liver is a large organ, herniation into the thorax may be a slow process and may occur after birth only with the onset of breathing. The lung problem reflects compression atelectasis rather than hypoplasia, and the right basal mass may present a confusing appearance on the chest radiograph of the newborn infant (Fig. 51–4). The right leaf of the diaphragm may appear elevated, as in eventration or paralysis of the diaphragm. Alternatively, the clinician may think that the patient has a right basal pneumonia or a pleural effusion; some patients have had a chest tube placed, which may injure the liver. The abdominal gas pattern on the right side may appear higher than usual and the lower edge of the liver more horizontal. Ultrasonography or a radionuclide liver scan usually indicates that the liver location is excessively high. There has been an unexplained association of this condition with group B streptococcal sepsis (Handa et al, 1992); it may be that increased negative pleural pressures and increased positive abdominal pressures encourage herniation into the chest.

### Eventration of the Diaphragm

Eventration of the diaphragm results from insufficient muscle development or the absence of phrenic nerves, so that the diaphragm is replaced by a fibrous sheet. An eventration may be localized or diffuse, and most cases of the latter type are unilateral, frequently on the left side. Many cases, especially those that are localized, produce no clinical signs. When eventration is severe, however, newborns have significant respiratory distress. There may be lung hypoplasia on the affected side and, if the mediastinum is shifted, even hypoplasia on the contralateral side. In addition, basal lung compression may cause atelectasis, poor drainage, and complicating bronchopneumonia. The diagnosis is suspected from undue elevation of the diaphragm

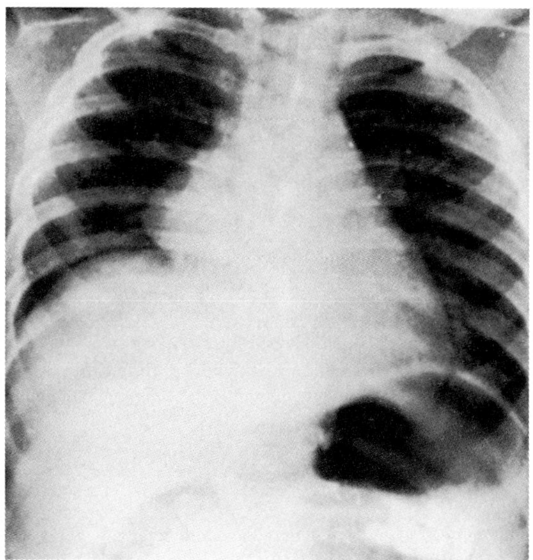

**FIGURE 51–5.** Eventration of the diaphragm in a 3-month-old asymptomatic infant; the right hemidiaphragm is moderately elevated.

seen on frontal and lateral chest radiographs and may be confirmed by fluoroscopy or ultrasound examination (Fig. 51–5). The major cause of confusion is a paralyzed diaphragm, but evidence for birth trauma or thoracotomy is absent in eventration. The diaphragm may show minimal motion during breathing, or the motion may be paradoxical, rising with inspiration and falling with expiration. In those cases in which signs are persistent, the treatment of choice is surgical plication (Goldstein and Reid, 1980; Wayne et al, 1974). Follow-up evaluation of patients with plicated diaphragms suggests that the functional outcomes are good in nearly all cases (Kizilcan et al, 1993).

## Paralysis of the Diaphragm

Diaphragmatic paralysis may occur in either of two clinical situations: after birth trauma or after thoracotomy.

### *Birth Trauma*

Although diaphragmatic paralysis sometimes is bilateral, most cases are unilateral, on the right side. The usual presentation is with respiratory distress, produced largely by overactivity of the normal hemidiaphragm. In cases of bilateral paralysis, however, there is cyanosis and a poor breathing effort that necessitates mechanical ventilation. The infants are usually large and have other signs of birth trauma. There is excessive stretching of the C3 to C5 nerve roots in the neck. The diaphragm is an especially important respiratory muscle in the newborn. Furthermore, during active sleep, the intercostals are inhibited, the supine position of the newborn pushes the paralyzed diaphragm upward, and the newborn is especially prone to muscle fatigue. The diagnosis is suggested on the chest radiograph if the right hemidiaphragm is two intercostal spaces higher than the left or if the left hemidiaphragm is one intercostal space higher than the right (Fig. 51–6). On fluoroscopy or ultrasound examination, the involved diaphragm shows either limited or paradoxical motion (Ambler et al, 1985). There may be associated basal atelectasis, which explains why some infants are markedly improved by nasal continuous positive airway pressure. When both hemidiaphragms are paralyzed, these infants require prolonged mechanical ventilation (Aldrich et al, 1980). Although many improve over 2 weeks, further improvement is possible over a period of 2 months. Once it is believed no further improvement will occur, and the patient cannot be weaned from ventilatory support, surgical plication of the diaphragm should be performed.

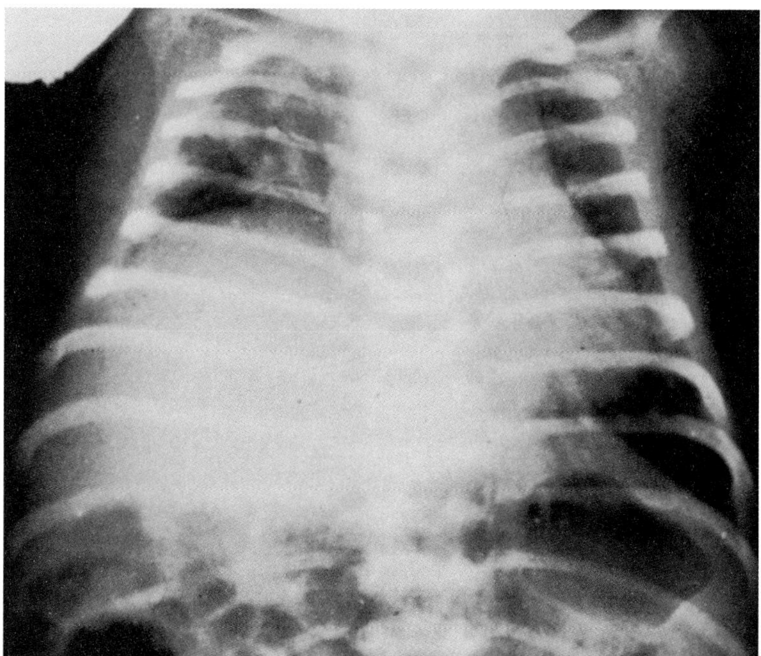

**FIGURE 51–6.** Right-sided diaphragmatic paralysis associated with a difficult delivery and a right-sided Erbs palsy; the right diaphragm is moderately elevated. The infant had tachypnea.

### Post-Thoracotomy

Diaphragmatic paralysis from phrenic nerve trauma is a known reason for failure to wean from mechanical ventilation after a thoracic operation, such as ligation of patent ductus arteriosus, creation of a systemic pulmonary shunt, or repair of a tracheoesophageal fistula. Management is similar to that for paralysis after birth trauma.

## REFERENCES

Adolph V, Flageole H, Perreault T, et al: Repair of congenital diaphragmatic hernia after weaning from extracorporeal membrane oxygenation. J Pediatr Surg 30:349, 1995.

Adzick NS: On the horizon: Neonatal lung transplantation. Arch Dis Child 67:455, 1992.

Adzick NS, Harrison MR, Glick PL, et al: Diaphragmatic hernia in the fetus: Prenatal detection and outcome in 94 cases. J Pediatr Surg 20:357, 1985.

Adzick NS, Vacanti JP, Lillehei CW, et al: Fetal diaphragmatic hernia: Ultrasound diagnosis and clinical outcome in 38 cases. J Pediatr Surg 24:654, 1989.

Albanese CT, Lopoo J, Goldstein RB, et al: Fetal liver position and perinatal outcome for congentital diaphragmatic hernia. Prenatal Diagnosis 18:1138, 1998.

Aldrich TK, Herman JH, Rochester DF: Bilateral diaphragmatic paralysis in the newborn infant. J Pediatr 97:988, 1980.

Allan LD, Irish MS, Glick PL: The fetal heart in diaphragmatic hernia. Clin Perinatol 23:795, 1996.

Ambler R, Gruenewald S, John E: Ultrasound monitoring of diaphragm activity in bilateral diaphragmatic paralysis. Arch Dis Child 60:170, 1985.

Antunes MJ, Greenspan JS, Cullen JA, et al: Prognosis with preoperative pulmonary function and lung volume assessment in infants with congenital diaphragmatic hernia. Pediatrics 96:1117, 1995.

Atkinson JB, Ford EG, Humphries B, et al: The impact of extracorporeal membrane support in the treatment of congenital diaphragmatic hernia. J Pediatr Surg 26:791, 1991.

Atkinson JB, Poon MW: ECMO and the management of congenital diaphragmatic hernia with large diaphragmatic defects requiring a prosthetic patch. J Pediatr Surg 27:754, 1992.

Azizkhan RG, Canfield J, Alford BA, et al: Pleuroperitoneal shunts in the management of neonatal chylothorax. J Pediatr Surg 18:842, 1983.

Baumgart S, Hirschl R, Butler SZ, et al: Diagnosis related criteria in the consideration of extracorporeal membrane oxygenation in neonates previously treated with high frequency jet ventilation. Pediatrics 89:491, 1992.

Baumgart S, Paul JJ, Huhta JC, et al: Cardiac malposition, redistribution of fetal cardiac output, and left heart hypoplasia reduce survival in neonates with congenital diaphragmatic hernia requiring extracorporeal membrane oxygenation. J Pediatr 133:57, 1998.

Bealer JF, Skarsgard ED, Hedrick MH, et al: The PLUG odyssey: Adventures in experimental fetal tracheal occlusion. J Pediatr Surg 30:361, 1995.

Beals DA, Schloo BL, Vacanti JP, et al: Pulmonary growth and remodeling in infants with high risk congenital diaphragmatic hernia. J Pediatr Surg 27:997, 1992.

Bohn DJ, Pearl R, Irish MS, Glick PL: Postnatal management of congenital diaphragmatic hernia. Clin Perinatol 23:843, 1996.

Bohn D, Tamura M, Perrin D, et al: Ventilatory predictors of pulmonary hypoplasia in congenital diaphragmatic hernia, confirmed by morphologic assessment. J Pediatr 111:423, 1987.

Boloker J, Bateman DA, Wung JT, et al: Congenital diaphragmatic hernia in 120 infants treated consecutively with permissive hypercapnea/spontaneous respiration/elective surgery. J Pediatr Surg 37:357, 2002.

Bratu I, Flageole H, Laberge JM, et al: Pulmonary structural maturation and pulmonary remodeling after reversible fetal ovine tracheal occlusion in diaphragmatic hernia. J Pediatr Surg 36:739, 2001.

Breaux CW, Rouse TM, Cain WS, Georgeson KE: Improvement in survival of patients with congenital diaphragmatic hernia utilizing a strategy of delayed repair after medical and/or extracorporeal membrane oxygenation stabilization. J Pediatr Surg 26:333, 1991.

Brodman RF: Congenital chylothorax: Recommendations for treatment. N Y State J Med 75:553, 1975.

Buettiker V, Hug MI, Burger R, et al: Somatostatin: A new therapeutic option for the treatment of chylothorax. Intensive Care Med 27:1083, 2001.

Burge DM, Atwell JD, Freeman NV: Could the stomach site help predict outcome in babies with left sided congenital diaphragmatic hernia diagnoses antenatally? J Pediatr Surg 24:567, 1989.

Cacciari A, Ruggeri G, Mordenti M, et al: High frequency oscillatory ventilation versus conventional mechanical ventilation in congenital diaphragmatic hernia. Eur J Pediatr Surg 11:3, 2001.

Cantrell JR, Haller JA, Ravitch MM: A syndrome of congenital defects involving the abdominal wall, sternum, diaphragm, pericardium and heart. Surg Gynecol Obstet 107:602, 1958.

Cartlidge PHT, Mann NP, Kapila L: Pre-operative stabilisation in congenital diaphragmatic hernia. Arch Dis Child 61:1226, 1986.

Charlton AJ, Bruce J, Davenport M: Timing of surgery in congenital diaphragmatic hernia: Low mortality after pre-operative stabilization. Anaesthesia 46:820, 1992.

Chernick V, Reed MH: Pneumothorax and chylothorax in the neonatal period. J Pediatr 76:624, 1970.

Chervenak FA, Isaacson G, Blakemore KJ, et al: Fetal cystic hygroma: Cause and natural history. N Engl J Med 309:822, 1983.

Cloutier R, Fournier L, Levasseur L: Reversion to fetal circulation in congenital diaphragmatic hernia: A preventable postoperative complication. J Pediatr Surg 18:551, 1983.

Crawford DC, Wright VM, Drake DP, Allan LD: Fetal diaphragmatic hernia: The value of fetal echocardiography in the prediction of postnatal outcome. Br J Obstet Gynaecol 96:705, 1989.

Cunnif C, Jones KL, Jones MC: Patterns of malformation in children with congenital diaphragmatic defects. J Pediatr 116:258, 1990.

D'Agostino JA, Bernbaum JC, Gerdes M, et al: Outcome for infants with congenital diaphragmatic hernia requiring extracorporeal membrane oxygenation: The first years. J Pediatr Surg 30:10, 1995.

Davis JT, Heistein JB, Castille RG, et al: Lateral thoracic expansion for Jeune's syndrome: Midterm results. Ann Thorac Surg 72:872, 2001.

Davis JT, Penney DP, Notter RH, et al: Lung injury in the neonatal piglet caused by hyperoxia and mechanical ventilation. J Appl Physiol 67:1007, 1989.

Devine PC, Malone FD: Noncardiac thoracic anomalies. Clin Perinatol 27:865, 2000.

Dhande V, Kattwinkel J, Alford B: Recurrent bilateral pleural effusions secondary to superior vena cava obstruction as a complication of central venous catheterization. Pediatrics 72:109, 1983.

DiFiore JW, Fauza DO, Slavin R, et al: Experimental fetal tracheal ligation reverses the structural and physiological effects of pulmonary hypoplasia in congenital diaphragmatic hernia. J Pediatr Surg 29:248, 1994.

Dillon PW, Cilley RE, Hudome SM, et al: Nitric oxide reversal of recurrent pulmonary hypertension and respiratory failure in an infant with CDH after successful ECMO therapy. J Pediatr Surg 30:743, 1995.
Dimmitt RA, Moss RL, Rhine WD, et al: Venoarterial versus venovenous extracorporeal membrane oxygenation in congenital diaphragmatic hernia; the Extracorporeal Life Support Organization Registry 1990-1999. J Pediatr Surg 36:1199, 2001.
Dutheil P, Leraillez J, Guillemette J, Wallach D: Generalized lymphangiomatosis with chylothorax and skin lymphangiomas in a neonate. Pediatr Dermatol 15:296, 1998.
Eddleman KA, Levine AB, Chitkara U, et al: Reliability of pleural fluid lymphocyte counts in the antenatal diagnosis of congenital chylothorax. Obstet Gynecol 78:530, 1991
Fauza DO, Wilson JM: Congenital diaphragmatic hernia and associated anomalies: Their incidence, identification, and impact on prognosis. J Pediatr Surg 29:1113, 1994.
Fernandez Alvarez JR, Kalache KD, Grauel EL: Management of spontaneous congenital chylothorax: Medium chain triglycerides versus total parenteral nutrition. Am J Perinatol 16:415, 1999.
Finer NN, Tierney AL, Hallgren R, et al: Neonatal congenital diaphragmatic hernia and extracorporeal membrane oxygenation. Can Med Assoc J 146:501, 1992.
Finer NN, Tierney A, Etches PC, et al: Congenital diaphragmatic hernia: Developing a protocolized approach. J Pediatr Surg 33:1331, 1998.
Geggel RL, Murphy JD, Langleben D, et al: Congenital diaphragmatic hernia: Arterial structural changes and persistent pulmonary hypertension after surgical repair. J Pediatr 107:457, 1985.
George K, Cooney TP, Chiu BK, et al: Hypoplasia and immaturity of the terminal lung unit (acinus) in congenital diaphragmatic hernia. Am Rev Respir Dis 136:947, 1987.
Glick PL, Irish MS, Holm BA (eds): New insights into the pathophysiology of congenital diaphragmatic hernia. Clin Perinatol 23, 1996.
Glick PL, Leach CL, Besner GE, et al: Pathophysiology of congenital diaphragmatic hernia: III. Exogenous surfactant therapy for the high risk neonate with CDH. J Pediatr Surg 27:866, 1992a.
Glick PL, Stannard VA, Leach CL, et al: Pathophysiology of congenital diaphragmatic hernia: II. The fetal lamb model is surfactant deficient. J Pediatr Surg 27:382, 1992b.
Goh DW, Drake DP, Brereton RJ, et al: Delayed surgery for congenital diaphragmatic hernia. Br J Surg 79:644, 1992.
Goldstein JD, Reid LM: Pulmonary hypoplasia resulting from phrenic nerve agenesis and diaphragmatic amyoplasia. J Pediatr 97:282, 1980.
Handa N, Suita S, Shono T, Kukita J: Right sided diaphragmatic hernia following group B streptococcal pneumonia and sepsis. J Pediatr Surg 27:764, 1992.
Hansen J, James S, Burrington J, Whitfield J: The decreasing incidence of pneumothorax and improving survival of infants with congenital diaphragmatic hernia. J Pediatr Surg 19:385, 1984.
Harrison MR, Adzick NS, Bullard K, et al: Correction of congenital diaphragmatic hernia in utero VII: A prospective trial. J Pediatr Surg 31:1637, 1997.
Harrison MR, Adzick NS, Estes JM, Howell LJ: A prospective study of the outcome for fetuses with diaphragmatic hernia. JAMA 271:382, 1994.
Harrison MR, Adzick NS, Flake AW, et al: Correction of congenital diaphragmatic hernia in utero VI: Hard earned lessons. J Pediatr Surg 28:1411, 1993a.
Harrison MR, Adzick NS, Flake AW, et al: Correction of congenital diaphragmatic hernia in utero VIII: Response of the hypoplastic lung to tracheal occlusion. J Pediatr Surg 31:1339, 1996.
Harrison MR, Adzick NS, Flake AW, Jennings RW: The CDH two-step: A dance of necessity. J Pediatr Surg 28:813, 1993b.
Harrison MR, Adzick NS, Longaker MT, et al: Successful repair in utero of a fetal diaphragmatic hernia after removal of herniated viscera from the left chest. N Engl J Med 322:1582, 1990.
Harrison MR, Mychaliska GB, Albanese CT, et al: Correction of congenital diaphragmatic hernia in utero IX: Fetuses with poor prognosis (liver herniation and low lung to head ratio) can be saved by fetoscopic temporary tracheal occlusion. J Pediatr Surg 33:1017, 1998.
Hasegawa S, Kohno S, Sugiyama T, et al: Usefulness of echocardiographic measurement of bilateral pulmonary artery dimensions in congenital diaphragmatic hernia. J Pediatr Surg 29:622, 1994.
Hatch EI, Kendall J, Blumhagen J: Stomach position as an in utero predictor of neonatal outcome in left sided diaphragmatic hernia. J Pediatr Surg 27:778, 1992.
Haugen SE, Linker D, Eik-Nes S, et al: Congenital diaphragmatic hernia: Determination of the optimal time for operation by echocardiographic monitoring of the pulmonary arterial pressure. J Pediatr Surg 26:560, 1991.
Hedrick MH, Estes JM, Sullivan KM, et al: Plug the lung until it grows (PLUG): A new method to treat congenital diaphragmatic hernia in utero. J Pediatr Surg 29:612, 1994.
Henneberg SW, Jepsen S, Andersen PK, Pedersen SA: Inhalation of nitric oxide as a treatment of pulmonary hypertension in congenital diaphragmatic hernia. J Pediatr Surg 30:853, 1995.
Jesudason EC, Connell MG, Fernig DG, et al: In vitro effects of growth factors on lung hypoplasia in a model of congenital diaphragmatic hernia. J Pediatr Surg 35:914, 2000.
Jeune N, Cararon B, Berand C, et al: Polychondrodystrophie avec blocage thoracique d'évolution fatale. Pediatrie 9:390, 1954.
Kamata S, Hasegawa T, Ishikawa S, et al: Prenatal diagnosis of congenital diaphragmatic hernia and perinatal care: Assessment of lung hypoplasia. Early Hum Dev 29:375, 1992.
Kanai M, Kitano Y, von Allmen D, et al: Fetal tracheal occlusion in the rat model of nitrofen induced congenital diaphragmatic hernia: Tracheal occlusion reverses the arterial structural abnormality. J Pediatr Surg 36:839, 2001.
Karamanoukian HL, Glick PL, Wilcox DT, et al: Pathophysiology of congenital diaphragmatic hernia: VIII. Inhaled nitric oxide requires exogenous surfactant therapy in the lamb model of congenital diaphragmatic hernia. J Pediatr Surg 30:1, 1995.
Karamanoukian HL, Glick PL, Zayek M, et al: Inhaled nitric oxide in congenital hypoplasia of the lungs due to diaphragmatic hernia or oligohydramnios. Pediatrics 94:715, 1994.
Kavanagh M, Battistini B, Jean S, et al: Effect of ABT-627 (A-147627), a potent ET(A) receptor antagonist, on the cardiopulmonary profile of newborn lambs with surgically induced diaphragmatic hernia. Br J Pharmacol 134:1679, 2001.
Keshen TH, Gursoy M, Shew SB, et al: Does extracorporeal membrane oxygenation benefit neonates with congenital diaphragmatic hernia? Application of a predictive equation. J Pediatr Surg 32:818, 1997.
Kieffer J, Sapin E, Berg A, et al: Gastro-esophageal reflux after repair of congenital diaphragmatic hernia. J Pediatr Surg 30:1330, 1995.
Kitano Y, Flake AW, Crombleholme TM, et al: Open fetal surgery for life threatening fetal malformations. Semin Perinatol 23:448, 1999.
Kizilcan F, Tanyel FC, Hicsonmez A, et al: The long term results of diaphragmatic plication. J Pediatr Surg 28:42, 1993.
Kobayashi H, Puri P: Plasma endothelin levels in congenital diaphragmatic hernia. J Pediatr Surg 29:1258, 1994.

Kling DE, Narra V, Islam S, et al: Decreased mitogen activated protein kinase activities in congenital diaphragmatic hernia associated pulmonary hypoplasia. J Pediatr Surg 36:1490, 2001.

Kohler E, Babbitt DP: Dystrophic thoraces and infantile asphyxia. Radiology 94:55, 1970.

Koot VCM, Bergmeijer JH, Bos AP, Molenaar JC: Incidence and management of gastroesophageal reflux after repair of congenital diaphragmatic hernia. J Pediatr Surg 28:48, 1993.

Lally KP, Breaux CW: A second course of extracorporeal membrane oxygenation in the neonate—is there a benefit? Surgery 117:175, 1995.

Lally KP, Paranka MS, Roden J, et al: Congenital diaphragmatic hernia: Stabilization and repair on ECMO. Ann Surg 216:569, 1992.

Langer JC, Filler RM, Bohn DJ, et al: Timing of surgery for congenital diaphragmatic hernia: Is emergency operation necessary? J Pediatr Surg 23:731, 1988.

Langham MR, Kays DW, Ledbetter DJ, et al: Congenital diaphragmatic hernia: Epidemiology and outcome. Clin Perinatol 23:671, 1996.

Lipschutz GS, Albanese CT, Feldstein VA, et al: Prospective analysis of lung to head ratio predicts survival in patients with prenatally diagnosed congenital diaphragmatic hernia. J Pediatr Surg 32:1634, 1997.

Longaker MT, Golbus MS, Filly RA, et al: Maternal outcome after fetal surgery: A review of the first 17 human cases. JAMA 265:737, 1991.

Lotze A, Knight GR, Andersen KD, et al: Surfactant (beractant) therapy for infants with congenital diaphragmatic hernia on ECMO: Evidence of persistent surfactant deficiency. J Pediatr Surg 29:407, 1994.

Lund DP, Mitchell J, Kharasch V, et al: Congenital diaphragmatic hernia: The hidden morbidity. J Pediatr Surg 29:258, 1994.

Mahieu-Caputo D, Sonigo P, Dommergues M, et al: Fetal lung volume measurement by magnetic resonance imaging in congenital diaphragmatic hernia. Br J Obstet Gynecol 108:863, 2001.

Maier HC, Bortone F: Complete failure of sternal fusion with herniation of pericardium. J Thorac Surg 18:851, 1949.

Marshall A, Sumner E: Improved prognosis in congenital diaphragmatic hernia: Experience of 62 cases over 2 year period. J R Soc Med 75:607, 1982.

Mellins RB, Levine OR, Fishman AP: Effect of systemic and pulmonary venous hypertension on pleural and pericardial fluid accumulation. J Appl Physiol 29:564, 1970.

Michalevicz D, Chaimoff C: Use of a Silastic sheet for widening the abdominal cavity in the surgical treatment of diaphragmatic hernia. J Pediatr Surg 24:265, 1989.

Miyazaki E, Ohshiro K, Taira Y, et al: Altered insulin-like growth factor I mRNA expression in human hypoplastic lung in congenital diaphragmatic hernia. J Pediatr Surg 33:1476, 1998.

Moise AA, Gest AL, Weickmann PH, et al: Reduction in plasma protein does not affect body water content in fetal sheep. Pediatr Res 29:623, 1991.

Morin L, Crombleholme TM, D'Alton ME: Prenatal diagnosis and management of fetal thoracic lesions. Semin Perinatol 18:228, 1994.

Moya FR, Thomas VL, Romaguera J, et al: Fetal lung maturation in congenital diaphragmatic hernia. Am J Obstet Gynecol 173:1401, 1995.

Muraskas JK, Husain A, Myers TF, et al: An association of pulmonary hypoplasia with unilateral agenesis of the diaphragm. J Pediatr Surg 28:999, 1993.

Muratore CS, Utter S, Jaksic T, et al: Nutritional morbidity in survivors of congenital diaphragmatic hernia. J Pediatr Surg 36:1171, 2001.

Mychaliska GB, Bullard KM, Harrison MR: In utero management of congenital diaphragmatic hernia. Clin Perinatol 23:823, 1996.

Mysore MR, Margraf LR, Jaramillo MA, et al: Surfactant protein A is decreased in a rat model of congenital diaphragmatic hernia. Am J Respir Crit Care 157:654, 1998.

Nagaya M, Akatsuka H, Kato J: Gastroesophageal reflux occurring after repair of congenital diaphragmatic hernia. J Pediatr Surg 29:1447, 1994.

Nakayama DK, Motoyama EK, Tagge EM: Effect of preoperative stabilization on respiratory system compliance and outcome in newborn infants with congenital diaphragmatic hernia. J Pediatr 118:793, 1991.

Neonatal Inhaled Nitric Oxide Study Group (NINOS): Inhaled nitric oxide and hypoxic respiratory failure in infants with congenital diaphragmatic hernia. Pediatrics 99:838, 1997.

Newman BM, Jewett TC, Lewis A, et al: Prosthetic materials and muscle flaps in the repair of extensive diaphragmatic defects: An experimental study. J Pediatr Surg 20:362, 1985.

Newman KD, Anderson KC, Van Meurs K, et al: Extracorporeal membrane oxygenation and congenital diaphragmatic hernia: Should any infant be excluded? J Pediatr Surg 25:1048, 1990.

Nguyen L, Guttman FM, DeChadarevian JP, et al: The mortality of congenital diaphragmatic hernia: Is total pulmonary mass inadequate, no matter what? Ann Surg 198:766, 1983.

Nio M, Haase G, Kennaugh J, et al: A prospective randomized trial of delayed versus immediate repair of congenital diaphragmatic hernia. J Pediatr Surg 29:618, 1994.

Njolstad PR, Reigstad H, Westby J, Espeland A: Familial non-immune hydrops fetalis and congenital pulmonary lymphangiectasia. Eur J Pediatr 157:498, 1998.

Nobuhara KK, Lund DP, Mitchell J, et al: Long term outlook for survivors of congenital diaphragmatic hernia. Clin Perinatol 23:873, 1996.

Oberkaid F, Danks DM, Mayne V, et al: Asphyxiating thoracic dysplasia: Clinical, radiological and pathological information on 10 patients. Arch Dis Child 52:758, 1977.

O'Rourke PP, Vacanti JP, Crone RK, et al: Use of the postductal $PaO_2$ as a predictor of pulmonary vascular hypoplasia in infants with congenital diaphragmatic hernia. J Pediatr Surg 23:904, 1988.

O'Toole SJ, Irish MS, Holm BA, Glick PL: Pulmonary vascular abnormalities in congenital diaphragmatic hernia. Clin Perinatol 23:781, 1996a.

O'Toole SJ, Karamanoukian HL, Morin FC III, et al: Surfactant decreases pulmonary vascular resistance and increases pulmonary blood flow in the fetal lamb model of CDH. J Pediatr Surg 31:507, 1996b.

O'Toole SJ, Karamanoukian HL, Irish MS, et al: Tracheal ligation: The dark side of in utero congenital diaphragmatic hernia treatment. J Pediatr Surg 32:407, 1997.

Paranka MS, Clark RH, Yoder BA, Null DM: Predictors of failure of high frequency oscillatory ventilation in term infants with severe respiratory failure. Pediatrics 95:400, 1995.

Piedboeuf B, Laberge JM, Ghitulescu G, et al: Deleterious effect of tracheal obstruction on type 2 pneumocytes in fetal sheep. Pediatr Res 41:473, 1997.

Porter HJ: Pulmonary hypoplasia. Arch Dis Child 81:F81, 1999.

Pranikoff T, Gauger PH, Hirschl RB: Partial liquid ventilation in newborn patients with congenital diaphragmatic hernia. J Pediatr Surg 31:613, 1996.

Prontera W, Jaeggi ET, Pfizenmaier M, et al: Ex utero intrapartum treatment (EXIT) of severe fetal hydrothorax. Arch Dis Child 86:F58, 2002.

Ramenofsky ML: The effects of intrapleural pressure on respiratory insufficiency. J Pediatr Surg 14:750, 1979.

Raphaely RC, Downes JJ: Congenital diaphragmatic hernia: Prediction of survival. J Pediatr Surg 8:815, 1973.

Reid IS, Hutcherson RJ: Long-term follow-up of patients with congenital diaphragmatic hernia. J Pediatr Surg 11:939, 1976.

Rodeck CH, Fisk NM, Fraser DI, et al: Long term in utero drainage of fetal hydrothorax. N Engl J Med 319:1135, 1988.

Ryan CA, Perreault T, Johnston-Hodgson A, Finer NN: Extracorporeal membrane oxygenation in infants with congenital diaphragmatic hernia and cardiac malformations. J Pediatr Surg 29:878, 1994.

Sabiston DC: The surgical management of congenital bifid sternum with partial ectopia cordis. J Thorac Surg 35:118, 1958.

Sakai H, Tamura M, Hosokawa Y, et al: Effect of surgical repair on respiratory mechanics in congenital diaphragmatic hernia. J Pediatr 111:432, 1987.

Samarakkody U, Klaassen M, Nye B: Reconstruction of congenital agenesis of hemidiaphragm by combined reverse latissimus dorsi and serratus anterior muscle flaps. J Pediatr Surg 36:1637, 2001.

Schmidt W, Harms E, Wolf D: Successful prenatal treatment of nonimmune hydrops fetalis due to congenital chylothorax: Case report. Br J Obstet Gynaecol 92:685, 1985.

Schnitzer JJ, Kikiros CS, Short BL, et al: Experience with abdominal wall closure for patients with congenital diaphragmatic hernia repaired on ECMO. J Pediatr Surg 30:19, 1995.

Schwartz SM, Vermilion RP, Hirschl RB: Evaluation of left ventricular mass in children with left sided congenital diaphragmatic hernia. J Pediatr 125:447, 1994.

Sharland GK, Lockhart SM, Heward AJ, Allan LD: Prognosis in fetal diaphragmatic hernia. Am J Obstet Gynecol 166:9, 1992.

Shehata SM, Mooi WJ, Okazaki T, et al: Enhanced expression of vascular endothelial growth factor in lungs of newborn infants with congenital diaphragmatic hernia and pulmonary hypertension. Thorax 54:427, 1999.

Shehata SM, Tibboel D, Sharma HS, et al: Impaired structural remodelling of pulmonary arteries with congenital diaphragmatic hernia: A histological study of 29 cases. J Pathol 189:112, 1999.

Shehata SM, Sharma HS, van der Staak FH, et al: Remodeling of pulmonary arteries in human congenital diaphragmatic hernia with or wihout extracorporeal membrane oxygenation. J Pediatr Surg 35:208, 2000.

Sigalet DL, Nguyen LT, Adolph V, et al: Gastroesophageal reflux associated with large diaphragmatic hernias. J Pediatr Surg 29:1262, 1994.

Sigalet DL, Tierney A, Adolph V, et al: Timing of repair of congenital diaphragmatic hernia requiring extracorporeal membrane oxygenation support. J Pediatr Surg 30:1183, 1995.

Smeltzer DM, Stickler GB, Fleming RE: Primary lymphatic dysplasia in children: Chylothorax, chylous ascites, and generalized lymphatic dysplasia. Eur J Pediatr 145:286, 1986.

Springer SC, Fleming D, Hulsey TC: A statistical model to predict nonsurvival in congenital diaphragmatic hernia. J Perinatol 22:263, 2002.

Steimle CN, Meric F, Hirschl RB, et al: Effect of extracorporeal life support on survival when applied to all patients with congenital diaphragmatic hernia. J Pediatr Surg 29:997, 1994.

Stenzl W, Rigler B, Tscheliessnigg KH, et al: Treatment of postsurgical chylothorax with fibrin glue. Thorac Cardiovasc Surg 31:35, 1983.

Stolar C, Dillon P, Reyes C: Selective use of extracorporeal membrane oxygenation in the management of congenital diaphragmatic hernia. J Pediatr Surg 23:207, 1988.

Stolar CJH, Levy JP, Dillon PW, et al: Anatomic and functional abnormalities of the esophagus in infants surviving congenital diaphragmatic hernia. Am J Surg 159:204, 1990.

Stringel G, Mercer S, Bass J: Surgical management of persistent postoperative chylothorax in children. Can J Surg 27:543, 1984.

Suda K, Bigras J, Bohn D, et al: Echocardiographic predictors of outcome in newborns with congenital diaphragmatic hernia. Pediatrics 105:1106, 2000.

Suen HC, Bloch KD, Donahue PK: Antenatal glucocorticoid corrects pulmonary immaturity in experimentally induced congenital diaphragmatic hernia in rats. Pediatr Res 35:523, 1994a.

Suen HC, Catlin EA, Ryan DP, et al: Biochemical immaturity of lungs in congenital diaphragmatic hernia. J Pediatr Surg 28:471, 1993.

Suen H, Losty P, Donahue P, et al: Combined antenatal thyrotrophin-releasing hormone and low-dose glucocorticoid therapy improves the pulmonary biochemical immaturity in congenital diaphragmatic hernia. J Pediatr Surg 29:359, 1994b.

Sullivan KM, Hawgood S, Flake AW, et al: Amniotic fluid phospholipid analysis in the fetus with congenital diaphragmatic hernia. J Pediatr Surg 29:1020, 1994.

Sylvester KG, Rasanen J, Kitano Y, et al: Tracheal occlusion reverses the high impedance to flow in the fetal pulmonary circulation and normalizes its physiological response to oxygen at full term. J Pediatr Surg 33:1071, 1998.

Tamura M, Tsuchida Y, Kawano T, et al: Piston pump type high frequency oscillatory ventilation for neonates with congenital diaphragmatic hernia: A new protocol. J Pediatr Surg 23:478, 1988.

Teramoto H, Puri P: Gene expression of insulin like growth factor-1 and epidermal growth factor is downregulated in the heart of rats with nitrofen induced diaphragmatic heria. Pediatr Surg Int 17:284, 2001.

Thebaud B, Barlier-Mur AM, Chailley-Heu B, et al: Restoring effects of vitamin A on surfactant synthesis in nitrofen induced congenital diaphragmatic hernia in rats. Am J Respir Crit Care Med 164:1083, 2001.

Thibeault DW, Zalles C, Wickstrom C: Familial pulmonary lymphatic hypoplasia associated with fetal pleural effusions. J Pediatr 127:979, 1995

Thibeault DW, Haney B: Lung volume, pulmonary vasculature, and factors affecting survival in congenital diaphragmatic hernia. Pediatrics 101:289, 1998

Tsang TM, Tam PKH, Dudley NE, Stevens J: Diaphragmatic agenesis as a distinct clinical entity. J Pediatr Surg 30:16, 1995.

vanden Staak FHJM, De Haan AFJ, Geven WB, et al: Improving survival for patients with high risk congenital diaphragmatic hernia by using extracorporeal membrane oxygenation. J Pediatr Surg 30:1463, 1995.

vanden Staak FHJ, Thiesbrummel A, de Haan AFJ, et al: Do we use the right entry criteria for extracorporeal membrane oxygenation in congenital diaphragmatic hernia? J Pediatr Surg 28:1003, 1993.

Van Meurs KP, Rhine WD, Benitz WE, et al: Lobar lung transplantation as a treatment for congenital diaphragmatic hernia. J Pediatr Surg 29:1557, 1994.

Van Meurs KP, Robbins ST, Reed VL, et al: Congenital diaphragmatic hernia: Long term outcome in neonates treated with extracorporeal membrane oxygenation. J Pediatr 122:893, 1993.

Vasquez WD, Cheu HW: Hemorrhagic complications and repair of congenital diaphragmatic hernias: Does timing of the repair make a difference? Data from the Extracorporeal Life Support Organization. J Pediatr Surg 29:1002, 1994.

Wayne ER, Campbell JB, Burrington JD, et al: Eventration of the diaphragm. J Pediatr Surg 9:643, 1974.

Weinstein S, Stolar CJH: Newborn surgical emergencies: Congenital diaphragmatic hernia and extracorporeal membrane oxygenation. Pediatr Clin North Am 40:1315, 1993.

Welch KJ: Chest wall deformities. In Holder TM, Ashcraft KW (eds): Pediatric Surgery. Philadelphia, WB Saunders, 1980, p 162.

Wiener-Kronish JP, Berthiaume Y, et al: Pleural effusions and pulmonary edema. Clin Chest Med 6:509, 1985.

Wilcox DT, Glick PL, Karamanoukian H, et al: Pathophysiology of congenital diaphragmatic hernia: V. Effect of exogenous surfactant therapy on gas exchange and lung mechanics in the lamb congenital diaphragmatic hernia model. J Pediatr 124:289, 1994.

Wilcox DT, Glick PL, Karamanoukian H, et al: Perflubron associated gas exchange improves pulmonary mechanics, oxygenation, ventilation and allows nitric oxide delivery in the hypoplastic lung congenital diaphragmatic hernia lamb model. Crit Care Med 23:1858, 1995a.

Wilcox DT, Glick PL, Karamanoukian H, et al: Pathophysiology of congenital diaphragmatic hernia: XII. Amniotic fluid lecithin/sphingomyelin ratio and phosphatidylglycerol concentrations do not predict surfactant status in congenital diaphragmatic hernia. J Pediatr Surg 30:410, 1995b.

Wilcox DT, Irish MS, Holm BA, Glick PL: Prenatal diagnosis of congenital diaphragmatic hernia with predictors of mortality. Clin Perinatol 23:701, 1996a.

Wilcox DT, Irish MS, Holm BA, Glick PL: Pulmonary parenchymal abnormalities in congenital diaphragmatic hernia. Clin Perinatol 23:771, 1996b.

Wilson JM, Bower LK, Lund DP: Evolution of the technique of congenital diaphragmatic hernia repair on ECMO. J Pediatr Surg 29:1109, 1994a.

Wilson JM, Fauza DO, Lund DP, et al: Antenatal diagnosis of isolated congenital diaphragmatic hernia is not an indicator of outcome. J Pediatr Surg 29:815, 1994b.

Wilson JM, Lund DP, Lillehei CW, Vacanti JP: Congenital diaphragmatic hernia: Predictors of severity in the ECMO era. J Pediatr Surg 26:1028, 1991.

Wohl MEB, Griscou NT, Strieder DJ, et al: The lung following repair of congenital diaphragmatic hernia. J Pediatr 90:405, 1977.

Wung JT, Sahni R, Moffitt ST, et al: Congenital diaphragmatic hernia: Survival treated with very delayed surgery, spontaneous respiration, and no chest tube. J Pediatr Surg 30:406, 1995.

Yamamoto T, Koeda T, Tamura A, et al: Congenital chylothorax in a patient with 21 trisomy syndrome. Acta Paediatr Jpn 38:689, 1996.

# CARDIOVASCULAR SYSTEM

Editors: **ROBERTA A. BALLARD** and **GIL WERNOVSKY**

PART XI

CHAPTER 52

# Nomenclature and the Segmental Approach to Congenital Heart Disease

**Tal Geva**

The spectrum of congenital anomalies of the cardiovascular system is infinite, ranging from benign anatomic variations without clinical implications to complex and lethal anomalies. A comprehensive scheme for classification of congenital heart disease (CHD) based on clear and consistent nomenclature is therefore essential for diagnosis, management, and research. Since the publication of Maude Abbott's seminal *Atlas of Congenital Cardiac Disease* in 1936, many classification schemes have been proposed, each adding a building block to the knowledge and understanding of CHD. The goals of any classification system for CHD are (1) to provide a consistent nomenclature based on anatomic-morphologic features of the cardiac chambers; (2) to devise a systematic analytic approach that produces a specific and unique set of diagnoses for each congenital cardiac malformation; (3) to be applicable to all forms of CHD, including predictable cardiac malformations that have not yet been described; and (4) to promote understanding and exchange of data among clinicians and researchers.

This chapter describes a segment-by-segment approach to the classification and nomenclature of congenital anomalies of the heart and great vessels. This classification system, known as the *segmental approach to congenital heart disease*, was originally proposed by Van Praagh and his colleagues in the 1960s and early 1970s (Van Praagh, 1964, 1966, 1967). It has since been refined by its originators as well as by many other investigators in the fields of developmental biology and embryology, cardiology, cardiovascular surgery, pathology, radiology, and others (Anderson et al, 1984a, 1984b; de la Cruz and Nadal-Ginard, 1972; Freedom, 1984; Lev, 1966; Lev et al, 1971; Rao, 1981; Shinebourne et al, 1976; Stanger et al, 1977; Tynan et al, 1979; Van Praagh, 1984a, 1984b, 1985; Weinberg, 1986).

## SEGMENTAL ANALYSIS OF CONGENITAL HEART DISEASE

Segmental analysis of CHD is based on an understanding of the development, morphology, and segmental anatomy of the heart and great vessels. The cardiac segments are the anatomic and embryologic building blocks that form the mammalian heart (Fig. 52–1). The three *main segments* are (1) the atria, (2) the ventricles, and (3) the great arteries. There are two *connecting segments* between the main segments: (1) the atrioventricular (AV) canal and (2) the conus, or infundibulum. The AV canal consists of the AV valves (the mitral and tricuspid valves in normally formed hearts) and the atrioventricular septum. The infundibulum, or conus, is the connecting segment between the ventricles and the great arteries. In normally formed hearts, the infundibulum consists of a circumferential subpulmonary myocardium with muscular separation between the pulmonary and tricuspid valves and partial absence of the subaortic infundibular myocardium that results in fibrous continuity between the aortic and mitral valves.

The fundamental principle of the segmental approach to CHD is to analyze each component of the heart in a sequential, step-by-step fashion. First, the anatomic pattern (i.e., situs) of the abdominal and thoracic organs is defined and the position of the heart is described. Then, each of the main cardiac segments is examined, described, and assigned a designation based on its unique morphologic features, independent of neighboring segments (Fig. 52–2). For example, each ventricle is defined according to its intrinsic morphology and not by the entering AV valve or the exiting great artery.

Analysis of the main cardiac chambers—atria, ventricles, and great arteries—involves two steps. First, the *identity* of the chamber or great vessel is defined according to its morphology and intrinsic myocardial architecture. For example, the right and left atria are so designated according to their morphology, not according to their spatial location. Second, the *situs* of the cardiac segment is determined. In the case of the atria, there are three possible configurations: situs solitus (normal), situs inversus, and situs ambiguus (indeterminate).

Once the three main cardiac chambers are characterized according to their unique morphologic features, the connecting segments are analyzed and defined. Finally, a complete set of diagnostic categories is formulated by combining the five cardiac segments and all associated cardiovascular anomalies, as described in the following section.

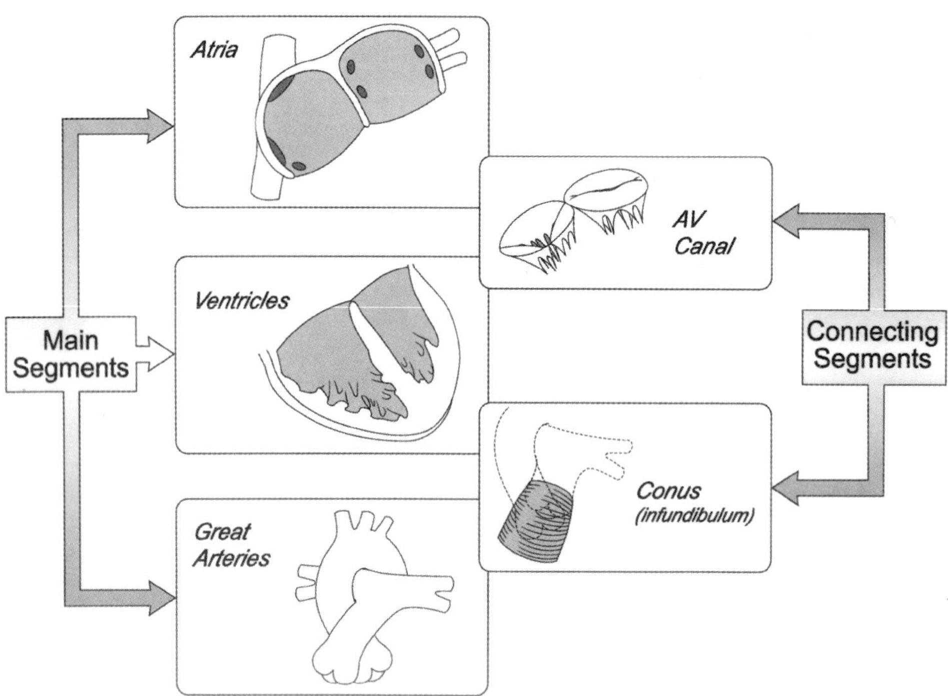


**FIGURE 52–1.** Anatomic segments of the heart. The three main cardiac segments are the atria, ventricles, and great arteries. There are two connecting segments: the atrioventricular (AV) canal (including the AV valves and the interatrial and interventricular components of the AV canal septum) and the conus (or infundibulum). The connecting segments may be viewed as multidirectional joints between the main cardiac segments, allowing infinite possibilities of AV and ventriculoarterial alignments. Essential to the segmental approach to congenital heart disease is that each cardiac segment must be analyzed separately and independent of adjacent segments.

## STEP-BY-STEP SEGMENTAL ANALYSIS

The segmental approach to CHD comprises ten steps, each focusing on a specific anatomic-morphologic component, as follows.

**1. Thoracoabdominal Situs** (Fig. 52–3)
Before the intracardiac anatomy is considered, the situs of the thoracic and abdominal organs is determined to provide an anatomic framework for further analysis. Normally, the visceral organs are "lateralized." In other words, the pattern of anatomic organization of the abdominal organs, tracheobronchial tree, and lungs is asymmetrical. In *situs solitus*, the spleen, pancreas, stomach, and sigmoid colon are left-sided; the liver, cecum, and appendix are right-sided; the left lung is bilobed; the left main bronchus is longer and more horizontal compared with the right main bronchus, and the right lung is trilobed. In visceral *situs inversus*, the spatial organization of the abdominal and thoracic organs is mirror-imaged. In other words, there is complete left-right reversal of the position and orientation of the organs. It is worth noting that in visceral situs inversus, the pattern of anatomic organization is asymmetrical as it is in situs solitus. In *situs ambiguus*, the spatial position and orientation of the abdominal and thoracic organs are abnormally symmetrical and inconsistent. For example, the spleen may be absent, the liver may be midline, both lungs may be bilobed or trilobed, and the bronchi may be similar to each other in length and orientation. Situs ambiguus is typically associated with heterotaxy syndrome, a condition characterized by partial or complete lack of lateralization of the visceral organs, splenic anomalies, congenital heart disease, and extracardiac anomalies. In many patients with heterotaxy syndrome, visceral situs cannot be clearly designated as solitus or inversus—hence the term *situs ambiguus* is used. However, the anatomic organization of the visceral organs in these patients is often partially lateralized, allowing for determination of a "predominant situs." For example, when the stomach is right-sided and the inferior vena cava is left-sided, the predominant abdominal situs is situs inversus, even though the liver may be midline. In such circumstances it is possible to assign a designation of "situs ambiguus, predominantly inversus" (or "predominantly solitus") for the visceral situs.

**2. Cardiac Position** (Fig. 52–4)
In levocardia, the heart is predominantly in the left hemithorax with a leftward apex. In dextrocardia, the heart is predominantly in the right hemithorax. Primary dextrocardia is defined as a condition in which the heart is in the right hemithorax due to a structural congenital heart defect. In primary dextrocardia the apex usually points to the right. Secondary dextrocardia is a condition in which the heart is either "pushed" or "pulled" toward the right hemithorax as a result of extracardiac abnormalities. Examples of conditions in which the heart is pushed toward the right hemithorax include left-sided tension pneumothorax, left congenital lobar emphysema, and left-sided diaphragmatic hernia. Conditions in which the heart is pulled toward the right hemithorax include hypoplasia and agenesis of the right lung. In secondary

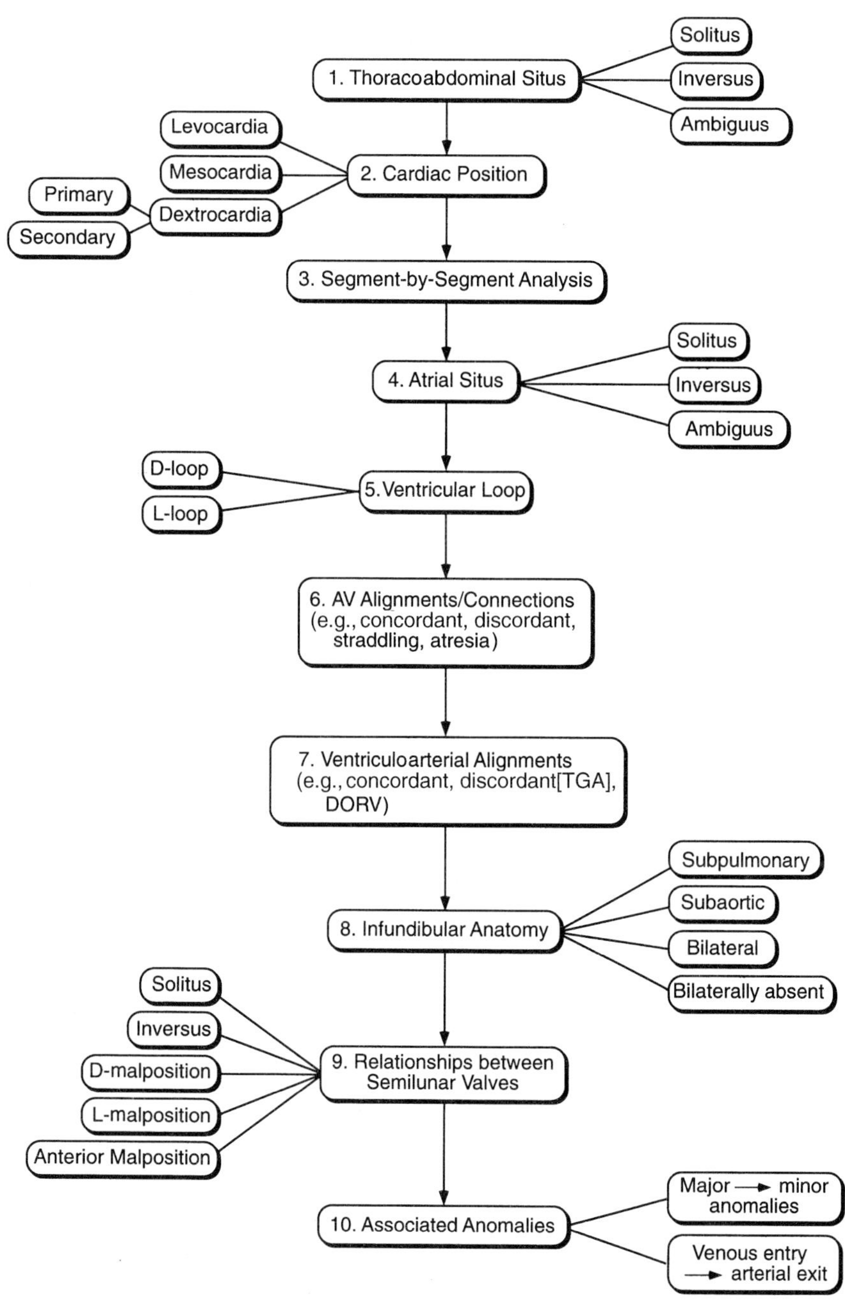


**FIGURE 52–2.** The ten steps of the segmental approach to diagnosis of congenital heart disease. Before analysis of intracardiac anatomy, the situs of the thoracic and abdominal organs and cardiac position within the thorax must be determined to provide an anatomic framework for further analysis (steps 1 and 2). In describing cardiac anatomy, the following three principles apply: (1) Each cardiac segment must be described in terms of its own unique anatomic features and not according to those of adjacent segments (steps 3–9). For example, the left ventricle is identified according to its internal morphology, particularly its smooth superior septal surface, and not according to the AV valve that connects it with the atria (this usually is the mitral valve but may be both the mitral and tricuspid valves, as in double-inlet left ventricle; it may be a common AV valve or even a tricuspid valve). (2) For each cardiac segment, both its situs and connections must be described specifically and not inferred from each other. (3) Associated malformations (step 10) may be described in order of their hemodynamic importance or in an anatomic order (progressing from the venous entry to the arterial exit of the heart).

dextrocardia, the cardiac apex may point to the left or anteriorly. In mesocardia, the heart is midline and the apex typically points anteriorly or inferiorly.

**3. Segment-by-Segment Analysis of Cardiac Anatomy** (see Fig. 52–2)

At this stage, the three main segments and the two connecting segments are analyzed individually (steps 4 through 9 following).

**4. Atrial Situs** (Fig. 52–5)

The first step in determining atrial situs is to identify the atria according to their morphologic characteristics (Table 52–1; see also Fig. 52–5A and B). The right atrium receives the major horn of the sinus venosus, including the superior vena cava, inferior vena cava, and the orifice of the coronary sinus (the cardiac termination of the left horn of the sinus venosus). The right atrial musculature includes the crista terminalis and tinea sagittalis (see Fig. 52–5A). The septal surface of the right atrium features the superior and inferior limbic bands of the fossa ovale. The right atrial appendage is typically broad-based, triangular, and anterior relative to the left atrial appendage (see Fig. 52–5B). In atrial situs solitus (see Fig. 52–5C), the right atrium is right-sided, and in atrial situs inversus, it is left-sided. The left atrium normally receives the pulmonary veins; its septum features septum

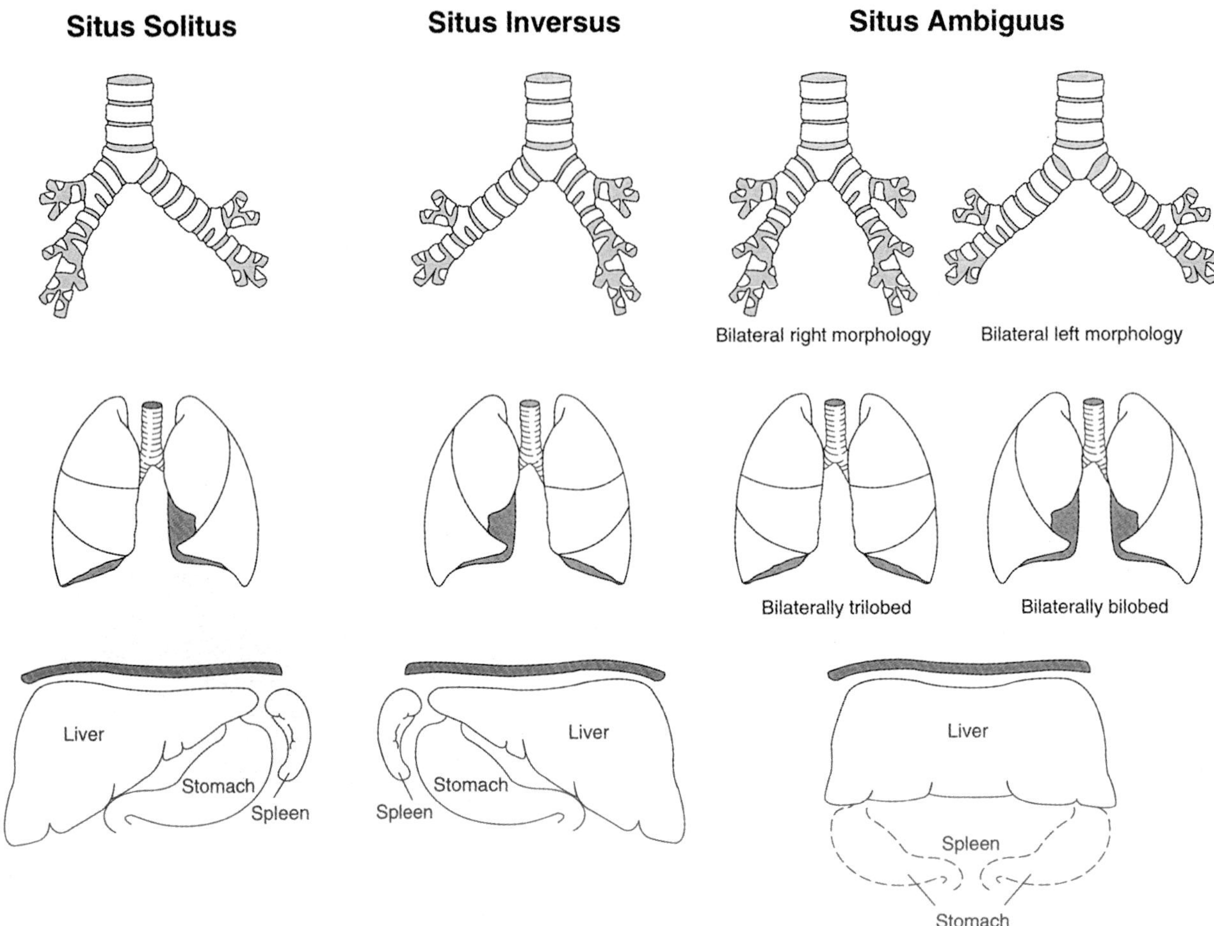


**FIGURE 52–3.** Thoracoabdominal situs. **Top panel,** The morphology of the tracheobronchial tree can be helpful in predicting atrial situs. In situs solitus, the right main bronchus is short and eparterial (its branch for the right upper lobe is over the second branch of the right pulmonary artery) and the left main bronchus is longer and hyparterial (it courses underneath the left pulmonary artery). In situs inversus, the anatomy is a mirror image of that seen in situs solitus. In situs ambiguus, the bronchi can have a bilaterally right or bilaterally left morphology. Bilaterally hyparterial left bronchial morphology can be seen in patients with heterotaxy syndrome and polysplenia, whereas bilaterally eparterial right bronchial morphology is seen in patients with heterotaxy syndrome and asplenia. **Middle panel,** Lung lobation also correlates with atrial situs. A bilobed left lung and a trilobed right lung are typical in situs solitus. In situs inversus, the right lung is bilobed and the left lung is trilobed. As with the tracheobronchial tree, in situs ambiguus the lungs may be bilaterally bilobed or bilaterally trilobed. **Lower panel,** In visceral situs solitus, the liver is right-sided and the stomach and spleen are left-sided. Incomplete lateralization of the abdominal organs with a midline liver and stomach may be seen in patients with heterotaxy syndrome. Splenic anomalies (asplenia, polysplenia, hyposplenia, and a single right-sided spleen) and complex cardiac anomalies are frequent. In patients with heterotaxy syndrome and visceral situs ambiguus, the disposition of the abdominal situs predicts atrial situs less reliably than does the bronchial anatomy.

primum (the flap valve of the foramen ovale) and a narrow-based, elongated posterior appendage. In atrial situs ambiguus, typically seen in patients with heterotaxy syndrome, the anatomic landmarks characteristic of the right and left atria are not sufficient to determine situs (either situs solitus or situs inversus). Often in this situation, the atria are in common, with absence (or presence of only remnants) of the atrial septum, the inferior vena cava is interrupted between the renal and hepatic segments, there are bilateral superior venae cavae, and the coronary sinus is unroofed. The atrial appendages may be quite similar to each other. Although the distribution of the pectinate muscle has been proposed as a useful marker of atrial identity (Uemura et al, 1995), imaging of the pectinate muscle in living patients has not been consistently achieved.

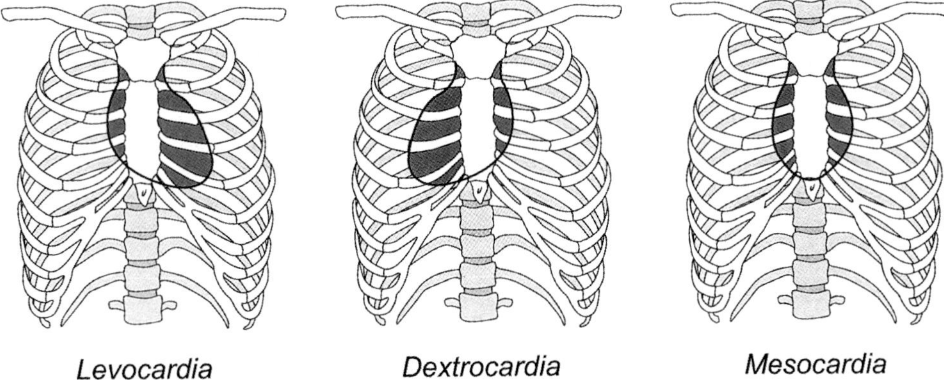


**FIGURE 52–4.** Cardiac position within the thorax. In levocardia, the heart is predominantly in the left hemithorax. In dextrocardia, the heart is predominantly in the right hemithorax. In mesocardia, the heart is midline and the apex typically points anteriorly or inferiorly.

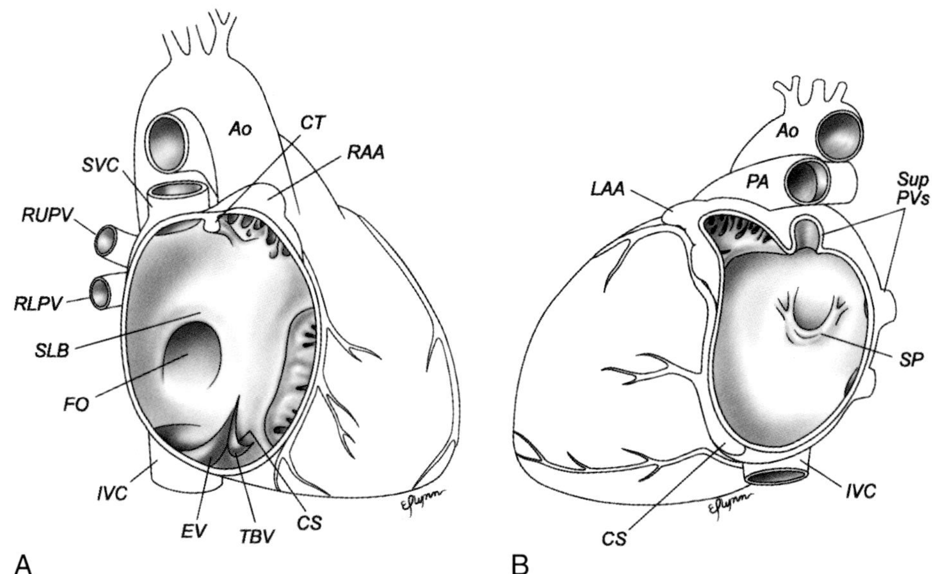


**FIGURE 52–5.** Atrial morphology and situs. **A,** Right atrial morphology: The right atrium (RA) can be divided into three components: 1. The *sinus venosus*, including the orifices of the inferior vena cava (IVC), superior vena cava (SVC), and coronary sinus (CS), which is characterized by its smooth surface (absence of muscular trabeculations). The sinus venosus is separated from the other components of the right atrium by remnants of the embryonic right venous valve system, which includes the thebesian valve (TBV) and the eustachian valve (EV). 2. The *right atrial appendage* (RAA), characterized by a broad-based triangular shape and coarse trabeculations (pectinate muscle). The crista terminalis (CT) is a prominent muscle bar that separates the sinus venosus component of the RA from the trabeculated right atrial appendage and is the site of the sinoatrial node. 3. The *interatrial portion of the AV canal*, which includes the base of the atrial septum and the tricuspid valve annulus. The fossa ovale (FO) forms the interatrial septum and is characterized by an oval-shaped muscular boundary termed *septum secundum*, or *limbus of the fossa ovale*, whereas the floor of the fossa is covered by septum primum. **B,** Left atrial morphology. Similar to the right atrium, the left atrium can also be divided into three components: 1. Pulmonary venous component. 2. Left atrial appendage (LAA), which is narrow-based and elongated. 3. AV canal region, which is bordered distally by the mitral valve annulus. Note the attachments of septum primum (SP) on the left atrial septal surface.

*Continued*

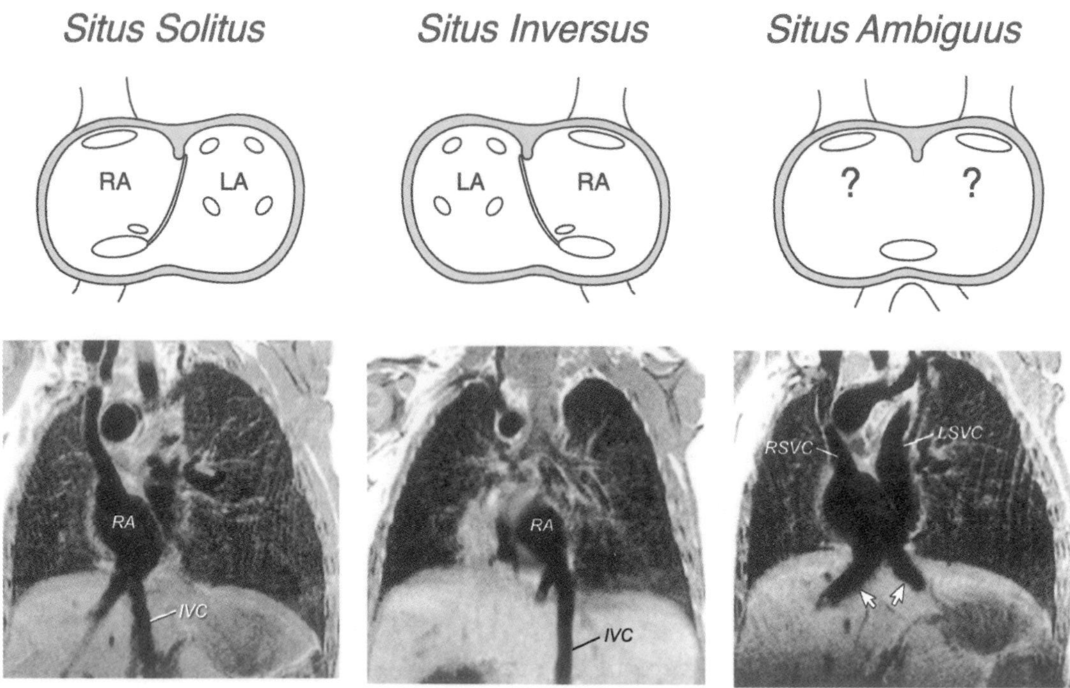


**FIGURE 52–5. Cont'd C,** Diagram of atrial situs. **Upper panel,** In *atrial situs solitus*, the right-sided right atrium receives the major horn of the sinus venosus, including the superior vena cava, inferior vena cava, and the orifice of the coronary sinus. The left-sided left atrium normally receives the pulmonary veins, its septum features septum primum (the flap valve of the foramen ovale) and a narrow-based, elongated posterior appendage (see Table 52–1). In *atrial situs inversus*, the right atrium is left-sided and the left atrium is right-sided. In *atrial situs ambiguus*, typically seen in patients with heterotaxy syndrome, the anatomic landmarks characteristic of the right and left atria are not sufficient to determine situs (either situs solitus or situs inversus). Often in this situation, the atria are in common, with absence (or presence of only remnants) of the atrial septum, the inferior vena cava may be interrupted between the renal and hepatic segments, there may be bilateral superior venae cavae and the coronary sinus may be unroofed. The atrial appendages may be quite similar to each other. **Lower panel,** Coronal plane spin echo MR images in patients with heterotaxy syndrome and atrial situs solitus *(left)*, atrial situs inversus *(middle)*, and atrial situs ambiguus *(right)*. *Ao, aorta; LSVC, left superior vena cava; PA, pulmonary artery; RA, right atrium; RLPV, right lower pulmonary vein; RSVC, right superior vena cava; RUPV, right upper pulmonary vein; SLB, superior limbic band of fossa ovale; Sup PVs, superior pulmonary veins.*

**TABLE 52–1**

**Morphologic Criteria for Identification of the Right Atrium and the Left Atrium**

| Anatomic Feature | Right Atrium | Left Atrium |
|---|---|---|
| Veins | Receives the major horn of the sinus venosus: IVC,* SVC,† CS | Normally receives all pulmonary veins‡ |
| Appendage | Broad-based, triangular, anterior | Narrow, finger-like, posterior |
| Septum | Septum secundum (limbus of the fossa ovale) | Septum primum (valve of the foramen ovale) |
| Musculature | Crista terminalis, tinea sagittalis | Thin, few trabeculations§ |

*In cases with interrupted IVC, the right atrium receives all hepatic veins and CS.

†The SVC is not a reliable marker of the right atrium because a persistent left superior vena cava may drain directly into the left atrium when the CS is unroofed. When the CS is unroofed and the IVC is interrupted, the shape, size, and location of the atrial appendages may be used for identification of atrial situs.

‡The pulmonary veins are not a reliable marker of the left atrium because of their potential for variable connections.

§When a persistent left SVC drains directly into the left atrium, a muscle bar similar to a crista terminalis may be present in the left SVC–left atrium junction.

CS, coronary sinus; IVC, inferior vena cava; SVC, superior vena cava.

**5. Ventricular Loop** (Fig. 52–6)

The first step in determining the ventricular loop (situs) is to identify the left and right ventricles. It is important to recognize that between the AV and the semilunar valves (what is generally considered the ventricular mass of the heart), there are three distinct chambers: the left ventricle, the right ventricular sinus, and the infundibulum (or conus) (Geva et al, 1998; Van Praagh and Van Praagh, 1966, 1967; Van Praagh et al, 1964). The infundibulum is normally well incorporated with the right ventricular sinus, so that their separate identities may be obscured (see Fig. 52–6A and B). However, these chambers have different embryologic and developmental origins. Moreover, in several congenital cardiac anomalies, the infundibulum

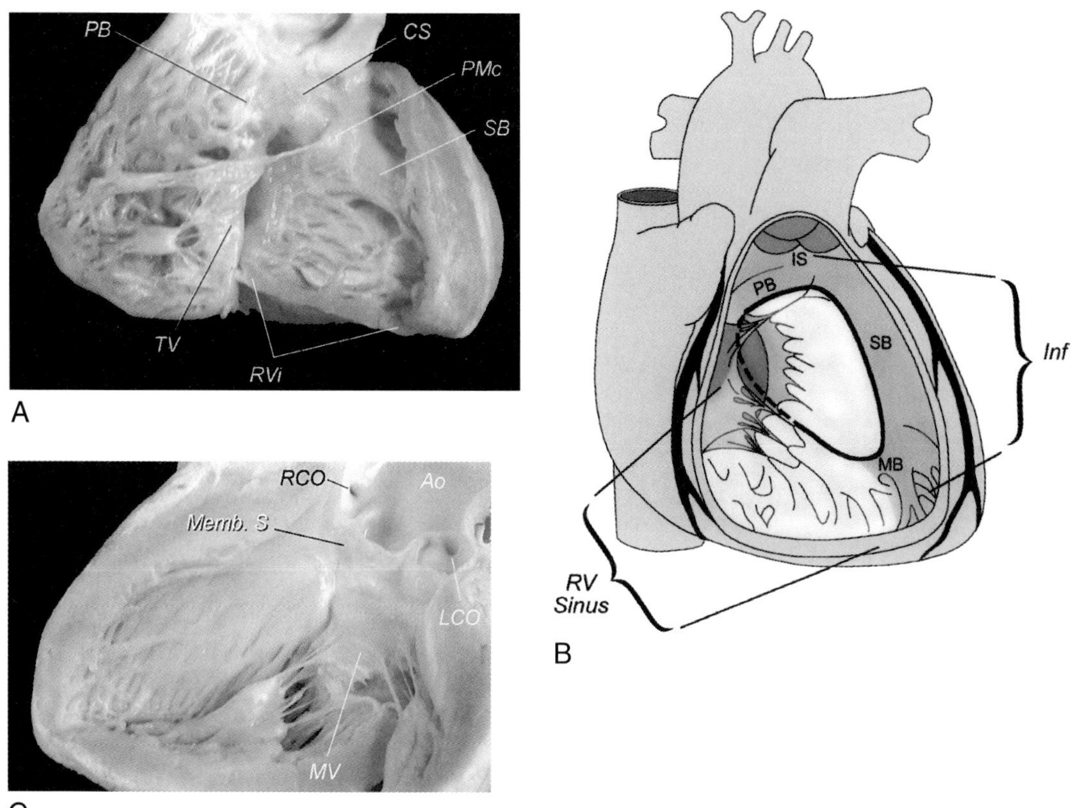


**FIGURE 52–6.** Ventricular morphology and situs. **A,** Right ventricular (RV) morphology. Note the coarse trabeculations and the chordal attachments of the tricuspid valve (TV) to the trabeculated septal surface. PB, parietal band; PMc, papillary muscle of the conus; RVi, right ventricular inflow (sinus). **B,** The normal right ventricle comprises two distinct chambers that are well incorporated into each other: the right ventricular (RV) sinus and the infundibulum (Inf). The boundary between the RV sinus and the infundibulum is termed the *proximal os infundibulum* (shown as a dark ring) and is composed of the parietal band (PB), infundibular septum (IS), septal band (SB), moderator band (MB), and the anterior papillary muscle of the tricuspid valve. The RV sinus may be subdivided into an AV canal portion (underneath the septal leaflet of the tricuspid valve) and the trabecular portion, which extends to the RV apex. The infundibulum may be subdivided into a distal (subpulmonary) portion, which includes the distal portion of septal band (SB), infundibular septum (IS), and parietal band (PB), and the proximal infundibulum, which is typically trabeculated and has its own apex adjacent to the RV sinus apex. **C,** Left ventricular morphology. The most reliable morphologic feature of the left ventricle is its smooth superior septal surface. In the normal left ventricle, the finely trabeculated apex (trabeculae carneae) are quite characteristic. However, in a markedly hypertrophied left ventricle, or in a double-inlet or common-inlet left ventricle, the apical trabeculations may be prominently hypertrophied (similar to the trabeculations seen in the right ventricle). In the normal left ventricle, the mitral valve (MV) attaches to two large groups of papillary muscles that attach to the left ventricular free wall. The aortic valve is in fibrous continuity with the mitral valve due to the absence of an intervening conal musculature in this region. More anteriorly, under the right coronary cusp of the aortic valve, conal musculature comprises the infundibular septum. Ao, aorta; LCO, left coronary orifice; Memb. S, membranous septum; RCO, right coronary orifice.

*Continued*

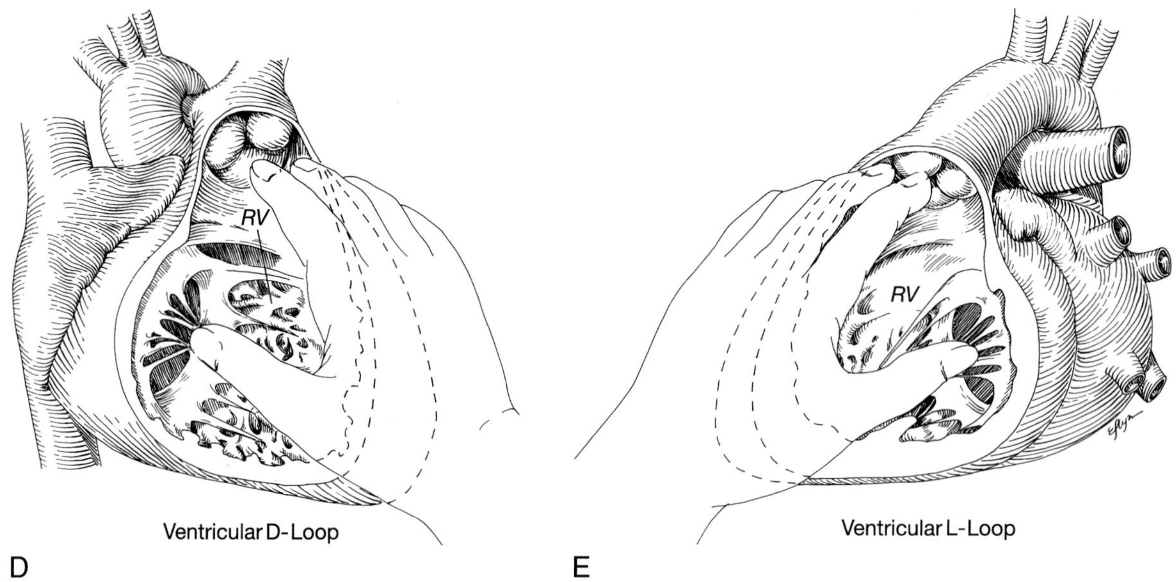


**FIGURE 52–6. Cont'd D,** Ventricular situs. In ventricular D-loop, the palmar aspect of the right hand is placed over the right ventricular septal surface with the thumb in the tricuspid valve, the fingers in the right ventricular outflow tract, and the dorsum of the right hand facing the right ventricular free wall. **E,** In ventricular L-loop, the palmar aspect of the left hand faces the right ventricular septal surface with the thumb in the tricuspid valve (or inflow), the fingers in the right ventricular outflow tract, and the dorsum of the left hand facing the right ventricular free wall. Using this principle, ventricular situs can be determined regardless of ventricular position in the chest. The same principle also applies to the left ventricle: A right-handed left ventricle will be L-looped and a left-handed left ventricle will be D-looped.

either is poorly incorporated with the right ventricular sinus (e.g., with double-chambered right ventricle [Wong et al, 1991]) or is completely dissociated from the right ventricular sinus and completely associated with the left ventricle (e.g., with anatomically corrected malposition of the great arteries and transposition of the great arteries with posterior aorta [Van Praagh and Van Praagh, 1967; Van Praagh et al, 1971]). The anatomic features of the left ventricle are illustrated in Figure 52–6C.

Once ventricular identity has been established on the basis of morphologic criteria, the type of ventricular loop can be determined (see Fig. 52–6D and E). The clinical relevance of the type of ventricular loop is that it determines the pattern of coronary artery distribution, the disposition of the conduction system, and the internal organization of the ventricular myocardium. Furthermore, ventricular L-loop is associated with increased risks of AV block (either congenital or acquired), Ebstein-like malformation of the left-sided tricuspid valve, and hypoplasia of the left-sided right ventricular sinus. Because the spatial position of the ventricles vary widely, a right-left location relative to each other cannot reliably be used to determine the ventricular loop. Instead, the principle of chirality is used. This method can be applied regardless of the spatial position of the ventricles and requires only the identification of the inflow and outflow tracts, and septal surface of one of the ventricles (Fig. 52–6D and E). The only circumstance in which the type of ventricular loop cannot be reliably determined is in an anatomically single right ventricle without a recognizable left ventricle or interventricular septum.

**6. Atrioventricular Alignments and Connections** (Fig. 52–7)

Once the identity and situs of the atria and the ventricles have been established, attention is then focused on the first connecting segment, the AV canal. Figure 52-7 illustrates several representative types of AV alignments and connections. However, it is important to recognize that these patterns are only examples of an anatomic continuum.

**7. Ventriculoarterial Alignments** (Fig. 52–8)

Next, the outflow of the heart is examined to determine from which cardiac chamber each great artery originates. Figure 52–8 illustrates several representative types of ventriculoarterial (VA) alignments. However, as is the case with AV alignments, it is important to recognize that these patterns are merely examples from a continuous anatomic spectrum.

**8. Type of Infundibulum (Conus)** (Fig. 52–9)

The infundibulum is the connecting segment between the ventricles and the great arteries. In normal anatomy, there

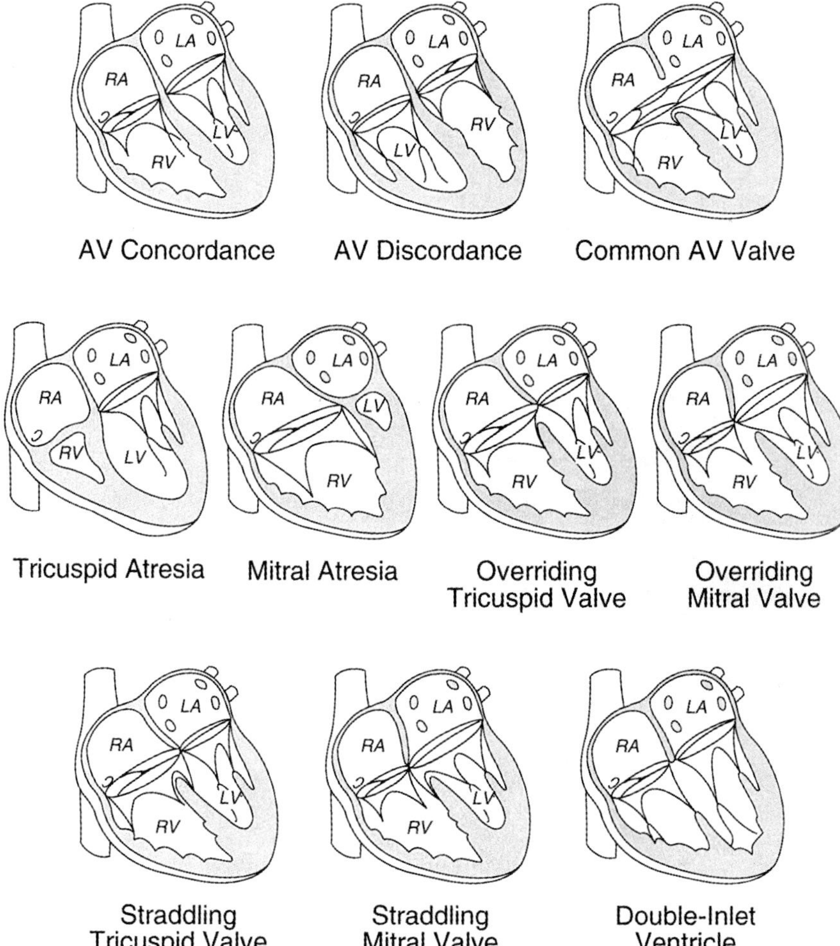


**FIGURE 52–7.** Diagram illustrating some of the possible atrioventricular (AV) alignments and connections. This step in the segmental approach to congenital heart disease follows identification of atrial and ventricular morphology and situs. LA, left atrium: LV, left ventricle; RA, right atrium; RV, right ventricle.

is a complete subpulmonary conus with muscular separation between the pulmonary and the AV valves (see Fig. 52–6A and B), whereas the subaortic conus is incomplete, allowing fibrous continuity between the left and noncoronary cusps of the aortic valve and the anterior leaflet of the mitral valve (see Fig. 52–6C). Part of the subaortic conus is normally present in the form of a conal septum represented by the myocardium that separates the anterolateral aspect of the left ventricular outflow tract (the myocardium under the right coronary cusp of the aortic valve) and the right ventricular outflow tract. In some patients, there is an increased distance between the left coronary cusp and the anterior mitral leaflet owing to elongation of the intervalvular fibrosa. In this circumstance, the aortic and mitral valves are said to have *fibrous contiguity*, as opposed to *fibrous continuity*.

Normal-type conus is termed *subpulmonary conus*, indicating the presence of a complete subpulmonary infundibular myocardium and partial absence of the subaortic infundibular free wall.

A *subaortic conus* is present when the aortic valve is supported by infundibular myocardium that completely separates it from the AV valve(s). The subpulmonary conus is incomplete with absence of infundibular myocardium between the pulmonary and AV valve(s). A subaortic conus is often found in transposition of the great arteries. However, it is important to recognize that (1) transposition of the great arteries is a specific type of VA alignment (which great artery originates from which ventricle) and is not defined by the type of conus, and that (2) any type of conus may be present in transposition of the great arteries and any other type of VA alignment (Pasquini et al, 1993).

*Bilateral conus* is present when both semilunar valves are completely separated from the AV valve(s) by infundibular myocardium. Although a bilateral conus is commonly associated with a double outlet right ventricle, it is important to recognize that (1) a double outlet right ventricle is a specific type of VA alignment (which great artery originates from which ventricle) and is not defined by the type of conus; and (2) any type of conus may be present in a double outlet right ventricle and any other type of VA alignment.

*Bilaterally absent conus* is the least common type of infundibulum. It is present when both semilunar valves are in direct fibrous continuity with the AV valve(s) as a result of absence of infundibular myocardium.

**9. Relationship between Semilunar Valves** (Fig. 52–10) This step in the segmental approach to congenital heart disease describes the spatial relationship between the

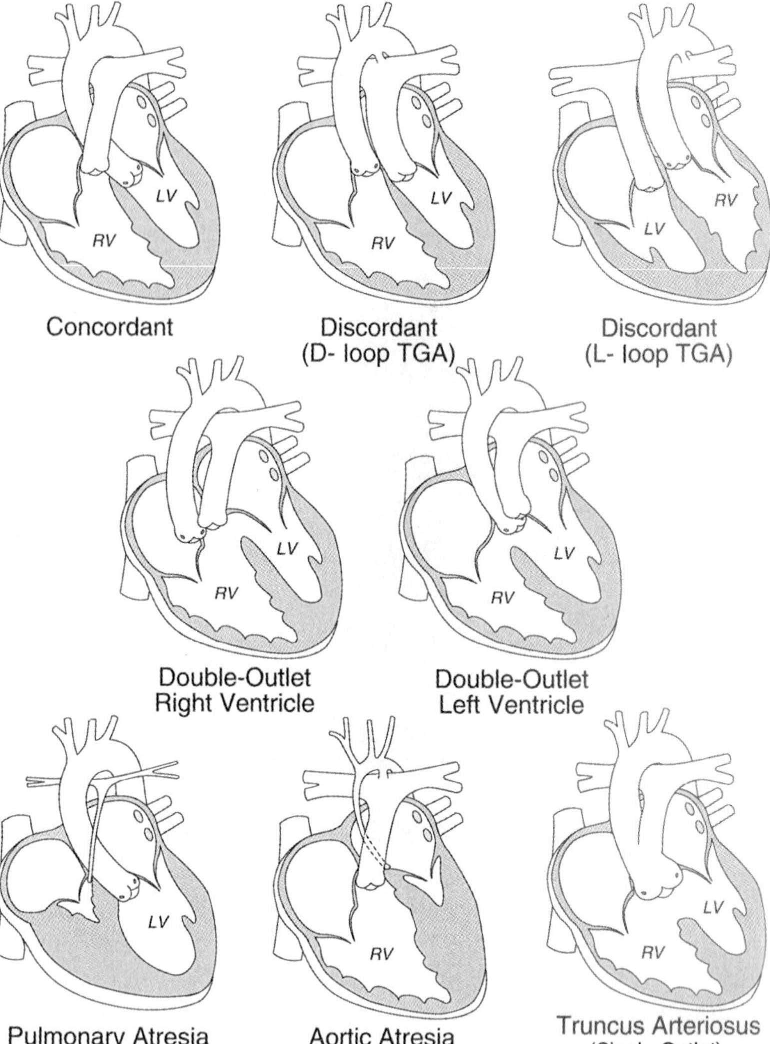


**FIGURE 52–8.** Diagram illustrating some of the possible ventriculoarterial (VA) alignments and connections. Note that the type of VA alignment is determined by which great artery arises entirely or predominantly from which ventricle. It is clinically impractical to accurately and reproducibly determine great arterial origin from either ventricle in terms of percent origin. Specifically, the so-called "50% rule" is not applicable in vivo. This is due to complex three-dimensional relations between the ventricles and the great arteries and the complex geometric nature of the ventricular septum and cardiac motion in systole and diastole and with respiration. LV, left ventricle; RV, right ventricle; TGA, transposition of great arteries.

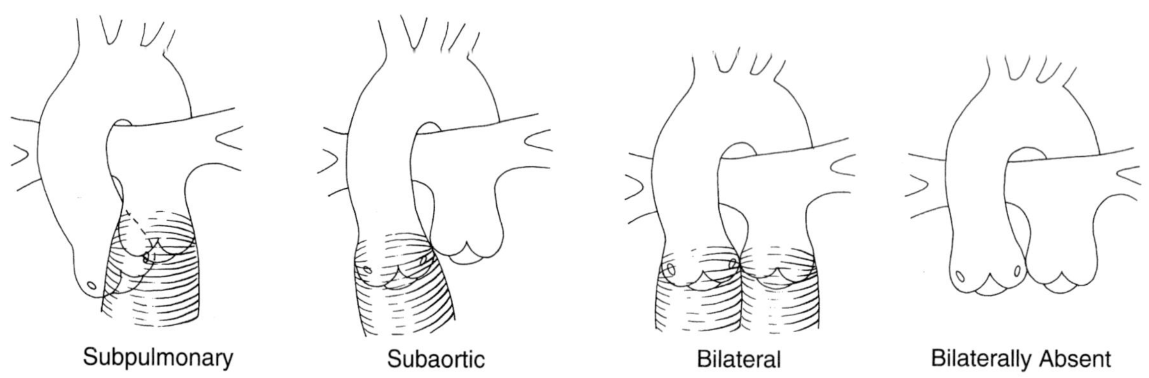


**FIGURE 52–9.** Type of infundibulum (conus). In general, there are four types of conus: 1. *subpulmonary*, with absence of subaortic infundibular free wall (found in the normal heart); 2. *subaortic*, with absence of subpulmonary infundibular free wall (often found in transposition of the great arteries); 3. b*ilateral conus* (commonly found in patients with a double-outlet right ventricle, but can be rarely found in patients with TGA and even in patients with normally related great arteries); and 4. b*ilaterally absent* (found in some patients with a double-outlet left ventricle).

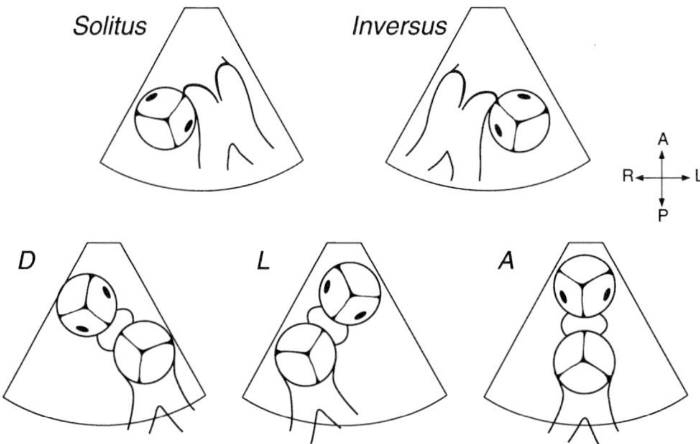


**FIGURE 52–10.** Relationship between semilunar valves. The diagram illustrates several common patterns as seen on a transthoracic echocardiographic parasternal short-axis view. It must be recognized, however, that the relationship depicted constitute samples from an anatomic continuum. A, anterior; R, right; L, left; P, posterior.

aortic and pulmonary valves. Although the spatial relationships between the semilunar valves are often associated with predictable patterns of VA alignments, there are many exceptions to these rules.

### 10. Associated Anomalies

Once the three main cardiac segments and the two connecting segments have been analyzed, all associated cardiovascular anomalies are systematically examined and described. To provide a logical and consistent description of all associated anomalies, they can be described either in order of their hemodynamic importance (from major to minor anomalies) or in an anatomic order (progressing from the venous entry to the arterial exit of the heart).

## CONCLUSIONS

The segmental approach to anatomic analysis of CHD allows an accurate description of all known forms of cardiac anomalies and can be applied to patients of all ages using diagnostic imaging modalities such as angiography, echocardiography, computed tomography, and magnetic resonance imaging. In rare circumstances when the morphology does not conform to a clearly defined diagnostic category, it is essential to provide an accurate detailed description of the anatomy using tools provided by the segmental approach to CHD.

## REFERENCES


Abbott ME: Atlas of Congenital Cardiac Disease. New York, American Heart Association, 1936.

Anderson RH, Becker AE, Freedom RM, et al: Sequential segmental analysis of congenital heart disease. Pediatr Cardiol 5:281-287, 1984a.

Anderson RH, Becker AE, Tynan M, et al: The univentricular atrioventricular connection: Getting to the root of a thorny problem. Am J Cardiol 54:822-828, 1984b.

de la Cruz MV, Nadal-Ginard B: Rules for the diagnosis of visceral situs, truncoconal morphologies, and ventricular inversions. Am Heart J 84:19-32, 1972.

Freedom RM: The "anthropology" of the segmental approach to the diagnosis of complex congenital heart disease. Cardiovasc Intervent Radiol 7:121-123, 1984.

Geva T, Powell AJ, Crawford EC, et al: Evaluation of regional differences in right ventricular systolic function by acoustic quantification echocardiography and cine magnetic resonance imaging. Circulation 98:339-345, 1998.

Lev M: Some newer concepts of the pathology of congenital heart disease. Med Clin North Am 50:3-14, 1966. .

Lev M, Liberthson RR, Golden JG, et al: The pathologic anatomy of mesocardia. Am J Cardiol 28:428-435, 1971.

Pasquini L, Sanders SP, Parness IA, et al: Conal anatomy in 119 patients with d-loop transposition of the great arteries and ventricular septal defect: An echocardiographic and pathologic study. J Am Coll Cardiol 21:1712-1721, 1993.

Rao PS: Dextrocardia: Systematic approach to differential diagnosis. Am Heart J 102:389-403, 1981.

Shinebourne EA, Macartney FJ, Anderson RH: Sequential chamber localization—logical approach to diagnosis in congenital heart disease. Br Heart J 38:327-340, 1976.

Stanger P, Rudolph AM, Edwards JE: Cardiac malpositions. An overview based on study of sixty-five necropsy specimens. Circulation 56:159-172, 1977.

Tynan MJ, Becker AE, Macartney FJ, et al: Nomenclature and classification of congenital heart disease. Br Heart J 41:544-553, 1979.

Uemura H, Ho SY, Devine WA, Anderson RH: Analysis of visceral heterotaxy according to splenic status, appendage morphology, or both. Am J Cardiol 76:846-849, 1995.

Van Praagh R: The segmental approach to diagnosis of congenital heart disease. In Birth Defects: Original Article Series. Baltimore, Williams & Wilkins, 1972, pp 4-23.

Van Praagh R: Diagnosis of complex congenital heart disease: Morphologic-anatomic method and terminology. Cardiovasc Intervent Radiol 7:115-120, 1984a.

Van Praagh R: The segmental approach clarified. Cardiovasc Intervent Radiol 7:320-325, 1984b.

Van Praagh R: The importance of segmental situs in the diagnosis of congenital heart disease. Semin Roentgenol 20:254-271, 1985.

Van Praagh R, Perez-Trevino C, Lopez-Cuellar M, et al: Transposition of the great arteries with posterior aorta, anterior pulmonary artery, subpulmonary conus and fibrous continuity between aortic and atrioventricular valves. Am J Cardiol 28:621-631, 1971.

Van Praagh R, Van Praagh S: Isolated ventricular inversion. A consideration of the morphogenesis, definition and diagnosis of nontransposed and transposed great arteries. Am J Cardiol 17:395-406, 1966.

Van Praagh R, Van Praagh S: Anatomically corrected transposition of the great arteries. Br Heart J 29:112-119, 1967.

Van Praagh R, Van Praagh, S, Vlad P, Keith JD: Anatomic types of congenital dextrocardia: Diagnostic and embryologic implications. Am J Cardiol 13:510-531, 1964.

Weinberg PM: Systematic approach to diagnosis and coding of pediatric cardiac disease. Pediatr Cardiol 7:35-48, 1986.

Wong PC, Sanders SP, Jonas RA, et al: Pulmonary valve–moderator band distance and association with development of double-chambered right ventricle. Am J Cardiol 68:1681-1686, 1991.

CHAPTER 53

# Embryology and Development of the Cardiovascular System

**Kathryn L. Maschhoff and H. Scott Baldwin**

The heart is the first organ to form in vertebrates, arising through a complex series of morphogenetic interactions involving cells from several embryonic origins. Long before it has obtained its final four-chambered adult form, the heart must function to support the rapidly growing embryo. The combination of the complex morphogenetic events necessary for cardiogenesis and the superimposed hemodynamic influences may contribute to the exquisite sensitivity of the developing heart to perturbations. This phenomenon is reflected in the estimated 10% incidence of severe cardiac malformations observed in spontaneously aborted fetuses and in the observation that approximately 1 in 100 children is born with congenital heart disease (CHD), which remains the leading cause of noninfectious death in the first year of life.

## MYOCYTE SPECIFICATION AND FORMATION OF THE PRIMITIVE HEART TUBE

Beginning soon after gastrulation (about embryonic day 20 in humans), progenitor cells within the anterior lateral plate mesoderm become committed to a cardiogenic fate in response to an inducing signal thought to emanate from the adjacent endoderm (Schultheiss et al, 1995). This heart-forming region of the developing embryo is primarily restricted to a crescent-shaped region of splanchnic mesoderm lateral and rostral to the forming foregut invagination. The specific signaling molecule(s) responsible for cardiogenic commitment remains to be identified, although bone morphogenetic proteins (BMPs) and fibroblast growth factor 8 (FGF-8) appear to be crucial for this step (Alsan and Schultheiss, 2002; Schultheiss et al, 1995). Cardiac precursors form a bilaterally symmetrical cardiogenic "field," or cardiogenic crest (Redkar et al, 2001).

In *drosophila*, formation of the dorsal vessel, which functions as a heart, is dependent on tinman, a member of the homeodomain family of proteins that were initially described to play a role in establishing regional identity of cells and organs during embryogenesis. The expression pattern of *NKX2.5*, a member of the *NKX2* homeodomain family (the vertebrate homologues of tinman), overlaps (but does not entirely coincide with) the crescent-shaped heart-forming region. Unlike tinman, *NKX2.5* is not required for cardioblast specification. However, *NKX2.5* does have a role in cardiac development. In humans, several families with atrial septal defects, and conduction abnormalities have heterozygous mutations in *NKX2.5* (Schott et al, 1998), and sporadic cases of a wide variety of congenital heart defects also are associated with heterozygous mutations in *NKX2.5* (Benson et al, 1999; Goldmuntz et al, 2001; Kasahara et al, 2000; Tanaka et al, 1999). A recently identified transcription factor called myocardin activates the transcription of a variety of cardiac genes, including *NKX2.5*, and appears to play a crucial role in early differentiation of cardiomyocytes (Wang et al, 2001).

Simultaneously with myocardial differentiation, endocardial differentiation begins in the adjacent splanchnopleuric mesoderm. The endocardium arises almost exclusively by a process known as *vasculogenesis*, the de novo organization of blood vessels by in situ differentiation of endothelial cells from mesoderm. Late in the third week, as the embryo folds, the parallel cardiac primordia fuse at the midline to form the primitive cardiac tube (DeHaan, 1965; Rosenquist and DeHaan, 1966). It has generally been stated that two separate endothelial tubes develop in the lateral body folds and then "fuse" in the midline to form the single heart (O'Rahilly and Muller, 1987). However, a close analysis of mouse heart tube formation suggests that endothelial cells of the precardiac mesoderm organize into an extensive vascular plexus, which then undergoes extensive remodeling during approximation of the lateral body folds to form a single endothelial channel (DeRuiter et al, 1992). The result is a straight heart tube with an outer myocardium and an inner endocardium separated by an extracellular matrix (ECM) known as the *cardiac jelly*.

## CARDIAC CHAMBER FORMATION

The primitive heart begins to beat by 4 weeks. The flow of blood is initially an ebb and flow but soon becomes unidirectional. As the straight heart tube takes shape, four distinct tubular segments form in a temporal sequence along the anteroposterior (AP) axis (Fig. 53–1). The primitive right and left ventricles are the first to be distinguished, followed by the atrioventricular canal segment. The sinoatrial segment forms most caudally and has distinct left-right asymmetry, with the right and left limbs of this segment later contributing to the right and left atria, respectively. The conotruncus is the last segment to form and lies in the most anterior portion of the heart tube. This patterning of the heart along the AP axis to form the conotruncus, ventricles, and atria is set up in the bilaterally symmetrical cardiac primordia before formation of the primitive heart tube (Yutzey and Bader, 1995).

Atrial and ventricular cardiac myocytes express distinct subsets of cardiac muscle genes that confer the contractile, electrophysiologic, and pharmacologic properties unique to each chamber (Lyons, 1994). For example, two related transcription factors, *dHAND* (Srivastava et al, 1995) and *eHAND* (Cserjesi et al, 1995), exhibit a complementary expression pattern in the primitive right and left ventricle segments, respectively (Srivastava et al, 1997; Thomas et al, 1998). Deletion of the *dHAND* gene in mice results in hypoplasia of the right ventricle segment, suggesting

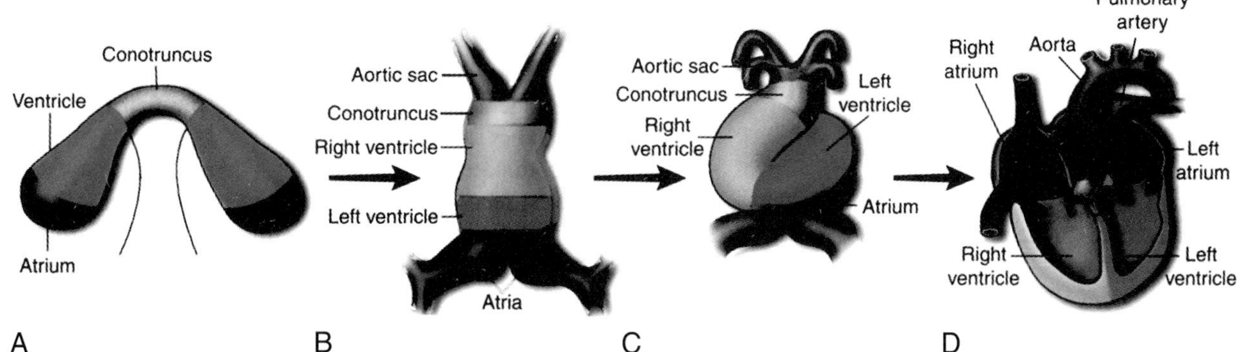


**FIGURE 53–1.** (See also Color Plate 53–1.) Schematic diagram of cardiogenesis. Bilaterally symmetrical cardiac progenitor cells (**A**) are prepatterned to form distinct regions of the heart, as shown in color-coded fashion. The precardiac mesodermal cells give rise to a linear heart tube (**B**), which forms a rightward loop (**C**) and begins to establish the spatial orientation of the four-chambered mature heart (**D**). *(Adapted from Srivastava D, and Olson EN: Knowing in your heart what's right. Trends Cell Biol. 7:447, 1997.)*

that a single gene defect can result in specific ablation of an entire chamber of the heart (Srivastava et al, 1997).

Development of the ventricles is affected by hemodynamic influences in the developing embryo. In chick embryos, reduction of left ventricular preload by ligation of the left atrium results in marked hypoplasia of the left ventricle (Sedmera et al, 1999, 2002). The hypoplasia was accompanied (and probably caused) by a decrease in cardiomyocyte proliferation in the trabeculae and compact myocardium of the left ventricle. Thus, adequate loading is crucial for normal ventricular morphogenesis as well as proper formation of the atrioventricular and semilunar valves (Hove et al, 2003). It is not yet known how the mechanical stimulus is translated into changes in cell division, but the finding that FGF-2 is decreased after left atrial ligation implicates changes in the levels of key growth factors in normal cardiac chamber growth as well as in the pathogenesis of hypoplastic left heart syndrome (HLHS).

After the initial morphogenetic cues have resulted in a four-chambered heart, the individual chambers continue to grow and develop. The myocardium of the ventricles becomes trabeculated, a feature that enables the myocardium to increase its mass before the establishment of the coronary circulation. As development progresses, the outer layer of the myocardium becomes compacted and the trabecular portion becomes more solid. Genes involved in the regulation of both of these processes, trabeculation and compaction, have been identified. Mice homozygous for a null mutation in the retinoid X receptor-α gene (*RXRA*) display ventricular chamber hypoplasia and have a defect in compaction of the myocardium (Chen et al, 2002; Sucov et al, 1994), similar to what has been referred to as "spongy" myocardium in children with noncompaction of the ventricular wall (Angelini et al, 1999). A similar phenotype is seen in mice carrying mutations in the N-*myc*, *VCAM1*, *TEF1*, and neurofibromatosis (*NF1*) genes. Mice deficient for the peptide growth factor neuregulin-1 (expressed in the endocardium) or for its receptors, the *ErbB2/ErbB4* complex (expressed in the myocardium), fail to undergo ventricular trabeculation (Gassmann et al, 1995; Kramer et al, 1996; Lee et al, 1995; Meyer and Birchmeier, 1995). Thus, the neuregulin-signaling pathway between the endocardium and myocardium is a very specific and essential step in ventricular morphogenesis.

## CARDIAC LOOPING AND ESTABLISHMENT OF LEFT-RIGHT CARDIAC ASYMMETRY

Cardiac looping is central to proper alignment of the heart and begins with rightward looping of the heart tube, with the caudal portion of the tube moving to a more anterior and dorsal position. The cellular mechanisms that drive cardiac looping remain poorly understood, but it has been postulated that differential rates of proliferation of cardioblasts, regional differences in intracardiac actin bundles, or altered cell adhesion across the heart tube may be involved. Abnormalities in the process of cardiac looping probably underlie a number of congenital heart defects. Folding of the heart tube positions the inflow cushions adjacent to the outflow cushions and involves extensive remodeling of the inner curvature of the looped heart tube. In the primitive looped heart, the segments of the heart are still in a linear pattern and must be repositioned considerably for alignment of the atrial chambers with the appropriate ventricles, and of the ventricles with the aorta and pulmonary arteries. Looping begins to convert the "in series" heart to an "in parallel" arrangement. Blood streams from the right and left horns of the sinus venosus spiral around each other as they pass through the ventricles and outflow tract. As a result of this spiral streaming, blood from the left ventricle passes to the left fourth aortic arch, whereas the right ventricular output passes to the left sixth aortic arch. As the developing venous system remodels, the systemic venous return comes to flow exclusively into the right atrium. The atrioventricular canal, which originally connects the left atrium and left ventricle, comes to open, by a mechanism that is not yet clear, into both atria. The atrioventricular septum (AVS) begins to divide the common atrioventricular canal (AVC) into a right and a left AVC, and subsequently shifts to the right to position the AVS over the muscular ventricular septum. This allows the right AVC and the left AVC to be aligned with the right and the left ventricles, respectively. Simultaneously, the conotruncal region becomes divided into the aorta and pulmonary trunks as the conotruncus moves toward the left side of the heart such that the conotruncal septum is positioned over the AVS. The rightward shift of the AVS and the leftward shift of the conotruncus convert the single-inlet, single-outlet heart into a four-chambered heart that has separate atrial inlets and ventricular outlets (Mjaatvedt et al, 1999).

Arrest or incomplete movement of the AVS or conotruncus might result in malalignment of the inflow and outflow tracts. Failure of the AVS to shift to the right would result in communication of the right and left AVCs with the left ventricle, a condition known as double-inlet left ventricle (DILV). Incomplete shifting may be the basis for "unbalanced" AVC defects in which the right AVC only partly communicates with the right ventricle. Similarly, if the conotruncal septum fails to shift to the left, both the aorta and pulmonary artery would arise from the right ventricle, causing a double-outlet right ventricle (DORV). From this embryologic perspective, it is not surprising that DOLVs and DILVs are rarely, if ever, seen clinically, whereas any abnormality in cardiac looping can be associated with DILV or DORV.

Although the molecular basis for the process of cardiac looping is unknown, the pathways that control the direction of cardiac looping along the left-right axis have recently been elucidated. The heart is the first organ to break the bilateral symmetry present in the early embryo, and the direction of its looping reflects a more global establishment of left-right asymmetry throughout the embryo that affects the visceral organs, including the lungs, liver, spleen, and gut. Initial clues to the origin of left-right asymmetry came from clinical studies describing a condition known as Kartagener syndrome in which affected persons have situs inversus totalis, with mirror-image reversal of all organs. Men with Kartagener syndrome also are infertile secondary to immotility of sperm and subsequently both men and women were found to have immotile cilia (Ajzelius, 1976). Recently, a mechanism for a link between ciliary beating and left-right asymmetry has become clear. A region of the early symmetrical embryo known as the *node* contains ciliary processes that beat in a vortical fashion in a counterclockwise direction. The ciliary beating generates a leftward flow of fluid that moves morphogens to the left side of the embryo (Essner et al, 2002; Nonaka et al, 1998, 2002; Okada et al, 1999; Wagner and Yost, 2000). The resultant asymmetrical distribution of morphogens sets up an asymmetrical cascade of signaling molecules, resulting in left- and right-sided programs of gene expression that ultimately control asymmetrical development of the visceral organs (reviewed in Mercola, 1999; Mercola and Levin, 2001). Not all components of the cascade are evolutionarily conserved; however, in all species observed to date, the cascade culminates in left-sided expression of nodal, a transcription factor that induces rightward looping of the midline heart tube, the first overt sign of embryonic left-right asymmetry. Ultimately, the nodal-dependent pathway results in expression of a homeodomain protein, Ptx2, on the left side of the visceral organs and repression of Ptx2 on the right. Asymmetrical expression of Ptx2 appears to be sufficient for establishing the left-right asymmetry of the heart, lungs, and gut.

Disorders of asymmetry have significant clinical implications. Patients with situs inversus totalis have a well-coordinated reversal of asymmetry and thus have a low incidence of defects in visceral organogenesis. However, the majority of patients with defects have visceroatrial heterotaxy and thus have randomization of cardiac, pulmonary, and gastrointestinal situs. Heterotaxy almost always results in complex congenital heart defects. Often either the right or the left side predominates, with patients having either bilateral right-sidedness (asplenia syndrome) or bilateral left-sidedness (polysplenia syndrome). Mutations in pathway members are found in some patients with heterotaxy (Kosaki and Casey, 1998; Kosaki et al, 1999; Maeyama et al, 2001). Familial cases of heterotaxy also have led to identification of mutations in a zinc-finger transcription factor, *ZIC3*, that result in axis abnormalities (Gebbia et al, 1997).

## SEPTATION AND VALVULOGENESIS

### Formation of the Endocardial Cushions

The initial event in cardiac septation is the formation of the endocardial cushions (EDCs), regional swellings of extracellular matrix that provide valvelike function in the primitive heart, and are the primordia of the atrioventricular, conotruncal, and interventricular septa, as well as the atrioventricular and semilunar valves. Formation of the endocardial cushions begins with expansion of the extracellular matrix, known as the cardiac jelly, in the atrioventricular junction and outflow tract regions of the heart tube. Components of the cardiac jelly, which separates the endocardium and the myocardium, are synthesized primarily by the myocardium, with some contribution from the endocardium. In response to signals from the myocardium, including proteins in the transforming growth factor-β (TGF-β) signaling pathway (Nakajima et al, 2000), some endocardial cells in the atrioventricular junction and outflow regions undergo a transition to a mesenchymal phenotype—a process termed epithelial-mesenchymal transformation (EMT). They then delaminate from the endocardial surface and migrate into the extracellular matrix. The ability to induce EMT in endocardial cells is restricted to myocardium in the regions of the developing endocardial cushions. Similarly, endocardial cells in the regions of the cushions are unique in their ability to respond to signals produced by the atrioventricular and outflow tract (OFT) myocardium (Eisenberg and Markwald, 1995; Mjaatvedt et al, 1999).

Following EMT, the cushion mesenchyme expands as the endocardium-derived mesenchymal cells proliferate. As they leave the zone of proliferation and migrate toward the myocardium, mesenchymal cells down-regulate genes associated with proliferation and begin to differentiate. Finally, as the cushions remodel to form the septa and valves, some cushion cells undergo apoptosis. Thus, morphogenesis of the endocardial cushions appears to be the result of a carefully orchestrated sequence of cell proliferation, differentiation, and cell death (Zhao and Rivkees, 2000).

## Atrioventricular Canal Septation and Atrioventricular Valve Formation

Septation of the atria begins at the end of the fourth week of gestation, when the septum primum begins to grow down from the roof of the atrium, extending into the atrium from the superioposterior wall (Fig. 53–2A). During the fifth week, the free edge of the septum primum grows caudally toward the atrioventricular canal, diminishing the size of the foramen connecting the atria, the ostium primum. By the end of the sixth week, the septum primum has fused with the superior and inferior endocardial cushions, which fuse to form the atrioventricular septum, to divide the atrioventricular canal into the right (tricuspid) and left (mitral) inlets. Fusion of the septum primum with the atrioventricular cushions results in obliteration of the ostium primum. Prior to closure of the ostium primum, apoptosis near the superior edge of the septum primum results in small perforations that coalesce to form the ostium secundum, which allows continued right-to-left shunting of blood. While the septum primum is forming, the septum secundum begins to grow from the ceiling of the right atrium, just adjacent to the septum primum (see Fig. 53–2B). In contrast with the septum primum, the septum secundum is thick and muscular. Growth of the septum secundum stops short of the floor of the right atrium, resulting in the foramen ovale. For the remainder of fetal life, blood flows from the right atrium to the left atrium through two staggered openings, the foramen ovale, near the floor of the right atrium, and the foramen secundum, near the roof of the left atrium (see Fig. 53–2C).

Septation of the atria and the atrioventricular canal occurs simultaneously with the shift of the atrioventricular canal to the right, so that at the time of septation, the resulting atrioventricular channels are aligned with their respective atria and ventricles (Fig. 53–3). The mechanism by which the atrioventricular canal, which originally connects the left atrium and left ventricle, comes to open into both atria is not yet clear. Analysis of the developing human heart suggests that the inlet portion of the right ventricle is derived from the embryonic right (outlet) ventricle (Lamers et al, 1992). The atrioventricular valves themselves are derived in equal proportions from endocardial cushion tissue and ventricular myocardium (Lamers et al, 1995).

Defects in atrioventricular septation—atrioventricular septal defect (AVSD)—occur in 7.3% of human congenital heart malformations. The most common association with AVSD is trisomy 21. Because of synteny between human chromosome 21 and the distal region of mouse chromosome 16, the trisomy 16 mouse has been used as an animal model of the heart defects seen in trisomy 21. The atrioventricular canal defects (AVCDs) in these mice appear to result from inadequate remodeling of the inner curvature of the heart, which results in failure of the atrioventricular junction to expand to the right (Webb et al, 1999). In addition, these embryos exhibit variability in the connection of the primary atrial cardiac segment to the body (known as the dorsal mesocardium). A derivative of the dorsal mesocardium, the spina vestibuli, fails to undergo the forward growth required for proper division of the atrioventricular canal.

Atrial septal defects (ASDs), ventricular septal defects (VSDs), and AVCDs have been seen as components of several disorders with mendelian inheritance. One such autosomal dominant disorder, Holt-Oram syndrome, is characterized by congenital heart defects, most often ASDs and VSDs, and characteristic upper limb malformations. Holt-Oram syndrome is caused by mutations in Tbx5, a member of the T-box family of transcription factors (Li et al, 1997b). Of interest, overexpression of Tbx5 in mouse or chick embryos results in cardiac defects similar to those seen with Holt-Oram syndrome, suggesting that normal embryogenesis requires precise regulation of Tbx5 dosage (Liberatore et al, 2000). As mentioned previously, mutations in *NKX2.5* can result in ostium secundum ASDs (which probably results from incomplete coverage of the ostium secundum by the septum primum) (Schott et al, 1998). AVSDs are commonly seen with heterotaxy syndromes. AVCDs are the most frequent defects seen in the asplenia (Ivemark) syndrome (i.e., right isomerism) and are seen as a component of the complex malformations seen with polysplenia (Pierpont et al, 2000). Clearly, an understanding of development of the atrioventricular region of the heart will provide insight into the etiology of a common class of congenital cardiac malformations.

## Conotruncal and Aortic Arch Development

Congenital cardiac defects involving the cardiac outflow tract, aortic arch, ductus arteriosus, and proximal pulmonary arteries account for 15% to 20% of all cases of CHD. The cardiac outflow tract, which arises from the primitive right ventricle, can be divided into the muscularized conus and the adjacent truncus arteriosus, collectively termed the conotruncus. The conotruncus shifts to the left to override the forming ventricular septum. As development proceeds, endocardial ridges grow from opposite sides of the conotruncus and meet in the middle to form the conotruncal septum. The endocardial ridges grow in a spiral configuration, placing the aorta in a more dorsal and leftward position and the pulmonary artery in a more ventral and rightward location (Fig. 53–4). The septum splits to divide the truncus arteriosus into the ascending aorta and the pulmonary trunk. Finally, fusion of the endocardial ridges with the inferior endocardial cushion and the muscular interventricular septum results in complete separation of the aortic and pulmonary outflow tracts.

Proper spiraling is crucial for the normal alignment of the aorta and pulmonary artery to the left and right ventricles, respectively. For example, in tetralogy of Fallot (TOF), the conotruncal septum forms, but because of malalignment of the great vessels, the conotruncal septum and aorta are shifted to the right and anterior. This malalignment results in an overriding aorta. Additionally, the failure of the conotruncal septum to connect to the muscular ventricular septum results in a ventricular septal defect that, unlike muscular VSDs, does not close spontaneously after birth.

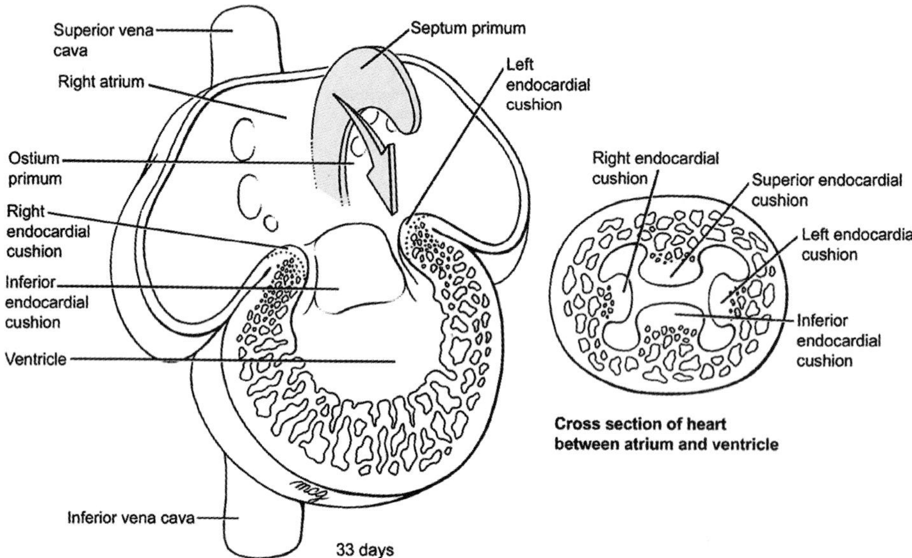


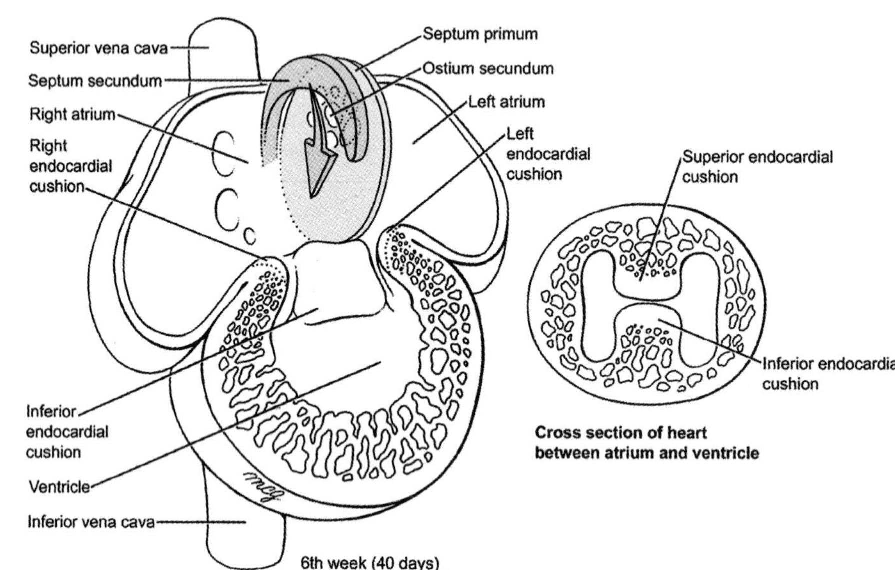


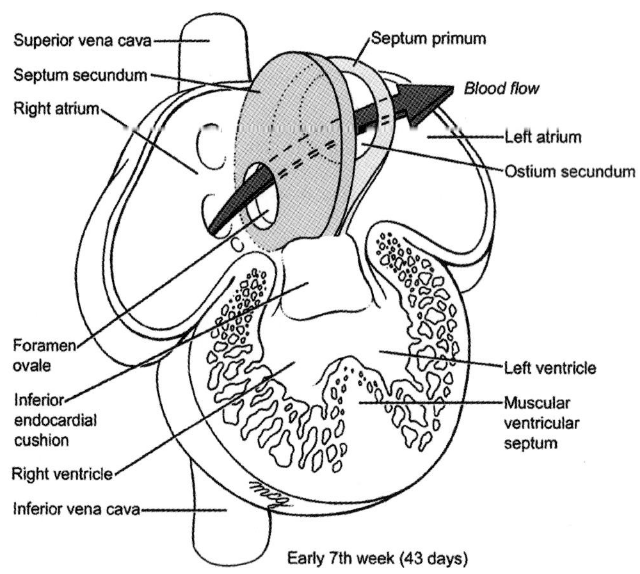


**FIGURE 53–2.** (See also Color Plate 53–2.) Septation of the atria. **A,** Atrial septation begins during the fifth week, when the septum primum forms from the roof of the atrium and grows toward the atrioventricular canal, which is being divided into right and left orifices by the superior and inferior endocardial cushions. **B,** During the sixth week, the septum primum fuses with the superior and inferior endocardial cushions, and the septum secundum grows from the roof of the right ventricle. The ostium secundum forms when small openings in the septum primum coalesce. **C,** Definitive fetal separation of the atria. *(From Larsen WJ: Development of the human heart. In Larsen WJ [ed]: Human Embryology. New York, Churchill Livingstone, 1977, pp 151-188.)*

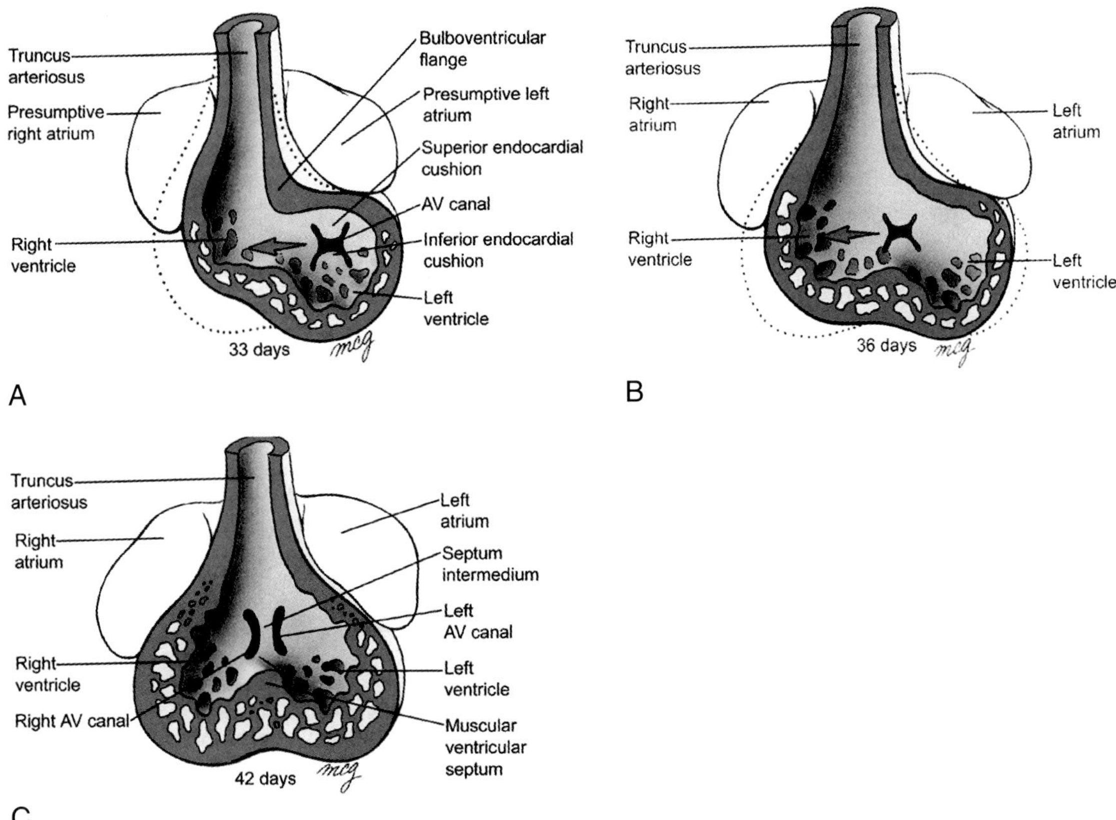


**FIGURE 53–3.** (See also Color Plate 53–3.) Realignment of the heart from 33 days (**A**) through 36 days (**B**), and 42 days (**C**). Remodeling of the heart during the fifth and sixth week, results in progressive alignment of the developing left atrioventricular canal with the left atrium and ventricle and the right atrioventricular canal with the right atrium and ventricle. **A,** The atrioventricular canal initially opens into the presumptive left ventricle. **B,** The atrioventricular can shifts to the right, so that it will overlie the developing ventricular septum. **C,** The single atrioventricular canal is divided into right and left atrioventricular canals. *(From Larsen WJ: Development of the human heart. In Larsen WJ [ed]: Human Embryology. New York, Churchill Livingstone, 1977, pp 151-188.)*

The aortic sac lies distal to the conotruncus and gives rise to six bilaterally symmetrical vessels known as aortic arch arteries. The aortic arch arteries arise sequentially along the AP axis, each traversing a pharyngeal arch before joining the paired dorsal aortas. The first and second arch arteries involute, and the fifth arch arteries do not fully form. The third, fourth, and six arch arteries undergo extensive remodeling to ultimately form distinct regions of the mature aortic arch and proximal pulmonary arteries. A majority of the right-sided dorsal aorta and aortic arch arteries undergo programmed cell death, leading to a left-sided aortic arch. The third aortic arch artery contributes to the proximal carotid arteries and right subclavian artery. The left fourth aortic arch artery forms the transverse aortic arch between the left common carotid and left subclavian arteries. Finally, the sixth arch artery contributes to the proximal pulmonary artery and the ductus arteriosus (Van Mierop and Kutsche, 1986). Extrapolating from their embryologic origins, it is believed that aberrant right subclavian arteries and other subtle arch anomalies are the results of third aortic arch defects; interrupted aortic arch of fourth arch defects; and patent ductus arteriosus and proximal pulmonary artery hypoplasia/discontinuity of defects in sixth arch artery development.

One intriguing feature of cardiac development is the involvement of cells that originate outside the heart and migrate in during cardiogenesis. Two such in-migrating cell populations are the cardiac neural crest cells and cells from the secondary or anterior heart-forming region. Prior to septation of the conotruncus, neural crest cells migrate from a portion of the dorsal neural tube (from the posterior rhombencephalon) into pharyngeal arches 3, 4, and 6, where they are required for proper remodeling of the aortic arch arteries (Fig. 53–5). Some of these cells continue to migrate to the outflow tract of the developing heart, where they become incorporated into the aorticopulmonary septum and the conotruncal cushions (Epstein et al, 2000; Jiang et al, 2000; Phillips et al, 1987; Waldo and Kirby, 1993). Recently, a subpopulation of precursor cells identified in the pharyngeal mesoderm anterior to the heart tube have been shown to give rise to the myocardium of the arterial pole of the heart (Kelly and Buckingham, 2002). The observation that the outflow tract of the heart is derived primarily from the latter addition of these "extracardiac" cell populations provides potential new insights to the potential origin of and accentuated frequency of congenital defects in this region of the heart.

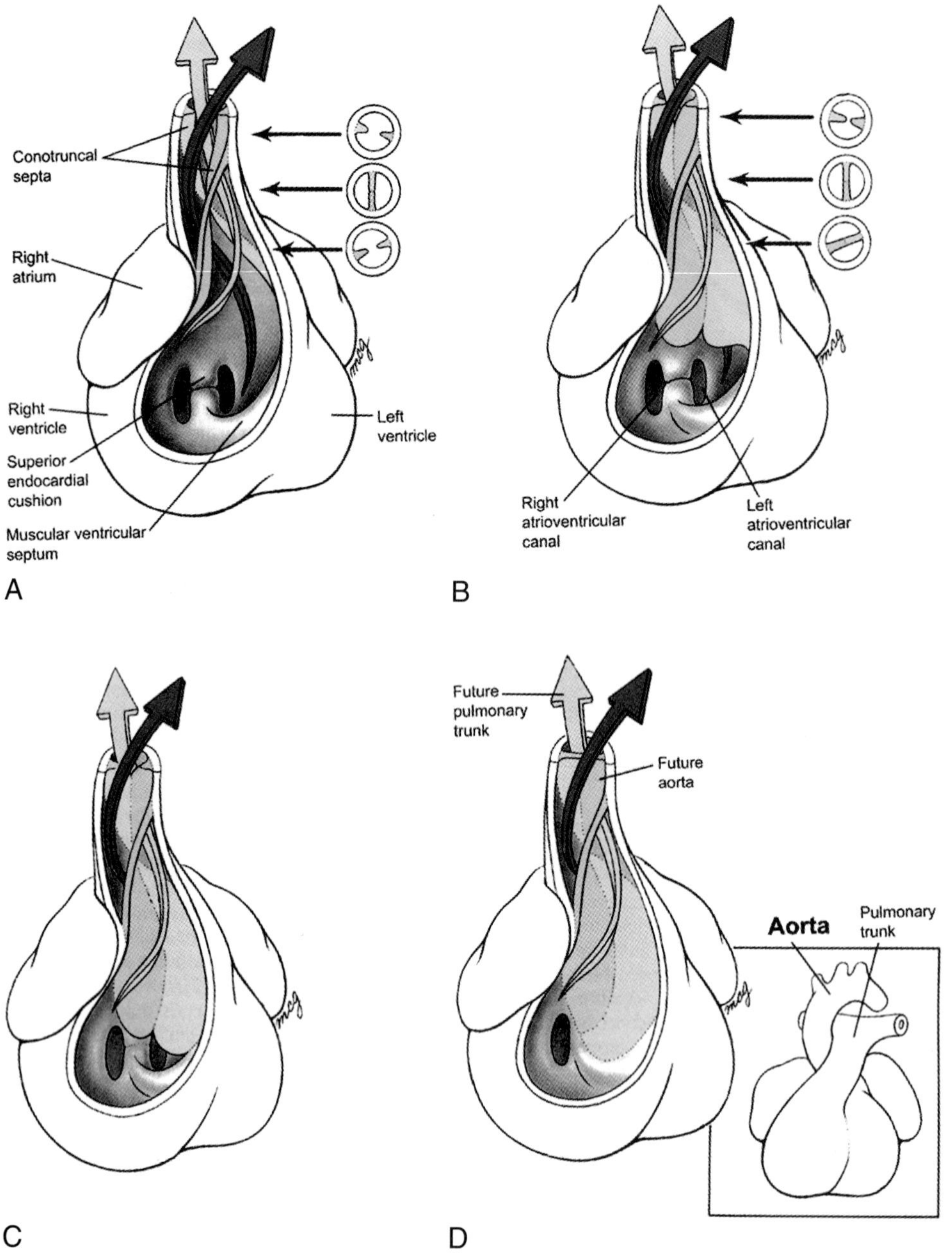

**FIGURE 53–4.** (See also Color Plate 53–4.) Septation of the cardiac outflow tract. During the fifth week, the right and left conotruncal swellings grow out of the wall of the outflow tract in a spiral configuration (**A**), fusing where they meet (**B**). By the ninth week, the inferior portion of the conotruncal swellings has grown onto and fuses with the muscular ventricular septum and the inferior endocardial cushion (**C** and **D**). *(From Larsen WJ: Development of the human heart. In Larsen WJ [ed]: Human Embryology. New York, Churchill Livingstone, 1977, pp 151-188.)*

One of the most common chromosomal anomaly syndromes is the 22q11 deletion spectrum (22q11 DS) comprising the DiGeorge, CATCH22, and velocardiofacial (VCFS) syndromes. Because the structures affected—namely, the thymus gland, parathyroid glands, branchial arch arteries, face, and conotruncal region of the heart—are all derived in part from the cranial neural crest, it has been postulated that haploinsufficiency for one or more genes in this region disrupts development of neural crest cells or that of the cells with which they interact in the developing pharyngeal arches (Van Mierop and Kutsche, 1986). The similarity between the phenotype of the 22q11DS and those produced by neural crest ablation in the chicken or by natural or induced mutations of mouse genes important for neural crest development supports this hypothesis. The genes within the 22q11 deletion interval have been completely mapped and sequenced. Much of the corresponding region on mouse chromosome 16 (the murine DiGeorge chromosomal region, or mudgcr) has been mapped as well (Botta et al, 1997; Galili et al, 1997; Lund et al, 1999). Recently, haploinsufficiency of one gene in the DiGeorge critical region, *Tbx1*, has been shown to result in many of the features of DiGeorge syndrome in mice (Jerome and Papaioannou, 2001; Lindsay et al, 2001; Merscher et al, 2001; Vitelli et al, 2002). *Tbx1* is not expressed in neural crest cells and is not required for migration of neural crest cells into the pharyngeal arches and conotruncus. Rather, it is expressed in pharyngeal endoderm and mesoderm, where it is involved in signaling pathways that regulate normal differentiation of neural crest cell derivatives (Kochilas et al, 2002). *Tbx1*-mediated neural crest cell differentiation is not required for formation of

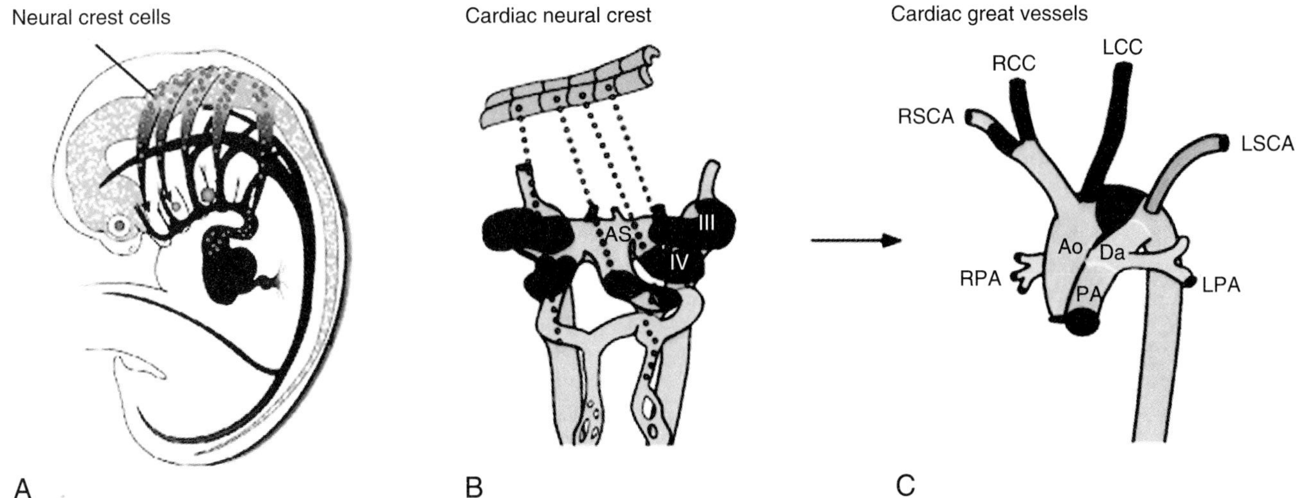


**FIGURE 53–5.** (See also Color Plate 53–5.) Contribution of neural crest cells to aortic arch selection and conotruncal development. **A,** Between the fifth and sixth week, neural crest cells migrate from the hindbrain through pharyngeal arches 4 and 6, then invade the truncus arteriosus to form the conotruncal septa. **B,** Neural crest cells are required for normal remodeling of the pharyngeal arch arteries to the adult configuration (**C**). Ao, aorta; Da, ductus arteriosus; LCC, left common carotid artery; LPA, left pulmonary artery; LSCA, left subclavian artery; PA, pulmonary artery; RCC, right common carotid artery; RPA, right pulmonary artery; RSCA, right subclavian artery.

the aortic arch arteries, which initially develop normally in the absence of neural crest cells. Instead, the aortic arch defects seen with Tbx1 deficiency appear to result from inappropriate regression of aortic arch segments and may be directly related to abnormalities in formtion of the early vasculature (Stalmans et al, 2003).

The genetic etiology for conotruncal defects associated with syndromes other than DiGeorge syndrome/VCFS is beginning to be elucidated. The Notch signaling pathway has become a prominent focus in this regard. Initial studies on the genetic etiology of Alagille syndrome, an autosomal dominant disorder involving biliary atresia and conotruncal defects, has revealed an unsuspected role in cardiogenesis for a previously known molecular pathway. Linkage analysis and subsequent DNA sequencing in large kindreds with Alagille syndrome identified mutations in Jagged 1, a secreted ligand for the transmembrane receptor Notch (Li et al, 1997a; Oda et al, 1997). Further analyses of nonsyndromic patients with similar cardiac defects have identified previously unsuspected mutations in Jagged 1 as well (Krantz et al, 1999). In mice, heterozygous mutations in both Jagged 1 and Notch 2 result in a spectrum of conotruncal defects (McCright et al, 2002). Of interest, other members of the Notch signaling pathway, the HRT family of basic helix-loop-helix (bHLH) transcription factors, have very distinct chamber-specific expression patterns: HRT1 is expressed in the atrial precursors, whereas HRT2 is expressed in the future ventricular cells. HRT proteins are involved in transduction of Notch signals, which are involved in establishing defined regions of gene expression (Greenwald, 1998). HRT2 inactivation in mice results in a phenotype similar to tetralogy of Fallot, one of the most common conotruncal defects (Donovan et al, 2002; Gessler et al, 2002). Finally, FGF8 has been implicated as a potential "modifying" factor in the development of DiGeorge syndrome (Abu-Issa et al, 2002; Frank et al, 2002).

## Semilunar Valve Formation

The anlage of the semilunar valve leaflets is provided by three pairs of mesenchymal swellings or endocardial cushions: two from the developing conotruncal ridges and one that grows directly from the wall of the truncus. These endocardial cushions are subsequently "remodeled" to provide true valve leaflets. The mechanisms of this remodeling, however, are not well defined. The critical initial event in the formation of valve cusps appears to be a restricted proliferation of endothelium overlying the conotruncal ridges on the arterial face of the OFT. This proliferation results in a thickened endothelial ridge that protrudes into the lumen of the OFT. Subsequently, there is a gradual expansion of this ridge, combined with excavation in the arterial face, which results in formation of the sinuses of Valsalva and development of a valve cusp. During this process, there appears to be a tightly regulated balance between endothelial proliferation and endothelial cell death in the expanding endothelial ridge, and it is postulated that these processes are regulated by interactions with the underlying mesenchyme (Hurle et al, 1980; Maron and Hutchins, 1974). The balance between endothelial proliferation and cell death does not appear to be a characteristic of mitral or tricuspid valve histogenesis, which involves formation of a leaflet but does not require development of a valve cusp or sinus.

Little is known about the molecular mechanisms directing semilunar valve development. Several genes have been identified that are required for formation of the semilunar but not atrioventricular valves. NFATc, or NFAT2 (for nuclear factor of activated T cells) (de la Pompa et al, 1998; Ranger et al, 1998), is preferentially expressed by endocardial cells. Null mutations result in complete absence of aortic and pulmonary valve formation. Similarly, a null mutation in the *Sox4* gene (a member of the Sox, or Sry-box, family of transcription factors) results in OFT defects, including truncus arteriosus and abnormal semilunar valve formation (Schilham et al, 1996; Ya et al, 1998), and mutations in the protein tyrosine phosphatase SHP-2 have been associated with abnormalities in pulmonary valve formation associated with Noonan syndrome (Tartaglia et al, 2001, 2002). The downstream targets of these transcription factors and signaling molecules are not yet known; identification of these targets will be an important step in understanding normal and abnormal semilunar valve formation.

## THE EPICARDIUM AND CORONARY VASCULATURE

The origin of coronary vascular endothelium and formation of the coronary vessels has been areas of intense investigation. Several theories ranging from the sprouting of vessels from the aorta into developing myocardium to outgrowth of the endocardial lining of the heart to the epicardial vessels have evolved to explain coronary morphogenesis. Recently, several investigators have demonstrated that the coronary vessels are derived from the epicardium itself. The epicardium originates as a villous projection of mesothelial cells in the area of the sinus venosus. These cells contact the dorsal heart in the region of the atrioventricular junction and subsequently migrate across this bridge to form a cellular monolayer that ultimately covers the surface of the heart. After migration over the surface of the heart, some epicardial cells undergo EMT and invade the extracellular matrix of the underlying subepicardium. Some of these mesenchymal cells become incorporated into the developing coronary endothelial plexus (Dettman et al, 1998; Perez-Pomares et al, 1998; Vrancken Peeters et al, 1999). Epicardially-derived cells (EPDCs) also have been found in the atrioventricular cushions, the myocardial wall, and the fibrous skeleton of the heart. In addition to being the source of coronary blood vessels, the epicardium is probably an important source of growth factors and morphogens, such as retinoic acid, which are required for normal growth and development of the myocardium; disruption of retinoic acid signaling from the epicardium to the myocardium results in thinning of the compact layer of the myocardium (Tran and Sucov, 1998; Xavier-Neto et al, 2000).

Whereas distal coronary development occurs by vasculogenesis, proximal coronary artery morphogenesis appears to result from an angiogenic process. Traditionally, the proximal coronary arteries were described as an outgrowth from the aorta to the epicardial surface of the heart; however, several investigators have recently shown that in fact the angiogenic process is in the reverse direction. Angiogenic sprouts from the subepicardial endothelial plexus form endothelial strands that grow into the aorta and develop multiple communications with all three cusps of the developing aortic valve (Waldo et al, 1990). These observations have obvious implications for determining the factors that direct coronary artery anatomy in CHDs.

## THE CONDUCTION SYSTEM

Although many human congenital heart defects are accompanied by electrophysiologic abnormalities, relatively little is known about development of the cardiac conduction system. Polarity of the vertebrate heart is established early in development, with both the dominant pacemaker activity and the highest beat frequency found at the posterior (atrial) end of the developing cardiac tube. Electrical activity of the primitive heart tube is characterized by slow conduction of the impulse, resulting in a slow peristaltic contraction. As the atrial and ventricular chambers of the heart develop, they begin to contract synchronously and sequentially, resulting in an adult-type electrocardiogram (ECG). Initiation of impulses from a sinoatrial "pacemaker" and delay of conduction through the atrioventricular canal are evident before the appearance of morphologically identifiable sinoatrial and atrioventricular nodes at approximately 5 weeks in the human heart.

Because cells of the conducting system express proteins commonly associated with neural crest cells, such as HNK-1, it had been theorized that the conducting system was derived from in-migrating neural crest cells. However, recent studies have shown that cells of the ventricular conducting system are in fact derived from local recruitment of differentiated ventricular myocytes (Cheng et al, 1999). In avian embryos, only myocytes located adjacent to the developing coronary vasculature are recruited to become conducting cells, suggesting that differentiation occurs in response to signals, from the arterial bed (Gourdie et al, 1995; Hyer et al, 1999). One candidate signal is endothelin-1, which is produced by the developing coronary vasculature in response to blood flow and is able to induce a Purkinje cell phenotype in cardiomyocytes (Takebayashi-Suzuki et al, 2000). A role for the coronary vasculature in mammalian cardiac conduction system development is not as clear. In mammals, in contrast with the chick, the peripheral Purkinje fiber network is largely confined to the subendocardial myocardium, and periarterial fibers have not been clearly documented. In the developing mouse heart, most Purkinje fibers are subendocardial and appear to be derived form the trabeculated myocardium (Rentschler et al, 2001). Indeed, development of the ventricular conduction system appears to require signals from the endocardium. Neuregulin-1, which is required for formation of the trabeculated myocardium, is able to induce at least some features of a conducting phenotype in murine cardiomyocytes (Rentschler et al, 2002). The roles of hemodynamic and endocardial signaling in development of the human conduction system remain to be elucidated. However, these seminal observations pave the way for a more detailed evaluation of the factors that regulate normal and potentially abnormal development of the conduction system.

## FUTURE DIRECTIONS

Development of the cardiovascular system represents a complicated interplay between developing form and function. There has been an explosion in the identification of potential candidate genes regulating these processes, and the initial translation of basic observations from animal models to clinical relevance is well under way. However, much still needs to be done, particularly in defining the signaling cascades that lead to specific forms of congenital heart diseases. Thus, cardiac morphogenesis provides a fertile field for future investigation by collaborative teams of both basic and clinical scientists.

## REFERENCES


Abu-Issa R, Smyth, G, Smoak I, et al: Fgf8 is required for pharyngeal arch and cardiovascular development in the mouse. Development 129:4613-4625, 2002.

Ajzelius BA: A human syndrome caused by immotile cilia. Science 193:317-319, 1976.

Alsan BH, Schultheiss TM: Regulation of avian cardiogenesis by Fgf8 signaling. Development 129:1935-1943, 2002.

Angelini A, Melacini P, Barbero F, Thiene G: Evolutionary persistence of spongy myocardium in humans. Circulation 99:2475, 1999.

Benson DW, Silberbach GM, Kavanaugh-McHugh A, et al: Mutations in the cardiac transcription factor *NKX2.5* affect diverse cardiac developmental pathways. J Clin Invest 104:1567-1573, 1999.

Botta A, Lindsay EA, Jurecic V, Baldini A: Comparative mapping of the DiGeorge syndrome region in the mouse shows inconsistent gene order and differential degree of gene conservation [published erratum appears in Mamm Genome 9:344, 1998]. Mamm Genome 8:890-895, 1997.

Chen TH, Chang TC, Kang JO, et al: Epicardial induction of fetal cardiomyocyte proliferation via a retinoic acid–inducible trophic factor. Dev Biol 250:198-207, 2002.

Cheng G, Litchenberg WH, Cole GJ, et al: Development of the cardiac conduction system involves recruitment within a multipotent cardiomyogenic lineage. Development 126:5041-5049, 1999.

Cserjesi P, Brown D, Lyons GE, Olson EN: Expression of the novel basic helix-loop-helix gene eHAND in neural crest derivatives and extraembryonic membranes during mouse development. Dev Biol 170:664-678, 1995.

de la Pompa JL, Timmerman LA, Takimoto H, et al: Role of the NF-ATc transcription factor in morphogenesis of cardiac valves and septum. Nature 392:182-186, 1998.

DeHaan RL: Morphogenesis of the vertebrate heart. In DeHaan RL, Ursprung H (eds): Organogenesis. New York, Holt, Rinehart and Winston, 1965, pp 377-420.

DeRuiter MC, Poelmann RE, VanderPlas-de Vries I, et al: The development of the myocardium and endocardium in mouse embryos. Fusion of two heart tubes? Anat Embryol (Berl) 185:461-473, 1992.

Dettman RW, Denetclaw W Jr, Ordahl CP, Bristow J: Common epicardial origin of coronary vascular smooth muscle, perivascular fibroblasts, and intermyocardial fibroblasts in the avian heart. Dev Biol 193:169-181, 1998.

Donovan J, Kordylewska A, Jan YN, Utset MF: Tetralogy of Fallot and other congenital heart defects in Hey2 mutant mice. Curr Biol 12:1605-1610, 2002.

Eisenberg LM, Markwald RR: Molecular regulation of atrioventricular valvuloseptal morphogenesis. Circ Res 77:1-6, 1995.

Epstein JA, Li J, Lang D, et al: Migration of cardiac neural crest cells in Splotch embryos. Development 127:1869-1878, 2000.

Essner JJ, Vogan KJ, Wagner MK, et al: Conserved function for embryonic nodal cilia. Nature 418:37-38, 2002.

Frank DU, Fotheringham LK, Brewer JA, et al: An Fgf8 mouse mutant phenocopies human 22q11 deletion syndrome. Development 129:4591-4603, 2002.

Galili N, Baldwin HS, Lund J, et al: A region of mouse chromosome 16 is syntenic to the DiGeorge, velocardiofacial syndrome minimal critical region. Genome Res 7:399, 1997.

Gassmann M, Casagranda F, Orioli D, et al: Aberrant neural and cardiac development in mice lacking the ErbB4 neuregulin receptor. Nature 378:390-394, 1995.

Gebbia M, Ferrero GB, Pilia G, et al: X-linked situs abnormalities result from mutations in *ZIC3*. Nat Genet 17:305-308, 1997.

Gessler M, Knobeloch KP, Helisch A, et al: Mouse gridlock: No aortic coarctation or deficiency, but fatal cardiac defects in Hey2-/- mice. Curr Biol 12:1601-1604, 2002.

Goldmuntz E, Geiger E, Benson DW: *NKX2.5* mutations in patients with tetralogy of Fallot. Circulation 104: 2565-2568, 2001.

Gourdie RG, Mima T, Thompson RP, Mikawa T: Terminal diversification of the myocyte lineage generates Purkinje fibers of the cardiac conduction system. Development 121:19,1423-1431, 95.

Greenwald I: LIN-12/Notch signaling: Lessons from worms and flies. Genes Dev 12:1751-1762, 1998.

Hove JR, Koster RW, Forouhar AS, et al: Intracardiac fluid forces are an essential epigenetic factor for embryonic cardiogenesis. Nature 421:172-177, 2003.

Hurle JM, Colvee E, Blanco AM: Development of mouse semilunar valves. Anat Embryol 160:83-91, 1980.

Hyer J, Johansen M, Prasad A, et al: Induction of Purkinje fiber differentiation by coronary arterialization. Proc Natl Acad Sci U S A 96:13214-13218, 1999.

Jerome LA, Papaioannou VE: DiGeorge syndrome phenotype in mice mutant for the T-box gene, *Tbx1*. Nat Genet 27:286-291, 2001.

Jiang X, Rowitch DH, Soriano P, et al: Fate of the mammalian cardiac neural crest. Development 127:1607-1616, 2000.

Kasahara H, Lee B, Schott JJ, et al: Loss of function and inhibitory effects of human CSX/*NKX2.5* homeoprotein mutations associated with congenital heart disease. J Clin Invest 106:299-308, 2000.

Kelly RG, Buckingham ME: The anterior heart-forming field: Voyage to the arterial pole of the heart. Trends Genet 18:210-216, 2002.

Kochilas L, Merscher-Gomez S, Lu MM, et al: The role of neural crest during cardiac development in a mouse model of DiGeorge syndrome. Dev Biol 251:157-166, 2002.

Kosaki K, Casey B: Genetics of human left-right axis malformations. Semin Cell Dev Biol 9:89-99, 1998.

Kosaki R, Gebbia M, Kosaki K, et al: Left-right axis malformations associated with mutations in *ACVR2B*, the gene for human activin receptor type IIB. Am J Med Genet 82:70-76, 1999.

Kramer R, Bucay N, Kane DJ, et al: Neuregulins with an Ig-like domain are essential for mouse myocardial and neuronal development. Proc Natl Acad Sci U S A 93:4833-4838, 1996.

Krantz ID, Smith R, Colliton R, et al: Jagged1 mutations in patients ascertained with isolated congenital heart defects. Am J Med Genet 84:56-60, 1999.

Lamers WH, Viragh S, Wessels A, et al: Formation of the tricuspid valve in the human heart. Circulation 91:111-121, 1995.

Lamers WH, Wessels A, Verbeek FJ, et al: New findings concerning ventricular septation in the human heart: Implications for maldevelopment. Circulation 86:1194-1205, 1992.

Lee KF, Simon H, Chen H, et al: Requirement for neuregulin receptor erbB2 in neural and cardiac development. Nature 378:394-398, 1995.

Li L, Krantz ID, Deng Y, et al: Alagille syndrome is caused by mutations in human *Jagged1*, which encodes a ligand for *Notch1*. Nat Genet 16:243-251, 1997a.

Li QY, Newbury-Ecob RA, Terrett JA, et al: Holt-Oram syndrome is caused by mutations in *TBX5*, a member of the *Brachyury* (T) gene family. Nat Genet 15:21-29, 1997b.

Liberatore CM, Searcy-Schrick RD, Yutzey KE: Ventricular expression of tbx5 inhibits normal heart chamber development. Dev Biol 223:169-180, 2000.

Lindsay EA, Vitelli F, Su H, et al: Tbx1 haploinsufficiency in the DiGeorge syndrome region causes aortic arch defects in mice. Nature 410:97-101, 2000.

Lund J, Roe B, Chen F, et al: Sequence-ready physical map of the mouse chromosome 16 region with conserved synteny to the human velocardiofacial syndrome region on 22q11.2. Mamm Genome 10:438-443, 1999.

Lyons G: In situ analysis of the cardiac muscle gene program during embryogenesis. Trends Cardiovasc Med 4:70-77, 1994.

Maeyama K, Kosaki R, Yoshihashi H, et al: Mutation analysis of left-right axis determining genes in NOD and ICR, strains susceptible to maternal diabetes. Teratology 63:119-126, 2001.

Maron BJ, Hutchins GM: The development of the semilunar valves in the human heart. Am J Pathol 74:331-344, 1974.

McCright B, Lozier J, Gridley T: A mouse model of Alagille syndrome: Notch2 as a genetic modifier of Jag1 haploinsufficiency. Development 129:1075-1082, 2002.

Mercola M: Embryological basis for cardiac left-right asymmetry. Semin Cell Dev Biol 10:109-116, 1999.

Mercola M, Levin M: Left-right asymmetry determination in vertebrates. Annu Rev Cell Dev Biol 17:779-805, 2001.

Merscher S, Funke B, Epstein JA, et al: TBX1 is responsible for cardiovascular defects in velo-cardio-facial/DiGeorge syndrome. Cell 104:619-629, 2001.

Meyer D, Birchmeier C: Multiple essential functions of neuregulin in development. Nature 378:386-390, 1995.

Mjaatvedt CH, Yamamura H, Wessels A, et al: Mechanisms of Segmentation, Septation, and Remodeling of the Tubular Heart: Endocardial Cushion Fate and Cardiac Looping in Heart Development. London, Academic Press, 1999.

Nakajima Y, Yamagishi T, Hokari S, Nakamura H: Mechanisms involved in valvuloseptal endocardial cushion formation in early cardiogenesis: Roles of transforming growth factor (TGF)-beta and bone morphogenetic protein (BMP). Anat Rec 258:119-127, 2000.

Nonaka S, Shiratori H, Saijoh Y, Hamada H: Determination of left-right patterning of the mouse embryo by artificial nodal flow. Nature 418:96-99, 2002.

Nonaka S, Tanaka Y, Okada Y, et al: Randomization of left-right asymmetry due to loss of nodal cilia generating leftward flow of extraembryonic fluid in mice lacking KIF3B motor protein. Cell 95:829-837, 1998.

O'Rahilly R, Muller F: Developmental stages in human embryos. Carnegie Inst Washington Contrib Embryol 637:93-104, 1987.

Oda T, Elkahloun AG, Pike BL, et al: Mutations in the human *Jagged1* gene are responsible for Alagille syndrome. Nat Genet 16:235-242, 1997.

Okada Y, Nonaka S, Tanaka Y, et al: Abnormal nodal flow precedes situs inversus in *iv* and *inv* mice. Mol Cell 4:459-468, 1999.

Perez-Pomares JM, Macias, Garcia-Garrido L, Munoz-Chapuli R: The origin of the subepicardial mesenchyme in the avian embryo: An immunohistochemical and quail-chick chimera study. Dev Biol 200:57-68, 1998.

Phillips MT, Kirby ML, Forbes G: Analysis of cranial neural crest distribution in the developing heart using quail-chick chimeras. Circ Res 60:27-30, 1987.

Pierpont ME, Markwald RR, Lin AE: Genetic aspects of atrioventricular septal defects. Am J Med Genet 97:289-296, 2000.

Ranger AM, Grusby MJ, Hodge MR, et al: The transcription factor NF-ATc is essential for cardiac valve formation [see comments]. Nature 392:186-190, 1998.

Redkar A, Montgomery M, Litvin J: Fate map of early avian cardiac progenitor cells. Development 128:2269-2279, 2001.

Rentschler S, Vaidya DM, Tamaddon H, et al: Visualization and functional characterization of the developing murine cardiac conduction system. Development 128:1785-1792, 2001.

Rentschler S, Zander J, Meyers K, et al: Neuregulin-1 promotes formation of the murine cardiac conduction system. Proc Natl Acad Sci U S A 99:10464-10469, 2002.

Rosenquist GC, DeHaan RL: Migration of precardiac cells in the chick embryo: A radioautographic study. Carnegie Inst Washington Contrib Embryol 38:111-121, 1966.

Schilham MW, Oosterwegel MA, Moerer P, et al: Defects in cardiac outflow tract formation and pro-B-lymphocyte expansion in mice lacking Sox-4. Nature 380:711-714, 1996.

Schott JJ, Benson DW, Basson CT, et al: Congenital heart disease caused by mutations in the transcription factor *NKX2.5*. Science 281:108-111, 1998.

Schultheiss TM, Xydas S, Lassar AB: Induction of avian cardiac myogenesis by anterior endoderm. Development 121:4203-4214, 1995.

Sedmera D, Hu N, Weiss KM, et al: Cellular changes in experimental left heart hypoplasia. Anat Rec 267:137-145, 2002.

Sedmera D, Pexieder T, Rychterova V, et al: Remodeling of chick embryonic ventricular myoarchitecture under experimentally changed loading conditions. Anat Rec 254:238-252, 1999.

Srivastava D, Cserjesi P, Olson EN: A subclass of bHLH proteins required for cardiac morphogenesis. Science 270:1995-1999, 1995.

Srivastava D, Thomas T, Lin Q, et al: Regulation of cardiac mesodermal and neural crest development by the bHLH transcription factor, dHAND. Nat Genet 16:154-160, 1997.

Stalmans I, Lambrechts D, De Smet F, et al: VEGF: A modifier of the del22q11 (DiGeorge) syndrome? Nat Med 9:173-182, 2003.

Sucov HM, Dyson E, Gumeringer CL, et al: RXR alpha mutant mice establish a genetic basis for vitamin A signaling in heart morphogenesis. Genes Dev 8:1007-1018, 1994.

Takebayashi-Suzuki K, Yanagisawa M, Gourdie RG, et al: In vivo induction of cardiac Purkinje fiber differentiation by coexpression of preproendothelin-1 and endothelin-converting enzyme-1. Development 127:3523-3532, 2000.

Tanaka M, Chen Z, Bartunkova S, et al: The cardiac homeobox gene *Csx/Nkx2.5* lies genetically upstream of multiple genes essential for heart development. Development 126:1269-1280, 1999.

Tartaglia M, Kalidas K, Shaw A, et al: *PTPN11* mutations in Noonan syndrome: Molecular spectrum, genotype-phenotype correlation, and phenotypic heterogeneity. Am J Hum Genet 70:1555-1563, 2002.

Tartaglia M, Mehler EL, Goldberg R, et al: Mutations in *PTPN11*, encoding the protein tyrosine phosphatase SHP-2, cause Noonan syndrome. Nat Genet 29:465-468, 2001.

Thomas T, Yamagishi H, Overbeek PA, et al: The bHLH factors, dHAND and eHAND, specify pulmonary and systemic cardiac ventricles independent of left-right sidedness. Dev Biol 196:228-236, 1998.

Tran CM, Sucov HM: The *RXRalpha* gene functions in a non-cell-autonomous manner during mouse cardiac morphogenesis. Development 125:1951-1956, 1998.

Van Mierop LH, Kutsche LM: Cardiovascular anomalies in DiGeorge syndrome and importance of neural crest as a possible pathogenetic factor. Am J Cardiol 58:133-137, 1986.

Vitelli F, Morishima M, Taddei I, et al: *Tbx1* mutation causes multiple cardiovascular defects and disrupts neural crest and cranial nerve migratory pathways. Hum Mol Genet 11:915-922, 2002.

Vrancken Peeters MP, Gittenberger–de Groot AC, Mentink MM, Poelmann RE: Smooth muscle cells and fibroblasts of the coronary arteries derive from epithelial-mesenchymal transformation of the epicardium. Anat Embryol (Berl) 199:367-378, 1999.

Wagner MK, Yost HJ: Left-right development: The roles of nodal cilia. Curr Biol 10:R149-R151, 2000.

Waldo KL, Kirby ML: Cardiac neural crest contribution to the pulmonary artery and sixth aortic arch artery complex in chick embryos aged 6 to 18 days. Anat Rec 237:385-399, 1993.

Waldo KL, Willner W, Kirby ML: Origin of the proximal coronary artery stems and a review of ventricular vascularization in the chick embryo. Am J Anat 188:109-120, 1990.

Wang D, Chang PS, Wang Z, et al: Activation of cardiac gene expression by myocardin, a transcriptional cofactor for serum response factor. Cell 105:851-862, 2001.

Webb S, Anderson RH, Lamers WH, Brown NA: Mechanisms of deficient cardiac septation in the mouse with trisomy 16. Circ Res 84:897-905, 1999.

Xavier-Neto J, Shapiro MD, Houghton L, Rosenthal N: Sequential programs of retinoic acid synthesis in the myocardial and epicardial layers of the developing avian heart. Dev Biol 219:129-141, 2000.

Ya J, Schilham MW, de Boer PA, et al: Sox4-deficiency syndrome in mice is an animal model for common trunk. Circ Res 83: 986-994, 1998.

Yutzey KE, Bader D: Diversification of cardiomyogenic cell lineages during early heart development. Circ Res 77:216-219, 1995.

Zhao Z, Rivkees SA: Programmed cell death in the developing heart: Regulation by BMP4 and FGF2. Dev Dyn 217:388-400, 2000.

CHAPTER 54

# Echocardiography in the Neonatal Intensive Care Unit

Jack Rychik and Meryl S. Cohen

*Echocardiography* is the application of ultrasound in evaluation of the cardiovascular system. A variety of diagnostic modalities in echocardiography provide detailed, reliable, and reproducible information on cardiovascular form and function. Fine cardiac structures can be identified, with differentiation of abnormal from normal anatomy, using high-resolution two-dimensional echocardiography. Detailed measures of myocardial thickness and cavity dimensions can be obtained via M-mode echocardiography. Components of hemodynamics, such as blood flow velocity and spatial direction, can be used to derive pressure measurements by the use of Doppler echocardiography.

Echocardiography is a very useful tool in the evaluation of the infant in the neonatal intensive care unit (NICU). The information obtained is real-time, noninvasive, and acquired at the patient's bedside. Physiologic data points can be measured in a serial manner, which can be of great value in managing the sick neonate as conditions are explored and responses to management strategies are gauged. Echocardiography is important not only in the diagnostic evaluation of congenital heart disease but also in the overall assessment of the cardiovascular system in disorders unique to the newborn infant. This chapter reviews the basic principles of echocardiography and their applications in the infant in the NICU setting.

## BASIC PRINCIPLES AND INSTRUMENTATION OF ECHOCARDIOGRAPHY

Ultrasound energy is generated by the stimulation of piezoelectric crystals housed in a unit called a transducer. When ultrasound energy is transmitted into biologic tissue, the majority is absorbed; however, a small amount is reflected back to the transducer. Reflected energy is processed and an image created on a screen. Ultrasound scatter is greatest at the interfaces between biologic tissues of disparate densities. Hence, bone and air, when adjacent to soft tissues such as the heart, create poor acoustic windows for ultrasound transmission. Soft tissue and fluid are excellent media for ultrasound transmission and provide clear windows for cardiac imaging (Weyman, 1994).

The range of frequencies used for diagnostic assessment of biologic tissue is 2 to 10 MHz (1 MHz = 1 million cycles per second). Low-frequency ultrasound energy penetrates tissue better than high-frequency ultrasound; however, higher frequency ultrasound provides for greater spatial resolution of fine structures. This principle is dictated by a fundamental law of physics that defines the relation between ultrasound frequency and wavelength, in which

$$\text{velocity of sound in biologic tissue} = \text{ultrasound frequency} \times \text{wavelength}$$

An ultrasound wavelength distance is the physical limit beyond which two structures in space cannot be distinguished. Hence, the smaller the wavelength (i.e., the higher the frequency), the greater the ability to distinguish two points in space that are very close to each other.

Let us look at the following example. Two structures exist in space 0.5 mm apart from each other. The velocity of sound in biologic tissue is a constant at approximately 1540 meters/second. Applying a frequency of 2 MHz of ultrasound energy will result in a wavelength of 0.77 mm, whereas applying a frequency of 8 MHz of ultrasound energy will result in a wavelength of 0.19 mm. Hence, to the operator using the 2-MHz transducer, the two structures will not be distinguishable from each other and will appear as one, whereas the operator using the 8-MHz transducer will be able to differentiate between the structures with ease. Accordingly, higher frequencies, in the range of 5 MHz or greater, are always used in the neonatal setting, because penetration is less important in the small subject and the objective is to maximize fine structure resolution.

Technologic advancements in miniaturization have allowed for the development of tiny transducer housings and small footprints for the performance of surface echocardiography in the neonate. Similar technology has allowed for the development of transesophageal echocardiography (TEE), in which a small transducer can be introduced into the esophagus of an infant weighing as little as 2.5 to 3.0 kg. TEE is helpful in elucidating structures in the posterior mediastinum, such as pulmonary veins, and in overcoming acoustic impediments at the surface such as air and bone (Randolph et al, 2002). Most important, TEE has allowed for imaging to take place during interventional procedures in the operating room or catheterization laboratory by eliminating the need to place a transducer directly on the chest or abdomen, thereby avoiding potential interference in the operative field. Interventional procedures can be guided by TEE imaging with immediate feedback provided and overall outcome improved. Recently, ultrasound transducer technology has been incorporated into the tips of catheters, allowing for intracardiac imaging (Li et al, 2002). These catheter-based ultrasound devices probably herald the development of TEE for tiny premature infants in the future (Bruce et al, 2002).

### How to Perform the Neonatal Echocardiogram

A systematic and standardized approach is important in performing the echocardiogram in the neonate. Follow-up echocardiographic studies may be curtailed and limited

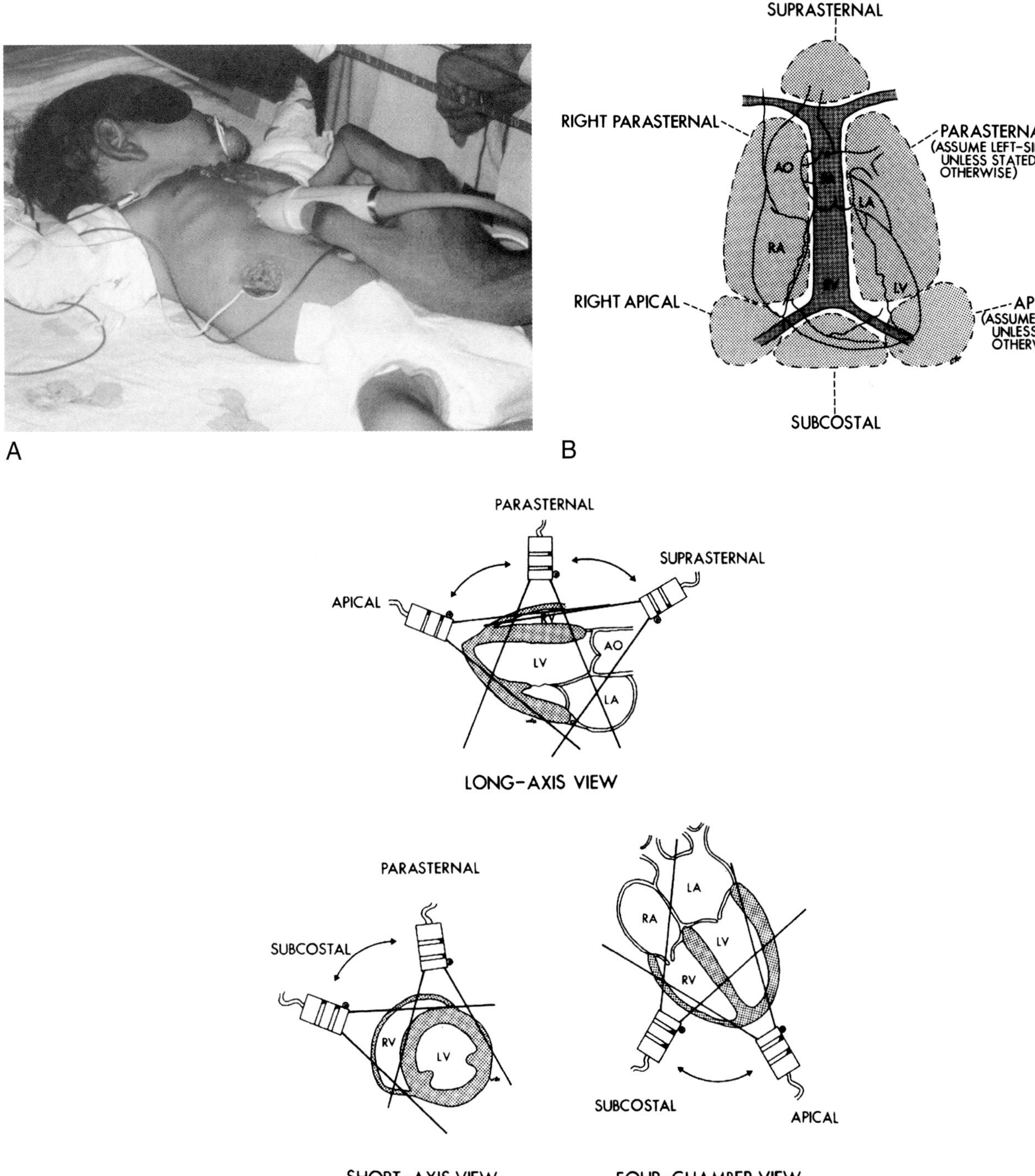


**FIGURE 54–1. A,** Demonstration of position of ultrasound transducer utilizing the subcostal approach in a neonate. **B,** By moving the transducer to multiple windows surrounding the heart, echocardiographic two-dimensional tomographic imaging provides for a three-dimensional look at the heart via "mental reconstruction" once each of the corresponding windows has been examined. **C,** Long-axis, short-axis, and four-chamber views of the heart contribute to visualization of the overall detail of complex cardiac anatomy. *(**B** and **C**, Courtesy of the American Society of Echocardiography.)*

in scope; however, initial evaluation should be complete and include investigation of all aspects of the heart and great vessels using two-dimensional, Doppler, color Doppler, and M-mode imaging. More than a dozen sweeps and views through numerous windows and from various angles are used to create a complete picture of the heart and great vessels (Fig. 54–1). The technique of subcostal (subxiphoid) two-dimensional sweep imaging with tomographic cuts of the heart provides for a three-dimensional (3D) look at cardiac structures via "mental reconstruction" once each of the corresponding windows has been examined. Usefulness of subcostal imaging is unique to neonates and pediatric patients, as the liver acts to enhance acoustic transmission and the heart is only a short distance away in the young subject.

Although echocardiography is considered a noninvasive diagnostic test, care should be taken during the performance of the echocardiogram, particularly in small, premature infants. Often, sedation is necessary to obtain patient compliance, so that continuing assessment during the procedure and monitoring thereafter are essential. Application of cold ultrasound gel and exposure to air may cause temperature instability. Applying pressure on the abdomen during subcostal imaging or extending the neck during suprasternal imaging may cause destabilization of the patient. Either the person performing the echocardiogram or another assigned person should monitor heart rate, blood pressure, and ventilatory parameters during the procedure in unstable, ill infants.

## MODALITIES OF ECHOCARDIOGRAPHY AND THEIR APPLICATIONS

### M-Mode Echocardiography

The earliest form of echocardiographic imaging, M-mode echocardiography, displays fine detail of cardiac structure along a time line. A single thin plane of ultrasound energy is focused onto a targeted region of the heart. All structures within the targeted plane of insonation are then displayed in real time as they change during various portions of the cardiac cycle.

M-mode echocardiography is commonly used for measurement of myocardial wall thickness and cavity dimensions and is useful in estimating ventricular cavity size for calculation of the ventricular *shortening fraction*— an estimate of ventricular function. By angling the plane of insonation through the short axis of the left ventricle at the level of the tips of the papillary muscles, the clinician can obtain an M-mode display of the change in ventricular cavity dimension over time (Fig. 54–2). The ratio of the difference between left ventricle end-diastolic dimension (LVEDD) and left ventricle end-systolic dimension (LVESD) to the left ventricle end-diastolic dimension is the shortening fraction [(LVEDD − LVESD)/LVEDD × 100 = %SF]. The normal range is 28% to 38%, which correlates with a ventricular volumetric ejection fraction ratio of 55% to 65%, suggesting normal ventricular function. Interpretation of the %SF must also take into account the over-

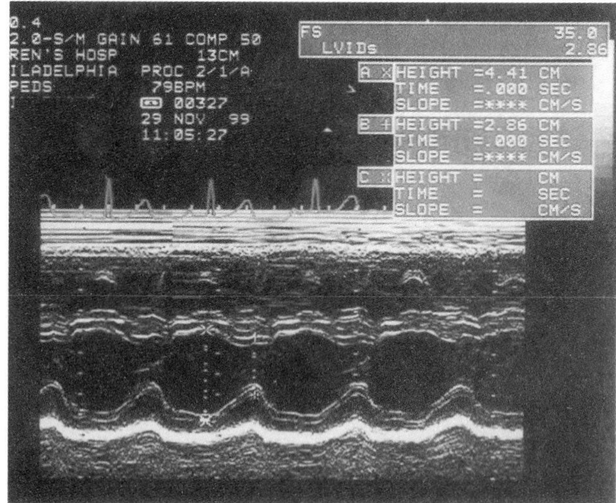


**FIGURE 54–2.** (See also Color Plate 54–2.) M-mode tracing of the left ventricle dimensions over time obtained in the short-axis view. The electrocardiographic tracing helps identify the timing of the cardiac cycle as systolic or diastolic. Measurement A demonstrates the left ventricle end-diastolic dimension, and measurement B, the left ventricle end-systolic measurement. The shortening fraction is calculated at 35%.

all dimensions of the left ventricle. For example, an infant with a volume load due to mitral regurgitation or a large patent ductus arteriosus (PDA) may have a normal %SF but may have a dilated, enlarged left ventricle for age. The %SF also can be helpful in investigating the cause of hypotension in infants. With hypotension due to myocardial dysfunction, the infant will have a dilated left ventricle and diminished %SF. With hypotension due to vasodilatation, such as seen in various conditions of sepsis, the infant may have a normal or hyperdynamic %SF, often exceeding 40%. Volume-depleted infants will exhibit a normal %SF but a small left ventricular cavity size.

Although it is the most commonly used technique for determination of ventricular function, the M-mode measurement of %SF has a number of limitations. It provides for only a single-plane assessment of ventricular contraction and is invalid in conditions in which there is wall motion abnormality. Paradoxical movement of the ventricular septum away from the posterior wall during systole may create a spuriously low %SF value. Hence, %SF measures may be difficult to interpret in the presence of right bundle branch block, right ventricle dilatation due to atrial septal defect, frequent premature ventricular contractions, or complete heart block.

### Two-Dimensional Echocardiography

Development of phased-array transducers has allowed for sector scanning and the display of two-dimensional images. This is the most commonly applied modality of echocardiography and is used primarily for determination of anatomic structure (Fig. 54–3).

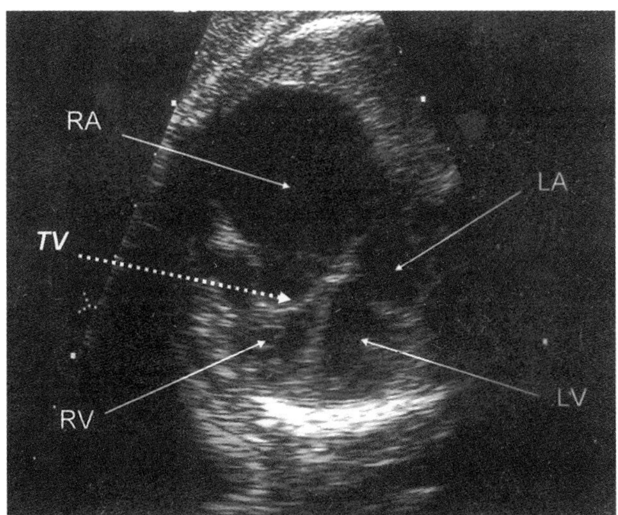


**FIGURE 54–3.** A two-dimensional echocardiographic image from an infant with Ebstein anomaly of the tricuspid valve. This apical view demonstrates the detail of anatomy that is obtainable with two-dimensional imaging. *Arrow* points to the apically displaced tricuspid valve, classically seen in Ebstein anomaly. LA, left atrium; LV, left ventricle; RA, right atrium; RV, right ventricle; TV, tricuspid valve.

## Doppler Echocardiography

Application of the Doppler principle allows for determination of the velocity and direction of moving objects. Because blood and myocardial tissue both are in motion throughout the cardiac cycle, either can be assessed by Doppler echocardiography. Doppler imaging can be performed in a number of ways. In pulsed wave Doppler echocardiography, transducer crystals alternately fire pulses of energy and then "listen" for reflected signal return. This mode allows for determination of spatial signal position but limits the ability to measure increased velocities. In continuous wave Doppler echocardiography, half of the transducer crystals fire continuously while the other half "listen" continuously. This mode allows for unambiguous assessment of increased velocities but limits the ability to pinpoint precise spatial position of these velocities. In combination, pulsed wave and continuous wave Doppler modes provide a complete picture of blood flow direction and velocity (Fig. 54–4).

Color Doppler echocardiography utilizes pulsed wave principles to create a two-dimensional sector display of all velocities within a given region of interest. A sector within a two-dimensional image is identified and pixels of color are displayed overlying the area of interrogation. Each color pixel reflects the direction of motion; the shade of color reflects the velocity. By convention, "warm" colors such as red and orange designate direction of flow toward the transducer, and "cold" colors such as blue and white designate flow away from the transducer. Recently, Doppler techniques have been applied to tissue motion of the myocardium.

Although tissue signals move at much lower velocities than blood signals, determination of Doppler-derived tissue velocities can aid in understanding complex states of systolic and diastolic dysfunction. Distinct patterns of

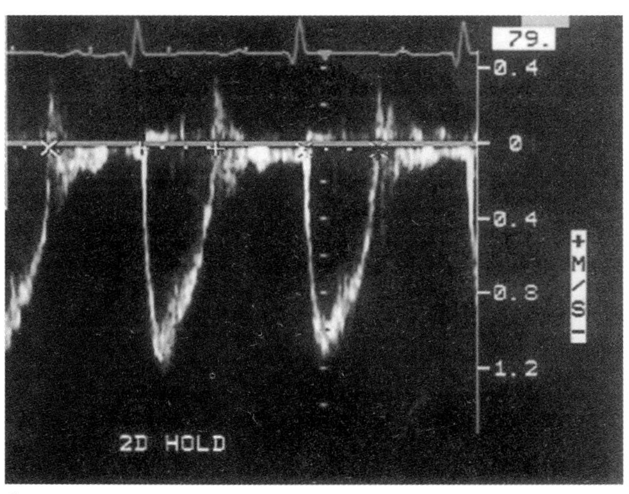


A

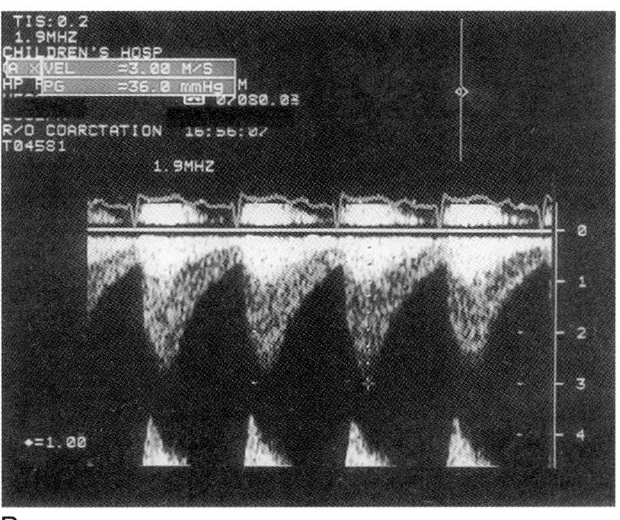


B

**FIGURE 54–4.** (See also Color Plate 54–4.) **A,** Example of a pulsed wave Doppler signal. Time is on the *x*-axis, and velocity is in meters/second on the *y*-axis. Note the central clearing of the signal, with a fine envelope displayed. The maximal velocity is approximately 1 meter/second. **B,** Example of a continuous wave Doppler signal. Note the filling-in of the signal envelope. The peak velocity is 3 meters/second. This pattern is classic for coarctation of the aorta: There is a run-off of the Doppler signal into diastole, with a double-peak envelope (a smaller peak at 1 meter/second within the larger peak of 3 meters/second). This latter feature reflects the fact that continuous wave Doppler cannot distinguish between the lower velocities proximal to the coarctation from the elevated velocities just distal to the coarctation; hence, both velocities are displayed as a single signal, one overlaid on the other.

normal and abnormal motion of various myocardial segments have been described.

Data derived from Doppler echocardiography are used to provide physiologic information. Utilizing the principles of flow hydraulics across a tubular system with discrete narrowing, velocity data can be translated into pressure data via modification of the Bernoulli equation (Fig. 54–5), in which

$$P_1 - P_2 = 4 \times (V_2 - V_1)^2$$

Normal velocities in the heart are rarely greater than 1 meter/sec. Velocities proximal to areas of narrowing are typically less than 1 meter/sec, and can often be ignored. Hence, the equation can be simplified to

$$\text{pressure change} = 4 \times \text{Vmax}^2$$

This principle can be applied in a variety of clinical settings. For example, in the presence of tricuspid regurgitation (TR), the peak right ventricle pressure (which will equal the pulmonary artery pressure in the absence of pulmonary stenosis) can be estimated by measuring the regurgitant jet peak velocity. A TR peak velocity of 2 meters/second suggests a right ventricle pressure of 16 mm Hg ($4 \times (2)^2$) greater than the right atrial pressure. One must remember that the Bernoulli equation provides for the pressure difference between two chambers; hence, to assess the absolute pressure in the right ventricle, the right atrial pressure must be added to the difference between the right atrium and right ventricle pressures as measured by the TR jet. In infants and children, right atrial pressure is estimated to be between 3 and 10 mm Hg, with 5 mm Hg typically chosen as an estimated guess. Hence, in the foregoing example, the patient would have a right ventricle pressure of 21 mm Hg, which is within normal limits. Alternatively, an infant with severe chronic lung disease may have a TR peak jet of 4 meters/second. This would translate to a pressure estimate of 64 mm Hg ($4 \times (4)^2$); 64 mm Hg added to the estimated right atrial pressure of 5 mm Hg gives a right ventricle pressure of 69 mm Hg, which suggests pulmonary hypertension. The Bernoulli equation also is commonly used to assess pressure gradients across stenotic valves such as in valvar aortic or pulmonic stenosis. Using the maximum velocity across the stenotic valve, the clinician can derive the "peak instantaneous" gradient across the outflow tract.

Bernoulli Equation

$$P_1 - P_2 = 4 \times (V_2 - V_1)^2$$

*If $V_1 < 1$ m/sec, then*

$$\text{Pressure change} = 4 \times V_{max}^2$$

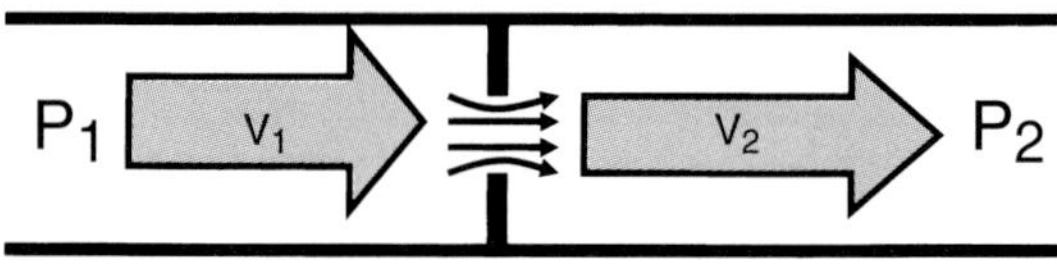


*Direction of flow in a closed system* →

**FIGURE 54–5.** Bernoulli equation of flow dynamics describes the relationship between pressure differences and velocity differences across an area of narrowing in a closed fluid system. $P_1$, proximal pressure; $P_2$, downstream distal pressure; $V_1$, proximal velocity; $V_2$, distal downstream velocity.

### Three-Dimensional Echocardiography

Integration of multiplanar image data into a real-time 3D display has been a goal of echocardiography for many years. Recently, early systems have been developed that are capable of displaying 3D echocardiographic images. Benefits of 3D echocardiography include an improved way of identifying the spatial relationship of adjacent structures and providing rapid data acquisition times for a large amount of image data. Although in its infancy, 3D echocardiography promises to become an important modality as technologic advances continue.

## LIMITATIONS OF ECHOCARDIOGRAPHY

Although an extremely useful tool that has revolutionized the approach to diagnostic evaluation of the cardiovascular system in the neonate, echocardiography has a number of limitations:

- *Discrepancy between "echo-derived" and "catheter-derived" gradients.* Doppler echocardiography measures the "peak instantaneous" pressure difference at any point in time during flow across a stenotic valve. In the case of a stenotic aortic valve, this may occur during the upstroke of systole, not at the peak of systole. Catheter-based measures of pressure are taken at the peak of systole; hence, echo-derived pressure gradients do not equal, and usually exceed, catheter-derived measures. This discrepancy does not invalidate the measures of either modality but rather highlights the point that they are measures of gradients occurring during two different points in systole. Historically, clinical decision making has been based on catheter-derived information; therefore, echocardiographically derived data should be interpreted in this light. Other factors that may have an impact on differences in echocardiographic versus catheter-based gradients are level of sedation, hydration status, medications (inotropes), and ventilatory strategy.
- *Stress of the test.* Lengthy environmental exposure, temperature instability, and pressure application on the chest or abdomen during transducer contact may result in stress for the premature or hemodynamically unstable infant, often necessitating termination of the procedure or limiting the scope of the ultrasound evaluation.
- *Inadequate visualization of structures.* Lung disease and air trapping can cause acoustic impedance, limiting the ability to visualize structures.
- *Inadequate Doppler signal for velocity measurement.* Small blood volumes in small structures may at times not be seen with echocardiography. Examples are coronary arteries in the very small, premature infant and pulmonary

vein flow in patients with severe lung disease, in whom pulmonary blood flow may be limited. Identification of pulmonary venous anatomy and flow in infants on extracorporeal membrane oxygenation also may be difficult owing to blood volume bypass of the pulmonary circulation. TEE may be indicated in these patients.

## INDICATIONS FOR ECHOCARDIOGRAPHY IN THE NEONATE

### Suspected Congenital Heart Disease

Echocardiography is the primary imaging modality used to diagnose congenital heart disease. Information concerning structure and physiology can be obtained, thereby obviating the need for further invasive diagnostic tests. Data obtained from echocardiography are frequently sufficient for the development of a surgical plan and management strategy for most forms of congenital heart disease (Tworetzky et al, 1999). Detailed review of the application of echocardiography in congenital heart disease is beyond the scope of this chapter and is covered elsewhere (see Snider and Serwer, 1990).

### Assessment of the Ductus Arteriosus

Before the routine use of echocardiography, a hemodynamically significant PDA was diagnosed clinically by the presence of a heart murmur, hyperdynamic precordium, bounding and palmar pulses, need for increased ventilatory support, and radiographic evidence of cardiomegaly with increased pulmonary vascular markings. Unfortunately, the cardiac examination of a critically ill premature infant can be difficult and unreliable. Thus in the present era, a complete transthoracic echocardiogram is recommended before medical or surgical treatment of PDA (Fig. 54–6).

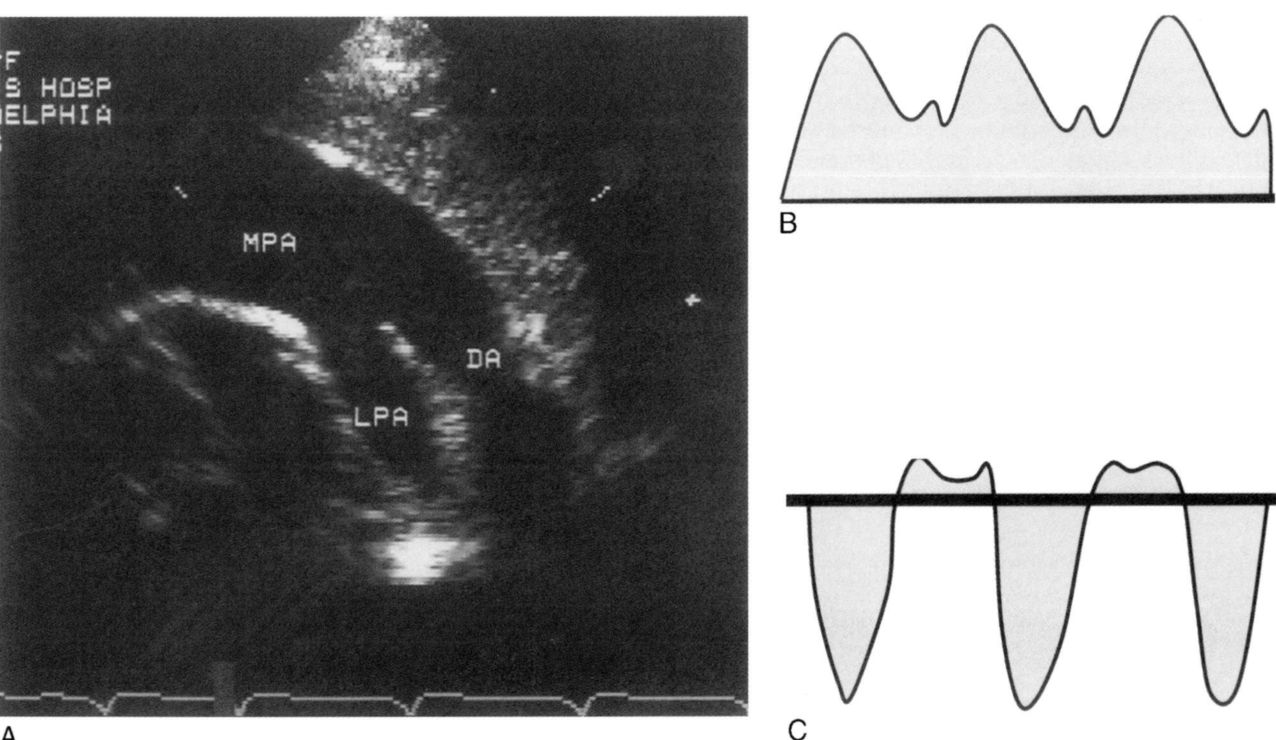


**FIGURE 54–6.** **A,** Two-dimensional echocardiographic image of a large ductus arteriosus, high parasternal view. DA, ductus arteriosus; LPA, left pulmonary artery; MPA, main pulmonary artery. **B,** Schematic of the Doppler flow pattern seen in a neonate with a patent ductus arteriosus and normal pulmonary vascular resistance and left-to-right shunting. Note that all of the flow is above the baseline and, on the high parasternal view, is directed toward the MPA from the aorta. **C,** Schematic of the Doppler flow pattern seen in a neonate with a patent ductus arteriosus and right-to-left shunting in systole and left-to-right shunting in diastole. Flow is below the baseline away from the MPA toward the descending aorta in systole (antegrade) and above the baseline back toward the MPA from the descending aorta (retrograde) in diastole. This pattern is classically seen in critical left-sided congenital heart disease in which ductal support for systemic perfusion is required (hypoplastic left heart syndrome, critical coarctation of the aorta) and in severe pulmonary hypertension of the newborn.

The echocardiogram is important not only to confirm the presence of a PDA but also to ensure that other important structural heart defects are not present. Premature infants with critical left-sided obstructive lesions (e.g., hypoplastic left heart syndrome, critical aortic stenosis, coarctation of the aorta) or right-sided obstructive lesions (e.g., tetralogy of Fallot with pulmonary atresia, pulmonary atresia with intact ventricular septum, tricuspid atresia) rely on a PDA for survival until surgical intervention.

Echocardiographic assessment of the PDA also can be useful in determining the size of the ductus and the impact of the patency on the cardiovascular status of the neonate. Flow across the ductus arteriosus can be purely left to right, purely right to left as seen in association with severe pulmonary hypertension, or bidirectional, with right-to-left flow in systole and left-to-right flow in diastole, as seen in some patients with pulmonary hypertension and in infants with ductus-dependent systemic circulation with normal pulmonary artery pressure (Cloez et al, 1986). When there is isolated left-to-right flow through a PDA, the peak systolic pressure gradient from the aorta to the pulmonary artery (as measured by the modified Bernoulli equation) can be used as a rough estimate of pulmonary artery pressure, if the systolic blood pressure is simultaneously measured (Musewe et al, 1990). However, this method does have limitations and tends to underestimate the true pulmonary artery pressure (Snider, 1990).

PDA closure with indomethacin therapy occurs in approximately 85% of cases (Gersony et al, 1983); however, reopening of the ductus after successful pharmacologic closure has been reported in up to 25% of premature infants so treated (Weiss et al, 1995). In such cases, surgical ligation of the PDA is recommended. Determination of aortic arch "sidedness" via echocardiography is important when surgical thoracotomy is planned (Murdison et al, 1990). Although the majority of patients have a left aortic arch with a left-sided ductus arteriosus, so that surgical access is through a left thoracotomy, there are cases of right aortic arch, right-sided PDA, and/or vascular ring in the premature infant. Identification of one of these findings will alter the surgeon's approach to ductal ligation.

## Evaluation of Pulmonary Hypertension in the Newborn

Infants with persistent pulmonary hypertension of the newborn (PPHN) have severe vasoconstriction of the pulmonary vasculature resulting in elevation of pulmonary artery pressure and pulmonary vascular resistance with normal left atrial pressure. Right-to-left shunting is therefore observed at the level of the ductus arteriosus and foramen ovale (hence the other common term for this disorder—"persistent fetal circulation"). In infants with PPHN, transthoracic echocardiography determines if the heart is structurally normal, demonstrates atrial and ductal level shunting (by color flow mapping), and can provide an estimate of pulmonary artery pressure by measuring the velocity of the tricuspid regurgitation jet, if present. The appearance of the Doppler pattern sampled in the branch pulmonary artery also may provide information about the peripheral vascular resistance and potential response to supplemental oxygen (Fig. 54–7). The velocity of ductal flow also has been used to estimate pulmonary artery pressure. With unidirectional shunting at the ductus, the peak velocity of ductal flow has been correlated with pulmonary artery pressure estimated from the tricuspid regurgitation jet. In addition, with bidirectional shunting at the ductus, duration of right-to-left flow of at least 60% has been associated with systemic level pulmonary artery pressure and resistance and signifies severe PPHN (Musewe et al, 1990). Although some infants may normally exhibit a very short duration of right-to-left shunting early in systole, the presence of right-to-left systolic shunting of significant duration at the ductus arteriosus suggests critical left-sided congenital heart disease or PPHN. When such right-to-left shunting is present, closure of the ductus arteriosus should not be undertaken.

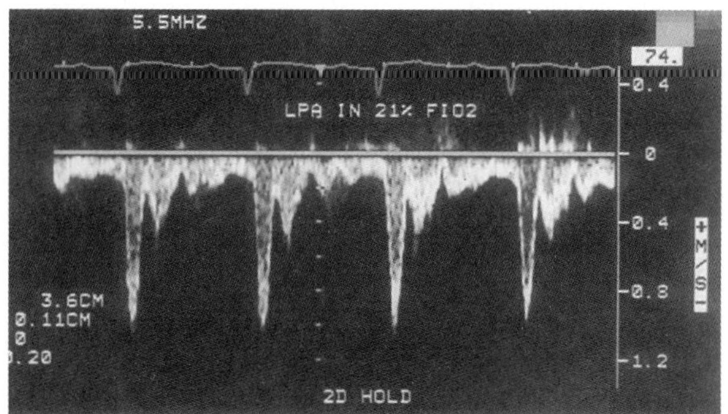


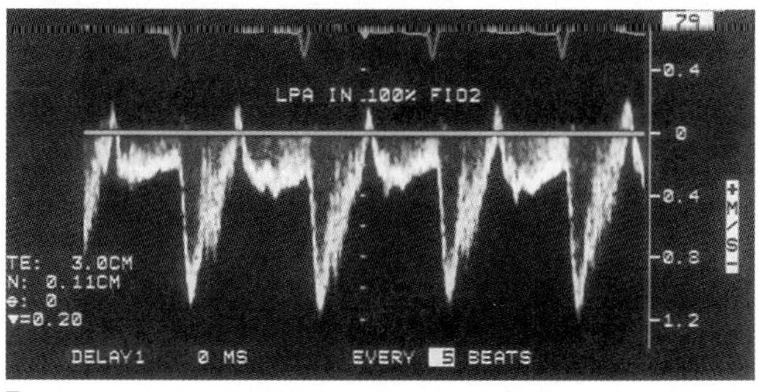


**FIGURE 54–7.** (See also Color Plate 54–7.) **A,** Doppler flow pattern obtained in the left pulmonary artery of an infant with severe pulmonary hypertension breathing room air (21%). **B,** Doppler flow pattern obtained in the same left pulmonary artery after the addition of supplemental oxygen (100%). Note the increase in area under the Doppler flow envelope with increased flow in both systole and diastole, reflecting pulmonary vasodilatation.

In addition to the assessment of pulmonary artery pressure, echocardiography may be used to assess ventricular function in the infant with PPHN. Neonates with PPHN typically have cardiac dysfunction affecting the right ventricle (Valdes-Cruz et al, 1981). However, the left ventricle can be involved as well, with evidence of myocardial ischemia, abnormal electrocardiogram, and mitral regurgitation (Riemenschneider et al, 1976). Although the etiology of cardiac dysfunction in PPHN is unclear, prenatal constriction of the ductus arteriosus has been suggested as a possible mechanism (Fox et al, 1977; Morin, 1989).

Extracorporeal membrane oxygenation (ECMO) is often utilized to treat infants with severe PPHN whose hypoxemia does not respond to routine methods of mechanical ventilatory support and pulmonary vasodilation. In the decision-making process, an echocardiogram is often crucial to confirm the diagnosis of PPHN and, more important, to rule out congenital heart defects that may mimic PPHN. Many forms of structural heart disease can manifest with severe hypoxemia and pulmonary artery hypertension, which can mimic PPHN. The common finding in these defects is impediment to pulmonary venous return to the left atrium (Long, 1984). Such lesions include total anomalous pulmonary venous connection (TAPVC) with obstruction, cor triatriatum, transposition of the great arteries with intact atrial septum, and hypoplastic left heart syndrome with intact atrial septum. TAPVC can be extremely difficult to diagnose by echocardiography, particularly in the critically ill neonate. TAPVC results in significantly diminished pulmonary blood flow; therefore, it is often difficult to confirm the pulmonary venous connections by noninvasive methods (Kimball et al, 1989). Also, if a patient is on ECMO support before echocardiographic evaluation, diagnosis of TAPVC can be even more challenging, because the volume of blood traversing the pulmonary circulation is markedly diminished. If TAPVC is suspected but not well seen on transthoracic echocardiography, TEE may be useful. Cardiac catheterization is recommended to make the diagnosis if findings of noninvasive methods are inconclusive. Causes for difficulties in circuit flow dynamics while the infant is receiving ECMO often can be elucidated by an echocardiogram. Visualizing an obstructive cannula position, either in the atria or aorta, may explain impaired flow.

Echocardiography can also be useful to document progressive improvement in the patient with PPHN. Aggressive treatment with oxygen, nitric oxide, and other pulmonary vasodilators can be avoided if echocardiography demonstrates a lesser degree of right-to-left or exclusively left-to-right shunting within the heart. Documentation of closure of the PDA also is important because once the ductus is closed, the patient is no longer relying on the right ventricle to augment cardiac output to the systemic circulation. In addition, if tricuspid regurgitation is present, echocardiography can be used to serially monitor the systolic pressure in the pulmonary artery.

## Transitory Myocardial Ischemia of the Newborn

Transitory myocardial ischemia (TMI) occurs in association with severe perinatal asphyxia and may manifest with tachycardia, tachypnea, poor perfusion, and heart murmur (Barberi et al, 1999; Fox et al, 1977). This clinical presentation is often difficult to distinguish from critical left heart obstruction (i.e., critical coarctation of aorta, hypoplastic left heart syndrome). Typical echocardiographic findings include diminished ventricular function (including wall motion abnormalities), atrioventricular valve regurgitation (most commonly tricuspid regurgitation), and in rare cases, echobright areas within the myocardium consistent with infarction. For the majority of infants with TMI, the cardiac abnormalities are temporary, with return of ventricular function and valve competence to normal within days of birth.

## Assessment of the Neonate with Extracardiac Anomalies

A variety of extracardiac anomalies and conditions are associated with congenital heart disease (Table 54–1). When these anomalies or conditions are suspected or known, an echocardiographic assessment is usually warranted. Confirmation of absence of structural heart disease can be extremely helpful to the neonatologist, the anesthesiologist, and the pediatric surgeon, whereas presence of a congenital heart defect may alter the management strategy and clinical course of the infant. Identification of a significant congenital heart defect in combination with an extracardiac anomaly may require attention to specific details at the

**TABLE 54–1**

**Indications for Echocardiographic Evaluation in the Neonate**

| Conditions Associated with Congenital Heart Defects | |
|---|---|
| *Syndromes* | *Non-Syndromes* |
| Trisomies 13, 18, 21 | Congenital diaphragmatic hernia |
| VACTER association | Gastroschisis |
| CHARGE association | Omphalocele |
| Holt-Oram syndrome | Tracheoesophageal fistula |
| Goldenhar syndrome | Absence of radius |
| Cornelia de Lange syndrome | |
| Turner syndrome | |
| Noonan syndrome | |
| Williams syndrome | |
| Infantile Marfan syndrome | |
| ***Conditions Associated with Impact on Cardiovascular System*** | |
| Congenital diaphragmatic hernia | |
| Sacrococcygeal teratoma | |
| Twin-twin transfusion syndrome | |
| Arteriovenous malformation | |
| Perinatal asphyxia | |
| Severe anemia | |

CHARGE, coloboma, heart disease, retarded growth/development and/or central nervous system anomalies, genital hypoplasia, ear anomalies and/or deafness; VACTER, vertebral abnormalities, anal atresia, cardiac abnormalities, tracheo-esophageal fistula and/or esophageal atresia, renal agenesis/dysplasia.

time of echocardiographic evaluation. One such extra cardiac anomaly is congenital diaphragmatic hernia (CDH).

CDH is frequently associated with congenital heart disease (prevalence of 10% to 35% of infants with CDH) (Greenwood et al, 1976; Ryan et al, 1994), and the combination frequently is lethal (Cohen et al, 2002). Patients with CDH often have hypoxemia; it is therefore important to distinguish between the cyanosis of severe lung hypoplasia (with PPHN) and that of cyanotic heart disease (e.g., tetralogy of Fallot, pulmonary atresia). If the heart is structurally normal, echocardiography can help in the assessment of the severity of the CDH. Assessment of pulmonary artery pressure and intracardiac shunting (as described for PPHN) can be useful for prognostic purposes. Left ventricular hypoplasia occurs commonly in patients with CDH. This association may be related to prenatal factors such as mechanical compression of the left ventricle by abdominal contents, diminished flow across the foramen ovale, or diminished pulmonary venous return secondary to lung hypoplasia. The degree of left ventricular hypoplasia is a predictor of mortality in infants with left-sided CDH (Baumgart et al, 1998; Schwartz et al, 1994; Seibert et al, 1984). Infants with CDH in association with left ventricular hypoplasia are more likely to require ECMO support after birth. Echocardiographic measurements of mitral annulus, left ventricular length, and aortic dimensions can help establish the viability of the left ventricle as a systemic ventricle in patients with CDH.

## FETAL ECHOCARDIOGRAPHY

Echocardiographic techniques have been applied to the developing human fetal cardiovascular system. Excellent images of fetal cardiac anatomy and flow dynamics can be obtained as early as 16 weeks of gestation. Prenatal detection of congenital heart disease has been shown to improve outcome in the postnatal state by reducing postnatal acidosis and mortality (Tworetzky et al, 2001; Verheijen et al, 2001). Indications for fetal echocardiography can be separated into maternal and fetal and are listed in Table 54–1. Application of Doppler echocardiography in the fetus has been helpful in diagnosing and monitoring a variety of disorders. Evaluation of blood flow patterns in the fetal ductus venosus, umbilical vein, and umbilical artery can provide important information on fetal cardiovascular status and condition of the placenta (Hecher et al, 1995).

Fetal echocardiography can be used to monitor the development and progression of congenital heart disease. Various forms of obstructive disease have been observed to progress in severity, or to evolve into a new category of anomaly, over the period from the second to the third trimester (Hornberger et al, 1995). Moderate forms of pulmonic stenosis may progress to severe stenosis or valvar atresia. Left-sided heart disease such as aortic stenosis diagnosed at 18 weeks of gestation may progress to hypoplastic left heart syndrome, with "arrest" of left ventricular development at 30 weeks of gestation, when flow traversing the left ventricle is impeded. Factors that dictate the presence and rate of progression of congenital heart disease in utero have not yet been determined.

## REFERENCES

Barberi I, Calabro MP, Cordaro S, et al: Myocardial ischemia in neonates with perinatal asphyxia: Electrocardiographic, echocardiographic and enzymatic correlations. Eur J Pediatr 158:742-747, 1999.

Baumgart S, Paul JJ, Huhta JC, et al: Cardiac malposition, redistribution of fetal cardiac output, and left ventricular hypoplasia reduce survival in neonates with congenital diaphragmatic hernia requiring extracorporeal membrane oxygenation. J Pediatr 133:57-62, 1998.

Bruce CJ, O'Leary P, Hagler DJ, et al: Miniaturized transesophageal echocardiography in newborn infants. J Am Soc Echocardiogr 15:791-797, 2000.

Cloez JL, Isaaz K, Pernot C: Pulsed Doppler flow characteristics of ductus arteriosus in infants with associated congenital anomalies of the heart or great arteries. Am J Cardiol 57:845, 1986.

Cohen MS, Rychik J, Bush DM, et al: Influence of congenital heart disease on survival in children with congenital diaphragmatic hernia. J Pediatr 141:25-30, 2002.

Fox W, Gewitz M, Dinwiddie R, et al: Pulmonary hypertension in the perinatal aspiration syndromes. Pediatrics 59:205-211, 1977.

Gersony WM, Peckham GJ, Ellison RC, et al: Effects of indomethacin in premature infants with patent ductus arteriosus: Results of a national collaborative study. J Pediatr 102:895-906, 1983.

Greenwood RD, Rosenthal A, Nadas AS: Cardiovascular abnormalities associated with congenital diaphragmatic hernia. Pediatrics 57:92-97, 1976.

Hecher K, Campbell S, Doyle P, et al: Assessment of fetal compromise by Doppler ultrasound investigation of the fetal circulation: Arterial, intracardiac, and venous blood flow velocity studies. Circulation 91:129-138, 1995.

Hornberger LK, Sanders SP, Rein AJ, et al: Left heart obstructive lesions and left ventricular growth in the midtrimester fetus: A longitudinal study. Circulation 92:1531-1538, 1995.

Kimball TR, Weiss RG, Meyer RA, et al: Color flow mapping to document normal pulmonary venous return in neonates with persistent pulmonary hypertension being considered for extracorporeal membrane oxygenation. J Pediatr 114:433-437, 1989.

Li P, Dairywala IT, Liu Z, et al: Anatomic and hemodynamic imaging using a new vector phase-array intracardiac catheter. J Am Soc Echocardiogr 15:349-355, 2002.

Long W: Structural cardiovascular abnormalities presenting as persistent pulmonary hypertension of the newborn. Clin Perinatol 11:601-626, 1984.

Morin FC: Ligating the ductus arteriosus before birth causes persistent pulmonary hypertension in the newborn lamb. Pediatr Res 25:245-250, 1989.

Murdison KA, Andrews BA, Chin AJ: Ultrasonographic display of complex vascular rings. J Am Coll Cardiol 15:1645-1653, 1990.

Musewe NN, Poppe D, Smallhorn JF, et al: Doppler echocardiographic measurement of pulmonary artery pressure from ductal Doppler velocities in the newborn. J Am Coll Cardiol 15:446-456, 1990.

Randolph GR, Hagler DJ, Connolly HM, et al: Intraoperative transesophageal echocardiography during surgery for congenital heart defects. J Thorac Cardiovasc Surg 124:1176-1182, 2002.

Riemenschneider T, Nielson J, Ruttenberg H, Jaffe R: Disturbances of the transitional circulation: Spectrum of pulmonary hypertension and myocardial dysfunction. J Pediatr 89:622-625, 1976.

Ryan CA, Perreault T, Johnston-Hodgson A, Finer NN: Extracorporeal membrane oxygenation in infants with congenital

diaphragmatic hernia and cardiac malformations. J Pediatr Surg 29:878-881, 1994.
Schwartz SM, Vermillion RP, Hirschl RB: Evaluation of left ventricular mass in children with left-sided congenital diaphragmatic hernia. J Pediatr 125:447-451, 1994.
Seibert JR, Haas JE, Beckwith JB: Left ventricular hypoplasia in congenital diaphragmatic hernia. J Pediatr Surg 19:567-571, 1984.
Snider AR: The ductus arteriosus: A window for assessment of pulmonary artery pressure? J Am Coll Cardiol 15:457, 1990.
Snider AR, Serwer GA: Echocardiography in Pediatric Heart Disease. Chicago, Year Book Medical Publishers, 1990.
Tworetzky W, McElhinney DB, Brook MM, et al: Echocardiographic diagnosis alone for complete repair of major congenital heart defects. J Am Coll Cardiol 33:228-233, 1999.
Tworetzky W, McElhinney DB, Reddy VM, et al: Improved surgical outcome after fetal diagnosis of hypoplastic left heart syndrome. Circulation 103:1269-1273, 2001.
Valdes-Cruz L, Dudell G, Ferrara A: Utility of M-mode echocardiography for early identification of infants with persistent pulmonary hypertension of the newborn. Pediatrics 68:515-525, 1981.
Verheijen PM, Lisowski LA, Stoutenbeek P, et al: Prenatal diagnosis of congenital heart disease affects preoperative acidosis in the newborn patient. J Thorac Cardiovasc Surg 121:798-803, 2001.
Weiss H, Cooper B, Brook M, et al: Factors determining reopening of the ductus arteriosus after successful clinical closure with indomethacin. J Pediatr 127:466-471, 1995.
Weyman AE (ed): Principles and Practice of Echocardiography, 2nd ed. Philadelphia, Lea & Febiger, 1994.

CHAPTER 55

# Stabilization and Transport of the Neonate with Congenital Heart Disease

**Bradley S. Marino and Gil Wernovsky**

Once a diagnosis of congenital heart disease is suspected, the neonate must be stabilized and arrangements made for a complete evaluation to delineate the anatomic abnormalities. Such evaluation may necessitate transport of the neonate to an intensive care unit at another medical center where a pediatric cardiologist and a pediatric cardiothoracic surgeon are available (Castañeda et al, 1989). The initial hours after diagnosis are crucial in the outcomes of these neonates, as increasing numbers of short- and long-term outcome studies have revealed that the preoperative status of the patient is a major factor in determining mortality risk (Mahle et al, 2000), length of hospital stay (Wernovsky et al, 2000a), and long-term neurologic and developmental outcomes (Mahle and Wernovsky, 2000; Mahle et al, 2000; Wernovsky et al, 2000b). The most important aspects of stabilization and transport are the initial resuscitation, airway management, vascular access, the judicious use of supplemental oxygen, prostaglandin $E_1$ ($PGE_1$) therapy, inotropic support, and the specifics surrounding the transportation of the neonate.

## STABILIZATION

### Initial Resuscitation

For the neonate who presents with hypoxemia unresponsive to supplemental oxygen, congestive heart failure, or shock, simultaneous attention is devoted to the basics of advanced life support and to maintenance of a patent ductus arteriosus. If necessary, a stable airway must be maintained, allowing for adequate alveolar oxygenation and ventilation. In neonates critically ill with congenital heart disease, intubation should be performed following premedication with sedation (with a narcotic or benzodiazepine), preferably with neuromuscular blockade in most cases (as discussed subsequently). Reliable venous access is essential; the umbilical vein should be used if patent. An arterial line assists in monitoring the blood pressure, acid-base status, and oxygenation of the patient. In the neonate, arterial access can be most reliably obtained through the umbilical artery. Volume resuscitation, inotropic support, and correction of metabolic acidosis are required to maximize cardiac output and tissue perfusion.

Blood glucose level and ionized calcium level should be checked to determine if hypoglycemia or hypocalcemia is present. In the initial evaluation of a newborn with cyanosis or circulatory collapse, a sepsis work-up usually is performed, and the patient is started on appropriate antibiotics.

### Airway Management and Supplemental Oxygen

In general, if respiratory distress or profound hypoxemia is present, the infant should be sedated, paralyzed, intubated, and mechanically ventilated. Although intubation may be "successfully" carried out without sedation and neuromuscular blockade, there are compelling reasons to intubate with the aid of these agents in patients with congenital heart disease. First, the increased secretion of catecholamines with intubation may result in significant dysrhythmias in the at-risk myocardium. Second, vagally mediated bradycardia from hypoxemia, hypercapnia, or laryngeal stimulation may lead to asystole in these neonates, who have little reserve. Finally, sedation and neuromuscular blockade will reduce whole-body oxygen consumption, raising the mixed venous oxygen saturation and improving oxygen delivery. Premedication with atropine 0.02 mg/kg usually is employed to blunt the vagal effects of laryngoscopy. Fentanyl (1 to 2 μg/kg) or midazolam (0.05 to 0.1 mg/kg) may be given, with titration of dose to effect. Chest wall rigidity may occur in the neonate with even low-dose fentanyl, and neuromuscular blockade may be necessary to obtain adequate ventilation. The neonate who has tolerated $PGE_1$ with stable hemodynamics and little to no apnea may usually be safely transported with a natural airway and spontaneous breathing.

Supplemental oxygen is a potent pulmonary vasodilator and may adversely affect the physiology in neonates with a single ventricle, as well as those with two ventricles with unrestrictive ventricular or great vessel communication (see Chapter 57, on congenital heart disease). An excess of oxygen will decrease pulmonary vascular resistance and increase the pulmonary blood flow at the expense of systemic blood flow. Rather than being managed according to "rules" dictating the concentration of supplemental oxygen, the child with suspected congenital heart disease should receive supplemental oxygen via a nasal cannula or face mask to titrate the peripheral oxygen saturation to 80% to 85%. With a normal hemoglobin level and cardiac output, an oxygen saturation of 80% to 85% will provide adequate oxygen content in the blood and adequate oxygen delivery.

The goal of ventilation generally is to "normoventilate" the neonate with congenital heart disease (to achieve a $P_{CO_2}$ of 35 to 40 mm Hg). In both the two-ventricle neonate with unrestrictive ventricular or great vessel communication and the neonate with a single ventricle, hyperventilation will decrease pulmonary vascular resistance and increase the pulmonary blood flow at the expense of systemic blood flow.

### Prostaglandin $E_1$ Therapy

The neonate who "fails" the hyperoxia test without an obvious pulmonary etiology, who has an "equivocal" result on the hyperoxia test but has other signs or symptoms of congenital heart disease, or who presents in shock within the first 3 weeks of life is highly likely to have complex congenital heart disease. Such neonates are likely to have congenital lesions that depend on blood flow through a patent ductus arteriosus for pulmonary blood flow or systemic blood flow, or they may need a patent ductus arteriosus to promote intercirculatory mixing (Freed et al, 1981). The administration of $PGE_1$ will open the ductus arteriosus and, depending on the lesion, increase pulmonary blood flow, systemic blood flow, or intercirculatory mixing. In patients with ductus-dependent pulmonary blood flow, as the ductus becomes large and non-restrictive, hypoxemia is lessened, and any metabolic acidosis that resulted from severe hypoxemia is corrected. In patients with ductus-dependent systemic flow and shock, resuscitation of the infant will not be successful until the ductus is opened. In neonates with transposition of the great arteries, maintenance of a patent ductus arteriosus improves intercirculatory mixing (Paul and Wernovsky, 1995; Wernovsky and Jonas, 1998).

The timing of diagnosis and the degree of ductal patency determine the dose of $PGE_1$. A dose of 0.01 to 0.025 μg/kg/minute usually is sufficient for stabilization of neonates with an echocardiographically demonstrated patent ductus arteriosus, as well as for those with a prenatal diagnosis in whom $PGE_1$ is given in the delivery room. Neonates presenting with significant ductal restriction may require doses of $PGE_1$ as high as 0.1 μg/kg/minute. Rarely, an older neonate (1 to 2 weeks of age) may require a higher dose of $PGE_1$ to initially reopen the ductus. Once a therapeutic effect has been achieved, the dose may often be decreased to as low as 0.01 μg/kg/minute without loss of therapeutic effect. The response to $PGE_1$ is often immediate if patency of the ductus is important for the hemodynamic state of the infant. Failure to respond to $PGE_1$ may mean that the initial diagnosis is incorrect; that the ductus is unresponsive to $PGE_1$ (which occurs in the older infant); that the ductus is absent; or that there is obstruction to pulmonary venous return.

Rarely, the patient with congenital heart disease may become progressively more unstable after the institution of $PGE_1$ therapy. This clinical deterioration after the institution of $PGE_1$ is an important diagnostic finding that identifies the congenital heart defect as involving obstructed blood flow out of the pulmonary veins or left atrium. Lesions with impairment of blood flow out of the left atrium include:

1. Hypoplastic left heart syndrome with a restrictive foramen ovale or intact atrial septum
2. Other variants of mitral atresia with a restrictive foramen ovale
3. Transposition of the great arteries with an intact ventricular septum and a restrictive foramen ovale
4. Total anomalous pulmonary venous return with obstruction of the common pulmonary vein

If there is clinical deterioration despite $PGE_1$ therapy, then plans for urgent echocardiography and interventional catheterization or cardiac surgery should be made.

$PGE_1$ administered as a continuous intravenous infusion is associated with adverse reactions that must be anticipated. Adverse reactions are more common in premature and/or low-birth-weight infants. Common side effects from $PGE_1$ administration are delineated in Table 55–1.

Apnea and hypotension are two clinically significant side effects of $PGE_1$ that seem to be dose dependent. Apnea resulting from $PGE_1$ therapy typically occurs within the first hours of administration but may occur *at any time* during administration of the drug. Therefore, after institution of $PGE_1$ therapy, infants require continuous cardiorespiratory monitoring. For those neonates with apnea in whom transport to another facility is planned, consideration should be made for control of the airway and mechanical ventilation before transport. Factors that influence the decision for intubation are the severity of hypoxemia and hemodynamic instability, gestational age of the patient, transport distance, and the skill of the transport team in urgent intubation.

The most undesirable side effect of $PGE_1$ is peripheral vasodilatation, which is manifested as hypotension and/or cutaneous flushing (Lewis et al, 1981). The infant presenting in shock is more likely to need a higher dose of $PGE_1$. Due to this phenomenon, a separate intravenous line should be secured for volume administration in infants receiving $PGE_1$, especially if transport will be required. If hypotension is noted, a 10 to 20 mL/kg bolus of normal saline, lactated Ringer's solution, or 5% albumin generally will normalize the infant's blood pressure. Serum ionized calcium levels also should be checked and should be normalized if low. If volume resuscitation does not correct hypotension induced by $PGE_1$, then dopamine 3 to 5 μg/kg/minute may be given to counter the vasodilatory effects. It is prudent to remeasure arterial blood gases and

**TABLE 55–1**

**Potential Side Effects of Prostaglandin $E_1$: Frequency and Birth Weight**

| Effect(s) | >2.0 kg | <2.0 kg |
|---|---|---|
| *Cardiovascular*: hypotension, rhythm disturbance, peripheral vasodilation | 16% | 36% |
| *Central nervous system*: seizure, temperature elevation | 16% | 16% |
| *Respiratory*: apnea, hypoventilation | 10% | 42% |
| *Metabolic*: hypoglycemia, hypocalcemia | 3% | 5% |
| *Infectious*: sepsis, wound infections | 3% | 10% |
| *Gastrointestinal*: diarrhea, necrotizing enterocolitis | 4% | 10% |
| *Hematologic*: DIC, hemorrhage, thrombocytopenia | 3% | 5% |
| *Renal*: renal failure, renal insufficiency | 1% | 3% |

DIC, disseminated intravascular coagulopathy.

Data from Lewis AB, Freed MD, Heymann MA, et al: Side effects of therapy with prostaglandin $E_1$ in infants with critical congenital heart disease. Circulation 64:893-898, 1981.

to reassess the infant's capillary refill and vital signs within 15 to 30 minutes of starting the $PGE_1$ infusion.

### Vascular Access

Umbilical venous (UVC) and umbilical arterial (UAC) catheters are useful in the stabilization, transport, and preoperative and postoperative management of neonates with congenital heart disease. The UVC should be located centrally in the right atrium. There is controversy over the optimal placement of the UAC. The UAC may be placed in a "high" position, with the tip in the thoracic aorta above the diaphragm (T4 to T10), or may be placed in a "low" position just distal to the take-off of the renal arteries (L3 to L4). Theoretically, high catheter placement may increase the risk of stroke or necrotizing enterocolitis, whereas low catheter placement may be associated with increased vascular complications; case-control studies of umbilical line complications in neonates with congenital heart disease have reported conflicting results. Other than in anecdotal reports, the risk-benefit relation for use of umbilical lines in full-term neonates, or in the neonate with a ductus-dependent circulation, has not been well delineated.

### Inotropic Agents

For the neonate or infant in cardiogenic shock, a continuous infusion of an inotropic agent may improve myocardial contractility and thereby enhance tissue perfusion of the vital organs and peripheral tissues. Care should be taken to replete the intravascular volume before institution of vasoactive agents.

The sympathomimetic amines are the inotropic agents most commonly used for hemodynamic stabilization. Sympathomimetic amines may be endogenous—dopamine and epinephrine—or synthetic—dobutamine and isoproterenol. Dopamine and dobutamine are recommended for the neonate with hypotension and tachycardia, as these agents have less chronotropic properties in low doses. *Dopamine* is a precursor of norepinephrine and stimulates dopaminergic, $beta_1$-adrenergic, and alpha-adrenergic receptors in a dose-dependent manner. Dopamine improves myocardial contractility, thereby increasing stroke volume, cardiac output, and mean arterial pressure, as well as urine output, with a low incidence of side effects at doses of less than 10 μg/kg/minute. *Dobutamine*, an analogue of dopamine, stimulates $beta_1$ receptors predominantly, with relatively weak $beta_2$ receptor– and alpha receptor–stimulating activity. In comparison with dopamine, dobutamine lacks renal vasodilating properties and does not depend on norepinephrine release from peripheral nerves for its effect. Data concerning the use of dobutamine in neonates are sparse, although clinical experience has been favorable. A combination of low-dose dopamine, up to 5 μg/kg/minute, and dobutamine, up to 10 μg/kg/minute, may be used to minimize the potential peripheral vasoconstriction induced by high doses of dopamine while maximizing the dopaminergic effects on renal perfusion.

Isoproterenol and epinephrine have been clinically utilized in neonates with hypotension and a normal or low heart rate, as these agents have both inotropic and chronotropic effects. *Isoproterenol* stimulates both $beta_1$ and $beta_2$ receptors. In comparison with dobutamine, it has a greater chronotropic effect and a stronger vasodilatory effect via its $beta_2$ mechanism. Because of its strong chronotropic effect, it should be started at a low dose, which is increased slowly, titrated to effect. Chronotropic effects appear before inotropic effects in responsive hearts, and isoproterenol can produce tachyarrhythmias. The heart usually accommodates quickly to the chronotropic properties, allowing the dose to be raised further for inotropic needs. The recommended starting dose for isoproterenol is 0.05 μg/kg/minute. *Epinephrine* has $alpha_1$, $alpha_2$, $beta_1$, and $beta_2$ effects. It is most commonly used when the previously listed inotropic infusions at high doses and in combination fail to produce the desired cardiac response. The recommended starting dose is 0.05 μg/kg/minute. Adverse reactions to the sympathomimetic amines include tachycardia, atrial and ventricular arrhythmias, and increased afterload due to peripheral vasoconstriction. Tachycardia increases myocardial oxygen consumption, whereas atrial and ventricular arrhythmias and peripheral vasoconstriction decrease cardiac output.

## TRANSPORT

After resuscitation and stabilization are complete, the neonate with suspected congenital heart disease may need to be transferred to an institution with an intensive care unit that provides subspecialty care in pediatric cardiology and pediatric cardiothoracic surgery. A successful transport involves two transitional phases of care for the neonate: (1) from the referring hospital staff to the transport team and (2) from the transport staff to the accepting hospital staff. The need for accurate, detailed, and complete communication of information between the respective teams cannot be overemphasized. If possible, the pediatric cardiologist and/or surgeon at the accepting hospital should be included in formulating the transport management plan while the neonate is still at the referring hospital.

Reliable vascular access should be secured for the neonate receiving continuous infusions of $PGE_1$ or inotropic agents during transport. Some neonates receiving a $PGE_1$ infusion will be intubated for transport (see earlier). All intubated patients should have gastric decompression by nasogastric tube or orogastric tube and should not receive anything by mouth or nasogastric tube.

Acid-base status, oxygen delivery, temperature, and serum glucose should be evaluated before transport. Although some patients with structurally normal hearts are transported receiving supplemental oxygen at or near 100%, this is not the inspired oxygen concentration of choice for most neonates with congenital heart disease. Enough oxygen should be used to maintain an oxygen saturation of 80% to 85% (see Chapter 57). This management decision for transport is particularly important in infants with ductus-dependent systemic or pulmonary blood flow and complete intracardiac mixing with single-ventricle physiology, and emphasizes the need to consult with a pediatric cardiologist before transport of the infant for optimal in-transport care.

In neonates, hypotension is a late finding in shock. More sensitive signs of impending decompensation include persistent tachycardia, poor tissue perfusion, and metabolic acidosis. Treatment of shock should occur before transport during the stabilization phase of management. Before the patient leaves the referring hospital, the hemodynamic status (capillary refill, heart rate, systemic blood pressure, and acid-base status) should be reassessed and relayed to the receiving hospital.

Before transfer, the calcium and glucose status of the neonate should be evaluated. In particular, neonates with conotruncal anomalies have an increased frequency of 22q11 deletion (Goldmuntz et al, 1998), thymic and parathyroid hypoplasia, and problems with calcium homeostasis resulting in hypocalcemia. The neonatal myocardium may be more dependent on calcium for inotropy than the adult myocardium, and ionized calcium levels of less than 1.0 mg/dL may have a significant negative impact on neonatal myocardial contractility. If the ionized calcium concentration is less than 1.0 mg/dL, 50 to 100 mg/kg of calcium gluconate may be given intravenously.

## SUMMARY

The stabilization and transport of the neonate with known or suspected critical congenital heart disease have significant impacts on the child's preoperative condition, potentially contributing to the risk for long-term morbidity. Critical factors in stabilization include the initial resuscitation, airway management, vascular access, and the judicious utilization of oxygen, $PGE_1$, and inotropic support. The key to successful transport that will minimize morbidity risk for the infant is accurate detailed communication among the respective staffs of the referring hospital, transport team, and accepting hospital.

## REFERENCES

Castañeda AR, Mayer JE Jr, Jonas RA, et al: The neonate with critical congenital heart disease: Repair—a surgical challenge. J Thorac Cardiovasc Surg 98:869-875, 1989.

Freed MD, Heymann MA, Lewis AB, et al: Prostaglandin $E_1$ in infants with ductus arteriosus–dependent congenital heart disease. Circulation 64:899-905, 1981.

Goldmuntz E, Clark BJ, Mitchell LE, et al: Frequency of 22q11 deletions in patients with conotruncal defects. J Am Coll Cardiol 32:492-498, 1998.

Lewis AB, Freed MD, Heymann MA, et al: Side effects of therapy with prostaglandin $E_1$ in infants with critical congenital heart disease. Circulation 64:893-898, 1981.

Mahle WT, Clancy RR, Moss E, et al: Neurodevelopmental outcome and lifestyle assessment in school-age and adolescent children with hypoplastic left heart syndrome. Pediatrics 105:1082-1089, 2000.

Mahle WT, Wernovsky G: Neurodevelopmental outcomes after complex infant heart surgery. ACC Curr J Rev 9:93-97, 2000.

Paul MH, Wernovsky G: Transposition of the great arteries. In Emmanouilides GC, Riemenschneider TA, Allen HD, Gutgesell HP (eds): Moss and Adams' Heart Disease in Infants, Children, and Adolescents, Including the Fetus and Young Adult. Baltimore, Williams & Wilkins, 1995, pp 1154-1225.

Wernovsky G, Jonas RA: 1998, Transposition of the great arteries. In Chang AC, Hanley FL, Wernovsky G, Wessel DL (eds): Pediatric Cardiac Intensive Care. Baltimore, Williams & Wilkins, 1998, pp 289-301.

Wernovsky G, Mayer JE, Jonas RA, et al: Factors influencing early and late outcome of the arterial switch operation for transposition of the great arteries. J Thorac Cardiovasc Surg 109:289-302, 2000a.

Wernovsky G, Stiles KM, Gauvreau K, et al: Cognitive development after the Fontan operation. Circulation 102:883-889, 2000b.

CHAPTER

# 56

# Patent Ductus Arteriosus in the Premature Infant

Ronald I. Clyman

The ductus arteriosus represents a persistence of the terminal portion of the sixth branchial arch. During fetal life, the ductus arteriosus serves to divert blood away from the fluid-filled lungs toward the descending aorta and placenta. After birth, constriction of the ductus arteriosus and obliteration of its lumen result in separation of the pulmonary and systemic circulations. In the full-term infant, obliteration of the ductus arteriosus takes place through a process of vasoconstriction and anatomic remodeling. In the preterm infant, the ductus arteriosus frequently fails to close. The clinical consequences of a patent ductus arteriosus (PDA) are related to the magnitude of the left-to-right shunt through the patent ductus with its associated change in blood flow to the lungs, kidneys, and intestine.

## REGULATION OF DUCTAL CLOSURE

In the full-term infant, closure of the ductus arteriosus occurs in two phases: (1) "functional" closure of the lumen within the first hours after birth by smooth muscle constriction and (2) "anatomic" occlusion of the lumen over the next several days due to extensive neointimal thickening and loss of smooth muscle cells from the inner muscle media.

### Functional Closure

The initial functional constriction of the ductus depends on alterations in the balance between dilating and contracting forces. The ductus arteriosus normally has a high level of intrinsic tone during fetal life (Kajino et al, 2001). After delivery, an increase in arterial $PaO_2$ plays an additional important role in ductus arteriosus constriction (Kennedy and Clark, 1942). Oxygen's mechanism of action is still unknown. Although neural and hormonal factors possibly contribute to ductus closure under physiologic conditions, they do not mediate oxygen-induced vessel closure. A cytochrome P-450 hemoprotein that is located in the plasma membrane of the vascular smooth muscle cells appears to act as a receptor in the oxygen-mediated contractile pathway (Coceani et al, 1989b, 1994). Oxygen inhibits $K^+$ channels (Michelakis et al, 2000; Reeve et al, 2001), which in turn causes membrane depolarization, an increase in smooth muscle intracellular calcium (Nakanishi et al, 1993), and formation of the potent vasoconstrictor endothelin-1 (Coceani et al, 1989a). However, the role of endothelin-1 in postnatal ductus closure or as a mediator of oxygen-induced ductus constriction has been questioned (Coceani et al, 1999; Fineman et al, 1998; Michelakis et al, 2000). Similarly, the mechanisms that alter membrane potential are still uncertain (Clyman et al, 1988; Reeve et al, 2001).

The fetal ductus also produces several vasodilators that oppose the ability of the intrinsic tone and oxygen to constrict the vessel. Vasodilator prostaglandins (PGs), $PGE_2$ and $PGI_2$, play significant roles in maintaining ductus patency during fetal and neonatal life. $PGE_2$ appears to be the most important prostanoid regulating ductus patency because it is the most potent prostaglandin produced by the ductus (Clyman et al, 1978; Coceani et al, 1978). The response of the ductus to $PGE_2$ is unique among blood vessels in that it is extraordinarily sensitive to this vasodilating substance. Inhibition of prostaglandin synthesis, by inhibiting the enzyme cyclooxygenase, produces constriction of the fetal ductus (Moise et al, 1988). Both isoforms of cyclooxygenase—COX-1 and COX-2—are expressed in the ductus arteriosus (Takahashi et al, 2000), and both nonselective (e.g., indomethacin) and selective cyclooxygenase inhibitors constrict the DA. The DA also produces a nitric oxide (NO)–like vasodilator. Competitive inhibitors of nitric oxide synthase (NOS) constrict the newborn ductus, both in vivo and in vitro (Clyman et al, 1998; Seidner et al, 2001).

Following delivery there are several events that promote ductus constriction in the full-term newborn: (1) an increase in arterial $Po_2$, (2) a decrease in blood pressure within the ductus lumen (due to the postnatal decrease in pulmonary vascular resistance), (3) a decrease in circulating $PGE_2$ (due to the loss of placental prostaglandin production and the increase in prostaglandin removal by the lung), and (4) a decrease in the number of $PGE_2$ receptors in the ductus wall (Bouayad et al, 2001). These factors promote ductus constriction after birth. In contrast with the full-term ductus, the premature ductus is less likely to constrict after birth. The intrinsic tone of the extremely immature ductus (at $< 70\%$ of full gestation) is decreased compared with the ductus at term (Kajino et al, 2001). In addition, there is an increased sensitivity of the immature ductus to the vasodilating effects of $PGE_2$ and NO (Clyman et al, 1998). Inhibitors of prostaglandin production such as indomethacin, ibuprofen, and mefenamic acid have proved to be effective agents in promoting ductus closure. It follows that drugs interfering with NO synthesis or function also could become useful adjuncts, especially in cases in which indomethacin has proved to be ineffective (Seidner et al, 2001).

The endogenous factors that alter the ability of the preterm ductus to constrict with advancing gestation are unknown. Recently, prenatal administration of vitamin A has been shown to increase both the intracellular calcium response and the contractile response of the preterm ductus to oxygen (Wu et al, 2001). Elevated cortisol concentrations in the fetus have been found to decrease the sensitivity of the ductus to $PGE_2$ (Clyman et al, 1981a); consistent with these findings, prenatal administration of glucocorticoids causes a significant reduction in the incidence of PDA in premature humans and animals (Clyman et al, 1981b; Collaborative Group on Antenatal Steroid Therapy, 1985; Momma et al, 1981; Thibeault et al, 1978; Waffarn et al, 1983). The postnatal administration of glucocorticoids also has been shown to reduce the incidence of PDA (Early postnatal dexamethasone therapy, 2001). However, postnatal glucocorticoid treatment also seems to increase the incidence of several of the other neonatal morbidities (Early postnatal dexamethasone therapy, 2001).

### Anatomic Closure

In normal, full-term animals, loss of responsiveness to $PGE_2$ shortly after birth prevents the ductus arteriosus from reopening once it has constricted. This is accompanied by rapid histologic changes that ultimately lead to obliteration of the vessel lumen and loss of smooth muscle cells from the inner muscle media. The loss of vasodilator regulation of the ductus and the "anatomic" remodeling that leads to permanent ductus closure both appear to be related to the intensity of the initial ductus constriction. Constriction produces ischemic hypoxia of the vessel wall (Clyman et al, 1999). In the full-term newborn ductus, the ischemic hypoxia that accompanies constriction is due to a marked reduction in intramural vasa vasorum flow. Profound ductus wall hypoxia occurs even before luminal flow has been eliminated (Kajino, 2001). Loss of vasa vasorum flow produces a threefold increase in the diffusion distance for oxygen across the ductus wall.

Following delivery, the profound ductus wall hypoxia inhibits local production $PGE_2$ and NO, produces smooth muscle apoptosis, and induces local production of growth factors such as transforming growth factor-β (TGF-β) and vascular endothelial growth factor (VEGF), which play early roles in ductus remodeling. Experimental genetic models that alter the ability of the ductus to contract at term also prevent the normal histologic changes that occur after birth (Loftin et al, 2001; Mason et al, 1999; Nguyen et al, 1997).

In preterm infants, the ductus frequently remains open for many days after birth. Even when it does constrict, the premature ductus frequently fails to develop profound hypoxia and to undergo anatomic remodeling. Therefore, the immature ductus is susceptible to vessel reopening. When the ductus arteriosus reopens after initial successful closure, the most frequent cause is the effects of endogenous $PGE_2$. Consequently, in 70% of cases of ductal reopening, the ductus can be closed again with a second course of indomethacin. However, the relative importance of the two vasodilators, $PGE_2$ and NO, also can change after birth. Both the flow of oxygenated arterial blood through the narrowed ductus lumen (with its increased shear stress) and the ingrowth of vasa vasorum (which contain NOS), increase the amount of NO produced within the ductus wall. As NO production increases in the ductus, it is likely that ductus patency becomes less dependent on prostaglandin generation. With increasing ductal dependency on NO, inhibitors of prostaglandin production (such as indomethacin) would become less likely to produce ductus constriction. These findings fit with clinical observations that indomethacin is much more likely to achieve ductus closure if given on the first day after birth; its effectiveness wanes with increasing postnatal age (Clyman, 1996; Schmidt et al, 2001) (see later). In premature baboons, the combined use of an NOS inhibitor and indomethacin produces a much greater degree of ductus constriction than is achieved with indomethacin alone (Seidner et al, 2001). It follows that drugs interfering with NO synthesis could become a useful adjunct, especially in cases in which indomethacin has proved to be ineffective.

Preterm infants seem to require more ductus constriction to produce the same level of wall hypoxia as that found at term. In contrast with the full-term ductus, the thin-walled preterm ductus does not depend on intramural vasa vasorum to provide oxygen and nutrients to its wall. As a result, the preterm ductus requires complete obstruction of luminal flow before it can develop the same degree of hypoxia as that found at term. If this degree of hypoxic ischemia can be induced in the preterm ductus, then most of the anatomic changes seen at term will occur (Kajino et al, 2001; Seidner et al, 2001).

## HEMODYNAMIC AND PULMONARY ALTERATIONS

The pathophysiologic features of a PDA depend both on the magnitude of the left-to-right shunt and on the cardiac and pulmonary responses to shunting. There are important differences between immature and mature infants in the heart's ability to handle a volume load. Immature infants have less cardiac sympathetic innervation. Before term, the myocardium has more water and less contractile mass. Therefore, in the immature fetus the ventricles are less distensible than at term and also generate less force per gram of myocardium (even though they have the same ability to generate force per sarcomere as the ventricles in more mature infants) (Friedman, 1972). The relative lack of left ventricular distensibility in immature infants is more a function of the ventricle's tissue constituents than of poor muscle function. As a result, left ventricular distention secondary to a large left-to-right PDA shunt may produce a higher left ventricular end-diastolic pressure at smaller ventricular volumes. The increase in left ventricular pressure increases pulmonary venous pressure, causing pulmonary congestion.

Studies in preterm lamb and human newborns (Clyman et al, 1987; Shimada et al, 1994) have shown that despite these limitations, preterm newborns are able to increase left ventricular output and maintain their "effective" systemic blood flow, even with left-to-right PDA shunts equal to 50% of left ventricular output. With shunts greater than 50% of left ventricular output, "effective" systemic blood flow falls, despite a continued increase in left ventricular output. The increase in left ventricular output associated with PDA is accomplished not by an increase in heart rate but by an increase in stroke volume (Clyman et al, 1987; Shimada et al, 1994). Stroke volume increases primarily as a result of the simultaneous decrease in afterload resistance on the heart and the increase in left ventricular preload. Despite the ability of the left ventricle to increase its output in the face of a left-to-right ductus shunt, blood flow distribution is significantly rearranged. This redistribution of systemic blood flow occurs even with small shunts (Clyman et al, 1987). Blood flow to the skin, bone, and skeletal muscle is most likely to be affected by the left-to-right ductus shunt. The next most likely organs to be affected are the gastrointestinal tract and kidneys. These organs receive decreased blood flow as a result of a combination of decreased perfusion pressure (due to a drop in diastolic pressure) and localized vasoconstriction. These organs may experience significant hypoperfusion before there are any signs of left ventricular compromise (Meyers et al, 1990; Shimada et al, 1994). This decrease in organ perfusion contributes to some of the morbid conditions caused by PDA: necrotizing enterocolitis (NEC) and decreased glomerular filtration rate (Cassady et al, 1989; Clyman, 1996).

The decreased ability of the preterm infant to maintain active pulmonary vasoconstriction (Lewis et al, 1976) may be responsible in part for the earlier clinical manifestation of a "large" left-to-right PDA shunt (Gersony et al, 1983; Jacob et al, 1980). In addition, therapeutic maneuvers (e.g., surfactant replacement) that lead to a more rapid drop in pulmonary vascular resistance can exacerbate the magnitude of left-to-right shunt in preterm infants with respiratory distress syndrome (RDS), leading to pulmonary hemorrhage (Alpan and Clyman, 1995; Raju and Langenberg, 1993). Although the mechanisms responsible for pulmonary hemorrhage after surfactant are uncertain, a retrospective cohort study found that a clinically detectable PDA was associated with the onset of the hemorrhage (Garland et al, 1994). Early ductus closure has been shown to decrease the incidence of significant pulmonary hemorrhage (Clyman, 1996; Domanico et al, 1994).

A wide-open ductus arteriosus exposes the pulmonary vasculature to systemic blood pressure, and when pulmonary vascular resistance is less than systemic vascular resistance, to increased pulmonary blood flow. Because the premature infant with RDS frequently has low plasma oncotic pressure and may have increased capillary permeability, increases in pulmonary microvascular pressure increase interstitial and alveolar lung fluids. If plasma proteins leak into the alveolar space, surfactant function will be inhibited and pulmonary compliance will fall (Ikegami et al, 1983). The increased fraction of inspired oxygen ($F_{IO_2}$) and mean airway pressures required to overcome these early changes in compliance may explain why a persistent PDA increases the risk of developing chronic lung disease (Brown, 1979; Clyman, 1996; Cotton et al, 1978).

In the preterm infant, there is a delicate balance between PDA-induced lung fluid filtration and lung lymphatic fluid reabsorption. A PDA that closes by 72 hours after birth usually has no effect on the newborn's respiratory condition (Alpan et al, 1989; Clyman, 1996; Krauss et al, 1989; Pérez Fontán et al, 1987; Shimada et al, 1989). However, if PDA persists for longer than 72 hours or if lymphatic drainage is impaired (as it is in the presence of pulmonary interstitial emphysema or fibrosis), the likelihood of edema increases dramatically. In infants with a persistent PDA, pulmonary edema and alterations in pulmonary mechanics usually develop at 7 to 10 days after birth. In these infants, improvement in lung compliance occurs following closure of the PDA (Clyman, 1996; Gerhardt and Bancalari, 1980; Johnson et al, 1978; Naulty et al, 1978; Stefano et al, 1991; Yeh et al, 1981).

## DIAGNOSIS

The combination of two-dimensional echocardiographic visualization of the ductus with either pulsed wave, continuous wave, or color Doppler measurements appears to be not only very sensitive but also specific for identifying ductus patency (Drayton and Skidmore, 1987; Gentile et al, 1981; Huhta et al, 1984; Mellander et al, 1987; Stevenson et al, 1980). This combination may also be useful in determining pressure gradients across the ductus (see also Chapter 53) (Musewe et al, 1987). Unfortunately, determining the size of the lumen of the ductus arteriosus and the magnitude of the Doppler signal from the shunt give only qualitative measures of the size of the shunt. M-mode measurements of LA:Ao ratio (diameter of the left atrium to that of the aortic root) of greater than 1.4 (Johnson et al, 1983), Doppler-derived measurements of cardiac output (Walther et al, 1989), and/or evidence of diastolic retrograde flow in the descending aorta help to determine when moderate-to-large PDA shunts are present (Ellison et al, 1983; Evans and Iyer, 1994; Iyer and Evans, 1994; Mellander et al, 1987; Serwer et al, 1982).

Clinical signs of a PDA usually appear later than echocardiographic signs but have a higher correlation with the development of PDA-associated neonatal morbidity. Ellison and colleagues (1983) attempted to evaluate several commonly used criteria for diagnosing a large left-to-right shunt through the ductus arteriosus by noting the occurrence of each sign both before and 36 to 48 hours after surgical ligation (Fig. 56–1). No single criterion alone sufficed as an indicator of PDA. Certain signs, such as continuous murmur or hyperactive left ventricular impulse, were specific for PDA but lacked sensitivity; conversely, ventilatory support criteria were very sensitive but lacked specificity. On the other hand, the appearance of three or more of these clinical signs—systolic murmur, hyperdynamic precordial impulse, full pulses, widened pulse pressure and/or worsening respiratory status—correlated well with the subsequent development of PDA-related morbidity (see "Treatment" later).

## INCIDENCE

Pulsed Doppler echocardiographic assessments of full-term infants indicate that functional closure of the ductus has occurred in almost 50% by 24 hours, in 90% by 48 hours, and in all by 72 hours. The rate of ductus closure is delayed in preterm infants; however, in essentially all healthy preterm infants of 30 weeks of gestation or greater, ductus closure will have occurred by the fourth day after birth (Table 56–1). RDS also delays ductus closure; however, in most infants of 30 weeks of gestation or greater, the actual impact of RDS on ductal shunting may be less than has been commonly assumed (see Table 56–1). On the other hand, preterm infants of less than 30 weeks of gestation with severe respiratory distress have a high incidence of persistent PDA (see Table 56–1).

The introduction of exogenous surfactant therapy has altered both the incidence and the presentation of PDA. Although surfactant has no effect on the contractile behavior of the ductus, its effects on pulmonary vascular

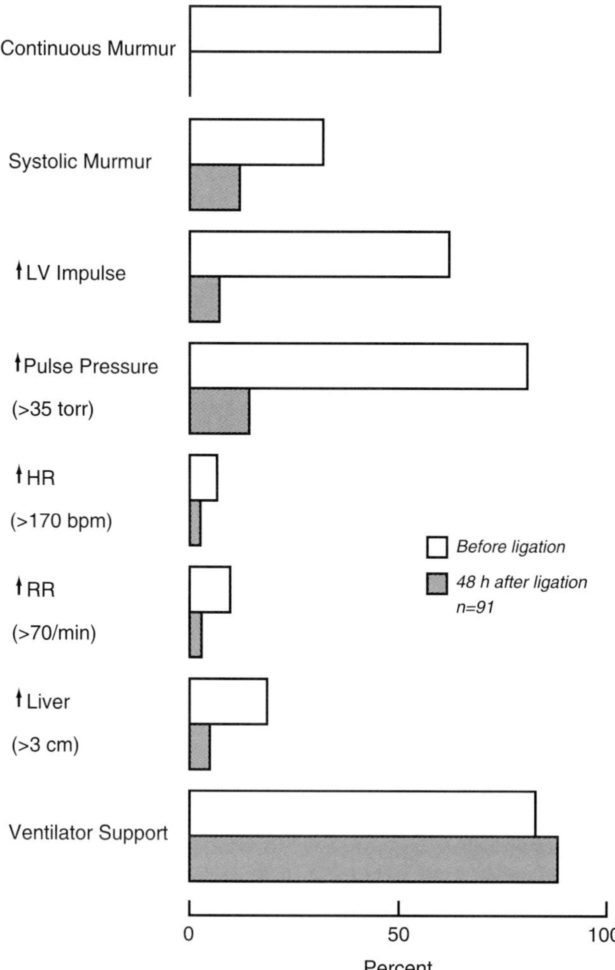


**FIGURE 56–1.** Clinical signs associated with a patent ductus arteriosus. *(Data from Ellison RC, Peckham GJ, Lang P, et al: Evaluation of the preterm infant for patent ductus arteriosus. Pediatrics 71:364-372, 1983.)*

resistance lead to earlier clinical manifestation of the left-to-right shunt in preterm animals (Clyman et al, 1982; Shimada et al, 1989) and humans (Alpan and Clyman, 1995; Kaapa et al, 1993; Reller et al, 1991, 1993). Infants who receive excessive fluid administration during the first days of life also are more likely to develop a clinically symptomatic PDA (Bell and Acarregui, 2001).

## TREATMENT

In some centers, conservative measures including fluid restriction, diuretics, and digitalis have been advocated to treat the symptoms associated with a PDA. Although excessive fluid administration has been associated with an increased incidence of PDA (Bell and Acarregui, 2001), fluid restriction is unlikely to cause ductus closure (Green et al, 1980). In addition, the combination of fluid restriction and diuretics frequently leads to electrolyte abnormalities, dehydration, and, most important, caloric deprivation. Digitalis would not be expected to be very useful because myocardial contractility is increased rather than reduced in infants with PDA. Moreover, there may be an interaction between digoxin and indomethacin that increases the patient's susceptibility to the toxic effects of digoxin (Berman et al, 1978; Koren et al, 1984; Wilkerson and Glenn, 1977).

The addition of positive end-expiratory pressure has been found to be useful in managing infants with a PDA. When end-expiratory pressure is added, the degree of left-to-right shunting through the ductus arteriosus decreases; as a result, effective systemic blood flow increases (Cotton et al, 1980). A low hematocrit has been shown to aggravate left-to-right shunting by lowering the resistance to blood flow through the pulmonary vascular bed (Lister et al, 1982). Higher hematocrits diminish excessive shunting through the PDA and help ensure adequate systemic oxygen delivery when perfusion is limited. Similarly, demands on left ventricular output should be minimized in infants with PDA by maintaining adequate oxygenation and by keeping the patient in a neutral thermal environment. Nevertheless, such therapies usually only delay, rather than prevent, the ultimate need for PDA closure.

Cotton and associates (1978) demonstrated that failure of the ductus to close after significant clinical symptoms of cardiovascular compromise have developed (approximately 7 to 10 days after birth) significantly increases the neonatal morbidity risk. Ligation of a symptomatic PDA

**TABLE 56–1**

**Incidence of Patent Ductus Arteriosus with Postnatal Age***

| | Incidence (%) | | | | | | | |
|---|---|---|---|---|---|---|---|---|
| | 0-24 hr | | 24-48 hr | | 48-72 hr | | 72-96 hr | |
| ***Gestation (wk)*** | ***Healthy*** | ***RDS*** | ***Healthy*** | ***RDS*** | ***Healthy*** | ***RDS*** | ***Healthy*** | ***RDS*** |
| >40 | 55 | | 0 | | 0 | | 0 | |
| 38-40 | 85 | | 50 | | 5 | | 0 | |
| 34-37 | 96 | | 42 | | 12 | | 4 | |
| 30-33 | 87 | 87 | 31 | 56 | 13 | 25 | 0 | 11 |
| ≤29 | 80 | 88 | 40 | 84 | 20 | 77 | 7 | 65 |

*Hours of postnatal life.

RDS, respiratory distress syndrome.

Data from the following references: Dudell and Gersony, 1984; Gentile et al, 1981; Hammerman et al, 1986; Reller et al, 1993.

in premature infants now can be done in the neonatal intensive care unit, with low mortality and morbidity rates (Mikhail et al, 1982; Wagner et al, 1984). However, respiratory compromise, blood pressure fluctuations, intracranial hemorrhage, infection, chylothorax, recurrent laryngeal nerve paralysis, and death are still significant risks among infants of less than 28 weeks of gestation.

Inhibition of prostaglandin synthesis with nonselective cyclooxygenase (COX-1 and COX-2) inhibitors (such as indomethacin and ibuprofen) appears to be an effective alternative to surgical ligation (Gersony et al, 1983). At this time, indomethacin is the only nonselective cycloooxygenase inhibitor approved for the treatment of PDA. Its efficacy and toxicity have been explored extensively, and it appears comparable to surgical ligation in preventing the complications associated with PDA: bronchopulmonary dysplasia (BPD), NEC, and intolerance of enteral feedings (Gersony et al, 1983). In most intensive care nurseries, indomethacin has replaced surgery as the preferred therapy for persistent PDA. However, indomethacin has been associated with several adverse effects in the newborn: alterations in renal function (Betkerur et al, 1981; Gersony et al, 1983), NEC, and gastrointestinal hemorrhage (Rennie et al, 1986). Indomethacin produces significant reductions in renal (Pezzati et al, 1999; Rennie et al, 1986) and mesenteric (Coombs et al, 1990; Van Bel et al, 1990) blood flow, which may play a role in the pathogenesis of adverse effects. Indomethacin also reduces cerebral blood flow velocity (Austin et al, 1992; Edwards et al, 1990; Laudignon et al, 1988; Patel et al, 2000; Pryds et al, 1988; Van Bel et al, 1989) and cerebral oxygenation (McCormick et al, 1993; Patel et al, 2000), which could lead to cerebral ischemia; however, indomethacin has not been shown to have a negative impact on neurodevelopmental outcome (Couser et al, 2000; Merritt et al, 1982; Peckham et al, 1984; Yeh et al, 1982). Unlike its effects on the ductus arteriosus, indomethacin's action on these other organ systems may not be due entirely to its inhibition of prostaglandin synthesis (Chemtob et al, 1991; Malcolm et al, 1993; Speziale et al, 1999). Indomethacin also has effects on lipoxygenase activity and on histamine and endothelin release (Docherty and Wilson, 1987; Konig et al, 1987; Therkelsen et al, 1994), although the relevance of these effects to observed neonatal morbidity is still unknown.

Ibuprofen, another nonselective cyclooxygenase inhibitor, also has been shown to close the ductus arteriosus in animals (Coceani et al, 1979). However, ibuprofen does not appear to affect mesenteric blood flow (Malcolm et al, 1993; Pezzati et al, 1999; Speziale et al, 1999) and has less of an effect on renal perfusion than indomethacin (Malcolm et al, 1993; Pezzati et al, 1999; Speziale et al, 1999). Similarly, ibuprofen does not decrease cerebral blood flow and may even extend its autoregulatory range (Chemtob et al, 1990; Mosca et al, 1997; Patel et al, 2000; Speziale et al, 1999). Animal studies suggest that ibuprofen may even have cytoprotective effects in the intestinal tract (Grosfeld et al, 1983). Early clinical trials have shown that ibuprofen is as effective as indomethacin for treatment of PDA but is associated with a significantly lower incidence of renal toxicity (Van Overmeire et al, 2000).

## Indomethacin

### Dose

Although there may be general consensus regarding the efficacy of indomethacin for the treatment of PDA, questions about proper dosage, treatment duration, and optimal timing of treatment remain quite controversial. Indomethacin's plasma clearance depends on postnatal age (Brash et al, 1981; Smith et al, 1984; Thalji et al, 1980; Yaffe et al, 1980; Yeh et al, 1989). Therefore, a dosage regimen recommended for infants at the end of the first week (when the half-life of the drug is 21 hours) (Yaffe et al, 1980; Yeh et al, 1989) may lead to elevated and prolonged plasma concentrations when this agent is used in infants on day 1 (when the half-life is 71 hours) (Smith et al, 1984). Conversely, a single loading dose of indomethacin (0.2 mg/kg), without subsequent maintenance doses, can be effective in preventing clinical symptoms associated with a PDA when administered within the first 24 hours following delivery (Krueger et al, 1987). Many variations in dosage regimens have been reported. Table 56–2 outlines one successful approach. Serious side effects are uncommon with these doses; however, oliguria and dilutional hyponatremia are frequent and may necessitate interruption of a full course of treatment. Isolated bowel perforation is unusual (although the incidence has been shown to increase markedly if indomethacin and stress doses of glucocorticoids are administered concurrently) (Early postnatal dexamethasone therapy, 2001). There is no clear evidence that the incidence or severity of NEC is affected by indomethacin treatment.

### Duration

Prostaglandin production is only transiently suppressed following indomethacin therapy. Within 6 to 7 days following completion of therapy, circulating prostaglandin $E_2$ concentrations return to the normal range (Seyberth et al, 1982). This interval may not allow enough time for anatomic remodeling of the ductus in the most immature infants. A prolonged maintenance course of low-dose indomethacin (0.1 mg/kg every 24 hours for 5 to 7 days) appears to both increase the success of the initial closure rate and decrease the relapse rate when compared with a shorter course (two or three doses over 24 hours) (Hammerman and Aranburo, 1990; Rennie and Cooke, 1991; Rhodes et al, 1988). This dosage regimen still needs further evaluation because, in some reports (Rennie and Cooke, 1991; Rhodes et al, 1988), a higher mortality rate was observed in the infants receiving prolonged maintenance indomethacin.

In addition to its effects on the ductus, indomethacin also is associated with vasoconstriction of other vascular beds (e.g., cerebral, mesenteric, renal). Prolonging the rate of indomethacin infusion (20 to 30 minutes) alleviates some of the drop in organ blood flow (Colditz et al, 1989); a continuous indomethacin infusion, of the same total daily dose, appears to decrease indomethacin's detrimental effects even further (Hammerman et al, 1995).

**TABLE 56-2**

**Dosage Schedule for Indomethacin in Premature Infants with Patent Ductus Arteriosus**

| | | IV Dose (mg/kg)* | | | |
|---|---|---|---|---|---|
| | | Time after Initial Dose | | | |
| **Age at Onset of Treatment** | **Initial Dose** | **12** | **24** | **36** | **48** |
| Infants <1200 g | | | | | |
| <24 hours | 0.2 | | 0.1 | | 0.1 |
| >48 hours | 0.2 | 0.1 | | 0.1 | |
| Infants ≥1200 g | | | | | |
| >48 hours | 0.2 | 0.2 | | 0.2 | |

*Three doses of indomethacin usually are given by intravenous (*never* intra-arterial) administration over 20-30 minutes.

### Timing

The postnatal age at which indomethacin is administered plays an important role in determining its effectiveness. Several investigators have suggested that the relative ineffectiveness of indomethacin in treating infants of advanced postnatal age may be due to rapid drug clearance with a resultant inability to maintain "desired" plasma concentrations (Brash et al, 1981; Thalji et al, 1980). However, even when indomethacin concentrations have been maintained in the "desired" range, the drug's ability to produce ductus closure remains inversely proportional to the postnatal age at the time of treatment (Achanti et al, 1986; Rennie et al, 1986; Rheuban et al, 1987). With advancing postnatal age, dilator prostaglandins play a lesser role in maintaining ductus patency (see earlier). As a result, indomethacin becomes less effective in producing PDA closure (Achanti et al, 1986). It appears that in some situations, prostaglandins may not be the dominant factor maintaining ductus patency (Cotton et al, 1991).

A second type of indomethacin treatment failure is found in patients in whom the ductus initially constricts following treatment with indomethacin, only to reopen several days later. Recurrence of a symptomatic PDA after initial successful treatment is independent of initial plasma indomethacin concentrations (Brash et al, 1981; Gersony et al, 1983; Ramsey et al, 1987). The rate of reopening, which is greatest among the most immature infants, appears to be related to the timing of treatment with indomethacin and the completeness of initial ductus closure after treatment (Clyman, 1996; Narayanan et al, 2000). Permanent anatomic closure requires tight constriction of the ductus lumen and the development of ductus wall hypoxia (see earlier). Infants delivered at less than 28 weeks of gestation, with a clinically closed ductus following indomethacin treatment, will experience reopening of the ductus with development of clinical symptoms if there is any evidence of luminal patency on the Doppler examination performed at the end of indomethacin treatment. Even when there is echocardiographic evidence of ductus closure, the ductus fails to remodel in a significant number of infants. The more immature the ductus is, the greater the chance of ductus reopening: 23% of infants who were delivered before 26 weeks of gestation demonstrate reopening in spite of echocardiographic evidence of closure; in contrast, only 9% of those who were delivered between 26 and 27 weeks of gestation demonstrate reopening if the ductus is found after indomethacin treatment to be closed by echocardiography. Early treatment leads to a higher rate of permanent ductus closure. This is due to the greater degree of initial ductus constriction in the early treatment group (Narayanan et al, 2000).

Although indomethacin treatment is most effective when given within the first 24 to 48 hours after delivery, is that necessarily the best time to administer it? Among infants born at 32 weeks of gestation, 90% of those with severe respiratory distress will have echocardiographic evidence of a PDA during the first 24 hours; however, only 40% will subsequently develop symptoms of a hemodynamically large left-to-right shunt that will require intervention with indomethacin or surgery. If this group of infants had been treated during the first 24 hours after delivery, approximately 60% would have been treated unnecessarily. Therefore, such an aggressive approach to therapy can be justified only if early treatment can be demonstrated to significantly alter outcome in these infants. If a group of infants who have a high chance (>50%) of developing a persistent PDA can be identified, then treating the PDA in the first days after delivery will significantly reduce the risk of long-term pulmonary morbidity, pulmonary hemorrhage, NEC, and the ultimate need for surgical ligation (Clyman, 1996). For example, infants who weigh less than 1000 g at birth and who develop a murmur, even without other signs of a PDA, are at high risk (80%) for developing persistent, large PDA shunts. It seems appropriate to treat these very low-birth-weight (VLBW) infants when their PDA first becomes apparent, and before signs of a large shunt become evident (Mahony et al, 1982).

Although prophylactic indomethacin (treatment within 18 hours of birth) reduces the chances of developing a symptomatic PDA, this approach does not appear to offer any additional advantage in reducing pulmonary morbidity risk or decreasing the risk of NEC when compared with an approach that waits for the first symptoms of PDA to appear (around day 3) before initiation of treatment (Clyman, 1996; Schmidt et al, 2001). However, in certain circumstances, administration of prophylactic indomethacin may be the most appropriate strategy to follow—for example, in identified populations of infants in which (1) either the incidence of grade III or IV intracranial hemorrhage or of severe pulmonary hemorrhage is high (>10%) or (2) indomethacin failure, with the need for surgical ligation, is frequent (>30%) (Clyman, 1996).

### Indomethacin and Intracranial Hemorrhage

Previous studies have shown that indomethacin decreases cerebral blood flow, decreases reactive postasphyxia cerebral hyperemia, accelerates maturation of the germinal matrix microvasculature, and decreases the incidence of intracranial hemorrhage (ICH) in experimental animals (Dahlgren et al, 1981; Ment et al, 1983, 1992). The effects of indomethacin on ICH do not appear to be due to its effects on ductus patency (Ment et al, 1985, 1988). Because most intracranial hemorrhages occur within the first 3 days after birth, one would expect to see beneficial effects only when indomethacin is given in a *prophylactic* strategy (within the first 18 hours after birth). When prophylactic indomethacin is given to infants with normal findings on an echoencephalogram, there is a significant reduction in the incidence of all grades (I to IV) as well as the most severe grades (III and IV) of ICH. The dramatic effect of prophylactic indomethacin in infants with known, *normal* echoencephalographic findings is somewhat tempered when prophylactic indomethacin is administered to populations in which the prior ICH status is unknown. Between 30% and 50% of infants who ultimately develop an ICH have evidence of an ICH on their screening pre-indomethacin echoencephalogram. When indomethacin is administered prophylactically, without knowledge of prior ICH status, there is no longer a difference in the overall incidence of ICH; however, there is still a significant reduction in the incidence of severe (grades III and IV) ICH (Clyman, 1996).

The long-term effects of prophylactic indomethacin on cerebral function have not been fully evaluated. On evaluation at a corrected age of 18 months, there does not appear to be any change in the incidence of neurosensory impairment in infants who received indomethacin prophylaxis at birth (Schmidt et al, 2001).

### Contraindications to the Use of Indomethacin

#### *Poor Renal Function*

Many clinicians do not use indomethacin if a neonate's serum creatinine is above 1.8 to 2.0 mg/dL, or if urine output is below 1 mL/kg/hour. The reasoning behind this is that indomethacin may decrease urine output further and cause significant water and electrolyte problems. Whether indomethacin administered to a patient with moderate renal failure damages the kidney is uncertain; nevertheless, it is prudent to withhold indomethacin in infants who have significant renal failure. In some infants, administration of indomethacin is followed by a markedly decreased urine output which must be allowed for when replacing fluid and electrolyte losses. Neither dopamine nor furosemide is able to minimize the renal side effects (Baenziger et al, 1999; Brion and Campbell, 2001; Fajardo et al, 1992).

#### *Bleeding Disorders and Thrombocytopenia*

Frank renal or gastrointestinal bleeding is a contraindication to the use of indomethacin. ICH, however, is not a contraindication to the use of this drug (Ment et al, 1994). As mentioned previously, indomethacin may actually decrease the incidence of ICH.

Indomethacin impairs platelet function for 7 to 9 days (Friedman et al, 1978). Usually, this impairment has not been clinically relevant; however, it is customary to withhold indomethacin if platelet counts are less than 50,000/mm$^3$, even in the absence of overt bleeding.

#### *Necrotizing Enterocolitis*

If infants have signs of early necrotizing enterocolitis (NEC), indomethacin is usually contraindicated. Part of the rationale for this is that the NEC may be due to bowel ischemia secondary to PDA shunting, and indomethacin may further decrease blood flow to the bowel.

#### *Sepsis*

Indomethacin should not be used if sepsis is strongly suspected because it impairs white blood cell motility.

## SUMMARY

The clinical consequences of PDA are related to the degree of left-to-right shunting with its associated increase in blood flow to the lungs and decrease in blood flow to the kidneys and intestines. Treatment with indomethacin is effective in closing a PDA, particularly when given within the first few days after birth.

The current use of exogenous surfactant has caused the symptomatic PDA to present earlier than it did during the presurfactant era. The presence of a large, symptomatic PDA that persists through the end of the first week after birth increases the likelihood of pulmonary morbidity, pulmonary hemorrhage, NEC, and the ultimate need for surgical ligation. Early treatment of a clinically symptomatic PDA, in the first days after delivery, will reduce the risk of developing these morbidities if the group of infants treated has a high chance (>50%) of developing a persistent PDA. Several centers have noted that VLBW infants who develop murmurs, even without other signs of a ductus, are at high risk (80%) for developing persistent, large PDA shunts (Mahony et al, 1982, 1985). It seems appropriate to treat these VLBW infants when their PDA first becomes apparent and before signs of a large shunt are evident.

Although prophylactic indomethacin (treatment within 18 hours of birth) reduces the chances of development of a symptomatic PDA, this approach does not appear to offer any additional advantage in reducing pulmonary morbidity or NEC when compared with early symptomatic treatment. This finding is not surprising in light of the fact that less than 40% of the placebo-treated infants in the prophylactic trials ever developed a symptomatic PDA requiring treatment. On the other hand, administration of prophylactic indomethacin may be the most appropriate strategy to follow in certain populations of infants in which either the incidence of grade III or IV ICH (>10%) or of severe pulmonary hemorrhage (>10%) is high or indomethacin failure, with the need for surgical ligation, is frequent (>30%).

## REFERENCES


Achanti B, Yeh TF, Pildes RS: Indomethacin therapy in infants with advanced postnatal age and patent ductus arteriosus. Clin Invest Med 9:250-253, 1986.

Alpan G, Clyman RI: Cardiovascular effects of surfactant replacement with special reference to the patent ductus arteriosus. In Robertson B, Taeusch HW (eds): Surfactant Therapy for Lung Disease: Lung Biology in Health and Disease, vol 84. New York, Marcel Dekker, 1995, pp 531-545.

Alpan G, Mauray F, Clyman RI: Effect of patent ductus arteriosus on water accumulation and protein permeability in the premature lungs of mechanically ventilated premature lambs. Pediatr Res 26:570-575, 1989.

Austin NC, Pairaudeau PW, Hames TK, Hall MA: Regional cerebral blood flow velocity changes after indomethacin infusion in preterm infants. Arch Dis Child 67:851-854, 1992.

Baenziger O, Waldvogel K, Ghelfi D, et al: Can dopamine prevent the renal side effects of indomethacin? A prospective randomized clinical study. Klin Padiatr 211:438-441, 1999.

Bell EF, Acarregui MJ: Restricted versus liberal water intake for preventing morbidity and mortality in preterm infants (Cochrane Review). Cochrane Database Syst Rev 3, 2001.

Berman W Jr, Dubynsky O, Whitman V, et al: Digoxin therapy in low-birth-weight infants with patent ductus arteriosus. J Pediatr 93:652-655, 1978.

Betkerur MV, Yeh TF, Miller K, et al: Indomethacin and its effect on renal function and urinary kallikrein excretion in premature infants with patent ductus arteriosus. Pediatrics 68:99-102, 1981.

Bouayad A, Kajino H, Waleh N, et al: Characterization of $PGE_2$ receptors in fetal and newborn lamb ductus arteriosus. Am J Physiol Heart Circ Physiol 280: H2342-H2349, 2001.

Brash AR, Hickey DE, Graham TP, et al: Pharmacokinetics of indomethacin in the neonate. N Engl J Med 305:67-72, 1981.

Brion LP, Campbell DE: Furosemide for symptomatic patent ductus arteriosus in indomethacin-treated infants (Cochrane Review). Cochrane Database Syst Rev 3, 2001.

Brown E: Increased risk of bronchopulmonary dysplasia in infants with patent ductus arteriosus. J Pediatr 95:865-866, 1979.

Cassady G, Crouse DT, Kirklin JW, et al: A randomized, controlled trial of very early prophylactic ligation of the ductus arteriosus in babies who weighed 1000 g or less at birth. N Engl J Med 320:1511-1516, 1989.

Chemtob S, Beharry K, Barna T, et al: Differences in the effects in the newborn piglet of various nonsteroidal antiinflammatory drugs on cerebral blood flow but not on cerebrovascular prostaglandins. Pediatr Res 30:106-111, 1991.

Chemtob S, Laudignon N, Beharry K, et al: Effects of prostaglandins and indomethacin on cerebral blood flow and cerebral oxygen consumption of conscious newborn piglets. Dev Pharmacol Ther 14:1-14, 1990.

Clyman RI: Commentary: Recommendations for the postnatal use of indomethacin. An analysis of four separate treatment strategies. J Pediatr 128:601-607, 1996.

Clyman RI, Ballard PL, Sniderman S, et al: Prenatal administration of betamethasone for prevention of patent ductus arteriosus. J Pediatr 98: 123-126, 1981b.

Clyman RI, Chan CY, Mauray F, et al: Permanent anatomic closure of the ductus arteriosus in newborn baboons: The roles of postnatal constriction, hypoxia, and gestation. Pediatr Res 45:19-29, 1999.

Clyman RI, Jobe A, Heymann MA, et al: Increased shunt through the patent ductus arteriosus after surfactant replacement therapy. J Pediatr 100:101-107, 1982.

Clyman RI, Mauray F, Heymann MA, Roman C: Cardiovascular effects of a patent ductus arteriosus in preterm lambs with respiratory distress. J Pediatr 111:579-587, 1987.

Clyman RI, Mauray F, Roman C, et al: Effects of antenatal glucocorticoid administration on the ductus arteriosus of preterm lambs. Am J Physiol 241:H415-H420, 1981a.

Clyman RI, Mauray F, Roman C, Rudolph AM: $PGE_2$ is a more potent vasodilator of the lamb ductus arteriosus than either $PGI_2$ or 6 keto $PGF_{1a}$. Prostaglandins 16:259-264, 1978.

Clyman RI, Saugstad OD, Mauray F: Oxygen metabolites stimulate prostaglandin $E_2$ production and relaxation of the ductus arteriosus. Clin Res 36:228A, 1988.

Clyman RI, Waleh N, Black SM, et al: Regulation of ductus arteriosus patency by nitric oxide in fetal lambs: The role of gestation, oxygen tension and vasa vasorum. Pediatr Res 43:633-644, 1998.

Coceani F, Armstrong C, Kelsey L: Endothelin is a potent constrictor of the lamb ductus arteriosus. Can J Physiol Pharmacol 67:902-904, 1989a.

Coceani F, Bodach E, White E, et al: Prostaglandin $I_2$ is less relaxant than prostaglandin $E_2$ on the lamb ductus arteriosus. Prostaglandins 15:551-556, 1978.

Coceani F, Kelsey L, Ackerley C, et al: Cytochrome P450 during ontogenic development: Occurrence in the ductus arteriosus and other tissues. Can J Physiol Pharmacol 72:217-226, 1994.

Coceani F, Liu Y, Seidlitz E, et al: Endothelin A receptor is necessary for $O_2$ constriction but not closure of ductus arteriosus. Am J Physiol 277:H1521-H1531, 1999.

Coceani F, White E, Bodach E, Olley PM: Age-dependent changes in the response of the lamb ductus arteriosus to oxygen and ibuprofen. Can J Physiol Pharmacol 57:825-831, 1979.

Coceani F, Wright J, Breen C: Ductus arteriosus: Involvement of a sarcolemmal cytochrome P-450 in $O_2$ constriction? Can J Physiol Pharmacol 67:1448-1450, 1989b.

Colditz P, Murphy D, Rolfe P, Wilkinson AR: Effect of infusion rate of indomethacin on cerebrovascular responses in preterm neonates. Arch Dis Child 64:8-12, 1989.

Collaborative Group on Antenatal Steroid Therapy: Prevention of respiratory distress syndrome: Effect of antenatal dexamethasone administration. Publication No 85–2695. Bethesda, MD, National Institutes of Health, 1985.

Coombs RC, Morgan MEI, Durin GM, et al: Gut blood flow velocities in the newborn: Effects of patent ductus arteriosus and parenteral indomethacin. Arch Dis Child 65:1067-1071, 1990.

Cotton RB, Haywood JL, FitzGerald GA: Symptomatic patent ductus arteriosus following prophylactic indomethacin: A clinical and biochemical appraisal. Biol Neonate 60:273-282, 1991.

Cotton RB, Lindstrom DP, Kanarek KS, et al: Effect of positive-end-expiratory pressure on right ventricular output in lambs with hyaline membrane disease. Acta Paediatr Scand 69:603-606, 1980.

Cotton RB, Stahlman MT, Berder HW, et al: Randomized trial of early closure of symptomatic patent ductus arteriosus in small preterm infants. J Pediatr 93:647-651, 1978.

Couser RJ, Hoekstra RE, Ferrara TB, et al: Neurodevelopmental follow-up at 36 months' corrected age of preterm infants treated with prophylactic indomethacin. Arch Pediatr Adolesc Med 154:598-602, 2000.

Dahlgren N, Nilsson B, Sakabe T, Siesjo BK: The effect of indomethacin on cerebral blood flow and oxygen consumption in the rat at normal and increased carbon dioxide tensions. Acta Physiol Scand 111:475-485, 1981.

Docherty JC, Wilson TW: Indomethacin increases the formation of lipoxygenase products in calcium ionophore–stimulated human neutrophils. Biochem Biophys Res Commun 148:534-538, 1987.

Domanico RS, Waldman JD, Lester LA, et al: Prophylactic indomethacin reduces the incidence of pulmonary hemorrhage and patent ductus arteriosus in surfactant-treated infants <1250 grams. Pediatr Res 35:331A, 1994.

Drayton MR, Skidmore R: Ductus arteriosus blood flow during first 48 hours of life. Arch Dis Child 62:1030-1034, 1987.

Dudell GG, Gersony WM: Patent ductus arteriosus in neonates with severe respiratory disease. J Pediatr 104:915-920, 1984.

Early postnatal dexamethasone therapy for the prevention of chronic lung disease. Pediatrics 108:741-748, 2001.

Edwards AD, Wyatt JS, Richardson C, et al: Effects of indomethacin on cerebral haemodynamics in very preterm infants. Lancet 335:1491-1495, 1990.

Ellison RC, Peckham GJ, Lang P, et al: Evaluation of the preterm infant for patent ductus arteriosus. Pediatrics 71:364-372, 1983.

Evans N, Iyer P: Assessment of ductus arteriosus shunt in preterm infants supported by mechanical ventilation: Effect of interatrial shunting. J Pediatr 125:778-785, 1994.

Fajardo CA, Whyte RK, Steele BT: Effect of dopamine on failure of indomethacin to close the patent ductus arteriosus. J Pediatr 121:771-775, 1992.

Fineman JR, Takahashi Y, Roman C, Clyman RI: Endothelin-receptor blockade does not alter closure of the ductus arteriosus. Am J Physiol 275:H1620-H1626, 1998.

Friedman WF: The intrinsic physiologic properties of the developing heart. In Friedman WF, Lesch M, Sonnenblick EH (eds): Neonatal Heart Disease. New York, Grune & Stratton, 1972, pp 21-49.

Friedman Z, Whitman V, Maisels MJ, et al: Indomethacin disposition and indomethacin-induced platelet dysfunction in premature infants. J Clin Pharmacol 18:272-279, 1978.

Garland J, Buck R, Weinberg M: Pulmonary hemorrhage risk in infants with a clinically diagnosed patent ductus arteriosus: A retrospective cohort study. Pediatrics 94:719-723, 1994.

Gentile R, Stevenson GM, Dooley T, et al: Pulsed Doppler echocardiographic determination of time of ductal closure in normal newborn infants. J Pediatr 98:443-448, 1981.

Gerhardt T, Bancalari E: Lung compliance in newborns with patent ductus arteriosus before and after surgical ligation. Biol Neonate 38:96-105, 1980.

Gersony WM, Peckham GJ, Ellison RC, et al: Effects of indomethacin in premature infants with patent ductus arteriosus: Results of a national collaborative study. J Pediatr 102:895-906, 1983.

Green TP, Thompson TR, Johnson D, Lock JE: Fluid administration and the development of patent ductus arteriosus. N Engl J Med 303:337-338, 1980.

Grosfeld JL, Kamman K, Gross K, et al: Comparative effects of indomethacin, prostaglandin E1, and ibuprofen on bowel ischemia. J Pediatr Surg 18:738-742, 1983.

Hammerman C, Aranburo MJ: Prolonged indomethacin therapy for the prevention of recurrences of patent ductus arteriosus. J Pediatr 117:771-776, 1990.

Hammerman C, Strates C, Valaitis S: The silent ductus: Its precursors and its aftermath. Pediatr Cardiol 7:121-127, 1986.

Hammerman C, Glaser J, Schimmel MS, et al: Continuous versus multiple rapid infusions of indomethacin: Effects on cerebral blood flow velocity. Pediatrics 95:244-248, 1995.

Huhta JC, Cohen M, Gutgesell HP: Patency of the ductus arteriosus in normal neonates: Two dimensional echocardiography vs Doppler assessment. J Am Coll Cardiol 4:561-564, 1984.

Ikegami M, Jacobs H, Jobe A: Surfactant function in respiratory distress syndrome. J Pediatr 102:443-447, 1983.

Iyer P, Evans N: Re-evaluation of the left atrial to aortic root ratio as a marker of patent ductus arteriosus. Arch Dis Child 70:F112-F117, 1994.

Jacob J, Gluck G, DiSessa T, et al: The contribution of PDA in the neonate with severe RDS. J Pediatr 96:79-87, 1980.

Johnson DS, Rogers JH, Null DM, DeLemos RA: The physiologic consequences of the ductus arteriosus in the extremely immature newborn. Clin Res 26:826A, 1978.

Johnson GL, Breart GL, Gewitz MH, et al: Echocardiographic characteristics of premature infants with patent ductus arteriosus. Pediatrics 72:864-871, 1983.

Kaapa P, Seppanen M, Kero P, Saraste M: Pulmonary hemodynamics after synthetic surfactant replacement in neonatal respiratory distress syndrome. J Pediatr 123:115-119, 1993.

Kajino H, Chen YQ, Seidner SR, et al: Factors that increase the contractile tone of the ductus arteriosus also regulate its anatomic remodeling. Am J Physiol 281:R291-R301, 2001.

Kennedy JA, Clark SL: Observations on the physiological reactions of the ductus arteriosus. Am J Physiol 136:140-147, 1942.

Konig W, Brom J, Schonfeld W, et al: Effect of tenoxicam and indomethacin on the release of histamine, prostaglandin E2 and leukotrienes from various cells. Arzneimittelforschung 37:296-299, 1987.

Koren G, Zarfin Y, Perlman M, MacLeod SM: Effects of indomethacin on digoxin pharmacokinetics in preterm infants. Pediatr Pharmacol 4:25-30, 1984.

Krauss AN, Fatica N, Lewis BS, et al: Pulmonary function in preterm infants following treatment with intravenous indomethacin. Am J Dis Child 143:78-81, 1989.

Krueger E, Mellander M, Bratton D, Cotton R: Prevention of symptomatic patent ductus arteriosus with a single dose of indomethacin. J Pediatr 111:749-754, 1987.

Laudignon N, Chemtob S, Bard H, Aranda JV: Effect of indomethacin on cerebral blood flow velocity of premature newborns. Biol Neonate 54:254-262, 1988.

Lewis AB, Heymann MA, Rudolph AM: Gestational changes in pulmonary vascular responses in fetal lambs in utero. Circ Res 39:536-541, 1976.

Lister G, Hellenbrand WE, Kleinman CS, Talner NS: Physiologic effects of increasing hemoglobin concentration in left-to-right shunting in infants with ventricular septal defects. N Engl J Med 306:502-506, 1982.

Loftin CD, Trivedi DB, Tiano HF, et al: Failure of ductus arteriosus closure and remodeling in neonatal mice deficient in cyclooxygenase-1 and cyclooxygenase-2. Proc Natl Acad Sci U S A 98:1059-1064, 2001.

Mahony L, Caldwell RL, Girod DA, et al: Indomethacin therapy on the first day of life in infants with very low birth weight. J Pediatr 106:801-805, 1985.

Mahony L, Carnero V, Brett C, et al: Prophylactic indomethacin therapy for patent ductus arteriosus in very low-birth-weight infants. N Engl J Med 306:506-510, 1982.

Malcolm DD, Segar JL, Robillard JE, Chemtob S: Indomethacin compromises hemodynamics during positive-pressure ventilation, independently of prostanoids. J Appl Physiol 74:1672-1678, 1993.

Mason CA, Bigras JL, O'Blenes SB, et al: Gene transfer in utero biologically engineers a patent ductus arteriosus in lambs by arresting fibronectin-dependent neointimal formation. Nat Med 5:176-182, 1999.

McCormick DC, Edwards AD, Brown GC, et al: Effect of indomethacin on cerebral oxidized cytochrome oxidase in preterm infants. Pediatr Res 33:603-608, 1993.

Mellander M, Larsson LE, Ekström-Jodal B, Sabel KG: Prediction of symptomatic patent ductus arteriosus in preterm infants using Doppler and M-mode echocardiography. Acta Paediatr Scand 76:553-559, 1987.

Ment LR, Duncan CC, Ehrenkranz RA, et al: Randomized indomethacin trial for prevention of intraventricular hemorrhage in very low birth weight infants. J Pediatr 107:937-943, 1985.
Ment LR, Duncan CC, Ehrenkranz RA, et al: Randomized low-dose indomethacin trial for prevention of intraventricular hemorrhage in very low birth weight neonates. J Pediatr 112:948-955, 1988.
Ment LR, Oh W, Ehrenkranz RA, et al: Low-dose indomethacin therapy and extension of intraventricular hemorrhage: A multicenter randomized trial. J Pediatr 124:951-955, 1994.
Ment LR, Stewart WB, Ardito TA, et al: Indomethacin promotes germinal matrix microvessel maturation in the newborn beagle pup. Stroke 23:1132-1137, 1992.
Ment LR, Stewart WB, Scott DT, Duncan CC: Beagle puppy model of intraventricular hemorrhage: randomized indomethacin prevention trial. Neurology 33:179-184, 1983.
Merritt TA, White CL, Coen RW, et al: Preschool assessment of infants with a patent ductus arteriosus: Comparison of ligation and indomethacin therapy. Am J Dis Child 136:507-512, 1982.
Meyers R, Alpan G, Clyman RI: Effect of patent ductus arteriosus and indomethacin on intestinal blood flow in the newborn lamb. Pediatr Res 27:216A, 1990.
Michelakis E, Rebeyka I, Bateson J, et al: Voltage-gated potassium channels in human ductus arteriosus. Lancet 356:134-137, 2000.
Mikhail M, Lei W, Toews W, et al: Surgical and medical experience with 734 premature infants with patent ductus arteriosus. J Thorac Cardiovasc Surg 83:349-357, 1982.
Moise KJ Jr, Huhta JC, Sharif DS, et al: Indomethacin in the treatment of preterm labor: Effects on the fetal ductus. N Engl J Med 319:327-331, 1988.
Momma K, Mishihara S, Ota Y: Constriction of the fetal ductus arteriosus by glucocorticoid hormones. Pediatr Res 15:19-21, 1981.
Mosca F, Bray M, Lattanzio M, et al: Comparative evaluation of the effects of indomethacin and ibuprofen on cerebral perfusion and oxygenation in preterm infants with patent ductus arteriosus. J Pediatr 131:549-554, 1997.
Musewe NN, Smallhorn JF, Benson LN, et al: Validation of Doppler-derived pulmonary arterial pressure in patients with ductus arteriosus under different hemodynamic states. Circulation 76:1081-1091, 1987.
Nakanishi T, Gu H, Hagiwara N, Momma K: Mechanisms of oxygen-induced contraction of ductus arteriosus isolated from the fetal rabbit. Circ Res 72:1218-1228, 1993.
Narayanan M, Cooper B, Weiss H, Clyman RI: Prophylactic indomethacin: Factors determining permanent ductus arteriosus closure. J Pediatr 136:330-337, 2000.
Naulty CM, Horn S, Conry J, Avery GB: Improved lung compliance after ligation of patent ductus arteriosus in hyaline membrane disease. J Pediatr 93: 682-684, 1978.
Nguyen M, Camenisch T, Snouwaert JN, et al: The prostaglandin receptor EP4 triggers remodelling of the cardiovascular system at birth. Nature 390:78-81, 1997.
Patel J, Roberts I, Azzopardi D, et al: Randomized double-blind controlled trial comparing the effects of ibuprofen with indomethacin on cerebral hemodynamics in preterm infants with patent ductus arteriosus [see comments]. Pediatr Res 47:36-42, 2000.
Peckham GJ, Miettinen OS, Ellison RC, et al: Clinical course to 1 year of age in premature infants with patent ductus arteriosus: Results of a multicenter randomized trial of indomethacin. J Pediatr 105:285-291, 1984.
Pérez Fontán JJ, Clyman RI, Mauray F, et al: Respiratory effects of a patent ductus arteriosus in premature newborn lambs. J Appl Physiol 63:2315-2324, 1987.
Pezzati M, Vangi V, Biagiotti R, et al: Effects of indomethacin and ibuprofen on mesenteric and renal blood flow in preterm infants with patent ductus arteriosus. J Pediatr 135:733-738, 1999.
Pryds O, Greisen G, Johansen KH: Indomethacin and cerebral blood flow in premature infants treated for patent ductus arteriosus. Eur J Pediatr 147:315-316, 1988.
Raju TNK, Langenberg P: Pulmonary hemorrhage and exogenous surfactant therapy—a meta-analysis. J Pediatr 123:603-610, 1993.
Ramsey JM, Murphy DJ, Vick GW III, et al: Response of the patent ductus arteriosus to indomethacin treatment. Am J Dis Child 141:294-297, 1987.
Reeve HL, Tolarova S, Nelson DP, et al: Redox control of oxygen sensing in the rabbit ductus arteriosus. J Physiol 533:253-261, 2001.
Reller MD, Buffkin DC, Colasurdo MA, et al: Ductal patency in neonates with respiratory distress syndrome. A randomized surfactant trial. Am J Dis Child 145:1017-1020, 1991.
Reller MD, Rice MJ, McDonald RW: Review of studies evaluating ductal patency in the premature infant. J Pediatr 122:S59-S62, 1993.
Rennie JM, Cooke RWI: Prolonged low dose indomethacin for persistent ductus arteriosus of prematurity. Arch Dis Child 66:55-58, 1991.
Rennie JM, Doyle J, Cooke RWI: Early administration of indomethacin to preterm infants. Arch Dis Child 61:233-238, 1986.
Rheuban KS, Everett AD, Zellers TM, et al: Ductus arteriosus closure rates and indomethacin levels in premature infants. Pediatr Res 21:387A, 1987.
Rhodes PG, Ferguson MG, Reddy NS, et al; Effects of prolonged versus acute indomethacin therapy in very low birth weight infants with patent ductus arteriosus. Eur J Pediatr 147:481-484, 1988.
Schmidt B, Davis P, Moddemann D, et al: Long-term effects of indomethacin prophylaxis in extremely low-birth-weight infants. N Engl J Med 344:1966-1972, 2001.
Seidner SR, Chen Y-Q, Oprysko PR, et al: Combined prostaglandin and nitric oxide inhibition produces anatomic remodeling and closure of the ductus arteriosus in the premature newborn baboon. Pediatr Res 50:365-373, 2001.
Serwer GA, Armstrong BE, Anderson PA: Continuous wave Doppler ultrasonographic quantitation of patent ductus arteriosus flow. J Pediatr 100:297-299, 1982.
Seyberth HW, Müller H, Wille L, et al: Recovery of prostaglandin production associated with reopening of the ductus arteriosus after indomethacin treatment in preterm infants with respiratory distress syndrome. Pediatr Pharmacol 2:127-141, 1982.
Shimada S, Kasai T, Konishi M, Fujiwara T: Effects of patent ductus arteriosus on left ventricular output and organ blood flows in preterm infants with respiratory distress syndrome treated with surfactant. J Pediatr 125: 270-277, 1994.
Shimada S, Raju TNK, Bhat R, et al: Treatment of patent ductus arteriosus after exogenous surfactant in baboons with hyaline membrane disease. Pediatr Res 26:565-569, 1989.
Smith M, Setzer ES, Garg DC, Goldberg RN: Pharmacokinetics of prophylactic indomethacin in very low birthweight premature infants. Pediatr Res 18:161A, 1984.
Speziale MV, Allen RG, Henderson CR, et al: Effects of ibuprofen and indomethacin on the regional circulation in newborn piglets. Biol Neonate 76:242-252, 1999.
Stefano JL, Abbasi S, Pearlman SA, et al: Closure of the ductus arteriosus with indomethacin in ventilated neonates with respiratory distress syndrome: Effects of pulmonary compliance and ventilation. Am Rev Respir Dis 143:236-239, 1991.
Stevenson JG, Kawabori I, Guntheroth WG: Pulsed Doppler echocardiographic diagnosis of patent ductus arteriosus: Sensitivity, limitations and technical features. Cathet Cardiovasc Diagn 6:255-263, 1980.
Takahashi Y, Roman C, Chemtob S, et al: Cyclooxygenase-2 inhibitors constrict the fetal lamb ductus arteriosus both in

vitro and in vivo. Am J Physiol Regul Integr Comp Physiol 278:R1496-R1505, 2000.

Thalji AA, Carr I, Yeh TF, et al: Pharmacokinetics of intravenously administered indomethacin in premature infants. J Pediatr 97:995-1000, 1980.

Therkelsen K, Jensen KA, Freundlich M, et al: Endothelin-1 and cerebral blood flow: Influence of hypoxia, hypercapnia and indomethacin on circulating endothelin levels in healthy volunteers. Scand J Clin Lab Invest 54:441-451, 1994.

Thibeault DW, Emmanouilides GC, Dodge ME: Pulmonary and circulatory function in preterm lambs treated with hydrocortisone in utero. Biol Neonate 34:238-247, 1978.

Van Bel F, Van de Bor M, Stijnen T, et al: Cerebral blood flow velocity changes in preterm infants after a single dose of indomethacin: Duration of its effect [see comments]. Pediatrics 84:802-807, 1989.

Van Bel F, Van Zoeren D, Schipper J, et al: Effect of indomethacin on superior mesenteric artery blood flow velocity in preterm infants. J Pediatr 116:965-970, 1990.

Van Overmeire B, Smets K, Lecoutere D, et al: A comparison of ibuprofen and indomethacin for closure of patent ductus arteriosus. N Engl J Med 343:674-681, 2000.

Waffarn F, Siassi B, Cabal L, Schmidt PL: Effect of antenatal glucocorticoids on clinical closure of the ductus arteriosus. Am J Dis Child 137:336-338, 1983.

Wagner HR, Ellison RC, Zierler S, et al: Surgical closure of patent ductus arteriosus in 268 preterm infants. J Thorac Cardiovasc Surg 87:870-875, 1984.

Walther FJ, Kim DH, Ebrahimi M, Siassi B: Pulsed Doppler measurement of left ventricular output as early predictor of symptomatic patent ductus arteriosus in very preterm infants. Biol Neonate 56:121-128, 1989.

Wilkerson RD, Glenn TM: Influence of nonsteroidal antiinflammatory drugs on ouabain toxicity. Am Heart J 94:454-459, 1977.

Wu GR, Jing S, Momma K, Nakanishi T: The effect of vitamin A on contraction of the ductus arteriosus in fetal rat. Pediatr Res 49:747-754, 2001.

Yaffe SJ, Friedman WF, Rogers D, et al: The disposition of indomethacin in premature babies. J Pediatr 97:1001-1006, 1980.

Yeh TF, Achanti B, Jain R, et al: Indomethacin therapy in premature infants with PDA-determination of therapeutic plasma levels. Dev Pharmacol Ther 12:169-178, 1989.

Yeh TF, Goldbarg HR, Henek T, et al: Intravenous indomethacin therapy in premature infants with patent ductus arteriosus: Causes of death and one-year follow-up. Am J Dis Child 136:803-807, 1982.

Yeh TF, Thalji A, Luken L, et al: Improved lung compliance following indomethacin therapy in premature infants with persistent ductus arteriosus. Chest 80:698-700, 1981.

CHAPTER

# 57

# Common Congenital Heart Disease: Presentation, Management, and Outcomes

**Gil Wernovsky and Peter J. Gruber**

Cardiac anomalies resulting in congenital heart disease (CHD) constitute the most common birth defect, occurring in nearly 1 in 100 live births. The normal and abnormal formation of the heart during pregnancy, as well as a system of nomenclature for categorizing the multitude of congenital defects of the heart, are discussed in Chapters 52 and 53.

This chapter focuses on the common features of the *neonatal* presentation of CHD, as well as initial stabilization, management, and current data on short- and mid-term outcomes. For a complete compendium of CHD, the reader is referred to extensive texts dedicated solely to congenital and acquired heart disease (Allen et al, 2001; Braunwald, 1997; Fyler, 1992a; Moller and Hoffman, 2000) and its management (Castañeda et al, 1994; Chang et al, 1998; Gravlee et al, 2002; Litwin, 1996; Mavroudis and Backer, 1994).

## GENERAL CONSIDERATIONS

### Epidemiology

The prevalence of structural heart disease in the first year of life confirmed by noninvasive imaging is 6 to 8 cases per 1000 live births. When cases diagnosed solely by clinical means are included, the prevalence is 8 to 10 cases per 1000 live births. The prevalence has been relatively constant over the years and in different areas around the world. Table 57–1 summarizes and compares prevalence data from several large population-based studies. Data from the New England Regional Infant Cardiac Program suggest that approximately 3 infants per 1000 live births have heart disease that results in death or necessitates cardiac catheterization or surgery during the first year of life (Fyler, 1980). A majority of these infants with congenital heart disease are identified by the end of the neonatal period (Fyler, 1980). The most common congenital heart lesions manifesting in the first weeks of life are summarized in Table 57–2. Advances in diagnostic imaging, cardiac surgery, and intensive care have reduced the operative risks for many complex lesions; the hospital mortality rate following all forms of neonatal cardiac surgery has significantly decreased since the early 1990s.

### Effects of the Transitional Circulation in Neonates with Congenital Heart Disease

In the *normal* newborn, a series of rapid physiologic changes occur at birth and in the subsequent days. Separation from the low-resistance placenta results in an increase in systemic vascular resistance (SVR) to which the systemic (usually left) ventricle needs to adapt. Expansion of the lungs and exposure to oxygen (usually 21%, but occasionally increased with supplemental oxygen in the delivery room) result in a decrease in pulmonary vascular resistance (PVR), resulting in an increase in pulmonary blood flow (PBF) and increased left atrial return via the pulmonary veins. This increase in left atrial pressure and volume tends to close the flap valve of the foramen ovale. In most cases the ductus arteriosus constricts and closes within the first hours to days of life. In the normal heart, these physiologic and anatomic changes result in an effective separation of systemic and pulmonary venous returns, with the elimination of hypoxemia and the establishment of an "series" circulation. Over the subsequent days to weeks, there is a further fall in PVR, improved left ventricular compliance, and increased cardiac output and ventricular reserve. Hematocrit falls (physiologic anemia), which further reduces PVR by virtue of decreased blood viscosity. These physiologic changes are well suited to the transition from fetal to adult circulation.

However, in the newborn with undiagnosed CHD, it is these very changes that typically result in the signs and symptoms of a cardiac malformation. Despite the multiple anatomic variations of CHD, the newborn with CHD—even that due to very complex lesions—typically presents in one of three ways: (1) with cyanosis (the visible sign of hypoxemia); (2) with congestive heart failure (CHF), occasionally in its most severe form of circulatory collapse; or (3) as an asymptomatic or minimally symptomatic newborn with a heart murmur. As is discussed in more detail in subsequent sections on individual lesions, the *fall in PVR* is particularly deleterious in a majority of cases of CHD—those with anatomic connections between the systemic and the pulmonary circuits (e.g., ventricular septal defects [VSDs] and CHD with connections between the pulmonary arteries and aorta, such as a patent ductus arteriosus or truncus arteriosus). In addition, *closure of the ductus arteriosus* is particularly deleterious in patients with duct-dependent PBF or systemic blood flow (SBF), including virtually all patients with single ventricle, as well as those with coarctation of the aorta and interruption of the aortic arch. In these lesions, the open ductus constitutes the proverbial double-edged sword: Although necessary to perfuse the systemic or pulmonary vascular bed, the connection between the systemic and the pulmonary circuits typically results in a "steal" of systemic cardiac output into the lower-resistance pulmonary vascular bed in diastole, resulting in decreased oxygen delivery, a widened pulse pressure, and decreased overall organ perfusion.

### Mimicking the Fetal Circulation

Because in most cases, CHD is associated with stable physiology in utero, the basic principle of initial stabilization in critical CHD is to mimic the fetal circulation by providing $PGE_1$ to maintain ductal patency, keeping PVR high, keeping SVR low, providing adequate mixing at the atrial level if necessary, and minimizing whole-body oxygen consumption. Following this initial stabilization, however, prompt surgical intervention usually is necessary; although

**TABLE 57–1**

**Prevalence of Congenital Heart Disease: Summary of Data from Population-Based Studies**

| Feature | Study: Baltimore Washington Infant Study (Ferencz, 1985) | New England Regional Infant Cardiac Program (Fyler, 1980) | Carlgren (1987) | Dickinson et al (1981) | Laursen (1980) | Total | |
|---|---|---|---|---|---|---|---|
| Years of study | 1981-1982 | 1969-1977 | 1941-1950 | 1960-1969 | 1963-1973 | | |
| Reference population | Resident births, Maryland, Washington, DC Metropolitan area | Resident births, 6 New England States | Resident births, Gothenburg, Sweden | Resident births, Liverpool, England | Live births Denmark | | |
| Birth Cohort: length of follow-up | 1 yr | 1 yr | 7-16 yr | 3-12 yr | Birth–15 yr | | |
| No. of congenital heart disease cases | 664 | 2251 | 369 | 884 | 5249 | 9417 | |
| No. of live births | 179,697 | 1,528,686 | 58,105 | 160,480 | ~855,000 | ~2,781,968 | |
| **Cardiac Lesion** | **Prevalence per 1000 Live Births** | | | | | **Mean** | **Approximate No. of Affected Infants per Live Births** |
| **Conotruncal and Major Septation Defects** | | | | | | | |
| Transposition of great arteries | 0.211 | 0.215 | 0.379 | 0.27 | 0.29 | 0.273 | 1/3500 |
| Tetralogy of Fallot | 0.252 | 0.214 | 0.31 | 0.32 | 0.36 | 0.293 | 1/3500 |
| Truncus arteriosus | 0.056 | 0.034 | 0.069 | 0.06 | 0.09 | 0.062 | 1/16,000 |
| Endocardial cushion defect | 0.352 | 0.118 | 0.172 | 0.13 | 0.15 | 0.186 | 1/5500 |
| Total anomalous pulmonary venous return | 0.053 | 0.058 | 0.052 | 0.07 | | 0.066 | 1/15,000 |
| **Single-Ventricle Defects** | | | | | | | |
| Tricuspid atresia | 0.039 | 0.057 | 0.086 | 0.09 | 0.05 | 0.064 | 1/15,500 |
| Pulmonary atresia | 0.053 | 0.071 | 0.069 | 0.04 | 0.04 | 0.061 | 1/16,500 |
| Hypoplastic left heart syndrome | 0.257 | 0.164 | 0.103 | 0.16 | 0.18 | 0.175 | 1/5500 |
| **Valve and Vessel Lesions** | | | | | | | |
| Pulmonic stenosis | 0.139 | 0.073 | 0.275 | 0.42 | 0.36 | 0.263 | 1/4000 |
| Aortic stenosis | 0.111 | 0.041 | 0.344 | 0.28 | 0.29 | 0.213 | 1/4500 |
| Coarctation of aorta | 0.239 | 0.185 | 0.62 | 0.35 | 0.43 | 0.365 | 1/2500 |
| **Shunt Lesions** | | | | | | | |
| Ventricular septal defect (requiring closure) | 0.853 | 0.379 | 1.699 | 1.8 | 1.48 | 1.244 | 1/1000 |
| Atrial septal defect | 0.317 | 0.073 | 0.241 | 0.32 | 0.58 | 0.306 | 1/3000 |
| Patent ductus arteriosus | 0.039 | 0.138 | 0.602 | 0.65 | 0.77 | 0.45 | 1/2000 |
| Rate of confirmed congenital heart disease/1000 live births | 3.7 | 2.03 | 4 | 3.75 | 4.4 | 3.56 | |

**TABLE 57–2**

**Most Common Congenital Heart Lesions Manifesting in the First Month of Life* (Frequency Distribution Based on Age at Diagnosis)**

| Age at Diagnosis | | |
|---|---|---|
| **0-6 Days (n = 1603)** | **7-13 Days (n = 311)** | **14-28 Days (n = 306)** |
| D-TGA (15%) | Coarctation (20%) | VSD (18%) |
| HLHS (12%) | VSD (14%) | TOF (17%) |
| TOF (8%) | HLHS (9%) | Coarctation (12%) |
| Coarctation (7%) | D-TGA (8%) | D-TGA (10%) |
| VSD (6%) | TOF (7%) | PDA (5%) |
| Other (52%) | Other (42%) | Other (38%) |

*These six lesions account for ~50% of cases of congenital heart disease that manifests in the first month of life.

HLHS, hypoplastic left heart syndrome; PDA, patent ductus arteriosus; TGA, transposition of the great arteries; TOF, tetralogy of Fallot; VSD, ventricular septal defect.

prostaglandin therapy may maintain patency of the ductus for a considerable period of time, long-term medical management cannot overcome the principal physiologic change of the transitional circulation, namely, the expected fall in PVR.

## PHYSIOLOGIC CATEGORIZATION OF CONGENITAL HEART DISEASE

Although the different anatomic variations of CHD are many, the physiologic manifestations in the newborn period are much more limited. Two basic principles apply:

1. Anatomic connections of large enough size between the two atria (e.g., atrial septal defect [ASD]), ventricles (e.g., VSD), or great vessels (e.g., ductus arteriosus) will equalize the pressures on both sides of the defect.
2. Blood flow will be toward the pathway of lower resistance.

### Pulmonary Hypertension

Pulmonary hypertension—defined strictly as elevated pressure in the pulmonary artery—will result from any nonrestrictive communication at the ventricular or great vessel level. Unfortunately, the term *pulmonary hypertension* frequently is mistakenly used in the neonatal intensive care unit (NICU) to mean "elevated pulmonary vascular resistance"; in fact, however, the terms are not synonymous, as they refer to very different physiologic states. For example, the child with a congenital heart defect such as a large VSD or patent ductus arteriosus will have systemic pressure in the pulmonary artery because of the transmitted systemic pressure into the pulmonary vascular bed. However, the net shunt will be from left to right, and the baby will have symptoms of CHF. This clinical scenario should be distinguished from that in the child with pulmonary hypertension secondary to severely elevated PVR (e.g., congenital diaphragmatic hernia, meconium aspiration, idiopathic pulmonary hypertension of the newborn [PPHN]), in whom the direction of shunt at the ductus is right to left, resulting in hypoxemia rather than CHF. Both cases demonstrate elevated pulmonary artery pressures—"pulmonary hypertension"—but the physiologic sequelae are very different. Care should be taken to accurately describe a patient with pulmonary hypertension as having either low PVR (as in most cases of CHD) or high PVR (as in most cases of lung disease).

### Series Circulation: Shunt Physiology

In the absence of associated obstructive lesions, newborns with septal defects or connections between the great vessels will have blood flow shunted from the systemic circulation into the pulmonary circulation. This resultant "left-to-right" shunt results in a higher PBF (Qp) than SBF (Qs). The magnitude of left-to-right shunt is typically expressed as the ratio of SBF to PBF (Qp:Qs). As PVR falls, an increasing amount of SBF is shunted into the pulmonary circulation, resulting in a volume load in the pulmonary circuit. Compensatory mechanisms to increase SBF occur, including increase in heart rate, increase in stroke volume, and increase in renin and aldosterone production with resultant salt and water retention. The clinical manifestations include tachypnea, tachycardia, and other signs of CHF.

### Single-Ventricle Physiology

Atresia of an atrioventricular (AV) or semilunar valve results in a physiologic state in which there is complete mixing of the systemic and pulmonary venous circulations. In addition, in some children, there is borderline hypoplasia of an AV valve, outflow tract, or ventricle; in such cases, a separated two-ventricle circulation is ultimately possible. In each of these situations, there is essentially complete mixing of the systemic and pulmonary venous return, typically at the ventricular and/or atrial level (Fig. 57–1). A consequence of the mixing is that the ventricular output must be divided between the pulmonary and systemic arterial circuits: the two parallel circuits. In this situation the pulmonary artery and the aortic oxygen saturations are equal, and the ventricular output is the sum of the PBF (Qp) and the SBF (Qs). The proportion of the ventricular output that goes to the pulmonary or systemic vascular bed is determined by the relative resistance to flow into the two circuits.

In almost all hearts with single-ventricle physiology, one of the two outflows (pulmonary artery or aorta) is obstructed. It is extremely rare to have no outflow obstruction or to have obstruction to the pulmonary *and* the systemic circuits. As a result, patients generally fall into two distinct categories: those with obstructed pulmonary outflow and those with obstructed systemic outflow.

Resistance to *pulmonary* flow is determined by

- the degree of subvalvar or valvar pulmonary stenosis
- the pulmonary arteriolar resistance
- the pulmonary venous and left atrial pressure
- the size of the ductus arteriosus

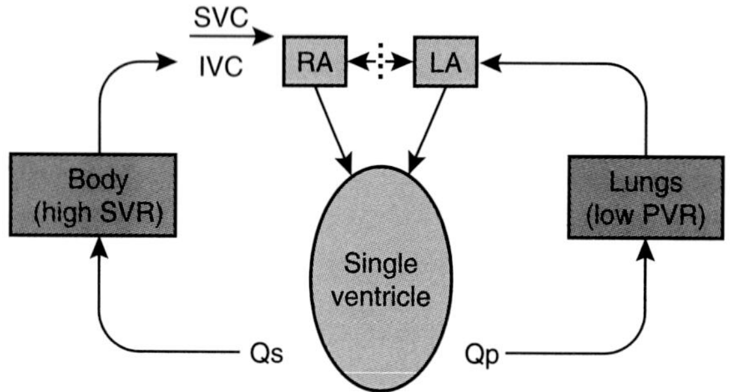


**FIGURE 57–1.** Single-ventricle physiology. This physiologic variant occurs in several heterogeneous forms of congenital heart disease in which there is complete mixing of the systemic and pulmonary venous returns at the atrial or ventricular level. The ventricular output is divided between the systemic and the pulmonary arterial circulations; the relative distribution is dependent on the relative resistances of the systemic and pulmonary vascular beds, as well as the presence of any anatomic obstruction (see text). IVC, inferior vena cava; LA, left atrium; PVR, pulmonary vascular resistance; Qp, pulmonary blood flow; Qs, systemic blood flow; RA, right atrium; SVC, superior vena cava; SVR, systemic vascular resistance.

The left atrial pressure is determined by the volume of the PBF entering the left atrium and the degree of obstruction to outflow through the left AV valve and atrial septum.

Resistance to *systemic* flow is determined by

- the degree of subaortic or aortic valvar stenosis, arch hypoplasia, or coarctation
- the SVR
- the size of the ductus arteriosus

### *Balancing the Parallel Circulations*

In managing the neonate with single-ventricle physiology, the goal is to balance the ventricular output between the systemic and the pulmonary vascular beds in such a way as to provide for adequate oxygen delivery to prevent acidosis, while minimizing volume load to the single ventricle. Assuming a pulmonary venous saturation of 95% to 100% and a mixed venous oxygen saturation of 55% to 60%, an arterial oxygen saturation of 75% to 80% represents a Qp:Qs of approximately 1.0. This typically results in ventricular volume overload that is twice normal (the ventricle must pump the Qp *plus* the Qs), with minimal AV valve regurgitation and normal systemic blood flow and oxygen delivery.

### *The Transitional Circulation in the Patient with Single Ventricle*

After birth, there is a fall in PVR and a relative increase in the proportion of PBF from the combined ventricular output. As the PVR continues to fall with time, an increasing proportion of the combined ventricular output is committed to the lungs. The normal homeostatic mechanisms to improve systemic output result in an increased stroke volume and an increase in heart rate.

However, the normal fall in PVR over the first few hours to days of life, in the absence of a significant obstruction to PBF, gradually results in elevated PBF at the expense of SBF. As Qp:Qs approaches 2.0, the single ventricle becomes progressively volume overloaded, with mildly elevated end-diastolic and atrial pressures. The neonate may show signs of respiratory distress. The greater proportion of pulmonary venous return in the mixed ventricular blood results in an elevated systemic arterial oxygen saturation (approximately 85% to 90%), and visible cyanosis may be mild or absent.

Before surgical intervention, a number of ventilatory and pharmacologic maneuvers may be employed to "balance" the circulation (to achieve Qp:Qs of approximately 1), resulting in adequate oxygen delivery and SBF. However, in many of these patients, ventilatory and pharmacologic management only temporizes the need for surgical intervention. Cases of "unbalanced" single-ventricle physiology may be divided into two physiologic extremes: (1) inadequate PBF, which results in hypoxemia, and (2) excessive PBF, which results in CHF.

### *Inadequate Pulmonary Blood Flow*

The newborn with single-ventricle physiology and an inadequate oxygen saturation (less than 65%) may have limited PBF as a result of (1) intracardiac obstruction (e.g., severe valvar and/or subvalvar pulmonic stenosis); (2) a restrictive ductus arteriosus in lesions with "duct-dependent" PBF; (3) elevated PVR; or (4) obstruction to pulmonary venous outflow causing pulmonary venous hypertension and secondary pulmonary arteriolar hypertension.

Management strategies to improve PBF in this setting should be tailored to the underlying anatomic or pathophysiologic abnormality resulting in the decreased PBF. For example, in patients with *intracardiac obstruction* to PBF, maneuvers may be performed to increase blood pressure and SVR (e.g., increasing inotropic infusions), "forcing" more blood through the obstructed intracardiac pulmonary outflow. Interventional procedures such as pulmonary valve dilation may also be considered in this group of patients. Patients who are hypoxemic as a result of an obstructive left-sided AV valve and restrictive ASD may undergo transcatheter dilation of the atrial septum. Patients thought to be hypoxemic due to elevated PVR should undergo ventilatory maneuvers to decrease PVR (e.g., increased $FIO_2$, hyperventilation/induction of alkalosis, administration of nitric oxide). Most intravenous pulmonary vasodilators are nonspecific and result in unpredictable changes in the PVR and SVR.

### *Excessive Pulmonary Blood Flow*

A more common scenario in nonoperated patients with single ventricle is progressively increasing PBF at the expense of SBF. When the imbalance is severe, systemic hypoperfusion, metabolic acidosis, and shock may result. Once presence of a patent ductus arteriosus is confirmed, maneuvers to minimize SVR and maximize PVR should be employed. Hypotensive patients with a relatively high arterial oxygen saturation (i.e., less than 90%) generally have a severe "steal" of the combined ventricular output into the pulmonary vascular circuit. In these "overcirculated" patients, excessive inotropic support (particularly at alpha doses) should be minimized, and afterload reduction (e.g., sodium nitroprusside) may be especially helpful in patients with elevated SVR and an adequate blood pressure.

It is important to emphasize that many patients with single-ventricle physiology and "high" arterial oxygen saturations actually have *decreased* oxygen delivery to the tissues. The increased oxygen content comes at the expense of a relative reduction of SBF, which results in inadequate tissue perfusion, metabolic acidosis, and low cardiac output. In addition, ventricular wall tension and oxygen consumption are increased in the dilated, volume-overloaded single ventricle, potentially contributing to myocardial dysfunction and AV valve regurgitation. A progressive metabolic acidosis, even if mild, is a worrisome sign in these patients and requires prompt evaluation and management.

Maneuvers to increase PVR have been shown to be clinically effective in reducing excessive PBF. Supplemental inspired nitrogen or supplemental $CO_2$ may be used to elevate PVR by inducing alveolar hypoxia (Tabbutt et al, 2001). The hematocrit should be maintained at greater than 40% to 45%, as the increased viscosity also may serve to elevate PVR. Intubation and mechanical ventilation with sedation, paralysis, and permissive hypoventilation can be used to elevate the $P_{CO_2}$ to the range of 40 to 50 mm Hg. Metabolic acidemia should be corrected with sodium bicarbonate.

It is important to emphasize that preoperative patients with marked overcirculation and systemic hypoperfusion should not undergo a lengthy period of "medical management" of their unstable physiology. If a patient requires intubation and sedation to maintain adequate SBF, relatively urgent surgical management is indicated to achieve a more favorable physiology.

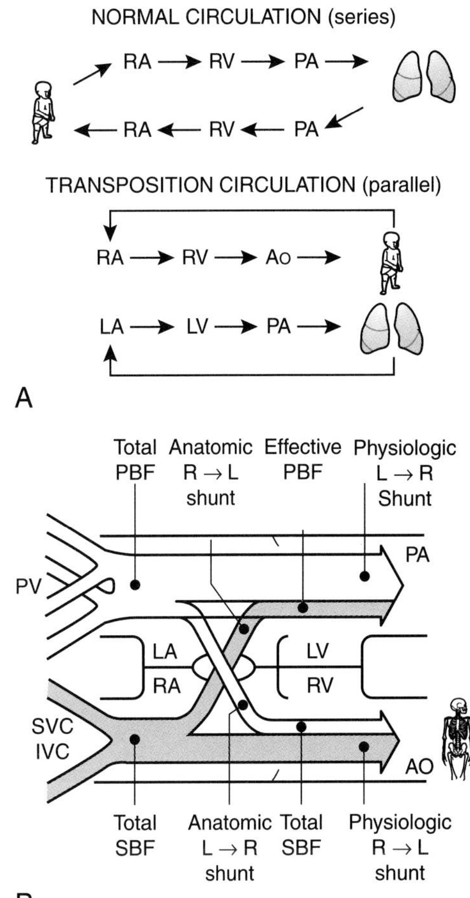


**FIGURE 57–2.** **A,** Comparison of the series circulation in the normal newborn with the parallel circulation in transposition of the great arteries (TGA). In TGA, survival after birth is dependent on mixing at either the atrial, ventricular, or great vessel level. **B,** Relative distribution of total and effective flows through the pulmonary and systemic arterial circulations in TGA. See text for details. Ao, aorta; IVC, inferior vena cava; LA, left atrium; LV, left ventricle; PA, pulmonary artery; PBF, pulmonary blood flow; RA, right atrium; RV, right ventricle; PV, pulmonary veins; SBF, systemic blood flow; SVC, superior vena cava. *(From Wernovsky G: Transposition of the great arteries. In Allen HD, Gutgesell HP, Clark EB, Driscoll DJ [eds]: Moss and Adams' Heart Disease in Infants, Children, and Adolescents: Including the Fetus and Young Adult, 6th ed. Philadelphia, Lippincott Williams & Wilkins, 2001, pp 1027-1084.)*

## Transposition Physiology

The dominant physiologic abnormalities in the newborn with transposition of the great arteries (TGA) are a deficiency of oxygen supply to the tissues and an excessive right and left ventricular workload. The systemic and the pulmonary circulations function in parallel rather than in series; hence, the greatest portion of the output of each ventricle is recirculated to that ventricle (Fig. 57–2). In TGA with intact ventricular septum (TGA/IVS), only a relatively small proportion of blood is exchanged by intercirculatory mixing between the two circulations; consequently, only a small proportion of the effective circulation reaches the appropriate vascular bed. The systemic and the pulmonary arterial oxygen saturations are thus dependent on one or more of the following locations for this exchange: *atrial* (patent foramen ovale, ASD); *ventricular* (VSD), and/or *great vessel* (patent ductus arteriosus, bronchopulmonary collateral circulation).

The net volume of blood passing from the pulmonary circulation (left atrium, left ventricle, pulmonary arteries) to the systemic circulation (right atrium, right ventricle, aorta) represents the anatomic *left-to-right* shunt and is the *effective* SBF (i.e., oxygenated pulmonary venous return perfusing the systemic capillary bed). Conversely, the net volume of blood passing from the systemic circulation to the pulmonary circulation represents the anatomic *right-to-left shunt* and is the *effective* PBF (systemic venous return perfusing the pulmonary capillary bed). The effective PBF, effective SBF, and net anatomic right-to-left and left-to-right shunts all are equal to each other. This volume is the *intercirculatory mixing*, which in TGA is the flow on which survival depends. The net volume exchanged between systemic and pulmonary circulations must be equal over a given short interval of time, because any major differences will result in a depletion of the blood volume of one circulation at the expense of overloading the other.

The volumes of anatomic right-to-left and left-to-right shunted blood (i.e., effective blood flow) that participate in functional gas exchange at the pulmonary and the systemic capillary levels are relatively small in comparison with the large volumes of blood *circulating* (total SBF and PBF) or *recirculating* (physiologic left-to-right and right-to-left shunt flows) within each circulation. The physiologic left-to-right shunt represents the volume of the pulmonary venous blood recirculating through the lungs without having passed through the body, and the physiologic right-to-left shunt is the volume of systemic venous blood reentering the systemic circulation without having passed through the lungs (Paul and Wernovsky, 1995) (see Fig. 57–2B).

The extent of intercirculatory mixing in TGA depends on the number, size, and position of the anatomic communications, and on the total blood flow through the pulmonary circuit. In the neonate with an intact ventricular septum and a closed or closing ductus arteriosus, severe hypoxemia secondary to inadequate mixing at the foramen ovale level is usually present. When the interatrial or interventricular shunting sites are of adequate size, the level of arterial oxygen saturation is influenced primarily by the pulmonary-to-systemic flow ratio, with a high PBF resulting in relatively high arterial oxygen saturation, as long as the ventricles can adequately maintain the high-output state (Wernovsky and Jonas, 1998). If the PBF is decreased by subpulmonary or pulmonary stenosis or elevated PVR, the arterial oxygen saturation will be lowered in spite of adequately sized anatomic shunting sites.

The physiologic mechanisms that precisely control the equalization of interchange between the two circulations remain speculative. The shunting patterns appear to be determined by local pressure gradients, which in turn are influenced by respiratory cycle phase, compliance of the cardiac chambers, heart rate, and the volume of blood flow and the vascular resistance in each of the circulations. With TGA/IVS, the interatrial shunt is from right atrium to left atrium during ventricular diastole, because left ventricular resistance to filling is less than right ventricular. The shunt is from left atrium to right atrium in ventricular systole, because the left atrium is less distensible than the right, and the net pressure in the left atrium is higher during ventricular systole. The pattern is affected by respiration, with the interatrial right-to-left (systemic-to-pulmonary) shunt increasing during inspiration, when the systemic venous return increases and pulmonary venous return decreases. The effects on intercirculatory mixing from positive pressure mechanical ventilation have not been fully studied.

### *Management of Profound Hypoxemia*

In neonates with TGA/IVS, the combination of a very low arterial $PO_2$ (i.e., less than 20 mm Hg), an elevated $PCO_2$ (despite adequate chest motion and ventilation), and metabolic acidosis (with or without pulmonary edema on the chest radiograph) constitutes a marker for severely decreased effective pulmonary and systemic arterial flows ("poor mixing") and requires urgent attention. The initial management of the severely hypoxemic patient with TGA includes (1) ensuring adequate mixing between the two parallel circuits and (2) maximizing the mixed venous oxygen saturation.

Once the diagnosis of TGA is made, maintaining patency of the ductus arteriosus with prostaglandin $E_1$ ($PGE_1$) will increase PBF and intercirculatory mixing, if PVR is lower than SVR *and* there is an atrial communication. In patients in whom the ductus arteriosus does not respond to prostaglandin infusion with an increased arterial oxygen saturation, the foramen ovale should be emergently enlarged by balloon atrial septostomy, and ventilatory maneuvers should be utilized to decrease PVR and to increase PBF. Balloon atrial septostomy remains an elective procedure in patients with adequate oxygen delivery. Many practitioners find it helpful to perform a balloon atrial septostomy—even in the stable patient on prostaglandin—so that $PGE_1$ can be discontinued and surgery can take place on a more elective basis.

Even after performance of corrective maneuvers as described, some patients remain hypoxemic despite an open ductus, an adequate-size atrial communication, and hyperventilation. In these patients, it is important to emphasize that a large proportion of SBF is the *recirculated* systemic venous return. In the presence of poor mixing, significant improvements in oxygen delivery can be achieved by increasing the mixed venous oxygen saturation, which is the major determinant of systemic arterial oxygen saturation. Maneuvers include decreasing oxygen consumption (with muscle relaxants, sedation, or mechanical ventilation) and improving oxygen delivery (by increasing cardiac output with inotropic agents or increasing oxygen-carrying capacity by treating anemia). Coexisting causes of pulmonary venous desaturation (e.g., pneumothorax) should be identified and treated. Increasing the fraction of inspired oxygen to 100% will have little effect on the arterial $PO_2$, unless this serves to lower PVR and increases total PBF.

### Summary

Three mutually exclusive physiologic states, as detailed, may occur in neonates with CHD: shunt physiology, single-ventricle physiology, and transposition physiology. They can easily be distinguished and categorized by the relationship of the pulmonary artery and aortic oxygen saturations. In shunt physiology, and in the normal heart, the pulmonary artery oxygen saturation is *less than* the aortic oxygen saturation. In single-ventricle physiology, the pulmonary artery oxygen saturation is *equal to* the aortic oxygen saturation, and in transposition physiology, the pulmonary artery oxygen saturation is *greater than* the aortic oxygen saturation.

## BASIC PRINCIPLES OF CARDIAC SURGERY

Surgery for congenital heart disease encompasses a broad variety of procedures specifically tailored to each disease process. Some can be accomplished through relatively simple surgical manipulations such as with ligation of a patent ductus arteriosus. However, other malformations require highly invasive procedures with complex modes of physiologic support. A balance must be drawn between appropriate anatomic repair and the child's physiologic condition at the time of surgery. In contemporary practice, one usually proceeds toward complete repair of an anatomic defect, even as early as the immediate neonatal period. However, staged repair is occasionally employed for children in marginal physiologic condition or those with lesions for which a staged operative approach is by now standard, for example, for various forms of single ventricle.

The term *closed procedures* refers to those surgical procedures in which the heart is not opened, and more commonly in which cardiopulmonary bypass is not used. Surgical repairs that can be performed via a closed procedure commonly include ligation of patent ductus arteriosus, repair of juxaductal aortic coarctation, pulmonary artery banding, and a variety of systemic-to-pulmonary artery shunt procedures. In general, *"open" procedures* require the use of cardiopulmonary bypass. This modality allows complete cardiopulmonary support of the patient while isolating the heart for repair. Closure of intracardiac defects and/or repair of great vessel abnormalities usually requires the use of cardiopulmonary bypass to provide adequate intracardiac exposure while maintaining support of other organs. Deep hypothermic circulatory arrest (DHCA) is a mode of protection that temporarily interrupts all organ perfusion. This is occasionally necessary because of either patient size or the need to reconstruct the aortic arch. With increasing frequency, centers are using selective cerebral perfusion, such that DHCA is not strictly necessary. However, at present, an advantage of selected perfusion over circulatory arrest, or vice versa, has not been identified.

For most open procedures, the surgical incision consists of a full, vertical midline sternotomy between the sternal notch and xiphoid process. Dissection is carried down to the sternum, which is opened with either a sternal saw or an electric cautery. A sternal retractor is placed, and the thymus typically is removed in its entirety, enhancing visualization of great vessels. It is important on removal of the thymus to avoid injury to the phrenic nerves, which are tethered near the pleural reflections. The pericardium is opened in a vertical fashion and suspended. It is important at this point to pause and perform an examination of the mediastinal contents. Despite the accuracy of modern imaging techniques, the surgeon occasionally may be surprised by the presence of additional abnormalities. In particular, the unexpected presence of a left superior vena cava can considerably alter the operative and/or cannulation strategy.

The type of cannulation performed depends entirely on the type of procedure to be performed (Fig. 57–3). The principle is to remove blood from the venous system, oxygenate the blood in the bypass machine, and replace

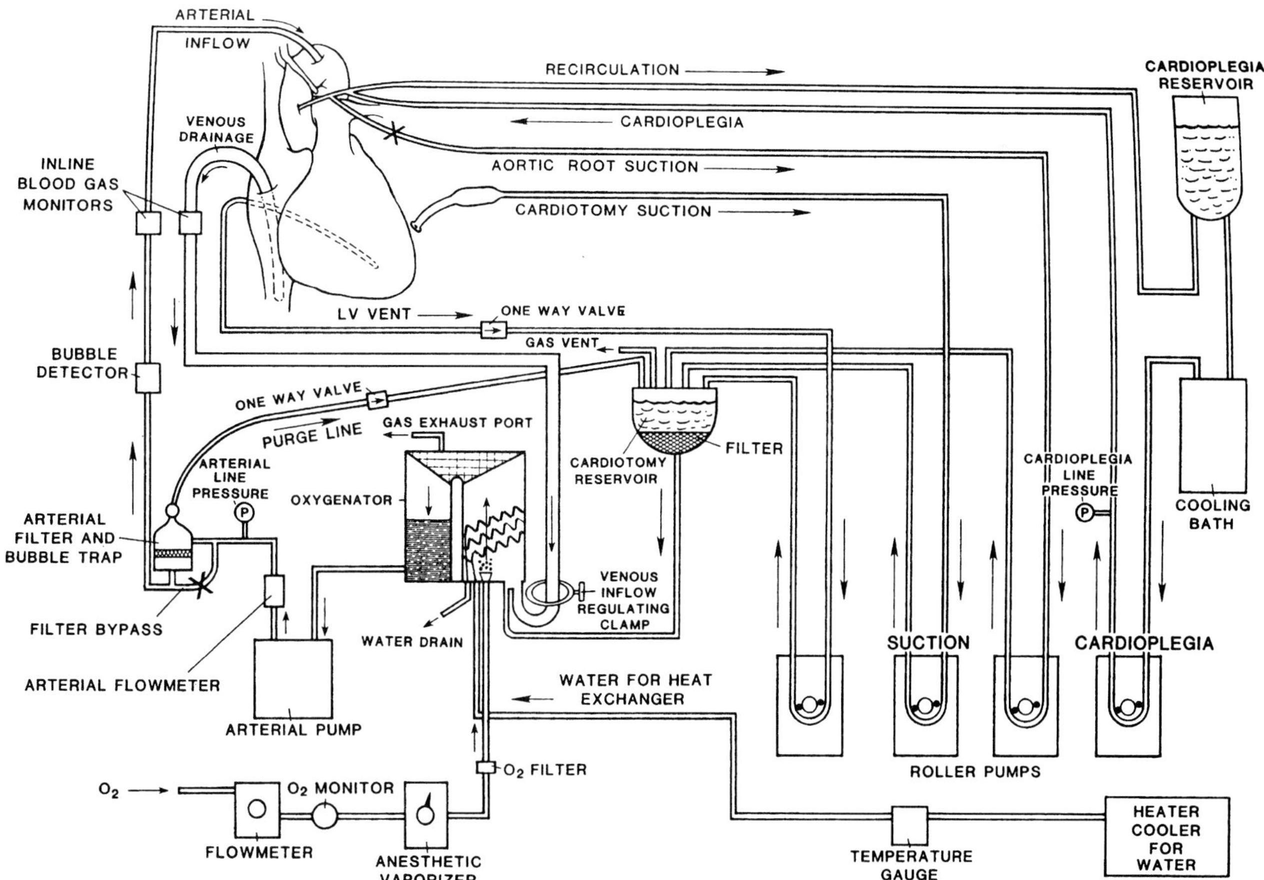


**FIGURE 57–3.** Cardiopulmonary bypass circuit. See text for details. *(From Gravlee GP, Davis RF, Kurusz M, et al: Cardiopulmonary Bypass: Principles and Practice. Baltimore, Lippincott Williams & Wilkins, 2002.)*

the blood into the arterial system. Generally, venous cannulation is performed in one of two ways. Either a single cannula is placed into the right atrial appendage for common atrial drainage, or the superior and the inferior venae cavae are cannulated separately, providing intracardiac isolation. This decision is determined by the need to visualize the inside of the heart or by whether DHCA will be performed. If DHCA is to be used, the cannulae will eventually be removed. Thus, a single atrial cannula is utilized. If bypass is to be continued, however (as in a majority of cases), bicaval cannulation is easily performed. This allows isolation of venous drainage from both the upper and the lower portions of the body, providing a bloodless intracardiac operative field. Arterial cannulation usually is performed in the ascending aorta near the base of the innominate artery. In newborns with a small ascending aorta and/or systemic perfusion maintained through the ductus arteriosus, arterial cannulation is performed through the pulmonary root. with systemic perfusion being maintained through a systemic-to-pulmonary communication, usually a ductus arteriosus.

Heparinization is a critical component of cardiopulmonary bypass. The profoundly procoagulant nature of the bypass circuit requires the use of an anticoagulant. Development of an effective and reversible method to prevent blood clotting began in 1916 with accidental discovery of heparin by a medical student. Twenty years of purification, characterization, and trials resulted in its routine incorporation into regimens requiring an anticoagulant. Although heparin's endogenous physiologic role is not clear, its ability to antagonize antithrombin III, thrombin, and other factors allow its routine use for anticoagulation during cardiopulmonary bypass. There is considerable variability in patient response to heparin; therefore, intraoperative dosing is dependent on on the activated clotting time (ACT). In general, ACT of greater than 300 seconds is required before the safe initiation of cardiopulmonary bypass. Intravenous heparin has a number of side effects including serotonin release, platelet release, rare instances of pulmonary edema, heparin-induced thrombocytopenia, and anaphylaxis. ACT is intermittently monitored during the procedure with heparin redosing to ensure appropriate anticoagulation during the procedure. Neutralization of heparin at the completion of cardiopulmonary bypass commonly is performed with administered protamine, a polyanionic protein derived from salmon sperm. Heparin binds to protamine to produce a stable precipitate, thus neutralizing its anticoagulant effect; reversal usually is prompt and complete. Adverse responses to protamine are rare but include severe pulmonary vasoconstriction.

A basic principle of cardiopulmonary bypass management is to minimize the patient's response to a controlled state of shock. Protection of the heart occurs primarily through two mechanisms: unloading the heart to reduce work and cooling to reduce metabolic rate. The vast majority of energy saved is due to arrest of the heart. Hypothermia reduces the metabolic rate and oxygen consumption approximately 5% per degree Celsius. Most procedures utilizing cardiopulmonary bypass and cardiac arrest are performed between 28° and 32° C. However, in those employing DHCA the body is cooled to a temperature of 16° to 18° C. With increasing frequency, studies are identifying a variety of adverse short- and long-term neurologic effects of cardiopulmonary bypass. DHCA "safe" times are dependent on patient temperature. Arrest times of 10 to 15 minutes can be obtained with moderate hypothermia to 28° C, while arrest times of 45 minutes can generally be obtained safely with patient temperatures of approximately 18° C (Wypij et al, 2003). Cooling to below a temperature of 14° C results in irreversible pulmonary injury.

Myocardial protection is enhanced by cardioplegia, in which a solution is delivered to the heart that results in (1) mechanical arrest, (2) cooling, and (3) metabolic replenishment. Cardioplegia strategies are institutionally based, with good data to support the use of both crystalloid-based and blood-based cardioplegic solutions. In general the simplest, most reproducible procedure is best. The cardioplegic solution usually is injected into the aortic root after the aorta is cross-clamped proximal to the aortic cannula. The clamp separates the heart from warm blood and allows antegrade instillation of cold cardioplegic solution into the coronary arteries. Although this method is adequate in the vast majority of cases, in other cases in which the patient has an incompetent aortic valve or stenotic proximal coronary arteries, alternative methods of cardioplegia delivery are required. Instillation of the solution can be done either in retrograde fashion through the coronary sinus or via direct cannulation of the coronary orifices. In general, a streamlined, reproducible system is usually the best route.

Myocardial injury during cardiopulmonary bypass is due to a number of factors, but it is largely on reperfusion that injury begins. Oxygen radicals are produced through a number of mechanisms including lipid peroxidation, oxidation of catecholamines, and xanthine oxidase pathways. However, the major source is through superoxide and hydrogen peroxide production by activated neutrophils. These neutrophils are stimulated by the complement cascade among other signals, which in turn is activated by the cardiopulmonary bypass circuit. Modulation of these oxygen radicals has been an area of intense investigation since the late 1980s, with disappointingly little progress. Manifestations of reperfusion injury include arrhythmia, myocardial dysfunction, cardiac necrosis, capillary leak, and nitric oxide–mediated endothelial dysfunction.

The neonatal heart differs considerably from that of the older child and adult with respect to the response to myocardial protection with cardioplegia. In general, the young heart has a denser structure than the adult heart, resulting in a less compliant myocardium with less preload reserve. Additionally, the immature heart relies more heavily on active glucose metabolism than on fatty acid metabolism. Calcium stores also are less, resulting in a relative protection during ischemia and reperfusion. Many children with CHD have chronic hypoxemia, which mitigates the recovery of systolic and diastolic function after a period of ischemic arrest and reperfusion. Volume loads associated with intracardiac shunts may progress to the point of hypertrophy or dilation and compromise ventricular function, posing additional stresses. The presence of systemic-pulmonary collaterals in some children with CHD complicates myocardial protection, with warming and "washout" of the initial cardioplegic solution. A combination of strategies such as hypothermia or reinstillation of cardioplegic solution can alleviate this difficulty.

Cardiopulmonary bypass can have profound effects on other organ systems. Striking morphologic changes in the lung are noted following cardiopulmonary bypass, including intra-alveolar edema and hemorrhagic atelectasis. Mechanical alterations such as atelectasis, diaphragmatic cooling, and airway compression are controlled by anesthetic attention. Microemboli, an inflammatory response, and lung hypoxia all contribute to decrease gas transfer and to alter mechanical properties. Use of blood filtration and membrane oxygenators and careful management of pulmonary vascular distention have helped to reduce the severity of acute lung injury. The use of adjunctive pharmacologic strategies has not resulted in a significant improvement.

Abnormalities in renal function following cardiopulmonary bypass are common, with severe renal failure occurring in up to 5% of all children following cardiac surgery. Multiple studies suggest that creatinine clearance is reduced following cardiopulmonary bypass (Dittrich et al, 2002; Hoffman et al, 2003). Although most of these children recover renal function, some require dialysis or other forms of renal replacement therapy. Among the factors contributing to perioperative renal dysfunction are diminished renal blood flow, nephrotoxic drugs, and hypothermia, especially in combination with hemoconcentration. Hemodilution is one of the most important factors in protecting renal function during cardiopulmonary bypass through its ability to increase renal plasma flow. As in other organ systems, microemboli have the capacity to impede renal function.

Metabolic and splanchnic visceral effects of cardiopulmonary bypass also follow the concepts outlined for other organ systems. Microemboli, hypercalcemia, metabolic substrate loss, and hypoperfusion contribute to visceral malfunction. Although these alterations are largely invisible at the time of surgery, they may become major complicating factors in the early postoperative period.

The neurologic effects of cardiopulmonary bypass have been the focus of significant interest over the last decade or more and are discussed in detail in Chapter 60. Much of the available data are from studies in adults with multiple comorbid conditions, making comparisons with newborn cardiopulmonary bypass difficult. Severe CNS damage secondary to stroke has a low (1% to 5%) but constant incidence following cardiac surgery. In adults, subtle CNS damage was overlooked for a number of years before more sensitive neuropsychological assessment offered a method for detecting subtle changes. These changes may become apparent only during more detailed and serial testing; with use of these methods, greater than 30% of adult patients are demonstrated to have neuropsychological defects a month or later following cardiac surgery. Current data from longitudinal studies following newborn cardiac surgery, reveal that, in general, most school-age survivors have cognitive abilities within the normal range, but nonverbal learning disabilities, attention-deficit hyperactivity disorder, and speech and language delays are common.

## PRINCIPLES OF POSTOPERATIVE CARE

### The Systematic Approach to the Patient

The heterogeneous nature of CHD, combined with the significant interpatient variability in the responses to anesthesia, surgery, and cardiopulmonary bypass, requires that a systematic but individualized approach be used for each patient. Because each patient is slightly different, we discourage "protocol" management in the strictest sense; however, a number of general principles should be followed in all children, especially the neonate. These principles include a constant evaluation of the surgical repair (including potential anatomic, electrophysiologic, and hemodynamic sequelae), the necessary inotropic support and afterload reduction necessary to maintain hemodynamic homeostasis, optimization of mechanical ventilation to reduce pulmonary trauma or hemodynamic impairment, analgesia and sedation, nutritional support, screening for infection, and assessment of secondary organ dysfunction.

### Assessment of the Repair

Perhaps the most important principle of postoperative care is that if the clinical or laboratory findings are at odds with the expected course of recovery, the care team should suspect a problem with either an inaccurate (or incomplete) diagnosis or an imperfect repair. All too often, appropriate interventions for significant residual anatomic defects are delayed as caregivers treat nonspecific states such as "low cardiac output syndrome," "pulmonary hypertension," or "sepsis."

With the advent of portable echocardiography and sophisticated bedside and intracardiac monitoring, frequent, minimally invasive assessment of the repair is possible at the bedside. A checklist should be developed for each repair, reviewing the planned surgical procedure and assessing for possible anatomic or electrophysiologic residual problems. Such problems generally fall into four broad categories: residual shunts, valvular regurgitation, residual obstruction to SBF or PBF, and arrhythmias. Shortly after arrival of the infant in the intensive care unit, the postoperative team should have ascertained, in detail, the preexisting anatomic defect, the surgical procedure used in the operating room, and the results of intraoperative studies such as hemodynamic measurements or echocardiography.

### Monitoring

Accurate measurement of systemic and pulmonary artery pressures, ventricular filling pressures, urine output, alveolar gas exchange, cardiac output, SVR, and PVR allows for precise pharmacologic and ventilatory support in the perioperative period. The neonate in particular demonstrates wide swings in physiologic variables such as heart rate, temperature, glucose metabolism, SVR, and PVR, compared with those in adults, and frequently requires *more* physiologic monitoring, not less, despite the small size of the patient. Use of a variety of invasive catheters has become the mainstay of postoperative care. Invasive monitoring catheters have two general functions: (1) assessment of the surgical repair and (2) ongoing assessment of hemodynamics. However, although these catheters are generally safe (Gold et al, 1986), they are associated with a number of risks, and their use should be determined on an individual basis.

In general, most patients are monitored in the perioperative period using arterial and urinary catheters, electrocardiographic monitoring, pulse oximetry, and intracardiac monitoring catheters. Following surgery, one to three right atrial (RA) catheters typically are placed through the RA appendage (frequently in the site used for venous cannulation on cardiopulmonary bypass), and a left atrial (LA) catheter may be placed into the right superior pulmonary vein or LA appendage. If necessary (see later), a pulmonary artery catheter is inserted through a pursestring suture in the right ventricular outflow tract, and possibly a single-lumen pressure catheter or a double-lumen catheter with a thermistor for measurement of cardiac output and core temperature.

RA catheters are used to assess the central venous pressure and for measurement of RA oxygen saturation. The RA saturation may not truly reflect the "mixed venous" saturation if the tip of the catheter is close to the renal vein flow (when it will be falsely high) or coronary sinus ostium or hepatic venous flow (when it will be falsely low); x-ray confirmation of tip position is important in correctly interpreting the data. Saline contrast injections through the RA catheter during echocardiography may detect right-to-left intracardiac shunting. RA catheters may be used for delivery of vasoactive and inotropic medications and also may be used for parenteral nutrition. This is particularly important in the low-birth-weight neonate, in whom nutritional reserve is minimal and in whom full caloric enteral feedings may be weeks away from surgery.

LA catheters provide indirect data on the function of the systemic ventricle and may be used for contrast (saline) injections during echocardiography to detect residual left-to-right shunts. Inspection of the pressure tracing allows assessment of the function of the systemic AV valve and may be helpful in distinguishing among various arrhythmias with loss of AV synchrony. The LA catheter is usually removed on the first or second postoperative day; RA catheters may be left in place for up to 2 weeks (or longer) if necessary. Complications with use of these catheters (occurring in approximately 1% in the pediatric population) include bleeding, entrapment, fragmentation, vessel perforation, transient arrhythmias, and infection (Gold et al, 1986)

Continuous monitoring of pulmonary artery pressure is helpful in a small number of patients at risk for reactive pulmonary hypertension following surgical repair of certain congenital lesions (e.g., truncus arteriosus, AV canal, obstructed total anomalous pulmonary venous connection, mitral stenosis). Use of a pulmonary artery catheter also allows for continuous assessment of the effects of respiratory and pharmacologic manipulations on the pulmonary vascular bed.

Continuous monitoring of intra-arterial systemic pressure is routinely employed. Blood pressure measurements by cuff and auscultation are unreliable in an unstable child, and automated Doppler techniques lack accuracy and reliability during low-flow states. Arterial catheters allow for beat-to-beat analysis of the arterial waveform, which can provide insight into specific disease states such as cardiac tamponade (narrow pulse pressure with pulsus paradoxicus) or a large run-off lesion such as a Blalock-Taussig shunt or aortic regurgitation (widened pulse pressure). Pronounced phasic variations in a patient receiving positive pressure ventilation, coupled with low atrial pressures, are typical for significant hypovolemia. The umbilical artery is the most frequently used site for arterial access in neonates.

### Other Monitoring

Continuous monitoring of the heart rate and QRS morphology is standard practice in most intensive care units. Indwelling urinary (Foley) catheters are useful for continuous, hourly assessment of urine output. Transcutaneous oxygen saturation monitors aid in the management of any patient with unstable respiratory status or labile PVR with intracardiac shunting. These monitors are particularly useful in cases in which parallel pulmonary and systemic circulations are supplied by a single ventricle, because variations in SVR and PVR may occur rapidly, with resulting changes in arterial saturation. Also, alterations in arterial oxygen saturation due to pneumothorax, unrecognized extubation, or ventilator failure are rapidly identified. Failure to obtain an adequate signal may be a sign of inadequate peripheral perfusion. Continuous monitoring of the mixed venous oxygen saturation by means of intravascular catheters specifically designed for this use (Oximetric, Abbott Laboratories, Chicago, IL) has been used with increasing frequency, especially in neonates with single ventricle. Finally, there is growing experience with intra-arterial sensors that provide continuous, real time assessment of blood gas data, temperature, and indices of base deficit (Neotrend, Diametrics Corporation, St. Paul, MN), even in low-birth-weight babies. These types of catheters are particularly beneficial in the postoperative low-birth-weight cardiac patient, who requires frequent laboratory assessments but has a more limited blood volume (see Chapter 59).

Temporary epicardial pacing wires are typically placed on the anterior surface of the right ventricle and, with increasing frequency, on that of the right atrium as well. Atrial wires may be used to increase heart rate (in the presence of sinus node dysfunction) while still allowing the ventricles to contract through the AV node and the normal His-Purkinje system. Rapid atrial pacing, occasionally with interposed premature beats, is very effective in converting many types of supraventricular tachycardia to normal sinus rhythm at the bedside, without the need for synchronized direct current (DC) cardioversion. In addition to the therapeutic uses, epicardial atrial wires may be used to record both unipolar and bipolar atrial electrograms for diagnostic purposes. Epicardial ventricular wires are useful in cases of AV node disease (complete heart block), although cardiac output may not be as effective when the ventricles contract dysynchronously (i.e., with the right ventricle contracting before contraction of the left ventricle, rather than through the His-Purkinje system) and without AV synchrony. Dual-chamber pacing is particularly useful in cases of complete heart block. In patients at risk for complete heart block, the temporary wires should be checked for threshold and sensitivity after arrival in the intensive care unit, and a temporary pacemaker should be at the bedside.

### The First 24 Hours after Cardiopulmonary Bypass

The first night after surgery utilizing cardiopulmonary bypass is a period of potentially significant hemodynamic lability. Compared with older children, the neonate is at particular risk because of limited myocardial and pulmonary reserve, immature organ systems, a more severe postoperative (dilutional) coagulopathy and an increased propensity for nosocomial complications of infection, vascular compromise, and central nervous system (CNS) injury. Multiple studies have shown a predictable and reproducible decrease in cardiac output (Hesz and Clark, 1988; Hoffman et al, 2003; Pesonen et al, 1999), thyroid function (Bettendorf et al, 2000), pulmonary function (Nagashima et al, 2000), and renal function (Hoffman et al, 2003), accompanied by increases in PVR and SVR (Hesz and Clark, 1988), complement activation, troponin (Hauser et al, 2001) and endothelin release, and capillary leak resulting in tissue edema and organ dysfunction. These abnormalities peak nearly simultaneously between 6 and 18 hours after surgery, which makes the neonate most vulnerable in the middle of the first night following surgery. In view of this predictable scenario, proactive steps can be taken to minimize the potential risk, including the routine use of inotropic support and afterload reduction (Hoffman et al, 2003; Tweddell et al, 1999), intermittent or continuous neuromuscular blockade, and analgesia, and minimization of stressful procedures during the most at-risk period (such as bathing, suctioning, and handling). It is emphasized, however, that this period of vulnerability is self-limited, and in most neonates, support can be rapidly weaned and discontinued within 24 hours or so of surgery, especially invasive monitoring and mechanical ventilation. A prolonged "weaning" strategy is typically not necessary on physiologic grounds, and longer periods of intensive care, invasive monitoring, and mechanical ventilation expose the neonate to potential nosocomial complications and infections. In the neonate with no other organ dysfunction except the transient effects from the surgical procedure and cardiopulmonary bypass, this "de-intensification" may usually be accomplished with a day or so of surgery. A slightly longer period of mechanical ventilation may be beneficial in neonates with more significant capillary leak and chest wall edema, until adequate diuresis is achieved.

## CONGENITAL LESIONS WITH A PREDOMINANT LEFT-TO-RIGHT SHUNT

### Ventricular Septal Defect

VSD is the most common form of CHD, occurring in isolation in 1/280 live births, and is a common component of more complex lesions discussed elsewhere in this chapter (e.g., tetralogy of Fallot, truncus arteriosus, interrupted aortic arch). VSDs may occur anywhere in the ventricular septum and usually are classified by their location (Fig. 57–4). Defects in the membranous septum are the most common type. The diagnosis of VSD usually is initially suspected on the basis of findings on physical examination of the infant: A harsh murmur develops as PVR falls and a pressure gradient develops across the defect. Echocardiography confirms the diagnosis and localizes the defect in the ventricular septum

VSD is the most common cause of CHF beyond the initial neonatal period. Moderate to large VSDs become hemodynamically significant in the first 4 to 6 weeks of life as the PVR decreases and PBF increases as a result of a left-to-right shunt across the defect. In neonates with an isolated VSD, even if large, development of symptoms of CHF is unusual, as PVR remains modestly elevated and the degree of left-to-right shunting generally is well tolerated. If CHF is present in a neonate with a VSD, additional investigations are indicated to rule out coexisting anatomic abnormalities, such as left ventricular outflow tract obstruction, coarctation of the aorta, or patent ductus arteriosus. (In premature infants, who have a lower initial PVR, clinical symptoms of heart failure may develop earlier and duration of necessary mechanical ventilation may be longer than in term infants with the same-size defect.)

Only a minority of all patients with isolated VSDs ever become clinically symptomatic. Medical management of CHF includes digoxin, diuretics, afterload reduction (typically with an angiotensin-converting enzyme inhibitor), and caloric supplementation. Growth failure is the most common symptom of CHF not fully compensated by medical management. When it occurs, failure to thrive is an indication for surgical repair of the defect, rather than prolonged medical management.

#### *Spontaneous Closure of Ventricular Septal Defect*

Depending on the anatomic location, a large number of VSDs may undergo spontaneous closure in infancy and childhood. In particular, defects in the membranous septum (see Fig. 57–4B) may become smaller or even close completely as a result of overlying tissue from the septal leaflet of the tricuspid valve. Defects in the muscular septum (see Fig. 57–4D) also may become smaller with time. Because a large number of VSDs (as many as 50% of such defects, depending on the anatomic type) may close spontaneously in infancy, and symptoms are rare in the first month of life, surgery—if necessary—usually is deferred beyond the neonatal period. As a general guideline, defects that are less than half the size of the aortic valve in the membranous or muscular septum generally are followed conservatively through infancy, as partial or complete closure is likely, and surgery can be avoided in many cases. However, malalignment defects (such as seen in tetralogy of Fallot or interrupted aortic arch), or defects in the inlet (or AV canal) portion (see Fig. 57–4C) of the ventricular septum *never* close spontaneously, and if this diagnosis is made in the neonatal period, surgery will be

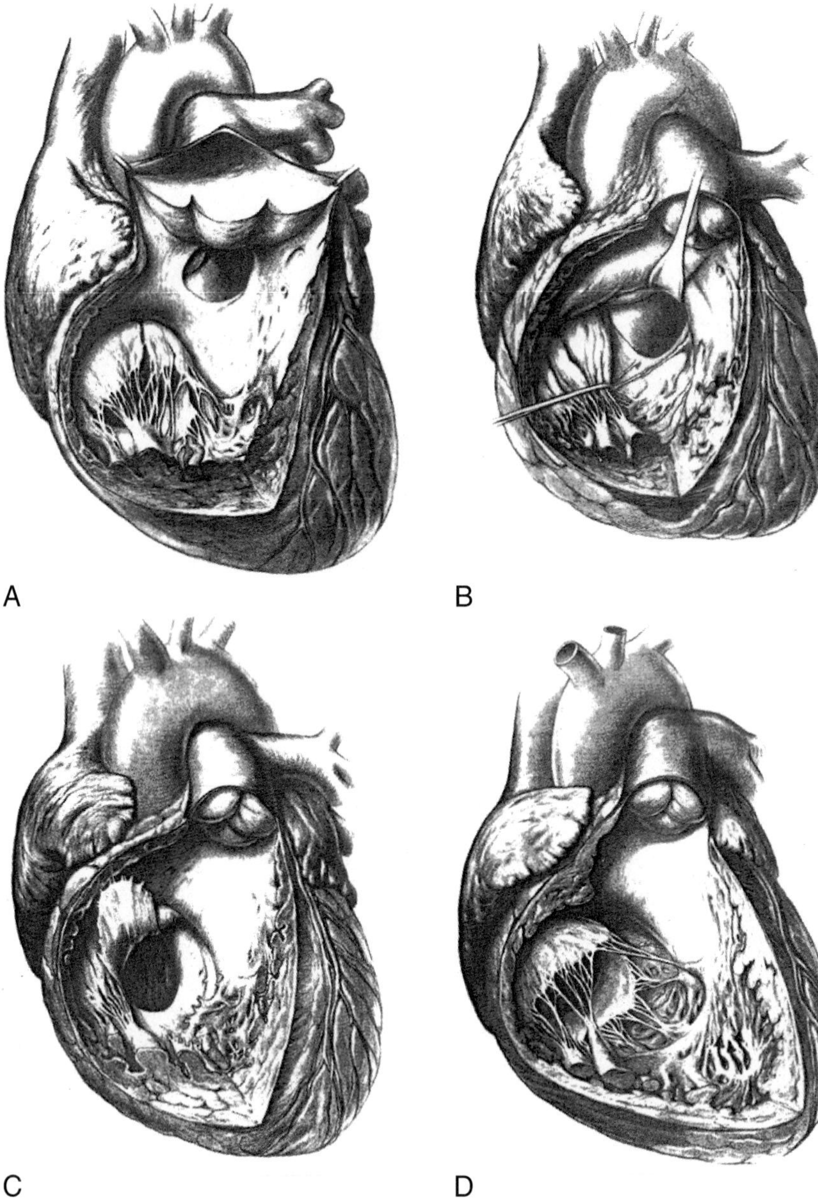

A

B

C

D

**FIGURE 57–4.** Anatomic varieties of ventricular septal defect: **A,** subpulmonary defect; **B,** membranous defect; **C,** inlet (atrioventricular canal type) defect; **D,** apical muscular defects. *(From Mavroudis C, Backer CL: Pediatric Cardiac Surgery. St. Louis, Mosby–Year Book, 1994.)*

inevitable. The timing of surgery will be determined by the clinical status of the patient. Finally, defects in the infundibular septum ("subpulmonary" defects; see Fig. 57–4A) may undergo spontaneous "closure," although this is usually due to prolapse of one of the cusps of the aortic valve, leading to aortic insufficiency. Therefore, surgery frequently is recommended in early childhood for children with a subpulmonary VSD and signs of aortic valve prolapse with aortic regurgitation.

### *Surgical Closure of Ventricular Septal Defect*

Surgical closure of VSDs is done utilizing cardiopulmonary bypass; the surgical exposure is dictated by the location of the VSD and the presence of associated defects. In most cases, the VSD can be repaired by performing an atriotomy and closing the defect through the tricuspid valve. VSDs located under the pulmonary valve (e.g., "supracristal" VSDs, subpulmonary VSDs) may be closed via a small pulmonary arteriotomy, with the operator working through the pulmonary valve. Occasionally, a ventriculotomy is necessary to gain adequate exposure to the VSD, especially of the muscular variety.

Surgical mortality rate for isolated VSDs at present is approximately 1%. Postoperative morbidity includes junctional ectopic tachycardia, and bundle branch block; permanent complete heart block is rare. Residual VSDs are fairly common on intraoperative transesophageal echocardiography; these small VSDs, if less than 3 mm, rarely are hemodynamically significant, and reoperation rarely is required. Reoperation following VSD closure is uncommon; indications include pacemaker implantation (in approximately 1% of cases), residual VSD (in approximately 1%), or the late development of a subaortic membrane or aortic regurgitation (in less than 5%).

### Complete Common Atrioventricular Canal

Complete common AV canal (CAVC) occurs in nearly 1/5000 live births. Although there are many anatomic variations, the most common form consists of a combination of defects in the (1) endocardial portion of the atrial septum and (2) the inlet portion of the ventricular septum and (3) a common, single AV valve. In the immediate neonatal period, affected infants may present with mild cyanosis as a result of the large intracardiac communications and the relatively high PVR. If the defect is not detected in the neonatal period, however, these infants typically present early in infancy with CHF because of the large left-to-right shunt, which increases as the PVR falls; symptoms of CHF may be present earlier if there is associated regurgitation of the common AV valve. Patients with CAVC have a characteristic finding on the electrocardiogram (ECG) of a "superior axis," and the diagnosis can be made conclusively with echocardiography.

In the absence of associated right ventricular outflow tract obstruction, pulmonary artery pressures are at systemic levels, and pulmonary vascular resistance may remain elevated, particularly in patients with trisomy 21 (nearly 70% of infants with CAVC have trisomy 21). Given the high association of CAVC with trisomy 21, a careful evaluation of phenotype—including a possible karyotype—should be considered in patients with CAVC.

The great majority of patients with CAVC will require medical treatment for symptomatic CHF with digoxin and diuretics, though prolonged medical therapy in patients with failure to thrive and symptomatic heart failure is not warranted. Complete surgical repair is undertaken electively in 3 to 6 months, with earlier repair in symptomatic patients. In the "transitional" form of AV canal, the VSD component may be partially, or nearly completely, covered by AV valve tissue, resulting in less left-to-right shunting, lower pulmonary artery pressure, and minimal symptoms. In these patients, elective repair takes place in the asymptomatic patient in the first few years of life.

#### *Surgical Repair of Common Atrioventricular Canal*

Repair of CAVC is done utilizing cardiopulmonary bypass in all cases (Fig. 57–5). The atrial and ventricular defects are closed—with either one or two separate patches—and the AV valve is reconstructed and resuspended on the VSD portion of the patch. Surgical mortality rate is low (less than 5%) in general but is higher in cases with significant AV valve regurgitation or in those patients with associated lesions (Castañeda et al, 1994). Postoperative complications include arrhythmias (sinus node dysfunction, junctional ectopic tachycardia, complete heart block [occurring in approximately 1% of cases]), AV valve regurgitation, and subaortic obstruction. Reoperation for hemodynamically significant AV valve regurgitation may be necessary in 5% to 10% of patients; surgical options at that time include valvuloplasty and valve replacement.

### Truncus Arteriosus

Truncus arteriosus is a relatively rare form of CHD, occurring in 1/16,000 live births. Truncus arteriosus (Fig. 57–6) consists of a single great artery arising from the heart that gives rise to (in order) the coronary arteries, the pulmonary arteries, and the brachiocephalic arteries. The truncal valve is often anatomically abnormal (only 50% are tricuspid) and is frequently thickened, stenotic, and/or regurgitant. A coexisting VSD is present in greater than 98% of cases. The aortic arch is right sided in approximately a third of cases; other arch anomalies such as hypoplasia, coarctation, and interruption are seen in 10% of cases. Extracardiac anomalies are present in 20% to 40% of cases. Recently, microdeletion of chromosome 22 (22q11 deletion—DiGeorge syndrome, velocardial facial syndrome, and so on) has been noted in as many as a third of patients with truncus arteriosus

The overwhelming majority of infants with truncus arteriosus present with symptoms of CHF in the first weeks of life as PVR falls. The infants may be somewhat cyanotic, but CHF symptoms and signs usually are dominant. In contrast with VSD and CAVC, discussed earlier, CHF occurs earlier and may be more severe, possibly because of the direct connection of the pulmonary arteries to the aorta. In the absence of stenosis at the origins of the pulmonary arteries, the PBF is significantly increased, the pulse pressure is wide, and significant pulmonary hypertension is present. CHF may be more severe, or manifest even earlier, if there is significant stenosis and/or regurgitation of the truncal valve.

The natural history of truncus arteriosus is quite bleak. If the defect is left unrepaired, only 15% to 30% of affected infants survive the first year of life. Furthermore, among survivors of the immediate neonatal period, the occurrence of accelerated irreversible pulmonary vascular disease is common, making surgical repair in the neonatal period (or as soon as the diagnosis is made) the treatment of choice. "Medical management" of heart failure should be considered only a temporizing measure until surgical correction can be accomplished.

#### *Surgical Correction of Truncus Arteriosus*

Repair is performed utilizing cardiopulmonary bypass (see Fig. 57–6). For unclear reasons, neonates with truncus arteriosus seem to be particularly prone to ventricular fibrillation on opening of the sternum. The pulmonary arteries are removed from the common trunk, and the resultant defect in the aorta is closed either directly or with a patch. Care is taken to inspect and avoid the origin of the left coronary artery, which typically arises near the pulmonary arteries. A ventriculotomy is made to expose the VSD for closure, and to provide the location for the proximal placement of a right ventricle–to–pulmonary artery conduit. The distal end of the conduit, usually homograft, is anastomosed to the pulmonary bifurcation. Surgical mortality rate ranges from 10% to 15%, with increased risk present in older patients, those with abnormal truncal valves, DiGeorge syndrome, or associated obstruction of the aortic arch. Early postoperative complications include ventricular arrhythmias (in approximately

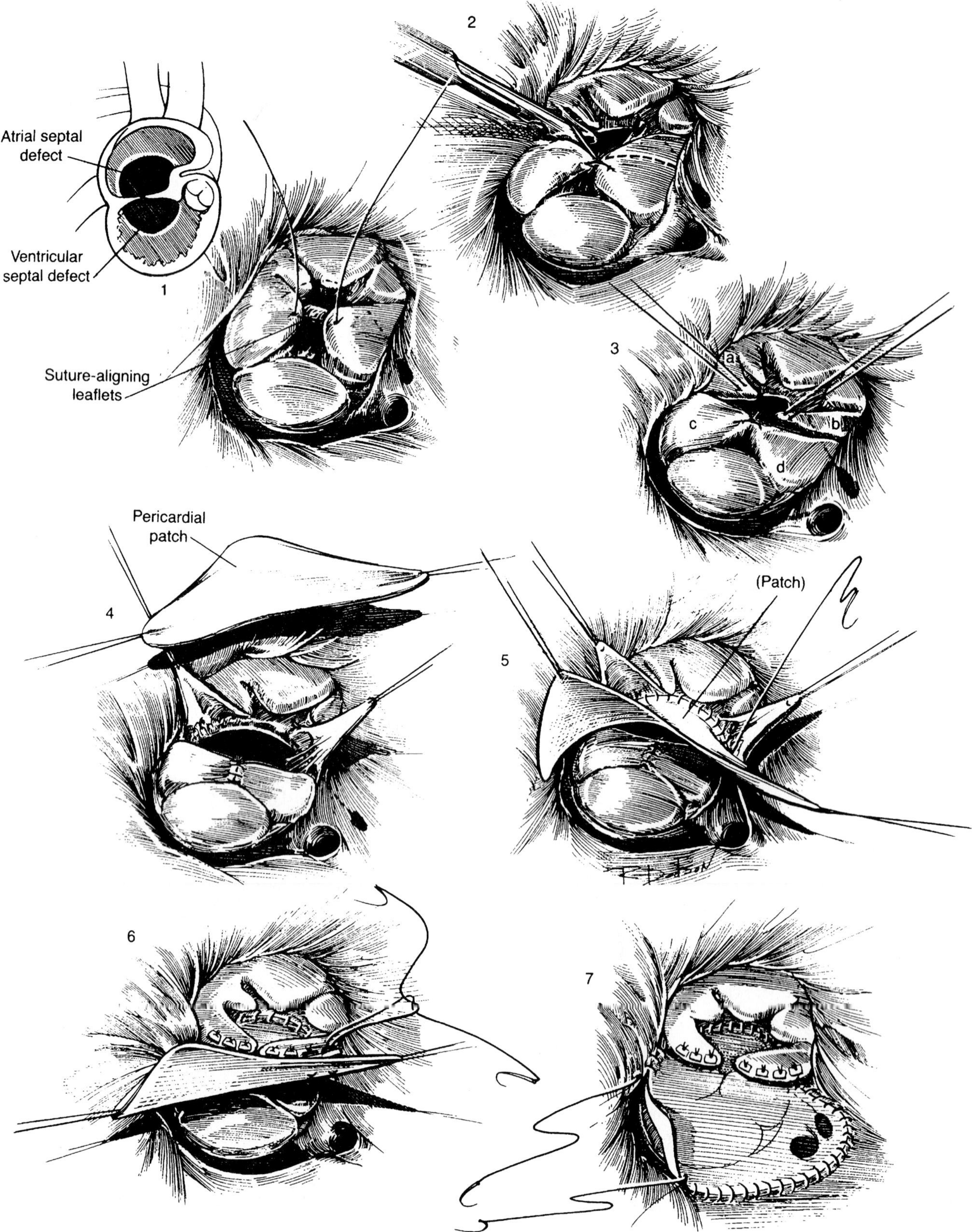


**FIGURE 57–5.** Anatomy and repair of complete common atrioventricular canal (CAVC) defect. Complete CAVC comprises both atrial and ventricular septal defects in addition to the common AV valve. Repair of this complex lesion through the right atrium entails creation of separate right and left AV valves (1 to 3), repair of the ventricular component of the defect (4 to 6), and closure of the atrial defect (6, 7). *(From Castañeda AR, Jonas RA, Mayer JE Jr, Hanley FL: Cardiac Surgery of the Neonate and Infant. Philadelphia, WB Saunders, 1994.)*

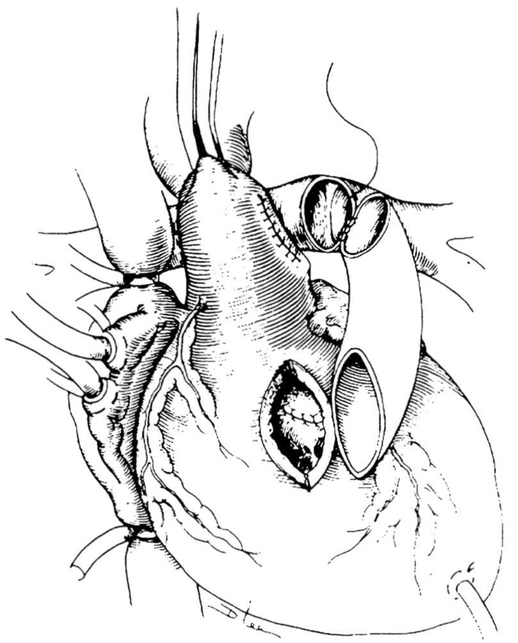

**FIGURE 57–6.** Anatomy and repair of truncus arteriosus. After the branch pulmonary arteries are removed from the common trunk (and the resulting aortic defect is closed), a ventriculotomy is performed. The ventricular septal defect is closed through this incision, and a conduit is placed from the right ventricle to the pulmonary arteries. *(From Behrendt DM, Dick M: Truncus repair with a valveless conduit in neonates. J Thorac Cardiovasc Surg 110:1148-1150, 1995).*

30% of cases), pulmonary hypertensive "crises," complete heart block (in 2% to 3%), conduit obstruction, and truncal ("neoaortic") valve stenosis and/or insufficiency. If the patient has 22q11 deletion, associated metabolic (hypocalcemia), infectious (immunodeficiency), feeding (palatal abnormalities and esophageal dysmotility), and CNS complications may occur as well. Late reoperations are necessary in nearly 100% of operative survivors, principally for conduit revision, but occasionally for neoaortic valve replacement.

### Atrial Septal Defect

ASDs are one of the more common types of CHD, occurring in 1/1000 live births and appearing in association with many other types of more complex CHD. Because the anatomic communication is at the atrial rather than the ventricular level, the fall in PVR has little initial effect on the degree of left-to-right shunting through the defect. The magnitude of left-to-right shunt is determined principally by the relative *compliance* of the two ventricles, rather than their afterload. As the normal newborn right ventricular hypertrophy regresses, typically in the first 3 to 6 months of life, there is a progressive left-to-right shunt at the atrial level. This left-to-right shunt only rarely causes symptoms of CHF, even if left unrepaired into adult life. If symptoms of CHF are present in patients with ASD, and/or there is a very large left-to-right shunt, presence of additional problems in the left side of the heart, such as mitral hypoplasia or stenosis or left ventricular hypoplasia, should be considered.

ASDs are characterized by their location in the atrial septum (Fig. 57–7). Secundum-type ASDs may spontaneously close in the first few years of life, and symptoms are rare; therefore, these defects generally are not surgically repaired before 2 to 3 years of age. Sinus venous defects (typically associated with anomalous right upper pulmonary venous return) and ostium primum defects do not undergo spontaneous closure, and surgical repair typically is electively performed in the first few years of life. The surgical mortality rate is quite low (less than 1%), and postoperative complications are uncommon. Arrhythmias may develop later in adult life.

## CONGENITAL LESIONS WITH DUCT-DEPENDENT SYSTEMIC BLOOD FLOW

Commonly referred to as *left-sided obstructive lesions*, congenital lesions with duct-dependent systemic blood flow constitute a group of defects involving hypoplasia of left-sided structures of the heart: critical aortic stenosis, isolated coarctation of the aorta, interruption of the aortic arch, and hypoplastic left heart syndrome (HLHS). These four lesions on the "left side" of the heart share the common presentation of CHF and or shock/circulatory collapse on closure or constriction of the ductus arteriosus. Of the four, critical aortic stenosis usually manifests shortly after birth, with signs of CHF, a gallop rhythm, murmur, and poor perfusion. In the other three left-sided lesions—coarctation of the aorta, interruption of the aortic arch, and HLHS—the most common clinical presentation is the following: A previously well newborn, frequently discharged as "healthy" from the term nursery, presents with poor feeding, poor pulses, tachycardia, perhaps an ashen appearance, or even full cardiac arrest in the first 1 to 2 weeks of life. In many ways, this presentation may mimic that in bacterial sepsis, but it is important to remember that bacterial sepsis in the full-term, noninstrumented newborn beyond the first 24 hours of life is a rare event, occurring in perhaps 1/3000 live births. In contrast, left-sided heart disease occurs in approximately 1/1000 live births, making the presentation of circulatory failure/shock in the first weeks of life three times more likely to be due to heart disease, rather than to sepsis, in the current era (Platt and O'Brien, 2003).

Although all infants with significant left-sided lesions and duct-dependent systemic blood flow require prostaglandin-maintained patency of the ductus arteriosus as part of the initial management, additional care varies somewhat with each lesion.

### Critical Aortic Stenosis

Morphologic abnormalities of the aortic valve may range from a bicuspid, nonobstructive functionally normal valve to a unicuspid, markedly deformed, and severely obstructive valve that greatly limits systemic cardiac output from the left ventricle. By convention, "critical" aortic stenosis is present if the systemic blood flow is dependent on patency of the ductus arteriosus, regardless of the measured

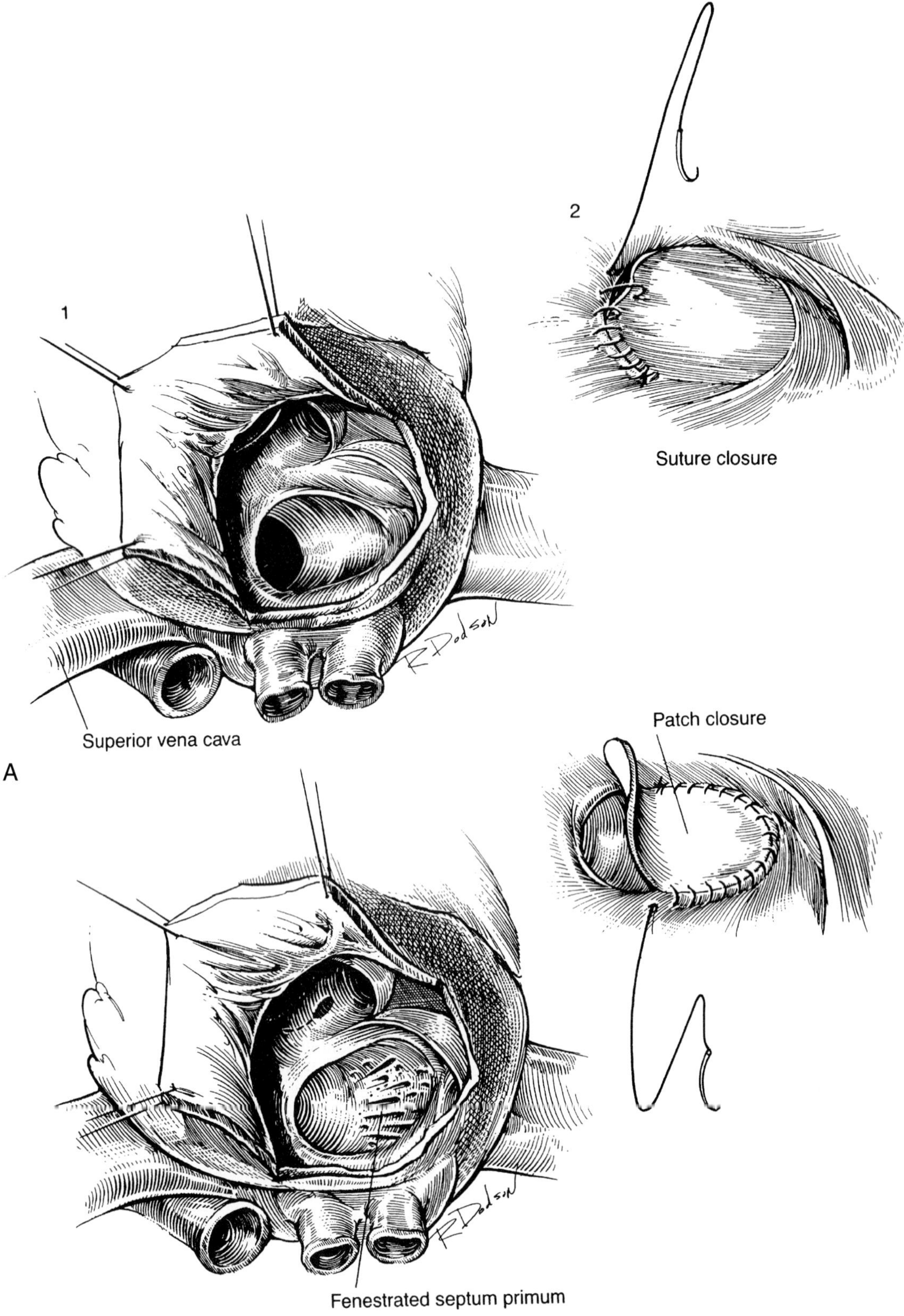


**FIGURE 57–7.** Anatomy and repair of atrial septal defects. **A,** Closure of a patent foramen ovale. **B,** Patch closure of ostium secundum atrial septal defect with fenestrated septum primum. *(From Castañeda AR, Jonas RA, Mayer JE Jr, Hanley FL: Cardiac Surgery of the Neonate and Infant. Philadelphia, WB Saunders, 1994.)*

gradient across the valve. Critical aortic stenosis results from severe anatomic obstruction with accompanying left ventricular failure and/or shock. Because of the severe left ventricular dysfunction, it is not uncommon for the output across the dysplastic aortic valve to be severely reduced. Because of the low-flow state, Doppler-measured gradients may be low—at times only 10 to 30 mm Hg—with this low value greatly underestimating the severity of the anatomic obstruction. In the presence of adequate left ventricular function, the degree of aortic stenosis is *severe* if the peak systolic gradient from left ventricle to ascending aorta is at least 60 mm Hg, *moderate* if the gradient is between 30 and 60 mm Hg, and *mild* if the gradient is less than 30 mm Hg.

Patients with critical aortic stenosis have severe obstruction present in utero (usually due to a unicuspid, plate-like valve) (Fig. 57–8), with resultant left ventricular hypertrophy and, frequently, endocardial fibroelastosis. Associated left-sided abnormalities such as mitral valve disease and coarctation are not uncommon. Following closure of the ductus, the left ventricle must supply all of the systemic cardiac output. In cases of severe myocardial dysfunction, clinical CHF or shock will become apparent.

Initial management of the severely affected infant includes treatment of shock, provision of stable vascular access, airway management and mechanical ventilation, sedation and muscle paralysis, inotropic support, and institution of $PGE_1$ therapy. Positive end-expiratory pressure is helpful to overcome pulmonary venous desaturation from pulmonary edema secondary to left atrial hypertension. For a patient with critical aortic stenosis to benefit from a $PGE_1$ infusion, however, there must be a small patent foramen ovale to allow "effective" SBF (pulmonary venous return) to cross the atrial septum and ultimately enter the systemic vascular bed through the ductus. If the atrial septum is severely restrictive or intact, there will be no way for pulmonary venous return to reach the tissues, and profound metabolic acidosis will result; even a $PGE_1$ infusion to ensure a patent ductus arteriosus will not suffice to stabilize the patient. In such cases, urgent balloon valvuloplasty, as well as a limited balloon atrial septostomy, may be necessary. Inspired oxygen should be limited to an $FIO_2$ of 50% to 60% unless severe hypoxemia is present.

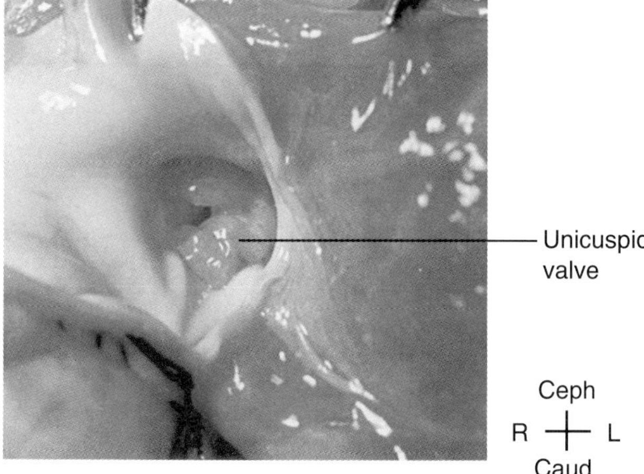


**FIGURE 57–8.** (See also Color Plate 57–8.) Congenital aortic stenosis. Frontal view through opened aorta demonstrates stenotic and dysmorphic aortic valve with commissural fusion. *(From Litwin SB: Color Atlas of Congenital Heart Surgery. St. Louis, Mosby, 1996.)*

Following anatomic definition of left ventricular size and of mitral valve and aortic arch anatomy by echocardiography, cardiac catheterization or surgery should be performed as soon as possible to accomplish aortic valvotomy. With either type of therapy, outcome will depend largely on (1) the degree of relief of the obstruction, (2) the degree of aortic regurgitation, (3) presence of associated cardiac lesions (especially left ventricular size), and (4) the severity of end-organ dysfunction secondary to the initial presentation (e.g., necrotizing enterocolitis, renal failure). The initial results from balloon valvuloplasty for critical aortic stenosis have been variable, mainly owing to the associated anatomic and physiologic variables rather than to technical aspects of the procedure. Some investigators have recently advocated a more radical surgical approach for the neonate with critical or severe aortic stenosis: a Ross procedure in the neonatal period (Ohye et al, 2001). In this surgical procedure, the diseased aortic valve is excised, typically with an annulus-enlarging procedure such as a Konno procedure; the patient's anatomic pulmonary valve is inserted in the aortic position; and a homograft is placed *in situ* in the pulmonary position (Fig. 57–9). Short-term results in well-selected patients have been acceptable, although long-term results of the anatomic pulmonary valve in the systemic position are currently unknown, and reoperation to replace the right-sided homograft is inevitable.

Critical aortic stenosis is a lifelong disease—all patients require lifelong follow-up and endocarditis prophylaxis. Restenosis or progressive regurgitation is common, and multiple procedures in childhood frequently are necessary.

### "Noncritical" Aortic Stenosis

Patients with less severe forms of aortic stenosis—namely, those in whom the ductus is not necessary for systemic perfusion and in whom left ventricular function is for the most part preserved—have a significantly better prognosis. Balloon valvuloplasty has become the procedure of choice and frequently is the only procedure necessary throughout infancy and childhood (Egito et al, 1997; Freedom et al, 2000; Rome, 1995).

### Coarctation of the Aorta

Coarctation of the aorta, present in approximately 1 in 2500 infants, is an anatomic narrowing of the descending aorta, most commonly at the site of insertion of the ductus arteriosus (i.e., "juxtaductal"). Additional cardiac abnormalities are common, including bicuspid aortic valve (which occurs in 80% of patients) and VSD (which occurs in 40% of patients). In addition, hypoplasia and obstruction of other left-sided structures including the mitral valve, the left ventricle, and the aortic valve are not uncommon and must be looked for during the initial echocardiographic evaluation.

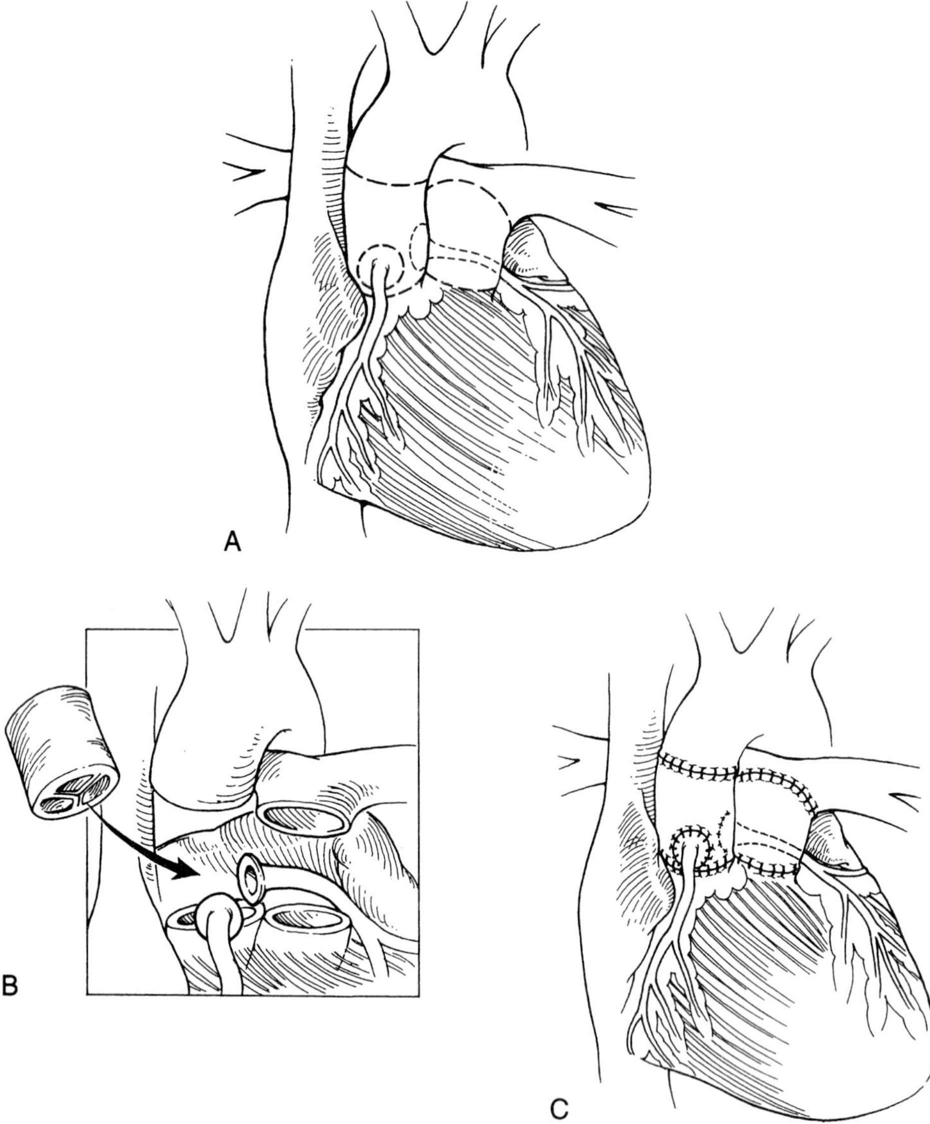


**FIGURE 57–9.** Ross procedure: "Autograft" aortic valve replacement. **A,** *Dotted lines* depict surgical incisions around coronary arteries, aorta, and pulmonary artery. **B,** The patient's native pulmonary valve ("autograft") is removed from the pulmonary position. Following removal of the coronary arteries from the diseased native aortic valve root, the aortic valve is removed and replaced by the autograft. **C,** Completed repair, with reimplanted coronary arteries. A cadaveric homograft valve is inserted in the pulmonary position in situ. *(From Chang AC, Burke RP: Left ventricular outflow tract obstruction. In Chang AC, Hanley FH, Wernovsky G, Wessel DL [eds]: Pediatric Cardiac Intensive Care. Baltimore, Williams & Wilkins, 1998, pp 233-256.)*

In utero, systemic blood flow to the lower body is via the patent ductus arteriosus. Following ductal closure, in the newborn with a critical coarctation, the left ventricle must suddenly generate adequate pressure and volume to pump the entire cardiac output past a significant point of obstruction. This sudden pressure load may be poorly tolerated by the neonatal myocardium, and the neonate may become rapidly and critically ill because of myocardial dysfunction and/or lower body hypoperfusion.

As in critical aortic stenosis, initial management of the severely affected infant includes treatment of shock, provision of stable vascular access, airway management and mechanical ventilation, moderate supplemental oxygen, sedation and muscle paralysis, inotropic support, and institution of $PGE_1$ therapy. Positive end-expiratory pressure is helpful to overcome pulmonary venous desaturation from pulmonary edema secondary to left atrial hypertension. In some infants, $PGE_1$ is unsuccessful in opening the ductus, and urgent surgical intervention is necessary after a brief period of resuscitation. In less severely affected newborns, especially those who are diagnosed before significant myocardial dysfunction or end-organ damage has occurred, low-dose inotropic support and a $PGE_1$ infusion may be all that is necessary until surgical intervention can be undertaken.

In symptomatic infants with coarctation, surgical repair is performed as soon as the child has been resuscitated and medically stabilized. Usually the procedure is performed through a left lateral thoracotomy incision. In most cases, the coarctation is resected, and the proximal and distal ends of the aorta are anastomosed to each other. The proximal incision may be extended on the underside of the aorta to manage areas of proximal hypoplasia ("extended end-to-end" anastomosis; Fig. 57–10). In infants with symptomatic coarctation and a large, coexisting VSD, consideration should be given to repair of both defects in the initial procedure via a median sternotomy. The surgical mortality rate for isolated coarctation repair is less than 5% and higher if additional defects are repaired simultaneously using cardiopulmonary bypass. Balloon dilation of native coarctation is not routinely done because of the high incidence of restenosis and aneurysm

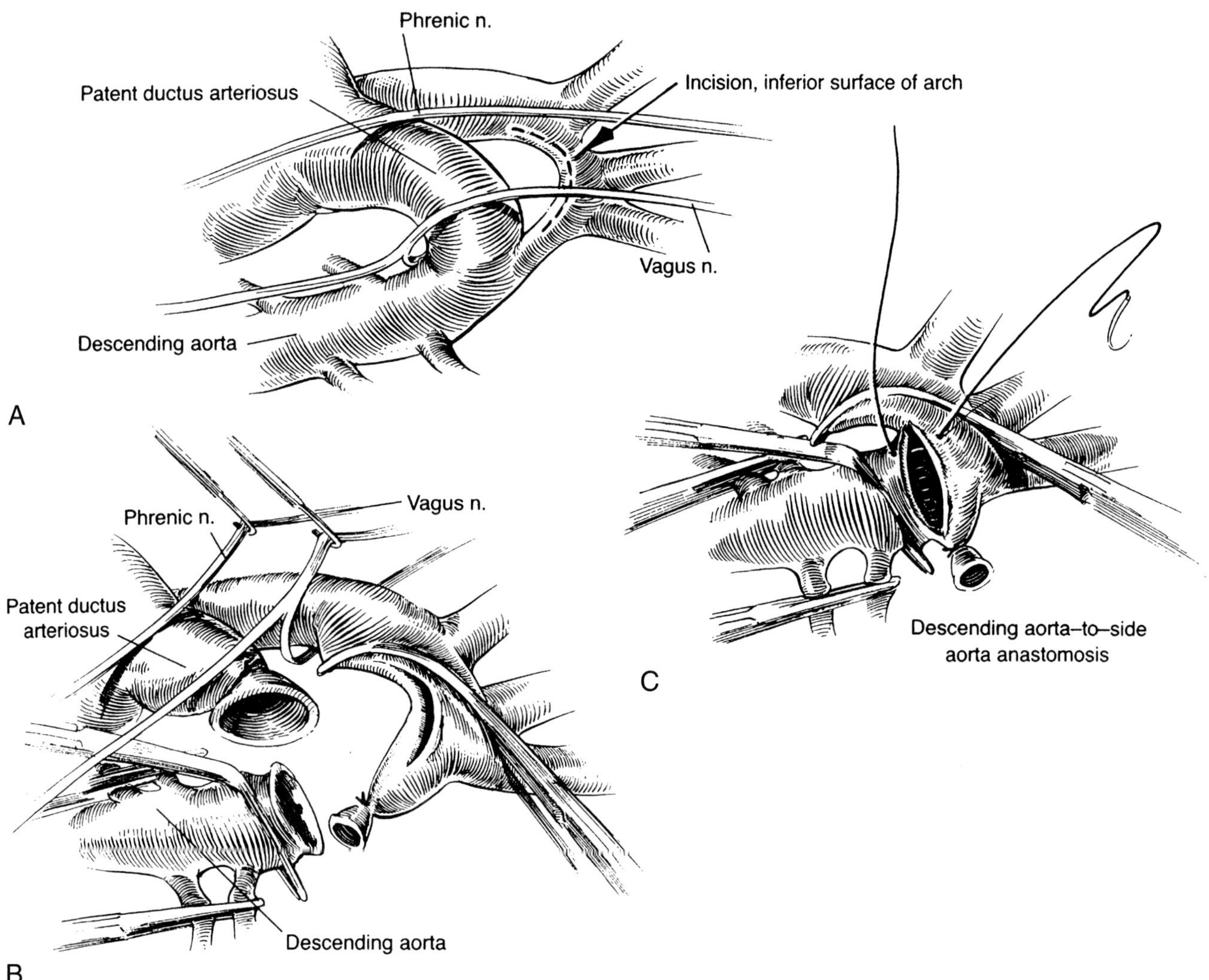


**FIGURE 57–10.** View through left lateral thoracotomy of the anatomy and repair of aortic coarctation. **A,** *Dotted line* depicts the surgical incision; important vascular and nerve landmarks are shown. **B,** The ductus arteriosus is divided and the proximal end is ligated. The coarctation segment and any residual ductal tissue in the descending aorta are resected. An incision in the undersurface of the transverse aortic arch is made. **C,** The descending aorta is brought superiorly and anastomosed to the undersurface of the aortic arch. *(From Castañeda AR, Jonas RA, Mayer JE Jr, Hanley FL: Cardiac Surgery of the Neonate and Infant. Philadelphia, WB Saunders, 1994.)*

formation, especially given the safe and effective surgical alternative.

Recoarctation occurs in 10% to 15% of children, especially if the repair is undertaken in the early newborn period (most likely due to the fact that early repair is necessary in the most severe forms of coarctation). Recoarctation is very effectively managed with balloon angioplasty.

## Interrupted Aortic Arch

Interrupted aortic arch is present in approximately 1/30,000 live births. Although this lesion is similar in many respects to severe coarctation of the aorta, there are a few notable exceptions. The clinical presentation—shock or severe CHF in the first 2 weeks of life—is remarkably similar. Interrupted aortic arch, however, is not a lesion isolated to the great vessels but is a complex conotruncal defect that occurs in most cases as a result of posterior malalignment of the infundibular septum with the muscular septum—almost a "mirror image" of tetralogy of Fallot, in which there is anterior malalignment. (Also as in tetralogy of Fallot, microdeletion of chromosome 22 is common.) The posterior malalignment results in a narrowed left ventricular outflow tract, sometimes nearly atretic. It is thought that this severe obstruction in utero results in decreased growth, hypoplasia, and eventual interruption of the distal aortic arch. Thus, in addition to the VSD and narrowed subaortic area, there is complete atresia of a segment of the aortic arch. There are three anatomic subtypes of interrupted aortic arch based on the location of the interruption: type A, distal to the left subclavian artery; type B, between the left subclavian artery and the left carotid artery; and type C, between the innominate artery and the left carotid artery. (Fig. 57–11). Type B is the most common variety. In up to 50% of cases of type B interruption, the right subclavian artery arises aberrantly from the descending aorta *below* the ductus. Thus, all four extremities have equal pressure, even in the presence of ductal constriction or, following repair, making assessment for recoarctation impossible by blood pressure measurements alone.

Infants with interrupted aortic arch are completely dependent on a patent ductus arteriosus for lower body blood flow; thus, they become critically ill when the ductus closes. Immediate management is similar to that described for coarctation; $PGE_1$ infusion is essential. All other resuscitative measures will be ineffective if blood flow to the lower body is not restored. Oxygen saturations should be measured in the upper body; pulse oximetry readings in the lower body are reflective of the pulmonary artery oxygen saturation, which typically is lower than that distributed to the CNS and coronary arteries. (However, as mentioned previously, those patients with an aberrant right subclavian artery from the descending aorta may have low oxygen saturations in all four extremities, and ear oximetry may be the only location to determine oxygen delivery to the CNS.) High concentrations of inspired oxygen may result in low PVR, a large left-to-right shunt, and a "run-off" during diastole from the lower body into the pulmonary circulation. Inspired oxygen levels should therefore be minimized, aiming for normal (95%) oxygen saturations in the *upper* body.

Surgical reconstruction should be performed as soon as metabolic acidosis (if present) has resolved, end-organ dysfunction is improving, and the patient is hemodynamically stable. The repair typically entails a corrective approach via a median sternotomy, with the method of arch reconstruction based on the distance between the interrupted segments (short: direct anastomosis [Fig. 57–12]; long: tissue-to-tissue connection with homograft patch augmentation—jump grafts are rarely used), and closure of the VSD. A staged approach (arch reconstruction and a pulmonary artery band via a lateral thoracotomy) generally is not recommended and typically is reserved for patients with multiple VSDs. The surgical mortality rate is less than 10% but higher in patients with multiple anomalies, severe left ventricular outflow tract obstruction, low birth weight, multiple VSDs, or end-organ dysfunction. Repeat operation is necessary in approximately 25% of patients for progressive subaortic obstruction in childhood (Gaynor et al, 2000; Monro et al, 2003), and approximately 10% to 15% of infants require balloon angioplasty of the arch reconstruction for recurrent obstruction.

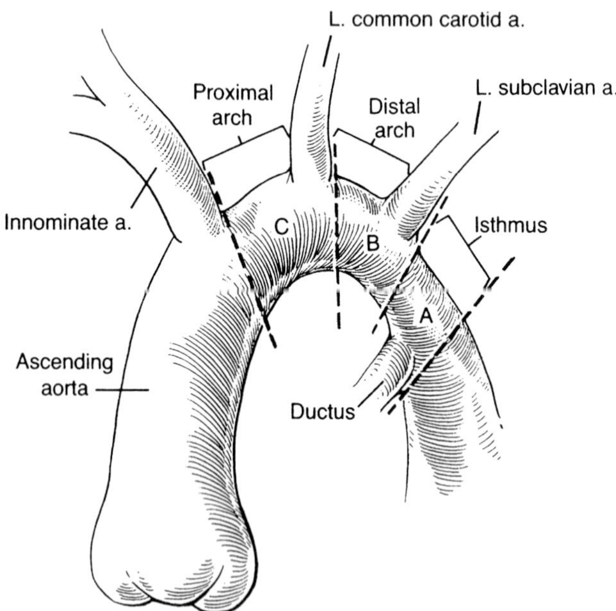


**FIGURE 57–11.** Anatomic classification of interrupted aortic arch. *Dashed lines* indicate the potential areas of discontinuity (interruption) in the aortic arch. See text for details. *(From Castañeda AR, Jonas RA, Mayer JE Jr, Hanley FL: Cardiac Surgery of the Neonate and Infant. Philadelphia, WB Saunders, 1994.)*

## Hypoplastic Left Heart Syndrome

HLHS is a fairly common, heterogeneous group of anatomic abnormalities in which there is a small or absent left ventricle with hypoplastic or atretic mitral and aortic valves. The incidence is 1/5500 live births, although a greater number of children with similar or related conditions are managed in a similar fashion. Although a genetic etiology has not yet been elucidated, there are increasing reports of HLHS occurring in families with other members affected with left-sided disease, such as a bicuspid aortic valve. HLHS is rare in trisomy 21 but has been reported in other trisomies such as 13 and 18, as well as in Turner syndrome.

Single-ventricle physiology and management strategies to optimize systemic oxygen delivery are discussed in detail earlier in this chapter. The presentation of HLHS typically is (1) *prenatal diagnosis*, in which an expectant team of caregivers manages a metabolically stable neonate; (2) *mild CHF* ± cardiac murmur, with no end-organ dysfunction; or (3) profound *circulatory collapse* and multiorgan system failure. In this last presentation, a sudden deterioration takes place with rapidly progressive CHF and shock as the ductus arteriosus constricts. There is decreased systemic perfusion and greatly increased PBF, largely independent of the level of pulmonary vascular resistance. The peripheral pulses are weak to absent. Renal, hepatic, coronary, and CNS perfusion are compromised, possibly resulting in acute tubular necrosis, necrotizing enterocolitis, or cerebral infarction or hemorrhage. A vicious circle also may result from inadequate retrograde perfusion of the ascending aorta (coronary artery blood supply), with further myocardial dysfunction and continued compromise of coronary blood flow. The pulmonary-to-systemic flow ratio approaches infinity as SBF nears zero. Thus, a paradoxical presentation results: a profound metabolic acidosis in the face of a relatively high $Po_2$ (70 to 100 torr). At the initial presentation, sepsis is frequently suspected before the diagnosis of CHD is made.

Arterial blood gas values may represent the single best indicator of hemodynamic stability and adequacy of systemic oxygen delivery. Although "low" arterial saturation (approximately 75% to 80%) with a normal pH and $CO_2$ indicates an acceptable balance of SBF and PBF with adequate periph-

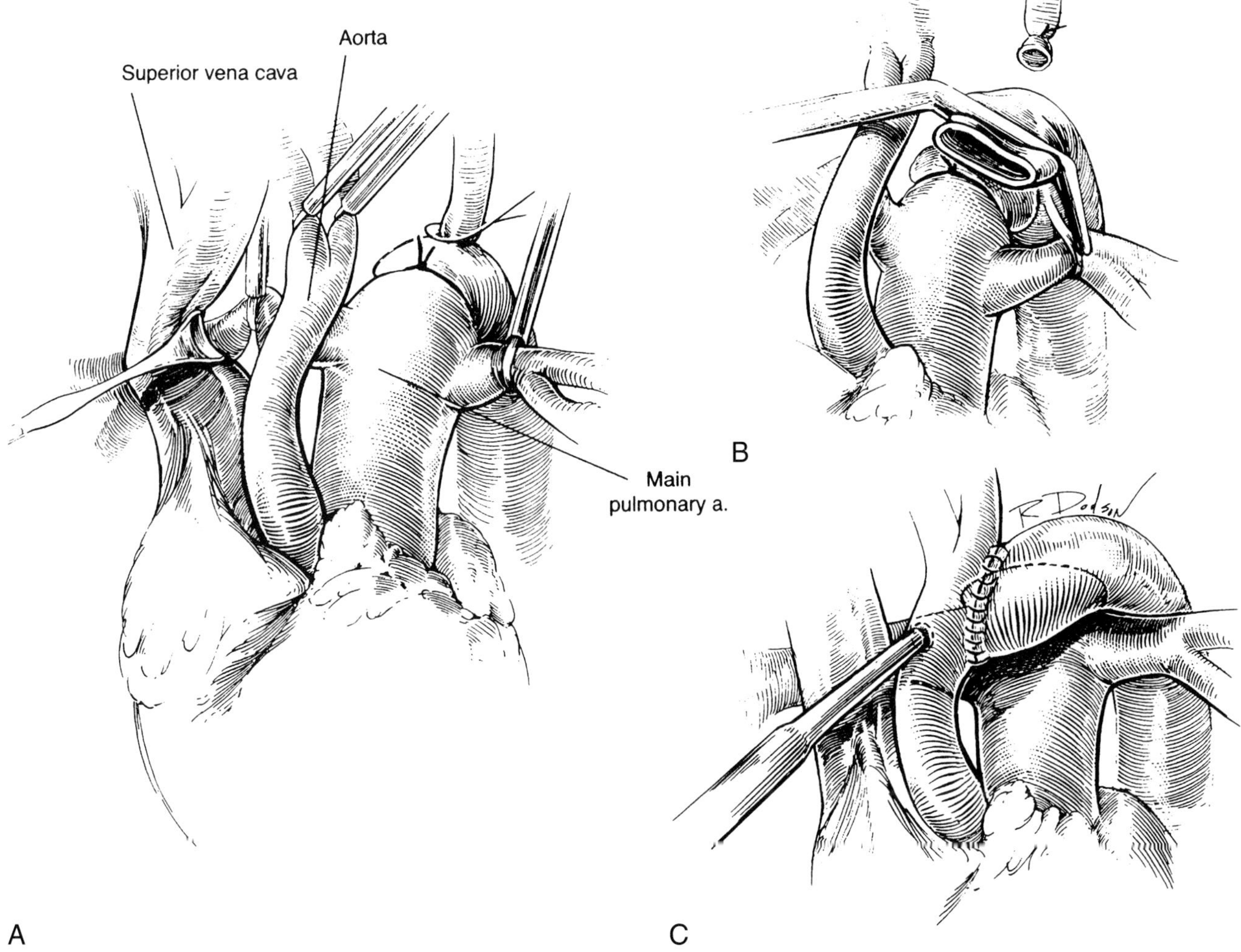


**FIGURE 57–12.** Surgical repair of interrupted aortic arch, type B. **A,** The descending aorta is cannulated for cardiopulmonary bypass distal to the ductus arteriosus, and the branch pulmonary arteries are snared. **B,** To adequately mobilize the descending aorta, the left subclavian artery may need to be divided. Following resection of the ductus arteriosus, the proximal (pulmonary artery) end is oversewn. **C,** The distal descending aorta is anastomosed directly to the ascending aorta. An alternative strategy is anastomosis of the left subclavian and left common carotid arteries combined with homograft patch augmentation of the inferior surface of the arch. Ventricular septal defect closure, when present, is also performed (not shown). *(From Castañeda AR, Jonas RA, Mayer JE Jr, Hanley FL: Cardiac Surgery of the Neonate and Infant. Philadelphia, WB Saunders, 1994.)*

eral perfusion, elevated oxygen saturation (greater than 90%) *with acidosis* represents significantly increased pulmonary and decreased systemic flows, with probable myocardial dysfunction and secondary effects on other organ systems.

### *Oxygen*

In general, supplemental oxygen should be avoided in the preoperative infant with HLHS. Oxygen will act as a pulmonary vasodilator, decreasing PVR and increasing Qp:Qs. The presence of a lung pathologic process (e.g., atelectasis, meconium aspiration, pneumonia) or of a restrictive ASD may result in an increased oxygen requirement. In the absence of lung disease or a restrictive ASD, most preoperative infants with HLHS have increased PBF with a room air oxygen saturation of 85% to 95% ($PaO_2$ of 45 to 50 mm Hg). Patients with a mildly restrictive atrial septum and/or elevated PVR will have oxygen saturations in the high 70s to low 80s. Although the temptation may be to increase the inspired oxygen, the low arterial oxygen saturation actually represents the best balance between Qp and Qs, increasing the supplemental oxygen may paradoxically decrease oxygen delivery to the tissues.

### *Indications for Treatment of a "High" Oxygen Saturation*

The clinically stable infant may tolerate significantly increased PBF in the preoperative period without significant intervention or obvious untoward effects. When the diagnosis of HLHS is made early, before onset of significant ductal constriction and a low-flow state, acidosis usually is avoided, and intubation may not be needed; the infant often may tolerate mild pulmonary overcirculation on low doses of $PGE_1$ (0.01 to 0.025 μg/kg/minute). Such infants often have a mild degree of restriction at the atrial septum, the left atrial hypertension keeping PVR a bit elevated and limiting Qp to some degree, and although tachypneic (respiratory rates of 60 to 80/minute), and well oxygenated ($SaO_2$ greater than 90%; $PaO_2$ 40 to 50 mm Hg), they remain clinically stable with minimal intervention. This group of patients maintains adequate SBF despite increased PBF, and further interventions to achieve some arbitrary $PO_2$—such as intubation and/or supplemental inspired gases—may not achieve improved patient stability and in fact may increase the potential for iatrogenic complications. In short, the neonate without significant CHF, acidosis, or progressive respiratory distress does not necessarily require significant therapy to treat a "high" $PO_2$.

Two subsets of infants with HLHS require aggressive preoperative management of the balance between their PBF and SBF: (1) those who are diagnosed late, following ductal constriction with circulatory collapse, and (2) those with clinically significant pulmonary overcirculation, independent of the timing of diagnosis.

### *Presentation in Shock*

Infants presenting with inadequate systemic cardiac output due to either ductal constriction with severe pulmonary overcirculation have depressed cardiac function, often with significant tricuspid insufficiency, profound metabolic acidosis, usually some degree of hepatic and renal failure, and occasionally bowel ischemia or disseminated intravascular coagulopathy. These infants require rapid and aggressive resuscitation. $PGE_1$ infusion must be initiated and the dose adjusted for the degree of ductal patency (confirmed by echocardiography). Dopamine at 3 to 5 μg/kg/minute will help augment overall cardiac output. Sedation, paralysis, and endotracheal intubation will allow for controlled ventilation and minimize systemic oxygen consumption. If normoventilation with 21% $FIO_2$ results in unacceptable pulmonary overcirculation, the addition of inspired $CO_2$ (20 mm Hg) has been shown to improve systemic oxygen delivery (see later). Most commonly, infants with HLHS presenting in shock benefit from recovery of end-organ function before proceeding to the operating room for surgical reconstruction or transplantation. Infants with persistent metabolic acidosis despite resuscitative efforts should be evaluated by echocardiogram for adequate ductal patency. Rarely, in a preoperative infant with HLHS, medically refractory pulmonary overcirculation persists, necessitating urgent stage I reconstruction.

### *Hypotension*

Although mild preoperative hypotension is common and frequently is thought to be caused by increased PBF at the expense of systemic flow, other causative disorders play a role as well. $PGE_1$ is a potent pulmonary and systemic vasodilator, and adequate volume resuscitation is indicated after the institution of $PGE_1$ therapy. It is important for the clinician to remember the neonatal myocardium's sensitivity to intracellular calcium and glucose, and serum levels of both should be monitored periodically. Myocardial dysfunction may coexist, and although small to moderate doses of inotropic agents frequently are beneficial, large doses of these agents may have a deleterious effect, depending on the relative effects on the systemic and pulmonary vascular beds. Preferential selective elevations of systemic vascular tone will secondarily increase PBF, and careful monitoring of mean arterial blood pressure and arterial oxygen saturation is warranted. Tricuspid regurgitation from an anatomically abnormal valve or secondary to ventricular dysfunction may contribute as well, and low doses of phosphodiesterase inhibitors such as milrinone—which may seem counterintuitive for the mildly hypotensive patient—may actually improve overall tissue perfusion and oxygen delivery. Finally, patients with refractory hypotension despite implementation of all of the foregoing measures should undergo echocardiography to confirm that the ductus remains widely patent and nonrestrictive; occasionally, inadvertent or unrecognized problems with $PGE_1$ administration result in a constricting ductus.

### *Inspired Gases*

The use of inspired gas mixtures to balance PBF and SBF in preoperative infants with HLHS or other single-ventricle physiologic defect is a topic of interest and controversy (Keidan et al, 2003; Tabbutt et al, 2001; Wessel, 1996). Several retrospective case reports and small series support the use of inspired $CO_2$ (14 to 35 mm Hg) to induce hypercarbia to stabilize preoperative infants with HLHS. Similarly, reports of small series of preoperative infants with HLHS have demonstrated clinical improvement or aortic Doppler measurements suggestive of lower Qp:Qs with increasing inspired nitrogen (to achieve 14% to 19% $FIO_2$) to induce alveolar hypoxia.

Until recently, prospective, controlled data comparing hypoxia and hypercarbia were limited to studies in shunt-dependent, single-ventricle animal models. The most elegant model is that of Reddy and colleagues (1996), who created a fetal sheep model of single ventricle. Two to three days after delivery, the lambs were anesthetized, intubated, and ventilated and underwent median sternotomy with ligation of the patent ductus arteriosus and placement of vascular pressure and flow probes. With use of both induced alveolar hypoxia and increased inspired $CO_2$, Qp:Qs was significantly decreased in both conditions compared with baseline. Tabbutt and associates (2001) recently compared the effects of hypoxia, achieved by adding increased inspired nitrogen (to achieve $FIO_2$ of 17%), with those of hypercarbia, achieved by adding increased inspired $CO_2$ (20 mm Hg inspired $CO_2$), in preoperative infants with HLHS under conditions of anesthesia, paralysis, and fixed minute ventilation. In this prospective, crossover study, systemic venous, arterial, and mixed cerebral oxygen saturations were measured, with each condition compared with baseline values in room air. Both inspired nitrogen (hypoxia) and $CO_2$ (hypercarbia) decreased Qp:Qs, although the decrease did not reach significant significance for hypoxia ($P$ = .056). Under these conditions of anesthesia and fixed mechanical ventilation, however, only hypercarbia increased cardiac output and mixed cerebral oxygenation.

In our practice at The Children's Hospital of Philadelphia, we tend to not use inspired gases preoperatively in most circumstances. If a child has significantly increased PBF but adequate SBF and oxygen delivery without acidosis, and is otherwise a good candidate for surgery, surgery is undertaken as soon as medically and logistically possible. However, for the neonate presenting with circulatory collapse and pulmonary overcirculation who is already intubated and mechanically ventilated, inspired $CO_2$ is utilized until surgery is undertaken. In these situations, minute ventilation is kept fixed, and $CO_2$ is added to the inspiratory limb of the ventilator to achieve an arterial $P_{CO_2}$ of approximately 55 mm Hg, with a normal pH. Although increased inspired $CO_2$ has been shown to improve oxygen delivery in the anesthetized infant under conditions of controlled ventilation, similar studies have not yet been reported in the spontaneously breathing infant. The increased oxygen consumption associated with the $CO_2$-induced tachypnea could potentially negate the benefits observed in the anesthetized patient. Thus, for patients in whom surgery must be delayed and there is clinically significant pulmonary over circulation with low systemic blood flow, inspired nitrogen may be utilized in the spontaneously breathing patient, and inspired $CO_2$ reserved for the mechanically ventilated patient, until surgery is undertaken. Between January 2001 and December 2002, 106 newborns underwent stage I reconstruction; 5 received supplemental inspired $CO_2$ and 4 received supplemental nitrogen.

### *Restrictive Atrial Septum*

In contrast, a severely restrictive atrial septum limits outflow from the pulmonary veins and, if coupled with mitral atresia, results in profound left atrial outlet obstruction, pulmonary hypertension, and hypoxemia following birth. The newborn with HLHS and an intact atrial septum will be difficult to manage immediately following birth; however, if the intact atrial septum is suspected prenatally, delivery of the infant should take place at the delivery center associated with the surgical referral center and with a surgical team or catheterization laboratory team available. The infant should be intubated, umbilical access obtained, and $PGE_1$ infusion initiated in the delivery room, followed by direct transportation to the operating room or catheterization laboratory where the planned septectomy or catheter intervention is to be performed. In the absence of a prenatal diagnosis, the clinical scenario is identical to that in obstructed total anomalous pulmonary venous return or severe "lung disease." From a management standpoint, the strategy is quite similar: intubation, positive end-expiratory pressure, supplemental oxygen as needed to maintain an oxygen saturation of approximately 80%, umbilical access, inotropic support, isotonic volume as necessary, and base replacement.

Anticipation of the potential diagnosis of CHD is critical. Having an echocardiographer, catheterization team, and operating room (OR) team available when the patient arrives at the tertiary care center provides the best chance of survival. On arrival of an infant in extremis with a clinical picture of obstructed pulmonary venous return but without a definitive diagnosis, obtaining a brief echocardiogram is of utmost importance. Obstructed pulmonary veins can be stabilized only with venovenous extracorporeal membrane oxygenation (ECMO) or corrective surgery. HLHS with intact atrial septum is best stabilized by septectomy (in the operating room or catheterization laboratory) or palliative surgery. Neck cannulation for venoarterial ECMO for unrepaired HLHS is impossible due to the size of the diminutive aorta and requires transthoracic cannulation with ligation of the patent ductus arteriosus to provide adequate SBF.

Unfortunately, the association of a severely restrictive or intact atrial septum with HLHS carries a significantly worse short- and long-term prognosis compared with other forms of HLHS, mainly because of the secondary changes that occur in the pulmonary vascular bed from in utero obstruction of pulmonary venous outflow (Rychik et al, 1999) The pulmonary vascular tree is abnormal in all patients with HLHS: There is an increase in the number of arteries per unit area of lung, and the arteries themselves have a considerable increase in muscularity. Increased medial arterial wall thickness is present, as well as extension of muscle into smaller and more peripheral arteries than is normal. These abnormalities may explain the predilection toward extreme sensitivity of the pulmonary vascular bed to vasoactive agents. The pulmonary veins are typically dilated, with thickened walls. The degree of restriction at the atrial level influences the histopathologic findings within the pulmonary vascular tree. Increased arterial tortuosity and arteriopathy consistent with grade III Heath-Edwards classification have been noted in patients with a severely restrictive (or absent) ASD. Marked thickening of the pulmonary veins with the appearance of multiple elastic laminae—so-called arterialization of the pulmonary veins—has been noted in patients with intact atrial septum (Rychik et al, 1999). Impediment to drainage from the left atrium in utero may be the reason for development of the histopathologic features seen in the pulmonary veins of infants with intact atrial septum. These pulmonary venous abnormalities further contribute to the pathophysiology once these infants are born and may explain why most of them continue to do poorly, with a high mortality rate despite creation of a large and effective interatrial communication at birth. Even if the newborn survives stage I reconstruction (for which the mortality rate is greater than 50% among those with an intact atrial septum), the underlying pulmonary vascular pathology may preclude a later Fontan procedure.

### *Surgical Therapy for Hypoplastic Left Heart Syndrome*

Although medical stabilization is important in the overall outcome in these children, ultimately surgical therapy is necessary for survival. After a period of medical stabilization and support to allow recovery of ischemic organ system injury (particularly of the kidneys, the liver, the CNS, and the heart itself), surgical relief of left-sided obstruction is required. The surgical management of HLHS remains controversial; surgical intervention involves either staged reconstruction (with a neonatal Norwood procedure followed by a staged

Fontan operation later in childhood) or neonatal cardiac transplantation. Recent results from both reconstructive surgery and transplantation have vastly improved the outlook for infants born with this previously 100% fatal condition (Bailey et al, 1993; Gaynor et al, 2002; Mahle et al, 2000).

### *Stage I Reconstruction*

The first stage reconstruction for HLHS with the classic Norwood operation (Fig. 57–13) is typically performed with a median sternotomy incision and use of DHCA, although some groups have recently utilized selective

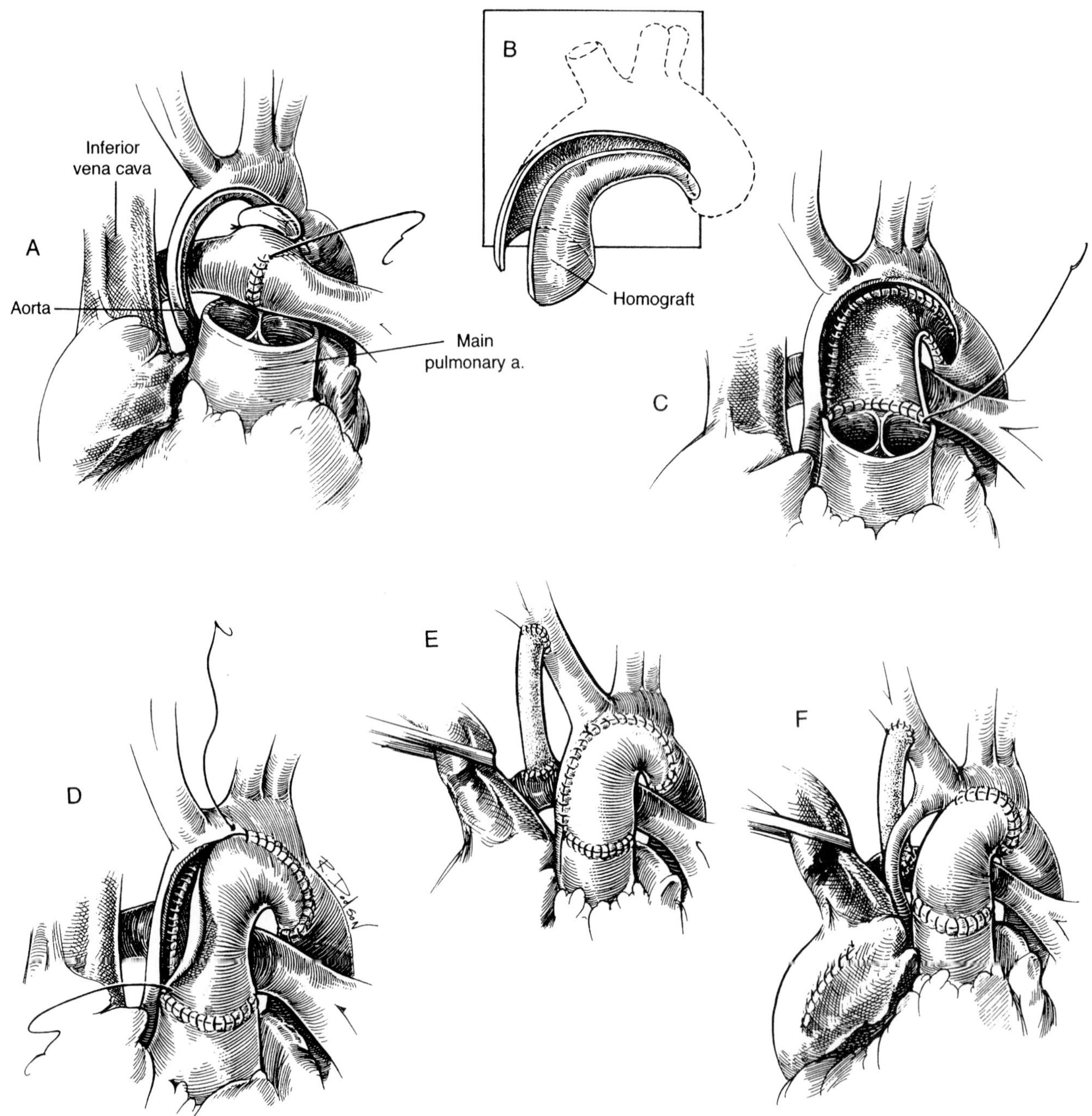


**FIGURE 57–13.** Stage I reconstruction for hypoplastic left heart syndrome: Classic Norwood procedure. **A,** The main pulmonary artery is transected, and the distal end oversewn. The ductus arteriosus is ligated, and an incision is made from the proximal ascending aorta around the aortic arch to the level of the ductus. **B,** A pulmonary homograft is utilized to create a patch to reconstruct the neoaorta. **C** and **D,** This homograft patch is used to connect the proximal main pulmonary artery and pulmonary (neoaortic) valve to the ascending aorta and transverse arch. **E,** A modified Blalock-Taussig shunt is placed from the base of the innominate artery to the right pulmonary artery. **F,** An alternative technique utilizing a circumferential tube graft from the proximal main pulmonary artery to the distal transverse aortic arch. *Not shown*: Atrial septectomy is performed to provide unobstructed egress from the pulmonary veins to the right ventricle. *(From Castañeda AR, Jonas RA, Mayer JE Jr, Hanley FL: Cardiac Surgery of the Neonate and Infant. Philadelphia, WB Saunders, 1994.)*

cerebral perfusion during cardiopulmonary bypass. The main pulmonary artery is transected just proximal to the branch pulmonary arteries, and the defect in the distal pulmonary arteries is closed. The pulmonary valve and proximal pulmonary artery become the systemic outflow, after anastomosis to the reconstructed aortic arch, usually following augmentation with pulmonary artery homograft. An atrial septectomy is performed to ensure adequate pulmonary venous outflow, and a shunt is created to provide PBF. Classically, this is a modified Blalock-Taussig shunt from the base of the innominate artery. Recently, there has been interest in creation of the shunt from the right ventricular infundibulum to the central pulmonary arteries, popularized by Sano and colleagues (2003) and others (Mahle et al, 2003; Malec et al, 2003; Pizarro et al, 2003) (Fig. 57–14). The theoretical advantages of a right ventricle–pulmonary artery shunt are a higher postoperative diastolic pressure (Pizarro et al, 2003), improved coronary artery flow, pulsatile end-organ perfusion, and improved growth of the central pulmonary arteries (Maher et al, 2003). However, this technical modification employs a small incision in the systemic right ventricle, and the long-term effects on ventricular function and/or arrhythmia are unknown. Follow-up studies examining the theoretical advantages of the right ventricle–pulmonary artery conduit modification are under way but short-term in duration. Decades of follow-up study are likely to be necessary to determine the better overall surgical strategy to be used in the neonatal period.

The surgical results of first-stage reconstruction for HLHS have progressively improved after the initial successes reported in the early 1980s. In the current era, it is increasingly recognized that there are "standard-risk" and "high-risk" patients; risk factors for first-stage operation include low birth weight (less than 2.5 kg) and the association of other cardiac (e.g., severe tricuspid regurgitation, intact atrial septum) or genetic anomalies. Standard-risk patients have an approximately 5% to 10% mortality risk, whereas infants with additional risk factors have incrementally increased risk (Gaynor et al, 2002) There is an approximately 5% to 10% interstage mortality rate (Mahle et al, 2001), but recent success with home monitoring programs may reduce this risk (Ghanayem et al, 2003). The expected operative mortality risks for the second (superior cavopulmonary connection) and third (Fontan operation) procedures are currently in the range of 1% to 2%. Thus, a majority of the deaths that occur in newborns with HLHS are concentrated in the newborn and early infancy period: from birth through the second-stage operation.

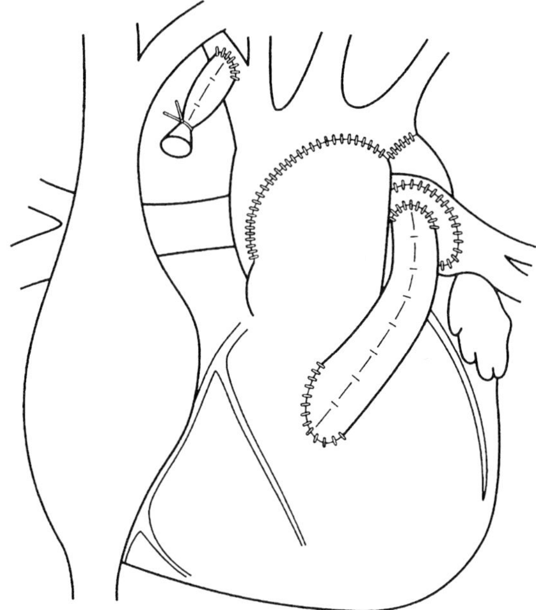

**FIGURE 57–14.** Right ventricle–pulmonary artery (RV-PA), or Sano, modification of stage I reconstruction. The arch repair is similar to that shown in Figure 57–13. The Blalock-Taussig shunt is replaced with a Gore-Tex tube inserted from the right ventricle to the main pulmonary artery. *(From Sano S, Ishino K, Kawada K, et al: Right ventricle–pulmonary artery shunt in first-stage palliation of hypoplastic left heart syndrome. J Thorac Cardiovasc Surg 126:504-510, 2003.)*

### *Infant Heart Transplantation*

In recent years, heart transplantation survival has improved in children and remains an important surgical option for patients with acquired and congenital forms of heart disease in whom medical and surgical treatment schemes are exhausted (Bailey et al, 1993). In neonates, HLHS remains the most common indication for heart transplantation either as initial therapy or as a treatment for those patients in whom surgical reconstruction has failed. The overall survival rate for pediatric cardiac transplantation worldwide is 73% at 1 year and 70% at 4 years after transplantation (Wernovsky and Chrisant, 2004). The biggest drawback to the routine use of transplantation as primary therapy for HLHS is a lack of donors. Even with most centers in North America performing staged reconstruction as primary therapy, thus limiting the number of babies with HLHS waiting for an organ at any given time (approximately 2000 neonates are born each year with HLHS, with approximately 200 neonatal and infant heart transplantations annually), approximately 25% to 30% of children never receive a transplant because of a limited donor supply. Risk factors for early death after transplantation in children (for any underlying cause) include CHD, pretransplantation use of a ventricular assist device, younger age, requirement for intensive care, retransplantation procedure, and performance of transplantation in a low-volume center.

The surgical technique for implantation of a donor heart in a newborn with HLHS is relatively straightforward; the primary technical consideration is reconstruction of the aortic arch. The procedure is a bit more technically demanding if prior stage I reconstruction has been performed (Fig. 57–15). Several reconstructive techniques have been used; however, in a majority of cases, the donor aorta is harvested with a greater length than is typical and the undersurface of the arch of the donor aorta is utilized to reconstruct the aortic arch in the recipient after ligation or excision of the diminutive ascending aorta, which functions as a common coronary artery in patients with aortic atresia and HLHS. The remainder of the implantation of the donor heart involves standardized techniques including anastomosis of the donor left atrium and recipient left atrium and anastomosis of the pulmonary trunk to the pulmonary bifurcation in the recipient. The right atrium can

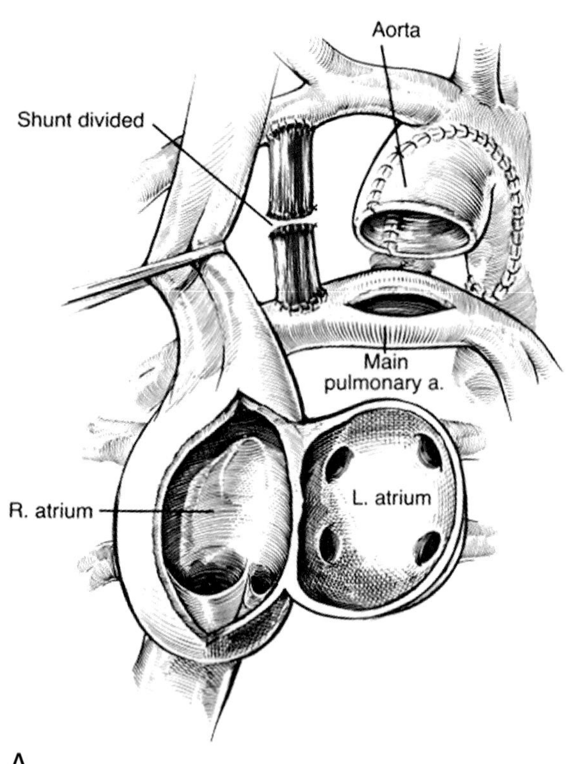


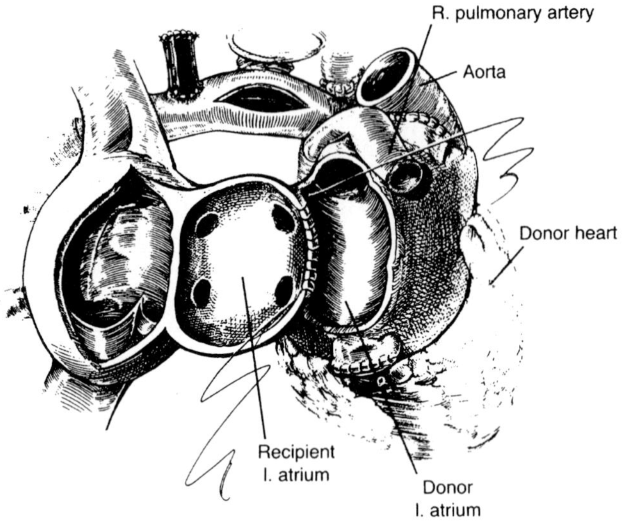


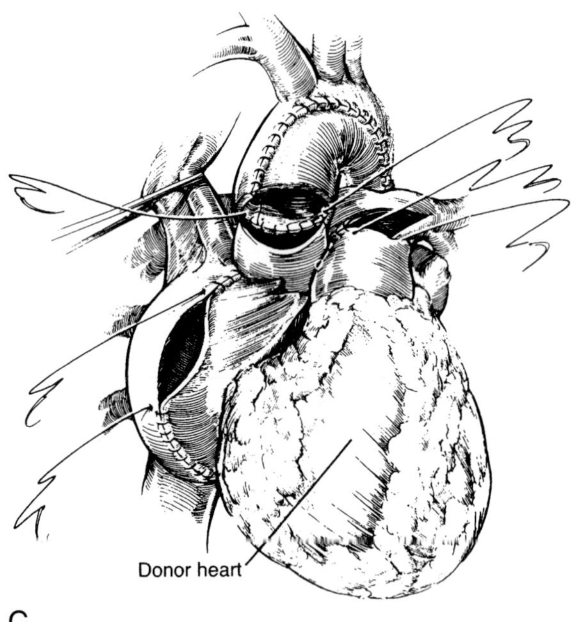


**FIGURE 57–15.** Cardiac transplantation following stage I reconstruction. **A,** Donor heart site following cardiectomy and division of the Blalock-Taussig shunt. The left atrium is typically small. **B,** The left atrial connection is started; the donor branch pulmonary arteries have been harvested to be used in the recipient for pulmonary arterioplasty. **C,** Completed transplantation procedure with aortic, pulmonary, and right atrial anastomoses. *(From Castañeda AR, Jonas RA, Mayer JE Jr, Hanley FL: Cardiac Surgery of the Neonate and Infant. Philadelphia, WB Saunders, 1994.)*

be connected by either a cuff of right atrium of the recipient left in place or by utilizing bicaval anastomoses. Because implantation of a donor heart in HLHS requires arch reconstruction, residual coarctation or subsequent development of stenosis at the anastomotic site is possible; either may be treated with balloon angioplasty.

Rejection of the graft can occur at any time (hyperacute, acute, and chronic); nearly 75% of children will have at least one episode of rejection. Infectious complications are common, occur most often in the immediate period after transplantation, and are a major cause of early morbidity and death, especially in the first year after transplantation. Longer-term sequelae include lymphoproliferative disease (in 2% to 10% of cases, possibly more in younger recipients) and graft vasculopathy (in 8% to 10%).

### *Transplantation Versus Staged Reconstruction*

As mentioned previously, the management of HLHS from a surgical perspective remains highly controversial. At present, the overall mortality risks are very similar, if one assumes continued organ availability at the current rate and no significant shift in the percentage of centers that adopt one or another strategy.

However, if transplantation is performed as an "intent to treat" strategy at more centers, and the donor supply does not change, the pretransplantation mortality rate will invariably increase. Thus, the optimal strategy will depend on the long-term mortality risks and morbidity associated with each strategy. Certain morbid conditions are inherent to transplantation (immunosuppression, lymphoproliferative disease, graft vasculopathy), and others are inherent to staged reconstruction culminating in a Fontan operation (arrhythmias, protein-losing enteropathy, thromboembolism). A number of such comorbid conditions, however, occur with nearly identical frequency with *either* strategy, including growth retardation, exercise limitations, chronic medication use, developmental delay, and psychological factors related to a "chronic" disease. Further research is necessary to determine which strategy is ideal for individual patients and their families (Wernovsky and Chrisant, 2004).

## LESIONS WITH DUCT-DEPENDENT PULMONARY BLOOD FLOW

### Tricuspid Atresia

Tricuspid atresia involves complete absence of the tricuspid valve and thus no direct communication from right atrium to right ventricle. The right ventricle may be severely hypoplastic or completely absent. An atrial-level communication is necessary for blood to exit the right atrium; there is an obligatory right-to-left shunt at this level. More than 90% of patients have an associated VSD, allowing blood to pass from the left ventricle to the right ventricle and its associated great vessel. In patients with normally related great arteries, accounting for 70% of cases of tricuspid atresia (Fig. 57–16A, B), PBF is derived from the right ventricle; if the right ventricle (or its connection with the left ventricle via a VSD) is severely diminutive, the PBF may be duct dependent; closure of the ductus leads to profound hypoxemia and acidosis. In the remaining 30% of cases, the great arteries are transposed (see Fig. 57–16C, D), with the aorta aligned with the small right ventricle. In these cases with transposition and tricuspid atresia, the VSD usually is smaller than the aorta, and the newborn may have limited SBF in the absence of a patent ductus arteriosus. Many patients have an associated coarctation as well.

Immediate medical management is aimed primarily at maintenance of adequate PBF. In the usual case of severe pulmonary stenosis and limited PBF, $PGE_1$ infusion maintains PBF via the ductus arteriosus. Surgical creation of a more permanent source of PBF (usually via a Blalock-Taussig shunt) is undertaken as soon as possible. More complex cases (e.g., with transposition) may require more extensive palliative procedures (Daebritz et al, 2000) similar to stage I reconstruction for HLHS.

### Ebstein Anomaly

Ebstein anomaly is an uncommon (1/25,000 live births) but grave anatomic lesion when presenting in the neonatal period (Knott-Craig et al, 2000). Anatomically, there is "downward displacement" of the tricuspid valve into the body of the right ventricle (Fig. 57–17). The tricuspid valve is frequently regurgitant resulting in marked right atrial enlargement, cardiomegaly, and CHF in utero; the resultant inadequate forward flow from the right ventricle (to the ductus arteriosus and placenta) results in hydrops fetalis, with a high rate of fetal demise. Following birth, right ventricular afterload increases further (temporarily, following removal from the placenta), and although PVR remains high, there is greatly diminished forward flow from the right ventricle, a large right-to-left shunt at the atrial level, and profound hypoxemia, acidosis, and CHF.

Medical management is aimed at supporting the neonate through the initial period of the transitional circulation. $PGE_1$ is used to maintain a patent ductus arteriosus while other measures aimed at decreasing PVR and

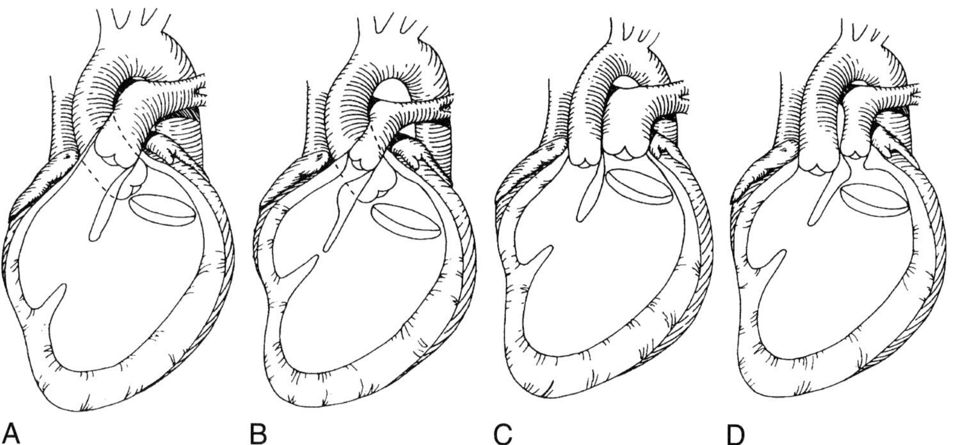


**FIGURE 57–16.** Anatomic variants in tricuspid atresia. **A,** Normally related great vessels with a large ventricular septal defect (VSD) and normal-sized pulmonary arteries (PAs). **B,** Normally related great vessels with a small VSD and PAs. **C,** Transposed great arteries (left ventricle aligned with the PA, right ventricle with the aorta) with a relatively small VSD and aorta. Many patients with this variant have coarctation as well (see text). **D,** Transposed great vessels with a VSD, subpulmonary obstruction, and small PAs. *(From Fyler DC: Tricuspid atresia. In Fyler DC [ed]: Nadas' Pediatric Cardiology. Philadelphia. Hanley & Belfus, 1992b, pp 659-667.)*

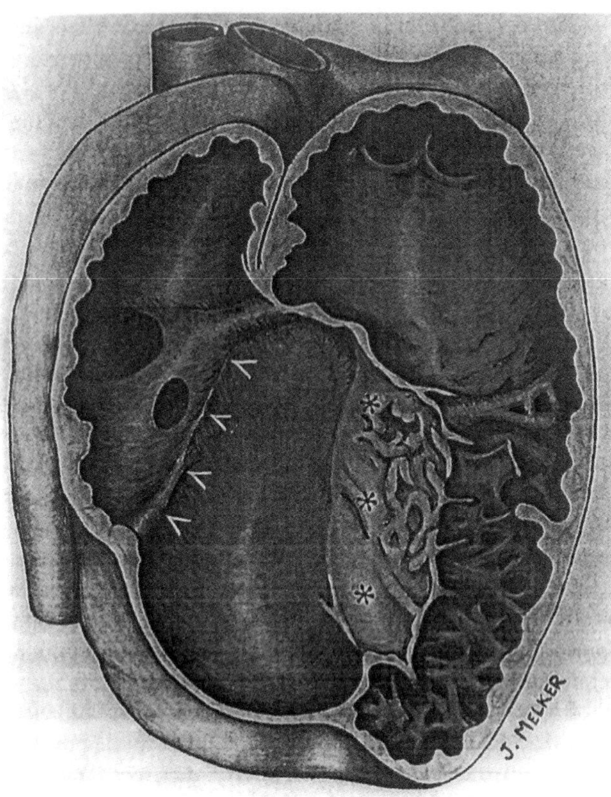


**FIGURE 57–17.** Inferior displacement of tricuspid valve leaflet (*) into the right ventricular cavity. The *white arrowheads* indicate the normally positioned tricuspid valve annulus. The area between the true annulus and the displaced valve leaflet is considered "atrialized". *(From Epstein ML: Congenital stenosis and insufficiency of the tricuspid valve. In Allen HD, Gutgesell HP, Clark EB, Driscoll DJ [eds]: Moss and Adams' Heart Disease in Infants, Children and Adolescents: Including the Fetus and Young Adult. Philadelphia, Lippincott Williams & Wilkins, 2001, pp 810-819.)*

promoting antegrade PBF are employed (such as a high level of supplemental oxygen and maintaining a mild respiratory alkalosis). Recently, nitric oxide has been utilized with limited success (Atz et al, 2003). Following a few days of medical management, a trial of discontinuing $PGE_1$ may be considered. Weaning from nitric oxide and/or $PGE_1$ may take 2 to 3 weeks. Weaning may be unsuccessful in some infants, who then may require a systemic-to-pulmonary shunt or more aggressive surgical reconstruction with a high mortality risk (Knott-Craig et al, 2000).

An important contributor to the high mortality rate in the neonate with severe Ebstein anomaly is the associated pulmonary hypoplasia (due to the massive enlargement of the right side of the heart in utero) (Fig. 57–18). The prognosis for neonates presenting with profound cyanosis due to Ebstein anomaly has been very guarded (Epstein, 2001; Knott-Craig et al, 2000). Surgical options are controversial and generally reserved for the severely symptomatic child. Systemic-to-pulmonary shunts have been used with limited success, and complicated neonatal tricuspid repairs have not been particularly successful. Further complicating the medical condition, Ebstein anomaly is associated with Wolff-Parkinson-White syndrome and supraventricular tachycardia in up to 50% of cases.

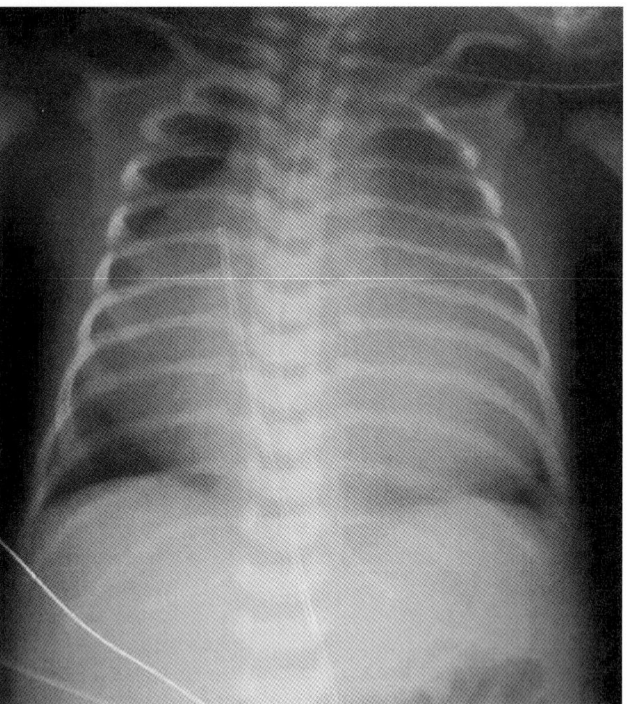

**FIGURE 57–18.** Chest radiograph in a 1-day-old newborn with Ebstein anomaly of the tricuspid valve. Note the massive cardiomegaly and relative pulmonary oligemia and hypoplasia.

## Pulmonary Atresia with Ventricular Septal Defect

Pulmonary atresia with VSD (PA/VSD) is sometimes also known as *tetralogy of Fallot with pulmonary atresia* (TOF/PA), as the VSD is almost always of the malalignment type with severe obstruction of the right ventricular outflow tract (tetralogy of Fallot with pulmonary stenosis is discussed later in this chapter). PA/VSD (or, alternatively, TOF/PA) is a heterogeneous anomaly with respect to the source(s) of PBF. Inside the heart, there is typically one VSD; the ventricles are of normal size, and there usually is a severely hypoplastic infundibulum with complete atresia of the pulmonary valve. The pulmonary vascular bed architecture is much more variable, ranging from normal-sized pulmonary arteries supplied by the ductus arteriosus, to diminutive pulmonary arteries and a small ductus, to discontinuous pulmonary arteries supplied by bilateral ductus, to virtually absent central pulmonary arteries with the PBF supplied by multiple aortopulmonary collateral arteries (MAPCAs) (Fig. 57–19).

Initial management is based on the source of PBF, as well as the size and branching pattern of the distal pulmonary arteries. In cases with a patent ductus arteriosus and normal branch pulmonary arteries, newborn surgery may consist of a systemic-pulmonary artery shunt followed by eventual shunt takedown, VSD closure, and placement of a right ventricular–pulmonary artery conduit (sometimes considered to be a Rastelli procedure); alternatively, the complete repair may be done in the neonatal period (Fig. 57–20). Complete repair in the neonate usually is dependent on good-sized pulmonary arteries and an adequately developed infundibulum to allow transannular patch

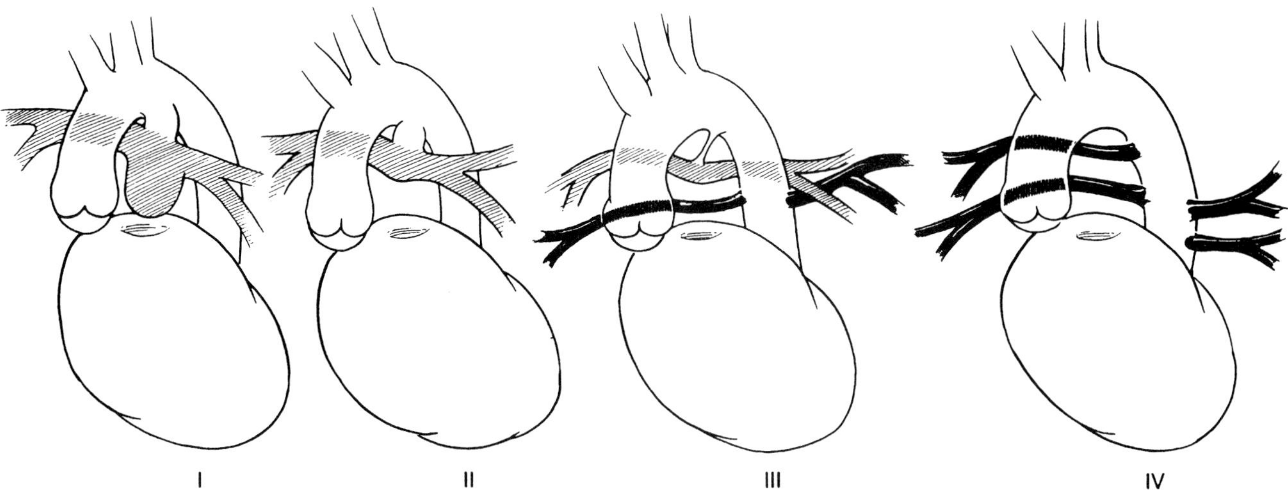


**FIGURE 57–19.** Variability in the pulmonary artery architecture in tetralogy of Fallot with pulmonary atresia (pulmonary atresia with ventricular septal defect). In types I and II, the pulmonary arteries are well developed and supplied by a single source, the ductus arteriosus. In type III, the ductus supplies small central pulmonary arteries and is either absent or diminutive. In type IV, there are no mediastinal pulmonary arteries, and aortopulmonary collateral arteries supply all bronchopulmonary segments. *(From Castañeda AR, Jonas RA, Mayer JE Jr, Hanley FL: Cardiac Surgery of the Neonate and Infant. Philadelphia, WB Saunders, 1994.)*

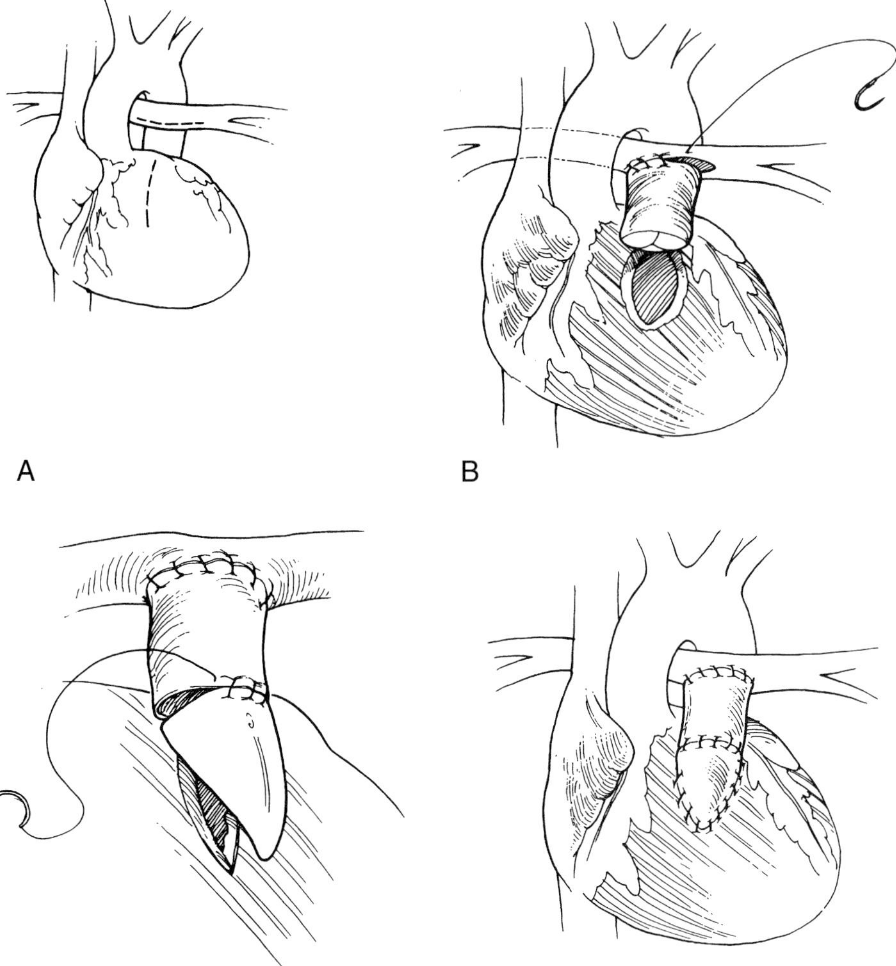


**FIGURE 57–20.** Repair of pulmonary atresia with ventricular septal defect and normal pulmonary arteries. **A,** *Dotted lines* depict the location of the ventriculotomy and pulmonary arteriotomy. **B,** The ventricular septal defect is closed through the ventriculotomy, and a valved homograft conduit is anastomosed to the distal pulmonary arteries and superior aspect of the ventriculotomy. **C** and **D,** A "hood" of pericardium is used to complete the repair. *(From Spray TL, Wernovsky G: Right ventricular outflow tract obstruction. In Chang AC, Hanley FH, Wernovsky G, Wessel DL [eds]: Pediatric Cardiac Intensive Care. Baltimore, Williams & Wilkins, 1998, pp 257-270.)*

placement and the absence of a conduit. In cases with diminutive pulmonary arteries and MAPCAs, amalgamation of the multiple mediastinal vessels into a common confluence ("unifocalization") may be considered, with placement of a right ventricle–to–pulmonary artery conduit. If the branch pulmonary arteries are too hypoplastic to accept the full cardiac output without unacceptable pulmonary hypertension, the VSD may be left open until the branch pulmonary arteries can undergo angioplasty ("rehabilitation") to increase the total cross-sectional area (Fig. 57–21).

The long-term outcomes are highly dependent on the status of the pulmonary vascular bed at birth. If the pul-

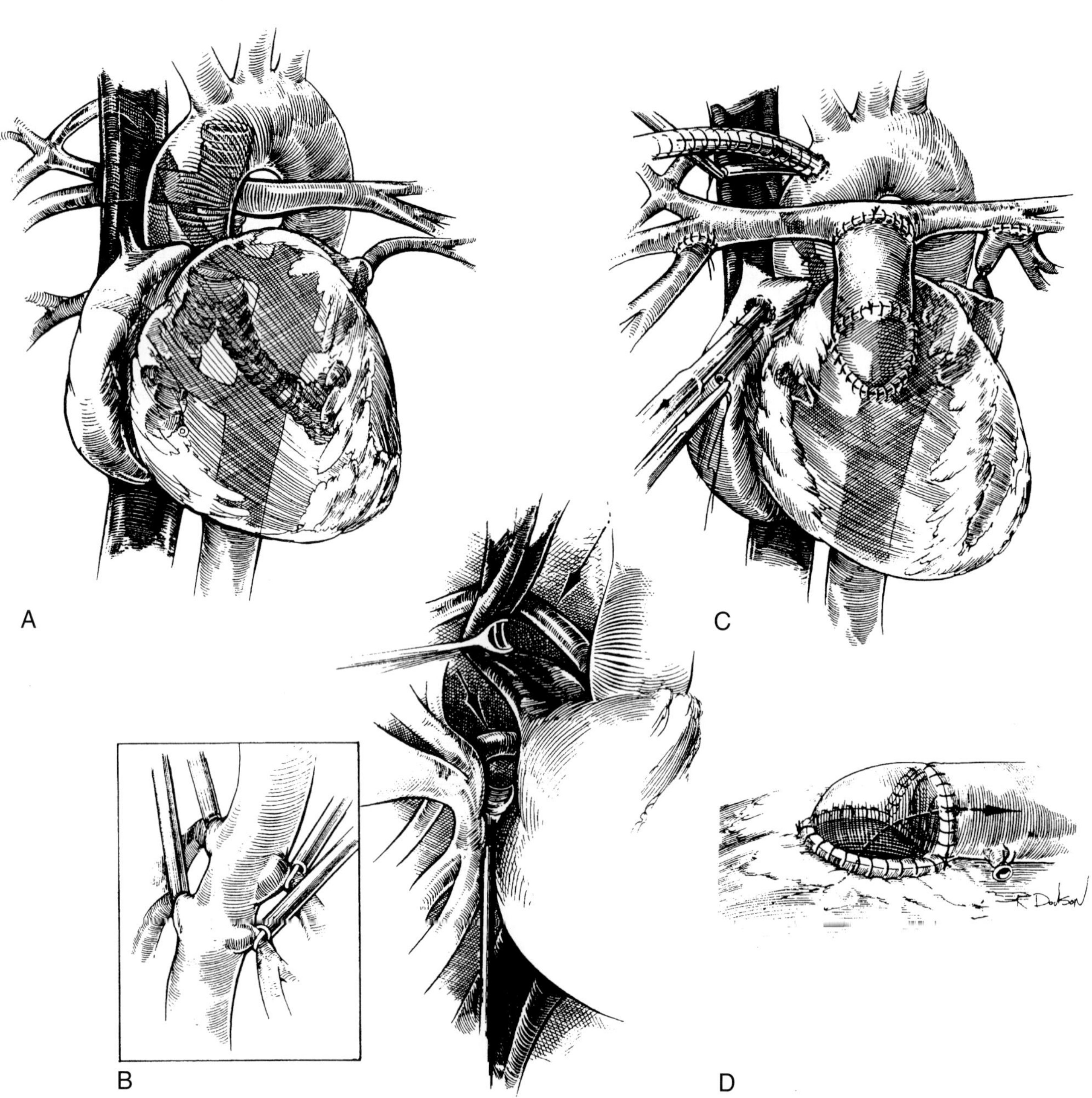


**FIGURE 57–21.** Example of complete repair of pulmonary atresia with multiple aorticopulmonary collaterals. **A,** Three large aorticopulmonary collaterals are seen arising from the descending aorta behind the heart. **B,** In some cases a preliminary thoracotomy may be necessary to identify posterior collaterals to either temporarily or permanently interrupt these vessels *(inset)*. **C,** Following cannulation for bypass, the three collaterals are unifocalized to the true mediastinal pulmonary arteries. The operation is completed by performing a ventriculotomy to close the ventricular septal defect (see also Fig. 57–20) and interposing a valved homograft from the ventriculotomy to the unifocalized pulmonary arteries. **D,** The proximal conduit anastomosis is augmented with a pericardial hood. *(From Castañeda AR, Jonas RA, Mayer JE Jr, Hanley FL: Cardiac Surgery of the Neonate and Infant. Philadelphia, WB Saunders, 1994.)*

monary arteries are essentially normal in size, the long-term outcomes are highly similar to those for "straightforward" tetralogy of Fallot. If there are diminutive pulmonary arteries, or MAPCAs, the prognosis is much more guarded (Permut et al, 1994; Rome et al, 1993).

## Pulmonary Atresia with Intact Ventricular Septum

Sometimes referred to as "hypoplastic right heart syndrome," pulmonary atresia with an intact ventricular septum is a heterogeneous disease. In all cases, there is absent antegrade flow from the right ventricle to the pulmonary arteries, with PBF supplied by a ductus arteriosus after birth. Right-sided hypoplasia is present in variable degrees, ranging from a nearly normal-sized right ventricle and tricuspid valve to severe hypoplasia (virtual atresia) of the tricuspid valve and a diminutive, muscle-bound right ventricle (Fig. 57–22). In the most severe cases, coronary artery blood flow is derived not from the aortic root but from the hypertensive, muscle-bound right ventricle (Fig. 57–23). These abnormal connections between the right ventricular sinus and coronary arteries develop in the fetus, possibly because of the suprasystemic pressure generated by the right ventricle during systole. Very abnormal coronary sinusoids, and even areas of complete coronary interruption, may be present at birth. These abnormal connections may represent the predominant source of coronary blood flow to the myocardium. In these cases with so-called right ventricle–dependent coronary circulation, relieving the pulmonary outflow tract obstruction would result in a fall in right ventricular pressure and hence coronary insufficiency and myocardial ischemia or infarction (Giglia et al, 1992).

Although the cornerstone of initial management is prostaglandin infusion to maintain ductal patency, a more permanent and reliable form of PBF must be surgically created for the infant to survive. Surgical management is often preceded by catheterization to define the coronary artery anatomy. In patients with right ventricle–dependent coronary arteries, creation of a systemic-to-pulmonary shunt is the typical initial surgical procedure in the neonate, with postoperative management similar to that with other forms of single-ventricle disorders. This procedure is followed by further staged reconstruction culminating in either a Fontan operation or cardiac transplantation.

In patients without significant coronary abnormalities, however, PBF is established by creating an outflow for the right ventricle by catheterization (valvoplasty, after valve perforation), surgical pulmonary valvotomy or right ventricular outflow tract augmentation. If surgery is performed, a systemic-to-pulmonary artery shunt (most often a Blalock-Taussig shunt) is constructed to also augment PBF (Fig. 57–24). Following this procedure, the patient may develop

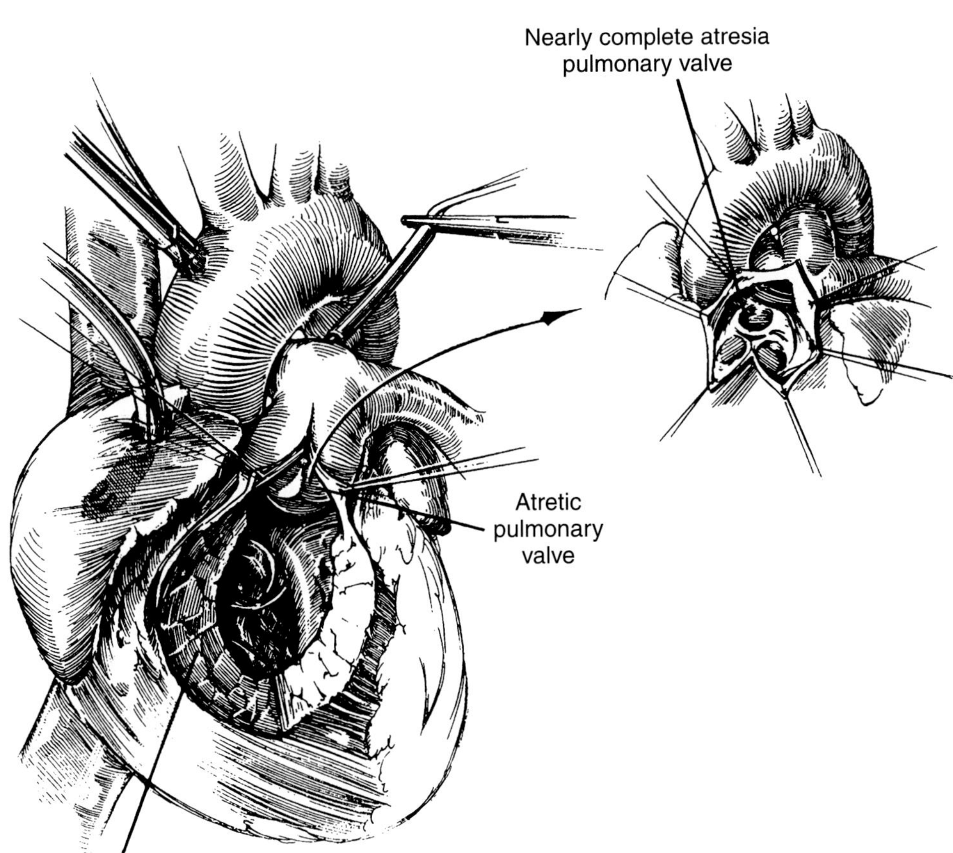


**FIGURE 57–22.** Exposure of the hypertrophied, diminutive right ventricle in pulmonary atresia with an intact ventricular septum. The *inset* shows the diminutive pulmonary valve with abnormal tissue and commissural fusion. *(From Castañeda AR, Jonas RA, Mayer JE Jr, Hanley FL: Cardiac Surgery of the Neonate and Infant. Philadelphia, WB Saunders, 1994.)*

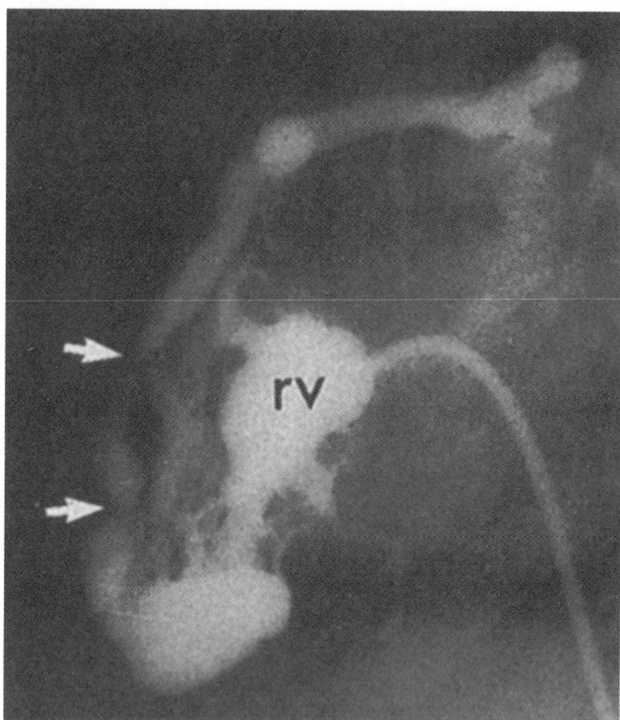


**FIGURE 57–23.** Lateral angiogram from a newborn with pulmonary atresia and intact ventricular septum. Following injection of contrast through the hypertrophied and diminutive right ventricle (RV), there is retrograde filling of tortuous coronary arteries through sinusoidal connections to the RV *(arrows)*.

low cardiac output, either from unrecognized coronary abnormalities or from a "circular shunt" (see Fig. 57–24).

Surgical mortality risk is highly dependent on the heterogeneous anatomy of this disease, in particular, the presence or absence of coronary abnormalities; the presence of sinusoidal connections between the right ventricle and the coronary arteries is associated with poorer long-term survival. In cases with adequate coronary arteries and minimal right ventricular hypoplasia, however, the prognosis is considerably more favorable. If the right ventricular outflow tract obstruction is adequately relieved and the tricuspid valve and right ventricle are of "adequate" size, within 2 to 3 months hypertrophy regresses, compliance improves, and the right ventricle can increase its contribution to PBF. At this time, the shunt can be closed surgically (or coil-embolized in the catheterization laboratory), and any residual shunting at the atrial level can be closed with either surgical or transcatheter techniques, resulting in a normal "series" circulation.

### "Critical" Pulmonary Stenosis

In contrast with pulmonary atresia with intact ventricular septum, isolated pulmonary valve stenosis (Fig. 57–25) typically coexists with a normal-sized right ventricle and tricuspid valve and normal distal pulmonary arteries. By convention, "critical" pulmonary stenosis is the terminology used when adequate oxygenation cannot be achieved without patency of the ductus arteriosus. Prostaglandin therapy may be necessary in some cases of severe hypoxemia. "Noncritical" pulmonary stenosis may result in very high (e.g., suprasystemic) right ventricular pressures, and there may even be a component of right-to-left atrial shunting and hypoxemia, but PBF is not completely dependent on the ductus. In most cases of severe or critical obstruction, right ventricular hypertrophy is considerable, and the noncompliant right ventricle creates a preferential right-to-left shunt at the atrial level, resulting in arterial hypoxemia. Balloon valvuloplasty has become the procedure of choice in this disease, with excellent short- and mid-term results (Planche et al, 1988). It is important to emphasize that in most cases of critical pulmonary stenosis, even after the valvar obstruction is relieved, there is persistent right-to-left atrial shunting and hypoxemia. However, regression of hypertrophy will occur over the next 3 to 6 months, and atrial-level shunting will decrease over time.

## OTHER COMMON LESIONS MANIFESTING IN THE NEONATAL PERIOD

### Heterotaxy Syndrome

Arguably, there is no more confusing nomenclature than that associated with the heterotaxy syndrome, and there is no larger group of heterogeneous congenital heart lesions. Alternatively, this group of structural heart lesions has been called *atrial isomerism* and *asplenia* or *polysplenia syndrome* (Fig. 57–26). It is beyond the scope of this chapter to detail all of the subtleties of the multiple anatomic variants and the corresponding surgical strategies for correction; the reader is referred to more comprehensive texts in cardiology and cardiac surgery (Allen et al, 2001; Fyler, 1992a).

This group of rare lesions (1/10,000 live births) (Lin et al, 2002) shares the common abnormality of failure of "right-left" differentiation, leading to ambiguities of atrial and visceral "sidedness," abnormalities of the conduction system, and characteristic anomalies of systemic and pulmonary venous return. Reported risk factors have included a family history of malformations, maternal diabetes, maternal cocaine use, and genetic microdeletions (Kuehl and Loffredo, 2002, Lin et al, 2002). Although some cases have trivial abnormalities of systemic venous return (e.g., bilateral superior venae cavae) and abdominal positioning abnormalities, a majority of cases have a functional single ventricle. These are usually of right ventricular morphology, with an endocardial cushion defect and a common AV valve. The conduction system frequently is abnormal, with dual sinus and/or AV nodes, and supraventricular tachycardia, sinus node dysfunction, or AV block may occur. The branching pattern of the pulmonary arteries and bronchi is variable and generally assumes one of two forms: bilateral right-sidedness (asplenia) with an eparterial bronchus and first branch of the pulmonary artery to the upper lobe or bilateral left-sidedness (polysplenia) with bronchi below the pulmonary artery at the hilum and bilateral, bilobate lungs. Frequently there is obstruction to PBF, as a result of muscular subvalvar pulmonary

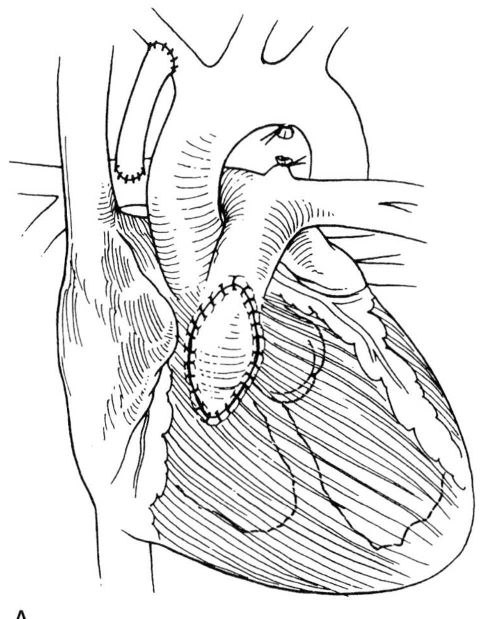

A

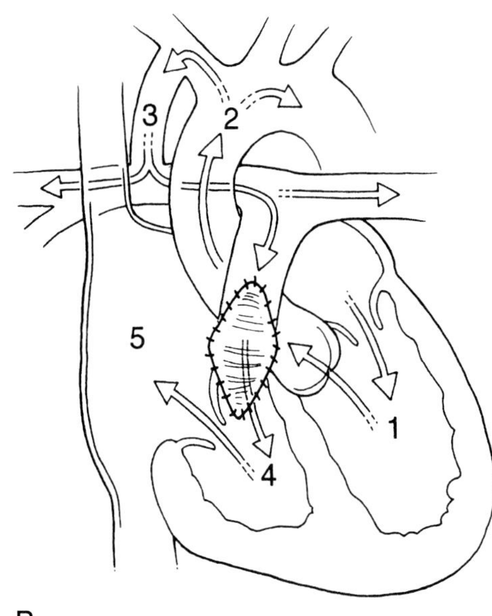


B

**FIGURE 57–24.** **A,** Newborn surgical palliation for pulmonary atresia with intact ventricular septum and normal coronary arteries. A right ventricular outflow tract patch is placed, the ductus is ligated and divided, and a modified Blalock-Taussig (BT) shunt is placed. **B,** Circular shunting following palliative surgery. Presence of a BT shunt in combination with obligate pulmonary insufficiency, associated tricuspid valve insufficiency, and atrial septal defect can result in flow patterns as shown *(arrows)* in this diagram. Blood from the left atrium enters the left ventricle (1) and the aorta (2) and then passes through the BT shunt (3) into the pulmonary artery, then retrograde across the right ventricular outflow tract (4) and retrograde across the tricuspid valve into the right atrium (5), and then across the right atrium back to the left atrium. See text for details *(From Wernovsky G, Hanley FL: Pulmonary atresia with intact ventricular septum. In Chang AC, Hanley FL, Wernovsky G, Wessel DL [eds]: Pediatric Cardiac Intensive Care. Baltimore, Williams & Wilkins, 1998, pp 265-270.)*

stenosis or plate-like valvar atresia, and prostaglandin therapy may be necessary to maintain ductal patency before placement of a Blalock-Taussig shunt. Although a majority of neonates with heterotaxy have obstruction to PBF, some may have obstruction to SBF, with subaortic obstruction and/or coarctation, necessitating neonatal palliation similar to that for HLHS.

Splenic function (even in *polysplenia syndrome*) is typically abnormal and can be diagnosed by the presence of an increased number of Howell-Jolly bodies in the routine blood smear. There is no strong evidence to support treatment for heterotaxy patients similar that for patients with functional asplenia from other medical or surgical conditions; nevertheless, many practitioners maintain patients with heterotaxy on life-long ampicillin, and immunization against encapsulated organisms is considered important.

Main pulmonary artery
Valve
Ceph
R L
Caud

**FIGURE 57–25.** (See also Color Plate 57–25.) Exposure of a severely stenotic pulmonary valve through a pulmonary arteriotomy. *(From Litwin SB: Color Atlas of Congenital Heart Surgery. St. Louis, Mosby, 1996.)*

### Total Anomalous Pulmonary Venous Return

Total anomalous pulmonary venous return occurs in 1/15,0000 live births. This condition is characterized by failure of incorporation of the common pulmonary vein/venous confluence into the posterior aspect of the left atrium. The fetal (and postnatal) pulmonary venous return is thus directed to the systemic venous circulation through a number of potential vestigial venous structures, with complete mixing of pulmonary and systemic venous returns. The anomalous connections of the pulmonary veins may be (1) supracardiac (usually into the right superior vena cava or to the innominate vein via a persistent vertical vein), (2) cardiac (usually to the right atrium or

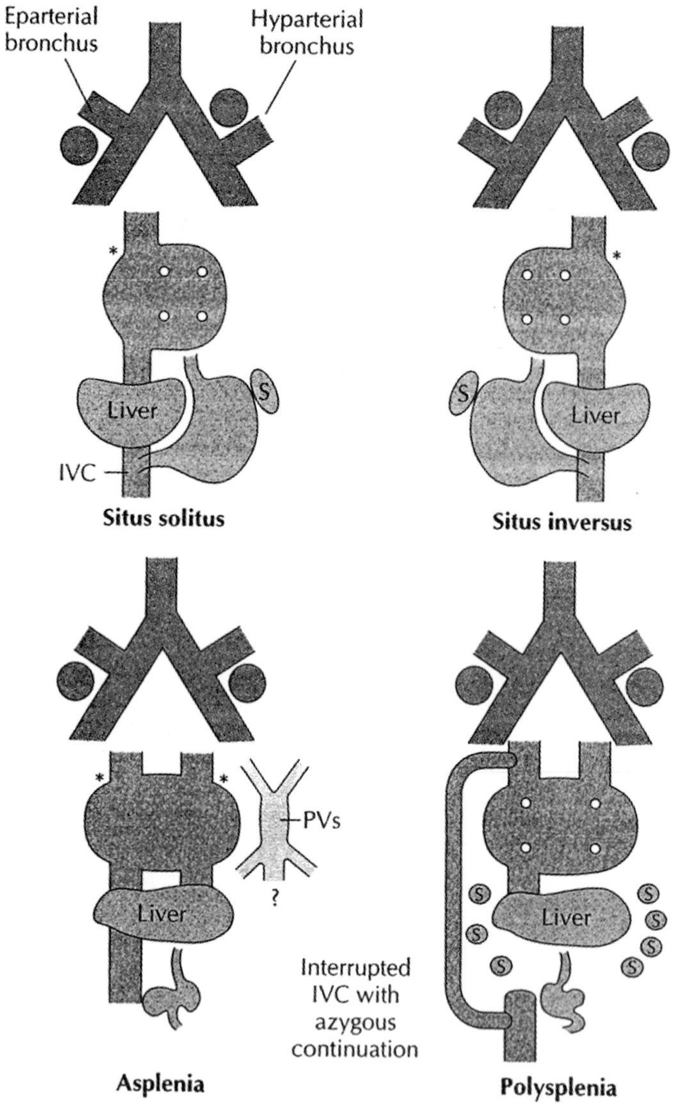

**FIGURE 57–26.** Situs and looping abnormalities: "Heterotaxy syndrome." See text for details. IVC, inferior vena cava; PVs, pulmonary veins; S, spleen. *(From Lacro RV: Genetics, teratology, and syndromes of congenital heart disease. In Braunwald E [ed]: Atlas of Heart Diseases. Philadelphia, Mosby–Year Book, 1997, pp 2.1-2.12.)*



coronary sinus), (3) infracardiac (usually into the portal system), or (4) mixed drainage (Fig. 57–27). Filling of the left ventricle is thus dependent on an obligate shunt through the patent foramen ovale into the left heart to provide adequate cardiac output.

Patients may be physiologically categorized as either those with no obstruction to pulmonary venous return or those with anatomic narrowing of the connection or pathway of the pulmonary venous confluence to the systemic venous circulation. In those with no obstruction (or only a mild degree of obstruction), there may be no symptoms or visible cyanosis, with many neonates escaping recognition of their condition until later in infancy. However, in patients with obstruction of pulmonary venous return, findings include severe pulmonary venous hypertension, severe restriction to antegrade PBF, pulmonary hypertension, and profound hypoxemia. Most of these cases will have an obstructed pathway from the pulmonary venous chamber inferiorly below the diaphragm through the liver (subdiaphragmatic type) or from the pulmonary venous chamber superiorly, with narrowing between the bronchus and pulmonary artery (supracardiac type). In patients with moderate obstruction, there is adequate PBF and mixing of systemic and pulmonary venous returns to achieve adequate oxygen delivery to the tissues. Many of these patients will benefit from supplemental oxygen, mechanical ventilation with positive end-expiratory pressure, and sedation to reduce oxygen consumption.

In cases of severe obstruction with significantly reduced PBF, the diagnosis may be difficult to make noninvasively by echocardiography. In these cases, the pulmonary veins may be small, and when little flow is present, they are difficult to visualize with color Doppler. In addition, the congested appearance of the lungs on radiographs and a right-to-left shunt at the ductus arteriosus may suggest lung disease with elevated PVR as the etiology of hypoxemia. Many neonates are so severely ill from profound hypoxemia that they are initially treated with ECMO before definitive diagnosis of obstructed pulmonary venous return. Even in the current era of prostaglandin therapy, echocardiography, improved ventilatory support, and advanced medical intensive care,

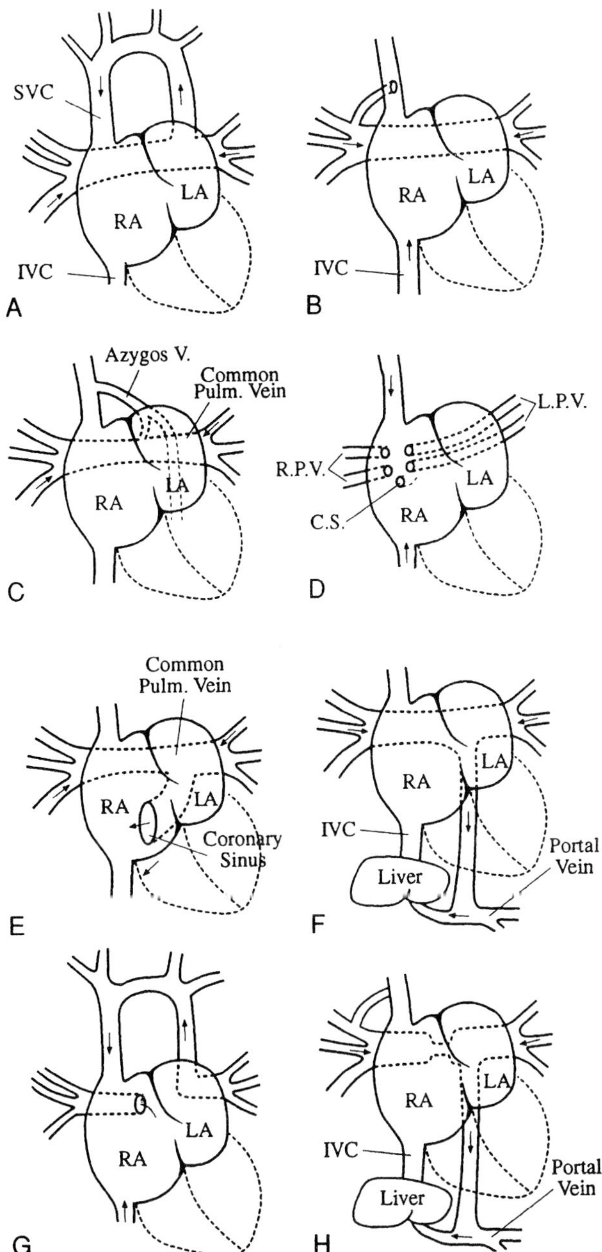


**FIGURE 57–27.** Anatomic varieties of total anomalous pulmonary venous return: **A-C,** supracardiac; **D** and **E,** cardiac; **F,** infracardiac; **G** and **H,** mixed. See text for details. C.S., coronary sinus; IVC, inferior vena cava; LA, left atrium; L.P.V., left pulmonary vein; RA, right atrium; R.P.V., right pulmonary vein; SVC, superior vena cava. *(From Eimbcke F, Enriquez G, Gomez O, Zilleruelo R: Total anomalous pulmonary venous connection. In Moller JH, Hoffman JIE [eds]: Pediatric Cardiovascular Medicine. Philadelphia, Churchill Livingstone, 2000, pp 409-420.)*

severely obstructed total anomalous pulmonary venous return represents one of the few remaining congenital heart lesions that may require emergent, "middle of the night" surgical intervention. Severe obstruction represents a surgical emergency, with minimal beneficial effects from medical management. Although $PGE_1$ will maintain ductal patency, the limitation of PBF in these patients is due *not* to limited antegrade flow into the pulmonary circuit but rather to outflow obstruction at the pulmonary veins. Early recognition of the problem and prompt surgical intervention are necessary for the infant to survive.

Whether or not obstruction to pulmonary venous return exists, in virtually all cases there is a common pulmonary venous confluence behind the left atrium. Surgical repair consists of a direct anastomosis of this chamber to the left atrium, with division and/or ligation of the accessory venous connection to the systemic venous return (Fig. 57–28). Surgical mortality risk is principally dependent on the anatomic and physiologic variability in this disease; the surgical mortality rate is less than 5% in patients with uncomplicated, unobstructed anatomy, and incrementally higher in cases of complex connections and/or obstruction. In cases with severe preoperative obstruction, the postoperative course is frequently marked by pulmonary vascular lability, right ventricular hypertension, and low cardiac output syndrome.

Late pulmonary venous obstruction may occur in upwards of 20% of cases (especially if obstruction exists at presentation) and, if present, is very difficult to treat surgically. Pulmonary venous hypoplasia, in addition to suture line narrowing, complicates many of these cases (Kirshbom et al, 2002). In addition, interventional catheterization procedures to dilate the confluence or to place expandable stents also have been met with little success. Lung transplantation may need to be considered in some cases. In children in whom late obstruction does not develop, functional outcomes are good, with little limitation to daily activities and no need for frequent follow-up or long-term medications.

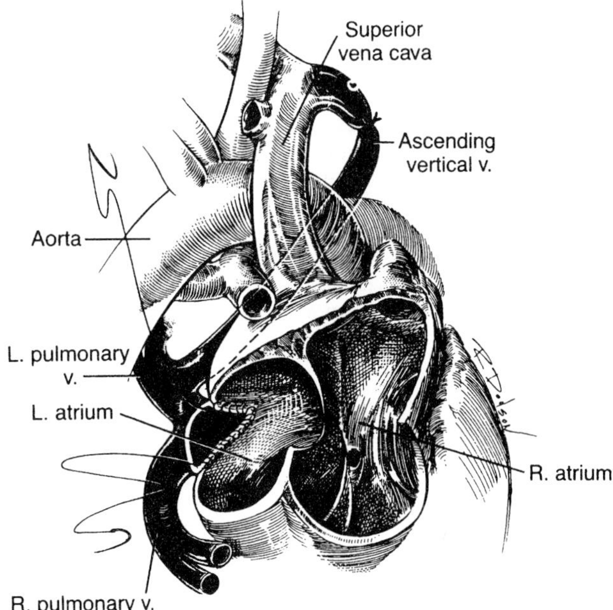


**FIGURE 57–28.** Repair of supracardiac total anomalous pulmonary venous return by connecting the horizontal pulmonary venous confluence into the left atrium. *(From Castañeda AR, Jonas RA, Mayer JE Jr, Hanley FL: Cardiac Surgery of the Neonate and Infant. Philadelphia, WB Saunders, 1994.)*

### Transposition of the Great Arteries

TGA occurs in approximately 1/3500 live births, is more frequent in males, and is not typically associated with additional noncardiac anomalies or genetic syndromes. *Transposition* is defined as an aorta arising from the morphologically right ventricle and the pulmonary artery from the morphologically left ventricle. About half of the patients have an associated VSD, and perhaps 10% have either obstruction to systemic blood flow (usually coarctation) or obstruction to PBF (usually subpulmonary and valvar pulmonary stenosis).

In the usual arrangement this creates a situation of "parallel circulations" with systemic venous return being pumped via the aorta back to the systemic circulation, and pulmonary venous return being pumped via the pulmonary artery to the pulmonary circulation. Following separation from the placenta, neonates with transposition are dependent on mixing between the parallel systemic and pulmonary circulations in order for them to survive. In patients with an intact ventricular septum, this communication exists through the patent ductus arteriosus and the patent foramen ovale. These patients are usually clinically cyanotic within the first hours of life, leading to early diagnosis of TGA. Those infants with an associated VSD typically have somewhat improved mixing between the systemic and pulmonary circulations and may not be as severely cyanotic. See the earlier sections on the transitional circulation and the physiologic classification of heart disease for a full description of transposition physiology, mixing, and initial management.

In the current era, definitive management in patients with two normal-sized ventricles and no obstruction to PBF is surgical correction with an arterial switch operation in the early neonatal period (Wernovsky and Freed, 1997; Wernovsky et al, 1995) (Fig. 57–29). In uncomplicated cases, the surgical mortality rate is less than 5%, with higher risk in patients with low birth weight, additional cardiac anomalies (e.g., coarctation, dextrocardia), and/or abnormal coronary artery origins or distribution. The postoperative course is frequently marked by a transient period of low cardiac output, and the multiple suture lines at systemic pressure are at risk for bleeding. Mid-term

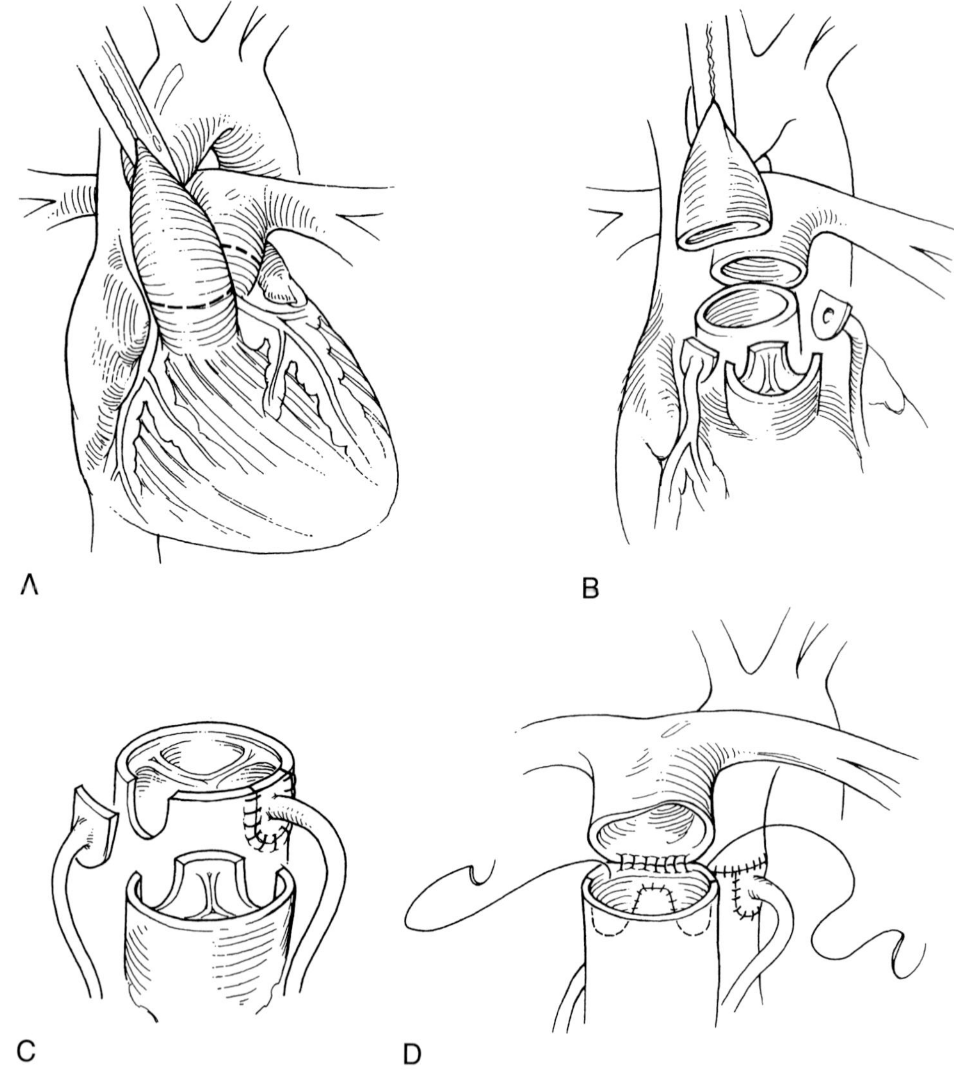


**FIGURE 57–29.** Repair of *d*-transposition of the great arteries by the arterial switch procedure. **A,** The *dashed lines* depict the planned location of transection of the great vessels. **B,** The coronary arteries are removed with surrounding aortic wall as "buttons." **C,** Following a counterincision in the neoaorta, the coronary buttons are translocated to the posterior semilunar root. **D,** The Lecompte maneuver brings both pulmonary arteries anterior to the neoaorta. The aortic suture line is completed, incorporating the coronary buttons. The coronary donor sites are filled in with patches of autologous pericardium, and the pulmonary anastomosis is completed. *(From Wernovsky G, Jonas RA: Transposition of the great arteries. In Chang AC, Hanley FL, Wernovsky G, Wessel DL [eds]: Pediatric Cardiac Intensive Care. Baltimore, Williams & Wilkins, 1998, pp 289-301.)*

follow-up studies (Haas et al, 1999; Hovels-Gurich et al, 2003; Hutter et al, 2002; Wernovsky et al, 1995; Williams et al, 2003) reveal a late reintervention rate of 10% to 15%, typically for supravalvar pulmonary stenosis. Rarely, late deaths have occurred, presumably from coronary events. As the earliest survivors of this operation now are approaching young adulthood, there is a growing recognition of late dilation of the neoaortic root and neoaortic regurgitation in as many as 50% of patients.

### Tetralogy of Fallot

Originally described in the early 19th century, tetralogy of Fallot remains one of the most common and well-described congenital heart lesions. Fallot originally recognized the common association of VSD, subvalvar and valvar pulmonary stenosis, right ventricular hypertrophy, and a location of the aortic root so that it appeared to "override" the ventricular septum (Fig. 57–30). Current thinking is that this constellation of morphologic observations results from a single anatomic defect: anterior deviation of the infundibular septum. This "malalignment" of the infundibular (or conal) septum with the muscular septum results in incomplete separation of the right and left ventricles (VSD), a narrowed right ventricular outflow tract (subvalvar obstruction to PBF), and an aortic valve that is more rightward and anterior than usual, thus "overriding" the muscular ventricular septum. Right ventricular hypertrophy develops not because of the obstruction to PBF but from the fact that the VSD is nonrestrictive, thus maintaining systemic-level pressure in the right side of the heart. The severity of pulmonary obstruction is variable, but all patients with tetralogy of Fallot will have right ventricular hypertrophy, even in the face of relatively mild pulmonary stenosis.

Most children with tetralogy of Fallot are asymptomatic and present in the early newborn period with a harsh murmur across the right ventricular outflow tract. Rarely, obstruction to PBF is quite severe, resulting in visible cyanosis; rare patients have such severe obstruction to PBF that they require stabilization with $PGE_1$. In these children, management options include palliation with a systemic-to-pulmonary shunt (e.g., modified Blalock-Taussig shunt) and complete anatomic correction in the newborn period. In older children without significant hypoxemia or symptoms, elective repair in the first 6 months of life is recommended (Fig. 57–31).

Surgical mortality risk is quite low (1% to 2%) in patients without additional comorbid conditions (e.g., prematurity) (Hirsch et al, 2000). Reintervention is uncommon in childhood, usually being limited to angioplasty of

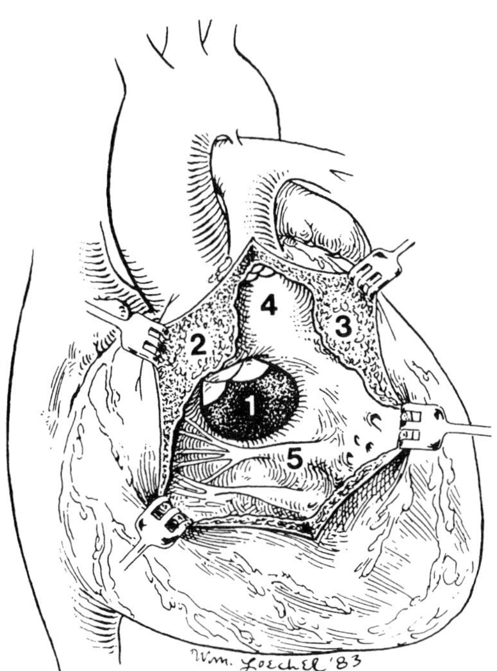


**FIGURE 57–30.** Anatomy of tetralogy of Fallot. Principal anatomic components include malalignment ventricular septal defect with aortic override (1), obstruction of the right ventricular outflow tract (2, 3) with pulmonary stenosis (4) and right ventricular hypertrophy (5). *(From Mavroudis C, Backer CL: Pediatric Cardiac Surgery. St. Louis, Mosby–Year Book, 1994.)*

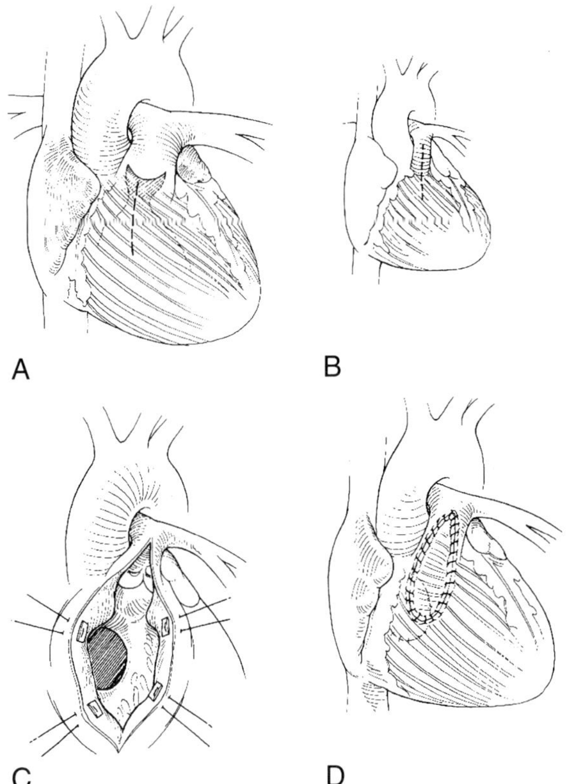


**FIGURE 57–31.** Repair of tetralogy of Fallot. **A,** *Dashed line* depicts non-transannular incision, used when the pulmonary valve and annulus are of adequate size. **B,** A transannular incision *(dashed line)* is used when there is annular hypoplasia. **C,** An example of transventricular exposure of the ventricular septal defect (VSD). Alternatively, the VSD may be closed via a right atriotomy through the tricuspid valve. **D,** External view of patch closure of the transannular incision. *(From Spray TL, Wernovsky G: Right ventricular outflow tract obstruction. In Chang AC, Hanley FH, Wernovsky G, Wessel DL [eds]: Pediatric Cardiac Intensive Care. Baltimore, Williams & Wilkins, 1998, pp 257-270.)*

narrowing in the branch pulmonary arteries or surgical closure of residual VSD (Kaulitz et al, 2001). Increasingly, as these patients enter adulthood, pulmonary valve replacement is becoming necessary to correct right ventricular dilation and/or dysfunction (Ternestedt et al, 2001; Warner et al, 2003).

### Tetralogy of Fallot with Absent Pulmonary Valve

Alternatively called *absent* (or *dysplastic*) *pulmonary valve syndrome*, tetralogy of Fallot with absent pulmonary valve (TOF/APV) represents a spectrum of conditions in which there is an abnormally formed pulmonary valve with varying degrees of (1) annular hypoplasia, (2) valvar stenosis, and, most significant, (3) pulmonary regurgitation. Virtually all reported cases are associated with a malalignment type of VSD morphologically identical to that seen in tetralogy of Fallot (hence the term *TOF/APV*), but rare cases with intact ventricular septum have been reported. The principal hemodynamic burden to the fetus in this lesion is pulmonary regurgitation. The regurgitant fraction increases right ventricular volume work and results in aneurysmal dilation of the branch pulmonary arteries with abnormal muscularization of branch pulmonary arteries and the large and small airways (Fig. 57–32).

There are two distinctly different groups of patients with TOF/APV, with minimal overlap: (1) severely symptomatic neonates with hypoxemia and respiratory distress and (2) relatively asymptomatic neonates and young infants with a cardiac murmur and mild hypoxemia (McDonnell et al, 1999). In the severely affected neonate, signs and symptoms related to the intracardiac pathology are worsened by coexisting *airway compression*, which manifests as hyperinflation, $CO_2$ retention, hypoxemia, and respiratory distress. It is sometimes difficult to determine whether the hypoxemia is due principally to intracardiac right-to-left shunting from severe right ventricular outflow obstruction or to intrapulmonary shunting from the airway disease. (In most cases, the hypoxemia results from a combination of these factors.) Because of the extrinsic airway compression, intubation and mechanical ventilation frequently do not improve the gas exchange and abnormal respiratory mechanics; a long expiratory phase, increased positive end-expiratory pressure, and occasionally prone positioning may be necessary. However, urgent surgery often is required in these patients.

In both the severely symptomatic neonate and the minimally symptomatic infant, surgery consists of VSD closure, plication of the pulmonary arteries, relief of the right ventricular outflow tract obstruction, and in most cases, insertion of a valve or monocusp in the right ventricular outflow tract (Fig. 57–33). The mortality risk and both short- and long-term outcomes are related principally to the severity of pulmonary artery dilation and airway compression; severely affected neonates have a high mortality risk, and most of the survivors require long-term mechanical ventilation, progressing to tracheostomy and home ventilation and/or airway stenting in some (Dodge-Khatami et al, 1999; McDonnell et al, 1999). In contrast, children with less significant pulmonary artery dilation and airway symptoms have a low mortality risk and a long-term course similar to that in tetralogy of Fallot.

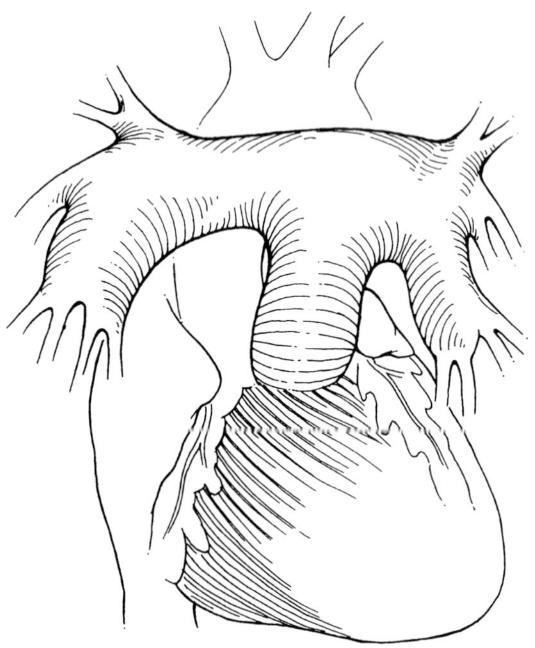

**FIGURE 57–32.** Tetralogy of Fallot with absent pulmonary valve is marked by severe dilatation of the main and branch pulmonary arteries, frequently with associated bronchial compression and large and small airway disease. The intracardiac anatomy is usually similar to that in standard tetralogy of Fallot. *(From Spray TL, Wernovsky G: Right ventricular outflow tract obstruction. In Chang AC, Hanley FH, Wernovsky G, Wessel DL [eds]: Pediatric Cardiac Intensive Care. Baltimore, Williams & Wilkins, 1998, pp 257-270.)*

### Aorticopulmonary Window

*Aorticopulmonary window* is defined as a connection between the ascending aorta and main pulmonary artery; the presence of two separate semilunar valves separates this disease from truncus arteriosus. Aorticopulmonary window is a rare disease sometimes associated with 22q deletion syndrome. More than 50% of the patients have associated lesions, especially ASDs and VSDs, or, more rarely, interruption of the aortic arch distal to the left subclavian artery (type A) with an associated VSD.

The developmental mechanisms leading to aorticopulmonary window are not clear. Anatomic classification of aorticopulmonary window depends on the location of the defect with respect to the semilunar valves. A proximal defect, type 1, occurs just above the sinuses of Valsalva leaving essentially no inferior rim. Distal defects, type 2, are located in the upper ascending aorta and have little upper rim but a well-formed inferior rim, whereas total defects, type 3, have neither upper nor lower rims, with near-complete absence of aorticopulmonary separation.

Affected infants usually demonstrate symptoms of CHF in the first few weeks of life following a fall in PVR. The anatomic communication typically is large and unrestrictive, with a resultant large left-to-right shunt and transmitted pulmonary hypertension; if the defect is left unrepaired, irreversible pulmonary vascular obstructive

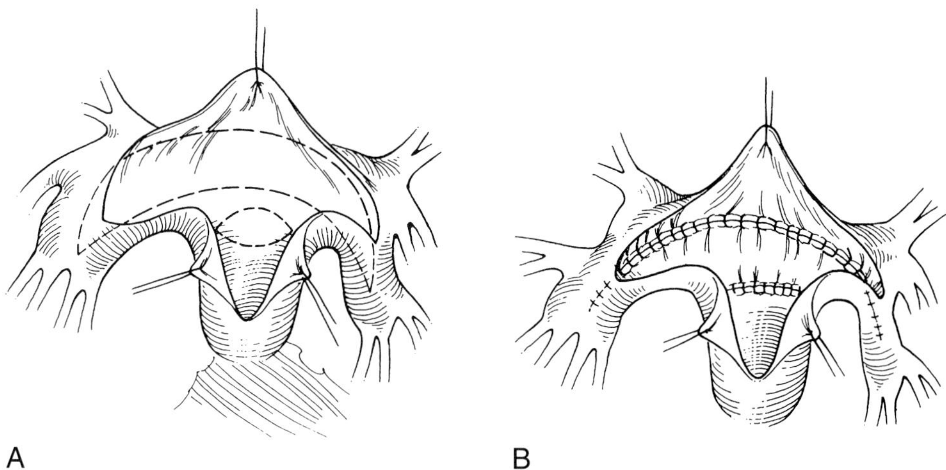


**FIGURE 57–33.** Repair of tetralogy of Fallot with absent pulmonary valve, along with closure of the ventricular septal defect and establishment of continuity between the right ventricle and pulmonary arteries. An important component of repair for tetralogy of Fallot with absent pulmonary valve is plication of the redundant pulmonary arteries. **A,** *Upper dashed line* depicts area of posterior pulmonary arterioplasty. **B,** Completed posterior suture line, prior to anterior pulmonary arterioplasty. *(From Spray TL, Wernovsky G: Right ventricular outflow tract obstruction. In Chang AC, Hanley FH, Wernovsky G, Wessel DL [eds]: Pediatric Cardiac Intensive Care. Baltimore, Williams & Wilkins, 1998, pp 257-270.)*

disease may result. Physiologically, this lesion is much like a patent ductus arteriosus, although the shunt is usually larger. The anatomic diagnosis is usually straightforward by echocardiography; catheterization is rarely necessary for anatomic diagnosis alone. Preoperative management should address the risks of pulmonary hypertension. Repair should be done in most cases shortly after the diagnosis is made. Intermediate forms can sometimes be repaired via catheter-based device closure, although most defects are repaired by surgery. Surgical repair usually is uncomplicated and typically involves patch closure of the defect (Backer and Mavroudis, 2002). The mortality rate is low in the absence of complicated comorbid conditions (Fig. 57–34).

### Vascular Rings and Pulmonary Artery Sling

Abnormalities of branching of the aortic arch vessels may cause compression of the airway and/or esophagus. In the most common form of vascular ring, there is a right-sided aortic arch, but the first branch is not a left innominate artery but an isolated left common carotid artery. The left subclavian artery arises from the descending aorta, passing behind the esophagus. The ligamentum arteriosum connects the posterior left subclavian artery to the anterior left pulmonary artery, "completing" the ring. The second most common variety is a double aortic arch (Fig. 57–35). Pulmonary artery sling is a very rare condition that results from an abnormal origin and course of the left pulmonary artery (LPA). In LPA sling, the artery initially proceeds directly posteriorly and then proceeds leftward in between the trachea and esophagus (Fig. 57–36). Complete cartilaginous rings may be present in the area where the LPA crosses behind the trachea, adding a fixed component of airway obstruction to the dynamic airway compression due to the LPA abnormality. The presentation is variable and related to the degree of airway compression; additional intracardiac pathology is very rare. In the absence of tracheal rings, repair typically is performed by division of the LPA followed by reimplantation anterior to the airway. However, if tracheal rings are present in association with an abnormal airway diameter, repair is much more extensive and complicated. In these cases, either the airway is transected with removal of the rings and end-to-end anastomosis (similar to repair for coarctation of the aorta), or a posterior incision is made in the airway followed by patch augmentation using gluteraldehyde-treated pericardium or artificial material over the posterior portion of the airway. Depending on the anatomy and geometry of the repair, the LPA may not require division but is brought anterior to the reconstructed airway (Bove et al, 2001; van Son et al, 1999) (Fig. 57–37).

If tracheal rings do not complicate the sling, the long-term outcomes are very good, with rare patients requiring balloon angioplasty of the origin of the LPA for late postoperative stenosis. However, if tracheal surgery is necessary, the long-term outcomes are much more variable and complicated and depend primarily on the length and caliber of the reconstructed airway, and whether airway scarring complicates long-term growth.

### Double-Outlet Right Ventricle

The term *double-outlet right ventricle* (DORV) (Fig. 57–38) refers to a heterogeneous group of lesions that share two principal characteristics: (1) both the aorta and pulmonary artery arise from the right ventricle, and (2) a muscular conus or infundibulum below each great artery connects it to the right ventricle. It is beyond the scope of this chapter to describe the multiple different anatomic subtleties of this

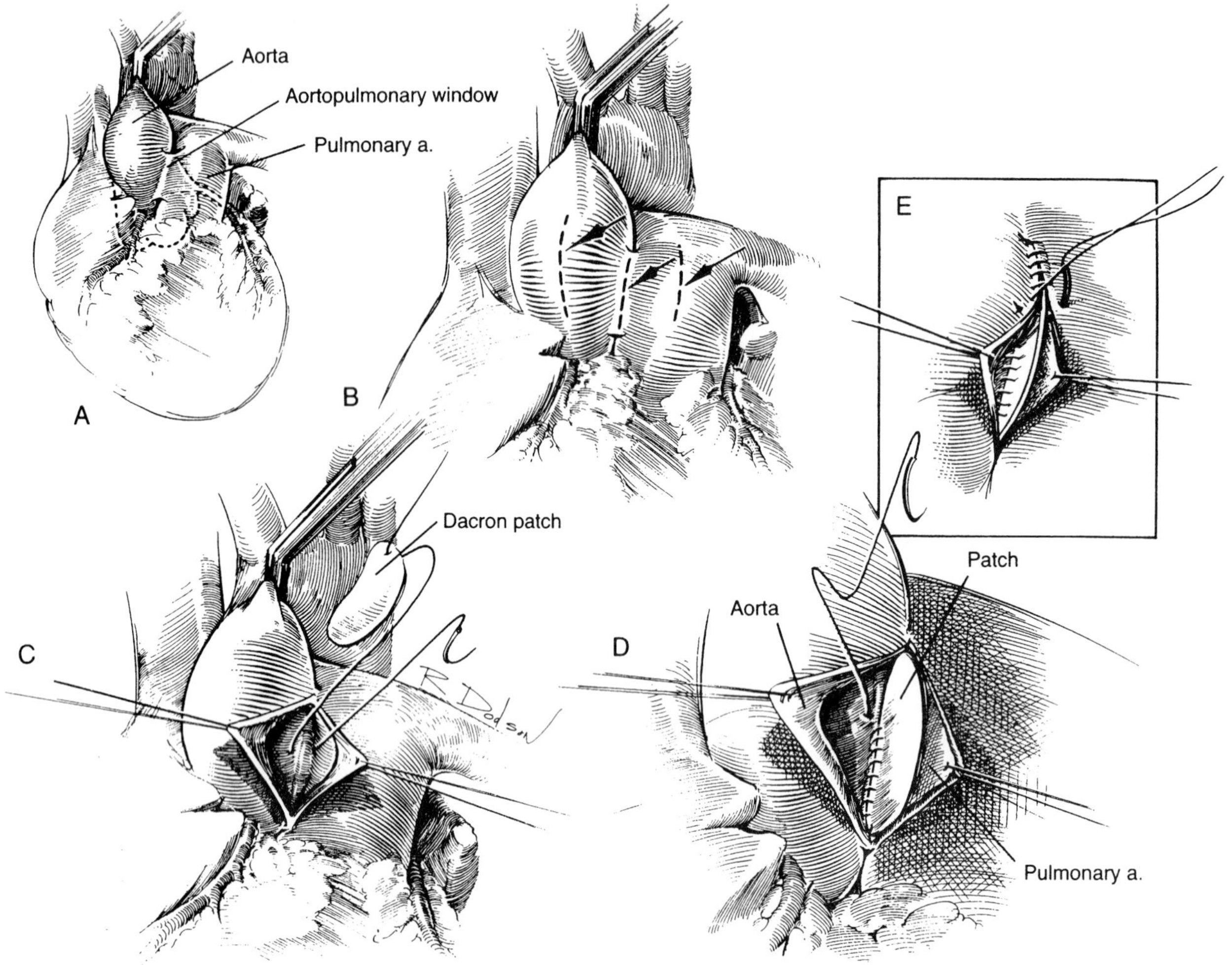

Aorta
Aortopulmonary window
Pulmonary a.
A
B
E
Dacron patch
C
Patch
Aorta
D
Pulmonary a.

**FIGURE 57–34.** Aortopulmonary window. **A,** Surface view. **B,** *Dashed lines* depict possible surgical incision lines based on individual anatomic variation. **C-E,** Patch closure of the defects. Care must be taken to avoid the coronary arteries. *(From Castañeda AR, Jonas RA, Mayer JE Jr, Hanley FL: Cardiac Surgery of the Neonate and Infant. Philadelphia, WB Saunders, 1994.)*

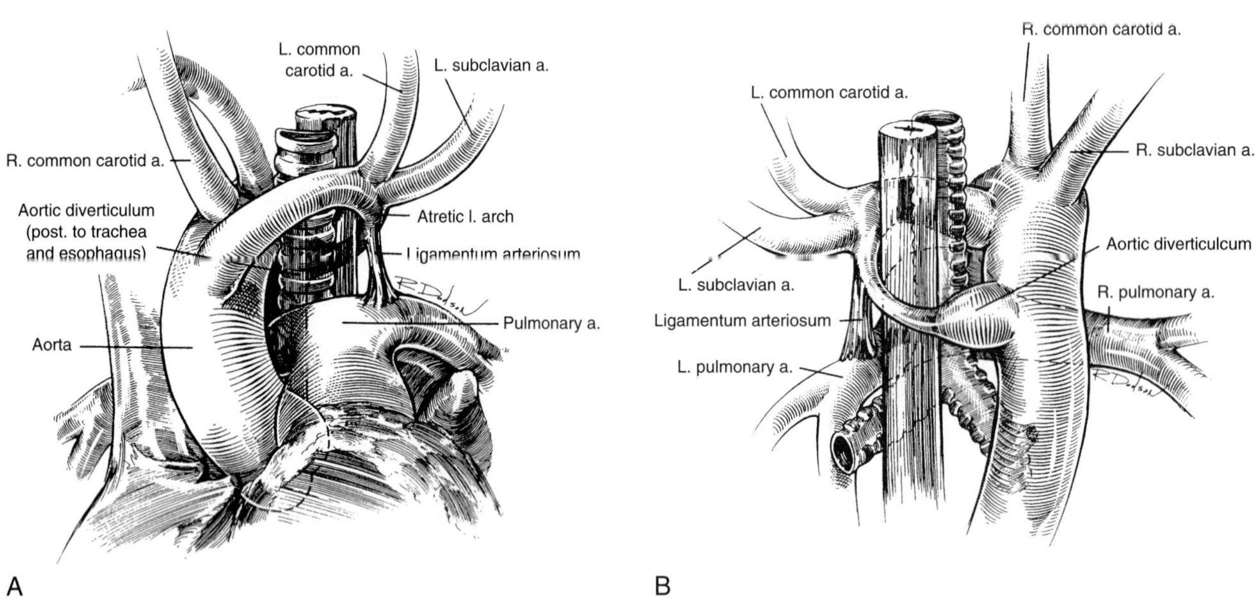


**FIGURE 57–35.** Vascular ring caused by a double aortic arch. **A,** Anteroposterior view; **B,** Posteroanterior view. The most common form of double aortic arch consists of a dominant, posterior right aortic arch and a smaller, anterior arch, usually in combination with a left ligamentum arteriosum. The ligamentum arteriosum contributes to the compression from the ring. *(From Castañeda AR, Jonas RA, Mayer JE Jr, Hanley FL: Cardiac Surgery of the Neonate and Infant. Philadelphia, WB Saunders, 1994.)*

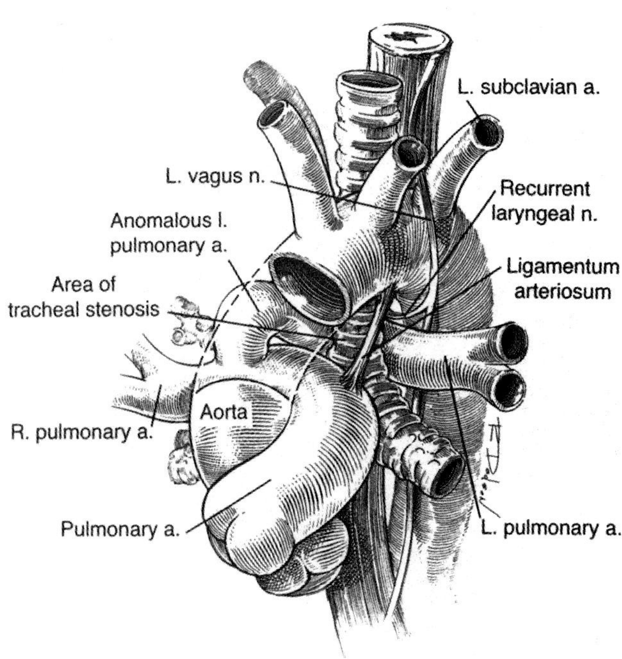


**FIGURE 57–36.** Anatomy of pulmonary artery sling. The left pulmonary artery passes behind the trachea, frequently resulting in tracheal compression.

lesion; entire book chapters and reviews have been dedicated to this one anatomic diagnosis alone (Anderson et al, 1996; Stellin et al, 1991). However, it is useful to characterize DORV into a classification scheme that is related to surgical management and outcome. Some patients have one functional ventricle and are managed with staged reconstruction similar to that for HLHS; these patients typically have a small or atretic mitral valve, a restrictive ASD, a small left ventricle connected to the right ventricle through a VSD, and a high prevalence (perhaps 20% to 25%) of an associated left superior cava to the coronary sinus.

In a larger group of patients with non–single-ventricle physiology, DORV typically is divided into four types related to the location of the VSD vis-à-vis the great arteries and the relationship of the great arteries to each other.

1. In DORV of the *tetralogy* type, the great vessels are normally related to each other, with the aorta–pulmonary artery conotruncus "pulled" anterior and rightward over the right ventricle. The VSD directs blood primarily toward the aorta (subaortic VSD); the pulmonary artery and its supporting conus are typically smaller than the aorta, and the physiology and repair are similar to those in tetralogy of Fallot.
2. In DORV of the *transposition* type, the great vessel relationship is more similar to that in transposition of the great arteries, with the aorta anterior to or directly to

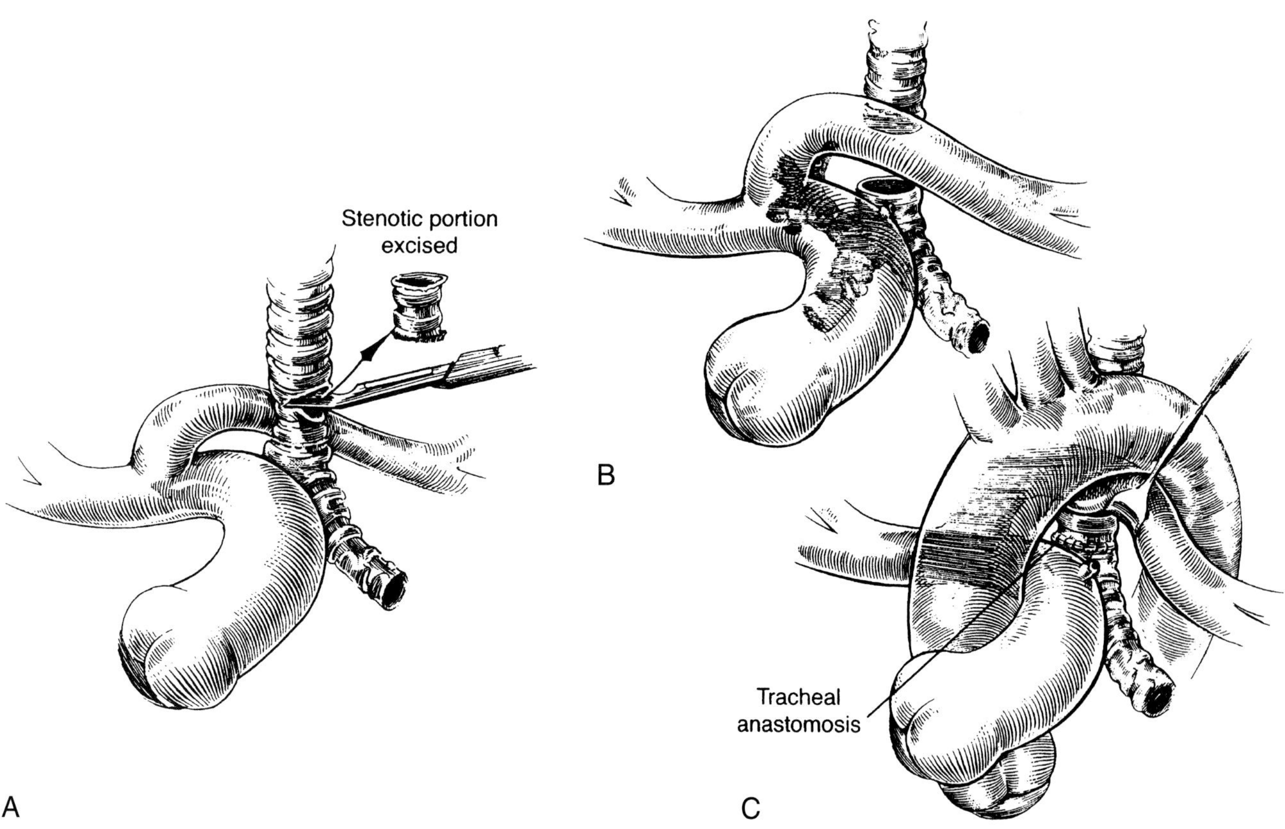


**FIGURE 57–37.** Repair of pulmonary artery sling associated with tracheal stenosis. **A,** The stenotic tracheal segment is resected. **B,** The left pulmonary artery is brought anterior to the tracheal reconstruction. **C,** Completion of the tracheal suture line. *(From Castañeda AR, Jonas RA, Mayer JE Jr, Hanley FL: Cardiac Surgery of the Neonate and Infant. Philadelphia, WB Saunders, 1994.)*

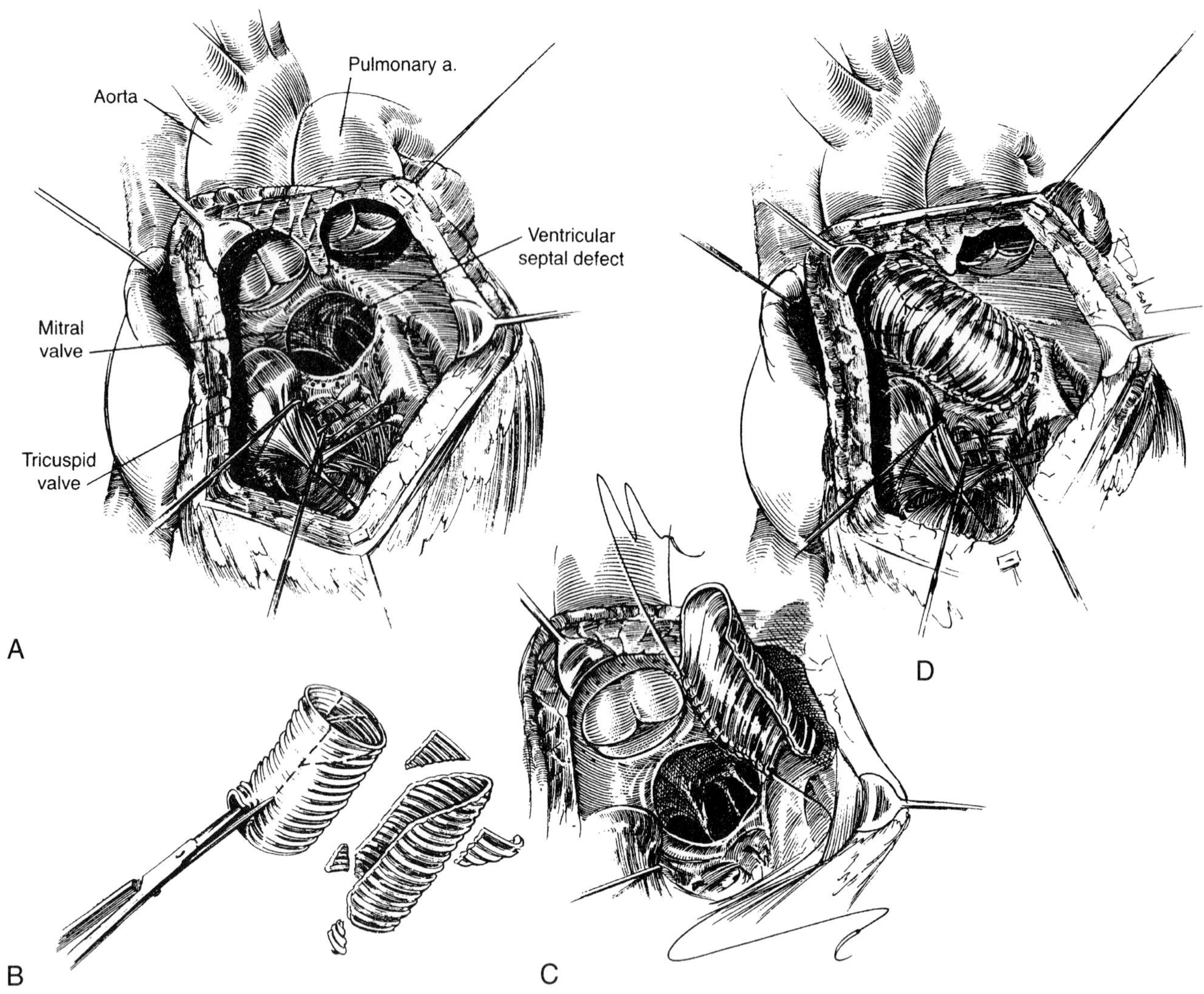


**FIGURE 57–38.** Double-outlet right ventricle with "doubly committed" ventricular septal defect (VSD) (see text). **A,** The *dotted line* depicts the location of the synthetic baffle that will direct blood from the left ventricle through the VSD to the aorta. **B,** Construction of the baffle. **C,** Beginning of suture line around the superior rim of the VSD. **D,** Completed intracardiac baffle ("tunnel"). The right ventriculotomy is then closed, typically with a patch of material to enlarge the right ventricular–to–pulmonary artery pathway. *(From Castañeda AR, Jonas RA, Mayer JE Jr, Hanley FL: Cardiac Surgery of the Neonate and Infant. Philadelphia, WB Saunders, 1994.)*

the right of the pulmonary artery. Again, the aorta–pulmonary artery conotruncus sits directly over the right ventricle, but in contrast with the tetralogy type of DORV, the VSD directs blood toward the pulmonary artery (subpulmonary VSD); the aorta and its supporting conus are typically smaller than the pulmonary artery, and the physiology and repair are similar to those in transposition of the great arteries. An associated coarctation is present in up to 25% of patients with DORV of the transposition type. The so-called Taussig-Bing malformation fits into this variety of DORV, with side-by-side great arteries (with the aorta more rightward), a subpulmonary VSD, and arch hypoplasia.

3. In DORV with a *"doubly committed"* VSD, a large VSD is present below *both* great arteries, with variable physiology depending on the relative degrees of obstruction from the subaortic or subpulmonary infundibulum or conus. Surgical repair in this subgroup must be customized in order to baffle the VSD to one of the great vessels without causing obstruction to the other. If the VSD is more easily "connected" to the pulmonary artery, an arterial switch operation may be necessary as well. If the VSD is more easily "directed" to the aorta, unobstructed flow to the pulmonary arteries may be achieved only with a right ventricle–to–pulmonary artery conduit.
4. Finally, the least common variety of DORV with two ventricles is that associated with a VSD that is *remote* from both great vessels, most typically in the inflow or posterior portion of the ventricular septum. Although there are two anatomically normal ventricles, this uncommon anatomy is most frequently palliated with a single-ventricle approach. Because the VSD is posterior, and both great vessels are anterior over the right ventricle

(typically with interposed chordae of the tricuspid valve), the only effective way to separate the circulation is by means of a Fontan operation. As this is not possible in the newborn period, a pulmonary artery band may be necessary to limit PBF and pressure in the newborn period, followed by staged reconstruction toward a Fontan operation.

The long-term outlook for most patients with DORV is good (Brown et al, 2001), with early and late postoperative sequelae principally related to the type of repair that is possible, which is determined by the location of the VSD and the interrelationship of the great vessels.

## REFERENCES


Allen HD, Gutgesell HP, Clark EB, Driscoll DJ: Heart Disease in Infants, Children, and Adolescents. Philadelphia, Lippincott Williams & Wilkins, 2001.

Anderson RH, Ho SY, Wilcox BR: The surgical anatomy of ventricular septal defect: Part 4. Double outlet ventricle. J Cardiac Surg 11:2-11, 1996.

Atz AM, Munoz RA, Adatia I, Wessel DL: Diagnostic and therapeutic uses of inhaled nitric oxide in neonatal Ebstein's anomaly. Am J Cardiol 91:906-908, 2003.

Backer CL, Mavroudis C: Surgical management of aortopulmonary window: A 40-year experience. Eur J Cardiothorac Surg 21:773-779, 2002.

Bailey LL, Gundry S, Razzouk A, et al: Bless the babies: One hundred fifteen late survivors of heart transplantation during the first year of life. J Thorac Cardiovasc Surg 105:805-815, 1993.

Behrendt DM, Dick M: Truncus repair with a valveless conduit in neonates. J Thorac Cardiovasc Surg 110:1148-1150, 1995.

Bettendorf M, Schmidt KG, Grulich-Henn J, et al: Tri-iodothyronine treatment in children after cardiac surgery: A double-blind, randomised, placebo-controlled study. Lancet 356:529-534, 2000.

Bove T, Demanet H, Casimir G, et al: Tracheobronchial compression of vascular origin—Review of experience in infants and children. J Cardiovasc Surg 42:663-666, 2001.

Braunwald E: Atlas of Heart Diseases. Philadelphia, Current Medicine, 1997.

Brown JW, Ruzmetov M, Okada Y, et al: Surgical results in patients with double outlet right ventricle: A 20-year experience. Ann Thorac Surg 72:1630-1635, 2001.

Carlgren LE, Ericson A, Källén B: Monitoring of congenital cardiac defects. Pediatr Cardiol 8: 247-256, 1987.

Castañeda AR, Jonas RA, Mayer JE Jr, Hanley FL: Cardiac Surgery of the Neonate and Infant. Philadelphia, WB Saunders, 1994.

Chang AC, Burke RP: Left ventricular outflow tract obstruction. In Chang AC, Hanley FH, Wernovsky G, Wessel DL (eds): Pediatric Cardiac Intensive Care. Baltimore, Williams & Wilkins, 1998, pp 233-256.

Chang AC, Hanley FL, Wernovsky G, Wessel DL: Pediatric Cardiac Intensive Care. Baltimore, Williams & Wilkins, 1998.

Daebritz SH, Nollert GDA, Zurakowski D, et al: Results of Norwood stage I operation: Comparison of hypoplastic left heart syndrome with other malformations. J Thorac Cardiovasc Surg 119:358-367, 2000.

Dickinson DF, Arnold RA, Wilkinson, JL: Congenital heart disease among 160, 480 liveborn children in Liverpool 1960 to 1969. Implications for surgical treatment. Br Heart J 46:55-62, 1981.

Dittrich S, Priesemann M, Fischer T, et al: Circulatory arrest and renal function in open-heart surgery on infants. Pediatr Cardiol 23:15-19, 2002.

Dodge-Khatami A, Backer CL, Holinger LD, et al: Complete repair of tetralogy of Fallot with absent pulmonary valve including the role of airway stenting. J Cardiac Surg 14:82-91, 1999.

Egito EST, Moore P, O'Sullivan J, et al: Transvascular balloon dilation for neonatal critical aortic stenosis: Early and midterm results. J Am Coll Cardiol 29:442-447, 1997.

Eimbcke F, Enriquez G, Gomez O, Zilleruelo R: Total anomalous pulmonary venous connection. In Moller JH, Hoffman JIE (eds): Pediatric Cardiovascular Medicine. Philadelphia, Churchill Livingstone, 2000, pp 409-420.

Epstein ML: Congenital stenosis and insufficiency of the tricuspid valve. In Allen HD, Gutgesell HP, Clark EB, Driscoll DJ (eds): Moss and Adams' Heart Disease in Infants, Children and Adolescents: Including the Fetus and Young Adult. Philadelphia, Lippincott Williams & Wilkins, 2001, pp 810-819.

Ferencz C, Rubin JD, McCarter RJ, et al: Congenital heart disease: Prevalence at livebirth. The Baltimore-Washington Infant Study. Am J Epidemiol 121:31-36, 1985.

Freedom RM, Lock J, Bricker JT: Pediatric cardiology and cardiovascular surgery: 1950-2000. Circulation 102:58-68, 2000.

Fyler DC: Report of the New England Regional Infant Cardiac Program. Pediatrics 65 (suppl):377, 1980.

Fyler DC (ed): Nadas' Pediatric Cardiology. Philadelphia, Hanley & Belfus, 1992a.

Fyler DC: Tricuspid atresia. In Fyler DC (ed): Nadas' Pediatric Cardiology. Philadelphia. Hanley & Belfus, 1992b, pp 659-667.

Gaynor JW, Mahle WT, Cohen MI, et al: Risk factors for mortality after the Norwood procedure. Eur J Cardiothorac Surg 22:82-89, 2002.

Gaynor JW, Wernovsky G, Rychik J, et al: Outcome following single-stage repair of coarctation with ventricular septal defect. Eur J Cardiol Surg 18:62-67, 2000.

Ghanayem NS, Hoffman GM, Mussatto KA, et al: Home surveillance program prevents interstage mortality after the Norwood procedure. J Thorac Cardiovasc Surg 126:1367-1377, 2003.

Giglia TM, Mandell VS, Connor AR, et al: Diagnosis and management of right ventricle–dependent coronary circulation in pulmonary atresia with intact ventricular septum. Circulation 86:1516-1628, 1992.

Gold JP, Jonas RA, Lang P, et al: Transthoracic intracardiac monitoring lines in pediatric surgical patients: A ten-year experience. Ann Thorac Surg 42:185-191, 1986.

Gravlee GP, Davis RF, Kurusz M, et al: Cardiopulmonary Bypass: Principles and Practice. Baltimore, Lippincott Williams & Wilkins, 2002.

Haas F, Wottke M, Poppert H, Meisner H: Long-term survival and functional follow-up in patients after the arterial switch operation. Ann Thorac Surg 68:1692-1697, 1999.

Hauser M, Bengel FM, Kuhn A, et al: Myocardial blood flow and flow reserve after coronary reimplantation in patients after arterial switch and Ross operation. Circulation 103:1875-1880, 2001.

Hesz N, Clark EB: Cognitive development in transposition of the great vessels. Arch Dis Child 63:198-200, 1988.

Hirsch JC, Mosca RS, Bove EL: Complete repair of tetralogy of Fallot in the neonate—Results in the modern era. Ann Surg 232:508-514, 2000.

Hoffman TM, Wernovsky G, Atz AM, et al: Efficacy and safety of milrinone in preventing low cardiac output syndrome in infants and children after corrective surgery for congenital heart disease. Circulation 107:996-1002, 2003.

Hovels-Gurich HH, Seghaye MC, et al: Long-term results of cardiac and general health status in children after neonatal arterial switch operation. Ann Thorac Surg 75:935-943, 2003.

Hutter PA, Kreb DL, Mantel SF, et al: Twenty-five years' experience with the arterial switch operation. J Thorac Cardiovasc Surg 124:790-797, 2002.

Kaulitz R, Jux C, Bertram H, et al: Primary repair of tetralogy of Fallot in infancy—the effect on growth of the pulmonary arteries and the risk for late reinterventions. Cardiol Young 11: 391-398, 2001.

Keidan I, Mishaly D, Berkenstadt H, Perel A: Combining low inspired oxygen and carbon dioxide during mechanical ventilation for the Norwood procedure. Paediatr Anaesth 13:58-62, 2003.

Kirshbom PM, Myung RJ, Gaynor JW, et al: Preoperative pulmonary venous obstruction affects long-term outcome for survivors of total anomalous pulmonary venous connection repair. Anna Thorac Surg 74:1616-1620, 2002.

Knott-Craig CJ, Overholt ED, Ward KE, Razook JD: Neonatal repair of Ebstein's anomaly: Indications, surgical technique, and medium-term follow-up. Ann Thorac Surg 69:1505-1510, 2000.

Kuehl KS, Loffredo C: Risk factors for heart disease associated with abnormal sidedness. Teratology 66:242-248, 2002.

Lacro RV: Genetics, teratology, and syndromes of congenital heart disease. In Braunwald E (ed): Atlas of Heart Diseases. Philadelphia, Mosby–Year Book, 1997, pp 2.1-2.12.

Laursen HB: Some epidemiological aspects of congenital heart disease in Denmark. Acta Paediatr Scand 69:619-624,1980.

Lin AE, Ticho BS, Weston WL, Holmes LB: Heterotaxy: Associated conditions and hospital-based prevalence in newborns. Genet Med 2:157-172, 2002.

Litwin SB: Color Atlas of Congenital Heart Surgery. St. Louis, Mosby, 1996.

Maher KO, Pizarro C, Gidding SS, et al: Hemodynamic profile after the Norwood procedure with right ventricle to pulmonary artery conduit. Circulation 108:782-784, 2003.

Mahle WT, Cuadrado AR, Tam VKH: Early experience with a modified Norwood procedure using right ventricle to pulmonary artery conduit. Ann Thorac Surg 76:1084-1088, 2003.

Mahle WT, Spray TL, Gaynor JW, Clark BJ III: Unexpected death after reconstructive surgery for hypoplastic left heart syndrome. Ann Thorac Surg 71:61-65, 2001.

Mahle WT, Spray TL, Wernovsky G, et al: Survival after reconstructive surgery for hypoplastic leftheart syndrome. A 15-year experience from a single institution. Circulation 102:136-141, 2000.

Malec E, Januszewska K, Kolcz J, Mroczek T: Right ventricle–to–pulmonary artery shunt versus modified Blalock-Taussig shunt in the Norwood procedure for hypoplastic left heart syndrome—influence on early and late haemodynamic status. Eur J Cardiothorac Surg 23:728-734, 2003.

Mavroudis C, Backer CL: Pediatric Cardiac Surgery. St. Louis, Mosby–Year Book, 1994.

McDonnell BE, Raff GW, Gaynor JW, et al: Outcome after repair of tetralogy of Fallot with absent pulmonary valve. Ann Thorac Surg 67:1391-1395, 1999.

Moller JH, Hoffman JIE: Pediatric Cardiovascular Medicine. Philadelphia, Churchill Livingstone, 2000.

Monro JL, Alexiou C, Salmon AP, Keeton BR: Reoperations and survival after primary repair of congenital heart defects in children. J Thorac Cardiovasc Surg 126:511-520, 2003.

Nagashima M, Imai Y, Seo K, et al: Effect of hemofiltrated whole blood pump priming on hemodynamics and respiratory function after the arterial switch operation in neonates. Ann Thorac Surg 70:1901-1906, 2000.

Ohye Rg, Gomez CA, Ohye BJ, et al: The Ross/Konno procedure in neonates and infants: Intermediate-term survival and autograft function. Ann Thorac Surg 72:823-830, 2001.

Paul MH, Wernovsky G: Transposition of the great arteries. In Emmanouilides GC, Riemenschneider TA, Allen HD, Gutgesell HP (eds): Moss and Adams' Heart Disease in Infants, Children, and Adolescents, Including the Fetus and Young Adult. Baltimore, Williams & Wilkins, 1995, pp 1154-1225.

Permut LC, Laks H, Aharon A: Surgical management of pulmonary atresia with ventricular septal defect and multiple aortopulmonary collaterals. Isr J Med Sci 30:215-224, 1994.

Pesonen EJ, Peltola KI, Korpela RE, et al: Delayed impairment of cerebral oxygenation after deep hyothermic circulatory arrest in children. Ann Thorac Surg 67:1765-1770, 1999.

Pizarro C, Malec E, Maher KO, et al: Right ventricle to pulmonary artery conduit improves outcome after stage I Norwood for hypoplastic left heart syndrome. Circulation 108:155-160, 2003.

Planche C, Bruniaux J, Lacour-Gayet F, et al: Switch operation for transposition of the great arteries in neonates: A study of 120 patients. J Thorac Cardiovasc Surg 96:354-363, 1988.

Platt JS, O'Brien WF: Group B streptococcus: Prevention of early-onset neonatal sepsis. Obstet Gynecol Surv 58:191-196, 2003.

Reddy VM, Liddicoat JR, Fineman JR, et al: Fetal model of single ventricle physiology: Hemodynamic effects of oxygen, nitric oxide, carbon dioxide, and hypoxia in the early postnatal period. J Thorac Cardiovasc Surg 112:437-449, 1996.

Rome JJ: The role of catheter-directed therapies in the treatment of congenital heart-disease. Ann Rev Med 46:159-168, 1995.

Rome JJ, Mayer JE, Castañeda AR, Lock JE: Tetralogy of Fallot with pulmonary atresia: Rehabilitation of diminutive pulmonary arteries. Circulation 88 (part 1):1691-1698, 1993.

Rychik J, Rome JJ, Collins MH, et al: The hypoplastic left heart syndrome with intact atrial septum: Atrial morphology, pulmonary vascular histopathology and outcome. J Am Coll Cardiol 34:554-560, 1999.

Sano S, Ishino K, Kawada K, et al: Right ventricle–pulmonary artery shunt in first-stage palliation of hypoplastic left heart syndrome. J Thorac Cardiovasc Surg 126:504-510, 2003.

Spray TL, Wernovsky G: Right ventricular outflow tract obstruction. In Chang AC, Hanley FH, Wernovsky G, Wessel DL (eds): Pediatric Cardiac Intensive Care. Baltimore Williams & Wilkins, 1998, pp 257-270.

Stellin G, Ho SY, Anderson RH, et al: The surgical anatomy of double-outlet right ventricle with concordant atrioventricular connection and noncommitted ventricular septal defect. J Thorac Cardiovasc Surg 102:849-855, 1991.

Tabbutt S, Ramamoorthy C, Montenegro LM, et al: Impact of inspired gas mixtures on preoperative infants with hypoplastic left heart syndrome during controlled ventilation. Circulation 104:I159-I164, 2001.

Ternestedt BM, Wall K, Oddsson H, et al: Quality of life 20 and 30 years after surgery in patients operated on for tetralogy of Fallot and for atrial septal defect. Pediatr Cardiol 22:128-132, 2001.

Tweddell JS, Hoffman GM, Fedderly RT, et al: Phenoxybenzamine improves systemic oxygen delivery after the Norwood procedure. Ann Thorac Surg 67:161-167, 1999.

van Son JAM, Hambsch J, Haas GS, et al: Pulmonary artery sling: Reimplantation versus antetracheal translocation. Ann Thorac Surg 68:989-994, 1999.

Warner KG, O'Brien PKH, Rhodes J, et al: Expanding the indications for pulmonary valve replacement after repair of tetralogy of Fallot. Ann Thorac Surg 76:1066-1071, 2003.

Wernovsky G: Transposition of the great arteries. In Allen HD, Gutgesell HP, Clark EB, Driscoll DJ (eds): Moss and Adams' Heart Disease in Infants, Children, and Adolescents: Including the Fetus and Young Adult, 6th ed. Philadelphia, Lippincott Williams & Wilkins, 2001, pp 1027-1084.

Wernovsky G, Chrisant MRK: Long term follow-up after staged reconstruction or transplantation for patients with functionally univentricular heart. Cardiol Young, 14 (supp I):115-126, 2004.

Wernovsky G, Freed MD: Transposition of the great arteries: The arterial switch operation—results and outcome. In Freedom RA (ed): Congenital Heart Disease. Philadelphia, Current Science, 1997.

Wernovsky G, Hanley FL: Pulmonary atresia with intact ventricular septum. In Chang AC, Hanley FL, Wernovsky G,

Wessel DL (eds): Pediatric Cardiac Intensive Care. Baltimore, Williams & Wilkins, 1998, pp 265-270.

Wernovsky G, Jonas RA: Transposition of the great arteries. In Chang AC, Hanley FL, Wernovsky G, Wessel DL (eds): Pediatric Cardiac Intensive Care. Baltimore, Williams & Wilkins, 1998, pp 289-301.

Wernovsky G, Mayer JE Jr, Jonas RA, et al: Factors influencing early and late outcome of the arterial switch operation for transposition of the great arteries. J Thorac Cardiovasc Surg 109:289-302, 1995.

Wessel DL: Commentary: Simple gases and complex single ventricles. J Thorac Cardiovasc Surg 112:655-657, 1996.

Williams WG, McCrindle BW, Ashburn DA, et al: Outcomes of 829 neonates with complete transposition of the great arteries 12–17 years after repair. Eur J Cardiothorac Surg 24:1-9, 2003.

Wypij D, Newburger JW, Rappaport LA, et al: The effect of duration of deep hypothermic circulatory arrest in infant heart surgery on late neurodevelopment: The Boston Circulatory Arrest Trial. J Thorac Cardiovasc Surg 126:1397-1403, 2003.

CHAPTER

# 58

# Arrhythmias in the Fetus and Newborn

**Mitchell I. Cohen and Roy Jedeikin**

Brady- and tachyarrhythmias may occur at any point during the perinatal period. This chapter reviews those arrhythmias occurring during fetal and early neonatal life.

Although the atrioventricular (AV) node and the His bundle develop as separate entities, they appear to join by the eighth week of gestation. By week 16 the conduction system of the fetus is fully developed and sinus rhythm can be detected on screening fetal echocardiograms. Although changes in the heart rate are seen throughout gestation, by the third trimester heart rates typically range from 120 to 160 beats/minute. Bradycardia is defined as a rate of less than 100 beats/minute, and tachycardia as a rate greater than 180 beats/minute. Fetal arrhythmias may develop at any time after the conduction system has completed development, although they are typically seen after 22 weeks of gestation.

Fetal arrhythmias are often the same arrhythmias that are seen in postnatal life. These include, but are not limited to, premature atrial and ventricular beats, automatic tachycardias (e.g., sinus tachycardia), reentrant tachycardias (e.g., supraventricular tachycardia [SVT] or ventricular tachycardia [VT]), and associated bradycardia in the form of either sinus node dysfunction or AV block. It is estimated that the incidence of fetal arrhythmias is 1% to 2% (Clavin et al, 1992). Arrhythmias in the developing fetus may be completely benign, without any hemodynamic sequelae, or in 6% to 7% of fetuses result in significant cardiovascular decompensation, hydrops, and possibly intrauterine death (Allen et al, 1983; Kleinman, 1987; Reed, 1989). Although a majority of fetal arrhythmias are nonsustained events, such as premature atrial depolarizations, they may be associated with underlying congenital heart disease. Additionally, both brady- and tachyarrhythmias may represent underlying noncardiac pathology such as maternal drug abuse or placental insufficiency.

## ASSESSMENT OF FETAL ARRHYTHMIAS

Fetal echocardiography can be performed as early as 16 weeks of gestation and is used to assess structural, functional, and rhythm abnormalities of the fetal heart. Examination techniques have been well described (Cyr et al, 1986; Silverman and Globus, 1985), with emphasis on the importance of a systematic approach to the echocardiographic assessment of the cardiac anatomy. The segmental approach to the anatomic integrity of the fetal heart is the mainstay of accurate and complete diagnosis of fetal cardiac abnormalities (see Chapter 52).

Fetal echocardiography using M-mode (Fig. 58–1) and Doppler (Fig. 58–2) techniques has been well described in the evaluation of fetal cardiac arrhythmias (Allen et al, 1983; Kleinman et al, 1995; Silverman et al, 1988). These modalities allow assessment of atrial rate, ventricular rate, and the AV relationship to help define the exact type of dysrhythmia present.

More recently, tissue Doppler imaging in fetal cardiac arrhythmias has been used as a methodology allowing simultaneous recording and analysis of mechanical activity of the atrial and ventricular tissues at high temporal and spatial resolution (Rein et al, 2002).

Congenital complete heart block (CCHB) in the setting of maternal collagen vascular disease is associated with significant morbidity and mortality (Groves et al, 1996; Jaeggi, et al, 2002; Michaelsson and Engle, 1972; Schmidt et al, 1991). The diagnosis in utero of AV dissociation can be well established by using current Doppler and M-mode techniques (Fig. 58–3). It is known that once autoimmune CCHB has been established, this process is irreversible. Case reports have suggested that maternal steroid and other therapies may reduce the development of permanent injury to the AV node in these high-risk fetuses (Theander et al, 2000; Yamada et al, 1999).

Doppler echocardiography can now be used to estimate the P-R interval (mechanical interval [MI]). Normal measurement data indicate that in the unaffected fetus this interval is less than 150 msec; intervals longer than 150 msec suggest first-degree AV block (Glickstein et al, 2000). The MI can be obtained by placing the Doppler signal in the area between the aortic and the mitral valves. The MI is the interval from the onset of the atrial contraction (A-wave) to the onset of the ventricular contraction (V-wave) in the left ventricular outflow tract (see Fig. 58–2). Another tool to assess AV temporal relationships is the simultaneous recording of Doppler flow signals in the superior vena cava (retrograde A-wave flow during atrial systole) and the ascending aorta/antegrade ejection (V-wave) (Andelginfer et al, 2001). With systematic utilization of these physiologic/mechanical principles, electrical disturbances of the fetal heart can be defined, allowing appropriate in utero diagnosis and therefore appropriate treatment strategies.

## FETAL BRADYCARDIA

### Premature Atrial and Ventricular Ectopy

Irregularity is frequently seen during the third trimester of pregnancy and typically is a result of either premature atrial or ventricular contractions. Premature atrial contractions (PACs) are generally considered a benign entity, provided that there is no evidence of structural heart disease and that the premature beats do not initiate a sustained reentrant tachycardia. If a PAC occurs prior to ventricular myocardial recovery (early diastole), the PAC is unable to depolarize the ventricle and will reset the sinus node (blocked PAC). Care must be taken to ensure that blocked premature atrial beats are not mistaken for complete AV block. Although atrial ectopy is considered to have a

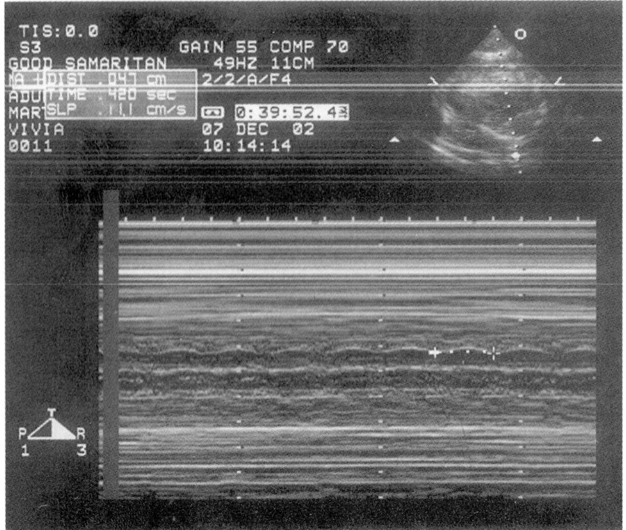


**FIGURE 58–1.** M-mode echocardiogram demonstrating ventricular wall motion. Hatch marks represent a ventricular cycle length of 420 msec (143 beats/minute).

benign prognosis, it is crucial that blocked PACs are *not* falsely identified as sinus bradycardia, a potentially more ominous sign of fetal demise necessitating early delivery. A small percentage of fetuses with isolated atrial ectopy may develop an in utero or postnatal form of SVT such as atrial flutter or orthodromic reentrant SVT. Our practice has been to closely follow newborns with isolated premature atrial beats for the first few months of life to be certain that there has not been a progression to a more sustained dysrhythmia warranting antiarrhythmic therapy.

Premature ventricular contractions (PVCs) are less frequently seen than their atrial counterpart; in isolation they also are thought to carry a benign prognosis. Associated conditions such as the long Q-T syndrome, congenital heart disease, or electrolyte abnormalities should be excluded if PVCs are identified. Neither atrial nor ventricular ectopy necessarily signifies fetal distress, and delivery should not be expedited on the basis of these findings. Frequent monitoring of fetal heart tones, for both PACs and PVCs, should be performed bimonthly by the obstetrician to be certain that progression of the arrhythmia, albeit rare, has not taken place. If there is any concern that a fetus is developing sustained or nonsustained episodes of SVT, follow-up discussions with the pediatric cardiologist are warranted.

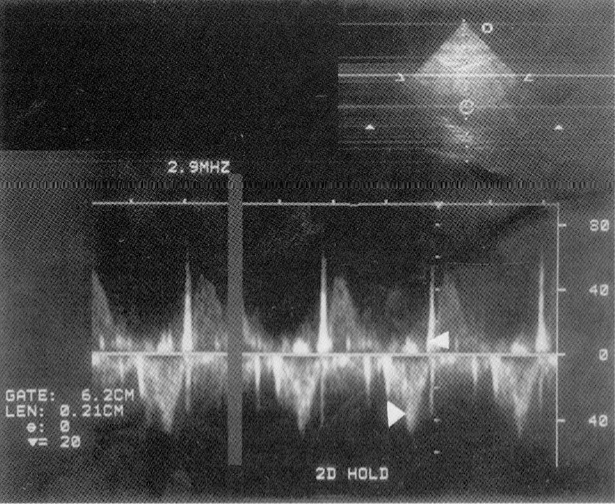


**FIGURE 58–2.** Doppler waveforms demonstrating atrioventricular synchrony. Mitral inflow (atrial systole) is shown below baseline, and left ventricular outflow tract (ventricular systole) signal is above baseline. Mechanical interval (MI) is shown between the two *arrows*.

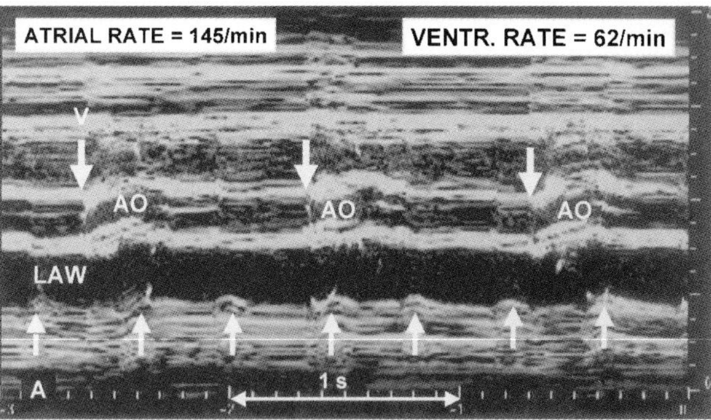


**FIGURE 58–3.** M-mode echocardiogram demonstrating complete heart block with dissociation between atria (left atrial wall motion, *upward arrows*) and ventricular systole (aortic valve opening, *downward arrows*).

## Fetal Heart Block

Congenital complete heart block (CCHB) is often detected by evaluation of a slow heart rate on a routine obstetric examination. Congenital complete heart block results from complete discontinuity between the atrium and the ventricle, with the atrial rate exceeding the ventricular rate (see Fig. 58–3). The QRS complexes are almost always narrow and normal. The Q-T interval may be prolonged. The incidence of CCHB is approximately 1 in every 15,000 to 20,000 live births (Michaelsson and Engle, 1972). In a study from Finland, Siren and colleagues (1998) found that the incidence during the last decade has increased to 1 in 11,000 births. This increase may be secondary to improved diagnostic capabilities as well as more effective antenatal care. Alternatively, the increase may reflect a higher obstetric success rate among gravid mothers with known connective tissue disorders.

Congenital AV block has been associated with structural heart defects in approximately 50% of cases (Schmidt et al, 1991). The etiology of the AV block probably resides in both the abnormal position and course of the conduction tissue. Malformations that are typically associated with CCHB include L-transposition of the great arteries (L-TGA), left atrial isomerism typically with AV septal defects, and other forms of AV discordance. However, in the absence of structural heart defects, CCHB is typically associated with maternal connective tissue disorders.

## Isolated Congenital Complete Heart Block

Although Stokes-Adams attacks were originally described by Morquio in 1901, it was not until the 1960s that the association of CCHB with maternal systemic lupus erythematosus (SLE) became well recognized (Hull et al, 1966; McCue et al, 1977). The pathogenesis of lupus-associated CCHB results from transplacental transfer of maternal antibodies (IgG Ro [SS-A] and IgG La [SS-B]), which initiates an inflammatory reaction within the AV node proper, resulting in tissue necrosis and fibrous replacement (Thomas et al, 1996). The majority of cases of CCHB are detected between 16 and 23 weeks of gestation coincident with the placental transfer of these antibodies. Congenital AV block associated with maternal connective tissue disorders is often complete, though cases of incomplete or transient AV block have been reported (Esscher and Scott, 1979).

Aside from transplacental AV node disruption, maternal antibodies may also cause an immunomyocarditis and dilated cardiomyopathy (Scott et al, 1983; Udink ten Cate et al, 2001). Whereas only 1% of fetuses born to mothers with maternal SLE develop CCHB, nearly 100% of the affected fetuses are positive for anti-Ro (SS-A) antibodies (Buyon et al, 1993). However, of pregnancies in mothers who are known to be anti-Ro positive, only 5% will result in a fetus with CCHB (Jones, 1994). Aside from maternal SLE, other maternal connective tissue disorders (e.g., Sjögren's syndrome) may result in CCHB. Of interest, despite the association of maternal connective tissue disorders with CCHB, most mothers are asymptomatic, without clinical evidence of a rheumatologic process, and the maternal diagnosis is often made retrospectively after the fetus is found to have high-grade AV block. Risk factors associated with the development of fetal heart block include (1) prior pregnancy resulting in CCHB, (2) a direct relationship between CCHB and titers of anti-SS-A, (3) presence of both maternal anti-SS-A and anti-SS-B antibodies, and (4) HLA-DR3-positive haplotype (Olah and Gee, 1991). As reported in the Association of European Pediatric Cardiologists Collaborative Study, of the 67 children with CCHB whose mothers had documented connective tissue disorders, 22 other siblings were affected (Cyr et al, 1986). Prior pregnancy resulting in fetal CCHB appears to be the single greatest risk factor (approximately 30%) for third-degree AV block in babies born subsequently (Waltuck and Buyon, 1994). Finally, the in utero environment or actual timing of transplacental antibody transference may also play a large role in the development of CCHB.

Outcome in the fetus with isolated CCHB appears to be directly related to the heart rate. Of fetuses with a heart rate less than or equal to 50 beats/minute, nearly 45% succumb to an intrauterine death; of the remaining patients, almost all require pacemaker implantation (Groves et al, 1996). In comparison, among fetuses with heart rates greater than 60 beats/minute, the mortality rate is only 6%, with few (3/16, or 18.8%) requiring a pacemaker (Groves et al, 1996). Fetuses with heart rates between 51 and 60 beats/minute tend to have an intermediate mortality rate (27%). Although heart rates generally remain stable during fetal life, a decline of more than 5 beats/minute portends a poorer prognosis (Groves et al, 1996).

## Congenital Complete Heart Block with Structural Heart Disease

The second possible cause of in utero congenital complete AV block relates to the malposition of the normal AV nodal conduction tissue secondary to underlying structural heart disease. Approximately 50% of fetuses with congenital heart block have structural heart disease, the most common forms of which are congenitally corrected transposition of the great arteries (L-TGA), left atrial isomerism, and atrioventricular septal defects (Reed, 1989). Third-degree AV block is present at birth in approximately 5% to 10% of patients with L-TGA, although it develops insidiously at a rate of approximately 2% per year or may occur during surgical correction of an associated lesion such as a ventricular septal defect (Friedberg and Nadas, 1970; Huhta et al, 1983). The etiology of CCHB in L-TGA relates to the anterior malposition of the AV node, which places the conduction system at high risk as the penetrating bundles encircle the subpulmonary (left ventricular [LV]) outflow tract. An alternative explanation may relate to abnormal development of the central fibrous body or a lack of union between the AV node and penetrating bundle (Lev, 1972). The clinical outcome of congenital heart block diagnosed in utero carries a poorer prognosis with concomitant congenital heart disease (CHD). In a multicenter study of 55 fetuses with CCHB (29 structural, 26 isolated), intrauterine death occurred in 7 (24%) with heart disease and 3 (11%) without associated congenital heart defects (Schmidt et al, 1991). Similarly, the incidence of neonatal death was quite high in the group with heart disease: Among infants born alive with CCHB/CHD, the mortality rate was 4/29 (13.8%); among those born alive with isolated CCHB, it was 22/26 (84.6%) (Schmidt et al, 1991). The surviving neonates with CCHB tended to have higher resting ventricular rates than nonsurvivors (68 ± 8 versus 53 ± 8 beats/minute) (Schmidt et al, 1991).

## Diagnosis of Fetal Heart Block

In order to maintain cardiac output, the fetus adapts to marked bradycardia with ventricular dilatation and an augmented stroke volume. Failure of the fetus to maintain an acceptable cardiac output in light of these hemodynamic perturbations results in congestive heart failure and hydrops fetalis. The degree of bradycardia appears to be directly related to the development of hydrops. Nearly 85% of fetuses having rates of less than 55 beats/minute exhibit signs of hydrops such as ascites, anasarca, pleural effusions, tricuspid regurgitation, and/or hepatopathy (Schmidt et al, 1991). Fetal electrocardiography, either through transabdominal auscultation or via electrodes placed directly on the fetal scalp, has largely been abandoned since the advent of fetal echocardiography. Fetal echocardiography allows for a noninvasive assessment of the heart's rate and rhythm by timing mitral valve opening with ventricular contractions. Fetuses can be followed noninvasively by echocardiography with particular attention to not only the junctional/ventricular escape rate but also, of more importance, clinical manifestations such as fetal growth, presence or absence of hydrops, and any associated malformations. Surface electrocardiography is all that is required to make the diagnosis postnatally.

### Management of Fetal Heart Block

Treatment for CCHB varies. In utero treatments for CCHB are designed not only to reduce the symptoms of congestive heart failure but to achieve a more stable intrauterine environment conducive to a successful term pregnancy. Therapeutic options include (1) sympathomimetics, (2) plasmapharesis, (3) steroids, (4) premature delivery, and (5) fetal pacing.

Sympathomimetics, either oral or intravenous, have had occasional anecdotal success in raising the fetal heart rate in both hydropic and nonhydropic fetuses (Groves et al, 1995; Yoshida et al, 2001). However, to date, there have been no controlled or large studies evaluating this therapy. Although plasmapharesis has been successful in reducing the maternal antibody load, there has been only one documented case reversing complete heart block (Kaaja et al, 1991). Both betamethasone and dexamethasone can cross the placenta and suppress the symptoms of hydrops, ascites, and effusions but, as with plasmapharesis, do not reverse the heart block. However, there is evidence that early (at approximately 20 to 23 weeks of gestation) use of dexamethasone (4 mg PO daily) in mothers carrying a fetus with CCHB may improve fetal cardiac contractility by reversing the often associated myocarditis component of this disease process (Copel et al, 1995). Additionally, anecdotal experience has illustrated rare cases of conversion from incomplete AV block (Wenckebach or 2:1 AV block) to sinus rhythm (Theander et al, 2000; Yamada et al, 1999). Fetal echocardiography can measure the mechanical P-R interval and may offer an avenue for institution of prophylactic therapy prior to the development of complete heart block. Studies are currently in progress to decide if early use of steroids in pregnancies with high-risk fetuses, before the development of CCHB, can in actuality prevent the progression to complete heart block. As a last resort, expedited delivery can be considered, although this approach carries significant morbidity and mortality risks, especially in the premature neonate. Although pacemaker implantation has been reported in a few fetuses with severe hydrops, the technique is currently not available in the majority of centers and is in essence experimental (Carpenter et al, 1986). Direct pacing is generally performed via a maternal transabdominal approach; lead dislodgement is likely to result from fetal movement. In addition, the possibility of pacemaker-mediated infection is a consideration (Silverman et al, 1997; Walkingshaw et al, 1994).

The prognosis for the fetus with structural heart disease is much poorer, with an estimated 80% to 90% mortality rate, with death occurring either in utero or during the first year of life (Machado et al, 1987; Schmidt et al, 1991). Fetal heart rates of less than 55 beats/minute in the cohort with structural heart disease carry an excessively high mortality rate; therefore, this group would be likely to benefit the most from in utero pacing (Schmidt et al, 1991). In most clinical settings, single-ventricle heart disease and congenital AV block are universally fatal even with the institution of pacing in the first hours of life. Postnatal CCHB therapy is discussed later (see Neonatal Bradycardia).

## FETAL TACHYCARDIA

### Fetal Supraventricular Tachycardia

The types of fetal tachycardia are comparable with those found in neonates and include both supraventricular tachycardia (SVT) and ventricular tachycardia (VT). SVT using an accessory bypass tract between the atrium and ventricle is the most common form of fetal tachycardia, with heart rates generally between 240 and 300 beats/minute. The tachycardia circuit tends to be orthodromic, with normal antegrade AV nodal conduction and retrograde conduction via the bypass tract. M-mode echocardiography will show equal atrial and ventricular rates exceeding 200 beats/minute with a fixed relationship (Fig. 58–4). Hydrops in association with reentrant SVT has been reported in 50% of fetuses (Machado et al, 1987; Walkingshaw et al, 1994). The development of nonimmune hydrops fetalis probably relates to several factors: the ventricular rate (Van Engelen et al, 1994), the length of time the fetus has been in the abnormal rhythm, and the onset of SVT at an earlier gestational age (Naheed et al, 1996).

The second most common form of SVT seen in fetuses is atrial flutter. Atrial tachycardias originate in the atrium without either the AV node or ventricle needed to complete the circuit. Because fetuses have rapid AV nodal conduction, 1:1 conduction with ventricular rates of 350 to 480 beats/minute can be seen (Lisowski et al, 2000). More commonly, however, AV nodal block results in either 2:1 conduction (Fig. 58–5) or a Wenckebach pattern. Automatic atrial tachycardia with a classic "warm-up" and "cool-down" phase is similar to sinus tachycardia and can also be seen in fetuses at any point in the second or third trimester. Although less common than atrial flutter, automatic atrial

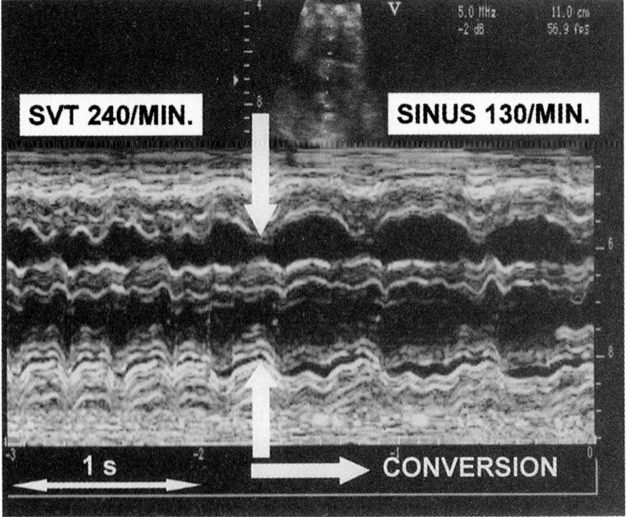


**FIGURE 58–4.** M-mode echocardiogram demonstrating ventricular wall motion at a rate of 240 beats/minute, with spontaneous conversion *(arrows)* to a physiologic rate of 130 beats/minute.

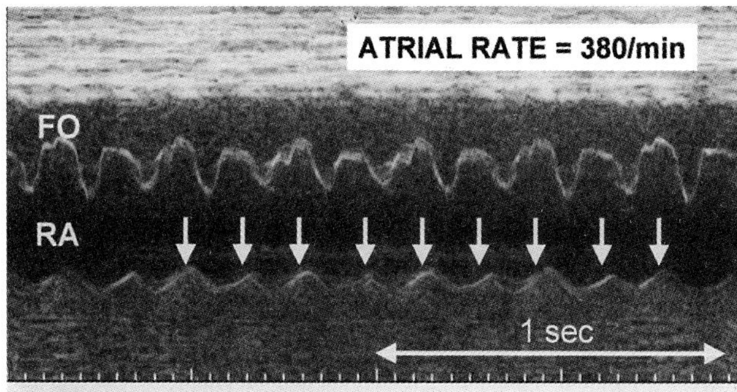


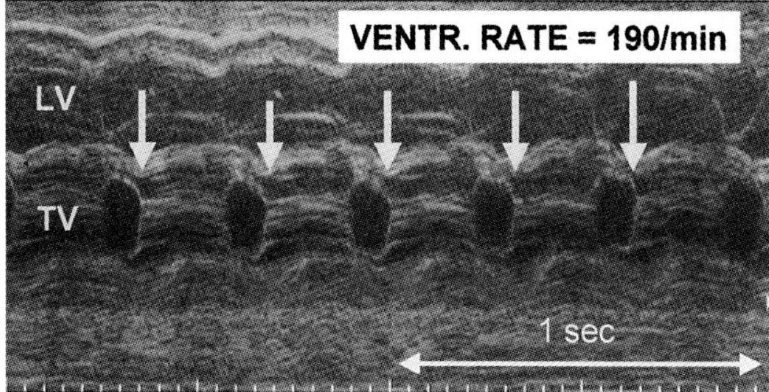


**FIGURE 58–5. Upper panel,** Atrial wall motion at a rate of 380 beats/minute. FO, foramen ovale; RA, right atrial wall. **Lower panel,** Ventricular response at 190 beats/minute consistent with 2:1 AV node conduction. LV, left ventricle; TV, tricuspid valve.

tachycardias (ectopic or chaotic) tend to be incessant and more difficult to control with primary drug therapy. As with all forms of SVT, fetuses may exhibit no signs of heart failure or have marked ascites, skin edema, effusions, or abnormal umbilical venous pulsations with imminent fetal demise. The development of hydrops is known to decrease the effectiveness of antiarrhythmic therapy and to increase the mortality rate.

## Management of Fetal Supraventricular Tachycardia

Management of the fetus with SVT should be based on the gestational age, frequency of the dysrhythmia, and the presence or absence of hydrops. Although management strategies vary by center, there are generally four approaches to management of fetal SVT: (1) observation, (2) expedited delivery of the fetus, (3) maternal drug therapy, and (4) fetal therapy. Observation is generally reserved for term or near-term fetuses or in those experiencing nonsustained bouts of SVT without any compromise. Expedited delivery is a reasonable consideration in the term neonate, thus avoiding the potential side effects of many of the antiarrhythmic agents. Delivery of the preterm fetus with SVT has been met with a high incidence of complications related to the prematurity, including lung disease, intraventricular hemorrhage, necrotizing enterocolitis, and sepsis (Hansmann et al, 1991; Maxwell et al, 1988).

The rationale in treating fetal SVT is to prevent the development of hydrops and fetal death. The exact timing of drug initiation (Table 58–1) or early delivery needs to be individually tailored. Fetuses without hydrops and intermittent tachycardia can be closely followed for development of hydrops or sustained arrhythmia. However, it is unknown which arrhythmia will become sustained and what interval may elapse before hydrops ensues. For fetuses with a nonhydropic clinical picture and a sustained dysrhythmia, drug therapy should be initiated unless the pregnancy is full term and the mother can be considered for early delivery. In all fetuses with a documented sustained arrhythmia and even in those with frequent intermittent tachyarrhythmias, weekly follow-up with particular attention to fetal well-being should be considered as part of routine obstetric care. If a sustained arrhythmia results in nonimmune hydrops, the fetus is at high risk for demise, and drug therapy or delivery needs to be implemented.

The treatment of fetal tachycardia requires the use of the mother as the vehicle to deliver therapy to the patient. Effectiveness of drug therapy requires successful transplacental absorption, stability of fetal and maternal hemodynamics, and knowledge of the actual mechanism of the arrhythmia (automatic versus reentrant). Fetal pharmacokinetics of drug absorption, distribution, metabolism, and elimination is variable and different from that in adults. Second, the placenta may be a barrier to successful drug delivery, and the actual antiarrhythmic concentration in the maternal serum is not necessarily reflective of fetal levels. Once cardiac failure develops, the success of fetal drug delivery diminishes because of poorer placental transfer and fetal absorption. In multiple studies, the presence or absence of fetal hydrops has consistently been the single greatest predictor of survival, with a nonhydropic fetal mortality rate between zero and 4% and a mortality rate in hydropic fetuses of 13% to 35% (Frohn-Mulder et al, 1995; Hansmann et al, 1991; Maxwell et al, 1988; Simpson and Sharland, 1998; Van Engelen et al, 1994).

In the nonhydropic infant, digoxin is the first-line agent and has achieved excellent safety and efficacy. Digoxin levels may be decreased by as much as 50% in the hydropic fetus, which may warrant an alternative treatment strategy (Younis and Granat, 1987). Maternal digoxin may be administered via either an oral or an intravenous route. The advantage of intravenous administration is the rapidity with which the fetus typically responds to the medication, but use of this route requires that the mother be hospitalized. Oral administration is generally more convenient, but therapy given by this route should continue for at least 1 or 2 weeks before it is deemed a failure. Using ultrasound guidance, direct administration of the drug to the fetus by an intramuscular, intraperitoneal, intra-amniotic, or umbilical venous route has been previously described (Hallak et al, 1991; Weiner and Thompson, 1988; Wiggins et al, 1986). As a result of the increased volume of distribution, maternal drug levels in the high range (1.5 to 2.5 ng/mL) are generally required. Such levels can typically be achieved with a maternal loading dose of 1 to 2 mg and a maintenance dose between 0.5 and 1.0 mg daily. If digoxin is unsuccessful, a combination of digoxin and verapamil has been reported to give 91% efficacy; however, side effects of both hypotension and asystole have made this treatment less frequently utilized in recent years (Hansman et al, 1991). Flecainide also has been used, but in view of the potential for proarrhythmic side effects, our approach has been to reserve this therapy for fetuses with SVT-related hydrops.

**TABLE 58–1**

**Drugs Used in the Treatment of Fetal Arrhythmias**

| Medication | Maternal Dose | Fetal/Maternal Plasma Ratio | Adverse Effects | Comments |
|---|---|---|---|---|
| Digoxin | 0.5-1 mg/day (M serum levels 1.5-2.5 ng/mL) | 0.1-0.9 | Safe | Adjust dose on basis of serum levels |
| Procainamide | 3-6 g/day | 0.3-1.3 | Proarrhythmia (F), uterine contractions, preterm labor, Q-T prolongation (M/F) | Adjust dose on basis of serum procainamide, NAPA levels |
| Propranolol | 40-320 mg/day | 0.2-1.3 | Hypoglycemia (F), IUGR, myocardial depression (F), respiratory depression (F), hyperbilirubinemia (F) | Serum levels not readily available |
| Lidocaine | 1 mg/kg/dose (bolus); 20-40 μg/kg/min (infusion) | | Safe | Adjust dose on basis of serum levels; lower dose if Cr elevated |
| Flecainide | 100-450 mg/day | 0.5-0.8 | (?)Proarrhythmia (M), fetal demise, Q-T prolongation (M/F) | No intravenous form |
| Sotalol | 80-320 mg/day | 0.5-1.0 | Q-T prolongation (M/F) | More effective for atrial flutter than for AV reciprocating SVT |
| Amiodarone | *Load*: 600 mg infused over 6 hr *Maintenance*: 800 mg/day | 0.1-0.4 | IUGR, prematurity, thyroid dysfunction (F), Q-T prolongation (M/F) neurologic dysfunction (F) | Direct fetal delivery may be required secondary to prolonged oral loading, slow clearance |

AV, atrioventricular; F, fetal; Cr, creatinine; IUGR, intrauterine growth restriction; M, maternal; NAPA, *N*-acetyl-procainamide; SVT, supraventricular tachycardia.

Data from Ito S, Magee L, Smallhorn J: Drug therapy for fetal arrhythmias. Clin Perinatol 21:543-572, 1994; Simpson JM, Sharland GK: Fetal tachycardias: Management and outcome of 127 consecutive cases. Heart 79:576-581, 1998; Tanel RE, Rhodes LA: Fetal and neonatal arrhythmias. Clin Perinatol 28:187-208, 2001.

In the hydropic fetus, isolated use of digoxin has had limited efficacy (10% to 20%); this result may be related to poor absorption across the placenta (Frohn-Mulder et al, 1995; Hansmann et al, 1991; Simpson and Sharland, 1998; Van Engelen et al, 1994). Direct fetal therapy with intraumbilical adenosine has been used to successfully terminate SVT (Friedman et al, 1993). Although the half-life of adenosine is quite short, a dose-dependent constriction of placental blood flow has been reported, which urges caution with this therapy (Omar et al, 1996).

Flecainide has been used extensively as a second-line agent for treatment of fetal arrhythmias. Flecainide is a class IC antiarrhythmic drug that blocks conduction through sodium channels with little to no effect on the refractory properties of the tissue. Flecainide is typically given by the oral route, with a maternal-to-fetal placental transference of 65% to 95% (Allan et al, 1991; Wren and Hunter, 1988). Although there are no known teratogenic side effects of flecainide, caution must be exercised because of the potential for fetal proarrhythmic effects. A decrease in heart rate variability occurs with flecainide and appears to be dose-related (Van Gelder-Hasker et al, 1995). The typical starting dose for oral flecainide is 200 to 300 mg/day; with adequate control of the SVT, the fetus can be weaned to the lowest possible dose with continued efficacy.

Although amiodarone (class III) is an effective antiarrhythmic agent, reports of thyroid gland suppression and neurologic motor delay make this drug less appealing (Magee et al, 1995; Plomp et al, 1992).

Sotalol is a potent β-blocking agent with additional class III antiarrhythmic properties (increases the action potential duration). Sotalol appears to have minimal negative inotropic effects with excellent transplacental properties. In a recent multicenter study, regimens using sotalol and the combination of sotalol and digoxin were very successful in fetuses with atrial flutter (Oudjik et al, 2001). The conversion rate was 80%, with a relatively low recurrence rate. However, the results with sotalol in the treatment of fetal SVT were not as promising, with only 6 of 10 fetuses converting to sinus rhythm, but more alarming was the intrauterine demise of three fetuses. All of the intrauterine deaths occurred within the first week of therapy, bringing into question the known proarrhythmic side effects of this medication (Oudjik et al, 2001). Other drugs utilized in the treatment of fetal SVT with hydrops include propranolol, verapamil, and procainamide (Teuscher et al, 1978; Wolff et al, 1980).

Failure of either oral or intravenous maternal drug therapy to convert the fetal heart to sinus rhythm warrants consideration of direct fetal therapy by an intraumbilical, intramuscular, intraperitoneal, or intracardiac approach.

This more aggressive approach avoids the need for transplacental absorption but carries a significant risk to both the fetus and the mother. It is important to remember that infusion of a drug directly into the fetal circulation still mandates a background level of drug (achieved with maternal oral or intravenous administration) to avoid recurrences of SVT once the direct fetal dose is diminished. Finally, direct overdrive fetal pacing is potentially possible either by transventricular puncture (Strasburger et al, 1986) or through the umbilical vein. The potential hazards of this more aggressive approach include wire dislodgement, infection, premature labor, and degeneration of a reentrant SVT into atrial fibrillation.

### Fetal Ventricular Tachycardia

The prenatal diagnosis of VT is rare in the fetus. The importance of diagnosing VT rests in the coexistent association of structural heart defects, ventricular dysfunction, and ventricular tumors. VT does not require the atrium or the AV node as part of the circuit and is typically diagnosed by M-mode demonstration of AV dissociation with the ventricular rate exceeding the atrial rate. Congenital junctional ectopic tachycardia cannot be distinguished from VT, although it is exceedingly rare. Treatment for VT is relatively similar to SVT management, with the exception of the need to avoid digoxin. In addition to beta-blockers, procainamide and intravenous lidocaine can be used, although levels need to be closely followed in the latter two choices.

## NEONATAL BRADYCARDIA

Bradyarrhythmias in the neonate are similar to those in the fetus. Either sinus or AV node dysfunction may cause neonatal bradycardia. As in the fetus, bradycardia may be associated with structural heart defects ranging from simple septal defects to complex single-ventricle lesions. Symptoms related to marked bradycardia in the infant include poor growth, feeding intolerance, dyspnea, and on rare occasions syncope. Congenital complete heart block in the neonate (Fig. 58–6) is typically a result of transplacental passage of anti-Ro and anti-La antibodies with concomitant fibrosis of the AV nodal conduction system. This process is not reversible after birth, and the typical decision for the managing physician is not *if* to pace but *when* to pace. Alternatively, congenital heart block may be seen in association with structural heart defects such as L-transposition of the great vessels, heterotaxy syndrome, or atrioventricular septal defects (Fig. 58–7).

Guidelines from the American College of Cardiology and the American Heart Association recommend permanent pacemaker implantation for infants with congenital third-degree AV block with a ventricular rate of less than 50 to 55 beats/minute or with congenital heart disease and a ventricular rate of less than 70 beats/minute (Gregoratos et al, 1998). However, more often than not, the decision regarding pacing is very difficult, as in an infant with a structurally normal heart and a ventricular rate of 59 beats/minute, or with a rate of 72 beats/minute in association with heart disease. Aside from the ventricular rate, several reviews of CCHB have identified a wide escape rhythm, prolonged Q-T, cardiomegaly, right atrial enlargement, ventricular dysfunction, and ventricular ectopy as risk factors that might prompt consideration for early permanent pacing (Gregoratos et al, 1998; Michaelsson et al, 1995; Pinsky et al, 1982; Sholler and Walsh, 1989). Despite the early institution of pacing, some infants with CCHB develop a cardiomyopathy, and it is critical that patients be followed closely not only for rate assessment but for overall myocardial performance (Moak et al, 2001; Udink ten Cate et al, 2001).

Isolated atrial premature depolarizations are frequently seen in the newborn period and typically require no treatment. They may be blocked within the AV node resulting in a pause, conduct normally, or aberrantly conduct. The development of symptoms in affected infants is unlikely, although a small percentage will go on to have SVT or atrial flutter. Drug therapy is not required to treat isolated benign premature atrial beats.

Idiopathic long Q-T syndrome is a rare disorder that may lead to syncope, seizures, and sudden death. The long Q-T syndrome is an abnormality in ventricular repolarization secondary to an abnormal sodium or potassium ion channel. Patients with long Q-T syndrome are at risk for the development of life-threatening ventricular arrhythmias (e.g., torsade de pointes). As a result of the findings of the International Study of the Pediatric Electrophysiology Group, in which sudden death was the presenting

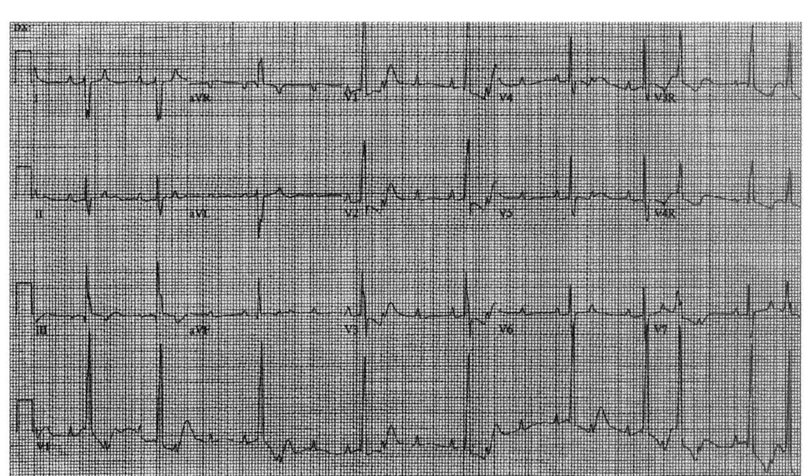

**FIGURE 58–6.** A 12-lead electrocardiogram demonstrating complete heart block with atrioventricular dissociation. Evidence of right atrial enlargement and right ventricular hypertrophy with a strain pattern and isolated premature ventricular complexes are also noted.

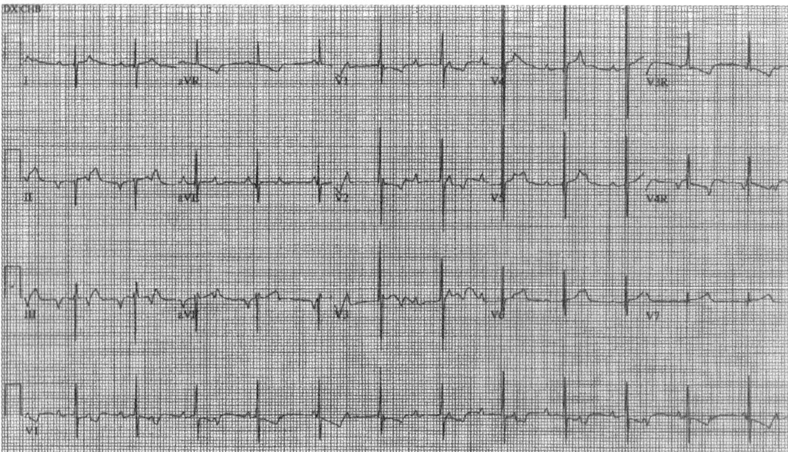

**FIGURE 58–7.** A 12-lead electrocardiogram demonstrating complete heart block with atrioventricular dissociation. Note the presence of a left superior axis and an abnormal P wave axis consistent with heterotaxy syndrome.

symptom in 9% of children without any preceding symptoms, prophylactic therapy with beta-blockers is now standard (Garson et al, 1993). Congenital long Q-T syndrome is associated with neonatal sinus bradycardia, and there is now some clinical evidence that this may be associated with sudden infant death syndrome (Hofbeck et al, 1997; Schwartz et al, 1998). Congenital long Q-T syndrome has also been seen as a presentation with bradycardia secondary to 2:1 AV nodal conduction (Fig. 58–8). A careful family history with particular attention to sudden death, near drowning, and seizures should be obtained in all neonates with bradycardia and/or ventricular ectopy.

## NEONATAL TACHYCARDIA

### Neonatal Supraventricular Tachycardia

Rate alone is insufficient to diagnose a tachydysrhythmia. Neonates can have sinus tachycardia with rates of 230 to 240 beats/minute secondary to pain, fever, anemia, hyperthyroidism, infection, or related to intravenous inotropic medication. Interpretation of the electrocardiogram should be performed methodically, with careful attention to regularity, P wave axis, and the relationship of each P wave to QRS complex. Although supraventricular tachycardias are typically narrow-complex, it is not unusual for the first few beats to demonstrate aberrancy before narrowing of complexes. Our general approach has been to obtain an echocardiogram in all neonates presenting with sustained SVT or VT, as 25% of infants may have associated structural heart disease.

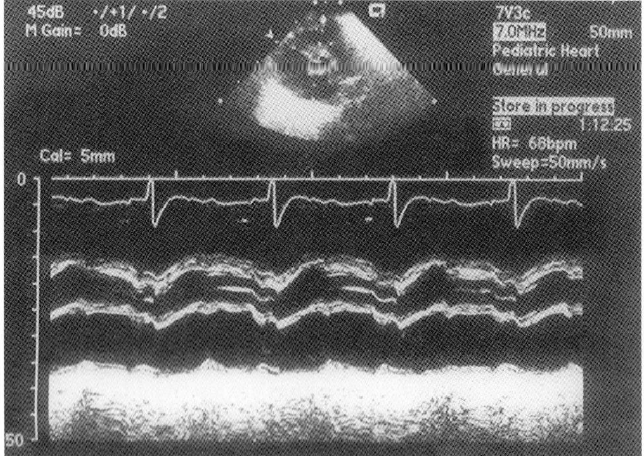


**FIGURE 58–8.** M-mode echocardiogram and postnatal electrocardiogram depict prolonged Q-T interval (580 msec) with 2:1 AV conduction in a 1-day-old infant with a history of fetal bradycardia.

The clinical presentation of the newborn with either SVT (Fig. 58–9) or VT generally depends not only on the tachycardia rate but also the duration of tachycardia and on the presence of any associated structural heart defects that may further compromise systemic output. Newborns with sustained SVT or VT may present with irritability, feeding intolerance, pallor, diaphoresis, tachypnea, decreased urine output, or shock. The mechanisms of SVT that are seen in the newborn are similar to the fetus, although diagnosis is easier because direct electrocardiographic analysis can be performed on the patient, as well as assessment of therapeutic vagal maneuvers.

SVTs may be reentrant or automatic. Reentrant arrhythmias generally manifest with a sudden onset and termination. These types of tachycardia respond well to maneuvers that block the AV node and interrupt the circuit, such as administration of adenosine or digoxin. The most common form of reentry in the newborn involves an accessory bypass tract. If the bypass tract has the potential to conduct antegrade, the diagnosis is Wolff-Parkinson-White (WPW) syndrome (Fig. 58–10). Anatomic lesions such as Ebstein's anomaly of the tricuspid valve, ventricular inversion, and hypertrophic cardiomyopathy can be associated with WPW syndrome; therefore, all newborns with WPW syndrome should undergo a screening echocardiogram. If, however, the bypass tract conducts only in retrograde fashion, the accessory pathway is "concealed" and does not have the typical delta wave on the resting electrocardiogram. During orthodromic SVT, no distinction can be seen on the electrocardiogram between these two types of dysrhythmia. The mechanism of the tachycardia appears to be antegrade conduction through the AV node and His-Purkinje system with retrograde conduction via the bypass tract. Occasionally, patients with WPW syndrome can have antegrade conduction via the accessory pathway with retrograde AV nodal

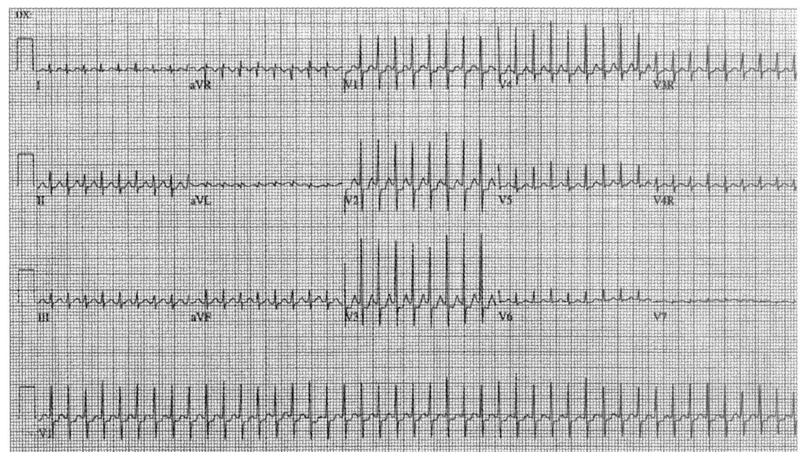

**FIGURE 58–9.** A 15-lead electrocardiogram demonstrating a narrow-complex tachycardia with a ventricular rate of 265 beats/minute. Note absence of P wave secondary to rapid retrograde conduction.

conduction (antidromic SVT). In this instance, unlike in the former, the tachycardia is of the wide-complex type and is indistinguishable from VT. In AV reciprocating (narrow-complex) SVT, the onset and termination are sudden and characterized by a fairly fixed heart rhythm with rates between 240 and 300 beats/minute, with often unidentifiable P waves, as they are superimposed upon the T wave.

AV nodal reentrant tachycardia is rarely seen in neonates and more commonly diagnosed in adolescents and young adults. Another form of reentrant SVT is permanent junctional reciprocating tachycardia (PJRT), which tends to be slower (less than 200 beats/minute) and incessant. The electrocardiogram typically demonstrates a narrow-complex tachycardia, with easily identifiable P waves secondary to the long R-P interval from the slowly conducting retrograde limb of the circuit (Fig. 58–11). Because of the incessant nature of PJRT, infants may present with a dilated cardiomyopathy and congestive heart failure.

## Management of Neonatal Supraventricular Tachycardia

The treatment of reentrant SVT entails both acute therapy and more long-term treatment (Table 58–2). Acute treatments can be broken down into (1) reflex vagal maneuvers, (2) drug therapy, and (3) electrical conversion. Vagal maneuvers transiently block AV conduction by upregulating parasympathetic (vagal) input and terminating the tachycardia. Our general approach in the neonate is to use a bag filled with a water-ice mixture, or a bag of frozen vegetables (e.g., peas), to cover the forehead to the brim of the nose. Rectal stimulation is another successful vagal modality that has been used for reentrant SVT. If the tachycardia terminates and returns almost immediately, additional vagal maneuvers will be no more effective, and in essence the patient needs to begin an antiarrhythmic medication. In our experience, vagal maneuvers are safe and effective, although of somewhat limited effectiveness in patients with high levels of circulating catecholamines. Although numerous antiarrhythmic medications including digoxin, beta-blockers, procainamide, amiodarone, flecainide, and sotalol have been utilized for the acute treatment of neonatal SVT, adenosine is the most effective short-term pharmacologic agent available. Adenosine given in rapid intravenous bolus form (100 to 300 μg/kg) blocks AV nodal conduction and effectively stops the reentrant circuit. Side effects of adenosine include flushing, chest discomfort, bronchospasm, and rarely induction of atrial fibrillation. In patients with low cardiac output and poor systemic blood flow, a higher dose of adenosine may be required to circumvent the rapid metabolism in the vascular endothelium and erythrocytes.

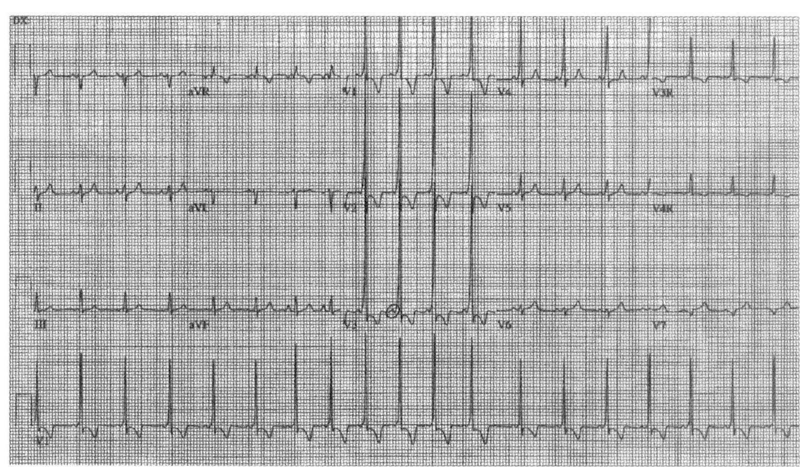

**FIGURE 58–10.** Electrocardiogram from a newborn with Wolff-Parkinson-White (WPW) syndrome. During sinus rhythm there is a short P-R interval, with obvious delta waves in leads $V_1$-$V_3$ *(circle)*.

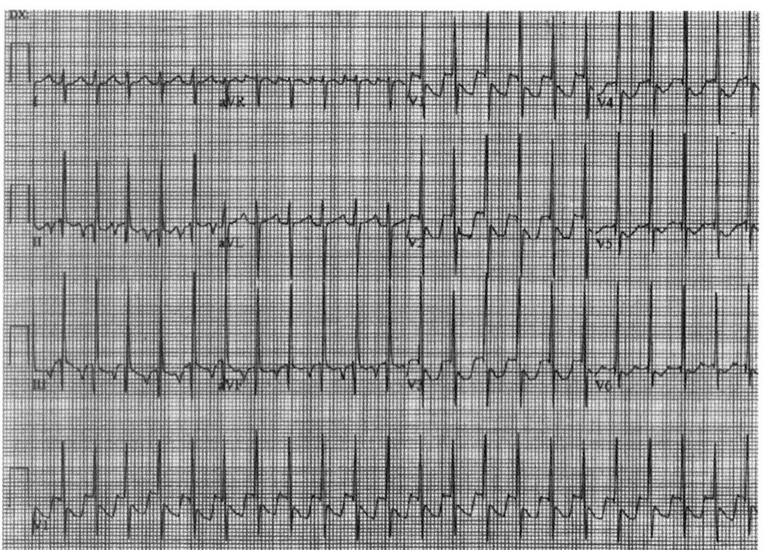

**FIGURE 58–11.** Narrow-complex tachycardia (permanent junctional reciprocating tachycardia) with a long R-P interval and classically inverted P waves in the inferior leads (II, III, aVF).

Direct current cardioversion should be reserved for the hemodynamically compromised (hypotensive) neonate. Transesophageal overdrive atrial pacing has also been shown to be highly efficacious and safe in neonates, with an excellent conversion rate (Schwartz et al, 1998).

Once the acute tachycardia has been terminated, prophylactic antiarrhythmic therapy is prescribed for most infants, given the high recurrence risk of AV reciprocating tachycardias in the first year of life (Benson et al, 1987; Perry and Garson, 1990). In fact, Perry and Garson (1990) reported that of infants presenting with WPW syndrome prior to 2 months of age, 93% experienced disappearance of the tachycardia, although 31% had recurrent SVT at an average age of 8 years. This finding was corroborated by Wu and associates (1994); in their study, 40% of children who presented with SVT in infancy were still symptomatic by age 5 years. Although digoxin has often been considered the first-line antiarrhythmic, its use in patients with WPW syndrome is controversial and potentially contraindicated. Digoxin may impair AV nodal conduction and enhance more rapid antegrade bypass conduction, and even ventricular fibrillation.

Digoxin is generally regarded as a safe and effective antiarrhythmic medication, but the dose must be decreased in the premature neonate and in patients with renal insufficiency. Beta-blockers (e.g., propranolol) can be used safely in the neonate with SVT, especially if the WPW pattern is seen on the resting electrocardiogram. Because of the potential hypoglycemic effect of beta-blockers, our recommendation is to usually give the medication during or shortly after a feeding. Beta-blockers act as competitive antagonists at catecholamine-binding sites and slow AV nodal conduction. Beta-blockers may also impair myocardial contractility and should be used with caution in the newborn with depressed ventricular function. Beyond digoxin and/or beta-blockers, drug therapy should be individualized and often varies depending on the practitioner. Whereas verapamil is an excellent drug in older children, it should be *avoided* in neonates because of its potent negative inotropic effect (Epstein et al, 1985). Procainamide is a class IA antiarrhythmic medication that has been used extensively in the treatment of neonatal SVT. Procainamide is a negative inotrope and has vasodilating properties, especially during the intravenous loading infusion. The bolus (5 to 15 mg/kg) is generally given over 30 to 45 minutes; adjustments in the bolus infusion rate and need for additional volume should be individualized according to the patient's cardiac status. Amiodarone is a class III drug that is also effective in the treatment of neonatal SVT. The intravenous dose is usually 5 mg/kg given over 30-60 minutes, with close observation needed secondary to potential hypotension from acute vasodilatation. Chronic oral amiodarone has a rather extended half-life, and in our experience, 2 to 3 weeks or longer may be needed to achieve full therapeutic levels in newborns. Side effects of amiodarone include photosensitivity, hypothyroidism, hyperthyroidism, hepatitis, and proarrhythmia.

If available, overdrive esophageal atrial pacing can be effective in terminating AV reciprocating tachycardias. A flexible 4 or 5 F lead can be advanced into the nares and situated in the esophagus posterior to the left atrium. Electrical stimulation allows capture of the left atrial myocardium, and pacing slightly faster than the atrial rate should terminate the dysrhythmia. Sedation with a medication such as midazolam is usually helpful. As with any attempt at atrial pacing, there is the potential for initiating atrial fibrillation, which would require an alternative treatment strategy and possible direct current cardioversion. Finally, direct current cardioversion should be readily available if the patient is hemodynamically unstable or is resistant to medications, or if overdrive esophageal pacing fails to correct the dysrhythmia. Synchronized cardioversion (using 0.25 to 2 J/kg) is recommended for patients with an organized reentrant tachycardia, whereas asynchronous defibrillation should be performed in the pulseless patient or if the rhythm is disorganized. Sedation, if not general anesthesia, is always warranted for an elective cardioversion/defibrillation. Radiofrequency ablation is used infrequently in infants and is more commonly reserved for older children and adolescents.

Atrial flutter represents another form of SVT seen in infants and results from a single reentrant focus in the

**TABLE 58–2**

**Drugs Used in the Treatment of Neonatal Arrhythmias**

| Medication (Class) | Route of Metabolism/ Excretion | Oral Dose | IV Dose | Therapeutic Level | Common Adverse Effects |
|---|---|---|---|---|---|
| Adenosine | RBCs, vascular endothelium | | 0.05 mg/kg; may increase to 0.25 mg/kg if no effect (IV push) | | Hypotension, flushing, chest pain, heart block, Afib |
| Digoxin | Renal | *Load*: Preterm: 20 μg/kg in 3 doses; full-term: 30 μg/kg in 3 doses<br>*Maintenance*: Preterm: 5-7.5 μg/kg div q12h; full-term: 6-10 μg/kg div q12h | 75%-80% oral dose<br>*Load*: Preterm: 15 μg/kg in 3 doses; full term 20 μg/kg in 3 doses<br>*Maintenance*: Preterm: 3-4 μg/kg div q12h; full-term: 6-8 μg/kg div q12h | 0.8-2.0 ng/mL | AV, SA block, bradycardia, nausea/ vomiting, toxicity with hypocalcemia or K abnormality |
| Procainamide (IA) | Renal, hepatic | 15-50 mg/kg/day in 4-8 div doses | *Load*: 3-6 mg/kg/dose over 5 minutes; repeat dose over 10 minutes up to a maximum of 15 mg/kg.<br>*Maintenance*: 20-80 μg/kg/min | Procainamide, NAPA levels = 10-20 μg/mL | Hypotension, AV block, nausea/ vomiting, lupus-like syndrome |
| Disopyramide (IA) | Renal, hepatic | 3.5-7.5 mg/kg q6h | | 2-5 μg/mL | Negative inotropy, AV block, anti-cholinergic effects, hypoglycemia, ventricular arrhythmias |
| Lidocaine (IB) | Renal, hepatic | | 1 mg/kg/dose (bolus); 20-50 μg/kg/min (infusion); decrease with hepatic or renal dysfunction | 2-5 μg/mL | Hypotension, heart block, CNS effects, respiratory depression |
| Mexilitine (IB) | Hepatic | 1.4-5 mg/kg/dose q8h | | 0.5-2.0 g/L | CNS effects, nausea/vomiting, bradycardia, hepatopathy |
| Flecainide (1C) | Renal, hepatic | 0.3-2 mg/kg q8h; decrease with hepatic or renal dysfunction | | 0.2-1.0 μg/mL | Bradycardia, conduction block, VT, nausea, CHF; avoid in CHD |
| Propranolol (II) | Hepatic | 0.25 mg/kg/dose q6-8h, usual dosage range 2-4 mg/kg/day divided q6-q8h | 0.01 mg/kg over 10 min; repeat q6-8h, may increase slowly to 0.15 mg/kg/dose q6-8h | | Hypotension, bradycardia, conduction block, hypoglycemia, bronchospasm, weakness |
| Esmolol (II) | RBC esterases | | *Load*: 100-500 μg/kg/min over 1 min<br>*Maintenance*: 40-300 g/kg/min | | Same as for propranolol |
| Sotalol (II/III) | Renal | 20-120 mg/m$^2$ BSA q12h | | | Bradycardia, conduction block, VT/torsades, nausea, CHF |
| Amiodarone (III) | Hepatic | 5 mg/kg q12h for 7 days, then 2-5 mg/kg/day; decreased with liver dysfunction | 5 mg/kg/dose over 30 min; may repeat up to 15 mg/kg on day 1<br>*Maintenance*: 3-10 μg/kg/min | Follow reverse $T_3$ | Thyroid/ hepatic dysfunction, AV block, hypotension, corneal deposits, proarrhythmia |

Afib, atrial fibrillation; AV, atrioventricular; BSA, body surface area; CHD, congenital heart disease; CHF, congestive heart failure; CNS, central nervous system; IV, intravenous; NAPA, *N*-acetyl-procainamide; RBC, red blood cell; SA, sinoatrial; $T_3$, triiodothyronine; VT, ventricular tachycardia.

atrium, typically around vena caval orifices or the tricuspid valve. Atrial rates in the newborn will range from 240 to 360 beats/minute, and the typical "saw-toothed" P wave pattern will be seen in the inferior leads. Typically, AV nodal conduction block allows for 2:1 conduction and better-tolerated hemodynamics. Newborn atrial flutter is not typically associated with structural heart defects (occurring in approximately 8% of cases by report) but can on occasion be seen in the setting of systemic illness, with the presence of a central venous catheter, or in association with a rare defect, septum primum aneurysm (Mendelsohn et al, 1991; Moller et al, 1969; Rice et al, 1988). Atrial flutter, like the other reentrant forms of SVT, responds well to overdrive esophageal pacing and, in addition, may spontaneously resolve. Results on long-term follow-up evaluation of neonates with isolated atrial flutter are exceedingly promising, and often acute and chronic digoxin therapy is probably unnecessary. If the diagnosis cannot be made by a standard 12-lead electrocardiogram, either an esophageal recording or administration of intravenous adenosine during recording of the 12-lead electrocardiogram may be used for diagnostic purposes. Intravenous adenosine will block the AV node, and if atrial flutter is present, will unmask the typical flutter pattern.

Automatic atrial tachycardias are a result of enhanced automaticity resulting from a microfocus within the atrial wall itself. The rate of automatic ectopic atrial tachycardia (EAT) is faster than the sinus rate but may vary among patients and even within an individual patient. A characteristic feature of EAT is a "warm-up" and a "cool-down" phase, without the need for either the AV node or the ventricle to contribute to the circuit. Variable degrees of AV block may be seen, and patients typically have no evidence of structural heart disease, although they may present with or develop a dilated cardiomyopathy (Garson et al, 1990). Chaotic atrial tachycardia is a similar automatic atrial rhythm that typically has a minimum of three P wave morphologies and tends to be more incessant than EAT. Automatic tachycardias do not respond to typical vagal maneuvers, adenosine, or diect current cardioversion. Medical therapy for patients with automatic atrial tachycardias usually revolves around ventricular rate control rather than termination of the tachycardia. Although digoxin and beta-blockers remain first-line agents for the treatment of EAT/CAT, better control seems to occur with amiodarone or flecainide (Garson et al, 1990; Von Bernuth et al, 1992). Often, combination drug therapy is required. Pacing to achieve 2:1 block will result in a slower ventricular response but is a more invasive strategy.

## Neonatal Ventricular Tachycardia

VT and accelerated ventricular rhythm are uncommon in newborns, although they may be related to a number of causes including right- or left-sided cardiac obstructive lesions, myocarditis, electrolyte abnormalities, cardiac tumors, or proarrhythmia from a variety of antiarrhythmic medications (Fig. 58–12). Although the prognosis is generally good in the infant with a structurally normal heart (Pfammater and Paul, 1999), cases of deterioration to ventricular fibrillation and sudden death have been seen in those with the long Q-T syndrome (Pfammater and Paul, 1999) or cardiac hamartomas. Pfammatter and associates observed that infants with VT tend to be less symptomatic than older children and have nearly a 90% spontaneous resolution rate. VT associated with a left bundle branch pattern (originating from the right ventricle) carries a more favorable prognosis than that for right bundle branch (left ventricular origin) VT (Pfammater and Paul, 1999). Accelerated ventricular rhythm (more than 20% above the sinus rate) in infants younger than 1 month of age usually portends an excellent prognosis, and antiarrhythmic therapy is probably not warranted (Van Hare and Stanger, 1991). In our experience, PVCs in healthy newborns typically resolve by 12 weeks of age and do not require treatment once the presence of a structurally normal heart and normal QTc interval and the absence of symptoms have been confirmed. Both isolated PVCs and idiopathic neonatal VT probably result from developmental factors related to the autonomic nervous system.

It is important that all neonates presenting with ventricular ectopy or VT, especially if polymorphic, be evaluated for possible long Q-T syndrome. A careful family history should be obtained, with particular attention to syncope, deafness, seizures, drowning, or sudden death. The QTc should be measured on the electrocardiogram in

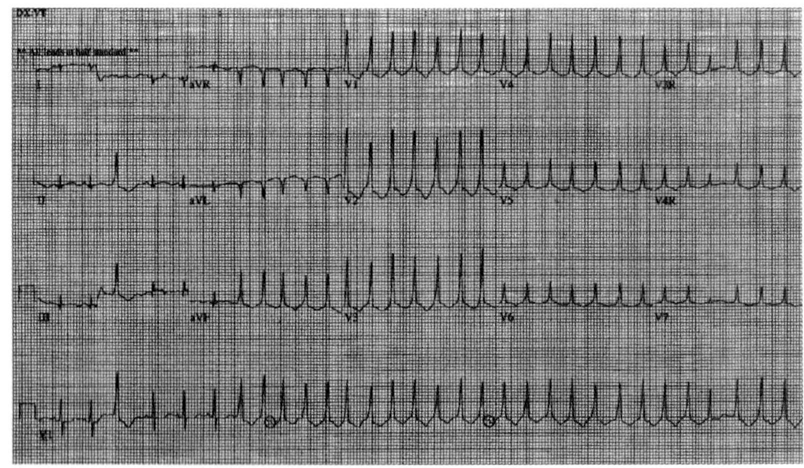


**FIGURE 58–12.** Onset of a wide-complex tachycardia (ventricular tachycardia) slightly faster than the sinus rate. Atrioventricular dissociation is seen during ventricular tachycardia (*circled* P waves).

a region (typically lead II) free of PVCs. Normal values for children are less than 450 msec.

### Management of Neonatal Ventricular Tachycardia

The therapies discussed for treating SVT can be used in managing patients with VT, with the sole exception of the need to avoid digoxin and adenosine. Degeneration to ventricular fibrillation has been reported in patients being digitalized for presumptive SVT with aberrancy, when in reality the underlying rhythm was VT. Intravenous lidocaine (bolus dose of 1 mg/kg; infusion of 20 to 50 μg/kg/minute) is effective in the treatment of neonatal VT, with good results. In the setting of renal failure, the dosing of lidocaine needs to be adjusted on the basis of the creatinine clearance. Amiodarone, procainamide, and beta-blockers are also effective in the treatment of neonatal VT. Calcium channel blockers in newborns should be avoided because of the potential for hypotension, myocardial depression, and even cardiac arrest. As in any patient presenting with an arrhythmia and hemodynamic instability, cardioversion (1 to 2 J/kg) and airway control should be considered as first-line therapy. Because VT can degenerate into ventricular fibrillation, it is important that *any* neonate presenting with a wide-complex tachycardia be treated first and foremost as having VT. More often than not, a wide-complex tachycardia is VT, and error typically occurs if the patient is wrongly and prematurely diagnosed as having SVT with aberrancy.

## CONCLUSIONS

In general, fetal and neonatal arrhythmias encompass a broad spectrum ranging from benign isolated atrial ectopy to malignant polymorphic ventricular tachycardia. The management of the fetus or newborn with an arrhythmia depends on a host of factors related to the type of dysrhythmia, ventricular rate, the presence of any associated structural cardiac defect, and also the overall clinical status of the patient. Many medications are available to the fetus via delivery to the mother as well as to the newborn. In the absence of congenital heart defects, most newborn tachy- and bradyarrhythmias are well tolerated and can be managed medically. Finally, most arrhythmias seen in newborns spontaneously resolve within the first year of life and carry an excellent long-term prognosis.

## REFERENCES


Allan LD, Chita SK, Sharland GK, et al: Flecainide in the treatment of fetal tachycardias. Br Heart J 65:46-48, 1991.

Allen LD, Anderson RH, Sullivan ID, et al: Evaluation of fetal arrhythmias by echocardiography. Br Heart J 50:240-245, 1983.

Andelginfer G, Fouron JC, Sonesson SE, et al: Reference values for time intervals between atrial and ventricular contractions of the fetal measured by two Doppler techniques. Am J Cardiol 88(12):1433-1436, 2001.

Benson DW Jr, Dunnigan A, Benditt DG: Follow-up evaluation of infant paroxysmal atrial tachycardia. Transesophageal study. Circulation 75:542-549, 1987.

Buyon JP, Winchester RJ, Slade SG, et al: Identification of mothers at risk for congenital heart block and other neonatal lupus syndromes in their children: Comparison of enzyme-linked immunosorbent assay and immunoblot for measurement of anti-SS-A/Ro and anti-SS-B-La antibodies. Arthritis Rheum 36:1263-1273, 1993.

Carpenter Jr RJ, Strasburger JF, Garson A Jr, et al: Fetal ventricular pacing for hydrops secondary to complete atrioventricular block. J Am Coll Cardiol 8:1434-1436, 1986.

Clavin SE, Gaziano EP, Bendel RP, et al: Evaluation of fetal cardiac arrhythmias. Ultrasound findings and neonatal outcome. Minn Med 75:29-31, 1992.

Copel JA, Buyon JP, Kleinman CS: Successful in utero therapy of fetal heart block. Am J Obstet Gynecol 173:1384-1390, 1995.

Cyr DR, Guntheroth WO, Mack LA, et al: A systematic approach to fetal echocardiography using real time two-dimensional sonography. J Ultrasound Med 5:343-350, 1986.

Epstein ML, Kiel EA, Victoria BE: Cardiac decompensation following verapamil therapy in infants with supraventricular tachycardia. Pediatrics 75:737-740, 1985.

Esscher E, Scott JS: Congenital heart block and maternal systemic lupus erythematosus. Br Med J 1:1235-1238, 1979.

Friedberg DZ, Nadas AS: Clinical profile of patients with congenital corrected transposition of the great arteries. N Engl J Med 282:1053-1059, 1970.

Friedman AH, Copel JA, Kleinman CS: Fetal echocardiography and fetal cardiology: Indications, diagnosis, and management. Semin Perinatol 17:76-88, 1993.

Frohn-Mulder IM, Stewart PA, Witsenberg M, et al: The efficacy of flecainide versus digoxin in the management of fetal supraventricular tachycardia. Prenat Diag 15:1297-1302, 1995.

Garson A Jr, Dick M II, Fournier A, et al: The long QT syndrome in children: An international study of 287 patients. Circulation 87:1866-1872, 1993.

Garson A Jr, Gillette PC, Moak JP: Supraventricular tachycardia due to multiple atrial ectopic foci: A relatively common problem. J Cardiovasc Electrophysiol 1:132-138, 1990.

Glickstein JS, Buyon J, Friedman D: Pulsed Doppler echocardiographic assessmet of the fetal PR interval. Am J Cardiol 86(2):236-239, 2000.

Gregoratos G, Cheitlin MD, Conill A, et al: ACC/AHA Guidelines for implantation of cardiac pacemakers and antiarrhythmia devices. J Am Coll Cardiol 31:1175-1209, 1998.

Groves ANM, Allan LD, Rosenthal E: Outcome of isolated congenital complete heart block diagnosed in utero. Heart 75: 190-194, 1996.

Groves, ANM, Allan LD, Rosenthal E: Therapeutic trial of sympathomimetics in three cases of complete heart block in the fetus. Circulation 92:3394-3396, 1995.

Hallak M, Neerhof MG, Perry R, et al: Fetal supraventricular tachycardia and hydrops fetalis: Combined intensive, direct, and transplacental therapy. Obstet Gynecol 78:523-525, 1991.

Hansmann M, Gembruch U, Bald R, et al: Fetal arrhythmias: Transplacental and direct treatment of the fetus—a report of sixty cases. Ultrasound Obstet Gynecol 1:162-170, 1991.

Hofbeck M, Ulmer H, Beinder E, et al: Prenatal findings in patients with prolonged QT interval in the neonatal period. Heart 77:198-204, 1997.

Huhta JC, Maloney JD, Ritter DG, et al: Complete atrioventricular block in patients with atrioventricular discordance. Circulation 67:1374-1377, 1983.

Hull D, Binns BAO, Joyce D: Congenital heart block and widespread fibroelastosis due to maternal lupus erythematous. Arch Dis Child 41:688-690, 1966.

Jaeggi ET, Hamilton RM, Silverman ED, et al: Outcome of children with fetal, neonatal, and childhood diagnosis of isolated congenital atrioventricular block. A single institution's experience of 30 years. J Am Coll Cardiol 2002;39(1):130-137.

Jones WR: Autoimmune disease and pregnancy. Aust N Z J Obstet Gynaecol 34:251-258, 1994.

Kaaja R, Julkunen H, Ammala H, et al: Congenital heart block: Successful prophylactic treatment with intravenous gamma globulin and corticosteroid therapy. Am J Obstet Gynecol 165:1333-1334, 1991.

Kleinman CS: Combined echocardiographic and Doppler assessment of fetal congenital atrioventricular block. Br J Obstet Gynaecol 94:967, 1987.

Kleinman CS, Copel JH, Weinstein EM, et al: Treatment of fetal supraventricular tachyarrhythmias. J Clin Ultrasound 13: 265-273, 1995.

Lev M: Pathogenesis of congenital atrioventricular block. Prog Cardiovasc Disease 25:145-162, 1972.

Lisowski LA, Verheijen PM, Benatar AA, et al: Atrial flutter in the perinatal age group: Diagnosis, management, and outcome. J Am Coll Cardiol 35:771-777, 2000.

Machado MVL, Chita SC, Allan LD: Acceleration time in the aorta and pulmonary artery measured by Doppler echocardiography in the midtrimester normal human fetus. Br Heart J 58:15-18, 1987.

Magee LA, Downar E, Sermer M, et al: Pregnancy outcome after gestational exposure to amiodarone in Canada. Am J Obstet Gynecol 172:1307-1311, 1995.

Maxwell DJ, Crawford DC, Curry PVM, et al: Obstetric importance, diagnosis, and management of fetal tachycardias. BMJ 297:107-110, 1988.

McCue CM, Mantakas ME, Tingelstad JB, et al: Congenital heart block in newborns of mothers with connective tissue disease. Circulation 56:82-90, 1977.

Mendelsohn A, Dick M III, Serwer GA: Natural history of isolated atrial flutter in infancy. J Pediatr 119:386-391, 1991.

Michaelsson M, Engle MA: Congenital complete heart block: An international study of the natural history. Cardiovasc Clin 4:85-101, 1972.

Michaelsson M, Jonson A, Riesenfeld T: Isolated congenital complete atrioventricular block in adult life: A prospective study. Circulation 91:442-449, 1995.

Moak JP, Barron KS, Hougen TJ: Congenital heart block: Development of late-onset cardiomyopathy, a previously under appreciated sequelae. J Am Coll Cardiol 37:238-242, 2001.

Moller JH, Davachi F, Anderson RC: Atrial flutter in infancy. J Pediatr 75:643-51, 1969.

Morquio L: Sur un maladie infantile et familiale caracteristique et la morte subite. Arch Med Enfantes 4:467-475, 1901.

Naheed ZJ, Strasburger JF, Deal BJ, et al: Fetal tachycardia: Mechanisms and predictors of hydrops fetalis. J Am Coll Cardiol 27:1736-1740, 1996.

Olah KS, Gee H: Fetal heart block associated with maternal anti-Ro (SS-A) antibody: Current management: A review. Br J Obstet Gynaecol 98:751-755, 1991.

Omar HA, Rhodes LA, Ramirez R, et al: Alteration of human placental vascular tone by antiarrhythmic medications in vitro. J Cardiovasc Electrophysiol 7:1197-1203, 1996.

Oudjik MA, Michon MM, Kleinman CS, et al: Sotalol in the treatment of fetal dysrhythmias. Circulation 101:2721-2726, 2001.

Perry JC, Garson A Jr: Supraventricular tachycardia due to Wolff-Parkinson-White syndrome in children: early disappearance and late recurrence. J Am Coll Cardiol 16:1215-1220, 1990.

Pfammatter JP, Paul T: Idiopathic ventricular tachycardia in infancy and childhood. A multicenter study on clinical profile and outcome. J Am Coll Cardiol 33:2067-2072, 1999.

Pinsky WW, Gillette PC, Garson A Jr, McNamara DG: Diagnosis, management, and long-term results of patients with congenital complete atrioventricular block. Pediatrics 69:728-733, 1982.

Plomp TA, Vulsma T, de Vijlder JL: Use of amiodarone during pregnancy. Eur J Obstet Gynecol Reprod Biol 43:201-207, 1992.

Reed KL: Fetal arrhythmias: Etiology, diagnosis, pathophysiology, and treatment. Semin Perinatol 13:294, 1989.

Rein AJ, O'Donnell C, Geva T, et al: Use of tissue velocity imaging in the diagnosis of fetal cardiac arrhythmias. Circulation 106(14):1827-1833, 2002.

Rhodes LA, Walsh EP, Saul JP: Conversion of atrial flutter in pediatric patients by transesophageal atrial pacing: A safe, effective, minimally invasive procedure. Am Heart J 130:323-327, 1995.

Rice MJ, McDonald RW, Reller MD: Fetal arrhythmias: A cause of fetal arrhythmias. J Am Coll Cardiol 12(5):1292-1297, 1988.

Schmidt KG, Ulmer HE, Silverman NH, et al: Perinatal outcome of fetal complete atrioventricular block: A multicenter experience. J Am Coll Cardiol 17:1360-1366, 1991.

Schwartz PJ, Stramba-Badiale M, Segantini A, et al: Prolongation of the QT interval and the sudden infant death syndrome. N Engl J Med 338:1709-1714, 1998.

Scott JS, Maddison PJ, Taylor PV, et al: Connective-tissue disease, antibodies to ribonucleoprotein, and congenital heart block. N Engl J Med 309:209-212, 1983.

Sholler GF, Walsh EP: Congenital complete heart block in patients without anatomic cardiac defects. Am Heart J 118:1193-1198, 1989.

Silverman NH, Enderlein MA, Stanger P, et al: Recognition of fetal arrhythmias by echocardiography. J Clin Ultrasound 13: 255-263, 1988.

Silverman NH, Golbus MS. Echocardiographic techniques for assessing normal and abnormal fetal cardiac anatomy. J Am Coll Cardiol 5(suppl):20S-29S, 1985.

Silverman NH, Kohl T, Harrison MR, et al: Experimental surgery in the animal model and in the human fetus. Paper presented at the Second World Congress of Pediatric Cardiology and Cardiac Surgery, Honolulu, Hawaii, 1997, 106.

Simpson JM, Sharland GK: Fetal tachycardias: Management and outcome of 127 consecutive cases. Heart 79:576-581, 1998.

Siren MK, Julkunen H, Kaaja R: The increased incidence of isolated congenital heart block in Finland. J Rheumatol 25: 1262-1264, 1998.

Strasburger JF, Carpenter R, Garson A, et al: Fetal transthoracic pacing for advanced hydrops fetalis secondary to complete atrioventricular block. J Am Coll Cardiol 8:1434-1436, 1986.

Teuscher A, Bossi E, Imhof P, et al: Effect of propranolol on fetal tachycardia in diabetic pregnancy. Am J Cardiol 42: 304-307, 1978.

Theander E, Brucato A, Gudmundsson S, et al: Primary Sjögren's syndrome—treatment of fetal incomplete atrioventricular block with dexamethasone. J Rheumatol 28(2):373-376, 2001.

Thomas J, Edwards M, Park W, et al: Apoptosis as a possible cause of gradual development of complete heart block and fatal arrhythmias associated with absence of the AV node, sinus node, and internodal pathways. Circulation 93:1424-1438, 1996.

Udink ten Cate FEA, Breur JMPJ, Cohen MI, et al: Dilated cardiomyopathy in isolated congenital complete atrioventricular block: Early and long-term risk in children. J Am Coll Cardiol 37:1129-1134, 2001.

Van Engelen AD, Weijtens O, Brenner JL, et al: Management, outcome and follow-up of fetal tachycardia. J Am Coll Cardiol 24:1371-1375, 1994.

Van Gelder-Hasker MR, de Jong CL, de Vries JI, van Geijn HP: The effect of flecainide acetate on fetal heart rate variability: A case report. Obstet Gynecol 86:667-669, 1995.

Van Hare GF, Stanger P: Ventricular tachycardia and accelerated ventricular rhythm presenting in the first month of life. Am J Cardiol 67:42-45, 1991.

Von Bernuth G, Engerlhardt W, Kramer HH, et al: Atrial automatic tachycardia in infancy and childhood. European Heart J 13:1410-1415, 1992.

Walkingshaw SA, Welch CR, McCormack J, et al: In utero pacing for fetal congenital heart block. Fetal Diagn Ther 9: 183-185, 1994.

Waltuck J, Buyon JP: Autoantibody-associated congenital heart block: Outcome in mothers and children. Ann Intern Med 120:544-551, 1994.

Weiner CP, Thompson MIB: Direct treatment of fetal supraventricular tachycardia after failed transplacental therapy. Am J Obstet Gynecol 158:570-573, 1988.

Wiggins JW, Bowes W, Clewell W, et al: Echocardiographic diagnosis and intravenous digoxin management of fetal tachyarrhythmias and congestive heart failure. Am J Dis Child 140:202-204, 1986.

Wolff F, Breuker KH, Schlensker KH, Bolte A: Prenatal diagnosis and therapy of fetal heart rate anomalies: With a contribution on the placental transfer of verapamil. J Perinatol 8:203-208, 1980.

Wren C, Hunter S: Maternal administration of flecainide to terminate and suppress fetal tachycardia. BMJ 296:249-251, 1988.

Wu MHm, Chang YC, Lin JL, et al: Probability of supraventricular tachycardia recurrence in pediatric patients. Cardiology 85:284-289, 1994.

Yamada H, Kato EH, Ebina Y, et al: Fetal treatment of congenital heart block ascribed to anti-SSA antibody: Case reports with observation of cardiohemodynamics and review of the literature. Am J Reproduct Immunol 42:226-232, 1999.

Yoshida H, Iwamoto M, Sakakibara H, et al: Treatment of fetal congenital heart block with maternal administration of betasympathomimetics (terbutaline): A case report. Gynecol Obstet Invest 52(2):142-144, 2001.

Younis JS, Granat M: Insufficient transplacental digoxin transfer in severe hydrops fetalis. Am J Obstet Gynecol 157:1268-1269, 1987.

CHAPTER 59

# Management of Congenital Heart Disease in the Low-Birth-Weight Infant

Gil Wernovsky, Anne M. Ades, and Thomas L. Spray

Low birth weight may coexist in upward of 35% of neonates with critical congenital heart disease (CHD) (Levin et al, 1975), either associated with prematurity or secondary to other factors that make the neonate small for gestational age. The optimal management strategy for these newborns is controversial and has not been fully evaluated.

## GENERAL CONSIDERATIONS IN MANAGEMENT

The preterm low-birth-weight (LBW) neonate with associated complex CHD presents many intricate clinical problems in management, more so than either the preterm neonate without complex heart disease or the term neonate with a complex cardiac malformation. Therapies utilized for the preterm neonate without heart disease frequently need to be altered in the presence of heart disease, and those needed for management of heart disease may need to be altered because of prematurity. Optimal management requires a collaborative approach among many disciplines, including input from neonatologists, cardiologists, surgeons, anesthesiologists, perfusionists, and nurses.

The goals of therapy should be as follows:

1. Initial stabilization, including establishment of reliable vascular access
2. Determination of a complete anatomic diagnosis noninvasively, with minimal stress to the infant
3. Monitoring of the physiology associated with the transition from in utero to ex utero life, which may be more problematic in the preterm infant
4. Evaluation of the newborn for additional congenital defects
5. Early surgical correction of the cardiac defect when technically and logistically possible
6. Establishment of enteral feedings and removal of invasive support and monitoring as rapidly as possible, to minimize hospital-related morbidity

In the past, therapeutic plans for preterm or small-for-gestational age (SGA) neonates with complex heart disease relied on a "conservative" medical approach to attain those goals. It is important to recognize that the secondary effects of uncorrected CHD in the preterm infant may be more severe than in a full-term infant with the same lesions. For example, lesions associated with increased pulmonary blood flow may complicate lung disease of prematurity, and hypoxemia secondary to intracardiac right-to-left shunting may be more deleterious to the immature central nervous system (CNS). In addition, low systemic blood flow may result in an increased risk of significant renal impairment or of necrotizing enterocolitis (NEC) in the preterm infant. Anecdotally, we have found that the hypertrophic response to pressure and volume overload in the postnatal preterm infant appears to be more severe than in the full-term child with the same lesion. With recent technical improvements in cardiopulmonary bypass, anesthesia, and neonatal intensive care, as well as improved (and perhaps more aggressive) surgical techniques, correction of abnormal cardiac anatomy can now be accomplished at an earlier postnatal age and smaller weight. Of importance, this approach restores a more normal cardiac physiology as early as possible, minimizing the secondary effects of the abnormal physiology associated with the CHD, such as increased pulmonary blood flow, pulmonary hypertension, hypoxemia, low systemic blood flow as well as low myocardial pressure, and/or volume overload. In turn, this may shorten hospital length of stay and diminish associated morbidity.

We believe that postponing surgery while waiting for an LBW neonate to gain weight and grow to a desired—though clearly arbitrary—size is an approach not worth taking in the great majority of cases. The requisite stay in the intensive care unit (ICU) for the infant with unrepaired CHD is associated with significant morbidity, and the eventual repair may be no easier from a technical perspective. In fact, the secondary effects of long-standing CHD on the lungs, pulmonary vasculature, and myocardium may render the infant *more* unstable following surgery. Finally, even in optimal circumstances, significant weight gain is rare with critical CHD, even in full-term neonates and infants.

However, it must be recognized that cardiac surgery in LBW neonates—especially procedures involving cardiopulmonary bypass (CPB)—has a complication rate that is significantly higher than in infants and older children, and the risk for mortality and morbidity increases with lower body weight (Heinle et al, 1997; Jacobs et al, 1998; Jonas et al, 1994; Reddy et al, 1999; Wernovsky et al, 2000a). The causes of this increased mortality and morbidity are multifactorial and may include the following:

- Technical issues related to small cardiac structures
- Technical issues related to cannulation for CPB
- Immaturity of organ systems, especially the lungs
- Decreased nutritional reserve
- Limited ability to increase cardiac output secondary to a relatively fixed stroke volume
- Increased risk of bleeding from an immature germinal matrix compounded by the dilutional coagulopathy and thrombocytopenia after CPB
- Increased risk of infection, including NEC
- Abnormal chest wall mechanics, especially after median sternotomy or thoracotomy

For all of these reasons, neonates with complex heart disease and low birth weight have been thought to be at too great a risk for surgery and traditionally have been managed "conservatively" with the hope of weight gain.

However, the rates of complications and of comorbid conditions that may occur in LBW newborns with critical CHD who do *not* undergo surgery—the effects of chronic hospitalization, intravenous access, abnormal cardiovascular physiology, and cardiopulmonary interaction—have not been reported. It is rare in surgical reports to include a consideration of preoperative mortality associated with the CHD. For example, studies that describe the mortality risk for a certain surgical procedure typically do not include the mortality rate for LBW newborns who died while waiting for surgery.

Thus, it is important to carefully categorize and describe critical CHD in the newborn, and to understand the natural history of the unrepaired state (see also Chapter 57). The largest groups of infants with these lesions are those with *duct-dependent pulmonary blood flow* (as in tricuspid atresia, pulmonary atresia, many forms of heterotaxy, and severe forms of tetralogy of Fallot), those with *duct-dependent systemic blood flow* (as in coarctation, hypoplastic left heart syndrome [HLHS], or interrupted aortic arch), or others in whom maintenance of a patent ductus arteriosus improves overall circulatory stability or oxygenation (as in most forms of transposition of the great arteries). The underlying pathophysiology in all of these lesions results in congestive heart failure (CHF), hypoxemia, or both. In these newborns, intravenous prostaglandin is necessary for maintenance of ductus patency, with the attendant risks of infection, apnea, vasodilatation, seizures, and NEC. The benefit of waiting for surgery until some arbitrary weight has been achieved versus performing surgery at a lower body weight with increased risk (i.e., the risk benefit ratio) has not been evaluated. However, it is important to note that studies in LBW newborns with HLHS suggest that weight gain is *not* achieved with time (Weinstein et al, 1999).

Thus, in our center, we recommend cardiac surgery shortly after birth in *any* child with a duct-dependent lesion, essentially regardless of weight. This recommendation is based on the following considerations:

- The known complications of long-term prostaglandin use
- The morbidity associated with in-hospital intensive care
- The fact that weight gain is unlikely
- The abnormal physiology present in all of these children (volume overload, CHF, hypoxemia) with its significant but difficult-to-quantify secondary effects on the heart, pulmonary vasculature, mesenteric and renal circulations, and CNS

We believe it is likely that the *combined* risks associated with the unrepaired physiology, ICU-related complications, and eventual surgery (at a weight that is typically not much different from birth weight) are greater than the risks for mortality and morbidity with surgery shortly after birth. In addition, we recommend surgery for neonates with noncritical lesions that result in increased ventricular work—regardless of weight—at the first signs of CHF and failure to thrive. However, there are many issues that must be addressed and anticipated in this high-risk group of neonates.

A second large group of patients are those with large left-to-right shunt lesions and pulmonary hypertension, as with large ventricular septal defects, truncus arteriosus, complete atrioventricular canal, patent ductus arteriosus, and aortopulmonary window. Following the expected fall in pulmonary vascular resistance, pulmonary blood flow will increase, resulting in CHF, failure to thrive, and/or ventilator dependence. In essentially all of these children, the abnormal circulatory physiology results in increased total energy expenditure, making weight gain even in optimal conditions unlikely. Struggling to "get weight on the baby" may not be worth the risk. For example, a 1.9-kg baby with CHF who might only gain 10 to15 g/day (requiring high-caloric feeds, anticongestive medications, possible tube feedings, or even mechanical ventilation) will take 1 to 3 months to achieve a weight of 2.5 kg. The risks to the baby during that time may be considerable, especially if hospitalization is required, and include infection, long-standing increased pulmonary blood flow and pulmonary artery pressure (making the postoperative course *more* risky), and an uncertain promise of weight gain. Of importance, the relative risk for surgery for a baby of 1.9 kg who has *not* had a prolonged period of CHF versus that for a baby of 2.5 kg who has been in CHF for 2 additional months is unclear.

## SURGICAL ISSUES

As diagnostic, intensive care, and intraoperative cardiac surgical techniques have improved, the technical issues related to operating on LBW infants (with birth weights of <2.5 kg) have become less of a consideration. Philosophically, the surgical team may be faced with a decision to perform palliative procedures initially, followed by corrective surgery at a later date, or to proceed with corrective "open" procedures with use of CPB. In general, for the LBW infant, if palliative procedures can be performed to allow control of CHF without compromising the patient's nutrition or other organ systems, palliation may be preferable to an open repair with the attendant risks of CNS bleeding, hypoxemic-ischemic damage, and activation of the inflammation cascade.

"Closed" operations may include shunt placement, pulmonary arterial banding, coarctation repair, and ductus ligation. Although vessels are small, it is certainly possible to consider repair of coarctation of the aorta even in very small neonates weighing less than 1 kg. Ductus ligation has been performed frequently in newborns of this weight (Perez et al, 1998), and coarctation repair also can be performed with reasonable safety. As a practical matter, however, it is unusual to require coarctation repair in very small neonates with noncritical coarctation, in whom the blood pressure generally can be well controlled after ductal closure with antihypertensive medication until an older age and higher weight are achieved. In the presence of a coexisting ventricular septal defect, however, it may be necessary to address the distal aortic obstruction in addition to performing pulmonary artery banding at a very low weight to allow for satisfactory growth and development.

Lesions with duct-dependent pulmonary blood flow (e.g., severe forms of tetralogy of Fallot, pulmonary atresia with intact ventricular septum) may be treated temporarily by short-term prostaglandin infusion and placement of aortopulmonary artery shunts. In general, it is preferable to create an aortopulmonary shunt rather than to continue prostaglandin therapy indefinitely during postnatal life, because the long-term complications of intravenous access and continuous prostaglandin therapy are considerable. Shunts may be physiologically quite large in very small babies, and determining the appropriate size of the shunt is of prime importance. Generally, a modified Blalock-Taussig shunt 3 mm in diameter can be used for babies weighing 1 to 1.5 kg, and a 3.5-mm shunt may be adequate for babies weighing greater than 1.5 kg, with the length altered to allow for additional resistance in children at the lower end of that weight range. Central shunts may be more advisable for patients with suitable anatomy; however, a short central shunt may actually provide excessive pulmonary blood flow. To reemphasize, shunting in patients at a very low birth weight is a temporary palliative procedure to allow for weight gain and to avoid CPB, followed by either conversion to a complete repair in patients with two ventricles when the baby achieves an acceptable weight, or conversion to a cavopulmonary shunt in patients with a single ventricle at 4 to 6 months of age.

However, true "correction" of most cardiac defects in LBW infants requires the use of CPB. In these neonates, technical modifications related to cannulation and to bypass technique are necessary. Even with current miniaturization of CPB circuits, the relative volume of the circuit will dilute clotting factors in the very small infant to a significant degree. Addition of clotting factors to the bypass circuit may be necessary. Our current method for dealing with this problem is the use of fresh whole blood added to the bypass circuit, and following separation from CPB while in the ICU (Manno et al, 1991). Although significant hemodilution may be tolerated in older babies, the use of a very hemodiluted bypass prime in LBW babies adds to the difficulty in supplying adequate red cell mass after completion of the operation. Even with the use of modified ultrafiltration techniques (Skaryak et al, 1995), the hematocrit may not be able to be raised to a suitable level following the operation if severe hemodilution is used. Therefore, we prefer to use only moderate hemodilution in very small babies with use of modified ultrafiltration to eliminate as much free water as possible following the operation. This approach allows the venous pressures to be brought as low as possible, thereby providing "room" to infuse additional clotting factors after separation from the bypass circuit. If hemodilution is too great, it may not be possible to give clotting factors and blood following the operation without excessively raising venous pressures, which may contribute to intracranial bleeding and lead to hemodynamic instability.

It is important in LBW babies, especially premature infants, to maintain blood pressures in the lower range of normal. Particular care should be taken to prevent mean arterial pressure elevations during CPB in the heparinized patient. Hypertension in association with a post-bypass coagulopathy may result in generalized oozing at the intracardiac suture lines, but the combination of hypertension and coagulopathy may be particularly disastrous, given the increased risk of intracranial bleeding in the preterm neonate. We therefore institute systemic vasodilatation after weaning from bypass—typically with milrinone and/or sodium nitroprusside.

Because of the technical difficulties and size of bypass cannulae during CPB in very small babies, deep hypothermic circulatory arrest is frequently utilized. With circulatory arrest techniques, accurate repairs can be performed in even very small babies weighing less than 1 kg, but use of these techniques may increase the long-term risk of neurologic morbidity (see also Chapter 60) (Bellinger et al, 1999; Rappaport et al, 1998; Wernovsky et al, 2000b). Even in the absence of CHD, long-term follow-up evaluation of very LBW (VLBW) neonates has revealed an increased incidence of neurologic abnormalities; therefore, long-term follow-up is particularly warranted in this group of patients with CHD (Borowski et al, 1997; Vohr et al, 2000).

## RESULTS

An increasing number of studies are reviewing the overall surgical outcomes in LBW infants who have undergone cardiac operations (Beyens et al, 1998; Borowski et al, 1997; Bove and Lloyd, 1996; Chang et al, 1994; Malec et al, 2000; Numa et al, 1992; Pawade et al, 1993; Reddy and Hanley, 2000; Reddy et al, 1999; Rossi et al, 1998; Weinstein et al, 1999). The overall survival rate for infants undergoing corrective or palliative reconstruction for CHD in these series was 80% to 87% but was lower than for babies of normal weight with similar cardiac lesions. In addition, although most studies have confirmed the increased morbidity (and slightly greater early mortality) for surgery in infants in these weight ranges compared with that associated with surgery in babies of normal birth weight, the combined effect of prolonged attempts at weight gain on chronic morbidity would seem to favor primary repair in most patients, especially those with two-ventricle physiology. Even complex reconstructions such as the arterial switch repair and truncus arteriosus correction can be accomplished in very small babies with acceptable operative risk.

A major question is "How small is too small?" when complex palliative operations such as stage I reconstruction for HLHS are under consideration. Although early survival after the first stage of reconstructive surgery for HLHS has steadily improved, with rates now approaching 95% among standard-risk patients at our institution, early survival for HLHS remains significantly less than for other cardiac defects requiring neonatal surgery. In addition, low birth weight and being small for gestational age (below the 10th percentile for birth weight) are more common in these infants, and there is an increased incidence of extracardiac anomalies (Glauser et al, 1990), both increasing the surgical risk for stage I reconstruction. Only a few patients with HLHS have been included in previously published studies on the results of cardiac surgery in LBW infants (Beyens et al, 1998; Bove and Lloyd, 1996; Chang et al, 1994; Malec et al, 2000; Pawade et al, 1993; Rossi et al, 1998).

Not surprisingly, prematurity and low weight in infants with HLHS have been found to be risk factors associated with higher mortality (Jacobs et al, 1998; Razzouk et al, 1996; Weinstein et al, 1999). A review of overall surgical results for HLHS from Bove and Lloyd (1996) recognized low birth weight as a significant risk factor for in-hospital mortality. Because of these outcomes, some authors have suggested that LBW patients might best be referred for cardiac transplantation. However, in a Congenital Heart Surgeons Society study, low birth weight was found to be an incremental risk factor for death in both staged reconstruction and transplantation protocols (Jacobs et al, 1998), and in the largest series of infants receiving transplants reported from Loma Linda, the average weight was 3.7 kg and the smallest patient who underwent transplantation weighed 2.0 kg (Razzouk et al, 1996). Thus, the availability of hearts for VLBW babies is probably limited, and low birth weight may in fact be a contraindication to transplantation as the primary surgical strategy.

We have previously reported on the experience with 67 children weighing less than 2.5 kg undergoing first-stage reconstruction for HLHS between January 1, 1990, and December 31, 1997 (Weinstein et al, 1999). Mean age at surgery was 10.1 days, with a median of 8 days, and mean weight was 2.2 kg, with a median weight of 2.2 kg. Fourteen patients weighed less than 2.0 kg and two patients weighed less than 1.5 kg. Early mortality rate (death within 30 days or before hospital discharge) was 51%. No patient-, procedure-, or time-related variables correlated with increased mortality. However, there was a trend toward increased mortality with increased cardiopulmonary bypass time ($P = .08$) and decreased preoperative ventricular performance ($P = .1$). Babies in whom surgery was delayed did not experience a statistically significant increase in weight before the date of surgery, suggesting that delay in surgery to permit weight gain is not justified and exposes the patient to prolonged risks of pulmonary overcirculation, long-term mechanical ventilation, and other ICU-related complications.

We also recently retrospectively analyzed LBW infants with congenital heart disease who had cardiac surgery at our institution between July 2000 and July 2002. Patients were excluded if they had atrial or ventricular septal defects not requiring surgical closure during the initial hospitalization or isolated patent ductus arteriosus. Fifty-four LBW infants underwent cardiac surgery at our institution in the specified time period. For the overall population, the median gestational age and weight were 35 weeks and 2061 g, respectively. Thirteen infants (24%) were also small for gestational age. The median gestational age and weight of the SGA infants were 37 weeks and 1845 g, respectively. Nineteen (35%) of the patients had HLHS and its variants. Postoperative mortality rates were 25.9% (14/54) overall and 36.8% in patients with HLHS. There was no influence of SGA status ($P = .31$) or associated major congenital anomalies ($P = .53$) on mortality. Common postoperative morbidity included blood culture–positive sepsis (22.6%), proven NEC (5.7%), suspected NEC (15.1%), periventricular echodensities (37%), and severe intracranial hemorrhage (ICH) in 3.8% of infants.

## NUTRITION

During the third trimester of pregnancy, which is foreshortened in the preterm baby, the transplacental accretion rate of metabolic and growth fuels is incredibly high. It is extremely difficult to successfully reproduce this function of placental transfer in the extrauterine environment. The task of supplying fuel for growth becomes even more difficult when necessary limits are placed on the total amount of fluid that may be administered either parenterally or via the enteral route in these preterm neonates with CHD. In the neonate being enterally nourished, formula concentrated to a caloric density in excess of 30 calories per ounce is sometimes utilized for growth but may present a hyperosmolar load to the gastrointestinal tract or provide calories in a nonphysiologic distribution of protein, fat, and carbohydrate. Hyperosmolar feedings have been associated with an increased risk of NEC in the preterm neonate or, more rarely, in the neonate born at term who has decreased splanchnic blood flow from any cause, such as left-sided obstructive lesions (see later). If nutritional needs are met by the parenteral route, as is frequently the case in the preterm neonate with complex heart disease, administration of highly concentrated parenteral nutrition fluid into a large central vein is required, to maximize caloric administration while limiting infusion volumes.

When composing the parenteral nourishment, one must be aware of the increased risk of precipitation of its constituents when the solution is concentrated to the degree necessary for the fluid-restricted preterm neonate. Crucial for growth is administration of calories in the correct proportions of protein, lipid, and carbohydrates; also crucial but problematic can be intravenous access with a centrally placed catheter.

In the preoperative patient, the preferred method of placing central catheters is via the percutaneous route (peripherally inserted central catheters [PICCs], transumbilical lines), rather than operative placement of Broviac catheters; however, preterm neonates with central catheters placed by either route frequently have complicated hospital courses with catheter-related problems. In particular, thrombosis of central vessels or bacteremia is particularly problematic in patients awaiting cardiac surgery. Complications include nosocomially acquired bacteremia, thrombosis, sympathetic effusions, and rarely, perforation through a vessel wall. Hydrothorax, hemothorax, and pericardial effusions with or without tamponade are not rare events. The use of central catheters in VLBW neonates (<1500 g) *without* congenital heart disease is clearly associated with sepsis; upward of 20% of those neonates with central catheters in place have at least one episode of sepsis. This risk is likely to be higher in patients with CHD, especially in the postoperative period with increased numbers of monitoring and drainage catheters. Although hospital-acquired infections have been associated with a myriad of etiologic agents (e.g., sporadic reports of contaminated intravenous fluids, suction catheters, thermometers, use of artificial nails by caregivers, overuse of antimicrobial agents), the risk factors that repeatedly correlate with neonatal infection are (1) the use of central catheters and (2) the use of mechanical ventilation. Every attempt must be made to wean patients to spontaneous ventilation and to start enteral feeds as rapidly as possible to minimize these complications.

## MECHANICAL VENTILATION

Mechanical ventilation is frequently necessary in caring for the preterm neonate with complex CHD, especially in those babies with malformations that either produce or are associated with increased pulmonary blood flow or pulmonary venous engorgement of any cause. Such cardiac lesions are associated with decreased pulmonary compliance, compelling the most fragile babies to breathe with the greatest of effort and generate greater-than-normal inspiratory pressures. This increased work of breathing can be sustained for only a limited period without the use of mechanical ventilatory support. In addition, the chest wall and airways of these preterm neonates are far more compliant than their noncompliant lungs, further decreasing effective tidal volumes and minute ventilation. Dead space ventilation as a proportion of tidal volume increases, promoting further respiratory failure with the need for both endotracheal intubation and initiation of mechanical ventilation. Both of these interventions have been associated with lung inflammation and the subsequent release of inflammatory mediators, recently suggested as the initiating events in the etiology of the chronic lung disease affecting the lungs of preterm neonates known as bronchopulmonary dysplasia (BPD). In addition, the pulmonary toxicity of high concentrations of inspired oxygen in the pathogenesis of this disease should not be forgotten. The presence of BPD is likely to be detrimental to surgical outcomes. Whenever possible, early correction may be advantageous for these prematurely born neonates.

Following sternotomy or thoracotomy, intermittent positive-pressure ventilation is almost always necessary; preterm neonates in particular do not spontaneously ventilate well because of the added chest wall instability induced by the surgical approach. Even when pre-extubation cardiac and pulmonary parameters appear appropriate for a trial of extubation, re-intubation for respiratory failure in these children is not uncommon, being required in up to 25% of cases in our experience. This is in stark contrast to a low re-intubation rate for full-term neonates and infants (<5%) after similar cardiac surgical procedures. It is important to recognize and investigate the possibility of phrenic nerve injury contributing to the difficulty with attempts at extubation in these babies, especially following procedures with placement of a Blalock-Taussig shunt (deLeeuw et al, 1999), arch reconstruction, and/or hilar dissection of the pulmonary arteries (e.g., coarctation repair, stage I reconstruction for HLHS, arterial switch operation, repair or palliation of tetralogy of Fallot).

Preterm or LBW neonates may particularly benefit from nasal continuous positive airway pressure (CPAP) as a "wean" from continuous positive-pressure mechanical ventilation. Permissive hypercarbia is currently under research study in preterm neonates as a means of minimizing both "volutrauma" and "barotrauma"; although the evidence is not yet finalized, use of this modality may be an effective and safe way to decrease the incidence of BPD. If true, and *if the cardiac physiology does not preclude or contraindicate its use*, mechanical ventilation that produces $P_{CO_2}$ values of 50 to 55 mm Hg may be less detrimental to the pulmonary outcome in these neonates.

## NECROTIZING ENTEROCOLITIS

NEC is a disease of the neonate in which the mucosal barrier of the gut is typically damaged and breached by pathogenic enteric bacteria, resulting in intestinal injury that may progress to bowel necrosis, sepsis, and death. The risk of developing NEC is inversely related to gestational age at birth. In addition, CHD has been found in several studies to be a predisposing factor for the development of NEC in neonates born at or close to term (Martinez-Tallo et al, 1997; Wiswell et al, 1988). A recent report by McElhinney and colleagues (2000) described a cohort of 643 neonates with complex CHD admitted to our cardiac intensive care unit (CICU). The incidence of NEC in this cohort was 3.3%, which is substantially (10- to 100-fold) higher than the reported population-wide rates of 0.3/1000 to 3/1000 term newborns. In a case-control analysis of data for infants matched by diagnosis and age at admission to the CICU, risk factors for the development of NEC were prematurity (<36 weeks), episodes of poor systemic perfusion, and a maximum dose of prostaglandin of greater than 0.05 μg/kg/minute. By multivariable analyses, lesions with significant aortic "run-off" into the lungs (e.g., HLHS, truncus arteriosus, aortopulmonary window), lower gestational age, and episodes of low cardiac output (based on laboratory criteria suggesting end-organ damage) were found to be independently significant risk factors. Although prostaglandin use and, to a lesser extent, indwelling umbilical catheters and cardiac catheterization have been reported as probable causative factors for NEC, it may in fact be the underlying CHD and its management, rather than the prostaglandin or umbilical lines per se, that are most contributory. Thus, the LBW baby with CHD has two major risk factors for the development of NEC, adding to the surgical risk and overall morbidity. Strategies aimed at minimizing preoperative prostaglandin dose and maximizing preoperative and postoperative cardiac output and oxygen delivery and prompt surgical intervention in the neonate with high-risk anatomy may reduce these risks in the future.

## POSTOPERATIVE CONSIDERATIONS

Ideal postoperative care of the patient following either reparative or palliative operations requires a thorough understanding and systematic evaluation of the following:

1. The underlying anatomic defect
2. The pathophysiology of the preoperative state (including secondary effects on other organ systems from altered cardiac output preoperatively)
3. The anesthetic regimen used during surgery
4. CPB issues (e.g., duration of bypass and circulatory arrest, if utilized)
5. The details of the operative procedure and any concerns of the surgeon regarding the potential for residual defects
6. Data available from monitoring catheters, echocardiography, and cardiac catheterization

Optimal management of these critically ill children can best be achieved through a harmonious "team" approach, combining the expertise of cardiologists, cardiac surgeons, neonatologists, anesthesiologists, intensivists, nurses and respiratory therapists.

In general, when the clinical course, postoperative hemodynamic measurements, or laboratory data do not correspond to the expected postoperative recovery, it is prudent to suspect both the accuracy of the preoperative diagnosis and the adequacy of the surgical repair, rather than to presume that the preoperative diagnosis and surgical repair were entirely complete and that the patient is failing for some ill-defined reason (such as "low-cardiac output syndrome"). Decreased cardiac output does occur following CPB (Wernovsky et al, 1995) but usually can be anticipated and adequately managed (Hoffman et al, 2002). When significant residual anatomic defects are suspected, complete investigation, including echocardiography and/or catheterization, should be pursued. It is important to emphasize that echocardiography in the postoperative patient—particularly in the LBW neonate—is not entirely a benign, "noninvasive" procedure (see Chapter 54). Abnormal respiratory mechanics and changes in preload and afterload should be expected and anticipated during the study. A caregiver *not* involved in the performance or interpretation of the echocardiogram should be present to perform ongoing assessment of the baby's airway, ventilation, perfusion, and metabolic stability.

## Pain Control and Sedation

Stress responses to pain and other noxious stimuli are profound in even the youngest neonates, regardless of gestational age (Anand and Hickey, 1987). These hormonal and metabolic stress responses may have pathologic and deleterious consequences (Anand and Hickey, 1992), and the hypertensive sequelae of pain and agitation are to be particularly avoided (see earlier). Regardless of which medications are chosen, it is important on physiologic grounds alone to give children of all ages adequate anesthesia or analgesia for suppression of the responses to noxious stimulation. The neonate responds to stressful perioperative stimuli with altered hemodynamics and stress hormone levels (Anand and Hickey, 1987).

Evidence of the adverse cardiorespiratory effects of stress is provided in reports of bradycardia, hypoxia, systemic blood pressure lability, and increased intracranial pressure in newborns undergoing the stress of awake intubation. Patients with CHD who are recovering from surgical reconstruction are especially sensitive to stressful interventions and have marginal organ system reserves and insufficient compensatory mechanisms to respond adequately.

Evidence is accumulating that extending anesthesia for a short time in the immediate postoperative period may blunt the adverse hemodynamic lability and hormonal stress response and improve outcome without complicating or extending postoperative care (Wernovsky et al, 1995). The postoperative myocardium that has been exposed to the effects of CPB, aortic cross-clamping, deep hypothermia, or myocardial ischemic damage may not be capable of increasing stroke volume during a bradycardic episode or of maintaining cardiac output during an acute increase in afterload following surgical procedures. This is especially true if myocardial performance is impaired by a ventriculotomy as required for repair of a variety of CHDs. Therefore, we typically use intermittant neuromuscular blockade and analgesia with fentanyl (2 to 4 μg/kg/hour) for the first 12 to 24 hours following neonatal repairs that utilize CPB.

Wakefulness, agitation, and stress responses in mechanically ventilated children may increase the work of breathing, exacerbate asynchrony between patient and ventilator, and cause an increase in arterial $P_{CO_2}$. The associated decrease in pH significantly raises pulmonary vascular resistance (PVR) in children following CPB. Endotracheal suctioning causes sympathetic stimulation and marked elevation in PVR which can be attenuated by pretreatment with high doses of narcotic (Hickey et al, 1985). In an infant with a healthy heart and normal cardiovascular reserve, a painful or stressful stimulus may produce tachycardia, hypertension, and a transient decrease in arterial $P_{O_2}$ (Tanner et al, 1985). However, in a postoperative cardiac surgical patient, the tachycardia may evolve into a hemodynamically compromising tachyarrhythmia, and the hypertension may present a critical and intolerable increase in ventricular afterload or may complicate hemostasis. Hypoxia may be profound and prolonged if the child has cyanotic heart disease or experiences intermittent right-to-left shunting during periods of agitation, when intrathoracic pressure and right ventricular afterload are increased.

This sensitivity to stimuli and lability in hemodynamic response may be expressed as sudden death during the first postoperative night following apparently successful and uncomplicated congenital heart surgery. This appears to be especially true among patients with labile pulmonary artery hypertension and in palliated single-ventricle patients, in whom the balance between systemic and pulmonary vascular resistance plays an important role in hemodynamic stability.

## Monitoring

Accurate measurement of systemic and pulmonary arterial pressures, ventricular filling pressures, urine output, alveolar gas exchange, cardiac output, and systemic and pulmonary vascular resistances allows for precise pharmacologic and ventilatory support in the perioperative period. Monitoring techniques and risks and benefits are detailed in Chapter 57. In the LBW neonate undergoing cardiac surgery, invasive, transthoracic intracardiac monitoring is well tolerated and reduces the risk of central vein thrombosis associated with use of transcutaneous catheters in small babies. Because the LBW neonate has such wide swings in physiologic variables such as heart rate, blood pressure, temperature, and glucose metabolism, frequently *more* physiologic monitoring, not less, is required, despite the baby's small size. In particular, *continuous* monitoring of important hemodynamic and respiratory parameters is gaining widespread acceptance in postoperative cardiac patients. In addition to the routine use of systemic intra-arterial catheters, typically in the umbilical artery, there is growing experience with intra-arterial sensors that provide continuous, real-time assessment of blood gas data, temperature, and calculated base deficit (Neotrend, Diametrics Medical, St. Paul, Minnesota), even in LBW babies. These types of catheters are likely to be particularly beneficial in the LBW postoperative cardiac patient, who requires frequent laboratory assessments but has a more limited blood volume.

Finally, *cranial ultrasonography* should be performed in LBW babies preoperatively to identify intracranial hemorrhage, which may influence the timing of surgery or the CPB strategy. Cranial ultrasound examination also is useful to diagnose periventricular leukomalacia in this at-risk population. In premature infants, we also perform a postoperative head ultrasound examination 2 to 3 days after surgery in view of their increased risk of intracranial hemorrhage, or if there are neurologic or hematologic concerns.

## SUMMARY

LBW infants with CHD are likely to be at a higher risk for postoperative death and complications than that observed in their normal-sized counterparts owing to the combined effects of prematurity and of the unrepaired CHD on organ system function and technical issues related to the repair. However, current experience does not suggest that waiting until the baby attains an arbitrary weight before surgery significantly improves outcome. Survival rates for LBW infants undergoing complex repairs such as those for interruption of the aortic arch and HLHS are less than those for larger babies undergoing the same operation at the same institution; however, the absolute survival rates are still acceptable (given the alternative of death). Weight alone should therefore not be considered a contraindication to surgery for complex CHD. A careful investigation for the *cause* of the low birth weight must be undertaken (e.g., prematurity, intrauterine infections, multiple congenital anomalies, genetic syndromes) and appropriate options discussed and therapies initiated. The medical and surgical teams should collaborate to determine the optimal timing and type of surgery, with body weight being only of minor importance.

## REFERENCES


Anand KJS, Hickey PR: Pain and its effects in the human neonate and fetus. N Engl J Med 317:1321-1329, 1987.

Anand KJS, Hickey PR: Halothane-morphine compared with high-dose sufentanil for anesthesia and postoperative analgesia in neonatal cardiac surgery. N Engl J Med 326:1-9, 1992.

Bellinger DC, Wypij D, Kuban KCK, et al: Developmental and neurologic status of children at 4 years of age after heart surgery with hypothermic circulatory arrest or low-flow cardiopulmonary bypass. Circulation 100:526-532, 1999.

Beyens T, Biarent D, Bouton JM, et al: Cardiac surgery with extracorporeal circulation in 23 infants weighing 2500 g or less: Short and intermediate term outcome. Eur J Cardiothorac Surg 14:165-172, 1998.

Borowski A, Schickendantz S, Mennicken U, Korb H: Open heart interventions in premature low- and very-low-birth-weight neonates: Risk profile and ethical considerations. Thorac Cardiovasc Surg 45:238-241, 1997.

Bove E, Lloyd T: Staged reconstruction for hypoplastic left heart syndrome: Contemporary results. Ann Surg 224:387-395, 1996.

Chang AC, Hanley FH, Lock FE, et al: Management and outcome of low birth weight neonates with congenital heart disease. J Pediatr 124:461-466, 1994.

deLeeuw M, Williams JM, Freedom RM, et al: Impact of diaphragmatic paralysis after cardiothoracic surgery in children. J Thorac Cardiovasc Surg 118:510-517, 1999.

Glauser T, Rorke L, Weinberg P, Clancy R: Congenital brain anomalies associated with the hypoplastic left heart syndrome. Pediatrics 85:984-990, 1990.

Heinle JS, Diaz LK, Fox LS: Early extubation after cardiac operations in neonates and young infants. J Thorac Cardiovasc Surg 114:413-418, 1997.

Hickey PR, Hansen DD, Wessel DL, et al: Blunting of stress responses in the pulmonary circulation of infants by fentanyl. Anesth Analg 64:1137-1142, 1985.

Hoffman TM, Wernovsky G, Atz AM, et al: Efficacy and safety of milrinone in preventing low cardiac output syndrome in infants and children after corrective surgery for congenital heart disease. Circulation 107:996-1002, 2002.

Jacobs ML, Blackstone EH, Bailey LL, Congenital Heart Surgeons Society: Intermediate survival in neonates with aortic atresia: A multi-institutional study. J Thorac Cardiovasc Surg 116:417-431, 1998.

Jonas RA, Quaegebeur JM, Kirklin JW, et al: Outcomes in patients with interrupted aortic arch and ventricular septal defect. J Thorac Cardiovasc Surg 107:1099-1113, 1994.

Levin DL, Stanger P, Kitterman JA, Heymann MA: Congenital heart disease in low birth weight infants. Circulation 52: 500-503, 1975.

Malec E, Werynski P, Mroczek T, et al: Results of surgical treatment of congenital heart defects in infants below 2500 grams. Przegl Lek 57:187-190, 2000.

Manno C, Hedberg K, Kim H, et al: Comparison of the hemostatic effects of fresh whole blood, stored whole blood, and components after open heart surgery in children. Blood 77:930-936, 1991.

Martinez-Tallo E, Claure N, Bancalari E: Necrotizing enterocolitis in full-term or near-term infants; risk factors. Biol Neonate 71:292-298, 1997.

McElhinney DB, Hedrick HL, Bush DM, et al: Necrotizing enterocolitis in neonates with congenital heart disease: risk factors and outcomes. Pediatrics 106:1080-1087, 2000.

Numa A, Butt W, Mee RB: Outcome of infants with birthweight 2000 g or less who undergo major cardiac surgery. J Paediatr Child Health 28:318-320, 1992.

Pawade A, Waterson K, Laussen P, et al: Cardiopulmonary bypass in neonates weighing less than 2.5 kg: Analysis of the risk factors for early and late mortality: J Cardiovasc Surg 8:1-8, 1993.

Perez CA, Bustorff-Silva JM, Villasenor E, et al: Surgical ligation of patent ductus arteriosus in very low birth weight infants: Is it safe? Am Surg 64:1007-1009, 1998.

Rappaport LA, Wypij D, Bellinger DC, et al: Relation of seizures after cardiac surgery in early infancy to neurodevelopmental outcome. Circulation 97:773-779, 1998.

Razzouk AJ, Chinnock RE, Gundry SR, et al: Transplantation as a primary treatment for hypoplastic left heart syndrome: Intermediate-term results. Ann Thorac Surg 62:1-8, 1996.

Reddy VM, Hanley FH: Cardiac surgery in infants with very low birth weight. Semin Pediatr Surg 9:91-95, 2000.

Reddy VM, McElhinney DB, Sagrado T, et al: Results of 102 cases of complete repair of congenital heart defects in patients weighing 700 to 2500 grams. J Thorac Cardiovasc Surg 117: 324-331, 1999.

Rossi AF, Seiden HS, Sadeghi AM, et al: The outcome of cardiac operations in infants weighing two kilograms or less. J Thoracic Cardiovasc Surg 116:28-32, 1998.

Skaryak L, Kirshbom P, DiBernardo L, et al: Modified ultrafiltration improves cerebral metabolic recovery after circulatory arrest. J Thorac Cardiovasc Surg 109:744-752, 1995.

Tanner GE, Angers DG, Barash PG: Effect of left-to-right, mixed left-to-right, and right-to-left shunts on inhalational anesthetic induction in children. Anesth Analg 64:101-107, 1985.

Vohr BR, Wright LL, Dusick AM, et al: Neurodevelopmental and functional outcomes of extremely low birth weight infants in the National Institute of Child Health and Human

Development Neonatal Research Network, 1993-1994. Pediatrics 105:1216-1226, 2000.

Weinstein S, Gaynor JW, Bridges ND, et al: Early survival of infants weighing 2.5 kilograms or less undergoing first-stage reconstruction for hypoplastic left heart syndrome. Circulation 100[suppl II]: II-167–II-170, 1999.

Wernovsky G, Mayer JE, Jonas RA, et al: Factors influencing early and late outcome of the arterial switch operation for transposition of the great arteries. J Thorac Cardiovasc Surg 109:289-302, 2000a.

Wernovsky G, Stiles KM, Gauvreau K, et al: Cognitive development after the Fontan operation. Circulation 102:883-889, 2000b.

Wernovsky G, Wypij D, Jonas RA, et al: Postoperative course and hemodynamic profile after the arterial switch operation in neonates and infants: A comparison of low-flow cardiopulmonary bypass and circulatory arrest. Circulation 92:2226-2235, 1995.

Wiswell TE, Robertson CF, Jones TA, Tuttle DJ: Necrotizing enterocolitis in full-term infants: A case-control study. Am J Dis Child 142:535, 1988.

CHAPTER 60

# Long-Term Neurologic Outcomes in Children with Congenital Heart Disease

J. William Gaynor and Gil Wernovsky

An estimated 30,000 to 40,000 children are born in North America each year with congenital heart disease (CHD), and approximately one third require surgical intervention during the first year of life. In the past 2 decades, there has been a dramatic reduction in surgical mortality, which has been accompanied by increasing recognition of adverse neurodevelopmental sequelae in some children. Evaluation of preschool- and school-aged children following neonatal and infant repair of CHD demonstrates a pattern of neurodevelopmental sequelae characterized by mild cognitive impairment; expressive speech and language abnormalities; impaired visual-spatial and visual-motor skills; attention-deficit/hyperactivity disorder (ADHD); motor delays; and learning disabilities (Table 60–1). The need for early intervention, rehabilitative services, and special education reduces the quality of life for the children and their families, as well as resulting in significant costs to society.

Central nervous system (CNS) injury in children with CHD is a result of a complex interaction of patient-specific factors (diagnosis, genetic susceptibility) and environmental influences (cardiac surgery, socioeconomic status) (Table 60–2). The risk of a poor developmental outcome varies according to the specific cardiac defect. In addition, there is significant interindividual variation in developmental outcome, even among children with the same cardiac defect. Cerebral ischemia before, during, and after the surgical repair of CHD has been proposed to be a primary mechanism of CNS injury. However, many factors may contribute to neurologic dysfunction: congenital or acquired structural CNS abnormalities; hypoxemia and acidosis secondary to uncorrected CHD; and associated anomalies or genetic syndromes. Immaturity of the developing CNS also may be a factor. Perioperative events at the time of reconstructive surgery have been implicated as important factors in postoperative neurologic dysfunction. Factors that possibly contribute to intraoperative neurologic injury include the type of support during surgery (deep hypothermic circulatory arrest [DHCA] or continuous cardiopulmonary bypass [CPB]), use of hemodilution, the degree of cooling, and type of blood gas management. Hemodynamic instability with impaired cerebral perfusion in the postoperative period or fever with increased oxygen consumption may exacerbate cerebral injury. However, these potential risk factors do not fully explain either the high frequency or the pattern of neurodevelopmental dysfunction described following infant cardiac surgery, suggesting that other patient-specific factors may be important determinants of neurologic injury.

It may be very difficult to completely define the etiologic factors leading to CNS injury in patients with CHD. The neurologic sequelae of cardiac surgery can be subtle in very young infants. The full extent of an injury is often not fully recognized until long after the event, when certain cognitive and higher executive skills are required. Neurologic examination of neonates and infants is limited; and developmental testing, even at 1 year of age, has imprecise predictive value for long-term neurodevelopmental outcomes. Investigators have evaluated potential surrogate measures such as electroencephalographic monitoring and magnetic resonance imaging (MRI) of the brain. However, the predictive value of these tests in isolation for long-term neurodevelopmental outcome is uncertain. Examination of preschool- and school-aged children provides greater sensitivity and specificity in determination of neurologic defects and remains the standard for evaluation of the neurologic sequelae of infant cardiac surgery.

## GENETIC SUSCEPTIBILITY TO NEUROLOGIC INJURY AND DEVELOPMENTAL DYSFUNCTION

Intellectual development and cognitive function are highly heritable and probably are dependent on multiple genes, as well as on environmental factors. Numerous inherited defects or syndromes that are associated with compromised mental development and intellectual capacity (e.g., Down syndrome, Williams syndrome, DiGeorge syndrome) may have CHD as one of the phenotypic outcomes. Although the genetic basis for most cardiac defects has not been delineated, specific genetic anomalies have been implicated in the pathogenesis of some defects. For example, microdeletions of chromosome 22 are associated with DiGeorge syndrome and a variety of heart defects, including tetralogy of Fallot (TOF), truncus arteriosus, and interruption of the aortic arch. Developmental abnormalities are present in children with 22q11 microdeletions, even those with no cardiac abnormalities (Gerdes et al, 1999). Thus, children with cardiac defects and 22q11 microdeletions may be developmentally impaired independent of the cardiac defect and cardiac surgery. It may be difficult to separate the adverse developmental sequlae of an underlying genetic anomaly from those related to CHD and cardiac surgery.

Risk of disease or injury in response to an environmental stimulus is a complex interaction between genetic susceptibility and environmental exposures. Interindividual variation in "disease risk" and in the response to environmental factors is significant. The "risk" may be modified by age, gender, ethnicity, and the extent of exposure to environmental factors. Multiple genes are involved in determining an individual's response to a specific environmental factor. Interindividual variation in response to environmental exposures, such as cardiac surgery, probably is due in part to genetic polymorphisms. Common

**TABLE 60–1**

**Neurodevelopmental Sequelae of Congenital Heart Disease and Cardiac Surgery**

| |
|---|
| Cognitive impairment |
| Seizures |
| Gross and fine motor delays |
| Poor visual-motor integration |
| Poor oromotor control |
| Expressive speech and language abnormalities |
| Attention deficit/hyperactivity disorder |
| Learning disabilities |

genetic variants, often due to single nucleotide substitutions, occur with a frequency of greater than 1%. For a child with CHD, environmental factors include cardiac surgery, use of DHCA, need for repeated operations, and socioeconomic status. The role of genetic polymorphisms in determining susceptibility to CNS injury in children with CHD is not known. Recent studies suggest that polymorphisms of apolipoprotein E may be predictors of adverse neurodevelopmental sequelae following infant cardiac surgery (Gaynor et al, 2003). It is likely that multiple genes modulate the CNS response to CPB, DHCA, and other environmental factors modifying the risk and pattern of injury.

## NEUROLOGIC ABNORMALITIES IN CHILDREN WITH CONGENITAL HEART DISEASE PRIOR TO SURGERY

It has long been recognized that the neurologic status of newborns with CHD is frequently abnormal prior to open heart surgery. Gillon (1973) reported neurologic findings including tone abnormalities, abnormal posturing, weak cry, and poor coordination of suck, swallow, and breathing in many infants prior to open heart surgery. A recent study from Montreal Children's Hospital evaluated 56 consecutive neonates referred for open heart surgery (Limperopoulos et al, 1999). Neurobehavioral and neurologic abnormalities, including hypotonia, hypertonia, jitteriness, motor asymmetries, and absence of suck reflex, were noted in more than 50% of the patients before surgery. Preoperative seizures were present in three patients, 35% were microcephalic, and 12.5% were macrocephalic. Investigators at Boston Children's Hospital evaluated neurodevelopmental outcome in infants undergoing the arterial switch operation (Newburger et al, 1993). Definite neurologic abnormalities were found before surgery in 55 of 155 patients. In addition, the preoperative electroencephalogram (EEG) was abnormal in 59 of 134 patients, with seizures in 14 patients. Mahle and colleagues (2001b) at The Children's Hospital of Philadelphia evaluated infants with MRI of the brain before cardiac surgery. Periventricular leukomalacia was present in 4 of 24 infants preoperatively; cerebral infarctions were identified in two additional infants. Congenital CNS anomalies are sometimes present in children with CHD (Glauser et al, 1990). In addition, abnormal development of the heart and great vessels may alter cerebral flow patterns during in utero development, leading to abnormal development of the brain. Kochilas and colleagues (2001) at The Children's Hospital of Philadelphia demonstrated a significant correlation between smaller diameter of the ascending aorta in patients with hypoplastic left heart syndrome (HLHS) and the occurrence of microcephaly.

Hypoxemia, low cardiac output, and cardiac arrest in patients with uncorrected CHD may result in CNS ischemia and injury. Aisenberg and associates (1982) evaluated mental and motor development with 173 infants with uncorrected CHD. Developmental delay was present in 25% and was apparent as early as 2 months of age. Congestive heart failure and hypoxemia were risk factors for developmental delay. Kurth and associates (2001) from The Children's Hospital of Philadelphia used near infrared spectroscopy (NIRS) to evaluate cerebral oxygenation in 93 infants with heart defects prior to surgery. Decreased cerebral oxygenation was present in many patients, particularly infants with TOF and those with HLHS or other single-ventricle physiology. Very low cerebral oxygen saturations (<38%) were found in 13 patients, suggesting that patients with CHD are at risk for cerebral ischemia and CNS injury in the preoperative period.

**TABLE 60–2**

**Risk Factors for Neurodevelopmental Dysfunction**

| |
|---|
| **Preoperative** |
| Congenital central nervous system abnormalities |
| Genetic syndromes |
| Genetic susceptibility to cerebral ischemia/reperfusion injury |
| Cardiac diagnosis |
| Cardiac arrest |
| Low cardiac output |
| **Operative** |
| Cardiopulmonary bypass |
| Deep hypothermic circulatory arrest |
| **Postoperative** |
| Hypoxemia |
| Low cardiac output |
| Cardiac arrest |
| Postoperative seizures |
| **Other** |
| Chronic (preoperative/postoperative) hypoxemia |
| Lower socioeconomic status |

## MECHANISM OF CENTRAL NERVOUS SYSTEM INJURY DURING CARDIAC SURGERY

Even though there is increasing evidence of congenital CNS and neurologic abnormalities as well as preoperative CNS injury in children with CHD, most studies have focused on intraoperative management as the primary mechanism of CNS injury. Multiple factors may contribute to CNS injury during surgical repair including hypoxemia, cerebral hypoperfusion, and cerebral embolism (particulate and/or air). Cerebral ischemia occurring during surgical repair of CHD has been proposed to be a primary mechanism of CNS injury. Potential contributing factors include the type of support during surgery (DHCA or continuous CPB), use of hemodilution, the depth and rate of core cooling, and type of blood gas management. There has been particular interest in the type of support utilized during the cardiac repair. Use of CPB exposes the blood to the foreign surfaces of the bypass circuit, initiating a systemic inflammatory response characterized by neutrophil activation, complement activation, and increased circulating levels of inflammatory cytokines (du Plessis, 1999). This inflammatory response may result in increased capillary permeability, tissue edema, and organ dysfunction. When continuous CPB is utilized, perfusion to the body and brain is maintained. When DHCA is utilized, there is a period of obligate global cerebral ischemia followed by reperfusion. Use of DHCA provides a bloodless surgical field, facilitating meticulous completion of the repair, and decreases the duration of blood exposure to the bypass circuit, but at the cost of a period of global cerebral ischemia. Continuous CPB maintains perfusion to the brain and body but increases the duration of blood exposure to the bypass circuit, which may increase the severity of the inflammatory response. Use of continuous CPB avoids the period of cerebral ischemia but results in a greater increase in total body water and more severe dysfunction of other organs, such as the lungs (Skaryak et al, 1996; Wernovsky et al, 1995). Both continuous CPB and DHCA have been associated with perioperative CNS injury (Bellinger et al, 2003; Newburger et al, 1993).

## CENTRAL NERVOUS SYSTEM INJURY IN THE POSTOPERATIVE PERIOD

CNS injury may occur or be exacerbated in the postoperative period. Most studies have focused on the operating room as the site of CNS injury; however, events in the cardiac intensive care unit (CICU) may be as important. Cerebral ischemia can result from low cardiac output or severe hypoxemia. Postoperative hyperthermia may increase the metabolic needs of the brain, resulting in worsening CNS injury (Shum-Tim et al, 1998). In addition, postoperative cardiac arrest may result in significant CNS injury.

Especially following newborn and infant repairs, there is a predictable and reproducible fall in cardiac output (Wernovsky et al, 1995). This period of decreased oxygen delivery, usually within the first 24 hours after surgery, represents a particularly vulnerable time for the CNS, especially if associated with increased oxygen consumption (as with fever, pain, or agitation). At present, studies linking postoperative hemodynamic lability to long-term CNS outcomes are lacking. However, postoperative hypotension may lead to cerebral white matter injury characterized by periventricular leukomalacia (Galli et al, 2004).

## NEURODEVELOPMENTAL OUTCOME FOLLOWING REPAIR OF CONGENITAL HEART DISEASE

Only a few well-designed studies have prospectively evaluated neurologic outcome in children with CHD. A randomized trial at Boston Children's Hospital examined the incidence of acute neurologic injury, as well as late cognitive outcome, following repair of transposition of the great arteries (TGA) with or without a ventricular septal defect (VSD) (Newburger et al, 1993). Although this study has the advantage of a homogeneous patient population (TGA with or without VSD, 76% male, 89% Caucasian), the results cannot necessarily be extrapolated to patients with other cardiac defects or different ethnic origins. Children were randomized to an operative strategy of either predominantly DHCA or continuous low-flow CPB. However, even those patients randomized to predominantly continuous CPB did undergo a brief period of DHCA; thus, the study does not compare use of DHCA and no DHCA. Evaluation of acute neurologic injury included EEG monitoring and neurologic examination. There was a trend toward more frequent seizures as determined by continuous EEG monitoring within the first 48 hours after surgery in children assigned to DHCA; however, the difference was not significant ($P = .07$). Presence of an associated VSD was an independent risk factor for seizures. Abnormalities on neurologic examination at discharge from the hospital were common (possible, in 31% of patients; definite, in 20%); however, the incidence was not related to either treatment assignment or duration of DHCA.

Cognitive function and developmental outcomes for patients in the Boston Circulatory Arrest Study have been evaluated at 1, 4, and 8 years of age (Bellinger et al, 1995, 1999, 2003). Testing at 1 year included the Bayley Scales of Infant Development, neurologic examination, and MRI of the brain (Bellinger et al, 1995). The mean score on the Psychomotor Development Index (PDI) of the Bayley Scales for the entire cohort was 95 ± 15.5 (norm 100 ± 15). PDI scores were significantly lower among children assigned to DHCA than among those assigned to CPB, with a mean difference of 6.5 points. Longer duration of circulatory arrest also was associated with lower PDI scores. Of importance, presence of a VSD was an independent risk factor for a lower PDI score, with a similar mean difference between the two groups (6.6 points). The mean score on the Mental Development Index (MDI) of the Bayley Scales for the entire cohort was 105.1 ± 15 (norm 100). MDI scores tended to be lower among children assigned to DHCA; however, the difference did not reach statistical significance ($P = .1$) However, as with the PDI, presence of a VSD was an independent risk factor for a lower MDI score, with a mean difference between the groups of 8.6 points ($P = .004$) Developmental outcome was also assessed by the Fagan Test of Infant Development. Scores were not related to either treatment assignment or duration of circulatory arrest; however, presence of a VSD was associated with significantly lower scores. Neurologic examination revealed no significant differences between treatment groups. Preoperative factors including a low Apgar score at 5 minutes and younger gestational age, however, were independent risk factors for abnormalities on the neurologic examination. Occurrence of an EEG-confirmed seizure in the early postoperative period was associated with a mean reduction of 11.2 points on the PDI and with a higher risk of possible or definite abnormalities on MR imaging. Thus at 1 year of age, although use of DHCA was associated with a lower PDI score, factors related to preoperative status (Apgar scores, gestational age) and cardiac anatomy (TGA with an associated VSD) were independent predictors of adverse developmental outcomes. Because the children with an associated VSD were older at the time of surgery, it was not possible to separate the potential effects of older age at surgery and presence of a VSD. The authors noted that the "the ability to establish a safe threshold (for duration of DHCA) was limited by the modest effect of duration of circulatory arrest and by the considerable scatter in the data" (Bellinger et al, 1995).

The cohort was reevaluated at 4 years of age. Full-Scale, Verbal, and Performance IQs for the entire cohort were lower than population means; however, treatment group differences were not significant (Bellinger et al, 1999). Results were similar when the duration of DHCA replaced treatment group in the regression model. Social class and diagnosis accounted for more of the variation in IQ (24%) than did use of DHCA (3%). Presence of a VSD was an independent risk factor for lower Full-Scale IQ, Performance IQ, and Verbal IQ. Twenty-eight percent of the children had possible abnormalities on neurologic examination, and 30% had definite abnormalities. Abnormalities tended to be more common in the DHCA group, but the difference did not reach statistical significance. Assignment to DHCA was associated with significantly lower gross and fine motor function scores. Evaluation of language function revealed scores in the full cohort that were significantly below population means; however, treatment group differences were not significant for any language test. Speech evaluation demonstrated that assignment to the DHCA group was associated with a reduced ability to imitate oral movements and speech sounds. Apraxia of speech was more prevalent and more severe among children assigned to DHCA. Presence of a VSD was also significantly associated with apraxia of speech. Thus at 4 years of age cognitive, language, and motor performance for the entire cohort were significantly reduced relative to the general population. Use of a predominant strategy of DHCA was associated with worse motor function, but not with significantly worse IQ scores or worse overall neurologic status. As at the 1-year evaluation, the outcome for patients with an associated diagnosis of VSD was generally worse than that in patients with intact ventricular septum.

Results from the 8-year evaluation have recently been published. Full-Scale and Performance IQ scores for the entire cohort were slightly lower than population norms (Bellinger et al, 2003). There was no significant effect of assignment to DHCA or duration of DHCA on IQ. Scores of the entire cohort for memory, attention, and visual-spatial skills, as well as academic achievement, were lower than population means, and there was no treatment group effect. As at the 4-year evaluation, assignment to DHCA was associated with worse speech and fine motor function. Overall, there was a significant incidence of learning disabilities in both groups, and 43% received special education services. The investigators concluded that the treatment groups were similar in most aspects of neuropsychological and academic performance; however, performance was lower than in the general population. A substantial number of the patients are experiencing academic difficulties.

Cardiac diagnosis may have a significant impact on neurodevelopmental outcome and may modulate the effects of neuroprotective strategies. Presence of a VSD in patients undergoing the arterial switch procedure is a significant risk factor for poor developmental outcome (Bellinger et al, 1995, 1999; Newburger et al, 1993). At Boston Children's Hospital, developmental and neurologic outcomes were evaluated in infants undergoing repair of a variety of cardiac defects at less than 9 months of age who were randomized to either alpha-stat or pH-stat blood gas management strategy during deep hypothermic CPB (Bellinger et al, 2001). Children with TGA with or without VSD, TOF, isolated VSD, atrioventricular canal defect, truncus arteriosus, and total anomalous pulmonary venous return were enrolled. The use of either alpha-stat or pH-stat blood gas management strategy was not consistently related to either improved or impaired neurodevelopmental outcomes. There was no effect of treatment group on the PDI score. The MDI score, however, varied significantly depending on treatment group and diagnosis. For patients with TGA and TOF, use of pH-stat resulted in a slightly higher MDI, although the difference was not statistically significant. Of interest, in the VSD subgroup, the treatment effect was opposite with use of alpha-stat management, resulting in significantly improved scores. Cardiac diagnosis had a significant effect on outcomes: PDI and MDI scores were significantly higher in the TGA group compared with those noted for the other cardiac defects. A recent study at The Children's Hospital of Philadelphia evaluated the neuroprotective effect of allopurinol, a scavenger and inhibitor of oxygen free radical production, during infant cardiac surgery using DHCA (Clancy et al, 2001). A total of 318 infants (131 with HLHS) underwent surgery. Allopurinol provided significant neuroprotection only in patients with HLHS; no benefit was found in the non-HLHS patients. In the same cohort of patients, preoperative factors including cardiac diagnosis were evaluated as predictors of operative mortality (Clancy et al, 2000). Because of the number of different defects in these patients, they were grouped according to a classification based on anatomy and physiology: class I was defined as presence of two ventricles with no aortic arch obstruction; class II, two ventricles with aortic arch obstruction; class III, single ventricle with no arch obstruction; and class IV, single ventricle with arch obstruction. Patients with TOF, TGA, and VSD are grouped in class I, whereas patients with HLHS or variants are in class IV. This classification correlated significantly with operative mortality. Mortality rates for class I patients were 1%, compared with 10.7% for class II, and 25.5% for classes III and IV. These studies demonstrate that cardiac diagnosis has a significant impact on both operative mortality and neurodevelopmental outcome.

Previous studies have suggested that developmental outcome is worst for patients with complex cardiac defects, such as HLHS, who require multiple operations during infancy and early childhood. Rogers and colleagues at the Children's Hospital of Buffalo evaluated 11 survivors of staged repair for HLHS at a mean age of 38 months (Rogers et al, 1995). Seven children (64%) had major developmental disabilities and were considered to be mentally retarded. Two had severe cerebral palsy. Gross motor delays were present in five children (45%). At follow-up microcephaly was present in eight children (73%) and correlated with cognitive delay. More recent studies, however, suggest that developmental outcomes for these children have improved. Kern and associates (1998) at Columbia-Presbyterian Medical Center evaluated early neurodevelopmental outcome following stage I reconstruction for HLHS. Twelve patients who had undergone the Norwood procedure and subsequent surgery were evaluated along with a control group of children including siblings and first cousins. DHCA was utilized for the stage I reconstruction, with a mean duration of 56 minutes. The median scores for Full-Scale IQ were in the lower range of normal. Although scores for controls were generally higher than for patients, the differences between the two groups in intelligence testing did not reach statistical significance. The only statistically significant difference was in adaptive behavior, with the controls scoring higher. There was no correlation between neurologic outcome and bypass time, age at surgery, number of operations, or age at testing. Longer duration of DHCA was a risk factor for lower Full-Scale IQ. Eke and colleagues (1996) from Loma Linda evaluated the neurologic sequelae of DHCA in patients undergoing neonatal cardiac transplantation. The majority of these patients had HLHS. Developmental outcomes were evaluated using the Bayley Scales of Infant Development. There was no correlation between the duration of DHCA and neurodevelopmental outcome. Mahle and associates (2000a) at The Children's Hospital of Philadelphia evaluated neurodevelopmental outcomes in school-aged survivors of reconstructive surgery for HLHS. A majority of patients had IQ scores within the normal range; however, mean performance for the study group was lower than population norms. In a multivariable analysis, only the occurrence of a preoperative seizure predicted lower Full-Scale IQ. Duration of DHCA was not a predictor of lower IQ, although this lack of correlation may be due to the narrow spread of DHCA time in the study cohort. Scores on achievement tests (mathematics and reading) were lower than expected for the normal population. Nearly two thirds of the cohort had a clinical diagnosis of ADHD. Goldberg and colleagues (2000) evaluated neurodevelopmental outcome for children with functional single ventricle (both HLHS and non-HLHS) following completion of the Fontan procedure. Cognitive outcomes were assessed with the Wechsler Preschool and Primary Scale of Intelligence–Revised. Mean scores for the entire cohort were within the normal range for Full-Scale IQ, Verbal IQ, and Performance IQ. Scores for patients with HLHS were lower than for patients with other defects but were not significantly different from scores for the standard population. Use of DHCA was associated with lower scores. Because of the significant mortality previously associated with staged reconstructive surgery for HLHS, most of these studies evaluated relatively small numbers of young patients. In addition, these studies provide conflicting evidence concerning the significance of DHCA as a risk factor for adverse neurodevelopmental outcomes. Outcomes for these complex patients, overall, have improved in recent years, in terms of both mortality and neurodevelopmental outcome.

## Functional Status after Repair of Congenital Heart Disease

Most studies have focused on delineating cognitive impairments in children who have undergone repair of CHD; however, the impact on the child's functional status and on the child's caregivers has not been as carefully investigated. Developmental delay following cardiac surgery can impair a child's functional status, resulting in a considerable burden for family and caregiver. Limperopoulos and colleagues (2001) from Montreal Children's Hospital evaluated functional limitations and burden of care in 131 infants following surgical repair of CHD, using the WeeFIM (Functional Independence Measure), a pediatric functional assessment designed to assess and track levels of functional independence, and the Vineland Adaptive Behavior Scale. Only 21% of the patients were functioning within their appropriate age range. Moderate disability was noted in 37% and severe disability in 6%. Functional difficulties in daily living skills were documented in 40% of the patients, and greater than 50% had poor socialization skills. Factors that increased the risk of functional disabilities included microcephaly, longer duration of DHCA, longer length of stay in the intensive care unit, and maternal education.

## SUMMARY

Children with CHD constitute an at-risk population with a significant incidence of adverse developmental outcomes, particularly following surgical repair. Current techniques for developmental evaluation in neonates and infants are imprecise predictors of late outcomes. Evaluation of preschool- and school-aged children reveals a pattern of neurodevelopmental dysfunction characterized by mild cognitive impairment, motor dysfunction, impaired visual-spatial and visual-motor skills, and attention and academic difficulties. There are significant problems with expressive speech and language and a high incidence of learning disabilities. The factors resulting in CNS injury and developmental dysfunction in these children are not completely understood. Developmental dysfunction results from a complex interaction between patient-specific factors (genetic susceptibility, cardiac diagnosis) and environmental factors (preoperative events; techniques of support during surgical repair, including the use of DHCA; postoperative events; socioeconomic status). Previous studies have focused on the use of DHCA during the surgical repair as a risk factor for neurologic dysfunction. There is conflicting evidence concerning the significance of DHCA as a risk factor for adverse neurodevelopmental outcomes. However, these studies demonstrate that CPB alone (with or without use of DHCA) is associated with postoperative neurodevelopmental sequelae. Currently, reported risk factors do not adequately explain the pattern or incidence of CNS injury following cardiac surgery in infants, suggesting that other patient-specific factors may modulate the response to CHD and cardiac surgery, increasing the risk of adverse neurodevelopmental sequelae. Children with CHD are at risk for cerebral ischemia before, during, and after cardiac surgery; therefore, factors, that impair CNS recovery following ischemia may be important determinants of long-term neurologic outcome.

## REFERENCES

Aisenberg RB, Rosenthal A, Nadas AS, Wolff PH: Developmental delay in infants with congenital heart disease: Correlation with hypoxemia and congestive heart failure. Pediatr Cardiol 3:133-137, 1982.

Bellinger DC, Jonas RA, Rappaport LA, et al: Developmental and neurologic status of children after heart surgery with hypothermic circulatory arrest or low-flow cardiopulmonary bypass. N Engl J Med 332:549-555, 1995.

Bellinger DC, Wypij D, du Plessis AJ, et al: Developmental and neurologic effects of alpha-stat versus pH-stat strategies for deep hypothermic cardiopulmonary bypass in infants. J Thorac Cardiovasc Surg 121:374-383, 2001.

Bellinger DC, Wypij D, du Plessis AJ, et al: Neurodevelopmental status at eight years in children with dextro-transposition of the great arteries: The Boston Circulatory Arrest Trial. J Thorac Cardiovasc Surg 126:1385-1396, 2003.

Bellinger DC, Wypij D, Kuban KCK, et al: Developmental and neurological status of children at 4 years of age after heart surgery with hypothermic circulatory arrest or low-flow cardiopulmonary bypass. Circulation 100:526-532, 1999.

Clancy RR, McGaurn SA, Goin JE, et al: Allopurinol neurocardiac protection trial in infants undergoing heart surgery using deep hypothermic circulatory arrest. Pediatrics 108:61-70, 2001.

Clancy RR, McGaurn SA, Wernovsky G, et al: Preoperative risk-of-death prediction model in heart surgery with deep hypothermic circulatory arrest in the neonate. J Thorac Cardiovasc Surg 119:347-357, 2000.

DeMaso DR, Campis LK, Wypij D, et al: The impact of maternal perceptions and medical severity on the adjustment of children with congenital heart disease. J Pediatr Psychol 16: 137-149, 1991.

du Plessis AJ: Mechanisms of brain injury during infant cardiac surgery. Semin Pediatr Neurol 6:32-47, 1999.

Eke CC, Gundry SR, Baum MF, et al: Neurologic sequelae of deep hypothermic circulatory arrest in cardiac transplant infants. Ann Thorac Surg 61:783-788, 1996.

Galli KK, Zimmerman RA, Jarvik GP, et al: Periventricular leukomalacia is common following neonatal cardiac surgery. J Thorac Cardiovasc Surg 127:692-704, 2004.

Gaynor JW, Gerdes M, Zackai EH, et al: Apolipoprotein E genotype and neurodevelopmental sequelae of infant cardiac surgery. J Thorac Cardiovasc Surg 126:1736-1745, 2003.

Gerdes M, Solot C, Wang PP, et al: Cognitive and behavior profile of preschool children with chromosome 22q11.2 deletion. Am J Med Genet 85:127-133, 1995.

Gillon JE: Behavior of newborns with cardiac distress. Am J Nurs 73:254-257, 1973.

Glauser TA, Rorke LB, Weinberg PM, Clancy RR: Congenital brain anomalies associated with the hypoplastic left heart syndrome. Pediatrics 85:984-990, 1990.

Goldberg CS, Schwartz EM, Brunberg JA, et al: Neurodevelopmental outcome of patients after the fontan operation: A comparison between children with hypoplastic left heart syndrome and other funtional single ventricle lesions. J Pediatr 137: 646-652, 2000.

Kern JH, Hinton VJ, Nereo NE, et al: Early developmental outcome after the Norwood procedure for hypoplastic left heart syndrome. Pediatrics 102:1148-1152, 1998.

Kochilas L, Shores JC, Novello RT, et al: Aortic morphometry and microcephaly in the hypoplastic left heart syndrome. J Am Coll Cardiol 37:470A, 2001.

Kurth CD, Steven JM, Montenegro LM, et al: Cerebral oxygen saturation before congenital heart surgery. Ann Thorac Surg 72:187-192, 2001.

Limperopoulos C, Majnemer A, Shevell MI, et al: Neurologic status of newborns with congenital heart defects before open heart surgery. Pediatrics 103:402-408, 1999.

Limperopoulos C, Majnemer A, Shevell MI, et al: Functional limitations in young children with congenital heart defects after open heart surgery. Pediatrics 108:1325-1331, 2001.

Mahle WT, Clancy RR, Moss EM, et al: Neurodevelopmental outcome and lifestyle assessment in school-aged and adolescent children with hypoplastic left heart syndrome. Pediatrics 105:1082-1089, 2000a.

Mahle WT, Zimmerman RA, Nicolson SC, et al: Serial magnetic resonance imaging of the brain in newborns underoing congenital heart surgery. Circulation 104:2058, 2000b.

Newburger JW, Jonas RA, Wernovsky G, et al: Comparison of the perioperative neurologic effects of hypothermic circulatory arrest versus low-flow cardiopulmonary bypass in infant heart surgery. N Engl J Med 329:1057-1064, 1993.

Rogers BT, Msall ME, Buck GM: Neurodevelopmental outcome of infants with hypoplastic left heart syndrome. J Pediatr 126:496-498, 1995.

Shum-Tim D, Nagashima M, Shinoka T, et al: Postischemic hyperthermia exacerbates neurologic injury after deep hypothermic circulatory arrest. J Thorac Cardiovasc Surg 116:780-792, 1998.

Skaryak LA, Kirshbom PM, DiBernardo LR, et al: Low-flow cardiopulmonary bypass produces greater pulmonary dysfunction than circulatory arrest. Ann Thorac Surg 62:1284-1288, 1996.

Wernovsky G, Stiles KM, Gauvreau K, et al: Cognitive development after the Fontan operation. Circulation 102:883-889, 2000.

Wernovsky G, Wypij D, Jonas RA, et al: Postoperative course and hemodynamic profile after the arterial switch operation in neonates and infants: A comparison of low-flow cardiopulmonary bypass and circulatory arrest. Circulation 92:2226-2235, 1995.

# NEUROLOGIC SYSTEM

Editor: CHRISTINE A. GLEASON

CHAPTER 61

## Developmental Physiology of the Central Nervous System

Christine A. Gleason* and Stephen A. Back

Over the past several decades, numerous important advances have been made in neonatal cardiovascular and pulmonary medicine, which have dramatically improved survival of critically ill term and preterm infants. Attention has now turned increasingly toward improving the neurologic outcome of not only these critically ill high-risk infants but also those born with prenatal brain injuries, brain malformations, or neurodevelopmental disorders. In the first edition of this book, there was limited attention devoted to neonatal neurology. This eighth edition now features a comprehensive neurology section that, in addition to this introductory chapter, includes chapters devoted to neonatal neuroimaging; malformations and deformations of the developing brain; brain injury and neuroprotection; neuromuscular disorders; neonatal seizures and finally, risk assessment and neurodevelopmental outcomes. This introductory chapter provides an overview of central nervous system (CNS) physiology and a discussion of normal principles of regulation of cerebral blood flow (CBF) and energy metabolism. Chapter 63 discusses normal CNS developmental anatomy in the context of the associated major human brain malformations.

### CENTRAL NERVOUS SYSTEM VASCULAR DEVELOPMENT

The earliest parts of the nervous system are essentially avascular. Blood vessels form as a meshwork in the meninges before growing into the CNS from the pial surface in a caudal-to-rostral progression. The blood-brain barrier is essentially a function of capillary endothelial cell tight junctions and develops under the influence of astrocytes. Brain blood vessel formation and blood-brain barrier capacities are present early in the CNS, but maximal capillary sprouting occurs during the period of dendritic growth and glial cell proliferation.

The vascular development in the periventricular areas of the developing brain is particularly clinically relevant because the immature infant is susceptible to ischemic injury in the white matter around the ventricles and to hemorrhage in the germinal eminence region (part of the ventricular zone) (Takashima and Tanaka, 1978a, 1978b). The periventricular white matter may be particularly susceptible to ischemia or to reduced substrate supply because for a period of time it has a decreased density of blood vessels at the junction of penetrating vessels that extend downward from the cortex and deep white matter vessels that branch upward. This decreased density also is seen in the subcortical vessels at the depths of the sulci in the more mature infant. The conditions of periventricular leukomalacia and subcortical leukomalacia are well-known pathologic entities (Takashima and Tanaka, 1978a, 1978b).

The germinal eminence is supplied by striatal arteries through a dense capillary network that is particularly susceptible to hemorrhage in the preterm infant. The hemodynamics of this region and the biology of the maturation of its vessels are current research areas that continue to hold promise for prevention of intraventricular hemorrhage. Evidence suggests that maturation of vessels of the germinal eminence can be influenced by the postnatal environment and by agents such as indomethacin (Ment et al, 1991). Studies of the ultrastructural features of the blood-brain barrier in this region in an animal model also have suggested that postnatal endothelial basal lamina deposition occurs before tight junction formation and glial investiture and that basal lamina induction influences the latter two processes (Ment et al, 1995). In the human preterm infant less than 34 weeks of gestational age, the period of risk for germinal matrix and intraventricular hemorrhage is the first 3 to 4 postnatal days, regardless of gestational age (Ment et al, 1995). This finding suggests that postnatal induction of vascular maturation may occur at the same rate and over the same period of time in these infants.

### REGULATION OF CEREBRAL BLOOD FLOW AND ENERGY METABOLISM

Cerebral blood flow (CBF) is regulated by many systemic and local factors, including arterial blood pressure, intracranial pressure, arterial $O_2$ content, hematocrit, and arterial

*In writing this chapter, Dr. Gleason excerpted significant portions of the chapter titled "The Intrauterine Nervous System" by Jan Goddard-Finegold, MD, in the previous edition of this book, as well as portions of her own contribution to Arensman RM, Cornish D (eds): Extracorporeal Life Support. Boston, Blackwell Scientific Publications, 1993, pp 138-155.

$CO_2$ tension. Cerebral $O_2$ consumption (i.e., cerebral metabolic rate) ($CMRO_2$) is an important determinant of CBF; these variables are said to be "tightly coupled." Responsivity of the cerebral circulation to the aforementioned stimuli also is determined in part by $CMRO_2$.

CBF normally is regulated to maintain adequate oxygen and substrate delivery to the brain. When blood flow regulatory limits and oxygen extraction capabilities of the brain are exceeded, the brain suffers hypoxic damage. When abnormally low cerebral blood flow is the primary abnormality, then the brain suffers ischemic damage. In most clinical situations, both hypoxic and ischemic types of damage occur, although one type may predominate.

### Autoregulation

Cerebral autoregulation refers to the maintenance of constant CBF despite changes in cerebral perfusion pressure (Lassen and Christensen, 1976; Paulson et al, 1990). This autoregulatory range has both upper and lower limits; above or below these limits, CBF increases or decreases passively, along with changes in perfusion pressure. Cerebral autoregulation has been demonstrated in several species and across developmental stages, but the mechanism of this important phenomenon remains elusive. Current thinking supports the notion that autoregulation is mediated by a fine balance between endothelial cell–derived constricting and relaxing factors (Volpe, 2000). In adults, CBF remains constant over an autoregulatory range of mean blood pressures from 50 to 150 mm Hg (Paulson et al, 1990). In preterm fetal lambs, the range is lower and narrower (40 to 80 mm Hg), but more important, normal blood pressure is only 5 to 10 mm Hg above the lower limit of the autoregulatory curve (Papile et al, 1985).

Autoregulation of CBF is of considerable interest to neonatologists because of the many clinical circumstances under which it may be impaired, resulting in tissue hypoxia or hemorrhage, or both. Severe asphyxia, hypoxia, head trauma, and hypercapnic acidosis, even when relatively mild, have been shown to attenuate or even abolish autoregulation (Busija and Heistad, 1984; Jones et al, 1988; Tweed et al, 1986).

The Cushing phenomenon is characterized by increasing systemic arterial pressure, enough to maintain cerebral perfusion pressure when intracranial pressure rises. Harris and colleagues et al, (1989) have shown that this response is highly developed in fetal sheep, possibly as an adaptation to the rigors of head compression during labor. If the newborn human Cushing response is similarly well developed, then the newborn brain may be better able to preserve cerebral blood pressure when intracranial pressure (ICP) rises (as with postasphyxial cerebral edema).

### Response to Hypoxia

When arterial oxygen content ($CaO_2$) decreases, the brain responds by increasing CBF. This cerebral vasodilatory hypoxic effect is directly related to $CaO_2$ and not to arterial oxygen tension ($PaO_2$). Increased CBF preserves cerebral oxygen delivery ($CaO_2 \times$ CBF) and cerebral $O_2$ consumption [$(CaO_2 - CvO_2) \times$ CBF]. There is a limit beyond which CBF cannot increase, and then $O_2$ delivery falls. The brain must then increase $O_2$ extraction to maintain $CMRO_2$. There is a limit to this also (cerebral venous $PO_2$), and when this is reached, $CMRO_2$ falls and brain tissue hypoxia results.

Jones and colleagues (1981) studied hypoxic hypoxia in neonatal sheep and found that CBF correlates best with $CaO_2$; as $CaO_2$ decreases, CBF increases. Studies have shown similar cerebral hypoxic cerebral vasodilatory responses in fetal (Ashwal et al, 1981) and adult sheep (Koehler et al, 1984). Developmental differences have been noted, however, in the regional brain blood flow responses to hypoxia. Ashwal and associates (1981) demonstrated a hierarchy of responsivity in fetal sheep in which the brainstem is more responsive than the subcortex or cortex. Such a hierarchy has not been noted in more mature sheep. Studies in immature sheep (Gleason et al, 1990) have shown that cerebral $O_2$ delivery is not maintained during hypoxic hypoxia; therefore, fractional $O_2$ extraction must increase to maintain $CMRO_2$. This finding suggests that important regulatory mechanisms are not fully developed in the immature brain, so that it is more vulnerable to hypoxic injury.

Anemic hypoxia produces a rise in CBF similar to hypoxic hypoxia so that oxygen delivery is maintained despite reduced $CaO_2$ (Jones et al, 1981). Arterial $PaO_2$ changes little, if at all, in anemic hypoxia, and changes in blood viscosity alone are not sufficient to account for the increase. Patchy areas of tissue hypoxia, with some areas receiving only plasma, could produce cerebral vasodilation (Jones et al, 1988).

### Polycythemia/Hyperviscosity

Arterial $O_2$ content increases when hemoglobin concentration rises, as does whole blood viscosity. An increase in $CaO_2$ alone results in decreased CBF. The independent effect of hyperviscosity on decreasing CBF in polycythemic animals has been studied by Massik and colleagues (1987). In their study in lambs, methemoglobin was used to dissociate the effects of hematocrit and $CaO_2$ as the hematocrit was raised. Approximately 50% of the decrease in CBF associated with polycythemia could be attributed to hyperviscosity and the remainder to changes in $CaO_2$.

### Hyperoxia

Several studies have demonstrated a decrease in cerebral blood flow when $PaO_2$ is raised to relatively hyperoxic levels. Gleason and colleagues (1988) raised fetal $PaO_2$ from 20 to 73 mm Hg in fetal sheep and noted a 46% drop in CBF. Kennedy and associates (1971) showed a 20% to 30% decrease in CBF with extreme hyperoxia ($PaO_2$ of 349 mm Hg) in neonatal puppies; this CBF response disappeared by age 3 weeks. Rahilly (1980) demonstrated a 33% drop in cranial blood flow in term infants breathing 100% $O_2$, and Leahy and colleagues (1980) showed a 15% drop in CBF in preterm infants who received similar treatment. These results are not surprising when the curve for the CBF response to hyperoxia is placed along the inverse hyperbolic hypoxic response curve previously described by Jones and colleagues (1977) for fetal sheep. This potential decrease in CBF with increased $O_2$ is certainly an important consideration in the decision to use extracorporeal membrane oxygenation (ECMO) in a hypoxemic neonate, during which the carotid $PaO_2$ may be as high as 500 mm Hg, or in resuscitation of a newborn using 100% oxygen (Gleason, 1993).

### Alterations in Cerebral Oxygen Consumption

CBF normally is coupled with $CMRO_2$, such that when clinical conditions alter $CMRO_2$, CBF is adjusted appropriately (Siesjo, 1984). For example, barbiturate coma lowers $CMRO_2$; therefore, CBF is comparably reduced. Donegan and associates (1985) studied CBF autoregulation and hypoxic responses during pentobarbital-induced coma in newborn lambs. The CBF response to hypoxia was attenuated during coma, but only in proportion to the decrease in $CMRO_2$. Chronic narcotic infusions in ventilated sick preterm infants may induce a similar response.

Cerebral $O_2$ consumption increases during neuronal excitation such as seizures (Metzger, 1979; Plum and Duffy, 1975). Increased CBF mirrors the increased $CMRO_2$, but there may not be adequate $PO_2$. If seizure activity is sustained, the high metabolic rate and potentially maximal CBF may increase the brain's susceptibility to additional hypoxic-ischemic injury (Meldrum and Nilsson, 1976).

### Carbon Dioxide Reactivity

Changes in arterial $PCO_2$ induce significant cerebral vascular responses in developing animals. Hypercapnia is a potent cerebral vasodilator, and hypocapnia is a potent vasoconstrictor (Reivich et al, 1971; Volpe, 2000). Hypocapnia may occur clinically secondary to overventilation or may be induced intentionally, in an attempt to decrease pulmonary vascular resistance. Numerous studies have demonstrated a 30% to 40% reduction in CBF after 15 to 30 minutes of moderately severe hypocapnia ($PaCO_2$ of 15 to 25 mm Hg). A gradual increase in CBF during prolonged hypocarbia has been shown by Gleason and colleagues (1989) in newborn lambs, with CBF returning to baseline after 6 hours of hyperventilation. In these hyperventilated lambs and in a similar study of adult goats (Albrecht et al, 1987), significant cerebral hyperemia was noted after abrupt discontinuation of hyperventilation.

Animal studies by Delivoria-Papadopoulos and associates (1988) have suggested that severe hypocapnia ($PaCO_2$ less than 10 mm Hg) results in tissue ischemia. Additional clinical studies have shown abnormal electroencephalograms, auditory evoked responses, and abnormal neurodevelopmental outcomes associated with significant hypocarbia.

### Brain Energy Metabolism

Oxygen and glucose are the brain's primary energy fuels. Although the requirement for oxygen is absolute, other substrates can replace or augment glucose during special circumstances such as hypoglycemia or anoxia (Jones, 1979). When oxygen delivery to the brain is impaired and oxygen extraction capability is exceeded, tissue hypoxia occurs, and brain damage may be the result. The issue of whether or not newborns have decreased vulnerability or "resistance" to anoxic insult continues to be debated. Increased survivability after prolonged anoxia has been demonstrated in immature animals such as newborn rats, and there have been occasional anecdotal reports of this phenomenon in newborn infants, but whether or not such increased survivability reflects resistance of the *brain* to anoxia is debatable. Nevertheless, immature animals do have better survival, and this has been variously attributed to (1) lower cerebral $O_2$ consumption, (2) predominance of anaerobic metabolism as an energy source, or (3) circulatory adaptations in immature animals, such as greater stores of cardiac glycogen that enable the heart to sustain the cerebral circulation. None of these possible mechanisms accounts for increased survival in all species, and none has been definitely proved to be important exclusively in immature animals (Jones, 1979; Gleason, 1993).

Hypoglycemia occurs quite commonly in sick newborn infants, although the associated physiologic conditions vary considerably. Poor glycogen stores, increased glucose demands, hyperinsulinism, and poor glucose intake are among the more common of these conditions. Cerebral effects of hypoglycemia may depend in part on the cerebral effects of the associated physiologic conditions. Alternative oxidative substrates are available to the brain, including ketone bodies, lactate, amino acids, and lipids. Owen and colleagues (1967) showed that cerebral ketone body consumption accounts for 50% of cerebral $O_2$ consumption in obese adults who are starved for 5 to 6 weeks. Hypoglycemia is associated with decreased cerebral glucose consumption but no change in cerebral $O_2$ consumption (Jones, 1979). Whether this response is adaptive or pathologic is not known.

### Metabolic Alkalosis/Acidosis

Cerebrovascular resistance is believed to be directly related to brain interstitial pH (Kontos et al, 1977). Biologic membranes are highly permeable to $CO_2$, so a change in $PaCO_2$ has an almost immediate effect on interstitial pH and, consequently, on CBF. In contrast, hydrogen and bicarbonate ions do not diffuse as easily through membranes. Therefore, induction of acute metabolic acidosis or alkalosis has not been shown to change CBF or autoregulation (Hermansen et al, 1984; Harper and Bell, 1963). During hypocapnia, addition of metabolic alkalosis does not alter CBF. However, during hypercapnia, bicarbonate infusion causes a significant decrease in CBF (Arvidsson et al, 1981), suggesting that hypercapnia alters the blood-brain permeability to ions. Such alterations in blood-brain barrier may also be associated with neonatal hypoxic/ischemic brain injury.

Sodium bicarbonate may be used clinically to correct metabolic acidosis in neonates. It is used with caution because of an earlier report linking its use with hypernatremia, intracranial hemorrhage, and acute secondary changes in arterial $PCO_2$ (Simmons et al, 1974). Such clinical studies are difficult to interpret because bicarbonate usually is given to treat metabolic acidosis that may be secondary to perinatal asphyxia, itself a major risk factor for intracranial hemorrhage. Laptook (1985) evaluated the cerebral effects of sodium bicarbonate (2 mEq/kg given over 3 minutes) administered to paralyzed newborn piglets to correct metabolic acidosis associated with hypoxemia. This investigator noted no alterations in brain blood flow or $O_2$ delivery. Constant $PaCO_2$ was maintained by increasing the ventilator rate during the bicarbonate infusion.

## SUGGESTED GUIDELINES FOR CEREBROVASCULAR AND METABOLIC CARE IN HIGH-RISK NEWBORNS

Guiding principles for the cerebrovascular and metabolic care of critically ill preterm and term infants may include the following:

1. Maintain stable blood pressure. Severe hypotension is clearly detrimental, but so are rapid increases in blood pressure in a pressure-passive circulation.
2. Maintain stable acid-base balance without rapid corrections.
3. Avoid severe hypoxemia.
4. Avoid marked hyperoxemia (i.e., consider effects of resuscitating with 100% oxygen).
5. Avoid sudden changes in $PaCO_2$.
6. Correct significant anemia or polycythemia; if chronic, correct slowly.
7. Consider cerebrovascular and metabolic effects of any new (and existing) drug therapies. Use the lowest effective dose for the shortest period of time.
8. Maintain euglycemia.

## REFERENCES


Albrecht RF, Miletich DJ, Ruttle M: Cerebral effects of extended hyperventilation in unanesthetized goats. Stroke 18:649, 1987.

Arvidsson S, Haggendal E, Winso I: Influence on cerebral blood flow of infusion of sodium bicarbonate during respiratory acidosis and alkalosis in the dog. Acta Anaesth Scand 25:146, 1981.

Ashwal S, Majcher JS, Longo LD: Patterns of fetal lamb regional cerebral blood flow during and after prolonged hypoxia: Studies during the posthypoxic recovery period. Am J Obstet Gynecol 139:365, 1981.

Busija DW, Heistad DD: Factors involved in the physiological regulation of the cerebral circulation. Rev Physiol Biochem Pharmacol 101:161, 1984.

Delivoria-Papadopoulos M, Wagerle LC, Cahillane G, et al: Cerebral oxygenation and membrane dysfunction following hyperventilation in newborn (NB) piglets [abstract]. Pediatr Res 23:231A, 1988.

Donegan JH, Traystman RJ, Koehler RC, et al: Cerebrovascular hypoxic and autoregulatory responses during reduced brain metabolism. Am J Physiol 249:H421, 1985.

Gleason CA: ECMO and the brain. In Arensman RM, Cornish JD (eds): Extracorporeal Life Support. Boston, Blackwell Scientific Publications, 1993, pp 138-155.

Gleason CA, Hamm C, Jones MD Jr: Effect of acute hypoxemia on brain blood flow and oxygen metabolism in immature fetal sheep. Am J Physiol 258:H1064, 1990.

Gleason CA, Jones MD Jr, Traystman RJ: Fetal cerebral responses to ventilation and oxygenation in utero. Am J Physiol 255:R1049, 1988.

Gleason CA, Short BL, Jones MD Jr: Cerebral blood flow and metabolism during and after prolonged hypocapnia in newborn lambs. J Pediatr 155:309, 1989.

Harper AM, Bell RA: The effect of metabolic acidosis and alkalosis on the blood flow through the cerebral cortex. J Neurol Neurosurg Psychiat 26:341, 1963.

Harris AP, Koehler RC, Gleason CA, et al: Cerebral and peripheral circulatory responses to intracranial hypertension in fetal sheep. Circ Res 64:991, 1989.

Hermansen MC, Kotagal UR, Kleinman LI: The effect of metabolic acidosis upon autoregulation of cerebral blood flow in newborn dogs. Brain Res 324:101, 1984.

Jones MD Jr: Energy metabolism in the developing brain. Semin Perinatol 3:121, 1979.

Jones MD Jr, Koehler RC, Traystman RJ: Regulation of cerebral blood flow in the fetus, newborn, and adult. In Guthrie RD (ed): Neonatal Intensive Care. New York, Churchill Livingstone, 1988.

Jones MD Jr, Sheldon RE, Peeters LL, et al: Fetal cerebral oxygen consumption at different levels of oxygenation. J Appl Physiol Respir Environ Exercise Physiol 43:1080, 1977.

Jones MD Jr, Traystman RJ, Simmons MA, et al: Effects of changes in arterial $O_2$ content on cerebral blood flow in the lamb. Am J Physiol 240:H209, 1981.

Kennedy C, Grave GD, Jehle JW: Effect of hyperoxia on the cerebral circulation of the newborn puppy. Pediatr Res 5:659, 1971.

Koehler RC, Traystman RJ, Zeger S, et al: Comparison of cerebrovascular response to hypoxic and carbon monoxide hypoxia in newborn and adult sheep. J Cereb Blood Flow Metab 4: 115, 1984.

Kontos HA, Raper AJ, Patterson JL: Analysis of vasoactivity of local pH, $PCO_2$ and bicarbonate on pial vessels. Stroke 8:358, 1977.

Laptook AR: The effects of sodium bicarbonate on brain blood flow and $O_2$ delivery during hypoxemia and academia in the piglet. Pediatr Res 19:815, 1985.

Lassen NA, Christensen MS: Physiology of cerebral blood flow. Br J Anesth 48:719, 1976.

Leahy FAN, Cates D, MacCallum M, et al: Effect of $CO_2$ and 100% $O_2$ on cerebral blood flow in preterm infants. J Appl Physiol: Respir Environ Exercise Physiol 48:468, 1980.

Levasseur JE, Wei EP, Kontos HA, et al: Responses of pial arterioles after prolonged hypercapnia and hypoxia in the awake rabbit. J Appl Physiol Respir Environ Exercise Physiol 46:89, 1979.

Massik J, Tang Y-L, Hudak ML, et al: Effect of hematocrit on cerebral blood flow with induced polycythemia. J Appl Physiol 62:1090, 1987.

Meldrum BS, Nilsson B: Cerebral blood flow and metabolic rate early and late in prolonged epileptic seizures induced in rats by bicuculline. Brain 99:523, 1976.

Ment LR, Stewart WB, Ardito TA, et al: Beagle pup germinal matrix maturation studies. Stroke 2:390, 1991.

Ment LR, Stewart WB, Ardito TA, et al: Germinal matrix microvascular maturation correlates inversely with the risk period for neonatal intraventricular hemorrhage. Dev Brain Res 84:142, 1995.

Metzger H: Effects of direct stimulation on cerebral cortex oxygen tension level. Microvascular Res 17:80, 1979.

Owen OE, Morgan AP, Kemp HG, et al: Brain metabolism during fasting. J Clin Invest 46:1589, 1967.

Papile LA, Rudolph AM, Heymann MA: Autoregulation of cerebral blood flow in the preterm fetal lamb. Pediatr Res 19:159, 1985.

Paulson OB, Strandgaard S, Edvinsson L: Cerebral autoregulation. Cerebrovasc Brain Metab Rev 2:161, 1990.

Plum F, Duffy TE: The couple between cerebral metabolism and blood flow during seizures. In Ingvar DH, Lassen NA (eds):

Brain Work. Proceedings of the Alfred Benzon Symposium VIII. Copenhagen, Munksgaard, 1975.

Rahilly PM: Effects of 2% carbon dioxide, 0.5% carbon dioxide and 100% oxygen on cranial blood flow of the human neonate. Pediatrics 66:685, 1980.

Reivich M, Brann AW Jr, Shapiro H, et al: Reactivity of cerebral vessels to $CO_2$ in the newborn rhesus monkey. Eur Neurol 6:132, 1971.

Rosenberg AA, Jones MD Jr, Traystman RJ, et al: Response of cerebral blood flow to changes in $PCO_2$ in fetal newborn, and adult sheep. Am J Physiol 242:H862, 1982.

Siesjo BK: Cerebral circulation and metabolism. J Neurosurg 60:883, 1984.

Simmons MA, Adcock EW III, Bard H, et al: Hypernatremia and intracranial hemorrhage in neonates. N Engl J Med 291:6, 1974.

Takashima S, Tanaka K: Development of cerebral architecture and its relationship to periventricular leukomalacia. Arch Neurol 35:11, 1978a.

Takashima J, Tanaka K: Microangiography and vascular permeability of the subependymal matrix in the premature infant. Can J Neurol Sci 5:45, 1978b.

Tweed A, Cote J, Lou H, et al: Impairment of cerebral blood flow autoregulation in the newborn lamb by hypoxia. Pediatr Res 20:516, 1986.

Volpe JP: Neurology of the Newborn. Philadelphia, WB Saunders, 2000.

CHAPTER

# 62

# Neonatal Neuroimaging

**Richard L. Robertson and George A. Taylor**

## ULTRASONOGRAPHY

### Anatomic (Gray Scale) Sonography

*Ultrasonography* (US) became a viable tool for imaging the neonatal brain in the late 1970s with the development of real-time capabilities (Pape et al, 1979). Subsequent advances in ultrasound technology have dramatically improved our ability to visualize normal structures and abnormalities in the neonatal brain. As a result, US continues to be an integral part of caring for the critically ill neonate.

Diagnostic ultrasound relies on the transmission and reflection of high-frequency sound waves into tissues. The speed and reflectivity of sound differ among various tissues, resulting in acoustic interfaces that can be used to create images of anatomic structures. By convention, tissues with high reflectance, such as clotted blood, are bright, and those with low reflectance, such as cerebrospinal fluid (CSF) or moving blood, are dark. Thick bone and air significantly interfere with the transmission of sound into deeper tissues. Consequently, cranial US requires a coupling agent (gel) between the transducer and the skin to eliminate as much intervening air as possible and most often is performed through an open fontanel.

### Doppler Sonography

Continuous wave and pulsed wave Doppler techniques have been used for decades to sample hemodynamics in specific intracranial vessels. The resistive index (RI) and mean blood flow velocity over time (time-averaged velocity) are the most commonly used spectral Doppler measures for monitoring intracranial hemodynamics. The easiest and most reproducible are measures of pulsatility, which are relatively insensitive to differences in angle of insonation and correlate well with acute changes in intracerebral perfusion pressure. However, many factors other than cerebrovascular resistance may affect the RI in an intracranial vessel, including the presence of a patent ductus arteriosus, alterations in heart rate and cardiac output, and the amount of pressure applied on the fontanel during scanning (Perlman et al, 1981; Taylor, 1992a; Taylor et al, 1989).

Although reproducible and easy to obtain, the RI is only a weak predictor of cerebrovascular resistance under most physiologic conditions. Mean blood flow velocity measures are the most informative indices of cerebral blood flow (CBF). A strong correlation has been demonstrated between mean blood flow velocity and changes in global CBF under a variety of clinical and experimental conditions (Taylor et al, 1990).

Before 1989, the exact origin of the Doppler signal could not be determined because of the inability to resolve most intracranial vessels with gray scale sonography. The introduction of color Doppler technology made imaging and reliable hemodynamic sampling of the intracranial vasculature routinely possible in the normal newborn (Dean and Taylor, 1995; Mitchell et al, 1988, 1989; Taylor, 1992b). Standard color Doppler sonography is based on an estimate of the mean frequency shift created by the movement of red blood cells at different velocities within the tissue or blood vessel being examined. Flow is generally depicted as variations of red or blue color, depending on the degree of shift from the baseline frequency, and on the direction of the moving red cells.

### Equipment and Scanning Technique

#### Transducers

In the premature infant, transducers operating at a higher frequency range (7 to 10 MHz) are recommended because of their higher spatial resolution. Lower-frequency transducers (3.5 to 5 MHz) are often used in larger infants to obtain adequate sound penetration. Sector transducers with a 120-degree imaging field are most useful for imaging through the anterior and posterior fontanels.

#### Scanning Technique

For sonographic examination of the neonatal brain, standardized coronal and sagittal images are obtained through the anterior fontanel. Coronal images are obtained by placing the transducer transversely across the fontanel and sweeping it in an anteroposterior direction to cover the entire brain (Fig. 62–1). The transducer should be carefully held to produce symmetrical imaging of both hemispheres.

At least six angled images are obtained. The most anterior image is anterior to the frontal horns of the lateral ventricles at the level of the orbits. The frontal lobes and anterior portion of the interhemispheric fissure can be visualized. The second image is obtained through the anterior horns of the lateral ventricles at the level of the suprasellar cistern. This structure has the appearance of an echogenic five-pointed star. The hypoechoic caudate nucleus can be seen inferior and lateral to the comma-shaped lateral ventricles. The ventricles are separated from each other by the centrally positioned cavum of the septum pellucidum. Basal ganglia, frontal and temporal lobes, insula, and T-shaped sylvian fissure can be identified in this plane. The next image is obtained more posteriorly through the body of the lateral ventricles at the level of the paired foramina of Monro and brainstem. The anterior portion of the choroid plexus can identified as three small echogenic structures along the inferomedial aspect of the lateral ventricles, and paired thalami can be seen lateral to the third ventricle. Lateral and superior to the lentiform nuclei is a region of the deep white matter called the

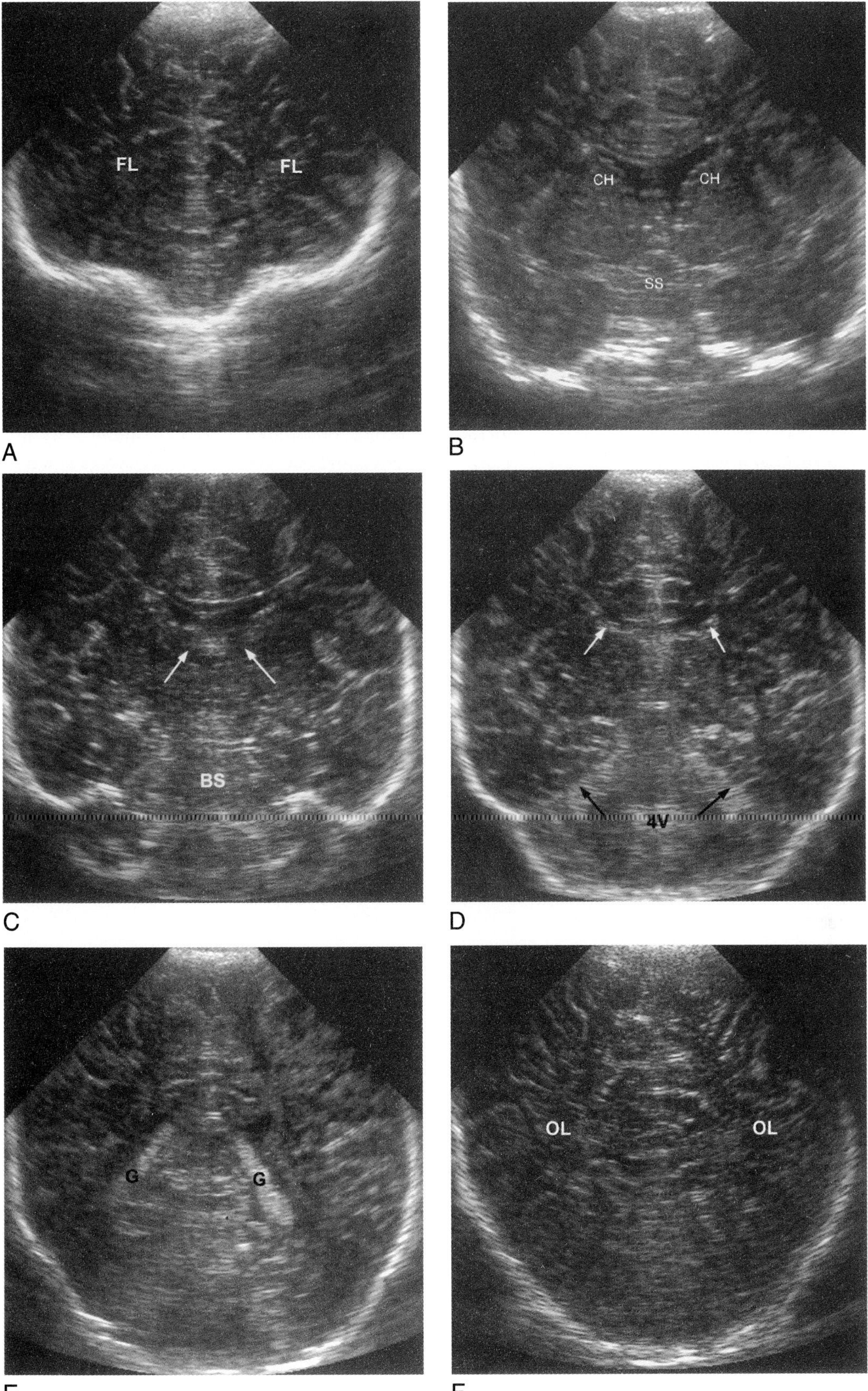


**FIGURE 62–1.** Standard coronal planes of cranial sonography performed through the anterior fontanel. **A,** Plane 1 is angled anteriorly to include the frontal lobes (FL) and orbits. **B,** Plane 2 demonstrates the caudate heads (CH) and the suprasellar cistern (SS). **C,** Plane 3 passes through the foramina of Monro *(arrows)* and the brainstem (BS). **D,** Coronal plane 4 shows the rounded echogenic choroid plexus within the body of the lateral ventricles *(white arrows)*, the fourth ventricle (4V) and the tentorium *(black arrows)*. **E,** Plane 5 includes the glomus (G) of the choroid plexus in the trigones of the lateral ventricles. **F,** Plane 6 is angled posteriorly to include the occipital lobes (OL).

centrum semiovale. The fourth image is obtained with the transducer angled slightly more posteriorly. At this level, the lateral ventricles have a more rounded appearance, and the choroid plexus is seen as a more prominent echogenic structure along the floor of the ventricles. The confluence of frontal, parietal, and temporal lobes can be seen as well as the echogenic tentorium cerebelli and the anterior portion of the cerebellum and fourth ventricle. The transducer sweep is continued posteriorly until the prominent paired echogenic structures of the glomus of the choroid plexus are seen in the atrium of the lateral ventricles. The parietal and posterior aspects of the temporal lobe and sylvian fissure can be visualized, along with the echogenic cerebellum inferiorly. The last coronal image is obtained posterior to the lateral ventricles. The posterior aspect of the interhemispheric fissure and the occipital lobes are seen on this view.

Sagittal images are obtained by placing the transducer longitudinally along the anterior fontanel (Fig. 62–2). A total of five images are usually obtained, one along the midline and two on each side by angling the transducer laterally. True midline can be established by identifying the curved corpus callosum and echogenic cerebellar vermis on the same imaging plane. The cingulate gyrus can be seen as an undulating echogenic line superior to the corpus callosum. The medial aspect of the paired thalamic nuclei, the tectum of the midbrain, and fourth ventricle can be identified on this image. The transducer is swept laterally approximately 10 degrees to show the body of the lateral ventricle. Because the lateral ventricles are not located in a straight anteroposterior line, the transducer must be slightly angled so that the posterior aspect of the probe is positioned more laterally than its anterior aspect. The echogenic choroid plexus is C-shaped and cups the

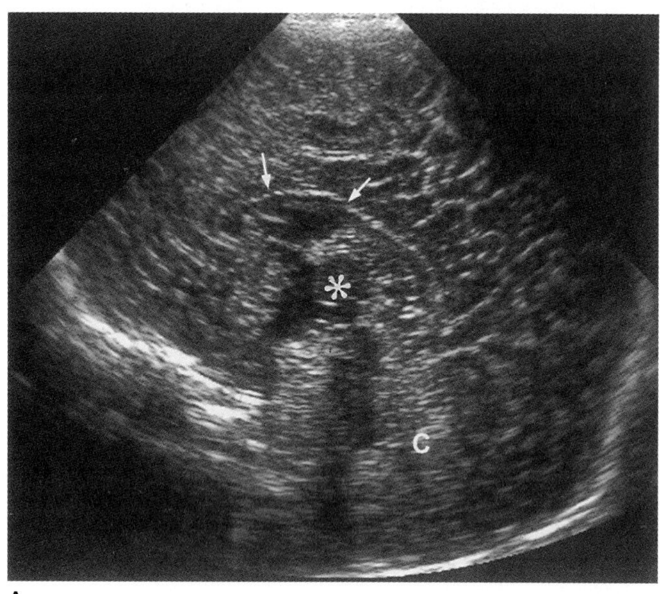


A

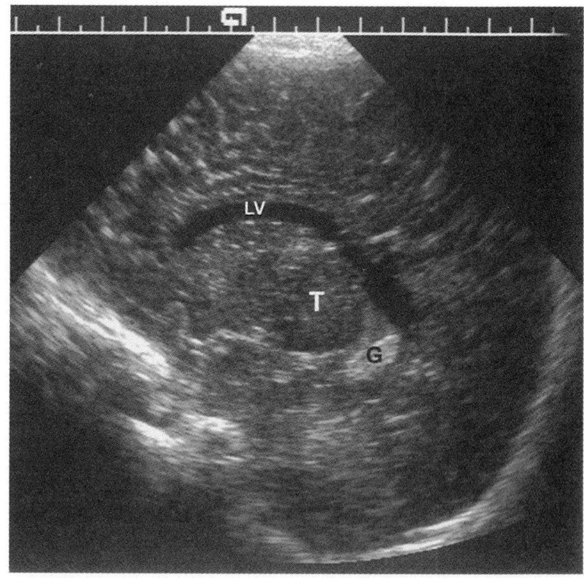


B

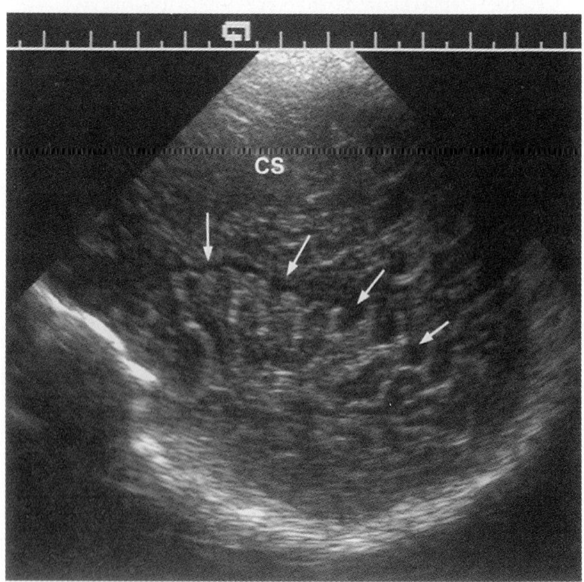


C

**FIGURE 62–2.** Standard sagittal planes of cranial sonography performed through the anterior fontanel. **A,** The midline sagittal image demonstrates the corpus callosum *(arrows)*, interthalamic adhesion (*), and cerebellar vermis (C). **B,** The first off-midline sagittal image is angled to illustrate the body of the lateral ventricle (LV), the glomus (G) of the choroid plexus in the trigone of the lateral ventricle, and the thalamus (T). **C,** The far-lateral sagittal image includes the sylvian fissure *(arrows)*.

thalamus like a baseball in a catcher's mitt. Its superior limb extends anteriorly to the caudothalamic notch immediately posterior to the head of the caudate nucleus. Its inferior limb extends well into the temporal horn. The second angled sagittal image is obtained with the transducer angled lateral to the body of the lateral ventricle. The centrum semiovale is well shown, and the sylvian fissure can be seen separating the parietal and temporal lobes (Naidich and Yousefzadeh, 1986; Siegel, 2001).

### Clinical Indications

The most common indication for cranial US in the newborn is screening for suspected intracranial hemorrhage and periventricular leukomalacia (PVL) in the premature infant. Once either is detected, US is an excellent method for monitoring the progression or resolution of the pathologic process as well as for detecting the attendant complications of ventricular dilatation and progressive hydrocephalus. Sonography also is a very useful tool in the identification of focal infarction and hemorrhagic lesions in the term or near-term infant, as well as congenital midline anomalies, cystic lesions, vascular malformations, and intracranial calcifications, and in the definition of extra-axial fluid collections. The portable, noninvasive nature of cranial US allows for the cribside identification of many important lesions on an urgent basis without need for transport of the unstable or critically ill newborn. A more definitive characterization of a sonographic finding or suspected lesion can be performed subsequently with magnetic resonance imaging (MRI) or computed tomography (CT) once the infant is more stable.

## COMPUTED TOMOGRAPHY

CT uses a narrowly collimated x-ray beam in conjunction with a digital detector array to produce a cross-sectional anatomic image (Boyd, 1995) (Fig. 62–3). Although employing ionizing radiation, current-generation CT scanners effectively limit exposure to the immediate volume of interest (Raj et al, 2000). Tissue contrast in CT is dependent on differential attenuation of the x-ray beam. Tissues with high electron density, such as bone, markedly attenuate the beam, whereas brain and other soft tissues absorb fewer photons. Relative tissue densities on CT images are, by convention, measured in Hounsfield units (HU). After acquisition of the digital data, the images can be adjusted to emphasize different tissues such as bone or soft tissue.

### Techniques

CT images are typically acquired in either the axial or the coronal plane. In most systems, the patient lies supine on a specialized scan table while the x-ray tube and detector array are rotated through a 360-degree arc. The scan table is then advanced several millimeters, and the next image slice is obtained. For certain indications, the images may be acquired in a spiral (helical) or volumetric fashion with continuous rotation of the x-ray tube–detector array and uninterrupted scan table advancement.

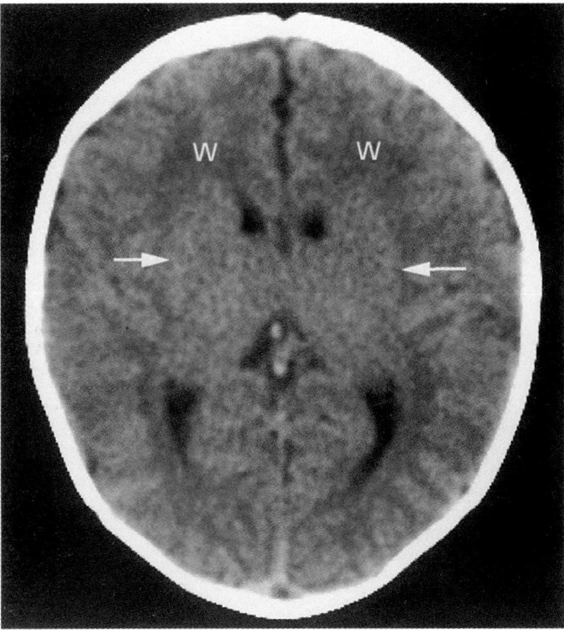


**FIGURE 62–3.** Axial computed tomographic image in a normal term newborn. Unmyelinated white matter is characterized by low density (W), while cortex and deep gray matter *(arrows)* are slightly denser.

Brain CT in the newborn is usually performed without the administration of intravenous contrast. Intravenous contrast may be used in CT for the evaluation of blood brain barrier breakdown and as a blood pool agent for vascular imaging. Most often, however, the relevant clinical questions regarding the presence of tumors, infections, vascular malformations, and vascular patency can be answered without the use of contrast or are more fully evaluated with MRI (Cowan and MacDonald, 1999; Haring et al, 1999).

### Clinical Indications

Brain CT is most often requested in the newborn to evaluate potential causes of an acute change in neurologic status. In the neonate, neurologic manifestations of intracranial abnormalities are often nonspecific and/or nonlocalizing (Rivkin, 1997; Robertson and Robson, 2001). In this setting, CT may demonstrate a variety of underlying abnormalities including intracranial hemorrhage, hypoxic-ischemic brain injury, focal infarction, posthemorrhagic hydrocephalus, vascular anomalies and malformations, infections, tumors, and certain of the phakomatoses. CT is particularly useful for the detection of acute hemorrhage, calcification or mineralization, and mass lesions.

US, because the equipment is portable and the examination can be performed at the bedside and does not utilize ionizing radiation, is the preferred method for evaluating many suspected central nervous system (CNS) disorders in the neonate. CT examination of the brain is usually obtained to clarify findings seen with US (e.g., hemorrhage versus edema) and to evaluate regions of the brain that are poorly seen with US owing to lack of an adequate acoustic

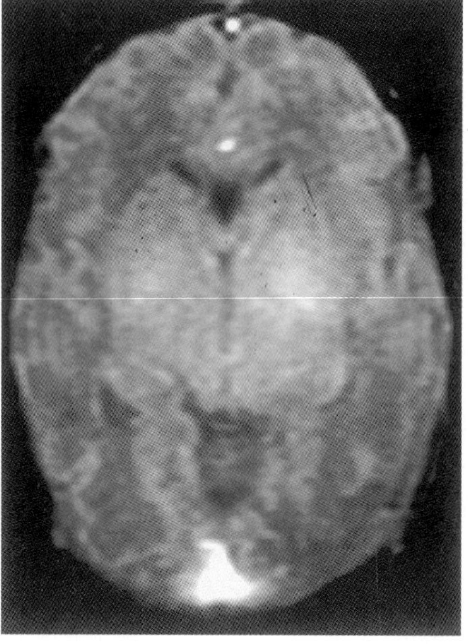


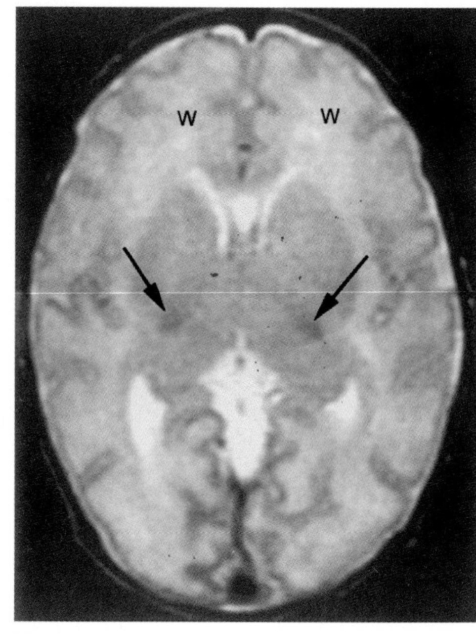


**FIGURE 62–4.** Axial images in a normal 34-week-gestation preterm neonate. **A,** Unmyelinated subcortical white matter appears hypointense (dark) on T1-weighted imaging, while the cortical and deep gray matter exhibit higher signal intensity. **B,** Unmyelinated subcortical white matter (W) appears markedly hyperintense (bright) on the T2-weighted fast spin echo image, while areas of early myelination, such as in the lateral thalamus *(arrows)*, are of lower signal intensity. Loss of this focus of hypointensity is one of the earliest indicators of hypoxic-ischemic injury on T2-weighted images.

window (e.g., peripheral cortex) (Barnes and Taylor, 1998). Because the majority of CT scanners are not portable, the neonate must be transferred to the imaging suite for evaluation. Monitoring and support equipment can be brought into the imaging suite without the restrictions inherent with MRI. In recent years, however, MRI, because of its superior tissue contrast, multiplanar capabilities, available functional information, and lack of ionizing radiation, has largely supplanted CT as an adjunct to US for the evaluation of the newborn brain (Robertson et al, 2003).

## MAGNETIC RESONANCE IMAGING

MRI is an established technique based on the principles of nuclear MR. Clinical MRI uses a nonionizing radiofrequency (RF) pulse to interrogate the properties of water protons in an applied external magnetic field (Balter, 1987; Mulkern and Chung, 2000). The behavior of the protons is determined by both the applied external magnetic field and the local magnetic field produced by neighboring protons. Image signal intensity (brightness) is related to the overall water content of the tissue as well as the inherent tissue properties: T1, T2, proton flow, proton diffusion, paramagnetism, magnetic susceptibility, and chemical shift (Barnes and Taylor, 1998). MR contrast is determined by the relative emphasis (i.e., weighting) placed on these various factors during image acquisition (Figs. 62–4, 62–5, and 62–6). The manipulation of multiple tissue properties in MRI provides greater flexibility in imaging than is available with the single tissue property used in US (acoustic impedance) or CT (x-ray attenuation). MR images may be obtained in any desired anatomic plane without repositioning the patient. With few exceptions (e.g., Sturge-Weber syndrome, tumor), neonatal brain MRI does not require the use of intravenous contrast.

### Techniques

#### Anatomic Magnetic Resonance Imaging

In general, conventional MR spin echo imaging is not as rapid as US or CT. In recent years, however, a number of fast imaging pulse sequences such as fast spin echo and fast spoiled gradient-recalled imaging have

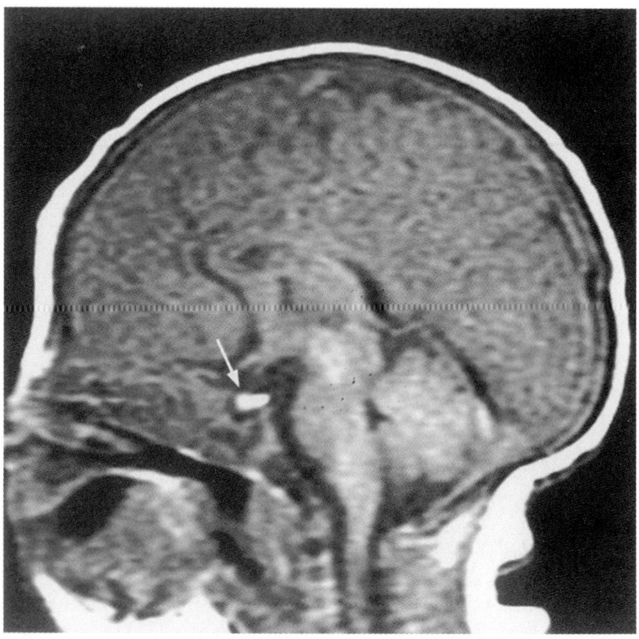

**FIGURE 62–5.** Midline sagittal T1-weighted image from a normal term neonate. Midline structures such as the corpus callosum, brainstem, and cerebellar vermis are well seen in the newborn. Of note, the pituitary *(arrow)* is diffusely hyperintense owing to hormonal activity.

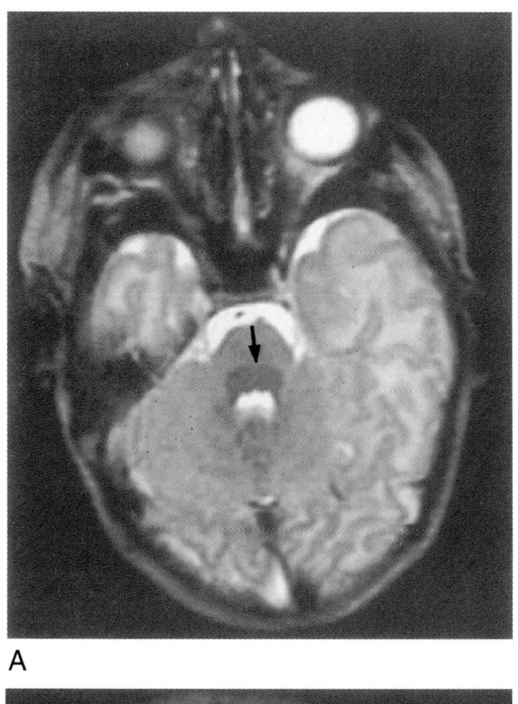
A

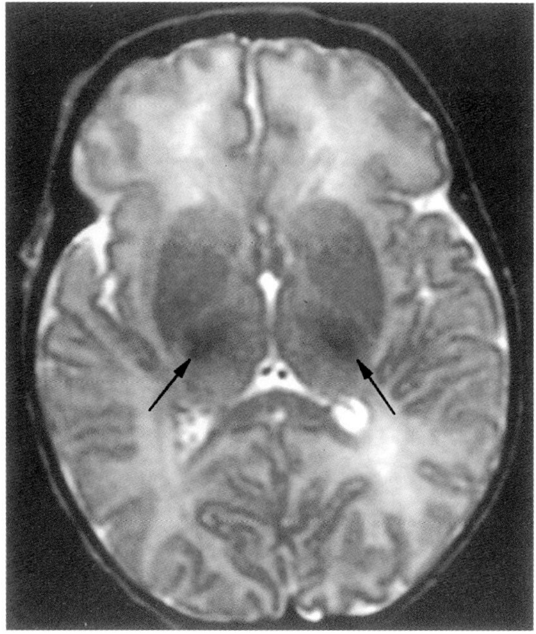
B

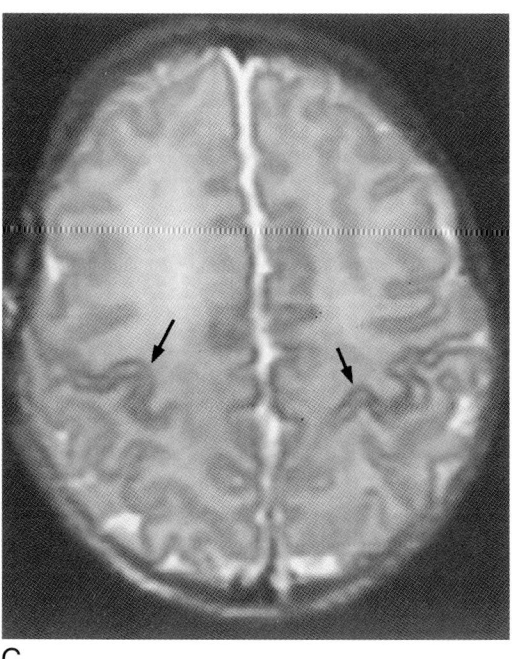
C

**FIGURE 62–6.** Axial fast spin echo T2-weighted images of the brain obtained at multiple levels in a normal term neonate. **A,** Unlike with computed tomography, magnetic resonance images obtained through the posterior fossa are free from artifact from the skull base. Early myelination, indicated by hypointensity, is evident in the dorsal pons *(arrow)*. **B,** As in the preterm infant (see Fig. 62–4B), at the level of the basal ganglia and thalami, early myelination is present in the lateral thalamus and posterior limb of the internal capsule *(arrows)*. Unmyelinated white matter is still markedly hyperintense (bright) in the normal term newborn. **C,** On images obtained at the level of the centrum semiovale, the rolandic cortex is easily identified by its low signal intensity *(arrows)* owing to early myelination.

been developed (see Figs. 62–4*B* and 62–6). The use of these techniques does help to minimize the examination time while preserving tissue contrast but still requires that the patient remain motionless for 2 to 3 minutes at a time. Consequently, sedation or anesthesia is often required to perform an adequate examination in the newborn.

MR angiography (MRA) and MR venography (MRV) may be used to demonstrate the intracranial arteries and veins of the neonatal brain without the use of intravenous contrast. The most commonly used sequence is a gradient-echo sequence in which stationary tissues are repeatedly excited with RF pulses at short intervals. Because of the long T1 of the brain, the protons are unable to regain longitudinal magnetization between RF pulses, and their signal is suppressed. The protons in inflowing blood have not experienced the previous RF pulses and can give back signal. This is termed the *time-of-flight* (TOF) *effect* and is the basis for the most commonly used MR technique for the depiction of blood flow.

### Functional Magnetic Resonance Imaging

In addition to the anatomic information available with standard MRI sequences, functional information may be obtained with newer MRI techniques such as diffusion-weighted MRI (Fig. 62–7), perfusion MRI, brain activation

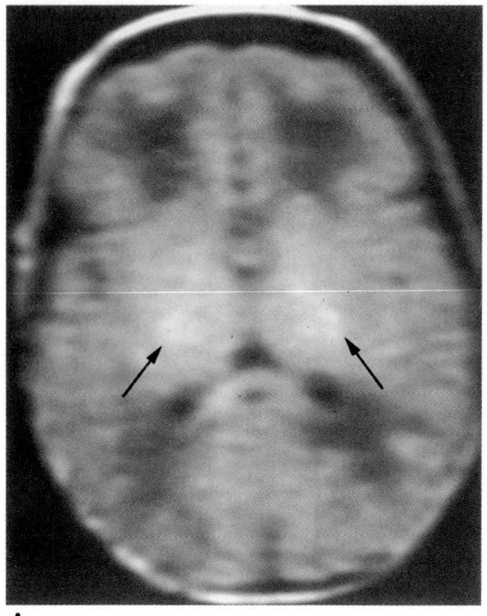


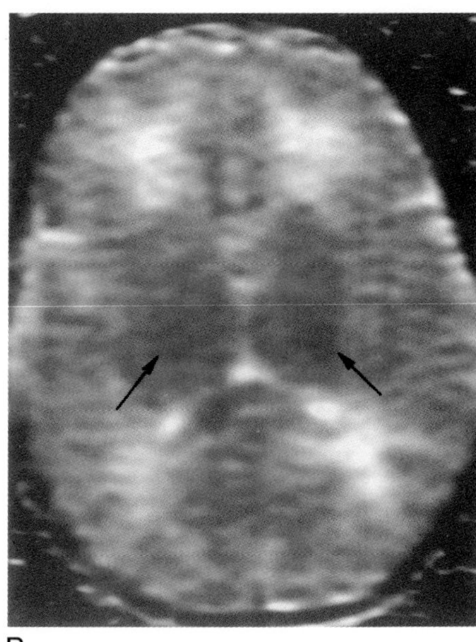


**FIGURE 62–7.** Axial line scan diffusion-weighted imaging in a normal term newborn. **A,** Isotropic diffusion- weighted image at the level of the basal ganglia. Unmyelinated white matter has very low signal intensity owing to the rapid diffusion of water in these regions, while areas that have already begun to myelinate, such as the lateral thalamus and posterior limb of the internal capsule *(arrows)*, have more restricted diffusion and increased signal. **B,** Corresponding processed apparent diffusion coefficient (ADC) map. These maps are produced to limit T2 effects in the images. Areas with relatively restricted molecular diffusion are, by convention, depicted as lower pixel values *(arrows)*.

MRI, and MR spectroscopy (MRS) (Fig. 62–8) (Barkovich et al, 1999; Huppi and Inder, 2001; Robertson et al, 2000a; Warach et al, 1996). These newer sequences have been made possible in large part by the development of ultrafast imaging such as echo planar MRI and the improved uniformity of the magnetic field available with newer MR scanners. Used in adults and older children for several years, functional techniques are now being applied in the newborn.

### *Diffusion Imaging*

Initially popularized for its usefulness in the evaluation of acute stroke in adults, diffusion imaging (DI) is now widely utilized to evaluate the neonatal brain (Robertson et al, 1999; Rutherford et al, 1995). In newborns, DI has been used to study normal brain myelination as well as ischemic and nonischemic CNS disorders. The immature brain is characterized by a high water content and relatively rapid molecular diffusion (Robertson and Robson, 2001; Robertson et al, 1999, Sakuma et al, 1991) (see Fig 62–7). The bulk of the water in the neonatal brain is within the extracellular space (Barlow et al, 1961). As the brain matures, a gradual decline in the extracellular volume fraction occurs owing to the hydrophobic nature of myelin. Myelin also impairs the exchange of water molecules across the cell membrane. Because the movement of water within the cell is limited by its interaction with intracellular structures and the cell membrane, the apparent diffusion coefficient (ADC) of intracellular water is lower than that of extracellular water. Consequently, the ADC of myelinated white matter is lower than that of unmyelinated white matter. In addition, because of cellular structure, the direction of movement of intracellular water is preferentially along the length of the axon rather than perpendicular to it. Therefore, the relative anisotropy (RA), a measure of the inequality of diffusibility in different directions, increases as the proportion of intracellular water increases (Takeda et al, 1997; Toft et al, 1996).

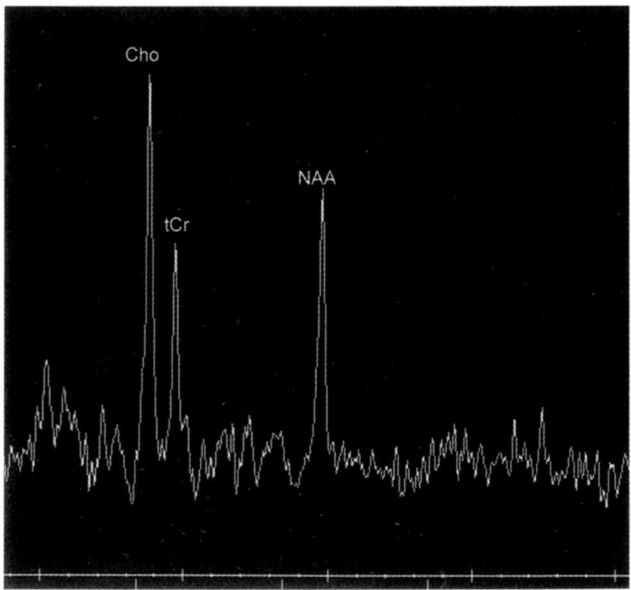


**FIGURE 62–8.** Single-voxel proton spectroscopy of the brain from a normal term neonate. The spectra were obtained with an echo time of 144 msec. Three prominent peaks are identified: At 3.2 ppm is choline (Cho). Choline compounds are involved in the metabolism of membrane lipids. At 3.0 ppm is total creatine (tCr). Creatine and phosphocreatine are involved in ATP metabolism. At 2.0 ppm is *N*-acetyl aspartate (NAA). NAA is an intracellular compound found primarily in neurons. Note that lactate, which would appear, if present, as an inverted doublet at 1.3 ppm, is not seen in the normal newborn.

### *Perfusion Imaging*

To date, performing perfusion MRI of the brain in the newborn has been relatively unsuccessful. Implementing contrast bolus tracking (Kucharczyk et al, 1993), the most common perfusion MRI technique, has been difficult because of the small volume of contrast that can be used in the newborn and the lack of adequate intravenous access to permit administration of a compact contrast bolus. The use of spin-tagging methods that do not require the administration of an exogenous contrast agent (Alsop and Detre, 1996; Kim and Tsekos, 1997) has been equally challenging.

### *Brain Activation Imaging*

MR brain activation studies have been performed successfully in the neonate, albeit in limited scope (Anderson et al, 2001; Benaron et al, 2000; Born et al, 1998). The use of MRI to indirectly demonstrate cortical activation is based on the observation that regional blood flow varies with neuronal activity. That is, in areas of the brain that are activated, there is an increase in blood flow, while the oxygen extraction fraction remains constant. Consequently, there is an increase in the local concentration of oxyhemoglobin and a decrease in the local concentration of deoxyhemoglobin (Buchbinder and Cosgrove, 1998). Deoxyhemoglobin has susceptibility effects that cause minor perturbations in the magnetic field, leading to signal loss. The increase in oxyhemoglobin that accompanies brain activation causes a local increase in signal intensity. These changes form the basis of the MRI technique called blood oxygenation level–dependent (BOLD) imaging, the MRI sequence most often used to assess brain activation. Because the signal changes associated with brain activation are quite small, a number of images can be averaged together to produce a composite view of cortical activation. Typically, therefore, BOLD imaging requires that the subject cooperate with repetitive tasks to demonstrate brain activation. Because the neonate is unable to perform such tasks, only those stimuli that produce an involuntary response, such as visual cortical activation with strobe light flashes, may be tested. Despite these limitations, the use of BOLD MRI to evaluate neonatal brain activation is an active area of research (Anderson et al, 2001; Benaron et al, 2000; Born et al, 1998).

### *Magnetic Resonance Spectroscopy*

Proton MRS exploits the minute differences in magnetic moments of hydrogen atoms reflecting differences in their local chemical environment to produce spectra characteristic of a variety of metabolites (Keevil et al, 1998) (see Fig. 62–8). Because of its ability to detect abnormal metabolites and metabolic ratios, MRS is becoming popular in the MR assessment of a number of processes affecting the newborn (Vigneron et al, 2001).

With most proton MRS techniques, the signal from water protons must be suppressed in order to demonstrate biologically interesting metabolites that are present in very small quantities. This requires a very homogeneous magnetic field that is generally found only in newer and higher- field-strength MR systems. Because of the tiny amount of signal emanating from the metabolites of interest, relatively large voxels (1 to 2 cc) must be acquired to obtain adequate signal intensity. MRS may be performed using single voxels, which sample a small region of the brain, or multiple voxels, by which many areas may be interrogated during a single acquisition (Vigneron et al, 2001). Typically, single-voxel MRS provides higher quality spectra than those available with multiple-voxel techniques.

Three metabolites are most apparent in the normal neonatal brain: choline (3.2 ppm), total creatine (3.0 ppm), and *N*-acetyl aspartate (NAA) (2.0 ppm) (Heerschap and van den Berg, 1994). Choline compounds are central in the metabolism of membrane lipids and tend to be elevated in processes that result in rapid cell turnover. As a consequence of membrane development during myelination, choline tends to be relatively increased in the normal newborn brain. The creatine peak consists of creatine and phosphocreatine, which serve as a reserve for high-energy phosphates in neurons and also as an ATP/ADP buffer. Total creatine tends to remain relatively constant in most intracranial processes (Govindaraju et al, 2000). NAA is an intracellular compound found primarily in neurons, although its biologic function is largely unknown (Miller, 1991). NAA is present in smaller quantities in the neonate than in the older child or adult.

Lactate is a terminal product of glycolysis. The tissue concentration of lactate can vary from minute to minute, depending upon the status of a number of major metabolic pathways. Lactate is not demonstrated on MRS in the normal newborn brain but may be seen as a prominent doublet at 1.3 ppm in certain pathologic conditions such as infarction. Depending on the parameters chosen for imaging, the lactate peaks may project above or below the baseline.

## Fetal Magnetic Resonance Imaging

The recent development of ultrafast MR sequences such as single-shot fast spin echo and echo planar imaging has allowed the use of MRI to evaluate fetal abnormalities (Girard et al, 2001; Levine, 2001a, 2001b; Whitby et al, 2001) (Fig. 62–9). These studies do not require the use of sedation or anesthesia and provide reproducible and reliable images of the fetus from the late second trimester to term. To date, no known effects harmful to the developing fetus have been documented using clinical MR scanners at or below 1.5 tesla (T) (Myers et al, 1998; Baker et al, 1994). Gadolinium contrast agent is not given, as transplacental passage of the agent occurs and its toxic effects on the fetus are not fully known.

Although US remains the study of choice for screening for fetal anomalies of the CNS, MRI is becoming widely utilized to further characterize suspicious findings on prenatal US. Additionally, MRI may be useful when oligohydramnios or a difficult fetal lie (e.g., fetal head engaged in maternal pelvis) makes US examination of the fetal CNS suboptimal (Hubbard and States, 2001).

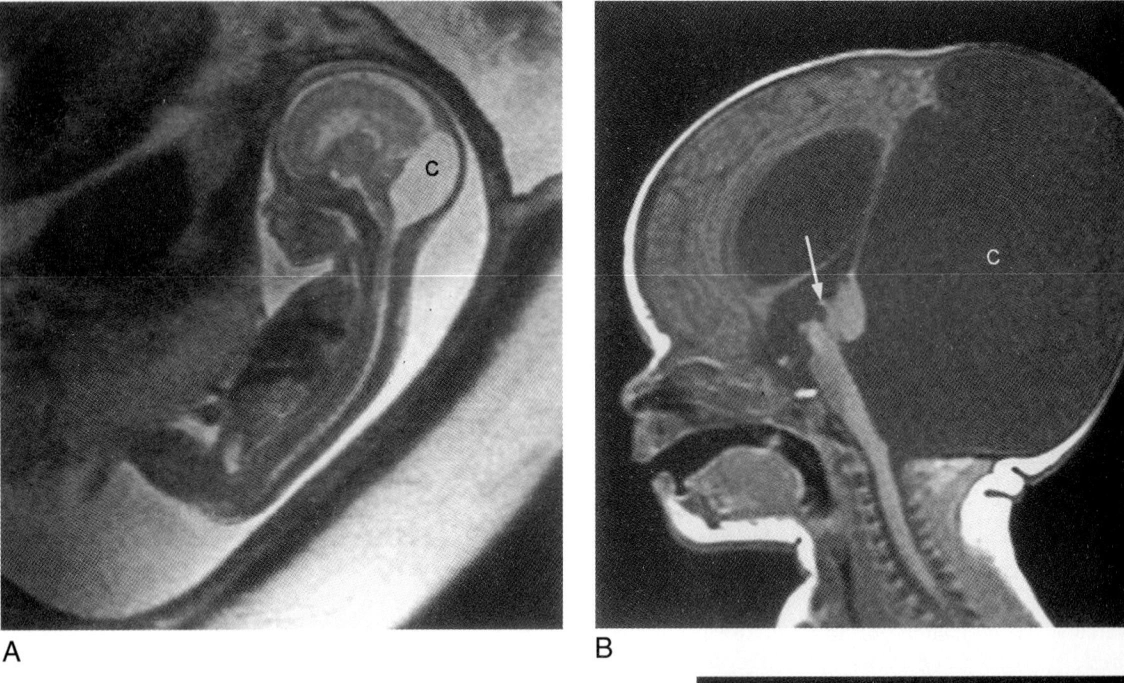


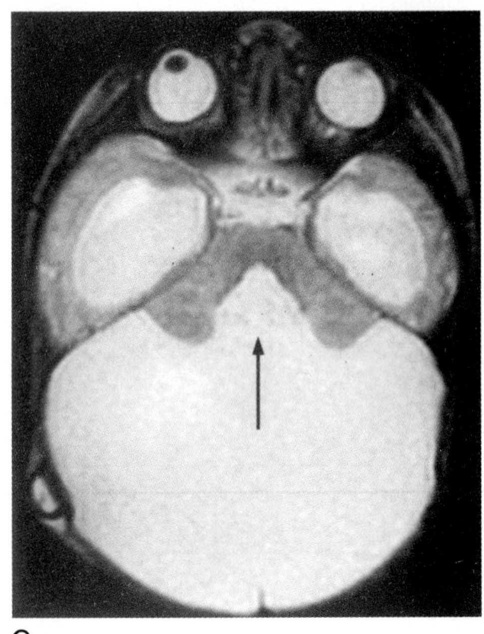


**FIGURE 62–9.** Fetal and postnatal magnetic resonance (MR) images from an infant with Dandy-Walker malformation. **A,** Sagittal single-shot fast spin echo T2-weighted fetal MR image obtained at 19.5 weeks of gestation. A large posterior fossa cystic malformation (C) is clearly demonstrated. Axial images (not shown) confirmed absence of the cerebellar vermis. **B,** Postnatal sagittal T1-weighted image shows enlargement of the posterior fossa cyst (C). There is dilatation of the lateral and third ventricles due to aqueductal stenosis indicated by elevation of the tectum *(arrow)*. **C,** Absence of the cerebellar vermis is apparent on the axial T2-weighted image *(arrow)*.

US and MRI are complementary imaging methods in the evaluation of high-risk pregnancy. When a CNS anomaly is suspected on US, MRI may demonstrate additional findings that can alter patient counseling (Levine et al, 1997). In a recent study, MRI demonstrated additional findings not seen on US. These findings included agenesis of the corpus callosum, cerebellar hypoplasia, cortical cleft, polymicrogyria, porencephaly, and partial agenesis of the septum pellucidum (Levine et al, 1997). Other structural anomalies such as Dandy-Walker malformation, aqueductal stenosis, hydrocephalus, Chiari malformation and vascular malformations are also readily demonstrated with MRI (Chi et al, 1977; Hubbard and States, 2001).

## Clinical Indications

MRI may be performed for clarification of known or suspected structural abnormalities or to investigate the cause of an acute change in neurologic status. Unlike US, which can be performed at the patient's bedside, MRI necessitates transporting the infant to the MRI suite. In most centers, the MRI suite is remote from the neonatal intensive care unit. Minimizing stress on the infant and ensuring patient stability during transport and MR scanning must therefore be carefully attended to. The MRI suite must be kept cool to avoid overheating of the equipment, so hypothermia in the newborn is also a concern.

Although not widely available at present, MR-compatible incubators have recently been developed and may be helpful in decreasing the stress of the MR examination for the neonate.

The requirement of a strong, homogeneous magnetic field to perform MRI places additional constraints on neonatal imaging. Supportive equipment (e.g., anesthesia ventilatory equipment, intravenous pumps, monitoring equipment) placed in the MR scanning room must be nonferromagnetic. Indwelling ferromagnetic metallic or electrical devices constitute a contraindication to MRI (Bhachu and Kanal, 2000; Ho, 2001).

## IMAGING APPLICATIONS

### Normal Preterm versus Term Infants

The most obvious difference between the preterm and the term neonatal brain is relative maturation of the sulcal/gyral architecture. As with fetal imaging, preterm infants studied at 25 weeks of gestational age equivalent will show a very smooth cortical mantle with a largely uncovered sylvian fissure and very few developed gyri. At this age, demonstration of lissencephaly and of some localized anomalies of cortical development is not possible with US and may be difficult with more advanced imaging techniques as well. Cortical maturation proceeds in a predictable fashion and should attain a fully developed secondary sulcal/gyral pattern by 40 to 44 weeks of gestational age (Chi et al, 1977). On US, gyri are depicted as linear echoes that increase in length, undulation, and branching as the infant matures.

A prominent feature of both the preterm and the term neonatal brain is the very high water content of the unmyelinated subcortical white matter. In the premature infant, there is little difference in echogenicity between gray and white matter until beyond 32 to 34 weeks of gestation. In the near-term infant, the cortical ribbon is hypoechoic in relation to the underlying white matter. Beyond 40 weeks of gestation, the overall echogenicity of white matter structures increases markedly, and visualization of deeper structures may become more difficult. On CT, unmyelinated white matter is hypodense relative to cortex and deep central gray matter. On MRI, the high water content of unmyelinated white matter produces marked prolongation of T1 and T2, causing the white matter to be hypointense to gray matter on T1-weighted imaging and hyperintense to gray matter on T2-weighted imaging. This pattern is the inverse of signal intensities of gray and white matter present in the fully myelinated brains of older children and adults (Barkovich, 2000; Barkovich et al, 1988). Because many pathologic processes result in edema, seen as low density on CT studies and resulting in T1 and T2 prolongation on MR images, these lesions are especially difficult to see in the neonatal white matter.

### Intracranial Hemorrhage

Acute intracranial hemorrhage in the neonate may be epidural, subdural, subarachnoid, or parenchymal in location. Hemorrhages may be small and noted incidentally on imaging performed for other reasons or may be large and produce acute neurologic symptoms.

Small parturitional subdural hemorrhages are common even in the absence of a traumatic birth history and are often asymptomatic (Holden et al, 1999). Significant subdural hemorrhages are most frequently encountered in the setting of traumatic delivery or accidental trauma. Laceration of the falx cerebri or the tentorium cerebelli may produce large or rapidly expanding subdural hematomas. Larger subdural hematomas may be associated with acute or progressive symptoms of intracranial mass effect.

A small amount of parturitional subarachnoid bleeding is not uncommon. Subarachnoid hemorrhage with larger amounts of bleeding may occasionally occur in conjunction with vascular malformations. The most common symptomatic intracranial vascular malformation in the newborn is the Galenic malformation (Fig. 62–10). Although most newborns with Galenic malformations present with cardiopulmonary distress due to high-output cardiac failure resulting from arteriovenous shunts, massive subarachnoid bleeding may occasionally occur from either spontaneous or iatrogenic perforation of the varix or feeding arteries.

Parenchymal hemorrhage in the preterm infant occurs most often in or around the germinal matrix. Although its pathogenesis is multifactorial (Volpe, 2001), a common final pathway seems to be microscopic perivenular hemorrhage in the highly vascular germinal matrix (Ghazi-Birry et al, 1997). Rupture into the ventricular system frequently occurs. Further enlargement of the hematoma may lead to thrombosis or compression of the terminal veins in the region of residual germinal matrix at the caudothalamic groove (Fig. 62–11). Extension of the venous thrombosis can result in hemorrhagic venous infarction, which can be depicted with color Doppler techniques (Taylor, 1995, 1997).

The classification originally proposed by Papile and colleagues remains the most widely accepted method of grading the severity of intracranial hemorrhage in the preterm infant (Papile et al, 1983). Grade I consists of subependymal hemorrhage only (Fig. 62–12; see also Fig. 62–11). On US, grade I hemorrhages appear as bright echogenic foci in the subependymal area typically located in or anterior to the caudothalamic notch. Grade II is defined as subependymal and intraventricular hemorrhage without ventricular dilatation (Fig. 62–13). Grade III is the combination of subependymal and intraventricular hemorrhage with ventricular dilatation by clot (Fig. 62–14). Small choroid plexus hemorrhages may be difficult to distinguish from a normal "lumpy bumpy" choroid plexus, because both are brightly echogenic. Larger, acute intraventricular clots can be identified as echogenic irregular and asymmetrical masses. Poorly clotted blood will often result in a fluid-debris level within the ventricle that disappears when the baby is repositioned and blood is remixed with CSF. In critically ill premature infants it is important to distinguish progression of a grade II hemorrhage to grade III from the development of posthemorrhagic hydrocephalus. Both entities are associated with intraventricular clot and dilatation of the ventricular system. However, in grade III hemorrhage, the ventricle is

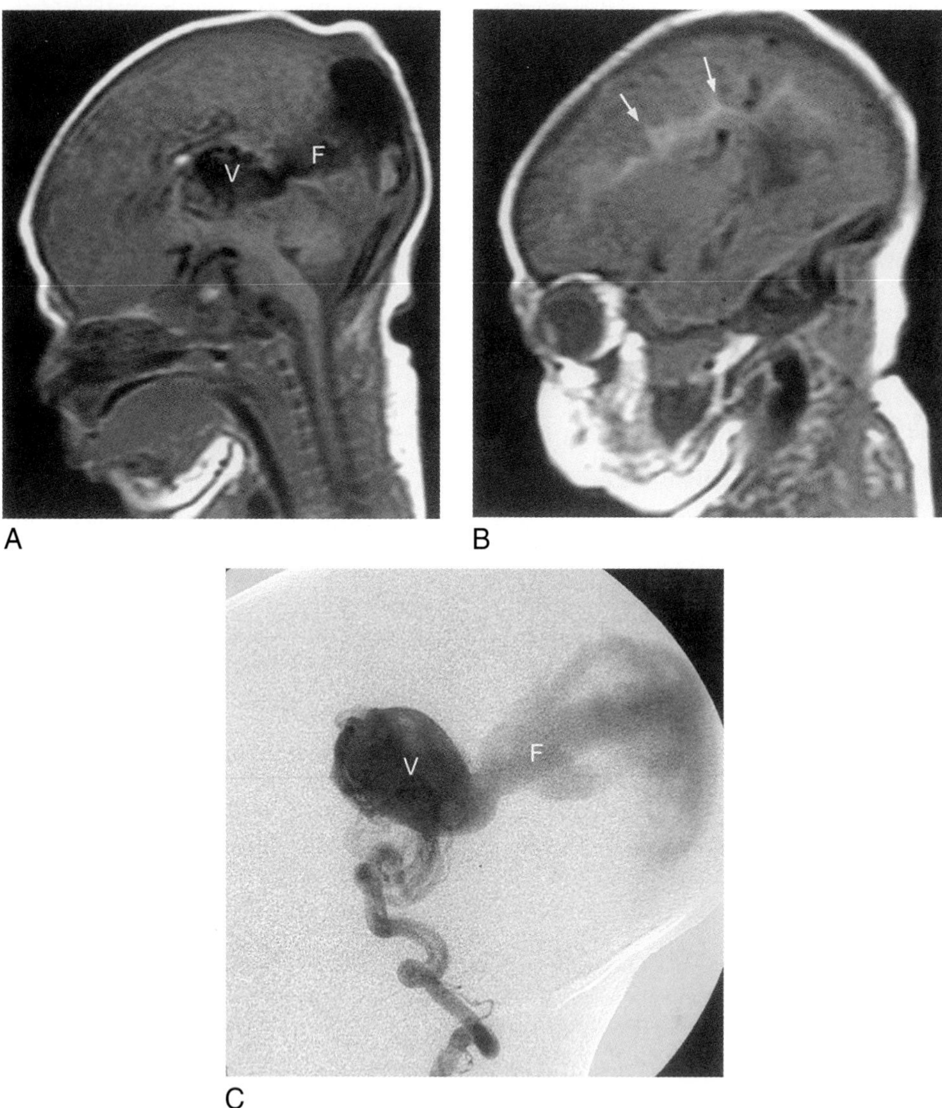


**FIGURE 62–10.** The patiemt was a neonate with congestive heart failure due to a Galenic arteriovenous malformation (also called vein of Galen aneurysm). **A,** Midline sagittal T1-weighted magnetic resonance (MR) image shows a signal void within the median prosencephalic vein (V), the embryologic precursor to the vein of Galen, and the persistent falcine sinus (F). **B,** Parasagittal T1-weighted MR image shows hyperintensity of the subcortical white matter *(arrows)* due to chronic ischemic injury. **C,** Selective vertebral artery conventional angiogram performed as part of a transcatheter therapeutic procedure shows flow within the varix (V) and draining sinus (F). Note that although the feeding arteries are markedly dilated owing to the massive intracranial flow that is present, all of the blood flow is diverted through the fistulas, and there are no brain parenchymal branches filling. This "steal" phenomenon produces the ischemic changes that can be demonstrated with computed tomography and MR imaging.

almost completely distended by clot, whereas the ventricle in posthemorrhagic hydrocephalus is often primarily distended with CSF. The size of the obstructing intraventricular clot may be relatively small. The distinction is important because vntricular dilatation caused by increasing hemorrhage may have therapeutic implications different from those associated with posthemorrhagic hydrocephalus. Grade IV includes all findings seen in grade III plus intraparenchymal blood. The intraparenchymal hematoma will appear brightly echogenic on US and is often associated with a mass effect on surrounding structures (Fig. 62–15A). Within 7 to 10 days it will develop a hypoechoic center and echogenic rim. Over time, hematomas further resolve by liquefaction, resulting in cystic lesions of varying sizes (Fig. 62–15B).

In the term infant, lobar parenchymal and subpial hemorrhages are occasionally encountered (Koenigsberger, 1999) (Fig. 62–16). These hemorrhages appear to occur spontaneously in the first few days of life in otherwise healthy babies.

Color Doppler US may be used to characterize extracerebral fluid collections as subarachnoid, subdural, or

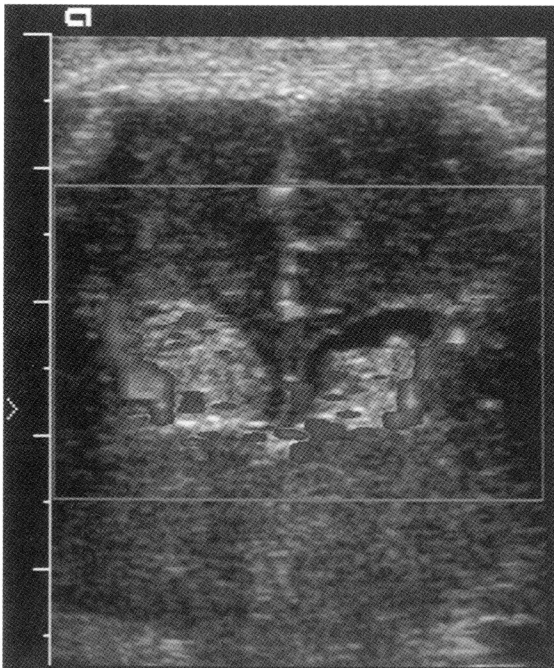

**FIGURE 62–11.** (See also Color Plate 62–11.) Coronal color Doppler image of bilateral grade I germinal matrix hemorrhages. The hemorrhages are echogenic. Although flow is confirmed within the terminal veins *(blue)*, the veins are laterally displaced by the subependymal hemorrhages.

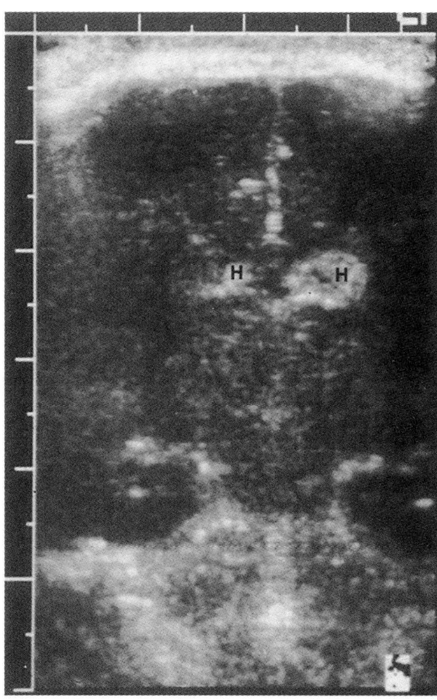


**FIGURE 62–13.** Coronal ultrasound study of bilateral grade II intracranial hemorrhage in the preterm neonate. Echogenic subependymal hemorrhages (H) are seen extending into the lateral ventricles. There is no hydrocephalus.

combined. Because superficial cortical blood vessels lie within the pia-arachnoid, fluid in this (subarachnoid) space lifts the cortical vessels away from the brain surface, while fluid in the subdural space approximates cortical vessels to the brain surface and is separated from these vessels by a thin membrane (Fig. 62–17). Correlation with MRI and CT suggests that color Doppler is reliable in making this differentiation (Chen et al, 1996).

Suspected intracranial hemorrhage is one of the most common reasons to obtain a brain CT in the neonate. On CT, acute hemorrhage appears hyperdense relative to the brain parenchyma (Fig. 62–18). Of note, the dural venous sinuses and cortical veins appear relatively dense during the

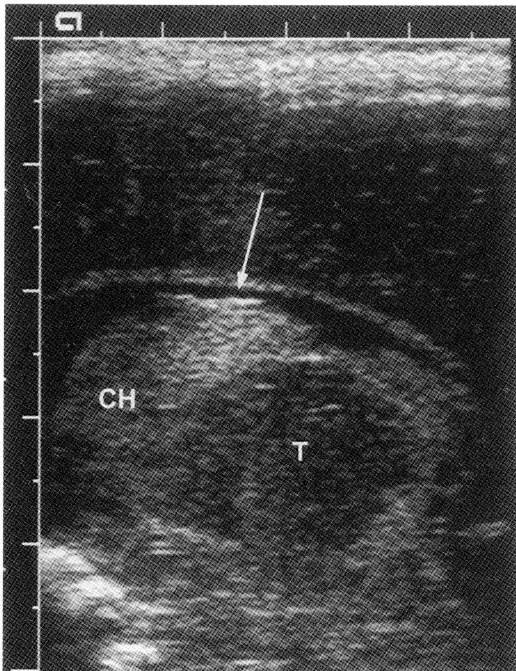


**FIGURE 62–12.** Sagittal ultrasound study of grade I germinal matrix hemorrhage. Echogenic hemorrhage *(arrow)* is seen at the caudothalamic notch situated between the caudate head (CH) anteriorly and the thalamus (T) posteriorly.

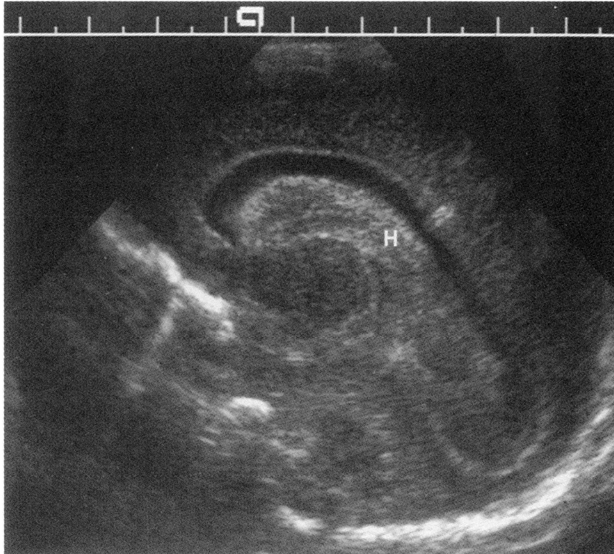


**FIGURE 62–14.** Sagittal ultrasound study of grade III intracranial hemorrhage. The lateral ventricle is moderately dilated and filled with echogenic blood (H).

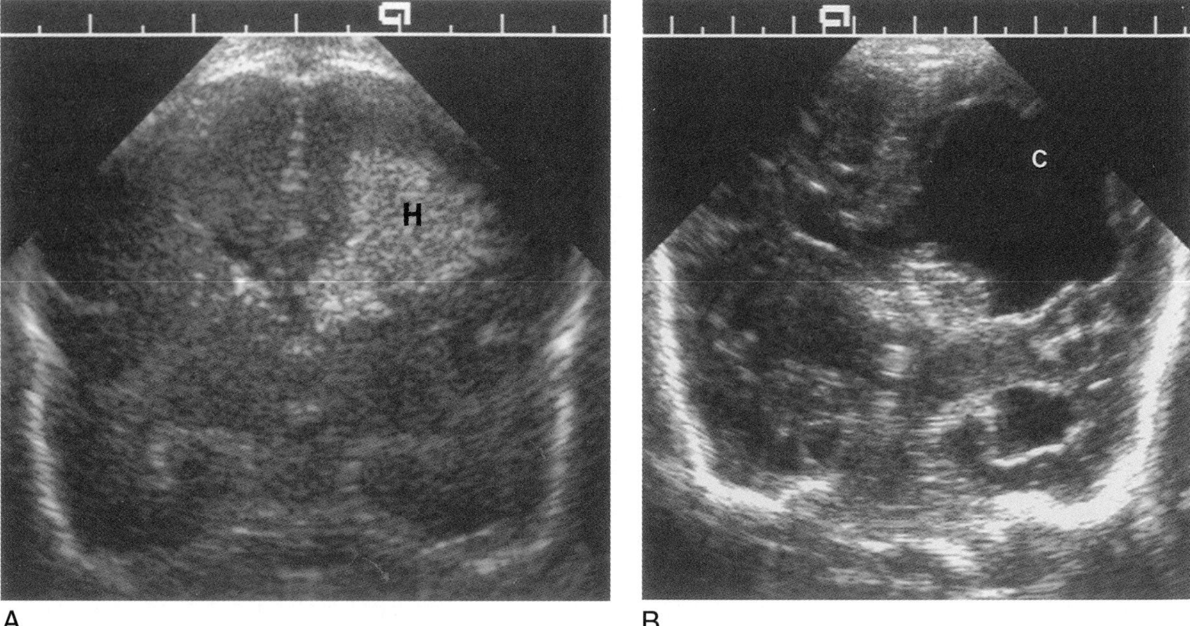


**FIGURE 62–15.** Coronal ultrasound study of grade IV intracranial hemorrhage. **A,** Initially the parenchymal hemorrhage (H) is echogenic. **B,** As the hematoma ages, liquefaction occurs and the hematoma becomes echolucent with the development of a porencephalic cyst (C).

first few days of life owing to high hematocrit levels. This normal density of the venous structures should not be mistaken for subdural bleeding or dural venous sinus thrombosis on CT. As blood ages, the density of the clot will decrease. In the chronic phase, sites of extra-axial or parenchymal hemorrhage have decreased density relative to the brain parenchyma. Parturitional subdural hemorrhages are typically completely resolved by 6 to 8 weeks of life.

In general, MRI is considered to be less sensitive for the detection of acute intracranial hemorrhage than CT. However, in the newborn, all significant hemorrhages seen on CT are usually demonstrated by MRI (Blankenberg et al, 2000;

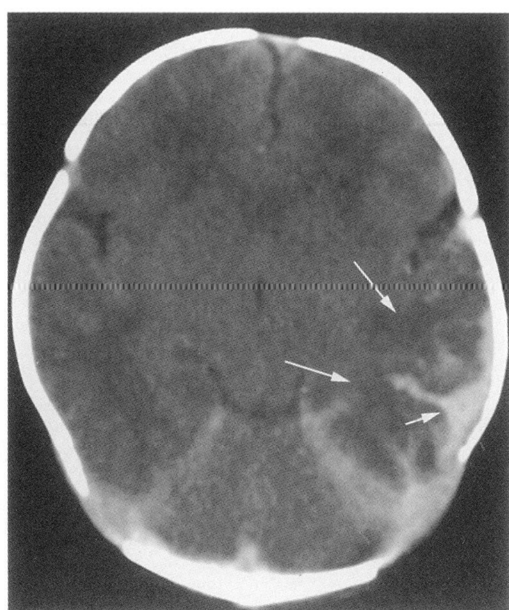

**FIGURE 62–16.** The patient was a term neonate with uneventful delivery who developed seizures on the third day of life. Unenhanced brain computed tomography scan shows parenchymal and subpial hemorrhage *(short arrow)* in the left temporal lobe. Surrounding low-density edema is also present *(long arrows)*.

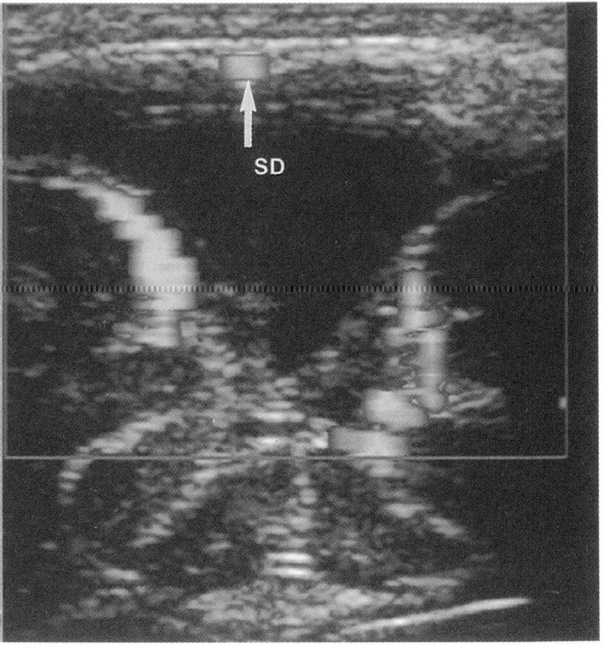


**FIGURE 62–17.** (See also Color Plate 62–17.) Coronal color Doppler ultrasound study shows that the vessels (color) are displaced toward the brain parenchyma by the subdural fluid (SD). Note flow in the superior sagittal sinus *(arrow)*.

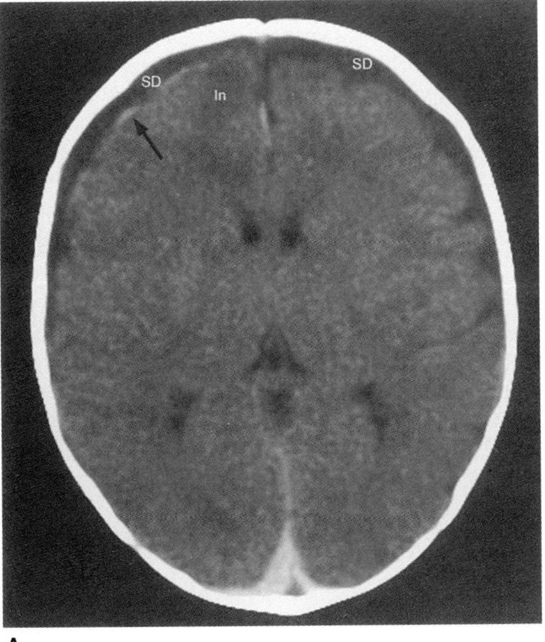


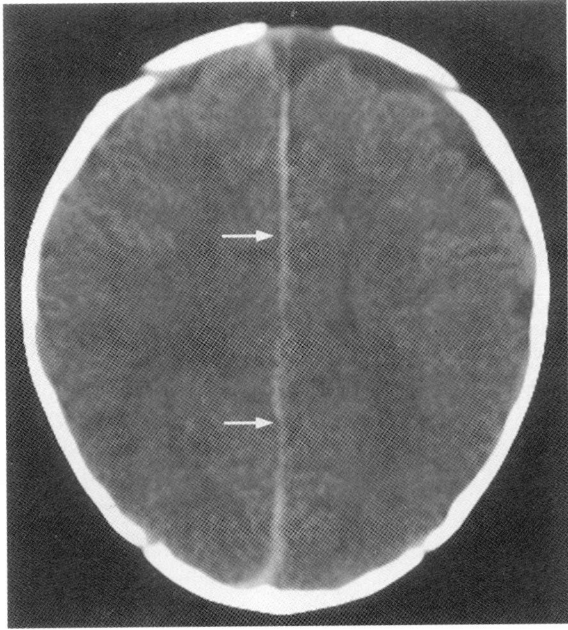


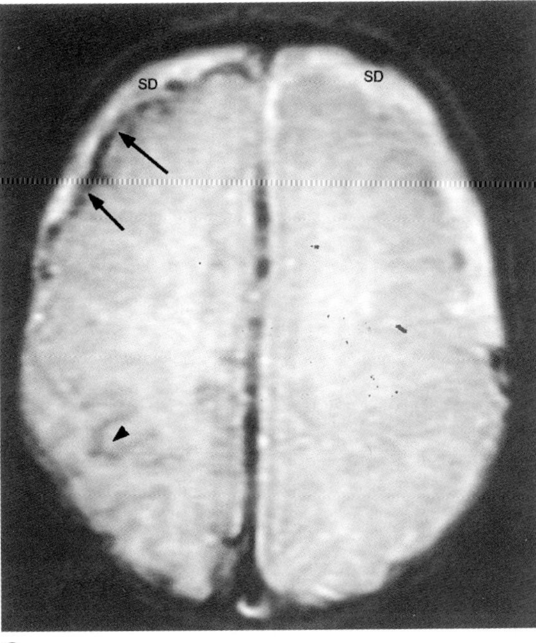


**FIGURE 62–18.** The patient was a neonate hospitalized with obtundation following nonaccidental injury. **A,** Axial noncontrast computed tomography (CT) study obtained at the level of the basal ganglia shows a mixed-density acute subdural collection (SD) with hyperdense clot adjacent to the brain *(arrow)* and superficial low-density subdural fluid. A small hypodense parenchymal infarction (In) is also present. **B,** Axial CT study obtained at the level of the centrum semiovale shows a hyperdense acute interhemispheric-subdural hematoma *(arrows)*. **C,** Corresponding axial gradient-echo magnetic resonance image shows a mixed-intensity subdural collection with hypointense clot *(arrows)* adjacent to the brain and hyperintense supernatant (SD). A small amount of subarachnoid blood is also present *(arrowhead)*.

Robertson et al, 2003). On MRI, the signal intensity of blood varies with age.

Although the timing for the development of the various stages of hemorrhage in the newborn may differ from that in the adult, the signal intensity changes are similar. With hyperacute hemorrhage, unclotted blood appears similar to free fluid (i.e., low signal intensity on T1-weighted images and high signal intensity on T2-weighted images). Within hours, oxyhemoglobin is converted to deoxyhemoglobin. Deoxyhemoglobin within the red blood cells causes susceptibility artifact that produces low signal intensity on T2-weighted images (see Fig. 62–18). Over the first several days, deoxyhemoglobin is converted to methemoglobin, which results in high signal intensity on T1-weighted images and low signal intensity on T2-weighted images. Subsequently, the red blood cells lyse, and an increase in signal intensity is observed on the T2-weighted images. Chronically, hemosiderin staining occurs, which appears dark on both T1-weighted and T2-weighted images.

The administration of contrast agent is not usually required in the MR investigation of hemorrhage, except in the rare case of suspected underlying tumor. When tumor is present, it is imperative that spinal imaging also be performed because most brain tumors discovered in the newborn period have a propensity to seed the CSF.

### Neonatal Cerebral Infarction

Neonatal cerebral infarction is a common cause of infant morbidity and mortality (Rivkin, 1997; Volpe, 2001). Infarctions in the newborn may be due to global transient decreases in blood flow or in oxygen delivery to the brain (hypoxic-ischemic injury) (Fig. 62–19) or to focal arterial or venous occlusions (Figs. 62–20, 62–21, and 62–22). Hypoxia-ischemia tends to produce bilaterally symmetrical lesions, whereas arterial or venous occlusions are associated with focal or asymmetrical multifocal areas of infarction. A variety of imaging appearances of infarction may be observed at a given postnatal age, and lack of specificity in the clinical presentation may further complicate the interpretation of the imaging (Robertson and Robson, 2001).

In the term infant, the vascular border-zone territories are in a parasagittal location, anteriorly between the major branches of the anterior and middle cerebral arteries and posteriorly between the branches of the anterior, middle, and posterior cerebral arteries. In our experience,

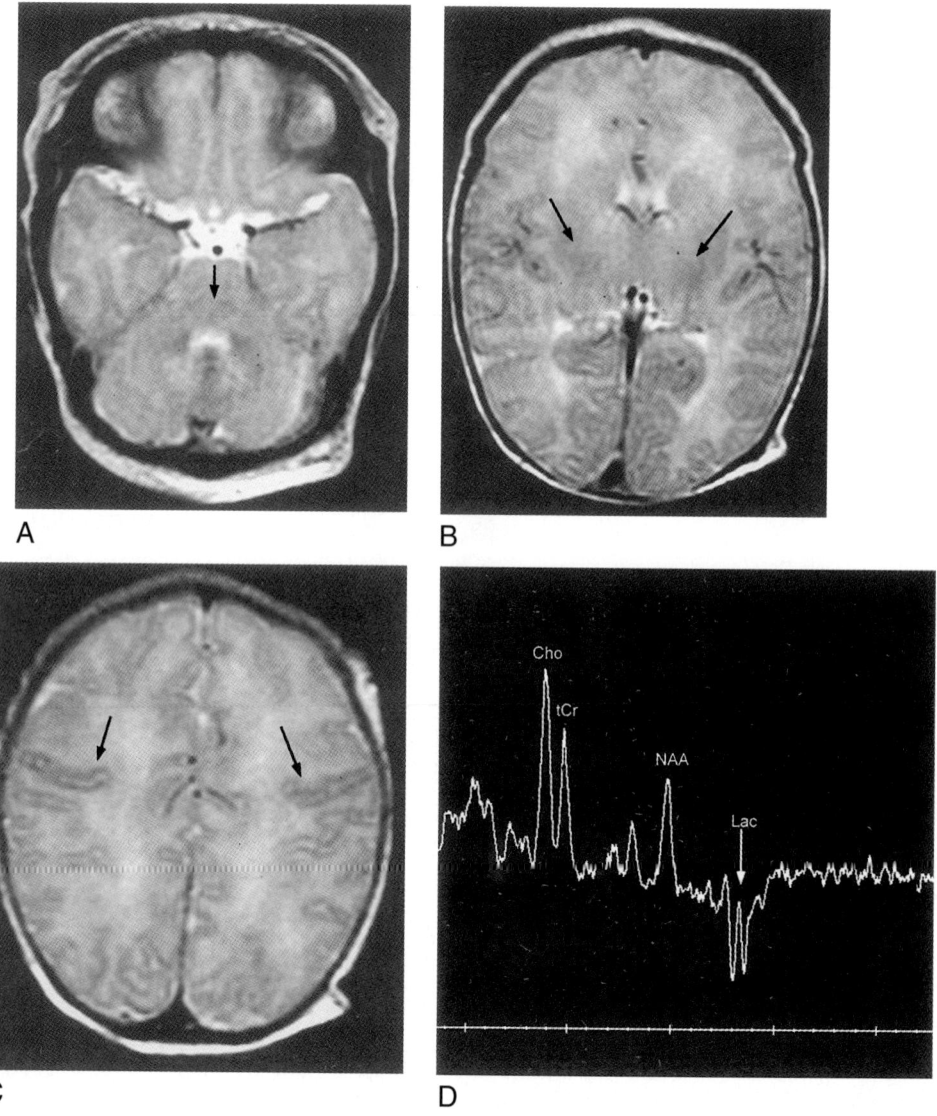


**FIGURE 62–19.** Magnetic resonance images obtained at 24 hours of life in a neonate with profound hypoxic-ischemic brain injury. Compare with normal T2-weighted and diffusion images (see Figs. 62–6 and 62–7). **A, B, C,** T2-weighted images demonstrate edema with loss of normal hypointensity *(arrows)* in the dorsal pons *(arrow)* (**A**), the lateral thalami and internal capsule *(arrows)* (**B**), and perirolandic cortex *(arrows)* (**C**). **D,** Single-voxel spectroscopy obtained from the left basal ganglia demonstrates a prominent lactate doublet (Lac). The peaks project below the baseline because of the echo time used (TE = 144 ms). Cho, choline; NAA, *N*-acetyl aspartate; tCr, total creatine.

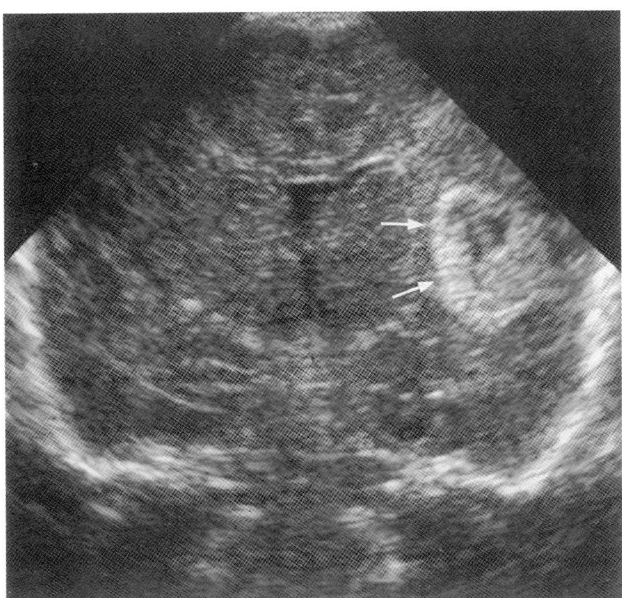

**FIGURE 62–20.** Coronal ultrasound image shows an echogenic left middle cerebral artery distribution infarction *(arrows)*.

border-zone ischemic injury in the term neonate most often occurs in conjunction with deep central gray and white matter injury in cases of profound hypoxia-ischemia.

Profound hypoxia-ischemia in the preterm or term infant tends to affect those regions of the brain with the greatest metabolic requirements. These include areas with high concentrations of excitatory neurotransmitters or regions that are actively myelinating (Rivkin, 1997; Volpe, 1997). The dorsal brainstem, thalami, posterior portions of basal ganglia, posterior limb of internal capsule, corona radiate, and mesial temporal lobes are especially susceptible to injury (see Fig. 62–19). The medial portions of the cerebellar hemispheres and cerebellar vermis are also commonly affected. Areas of the brain with lower energy requirements, such as unmyelinated white matter and cortex tend to be relatively spared unless the ischemia is particularly severe. Following severe hypoxia-ischemia, the pattern of tissue injury is variable. In some infants, a deep central gray matter distribution of injury with relative preservation of the cortex and subcortical white matter is present (Roland et al, 1998). In other infants, there is widespread necrosis, ultimately producing a pattern of cystic encephalomalacia. The deep central pattern of injury is associated with a variable outcome, whereas widespread encephalomalacia more consistently portends a poor prognosis.

On cranial US, ischemic areas of thalamus and basal ganglia may appear focally or diffusely echogenic. US findings may be quite variable in time of onset and are insensitive to the extent of injury compared to CT or MRI.

In the first few hours following hypoxia-ischemia, brain CT findings are usually normal. Depending on the severity of the insult, changes may begin to be apparent in 24 to 48 hours. In severe hypoxia-ischemia, the thalami and basal ganglia develop low density. The cortical ribbon may become indistinct or even indistinguishable from the subcortical white matter. A subset of babies with hypoxia-ischemia will develop mineralization and hypermyelination in the deep gray matter structures, producing hyperdensity in these structures, an appearance termed *status marmoratus*.

Although there is considerable variability in the MR appearance of hypoxia-ischemia, some general trends may be observed (Johnson et al, 1999; Robertson et al, 1999; Rutherford et al, 1995; Wolf et al, 2001). By 15 to 18 hours

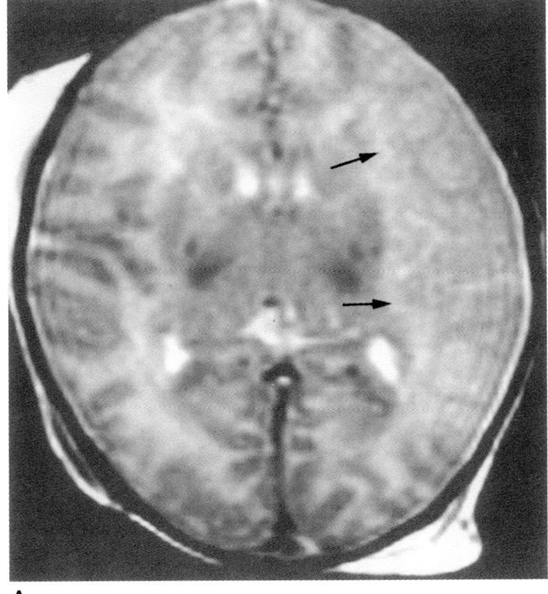

A

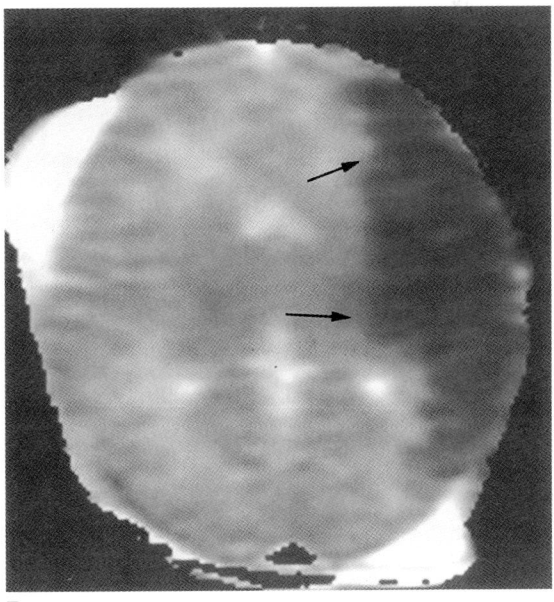

B

**FIGURE 62–21.** Magnetic resonance imaging of a focal left middle cerebral artery infarction in a 24-hour-old neonate. **A,** Axial T2-weighted image shows edema and loss of the cortical ribbon in the left middle cerebral artery territory *(arrows)*. **B,** Apparent diffusion coefficient (ADC) map shows very restricted diffusion (hypointensity) in the area of infarction *(arrows)*.

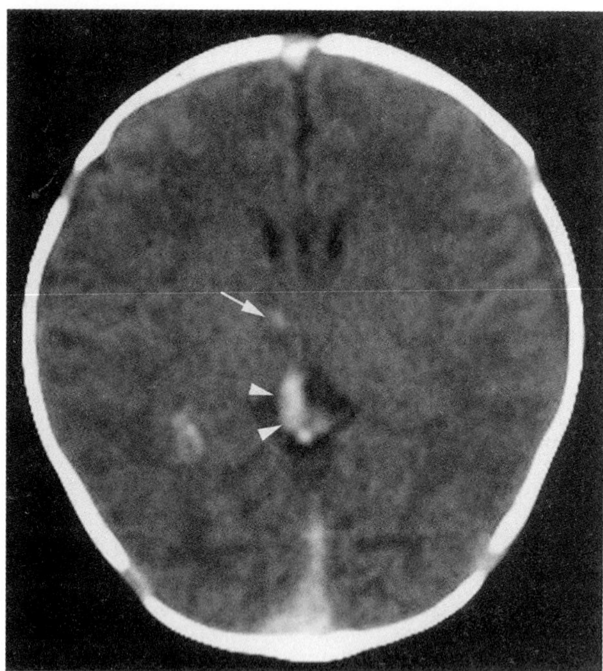

**FIGURE 62–22.** The patient was a newborn with sagittal sinus, straight sinus, and right internal cerebral vein thrombosis and right thalamic hemorrhagic venous infarction. An axial, non–contrast-enhanced CT scan shows high-density clot *(arrowheads)* in the right internal cerebral vein and a small hemorrhagic infarction *(arrow)* in the right thalamus.

following the ischemic event, the diffusion-weighted imaging is often normal. At this time, T1- and T2-weighted sequences typically also fail to show any abnormality. Progressively over the next 24 to 48 hours, restricted diffusion develops within the regions of the brain with the highest metabolic requirements (Robertson and Robson, 2001). During this time, the T1- and T2-weighted images also become abnormal (Barkovich et al, 1995). Toward the end of the first week, it is not uncommon to demonstrate restricted diffusion in the subcortical white matter in areas that on early examinations showed normal or even increased diffusion (Robertson et al, 1999). These white matter regions typically show hyperintensity on T2-weighted sequences in advance of the development of restricted diffusion. By 10 to 14 days, the diffusion abnormalities typically normalize, and ultimately, increased diffusion may be present. Chronically, T1-weighted and T2-weighted sequences show areas of signal abnormalities related to gliosis, mineralization, or hypermyelination associated with variable tissue loss.

MRS also has been used to evaluate neonates with hypoxia-ischemia (Barkovich et al, 1999; Cady, 2001; Groenendaal et al, 2001). The observed changes on MRS in newborns with hypoxia-ischemia include the presence of lactate, indicating energy failure, and a decrease in NAA, suggesting decreased neuronal density or activity (see Fig. 62–19). The demonstration of lactate requires the use of a long echo sequence (e.g., echo time [TE] of 135 msec or 270 msec). On the 135- msec TE acquisition, lactate is seen as a doublet peak projecting below the baseline at 1.3 ppm (lactate peaks project above the baseline at the 270-msec TE). Lactate is evident within the first few hours following onset of hypoxia-ischemia. The amount of lactate slowly diminishes over the ensuing several days. Occasionally, elevation of lactate levels will recur several weeks after the insult (Hanrahan et al, 1998). The etiology of this delayed appearance of lactate is uncertain, but it may be due to the production of lactate by macrophages moving into the area of infarction as part of the reparative process. Studies have shown that the presence of lactate within the basal ganglia or as a delayed finding is associated with an abnormal neurologic outcome at 1 year of age (Barkovich et al, 1999; Hanrahan et al, 1998).

Focal infarctions most often occur in a middle cerebral artery distribution (de Vries et al, 1997, 1999; Sreenan et al, 2000) (see Figs. 62–20 and 62–21). Focal infarcts may be small and involve the cortex only, or they may involve the subcortical white matter and basal ganglia. Infarcts that are confined to the cortex tend to carry a relatively good prognosis. Lesions also involving the internal capsule and basal ganglia are usually associated with a persistent hemiparesis (de Vries et al, 1999; Mercuri et al, 1999).

Sonographically, focal infarcts initially manifest as geographic areas of increased echogenicity, followed by progressively increased echogenicity and loss of gyral and sulcal definition (see Fig. 62–20). Mass effect and effacement of the ventricular system are often present. Initially there is diminished flow demonstrated on duplex and color Doppler US. Over time, increased flow in the surrounding tissues consistent with "luxury perfusion" can be seen on color Doppler US (Fig. 62–23) (Hernanz-Schulman et al, 1988; Taylor, 1994).

On CT, focal infarcts appear as localized regions of hypodensity with loss of the cortical ribbon. Hemorrhagic conversion of an arterial infarction in the newborn is uncommon.

On MRI, focal infarcts are seen as regions of low signal intensity on T1-weighted sequences and high signal intensity on T2-weighted sequences (see Fig. 62–21). Signal alterations occur earlier and more consistently on both diffusion and conventional MRI in focal infarctions than in hypoxia-ischemia (Robertson et al, 1999).

Unlike imaging in hypoxia-ischemia, even on the first day of life, the diffusion and the conventional imaging will typically demonstrate focal infarctions (Robertson et al, 1999). Also unlike hypoxia-ischemia, focal infarctions in the neonate do not usually show an increase in extent on follow-up imaging. The diffusion abnormality tends to normalize by 10 to 14 days. Atrophic changes are generally apparent on follow-up T1- and T2-weighted images; however, the degree of accompanying gliosis is variable. At times, chronic infarcts may appear simply as focally prominent sulci.

## Periventricular Leukomalacia

In the premature infant, periventricular leukomalacia (PVL) is the most common form of hypoxic-ischemic brain injury (Inder et al, 1999; Volpe, 1997). PVL is characterized by focal necrotic lesions in the periventricular white matter, optic radiations, and acoustic radiations and less prominent, more diffuse cerebral white matter injury.

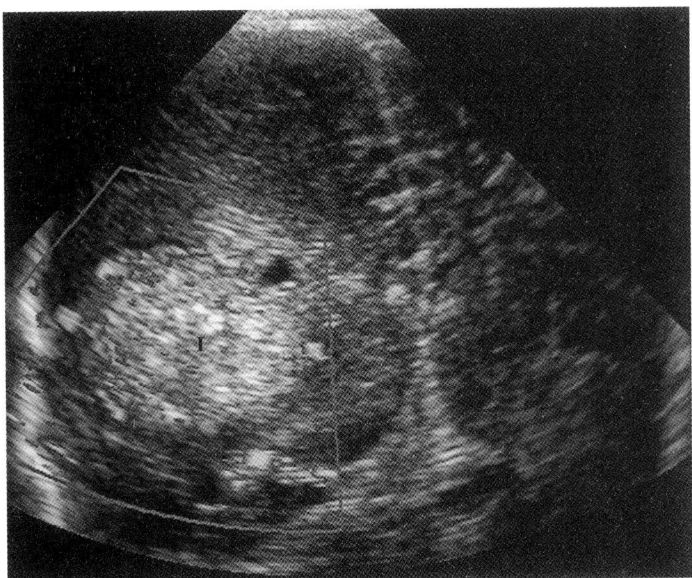


**FIGURE 62–23.** (See also Color Plate 62–23.) The patient was a neonate with a focal right occipital infarction with surrounding "luxury perfusion." A coronal ultrasound image obtained through the anterior fontanel shows a hyperechoic right occipital infarction (I) surrounded by increased flow on color Doppler examination.

In the premature infant, these sites have in common their location in vascular border zones, lying between the long penetrating branches of the middle, anterior, and posterior cerebral arteries that pierce the cortex from the pial surface and the basal penetrating vasculature (e.g., lenticulostriate and choroidal vessels) (Shuman and Selednik, 1980; Volpe, 2001). As the fetus or infant approaches term, there is a gradual shift in these border zone territories toward a parasagittal location. Neuropathologically, PVL is characterized in the acute phase by coagulation necrosis and neuroaxonal swelling (Volpe, 2001). A variable amount of hemorrhage may be present. In the subacute stage, cysts may form in the larger lesions. Ultimately, astrogliosis develops and the cysts become less apparent.

The US appearance of the brain may be normal within the first 2 weeks after the inciting ischemic event. After 10 to 14 days, the echogenicity of affected areas of deep white matter increases. These areas of abnormality may be focal or diffuse, symmetrical or asymmetrical. They are typically located along the trigones of the lateral ventricles but can involve extensive areas of white matter. The differentiation between ischemic and hemorrhagic lesions may be difficult. However, PVL is seldom associated with mass effect and displacement of surrounding structures. Cystic encephalomalacia appears in the areas of increased echogenicity within 2 to 3 weeks after the initial insult (Fig. 62–24). These are characterized by cysts ranging between 1 mm and 2 to 3 centimeters in size. They may be single or multiple and may occasionally communicate with the ventricular system. Focal or hemispheric atrophy is the final stage of PVL and is characterized by dilatation of the ipsilateral ventricle and prominence of the sulci and interhemispheric fissure (Schellinger et al, 1984).

Ischemic white matter lesions, including those due to PVL, are difficult to detect in the neonate using either CT or MRI owing to the inherent high water content of unmyelinated white matter. On CT, even relatively large cysts may be inapparent. Occasionally, the cystic areas may appear slightly more lucent (hypodense) than the surrounding parenchyma. Acute hemorrhagic lesions are hyperdense. The cystic phase of PVL is also difficult to identify on MRI, as the cysts are characterized by long T1 (hypointensity) and long T2 (hyperintensity), similar to normal unmyelinated white matter. Hemorrhagic lesions appear as foci of hyperintensity on T1-weighted sequences and hypointensity on T2-weighted sequences (Fig. 62–25). To date, there has been little published about the DI appearance of PVL; however, PVL has been reported to show restricted diffusion in the acute phase (Inder et al, 1999).

## Congenital Malformations

Although use of cranial sonography is limited by the availability of an acoustic window, many structural anomalies

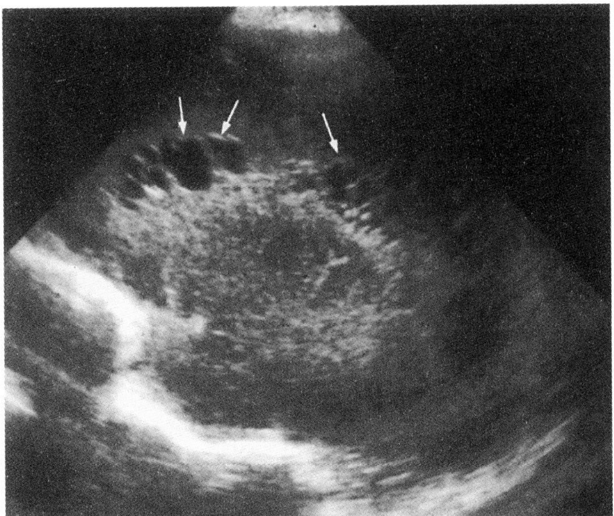

**FIGURE 62–24.** Sagittal ultrasound image of cystic periventricular leukomalacia demonstrates multiple echolucent periventricular cysts *(arrows)* involving the frontal, parietal, and occipital white matter.

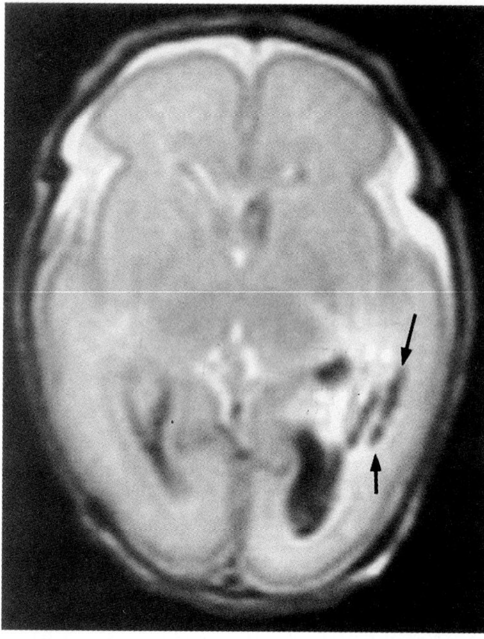

**FIGURE 62–25.** Axial T2-weighted magnetic resonance image from a 26-week-gestation premature infant. Hemorrhagic PVL is indicated by periventricular hypointensity *(arrows)*. Intraventricular hypointense hemorrhage is also present in this neonate.

of the brain can be well characterized by this portable technique, especially in the unstable neonate. However, for most congenital anomalies, MRI has become the most definitive imaging examination (Barkovich, 1988). The multiplanar capability and inherent high tissue contrast of MRI make it superior to CT for the delineation of most congenital malformations. Additionally, unlike CT, MR images are not degraded by artifact from bone. Therefore, MRI is able to provide a detailed evaluation of the regions of the supratentorial brain near the skull base and the posterior fossa.

For most congenital brain malformations, standard T1-weighted and T2-weighted images are sufficient to characterize the anomaly with MRI. Multiplanar conventional imaging is usually all that is required to characterize disorders of structural development including the holoprosencephaly spectrum, malformations of the corpus callosum, leptomeningeal malformations, and posterior fossa malformations (Dodge and Dobyns, 1995; Lena et al, 1995; Rubinstein et al, 1996; Smith et al, 1996) (see Fig. 62–9). The intracranial findings associated with the most common anomaly of neural tube closure, the Chiari II malformation, also can be documented with multiplanar T1-weighted and T2-weighted MRI using a standard head coil. Intravenous contrast is not usually required for the MR evaluation of congenital brain anomalies.

Although CT is not considered the imaging modality of choice for most congenital brain malformations, it may be used to assess bone integrity and to search for parenchymal calcifications. CT is useful in the assessment of scalp lesions and for calvarial or skull base defects in the setting of certain intracranial lesions such as cephaloceles and dermoids (Ruge et al, 1988). Sutural synostosis, although rarely presenting in the newborn, is best assessed with three-dimensional (3D) CT. Cutis aplasia may require CT evaluation to determine the extent of underlying bone deficiency (Madsen et al, 1998).

High-resolution CT is useful for anatomic delineation of facial and temporal bone lesions (Vanzieleghem et al, 2001). Choanal atresia, especially if bilateral, may require urgent CT assessment. Nasal pits or dermoids are typically evaluated using a combination of high-resolution CT for bone detail and MRI for soft tissue extent of the lesion (Lusk and Lee, 1986). Most temporal bone anomalies do not require intervention during the neonatal period; therefore, CT studies are usually deferred until later in infancy.

## Vascular Malformations

Vascular malformations are classified on the basis of hemodynamics as high-flow or low-flow anomalies (Meyer et al, 1991). High-flow lesions include arteriovenous fistula (AVF), with direct, macroscopic connections between arteries and veins, and arteriovenous malformation (AVM), with a meshwork of dysplastic vessels termed a "nidus" interposed between the supplying artery and draining vein. Low-flow vascular malformations include cavernous malformation, developmental venous anomaly (DVA), and capillary telangiectasia. Both high- and low-flow intracranial vascular malformations may be present in the newborn; however, it is typically the high-flow lesions that are likely to be symptomatic during the neonatal period.

Many high-flow vascular malformations are now diagnosed in utero using fetal US or MRI. A majority of high-flow vascular malformations manifest in the neonate with symptoms related to high-output cardiac failure (Lasjaunias et al, 1986, 1989). CT and postnatal MRI are not typically required to diagnose the presence of the malformation but may provide useful information with respect to prognosis. In high-flow lesions, blood flow is diverted away from the brain parenchyma and through the shunt(s), so that ischemic brain injury may result (see Fig. 62–10).

The presence of encephalomalacia and parenchymal calcification on CT indicates chronic ischemic injury and is associated with a poor neurologic outcome (Brunelle, 1997). CT angiography (CTA) and CT venography (CTV) may occasionally be performed to characterize the arterial supply and size of shunts prior to intervention.

MRI is performed less frequently than CT in neonates with high-flow vascular anomalies because of the hemodynamic instability of many of the infants. MRI will show changes similar to those seen with CT including parenchymal ischemic changes (see Fig. 62–10B). MRA/MRV can be used in a similar fashion to that for CTA/CTV to characterize the vascular anomaly. However, MRA/MRV is prone to signal loss related to turbulent flow and may therefore be less reliable than CTA/CTV in high-flow lesions.

Conventional catheter angiography is usually performed as a part of a planned endovascular approach to therapy. Subselective vascular injections are used to carefully define the anatomy of the arteriovenous shunts. The choice of embolic material employed depends on the nature and location of the shunts. Sonography with color and duplex Doppler techniques may be used as an adjunct to monitor changing cerebral hemodynamics and complications during endovascular procedures.

Low-flow intracranial vascular anomalies are occasionally encountered as incidental findings on brain CT and MRI in the newborn. Hemorrhage due to low-flow vascular anomalies is exceedingly rare in the neonate.

## Hydrocephalus

Hydrocephalus is one of the most common reasons to perform brain imaging in the newborn. Hydrocephalus is nearly always due to an obstruction of CSF resorption. The blockage may occur within the ventricles or in the extracerebral CSF spaces. Hydrocephalus due to the overproduction of CSF is exceedingly rare but may occasionally occur with choroid plexus papilloma (Fig. 62–26).

Hydrocephalus may be either congenital or acquired. Congenital causes of hydrocephalus include Chiari II malformation, aqueductal stenosis, encephalocele, universal

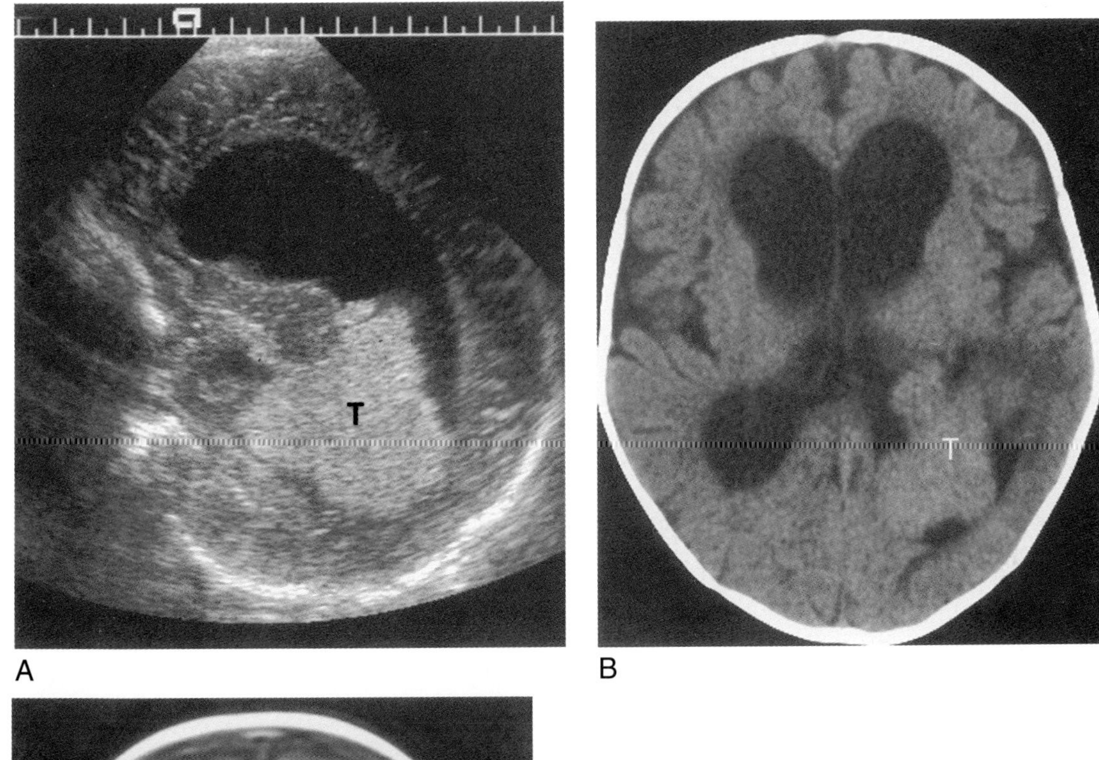


**FIGURE 62–26.** The patient was an infant with macrocrania due to hydrocephalus caused by a choroid plexus papilloma. **A,** Sagittal ultrasound study shows an echogenic mass (T) in the trigone of the left lateral ventricle with associated hydrocephalus. **B,** Axial noncontrast computed tomographic study shows an isodense mass (T) filling the trigone of the left lateral ventricle. The lateral ventricles are dilated bilaterally without an obvious cause of obstruction. **C,** Contrast-enhanced T1-weighted magnetic resonance image shows intense enhancement of the tumor (T) typical of choroid plexus papilloma.

craniosynostosis, and skull base dysplasia with jugular venous stenosis as in Crouzon syndrome (McLone and Naidich, 1992; Naidich et al, 1992; Robson et al, 2000). Acquired hydrocephalus may be due to hemorrhage, infection, mass effect from tumor, or venous hypertension (Brann et al, 1990; Hedlund and Boyer, 1999; Lasjaunias et al, 1989).

Sonography plays an important role in the evaluation of posthemorrhagic hydrocephalus (Fig. 62–27). The goals of the US examination are to determine the presence and severity of ventricular dilatation, to identify the location and cause of obstruction (ependymitis versus clot), to monitor the adequacy of treatment, and to identify potential complications of therapy. The evaluation of the ventricular system in the neonate should include standardized measurements of the lateral ventricles. Although the atria dilate early in the course of ventriculomegaly, measurements of the lateral ventricles on parasagittal images are the most variable in clinical practice (Shackleford, 1986). We use the maximal width of the frontal horns measured at the level of the foramen of Monro to follow ventricular size. This measurement was chosen because it uses reproducible landmarks that are not affected by angulation of the transducer and provide independent measures of each lateral ventricle. In our experience, it provides the most useful measurement in monitoring change in ventricular size.

In general, dilatation tends to be greatest in the ventricle just proximal to the point of obstruction to flow. For example, the normal aqueduct of Sylvius is a narrow passage and often not clearly visible on US. It typically does not become distended by clot. However, when an obstruction to CSF flow exists at the level of the fourth ventricle or beyond, the aqueduct may become markedly distended and is then easily depicted (Taylor, 2001) (Fig. 62–28). Early detection of a dilated fourth ventricle may have important therapeutic implications, especially when accompanied by clot or absence of CSF in the cisterna magna. This combination of findings strongly suggests the presence of a blockage to CSF flow into the spinal subarachnoid space (Hall et al, 1992) and the probable failure of serial lumbar punctures as a therapeutic option.

As the intracranial pressure (ICP) rises, arterial flow tends to be more affected during diastole than during systole, resulting in an elevated pulsatility of flow. Seibert and colleagues (1989) have shown that increasing resistive index (RI) on pulsed Doppler interrogation correlates well with elevation in ICP in an animal model of acute hydrocephalus. They and others also have shown a significant drop in pulsatility following ventricular tapping and shunting in infants with hydrocephalus (Bada et al, 1982). However, elevated ICP may not always be present in infants with ventricular dilatation, and the RI may be well within the normal range. Doppler examination of the anterior or middle cerebral artery during fontanel compression may be useful in the early identification of infants with abnormal intracranial compliance prior to the development of increased ICP as shown by elevated baseline RI (Taylor et al, 1994). According to the Monro-Kellie hypothesis, the volume of brain, CSF, blood, and other intracranial components is constant (Bruce et al, 1977). During graded fontanel compression in normal infants, CSF or blood can be readily displaced in order to compensate for the small

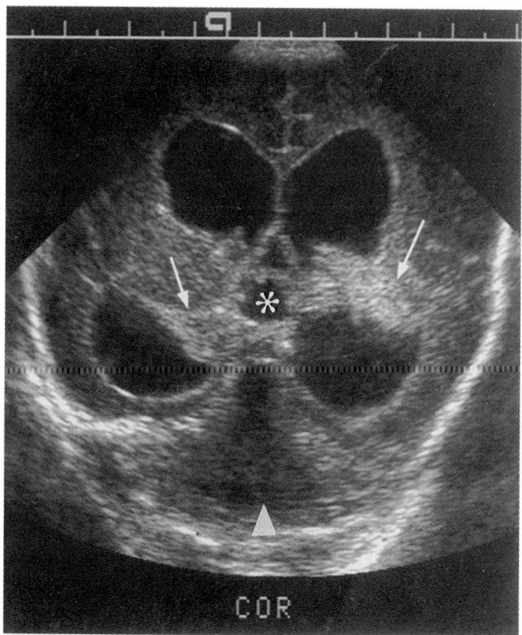


**FIGURE 62–27.** Coronal ultrasound study of posthemorrhagic hydrocephalus obtained through the anterior fontanel. Adherent, nondependent echogenic clot *(arrows)* is present within the dilated lateral ventricles. The absence of positional change in location of the echogenic material helps to differentiate blood clot from debris in ventriculitis. Note the dilated third ventricle (*) and fourth ventricle *(arrowhead)*.

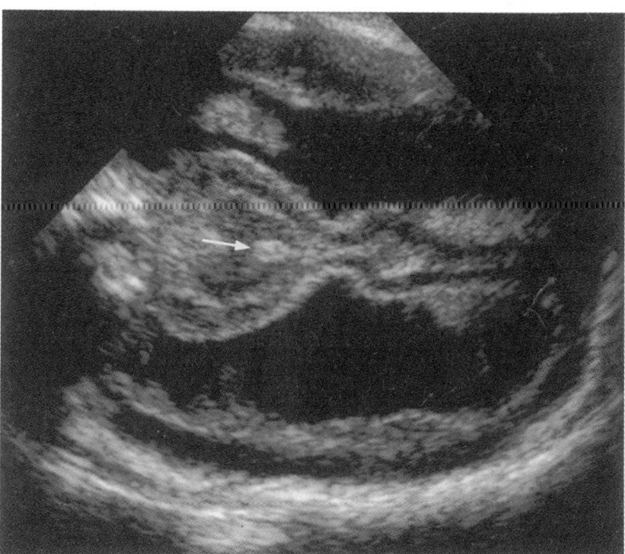

**FIGURE 62–28.** Axial ultrasound image from an infant with posthemorrhagic hydrocephalus. Due to obstructing clot at the level of the aqueduct of Sylvius *(arrow)*, the lateral ventricles and upper aqueduct are distended.

increase in volume delivered by compression of the anterior fontanel, resulting in no increase in ICP. In infants with hydrocephalus however, the increase in intracranial volume with fontanel compression is translated into a transient increase in ICP and an acute increase in arterial pulsatility (Fig. 62–29). Serial examinations using this technique can also be used to follow an individual infant's ability to compensate for minor changes in intracranial volume and thus serve as a noninvasive indirect measure of intracranial compliance (Taylor and Madsen, 1996).

In our experience, transient (3 to 5 seconds) fontanel compression is a safe and well-tolerated procedure, even in critically ill premature infants. However, prolonged compression of the fontanel should be avoided. Pressure should be immediately released if heart rate significantly decreases during Doppler examination. In addition, the presence of reversed flow during diastole in a Doppler study obtained without fontanel compression is strongly suggestive of elevated ICP, and fontanel compression is not necessary or recommended in these patients.

Imaging of hydrocephalus is carried out prior to shunting to determine the cause of ventricular dilatation, to identify the site of obstruction, and to differentiate hydrocephalus from other intracranial abnormalities, such as holoprosencephaly and hydranencephaly, that may mimic severe hydrocephalus. Following shunt placement, imaging is carried out to evaluate ventricular decompression and shunt position, and to assess for the presence of surgical complications and for the development of extra-axial collections.

MRI is the preferred examination for preoperative assessment of hydrocephalus. Thin-section T1- or T2-weighted images are useful in demonstrating stenosis of the aqueduct of Sylvius. On MRI, the findings in aqueductal stenosis include loss of the normal signal void within the aqueduct and elevation of the superior tectal plate (see Fig. 62–9). Occasionally, high signal intensity suggesting gliosis is seen in the periaqueductal gray matter. Tectal tumors are rarely encountered in neonates. CSF flow studies may be performed to corroborate lack of flow within the aqueduct in equivocal cases. Use of contrast media may be required to evaluate congenital tumors causing hydrocephalus and to search for leptomeningeal metastatses.

## Neonatal Infection

Congenital cytomegalovirus (CMV) infection is associated with anomalies of cortical development, diminished white matter volume, delayed myelination, variably small cerebella, parenchymal calcification, and mild ventriculomegaly (Barkovich and Lindan, 1994).

Whereas both US and CT may demonstrate parenchymal calcifications, multiplanar MRI provides superior delineation of the anomalies associated with congenital CMV infection of the CNS. Conventional imaging including coronal T2-weighted images is useful in defining the anatomic abnormalities. The DI characteristics of congenital CMV affecting the brain have not been reported. We have noted increased diffusion in the regions of delayed

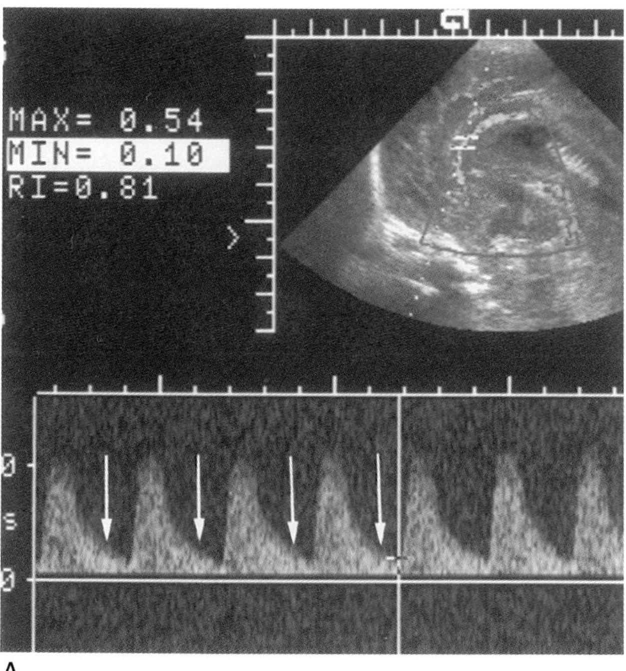


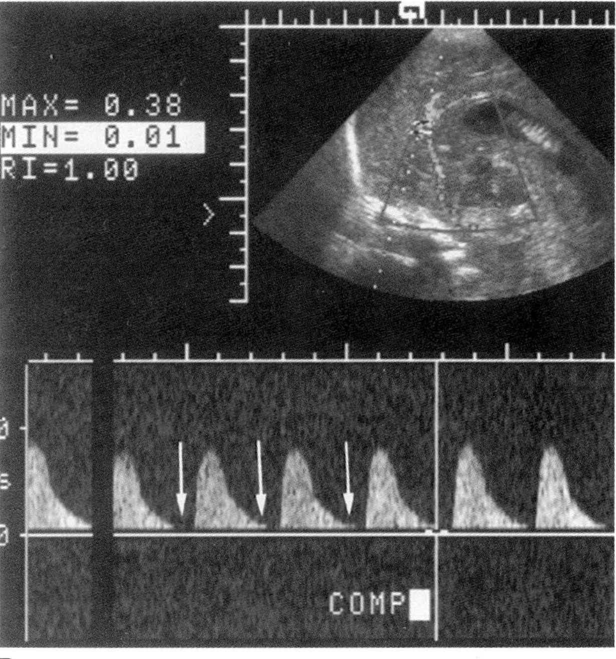


**FIGURE 62–29.** Positive Doppler ultrasound compression study in hydrocephalus. **A,** Baseline examination of blood flow within the anterior cerebral artery without fontanel compression shows a low resistance pattern with flow during both systole and diastole (resistive index = 0.81). **B,** Examination during transient compression of the anterior fontanel using the ultrasound transducer results in a loss of diastolic flow resulting from increased intracranial pressure (resistive index = 1.0).

myelination. DI findings have otherwise been unremarkable. Findings on high-resolution temporal bone MRI performed in infants with associated hearing loss are typically normal.

Neonatal herpes simplex virus (HSV) infection may involve any region of the brain and is typically multifocal (unlike HSV infection in adults, which has a predilection for the temporal lobes) (Schlesinger et al, 1995).

Brain CT in HSV infection usually shows multifocal low density in the cortex and subcortical white matter. Occasionally, petechial hemorrhage may occur. Conventional MRI demonstrates multiple areas of cortical and deep gray matter of low signal intensity on T1-weighted images and high signal intensity on T2-weighted images (Fig. 62–30). Hemorrhage produces shortening of T1 (hyperintensity) and T2 (hypointensity). On DI, sites of involvement typically have restricted diffusion during the acute phase of the illness. The restricted diffusion is presumably due to necrosis.

Congenital human immunodeficiency virus (HIV) infection has become a significant public health problem over the last two decades. However, despite the fact that more than 90% of all childhood HIV infections are due to in utero transmission, neurologic and imaging manifestations of HIV infection in the neonatal period are rare (Volpe, 1995). To date, we have not observed imaging abnormalities in newborns with known HIV infection.

Neonatal bacterial CNS infections are rarely associated with imaging abnormalities. Some bacteria such as *Citrobacter* species, *Serratia marcescens, Proteus, Pseudomonas aeruginosa*, and members of family Enterobacteriaceae produce parenchymal necrosis and abscess formation (Fig. 62–31). Thrombosis of cortical and subependymal veins may also occur. By both CT and MRI, leptomeningeal enhancement may be seen following the administration of intravenous contrast. If cerebritis develops, the cortex and subcortical white matter may be seen as areas of low density on CT and of increased signal intensity on T2-weighted MRI. Abscesses are demonstrated as rim-enhancing lesions on both CT and MRI. These lesions, along with the surrounding hyperemia, can also be well demonstrated by cranial US. The DI appearance of abscesses in neonates has not been reported. Widespread malacic changes may be seen on late follow-up imaging after necrotizing CNS infections.

## Neonatal Brain Tumors

Brain tumors are rare in the newborn. When they occur, they are most often supratentorial, large, high-grade lesions such as primitive neuroepithelial tumors and choroid plexus carcinoma (Fig. 62–32).

The imaging appearance of brain tumors is variable depending on the cellularity of the lesion and the presence or absence of necrosis (Klisch et al, 2000) (see Fig. 62–32). Low-grade, less cellular tumors tend to have low density on CT, high signal intensity on T2-weighted

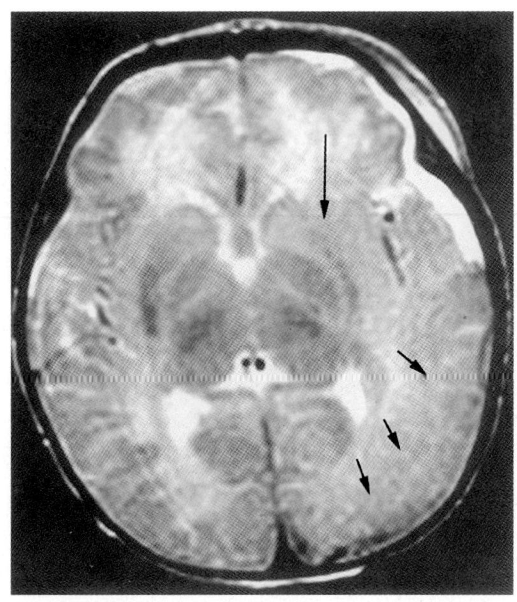
A

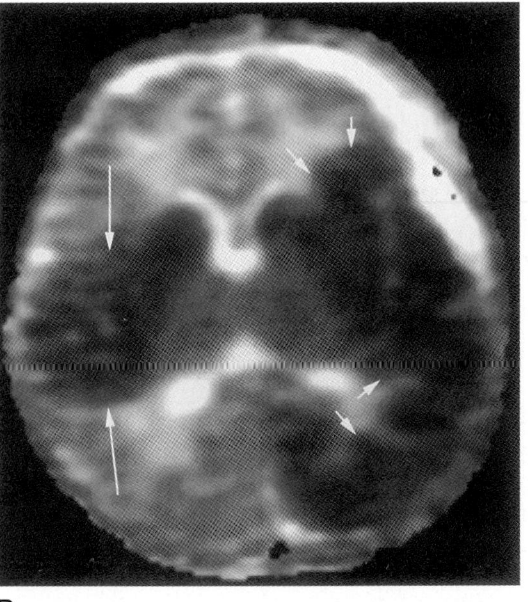
B

**FIGURE 62–30.** Magnetic resonance images from a term neonate with herpes simplex virus (HSV) encephalitis. **A,** Axial T2-weighted image shows high signal intensity in the left basal ganglia *(long arrow)* and loss of the cortical ribbon in the left cerebral hemisphere *(short arrows)*. Unlike HSV infection in adults, neonatal herpes is not confined to the temporal and subfrontal lobes, and basal ganglia involvement is common. **B,** Apparent diffusion coefficient (ADC) map from the same examination shows extensive restricted diffusion (hypointensity) involving the areas on the left seen on the T2-weighted images *(short arrows)* and additional right hemispheric cortical *(long arrows)* and deep gray matter involvement.

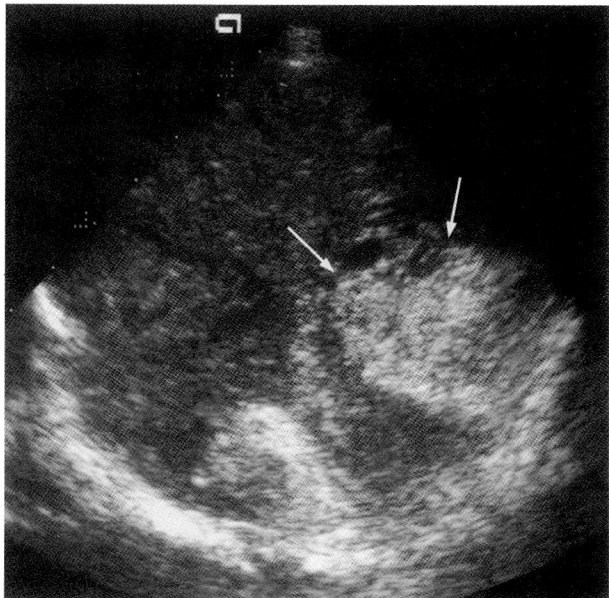

**FIGURE 62–31.** Ultrasound study of abscess due to *Citrobacter* infection. A large echogenic mass/abscess *(arrows)* is clearly demonstrated. Abscess formation is most often associated with bacterial infections such as that due to *Citrobacter* species that cause parenchymal necrosis.

MRI, and increased diffusion relative to normal brain. High-grade, densely cellular tumors generally are hyperdense on CT and of low signal intensity on T2-weighted MRI and have decreased diffusion relative to normal brain. Enhancement of the tumors is variable but tends to increase with increasing malignancy of the tumor. Important exceptions to this general rule are pilocytic astrocytoma and choroid plexus papilloma (see Fig. 62–26), which, despite their low grade, tend to avidly enhance following contrast administration.

Malformative masses such as dermoid, epidermoid, and teratoma are occasionally detected in the neonate (Fig. 62–33) (Haddad et al, 1991). These lesions may be associated with other markers of cerebral dysgenesis such as anomalies of the corpus callosum or pericallosal lipoma. A dermal sinus tract is often present in association with midline cysts.

Malformative masses often have a characteristic appearance on imaging owing to the presence of fat and/or calcification within the lesion (Smirniotopoulos and Chiechi, 1995). Both dermoid and epidermoid tend to be of low density on CT. Calcification is sometimes seen within the cyst wall. Teeth formed within a teratoma will produce dense calcification on CT, whereas foci of fat have very low density, comparable to that of subcutaneous fat. CT is also used to document associated bone defects that accompany dermal sinus tracts.

On MRI, epidermoids tend to be similar to CSF in signal intensity on T1- and T2-weighted sequences. Occasionally, the cyst wall may enhance following intravenous contrast administration. Dermoid cysts containing fat have high signal intensity on T1-weighted sequences. High-resolution MRI may occasionally be required to demonstrate an associated dermal sinus tract. Teratomas may have foci of fat that produce high signal intensity on T1-weighted sequences. Calcifications appear as rounded signal voids on both T1-weighted and T2-weighted sequences.

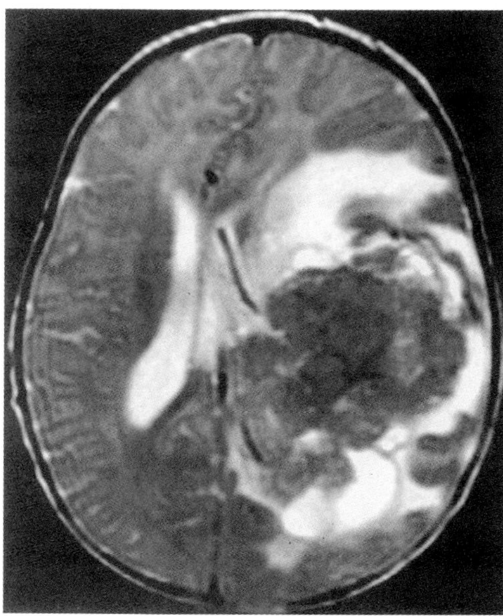

**FIGURE 62–32.** The patient was a 1-month-old infant with choroid plexus carcinoma. A large left hemispheric mass with regions hypointensity densely cellular tumor is evident on T2-weighted magnetic resonance image.

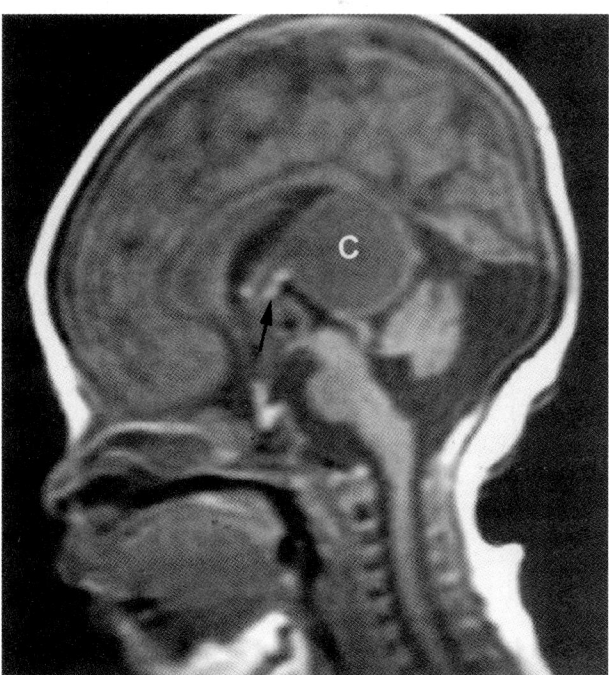


**FIGURE 62–33.** The patient was a neonate with a pineal region teratoma. Sagittal T1-weighted image shows a large cystic lesion (C). The mass contains a small amount of high signal intensity *(arrow)* due to the presence of fat, which strongly suggests the diagnosis of teratoma.

### Hypoglycemia and Hyperbilirubinemia

Severe perinatal hypoglycemia may result in energy exhaustion and parenchymal infarction in the neonate. In severe hypoglycemia, diffuse cortical and subcortical white matter damage may be evident, with the parietal and occipital lobes most severely affected (Barkovich et al, 1998). Globus pallidus injury has been observed in patients with the most severe cortical injury (Barkovich et al, 1998).

Initially, on CT and MRI, cortical edema is present within the parietal and occipital regions of the cortex (Fig. 62–34). As with other causes of infarction, restricted diffusion is usually observed acutely (Barkovich et al, 1998). Chronically, tissue loss is present in the areas that earlier showed edema and restricted diffusion (Sugama et al, 2001). In newborns, severe hyperbilirubinemia and consequent kernicterus may develop. The findings on brain MRI in patients with kernicterus are characteristic. Unlike hypoxia-ischemia, which tends to primarily affect the putamen and thalamus, hyperbilirubinemia selectively affects the globus pallidus. Recently, it has been suggested that the high resting neuronal activity in the globus pallidus might make it more vulnerable to less intense, subacute oxidative stresses from mitochondrial toxins such as bilirubin (Johnston and Hoon, 2000).

The imaging findings in kernicterus are most apparent on MRI, with hyperintensity at the posterior margin or throughout the globi pallidi on T2-weighted sequences (Sugama et al, 2001).

### Neurocutaneous Disorders

Of the phakomatoses, the two for which imaging is most commonly required in the neonate are tuberous sclerosis and Sturge-Weber syndrome. Because the outwardly apparent clinical features of tuberous sclerosis, such as adenoma sebaceum, are not usually apparent until late childhood or adulthood, early brain imaging is most often requested when cardiac tumors are identified on prenatal US or when there is a positive family history. The intracranial manifestations of tuberous sclerosis include cortical tubers, subependymal hamatomas, subependymal giant cell tumors, and abnormal neuronal and glial cells in the white matter.

On brain CT in the neonate, there is variable calcification of subependymal nodules that appear as small nodular densities projecting into the lateral ventricles (Griffiths and Martland, 1997) (Fig. 62–35). The appearance may be similar to that of periventricular calcifications seen with congenital infections such as with CMV but can be differentiated from the latter on the basis of the projection of the lesions into the lateral ventricles and demonstration of cortical tubers. White matter abnormalities are extremely difficult to demonstrate owing to the normal low density of unmyelinated neonatal white matter. Likewise, cortical tubers, which are not usually calcified in the newborn, may be difficult to demonstrate with CT, as the affected gyri may simply appear mildly broadened.

On brain MRI in the newborn, subependymal hamartomas may be quite subtle in appearance and must be carefully searched for. The cortical lesions of tuberous sclerosis have variable signal intensity. Cortical tubers appear may appear hyperintense or hypointense to unmyelinated white matter on T1-weighted images. The cortical tubers may be difficult to identify on T2-weighted images in the neonate, as their signal intensity is often similar to that of the unmyelinated subcortical white matter (see Fig. 62–35).

Sturge-Weber syndrome (i.e., encephalotrigeminal angiomatosis) is a neurocutaneous disorder comprising a capillary malformation in the distribution of branches of the trigeminal nerve and an intracranial leptomeningeal

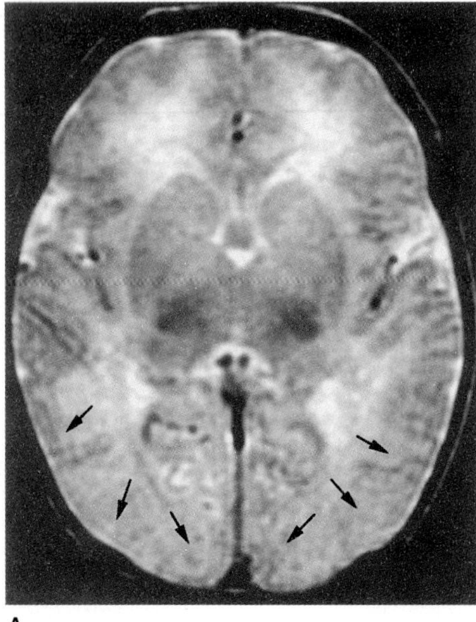


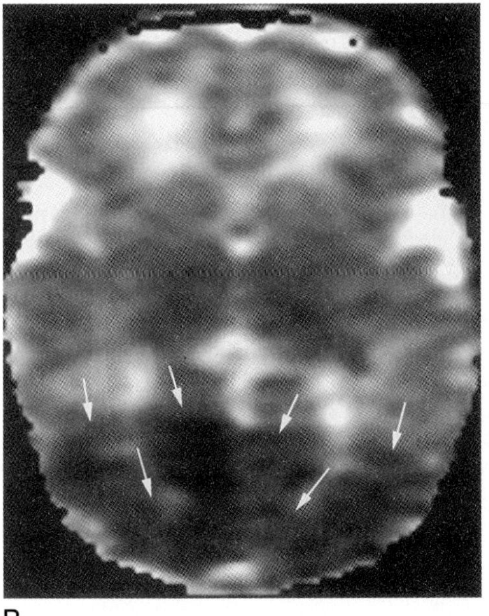


**FIGURE 62–34.** Term newborn with marked hypoglycemia and seizures. **A,** Bilaterally symmetric loss of the cortical ribbon is apparent in the parietal and occipital lobes on T2-weighted imaging *(arrows)*. **B,** Decreased ADC values are present in corresponding regions of the parietal and occipital cortex *(arrows)*.

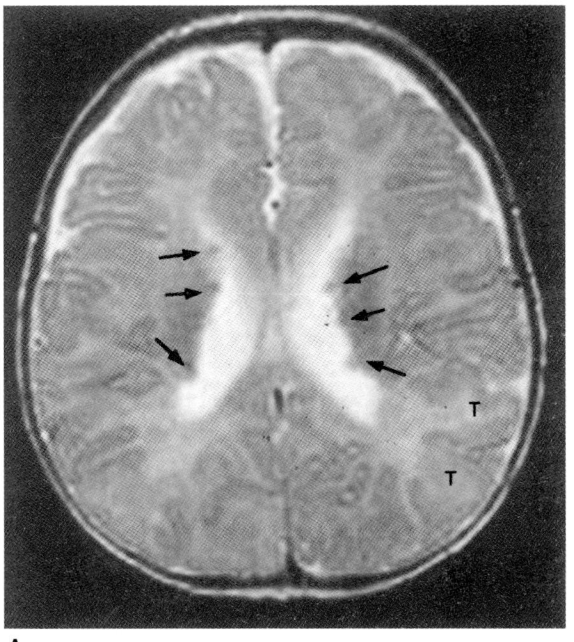


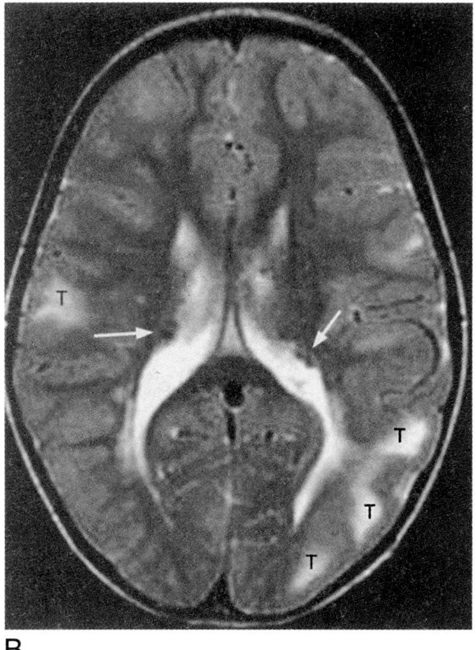


**FIGURE 62–35.** The patient was a term neonate with cardiac rhabdomyomas. **A,** Axial T2-weighted magnetic resonance (MR) image obtained at 2 weeks of age shows subependymal nodules *(arrows)* indicative of tuberous sclerosis. Note that the cortical tubers (T) may be difficult to see in the newborn. **B,** Follow-up T2-weighted MR image in the same child at 5 years of age shows hypointense subependymal nodules *(arrows)*. The cortical tubers (T) are now much more obvious.

capillary-venous malformation. Clinically, patients present with a "port-wine facial nevus" and seizures (Pascual-Castroviejo et al, 1993).

On brain CT, Sturge-Weber syndrome in the newborn may be difficult to detect. Gyral calcification, a radiographic hallmark of this disorder, may or may not be present. Even when this abnormality is present, the extent of the calcification may not reflect the entire distribution of the vascular malformation. The choroid plexus is typically enlarged on the side of the malformation, and enlarged medullary veins are seen following the administration of intravenous contrast. Hemiatrophy of the brain and overgrowth of the skull often are not apparent in the newborn.

Contrast-enhanced brain MRI is considered the imaging modality of choice for evaluation of Sturge-Weber syndrome (Elster and Chen, 1990; Pascual-Castroviejo et al, 1993). T1-weighted imaging following the administration of intravenous gadolinium provides the best depiction of the extent of the vascular anomaly (Fig. 62–36). Although gradient echo MRI may be less sensitive than CT for the demonstration of gyral calcification, it is often useful in demonstrating the presence of cortical mineralization.

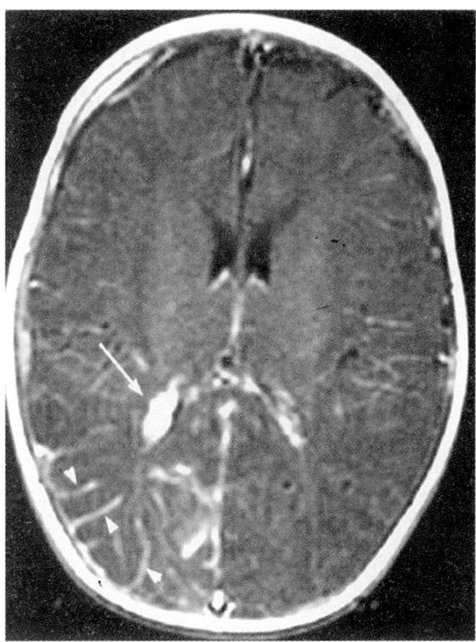

**FIGURE 62–36.** The patient was a term neonate with seizures and facial capillary nevus. Axial T1-weighted post–gadolinium magnetic resonance image demonstrates asymmetrical leptomeningeal enhancement *(arrowheads)* in the right parietal and occipital lobes due to the presence of the leptomeningeal capillary-venous malformation that defines Sturge-Weber syndrome. The choroid plexus ipsilateral *(arrow)* to the leptomeningeal anomaly is typically enlarged. Note that the brain is not yet atrophic in the area of the malformation.

## ADVANTAGES AND DISADVANTAGES OF NEUROIMAGING TECHNIQUES

### Ultrasonography

The most significant advantages of US are its portability, lack of ionizing radiation, relative availability and affordability, and ability to depict hemodynamics of blood flow in real time. The most serious disadvantages are its relative lack of spatial resolution compared with CT and MRI, the need for an acoustic window, its operator dependence, and the nonspecificity of many US findings. In addition, the differentiation between bland and hemorrhagic lesions is often difficult, and it is an insensitive tool for the diagnosis of neuronal migration disorders and diffuse neuronal injury.

### Computed Tomography

Advantages of CT include availability, compatibility with life support systems, rapid image acquisition, and relative lack of operator dependency.

Unfortunately, CT offers more limited soft tissue contrast than that provided by MRI and is prone to beam-hardening artifact from the skull base such that there is limited detail of the posterior fossa and temporal lobes. In addition, imaging can be acquired only in the axial or coronal plane. The risks associated with exposure to ionizing radiation from CT have come under increased scrutiny (Brenner et al, 2001; Huda et al, 2001). It appears that the long-term risk of malignancy due to x-ray exposure may be greatest in the newborn and gradually diminishes with age (Brenner et al, 2001). The risk associated with neonatal brain CT, however, is largely theoretical, and the decision to perform CT for neonatal brain CT should be made on a case-by-case basis, with recognition of the potentially significant medical benefit of performing the study compared with a small theoretical risk of the development of malignancy over the patient's lifetime. When appropriate, it may be prudent to consider using MRI or US, because neither employs ionizing radiation.

Although most brain CT studies in the neonate do not require the administration of intravenous contrast, occasionally, as with suspected dural venous sinus thrombosis, contrast may be of benefit. Because the primary route of contrast excretion is via the kidney, the renal status must be considered in the newborn, just as in the older child or adult. Typically, nonionic contrast is used to decrease the side effects related to the high osmolality of the ionic agents.

### Magnetic Resonance Imaging

Advantages of MRI include superior image detail compared with CT and US and the possibility of evaluating multiple tissue parameters. As with US, MRI does not carry the theoretical risks associated with the use of ionizing radiation. In addition, both anatomic and functional information may be obtained from MRI during the same examination. Moreover, MRI offers improved delineation of the posterior fossa structures without significant artifact from the skull base as occurs with CT, and without the need for an appropriate acoustic window as is essential with US.

The single biggest disadvantage of MRI is the requirement for a strong magnetic field. As a result, the MRI examination room must be magnetically shielded, and all equipment entering the room must be nonferromagnetic. For these reasons, the imaging of the ill neonate can be difficult. Additionally, because of the relatively long time of image acquisition, sedation or anesthesia is often required. However, generally, the additional information obtained with MRI over CT warrants the added inconvenience of the examination, provided that the imaging suite and personnel are equipped to handle the unique requirements of neonatal brain MRI.

## SUMMARY OF NEUROIMAGING PRACTICE GUIDELINES

A multidisciplinary group has reviewed the literature and established guidelines for neuroimaging in the neonate (Ment et al, 2002). This practice parameter is endorsed by the American Academy of Pediatrics, the American Society of Pediatric Neuroradiology, and the Society for Pediatric Radiology. The paractice parameter recommendations for imaging of the preterm neonate are that routine cranial US screening be performed in all infants born at less than 30 weeks of gestational age once between days 7 and 14 of life and repeated between 36 and 40 weeks of postmenstrual age. For term infants, the recommendations are that noncontrast CT be performed to detect hemorrhagic lesions in the encephalopathic newborn with a history of birth trauma, low hematocrit, or coagulopathy. If CT is inconclusive, then MRI should be performed between days 2 and 8 of life to assess the location and extent of injury. This practice parameter reflects a review of available literature.

Of interest, the potential late untoward effects of radiation used for diagnostic CT scanning have recently been highlighted (Donnelly and Frush, 2001). The theoretical risk of malignancy related to exposure to ionizing radiation is highest in the neonate. Given that significant intracranial hemorrhage is detected by MRI as well as by CT, an argument can be made for eliminating CT for the evaluation of the encephalopathic term neonate, thereby avoiding the potential risks of ionizing radiation altogether (Robertson et al, 2003). CT is superior to MRI, and remains the study of choice, for the detection of parenchymal calcification and demonstration of bone abnormalities.

## REFERENCES

Alsop DC, Detre JA: Reduced transit-time sensitivity in noninvasive magnetic resonance imaging of human cerebral blood flow. J Cereb Blood Flow Metab 16:1236-1249, 1996.

Anderson AW, Marois R, Colson ER, et al: Neonatal auditory activation detected by functional magnetic resonance imaging. Magn Reson Imaging 19:1-5, 2001.

Bada HS, Miller JE, Menke JA, et al: Intracranial pressure and cerebral arterial pulsatile flow measurement in neonatal intraventricular hemorrhage. J Pediatr 100:291-296, 1982.

Baker PN, Johnson IR, Harvey PR, et al: A three-year follow-up of children imaged in utero with echo-planar magnetic resonance. Am J Obstet Gynecol 170:32-33, 1994.

Balter S: An introduction to the physics of magnetic resonance imaging. Radiographics 7:371-383, 1987.

Barkovich AJ: Techniques and methods in pediatric magnetic resonance imaging. Semin Ultrasound CT MR 9:186-191, 1988.

Barkovich AJ: Concepts of myelin and myelination in neuroradiology. AJNR Am J Neuroradiol 21:1099-1109, 2000.

Barkovich AJ, Ali FA, Rowley HA, et al: Imaging patterns of neonatal hypoglycemia. AJNR Am J Neuroradiol 19:523-528, 1998.

Barkovich AJ, Baranski K, Vigneron D, et al: Proton MR spectroscopy for the evaluation of brain injury in asphyxiated, term neonates. AJNR Am J Neuroradiol 20:1399-1405, 1999.

Barkovich AJ, Kjos BO, Jackson DE Jr, et al: Normal maturation of the neonatal and infant brain: MR imaging at 1.5 T. Radiology 166:173-180, 1988.

Barkovich AJ, Westmark K, Partridge C, et al: Perinatal asphyxia: MR findings in the first 10 days. AJNR Am J Neuroradiol 16:427-438, 1995.

Barlow CF, Domek NS, Boldberg MA, et al: Extracelluar brain space measured by $^{35}S$ sulfate. Archives of Neurology 5:102-110, 1961.

Barnes PD, Taylor GA: Imaging of the neonatal central nervous system. Neurosurg Clin N Am 9:17-47, 1998.

Benaron DA, Hintz SR, Villringer A, et al: Noninvasive functional imaging of human brain using light. J Cereb Blood Flow Metab 20:469-477, 2000.

Bhachu DS, Kanal E: Implantable pulse generators (pacemakers) and electrodes: Safety in the magnetic resonance imaging scanner environment. J Magn Reson Imaging 12:201-204, 2000.

Born P, Leth H, Miranda MJ, et al: Visual activation in infants and young children studied by functional magnetic resonance imaging. Pediatr Res 44:578-583, 1998.

Boyd DP: Computed tomography: Physics and instrumentation. Acad Radiol 2(Suppl 2):S138-S140, 1995.

Brann BS, Qualls C, Papile L, et al: Measurement of progressive cerebral ventriculomegaly in infants after grades III and IV intraventricular hemorrhages. J Pediatr 117:615-621, 1990.

Brenner D, Elliston C, Hall E, et al: Estimated risks of radiation-induced fatal cancer from pediatric CT. AJR Am J Roentgenol 176:289-296, 2001.

Bruce DA, Berman WA, Schut L: Cerebrospinal fluid pressure monitoring in children: Physiology, pathology and clinical usefulness. Adv Pediatr 24:233-290, 1977.

Brunelle F: Arteriovenous malformation of the vein of Galen in children. Pediatr Radiol 27:501-13, 1997.

Buchbinder BR, Cosgrove GR: Cortical activation MR studies in brain disorders. Magn Reson Imaging Clin N Am 6:67-93, 1998.

Cady EB: Magnetic resonance spectroscopy in neonatal hypoxic-ischaemic insults. Childs Nerv Syst 17:145-149, 2001.

Chen CY, Chou TY, Zimmerman RA, et al: Pericerebral fluid collection: Differentiation of enlarged subarachnoid spaces from subdural collections with color Doppler US. Radiology 201:389-392, 1996.

Chi JG, Dooling EC, Gilles FH: Gyral development of the human brain. Ann Neurol 1:86-93, 1977.

Cowan I, MacDonald S: How useful is contrast enhancement after a normal unenhanced computed tomography brain scan? Australas Radiol 43:448-450, 1999.

de Vries LS, Groenendaal F, Eken P, et al: Infarcts in the vascular distribution of the middle cerebral artery in preterm and fullterm infants. Neuropediatrics 28:88-96, 1997.

de Vries LS, Groenendaal F, van Haastert IC, et al: Asymmetrical myelination of the posterior limb of the internal capsule in infants with periventricular haemorrhagic infarction: An early predictor of hemiplegia. Neuropediatrics 30:314-319, 1999.

Dean LM, Taylor GA: The intracranial venous system in infants: Normal and abnormal findings on duplex and color Doppler sonography. AJR Am J Roentgenol 164:151-156, 1995.

Dodge NN, Dobyns WB: Agenesis of the corpus callosum and Dandy-Walker malformation associated with hemimegalencephaly in the sebaceous nevus syndrome. Am J Med Genet 56:147-150, 1995.

Donnelly LF, Frush DP: Minimizing fallout from recent articles on radiation dose and pediatric CT. Pedatr Radiol 176:389-391, 2001.

Elster AD and Chen MY: MR imaging of Sturge-Weber syndrome: Role of gadopentetate dimeglumine and gradient-echo techniques. AJNR Am J Neuroradiol 11:685-689, 1990.

Ghazi-Birry HS, Brown WR, Moody DM, et al: Human germinal matrix: Venous origin of hemorrhage and vascular characteristics. AJNR Am J Neuroradiol 18:219-229, 1997.

Girard N, Raybaud C, Gambarelli D, et al: Fetal brain MR imaging. Magn Reson Imaging Clin N Am 9:19-56, vii, 2001.

Govindaraju V, Young K, Maudsley AA: Proton NMR chemical shifts and coupling constants for brain metabolites. NMR Biomed 13:129-153, 2000.

Griffiths PD and Martland TR: Tuberous sclerosis complex: The role of neuroradiology. Neuropediatrics 28:244-252, 1997.

Haddad SF, Menezes AH, Bell WE, et al: Brain tumors occurring before 1 year of age: A retrospective review of 22 cases in an 11-year period (1977-1987). Neurosurgery 29:8-13, 1991.

Hall TR, Choi A, Schellinger D, et al: Isolation of the fourth ventricle causing transtentorial herniation: neurosonographic findings in premature infants. AJR Am J Roentgenol 159:811-815, 1992.

Hanrahan JD, Cox IJ, Edwards AD, et al: Persistent increases in cerebral lactate concentration after birth asphyxia. Pediatr Res 44:304-311, 1998.

Haring HP, Dilitz E, Pallua A, et al: Attenuated corticomedullary contrast: An early cerebral computed tomography sign indicating malignant middle cerebral artery infarction. A case-control study. Stroke 30:1076-1082, 1999.

Hedlund GL, Boyer RS: Neuroimaging of postnatal pediatric central nervous system infections. Semin Pediatr Neurol 6:299-317, 1999.

Heerschap A and van den Berg PP: Proton magnetic resonance spectroscopy of human fetal brain. Am J Obstet Gynecol 170:1150-1151, 1994.

Hernanz-Schulman M, Cohen W, Genieser NB: Sonography of cerebral infarction in infancy. AJR Am J Roentgenol 150:897-902, 1988.

Ho HS: Safety of metallic implants in magnetic resonance imaging. J Magn Reson Imaging 14:472-7, 2001.

Holden KR, Titus MO, Van Tassel P: Cranial magnetic resonance imaging examination of normal term neonates: A pilot study. J Child Neurol 14:708-710, 1999.

Hubbard AM, States LJ: Fetal magnetic resonance imaging. Top Magn Reson Imaging 12:93-103, 2001.

Huda W, Chamberlain CC, Rosenbaum AE, et al: Radiation doses to infants and adults undergoing head CT examinations. Med Phys 28:393-9, 2001.

Huppi PS, Inder TE: Magnetic resonance techniques in the evaluation of the perinatal brain: recent advances and future directions. Semin Neonatol 6:195-210, 2001.

Inder T, Huppi PS, Zientara GP, et al: Early detection of periventricular leukomalacia by diffusion-weighted magnetic resonance imaging techniques. J Pediatr 134:631-634, 1999.

Johnson AJ, Lee BC, Lin W: Echoplanar diffusion-weighted imaging in neonates and infants with suspected hypoxic-ischemic injury: Correlation with patient outcome. AJR Am J Roentgenol 172:219-226, 1999.

Johnston MV, Hoon AH, Jr.: Possible mechanisms in infants for selective basal ganglia damage from asphyxia, kernicterus, or mitochondrial encephalopathies. J Child Neurol 15:588-591, 2000.

Keevil SF, Barbiroli B, Brooks JC, et al: Absolute metabolite quantification by in vivo NMR spectroscopy: II. A multicentre trial of protocols for in vivo localised proton studies of human brain. Magn Reson Imaging 16:1093-1106, 1998.

Kim SG, Tsekos NV: Perfusion imaging by a flow-sensitive alternating inversion recovery (FAIR) technique: application to functional brain imaging. Magn Reson Med 37:425-435, 1997.

Klisch J, Husstedt H, Hennings S, et al: Supratentorial primitive neuroectodermal tumours: Diffusion-weighted MRI. Neuroradiology 42:393-398, 2000.

Koenigsberger MR: [Complications of intracranial hemorrhage in full term newborns]. Rev Neurol 29:247-249, 1999.

Kucharczyk J, Vexler ZS, Roberts TP, et al: Echo-planar perfusion-sensitive MR imaging of acute cerebral ischemia. Radiology 188:711-717, 1993.

Lasjaunias P, Manelfe C, Chiu M: Angiographic architecture of intracranial vascular malformations and fistulas—pretherapeutic aspects. Neurosurg Rev 9:253-263, 1986.

Lena G, van Calenberg F, Genitori L, et al: Supratentorial interhemispheric cysts associated with callosal agenesis: Surgical treatment and outcome in 16 children. Childs Nerv Syst 11:568-573, 1995.

Levine D: Fetal magnetic resonance imaging. Top Magn Reson Imaging 12:1-2, 2001a.

Levine D: Ultrasound versus magnetic resonance imaging in fetal evaluation. Top Magn Reson Imaging 12:25-38, 2001b.

Levine D, Barnes PD, Madsen JR, et al: Fetal central nervous system anomalies: MR imaging augments sonographic diagnosis. Radiology 204:635-642, 1997.

Lusk RP, Lee PC: Magnetic resonance imaging of congenital midline nasal masses. Otolaryngol Head Neck Surg 95:303-306, 1986.

Madsen JR, Robertson RL, Bartlett R: Surgical management of cutis aplasia with high-flow sinus pericranii. Pediatr Neurosurg 28:79-83, 1998.

McLone DG, Naidich TP: Developmental morphology of the subarachnoid space, brain vasculature, and contiguous structures, and the cause of the Chiari II malformation. AJNR Am J Neuroradiol 13:463-482, 1992.

Ment LR, Bada HS, Barnes P, et al: Practice parameter: Neuroimaging of the neonate. Neurology 58:1726-1738, 2002.

Mercuri E, Rutherford M, Cowan F, et al: Early prognostic indicators of outcome in infants with neonatal cerebral infarction: a clinical, electroencephalogram, and magnetic resonance imaging study. Pediatrics 103:39-46, 1999.

Meyer JS, Hoffer FA, Barnes PD, et al: Biological classification of soft-tissue vascular anomalies: MR correlation. AJR Am J Roentgenol 157:559-564, 1991.

Miller BL: A review of chemical issues in 1H NMR spectroscopy: *N*-acetyl-L-aspartate, creatine and choline. NMR Biomed 4:47-52, 1991.

Mitchell DG, Merton D, Needleman L, et al: Neonatal brain: color Doppler imaging. Part I. Technique and vascular anatomy. Radiology 167:303-306, 1988.

Mitchell DG, Merton DA, Mirsky PJ, et al: Circle of Willis in newborns: Color Doppler imaging of 53 healthy full-term infants. Radiology 172:201-205, 1989.

Morris MW, Smith S, Cressman J, et al: Evaluation of infants with subdural hematoma who lack external evidence of abuse. Pediatrics 105:549-553, 2000.

Mulkern RV, Chung T: From signal to image: Magnetic resonance imaging physics for cardiac magnetic resonance. Pediatr Cardiol 21:5-17, 2000.

Myers C, Duncan KR, Gowland PA, et al: Failure to detect intrauterine growth restriction following in utero exposure to MRI. Br J Radiol 71:549-551, 1998.

Naidich TP, Altman NR, Braffman BH, et al: Cephaloceles and related malformations. AJNR Am J Neuroradiol 13:655-690, 1992.

Naidich TP and Yousefzadeh DK: Sonography of the normal neonatal head. Supratentorial structures: State-of-the-art imaging. Neuroradiology 28:408-427, 1986.

Pape KE, Blackwell RJ, G C, et al: Neonatal brain scanning with real-time ultrasound [abstract]. Pediatr Res 5:528, 1979.

Papile LA, Munsick-Bruno G, Schaefer A: Relationship of cerebral intraventricular hemorrhage and early childhood neurologic handicaps. J Pediatr 103:273-277, 1983.

Pascual-Castroviejo I, Diaz-Gonzalez C, Garcia-Melian RM, et al: Sturge-Weber syndrome: Study of 40 patients. Pediatr Neurol 9:283-288, 1993.

Perlman JM, Hill A, Volpe JJ: The effect of patent ductus arteriosus on flow velocity in the anterior cerebral arteries: Ductal steal in the premature newborn infant. J Pediatr 99:767-771, 1981.

Raj P, Stansbie JM, Phelps PD: Minimising radiation dose to the lens in axial computed tomography of the temporal bone. Rev Laryngol Otol Rhinol (Bord) 121:83-85, 2000.

Rivkin MJ: Hypoxic-ischemic brain injury in the term newborn. Clin Perinatol 24:607-625, 1997.

Robertson NJ, Kuint J, Counsell TJ, et al: Characterization of cerebral white matter damage in preterm infants using $^{1}$H and $^{31}$P magnetic resonance spectroscopy. J Cereb Blood Flow Metab 20:1446-1456, 2000.

Robertson RL, Ben-Sira L, Barnes PD, et al: MR line-scan diffusion-weighted imaging of term neonates with perinatal brain ischemia. AJNR Am J Neuroradiol 20:1658-1670, 1999.

Robertson RL, Robson CD: Diffusion Imaging in Neonates. Neuroimag Clin N Am 12:55-70, 2002.

Robertson RL, Robson CD, Antiles S, et al: CT versus MR in neonatal brain imaging at term. Pediatric Radiology 33:442-449, 2003.

Robson CD, Mulliken JB, Robertson RL, et al: Prominent basal emissary foramina in syndromic craniosynostosis: Correlation with phenotypic and molecular diagnoses. AJNR Am J Neuroradiol 21:1707-1717, 2000.

Roland EH, Poskitt K, Rodriguez E, et al: Perinatal hypoxic-ischemic thalamic injury: Clinical features and neuroimaging. Ann Neurol 44:161-166, 1998.

Rubinstein D, Cajade-Law AG, Youngman V, et al: The development of the corpus callosum in semilobar and lobar holoprosencephaly. Pediatr Radiol 26:839-844, 1996.

Ruge JR, Tomita T, Naidich TP, et al: Scalp and calvarial masses of infants and children. Neurosurgery 22:1037-1042, 1988.

Rutherford MA, Pennock JM, Schwieso JE, et al: Hypoxic ischaemic encephalopathy: Early magnetic resonance imaging findings and their evolution. Neuropediatrics 26:183-191, 1995.

Sakuma H, Nomura Y, Takeda K, et al: Adult and neonatal human brain: Diffusional anisotropy and myelination with diffusion-weighted MR imaging. Radiology 180:229-233, 1991.

Schellinger D, Grant EG and Richardson CJ: Cystic periventricular leukomalacia: Sonographic and CT findings. AJNR Am J Neuroradiol 5:439-445, 1984.

Schlesinger Y, Buller RS, Brunstrom JE, et al: Expanded spectrum of herpes simplex encephalitis in childhood. J Pediatr 126:234-241, 1995.

Seibert JJ, McCowan TC, Chadduck WM, et al: Duplex pulsed Doppler US versus intracranial pressure in the neonate: Clinical and experimental studies. Radiology 171:155-159, 1989.

Shackleford GD: Neurosonography of hydrocephalus in infants. Neuroradiology 28:452-462, 1986.

Shuman RM, Selednik LJ: Periventricular leukomalacia. A one year autopsy study. Arch Neurol 37:231-235, 1980.

Siegel MJ: Brain. In Siegel MJ (Ed) Pediatric Sonography. Philadelphia, Lippincott Williams & Wilkins, 2001, pp 41-121.

Smirniotopoulos JG, Chiechi MV: Teratomas, dermoids, and epidermoids of the head and neck. Radiographics 15:1437-1455, 1995.

Smith CD, Ryan SJ, Hoover SL, et al: Magnetic resonance imaging of the brain in Aicardi's syndrome. Report of 20 patients. J Neuroimaging 6:214-221, 1996.

Sreenan C, Bhargava R, Robertson CM: Cerebral infarction in the term newborn: Clinical presentation and long-term outcome. J Pediatr 137:351-355, 2000.

Sugama S, Soeda A, Eto Y: Magnetic resonance imaging in three children with kernicterus. Pediatr Neurol 25:328-331, 2001.

Takeda K, Nomura Y, Sakuma H, et al: MR assessment of normal brain development in neonates and infants: Comparative study of T1- and diffusion-weighted images. J Comput Assist Tomogr 21:1-7, 1997.

Taylor GA: Effect of scanning pressure on intracranial hemodynamics during transfontanellar duplex US. Radiology 185: 763-766, 1992a.

Taylor GA: Intracranial venous system in the newborn: Evaluation of normal anatomy and flow characteristics with color Doppler US. Radiology 183:449-452, 1992b.

Taylor GA: Alterations in regional cerebral blood flow in neonatal stroke: Preliminary findings with color Doppler sonography. Pediatr Radiol 24:111-115, 1994.

Taylor GA: Effect of germinal matrix hemorrhage on terminal vein position and patency. Pediatr Radiol 25(Suppl 1):S37-S40, 1995.

Taylor GA: New concepts in the pathogenesis of germinal matrix intraparenchymal hemorrhage in premature infants. AJNR Am J Neuroradiol 18:231-232, 1997.

Taylor GA: Doppler of the neonatal and infant brain. In Rumack CM, Wilson SR, Charboneau JW (eds): Diagnostic Ultrasound. St Louis, Mosby, 1998, pp 1503-1525.

Taylor GA: Sonographic assessment of posthemorrhagic ventricular dilatation. Radiol Clin North Am 39:541-551, 2001.

Taylor GA and Madsen JR: Neonatal hydrocephalus: Hemodynamic response to fontanel compression—correlation with intracranial pressure and need for shunt placement. Radiology 201:685-689, 1996.

Taylor GA, Martin GR, Short BL: Cardiac determinants of cerebral blood flow during extracorporeal membrane oxygenation. Invest Radiol 24:511-516, 1989.

Taylor GA, Phillips MD, Ichord RN, et al: Intracranial compliance in infants: Evaluation with Doppler US. Radiology 191:787-791, 1994.

Taylor GA, Short BL, Walker LK, et al: Intracranial blood flow: quantification with duplex Doppler and color Doppler flow US. Radiology 176:231-236, 1990.

Toft PB, Leth H, Peitersen B, et al: The apparent diffusion coefficient of water in gray and white matter of the infant brain. J Comput Assist Tomogr 20:1006-1011, 1996.

Vanzieleghem BD, Lemmerling MM, Vermeersch HF, et al: Imaging studies in the diagnostic workup of neonatal nasal obstruction. J Comput Assist Tomogr 25:540-549, 2001.

Vigneron DB, Barkovich AJ, Noworolski SM, et al: Three-dimensional proton MR spectroscopic imaging of premature and term neonates. AJNR Am J Neuroradiol 22:1424-1433, 2001.

Volpe JJ: Neurology of the Newborn, 4th ed. Philadelphia, WB Saunders, 2001.

Volpe JJ: Brain injury in the premature infant. Clin Perinatol 24:567-587, 1997.

Warach S, Dashe JF, Edelman RR: Clinical outcome in ischemic stroke predicted by early diffusion-weighted and perfusion magnetic resonance imaging: A preliminary analysis. J Cereb Blood Flow Metab 16:53-59, 1996.

Whitby E, Paley MN, Davies N, et al: Ultrafast magnetic resonance imaging of central nervous system abnormalities in utero in the second and third trimester of pregnancy: Comparison with ultrasound. Br J Obstet Gynaecol 108:519-526, 2001.

Wolf RL, Zimmerman RA, Clancy R, et al: Quantitative apparent diffusion coefficient measurements in term neonates for early detection of hypoxic-ischemic brain injury: Initial experience. Radiology 218:825-833, 2001.

CHAPTER 63

# Congenital Malformations of the Central Nervous System

**Stephen A. Back**

During the formation of the fetal central nervous system (CNS), developmental processes may be interrupted by deleterious intrinsic or extrinsic insults that result in CNS malformations. The origins and consequences of these disorders are best understood within the context of normal CNS development. Accordingly, for each of the major developmental processes, this chapter reviews the sequence of events and examines the associated CNS malformations that are more commonly encountered in the clinical practice of neonatal medicine. The peak timing of these events during fetal gestation is summarized in Table 63–1.

Remarkable progress in basic developmental neurobiology in the last decade has translated into rapid advances in our understanding of the molecular and genetic basis of many of these previously perplexing disorders. Although a majority of these disorders arise from adverse events that occur during the early phases of pregnancy, these new insights begin to provide a more rational basis for the assessment of prognosis, as well as for the management of future pregnancies.

A true CNS malformation may be multifactorial in origin and results when a disruption occurs in an intrinsic developmental process. Acquired defects occur when an already normally formed brain is injured by a secondary process, such as vascular compromise, hypoxia-ischemia, infection, toxic exposure, physical compression, or trauma. The nature of acquired malformations is closely related to the stage of development at which the injury occurs, as well as the duration of the insult. Although acquired lesions are usually *encephaloclastic* in nature, which means that destruction of normal brain tissue has occurred, they can resemble primary developmental lesions in some cases (Roessmann, 1995).

## PRIMARY AND SECONDARY NEURAL TUBE FORMATION (NEURULATION)

The earliest developmental stages include the one-celled embryo, the cleaving embryo, the blastocyst, the process of implantation and development of the amniotic cavity and umbilical vesicle, the formation of chorionic villi, and the formation of axial features (right and left sides, rostral and caudal ends). All of these events occur during the first 14 postconceptional days. At 16 days, the site of the future neural plate can be defined by autoradiographic means, and at about 18 days, the neural groove can be seen (England, 1988; O'Rahilly and Muller, 1994).

Neural tube formation, or neurulation, occurs through an inductive process that stimulates the dorsal aspect of the embryo to form the brain and spinal cord. Initial events involve formation of the brain and much of the spinal cord, with the exception of the sacral-coccygeal segments (primary neurulation). Later in embryogenesis, the lower sacral segments of the spinal cord are formed (secondary neurulation). Disruption of primary neurulation and of secondary neurulation results in distinctly different malformations that are considered separately.

### Primary Neural Tube Formation

The process of primary neural tube formation involves the formation of the brain and spinal cord, with the exception of the most caudal (sacral-coccygeal) segments of the spinal cord. Primary neurulation spans from 18 days of gestation to the end of the fourth gestational week. Initially, an area of thickened neuroectoderm, the neural plate, is formed after induction by the underlying notochord and chordal mesoderm (Fig. 63–1). At 20 to 21 days, the neural groove forms in the midline, with a neural fold on either side. Areas destined to become the forebrain, midbrain, and hindbrain can be identified at this early stage. By day 22, the neural folds are beginning to fuse to form the neural tube and central canal (England, 1988; O'Rahilly and Muller, 1994).

### Neural Tube Closure and Neural Crest Migration

Primary neurulation concludes with a series of critical events that result in closure of the neural tube. The neural folds fuse first in the nascent occipitocervical region. Current studies no longer support the "zipper concept" of closure of the neural tube. Rather, fusion occurs at multiple closure sites, with the closure of the cranium being the most complex. Inbred strains of mice show differences in the timing of the various closure sites and in the exact locations and sequences of closure, all of which are dependent on different, specific genes (Van Allen et al, 1993). Analysis of the locations where human anterior neural tube defects occur supports the notion that anterior neural tube closure proceeds simultaneously at multiple sites (Golden and Chernoff, 1995). Disturbances in human neural tube closure appear to occur by failure of closure at one or more sites or by defective fusion between two adjacent sites of closure.

By day 24 to 25, fusion progresses rostrally to the level of the colliculi, and fusion continues rostrally and caudally until only the anterior neuropore and the posterior neuropore are open (Fig. 63–2). By day 25, the anterior neuropore has closed; by day 26, the posterior neuropore has closed at the site corresponding to around S2 (O'Rahilly and Muller, 1994). The skull, vertebrae, and dura form through interactions between the neural tube and the adjacent mesoderm. As the rostral parts of the neural folds fuse, the neural crest is formed from ectodermal cells on both sides of the neural tube. The neural crest cells migrate shortly after neural tube closure. They give rise to sensory, sympathetic, and parasympathetic ganglia; chromaffin cells of the adrenal medulla; skin melanocytes; enteric neurons in the

**TABLE 63–1**

**Timing of the Major Gestational Events in Human Brain Development and Representative Examples of Significant Related Disorders**

| Major Developmental Event | Window in Development |
|---|---|
| **Primary Neurulation**<br>Craniorachischisis totalis, anencephaly, encephalocele, myeloschisis, myelomeningocele/Arnold-Chiari malformation | 3-4 weeks |
| **Prosencephalic Development**<br>Holoprosencephaly, agenesis of the corpus callosum, agenesis of septum pellucidum/septo-optic dysplasia | 4-8 weeks |
| **Hindbrain Development**<br>Dandy-Walker malformation, malformations associated with cerebellar vermis hypoplasia, malformations associated with the molar tooth sign (Joubert syndrome) | 3-12+ weeks |
| **Neuronal Proliferation**<br>Micrencephaly (micrencephaly vera, radial microbrain), human autosomal recessive primary micrencephaly 1-5, macrencephaly, hemimegalencephaly | 8-12 weeks |
| **Neuronal Migration**<br>Schizencephaly, polymicrogyria, lissencephaly/pachygryria, lissencephaly with cerebellar hypoplasia, cobblestone complex syndromes, neuronal heterotopia, cortical dysplasia | 8-16 weeks |

gastrointestinal tract; and facial connective tissue (O'Rahilly and Muller, 1994).

### Secondary Neural Tube Formation and Caudal Regression

The process of secondary neural tube formation occurs approximately between gestational days 30 and 50, during which vacuoles form in a caudal cell mass that surrounds the lower neural tube. The vacuoles coalesce and connect with the central canal of the already present neural tube. At postconceptional days 41 to 51, the caudalmost part of the neural tube and central canal begins to regress as the tail of the embryo disappears. Atrophy of the caudal neural tube results in formation of a fibrous strand called the filum terminale, which is present throughout life. As the vertebral bodies grow, the end of the central canal (the conus medullaris) becomes placed higher in the vertebral column, eventually reaching the L1 to L2 level (usually by 2 weeks postnatally). This may be due to proportionately greater lengthening of the spinal vertebrae compared with the spinal cord (England, 1988; O'Rahilly and Muller, 1994).

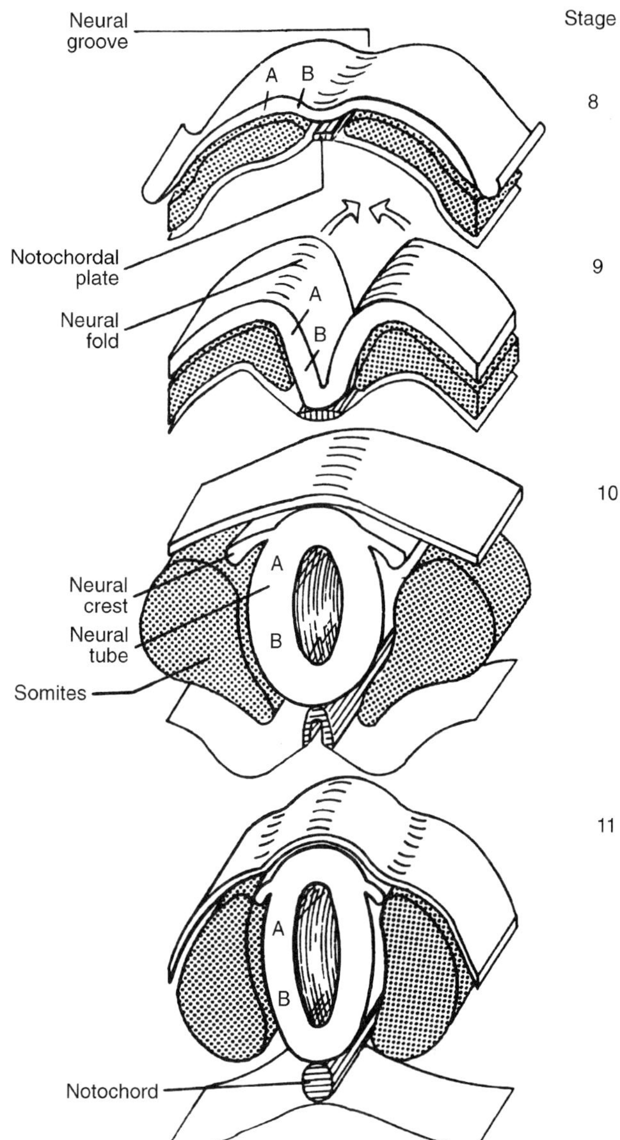


**FIGURE 63–1.** Formation of the neural tube. *(From O'Rahilly R, Muller F: The Embryonic Human Brain. New York, Wiley-Liss, 1994, p 41.)*

Disorders of secondary neurulation give rise to several clinically significant occult dysraphic states, discussed later on.

## Neural Tube Defects

Neural tube defects result from a failure of primary neural tube closure during the fourth week of human gestation (Roessmann, 1995). Most of these defects are related to some degree of failure of anterior or posterior neuropore closure. On the clinical spectrum of brain malformations associated with disrupted *anterior* neuropore closure, anencephaly represents the most profound defect, with encephaloceles of decreasing severity accounting for the remainder of such malformations. Myeloschisis and myelomeningoceles with the associated Arnold-Chiari malformations are the spinal cord defects associated with failure of *posterior* neuropore closure. In addition, craniorachischis totalis is a

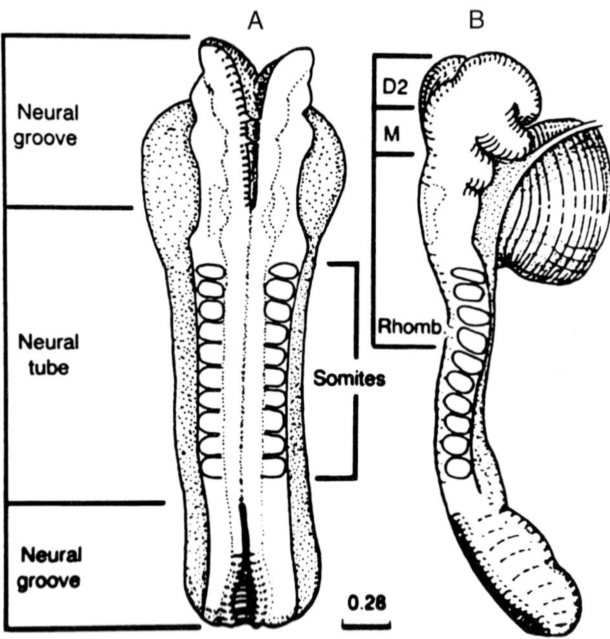


**FIGURE 63–2.** Positions of anterior and posterior neuropores. *(From O'Rahilly R, Muller F: The Embryonic Human Brain. New York, Wiley-Liss, 1994, p 45.)*

severe malformation of the brain and spinal cord involving essentially *complete* failure of neural tube closure; it usually results in spontaneous abortion during embryogenesis or early fetal development. Similarly, myeloschisis commonly results in stillbirth, as a result of extensive malformation of large portions of the spinal cord. Other neural tube defects result in malformations of the CNS and the overlying axial skeleton, meninges, and skin that are associated with various degrees of viability in the newborn period.

### Epidemiology

Neural tube defects remain one of the most common congenital malformations encountered in newborns, despite a recent decline in prevalence. Because many congenital malformations occur during embryonic development, incidence data are essentially impossible to ascertain. Nevertheless, it is clear that the prevalence of neural tube defects varies widely and is particularly influenced by race, ethnicity, geographic area, and socioeconomic status (Frey and Hauser, 2003). In the United States, for example, the risk for neural tube defects is higher for Hispanics but lower for African Americans. Geographically, one of the higher prevalence rates occurs in the United Kingdom, where distinct geographic gradients also exist within this region. It should also be noted that once a woman has had a pregnancy complicated by a neural tube defect, the risk of recurrence may be disproportionately higher with each subsequent preganancy. For unclear reasons, after the first affected pregnancy, this risk increases to become markedly higher than the baseline risk for the relevant general population. In fact, the risk may nearly triple after each subsequent pregnancy (Elwood et al, 1992).

Superimposed on these factors has been a marked decline in prevalence at birth of both anencephaly and spina bifida. In 1960, the prevalence for England and Wales was about 6 in 1000 births; in 1990, this rate dropped to about 1 in 1000. The lower occurrence rates reflect two major interventions: in utero diagnosis with termination of affected pregnancies and maternal periconceptional folate therapy. The latter is estimated to prevent approximately 60% to 70% of neural tube defects (Castilla et al, 2003; Czeizel and Dudas, 1992; Frey and Hauser, 2003; MRC Vitamin Study Research Group, 1992; Oakley et al, 1994; Smithells et al, 1981). The mechanisms by which folate is involved in neural tube closure are currently unclear. There are approximately 150 known genes involved in folic acid metabolism and transport that are under investigation (Juriloff and Harris, 2000).

### Etiology

The etiology of neural tube defects is complex and clearly multifactorial. Genetic and environmental factors operate independently to determine individual and population risk. Although numerous genetic syndromes are associated with neural tube defects, affected pregnancies uncommonly come to term, and such syndromes appear to constitute a very small percentage of all cases (Hall and Solehdin, 1998). An independent role for genetic factors is supported by a particular mouse model of neural tube defects, the curly tail *(ct)* variant. The responsible *ct* gene localizes to the distal arm of chromosome 4 and has at least three modifier loci that influence the incidence of neural tube defects (Neumann et al, 1994). Among the numerous environmental risk factors that have been studied, the most prominent include maternal febrile illness, maternal heat exposure in the first trimester (e.g., sauna or hot tub use), lower socioeconomic status, dietary factors (prenatal tea but not caffeine consumption), and prenatal exposure to a number of drugs including antiepileptic medications (Frey and Hauser, 2003). Valproate and carbamazepine both are associated with an increased risk of neural tube defects (Jones et al, 1989; Yerby, 2003).

## Disorders of Primary Neurulation

### Anencephaly

Anencephaly comprises roughly more than half of all human neural tube defects. As an early neurulation defect, it occurs no later than 24 days of gestation. Anencephaly is the most severe and common of the disorders of anterior neural tube closure (Fig. 63–3). Both anencephaly and occipital encephaloceles (see later) affect girls more often than boys. A majority of infants are stillborn. Moreover, it is uniformly lethal within the first 2 months of life in the roughly 25% of cases with survival into the neonatal period (Baird and Sadovnick, 1984; Peabody et al, 1989). The duration of survival is critically related to intensive care support. Without intensive care, survival has not been reported beyond 14 days of life. Survival is related in part to persistence of rudimentary brainstem function. This finding is inconsistent with the diagnosis of brain death in the United States, which is a requirement for organ donation (AAP Committee on Bioethics, 1992; McAbee et al, 2000).

Anencephaly most commonly involves the forebrain and upper brainstem, which accounts for the devastating outcome. It is characterized by absence of the calvaria, with

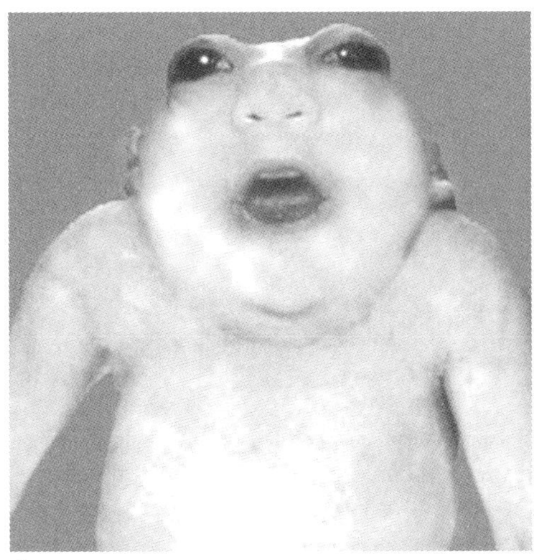

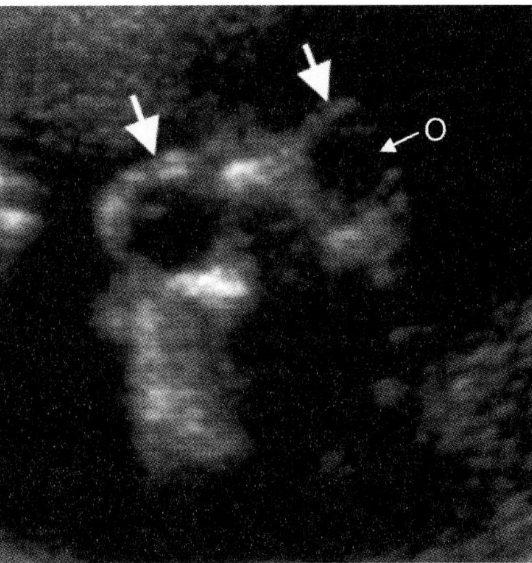


A B

**FIGURE 63–3.** **A,** An anencephalic infant. **B,** Ultrasonogram of anencephaly. Note the absence of the normal cranial structures *(large arrows)* superior to the orbits (O). *(Courtesy of Dr. Marjorie Grafe, Department of Pathology, Oregon Health & Science University.)*

replacement of the intracranial contents by vascularized, disorganized glial tissue (area cerebrovasculosa) (Menkes, 1991; Roessmann, 1995). The hypothalamus and cerebellum usually are malformed, the anterior lobe of the pituitary is present, and the internal carotid arteries are hypoplastic, which may be secondary to abnormal brain formation. Because the anencephalic fetus experiences a period of exencephaly, in which the brain tissue extrudes through the unformed calvaria and then is degraded by exposure to the amniotic fluid, some investigators have hypothesized that the primary defect is the abnormal skull formation. In some cases of anencephaly, remnants of calvarial bones are present, with normal brain under the protective bones (Roessmann, 1995).

Anencephaly can be diagnosed by fetal ultrasound examination (see Fig. 63-3B) in the second trimester of gestation (Crane, 1992; Goldstein and Filly, 1988). Polyhydramnios is frequently associated. Anencephaly also may be suggested by increased levels of alpha-fetoprotein (AFP) in maternal serum. AFP is the major serum protein in the early embryo and is fetus specific. It normally passes from the fetal serum into fetal urine and then into amniotic fluid; in the amniotic fluid, it is swallowed by the fetus and metabolized in the fetal gastrointestinal tract (Brock, 1976). In anencephaly, open spina bifida, and open encephalocele, there is leakage of fetal serum directly into the amniotic fluid, and levels of AFP as well as of maternal serum protein are elevated in the amniotic fluid. By contrast, when a neural tube defect is closed (i.e., covered by intact skin), the AFP level is not elevated. This occurs in about 5% of neural tube defects (Milunsky et al, 1980).

### Encephalocele

In contrast with anencephaly, encephalocele appears to arise from a restricted rather than diffuse failure of anterior neuropore closure around 26 days of gestation. Encephalocele typically manifests as a cranial defect through which brain tissue protrudes. Less severe defects may result with later onset. These include cranium bifidum, in which there is a failure of midline fusion of the skull, and cranial meningoceles, which contain meningeal but not neural tissue. In up to 80% of cases, encephaloceles occur in the occipital region (Fig. 63–4), with the remainder in the parietal, frontonasal, intranasal, and nasopharyngeal regions. Although the precise pathogenetic mechanism remains unclear, geographic or ethnic-genetic factors appear to influence the location of the lesion. Frontal encephaloceles are more prevalent in Southeast Asia, for example, whereas lesions that involve the occipital lobe are more common in Western populations. A role for genetic factors is supported by the presence of encephalocele in a number of autosomal recessive syndromes (e.g., Meckel syndrome, Walker-Warburg syndrome). Overall, about one half of infants with encephaloceles have other major congenital anomalies that include microcephaly, arhinencephaly, anophthalmia, cleft lip or palate, craniosynostosis, complex congenital heart disease, and other systemic abnormalities (Brown and Sheridan-Pereira, 1992).

Encephaloceles also are associated with various other CNS defects that influence the severity of the outcome as well as the surgical management. These defects include anomalous draining veins, as well as hydrocephalus, which is observed in up to 50% of cases (Diebler and Dulac,

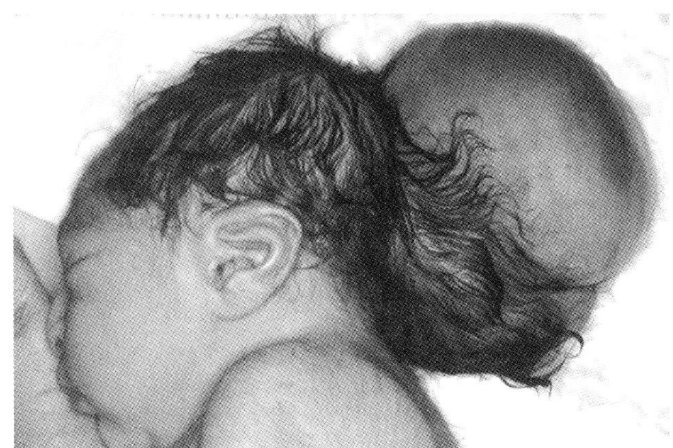

**FIGURE 63–4.** Newborn infant with a large occipital encephalocele. *(Courtesy of Dr. Marjorie Grafe, Department of Pathology, Oregon Health & Science University.)*

1987; Menkes, 1991). The occurrence of lower occipital lobe encephalocele with skull base defects and malformations of the cerebellum and lower brainstem defines Chiari type III malformations (see later discussion of Chiari type II malformations that occur in association with myelomeningocele). Partial or complete agenesis of the corpus callosum and subependymal nodular heteropias are other frequently associated CNS malformations, as discussed later.

Evaluation of the infant with an encephalocele can be aided by transillumination, skull radiography, cranial ultrasonography, computed tomography (CT) scanning, and magnetic resonance imaging (MRI). Decisions about the appropriate modality depend on the individual cases and whether other cerebral anomalies or hydrocephalus is suspected. Frontonasal encephaloceles pulse or bulge with brief bilateral jugular vein compression, indicating communication with the subarachnoid space. Nasal gliomas, dermoids, and teratomas all can occur in the same region. Intranasal encephalocele should be suspected when an intranasal mass is found in a child with a broad nasal bridge and widely spaced eyes. Some affected children may also present with recurrent meningitis (Menkes, 1991). Basal encephaloceles are not usually diagnosed until childhood and can be located in the nasopharynx, sphenoid sinus, or posterior orbit.

In a majority of patients, neurosurgical management is indicated early in life. Large lesions or other severe CNS anomalies, however, may preclude intervention. Early intervention is imperative for those infants at high risk for meningitis because their lesions externally communicate and leak cerebrospinal fluid (CSF). Survival and outcome remain difficult to predict owing to the variability of presentation and surgical selection bias. One study of a series of children with encephalocele reported an overall mortality rate of 29% (45% in infants with posterior defects; 0% in infants with anterior defects) (Brown and Sheridan-Pereira, 1992). Neurologic deficits were severe in 33% of survivors with anterior defects and in 33% of survivors with posterior defects. Mild neurologic deficits were found in 17% of survivors of anterior defects and in 50% of survivors of posterior defects.

## Myeloschisis

Myeloschisis may be regarded as being at the more severe end of the spectrum of malformations of the spinal cord that arise from failure of posterior neuropore closure no later than 24 days of gestation. Hence, myeloschisis arises from an extensive failure of posterior neuropore closure, whereas myelinomeningocele (described next) arises from more restricted disturbances in posterior neuropore closure. Myeloschisis manifests as a severely malformed spinal cord that comprises an exposed primitive neural plate-like structure that lacks overlying vertebrae and skin. At the level of the malformed upper cervical cord, there often may be associated malformations of the base of the skull that result in retroflexion of the head on the cervical spine (iniencephaly). Not unexpectedly, a majority of infants with myeloschisis are stillborn.

## Myelomeningocele

Myelomeningocele and other associated malformations of the spinal cord arise from restricted failure of posterior neuropore closure probably no later than day 26 of gestation. The incidence of myelomeningocele in the United States is about 0.2 to 0.4 per 1000 live births (Yen et al, 1992). Spinal cord malformations involving the meninges include myelomeningocele and meningocele. *Myelomeningocele* is characterized by herniation of the meninges and spinal cord at the site of the defect. Myelomeningoceles are usually "exposed" lesions on the back without vertebral or dermal covering (Fig. 63–5), unless a lipoma overlies the defect (i.e., a lipomyelomeningocele) (Menkes, 1991). A *meningocele* is a restricted herniation of the meninges at the defect site, which usually is covered by skin; neurologic function is often normal. Myelomeningoceles are about four times more common than meningoceles (Friede, 1989; Menkes, 1991). These lesions most often occur in the lumbar or lumbosacral region (in 69% of cases), which supports the concept that the site of final closure of the posterior neuropore is in the lumbar region.

Myelomeningocele is rarely an isolated malformation; rather, it usually is accompanied by other clinically significant CNS abnormalities. Of major importance is hydrocephalus, which is frequently associated with the Arnold-Chiari II malformation (discussed next). Hydrocephalus is not universal, and its development in myelomeningocele correlates with the site of the lesion. Hydrocephalus develops

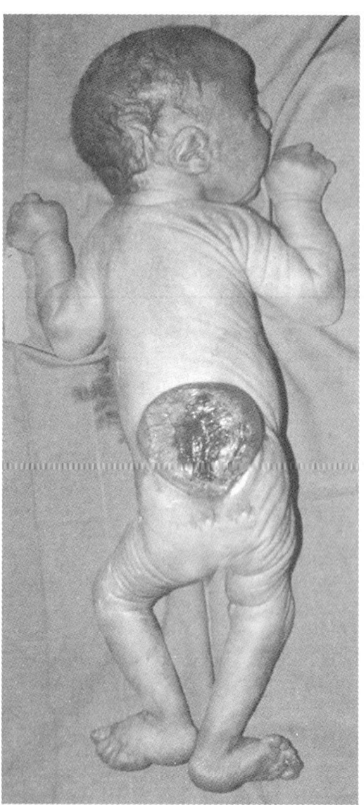

**FIGURE 63–5.** Newborn infant with a large thoracolumbar myelomeningocele. The infant demonstrated weakness of the distal musculature in the lower extremities. *(Courtesy of Dr. Marjorie Grafe, Department of Pathology, Oregon Health & Science University.)*

in 60% of patients with occipital, cervical, thoracic, or sacral lesions, whereas it develops in 90% of those with thoracolumbar, lumbar, or lumbosacral lesions (Lorber, 1961). Increased intracranial pressure is present in about 15% of newborns with myelomeningocele. In some infants, there are no signs of increased pressure because of decompression due to leakage of CSF from the myelomeningocele (Stein and Schut, 1979). In these infants, hydrocephalus and increased pressure may become evident later after surgical closure of the myelomeningocele. In most infants with hydrocephalus, an abnormal increase in head circumference occurs within a month after birth (Stein and Schut, 1979).

As in anencephaly, presence of an open myelomeningocele is suspected following detection of an elevation in alpha-fetoprotein (AFP) in maternal serum and can be confirmed by fetal ultrasound examination or MRI. Another marker, amniotic fluid acetylcholinesterase, is also used to diagnose neural tube defects in utero, along with amniotic AFP, which increases the sensitivity of the screen when the maternal serum AFP level is questionable or high (Cuckle, 1994). Other causes of a high maternal serum AFP include contamination of the amniotic fluid by fetal blood, which may occur in cases of esophageal and duodenal atresia, annular pancreas, omphalocele, gastroschisis, congenital nephrosis, polycystic kidneys, renal agenesis, or fetal demise. Elevation of maternal serum AFP also may be related to a multiple gestation pregnancy (Brock, 1976). The optimal time for determination in maternal serum is at 16 to 18 weeks of gestation and in amniotic fluid at 14 to 16 weeks of gestation.

Clinical management of the newborn with a neural tube defect must be individualized. In the past, selective aggressive treatment was instituted for infants anticipated to have a better outcome. At present, aggressive surgical therapy is advocated for most infants; to date, this approach has resulted in better outcomes as demonstrated by increased cognitive abilities, increased ambulation, a lower incidence of incontinence, and a lower mortality rate (Hunt and Holmes, 1975; McLone, 1992; Stein et al, 1975).

## Arnold-Chiari Malformation

The Arnold-Chiari malformation occurs in at least 95% of children with a myelomeningocele that includes a lumbar lesion (Fig. 63–6). This malformation results in two serious complications—hydrocephalus and brainstem dysfunction—that are a significant cause of morbidity and death in infants with a myelomeningocele. The clinical sequelae with this class of malformations are best understood in the context of the principal types of associated anatomic abnormalities. Hindbrain malformations involve both the brainstem and the cerebellum. Brainstem abnormalities include downward herniation of the medulla and the fourth ventricle through the foramen magnum into the upper cervical canal, which results in obstruction of the fourth ventricle and compression of the upper cervical cord. The resultant downward stretch of the cervical roots causes them to project cranially to their foramina rather than to follow their normal lateral or descending course. The caudal displacement of the brainstem thins and elongates the lower pons and upper medulla, which may compress brainstem nuclei as well as

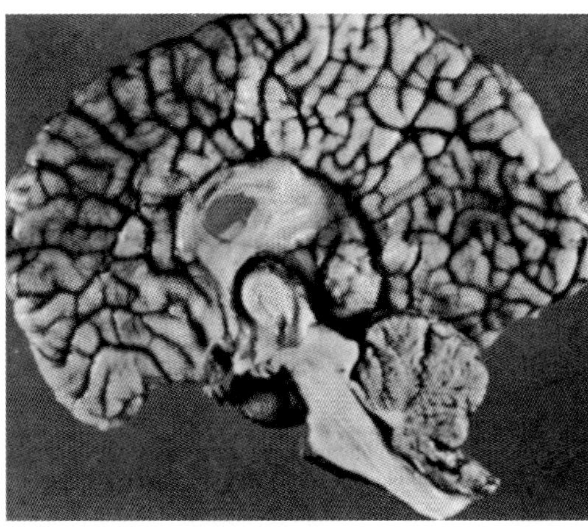

**FIGURE 63–6.** Arnold-Chiari malformation seen in association with a thoracolumbar myelomeningocele. This defect is one of elongation of the lower brainstem with downward displacement of the inferior part of the vermis of the cerebellum. The tectal plate is beaked, and the massa intermedia is enlarged. Note that polymicrogyria also is present in this particular case.

compromise the roots of the cranial nerves (Blaauw, 1971; Friede, 1989; Naidich et al, 1980). The herniation of the cerebellar tonsils through the foramen magnum and flattening of the lower cerebellar hemispheres are frequently associated with the caudal displacement of the brainstem. A variety of bone malformations are observed that include enlargement of the foramen magnum, defects of the occiput, and anomalies of the cervical vertebrae. Finally, cortical neuronal migration abnormalities (cerebral cortical dysplasia or polymicrogyria) are frequently associated with Chiari malformations and may account for cognitive deficits and epilepsy seen in some patients.

It follows from this constellation of hindbrain abnormalities that hydrocephalus is commonly associated with Chiari malformations. The hydrocephalus may arise from compression of the fourth ventricle or obstruction of CSF outflow through the foramen magnum. In addition, many patients also have aqueductal stenosis or, uncommonly, aqueductal atresia (Gilbert et al, 1986; Peach, 1965; Stein and Schut, 1979). A less well-recognized but potentially fatal complication of hindbrain abnormalities is primary dysfunction of the brainstem. This deficit can manifest as apneic episodes with cyanosis, vocal cord paralysis with laryngeal stridor, or feeding disturbances that result in aspiration related to reflux. Ventilatory disturbances may be either obstructive or central and thus prominent during sleep. These disturbances may be identified by polysomnography and pulmonary function studies (Kirk et al, 1999).

## Occult Spinal Dysraphisms

Occult spinal dysraphic states are the result of defects in caudal neural tube formation (i.e., secondary neurulation). As discussed previously, development of the sacral and coccygeal segments of the spinal cord involves a process of canalization and caudal regression of the distal neural tube. In contrast with defects in primary neural tube formation, these defects thus uniformly localize to the distal cord and are closed defects with an intact dermal covering. In some instances, these defects are truly occult, without any overlying abnormalities of the skin, and may go undetected until the affected person becomes symptomatic. In a majority of newborn infants so affected, however, a lumbosacral midline cutaneous lesion may indicate an occult spinal dysraphism (Fig. 63–7). These lesions include abnormal hair tufts, hemangiomas, pigmented spots, skin tags, aplasia cutis congenita, cutaneous dimples or tracts, and a subcutaneous mass (Albright et al, 1989; Hall et al, 1981; Scatliff et al, 1989).

The spinal cord lesions associated with occult dysraphisms include myelocystocele; diastematomyelia-diplomyelia; meningocele-lipomeningocele; lipoma, teratoma, and other tumors; dermal sinus with or without dermoid or epidermoid cyst formation; and tethered cord (Anderson, 1975; Menkes, 1991) (Fig. 63–8). More severe lesions include neurenteric cyst, anterior meningocele, and the caudal regression syndrome (dysraphia of sacrum and coccyx, atrophy of muscles and bones of the legs, fusion of spinal nerves and sensory ganglia, and/or agenesis of the distal spinal cord) (Towfighi and Housman, 1991). Infants of diabetic mothers are at increased risk for these lesions as well as for more severe neural tube defects (Becerra et al, 1990).

Regardless of the caudal neural tube malformation, an almost invariable feature is an abnormal conus with a thickened filum. The movement of the filum is commonly restricted or "tethered" by fibrous bands or masses (e.g., a lipoma or teratoma). Consequently, during growth of the lower spinal cord, progressive functional impairment can occur as the cord is stretched against the fixed filum. Neurologic impairment rarely manifests in the newborn period. Deficits related to these lesions that occur in infancy and childhood include delay in walking, disturbed sphincter control, anatomic abnormalities of the feet or legs, and pain in the back or legs. Gait and sphincter abnormalities, foot deformities, and scoliosis are more common in older patients. Recurrent meningitis and rapid loss of function are rare but serious presentations. In the newborn period, diagnostic evaluation for occult dysraphisms is indicated because early surgical intervention now carries a low risk of morbidity and can preclude sudden neurologic deterioration and the development of permanent deficits (Gower et al, 1988; Scatliff et al, 1989). Such evaluation may be facilitated by spinal radiography or CT, which may detect vertebral anomalies; spinal ultrasonography, which permits a dynamic evaluation of lower spinal cord mobility; and MRI to define structural anomalies of the cord.

## Disorders of Neural Crest Migration

As the neural tube closes during weeks 3 to 4 of gestation, the neural crest cells become isolated between the neural tube and the posterior ectoderm (Reznik and Pierard, 1995). This layer differentiates into cephalic and truncal neural crests. The cephalic neural crest forms the trigeminal neural crest, the facial-auditory neural crest, and the glossopharyngeal and vagal neural crest. These structures give rise to the cranial nerves and their sensory ganglia as well as to parts of the branchial arches (Reznik and Pierard, 1995). The truncal neural crest becomes fragmented along with the truncal somites. After the neural crest anlagen

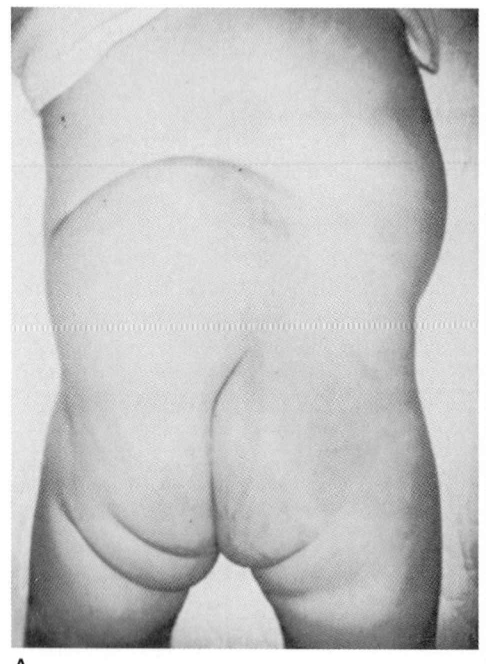
A

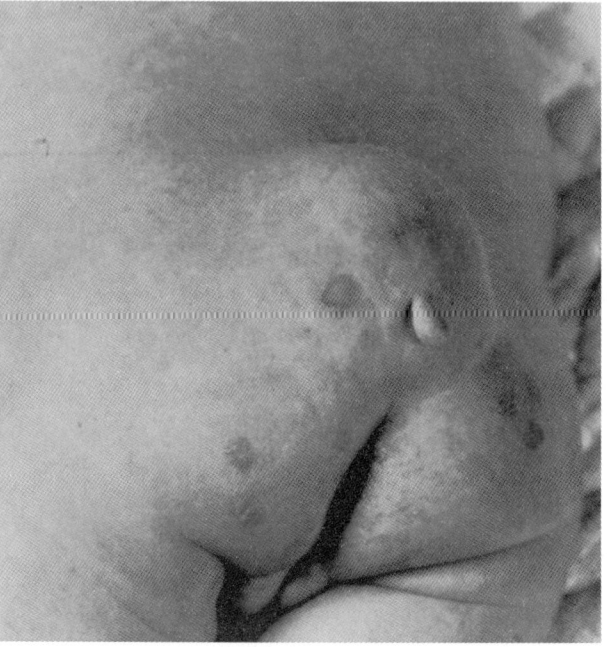
B

**FIGURE 63–7.** **A** and **B,** Two examples of lipomeningocele. Each manifested in the left buttock as a firm, well-circumscribed, lobulated tumor that became tense when the infant cried. Over the surface of the lesion in **B** are some macular erosions and a congenital skin tag and dimple. This last feature may be a pilonidal dimple displaced by the tumor.

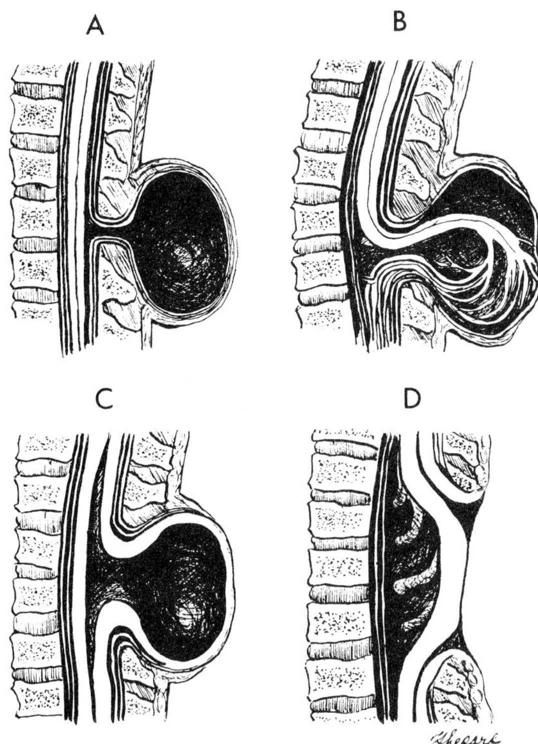


**FIGURE 63–8.** Diagram of meningoceles. **A,** Meningocele: Through the bone defect (spina bifida), the meninges herniate to form a cystic sac filled with cerebrospinal fluid. The spinal cord does not participate in the herniation and may or may not be abnormal. **B,** Myelomeningocele. Spina bifida with myelomeningocele; the spinal cord is herniated into the sac and ends there or may continue in an abnormal way further downward. **C,** Myelocystocele or syringomyelocele: The spinal cord shows hydromyelia; the posterior wall of the spinal cord is attached to the ectoderm and undifferentiated. **D,** Myelocele: The spinal cord is araphic; a cystic cavity is in front of the anterior wall of the spinal cord. *(From Benda CE: Developmental Disorders of Mentation and Cerebral Palsies. New York, Grune & Stratton, 1952.)*

is formed, neural crest cells migrate throughout the entire embryo. Migration is rostrocaudal, along the medial axis of the embryo (LeDouarin, 1982). After migration is accomplished, the neural crest cells are located in four areas: (1) nervous system: meningioblasts, Schwann cells, ganglion and paraganglion cells (including enteric ganglion cells of the digestive tract); (2) endocrine system: chromaffin cells of the adrenal medulla and several types of endocrine and paraendocrine cells; (3) melanoblasts in all tissues except the retina; and (4) the skeletal system of the head, face, and neck. Abnormalities thus can arise with the migration or differentiation of the neural crest cells, or neural crest derivatives may develop tumors (Jacobson, 1991; Reznik and Pierard, 1995).

Disorders thought to arise from abnormalities of neural crest formation, migration, proliferation, or differentiation include the LEOPARD (*l*entigines, *e*lectrocardiographic abnormalities, *o*cular hypertelorism, *p*ulmonary stenosis, *a*bnormal genitalia, *r*etardation of growth, *d*eafness) syndrome; multiple lentigines syndrome; NAME (*n*evi, *a*trial myxoma, *m*yxoid neuroma, *e*phelides) syndrome; LAMB (*l*entigines, *a*trial myxoma, *m*ucocutaneous myxomas, *b*lue nevi) syndrome; and Peutz-Jeghers-Touraine syndrome (Table 63–2).

Tumors derived from neural crest cells include those arising from Schwann cells, perineural cells, or fibrocytes; from neural sense organs; from ganglionic or neuroendocrine cells; and from melanogenic cells (Louis and von Deimling, 1995; Reznik and Pierard, 1995). Neuroblastoma is a neuroectodermal tumor that occurs mostly in children. It usually arises from the adrenal gland but can arise from sympathetic ganglia, the neuroendocrine system, or the ovary (Reznik and Pierard, 1995). It is sometimes seen in association with neurofibromatosis. Cutaneous metastases from neuroblastoma can occur as multiple skin nodules and have been seen in the newborn.

Hirschsprung disease is a disorder of neural crest stem cells that occurs in 1 in 5000 births. It is characterized by absence of hindgut intramural ganglion cells, which causes intestinal obstruction in the neonatal period. A gene associated with some cases of Hirschsprung disease has been mapped to chromosome 10 and localized to the *RET* proto-oncogene (Edery et al, 1994; Romeo et al, 1994; Yin et al, 1994). Mutations that affect the RET protein also occur in patients with multiple endocrine neoplasia type 2A (Donis-Keller et al, 1993; Mulligan et al, 1993).

## PROSENCEPHALIC CLEAVAGE AND RELATED EVENTS

### Normal Prosencephalic Development

The prosencephalon refers embryologically to the telencephalon and the diencephalon, the future forebrain. The telencephalon gives rise to the cerebral hemispheres. The diencephalon gives rise to the thalamus and hypothalamus. The major period for prosencephalic development is during the second and third months of gestation. The beginning of prosencephalic development occurs shortly after the closure of the anterior neuropore. The prosencephalon essentially arises through developmental processes that induce the bifurcation of the rostal extent of the fluid-filled neural tube to form the right and left forebrain structures (Rubenstein and Beachy, 1998). This process involves the duplication of structures along the midline. It should be emphasized that the inductive processes that direct forebrain development also control craniofacial development. Hence, disruption of prosencephalic development is frequently associated with midline anomalies of both the forebrain and the face that result from a failure to cleave the neural tube.

During the fifth to sixth weeks of development, the ultimate structure of the forebrain is defined by the sequential cleavage of the forebrain along three major planes. As the anterior neuropore is closing, the first major event is formation of the optic vesicles and nasal placodes, separated along the *horizontal* plane, which will give rise to the neural and craniofacial structures of the visual and olfactory systems, respectively. Shortly thereafter, when the embryo has reached a length of about 5 mm, both neuropores have closed, thus isolating the developing ventricular system from the amniotic fluid. At this time, the retinal and lens placodes are developing. Separately, in the brainstem, the cerebellum begins to

**TABLE 63–2**

**Disorders of Neural Crest Formation, Migration, Proliferation, or Differentiation**

| Syndrome/ Disorder | Defining Features | | | | | | |
|---|---|---|---|---|---|---|---|
| LEOPARD | Multiple lentigines | Electrocardiographic defects | Ocular hypertelorism | Pulmonary stenosis | Genital abnormalities | Growth retardation | Sensorineural deafness |
| Multiple lentigines | Cutaneous pigmented macules | Obstructive cardiomyopathy | Genital abnormalities | Delayed puberty | Sensorineural hearing loss | Hypertelorism and skeletal abnormalities | Growth retardation |
| NAME | Cutaneous nevi | Atrial myxoma | Myxoid neurofibromas | Ephelides | | | |
| LAMB | Lentigines | Atrial myxoma | Mucocutaneous myxoma | Blue nevi | | | |
| Peutz-Jeghers-Touraine | Mucocutaneous lentigines | Gastrointestinal polyposis | Schwannoma of the gut; acoustic neurinomas | Increased risk of malignancies | | | |

form at this time, as well as some somatic and visceral efferent nuclei, the common afferent tract, and the ganglia for most of the cranial nerves.

At about day 32 of gestation, when the embryo is 5 to 7 mm long, the second major event in forebrain development occurs when the forebrain is cleaved in the *sagittal* plane to give rise to the paired cerebral hemispheres, lateral ventricles, and basal ganglia. Specific areas, such as the hypothalamic, amygdaloid, hippocampal, and olfactory regions, can be defined. Shortly thereafter, the third major event in forebrain development occurs when the forebrain is cleaved in the *coronal* or *transverse* plane to separate the telencephalon from the diencephalon, thus defining the epithalamus, subthalamus, and hypothalamus.

During the remainder of the second and third months of gestation, the subsequent events in forebrain development occur along the midline to generate three major structures: the corpus callosum, the optic nerve/chiasm, and the hypothalamus. Disturbances in the formation of these midline structures, in particular, the corpus callosum and the optic chiasm, are reflected in abnormal axon "path-finding" to the midline and the failure of hemispheric and optic fibers to cross to the opposite hemisphere.

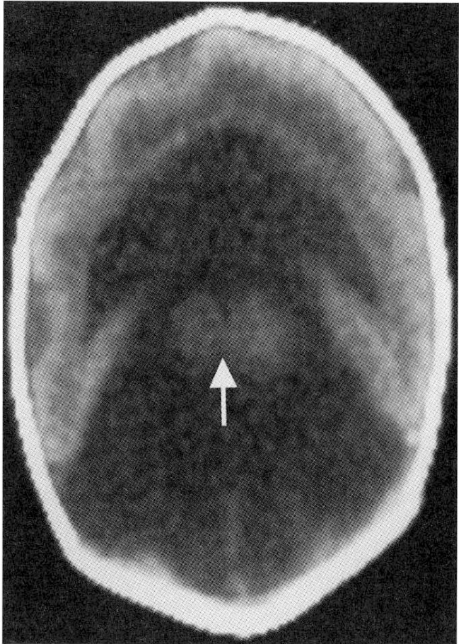

**FIGURE 63–9.** Holoprosencephaly: Computed tomography scan. Note the single central ventricular cavity with no division of the hemispheres. There is agenesis of the corpus callosum, and the thalami are fused *(arrow)*. *(Courtesy of Dr. Thomas Koch, Department of Pediatrics, Oregon Health & Science University.)*

## Disorders of Structures Derived from the Prosencephalon

### Holoprosencephaly

Holoprosencephaly is the most common human brain malformation (Barr and Cohen, 1999; Norman et al, 1995a). It has a prevalence of 1/250 in the developing embryo and occurs in 1 in 10,000 to 1 in 20,000 live births. This defect involves a variable degree of incomplete cleavage of the prosencephalon along one or more of its three major planes. The spectrum includes alobar, semilobar, and lobar types. All three types have the unifying diagnostic feature of a single ventricle that is readily visualized by cranial ultrasonography, CT, or MRI (Fig. 63–9). In *alobar* holoprosencephaly (Fig. 63–10), a single anterior ventricle is contained within a holosphere (i.e., there is a complete lack of separation of the prosencephalon into two distinct hemispheres, manifesting as the absence of the interhemispheric fissure). There is agenesis of the corpus callosum, the thalami usually are fused, and the basal ganglia are a single mass. Milder presentations involve partially formed hemispheres—*semilobar* holoprosencephaly—and *lobar* forms in which the distinct hemispheres can be distinguished. Arhinencephaly, absence of the olfactory bulbs and tracts, always accompanies holoprosencephaly but can exist as an isolated lesion, in which case it usually is found incidentally at autopsy. Craniofacial anomalies range from cyclopia (a single central eye) with a nose-like structure (proboscis) above the eye, to cebocephaly (a flattened single nostril situated centrally between the eyes), to median cleft lip. Mildly affected infants may display a single central incisor or hypotelorism. Survival correlates with the severity of the brain malformations. Severely affected infants often are stillborn or rarely survive beyond the first year of life.

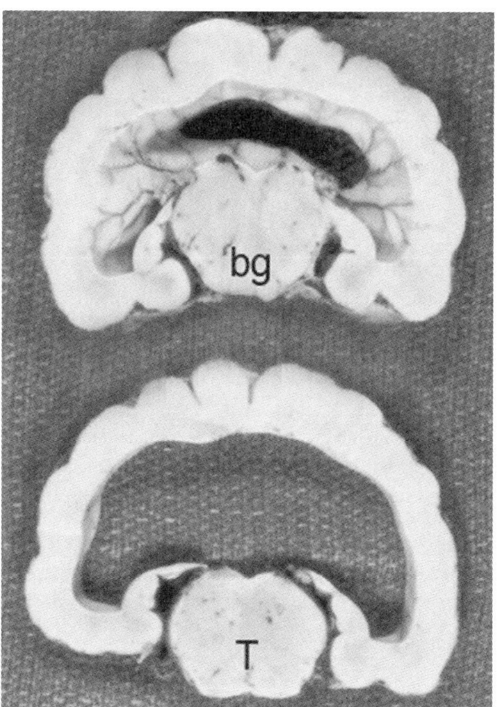


**FIGURE 63–10.** Alobar holoprosencephaly. Coronal sections demonstrate a single anterior ventricle. Note the complete lack of separation of the forebrain into two distinct hemispheres. There is agenesis of the corpus callosum, the basal ganglia are a single mass (bg), and the thalami (T) usually are fused. *(Courtesy of Dr. Marjorie Grafe, Department of Pathology, Oregon Health & Science University.)*

### Clinical Features

The degree of neurologic impairment is variable and directly reflects the severity of the cerebral malformation. In general, less severe pathology is associated with milder clinical deficits. These may include frequent apneic episodes that occur in association with intractable epilepsy or stimulus-sensitive tonic spasms. Autonomic dysfunction can manifest as temperature instability and hypothermia. Electrolyte dyscrasias, particularly hypernatremia or hyponatremia, occur in the setting of diabetes insipidus or inappropriate secretion of antidiuretic hormone, or both (Hasegawa et al, 1990). Failure to thrive occurs in association with impaired suck and swallow and may necessitate nasogastric or gastric tube feeding. Abnormalities of other organ systems, particularly cardiac, genitourinary, and gastrointestinal, occur commonly, even in cases without chromosomal anomalies.

Microcephaly is the norm. The spectrum of cognitive impairment correlates with the severity of the brain malformations. Less severely affected infants may display an apparently normal repertoire of behaviors, but closer examination reveals that these are often stereotypic and not stimulus-sensitive. Primitive reflexes may be persistent as well, and a social smile fails to develop.

### Etiology and Epidemiology

The etiology of holoprosencephaly clearly is multifactorial, and both genetic and environmental factors appear to contribute to the extremely variable spectrum of forebrain and craniofacial malformations (Golden, 1998; Muenke and Beachy, 2000; Norman et al, 1995a). It has been appreciated for over a century that a wide variety of environmental insults (e.g., ethanol, vitamin A toxicity related to elevated retinoic acid levels) applied experimentally can produce cyclopia during the early phase of gastrulation in vertebrate embryos. Maternal diabetes mellitus increases the risk for holoprosencephaly about 200-fold, to approximately 1% to 2% of all pregnancies.

The most common chromosomal disorders that manifest with holoprosencephaly are trisomies 13 and 18. At least 25 rare genetic syndromes are associated with holoprosencephaly and account for roughly 15% to 25% of cases. The most notable are the Smith-Lemli-Opitz, Rubenstein-Taybi, and Pallister-Hall syndromes (Muenke and Beachy, 2000), because the specific defects in these syndromes all appear to be related in part to disturbances in signaling via the Sonic hedgehog (Shh) pathway, discussed later on.

Holoprosencephaly is characterized by extreme intrafamilial variability. Asymptomatic or mildly affected family members may carry a deletion for a gene associated with holoprosencephaly, whereas in a subsequent generation, offspring with the same gene may be severely affected. One explanation for these paradoxical observations comes from recent studies supporting that the mode of inheritance for holoprosencephaly is most compatible with multigenic transmission (Ming and Muenke, 2002). Several mouse models of holoprosencephaly exist in which mutations in two distinct genes are required, whereas a mutation in only one gene results in an apparently normal phenotype. Several affected patients have been identified in whom abnormal alleles for two separate genes were identified. Of interest, in these cases, a phenotypically normal parent carried a mutation for one gene but not the other (Nanni et al, 1999; Roessler et al, 1996). Hence, the severity of expression of the holoprosencephaly phenotype throughout a given family may be influenced by the additive contributions from multiple environmental/teratogenic and genetic factors, which may be weighted differently in each affected family member.

### Related Molecular Genetic Events

It was recognized decades ago that experimental ablation of the prechordal mesoderm, a mesodermal cell group under the ventral forebrain, disrupted the formation of the chiasmatic plate and optic vesicles and produced cyclopia. It was proposed that the prechordal plate induced the formation of ventral forebrain structures and directed the segmentation of the developing optic fields. Only recently has this complex picture begun to be clarified by the identification of eight genes expressed in the prechordal plate that directly or indirectly regulate the development of the ventral forebrain. All of these genes were identified in chromosomal regions with known deletions associated with holoprosencephaly. The complexity of the signaling pathways that regulates prosencephalic development is suggested by the fact that mutations in these eight genes account for only approximately 15% to 20% of the holoprosencephaly cases studied with normal karyotypes.

Sonic hedgehog (Shh) is a signaling molecule secreted in the prechordal mesoderm that directs early embryonic patterning of the ventral forebrain. Mutations of the gene for Shh were the first identified to cause human holoprosencephaly (Nanni et al, 1999; Roessler et al, 1996). *SHH* mutations appear to occur more frequently than do mutations of other genes and have been identified in both sporadic and familial cases. Subsequently, mutations in other genes in the Shh signaling pathway also were identified, underscoring the importance of defects in Shh signaling in the pathogenesis of holoprosencephaly (Muenke and Beachy, 2000). These include mutations in the receptor for Shh (Patched) and in the Gli family of zinc finger transcription factor that mediate Shh signaling downstream of the Patched receptor. Mutations in *GLI3* are associated with human disease.

The signaling activity of Shh is regulated both by initial enzymatic processing of a precursor protein and by lipid modifications that involve the coupling of cholesterol and palmitate to Shh. The role of these lipid modifications is unclear, but they may serve to limit the diffusion of Shh, thereby controlling the sites in the embryonic ventral forebrain where Shh biologic actions occur. The importance of these lipid modifications is suggested by an apparent association between holoprosencephaly and some cases of Smith-Lemli-Opitz syndrome, which arises from a defect in the terminal step in cholesterol biosynthesis (7-dehydrocholesterol reductase); approximately 5% of cases of this syndrome manifest with cerebral malformations in the spectrum of holoprosencephaly. Of interest, two plant alkaloids—cyclopamine and jervine—have been identified that caused epidemics of cyclopia in sheep that ingested plants rich in these compounds. Both compounds alter Shh signaling pathway by inhibition of cholesterol biosynthesis. Such findings support that the interactions of multiple environmental/teratogenic and genetic variables are likely to account for the considerable heterogeneity in the phenotypic expression of holoprosencephaly within families and populations.

## Agenesis of the Corpus Callosum

Although sometimes found at autopsy as an incidental finding in otherwise asymptomatic persons, agenesis of the corpus callosum is not a discrete entity (Fig. 63–11). Rather, it is a nonspecific feature of at least 70 conditions and is associated with a wide variety of CNS malformations (Norman et al, 1995a). The corpus callosum is absent, for example, in alobar holoprosencepaly. Agenesis of the corpus callosum frequently is found in association with abnormalities of chromosomes 8, 11, 13 to 15, and 18 (Jeret et al, 1987). Agenesis of the corpus callosum also is variably found in fetal alcohol syndrome, Dandy-Walker syndrome, and Leigh disease and in association with the Arnold-Chiari type II malformation. Other CNS lesions are common in patients with agenesis of the corpus callosum (occurring in 29% to 80% of such patients) (Jeret et al, 1987; Parrish et al, 1979).

Agenesis of the corpus callosum may be difficult to distinguish from conditions in which dysgenesis, hypoplasia, or destructive lesions have occurred. The anatomic features of true agenesis of the corpus callosum include abnormal gyration of the medial portion of each hemisphere, eversion of the cingulate gyri, and sulcation that is perpendicular to the long axis of the hemisphere (Barkovich and Norman, 1988). The external angles of the lateral ventricle are oriented parallel and upward, toward the vertex, and the fornices are widely separated (Fig. 63–12). When present, a useful distinguishing feature is Probst's bundles, which are fiber bundles that run parallel to the ventricle and carry callosal fibers in an anterior-to-posterior direction. Agenesis of the corpus callosum can be total or partial; when it is partial, the splenium is involved, and the genu remains intact (Roessmann, 1995; Schaefer, 1991). Other, less frequently associated pathologic findings are neuronal migration abnormalities (neuronal heterotopias, lissencephaly, pachygryia, and schizencephaly), hydrocephalus related to ventricular obstruction by a midline dorsal cyst of the third ventricle (Jeret et al, 1987) and tumors (Tagawa et al, 1989).

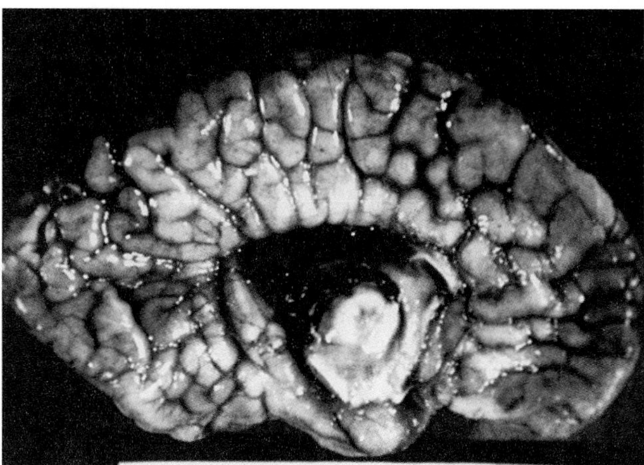

**FIGURE 63–11.** Agenesis of the corpus callosum. *(Courtesy of Dr. Dawna L. Armstrong, Department of Pathology, Texas Children's Hospital.)*

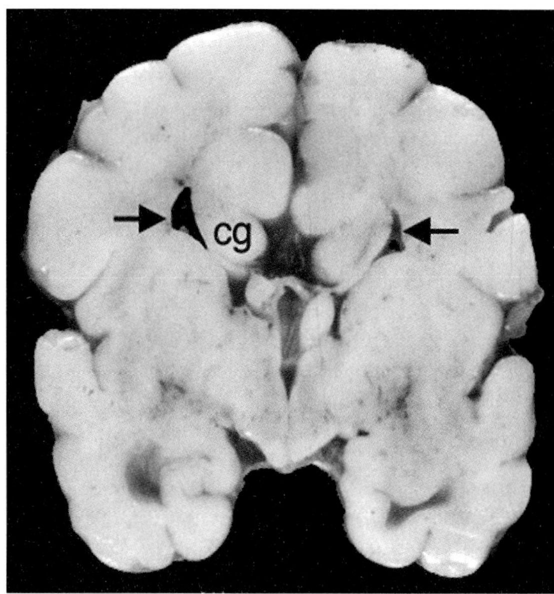


**FIGURE 63–12.** Agenesis of the corpus callosum. Note the eversion of both of the cingulate gyri (cg). The lateral ventricles are oriented parallel and pointed upward toward the vertex *(arrows)*. Probst's bundles are not apparent in this immature brain. *(Courtesy of Dr. Marjorie Grafe, Department of Pathology, Oregon Health & Science University.)*

Four syndromes are characterized by agenesis of the corpus callosum: Aicardi, acrocallosal, Andermann, and Shapiro syndromes (Jeret et al, 1987). The Aicardi syndrome is notable for the association of complete or partial agenesis of the corpus callosum with severe epilepsy, mental retardation, and ocular lesions (optic coloboma, micro-opthalmia, chorioretinal lacunae) in girls (Aicardi et al, 1965). The inheritance pattern is proposed as X-linked dominant, with lethality in males. Nonrandom X-inactivation in lymphocytes has been noted to correlate with the severity of the neurologic symptoms (Neidich et al, 1990). The prominence of intractable seizure types, particularly infantile spasms, is related to neuronal migration abnormalities. These are primarily periventricular nodular heterotopias and polymicrogyria.

## Agenesis of the Septum Pellucidum and Septo-optic Dysplasia

Agenesis of the septum pellucidum frequently acompanies optic nerve hypoplasia and agenesis or thinning of the corpus callosum (Mott et al, 1992; Williams et al, 1993). This triad, known as *septo-optic dysplasia*, is clinically associated with pituitary dwarfism and other forms of hypothalamic-pituitary dysfunction. Although agenesis of the septum pellucidum is never an isolated finding, optic nerve hypoplasia can occur unilaterally or bilaterally without other associated lesions (Barkovich and Norman, 1989; Ouvrier and Billson, 1986; Zeki et al, 1992). Frequently, other cerebral abnormalities are present, including schizencephaly and absence of the pituitary infundibulum. Children with septo-optic dysplasia are blind or have reduced vision and nystagmus. Their neurodevelopmental prognosis has been controversial. In earlier studies, cerebral palsy was found in 57%, mental retardation in 71%, epilepsy in 37%, and behavior problems in 20% of children with septo-optic dysplasia (Acers, 1981; Margalith et al, 1984). A more recent neurodevelopmental study of seven children with unilateral or bilateral optic nerve hypoplasia, whose only other documentable CNS abnormality was absence of the septum pellucidum, found normal cognitive development, intact neurologic status, normal language development, and age-appropriate behavior in six of the seven (Williams et al, 1993). Thus, the abnormalities found in many patients with septo-optic dysplasia are probably due to other associated brain lesions.

The cavum septi pellucidi is an opening formed by the separation of the lamellae of the septum pellucidum; the lamellae fuse as the fetal brain matures. The cavum septi pellucidi may persist into extrauterine life, especially in preterm infants. Mott and associates (1992) have documented the presence of a cavum septi pellucidi in all infants born at less than 36 weeks of gestation routinely studied by cranial sonographic examination. A cavum septi pellucidi was present in 36% of term newborns in the series reported by these investigators.

## DEVELOPMENT OF POSTERIOR FOSSA STRUCTURES

### Normal Hindbrain Development

Malformations of the posterior fossa constitute an embryologically diverse group of disorders. Because these disorders frequently are associated with compromise to vital functions of the brainstem, clinical management may focus on concerns for apnea and hydrocephalus, for example. Controversies will undoubtedly persist regarding the appropriate classification of these disorders until such time as the molecular genetic basis is further resolved.

The onset of development of posterior fossa structures occurs shortly after closure of the neural tube and coincides with the onset of prosencephalic development. At this time, the primary brain vesicles of the primitive hindbrain (rhombencephalon) emerge distal to the prosencephalon along an anterior-posterior axis. The midbrain derives from the mesencephalon and is embryologically distinct from the rhombencephalon, from which the major hindbrain structures derive (cerebellum, pons [metencephalon], and medulla [myelencephalon]). At 3 to 5 weeks of gestation, the rhombencephalon can be identified between the cranial and cervical flexures of the neural tube. Eight distinct rhombomeres have been defined in the rhombencephalon. Rhombomere 1 gives rise to the cerebellum, and rhombomeres 2 to 8 give rise to the pons, medulla, and cranial nerves V to X.

## Malformations with Major Cerebellar Involvement

### Dandy-Walker Malformation

Of the cerebellar malformations associated with significant posterior fossa CSF collections, the protoype is the Dandy-Walker malformation (DWM). A number of other posterior fossa malformations share similar embryologic derivatives or similar anatomic features with DWM (Fig. 63–13). These include several syndromes of cerebellar vermis hypoplasia and dysplasia, syndromes that involve diffuse cerebellar hypoplasia, and syndromes with normal cerebellar size and architecture but with a large posterior fossa fluid collection that does not communicate with the fourth ventricle (e.g., mega cisterna magna, arachnoid cyst) (Altman et al, 1992; Niesen, 2002; Parisi and Dobyns, 2003; Patel and Barkovich, 2002). Moreover, numerous chromosomal anomalies, such as trisomies 9, 13 and 18, manifest with DWM. This malformation also has been described in association with a variety of genetic syndromes. One such is the Walker-Warburg syndrome,

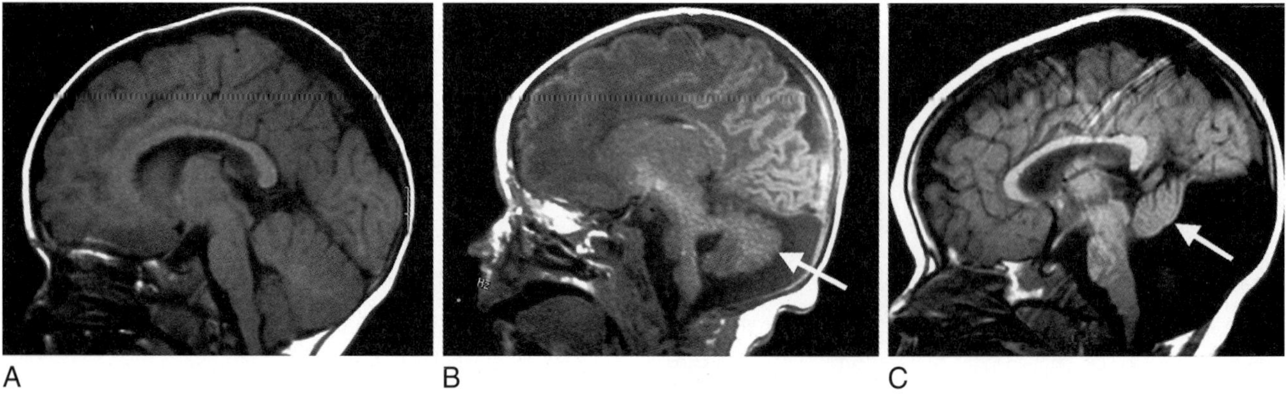


**FIGURE 63–13.** Dandy-Walker malformation (DWM). Sagittal magnetic resonance images (MRI) from a normal brain (**A**), a child with Joubert syndrome (**B**), and a child with DWM (**C**) illustrate that features of the hindbrain malformations seen in DWM overlap with those of other disorders. Note the presence of cerebellar vermis hypoplasia *(arrow)* in both **B** and **C**. By contrast, the patient with Joubert syndrome (**B**) has only a slightly enlarged fourth ventricle, whereas in DWM (**C**) the fourth ventricle is massively dilated. *(Courtesy of Dr. Joseph G. Gleeson, Department of Neurology, University of California, San Diego, School of Medicine; and Dr. William B. Dobyns, The University of Chicago School of Medicine.)*

which is characterized by not only extensive brainstem and cerebellar hypoplasia but also ocular anomalies, congenital muscular dystrophy, cortical migration abnormalities, and encephalocele. These associations have led to a variety of attempts for unifying classification schemes under the rubric of "DWM and its variants." Because the molecular mechanisms that underlie these malformations are mostly unknown, there is currently no basis for linking them as a spectrum. It should be emphasized that a more unfavorable outcome is related to the extent of other posterior fossa and CNS malformations. Hence, when "DWM" is diagnosed, the prenatal and postnatal management and prognosis depends on precise definition of the particular anatomic abnormalities present. High-resolution MRI is particularly valuable for definition of associated CNS malformations. The most clinically significant defects are agenesis of the corpus callosum and cerebral neuronal migration disturbances (polymicrogyria and heterotopias).

Precise estimates of the incidence of DWM are clearly affected by the lack of agreement regarding the definition of DWM. Nevertheless, DWM appears to occur in at least 1 in 5000 live born infants (Parisi and Dobyns, 2003). The invariant features of DWM are aplasia or hypoplasia of the vermis of the cerebellum, cystic dilation of the fourth ventricle, and enlargement of the posterior fossa with upward displacement of the lateral sinuses, tentorium, and torcular (Benda, 1954; D'Agostino, 1963; Friede, 1989; Hart et al, 1972). The enlargement of the posterior fossa and displacement of its contents are related to communication of the fourth ventricle with a retrocerebellar cyst, which may be of considerable size. Communicating hydrocephalus with dilated lateral ventricles also is a common feature and may manifest in the neonatal period with macrocephaly. In fact, a majority of cases of DWM manifest with symptoms related to hydrocephalus (Costa and Hauw, 1995; Hart et al, 1972). There is no general agreement regarding the optimal management of hydrocephalus in DWM, which usually involves some combination of ventricular or posterior fossa shunt placement. Other prominent pathoneurologic features include ataxia, nystagmus, apnea, cranial neuropathies, and developmental delay.

### Syndromes Associated with the Molar Tooth Sign

Abnormalities of the cerebellum also are found in Joubert syndrome, which is the most extensively studied of several uncommon autosomal recessive cerebello-oculorenal syndromes associated with the molar tooth sign (MTS) (Parisi and Dobyns, 2002). The cerebellar lesion usually involves complete or partial agenesis of the vermis (see Fig. 63-13B), but there may also be dysplasia of the dentate nucleus, cerebellar heterotopias, anomalies of brainstem nuclei, and absence of decussation of the pyramidal tracts (Curatolo et al, 1980). The lesion responsible for the MTS is defined as the triad of cerebellar vermis hypoplasia and two mid–hind brain malformations (an abnormally deep interpeduncular fossa and elongated cerebellar peduncles). When viewed on axial MRI studies (Fig. 63–14), the brainstem malformations have the distinctive appearance of a molar tooth. The most prominent clinical features of Joubert syndrome are hypotonia, abnormal eye movements (horizontal nystagmus and oculomotor apraxia), ataxia, abnormal breathing patterns (periods of hyperpnea alternating with apnea), and cognitive delays/mental retardation (Joubert et al, 1969). Variable features of Joubert syndrome include occipital encephalocele, microcephaly, low-set ears, polydactyly, and pigmentary retinopathy (Egger et al, 1982; Friede and Boltshauser, 1978). Renal disease in Joubert syndrome includes cystic dysplasia of the kidneys and juvenile nephronophthisis. The latter is a form of medullary cystic renal disease that progresses to chronic renal failure (Satran et al, 1999).

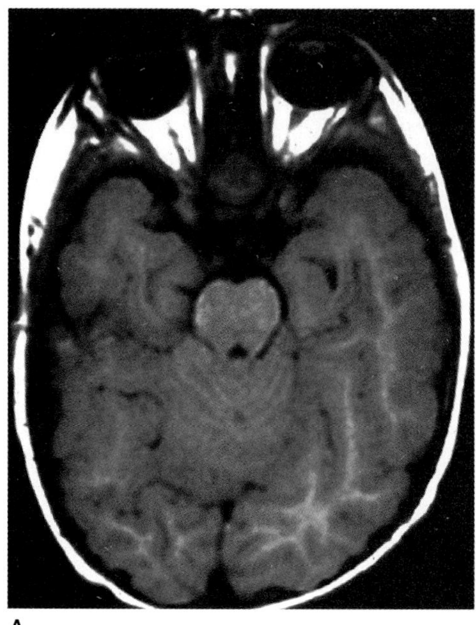
A

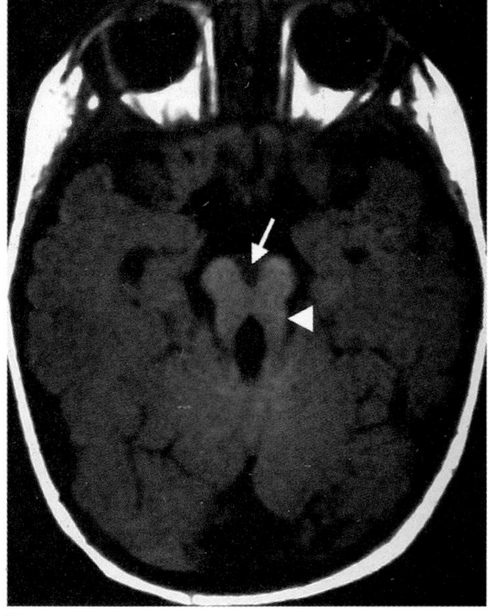
B

**FIGURE 63–14.** Molar tooth sign (MTS). Compare the axial magnetic resonance image of a normal brain (**A**) with that of the brain of a child with Joubert syndrome (**B**). Note two key features of the MTS: a deepened interpeduncular fossa *(arrow)* and the elongated superior cerebellar peduncles *(arrowhead)*. The third feature, cerebellar vermis hypoplasia, is seen in Figure 63–13B. *(Courtesy of Dr. Joseph G. Gleeson, Department of Neurology, University of California, San Diego, School of Medicine.)*

## CENTRAL NERVOUS SYSTEM DEVELOPMENT IN THE POSTEMBRYONIC PERIOD

### Normal Development of the Cortical Plate

#### *Proliferative Events*

Four transient tangential layers form during the process of cerebral cortical development. From the ventricle to the brain surface, these layers are the ventricular, subventricular, intermediate, and marginal zones. Initially, the nascent cortical plate derives from the *ventricular zone* (VZ). The VZ is the site of earliest proliferation of neuronal and radial glial progenitor cells in the wall of the neural tube. As the cerebral wall expands, the *subventricular zone* becomes a secondary site of later neuronal and glial proliferation. These proliferative events occur roughly between 4 and 16 weeks of gestation. Peak cell proliferation occurs around 8 to 16 weeks. This coincides with the appearance and expansion of the cortical plate, which appears when the embryo is about 22 to 24 mm long, at about 52 days.

The initial cycles of neural progenitor profileration in the VZ result in the symmetrical expansion of the stem cell pool such that each mitotic event results in the generation of two additional stem cells (Caviness et al, 1995; Rakic, 1995). This process determines the total pool of stem cells, or so-called proliferative units, from which the cortical plate will form. Once the generation of this stem cell pool stabilizes, a second phase of proliferation begins during which individual stem cell clones begin to divide asymmetrically. During this phase of clonal expansion, each mitotic division generates an additional stem cell and another neuronal cell that withdraws from the cell cycle. The latter postmitotic neuron then begins migration from the VZ to the outer wall of the neural tube. Hence, this second phase of asymmetrical cell division results in the expansion of each individual stem cell clone or proliferative unit. Eventually, this phase results in a proportionately larger number of postmitotic cells that all derive from the same proliferative unit.

#### *Migrational Events*

Rakic (1998) first proposed that the postmitotic neurons that derive from an individual clonal population in the VZ migrate together along the same radial glial fiber to generate individual columns of cells within the cortical plate. The radial glial processes extend from the VZ to the outer wall of the neural tube and serve as a scaffold to guide the migration of individual clones of postmitotic neurons to form the preplate. Migration of neurons from the VZ occurs in an "outside-in" fashion, such that the neurons farthest from the ventricle migrate first and those closest to the ventricle migrate last.

As neuronal migration proceeds, the preplate is split by the arrival of subsequent populations of neuronal progenitors that will form the cortical plate. The cortical plate ultimately gives rise to cortical layers IIB to IV. The splitting of the preplate results in the formation of the *marginal zone* (future cortical layer I) and the subplate, which resides between the *intermediate zone* (the future cerebral white matter) and the bottom of the cortical plate (Marin-Padilla, 1988, 1998). The Cajal-Retzius neurons of the marginal zone and the subplate neurons play critical roles in neuronal migrations, as discussed later.

As neuronal migration progresses, each subsequent group of neurons migrates past the neurons that migrated earlier. Hence, the earliest neurons to migrate eventually reside in the deepest cortical layer. Because the last neurons to migrate are closest to layer 1, the cortical layers are thereby formed in an "inside-out" sequence. The major events involved in formation of the cortical layers are occurring between approximately 7 and 11 weeks.

#### *Subplate Neurons and Establishment of Thalamocortical Connections*

As emphasized previously, the cortical plate develops from within the preplate. The preplate consists of the earliest-generated neurons and a plexus of nerve fibers. With subsequent waves of neuronal migration, the preplate is split into the marginal zone (i.e., a superplate) and a subplate. Hence, the cells in these layers are among the earliest-generated neurons. In the second trimester, two subcortical afferent systems are present in the subplate (Allendoerfer and Shatz, 1994): thalamocortical fibers and basal forebrain fibers, which remain in the subcortical region for a period of time before their fibers penetrate the cortical plate. The neurons of layer IV in the cortex receive their predominant ascending inputs from the thalamus. Of interest, however, the thalamic axons are present in the cortex long before the layer IV neurons have reached the cortical plate. These axons reside in the subplate for a period of weeks in proximity to postmitotic neurons in the subplate. Most of these early-maturing subplate neurons undergo programmed cell death after the thalamic axons have grown into the cortical plate (Chun et al, 1987).

Hence, subplate neurons transiently appear during a critical window in development, and few are present in the adult neocortex. In humans, the subplate achieves its peak size by 24 weeks of gestational age and declines thereafter (Kostovic and Rakic, 1990). The hypothesis that these subplate neurons play a critical role in thalamocortical development by guiding thalamic axons into the cortical plate has been substantiated by studies showing that deletion of the early subplate neurons prevents the thalamic axons from innervating the cortex. Thus, the transient subplate neurons play an important role in establishing both thalamocortical and corticocortical connections (Ghosh et al, 1990; Kanold et al, 2003).

## Disorders of Neuronal Proliferation

### Micrencephaly

*Micrencephaly* is a disorder in which the primary defect is a marked reduction in the size of the brain or of the cerebral hemispheres. *Microcephaly* denotes a small cranial vault (less than 2 standard deviations below normative curves for age) that is associated with either micrencephaly or acquired brain atrophy (e.g., multicystic encephalopathy, hydranencephaly, diffuse cortical atrophy). Until recently, micrencephaly was considered to be an isolated defect of either decreased neuronal proliferation or increased apoptosis (programmed cell death). Representative examples are radial microbrain and "microencephaly vera," discussed next (Evrard et al, 1989; Rakic, 1988). However, MRI studies have begun to define greater heterogeneity in the types of malformations that are associated with micrencephaly (Barkovich et al, 2001). Associated malformations include simplified gyral patterns, microlissencephaly with thickened cortical gray matter, and polymicrogyria (Barkovich et al, 1998; Peiffer et al, 1999; Sztriha et al, 1998). The association of micrencephaly with features of cortical neuronal migration abnormalities suggests overlap in the mechanisms that direct neuronal proliferation and migration in humans.

Two subgroups of isolated micrencephaly, *radial microbrain* and *"micrencephaly vera,"* provide insight into mechanisms of isolated disturbances of neuronal proliferation. Radial microbrain appears to be related to a reduced number of proliferative units. By contrast, "microencephaly vera" appears to be related to a reduced size of proliferative units (Evrard et al, 1989; Rakic, 1988). Radial microbrain is a rare familial condition characterized by a normal gyral and cortical lamination pattern but an abnormal number of cortical neuronal columns. Because the number of cells per column is normal, this implies that the defect resides in early neural stem cell division with an impact on the ultimate number of "proliferative units" available to generate the cortical columns.

"Micrencephaly vera" describes a variety of conditions with small brain size in which the underyling etiology may be related to a disturbance in neuronal proliferation. Cases of autosomal recessive "micrencephaly vera" demonstrate a simplified gyral pattern. The number of cortical neuronal columns is normal, but the cell number in each column is reduced (Evrard et al, 1989). This constellation of findings is most likely to occur between 6 and 18 weeks of gestation, when later proliferative events occur.

The etiology of micrencephaly includes diverse factors. Irradiation before 18 weeks of gestation is a well-known teratogenic factor that can produce micrencephaly. Exposure to alcohol and cocaine during this time also can result in micrencephaly (Gieron-Korthals et al, 1994; Peiffer et al, 1979). Maternal hyperphenylalaninemia also has been associated with these defects in nonphenylketonuric offspring (Lenke and Levy, 1980; Waisbren and Levy, 1990). Autosomal dominant, autosomal recessive, and X-linked recessive inheritance patterns have been described (Robain and Lyon, 1972; Warkany et al, 1981).

Recently, at least five genetic loci for human autosomal recessive primary micrencephaly (MCPH) have been mapped (Mochida and Walsh, 2001). All result in a small but structurally normal-appearing brain and a similar degree of mental retardation without other neurologically distinguishing features. The most prevalent is MCPH5, for which the defect was recently shown to involve protein-truncating mutations in the *ASPM* gene. *ASPM* (*a*bnormal, *sp*indle-like, *m*icrocephaly-associated) encodes a human microtubule-associated protein required for normal mitotic spindle function in embryonic neuronal stem cells (Bond et al, 2003). Of interest, some deletions that were sufficient to cause MCPH5 mapped to a region of *ASPM* that contains a series of repeated calmodulin-binding "IQ" (intelligence quotient) domains (Bond et al, 2002). The number of these "IQ" repeats varies between species and is directly proportional to the ultimate size of the protein. Whereas the *Drosophila* homologue contains only 24 "IQ" repeats, the mouse has 61 and the human *ASPM* gene contained the highest number, 74. Although the function of the large insertion encoded by these IQ repeats is unknown, a direct correlation was established between the size of the IQ domain and brain size during evolution. The distribution and timing of appearance of Aspm to proliferative regions of the developing murine CNS before and after birth indicate that it is required for normal neurogenesis and determination of brain size.

## Macrencephaly

Macrencephaly refers to a diverse group of conditions characterized by a large brain. Although it has been hypothesized that macrencephaly is related to an aberrant increase in neuronal proliferation, quantitative neuropathologic studies are lacking. Macrencephaly manifests most commonly as an isolated finding in familial (autosomal dominant or autosomal recessive) and sporadic cases. Among the other diverse conditions that are associated with macrencephaly are chromosomal disorders (fragile X syndrome and Klinefelter syndrome) and neuroendocrine disorders related to a generalized disturbance in growth (Beckwith-Wiedemann syndrome, cerebral gigantism, and achondroplasia) (DeMyer, 1972; Dodge et al, 1983).

At birth, the head circumference in about half of the cases is greater than that for the 90th percentile. The diagnosis of autosomal dominant macrencephaly is greatly favored by the finding of a large head circumference (macrocephaly) in either parent. Autosomal dominant inheritance generally is associated with a more favorable outcome, whereas the rare cases of autosomal recessive inheritance commonly are associated with mental retardation and epilepsy. One generally benign form of autosomal dominant macrencephaly is accompanied by extracerebral fluid collections that enlarge the subarachnoid spaces (Alvarez et al, 1986). Erroneously referred to as "external hydrocephalus," this condition rarely constitutes an indication for placement of a shunt to drain the fluid. Rather, the initial acceleration in head circumference generally arrests spontaneously by around the first year of life; thereafter, the fluid collections decrease in amount. These fluid collections appear to be related to an imbalance in CSF generation at birth related to developmental immaturity of the subarachnoid granulations that resorb this fluid (Barlow, 1984; Neveling and Truex, 1983).

Hemimegalencephaly (Fig. 63–15) refers to a rare malformation consisting of unilateral macrencephaly related to enlargement of some portion of one cerebral hemisphere and accompanied by increased cortical thickness and abnormal cortical gyration (Robain et al, 1972). The primary defect is unknown. The pathologic features include apparent disturbances in astroglia proliferation and morphology as well as neuronal heterotopias in subcortical white matter (DeRosa et al, 1992). The usual onset for intractable epilepsy is in the neonatal period (Ohtsuka et al, 1999). A markedly improved outcome may be achieved in selected patients after hemispherectomy performed as early as the neonatal period (Battaglia et al, 1999).

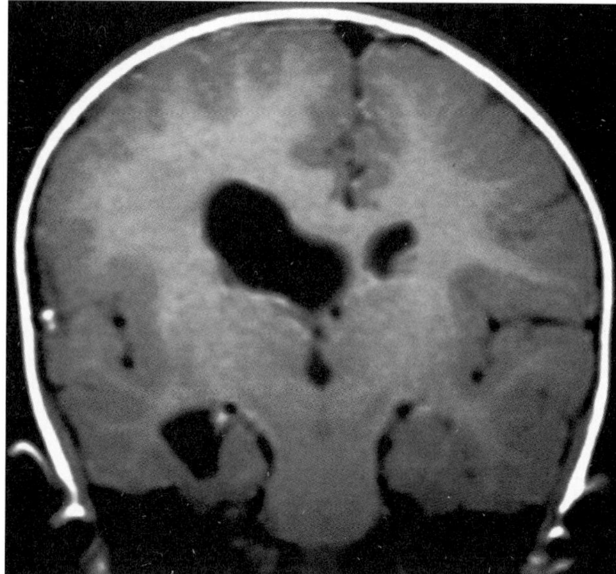

**FIGURE 63–15.** Hemimegalencephaly: Magnetic resonance image. Note the marked asymmetry of the two cerebral hemispheres, with the pronounced enlargement on the left. *(Courtesy of Dr. Martin Salinsky, Department of Neurology, Oregon Health & Science University.)*

## Disorders of Neuronal Migration

Neuronal migration disorders are characterized anatomically by defects in the lamination of the cerebral cortex. Most of these defects are related to some degree of failure of neurons to migrate to their appropriate target positions within the normal six layers of the developing cerebral cortex. The clinical spectrum of brain malformations associated with disrupted neuronal migration ranges from complete focal agenesis of an entire region of the cerebral cortex in schizencephaly to more subtle abnormalities in which heterotopic clusters of neurons are retained in abnormal locations within the subcortical white matter (see Table 63–1). In many disorders, there are prominent disturbances in the formation of the cortical surface that manifest as gyral abnormalities. At one end of the spectrum of these abnormalities is complete absence of gyri, with a smooth cortical surface (lissencephaly); at the other end is an excess of small gyral convolutions (polymicrogyria). The fact that these gyral abnormalities often are accompanied by other malformations, such as hypoplasia or agenesis of the corpus callosum, points to a complex interplay between the mechanisms that determine neuronal migration and axon path-finding. This is consistent with the fact that the timing of neuronal migration and that of midline prosencephalic development overlap. Hence, disturbances in neuronal migration would be anticipated to have a deleterious impact on the axonotropic signaling required for establishment of interhemispheric and intrahemispheric cortical connections.

### Schizencephaly

Schizencephaly ("split brain") is characterized by severe focal malformations of the cerebral cortex that result in complete agenesis of all layers of the cortical wall. The resultant defect is a cleft in the cerebral cortex in one or both hemispheres, which thus connects the lateral ventricle with the extracerebral space (Fig. 63–16). When the defect is wide (separated-lip schizencephaly), the malformation may be confused with a lesion due to a severe destructive process. However, a feature of schizencephaly that differentiates it from an encephaloclastic lesion (e.g., hydrancephaly, porencephaly) is that on histologic examination, the cleft has features of a migrational disturbance, such as large neuronal heterotopias bordered by adjacent polymicrogyria. When the defect is narrow (closed-lip schizencephaly), it has the appearance of a narrow groove in the cortical mantle. The morphologic features of schizencephalic clefts by neuroimaging are best delineated by MRI, which has demonstrated the common occurrence of subependymal heterotopias and polymicrogyria and the universal finding of diminished volume of the cerebral white matter (Hayashi et al, 2002a). In addition, a wide range of anomalies related to disturbances of prosencephalic development may occur in association with schizencephaly.

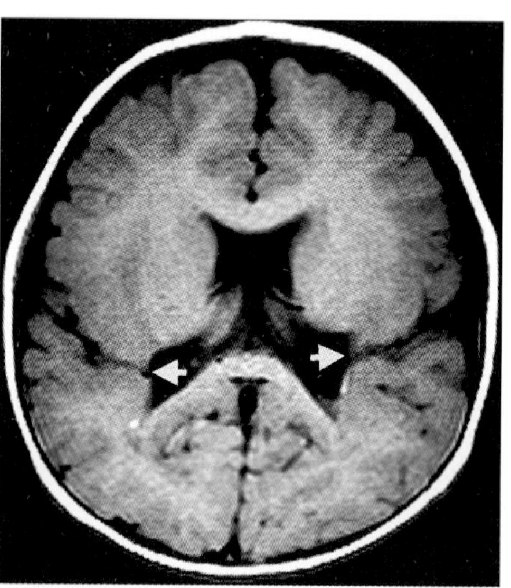

A

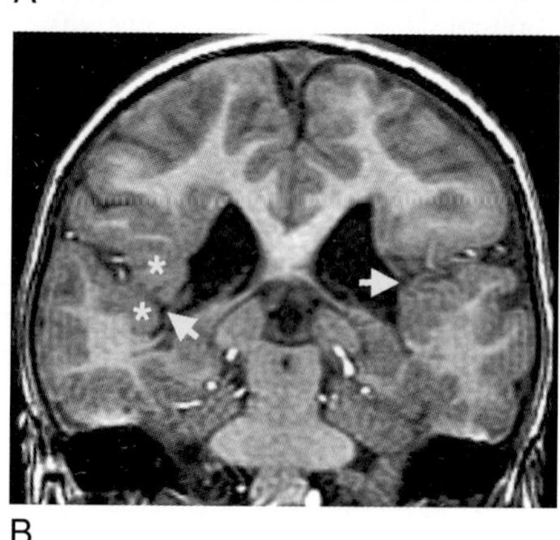

B

**FIGURE 63–16.** Bilateral open-lip schizencephaly: Magnetic resonance images. **A,** Axial T1-weighted image. Note that the bilateral clefts *(arrows)* extend to the lateral ventricles. **B,** Coronal T1-weighted image. Note that the clefts *(arrows)* are lined with gray matter (*). *(Courtesy of Dr. A. James Barkovich, Department of Radiology, University of California, San Francisco, School of Medicine.)*

These include holoprosencephaly, agenesis of the corpus callosum, and agenesis of the septum pellucidum.

Schizencephaly occurs with a wide range of clinical severity that is related to the size and distribution of the cerebral clefts and the extent of associated malformations (Barkovich and Kjos, 1992; Packard et al, 1997). Significant cognitive impairment is almost universal with bilateral anomalies but occurs in a minority of cases with unilateral lesions. Motor disturbances are common with both unilateral and bilateral lesions; this finding may be related in part to the predilection for frontal lesions. A wide variety of seizure types, including partial epilepsies, are common (Guerrini and Carrozzo, 2001). Hydrocephalus is seen almost exclusively with separated-lip lesions.

Of interest, in one large series, schizencephaly involved predominantly the regions of the rolandic and sylvian fissures in the frontal cortex (Barkovich and Kjos, 1992). The basis for this predilection is suggested by rare familial cases of severe separated-lip schizencephaly associated with mutations in the human homeobox gene *EMX2* (Granata et al, 1997). In mice, *Emx2* and the *Pax6* homeobox genes are expressed in opposing anterior-to-posterior gradients in the cortical ventricular zone. Multiple studies support that these Emx2 and Pax6 countergradients intrinsically specify the size of anterior and posterior cortical areas (Monuki and Walsh, 2001). Mutations in *Emx2* result in disturbances in neuronal migration via radial glial fibers and cause shifts in the regionalization of cerebral cortex such that anterior lateral cortical areas are expanded, whereas posteromedial areas are reduced in size (Bishop et al, 2000, Mallamaci et al, 2000). Other potential etiologic factors in schizencephaly are suggested by both experimental and clinical findings in schizencephaly following fetal viral infection of the CNS (Iannetti et al, 1998; Takano et al, 1999).

## Polymicrogyria

Polymicrogyria constitutes a heterogeneous group of malformations with multiple potential etiologic factors. The unifying feature is an excess number of small convolutions on the cortical surface (Fig. 63–17). The cortical mantle is thin and excessively folded and may contain multiple fused gyri. Histopathologic studies have defined two major types of polymicrogyria, layered and unlayered, each characterized by an abnormal cortical lamination pattern. In contrast with the normal six-layered cerebral cortex, *layered polymicrogyria* comprises four distinct cortical layers. This "classic" form is not associated with other migrational abnormalities but often is more diffusely localized adjacent to regions of encephalomalacia related to infection (e.g., toxoplasmosis, cytomegalovirus infection) or ischemia with cortical laminar necrosis.

*Unlayered polymicrogyria* is characterized by a markedly disorganized cortex that lacks distinct cortical layers. The timing of appearance of this form appears to be no later than 4 to 5 months of gestation. Unlayered polymicrogyria is associated with other migrational disturbances, particularly subcortical nodular heterotopias, lissencephaly, and schizencephaly. A genetic basis is suggested by syndrome associations (e.g., Zellweger syndrome, Miller-Dieker syndrome), familial transmission, and sporadic cases with X-linked, autosomal recessive and autosomal dominant inheritance patterns (Barkovich et al, 1999; Ross and Walsh, 2001). Several syndromes of bilateral polymicrogyria have been mapped to specific genetic loci (Chang et al, 2003; Villard et al, 2002).

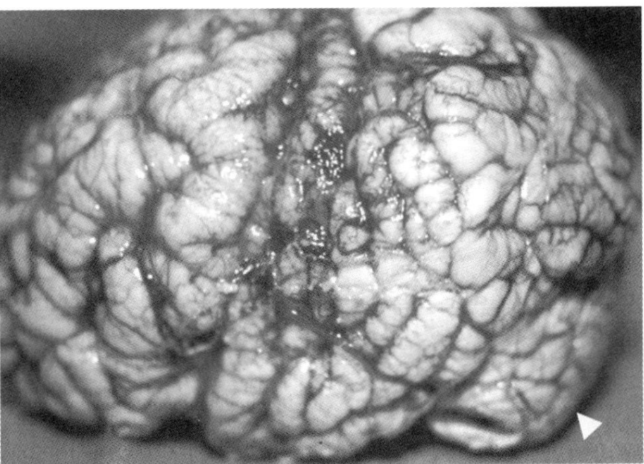

**FIGURE 63–17.** Polymicrogyria. Much of the cerebral cortex in this photograph shows the irregular, "cobblestone" appearance of polymicrogyria. More normal gyri are present at the frontal pole *(lower left)*. The cerebellum is indicated at lower right *(arrowhead)*. *(Courtesy of Dr. Marjorie Grafe, Department of Pathology, Oregon Health & Science University.)*

Delineation of the spectrum of CNS malformations associated with polymicrogyria has been greatly advanced by MRI. Of importance, if thick sections (thicker than 4 mm) are imaged, these anomalies may resemble focal pachygyria owing to signal averaging from the microgyri. Four subtypes have been identified by high-resolution MRI with thin sections: isolated polymicrogyria, an association with localized megalencephaly, subcortical heterotopias, or schizencephaly (Hayashi et al, 2002b). Polymicrogyria shows a strong predilection for the sylvian fissure and adjacent regions of frontal and parietal cortex, whereas the cingulate cortex, striate cortex, gyrus rectus, and hippocampus are spared. A further defining feature is often a decrease in cerebral white matter volume adjacent to the regions of dysplastic cortex.

The clinical features of patients with polymicrogyria are variable and relate in part to the distribution of cortical dysplasia. Several familial syndromes of bilateral polymicrogyria encompass much of the spectrum of clinical findings (Barkovich et al, 1999). Epilepsy, notably partial complex seizures and multiple generalized seizure types, is common but may be delayed in onset beyond the neonatal period. In bilateral frontoparietal polymicrogyria, consistent findings include global developmental delay, dysconjugate gaze/esotropia, and bilateral pyramidal and cerebellar motor signs (Chang et al, 2003). The perisylvian cortex is devoted to control of the mouth and the motor programs of language. Dysarthria, language delay, abnormal tongue movements, dysphagia, and severe seizures are features of familial syndromes with bilateral polymicrogyria of the perisylvian cortex. Discoordination of suck and swallow is common in the neonate (Guerriero et al, 2000).

## Lissencephaly and Pachygyria

The lissencephalies are a class of neuronal migrational disorders characterized by a paucity or absence of gyri *(agyria)*, which gives the cortical surface a smooth or nearly smooth appearance (Kato and Dobyns, 2003). In most patients, lissencephaly is characterized by an abnormally thick cortex and disturbances in the organization of the cortical layers that may be accompanied by diffuse neuronal heterotopias (Fig. 63–18). The spectrum of gyral malformations includes *pachygyria*, characterized by regions of cortex with a reduced number of coarse, broadened gyri, and *subcortical band heterotopia* ("double cortex"), in which a circumferential band of heterotopic neurons resides within the subcortical white matter directly beneath a relatively normal cortex.

The classification of the lissencephalies has undergone major revision to reflect the rapidly evolving understanding of the molecular basis of these disorders (Barkovich et al, 2001). A majority of cases are subsumed under the *classic lissencephaly/subcortical band heteropia spectrum* (previously type 1). At present, five genes are known to cause or contribute to lissencephaly in humans (Kato and Dobyns, 2003). Two of these genes, *LIS1* and *DCX*, account for a majority of cases of classic lissencephaly. Mutations of the *LIS1* gene were first detected in the Miller-Dieker syndrome (severe lissencephaly and distinct craniofacial abnormalities) after indentification of chromosome 17p13.3 deletions in greater than 90% of these patients (Ledbetter et al, 1992). This syndrome is always associated with a more severe lissencephaly phenotype, which appears to reflect the fact that the 17p deletion also contains the 14–3–3ϵ gene, which also is implicated in neuronal migration. Subsequent studies determined that sporadic cases of isolated lissencephaly were caused by *LIS1* mutations as well. *LIS1* encodes a noncatalytic subunit of a ubiquitously expressed enzyme, platelet-activating factor acetylhydrolase. The mechanisms by which *LIS1* mutations disrupt neuronal migration relate in part to its roles in cell motility as well as mitosis (neurogenesis). The *DCX* gene was first demonstrated to cause X-linked lissencephaly and subcortical band heteropia. *DCX* encodes the doublecortin protein, which is a neuron-specific protein that functions in part in microtubule polymerization and may interact with LIS-1 (des Portes et al, 1998; Gleeson et al, 1998). Mutations in the *ARX* gene result in another form of X-linked lissencephaly with abnormal genitalia, further characterized by abnormal basal ganglia, often with small cysts, immature white matter, and agenesis of the corpus callosum (Kitamura et al, 2002). *ARX* is a homebox gene specifically expressed in forebrain interneurons and the male gonads, where it directs differentiation of the testes. ARX functions in proliferation of neuronal progenitors and in differentiation and migration of interneurons.

LIS-1, doublecortin, and other genes implicated in neuronal migration encode proteins that appear to interact via functionally complex signaling mechanisms to modulate alterations in cell shape at the level of the actin and microtubule-based cytoskeleton (Ross and Walsh, 2001). It is thus not surprising that LIS-1 and DCX mutations are associated with considerable variation in the phenotypic expression of classic lissencephaly. Six distinct grades of morphologic severity have been defined that overlap among agyria, pachygyria, and subcortical band heteropia (Kato and Dobyns, 2003). The most severe form (grade 1) usually is associated with either the Miller-Dieker syndrome or a severe mutation of *DCX*. Moreover, the gyral malformations associated with *LIS1* mutations are more pronounced posteriorly than anteriorly, whereas the gradient of injury is reversed (more pronounced anteriorly than posteriorly) with *DCX* mutations. The picture is further complicated in X-linked dominant lissencephaly insofar as males and females typically display different phenotypes related to *DCX* mutations. Owing to hemizygosity for *DXC* on the X chromosome, males often display severe lisssencephaly resembling that seen in *LIS1* mutations. Because of lyonization (random X-inactivation), females typically display the subcortical band heteropia phenotype (Fig. 63–19). However, when mosaicism for the aberrant

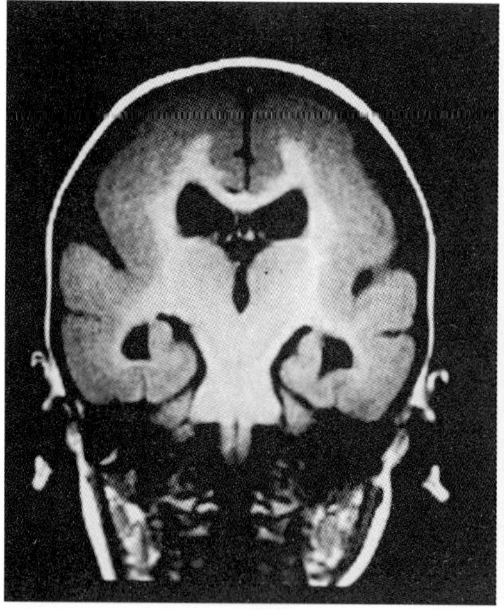


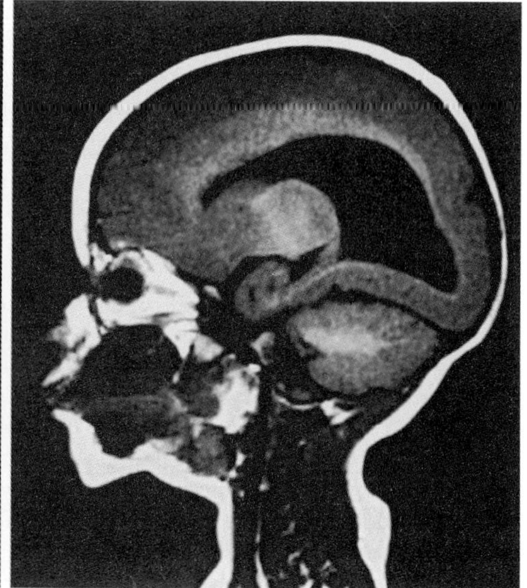


**FIGURE 63–18.** T1-weighted magnetic resonance images of the brain of a child with classic lissencephaly. **A,** Coronal view. **B,** Sagittal view. Note the pronounced thickening of the cerebral cortex and the striking reduction in cortical gyration. *(Courtesy of Dr. C. McCluggage, Department of Radiology, Texas Children's Hospital.)*

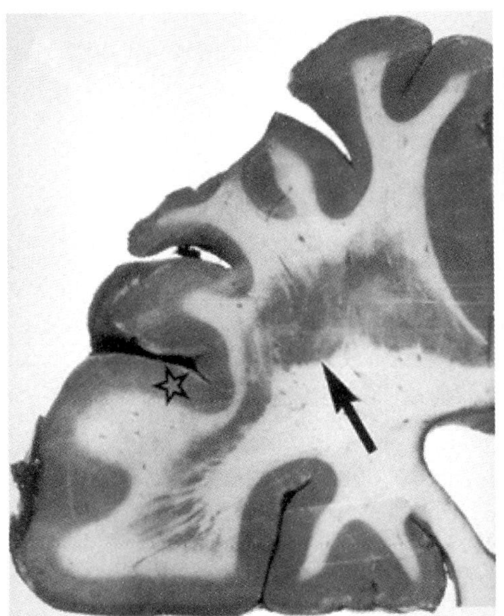


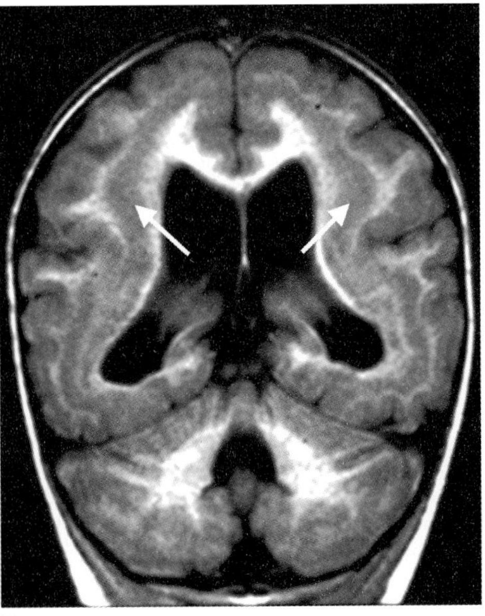


**FIGURE 63–19.** Subcortical band heteropia in two female patients diagnosed with a *DCX* mutation. **A,** This histologic specimen demonstrates the presence of a broad band of heterotopic gray matter *(arrow)* that is situated within the cerebral white matter and distinct from the cerebral cortex, *(star)*. **B,** T1-weighted axial magnetic resonance image demonstrates the circumferential nature of the subcortical band heteropia *(arrows)*. *(Courtesy of Dr. Joseph G. Gleeson, Department of Neurology, University of California, San Diego, School of Medicine; M. Elizabeth Ross, Department of Neurology, University of Minnesota; Christopher A. Walsh, Department of Neurology, Harvard Medical School.)*

*DCX* allele predominates, some *DCX* females can display severe lissencephaly.

Although predictions of genotype are not readily feasible on the basis of the pattern of malformations present, clinical features more consistently correlate with the lesions present. Superior definition of malformations is achieved by MRI. In the newborn, the typical presentation of isolated lissencephaly is pronounced hypotonia accompanied by a lack of motor activity. Only later in the first year may spasticity develop. Depending on the nature of the *LIS1* mutation on chromosome 17, craniofacial anomalies can be subtle (bitemporal hollowing and a small jaw) or may entail the full expression of the Miller-Dieker syndrome (Dobyns et al, 1984). Head circumference is typically normal at birth, but progressive microcephaly evolves during the first year of life. Although neonatal seizures may occur, severe myoclonic epilepsy typically develops in the latter half of the first year (e.g., infantile spasms, Lennox-Gastaut syndrome) (Gerrini and Carrozzo, 2002). Isolated lissencephaly carries poor long-term prognosis dominated by mental retardation, spastic quadriparesis, and epilepsy. The severity of clinical deficits is typically less for infants with focal pachygyria. Patients with subcortical band heteropia are much less affected than those with isolated lissencephaly. Although potential sequelae include development of seizures and cognitive impairment, roughly 25% of patients have normal or near-normal intelligence. Neurologic deficits roughly correlate with the thickness and extent of the subcortical band (Dobyns et al, 1996).

### Lissencephaly with Cerebellar Hypoplasia

Lissencephaly with cerebellar hypoplasia (LCH) encompasses six broad classes (designated a to f) of malformations that have in common a lissencephaly spectrum of agyria-pachygyria plus some degree of cerebellar hypoplasia (Barkovich et al, 2001; Kato and Dobyns, 2003; Ross et al, 2001). Individual classes are defined on the basis of additional malformations (e.g., brainstem hypoplasia, agenesis of the corpus callosum). The prototype for these disorders is LCHb, in which lissencephaly is accompanied by severe global cerebellar hypoplasia and a very malformed hippocampus. The lissencephaly is characterized by a moderately thick cortex with an anterior-to-posterior decreasing gradient of severity. Several patients with LCHb have proven mutations in the *RELN* gene, which encodes reelin, a large extracellular matrix protein (Hong et al, 2000; Ross and Walsh, 2001). This is a notable finding, because the mouse homologue of the *RELN* gene has been shown to account for the phenotype of the reeler mouse, a severely ataxic mutant mouse strain in which the cerebral cortex and cerebellar cortex display an inversion of the normal mammalian "inside-out" laminar organization pattern (Rakic and Caviness, 1995). A role for reelin in neuronal migration is supported by the observation that it is secreted by the Cajal-Retzius cells of the embryonic preplate as well as cerebellar external granule cell layer neurons and pioneering cells of the hippocampus. The distribution pattern of reelin is thus consistent with the pattern of malformations seen in LCHb. Functionally, reelin activates a signal transduction pathway via two distinct membrane-associated lipoproteins, the apolipoprotein $E_2$ and the very-low-density lipoprotein receptors. These receptors direct the phosphorylation of mDab1, which on activation participates in actin polymerization, an integral event in cell migration. Of interest, abnormalities very similar to those in the reeler mouse are observed in mutant mouse strains with disruptions of mDab1 or both lipoprotein receptors.

### Cobblestone Complex Syndromes

The cobblestone complex syndromes are included here because they all involve abnormal neuronal migration and were previously classified with type II lissencephaly (Barkovich et al, 2001). Three congenital muscular dystrophy syndromes are represented: Walker-Warburg syndrome, muscle-eye-brain disease, and Fukuyama congenital muscular dystrophy. The isolated cobblestone complex malformation without retinal or muscle involvement is rare. The neuronal migration anomaly in the cobblestone complex arises as a result of failure of early migrating neurons to arrest at the marginal zone (the future layer I of the cerebral cortex). Rather, these heterotopic neurons migrate further through a defective glia-limiting membrane into the leptomeninges, which thicken and adhere to the cortical surface—hence the term *cobblestone lissencephaly*. These collections of leptomeningeal neurons can be sufficiently large to obliterate the subarachnoid spaces, with resultant communicating hydrocephalus related to disruption of CSF resorption. The organization of the cerebral cortex is markedly more abnormal than in classic lissencephaly and is characterized by large ectopic clusters of neurons with no discernible lamination pattern.

*Walker-Warburg syndrome* is the most severe of the three cobblestone complex congenital muscular dystrophy syndromes (Warburg, 1987). Several clinical features distinguish this entity from classic lissencephaly. Macrocephaly commonly is present at birth or develops in the first year of life. The macrocephaly typically is related to communicating hydrocephalus, as well as dilation of the third and fourth ventricles when a retrocerebellar cyst is present (see later). In addition to lissencephaly, cerebellar/hindbrain and oculoretinal malformations and congenital muscular dystrophy also are universal and required for the diagnosis. Cerebellar malformations are discussed earlier, in the context of DWM, and include midline cerebellar hypoplasia and retrocerebellar cyst. Protrusions of the retrocerebellar cyst through a skull defect can result in a posterior encephalocele. Ocular anomalies include retinal detachment, optic nerve hypoplasia, microphthalmia, and colobomas. The muscular weakness is typically severe and is associated with elevated serum creatine kinase. The prognosis for survival beyond the first year is poor. This complex constellation of features may be recalled by the eponym CHARM + E (*c*erebellar *h*ydrocephalus, *a*gyria, *r*etinal, *m*uscle, *e*ncephalocele) (Volpe, 2000).

The spectrum of brain malformations in *muscle-eye-brain disease* is generally less severe than in Walker-Warburg syndrome. These include milder lissencephaly with frontal pachgyria and less severe occipital gyral dysplasia. Midline cerebellar hypoplasia is more variable, and the retrocerebellar cyst and encephalocele are not seen. Ocular abnormalities include retinal and optic nerve hypoplasia, cataracts, and glaucoma.

The cobblestone complex malformations are generally the least severe in *Fukuyama congenital muscular dystrophy* (FCMD), and the eye abnormalities are minor or do not occur (Fukuyama et al, 1984). The cortical dysplasia in FCMD, however, is sufficiently severe to produce severe mental retardation in at least half of the patients. Hence, it can be difficult clinically to distinguish between patients with severe FCMD and those with mild Walker-Warburg syndrome.

Despite overlap in their clinical features, current data indicate that the cobblestone complex muscular dystrophy syndromes are genetically distinct autosomal recessive disorders (Cormand et al, 2001). Emerging evidence suggests that these disorders belong to a new class of glycosylation-deficient muscular dystrophies that are related to mutations in enzymes that catalyze the post-translational *O*-glycosylation of a small number of mammalian glycoproteins (Grewal and Hewitt, 2003). Point mutations in POMT1, a putative *O*-mannosyltransferase, account for approximately 20% of cases of Walker-Warburg syndrome (Beltran-Valero de Barnabe et al, 2002). The defect in muscle-eye-brain disease is in *POMGnT1*, the gene for a definitive mannosyltransferase, *O*-linked mannose β1,2-*N*-acetylglucosaminyltransferase-1 (Taniguchi et al, 2003). The defect in FCMD resides in the protein fukutin (Kobayashi et al, 2000), a putative phospholigand transferase that shares homology with microbial proteins involved in mannosyl phosphorylation. Hence, the preponderance of data suggests that the overlapping clinical phenotypes for the three cobblestone complex muscular dystrophies are related to defects in a common glycosylation pathway that involves *O*-mannosylation of proteins.

## Neuronal Heterotopia

Heterotopia are displaced collections of neurons that have failed to complete their normal migration from the ventricular zone. They are most commonly observed in periventricular white matter, where they are nodular collections of cells ("periventricular nodular heterotopia") (Fig. 63–20), or in the subcortical white matter, where they may be nodular or diffuse (Fig. 63–21). Heterotopia are in fact a feature of virtually all of the migrational disorders. In addition, they are often the primary migrational disturbance associated with a wide range of disorders. These include metabolic disorders, fetal toxic exposures,

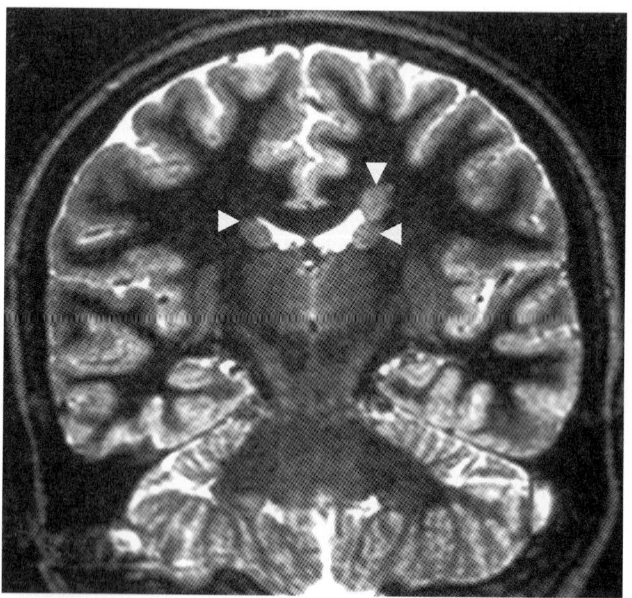

**FIGURE 63–20.** Magnetic resonance imaging scan of brain in periventricular nodular heterotopia. Three discrete periventricular nodular masses *(arrowheads)* are visualized adjacent to the lateral ventricles in this T2-weighted coronal image. Note the otherwise normal convolutional pattern of the cerebral cortex. *(Courtesy of Dr. Martin Salinsky, Department of Neurology, Oregon Health & Science University.)*

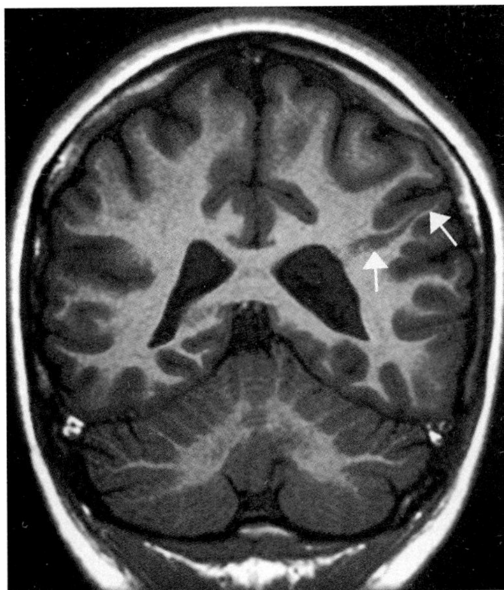

**FIGURE 63–21.** Subcortical white matter heterotopia: Magnetic resonance imaging scan. This T1-weighted coronal image shows a diffuse stream of heterotopic gray matter *(arrows)* that spans from near the ventricular surface to the cerebral cortex. The appearance of this focal disturbance of neuronal migration suggests that the neurons were "hung up" in their migration from the ventricular surface to the cerebral cortex. *(Courtesy of Dr. Martin Salinsky, Department of Neurology, Oregon Health & Science University.)*

and neurocutaneous, multiple congenital, and chromosomal syndromes (Volpe, 2000). Hence, the clinical significance of heterotopic neurons in these conditions may be as an overt sign of a more serious underlying neurologic condition.

As isolated disorders, the heterotopias are clinically and pathologically less severe than the subcortical band heterotopias, separate disorders that are variously expressed in the spectrum of classic lissencephaly, discussed earlier. The isolated heteropias are classified with regard to a primary periventricular (subependymal), subcortical white matter, or marginal (superficial cortical/leptomeningeal) site of pathology (Barkovich et al, 2001). Typically, superficial cortical neuronal heterotopias are incidental finding at autopsy. However, glial-neuronal heteropias that infiltrate the leptomeninges occur in association with fetal exposure to teratogens such as methylmercury (Choi et al, 1978) or as seen in the fetal alcohol syndrome (Norman et al, 1995b).

The most well-characterized isolated heterotopia syndrome is the bilateral periventricular nodular heterotopia (BPNH) syndrome (Ross and Walsh, 2001). The BPNH syndrome is inherited as an X-linked dominant disorder that therefore occurs in females and usually is embryonic lethal in males. A familial syndrome exists in which the typical presentation is one of epilepsy associated with normal intelligence. The milder phenotype in females relates to apparent X-inactivation, in which silencing of the normal allele has occurred in the heterotopic neurons. The gene defect in BPNH involves filamin 1 (FLN-1), an actin cross-linking phosphoprotein that appears to function in the actin remodeling required for cell migration out of the ventricular zone (Fox et al, 1998).

Focal cortical dysplasias are commonly associated with subcortical neuronal heterotopias. They are characterized by focal gyral abnormalities in which a normal cortical lamination pattern is lacking. These lesions may have the appearance of focal polymicrogyria or pachygyria. Although the origin of these lesions is unclear, they are composed mostly of ectopic neurons that express glutamatergic markers (Crino et al, 2001). This finding has led to the speculation that cortical dysplasias derive from single clones of ventricular zone progenitors that normally are destined to generate a cortical column of glutamatergic projection neurons (Monuki and Walsh, 2001).

The development of high-resolution MRI has greatly advanced the detection of neuronal heterotopias and cortical dysplasias. Such studies, together with autopsy findings, support the notion that subtle migrational dysplasias are not uncommon and may be present in virtually all of us. The application of positron emission tomography has also greatly facilitated the detection of heterotopias and other cortical dysplasias that may be undetected by MRI (Juhasz et al, 2003). Such imaging studies have demonstrated the role of these lesions in the pathogenesis of a variety of medication-resistant seizure disorders that may be controlled by surgical resection (Guerrini and Carrozzo, 2002; Russo et al, 2003).

It is clear that the evolutionary pressures that led to the enormous expansion of the human cerebral cortex required more elaborate genetic programs, at times unique to human development (Gupta et al, 2002). Remarkably, the study of human brain malformations has now become a critical interface between developmental molecular neurobiology and neonatal medicine that is unraveling the intricate mechanisms that determine the development of the human brain.

## REFERENCES

AAP Committee on Bioethics: Infants with anencephaly as organ sources: Ethical considerations. Pediatrics 89:1116, 1992.

Acers TE: Optic nerve hypoplasia: Septo-optic-pituitary dysplasia syndrome. Trans Am Ophthalmol Soc 79:425, 1981.

Aicardi J, Lefebvre JJ, Lerique-Koechlin A: A new syndrome: Spasms in flexion, callosal agenesis, ocular abnormalities. Electroencephalogr Clin Neurophysiol 19:609-610, 1965.

Albright AL, Gartner JC, Wiener ES: Lumbar cutaneous hemangiomas as indicators of tethered spinal cords. Pediatrics 83:977, 1989.

Allendoerfer KL, Shatz CJ: The subplate, a transient neocortical structure: Its role in the development of connections between thalamus and cortex. Annu Rev Neurosci 17:185-218, 1994.

Altman NR, Naidich TP, Braffman BH: Posterior fossa malformations. AJNR Am J Neuroradiol 13:691, 1992.

Alvarez LA, Maytal J, Shinnar S: Idiopathic external hydrocephalus: Natural history and relationship to benign familial macrocephaly. Pediatrics 77:901-907, 1986.

Anderson FM: Occult spinal dysraphism: A series of 73 cases. Pediatrics 55:826, 1975.

Baird PA, Sadovnick AD: Survival in infants with anencephaly. Clin Pediatr (Phila) 23:268-271, 1984.

Barkovich AJ, Ferriero DM, Barr RM, et al: Microlissencephaly: A heterogeneous malformation of cortical development. Neuropediatr 29:113-119, 1998.

Barkovich AJ, Hevner R, Guerrini R: Syndromes of bilateral symmetrical polymicrogyria. AJNR Am J Neuroradiol 20: 1814-1821, 1999.

Barkovich AJ, Kjos BO: Schizencephaly: Correlation of clinical findings with MR characteristics. Am J Neuroradiol 13:85-94, 1992.

Barkovich AJ, Kuzniecky RI, Jackson GD, et al: Classification system for malformations of cortical development update 2001. Neurology 57:2168-2178, 2001.

Barkovich, AJ, Norman D: Anomalies of the corpus callosum: Correlation with further anomalies of the brain. AJNR Am J Neuroradiol 9:493-501, 1988.

Barkovich AJ, Norman D: Absence of the septum pellucidum: A useful sign in the diagnosis of congenital brain malformations. Am J Radiol 152:353, 1989.

Barlow CF: CSF dynamics in hydrocephalus with special attention to external hydrocephalus. Brain Dev 6:119-127, 1984.

Barr M Jr, Cohen MM Jr: Holoprosencephaly survival and performance. Am J Med Genet 89:116-120, 1999.

Battaglia D, Di Rocco C, Iuvone L, et al: Neuro-cognitive development and epilepsy outcome in children with surgically treatable hemimegalencephaly. Neuropediatrics 30:307-313, 1999.

Becerra JE, Khoury MJ, Cordero JF, et al: Diabetes mellitus during pregnancy and the risks for specific birth defects: A population-based case-control study. Pediatrics 85:1, 1990.

Beltran-Valera de Bernabe D, Currier S, Steinbrecher A, et al: Mutations in the *O*-mannosyltransferase gene *POMT1* give rise to the severe neuronal migration disorder Walker-Warburg syndrome. Am J Hum Genet 71:1033-1043, 2002.

Benda CE: The Dandy-Walker syndrome or the so-called atresia of the foramen of Magendie. J Neuropathol Exp Neurol 13:14, 1954.

Bishop KM, Goudreau G, O'Leary DD: Regulation of area identity in the mammalian neocortex by Emx2 and Pax6. Science 288:344-349, 2000.

Blaauw G: Defect in posterior arch of atlas in myelomeningocele. Dev Med Child Neurol 13 (suppl 25):113, 1971.

Bond J, Roberts E, Mochida G, et al: *ASPM* is a major determinant of cerebral cortical size. Nat Genet 32:316-320, 2002.

Bond J, Scott S, Hampshire DJ, et al: Protein-truncating mutations in *ASPM* cause variable reduction in brain size. Am J Hum Genet 73:1170-1177, 2003.

Brock DJ: Mechanisms by which amniotic-fluid alpha-fetoprotein may be increased in fetal abnormalities. Lancet 2:345, 1976.

Brown MS, Sheridan-Pereira M: Outlook for the child with a cephalocele. Pediatrics 90:914, 1992.

Castilla EE, Orioli IM, Lopez-Camelo JS, et al: Preliminary data on changes in neural tube defect prevalence rates after folic acid fortification in South America. Am J Med Genet 123A: 123, 2003.

Caviness VS, Takahashi T, Nowakowski RS: Numbers, time and neocortical neuronogenesis: A general developmental and evolutionary model. Trends Neurosci 18:379-383, 1995.

Chang BSS, Piao X, Bodell A, et al: Bilateral frontoparietal polymicrogyria: Clinical and radiological features in 10 families with linkage to chromosome 16. Ann Neurol 53:596-606, 2003.

Choi BH, Lapham LW, Amin-Zaki L, et al: Abnormal neuronal migration, deranged cerebral cortical oganization, and diffuse white matter astrocytosis of human fetal brain: A major effect of methylmercury poisoning in utero. J Neuropathol Exp Neurol 37:719, 1978.

Chun JJ, Nakamura MJ, Shatz CJ: Transient cells of the developing mammalian telencephalon are peptide-immunoreactive neurons. Nature 325:617-620, 1987.

Cormand B, Pikho H, Bayes M, et al: Clinical and genetic distinction between Walker-Warburg syndrome and muscle-eye-brain disease. Neurology 36:1054-69, 2001.

Costa C, Hauw JJ: Pathology of the cerebellum, brainstem, and spinal cord. In Duckett S (ed): Pediatric Neuropathology. Baltimore, Williams & Wilkins, 1995, pp 217-239.

Crane JP: Sonographic detection of neural tube defects. In Elias S, Simpson JL (eds): Maternal Serum Screening for Fetal Genetic Disorders. New York, Churchill-Livingstone, 1992, pp 59B74.

Crino PB, Duhaime AC, Baltuch G, White R: Differential expression of glutamate and GABA-A receptor subunit mRNA in cortical dysplasia. Neurology 56:906-913, 2001.

Cuckle HS: Screening for neural tube defects. In Bock G, Marsh J (eds): Neural Tube Defects. Ciba Foundation Symposium 181. Chicester, John Wiley & Sons, 1994, pp 253-267.

Curatolo P, Mercuri S, Cotroneo E: Joubert syndrome: A case confirmed by computerized tomography. Dev Med Child Neurol 22:362, 1980.

Czeizel AE, Dudas I: Prevention of the first occurrence of neural tube defects by periconceptional vitamin supplementation. N Engl J Med 317:1832, 1992.

D'Agostino AN, Kernohan JW, Brown JR: Dandy-Walker syndrome. J Neuropathol Exp Neurol 22:450, 1963.

DeMyer W: Megalencephaly in children: Clinical syndromes, genetic patterns, and differential diagnosis from other causes of megalocephaly. Neurology 22:634, 1972.

des Portes V, Pinaard JM, Billuart P: A novel CNS gene required for neuronal migration and involved in X-linked subcortical laminar heterotopia and lissencephaly syndrome. Cell 92:51-61, 1998.

DeRosa MJ, Secor DL, Barsom M, et al: Neuropathological findings in surgically treated hemimegalencephaly—immunohistochemical, morphometric, and ultrastructural study. Acta Neuropathol 84:250-260, 1992.

Diebler C, Dulac O: Pediatric Neurology and Neuroradiology. Berlin, Springer-Verlag, 1987, pp 51-57.

Dobyns WB, Stratton RF, Greenberg F: Syndromes with lissencephaly: I. Miller-Dieker and Norman-Roberts syndromes and isolated lissencephaly. Am J Med Genet 18:509, 1984.

Dobyns WB, Andermann E, Anderman F, et al: X-linked malformations of neuronal migration. Neurology 47:331-339, 1996.

Dodge PR, Holmes SJ, Sotos JF: Cerebral gigantism. Dev Med Child Neurol 25:248, 1983.

Donis-Keller H, Dou S, Chi D, et al: Mutations in the *RET* proto-oncogene are associated with MEN 2A and FMTC. Hum Mol Genet 2:851, 1993.

Edery P, Lyonnet S, Mulligan LM, et al: Mutations of the *RET* proto-oncogene in Hirschsprung's disease. Nature 367:378, 1994.

Egger J, Bellman MM, Ross EM, et al: Joubert-Boltshauser syndrome with polydactyly in siblings. J Neurol Neurosurg Psychiatry 45:737, 1982.

Elwood JM, Little J, Elwood JH: Epidemiology and Control of Neural Tube Defects. New York, Oxford University Press, 1992.

England MA: Normal development of the central nervous system. In Levene MI, Bennett MJ, Punt J (eds): Fetal and Neonatal Neurology and Neurosurgery. Edinburgh, Churchill-Livingstone, 1988, pp 3-31.

Evrard P, Kadhim HJ, de Saint-Georges P, et al: Abnormal development and destructive processes of the human brain during the second half of gestation. In Evrard P, Minkowski A (eds): Developmental Neurobiology. Nestle Nutrition Workshop Series, 12. New York, Raven Press, 1989, pp 1-12.

Fox JW, Lamperti ED, Eksioglu YZ, et al: Mutations in filamin 1 prevent migration of cerebral cortical neurons in human periventricular heterotopia. Neuron 21:1315-1325, 1998.

Frey L, Hauser WA: Epidemiology of neural tube defects. Epilepsia 44 (suppl 3):4, 2003.

Friede RL: Developmental Neuropathology, 2nd ed. New York, Springer-Verlag, 1989.

Friede RL, Boltshauser E: Uncommon syndromes of cerebellar vermis aplasia: I. Joubert syndrome. Dev Med Child Neurol 20:758, 1978.

Fukuyama YM, Ohsawa M, Suzuki H: Congenital progressive muscular dystrophy of the Fukuyama type: Clinical genetic and pathologic considerations. Brain Dev 3:1, 1984.

Ghosh A, Antonini A, McConnell SK, et al: Requirement for subplate neurons in the formation of thalamocortical connections. Nature 347:179, 1990.

Gieron-Korthals MA, Helal A, Martinez CR: Expanding spectrum of cocaine induced central nervous system malformations. Brain Dev 16:253, 1994.

Gilbert JN, Jones KL, Rorke LB, et al: Central nervous system anomalies associated with meningomyelocele, hydrocephalus, and the Arnold-Chiari malformation: Reappraisal of theories regarding the pathogenesis of posterior neural tube closure defects. Neurosurgery 18:559, 1986.

Gleeson JG, Allen KM, Fox JW: Doublecortin, a brain-specific gene mutated in human X-linked lissencephaly and double cortex syndrome, encodes a putative signaling protein. Cell 92:63-72, 1998.

Golden JA: Holoprosencephaly: A defect in brain patterning. J Neuropath Exp Neurol 57:991-999, 1998.

Golden JA, Chernoff GF: Multiple sites of anterior neural tube closure in humans: Evidence from anterior neural tube defects (anencephaly). Pediatrics 95:506, 1995.

Goldstein RB, Filly RA: Prenatal diagnosis of anencephaly: spectrum of sonographic appearances and distinction from the amniotic band syndrome. AJR Am J Roentgenol 151:547, 1988.

Gower DJ, Del Curling O, Kelly DLJ, et al: Diastematomyelia: A 40-year experience. Pediatr Neurosci 14:90, 1988.

Granata T, Farina L, Faiella A, et al: Familial schizencephaly associated with *EMX2* mutation. Neurology 48:1403-1406, 1997.

Grewal PK, Hewitt JE: Glycolylation defects: A new mechanism for muscular dystrophy? Hum Mol Genet 12 (rev issue 2): R259-R264, 2003.

Guerriero MM, Anderman F, Guerrini R, et al: Familial perisylvian polymicrogyria: A new familial syndrome of cortical maldedevelopment. Ann Neurol 48:39-48, 2000.

Guerrini R, Carrozzo R: Epilepsy and genetic malformations of the cerebral cortex. Am J Med Genet 106:160-173, 2002.

Gupta A, Tsai LH, Wynshaw-Boris A: Life is a journey: A genetic look at neocortical development. Nat Rev Genet. 3:342-355, 2002.

Hall DE, Udvarhelyi GB, Altman J: Lumbosacral skin lesions as markers of occult spinal dysraphism. JAMA 246:2606, 1981.

Hall JG, Solehdin F: Genetics of neural tube defects. MRRD Res Rev 4:269, 1998.

Hart MN, Malamud N, Ellis WG: The Dandy-Walker syndrome: A clinico-pathological study based on 28 cases. Neurology 22:771, 1972.

Hasegawa Y, Hasegawa T, Yokoyama T, et al: Holoprosencephaly associated with diabetes insipidus and syndrome of inappropriate secretion of antidiuretic hormone. J Pediatr 117:756, 1990.

Hayashi N, Tsutsumi Y, Barkovich AJ: Morphological features and associated anomalies of schizencephaly in the clinical population: Detailed analysis of MR images. Neuroradiology 44: 418-427, 2002a.

Hayashi N, Tsutsumi Y, Barkovich AJ: Polymicrogyria without porencephly/schizencephaly. MRI analysis of the spectrum and prevalence of macroscopic findings in the clinical population. Neuroradiology 44:647-655, 2002b.

Hong SE, Shugart YY, Huang DT, et al: Autosomal recessive lissencephaly with cerebellar hypoplasia is associated with human *RELN* mutations. Nat Genet 26:93-96, 2000.

Hunt GM, Holmes AE: Some factors relating to intelligence in treated children with spina bifida cystica. Dev Med Child Neurol 17 (suppl):65, 1975.

Iannetti P, Nigro G, Spalice A, et al: Cytomegalovirus infection and schizencephaly: Case reports. Ann Neurol 43:123-127, 1998.

Jacobson M: Developmental Neurobiology. New York, Plenum Press, 1991.

Jeret JS, Serur D, Wisniewski KE, et al: Clinicopathological findings associated with agenesis of the corpus callosum. Brain Dev 9:255, 1987.

Jones KL, Lacro RV, Johnson KA, et al: Pattern or malformations in the children of women treated with carbamazepine during pregnancy. N Engl J Med 320:1661, 1989.

Joubert M, Eisenring JJ, Robb JP, Andermann F: Familial agenesis of the cerebellar vermis: A syndrome of episodic hyperpnea, abnormal eye movements, ataxia, and retardation. Neurology 19:813, 1969.

Juhasz C, Chugani DC, Muzik O, et al: Alpha-methyl-L-tryptophan PET detects epileptogenic cortex in children with intractable epilepsy. Neurology 60:960-968, 2003.

Juriloff DM, Harris MJ: Mouse models of neural tube closure defects. Hum Mol Genet 9:993, 2000.

Kanold PO, Kara P, Reid RC, Shatz CJ: Role of subplate neurons in functional maturation of visual cortical columns. Science 301:521-525, 2003.

Kato M, Dobyns WB: Lissencephaly and the molecular basis of neuronal migration. Hum Mol Genet 12 (rev issue 1): R89-R96, 2003.

Kirk VG, Morielli A, Brouillette RT: Sleep-disordered breathing in patients with myelomeningocele: The missed diagnosis. Dev Med Child Neurol 41:40-43, 1999.

Kitamura K, Yanazawa M, Sugiyama N, et al: Mutation of *ARX* causes abnormal development of forebrain and testes in mice and X-linked lissencephaly with abnormal genitalia in humans. Nat Genet 32:359-369, 2002.

Kobayashi K, Nakahori Y, Miyake M, et al: An ancient retrotransposal insertion causes Fukuyama-type congenital muscular dystrophy. Nature 394:388-392, 2000.

Kostovic I, Rakic P: Developmental history of the transient subplate zone in the visual and somatosensory cortex of the macaque monkey and human brain. J Comp Neurol 297:441-470, 1990.

Ledbetter SA, Kuwano A, Dobyns WB, et al: Microdeletions of chromosome 17p13 as a cause of isolated lissencephaly. Am J Hum Genet 50:182, 1992.

LeDouarin NM: The Neural Crest. New York, Cambridge University Press, 1982.

Lenke RR, Levy HL: Maternal phenylketonuria and hyperphenylalanemia: An international survey of the outcome of untreated and treated pregnancies. N Engl J Med 303:1202, 1980.

Lorber J: Systematic ventriculographic studies in infants born with meningomyelocele and encephalocele. Arch Dis Child 36:381, 1961.

Louis DN, von Deimling A: Hereditary tumor syndromes of the nervous system: Overview and rare syndromes. Brain Pathol 5:145, 1995.

Mallamaci A, Mercurio S, Muzio L, et al: The lack of EMX2 causes impairment of reelin signaling and defects in neuronal migration in the developing cerebral cortex. J Neurosci 20:1109-18, 2000.

Margalith D, Jan JE, McCormick AQ, et al: Clinical spectrum of congenital optic nerve hypoplasia: A review of 51 patients. Dev Med Child Neurol 26:311, 1984.

Marin-Padilla M: Early ontogenesis of the human cerebral cortex. In Peters A, Jones EG (eds): Cerebral Cortex: Vol 7. Development and Maturation of Cerebral Cortex. New York, Plenum Press, 1988, pp 1-30.

Marin-Padilla M: Cajal-Retzius cells in the development of the neocortex. Trends Neurosci 21:64-71, 1998.

McAbee GN, Chan A, Erde EL: Prolonged survival with hydrancephaly: Report of two patients and literature review. Pediatr Neurol 23:80, 2000.

McLone DG: Continuing concepts in the management of spina bifida. Pediatr Neurosurg 18:254, 1992.

Menkes JH: Malformations of the central nervous system. In Taeusch HW, Ballard RA, Avery ME (eds): Diseases of the Newborn, 6th ed. Philadelphia, WB Saunders, 1991, pp 426-445.

Milunsky A, Alpert E, Neff RK, et al: Prenatal diagnosis of neural tube defects: IV. Maternal serum alpha-fetoprotein screening. Obstet Gynecol 55:60, 1980.

Ming JE, Muenke M: Multiple hits during early embryonic development: Digenic diseases and holoprosencephaly. Am J Hum Genet 71:1017-1032, 2002.

Mochida GH, Walsh CA: Molecular genetics of human microcephaly. Curr Opin Neurol 14:151-156, 2001.

Monuki ES, Walsh CA: Mechanisms of cerebral cortical patterning in mice and humans. Nature Neurosci Suppl 4:1199-1206, 2001.

Mott SH, Bodensteiner JB, Allen WC: The cavum septi pellucidi in term and preterm newborn infants. J Child Neurol 7:35, 1992.

MRC Vitamin Study Research Group: Prevention of neural tube defects: Results of the MRC Vitamin Study. Lancet 338:132, 1992.

Muenke M, Beach PA: Genetics of ventral forebrain development and holoprosencephaly. Curr Opin Genet Dev 10:262-269, 2000.

Muller F, O'Rahilly R: The human chondrocranium at the end of the embryonic period proper, with particular reference to the nervous system. Am J Anat 159:33-58, 1980.

Mulligan LM, Kwok JB, Healey CS, et al: Germ-line mutations of the *RET* proto-oncogene in multiple endocrine neoplasia type 2A. Nature 363:458, 1993.

Nagano T, Yoneda T, Hatanaka Y, et al: Filamin A-interacting protein (FLIP) regulates cortical cell migation out of the ventricular zone. Nat Cell Biol 4:495-501, 2002.

Naidich TP, Pudlowshi RM, Naidich JB: Computed tomographic signs of Chiari II malformation: II. Midbrain and cerebellum. Radiology 134:391, 1980.

Nanni L, Ming JE, Bocian M, Steinhaus K, et al: The mutational spectrum of the Sonic Hedgehog gene in holoprosencephaly: *SHH* mutations cause a significant proportion of autosomal dominant holoprosencephaly. Hum Mol Genet 8:2479-2488, 1999.

Neidich JA, Nussbaum RL, Packer RJ, et al: Heterogeneity of clinical severity and molecular lesions in Aicardi syndrome. J Pediatr 116:911-917, 1990.

Neumann PE, Frankel WN, Letts VA, et al: Multifactorial inheritance of neural tube defects: Localization of the major gene and recognition of modifiers in *ct* mutant mice. Nat Genet 6:357, 1994.

Neveling EA, Truex RC: External obstructive hydrocephalus: A study of clinical and developmental aspects in ten children. J Neurosurg Nurs 15:255-260, 1983.

Niesen CE: Malformations of the posterior fossa: Current perspectives. Semin Pediatr Neurol 9:320-334, 2002.

Norman MG, McHillivray B, Kalousek DK, et al: Holoprosencephaly: Defects of the mediobasal prosencephalon. In Congenital Malformations of the Brain: Pathological, Embryological, Clinical, Radiological and Genetic Aspects. New York, Oxford University Press, 1995a, pp 187-221.

Norman MG, McHillivray B, Kalousek DK, et al: Causes of malformations. In Congenital Malformations of the Brain: Pathological, Embryological, Clinical, Radiological and Genetic Aspects. New York, Oxford University Press, 1995b, pp 94-96.

Oakley GP, Erickson JD, James LM, et al: Prevention of folic acid–preventable spina bifida and anencephaly. In Bock G, Marsh J (eds): Neural Tube Defects. CIBA Foundation Symposium 181. Chicester, John Wiley & Sons, 1994, pp 212-231.

Ohtsuka Y, Ohno S, Oka E: Electroclinical characteristics of hemimegalencephaly. Pediatr Neurol 20:390-393, 1999.

O'Rahilly R, Muller F: The Embryonic Human Brain: An Atlas of Developmental Stages. New York, Wiley-Liss, 1994.

Ouvrier R, Billson F: Optic nerve hypoplasia: A review. J Child Neurol 1:181, 1986.

Packard AM, Miller VS, Delgado MR: Schizencephaly: Correlation of clinical findings and radiologic features. Neurology 48:1427-1434, 1997.

Parisi MA, Dobyns WB: Human malformations of the midbrain and hindbrain: A review and proposed classification scheme. Mol Genet Metabol 80:36-53, 2003.

Parrish ML, Roessmann U, Levinsohn MW: Agenesis of the corpus callosum: A study of the frequency of associated malformations. Ann Neurol 6:349, 1979.

Patel S, Barkovich AJ: Analysis and classification of cerebellar malformations. AJNR Am J Neuroradiol 23:1074-1087, 2002.

Peabody JL, Emery JR, Ashwal S: Experience with anencephalic infants as prospective organ donors. N Engl J Med 321: 344-350, 1989.

Peach B: Arnold-Chiari malformation: Anatomic features in 20 cases. Arch Neurol 12:613, 1965.

Peiffer, Singh N, Leppert M, et al: Microlissencephaly with simplified gyral pattern in six related children. Am J Med Genet 84:137-144, 1999.

Peiffer J, Majewski F, Fischbach H: Alcohol embryo and fetopathy: Neuropathology of 3 children and 3 fetuses. J Neurol Sci 41:125, 1979.

Rakic P: A small step for the cell, a giant leap for mankind: A hypothesis of neocortical expansion during evolution. Trends Neurosci 838, 1995.

Rakic P: Specification of cerebral cortical areas. Science 241:170-176, 1988.

Rakic P, Caviness VS: Cortical development: View from neurological mutants two decades later. Neuron 14:1101-1104, 1995.

Reznik M, Pierard GE: Neurophakomatoses and allied disorders. In Duckett S (ed): Pediatric Neuropathology. Baltimore, Williams & Wilkins, 1995, pp 734-755.

Robain O, Lyon G: Familial microcephalies due to cerebral malformation: Anatomical and clinical study. Acta Neuropathol 20:96, 1972.

Roessler E Belloni E, Gaudenz K, et al: Mutations in the human Sonic Hedgehog gene cause holoprosencephaly. Nat Genet 14:357-360, 1996.

Roessmann U: Congenital malformations. In Duckett S (ed): Pediatric Neuropathology. Baltimore, Williams & Wilkins, 1995, pp 123-149.

Romeo G, Ronchetto P, Luo Y, et al: Point mutations affecting the tyrosine kinase domain of the RET proto-oncogene in Hirschsprung's disease. Nature 367:377, 1994.

Ross ME: Full circle to cobbled brain. Nature 418:376-377, 2002.

Ross ME, Swanson K, Dobyns WB: Lissencephaly with cerebellar hypoplasia (LCH): A heterogeneous group of cortical malformations. Neuropediatrics 32:56-263, 2001.

Ross ME, Walsh CA: Human brain malformations and their lessons for neuronal migration. Annu Rev Neurosci 24:1041-1070, 2001.

Rubenstein JL, Beachy PA: Patterning of the embryonic forebrain. Curr Opin Neurobiol 8:18-26, 1998.

Russo GL, Tassi L, Cossu M, et al: Focal cortical resection in malformations of cortical development. Epilept Disord Suppl 2:S115-S123, 2003.

Satran D, Pierpont ME, Dobyns WB: Cerebello-oculo-renal syndromes including Arima, Senior-Loken and COACH syndromes: More than just variants of Joubert syndrome. Am J Med Genet 86:459-469, 1999.

Scatliff JH, Kendall BE, Kingsley DP, et al: Closed spinal dysraphism: Analysis of clinical, radiological, and surgical findings in 104 consecutive patients. AJNR Am J Neuroradiol 10:269, 1989.

Schaefer GB: Partial agenesis of the corpus callosum: Correlation between appearance, imaging, and neuropathology. Pediatr Neurol 7:39, 1991.

Smithells RW, Sheppard S, Schorah CJ, et al: Apparent prevention of neural tube defects by periconceptional vitamin supplementation. Arch Dis Child 56:911, 1981.

Stein SC, Schut L: Hydrocephalus in myelomeningocele. Childs Brain 5:413, 1979.

Stein SC, Schut L, Ames MD: Selection of early treatment of myelomeningocele: A retrospective analysis of selection procedures. Dev Med Child Neurol 17:311, 1975.

Sztriha L, Al-Gazali L, Varady E, et al: Microlissencephaly. Pediatr Neurol 18:362-365, 1998.

Tagawa T, Mimaki T, Ono J, et al: Aicardi syndrome associated with an embryonal carcinoma. Pediatr Neurol 5:45-47, 1989.

Takano T, Takikita S, Shimada M: Experimental schizencephaly induced by Kilham strain of mumps virus: Pathogenesis of cleft formation. Neuroreport 10:3149-3154, 1999.

Taniguchi K, Kobayashi K, Saito K, et al: Worldwide distribution and broader clinical spectrum of muscle-eye-brain disease. Hum Mol Genet 12:527-524, 2003.

Towfighi J, Housman C: Spinal cord abnormalities in caudal regression syndrome. Acta Neuropathol (Berlin) 81:458, 1991.

Van Allen MI, Kalousek DK, Chernoff GF, et al: Evidence for multi-site closure of the neural tube in humans. Am J Med Genet 47:723, 1993.

Villard L, Nguyen K, Cardoso C, et al: A locus for bilateral perisylvian polymicrogyria maps to Xq28. Am J Hum Genet 70:1003-1008, 2002.

Volpe JJ: Neurology of the Newborn, 4th ed. Philadelphia, WB Saunders, 2000, pp 1-99.

Waisbren SE, Levy HL: Effects of untreated maternal hyperphenylalanemia on the fetus: Further study of families identified by routine cord blood screening. J Pediatr 116:926, 1990.

Warburg M: Ocular malformations and lissencephaly. Eur J Pediatr 146:450, 1987.

Warkany U, Lemire RJ, Cohen MM Jr: Mental Retardation and Congenital Malformations of the Nervous System. Chicago, Year Book Medical Publishers, 1981.

Williams J, Brodsky MC, Griebel M, et al: Septo-optic dysplasia: The clinical insignificance of an absent septum pellucidum. Dev Med Child Neurol 35:490, 1993.

Yen IH, Khoury MJ, Erickson JD, et al: The changing epidemiology of neural tube defects in the United States, 1968-1989. Am J Dis Child 146:857, 1992.

Yerby MS: Clinical care of pregnant women with epilepsy: Neural tube defects and folic acid supplementation. Epilepsia 44 (suppl 3):33, 2003.

Yin L, Barone V, Seri M, et al: Heterogeneity and low detection rate of *RET* mutations in Hirschsprung disease. Eur J Hum Genet 2:272, 1994.

Zeki SM, Hollman AS, Dutton GN: Neuroradiological features of patients with optic nerve hypoplasia. J Pediatr Ophthalmol Strabismus 29:107, 1992.

CHAPTER

# 64

# Central Nervous System Injury and Neuroprotection

Ashima Madan, Shannon E. G. Hamrick, and Donna M. Ferriero

## INJURY AND PROTECTION IN THE DEVELOPING NERVOUS SYSTEM

Injury in the developing brain from ischemia results in a variety of pathologic patterns based on age at the time of insult, severity of the insult, mechanism of the insult, and the selective vulnerability of populations of cells undergoing active metabolic change. The most common type of injury in the preterm brain is intraventricular hemorrhage (IVH) from germinal matrix bleeding. IVH is a common injury in the premature brain due to perturbations of circulatory factors affecting the venous system. Hypoxic-ischemic injury results in periventricular leukomalacia (PVL) in the premature brain, whereas in the term brain, the deep gray matter is more likely to be affected. A variety of patterns of cortical and subcortical parenchymal injuries can be seen, depending on how the arterial supply is disrupted. Stroke from arterial or venous (sinovenous thrombosis) causes can occur at any time in the perinatal period. A number of traumatic injuries also can occur in the neonatal period, including damage to the calvaria, cranial nerves, spinal cord, and peripheral nerves. The ability to protect against these varied types of ischemic injuries will depend on accurate diagnosis, careful early management, and the development of age-appropriate therapies.

### Intraventricular and Periventricular Hemorrhage in the Preterm Infant

#### Pathogenesis

IVH originates in the subependymal germinal matrix. Cortical neuronal and glial cell precursors develop from the germinal matrix and adjacent ventricular germinal zone during the late second and early third trimesters. The subependymal germinal matrix is a highly vascularized region whose arterial supply is derived from the anterior and middle cerebral arteries as well as the anterior choroidal artery. These arteries feed an elaborate capillary network of thin-walled vessels that is continuous with a deep venous system that terminates in the vein of Galen. The terminal, choroidal, and thalamostriate veins course anteriorly to form the internal cerebral vein, which courses posteriorly to join the vein of Galen, thus leading to a U-shaped turn in the direction of blood flow. Involution of the germinal matrix occurs with advancing gestation.

The predisposition of the premature infant to IVH probably is due to several factors. A pressure-passive state exists due to the lack of autoregulation of cerebral blood flow in the cerebral arterioles in the premature brain. In the presence of a highly vascularized subependymal germinal matrix, the lack of a supporting basement membrane in the blood vessels of the germinal matrix and an increased amount of fibrinolytic activity in the germinal matrix region also predispose to the development of IVH. Extravascular tissue pressure decreases in the first few days of extrauterine life, and in the setting of elevation of venous pressure or an increase in fluctuations in cerebral blood flow velocity from a variety of factors (respiratory distress, pneumothorax, asphyxia, myocardial failure, patent ductus arteriosus, hypotension, hypothermia, hyperosmolarity), IVH may occur (Ment and Schneider, 1993).

IVH has been produced experimentally after hypotension followed by reperfusion (Goddard-Finegold et al, 1982; Ment et al, 1982), and infants with IVH are more likely to have had an early period of prolonged hypotension followed by an increase in blood pressure (Miall-Allen and Whitelaw, 1987; Miall-Allen et al, 1987). Hypertension associated with seizures, attempts at intubation, and suctioning also can lead to IVH. Even gavage feeding can lead to changes in cerebral hemodynamics as measured by near-infrared spectroscopy (NIRS) (Mischel et al, 1997). Disturbances in coagulation from various causes can lead to IVH. In rare cases, hemorrhage can result from a congenital arteriovenous malformation, a ruptured aneurysm, or small hemangiomas or papillomas of the choroid plexus (Schum et al, 1979). Table 64–1 lists the different factors that may interact in an individual case to produce IVH.

Cellular injury in infants with grade III or IV IVH may occur from ischemic injury that may precede IVH, from a decrease in cerebral blood flow to the region of the intraparenchymal bleed, or from increased intracranial pressure, as well as vasospasm and from post-hemorrhagic hydrocephalus. These conditions are associated with periventricular white matter injury and pontine neuronal necrosis (Volpe, 2001b). In this setting, venous infarction leads to neuronal as well as oligodendroglial cell death (Craig et al, 2003).

#### Site, Incidence, and Timing of Hemorrhage

In preterm infants, germinal matrix hemorrhage is most commonly seen at the junction of the terminal, choroidal, and thalamostriate veins in the germinal matrix over the body of the caudate nucleus at the level of the foramen of Monro. Parenchymal hemorrhage occurs most commonly in the frontoparietal region, in approximately 15% of cases, and is thought to be not an extension of the IVH but rather a separate process, a hemorrhagic infarction. The hemorrhage is more often unilateral or, in less than 30% of cases, asymmetrically bilateral.

The incidence and severity of IVH increase with decreasing gestation. It occurs in approximately 4.6% of term newborns and was previously reported to occur in

**TABLE 64–1**

**Pathogenetic Factors Leading to Intraventricular Hemorrhage**

| |
|---|
| Increase in cerebral blood flow |
| Fluctuation in cerebral blood flow |
| Increase in cerebral venous pressure |
| Endothelial injury |
| Vulnerable germinal matrix capillaries |
| Coagulation disturbances |
| Increased fibrinolysis |

40% to 60% of very low-birth-weight (VLBW) infants (less than 1500 g). An overall reduction of IVH in this population to 15% to 20% has been observed in the past decade (Paneth et al, 1993; Vohr et al, 2000). Although there has been a gradual decline in the incidence of all grades of IVH, the increased survival of VLBW infants has resulted in an increase in the absolute number of infants with IVH. The risk period for the occurrence of IVH is highest in the first 3 or 4 days of life. Hemorrhage is rarely seen at birth, although it has been reported as early as within the first hour of age (Ment et al, 1984). Antenatal hemorrhages can occur, especially in the setting of neonatal alloimmune thrombocytopenia. Twenty-five percent of hemorrhages occur by the sixth hour and 50% of hemorrhages occur during the first 24 hours of life. Less than 5% of infants develop IVH after the fourth or fifth day of life (Ment and Schneider, 1993). Extension of the hemorrhage may occur over the first few days secondary to events leading to alteration in cerebral blood flow.

## Clinical Presentation

The clinical presentation of IVH in the newborn depends on the extent of the hemorrhage and may vary from asymptomatic to a sudden and catastrophic deterioration that manifests with neurologic signs such as stupor or coma, fixed pupils, seizures, decerebrate posturing, or apnea. A full fontanel along with drops in hematocrit, hyperglycemia, hyperkalemia, hypotension, and bradycardia herald an IVH. Inappropriate secretion of antidiuretic hormone may also be present. The more common presentation, however, is that of a gradual clinical deterioration with an altered level of consciousness, hypotonia, abnormal extremity or eye movements. In 25% to 50% of cases, clinical correlation is lacking (Dubowitz et al, 1998).

## Screening for Intraventricular Hemorrhage

A practice parameter published jointly by the American Academy of Pediatrics, the American Society of Pediatric Neuroradiology and the Society for Pediatric Radiology recommends routine screening with cranial ultrasonography for all infants of less than 30 weeks of gestation between 7 and 14 days of age. A repeat ultrasound examination is recommended between 36 and 40 weeks of postmenstrual age (Ment et al, 2002). Insufficient evidence exists at present to recommend routine magnetic resonance imaging (MRI) screening of all LBW infants with abnormal findings on head ultrasound examination (Ment et al, 2002). However, considerable advances in the field of MRI in premature infants have been made recently (Miller et al, 2002a). Several studies have focused on determining the spectrum of white matter injury detected by MRI and its effect on neurodevelopment (Groenendaal et al, 1997; Huppi et al, 1998; Inder et al, 1999; Maalouf et al, 1999, 2001; Ment et al, 2002; van Wezel-Meijler et al, 1998). It is now becoming clear that lesions that affect developmental outcome and that are not present on cranial ultrasound images can be detected by MRI. Therefore, we recommend that an MRI study be considered in all extremely low-birth-weight (ELBW) infants at 36 to 40 weeks of postmenstrual age if clinical suspicion for parenchymal brain injury exists.

## Grading of Intraventricular Hemorrhage

Ultrasound examination is a reliable and sensitive technique for evaluating the severity of IVH in the newborn nursery (Pape et al, 1979, 1983). Papile and associates (1978) adapted the standard grading system originally applied to computed tomographic images of IVH to ultrasound images and classified IVH into four different grades of severity depending on the location and extent of the bleed (Fig. 64–1; Table 64–2). Outcome studies performed over the past decade use this system for classification. In

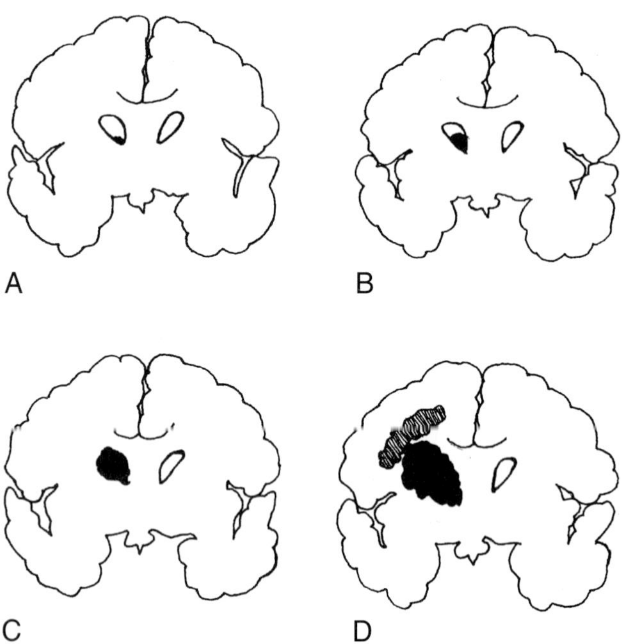


**FIGURE 64–1.** Illustration of intraventricular hemorrhage (IVH) grades as determined by degree of hemorrhage (see Table 64–2). **A,** Grade I hemorrhage involves less than 10% of the ventricular volume in the lateral ventricles; **B,** grade II hemorrhage involves 10% to 50%; **C,** grade III involves greater than 50% of the ventricular volume and is often associated with some ventricular dilatation; and **D,** grade IV (Papile et al, 1978) or unclassified (Volpe, 2001) is associated with parenchymal echodensities on head ultrasound study, indicating parenchymal infarction.

**TABLE 64–2**

**Grading of Intraventricular Hemorrhage (IVH) by Cranial Ultrasound Findings**

| Papile | Grading System | Volpe | Grading System* |
|---|---|---|---|
| I | Subependymal hemorrhage with minimal or no intraventricular hemorrhage | I | Germinal matrix hemorrhage <10% IVH |
| II | Definite intraventricular hemorrhage without distention of the ventricles | II | IVH 10%-50% |
| III | Enlargement of the ventricles secondary to distention with blood | III | IVH >50%, usually with distention of lateral ventricle |
| IV | Extension of the hemorrhage into the parenchyma along with intraventricular hemorrhage and enlargement | Separate notation | Periventricular echodensity signifying parenchymal lesion |

*By cranial ultrasound

IVH, intraventricular hemorrhage

the preferred grading system used by Volpe (2001b), the presence of intracerebral hemorrhage or parenchymal lesions is mentioned separately and not designated as grade IV. This system relies on the head ultrasound examination as the diagnostic measure and more accurately defines IVH based on the extent of the ventricular hemorrhage. Because parenchymal involvement is a distinct process, it is not included in the continuous grading (see Table 64–2).

### Outcome and Prognosis

Grade I hemorrhage and grade II hemorrhage generally are followed by resolution. Grade III hemorrhage evolves over a period of 1 to 3 weeks and in some cases produces a fibrotic reaction that obliterates the subarachnoid space and leads to ventricular dilatation and hydrocephalus. Traditional clinical criteria of increasing ventricular dilatation such as rapid head growth, full anterior fontanel, and separated cranial sutures often appear days or even weeks after the dilatation begins. This delayed appearance is due to the presence of a large subarachnoid space as well as the paucity of myelin in premature infants. In 15% of cases of IVH, areas of periventricular hemorrhagic involvement are noted (Volpe, 2001b). This finding is believed to be due to an independent venous infarct of the periventricular white matter and not a direct extension of the IVH into the parenchyma (Volpe, 2001b). Intraparenchymal hemorrhage is followed in 1 to 8 weeks by tissue destruction and formation of a porencephalic cyst. Outcomes vary between studies, but in general, mortality rates are not significantly increased in infants with a grade I or II hemorrhage. Grades III and IV are associated with increased mortality, with mortality rates in neonates suffering hemorrhagic infarction approaching 50% (Vohr et al, 2000; Whitelaw, 2001).

Several studies have focused on the relationship between IVH and subsequent neurologic dysfunction. Again, grade I IVH and grade II IVH are not associated with significant morbidity. However, grade III is associated with neurologic sequelae in 35% of infants, and grade IV is associated with sequelae in as many as 90% of affected infants (Whitelaw, 2001). The severity of neurologic sequelae such as seizures, severe motor handicap, and severe hearing and vision impairment increases in infants with grade III or IV hemorrhage in whom persistent ventriculomegaly develops. The presence of hydrocephalus with or without shunting at term increases the odds of a poor neurodevelopmental outcome. Vohr and colleagues (2000), in a longitudinal study of 90 preterm infants with birth weights of less than 1750 g, reported that by 2 years of age, only infants with grade III and grade IV differed in neurologic examination findings from the term control infants. Unlike motor function, cognitive function as assessed by the Bayley scores deteriorates in the first 18 months of life. Infants with grade I and grade II IVH have lower scores than those infants with no IVH or normal term infants. Follow-up studies have shown that the degree of IVH at birth and the presence of ventriculomegaly are predictors of neurologic status at 5 years (Lowe and Papile, 1990; Ment et al, 1999; Vohr et al, 1992, 1999). Data suggest that even infants with lesser degrees of hemorrhage are at risk for cognitive difficulties possibly related to under-recognized white and gray matter injury (Inder, 1999).

### Prevention

Prevention of preterm birth is the most effective method of eliminating IVH. In the event of preterm labor it is advisable that the infant be born at a center specializing in high-risk deliveries. The risk of IVH is higher in infants who are transported after birth. Adequate management of labor and delivery is essential. Appropriate resuscitation of the preterm infant and vigilance in avoiding hyperventilation and low $P_{CO_2}$ or hypoxia, maintaining adequate mean arterial pressure, and avoiding elevations in cerebral blood flow by excessive handling or tracheal suctioning are vital. Prevention of pneumothorax and acidosis and avoidance of rapid infusions of sodium bicarbonate or volume expanders also are critical. Due to the increased risk of neurodevelopmental sequelae in infants with IVH, several clinical trials have studied the effects of different pharmacologic interventions to reduce the incidence of IVH. Muscle paralysis causes a decrease in the fluctuations of cerebral blood flow velocity, and a controlled prospective study of short-term paralysis showed reduction in IVH in the paralyzed group (Perlman et al, 1985). Several clinical trials have been done to evaluate the role of prolonged neuromuscular paralysis in preterm infants. A meta-analysis of five trials concluded that although neuromuscular paralysis with pancuronium may help decrease IVH and pneumothorax in asynchronously breathing infants, its routine use cannot be recommended because of concerns about safety and long-term pulmonary and neurologic effects. (Cools and Offringa, 2000).

A low mean arterial blood pressure (MAP) and an increase in fluctuation of blood pressure have been associated with an increased risk of IVH. Close monitoring of the MAP is recommended; however, there is no evidence suggesting that pharmacologic manipulation of the MAP (e.g., with pressors, steroids, or volume expanders) to achieve a set goal (e.g., MAP >30 mm Hg) alters the incidence of IVH or improves neonatal outcome. Antenatal phenobarbital administration was shown in early studies to be beneficial by preventing fluctuations in blood pressure (Donn et al, 1981). Subsequently, the results of a large multicenter trial testing the effect of antenatal administration of phenobarbital (10 mg/kg) to 610 women on the frequency of IVH in infants between 24 and 33 weeks of age showed no decrease in IVH in infants born to mothers treated with phenobarbital (Kaempf et al, 1990). Although additional studies showed some benefit for higher grades of hemorrhage, there was no significant difference in neurologic outcome in the treated population (Shankaran et al, 1996). Postnatal administration of phenobarbital has also not been shown to be effective (Kuban et al, 1986).

Pharmacologic doses of vitamin E, an antioxidant, were associated with a reduction in the incidence of IVH in LBW infants when given intramuscularly (Speer et al, 1984). However, following reports of the association of such large doses of vitamin E with sepsis and necrotizing enterocolitis, its use for prevention of IVH was curtailed (Finer et al, 1984; Johnson et al, 1985).

Indomethacin, a prostaglandin synthetase inhibitor, had originally been shown to decrease the incidence of IVH in infants weighing less than 1250 g (Ment et al, 1985). In a subsequent study of 431 infants, low-dose indomethacin (0.1 mg/kg) given intravenously (IV) at 6 to 12 hours of age and every 24 hours for a total of three doses decreased the incidence and severity of IVH (Ment et al, 1994). Follow-up studies at 4.5 years of age showed no adverse effect of indomethacin on neurodevelopmental function (Ment et al, 2000). However, indomethacin is not without short-term serious side effects. A meta-analysis of 16 studies demonstrated an increase in renal complications and necrotizing enterocolitis to achieve only a slight reduction in grade III or IV IVH (Fowlie, 1996). A more recent study on the long-term effects of indomethacin prophylaxis in extremely LBW infants showed no improvement in the rate of survival without neurosensory impairment at 18 months, despite the reduction in severe IVH (Schmidt et al, 2001).

Ethamsylate, an inhibitor of prostacyclin synthesis used to reduce capillary bleeding in surgery, has been shown in a multicenter randomized controlled trial to reduce the severity and overall incidence of IVH (Benson et al, 1986). Use of antenatal steroids (Canterino et al, 2001; Elimian et al, 2000; Smith et al, 2000) and surfactant replacement therapy have been shown to decrease the incidence of IVH as well as neonatal mortality in LBW infants (Soll and Dargaville, 2000). The increase in IVH reported with surfactant administration may occur as a result of the mode of instillation (Cowan et al, 1991; Hellstrom-Westas et al, 1991, 1992). A significant drop in MAP and cerebral blood flow volume can occur during surfactant administration; attention should be paid to the speed and volume of instillation.

Several studies have been done to evaluate the early use of high-frequency oscillatory ventilation (HFOV) versus conventional ventilation for infants with respiratory distress syndrome. Some of these studies have shown an increased incidence of IVH with HFOV (HIFI Study Group, 1989; Castro et al, 2000; Moriette et al, 2001). Other studies did not find an increase in IVH (Keszler et al, 1997).

It is important to avoid both hypocarbia ($P_{CO_2}$ <30 mm Hg) or hypercarbia ($P_{CO_2}$ >55 mm Hg) because of effects on cerebral blood flow. Hypocarbia is associated with hypotension as well as an acute decrease in cerebral blood flow. Avoiding low $P_{CO_2}$ has been shown to be neuroprotective in animal studies (Sola et al, 1983; Vannucci et al, 1995). Although the effect of low $P_{CO_2}$ levels has not been systematically studied in preterm infants, low levels have been shown to be deleterious in term infants with pulmonary hypertension (Ferrara et al, 1984). Hypercarbia leads to increases in cerebral blood flow, which in the presence of other therapies aimed at increasing blood pressure, may be damaging to the central nervous system (CNS).

Free radicals and iron have been shown to be damaging to oligodendrocytes in both cell culture and animal studies (Back et al, 1998; Dommergues et al, 1998). Also, iron-chelating agents such as deferoxamine have been shown to be neuroprotective (Sarco et al, 2000). It may be wise to prevent iron overload during the period of critical cortical development (Gressens et al, 2002). Similarly, avoiding hyperoxia is important to prevent free radical injury.

Several of the medications that are used frequently in LBW infants may have effects on neurodevelopment. The long-term neurodevelopmental effects of theophylline and caffeine, which are frequently used to prevent apnea in preterm infants, have not been studied. Postnatal steroid use in preterm infants has been found to be associated with an increased risk of PVL and poor neurodevelopment (Merz et al, 1999; Murphy et al, 2001). Pain medications such as morphine, fentanyl, and midazolam are often used for analgesia in ventilated preterm infants. However, there is increasing concern regarding the potential detrimental effects of this practice on the developing brain. Recently, Simons and colleagues (2003) found that routine morphine infusion in ventilated preterm newborns had no measurable analgesic effect and no beneficial effect on neurodevelopment. More controlled studies are needed comparing the efficacy and safety of different analgesic practices in the preterm population.

## Management

Infants with birth weights of less than 1500 g or gestational age of less than 32 weeks should have a screening ultrasound performed to detect IVH. A scan on the fourth postnatal day detects 90% of lesions. Because extension of the bleed sometimes occurs over the next few days, a repeat ultrasound examination after 5 days is necessary to establish the extent of the bleed.

The decision to continue intensive care support depends on the severity of the bleed as assessed by head ultrasound examination as well as the infant's gestational age and clinical condition. Parents should be informed regarding the presence of IVH and the prognosis of the infant.

The acute management is mainly supportive and requires control of ventilation, maintenance of a normal metabolic status and optimal nutritional state, and avoidance of seizures. Systemic blood pressure should be maintained with cautious attention to the rate of administration of fluid. Consideration of the aforementioned risk factors is important to prevent ischemic infarction.

Of the infants in whom enlargement of the ventricles occurs, approximately 50% develop rapidly progressive ventricular dilatation over the next 4 to 8 weeks. Regular measurement of head circumference and examination of the fontanel and clinical status are recommended in the first 4 weeks in cases of slowly progressive hydrocephalus. Serial lumbar puncture or use of carbonic anhydrase inhibitors has been recommended by some clinicians. A recent randomized controlled trial of the combined use of furosemide and acetazolamide in 177 infants with posthemorrhagic hydrocephalus concluded that this treatment is ineffective in decreasing the need for shunt placement and is associated with increased risk of a poor neurologic outcome (Kennedy et al, 2001). Use of streptokinase immediately after an IVH with development of posthemorrhagic hydrocephalus has been advocated by some to be beneficial. However, the studies to date have been too small to allow reasonable conclusions (Haines and Lapointe, 1999; Luciano et al, 1998; Whitelaw, 2001).

In infants with rapidly progressive hydrocephalus that does not respond to serial lumbar punctures, placement of an external ventriculostomy is necessary as a temporizing measure. Placement of a ventriculoperitoneal shunt that diverts cerebrospinal fluid (CSF) from the lateral ventricles to the peritoneal cavity in a premature infant is problematic due to the risk of skin breakdown, shunt obstruction, and/or infection. However, some centers are placing subgaleal shunts as a temporizing measure in these infants; these shunts may be associated with significantly fewer complications (Fulmer et al, 2000).

## Hypoxic-Ischemic Reperfusion Injury in the Newborn

Perinatal hypoxic-ischemic reperfusion (HI-R) injury may result in neonatal hypoxic-ischemic encephalopathy (HIE), which is a significant cause of neonatal morbidity and mortality and can lead to severe long-term neurologic deficits. The incidence of HIE is approximately 6 in 1000 term infants, with the incidence of death or severe neurologic deficit being 1 in 1000 (Levene and Evans, 1985). Much of our understanding concerning the effects of hypoxic-ischemic injury in the newborn brain has been derived from studies done in experimental models in animals.

### Etiology

Hypoxia-ischemia results when the decrease in cerebral perfusion is severe enough to overcome the ability of tissue to extract oxygen from the blood, thereby leading to a mismatch between cerebral blood flow and oxidative metabolism. Although the final pathways leading to cerebral brain death are remarkably similar regardless of the instigating event, the extent, location, and evolution of cell death probably are determined by the nature of the insult. The etiology of HIE is multifactorial. In a study of risk factors for neonatal encephalopathy, antepartum risk factors such as maternal hypotension, infertility treatment, and thyroid disease were present in 69% of the cases; both antepartum and intrapartum risk factors were present in 24%; and a history of an intrapartum event such as maternal fever, difficult forceps delivery, breech extraction, cord prolapse, or abruptio placentae was present in 5% of the cases (Badawi et al, 1998). Postnatal events such as severe respiratory distress or congenital heart disease, sepsis, and shock are responsible for fewer than 10% of cases of HIE.

### Clinical Signs and Symptoms

The clinical signs and symptoms depend on the severity, timing, and duration of the insult. The infant's gestational age needs to be taken into consideration in the evaluation. Symptoms usually evolve over a period of 72 hours (Sarnat and Sarnat, 1976) (Table 64–3).

During the first 12 hours after birth, the signs and symptoms are secondary to cerebral hemisphere depression, although signs of brainstem involvement may be present. During this period the infant is not easily arousable. This alteration in consciousness is attributed to the involvement of the cerebral hemispheres, the reticular activating system, or the thalamus. Periodic breathing with apnea or bradycardia is usually present. The infant has intact pupillary responses and may have spontaneous eye movements, depending on involvement of cranial nuclei 3, 4, and 6. Cerebral cortical or cerebellar cortical involvement may manifest as hypotonia with decreased movement or as jitteriness or seizure activity, which is seen in 50% of severely affected infants by 6 to 12 hours after birth. The Moro, grasp, and suck and swallow reflexes may be absent or depressed. In cases of severe asphyxia, seizures may be seen within 2 to 3 hours following the insult. Seizure activity in a term infant can be multifocal or focal in nature. Subtle seizures may also manifest as ocular movements such as tonic horizontal deviation of the eyes or sustained eye opening or blinking; orolingual movements such as tongue or lip smacking or sucking, or rowing or bicycling movements of the extremities, or as recurrent apnea (Mizrahi and Kellaway, 1987).

During the 12- to 24-hour period after the injury, there is an apparent increase in the level of alertness, but this is not associated with other signs of improvement in neurologic function. This period is accompanied by seizures in 15% to 20% of infants, apneic episodes in 50%, and jitteriness as well as weakness in the proximal limbs in 35% to 50%. The Moro reflex is exaggerated, the infant's cry is shrill and monotonous, and the deep tendon reflexes are exaggerated.

**TABLE 64–3**

**Clinical Staging of Hypoxic-Ischemic Encephalopathy**

| Factor | Stage 1 | Stage 2 | Stage 3 |
|---|---|---|---|
| Level of consciousness | Alert | Lethargy | Coma |
| Muscle tone | Normal | Hypotonia | Flaccidity |
| Tendon reflexes | Normal/increased | Increased | Depressed/absent |
| Myoclonus | Present | Present | Absent |
| Complex reflexes | | | |
| Sucking | Active | Weak | Absent |
| Moro | Exaggerated | Incomplete | Absent |
| Grasping | Normal/exaggerated | Exaggerated | Absent |
| Oculocephalic (doll's eyes) | Normal | Overreactive | Reduced/absent |

Data from Sarnat NB, Sarnat MS: Neonatal encephalopathy following distress. Arch Neurol 33:696-705, 1976.

After 24 to 72 hours the infant's level of consciousness deteriorates. This is followed by respiratory arrest and signs of brainstem dysfunction such as loss of responsiveness to the doll's eyes maneuver, fixed and dilated pupils, and sometimes death. Infants who survive until 72 hours continue in stupor with disturbed suck, swallow, and gag reflexes; hypotonia; and weakness of the proximal limbs and especially facial and bulbar musculature.

## Diagnosis

The diagnosis of HIE is made through a careful history, laboratory studies, and neurologic examination. Metabolic abnormalities, cerebral dysgenesis, and infection all can mimic HIE. There is sometimes a history of intrauterine distress, as evidenced by abnormalities on the fetal heart tracing, passage of meconium, or a history of difficult labor or delivery with a decrease in placental or fetal blood flow. A history of a difficult resuscitation that includes the use of cardiopulmonary resuscitation, medications in the delivery room, and intubation and assisted ventilation at birth and low extended Apgar scores after 5 minutes of age are associated with HIE. Presence of jitteriness, seizures, apneic episodes, or abnormal cry is suggestive of injury.

The neurologic examination provides important information for prognosis. Laboratory tests can be helpful in diagnosing HIE. Metabolic complications such as hypoglycemia, hypocalcemia, hyponatremia, hypoxemia, and acidosis are frequently seen. The nucleated red blood cell count may be elevated on review of the complete blood count. Several other metabolic parameters such as serum brain-specific creatine kinase (BB fraction), serum hypoxanthine, and serum lactate also are elevated. Lumbar puncture should be performed if the history is not consistent with perinatal distress, to rule out conditions that may mimic HIE. Lumbar puncture should be used to measure cell count, protein and glucose levels, and ratio of lactate to pyruvate, as well as brain-specific creatine kinase. A CSF protein level above 150 mg/dL is considered abnormal. Urinary lactate-to-creatine ratios have been shown to be elevated in asphyxiated infants (Huang et al, 1999).

Changes on the electroencephalogram (EEG) can be helpful in determining the severity of the insult. The initial change is a suppression of amplitude and frequency. This is followed after 24 hours by a periodic pattern that consists of periods of greater voltage suppression interspersed with bursts of sharp and slow waves. Subsequently, a "burst suppression" pattern with fewer bursts and more severe voltage depression is seen, followed by an isoelectric tracing. The EEG is helpful in supporting the diagnosis of HIE, and amplitude-integrated electroencephalography has been used in both animal and human studies as an aid to identify newborns moderately to severely compromised by hypoxic-ischemic injury (al Naqeeb et al, 1999; Toet et al, 1999). Obtaining an EEG is critically important after phenobarbital administration because this drug causes electroclinical dissociation (Biagioni et al, 1998).

Neuroimaging has become increasingly useful for the accurate diagnosis of HIE. Computed tomography (CT) often is not helpful in making a diagnosis because it is insensitive to changes in water content. Also, especially in the posterior fossa, injury can be obscured by bone artifact. CT is best used to determine the extent of bleeding in an emergency situation when MRI is not available.

MRI has proved to be a sensitive technique to determine injury in both the premature and term brain. In the term infant, absence of signal in the posterior limb of the internal capsule (PLIC) is strongly associated with poor neurologic outcome (Rutherford et al, 1995). Newer techniques such as diffusion tensor imaging (DTI) have been shown to be helpful in defining areas of the brain at risk for damage (Barkovich et al, 2001; Huppi et al, 2001). DTI can also be used to monitor normal development of pathways using the apparent diffusion coefficient (ADC) and anisotropy in certain regions (Miller et al, 2002c). In a comparison of head ultrasound examination with MRI, MRI was more sensitive in identifying PVL (Rijn et al, 2001).

Ultrasonography is extremely useful for imaging the unstable patient if performed with high-resolution transducers (de Vries et al, 1997). Injury to the basal ganglia, periventricular echodensities, and presence of focal or multifocal ischemic parenchymal lesions suggest neurologic deficits.

Ultrasound is insensitive to cortical damage; therefore, in term infants, ultrasound findings may under-represent the extent of the lesion.

Proton magnetic resonance spectroscopy (MRS) also has been useful for depicting age-dependent changes in preterm infants and can be a powerful tool for diagnosing early damage in both preterm and term infants (Vigneron et al, 2001). MRS provides a quantitative in vivo measure of brain biochemistry. At long echo times, it can measure resonance intensities for *N*-acetyl aspartate (NAA), creatine (Cr), and phosphocreatine, choline (Cho), and lactate. The measure of NAA in reference to baseline Cr or Cho has provided a sensitive indicator of neuronal integrity, whereas lactate has indicated the presence of oxidative stress or ongoing injury. MRS is now being used more extensively to identify areas at risk in perinatal HIE (Holshouser et al, 2000).

NIRS is a noninvasive technique that holds promise in the future. It can be used at the bedside to provide information regarding cerebral oxygen delivery. However, this modality is not quantitative and is not available at many centers.

## Patterns of Injury and Pathology

The mechanism of injury can be one of several types. Different patterns of injury may result, depending on the duration and severity of the insult.

### *Global Ischemia*

Global hypoxia-ischemia develops when the oxygen requirements for cerebral metabolism are unable to be met by cerebral perfusion pressure, as is seen with a decrease in cerebral arterial pressure or an increase in cerebral venous pressure. Although the injury may be transient, it sets into motion a cascade of events that ultimately lead to neuronal death. The duration of the insult necessary to produce brain injury is inversely proportional to the gestational age of the fetus. The extent and location of the injury can be patchy bilaterally or diffuse involving the entire cortex. The latent period to neuronal cell death produced by a global insult can range from hours to days and is determined by a complex interaction among various vascular, cellular, and metabolic factors (see later). A detailed understanding of these mechanisms is necessary for determination of appropriate timing for therapeutic intervention.

### *Focal or Partial Ischemia*

Focal ischemia occurs when the artery or venous supply to a region is compromised. The degree of injury is dependent on the collateral blood supply to this region. The injured region typically consists of a central dense region of ischemia that undergoes rapid cell death—the *core*—surrounded by a region of evolving cell injury—the *penumbra*. The cells in the penumbral region initially are sustained by anaerobic glycolysis. However, within hours the injury becomes irreversible, thus bringing the penumbra into the gradually enlarging area of infarction. This period of delay in cell death provides an opportunity for therapeutic intervention and prevention of further cell damage. Partial asphyxia without acidosis, as occurs in response to impairment of placental gas exchange by uterine contractions, maternal hypotension, or impairment in maternal placental circulation, can produce either a widespread cerebral cortical necrosis or a more focal injury to the posterior parietal parasagittal regions. Partial asphyxia with acidosis has been shown to cause white matter injury.

Cerebral blood flow is closely autoregulated over a wide range of systemic blood pressure by either vasoconstriction or dilatation of cerebral arterioles. However, this mechanism is imperfect in the newborn. Therefore, rapid changes in cerebral perfusion pressure can occur in response to changes in systemic blood pressure, as well as changes in cerebral $Pa{O_2}$ and $Pa{CO_2}$. Injury typically tends to occur in the watershed regions, which in the term newborn are located in the parasagittal regions of the cerebral cortex. The periventricular white matter is the most vulnerable region in preterm newborns.

Certain portions of the brain such as the basal ganglia, the thalamus, and the brainstem nuclei are more prone to injury by virtue of either increased myelination or metabolism or the presence of glutamate-responsive receptors and increased glutaminergic synapses. The major patterns of neuropathologic injury are as follows: selective neuronal necrosis, parasagittal lesions, status marmoratus of the basal ganglia and thalamus, focal or multifocal necrosis, pontosubicular necrosis, spinal cord ischemic infarction, and periventricular leukomalacia.

*Selective neuronal necrosis* can involve specific regions of the cortex, thalamus, brainstem, cerebellum, or hippocampus. An acute global injury such as is seen with uterine rupture or cord prolapse causes injury to the basal ganglia, thalamus, and brainstem, whereas a prolonged partial injury affects mainly the cortex and subcortical white matter. Damage is more extensive in the posterior parietal-occipital region than in the anterior cortical areas. Clinical signs in the infant relate to the site of injury. Seizures are a feature of cortical injury, whereas irritability, posturing, and brainstem dysfunction are seen with infarcts affecting the basal ganglia and thalamus. Long-term sequelae of such an injury include cerebral atrophy and multicystic encephalomalacia.

Clinical features of *parasagittal injury* include hypotonia and weakness, especially in the upper trunk. Cortical infarcts usually occur in the watershed region supplied by the most peripheral branches of the anterior, middle, and posterior cerebral arteries.

*Status marmoratus* refers to the marbled appearance of the basal ganglia, thalamus, and cerebral cortex in response to the injury. This appearance results from gross shrinkage of the striatum and defects in myelination. It may relate to the type of insult or the density of glutaminergic receptors in the basal ganglia (Johnston, 1995). Although the clinical correlate of this condition in the newborn is not well defined, it is seen in children with choreoathetoid cerebral palsy.

*Focal* and *multifocal cerebral necroses* occur secondary to an embolus or thrombus (see "Perinatal Stroke"). There are often underlying problems such as thrombophilias, maternal idiopathic thrombocytopenic purpura (ITP), vascular maldevelopment, or history of maternal cocaine use. Infants may present with unilateral, focal seizures or display asymmetrical motor function, or they may be asymptomatic. In some circumstances, lesions may involve the brain stem (*pontosubicular necrosis*) or the cerebellum. Babies with pontosubicular necrosis have impairment of the cranial nerve nuclei and will exhibit ptosis and facial diparesis.

*Spinal cord ischemia* is not uncommon following HI-R injury. In patients with hyporeflexia or areflexia, spinal cord pathology should be considered. Ischemic necrosis occurs in spinal cord gray matter. (Clancy et al, 1989).

*Periventricular leukomalacia* (PVL) is a form of white matter injury that occurs at the arterial end zones in premature infants. The pathologic features of PVL consist of a focal, deep component that is characterized by localized necrosis and cyst formation, as well as a less severe diffuse injury to the oligodendroglial cell precursors that is much more difficult to visualize on cranial ultrasound examination. The focal component of PVL occurs mainly in the regions that are in the end zones of the long penetrating arteries, whereas the diffuse component occurs mainly in the regions bordering the areas between the long penetrating arteries. Together with periventricular hemorrhagic infarction, a complication of IVH, and focal periventricular white matter injury (Miller et al, 2002c), these conditions result in severe spastic motor deficits and other developmental and cognitive disabilities in up to 50% of affected children (Volpe, 1997). Asphyxia, sepsis, recurrent episodes of apnea, seizures, and prolonged ventilation all are conditions that may predispose the premature infant to develop PVL. Hypotension frequently accompanies all of these conditions. It is hypothesized that oxidative stress is the major cause of PVL in the setting of ischemia (Volpe, 2001b). Newer theories of the pathogenesis of white matter injury implicate several other mechanisms besides hypoxic-ischemic events (Nelson and Ellenberg, 1986). Prenatal or perinatal factors such as thyroid hormone deficiency, growth factor deficiency, genetic factors, maternal infections, and free radicals may lead to an increase in cytokine production (Gressens et al, 2002). Studies in animal models have shown that cytokine exposure followed by an insult can produce white matter damage, whereas cytokine exposure alone does not cause injury; this finding suggests a "two-hit mechanism" in which injurious factors after birth could exacerbate the damaging events that originated in utero (Dammann et al, 2002; Dommergues et al, 1998).

The cellular target in white matter injury is unknown. It has been suggested that late oligodendrocyte progenitors that populate human cerebral white matter during the high-risk period for PVL are the major target of ischemic, free radical, or cytokine injury (Back and Volpe, 1997; Back et al, 2001, 2002). In addition, recent data suggest vulnerability of the subplate neurons as well (McQuillen et al, 2003). Tissue damage is associated with proliferation of astrocytes and microglial cells in areas of subcortical degeneration. PVL may be associated with hemorrhage into the lesion in some cases and may be unilateral or asymmetrical. This condition is often confused with the hemorrhage observed after IVH. The severity of injury in PVL can range from small areas of focal necrosis to diffuse involvement leading to cavitations over a period of 2 to 4 weeks (cystic leukomalacia). The head ultrasound study sometimes misses the lesions seen on MRI (Fig. 64–2). Clinical features in the premature infant may involve impairment of gaze and hearing, weakness, or altered muscle tone. Long-term problems may include spastic diplegia and visual and auditory impairment.

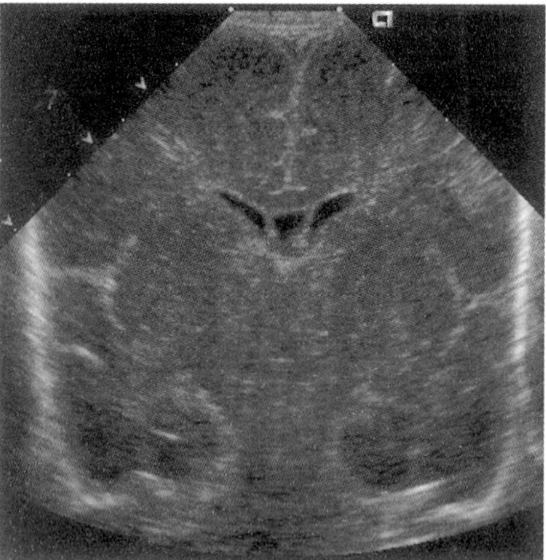


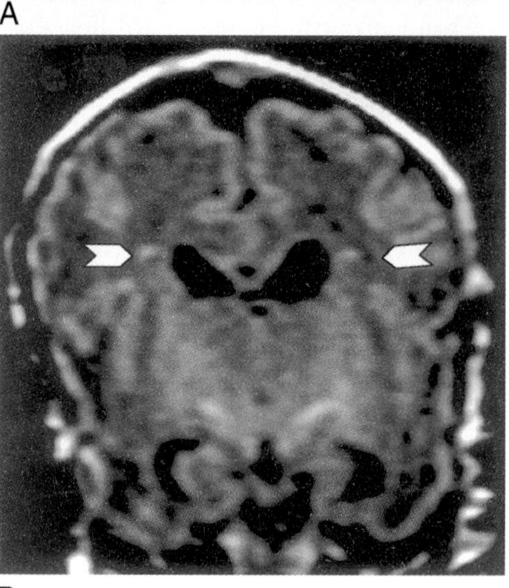


**FIGURE 64–2.** **A,** Head ultrasound image with no evidence of periventricular leukomalacia. **B,** Abnormalities are well seen on T1-weighted magnetic resonance image (*arrows*) in the same patient.

Maintenance of cerebral perfusion is key for prevention of PVL. Also important is avoidance of factors that lead to cerebral ischemia such as marked hypocapnia or hypotension. In the future, use of free radical scavengers, antiapoptotic agents, or amino-3-hydroxy-5-methyl-4-isoxazolepropionic acid (AMPA) antagonists, or combinations of therapies, may be effective at preventing PVL (Volpe, 2001a).

## Pathogenesis

Studies in animal models of asphyxia have shown that although the newborn can survive an asphyxial insult better than the mature animal, the brain is still injured. The immature brain is more susceptible to hypoxic ischemic injury for several reasons, including immaturity of vascular regulation, along with maturational differences in metabolic oxidative function between the newborn and adult brain (Ferriero, 2001).

Asphyxia leads to a redistribution of cardiac output, with a 30% to 175% increase in cerebral blood flow. Because cerebral vasoautoregulation is compromised, the cerebral arterioles are unable to respond appropriately in response to the alteration in blood flow or hypercapnia. Continued asphyxia leads ultimately to a fall in cardiac output, hypotension, and thus a fall in cerebral perfusion. Cerebral edema can further compromise cerebral blood flow and set into motion a cascade of events that leads to necrosis.

Although overall cerebral $O_2$ demands are lower in the infant than in the adult, cerebral oxidative metabolism is considerably increased in areas of active neural development that are associated with either synapse formation or activation of enzymes required for ion homeostasis. Glucose is the primary source of energy in cerebral metabolism and although the newborn brain is capable of utilizing alternative energy substrates such as ketones, lactate, and free fatty acids, glucose uptake mechanisms are relatively underdeveloped (Cremer et al, 1979; Gregoire et al, 1978). Absence of energy stores makes the brain dependent on sustained perfusion. Animal studies have shown that this impaired uptake of glucose can impair cerebral metabolism even prior to oxygen depletion (Yager et al, 1996).

Vasoautoregulation in response to increased cerebral blood pressure or flow is relatively underdeveloped in the newborn, thus rendering the infant more vulnerable to ischemic events. The gradual increase in vascularity of the developing brain leads to the creation of "watershed areas" (i.e., areas not well vascularized). These regions are more vulnerable to global ischemic events. These global events lead to patterns of focal injury that are dependent on maturational processes. The similarities between processes essential for brain development and those mediating cellular injury make the immature brain particularly vulnerable to ischemic insult. These similarities include an increased density of glutamate receptors, an increase in glutaminergic synapses in particular regions of the immature brain, and enhanced accumulation of cytosolic calcium after activation of the glutamate receptor. It has been shown that there are proportionately more glutamate receptors in the immature rat brain than in the mature rat brain and that the developing rat brain is much more sensitive to injury than the newborn or adult brain (Yager et al, 1996). HI-R injury triggers a complex series of cellular events that evolve rapidly through amplifying cascades, eventually leading to severe cerebral damage. A gradual or sudden decrease in cerebral oxygen and energy substrates initially leads to synaptic inactivation, which is a reversible and adaptive response to HI-R injury. Decreased cerebral energy stores lead to membrane pump failure and the subsequent inability to maintain normal ion gradients (Fig. 64–3). This is followed by neuronal membrane depolarization and release of neurotransmitters such as glutamate, which increase cytosolic calcium and induce destructive enzymes and free radicals. Reoxygenation after the ischemic episode plays a significant role in cellular injury. The pathogenesis of HI-R injury can be divided arbitrarily into four phases (Table 64–4; see also Fig. 64–1):

1. A decrease in cerebral energy and membrane depolarization
2. A phase of increased release of neurotransmitters and neuronal damage
3. A period of reperfusion
4. A final phase of irreversible cell death

**Decrease in Cerebral Energy and Membrane Depolarization.** HI-R injury is followed by a depression of brain function that probably is a protective mechanism to preserve energy. In the normal state, glucose and oxygen are the main requirements for brain energy production, which occurs by oxidative phosphorylation. Glucose is taken up by a carrier-mediated diffusion process and phosphorylated to glucose-6-phosphate, the major portion of which enters the glycolytic pathway to form pyruvate. Pyruvate enters the mitochondria and is converted to acetyl coenzyme A (acetyl CoA); acetyl CoA enters the citric acid cycle and undergoes oxidation to $CO_2$. The electrons generated get transported through several carrier proteins such as (reduced) nicotinamide adenine dinucleotide (NADH) within the mitochondria. NADH couples to molecular oxygen and forms ATP through phosphorylation of ADP by adenine kinase. Phosphocreatine also can serve as a store of energy that can transfer phosphorus to generate ATP. HI-R injury is followed by a decrease in brain glucose and ATP. Anaerobic glycolysis is much less efficient at ATP production. Aerobic glycolysis generates 38 moles of ATP per mole of glucose, compared with 2 moles of ATP produced by anaerobic glycolysis.

A decrease in ATP affects the $Na^+$,$K^+$-ATPase pump that helps to maintain the state of polarization of the neuronal membrane. A failure of the pump leads to an influx of sodium into the cell and potassium outside the cell. Associated glial uptake of sodium and water leads to astrocytic swelling that in turn decreases diffusion of oxygen and glucose to the neurons.

Accumulation of lactate secondary to anaerobic glycolysis leads to tissue acidosis, which inhibits both vascular autoregulation and phosphfructokinase, the rate-limiting enzyme in glycolysis. In immature animals hypoglycemia has been shown to be damaging; pretreating animals with glucose decreases the impact of the injury when given prior to, but not during, the injury (Sheldon et al, 1992; Vannucci and Vannucci, 2000). This is in contrast to the effect of glucose administration in mature animals.

**Increased Release of Neurotransmitters and Neuronal Damage.** There is sufficient evidence that excitatory neurotransmitters play a major role in HI-R injury. Under normal conditions there is a balance between excitatory neurotransmitters such as acetylcholine, dopamine, serotonin, glutamate, and aspartate and inhibitory agents such as glycine and gamma-aminobutyric acid (GABA). Neuronal injury is initiated by release of glutamate and other excitatory neurotransmitters from the presynaptic neurons. Initially the decrease in energy supply decreases ATP-dependent exocytosis of glutamate and decreases activity of glutamate synthetase, the enzyme responsible

**Hypoxic-Ischemic Insult**

*Decrease in cerebral ATP*

*Synaptic inactivation*

- *Inactivation of $N_A{}^+$,$K^+$-ATPase membrane pumps*
- *Ion gradients not maintained*
- *Membrane depolarization*
- *Release of neurotransmitters and glutamate*

Postsynaptic receptor

*NMDA* AMPA *Metabotropic*

Increased Na influx

*Release of Mg block of ion channel* Membrane depolarization

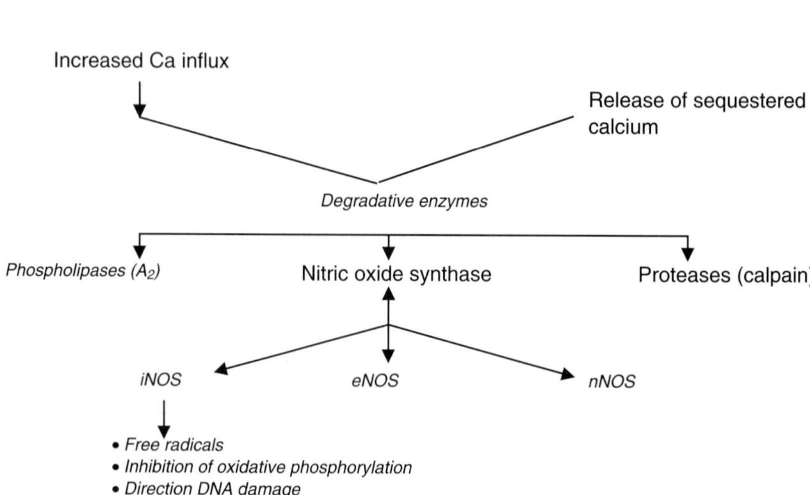


**FIGURE 64–3.** Flow diagram of events occurring after hypoxic-ischemic/reperfusion injury leading to energy depletion, membrane polarization, neurotransmitter release, calcium influx, and intracellular enzymatic activation leading to cell death.

**TABLE 64–4**

**Phases of Injury During Reperfusion**

| Phases of Injury During Reperfusion |
|---|
| **First Phase** |
| Cerebral energy metabolism restored over 30 minutes |
| Resolution of acute cellular hypoxic depolarization and cell swelling |
| **Latent Phase** |
| Near-normal oxidative cerebral metabolism |
| Depressed electroencephalogram and reduced blood flow |
| **Secondary Energy Failure** |
| Inhibition of oxidative phosphorylation |
| Cytotoxic edema leading to delayed seizures |

for converting glutamate to nontoxic glutamine. Subsequently, glutamate release occurs by both a reversal of normal glutamate uptake mechanisms by the nerve terminals and glia and membrane leakage. A secondary increase in glutamate occurs during the phase of reoxygenation.

Glutamate receptors are of three subtypes: the *N*-methyl-D-aspartate receptor (NMDA), the AMPA receptor, and the G protein–associated metabotropic receptor. The NMDA receptor is a postsynaptic receptor that is activated by glutamate and has been shown to play an important role in normal brain development including neuronal survival, differentiation, arborization of dendrites, growth of axons, and development of synapses. The expression of NMDA receptor subtypes as well as the subunit composition of the glutamate receptors changes with maturation (Johnston, 1995; MacDonald and Nowak, 1990). The density of receptors is higher in regions of active development, and the different subtypes vary in different regions of the brain at different gestational ages. Several features in the subunit composition of the immature NMDA receptor result in enhanced opening and influx of calcium into the ion channels (Andersen et al, 1995; Ben-Ari et al, 1988; Morrisett et al, 1990). Thus, neuroprotective interventions that act at the level of the glutaminergic receptors may disturb normal brain development.

Activation of any of the three subtypes of glutamate-activated postsynaptic neuron receptors leads to an influx of calcium into the postsynaptic neurons. Activation of the NMDA receptor releases the magnesium block within the ion channel and leads to the entry of calcium into the ion channel. Activation of the AMPA receptor mediates fast excitatory neurotransmission by triggering an influx of sodium. The resulting membrane depolarization opens calcium channels and releases the magnesium block of the NMDA channel, thereby leading to cytosolic accumulation of calcium. Activation of the metabotropic receptor results in the generation of inositol triphosphate, which triggers release of sequestered calcium.

The increase in intracellular calcium sets into motion an irreversible cascade of events that leads to cell injury. Calcium activates several degradative enzymes such as phospholipases, proteases, and endonucleases. Activated phospholipases such as phospholipase $A_2$ hydrolyze membrane phospholipid, thereby releasing free fatty acids such as arachidonic acid. Arachidonic acid can mediate injury by several mechanisms, including increased release of glutamate, uncoupling of oxidative phosphorylation, and inactivation of membrane $Na^+,K^+$-ATPase. Proteases degrade cytoskeletal and other proteins. Cyclooxygenase stimulates production of arachidonic acid and prostaglandins. Enzyme activation as well as activation of xanthine and prostaglandins generate free radicals that perpetuate the injury by lipid membrane peroxidation. Hypoxic-ischemic injury also leads to a change in iron homeostasis. Iron is usually maintained in a nontoxic "ferric" state but is reduced into the injurious "ferrous" form, which can react with oxygen-reactive species to propagate further injury.

Nitric oxide synthase (NOS), one of the enzymes that are released during HI-R injury, has been identified as a mediator of cellular injury. It has multiple and complex biologic functions and converts L-arginine to nitric oxide (NO). Several lines of evidence support the role of NO in hypoxic-ischemic injury. Studies in transgenic mice that are deficient for the *nNOS* gene showed that these mice had a decreased propensity for brain injury compared with that in their wild-type littermates (Ferriero et al, 1996). Also, expression of nNOS protein in the developing brain correlates with regions of vulnerability to hypoxic injury (Black et al, 1995). NOS exists in three different isoforms—eNOS (endothelial), iNOS (inducible), and nNOS (neuronal). The increase in NOS in HI-R injury occurs in two phases. The initial decrease in cerebral perfusion leads initially to a rapid increase in the eNOS and nNOS isoforms, followed by a sustained increase in NO. A subsequent increase in the iNOS isoform occurs several hours after the injury in response to inflammatory mediators such as lipopolysaccharides and cytokines. It is hypothesized that NO generated by different isoforms of NOS either can be beneficial by causing vasodilatation and inhibition of leukocyte and platelet activation or can mediate injury. NO causes cellular injury by various mechanisms: combining with superoxide to form a peroxynitrite radical that causes lipid peroxidation, generating of free radicals by stimulation of cyclooxygenase activity, direct DNA damage, and participating in the neurotransmitter response by reentering the presynaptic neuron and further increasing release of glutamate.

Membrane peroxidation and ATP breakdown lead to the accumulation of free fatty acids, adenine nucleotides, and hypoxanthine in endothelial cells as well.

**Phase of Reperfusion.** During the immediate period of return of cerebral circulation and reoxygenation, there is a resolution of the acute cellular hypoxic depolarization and cellular edema, with a restoration of cellular energy metabolism over the next 30 minutes. This is followed by a latent phase with near-normal oxidative cerebral energy metabolism as seen by MRS. However, EEG activity is blunted and cerebral blood flow is decreased during this period. The phase of delayed cerebral energy depletion follows subsequently, with clinical deterioration, delayed seizures, and cytotoxic edema as well as a release of excitatory neurotransmitters. This phase may last for 6 to 15 hours prior to neuronal death and therefore offers a therapeutic window. These delayed forms of neuronal injury have clinical correlates in the seizure activity that is seen after a latent period of 6 to 12 hours in HIE as well as the secondary deterioration seen after 24 hours in asphyxiated newborns. The exact mechanism responsible for the delayed injury is the subject of intense research. The overall effect of post–HI-R injury changes is to cause an augmentation of calcium influx and perpetuation of the injury.

NO may mediate both the initial reperfusion by vasodilatation and the later mitochondrial enzyme inhibition. During the initial period of reperfusion there is a clearance of glutamate (Takahashi et al, 1997). Several mechanisms that have been proposed to explain the ultimate increase in calcium influx and perpetuation of injury have been the subject of recent reviews (Inder and Volpe, 2000; White et al, 2000). Some of the mechanisms proposed include a long-term potentiation of NMDA receptors to low levels of extracellular glutamate, which can then lead to an exaggerated calcium influx, an impairment of the $Na^+$, $K^+$-ATPase pump from delayed energy failure (Obrenovitch and Urenjak, 1997), and enhanced release of glutamate by NO. Generation of free radicals during this phase occurs by two methods: free fatty acids enter the cyclooxygenase pathway and generate arachidonic acid and prostaglandins, and xanthine oxidase converts hypoxanthine to uric acid. Free radicals activate adhesion molecules in platelets and leukocytes, which increases occlusion of the microvasculature, thereby perpetuating injury.

**Phase of Irreversible Cell Death.** HIE results in two major forms of cell death: necrosis and apoptosis. *Apoptosis* refers to programmed cell death, a mechanism that is ongoing during the process of brain maturation. Apoptotic cells are characterized by nuclear shrinkage, chromatin condensation, and DNA fragmentation. Necrotic cells are characterized by cellular swelling, fracture of cell membranes, and an inflammatory cellular reaction. It is hypothesized that a severe insult leads to necrosis, as is seen in the central area of injury, whereas a longer duration of a less severe injury may lead to apoptosis, as seen in the penumbra. In the immature brain, a third pathologic form of injury has been described: the apoptotic-necrotic continuum (Portera-Cailliau et al, 1997). This particular pattern may represent the predominant form of injury (Northington et al, 2001a, 2001b). It has recently been shown in animal models that there is a prolonged period of delayed cell death due to apoptosis (Nakajima et al, 2000; Northington et al, 2001a, 2001b). This exciting finding suggests that there is a prolonged window of opportunity for interventional strategies.

Apoptotic cell death is a highly regulated process that in most cases requires activation of caspases, a superfamily of cysteine aspartyl–specific proteases (Kumar, 1995). Several of the 14 known mammalian caspases are involved in initiation of the apoptotic cascades; other caspases are responsible for the execution of apoptosis. Caspase-3, an executional caspase, appears to play a central role in apoptosis in a wide variety of cells (Marks and Berg, 1999). Activation of caspase-3 occurs through at least two distinct caspase cascades and requires cleavage of its proenzyme. The level of inactive caspase-3 in normal forebrain tissue gradually declines from a high level in P7 rat pups to a very low level in adult rats (Hu et al, 2000). The involvement of caspase-3 in cell death after hypoxia-ischemia also diminishes on brain maturation (Hu et al, 2000).

## Management

The immediate management of HIE requires securing an appropriate airway and maintaining adequate circulation. Cerebral edema resulting from hypoxia-ischemia is maximal between 36 and 96 hours and can impair cerebral blood flow secondary to increased vascular pressure. There is no consensus regarding the need to treat cerebral edema aggressively, as its role in producing neurologic sequelae is debatable. Although steroids have been shown to be beneficial in vasogenic cerebral edema, most investigators agree that corticosteroids are not beneficial for cerebral edema arising from hypoxic-ischemic injury. Attempts to decrease intracranial pressure by controlled hyperventilation ($Pa{CO_2}$ of 20 to 25 mm Hg) as well as the use of furosemide or mannitol may actually be harmful (Collins et al, 2001). Seizure activity should be controlled to limit further compromise of neurologic status, and electroencephalography should be used to monitor for subclinical seizures. Multiorgan function must be monitored carefully. Maintenance of adequate cerebral perfusion is necessary and inotropic agents need to be used in cases of myocardial dysfunction. It is important to avoid both systemic hypotension and hypertension. Infants with hypoxic-ischemic injury can develop hyponatremia from syndrome of inappropriate secretion of antidiuretic hormone (SIADH). Hypoglycemia in an immature animal model during the evolution of HIE has been found to aggravate the insult (Sheldon et al, 1996). Therefore, fluid overload should be avoided, and serum glucose and electrolytes should be monitored closely.

## Prognosis

Predicting the neurodevelopmental outcome for the asphyxiated newborn is extremely difficult. Explanations for the lack of predictive success include functional and anatomic plasticity, interindividual variability for the same insult, differences in provision of services, and differences in socioeconomic status (Shevell et al, 1989). Outcome of HIE depends on the severity of the injury and the degree of brain damage. Some investigators have suggested that there is a threshold of injury beyond which the brain is damaged. Several factors such as maturity of the infant, placental-fetal blood flow, energy reserves, or presence of cerebral anomalies can affect the final outcome. It is often difficult to determine the duration of the insult because the vast majority of insults occurs in utero and because adequate fetal surveillance is difficult. Certain clinical factors as well as the results of brain imaging studies can help identify infants with a poor prognosis (Barkovich et al, 1995; Biagioni et al, 2001).

### *Clinical Factors*

The Apgar score is not a good predictor of outcome. This measure is affected by the use of maternal drugs or anesthesia, and by the vagal-induced respiratory depression that occurs from the use of suction catheters or from oropharyngeal secretions. There is also considerable variation among personnel in assigning the Apgar score, and all of the five different parameters that compose the Apgar score are not equally weighted for neurologic outcome. Although the Apgar score at 1 minute is not predictive of a poor outcome, the predictive ability does increase with a continued depressed score with increasing age of the infant. It has been shown that infants with Apgar scores of less than 6 at 5 minutes are three times more likely to have abnormalities on neurologic examination than are infants with scores greater than 6 (Levene et al, 1986). However, if the infant shows no neurologic symptoms in the perinatal period, the outcome is often normal. Ekert and colleagues (1997) built a model to predict severe adverse outcome within 4 hours of birth in neonates with HIE and found that delayed onset of breathing, need for chest compressions, and seizures had a sensitivity of 85% and specificity of 68%. In a population-based case-control study using these and expanded criteria in 84 children with spastic cerebral palsy, only 18 had 5-minute Apgar scores of less than 6, 20 required ventilation in the delivery room, and only 5 had initial pH of less than 7.00. Only 3 children had all three signs, and these 3 had neonatal seizures (Nelson and Grether, 1999).

The severity of the neurologic symptoms is helpful in assessment of the prognosis. The incidence of long-term problems is low in infants with mild HIE (Robertson and Finer, 1985). Infants with moderate encephalopathy have an abnormal outcome in 20% to 40% of cases, whereas infants with severe encephalopathy either die in the first 3 days of life or have severe deficits. Sarnat scores are a commonly used indicator of HIE and show similar predictive ability for which infants are at risk for sequelae (Volpe, 2001b). Hypotonia with depressed primitive reflexes or episodes of recurrent apnea indicate a poor outcome. The presence of seizures is perhaps the best clinical indicator of adverse outcome, especially if seizure activity occurs in the first 12 hours of life or if they are difficult to control (see Miller et al, 2002d).

The duration of the neurologic abnormalities is usually helpful in predicting long-term neurologic disability. In two separate studies, normal examination findings at 1 week of age and at 2 weeks of age correlated with a good outcome (Robertson and Finer, 1985; Sarnat and Sarnat, 1976). Other clinical tools used include the presence of impairment of other organ systems and the Score for Neonatal Acute Physiology-Perinatal Extension (SNAP-PE) score, a physiologic assessment done within the first 24 hours of life (Newton et al, 2001). As with other clinical measures, neither of these tools is able to prognosticate outcome in the moderately asphyxiated newborn.

### *Brain Imaging Findings*

**Electroencephalography.** The rate of recovery of the EEG to normal baseline activity and the severity of neonatal encephalopathy can be helpful in establishing the neurologic prognosis (Biagioni et al, 2001).

**Evoked Potentials.** Ideally, evoked potentials would be done for pathways selectively vulnerable to HIE. A substantial HI-R event that results in the absence of visual or auditory waveforms is strongly predictive of significant abnormalities (McCulloch et al, 1991; Taylor and McCulloch, 1992).

**Magnetic Resonance Imaging.** MRI has been shown in a variety of studies to be useful in predicting outcome in neonates with HIE (Barkovich et al, 1998; Biagioni et al, 2001; Ment et al, 2002; Rutherford et al, 1994). In particular, absence of the signal in the posterior limb of the internal capsule has been associated with poor neurodevelopmental outcome. A joint statement from the American Academy of Pediatrics, the American Society of Pediatric Neuroradiology, and the Society for Pediatric Radiology recommends that a noncontrast CT study be performed to detect hemorrhagic lesions in term infants with encephalopathy and a birth history of trauma, coagulopathy, or low hematocrit. If the CT findings are inconclusive, MRI is recommended between days 2 and 8 to assess location and extent of injury (Ment et al, 2002). Because the CT scan does not compare favorably with MRI for confirming the diagnosis of hypoxic-ischemic injury or for providing prognostic information, Miller and colleagues (2002a) recommend that an MRI study be performed in the first week of life for establishing the diagnosis in an encephalopathic newborn (Fig. 64–4A).

**Magnetic Resonance Spectroscopy.** MRS has been shown to correlate with neurologic outcome and may be more sensitive in identifying injury and metabolic disturbances from seizures than standard imaging (Miller et al, 2002b) (see Fig. 64–4B). Abnormalities seen on MRS have been highly significantly associated with both neurologic and cognitive outcomes. Both high lactate and low NAA levels have been associated with persistent injury (Barkovich et al, 2001; Miller et al, 2002d). Study results have varied in accordance with the timing of the scan in relation to the injury. It has been reported that the lactate level of the injured brain increases within the first 24 hours and remains elevated thereafter, presumably due to energy failure and the necessity to metabolize glucose anaerobically (Hanrahan et al, 1996; Penrice et al, 1996). However, the NAA level does not diminish significantly until sometime beyond 48 hours (Penrice et al, 1997). The precise time at which NAA begins to diminish in asphyxiated neonates is not precisely known.

### Outcome

The outcome for ischemic injury differs substantially for the preterm infant and the term infant. Although more preterm infants survive the insult than term infants, preterm survivors are affected with more neurodevelopmental disabilities. In a recent study of extremely preterm children, 49% had disabilities, with 23% meeting criteria for severe disabilities (Wood et al, 2000). In term babies with neonatal encephalopathy, the presence of seizures and the severity and duration of encephalopathic state are predictors of poor outcome (Robertson et al, 1989; Thornberg et al, 1995). Infants with mild neonatal encephalopathy syndromes have no deficits, whereas those with severe encephalopathy die or are severely impaired with spastic quadriparesis, cortical visual impairment, and seizure disorders. Those with moderate degrees of encephalopathy can be normal to severely abnormal, depending on the pattern of injury seen on MRI and MRS and the persistence of EEG abnormalities (Barkovich et al, 2001; Biagioni et al, 2001). The neurologic examination at 3 months may be a good prognostic indicator (Hajnal et al, 1999).

## Perinatal Stroke

Perinatal strokes are arterial in nature (Fig. 64–5), but this section also includes venous infarction and sinovenous thrombosis in the term infant. Perinatal stroke is defined as an ischemic event that occurs between 28 weeks of gestation and 7 days of age and includes in utero strokes. The term *neonatal stroke* is reserved for events occurring between birth and the end of the first month of life. It is difficult to establish the exact prevalence of perinatal stroke. Using studies of children with neonatal seizures, prevalence has been estimated to be roughly 12% of neonates of greater than 31 weeks of gestation with seizures (Lynch et al, 2002). This rate translates to a prevalence of perinatal stroke of 24.7/100,000 per year in infants of greater than 31 weeks of gestation and is similar to the estimated prevalence of 28.6/100,000 live births reported by Perlman (1994). On the basis of these estimates, perinatal stroke is recognized in approximately 1/4000 live births. However, there is a subgroup of neonates who do not present with evidence of injury until late infancy because the neurologic examination findings are normal in the newborn period. These infants present later with pathologic early hand preference and/or seizures (Golomb et al, 2001). Stroke in the newborn has a male predominance,

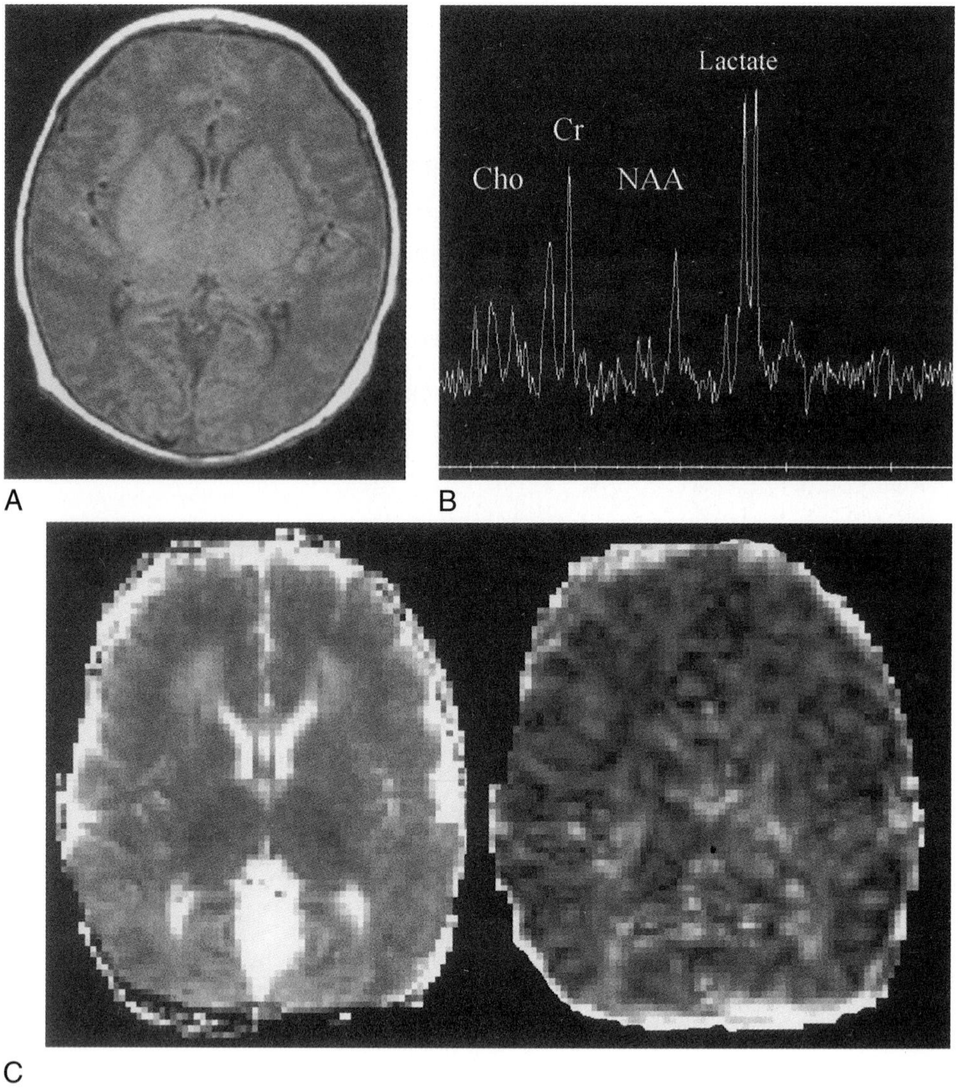

**FIGURE 64–4.** Magnetic resonance (MR) spectra and diffusion-weighted images obtained on day 2 of life in a term infant with moderate hypoxic-ischemic encephalopathy. **A,** MR image shows loss of signal intensity in the posterior limb of the internal capsule. **B,** The MR spectra show elevated lactate and decreased *N*-acetyl aspartate (NAA) peaks in the basal ganglia in that area; **C,** diffusion-weighted images show restricted diffusion on the apparent diffusion coefficient (ADC) image (*left*) and loss of anisotropy (*right*).

and there is a tendency toward left-sided lesions (Golomb et al, 2001; Trauner et al, 1993). It is unclear why there is a gender difference.

The United States infant mortality rate for years 1995 to 1998 due to stroke (ICD-9 CM 430-437) is 5.33/100,000 per year, perinatal mortality is 2.21/100,000, and neonatal mortality is 3.49/100,000 live births per year (Lynch and Nelson, 2001). The National Hospital Discharge Survey, from 1980 through 1998, determined that for infants younger than 30 days of age, the in-hospital mortality rate for neonatal stroke was 10.1%, or 2.67/100,000 live births (Lynch and Nelson, 2001; Lynch et al, 2002).

## Cerebral Venous Thrombosis

Sinovenous thrombosis (SVT) is an important cause of stroke in the neonate. It is being increasingly diagnosed in recent years, probably reflecting the use of more sensitive neuroimaging techniques. In a retrospective series of children with abnormal imaging studies suggestive of SVT, 61% were neonates (Carvalho et al, 2001). The Canadian Pediatric Ischemic Stroke Registry (CPISR) identified 0.67 cases per 100,000 per year, with neonates the most commonly affected (43%) (deVeber and Andrew, 2001). Risk factors are similar to those for ischemic stroke, with thrombophilias, asphyxial stress, dehydration, and infection being more common in the neonate. Often, more than one risk factor is present (Wu et al, 2003).

Neonates present with seizures as the most common sign. The head ultrasound examination often reveals an intraventricular hemorrhage. Further neuroimaging with MRI and MR venography will reveal the site of the venous thrombosis and may also show other parenchymal abnormalities, such as thalamic hemorrhage (Wu et al, 2003) (Fig. 64–6).

### Risk Factors

A number of different types of studies of infants with perinatal stroke has found an association with cardiac disorders, blood disorders, infection, trauma, drugs,

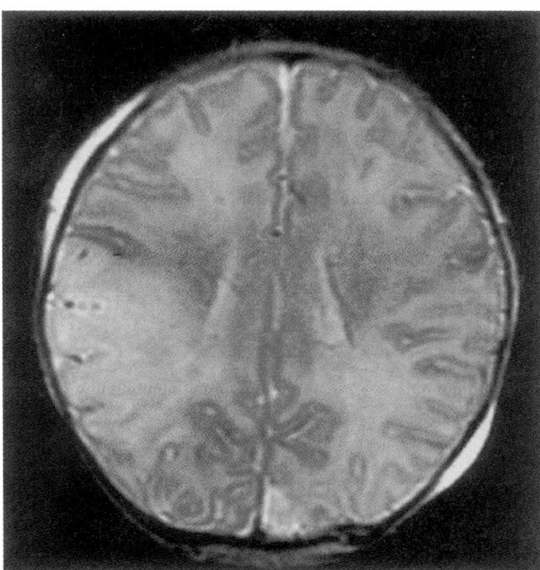

**FIGURE 64–5.** Brain magnetic resonance T2-weighted image in term neonate who suffered ischemic arterial stroke. Increased signal intensity is seen in the right parietal and frontal areas and the left posterior parietal region.

maternal and placental disorders, and perinatal asphyxia. In some studies, the occurrence of multiple risk factors has been noted, especially blood disorders and asphyxial stress (Golomb et al, 2001; Wood et al, 2000).

#### Outcome

A review of the literature for case reports, series, and case-control studies of perinatal or neonatal stroke, which included 572 infants with perinatal stroke, revealed that 40% of infants with perinatal stroke were neurologically normal, 56% were abnormal (having neurologic or cognitive abnormalities), and 3.0% had died by the outcome evaluation period (Lynch et al, 2002). A similar review concluded that more than 50% of children with neonatal stroke appear normal by 12 to 18 months of age (de Vries et al, 1997). In the CPISR, the recurrence rate among children with neonatal stroke was 3% to 5%, and among survivors, outcome was normal in 33% (deVeber and Andrew, 2001). In one case series of 24 infants with MRI-confirmed cerebral infarction, 64% of the neonates had neurodevelopmental sequelae. The presence of prothrombotic disorders, especially presence of factor V Leiden, was associated with poor outcome in term infants (Mercuri, 2001).

The neurodevelopmental outcome of neonates with SVT is reported to be normal in 77% to 82%. Presence of venous infarction and refractory seizures has been associated with neurologic sequelae. (Carvalho et al, 2001; deVeber and Andrew, 2001; Shevell et al, 1989; Wu et al, 2003).

#### Management

The use of anticoagulation therapy for the newborn is undetermined. It is difficult to extrapolate from adult or even non-neonatal pediatric studies. However, the CPISR data suggest that anticoagulant therapy is not associated with serious hemorrhage in selected patients. Its use in neonates awaits further evaluation.

## Perinatal Trauma

Injuries of the cranial structures and the brain can occur secondary to trauma during the process of birth. Perinatal trauma can result from various causes in utero, during labor, and postnatally. The nature of the trauma can be either mechanical or vascular. Embolism and thrombosis can result from placental infarcts or absorption of material from a macerated twin fetus, or with disorders of coagulation or sepsis. Mechanical trauma can cause injury to both cranial and extracranial structures as well as the spinal cord and peripheral nerve structures.

### Mechanical Trauma

Mechanical trauma can result in damage to either extracranial structures, cranial structures, intracranial structures, spinal cord, or peripheral nerves. Extracranial injury can present as molding of the head and caput succedaneum, subgaleal hemorrhage, or cephalohematoma.

#### *Scalp Electrode Injury*

Use of scalp electrodes for fetal monitoring has increased, along with fetal blood sampling for blood gas measurement. The site of insertion can become a site of infection or bleeding. Although generally benign, such lesions are associated with infection in 1% of cases, and in rare cases (usually in premature infants) they can cause severe bleeding leading to hypotension.

#### *Molding of the Head and Caput Succedaneum*

Molding of the head is frequently seen in the newborn delivered either vaginally or by cesarean section. It refers to the asymmetrical shape of the head that results from mechanical pressure exerted during passage through the birth canal or during extraction by cesarean section. *Caput succedaneum* refers to the edematous soft tissue swelling that is often associated with bruising over the molded region. Although this condition is generally benign and resolves with time, abrasions over the area can become infected, and hyperbilirubinemia may develop with resolution of bruising (Fig. 64–7).

#### *Subgaleal Hemorrhage*

In certain cases the trauma may be severe enough to cause a subgaleal hemorrhage, which consists of extension of the bleeding beneath the scalp aponeurosis to the nape of the neck. This condition needs to be recognized immediately because it can lead to severe blood loss and shock. The coagulation status should be evaluated, as subgaleal hemorrhage may be a presenting sign of hemophilia, hemorrhagic disease of the newborn, or other coagulation disorders. A CT scan or MRI is indicated, especially in

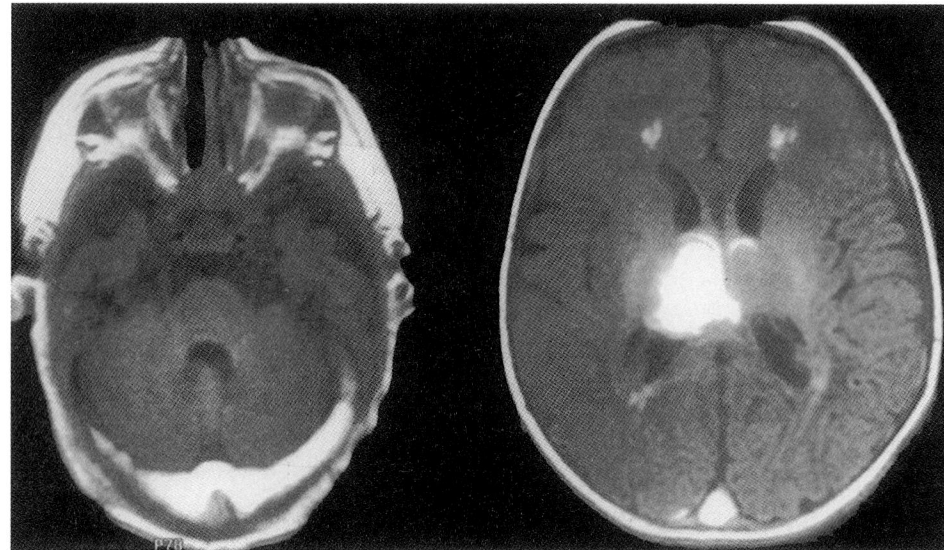


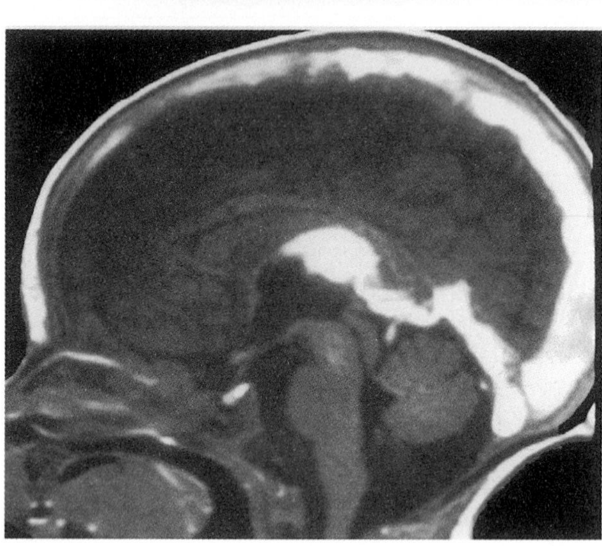


**FIGURE 64–6.** Brain magnetic resonance images of sinovenous thrombosis with thalamic infarction in a term neonate. **A,** Right thalamic infarction and hemorrhage seen on axial T1-weighted MR image; **B,** thrombosis of entire venous system seen on sagittal T1-weighted MR image.

conditions associated with an enlarging swelling, altered mental status, or decreasing hematocrit. Maintenance of the circulatory status of the infant is critical and may require use of packed cells or plasma to correct hypovolemia and any coagulopathy. Occasionally, severe trauma can lead to tearing of either the tentorium or the falx cerebri. A subdural hematoma may occur in cases with venous lacerations.

### Cephalohematoma

Hemorrhage beneath the subperiosteum of the scalp leading to an elevation in usually the parietal region of the skull is called a *cephalohematoma*. It is distinguished from a caput as follows: it does not cross suture lines, it manifests as a firmer swelling that does not transilluminate, and it has a well-defined edge. Rarely, it is seen in the occipital region as a soft swelling that needs to be distinguished from an encephalocele. The incidence of cephalohematoma is estimated to be 1.5% to 2.5% of all deliveries. It is seen twice as frequently in male infants and presents bilaterally in 15% of patients. Linear fractures are seen in 5% of unilateral lesions and in 18% of bilateral lesions.

A cephalohematoma generally resolves over a period of 2 to 8 weeks. It often leaves behind a sharp palpable ridge due to calcium deposition. Resorption of the extravasated blood can lead to hyperbilirubinemia, and infants should be observed for jaundice. A severe bleed can lead to anemia. Infection of the mass with formation of an abscess and associated osteomyelitis can occur in rare cases. It should be suspected in the event of an enlarging mass manifesting with fever and laboratory results suggestive of an infection. Needle aspiration may be necessary to establish a diagnosis, although this should not be performed in all cases of cephalohematoma due to the risk of introducing an infection.

A skull radiograph or a CT scan is indicated in cases in which a fracture is suspected. Hyperostosis and thickening of the parietal region, calcium deposition, or cystic defects within the hematoma may be seen on neuroimaging studies.

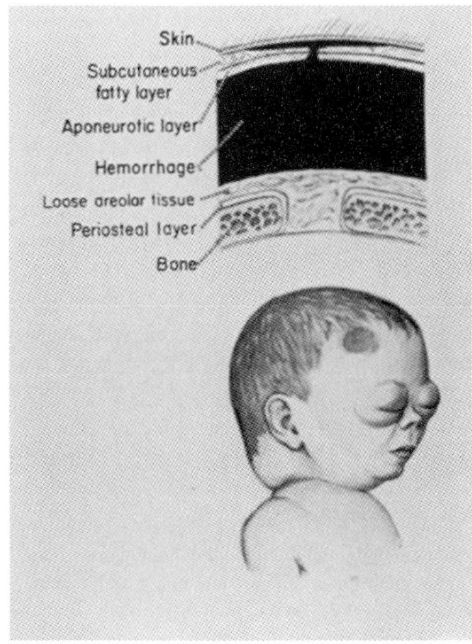


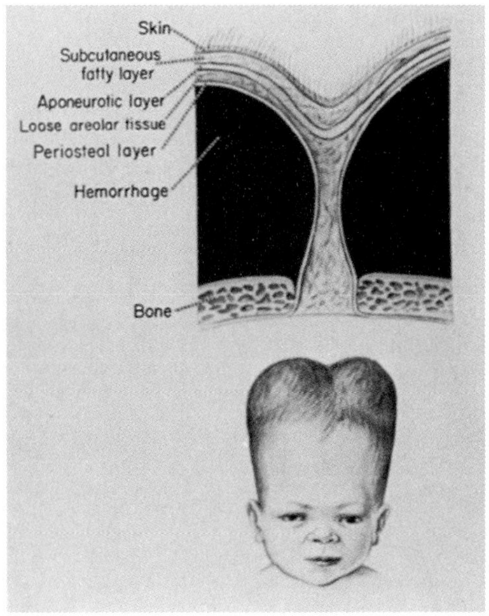


**FIGURE 64–7.** **A,** Location of edema and hemorrhage seen with a caput succedaneum. **B,** Location of hemorrhage seen with a cephalohematoma.

## Skull Fractures

Several features of the skull of the newborn make it less likely to sustain fractures, even in the presence of considerable pressure during the process of birth. The presence of unossified sutures and decreased mineralization make the neonatal skull less rigid and more amenable to temporary distortion. However, fractures do occur in deliveries, especially those associated with forceps or blunt abdominal trauma to the mother. Fractures can also occur simply from pressure of the head against the sacral promontory during delivery from forceful uterine contractions.

Fractures may be linear or depressed and usually occur in the frontal or parietal region. Linear fractures are more common and if nondisplaced usually do not pose a problem and do not need treatment. They are seen as a linear region of decreased density on a skull radiograph.

Depressed skull fractures associated with application of pressure over the parietal region are seen on the anteroposterior skull radiograph as a linear region of increased density. These may not be visualized on the lateral film. A depressed fracture can serve as a focus for seizure activity, and it is therefore recommended that the region be elevated by a surgical procedure.

## Subdural Hemorrhage

The dura mater, the outer meningeal layer, lies immediately below the bony layer of the skull and contains several blood vessels. It also encloses the major sinuses between its two layers. Severe compression and stretching can lead to tears of the falx cerebri or the tentorium cerebelli, especially at the site at which the falx meets the tentorium. Risk factors include macrosomia, cephalopelvic disproportion, shoulder dystocia, forceps delivery, and premature delivery. Hemorrhage can occur by injury to the dural sinuses, the major cerebral veins, or the vein of Galen. Injury of the superficial cerebral veins leads to hemorrhage over the cerebrum. Injury to the straight sinus or the vein of Galen can cause extension of a subdural hemorrhage from the base of the brain into the posterior fossa. Damage to the sagittal sinus from overriding parietal bones, and damage to the occipital sinus in conditions leading to separation of the squamous from the lateral parts of the occipital bone, can be seen with breech presentation.

A subdural hemorrhage should be suspected in cases in which there is a history of trauma or a difficult delivery with development of focal cerebral signs such as unequal pupils, deviation of the eyes, or hemiparesis. Symptoms may present over a period of a few hours to days. Often the infant presents with nonspecific signs such as pallor, lethargy, irritability, and a decreased Moro response. A bulging anterior fontanel may be the sign of an acute bleed. Posterior fossa hemorrhages, which can be accompanied by cerebellar hemorrhages or IVH, may manifest later with opthisotonos, apnea and bradycardia, altered mental status, and seizures. Pressure on the fourth ventricle can lead to signs of increased intracranial pressure and apnea.

Ultrasonography is inadequate for demonstrating the presence of a subdural bleed. Either CT or MRI is a more appropriate imaging study for this purpose and should be undertaken immediately once the diagnosis is suspected.

No surgical treatment is recommended in asymptomatic cases. Evacuation of a posterior fossa bleed can sometimes be lifesaving, although surgical evacuation is not effective in the case of a large subdural hemorrhage. Close monitoring is necessary to detect signs of deterioration in neurologic status. Presence of increased intracranial pressure may require a subdural tap or placement of a subdural shunt.

### Subarachnoid Hemorrhage

Subarachnoid hemorrhage occurs as a result of damage to veins traversing the subarachnoid space. This type of injury is fairly common and may manifest as seizures. Diagnosis is suspected when frank blood or blood-tinged fluid is obtained on lumbar puncture. No treatment is needed, as the condition usually resolves spontaneously.

### Spinal Cord Injury

Spinal cord injury was first described in the 1800s and is a relatively rare event now because of improved obstetric practices. In a review of studies of cerebral palsy, spinal cord injury was noted to account for just 0.6% of injuries. It is most commonly associated with breech delivery and occurs secondary to either a lateral or longitudinal stretching force or torsion of the neck during delivery. It can also be seen in premature infants as a result of extension of an intracranial hemorrhage. Damage occurs to the cord, the covering meninges, nerve roots, and blood vessels.

The pathologic findings may include laceration of the cord, epidural hemorrhage, laceration of the dura with a subdural hemorrhage, and tears of the nerve roots, as well as focal hemorrhages within the cord.

Most patients with a severe spinal cord injury do not survive. The cervical and upper thoracic segments of the spine are most commonly affected. The condition should be suspected in any infant with a breech presentation who has poor muscle tone and flaccid weakness of the extremities. The presentation in many cases is that of spastic paraparesis with respiratory depression and hypotonia. There is often involvement of both the motor and the sensory systems. Urinary retention and abdominal distention with paradoxical respirations may be present. The neurologic examination is significant for an absence of sensation below the level of the injury. This can manifest as reduced skin temperature and decreased tendon reflexes in the acute phase, followed by the appearance of triple-flexion withdrawal movements.

The differential diagnosis includes neuromuscular disorders such as spinal muscular atrophy, congenital myasthenia gravis, and a tumor of the cervical or lumbar region of the cord. Spinal muscular atrophy is usually not associated with loss of sensation or bladder control. A tumor of the spinal cord is usually associated with midline skin abnormalities such as dimpling, hemangioma, or tufts of hair.

Treatment is usually supportive and may require intubation for respiratory support. No specific treatment is available. Most cases are severe and irreversible, although milder degrees of injury are potentially reversible.

### Cranial Nerve Injury

#### *Facial Nerve Injury*

Facial nerve injury is the most common cranial nerve injury seen secondary to birth trauma. Contrary to common belief, forceps application is not associated with an increased incidence of facial nerve palsy. The site of injury and the precise timing of injury are controversial. The nerve is most commonly injured at the point where it emerges from the stylomastoid foramen, and the lesion is therefore similar to a lower motor neuron lesion. The signs and symptoms include difficulty in closing the eyelid on the affected side, loss of the normal nasolabial fold, and an asymmetrical crying facies. The forehead is spared, as it is innervated by the opposite facial nerve. The injury occurs as a result of compression of the nerve against the sacral promontory especially in cases in which presentation of the fetal head leads to compression of the mandible and the neck against the shoulder. Usually, compression of the nerve occurs after it has exited the mastoid canal, although occasionally the portion within the mastoid can also be affected.

Nerve excitability or conduction tests are not usually recommended unless there is no improvement over 3 to 4 days. Most lesions begin to resolve after 1 week. Nerve excitability tests are usually helpful in distinguishing partial from complete denervation. In the case of partial injury, nerve stimulation can lead to some muscular contraction. However, the lack of response to nerve stimulation does not necessarily predict a poor outcome. A neurology consultation should be obtained in cases that do not show resolution within a few weeks. Methyl cellulose eye drops should be used on the affected side to prevent irritation from dryness of the conjunctiva. In severe cases, surgery may be necessary to repair a severed nerve.

#### *Congenital Hypoplasia of the Depressor Anguli Oris Muscle*

Congenital hypoplasia of the depressor anguli oris muscle is not due to perinatal trauma but is included here for differential diagnosis purposes. In affected infants, unilateral congenital absence of the depressor anguli oris muscle leads to an inability of contraction and eversion of the lower lip on the same side during crying episodes. The infant thus appears to have an asymmetrical face while crying. The condition becomes less prominent with age, as episodes of crying are reduced in the older child. This condition can occur as an isolated anomaly or be associated with other anomalies. In a review of 41 infants with the condition, 27 had associated genitourinary, respiratory, or cardiovascular abnormalities (Pape and Pickering, 1972). Congenital heart disease, especially ventricular septal disease, is the most common associated anomaly.

#### *Injury to Other Cranial Nerves*

Injury of other cranial nerves secondary to birth injury is rare. Transient ptosis may be seen as a result of damage to the oculomotor nerve. Unilateral as well as bilateral optic nerve atrophy has been reported to occur from orbital fracture.

### Peripheral Nerve Injury

#### *Brachial Plexus Injury*

Injury to the brachial plexus usually results from the prolonged delivery of a macrosomic infant. Traction of the shoulder in a breech presentation as well as turning away of the head in a difficult vertex presentation leads to stretching of the plexus. In the mildest cases, nerves C5 and C6 are affected, followed by additional nerves in more severe cases. The nerve is compressed within the nerve sheath from hemorrhage and edema. In severe cases there may be avulsion of the nerve from the spinal cord. Improvement in obstetric care has resulted in a decrease in incidence of this condition.

In most cases, the condition is unilateral; it is located on the right twice as often as on the left. *Erb-Duchenne paralysis* refers to the paralysis of the upper brachial plexus involving nerves C5 and C6. Weakness of the deltoid, biceps, brachioradialis, and supinator muscles leads to the classic clinical picture in which the infant holds the affected arm in a position of tight adduction and internal rotation of the shoulder along with extension and pronation of the elbow. Involvement of C7 can lead to a weakness of the extensors and exaggerated flexion of the wrist. The Moro reflex is asymmetrical and absent on the affected side, and the biceps reflex is weak or absent. The grasp reflex is usually present. The injury may be associated with a fracture of the clavicle or humerus, displacement of the radial head, or shoulder dislocation. Injury of C4 can lead to phrenic nerve paralysis, which manifests with rapid, shallow breathing and decreased movement of the diaphragm on the affected side.

*Klumpke paralysis* results from injury to the lower brachial plexus and accounts for 2.5% of cases of brachial plexus injury. It is associated with weakness of the flexor muscles of the wrist as well as the intrinsic muscles of the hand. The grasp reflex is absent, and there may be loss of sensation over the hand. Involvement of the cervical sympathetic nerves can lead to unilateral miosis (Horner syndrome). Complete paralysis of the arm is seen in cases in which the entire brachial plexus is damaged.

The diagnosis can be made on the basis of the history of difficult delivery, posture of the affected arm, and the loss of voluntary and reflex movements. Radiographic examination performed with fluoroscopy or ultrasonography can help make the diagnosis of phrenic nerve injury. Radiographic studies can also detect any associated fractures or dislocations. Use of somatosensory evoked potentials may help to distinguish completed avulsion at the spinal cord from a more distal lesion. MRI also can be used to demonstrate root avulsion. The extent of denervation can be demonstrated by performing an EEG 2 to 3 weeks after the injury.

The treatment is mainly supportive and consists of physical therapy to avoid the development of contractures. The arm should be positioned in a natural position and not be overimmobilized. Passive exercises should be started 1 week after birth. The timing of recovery is dependent on the extent of the lesion. In mild partial plexus injury and Erb-Duchenne injury, improvement is seen by 1 or 2 weeks after birth, and recovery is complete by 1 to 18 months. Prognosis is poorer in Klumpke paralysis and in cases of complete plexus damage. Recovery is rarely complete in these infants, and sequelae may include muscle atrophy and contractures. Return of neuromuscular function is not always associated with return of normal movements of the extremities due to early deprivation of sensorimotor function.

### *Sciatic Nerve Palsy*

Sciatic nerve palsy is usually iatrogenic from injection of medications into the umbilical artery or from an inappropriate injection into the gluteal muscle. Direct injury to the sciatic nerve may result, or more commonly, ischemic sciatic neuropathy can result from spasm or occlusion of the inferior gluteal artery. The weakness may be mild, affecting only dorsiflexion of the foot, or may be severe enough to result in extensive weakness and atrophy of the muscles of the thigh and below the knee. Ischemic neuropathy is sometimes associated with signs of vascular insufficiency in the regions of the buttocks and the lower limb.

Prompt recognition of this condition is important for institution of physical therapy and measures to avoid joint contractures. Surgical resection of the affected nerve segment may be necessary in cases without any improvement over a period of 6 months. Permanent sequelae such as weakness and atrophy are common in cases of sciatic nerve injury.

## STRATEGIES FOR NEUROPROTECTION IN CENTRAL NERVOUS SYSTEM INJURY

Considerable advances have been made in recent years in elucidating the cellular and vascular mechanisms of hypoxic-ischemic brain injury. Anticipation and prevention of conditions that cause HIE constitute the best neuroprotective strategy. However, until such time as appropriate techniques to detect imminent fetal hypoxia become available, the best method is to target post injury sequelae. Several agents are currently being explored. Many of these potential strategies have been studied in animal or adult models of disease. Extrapolating the effects of these studies to the human newborn is difficult because the mechanism of injury in experimental animal models is not necessarily similar to that in infants, and several features of the newborn developing brain make it uniquely more susceptible to injury than the adult brain. Therefore, these therapies must be tested in the neonatal population (Table 64–5).

Because infants with mild HIE usually do not suffer long-term neurologic consequences and because severe injury leads to a devastating outcome, most therapies should be directed at infants with moderate- to severe-intensity insults. Early identification of infants with a moderately severe insult is necessary in order to initiate appropriate therapy within the narrow therapeutic window. The lack of sophistication of the current technology compromises our ability to make an early diagnosis and intervene earlier in cases of HI-R injury (Nelson and Grether, 1999).

In addition to our lack of ability to select neonates for neuroprotective therapies, interruption of the injurious events by neuroprotective agents may also simultaneously affect normal developmental processes. Another important issue relates to the route and timing of intervention. Administration of medications to the mother at the time of identification of fetal distress may adversely affect the mother and the process of labor. Asphyxia in neonates is often associated with multiorgan dysfunction, which can

**TABLE 64-5**

**Possible Neuroprotective Strategies**

- Hypothermia
- Adenosine
- Glutamate receptor antagonists
  - NMDA receptor antagonists
    - Glutamate-binding site
    - Glycine, phencyclidine, magnesium-binding sites
  - AMPA receptor antagonists
- Erythropoietin
- GABA antagonists
- Calcium channel blockers
- Nitric oxide synthase inhibitors
- Other free radical inhibitors
  - Allopurinol
  - Vitamin E
  - Lazaroids
- Metalloporphyrins
- Desferoxamine
- Growth factors
- Caspase inhibitors

AMPA, amino-3-hydroxy-5-methyl-4-isoxazole propionic acid; GABA, gamma-aminobutyric acid; NMDA, *N*-methyl-D-aspartate.

affect the pharmacokinetics of drug therapies. Side effects of these agents can include hypotension and cardiac depression, exacerbating the initial injury by reducing cerebral perfusion pressure.

Given the complexity of cellular events triggered by HI-R injury, it is most likely that a multi-tiered approach will be more effective than a single drug in achieving neuroprotection. However, such an approach will need to take several factors into consideration. An ideal neuroprotective agent can cross the blood-brain barrier and accumulate in sufficient quantities at the site of action, has minimal side effects so as not to further extend the injury, does not inhibit the normal processes of maturation, and preferably has a long therapeutic window of action with no drug interactions.

Several strategies for neuroprotection exert their effects at different stages of the cascade of events that is initiated after injury. These strategies include methods to reduce depletion of ATP stores, both in cases in which hypoxic-ischemic insult is predictable and in the early postinsult phase, to reduce membrane depolarization, to inhibit glutamate release, to inhibit accumulation of intracellular calcium, to block glutamate-responsive NMDA and AMPA receptors, to prevent release of degradative enzymes, to sequester free radicals, to use thrombolytic agents, and to prevent the reperfusion injury by inhibition of xanthine oxidase. The following discussion examines some of these methods in more detail.

## Maintaining Energy Stores

Prevention of depletion of cerebral energy stores is a strategy that can be utilized in cases in which injury is anticipated (e.g., cardiac surgery requiring placement of the infant on cardiopulmonary bypass). It is recommended that seizures and conditions that exacerbate energy depletion, such as hyperthermia, be avoided in cases of HI-R injury.

## Hypothermia

Mild sustained hypothermia is one of the most exciting and viable neuroprotective strategies for limiting neonatal HI-R injury to emerge from the laboratory in recent years. Cerebral metabolism after the initial phase of energy failure during asphyxia may recover in a latent phase but then deteriorate in a secondary phase of brain injury 6 to 15 hours later. In studies in cell culture and in vivo models of focal and global cerebral ischemias in both adults and immature animals, hypothermia has been shown to have a neuroprotective effect (Coimbra and Wieloch, 1994; Colbourne and Corbett, 1994; Sirimanne et al, 1996). Experimental studies in animal models have shown that moderate hypothermia established within 30 minutes after the HI-R injury is neuroprotective (Edwards et al, 1995; Haaland et al, 1997; Thoresen et al, 1995, 1996). These and other studies have shown that hypothermia inhibits early events as well as later events such as secondary energy failure and apoptosis. Studies in fetal sheep have shown that prolonged cerebral cooling starting 5.5 hours but not 8.5 hours after cerebral ischemia may still be associated with neuronal rescue (Gunn et al, 1997).

The possible mechanisms by which hypothermia helps in neuroprotection are inhibition of glutamate release, decreased metabolism and energy conservation, decreased metabolic acidosis, decreased free radical generation, prevention of energy failure and apoptosis, and inhibition of effects of adhesion molecules at the microvascular level, thereby inhibiting the breakdown of the blood-brain barrier and reducing brain edema. Some studies indicate that hypothermia delays but does not prevent the cellular or vascular outcome of HIE. However, even delaying onset of damage can be helpful in prolonging the therapeutic window for other therapies to take effect.

Hypothermia was first reported in the therapy of infants after perinatal asphyxia in 1959, but these experiments did not have a group of control infants (Westin et al, 1959). The adverse consequences of hypothermia and the importance of maintaining infants in a normothermic environment are well known. Metabolic, cardiovascular, pulmonary, coagulation, and immunologic disturbances all have been reported with hypothermia. A prospective randomized trial conducted to identify the adverse effects of hypothermia showed that selective head cooling was safe, with minimal systemic toxicity (Gunn et al, 1998). Mild hypothermia in this study was induced by application of a water-cooled coil to the infant's head, thereby lowering the cranial temperature to 34.5° C for 72 hours within 2 to 5 hours after the injury. Rectal temperature was maintained up to 35.7° C. The results of this and other studies led to the initiation of a multicenter clinical trial for neuroprotective efficacy. Although hypothermia holds much promise as a treatment modality for HI-R, several details regarding detection of early injury, timing and duration of the treatment, technique of head cooling, combination with other therapies, and whole-body cooling versus head cooling will need to be determined before it can be used routinely in infants.

### Pharmacologic Adenosine

Adenosine is an inhibitory agent that is endogenously produced. It acts on the presynaptic and postsynaptic $A_1$ receptors that colocalize with the NMDA receptors, inhibiting release of glutamate and glycine and delaying the onset of depolarization (de Mendonca et al, 2000). Although adenosine and its analogues may mediate neuroprotective actions at a number of cellular or vascular sites, side effects associated with its use such as hypotension and generation of free radicals may limit its application in HI-R.

### Inhibition of Glutamate Release

Prevention of glutamate release can occur by blocking presynaptic voltage-dependent sodium channels and stimulating presynaptic adenosine receptors. Prevention of sodium accumulation inhibits the reversal of the glutamate uptake carrier mechanism that is induced by ischemia. The $Na^+$,$K^+$-ATPase pump that maintains ionic gradients uses considerable energy. Inhibition of sodium influx also helps to decrease energy consumption. Agents that have been found to be beneficial in adults include phenytoin and lamotrigine. Phenytoin has been shown in some studies to be protective only when used prior to the injury; other studies have described protection when the drug is given soon after the injury (Hayakawa et al, 1994; Stanton and Moskal, 1991; Vartanian et al, 1996). Although it is able to cross the fetal blood-brain barrier, its role as a neuroprotective agent in neonates with HI-R is unclear.

### Glutamate Receptor Antagonists

Glutamate receptor antagonists can be broadly divided into two types: agents that block the NMDA receptor and those that block the AMPA receptor. Antagonists of the NMDA receptor act either by competitive antagonism at the glutamate-binding site or by noncompetitive antagonism at the glycine-, phencyclidine (PCP)-, and magnesium-binding sites. Competitive antagonists such as CGS-19755 have been shown to have limited clinical utility because of poor penetration of the blood-brain barrier.

Noncompetitive antagonists acting at the NMDA receptor have been shown to be effective in adult models of focal ischemia, with a therapeutic window as long as 3 hours. However, these are not as effective in global ischemia. Dizocilpine (MK-801), the most widely used NMDA blocker in experimental models, was shown to be protective in the newborn beagle puppy model (Ment et al, 1989). It also has been shown to be protective in the rat but not the piglet model (LeBlanc et al, 1993). In the rat model it reduced the infarct volume by 50% to 70%, with a post-therapeutic window of 2 hours. However, it has a low therapeutic index and steep dose-response curve. There are no published data on the use of this agent in humans. A more recent report described apoptosis in the immature P7 rat brain after injection of the antagonist even in the absence of injury (Ikonomidou et al, 1999).

Dextromethorphan is a widely used antitussive agent and a competitive NMDA receptor blocker that is able to cross the blood-brain barrier. It has several side effects, however, and is unlikely to be useful in neonates.

Magnesium, which has been used for several years to treat preeclampsia and whose effects on the fetus and newborn are well known, has shown mixed results in regard to neuroprotection (Galvin and Oorschot, 1998; MacDonald and Nowak, 1990). It is hypothesized to work by blockade of the immature NMDA ion channel as well as inhibition of neurotransmitter release and induction of NOS. In a study evaluating two different doses of magnesium sulfate in a group of full-term infants with Apgar scores of less than 6 at 10 minutes within 12 hours after delivery, even the lower dose of 250 mg/kg resulted in respiratory depression and hypotension (Levene et al, 1995). Maternal $MgSO_4$ does not reduce the risk of neonatal white matter damage, IVH, or ventriculomegaly (Leviton et al, 1997), and $MgSO_4$ during labor does not reduce the risk of cerebral palsy in infants with birth weights of less than 2000 g (Paneth et al, 1997).

In contrast to NMDA antagonists, AMPA receptor antagonists protect against global ischemic insults in adult models of ischemia, with a therapeutic window of as long as 12 hours (Li and Buchan, 1993). AMPA receptors are activated in the postischemic phase of injury. Antagonists to these receptors decrease glucose metabolism and increase brain-derived neurotrophic factor (BDNF), thereby promoting neuronal protection.

Erythropoietin has been shown in cell culture experiments to reduce neuronal cell death from oxygen-glucose deprivation and to attenuate the neurotoxic effect of AMPA. It has been used extensively in premature infants to treat anemia and has not been shown to have any major side effects (Ohls, 2000).

### Calcium Entry Blockade by Gamma-Aminobutyric Acid

Activation of the postsynaptic GABA receptor, an inhibitory receptor, stimulates entry of chloride and hyperpolarization of the neuronal cell membrane. Stimulation of these receptors by agents during the ischemic phase can prevent entry of calcium into the postsynaptic neuron. Stimulation during the postischemic phase can reduce the energy expended by the $Na^+$,$K^+$-ATPase pump and thus stabilize the cell membrane. Agents in this group include benzodiazapines, GABA uptake inhibitors (tiagabine), and inhibitors of GABA transaminase (vigabatrin). These drugs have shown mixed results in animal studies, and it is unclear if they will be of any use in the neonate because the inhibitory systems in the newborn brain are underdeveloped (Sternau et al, 1989).

### Calcium Channel Blockers

Calcium channel blockers exert their effects at both their neuronal and vascular targets by inhibition of calcium influx into the cell. Large clinical trials in adults as well as a meta-analysis of nimodipine use have not been successful due to a narrow therapeutic window (Di Mascio et al, 1994). Nicardipine was tested in four full-term newborns but was found to be associated with severe hypotension (Levene et al, 1990). Flunarizine pretreatment has been shown to decrease dopamine release during hypoxia and to reduce infarct size in the Rice-Vannucci rat model (Gunn et al, 1989; Silverstein et al, 1986). Nonselective agents such as dihydropyridines also can cause hypotension. Newer neuron-specific calcium channel blockers seem more promising.

### Enzyme Inhibition

Inhibition of activation of enzymes such as calpain, a proteolytic agent that affects membrane proteins, as well as cyclooxygenase, xanthine oxidase, and NOS, is a potential therapeutic strategy.

NOS inhibitors have been studied in animal models of global and focal ischemia. Inhibition of NOS is complicated by the presence of three different isoforms, with differences in the timing of NOS inhibition, duration of treatment, and degree of effective binding to NOS. Increased understanding of the actions of the different isoforms, the stimuli that induce them, and their duration of action will help in designing newer and more focused treatment methods using these agents. In a study in the neonatal rat, $N^G$-nitro-L-arginine (NO-Arg) showed efficacy if the drug was administered prior to the insult, but not afterward (Hamada et al, 1994). Similar results were obtained by Trifiletti (1992), who showed that documented inhibition of NOS with NO-Arg 15 hours before the onset of the hypoxic-ischemic insult provided almost complete protection against neuronal damage. In a post-treatment study in fetal sheep, Marks and colleagues (1996) showed that a continuous infusion of NO-Arg at a dose of 50 mg/kg instituted 2 hours after a 30-minute in utero ischemic insult delayed the increase in cerebral blood volume but did not decrease the extent of cerebral injury. Better protection has been achieved with the use of more selective neuronal NOS inhibitors, but the timing of administration is critical for protection (Groenendaal et al, 1999; Hamada et al, 1994; Muramatsu et al, 2000).

At present, no NOS inhibitors have been approved for use in humans.

### Inhibition of Other Free Radicals

Free radicals can be produced by different mechanisms. Endogenously occurring enzymes such as superoxide dismutase (SOD), catalase, and glutathione help in decreasing production of free radicals. In a murine model, transgenic mice that overexpress SOD showed less injury than wild-type mice in adult animals but more injury in immature animals (Ditelberg et al, 1996). Exogenous SOD has been of limited effectiveness due to its inability to penetrate lipid membranes and its short half-life. Lazaroids are a new class of lipophilic steroids that inhibit lipid peroxidation selectively without any effect on glucose metabolism. However, a randomized trial in adults treated within 6 hours of a stroke with tirilazad, a lazaroid medication that had been shown in animal models of focal ischemia to help decrease the size of the infarct, failed to show any improvement (RANTTAS investigators, 1996).

Metalloporphyrins have been shown in in vitro experiments with hippocampal cells to be neuroprotective via direct neural effects (Panizzon et al, 1996).

Allopurinol has been shown to be neuroprotective in some animal studies, but when this drug was administered to severely asphyxiated neonates, there was no significant improvement in outcome despite documented decrease in oxidative stress (Van Bel et al, 1998; Veen et al, 1999). It acts primarily by inhibiting xanthine oxidase and by decreasing synthesis of uric acid. However, the mechanism of action is not completely clear, because the doses needed are higher than those required to block xanthine oxidase. Allopurinol may act by preventing the release of lysosomal enzymes, by chelating iron or copper, or by scavenging hydroxyl radicals. Allopurinol did not further improve outcome when used in combination with other scavengers such as deferoxamine (DFO) or indomethacin in animal models (Shadid et al, 1998).

### Hypoxic Preconditioning and Deferoxamine

Hypoxic preconditioning has been shown in both hippocampal cells and in the Rice-Vannucci neonatal rat model to activate protective mechanisms, possibly by triggering expression of gene products or deoxygenation of a heme moiety. Levels of a hypoxia-inducible transcription factor (HIF-1) are elevated in the penumbra in neonatal rats treated with hypoxia preconditioning (Bergeron et al, 2000). Pretreatment of animals with either cobalt chloride or DFO before injury was found to provide a 75% or 56% degree of protection, respectively. Other studies in the ischemic gerbil model (Patt et al, 1990), as well as in the neonatal rat, mouse, and lamb models, have shown decreased injury with use of DFO (Groenendaal et al, 2000; Kompala et al, 1986; Palmer et al, 1994; Sarco et al, 2000). DFO may act by iron chelation or by inducing HIF-1, or by other mechanisms. Although it has not been tested in human trials, it is a good candidate for clinical trials in neonates, as it has been studied extensively in clinical situations requiring iron chelation.

### Growth Factors

Genes up-regulated by stress, such as those that induce growth and differentiation including brain-derived neurotrophic factor (BDNF) and insulin-like growth factor (IGF), have been shown to be neuroprotective in animal models (Han and Holtzman, 2000). IGF-1 administered shortly after an injury is neuroprotective in the modified Levine adult rat model (Guan et al, 2000; Sizonenko et al, 2001).

### Caspase Inhibitors

Use of relatively specific inhibitors of apoptosis—caspase inhibitors—in immature animals significantly decreases brain injury, with the neuroprotective effect being dependent on the drug used (Cheng et al, 1998). Evidence suggests that although some of the cell death in the adult brain following ischemia is apoptotic and caspase dependent, apoptotic-like death is particularly prominent in the neonatal brain after hypoxic and ischemic insults including hypoxia-ischemia (Cheng et al, 1997; Ferrer et al, 1997). This finding, coupled with the prolonged evolution of cell death after HI-R injury, provides new opportunities for intervention.

### Combination Regimens

Due to the complexity of the pathways involved in cell death, it is likely that more than one method or agent will be needed to stop the cascade of deleterious events. Modalities that reduce cellular metabolic demands (hypothermia) coupled with agents that reduce oxidative stress (scavengers) and inhibit cell death (caspase inhibitors) might provide the best results.

## SUMMARY

The past decade has seen an explosion of information regarding the pathophysiology of ischemic and traumatic injuries to the developing nervous system. The realization that the immature brain has different pathogenetic mechanisms in response to these insults has led investigators to think differently about designing therapies for the immature brain. With the continued investigations regarding the mechanisms of cell death in the immature brain, the development of age-appropriate neuroprotective strategies is not far behind.

## REFERENCES


al Naqeeb N, Edwards AD, Cowan FM, et al: Assessment of neonatal encephalopathy by amplitude-integrated electroencephalography. Pediatrics 103:1263-1271, 1999.

Andersen DL, Tannenberg AE, Burke CJ, et al: Developmental rearrangements of cortical glutamate-NMDA receptor binding sites in late human gestation. Brain Res Dev Brain Res 88:178-185, 1995.

Back SA, Gan X, Li Y, et al: Maturation-dependent vulnerability of oligodendrocytes to oxidative stress-induced death caused by glutathione depletion. J Neurosci 18:6241-6253, 1998.

Back SA, Han BH, Luo NL, et al: Selective vulnerability of late oligodendrocyte progenitors to hypoxia-ischemia. J Neurosci 22:455-463, 2002.

Back SA, Luo NL, Borenstein NS, et al: Late oligodendrocyte progenitors coincide with the developmental window of vulnerability for human perinatal white matter injury. J Neurosci 21:1302-1312, 2001.

Back SA, Volpe JJ: Cellular and molecular pathogenesis of periventricular white matter injury. Ment Retard Dev Disabil Res Rev 3:96-107, 1997.

Badawi N, Kurinczuk JJ, Keogh JM, et al: Intrapartum risk factors for newborn encephalopathy: The Western Australian case-control study. BMJ 317:1554-1558, 1998.

Barkovich AJ, Hajnal BL, Vigneron D, et al: Prediction of neuromotor outcome in perinatal asphyxia: Evaluation of MR scoring systems. AJNR Am J Neuroradiol 19:143-149, 1998.

Barkovich AJ, Westmark K, Partridge C, et al: Perinatal asphyxia: MR findings in the first 10 days. AJNR Am J Neuroradiol 16:427-438, 1995.

Barkovich AJ, Westmark KD, Bedi HS, et al: Proton spectroscopy and diffusion imaging on the first day of life after perinatal asphyxia: Preliminary report. AJNR Am J Neuroradiol 22:1786-1794, 2001.

Ben-Ari Y, Cherubini E, Krnjevic K: Changes in voltage dependence of NMDA currents during development. Neurosci Lett 94:88-92, 1988.

Benson JW, Drayton MR, Hayward C, et al: Multicentre trial of ethamsylate for prevention of periventricular haemorrhage in very low birthweight infants. Lancet 2:1297-1300, 1986.

Bergeron M, Gidday JM, Yu AY, et al: Role of hypoxia-inducible factor-1 (HIF-1) in hypoxia-induced ischemic tolerance in neonatal rat brain. Ann Neurol 48:285-296, 2000.

Biagioni E, Ferrari F, Boldrini A, et al: Electroclinical correlation in neonatal seizures. Eur J Paediatr Neurol 2:117-125, 1998.

Biagioni E, Mercuri E, Rutherford M, et al: Combined use of electroencephalogram and magnetic resonance imaging in full-term neonates with acute encephalopathy. Pediatrics 107:461-468, 2001.

Black SM, Bedolli MA, Martinez S, et al: Expression of neuronal nitric oxide synthase corresponds to regions of selective vulnerability to hypoxia-ischaemia in the developing rat brain. Neurobiol Dis 2:145-155, 1995.

Canterino JC, Verma U, Visintainer PF, et al: Antenatal steroids and neonatal periventricular leukomalacia. Obstet Gynecol 97:135-139, 2001.

Carvalho KS, Bodensteiner JB, Connolly PJ, et al: Cerebral venous thrombosis in children. J Child Neurol 16:574-580, 2001.

Castro A, Bogido M, Sola A: Does "routine" early use of high-frequency ventilation add benefits to VLBW with lung disease? J Invest Med 48:26A, 2000.

Cheng EH, Kirsch DG, Clem RJ, et al: Conversion of Bcl-2 to a Bax-like death effector by caspases. Science 278:1966-1968, 1997.

Cheng Y, Deshmukh M, D'Costa A, et al: Prominent apoptosis in neonatal hypoxia-ischemia: Caspase inhibitor affords neuroprotection with delayed administration in a rat model of neonatal hypoxic-ischemic brain injury [see comments]. J Clin Invest 101:1992-1999, 1998.

Clancy RR, Sladky JT, Rorke LB: Hypoxic-ischemic spinal cord injury following perinatal asphyxia. Ann Neurol 25:185-189, 1989.

Coimbra C, Wieloch T: Moderate hypothermia mitigates neuronal damage in the rat brain when initiated several hours following transient cerebral ischemia. Acta Neuropathol (Berl) 87:325-331, 1994.

Colbourne F, Corbett D: Delayed and prolonged post-ischemic hypothermia is neuroprotective in the gerbil. Brain Res 654:265-272, 1994.

Collins MP, Lorenz JM, Jetton JR, et al: Hypocapnia and other ventilation-related risk factors for cerebral palsy in low birth weight infants. Pediatr Res 50:712-719, 2001.

Cools F, Offringa M: Neuromuscular paralysis for newborn infants receiving mechanical ventilation. Cochrane Database Syst Rev 312:CD002773, 2000.

Cowan F, Whitelaw A, Wertheim D, et al: Cerebral blood flow velocity changes after rapid administration of surfactant [see comments]. Arch Dis Child 66:1105-1109, 1991.

Craig A, Ling Luo N, Beardsley DJ, et al: Quantitative analysis of perinatal rodent oligodendrocyte lineage progression and its correlation with human. Exp Neurol 181:231-240, 2003.

Cremer JE, Cunningham VJ, Pardridge WM, et al: Kinetics of blood-brain barrier transport of pyruvate, lactate and glucose in suckling, weanling and adult rats. J Neurochem 33:439-445, 1979.

Dammann O, Kuban KC, Leviton A: Perinatal infection, fetal inflammatory response, white matter damage, and cognitive limitations in children born preterm. Ment Retard Dev Disabil Res Rev 8:46-50, 2002.

de Mendonca A, Sebastiao AM, Ribeiro JA: Adenosine: Does it have a neuroprotective role after all? Brain Res Brain Res Rev 33:258-274, 2000.

de Vries LS, Groenendaal F, Eken P, et al: Infarcts in the vascular distribution of the middle cerebral artery in preterm and fullterm infants. Neuropediatrics 28:88-96, 1997.

deVeber G, Andrew M: Cerebral sinovenous thrombosis in children. N Engl J Med 345:417-423, 2001.

Di Mascio R, Marchioli R, Tognoni G: From pharmacological promises to controlled clinical trials to meta-analysis and back: The case of nimodipine in cerebrovascular disorders. Clin Trials Metaanal 29:57-79, 1994.

Ditelberg JS, Sheldon RA, Epstein CJ, et al: Brain injury after perinatal hypoxia-ischemia is exacerbated in copper/zinc superoxide dismutase transgenic mice. Pediatr Res 39:204-208, 1996.

Dommergues MA, Gallego J, Evrard P, et al: Iron supplementation aggravates periventricular cystic white matter lesions in newborn mice. Eur J Paediatr Neurol 2:313-318, 1998.

Donn SM, Roloff DW, Goldstein GW: Prevention of intraventricular haemorrhage in preterm infants by phenobarbitone. A controlled trial. Lancet 2:215-217, 1981.

Dubowitz L, Mercuri E, Dubowitz V: An optimality score for the neurologic examination of the term newborn. J Pediatr 133:406-416, 1998.

Edwards AD, Yue X, Squier MV, et al: Specific inhibition of apoptosis after cerebral hypoxia-ischaemia by moderate post-insult hypothermia. Biochem Biophys Res Commun 217:1193-1199, 1995.

Ekert P, Perlman M, Steinlin M, et al: Predicting the outcome of postasphyxial hypoxic-ischemic encephalopathy within 4 hours of birth. J Pediatr 131:613-617, 1997.

Elimian A, Verma U, Visintainer P, et al: Effectiveness of multidose antenatal steroids. Obstet Gynecol 95:34-36, 2000.

Ferrara B, Johnson DE, Chang PN, et al: Efficacy and neurologic outcome of profound hypocapneic alkalosis for the treatment of persistent pulmonary hypertension in infancy. J Pediatr 105:457-461, 1984.

Ferrer I, Pozas E, Lopez E, et al: Bcl-2, Bax and Bcl-x expression following hypoxia-ischemia in the infant rat brain. Acta Neuropathol (Berl) 94:583-589, 1997.

Ferriero DM: Oxidant mechanisms in neonatal hypoxia-ischemia. Dev Neurosci 23:198-202, 2001.

Ferriero DM, Holtzman DM, Black SM, et al: Neonatal mice lacking neuronal nitric oxide synthase are less vulnerable to hypoxic-ischemic injury. Neurobiol Dis 3:64-71, 1996.

Finer NN, Peters KL, Hayek Z, et al: Vitamin E and necrotizing enterocolitis. Pediatrics 73:387-393, 1984.

Fowlie PW: Prophylactic indomethacin: Systematic review and meta-analysis. Arch Dis Child Fetal Neonatal Ed 74:F81-87, 1996.

Fulmer BB, Grabb PA, Oakes WJ, et al: Neonatal ventriculosubgaleal shunts. Neurosurgery 47:80-83; discussion 83-84, 2000.

Galvin KA, Oorschot DE: Postinjury magnesium sulfate treatment is not markedly neuroprotective for striatal medium spiny neurons after perinatal hypoxia/ischemia in the rat. Pediatr Res 44:740-745, 1998.

Goddard-Finegold J, Armstrong D, Zeller RS: Intraventricular hemorrhage, following volume expansion after hypovolemic hypotension in the newborn beagle. J Pediatr 100:796-799, 1982.

Golomb MR, MacGregor DL, Domi T, et al: Presumed pre- or perinatal arterial ischemic stroke: Risk factors and outcomes. Ann Neurol 50:163-168, 2001.

Gregoire NM, Gjedde A, Plum F, et al: Cerebral blood flow and cerebral metabolic rates for oxygen, glucose, and ketone bodies in newborn dogs. J Neurochem 30:63-69, 1978.

Gressens P, Rogido M, Paindaveine B, et al: The impact of neonatal intensive care practices on the developing brain. J Pediatr 140:646-653, 2002.

Groenendaal F, de Graaf RA, van Vliet G, et al: Effects of hypoxia-ischemia and inhibition of nitric oxide synthase on cerebral energy metabolism in newborn piglets. Pediatr Res 45:827-833, 1999.

Groenendaal F, Shadid M, McGowan JE, et al: Effects of deferoxamine, a chelator of free iron, on NA(+), K(+)-ATPase activity of cortical brain cell membrane during early reperfusion after hypoxia-ischemia in newborn lambs. Pediatr Res 48:560-564, 2000.

Groenendaal F, van der Grond J, Eken P, et al: Early cerebral proton MRS and neurodevelopmental outcome in infants with cystic leukomalacia. Dev Med Child Neurol 39:373-379, 1997.

Guan J, Bennet TL, George S, et al: Selective neuroprotective effects with insulin-like growth factor-1 in phenotypic striatal neurons following ischemic brain injury in fetal sheep. Neuroscience 95:831-839, 2000.

Gunn AJ, Gluckman PD, Gunn TR: Selective head cooling in newborn infants after perinatal asphyxia: A safety study. Pediatrics 102:885-892, 1998.

Gunn AJ, Gunn TR, de Haan HH, et al: Dramatic neuronal rescue with prolonged selective head cooling after ischemia in fetal lambs. J Clin Invest 99:248-256, 1997.

Gunn AJ, Mydlar T, Bennet L, et al: The neuroprotective actions of a calcium channel antagonist, flunarizine, in the infant rat. Pediatr Res 25:573-576, 1989.

Haaland K, Loberg EM, Steen PA, et al: Posthypoxic hypothermia in newborn piglets. Pediatr Res 41:505-512, 1997.

Haines SJ, Lapointe M: Fibrinolytic agents in the management of posthemorrhagic hydrocephalus in preterm infants: The evidence. Childs Nerv Syst 15:226-234, 1999.

Hajnal BL, Sahebkar-Moghaddam F, Barnwell AJ, et al: Early prediction of neurologic outcome after perinatal depression. Pediatr Neurol 21:788-793, 1999.

Hamada Y, Hayakawa T, Hattori H, et al: Inhibitor of nitric oxide synthesis reduces hypoxic-ischemic brain damage in the neonatal rat. Pediatr Res 35:10-14, 1994.

Han BH, Holtzman DM: BDNF protects the neonatal brain from hypoxic-ischemic injury in vivo via the ERK pathway. J Neurosci 20:5775-5781, 2000.

Hanrahan JD, Sargentoni J, Azzopardi D, et al: Cerebral metabolism within 18 hours of birth asphyxia: A proton magnetic resonance spectroscopy study. Pediatr Res 39:584-590, 1996.

Hayakawa T, Hamada Y, Maihara T, et al: Phenytoin reduces neonatal hypoxic-ischemic brain damage in rats. Life Sci 54:387-392, 1994.

Hellstrom-Westas L, Bell AH, Skov L, et al: Cerebroelectrical depression following surfactant treatment in preterm neonates. Pediatrics 89:643-647, 1992.

Hellstrom-Westas L, Rosen I, Svenningsen NW: Cerebral function monitoring during the first week of life in extremely small low birthweight (ESLBW) infants. Neuropediatrics 22:27-32, 1991.

HIFI Study Group: High-frequency oscillatory ventilation compared with conventional mechanical ventilation in the treatment of respiratory failure in preterm infants. The HIFI Study Group. N Engl J Med 320:88-93, 1989.

Holshouser BA, Ashwal S, Shu S, et al: Proton MR spectroscopy in children with acute brain injury: Comparison of short and long echo time acquisitions. J Magn Reson Imaging 11:9-19, 2000.

Hu BR, Liu CL, Ouyang Y, et al: Involvement of caspase-3 in cell death after hypoxia-ischemia declines during brain maturation. J Cereb Blood Flow Metab 20:1294-1300, 2000.

Huang CC, Wang ST, Chang YC, et al: Measurement of the urinary lactate:creatinine ratio for the early identification of newborn infants at risk for hypoxic-ischemic encephalopathy. N Engl J Med 341:328-335, 1999.

Huppi PS, Murphy B, Maier SE, et al: Microstructural brain development after perinatal cerebral white matter injury assessed by diffusion tensor magnetic resonance imaging. Pediatrics 107:455-460, 2001.

Huppi PS, Warfield S, Kikinis R, et al: Quantitative magnetic resonance imaging of brain development in premature and mature newborns. Ann Neurol 43:224-235, 1998.

Ikonomidou C, Bosch F, M. M, et al: Blockade of NMDA receptors and apoptotoic neruodegeneration in the developing brain. Science 283:70-74, 1999.

Inder TE, Huppi PS, Warfield S, et al: Periventricular white matter injury in the premature infant is followed by reduced cerebral cortical gray matter volume at term. Ann Neurol 46:755-760, 1999.

Inder TE, Volpe JJ: Mechanisms of perinatal brain injury. Semin Neonatol 5:3-16, 2000.

Johnson L, Bowen FW, Jr., Abbasi S, et al: Relationship of prolonged pharmacologic serum levels of vitamin E to incidence of sepsis and necrotizing enterocolitis in infants with birth weight 1,500 grams or less. Pediatrics 75:619-638, 1985.

Johnston MV: Neurotransmitters and vulnerability of the developing brain. Brain Dev 17:301-306, 1995.

Kaempf JW, Porreco R, Molina R, et al: Antenatal phenobarbital for the prevention of periventricular and intraventricular hemorrhage: A double-blind, randomized, placebo-controlled, multihospital trial [see comments]. J Pediatr 117:933-938, 1990.

Kennedy CR, Ayers S, Campbell MJ, et al: Randomized, controlled trial of acetazolamide and furosemide in posthemorrhagic ventricular dilation in infancy: Follow-up at 1 year. Pediatrics 108:597-607, 2001.

Keszler M, Modanlou HD, Brudno DS, et al: Multicenter controlled clinical trial of high-frequency jet ventilation in preterm infants with uncomplicated respiratory distress syndrome. Pediatrics 100:593-599, 1997.

Kompala SD, Babbs CF, Blaho KE: Effect of deferoxamine on late deaths following CPR in rats. Ann Emerg Med 15:405-407, 1986.

Kuban KCK, Leviton A, Krishnamoorthy KS, et al: Neonatal intracranial hemorrhage and phenobarbital. Pediatrics 77:443-450, 1986.

Kumar S: ICE-like proteases in apoptosis. Trends Biochem Sci 20:198-202, 1995.

LeBlanc MH, Huang M, Vig V, et al: Glucose affects the severity of hypoxic-ischemic brain injury in newborn pigs. Stroke 24:1055-1062, 1993.

Levene M, Blennow M, Whitelaw A, et al: Acute effects of two different doses of magnesium sulphate in infants with birth asphyxia. Arch Dis Child Fetal Neonatal Ed 73:F174-177, 1995.

Levene MI, Evans DH: Medical management of raised intracranial pressure after severe birth asphyxia. Arch Dis Child 60:12-16, 1985.

Levene MI, Gibson NA, Fenton AC, et al: The use of a calcium-channel blocker, nicardipine, for severely asphyxiated newborn infants. Dev Med Child Neurol Suppl 32:567-574, 1990.

Levene MI, Sands C, Grindulis H, et al: Comparison of two methods of predicting outcome in perinatal asphyxia. Lancet 1:67-69, 1986.

Leviton A, Paneth N, Susser M, et al: Maternal receipt of magnesium sulfate does not seem to reduce the risk of neonatal white matter damage. Pediatrics 99:E2, 1997.

Li H, Buchan AM: Treatment with an AMPA antagonist 12 hours following severe normothermic forebrain ischemia prevents CA1 neuronal injury. J Cereb Blood Flow Metab 13:933-939, 1993.

Lowe J, Papile L: Neurodevelopmental performance of very-low-birth-weight infants with mild periventricular, intraventricular hemorrhage. Outcome at 5 to 6 years of age. Am J Dis Child 144:1242-1245, 1990.

Luciano R, Tortorolo L, Chiaretti A, et al: Intraventricular streptokinase infusion in acute post-haemorrhagic hydrocephalus. 24:526-529, 1998.

Lynch JK, Hirtz DG, DeVeber G, et al: Report of the National Institute of Neurological Disorders and Stroke Workshop on Perinatal and Childhood Stroke. Pediatrics 109:116-123, 2002.

Lynch JK, Nelson KB: Epidemiology of perinatal stroke. Curr Opin Pediatr 13:499-505, 2001.

Maalouf EF, Duggan PJ, Counsell SJ, et al: Comparison of findings on cranial ultrasound and magnetic resonance imaging in preterm infants. Pediatrics 107:719-727, 2001.

Maalouf EF, Duggan PJ, Rutherford MA, et al: Magnetic resonance imaging of the brain in a cohort of extremely preterm infants. J Pediatr 135:351-357, 1999.

MacDonald JF, Nowak LM: Mechanisms of blockade of excitatory amino acid receptor channels. Trends Pharmacol Sci 11:167-172, 1990.

Marks KA, Mallard CE, Roberts I, et al: Nitric oxide synthase inhibition attenuates delayed vasodilation and increases injury after cerebral ischemia in fetal sheep. Pediatr Res 40:185-191, 1996.

Marks N, Berg MJ: Recent advances on neuronal caspases in development and neurodegeneration. Neurochem Int 35:195-220, 1999.

McCulloch DL, Taylor MJ, Whyte HE: Visual evoked potentials and visual prognosis following perinatal asphyxia. Arch Ophthalmol 109:229-233, 1991.

McQuillen PS, Sheldon RA, Shatz CJ, et al: Selective vulnerability of subplate neurons after early neonatal hypoxia-ischemia. J Neurosci 23:3308-3315, 2003.

Ment LR, Bada HS, Barnes P, et al: Practice parameter: Neuroimaging of the neonate: Report of the Quality Standards Subcommittee of the American Academy of Neurology and the Practice Committee of the Child Neurology Society. Neurology 58:1726-1738, 2002.

Ment LR, Duncan CC, Ehrenkranz RA, et al: Intraventricular hemorrhage in the preterm neonate: timing and cerebral blood flow changes. J Pediatr 104:419-425, 1984.

Ment LR, Duncan CC, Ehrenkranz RA, et al: Randomized indomethacin trial for prevention of intraventricular hemorrhage in very low birth weight infants. J Pediatr 107:937-943, 1985.

Ment LR, Oh W, Ehrenkranz RA, et al: Low-dose indomethacin and prevention of intraventricular hemorrhage: A multicenter randomized trial [see comments]. Pediatrics 93:543-550, 1994.

Ment LR, Schneider K: Intraventricular hemorrhage of the preterm infant. Semin Neurol 13:40-47, 1993.

Ment LR, Stewart WB, Duncan CC, et al: Beagle puppy model of intraventricular hemorrhage. J Neurosurg 57:219-223, 1982.

Ment LR, Stewart WB, Petroff OA, et al: Beagle puppy model of perinatal asphyxia: Blockade of excitatory neurotransmitters. Pediatr Neurol 5:281-286, 1989.

Ment LR, Vohr B, Allan W, et al: The etiology and outcome of cerebral ventriculomegaly at term in very low birth weight preterm infants. Pediatrics 104:243-248, 1999.

Ment LR, Vohr B, Allan W, et al: Outcome of children in the indomethacin intraventricular hemorrhage prevention trial. Pediatrics 105:485-491, 2000.

Mercuri E: Early diagnostic and prognostic indicators in full term infants with neonatal cerebral infarction: An integrated clinical, neuroradiological and EEG approach. Minerva Pediatr 53:305-311, 2001.

Merz U, Peschgens T, Kusenbach G, et al: Early versus late dexamethasone treatment in preterm infants at risk for chronic lung disease: A randomized pilot study. Eur J Pediatr 158:318-322, 1999.

Miall-Allen VM, de Vries LS, Whitelaw AG: Mean arterial blood pressure and neonatal cerebral lesions. Arch Dis Child 62:1068-1069, 1987.

Miall-Allen VM, Whitelaw AG: Effect of pancuronium and pethidine on heart rate and blood pressure in ventilated infants. Arch Dis Child 62:1179-1180, 1987.

Miller S, Ferriero D, Barkovich AJ, et al: Practice parameter: Neuroimaging of the neonate: Report of the Quality Standards Subcommittee of the American Academy of Neurology and the Practice Committee of the Child Neurology Society. Neurology 59:1663; author reply 1663-1664, 2002a.

Miller SP, Newton N, Ferriero DM, et al: MRS predictors of 30-month outcome following perinatal depression: Role of socioeconomic factors. Pediatr Res 52:71-77, 2002b.

Miller SP, Vigneron DB, Henry RG, et al: Serial quantitative diffusion tensor MRI of the premature brain: Development in newborns with and without injury. J Magn Reson Imaging 16:621-632, 2002c.

Miller SP, Weiss J, Barnwell A, et al: Seizure-associated brain injury in term newborns with perinatal asphyxia. Neurology 58:542-548, 2002d.

Mischel R, Tureen J, Baserga M, et al: Effect of gavage feeding on cerebral hemodynamics, oxygenation, and metabolism in the premature neonate determined by near-infrared spectroscopy. J Investig Med 45:149A, 1997.

Mizrahi EM, Kellaway P: Characterization and classification of neonatal seizures. Neurology 37:1837-1844, 1987.

Moriette G, Paris-Llado J, Walti H, et al: Prospective randomized multicenter comparison of high-frequency oscillatory ventilation and conventional ventilation in preterm infants of less than 30 weeks with respiratory distress syndrome. Pediatrics 107:363-372, 2001.

Morrisett RA, Chow CC, Sakaguchi T, et al: Inhibition of muscarinic-coupled phosphoinositide hydrolysis by *N*-methyl-D-aspartate is dependent on depolarization via channel activation. J Neurol 54:1517-1525, 1990.

Muramatsu K, Sheldon RA, Black SM, et al: Nitric oxide synthase activity and inhibition after neonatal hypoxia-ischemia in the mouse. Brain Res Dev Brain Res 123:119-127, 2000.

Murphy BP, Inder TE, Huppi PS, et al: Impaired cerebral cortical gray matter growth after treatment with dexamethasone for neonatal chronic lung disease. Pediatrics 107:217-221, 2001.

Nakajima W, Ishida A, Lange MS, et al: Apoptosis has a prolonged role in the neurodegeneration after hypoxic ischemia in the newborn Rat. J Neurosci 20:7994-8004, 2000.

Nelson KB, Ellenberg JH: Antecedents of cerebral palsy. Multivariate analysis of risk. N Engl J Med 315:81-86, 1986.

Nelson KB, Grether JK: Selection of neonates for neuroprotective therapies: One set of criteria applied to a population. Arch Pediatr Adolesc Med 153:393-398, 1999.

Newton NR, Miller SP, Ferriero DM, et al: SNAP-PE as a Predictor of Neurodevelopmental Outcome at 1 and 2.5 Years of Age Following Perinatal Depression. Pediatr Res 49:310A, 2001.

Northington FJ, Ferriero DM, Flock DL, et al: Delayed neurodegeneration in neonatal rat thalamus after hypoxia-ischemia is apoptosis. J Neurosci 21:1931-1938, 2001a.

Northington FJ, Ferriero DM, Graham E, et al: Early neurodegeneration after hypoxia-ischemia in neonatal rat is necrosis while delayed neuronal death is apoptosis. Neurobiol Dis 8:207-219, 2001b.

Obrenovitch TP, Urenjak J: Is high extracellular glutamate the key to excitotoxicity in traumatic brain injury? J Neurotrauma 14:677-698, 1997.

Ohls RK: The use of erythropoietin in neonates. Clin Perinatol 27:681-696, 2000.

Palmer C, Roberts RL, Bero C: Deferoxamine posttreatment reduces ischemic brain injury in neonatal rats. Stroke 25:1039-1045, 1994.

Paneth N, Jetton J, Pinto-Martin J, et al: Magnesium sulfate in labor and risk of neonatal brain lesions and cerebral palsy in low birth weight infants. The Neonatal Brain Hemorrhage Study Analysis Group. Pediatrics 99:E1, 1997.

Paneth N, Pinto-Martin J, Gardiner J, et al: Incidence and timing of germinal matrix/intraventricular hemorrhage in low birth weight infants. Am J Epidemiol 137:1167-1176, 1993.

Panizzon KL, Dwyer BE, Nishimura RN, et al: Neuroprotection against CA1 injury with metalloporphyrins. Neuroreport 7:662-666, 1996.

Pape KE, Bennett-Britton S, Szymonowicz W, et al: Diagnostic accuracy of neonatal brain imaging: A postmortem correlation of computed tomography and ultrasound scans. J Pediatr 102:275-280, 1983.

Pape KE, Blackwell RJ, Cusick G, et al: Ultrasound detection of brain damage in preterm infants. Lancet 1:1261-1264, 1979.

Pape KE, Pickering D: Asymmetric crying facies: An index of other congenital anomalies. J Pediatr 81:21-30, 1972.

Papile LA, Burstein J, Burstein R, et al: Incidence and evolution of subependymal and intraventricular hemorrhage: A study of infants with birth weights less than 1,500 gm. J Pediatr 92:529-534, 1978.

Patt A, Horesh IR, Berger EM, et al: Iron depletion or chelation reduces ischemia/reperfusion-induced edema in gerbil brains. J Pediatr Surg 25:224-227; discussion 227-228, 1990.

Penrice J, Cady EB, Lorek A, et al: Proton magnetic resonance spectroscopy of the brain in normal preterm and term infants, and early changes after perinatal hypoxia-ischemia. Pediatr Res 40:6-14, 1996.

Penrice J, Lorek A, Cady EB, et al: Proton magnetic resonance spectroscopy of the brain during acute hypoxia-ischemia and delayed cerebral energy failure in the newborn piglet. Pediatr Res 41:795-802, 1997.

Perlman JM, Goodman S, Kreusser KL, et al: Reduction in intraventricular hemorrhage by elimination of fluctuating cerebral blood-flow velocity in preterm infants with respiratory distress syndrome. N Engl J Med 312:1353-1357, 1985.

Perlman JM, Rollins NK, Evans D: Neonatal stroke: Clinical characteristics and cerebral blood flow velocity measurements. Pediatr Neurol 11:281-284, 1994.

Portera-Cailliau C, Price DL, Martin LJ: Excitotoxic neuronal death in the immature brain is an apoptosis-necrosis morphological continuum. J Comp Neurol 378:70-87, 1997.

RANTTAS investigators: A randomized trial of tirilazad mesylate in patients with acute stroke (RANTTAS). Stroke 27:1453-1458, 1996.

Rijn AM, Groenendaal F, Beek FJ, et al: Parenchymal brain injury in the preterm infant: Comparison of cranial ultrasound, MRI and neurodevelopmental outcome. Neuropediatrics 32:80-89, 2001.

Robertson CM, Finer NN: Term infants with hypoxic-ischemic encephalopathy: Outcome at 3.5 years. Dev Med Child Neurol 27:473-484, 1985.

Robertson CM, Finer NN, Grace MG: School performance of survivors of neonatal encephalopathy associated with birth asphyxia at term. J Pediatr 114:753-760, 1989.

Rutherford MA, Pennock JM, Dubowitz LM: Cranial ultrasound and magnetic resonance imaging in hypoxic-ischaemic encephalopathy: A comparison with outcome. Dev Med Child Neurol 36:813-825, 1994.

Rutherford MA, Pennock JM, Schwieso JE, et al: Hypoxic ischaemic encephalopathy: Early magnetic resonance imaging findings and their evolution. Neuropediatrics 26:183-191, 1995.

Sarco D, Becker J, Palmer C, et al: The neuroprotective effect of deferoxamine in the hypoxic-ischemic immature mouse brain. Neurosci Lett 282:113-116, 2000.

Sarnat HB, Sarnat MS: Neonatal encephalopathy following fetal distress: A clinical and electroencephalographic study. Arch Neurol 33:696-705, 1976.

Schmidt B, Davis P, Moddemann D, et al: Long-term effects of indomethacin prophylaxis in extremely-low-birth-weight infants. Trial of Indomethacin Prophylaxis in Preterms Investigators. N Engl J Med 344:1966-1972, 2001.

Schum TR, Meyer GA, Grausz JP, et al: Neonatal intraventricular hemorrhage due to an intracranial arteriovenous malformation: A case report. Pediatrics 64:242-244, 1979.

Shadid M, Moison R, Steendijk P, et al: The effect of antioxidative combination therapy on post hypoxic-ischemic perfusion, metabolism, and electrical activity of the newborn brain. Pediatr Res 44:119-124, 1998.

Shankaran S, Woldt E, Nelson J, et al: Antenatal phenobarbital therapy and neonatal outcome. II: Neurodevelopmental outcome at 36 months. Pediatrics 97:649-652, 1996.

Sheldon RA, Chuai J, Ferriero DM: A rat model for hypoxic-ischemic brain damage in very premature infants. Biol Neonate 69:327-341, 1996.

Sheldon RA, Partridge JC, Ferriero DM: Postischemic hyperglycemia is not protective to the neonatal rat brain. Pediatr Res 32:489-493, 1992.

Shevell MI, Silver K, O'Gorman AM, et al: Neonatal dural sinus thrombosis. Pediatr Neurol 5:161-165, 1989.

Silverstein FS, Buchanan K, Hudson C, et al: Flunarizine limits hypoxia-ischemia induced morphologic injury in immature rat brain. Stroke 17:477-482, 1986.

Simons SH, van Dijk M, van Lingen RA, et al: Routine morphine infusion in preterm newborns who received ventilatory support. JAMA 290:2419-2427, 2003.

Sirimanne ES, Blumberg RM, Bossano D, et al: The effect of prolonged modification of cerebral temperature on outcome after hypoxic-ischemic brain injury in the infant rat. Pediatr Res 39:591-597, 1996.

Sizonenko SV, Sirimanne ES, Williams CE, et al: Neuroprotective effects of the N-terminal tripeptide of IGF-1, glycine-proline-glutamate, in the immature rat brain after hypoxic-ischemic injury. Brain Res 922:42-50, 2001.

Smith LM, Qureshi N, Chao CR: Effects of single and multiple courses of antenatal glucocorticoids in preterm newborns less than 30 weeks' gestation. J Matern Fetal Med 9:131-135, 2000.

Sola A, Spitzer AR, Morin FC, 3rd, et al: Effects of arterial carbon dioxide tension on the newborn lamb's cardiovascular responses to rapid hemorrhage. Pediatr Res 17:70-76, 1983.

Soll RF, Dargaville P: Surfactant for meconium aspiration syndrome in full term infants. Cochrane Database Syst Rev 2, 2000.

Speer ME, Blifeld C, Rudolph AJ, et al: Intraventricular hemorrhage and vitamin E in the very low-birth-weight infant: Evidence for efficacy of early intramuscular vitamin E administration. Pediatrics 74:1107-1112, 1984.

Stanton PK, Moskal JR: Diphenylhydantoin protects against hypoxia-induced impairment of hippocampal synaptic transmission. Brain Res 546:351-354, 1991.

Sternau LL, Lust WD, Ricci AJ, et al: Role for gamma-aminobutyric acid in selective vulnerability in gerbils. Stroke 20:281-287, 1989.

Takahashi M, Billups B, Rossi D, et al: The role of glutamate transporters in glutamate homeostasis in the brain. J Exp Biol 200:401-409, 1997.

Taylor MJ, McCulloch DL: Visual evoked potentials in infants and children. J Clin Neurophysiol 9:357-372, 1992.

Thoresen M, Bagenholm R, Loberg EM, et al: Posthypoxic cooling of neonatal rats provides protection against brain injury. Arch Dis Child Fetal Neonatal Ed 74:F3-9, 1996.

Thoresen M, Penrice J, Lorek A, et al: Mild hypothermia after severe transient hypoxia-ischemia ameliorates delayed cerebral energy failure in the newborn piglet. Pediatr Res 37:667-670, 1995.

Thornberg E, Thiringer K, Odeback A, et al: Birth asphyxia: Incidence, clinical course and outcome in a Swedish population. Acta Paediatr 84:927-932, 1995.

Toet MC, Hellstrom-Westas L, Groenendaal F, et al: Amplitude integrated EEG 3 and 6 hours after birth in full term neonates with hypoxic-ischaemic encephalopathy. Arch Dis Child Fetal Neonatal Ed 81:F19-23, 1999.

Trauner DA, Chase C, Walker P, et al: Neurologic profiles of infants and children after perinatal stroke. Pediatr Neurol 9:383-386, 1993.

Trifiletti RR: Neuroprotective effects of NG-nitro-L-arginine in focal stroke in the 7-day-old rat. Eur J Pharmacol 218:197-198, 1992.

Van Bel F, Shadid M, Moison RM, et al: Effect of allopurinol on postasphyxial free radical formation, cerebral hemodynamics, and electrical brain activity. Pediatrics 101:185-193, 1998.

van Wezel-Meijler G, van der Knaap MS, Sie LT, et al: Magnetic resonance imaging of the brain in premature infants during the neonatal period: Normal phenomena and reflection of mild ultrasound abnormalities. Neuropediatrics 29:89-96, 1998.

Vannucci RC, Towfighi J, Heitjan DF, et al: Carbon dioxide protects the perinatal brain from hypoxic-ischemic damage: An experimental study in the immature rat. Pediatrics 95:868-874, 1995.

Vannucci RC, Vannucci SJ: Glucose metabolism in the developing brain. Semin Perinatol 24:107-115, 2000.

Vartanian MG, Cordon JJ, Kupina NC, et al: Phenytoin pretreatment prevents hypoxic-ischemic brain damage in neonatal rats. Brain Res Dev Brain Res 95:169-175, 1996.

Veen S, de HMJJ, Martens SE, et al: Allopurinol (ALLO) treatment following severe asphyxia: Follow-up at 2 years of age. Pediatr Res 45:230A, 1999.

Vigneron DB, Barkovich AJ, Noworolski SM, et al: Three-dimensional proton MR spectroscopic imaging of premature and term neonates. AJNR Am J Neuroradiol 22:1424-1433, 2001.

Vohr B, Allan WC, Scott DT, et al: Early-onset intraventricular hemorrhage in preterm neonates: Incidence of neurodevelopmental handicap. Semin Perinatol 23:212-217, 1999.

Vohr B, Garcia Coll C, Flanagan P, et al: Effects of intraventricular hemorrhage and socioeconomic status on perceptual, cognitive, and neurologic status of low birth weight infants at 5 years of age. J Pediatr 121:280-285, 1992.

Vohr BR, Wright LL, Dusick AM, et al: Neurodevelopmental and functional outcomes of extremely low birth weight infants in the National Institute of Child Health and Human Development Neonatal Research Network, 1993-1994. Pediatrics 105:1216-1226, 2000.

Volpe JJ: Brain injury in the premature infant—from pathogenesis to prevention. Brain Dev 19:519-534, 1997.

Volpe JJ: Neurobiology of periventricular leukomalacia in the premature infant. Pediatr Res 50:553-562, 2001a.

Volpe JJ: Neurology of the Newborn (4th ed). Philadelphia, WB Saunders, 2001b.

Westin B, Miller JA, Jr., Nyberg R, et al: Neonatal asphyxia pallida treated with hypothermia alone or with hypothermia and transfusion of oxygenated blood. Surgery 45:868, 1959.

White BC, Sullivan JM, DeGracia DJ, et al: Brain ischemia and reperfusion: Molecular mechanisms of neuronal injury. J Neurol Sci 179:1-33, 2000.

Whitelaw A: Intraventricular haemorrhage and posthaemorrhagic hydrocephalus: Pathogenesis, prevention and future interventions. Semin Neonatol 6:135-146, 2001.

Wood NS, Marlow N, Costeloe K, et al: Neurologic and developmental disability after extremely preterm birth. EPICure Study Group. N Engl J Med 343:378-384, 2000.

Wu YW, Hamrick SE, Miller SP, et al: Intraventricular hemorrhage in term neonates caused by sinovenous thrombosis. Ann Neurol 54:123-126, 2003.

Yager JY, Shuaib A, Thornhill J: The effect of age on susceptibility to brain damage in a model of global hemispheric hypoxia-ischemia. Brain Res Dev Brain Res 93:143-154, 1996.

CHAPTER

# 65

# Neonatal Neuromuscular Disorders

Harvey B. Sarnat and Laura Flores-Sarnat

Many primary myopathies and neuropathies are already expressed in the neonatal period, whereas others, even if not yet clinically evident, may be diagnosed by proper testing if suspected because of an affected sibling or other family history of genetic disease. It is not necessary to defer investigations to an older age when the disease becomes more obvious clinically, if early diagnosis is desired for prognosis, management, and genetic counseling.

## ONTOGENY OF STRIATED MUSCLE

Interpretation of the neonatal muscle biopsy and of the clinical presentation of myopathies, in both preterm and term neonates, requires an understanding of the embryonic and fetal development of muscle. These features are detailed elsewhere (Sarnat, 1998) but are here briefly summarized.

All skeletal muscles of the extremities develop from two sources: The myocytes themselves are derived from the segmental myotomes, whereas all other tissues of the muscle—the connective tissue, blood vessel walls, nerve sheaths, tendons, and fascia—are derived from the superficial of the two sheets of lateral mesoderm. The medial mesoderm is the somites that contain the myotomes and dermatomes; the intermediate mesoderm gives rise to the kidneys; the deeper sheet of lateral mesoderm becomes the omenta and peritoneum.

*Myoblasts* differ from undifferentiated mesenchymal cells by their formation of filaments of actin and myosin, a process that begins at 5 to 8 weeks of gestation. The *myotubular stage* of muscle development in the human encompasses weeks 8 to 15 of gestation. Myotubes are formed by the fusion of myoblasts and by the organization of their interdigitating filaments to form parallel arrays in bundles (myofibrils) and periodic Z-bands and M-bands that create the repeating sarcomeres of mature muscle. Myotubes still differ from mature muscle in other ways. The nuclei and mitochondria are concentrated in rows in the centers of the fiber, surrounded by the "tube" of myofibrils. Myotubes also have many ribosomes, unlike more mature muscle, which has few.

Between 15 and 20 weeks of gestation, the central nuclei of myotubes "migrate" to the peripheral, subsarcolemmal position of mature muscle. The mitochondria become redistributed from the central core between nuclei to the intermyofibrillar sarcoplasm throughout the myofiber and to the subsarcolemmal region. A regression of vimentin intermediate filaments allows this cytoarchitectural reorganization by no longer holding the nuclei and mitochondria in the central core of the myofiber (Sarnat, 1990). The period of 20 to 28 weeks of gestation is the histochemical stage of development, when myofibers differentiate their slow- or fast-twitch characteristics that correspond in histochemical stains of the muscle biopsy to type I or type II fibers. Early in this period, nearly all fibers closely resemble type II. By 24 weeks, about 10% of the fibers are larger than the rest; these fibers are uniformly scattered without grouping and stain as type I fibers. Subsequently, more small type II fibers become converted to type I until the ratio is about equal in most muscles by 28 weeks. The population of type II fibers also grows in size so that the two types are no longer distinguished by size. The differentiation of fiber types depends on innervation and not independent genetic programming.

At 30 weeks, the transverse tubules and terminal cisternae of the sarcoplasmic reticulum (triads) change their orientation from parallel to perpendicular to the long axis of the myofiber. The alignment of Z-bands of adjacent myofibrils also is a late development, at about 30 weeks. The mean myofibril diameter in full-term neonatal muscle is 15 μm; the adult diameter of 65 μm is not achieved until about 13 years of age.

The sarcolemmal and basement and nuclear membrane proteins of striated muscle fibers, including those defective in various muscular dystrophies, are demonstrated at 9 to 11 weeks of gestation. During this same period, innervation of the muscle from axons of motor neurons takes place. Initially, myofibers are innervated by several axons, but later, only one persists in the center of the fiber, and all others retract. The postsynaptic membrane of the neuromuscular junction continues to acquire more complexity of folding and specialization of the membrane throughout gestation and in the postnatal period.

The most important intermediate-filament proteins of muscle during development are vimentin and desmin. They are in highest concentration in myotubes and then diminish until vimentin disappears completely by 36 weeks of gestation, whereas desmin persists in very low concentration even in adult muscle. Desmin forms links between the Z-bands of adjacent myofibrils so that they are aligned. One or both of these intermediate-filament proteins retain high fetal concentrations after birth in several congenital myopathies.

Four principal genes are essential to myodifferentiation, each having a basic helix-loop-helix transcription factor. The earliest-expressed gene to signal myoblast differentiation is *myoblast factor 5* (*MYF5*), on chromosome 12; *myogenin*, on chromosome 1, promotes the fusion of myoblasts to form myotubes; herculin (*MRF4/6*), essential for myotube conversion to myofibers, is on chromosome 12; *MyoD1* is so potent a gene of myoblast differentiation that, in cell culture, it can cause the transformation of partially differentiated nonmuscular cells of mesodermal lineage, such as fibroblasts and chondroblasts, into muscle. It is localized on chromosome 11, very near to the domain for rhabdomyosarcoma. *Pax-3* is redundant with *MYF5* and, in the absence of *MYF5*, can activate *MyoD1*. Upregulation of *Pax-3* results in precocious differentiation of muscle. Another gene, called *myostatin*, is expressed after the myogenic genes and functions as a negative regulator of muscle differentiation, by inhibiting the shift from proliferation to differentiation of myoblasts, but does not affect mitosis or cause apoptotic cell death.

Regenerating muscle recapitulates the stages of embryonic and fetal myogenesis.

## ONTOGENY OF PERIPHERAL NERVE

The embryology of peripheral nerve begins with the migration of the neural crest cells, which include precursors of Schwann cells, and lateral mesodermal components that contribute connective tissue portions of the nerve in preparation for the arrival of the growing axon of motor neurons or dendrite of sensory neurons. The ontogeny of nerve in the fetal period was demonstrated and reviewed by Hasan and associates (1993) and Teixeira and colleagues (1999). Immature unmyelinated axons and early myelinating axons contain more microtubules than neurofilaments, but this ratio becomes reversed with maturation so that neurofilaments predominate in mature axons. Cross-linkages between neurofilaments begin to form before midgestation and progressively increase with phosphorylation throughout the remainder of fetal life. Growth in axonal diameter, as well as in length, continues in the postnatal period.

Initially, all axons of peripheral nerve are unmyelinated and variable in diameter, and as many as 25 may be enclosed by a single Schwann cell. The mean axonal diameter increases in inverse relation to the decreasing ratio of axons per Schwann cell as the nerve matures. Myelination occurs only in Schwann cells that enclose a single axon, although occasionally two axons may be myelinated by one Schwann cell. Axonal diameter is inversely related to the number of axons per Schwann cell. Myelin sheaths initially are thin, and the number of whorls of Schwann cell cytoplasm increases. Nodes of Ranvier (gaps between myelin formed by adjacent Schwann cells that are important for saltatory conduction of depolarization or action potentials) and Schmidt-Lanterman clefts (normal discontinuities in the myelin) are formed from the onset of myelination. The number of myelinated axons increases, and the emergence of two distinct populations of large and small myelinated axons is a relatively late event, this bimodal distribution occurring at about 37 to 38 weeks of gestation. Fibers that persist as unmyelinated axons at maturity also decrease in their ratio to enclosing Schwann cells, so that at birth no more than four unmyelinated axons per Schwann cell are found, as in the adult.

As with muscle, the development of nerve is highly genetically programmed, and several genes are recognized that are essential to normal development. *Desert hedgehog* (*DHH*) is key to the differentiation of Schwann cells. *EGR2* (human homologue of *Krox-20* in the mouse) is necessary for the maintenance of myelin, but *peripheral myelin protein-22* (*PMP22*) is the regulator of the initiation of myelin, and *myelin protein zero* (*MPZ*) is the major determinant of myelin structure including periodicity of the concentric whorls. *EGR3* is needed for the maintenance of axoplasm. *PMP22* and *PMZ* are mutated in most of the hereditary sensory-motor neuropathies, whereas *EGR2* is deficient in at least one form of congenital insensitivity to pain.

## MUSCULAR DYSTROPHIES

The *muscular dystrophies* are a group of unrelated diseases that may be defined and distinguished from all other neuromuscular diseases by four obligatory criteria: (1) primary myopathy, (2) genetic determination, (3) progressive course, and (4) degeneration of myofibers noted at some stage in the disease, although not always demonstrated in the neonatal muscle biopsy. Several distinct diseases are known, and the molecular genetic basis, as well as the pattern of inheritance, is now known for a majority of them. Table 65–1 summarizes the genetic data for the most frequent disorders that may present in the neonatal period.

### Duchenne Muscular Dystrophy

Duchenne muscular dystrophy is inherited as an X-linked recessive trait and is the most frequent muscular dystrophy, with an incidence of 1:3000 liveborn male infants, affecting all racial and ethnic groups throughout the world. The defective gene at the Xp21.2 locus is the largest known gene, and it programs a sarcolemmal protein known as *dystrophin*. Clinical myopathic features often are not yet expressed at birth, but some infants may already show generalized weakness and hypotonia. Calf pseudohypertrophy is not yet present in neonates. Cardiomyopathy is rare in early infancy but common at older ages. The serum creatine kinase (CK) level is always extremely elevated in Duchenne dystrophy at all ages. Therefore, if the diagnosis is suspected in an asymptomatic male infant because of an affected brother or male maternal cousin, determination of the serum CK (after 5 days of age to allow for the transient rise due to birth trauma) may be performed as a screening test; in affected infants, serum CK is already in the range of several thousand IU/L. The diagnosis is confirmed by polymerase chain reaction (PCR) genetic blood testing, but false-negative results are obtained in one third of boys with Duchenne muscular dystrophy. In those cases, the muscle biopsy is definitively diagnostic, even in presymptomatic stages in the neonatal period. The dystrophin abnormality may be demonstrated in myofibers by immunocytochemical studies or immunofluorescence of biopsy tissue, and different portions of the protein may be studied individually (C-terminus, N-terminus, and rod domain). Fetal muscle biopsy before midgestation was briefly advocated, shortly before the genetic defect was demonstrated (Kuller et al, 1992), but prenatal diagnosis using chorionic villi is now available, so that fetal muscle biopsy in this disease is now of historical interest only.

Male infants with Becker muscular dystrophy are not symptomatic in the neonatal period and have normal findings on neuromuscular examination, but if the diagnosis is suspected because of a previously affected brother, it may be confirmed by high serum CK after 5 days of age, by the PCR marker in blood, or by neonatal muscle biopsy showing defective dystrophin in myofibers.

**TABLE 65–1**

**Genetic Myopathies Symptomatic in the Newborn**

| Disease | Transmission | Locus | Gene | Transcription Product |
|---|---|---|---|---|
| **Muscular Dystrophies** | | | | |
| Muscle-eye-brain | AR | 1p3 | *MEB* | OMGnT |
| Duchenne (neonatal) | XR | Xp21.2 | (Dystrophin) | Dystrophin |
| Facioscapulohumeral | AD | 4q35 | *FSHD* | |
| Myotonic, neonatal form | AD (M) | 19q13 | *DMPK* | Myotonin protein kinase |
| **Congenital Myopathies** | | | | |
| Congenital fiber-type disproportion | AR, sporadic | ? | ? | None known |
| Nemaline rod | AD | 1q21-q23 | *NEM1* (*TPM3*) | α-Tropomyosin |
| | AR | 2q21.2-q22 | *NEM2* | Nebulin |
| | AD, AR | 1q42.1 | *NEM3* (*ACTA1*) | α-Actin |
| | AD | 9p13 | *NEM4* (*TPM2*) | Tropomyosin |
| | AR | 19q13 | *NEM5* (*TNNT1*) | Troponin-T |
| Infantile myofibrillar | AR, AD | ? | ? | ? |
| X-linked myotubular | XR | Xq28 | *MTMX* | Myotubularin |
| Central core | AD | 19q13.1 | *RYR1* | Ryanodine receptor |
| Myotonia congenita: Thomsen disease, Becker disease | AD, AR | 7q35 | *CLC1* | Muscle chloride channel protein |
| **Glycogenoses with Myopathy** | | | | |
| Glycogen storage disease type II (Pompe disease) | AR | 17q23 | *GAA* | α-Glucosidase (acid maltase) |
| Glycogen storage disease type V (McArdle disease, neonatal form) | AR | 11q13 | *PYGM* | Myophosphorylase |
| **Spinal Muscular Atrophy** (motor neuron disease, not a myopathy) | | | | |
| Type 1: Werdnig-Hoffmann | AR | 5q11-q13 | *SMN/NAIP* | Neuronal apoptosis inhibitory protein |

AD, autosomal dominant; AR, autosomal recessive; M, maternal; XR, X-linked recessive.

## Emery-Dreifuss Muscular Dystrophy

Emery-Dreifuss muscular dystrophy is not usually symptomatic in the neonatal period, but the severe cardiomyopathy and cardiac conduction defects sometimes appear surprisingly early in infancy or even in the first days of life, before the generalized myopathy is evident. The X-linked recessive form of this disease is due to a defective protein called *emerin*. An autosomal dominant form of the disease is due to another defective protein, *lamin*, of which three varieties have been distinguished. Both emerin and lamin are proteins of the nuclear, rather than the sarcolemmal, membrane, and both may be demonstrated by immunocytochemical studies on muscle biopsy tissue.

## Congenital Muscular Dystrophy

*Congenital muscular dystrophy* refers to a group of disorders that usually manifest in the neonatal period with variable congenital contractures, generalized hypotonia and weakness, often facial weakness, and sometimes dysphagia and respiratory insufficiency. The muscle biopsy specimen is characteristic and shows extensive endomysial connective tissue proliferation but only minimal cytoarchitectural changes in myofibers or fiber necrosis. *Merosin* (the α2 chain of laminin that connects the sarcolemma to the basal lamina or basement membrane) is not expressed on immunocytochemistry studies in half of the cases, and electron microscopy demonstrates absence of the basal lamina, but there is little clinical correlation of the severity of the myopathy with the presence or absence of merosin. Many cases of congenital muscular dystrophy are associated with cerebral malformations, usually pachygyria, and imaging of the brain is indicated if this diagnosis is established from the muscle biopsy. Some genetic diseases that regularly include congenital muscular dystrophy and cerebral dysgenesis are Fukuyama muscular dystrophy (the second most common muscular dystrophy in Japan after Duchenne dystrophy, but rare in other populations), Walker-Warburg syndrome of type 2 lissencephaly, and muscle-eye-brain disease of Santavuori (Fukuyama et al, 1997; Muntoni, 2002).

### Myotonic Muscular Dystrophy, Neonatal Form

The neonatal form of myotonic muscular dystrophy differs from the adult form both clinically and pathologically. Findings in the neonatal period include generalized weakness, hypotonia, often contractures ranging from clubfoot to more extensive arthrogryposis involving the cervical spine, characteristic facial weakness associated with a high-arched palate, inverted V–shaped upper lip, dolichocephaly, dysphagia, and respiratory insufficiency (Sarnat et al, 1976). Myotonia is not expressed in neonates. Smooth muscle also is involved, and affected infants have poor peristalsis, inability to expel meconium or later stool, and often abdominal distention due to gas in the stomach and intestines that impinges on the diaphragm from below, further compromising respiratory effort. Congenital cataracts are found in a minority. Cardiac conduction defects may occur. On pathologic examination, the muscle shows either congenital muscle fiber-type disproportion (Agrov et al, 1980) or arrest of maturation in various stages of development, with myoblasts, myotubes, histochemically undifferentiated myofibers and mature neonatal myofibers all mixed in the same fascicles (Iannaccone et al, 1986; Sahgel et al, 1983; Sarnat and Silbert, 1976). Immature features are confirmed ultrastructurally. Muscle spindles also are abnormal in myotonic dystrophy, unlike in most other myopathies.

Although myotonic dystrophy is an autosomal dominant trait, the mother is the transmitting parent in 94% of cases (Harper, 1992). The reason for the maternal predominance is not due to hormonal factors but is genetic. The triplet expansion (CTG codon) of the myotonic dystrophy gene that encodes a serine-threonine kinase (*DMPK*) on chromosome 19q13 is many times greater in affected neonates than in the usual childhood or adult presentation of the disease, sometimes with as many as 2000 repeats (normal allele shows 5 to 37 repeats, with the usual adult form of myotonic dystrophy typically showing 50 to 500 repeats) (Hofman-Padvanyi et al, 1993). The female locus is more unstable than the male locus—hence the predominance of maternal transmission (Mulley et al, 1993). There is no gender predominance among affected neonates, however. The genetic anticipation phenomenon may be seen in myotonic dystrophy (Harper, 1992).

In pregnancy, myotonic mothers often show worsening of their disease and have a high rate of fetal loss or premature birth. Prolonged labor is not frequent, but contractions may be ineffective, and intrapartum asphyxia of the fetus is an additional risk (Sarnat et al, 1976).

In suspected neonatal myotonic dystrophy, the investigation should begin with examination of the mother and then proceed in the infant to include assay for the molecular genetic marker in blood, electrocardiography (ECG), slit-lamp examination of the lens of the eye, and muscle biopsy if the blood marker assay is inconclusive. Electromyography (EMG) is of very limited value. Serum CK is normal or only mildly elevated.

### Facioscapulohumeral Muscular Dystrophy

Facioscapulohumeral muscular dystrophy is inherited as an autosomal dominant trait. The disease usually becomes symptomatic in childhood or adolescence but shows a propensity for the genetic phenomenon of *anticipation*, and neonates may sometimes be symptomatic or even severely affected. Facial muscles and sometimes extraocular muscles are affected. The atrophy or hypoplasia of the orbicularis oris muscle gives the mouth an unusual shape, with protruding and turned-out lips exposing mucosal surfaces; this is unlike the inverted V–shaped mouth of neonatal myotonic dystrophy and nemaline rod disease. Shoulder girdle and parascapular muscles are thin and weak. Dysphagia may be a feature. Assay for a molecular marker in blood to demonstrate the defective *FSHD* gene at the 4q35 locus is available. Findings on neonatal EMG are nonspecifically myopathic, and the muscle biopsy shows endomysial connective tissue proliferation, hypertrophic type II fibers as well as atrophic fibers of both types, little or no myofiber necrosis, and, in many cases, lymphocytic infiltrates in perivascular and interstitial spaces that may be confused with an inflammatory autoimmune myopathy. Steroid treatment is ineffective, despite the presence of lymphocytic "inflammation."

### Limb-Girdle Muscular Dystrophies

Limb-girdle muscular dystrophies, a mixed group of diseases with a variety of genetic defects often due to sarcoglycanopathies, dysferlinopathies, or caveolin-3 deficiency, rarely produce clinical manifestations in infancy and are not evident in the neonatal period.

## CONGENITAL MYOPATHIES

*Congenital myopathy* is a generic term that refers to any of a group of mainly nonprogressive, non-necrotizing myopathies, most of which are genetically determined and others of which are sporadic. Most are characterized by structural alterations in myofibers, such as rod-like inclusions or internal sarcolemmal nuclei; additional findings include abnormalities in relative growth, differentiation, and ratio of fiber types within the muscle. The diagnosis is usually established by muscle biopsy. More genetic markers in blood are becoming available for some, however, and clinical features including phenotype may be suggestive of a diagnosis, to justify muscle biopsy. Congenital myopathies may be thought of as "developmental disorders" of striated muscle.

*Amyoplasia*, a term that technically denotes absence of muscle, is sometimes misused in reference to disappearance of muscle as a result of chronic neurogenic atrophy, as in severe spinal muscular atrophy (SMA) or the *Pena-Shokeir syndrome* with motor neuron involvement, but this usage is incorrect. The lack of differentiation of muscle does occur on a genetically programmed basis and may be divided into *segmental amyoplasia*, *generalized amyoplasia*, and *focal amyoplasia* of specific muscles.

The prototype of segmental amyoplasia is sacral agenesis, which most often occurs in infants of diabetic mothers. Not only do the bony and cartilaginous elements of the lower spine (sacrum and often lumbar and even lower thoracic vertebrae) fail to form, but the associated somites including the myotomes are incomplete or totally aplastic, resulting in absence of muscle formation in those segments, particularly muscles of the lower legs innervated by sacral roots. The spinal cord also is severely dysplastic at the sacral levels due to failure of induction by the defective or absent notochord, so that the *Sonic hedgehog* gene needed for motor neuron differentiation is not expressed. Despite the absence of myofibers in muscles such as the peroneus longus, gastrocnemius, and soleus, the connective tissue components and blood vessels, which are derived from lateral mesoderm, are present, and adipose tissue replaces the myofibers (Sarnat, 1992).

The selective agenesis of individual muscles may also be classified under the rubric of segmental amyoplasia, but these abnormalities are not field effects as with sacral agenesis. An example is the absence of the pectoralis major in the Poland anomalad. Another example is the isolated agenesis of the depressor angularis oris muscle on one side only, which gives the neonate an asymmetrical mouth when crying and may be confused with facial nerve palsy. Yet another example, of no clinical importance, is the congenital absence of the flexor palmaris longus muscle of the forearm, which is absent in one third of all normal persons; in this case, other flexors of the wrist easily compensate for the lack of function.

Generalized amyoplasia, which involves the diaphragm and other muscles of respiration and of deglutition as well as those of the spine and extremities, is incompatible with life and usually results in sponaneous fetal death at the end of the first trimester of gestation. The cause is probably a deletion of or mutation in one of the essential myogenic genes (see earlier), although this hypothesis is not yet proved. *Pax-3* and *Myf-5* are redundant together; in the chick and rat, mutations in *Pax-3* with lack of expression result in severe amyoplasia, whereas underexpression of *Myf-5* results only in hypoplasia with some muscular development. At autopsy, the affected human fetus with generalized amyoplasia shows arthrogryposis and only rudimentary striated muscle formation throughout the body, although cardiac and smooth muscles are developed. The *fetal akinesia sequence* may be a form of generalized amyoplasia.

## Congenital Muscle Fiber-Type Disproportion

Congenital muscle fiber-type disproportion (CMFTD) is both an isolated congenital myopathy and also a syndrome associated with a variety of unrelated other congenital myopathies, with systemic metabolic diseases, or with central nervous system (CNS) malformations. CMTFD is a muscle biopsy diagnosis that refers to disproportion in (1) the ratio and (2) the size of the two principal histochemical types of myofibers. Type I fibers are uniformly smaller than type II fibers and more numerous, with a predominance of 80% or more (Brooke, 1973; Iannaccone et al, 1983; Sarnat, 1994). Degenerative changes are rare, but some cases show myofibrillar lysis (Barth et al, 1998).

When CMFTD occurs as an *isolated congenital myopathy*, affected patients already have a characteristic phenotype at birth, and the muscle biopsy also is diagnostic in the neonatal period. The appearance of these infants is nearly identical to those with nemaline rod disease and also resembles the neonatal form of myotonic dystrophy. Craniofacial anomalies include a dolichocephalic head shape, high-arched palate, and facial weakness (Baccetti et al, 1997); generalized hypotonia, weakness, and thin muscle bulk in the trunk and extremities are other features. Congenital contractures such as clubfoot occur in a few patients, and some have congenital subluxation of the hip, but most do not have contractures, and arthrogryposis multiplex congenita is rare. Affected infants may have dysphagia and require feeding by gavage. Mild ptosis is sometimes seen, but extraocular movements usually are not impaired, although a few infants with ophthalmoplegia have been reported (Owen et al, 1981). Cardiac involvement or anomalies are found in a minority of cases (Barth et al, 1998). Respiratory failure is exceptional (Mizuno and Komiya, 1990). Severe insulin-resistant diabetes mellitus occurs rarely (Vestergaard et al,1995).

Both genders are affected equally; presence of the disorder in siblings (Barth et al, 1998; Eisler and Wilson 1978; Fardeau et al, 1975; Gerdes et al, 1994; Jaffe et al, 1988; Marolda, 1992) and identical twins (Curless and Nelson 1977) suggests an autosomal recessive inheritance, but other affected families appear to have an autosomal dominant trait (Kim et al, 2000). No defective genes are yet demonstrated; thus, no genetic markers in blood are available, although a chromosomal translocation was discovered in one family (Gerdes et al, 1994). The serum CK is normal, and the EMG and nerve conduction velocity (NCV) studies also show no specific alterations. The clinical course is that of a nonprogressive congenital myopathy, with persistent hypotonia, weakness, and developmental delay for gross motor skills in particular.

CMFTD also occurs in the context of other congenital neuromuscular diseases that also are evident in the neonate. *Nemaline rod myopathy*, both the autosomal dominant and recessive forms, shows CMFTD as an associated finding in the muscle biopsy (see later). In globoid cell leukodystrophy (Krabbe disease, severe infantile form), CMFTD is seen in muscle biopsy tissue earlier than the neurogenic atrophy of progressive neuropathy is expressed (Dehkharghani et al, 1978; Marjanoic et al, 1996; Martin et al, 1976). CMFTD also is a feature of some cases of the severe neonatal form of myotonic muscular dystrophy (see earlier). It is reported rarely in infants with Emery-Dreifuss muscular dystrophy, but whether it appears in neonates with this myopathy is unknown. CMFTD is a feature of the *rigid spine syndrome* (Goebel et al, 1977; Seay et al, 1977), associated with a mutation of the *SEPN1* gene at 1p3 (Muntoni, 2002); this disorder may also involve interneurons in the ventral horns of the spinal cord.

CMFTD occurs inconstantly, in the neonatal period, in many systemic metabolic diseases including glycogenosis II (Pompe disease), III (Cori-Forbes disease), and X (phosphorylase-B kinase deficiency); multiple sulfatase deficiency; phosphoglyceromutase deficiency; mitochondrial cytopathies; and congenital hypothyroidism. It also is found in some cases of fetal alcohol syndrome (Martin et al, 1976) and in oculocerebrorenal disease of Lowe (Kohyama et al, 1989). In these disorders, CMFTD often is incomplete and does not involve all fascicles, or the type I predominance is not as massive as in the pure congenital myopathy.

CMFTD also is found in some infants with diffuse hypotonia due to cerebellar hypoplasia or other posterior fossa malformations, as a suprasegmental effect on the motor neurons during fetal life (Nakagawa et al, 1996; Sarnat, 1985, 1986). A magnetic resonance imaging (MRI) study of the brain should be considered in the clinical investigation of CMFTD.

If the diagnosis of CMFTD is made on the basis of neonatal muscle biopsy findings, therefore, the clinician should not accept this as a definitive diagnosis but should recognize the need to look further for an associated condition responsible for this unique developmental pattern.

## Nemaline Rod Myopathy

The phenotype of nemaline rod myopathy is virtually identical to that described for CMFTD but is often more severe, particularly in terms of respiratory insufficiency and dysphagia. Other children with nemaline myopathy have little or no problem with respiration or swallowing in the neonatal period, but all show diffuse muscular hypotonia and weakness. Nemaline rods are seen in muscle biopsy tissue as rod-shaped structures within the myofibrils that represent excessive Z-band material and that have the same ultrastructural periodicity as that of the Z-band. The diagnosis can be established by muscle biopsy in the neonatal period (Shimomura et al, 1989). CMFTD is an integral part of the histopathologic pattern in infancy, and myofiber degeneration does not occur. Both autosomal dominant and autosomal recessive mendelian patterns are well documented, and five genes are now identified in various cases. Loci for autosomal dominant forms are at 1q21-q23 and 9p13, which both encode *α-tropomyosin* (Laing et al, 1995), and 1q42.1, which encodes *α-actin* (Nowak et al, 1999). The locus in the most frequent autosomal recessive form is 2q21.2-q22, encoding *nebulin*, a very large molecule of the Z-band of muscle (Pelin et al, 1999; Wallgren-Pettersson et al, 1995), 19q13 that encodes troponin-$T_1$ and another autosomal recessive form is at the same *α-actin* locus as that of the autosomal dominant gene encoding this protein, 1q42.1.

## X-Linked Recessive Myotubular Myopathy

Male infants with X-linked recessive myotubular myopathy exhibit severe involvement at birth, often with respiratory failure and dysphagia in addition to generalized hypotonia, weakness, and undescended testes; the condition often progresses to neonatal death (Barth et al, 1975; Sarnat, 1990, 1994). They do not, however, have the craniofacial characteristics of CMFTD, nemaline rod myopathy, and myotonic dystrophy. Cardiac involvement is exceptional but is reported. The defective gene (*MTMX*), at the Xq28 locus, produces a defective form of a protein called *myotubularin* (Laporte et al, 1997). A genetic blood test is available, and the muscle biopsy also is diagnostic. Internal nuclei, a central core location of mitochondria, and persistently high concentrations of desmin and vimentin are suggestive of fetal myotubes, but these fibers are not true arrested myotubes and show histochemical differentiation and ultrastructural features of much more mature myofibers.

## Other Centronuclear Myopathies

Some nonprogressive congenital myopathies presenting in the neonatal period, as well as some that do not become symptomatic until later, are characterized histopathologically by rows of central nuclei in myofibers resembling those of X-linked myotubular myopathy, but genetic tests prove that that are not due to a defective *MTMX* gene. The inheritance of these disorders may be autosomal recessive or autosomal dominant, or they may be sporadic. Some are associated with CMFTD, and it is uncertain whether the central nucleation of the CMFTD is the primary or most important feature; the clinical manifestations are usually more severe than in isolated CMFTD (Sarnat, 1994). These diseases are not as well understood as some of the other congenital myopathies, but in general hypotonia, developmental delay, weakness and thin muscle mass are the characteristic features, with or without facial involvement and dysphagia.

## Central Core Disease

Central core disease is a myopathy with the same genetic mutation at 19q13.1 as in malignant hyperthermia, with both autosomal dominant and autosomal recessive forms determined at this same locus. The gene encodes a tetramer "ryanodine" receptor to a calcium channel of the sarcoplasmic reticulum within the myofiber. The central cores are longitudinal columns of disorganized myofibrils in the centers of myofibers, seen in muscle biopsy tissue by both light and electron microscopy. Histochemically, these patients have a massive type I myofiber predominance, or almost no type II fibers are differentiated. Most infants are not symptomatic in the neonatal period, or the manifestations are nonspecific myopathic features of hypotonia and weakness. Some, however, have congenital contractures and dislocations of the hips and knees, kyphoscoliosis, and pes cavus. Malignant hyperthermia is precipitated by exposure to anesthetic drugs and may be prevented by pretreatment with dantrolene sodium.

A morphologically similar but unrelated disorder, *multicore* or *minicore myopathy*, manifests shortly after birth with generalized hypotonia and weakness (Panegyres and Kakulas, 1991). The diagnosis rests on muscle biopsy.

## Infantile Myofibrillar Myopathy

Infantile myofibrillar myopathy is a congenital myopathy characterized pathologically by sarcomeres of disorganized myofilaments and fragmented Z-bands within myofibrils in which other sarcomeres show normal structure. Some infants exhibit severe involvement at birth and have respiratory failure and dysphagia in addition to generalized weakness and hypotonia. Autosomal recessive transmission is suspected, but the chromosomal locus and gene are not yet identified. The diagnosis is established by muscle biopsy. Serum CK is normal, and genetic markers are not available.

## Proteus Syndrome Myopathy

The Proteus syndrome is a sporadic disorder of cellular growth involving many tissues of the body and often producing grotesque, asymmetrical malformations. The muscle in Proteus syndrome shows features of a "muscular dysgenesis" with abnormal structure of sarcomeres that do not correspond to normal anatomic boundaries, but it is not a neoplastic condition (Sarnat et al, 1993).

### Myotonia Congenita

Myotonia congenita is a nonprogressive myopathy. Both the autosomal dominant form (Thomsen disease) and the autosomal recessive form (Becker disease) of this disorder are due to a genetic (*CLC1* gene) abnormality in the same chloride channel in muscle, both at the 7q35 locus. Generalized muscular pseudohypertrophy is an important clinical characteristic and sometimes can be seen even in the neonate, although myotonia is not expressed in infancy and the weakness may be subtle. This disease is unrelated to myotonic muscular dystrophy or to Becker muscular dystrophy.

## INFLAMMATORY AND AUTOIMMUNE MYOPATHIES

Autoimmune diseases causing myositis are extremely rare at birth, in large part because of the immaturity of the immune system and lack of time for autoantibodies to develop. Inflammation in the neonatal muscle biopsy probably is a form of facioscapulohumeral muscular dystrophy, but a few cases have been reported as neonatal myositis and not genetic dystrophy.

## EXTRAMEDULLARY HEMATOPOIESIS IN MUSCLE

Extramedullary hematopoiesis may occur in the muscles of normal, as well as abnormal, neonates, similar to hematopoiesis in the liver. This is a benign, transitory, asymptomatic condition that is occasionally seen as an incidental finding in neonatal muscle biopsy specimens. It must be distinguished from inflammation and not treated with steroids.

## METABOLIC AND ENDOCRINE MYOPATHIES

Congenital hypothyroidism (cretinism) is associated with diffuse muscular hypotonia and weakness and often an enlarged tongue. In one form, *Kocher-Debré-Sémélaigne syndrome*, generalized muscular hypertrophy and weakness are seen. Muscle biopsy is not needed for diagnosis if the condition is recognized clinically, but if performed before the diagnosis is established, it shows a variety of abnormalities including, at times, CMFTD (Mastaglia et al, 1989). Myopathy also may accompany adrenocortical insufficiency in the neonate. Vitamin E (α-tocopherol) deficiency can cause myopathy, and neonates on prolonged total parenteral nutrition (TPN) suffered this complication before vitamin E was regularly added to the TPN composition. Infants with *Prader-Willi syndrome* have diffuse and severe hypotonia. They do not require muscle biopsy for diagnosis if the deletion at 15q11-q13 is confirmed by fluorescence in situ hybridization (FISH) analysis of blood, but the muscle histopathologic findings are abnormal and include excessive perimysial fat, a feature shared with infants of diabetic mothers, patients with congenital hypothyroidism, spinal muscular atrophy, and occasionally, infants on chronic parenteral nutrition.

Mitochondrial cytopathies are now recognized as an important category of systemic metabolic disease that affects striated muscle and the nervous system. The muscle biopsy specimen is an excellent source of tissue for mitochondrial study because of the large number of mitochondria and their large size in muscle. Some of the classical histopathologic features in older children and adults, such as ragged red fibers and paracrystalline inclusion-like structures in mitochondria seen by electron microscopy, are not formed in neonates, but many other abnormalities are present at birth. These include the absence of cytochrome-*c* oxidase from scattered myofibers, ultrastructural alterations in cristae, and deficiencies in respiratory chain enzymatic activities and point mutations in mitochondrial DNA. One limitation of biochemical analysis of muscle for mitochondrial studies in the newborn is the small volume of tissue that can be taken in a neonatal muscle biopsy. Nevertheless, at times it may be useful to study neonatal muscle if the diagnosis cannot be provided from markers in blood. It is useful in the diagnosis of Leigh encephalopathy, the most frequent mitochondrial cytopathy of early infancy.

## SPINAL MUSCULAR ATROPHY

Spinal muscular atrophy (SMA) is a progressive degenerative disease of spinal and brainstem motor neurons that begins in fetal life and continues postnatally. The etiology is a pathologic continuation of a process of programmed cell death that is normal in embryonic life. A surplus of motor neuroblasts and other neurons is generated from primitive neuroectoderm, but only about half survive and mature to become neurons; the excess cells have a limited life cycle and degenerate. If the process that arrests physiologic cell death fails to intervene by a certain stage, neuronal death may continue. The *survivor motor neuron* (*SMN*) gene arrests apoptosis (programmed cell death) of motor neuroblasts (Roy et al, 1995). Unlike most genes that are highly conserved in evolution, *SMN* is a unique mammalian gene not identified in other animals.

SMA is clinically divided into three forms by presentation: type 1 is *Werdnig-Hoffmann disease*, a severe disorder expressed at birth and associated with death by age 2 years in 75% of affected children; type 2 is a milder form that also may show diffuse hypotonia, weakness, and areflexia in the neonatal period or early infancy, associated with a less rapidly progressive course and longer survival into childhood; and type 3 is *Kugelberg-Welander disease*, having the slowest course and compatible with survival well into adult life and not symptomatic in infancy. The cardinal clinical features of SMA type 1 in the neonatal period are severe generalized hypotonia and weakness, a thin muscle mass, absence of tendon stretch reflexes, and involvement of the tongue, face, and jaw muscles with selective sparing of extraocular muscles and sphincters. Infants who are symptomatic at birth may have respiratory distress and are unable to feed. Congenital contractures, ranging from simple clubfoot to generalized arthrogryposis, are present in about 10% of severely involved neonates. Infants lie flaccid with little movement and are unable to overcome gravity. They lack head control. Fasciculations are a specific clinical sign of denervation of muscle. They are best observed in the tongue, where almost no subcutaneous connective tissue separates the muscular layer from the epithelium. If the intrinsic lingual muscles are contracted, such as in crying or when the tongue protrudes, fasciculations are more difficult to see than when the tongue is relaxed. The heart is not involved in SMA. Neonates and infants with SMA are alert and show normal social responses, unlike infants with encephalopathy at birth, and there are no signs of CNS disease except for motor neuron involvement.

The simplest, most definitive diagnostic test is a molecular genetic marker in blood for the *SMN* gene. The serum CK level may be normal but more commonly is mildly elevated in the hundreds. Results of motor nerve conduction studies are normal, at times an important feature distinguishing SMA from congenital peripheral neuropathies. EMG shows fibrillation potentials and other signs of denervation of muscle, but findings are often nonspecific in neonates. Muscle biopsy tissue in SMA reveals a characteristic pattern of perinatal denervation that is unlike that of mature muscle. Groups of giant type I fibers are mixed with fascicles of severely atrophic fibers of both histochemical types. Scattered immature myofibers resembling myotubes also are demonstrated. The muscle biopsy does not distinguish between type 1 and type 2 SMA. Sural nerve biopsy is not required, but often shows giant unmyelinated axons and other changes. At autopsy, mild degenerative changes are seen in sensory neurons of dorsal root ganglia and in somatosensory nuclei of the thalamus, but these alterations are not detected by clinical or electrophysiologic examination.

Molecular genetic diagnosis by DNA probes in blood samples or in muscle biopsy or chorionic villi tissues are available not only for diagnosis in suspected cases but also for prenatal diagnosis. Most cases are inherited as an autosomal recessive trait. The incidence of SMA is 10 to 15 cases in 100,000 live births; it affects all ethnic groups and is the second most common neuromuscular disease following Duchenne muscular dystrophy. The incidence of heterozygosity for autosomal recessive SMA is 1:50. The genetic locus for all three of the common forms of SMA is on chromosome 5, a deletion at the 5q11-q13 locus, indicating that they are variants of the same disease rather than different diseases. The affected gene is called *survival motor neuron* (*SMN*) and contains 8 exons that span 20 kilobases, with telomeric and centromeric exons that differ only by 5 base pairs and produce a transcript encoding 294 amino acids. Another gene, the *neuronal apoptosis inhibitory gene* (*NAIP*), is located next to the *SMN* gene, and in many cases there is an inverted duplication with two copies, telomeric and centromeric, of both genes; isolated mutations or deletions of *NAIP* do not produce clinical SMA. Infrequent families with autosomal dominant inheritance are described, and a rare X-linked recessive form is reported. Carrier testing by dosage analysis is available.

## NON–SPINAL MUSCULAR ATROPY MOTOR NEURON DISEASES

Motor neuron diseases that are not hereditary SMAs are rare in neonates. The Pena-Shokeir sequence has two forms. One is associated with arthrogryposis and a progressive motor neuron degeneration closely resembling SMA but with normal *SMN* gene expression; this disorder often can be recognized clinically by the associated pulmonary hypoplasia (Hageman et al, 1987). The Marden-Walker syndrome is another arthrogrypotic disorder involving progressive motor neuron degeneration beginning before birth, but with anomalies of several organ systems. *Pontocerebellar hypoplasias* are progressive degenerative diseases of the CNS, transmitted as autosomal recessive traits, that begin in fetal life; one form also involves motor neuron degeneration resembling an SMA, but the *SMN* gene on chromosome 5 is normal (Barth, 1993).

Involvement of motor neurons is a feature of several metabolic diseases of the nervous system, such as gangliosidosis (Tay-Sachs disease), ceroid lipofuscinosis (Batten disease), and glycogen storage disease type II (Pompe disease), but the signs of denervation may be minor or obscured by the more prominent involvement of other parts of the CNS or of muscle.

Enteroviral infections may specifically target motor neurons and include *poliovirus*, *echovirus*, and *coxsackievirus* infections; maternal infections with these viruses affect the fetus and neonate rarely. The clinical picture is that of diffuse flaccid paralysis and may include dysphagia, but symptoms of diffuse meningoencephalitis also may be present, distinguishing it from spinal muscular atrophy. Specific PCR tests and viral cultures of cerebrospinal fluid are diagnostic. West Nile virus involves motor neurons, but this infection has not been reported in neonates.

## CONGENITAL HEREDITARY NEUROPATHIES

Some hereditary motor-sensory neuropathies (HMSNs) manifest at birth. Congenital insensitivity to pain may be due to a congenital hypomyelinating neuropathy, for example. Neuropathies symptomatic at birth often have a component of autonomic dysfunction, such as with familial dysautonomia type 3 (Riley-Day syndrome, localized to 9q31). The majority of HMSNs have a known genetic basis, largely related to mutations in genes that program peripheral nerve development (see "Ontogeny of Peripheral Nerve," earlier), but the genetic relations in these diseases are complex. Molecular genetic diagnosis from blood is confirmatory in most cases, but if not, sural nerve biopsy often can determine the nature of the neuropathy. Prenatal testing also is available. Most HMSNs are not clinically symptomatic in the neonatal period.

## ARTHROGRYPOSIS MULTIPLEX CONGENITA

*Arthrogryposis multiplex congenita* is a descriptive term that implies multiple congenital contractures and is not a diagnosis. The specific etiologic disorder may vary from motor neuron diseases such as SMA to congenital myopathies and muscular dystrophies and, rarely, congenital myasthenia gravis. Arthrogyposis also may be secondary to CNS malformations, bone dysplasias, and even mechanical factors such as immobilization of the fetus in utero secondary to oligohydramnios or bicornuate uterus. A form of arthrogryposis occurs without evident neuromuscular, neurologic, or systemic disease. Simple clubfoot deformities are not arthrogryposis.

## TORTICOLLIS

Isolated contracture of the sternocleidomastoid muscle (SCM) with obligate head turning to one side may be due to a lesion of one SCM, as with a hematoma in the muscle due to traumatic birth injury or with anomalous absence of one SCM, or may be due to a lesion of the spinal accessory nerve (cranial nerve XI) to one SCM muscle. This nerve is unique in passing through the belly of the clavicular head to innervate the sternal head of the muscle (Sarnat and Morrissey, 1981). Torticollis also may be due to CNS lesions. Occasionally, it appears to simply be the functional result of an unusual position in utero; in such cases it responds well to gentle physiotherapy.

## CONGENITAL, NEONATAL, AND FAMILIAL MYASTHENIA GRAVIS

Infants born to myasthenic mothers may have respiratory insufficiency, inability to suck or swallow, and generalized hypotonia and weakness. They may show little spontaneous motor activity for several days to weeks. Some require ventilatory support and feeding by gavage during this period. After the abnormal antibodies disappear, the infants have normal strength and are not at increased risk for developing myasthenia gravis in later childhood. The syndrome of *transient neonatal myasthenia gravis* is to be distinguished from a rare, and often hereditary, *congenital myasthenia gravis* not related to maternal myasthenia that is nearly always a permanent disorder without spontaneous remission (Engel et al, 2000). Apnea and hypoventilation in sleep may be serious complications (Iannaccone et al, 2000). Three *presynaptic* congenital myasthenic syndromes are recognized, all inherited as autosomal recesssive traits, but their molecular genetic basis remains undeciphered (Walls et al, 1993). An additional *synaptic* form is caused by absence of marked deficiency of acetylcholinesterase (AChE) in the synaptic basal lamina. *Postsynaptic* forms of congenital myasthenia are due to mutations in acetylcholine receptor (AChR) subunit genes that alter the synaptic response to ACh. An abnormality of the AChR channels appearing as high conductance and excessively fast closure may be due to a point mutation in a subunit of the receptor affecting a single amino acid residue. Neonates with congenital myasthenia gravis do not experience myasthenic crises or exhibit elevations of anti-ACh antibodies in plasma.

Infantile botulism is an important consideration in the differential diagnosis if signs and symptoms suggestive of congenital myasthenia gravis manifest in early infancy (Schreiner et al, 1991). This diagnosis would be most likely if the delivery had been performed at home or under less than sterile conditions, or if the neonate had been given contaminated honey on a pacifier or in a bottle of formula.

### *Laboratory Findings and Diagnosis*

Myasthenia gravis is one of the few neuromuscular diseases in which EMG is more specifically diagnostic than a muscle biopsy. A decremental response is seen in response to repetitive nerve stimulation; the muscle potentials diminish rapidly in amplitude until the muscle becomes refractory to further stimulation. Motor NCV remains normal. This unique EMG pattern is the electrophysiologic correlate of the fatigable weakness observed clinically and is reversed after a cholinesterase inhibitor is administered. A myasthenic decrement may be absent or difficult to demonstrate in muscles that are not involved clinically. This feature may be confusing in early cases or in patients showing only weakness of extraocular muscles.

*Anti-ACh receptor antibodies* should be assayed in the plasma but are inconsistently demonstrated. About one third of adolescents show elevations, but anti-ACh receptor antibodies are only occasionally demonstrated in the plasma of prepubertal children. Other serologic markers of autoimmune disease, such as antinuclear antibodies and abnormal immune complexes, should also be sought. If assays for these markers are positive, more extensive autoimmune disease involving vasculitis or tissues other than muscle is likely. A thyroid profile should always be examined. The serum CK level is normal in myasthenia gravis. An enlarged thymus is not seen in neonates. Muscle biopsy is not indicated.

Edrophonium should not be given to young infants because cardiac arrhythmias may result. An alternative agent with fewer cardiogenic side effects is intramuscular neostigmine. If the initial test dose of 0.04 mg/kg produces negative results, the infant may be retested 4 hours later with 0.08 mg/kg. A maximal effect occurs in 20 to 40 minutes. Because of muscarinic side effects, 0.01 mg/kg of atropine may be given just before the prostigmine.

Recommendations on the use of cholinesterase inhibitors as a diagnostic test for myasthenia gravis in neonates include the following:

1. Ideally, the test should measure a specific fatigable weakness, such as ptosis of the eyelids, dysphagia, or inability of cervical muscles to support the head; in nonspecific generalized weakness without cranial nerve motor deficits, results are more difficult to assess, but generalized weakness may be a criterion at times.
2. An intravenous infusion should be started as a rapid route for medications in the event of an adverse effect of the test medication.
3. ECG monitoring is recommended during testing.
4. Pretreatment with *atropine sulfate* to block the muscarinic effects (abdominal distention, diarrhea, profuse tracheal secretions) of the test medication may be given, although this is not essential, but this drug should be available at the bedside in a prepared syringe. If needed, it should be administered intravenously in a dose of 0.1 mg/kg.
5. *Edrophonium is not recommended for use in infants*; its effect is too brief for objective assessment, and an

increased incidence of acute cardiac arrhythmias is reported in infants, especially neonates.

6. *Prostigmine methylsulfate* (Neostigmine) is administered *intramuscularly* in a dose of 0.04 mg/kg; if the result is negative or equivocal, another dose of 0.04 mg/kg may be administered 4 hours after the first dose. The peak effect is seen in 20 to 40 minutes. Intravenous administration is not recommended because of the risk of arrhythmia.

## INVESTIGATION OF NEUROMUSCULAR DISEASES IN THE NEONATE

Investigation of myopathies and neuropathies in the neonatal period is generally as reliable as at older ages, although in some diseases, EMG or muscle biopsy features may not develop until the pathologic process has progressed further.

### Genetic Markers

Assays for genetic markers in blood are available for many of the muscular dystrophies, SMA, and many hereditary neuropathies and are already diagnostic at birth. A positive result may confirm a diagnosis without the need for more invasive procedures such as muscle biopsy. These tests are expensive, however, and many health insurance plans in the United States do not include them; this may be a limiting economic factor.

### Serum Creatine Kinase

Serum CK (formerly creatine phosphokinase [CPK]) is not a general screening test for neuromuscular diseases and is normal in most congenital myopathies and neuropathies and normal or only mildly elevated in SMA. It is greatly elevated to levels of several thousand IU/L even at birth in all male infants affected with Duchenne muscular dystrophy, even if they are clinically asymptomatic at this stage; thus, it is a reliable and inexpensive screen for this disease if the family history suggests an increased risk. In other muscular dystrophies, including congenital muscular dystrophy and neonatal myotonic dystrophy, the CK is normal or only mildly to moderately increased in neonates. The serum CK of normal infants is less than 160 IU/L and often is elevated to as much as five times normal soon after birth, as a result of the normal trauma of delivery with stretch and compression of muscles, and returns to normal within 5 days. An elevated CK in infants younger than 5 days of age should be interpreted with great caution, and the test should be repeated in a few days.

### Blood Studies of Metabolic Products and Endocrine Function

Blood studies of metabolic products and endocrine function may be indicated in some cases. Examples are lactate and pyruvate in mitochondrial cytopathies, thyroid-stimulating hormone and thyroxine ($T_4$) for suspected hypothyroid myopathy, and serum amino acids if a systemic metabolic disease that may also produce muscular hypotonia and weakness is suspected.

### Nerve Conduction Velocities

The conduction velocity of motor and sensory nerves, such as the peroneal, ulnar, and median nerves, is about half the velocity of adults at birth (average 24 m/sec in the term neonate versus 48 m/sec in the adult, the adult velocity being achieved at about 2 years of age). The results of NCV studies are inherently not as precise as in the adult because the distance over which the conduction is measured (e.g., ankle to hip) is very short in neonates. Nevertheless, if a neonatal polyneuropathy is suspected, this test is both feasible and confirmatory even at birth. More than 80% of the largest conducting axons must be impaired before a reduction in conduction velocity is shown electrophysiologically; thus, a normal result does not exclude neuropathy.

### Electromyography

EMG is generally not very useful in early infancy, both because of technical limitations and because of difficulty in interpretation. Some diagnostic features, such as myotonia, are not yet expressed at this age. If a myopathic or a neurogenic pattern is shown, it does not specify the type of myopathy or neuropathy and usually does not preclude the need for other tests, including the muscle biopsy, which provides the same information and much more. EMG should not be ordered routinely for all infants with suspected neuromuscular disease. Myasthenic decremental responses to repetitive nerve stimulation, as a specialized EMG technique that is not routinely done, may sometimes be demonstrated.

### Muscle Biopsy

Muscle biopsy is the most specific diagnostic test for most neuromuscular diseases, with a few exceptions such as myasthenia gravis and some endocrine myopathies. If molecular genetic analysis of blood does not provide confirmation of a suspected hereditary disease, muscle biopsy often is more specific (e.g., one third of assays for genetic PCR blood markers for Duchenne dystrophy are falsely negative, but the demonstration of deficient dystrophin in the muscle biopsy is 100% reliable). It was shown in 1978 that the muscle biopsy is as diagnostic in the neonatal period as in older children; therefore, definitive diagnosis should not be deferred (Sarnat, 1978). A quarter-century later, this is even more true, because in addition to the traditional histochemical stains used in 1978, many immunohistochemical markers for proteins of the sarcolemma region and nuclear membranes are now available to precisely diagnose the type of muscular dystrophy, as well as studies of muscle tissue to diagnose mitochondrial cytopathies that have been developed only in the past decade.

The muscle biopsy requires a highly specialized and complex pathological preparation that includes frozen sections for histochemistry, fixation for possible electron microscopy, and separate frozen tissue for biochemical analysis as needed, and also a pathologist who is experienced and skilled with interpretation of neonatal muscle biopsies and normal maturation patterns. If the tissue cannot be properly processed and interpreted at the hospital where the infant is admitted, arrangements should be made for transfer of the infant or for having the tissue properly fixed or frozen and sent to another medical center with this specialized type of laboratory.

The vastus lateralis (quadriceps femoris) muscle is generally the best muscle to biopsy because it is a proximal large muscle that shows all of the features of generalized myopathies and neuropathies and is not traversed by major blood vessels or nerves that could become damaged. The laboratory should be given advance notice to prepare to receive the specimen. The biopsy itself is a simple surgical procedure that can be done at the bedside or in an isolette with the use of local anesthesia and femoral nerve block (regional anesthesia); a general anesthetic is almost never required.

## Sural Nerve Biopsy

Sural nerve biopsy may be diagnostic of hereditary neuropathies even in the neonate, but patients should be selected carefully. As with muscle biopsy, considerable specialized tissue preparation and interpretation are required. The sural nerve is a pure sensory nerve, and biopsy specimens usually are taken from behind the lateral malleolus of the ankle, where the nerve is superficial, easy to find, and functions only to innervate a small sensory cutaneous zone on the lateral side of the foot. If the surgery is performed carefully so that internal scarring is minimal, the nerve often regenerates at this distal site. Care should be taken to not stretch or crush the nerve during biopsy, as the tissue is delicate and artifacts are more easily introduced by trauma to nerve than to muscle.

## Cardiac Evaluation

Cardiac evaluation, including ECG and echocardiography, sometimes is indicated in diseases in which cardiac muscle or conduction may be involved, such as Duchenne and myotonic muscular dystrophies, even if the infant is clinically asymptomatic for cardiovascular disease. Pediatric cardiology consultation may be useful in selected cases.

## Central Nervous System Evaluation

CNS evaluation, including imaging studies and EEG, may be indicated in some cases, particularly in congenital muscular dystrophy, which often is associated with cerebral malformations such as pachygyria, or in CMFTD that may be secondary to cerebellar hypoplasia.

## REFERENCES


Agrov Z, Gardner-Medwin D, Johnson MA, Mastaglia FL: Congenital myotonic dystrophy: Fiber type abnormalities in two cases. Arch Neurol 37:693-696, 1980.

Baccetti T, Defraia E, Donati MA: Craniofacial abnormalities associated with congenital fiber type disproportion myopathy. J Clin Ped Dent 21:167-171, 1997.

Barth PG: Pontocerebellar hypoplasias: An overview of a group of inherited neurodegenerative disorders with fetal onset. Brain Dev 15:411-422, 1993.

Barth PG, van Wijngaarden GK, Bethlem J: X-linked myotubular myopathy with fatal neonatal asphyxia. Neurology 25:531-536, 1975.

Barth PG, Wanders RJ, Ruitenbeek W, et al: Infantile fibre-type disproportion, myofibrillar lysis and cardiomyopathy: A disorder in three unrelated Dutch families. Neuromusc Disord 8:296-304, 1998.

Brett FM, Costigan D, Farrell MA, et al: Merosin-deficient congenital muscular dystrophy and cortical dysplasia. Eur J Paed Neurol 2:77-82, 1998.

Brooke MH: Congenital fiber type dysproportion. In Kakulas BA (ed): Clinical Studies in Myology. Amsterdam, Excerpta Medica, 1973, pp 147-159.

Curless RG, Nelson MB: Congenital fiber-type disproportion in identical twins. Ann Neurol 2:455-459, 1977.

Dehkharghani F, Sarnat HB, Brewster MA, Roth SI: Congenital muscle fiber type disproportion in Krabbe's leukodystrophy. Arch Neurol 38:585-587, 1981.

Eisler T, Wilson JH: Muscle fiber-type disproportion: Report of a family with symptomatic and asymptomatic members. Arch Neurol 35:823-826, 1978.

Engel AG, Olino K, Stans AA: Congenital myasthenic syndromes. In Deymeer F (ed): Neuromuscular Disorders: From Basic Mechanisms to Clinical Management. Basel, Karger, 2000. Monogr Clin Neurosci 18:96-112, 2000.

Fardeau M, Harpey JP, Caille B: [Congenital disproportion of various types of size of type I fibers. Morphological documents in the same family]. Rev Neurol (Paris) 131:745-766, 1975.

Fukuyama Y, Osawa M, Saito K: Congenital Muscular Dystrophies. Amsterdam, Elsevier, 1997.

Gerdes AM, Petersen MH, Schroder HD, et al: Congenital myopathy with fiber type disproportion: A family with a chromosomal translocation t(10:17) may indicate candidate gene regions. Clin Genet 45:11-16, 1994.

Goebel HH, Lenard HG, Görke W, Kunze K: Fibre type disproportion in the rigid spine syndrome. Neuropädiatrie 8:467-477, 1977.

Hageman G, Willemse J, van Ketel BA, et al: The heterogeneity of the Pena-Shokeir syndrome. Neuropediatrics 18:45, 1987.

Harper PS, Harley HG, Reardon W, Shaw DJ: Anticipation in myotonic dystrophy: New light on an old problem. Am J Hum Genet 51:10-16, 1992.

Hasan SU, Sarnat HB, Auer RN: Vagal nerve maturation in the fetal lamb: An ultrastructural and morphometric study. Anat Rec 237:527-537, 1993.

Hofmann-Radvanyi H, Lavedan C, Rabes JP, et al: Myotonic dystrophy: Absence of CTG enlarged transcript in congenital forms, and low expression of the normal allele. Hum Mol Genet 2:1263-1266, 1993.

Iannaccone ST, Bove KE, Vogler CA, Buchino JJ: Type I fiber size disproportion: Morphometric data from 37 children with myopathic, neuropathic, or idiopathic hypotonia. Pediatr Pathol 7:395-419, 1987.

Iannaccone ST, Bove KE, Vogler CA, et al: Muscle maturation delay in infantile myotonic dystrophy. Arch Pathol Lab Med 110:405-41, 19861.

Iannaccone ST, Mills JK, Harris KM, et al: Congenital myasthenic syndrome with sleep hypoventilation. Muscle Nerve 23:1129-1132, 2000.

Jaffe M, Shapira J, Borochowitz Z: Familial congenital fiber type disproportion (CFTD) with an autosomal recessive inheritance. Clin Genet 33:33-37, 1988.

Kim WK, Choi BO, Cheon HY, et al: Muscle fiber-type disproportion with an autosomal dominant inheritance. Yonsei Med J 41:281-284, 2000.

Kohyama J, Niimura F, Kawashima K, et al: Congenital fiber type disproportion myopathy in Lowe syndrome. Pediatr Neurol 5:373-376, 1989.

Kuller JA, Hoffman EP, Fries MH, et al: Prenatal diagnosis of Duchenne muscular dystrophy by fetal muscle biopsy. Hum Genet 90:34-40, 1992.

Laing NG, Wilton SD, Akkari FA, et al: A mutation in the α-tropomyosin gene *TPM3* associated with autosomal dominant nemaline myopathy NEM1. Nat Genet 9:75-79, 1995.

Laporte J, Guiraud-Chaumeil C, Vincent M-C, et al: Mutations in the *MTM1* gene implicated in X-linked myotubular myopathy. Hum Mol Genet 6:1505-1510, 1997.

Marjanovic B, Cvetkovic D, Dozic S, et al: Association of Krabbe leukodystrophy and congenital fiber type disproportion. Pediatr Neurol 15:79-82, 1996.

Marolda M: Congenital fiber type disproportion in two sisters: A clinical and histopathological study. Acta Neurol (Napoli) 14:398-407, 1992.

Martin JJ, Clara R, Ceutrerick C, Joris C: Is congenital fibre type disproportion a true myopathy? Acta Neurol Belg 76:335-344, 1976.

Mastaglia FL, Ojeda VJ, Sarnat HB, Kakulas BA: Myopathies associated with hypothyroidism: A review based upon 13 cases. Austr N Z J Med 53:93-101, 1989.

Mizuno Y, Komiya K: A serial muscle biopsy study in a case of congenital fiber-type disproportion associated with progressive respiratory failure. Brain Dev 12:431-436, 1990.

Mulley JC, Staples A, Donnelly A, et al: Explanation for exclusive maternal origin for congenital form of myotonic dystrophy. Lancet 341:236-237, 1993.

Muntoni F: Gene table: Congenital muscular dystrophies. Eur J Paed Neurol 6:79, 2002.

Nakagawa E, Ozawa M, Yamanouchi H, et al: Severe central nervous system involvement in a patient with congenital fiber-type disproportion myopathy. J Child Neurol 11:71-73, 1996.

Nowak KJ, Wattanasirichaigoon D, Goebel HH, et al: Mutations in the skeletal muscle α-actin gene in patients with actin myopathy and nemaline myopathy. Nat Genet 23:208-212, 1999.

Owen JS, Kline LB, Oh SJ, et al: Ophthalmoplegia and ptosis in congenital fiber type disproportion. J Pediatr Ophthal Strabis 18:55-60, 1981.

Panegyres PK, Kakulas BA: The natural history of minicore-multicore myopathy. Muscle Nerve 14:411-415, 1991.

Pelin K, Hilpela P, Donner E, et al: Mutations in the nebulin gene associated with autosomal recessive nemaline myopathy. Proc Natl Acad Sci U S A 96:2305-2310, 1999.

Roy N, Mahedevan N, McLean M, et al: The gene for neuronal apoptosis inhibitory protein is partially deleted in individuals with spinal muscular atrophy. Cell 80:167-178, 1995.

Sahgal V, Bernes S, Sahgal S, et al: Skeletal muscle in preterm patients with congenital myotonic dystrophy: Morphologic and histochemical study. J Neurol Sci 59:47-55, 1983.

Sarnat HB: Diagnostic value of the muscle biopsy in the neonatal period. Am J Dis Child 132:782-785, 1978.

Sarnat HB: Le cerveau influence-t-il le développement musculaire du foetus humain? Mise en évidence de 21 cas. Can J Neurol Sci 12:111-120, 1985.

Sarnat HB: Cerebral dysgeneses and their influence on fetal muscle development. Brain Dev 8:495-499, 1986.

Sarnat HB: Myotubular myopathy: Arrest of morphogenesis of myofibres associated with persistence of fetal vimentin and desmin: Four cases compared with fetal and neonatal muscle. Can J Neurol Sci 17:1009-1123, 1990.

Sarnat HB: Cerebral Dysgenesis. Embryology and Clinical Expression. New York, Oxford University Press, 1992, pp 92-98.

Sarnat HB: New insights into the pathogenesis of congenital myopathies. J Child Neurol 9:193-201, 1994.

Sarnat HB: Ontogenesis of striated muscle. In Polin RA, Fox WW (eds): Fetal and Neonatal Physiology, vol 2, 2nd ed. Philadelphia, WB Saunders, 1998, pp 2226-2247.

Sarnat HB, Diadori P, Trevenen CL: Myopathy of the Proteus syndrome: Hypothesis of muscular dysgenesis. Neuromusc Disord 3:293-301, 1993.

Sarnat HB Morrissy RT: Idiopathic torticollis: Sternocleidomastoid myopathy and accessory neuropathy. Muscle Nerve 4:374-380, 1981.

Sarnat HB, O'Connor T, Byrne PA: Clinical effects of myotonic dystrophy on pregnancy and the neonate: Arch Neurol 33:459-465, 1976.

Sarnat HB, Roth SI, Jiménez JF: Neonatal myotubular myopathy: Neuropathy and failure of postnatal maturation of fetal muscle. Can J Neurol Sci 8:313-320, 1981.

Sarnat HB, Silbert SW: Maturational arrest of fetal muscle in neonatal myotonic dystrophy: A pathologic study of four cases. Arch Neurol 33:466-474, 1976.

Schreiner MS, Field E, Ruddy R: Infant botulism: A review of 12 years' experience at the Children's Hospital of Philadelphia. Pediatrics 87:159, 1991.

Seay AR, Ziter FA, Petajan JH: Rigid spine syndrome: A type I fiber myopathy. Arch Neurol 34:119-122, 1977.

Shimomura C, Nonaka I: Nemaline myopathy: Comparative muscle histochemistry in the severe neonatal, moderate congenital and adult-onset forms. Pediatr Neurol 5:25-31, 1989.

Teixeira FJ, Aranda F, Becker LE: Postnatal maturation of phrenic nerve in children. Pediatr Neurol 8:450-454, 1992.

Vestergaard H, Klein HH, Hansen T, et al: Severe insulin-resistant diabetes mellitus in fiber type disproportion myopathy. J Clin Invest 95:1925-1932, 1995.

Wallgren-Pettersson C, Avela K, Marchand S, et al: A gene for autosomal recessive nemaline myopathy assigned to chromosome 2q by linkage analysis. Neuromusc Disord 5:441-443, 1995.

Walls TJ, Engel AG, Nagel AS, et al: Congenital myasthenic syndrome associated with paucity of synaptic vesicles and reduced quantal release. Ann N Y Acad Sci 681:461-468, 1993.

CHAPTER

# 66

# Neonatal Seizures

Mark S. Scher

Neonatal seizures are one of the few neonatal neurologic conditions that require immediate medical attention. Although prompt diagnostic and therapeutic interventions are needed, multiple challenges impede the physician's evaluation of the newborn with suspected seizures (Table 66–1) (Scher, 1989, 1997a, 2001b, 2002). Clinical and electroencephalographic manifestations of neonatal seizures vary dramatically from those in older children, and seizure recognition remains the foremost challenge to overcome. This dilemma is underscored by the brevity and subtlety of the clinical repertoire of the neonatal neurologic examination. Environmental restrictions in an intensive care setting—the sick infant may be confined to an isolette, intubated, and attached to multiple catheters—limit accessibility by caregivers. Medications alter arousal and muscle tone and limit the clinician's ability to detect clinical neurologic signs reflective of the underlying disease state. Brain injury from antepartum factors may precipitate neonatal seizures as part of an encephalopathic clinical picture during the intrapartum and neonatal periods (Scher, 1994), well beyond when brain injury occurred. Overlapping medical conditions from fetal through neonatal periods must be factored into the most appropriate etiologic algorithm that explains seizure expression before application of the most accurate prognosis. Medication options that effectively treat seizures remain elusive and may need to be designed and utilized on the basis of the underlying diagnosis (Scher, 2001a). This chapter presents issues regarding recognition, differential diagnosis, prognosis, and treatment of neonatal seizures, in the context of current neurobiologic and pathophysiologic explanations or causes for neonatal seizures and consequential brain injury.

## DIAGNOSTIC DILEMMAS: CLINICAL VERSUS ELECTROENCEPHALOGRAPHIC CRITERIA

Because neonatal seizures are generally brief and subtle in clinical appearance, unusual behaviors may be difficult to recognize and classify. The most common practice in many neonatal intensive care units (NICUs) is to rely on clinical behaviors to identify seizures, without confirmation by electroencephalogram (EEG). Motor or autonomic behaviors, however, may represent normal gestational age- and state-specific behaviors in healthy infants or, alternatively, nonepileptic paroxysmal conditions in encephalopathic infants. Medical personnel also vary significantly in their ability to recognize suspicious behaviors; this variability will contribute to overdiagnosis or underdiagnosis. Therefore, confirmation of suspicious clinical events as seizures using coincident electroencephalographic recordings is now strongly recommended. Using either routine electroencephalographic studies (Glauser, 1992) or continuous synchronized video-EEG-polygraphic recordings (Mizrahi and Kellaway, 1998), more reliable start and end points of electrographically confirmed seizures can be established before decisions are made regarding treatment intervention. Rigorous physiologic monitoring of non–central nervous system (CNS) measures also assists in the recognition and management of seizures.

### Clinical Seizure Criteria

The International League Against Epilepsy's classification adopted by the World Health Organization still considers neonatal seizures within an unclassified category (Commission, 1981). A more recent classification scheme suggests a stricter distinction of clinical seizure (nonepileptic) events from electrographically confirmed (epileptic) seizures with respect to possible treatment interventions (Mizrahi and Kellaway, 1998). Continued refinement using novel seizure classifications is needed to reconcile disagreements between clinical and EEG criteria, which impede a correct seizure diagnosis.

Several caveats useful in the evaluation for suspected neonatal seizures are listed in Table 66–2.

Clinical criteria for neonatal seizure diagnosis were historically subdivided into five categories: focal clonic, multifocal or migratory clonic, tonic, myoclonic, and subtle seizures (Volpe, 2001). A more recent classification expands these clinical subtypes, adopting a strict temporal occurrence of specific clinical events with coincident electrographic seizures, to distinguish neonatal clinical "nonepileptic" seizures from "epileptic" seizures (Mizrahi and Kellaway, 1998) (Table 66–3).

### Subtle Seizure Activity

Subtle seizure activity—now termed *motor automatisms* and *buccolingual movements*—is the most frequently observed category of neonatal seizures. Before a seizure evaluation is initiated, the normal occurrence of alterations in cardiorespiratory regularity, body movements, and other behaviors during active sleep (rapid eye movement [REM] sleep), quiet sleep (non-REM [NREM] sleep), or waking states should be appreciated (DaSilva et al, 1998; Scher, 1996). In any event, paroxysmal activity that interrupts the expected behavioral repertoire of the newborn infant and appears stereotypic or repetitive should heighten the clinician's level of suspicion for seizures. Repetitive buccolingual movements, orbital-ocular movements, unusual "bicycling" or "pedaling," and autonomic signs are examples of this seizure category (Fig. 66–1). Periodic alterations in heart rate, blood pressure, or oxygenation or other autonomic signs are particularly helpful clues to seizure activity during pharmacologic paralysis for ventilatory care. Autonomic expressions, however, also are intermixed with somatic findings. Isolated autonomic signs such as apnea are rarely associated with coincident electrographic

**TABLE 66-1**

**Dilemmas Regarding Neonatal Seizures**

*Diagnostic choices*—reliance on clinical vs. electroencephalographic criteria
*Etiologic explanations*—multiple prenatal/neonatal conditions with variable times of onset and duration
*Treatment decisions*—who, when, how, and for how long?
*Prognostic questions*—consider mechanisms of injury based on underlying disorder vs. intrinsic vulnerability of the immature brain to prolonged seizures

**TABLE 66-2**

**Caveats Concerning Recognition of Neonatal Seizures**

- Stereotypic behaviors occur in association with normal neonatal sleep or waking states, medication effects, and gestational maturity.
- Any abnormal repetitive activity may be a clinical seizure if out of context for expected neonatal behavior.
- Document coincident electrographic seizures with the suspected clinical event.
- Abnormal behavioral phenomena with inconsistent relationships with coincident electroencephalographic seizures suggest a subcortical seizure focus.
- Nonepileptic pathologic movement disorders are independent of the seizure state.

seizures (Fenichel et al, 1979). Synchronized video-EEG-polygraphic recordings are now preferred to document temporal relationships between clinical and electrographic events (Mizrahi and Kellaway, 1998; Scher, 1997a, 2001b). Despite the "subtle" expression of this seizure category, affected children may suffer significant brain injuries.

## Clonic Seizures

Rhythmic movements of body parts that consist of a rapid flexion phase followed by a slower extensor movement may be *clonic seizures*, to be distinguished from the symmetrical "to-and-fro" movements of nonepileptic tremulousness or jitteriness (Scher, 2001b). Gentle flexion of the affected body part easily suppresses the tremor, whereas clonic seizures persist. Clonic movements can involve face, arm, leg, or respiratory or pharyngeal muscles (Fig. 66–2A and B). Generalized clonic activities also can occur but rarely consist of the classic tonic followed by clonic phases, characteristic of the generalized motor seizure noted in older children and adults. Focal clonic and hemiclonic seizures have been described with localized brain injury, usually from cerebrovascular lesions (Clancy et al, 1985; Levy et al, 1985; Scher et al, 1986), but also can be seen with generalized or multifocal brain abnormalities. As with older patients, focal seizures in the neonate can be followed by transient motor weakness, historically referred to as a transient Todd's paresis or paralysis, characterized by a more persistent hemiparesis over days to weeks. Clonic movements without EEG-confirmed seizures have been described in neonates with normal electroencephalographic background rhythms, in whom neurodevelopmental outcome can be normal (Rose and Lombroso, 1970). The less experienced clinician may misclassify myoclonic as clonic movements.

## Multifocal (Fragmentary) Clonic Seizures

The word *fragmentary* was historically applied to distinguish multifocal clonic seizures from the more classic generalized tonic-clonic seizure seen in the older child. Multifocal or migratory clonic activities spread over body parts in either a random or an anatomically appropriate fashion. Seizure movements may alternate from side to side and appear asynchronously between the two halves of the child's body. Multifocal clonic seizures may be misclassified as myoclonic seizures, and video-EEG documentation helps with proper identification. Neonates with this seizure description often suffer death or significant neurologic morbidity (Rose and Lombroso, 1970).

## Tonic Seizures

*Tonic seizure* refers to a sustained flexion or extension of axial or appendicular muscle groups (Fig. 66–3). Tonic movements of a limb or sustained head or eye turning may also be noted. Documentation of tonic activity during coincident electroencephalographic recording is needed, because 30% of such movements lack a temporal correlation with electrographic seizures (Kellaway and Hrachovy, 1983). Such nonepileptic activity is referred to as "brainstem release" resulting from functional decortication after severe neocortical dysfunction or damage. Extensive neocortical damage or dysfunction permits the emergence of uninhibited subcortical expressions of extensor movements (Sarnat, 1984). Tonic seizures may also be misidentified when nonepileptic movement disorders consisting of dystonia are more appropriate behavioral descriptions. Both tonic movements and dystonic posturing may simultaneously occur in the same neonate.

## Myoclonic Seizures

Myoclonic movements are rapid, isolated jerks that can be generalized, multifocal, or focal in an axial or appendicular distribution. Myoclonus lacks the slow return phase of the clonic movement complex. Healthy preterm infants commonly exhibit myoclonic movements without seizures or a brain disorder. An EEG, therefore, is recommended to confirm the coincident appearance of electrographic discharges with these movements (Fig. 66–4A). Pathologic myoclonus in the absence of electrographically confirmed seizures also can occur in severely ill pre-term or full-term infants after severe brain dysfunction or damage (Scher, 1985). As with older children and adults, myoclonus may reflect injuries at multiple levels of the neuraxis, from spinal cord to brainstem to cortical regions. Stimulus-evoked myoclonus with either single coincident spike discharges or sustained electrographic seizures has been reported

TABLE 66-3

**Classification and Clinical Characteristics of Neonatal Seizures***

| Seizure Class | Characterization |
|---|---|
| Focal clonic | Repetitive, rhythmic contracts of muscle groups of the limbs, face, or trunk<br>May be unifocal or multifocal<br>May occur synchronously or asynchronously in muscle groups on one side of the body<br>May occur simultaneously but asynchronously on both sides<br>Cannot be suppressed by restraint<br>*Pathophysiology*: epileptic |
| Focal tonic | Sustained posturing of single limbs<br>Sustained asymmetrical posturing of the trunk<br>Sustained eye deviation<br>Cannot be provoked by stimulation or suppressed by restraint<br>*Pathophysiology*: epileptic |
| Generalized tonic | Sustained symmetrical posturing of limbs, trunk, and neck<br>May be flexor, extensor, or mixed extensor/flexor<br>May be provoked or intensified by stimulation<br>May be suppressed by restraint or repositioning<br>*Presumed pathophysiology*: nonepileptic |
| Myoclonic | Random, single, rapid contractions of muscle groups of the limbs, face, or trunk<br>Typically not repetitive or may recur at a slow rate<br>May be generalized, focal, or fragmentary<br>May be provoked by stimulation<br>*Presumed pathophysiology*: may be epileptic or nonepileptic |
| Spasms | May be flexor, extensor, or mixed extensor/flexor<br>May occur in clusters<br>Cannot be provoked by stimulation or suppressed by restraint<br>*Pathophysiology*: epileptic |
| Motor automatisms | |
| Ocular signs | Random and roving eye movements or nystagmus (distinct from tonic eye deviation)<br>May be provoked or intensified by tactile stimulation<br>*Presumed pathophysiology*: nonepileptic |
| Oral-buccal-lingual movements | Sucking, chewing, tongue protrusions<br>May be provoked or intensified by stimulation<br>*Presumed pathophysiology*: nonepileptic |
| Progression movements | Rowing or swimming movements<br>Pedaling or bicycling movements of the legs<br>May be provoked or intensified by stimulation<br>May be suppressed by restraint or repositioning<br>*Presumed pathophysiology*: nonepileptic |
| Complex purposeless movements | Sudden arousal with transient increased random activity of the limbs<br>May be provoked or intensified by stimulation<br>*Presumed pathophysiology*: nonepileptic |

*Mizrahi EM, Kellaway P: Diagnosis and Management of Neonatal Seizures. Lippincott-Raven, Philadelphia, 1998, pp 1-155.

(Scher, 1997b). An extensive evaluation must be initiated to exclude metabolic, structural, and genetic causes. Rarely, healthy sleeping neonates exhibit abundant myoclonus that subsides on arousal to the waking state (Resnick et al, 1986); this entity is termed benign *sleep myoclonus of the newborn*.

## Nonepileptic Behaviors of Neonates

Nonepileptic neonatal movement repertoires continue to challenge the physician's attempt to accurately diagnose seizures. Coincident synchronized video-EEG-polygraphic recordings are now suggested to confirm the temporal relationships between the suspicious clinical phenomena and electrographic expression of seizures (Mizrahi and Kellaway, 1998; Scher, 1997a, 2001b).

## Tremulousness or Jitteriness without Coincident Electrographic Seizures

Tremors are frequently misidentified as clonic activity by inexperienced medical personnel. The flexion and extension phases of tremor are equal in amplitude, unlike the unequal phases of clonic movements. Children are generally alert or hyperalert but may also appear somnolent or lethargic as part of an encephalopathy. Passive flexion and repositioning of the affected tremulous body part will diminish or eliminate the movement. Such movements

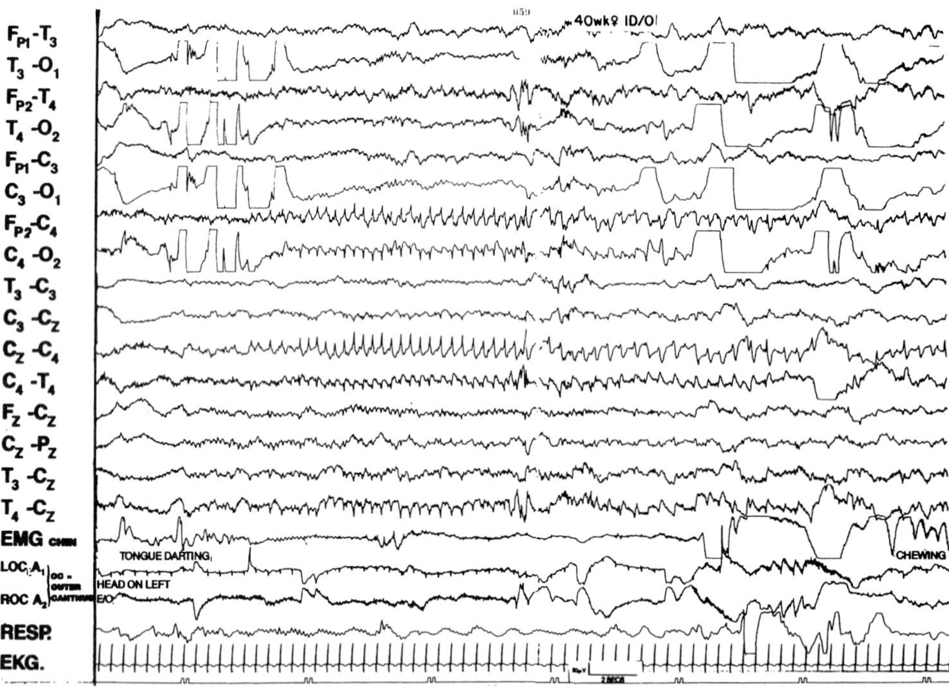


**FIGURE 66–1.** Segment of electroencephalogram (EEG) from a 40-week-gestation, 1-day-old female infant following severe asphyxia resulting from rupture of velamentous insertion of the umbilical cord during delivery. An electrical seizure in the right central/midline region is recorded coincident with buccolingual and eye movements (see comments and eye channels on record). *(From Scher MS, Painter MJ: Electrographic diagnosis of neonatal seizures: Issues of diagnostic accuracy, clinical correlation and survival. In Wasterlain CG, Vert P [eds]: Neonatal Seizures. New York, Raven Press, 1990, p 17.)*

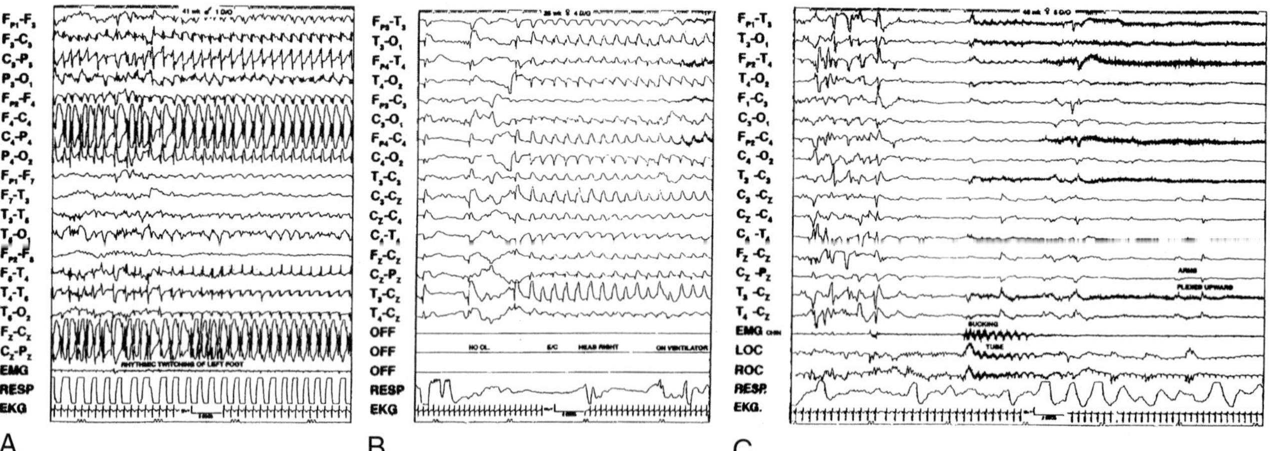


**FIGURE 66–2. A,** Segment of electroencephalogram (EEG) from a 41-week-gestation, 1-day-old male infant with an electroclinical seizure characterized by rhythmic clonic movements of the left foot coincident with bihemispheric electrographic discharges of higher amplitude in the right hemisphere. This seizure was documented prior to administration of antiepileptic medication. **B,** Segment of EEG from a 25-week-gestation, 4-day-old female infant with an electrographic seizure without clinical accompaniments. **C,** Segment of EEG from a 40-week-gestation, 6-day-old infant with stereotypic flexion posturing in the absence of electrographic seizures (note muscle artifact). *(From Scher MS: Pediatric electroencephalography and evoked potentials. In Swaiman KS [ed]: Pediatric Neurology: Principles and Practice. St. Louis, CV Mosby, 1999, p 164.)*

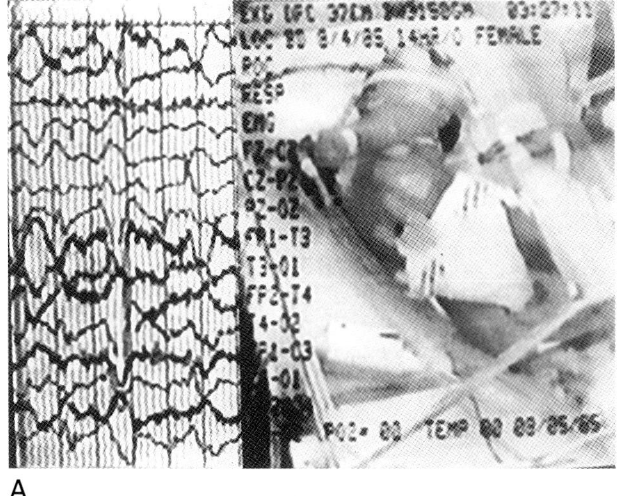
A

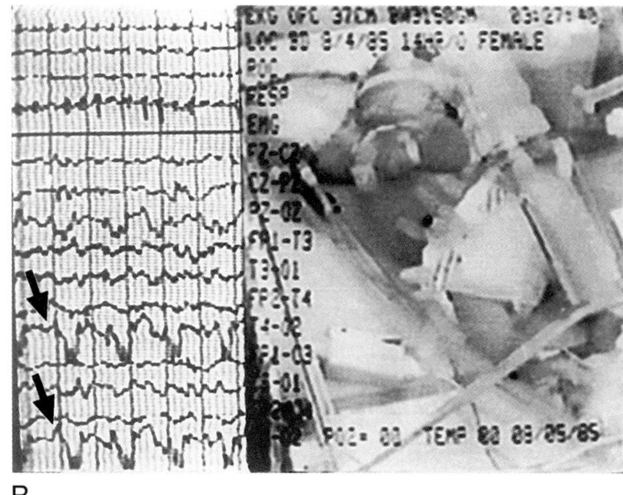
B

**FIGURE 66–3.** **A,** Segment of a synchronized video-electroencephalographic recording from a 37-week-gestation, 1-day-old female infant who suffered asphyxia demonstrates prominent opisthotonos with left arm extension in the absence of coincident electrographic seizure activity. **B,** Synchronized video-electroencephalographic recording from the same patient as in **A,** documenting electrographic seizure in the right posterior quadrant (*arrows*), following cessation of left arm tonic movements and persistent opisthotonos. *(From Scher MS, Painter MJ: Controversies concerning neonatal seizures. In Pellock JM [ed]: Seizure Disorders. Pediatr Clin North Am 36:292, 1989.)*

usually are spontaneous but can be provoked by tactile stimulation. This movement may also appear asymmetrical, with decreased expression in a weak limb following a brain injury or peripheral neuropathy. Metabolic or toxin-induced encephalopathies including those due to mild asphyxia, drug withdrawal, hypoglycemia or hypocalcemia, intracranial hemorrhage, hypothermia, and growth restriction are common clinical scenarios in which tremulous movements occur. Neonatal tremors generally diminish with increasing postconceptional age, spontaneously resolving over days to weeks, with normal neurologic outcome (Parker et al, 1990).

## Neonatal Myoclonus without Coincident Electrographic Seizures

Myoclonic movements can be bilateral and synchronous or asymmetrical and asynchronous in appearance. Benign myoclonic activity occurs more frequently during active (REM) sleep and is more predominant in the preterm infant (Hakamada et al, 1981; Scher, 1996), as well as rarely in healthy full-term infants; movements are not stimulus sensitive, have no coincident electrographic seizure correlates, are not associated with EEG background abnormalities, and are suppressed during wakefulness. Benign neonatal sleep myoclonus must be a diagnosis of exclusion.

Infants with severe CNS dysfunction may present with nonepileptic spontaneous or stimulus-evoked pathologic myoclonus (see Fig. 66–4B). Neonates with different forms of metabolic encephalopathies such as glycine encephalopathy, cerebrovascular lesions, brain infections, or congenital malformations can present with nonepileptic pathologic myoclonus (Scher, 1985, 1997b). Encephalopathic neonates may respond to tactile or painful stimulation by either isolated focal, segmental, or generalized myoclonic movements. Rarely, cortically generated spike or sharp wave discharges, as well as seizures, also may be noted on the electroencephalographic recordings that are coincident with these myoclonic movements. Medication-induced myoclonus as well as other stereotypic movements also have been described (Sexson et al, 1995); these abnormalities resolve when the drug is withdrawn.

## Neonatal Dyskinesias: Dystonia or Choreoathetosis without Coincident Electrographic Seizures

Dystonia and choreoathetosis are commonly occurring movement disorders that are often misdiagnosed as seizures. These nonepileptic movement disorders are associated with either acute or chronic disease states involving basal ganglia structures, or the extrapyramidal pathways that innervate these regions. Antepartum or intrapartum adverse events such as severe asphyxia can damage the basal ganglia (i.e., status marmoratus) (Volpe, 2001); rarely, specific inherited metabolic diseases (Barth, 1992) (e.g., glutaricaciduria) also can injure these structures. Sustained posturing or dystonia also may reflect lack of functional inhibition of subcortical motor pathways due to disease or malformation of neocortex (Sarnat, 1984) (see Fig. 66–2C). Documentation of electrographic seizures by coincident video-EEG-polygraphic recordings will help avoid misdiagnosis and inappropriate treatment (see Fig. 66–3A and B)

## Electrographic Seizure Criteria

Over the last several decades, electrographic/polysomnographic studies have become invaluable tools for the assessment of suspected seizures (Mizrahi and Kellaway,

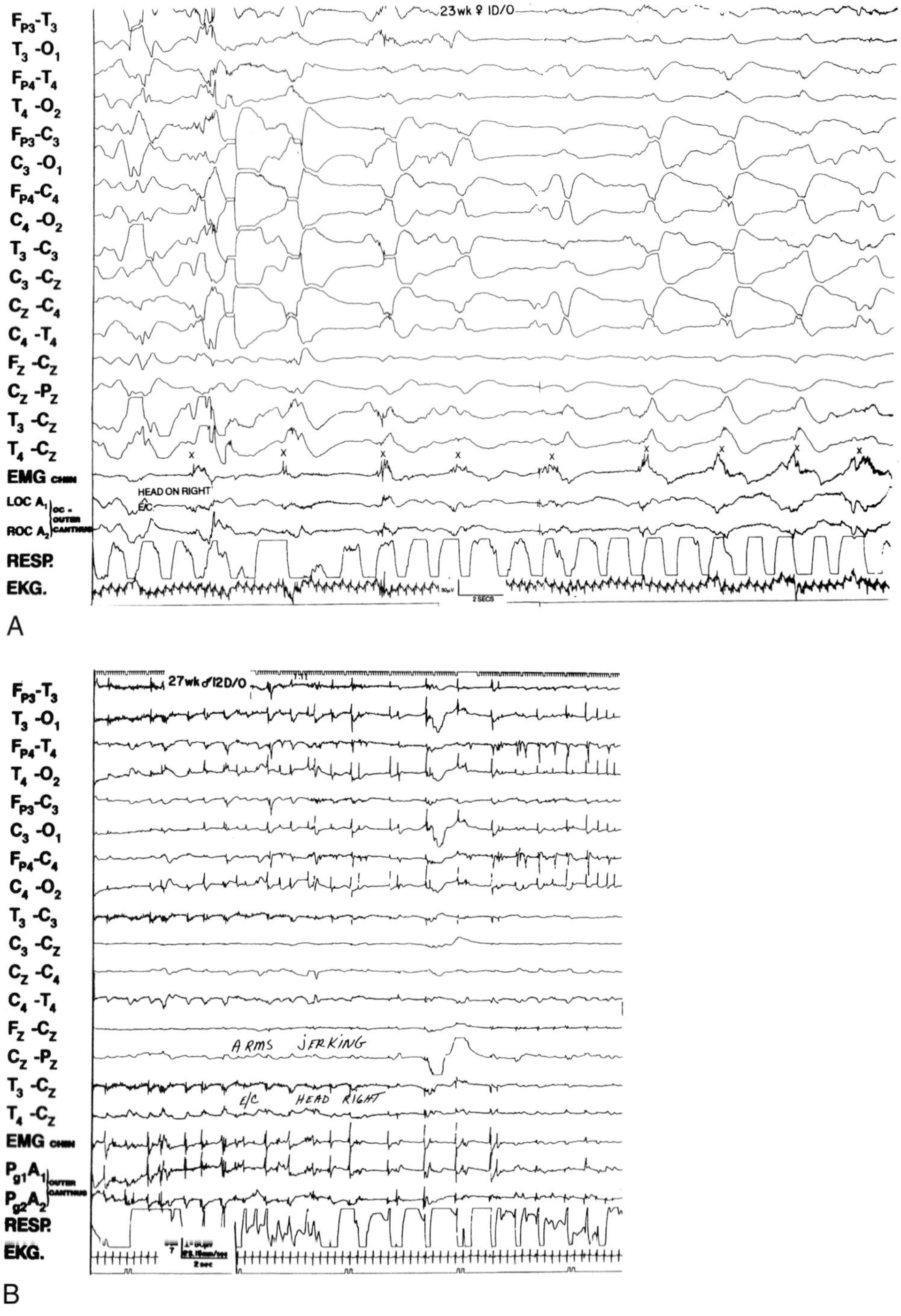

**FIGURE 66–4. A,** Segment of an electroencephalogram (EEG) from a 23-week-gestation, 1-day-old female infant with grade III intraventricular hemorrhage and progressive ventriculomegaly. An electroclinical seizure is noted with coincident with myoclonic movements of the diaphragm (*x marks*). **B,** Segment of an EEG from an encephalopathic 27-week-gestation, 12-day-old male infant with herpes encephalitis who exhibits nonepileptic multifocal myoclonus (myogenic potentials as electroencephalographic artifacts). (**A,** *From Scher MS: Pathological myoclonus of the newborn: Electrographic and clinical correlations. Pediatr Neurol 1:342-348, 1985, with permission.)*

1998; Pope et al, 1992; Scher, 1999, 2001b). Technical and interpretive skills for assessment of normal and abnormal neonatal EEG sleep patterns must be mastered to develop a confident visual analysis style for seizure recognition. Corroboration with the EEG technologist is always an essential part of the diagnostic process, because physiologic and nonphysiologic artifacts can masquerade as electrographic seizures. The physician also must anticipate expected behaviors for the child for gestational maturity, medication use, and state of arousal, in the context of potential artifacts.

As with the epileptic older child and adult, it is generally accepted that the neonatal epileptic seizure is a clinical paroxysm of altered brain function with the simultaneous presence of an electrographic event on an EEG recording. For assessment of the suspected clinical event in the neonate, synchronized video-EEG-polygraphic monitoring is a useful tool to distinguish an epileptic from a nonepileptic event. Single-channel computerized devices for continuous prolonged monitoring (Hellström-Westas, 1992) may fail to detect focal or regional seizures if the single-channel recording is distant from the brain region involved with seizure expression. Neonatal electrographic seizures commonly arise focally from a single brain region. One brain study described 56% of neonatal seizures presenting in a single location, with the remainder occurring in multiple locations (Bye and Flanagan, 1995).

## Ictal Electroencephalographic Patterns: A More Reliable Marker for Seizure Onset, Duration, and Severity

Neonatal electroencephalographic seizure patterns commonly consist of a repetitive sequence of waveforms that evolve in frequency, amplitude, electrical field, and/or morphology. Four types of ictal patterns have been described: focal ictal patterns with normal backgrounds, focal patterns with abnormal backgrounds, multifocal ictal patterns, and focal monorhythmic periodic patterns of various frequencies (Scher, 2001b). It is generally suggested that a minimal duration of 10 seconds for the evolution of discharges is required to distinguish electrographic seizures from repetitive but nonictal epileptiform discharges (Bye and Flanagan, 1995; Clancy and Legido, 1987; Scher et al, 1993) (see Fig. 66–1). Clinical neurophysiologists alternatively classify brief or prolonged repetitive discharges that lack this electrographic evolution as nonictal abnormal epileptiform patterns, which does not conform to the seizure definition.

For the older patient, status epilepticus is defined as at least 30 minutes of continuous seizures or two consecutive seizures with an interictal period during which the patient fails to return to full consciousness. This definition, however, does not easily apply to the neonate because levels of arousal are difficult to assess, particularly if sedative medications are given. Neonatal status epilepticus was reported in one third of full-term infants and in 20% of the total cohort of preterm and full-term infants (Scher et al, 1993) using a definition of status epilepticus as continuous seizure activity for 30 minutes or 50% of the recording time. If clinicians relied only on clinical criteria, status epilepticus would be underdiagnosed. Without EEG confirmation, the underdiagnosis of status epilepticus would contribute to brain injury, as discussed later in the section "Effects of Neonatal Seizures on Brain Development: Consequences of Underdiagnosis."

Uncoupling of the clinical and electrographic expressions of neonatal seizures after antiepileptic medication administration also contributes to the underestimation of the true seizure duration and frequency of status epilepticus (Fig. 66–5). One study estimated that 25% of neonates expressed persistent electrographic seizures despite resolution of their clinical seizure behaviors after receiving one or more antiepileptic medications (Scher et al, 1994); this phenomenon is termed *electroclinical uncoupling*.

The neonate may alternately express or sustain repetitive or periodic discharges greater than 10 seconds in duration that do not satisfy the electrographic criteria for seizures. The same neonate may express both periodic discharges and electrographic seizures at other times during the same EEG recording (Scher and Beggarly, 1989).

At the opposite end of the spectrum from periodic discharges, brief rhythmic discharges that are less than 10 seconds in duration also do not satisfy electroencephalographic criteria for seizures. Some neonates with electrographic seizures also may exhibit these brief discharges. Both periodic and brief discharges are associated with compromised neurodevelopmental outcome (Oliveira et al, 2000; Scher and Beggarly, 1989).

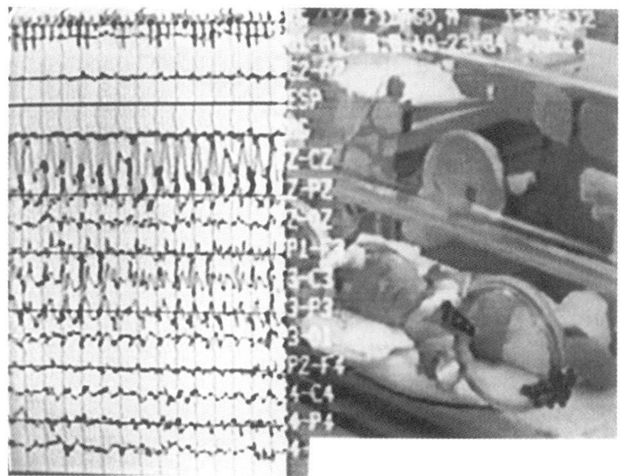

**FIGURE 66–5.** Segment of a synchronized video-electroencephalographic recording from a 40-week-gestation, 1-day-old male infant with electrographic status epilepticus noted in the left central/midline regions, after antiepileptic medication administration. Focal right shoulder clonic activity was only intermittently noted, while continuous electrographic seizures were documented mostly without clinical expression. This phenomenon of uncoupling of electrical and clinical seizure activities is associated with antiepileptic drug administration (see text). *(From Scher MS, Painter MJ: Controversies concerning neonatal seizures. In Pellock JM [ed]: Seizure Disorders. Pediatr Clin North Am 36:290, 1989.)*

## Subcortical Seizures versus Nonictal Functional Decortication

Experimental animal models offer conflicting evidence regarding suspicious clinical events for which coincident electrographic confirmation of seizures is absent (Scher, 2001b). Most neurologists prefer documentation of an ictal pattern by surface EEG electrodes before diagnosing a seizure. However, subcortical seizures with or without intermittent propagation to the surface may also occur. Electroclinical disassociation (ECD) is one proposed mechanism by which subcortical neonatal seizures intermittently appear on surface-recorded electroencephalographic studies (Biagioni et al, 1998; Weiner et al, 1991). ECD is defined as a reproducible clinical event that occurs both with and without coincidental electrographic seizures documented in one study as 34% of 51 neonates (Weiner et al, 1991). A clinical seizure precedes the electrographic expression, suggesting a subcortical onset before propagation to the cortical surface.

Some investigators have proposed a nonictal "brainstem release" phenomenon that explains suspicious clinical events that never have coincident EEG seizures expressed on surface recording (Mizrahi and Kellaway, 1998). These authors argue, for example, that motor automatisms have an inconsistent relationship with coincident EEG seizure activity. They alternatively speculate that functional nonictal decortication resulting from neocortical damage best explains these movements, without diagnosing epileptic seizures (Kellaway and Hrachovy, 1983).

This dilemma should encourage the clinician to use the EEG as a neurophysiologic yardstick by which more exact seizure start and end points can be assigned, before offering pharmacologic treatment with antiepileptic drugs (AEDs). Neonates can exhibit electrographic seizures that will go undetected unless electroencephalographic studies are utilized (O'Meara et al, 1995; Scher et al, 1993) (Fig. 66–6; see also Fig. 66–5). For example, in neonates who have been pharmacologically paralyzed for ventilatory assistance or in those who have received AEDs, clinical expression of seizures will be suppressed. In one cohort of 92 infants, 60% were pretreated with antiepileptic medications, and 50% of the cohort had electrographic seizures with no clinical accompaniment. Both clinical and electrographic seizure criteria were noted for 45% of 62 preterm infants and 53% of 30 full-term infants. Seventeen infants were pharmacologically paralyzed when the electrographic seizure was first documented. In a more recent cohort of 60 infants who were not pretreated with antiepileptic medications, 7% of infants had only electrographic seizures prior to AED administration (Scher et al, 1994), and 25% expressed electroclinical uncoupling after AED use.

Both overestimation and underestimation of neonatal seizure incidences are reported, depending on whether clinical or electrical criteria are used. Based on clinical criteria, seizure incidences ranged from 0.5% in term infants to 22.2% in preterm neonates (Lanska et al, 1995, 1996; Ronen et al, 1999; Seay and Bray, 1977). Discrepancies in incidence estimates reflect varying postconceptional ages of the study populations chosen, interobserver variability, and the hospital setting in which the diagnosis was made. Hospital-based studies, which will include a greater incidence of high-risk deliveries, generally report a higher seizure incidence. Population studies that include less medically fragile infants from general nurseries report lower percentages. Incidence figures based only on clinical criteria without electroencephalographic confirmation include "false positives," consisting of cases in which the neonates had either normal or nonepileptic pathologic neonatal behaviors. Conversely, the lack of electrographic seizures may include a subset of "false negatives," in which the infants express seizures only from subcortical brain regions, without propagation to the cortical surface. Consensus between clinical and electroencephalographic criteria, therefore, is still needed to reach the best incidence estimate.

### Interictal Electroencephalographic Abnormalities

Besides use of the EEG to diagnose seizures, documentation of interictal EEG abnormalities is extremely useful for patient management and prognosis. Interictal EEG findings are not pathognomonic for particular etiologic disorders, mechanisms, or timing (Scher, 1994). The clinician must integrate historical, physical examination, and laboratory findings with the electrographic interpretation of both seizure and nonseizure pattern findings for the particular child. The depth and the severity of neonatal brain disorders, as measured by the markedly abnormal interictal findings, help to predict subsequent development of seizures (Laroia et al, 1998). Serial electroencephalographic studies help the clinician to predict long-term outcome (see later section on prognosis).

## DIAGNOSTIC DILEMMAS: IDENTIFYING CAUSES FOR SEIZURES

Diverse medical conditions in the newborn can be associated with seizure activity (Adamson et al, 1995; Kellaway and Hrachovy, 1983) (Table 66–4). Asphyxia is traditionally introduced as the representative etiologic disorder that exemplifies when seizures may occur. The asphyxial con-

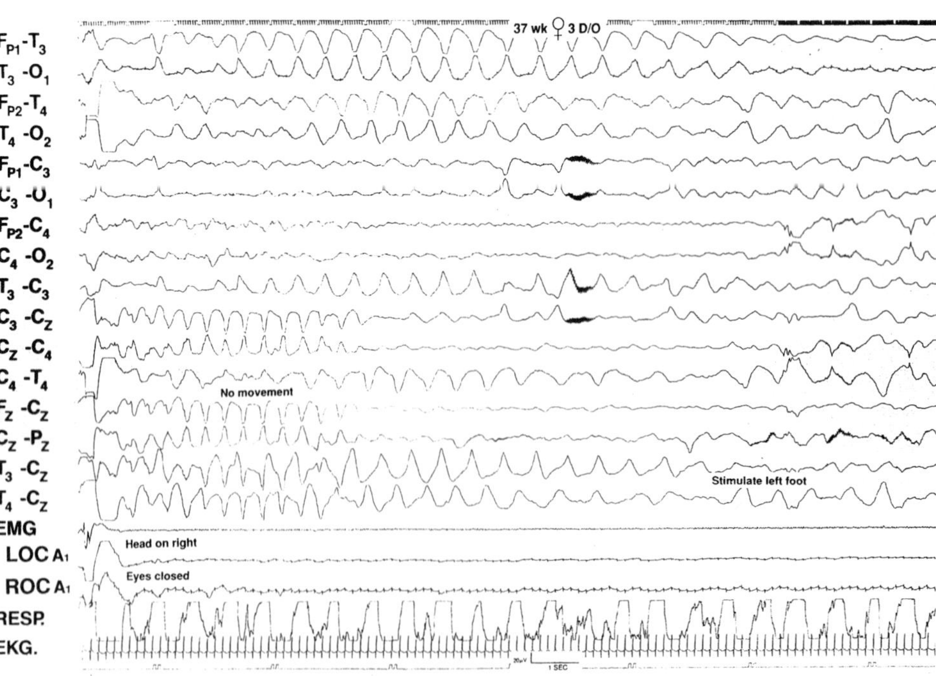


**FIGURE 66–6.** Segment of a synchronized video-electroencephalographic recording from a 37-week-gestation, 3-day-old female infant who was pharmacologically paralyzed for ventilatory care. A seizure is noted in the right posterior quadrant and midline. *(From Scher MS, Painter MJ: Controversies concerning neonatal seizures. In Pellock JM [ed]: Seizure Disorders. Pediatr Clin North Am 36:287, 1989.)*

**TABLE 66–4**

**Differential Diagnosis of Neonatal Seizures***

| | |
|---|---|
| **Metabolic** | Congenital infections |
| Hypoxia-ischemia (i.e., asphyxia) | Herpes simplex |
| Hypoglycemia | Syphilis |
| Hypocalcemia | Cytomegalovirus infection |
| Hypomagnesemia | Coxsackie virus meningoencephalitis |
| Hypoglycemia | Toxoplasmosis |
| Glycogen storage disease | Acquired immunodeficiency syndrome (AIDS) |
| Galactosemia | Brain abscess |
| **Idiopathic** | **Brain anomalies** (i.e., cerebral dysgenesis from either congenital or acquired causes) |
| Hypomagnesemia | **Drug withdrawal or toxins** |
| Infant of a diabetic mother | Prenatal exposure to substances of abuse—methadone, heroin, barbiturate, cocaine |
| Neonatal hypoparathyroidism | Prescribed medications—propoxyphene, isoniazid |
| Maternal hyperparathyroidism | Local anesthetics |
| High phosphate load | **Hypertensive encephalopathy** |
| Other electrolyte imbalances | **Amino acid metabolism** |
| Hypernatremia | Branched-chain amino acidopathies |
| Hyponatremia | Urea cycle abnormalities |
| **Intrauterine growth restriction** | Nonketotic hyperglycinemia |
| **Infant of a diabetic mother** | Ketotic hyperglycinemia |
| **Intracranial hemorrhage** | **Familial seizures** |
| Subarachnoid hemorrhage | Neurocutaneous syndromes |
| Subdural/epidural hematoma | Tuberous sclerosis |
| Intraventricular hemorrhage | Incontinentia pigmenti |
| **Cerebrovascular lesions** (other than trauma) | Autosomal dominant neonatal seizures |
| Cerebral infarction (thrombotic vs. embolic causes) | **Selected genetic syndromes** |
| Ischemic vs. hemorrhagic lesions | Zellweger syndrome |
| Cortical vein thrombosis | Neonatal adrenoleukodystrophy |
| Circulatory disturbances from hypoperfusion | Smith-Lemli-Opitz syndrome |
| **Trauma** | |
| **Infections** | |
| Bacterial meningitis | |
| Viral encephalitis | |

*Etiology independent of timing from fetal to neonatal periods.

Adapted from Scher MS: Neonatal seizures: An expression of fetal or neonatal brain disorders. In Stevenson DK, Benitz WE, Sunshine P (eds): Fetal and Neonatal Brain Injury: Mechanisms, Management and the Risks of Practice, 3rd ed. Cambridge, UK, Cambridge University Press, 2002, pp 735-784.

dition, however, encompasses heterogeneous conditions associated with hypoxia-ischemia, which may lead to seizures over a variable timeline encompassing antepartum, intrapartum, and neonatal periods.

Neonatal seizures are not disease specific and can be associated with a variety of medical conditions occurring before, during, or after parturition. Seizures may occur as part of an asphyxial brain disorder that is expressed after birth (i.e., hypoxic-ischemic encephalopathy). Alternatively, neonatal encephalopathies may represent other etiologic disorders with incidental asphyxia. Finally, seizures can present as an isolated clinical sign secondary to a remote antepartum asphyxial stress without other signs of a postnatal encephalopathy. A logistic model developed to predict seizures emphasizes the accumulation of both antepartum and intrapartum factors that increase the likelihood of neonatal seizure occurrence in the context of asphyxia (Patterson et al, 1989). Although separately these same factors have low positive predictive values, a significant cumulative risk profile results when maternal anemia, vaginal bleeding, asthma, meconium-stained amniotic fluid, abnormal fetal presentation, fetal distress, and shoulder dystocia all are considered. Another study of 40 neonates with clinical seizures indicated that only 37.5% of the seizures were associated with asphyxia, whereas a majority of term infants had early-onset seizures due to malformation, stroke, infection, or hemorrhage (Lien et al, 1995).

## Hypoxia-Ischemia

Hypoxia-ischemia or asphyxia is nonetheless traditionally considered the most common cause of neonatal seizures (Brown et al, 1972, 1974, 1983; Sarnat and Sarnat, 1976; Volpe, 2001). However, infants can suffer asphyxia before as well as during parturition, and 10% of neonatal asphyxia cases also result from postnatal causes (Volpe, 2001). When asphyxia is suspected during the labor and delivery process, biochemical confirmation is required. This metabolic definition of asphyxia represents the cardinal feature of hypoxic-ischemic encephalopathy (HIE).

The American College of Obstetrics and Gynecology (ACOG) initially published guidelines that suggest four cardinal criteria to define postasphyxial neonatal encephalopathy—that is, HIE—after significant clinical depression noted at birth (ACOG, 1992). These four criteria include:

1. Profound metabolic or mixed acidemia with a pH of less than 7.00 in umbilical cord blood
2. Persistence of an Apgar score of 0 to 3 for longer than 5 minutes
3. Neonatal neurologic sequelae (i.e., seizures, coma, and hypotonia)
4. Multiorgan system dysfunction (i.e., significant cardiovascular, gastrointestinal, hematologic, pulmonary, and renal involvement)

More recent guidelines have been published which suggest stricter criteria which include the four cardinal criteria as well as four collective criteria. Clinicians now recognize antepartum (as well as peripartum reasons) for HIE (ACOG, 2003).

## Other Causes of Neonatal Encephalopathy

Diverse etiologic disorders and conditions occurring in the antepartum, intrapartum, and neonatal periods may cause neonatal encephalopathies, with or without accompanying seizures. Children certainly may exhibit altered arousal and muscle tone, as well as seizures, without meeting the suggested criteria for HIE from intrapartum causes (ACOG, 2003). These children can appear neurologically abnormal based on antepartum conditions involving maternal, placental, or fetal diseases (Adamson et al, 1995).

A case-control study of term infants with clinical seizures reported a fourfold increase in the risk of unexplained early-onset seizures after intrapartum fever (Lieberman et al, 2000). All known causes of seizures were eliminated including meningitis and sepsis. Compared with 152 controls, the 38 newborns experienced intrapartum fever as an independent risk factor on logistic regression analysis that predicted seizures. The authors speculated on the role of circulating maternal cytokines that triggered "physiologic events" contributing to neonatal encephalopathy seizures, which did not occur from asphyxia.

Postnatal medical illnesses also cause or contribute to asphyxia-induced brain injury and seizures without intrapartum HIE. Persistent pulmonary hypertension of the newborn (PPHN), cyanotic congenital heart disease, sepsis, and meningitis are several examples. In one hospital-based study conducted over a 14-year period, 62 of 247 infants presented with EEG-confirmed seizures after an uneventful delivery without fetal distress during labor or neonatal depression at birth. Twenty of these 62 infants (32%) later presented with postnatal onset of pulmonary disease, sepsis, or meningitis (Scher et al, 1994).

Placental findings may reflect chronic disease states at antepartum time points with or without metabolic acidosis and evolving HIE after birth (Scher, 2002). Although meconium passage more commonly occurs in otherwise healthy newborns, meconium-stained skin also may be associated with meconium-laden macrophages within placental membranes in the depressed newborn. Meconium staining through the chorionic to amnion layers suggests a longer-standing asphyxial stress over a 4- to 6-hour period, which may precede the labor period.

Placental weights below the 10th or above the 90th percentile suggest chronic perfusion abnormalities to the fetus over weeks. Microscopic evidence of lymphocytic infiltration, altered villous maturation, chorangiosis, and erythroblastic proliferation of villi of the placenta supports chronic asphyxial stresses to the fetus. In a study of preterm and full-term neonates (23 to 42 weeks of chronologic age) with electrographically confirmed seizures, a significant association between seizures and chronic (with or without acute) placental lesions was noted by calculated odds-risk ratios, increasing to a factor of 12.1 ($P < .003$) by term age. In contrast, odds ratios were not significant for infants with seizures and exclusively acute placental lesions, presumably from events closer to labor and delivery (Scher et al, 1998).

Clinical examination findings in the depressed neonate with suspected HIE may reflect antepartum disease states rather than evolving HIE (Ajayi et al, 1998). Intrauterine growth restriction, hydrops fetalis, and joint contractures (including arthrogryposis) are findings that suggest intrauterine disease conditions associated with antepartum disease states. Later intrapartum fetal distress with or without asphyxia and neonatal depression also may occur with subsequent neonatal seizures (Scher, 2001a, 2001c). Hypertonicity, often with cortical thumbs (i.e., severely adducted across closed palms), in a depressed child who then rapidly recovers over hours after a successful resuscitative effort also suggests a longer-standing fetal brain disorder. Sustained hypotonia and unresponsiveness for 3 to 7 days constitute the expected clinical repertoire of HIE after an intrapartum asphyxial stress, either with or without coincident brain injury. In encephalopathic newborns, depressed arousal and hypotonia nonetheless also may reflect an antepartum disease process with neonatal dysfunction or superimposed injury after a stressful intrapartum period. For example, this was described in 10 of 20 neurologically depressed infants with electrographic seizures and isoelectric interictal EEG pattern abnormalities, who were comatose and flaccid for days, requiring ventilator assistance after difficult deliveries (Barabas et al, 1993). All children appeared neurologically depressed after asphyxial stress during the intrapartum period (i.e., depressed Apgar scores and metabolic acidosis). Evidence of fetal brain injury from pre-existing maternal-placental diseases was documented by evidence of chronic brain lesions on neuroimaging studies and/or neuropathologic postmortem findings. Although intrapartum asphyxial stress may worsen brain injury in some children, it was impossible to differentiate the neonatal encephalopathy from pre-existing antepartum brain injury for these 10 children.

## Hypoglycemia

*Hypoglycemia* is generally defined as glucose levels of less than 20 mg/dL in preterm infants and less than 30 mg/dL in term infants (Cornblath and Schwartz, 1967; Milner, 1972). No clear consensus exists concerning a direct cause and effect for hypoglycemia with seizure occurrence (Sencor, 1973). Methods of glucose determination (i.e., dextrose stick versus serum sampling) will affect the accuracy of the value. Also, associated disturbances may coexist, such as hypocalcemia, craniocerebral trauma, cerebrovascular lesions, and asphyxia, which may contribute to lowering the threshold for seizures. Infants born to diabetic or pre-eclamptic mothers, particularly those who were small for gestational age, also are at risk for hypoglycemia. Jitteriness, apnea, and altered tone are clinical signs that may appear in children with hypoglycemia, but they are not representative of a seizure state. Cerebrovascular lesions in posterior brain regions have been reported in children who suffer hypoglycemia (Griffiths and Laurence, 1974). Vulnerability of brain to ischemic insults is enhanced by concomitant hypoglycemia, as reported in mature animals (Siemkowicz and Hansen, 1978) and neonatal infants (Griffiths and Laurence, 1974).

## Hypocalcemia

Total serum calcium levels of less than 7.5 mg/dL in preterm and less than 8 mg/dL in the term infant generally define hypocalcemia. The ionized fraction is a more sensitive indicator of seizure vulnerability. As with hypoglycemia, the exact level of hypocalcemia at which seizures occur is debatable. An ionized fraction of 0.6 or less may have a more predictable association with the occurrence of seizures. Late-onset hypocalcemia due to use of high-phosphate infant formula has been previously cited as a common cause of seizures (Keen and Lee, 1973; McInterny and Schubert, 1969; Rose and Lombroso, 1970). However, hypocalcemia now more commonly occurs in infants with trauma, hemolytic disease, or asphyxia and may coexist with hypoglycemia or hypomagnesemia. Rarely, congenital hypoparathyroidism occurring in association with other genetic abnormalities such as DiGeorge syndrome (i.e., velocardiofacial syndrome, with a 22q11 deletion associated with cardiac and brain anomalies) must be considered. Affected infants may have severe congenital heart disease, as well hypoparathyroid state with hypocalcemia and hypomagnesemia, which precipitates seizures (Lynch and Rust, 1994). Hypocalcemia of unknown etiology in infants also may be the result of maternal hypercalcemia. Ascertainment of the mother's calcium status should be considered, because maternal hypercalcemia can suppress fetal parathyroid development.

## Hyponatremia and Hypernatremia

*Hyponatremia* is a metabolic disturbance that may result from inappropriate secretion of antidiuretic hormone following severe brain trauma, infection, or asphyxia (Volpe, 2001) but is an uncommon isolated cause of neonatal seizures. *Hypernatremia* also is a rare cause of seizures, usually associated with congenital adrenal abnormalities or iatrogenic disturbance of serum sodium balance, from the use of intravenous fluids with high concentrations of sodium.

## Cerebrovascular Lesions

Hemorrhagic or ischemic cerebrovascular lesions are associated with neonatal seizures, on either an arterial or a venous basis (Clancy et al, 1985; Levy et al, 1985; Ment et al, 1984; Rivkin et al, 1992; Scher et al, 1986, 1989). Intraventricular or periventricular hemorrhage (IVH or PVH) is the most common intracranial hemorrhagic lesion in the preterm infant and has been associated with seizures in as much as 45% of a preterm population with EEG-confirmed seizures (Scher et al, 1993). In a cohort of newborns with clinical seizures, IVH was the predominant cause of seizures in preterm infants of less than 30 weeks of gestational age (Sheth et al, 1999). Intracranial hemorrhage is usually expected within the first 72 hours of life of the preterm infant. Although IVH-PVH may occur in otherwise asymptomatic infants, the neonate with a catastrophic deterioration of clinical status will exhibit signs of apnea, bulging fontanel, hypertonia, and seizures (Volpe, 2001). Seventeen percent of preterm infants with IVH may have acute seizures during the first month of life; 10% of one cohort suffered remote seizures (after hospital discharge) (Strober et al, 1997). Full-term infants present less commonly with IVH, which usually originates from the choroid plexus or thalamus.

Another site of intracranial hemorrhage is the subarachnoid space; hemorrhage in this location may result in seizures but generally is associated with a more favorable outcome. Subdural hematoma, whether spontaneous or with craniocerebral trauma, should always be considered, particularly when focal trauma to the face, scalp, or head has occurred; simultaneous occurrences of cerebral contusion and infarction also should be considered.

Cerebral infarction has been described in neonates with seizures and can result from events during the antepartum, intrapartum, or neonatal period. Either preterm or term neonates with infarction also may present without seizure expression (DeVries et al, 1997). Seizures also can occur in otherwise healthy infants, suggesting an antepartum occurrence of cerebral infarction (Mercuri et al, 1995; Scher et al, 1991). Aggressive use of neuroimaging during the antepartum period by fetal sonography or magnetic resonance (MR) techniques, or within the first days after birth, may document remote brain lesions (Scher, 2001a, 2001c). In a group of 62 healthy infants with electrographic seizures after an uneventful delivery, 23 (37%) had cerebrovascular lesions, 18 of whom had ischemic brain lesions (Scher et al, 1995). Destructive lesions such as evolving porencephaly require approximately 5 to 7 days before becoming radiographically evident. The occurrence of injury during more recent intrapartum or neonatal periods can be supported by the presence of early cerebral edema using diffusion-weighted MR images (Forbes et al, 2000). Cerebral infarction also may occur during the postnatal period from asphyxia, polycythemia, dehydration, or coagulopathy.

PPHN with severe and recurrent hypoxia also can be associated with cerebrovascular lesions and seizures (Scher et al, 1986) (Fig. 66–7A and B). Certain infants with PPHN will require extracorporeal membrane oxygenation (ECMO) to treat severe forms of this pulmonary disease, which does not respond to traditional ventilatory therapy. Radiographic documentation of brain lesions is needed before initiation of ECMO, because the anticoagulation required for ECMO may convert "bland" or ischemic infarctions to hemorrhagic forms, with greater risk for cerebral edema and herniation. Although meconium aspiration syndrome has historically been identified with an intrapartum/neonatal presentation of PPHN, in most affected children this lung disease generally is secondary to antepartum maternal/fetal or placental conditions that predispose the fetus to thickening of the muscular layers of the pulmonary arteries in utero, with resultant sustained increased pulmonary vascular resistance after birth (Benitz et al, 1997).

Cerebral infarction in the venous distribution of the brain may also lead to neonatal seizures (Rivkin et al, 1992; Shevell et al, 1989). Lateral or sagittal sinus thrombosis after coagulopathy can occur secondary to systemic infection, polycythemia, or dehydration. Venous infarction within the deep white matter of the preterm infant's brain also occurs in association with IVH.

## Infection

CNS infections during the antepartum or postnatal period can be associated with neonatal seizures (Kairam and DeVivo, 1981). A specific group of congenital infections— toxoplasmosis, rubella, cytomegalic inclusion disease, and herpes (the TORCH infections)—can produce severe encephalopathic damage that results in seizures, as well as more diffuse brain disorders. Other congenital infections include those due to enteroviruses and parvoviruses. Specific infections—for instance, neonatal herpes encephalitis—may be associated with severe EEG pattern abnormalities (Mizrahi and Tharp, 1982). Rubella, toxoplasmosis, and cytomegalic inclusion disease each also can lead to devastating encephalitis, usually manifesting with microcephaly, jaundice, body rash, hepatosplenomegaly, and/or chorioretinitis. Increasing lethargy and obtundation with or without seizures may suggest the subacute presentation of encephalitis during the postnatal period. Serial cerebrospinal fluid (CSF)

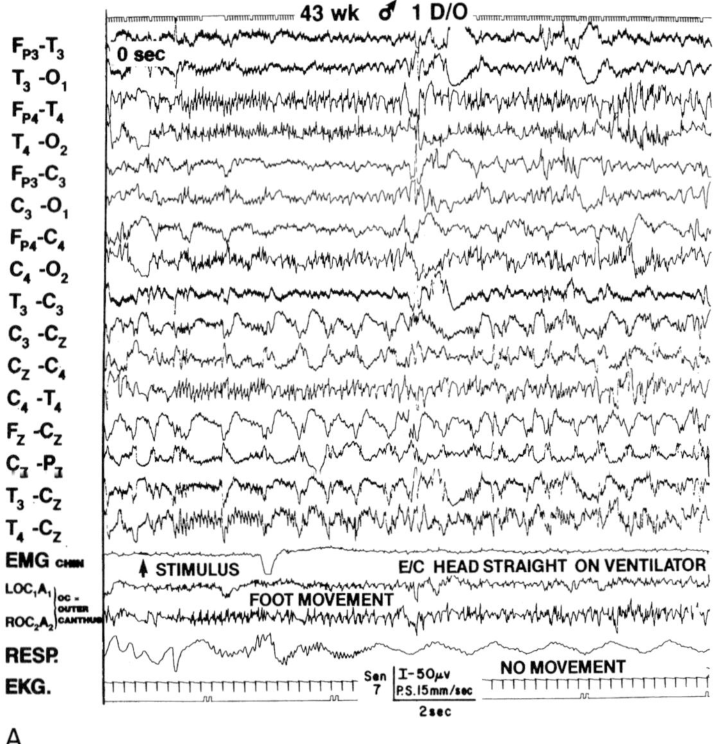


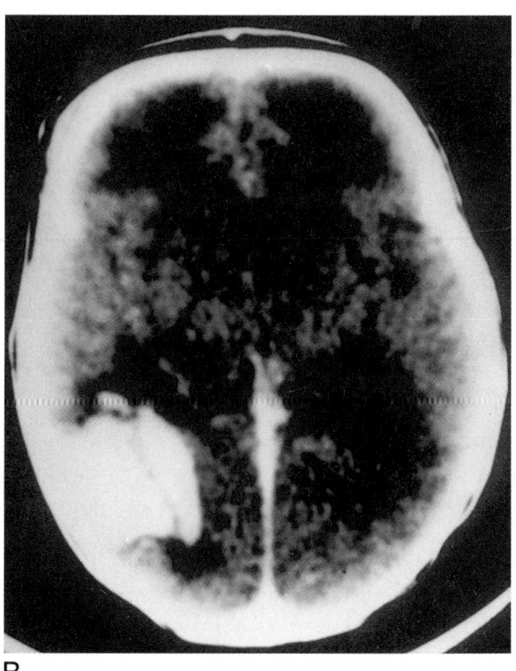


**FIGURE 66–7. A,** Segment of an electroencephalographic recording from a 43-week-gestation, 1-day-old male infant with a stimulus-evoked electrographic seizure (*arrow*) in the right temporal region, without clinical accompaniments. The child required ventilatory care for persistent pulmonary hypertension of the neonate (see text). **B,** Computed tomography scan on day 6 from the patient in **A,** documenting a hemorrhagic infarction in the right posterior quadrant with surrounding edema. *(From Scher MS, Klesh KW, Murphy TF, Guthrie RD: Seizures and infarction in neonates with persistent pulmonary hypertension. Pediatr Neurol 2:332-339, 1986, with permission.)*

analyses document progressively increasing protein levels and/or pleocytosis.

Bacterial infections from either gram-negative or gram-positive organisms, acquired in utero or postnatally, also are associated with neonatal seizures. Infection with some organisms, such as *Escherichia coli*, group B streptococci, *Listeria monocytogenes*, and *Mycoplasma*, may produce severe leptomeningeal infiltration, with possible abscess formation and cerebrovascular occlusions. A high percentage of survivors suffers significant neurologic sequelae.

## Central Nervous System Malformations

Disorders occurring during the stages of induction, segmentation, proliferation, migration, myelination, and synaptogenesis can contribute to brain malformations. The neonate with such malformations is at increased risk for seizures in association with the stress experienced around the time of birth (Palmini et al, 1994), which presumably lowers seizure thresholds. Brain anomalies may occur as a result of either genetic causes from conception and/or acquired defects early during gestation. Specific dysgenesis syndromes, such as holoprosencephaly and lissencephaly, can be associated with characteristic facial or body anomalies. Cytogenetic studies may document trisomies or deletion defects. Unfortunately, infants may lack physical clues to the presence of a brain malformation. Therefore, a high index of clinical suspicion for this entity is warranted in evaluating neonates with persistent seizures. In one study, 9% of 356 infants who presented with neonatal seizures were found to have brain malformations (Sheth et al, 1999). Neuroimaging, preferably with MR techniques, documents brain dysgenesis in children who may also express severe electrographic disturbances including seizures. Focal or regional brain malformations are rare causes of early-onset epilepsy in neonates and young infants (Aicardi, 1985; Ohtahara, 1978). Functional imaging studies such as positron emission tomography scans (Chugani et al, 1994) may identify localized areas of altered brain metabolism, which can assist in a neurosurgical approach to seizure management, even in young children who fail to respond to AED maintenance (Pedespan et al, 1995).

## Inborn Errors of Metabolism

Inherited biochemical abnormalities are rare causes of neonatal seizures (Scher, 2001b). Intractable seizures associated with elevated lactate and pyruvate levels in blood and CSF may reflect specific inborn errors of metabolism. Dysplastic or destructive brain lesions, as documented on neuroimaging, may be associated with specific biochemical defects, such as glycine encephalopathy or branched-chain aminoacidopathies. Pregnancy, labor, and delivery histories for affected infants are commonly uneventful. The emergence of food intolerance and also increasing lethargy, stupor, coma, and seizures are early indications of an inborn metabolic disturbance during the first few days of life. The newborn with an inherited metabolic disorder may initially present as a neurologically depressed and hypotonic child with asphyxia and seizures (Barth, 1992). Some children respond to specific dietary therapies, including vitamin supplementation (Painter et al, 1984), depending on the enzymatic defect. Specific urea cycle defects such as carbamoylphosphate synthetase deficiency may manifest as coma and seizures during the first 2 days of life, with marked elevations in plasma ammonia levels. Affected infants may respond to aggressive treatment with exchange transfusion, dialysis, and appropriate dietary adjustments.

Vitamin $B_6$ or pyridoxine dependency is a rare cause of neonatal seizures (Bejsovec et al, 1967; Clarke et al, 1979). Pyridoxine acts as a cofactor in gamma-aminobutyric acid synthesis, and its absence or paucity promotes seizures. The mother occasionally reports paroxysmal fetal movements (Oslovich and Barrington, 1996). The infant who is unresponsive to conventional antiepileptic medications should promptly receive an intravenous injection of 50 to 500 mg of pyridoxine, preferably with concomitant EEG monitoring. Termination of the seizure within minutes to hours as well as resolution of EEG background disturbances suggests a pyridoxine-dependent seizure state. Prophylactic doses of pyridoxine may be needed to achieve and maintain seizure control.

Other rare causes of seizures include disorders of carbohydrate metabolism with coincident hypoglycemia (Scher, 2002) as well as peroxisomal disorders such as neonatal adrenoleukodystrophy or Zellweger syndrome. A defect in a glucose transporter protein necessary to move glucose across the blood-brain barrier also has been reported, which results in hypoglycorrhachia and seizures (DeVivo et al, 1991). Affected children may achieve seizure control with a ketogenic diet but nonetheless suffer delayed development.

Molybdenum cofactor deficiency and isolated sulfite oxidase deficiences are other rare metabolic defects that cause neonatal seizures and associated destructive changes on neuroimaging, which may resemble findings in cerebrovascular disease or asphyxia (Slot et al, 1993).

## Drug Withdrawal and Intoxication

Newborns born to mothers with a history of prenatal substance abuse may be at increased risk for neonatal seizures (Herzlinger et al, 1977; Zelson et al, 1971). Exposure to barbiturates, alcohol, heroin, cocaine, or methadone commonly results in neurologic abnormalities that include tremors and irritability. Withdrawal symptoms, in addition to seizures, may occur as long as 4 to 6 weeks after birth (Kandall and Garner, 1974); electroencephalographic studies are useful to corroborate such movements with coincident electrographic seizures. Certain drugs such as short-acting barbiturates may be associated with seizures within the first several days of life (Bleyer and Marshall, 1972). Seizures may occur directly after substance withdrawal or may be associated with longer-standing uteroplacental insufficiency, promoted by chronic substance use and poor prenatal health maintenance by the mother. Careful review of placental/cord specimens may reveal chronic or acute pathologic lesions that contribute to antepartum or intrauterine asphyxia.

Inadvertent fetal injection with a local anesthetic agent during delivery may induce intoxication, which is a rare cause of seizures (Dodson, 1976; Hillman et al, 1979). Patients present during the first 6 to 8 hours of life with apnea, bradycardia, and hypotonia and are comatose, without brainstem reflexes. If the obstetric history indicates pudendal administration of an anesthetic to the mother, a careful examination of the child's scalp or body for puncture marks is indicated. Determination of plasma levels of the suspected anesthetic agent will establish the diagnosis. Treatment consists of ventilatory support and removal of the drug by therapeutic diuresis, acidification of the urine, or exchange transfusion. Antiepileptic medications are rarely indicated.

### Progressive Neonatal Epileptic Syndromes

Progressive epileptic syndromes rarely manifest during the first month of life (Mizrahi and Clancy, 2000). These children usually exhibit myoclonic or migratory seizures that are poorly controlled by antiepileptic medications, with brain malformations often demonstrable on brain imaging (Ekert et al, 1997; Ohtahara, 1978). These neonatal epileptic syndromes are termed *early myoclonic encephalopathy* or *early infantile epileptic encephalopathy* (Ohtahara syndrome), and the EEG commonly documents burst suppression or markedly disorganized background rhythms. Rarely, an idiopathic group of neonates with localization-related or partial seizures without neuroimaging abnormalities presents with intractable epilepsy (Natsume et al, 1996).

With neurocutaneous syndromes such as incontinentia pigmenti and tuberous sclerosis, symptomatic epilepsy during the neonatal period may be the presenting clinical manifestation of either of these genetic disorders. Incontinentia pigmenti is accompanied by a vesicular crusting rash, which initially mimics a herpetic infection. Seizures may or may not be present. The skin lesions evolve into lightly pigmented, raised sebaceous lesions in older infants and children. Tuberous sclerosis also rarely manifests with skin lesions in the newborn period. Hypopigmented lesions, initially noted under ultraviolet light, usually appear later during infancy. Two fetal presentations of tuberous sclerosis are that of the more common cardiac tumor, usually a rhabdomyoma, and rarely that of a congenital brain tumor, both noted on fetal sonography. Neonatal seizures also may be the presenting feature (Miller et al, 1998), with documentation of intracranial lesions on postnatal neuroimaging.

### Benign Familial Neonatal Seizures

The autosomal dominant form of neonatal seizures is a rare genetic epilepsy that should be considered in the context of a positive family history (Bjerre and Corelius, 1978; Petit and Fenichel, 1980; Ryan et al, 1991). Exclusion of infectious, metabolic, toxic, or structural causes needs to be completed before this entity is considered in the diagnosis. The genetic defect was first described on chromosome 20q, specifically at the D20S19 and D20S20 loci, as well as a locus EBN2 on chromosome 8q24. By positional cloning, a potassium channel gene (*KCNQ2*) located on 20q13.3 was first isolated and found to be expressed in the brain (Bjerre and Corelius, 1978). A second potassium channel gene (*KCNQ3*) also has been described and may explain the variability in phenotypic expression of seizures and outcome (Leppert and Singh, 1999). Recently, mutations in ion channels also have been implicated in Jervell and Lange-Nielsen syndrome, whose symptoms include congenital deafness and cardiac arrhythmias (Jentsch et al, 2000). Infant outcomes range from excellent to guarded, depending on the persistence of seizures beyond the neonatal period. Response to antiepileptic medication is generally good, although some clinicians describe variable success. Further studies are needed to clarify the relationship between phenotypic and genotypic expressions of this disorder.

## SEIZURES REFLECTING FETAL OR NEONATAL BRAIN DISORDERS: GUIDE TO DIFFERENTIAL DIAGNOSIS

The neurologist must place EEG-confirmed seizures in the context of historical, clinical, and laboratory evidence to determine both the pathogenesis and timing of a brain disorder. Seizures occurring in neonates who have experienced asphyxia support either acute intrapartum events or antepartum disease processes, or both. Does the child with seizures also have clinical and laboratory signs of evolving cerebral edema? The presence of a bulging fontanel with neuroimaging evidence of increased intracranial pressure and cerebral edema (i.e., obliterated ventricular outline and abnormal diffusion-weighted MR images), hyponatremia, and increased urine osmolality (i.e., the syndrome of inappropriate secretion of antidiuretic hormone) more strongly suggest a more recent asphyxial disease process, in or around the intrapartum period, causing acute or subacute cerebral edema.

Alternatively, failure to document evolving cerebral edema during the first 3 days after asphyxia or documentation of encephalomalacia or cystic brain lesions on neuroimaging shortly after birth (even in the encephalopathic newborn) suggests a more chronic disease process with remote antepartum brain injury. Liquefaction necrosis requires 2 weeks or longer after a presumed asphyxial event to produce a cystic cavity (Friede, 1975), before becoming visible on neuroimaging.

Isolated seizures in an otherwise asymptomatic neonate also suggest a disease process that occurred during either the postnatal or the antepartum period. Neonates present with seizures as a result of postnatal illnesses from intracranial infection, cardiovascular lesions, drug toxicity, or inherited metabolic diseases. Children with antepartum injuries may express isolated seizures after in utero cerebrovascular injury secondary to thrombolytic and/or embolic disease of the mother, placenta, or fetus. Fetal injury alternatively may occur after ischemia-hypoperfusion events from circulatory disturbances such as maternal shock, chorioamnionitis, or placental fetal vasculopathy (Miller, 2000).

Only a fraction of neonates with cerebrovascular disease present with neonatal seizures (DeVries et al, 1997). Why some children remain asymptomatic until later during childhood is unknown. Neonatal expression of seizures may reflect superimposed stress during parturition, which lowers seizure threshold in susceptible brain regions that have been previously damaged.

Following a careful review of the medical histories of the mother, fetus, and newborn, determination of serum glucose, electrolytes, ammonia, lactate, pyruvate, magnesium, calcium, and phosphorus levels may diagnose correctable metabolic conditions in newborns with seizures who will not require antiepileptic medications. CSF analyses including cell count, protein, glucose, lactate, pyruvate, amino acids, and culture studies are performed to assess for CNS infection, intracranial hemorrhage, and metabolic disease. Alternatively, metabolic acidosis on serial arterial blood gas determinations may suggest an inherited metabolic disease, particularly if intrapartum asphyxia was not judged to be severe. Absence of multiorgan dysfunction may alert the clinician to other potential causes of seizures besides intrapartum asphyxia. Signs of chronic in utero stress such as growth restriction, early hypertonicity after neonatal depression, joint contractures, or elevated nucleated red blood cell values all suggest longer-standing antepartum stress to the fetus. Genetic or syndromic conditions may contribute to the expression of neonatal encephalopathies independent of asphyxial injury (Felix et al, 2000). Careful review of placental and cord specimens also can be extremely useful to help time a brain insult. Neuroimaging, preferably using MR techniques, can locate, grade the severity of, and possibly time an insult (Leth et al, 1997) (i.e., using diffusion-weighted images). Ancillary studies may also include measurement of long-chain fatty acid and chromosomal/DNA analyses, as deemed necessary by family and clinical history. Finally, serum and urine organic acid and amino acid determinations may be needed to delineate a specific biochemical disorder for the child with a persistent metabolic acidosis. Lysosomal enzyme studies also are occasionally considered to diagnose specific enzymatic deficiencies in children with neonatal seizures.

## CHALLENGES REGARDING PROGNOSTIC ASSESSMENTS

The mortality rate among infants who present with clinical neonatal seizures has declined from 40% to 15% (Volpe, 2001). Studies of EEG-confirmed seizures documented mortality rates of 50% in preterm and 40% in full-term infants during the 1980s (Scher and Painter, 1990; Scher et al, 1993), with the mortality rate dropping below 20% in the 1990s in the same obstetric center (Scher, 1997a). The incidence of adverse neurologic sequelae, however, remains high; approximately two thirds of survivors are so affected. Even if major neurodevelopmental sequelae such as motor deficits and mental retardation were avoided in survivors after neonatal seizures, subtle neurodevelopmental vulnerability may manifest in late teenage years as specific learning difficulties or poor social adjustment (Temple et al, 1995), underscoring more recent experimental findings of long-term deficits in animal populations (Holmes and Ben-Ari, 2001).

Prediction of outcome should also consider the etiologic disorder for the seizures, such as severe asphyxia, significant craniocerebral trauma, and brain infections. More accurate imaging procedures (magnetic resonance imaging [MRI] in particular) have increased our awareness of destructive and congenital brain lesions with a higher risk for compromised outcome.

Interictal EEG pattern abnormalities are also extremely helpful in predicting neurologic outcome in the neonate with seizures (Bye et al, 1997; Monod et al, 1972; Sinclair et al, 1999; Tharp et al, 1981). Major background disturbances such as burst suppression are highly predictive of poor outcome, particularly when persistent abnormalities are still present on serial electroencephalographic studies into the second week of life. Seizure patterns alone, however, are not accurate to predict outcome, unless quantified to high numbers, long durations, and multifocal distribution (McBride et al, 2000). In one study, normal findings on interictal EEGs were associated with an 86% chance of normal development at 4 years of age in 139 neonates with seizures (Rose and Lombroso, 1970); by contrast, neonates with markedly abnormal EEG background disturbances had only a 7% chance for normal outcome. Another study (Rowe et al, 1985) reported outcome in term and preterm infants with seizures, concluding that the EEG background was more predictive of outcome than the presence of isolated sharp wave discharges. Even severe electroencephalographic abnormalities on single-channel spectral EEG recordings after asphyxia carry a higher risk for sequelae (Hellström-Westas, 1992).

Neonates with seizures have an increased risk for epilepsy during childhood (Watanabe et al, 1982). On the basis of clinical seizure criteria, 20% to 25% of neonates with seizures later develop epilepsy (Holden et al, 1982). Excluding febrile seizures, the prevalence of epilepsy by 6 to 7 years of age is estimated to be between 15% and 30%, based on EEG-confirmed seizures for an inborn hospital population; two thirds of this cohort were preterm neonates (Scher et al, 1993). These findings are in contrast with an incidence of 56% with epilepsy for an exclusively outborn neonatal population of primarily full-term newborns with seizures (Clancy and Legido, 1991). Epilepsy risk therefore reflects selection bias of specific study groups, as well as referral patterns in different hospital settings.

## DIAGNOSTIC DILEMMAS REGARDING TREATMENT CHOICES

### Corrective Therapies

Rapid infusion of glucose or other supplemental electrolytes should be initiated before antiepileptic medications are considered. Hypoglycemia can be readily corrected by intravenous administration of 5 to 10 mg/kg of a 10% to 15% dextrose solution, followed by an infusion of 8 to 10 mg/kg/minute. Persistent hypoglycemia may require more hypertonic glucose solutions. Rarely, prednisone, 2 mg/kg/day, may be needed to establish a glucose level within the normal range (Scher, 2001b).

Hypocalcemia-induced seizures should be treated with an intravenous infusion of 200 mg/kg of calcium gluconate. This dosage should be repeated every 5 to 6 hours over the first 24 hours. Serum magnesium concentrations also should be measured, because hypomagnesemia may accompany hypocalcemia; 0.2 mg/kg of magnesium sulfate should be given by intramuscular injection (Scher, 2001b).

Disorders of serum sodium are rare causes of neonatal seizures. Either fluid restriction or replacement with hypotonic solutions is generally the mode of therapy for correcting sodium dysmetabolism.

Pyridoxine dependency requires the injection of 50 to 500 mg of pyridoxine during a seizure with coincident EEG monitoring. A beneficial pyridoxine effect occurs either immediately or over the first several hours. A daily dose of 50 to 100 mg of pyridoxine should then be administered (Scher, 2001b).

## Antiepileptic Medications

If the decision to treat neonates with AEDs is reached, important questions must be addressed with respect to who should be treated, when to begin treatment, which drug to use, and for how long. Some clinicians suggest that only neonates with clinical seizures should receive medications; brief electrographic seizures need not be treated. Others suggest more aggressive treatment of electrographic seizures, because uncontrolled seizures potentially have an adverse effect on immature brain development (Dwyer and Wasterlain, 1982; Wasterlain, 1997). Others warn that early administration of an AED, such as phenobarbital, even before signs of HIE appear, may have adverse effects on outcome in term infants (Ajayi et al, 1998).

Phenobarbital and phenytoin, nonetheless, remain the most widely used AEDs; use of benzodiazepines, primidone, and valproic acid has been anecdotally reported (Scher, 2001b). The half-life of phenobarbital ranges from 45 to 173 hours in the neonate (Lockman et al, 1979; Painter et al, 1978, 1981); the initial loading dose is recommended at 20 mg/kg, with a maintenance dose of 3 to 4 mg/kg/day. Therapeutic levels are generally suggested to be between 16 and 40 μg/mL; however, there is no consensus with respect to drug maintenance.

The preferred loading dose of phenytoin is 15 to 20 mg/kg (Painter et al, 1978, 1981). Serum levels of phenytoin are difficult to maintain because this drug is rapidly redistributed to body tissues. Blood levels cannot be well maintained using an oral preparation. A water-soluble form, fosphenytoin, may be administered at the same loading dose. This specific agent has less harmful effects on the vein where it is injected.

Benzodiazepines also may be used to control neonatal seizures. The drug most widely used is diazepam. One early study suggests a half-life of 54 hours in preterm infants to 18 hours in full-term infants (Smith and Misoh, 1971). Intravenous administration is recommended because the drug is slowly absorbed after an intramuscular injection. Diazepam is highly protein bound; alteration of bilirubin binding is low. Recommended intravenous doses for acute management should begin at 0.5 mg/kg. Deposition into muscle precludes its use as a maintenance antiepileptic medication, because profound hypotonia and respiratory depression may result, particularly if barbiturates also have been administered.

## Efficacy of Treatment

Conflicting studies report varying efficacy with phenobarbital or phenytoin. Most studies only apply a clinical end point to seizure cessation. One study (Painter et al, 1978) found that only 36% of neonates with clinical seizures responded to phenobarbital; another study noted cessation of clinical seizures with phenobarbital in only 32% of neonates (Lockman et al, 1979). With doses as high as 40 mg/kg (Gal et al, 1982), the rate of clinical seizure control was reported to be 85%. A more recent study reported that the earlier administration of high-dose phenobarbital in a group of asphyxiated infants was associated with a 27% reduction in clinical seizures and better outcomes than in a group of infants who did not receive high dosages (Hall et al, 1998). However, coincident electroencephalographic studies are now suggested to verify the resolution of electrographic seizures. A recent report suggests that 25% of neonates have persistent electrographic seizures after suppression of clinical seizure behaviors following drug administration (Scher et al, 1994). With use of the EEG to judge cessation of seizures, neither phenobarbital nor phenytoin was effective in controlling seizure activity (Painter et al, 1999).

The use of free or drug-bound fractions of AEDs has been suggested to better assess both efficacy and potential toxicity of these drugs in pediatric populations (Painter et al, 1987). Drug binding in neonates with seizures has only recently been reported and can be altered in a sick neonate with organ dysfunction. Toxic side effects may result from elevated free fractions of a drug, which may adversely affect cardiovascular and respiratory functions. To guard against untoward effects, evaluation of treatment and efficacy must take into account both total and free AED fractions, in the context of the newborn's progression or resolution of systemic illness.

Newer anticonvulsant alternatives to treat seizures are being suggested, with *N*-methyl-D-aspartate (NMDA) antagonists such as topiramate (Jensen, 1999) developed from experimental models of hypoxia-induced seizure activity in immature brain. Such models provide data regarding pharmacologic and physiologic characteristics of neuronal responses to an asphyxial stress, which causes excessive release of excitotoxic neurotransmitters (Jensen and Wang, 1996) such as glutamate. Specific cell membrane receptors termed *metabotropic glutamate receptors* (MGluRs) are sensitive to extracellular glutamate release and may play a role in epileptogenesis and seizure-induced brain damage (Aronica et al, 1997). Investigation of subclasses of MGluRs will lead to development of novel drugs that block these membrane receptors as the mode of treatment for neonatal seizures (Lie et al, 2000).

## Discontinuation of Drug Use

The clinician's decision to maintain or discontinue AED use is also uncertain. Discontinuation of drugs before discharge from the NICU is generally recommended, because then clinical assessments of arousal, tone, and behavior will not be hampered by medication effect. However, newborns with congenital or destructive brain lesions on neuroimaging or those with persistently abnormal findings on neurologic examination at the time of discharge may require a slower taper off medication over several weeks or months. In most children with neonatal seizures, the seizures rarely reoccur during the first 2 years of life, and prophylactic AED administration need not be maintained past 3 months of age, even in the child at risk. This recommendation is supported by a recent study suggesting a low risk of seizure reoccurrence after early withdrawal of AED therapy in the neonatal period (Hellström-Westas et al, 1995). Also, older infants who present with specific epileptic syndromes, such as infantile spasms, will not respond to the conventional AEDs that were initially begun during the neonatal period. This honeymoon period without seizures commonly persists for many years in most children, before isolated or recurrent seizures appear.

The potential for damage to the developing CNS from AEDs also emphasizes the need to consider early discontinuation of these agents in the newborn period. Adverse effects on the morphology and metabolism of neuronal cells have been extensively reported from collective research performed over the last several decades (Mizrahi, 1999).

## EFFECTS OF NEONATAL SEIZURES ON BRAIN DEVELOPMENT: CONSEQUENCES OF UNDERDIAGNOSIS

Embedded within the controversy regarding how to diagnose neonatal seizures (i.e., clinical versus electroencephalographic) is the association of repetitive or prolonged seizures with brain damage and altered brain development. Linked to the clinician's concern for seizure duration is an appreciation of the diverse neuropathologic processes and etiologic disorders that cause neonatal seizures and have neurologic sequelae (Lien et al, 1995). CNS infections and severe asphyxia are two etiologic disorders that exemplify underlying pathophysiologic mechanisms responsible for brain damage in neonates independent of seizure expression.

Adverse effects of the seizure state on the developing brain (Holmes and Ben-Ari, 2001) have been recently reviewed. Seizures can disrupt a cascade of biochemical and molecular pathways that normally are responsible for the plasticity or activity-dependent development of the maturing nervous system. Depending on the degree of brain immaturity, seizures may disrupt the processes of cell division, migration, and myelination; sequential expression of receptor formation; and stabilization of synapses—each of which contributes to the risk of neurologic sequelae, to varying degrees (Holmes et al, 1998).

Experimental models of seizures in immature animals suggest comparatively less vulnerability to seizure-induced brain injury than in mature animals (Huang et al, 1999). In adult animals, seizures alter growth of hippocampal granule cells and of axonal and mossy fibers, resulting in long-term deficits in learning, memory, and behavior. A single prolonged seizure in an immature animal, on the other hand, results in less cell loss or fiber sprouting and consequentially fewer deficits in learning memory and behavior. Resistance to brain damage, from prolonged seizure activity, however, is age specific, as evidenced by increased cell damage after only 2 weeks of age (Sankar et al, 2000). A recent study examined developmental changes in epileptiform activity in neocortical preparations in four different age groups and using four different pharmacologic models. The study confirmed that there are definite age-dependent differences in susceptibility to epileptiform activity in the neocortex. These developmental changes seem to relate to intrinsic network properties of the neocortex that are independent of ontogenetic differences in any specific neurotransmitter system (Wong and Yamada, 2001).

Repetitive or prolonged neonatal seizures alternatively can increase the susceptibility of the developing brain to suffer subsequent seizure-induced injury during adolescence or early adulthood, by altering neuronal connectivity rather than increasing cell death (Holmes and Ben-Ari, 2001; Holmes et al, 1998; Koh et al, 1999; Schmid et al, 1999). Neonatal animals subjected to status epilepticus have reduced seizure thresholds at later ages and demonstrate impairments of learning, memory, and activity levels after suffering seizures as adults. Proposed mechanisms of injury also include reduced neurogenesis in the hippocampus, for example, possibly because of ischemic-induced apoptosis, as well as necrotic pathways (McCabe et al, 2001). Other suggested mechanisms of injury include effects of nitric oxide synthase inhibition on cerebral circulation, which then contributes to ischemic injury (Takei et al, 1999). Neonatal seizures, therefore, may initiate a cascade of diverse changes in brain development that become maladaptive at older ages and increase the risk of subsequent damage after subsequent insults. Destructive mechanisms such as mossy fiber sprouting in the hippocampus or increased neuronal apoptosis may explain mutually exclusive pathways by which the immature brain suffers altered connectivity and reduced cell number, which is then "primed" for later seizure-induced cell loss at older ages.

The critical duration of seizures, whether cumulative or continuous, remains elusive with respect to resultant brain injury. Given that as many as one third of full-term infants experience electrographic seizures that satisfy a definition of status epilepticus (Scher et al, 1993), EEG documentation appears crucial to assign seizure duration. A recent study in 10-day-old rat pups indicated that prolonged seizures for 30 minutes after asphyxia resulted in exacerbation of brain injury specific to the hippocampus, while sparing the neocortex. Prolonged neonatal seizures do worsen damage incurred by an already compromised brain (Wirrell et al, 2001) in a region-specific manner. In a neonatal rodent model of brief recurrent seizures, Landrot and colleagues (2001) demonstrated increased mossy fiber sprouting in the granule cells of the hippocampus, which correlated with impaired cognition and reduced EEG power spectra during adolescence. A companion study from the same laboratory demonstrated alterations in cognition and seizure susceptibility within 2 weeks of the last seizure before the adult pattern of mossy fiber distribution is achieved. Therefore, therapeutic strategies to alter the adverse outcomes of neonatal seizures must be initiated during or shortly after the seizures.

The overlapping effects of brain dysgenesis or injury from specific etiologic disorders versus seizure-induced brain damage make it difficult to differentiate pre-existing brain lesions from the direct injurious effects of seizures themselves. The use of microdialysis probes in white and gray matter of piglet brains subjected to hypoxia indicates elevated lactate-pyruvate ratios after hypoxia but no direct association with seizure activity (Thoresen et al, 1998). These findings support the conclusion that seizures themselves may not always be injurious to brain.

The dearth of well-designed clinical investigations of outcome after neonatal seizures in humans unfortunately does not permit confirmation of these experimental findings. Better definitions of neonatal seizure severity, including electrographic expression and seizure duration, are required to help resolve this controversy. A recently published investigation in human newborns with perinatal asphyxia suggests that seizure severity is independently associated with brain injury, as measured by MR spectroscopy (Miller et al, 2002), but not all subjects had electrographic confirmation of seizures.

Aggressive use of antiepileptic medications without electroencephalographic confirmation contributes to the inaccurate estimate of seizure severity in neonates and possible medication-induced brain injury. Intractable seizures generally require the use of multiple antiepileptic medications, which may still not effectively control seizures (Painter et al, 1999). Drugs also may impede the clinician's ability to recognize persistent seizures, because of the uncoupling phenomenon in which the clinical expression is suppressed while the electrical expression of seizures continues. Clinical definitions of seizure occurrence and duration consequently underestimate seizure severity, which may be associated with increased risk for brain damage (Ekert et al, 1997). AED use also has secondary harmful effects on cardiac and respiratory functions, with resultant circulatory disturbances that will contribute to brain injury because of hypoperfusion (Lien et al, 1995). Finally, AED use may have teratogenetic effects on brain development with exposure over long periods of time.

## REFERENCES


Adamson SJ, Alessandri LM, Badawi N, et al: Predictors of neonatal encephalopathy in full term infants. BMJ 311:598-602, 1995.

Aicardi, J: Early myoclonic encephalopathy. In Roger J, Dravet D, Bureau M, et al (eds): Epileptic Syndromes in Infancy, Childhood, and Adolescence. London, J Libbey Eurotext, 1985, pp 12-22.

Ajayi OA, Oyaniyi OT, Chike-Obi UD, et al: Adverse effects of early phenobarbital administration in term newborns with perinatal asphyxia. Trop Med Int Health 3:592-595, 1998.

American College of Obstetrics and Gynecology (ACOG) Technical Bulletin #163. Neonatal Encephalopathy and Cerebral Palsy. January 2003, pp 1-85.

Aronica EM, Gorter JA, Paupard MC, et al: Status epilepticus-induced alterations in metabotropic glutamate receptor expression in young and adult rats. J Neurosci 17:8588-8595, 1997.

Barabas RE, Barmada MA, Scher MS: Timing of brain insults in severe neonatal encephalopathies with an isoelectric EEG. Pediatr Neurol 9:39-44, 1993.

Barth PJ: Inherited progressive disorders of the fetal brain: a field in need of recognition. In Fukuyama Y, Suzuki Y, Kamoshita S, Casear P (eds): Fetal and Perinatal Neurology. Basel, Karger, 1992, pp 299-313.

Bejsovec M, Kulenda Z, Ponca E: Familial intrauterine convulsions in pyridoxine dependency. Arch Dis Child 42:201-207, 1967.

Benitz WE, Rhine WD, VanMeurs KP: Persistent pulmonary hypertension of the newborn. In Stephenson DK, Sunshine P (eds): Fetal and Neonatal Brain Injury. Oxford, Oxford Medical Publications, 1997, pp 564-582.

Bergman I, Painter MJ, Hirsh RP, et al: Outcome in neonates with convulsions treated in an intensive care unit. Ann Neurol 14:642-647, 1983.

Biagioni E, Ferrari F, Boldrini A, et al: Electroclinical correlation in neonatal seizures. Eur J Paediatr Neurol 2:117-125, 1998.

Bjerre I, Corelius E: Benign familial neonatal convulsions. Acta Paediatr Scand 57:557-561, 1978.

Bleyer WA, Marshall RE: Barbiturate withdrawal syndrome in a passively addicted infant. JAMA 221:185-186, 1972.

Bye AME, Cunningham CA, Chee KY, et al: Outcome of neonates with electrographically identified seizures, or at risk of seizures. Pediatr Neurol 16:225-231, 1997.

Bye AME, Flanagan D: Spatial and temporal characteristics of neonatal seizures. Epilepsia 36:1009-1016, 1995.

Chugani HT, Rintahaka PJ, Shewmon DA: Ictal patterns of cerebral glucose utilization in children with epilepsy. Epilepsia 35:813-822, 1994.

Clancy R, Legido A: The exact ictal and interictal duration of electroencephalographic neonatal seizures. Epilepsia 28: 537-541, 1987.

Clancy R, Malin S, Laraque D, et al: Focal motor seizures heralding a stroke in full-term neonates. Am J Dis Child 139:601-606, 1985.

Clancy RR, Legido A: Postnatal epilepsy after EEG-confirmed neonatal seizures. Epilepsia 32:69-76, 1991.

Clarke TA, Saunders BS, Feldman B: Pyridoxine-dependent seizures requiring high doses of pyridoxine for control. Am J Dis Child 133:963-965, 1979.

Commission on Classification and Terminology of the International League Against Epilepsy: Proposal for revised clinical and electroencephalographic classification of epileptic seizures. Epilepsia 22:489-501, 1981.

Cornblath M, Schwartz R: Disorders of Carbohydrate Metabolism in Infancy. Philadelphia, WB Saunders, 1967, pp 33-54.

DaSilva O, Guzman GMC, Young GB: The value of standard electroencephalograms in the evaluation of the newborn with recurrent apneas. J Perinatol 18:377-380, 1998.

DeVivo DC, Trifiletti RR, Jacobson RI, et al: Defective glucose transport across the blood-brain barrier as a cause of persistent hypoglycorrhachia, seizures, and developmental delay. N Engl J Med 325:703-709, 1991.

DeVries LS, Groenendaal F, Eken P, et al: Infarcts in the vascular distribution of the middle cerebral artery in preterm and full-term infants. Neuropediatrics 28:88-96, 1997.

Dodson WE: Neonatal drug intoxication: Local anesthetics. Pediatr Clin North Am 23:399-411, 1976.

Dwyer BE, Wasterlain CG: Electroconvulsive seizures in the immature rat adversely affect myelin accumulation. Exp Neurol 78:616-628, 1982.

Felix JF, Badawi N, Kuringzuk JJ, et al: Birth defects in children with newborn encephalopathy. Dev Med Child Neurol 42: 803-808, 2000.

Fenichel GM, Olson BJ, Fitzpatrick JE: Heart rate changes in convulsive and nonconvulsive apnea. Ann Neurol 7:577-582, 1979.

Forbes KPN, Pipe JG, Byrd R: Neonatal hypoxic-ischemic encephalopathy: Detection with diffusion-weighted MRI imaging. AJNR Am J Neuroradiol 21:1490-1496, 2000.

Friede RL: Porencephaly, hydranencephaly, multilocular cystic encephalopathy. In Friede RL: Developmental Neuropathology. New York, Springer-Verlag, 1975, pp 102-113.

Gal P, Toback J, Boer HR, et al: Efficacy of phenobarbital monotherapy in treatment of neonatal seizures: Relationship of blood levels. Neurology 32:1401-1404, 1982.

Glauser TA, Clancy RR: Adequacy of routine EEG examinations in neonates with clinically suspected seizures. J Child Neurol 7:215-220, 1992.

Griffiths AD, Laurence KM: The effect of hypoxia and hypoglycemia on the brain of the newborn human infant. Dev Med Child Neurol 16:308-319, 1974.

Hakamada S, Watanabe K, Hara K, et al: Development of motor behavior during sleep in newborn infants. Brain Dev. 3:345-350, 1981.

Hall RT, Hall FK, Daily DK: High-dose phenobarbital therapy in term newborn infants with severe perinatal asphyxia: A randomized, prospective study with three-year follow-up. J Pediatr 132:345-348, 1998.

Hellström-Westas L: Comparison between tape recorded and amplitude integrated EEG monitoring in sick newborn infants. Acta Pediatr 81:812-819, 1992.

Hellström-Westas L, Blennow G, Lindroth M, et al: Low risk of seizure recurrence after early withdrawal of antiepileptic treatment in the neonatal period. Arch Dis Child 72:F97-F101, 1995.

Herzlinger RA, Kandall SR, Vaughn HG: Neonatal seizures associated with narcotic withdrawal. J Pediatr 92:638-641, 1977.

Hillman LS, Hillman RE, Dodson WE: Diagnosis, treatment, and follow-up of neonatal mepivacaine intoxication secondary to paracervical and pudendal blocks during labor. J Pediatr 94:472-477, 1979.

Holden KR, Mellits ED, Freeman JM: Neonatal seizures. I: Correlation of prenatal and perinatal events with outcomes. Pediatrics 70:165-176, 1982.

Holmes GL: Diagnosis and management of seizures in childhood. In Markowitz M (ed): Major Problems in Clinical Pediatrics, Philadelphia, WB Saunders, 1987, pp 237-261.

Holmes GL, Ben-Ari Y: The neurobiology and consequences of epilepsy in the developing brain. Pediatr Res 49:320-325, 2001.

Holmes GL, Gairsa JL, Chevassus-Au-Louis N, Ben-Ari Y: Consequences of neonatal seizures in the rat: Morphological and behavioral effects. Ann Neurol 44:845-857, 1998.

Huang L-T, Cilio MR, Silveira DC, et al: Long-term effects of neonatal seizures: A behavioral, electrophysiological, and histological study. Dev Brain Res 118:99-107, 1999.

Jensen FE: Acute and chronic effects of seizures in the developing brain: Experimental models. Epilepsia 40:S51-S58, 1999.

Jensen FE, Wang C: Hypoxia-induced hyperexcitability in vivo and in vitro in the immature hippocampus. Epilepsy Res 26:131-140, 1996.

Jentsch TJ, Schroeder BC, Kubisch C, et al: Pathophysiology of KCNQ channels: Neonatal epilepsy and progressive deafness. Epilepsia 41:1068-1069, 2000.

Kairam R, DeVivo DC: Neurologic manifestations of congenital infection. Clin Perinatol 8:455-465, 1981.

Kandall SR, Garner LM: Late presentation of drug withdrawal symptoms in newborns. Am J Dis Child 127:58-61, 1974.

Keen JH, Lee D: Sequelae of neonatal convulsions: Study of 112 infants. Arch Dis Child 48:541-542, 1973.

Kellaway P, Hrachovy RA: Status epilepticus in newborns: A perspective on neonatal seizures. In Delgado-Escueta AV, Wasterlain CG, Treiman DM, Porter RJ (eds): Status Epilepticus: Mechanisms of Brain Damage and Treatment. New York, Raven Press, 1983, pp 93-99.

Koh S, Storey TW, Santos TC, et al: Early-life seizures in rats increase susceptibility to seizure-induced brain injury in adulthood. Neurology 53:915-921, 1999.

Landrot DR, Minokosh M, Silver DA, et al: Recurrent neonatal seizures: Relationship of pathology to the electroencephalogram and cognition. Dev Brain Res 129:27-38, 2001.

Lanska MJ, Lanska DJ, Baumann RJ, et al: A population-based study of neonatal seizures in Fayette County, Kentucky. Neurology 45:724-732, 1995.

Lanska MJ, Lanska DJ, Baumann RJ, et al: Interobserver variability in the classification of neonatal seizures based on medical record data. Pediatr Neurol 15:120-123, 1996.

Laroia N, Guillet R, Burchfiel J, et al: EEG background as predictor of electrographic seizures in high-risk neonates. Epilepsia 39:545-551, 1998.

Leppert M, Singh N: Benign familial neonatal epilepsy with mutations in two potassium channel genes. Curr Opin Neurol 12:143-147, 1999.

Leth H, Toft PM, Herning M, et al: Neonatal seizures associated with cerebral lesions shown by magnetic resonance imaging. Arch Dis Child Fetal Neonatal Ed 77:F105-F110, 1997.

Levy SR, Abroms IF, Marshall PC, et al: Seizures and cerebral infarction in the full-term newborn. Ann Neurol 17:366-370, 1985.

Lie AA, Becker A, Behle K, et al: Up-regulation of the metabotropic glutamate receptor mGluR4 in hippocampal neurons with reduced seizure vulnerability. Ann Neurol 47:26-35, 2000.

Lieberman E, Eichenwald E, Mathur G, et al: Intrapartum fever and unexplained seizures in term infants. Pediatrics 106:983-988, 2000.

Lien JM, Towers CV, Quilligan EJ, et al: Term early-onset neonatal seizures: Obstetric characteristics, etiologic classifications, and perinatal care. Obstet Gynecol 85:163-169, 1995.

Lockman LA, Kriel R, Zaske D, et al: Phenobarbital dosage for control of neonatal seizures. Neurology 29:1445-1449, 1979.

Lynch BJ, Rust RS: Natural history and outcome of neonatal hypocalcemic and hypomagnesemic seizures. Pediatr Neurol 11:23-27, 1994.

McBride M, Laroia N, Guillet R: Electrographic seizures in neonates correlate with poor neurodevelopmental outcome. Neurology 55:506-513, 2000.

McCabe BK, Silveira DC, Cilio MR, et al: Reduced neurogenesis after neonatal seizures. J Neurosci 21:2094-2103, 2001.

McInterny JK, Schubert WK: Prognosis of neonatal seizures. Am J Dis Child 117:261-264, 1969.

Ment LR, Duncan CC, Ehrenkranz RA: Perinatal cerebral infarction. Ann Neurol 16:559-568, 1984.

Mercuri E, Cowan F, Rutherford M, et al: Ischaemic and haemorrhagic brain lesions in newborns with seizures and normal Apgar scores. Arch Dis Child 73:F67-F74, 1995.

Miller SP, Tasch T, Sylvain M, et al: Tuberous sclerosis complex and neonatal seizures. J Child Neurol 13:619-623, 1998.

Miller SP, Weiss J, Barwell A, et al: Seizure-associated brain injury in term newborns with perinatal asphyxia. Neurol 58:542-548, 2002.

Miller V: Neonatal cerebral infarction. Semin Pediatr Neurol 7:278-288, 2000.

Milner RDG: Neonatal hypoglycemia: A critical reappraisal. Arch Neurol 47:679-682, 1972.

Mizrahi EM: Acute and chronic effects of seizures in the developing brain: Lessons from clinical experience. Epilepsia 40:S42-S50, 1999.

Mizrahi EM, Clancy RR: Neonatal seizures: Early-onset seizure syndromes and their consequences for development. Ment Retard Dev Disabil Res Rev 6:229-241, 2000.

Mizrahi EM, Kellaway P: Characterization and classification of neonatal seizures. Neurology 37:1837-1844, 1987.

Mizrahi EM, Kellaway P: Diagnosis and Management of Neonatal Seizures. Lippincott-Raven, Philadelphia, 1998, pp 1-155.

Mizrahi EM, Tharp BR. Characteristic EEG pattern in neonatal herpes simplex encephalitis. Neurology 32:1215-1220, 1982.

Monod N, Pajot N, Guidasci S: The neonatal EEG: Statistical studies and prognostic value in full-term and preterm babies. Electroencephalogr Clin Neurophysiol 32:529-544, 1972.

Natsume J, Watanabe K, Negoro T, et al: Cryptogenic localization-related epilepsy of neonatal onset. Seizure 5:317-319, 1996.

O'Meara WM, Bye AME, Flanagan D: Clinical features of neonatal seizures. J Pediatr Child Health 31:237-240, 1995.

Ohtahara S: Clinico-electrical delineation of epileptic encephalopathies in childhood. Asian Med J 21:7-17, 1978.

Oliveira AJ, Nunes ML, Haertel LM, et al: Duration of rhythmic EEG patterns in neonates: New evidence for clinical and prognostic significance of brief rhythmic discharges. Clin Neurophysiol 111:1646-1653, 2000.

Oslovich H, Barrington K: Prenatal ultrasound diagnosis of seizures. Am J Perinatol 13:499-501, 1996.

Painter MJ, Bergman I, Crumrine PK: Neonatal seizures. In Pellock MJ, Myer EC (eds): Neurologic Emergencies in Infancy and Childhood. New York, Harper & Row, 1984, pp 17-35.

Painter MJ, Minnigh B, Mollica L, et al: Binding profiles of anticonvulsants in neonates with seizures. Ann Neurol 22:413-420, 1987.

Painter MJ, Pippenger C, McDonald H, et al: Phenobarbital and diphenylhydantoin levels in neonates with seizures. J Pediatr 9:315-319, 1978.

Painter MJ, Pippenger C, Wasterlain C, et al: Phenobarbital and phenytoin in neonatal seizures, metabolism, and tissue distribution. Neurology 31:1107-1112, 1981.

Painter MJ, Scher MS, Alvin J, et al: A comparison of the efficacy of phenobarbital and phenytoin in the treatment of neonatal seizures. N Engl J Med 341:485-489, 1999.

Palmini A, Andermann E, Andermann F: Prenatal events and genetic factors in epileptic patients with neuronal migration disorders. Epilepsia 35:965-973, 1994.

Parker S, Zuckerman B, Bauchner H, et al: Jitteriness in full-term neonates: Prevalence and correlates. Pediatrics 85:17-23, 1990.

Patterson CA, Graves WL, Bugg G, et al: Antenatal and intrapartum factors associated with the occurrence of seizures in the term infant. Obstet Gynecol 74:361-365, 1989.

Pedespan JM, Loiseau H, Vital A, et al: Surgical treatment of an early epileptic encephalopathy with suppression-bursts and focal cortical dysplasia. Epilepsia 36:37-40, 1995.

Petit RE, Fenichel GM: Benign familial neonatal seizures. Arch Neurol l37:47-48, 1980.

Pope SS, Stockard JE, Bickford RG: Atlas of Neonatal Electroencephalography. New York, Raven Press, 1992.

Resnick TJ, Moshé SL, Perotta L, et al: Benign neonatal sleep myoclonus: Relationship to sleep states. Arch. Neurol. 43: 266-268, 1986.

Rivkin MJ, Anderson ML, Kaye EM: Neonatal idiopathic cerebral venous thrombosis: An unrecognized cause of transient seizures or lethargy. Ann Neurol 32:51-56, 1992.

Ronen GM, Penney S, Andrews W: The epidemiology of clinical neonatal seizures in Newfoundland: A population-based study. J Pediatr 134:71-75, 1999.

Rose AL, Lombroso CT: A study of clinical, pathological, and electroencephalographic features in 137 full-term babies with a long-term follow-up. Pediatrics 45:404-425, 1970.

Rowe RJ, Holmes GL, Hafford J, et al: Prognostic value of electroencephalogram in term and preterm infants following neonatal seizures. Electroencephalogr Clin Neurophysiol 60:183-196, 1985.

Ryan SG, Wiznitzer M, Hollman C, et al: Benign familial neonatal convulsions: Evidence for clinical and genetic heterogeneity. Ann Neurol 29:469-473, 1991.

Sankar R, et al: Epileptogenesis after status epilepticus reflects age- and model-dependent plasticity. Ann Neurol 48:580-589, 2000.

Sarnat HB, Sarnat MS: Neonatal encephalography following fetal distress: A clinical and encephalographic study. Arch Neurol 33:696-705, 1976.

Sarnat HB: Anatomic and physiologic correlates of neurologic development in prematurity. In Sarnat HB (ed): Topics in Neonatal Neurology. Orlando, Grune & Stratton, 1984, pp 1-25.

Scher MS: Electroencephalography of the newborn: Normal and abnormal features. In Niedermeyer E, Da Silva L (eds): Electroencephalography, 4th ed. Baltimore, Williams & Wilkins, 1999, pp 869-946.

Scher MS: Fetal and neonatal neurologic consultations: Identifying brain disorders in the context of fetal-maternal-placental disease. Semin Pediatr Neurol 8:55-73, 2001a.

Scher MS: Neonatal encephalopathies as classified by EEG-sleep criteria: Severity and timing based on clinical/pathologic correlations. Pediatr Neurol 11:189-200, 1994.

Scher MS: Neonatal seizures: Seizures in special clinical settings. In Wyllie E (ed): The Treatment of Epilepsy: Principles and Practices, 3rd ed. Baltimore, Lippincott Williams & Wilkins, 2001b, pp 577-600.

Scher MS: Normal electrographic-polysomnographic patterns in preterm and full-term infants. Semin Pediatr Neurol 3:12, 1996.

Scher MS: Pathologic myoclonus of the newborn: Electrographic and clinical correlations. Pediatr Neurol 1:342-348, 1985.

Scher MS: Perinatal asphyxia: Timing and mechanisms of injury relative to the diagnosis and treatment of neonatal encephalopathy. Curr Neurol Neurosci Rep 1:175-184, 2001c.

Scher MS: Seizures in the newborn infant: Diagnosis, treatment and outcome. Clin Perinatol 24:735-772, 1997a.

Scher MS: Stimulus-evoked electrographic patterns in neonates: Abnormal form of reactivity. Electroenceph Clin Neurophysiol 103:679-691, 1997b.

Scher MS: Neonatal seizures: An expression of fetal or neonatal brain disorders. In Stevenson DK, Benitz WE, Sunshine P (eds): Fetal and Neonatal Brain Injury: Mechanisms, Management and the Risks of Practice, 3rd ed. Cambridge, Cambridge University Press, 2002, pp 735-784.

Scher MS, Alvin J, Gaus L, et al: Uncoupling of electrical and clinical expression of neonatal seizures after antiepileptic drug administration. Pediatr Neurol 11:83, 1994.

Scher MS, Aso K, Beggarly ME, et al: Electrographic seizures in preterm and full-term neonates: Clinical correlates, associated brain lesions, and risk for neurological sequelae. Pediatrics 91:128-134, 1993.

Scher MS, Beggarly M: Clinical significance of focal periodic patterns in the newborn. J Child Neurol 4:175-185, 1989.

Scher MS, Belfar H, Martin J, et al: Destructive brain lesions of presumed fetal onset: Antepartum causes of cerebral palsy. Pediatrics 88:898-906, 1991.

Scher MS, Hamid MY, Steppe DA, et al: Ictal and interictal durations in preterm and term neonates. Epilepsia 34:284-288, 1993.

Scher MS, Klesh KW, Murphy TF, et al: Seizures and infarction in neonates with persistent pulmonary hypertension. Pediatr Neurol 2:332-339, 1986.

Scher MS, Painter MJ: Controversies concerning neonatal seizures. In Pellock JM (ed): Seizure Disorders. Pediatr Clin North Am 36:281-310, 1989.

Scher MS, Painter MJ: Electrographic diagnosis of neonatal seizures: Issues of diagnostic accuracy, clinical correlation and survival. In Wasterlain CG, Vert P (eds): Neonatal Seizures. New York, Raven Press, 1990.

Scher MS, Trucco J, Beggarly ME, et al: Neonates with electrically-confirmed seizures and possible placental associations. Pediatr Neurol 19:37-41, 1998.

Schmid R, Tandon P, Stafstrom CE, Holmes G: Effects of neonatal seizures on subsequent seizure-induced brain injury. Neurology 53:1754-1761, 1999.

Seay AR, Bray PF: Significance of seizures in infants weighing less than 2500 grams. Arch Neurol 34:381-382, 1977.

Sencor B: Neonatal hypoglycemia. N Engl J Med 289:790-793, 1973.

Sexson WR, Thigpen J, Stajich GV: Stereotypic movements after lorazepam administration in premature neonates: A series and review of the literature. J Perinatol 15:146-199, 1995.

Sheth RD, Hobbs GR, Mullett M: Neonatal seizures: Incidence, onset, and etiology by gestational age. J Perinatol 19:40-43, 1999.

Shevell MI, Silver K, O'Gorman AM et al: Neonatal dural sinus thrombosis. Pediatr Neurol 5:161-165, 1989.

Siemkowicz E, Hansen AJ: Clinical restitution following cerebral ischemia in hypo-, normo-, and hyperglycemic rats. Acta Neurol Scand 58:1-9, 1978.

Sinclair DB, Campbell M, Byrne P, et al: EEG and long-term outcome of term infants with neonatal hypoxic-ischemic encephalopathy. Clin Neurophysiol 110:655-659, 1999.

Slot HM, Overwg-Plandsoen WC, Baker HD, et al: Molybdenum-cofactor deficiency: An easily missed cause of neonatal convulsions. Neuropediatrics 24:139-142, 1993.

Smith BI, Misoh RE: Intravenous diazepam in the treatment of prolonged seizure activity in neonates and infants. Dev Med Child Neurol 13:630-634, 1971.

Strober JB, Bienkowski RS, Maytal J: The incidence of acute and remote seizures in children with intraventricular hemorrhage. Clin Pediatr 36:643-648, 1997.

Takei Y, Takashima S, Ohyu J, et al: Effects of nitric oxide synthase inhibition on the cerebral circulation and brain damage during kainic acid–induced seizures in newborn rabbits. Brain Dev 21:253-259, 1999.

Temple CM, Dennis J, Carney R, et al: Neonatal seizures: Long-term outcome and cognitive development among "normal" survivors. Dev Med Child Neurol 37:109-118, 1995.

Tharp BR, Cukier F, Monod N: The prognostic value of the electroencephalogram in premature infants. Electroencephalogr Clin Neurophysiol 51:219, 1981.

Thoresen M, Hallström ASA, Whitelaw A, et al: Lactate and pyruvate changes in the cerebral gray and white matter during posthypoxic seizures in newborn pigs. Pediatr Res 44:746-754, 1998.

Volpe JJ: Neurology of the Newborn, 4th ed. Philadelphia, WB Saunders, 2001, pp 178-214.

Wasterlain CG: Controversies in epilepsy: Recurrent seizures in the developing brain are harmful. Epilepsia 38:728-734, 1997.

Watanabe K, Kuroyanagi M, Hara K, et al: Neonatal seizures and subsequent epilepsy. Brain Dev 4:341-346, 1982.

Weiner SP, Painter MJ, Scher MS: Neonatal seizures: Electroclinical disassociation. Pediatr Neurol 7:363-8, 1991.

Wirrell EC, Armstrong EA, Osman LO, et al: Prolonged seizures exacerbate perinatal hypoxic-ischemic brain damage. Pediatr Res 50:445-454, 2001.

Wong M, Yamada KA: Developmental characteristics of epilepiform activity in immature rat neocortex: A comparison of four in vitro seizure models. Dev Brain Res 128:113-120, 2001.

Zelson C, Rubio E, Wasserman E: Neonatal narcotic addiction: 10 year observation. Pediatrics 48:178-189, 1971.

CHAPTER

# 67

# Risk Assessment and Neurodevelopmental Outcomes

Marilee C. Allen

## RISK OF NEURODEVELOPMENTAL DISABILITY

"Will my child survive?" "What kind of life will my child have?" These are the two questions most frequently asked by parents of infants in a neonatal intensive care unit (NICU). As difficult as it is to predict survival of a sick or very preterm infant, it is far more difficult to answer questions regarding quality of life for the infant who survives. How much recovery will there be? Will the child develop further complications? Most important, how will this early illness influence the child's neurologic, sensory, and cognitive development?

Only a few conditions (e.g., some chromosome disorders, dysmorphic syndromes, brain malformations) carry certain knowledge of disability, and many of these are associated with shortened life span. For most conditions requiring neonatal intensive care, it is difficult to define the full extent (if any) of damage to or malformation of the infant's organ systems. In addition, the newborn has a remarkable potential for recovery. Few factors hindering or contributing to this recovery have been identified. Predicting the outcome for individual children is therefore difficult.

How is quality of life defined? What is abnormal outcome? The World Health Organization has differentiated among the words *impairment*, *disability*, and *handicap* (International Classification of Impairments, Disabilities, and Handicaps, 1980). An *impairment* is a structural, psychological, or physical abnormality; a *disability* is a restriction or inability to perform normally due to impairment; and a *handicap* is a disadvantage in society due to a disability. Most commonly, *high risk* refers to likelihood of neurodevelopmental disability, which is a group of interrelated, chronic, nonprogressive disorders of the central nervous system (CNS) caused by injury to or malformation of the developing brain. They form a spectrum ranging from cerebral palsy (motor impairment) and mental retardation (cognitive impairment), to sensory impairment, to the more subtle disorders of CNS function (Table 67–1). These more subtle disorders of higher cortical function include language disorder, visual-perceptual problems, learning disability, minor neuromotor dysfunction, attention deficits, hyperactivity, and behavioral problems. They have a lesser severity and a higher prevalence in the general population than is the case for the major disabilities (i.e., cerebral palsy and mental retardation).

Although preterm infants and sick full-term infants have an increased risk of neurodevelopmental disabilities compared with the general population, most do not develop major disability and are quite functional. Most children with disability manifest initial developmental delay. However, children may have functional limitations without delay in milestone attainment. A preterm infant who was born at 27 weeks of gestation and had a right intraparenchymal hemorrhage had no delays when seen at 14 months in neonatal follow-up. He walked independently, had a right pincer grasp, and said his first meaningful word. On careful inspection, however, circumduction of the left foot was evident on walking, with only a raking grasp with the left hand. Findings on examination—a tight left heel cord and increased tone on pronation and supination of the left arm—were consistent with a left spastic hemiplegia. Children with complex medical conditions may initially demonstrate developmental delay but not have long-term disability. An infant with chronic lung disease and mild hypotonia who is not rolling over by 6 months has delayed development and is at risk for motor and language impairment. However, his rate of development may increase as his lung disease resolves, and he may have much milder impairment than expected or even no impairment.

A large number of perinatal and demographic risk factors, with differing capacities to predict neurodevelopmental disabilities, have been identified. They are best grouped by category (Table 67–2). Socioeconomic status is strongly related to cognition but has little effect on cerebral palsy (except as it may be related to preterm birth, intrauterine growth restriction, and other biologic risk factors) (Aylward, 2002; Hack et al, 1995; Ornstein et al, 1991). A number of obstetric conditions (e.g., abruptio placentae, maternal antepartum hemorrhage, fetal distress during labor) may be catastrophic, but prompt intervention may circumvent death or disability. Neonatal conditions (e.g., encephalopathy) are better predictors of outcome than either preceding obstetric conditions or measures of the infant's condition at the time of birth (e.g., Apgar scores, need for resuscitation) (Nelson, 2002; Weisglas-Kuperus et al, 1992). The more severe the encephalopathy, abnormalities on examination, or neuroimaging abnormalities, the higher the risk of disability (Allen and Capute, 1989; Aziz et al, 1995; Robertson et al, 1989; Rogers et al, 1994).

Multiple risk factors increase the risk of developmental disability, by either additive or multiplicative effects. The effects of prematurity and intrauterine growth restriction on cognition are greatest in infants born to parents of low socioeconomic status. Combining results of neuroimaging studies with neurodevelopmental examinations improves prediction of disability (Allen and Capute, 1989; Weisglas-Kuperus et al, 1992). Just as complications of prematurity increase with decreasing birth weight, incidence of neurodevelopmental disability also increases (Lemons et al, 2001; Vohr et al, 2000). However, the presence of multiple risk factors in the sickest infants makes it more difficult to attribute risk to individual factors.

TABLE 67–1

**Prevalence of Neurodevelopmental Disabilities in the General Population**

| Disability | Descriptor | Prevalence (%)* |
|---|---|---|
| Major disability | CP + MR† | 2-3 |
| Cerebral palsy | Motor impairment | 0.1-0.3 |
| Mental retardation | IQ‡ <70 | 1-2 |
| Mild mental retardation | IQ 50-70 | 1.5 |
| Severe mental retardation | IQ <50 | 0.5 |
| Sensory impairments | | |
| Visual impairment | Severe | 0.4-0.6 |
| Hearing impairment | Severe | 1.5-2.0 |
| Disorders of higher cortical function | | |
| Language delay/speech defects | | 4-11 |
| Learning disability | | 5-10 |
| Attention-deficit disorder | | 6-20 |
| Minor neuromotor dysfunction | | 5-15 |

*Prevalence figures adapted from Boyle CA, Decoufle P, Yeargin-Allsopp M: Prevalence and health impact of developmental disabilities in U.S. children. From Pediatrics, Vol 93, pages 399-403, 1994.

†CP + MR, cerebral palsy and mental retardation.

‡IQ, intelligence quotient (2 SD below the mean varies by test, may be 68 or 70).

Neither risk nor statistical association implies causation. Prematurity, intrauterine growth restriction, or poor respiratory effort at birth may be caused by a prenatal insult or malformation. An abnormal fetus may grow poorly, precipitate preterm delivery, fail to descend properly, need stimulation to breathe at birth or nipple feed poorly. All of these risk factors predict neurodevelopmental disability, but the etiology of the disability is the fetal abnormality, which often is difficult to detect. Recent population studies of children with cerebral palsy have reported an improved ability to determine probable causes for the cerebral palsy, with a decrease in unclassifiable causes from 38% to 27% in preterm infants and from 39% to 14% in term infants (Hagberg et al, 1996, 2001). In a comprehensive long-term follow-up study of preterm infants, Drillien and colleagues (1980) found that preterm infants "who showed no evidence of early intrauterine insult and who were neurologically normal in the first year of life were largely indistinguishable from control children reared in similar homes." This finding suggests that the causes and complications of prematurity are the etiologic disorders and conditions leading to disability.

TABLE 67–2

**Categories of Perinatal Risk Factors**

Background characteristics
- Socioeconomic status/social class, parental education, race

Obstetric/prenatal complications
- Maternal acute or chronic illness, maternal ingestion of drugs, congenital infection, multiple gestation, labor or delivery complications (e.g., abruptio placentae, cord prolapse), placental abnormalities

Physical characteristics
- Prematurity, postmaturity, small for gestational age/intrauterine growth restriction, gender, microcephaly, congenital anomalies, dysmorphic features

Condition at birth
- Apgar scores, cord pH, meconium staining, need for and response to resuscitation

Neonatal complications
- Hypoxia, acidosis, hypotension/shock, apnea and bradycardia, chronic lung disease, sepsis, meningitis, seizures, hypoxic-ischemic encephalopathy

Measures of central nervous system structure and function
- Intraventricular hemorrhage, intraparenchymal hemorrhage, ventricular dilation, cortical atrophy, intraparenchymal cysts or echodensities (Periventricular leukomalacia), burst-suppression pattern on electroencephalogram, abnormal neonatal neurodevelopmental examination

Studies of risk factors can provide important insights into causes of neurodevelopmental disability (Allen, 2002; Nelson, 2002; O'Shea, 2002). More than half of children with cerebral palsy are full-term, half of which have prenatal causes for their cerebral palsy, including intrauterine infection, coagulopathy, placental pathology, and death of a co-twin (Cummins et al, 1993; Hagberg et al, 1996, Nelson, 2002). Among preterm children with cerebral palsy, perinatal and neonatal etiologic disorders are more frequent than prenatal causes (61% versus 12%) (Hagberg et al, 2001). Strong evidence links cerebral palsy in preterm infants to ischemic and/or cytokine-mediated brain injury, with perhaps also a role for insufficient levels of developmentally regulated neuroprotective substances (e.g., thyroxine, hydrocortisone) (O'Shea, 2002).

Although risk factors cannot diagnose neurodevelopmental disability, the absence of significant risk factors is reassuring. All children should have their development monitored during infancy and childhood because of a baseline incidence of neurodevelopmental disability (see Table 67–1). Nevertheless, absence of significant risk factors and normal findings on neuroimaging studies and on neurodevelopmental examinations can be used to help alleviate parental anxiety related to having an infant in a NICU.

Mildly increased risk should be acknowledged but should also be put into perspective for parents. Parents of infants with significant or multiple risk factors should be offered focused neurodevelopmental follow-up evaluation and support, especially during critical early years. A comprehensive, developmentally based, family-oriented follow-up clinic ensures early diagnosis of neurodevelopmental disability, helps to shape early intervention strategies to meet the infant's and family's evolving needs, and provides parents with continuity and ongoing support during a very difficult period of uncertainty and adjustment.

Uncertainty regarding a child's outcome is difficult for both parents and professionals. The clinician can describe to parents the range of possible outcomes and estimate their likelihood for a given infant, based on a knowledge of the literature and experience. Helping parents to recognize and cope with parental fears allows development of a realistic plan for the future, including identifying family support systems, early intervention strategies, and community resources.

## NEURODEVELOPMENTAL OUTCOME

This section describes the outcome for several groups of high-risk infants cared for in the NICU. The reported incidences of disability differ from study to study because of a number of factors: variations in study criteria, ethnic and demographic composition of the populations, obstetric and neonatal care practices, follow-up rate, length of follow-up, and assessment methodologies. High follow-up rates are preferable but difficult to attain. Low follow-up rates raise concerns about bias—for example, whether infants lost to follow-up were more impaired or had fewer problems. One study found difficulty with follow-up to be associated with lower intelligence quotients (IQs), more disability, and single parents with less education (Callanan et al, 2001).

How the children are followed, and for how long, influences what neurodevelopmental disabilities are detected. Studies that evaluate infants up to 1 year focus on the major disabilities but are inadequate for assessing mild cerebral palsy, mild mental retardation, or borderline intelligence. Evaluating older children improves diagnostic accuracy but lowers follow-up rates, and socioeconomic factors play a role in cognition by the age of 2 years. Mild to moderate sensory impairments may be missed if specific evaluations of hearing and vision are not performed. Follow-up assessments from 2 to 6 years can detect minor neuromotor dysfunction, behavioral problems, attention deficits, and language delay. Questions about learning disability and other school-related problems, however, require follow-up to school age. Follow-up to adolescence and adulthood raises questions about functional abilities and quality of life.

Longitudinal studies have found an increased incidence of school problems the longer the period of follow-up evaluation (Aylward, 2002; Msall and Tremont, 2002). The younger child with more subtle impairments often has some ability to compensate for learning difficulties or inefficiencies. The child with subtle impairments may not demonstrate a learning disability until he or she reaches the higher grades, when the work becomes more complex, and efficiency becomes important in completing work and test-taking.

### Preterm Infants

Most preterm follow-up studies report outcomes related to birth weight because it is more reliably measured than gestational age ( Tables 67–3 and 67–4). Very low-birth-weight (VLBW) infants have birth weights below 1500 g (3 pounds 5 ounces), extremely low-birth-weight (ELBW) infants have birth weights below 1000 g (2 pounds 3 ounces), and incredibly low-birth-weight (ILBW) infants have birth weights below 750 to 800 g (1 pound 1 ounce).

#### Major Disability

Although preterm infants have a higher incidence of all neurodevelopmental disabilities than that reported for full-term infants, most preterm infants are free of major disability (cerebral palsy or mental retardation) (see Table 67–3). In a meta-analysis of 110 studies published between 1960 and 1990, the median incidence of cerebral palsy in VLBW infants was 7.7%, with a range of 0% to 50% (Escobar et al, 1991). Despite ongoing improvements in preterm survival, recent studies have not shown a consistent decrease: the prevalence for cerebral palsy has been 5% to 17% for infants with birth weights below 1000 g, 4% to 14% for infants with birth weights below 1500 g, 0.8% to 1.4% for infants with birth weights of 1500 to 2499 g, and 0.04% to 0.14% for infants with birth weights above 2500 g (Amiel-Tison et al, 2002; Bracewell and Marlow, 2002; Vohr et al, 2000).

One difficulty with reporting the incidence of cerebral palsy in these studies is variability in definition of cerebral palsy. The most common type of cerebral palsy in VLBW children is spastic diplegia, and it is frequently mild. There is no uniform agreement on whether the child with tight heel cords and hyperreflexia who toe-walks initially but walks independently by age 2 should be classified as having cerebral palsy (versus mild motor impairment, called here *minor neuromotor dysfunction*). Although some children require physical therapy and/or bracing (frequently, ankle-foot orthoses [AFOs]), the school and behavioral problems for which they are at higher risk may be far more devastating than their mild motor impairments (Bracewell and Marlow, 2002; Dammann et al, 1996; Khadilkar et al, 1993; Scottish Low Birthweight Study Group, 1992; Weisglas-Kuperus et al, 1994). Mild motor impairments at school age include asymmetries of leg or hand function and difficulties with balance, motor planning, and fine motor function.

Populations of preterm children demonstrate a normal range of intelligence, but VLBW and ELBW children tend to have mean IQs that are 4 to 10 points (or 0.3 to 0.6 standard deviation) below those of term children, even after adjustment for socioeconomic status and race (Aylward, 2002; Bhutta et al, 2002; Ornstein et al, 1991). The significance of a lower mean IQ is in the greater proportion of children with mental retardation, borderline intelligence, and low average intelligence who have difficulties

TABLE 67–3

**Neurodevelopmental Disability in Preterm Children**

| Study | Follow-up Age* | Follow-up No. | Cerebral Palsy (%) | Mental Retardation (%) | Hearing Loss (%) | Visual Impairment (%) | Learning Disability† (%) |
|---|---|---|---|---|---|---|---|
| **Gestational Age <33 wk** | | | | | | | |
| Roth et al, 1993 | 7-10 | 206 | 6 | 6 | 4 | 1 | 5 |
| Gross et al, 1992 | 4 | 125 | 9 | 9 | 1 | 1 | — |
| **Gestational Age <28 wk** | | | | | | | |
| Msall et al, 1992 | 4.4 | 149 | 9 | 15 | 0 | 1 | 51 |
| **Gestational Age <26 wk** | | | | | | | |
| Emsley, 1998 | 2-10 | 64 | 19 | 14 | 5 | 13 | 5 |
| **Birth Weight <1750 g** | | | | | | | |
| SLBSG, 1992 | 4.5 | 611 | 5 | — | 2 | 1 | — |
| **Birth Weight ≤1500 g** | | | | | | | |
| Zeben-van der Aa, 1989 | 2 | 944 | 6 | 6 | 0.1 | 0.1 | — |
| Grogaard et al, 1990 | 1.5 | 462 | 7.6 | 6.5 | 5.4 | 5.5 | — |
| Ross et al, 1991 | 7-8 | 88 | 14 | 8 | 1 | — | 48 |
| Hall et al, 1995 | 8 | 324 | — | — | — | — | |
| Ericson, 1998 | 18-19 | 260 | 7 | 2 | 7 | 15 | 65‡ |
| Hack, 2002 | 20 | 242 | 6 | 7 | 1 | 2 | 40 |
| **Birth Weight ≤1250 g** | | | | | | | |
| Thompson et al, 1993 | 2 | 96 | 6 | 4 | ?1 | 0 | — |
| Aziz et al, 1995 | 1 | 646 | 9 | 5 | 1 | 3 | — |
| Robertson et al, 1994 | 1 | 163 | 7 | 2 | 1 | 1 | — |
| **Brith Weight ≤1000 g** | | | | | | | |
| VICSG, 1991 | 8 | 88 | 9 | — | 6 | 11 | 23 |
| Teplin et al, 1991 | 6 | 28 | 11 | 14 | 7 | 12 | — |
| SMSG, 1994 | 2 | 429 | 9 | — | — | 4 | — |
| Halsey, 1996 | 7 | 54 | 9 | 6 | — | 2 | 50 |
| Saigal, 2000 | 12-16 | 150 | 13 | 22.5 | 1 | 9 | 58 |
| Vohr, 2000 | 1.5 | 1151 | 17 | 37 | 11 | 9 | — |
| **Birth Weight ≤750 g** | | | | | | | |
| Hack, 1996 | 1.7 | 114 | 10 | 20 | 6 | 2 | — |
| Hack, 2000a | 14 | 59 | — | — | 7 | 31 | 47 |

*Age in years at time of follow-up.

†Learning disability, required special education, or failed grade(s).

‡Completed less than 3 years of "gymnasium" (comparable with senior high school); this figure is higher than expected, by 15% (Ericson and Kallen, 1998).

SLBSG, Scottish Low Birthweight Study Group; SMSG, Survanta Multidose Study Group; VICSG, Victorian Infant Collaborative Study Group.

functioning at school and in society. Many VLBW and ELBW children with normal IQ scores have problems with attention, memory, complex verbal processing, visual-perceptual abilities, and/or executive function that interfere with school performance.

Preterm infants with lower birth weights or gestational ages have lower IQ scores and a higher incidence of neurodevelopmental disabilities (Aylward, 2002; Bhutta et al, 2002; Vohr et al, 2000). This is especially true for infants born at the lower limit of viability (see Table 67–4). Using birth weight criteria, the prevalence of disability in survivors ranges from 22% to 51% for ILBW infants with birth weights below 750 to 800 g and is as high as 69% for infants with birth weights below 500 g. Using gestational age criteria, the prevalence of disability in survivors ranges from 46% to 68% for infants born before 26 weeks of gestation and from 58% to 67% for infants born at 23 weeks of gestation. Cerebral palsy rates are a bit higher than in VLBW, ELBW, and more mature preterm infants. Cognitive impairment appears to be much more common in infants born at the lower limit of viability. Mental retardation occurs in 15% to 48% of ILBW infants and in 13% to 20% of preterm infants born before 26 weeks of gestation. Prevalence of borderline intelligence, when reported, ranges from 11% to 31%. Among children with birth weights of 500 g or less, or those born at or before 23 weeks of gestation, only 31% to 50% are normal when evaluated in the first few years. We expect that the prevalence of disabilities will increase further if these children are studied at later ages. Although survival has improved dramatically for these infants, disability rates have changed very little (Lorenz et al, 1998).

**TABLE 67–4**

**Neurodevelopmental Disability in Incredibly Low-Birth-Weight Children**

| Study | Follow-up Age* | Follow-up No. | Birth Years† | CP (%) | MR (%) | BIQ (%) | Deaf (%) | Blind (%) | Normal (%) |
|---|---|---|---|---|---|---|---|---|---|
| **Birth Weight 800 g** | | | | | | | | | |
| Hoffman et al, 1990 | 0.5-4 | 38 | 83-85 | 0 | — | 29 | — | — | 50 |
| LaPine et al, 1995 | 0.3-4 | 78 | 86-90 | — | — | — | 1 | 5 | 78 |
| Perlman et al, 1995 | 1.5 | 120 | 80-89 | 7 | 10 | — | 4 | 13 | 70 |
| O'Shea, 1997 | 1 | 61 | 84-89 | 20 | 20 | — | — | 0 | 72 |
| O'Shea, 1997 | 1 | 124 | 89-94 | 7 | 14 | — | — | 4 | 79 |
| Yeo, 1998 | 1.5 | 128 | 80-89 | — | — | — | 4 | 12 | — |
| Finnstrom, 1998 | 3 | | 118 | 90-92 | 8 | — | — | — | — |
| **Birth Weight 750 g** | | | | | | | | | |
| Ferrara et al, 1991 | 1 | 32 | 88-89 | 3 | — | — | — | 9 | 59 |
| Hack et al, 1994 | 6.7 | 68 | 82-86 | 9 | 21 | 29 | 1.5 | 6 | 50 |
| Robertson et al, 1994 | 2-3 | 63 | 90 | 5 | 15 | — | 5 | 10 | — |
| Hack, 1996 | 1.7 | 49 | 90-92 | 10 | 20 | — | 6 | 2 | 69 |
| Hack, 1999 | 1.7 | 43 | 93-95 | 16 | 48 | 18 | 10 | 2 | 49 |
| **Birth Weight ≤500 g** | | | | | | | | | |
| Sauve, 1998 | 1-3 | 13 | 83-94 | 38 | 61 | — | 8 | 15 | 31 |
| Vohr, 2000 | 1.5 | 14 | 93-94 | 29 | 31 | 15 | 7 | 21 | — |
| **Gestational Age <28 wk** | | | | | | | | | |
| Msall et al, 1992 | 4.4 | 153 | 83-86 | 5 | 10 | — | — | 1 | 24 |
| Doyle, 2001 | 5 | 221 | 91-92 | 11 | 15 | — | 1 | 2 | 82 |
| **GestationalAge <26-27 wk** | | | | | | | | | |
| Whyte et al, 1993 | 2 | 322 | 92-87 | 16 | 13 | 15 | 3 | 7 | 61 |
| Synnes et al, 1994 | 1.5 | 129 | 83-89 | 26 | 15 | — | 3 | 15 | 64 |
| Emsley, 1998 | 3-10 | 24 | 84-89 | 21 | 13 | — | 8 | 4 | 62 |
| Emsley, 1998 | 2-6 | 40 | 90-94 | 18 | 15 | — | 3 | 18 | 32 |
| Wood, 2000 | 2.5 | 283 | 95 | 18 | 19 | 11 | 3 | 2 | 49 |
| **Gestational Age <25 wk** | | | | | | | | | |
| Whyte et al, 1993 | 2 | 61 | 82-87 | 15‡ | 20 | — | 10 | 21 | 43 |
| Synnes et al, 1994 | 1.5 | 52 | 83-89 | 33 | 19 | — | 4 | 12 | 58 |
| Finnstrom, 1998 | 3 | 28 | 90-92 | 14 | — | — | — | — | 86 |
| **Gestational Age 23 wk** | | | | | | | | | |
| Whyte et al, 1993 | 2 | 12 | 82-87 | 16 | 8 | — | 0 | 11 | 50 |
| Synnes et al, 1994 | 1.5 | 9 | 83-89 | 33 | 11 | — | 0 | 22 | 33 |
| Wood, 2000 | 2.5 | 26 | 95 | 16 | 27 | 31 | — | — | 42 |

*Follow-up age: age at follow-up examination, either range or mean age at follow-up when range not given.

†Birth years: years during which study samples were born (e.g., 1974-1977).

‡Only severe cerebral palsy was reported.

BIQ, borderline intelligence [quotient]: with developmental or intelligence quotient 68-70 or 80-85, respectively; CP, cerebral palsy: sometimes reported as severe neurologic impairment; ILBW, incredibly low-birth-weight; MR, mental retardation: with developmental or intelligence quotient <68-70.

Any attempt to evaluate and predict outcomes at the lower limit of viability must take into account perinatal management strategies. Considerable variability exists in perceptions of viability, and in treatment strategies regarding mode of delivery, delivery room resuscitation, and initiation of neonatal intensive care. A study by Lorenz and colleagues (2001) compared outcomes in two regions in which systematically different management approaches were used. Infants born at 23 to 26 weeks of gestation in three counties of New Jersey were aggressively managed at birth, whereas the approach in the Netherlands focused on tocolysis and prevention of prematurity. In the Netherlands, infants born at 23 to 26 weeks of gestation were less likely to be delivered by cesarean section or offered neonatal intensive care (and intensive care was withdrawn in 20%). The more aggressive resuscitation approach resulted in 24.1 additional survivors and 7.2 cases of disabling cerebral palsy and required 1372 additional ventilator days per 100 live births.

Universal agreement is lacking about what role parents should play in these complex decisions, and about whether efforts to lower the limit of viability further should continue.

Clearly, these patients require a great deal of resources, not only at birth and in the neonatal period but also throughout infancy and childhood and even into adulthood. A more compelling goal would be to develop strategies that improve quality of life for them and their families.

### Sensory Impairments

Retinopathy of prematurity continues to be a cause of severe visual impairment, especially in the most immature and smallest preterm infants (see Tables 67–3 and 67–4). Myopia and strabismus are common in preterm infants and generally necessitate intervention. The incidence of hearing impairment in very preterm infants ranges from 1% to 11%, depending on the population and definitions used. Hearing impairment is important to diagnose as early as possible, before language acquisition. Many states have implemented universal hearing screening; all preterm NICU infants should have their hearing screened in the neonatal period.

### Function at School Age

Most (95%) VLBW children attend regular schools, but 10% to 48% of VLBW children and 20% to 50% of ELBW children have diagnosed learning disabilities, require special education, or fail grades (see Table 67–3). Despite normal intelligence, children with learning disabilities may have difficulties in processing complex language, in perceiving or copying symbols, or with the fine motor control involved in drawing and writing. When compared with full-term control subjects, VLBW, ELBW, and ILBW children have higher incidences of minor neuromotor dysfunction, language delay, visual-perceptual problems, reading disability, difficulties with arithmetic, and behavioral problems. These differences persist even when only preterm children with normal intelligence and no neurologic impairments are included in the data analysis (Grunau et al, 2002; Saigal et al, 2000). ILBW children had worse language processing, gross motor function, visual motor abilities, attention, academic achievement, behavior, and social skills than children with birth weight 750 to 1499 g or full-term controls (Hack et al, 1994; Saigal et al, 2000). There is no doubt that preterm children have more school difficulties and require more special education than is documented for full-term children from similar socioeconomic environments.

Visual-perceptual abnormalities, sensorimotor integration problems, and minor neuromotor dysfunction are often striking findings in preschool and school-age preterm children (Aylward, 2002; Bracewell and Marlow, 2002; Dammann et al, 1996; Drillien et al, 1980; Khadilkar et al, 1993; Roth et al, 2001; Saigal et al, 2000; Weisglas-Kuperus et al, 1994). Many preterm children have initial motor delays and persistent mild abnormalities on examination, including asymmetries, tight heel cords, and trunk and upper extremity hypotonia consistent with minor neuromotor dysfunction. Children who have neuromotor abnormalities during the first 1 to 2 years but do not develop cerebral palsy (called *transient dystonia* by Drillien and colleagues) have a high incidence of associated school and behavioral problems. In addition, subtle residual motor impairments can lead to day-to-day problems, including difficulties in dressing, cutting with scissors, using playground equipment, and writing. Difficulty in processing complex language makes it more difficult for a child to comprehend and follow school lessons or even directions. Preterm children have a higher incidence of attention deficit disorder and behavioral problems, which can further interfere with school functioning and interpersonal relationships. These and other functional impairments often are not adequately appreciated in preterm outcome studies, unless specifically looked for (Msall and Tremont, 2002). Studies of preterm adults continue to demonstrate a higher rate of impairments, lower IQ scores, and poorer academic achievement (Ericson and Kallen, 1998; Hack et al, 2002).

All of these subtle CNS abnormalities can have a devastating impact on self-esteem, peer relationships, and school performance. The goal of early recognition and intervention is to help the child to become more functional in his or her daily life. Alerting parents, teachers, and friends about a child's difficulties and frustrations, and the impact of these on the child's self-esteem, allows them to provide a more supportive environment. By helping to maintain a child's self-esteem and improving the child's ability to cope with the demands of school and playground, many secondary social and emotional problems can be prevented or ameliorated. Hack and colleagues (2002) found lower rates of drug and alcohol abuse, police contact, and pregnancy in preterm adults compared with full-term peers and raised the question of whether they have a closer and more supportive relationship with their parents.

## Small-for-Gestational-Age Infants

The term *small for gestational age* is an arbitrary classification that refers to an infant whose intrauterine growth is less than expected for gestational age at birth. It is, in fact, a heterogeneous category, with a wide range of causes, risk of perinatal complications, and outcomes (Allen, 1992). Small size at birth may be due to parental (especially maternal) small size; insult or injury to the fetus; fetal maldevelopment; or deprivation of supply of oxygen or nutrients due to placental insufficiency, maternal ingestion (e.g., cigarettes, alcohol, narcotics), or maternal illness. Magnitude of risk for death, perinatal complications, and neurodevelopmental disability varies with the cause of the intrauterine growth restriction (IUGR), the timing of the insult (if any), and the perinatal complications that the child encounters.

The small-for-gestational-age (SGA) infant whose mother is small is likely to be only mildly growth restricted and have no increased risk. With trisomy 18, poor fetal growth early in pregnancy is likely, with death within the first several months, or the affected child will develop multiple severe neurodevelopmental disabilities. The SGA infant with fetal alcohol syndrome has prenatal and postnatal growth deficiencies and an increased risk of congenital anomalies (e.g., characteristic facies, joint anomalies, ventricular septal defect) and CNS dysfunction (e.g., mild to moderate mental retardation, tremors, fine motor incoordination, hyperactivity). Uteroplacental insufficiency often manifests later in pregnancy (after 27 or 28 weeks of gestation) and often causes asymmetrical growth restriction with sparing of head growth. IUGR from uteroplacental insufficiency can be viewed as an adaptation to restricted supply of nutrients. Although it may be an effective human adaptation to adverse intrauterine circumstances, there are consequences to this strategy: increased risk of perinatal complications that can affect survival and outcome (e.g., perinatal asphyxia, hypoglycemia), of hypertension later in life, of short stature, and of disability (Allen, 1992; Hollo et al, 2002; Low et al, 1992; Paz et al, 1995; Pena et al, 1988; Pryor et al, 1995; Strauss, 2000, Wocadlo and Rieger, 1994).

Studies that report developmental outcome of SGA infants generally exclude infants with congenital anomalies, genetic syndromes, or congenital infections. They follow primarily infants with placental insufficiency or unknown cause of IUGR, and they distinguish between the full-term and the preterm SGA infant. Although retrospective studies of children with disability find a higher-than-expected proportion who were SGA infants, prospective studies find only a higher incidence of academic failure (as high as 25% versus 14%) and behavior problems in full-term SGA children than in full-term appropriate-for-gestational age (AGA) children (Hollo et al, 2002; Larroque et al, 2001; Low et al, 1992; Paz et al, 1995). Lower mean IQ scores have been found in some samples of full-term SGA children, but this is not a consistent finding in IUGR infants born to mothers with pregnancy-induced hypertension and in IUGR adults (Goldenberg et al, 1996; McCowan et al, 2002, Paz et al, 1995, 2001; Pryor et al, 1995). Full-term IUGR adolescents and adults report greater disadvantage when it comes to school failures and dropout, job status, and income (Larroque et al, 2001; Paz et al, 1995; Strauss, 2000).

The preterm SGA infant has the disadvantages of both prematurity and IUGR, but it is difficult to determine how much IUGR further increases the preterm infant's risk of neurodevelopmental disability (Pena et al, 1988; Robertson et al, 1990; Thompson et al, 1993; Wocadlo and Rieger, 1994). Preterm SGA infants have more severe IUGR than that noted in full-term SGA infants because they already manifest significant growth restriction at the time of their preterm birth. Most preterm SGA children have normal intelligence, but their mean IQ is lower than that of full-term AGA and SGA children and sometimes even preterm AGA children (depending on whether controls are matched for birth weight or gestational age) (Table 67–5). Major disability occurs in 7% to 23% of preterm SGA children. Learning disabilities occur in 36% to 50% of preterm SGA children at 8 to 11 years, and preterm SGA children are more hyperactive than preterm AGA and full-term controls (Low et al, 1992; Robertson et al, 1990). The most striking finding of these studies is that all preterm groups, whether SGA or AGA, scored worse than full-term control groups on measures of growth, intellectual function, visual-motor integration abilities, reading, arithmetic, and behavior. This finding highlights the importance of long-term follow-up evaluation to school age for children with prematurity or IUGR.

## Sick Full-Term Infants

The full-term infant may require neonatal intensive care for a variety of reasons, including complications of IUGR, perinatal asphyxia, maternal substance abuse, congenital anomalies, or infection. It is most difficult to predict outcome in infants with poorly understood illness: the newborn with sluggish but eventually good response in the delivery room, the newborn who appears septic but has negative culture results, the newborn who does not feed well initially, and others with undefined illness. Under most circumstances, these children will do well, but for some, initial illness may be a sign of a CNS disorder or systemic illness that contributes to abnormal outcome. Maternal drug use, infection, or congenital anomalies may underlie conditions that require neonatal intensive care, thereby adding to risk for disability.

One recurring scenario in the NICU is that of the full-term infant who has either subtle or florid signs of neonatal

**TABLE 67–5**

**Neurodevelopmental Outcome in Preterm Infants Small for Gestational Age (SGA) Versus Appropriate for Gestational Age (AGA)**

| | | | | | AGA Infants Matched for: | | | |
|---|---|---|---|---|---|---|---|---|
| | Follow-up | | SGA Infants | | Birth Weight | | Gestational Age | |
| Study | Age (Years) | No. | MD (%) | DQ/IQ | MD (%) | DQ/IQ | MD (%) | DQ/IQ |
| Pena et al, 1988 | 0.8/1* | 35 | 23 | 88 | 26 | 88 | 5 | 99† |
| Robertson et al, 1990 | 8 | 36 | 17 | 102 | 22 | 102 | 14 | 101 |
| Sung et al, 1993 | 3 | 27 | 7 | 87 | 4 | 82 | 26 | 102† |
| Wocadlo and Rieger, 1994 | 1 | 18 | 22 | — | 22 | — | — | — |
| Amin, 1997 | 3 | 52 | 15 | 95 | 15 | 94 | 16 | 98 |

*0.8/1: DQ at 40 weeks from term: neurologic outcome determined at 1 year from term.

†Significantly different from SGA infants, at least at $P < .05$ level.

MD, major disability or neurologic impairment, as defined by authors; generally cerebral palsy and mental retardation and occasionally includes severe sensory impairment.

DQ/IQ, mean developmental quotient (DQ) or intelligence quotient (IQ).

encephalopathy (see Chapter 64). Increasing attention to the difficulties of defining encephalopathy has led to an appreciation of the complexities of determining causes, effects, and outcomes (Dixon et al, 2002; Ekert et al, 1997; Ishikawa et al, 1987; Jongeling et al, 2002; Leviton and Nelson, 1992; Mercuri et al, 1999; Nelson and Leviton, 1991; Rutherford et al, 1994; Shalak et al, 2003; Thompson et al, 1997). We used the term *hypoxic-ischemic encephalopathy* (HIE) in the past, but this term described the clinical picture of the encephalopathic infant with hyperexcitability or lethargy leading to coma and often neonatal seizures. Thus, "HIE" implied that we knew the cause, but the reality is that many of these infants did not have a clear history of an asphyxiating insult. They may have had low Apgar scores or low cord pH or may have required resuscitation at delivery, but these findings indicate infant response, not the nature of the insult. Accordingly, the more neutral term *neonatal encephalopathy* is preferred.

Severity of neonatal encephalopathy is the best predictor of neurodevelopmental outcome (Dixon et al, 2002; Ekert et al, 1997; Ishikawa et al, 1987; Jongeling et al, 2002; Mercuri et al, 1999; Robertson et al, 1989; Rutherford et al, 1994; Yeo and Tudehope, 1994). Infants with severe encephalopathy die or develop major disabilities. Major disabilities tend to be severe and multiple, including severe mental retardation, spastic quadriplegia or mixed cerebral palsy, microcephaly, seizure disorder, cortical blindness, and/or hearing impairment. Children with moderate encephalopathy have an increased incidence (21% to 46%) of major disabilities. Many without major disabilities have lower scores on tests of intelligence, visual-motor integration, vocabulary, reading, spelling, and arithmetic than such scores achieved by either healthy peers or children with mild encephalopathy. Findings of abnormalities on physical examination, neuroimaging studies (especially magnetic resonance imaging [MRI]), and electroencephalography (EEG) can be helpful in predicting neurodevelopmental outcome for infants with neonatal encephalopathy.

Infants with persistent pulmonary hypertension have a higher risk of major disability (13% to 24%), mild impairments (minor neuromotor dysfunction, borderline intelligence, and attention problems in up to 30%), and hearing impairment (Marron et al, 1992; Walsh-Sukys et al, 1994). The hearing loss can be progressive, which highlights the need for serial audiologic evaluations in addition to neurodevelopmental follow-up evaluation in this population. Likewise, neonates treated with extracorporeal membrane oxygenation (ECMO) have a variety of life-threatening conditions that carry an increased risk of neurodevelopmental disability (Bernbaum et al, 1995; Bulas et al, 1995; Lago et al, 1995; Revenis et al, 1992; Robertson et al, 1995; Stolar et al, 1995). From 2% to 26% of survivors of ECMO develop major disability, and 3% to 21% develop hearing impairment. Mild disability, including borderline intelligence, language delay, visual impairment, and minor neuromotor dysfunction, occurs in 8% to 49%. Glass and colleagues (1995) found that 5-year-old ECMO survivors had an 11% incidence of mental retardation (1% profound mental retardation), 5% cerebral palsy (most had mild cerebral palsy), 2% severe learning disabilities, and a lower mean IQ than that in 37 healthy control children (96 versus 115, $P < .001$). Adverse neurodevelopmental outcome was associated with lower birth weight, sepsis, congenital diaphragmatic hernia, and abnormal findings on neuroimaging studies.

Infants with congenital anomalies have an increased risk of neurodevelopmental disability. Children with hypoplastic left heart syndrome, for example, can have cognitive, adaptive and behavioral abnormalities related to maldevelopment, hypoxia/ischemia, and a prolonged circulatory arrest time during cardiac surgery (Ikle et al, 2003; Kern et al, 1998; Rogers et al, 1995). Much more research is needed to understand the scope of neurodevelopmental deficits in NICU infants with these and other congenital anomalies.

## HEALTH AND GROWTH

Although NICU infants are much improved at the time of discharge, many have lingering medical problems that require close follow-up evaluation by their primary care providers. They remain vulnerable to infections, further complications, difficulty feeding, and poor growth. Rehospitalization for illness (especially respiratory illness) or surgery (e.g., umbilical hernia repair, gastrostomy, Nissen fundoplication) is common (Combs-Orme et al, 1988; Lefebvre et al, 1988; Survanta Multidose Study Group, 1994; Teplin et al, 1991).

Adequate nutrition is essential for growth of the developing infant, especially for brain growth. Good weight gain, linear growth, and head growth are good measures of nutrition. Preterm infants are frequently below the 5th percentile for chronologic age, but they should grow along their own parallel curve, and some growth curves specific to LBW infants have been developed (Casey et al, 1991). Although most infants catch up in their growth within several years, some infants with extreme prematurity, IUGR, severe neonatal illness, or syndromes such as fetal alcohol syndrome always remain small for their age.

Infants who exhibit significant deviation below normal on growth curves should be evaluated for undetected or inadequately treated gastrointestinal, pulmonary, urologic, or cardiac conditions. Gastroesophageal reflux can lead to discomfort from esophagitis, irritability, extensor posturing, and poor growth. Some children with genetic syndromes or who were critically ill as newborns demonstrate decreased appetite, food refusal, and poor growth. Oromotor dysfunction, with poorly coordinated suck and swallow, must be considered in NICU newborns with poor growth, food refusal behaviors, or neurologic abnormalities. Infants with chronic lung disease or congestive heart failure may tire with feedings and require frequent interruptions because of exercise intolerance.

An oromotor evaluation by an occupational therapist or speech pathologist may include a radiographic swallow study to pinpoint the problem, to determine if oral feeding is safe, and to assess how the infant handles liquids versus solid foods. The cause of the feeding problem determines treatment: positioning, thickening liquids, medications, and possibly surgery for infants with gastroesophageal reflux; calorically dense food for poor appetite and growth; behavior management program for food refusal behavior not due to organic causes; supplemental oxygen for children with intermittent hypoxia; and gastrostomy for children who chronically aspirate, have severe oromotor dysfunction, or demonstrate food refusal unresponsive to behavioral interventions. Children fed totally or primarily by gastrostomy require an oromotor stimulation program to maintain feeding skills and prevent oromotor hypersensitivity. When NICU infants are discharged with gastrostomy, continuous feedings, special formulas, or dietary supplements, they require specific nutritional or gastrointestinal follow-up evaluation to address changing needs and parental concerns.

Chronic lung disease (i.e., bronchopulmonary dysplasia) occurs in 11% to 40% of VLBW preterm infants, 7% to 9% of more mature preterm infants, 7% to 35% of full-term infants with persistent pulmonary hypertension, 15% to 40% of infants treated with ECMO, and 63% of infants with congenital diaphragmatic hernia (Bernbaum et al, 1995; Ferrara et al, 1991; Glass et al, 1995; Hack et al, 1994; Revenis et al, 1992; Survanta Multidose Study Group, 1994; Walsh-Sukys et al, 1994). These children are vulnerable to respiratory infections, and they frequently require bronchodilators, oxygen supplement, or diuretics. The experienced clinician uses clinical history, physical examination, evidence of growth, signs of exercise intolerance, and pulse oximetry (especially during feeding and sleep) in making decisions regarding tapering oxygen supplements and diuretics. Infants who are well oxygenated at rest may be relying on their reserves and have difficulties when nipple feeding or sleeping. Some infants with chronic lung disease have transient increases in oxygen requirements during periods of accelerated growth.

Developmental interventions for medically fragile infants should be home based whenever possible to reduce the risks of infection. Infants should be shielded from friends and family with infectious illnesses. Therapists who provide early intervention should be skilled in working with these infants, should recognize the signs of exercise intolerance or increasing distress, and should be trained in how to respond promptly in an emergency (e.g., cardiopulmonary resuscitation training). Infants on supplemental oxygen may need an increase in oxygen when handled.

Preterm infants and other high-risk infants need the protection from childhood illnesses that is conferred by immunization. Immunizations should be given according to the recommended schedule (Saari et al, 2003). Even in extremely preterm infants, full doses appropriate for chronologic age should be used. Infants who are still in the NICU or who are immunocompromised (or whose family includes an immunocompromised person) should not be given live viral vaccines. Pertussis protection should be deferred only for infants with signs of neurologic deterioration or uncontrolled seizure disorder, although it may be postponed pending diagnostic evaluation in a child with recent onset of seizures.

## FOLLOW-UP EVALUATION OF THE HIGH-RISK INFANT

The high-risk NICU infant's medical problems, increased risk of neurodevelopmental disability, and uncertainty regarding outcome necessitate long-term follow-up evaluation.

### Importance of Discharge Planning

Good discharge planning aims to smooth the infant's transition from hospital to home and to provide the health care, developmental, and parental supports needed by the infant and family. A parent conference that reviews the infant's hospital course and plans for discharge provides an opportunity to discuss the infant's risk status, to assess the parent's understanding, to appreciate the infant's progress, and to begin to make plans for discharge home. In the review of the infant's various risk factors, an honest but sensitive discussion puts the infant's risk for neurodevelopmental disabilities into perspective, giving the range of possible outcomes. Parents should be reassured whenever possible, given the opportunity to hope, and provided with perspective on their infant's risks.

Discharge teaching includes well-baby care (for first-time parents); techniques of cardiopulmonary resuscitation (useful for all parents); use of any special equipment or medication; and recommendations regarding infant car seats, bedding, feeding, positioning, and handling. Plans for follow-up care after hospital discharge should address both the infant's and the family's special needs. All infants discharged from a NICU should have a designated primary care provider who can follow the infant closely and address the infant's special needs as they emerge. Preterm infants with retinopathy of prematurity, incompletely vascularized retinas, congenital infection, or cortical abnormalities require ophthalmologic follow-up evaluation. Infants who failed or did not receive audiologic screening require audiologic follow-up evaluation. Infants with specific medical conditions may require pediatric surgical, pulmonary, gastrointestinal, nutritional, cardiologic, neurologic, orthopedic, or other subspecialty follow-up evaluations.

### Comprehensive Developmental Follow-up Evaluation

Criteria for referral of high-risk NICU infants for comprehensive developmental follow-up vary widely, based on available resources, funding, geography, and family needs. Ideally, all NICU infants should be viewed as high risk and offered comprehensive developmental follow-up evaluations through school age. Incentives for families to return for follow-up evaluations encourage high follow-up rates, thereby providing NICUs with accurate outcome data for specific conditions. Close relationships between a NICU follow-up clinic and community health, educational, and social services promote coordination of intervention services based on the child's and family's needs. Limited resources and funding, organizational difficulties, and time constraints all interfere with ideal comprehensive, coordinated, family-focused follow-up and intervention efforts. Although often considered dispensable, developmental follow-up evaluations and early intervention should be viewed as an essential part of the continuum of care provided to high-risk infants and their families.

The goals of comprehensive, coordinated developmental follow-up are to help the family optimize the child's growth and development; to help integrate the child into the family, school, and community; and to intervene when possible to reduce future medical, social, and emotional costs. These goals are promoted by the recognition that each child is an individual with unique qualities, strengths, impairments, and abilities, and that each family differs in background, social supports, finances, and personal coping mechanisms.

Follow-up is a dynamic process that evolves as the child grows, develops, and increasingly interacts with his or her environment. Recognition of impairments, disabilities, and handicaps relies on parental reports, an appreciation of individual variability in the normal pattern of development over time, and the examiner's assessment skills and ability to determine the significance of abnormalities or deviations from the normal pattern. Once recognized, problems should be discussed with parents, including a nonmedical definition of specific diagnoses (e.g., cerebral palsy, learning disability) and identification of specific intervention strategies.

Assessing the development of the high-risk infant relies on the basic tools of medicine: the history and the physical examination. The focus of the developmental history is to obtain information about the infant's behavior (e.g., sleep, feeding, temperament, behavior problems) and developmental milestone acquisition. The physical examination is expanded to a neurodevelopmental examination that includes an assessment of posture, muscle tone, reflexes, and functional abilities.

The developmental milestones should be viewed in terms of the major streams of development: gross motor, fine motor, adaptive, and language abilities (Tables 67–6 and 67–7). Gross and fine motor abilities are used to assess motor development and to screen for cerebral palsy and minor neuromotor dysfunction. Children with cerebral palsy generally have significant motor delay and persistent neuromotor abnormalities. Children with minor neuromotor dysfunction have milder or no delay and mild neuromotor abnormalities on examination. Delay in adaptive, or self-help, skills may be seen with mental retardation, cerebral palsy, minor neuromotor dysfunction, or environmental or behavioral causes (e.g., the child's mother did not introduce a fork or took it away). Delay in language abilities can signal mental retardation, hearing impairment, or language disorder and requires an audiologic evaluation.

Assessing milestone acquisition in preterm infants raises the controversial question of whether to correct for the degree of prematurity. This issue is most important early in life and in extremely preterm infants. Consider

**TABLE 67–6**

**Gross and Fine Motor Milestone Attainment**

| Milestone | Motor Milestone Attainment (in months) | |
|---|---|---|
| | **Mean Age*** | **Delay Criterion†** |
| **Gross Motor Abilities** | | |
| Roll over prone to supine | 3.6 | 5.5 |
| Roll over supine to prone | 4.8 | 7.25 |
| Sit with arm support‡ | 5.3 | 8.0 |
| Sit without arm support§ | 6.3 | 9.5 |
| Creep‖ | 6.7 | 10.25 |
| Come to sit¶ | 7.5 | 11.25 |
| Crawl** | 7.8 | 11.75 |
| Pull to stand on furniture | 8.1 | 12.25 |
| Cruise†† | 8.8 | 13.25 |
| Walk independently | 11.7 | 17.25 |
| Walk backwards | 14.3 | |
| Run | 14.8 | |
| **Fine Motor Abilities** | | |
| Unfisted | 3 | |
| Brings hands to midline | 3 | |
| Unilateral reach and grasp | 4 | |
| Transfers object from hand to hand | 5 | |
| Raking grasp | 6 | |
| Three-finger grasp (picks up pellets) | 8 | |
| Mature pincer grasp | 11 | |
| Good voluntary release | 12 | |

*Gross motor milestone mean ages of attainment from a longitudinal study of 381 normal full-term children, followed from birth to 2 years (Capute et al, 1985).

†Delay criteria from Allen and Alexander, 1994.

‡*Sit with arm support* uses arms to maintain balance in sitting but not propped up with pillows.

§*Sit without arm support* means good independent sitting, without using arms for balance.

‖*Creep* means pulling self forward on abdomen, using arms and legs for propulsion.

¶*Come to sit* means independently getting into a sitting position from supine or prone, without pulling up on furniture.

***Crawl* means good reciprocal crawl, up on hands and knees.

††*Cruise* means walking holding onto furniture.

**TABLE 67–7**

**Language Milestone Attainment**

| Milestone | Milestone Attainment: Mean Age (mo) | Standard Deviation |
|---|---|---|
| Alert to sound* | 0.25 | 0.3 |
| Social smile* | 1.2 | 0.5 |
| Coo (musical vowel sounds) | 1.5 | 0.6 |
| Orient (turn) to voice* | 2.8 | 1.2 |
| Say "ah-goo" | 4.0 | 1.6 |
| Make raspberry (razz, "Bronx cheer") | 4.4 | 1.6 |
| Babble (repetitive consonant sound) | 6.3 | 1.4 |
| "Mama"/"Dada" indiscriminately | 7.7 | 1.7 |
| Gesture language (e.g., peekaboo)* | 8.6 | 1.5 |
| "Dada" discriminately | 10.5 | 2.5 |
| "Mama" discriminately | 11.1 | 2.7 |
| Follow one-step command with gesture* | 11.1 | 1.7 |
| First meaningful word (not a name) | 11.3 | 2.3 |
| Immature jargon (no words) | 12.2 | 2.1 |
| Second meaningful word (no names) | 12.4 | 2.2 |
| Third meaningful word (no names) | 13.2 | 2.2 |
| Follow one-step command without gesture* | 13.6 | 2.1 |
| Use four to six words (not including names) | 14.7 | 2.5 |
| Mature jargon (includes words) | 16.5 | 2.9 |
| Point to five body parts when asked* | 16.7 | 2.8 |
| Use 7- to 10-word vocabulary | 16.9 | 2.9 |
| Use novel two-word combinations | 19.2 | 3.0 |
| Use two- to three-word sentences | 20.9 | 3.0 |
| Use 50-word vocabulary | 20.9 | 3.2 |

*Receptive language milestones; the remainder are expressive language milestones.

Data from Clinical Linguistic and Auditory Milestone Scale (CLAMS), Capute and Accardo (1978), and Capute et al (1986a).

the following example: An infant born at 27 weeks of gestation is now 6 months old and not yet rolling over but plays with her hands in midline, and can support herself on her forearms in prone position (see Table 67–6). Her motor quotient (i.e., developmental age divided by chronologic age) is 50 (i.e., 50% of normal—therefore delayed). If one corrects for degree of prematurity (using her term age equivalent/adjusted age/corrected age), her motor quotient is 100 (i.e., normal). Her developmental status at this age is determined by whether one corrects for degree of prematurity. At 5 years, correction is no longer important, because children between 57 and 60 months of age do not significantly differ.

When considering correction for degree of prematurity, the clinician should evaluate each stream of development separately because they may differ in responsiveness to environmental stimulation. Earlier exposure to the extrauterine environment may have greater effect on the development of language than on motor development. Language, a component of cognition, may be accelerated by early extrauterine experience (Eilers et al, 1993).

Traditionally, psychologists do correct for degree of prematurity in preterm infants when assessing cognition. They do not agree on full versus partial correction or on how long to correct: for 1 year, 2 years, or indefinitely (Allen, 2002; Aylward, 2002). There is some concern that correcting for degree of prematurity overestimates a child's cognitive abilities and may fail to identify those infants who would benefit from early intervention (Den Ouden et al, 1991; Thompson et al, 1993). Nevertheless, most agree to correct for degree of prematurity for at least 2 years. This issue is important early in infancy and with the most immature infants, but it influences outcomes until 8.5 years (Rickards et al, 1989). Preterm children with language or cognitive abilities consistently below their age corrected for degree of prematurity should be referred for multidisciplinary evaluation and early intervention.

Using age at attainment of the motor milestones is a quick, practical, and inexpensive method of identifying infants at highest risk of having cerebral palsy (Allen and Alexander, 1994, 1997). It is most effective when a history of motor milestone attainment is obtained at each child care visit, when correction for degree of prematurity is done, and when 50% delay criteria are used (see Table 67–7). Infants identified as demonstrating motor delay warrant a comprehensive neurodevelopmental examination, multidisciplinary evaluation, and often referral for physical and occupational therapy.

Language assessments such as the Clinical Linguistic and Auditory Milestone Scale (CLAMS) (see Table 67–7) can be used to follow language development and to screen for cognitive delays (Capute and Accardo, 1978; Capute et al, 1986a, 1986b; Rossman et al, 1994; Wachtel et al, 1994). Infants identified as having language delays should then be referred for both hearing assessment and neuropsychological testing. Many follow-up clinics rely on neuropsychologists to assess the cognition of high-risk infants, either with sequential assessments or with one or two carefully timed assessments (e.g., at 12, 18, or 24 months). A number of frequently used cognitive tests developed for use in infants and children are listed in Table 67–8.

## Referral for Multidisciplinary Evaluation and Early Intervention Services

Infants with identified developmental delays should be referred for a multidisciplinary evaluation that assesses all aspects of development. Brain injury is more likely to be diffuse than focal, and more than one stream of development may be affected. Although the most obvious abnormality is identified first, this may not be the most disabling of the child's problems. A preterm infant who presents with delayed walking and tight heel cords may be diagnosed with mild spastic diplegia. This child has an excellent prognosis for walking, running, and good motor function. Problems associated with cerebral palsy (e.g., learning disability, myopia, attention deficit) may have far more impact on the child's quality of life and adult functioning than will the presenting motor impairment.

Part H of Public Law (PL) 99-157 passed by the U.S. Congress in 1986, followed by the Individuals with Disabilities Education Act (IDEA, PL 101-476 and PL 102-119) in 1990, encouraged and then required states to provide a comprehensive, coordinated interagency system of early intervention services for infants and toddlers with developmental delays and with conditions that lead to developmental delays (e.g., Down syndrome, fetal alcohol syndrome). Some states also provide services for high-risk infants and their families. Infants may be referred by NICUs, NICU follow-up clinics, pediatricians, or families. Each child who is referred is entitled to a multidisciplinary assessment and a service coordinator to help coordinate the assessment and services. If the child is eligible for the program, the parents, service coordinator, and multidisciplinary team devise an individualized family service plan (IFSP) that identifies the child's and family's needs and what services will be used to address these needs. This program recognizes the importance of (1) viewing each child as a unique individual, (2) evaluating not only needs but also strengths, (3) including the family in the planning process, and (4) coordinating all intervention services.

Early intervention strategies minimize secondary complications and provide much-needed parental support in coping with disability or uncertainty. The choice of interventions is determined by the individual child's developmental profile and health, the needs of the family, and available resources. Programs or services that enable the family to meet the child's needs better (e.g., drug counseling, transportation, parent support groups) also are identified.

Although a number of studies have demonstrated beneficial effects of early intervention programs, there is no proof that early intervention prevents neurodevelopmental disability (Achenbach et al, 1993; Bennett and Guralnick, 1991; Brooks-Gunn et al, 1994; Infant Health and Developmental Program, 1990; Palmer et al, 1988; Piper et al, 1986; Ramey et al, 1992; Rothberg et al, 1991). One difficulty lies with the use of the global term *early intervention*, which covers many different intervention strategies. Early intervention can be as nonspecific as providing social work support and parent classes

**TABLE 67–8**

**Cognitive Tests for Infants and Children**

| Test | Age Range | Score | Reference |
|---|---|---|---|
| Bayley Scales of Infant Development—Second Edition (BSID-II) | 1-42 mo | MDI* | Bayley, 1993 |
| Clinical Adaptive Text/Clinical Linguistic and Auditory Milestone Scale (CAT/CLAMS) | Newborn–35 mo | CAT DQ†<br>CLAMS DQ† | Capute and Accardo, 1978<br>Capute et al, 1986a<br>Wachtel et al, 1994 |
| Gesell Developmental Schedules (Gesell) | 1-36 mo | DQ† | Knoblach et al, 1980 |
| Stanford-Binet Intelligence Scale—Fourth Edition | 2 yr–adult | Composite score | Thorndike et al, 1986 |
| McCarthy Scales of Children's Abilities | 2.5-3.5 yr | GCI‡ | McCarthy, 1972 |
| Kaufman Assessment Battery for Children (K-ABC) | 2.5-12 yr | Composite score | Kaufman |
| Wechsler Preschool and Primary Scale of Intelligence—Revised (WPPSI-R) | 3-7.25 yr | FS IQ VIQ, PIQ§ | Wechsler, 1989 |
| Wechsler Intelligence Scale for Children—Third Edition (WISC-III) | 6-16 yr | FS IQ VIQ, PIQ§ | Wechsler, 1993 |

*MDI, mental developmental index. The Bayley also has a motor and behavior scale.

†DQ, developmental quotient, including both a CLAMS DQ and CAT DQ.

‡GCI, general cognitive index, a composite of the verbal, perceptual/performance, and quantitative scales.

§FS IQ, full-scale intelligence quotient; VIQ, verbal intelligence quotient; PIQ, performance intelligence quotient. The Wechsler tests have 13 subtests that compose its verbal and performance scales, and these two scales are combined to give the full-scale IQ.

on infant development or as specific as a physical therapy intervention aimed at facilitating coming to a sitting position from supine in a child with the prerequisite skills and postural reactions. Early intervention for a child with severe spastic quadriplegia would include recommendations for positioning and handling the child and providing adaptive equipment for sitting, traveling, eating, and communication. Designing good intervention trials that evaluate the efficacy of specific intervention strategies is complicated by the fact that each person is so unique. This makes it difficult to define study sample criteria and outcomes and to match disabled children for randomization.

Nevertheless, each intervention strategy must be evaluated for efficacy in a well-defined population. Both hearing and visual impairments are responsive to early intervention services that can dramatically improve the child's functioning and quality of life, especially if begun early. Infants with severe hearing impairments may benefit from wearing hearing aids, learning to respond to and to use sign language, specific educational interventions using multiple sensory modalities and parental support. Studies have shown that a focused educational intervention for preterm infants has beneficial initial effects on cognition and behavior, although long-term benefits have not been proved (Achenbach et al, 1993; Brooks-Gunn et al, 1994; Infant Health and Developmental Program, 1990; Ramey et al, 1992). Few early intervention studies have evaluated whether there is an effect on function at school or at home. These functional abilities may be not only the most responsive to early intervention but also the most important outcome variables. Studies have been limited to short-term interventions. It stands to reason that most benefit can be derived from long-term, continuous interventions.

## SUMMARY

Although children who required neonatal intensive care have a higher incidence of neurodevelopmental disabilities and health sequelae, most survivors are healthy and function well. The likelihood, type, and severity of disability vary with the condition requiring neonatal intensive care, with various perinatal and demographic risk factors, and perhaps with availability of developmental supports for the child and social supports for the family. It is impossible to diagnose neurodevelopmental disabilities with certainty in the neonatal period. Absence of risk factors and neurologic abnormalities is reassuring. Multiple or severe risk factors can identify infants at high risk for disability.

The uncertainty regarding an infant's outcome and the dynamic nature of early infant and child development necessitate careful medical and developmental follow-up evaluation of high-risk NICU infants during infancy and childhood. Survival is not the only goal of neonatal intensive care. Because the NICU is but the first step in an infant's life, follow-up (or perhaps follow-through) is an important component of the continuum of care that should be offered to high-risk infants. The goals of follow-up are to assist the family to optimize the child's growth and development so that the child is as functional as possible and to help integrate the child into the family, school, and community.

## REFERENCES

Achenbach TM, Howell CT, Aoki MF, et al: Nine-year outcome of the Vermont Intervention Program for Low Birthweight Infants. Pediatrics 91:45, 1993.

Allen MC: Developmental implications of intrauterine growth retardation. Infants Young Child 5:13, 1992.

Allen MC: The high-risk infant. Pediatr Clin North Am 40:479, 1993.

Allen MC: Preterm outcomes research: A critical component of neonatal intensive care. Ment Retard Dev Disabil Res Rev 8:221, 2002.

Allen MC, Alexander GR: Gross motor milestones in preterm infants: Correction for degree of prematurity. J Pediatr 116:955, 1990.

Allen MC, Alexander GR: Using gross motor milestones to identify very-preterm infants at risk for cerebral palsy. Dev Med Child Neurol 34:226, 1992.

Allen MC, Alexander GR: Screening for cerebral palsy in preterm infants: Delay criteria for motor milestone attainment. J Perinatol 14:190, 1994.

Allen MC, Alexander GR: Using motor milestones as a multistep process to screen preterm infants for cerebral palsy. Dev Med Child Neurol 39:12, 1997.

Allen MC, Capute AJ: Neonatal neurodevelopmental examination as a predictor of neuromotor outcome in premature infants. Pediatrics 83:498, 1989.

Allen MC, Donohue PK, Dusman AE: The limit of viability: Neonatal outcome of infants born at 22-25 weeks' gestation. N Engl J Med 329:1597, 1993.

American Academy of Pediatrics: 1994 Red Book: Report of the Committee on Infectious Diseases. Elk Grove Village, Ill, American Academy of Pediatrics, 1994.

Amiel-Tison C, Allen MC, Lebrun F, Rogowski, J: Macropreemies: Underprivileged newborns. Ment Retard Dev Disabil Res Rev 8:281, 2002.

Aylward GP: Cognitive and neuropsychological outcomes: More than IQ scores. Ment Retard Dev Disabil Res Rev 8:234, 2002.

Aylward GP, Pfeiffer SI, Wright A, et al: Outcome studies of low-birth-weight infants published in the last decade: A meta-analysis. J Pediatr 115:515, 1989.

Aziz K, Vickar DB, Sauve RS, et al: Province-based study of neurologic disability of children weighing 500 through 1249 g at birth in relation to neonatal cerebral ultrasound findings. Pediatrics 95:837, 1995.

Bayley N: The Bayley Scales of Infant Development—Second Edition Manual. San Antonio, TX, Psychological Corporation, 1993.

Bennett FC, Robinson NM, Sells CJ: Growth and development of infants weighing less than 800 g at birth. Pediatrics 71:319, 1983.

Bennett RC, Guralnick MJ: Effectiveness of developmental intervention in the first five years of life. Pediatr Clin North Am 38:1513, 1991.

Bernbaum J, Schwartz IP, Gerdes M, et al: Survivors of extracorporeal membrane oxygenation at 1 year of age: The relationship of primary diagnosis with health and neurodevelopmental sequelae. Pediatrics 96:907, 1995.

Bhushan V, Paneth N, Kiely JL: Impact on improved survival of very-low-birth-weight infants on recent secular trends in the prevalence of cerebral palsy. Pediatrics 91:1094, 1993.

Bhutta AT, Cleves MA, Casey PH, et al: Cognitive and behavioral outcomes of school-aged children who were born preterm: A meta-analysis. JAMA 288:728, 2002.

Bifano EM, Pfannenstiel A: Duration of hyperventilation and outcome in infants with persistent pulmonary hypertension. Pediatrics 81:657, 1988.
Blair E, Stanley F: Intrapartum asphyxia: A rare cause of cerebral palsy. J Pediatr 112:515, 1988.
Bracewell M, Marlow N: Patterns of motor disability in very preterm children. Ment Retard Dev Disabil Res Rev 8:241, 2002.
Britton SG, Fitzhardinge PM, Ashby S: Is intensive care justified for infants weighing less than 801 gm at birth? J Pediatr 99:937, 1981.
Brooks-Gunn J, McCarton CM, Casey PH, et al: Early intervention in low-birth-weight premature infants: Results through age 5 years from the Infant Health and Development Program. JAMA 272:1257, 1994.
Buckwald S, Zorn WA, Egan EA: Mortality and follow-up data for neonates weighing 500 to 800 g at birth. Am J Dis Child 138:779, 1984.
Bulas DI, Glass P, O'Donnell RM, et al: Neonates treated with ECMO: Predictive value of early CT and US neuroimaging findings on short-term neurodevelopmental outcome. Radiology 195:407, 1995.
Callanan C, Doyle L, Rickards A, et al: Children followed with difficulty: How do they differ? J Paediatr Child Health 37:152, 2001.
Capute AJ, Accardo PJ: Linguistic and auditory milestones during the first two years of life: A language inventory for the practitioner. Clin Pediatr 17:847, 1978.
Capute AJ, Accardo PJ (eds): Developmental Disabilities in Infancy and Childhood, vols I and II, 2nd ed. Baltimore, Paul H. Brookes Publishing, 1996.
Capute AJ, Palmer FB, Shapiro BK, et al: Clinical Linguistic and Auditory Milestone Scale: Prediction of cognition in infancy. Dev Med Child Neurol 28:762, 1986a.
Capute AJ, Shapiro BK, Palmer FB, et al: Normal gross motor development: The influences of race, sex, and socioeconomic status. Dev Med Child Neurol 27:635, 1985.
Capute AJ, Shapiro BK, Wachtel RC, et al: The Clinical Linguistic and Auditory Milestone Scale (CLAMS): Identification of cognitive defects in motor delayed children. Am J Dis Child 140:694, 1986b.
Casey PH, Kraemer HC, Bernbaum J, et al: Growth status and growth rates of a varied sample of low-birth-weight, preterm infants: A longitudinal cohort from birth to three years of age. J Pediatr 119:599, 1991.
Combs-Orme T, Fishbein J, Summerville C, Evans MG: Rehospitalization of very-low-birth-weight infants. Am J Dis Child 142:1109, 1988.
Cummins SK, Nelson KB, Grether JK, et al: Cerebral palsy in four northern California counties: Births 1983 through 1985. J Pediatr 123:230, 1993.
Dammann O, Walther H, Allers B, et al: Development of a regional cohort of very-low-birth-weight children at six years: Cognitive abilities are associated with neurological disability and social background. Dev Med Child Neurol 38:97, 1996.
Den Ouden L, Rijken M, Brand R, et al: Is it correct to correct? Developmental milestones in 555 "normal" preterm infants compared with term infants. J Pediatr 118:399, 1991.
Dixon G, Badawi N, Kurinczuk JJ, et al: Early developmental outcomes after newborn encephalopathy. Pediatrics 109:26, 2002.
Drillien CM, Thomson AJM, Burgoyne K: Low-birthweight children at early school-age: A longitudinal study. Dev Med Child Neurol 22:26, 1980.
Dubowitz LMS, Dubowitz V, Palmer PG, et al: Correlation of neurologic assessment in the preterm newborn infant with outcome at 1 year. J Pediatr 105:452, 1984.
Eilers RE, Oller DK, Levine S, et al: The role of prematurity and socioeconomic status in the onset of canonical babbling in infants. Inf Behav Dev 16:297, 1993.
Ekert P, Perlman M, Steinlin M, et al: Predicting the outcome of postasphyxial hypoxic-ischemic encephalopathy within 4 hours of birth. J Pediatr 131:613, 1997.
Ellenberg JH, Nelson KB: Cluster of perinatal events identifying infants at high risk for death or disability. J Pediatr 113:546, 1988.
Ericson A, Kallen B: Very low birthweight boys at the age of 19. Arch Dis Child Fetal Neonatal Ed 78:F171, 1998.
Escobar GJ, Littenberg B, Petitti DB: Outcome among surviving very-low-birth-weight infants: A meta-analysis. Arch Dis Child 66:204, 1991.
Fawer C, Diebold P, Calame A: Periventricular leucomalacia and neurodevelopmental outcome in preterm infants. Arch Dis Child 62:30, 1987.
Ferrara TB, Hoekstra RE, Couser RJ, et al: Effects of surfactant therapy on outcome of infants with birth weights 600 to 750 g. J Pediatr 119:455, 1991.
Fitzhardinge PM, Steven EM: The small-for-date infant: II. Neurological and intellectual sequelae. Pediatrics 49:50, 1972.
Forfar JO, Hume R, McPhail FM, et al: Low birth weight: A 10-year outcome study of the continuum of reproductive casualty. Dev Med Child Neurol 36:1037, 1994.
Freeman JM: Prenatal and Perinatal Factors Associated with Brain Disorders. National Institutes of Health Publication No. 85-1149. Bethesda, Md, US Department of Health and Human Services, 1985.
Glass P, Wagner AE, Papero PH, et al: Neurodevelopmental status at age five years of neonates treated with extracorporeal membrane oxygenation. J Pediatr 127:447, 1995.
Goldenberg RL, Dubard MB, Cliver SP, et al: Pregnancy outcome and intelligence at age five years. Am J Obstet Gynecol 175:1511, 1996.
Grogaard JB, Lindstrom DP, Parker RA, et al: Increased survival rate in very-low-birth-weight infants (1500 g or less): No association with increased incidence of handicaps. J Pediatr 117:139, 1990.
Gross SJ, Slagle TA, D'Eugenio DB, et al: Impact of a matched term control group on interpretation of developmental performance in preterm infants. Pediatrics 90:681, 1992.
Grunau RE, Whitfield MF, Davis C: Pattern of learning disabilities in children with extremely low birth weight and broadly average intelligence. Arch Pediatr Adolesc Med 156:615, 2002.
Hack M, Fanaroff AA: Outcome of extremely low-birth-weight infants between 1982 and 1988. N Engl J Med 321:1642, 1989.
Hack M, Flannery DJ, Schluchter M, et al: Outcomes in young adulthood for very-low-birth-weight infants. N Engl J Med 346:149, 2002.
Hack M, Taylor HG, Klein N, et al: School-age outcomes in children with birth weights under 750 g. N Engl J Med 331:753, 1994.
Hagberg B, Hagberg G, Olow I, et al: The changing panorama of cerebral palsy in Sweden. VII. Prevalence and origin in the birth year period 1987-1990. Acta Paediatr 85:954, 1996.
Hagberg B, Hagberg G, Beckung E, et al: Changing panorama of cerebral palsy in Sweden. VIII. Prevalence and origin in the birth year period 1991-1994. Acta Paediatr 90, 271, 2001.
Hall A, McLeod A, Counsell C, et al: School attainment, cognitive ability, and motor function in a total Scottish very-low-birth-weight population at eight years: A controlled study. Dev Med Child Neurol 37:1037, 1995.
Hendricks-Munoz KD, Walton JP: Hearing loss in infants with persistent fetal circulation. Pediatrics 81:650, 1988.
Hirata T, Epcar JT, Walsh A, et al: Survival and outcome of infants 501 to 750 gm: A six-year experience. J Pediatr 102:741, 1983.
Hoffman EL, Bennett FC: Birth weight less than 800 g: Changing outcomes and influences of gender and gestation number. Pediatrics 86:27, 1990.

Hofkosh D, Thompson AE, Nozza RJ, et al: Ten years of extracorporeal membrane oxygenation: Neurodevelopmental outcome. Pediatrics 87:549, 1991.

Hollo O, Rautava P, Korhonen T, et al: Academic achievement of small-for-gestational-age children at age 10 years. Arch Pediatr Adolesc Med 156:179, 2002.

Hunt JV, Tooley WH, Harvin D: Learning disabilities in children with birth weight 1500 g. Semin Perinatol 6:280, 1982.

Ikle L, Hale K, Fashaw L, et al: Developmental outcome of patients with hypoplastic left heart syndrome treated with heart transplantation. J Pediatr 142:20, 2003.

Infant Health and Developmental Program: Enhancing the outcomes of low-birth weight, premature infants: A multisite, randomized trial. JAMA 263:3035, 1990.

International Classification of Impairments, Disabilities, and Handicaps. Geneva, World Health Organization, 1980.

Ishikawa T, Ogawa Y, Kanayama M, et al: Long-term prognosis of asphyxiated full-term neonates with CNS complications. Brain Dev 9:48, 1987.

Ishizuka Y: Long-term survival of infants born less than 500 g or less than 24 weeks' gestation [in Japanese]. J Jpn Pediatr Soc 94:841, 1990.

John E, Roberts V, Burnard ED: Persistent pulmonary hypertension of the newborn treated with hyperventilation: Clinical features and outcome. Aust Paediatr J 24:357, 1988.

Jongeling BR, Badawi N, Kurinczuk JJ, et al: Cranial ultrasound as a predictor of outcome in term newborn encephalopathy. Pediatr Neurol 26:37, 2002.

Kaufman AS, Kaufman NL: Kaufman Assessment Battery for Children (K-ABC). Circle Pines, MN, American Guidance Service Publishing. www.agsnet.com/assessments/bibliography/kabc.asp

Keith CG, Doyle LW: Retinopathy of prematurity in extremely low-birth-weight infants. Pediatrics 95:42, 1995.

Kern JH, Hinton VJ, Nereo NE, et al: Early developmental outcome after the Norwood procedure for hypoplastic left heart syndrome. Pediatrics 102:1148, 1998.

Khadilkar V, Tudehope D, Burns Y, et al: The long-term neurodevelopmental outcome for very-low-birth-weight (VLBW) infants with "dystonic" signs at 4 months of age. J Pediatr Child Health 29:415, 1993.

Kitchen WH, Ford GW, Doyle LW, et al: Health and hospital readmissions of very-low-birth-weight and normal-birth-weight children. Am J Dis Child 144:213, 1990.

Kitchen WH, Ford GW, Rickards AL, et al: Children at birth weight <1000 g: Changing outcome between ages 2 and 5 years. J Pediatr 110:283, 1987.

Kitchen WH, Rickards A, Ryan MM, et al: Improved outcome to two years of very-low-birth-weight infants: Fact or artifact? Dev Med Child Neurol 28:479, 1986.

Kitchen WH, Ryan MM, Rickards A, et al: A longitudinal study of very-low-birth-weight infants: IV. An overview of performance at eight years. Dev Med Child Neurol 22:172, 1980.

Klein N, Hack M, Gallagher J, et al: Preschool performance of children with normal intelligence who were very-low-birth-weight infants. Pediatrics 75:531, 1985.

Knoblach H, Stevens F, Malone A: Manual of Developmental Diagnosis: The Administration and Interpretation of the Revised Gesell and Amatruda Developmental and Neurologic Examination. New York, Harper & Row, 1980.

Kuban KCK, Leviton A: Cerebral palsy. N Engl J Med 330:188, 1994.

Lago P, Rebsamen S, Clancy RR, et al: MRI, MRA, and neurodevelopmental outcome following neonatal ECMO. Pediatr Neurol 12:294, 1995.

LaPine TRL, Jackson JC, Bennett FC: Outcome of infants weighing less than 800 g at birth: 15 years' experience. Pediatrics 96:479, 1995.

Largo RH, Molinari L, Rinto LC, et al: Language development of term and preterm children during the first five years of life. Dev Med Child Neurol 28:333, 1986.

Larroque B, Bertrais S, Czernichow P, et al: School difficulties in 20-year-olds who were born small for gestational age at term in a regional cohort study. Pediatrics 108:111, 2001.

Lefebvre F, Bard H, Veilleux A, et al: Outcome at school age of children with birth weights of 1000 g or less. Dev Med Child Neurol 30:170, 1988.

Leijon I, Billstrom G, Lind I: An 18-month follow-up study of growth-retarded neonates: Relation to biochemical tests of placental function in late pregnancy and neurobehavioural condition in the newborn period. Early Hum Dev 4:271, 1980.

Lemons JA, Bauer CR, Oh W, et al: Very low birth weight outcomes of the National Institute of Child Health and Human Development Neonatal Research Network, January 1995 through December 1996. NICHD Neonatal Research Network. Pediatrics 107:E1, 2001.

Leonard CH, Clyman RI, Piecuch RE, et al: Effect of medical and social risk factors on outcome of prematurity and very low birth weight. J Pediatr 116:620, 1990.

Leviton A, Nelson KB: Problems with definitions and classifications of newborn encephalopathy. Pediatr Neurol 8:85, 1992.

Lloyd BW, Wheldall K, Perks D: Controlled study of intelligence and school performance of very-low-birth-weight children from a defined geographical area. Dev Med Child Neurol 30:36, 1988.

Lorenz JM, Wooliever DE, Jetton JR, et al: A quantitative review of mortality and developmental disability in extremely premature newborns. Arch Pediatr Adolesc Med 152:425, 1998.

Lorenz JM, Paneth N, Jetton JR, et al: Comparison of management strategies for extreme prematurity in New Jersey and the Netherlands: Outcomes and resource expenditure. Pediatrics, 108:1269, 2001.

Louhiala P: Risk indicators of mental retardation: Changes between 1967 and 1981. Dev Med Child Neurol 37:631, 1995.

Low JA, Galbraith RS, Muir D, et al: Intrauterine growth retardation: A preliminary report of long-term morbidity. Am J Obstet Gynecol 130:534, 1978.

Low JA, Galbraith RS, Muir D, et al: Intrauterine growth retardation: A study of long-term morbidity. Am J Obstet Gynecol 142:670, 1982.

Low JA, Handley-Derry MH, Burke SO, et al: Association of intrauterine fetal growth retardation and learning deficits at age 9 to 11 years. Am J Obstet Gynecol 167:1499, 1992.

Marlow N, Roberts BL, Cooke RWI: Motor skills in extremely low-birth-weight children at the age of 6 years. Arch Dis Child 64:839, 1989.

Marron MJ, Crisafi MA, Driscoll JM Jr, et al: Hearing and neurodevelopmental outcome in survivors of persistent pulmonary hypertension of the newborn. Pediatrics 90:392, 1992.

Matilainen R, Heinonen K, Siren-Tiusanen H, et al: Neurodevelopmental screening of in utero growth-retarded prematurely born children before school age. Eur J Pediatr 146:453, 1987.

Mauk JE, Ting RY: Correction for prematurity: How much, how long? Am J Dis Child 141:373, 1987.

McCarthy DA: Manual for the McCarthy Scales of Children's Abilities. New York, Psychological Corporation, 1972.

McCormick MC, Workman-Daniels K, Brooks-Gunn J: The behavioral and emotional well-being of school-age children with different birth weights. Pediatrics 97:18, 1996.

McCowan LM, Pryor J, Harding JE: Perinatal predictors of neurodevelopmental outcome in small-for-gestational-age children at 18 months of age. Am J Obstet Gynecol 186:1069, 2002.

Mercuri E, Guzzetta A, Haataja L, et al: Neonatal neurological examination in infants with hypoxic ischaemic encephalopathy: Correlation with MRI findings. Neuropediatrics 30:83, 1999.

Miller G, Dubowitz LMS, Palmer P: Follow-up of pre-term infants: Is correction of the developmental quotient for prematurity helpful? Early Hum Dev 9:137, 1984.

Msall ME, Buck GM, Rogers BT, et al: Kindergarten readiness after extreme prematurity. Am J Dis Child 146:1371, 1992.

Msall ME, Tremont MR: Measuring functional outcomes after prematurity: Developmental impact of very low birth weight and extremely low birth weight status on childhood disability. Ment Retard Dev Disabil Res Rev 8:258, 2002.

Mullen EM: Mullen Scales of Early Learning: AGS Edition. Circle Pines, MN, American Guidance Service Publishing. www.agsnet.com/Group.asp?nGroupInfoID = a11150

Neligan GA: Born too soon or born too small: A follow-up study to seven years of age. Clinics in Developmental Medicine. London, Spastics International Medical Publications, 1976.

Nelson KB: The epidemiology of cerebral palsy in term infants. Ment Retard Dev Disabil Res Rev 8:146, 2002.

Nelson KB, Leviton A: How much of neonatal encephalopathy is due to birth asphyxia? Am J Dis Child 145:1325, 1991.

Nishida H: Outcome of infants born preterm, with special emphasis on extremely low-birth-weight infants. Bailliere's Clin Obstet Gynaecol 7:611, 1993.

Nwaesei CG, Young DC, Byrne JM, et al: Preterm birth at 23 to 26 weeks' gestation: Is active obstetric management justified? Am J Obstet Gynecol 157:890, 1987.

O'Shea TM: Cerebral palsy in very preterm infants: New epidemiological insights. Ment Retard Dev Disabil Res Rev 8:135, 2002.

Ornstein M, Ohlsson A, Edmonds J, et al: Neonatal follow-up of very low birthweight/extremely low birthweight infants to school age: A critical overview. Acta Paediatr Scand 80:741, 1991.

Palisano RJ: Use of chronological and adjusted ages to compare motor development of healthy preterm and fullterm infants. Dev Med Child Neurol 28:180, 1986.

Palmer FB, Shapiro BK, Wachtel RC, et al: The effects of physical therapy on cerebral palsy: A controlled trial in infants with spastic diplegia. N Engl J Med 318:803, 1988.

Parkinson CE, Scrivener R, Graves L, et al: Behavioural differences of school-age children who were small-for-dates babies. Dev Med Child Neurol 28:498, 1986.

Parkinson CE, Wallis S, Harvey D: School achievement and behaviour of children who were small-for-dates at birth. Dev Med Child Neurol 23:41, 1981.

Paz I, Gale R, Laor A, et al: The cognitive outcome of full-term small for gestational age infants at late adolescence. Obstet Gynecol 65:452, 1995.

Pena IC, Teberg AJ, Finello KM: The premature small-for-gestational-age infant during the first year of life: Comparison by birth weight and gestational age. J Pediatr 113:1066, 1988.

Perlman M, Claris O, Hao Y, et al: Secular changes in the outcomes to eighteen to twenty-four months of age of extremely low-birth-weight infants, with adjustment for changes in risk factors and severity of illness. J Pediatr 126:75, 1995.

Piper MC, Kunos I, Willis DM, et al: Early physical therapy effects on the high-risk infant: A randomized, controlled trial. Pediatrics 78:216, 1986.

Pryor J, Silva PA, Brooke M: Growth, development and behaviour in adolescents born small-for-gestational-age. J Paediatr Child Health 31:403, 1995.

Ramey CT, Bryant DM, Wasik BH, et al: Infant health and development program for low-birth-weight, premature infants: Program elements, family participation, and child intelligence. Pediatrics 89:454, 1992.

Regev R, Dolfin T, Ben-nun Y, et al: Survival rate and two-year outcome in very-low-birth-weight infants. Isr J Med Sci 31:309, 1995.

Revenis ME, Glass P, Short BL: Mortality and morbidity rates among lower-birth-weight infants (2000 to 2500 g) treated with extracorporeal membrane oxygenation. J Pediatr 121:452, 1992.

Rickards AL, Kitchen WH, Doyle LW, et al: Correction of developmental and intelligence test scores for premature birth. Aust Paediatr J 25:127, 1989..

Robertson C, Sauve RS, Christianson HE: Province-based study of neurologic disability among survivors weighing 500 through 1249 g at birth. Pediatrics 93:636, 1994.

Robertson CM, Finer NN, Sauve RS, et al: Neurodevelopmental outcome after neonatal extracorporeal membrane oxygenation. Can Med Assoc J 152:1981, 1995.

Robertson CMT, Etches PC, Kyle JM: Eight-year school performance and growth of preterm, small-for-gestational-age infants: A comparative study with subjects matched for birth weight or for gestational age. J Pediatr 116:19, 1990.

Robertson CMT, Finer NN: Term infants with hypoxic-ischemic encephalopathy: Outcome at 3–5 years. Dev Med Child Neurol 27:473, 1985.

Robertson CMT, Finer NN, Grace MGA: School performance of survivors of neonatal encephalopathy associated with birth asphyxia at term. J Pediatr 114:753, 1989.

Rogers B, Msall M, Owens T, et al: Cystic periventricular leukomalacia and type of cerebral palsy in preterm infants. J Pediatr 125:S1, 1994.

Rogers BT, Msall ME, Buck GM, et al: Neurodevelopmental outcome of infants with hypoplastic left heart syndrome. J Pediatr 126:496, 1995.

Ross G, Lipper EG, Auld PAM: Social competence and behavior problems in premature children at school age. Pediatrics 86:391, 1990.

Ross G, Lipper E, Auld PAM: Educational status and school-related abilities of very-low-birth-weight premature children. Pediatrics 88:1125, 1991.

Rossman MJ, Hyman SL, Rorabaugh ML, et al: The CAT/CLAMS assessment for early intervention services. Clin Pediatr 33:404, 1994.

Roth SC, Baudin F, McCormick DC, et al: Relation between ultrasound appearance of the brain of very-preterm infants and neurodevelopmental impairment at eight years. Dev Med Child Neurol 35:755, 1993.

Roth S, Wyatt J, Baudin J, et al: Neurodevelopmental status at 1 year predicts neuropsychiatric outcome at 14-15 years of age in very preterm infants. Early Hum Dev 65:81, 2001.

Rothberg AD, Goodman M, Jacklin LA, et al: Six-year follow-up of early physiotherapy intervention in very-low-birth-weight infants. Pediatrics 88:547, 1991.

Rutherford MA, Pennock JM, Dubowitz LMS: Cranial ultrasound and magnetic resonance imaging in hypoxic-ischemic encephalopathy: A comparison with outcome. Dev Med Child Neurol 36:813, 1994.

Saari TN, American Academy of Pediatrics Committee on Infectious Diseases: Immunization of preterm and low birth weight infants. Pediatrics 112:193, 2003.

Sabel KG, Olegard E, Victorin L: Remaining sequelae with modern prenatal care. Pediatrics 57:652, 1976.

Saigal S, Hoult LA, Streiner DL, et al: School difficulties at adolescence in a regional cohort of children who were extremely low birth weight. Pediatrics 105:325, 2000.

Saigal S, Rosenbaum P, Stoskopf B, et al: Follow-up of infants 501- to 1500-gm birth weight delivered to residents of a geographically defined region with perinatal intensive care facilities. J Pediatr 100:606, 1982.

Saigal S, Rosenbaum P, Stoskopf B, et al: Outcome in infants 501- to 1000-gm birth weight delivered to residents of the McMaster Health Region. J Pediatr 105:969, 1984.

Saigal S, Rosenbaum P, Stoskopf B, et al: Comprehensive assessment of the health status of extremely low-birth-weight children at eight years of age: Comparison with a reference group. J Pediatr 125:411, 1994.

Saigal S, Szatmari P, Rosenbaum P, et al: Intellectual and functional status at school entry of children who weighed 1000 g or less at birth: A regional perspective of births in the 1980s. J Pediatr 116:409, 1990.

Saigal S, Szatmari P, Rosenbaum P, et al: Cognitive abilities and school performance of extremely low-birth-weight children and matched term control children at age 8 years: A regional study. J Pediatr 118:751, 1991.

Schumacher RE, Palmer TW, Roloff DW, et al: Follow-up of infants treated with extracorporeal membrane oxygenation for newborn respiratory failure. Pediatrics 87:451, 1991.

Scottish Low Birthweight Study Group: The Scottish low birthweight study: I. Survival, growth, neuromotor and sensory impairment. Lancet 1:675, 1992.

Sell EF, Gaines JA, Gluckman C, et al: Persistent fetal circulation. Am J Dis Child 139:25, 1985.

Shalak LF, Laptook AR, Velaphi SC, et al: Amplitude-integrated electroencephalography coupled with an early neurologic examination enhances prediction of term infants at risk for persistent encephalopathy. Pediatrics 111:351, 2003.

Siegel LS: Correction for prematurity and its consequences for the assessment of the very-low-birth-weight infant. Child Dev 54:1176, 1983.

Skouteli HN, Eubowitz LMS, Levene MI, et al: Predictors for survival and normal neurodevelopmental outcome of infants weighing less than 1001 g at birth. Dev Med Child Neurol 27:588, 1985.

Stewart A, Hope PL, Hamilton P, et al: Prediction in very-preterm infants of satisfactory neurodevelopmental progress at 12 months. Dev Med Child Neurol 30:53, 1988.

Stewart AL, Reynolds EOR, Hope PL, et al: Probability of neurodevelopmental disorders estimated from ultrasound appearance of brains of very-preterm infants. Dev Med Child Neurol 29:3, 1987.

Stolar CJH, Crisafi MA, Driscoll YT: Neurocognitive outcome for neonates treated with extracorporeal membrane oxygenation: Are infants with congenital diaphragmatic hernia different? J Pediatr Surg 30:366, 1995.

Strauss RS: Adult functional outcome of those born small for gestational age: Twenty-six-year follow-up of the 1970 British Birth Cohort. JAMA 283:625, 2000.

Sung IK, Vohr B, Oh W: Growth and neurodevelopmental outcome of very-low-birth-weight infants with intrauterine growth retardation: Comparison with control subjects matched by birth weight and gestational age. J Pediatr 123:618, 1993.

Survanta Multidose Study Group: Two-year follow-up of infants treated for neonatal respiratory distress syndrome with bovine surfactant. J Pediatr 124:962, 1994.

Synnes AR, Ling EWY, Whitfield MF, et al: Perinatal outcomes of a large cohort of extremely low-gestational-age infants (23 to 28 completed weeks of gestation). J Pediatr 125:952, 1994.

Taylor GA, Fitz CR, Glass P, et al: CT of cerebrovascular injury after neonatal extracorporeal membrane oxygenation: Implications for neurodevelopmental outcome. AJR Am J Roentgenol 153:121, 1989.

Teplin SW, Burchinal M, Johnson-Martin N, et al: Neurodevelopmental, health, and growth status at age 6 years of children with birth weights less than 1001 g. J Pediatr 118:768, 1991.

Thompson CM, Buccimazza SS, Webster J, et al: Infants of less than 1250-g birth weight at Groote Shuur Hospital: Outcome at 1 and 2 years. Pediatrics 91:961, 1993.

Thompson CM, Puterman AS, Linley LL, et al: The value of a scoring system for hypoxic ischaemic encephalopathy in predicting neurodevelopmental outcome. Acta Paediatr 86:757, 1997.

Thorndike RL, Hagen EP, Sattler JM: Guide for Administering and Scoring the Stanford-Binet Intelligence Scale, 4th ed. Chicago, Riverside, 1986.

van Zeben-van der Aa TM, Verloove-Verhorick SP, Brand R, et al: Morbidity of very-low-birth-weight infants at corrected age of two years in a geographically defined population. Lancet 1:253, 1989.

Victorian Infant Collaborative Study Group: Eight-year outcome in infants with birth weight of 500 to 999 g: Continuing regional study of 1979 and 1980 births. J Pediatr 118:761, 1991.

Vohr BR, Wright LL, Dusick AM, et al: Neurodevelopmental and functional outcomes of extremely low birth weight infants in the National Institute of Child Health and Human Development Neonatal Research Network, 1993-1994. Pediatrics 105:1216, 2000.

Vohr B, Coll CG, Flanagan P, et al: Effects of intraventricular hemorrhage and socioeconomic status on perceptual, cognitive, and neurologic status of low-birth-weight infants at 5 years of age. J Pediatr 121:280, 1992.

Vohr BR, Garcia-Coll CT: Neurodevelopmental and school performance of very-low-birth-weight infants: A seven-year longitudinal study. Pediatrics 76:345, 1985.

Vohr BR, Oh W: Growth and development in preterm infants small for gestational age. J Pediatr 103:941, 1983.

Wachtel RC, Shapiro BK, Palmer FB, et al: A tool for the pediatric evaluation of infants and young children with developmental delay. Clin Pediatr 33:410, 1994.

Walker EM, Patel NB: Mortality and morbidity in infants born between 20 and 28 weeks' gestation. Br J Obstet Gynaecol 94:670, 1987.

Walsh-Sukys MC, Bauer RE, Cornell DJ, et al: Severe respiratory failure in neonates: Mortality and morbidity rates and neurodevelopmental outcomes. J Pediatr 125:104, 1994.

Warshaw JB: Intrauterine growth retardation: Adaptation or pathology? Pediatrics 76:998, 1985.

Wechsler D: Manual for the Wechsler Preschool and Primary Scale of Intelligence. New York, Psychological Corporation, 1989.

Wechsler D: Manual for the Wechsler Intelligence Scale for Children–III. New York, Psychological Corporation, 1993.

Weisglas-Kuperus N, Baerts W, Fetter WPF, et al: Neonatal cerebral ultrasound, neonatal neurology, and perinatal conditions as predictors of neurodevelopmental outcome in very-low birth-weight infants. Early Hum Dev 31:131, 1992.

Weisglas-Kuperus N, Baerts W, Fetter WPF, et al: Minor neurological dysfunction and quality of movement in relation to neonatal cerebral damage and subsequent development. Dev Med Child Neurol 36:727, 1994.

Weisglas-Kuperus N, Baerts W, Smrkovsky M, et al: Effects of biological and social factors on the cognitive development of very-low-birth-weight children. Pediatrics 92:658, 1993.

Westwood M, Kramer MS, Munz D, et al: Growth and development of full-term nonasphyxiated small-for-gestational-age newborns: Follow-up through adolescence. Pediatrics 71:376, 1983.

Whyte HE, Fitzhardinge PM, Shennan AT, et al: Extreme immaturity: Outcome of 568 pregnancies of 23 to 26 weeks' gestation. Obstet Gynecol 82:1, 1993.

Wildin SR, Landry SH, Zwischenberger JB: Prospective, controlled study of developmental outcome in survivors of extracorporeal membrane oxygenation: The first 24 months. Pediatrics 93:404, 1994.

Wocadlo C, Rieger I: Developmental outcome at 12 months corrected age for infants born less than 30 weeks' gestation: Influence of reduced intrauterine and postnatal growth. Early Hum Dev 39:127, 1994.

Yeo CL, Tudehope DI: Outcome of resuscitated apparently stillborn infants: A ten-year review. J Paediatr Child Health 30:129, 1994.

PART XIII

# NUTRITION

Editor: ROBERTA A. BALLARD

CHAPTER 68

## Enteral Nutrition for the High-Risk Neonate

Richard J. Schanler

In the neonatal period, high-risk premature infants have greater nutritional needs to achieve optimal growth than at any time in life. The circumstance of preterm delivery results in decreased nutrient deposition in the infant. The medical condition of these infants also imposes additional burdens on nutrient supply. Impediments to growth include the stress of common pathophysiologic events (hypertension, hypoxia, acidosis, infection, surgical intervention) and their therapies (corticosteroids), as well as physiologic immaturity (decreased gastrointestinal motility and delayed enzyme expression). There is also the fear, despite the lack of evidence-based data, that aggressive feeding may produce pathologic conditions such as feeding intolerance and necrotizing enterocolitis (NEC), and that some nutritional regimens may produce toxic effects on organ development. Finally, intense support is needed to correct growth restrictions present at birth and to continue appropriate weight gain, which is nearly double that in a term infant. Thus, the premature infant requires specialized nutritional support to meet these great demands for growth.

Special considerations regarding nutrient needs of premature infants arise at birth. Because of limited body stores, increased expenditure, severity of illness, and/or immaturity and inability to tolerate enteral feedings, premature infants are given parenteral nutrient mixtures immediately from birth. Enteral feedings are often precluded because of the multiplicity of medical problems, but gastrointestinal priming with minimal quantities of milk is used to stimulate intestinal function. As the infant matures physiologically and the medical condition stabilizes, parenteral nutrition is slowly replaced with enteral nutrition. This chapter describes the enteral nutrition support for high-risk neonates.

### GOALS FOR NUTRITIONAL SUPPORT

The nutritional reference standard for the term newborn is the exclusively breast-fed infant. A similar standard is not available for premature infants. Instead, the reference standard for the premature infant is the estimated nutrient intrauterine accretion rate achieved at corresponding stages during the last trimester of pregnancy. Data derived from the chemical analyses of fetal cadavers have been used to construct normative curves of net nutrient deposition or retention during the last trimester of pregnancy. From analyses of smoothed curves, these data have been computed on a daily basis per kilogram of body weight (Table 68–1). Although the original data were derived from human fetal cadaver analyses, the data for several minerals have been corroborated by noninvasive neutron activation techniques (Ellis et al, 1993).

The intrauterine accretion data provide a reference for nutrient deposition. In the absence of direct experimental verification, one way to determine the advisable intake for a particular nutrient is to use the factorial approach (Table 68–2). This method includes a summation of the quantity of the nutrient deposited and an estimate of nutrient losses. For infants receiving parenteral nutrition only, the advisable intake includes estimates of nutrient deposition, cutaneous and urinary losses, and an additional allowance to account for variability. For enteral nutrition, the factorial approach is amended to account also for the bioavailability of the particular nutrient. The intrauterine data also provide a minimal estimate of the postnatal rate of weight gain and incremental increases in length and head circumference that parallel the growth of the last-trimester fetus (Table 68–3).

### GASTROINTESTINAL PRIMING

The lack of enteral nutrients poses several problems for the development of the intestinal tract. In several animal species, the absence of enteral nutrients is associated with diminished intestinal growth, atrophy of intestinal mucosa, delayed maturation of intestinal enzymes, and increases in permeability and bacterial translocation. A lack of enteral nutrients also affects intestinal motility, perfusion, and hormonal responses. The hormonal response to feeding premature infants has been evaluated by measuring the plasma concentrations of a variety of gastrointestinal hormones in response to milk feeding during the first week after birth (Lucas et al, 1986). Significant hormonal surges were noted after milk feeding, but no response was observed in the absence of feeding. The responses to feeding were observed in both healthy premature infants and those with respiratory distress. In further investigations, it was observed that hormonal surges of gastrin, gastric inhibitory polypeptide (GIP), and enteroglucagon occurred after the feeding of small quantities of milk (24 mL), but

**TABLE 68-1**

**Estimated Intrauterine Nutrient Accretion Rates**

| Nutrient* | Units/kg/day |
|---|---|
| Calcium (mg) | 105 |
| Copper (μg) | 50 |
| Magnesium (mg) | 2.7 |
| Nitrogen (mg) | 325 |
| Phosphorus (mg) | 70 |
| Potassium (mEq) | 0.7 |
| Sodium (mEq) | 1.2 |
| Zinc (μg) | 240 |

*Values averaged from last trimester, adjusted for body weight.

motilin surges were not observed until the cumulative milk intake was 700 mL (Lucas et al, 1986).

The foregoing observations prompted prospective randomized clinical studies of the effects of small volumes of milk given as early minimal enteral feeding, or trophic feeding, in premature infants. When studied in the first or second week after birth, infants who received "early" milk feedings had a better feeding tolerance when feedings were advanced, required a shorter duration of parenteral nutrition, and had a lower incidence of conjugated hyperbilirubinemia compared with similar infants given only parenteral nutrition during the same interval (Dunn et al, 1988; Stagle and Gross, 1988). Probably because of better tolerance to feeding, premature infants receiving the trophic feedings had cumulatively greater milk intakes, which were associated with lower serum alkaline phosphatase activity (Dunn et al, 1988). The lower alkaline phosphatase activity, primarily of bone origin, was observed for 14 weeks, well beyond the initial intervention in the first week. Significant stimulation of gastrointestinal hormones, such as gastrin and GIP, also was reported following the early feeding of small quantities of milk (Meetze et al, 1992). Intestinal motility patterns matured more rapidly in premature infants receiving early enteral feeding (Berseth, 1992). Subsequent investigations demonstrated that trophic feeding was associated with greater absorption of calcium and phosphorus, greater lactase activity, and reduced intestinal permeability (Schanler et al; Shulman et al, 1998a, 1998b). The meta-analysis of several studies of gastrointestinal priming indicated that its use was associated with a shorter time to regain birth weight, fewer days when feeding was withheld, and a shorter duration of hospitalization but no increase in the incidence of NEC (Table 68–4). Noteworthy in the studies of minimal enteral nutrition is that the subject population consisted of premature infants selected because they had the greatest risk of feeding intolerance and NEC. Feedings were administered during mechanical ventilation and while umbilical arterial and venous catheters were in place (Davey et al, 1994; Dunn et al, 1988; Slagle and Gross, 1988). The infants also had the usual pathologic conditions of patent ductus arteriosus, intraventricular hemorrhage, and systemic hypotension. These data suggest that by the end of the first week after birth, and in the absence of evidence of cardiovascular instability (severe acidosis, hypotension, hypoxemia), small volumes of milk can be administered to premature infants. In general, for infants who are ill, the small volumes of 10 to 20 mL/kg/day continue for approximately 4 to 7 days before there is any consideration of advancing the milk volume (Schanler et al, 1999a). The decision for advancement of feedings, however, is made after clinical feeding tolerance is proved and clinical stability is achieved.

**TABLE 68-2**

**Estimating Optimal Nutrient Intake: Factorial Approach**

| Example: Calcium | |
|---|---|
| Net calcium deposition | 105 mg/kg/day |
| Urinary losses | 5 mg/kg/day |
| Cutaneous losses | 2 mg/kg/day |
| Subtotal | 112 mg/kg/day |
| Net absorption | 50% |
| Variability | 10% |
| Total | 246 mg/kg/day |

Thus, by adding deposition and losses and accounting for absorption and variability coefficients, the advisable calcium intake for a particular formula is 246 mg/kg/day.

**TABLE 68-3**

**Growth Guidelines**

| | |
|---|---|
| Weight gain | >15 g/kg/day for infants <2.0 kg<br>>20 g/day for infants >2.0 kg |
| Length gain | 0.7-1.0 cm/wk |
| Head circumference gain | 0.7-1.0 cm/wk |

**TABLE 68-4**

**Advantages of Gastrointestinal Priming**

Shortens time to regain birth weight
Improves feeding tolerance
Reduces duration of parenteral nutrition
Enhances enzyme maturation
Reduces intestinal permeability
Improves gastrointestinal motility
Matures hormone responses
Improves mineral absorption, mineralization
Lowers incidence of cholestasis
Reduces duration of phototherapy
Earlier use of mother's milk
Mother begins milk expression earlier
Infant receives more mother's milk
Psychological advantage for mother
Safety

## ENTERAL NUTRITION

### Energy

The energy needs of the neonate are derived from a computation of the energy expenditure, energy storage (growth), and energy losses. Energy expenditure consists of the energy needed to cover the resting metabolic rate, activity, thermoregulation, new tissue synthesis, and thermic effect of feeding. Energy storage consists of the energy (fat and lean mass) deposited for growth. Energy losses usually are due to incomplete absorption of nutrients and are greater in premature infants than in term infants or adults (Groh-Wargo, 2000).

The daily energy needs for the growing premature infant are summarized in Table 68–5. The values are not absolute. The range in resting energy expenditure has been reported from 49 to 60 kcal/kg/day at 8 to 63 days of postnatal age (Sinclair, 1978). When nourished parenterally, the premature infant has less fecal energy loss, generally fewer episodes of cold stress, and somewhat lesser activity so that the actual energy needs for growth are lowered to approximately 80 to 100 kcal/kg/day. In circumstances of chronic disease, such as bronchopulmonary dysplasia, the resting energy expenditure rises significantly (Weinstein and Oh, 1981; Yunis and Oh, 1989). Total energy needs in premature infants with bronchopulmonary dysplasia are increased because of greater energy expenditure, activity, and fecal energy losses. It is not surprising to find that these infants may require 150 kcal/kg/day to achieve weight gain.

After protein and essential fatty acid needs are met, the remaining energy needs are divided equally between fat and carbohydrate. A balanced distribution of fat and carbohydrate calories is appropriate to avoid potential effects on respiratory metabolism, especially in infants who are ill. A distribution of calories favoring glucose (and thus lower in fat) or a surplus of glucose calories such that glucose is converted to fat will increase the production of carbon dioxide, increase alveolar minute ventilation, and raise the respiratory quotient and may increase oxygen consumption (Bresson et al, 1991; Piedboeuf et al, 1991). In addition, a balanced distribution of glucose-lipid calories favors protein accretion, whereas glucose-only solutions are associated with protein oxidation and poor nitrogen utilization (Salas-Salvadó et al, 1993). Daily monitoring of the intakes for all energy sources is essential to ensure a relatively balanced distribution of calories derived from glucose and fat.

**TABLE 68–5**

**Partition of Energy Needs for Growing Premature Infants**

| Component | kcal/kg/day |
|---|---|
| Resting energy expenditure | 50 |
| Intermittent activity (+30% above resting) | 15 |
| Occasional cold stress (thermoregulation) | 10 |
| Thermic effect of feeding (synthesis) | 8 |
| Fecal loss (10% of intake) | 12 |
| Growth allowance (energy storage) | 25 |
| Total | 120 |

### Protein

#### *Milk Composition*

In the first few weeks after birth, the protein content of milk from mothers who deliver premature infants (preterm milk) is greater than that of milk obtained from women delivering term infants (term milk) (Atkinson et al, 1978). The protein content of both milks declines over time, such that beyond 2 weeks it levels off to that of what we call mature milk. The quality of protein—the proportion of whey and casein—in human milk is particularly suitable for the premature infant. Human milk contains 70% whey and 30% casein, whereas bovine milk contains 18% whey and 82% casein. A whey- and/or casein-dominant commercial formula, therefore, refers to these proportions of bovine milk. The whey fraction of milk consists of soluble proteins that are digested more easily. Human milk and then whey-dominated bovine milk, in that order, promote more rapid gastric emptying than occurs with casein-dominated milk (Billeaud et al, 1990). Elevated concentrations of potentially toxic amino acids (phenylalanine, methionine, and tyrosine) are reported in premature infants fed formulas with high casein content (Gaull et al, 1977; Rassin et al, 1977). Hepatic enzyme immaturity may explain the higher plasma amino acid concentrations. Because we infer that elevations of particular amino acids may be toxic to brain development, there may be a concern when premature infants are fed a casein-dominant milk, especially at a high protein intake.

The compositions of the whey fractions of human and bovine milks differ significantly. The major human whey protein is α-lactalbumin, a nutritional protein for the infant and a component of mammary gland lactose synthesis. Lactoferrin, lysozyme, and secretory immunoglobulin A (sIgA) are specific human whey proteins that are particularly resistant to hydrolysis, and, as such, line the gastrointestinal tract to play a primary role in host defense (Schanler et al, 1986). These proteins, therefore, may be suitable for the premature infant who is exposed to multiple pathogens in the nursery environment. The three host defense proteins are present in only trace quantities in bovine milk. The major whey protein in bovine milk is β-lactoglobulin, the protein often blamed for bovine milk protein allergy and colic (Savilahti and Kuitunen, 1992).

The major amino acid for the fetus and in human milk is glutamine, which is not found in commercial formula because of problems with stability of the free amino acid. Glutamine, however, is an important amino acid for cell growth, specifically intestinal epithelial growth; has a role in immune function; and is a precursor in glutathione synthesis. When commercial formula was supplemented with glutamine under experimental conditions, premature infants had better feeding tolerance and a significantly lower incidence of sepsis than were found in infants fed unsupplemented formula (Neu et al, 1997). Further research efforts are under way to define how to supply this amino acid if human milk is not fed to premature infants.

### Protein Needs

The quantity and quality of protein needed for premature infants have been investigated (Raiha et al, 1976). Formulas providing protein intakes of 2.25 and 4.50 g/kg/day as either whey- or casein-dominant preparations and pasteurized human milk with a protein intake of approximately 1.6 g/kg/day were compared. Although absolute growth rates reportedly were similar during the in-hospital study, hospitalization periods were longer for the infants fed human milk, suggesting a slower rate of weight gain than that of infants fed formula (Gaull et al, 1977; Rassin et al, 1977). Those infants receiving protein intakes of 4.5 g/kg/day, as well as infants given casein-dominant milk, had more abnormalities in plasma amino acids and protein indices of nutritional status (elevated blood concentrations of urea nitrogen and ammonia, acidosis, lethargy, and fever) suggesting excessive protein intake (Moro et al, 1989). Although generally considered an excessive protein intake, 4.5 g/kg/day was provided, with relatively low energy (115 kcal/kg/day) and mineral intakes. Some investigators comment that the low energy and mineral intakes may have limited the ability to utilize the protein and that such protein intakes may be appropriate if the total diet is adjusted.

The appropriate protein intake for premature infants has been defined further from evaluations of weight gain, nitrogen retention, and serum biochemical indicators of protein nutritional status (Kashyap et al, 1986, 1988). Protein intakes of 2.2 and 2.8 g/kg/day resulted in lower serum indices, weight gain, and nitrogen retention, and intakes of 3.8 g/kg/day appeared to be somewhat excessive. Therefore, protein intakes of approximately 3.5 g/kg/day at 120 kcal/kg/day seem appropriate for the otherwise normal premature infant (Kashyap et al, 1986).

An alternative way to compute the protein needs of the premature infant is to use the factorial approach to add the needs for tissue deposition, derived from intrauterine accretion rates of 1.8 to 2.2 g/kg/day, to the postnatal losses of protein from the skin (approximately 0.2 g/kg/day) and the urine (1.0 g/kg/day). As approximately 85% of the protein is absorbed, the calculated enteral protein intake is 3.5 to 4.0 g/kg/day (Tables 68–6, 68–7, and 68–8).

The previously mentioned studies were conducted using formulations with whole or intact protein. Although fetal nitrogen uptake is composed primarily of amino acids, no data suggest that postnatal formulations include hydrolyzed protein formulations or free amino acids. Whey-dominant protein formulations are well absorbed, and hydrolyzed protein formulations, usually casein-derived, for the otherwise healthy premature infant are not indicated (Table 68–9).

Protein needs should be considered in conjunction with energy. Protein synthesis requires energy. If energy intake is inadequate, protein synthesis may be depressed and amino acid oxidation increases (Groh-Wargi, 2000). Protein retention, or balance, generally is a function of protein intake if energy intake is inadequate (Zlotkin et al, 1981). Excessive protein intake is more of a risk if energy intake is limited.

### Human Milk Protein Needs

The aforementioned studies demonstrated that the lowest plasma concentrations of amino acids, albumin, and urea nitrogen and the slowest rates of weight gain were found in human milk–fed premature infants (Kashyap et al, 1990; Raiha et al, 1976). These observations suggest that after the first 2 weeks of feeding, the lower protein intakes in human milk–fed infants may become a concern. To meet protein needs, the human milk–fed premature infant needs a protein supplement (see Table 68–7). Growth rates and serum protein and urea nitrogen concentrations in premature infants increase when human milk is fortified with protein to achieve a protein intake of at least 3 to 3.5 g/kg/day (Polberger et al, 1989). This range of protein intake is adequate if no protein deficit has arisen as a result of a prolonged or deficient parenteral nutrition phase. Even greater intakes of protein may be necessary for premature infants to allow for catch-up protein nutritional support. Thus, intakes closer to 4 g/kg/day, with adequate energy and mineral intakes, often may be indicated.

## Fat

### Milk Composition

The lipid system in human milk is structured in a way that facilitates fat digestion and absorption. In human milk, fat exists as organized fat globules containing an outer protein coat and an inner lipid core. The type of fatty acids (high palmitic 16:0, oleic 18:1, linoleic 18:2ω-6, and linoleic 18:3ω-3), their distribution on the triglyceride molecule (16:0 at the 2 position of the molecule), and the presence of bile salt–stimulated lipase (Jensen and Jensen, 1992) are important components of the lipid system in human milk. Because the lipase is heat labile, the superior fat absorption from human milk is reported only when unprocessed milk is fed (Jensen and Jensen, 1992).

The most variable nutrient component in human milk is fat, the major energy source, comprising nearly 50% of the calories. The fat content of human milk varies among women, changes during the day, rises slightly during lactation, and increases dramatically within a single milk expression (Table 68–10) (Neville et al, 1984). The variability in total fat content is unrelated to maternal dietary fat intake. Because it is not homogenized, the fat separates out of human milk on standing. The separated fat may adhere to collection containers, feeding tubes, and syringes. The loss of fat, therefore, robs the premature infant of needed energy. The greatest losses of fat occur in continuous milk infusion systems. Care should be taken in using the continuous milk infusion system to ensure the inclusion of only a short length of tubing. If the system contains a cassette interface, much of the fat will be lost when the tubing system is changed. Milk infusion systems that use a syringe and a small infusion pump, in which the syringe is oriented upright, will allow more complete delivery of fat (Greer et al, 1984).

**TABLE 68-6**

**Consensus on Enteral Fluid, Energy, and Nutrient Intakes for Stable, Growing Extremely Low-Birth-Weight (ELBW) and Very Low-Birth-Weight (VLBW) Premature Infants**

| | Units/kg/day (except as noted) | |
|---|---|---|
| **Component (units)** | **ELBW** | **VLBW** |
| Water (mL) | 160-220 | 135-190 |
| Energy (kcal) | 130-150 | 110-130 |
| Protein (g) | 3.8-4.4 | 3.4-4.2 |
| Fat (g) | 6-8 | 5-7 |
| Carbohydrate (g) | 9-20 | 7-17 |
| Vitamin A (IU) | 700-1500 | 700-1500 |
| Vitamin D (IU) | 400 IU/day | 400 IU/day |
| Vitamin E (IU) | 6-12 | 6-12 |
| Vitamin K* (μg) | 8-10 | 8-10 |
| Thiamine (vitamin $B_1$) (μg) | 180-240 | 180-240 |
| Riboflavin (vitamin $B_2$) (μg) | 250-360 | 250-360 |
| Pyridoxine (vitamin $B_6$) (μg) | 150-210 | 150-210 |
| Vitamin $B_{12}$ (μg) | 0.3 | 0.3 |
| Niacin (mg) | 3.6-4.8 | 3.6-4.8 |
| Folic acid (μg) | 25-50 | 25-50 |
| Sodium (mEq) | 3.0-7.0 | 3.0-7.0 |
| Potassium (mEq) | 2.0-3.0 | 2.0-3.0 |
| Chloride (mEq) | 3.0-7.0 | 3.0-7.0 |
| Calcium (mg) | 100-220 | 100-220 |
| Phosphorus (mg) | 60-140 | 60-140 |
| Magnesium (mg) | 8-15 | 8-15 |
| Iron (mg) | 2-4 | 2-4 |
| Zinc (μg) | 1000-3000 | 1000-3000 |
| Copper (μg) | 120 150 | 120 150 |
| Chromium (μg) | 0.1-2.25 | 0.1-2.25 |
| Manganese (μg) | 0.7-7.5 | 0.7-7.5 |
| Selenium (μg) | 1.3-4.5 | 1.3-4.5 |

*Vitamin K, 0.5-1.0 mg given at birth.

The following conversion factors are used:
- Calcium: 40 mg = 1 mmol = 2 mEq
- Phosphorus: 31 mg = 1 mmol
- Magnesium: 24 mg = 1 mmol = 2 mEq
- Sodium: 23 mg = 1 mmol = 1 mEq
- Potassium: 39 mg = 1 mmol = 1 mEq
- Chloride: 35 mg = 1 mmol = 1 mEq
- Vitamin A: 1 μg retinol = 3.33 IU vitamin A = 6μg beta-carotene = 1.83 μg retinyl palmitate = 1 retinol equivalent (RE)
- Vitamin E: 1 mg alpha-tocopherol = 1 IU vitamin E
- Vitamin D: 1 μg vitamin D (cholecalciferol) = 40 IU vitamin D (cholecalciferol)
- Niacin: 1 mg niacin = 1 niacin equivalent (NE) = 60 mg tryptophan

Data from Tsang RC, et al (eds): Nutrition of the Preterm Infant: Scientific Basis and Practical Guidelines. Cincinnati, Digital Educational Publishing, in press.

Manufacturers of infant formulas modify their fat blends to mimic the fat absorption from human milk. This accounts for the differences in the constituent fatty acids between human milk and cow's-milk based formulas. Generally, commercial formulations have a greater quantity of medium-chain fatty acids (MCFA) to compensate for the absence of lipase and the unique structure of triglycerides in human milk (Innis, 1992; Jensen and Jensen, 1992). In human milk, saturated fatty acids, particularly palmitic acid, are esterified in the 2 position of the triglyceride molecule. The end product of digestion of the triglyceride is a 2-monoglyceride and minimal free fatty acid. The 2-monoglyceride is absorbed better than the free fatty acid. This enhanced absorption is important because free palmitic acid has a great tendency to bind with minerals to form soaps. In that event, both fat and mineral absorption would be limited. Thus, the overall structure of human milk is designed to provide optimal fat and mineral absorption.

### *Essential Fatty Acids*

The essential fatty acids, linoleic and linolenic acids, are present in ample quantities in human milk and commercial formula. Without an adequate intake of these fatty acids, essential fatty acid deficiency (thrombocytopenia, dermatitis, increased infections, and delayed growth)

**TABLE 68–7**

**Nutrient Composition of Human Milk and Selected Human Milk Fortifiers**

| | Human Milk (1 wk) | Mature Human Milk (1 mo) | Mature Human Milk + Human Milk Fortifier* |
|---|---|---|---|
| Volume (mL) | 100 | 100 | 100 |
| Energy (kcal) | 67 | 67 | 80 |
| Protein (g) | 2.4 | 1.4 | 2.4 |
| Whey/casein (%) | 70/30 | 70/30 | 70/30 |
| Fat (g) | 3.8 | 4.0 | 4.1-4.8 |
| Medium-chain triglycerides (%) | 2 | 2 | 10-15 |
| Carbohydrate (g) | 6.1 | 6.6 | 6.9-8.2 |
| Lactose (%) | 100 | 100 | 80-85 |
| Calcium (mg) | 25 | 25 | 112-139 |
| Phosphorus (mg) | 14 | 13 | 61-78 |
| Magnesium (mg) | 3.1 | 3.1 | 4.0-9.8 |
| Sodium (mEq [mmol]) | 2.2 | 1.1 | 1.6-1.7 |
| Potassium (mEq [mmol]) | 1.8 | 1.5 | 2.1-3.0 |
| Chloride (mEq [mmol]) | 2.6 | 1.6 | 1.9-2.6 |
| Zinc (μg) | 500 | 340 | 1030-1320 |
| Copper (μg) | 80 | 64 | 104-230 |
| Vitamin A (IU) | 560 | 390 | 980-1305 |
| Vitamin D (IU) | 4 | 2 | 120-150 |
| Vitamin E (mg) | 1.0 | 1.1 | 4.2-5.5 |

*Enfamil Human Milk Fortifier (Mead Johnson Nutritionals, Evansville, Ind) and Similac Human Milk Fortifier (Ross Laboratories, Columbus, OH): 4 packets + 100 mL mature milk.

Data from Ross Products Division, Abbott Laboratories, Columbus, OH, 2003.

**TABLE 68–8**

**Nutrient Composition of Fortified Human Milk (FHM), "Preemie" Formula, Enriched Formula, and Term Formula**

| | FHM | Preemie | Enriched | Term |
|---|---|---|---|---|
| Volume (mL) | 100 | 100 | 100 | 100 |
| Energy (kcal) | 80 | 81 | 73 | 67 |
| Protein (g) | 2.4 | 2.2-2.4 | 1.9-2.1 | 1.4 |
| Whey/casein (%) | 70/30 | 60/40 | 50/50 | 60/40 |
| Protein calories (%) | 12 | 11-12 | 10-11 | 8 |
| Fat (g) | 4.1-4.8 | 4.1-4.4 | 3.9-4.1 | 3.6 |
| Medium-chain triglycerides (%) | 10-15 | 40-50 | 20-25 | 2 |
| Fat calories (%) | 47-50 | 46-47 | 48-49 | 48 |
| Carbohydrate (g) | 6.9-8.2 | 8.6-9.0 | 7.7 | 7.3 |
| Lactose (%) | 80-85 | 50 | 40-50 | 100 |
| Carbohydrate calories (%) | 39-42 | 42-44 | 41 | 43 |
| Calcium (mg) | 112 -139 | 133-146 | 78-90 | 53 |
| Phosphorus (mg) | 61-78 | 65-80 | 45-50 | 28-36 |
| Magnesium (mg) | 4.0-9.8 | 7.3-9.7 | 6.0-6.7 | 4.0-5.4 |
| Sodium (mEq [mmol]) | 1.6-1.7 | 1.5-2.0 | 1.1 | 0.8 |
| Potassium (mEq [mmol]) | 2.1-3.0 | 2.0-27 | 2.0-2.7 | 1.9 |
| Chloride (mEq [mmol]) | 1.9-2.6 | 1.9-2.0 | 1.6 | 1.2 |
| Zinc (μg) | 1030-1320 | 1200 | 900 | 500-680 |
| Copper (μg) | 104-230 | 100-200 | 90 | 50-60 |
| Vitamin A (IU) | 980-1305 | 1000 | 340 | 200 |
| Vitamin D (IU) | 120-150 | 120-200 | 52-60 | 40 |
| Vitamin E (mg) | 4.2-5.5 | 3.2-5.1 | 2.7-3.0 | 1.0-1.4 |
| Osmolality (mOsm/L) | 350 | 250-270 | 220-255 | 270 |
| Renal solute load (mOsm) | 14 | 15 | 13 | 9 |

*EHMF*: Enfamil Human Milk Fortifier (Mead Johnson Nutritionals, Evansville, Ind) and Similac Human Milk Fortifier (Ross Laboratories, Columbus, OH): 4 packets + 100 mL mature human milk. *Preemie*: Similac Special Care Advance with Iron (Ross) and Enfamil Premature LIPIL with Iron (Mead Johnson). *Enriched*: Similac NeoSure Advance (Ross) and Enfamil EnfaCare LIPIL (Mead Johnson). *Term*: Enfamil LIPIL with Iron (Mead Johnson) and Similac Advance with Iron (Ross).

Data from Ross Products Division, Abbott Laboratories, Columbus, OH, 2003.

**TABLE 68-9**

**Comparison of Selected Hydrolysate Formulas with Selected "Preemie," Enriched, and Term Formulas**

| | Hydrolysate | Hydrolysate | Preemie | Enriched | Term |
|---|---|---|---|---|---|
| Volume (mL) | 100 | 100 | 100 | 100 | 100 |
| Energy (kcal) | 67 | 81 | 81 | 73 | 67 |
| Protein (g) | 1.9 | 2.3 | 2.2-2.4 | 1.9-2.1 | 1.4 |
| Whey/casein (%) | 0/100* | 0/100* | 60/40 | 50/50 | 60/40 |
| Protein calories (%) | 11 | 11 | 11-12 | 10-11 | 8 |
| Fat (g) | 3.8 | 4.6 | 4.1-4.4 | 3.9-4.1 | 3.6 |
| Medium-chain triglycerides (%) | 55 | 55 | 40-50 | 20-25 | 2 |
| Fat calories (%) | 48 | 48 | 46-47 | 48-49 | 48 |
| Carbohydrate (g) | 6.9 | 8.3 | 8.6-9.0 | 7.7 | 7.3 |
| Lactose (%) | 0 | 0 | 50 | 40-50 | 100 |
| Carbohydrate calories (%) | 41 | 41 | 42-44 | 41 | 43 |
| Calcium (mg) | 78 | 94 | 133-146 | 78-90 | 53 |
| Phosphorus (mg) | 51 | 61 | 65-80 | 45-50 | 28-36 |
| Magnesium (mg) | 7.4 | 8.9 | 7.3-9.7 | 6.0-6.7 | 4.0-5.4 |
| Sodium (mEq [mmol]) | 1.4 | 1.7 | 1.5-2.0 | 1.1 | 0.8 |
| Potassium (mEq [mmol]) | 1.9 | 2.3 | 2.0-27 | 2.0-2.7 | 1.9 |
| Chloride (mEq [mmol]) | 1.6 | 1.9 | 1.9-2.0 | 1.6 | 1.2 |
| Zinc (μg) | 676 | 811 | 1200 | 900 | 500-680 |
| Copper (μg) | 51 | 61 | 100-200 | 90 | 50-60 |
| Vitamin A (IU) | 255 | 300 | 1000 | 340 | 200 |
| Vitamin D (IU) | 34 | 41 | 120-200 | 52-60 | 40 |
| Vitamin E (mg) | 2.7 | 3.2 | 3.2-5.1 | 2.7-3.0 | 1.0-1.4 |
| Osmolality (mOsm/L) | 320 | 380 | 250-270 | 220-255 | 270 |
| Renal solute load (mOsm) | 17 | 20 | 15 | 13 | 9 |

*Enfamil Pregestimil (Mead Johnson Nutritionals, Evansville, Ind) is a casein hydrolysate preparation. *Preemie*: Similac Special Care Advance with Iron (Ross Laboratories, Columbus, Ohio) and Enfamil Premature LIPIL with Iron (Mead Johnson). *Enriched*: Similac NeoSure Advance (Ross) and EnfaCare LIPIL (Mead Johnson). *Term*: Enfamil LIPIL with Iron (Mead Johnson) and Similac Advance with Iron (Ross).

Data from Ross Products Division, Abbott Laboratories, Columbus, OH, 2003.

develops in 1 week. Approximately 0.5 g/kg/day (~4% of total energy intake) of essential fatty acids will prevent the deficiency (Gutcher and Farrell, 1991). Derivatives of linoleic and linolenic acids are arachidonic acid (20:4ω-6) and docosahexaenoic acid (22:6ω-3). The very-long-chain polyunsaturated fatty acids (PUFA), which are found in human but not bovine milk, are components of phospholipids found in brain, retina, and red blood cell membranes (Clandinin et al, 1992; Uauy and Hoffman, 1991). Arachidonic and docosahexaenoic acids functionally have been associated with body growth, vision, and cognition (Carlson et al, 1993; Uauy and Hoffman, 1991). In addition, the fatty acids are integral parts of prostaglandin metabolism. When their diet was supplemented with PUFA, formula-fed premature infants had red blood cell concentrations of 22.6ω-3 paralleling those of similar infants fed human milk (Clandinin et al, 1992). Follow-up studies of such supplemented infants suggest improvements in visual acuity compared with unsupplemented infants, but of similar magnitude to that in infants fed human milk (Carlson et al, 1993). PUFA are now added to many commercial formulas.

**TABLE 68-10**

**Composition of Foremilk and Hindmilk**

| Component | Foremilk (units/dL) | Hindmilk (units/dL) |
|---|---|---|
| Energy (kcal) | 63 ± 11* | 82 ± 8 |
| Fat (g) | 2.9 ± 0.8 | 4.8 ± 0.9 |
| Total nitrogen (mg) | 210 ± 27 | 210 ± 32 |
| Calcium (mg) | 27 ± 4 | 27 ± 4.4 |
| Phosphorus (mg) | 15 ± 3 | 16 ± 3 |
| Zinc (μg) | 291 ± 88 | 275 ± 88 |
| Copper (μg) | 29 ± 1 | 27 ± 1 |
| Sodium (mEq) | 0.3 ± 0.1 | 0.3 ± 0.1 |
| Potassium (mEq) | 1.1 ± 0.1 | 1.1 ± 0.1 |

*Mean ± SD.

Data from Valentine CJ, Hurst NM, Schanler RJ: Hindmilk improves weight gain in low-birth-weight infants fed human milk. J Pediatr Gastroenterol Nutr 18:474-477, 1994.

### *Medium-Chain Fatty Acids*

The proportion of MCFA, here defined as carbon length 6:0 to 12:0, is less than 12% of total fatty acids in human milk but approaches 50% in preterm formulas (see Table 68–7). MCFA are not essential fatty acids. Previous reports suggested that MCFA were absorbed passively and to a greater extent than long-chain fatty acids (LCFA) and affected growth and mineral absorption positively (Roy et al, 1975; Tantibhedhyangkul and Hashim, 1978). Data comparing premature infants receiving MCFA at 42% versus 7% of total fatty acids in a crossover design demonstrated no differences in either absorption of fat or weight gain (Hamosh et al, 1989). Similarly, no differences in nitrogen retention, weight gain, and energy digestibility, expenditure, and storage were found in premature infants participating in a randomized, crossover study of formulas with MCFA at 46% versus 4% (Whyte et al, 1986). Other reports also confirm the lack of effect of MCFA on weight gain and mineral absorption compared with exclusively LCFA diets (Huston et al, 1983). When used in a high proportion, MCFA may be incompletely oxidized and contribute to increased urinary dicarboxylic acid excretion and metabolic inefficiency compared with LCFA (Rebouche et al, 1990; Wu et al, 1986). When added exogenously to milk, MCFA have been reported to adhere to feeding tubes, thereby diminishing fat delivery to the infant (Mehta et al, 1988). Thus, no compelling data exist to suggest that a high proportion of MCFA is needed for preterm formulas. Indeed, formulas containing a very high proportion of MCFA (>80%) may produce essential fatty acid deficiency if fed for a prolonged period of time.

#### *Hindmilk*

The variability in the fat content of human milk may be used to advantage in the premature infant. Most milk transfer during a feeding occurs in 10 to 15 minutes, but continued milk expression yields a milk with a progressively higher fat content—the hindmilk—than that of the earlier foremilk. The fat content of hindmilk may be 1.5- to 3-fold greater than that of foremilk. The use of hindmilk in selected cases may provide the premature infant with additional energy. Fractionation of each milk expression into two portions, foremilk and hindmilk, is practical if the mother's milk production is greater than that needed by the infant. The additional fat from hindmilk, resulting in increased energy intake, has been shown to improve body weight gain in premature infants (Valentine et al, 1994). The composition of foremilk and hindmilk has been examined (see Table 68–10). No differences between fractions were observed for the concentration of nitrogen, calcium, phosphorus, sodium, or potassium. Copper and zinc concentrations declined by approximately 5% from foremilk to hindmilk.

The differences between foremilk and hindmilk also should be considered in terms of the distribution of calories. Fat and protein compose 42% and 12%, respectively, of calories in foremilk and 55% and 9% of calories in hindmilk. Theoretically, the long-term feeding of hindmilk could exert a negative effect on protein status. A greater proportion of protein calories (10% to 12%) is recommended for premature infants. Usual commercial human milk fortifiers (Table 68–11; see also Table 68–7), when mixed with hindmilk, raise the proportion of protein calories in hindmilk to approximately 12%. Therefore, the use of hindmilk can be recommended for premature infants whose rate of weight gain is low (below 15 g/kg/day).

#### *Carnitine*

Carnitine is synthesized from lysine and methionine and serves as an important effector of fatty acid oxidation in the mitochondria. The provision of carnitine in the diet results in improved fatty acid oxidation (Bonner et al, 1995). Human milk contains abundant carnitine, and all infant formulas are supplemented with carnitine.

## Carbohydrate

The carbohydrate fraction of human milk is composed of lactose (90% to 95%) and oligosaccharides (5% to 10%). The lactose content of human milk rises from 55 g/L in colostrum to 70 g/L in mature milk. Studies in term infants demonstrate a small proportion of lactose in the feces; the presence of lactose is assumed to be a normal physiologic effect of feeding human milk. A softer stool consistency, more nonpathogenic bacterial fecal flora, and

**TABLE 68–11**

**Comparison of Selected Fortifiers for Human Milk***

| Nutritional Component | PrHM | EHMF | SHMF | SNC | Eo | SMAHMF | FM85 |
|---|---|---|---|---|---|---|---|
| Energy (kcal) | 70 | 81 | 81 | 74 | 84 | 84 | 88 |
| Fat (g) | 4.0 | 4.9 | 4.2 | 4.2 | 4.0 | 4.0 | 4.0 |
| Carbohydrate (g) | 7.0 | 7.2 | 8.6 | 7.6 | 9.8 | 9.4 | 10.6 |
| Protein (g) | 1.8 | 2.8 | 2.8 | 1.8 | 2.6 | 2.8 | 2.6 |
| Calcium (mg) | 22 | 141 | 141 | 98 | 72 | 112 | 73 |
| Phosphorus (mg) | 14 | 62 | 78 | 53 | 48 | 59 | 48 |
| Magnesium (mg) | 2.5 | 4.5 | 10.3 | 6.4 | 5.3 | 4.0 | 4.5 |
| Sodium (mEq) | 1.3 | 1.9 | 1.9 | 1.3 | 2.5 | 1.7 | 2.5 |
| Zinc (μg) | 320 | 1040 | 1310 | 780 | 320 | 450 | 320 |
| Copper (μg) | 60 | 104 | 230 | 133 | 60 | 60 | 60 |
| Vitamins | Yes | Multi | Multi | Multi | A,C,E,K | Multi | No |

*Prepared per 100 mL of preterm human milk (PrHM). Fortifiers: EHMF, Enfamil Human Milk Fortifier (Mead Johnson Nutritionals, Evansville, Ind); SNC, Similac Natural Care Advance (Ross), mixed 1:1 (vol:vol) with preterm human milk; SHMF, Similac Human Milk Fortifier (Ross Laboratories, Columbus, Ohio); Eo, Eoprotin (Milupa, Friedrichsdorf, Germany); SMAHMF, S-26 SMA Human Milk Fortifier (Wyeth Nutritionals International, Philadelphia, Pa); FM85, (Nestle, Vevey, Switzerland).

A,C,E,K, added vitamins A, C, E, K; Multi, added multivitamins: A, D, E, K, $B_1$, $B_2$, $B_6$, C, niacin, folate, $B_{12}$, pantothenate, biotin; No, no additional vitamins added.

Data from Ross Products Division, Abbott Laboratories, Columbus, OH, 2003.

improved absorption of minerals have been attributed to the presence of small quantities of unabsorbed lactose in feces (MacLean and Fink, 1980). Dietary lactose also has been associated with increased mineral absorption (Ziegler and Fomon, 1983). Theoretical concerns that lactose may not be digested adequately by premature infants of less than 34 weeks of postmenstrual age may be unfounded, as clinical studies indicate that they tolerate the feeding of lactose-containing milk. Premature infants absorb more than 90% of the lactose in human milk (Atkinson et al, 1981). The feeding of milk and, in particular, human milk to premature infants stimulates intestinal lactase activity compared with no feeding or formula feeding (Shulman et al, 1998a). Thus, early feeding of human milk also may be beneficial to promote better lactose utilization.

Because of conflicting data regarding lactose utilization by premature infants, and as a result of attempts to reduce the osmolality of the milk, preterm formulas contain a large proportion of carbohydrate as corn syrup solids (glucose polymers) (Ziegler and Fomon, 1983). The usual lactose-glucose polymer mixture is 50:50. Glucose polymers are well absorbed by premature infants.

## Calcium and Phosphorus

Calcium and phosphorus are primary components of the skeleton, accounting for 99% and 85%, respectively, of bone mass. The goal for premature infant nutrition is to achieve a bone mineralization pattern similar to that in the fetus, to avoid osteopenia and fractures. Preterm human milk contains approximately 250 mg/L and 140 mg/L, respectively, of calcium and phosphorus (Butte et al, 1984). In contrast, the calcium and phosphorus contents of enteral products designed for premature infants in the United States are significantly greater (see Tables 68–7 and 68–8). In human milk, calcium and phosphorus exist in ionized and complexed forms that are easily absorbed. Thus, in the design of commercial formulas, greater quantities of these minerals are added to compensate for their poorer bioavailability. However, distinct from the term infant, the premature infant requires significantly greater quantities of calcium and phosphorus than can be provided in human milk.

For the human milk–fed premature infant, calcium and phosphorus are deficient throughout lactation, and levels are far below those necessary to achieve respective intrauterine accretion rates (Schanler, 1991). Skeletal radiographs may reveal poor bone mineralization, rickets, and fractures in the premature infant fed human milk (Koo et al, 1988). Deficient intakes of calcium and phosphorus are associated with biochemical markers such as low serum and urine phosphorus concentrations, elevated serum alkaline phosphatase activity, and elevated serum and urine calcium concentrations (Atkinson et al, 1983). Usually, serum phosphorus concentrations are the best indicators of calcium and phosphorus status in human milk–fed premature infants (Aiken et al, 1993). Prolonged deficiency of these minerals tends to stimulate bone resorption to normalize serum calcium concentrations. This bone activity often is correlated with elevated serum alkaline phosphatase activity. It has been reported that a majority of premature infants who had an elevated serum alkaline phosphatase activity were those fed human milk (Lucas et al, 1989). Moreover, follow-up evaluations of the same infants at 9 and 18 months noted that linear growth was significantly lower in the group that had the higher serum activity of alkaline phosphatase in the neonatal period (Lucas et al, 1989). A high alkaline phosphatase value in the neonatal period is a negative predictor of height in 9- to 12-year-old adolescents (Fewtrell et al, 2000).

The supplementation of human milk with both calcium and phosphorus not only improves the net retention of both minerals but also improves bone mineral content (Horsman et al, 1989; Salle et al, 1986). Current management of human milk–fed premature infants emphasizes the need for supplements of both calcium and phosphorus (Schanler and Garza, 1987). A linear relationship exists between calcium (or phosphorus) intake and net retention in enterally fed premature infants (Schanler and Rifka, 1994). Premature infants receiving unfortified human milk never achieve intrauterine accretion rates for calcium and phosphorus. Intakes of approximately 200 and 100 mg/kg/day, respectively, of calcium and phosphorus can be achieved with the use of specialized human milk fortifiers and preterm formulas, thus making it possible to meet intrauterine estimates (see Tables 68–7, 68–8, and 68-11). However, term infant formulas and specialized (not "preterm") formulas provide inadequate quantities of calcium and phosphorus to meet the needs of growing premature infants (see Tables 68–8 and 68–9). Several factors affect the absorption of calcium and phosphorus, including postnatal age and intake of calcium, phosphorus, lactose, fat, and vitamin D. Vitamin D, however, is responsible for only a small component of calcium absorption in premature infants (Bronner et al, 1992).

The time to supply sufficient calcium and phosphorus stores for premature infants is during the initial hospitalization, before their discharge and the beginning of exclusive breast-feeding. However, because of the need for prolonged parenteral nutrition and the inability to provide "catch-up" quantities of calcium and phosphorus in milk, some infants may benefit from additional calcium and phosphorus after hospital discharge (see later section, "Postdischarge Nutrition").

## Magnesium

Approximately 60% of body magnesium is in bone. Preterm human milk contains approximately 30 mg/L of magnesium (Butte et al, 1984). The absorption of magnesium is significantly greater from unfortified human milk (73%) than from formula (48%) (Schanler and Refka, 1994). Net magnesium retention in human milk–fed premature infants meets intrauterine estimates. Thus, the data from balance studies and biochemical monitoring suggest that magnesium supplements are not needed for premature infants fed human milk (Schanler and Abrams, 1995). Similar studies in premature infants fed preterm formula indicate that, despite lower absorption compared with human milk, intrauterine estimates for magnesium accretion are surpassed.

## Trace Elements

### Zinc

Several factors affect the zinc needs of the enterally fed premature infant. Fetal accretion of zinc is approximately 0.85 mg/kg/day. Growth is a major determinant of zinc needs. The major excretory route is via the gastrointestinal tract. Infants with large gastrointestinal fluid losses may become zinc deficient. Premature infants receiving pooled pasteurized human milk (zinc intake of ~0.7 mg/kg/day) are in negative zinc balance for 60 days postnatally and never meet the intrauterine accretion rate (Dauncey et al, 1977). In contrast, intakes of 1.8 to 2 mg/kg/day are associated with a net retention of zinc that surpasses intrauterine accretion rates (Ehrenkranz et al, 1989; Schanler et al, 1999b; Tyrala, 1986). The classic signs of zinc deficiency include an erythematous skin rash involving perioral, perineal, and facial areas, as well as the extremities (Groh-Wargo, 2000). Although there are limitations to the assay, plasma zinc values lower than 50 μg/dL are highly suggestive of deficiency (Groh-Wargo, 2000). A very low serum alkaline phosphatase activity, a zinc-dependent enzyme, also is suggestive of deficiency. Reports of symptomatic zinc deficiency in unsupplemented human milk–fed premature infants serve as a reminder of the decline in milk zinc concentration as lactation advances. The infants reported to be zinc deficient were several months of age (Bilinski et al, 1987).

### Copper

No universally accepted methods exist to assess copper status clinically. Balance study data provide only an estimate of copper retention at one point in time. Premature infants receiving pooled pasteurized human milk (copper intakes of ~85 μg/kg/day) are in negative copper balance for 30 days postnatally and never meet the intrauterine accretion rate (Dauncey et al, 1977). Fortified human milk provides a copper intake of as much as 180 μg/kg/day, and balance study data surpass intrauterine accretion rates (Schanler et al, 1999b). Copper retention was quite variable in studies using formula providing intakes of 200 to 300 μg/kg/day (Schanler et al, 1999b; Tyrala, 1986). Several premature infants with those intakes, however, achieved the intrauterine accretion rate. Symptoms of copper deficiency include osteopenia, neutropenia, and hypochromic anemia. As copper is excreted in bile, cases of severe cholestasis warrant limiting copper intakes.

### Iron

The iron needs of the premature infant are determined by birth weight, initial hemoglobin, rate of growth, and magnitude of iron loss and/or volume of transfused blood (Groh-Wargo, 2000). Postnatal iron metabolism occurs in three phases. In the first phase, there is decreased erythropoiesis. The hemoglobin concentration declines to a nadir, "physiologic anemia of prematurity," which is at approximately 2 to 3 months of postnatal age. In the second phase, the hemoglobin rises as active red cell production is occurring. In this phase, iron is needed. The third phase is an exhaustion of iron stores, or "late anemia of prematurity," observed if iron supplementation is inadequate (Groh-Wargo, 2000).

The concentration of iron in human milk declines through lactation, from approximately 0.6 mg/L at 2 weeks to 0.3 mg/L after 5 months of lactation (Siimes et al, 1979). The absorption of iron is affected adversely by blood transfusion (Dauncey et al, 1978). Premature infants fed human milk are in negative iron balance, which, in the absence of transfusion, corrects with iron supplements (Dauncey et al, 1978). Iron absorption also appears to be facilitated by a modest degree of anemia (Moody et al, 1999). Thus, the usual recommendations for premature infants suggest delaying iron supplementation until 2 to 3 months of postnatal age, when hemoglobin concentrations are at a nadir (Lundström et al, 1977). However, the provision of small doses of iron at 2 mg/kg/day beginning 2 weeks postnatally has been demonstrated, in the absence of blood transfusions, to prevent the development of iron deficiency at 3 months of postnatal age (Lundström et al, 1977). When recombinant erythropoietin for the treatment of anemia of prematurity is used, higher doses of iron are needed, in the range of 6 mg/kg/day, to support the more rapid rate of erythropoiesis (Ehrenkranz et al, 1994).

Generally, ferrous sulfate (elemental iron, 2 mg/kg/day) drops are used in human milk–fed premature infants beginning soon after the achievement of complete enteral feedings. Formula-fed premature infants should receive iron-fortified formula from the onset of milk feeding.

### Sodium and Potassium

Premature infants generally need more sodium per unit of body weight than is needed by term infants (Groh-Wargo, 2000). This increased need is due to immature renal sodium conservation mechanisms. Sodium wasting is inversely related to gestational age. A comparison of sodium intakes of 2.9 and 1.6 mEq (mmol)/kg/day in premature infants suggested that the former intake provided more appropriate serum sodium concentrations (Roy et al, 1976). Hyponatremia also may occur in premature infants primarily fed human milk because the sodium content of preterm milk continues to decline through lactation (Roy et al, 1976). The need for these electrolytes may increase during or after diuretic usage.

## Vitamins

The fat-soluble vitamins A, D, E, and K are stored in the body, and large doses may result in toxicity. Water-soluble vitamins—thiamine, riboflavin, niacin, vitamin $B_6$, folate, vitamin $B_{12}$, pantothenic acid, biotin, and vitamin C—are not stored in the body, and excess intakes are excreted in the urine or bile (vitamin $B_{12}$). The intake of water-soluble vitamins, therefore, should be at frequent intervals to avoid deficiency states. Vitamin A and riboflavin concentrations decline in human milk under conditions of light exposure and after passage through feeding tubes (Bates et al, 1985). As a consequence of exposure to air, ascorbic acid concentrations are lower in pooled human milk (Heinonen et al, 1986). Supplementary vitamins are provided in human milk fortifiers and in preterm formulas (Schanler, 2002). There is no indication for additional multivitamin supplements for infants receiving adequate intakes of fortified human milk, preterm formula, or enriched formula. Once feedings in the premature infant change to unfortified human milk or standard formula, a multivitamin supplement should be added. The supplemental vitamins should be continued until the infant is consuming 300 kcal/day or weighs more than 2.5 kg.

## HUMAN MILK

The American Academy of Pediatrics acknowledges that human milk also is beneficial in the management of premature infants. The beneficial effects generally relate to improvements in host defenses, digestion and absorption of nutrients, gastrointestinal function, neurodevelopment, and maternal psychological well-being. However, the special needs of the premature infant that arise as a result of metabolic and gastrointestinal immaturity, immunologic compromise, and associated medical conditions must be considered so that adequate nutrition can be provided to meet the needs for intrauterine rates of growth and nutrient accretion. Human milk is capable of satisfying most of the needs of premature infants if careful attention is given to nutritional status.

### Benefits of Unfortified Human Milk

Clinical studies in nurseries throughout the world have suggested a decrease in the rate of a variety of infections, including sepsis, NEC, and urinary tract infection, in premature infants fed human milk compared with those fed formula (Contreras-Lemus et al, 1992; Narayanan et al, 1980).

NEC, the devastating acute intestinal inflammatory disease in premature infants, occurs less frequently when feedings consist of human milk than when formula is used. A large, nonrandomized study of hospitalized premature infants reported that the incidence of NEC was significantly lower in infants fed human milk, either exclusively or partially, compared with infants fed formula (Lucas and Cole, 1990). That study reported clinical cases as well as cases confirmed at surgery or autopsy, and in both circumstances, the incidence of NEC was significantly greater in premature infants solely fed formula. These data provide some encouragement for the potential prevention of NEC.

Specific factors such as sIgA, lactoferrin, lysozyme, oligosaccharides, cytokines (such as interkeukin-10 [IL-10]), enzymes (such as acetylhydolase), growth factors (such as epidermal growth factor), and cellular components may affect host defense mechanisms in the premature infant. One of the major protective effects of human milk in the infant operates through the enteromammary immune system. It is reasonable to expect that exposure of the mother to the environment of the neonatal nursery through skin-to-skin contact with her premature infant may be advantageous to the infant. In this manner, mothers potentially may be "induced" to make specific antibodies against the nosocomial pathogens in the nursery environment.

### Limitations in the Use of Unfortified Human Milk

A major impediment to advocating human milk for premature infants is the difficulty many mothers experience in providing sufficient quantities of milk. Several explanations have been given for the low milk production, including biologic immaturity of the mammary gland, maternal stress and/or illness, and difficulty maintaining a supply without a suckling infant. Another reason of concern is that nutrient intake is limited by the milk volume restrictions imposed on premature infants, because they cannot feed ad libitum and also because their medical condition warrants fluid restriction. The most compelling reason for concern is that nutrient intake is inadequate to meet the very great needs of the premature infant. Unfortified human milk may not supply sufficient quantities of nutrients for several reasons. Because of differences in the methods of milk expression and storage, the feeding of "spot" samples (individual samples of expressed milk from one or both breasts or milk partially expressed from one breast), the use of feeding tubes, and the differences in length of lactation, the macronutrient composition of human milk used in feeding premature infants varies greatly. Much of the variation in energy content, for example, is a result of differences in fat content of the unfortified milk (2.2 to 4.7 g/dL).

In addition, significant declines in the contents of protein and sodium occur through lactation (Schanler and Oh, 1980). The content of other nutrients (calcium, phosphorus) is too low to meet the great needs of the premature infant. Moreover, for technical reasons associated with the collection, storage, and delivery of milk to the infant, the quantity of available nutrients (fat, vitamin C, vitamin A, riboflavin) is decreased. Accordingly, it should not be a surprise that the inadequacies of calcium, phosphorus, protein, sodium, vitamins, and energy are observed in the premature infant fed unfortified human milk. Thus, the exclusive feeding of unfortified milk in premature infants, generally infants with birth weights less than 1500 g, has been associated with poorer rates of growth and nutritional deficits, during and beyond the period of hospitalization (Atkinson et al, 1981, 1983; Cooper et al, 1984; Gross, 1983; Kashyap et al, 1990).

### Human Milk Fortification

Growth and nutrient deficits in the premature infant can be corrected with the addition to human milk of multinutrient supplements or fortifiers (Greer and McCormick, 1988; Horsman et al, 1989; Polberger et al, 1989; Schanler et al, 1985a). Mineral supplementation during hospitalization prevents a decrease in linear growth and increases bone mineralization during and beyond the neonatal period (Abrams et al, 1989). Supplementation with both calcium and phosphorus results in normalization of biochemical indices of mineral status: serum calcium, phosphorus, and alkaline phosphatase activity and urinary excretion of calcium and phosphorus (Schanler and Garza, 1987). Sodium supplementation results in normalization of serum sodium (Kumar and Sacks, 1978). Protein and energy supplementation is associated with improved rates of weight gain and indices of protein nutritional status: blood urea nitrogen, serum albumin, and transthyretin (Kashyap et al, 1990; Polberger et al, 1989).

Current practice suggests the use of multinutrient fortification of human milk. Nutritional outcomes of feeding fortified milk in the United States indicate that premature infants receive less volume but greater intakes of proteins and minerals and experience greater gain in weight and increment in linear growth than is the case in infants fed unfortified human milk exclusively (Greer and McCormick, 1988; Lucas et al, 1996; Schanler and Abrams, 1995; Schanler et al, 1999b). Balance study data indicate that the use of fortified human milk results in net nutrient retention that approaches or is greater than expected intrauterine rates of accretion. Fat absorption with the use of some fortifiers, however, has been lower than expected (Schanler and Garza, 1987; Schanler et al, 1985b). Fat absorption may be augmented by newer human milk fortifiers that contain fat (Barrett-Reis et al, 2000).

Questions have been raised about whether the addition of bovine-derived human milk fortifiers affects feeding tolerance in premature infants. Gastric residual volumes often are used to assess feeding tolerance. When assessed throughout hospitalization, the use of fortified human milk was not associated with feeding intolerance, as manifested by abdominal distention, vomiting, changes in stool frequency, or volume of gastric aspirate (Lucas et al, 1996). Comparisons with preterm formula have been made, and no major differences in feeding tolerance have been attributed to human milk fortification (Moody et al, 2000; Schanler et al, 1999b).

A major concern with human milk fortification is that the added nutrients may affect the complex system of host defense. The effects of nutrient fortification on some of the general host defense properties of the milk have been evaluated (Jocson et al, 1997). Fortification did not affect the concentration of IgA. Bacterial colony counts do not increase with 24 hours of refrigerator storage of fortified human milk.

The relationship between the feeding of fortified human milk and the incidence of illness (infection and NEC) in premature infants has been examined. Human milk–fed infants had a 26% incidence of documented infection, compared with 49% in formula-fed infants (Hylander et al, 1998). The use of fortified human milk was not associated with an increased incidence of either confirmed infection or NEC, compared with control-supplemented human milk (Lucas et al, 1996). When these two events were combined, however, the group fed fortified human milk had more events than the control-supplemented group. Although it is difficult to conclude that the use of fortifiers is harmful, these data indicate the need for continued surveillance of these events (Schanler, 1996).

In a comparison of fortified human milk and preterm formula, premature infants fed exclusively fortified human milk had a significantly lower incidence of NEC and/or late-onset sepsis, fewer positive blood cultures, and less antibiotic usage than those fed preterm formula (Schanler et al, 1996b). Infants fed exclusively fortified human milk had more episodes of skin-to-skin contact with their mothers and a shorter duration of hospitalization. These data suggest that feeding premature infants fortified human milk can have a marked effect on the cost of medical care. The data further suggest that skin-to-skin contact may promote an enteromammary response in the premature infant. It may well become the practice to encourage mothers to practice skin-to-skin contact to enhance their capacity to synthesize specific factors that counter the pathogens in the nursery environment.

### Comparison of Human Milk Fortifiers

Human milk fortifiers are designed to be mixed with human milk. A variety of fortifiers are available globally, but no head-to-head comparison has been published. Most fortifiers are powdered nutrient preparations that contain protein, carbohydrate, calcium, phosphorus, magnesium, and sodium; the contents of zinc, copper, and vitamins are variable (see Table 68–11). Inherent in the design is the adequacy of the mother's milk production to meet the needs of the infant. The use of pasteurized donor human milk has not been advocated routinely because of concerns with contamination, lack of sufficient supply, and cost. If there is an inadequate amount of mother's milk, two options are currently available. One option is to alternate the feeding of fortified human milk with preterm formula, and a second option is to mix mother's milk with preterm formula.

One study examined the nutrient adequacy of a liquid human milk fortifier mixed 1:1 with human milk (Schanler et al, 1988). Nitrogen, energy, calcium, and phosphorus retentions were below intrauterine rates of accretion. More beneficial outcomes may be observed if preterm formula is alternately fed with fortified mother's milk.

## FEEDING TOLERANCE

Limitations in the ability to tolerate enteral feedings constitute a major problem for premature infants. Moreover, the infants' tolerance of enteral feeding is a primary concern of neonatologists because it affects their decision to initiate, advance, and discontinue feedings. Because of these concerns, feeding intolerance may be a major factor affecting the duration of hospitalization. The fetus experiences swallowing of amniotic fluid from early gestation, but postnatally, many premature neonates do not appear to share as "simple" a tolerance for enteral fluid, even diluted fluid mixtures. Several factors affect how feedings are tolerated: immature intestinal motility, digestive enzyme immaturity, medical complications, too great a volume intake, and hyperosmolar medications/feedings.

Despite its importance, universally agreed-upon criteria to judge feeding tolerance in premature infants are lacking. Clinical criteria of feeding intolerance (Table 68–12) generally include physical findings on examination, including abdominal distention and tenderness, presence or absence and quality of bowel sounds, and signs of residual gastric fluid aspirated from the feeding tube just prior to the next feeding, emesis, and changes in stool output

**TABLE 68-12**

**Potential Criteria Used to Assess Feeding Tolerance**

Abdominal distention
  With visible bowel loops
  Without visible bowel loops
Abdominal tenderness
Emesis
Gastric residual volume
  >2 mL/kg
  >50% of 3 hours of feeding
  Any change from previous pattern
Gastric residual characteristics
  Green, bilious
  Red, blood-tinged
Stool output
  Increased frequency
  Decreased frequency
Feeding withheld
  Document reasons feedings withheld
  Assess number of feedings withheld
Clinical condition
  Any worsening in previous medical condition

(Jadcherla and Kleigman, 2002). Occasional associated signs that may suggest intolerance to a feeding include increased episodes of apnea and bradycardia, diminished oxygen saturation (desaturation events), and lethargy.

The gastric residual volume, usually measured prior to the next feeding, is an indication of milk remaining in the stomach several hours after a feeding (Mihatsch et al, 2002). The gastric residual volume indicates the rapidity of gastric emptying and appears to be affected by any changes in the clinical condition that results in decreased gastric emptying. The nonspecific nature of this assessment is reflected in the fact that changes in the clinical examination may or may not be related to intestinal pathology. Gastric residual volume has been quantitated on the basis of body weight (for example, a volume of greater than 2 mL/kg per feeding is abnormal) or the volume of feeding (for example, greater than 50% of volume for 3 hours of feeding is abnormal) (Schanler et al, 1999a). Some premature infants have measurable gastric residual volumes before every feeding, whereas others never have any measurable volume. In the latter infants, therefore, any small change might indicate a change in feeding tolerance. Furthermore, gastric residual volume would be difficult to interpret in infants receiving continuous gastric milk infusions. Such is not always the case, as these infants generally empty their stomachs rapidly and should still be evaluated every 2 to 4 hours in a manner similar to that used for infants fed by the intermittent bolus technique (Schanler et al, 1999a).

Assessment of the quality of the gastric residual also has been discussed as a tool to determine feeding tolerance. Gastric residuals that are green or bilious could indicate intestinal obstruction but more often indicate overdistention of the stomach and retrograde reflux of bile into the stomach. A blood-tinged residual could indicate an inflammatory process but may indicate a slight mucosal irritation from the indwelling gastric tube.

Unfortunately, the aforementioned criteria have little prognostic significance. In one study, infants who had more gastric residuals and emesis episodes were just as likely to reach the milestone of full enteral tube feeding than infants who did not have any increases in these measurements (Moody et al, 2000).

Most clinicians use the pattern of the previously mentioned criteria, as opposed to a single measurement, as an aid to determine feeding status. In several instances, the infant's feedings may be withheld because of one or more of the aforementioned signs. Often a single feeding is discarded. Careful assessment and examination prior to the next feeding generally aid the decision to continue feedings. A withheld feeding, however, does not imply that further enteral feeding should be terminated. Too often, feedings are withheld for prolonged periods of time, which hastens the complications of parenteral nutrition and intestinal atrophy.

The evaluation of the infant with a large gastric residual, for example, would include the following considerations. Has the medical condition worsened, such that gastric emptying is delayed because of systemic disease? Is the infant's feeding tube in the correct location? If the feeding tube is high in the esophagus or is of too small a caliber, then swallowed air may not be evacuated. Large amounts of swallowed air may cause gastric overdistention with displacement of ingested milk, resulting in emesis and/or large residuals. Body positioning also may play a role. In some cases, gastric emptying is improved by placement of the infant in the prone position or in the right lateral decubitis position, rather than the supine position. At times, tolerance is corrected by lowering milk intake somewhat.

## FEEDING METHODS

Tube feeding is an essential tool in enteral nutrition because the premature infant may be unable to suck and/or coordinate suck-swallow-breathe. Tube feeding methods include continuous and intermittent bolus methods. Any of various approaches may be used including orogastric, nasogastric, transpyloric, and gastrostomy. The selection of practice relates to the duration of the proposed therapy: premature infants will eventually suckle, so a temporary oro(naso)gastric tube is used; infants with major congenital anomalies may require a semipermanent gastrostomy.

The bolus feeding method mimics the normal adult feed-fast routine and is associated with greater hormonal responses than those occurring with continuous infusions (Aynsley-Green et al, 1982). The bolus technique does not require an infusion pump. Differences between continuous and intermittent bolus methods have been evaluated. Premature infants had more feeding tolerance and a slower rate of weight gain with continuous infusion than with the bolus technique (Schanler et al, 1999a). Neither method enhanced nutrient absorption.

Occasionally, intolerance is observed in the bolus-fed premature infant. In some instances, duodenal motility decreases following the bolus feeding (DeVille et al,

1993). Giving a bolus feeding over a longer time interval, such as 30 to 120 minutes, results in a return of motility and improved tolerance.

Continuous infusion technique has been associated with increased nutrient absorption in infants with gastrointestinal disease (Parker et al, 1981). It seems prudent to use this method in infants who have had intestinal surgery and in infants receiving milk via a transpyloric tube. In some infants with persistent gastric residuals or emesis in the absence of an obvious intestinal pathologic process, the use of transpyloric feeding tubes has been successful.

## FEEDING ISSUES

Enteral feeding and concomitant use of an umbilical arterial catheter have been subjects of much concern. However, most infants had an indwelling catheter in the most recent studies of gastrointestinal priming, and no untoward events were reported (Dunn et al, 1988; Schanler et al, 1999a). Infants were no more likely to develop intolerance or NEC if they received enteral feedings while they had an umbilical arterial catheter in place than if they received enteral feedings 24 hours after the catheter was removed (Davey et al, 1994). Moreover, fewer evaluations for sepsis and less frequent use of central venous catheters were observed in the group receiving feedings while the catheter was in place. Thus, there appears to be no increased risk associated with enteral feeding while an umbilical arterial catheter is in place as long as the catheter is functioning optimally.

The use of diluted milks has been suggested for feeding premature infants. In one study, however, intestinal motility responses to feeding were initiated earlier and persisted longer following the use of full-strength formula than with use of one-third and two-thirds dilutions of the formula (Koenig et al, 1995). The use of water for enteral feeding also has been shown not to affect intestinal motility as compared with milk (Berseth et al, 1992). Thus, initiating feedings with full-strength milk appears to be tolerated and appropriate.

The advancement of daily feeding volumes also has been investigated, especially with respect to the development of NEC. When compared with matched case controls, infants with NEC were more likely to have received enteral nutrition with daily intakes greater than 20 mL/kg, averaging 46 mL/kg (McKeown et al, 1992). One study examined the morbidity of low-birth-weight infants whose daily increments in feeding volume were 15 or 35 mL/kg/day (Rayyis et al, 1999). In infants whose feedings were advanced rapidly, the duration of time to achieve full tube feeding and regain birth weight was shorter than in infants whose feedings were advanced slowly, and no difference in morbidity was noted.

## NUTRITIONAL ASSESSMENT

Neonatal nutritional assessment is an emerging interest that requires a knowledge of both nutritional biochemistry and neonatal medical conditions. The nutritionist is a key person to provide input on a daily basis that is compatible with the medical condition of the infant.

The nutritional status of the premature infant (Table 68–13) is monitored by daily assessments of fluid and energy intake and evaluation of the rate of growth in weight, length, and head circumference. Growth parameters are plotted on graph paper or a specific chart for premature infants' growth. The charts are helpful, but equally important is the computation of the weekly rate of growth (Usher and McLean, 1969) (see Table 68–3). Once the infant reaches a weight of 2.5 kg, a daily weight gain of 20 to 30 g/day is appropriate.

The nutritional status of the premature infant also is monitored by serial evaluations of biochemical indices. These assessments include serum calcium, phosphorus, and alkaline phosphatase activity to assess bone mineral status and albumin and urea nitrogen to assess protein status. If more specific indices of protein status are needed, as when additional protein supplementation is used, the serum prealbumin (transthyretin) is measured before and 1 week after the supplementation. Serum sodium, chloride, and bicarbonate are evaluated in infants receiving diuretics, those whose intakes are limited, or those with slow growth. The hemoglobin and reticulocyte counts are monitored to assess for anemia. Specific determinations of plasma zinc and copper are not routinely useful, but zinc may be measured in infants with unusual losses, such as after gastrointestinal surgery and from enterostomies. The pattern of changes in biochemical indices may be more reflective of nutritional status than are isolated values.

**TABLE 68–13**

**Nutritional Assessment of the Enterally Fed Premature Infant**

| Component Measured | Frequency |
|---|---|
| Fluid intake (mL/kg/day) | Daily |
| Parenteral intake | |
| Enteral intake | |
| Nutrient intake (units/kg/day) | Daily |
| Energy intake (kcal) | |
| Protein intake (g) | |
| Specific nutrient (unit) | |
| Anthropometry | |
| Body weight (g) | Same time each day |
| Length (cm) | Weekly |
| Head circumference (cm) | Weekly |
| Biochemical monitoring | |
| Hemoglobin, hematocrit | Weekly |
| Reticulocyte count | Weekly |
| Serum electrolytes | Twice weekly, then every 2 weeks* |
| Calcium, phosphorus | Twice weekly, then every 2 weeks |
| Alkaline phosphatase | Twice weekly, then every 2 weeks |
| Albumin, blood urea nitrogen | Twice weekly, then every 2 weeks† |
| Other assessments | |
| Renal ultrasound examination‡ | At 2 months of age |

*If infant is receiving human milk or diuretics.

†Add prealbumin if abnormal.

‡To evaluate for nephrocalcinosis.

Occasionally, renal ultrasound examination to determine the presence of nephrocalcinosis and wrist x-ray studies to identify rickets are warranted.

## POST-DISCHARGE NUTRITION

Some evidence suggests that the quality of early nutrition support has long-term implications for infant health and development. The goal of in-hospital nutritional support is to meet intrauterine rates of nutrient accretion. Accordingly, the premature infant should receive fortified human milk or preterm formula during the hospitalization period. Hospital discharge, however, frequently occurs before the completion of the intrauterine growth phase (up to approximately 36 weeks). Moreover, during hospitalization, despite what we may consider to be optimal nutrient support, growth deficits emerge, such that at discharge, the infant is well below the 10th percentile on corresponding growth charts (Wilson et al, 1997). Thus, concerns about nutrition support extend into the postdischarge period. Unfortunately, unlike in the term infant, whose needs are modeled after the healthy breast-fed infant, and the premature infant, whose needs are determined by the intrauterine growth model, there are no references to determine the nutritional needs of the premature infant at discharge.

Nutrition should be discussed at all times when discharge planning is done. Certain key questions need to be answered so that an appropriate nutritional plan can be devised. If the infant continues to manifest adequate weight gain on feedings of unfortified human milk or term infant formula taken ad libitum, then those diets can be recommended. In addition, if the prior biochemical model of nutritional status shows no unusual pattern suggesting nutrient inadequacy, then the routine diets can be recommended.

More often, especially in infants with bronchopulmonary dysplasia, adequate intake is not achieved, and biochemical markers of nutritional status reveal deficits. These infants cannot be discharged on the routine diets. If they are formula fed, enriched formulas will provide multinutrient needs (Carver et al, 2001) (see Table 68–8). In addition, these formulas can be concentrated to 24 to 30 kcal/ounce formulations to meet the needs for fluid restriction. The breast-feeding infant needs further attention. It may suffice to allow unrestricted breast-feeding but then to add 2 to 3 feedings of the enriched formula, prepared as 24 to 30 kcal/ounce formulations. In all cases, follow-up visits for assessment of nutritional status are recommended at 1 week and 1 month after discharge. Rates of growth should exceed 20 g/day for weight and 0.7 cm/week for length and head circumference increments. Biochemical monitoring to assess mineral and protein status is indicated at these follow-up visits (Hall, 2001).

## SUMMARY OF NUTRITIONAL SUPPORT

A comprehensive enteral nutrition pathway for premature infants has been described. The approach is multifaceted, beginning with minimal enteral, or trophic, feeding to enteral nutrition, and continuing to full enteral feeding and hospital discharge. This approach does not increase the risks already associated with prematurity. Indeed, the use of an aggressive approach to nutritional support has resulted in improved growth, with fewer infants falling below the 10th percentile on standard growth charts (Wilson et al, 1997). Although improvements are found in growth, no increase in sepsis or NEC is associated with the more aggressive approach to nutritional support (Wilson et al, 1997).

## SELECTED READINGS

American Academy of Pediatrics Work Group on Breastfeeding: Breastfeeding and the use of human milk. Pediatrics 100: 1035-1039, 1997.

Hambraeus L: Proprietary milk versus human breast milk in infant feeding: A critical appraisal from the nutritional point of view. Pediatr Clin North Am 24:17-35, 1977.

Hay WW Jr, Lucas A, Heird WC, et al: Workshop summary: Nutrition of the extremely low birth weight infant. Pediatrics 104:1360-1368, 1999.

Kuschel CA, Harding JE: Multicomponent fortified human milk for promoting growth in preterm infants. Cochrane Database Syst Rev CD003310(4), 2000.

Life Sciences Research Office, American Society for Nutritional Sciences: Nutrient requirements for preterm infant formulas. American Society for Nutritional Sciences, Washington, DC, 2001.

Schanler RJ: Special methods in feeding the preterm infant. In Tsang RC, Nichols BL (eds): Nutrition During Infancy. Philadelphia, Hanley & Belfus, 1988, pp 314-325.

Tyson JE, Kennedy KA: Minimal enteral nutrition for promoting feeding tolerance and preventing morbidity in parenterally fed neonates. Cochrane Database Syst Rev CD000504(2), 2000.

Ziegler EE, O'Donnell AM, Nelson SE, et al: Body composition of the reference fetus. Growth 40:329-341, 1976.

## REFERENCES

Abrams SA, Schanler RJ, Tsang RC, et al: Bone mineralization in former very low birth weight infants fed either human milk or commercial formula: One year follow-up observation. J Pediatr 114:1041-1044, 1989.

Aiken CGA, Sherwood RA, Lenney W: Role of plasma phosphate measurements in detecting rickets of prematurity and in monitoring treatment. Ann Clin Biochem 30:469-475, 1993.

Atkinson SA, Bryan MH, Anderson GH: Human milk: Difference in nitrogen concentration in milk from mothers of term and premature infants. J Pediatr 93:67-69, 1978.

Atkinson SA, Bryan MH, Anderson GH: Human milk feeding in premature infants: Protein, fat and carbohydrate balances in the first two weeks of life. J Pediatr 99:617-624, 1981.

Atkinson SA, Radde IC, Anderson GH: Macromineral balances in premature infants fed their own mothers' milk or formula. J Pediatr 102:99-106, 1983.

Aynsley-Green A, Adrian TE, Bloom SR: Feeding and the development of enteroinsular hormone secretion in the preterm infant: Effects of continuous gastric infusion of human milk compared with intermittent boluses. Acta Paediatr Scand 71:379-383, 1982.

Barrett-Reis B, Hall RT, Schanler RJ, et al: Enhanced growth of preterm infants fed a new powdered human milk fortifier: A randomized controlled trial. Pediatrics 106:581-588, 2000.

Bates CJ, Liu DS, Fuller NJ, et al: Susceptibility of riboflavin and vitamin A in breast milk to photodegradation and its implications for the use of banked breast milk in infant feeding. Acta Paediatr Scand 74:40-44, 1985.

Berseth CL: Effect of early feeding on maturation of the preterm infant's small intestine. J Pediatr 120:947-953, 1992.

Berseth CL, Nordyke CK, Valdes MG, et al: Responses of gastrointestinal peptides and motor activity to milk and water feedings in preterm and term infants. Pediatr Res 31:587-590, 1992.

Bilinski DL, Ehrenkranz RA, Cooley-Jacobs J, et al: Symptomatic zinc deficiency in a breast-fed, premature infant. Arch Dermatol 123:1221-1224, 1987.

Billeaud C, Guillet J, Sandler B: Gastric emptying in infants with or without gastro-oesophageal reflux according to the type of milk. Eur J Clin Nutr 44:577-583, 1990.

Bonner CM, DeBrie KL, Hug G, et al: Effects of parenteral L-carnitine supplementation on fat metabolism and nutrition in premature neonates. J Pediatr 126:287-292, 1995.

Bresson JL, Bader B, Rocchiccioli F, et al: Protein-metabolism kinetics and energy-substrate utilization in infants fed parenteral solutions with different glucose-fat ratios. Am J Clin Nutr 54:370-376, 1991.

Bronner F, Salle BL, Putet G, et al: Net calcum absorption in premature infants: Results of 103 metabolic balance studies. Am J Clin Nutr 56:1037-1044, 1992.

Butte NF, Garza C, Johnson CA, et al: Longitudinal changes in milk composition of mothers delivering preterm and term infants. Early Hum Dev 9:153-162, 1984.

Carlson SE, Werkman SH, Rhodes PG, et al: Visual-acuity development in healthy preterm infants: Effect of marine-oil supplementation. Am J Clin Nutr 58:35-42, 1993.

Carver JD, Wu PYK, Hall RT, et al: Growth of preterm infants fed nutrient-enriched or term formula after hospital discharge. Pediatrics 107:683-689, 2001.

Clandinin MT, Parrott A, Van Aerde JE, et al: Feeding preterm infants a formula containing $C_{20}$ and $C_{22}$ fatty acids simulates plasma phospholipid fatty acid composition of infants fed human milk. Early Hum Dev 31:41-51, 1992.

Contreras-Lemus J, Flores-Huerta S, Cisneros-Silva I, et al: Disminucion de la morbilidad en neonatos preterminos alimentados con leche de su propia madre. Biol Med Hosp Infant Mex 49:671-677, 1992.

Cooper PA, Rothberg AD, Pettifor JM, et al: Growth and biochemical response of premature infants fed pooled preterm milk or special formula. J Pediatr Gastroenterol Nutr 3:749-754, 1984.

Dauncey MJ, Davies CG, Shaw JCL, et al: The effect of iron supplements and blood transfusion on iron absorption by low birth weight infants fed pasteurized human breast milk. Pediatr Res 12:899-904, 1978.

Dauncey MJ, Shaw JCL, Urman J: The absorption and retention of magnesium, zinc, and copper by low birth weight infants fed pasteurized human breast milk. Pediatr Res 11:1033-1039, 1977.

Davey AM, Wagner CL, Cox C, et al: Feeding premature infants while low umbilical artery catheters are in place: A prospective, randomized trial. J Pediatr 124:795-799, 1994.

DeVille KT, Shulman RJ, Berseth CL: Slow infusion feeding enhances gastric emptying in preterm infants compared to bolus feeding. Clin Res 41:787A, 1993.

Dunn L, Hulman S, Weiner J, et al: Beneficial effects of early hypocaloric enteral feeding on neonatal gastrointestinal function: Preliminary report of a randomized trial. J Pediatr 112:622-629, 1988.

Ehrenkranz RA, Gettner PA, Nelli CM, et al: Zinc and copper nutritional studies in very low birth weight infants: Comparison of stable isotope extrinsic tag and chemical balance methods. Pediatr Res 26:298-307, 1989.

Ehrenkranz RA, Sherwonit EA, Nelli CM, et al: Recombinant human erythropoietin stimulates incorporation of absorbed iron into RBCs in VLBW infants. Pediatr Res 35:311A, 1994.

Ellis KJ, Shypailo RJ, Schanler RJ, et al: Body elemental composition of the neonate: New reference data. Am J Hum Biol 5:323-330, 1993.

Fewtrell MS, Cole TJ, Bishop NJ, et al: Neonatal factors predicting childhood height in preterm infants: Evidence for a persisting effect of early metabolic bone disease? J Pediatr 137:668-673, 2000.

Gaull GE, Rassin DK, Raiha NCR, et al: Milk protein quantity and quality in low-birthweight infants. III. Effects on sulfur amino acids in plasma and urine. J Pediatr 90:348-355, 1977.

Greer FR, McCormick A: Improved bone mineralization and growth in premature infants fed fortified own mother's milk. J Pediatr 112:961-969, 1988.

Greer FR, McCormick A, Loker J: Changes in fat concentration of human milk during delivery by intermittent bolus and continuous mechanical pump infusion. J Pediatr 105:745-749, 1984.

Groh-Wargo S: Recommended enteral nutrient intakes. In Groh-Wargo S, Thompson M, Cox JH, et al (eds): Nutritional Care for High-Risk Newborns, 3rd rev ed. Chicago, Precept Press, 2000, pp 231-263.

Gross SJ: Growth and biochemical response of preterm infants fed human milk or modified infant formula. N Engl J Med 308:237-241, 1983.

Gross SJ, David RJ, Bauman L, et al: Nutritional composition of milk produced by mothers delivering preterm. J Pediatr 96:641-644, 1980.

Gutcher GR, Farrell PM: Intravenous infusion of lipid for the prevention of essential fatty acid deficiency in premature infants. Am J Clin Nutr 54:1024-1028, 1991.

Hall RT: Nutritional follow-up of the breastfeeding premature infant after hospital discharge. Pediatr Clin North Am 48: 453-460, 2001.

Hamosh M, Bitman J, Liao TH et al: Gastric lipolysis and fat absorption in preterm infants: Effect of medium-chain triglyceride– or long-chain triglyceride–containing formulas. Pediatrics 83:86-97, 1989.

Heinonen K, Mononen I, Mononen T, et al: Plasma vitamin C levels are low in premature infants fed human milk. Am J Clin Nutr 43:923-924, 1986.

Horsman A, Ryan SW, Congdon PJ, et al: Bone mineral accretion rate and calcium intake in preterm infants. Arch Dis Child 64:910-918, 1989.

Huston RK, Reynolds JW, Jensen C, et al: Nutrient and mineral retention and vitamin D absorption in low-birth-weight infants: Effect of medium-chain triglycerides. Pediatrics 72:44-48, 1983.

Hylander MA, Strobino DM, Dhanireddy R: Human milk feedings and infection among very low birth weight infants. Pediatrics 102:e38, 1998.

Innis SM: Human milk and formula fatty acids. J Pediatr 120:S56-S61, 1992.

Jadcherla SR, Kleigman RM: Studies of feeding intolerance in very low birth weight infants: Definition and significance. Pediatrics 109:516-517, 2002.

Jensen RG, Jensen GL: Specialty lipids for infant nutrition. I. Milks and formulas. J Pediatr Gastroenterol Nutr 15:232-245, 1992.

Jocson MAL, Mason EO, Schanler RJ: The effects of nutrient fortification and varying storage conditions on host defense properties of human milk. Pediatrics 100:240-243, 1997.

Kashyap S, Forsyth M, Zucker C, et al: Effects of varying protein and energy intakes on growth and metabolic response in low birth weight infants. J Pediatr 108:955-963, 1986.

Kashyap S, Schulze K, Forsyth M, et al: Growth, nutrient retention, and metabolic response in low birth weight infants fed varying intakes of protein and energy. J Pediatr 113:713-721, 1988.

Kashyap S, Schulze KF, Forsyth M, et al: Growth, nutrient retention, and metabolic response of low-birth-weight infants fed supplemented and unsupplemented preterm human milk. Am J Clin Nutr 52:254-262, 1990.

Koenig WJ, Amarnath RP, Hench V, et al: Manometrics for preterm and term infants: A new tool for old questions. Pediatrics 95:203-206, 1995.

Koo WWK, Sherman R, Succop P, et al: Sequential bone mineral content in small preterm infants with and without fractures and rickets. J Bone Miner Res 3:193-197, 1988.

Kumar SP, Sacks LM: Hyponatremia in very low-birth-weight infants and human milk feedings. J Pediatr 93:1026-1027, 1978.

Lucas A, Bloom R, Aynsley-Green A: Gut hormones and "minimal enteral feeding." Acta Paediatr Scand 75:719-723, 1986.

Lucas A, Brooke OG, Baker BA, et al: High alkaline phosphatase activity and growth in preterm neonates. Arch Dis Child 64:902-909, 1989.

Lucas A, Cole TJ: Breast milk and neonatal necrotizing enterocolitis. Lancet 336:1519-1523, 1990.

Lucas A, Fewtrell MS, Morley R, et al: Randomized outcome trial of human milk fortification and developmental outcome in preterm infants. Am J Clin Nutr 64:142-151, 1996.

Lundström U, Siimes MA, Dallman PR: At what age does iron supplementation become necessary in low birthweight infants? J Pediatr 91:878-883, 1977.

MacLean WC, Fink, BB: Lactose malabsorption by premature infants: Magnitude and clinical significance. J Pediatr 97:383-388, 1980.

McKeown RE, Marsh D, Amarnath U, et al: Role of delayed feeding and of feeding increments in necrotizing enterocolitis. J Pediatr 121:764-770, 1992.

Meetze WH, Valentine C, McGuigan JE, et al: Gastrointestinal priming prior to full enteral nutrition in very low birth weight infants. J Pediatr Gastroenterol Nutr 15:163-170, 1992.

Mehta NR, Hamosh M, Bitman J, et al: Adherence of medium-chain fatty acids to feeding tubes during gavage. J Pediatr 112:474-476, 1988.

Mihatsch WA, von Schoenaich P, Fahnenstich H, et al: The significance of gastric residuals in the early enteral feeding advancement of extremely low birth weight infants. Pediatrics 109:457-459, 2002.

Moody GJ, Schanler RJ, Abrams SA: Utilization of supplemental iron by premature infants fed fortified human milk. Acta Paediatr 88:763-767, 1999.

Moody GJ, Schanler RJ, Lau C, et al: Feeding tolerance in premature infants fed fortified human milk. J Pediatr Gastroenterol Nutr 30:408-412, 2000.

Moro GE, Fulconis F, Minoli I, et al: Growth and plasma amino acid concentrations in very low birthweight infants fed either human milk protein fortified human milk or whey-predominant formula. Acta Paediatr Scand 78:18-22, 1989.

Narayanan I, Prakash K, Bala S, et al: Partial supplementation with expressed breast-milk for prevention of infection in low-birth-weight infants. Lancet 2:561-563, 1980.

Neu J, Roig JC, Meetze WH, et al: Enteral glutamine supplementation for very low birth weight infants decreases morbidity. J Pediatr 131:691-699, 1997.

Neville MC, Keller RP, Seacat J, et al: Studies on human lactation. I. Within-feed and between-breast variation in selected components of human milk. Am J Clin Nutr 40:635-646, 1984.

Parker P, Stroop S, Greene H: A controlled comparison of continuous versus intermittent feeding in the treatment of infants with intestinal disease. J Pediatr 99:360-364, 1981.

Piedboeuf B, Chessex P, Hazan J, et al: Total parenteral nutrition in the newborn infant: Energy substrates and respiratory gas exchange. J Pediatr 118:97-102, 1991.

Polberger SKT, Axelsson IA, Raiha NCR: Growth of very low birth weight infants on varying amounts of human milk protein. Pediatr Res 25:414-419, 1989.

Raiha NCR, Heinonen K, Rassin DK, et al: Milk protein quantity and quality in low-birth-weight infants. I. Metabolic responses and effects on growth. Pediatrics 57:659-674, 1976.

Rassin DK, Gaull E, Raiha NCR, et al: Milk protein quantity and quality in low-birth-weight infants. IV. Effects on tyrosine and phenylalanine in plasma and urine. J Pediatr 90:356-360, 1977.

Rayyis SF, Ambalavanan N, Wright L, et al: Randomized trial of "slow" versus "fast" feed advancements on the incidence of necrotizing enterocolitis in very low birth weight infants. J Pediatr 134:293-297, 1999.

Rebouche CJ, Panagides DD, Nelson SE: Role of carnitine in utilization of dietary medium-chain triglycerides by term infants. Am J Clin Nutr 52:820-824, 1990.

Roy CC, Ste-Marie M, Chartrand L, et al: Correction of the malabsorption of the preterm infant with a medium-chain triglyceride formula. J Pediatr 86:446-450, 1975.

Roy RN, Chance GW, Radde IC, et al: Late hyponatremia in very low birthweight infants. Pediatr Res 526-53l, 1976.

Salas-Salvadó J, Molina J, Figueras J, et al: Effect of the quality of infused energy on substrate utilization in the newborn receiving total parenteral nutrition. Pediatr Res 33:112-117, 1993.

Salle B, Senterre J, Putet G, et al: Effects of calcium and phosphorus supplementation on calcium retention and fat absorption in preterm infants fed pooled human milk. J Pediatr Gastroenterol Nutr 5:638-642., 1986.

Savilahti E, Kuitunen M: Allergenicity of cow milk proteins. J Pediatr 121:S12-S20, 1992.

Schanler RJ: Calcium and phosphorus absorption and retention in preterm infants. Exp Med 2:24-36, 1991.

Schanler RJ: Human milk fortification for premature infants. Am J Clin Nutr 64:249-250, 1996.

Schanler RJ: Water-soluble vitamins for premature infants. In Tsang RC, Koletzko B, Uauy R, Zlotkin, S (eds): Nutrition of the Preterm Infant: Scientific Basis and Practical Guidelines. Cincinnati, Digital Educational Publishing, in press.

Schanler RJ, Abrams SA: Postnatal attainment of intrauterine macromineral accretion rates in low birth weight infants fed fortified human milk. J Pediatr 126:441-447, 1995.

Schanler RJ, Abrams SA, Garza C: Bioavailability of calcium and phosphorus in human milk fortifiers and formula for very low birth weight infants. J Pediatr 113:95-100, 1988.

Schanler RJ, Garza C: Improved mineral balance in very low birth weight infants fed fortified human milk. J Pediatr 112:452-456, 1987.

Schanler RJ, Garza C, Nichols BL: Fortified mothers' milk for very low birth weight infants: Results of growth and nutrient balance studies. J Pediatr 107:437-445, 1985b.

Schanler RJ, Garza C, Smith E O: Fortified mothers' milk for very low birth weight infants: Results of macromineral balance studies. J Pediatr 107:767-774, 1985a.

Schanler RJ, Goldblum RM, Garza C, et al: Enhanced fecal excretion of selected immune factors in very low birth weight infants fed fortified human milk. Pediatr Res 20:711-715, 1986.

Schanler RJ, Oh W: Composition of breast milk obtained from mothers of premature infants as compared to breast milk obtained from donors. J Pediatr 96:679-68l, 1980.

Schanler RJ, Rifka M: Calcium, phosphorus, and magnesium needs for low birth weight infants. Acta Paediatr 83:111-116, 1994.

Schanler RJ, Shulman RJ, Lau C: Feeding strategies for premature infants: Beneficial outcomes of feeding fortified human milk *vs* preterm formula. Pediatrics 103:1150-1157, 1999b.

Schanler RJ, Shulman RJ, Lau C, et al: Feeding strategies for premature infants: Randomized trial of gastrointestinal priming and tube-feeding method. Pediatrics 103:434-439, 1999a.

Shulman RJ, Schanler RJ, Lau C, et al: Early feeding, feeding tolerance, and lactase activity in preterm infants. J Pediatr 133:645-649, 1998a.

Shulman RJ, Schanler RJ, Lau C, et al: Early feeding, antenatal glucocorticoids, and human milk decrease intestinal permeability in preterm infants. Pediatr Res 44:519-523, 1998b.

Siimes MA, Vuori E, Kuitunen P: Breast milk iron: A declining concentration during the course of lactation. Acta Paediatr Scand 68:29-31, 1979.

Sinclair JC: Energy balance of the newborn. In Sinclair JC (ed): Temperature Regulation and Energy Metabolism in the Newborn. New York, Grune & Stratton, 1978, pp 187-204.

Slagle TA, Gross SJ: Effect of early low-volume enteral substrate on subsequent feeding tolerance in very low birth weight infants. J Pediatr 113:526-531, 1988.

Specker BL, Greer F, Tsang RC: Vitamin D. In Tsang RC, Nichols BL (eds): Nutrition During Infancy. Philadelphia, Hanley & Belfus, 1988, pp 264-276.

Tantibhedhyangkul P, Hashim SA: Medium-chain triglyceride feeding in premature infants: Effects on calcium and magnesium absorption. Pediatrics 61:537-544, 1978.

Tyrala EE: Zinc and copper balances in preterm infants. Pediatrics 77:513-517, 1986.

Uauy R, Hoffman DR: Essential fatty acid requirements for normal eye and brain development. Semin Perinatol 15:449-455, 1991.

Usher R, McLean F: Intrauterine growth of live-born Caucasian infants at sea level: Standards obtained from measurements in 7 dimensions of infants born between 25 and 44 weeks of gestation. Pediatrics 74:901-910, 1969.

Valentine CJ, Hurst NM, Schanler RJ: Hindmilk improves weight gain in low-birth-weight infants fed human milk. J Pediatr Gastroenterol Nutr 18:474-477, 1994.

Weinstein MR, Oh W: Oxygen consumption in infants with bronchopulmonary dysplasia. J Pediatr 99:958-993, 1981.

Whyte RK, Campbell D, Stanhope R, et al: Energy balance in low birth weight infants fed formula of high or low medium-chain triglyceride content. J Pediatr 108:964-971, 1986.

Wilson DC, Cairns P, Halliday HL et al: Randomised controlled trial of an aggressive nutritional regimen in sick very low birth-weight infants. Arch Dis Child 77:F4-F11, 1997.

Wu PYK, Edmond J, Auestad N, et al: Medium-chain triglycerides in infant formulas and their relation to plasma ketone body concentrations. Pediatr Res 20:338-341, 1986.

Yunis KA, Oh W: Effects of intravenous glucose loading on oxygen consumption, carbon dioxide production, and resting energy expenditure in infants with bronchopulmonary dysplasia. J Pediatr 115:127-132, 1989.

Ziegler EE, Fomon SJ: Lactose enhances mineral absorption in infancy. J Pediatr Gastroenterol Nutr 2:288-294, 1983.

Zlotkin SH, Bryan MH, Anderson GH: Intravenous nitrogen and energy intakes required to duplicate in utero nitrogen accretion in prematurely born human infants. J Pediatr 99: 115-120, 1981.

CHAPTER

# 69

# Parenteral Nutrition

**Brenda B. Poindexter and Scott C. Denne**

Effective nutritional support of premature and critically ill infants is largely dependent on parenteral nutrition, especially in early postnatal life. In practice, the supply of nutrients to preterm neonates—especially extremely low-birth-weight (ELBW) infants—is rarely adequate, and these infants accumulate major deficits in the first 2 weeks after birth (Berry et al, 1997). A recent large multicenter study documented that 99% of ELBW infants were below the 10th percentile for weight after 10 weeks in the neonatal intensive care unit (NICU) (Lemons et al, 2001). However, growing evidence indicates that early use of parenteral nutrition may minimize protein losses and improve growth outcomes (Van Goudoever et al, 1995; Wilson et al, 1997). For example, Wilson and colleagues (1997), in a randomized clinical trial in 125 sick very low-birth-weight (VLBW) infants, demonstrated that early aggressive parenteral nutrition combined with early enteral feeding reduced growth failure without an increased incidence of adverse clinical consequences or metabolic derangements. Parenteral nutrition solutions, although still imperfect, have improved markedly from the early days of use, and complications are less common. At present, improved growth outcomes in preterm infants appear to require a more sustained effort at providing parenteral nutritional support, especially in early postnatal life. This means initiating parenteral nutrition within the first 24 hours, continuing until enteral nutrition supplies at least 75% of the total protein and energy requirements, and reinstituting parenteral nutrition quickly whenever enteral feeding is suspended.

## COMPONENTS OF PARENTERAL NUTRITION

### Protein

The initial goal of parenteral nutrition is to minimize losses and preserve existing body stores; this is particularly important for protein. Protein losses are significant in all neonates in the absence of amino acid intake, and these losses are the highest in the most immature neonates. For example, 26-week-gestation infants lose 1.5 g/kg/day of body protein; protein losses in term infants are approximately half that rate (0.7 g/kg/day) (Denne et al, 1996). These high rates of loss in extremely premature infants result in substantial protein deficits. If extremely premature infants are provided with no amino acid supply, they lose over 1.5% of their body protein per day when they should be accumulating protein at a rate of 2% per day. After only 3 days of no protein intake, a 10% protein deficit results.

Fortunately, there is good evidence that early amino acid intake can compensate for high rates of protein loss and thus preserve body protein, even at low caloric intakes (Kashyap and Heird, 1994; Rivera et al, 1993; Saini et al, 1989, Van Lingen et al, 1992). Amino acid intakes of 1.1 to 2.3 g/kg/day at caloric intakes of 30 to 50 kcal/kg/day change the protein balance from significantly negative to neutral or positive in sick VLBW infants (Rivera et al, 1993; Saini et al, 1989; Van Lingen et al, 1992). Additional studies carried out in ELBW infants in early neonatal life support this conclusion (Denne et al, 1996). Nevertheless, in multiple controlled trials evaluating the effect of early amino acid intake in premature infants, no differences in ammonia concentrations, acid-base status, or blood urea nitrogen (BUN) levels were observed between infants who received amino acids and those who did not (Paisley et al, 2000; Rivera et al, 1993; Saini et al, 1989; Van Lingen et al, 1992). The fact that BUN concentrations do not correlate with amino acid intake in multiple trials demonstrates that these levels in early postnatal life are related primarily to fluid status and that increased BUN levels should not be used as an indication of protein excess. These data indicate that providing parenteral amino acids at a rate of 1.5 to 2 g/kg/day as soon as possible after birth (within hours) can preserve limited body protein stores in sick premature and ELBW infants, even at low caloric intakes.

It is important to point out that even though parenteral amino acid administration is beneficial at low caloric intakes, increasing caloric intake is likely to improve protein accretion. Older studies in premature infants have suggested that increasing caloric intake from 50 to 80 kcal/kg/day can significantly improve protein balance (Pineault et al, 1988; Zlotkin et al, 1981a). Preliminary data in ELBW infants indicate that protein balances are not further improved when daily parenteral energy intake is increased from 70 kcal/kg to 90 kcal/kg (Poindexter et al, 2000). Therefore, currently available data suggest that 70 to 80 kcal/kg/day may be sufficient to maximize protein accretion. However, additional energy beyond this amount probably is necessary to produce appropriate fat accretion (see "Energy" section).

The ultimate goal of parenteral amino acid administration is to achieve the rate of fetal protein accretion. Based on a variety of studies measuring protein losses and balance, 3.5 to 4.0 g/kg/day of amino acids is a reasonable estimate of parenteral protein requirements in ELBW infants (Denne et al, 1996; Ziegler, 1994) (Table 69–1). Recent evidence suggests that up to 4.0 g/kg/day of amino acids is well tolerated by ELBW infants (Porcelli and Sisk, 2002). For premature infants with birth weights of over 1000 g, estimated parenteral protein requirements are 3.0 to 3.5 g/kg/day. Estimates for term infants are 2.5 to 3 g/kg/day. Parenteral amino acid intake recommendations for premature infants are shown in Table 69–1.

The composition of currently available amino acid solutions is shown in Table 69–2. These amino acid solutions were designed to mimic plasma amino acid concentrations in healthy 30-day-old breast-fed term infants (Trophamine) or fetal or neonatal cord blood amino acid concentrations (Primene). No convincing information exists

**TABLE 69–1**

**Suggested Daily Parenteral Intakes for ELBW and VLBW Infants**

| Component (units/kg/day) | ELBW | | | VLBW | | |
|---|---|---|---|---|---|---|
| | Day 0* | Transition† | Growing | Day 0* | Transition† | Growing |
| Energy (kcal) | 40-50 | 75-85 | 105-115 | 40-50 | 70-80 | 90-100 |
| Protein (g) | 2 | 3.5 | 3.5-4 | 2 | 3.0-3.5 | 3.0-3.5 |
| Glucose (g) | 7-10 | 8-15 | 13-17 | 7-10 | 8-15 | 13-17 |
| Fat (g) | 1 | 1-3 | 3-4 | 1 | 1-3 | 3 |
| Na (mEq) | 0-1 | 2-4 | 3-7 | 0-1 | 2-4 | 3-5 |
| Potassium K (mEq) | 0 | 0-2 | 2-3 | 0 | 0-2 | 2-3 |
| Chloride (mEq) | 0-1 | 2-4 | 3-7 | 0-1 | 2-4 | 3-7 |
| Calcium (mg) | 20-60 | 60 | 60-80 | 20-60 | 60 | 60-80 |
| Phosphorus (mg) | 0 | 45-60 | 45-60 | 0 | 45-60 | 45-60 |
| Magnesium (mg) | 0 | 3-7.2 | 3-7.2 | 0 | 3-7.2 | 3-7.2 |

*Recommended parenteral intakes on the first day of life.

†Period of transition to physiologic and metabolic stability. For most premature neonates, this occurs between 2 and 7 days.

ELBW, extremely low-birth-weight: <1000 g; VLBW, very low-birth-weight, <1500 g.

to support the superiority of one neonatal amino acid solution over another.

Although the current neonatal amino acid solutions represent a substantial advance over previous casein hydrolysates and early crystalline amino acid mixtures, specific deficiencies remain. Glutamine, an amino acid abundantly supplied by breast milk and potentially conditionally essential in premature infants, is not included in any available amino acid solution because of issues of stability. Tyrosine has very limited solubility, so little is included in current amino acid solutions. Trophamine contains a soluble derivative of tyrosine (*N*-acetyltyrosine), but this derivative appears to have poor bioavailability. A variety of studies in premature infants suggest that the tyrosine supply may not be optimal in current amino acid solutions (Brunton et al, 2000). Cysteine is not included in

**TABLE 69–2**

**Composition of Commercial Parenteral Amino Acid Solutions**

| Amino Acid* | Concentration: mg/dL | | | |
|---|---|---|---|---|
| | Aminosyn-PF (Abbott) | TrophAmine (B. Braun) | Primene (Baxter)† | Premasol (Baxter)† |
| Histidine | 312 | 480 | 380 | 480 |
| Isoleucine | 760 | 820 | 670 | 820 |
| Leucine | 1200 | 1400 | 1000 | 1400 |
| Lysine | 677 | 820 | 1100 | 820 |
| Methionine | 180 | 340 | 240 | 340 |
| Phenylalanine | 427 | 480 | 420 | 480 |
| Threonine | 512 | 420 | 370 | 420 |
| Tryptophan | 180 | 200 | 200 | 200 |
| Valine | 673 | 780 | 760 | 780 |
| Alanine | 698 | 540 | 800 | 540 |
| Arginine | 1227 | 1200 | 840 | 1200 |
| Proline | 812 | 680 | 300 | 680 |
| Serine | 495 | 380 | 400 | 380 |
| Taurine | 70 | 25 | 60 | 25 |
| Tyrosine | 44 | 240‡ | 45 | 240‡ |
| Glycine | 385 | 360 | 400 | 360 |
| Cysteine | — | <16 | 189 | <16 |
| Glutamic acid | 820 | 500 | 1000 | 500 |
| Aspartic acid | 527 | 320 | 600 | 320 |

*All amino acid mixtures shown are 10% solutions.

†Primene available in Canada; Premasol available in the United States.

‡Mixture of L-tyrosine and *N*-acetyltyrosine.

Data from the American Hospital Formulary Service: Drug Information. Bethesda, Md, 2000; Drug Product Database; and Premasol package insert (Baxter Healthcare Corporation, Deerfield, IL, 2003).

most amino acid solutions because it is not stable for long periods. However, a cysteine hydrochloride supplement that can be added to the parenteral nutrition solution just prior to delivery is commercially available. A number of studies have suggested that the addition of cysteine can improve protein accretion, although some conflicting information exists (Poindexter et al, 2000; Rivera et al, 1993; Zlotkin et al, 1981b). The addition of cysteine hydrochloride also improves the solubility of calcium and phosphorus in parenteral nutrition solutions and also may improve the status of the important antioxidant glutathione. For these reasons, the addition of cysteine hydrochloride (40 mg/g of amino acid, up to a maximum of 120 mg/kg) is recommended. Cysteine hydrochloride can result in a metabolic acidosis, but this possibility can be appropriately countered by the use of acetate in the parenteral nutrition solution as a buffer (Peters et al, 1997).

## Energy

The initial goal of parenteral nutrition in early postnatal life is to provide sufficient energy intake to at least match rates of energy expenditure in order to preserve body energy stores. Measures of energy expenditure in premature infants weighing greater than 1000 g have ranged between 45 and 70 kcal/kg/day, so an intake of 70 to 80 kcal/kg/day is a reasonable initial clinical goal to achieve neutral or slightly positive energy balance in these infants. Data assessing energy expenditure in ELBW infants are sparse, but preliminary information suggests that energy expenditure in these infants may be close to 80 kcal/kg/day (Carr et al, 2000). Although 80 kcal/kg/day is a reasonable clinical goal, because of glucose and lipid intolerance this intake may not be able to be achieved for a number of days after birth. Nevertheless, maximizing energy intake within the limits of glucose and lipid tolerance can minimize accumulating energy deficits.

To support normal rates of growth, a positive energy balance of 20 to 25 kcal/kg/day must be achieved (Denne, 2001). This requires 90 to 100 kcal/kg/day for preterm infants with birth weights of less than 1000 g and 105 to 115 kcal/kg/day for ELBW infants (see Table 69–1). A parenteral intake of 80 to 90 kcal/kg/day is most often sufficient for term infants. Most of the parenteral calories are best supplied by a balanced caloric intake of lipid and glucose. Parenteral energy requirements are less than those required for enteral nutrition because no energy is lost in the stools. Recommendations for parenteral energy intake are shown in Table 69–1.

## Glucose

Glucose is typically the first parenteral nutrient provided to the preterm infant, and glucose administration is begun minutes after birth in order to maintain glucose homeostasis and preserve endogenous carbohydrate stores. Although the precise definitions of hypoglycemia and hyperglycemia remain a topic of debate, maintaining glucose concentrations of above 40 mg/dL and below 150 to 200 mg/dL is a reasonable clinical goal (Cornblath et al, 2000). Hypoglycemia is easily avoided in preterm infants by maintaining a constant intravenous glucose delivery, but hyperglycemia is more often problematic, especially in ELBW weight infants shortly after birth. A recent study suggested that approximately 40% of sick VLBW infants experience at least one episode of hyperglycemia within the first week of life (Wilson et al, 1997).

Glucose infusion rate of 4 to 7 mg/kg/minute (70 to 110 mL/kg/day of 10% dextrose in water [$D_{10}W$]) is an appropriate starting point for most infants. This rate of glucose infusion approximates or slightly exceeds the rate of endogenous glucose release from the liver in term and premature infants with birth weights of greater than 1000 g; therefore, this rate of glucose infusion serves to preserve the limited carbohydrate stores in these infants. For ELBW weight infants, a rate of 8 to 10 mg/kg/minute is required to match endogenous glucose production (Hertz et al, 1993). Unfortunately, many infants will not tolerate this rate of glucose infusion for several days without hyperglycemia. Because ELBW infants often have fluid requirements in excess of 100 mL/kg/day, beginning with 5% dextrose is usually necessary to maintain glucose infusion rates in the range of 4 to 7 mg/kg in order to achieve glucose homeostasis.

A gradual increase in glucose intake over 2 to 7 days, up to 13 to 17 g/kg/day, is usually tolerated when the glucose is combined with amino acid intake. An infusion rate of 18 g/kg/day is a reasonable maximum for intravenous glucose delivery, as higher rates probably exceed the glucose oxidative capacity (Chessex et al, 1995; Jones et al, 1993). Exceeding glucose oxidative capacity will drive extensive lipogenesis, an energy-expensive process. Supplying appropriate amounts of glucose rarely requires glucose solution concentrations in excess of 12.5%, unless infants are fluid restricted. Recommendations for glucose intake during parenteral nutrition are provided in Table 69–1.

Some ELBW infants have difficulty tolerating even moderate rates of glucose delivery. This problem usually can be overcome by a temporary reduction in the glucose infusion rate. The use of insulin in this situation remains a controversial practice. Collins and associates (1991), in a small randomized controlled trial, demonstrated increased weight gain in infants who received insulin infusions. No differences in head circumference or length were observed between these infants and controls, suggesting that insulin may have produced increases in fat mass but not in lean tissue. Poindexter and colleagues (1998) evaluated the effect of insulin on protein metabolism using a euglycemic hyperinsulinemic clamp. Insulin infusion resulted in no improvement in protein balance and unexpectedly produced significant lactic acidosis. At present, the ability of exogenous insulin to produce appropriate growth and body composition in extremely premature infants is unclear, and exogenous insulin cannot be recommended in routine practice. Nevertheless, there are rare ELBW infants who remain hyperglycemic despite very low glucose infusion rates; these infants may require exogenous insulin beginning at 0.05 unit/kg/hour for a short period of time to produce normoglycemia.

Meeting the goal of 13 to 17 g/kg/day of intravenous glucose will result in a caloric intake of 45 to 60 kcal/kg/day, which is insufficient by itself to meet total energy needs. Intravenous lipids are necessary to supply the rest of the nonprotein calories. A balanced glucose and lipid approach to supplying nonprotein calories has a number of advantages: it better approximates the carbohydrate-to-fat ratio in enteral feedings, it may improve overall protein accretion, and it minimizes overall energy expenditure (Nose et al, 1987; Van Aerde et al, 1989).

## Lipids

Intravenous lipids are made up of triglycerides, phospholipids from egg yolk to emulsify, and glycerol, which is added to achieve isotonicity. Intravenous lipid solutions commercially available in the United States are derived from soybean oil (Intralipid) or a combination of soybean oil and safflower oil (Liposyn II); these solutions contain long-chain triglycerides. Some lipid preparations available in Europe include medium-chain triglycerides (Medialipid) and a combination of olive oil and soybean oil (Clinoleic). Differences in lipid source result in a slightly different fatty acid profile; the compositions of available intravenous lipid solutions are shown in Table 69–3. All available intravenous lipid products have a fatty acid profile substantially different from that of human milk. At present, there is not convincing information that any of the solutions produce clinically different outcomes. Some theoretical advantages exist for the use of medium-chain triglycerides, including more rapid hydrolysis. However, a recent study in preterm infants demonstrated that medium-chain triglyceride–containing lipid emulsions may not be as effective as long-chain triglyceride–containing emulsions in promoting protein accretion (Liet et al, 1999).

Intravenous lipid solutions contain lipid particles similar in size to endogenously produced chylomicrons. These particles are hydrolyzed by lipoprotein lipase into free fatty acids. Lipoprotein lipase activity and triglyceride clearance is reduced in preterm infants of less than 28 weeks of gestation (Brans et al, 1990). Although heparin can release lipoprotein lipase from the endothelium into the circulation, at present no evidence exists that this increases lipid utilization in preterm infants (Spear et al, 1988). In the absence of any information demonstrating clinical benefit of heparin administration, the routine addition of heparin in lipid infusions is not recommended.

Linoleic and linolenic acids cannot be endogenously synthesized and therefore are essential fatty acids for humans. Biochemical evidence of essential fatty acid deficiency may be noted in preterm infants within 72 hours of birth (Foote et al, 1991). Essential fatty acid deficiency can be avoided if 0.5 to 1.0 g/kg/day of intravenous lipid is provided. Additional intravenous lipid beyond these amounts is necessary if the energy requirements of preterm infants are to be met in early postnatal life.

The early administration of intravenous lipids to preterm infants has been the subject of discussion and debate; this debate has centered primarily on the acute metabolic effects of early intravenous lipids and the potential long-term consequences. Gilbertson and colleagues (1991) evaluated the short-term metabolic effects of early intravenous lipids in a randomized controlled trial. This study examined 29 infants requiring mechanical ventilation with an average gestational age of 28 weeks and an average birth weight of 1.1 kg. One group received intravenous lipid at 1.0 g/kg/day beginning on day 1; this was gradually increased to 3.0 g/kg/day by day 4. The control group received intravenous lipid only after day 8. There were no differences in $Po_2$, $Pco_2$, hyperglycemia, bilirubin concentrations, thrombocytopenia, or free fatty acid concentrations between the two groups. In addition, triglyceride concentrations were similar in both groups. Another trial using a slightly different study design produced similar results (Murdock et al, 1995). Current evidence strongly suggests that intravenous lipids can be administered to sick preterm infants in early postnatal life without causing acute metabolic derangements.

Concern about the long-term safety of early intravenous administration of lipids, particularly the possibility of an increase in mortality and bronchopulmonary dysplasia, was raised by some early observational studies. Subsequently, however, six randomized control trials have been performed evaluating this question, and none have demonstrated an increase in bronchopulmonary dysplasia or mortality in preterm infants who received early intravenous lipids. A meta-analysis of these studies confirmed this conclusion (Fox et al, 1998). In view of these data and of the essential fatty acid and caloric needs of sick premature infants, early intravenous lipid administration (on day 1 of life) is a recommended clinical practice.

**TABLE 69–3**

**Compositions of Commercial (20%) Intravenous Lipid Emulsions**

| Component | Intralipid | Liposyn-II | Medialipid | Clinoleic |
|---|---|---|---|---|
| TG (g/L) | 200 | 200 | 200 | 200 |
| PL (g/L) | 12 | 12 | 12 | 12 |
| Glycerol (g/L) | 22 | 25 | 25 | 22.5 |
| Fatty acids (%) | | | | |
| Octanoic acid C8 | — | — | 30 | — |
| Decanoic acid C10 | — | — | 20 | — |
| Palmitic acid C16:0 | 10 | 9 | 4.5 | 10.7 |
| Stearic acid C18:0 | 3 | 3 | 1.5 | 3 |
| Oleic acid C18:1 | 25 | 18 | 13 | 65 |
| Linoleic acid C18:2 | 54 | 66 | 27 | 17 |
| Linolenic acid C18:3 | 8 | 4 | 4 | 0.3 |

PL, phospholipids; TG, triglycerides.

The rate of intravenous lipid infusion is important, and plasma lipid clearance is improved when intravenous lipid is given as a continuous infusion over 24 hours (Putet, 2000). Lipid infusion rates in excess of 0.25 g/kg/hour are associated with decreases in $PO_2$ (Brans et al, 1986). Lipid infusion rates well under this value can easily be achieved in clinical practice if lipids are provided over 24 hours in an amount not exceeding 3 to 4 g/kg/day. This level of lipid intake is usually sufficient to supply the caloric needs of preterm infants (in combination with glucose) and is usually tolerated by premature infants. Triglyceride concentrations are most often used as an indication of lipid tolerance, and maintaining triglyceride concentrations below 150 to 200 mg/dL seems desirable. Recommendations for parenteral lipid intake are provided in Table 69–1.

Numerous studies have documented superiority of 20% over 10% lipid emulsions (Putet, 2000). Lipid clearance is improved with the 20% solutions because these solutions have half the amount of phospholipid emulsifier relative to the same amount of triglycerides. Phospholipids can combine with cholesterol to form lipoprotein X, which ultimately interferes with the clearance of infused triglycerides. Consequently, the use of 10% lipid emulsions should be avoided.

Concern has been expressed about the use of intravenous lipids in infants with hyperbilirubinemia, as free fatty acids may displace bilirubin from albumin-binding sites, potentially increasing the risk of kernicterus. In vitro studies have shown that no free bilirubin is released if the free fatty acid–to–serum albumin ratio is less than 4 (Thiessen et al, 1972). In vivo, free bilirubin is not generated until the molar ratio of free fatty acids to bilirubin exceeds 6 (Andrew et al, 1976). In clinical practice, free fatty acid–to–bilirubin ratios above 6 have not been measured, and a relationship between free fatty acid concentrations and unbound bilirubin has not been documented (Rubin et al, 1995). At present, withholding intravenous lipids from jaundiced premature infants does not seem warranted.

Intravenous lipid emulsions may undergo lipid peroxidation, with the formation of organic free radicals, potentially initiating tissue injury. Light, especially phototherapy, may play some role in increasing lipid peroxidation in intravenous lipid emulsions (Neuzil et al, 1995). However, multivitamin preparations included in the intravenous solutions are major contributors to a generation of peroxides, and lipid emulsions may have only a minor additive effect (Lavoie et al, 1997). On the basis of these findings, some clinicians protect intravenous lipid solutions from light, although the importance or efficacy of this practice is unclear.

Carnitine facilitates transport of long-chain fatty acids through the myocardial membrane and thereby plays an important role in their oxidation. Premature infants receiving parenteral nutrition have low carnitine levels, but the clinical significance of this finding remains uncertain. Meta-analysis of the studies evaluating carnitine supplementation in parenteral nutrition showed no evidence of effect on ketogenesis, lipid utilization, or weight gain (Cairns and Stalker, 2002). At present, insufficient information is available to support a recommendation for the routine supplementation of parenterally fed neonates with carnitine.

## Electrolytes, Minerals, Trace Elements, and Vitamins

Sodium needs are low in the first few days of life because of the expected free water diuresis. For ELBW infants, addition of sodium to the parenteral nutrition solution may not be necessary until about day 3 of life. It is, however, necessary to frequently measure sodium concentrations and water balance. After the initial diuresis, 2 to 4 mEq/kg/day is usually sufficient to maintain serum sodium in the normal range, but ELBW infants sometimes require higher sodium intakes to compensate for larger renal sodium losses. Chloride requirements follow the same time course as for sodium requirements and also are 2 to 4 mEq/kg/day. Once electrolytes are added to the parenteral nutrition solution, chloride intake should not be less than 1 mEq/kg/day, and all chloride should not be omitted when sodium bicarbonate or acetate is given to correct metabolic acidosis. Potassium requirements again are low on the first few days of life, and potassium should probably be omitted from parenteral solutions in ELBW infants until renal function is clearly established. Potassium intakes of 2 to 3 mEq/kg/day are usually adequate to maintain normal serum potassium concentrations.

Parenteral nutrition solutions usually require the addition of anions, as either acetate or chloride. In general, excess anions should be provided as acetate in order to prevent hyperchloremic metabolic acidosis. A randomized controlled trial demonstrated that acetate in parenteral nutrition solutions effectively ameliorates acidosis (Phelps and Cochran, 1989).

Supplying calcium and phosphorus in parenteral nutrition remains a significant clinical challenge because of limited solubility. It is currently not possible to supply enough calcium and phosphorus to support adequate bone mineralization in preterm infants using the solutions available in the United States. In other countries organophosphate preparations are available (e.g., glycerophosphate), and calcium and phosphorus can be supplied in parenteral nutrition solutions in amounts that approximate enteral intakes. Precipitation of calcium and phosphorus remains an issue in the United States, however, and the solubility of calcium and phosphorus in parenteral nutrition solutions depends on temperature, type and concentration of amino acid, glucose concentration, pH, type of calcium salt, sequence of addition of calcium and phosphorus to the solution, the calcium-to-phosphorus ratio, and the presence of lipid. Adding cysteine to parenteral nutrition solutions lowers the pH, which improves calcium and phosphorus solubility. Currently, recommendations are to use parenteral nutrition solutions containing 50 to 60 mg/dL of elemental calcium (12.5 to 15 mmol/L) and 40 to 47 mg/dL of phosphorus (12.5 to 15 mmol/L). At typical fluid intakes (100 to 150 mL/kg/day), this composition will provide 50 to 90 mg/kg/day of calcium and 40 to 70 mg/kg/day of phosphorus (Koo et al, 1993). A calcium-to-phosphorus ratio of 1.7:1 by weight (1.3:1 by molar ratio) appears to be optimal for bone mineralization.

In general, calcium and phosphorus should be added to parenteral nutrition solutions in early postnatal life. Magnesium also is a necessary nutrient and should be supplied at 3 to 7.2 mg/kg/day. Calcium, phosphorus, and magnesium serum concentrations should be frequently monitored.

Recommendations for trace elements for term and preterm infants are primarily derived from the American Society for Clinical Nutrition (ASCN) guidelines from 1988 (Greene et al, 1988). There is reasonable consensus that zinc should be included early in parenteral nutrition solutions (250 μg/kg/day for term infants, 400 μg/kg/day for preterm infants). Other trace elements probably are not needed until after the first 2 weeks of life.

The recommended intakes of trace elements for term and preterm infants are shown in Table 69–4. Zinc and copper are available in the sulfate form and can be added separately to parenteral solutions. Several pediatric trace metal solutions are available that contain zinc, copper, magnesium, and chromium in various proportions; these solutions are usually provided at 0.2 mL/kg/day. When trace metal solutions are used, additional zinc usually is needed to provide the recommended intake for preterm infants. Supplementation with selenium is suggested after 2 weeks of age, because preterm infants can become selenium deficient after 2 weeks of exclusive parenteral nutrition. In infants with cholestasis, copper and manganese should be discontinued, and chromium and selenium should be used with caution and in smaller amounts in infants with renal dysfunction. At present, parenteral iron is recommended only when preterm infants are nourished exclusively by parenteral solutions for the first 2 months of life.

The recommended intakes of vitamins for term and preterm infants on parenteral nutrition are shown in Table 69–5. Currently only one pediatric multivitamin preparation is available, and it is delivered with a standard dosage of 2 mL/kg/day (maximum 5 mL/day) in preterm infants and 5 mL/day in term infants. These dosages provide higher amounts of most of the B vitamins and lower amounts of vitamin A relative to the recommendations.

**TABLE 69–4**

**Recommended Parenteral Intake of Trace Elements for Term and Preterm Infants**

| Trace Element | Term (μg/kg/day) | Preterm (μg/kg/day) |
|---|---|---|
| Chromium* | 0.20 | 0.2 |
| Copper† | 20 | 20 |
| Iron‡ | — | — |
| Fluoride§ | — | — |
| Iodide | 1 | 1 |
| Manganese† | 1 | 1 |
| Molybdenum | 0.25 | 0.25 |
| Selenium* | 2 | 2 |
| Zinc‖ | 250 | 400 |

*Renal dysfunction can cause toxicity.

†Impaired biliary excretion can cause toxicity.

‡Recommendation is made with caution because of very limited experience with intravenous iron in infants and lack of a safe, acceptable intravenous preparation (estimated daily intravenous requirement is 100 μg/kg for term infants and 200 μg/kg for preterm infants).

§Because of a lack of information on the compatibility of fluoride with TPN and on the contamination level of fluoride in TPN solutions, firm recommendations cannot be made; with long-term TPN (longer than 3 months), a dosage of 500 μg/day may be important in preterm infants, who already have a higher incidence of subsequent dental caries.

‖The only trace element recommended on day 1 of parenteral nutrition. If the infant requires TPN for longer than 3 months, the dosage must be reduced to 100 μg/kg/day.

ASCN, American Society for Clinical Nutrition; TPN, total parenteral nutrition.

Data from the American Society for Clinical Nutrition, Subcommittee on Pediatric Parenteral Nutrient Requirements, from the Committee on Clinical Practice Issues: Am J Clin Nutr 48:1324-1343, 1988.

## Complications of Parenteral Nutrition

Although a wide variety of complications associated with parenteral nutrition were reported in the early days of use, most of these are now rare with current parenteral solutions. Many of the complications (electrolyte and glucose imbalance) can be prevented or corrected by manipulating the constituents of the infusate. The primary complications of parenteral nutrition as currently used are cholestasis and those related to the infusion catheter.

Cholestatic jaundice as a result of hepatic dysfunction is a well-recognized complication of parenteral nutrition. The initial histologic legion is cholestasis, both intracellular and intracanalicular, followed by portal inflammation and progressing to bile duct proliferation after several weeks of parenteral nutrition. With prolonged administration, portal fibrosis and ultimately cirrhosis may develop. There is very little recent information about the incidence of cholestasis in preterm infants. Older studies suggest that cholestasis may be more prevalent at lower birth weights, with approximately 50% of ELBW infants exhibiting cholestasis after 2 weeks of parenteral nutrition (Beale et al, 1979). The incidence of cholestasis in infants receiving parenteral nutrition for longer than 90 days is over 90% regardless of birth weight. At present, the risk of cholestasis appears to be highest in premature infants receiving exclusively parenteral nutrition for prolonged periods.

The precise cause of cholestasis is unknown and probably is multifactorial. Critically ill premature infants experience a variety of insults, including hypoxia, hemodynamic instability, and infection. A higher incidence of sepsis has been reported in infants affected by cholestasis. Perhaps an equally if not more important factor in the development of cholestasis is the prolonged lack of enteral nutrition; there is growing evidence that enteral feedings, even at low caloric intakes, can reduce the incidences of cholestasis.

The clinical manifestations of cholestasis are hyperbilirubinemia and jaundice, and histologic changes in the liver occur much earlier. A sensitive but nonspecific indicator of early cholestasis is an increase in gamma-glutamyltransferase (GGT) (Nanji and Anderson, 1985); elevations of hepatic transaminases—aspartate transaminase (AST) (serum glutamic-oxaloacetic transaminase [SGOT]) and alanine transaminase (ALT) (serum glutamate-pyruvate transaminase [SGPT])—occur later. Cholestasis most often resolves after discontinuation of parenteral nutrition and initiation of enteral feedings. Some rare instances of irreversible liver failure have been documented, but this seems to occur only after several months of use.

**TABLE 69-5**

**Recommended Parenteral Intake of Vitamins for Term and Preterm Infants**

| Vitamin | Term (daily dose) | | Preterm (dose/kg/day)* | |
|---|---|---|---|---|
| | Recommended | MVI-Pediatric (1 vial: 5 mL) | Recommended | MVI-Pediatric (40% of vial: 2 mL/kg/day) |
| **Fat-Soluble** | | | | |
| Vitamin A (IU) | 2300 | 2300 | 1640 | 920 |
| Vitamin D (IU) | 400 | 400 | 160 | 160 |
| Vitamin E (IU) | 7 | 7 | 2.8 | — |
| Vitamin K (μg) | 200 | 200 | 80[†] | 80 |
| **Water-Soluble** | | | | |
| Vitamin $B_6$ (μg) | 1000 | 1000 | 180 | 400 |
| Vitamin $B_{12}$ (μg) | 1 | 1 | 0.3 | 0.4 |
| Vitamin C (mg) | 80 | 80 | 25 | 32 |
| Biotin (μg) | 20 | 20 | 6 | 8 |
| Folic acid (μg) | 140 | 140 | 56 | 56 |
| Niacin (mg) | 17 | 17 | 6.8 | 6.8 |
| Pantothenate (mg) | 5 | 5 | 2 | 2 |
| Riboflavin (μg) | 1400 | 1400 | 150 | 560 |
| Thiamin (μg) | 1200 | 1200 | 350 | 480 |

*Maximum not to exceed dosage for term infant. *Note*: American Society for Clinical Nutrition (ASCN) recommendations (1988) currently are not achievable because no ideal intravenous vitamin preparation is available for preterm infants; 40% of a vial (2 mL/kg/day) of MVI-Pediatric (Armor, USA; Rorer, Canada) is the closest intake that can be achieved.

†This does not include the 0.5-1 mg of vitamin K to be given at birth, as recommended by the American Academy of Pediatrics.

Data from the American Society for Clinical Nutrition, Subcommittee on Pediatric Parenteral Nutrient Requirements, from the Committee on Clinical Practice Issues: Am J Clin Nutr 48:1324-1343, 1988.

Some infants with cholestasis will require continued parenteral nutrition. In these infants, the use of small-volume enteral feeding in combination with parenteral nutrition may stabilize or improve hepatic function. The use of phenobarbital and ursodeoxycholic acid has been shown to be beneficial in some studies of older children and adults. However, a recent study in preterm infants demonstrated that tauroursodeoxycholic acid did not prevent the development of parenteral nutrition–associated cholestasis and was ineffective in reducing cholestasis once it occurred (Heubi et al, 2002). At present, the routine use of ursodeoxycholic acid or phenobarbital in parenteral nutrition–associated cholestasis cannot be recommended.

Catheter-related complications remain an important problem with parenteral nutrition; the major complication is infection. Two of the most common bacterial pathogens are *Staphylococcus epidermidis* and *Staphylococcus aureus*. Fungal infections also occur, *Candida albicans* and *Malassezia furfur* being the most common agents. The incidence of sepsis during parenteral nutrition is higher at the lower gestational ages and also increases with the duration of parenteral nutrition. Parenteral nutrition–associated sepsis is likely to be a product of many factors, not the least of which is that the most immature and critically ill patients are most likely to receive parenteral nutrition for prolonged periods. In infants who have developed cholestasis while receiving parenteral nutrition, the rate of sepsis may be increased. The infusate itself also may play a role in the development of sepsis; an association has been reported between the use of intravenous lipid and coagulase-negative staphylococcal bacteremia and *M. furfur* fungemia (Freeman et al, 1990; Redline et al, 1985). At present, avoiding parenteral nutrition–associated infections is best accomplished by meticulous attention to sterile technique in catheter care and early initiation and advancement of enteral nutrition. Prophylactic low-dose vancomycin may diminish the incidence of parenteral nutrition–associated sepsis, but in view of concerns about toxicities and the potential for antibiotic resistance, this approach cannot be recommended (Craft et al, 2002).

Complications specifically related to the catheter also have been reported. Broviac catheters are difficult to place and are associated with thrombosis in neonates (Sadiq et al, 1987). In most NICUs, Broviac catheters have largely been replaced by small-bore Silastic catheters placed percutaneously. However, all central catheters, including the small-bore variety, have produced life-threatening complications. Pericardial tamponade and significant plural effusions are known complications of the use of central catheters in neonates (Aiken et al, 1992; Giacoia, 1991). Although these are uncommon events, clinical awareness and early recognition of these complications can prevent mortality.

## USE OF PARENTERAL NUTRITION IN THE NEONATAL INTENSIVE CARE UNIT: A PRACTICAL APPROACH

The preceding portion of this chapter has presented the scientific basis for recommendations regarding provision of parenteral nutrition to neonates. The following paragraphs present a practical approach to the administration of parenteral nutrition, with a particular emphasis on ELBW infants.

Every clinician caring for ELBW infants must recognize the urgent need to initiate intravenous amino acids shortly after birth. As mentioned previously, the ELBW infant loses 1.5% of total body protein each day that amino acids are withheld. Consequently, the goal of early parenteral nutrition should be to limit catabolism and preserve endogenous protein stores. Numerous studies have clearly demonstrated both the safety and efficacy of early amino acids in accomplishing this goal, even at low caloric intakes.

We recommend starting with a minimum of 1.5 to 2.0 g/kg/day of amino acids on the first day of life. This can be accomplished simply by adding one of the crystalline amino acid solutions designed for use in neonates (Aminosyn-PF, Primene, Premasol, or TrophAmine) to glucose to use as the initial maintenance fluid in ELBW infants. In infants with rapidly changing fluid, dextrose, and electrolyte needs, one approach is to give the amino acids in 5% dextrose at a volume of 60 to 80 mL/kg/day. Additional fluids with or without electrolytes and/or a higher concentration of dextrose can then be "Y'd in," with adjustments as needed for the individual infant's fluid, dextrose, and electrolyte requirements, eliminating the need to discard the bag of parenteral nutrition fluid for such changes in status. In nurseries with standard "hang times" for parenteral nutrition and/or those that outsource this aspect of patient care, bags with 5% dextrose and 1.5 to 2.0 g/kg/day of amino acids can be made in advance so that intravenous amino acids are not delayed in a newly admitted neonate. This mixture of glucose and amino acids can be given via a peripheral intravenous line, umbilical venous line, or percutaneous central venous catheter. Increased usage of percutaneously placed central venous catheters has certainly facilitated early and widespread usage of parenteral nutrition in premature infants. In our nursery, strong consideration is given to percutaneous central venous line placement in ELBW infants early in their postnatal course.

To meet growth requirements, 2.7 to 4.0 g/kg/day of amino acids is required. It is important to point out that such amounts are merely estimates, and protein requirements to sustain optimal growth in ELBW weight infants may be even higher. Once administration of amino acids is initiated, intake can be advanced to meet requirements for growth over a relatively short period. We typically advance amino acid intake by 1.0 g/kg/day until the goal is reached. No data are available, however, to support the clinical practice of slowly advancing amino acid intake over several days. It would be equally reasonable to initiate parenteral amino acids at 3.0 to 3.5 g/kg/day. Given the available data, we also recommend the addition of cysteine to the amino acid solution (40 mg/g of amino acids, to a maximum of 120 mg).

Glucose should be supplied in a quantity sufficient to maintain normal plasma glucose concentrations. As discussed previously, glucose production and utilization rates are highest in the most premature infants; their glucose needs are in the range of 6 to 8 mg/kg/minute, whereas the term infant's needs are approximately 3 to 4 mg/kg/minute. Giving 10% dextrose at 100 mL/kg/day provides a glucose infusion rate of 7 mg/kg/minute. Starting infants with birth weights less than 1000 g on 5% dextrose is likely to be prudent if their total fluid requirements are greater than 120 to 150 mL/kg/day.

Lipids should be started within the first 24 hours of life, usually at 1.0 g/kg/day. We typically start lipids at 1.0 g/kg/day and advance by 0.5 to 1.0 g/kg/day to a usual maximum of 3 g/kg/day while monitoring and maintaining serum triglycerides at less than 200 mg/dL. Given the numerous advantages over 10% solutions, 20% lipid emulsions should always be used. To facilitate clearance and to avoid impairment of oxygenation, lipids should be infused over a 24-hour period. There is currently no evidence to support the use of cyclic infusion in the acute setting of the NICU.

Caloric goals during parenteral nutrition are lower than with enteral feeds. To achieve optimal protein retention, approximately 80 to 90 kcal/kg/day is a reasonable goal. To optimize growth, somewhat higher caloric intakes may be necessary. The non-protein balance between carbohydrate and lipid should be approximately 60:40. These goals can usually be achieved using glucose solutions with concentrations no greater than 12.5% (Table 69–6).

There is a paucity of data related to monitoring laboratory tests during provision of parenteral nutrition. Suggested monitoring for infants receiving parenteral nutrition in our institution is shown in Table 69–7. All of these laboratory tests may not be appropriate in ELBW infants due to constraints related to blood sampling.

The use of parenteral nutrition should be accompanied by the early initiation of enteral feeds (within the first 1 to 3

**TABLE 69–6**

**Caloric Value of Parenteral Nutrition Solutions**

| Composition* | kcal/kg/day | % of Non-protein Calories |
|---|---|---|
| **Example 1** | | |
| Total fluids at 110 mL/kg/day | | |
| 10% dextrose | 37 | 55 |
| 3 g/kg/day lipid | 30 | 45 |
| 3.5 g/kg/day amino acids | 14 | — |
| Total | 81 | — |
| **Example 2** | | |
| Total fluids at 80 mL/kg/day | | |
| 12.5% dextrose | 34 | 53 |
| 3 g/kg/day lipid | 30 | 47 |
| 3.5 g/kg/day amino acids | 14 | — |
| Total | 78 | — |
| **Example 3** | | |
| Total fluids at 140 mL/kg/day | | |
| 12.5% dextrose | 60 | 67 |
| 3 g/kg/day lipid | 30 | 33 |
| 3.5 g/kg/day amino acids | 14 | — |
| Total | 104 | — |

*Dextrose: 3.4 kcal/g; protein: 4 kcal/g; lipid (20% emulsion): 10 kcal/g.

**TABLE 69-7**

**Suggested Monitoring During Parenteral Nutrition**

| Parameter | Frequency |
|---|---|
| Weight | Daily |
| Length and OFC | Weekly |
| Serum glucose | 1 ×/shift during week 1, then daily |
| Serum Na, K, Cl, BUN, Ca, P, Mg, hematocrit | 2-3 ×/week during week 1, then weekly |
| Alkaline phosphatase, ALT (SGPT), GGT, fractionated bilirubin | Weekly |

ALT; alanine transaminase; BUN, blood urea nitrogen; GGT, gamma-glutamyl transferase; OFC, occipitofrontal circumference; SGPT, serum glutamate-pyruvate transaminase.

days of life). Parenteral nutrition should be continued until enteral feedings are well established and providing approximately 100 to 110 kcal/kg/day, although availability of intravenous access may necessitate earlier termination of parenteral nutrition in some circumstances. As enteral feeds are advanced, the protein and lipid contents of the parenteral nutrition can be gradually decreased. In addition, careful and prompt attention to reinstitution of parenteral nutrition during episodes of intolerance of enteral feeds cannot be overemphasized. Infants with intolerance of enteral feeds in whom nothing-by-mouth (NPO) status is frequently necessary present an additional challenge. In such infants, it may be prudent to determine full-volume parenteral nutrition needs as for NPO status and to then run the parenteral nutrition solution at a lower rate if enteral feeds are administered. With this approach, if a change to NPO status becomes necessary after administration of the parenteral nutrition fluid has begun, the volume can be safely increased and caloric and protein intake is not compromised.

## REFERENCES


Aiken G, Porteous L, Tracy M, Richardson V: Cardiac tamponade from a fine Silastic central venous catheter in a premature infant. J Paediatr Child Health 28:325-327, 1992.

Andrew G, Chan G, Schiff D: Lipid metabolism in the neonate: The effect of intralipid infusion on plasma triglyceride and free fatty acid concentrations in the neonate. J Pediatr 88:273-279, 1976.

Beale EF, Nelson RM, Bucciarelli RL, et al: Intrahepatic cholestasis associated with parenteral nutrition in premature infants. Pediatrics 64:342-347, 1979.

Berry MA, Abrahamowicz M, Usher RH: Factors associated with growth of extremely premature infants during initial hopitalization. Pediatrics 100:640-646, 1997.

Brans Y, Dutton E, Andrew D: Fat emulsion tolerance in very low birth weight neonates: Effect on diffusion of oxygen in the lungs and on blood pH. Pediatrics 78:79-84, 1986.

Brans YW, Andrew DS, Carrillo DW, et al: Tolerance of fat emulsions in very low birthweight neonates: Effect of birthweight on plasma lipid concentrations. Am J Perinatol 7:114-117, 1990.

Brunton J, Ball R, Pencharz P: Current total parenteral nutrition solutions for the neonate are inadequate. Curr Opin Clin Nutr Metab Care 3:299-304, 2000.

Cairns P, Stalker D: Carnitine supplementation of parenterally fed neonates. Cochrane Database Syst Rev 3, 2002.

Carr BJ, Denne SC, Leitch CA: Total energy expenditure in extremely premature and term infants in early postnatal life. Pediatr Res 47:284A, 2000.

Chessex P, Belanger S, Piedboeuf B, Pineault M: Influence of energy substrates on respiratory gas exchange during conventional mechanical ventilation of preterm infants. J Pediatr 126:619-624, 1995.

Collins J, Hoppe M, Brown K, et al: A controlled trial of insulin infusion and parenteral nutrition in extremely low birth weight infants with glucose intolerance. J Pediatr 118:921-927, 1991.

Cornblath M, Hawdon J, Williams A, et al: Controversies regarding definition of neonatal hypoglycemia: Suggested operational thresholds. Pediatrics 105:1141-1145, 2000.

Craft A, Finer N, Barrington K: Vancomycin for prophylaxis against sepsis in preterm neonates. Cochrane Database Syst Rev 3, 2002.

Denne SC: Protein and energy requirements in preterm infants. Semin Neonatol 6:377-382, 2001.

Denne SC, Karn CA, Ahlrichs JA, et al: Proteolysis and phenylalanine hydroxylation in response to parenteral nutrition in extremely premature and normal newborns. J Clin Invest 97:746-754, 1996.

Foote KD, MacKinnon MJ, Innis SM: Effect of early introduction of formula vs fat-free parenteral nutrition on essential fatty acid status of preterm infants. Am J Clin Nutr 54:93-97, 1991.

Fox GF, Wilson DC, Ohlsson A: Effects of ealry versus late introduction of intravenous lipid to preterm infants on death and chronic lung disease: Results of meta-analysis. Pediatr Res 43:214A, 1998.

Freeman J, Goldmann D, Smith N, et al: Association of intravenous lipid emulsion and coagulase-negative staphylococcal bacteremia in neonatal intensive care units. N Engl J Med 323:301-308, 1990.

Giacoia GP: Cardiac tamponade and hydrothorax as complications of central venous parenteral nutrition in infants. JPEN J Parenter Enteral Nutr 15:110-113, 1991.

Gilbertson N, Kovar IZ, Cox DJ, et al: Introduction of intravenous lipid administration on the first day of life in the very low birth weight neonate. J Pediatr 119:615-623, 1991.

Greene HL, Hambidge KM, Schanler R, Tsang RC: Guidelines for the use of vitamins, trace elements, calcium, magnesium, and phosphorus in infants and children receiving total parenteral nutrition. Am J Clin Nutr 48:1324-1342, 1988.

Hertz DE, Karn CA, Liu YM, et al: Intravenous glucose suppresses glucose production but not proteolysis in extremely premature newborns. J Clin Invest 92:1752-1758, 1993.

Heubi J, Wiechmann D, Creutzinger V, et al: Tauroursodeoxycholic acid (TUDCA) in the prevention of total parenteral nutrition-associated liver disease. J Pediatr 141:237-242, 2002.

Jones M, Pierro A, Hammond P, et al: Glucose utilization in the surgical newborn infant receiving total parenteral nutrition. J Pediatr Surg 28:1121-1125, 1993.

Kashyap S, Heird WC: Protein Requirements of Low Birthweight, Very Low Birthweight, and Small for Gestational Age Infants. New York, Vevey/Raven Press, 1994.

Koo WK, Tsang RC: Calcium, magnesium, phosphorus, and vitamin D. In Tsang RC, Lucas A, Uauy R (eds): Nutritional Needs of the Preterm Infant: Scientific Basis and Practical Guidelines. Baltimore, Williams & Wilkins, 1993.

Lavoie J-C, Belanger S, Spalinger M, Chessex P: Admixture of a multivitamin preparation to parenteral nutrition: The major contributor to in vitro generation of peroxides. Pediatrics 99:E6, 1997.

Lemons JA, Bauer CR, Oh W, et al: Very low birth weight outcomes of the National Institute of Child Health and Human Development Neonatal Research Network, January 1995 through December 1996. Pediatrics 107:E1, 2001.

Liet JM, Piloquet H, Marchini JS, et al: Leucine metabolism in preterm infants receiving parenteral nutrition with medium-chain compared with long-chain triacylglycerol emulsions. Am J Clin Nutr 69:539-543, 1999.

Murdock N, Crighton A, Nelson L, Forsyth J: Low birthweight infants and total parenteral nutrition immediately after birth. II. Randomised study of biochemical tolerance of intravenous glucose, amino acids, and lipids. Arch Dis Child Fetal Neonatal Ed 73:8F-12F, 1995.

Nanji AA, Anderson FH: Sensitivity and specificity of liver function tests in the detection of parenteral nutrition-associated cholestasis. JPEN J Parenter Enteral Nutr 9:307-308, 1985.

Neuzil J, Darlow B, Inder T: Oxidation of parenteral lipid emulsion by ambient and phototherapy lights: Potential toxicity of routine parenteral feeding. J Pediatr 126:785-790, 1995.

Nose O, Tipton J, Ament M, Yabuuchi H: Effect of the energy source on changes in energy expenditure, respiratory quotient, and nitrogen balance during total parenteral nutrition in children. Pediatr Res 21:538-541, 1987.

Paisley JE, Thureen PJ, Baron KA, Hay WW: Safety and efficacy of low versus high parenteral amino acids in extremely low birth weight neonates immediately after birth. Pediatr Res 47:293A, 2000.

Peters O, Ryan SW, Matthew L, et al: Randomised controlled trial of acetate in preterm neonates receiving parenteral nutrition. Arch Dis Child 77:F12-F15, 1997.

Phelps SJ, Cochran EB: Effect of the continuous administration of fat emulsion on the infiltration of intravenous lines in infants receiving peripheral parenteral nutrition solutions. JPEN J Parenter Enteral Nutr 13:628-632, 1989.

Pineault M, Chessex P, Bisaillon S, Brisson G: Total parenteral nutrition in the newborn: Impact of the quality of infused energy on nitrogen metabolism. Am J Clin Nutr 47:298-304, 1988.

Poindexter B, Wright-Coltart S, Denne SC: The effect of *N*-acetyl tyrosine and cysteine in parenteral nutrition on protein metabolism in extremely low birth weight neonates. Pediatr Res 47:294A, 2000.

Poindexter BB, Karn CA, Denne SC: Exogenous insulin reduces proteolysis and protein synthesis in extremely low birth weight infants. J Pediatr 132:948-953, 1998.

Porcelli P, Sisk P: Increased parenteral amino acid administrations to extremely low-birth-weight infants during early postnatal life. J Pediatr Gastroenterol Nutr 34:174-179, 2002.

Putet G: Lipid metabolism of the micropremie. Clin Perinatol 27:57, 2000.

Redline RW, Redline SS, Boxerbaum B, Dahms BB: Systemic *Malassezia furfur* infections in patients receiving intralipid therapy. Hum Pathol 16:815-822, 1985.

Rivera A, Bell EF, Bier DM: Effect of intravenous amino acids on protein metabolism of preterm infants during the first three days of life. Pediatr Res 33:106-111, 1993.

Rubin M, Naor N, Sirota L, et al: Are bilirubin and plasma lipid profiles of premature infants dependent on the lipid emulsion infused? J Pediatr Gastroenterol Nutr 21:25-30, 1995.

Sadiq HF, Devaskar S, Keenan WJ, Weber TR: Broviac catheterization in low birth weight infants: Incidence and treatment of associated complications. Crit Care Med 15:47-50, 1987.

Saini J, Macmahon P, Morgan J, Kovar I: Early parenteral feeding of amino acids. Arch Dis Child 64:1362-1366, 1989.

Spear ML, Stahl GE, Hamosh M, et al: Effect of heparin dose and infusion rate on lipid clearance and bilirubin binding in premature infants receiving intravenous fat emulsions. J Pediatr 112:94-98, 1988.

Thiessen H, Jacobsen J, Brodersen R: Displacement of albumin-bound bilirubin by fatty acids. Acta Paediatr 61:285-288, 1972.

Van Aerde J, Sauer P, Pencharz P, et al: Effect of replacing glucose with lipid on the energy metabolism of newborn infants. Clin Sci 76:581-588, 1989.

Van Goudoever JB, Colen T, Wattimena JLD, et al: Immediate commencement of amino acid supplementation in preterm infants: Effect on serum amino acid concentrations and protein klinetics on the first day of life. J Pediatr 127:458-465, 1995.

Van Lingen RA, Van Goudoever JB, Luijendijk IHT, et al: Effects of early amino acid administration during total parenteral nutrition on protein metabolism in pre-term infants. Clin Sci 82:199-203, 1992.

Wilson DC, Cairns P, Halliday HL, et al: Randomised controlled trial of an aggressive nutritional regimen in sick very low birthweight infants. Arch Dis Child Fetal Neonatal Ed 177:4F-11F, 997.

Ziegler EE: Protein in premature feeding. Nutrition 10:69-71, 1994.

Zlotkin SH, Bryan MH, Anderson GH: Intravenous nitrogen and energy intakes required to duplicate in utero nitrogen accretion in prematurely born human infants. J Pediatr 99:115-120, 1981a.

Zlotkin S, Bryan M, Anderson H: Cysteine supplementation to cysteine-free intravenous feeding regimens in newborn infants. Am J Clin Nutr 34:914-923, 1981b.

# PART XIV

# GASTROINTESTINAL SYSTEM

Editor: ROBERTA A. BALLARD

CHAPTER 70

## Developmental Anatomy and Physiology of the Gastrointestinal Tract

Carol Lynn Berseth

### STRUCTURAL AND FUNCTIONAL DEVELOPMENT

The gastrointestinal tract is formed as a result of invagination and folding of the embryo as early as the fourth week of gestation. When the buccopharyngeal and cloacal membranes rupture, complete continuity is established between the primitive gastrointestinal tract and the exterior environment. A series of evaginations, elongations, and dilations result in the ultimate formation of the esophagus, stomach, duodenum, liver, and pancreas from the foregut; the jejunum, ileum, and ascending and transverse segments of the colon from the midgut; and the descending and rectosigmoid colon from the hindgut. As the gut rapidly elongates during the first trimester, it herniates into the umbilical cord. It reenters the abdominal cavity and rotates counterclockwise around the superior mesenteric artery, achieving its final position by 20 weeks of gestation (Fig. 70–1). All of the anatomic structures of the gastrointestinal tract are recognizable and well formed by the second trimester. Functional maturation of these structures, however, occurs well after anatomic maturation. Many functions are still immature at birth in the term infant and are not established until 2 to 4 years of age (Table 70–1).

As late as the 1980s, maturation and growth of the gastrointestinal tract were considered to be regulated by genetic endowment, the biologic clock, endogenous events such as the release of hormones, and exposure to exogenous factors such as amniotic fluid or enteral feedings. We now know that these four factors are reflective on a molecular level of various transcription events and intercellular crosstalk. The gastrointestinal tract also is in continuity with the intrauterine environment, as the fetal gut is bathed in amniotic fluid as early as 4 weeks of postconceptional age. By 20 weeks, 15 mL of amniotic fluid traverses the fetal gut; this volume rapidly increases to 400 to 500 mL by term. Amniotic fluid contains nutrients as well as hormones and growth factors that may provide stimulation for maturation. Functional maturation occurs along axes directed proximodistally and aborally. Concurrently, vascular and neural structures migrate along similar axes to support and regulate intestinal function. Vascular supply is provided by the celiac, superior mesenteric, and inferior mesenteric arteries. Enteric neurons are derived from neuroblasts that originate in the vagal region of the neural crest and migrate along the gastrointestinal tract with the descending fibers of the vagus nerve.

Because structural development appears to develop asynchronously with functional development, a brief review of structural development precedes a description of functional development for each anatomic entity discussed.

#### Oropharynx and Esophagus

Non-nutritive sucking begins at approximately 20 weeks of gestation (Herbst, 1983). It is characterized by mouthing movements that may or may not be coordinated with swallowing. Nutritive sucking, which does not appear until 32 to 34 weeks of gestation, consists of prolonged bursts of sucking that also contain swallows. Swallowing frequency is significantly lower in preterm infants whose postconceptional age is 30 to 35 weeks than in infants whose gestational age exceeds 35 weeks (Schrank et al, 1998), and maturation of various characteristics of sucking is related to gestational age rather than postnatal age (Gewolb, 2001). Such features include the percent of sucks that are part of "runs" of sucks, duration of sucking runs, and rate of sucking (Gewolb, 2001). Lau and coworkers (2000) have characterized sucking and swallowing in terms of maturation of function; they defined five distinct stages based on the presence or absence of suction and the rhythmicity of suction and expression of milk into the posterior pharynx. Using this staging system, they have shown that oral feeding performance improves as an infant matures from stage 1 to stage 5.

Superficial glands are present in the pharyngeal and esophageal mucosa by 20 weeks and squamous cells by 28 weeks. Mucous and lingual lipases also are secreted. The upper esophageal sphincter is present by 32 weeks. The neuroblasts and circular muscle throughout the body of the esophagus appear by the end of the first trimester, and esophageal peristalsis is present in the preterm infant.

#### Stomach

The structure of the stomach is well established by 6 weeks; the circular and longitudinal muscles appear by 9 weeks; and the endocrine, chief, mucous, and parietal

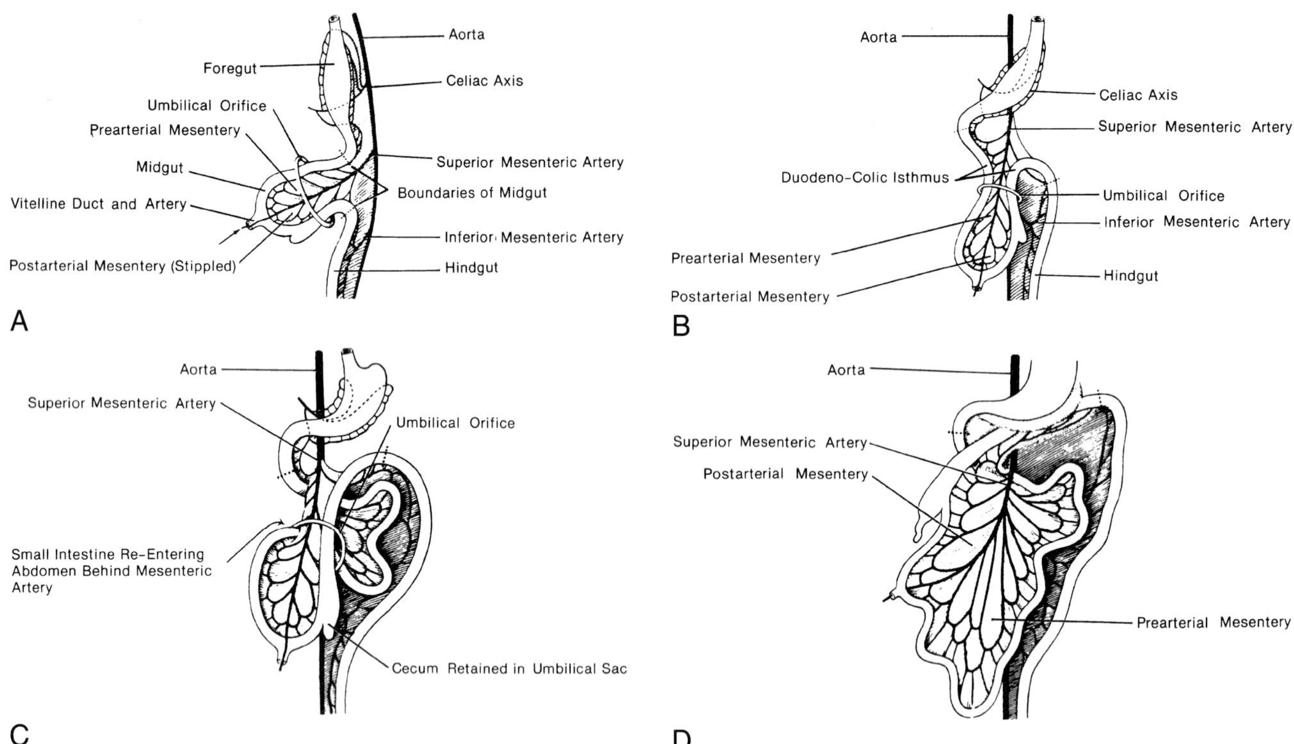


**FIGURE 70–1.** Diagram showing normal rotation of alimentary tract. **A,** Fifth week of intrauterine life *(lateral view)*. The foregut, midgut, and hindgut are shown with their individual blood supply supported by the common dorsal mesentery in the sagittal plane. The midgut loop has been extruded into the umbilical cord. **B,** Eighth week of intrauterine life *(anteroposterior view)*. The first stage of rotation is being completed. Note the narrow duodenocolic isthmus from which the midgut loop depends and the right-sided position of the small intestine and left-sided position of the colon. Maintenance of this position within the abdomen after birth is termed *nonrotation*. **C,** About the 10th week of intrauterine life, during the second stage of rotation *(anteroposterior view)*. The bowel in the temporary umbilical hernia is in the process of reduction; the most proximal part of the prearterial segment entering the abdomen to the right of the superior mesenteric artery is held forward close to the cecum and ascending colon, permitting the bowel to pass under it. As the coils of small intestine collect within the abdomen, the hindgut is displaced to the left and upward. **D,** Eleventh week of intrauterine life at the end of the second stage of rotation. From its original sagittal position, the midgut has rotated 270 degrees in a counterclockwise direction about the origin of the superior mesenteric artery. The essentials of the permanent disposition of the viscera have been attained. *(**A-D,** From Gardner CE Jr, Hart D: Arch Surg 29:942, 1934. Copyright 1934, American Medical Association.)*

cells appear by 12 weeks. By 16 weeks, all of these cells are secreting their respective substances: hydrochloric acid, intrinsic factor, pepsin, gastrin, and mucus. Although acid secretion is present shortly after birth in preterm and term infants, it is approximately 10% of that seen in adults. Adult values are achieved by 3 months of postnatal age. Acid secretion is less in preterm infants than in term infants (Fig. 70–2).

## Pancreas

The rotation and fusion of the dorsal and ventral buds of the pancreas are complete by 7 weeks. Differentiation of the endocrine and exocrine structure is present by 14 weeks. By 14 weeks, immunoreactive insulin is detected and pancreatic zymogen granules are present in the acini. By 16 weeks, amylase is present. Trypsin, lipase, and amylase are secreted into the duodenum by 31 weeks (Zoppi et al, 1972). Concentrations of these enzymes are lower in preterm than in term infants and, in turn, are significantly lower in term infants than in children (Fig. 70–3). Postnatally, trypsin increases in concentration, followed by chymotrypsin, carboxypeptidase, lipase, and amylase (Lebenthal and Lee, 1980). Postprandial release of these enzymes initially is blunted at birth and cannot be stimulated by specific nutrients. For example, high-protein diets can increase trypsin and lipase secretion, but a high-fat diet does not stimulate lipase secretion (Zoppi et al, 1972).

**TABLE 70–1**

**Anatomic and Functional Maturation of the Gastrointestinal Tract**

| Postconceptional Age (weeks) | | | | | |
|---|---|---|---|---|---|
| **15** | **20** | **25** | **30** | **35** | **40** |
| Mouth | Salivary glands | Swallow | Lingual lipase | *Sucking* | |
| Esophagus | Muscle layers present | Striated epithelium present | *Poor lower esophageal sphincter tone* | | |
| Stomach | Gastric glands present | G cells appear | *Gastric secretions present* | *Slow gastric emptying* | * |
| Pancreas | Exocrine and endocrine tissue differentiate | Zymogen present | *Reduced trypsin, lipase* | | * |
| Liver | Lobules form | *Bile secreted* | *Fatty acids absorbed* | | * |
| Intestine | Crypt and villus form | *Glucose transport present* | *Dipeptidase, sucrase, and maltase active* | *Lactase active* | |
| Colon | | Crypts and villi recede | | *Meconium passed* | |

*Full functional maturation occurs postnatally.

*Italics* indicate functional maturation.

## Liver

The liver is derived as an outbudding from the duodenum. The cranial portion of the bud differentiates into hepatic parenchyma, and the caudal portion, into the gallbladder. Lobules and bile canaliculi are present by 6 weeks; bile acids are synthesized by 12 to 14 weeks and are actively secreted by 22 weeks. There are qualitative and quantitative differences in bile acid synthesis in preterm infants. First, bile acid synthesis is decreased in the preterm infant compared with that in the term infant. Synthesis in the term infant, in turn, is approximately half of that seen in adults (Watkins et al, 1975) (Fig. 70–4). Similarly, bile acid pool size in preterm infants is approximately one-third that seen in term infants. Pool size in term infants, in turn, is approximately one-half that seen in adults. Hepatic hydroxylation is not fully developed

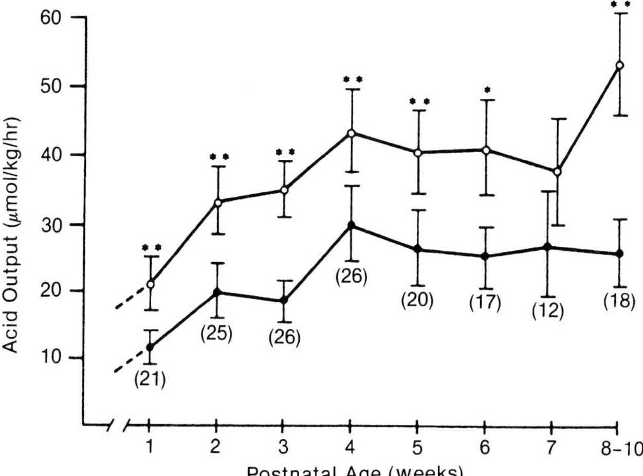


**FIGURE 70–2.** Basal acid output (○) and pentagastrin-stimulated acid output (●) in preterm infants. Number of subjects studied at each age is given in parentheses. $^{*}P < .05$. $^{**}P < .01$. *(From Hyman PE, Clarke DD, Everett SL: Gastric acid secretory function in preterm infants. J Pediatr 106:468, 1985.)*

in the fetus, and there is a decreased cholic acid–to–deoxycholic acid ratio. It also has been noted that atypical bile acids are present in the fetus; these are formed using fetal biosynthesis pathways. These compounds are not typically seen in adults and represent only a small percentage of bile acids by term (Nakagawa and Setchell, 1990). Degradation of bile salts also differs in preterm infants, in that preterm and term infants rely on taurine conjugation rather than glycine conjugation as in the adult. The active ileal transport mechanism of bile salts is present but immature (Heubi and Balistreri, 1980). Because hepatic uptake, secretion, and transport are not yet fully functional in the newborn, serum bile acid concentrations are elevated. These elevated levels persist for 6 to 8 weeks postnatally and slowly decline to adult values by 6 months (Suchy et al, 1981). Because hepatic processing of bile salts at multiple sites is immature, newborns are prone to develop cholestasis in response to stresses such as sepsis, mildly hepatotoxic drugs, or exposure to parenteral nutrition. This topic is reviewed in depth in Chapter 69.

## Small Intestine

By the time the intestine elongates, rotates, and returns to the abdominal cavity, the mucosal and muscular structures are well developed. The crypt and villus structure is present throughout. Because of rapid proliferation of epithelial tissue, the duodenum is transiently obstructed, but it is fully patent by 12 weeks. During the second trimester, the glycocalyx has appeared, and the brush border is structurally well defined. Endocrine cells are well established, and granules containing gastrin, secretin, cholecystokinin, motilin, serotonin, somatostatin, and substance P are present by 12 to 18 weeks. Gastrin, secretin, motilin, and gastrin inhibitory polypeptide are localized to duodenum and jejunum, whereas enteroglucagon, neurotensin, somatostatin, and vasoactive intestinal polypeptide are distributed throughout the intestines. Brush border

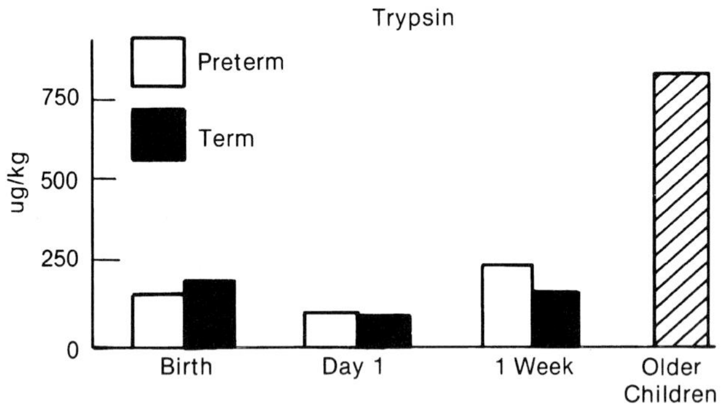


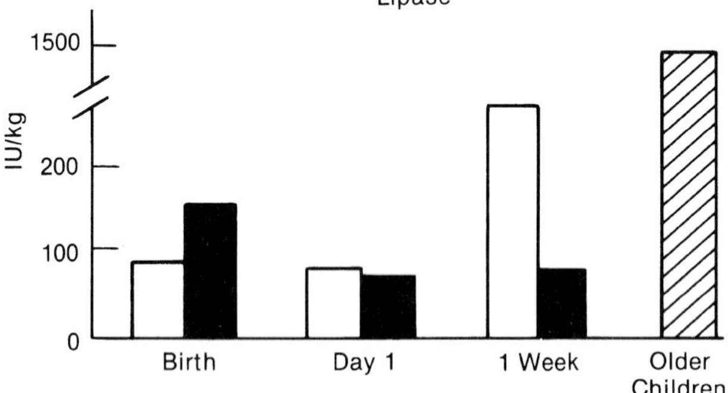


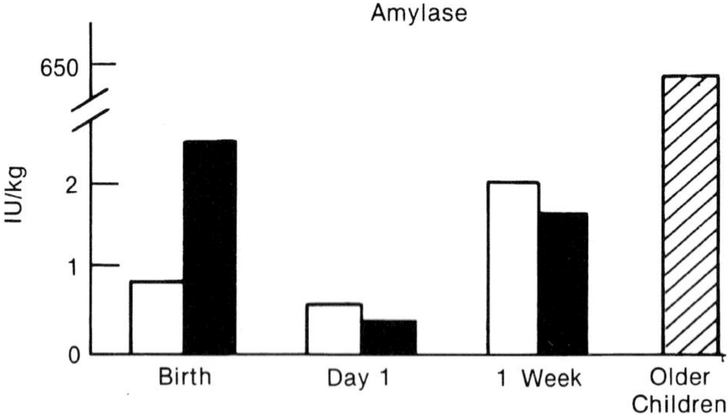


**FIGURE 70–3.** Pancreatic enzyme activity in preterm (32 to 34 weeks of gestational age) and full-term infants fed a balanced formula. Data represent mean values. *(Data from Zoppi G, Andreotti G, Pajno-Ferrara F, et al: Exocrine pancreas function in premature and term infants. Pediatr Res 6:880, 1972.)*

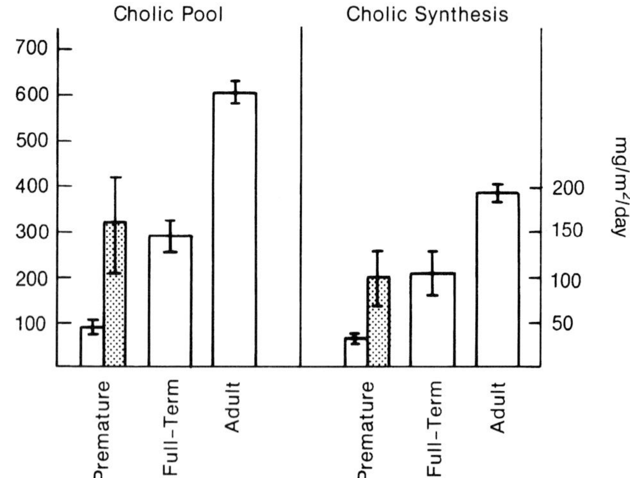


**FIGURE 70–4.** Comparison of bile acid pool size and synthesis rate in premature infants, full-term infants, and adults, corrected for body surface area. Shaded bars refer to premature infants whose mothers had received prenatal treatment with dexamethasone or phenobarbital. Data are means ± standard error (SE). *(Courtesy of Dr. John B. Watkins, Children's Hospital, Philadelphia. Values for premature infants are from Watkins JB, Szczepanik P, Gould JB, et al: Bile salt metabolism in the premature infant: Preliminary observations of pool size and synthesis rate following prenatal administration of dexamethasone and phenobarbital. Gastroenterology 69:706, 1975. Values for term infants are from Watkins JB, Ingall D, Szczepanik P, et al: Bile-salt metabolism in the newborn: Measurement of pool size and synthesis by stable isotope technique. N Engl J Med 288:431, 1973. Values for adults are from Vlahcevic et al, 1971.)*

membrane function, however, is immature. Although alpha-glucosidases, dipeptidases, and sucrase are functional by the end of the second trimester, lactase does not appear until 32 to 34 weeks of gestation. By 13 to 20 weeks of gestation, sucrase and maltase activities are 50% to 75% of those found in term infants and adults.

Lactase activity is present by 9 weeks (Fig. 70–5). By 24 weeks, however, lactase activity is still less than 25% of that found in term infants (Antonowicz et al, 1974; Auricchio et al, 1965). The abrupt rise in lactase activity that is noted to occur from 32 to 34 weeks of gestation coincides with an increase in lactase mRNA, implying that its delay in appearance is due to transcriptional control (Villa et al, 1992). When lactase first appears, its activity is distributed throughout the small intestine in a uniform manner. Shortly thereafter, a proximal gradient is established (Lacroix et al, 1984). Thus, lactase has been observed to be present in the colon at 13 to 20 weeks of gestation (Ménard and Pothier, 1987).

Sucrase and maltase also are present by 9 weeks of gestation. The activities of these enzymes achieve levels as high as 75% of those found in term infants by the end of the second trimester. Sucrase-isomaltase exists in a single high-molecular-weight form (Triadoru and Zweibaum, 1985). Glucoamylase, which is responsible for absorption of starches and glucose polymers, is present by the end of the second trimester, with activities approximately half those found at term (Antonowicz et al, 1974).

All of the numerous brush border peptidases, including alpha-glutamyl transpeptidase, aminopeptidase, oligoaminopeptidase, dipeptidylaminopeptidase IV, and carboxypeptidase, are present by the end of the second trimester. Thus, active glucose transport occurs by 10 weeks (Jirsova et al, 1996) and amino acid uptake by 12 weeks (Levin et al, 1968).

## Colon

The cecal dilation that forms the hindgut appears by 4 weeks, and by 12 weeks haustra and taeniae appear. When the rotation of the midgut is completed at 12 weeks, the cecum descends into the right iliac fossa. The rectum forms by 8 weeks, and formation of complete muscle layers and neural migration of ganglia cells are accomplished by 24 weeks. Morphologically, the premature colon

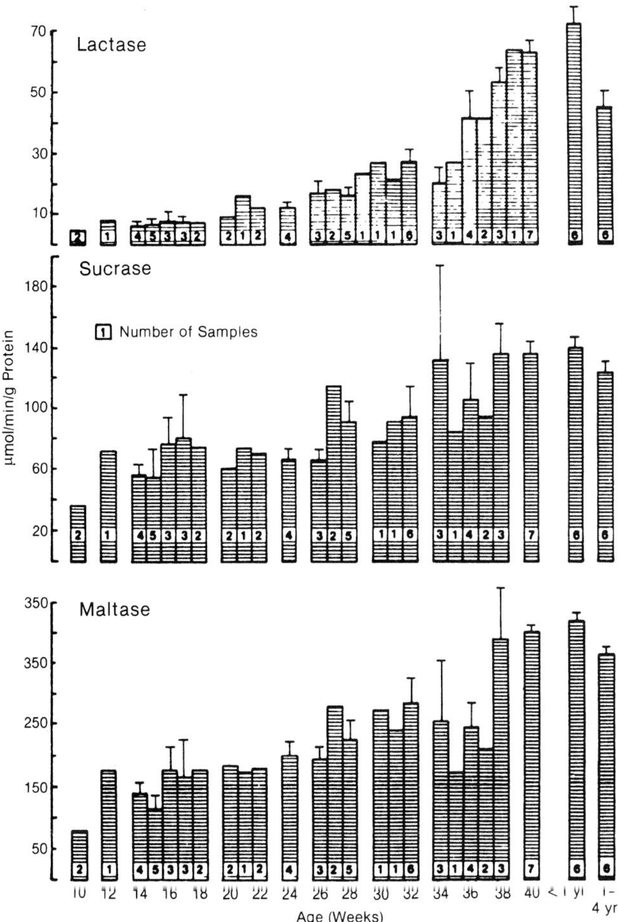


**FIGURE 70–5.** Developmental patterns of jejunal disaccharidase activities in human fetuses. *(From Antonowicz I, Lebenthal E: Developmental pattern of small intestinal enterokinase and disaccharidase activities in the human fetus. Gastroenterology 72:1301, 1977.)*

contains villi and crypts, and disaccharidase activities are present until 22 weeks of gestation. Although the villi and disaccharidase activities decrease and then disappear by term, sucrase and glucoamylase activities may still be present as late as 28 to 32 weeks of gestation (Raul et al, 1986).

## Gastrointestinal Hormones and Peptides

Numerous regulatory gut peptides are produced in the gastrointestinal tract. Several function as true hormones, including gastrin, cholecystokinin, motilin, pancreatic polypeptide, and somatostatin. Others have paracrine or neurocrine function, including gastric inhibitory polypeptide, bombesin, vasoactive intestinal polypeptide, neurotensin, enteroglucagon, and peptide YY. All of these peptides are present in the fetal intestine by the end of the first trimester. Adult distribution of these peptides may not be established until the end of the third trimester. All of these peptides have been identified in the plasma of preterm and term infants (Lucas et al, 1980). However, some concentrations are similar to those seen in adults, whereas others are lower or higher (Berseth, 1992). Earlier studies evaluated the plasma concentrations of peptides in the fasting state. Because several of these peptides function as true hormones, more recent studies have evaluated whether these peptides are released in response to feeding. It appears that these hormones are released in response to feeding (Berseth, 1998); however, their releases are limited in the newborn compared with the adult (Berseth et al, 1992; Lucas et al, 1980) (Fig. 70–6). With routine enteral feedings, release of these peptides becomes brisker and more intense over the first postnatal month (Berseth, 1992; Lucas et al, 1980).

# PROCESSING OF NUTRIENTS

## Digestion of Carbohydrates

Carbohydrates contribute approximately 40% of the caloric intake in healthy term infants. Lactose present in breast milk and formulas is the predominant source of carbohydrate. Some preterm formulas also contain glucose polymers. Although preterm infants have relatively low levels of lactase activity, they display normal growth with little diarrhea when they are fed lactose-containing milk and formula (MacLean and Fink, 1980). It is speculated that the relative absence of lactase activity is compensated for by the conversion of malabsorbed lactose by colonic bacteria to volatile organic acids, which are subsequently absorbed. It is not unusual, however, for stools of breast-fed preterm infants to contain disaccharides. Glucose polymers require amylase for hydrolysis. Because pancreatic amylase levels are quite low, these polymers probably are hydrolyzed by salivary amylase or absorbed directly at the mucosal level via mucosal glucoamylase, which has its maximal activity against polymers with chain lengths of 5 to 9 units (Kerzner et al, 1981). Once lactose and polycose are hydrolyzed to glucose, active glucose transport occurs by 17 weeks via two systems: a low-affinity, high-capacity sodium-glucose cotransport system found along the entire length of the intestines and a low-affinity, high-capacity system localized to the proximal small intestine (Malo, 1988).

## Digestion of Lipids

Fat provides 50% of the caloric intake of the newborn. Fat absorption is important not only for use in structural growth and cell membrane integrity but also in facilitating the absorption of fat-soluble vitamins. Fat processing has two components: (1) that occurring in the lumen of the intestine and (2) that occurring at the level of the mucosa. In the lumen, fats must be emulsified and hydrolyzed to form free fatty acids and monoglycerides. This process is achieved by bile acids and lipases, both of which are limited in amount or function (or both) in the preterm infant. Alternate mechanisms for fat hydrolysis appear to be present in the newborn. Lingual lipases and gastric lipases are present by 26 weeks of gestation. Serous glands located in the posterior third of the tongue produce lingual lipases, and non-nutritive sucking is a mechanism for its release. Lingual lipase tolerates the low gastric pH of 3.5 to 5.5. Gastric lipase, secreted by gastric glands, also contributes to luminal hydrolysis of fats in newborns (Cohen

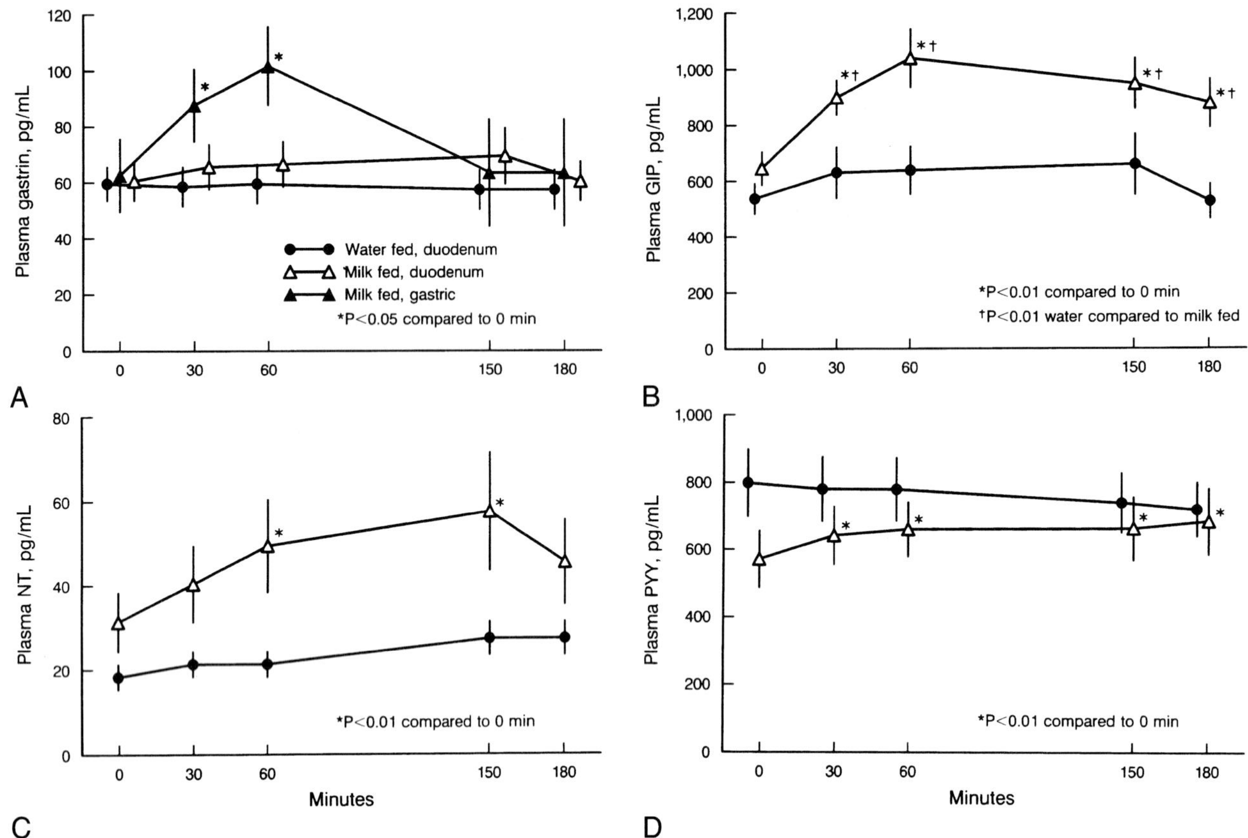


**FIGURE 70–6.** Plasma concentrations of four gastrointestinal peptides in response to a 2-hour slow infusion feeding. Values for infants fed water intraduodenally (●) and for infants fed formula intraduodenally (Δ) are plotted in **A** to **D**. Plasma concentrations of gastrin (**A**), gastric inhibitory polypeptide (GIP) (**B**), neurotensin (NT) (**C**), and peptide YY (PYY) (**D**) are similar during fasting and postprandial sampling. When infants were fed milk, plasma concentrations of gastrin did not increase with intraduodenal feeding. When feedings were given intragastrically, shown in **A** (▲), plasma gastric concentrations increased significantly over fasting values. *(Data summarized in Berseth CL, Nordyke CK, Valdes MG, et al: Responses of gastrointestinal peptides and motor activity to milk and water feedings in preterm and term neonates. Pediatr Res 31:587, 1992.)*

et al, 1971). Additional lipases also are present in breast milk. The major breast milk lipase is bile salt–stimulated lipase. In contrast to endogenous lipases, this lipase is capable of hydrolyzing all three ester bonds of triglycerides. A second lipase that resembles lipoprotein lipase also has been thought to be present in breast milk. Thus, it appears that these lipases substitute for the absence of pancreatic lipase. Furthermore, in contrast with pancreatic lipases, these three lipases function well in an environment that has low bile salt concentration, as is the case in the preterm infant. Because of decreased bile acid synthesis by the liver, intraluminal bile acid concentration in the preterm infant is 1 to 2 mmol/L (Katz and Hamilton, 1977), or approximately half of the critical micellar concentration required for adequate fat absorption. Thus, these alternate lipases appear to be well adapted for function in the immature environment of the gastrointestinal tract of the preterm infant.

There is also a relationship between intraluminal $Ca^{2+}$ concentration and fat absorption. In newborns, a high calcium intake impairs fat absorption, and for this reason the high calcium content of cow milk can cause malabsorption of fats (Hanna et al, 1970). Conversely, high fat intake may also impair $Ca^{2+}$ absorption. Therefore, the optimal relationship of dietary fat and calcium has not yet been identified for the preterm infant.

The source of dietary fat also influences absorption. Preterm infants digest and absorb fats derived from human milk better than formula-derived fats (Foman et al, 1970). Vegetable fats are absorbed better than animal fats. Unsaturated fats are absorbed better than saturated fats. Medium-chain and short-chain triglycerides are absorbed better than long-chain triglycerides (Roy et al, 1975).

Once the luminal phase of fat processing is completed, the mucosal phase of absorption must occur. The mucosal phase involves the passage of mixed micelles through the unstirred water layer at the mucosal cell surface. Monoglycerides and free fatty acids diffuse directly into the cells. Both of these processes appear to be well developed in the preterm infant. Thus, the inefficiency of fat absorption in the preterm infant, which ranges from 40% to 90%, largely reflects immaturity of intraluminal processing.

### Digestion of Proteins

Although proteins contribute less than 10% of ingested calories, they provide important "bricks" for the structure of somatic growth. Initial digestion of protein begins in the stomach, where dietary protein is denatured by gastric acid and cleaved to large polypeptides by pepsin. Because acid secretion is significantly lower in the preterm infant, it is not known how efficient this initial processing is. Gastric contents then are expelled into the upper intestine, where pancreatic proteases are capable of fairly efficient splitting of the peptides to oligopeptides and amino acids. As detailed previously, most of the brush border peptidases and cytosolic peptidases are well developed in the preterm infant, and the peptide transport system is efficient. In addition, there appears to be an alternate method for protein uptake in the intestine. Macromolecules can be actively taken up by pinocytosis by the neonatal intestine (Walker, 1978). In fact, preterm infants have been demonstrated to absorb intact lactoferrin of maternal origin (Hutchens et al, 1991).

## FACTORS INFLUENCING GASTROINTESTINAL FUNCTION

### Vascularization

Development of the mesenteric circulatory system parallels that of the intestine. Arterial supply occurs as a series of unpaired ventral outbuddings of vessels from the aorta to form the celiac axis, superior mesenteric artery, and inferior mesenteric artery. The celiac trunk originates at the level of T12 to L1, passes next to the median arcuate ligament of the diaphragm, and splits to form the splenic, left gastric, and hepatic arteries. Branches of the left gastric artery supply the lesser curvature and greater curvature of the stomach. Vessels from the hepatic artery supply the pancreas and duodenum. The superior mesenteric artery arises at L1 just caudal to the celiac trunk and supplies flow to the jejunum and ileum. Smaller branches form a series of arcades before entering the wall of the intestine. Therefore, collateral flow is considerable, and there are additional anastomoses with branches from the inferior mesenteric artery. The inferior mesenteric artery originates at L3 and supplies branches to the colon and rectum. Although rich collaterals are present throughout the gastrointestinal tract, watershed areas of marginal supply exist, as in the areas of the distal transverse colon and the upper rectum. In addition, the mucosa has the greatest need for vascular supply because of its high metabolic activity. Thus, it is the layer most sensitive to impairment of blood supply.

Regulation of mesenteric blood flow occurs at two points: the arteriole and the precapillary sphincter. Control is exerted on both intrinsic and extrinsic levels. Intrinsic control by local factors regulates blood flow in response to changes in arterial pressure and, consequently, tissue oxygenation. Vasodilation, for example, occurs in response to occlusion (reactive hyperemia) or feeding (functional hyperemia) and involves tonic changes at both the arteriolar and the precapillary levels. Extrinsic regulation is mediated by the splanchnic nerves by sympathetic input. In addition, circulating endogenous and exogenous factors, such as hormones, histamine, and prostaglandins, may modulate vascular tone. Two basic aspects of vascular regulation are the maintenance of basal vascular tone, or resistance, and vascular responses to stress.

It appears that postnatal change in intestinal basal vascular resistance in the neonate results from a transition from neonatal to a more mature pattern of regulation. All of the following information pertains to sheep and swine, which are considered to have postnatal maturation of vascular regulation that is similar to that found in humans. In the fetus, intestinal basal vascular resistance is higher than in the neonate. Blood flow—and its obligatory oxygen delivery—is twofold higher in the neonate than in the fetus (Edelstone and Holzman, 1983), and this change supports the intense metabolic activity in the neonate needed for nutrient absorption. Vascular resistance then increases during the second to fourth postnatal weeks, with a corresponding fall in blood flow and oxygen delivery (Reber et al, 2002).

Basal vascular resistance in the neonate is mediated by nitric oxide (NO), which in turn causes vasodilation and the myogenic response, and endothelin, both of which regulate vasoconstriction. Rates of NO production are high during the immediate neonatal period, but the role of NO in determining vascular tone lessens over the first postnatal month (Reber et al, 2000). The myogenic response refers to the onset of vasoconstriction in response to increases in intravascular pressure. It is mediated by vascular smooth muscle cell contracting in response to stretch via stimulation of a $Ca^{2+}$-induced phosphorylation of myosin light chain kinase (Davis and Hill, 1999). Endothelin, produced by the vascular endothelium, binds to endothelin A ($ET_A$) receptors and triggers vasoconstriction. As is the case for NO, endothelin production is high in the immediate neonatal period and declines thereafter (Nankervis and Nowicki, 2000).

These three mechanisms of regulation of intestinal vascular resistance dissipate by the end of the first postnatal month. Thereafter, intestinal growth causes increases surface area, which decreases vascular resistance, and extrinsic adrenergic innervation matures (Gootman et al, 1983).

The second set of mediators present in the gut vascular bed regulates vascular responses to hypoxemia and the presence of nutrients. In the intact animal, there appears to be a two-step response to hypoxemia. In response to modest hypoxemia ($PO_2$ of 50 mm Hg), the gut vascular bed dilates, increasing perfusion. In response to severe hypoxemia ($PO_2$ of <40 mm Hg), vasoconstriction, gut ischemia, and tissue hypoxia occur (Nowicki et al, 1988). Also present is a phenomenon called the *autoregulatory escape* (Shepherd and Granger, 1973). When gut blood flow is decreased by stimulating periarterial mesenteric nerves (i.e., the extrinsic system) or by infusion of norepinephrine, it is restored within minutes by the intrinsic regulation (Shepherd et al, 1973). This escape mechanism is present in newborn swine (Nowicki et al, 1991) and presumably in human newborns as well.

The presence of nutrients in the gut triggers the postprandial hyperemic response, which consists of brisk vasodilation and increased blood flow and oxygen delivery. This response occurs in neonatal swine (Crissinger and Burney,

1992) and also in pretem infants (Martinussen et al, 1996). In addition, studies involving small numbers of patients have suggested that drugs such as indomethacin or caffeine may cause reductions in the intensity of this response (Hoeker et al, 2002; Lane et al, 1999; Zhang et al, 1999).

## Motor Function and Neural Regulation

Motor activity is responsible for the forward movement of nutrients throughout the alimentary tract. For the infant to feed successfully, there must be coordinated sucking and swallowing, an ability to empty the stomach, coordinated propagation of nutrients through the intestine, and expulsion of waste products from the colon. All of these tasks are achieved by motor activity, which requires intact function of muscle, the nerves that regulate them, and the hormones that modulate their activity. Aboral movement of luminal contents requires the coordinated contractions of muscle, which in turn are regulated by the enteric nervous system (ENS), or nerves located in the gastrointestinal tract. The muscle layers of the alimentary tract are present by 14 weeks and the nerves and endocrine components by 20 to 24 weeks. Muscle mass is less in the preterm infant than in the term infant, however; thus, forcefulness of contraction also is less.

Control of gastrointestinal functions is provided primarily by the ENS. The ENS is a subsystem of the autonomic nervous system and is composed of complex neural circuits located within the gut wall. The basic unit of the ENS is the nerve cell, which functions by releasing neurotransmitters to other neurons or to effector cells (i.e., striated or smooth muscle). In general, the neurotransmitter acetylcholine is involved in excitatory synaptic events and norepinephrine in inhibitory synaptic events. Although the central nervous system and the ENS function in an integrated manner to regulate gastrointestinal events, the final common regulation for effectors is via the ENS. Thus, the ENS is capable of regulating gastrointestinal function independent of the central nervous system or spinal nerves.

The nerves that form the ENS are embryologically derived from cells that migrate from the vagal, truncal, and sacral regions of the neural crest. Cells from the vagal nerves populate the entire gastrointestinal tract, whereas those from the truncal nerves populate the foregut and those from the sacral nerves populate the distal gut. Neural crest cells first enter the outer gut mesenchyme and then later migrate to the mucosa. During this process of migration, neural cells proliferate. In addition, they are pluripotent and express catecholamines. When they reach the gut wall late in gestation, they differentiate into mature enteric neurons that no longer express catecholamines. The ENS consists of a variety of plexuses of nerve cell bodies and interneuronal circuits. The myenteric plexus is located between the longitudinal and circular muscle layers. The submucosal plexus is located between the (lamina) muscularis mucosae and the circular muscle layer. All of the differentiated neurons express serotoninergic and peptidergic neurotransmitters, such as serotonin, substance P, and neuropeptide Y. Finally, some of the neural crest cells and/or neuronal precursors cluster to form ganglia. The normal distribution of ganglion cells is present by 24 weeks. However, the density of these ganglia may change over the first several postnatal years (Wester et al, 1999).

Another structure formed during fetal life is the interstitial cell of Cajal. These are specialized cells that differentiate from muscle cells (Young, 1999). These cells are interspersed between muscle cells and and have intimate connections to neural cells, and they are responsible for maintaining the pacemaker function of the intestinal muscle. Thus, the denervated gut muscle has a basal contraction rate, as is the case for cardiac muscle. However, the coordination of this basal contraction is directly regulated by neural input. Fekete and colleagues (1995, 1996) have characterized the ontogeny of neural maturation in fetal tissues. At 10 weeks of postconceptional age, the circular muscle layer is formed, followed by the appearance of a primitive myenteric plexus and the longitudinal smooth muscle layer (Fekete et al, 1996). At 10 weeks, most neural cells in the gut myenteric plexus are still neuroblasts, with few specific contacts with muscle and few synaptic vesicles. By 18 weeks, however, both neuroblasts and ganglion cells are present. Neural cells have axoaxonic synapses and contain synaptic vesicles. Moreover, functional neural transmission appears to be present, as gut tissues display intense amine-specific fluorescence and nicotinamide adenine dinucleotide (NADH)-diaphorase staining, indicating that neurotransmitters are being produced (Fekete et al, 1995). Neurotransmitters are present by immunohistochemical staining by 24 weeks. The adult distribution along the length of the intestine of the transmitters may not be achieved until close to term.

Abnormalities in neural migration are reflected in clinical disease. Neural structures are abnormal in patients with Chagas disease, achalasia, chronic intestinal pseudo-obstruction, and Hirschsprung disease (Cohen, 1974; Schuffler and Jonah, 1982). Chemical ablation of myenteric neurons in rats results in hypertrophy of the longitudinal and circular muscle and, subsequently, enhanced myoelectric activity (Holle and Forth, 1990). In fetal sheep that have had artificial exteriorization of the bowel in utero to stimulate gastroschisis, profound disruption of the myenteric plexus occurs concurrently with the presence of highly disturbed motility (Holle and Forth, 1990). An absence of NO has been demonstrated among infants who have pyloric stenosis and Hirschsprung disease. NO is thought to provide inhibitory input to the ENS as a nonadrenergic, noncholinergic neurotransmitter. Hence, its absence results in increased muscle tone.

## Motility of the Digestive System

Sucking and swallowing involves the use of skeletal and smooth muscle. Maturation of sucking was reviewed earlier under "Esophagus." This section focuses on motor function in the gastrointestinal tract from the distal esophagus onward. The major limitation to enteral alimentation appears to be not digestion or absorption but the propulsion of chyme along the gastrointestinal tract. The human fetus can swallow as early at 17 weeks of gestation, and swallowing appears to play an important role in the regulation of amniotic fluid volume. For example, hydramnios is often seen in pregnancies in which fetal swallowing is impaired, such as when esophageal atresia or upper intestinal atresia is present. Exposure to factors in amniotic fluid appears to be important for gastrointestinal development. Mucosal maturation in the stomach is delayed in rabbit fetuses if the esophagus is ligated, and maturation returns to normal if the esophagus is exposed to amniotic fluid or epidermal growth factor.

Once milk or formula is ingested, it must be propelled distally past the lower esophageal sphincter into the stomach. The lower esophageal sphincter, which is responsible for preventing reflux of gastric content, is a 0.6- to 1-cm area of increased muscular tone located in the distal esophagus. Lower esophageal sphincter basal pressures range from 20 to 40 mm Hg in term infants and are as low as 5 mm Hg in infants born at 27 weeks of gestation (Newell et al, 1988). Coordinated activity constitutes a small proportion of the esophageal contractions in preterm infants (Omari et al, 1995); however, it does not appear that this is a limiting factor for the neonate ingesting formula or milk.

Motor activity in the preterm stomach and intestine has been extensively studied. The stomach fundus is responsible for dilation and accommodation of ingested milk or formula, and the antrum is responsible for mixing and expelling contents into the duodenum. Little is known about gastric accommodation. Zangen and colleagues (2001) have shown that compliance is increased in the newborn term stomach. Thus, accommodation is poor, but it improves rapidly within 24 to 48 hours. Gastric emptying requires that antral motor activity and duodenal motor activity be adequate and that their actions be coordinated. Antral motor activity is similar in the 24-week preterm infant and in the term infant (Ittman et al, 1992). Duodenal motor activity as well as its coordination with antral activity, however, differs in preterm and in term infants. The absence of coordination of antral and duodenal motor activity thus appears to reflect immaturity of duodenal function rather than of antral function. When term infants ingest a feeding, a brisk onset of duodenal contraction is noted. Approximately only 25% to 50% of preterm infants have this mature motor response to feeding (Al-Tawil and Berseth, 1996). Rather, in most preterm infants, duodenal contractions cease in response to a feeding. When this cessation of motor contractions occurs, gastric emptying is delayed (DeVille et al, 1998). Gastric emptying is delayed in the preterm infants compared with that seen in the term infants (Anderson and Berseth, 1996; Cavell, 1979). As in adults, meal composition also affects gastric emptying, with delay occurring as caloric density increases. Emptying also is delayed more with glucose or lactose than with glucose polymers and with long-chain triglycerides than with medium-chain triglycerides (Siegal et al, 1985). This last finding, however, has not been documented in preterm infants of fewer than 32 weeks of gestation.

McLain (1963), in one of the earliest studies of small bowel motility in human newborns, suggested that motility increases with advancing gestational age. Until 30 weeks, contrast material did not progress through the small intestine of the fetus; however, at 32 weeks, contrast material passed through the small bowel to the colon in 9 hours, compared with a transit time of 4.5 to 7 hours in term infants. More recent work has shown that transit times in the preterm infant may range from 0.5 to 7 days (Baker-Wills and Berseth, 1996).

In the adult, motor activity cycles through three patterns every 60 to 90 minutes. Often the muscle is still or quiescent for 10 to 20 minutes. This quiescence is then replaced by irregular contractions, which are replaced in turn by an episode of intense regular contractions that migrate distally through the bowel. This entire sequence of patterns is called the *interdigestive cycle* (Fig. 70–7). Complete interdigestive cycles are present in term infants (Amarnath et al, 1989). They are rarely seen in preterm infants, however. In extremely premature infants (24 to 28 weeks of gestation), unorganized irregular contractions are seen, and little quiescence is present (Berseth, 1992) (Fig. 70–8). In older preterm infants (28 to 32 weeks), motor quiescence begins to appear, and motor activity is organized into short bursts of phasic activity called *clusters* (Baker and Berseth, 1995). In more mature preterm infants (32 to 36 weeks), motor patterns become increasingly more organized, episodes of motor quiescence as well as clusters lengthen (Baker and Berseth, 1995), and migrating activity occasionally is seen (Berseth, 1992). Migrating motor complexes (MMCs), first seen around 33 weeks of gestation, are an interdigestive phenomenon that functions to sweep gut contents over long segments of intestine between meals. Eating inhibits this pattern, which initiates postprandial mixing-type contractions. In the term infant, the time between MMCs is 44 minutes, or about half the time observed in older children. The propagation rate, however, is 3.1 cm per minute in term infants, compared with 8.2 cm per minute for older children, and the duration is 10.9 minutes in infants, compared with 7.2 minutes for older children. Berseth (1992) has suggested that early feeding may be important in hastening the maturation of motility in preterm infants. In addition, she also has shown that the composition of feeding may alter motor

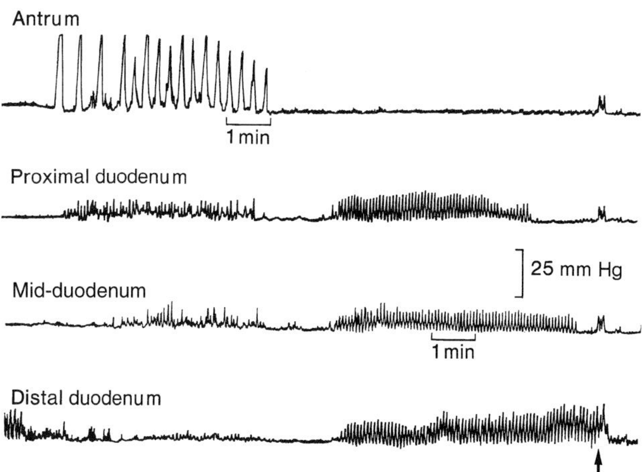


**FIGURE 70–7.** Migrating motor complex in a term infant. **Upper tracing,** Motor contractions recorded from the antrum. **Lower three tracings,** Motor contractions recorded from the duodenum. Phasic activity present in the antrum is temporally associated with the appearance of intense phasic activity that migrates distally to the three duodenal leads. *(From Ittman PI, Amarnath R, Berseth CL: Maturation of antroduodenal motor activity in preterm and term infants. Dig Dis Sci 37:14, 1992.)*

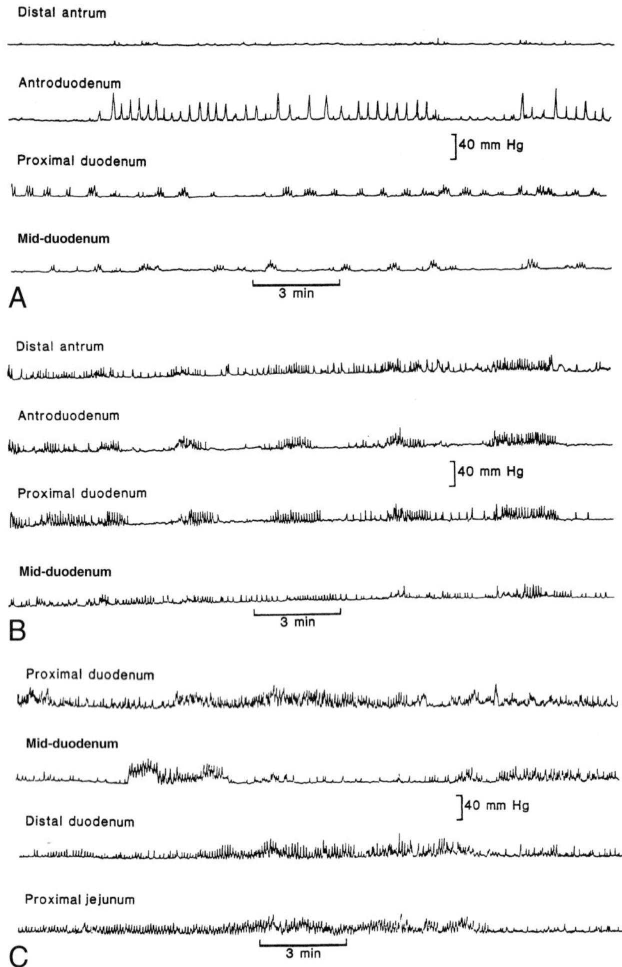


**FIGURE 70–8.** Serial gastrointestinal manometric tracings from an individual infant: **A,** at birth (32 weeks); **B,** at 2 weeks of postnatal age (34 weeks); and **C,** at 4 weeks of postnatal age (36 weeks). In **A,** clusters of phasic contractions occur in the two duodenal leads. Clusters are of short duration (approximately 0.75 minute), have low amplitude (approximately 12 mm Hg), and recur frequently. **B,** Two weeks later in the same infant, clusters are present in all leads. Individual clusters have a longer duration (approximately 2.5 minutes), have a higher amplitude (approximately 20 mm Hg), and recur less often. **C,** At 4 weeks of age, only one cluster can be displayed because its duration is now prolonged. *(From Berseth CL: Gestational evolution of small intestinal motility in preterm and term infants. J Pediatr 115:649, 1989.)*

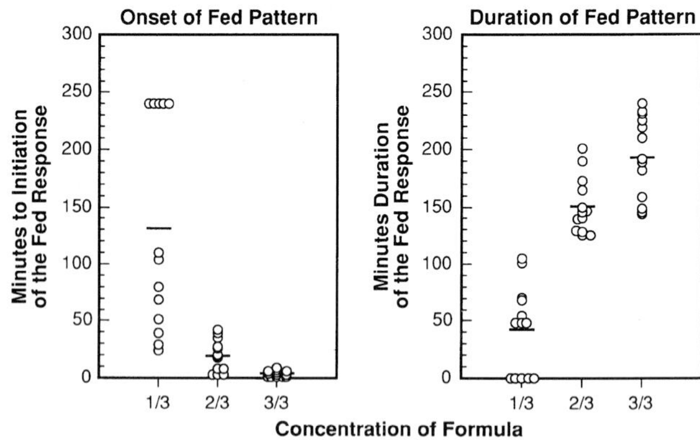


**FIGURE 70–9.** Motor activity responses to feeding formula diluted to one-third strength or two-thirds strength or full strength. **Left panel,** There is an increasing delay of the onset of the fed response as progressively more diluted formula is given ($r = .62$; $P < .01$). **Right panel,** The duration of the fed response is progressively longer as more concentrated formula is given ($r = .49$; $P < .01$). *(From Koenig WJ, Amarnath RP, Hench V, Berseth CL: Manometrics for preterm and term infants: A new tool for old questions. Pediatrics 95:203, 1995.)*

responses. For example, duodenal motor activity normally increases in response to feeding. When the preterm infant is fed diluted formula, motor responses are delayed in onset and are less intense (Fig. 70–9).

Just as gastric emptying can be affected by nutrient composition, small intestinal motor function can be influenced by many of the medications routinely given to preterm infants. For example, mydriatics used for routine screening eye examinations slow gastric emptying and cause significant feeding intolerance (Bonthala et al, 2000). Antenatal steroids may hasten maturation of motor patterns (Baker-Wills and Berseth, 1996). The chronic use of opioids, such as morphine, can change intestinal transit time (Berseth, 1996). In adults, the initiation of the MMC is triggered by the hormone motilin. This hormone is released in a cyclic fashion, with concentrations peaking every 60 to 90 minutes. The hormone binds to motilin receptors located in the distal antrum and proximal duodenum, which triggers the MMC. Plasma concentrations of motilin do not cycle in the neonate (Jadcherla et al, 1995), but administering low-dose erythromycin, which competitively binds to motilin receptors, triggers MMCs in preterm infants whose gestational ages exceed 31 weeks (Jadcherla et al, 1995). These findings are consistent with the conclusion that the absence of the cyclic release of the hormone motilin underlies the absence of the MMC in older preterm infants.

Colonic motility has not been studied in preterm infants. In a single study in preterm primates, colonic motor responses to feeding were less robust in preterm animals than in term animals (Cannon and Cheung, 1989). In children, colonic motor patterns are similar to those seen in adults (DiLorenzo et al, 1995).

Meconium is the thick black material that collects in the distal portion of the small intestine and colon of the fetus and consists of intestinal secretions, bile, desquamated cellular debris, and amniotic fluid. Ninety-four percent of newborns pass a meconium stool within 24 hours after birth. However, passage of meconium is often delayed in preterm infants with birth weights less than 1500 g (Wang and Huang, 1994). Meetze and colleagues (1993) have shown that passage of meconium may be delayed up to 10 days in infants with birth weights less than 1250 g.

## Host Defenses

Because the gut is in continuity with the neonatal environment, it is constantly exposed to antigens and bacteria. A complex series of host defenses, both immune and nonimmune in nature, are present in the newborn. The nonimmune system is also called the innate immune system, as it responds in a nonspecific fashion. The immune system is composed of specific humoral and cellular responses that are activated in response to specific antigens.

The innate immune system constitutes the first line of host defense in the neonate in that it prevents many potential antigens and organism from reaching the intestinal mucosa. The components of the innate system include physical barriers, cells, and chemical barriers.

First, intestinal motility is an important factor in moving nutrients aborally so that they do not have time to establish colonization in the lumen of the gut. As described in the previous section ("Motor Function and Neural Regulation"), the MMC, which is responsible for propelling luminal contents forward through the small intestine, often is absent in the preterm infant (Amarnath et al, 1989; Berseth, 1992). As a result, overall intestinal transit times are delayed in the preterm infant (Baker-Wills and Berseth, 1996; Berseth et al, 2003).

The release of gastric acid and pancreaticobiliary secretions also is an important component of the innate system. These secretions inhibit bacterial growth and activate proteolysis, which alters antigen structure. There are concerns that withholding enteral feedings in preterm infants results in a decreased release of these secretions and thereby may impair an important function of host defense in the preterm infant. Hyman and associates (1983) have confirmed that basal and maximal gastric acid production is significantly lower in unfed infants, and rates of infection are higher among infants whose gastric acid production is suppressed by histamine $H_2$ blockers (Beck-Sague et al, 1994).

Another physical barrier is created by mucus, which contains mucins, glycoproteins, inmunoglobulins, glycolipids, and albumin. These constituents form a protective gel over the surface of the intestine. Mucus presents a slippery surface that enhances forward propulsion of antigens and inhibits the diffusion of large molecules.

Cells that provide innate immune defense are the epithelial cells and other cells located close to them, including the goblet cells, the M cells, and subepithelial cells. The intestinal epithelial cells are closely approximated to one another by a series of tight junctions. These junctions allow for the physiologic passage of fluids and electrolytes but prevent the passage of larger proteins. In addition, microvilli form a physical barrier, as they prevent or retard the cellular penetration of large macromolecules and charged particles. In animals, glycosylation of the microvillus membrane glycoconjugates is not fully functional in neonates (Ozaki et al, 1989), which predisposes the neonate to increased pathologic bacterial colonization (Schiffrin et al, 1993). However, these findings have not been confirmed in human neonates. M cells are epithelial cells that lack well-developed microvilli, which permits macromolecular transport. They are present only in follicles that overlie lymphoid tissue and serve to deliver foreign antigens and microorganisms to the lymphoid tissue. Goblet cells are interspersed among the epithelial cells, and they secrete mucus.

Subepithelial cells include follicular dendritic cells, Peyer patches, and mast cells. Follicular dendritic cells, which are located in the lymphoid follicles, present antigens to T and B cells. Peyer patches, which are clusters of lymphoid tissue, are present by 19 weeks of gestation and become more abundant between 24 and 40 weeks (Cornes, 1965).

The immune system of host defense is composed of cellular components and secretory components. T cells, B cells, and macrophages are present in the fetal intestine by 20 weeks of gestation. Lymphocytes proliferate in response to a mitogen as early as 12 weeks, and M cells that specialize in the antigenic processing of macromolecules are present by 17 weeks. Antigenic stimulation of lymphoid tissues, however, cannot be demonstrated until 46 weeks. This deficiency is of most concern because the preterm gut absorbs macromolecules directly by pinocytosis. Although plasma immunoglobulin A (IgA) is relatively low in the newborn, secretory IgA is present by 22 weeks of gestation. The newborn intestine has few IgA-producing plasma cells, however, and when preterm infants are fed exogenous protein they are unable to form antibodies (Rieger and Rothberg, 1985).

When an antigen stimulates the host defense system, a variety of soluble proteins regulate growth and differentiation of lymphocytes. These proteins are called *cytokines* and include the interleukins (ILs), tumor necrosis factors, interferons, and platelet-activating factor. Cytokines play important roles in stimulating chemotaxis of netrophils, promotion of IgA expression, and epithelial cell proliferation after mucosal injury. When cultured fetal enterocytes (18 to 21 weeks) are stimulated by the general chemotoxin lipopolysaccharide, they release significantly greater amounts of the proinflammatory cytokine IL-8 (Nanthakumar et al, 2000), suggesting that there may be an imbalance of release of pro- and anti-inflammatory cytokines in response to a stimulus in the preterm infant.

A number of host defense functions appear to be mediated by enteral nutrients. Among those that have been recently studied are glutamine, arginine, long-chain fatty acids, nucleotides, and nutrients called probiotics and prebiotics.

Glutamine plays an important role in maintaining epithelial cell integrity, cell growth, and inflammatory responses. Glutamine and nucleotides appear to act in concert in regulating intestinal epithelial proliferation and differentiation and in this manner may play important roles in mounting inflammatory responses as well as active healing and recovery from insults. When the availability of glutamine is artificially reduced, intestinal cell growth is retarded; these results are reversed by adding nucleotide supplements (He et al, 1994). When endogenous glutamine synthesis is inhibited, small intestinal interepithelial junctional integrity is impaired (Wiess and associates, 1999). In vivo studies in neonatal rats show that feeding a diet that is glutamine deficient increases bacterial translocation (Neu, 2001). Finally, a randomized-masked trial was conducted in 68 very low-birth-weight infants during the first postnatal month. The incidence of sepsis was only 11% among infants who were given glutamine supplementation, compared with 30% in the control group, in which infants were given no supplement (Neu et al, 1997). These differences in outcome can effect a significant cost reduction (Dallas et al, 1998).

Another amino acid that has been investigated is arginine. This amino acid also plays an important role in immune function and growth. Plasma concentrations of arginine are lower among preterm infants who subsequently develop necrotizing enterocolitis (NEC) than among those who do not (Becker, 2000; Zamora, 1997). Arginine supplementation has been shown to reduce severity of NEC in piglets (DiLorenzo et al, 1995) and in human infants (Amin et al, 2002).

Recent studies also have evaluated the role of long-chain fatty acids (Caplan et al, 2001) and nucleotides (Pickering et al, 1998). Although some infant formulas are now supplemented with nucleotides, no large clinical trials have been performed to date in preterm infants. Another study demonstrated that formulas supplemented with egg phospholipid reduced the occurrence of NEC but not sepsis (Carlson et al, 1998).

Two classes of "nutrients" that recently have been shown to influence host defense are preobiotics and prebiotics. *Probiotics* are live organisms that can compete with and overgrow pathogenic organisms. The bowel flora of infants fed breast milk contains a predominance of bifidobacteria (Harmsen and Wildeboer-Veloo, 2000). Thus, researchers have speculated that colonizing the gut with these less pathogenic bactera may reduce the incidence of sepsis and necrotizing enterocolitis. The chronic administration of *Lactobacillus* GG reduces antibiotic-induced diarrhea in children (Vanderhoof et al, 1999; Arvola et al, 1999) and reduces the incidence of diarrhea in undernourished children (Oberhelman et al, 1999). Formula-fed infants given formula supplemented with *Bifidobacterium* had fecal pH and bacterial flora that were similar to those seen in breast fed infants (Pahwa and Mathur, 1987). Chronic administration of *Lactobacillus* results in colonization of the preterm gut (Millar, 1993; Reuman et al, 1986), and daily administration of *Lactobacillus* reduced the incidence of NEC in preterm infants in a recent study (Hoyos, 1999). Although the mechanism by which these probiotics achieve these outcomes is not yet known, studies in animals have shown that *Lactobacillus* modulates immune response and bowel flora (Schultz and Sartor, 2000) and reduces intestinal permeability in children who have Crohn's disease (Gupta et al, 2000). Other investigators hypothesize that probioticc bind competitively to epithelial receptors and essentially prevent pathogenic bacteria from establishing the first foothold in the process of translocation (Alvarez-Olmos and Oberhelman, 2001).

Several concerns limit the therapeutic use of probiotics. First, there is a need to establish the efficacy for each specific probiotic strain. Second, the quality control required in commercial preparation of therapeutic products is costly. Third, large clinical trials are needed to assess their efficacy and safety. Fourth, continuous administration is required to maintain colonization.

For these reasons, attention has shifted from probiotics to prebiotics. *Prebiotics* are defined to be nondigestible substrates that preferentially enhance the growth of nonpathogenic organisms. For example, breast milk contains galacto-oligosaccharides, which favor the growth of bifidobacteria. Fructo-oligosaccharides increase bifidobacterial counts and colonic metabolic activity in adults (Gibson et al, 1995).

## Gut Flora

The gut is sterile in utero, but colonization begins at birth. The pattern of bacterial growth reflects the maternal and neonatal environment, and enteric bacteria colonize the human infant in an oral-to-anal direction (Rotimi and Duerden, 1981). In healthy infants, aerobic organisms appear within a few hours. Anaerobic organisms are present by 24 hours and increase in number over the first 3 weeks (Cooperstock and Zedd, 1983). Because the route of access of organisms to the intestine is by ingestion, stools of breast milk–fed infants have a predominance of *Bifidobacterium*, whereas stools of formula-fed infants have a predominance of *Escherichia coli* and *Klebsiella* (Harmsen and Wildeboer-Veloo, 2000). These organisms are capable of metabolizing bile acids as well as nonabsorbed proteins, lipids, and carbohydrates and thus may potentially play an important role in further processing of nutrients in the preterm newborn. Consequently, alterations in gut flora due to certain drugs or to shortened bowel length may result in profound intestinal dysfunction.

## SELECTED READINGS

Back P, Walter K: Developmental pattern of bile acid metabolism as revealed by bile acid analysis of meconium. Gastroenterology 78:671, 1980.

## REFERENCES

Al-Tawil Y, Berseth CL: Gestational and postnatal maturation of duodenal motor responses to intragastric feeding. J Pediatr 129:374, 1996.

Alvarez-Olmos MI, Oberhelman RA: Prebiotic agents and infectious diseases: A modern perspective on a traditional therapy. Clin Infect Dis 32:1567, 2001.

Amarnath RP, Berseth CL, Malagelada J-R, et al: Postnatal maturation of small intestinal motility in preterm neonates. J Gastrointest Motil 1:138, 1989.

Amin HJ, Zamora SA, McMillan DD, et al: Arginine supplementation prevents necrotizing enterocolitis in the premature infant. J Pediatr 140:425, 2002.

Anderson CA, Berseth CL: Neither motor responses nor gastric emptying differ in response to formula temperature in preterm infants. Biol Neonate 70:265, 1996.

Antonowicz I, Chang SK, Grand RJ: Development and distribution of liposomal enzymes and disaccharidases in human fetal intestine. Gastroenterology 67:51, 1974.

Arvola T, Laiho K, Torkkeli S, et al: Prophylactic Lactobacillus GG reduces antibiotic-associated diarrhea in children with respiratory infections: a randomized study. Pediatrics 104:e64, 1999. Also available at: http://www.Pediatrics.org/cgi/content/full/104/5

Auricchio S, Rubino A, Mürset G: Intestinal glycosidase activities in the human embryo, fetus, and newborn. Pediatrics 3S:944, 1965.

Becker RM, Wu G, Galanko JA, et al: Reduced serum amino acid concentrations in infants with necrotizing enterocolitis. J Pediatr 137:785, 2000.

Baker J, Berseth CL: Postnatal change in inhibitory regulation of intestinal motor activity in human and canine neonates. Pediatr Res 38:133, 1995.

Baker-Wills E, Berseth CL: Antenatal steroids enhance maturation of small intestinal motor activity in preterm infants. Pediatr Res 39:193A, 1996.

Beck-Sague, CM, Azimi P, Fonseca SN, et al: Bloodstream infections in neonatal intensive care unit patients: results of a multicenter study. Pediatr Infect Dis J 13:1110, 1994.

Berseth CL: Chronic therapeutic morphine administration alters small intestinal motor patterns and gastroanal transit in preterm infants. Pediatr Res 39:305A, 1996.

Berseth CL: Effect of early feeding on maturation of the preterm infant's small intestine. J Pediatr 120:947, 1992.

Berseth CL: Selective nutrient feeding induces maturation of gastrointestinal hormone release in preterm infants. Pediatr Res 43:256A, 1998.

Berseth CL, Bisquera JA, Paje VU: Prolonging small feeding volumes early in life decreases the incidence of necrotizing enterocolitis in very low birth weight infants. Pediatrics 111:529, 2003.

Berseth CL, Nordyke CK, Valdes MG, et al: Responses of gastrointestinal peptides and motor activity to milk and water feedings in preterm and term neonates. Pediatr Res 31:587, 1992.

Bisset WM, Watt JB, Rivers RPA, et al: Ontogeny of fasting small intestinal motility in human infant. Gut 29:483, 1988.

Bonthala S, Musgrave V, Sparks J, Berseth CL: Mydriatics slow gastric emptying in preterm infants. J Pediatr 137:327, 2000.

Bryant MG, Buchan AM, Gregor M, et al: Development of intestinal regulatory peptides in the human fetus. Gastroenterology 83:47, 1982.

Cannon RA, Cheung AT: Development of methodology for recording colonic myoelectrical activity in the infant primate. Biomater Artif Cells Artif Organs 17:81, 1989.

Caplan MS, Russel T, Xiao Y, et al: Effect of polyunsaturated acid (PUFA) supplementation on intestinal inflammation and necrotizing enterocolitis (nec) in a neonatal rat model. Pediatr Res 49:647, 2001.

Carlson SE, Montalto MB, Ponder DL, et al: Lower incidence of necrotizing enterolcolitis in infants fed a preterm formula with egg phospholipids. Pediatr Res 44:491, 1998.

Cavell B: Gastric emptying in preterm infants. Acta Paediatr Scand 68:725, 1979.

Chappell JE, Clandinen MT, Kearney-Volpe C: Fatty acid balance studies in premature infants fed human milk or formula: Effect of calcium supplementation. J Pediatr 108:439, 1986.

Cohen M, Morgan GRH, Hofmann AF: Lipolytic activity of human gastric and duodenal juice against medium and long chain triglycerides. Gastroenterology 60:1, 1971.

Cohen S: Developmental characteristics of lower esophageal sphincter function: A possible mechanism for infantile cholasia. Gastroenterology 67:252, 1974.

Cohen S: Motor disorders of the esophagus. N Engl J Med 301:184, 1979.

Cooperstock MS, Zedd AJ: Intestinal flora of infants. In Hentgis D (ed): Human Intestinal Microflora in Health and Disease. New York, Academic Press, 1983, p 79.

Cornes JC: Number, size, and distribution of Peyer's patches in the human small intestine. Gut 6:225, 1965.

Crissinger KD, Burney DL: Influence of luminal nutrient composition on hemodynamics and oxygenation in developing piglet intestine. Pediatr Res 31:106A, 1992.

Dallas MJ, Bowling D, Roig JC, et al: Enteral glutamine supplementation for very-low-birth-weight infants decreases hospital costs. JPEN J Parenter Enteral Nutr 22:352, 1998.

Davis JM, Hill MA: Signaling mechanisms underlying the vascular myogenic response. Physiol Rev 79:387, 1999.

deBelle RC, Vaupshas V, Vitullo BB, et al: Intestinal absorption of bile salts: Immature development in the neonate. J Pediatr 94:472, 1979.

DeLeze G, Paumgartner G, Karlaganis G, et al: Bile acid pattern in human amniotic fluid. Eur J Clin Invest 8:41, 1978.

DiLorenzo C, Flores AF, Hyman PE: Age-related changes in colon motility. J Pediatr 127:593, 1995.

DeVille K, Baker JH, Al-Tawil Y, et al: Motor responses and gastric emptying in preterm infants fed formula with varying concentrations and rates of infusion. Am J Clin Nutr; 68:103, 1998.

Edelstone DI, Holzman IR: Fetal intestinal oxygen consumption at various levels of oxygenation. Am J Physiol 242:H50, 1983.

Ehrenkranz RA, Ackerman BA, Nelli CM, et al: Absorption of calcium in premature infants as measured with a stable isotope $^{46}$Ca extrinsic tag. Pediatr Res 19:178, 1985.

Ehrenkranz RA, Gettner PA, Nelli CM: Nutrient balance studies in premature infants fed premature formula or fortified preterm human milk. J Pediatr Gastroenterol Nutr 8:58, 1989.

Fekete E, Bendeczky I, Timmermans JP, et al: Sequential pattern of nerve-muscle contacts in the small intestine of developing human fetus. An ultrastructural and immunohistochemical study. Histol Histopath 11:845, 1996.

Fekete E, Resch BA, Benedeczky I: Histochemical and ultrastructural features of the developing enteric nervous system of the human foetal small intestine. Histol Histopathol 10:127, 1995.

Foman SJ, Ziegler EE, Thomas LN, et al: Excretion of fat by normal full-term infants fed various milks and formulas. Am J Clin Nutr 23:1299, 1970.

Gewolb IH, Vice FL, Schwietzer-Kenney EL, et al: Devlopmental patterns of rhythmic suck and swallow of preterm infants. Dev Med Child Neurol 43:22, 2001.

Gibson GR, Beatty ER, Want X, Cummings JH: Selective stimulation of bifidobacteria in the human colon by oligofructose and inulin. Gastroenterol 108:975, 1995.

Gootman P, Gootman N, Buchley B: Maturation of central autonomic control of the circulation. Fed Proc 42:1648, 1983.

Gupta P, Andrao H, Kirschner BS, Guandalini S: Is Lactobacillus GG helpful in children with Crohn's disease? Results of a preliminary open-label study. J Pediatr Gastroenterol Nutr 31:453, 2000.

Hamosh M: Lingual and breast milk lipases. Adv Pediatr 29:33, 1982.

Harmsen HJ, Wildeboer-Veloo: Analysis of intestinal flora development in breast fed and formula fed infants by molecular identification methods. J Pediatr Gastoenterol Nutr 30:61, 2000.

Hanna FM, Navarete DH, Hsu FA: Calcium–fatty acid absorption in term infants fed human milk and prepared formulas simulating human milk. Pediatrics 45:216, 1970.

He Y, Sanderson IR, Walker WA: Uptake, transport, and metabolism of exogenous nucleosides in intestinal epithelial cell cultures. J Nutr 124:1942, 1994.

Herbst JJ: Development of suck and swallow. J Pediatr Gastroenterol Nutr 2:S131, 1983.

Heubi JE, Balistreri WF: Bile salt metabolism in infants and children after protracted diarrhea. Pediatr Res 14:943, 1980.

Heubi JE, Fondacaro JD, Balistreri WF: Bile salt absorption in neonates. J Pediatr 95:1085, 1979.

Higashi A, Ikeda T, Iribe K, Matsuda I: Zinc balance in premature infants given the minimal dietary zinc requirement. J Pediatr 112:262, 1988.

Hoeker C, Nelle M, Roeschl J, et al: Caffeine impairs cerebral and intestinal blood flow velocity in preterm infants Pediatric 109:784, 2002.

Holle GE, Forth W: Myoelectric activity of small intestine after chemical ablation of myenteric neurons. Am J Physiol 258:G519, 1990.

Holzman IR, Tabata B, Edelstone DI: Effects of varying hematocrit on intestinal oxygen uptake in neonatal lambs. Am J Physiol 248:G432, 1985.

Hoyos AB: Reduced incidence of necrotizing enterocolitis associated with enteral administration of *Lactobacillus acidophilus* and *Bifidobacterium infantis* to neonates in an intensive care unit. Int J Inf Dis 3:197, 1999.

Hutchens TW, Henry JF, Yip TT, et al: Origin of intact lactoferrin and its DNA-binding fragments found in the urine of human milk fed preterm infants: Evaluation by stable isotope enrichment. Pediatr Res 29:243, 1991.

Hyman PE, Feldman EJ, Ament ME, et al: Effect of enteral feeding on the maintenance of gastric acid secretory function. Gastroenterol 84:341, 1983.

Ittman PI, Amarnath R, Berseth CL: Maturation of antroduodenal motor activity in preterm and term infants. Dig Dis Sci 37:14, 1992.

Jadcherla SR, Klee G, Berseth CL: Regulation of migrating motor complexes by motilin and pancreatic polypeptide in human neonates. Pediatr Res 96:331, 1995.

Jirsova V, Koldovsky O, Herrgova A, et al: The development of the functions of the small intestine of the human fetus. Biol Neonate 9:44, 1996

Katz L, Hamilton JR: Fat absorption in infants of birthweight less than 1300 gm. J Pediatr 90:431, 1977.

Kerzner B, Sloan HR, Haase GL, et al: The jejunal absorption of glucose oligomers in the absence of pancreatic enzymes. Pediatr Res 15:250, 1981.

Koo WWK, Tsang RC: Calcium, magnesium and phosphorus in nutrition during infancy. In Tsang RC, Nichols BS (eds): Nutrition During Infancy. Philadelphia, Hanley & Belfus, 1988, p 175.

Lacroix B, Kedinger M, Simon-Assman P, Haffen K: Early organogenesis of human small intestine: Scanning electron microscopy and brush border enzymology. Gut 25:925, 1984.

Lane AJ, Coombs RC, Eveans DH, Levin RJ: Effect of caffeine on neonatal splanchnic blood flow. Arch Dis Child Fetal Neonatal Ed 80:F128, 1999.

Langhendries JP, Detry J,VanHees J, et al: Effect of a fermented infant formula containing viable bifidobacteria on the fecal flora composition and pH of healthy full term infants. J Pediatr Gastroenterol Nutr 21:177, 1995.

Lau C, Alagugurusamy R, Schanler RJ, et al: Characterization of the developmental stages of sucking in preterm infants during bottle feeding. Acta Paediatr 89:846, 2000.

Lebenthal E, Lee PC: Development of functional responses in human exocrine pancreas. Pediatrics 66:556, 1980.

Levin RJ, Koldovsky O, Hoskova V, Uher J: Electrical activity across human fetal small intestine associated with absorption processes. Gut 9:206, 1968.

Lichtenberger LM, Johnson LR: Gastrin in the ontogenic development of the small intestine. Am J Physiol 227:390, 1974.

Lucas A, Bloom SR, Aynsley-Green A: Development of gut hormone responses to feeding in neonates. Arch Dis Child 55:678, 1980.

Lucas A, Bloom SR, Aynsley-Green A: Postnatal surges in plasma gut hormones in term and preterm infants. Biol Neonate 41:63, 1982.

MacLean WC, Fink BB: Lactase malabsorption by premature infants: Magnitude and clinical significance. J Pediatr 97:383, 1980.

Malo C: Kinetic evidence for heterogeneity in $Na^+$-D-glucose co-transport systems in the normal human fetal small intestine. Biochem Biophys Acta 938:181, 1988.

Martinussen M, Brubakk AM, Vik T, Yao AC: Mesenteric blood flow velocity and its relation to transitional circulatory adaptation in appropriate for gestational age preterm infants. Pediatr Res 39:275, 1996.

McLain CR Jr: Amniography studies of the gastrointestinal motility of the human fetus. Am J Obstet Gynecol 86:1079, 1963.

Meetze WH, Palazzolo VL, Bowling D, et al: Meconium passage in very-low-birth-weight infants. JPEN J Parenter Enteral Nutr 17:537, 1993.

Ménard D, Pothier P: Differential distribution of digestive enzymes in isolated epithelial cells from developing human fetal small intestine and colon. J Pediatr Gastroenterol Nutr 6:509, 1987.

Millar MR: Enteral feeding of premature infants with Lactobacillus GG. Arch Dis Child 69:483, 1993.

Motil KJ: Development of the gastrointestinal tract. In Wyllie R, Hyanes JS (eds): Pediatric Gastrointestinal Disease. Philadelphia, WB Saunders, 1993.

Nakagawa M, Setchell KDR: Bile acid metabolism in early life: Studies of amniotic fluid. J Lipid Res 31:1089, 1990.

Nankervis CA, Nowicki PT: Role of endothelin-1 in regulation of the postnatal intestinal circulation. Am J Physiol 278:G367, 2000.

Nankervis CA, Nowicki PT: Role of nitric oxide in regulation of vascular resistance in postnatal intestine. Am J Physiol 268: G949, 1995.

Nanthakumar NN, Fusunyan RD, Sanderson I, Walker WA: Inflammation in the developing human intestine: A possible pathophysiologic contribution to necrotizing enterocolitis. Proc Natl Acad Sci U S A 97:6043, 2000.

Neu J: Glutamine deprivation: Effect on the small intestinal barrier. FASEB J 15:A294, 2001.

Neu J, Roig JC, Meetze WH, et al: Enteral glutamine supplementation for very low birth weight infants decreases morbidity. J Pediatr 131:691, 1997.

Newell SJ, Sarkar PK, Durbin GM, et al: Maturation of the lower esophageal sphincter in the preterm baby. Gut 29:167, 1988.

Nowicki PT, Miller CE, Haun SE: Effects of arterial hypoxia and isoproterenol on in vitro postnatal intestinal circulation. Am J Physiol 255:H1144, 1988

Nowicki P, Miller C, Hayes J: Effect of sustained mesenteric nerve stimulation on intrinsic vascular oxygenation in developing swine. Am J Physiol 260:G333, 1991.

Oberhelman RA, Gilman RH, Sheen P, et al: A placebo-controlled trial of Lactobacillus GG to prevent diarrhea in undernourished Peruvian children. J Pediatr 134:15, 1999.

Omari TI, Miki K, Freaser R, et al: Esophageal body and lower esophageal sphincter function in healthy premature infants. Gastroenterol 109:1757, 1995.

Ozaki CK, Chu SW, Walker WA: Developmental changes in galactosyltransferase in the rat small intestine. Biochem Biophys Acta 991:243, 1989.

Pahwa A, Mathur BN: Assesssment of a bifidus-containing infant formula. Part II. Implantation of *Bifidobacterium bifidum*. Indian J Dairy Sci 40:364, 1987.

Pickering LK, Granoff DM, Eridkson JR, et al: Modulation of the immune system by human milk and infant formula containing nucleotides. Pediatrics 101:242, 1998.

Raul F, Lacroix B, Aprahamian M: Longitudinal distribution of brush border hydrolases and morphological maturation in the intestine of the preterm infant. Early Hum Dev 13:225, 1986.

Reber KM, Mager GM, Miller CE, et al: Relationship between flow rate and NO production in postnatal mesenteric arteries. Am J Physiol 280:G43, 2000.

Reber KM, Nankervis CA, Nowicki PT: Newborn intestinal circulation: Physiology and pathophysiology. Clin Perinatol 29:23, 2002.

Reuman PD, Duckworth DH, Smith KL, et al: Lack of effect of *Lactobacillus* on gastrointestinal bacterial colonization in premature infants. Pediatr Infect Dis 5:663, 1986.

Rieger CHL, Rothberg RM: Development of the capacity to produce specific antibody to an ingested food antigen in the premature infant. J Pediatr 87:515, 1985.

Rios E, Hunter RE, Cook J: The absorption of iron as supplements in infant cereal and infant formulas. Pediatrics 55:686, 1975.

Rotimi VO, Duerden BI: The bacterial flora in normal neonates. J Med Microbiol 14:51, 1981.

Roy CC, Ste-Marie M, Chartrand L, et al: Correction of the malabsorption of the preterm infant with a medium chain triglyceride formula. Pediatrics 86:446, 1975.

Ruger CHL, Rothberg RM: Development of the capacity to produce specific antibody to an ingested food antigen in the premature infant. J Pediatr 87:515, 1975.

Schiffrin EJ, Carter EA, Walker WA, et al: Influence of prenatal corticosteroids on bacterial colonization in the newborn rat. J Pediatr Gastroenterol Nutr 17:271, 1993.

Schrank W, Al-Sayed LE, Beahm PH, Thach BT: Feeding responses to free-flow formula in term and preterm infants. J Pediatr 132: 426, 1998.

Schuffler MD, Jonah A: Chronic idiopathic intestinal pseudo-obstruction caused by degenerative disorder of the myenteric plexus: The use of Smith's method to define neuropathy. Gastroenterology 82:476, 1982.

Schultz M, Sartor RB: Probiotics and inflammatory bowel diseases. Am J Gastroenterol 95:19, 2000.

Senterre J, Putet G, Salle B, et al: Effects of vitamin D and phosphorus supplementation on calcium retention in preterm infants fed banked human milk. J Pediatr 103:305, 1983.

Shaw JCL: Evidence of defective skeletal mineralization in low birth weight infants: The absorption of calcium and fat. Pediatrics 57:16, 1976.

Shepherd A, Granger J: Autoregulatory escape in the gut: A systems analysis. Gastroenterology 65:77, 1973.

Shepherd A, Mailman D, Burks T, Granger HJ: Effects of norepinephrine and sympathetic stimulation on extraction of oxygen and $^{86}$Rb in perfused canine small bowel. Circ Res 33:166, 1973.

Siegal M, Krantz B, Lebenthal E: Effect of fat and carbohydrate composition on the gastric emptying of isocaloric feedings in premature infants. Gastroenterology 89:785, 1985.

Simhon A, Douglas JR, Drasar BS, et al: Effect of feeding on infant's fecal flora. Arch Dis Child 57:54, 1982.

Strawczynski H, Beck IT, McKenna RD, et al: The behavior of the lower esophageal sphincter in infants and its relationship to gastroesophageal reflux. J Pediatr 64:17, 1964.

Suchy FJ, Balistreri WF, Heubi JE, et al: Physiologic cholestasis: Elevation of the primary serum bile acid concentrations in normal infants. Gastroenterology 80:1037, 1981.

Tantibhedhyangkal P, Hashim SA: Medium-chain triglyceride feeding in premature infants: Effects on calcium and magnesium absorption. Pediatrics 61:537, 1978.

Triadoru N, Zweibaum A: Maturation of sucrase-isomaltase complex in human fetal small and large intestine during gestation. Pediatr Res 19:136, 1985.

Vanderhoof JA, Whitney DB, Antonson DL, et al: *Lactobacillus* GG in the prevention of antibiotic-associated diarrhea in children. J Pediatr 135:564, 1999.

Villa M, Ménard D, Semenza G, Mantei N: Expression of the lactase enzymatic activity and mRNA in human fetal jejunum. FEBS Lett 301:202, 1992.

Voyer M, Davikis M, Artener I, et al: Zinc balances in preterm infants. Biol Neonate 42:87, 1982.

Walker WA: Antigen handling by the gut. Arch Dis Child 53:527, 1978.

Wang PA, Huang FY: Time of first defaecation and urination in very low birth weight infants. Eur J Pediatr 153:279, 1994.

Watkins JB, Szczepanik P, Gould JB, et al: Bile metabolism in the premature infant: Preliminary observations of pool size and synthesis rate following prenatal administration of dexamethasone and phenobarbital. Gastroenterology 69:706, 1975.

Weiss MD, DeMarco V, Strauss DM, et al: Glutamine synthetase: a key enzyme for intestinal epithelial differentiation. JPEN J Parenteral Enteral Nutr 23:140, 1999.

Wester T, O'Brian DS, Puri P: Notable postnatal alterations in the myenteric plexus of normal human bowel. Gut 44:666, 1999.

Worniak ER, Fenton TR, Milla PJ: The development of fasting small intestinal motility in human neonates. In Roman C (ed): Gastrointestinal Motility. London, Lancaster Press, 1983, p 265.

Young HM: Embryological origins of interstitial cells of Cajal. Microsc Res Tech 47:303, 1999.

Younoszai MK, Sapario RS, Laughlin M, et al: Maturation of jejunum and ileum in rats: Water and electrolyte transport during in vivo perfusion of hypertonic solutions. J Clin Invest 62:271, 1978.

Zamora SA, Amin HJ, McMillan DD, et al: Plasma L-arginine concentrations in premature infants with necrotizing enterocolitis. J Pediatr 131:226, 1997.

Zangen S, DiLorenzo C, Zangen T, et al: Rapid maturation of gastric relaxation in newborn infants. Pediatr Res 50:629, 2001.

Zhang J, Penny DJ, Kim NS, et al: Mechanisms of blood pressure increase induced by dopamine in hypotensive preterm infants. Arch Dis Child Fetal Neonatal Ed 81:F99, 1999.

Zoppi G, Andreotti G, Pajno-Ferrara F, et al: Exocrine pancreas function in premature and term infants. Pediatr Res 6:880, 1972.

CHAPTER 71

# Structural Anomalies of the Gastrointestinal Tract

**Carol Lynn Berseth and Dan Poenaru**

## DISORDERS OF THE TEETH, MOUTH, AND NECK

### Teeth

Infants may be born with one or more erupted teeth. These natal teeth should be extracted because their roots are poorly formed and they present a danger of aspiration when they loosen.

### Mouth

Tiny cystic lesions may be visible in the mouths of 80% of newborns. Those located on the hard palate on either side of the raphe are called *Epstein pearls*, and those located on the mandibular and maxillary alveolar ridges are called *Bohn nodules*. A *ranula* is a retention cyst of the sublingual salivary gland that presents as a pea-sized mass on the anterior floor of the mouth. Most cysts disappear within 1 month, but larger ones that interfere with feeding may require surgical excision.

Tumors of the mouth are rare in the newborn; however, when they are present, careful evaluation with computed tomgraphy (CT) is necessary to define the anatomy and to determine if a connection with the central nervous system is present. An *epignathus* is any type of growth that arises from the upper jaw or palate and projects from the mouth. Although most of these tumors are polyps, dermoids, or teratomas, they often cause respiratory or feeding difficulty. The definitive treatment is surgical removal.

*Congenital epulis* is a misnamed tumor that arises from the upper or lower jaw and projects into the mouth so that normal sucking is impaired. These tumors are covered with squamous epithelium and contain vascular connective tissue, large polyhedral round cells, and spindle-shaped cells (Langley and Davson, 1950), and they are considered to be benign. Histochemical staining of these tumors demonstrates that these tumor cells represent early mesodermal cells that express pericytic and myofibroblastic features (Damm et al, 1993).

Salivary gland lesions are rare in the newborn. Tumors or infection of the salivary gland (sialadenitis) may arise anywhere salivary gland tissue is present, including the floor of the mouth and the parotid regions. Hemangiomas are the most common tumors found in this region, and lymphangiomas are the second most common (Welch and Trump, 1979). Both of these benign lesions typically are confined to the intracapsular portion of the gland, although surface sentinel lesions may be present. Management consists of confirmation of a histologic diagnosis via open biopsy and long-term observation of the lesion. Juxtaparotid lymphangiomas that invade the gland should be locally excised. Suppurative parotitis may present during the first month of life and may involve one or both parotid glands. Pus may be expressed from the Stensen duct by putting gentle pressure on the gland. The infant may become septic; extension to the submaxillary gland is not uncommon. The offending organism is usually *Staphylococcus aureus* or *Escherichia coli*, but broad-spectrum antibiotic coverage is necessary until the organism has been identified and sensitivities have been established.

### Tongue

Aglossia congenita, or congenital absence of the tongue, has been described. Taste sensation is present, and these children can learn to speak. Ankyloglossia inferior ("tongue-tie") is common in newborns. The frenulum of the newborn is normally short, but this does not usually interfere with sucking and swallowing. Because the frenulum lengthens with postnatal age, it should not be cut unless inadequate bottle- or breast-feeding persists.

Ankyloglossia superior, attachment of the tongue to the roof of the mouth, is a rare anomaly that must be recognized at birth because respiratory obstruction may occur. Other lesions, such as micrognathia, macroglossia, and cleft palate, are frequently associated with this anomaly (Spivack and Bennett, 1968).

True macroglossia, or enlargement of the tongue, results in continuous protrusion of the tongue from the mouth, making feeding difficult and respiration noisy. Macroglossia often is present in infants who have Down syndrome or Beckwith-Wiedemann syndrome. Lymphangioma and idiopathic muscular hypertrophy are additional common causes of macroglossia. Characteristically, the gross appearance of a lymphangioma is that of a raised, firm mass in the tongue, which has a warty-looking surface. The treatment for lymphangioma is surgical removal, if possible, or reduction of the tumor bulk with reshaping of the tongue. Infants with idiopathic muscular hypertrophy should be treated conservatively because the relative size of the tongue often becomes smaller as the mandible grows postnatally.

Thyroid tissue may persist as a solid or cystic mass in the posterior midline of the tongue or under it. Because the presence of this mass represents a failure of migration of normal thyroid tissue, no other thyroid tissue may exist. A thyroid scan should be performed during evaluation of midline lingual tumors.

### Nasopharynx

Nasopharyngeal tumors are rare and are polyps, dermoids, or teratomas. Often these lesions are on a stalk and project into the mouth. Those not projecting externally may be palpated as movable, sausage-shaped masses in the pharynx. These lesions should be removed urgently because acute respiratory distress may occur if the nasopharynx is obstructed.

## Neck

Cystic hygroma is the most common lateral neck mass in the newborn (Fig. 71–1). Derived from lymphatic tissue, these multilobular, multicystic masses may rapidly enlarge and cause respiratory compromise. Magnetic resonance imaging (MRI) is useful in identifying their extent and ruling out intrathoracic extension. Excision is the treatment of choice, with sclerotherapy reserved for very large or recurrent tumors (Samuel et al, 2000). Prenatally diagnosed giant lymphangiomas impairing the airway may require removal using an "ex utero intrapartum technique" (the EXIT procedure) (Mychaliska et al, 1997).

Branchial cleft anomalies may manifest as skin tags, pits, sinuses, fistulas, or cysts in the preauricular and lateral cervical regions. Most are remnants of the second branchial cleft and pouch, and 10% to 15% occur bilaterally (Bill and Vadheim, 1955). Sinuses and fistulas may be discovered during the newborn period, but cysts require time to fill and usually are not recognized until childhood. Ultrasound or CT scan of the neck may be useful to define anatomic relationships, and surgical removal is the treatment of choice.

The so-called "sternomastoid tumor" can be seen and palpated within the body of the sternocleidomastoid muscle as a hard, smooth oval mass. Histopathologic study reveals that these lesions result from endomysial fibrosis and deposition of collagen and fibroblasts around individual muscle fibers that subsequently undergo atrophy. The cause is unknown, but the incidence is seven times higher following breech delivery (Ling and Low, 1973) and among infants who have had specific fetal positioning in utero (Rosegger and Steinwendner, 1992). Torticollis is not always present; instead, there may be rotation of the head to the side opposite the tumor. Cranial and facial asymmetry may also occur. In most infants, the lesion resolves within 6 to 12 months. Surgical correction is rarely indicated, in cases when severe hemihypoplasia develops (Wirth et al, 1992).

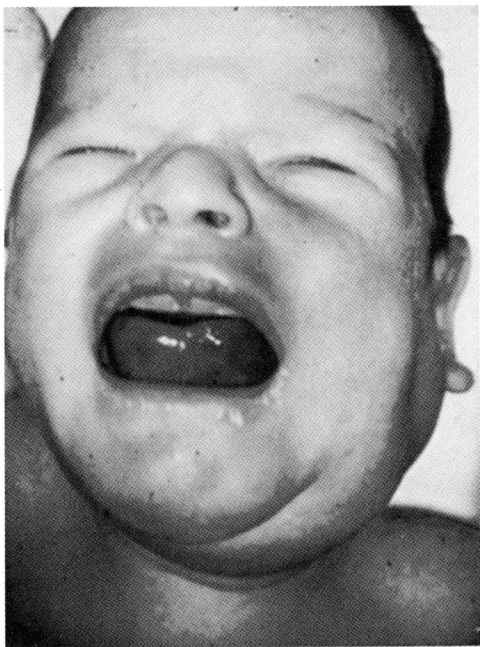

**FIGURE 71–1.** Hygroma of the neck and tongue.

Midline neck masses in newborns include cystic hygromas, hemangiomas, dermoid cysts, teratomas, goiter, ectopic thyroid tissue, and ectopic thymic tissue (Fig. 71–2). Goiters may be visible at birth and may be associated with hypothyroidism, hyperthyroidism, or euthyroidism. The second most common location for ectopic thyroid tissue is the anterior midline of the neck, just at or below the hyoid bone (Meyerowitz and Buchholz, 1969). Although this tissue may be easily mistaken for a thyroglossal duct cyst, such cysts are rarely present in the newborn. Before removal of ectopic thyroid tissue, it must be determined if this tissue is the infant's only functioning thyroid tissue.

Thymic tissue arises high in the cervical region of the embryo as two lateral buds. The buds migrate caudad and join in the anterior mediastinum. Abnormal migration results in ectopic location or cyst formation (or both); the aberrant tissue or cyst may manifest as a lateral or midline neck mass (Thompson and Love, 1972) and requires surgical removal.

# DISORDERS OF THE ESOPHAGUS

## Esophageal Atresia with Tracheoesophageal Fistula

### Definition

Esophageal atresia and tracheoesophageal fistula may occur as separate congenital defects, but more frequently they are seen together as a compound defect (Fig. 71–3). Esophageal atresia with distal tracheoesophageal fistula is by far the most common form, accounting for 85% of the cases.

### Epidemiology

The incidence of esophageal atresia with tracheoesophageal fistula (EA/TEF) ranges from 1/3000 to 1/4000 live births (Meyers, 1974; Raffensperger, 1990). Most series show a slight male predominance and an increased incidence in premature infants (Reckham, 1981). The role genetic factors play is unclear; however, this anomaly has been described in siblings as well as in identical twins (Hausmann et al, 1957; Woolley et al, 1961). In addition, two kindreds with autosomal dominant transmission have been reported (Pletcher et al, 1991).

### Etiology

The anomaly occurs before the eighth week of gestation, but the exact mechanism is unknown. The foregut divides into a ventral and a dorsal tube when the lateral walls invaginate, giving rise to the trachea and esophagus. When this process of division is abnormal or when there is compression of these primitive tubes by an extrinsic structure such as an anomalous blood vessel, esophageal atresia or tracheoesophageal fistula (or both) may result. Additional anomalies occur in a majority of these infants, as outlined later in the "Treatment" section.

### Diagnosis

Polyhydramnios is present in approximately one third of pregnant women carrying fetuses with esophageal atresia because the fetus is unable to swallow amniotic fluid.

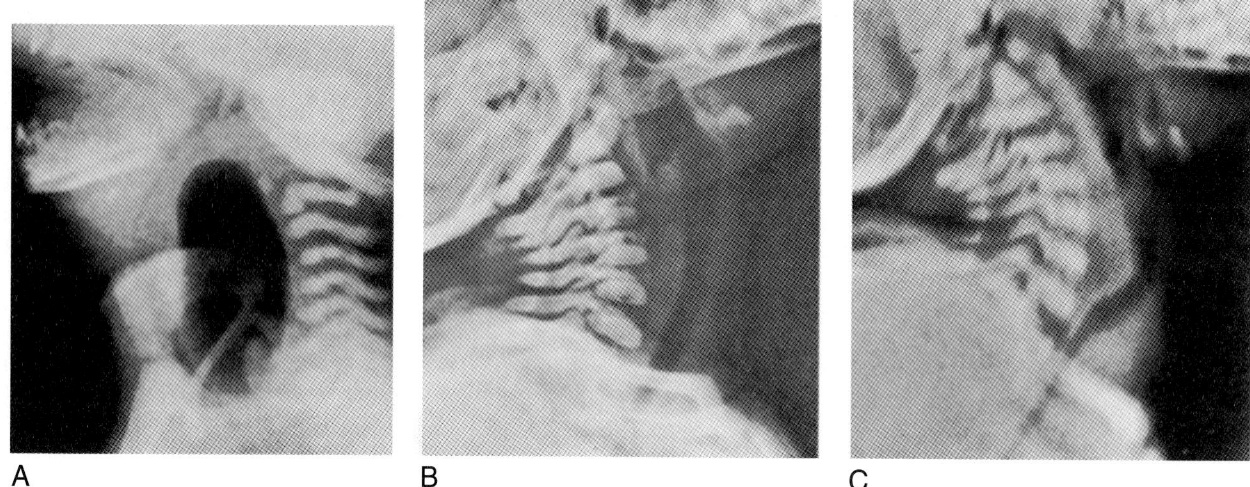


**FIGURE 71–2.** **A,** Lateral radiograph of the neck shows an air-containing cyst displacing the air passages and esophagus forward. **B,** Lateral view of the neck obtained with patient quiet demonstrates straight, unobstructed tracheal air column. **C,** Lateral view of the neck obtained with patient crying demonstrates mass lesion between the manubrium and the trachea, displacing the lower cervical trachea backward and moderately narrowing this portion of the trachea. *(From Thompson RE, Love WG: Persistent cervical thymoma apparent with crying. Am J Dis Child 124:761, 1972. Copyright 1972, American Medical Association.)*

Within hours after birth, these infants accumulate large amounts of oral secretions, which may precipitate coughing, choking, and respiratory distress. The infants vomit when they are fed, and in cases with a distal tracheoesophageal connection, abdominal distention may ensue as the intestine fills with air. The presence of a flat or gasless abdomen should suggest an isolated esophageal atresia without tracheoesophageal fistula (see Fig. 71–3B). Some patients with a gasless abdomen, however, may have a tracheoesophageal fistula that is partially obliterated and still requires surgical ligation (Goh et al, 1991). The most dramatic presentation of tracheoesophageal fistula occurs when the fistula is proximal to the esophageal atresia (see Fig. 71–3D, E, G). These infants develop life-threatening respiratory failure from aspiration almost immediately after birth.

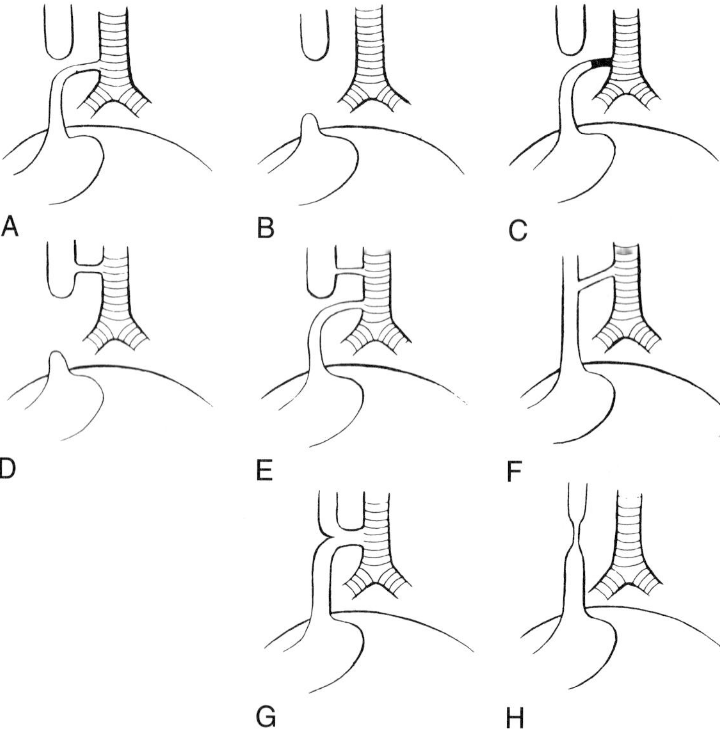


**FIGURE 71–3.** Types of tracheosophageal fistulas. **A** is overwhelmingly the most common, accounting for 85% of esophageal malformations. **B** is next most common and can be distinguished from **A** by the absence of air in the intestinal tract on radiograph. All the other types have been noted sporadically. *(From Avery ME, et al: The Lung and Its Disorders in the Newborn Infant, 4th ed. Philadelphia, WB Saunders, 1981.)*

Infants with the so-called H-type tracheoesophageal fistula (see Fig. 71–3F) usually do not develop symptoms in the newborn period. Instead, these infants frequently present with a history (over months to years) of mild respiratory distress related to feeding or recurrent pneumonias.

If a diagnosis of esophageal atresia is suspected, a soft 5 or 8 French feeding tube can be passed into the esophagus until it meets an obstruction. On occasion, the tube coils in a blind pouch, creating the false impression that the esophagus is patent. A plain film confirms the position of the tube and frequently demonstrates the presence of an air-filled upper esophageal pouch (Fig. 71–4). The presence of gas in the abdomen suggests that a distal tracheoesophageal fistula is present.

### Treatment

Preoperative care of the infant with esophageal atresia includes the insertion of a sump suction catheter into the proximal esophageal pouch for the continuous evacuation of secretions. The infant also should be placed in the upright position to decrease the reflux of gastric secretions through the fistula and into the lungs. Hydration is maintained by intravenous fluids, and surgical repair is undertaken when the infant's general condition permits. Thus, surgical repair in preterm infants may be delayed postnatally until the patient is clinically stable enough for surgery.

The preoperative pulmonary complications associated with EA/TEF occur because of aspiration of oral contents or reflux of gastric contents into the airway. Placing a Replogle tube with continuous suction into the proximal esophageal pouch can minimize the aspiration of saliva. Elevating the infant's head and minimizing any positive pressure ventilation can minimize reflux of gastric contents. If gastric distention, with reflux, becomes an important problem in the sick, small infant, a decompressive gastrostomy can be performed with local anesthesia at the bedside (Holder, 1993). If the fistula is large, there may be a significant loss of tidal volume if the infant requires positive pressure ventilation. This volume loss can usually be controlled by connecting the gastrostomy to a chest tube system under water seal (Fann et al, 1988). In extreme cases in which the infant may not tolerate a thoracotomy and definitive procedure, a Fogarty catheter can be passed with a bronchoscope to occlude the fistula (Filston et al, 1982).

Preoperative evaluation should include a search for additional anomalies, as they occur in 50% to 70% of patients with EA/TEF (Holder, 1993; Rowe et al, 1995; Rejjal, 1999). The VACTERL association is present in 25% to 30% of children with EA/TEF (Rowe et al, 1995). The VACTERL association, previously referred to as the VATER syndrome, consists of *v*ertebral anomalies, *a*nal agenesis (imperforate anus) (Figs. 71–5 and 71–6), *c*ardiac defects (most commonly patent ductus arteriosus, atrial septal defect, and ventricular septal defect), *t*racheo*e*sophageal fistula, *r*enal anomalies, and *l*imb anomalies (most often radial anomalies) (Corsello et al, 1993; Manning et al, 1986; Quan and Smith, 1973). Infants with EA/TEF and the VACTERL association tend to have higher proximal pouches, more complications, and a higher mortality rate than those in infants with isolated EA/TEF (Fig. 71–7) (Greenwood and Rosenthal, 1976; Holder, 1993; Touloukian and Keller, 1988; Weber et al, 1980). Cardiac defects often are repaired before the EA/TEF (Spitz, 1993). Gastrointestinal anomalies occur in 15% of patients (Rowe et al, 1995). Anal atresia is the most common gastrointestinal anomaly seen and requires a diverting colostomy at the time of the first general anesthetic procedure (Holder, 1993). Duodenal atresia also may occur (Holder, 1993).

The operative strategy is based on the anatomy and the presence of associated anomalies. Although it is preferable to correct the anomaly at the first anesthetic, staged procedures may be used in small infants (Alexander et al, 1993). In general, the infant who lacks significant associated anomalies and has a reasonably stable pulmonary status should undergo primary repair of the atresia and ligation of the fistula. To accomplish this, an extrapleural

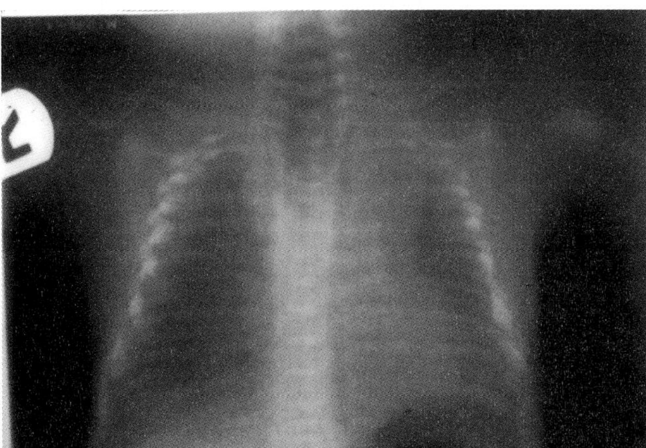

**FIGURE 71–4.** Anteroposterior view of the chest of a female infant with esophageal atresia and tracheoesophageal fistula. A large upper pouch is outlined by air and by a curled nasogastric tube. Air is seen within the abdomen.

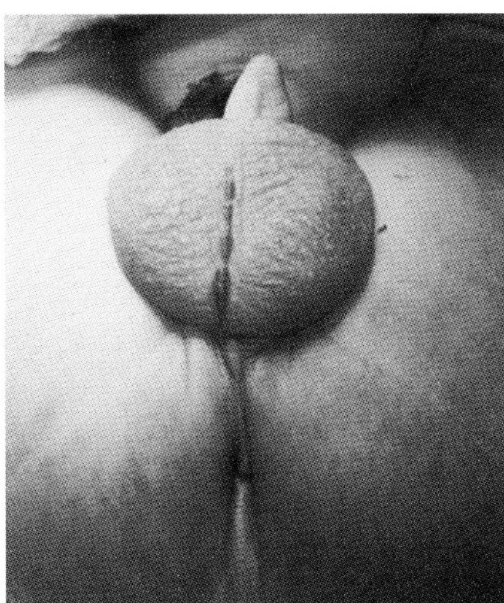

**FIGURE 71–5.** (See also Color Plate 71–5.) Perineum of male newborn with low imperforate anus and anocutaneous fistula. The fistula is seen as a dark meconium-filled track along the median raphe of the scrotum.

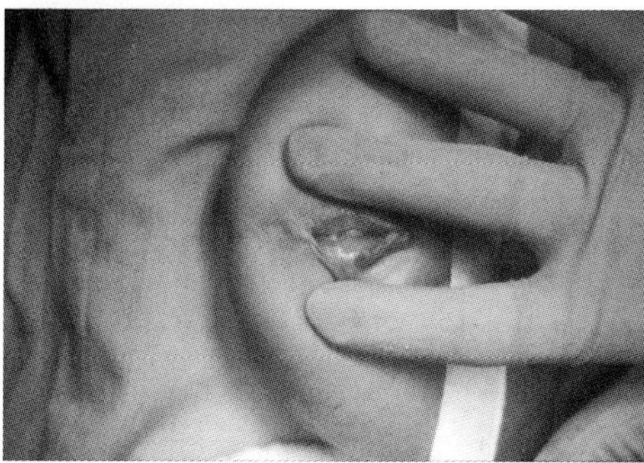

**FIGURE 71–6.** (See also Color Plate 71–6.) Perineum of female newborn with low imperforate anus and rectovestibular fistula. The fistula is evident as the meconium-stained site within the posterior vestibule.

or transpleural approach is used, the fistula is divided, and an anastomosis between the proximal and distal esophageal segments is achieved using an end-to-end anastomosis. Infants with the lowest probability of survival are likely to benefit from a staged approach. For infants with extreme pulmonary compromise or significant associated anomalies, an initial gastrostomy for decompression with later repair of the EA/TEF may be indicated.

Postoperative care consists of respiratory support, antibiotics, and intravenous nutritional support. Enteral feedings via a gastrostomy or a transpyloric tube may be started on the third or fourth postoperative day. These feedings initially are given by continuous infusion. Bolus feedings usually are introduced once full enteral alimentation is achieved, and oral feedings are started 7 to 10 days postoperatively after confirmation by radiographic contrast study that there are no esophageal anastomotic leaks. A recent study has questioned whether contrast studies are necessary for infants who remain free of clinical symptoms of postoperative complications (Yancher et al, 2001).

Five significant complications can occur after repair of EA/TEF: esophageal anastomotic leak, esophageal stricture, gastroesophageal reflux, recurrent fistula, and tracheal obstruction. The incidence of anastomotic leak is around 10% to 15% (Rowe et al, 1995). The diagnosis usually is made by noting the presence of saliva in the chest tube and is confirmed by a contrast swallow study (Rowe et al, 1995). The treatment is expectant, because most of these leaks close spontaneously (Rowe et al, 1995). A minor esophageal stricture is almost universal after repair of an EA/TEF. Significant strictures occur in 5% to 10% of infants (Rowe et al, 1995). The diagnosis is confirmed by barium swallow examination. Treatment is with esophageal dilatation, either with Jackson dilators or by balloon dilatation (Benjamin et al, 1993; Shah and Berman, 1993). Gastroesophageal reflux occurs in 40% to 70% of these children (Holder, 1993; Pieretii et al, 1974). Clinically significant tracheal obstruction may occur in as many as 25% of children with EA/TEF as a consequence of tracheomalacia (Corbally et al, 1993; Rowe et al, 1995). The onset of symptoms (cyanosis, bradycardia, and apnea, usually with or immediately after feeding) usually is in the months following repair of EA/TEF but may be in the immediate postoperative period (Holder, 1993). The diagnosis of tracheal obstruction due to tracheomalacia is made by bronchoscopy (Holder, 1993). In the child without significant distress, most symptoms subside over the first year or two of life (Holder, 1993). The surgical treatment of severe tracheomalacia is aortopexy, or suspension of the aorta (and therefore the anterior trachea) to the posterior surface of the sternum (Corbally et al, 1993; Holder, 1993). The incidence of recurrent fistula is probably less than 10% (Rowe et al, 1995). The tracheoesophageal fistula probably recurs in the immediate postoperative period, but the diagnosis may not be made for months or years. The manifestations of a recurrent fistula are the same as those of gastroesophageal reflux: aspiration, coughing with feeds, and recurrent pulmonary infections. Small fistulas may close spontaneously, but if a fistula persists for longer than 4 weeks, surgical closure is indicated (Rowe et al, 1995). Most surgeons prefer to wait 3 to 6 months after the initial EA/TEF repair, if possible, to decrease inflammation and edema (Holder, 1993).

### Prognosis

The overall survival rate in term infants without respiratory complications preoperatively approaches 95% (Holder and Ashcraft, 1970). Among premature infants or those with moderate to severe respiratory disease, survival is 85%. Infants with multiple anomalies or those with severe respiratory disease have a 75% survival rate.

Virtually all infants with esophageal atresia have residual problems with strictures and abnormal esophageal motility and swallowing. Esophageal strictures at the anastomotic site should be suspected if feeding difficulty develops, particularly after the third week. Repeated dilation may be necessary to relieve the stricture.

Gastroesophageal reflux occurs in up to 70% of patients after tracheoesophageal fistula repair (Roberts et al, 1980), owing to lower esophageal sphincter incompetence or abnormal motility in the body of the esophagus (Whitington et al, 1977). Medical therapy may be successful initially, but many patients require antireflux surgery.

## Tracheoesophageal Fistula without Esophageal Atresia

Only 5% of tracheoesophageal fistulas occur in the absence of esophageal atresia. Most of these fistulas are located superior to the second thoracic vertebra and can be repaired via a neck incision. Symptoms include coughing and cyanosis with feeding and recurrent episodes of pneumonia. If the diagnosis of tracheoesophageal fistula is suspected, oral feedings should be withheld and replaced by gavage feedings. A specialized contrast study is required to demonstrate the lesion, using a catheter gradually withdrawn through the esophagus (Fig. 71–8). If this is unsuccessful, simultaneous endoscopic examinations of the trachea and esophagus may be done; the injection of a small amount of methylene blue into the trachea and its subsequent appearance in the esophagus is diagnostic. The treatment involves surgical ligation of the fistula, usually performed through a right cervical approach.

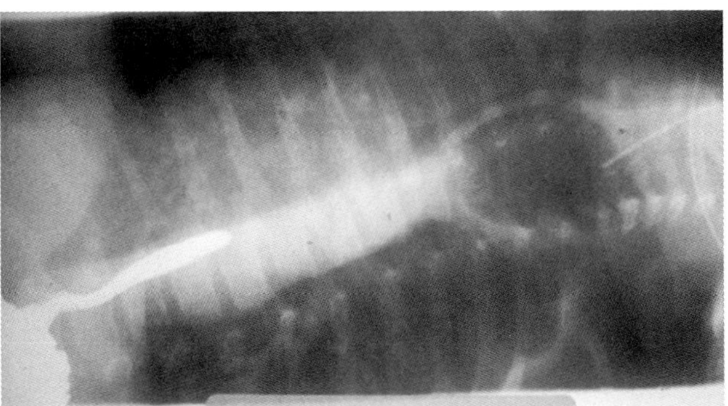

**FIGURE 71–7.** Anteroposterior view of chest of female newborn with isolated esophageal atresia. Air outlines the distended upper pouch; contrast material introduced via a gastrostomy fills the lower esophagus. There is a long gap in the esophagus, extending for more than the length of four vertebral bodies.

## Laryngotracheoesophageal Cleft

Laryngotracheoesophageal cleft is a communication of the larynx and trachea with the esophagus. The defect varies in length, with the shortest being the length of the arytenoid cartilages and the longest extending the entire length of the trachea (Fig. 71–9). These clefts form between the fifth and seventh weeks of gestation when there is a failure of the rostral advance and fusion of the lateral ridges of the laryngotracheal groove. One fifth of the clefts are associated with esophageal atresia and tracheoesophageal fistula. Clinical presentation occurs early in the newborn period and is similar to that for EA/TEF except that stridor also may be present. A carefully done esophageal dye study should establish the diagnosis. Tracheal spillover, however, may be misinterpreted to be due to the presence of a high H-type fistula or the presence of incoordination of the swallowing mechanism. Patients with clefts should undergo bronchoscopic evaluation with immediate surgical repair. A temporary tracheostomy is often placed because breakdown of the closure is common.

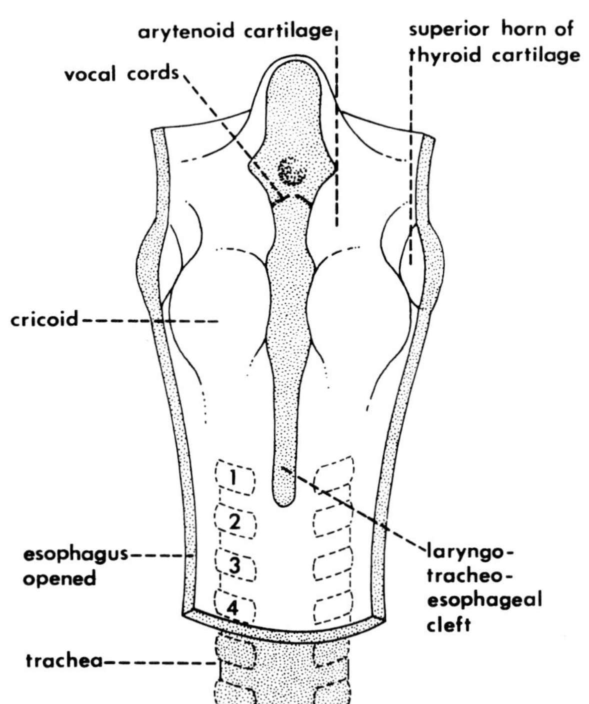


**FIGURE 71–9.** Illustration of the anatomy of a laryngotracheoesophageal cleft. *(From Burroughs N, Leape LL: Laryngotracheoesophageal cleft: Report of a case successfully treated and review of the literature. Pediatrics 53:517, 1974. Reproduced by permission of Pediatrics.)*

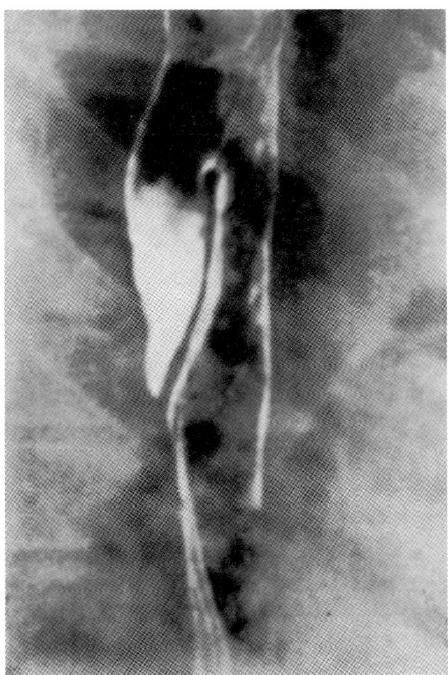

**FIGURE 71–8.** Radiograph after barium swallow, showing diverticulum before operation. The fistula is not demonstrated. *(From Robb D: Aust N Z J Surg 22:120, 1952.)*

## Congenital Esophageal Stenosis

Congenital esophageal stenosis is a very rare anomaly caused by inborn malformation of the esophageal wall musculature (Nihoul-Fekete et al, 1987). It may take the form of a membranous web or diaphragm or a fibromuscular thickening or may be secondary to tracheobronchial remnants in the wall of the esophagus. The last-named is the most common form and typically occurs in the distal esophagus. Most infants so affected are asymptomatic until solids are introduced into the diet; occasionally, the condition may manifest neonatally with severe regurgitation and respiratory distress syndrome. The diagnosis may be difficult to establish, although a contrast esophagogram will usually reveal the narrowing. Fibromuscular hypertrophy and occasionally webs can be treated with repeated dilatations; surgical resection is the treatment of choice for all other lesions. An antireflux procedure is added for distal lesions, and results are generally satisfactory.

## Esophageal Duplication Cysts

Esophageal duplications are very rare, representing 10% to 15% of all gastrointestinal duplications. The current hypothesis invokes formation of vacuoles during the early developmental obliteration of the esophageal lumen. If these vacuoles coalesce during recanalization, duplications are formed. The cysts are usually small and may be located anywhere in the posterior mediastinum or neck. Cysts often manifest asymptomatically during childhood, or with digestive or respiratory signs and symptoms even in the neonatal period (Stewart et al, 1993). Associated vertebral anomalies suggest the presence of a neurenteric cyst, which may have a connection to the spinal canal. Diagnosis is confirmed by CT, and treatment involves surgical excision.

## Cricopharyngeal Dysfunction

Some newborns aspirate at times despite having what appears to be a normal sucking and swallowing mechanism. If the problem is persistent, evaluation with a cineradiographic swallowing study is indicated. Diagnostic considerations include cricopharyngeal achalasia, familial dysautonomia, and myasthenia gravis. Cricopharyngeal achalasia is a rare disorder that may manifest as severe dysphagia in the newborn (Salib et al, 1999). Its treatment consists of a cricopharyngeal myotomy. Linde and Westover (1962) noted that infants with familial dysautonomia may have pharyngeal dysfunction at birth that causes chronic aspiration. In addition, poor esophageal peristalsis delays esophageal emptying.

## Rupture of the Esophagus

Esophageal perforation occurs in premature infants secondary to malpositioned endotracheal tubes as well as stiff nasogastric tubes (Krasna et al, 1987). Several newborns also have been described with spontaneous rupture of the esophagus. Hematemesis, hydropneumothorax, or both may be presenting manifestations. An esophagram can confirm the diagnosis, and urgent surgical repair is necessary.

# DISORDERS OF THE STOMACH

## Gastric Duplication

Gastric duplications are spherical or hollow tubular structures that (1) are lined by a mucosal layer composed of gastric, small bowel, or colonic epithelium; (2) contain a smooth muscle coat contiguous with the muscle of the stomach; and (3) are contiguous with the stomach wall. Most duplications do not communicate with the gastric lumen and are located along the greater curvature. Embryologically the lesion arises during the fourth week of gestation when normally the embryonic notochordal plates and endoderm separate. A band between them may cause a traction diverticulum, leading to gut cyst formation. In addition, associated anomalies occur in 50% of these patients, the most common being esophageal duplication and vertebral abnormalities. Infants may present with nonbilious vomiting or hematemesis (Holcomb et al, 1989). The treatment is complete surgical excision of the cyst.

## Congenital Gastric Outlet Obstruction

This rare condition may be caused by either a membrane or atresia, located in either the antrum or the pylorus. An incomplete web or diaphragm may also be present, causing partial obstruction. Maternal polyhydramnios occurs in half of the cases. The defect may be due to vascular compromise early in gestation, similar to that causing intestinal and colonic atresias. Associated anomalies are frequent, including epidermolysis bullosa (Okoye et al, 2000). The presence of a gasless abdomen on a plain film and the failure of contrast material to leave the stomach on an upper gastrointestinal series are suggestive of the diagnosis and warrant urgent operative intervention. Treatment involves excision of the defect with a pyloroplasty, but some patients may require a gastroduodenostomy.

## Pyloric Stenosis

### Definition and Epidemiology

Idiopathic hypertrophy of the pyloric muscle in early infancy results in partial gastric outlet obstruction. The incidence is 1/1000 to 3/1000 live births, and males are affected four times more often than females. Firstborns account for half of the cases. Whites are at greater risk than blacks (Laron and Horne, 1957). Premature infants are affected with the same frequency as term infants.

### Etiology

The exact cause of pyloric stenosis is unknown. Hereditary factors may play a role because there is a 7% incidence of pyloric stenosis among the siblings of affected patients.

### Diagnosis

Vomiting is the primary presenting symptom. It may occur from birth to 12 weeks, but most often the onset is between the third and the fifth weeks. In premature infants, the onset follows the same pattern postnatally, regardless of the postconceptual age. At first, vomiting may occur infrequently. With time, the frequency and volume of the emesis increase, and projectile vomiting develops. Weight loss, dehydration, and metabolic alkalosis may occur as a consequence of the vomiting. Gastric peristaltic waves may be seen passing obliquely from the left upper quadrant across the midline when the infant is fed. Jaundice may occasionally occur, but indirect hyperbilirubinemia recedes 5 to 10 days after pyloromyotomy. In most instances of pyloric stenosis, a definite tumor, or "olive," can be felt either in the epigastric area or just to the right of the midline in the right upper quadrant. Ultrasound examination is confirmatory, having replaced the upper gastrointestinal series as the diagnoatic modality of choice (Fig. 71–10) (Hallam et al, 1995).

### Treatment

The stomach should be decompressed, and dehydration and metabolic alkalosis should be corrected with intravenous fluids before surgery. Pyloromyotomy involves splitting the hypertrophied pyloric muscle, and may be performed through a periumbilical incision or laparoscopically (Shankar et al, 2000). Feedings may be resumed 6 to 12 hours after surgery and advanced toward a regular schedule.

### Prognosis

Surgery is curative. Complications may include incomplete pyloromyotomy and perforation.

## Pylorospasm

The diagnosis of infantile pylorospasm is made by radiographic or ultrasonographic evaluation, and it must be differentiated from pyloric stenosis (Cohen et al, 1998). Radiographically, infants with pylorospasm show a narrow distal antrum, but in contrast with pyloric stenosis, the caliber of the channels intermittently narrows and widens. Peristalsis is present in the affected area, and there are no features of muscular hypertrophy, as seen with pyloric stenosis. The cause of pylorospasm is unknown. Conservative medical management consisting of atropine sulfate given intravenously before meals may be more successful than metoclopramide in relieving the spasm. Pylorospasm usually is transient and resolves within 1 to 2 weeks.

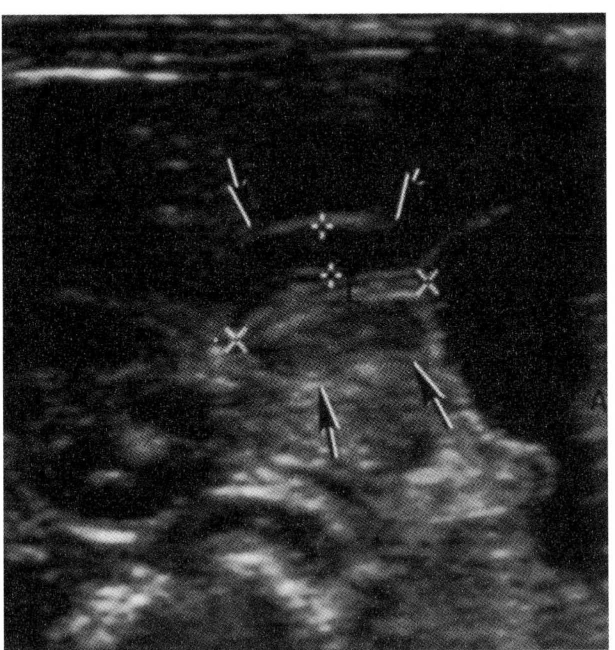

**FIGURE 71–10.** Ultrasonographic study of the right upper quadrant in a 1-month-old infant with a 1-week history of vomiting. The length (from + to +) of the pylorus is 18.4 mm (normal up to 16 mm), and wall thickness (H) is 4.5 mm (normal is up to 4.0 mm). The *arrows* outline the muscular wall and point to the lumen (L). A is the antral lumen. *(Courtesy of Dr. Ronald M. Cohen, Children's Hospital, Oakland, Calif.)*

## Peptic Ulcer Disease

### Definition and Epidemiology

Ulceration of the gastric or duodenal mucosa is rare in the newborn. Peptic ulcers may be classified as primary if they occur in otherwise healthy persons or secondary if they are seen in association with underlying systemic disorders. In the newborn, most ulcers are secondary and are found in the duodenum (Bell et al, 1981).

### Etiology

The cause of peptic ulcer disease is unknown but is probably multifactorial even in patients with secondary ulcers (Byrne, 1985). Genetic factors, emotional factors, dietary and environmental factors, the amount of hydrochloric acid, and local tissue resistance factors contribute to ulcer formation in the older child and adolescent. In the newborn, a breakdown of local tissue resistance plays the major role. Normally the mucosal cell is protected by a complex barrier, which includes gastric mucus, the secretion of bicarbonate by the mucosal cell, the *alkaline tide*, mucosal blood flow, and prostaglandins. Drugs, such as indomethacin, that block prostaglandin synthesis or conditions such as acidosis and shock, affect blood flow and bicarbonate production, which precipitates events that disrupt this barrier and thus permits mucosal cell destruction, inflammation, and ulcer formation to occur.

### Diagnosis

In the newborn, hematemesis, hematochezia, and perforation of the stomach or duodenum are presenting clinical manifestations. At times, the loss of blood may be considerable, causing a rapid drop in the hematocrit and the development of shock. At other times, bleeding may be gradual and recognized only by the presence of "coffee grounds" emesis or a Hemoccult-positive stool. In general, radiographic studies in the newborn are not useful in demonstrating the presence of ulceration or gastritis. Upper gastrointestinal fiberoptic endoscopy can be done in the smallest of infants and is therefore the modality of choice.

### Treatment

Blood loss into the gastrointestinal tract requires prompt and adequate replacement. A nasogastric tube should be passed and the stomach lavaged with room-temperature saline (Andrus and Ponsky, 1987). Antacid therapy and/or therapy with histamine $H_2$ blockers is then begun. If there is no further bleeding after 24 hours, feedings may be resumed. The antacids should be continued at the same dose and given 1 hour after each feeding for 6 to 8 weeks.

## Gastric Perforation

Spontaneous perforation of the stomach in the newborn occurs most often during the first few days of life (Fig. 71–11) (St.Vil et al, 1992). Perinatal stress leading to

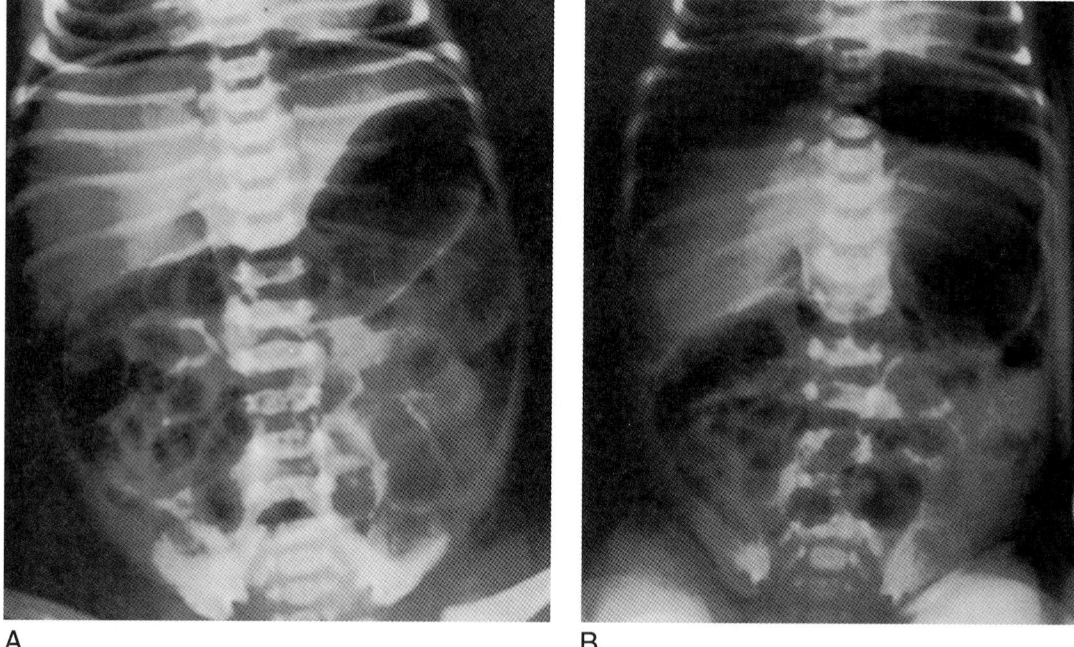


**FIGURE 71–11.** **A,** Anteroposterior view of abdomen obtained with the infant in the erect position at 72 hours of age. Air is present in the stomach and intestine, and there is a distinct impression that some of the air is outside the lumen of the bowel. A layer of air is clearly visible above the liver and below the diaphragm. **B,** Ten hours later. By now, there is a huge accumulation of air between the diaphragm and the liver.

localized ischemia appears to be the causative mechanism in most cases, although in others no cause can be identified. Potential causes include rapid overdistention, trauma from passage of a nasogastric tube, and spontaneous rupture of weak points in the gastric wall along the greater curvature where muscle is deficient.

Signs and symptoms that typically occur by the second to fifth day include refusal to suck, vomiting, and abdominal distention. Plain films of the abdomen show the presence of free air. Immediate decompression, fluid resuscitation, and broad-spectrum antibiotic administration should be followed by immediate surgical intervention to close the tear. Early recognition and treatment result in a high survival rate.

## DISORDERS OF THE INTESTINE

### Mechanical Obstruction

Complete or partial obstruction of the small bowel or colon is not unusual in the newborn. A variety of lesions, intrinsic or extrinsic, may be responsible (Table 71–1). Success or failure in terms of morbidity and mortality depends not so much on pinpointing the exact location of the lesion as on correctly diagnosing obstruction as the cause of the clinical symptoms and then instituting prompt operative intervention.

Vomiting, particularly of bile-stained material, with abdominal distention and the failure to pass meconium are highly suggestive of the presence of intestinal obstruction. If the obstruction is high or complete, symptoms start soon after birth. Vomiting of bile suggests that the lesion is located distal to the ampulla of Vater, whereas sporadic vomiting may be seen in patients with partial obstruction caused by malrotation, duplications, or annular pancreas. Abdominal distention may be present soon after birth, reaching a peak at 24 to 48 hours with visible peristaltic waves. Failure to pass meconium within 24 hours after birth suggests the presence of a colonic lesion. Infants with high obstruction or even those with obstruction as low as the ileum pass meconium, so this finding by

**TABLE 71–1**

**Causes of Intestinal Obstruction in the Newborn**

| Mechanical | | |
|---|---|---|
| **Congenital** | **Acquired** | **Functional** |
| Intrinsic | Necrotizing enterocolitis | Hirschsprung disease |
| Atresias | Intussusception | Meconium plug syndrome |
| Stenoses | Peritoneal adhesions | Ileus |
| Meconium ileus | | Peritonitis |
| Anorectal malformations | | |
| Enteric duplications | | |
| Extrinsic | | Intestinal pseudo-obstruction syndrome |
| Volvulus | | |
| Peritoneal bands | | |
| Annular pancreas | | |
| Cysts and tumors | | |
| Incarcerated hernias | | |

itself does not exclude obstruction. Prenatal diagnosis of gastrointestinal obstruction has been successful (Langer et al, 1989) and has become more common.

The initial radiographic studies should be plain films obtained with the infant in the supine and left lateral positions. Normally, air fills the stomach immediately after birth, the small bowel within 12 hours, and the colon within 24 hours. When obstruction exists, the air pattern stops abruptly at that point, leaving the remainder of the bowel airless. Obstruction at the pylorus produces one large bubble outlining the dilated stomach, whereas duodenal obstructions produce a "double-bubble" appearance (Fig. 71–12). Distal obstructions show a series of dilated, air- and fluid-filled loops of intestine. Obstruction resulting from meconium ileus is an exception in that air-fluid levels usually are not seen. In an incomplete obstruction, gas may be seen distal to dilated loops of bowel.

If the diagnosis is in doubt or a meconium plug is suspected, a contrast enema can be done. The finding of a microcolon is suggestive of small bowel atresia or meconium ileus. An upper gastrointestinal series is done only if the plain film and enema are nondiagnostic.

## Intrinsic Obstruction

### *Atresias*

#### Definition and Etiology

*Atresia*, complete obstruction of the lumen of the bowel, should be distinguished from *stenosis*, which is a narrowing of the lumen. Atresias account for one third of all intestinal obstructions in the newborn, occurring in 1 of every 1500 live births. Sites of occurrence, in order of frequency, are jejunoileal, duodenal, and colonic. Failure of the gut to recanalize during the eighth to tenth weeks of gestation seems to be the most likely cause for duodenal atresia. In the jejunum, ileum, and colon, vascular compromise early in gestation may be responsible for bowel atresias (Louw, 1966). Other potential causes in utero include incarceration of the physiologic umbilical hernia, localized volvulus, intussusception, focal peritonitis, and peritoneal band formation.

## Duodenal Atresia

Thirty percent of all atresias occur in the duodenum, and most are distal to the ampulla. Most infants with duodenal atresia also have other associated anomalies including Down syndrome, cardiovascular malformations, malrotation, esophageal atresia, small bowel lesions, and anorectal lesions (Dalla Vecchia et al, 1998). Annular pancreas also may be found but is often incidental and not the cause of the obstruction. Anatomically, duodenal atresia may occur in several forms (Fig. 71–13). Prenatal ultrasound diagnosis is becoming increasingly frequent (Stoll et al, 1996).

Bile-stained vomiting on the first day of life and a history of polyhydramnios are common presenting features. Abdominal distention is usually absent. Dehydration with a metabolic alkalosis rapidly ensues. The diagnosis may be made on plain abdominal films with the appearance of the "double bubble" sign (see Fig. 71–12).

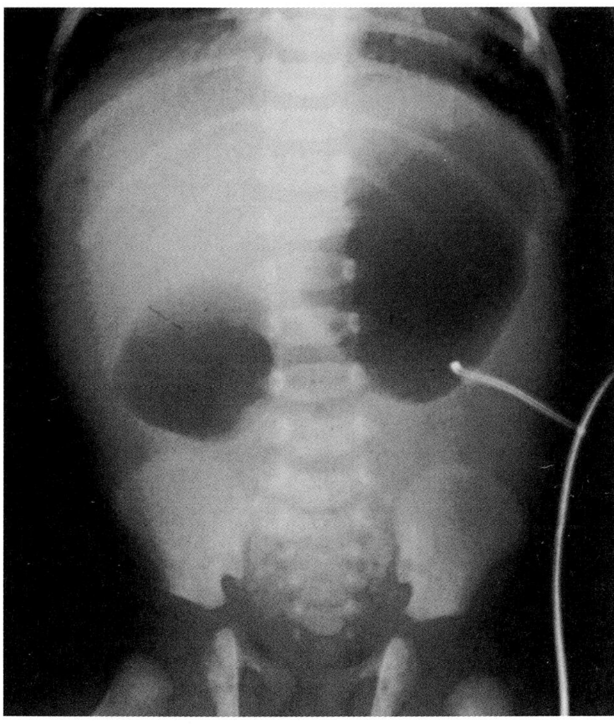

**FIGURE 71–12.** Abdominal film from a 12-hour-old infant with vomiting. A "double-bubble" sign is present. At laparotomy, duodenal atresia was found. *(Courtesy of Dr. Ronald M. Cohen, Children's Hospital, Oakland, Calif.)*

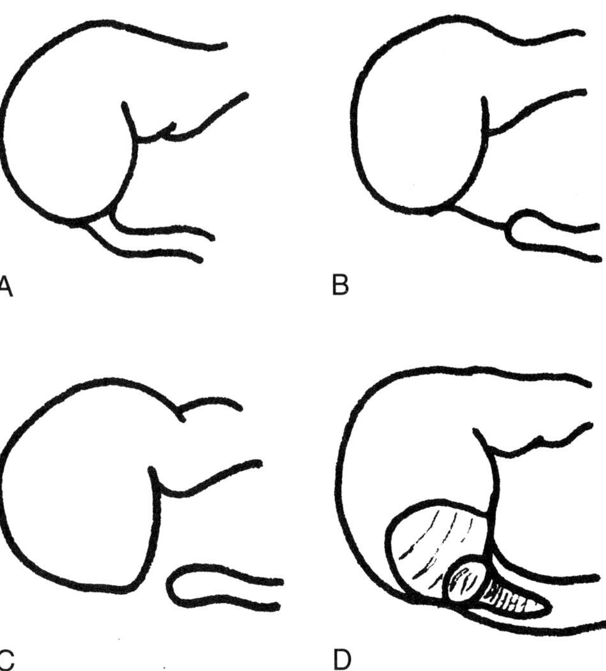


**FIGURE 71–13.** Forms of intrinsic duodenal obstruction. **A,** Duodenal atresia with continuity of the bowel wall. **B,** Duodenal atresia with a fibrous cord joining segments. **C,** Complete atresia with two separate segments. **D,** Windsock deformity.

Medical therapy consists of the passage of a nasogastric tube and correction of dehydration and electrolyte abnormalities. Prompt surgical intervention is necessary, although with a clear diagnosis, surgery may be delayed in very low birth-weight (VLBW) infants. Because of the high incidence of multiple atresias (15%), inspection of the entire bowel is carried out before bypassing the obstruction with a duodenoduodenostomy (Weber et al, 1986). An excessively distended proximal duodenum may need to be tapered as well, in an effort to reduce the duodenal dysmotility that often delays the start of normal feeds. The outcome for these infants generally is good but depends on their associated anomalies.

## Jejunoileal Atresia

Fifty percent of intestinal atresias occur in the jejunum or ileum. Associated extraintestinal anomalies, including gastroschisis, intrauterine volvulus, and meconium ileus, are infrequent (occurring in 7% of cases) (Dalla Vecchia et al, 1998). Atresias are thought to be most likely the result of a late intrauterine mesenteric vascular accident. They are equally distributed between the jejunum and ileum and are multiple in 10% to 20% of cases (Grosfeld et al, 1979). A useful classification is shown in Figure 71–14 (Grosfeld et al, 1979). Intestinal length may be significantly decreased in type IIIb atresias (so-called "apple peel" or "Christmas tree" deformity) and in type IV multiple atresias ("string of sausages" appearance). Prenatal ultrasound diagnosis is possible but is less accurate than in duodenal atresia.

Signs and symptoms of small bowel atresia include maternal polyhydramnios, bilious vomiting, abdominal distention (which may not become obvious until the second or third day of life), failure to pass meconium, and jaundice. Passage of meconium does not exclude an atresia, as 20% to 40% of newborns with the condition will pass some meconium. Plain abdominal radiographs show varying amounts of dilated, thumb-sized loops of bowel ("rule of thumb"), air-fluid levels, and absence of rectal gas (Fig. 71–15). Peritoneal calcification signifies the presence of meconium peritonitis, the result of a prenatal intestinal perforation. Contrast enema (usually using water-soluble contrast material) is the diagnostic test of choice. Contrast material may not reach the obstruction, but the appearance of a microcolon in the normal anatomic position is strong evidence that other lesions, such as malrotation, colonic atresia, and aganglionosis, are unlikely. Meconium ileus should be excluded by careful evaluation, as in most such cases the infant can be managed nonoperatively.

The type of surgical procedure depends on the lesion, but most often it involves resection of the atretic segment(s) with primary end-to-end anastomosis. Significant luminal discrepancies between the proximal and distal ends are addressed by amputation of large blind pouches, tapering enteroplasty, and/or end-to-oblique anastomosis. A certain degree of functional obstruction may still be encountered postoperatively, especially in proximal atresias. Prognosis is excellent, except with types IIIb and IV atresias, in which significant mesenteric defects may result in a short bowel syndrome.

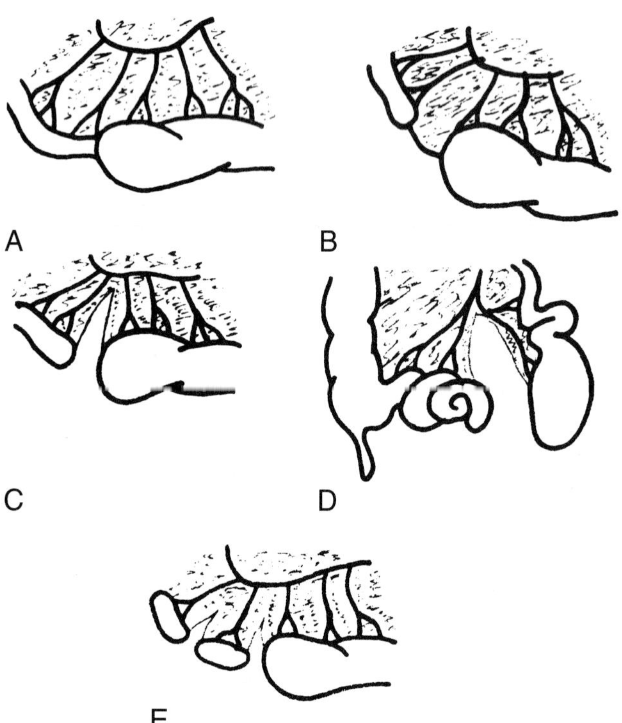


**FIGURE 71–14.** Classification of intestinal atresias. **A,** Mucosal atresia with intact bowel wall and mesentery. **B,** Blind ends joined by a fibrous cord. **C,** Blind ends separated by a mesenteric defect. **D,** Blind ends with the "apple peel" atresia. **E,** Multiple atresias.

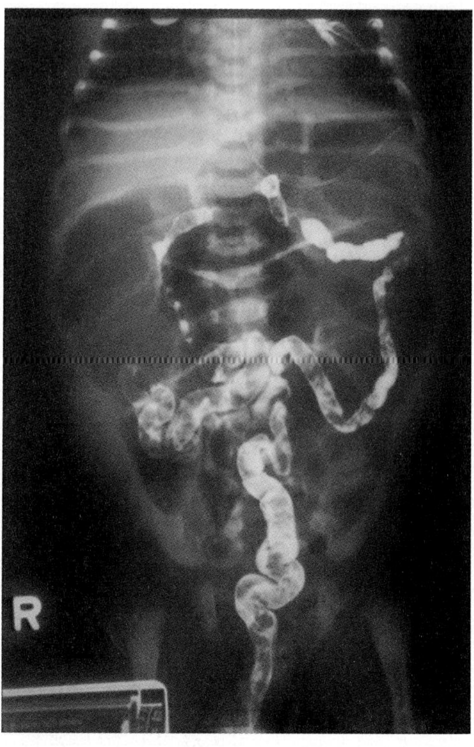


**FIGURE 71–15.** Anteroposterior view of abdomen of male newborn with intestinal atresia. Multiple dilated bowel loops are present. Rectal contrast shows microcolon.

## Colonic Atresia

Less than 10% of atresias occur in the colon, and stenosis is even less common. Associated anomalies may occur in one third of the infants. In up to 20% of cases, colonic atresia is accompanied by other intestinal atresias, and these must be sought carefully. Clinical signs and symptoms of colonic atresia include abdominal distention and vomiting beginning on the second or third day of life and failure to pass meconium. On plain radiographs, dilated loops of bowel are present, often with a distal cutoff. Pneumoperitoneum from intestinal perforation is found in 10% of cases. A contrast enema is essential for diagnosis, showing a distal microcolon. The preferred surgical approach involves resection of the atretic segment and primary anastomosis (Davenport et al, 1990). This approach has replaced various staging procedures in stable patients without peritonitis. Outcome generally is very good.

### *Meconium Ileus*

#### Definition and Etiology

*Meconium ileus* refers to an intraluminal intestinal obstruction produced by thick inspissated meconium. Ninety percent of patients with meconium ileus have cystic fibrosis (CF). Indeed, in 10% to 15% of cases of CF, the patient presents with meconium ileus. DNA markers for the CF gene have been identified and localized to chromosome 7 (Rommens et al, 1989; Mornet et al, 1988) showed different haplotypic variants for CF chromosomes in families with meconium ileus from those in families with no meconium ileus.

Severe pancreatic involvement is not a consistent finding in CF cases in which the patient presents with meconium ileus (Waters et al, 1990). In utero, some CF fetuses produce exceptionally viscid secretions from the mucous glands of the small intestine. The meconium formed is dry and contains higher-than-usual concentrations of protein, including albumin (Schwachmann and Antonowicz, 1981). The abnormal meconium adheres firmly to the mucosal surface of the distal small bowel, creating an intraluminal obstruction. Histologically, the goblet cells and mucous glands are prominent and distended with an eosinophilic material that merges with the intraluminal meconium for a cast of the crypts and villi. Proximal to the obstruction there may be intestinal muscular hypertrophy.

#### Diagnosis

Prenatal diagnosis of CF is possible (Lemna et al, 1990). A family history of CF should alert the clinician to the possibility of meconium ileus. In the simple form in which obstruction occurs in the middle and distal ileum without perforation and peritonitis, signs of obstruction appear within the first 48 hours in an otherwise healthy infant. Abdominal distention is noticed between 12 and 24 hours, after which vomiting occurs. No meconium is passed. Physical examinations may reveal firm palpable masses throughout the abdomen that are freely movable in any direction ("doughy abdomen"). Meconium ileus complicated by volvulus, atresias, meconium peritonitis, or pseudocyst formation is found in one third to one half of the patients (Rescorla and Grosfeld, 1993). Newborns with these complications present earlier than those with simple meconium ileus. They usually appear more ill, often with severe vomiting, signs of neonatal sepsis, and more marked distention causing respiratory distress.

Radiographic examination shows dilated loops of bowel. Fluid levels are inconspicuous because of the viscous nature of the meconium, which produces a coarse granular appearance ("ground-glass" appearance or "soap bubble" sign), typically in the right lower quadrant. The abdominal film may show, in addition to the distended gas-filled loops, intra-abdominal calcification indicative of meconium peritonitis (Fig. 71–16). The presence of air-fluid levels suggests the presence of jejunal or ileal atresia. The presence of a single grossly distended loop of bowel suggests the presence of postnatal volvulus. Perforations after birth result in free intraperitoneal air. Newborns suspected of having meconium ileus or with any other distal bowel obstruction should undergo a contrast enema study. In meconium ileus, this study typically shows a microcolon and obstruction by multiple filling defects in the terminal ileum.

All newborns with meconium ileus should be evaluated for CF. Boat and coworkers (1989) have reviewed the clinical, physiologic, and genetic aspects of CF. The identification and cloning of the primary CF gene and the ability to identify mutations causing CF have advanced

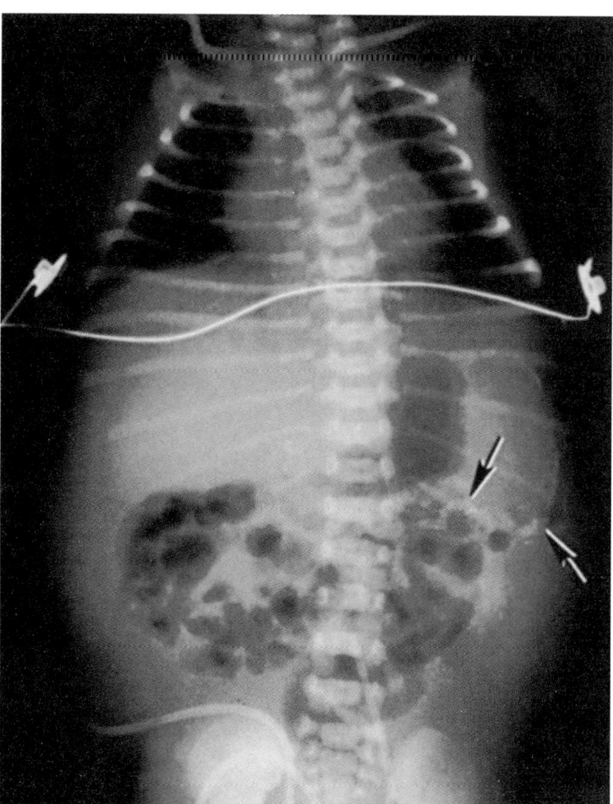

**FIGURE 71–16.** Ten-hour-old infant with ascites and abdominal calcification *(arrows)* secondary to meconium peritonitis. No gas is present in the rectum. The infant had ileal atresia, and a subsequent sweat chloride test was positive for cystic fibrosis. *(Courtesy of Dr. Ronald M. Cohen, Children's Hospital, Oakland, Calif.)*

the clinician's ability to provide accurate diagnosis as well as counseling (Kerem et al, 1989b; Lemna et al, 1990; Rommens et al, 1989).

### Treatment

In simple meconium ileus, approximately 60% of the infants have their obstruction successfully relieved by the diagnostic contrast enema, ideally using Gastrografin (Kao and Franken, 1995). Before the hyperosmolar enema is given, other complications, such as perforation, volvulus, or atresia, must be excluded. The hypertonic enema draws water into the intestinal tract, dislodging and breaking up the meconium. Because of rapid fluid shifts, great care must be taken to maintain fluid and electrolyte balance. Failure of the contrast to dislodge the inspissated meconium after two attempts is an indication for surgical intervention. If the enema is successful, acetylcysteine, 5 mL every 6 hours, may be given via a nasogastric tube to help complete the clean-out.

Surgical intervention in simple meconium ileus usually consists of enterotomy with acteylcysteine irrigation and immediate closure. Other procedures such as resection of the ileum, with or without construction of various defunctioning ileostomies, are rarely indicated (Rescorla and Grosfeld, 1993). Complicated meconium ileus always requires surgical intervention, and the choice of operative procedure depends on the pathologic findings.

### Prognosis

Operative mortality is minimal for simple meconium ileus. Perforation and electrolyte imbalance are the main complications of hyperosmolar enemas (Kao and Franken, 1995). Longer-term outcome is influenced by the severity of pulmonary involvement.

Meconium plug syndrome is a similar entity not related to CF. Affected infants present similarly clinically, yet on contrast enema the obstruction is colonic and uniformly relieved during the study. Because of the diagnostic similarity and the fact that some children with CF may present with this pattern, testing for CF is indicated in all newborns with meconium obstruction (Rosenstein, 1978).

## *Anorectal Malformations*

### Definition and Epidemiology

Anorectal anomalies occur in 1 of every 5000 births and are slightly more common in males (deVries and Cox, 1985). Associated anomalies occur in more than half of affected infants and are more frequent in "high" forms (see under "Etiology," next). Most frequent are vertebral, genitourinary, and gastrointestinal malformations (Kiely and Pena, 1998)

### Etiology

The proctoderm comprises the anus and a canal that extends cephalad a short distance to meet the blind end of the hindgut, which has simultaneously moved caudad. Around the seventh to eighth week of gestation these should make contact, separated only by an anal membrane. At the same time, the lower urinary tract develops alongside the lower intestinal tract, separated by the urorectal membrane. Anal malformations arise locally from maldevelopment within the proctoderm. Atresias, stenoses, and fistulas arise from imperfect resolution of the anorectal membrane with or without concomitant failure of the urorectal membrane to separate completely the rectal and genitourinary components.

Anorectal malformations have traditionally been classified on the basis of the level of the rectal pouch (above the levator sling, or "high," and below it, or "low") and the presence or absence of an associated fistula. This classification is, however, arbitrary and too simplistic. A descriptive listing of the anomalies as presented in Table 71–2 is therefore suggested (Pena, 1997). A fistula is present in 95% of the cases, either externally as an anocutaneous fistula or internally as a rectourethral or rectovesical fistula.

### Diagnosis and Treatment

Diagnosis is based on careful perineal examination, with imaging studies reserved for cases of diagnostic uncertainty and for evaluation of associated anomalies. The two key considerations in the assessment are the need for a colostomy and the presence of significant associated anomalies. The level of the defect may be clinically identifiable. Infants with low defects may have cutaneous fistulas, a bulging anal membrane, and well-formed buttocks. Females will pass meconium through a perineal, vestibular, or vaginal fistula, or the anomaly may manifest as a cloaca ("one-hole perineum") (see Fig. 71–6). Cutaneous fistulas in males may track along the midline raphe toward the penis, discharging a tiny epithelial "pearl" or a meconium drop (see Fig. 71–5). Finding meconium in the urine or air in the bladder may identify the presence of an internal fistula.

Plain abdominal radiographs may show progressive distal bowel obstruction. The traditional "invertogram" used to identify the distance between the rectal pouch and the skin has been replaced by a cross-table prone film obtained with the pelvis elevated, although this study should not be done in the first 24 hours of life, as the radiographic appearance may suggest a falsely increased gap (Kiely and Pena, 1998). Perineal ultrasound examination may prove to be more accurate than plain films. Abdominal ultrasonography, cardiac echography, and skeletal films may be required to rule out associated anomalies. The management of low defects includes several procedures aimed at restoring the anorectal canal, by "cut-back" of a cutaneous fistula, anal transposition, or limited posterior sagittal anorectoplasty (Kiely and Pena, 1998). High and so-called intermediate defects require an immediate colostomy, followed by elective repair. Before the final repair a distal colostogram allows the precise localization of the fistula. Although there are multiple approaches to the definitive correction of anorectal malformations, the aim of all is to close any fistula and then tunnel the rectal pouch through the anatomic sphincter muscle to the anoderm. The posterior sagittal anorectoplasty popularized by Pena has become the most frequent procedure worldwide (Kiely and Pena, 1998).

**TABLE 71-2**

**Anatomic Classification of Anorectal Malformations**

| | Lesion | Frequency (%) | | | Survival (%) |
|---|---|---|---|---|---|
| | | Overall | Male | Female | |
| Low (below the levator) | Anal stenosis | 8 | | | 100 |
| | Imperforate anal membrane | 6 | | | 95 |
| | Anal agenesis | 36 | | | 84 |
| | No fistula | 7 | 7 | 0 | |
| | Fistula | 29 | 8 | 21 | |
| | Anovulvar | | 1 | 14 | |
| | Anoperineal | | 8 | 7 | |
| High (above the levator) | Rectal agenesis | 47 | | | 72 |
| | No fistula | 13 | 11 | 2 | |
| | Fistula | 31 | 21 | 10 | |
| | Rectourethral | | 24 | | |
| | Rectovesical | | 1 | | |
| | Rectovaginal | | | 8 | |
| | Rectocloacal | | | 3 | |
| | Rectal atresia | 3 | 1 | 2 | 57 |
| Overall | | | | | 80 |

Data from Kiesewetter WB, Chang JHT: Imperforate anus: A five to thirty year follow-up perspective. Prog Pediatr Surg 10:81-90, 1977.

### Prognosis

Although the surgical mortality rate is low and primarily dependent on associated anomalies, functional long-term results are variable. Children born with low defects often will be chronically constipated; incontinence may occur in 30% to 35% of patients with high defects (Ditesheim and Templeton, 1987) Furthermore, quality of life correlates closely with whether continence can be established (Ditesheim and Templeton, 1987). Nevertheless, a majority of these children can be rendered functionally continent through a bowel management program, anorectal biofeedback, and antegrade enemas via a cecostomy in selected patients (Paidas, 1997).

## *Enteric Duplications*

Duplications of the gastrointestinal tract are relatively rare. Developmentally, the most favored hypothesis is the split notochord, resulting from adherence between ectoderm and endoderm in the neural plate (Pang et al, 1992),

Duplications may occur anywhere from the mouth to the rectum, although a majority are found in the small bowel. Associated anomalies, especially of the intestinal tract, are common. Duplications are generally located on the mesenteric side of the lumen, are lined by intestinal mucosa, and share a common wall and mesenteric blood supply with the adjacent intestine. Most duplications are spherical, presenting as cysts occasionally communicating with the main enteric lumen. Tubular duplications may involve long segments of bowel but are rare.

Many duplications manifest in the neonatal period, usually with obstructive signs in the presence of a palpable mass (Stringer and Spitz, 1995). Esophageal duplications may cause respiratory distress, whereas ectopic gastric tissue may cause rectal bleeding from peptic ulceration. Plain films of the abdomen may show displacement of adjacent viscera by a mass. Upper and/or lower gastrointestinal contrast studies may demonstrate a filling defect or, rarely, a communication between the cyst and normal bowel. Ultrasound diagnosis is possible both prenatally and postnatally, based on a characteristic appearance of the wall of the mass. CT or MRI is the modality of choice for imaging thoracic duplications.

The treatment of choice is surgical excision with primary anastomosis, although partial excision with destruction of residual enteric lining may be necessary for long tubular duplications (Stringer and Spitz, 1995).

## Extrinsic Obstruction

### *Malrotation and Midgut Volvulus*

### Presentation

Anomalies of intestinal rotation occur in 1/6000 live births. Malrotation of the gut occurs between the eighth and tenth weeks of gestation, when the elongating intestine returns to the abdominal cavity. If the mesenteric attachments do not develop properly, the midgut lies free, attached to the posterior abdominal wall at only two points: at the duodenum and at the proximal colon. It may therefore twist in either direction, but when volvulus occurs it is usually in the clockwise direction. Midgut volvulus may occur at any time postnatally, but 80% of cases are found in the neonatal period (Seashore and Touloukian, 1994)

The newborn with midgut volvulus presents with high intestinal obstructive symptoms, often in the first week of life. Sudden bilious vomiting with abdominal distention in a previously well newborn is particularly suspicious. Mesenteric vascular compromise of the midgut leads to rapidly progressive peritonitis, sepsis, and shock. Laboratory investigations usually reveal biochemical signs of visceral ischemia and sepsis.

Plain abdominal films may show a high intestinal obstruction, although the closed-loop obstruction produced may fail to show air-fluid levels, as the compromised bowel often is filled with fluid alone (Fig. 71–17). Findings on plain radiographs may therefore be variable and cannot be used to rule out a midgut volvulus. A "gasless abdomen" finding is particularly worrisome. The stable infant with suspected volvulus should undergo an urgent upper gastrointestinal contrast study to document the position of the duodenojejunal flexure and to identify any proximal obstruction. Ultrasound examination may reveal the "whirlpool sign" in an acute volvulus or may document the correct or reversed position of the superior mesentery artery and vein (Pracros et al, 1992). The infant with peritonitis and suspected midgut volvulus should be promptly resuscitated and taken for immediate laparotomy.

### Treatment

At laparotomy, the volvulus is reduced by counterclockwise rotation, and intestinal viability is carefully assessed. Frankly necrotic bowel is removed, followed by either primary anastomosis or stoma creation. A Ladd procedure also is carried out, including lysis of peritoneal bands, appendectomy, and replacement of the bowel in a malrotated position. Recurrent volvulus after this procedure is very unusual.

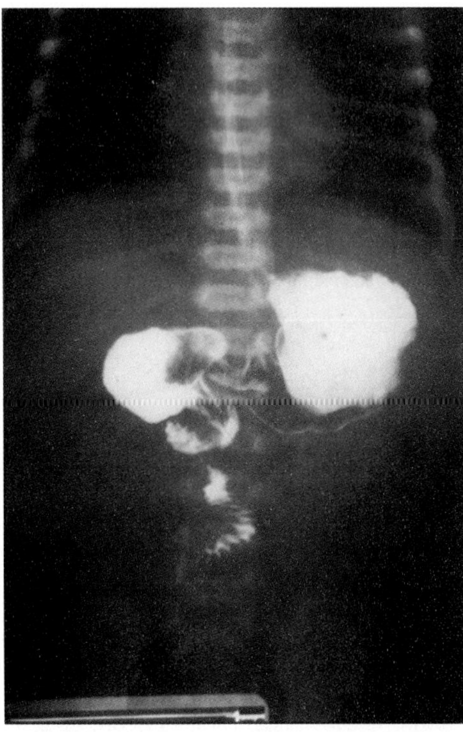

**FIGURE 71–17.** Anterposterior view of abdomen of male infant with midgut volvulus. The contrast material shows the duodenojejunal junction to be to the right of the spine, indicative of underlying malrotation. The proximal jejunum is obstructed in the "coil spring" appearance of acute midgut volvulus.

The infant with necrosis of the entire midgut presents a particularly challenging problem. A second-look laparotomy in 12 to 36 hours is often undertaken to assess intestinal viability. Options in the case of minimal intestinal recovery include short-gut protocols and bowel-lengthening procedures, intestinal transplantation, and compassionate care alone.

## *Intussusception*

*Intussusception* is the invagination of one loop of bowel into a loop distal to it. Although intussusception is a relatively common cause of intestinal obstruction in infants 6 to 18 months of age, it is very rare in neonates. Prenatal intussusception is responsible for some cases of intestinal atresia (Wang et al, 1998). In premature infants, intussusception may manifest without a specific leading point and with a picture mimicking that of necrotizing enterocolitis (Mooney et al, 1996). In the full-term newborn, a colonic leading point often is encountered (Wang et al, 1998).

Should a diagnosis of intussusception be entertained, ultrasound examination and/or contrast enema are indicated. Hydrostatic reduction is not usually successful in neonates, and therefore a laparotomy with operative reduction or resection is necessary.

## *Meconium Plug Syndrome*

Meconium plug syndrome originally was described as an intestinal obstruction in the newborn that is relieved by the passage of an inspissated gray plug of meconium from the distal colon (Ellis and Clatworthy, 1966). It was initially thought that the meconium itself was abnormal. However, this syndrome has come to be considered a form of colonic dysmotility without an abnormality of intramural ganglion cells. Affected infants pass no meconium for the first 24 to 48 hours of life, and eventually symptoms of distal intestinal obstruction develop. Contrast enema is both diagnostic and therapeutic.

## REFERENCES

### Mouth

Bill AH, Vadheim JL: Cysts, sinuses and fistulas of the neck arising from the first and second branchial clefts. Am Surg 142:904, 1955.

Chappuis JP: Current aspects of cystic lymphangioma in the neck. Arch Pediatr 1:186, 1994.

Damm DD, Cibull mL, Geissler RH, et al: Investigation into the histogenesis of congenital epulis of the newborn. Oral Surg Oral Med Oral Pathol 76:205, 1993.

Langley FA, Davson J: Epulis in the newborn. Arch Dis Child 25:89, 1950.

Ling CM, Low YS: Sternomastoid tumor and muscular torticollis. J Bone Joint Surg 55:236, 1973.

Meyerowitz BR, Buchholz RB: Midline cervical ectopic thyroid tissue. Surgery 65:358, 1969.

Mychaliska GB, Bealer JF, Graf JL, et al: Operating on placental support: The ex utero intrapartum treatment procedure. J Pediatr Surg 32:227, 1997.

Rosegger H, Steinwendner G: Transverse fetal position syndrome—a combination of congenital skeletal deformities in the newborn infant. Pediatr Padol 27:125, 1992.

Samuel M, McCarthy L, Boddy SA: Efficacy and safety of OK-432 sclerotherapy for giant cystic hygroma in a newborn. Fetal Diagn Ther 15:93, 2000.

Spivack J, Bennett JE: Glossopalatine ankylosis. Plast Reconstr Surg 42:129, 1968.

Thompson RE, Love WG: Persistent cervical thymoma apparent with crying. Am J Dis Child 124:761, 1972.

Welch KJ, Trump DS: The oropharynx and jaws. In Ravitch MM (ed): Pediatric Surgery. Chicago, Year Book Medical, 1979, p 308.

Wirth CJ, Hagena FW, Wuelker N, Siebert WE: Bi-terminal tenotomy for the treatment of congenital muscular torticollis. J Bone Joint Surg (Am) 74:427, 1992.

### Esophagus

Alexander F, Johanningman J, Martin L: Staged repair improves outcome of high-risk premature infants with esophageal atresia and tracheoesophageal fistula. J Pediatr Surg 28:151, 1993.

Benjamin B, Robb P, Glasson M: Esophageal stricture following esophageal atresia repair: Endoscopic assessment and dilatation. Ann Otol Rhinol Laryngol 102:332, 1993.

Corbally M, Spitz L, Kiely E, et al: Aortopexy for tracheomalacia in oesophageal anomalies. Eur J Pediatr Surg 3:264, 1993.

Corsello G, Maresi E, Corrao A, et al: VATER/VACTERL association: Clinical variability and expanding phenotype including laryngeal stenosis. Am J Med Genet 44:813, 1993.

Fann J, Hartmann G, Shocat S: “Waterseal” gastrostomy in the management of premature infants with tracheoesophageal fistula and pulmonary insufficiency. J Pediatr Surg 23:29, 1988.

Filston H, Chitwood WJ, Schkolne B, Blackmon L: The Fogarty balloon catheter as an aid to management of the infant with esophageal atresia and tracheoesophageal fistula complicated by severe RDS or pneumonia. J Pediatr Surg 17:149, 1982.

Goh DW, Brereton RJ, Spitz L: Esophageal atresia with obstructed tracheoesophageal fistula and gasless abdomen. J Pediatr Surg 26:160, 1991.

Greenwood RD, Rosenthal A: Cardiovascular malformations associated with tracheoesophageal fistula and esophageal atresia. Pediatrics 57:87, 1976.

Hausmann PF, Close AS, Williams LP: Occurrence of tracheoesophageal fistula in three consecutive siblings. Surgery 41:542, 1957.

Holder TM, Ashcraft KW: Esophageal atresia and tracheoesophageal fistula (collective review). Ann Thorac Surg 9:445, 1970.

Holder T: Esophageal atresia and tracheoesophageal malformations. In Ashcraft K, Holder T (eds): Pediatric Surgery. Philadelphia, WB Saunders 1993, p 249.

Krasna IH, Rosenfeld D, Benjamin BG, et al: Esophageal perforation in the neonate: An emerging problem in the nursery. J Pediatr Surg 22:784, 1987.

Linde LM, Westover JL: Esophageal and gastric abnormalities in dysautonomia. Pediatrics 29:303, 1962.

Manning P, Morgan R, Coran A, et al: Fifty years' experience with esophageal atresia and transesophageal fistula. Ann Surg 204:446, 1986.

Meyers NA: Oesophageal atresia: The epitome of modern surgery. Ann R Coll Surg Engl 54:312, 1974.

Nihoul-Fekete C, et al: Congenital esophageal stenosis: A review of 20 cases. Pediatr Surg Int 2:86, 1987.

Pieretii R, Shandling B, Stephens C: Resistant esophageal stenosis associated with reflux after repair of esophageal atresia. J Pediatr Surg 9:355, 1974.

Pletcher BA, Friedes JS, Breg WR, Touloukian RJ: Familial occurrence of esophageal atresia with and without tracheoesophageal fistula: Report of two unusual kindreds. Am J Med Genet 39:380, 1991.

Quan L, Smith DW: The VATER association: Vertebral defects, anal atresia, T-fistula with esophageal atresia, radial and renal dysplasia: A spectrum of associated defects. J Pediatr 104:7, 1973.

Raffensperger JG: Esophageal atresia and tracheoesophageal stenosis. In Raffensperger JG (ed): Swenson's Pediatric Surgery, 5th ed. Norwalk, Conn, Appleton & Lange, 1990, p 697.

Reckham PP: Infants with esophageal atresia weighing under 3 pounds. J Pediatr Surg 16:595, 1981.

Rejjal A: Congenital anomalies associated with esophageal atresia: Saudi Arabian experience. Am J Perinatol 16: 239, 1999.

Roberts CC, Herbst JJ, Jolley SG, et al: Evaluation of tests for gastroesophageal reflux in patients operated on for tracheoesophageal fistula. Pediatr Res 14:509, 1980.

Rowe M, O'Neill J Jr, Grosfeld J, et al: Congenital abnormalities of the esophagus. In Rowe M (ed): Essentials of Pediatric Surgery. St. Louis, Mosby–Year Book, 1995, p 397.

Salib SA, Aubert D, Valioulis I, de Billy B: Cricopharyngeal achalasia—a cause of major dysphagia in a newborn. A case report. Eur J Pediatr Surg 9:406, 1999.

Shah M, Berman W: Endoscopic balloon dilatation of esophageal strictures in children. Gastrointest Endosc 39:153, 1993.

Spitz L: Esophageal atresia and tracheoesophageal fistula in children. Curr Opin Pediatr 5:347, 1993.

Stewart RJ, Bruce J, Beasley SW: Oesophageal duplication cyst: Another cause of neonatal respiratory distress. J Paediatr Child Health. 29:391, 1993.

Touloukian R, Keller M: High proximal pouch esophageal atresia with vertebral, rib and sternal anomalies: An additional component to the VATER association. J Pediatr Surg 23:76, 1988.

Weber T, Smith W, Grosfeld J: Surgical experience in infants with the VATER syndrome. J Pediatr Surg 15:849, 1980.

Whitington PF, Shermeta DW, Eto DSY, et al: Role of lower esophageal sphincter incompetence in recurrent pneumonia after repair of esophageal atresia. J Pediatr 91:550, 1977.

Woolley MM, Chinnock RF, Paul RH: Premature twins with esophageal atresia and tracheoesophageal fistula. Acta Paediatr 50:423, 1961.

Yancher NL, Gordon R, Cooper M, et al: Significance of the clinical course and early upper gastrointestinal studies in predicting complications associated with repair of esophageal atresia. J Pediatr Surg 36: 15-22, 2001.

### Stomach

Andrus CH, Ponsky JL: The effects of irrigant temperature in upper gastrointestinal hemorrhage: A requiem for iced saline lavage. Am J Gastroenterol 82:1062, 1987.

Bell MJ, Keating JP, Ternberg JL, et al: Perforated stress ulcers in infants. J Pediatr Surg 16:998, 1981.

Byrne WJ: Diagnosis and treatment of peptic ulcer disease in children. Pediatr Rev 7:182, 1985.

Cohen HL, Zinn HL, Haller JO, et al: Ultrasonography of pylorospasm: Findings may simulate hypertrophic pyloric stenosis. J Ultrasound Med 17:705, 1998.

Hallam D, Hansen B, Bodner B, et al: Pyloric size in normal infants and infants suspected of having hypertropic pyloric stenosis. Acta Radiol 36:261, 1995.

Holcomb GW, Gheissari A, O'Neill JA Jr, et al : Surgical management of alimentary tract duplications. Ann Surg 209:167, 1989.

Laron Z, Horne LM: The incidence of infantile pyloric stenosis. Am J Dis Child 94:151, 1957.

Okoye BO, Parikh DH, Buick RG, Lander AD. Pyloric atresia: Five new cases, a new association, and a review of the literature with guidelines. J Pediatr Surg 35:1242, 2000

Shankar KR, Losty PD, Jones MO, et al: Umbilical pyloromyotomy—an alternative to laparoscopy? Eur J Pediatr Surg 11:8, 2001.

Shaw A, Blanc WA, Santulli TV, et al: Spontaneous rupture of the stomach: A clinical and experimental study. Surgery 58:561, 1965.

St.-Vil D, LeBouthillier G, Luks FI, et al: Neonatal gastrointestinal perforations. J Pediatr Surg 27:1340, 1992.

Wieczorek RL, Seidman I, Ranson JHC, et al: Congenital duplication of the stomach: Case report and review of the English literature. Am J Gastroenterol 79:597, 1984.

### Intestine

Boat TF, Welsh MJ, Beaudet AL, et al: Cystic fibrosis. In Scriver CR, Beaudet AL, Sly WS, et al (eds): The Metabolic Basis of Inherited Disease, 6th ed. New York, McGraw-Hill, 1989, p 2649.

Dalla Vecchia LK, Grosfeld JL, West KW, et al: Intestinal atresia and stenosis: A 25-year experience with 277 cases. Arch Surg 133:490, 1998.

Davenport M, Bianchi A, Doig CM, Gough DC: Colonic atresia: Current results of treatment. J Royal Coll Surg Edinb 35:25, 1990.

deVries PA, Cox KL: Surgery of anorectal anomalies. Surg Clin North Am 65:1139, 1985.

Ditesheim JA, Templeton JM: Short-term versus long-term quality of life in children following repair of high imperforate anus. J Pediatr Surg 22:581, 1987.

Ellis DG, Clatworthy HW: The meconium plug syndrome revisited. J Pediatr Surg 1:54, 1966.

Grosfeld JL, Ballantyne TVN, Shoemaker R: Operative management of intestinal atresia and stenosis based on pathologic findings. J Pediatr Surg 14:368, 1979.

Kao SCS, Franken EA Jr: Nonoperative treatment of simple meconium ileus: a survey of the Society for Pediatric Radiology. Pediatr Radiol 25:97, 1995.

Kerem E, Corey M, Levison H: Clinical and genetic comparisons of patients with cystic fibrosis, with or without meconium ileus. J Pediatr 114:767, 1989a.

Kerem BS, Rommens JM, Buchanan JA, et al: Identification of the cystic fibrosis gene: Genetic analysis. Science 245:1073, 1989b.

Kiely EM, Pena A: Anorectal malformations. In O'Neill JA, Rowe MI, Grosfeld JL, et al (eds): Pediatric Surgery, 5th ed. St Louis, Mosby, 1998, p 1425.

Langer JC, Adzick NS, Filly RA, et al: Gastrointestinal tract obstruction in the fetus. Arch Surg 124:1183, 1989.

Lemna WK, Feldman GL, Kerem B, et al: Mutation analysis for heterozygote detection and the prenatal diagnosis of cystic fibrosis. N Engl J Med 322:291, 1990.

Martin LW, Zerella JT: Jejunoileal atresia: A proposed classification. J Pediatr Surg 11:399, 1976.

Mooney DP, Steinthorsson G, Shorter NA: Perinatal intussusception in premature infants. J Pediatr Surg 31:695, 1996.

Mornet E, Serre JL, Farrell M: Genetic differences between cystic fibrosis with and without meconium ileus. Lancet 1:376, 1988.

Nguyen LT, Youssef S, Guttman FM, et al: Meconium ileus: Is a stoma necessary? J Pediatr Surg 21:766, 1986.

Paidas CN: Fecal incontinence in children with anorectal malformations. Semin Pediatr Surg 6:228, 1997.

Pang D, Dias MS, Mamdouha AB: Split cord malformation. Part I: A unified theory of embryogenesis for double spinal cord malformations. Neurosurg 31:451, 1992.

Pena A: Advances in anorectal malformations. Semin Pediatr Surg 6:165, 1997.

Rescorla FJ, Grosfeld JL: Contemporary management of meconium ileus. World J Surg 17:318, 1993.

Rosenstein BJ: Cystic fibrosis presenting with the meconium plug syndrome. Am J Dis Child 132:167, 1978.

Rommens JM, Zengerling S, Bums J: Identification and regional localization of DNA markers on chromosome 7 for cloning of the cystic fibrosis gene. Am J Hum Genet 43:645, 1989.

Schwachmann H, Antonowicz I: Studies on meconium. In Lebenthal E (ed): Textbook of Gastroenterology and Nutrition in Infancy. New York, Raven Press, 1981.

Seashore JH, Touloukian RJ: Midgut volvulus. An ever-present threat. Arch Pediatr Adolesc Med 148:43, 1994.

Stoll C, Alembik Y, Dott B, Roth MP. Evaluation of prenatal diagnosis of congenital gastrointestinal atresias. Eur J Epidem 12:611, 1996.

Stringer MD, Spitz L, Abel R, et al: Management of alimentary tract duplication in children. Br J Surg 82:74, 1995.

Wang NL, Yeh ML, Chang PY, et al: Prenatal and neonatal intussusception. Pediatr Surg Int 13:232, 1998.

Waters DL, Domey SF, Gaskin KJ, et al: Pancreatic function in infants identified as having cystic fibrosis in a neonatal screening program. N Engl J Med 322:303, 1990.

Weber TR, Lewis JE, Mooney D, Connors R: Duodenal atresia: A comparison of techniques for repair. J Pediatr Surg 21:1133, 1986.

Weber T, Smith W, Grosfeld J: Surgical experience in infants with the VATER syndrome. J Pediatr Surg 15:849, 1980.

CHAPTER

# 72

# Physiologic and Inflammatory Abnormalities of the Gastrointestinal Tract

Carol Lynn Berseth

## ASCITES AND PERITONITIS

### Ascites

Generalized abdominal enlargement may be due to intestinal distention, hepatomegaly, tumors, peritonitis, or ascites. Therefore, the presence or absence of each of these entities must be determined in evaluating the infant for suspected ascites. Imaging techniques such as radiography, ultrasonography, and computed tomography scanning may be useful in determining whether abdominal masses are present and in defining the type of ascites present. In addition, paracentesis to obtain peritoneal fluid for laboratory analysis provides additional clues to the cause of ascites. Most commonly, ascitic fluid in newborns is analyzed for content of red blood cells, white blood cells, protein, and fat, but additional analysis, as shown in Table 72–1, can be useful.

Ascites may be identified early in fetal life by obstetric ultrasound examination. Accumulation of fluid in the abdomen of the fetus may be so massive as to necessitate delivery by cesarean section. The presence of ascites may produce respiratory distress after birth (Fig. 72–1). Immediate paracentesis to aspirate ascitic fluid may be diagnostic as well as therapeutic. Ascites may be chylous, urinary, biliary, or pancreatic. It may be secondary to neonatal hydrops or congestive heart failure or caused by the rupture of a large ovarian cyst in the fetus during delivery. Although hyponatremia is found in 70% of these infants, electrolytes commonly are normal at birth because of the normalizing effect of the maternal-placental circulation. Postnatally, however, the presence of ascitic fluid containing high concentrations of urea, creatinine, and potassium triggers physiologic equilibration with the extracellular fluid, which may result in dramatic shifts of free water and solutes. Thus, sodium moves from the vascular compartment to the peritoneal cavity, causing hyponatremia.

#### Chylous Ascites

The most common type of neonatal ascites is chylous ascites, which occurs more often in males. In the newborn, chylous ascites usually is due to a congenital failure of the lymphatic channels to communicate (Cochran et al, 1985). The initial paracentesis may yield clear fluid, but after enteral feedings are initiated, subsequent paracenteses yield a milky fluid that is high in triglyceride content. Leukocyte counts also may be elevated, and protein content is variable. Because chylous ascites may accompany intestinal malrotation and incomplete volvulus, appropriate imaging should be done to rule out the presence of intestinal malrotation. Treatment consists of repeated paracentesis to relieve distention, which will avoid respiratory embarrassment. The use of a formula containing medium-chain triglycerides decreases the formation of chyle. If chyle formation persists despite the specialized formula, intravenous alimentation may be necessary. In most patients, the ascites remits spontaneously, and the prognosis is excellent.

#### Urinary Ascites

Urinary ascites accounts for 25% of all cases of neonatal ascites, and it is due to an obstructive uropathy. Posterior urethral valves are the most common cause (Mann et al, 1974), but other lesions that can cause urinary ascites include ureteroceles, urethral atresia, bladder neck obstruction, neurogenic bladder, and bladder hematoma. Although the most common cause of disruption of the urinary collecting system is the presence of a tear in the collecting system itself, most often located at the caliceal fornix, perforation of the bladder has also been described.

Paracentesis yields urine (i.e., fluid) containing elevated concentrations of urea, creatinine, and potassium and low-to-normal concentrations of sodium and chloride (Arnold, 1986). Evaluation should include an abdominal ultrasound study, intravenous pyelogram, and voiding cystourethrogram to characterize the abnormalities in the urinary tract and its collecting system. Surgical decompression of the urinary tract or definitive correction of the causative lesion should be performed with urgency. The immediate prognosis for these infants is excellent, and renal function in the neonatal period and infancy is excellent (Farhat et al, 2000). The long-term prognosis often is poor, however. In a recent report of outcomes in 10 consecutively treated infants, 7 progressed to end-stage renal disease by their preteen years (Roth et al, 2000).

#### Biliary Ascites

Biliary ascites is caused by spontaneous perforation of the biliary tree. In 68% of the cases, the perforation occurs in the main biliary tree. In the remainder, the perforation is located at the junction of the cystic and common ducts or in an accessory bile duct. Two clinical forms are apparent. In the acute form, the infant presents with abdominal distention, vomiting, absence of bowel sounds, and unstable vital signs. Clinical jaundice may not be present. In the more chronic form, which occurs in about 80% of reported cases, clinical jaundice appears early, followed by gradual abdominal distention. Paracentesis reveals fluid with a bilirubin content above 4 g/dL, and the diagnosis is confirmed by scintigraphy or sonography (Banani et al, 1993). Laparotomy with a biliary drainage procedure is essential for survival. Survival rate after surgery is 80%.

**TABLE 72-1**

**Laboratory Studies Useful in the Evaluation of Ascites**

| Routine | Special |
|---|---|
| Red cell count | Triglycerides |
| White cell count with differential | Amylase |
| Specific gravity | Bilirubin |
| Total protein | |
| Culture | |

### Pancreatic Ascites

Pancreatic ascites, an extremely rare lesion, may be the presenting manifestation of pancreatitis secondary to a pancreatic duct anomaly. Except for the presence of abdominal distention, infants are asymptomatic. The concentrations of amylase, fat, and protein in the ascitic fluid may be elevated. Urine and serum amylase levels may be normal. Most infants require a surgical drainage procedure.

### Ruptured Ovarian Cyst

Ahmed (1971) reported the complication of ruptured ovarian cyst in a review of newborns with ovarian cysts. The presenting symptoms at birth included ascites and hemoperitoneum.

### Peritonitis

Peritonitis in the newborn can be classified as either bacterial or chemical (Bell, 1985). Chemical peritonitis occurs as an inflammatory response to the presence of a caustic material. The two most common forms of chemical peritonitis are due to the presence of meconium and bile, respectively, as a result of spillage from the intestine and biliary tree.

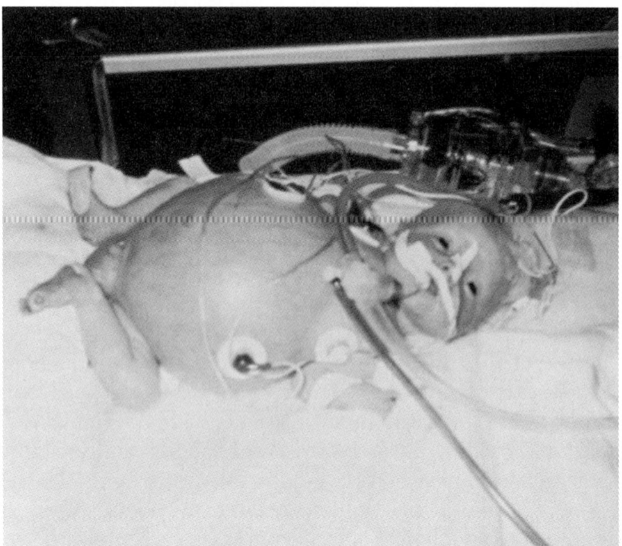

**FIGURE 72-1.** Full-term infant at 2 hours of age with massive ascites, which subsequently proved to be chylous. The distention was controlled with repeated paracentesis and an elemental diet. By 6 months of age, paracentesis was no longer necessary. At 13 months of age, the infant remains on an elemental diet and is growing and developing normally.

Meconium peritonitis may result from intestinal perforation that occurs in utero or shortly after birth. Most typically these cases of intestinal perforation are secondary to bowel obstruction; almost half are due to meconium ileus (Bell, 1985). Its presence is not commonly diagnosed prenatally (Yang et al, 1997), and at autopsy or surgery, the tear may be obvious or may have healed over. Although uncommon, other causes of meconium peritonitis are intussusception, volvulus, incarcerated internal hernia, imperforate anus, and meconium plugs.

Infectious peritonitis may be primary or secondary. Primary peritonitis occurs as a result of hematogenous or lymphatic spread, and secondary peritonitis occurs as a result of a primary abdominal catastrophe, such as necrotizing enterocolitis, appendicitis, biliary tract disease, rupture of a visceral abscess, or infection of indwelling foreign objects. Bacterial peritonitis in newborns is most commonly secondary. Thus, the organisms involved are mixed anaerobic and aerobic (Brook, 1989). The pathogenesis of peritonitis is multifactorial. First, many gut bacteria produce endotoxins, which activate inflammatory mediators such as tumor necrosis factor, interleukins, leukotrienes, and the complement system, all of which can cause increased vascular permeability and coagulation abnormalities. Anaerobes do not produce endotoxin but instead adhere to epithelial cells and produce exoenzymes such as hyaluronidase and protease. In addition, anaerobes possess capsules, which reduce the ability of immunoregulatory T cells to contain and compartmentalize infection. Moreover, there is a synergism of anaerobic and aerobic bacteria that is enhanced in the presence of irritants such as hemoglobin or bile. Finally, the exudation of intraperitoneal fluid that is triggered by these infections results in large fluid shifts, mechanical compromise of pulmonary function, and presence of a fibrinous glue, which may result in adherence of peritoneal surfaces to mesentery, resulting in abscess formation.

A new organism that has emerged as a causative agent of peritonitis is *Candida*, which is present in approximately 10% of cases of bowel perforation. Fungal peritonitis is more likely to occur in those infants who are extremely premature, require prolonged umbilical artery catheterization, have prolonged exposure to antibiotics, or require prolonged intubation (Karlowiez, 1993).

Management includes surgical drainage and antibiotics. Antifungal therapy also may be considered. In addition, aggressive rehydration and correction of electrolyte abnormalities must be provided. Mortality rates range from 33% to 80%, depending on the underlying cause (Bell, 1985).

## GASTROESOPHAGEAL REFLUX

### Physiology

Gastroesophogeal reflux (GER) refers to the retrograde movement of gastric contents into the distal esophagus. GER is a physiologic event that permits the clearance of air and other noxious materials from the stomach. Because gastric contents are acidic, and acidic material composes the wall of the air bubble cleared into the distal esophagus, mechanisms for returning acidic material to the stomach also must be present. Thus, these normal physiologic events require that the structures as well as the neural networks that mediate their function be intact and integrated. When this integrated system fails, acid reaches the distal esophagus, where it causes erosion. When this occurs, the patient is said to have gastroesophageal reflux disease (GERD). Many aspects of regulation of physiologic GER are limited in the neonate, but it remains unclear whether neonates have GER or GERD.

When food is ingested, swallowing triggers a series of sequential contractions that progress from the proximal esophagus to the distal esophagus, pushing the food bolus toward the stomach. The lower esophageal sphincter (LES) is a 1- to 2-cm segment of the distal esophagus that is identified functionally as an area of high pressure. Its primary function is to prevent reflux of gastric contents into the distal esophagus when active swallowing is not occurring. When a food bolus reaches the distal esophagus, interneuronal messages inhibit the tonic contraction of the LES. The LES relaxes and the food bolus is propelled into the stomach. The tone of the LES is further splinted by the diaphragmatic crura, which surround the LES like an elastic sling.

Only a minority of the peristaltic contractions in the esophagus of preterm infants are sequentially coordinated (Omari et al, 1995). In addition, the resting LES tone is low in the neonate, ranging from 5 to 10 mm Hg in the neonate, compared with 10 to 30 mm Hg in the adult (Novak, 1996). However, most infants with GERD have normal LES pressure (Kawahara et al, 1997). Factors other than intrinsic muscle tone affect LES pressure, including gastric distention, acute or chronic brain injury, position of the sphincter, angle of the indentation of the esophagus at entry of the stomach, and factors that alter sphincter circumference, such as edema, increases in intra-abdominal pressure, and delayed gastric emptying.

The diaphragmatic crura may offer limited splinting to the neonatal LES, as the LES is located 2 cm above the diaphragm for the first 6 postnatal months until it descends into the abdominal cavity (Moroz et al, 1976). Thus, when deep inspiration or straining causes increases in intra-abdominal pressure, this splinting mechanism may be limited in the neonate. Absence of the splinting mechanism may contribute to the high incidence of GERD among surviving infants with diaphragmatic hernia (Fasching et al, 2000).

Most episodes of physiologic GER occur during spontaneously during episodes of transient LES relaxation (TLESRs). It is thought that gastric distention triggers interneuronal pathways that trigger LES relaxation primarily to vent air (Cucchiara et al, 1998). Although LES relaxation can be triggered by swallows independently of peristaltic esophageal contractions, 82% of episodes of GER in preterm infants are associated with spontaneous TLESRs (Omari et al, 1998).

Once material has refluxed into the distal esophagus, mechanoreceptors and/or acid receptors trigger a series of peristaltic contractions in the distal esophagus to propel material back into the stomach. In addition, they trigger increased swallowing, which in turn provides a larger volume of saliva to buffer the acid (Helm et al, 1984). Thus, GERD may be the result of either increased GER or impaired clearance mechanisms.

### Presentation

In non-newborns, GER is clinically suspected when infants exhibit poor weight gain owing to regurgitation, nonspecific irritability, and apnea. Because of the use of parenteral nutrition to promote weight gain, neonates with GER rarely present with failure to thrive (Frakaloss et al, 1998). Newborns cannot verbalize pain; thus, GER also may manifest as recurrent fussiness, feeding aversion, bradycardia, or cyanotic episodes. However, many of these signs and symptoms are nonspecific, and trained observers cannot reliably identify the presence of GER using these indicators (Snel et al, 2000). GER occurs frequently in infants who have central nervous system abnormalities, bronchopulmonary dysplasia, cystic fibrosis, and esophageal atresia (Balson et al, 1998; Blecker et al, 1995; Dudley and Phelan, 1976; Lew et al, 1981). In addition, other neonatal intensive care unit (NICU) therapies may alter normal physiologic regulation and anatomic relationships to predispose the infant to developing GERD. Xanthines, used to treat apnea, reduce LES tone and increase gastric acid secretion (Berquist et al, 1984; Vandenplas et al, 1986). The use of gastric tubes may reduce LES pressure (Berezin et al, 1986). Increasing intra-abdominal pressure by delivering chest physiotherapy also may reduce LES pressure, increasing the occurrence of reflux (Newell et al, 1987). Infants spend considerably more time sleeping than do in children and adults, and LES basal pressure often falls during sleep (Sondheimer and Hoddes, 1992). There is also an association of GER with respiratory symptoms. GER occurs more commonly among infants with bronchopulmonary dysplasia and who have experienced acute life-threatening events (Gioffre et al, 1987; Veereman-Wauters et al, 1991). Moreover, the instillation of acidic agents into the distal esophagus can induce bronchospasm (Herve et al, 1986). The strong temporal association of GER and respiratory disease, however, has not been shown to be a causal one, and the mechanism for this association has not been delineated.

### Evaluation

Controversy currently surrounds issues related to diagnostic testing for GERD. Several techniques are available. Because of the limitations of the diagnostic techniques for newborns, many gastroenterologists proceed to a trial of therapy before extensive diagnostic studies are performed.

The barium swallow is the first study that should be done to evaluate GER. It is a poor method to demonstrate the presence of GER; rather it is used to confirm the presence of normal esophageal, gastric, and intestinal anatomy, because congenital anomalies in any of these structures may cause mild episodes of vomiting. Because this study is not performed under physiologic conditions (i.e., the patient is supine on a cold table, often crying or struggling, and provocative maneuvers such as abdominal compression may be used) and because the patient is monitored fluoroscopically for a brief period (generally <5 minutes), the frequency of GER demonstrated during these evaluations has little relationship with the presence of real reflux disease.

The pH probe is the most commonly used diagnostic test to evaluate GER. Testing is done by positioning a pH probe in the distal esophagus and measuring the frequency and duration of episodes of esophageal acidification over 18 to 24 hours. Placement of the probe is documented fluoroscopically or by estimation using the Strobel formula (Strobel et al, 1979). The neonatologist should be aware that interpretation of pH probe studies is limited by several factors. First, the ability to detect pH changes may be altered by the anatomic location of the probe. If the probe is located too proximally relative to the gastroesophageal junction, it may not detect reflux adequately; conversely, if it is located too distally, it inappropriately identifies the presence of acid. Second, the ability to detect acidosis up to 2 hours postprandially in infants is limited because milk buffers any acid contained in refluxate (Mitchell et al, 2001). As a result, as many as 85% of neonates may have false-negative studies (Hampton et al, 1990; Lee et al, 1999). Third, variability of infant position may alter variability of pH probe results (Hampton et al, 1990; Vandenplas and Sacre-Smits, 1985). The reflux index (RI), which consists of the sum of the periods in which pH is less than 4 as a percent of recording time, is the most widely used scoring system. An RI greater than 5% is abnormal in newborns (Vandenplas and Sacre-Smits, 1987).

Because all healthy persons have GER, a variety of techniques for scoring pH probe studies have been proposed (Orenstein et al, 1987a; Sutphen and Dillard, 1986; Vandenplas and Sacre-Smits, 1987). In general, the number of acid reflux episodes, the average duration of such episodes, and the overall proportion of time that the pH is less than 4 are quantified.

Esophagoscopy may be performed in larger neonates to visualize the distal esophagus and to obtain a biopsy specimen. A normal appearance does not exclude the presence of a histologic pathologic process (Biller et al, 1983). Acid exposure may cause basal zone hyperplasia and increased papillary length (Black et al, 1990).

Laryngoscopy and bronchoscopy may be helpful in evaluating infants with respiratory symptoms, as GER can occur in the absence of esophageal abnormalities (Blecker et al, 1995). Laryngoscopy may reveal the presence of vocal cord erosion or inflammation. Bronchoscopy may reveal the presence of milk-laden macrophages (Ahrens et al, 1999; Knauer-Fischer et al, 1999).

Technetium scintigraphy can be used to monitor for reflux, pulmonary aspiration, or both. Its ability to detect episodes is limited because it is performed during a single feeding and for a 2- to 3-hour postprandial period. Esophageal manometry rarely is used in the neonatal age group.

### Treatment

Conservative treatment to minimize GER includes positioning and dietary changes. A decade ago, infants with GER were positioned upright supine. This position for preterm newborns may place them at risk for airway obstruction if the head drops down on the chest (Orenstein et al, 1983). In a large controlled study, head elevation showed no benefit over the flat prone position (Orenstein, 1990). However, placing infants in the left lateral position may be safer and equally effective (Tobin et al, 1997). A supine position improves gastric emptying and decreases aspiration.

Because gastric distention may contribute to the occurrence of GER, infants may experience less GER if they are fed smaller volumes more frequently. Reflux occurs more typically postprandially, however, and the risk for GER may be increased with this practice. Another dietary manipulation is to add rice cereal to the milk. Although this measure does not reduce reflux, it does decrease emesis (Bailey et al, 1987; Orenstein et al, 1987b). Cow's milk protein allergy also can manifest with vomiting (see later section in this chapter). Thus, a 2-week trial of a hypoallergenic formula may be warranted (Iacono et al, 1996).

Transpyloric feeding can be used to provide enteral nutrition to premature infants who are not ready to feed orally and have GER associated with orogastric feeding. This feeding method may reduce symptoms sufficiently to allow enteral nourishment. Because GER in many healthy preterm infants is related to immaturity, the use of transpyloric feedings for 2 to 3 weeks may permit maturation to occur and avoid the complications that are associated with parenteral nutrition. The technique consists of placement of an unweighted Silastic tube in a transpyloric position under fluoroscopic guidance. This type of tube can be used without replacement for as long as 30 days. Milk is administered by slow continuous infusion.

Acid-suppressive agents may be used with or without prokinetics. Agents include histamine $H_2$ receptor antagonists, such as ranitidine or famotidine, and proton pump inhibitors. A randomized trial has shown $H_2$ receptor antagonists to be effective (Simeone et al, 1997). Trials using proton pump inhibitors, however, have not yet been done in neonates.

Prokinetic agents may enhance esophageal sphincter pressure and accelerate gastric emptying. However, no pharmacologic agent currently used can reduce the occurrence of transient LES relaxations. Bethanechol, a cholinergic drug, increases LES basal tone and overall forcefulness of esophageal peristalsis (Sondheimer and Arnold, 1986); however, it has not demonstrated consistent efficacy in clinical trials (Orenstein et al, 1986; Sondheimer et al, 1984), and it has a potential for exacerbating bronchospasm, which limits its use in infants with bronchopulmonary dysplasia. Metoclopramide, a dopamine antagonist, also increases gastric emptying and augments LES basal tone. Its efficacy is unknown, and it has been shown to increase episodes of reflux in one small trial (Machida et al, 1988). In addition, metoclopramide causes central nervous system side effects, an important limitation in infants recovering from respiratory distress syndrome who are trying to establish normal sucking skills (Putnam et al, 1992). Domperidone may be used as an alternative agent in countries where it is available, as central nervous system side effects are far less common with this drug. The U.S. Food and Drug Adminstration no longer approves cisapride, a noncholinergic nonantidopaminergic agent, for clinical use.

Surgical therapy is reserved for infants who have severe GER that results in recurrent pneumonia or life-threatening reactive airway disease, or has resulted in an acute life-threatening event (Ahrens et al, 1999; Orenstein, 2000). The most commonly used procedure is the Nissen fundoplication. Recent reports have shown that this procedure can be done laparoscopically (Esposito et al, 2001; Rothenberg, 1998). Kubiak and colleagues (1999) conducted a prospective follow-up evaluation of 66 infants to assess the efficacy of the procedure. They reported that improvement in clinical symptoms occurred in 90% of infants with isolated GER but in only 66% of infants who had primarily respiratory symptoms (i.e., apnea) and 58% of infants who had additional anomalies. In addition, 24 of their patients required revision of their fundoplication. Postoperative complications are common (Esposito et al, 2001; Subramaniam and Dickson, 2000; Wilkinson et al, 1987) and include failure of the wrap, overtightness of the wrap, and delayed gastric emptying. Because tincture of time provides improvement in GER in most patients, consideration should be given to the use of transpyloric feedings on a temporary basis in this population of infants to obviate the need for surgery.

## HIRSCHSPRUNG DISEASE

### Physiology

Hirschsprung disease, or congenital aganglionic megacolon, accounts for 20% to 25% of cases of neonatal intestinal obstruction. It is caused by agenesis of ganglion cells in the myenteric and submucosal plexuses. Recent data also suggest that the motility dysfunction is the result of reduced expression of the neuronal nitric oxide synthase gene at the messenger RNA level (Puri and Wester, 1998). The anus always is involved, with variable lengths of distal intestine affected. In 80% to 90% of the patients, involvement does not extend more proximally than the sigmoid colon, but in 8% to 10% of cases, the entire colon is involved. Because neural inhibitory input to affected areas is lacking, these areas of bowel are maintained in a tonic state, resulting in areas of functional intestinal obstruction.

It occurs in approximately one of 5000 births, with a 4:1 male-to-female incidence. Approximately 20% of infants with Hirschsprung disease have other, associated problems such as Down syndrome, Waardenburg syndrome, Smith-Lemli-Opitz syndrome, and central hypoventilation syndrome (Bonnet et al, 1996; Cass, 1990; Passarge, 1967; Rohrer et al, 2002).

Increasing evidence suggests that Hirschsprung disease may result from mutations in any of several genes, singly or in combination. Mutations of these genes may give dominant, recessive, or polygenic patterns of inheritance (Badner et al, 1990; Hofstra et al, 1997). Numerous genetic mutations have been identified to result in the common phenotype of Hirschsprung disease. Two groupings of genes, *RET/GDNF/NTN* and *EDNRB/EDN3/ECE-1*, are involved in signaling pathways, whereas another, *SOX10*, encodes a transcription factor. A truncating mutation of *SOX10* has been found in patients with Waardenburg syndrome with Hirschsprung disease (Touraine et al, 2000). From 30% to 50% of patients with familial Hirschsprung disease carry *RET* mutations, and 20% carry mutations in *EDNRB* (Chakravarti, 1996). In addition, Fujimoto and colleagues (1989) have shown that extracellular matrices in the human embryonic gut may influence final growth and maturation after neurons have completed migration and have "settled" in the gut.

### Presentation

Although Hirschsprung disease is congenital in etiology, only 15% of patients are actually diagnosed during the first month of life. Rather, a majority are diagnosed by 4 months, with some diagnoses delayed until early preschool age. During the newborn period, infants with Hirschsprung disease may pass their first meconium stool beyond 48 hours, have infrequent stooling, reluctance to feed, abdominal distention, or bilious vomiting. These signs and symptoms may be delayed in the preterm infant whose enteral feedings are initiated beyond the immediate newborn period. A small number of neonates will present with frank enterocolitis with diarrhea, dehydration, and shock.

Abdominal radiographs may demonstrate dilated gas- or fluid-filled loops of intestine. A barium enema may not be diagnostic in the newborn, as only 60% of studies will show the characteristic narrow rectosigmoid distal to a dilated sigmoid. The typical "transition zone" does not become apparent until the infant is 3 or 4 weeks of age. However, persistence of contrast in the rectosigmoid for more than 24 hours after the examination is highly suggestive of Hirschsprung disease. One should be aware that the barium enema is nondiagnostic in infants with total-colon Hirschsprung disease (De Campo et al, 1984).

The definitive diagnosis is made on rectal biopsy; suction biopsies performed at the bedside usually yield adequate specimens (Andrassy et al, 1981). A full-thickness biopsy at laparoscopy or laparotomy may be necessary in a small number of infants.

Hisrschsprung disease results from the absence of the intrinsic innervation of the distal colon, and both the myenteric and submucosal plexuses are absent. In contrast to the absence of the intrinsic innervation, the extrinsic innervation (i.e., the sympathetic and parasympathetic nerves derived from the spinal cord) may be increased as a result of the lack of feedback inhibition by the intrinsic nerves. These extrinsic neural trunks contain acetylcholinesterase, and staining for acetylcholinesterase has aided the accuracy of diagnosis, especially beyond 3 weeks of postnatal age, when the acetylcholinesterase-positive fibers have proliferated into the lamina propria. For the most accurate diagnosis, it is recommended that some diagnostic biopsy sections be stained with hematoxylin and eosin and some with acetylcholinesterase. Hirschsprung disease is diagnosed if neurons are absent in the hematoxylin and eosin–stained sections and the acetylcholinesterase stain is positive (Nakao et al, 2001).

### Treatment

Although the definitive treatment is surgical repair, there are three alternatives for initial treatment: rectal irrigation (Carcassonne et al, 1982), colostomy, and primary repair (Teitelbaum et al, 2000). Rectal irrigation may be used several times per day in patients whose aganglionic segments do not extend above the sigmoid. These irrigations decompress the intestine until further evaluation and growth are achieved in preparation for a definitive surgical repair. Alternatively, a colostomy is created proximal to the aganglionic segment, which is identified by perfoming serial biopsies. This procedure also permits decompression of the bowel and permits the infant to grow larger until a definitive repair can be done approximately 12 months later. As anesthetic techniques have improved, there has been a recent shift to attempt primary repair in the neonatal period, reserving the use of the colostomy for those patients who present with enterocolitis. In these latter patients, the colostomy permits the decompression of the bowel and permits time for the inflammatory changes from the enterocolitis to resolve.

Regardless, whether repair is done using two operations (i.e., the colostomy followed by a definitive repair) or one (i.e., primary repair), the classic operation for Hirschsprung disease consists of removal of the aganglionic segment and pulling the normally innervated bowel down to the anus. The major procedures are those of Swenson Duhamel, Soave-Boley, and Georgeson. For infants who have total colonic aganglionosis, total colectomy with creation of an ileostomy is usually performed. Regardless of the surgical technique used, infants may lose significant amounts of water and electrolytes postoperatively.

The most common cause of postoperative morbidity and mortality is the occurrence of enterocolitis (Reding et al, 1997). Infants with enterocolitis typically present with abdominal distention, diarrhea, and signs and symptoms of sepsis. Treatment includes rectal irrigations and antibiotics. Other complications that may occur are anal stricture, constipation, and cuff abscess.

### Prognosis

Although survival is excellent, long-term fecal continence may be problematic. Outcome is often related to the length of intestine affected (Reding et al, 1997). Outcome for total colonic aganglionosis is poor (Coran and Teitelbaum, 2000), as many of the affected infants will require multiple operations, experience poor growth, and fail to achieve fecal continence as adults (Tsuji et al, 1999).

## OTHER OBSTRUCTION SYNDROMES

The chronic idiopathic intestinal pseudo-obstruction syndrome comprises a group of motility disorders of both muscular and neurogenic origin, including the histologic entities called intestinal neuronal dysplasia (IND) and maturational arrest. Histologically, IND is characterized by hyperplasia of the enteric nerve plexuses, abnormal distribution of the neural elements, the presence of giant ganglia or etopic ganglia, and increased acetylcholinesterase activity (Puri and Wester, 1999). The presence of ganglioneuromas usually is associated with multiple endocrine neoplasia type IIB. Maturational arrest is characterized by hypoganglionosis and/or deficiency of neural and glial cell elements (Meier-Ruge et al, 1999). Patients may become symptomatic at any time, including during the neonatal period (Anuras et al, 1986). There is little correlation of clinical findings with histologic findings Symptoms include abdominal distention and vomiting. Prokinetics may provide some improvement. Laxatives and enemas may relieve symptoms due to IND or MA. In general, surgical intervention usually is not successful; however, internal sphincter myectomy may be helpful for some patients with IND (Dickson and Variend, 1983). Treatment consists of long-term parenteral nutritional support.

A variant of pseudo-obstruction is the megacystis–microcolon–intestinal hypoperistalsis syndrome, as described by Berdon and associates (1976). In newborns, this condition has been termed the "neonatal hollow visceral myopathy syndrome" by Puri and colleagues (1983), who also provided a review. Rarely seen in males, this disorder manifests in the newborn period with signs of a bowel obstruction. In addition, bilateral flank masses (hydronephrotic kidneys) and a single large midline abdominal mass (megacystis) suggest an obstructive uropathy. Ultrasound examination, voiding cystourethrogram, and barium enema are diagnostic. Surgical exploration usually reveals a massively dilated bladder and a short, malfixed small intestine with a microcolon. Adequate peristalsis never returns, so that long-term parenteral nutrition is necessary.

## COW'S MILK PROTEIN ALLERGY

### Definition

Cow's milk protein allergy (CMPA) has been defined as an adverse reaction occurring after the ingestion of cow's milk as a result of immunologic hypersensitivity to milk protein(s) (Hill et al, 1986). Adverse reactions may have a wide range of clinical manifestations, including gastrointestinal processes such as colitis and protein-losing enteropathy and more poorly defined symptoms including bronchitis, colic, and atopic dermatitis (Odze et al, 1995; Walther and Kootstra, 1983).

### Epidemiology

The frequency of CMPA ranges from 2% to 6% (Hill, 1996; Hill and Hosking, 1997; Host et al, 1988). It occurs more frequently in infants fed cow's milk or a cow's milk–based formula than in those fed human milk. Nonetheless, it does occur in approximately 0.5% of breast-fed infants (Jakobsson and Lindberg, 1979) because of maternal ingestion of cow milk protein and transfer of antigenic proteins to human milk (Host et al, 1988; Saarinen et al, 1999).

Although the specific cause of CMPA is unknown, it frequently displays a familial incidence (Cookeston, 1998). Several studies have also suggested that ingestion of cow's milk formula in the first weeks of life may increase the incidence of allergic symptoms (Host et al, 1988); however, this effect has not been confirmed by others (Lindfors and Enocksson, 1988). Acute infectious gastroenteritis also has been identified as a risk factor for developing CMPA (Cow's milk allergy [Italian Collaborative Study], 1988) because of the increased absorption of macromolecules during an acute infection (Stintzing et al, 1986).

### Differential Diagnosis

Symptoms of CMPA tend to be nonspecific. Approximately 50% to 60% of infants present with gastrointestinal or skin symptoms and 30% with respiratory symptoms (Sampson, 1997). The diagnosis of CMPA is confirmed when clinical improvement occurs when a milk-free diet is given and relapse occurs when a milk challenge is given (Goldman et al, 1963).

There are no specific biochemical tests for CMPA. Some investigators have found evaluation of immunoglobulins to be helpful but not diagnostic (Cow's milk allergy [Italian Collaborative Study], 1988). The presence of cow's milk–specific IgE and an index of lymphocyte stimulation with beta-lactoglobulin is the most sensitive (88%) and specific (67%) test for predicting whether a clinical reaction to cow's milk protein will occur (Tainio and Savilahti, 1990). Jejunal biopsies usually are not necessary to diagnose CMPA in newborns (Sumithran and Lyngkaran, 1977). If biopsy specimens are obtained, however, they demonstrate partial or total villus atrophy or an increase in the presence of eosinophils in the lamina propria, epithelial mucosa, or muscularis mucosae (Savilahti and Verkasalo, 1984). Biopsies may be useful to demonstrate the absence of parasites, ova, or crypt architectural abnormalities (Odze et al, 1995).

#### Management

The management of CMPA is the removal of cow's milk protein from the diet. Some clinicians advocate the use of soy protein–based formulas as an initial therapeutic approach (Businco et al, 1992). As many as 30% of infants who have CMPA, however, exhibit allergy to soy protein (Kleinman, 1992; Powell, 1978). Thus, it is currently recommended that soy-based formulas not be used in treatment of CMPA (American Academy of Pediatrics, 1983, 2000; Joint Statement of ESPACI and ESPGHAN, 1999).

*Hypoallergenic formulas* contain hydrolyzed protein to decrease their allergenic potential. Casein hydrolysate formulas are more extensively hydrolyzed and cause less allergic reactions (Businco et al, 1989; Wahn et al, 1992). On rare occasions, infants may remain allergic to these formulas, and an elemental diet consisting of free amino acids as the protein source may be needed (Odze et al, 1995).

Breast-fed infants with CMPA usually improve when dairy products are removed from the mother's diet (Barau and Dupont, 1994). If severe colitis persists in breast-fed infants, however, hypoallergenic or elemental formulas may be necessary. Sensitivity to cow's milk protein decreases with age. As many as 28% of children with CMPA are tolerant of milk protein by 2 years of age and 78% by 6 years of age (Bishop et al, 1990).

## PANCREAS-RELATED DISORDERS

### Shwachman Syndrome

Shwachman syndrome is characterized by pancreatic insufficiency, bone marrow dysfunction, and poor growth (Aggett et al, 1980; Mack, 1996). The defect appears to be with enzyme secretion and acinar function, not bicarbonate secretion and duct function (Hill et al, 1982). Thus, serum trypsinogen concentrations are low, resulting in steatorrhea (Ginzberg et al, 1999). The presence of neutropenia is almost universal, although the presence of neutropenia may be intermittent (Ginzberg et al, 1999). Infants also may have thrombocytopenia or anemia, and approximately 20% will have pancytopenia (Ginzberg et al, 1999). Skeletal anomalies often are present, especially of the rib cage. The cause of Shwachman syndrome is genetic, but the mode of inheritance is unknown. Clinically, affected infants present with neutropenia and failure to thrive. Although pancreatic enzyme replacement improves nutrition, most will have short stature. The mortality rate is high (30%) because of recurrent infections (Mack, 1996) and the risk for leukemia (Woods et al, 1981).

### Persistent Hyperinsulinemic Hypoglycemia of Infancy

Persistent hyperinsulinemic hypoglycemia of infancy (PHHI), or nesidioblastosis, typically manifests in a macrosomic infant who develops recurrent episodes of hyoglycemia. Aggressive glucose administration is required to maintain normoglycemia (Aynsley-Green et al, 1981). The diagnosis is made by confirming the presence of hyperinsulinemia when hypoglycemia is present. The diagnosis of PHHI requires the presence of an elevated insulin concentration concurrent with glucose less than 40 mg/dL on at least two or more occasions. (See Chapter 93 for a full discussion of this condition.)

## SELECTED READING

Biller JA, Winter HS, Grand RJ, et al: Are endoscopic changes predictive of histologic esophagitis in children? J Pediatr 103:215, 1983.

## REFERENCES

### Ascites and Peritonitis

Ahmed S: Neonatal and childhood ovarian cysts. J Pediatr Surg 6:702, 1971.

Arnold WC, Redman JF, Seibert JJ: Analysis of peritoneal fluid in urinary ascitis. South Med J 79:591, 1986.

Banani SA, Bahador A, Nezakatoo N: Idiopathic perforation of the extrahepatic bile duct in infancy: pahtogenesis, diagnosis, and management. J Pediatr Surg 28:950, 1993.

Bell MJ: Peritonitis in the newborn—current concepts. Pediatr Clin North Am 32:1181, 1985.

Brook I: A 12-year study of aerobic and anaerobic bacteria in intraabdominal and postsurgical abdominal wound infections. Surg Gynecol Obstet 169:387, 1989.

Cochran WJ, Klish WJ, Brown MR, et al: Chylous ascites in infants and children: A case report and literature review. J Pediatr Gastroenterol Nutr 4:668, 1985.

Farhat W, McLorie G, Capolicchio G, et al: Outcomes of primary valve ablation versus urinary tract diversion in patients with posterior urethral valves. Urology 56:653, 2000.

Karlowiez MG: Risk factors associated with fungal peritonitis in very low birth weight neonates with severe necrotizing enterocolitis: A case control study. Pediatr Infect Dis J 12:574, 1993.

Mann CM, Leape LL, Holder TM: Neonatal urinary ascites: A report of 2 cases of unusual etiology and a review of the literature. J Urol 111:124, 1974.

Roth KS, Carter WH Jr, Chan JC: Obstructive nephropathy in children: Long term progression after relief of posterior urethral valve. Pediatrics 107:1004, 2000.

Yang WT, Ho SY, Metrewdi C: Case report: Antenatal diagnosis of meconium peritonitis and subsequent evolving meconium pseudocyst formation without peritoneal calcification. Clin Radiol 52:477, 1997.

### Gastroesophageal Reflux


Ahrens, P, Heller K, Beyer P, et al: Antireflux surgery in children. Pediatr Pulmonol 28:89, 1999.

Ahrens P, Noll C, Ketz R, et al: Lipid-laden alveolar macrophages (LLAM): A useful marker of silent aspiration in children. Pediatr Pulmonol 28:83, 1999.

Bailey DJ, Andres JM, Danek GD, et al: Lack of efficacy of thickened feeding as treatment for gastroesophageal reflux. J Pediatr 110:187, 1987.

Balson BM, Kravityz EK, McGeady SJ: Diagnosis and treatment of gastroesophageal reflux in children and adolescents with severe asthma. Ann Allergy Asthma Immunol 81:159, 1998.

Berezin S, Schwartz SM, Halata MS, et al: Gastroesophageal reflux secondary to gastrostomy tube placement. Am J Dis Child 140:699, 1986.

Berquist WE, Rachelefsky GS, Rowshan N, et al: Quantitative gastroesophageal reflux and pulmonary function in asthmatic children and normal adults receiving placebo, theophylline, and metaproterenol sulfate therapy. J Allergy Clin Immunol 73:253, 1984.

Blecker U, dePont SM, Hauser B, et al: The role of "occult" gastroesophageal reflux in chronic pulmonary disease in children. Acta Gastroenterol Belg 58:348, 1995.

Black DD, Haggitt RC, Orenstein SR, et al: Esophagitis in infants. Morphometric histological diagnosis and correlation with measures of gastroesophageal reflux. Gastroenterology 98:1408, 1990.

Byrne WJ, Euler AR, Campbell M: Body position and esophageal sphincter pressure in infants. Am J Dis Child 136:523, 1982.

Cucchiara S, Staiano A, DiLorenzo C, et al: Pathophysiology of gastroesophageal reflux and distal esophageal motility in children with gastroesophageal reflux disease. J Pediatr Gastroenterol Nutr 7:830, 1988.

Dudley NE, Phelan PD: Respiratory complications in long-term survivors of esophageal atresia. Arch Dis Child 51:279, 1976.

Esposito C, Montupet P, Reinberg O: Laparoscopic surgery for gastroesophageal reflux disease during the first year of life. J Pediatr Surg 36:715, 2001.

Fasching, G, Huber, A, Uray, E, et al: Gastroesophageal reflux and diaphragmatic motility after repair of congenital diaphragmatic hernia. Eur J Pediatr Surg 10:360, 2000.

Frakaloss G, Burke G, Sanders MR: Impact of gastroesophageal reflux on growth and hospital stay in premature infants. J Pediatr Gastroenterol Nutr 26:146, 1998.

Gioffre RM, Burin S, Mitchell I: Antereflux surgery in infants with bronchopulmonary dysplasia. Am J Dis Child 141:648, 1987.

Hampton FJ, MacFadyen UM, Simpson H: Reproducibility of 24 hour esophageal pH studies in infants. Arch Dis Child 65:1249, 1990.

Helm JF, Dodds WJ, Pelc LR, et al: Effect of esophageal emptying and saliva on clearance of acid from the esophagus. N Engl J Med 310:284, 1984.

Herve P, Denjean A, Jian R, et al: Intraesophageal perfusion of acid increases the bronchomotor response to methacholine and to isocapnic hyperventilation in asthmatic patients. Am Rev Respir Dis 134:986, 1986.

Iacono G, Carroccio A, Cavataio F, et al: Gastroesophageal reflux and cow's milk allergy in infants: A prospective study. J Allergy Clin Immunol 97:822, 1996.

Kawahara H, Dent J, Davidson G: Mechanisms responsible for gastroesophageal reflux in children. Gastroenterol 113:399, 1997.

Knauer-Fischer S, Ratjen F: Lipid-laden macrophages in bronchoalveolar lavage fluid as a marker for pulmonary aspiration. Pediatr Pulmonol 217:419, 1999.

Kubiak R, Spitz L, Keily EM, et al: Effectiveness of fundoplication in early infancy. J Pediatr Surg 34:295, 1999.

Lee W, Beattie R, Meadows N, Walker-Smith J: Gastroesophageal reflux: Clinical profiles and outcome. J Paediatr Child Health 35:568, 1999.

Lew C, Keens T, O'Neal M, et al: Gastroesophageal reflux prevents recovery from bronchopulmonary dysplasia. Clin Res 29:149A, 1981.

Machida HM, Forbes DA, Gall DG, Scott RB: Metoclopramide in gastroesophageal reflux of infancy. J Pediatr 112:483, 1988.

Mitchell DJ, McClure BG, Tubman TRJ: Simultaneous monitoring of gastric and esophageal pH reveals limitations of conventional oesophageal pH monitoring in milk fed infants. Arch Dis Child 84:273, 2001.

Moroz SP, Esponoza J, Cumming WA, et al: Lower esophageal sphincter function in children with and without gastroesophageal reflux. Gastroenterology 71:236, 1976.

Newell SJ, Booth IW, Morgan MEI, et al: Gastroesophageal reflux in the pre-term infant. Pediatr Res 22:104, 1987.

Novak DA: Gastroesophageal reflux in the preterm infant. Clin Perinatol 23:305, 1996.

Omari TI, Barnett C, Snel A, et al: Mechanisms of gastroesophageal reflux in healthy preterm infants. J Pediatr 133:650, 1998.

Omari TI, Miki K, Fraser R, et al: Esophageal body and lower esophageal sphincter function in healthy premature infants. Gastroenterology 109:1757, 1995.

Orenstein SR: Management of supraesophageal complications of gastroesophageal reflux disease in infants and children. Am J Med 108(suppl 4a):139S, 2000.

Orenstein SR: Prone positioning in infant gastroesophageal reflux: Is elevation of the head worth the trouble? J Pediatr 117:184, 1990.

Orenstein SR, Klein HA, Rosenthal MS: Simultaneous comparison of pH probe and scintigraphy for gastroesophageal reflux (GER). Gastroenterology 92:1561, 1987a.

Orenstein SR, Lofton SW, Orenstein DM: Bethanechol for pediatric gastroesophageal reflux: A prospective, blind, controlled study. J Pediatr Gastroenterol Nutr 5:549, 1986.

Orenstein SR, Magill HL, Borrks P: Thickening of infant feedings for therapy of gastroesophageal reflux. J Pediatr 110:181, 1987b.

Orenstein SR, Whitington PF, Orenstein DM: The infant seat as treatment for gastroesophageal reflux. N Engl J Med 309:760, 1983.

Putnam PE, Orenstein SR, Wessel HB, et al: Tardive dyskinesia associated with use of metoclopramide in a child. J Pediatr 121:983, 1992.

Rothenberg SS: Experience with 220 consecutive laparoscopic Nissen fundoplications in infants and children. J Pediatr Surg 33:274, 1998.

Simeone D, Caria MC, Miele E, et al: Treatment of childhood peptic esophagitis: A double-blind placebo-controlled trial of nizatidine. J Pediatr Gastroenterol Nutr 25:51, 1997.

Snel A, Barnett CP, Cresp TL, et al: Behavior and gastroesophageal reflux in the premature neonate. J Pediatr Gastroenterol Nutr 30:3, 2000.

Sondheimer J, Arnold G: Early effects of bethanechol on the esophageal motor function of infants with gastroesophageal reflux. J Pediatr Gastroenterol Nutr 5:47, 1986.

Sondheimer JM, Hoddes E: Gastroesophageal reflux with drifting onset in infants: A phenomenon unique to sleep. J Pediatr Gastroenterol Nutr 15:418, 1992.

Sondheimer JM, Mintz HL, Michaels M: Bethanechol treatment of gastroesophageal reflux in infants: Effect on continuous esophageal pH records. J Pediatr 104:128, 1984.

Spitz L, Kirtane J: Results and complications of surgery for gastroesophageal reflux. Arch Dis Child 66:743, 1985.

Strobel CT, Byrne WJ, Ament ME, Euler AR: Correlation of esophageal lengths in children with height: Application to the Tuttle test without prior esophageal manometry. J Pediatr 49:81, 1979.

Subramaniam R, Dickson A: Long-term outcome of Boix-Ochoa and Nissen fundoplication in normal and neurologically impaired children. J Pediar Surg 35:1214, 2000.

Sutphen JL, Dillard VL: Effects of maturation and gastric acidity on gastroesophageal reflux in infants. Am J Dis Child 140:1062, 1986.

Tobin JM, McCloud P, Cameron DJ: Posture and gastro-oesophageal reflux: A case for left lateral positioning. Arch Dis Child 76:254, 1997.

Vandenplas Y, DeWolf D, Sacre L: Influence of xanthines on gastroesophageal reflux in infants at risk for sudden infant death syndrome. Pediatrics 77:807, 1986.

Vandenplas Y, Sacre-Smits L: Seventeen-hour continuous esophageal pH monitoring in the newborn: Evaluation of the influence of position in asymptomatic and symptomatic babies. J Pediatr Gastroenterol Nutr 4:356, 1985.

Vandenplas Y, Sacre-Smits L: Continuous 24-hour esophageal pH monitoring in 285 asymptomatic infants 0-15 months old. J Pediatr Gastroenterol Nutr 6:220, 1987.

Veereman-Wauters G, Bochner A, VanCaillie-Bertrand M: Gastroesophageal reflux in infants with a history of near miss sudden infant death syndrome. J Pediatr Gastroenterol Nutr 12:319, 1991.

Wilkinson JD, Dudgeon DL, Sondheimer JM: A comparison of medical and surgical treatment of gastroesophageal reflux in severely retarded children. J Pediatr 99:202, 1987.

### Hirschsprung Disease

Andrassy R, Issacs H, Weitzman J: Rectal suction biopsy for the diagnosis of Hirschsprung's disease. Ann Surg 193:419, 1981.

Angrist M, Bolk S, Thiel B, et al: Mutation analysis of the RET receptor kinase in Hirschsprung disease. Hum Mol Genet 4:821:830, 1995.

Anuras S, Metros FA, Soper RT, et al: Chronic intestinal pseudo obstruction in young children. Gastroenterology 91:62, 1986.

Badner JA, Sieber WK, Garver KL: A genetic study of Hirschsprung's disease. Am J Hum Genet 46:568, 1990.

Berdon WE, Baker DH, Blanc WA, et al: Megacystis-microcolon-intestinal hypoperistalsis syndrome: a new cause of intestinal obstruction in the newborn. Report of radiologic findings in five newborn girls. Am J Roentgenol 126:957, 1976.

Bonnet JP, Till M, Edery P, et al: Waardenburg-Hirschsprung disease in two sisters: A possible clue to the genetics of this association? Eur J Pediatr Surg. 6:245, 1996.

Byrne WJ, Cipil L, Ruler AR, et al: Chronic idiopathic intestinal pseudo-obstruction syndrome in children: Clinical characteristics and prognosis. J Pediatr 90:585, 1977.

Carcassonne M, Morrisson-Lacombe G, Letourneau JN: Primary corrective operation without decompression in infants less than three months of age with Hirschprung's disease. J Pediatr Surg 17:241, 1982.

Cass D: Aganglionosis: Associated anomalies. Paediatr Child Health 26:351, 1990.

Chakravarti A: Endothelin receptor–mediated signaling in Hirschsprung disease. Hum Mol Genet 5:303, 1996.

Coran AG, Teitelbaum DH: Recent advances in the management of Hirschrsprung's disease. Am J Surg 180:382, 2000.

De Campo J, Mayne V, Boldy D, et al: Radiological findings in total aganglionosis coli. Pediatr Radiol 14: 205, 1984.

Dickson JAS, Variend S: Colinic neuronal dysplasia. Acta Paediatr Scand 72:635, 1983.

Ditesheim JA, Templeton JM: Short-term versus long-term quality of life in children following repair of high imperforate anus. J Pediatr Surg 22:581, 1987.

Dow E, Cross S, Wolgemuth DJ, et al: Second locus for Hirschsprung disease/Waardenburg syndrome in a large Mennonite kindred. Am J Med Genet 53:75, 1994.

Fujimoto T, Hata J, Yokoyama S, et al: A study of the extracellular matrix protein as the migration pathway of neural crest cell for the gut: Analysis in human embryos with special reference to the pathogenesis of Hirschsprung's disease. J Pediatr Surg 24:550, 1989.

Hofstra RMW, Osinga J, Buys CHCM: Mutations in Hirschsprung disease: When does a mutation contribute to the phenotype? Europ J Hum Genet 5:180, 1997.

Joseph VT, Sim CK: Problems and pitfalls in the management of Hirschsprung's disease. J Pediatr Surg 23:398, 1988.

Meier-Ruge WA, Brunner LA, Engert J: A correlative morphometric and clinical investigation of hypoganglionosis of the colon in children. Eur J Pediatr Surg 9:67, 1999.

Nakao M, Suita S, Taguchi T, et al: Fourteen-year experience of acetylcholinesterase staining for rectal mucosal biopsy in neonatal Hirschsprung's disease. J Pediatr Surg 36:1357, 2001.

Passarge E: The genetics of Hirschspring's disease. Evidence for heterogeneous etiology and a study of sixty-three families. N Engl J Med 276:138, 1967.

Ponder BA: The gene causing multiple endocrine neoplasia type 2 (MEN 2). Ann Med 26:199, 1994.

Puri P, Lake BD, Gorman F, et al: Megacystis-microcolon-intestinal hypoperistalsis syndrome: a visceral myopathy. J Pediatr Surg 18:64, 1983.

Puri P, Wester T: Intestinal neuronal dysplasia. Semin Pediatr Surg 7:181, 1998.

Reding R, deVille de Goyet J, Gosseye S, et al: Hirschsprung's disease: A 20-year experience. J Pediatr Surg 32:1221, 1997.

Rohrer T, Trachsel D, Engelcke G, Hammer J: Congenital central hypoventilation syndrome associated with Hirschsprung's disease and neuroblastoma: Case of multiple neurocristopathies. Pediatr Pulmonol 33:71, 2002.

Sagel SD, Cohen H, Townsend SF: Neonatal Hirschsprung disease, dysautonomia, and central hypoventilation. Obstet Gynecol 93:834, 1999.

So HB, Schwartz DL, Becker JM, et al: Endorectal "pull-through" without preliminary colostomy in neonates with Hirschprung's disease. J Pediatr Surg 15:470, 1980.

Teitelbaum DH, Cilley RE, Sherman NJ, et al: A decade of experience with the primary pull-through for Hirschsprung disease in the newborn period. A multicenter analysis of outcomes. Ann Surg 232:372, 2000.

Touraine RL, Attie-Bitach T, Manceau E: Neurologic phenotype in Waardenburg syndrome type 4 correlates with novel *SOX10* truncating mutations and expression in developing brain. Am J Hum Genet 66:1496, 2000.

Tsuji H, Spitz L, Kiely EM, et al: Management and long-term follow-up of infants with total colonic aganglionosis. J Pediatr Surg 34:158, 1999.

Vintzileos AM, Eisenfeld LI, Herson VC, et al: Megacystis–microcolon–intestinal hypoperistalsis syndrome. Am J Perinatol 3:297, 1986.

### Cow's Milk Protein Allergy

American Academy of Pediatrics Committee on Nutrition: Hypoallergenic infant formulas. Pediatrics 106:346, 2000.

American Academy of Pediatrics Committee on Nutrition: Soy-protein formulas: Recommendations for use in infant feeding. Pediatrics 72:359, 1983.

Barau E, Dupont C: Allergy to cow's milk proteins in mother's milk or in hydrolyzed cow's milk infant formulas as assessed by intestinal permeability measurements. Allergy 49:295, 1994.

Bishop JM, Hill DJ, Hosking CS: Natural history of cow milk allergy: Clinical outcome. J Pediatr 116:862, 1990.

Businco L, Bruno G, Biampietro PG, Cantani A: Allergenicity and nutritional adequacy of soy protein formulas. J Pediatr 121:S21, 1992.

Businco L, Cantai A, Lohghi A, Giampietro PG: Anaphylactic reactions to a cow's milk whey protein hydrolysate (Alfa-Ré, Nestlé) in infants with cow's milk allergy. Ann Allergy 62:333, 1989.

Cow's milk allergy in the first year of life: An Italian Collaborative Study. Acta Paediatr Scand Suppl 348:1, 1988.

Cookeston WOCM: Genetic aspects of atopic allergy. Allergy 53:9, 1998.

Goldman AS, Anderson DW, Sellers WA, et al: Milk allergy: I. Oral challenge with milk and isolated milk proteins in allergic children. Pediatrics 32:425, 1963.

Hill DJ: Cow milk allergy in infancy and early childhood. Clin Exp Allergy 26:243, 1996.

Hill DJ, Firer MA, Shelton MJ, Hosking CS: Manifestations of milk allergy in infancy: Clinical and immunologic findings. J Pediatr 109:270, 1986.

Hill DJ, Hosking CS: Emerging disease profiles in infants and young children. Pediatr Allergy Immunol 10:21, 1997.

Host A, Husby S, Hansen L, Osterballe O: A prospective study of cow's milk allergy in exclusively breast fed infants. Incidence and pathogenic role of early inadvertant exposure to cow's milk formula and characterization of bovine milk protein in human milk. Acta Paediatr Scand 77:663, 1988.

Host A, Husby S, Hansen L, Osterballe O: Bovine beta-lactoglobulin in human milk from atopic and non-atopic mothers. Relationship to maternal intake of homogenized and nonhomogenized milk. Clin Exp Allergy 95:547, 1990.

Jakobsson I, Lindberg T: A prospective study of cow's milk protein intolerance in Swedish infants. Acta Paediatr Scand 68:853, 1979.

Joint Statement of ESPACI and ESPGHAN: Dietary products used in infants for treatment and prevention of food allergy. Arch Dis Child 81:80, 1999.

Kleinman RE: Cow milk allergy in infancy and hypoallergenic formulas. J Pediatr 121:LS116, 1992.

Lindfors A, Enocksson E: Development of atopic disease after early administration of cow milk formula. Allergy 43:11, 1988.

Odze RD, Wershel BK, Leichtner AM, Antonioli DA: Allergic colitis in infants. J Pediatr 126:163, 1995.

Powell GK: Milk- and soy-induced enterocolitis of infancy. Clinical features and standardization of challenge. J Pediatr 93:553, 1978.

Saarinen KM, Juntunen-Backman K, Jarvenpaa AL, et al: Supplementary feeding in maternity hospitals and the risk of cow's milk allergy: A prospective study of 6209 infants. J Allergy Clin Immunol 104:457, 1999.

Sampson HA: Immediate reactions to food in infants and children. In Metcalfe DD, Sampson HA, Simon RA (eds): Food Allergy: Adverse Reactions to Foods and Food Additives. Boston, Blackwell Scientific Publications, 1997, p 169.

Savilahti E, Verkasalo M: Intestinal cow's milk allergy: Pathogenesis and clinical presentation. Clin Rev Allergy 2:7, 1984.

Stintzing G, Johansen K, Magnusson KE, et al: Intestinal permeability in small children during and after rotavirus assessed with different-size polyethyleneglycols (PEG 400 and PEG 1000). Acta Paediatr Scand 75:1005, 1986.

Sumithran E, Lyngkaran N: Is jejunal biopsy really necessary in cow's milk protein intolerance? Lancet 1:1122, 1977.

Tainio VM, Savilahti E: Value of immunologic tests in cow milk allergy. Allergy 45:189, 1990.

Wahn U, Wahl R, Rugo E: Comparison of the residual allergenic activity of six different hydrolyzed protein formulas. J Pediatr 121:S80, 1992.

Walther FJ, Kootstra G: Necrotizing enterocolitis as a result of cow's milk allergy? Z Kinderchir 38:110, 1983.

#### Pancreas-Related Disorders

Aggett PJ, Cavanaugh NPC, Matthew DJ: Shwachman's syndrome. Arch Dis Child 55:331, 1980.

Aynsley-Green A, Polak JM, Bloom SR, et al: Nesidioblastosis of the pancreas: Definition of the syndrome and management of severe neonatal hyperinsulinemic hypoglycemia. Arch Dis Child 56:496, 1981.

Ginzberg H, Shin J, Ellis L, et al: Shwachman syndrome: Phenotypic manifestations of sibling sets and isolated cases in a large patient cohort are similar. J Pediatr 135:81, 1999.

Mack DR, Forstner GG, Wilschanski M: Shwachman syndrome: exocrine pancreatic dysfunction and variable phenotypic expression. Gastroenterology 111:1593, 1996.

Woods WG, Roloff JS, Lukens JN, et al: The occurrence of leukemia in patients with the Shwachman syndrome. J Pediatr 99:425, 1981.

CHAPTER 73

# Abdominal Wall Problems

Carol Lynn Berseth and Dan Poenaru

## DISORDERS OF THE UMBILICAL REGION

The umbilical region is the site of intricate, complex activity during embryonic life. Early in gestation, a widely open communication exists between the yolk sac and primitive gut. Later, the entire midgut passes through this communication to form a large physiologic umbilical hernia that persists in utero for several weeks. Thereafter, the gut returns to its position in the abdominal cavity. By the third trimester, the aperture around the vessels, omphalomesenteric (vitelline) duct, and urachus begins to narrow. After birth, the umbilical arteries contract, blood flow ceases, their intimal and medial layers undergo aseptic necrosis, and the stump separates. Alterations in this orderly but complex sequence of events result in serious congenital anomalies.

## UMBILICAL CORD LESIONS

### Noncoiled Umbilical Blood Vessels

The three vessels within the cord are coiled to form a helical structure. The number of twists can vary greatly (ranging from 0 to 40) and, rarely, reaches 380 per cord. Left-twisted vessels outnumber right-twisted vessels 7 to 1. Absence of any twists occurs in about 4% to 5% of pregnancies (Edmonds, 1954). The helical structure is identifiable by ultrasound examination by the end of the first trimester. Although how the vessels come to have this geometric arrangement has not been established, such a configuration—like that of a telephone cord—is more able to resist external compression, stretch or torsion, and the cord remains flexible (Strong et al, 1993). The absence of coils is associated with increased abnormalities that include single umbilical artery, trisomy 21, and coarctation of the aorta. Approximately 10% of infants without coils are stillborn, and the incidence of preterm birth is greater than expected.

### Single Umbilical Artery

Normally the umbilical cord is composed of two arteries and a vein. A single umbilical artery occurs in 1% of single births and in 7% of twin births. In approximately a third of these infants, gastrointestinal obstructive lesions and urogenital abnormalities are present. The presence of single umbilical artery is higher among aborted fetuses and thus is thought to be a marker for increased fetal risk (Persutte and Hobbins, 1995; Pierce, 2001). Among newborns with single umbilical artery, there is a higher incidence of poor fetal growth (Leung and Robinson, 1989) and a slightly increased risk for renal anomalies (Thummala et al, 1998) Therefore, the presence of a single umbilical artery warrants careful physical examination for other anomalies and consideration of further imaging after birth.

### Granuloma of the Umbilicus

If the separation of the umbilical stump is delayed beyond 5 to 8 days after birth, granulation tissue may be produced, delaying epithelialization. Granulomas must be differentiated from everted gastric or intestinal mucosa, which permits the entrance of a fine probe. Treatment for both is judicious desiccation with silver nitrate.

### Delay in Separation of the Cord

If the umbilical cord fails to separate after more than 14 days, investigation for a possible defect in neutrophil function and chemotaxis should be undertaken.

## ABDOMINAL WALL DEFECTS

### Umbilical Hernia

The umbilical ring is formed when the mesoderm of the muscle and fascia around the umbilical vessels and urachus contracts. Umbilical hernias are caused by failure of closure of the umbilical ring; unlike with omphaloceles, skin and subcutaneous tissue cover the defect. These lesions are found in 30% of African-American infants and in 4% of white infants; there is a high familial incidence. The condition is more common in low-birth-weight babies and in infants with Down syndrome.

The actual fascial defect varies in size, ranging from 1 to 4 cm in diameter. The sac may contain a loop of bowel that is easily pushed back into the abdomen, or some preperitoneal fat. Approximately 80% of these hernias close spontaneously by 3 to 4 years, and the risk of incarceration is exceedingly low (Fig. 73–1). Spontaneous closure is less likely in hernias with fascial defects greater than 1.5 cm. Surgical correction is therefore only indicated in large-defect hernias, in children over 4 to 6 years of age, or if symptoms occur (Poenaru et al, 2001) (Fig. 73–2).

### Omphalocele

#### Definition and Epidemiology

*Omphalocele* refers to a congenital defect in the formation of the umbilical portion of the abdominal wall that is larger than 4 cm in diameter (Table 73–1; Figs. 73–3, 73–4, and 73–5). The defect occurs in 1 in 6000 to 1 in 10,000 live births. Although many are isolated defects, some are part of a constellation of malformations (such as Beckwith-Wiedemann syndrome or trisomy 18), and a few cases are associated with maternal ingestion of valproic acid for seizure control (Boussemart et al, 1995). Omphalocele is also present in infants who have the OEIS complex, a constellation of anomalies that includes omphalocele, bladder exstrophy, imperforate anus, and spinal defects

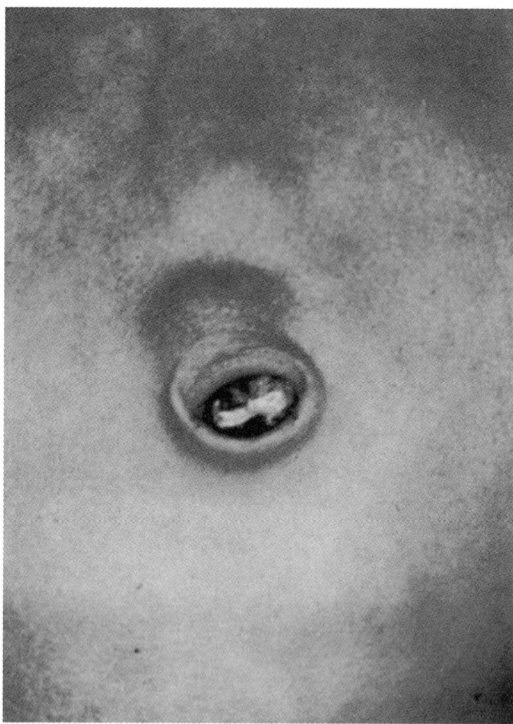

**FIGURE 73–1.** Two definite bulges are seen cephalad to the umbilicus, one above the other. Two distinct apertures could be felt in the midline. This finding represents a minor defect of the abdominal wall.

**TABLE 73–1**

**Characteristics of Gastroschisis and Omphalocele**

| Defect | Gastroschisis | Omphalocele |
|---|---|---|
| Covering sac | Absent | Present, but may be torn |
| Fascial defect | Small | Small or large |
| Cord attachment | Onto the abdominal wall | Onto the sac |
| Herniated bowel | Edematous | Normal |
| Prematurity (%) | 50-60 | 10-20 |
| Associated anomalies (%) | 10-15 | 45-55 |
| Gastrointestinal | 18 | 37 |
| Cardiac | 2 | 20 |
| Trisomy syndromes | — | 30 |
| Necrotizing enterocolitis (%) | 18 | Only if sac is ruptured |
| Malabsorption | Common | Only if sac is ruptured |

(Keppler-Noreuil, 2001.) Because of the nature of the developmental defect, all infants with omphalocele have malrotation.

### Etiology

Early in fetal life, the small intestine lies outside of the abdominal cavity. By the 10th week, the midgut returns to the abdomen, and the somatic layers of the cephalic, caudal, and lateral folds join to close the defect in the abdominal wall. For unknown reasons, this closure may not occur. Several types of omphalocele are recognized, based on the fold that fails to close. *Epigastric omphalocele* occurs when there is abnormal closure of the cephalic fold. Because these somites form the lower thoracic wall, failure of closure results in the Cantrell pentalogy, which includes cleft sternum, diaphragmatic defects, pericardial defects, cardiac anomalies, and omphalocele. *Classic omphalocele* occurs when there is an interruption in lateral fold development, resulting in an abdominal wall defect that lies between the epigastric and hypogastric regions. In addition to loops of bowel, liver also may herniate through the abdominal wall defect. The umbilicus arises from an anterior position on the omphalocele, and the muscular abdominal wall is normal. Failure in closure of the caudal fold results in a *hypogastric omphalocele*. Associated defects include bladder exstrophy and imperforate anus (Fig. 73–6).

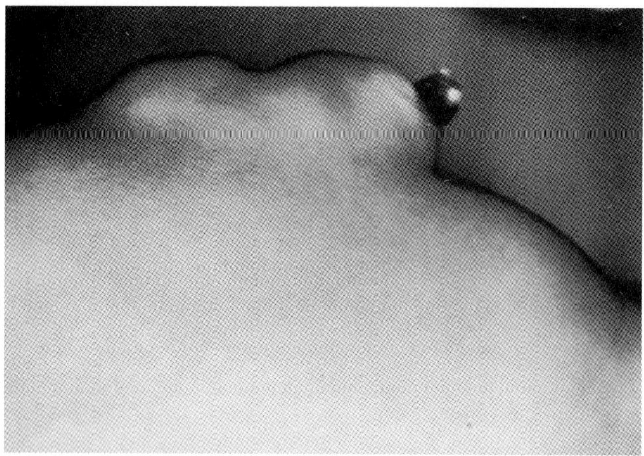

**FIGURE 73–2.** Large triangular herniation at and above the umbilicus. The bulge contained easily reducible bowel. A large aperture could be felt just above the umbilicus and a second, smaller one several centimeters above. Between them the rectus muscles were diastatic. This is a large defect of the abdominal wall demanding surgical closure.

### Diagnosis

Alpha-fetoprotein (AFP) is synthesized in the fetal liver and is excreted by the fetal kidneys. It also crosses the placenta and appears in the maternal circulation by 12 weeks of gestation. Maternal plasma levels of AFP are elevated when fetuses have neural tube defects, abdominal wall defects, or atresia of the duodenum or esophagus. Maternal serum AFP is used as a screening test although there is a 40% rate of false-positive results. Analysis of amniotic AFP and acetylcholinesterase-pseudocholinesterase can be sensitive in detecting abdominal wall defects, especially gastroschisis (Saleh et al, 1993; Saller et al, 1994). Human chorionic gonadotropin levels have shown promise in small series to detect abdominal wall defects (Schmidt et al, 1993).

Ultrasound evaluation is not useful during the first trimester because the midgut normally is herniated.

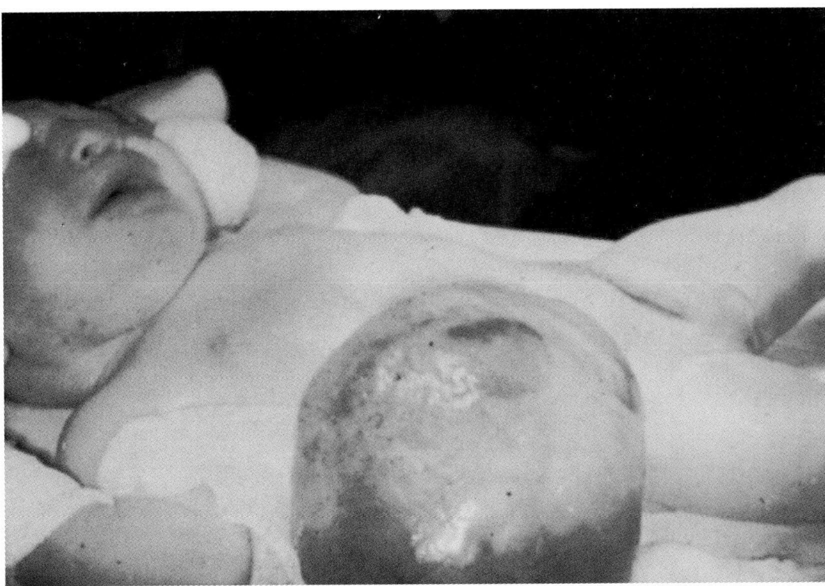

**FIGURE 73–3.** A mass is seen protruding from the umbilical region. No specific structure can be identified. It is covered by whitish, glistening membrane and obviously is an omphalocele.

Therefore, current recommendations are for use of this modality beyond 14 weeks (Cyr et al, 1986). The combined use of maternal serum AFP and ultrasound examination at 19 weeks has been shown in a series of 8000 patients to have excellent sensitivity in identifying abdominal wall defects (Luck, 1992). Once an abdominal wall defect has been identified, ultrasound examination often can distinguish omphalocele from gastroschisis. Because the association of cardiac anomalies and chromosomal disorders is high, fetal echocardiography and amniocentesis should also be performed. Vaginal delivery does not adversely affect outcome; therefore, the need for cesarean section should be based on obstetric indications alone (Lewis et al, 1990; Sipes et al, 1990). If not discovered prenatally, the diagnosis is obvious at birth. If the sac ruptures, the bowel loops may become edematous and matted together, mimicking gastroschisis.

### Treatment

The presence of exteriorized bowel results in heat loss and extravasation of fluid and provides a major portal of entry for bacteria. When the omphalocele is first seen, the sac should be kept moist by wrapping it with gauze sponges that have been soaked in warmed normal saline. A plastic covering is then wrapped around the defect to limit water and heat loss. Care should be taken to place the contents above the abdomen if the patient is prone, to prevent kinking of mesenteric vessels. Alternatively, the infant can be positioned on the side, with the exteriorized bowel in an anterior position. A nasogastric tube is passed to decrease the accumulation of air in the bowel. The infant should be given 1.5 times the maintenance intravenous fluid volume and broad-spectrum antibiotics. Thereafter, any inspection and manipulation of the abdominal contents should be done with sterile gloves.

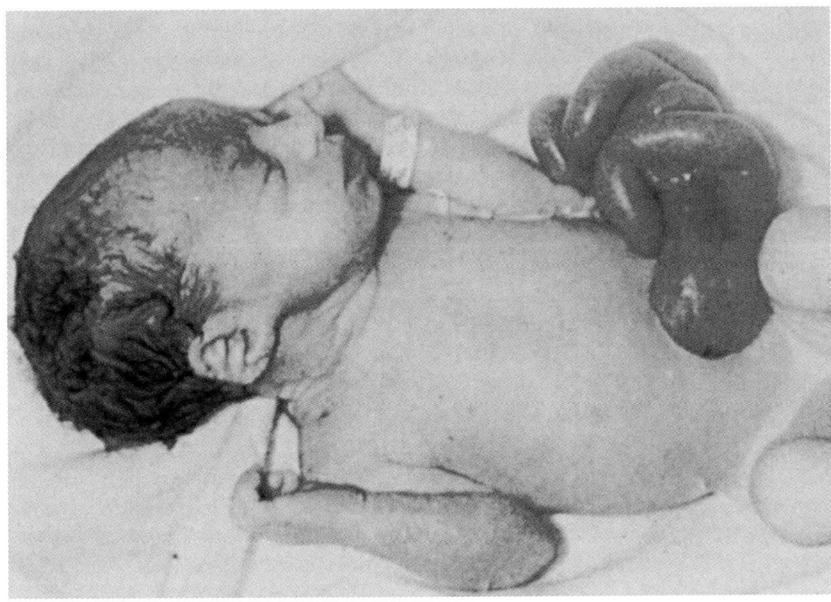

**FIGURE 73–4.** Omphalocele in which the containing amniotic-peritoneal membrane must have been torn away during the delivery. Loops of bowel lie free on the abdominal wall. *(Courtesy of Dr. Arnold Tramer, Baltimore, Maryland.)*

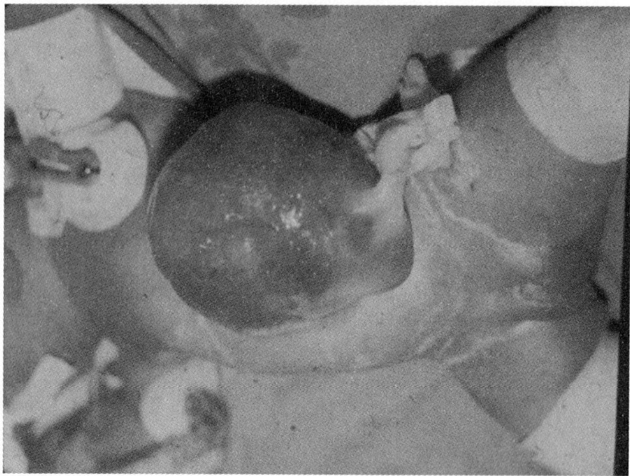

**FIGURE 73–5.** (See also Color Plate 73–5.) Male newborn with omphalocele. The fascial defect is large, situated at the base of the umbilical cord, covered by a glistening membrane and containing both liver and bowel.

Operative repair should be done as soon as possible, ideally within 2 to 4 hours of birth. Small defects can be closed with a single-stage repair. For larger defects, primary repair may cause respiratory failure and abdominal compartment syndrome because the abdominal cavity is too small to accommodate the bowel. Complications of compartment syndrome include renal failure, hypotension from vena cava compression, hepatic ischemia, and intestinal ischemia. In affected infants, a staged repair is performed using a prosthetic device called a *silo* to cover the defect. After the bowel is gradually pushed into the abdominal cavity over 7 to 10 days, finally closure can be achieved (Schuster, 1979).

Postoperatively, protracted ileus may occur, necessitating prolonged parenteral nutrition. Attention also must be directed to the diagnosis and management of associated anomalies.

### Prognosis

The mortality rate with associated heart disease is 80%. In the absence of heart disease, 70% to 90% of infants with omphalocele survive (Forrester and Merz, 1999; Kitchanan et al, 2000).

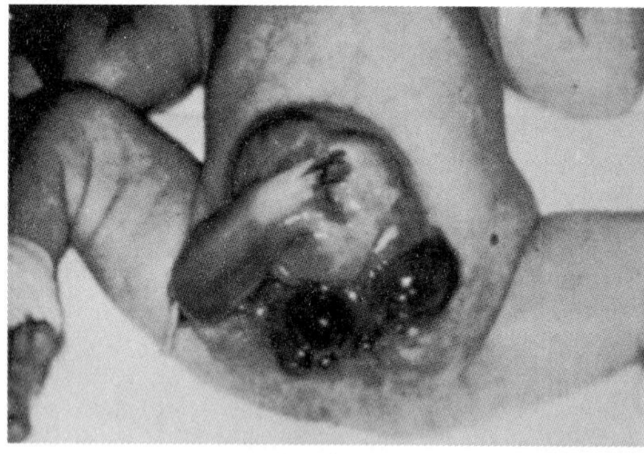

**FIGURE 73–6.** A combination of omphalocele and ectopia vesicae. The bright structure below the omphalocele is an everted, exstrophic bladder.

## Cord Hernia

A small omphalocele is called a *cord hernia*. By definition, the defect in the abdominal wall is less than 4 cm in diameter, and the exteriorized sac contains only loops of bowel (Figs. 73–7 and 73–8). This defect arises between the 8th and 10th weeks as a result of failure of closure of the umbilical ring. Cord hernias can be missed at birth, and the intestine can be injured by careless application of the cord clamp. Otherwise, these defects are easily managed by primary closure at birth and have an excellent outcome.

## Gastroschisis

### Definition and Epidemiology

Gastroschisis is the herniation of abdominal contents through an abdominal wall defect, usually occurring on the right side of a normally positioned umbilical cord (Fig. 73–9; see also Table 73–1). This lesion was traditionally less frequent than omphalocele, but its incidence appears to be increasing worldwide (Penman et al, 1998). The defect appears most common among young mothers and those of low gravidity (Yang et al, 1992). Associated anomalies are found in only 15% of patients, the vast majority being intestinal atresias (Snyder et al, 2001). Infants with gastroschisis tend to have intrauterine growth retriction (Forrester and Merz, 1999; Tan et al, 1996).

### Etiology

Although the cause of these lesions is not known, many investigators speculate that they may be of vascular origin. Intrauterine interruption of the omphalomesenteric artery has been proposed, an explanation that accounts for many of the clinically observed differences between this lesion and omphalocele (Hoyme et al, 1981).

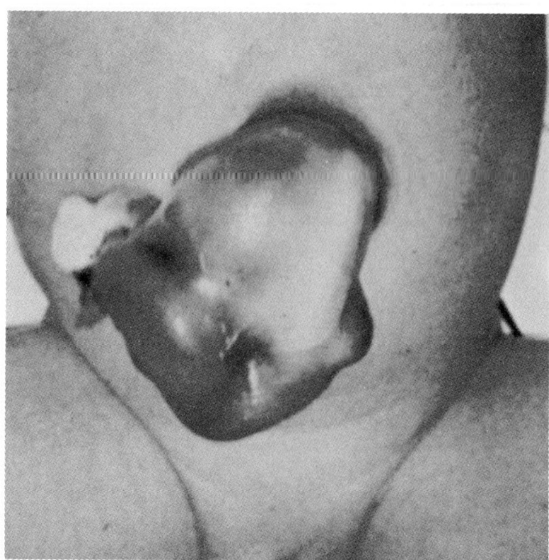

**FIGURE 73–7.** A comparatively small mass protrudes from the umbilical region, and a loop of bowel can be readily recognized running around its lower margin. The mass is completely covered by shiny transparent membrane—clearly an umbilical cord hernia.

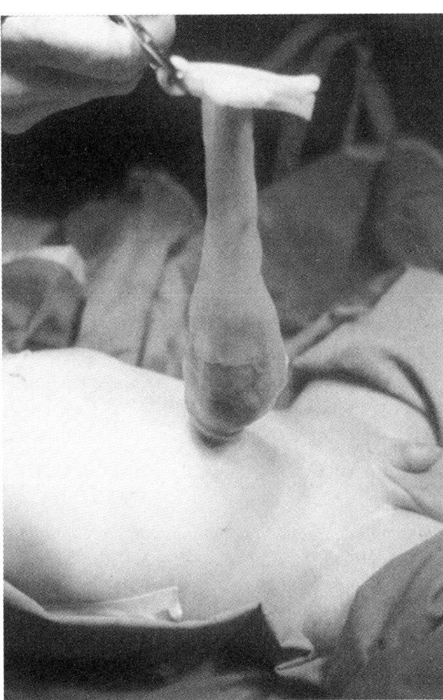

**FIGURE 73–8.** (See also Color Plate 73–8.) Hernia of the umbilical cord. This is in fact a small omphalocele, containing only bowel loops in a small sac within the umbilical cord.

### Diagnosis and Treatment

As described for omphalocele, gastroschisis can be correctly diagnosed prenatally. Because the peritoneal sac is absent, the fetal bowel is continuously bathed in amniotic fluid, which results in a significant intestinal "peel," causing poor intestinal motility. As with omphalocele, the need for cesarean section should be restricted to obstetric indications only, despite some isolated evidence that prelabor cesarean section results in better outcome because of the resulting absence of the fibrous peel (Moore et al, 1999).

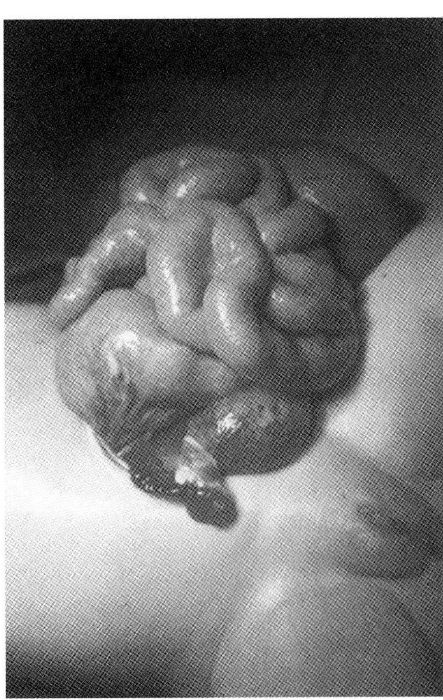

**FIGURE 73–9.** (See also Color Plate 73–9.) Female newborn with gastroschisis. The fascial defect is relatively small and situated to the right of the umbilical cord and contains exposed bowel (as well as an ovary in this instance).

The diagnosis is readily made at birth. The entire gastrointestinal tract usually is eviscerated, but unlike with omphalocele, the liver is not exteriorized. The intestinal loops usually are covered by a thick fibrous "peel," which makes them firm, often with a cauliflower-like appearance. Intestinal atresias may be apparent as well. Rare complications include intrapartum mesenteric disruption, prenatal volvulus, and closure of the abdominal wall defect around the exteriorized gut. All of these events can cause catastrophic intestinal loss.

As described for omphalocele, the bowel contents should be kept moist and relatively sterile at birth. A nasogastric tube is passed for decompression, and 1.5 times the maintenance intravenous fluid volume is given. Broad-spectrum antibiotics also should be started. Because the abdominal wall defect often is small, vascular compromise occurs more readily, and great care should be taken to position the infant and the exteriorized bowel to prevent kinking of mesenteric vessels. Unlike with omphalocele, primary closure is possible in 90% of patients, but larger defects may require staged repair. Postoperatively, prolonged ileus often occurs because of intestinal dysmorphology, which often includes the myenteric plexus. Affected infants are at increased risk for necrotizing enterocolitis (Oldham et al, 1988). Intestinal atresias usually are not repaired at the initial procedure because of the fibrous peel and therefore require repair at 3 to 4 weeks of age (Snyder et al, 2001).

### Prognosis

Mortality rates have decreased to 5% to 10% (Forrester and Merz, 1999; Kitchanan et al, 2000; Snyder, 1999). Postoperative recovery may be longer in infants undergoing repair of gastroschisis than in those undergoing repair of omphalocele. Enteral feedings may not be established until 2 months after operation, and some infants will require home parenteral nutrition (Molik et al, 2001). In spite of these initial feeding difficulties, most gastroschisis survivors maintain normal growth during infancy and childhood (Davies and Stringer, 1997).

## Prune-Belly Syndrome

*Prune-belly syndrome* refers to a triad of anomalies consisting of a deficiency of abdominal musculature, cryptorchidism, and urinary tract abnormalities. The most common urinary tract anomalies seen in this triad are megaloureter, cystic renal dysplasia, urethral obstruction, and megacystis (Lattimer, 1958). Malrotation occurs in 30% of the cases, and cardiac anomalies in 20%. The syndrome rarely occurs in females, and its exact cause is unknown. Theories include failure in the development of the abdominal wall between the sixth and eighth weeks of gestation and primary urethral obstruction with early bladder distention (Moerman et al, 1984). At birth, the defect is obvious on inspection. The abdomen is shapeless, and the skin hangs in wrinkled folds. There may be an open patent urachus, which by itself signals a poor prognosis. Of immediate concern is evaluation for and relief of urinary tract obstruction. Approximately 20% of patients with prune-belly syndrome die in the neonatal period from renal dysplasia or pulmonary hypoplasia, but of those who survive, 30% develop renal failure during childhood (Burbige et al, 1987). Surgical management of the genitourinary tract remains controversial, with advocates of both watchful waiting and major reconstruction. The latter should be performed only where specialized surgical and anesthesia expertise are available, as the surgery is challenging and postoperative complications are frequent (Snow and Duckett, 1987). The undescended testes are corrected in childhood for monitoring and psychological reasons.

### Inguinal Hernia

The gonads are formed during weeks 5 to 12 of gestation. The testes descend through the internal ring at 28 weeks. In the general population, inguinal hernias occur in 1% of all live births. The incidence of inguinal hernia in low-birth-weight and very low-birth-weight infants is as follows: with birth weights of 500 to 1000 g, 42%; with birth weights of 1000 to 1500 g, 10%; and with birth weights of 1500 to 2000 g, 3% (Peevy et al, 1986). With preterm delivery and the accompanying increase in intra-abdominal pressure, testicular descent and inguinal canal closure do not take place, thus explaining the increased incidence of inguinal hernia (Fig. 73–10).

Additional risk factors for inguinal hernias are cystic fibrosis, congenital dislocation of the hip, presence of a ventriculoperitoneal shunt, and abdominal wall defects. Incarceration and strangulation are common in infant hernias. The combined incidence of these complications appears to be as high as 30% (Rowe and Clatworthy, 1970), although it appears to be lower in preterm infants. Therefore, repeated examinations may be necessary, particularly if the infant's clinical status becomes unstable or if a tense, fluctuant scrotal mass or vomiting develops. Most of these incarcerated hernias may be reduced nonoperatively by placing the infant in the Trendelenburg position with sedation and application of an ice pack to the inguinal-scrotal area (Scherer and Grosfeld, 1993). Successful reduction should be followed by surgical repair in 24 to 48 hours (allowing for resolution of local edema). Failure of reduction necessitates immediate surgical repair.

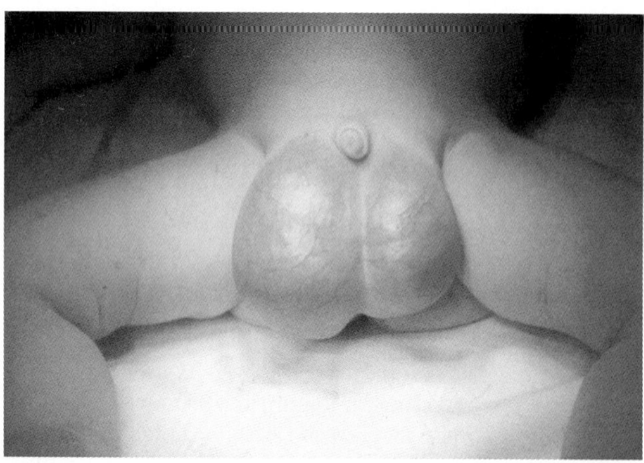

**FIGURE 73–10.** (See also Color Plate 73–10.) Large bilateral inguinal hernias in a previously premature infant.

Nonincarcerated hernias in infants require repair as soon as convenient, preferably within 1 to 2 weeks of diagnosis. Premature babies are best served with repair just before their discharge from the neonatal intensive care unit, or very soon afterward. Postoperative apnea is common in preterm infants, and postoperative overnight admission for apnea monitoring is therefore indicated for outpatients until 48 weeks of postconceptional age. The lowest incidence of apneas occurs with surgery performed using spinal block without sedation (Somri et al, 1998). Other specific postoperative complications include persistent scrotal swelling, recurrence, testicular atrophy, and injury to the vas deferens. Contralateral exploration is probably not indicated in most cases, as the actual risk of a metachronous hernia has been estimated at only 5% to 15% (Surana and Puri, 1993). The most common complication of operative repair is postoperative apnea.

### Hydrocele

A *hydrocele* is a collection of fluid in the scrotum without an obvious inguinal hernia. The typical hydrocele is noted at or shortly after birth as a unilateral or bilateral swelling in the scrotum, which may fluctuate in size.

The scrotum is enlarged, may be very tense with fluid, and usually is nontender, often with a bluish appearance; the inguinal canal is normal. Differentiation between hydrocele and hernia is critical and may be difficult in the infant. Transillumination is useful, but findings must be interpreted cautiously, as fluid or gas-filled bowel may transilluminate in small infants. An irreducible nontender groin or scrotal mass probably is a hydrocele.

The recommended management of a hydrocele is observation during the first 1 or 2 years of life, unless a hernia cannot be excluded. Hydroceles that persist or appear beyond that age are unlikely to resolve spontaneously, and affected infants should therefore undergo elective surgical repair.

## URACHAL LESIONS

The urachus is the remnant of the allantois that extends from the bladder portion of the cloaca to the umbilicus. The urachus may remain completely patent throughout its length or fail to obliterate (Fig. 73–11). All varieties of this defect are rare, and treatment is customized to each (Ney and Friedenberg, 1968).

### Completely Patent Urachus

A completely patent urachus manifests with the passage of urine from the umbilicus. Radiopaque contrast material injected into the orifice outlines the urachal tract and fills

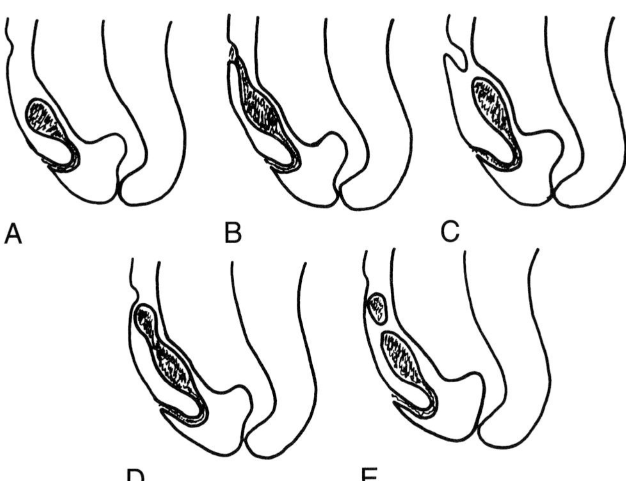


**FIGURE 73-11.** Urachal anomalies. **A,** Normal anatomy. **B,** Completely patent urachus. **C,** Blind external tract: urachal sinus. **D,** Blind internal tract: Bladder diverticulum. **E,** Urachal cyst.

the bladder. Treatment consists of surgical excision of the umbilicus along with the entire urachus and a small portion of the bladder. Results usually are good.

### *Blind External Type*

When only the distal end of the urachus fails to obliterate, a draining sinus results. Drainage of urine begins sometime after the cord separates. Treatment consists of surgical excision of the sinus tract.

### *Blind Internal Type*

Failure of obliteration of the proximal end of the urachus results in a bladder diverticulum. It produces no symptoms and may be coincidentally discovered on cystogram. Nothing needs to be done surgically.

### Urachal Cyst

Incomplete obliteration of the midportion of the urachus leads to the development of a urachal cyst. Cysts may present at birth or may grow slowly and become obvious at any time during infancy or childhood. The cysts frequently become infected. Ultrasound examination is diagnostic. Treatment involves surgical resection, which may be preceded by incision and drainage of the superimposed abscess.

## MALFORMATIONS OF THE OMPHALOMESENTERIC DUCT

In the developing embryo, the omphalomesenteric (vitelline) duct connects the yolk sac to the primitive midgut through the umbilical cord. In the normal course of ontogeny, the duct becomes obliterated and disappears. Under certain circumstances, all or portions of the duct may persist (Fig. 73–12). They may cause symptoms through drainage, infection, and intestinal obstruction. As with urachal remnants, presentation and management vary with each type (Moore, 1996).

### Patent Omphalomesenteric Duct

Patent omphalomesenteric duct is an enteroumbilical fistula, manifesting with the passage of meconium or fecal matter through the umbilicus. The condition may begin at birth or occur within 1 to 2 weeks. The most significant danger with this lesion is evagination (prolapse) of the small bowel through the umbilical orifice, with a significant increase in mortality. Once this lesion is diagnosed, it should be corrected by surgical excision of the umbilicus and the duct.

### Omphalomesenteric Sinus

Failure of distal closure of the omphalomesenteric duct leads to the formation of a sinus. Persistent watery discharge from the umbilical cord is the initial presentation. Examination of the umbilicus reveals a red nodule projecting from the base. Gentle massage results in the extrusion of mucus, which differentiates this lesion from an umbilical granuloma. Injection of radiopaque contrast material outlines the sinus tract. Treatment consists of surgical excision.

### Omphalomesenteric Duct Cyst

When the middle portion of the omphalomesenteric duct persists and eventually fills with secretions, a cyst forms. This lesion may be detected as an enlarging umbilical mass. Treatment consists of surgical excision.

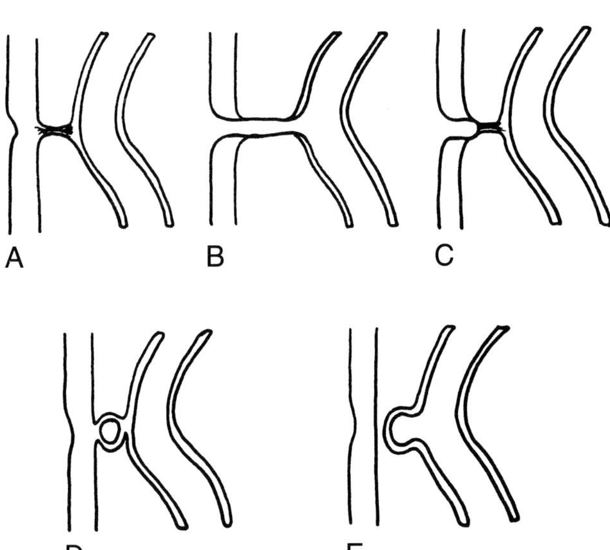


**FIGURE 73-12.** Omphalomesenteric (vitelline) duct anomalies. **A,** Normal anatomy. **B,** Patent omphalomesenteric duct. **C,** Blind external tract: umbilical sinus. **D,** Omphalomesenteric duct cyst. **E,** Blind internal tract: Meckel diverticulum.

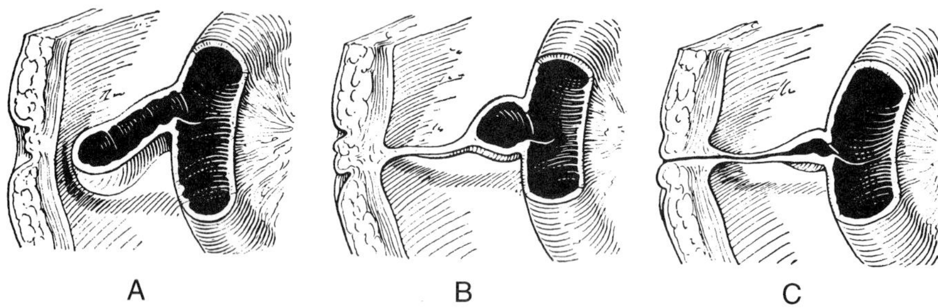


**FIGURE 73–13.** Meckel diverticulum of the ileum. **A,** Ordinary blind sac. **B,** Diverticulum continued to umbilicus as a cord. **C,** Diverticulum with fistulous opening of umbilicus. *(From Arey LB: Developmental Anatomy, 7th ed. Philadelphia, WB Saunders, 1974.)*

## Meckel Diverticulum

When the proximal, or intestinal, end of the omphalomesenteric duct fails to become obliterated completely, an outpouching of the ileum persists. The diverticulum may vary in size, shape, and point of attachment, although the junction usually lies at some point in the ileum. It must arise from the antimesenteric side of the bowel, a feature that distinguishes Meckel diverticulum from duplications. Its distal end usually lies free in the peritoneal cavity, but in some cases it is attached to the umbilicus by a fibrous cord and in a small minority remains patent to the umbilicus (omphalomesenteric fistula) (Fig. 73–13). Twenty percent of diverticula contain ectopic pancreatic or gastric tissue.

Meckel diverticulum manifests clinically with bowel obstruction, intestinal bleeding, inflammation, or perforation (St.-Vil et al, 1991). A pancreatic or gastric mass may act as a leading point to produce intussusception. Gastric mucosa may cause peptic ulceration and bleeding; the latter is almost always the presenting sign if Meckel diverticulum becomes symptomatic. The fibrous cord, if present, may produce intestinal obstruction. Rarely, inflammation of the diverticulum may lead to peritonitis.

The diagnostic test of choice for Meckel diverticulum is a technetium 99m pertechnetate scan ("Meckel scan"), which detects the ectopic gastric mucosa (Fig. 73–14). This test is most useful in patients presenting with rectal bleeding—the false-negative rate is high in patients with other symptoms. Treatment is reserved for symptomatic diverticula and those thought to contain ectopic tissue (Moore, 1996). Diverticulectomy can be performed by either laparotomy or laparoscopy (Huang and Lin, 1993).

### Incidence

A Meckel diverticulum can be discovered in 1.5% to 2% of all persons. Only a small proportion of these diverticula ever become symptomatic, and when they do, this usually happens beyond the age of 4 months. Only exceptionally do they cause illness in the neonatal period. Affected males outnumber females in a ratio of 3:1 to 5:1.

### Diagnosis

Hemorrhage from the bowel is the definitive sign of Meckel diverticulum. A few cases in older children and adults may produce the signs and symptoms of diverticulitis, but this condition has never been described in young infants. Hemorrhage is often sudden and catastrophic, causing a precipitous fall in the hematocrit and a shocklike state within a few hours. The first few stools passed may be composed almost entirely of unchanged blood; later, they become burgundy colored and then tarry. In other instances, bleeding is constant and occult. About

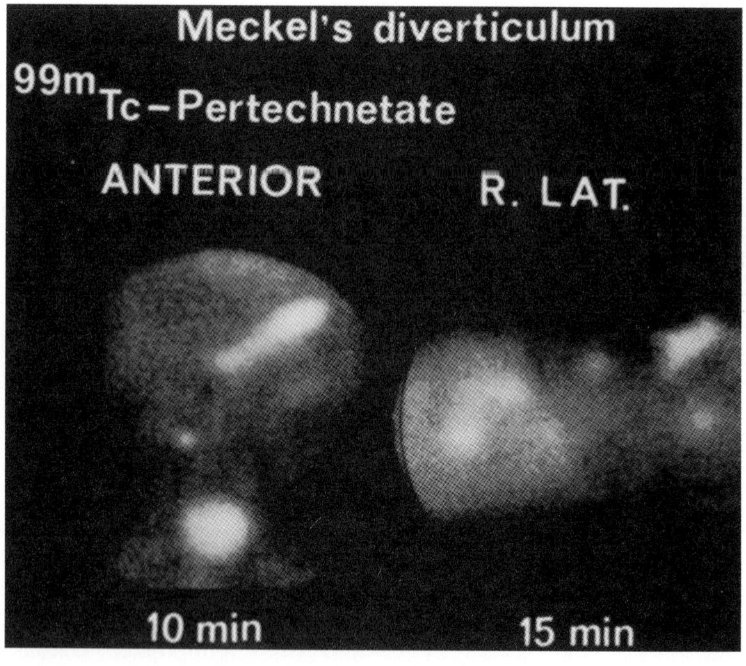


**FIGURE 73–14.** Anterior gamma camera view of the abdomen of a 2-year-old infant. Note the small, well-defined area of increased uptake located in the right lower quadrant. The stomach and bladder also are visualized. On the lateral view, some radioactivity is evident on the diaper as well. *(Courtesy of Dr. S. Treves, Children's Hospital, Boston, Massachussetts.)*

25% of persons with Meckel diverticulum present with intussusception.

Meckel diverticulum must be differentiated from other disorders that produce gross bleeding from the bowel: peptic ulcer, duplication, intestinal polyp, intussusception, and intestinal hemangioma. Fissure in ano, proctitis, and ulcerative colitis ordinarily do not lead to gross hemorrhage, blood loss being confined to the passage of bloody mucus or of stools containing a surface accumulation of blood. The most useful point in the differential diagnosis is that hematemesis usually coexists with rectal bleeding when peptic ulcer is present, whereas hematemesis rarely occurs with Meckel diverticulum. The mass of duplication is sometimes palpable.

Scans after intravenous injection of technetium-99 m pertechnetate are often, but not always, diagnostic of Meckel diverticulum because the technetium is concentrated in gastric mucosa. Pentagastrin or cimetidine is useful in enhancing the image of gastric mucosa on subsequent technetium scans (see Fig. 73–14).

### Treatment

Resuscitation and blood replacement therapy is the initial treatment regardless of the cause of bleeding. If bleeding ceases, careful observation for recurrence of bleeding is often all that is indicated, because peptic ulcer rarely recurs. A second episode of bleeding, however, strongly suggests that other diagnostic procedures may be needed, including endoscopy, laparoscopy, and laparotomy. If a diverticulum is discovered, it must be excised.

## SELECTED READING

Abrahamson J: Repair of inguinal hernias in infants and children. Clin Pediatr 12:617, 1973.

## REFERENCES

Adzick NS, Vacanti I, Lillehei CW, et al: Fetal hernia: Ultrasound diagnosis and clinical outcome in 38 cases. J Pediatr Surg 24:654, 1989.

Bloss RS, Aranda JV, Beardmore HE: Congenital diaphragmatic hernia: Pathophysiology and pharmacologic support. Surgery 89:518, 1981.

Boussemart T, Bonneau D, Levard G, et al: Omphalocele in a newborn baby exposed to sodium valproate in utero. Eur J Pediatr 154:220, 1995.

Burbige KA, Amodio J, Berdon WE, et al: Prune-belly syndrome: Thirty-five years of experience. J Urol 137:86, 1987.

Cyr DR, Mack LA, Schoenecker SA, et al: Bowel migration in the normal fetus: US detection. Radiology 161:119, 1986.

Davies BW, Stringer MD: The survivors of gastroschisis. Arch Dis Child 77:158, 1997.

Edmonds HW: The spiral twist of the normal umbilical cord in twins and singletons. Am J Obstet Gynecol 67:102, 1954.

Forrester MB, Merz RD: Epitdemiology of abdominal wall defects, Hawaii, 1986-1997. Teratology 60:117, 1999.

Glick PL, Harrison MR, Adzick NS, et al: The missing link in the pathogenesis of gastroschisis. J Pediatr Surg 20:406, 1985.

Goldfine C, Haddow JE, Knight GJ, et al: Amniotic fluid alphafetoprotein and acetylcholinesterase measurements in pregnancies associated with gastroschisis. Prenat Diagn 8:697, 1989.

Greenwood RD: Cardiovascular malformation associated with omphalocele. J Pediatr 85:818, 1974.

Harrison MR, Bjordal RL, Langmark F, et al: Congenital diaphragmatic hernia: The hidden mortality. J Pediatr Surg 13:227, 1978.

Hoyme HE, Higginbottom MC, Jones KL: The vascular pathogenesis of gastroschisis: Intrauterine interruption of the omphalomesenteric artery. J Pediatr 98:228, 1981.

Huang CS, Lin LH: Laparoscopic Meckel's diverticulectomy in infants: Report of three cases. J Pediatr Surg 28:1486, 1993.

Keppler-Noreuil KM: OEIS complex (omphalocele–exstrophy–imperforate anus–spinal defects: A review of 14 cases. Am J Med Genet 99:271, 2001.

Kitchanan S, Patole SK, Muller R, Whitehall JS: Neonatal outcome of gastroschisis and exomphalos: A 10-year review. J Paediatr Child Health 36:428, 2000.

Lassaletta L, Fonkalsrud EW, Tovar JA, et al: Management of umbilical hernias in infancy and childhood. J Pediatr 10:405, 1975.

Lattimer JK: Congenital deficiency of the abdominal musculature and associated genitourinary anomalies: A report of 22 cases. J Urol 79:343, 1958.

Leung AKC, Robinson WLM: Single umbilical artery. Am J Dis Child 143:108, 1989.

Lewis DF, Towers CV, Garita TJ, et al: Fetal gastroschisis and omphalocele: Is cesarean section the best method of delivery? Am J Obstet Gynecol 163:773, 1990.

Luck CA: Value of routine ultrasound scanning at 19 weeks: A four year study of 8849 deliveries. Br Med J 304:1474, 1992.

Meguid M, Canty T, Eraklis AJ: Complications of Meckel's diverticulum in infants. Surg Gynecol Obstet 139:541, 1974.

Moerman P, Fryns J, Goddeeris P, et al: Pathogenesis of the prune belly syndrome: A functional urethral obstruction caused by prostatic hypoplasia. Pediatrics 73:470, 1984.

Molik KA, Gingalewski CA, West KW, et al: Gastroschisis: A plea for risk categorization. J Pediatr Surg 36:51, 2001.

Moore TC: Omphalomesenteric duct malformations. Semin Pediatr Surg 5:116, 1996.

Moore TC, Collins DL, Catanzarite V, Hatch EI Jr: Pre-term and particularly pre-labor cesarean section to avoid complications of gastroschisis. Pediatr Surg Int 15:97, 1999.

Ney C, Friedenberg RM: Radiographic findings in anomalies of the urachus. J Urol 99:288, 1968.

Oldham KT, Coran AG, Drongowski RA, et al: The development of necrotizing enterocolitis following repair of gastroschisis: A surprisingly high incidence. J Pediatr Surg 23:945, 1988.

Paidas MJ, Crombleholme TM, Robertson FM: Prenatal diagnosis and management of the fetus with an abdominal wall defect. Semin Perinatol 18:196, 1994.

Peevy KJ, Speed FA, Hoff CJ: Epidemiology of inguinal hernia in preterm neonates. Pediatrics 77:246, 1986.

Penman DG, Fisher RM, Noblett HR, Soothill PW: Increase in incidence of gastroschisis in the south west of England in 1995. Br J Obstetr Gynaecol 105:328, 1998.

Persutte WH, Hobbins J: Single umbililical artery: A clinical enigma in modern prenatal diagnosis. Ultrasound Obstet Gynecol 6: 216-229, 1995.

Pierce BT, Dance VD, Wagner RK, et al: Perinatal outcome following fetal single umbilical artery diagnosis. J Matern Fetal Med 10:59, 2001.

Poenaru D and members of the Education Committee of the Canadian Association of Pediatric Surgeons: Consensus statement on umbilical conditions in children. Paed Child Health 6:312, 2001.

Rogers LW, Ostrow PT: The prune belly syndrome. J Pediatr 83:786, 1973.

Rowe MI, Clatworthy HW: Incarcerated and strangulated hernias in children. Arch Surg 101:136, 1970.

Saleh AA, Isada NB, Johnson MP, et al: Amniotic fluid acetylcholinesterase is found in gastroschisis but not omphalocele. Fetal Diagn Ther 8:168, 1993.

Saller DN, Canick JA, Palmoki GE, et al: Second-trimester maternal serum alpha-fetoprotein, unconjugated estriol, and hCG levels in pregnancies with ventral wall hernias. Obstet Gynecol 84:852, 1994.

Scherer LR III, Grosfeld JL: Inguinal and umbilical anomalies. Pediatr Clin North Am 40:1121, 1993.

Schmidt D, Rose E, Greenberg F: An association between fetal abdominal wall defects and elevated levels of human chorionic gonadotropin in mid-trimester. Prenat Diagn 13:9, 1993.

Schuster S: Omphalocele, hernia of the umbilical cord and gastroschisis. In Ravitch MM (ed): Pediatric Surgery. Chicago, Year Book Medical Publishers, 1979, p 778.

Sipes SL, Weiner CP, Sipes DR, et al: Gastroschisis and omphalocele: Does either antenatal diagnosis or route of delivery make a difference in perinatal outcome? Obstet Gynecol 76:195, 1990.

Snow BW, Duckett JW: Prune belly syndrome. In Gillenwater JY, et al (eds): Adult and Pediatric Urology. Chicago, Year Book Medical Publishers, 1987.

Snyder CL: Outcome analysis for gastroschisis. J Pediatr Surg 34:1253, 1999.

Snyder CL, Miller KA, Sharp RJ, et al: Management of intestinal atresia in patients with gastroschisis. J Pediatr Surg 36:1542, 2001.

Somri M, Gaitini L, Vaida S, et al: Postoperative outcome in high-risk infants undergoing herniorrhaphy: prospective comparison of spinal and general anesthesia. Anesthesiology 53:762, 1998.

St-Vil D, Brandt ML, Panic S, et al: Meckel's diverticulum in children: A 20-year review. J Pediatr Surg 26:1289, 1991.

Strong TH Jr, Elliott JP, Radin TG: Non-coiled umbilical blood vessels: A new marker for the fetus at risk. Obstet Gynecol 8:409, 1993.

Suita S, Nagasaki A: Urachal remnants. Semin Pediatr Surg 5:107, 1996.

Surana R, Puri P: Is contralateral exploration necessary in infants with unilateral inguinal hernia? J Pediatr Surg 28:1026, 1993.

Tan KH, Keiby MD, Whittle MJ, et al: Congenital anterior abdominal wall defects in England and Wales 1987-93: Retrospective analysis of OPCS data. BMJ 313:903, 1996.

Thummala MR, Raju TN, Langernberg P: Isolated single umbilical artery anomaly and the risk for congenital malformations: A meta-analysis. J Pediatr Surg 33:580, 1998.

West KN, Bengston K, Rescorla FJ, et al: Delayed surgical repair and ECMO improves survival in congenital diaphragmatic hernia. Am Surg 216:454, 1992.

Yang P, Beaty TH, Khoury MJ, et al: Genetic-epidemiologic study of omphalocele and gastroschisis: Evidence for heterogeneity. Am J Med Genetics 44:668, 1992.

CHAPTER 74

# Necrotizing Enterocolitis and Short Bowel Syndrome

**Carol Lynn Berseth and Dan Poenaru**

## NECROTIZING ENTEROCOLITIS

Necrotizing enterocolitis (NEC) is the most commonly occurring gastrointestinal emergency in preterm infants. With the advent of modern neonatology, its incidence has ranged from 10% to 25% over the past 3 decades or so. Signs or symptoms suggestive of NEC develop in approximately one third to one half of all very low-birth-weight infants; of these, approximately one third to one half eventually are given a diagnosis of NEC. Of the infants in whom NEC develops, approximately half require surgery. The mortality rate ranges from 25% to 30%. Of those who survive, approximately 25% experience long-term sequelae related to the gastrointestinal tract. In addition, these infants require longer hospitalizations than infants of similar maturity who do not have NEC (Bisquera et al, 2002) and have impaired neurodevolopmental outcomes (Sonntag et al, 2000). In the National Institute of Child Health and Human Development studies, NEC was a significant and independent predictor of neurodevelopmental morbidity (Vohr et al, 2000).

### Epidemiology and Pathogenesis

The incidence of NEC varies geographically and temporally. It typically occurs in a pattern of clustered cases. Although 10% of all cases of NEC occur in term infants, it is more commonly seen in preterm infants, particularly those with birth weights less than 1000 g. The incidence appears to be similar among male and female infants, but it is more common among black infants (Mizrahi et al, 1965; Wilson et al, 1983).

The age at onset of NEC is inversely related to gestational age, with a mean age of 3 to 4 days for term infants and 3 to 4 weeks for infants born at less than 28 weeks of gestation. NEC is 10 times more common in infants who have been fed than in those who have not received enteral nutrition, and it occurs more commonly among infants fed formula than among those fed breast milk. NEC, however, does occur in infants who have never been fed and in those who have received breast milk feedings.

NEC occurs in epidemics. Most neonatal intensive care units (NICUs) experience a low endemic incidence of NEC that is periodically punctuated by sporadic epidemics. A wide variety of organisms have been associated with these outbreaks, including *Klebsiella pneumoniae*, *Escherichia coli*, clostridia, coagulase-negative staphylococci, and rotavirus. Most typically, these outbreaks occur during times of nursery crowding, but it is not clear that NEC is caused by infectious agents. Although a single, clear-cut cause for NEC has not been identified, several contributing risk factors have been identified: bowel ischemia, immaturity of host defense, and enteral feedings.

#### *Bowel Ischemia*

The role of ischemia in the pathogenesis of NEC has been supported by reports of increased occurrences of NEC among infants who have low Apgar scores, umbilical vessel catheterization, polycythemia, and reduced aortic blood flow. It has been postulated that when the preterm infant is stressed by periods of hypoxia or hypotension, blood flow is redistributed via input from the adrenergic system away from the splanchnic bed. More recent evidence, however, suggests that these neurogenic events are transient and are reversed within 1 to 2 minutes by local vascular events called the *autoregulatory escape mechanism*, which restores intestinal tissue oxygenation. In fact, case-control studies have failed to confirm that hypoxic events occur any more frequently among infants im whom NEC develops than among those in whom it does not (Wilson et al, 1983).

Despite the lack of a direct causal relationship of hypoxia and NEC, regulation of vascular bed flow differs in preterm infants and in adults, and these unique differences may make the preterm intestine more vulnerable to hypoxia during the period of reperfusion that typically follows a period of ischemia. During reperfusion, oxygen free radicals are generated; these free radicals can cause the tissue damage that is typically seen in reperfusion injuries. These free radicals result from the enzymatic breakdown of hypoxanthine that accumulates during ischemia and from activated neutrophils that adhere to the gut microvasculature after ischemic injury.

The high tissue levels of xanthine that result from episodes of ischemia may contribute in part to NEC, but the occurrence of NEC also appears to be related to other vascular events that are related to the use of centrally placed vascular catheters. Vascular access in most preterm infants is achieved by the use of umbilical arterial or venous catheters. NEC also is seen among infants who have had umbilical catheters inserted to perform an exchange transfusion for hyperbilirubinemia or polycythemia. Increases in portal venous pressure that may occur during an exchange transfusion in term infants can result in a decrease in ileal and colonic blood flow (Touloukian et al, 1973). It is not clear whether this myogenic vasoconstriction occurs in preterm infants (Crissinger and Granger, 1989). Exchange transfusions, however, are no longer a common procedure in this population.

Umbilical arterial catheters may pose more serious risk to the intestinal vasculature. It has been suggested that embolization of catheters may result in embolization of mesenteric arteries.

Infusion of medications such as calcium may cause vasospasm in humans and frank intestinal necrosis in rabbits (Book and Herbst, 1980). Emboli, however, cannot be demonstrated to be present in the intestinal circulation of infants who have NEC (Tyson et al, 1976).

NEC also has been described among infants who have a patent ductus arteriosus (Ryder et al, 1980). In a randomized, control trial in infants whose birth weights were less than 1000 g, prophylactic closure of the ductus arteriosus by surgical ligation reduced the rate of NEC from 30% in the control group, compared with 8% in the early-closure group (Cassady et al, 1989). Meyers and colleagues (1991) have shown in a near-term fetal lamb model that the presence of a patent ductus arteriosus results in diminished intestinal blood flow. In spite of this observation, autoregulation prevented a decrease in intestinal oxygen consumption.

Other investigators have suggested that treatment for patent ductus arteriosus and not the presence of the patent ductus per se increases the risk for NEC (Grosfeld et al, 1996). NEC has been described to occur among infants who received indomethacin for treatment of a patent ductus arteriosus. It is speculated that indomethacin causes a generalized decrease in splanchnic bed flow that may compromise vascular supply to the distal ileum and colon. In a small descriptive study, administration of indomethacin caused a decrease in mean flow velocity in the superior mesenteric artery that was sustained for 12 hours after treatment (Van Bel et al, 1990). See also Chapter 56, Patent Ductus Arteriosus in the Preterm Infant.

As techniques for treatment for infants with cyanotic heart disease have improved, concerns regarding an increased risk for NEC among these infants have emerged (Martinez-Tallo et al, 1997; Polin et al, 1976). In a recent case-control analysis, McElhinney and associates (2000) showed that the risk of NEC among neonates with congenital heart disease was substantial, and it was highest among infants with hypoplastic left heart syndrome and truncus arteriosus or aortopulmonary window.

NEC also has an increased incidence among infants who are polycythemic (Leake et al, 1975). Polycythemia has been shown to cause a reduction in intestinal perfusion in swine (Nowicki et al, 1984) and intestinal necrosis in puppies (LeBlanc et al, 1984). It also has been shown that antenatal exposure to cocaine is associated with postnatal development of NEC. Cocaine may cause a generalized fetal hypoxia as a result of impaired uterine blood flow. It also can cause selective intestinal ischemia that is not reversed by the autoregulatory escape mechanism. Thus, cocaine-related NEC may be vascular in origin.

### *Host Defense Factors*

As reviewed in Chapter 70, host defenses in the preterm gastrointestinal tract are either absent or functionally immature. Because of the variety of agents that have been identified with outbreaks of NEC, it is unclear whether these organisms actually cause NEC or are agents of secondary infection. Although specific bacteria have been reported during some outbreaks of NEC, these same bacteria frequently can be cultured from unaffected infants.

Nevertheless, several immunologically based strategies have been employed to treat or prevent NEC. Several small studies have shown that the administration of oral antibiotics can reduce the incidence of NEC (Egan et al, 1976); however, there are concerns that liberal use of these medications may permit the overgrowth of resistant organisms. Other investigators have shown that the administration of oral immune globulin reduces the occurrence of NEC (Eibl et al, 1988), but this practice has not been validated by additional studies.

Other investigations have assessed whether mediators of inflammation contribute to the tissue damage of NEC. Platelet-activating factor, which is synthesized by white cells, stimulates the release of complement, oxygen radicals, catecholamines, prostaglandins, thromboxane, and leukotrienes. In animal models, the administration of exogenous platelet-activating factor causes neutrophil aggregation, platelet aggregation, systemic hypotension, and ischemic bowel necrosis. During artificially created episodes of ischemia/reperfusion of mesenteric circulation in animals, plasma platelet-activating factor levels increase, and severe bowel necrosis occurs. This sequence of events can be prevented if platelet-activating factor antagonists are administered (Kubes et al, 1990). Plasma platelet-activating factor concentrations are higher among infants who have NEC than in age-matched control infants (Caplan et al, 1990). Furthermore, providing enteral feedings results in increased levels of platelet-activating factor (MacKendrick et al, 1993b). The action of platelet-activating factor may be inhibited by the release of endogenous nitric oxide (MacKendrick, 1993a). Inducible nitric oxide messenger RNA (mRNA) expression is increased in stressed neonatal rats (Nadler, 2000).

In other recent studies, erythropoietin receptors have been identified on intestinal epithelium. Erthropoietin protects against programmed cell death in the intestinal epithelium (Juul, 1999), and the incidence of NEC is lower among preterm infants given recombinant erythropoietin for anemia of prematurity (4.6% versus 10.8% in age-matched controls) (Ledbetter and Juul, 2000). Using interleukin-8 (IL-8) as a marker for proinflammatory cytokine activation, Nanthakumar and colleagues (2000) showed that fetal intestinal epithelial cells and tissue make significantly more IL-8 in response to challenges by endotoxin and IL-1 than that made by more mature cells and tissues. These authors speculate that NEC may occur among preterm infants because their "over-response" triggers a brisk release of imflammatory mediators.

Nitric oxide also has been proposed to function as a mediator in NEC. Messenger RNA expression of intestinal trefoil factor, a small peptide that is secreted by goblet cells as a component of the mucosal barrier, does not emerge in the fetal rat until late gestation, and neonatal levels are lower than those seen in mature animals (Lin et al, 1999). Other mediators that are currently under investigation are tumor necrosis factor, endothelin-1, and prostaglandins.

Because NEC occurs less frequently among infants fed breast milk, and because breast-feeding appears to protect infants from a number of diseases (Schanler, 1999a), numerous investigators have attempted to delineate the factors in breast milk that contribute to neonatal host defense. As detailed in Chapter 68, breast milk contains immunoglobulins, leukocytes, and antibacterial agents. When neonatal rats were fed maternal milk, the incidence of NEC was significantly lower than that seen in neonatal rats fed artificial formula (Barlow et al, 1974). For breast milk to confer this protection from NEC, intact leukocytes had to be present in the milk. The protective effects conferred by the ingestion of breast milk also were reproduced by feeding the immunoglobulin fraction of breast milk alone. In a large prospective trial, infants fed formula had a 2.5-fold greater risk of developing NEC than that in infants fed breast milk. Furthermore, infants fed artificial formula supplemented by a preparation of human serum gamma immunoglobulin A (IgA) and IgG demonstrated a significant reduction in the incidence of NEC (Eibl et al, 1988). Thus, it appears that host defense conferred by feeding breast milk may provide some protection against the development of NEC (Schanler et al, 1999b). Additional research in this area is still needed, however, to elucidate the component(s) that confer this protection and the mechanism(s) whereby this protection is conferred.

### *Enteral Feeding*

Although NEC occurs in infants who have never been fed, its incidence is much higher among infants who have been fed than among those who have not. Earlier studies suggested that delaying the onset of the initiation of enteral feeding reduced the incidence of NEC (Lucas and Cole, 1990); however, more recent studies have not confirmed this observation. In fact, several randomized prospective studies have failed to show an increase in the occurrence of NEC among infants fed early (within the first postnatal week) compared with those whose feedings are initiated late (at 2 to 3 weeks of postnatal age) (Berseth, 1992; Dunn et al, 1988; La Gamma et al, 1985; Meetze et al, 1992). A retrospective study demonstrated that preterm infants who developed NEC had had their feeding volumes increased daily by 25 mL/kg per day or more (McKeown et al, 1992). However, a recent prospective trial failed to show a relationship between the incidence of NEC and two different increments of daily increase in feeding volume (Rayyis et al, 1999). Indeed, Owens and Berseth (1995) showed that the onset of NEC most commonly occurs when infants reach larger feeding volumes (i.e., those that exceed 100 mL/kg/day), regardless of the day of initiation of feeding or the rate of increasing feeding volume. On the other hand, the prolonged use of small enteral feeding volumes for the first 10 feeding days reduced the incidence of NEC compared with that in infants whose feeding volumes were increased daily by 20 mL/kg/day increments (Berseth et al, 2003). Because of the apparent protective effect of breast milk on the incidence of NEC, several studies have evaluated the use of additives for artificial formulas. Carlson and colleagues (1998), for example have shown that the addition of egg phospholipids to preterm formula reduced the incidence of NEC from 17.6% in a control group to 2.9%. In another trial, the addition of *Lactobacillus acidophilus* and *Bifidobacterium* significantly reduced the incidence of NEC in a treatment group compared with that in a historical control group (Hoyos, 1999). However, a prospective, randomized trial has not yet confirmed these findings. Other additives that have not been shown to be effective consistently include human IgA and IgG (Lawrence et al, 2001) and enteral antibiotics (Bury and Tudehope, 2001). See also Chapter 68, Enteral Nutrition for the High-Risk Neonate.

NEC has been linked to the use of hyperosmolar formulas (Abrams et al, 1975), and it is also important for the clinician to realize that the addition of medications such as theophylline, sodium bicarbonate, and calcium supplements as well as vitamins may significantly raise the osmotic loads of formulas (Ernst et al, 1983).

### Clinical Presentation

The clinical signs and symptoms of NEC are highly variable. In general, infants demonstrate gastrointestinal dysfunction, as reflected in the presence of abdominal distention, vomiting, bilious drainage from enteral feeding tubes, or hematochezia, and systemic illness, as reflected in temperature instability, apnea, lethargy, or hypotension (Fig. 74–1). Abdominal signs initially may be limited to distention and tenderness and then may progress to include palpable loops of bowel, fixed mass, abdominal wall erythema, and/or crepitus. The presentation of these signs and symptoms may be acute or insidious. Although a number of infants develop NEC within the first week of life, it also is a disease seen in the NICU graduate who has been transferred to the intermediate care nursery. Because the age at onset of NEC is inversely related to gestational age, clinicians must be exceedingly vigilant in assessing very preterm infants for a protracted postnatal period that may extend to 10 to 12 weeks. In addition, Owens and Berseth (1996) have noted that the clinical presentation in infants with birth weights less than 1500 g may differ from that in infants whose birth weights are 1501 to 2499 g (Table 74–1).

The initial evaluation of an infant who exhibits the signs or symptoms of NEC should include a radiographic examination of the abdomen, collection of body fluids for culture, a metabolic evaluation including electrolytes, and a complete blood count. As is the case in sepsis, white blood counts may be depressed or elevated, and thrombocytopenia commonly occurs in NEC. Hyponatremia and acidosis also commonly occur in NEC. The intestinal inflammatory process often causes shifts in body fluid distribution,

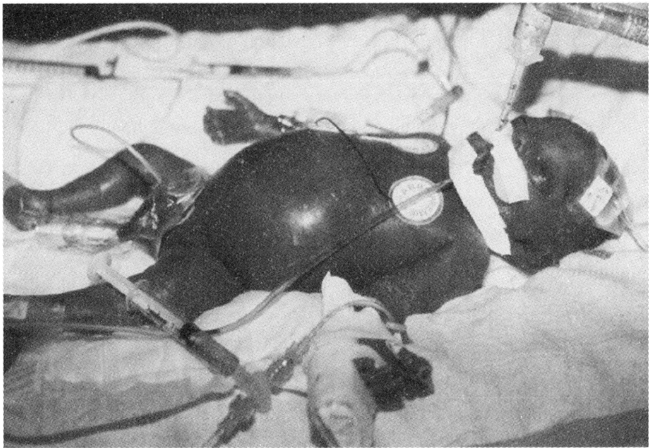

**FIGURE 74–1.** Clinical presentation of a preterm infant with necrotizing enterocolitis. This infant was born at 28 weeks of gestation and had been receiving enteral feedings for 1 week, when he developed acute abdominal distention, hematochezia, and vomiting. Note the discoloration of the skin overlying the abdomen. Also, this infant required endotracheal intubation because of respiratory compromise that occurred as a result of the upward pressure of the abdominal contents on the diaphragm. *(Courtesy of Dr. Lalo Cabrera-Meza, Baylor College of Medicine, Houston, Texas.)*

TABLE 74-1

**Clinical Presentation and Outcomes of Preterm Infants with Necrotizing Enterocolitis (NEC)***

| Characteristic | ≤1500 g | 1501-2499 g | P value |
|---|---|---|---|
| Number of patients | 95 | 46 | — |
| Birth weight (g) | 988 ± 29 | 1911 ± 46 | — |
| Postnatal day feeds begun | 13 ± 1 | 3 ± 1 | .0001 |
| Postnatal day of NEC diagnosis | 27 ± 2 | 9 ± 1 | .001 |
| Clinical findings: frequency† | | | |
| Positive blood culture | 62 (65%) | 10 (21%) | .001 |
| Feeding intolerance | 77 (81%) | 23 (50%) | .001 |
| Abnormal abdominal examination | 82 (86%) | 23 (50%) | .001 |
| Grossly bloody stools | 26 (27%) | 32 (70%) | .001 |
| Deaths | 26 (27%) | 3 (7%) | .05 |

*Values for birth weight, postnatal day of initiation of feeds, and postnatal day of NEC diagnosis are means ± standard error (SEM).

†Number of affected patients (%).

Data from Owens and Berseth, 1996.

resulting in hypotension and acid-base imbalance. In addition, inflammation and swelling of the abdominal contents can cause upward compression against the diaphragm, resulting in respiratory embarrassment. Thus, infants who are acutely ill may also require evaluation of respiratory status by laboratory and radiographic testing.

The severity of NEC is staged using criteria proposed by Bell and colleagues (1978) and later modified by Kliegman and associates (1982). These criteria are based on systemic signs, intestinal signs, and radiologic signs. As shown in Table 74–2, radiographic findings must be present to confirm a diagnosis of NEC.

TABLE 74-2

**Modified Bell's Staging Criteria for Necrotizing Enterocolitis**

| Stage | Systemic Signs | Intestinal Signs | Radiologic Signs | Treatment |
|---|---|---|---|---|
| I: Suspected | | | | |
| A | Temperature instability, apnea, bradycardia | Elevated pregavage residuals, mild abdominal distention, occult blood in stool | Normal or mild ileus | NPO, antibiotics × 3 days |
| B | Same as for IA | Same as for IA, plus gross blood in stool | Same as for IA | Same as for IA |
| II: Definite | | | | |
| A: Mildly ill | Same as for IA | Same as for I, plus absent bowel sounds, abdominal tenderness | Ileus, intestinal pneumatosis | NPO, antibiotics × 7-10 days |
| B: Moderately ill | Same as for I, plus mild metabolic acidosis, mild thrombocytopenia | Same as for I, plus absent bowel sounds, definite abdominal tenderness, abdominal cellulitis, right lower quadrant mass | Same as for IIA, plus portal vein gas, with or without ascites | NPO, antibiotics × 14 days |
| III: Advanced | | | | |
| A: Severely ill, bowel intact | Same as for IIB, plus hypotension, bradycardia, respiratory acidosis, metabolic acidosis, disseminated intravascular coagulation, neutropenia | Same as for I and II, plus signs of generalized peritonitis, marked tenderness, and distention of abdomen | Same as for IIB, plus definite ascites | NPO, antibiotics × 14 days, fluid resuscitation, inotropic support, ventilator therapy, paracentesis |
| B: Severely ill, bowel perforated | Same as for IIIA | Same as for IIIA | Same as for IIB, plus pneumoperitoneum | Same as for IIA, plus surgery |

NPO, nulla per os (nothing by mouth).

From Walsh MC, Kliegman RM, Fanaroff AA: Necrotizing enterocolitis: A practitioner's perspective. Pediatr Rev 9:225, 1988. Reproduced by permission of Pediatrics.

Nonspecific radiographic findings in suspected but unproven NEC are dilated bowel loops, bowel wall thickening, and increased peritoneal fluid. The diagnostic radiographic finding in NEC is the presence of intestinal pneumatosis. However, this radiographic feature is seen only in approximately 85% of infants subsequently proved to have NEC (Kliegman et al, 1982; Foglia, 1995). Intestinal pneumatosis is caused by the presence of hydrogen in the bowel wall as a byproduct of bacterial metabolism (Fig. 74–2A). Two radiographic patterns are commonly observed. More typically, there is a linear streak of gas within the bowel wall. This streaking may be visualized in a single discrete subserosal portion of the small intestine or may extend throughout the entire small and large intestine. The other pattern seen in NEC is a "bubbly gas" pattern in the submucosa similar to that seen in newborn infants who retain meconium in the intestine (see Fig. 74–2B). Because this pattern can be confused with that of retained meconium, it is less specific for NEC than is the linear streaking pattern. If gas is seen in the colon alone, the infant has a better prognosis than if the gas is seen in small bowel and colon (Leonidas et al, 1976). Portal venous gas may be an indicator of more severe disease because there is a 38% incidence of severe bowel necrosis, with mortality rates as high as 70%, associated with this finding (Grosfeld et al, 1991; Molik et al, 2001). If intestinal pneumatosis extends into the portal venous circulation, linear branching areas of radiolucency may appear overlying the liver (Fig. 74–3). Intraperitoneal fluid, with the associated displacement of intestinal loops to the central abdomen, usually is a sign of significant loss of integrity of the bowel wall, with impending or recent perforation (Foglia, 1995). If NEC progresses to bowel perforation, pneumoperitoneum may be identified. Most typically, free air is visualized on a cross-table lateral or right lateral decubitus film (Fig. 74–4A). Occasionally, free air can be visualized as a central periumbilical collection on an anteroposterior film—the "football sign" (see Fig. 74–4B).

## Treatment

### *Medical Management*

The medical management of NEC requires attention to acute care as well as long-term care. Acute care is focused on providing aggressive supportive care while attempting to limit the progression of disease. If the infant is receiving enteral nutrition, feedings should be discontinued and the stomach should be decompressed. Body fluids should be collected for culturing, and broad-spectrum antibiotic therapy should be initiated. Although NICUs may choose specific coverage based on their specific nursery flora, antibiotic coverage usually includes ampicillin or a cephalosporin and an aminoglycoside. In some nurseries, additional antistaphylococcal antibiotics may be given. In the event of bowel perforation, anaerobic coverage may be added by using clindamycin or detronidazole.

Because enteral nutrients generally are discontinued for 10 to 14 days, placement of central vascular lines often is necessary to deliver parenteral nutrition. Because NEC is an inflammatory process that results in substantial third space fluid loss, substantial volume support may be needed during the first 48 to 72 hours of treatment. In addition to the aggressive use of fluids and volume expanders such as albumin, pressor agents such as dopamine may be required to maintain the infant's blood pressure and peripheral perfusion. Because many infants with NEC develop apnea or respiratory compromise owing to abdominal distention and upward compression on the diaphragm, intubation and ventilatory support may be required. Frequent monitoring of blood gases assists in management decisions concerning ventilator support as well as fluid management.

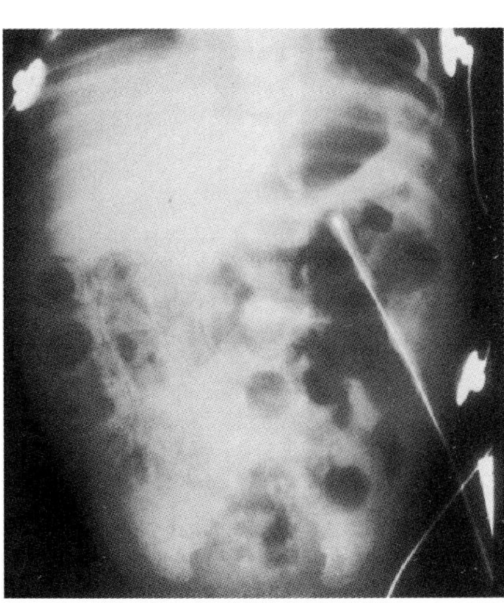
A

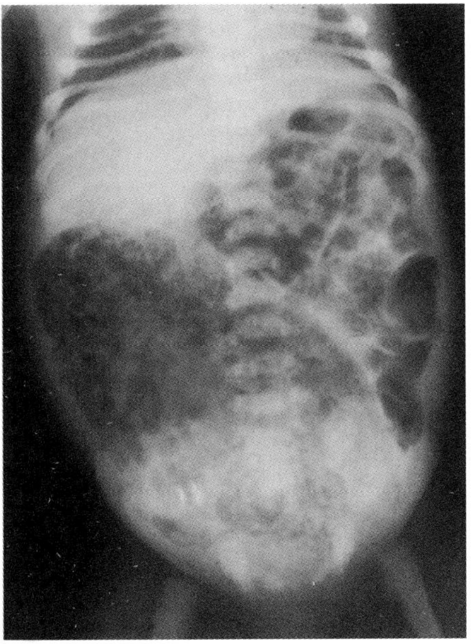
B

**FIGURE 74–2. A,** Typical abdominal radiographic appearance of intestinal pneumatosis seen in necrotizing enterocolitis: dark concentric rings around the bowel loops in the right upper quadrant. **B,** This radiograph displays the *bubbly gas* pattern occasionally seen in necrotizing enterocolitis. *(Courtesy of Dr. Lalo Cabrera-Meza, Baylor College of Medicine, Houston, Texas.)*

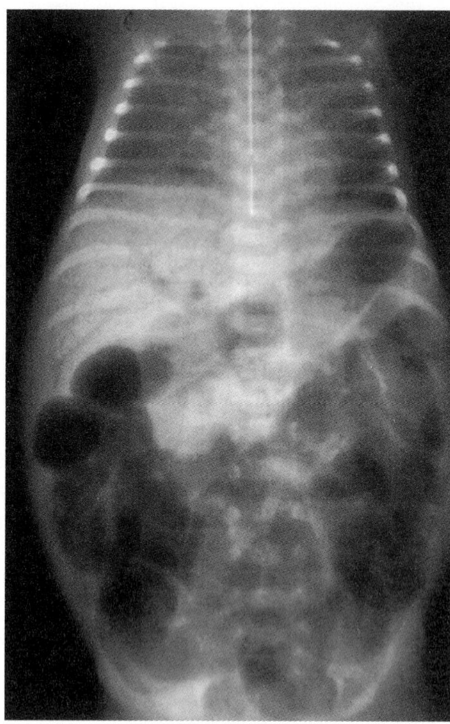

**FIGURE 74–3.** This radiograph displays the presence of portal gas, which is seen as linear dark streaks within the hepatic density. *(Courtesy of Dr. Lalo Cabrera-Meza, Baylor College of Medicine, Houston, Texas.)*

Radiographic evaluations should be repeated every 6 to 8 hours during the first 48 to 72 hours of the disease to assess whether the disease is progressing or to determine if pneumoperitoneum is present (Bisquera et al, 2002). Approximately one fourth to one half of infants with NEC require surgical intervention (Foglia, 1995; Janik and Ein, 1980; Kosloske, 1985).

NEC usually lessens in severity in 48 to 72 hours. Thereafter, infants typically are given antibiotics and parenteral nutrition for 10 to 14 days. Then enteral nutrition may be slowly reintroduced.

### *Surgical Management*

The most common indication for surgery is the presence of pneumoperitoneum. Other indications may be the presence of clinical deterioration despite aggressive medical therapy, the presence of portal vein gas, the presence of a fixed dilated loop of bowel on serial radiographs, and evidence of peritonitis and gangrenous bowel obtained by paracentesis (Koloske, 1994). In a study evaluating various clinical and radiologic criteria, Koloske found that pneumoperitoneum, portal vein gas, positive paracentesis, fixed loop, abdominal wall erythema, and palpable mass all are good indicators of intestinal gangrene. Preoperatively, the infant should undergo expeditious optimization of the clinical status, which may include bedside needle decompression of a tense pneumoperitoneum.

The goals of surgery are to resect necrotic bowel, to decompress the intestine, and to preserve as much bowel length as possible. The choice of procedures is based on the operative findings. The findings at surgery can be grouped into three general categories: (1) isolated perforation or localized NEC, (2) multiple localized areas of necrosis (with over 50% of gut viable), and (3) pan-necrosis (with less than 25% viable).

Isolated disease with limited necrosis or perforation is treated with resection of the affected area. The resected ends are brought out as stomas, usually at the ends of the abdominal incision. Occasionally, very limited NEC, with otherwise healthy-appearing bowel in a stable infant,

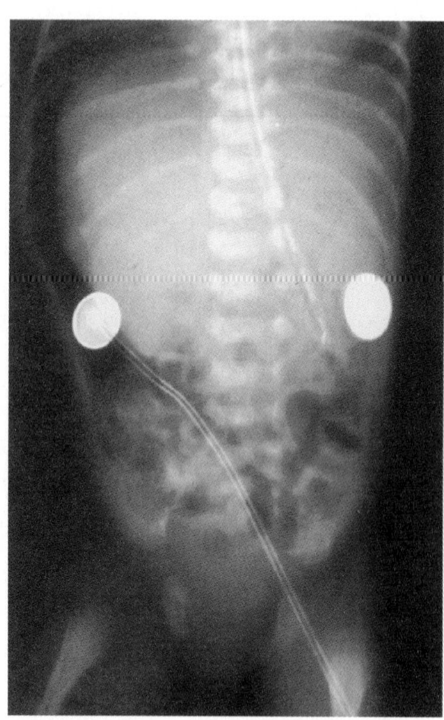

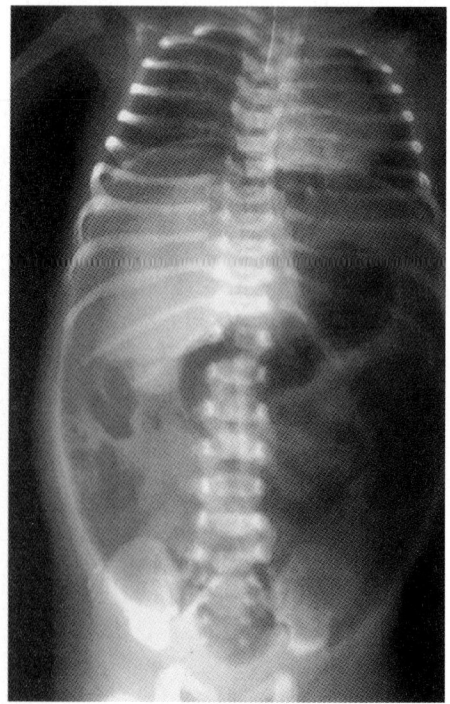

A B

**FIGURE 74–4.** **A,** This radiograph demonstrates intestinal perforation as displayed by the presence of a gas lucency that lies between the hepatic density and the outer abdominal wall. **B,** This radiograph is from another infant whose bowel is perforated. In **B,** air lies anterior to the loops of intestine as well as along the right abdominal wall, where it is displacing loops of bowel medially. *(Courtesy of Dr. Lalo Cabrera-Meza, Baylor College of Medicine, Houston, Texas.)*

may be treated with resection and primary anastomosis (Griffiths et al, 1989).

With multiple areas of necrosis, there are several operative approaches, depending on the overall condition of the infant and the extent of disease. If two or three isolated areas can be resected, the most proximal area of resection can be brought out as two stomas and the distal areas of resection anastomosed. In the case of more extensive disease, options include the "patch, drain, and wait" approach (Moore, 1989) and the "clip and drop-back" method (Vaughan et al, 1996).

Surgical options in the case of pan-necrosis include proximal diversion only, resection of all necrotic bowel, or simple abdominal closure and compassionate care. The last option is supported by the high mortality rate and uniform occurrence of short bowel syndrome associated with pan-necrosis.

In the unstable or very small newborn, another alternative is that of bedside peritoneal drainage. This procedure, originally advocated by Ein and colleagues (1990), consists of the placement of drains in the right lower quadrant (and sometimes the left). Peritoneal drainage appears to be a useful temporizing procedure in selected patients, with a majority still requiring an open surgical intervention. A recent meta-analysis of existing studies comparing peritoneal drainage and laparotomy showed no clear benefit for either approach, as well as a strong treatment bias for smaller infants to undergo drainage (Moss et al, 2001).

### Long-Term Complications

Approximately 75% of infants who develop NEC survive. Half of surviving infants incur a long-term complication. The two most common complications are intestinal strictures and short bowel syndrome.

Because NEC is an inflammatory process that involves all layers of the bowel, development of fibrosis is common during the healing phase. Strictures occur in infants who have been managed medically or surgically, with an incidence from 10% to 35% (Horowitz et al, 1995). Although NEC occurs most commonly in the distal ileum, strictures occur most commonly in the large bowel (Fig. 74–5), most often on the left side. These infants typically develop recurrent abdominal distention 2 to 3 weeks after recovery from NEC. The areas of stricture can be identified by barium enema examination. Surgical resection of the strictured areas is necessary. Because infants who have had surgical resection may also develop strictures, contrast studies are routinely performed in these patients before definitive reanastomosis of the bowel is performed so that areas of stricture can be resected at the time of surgery. Infants who have had conservatively treated NEC are often followed clinically without routine radiological studies.

Recurrent NEC occurs in about 5% of infants, usually a month after the initial episode. There are no identified risk factors for recurrence, and a nonoperative treatment is successful in most cases (Stringer et al, 1993).

Although the bowel may hypertrophy postoperatively after resection, infants may develop malabsorption owing to shortened bowel length. It is estimated that infants require a minimum of 25 to 40 cm of small intestine (Galea et al, 1992). As outlined in the next section, medical and surgical management must address issues related to malabsorption, bacterial overgrowth, and alterations in intestinal transit.

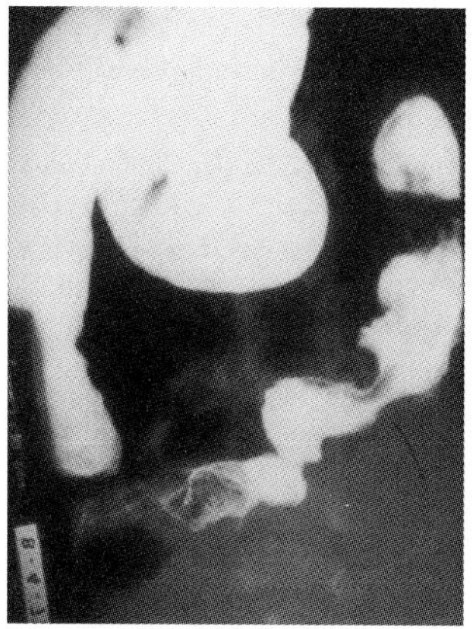
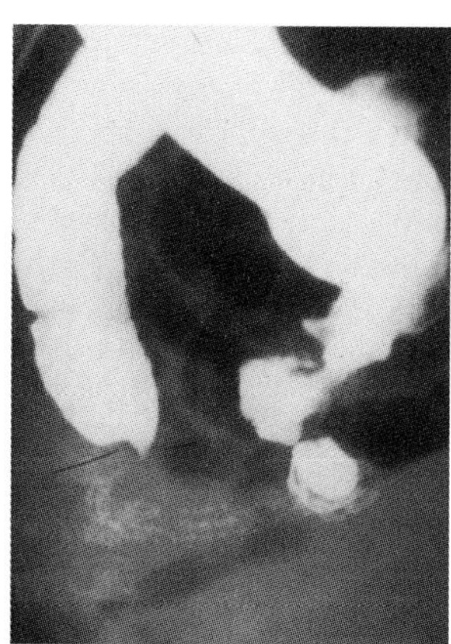

**FIGURE 74–5.** This barium study was obtained in an infant who had recovered from necrotizing enterocolitis and was experiencing intermittent episodes of abdominal distention when enteral feedings were given. Note that multiple areas of stricture are present. *(Courtesy of Dr. Lalo Cabrera-Meza, Baylor College of Medicine, Houston, Texas.)*

## SHORT BOWEL SYNDROME

The normal small intestine length in the term infant is 200 to 300 cm. The most common cause of short gut in the newborn is resection performed to treat NEC, midgut volvulus, or congenital anomalies such as jejunal or ileal atresia and gastroschisis. Thus, newborns most typically have a short gut characterized by losses of ileum and the ileocecal valve (ICV).

Reduction in bowel length results in loss of surface area for absorption of nutrients; thus, malnutrition and fluid electrolyte loss occur. Loss of the ICV results in greater disease because the absence of the valve permits colonic bacteria to reflux into the distal ileum and colonize it. Thus, outcome from intestinal resection depends on two factors: the length of bowel remaining and whether the ICV is intact. Despite many advances in neonatal care, the "traditional" limits of intestinal length as suggested by Wilmore (1972)—15 cm of intestine when the ileocecal valve is intact and 38 cm when it is absent—have not significantly changed. A more contemporary review identifies 25 cm of bowel with an intact ICV and 42 cm without an ICV as the minimum for successful survival and adaptation in full-term neonates (Galea et al, 1992). Premature neonates are capable of better adaptation, and lengths of 22 cm and 30 cm, respectively, apply. Instances of successful adaptation with shorter intestinal lengths have been reported, but constitute the exception rather than the rule (Dorney et al, 1985). As a result, the diagnosis of short bowel syndrome has become a functional one rather than an anatomic one based on gut length. Hence, patients are often identified as having short bowel syndrome if they require parenteral nutrition for more than 6 weeks (Sigalet, 2001; Vanderhoof and Langnas, 1997).

Intestinal adaptation after intestinal resection depends on several factors. First, the remaining bowel dilates, the mucosa hypertrophies, and functional absorptive capacity per length increases. These responses result in an increased absorption area per unit length of intestine. Second, as the infant grows in body length, the intestine elongates, increasing absorptive area. Third, adaptation occurs differently in ileum and jejunum. Ileal mucosa increases in size and function much more effectively than does jejunal mucosa (Dowling, 1982). Although ileal structures can perform jejunal functions, jejunal structures cannot perform ileal functions. Complete adaptation of all four of these aspects may not be completed for 2 years (Cooper et al, 1984; Grosfeld et al, 1986; Purdum and Kirby, 1991). Therefore, many neonatologists may be responsible for managing the care in only early stages of adaptation in an infant who develops short gut syndrome, and they must exercise restrained patience in caring for infants with this disease.

### Treatment

The first priority of treatment must be the provision of adequate calories for growth. This first must be achieved by using parenteral nutrition to establish positive nitrogen balance. Thereafter, clinical care for the newborn must address four issues: (1) malabsorption of nutrients and fluids, (2) gastric hypersecretion, (3) bacterial overgrowth, and (4) difficulties with intestinal adaptation.

Because bile salts and fat-soluble vitamins and trace minerals are absorbed in the distal ileum, infants with short bowel syndrome develop steatorrhea and specific vitamin and mineral deficiencies. Cholestyramine, an ion-exchange resin that binds bile salts, often is used to reduce steatorrhea. Although cholestyramine reduces steatorrhea, it does not reduce fat malabsorption, and attention should still be given to nutritional needs for fat. Fats can be given either parenterally or enterally. Deficiencies of vitamins A, D, E, K, and $B_{12}$ as well as zinc and magnesium all have been described in infants with short gut. Therefore, levels of all of these substrates should be monitored and supplemented appropriately.

Gastric acid hypersecretion occurs after intestinal resection in adults and children (Clark, 1984). Infants have limited gastric acid secretion, and it has not been confirmed that gastric acid hypersecretion occurs in preterm infants following resection. $H_2$ blockers and proton pump inhibitors, however, commonly are used to suppress acid secretion, to prevent low pH in the duodenum, which can inactivate pancreatic enzymes or impair micelle formation. Occasionally, somatostatin or its synthetic analogue octreotide may be used to reduce acid secretion (Schwartz and Kuenzler, 2001).

Bacterial overgrowth can occur intermittently as a result of reflux of colonic contents into the distal ileum in the absence of an ileocecal valve. Bacterial overgrowth also can occur as the result of the presence of hypotonic, dilated bowel segments or the presence of fistulas. Bacterial overgrowth can impair fat and vitamin $B_{12}$ absorption and depress mucosal levels of maltase, sucrose, lactase, and enterokinase (Gianella et al, 1974), resulting in malabsorption and profound diarrhea. Patients may require intermittent cyclic treatment with double-antibiotic regimens, such as metronidazole and trimethoprim-sulfamethoxazole or oral vancomycin and gentamicin, to suppress bacterial overgrowth and its attendant complications.

Finally, these patients require adequate long-term nutritional support. Most infants initially are supported by parenteral nutrition supplemented by additional fluid and electrolytes to overcome losses caused by malabsorption and those occurring via ostomy sites. Enteral feedings are exceedingly important in providing stimulation for intestinal growth and adaptation. In a recent retrospective review of patients with short bowel syndrome, Andorsky and colleagues (2001) showed that although remaining bowel length was the greatest predictor of required duration of parenteral nutrition, early enteral feeding also was associated with reduced duration of parenteral nutrition and a lower incidence of cholestasis. The physical presence of luminal nutrients stimulates mucosal growth. In addition, enteral nutrients stimulate the release of hormones and pancreatic biliary secretions, which also stimulate intestinal growth. Recently, investigators have studied the used of additives such as glutamine and insulin-like growth factor (IGF-1) to enhance mucosal growth, but results of these studies have been equivocal (Schwartz and Kuenzler, 2001). Enteral nutrients also may cause diarrhea, because mucosal hypoplasia may result in inadequate processing of enteral nutrients. Therefore, most infants initially are fed small volumes of elemental formulas that are lactose-free and contain medium-chain triglycerides. As adaptation occurs, more complex standard formulas can be used to stimulate mucosal hyperplasia better (Purdum and Kirby, 1991). Fluid and electrolyte losses via ostomy sites should be replaced, and reinfusion of ostomy losses into noncontiguous distal bowel segments prevents bowel atrophy while the patient is awaiting reanastomosis (Purdum and Kirby, 1991). The stool pH may be acidic if malabsorption, bacterial overgrowth, or both are present. Because acidic fecal material has a more rapid transit, the addition of sodium bicarbonate to feedings may be needed to maintain the stool pH above 6.

Although most infants can be managed medically until intestinal adaptation occurs, approximately 10% to 15% are dependent on total parenteral nutrition. Several surgical options are available for this group of patients. Techniques include reversal of a small segment of bowel to slow transit, tapering or plicating dilated loops of intestine to improve motility, and intestinal lengthening procedures such as Bianchi's isoperistaltic doubling (Bianchi, 1980) and Kimura's isolated segments technique (Vernon and Georgeson, 2001). Experience with these procedures remains limited, and their associated complication and failure rates are high; still, they constitute a less invasive option than intestinal transplantation.

Intestinal transplantation is becoming an increasingly viable option for selected patients. A recent review by one center reported a 3-year survival rate of 60% (Vennarecci et al, 2001). A significant shortage of appropriate donors has created long waiting lists, resulting in the death of many patients from complications of total parenteral nutrition–induced cholestasis while waiting for a donor. It is not surprising, therefore, that significant disagreement exists among neonatologists and pediatric gastroenterologists concerning the outcomes of various treatment options for patients and concerning the subspecialist who should discuss treatment options with families (Cooper et al, 1999). Thus, the care of these infants must be multidisciplinary in nature and should occur in an environment that fosters broad communication among subspecialists, nursing staff, and families.

## SELECTED READING

Book LS, Herbst JJ, Jung AL: Comparison of fast- and slow-feeding rate schedules to the development of necrotizing enterocolitis. J Pediatr 89:463, 1976.

## REFERENCES

### Necrotizing Enterocolitis

Abrams CA, Phillips LL, Berkowitz C, et al: Hazards of over-concentrated milk formula. JAMA 232:1136, 1975.

Barlow B, Santulli TV, Heird WC, et al: An experimental study of acute neonatal enterocolitis: The importance of breast milk. J Pediatr Surg 9:587, 1974.

Bell JM, Ternberg JL, Feigin RD, et al: Neonatal necrotizing enterocolitis: Therapeutic decisions based upon clinical staging. Ann Surg 187:1, 1978.

Berseth CL: Early feeding enhances maturation of the preterm small intestine. J Pediatr 120:947, 1992.

Berseth CL, Bisquera JA, Paje VU: Prolonging small feeding volumes early in life decreases the incidence of necrotizing enterocolitis in very low birth weight infants. Pediatrics 111:529, 2003.

Bisquera JA, Cooper TR, Berseth CL: Impact of necrotizing enterocolitis on length of stay and hospital charges. Pediatrics 109:423, 2002.

Book S, Herbst J: Intra-arterial infusions and intestinal necrosis in the rabbit: Potential hazards of umbilical artery injections of ampicillin, glucose, and sodium bicarbonate. Pediatrics 65:1145, 1980.

Bury RG, Tudehope D: Enteral antibiotics for preventing necrotizing enterocolitis in low birthweight or preterm infants. Cochrane Database Syst Rev CD000405(1), 2001.

Caplan MS, Sun XM, Hsueh W, et al: Role of platelet activating factor and tumor necrosis factor-alpha in neonatal necrotizing enterocolitis. J Pediatr 116:960, 1990.

Carlson SE, Montalto MB, Ponder DL, et al: Lower incidence of necrotizing enterocolitis in infants fed a preterm formula with egg phospholipids. Pediatr Res 44:491, 1998.

Cashore WJ, Peter G, Lauermann M, et al: Clostridia colonization and clostridial toxin in neonatal necrotizing enterocolitis. J Pediatr 98:308, 1981.

Cassady G, Crose DT, Kirklin JW, et al: A randomized, controlled trial of very early prophylactic ligation of the ductus arteriosus in babies who weighed 1000 g or less at birth. N Engl J Med 320:1511, 1989.

Cikrit D, Mastandrea J, Grosfeld JL, et al: Significance of portal vein in necrotizing enterocolitis: Analysis of 53 cases. J Pediatr Surg 20:425, 1985.

Cone TE: History of the Care and Feeding of the Premature Infant. New York, Little, Brown, 1985.

Crissinger K, Granger D: Mucosal injury induced by ischemia and reperfusion in the piglet intestine: Influences of age and feeding. Gastroenterology 97:920, 1989.

Crissinger K, Grisham J, Granger D: Developmental biology of oxidant-producing enzymes and antioxidants in the piglet intestine. Pediatr Res 25:612, 1989.

Dunn L, Hulman S, Weiner J, et al: Beneficial effects of early hypocaloric enteral feeding on neonatal gastrointestinal function: Preliminary report of a randomized trial. J Pediatr 112:622, 1988.

Edelson MB, Bagwell CE, Rozycki HJ: Circulating pro- and counterinflammatory cytokine levels and severity in necrotizing enterocolitis. Pediatrics 103:766, 1999.

Egan EA, Mantilla G, Nelson RM, et al: A prospective controlled trial of oral kanamycin in the prevention of neonatal necrotizing enterocolitis. J Pediatr 89:467, 1976.

Eibl M, Wolf HM, Furnkranz H, et al: Prevention of necrotizing enterocolitis in low birth weight infants by IgA-IgG feeding. N Engl J Med 319:1, 1988.

Ein S, Shandling B, Wesson D, Filler R: A 13 year experience with peritoneal drainage under local anesthesia for necrotizing enterocolitis perforation. J Pediatr Surg 25:1034, 1990.

Ernst JA, Williams JM, Glick MR, et al: Osmolality of substances used in the intensive care nursery. Pediatrics 72:347, 1983.

Foglia R: Necrotizing enterocolitis. Curr Probl Surg 32:757, 1995.

Galea MH, Holliday H, Carach R, Kapila L: Short-bowel syndrome: A collective review. J Pediatr Surg 27:592, 1992.

Gastinne H, Wolff M, Delatour F, et al: A controlled trial in intensive care units of selective decontamination of the digestive tract with nonabsorbable antibiotics. N Engl J Med 326:594, 1992.

Goldman HI: Feeding and necrotizing enterocolitis. Am J Dis Child 134:553, 1980.

Griffiths DM, Forbes DA, Pemberton PJ, Penn IA: Primary anastomosis for necrotizing enterocolitis: A 12-year experience. J Pediatr Surg 24:515, 1989.

Grosfeld JL, Chaet M, Molinari F, et al: Increased risk of necrotizing enterocolitis in premature infants with patent ductus arteriosus treated with indomethacin. Ann Surg 224:350, 1996.

Grosfeld J, Cheu H, Schletter M: Changing trends in necrotizing enterocolitis. Ann Surg 214:300, 1991.

Grulee CG, Sanford HN, Schwartz H: Breast and artificially fed infants: A study of the age incidence in the morbidity and mortality in twenty thousand cases. JAMA 104:1986, 1935.

Horwitz JR, Lallyy KP, Cheu HW, et al: Complications after surgical intervention for necrotizing enterocolitis: A multicenter review. J Pediatr Surg 30:994, 1995.

Hoyos AB: Reduced incidence of necrotizing enterocolitis associated with the administration of *Lactobacillus acidophilus* and *Bifidobacterium* to neonates in an intensive care unit. Int J Infect Dis 3:197, 1999.

Janik JS, Ein SH: Peritoneal drainage under local anesthesia for necrotizing enterocolitis (NEC) perforation: A second look. J Pediatr Surg 15:565, 1980.

Juul SE, Joyce AE, Zhao Y, et al: Why is erythropoietin present in human milk? Studies of erythropoietin receptors on enterocytes of human and rat neonates. Pediatr Res 46:263, 1999.

Kliegman RM, Hack M, Jones P, et al: Epidemiologic study of necrotizing enterocolitis among low-birth-weight infants: Absence of identifiable risk factors. J Pediatr 100:440, 1982.

Kosloske AM: Surgery of necrotizing enterocolitis. World J Surg 9:277, 1985.

Kosloske AM: Indication for operation in necrotizing enterocolitis revisited. J Pediatr Surg 29:663, 1994.

Kubes P, Ibbotson G, Russell J, et al: Role of platelet-activating factor in ischemia/reperfusion-induced leukocyte adherence. Am J Physiol 259:G300, 1990.

La Gamma EF, Ostertag SG, Birenbaum H: Failure of delayed oral feedings to prevent necrotizing enterocolitis. Am J Dis Child 139:385, 1985.

Lawrence G, Tudehope D, Baumann K, et al: Enteral human IgG for prevention of necrotising enterocolitis: Controlled, randomized trial. Lancet 357:2090, 2001.

Leake R, Thanopoulos B, Nielberg R: Hyperviscosity syndrome associated with necrotizing enterocolitis. Am J Dis Child 129:1192, 1975.

LeBlanc M, D'Cruz C, Pate K: Necrotizing enterocolitis can be caused by polycythemic hyperviscosity in the newborn dog. J Pediatr 105:804, 1984.

Ledbetter DJ, Juul SE: Erythropoietin and the incidence of necrotizing enterocolitis in infants with very low birth weight. J Pediatr Surg 35:178, 2000.

Leonard TJ, Johnson J, Pettett P: Critical evaluation of the persistent loop sign in necrotizing enterocolitis. Radiology 142:385, 1982.

Leonidas J, Hall R, Amoury R: Critical evaluation of the roentgen signs of neonatal enterocolitis. Ann Radiol 219:123, 1976.

Lin J, Holzman IR, Jiang P, Babyatsky MW: Expression of intestinal trefoil factor in developing rat intestine. Biol Neonate 76:92, 2000.

Lucas A, Cole TJ: Breast milk and neonatal necrotizing enterocolitis. Lancet 336:1519, 1990.

MacKendrick W, Caplan M, Hsueh W: Endogenous nitric oxide protects against platelet-activating factor–induced bowel injury in the rat. Pediatr Res 34: 222, 1993a.

MacKendrick W, Hill N, Hsueh W, et al: Increase in plasma platelet activating factor levels in enterally fed preterm infants. Biol Neonate 64:89, 1993b.

Martinez-Tallo E, Claure N, Bancalari E: Necrotizing enterocolitis in full-term or near-term infants: Risk factors. Biol Neonate 71:292, 1997.

McElhinney DB, Hedrick HL, Bush DM, et al: Necrotizing enterocolitis in neonates with congenital heart disease: Risk factors and outcomes. Pediatrics 106:1080, 2000.

McKeown RE, Marsh TD, Amaranth U, et al: Role of delayed feeding and of feeding increments in necrotizing enterocolitis. J Pediatr 121:764, 1992.

Meetze WH, Valentine C, McGuigan JE, et al: Gastrointestinal priming prior to full enteral nutrition in very low birth weight infants. J Pediatr Gastroenterol Nutr 15:163, 1992.

Meyers RL, Gad A, Lin E, Clyman RI: Patent ductus arteriosus, indomethacin, and intestinal distension: Effects on intestinal blood flow and oxygen consumption. Pediatr Res 29:569, 1991.

Mizrahi A, Barlow O, Berdon W, et al: Necrotizing enterocolitis in premature infants. J Pediatr 66:697, 1965.

Molik KA, West KW, Rescorla FJ, et al: Portal venous air: The poor prognosis persists. J Pediatr Surg 36:1143, 2001.

Moore T: The management of necrotizing enterocolitis by "patch, drain, and wait." Pediatr Surg Int 4:110, 1989.

Moss RL, Dimmitt RA, Henry MC, et al: A meta-analysis of peritoneal drainage versus lapartotomy for perforated necrotizing enterocolitis. J Pediatr Surg 36:1210, 2001.

Nadler EP, Dickinson E, Knisely A: Expression of inducible nitric oxide synthase and interleukin-12 in experimental necrotizing enterocolitis. J Surg Res 92:71, 2000.

Nanthakumar NN, Fusunyan RD, Sanderson I, Walker WA: Inflammation in the developing human intestine: A possible pathophysiologic contribution to necrotizing enterocolitis. Proc Natl Acad Sci USA 97:6043, 2000.

Nowicki P, Oh W, Yao A, et al: Effect of polycythemia on gastrointestinal blood flow and oxygenation in piglets. Am J Physiol 247:G220, 1984.

Owens L, Berseth CL: Clinical presentation of necrotizing enterocolitis (NEC) differs between very low birth weight (VLBW) and low birth weight (LBW) infants. J Clin Investigative Med 44:14A, 1996.

Owens L, Berseth C: Is there a volume threshold for enteral feeding and necrotizing enterocolitis? Pediatr Res 37:315A, 1995.

Pokorny WJ, Fowler CL: Isoperistaltic intestinal lengthening for short bowel syndrome. Surg Gynecol Obstet 172:39, 1991.

Polin RA, Pollack PF, Barlow B, et al: Necrotizing enterocolitis in term infants. J Pediatr 89:460, 1976.

Rayyis SF, Ambalavanan N, Wright L, Carlo WA: Randomized trial of "slow" versus "fast" feed advancements on the incidence of necrotizing enterocolitis in very low birth weight infants. J Pediatr 134:293, 1999.

Ricketts RR: The surgical role of paracentesis in the management of infants with necrotizing enterocolitis. Am Surg 52:61, 1986.

Ricketts RR: Surgical treatment of necrotizing enterocolitis and the short bowel syndrome. Clin Perinatol 21:14, 1994.

Ryder RW, Shelton JD, Guinan ME: Necrotizing enterocolitis: A prospective multicenter investigation. Am J Epidemiol 112:113, 1980.

Santulli TV, Schullinger JN, Heird WC, et al: Acute necrotizing enterocolitis in infancy: A review of 64 cases. Pediatrics 55:376, 1975.

Schanler RJ, Hurst NM, Lau C: The use of human milk and breastfeeding in premature infants. Clin Perinatol 26:379, 1999a.

Schanler RJ, Shulman RJ, Lau C: Feeding strategies for premature infants: Beneficial outcomes of feeding fortified human milk versus preterm formula. Pediatrics 103:1150, 1999b.

Schwartz MZ, Hayden CK, Richardson CJ, et al: A prospective evaluation of intestinal stenosis following necrotizing enterocolitis. J Pediatr Surg 17:764, 1982.

Smith MF, Borriello SP, Clayden GS, et al: Clinical and bacteriological findings in necrotizing enterocolitis: A controlled study. J Infect 2:23, 1980.

Sonntag J, Grimmer I, Scholz T, et al: Growth and neurodevelopmental outcome of very low birthweight infants with necrotizing enterocolitis. Acta Paediatr 89:528, 2000.

Stringer MD, Brereton RJ, Drake DP, et al: Recurrent necrotizing enterocolitis. J Pediatr Surg 28:979, 1993.

Touloukian R, Kadar A, Spencer R: The gastrointestinal complications of neonatal umbilical venous exchange transfusion: A clinical and experimental study. Pediatrics 51:36, 1973.

Tyson J, deSa D, Moore S: Thromboatheromatous complications of umbilical arterial catheterization in the newborn period. Arch Dis Child 51:744, 1976.

Van Bel F, Van Aoeren D, Schipper J, et al: Effect of indomethacin on superior mesenteric artery blood flow velocity in preterm infants. J Pediatr 116:965, 1990.

Vaughan WG, Grosfeld JL, West K, et al: Avoidance of stomas and delayed anastomosis for bowel necrosis: The "clip and drop-back technique." J Pediatr Surg 31:542, 1996.

Vohr BR, Wright LL, Dusick AM, et al: Neurodevelopmental and functional outcomes of extremely low birth weight infants in the National Institute of Child Health and Human Development Neonatal Research Network 1993-1994. Pediatrics 105:1216, 2000.

Walsh MC, Kliegman RM: Necrotizing enterocolitis: Treatment based on staging criteria. Pediatr Clin North Am 33:179, 1986.

Wilson R, delPortillo M, Schmidt E, et al: Risk factors for necrotizing enterocolitis in infants weighing more than 2,000 grams at birth: A case-controlled study. Pediatrics 71:19, 1983.

**Short Bowel Syndrome**

Andorsky DJ, Lund DP, Lillehei CW, et al: Nutritional and other postoperative management of neonates with short bowel syndrome correlated with clinical outcomes. J Pediatr 139:27, 2001.

Bianchi A: Intestinal loop lengthening—a technique of increasing small intestinal length. J Pediatr Surg 15:145, 1980.
Clark JH: Management of short bowel syndrome in the high-risk infant. Clin Perinatol 11:189, 1984.
Cooper A, Floyd TF, Ross AJ III, et al: Morbidity and mortality of short-bowel syndrome acquired in infants: An update. J Pediatr Surg 19:711, 1984.
Cooper TR, Garcia-Prats JA, Brody BA: Managing disagreements in the management of short bowel and hypoplastic left heart syndrome. Pediatrics 104:e48, 1999. Also available at: http://www.pediatrics.org/cgi/content/full/104/4/e48
Dorney SFA, Ament ME, Berquist WE, et al: Improved survival in very short small bowel infants with use of long-term parenteral nutrition. J Pediatr 107:521, 1985.
Dowling RH: Small bowel adaptation and its regulation. Scand J Gastroenterol 17:53, 1982.
Galea MH, Holliday H, Carach R, Kapila L: Short-bowel syndrome: A collective review. J Pediatr Surg 27:592, 1992.
Gianella RA, Rout WR, Toskes PP: Jejunal brush border injury and impaired sugar and amino acid uptake in the blind loop syndrome. Gastroenterology 67:965, 1974.
Grosfeld JL, Rescoria FJ, West KW: Short bowel syndrome in infancy and childhood: Analysis of survival in 60 patients. Am J Surg 151:41, 1986.
Purdum PP III, Kirby DF: Short-bowel syndrome: A review of the role of nutrition support. JPEN J Parenter Enteral Nutr 15:93, 1991.
Schwartz MZ, Kuenzler KA: Pharmacotherapy and growth factors in the treatment of short bowel syndrome. Semin Pediatr Surg 10:81, 2001.
Sigalet DL: Short bowel syndrome in infants and children: An overview. Semin Pediatr Surg 10:44, 2001.
Vanderhoof JA, Langnas AN: Short-bowel-syndrome in children and adults. Gastroenterology 113:1767, 1997.
Vennarecci G, Kato T, Misiakos EP, et al: Intestinal transplantation for short gut syndrome attributable to necrotizing enterocolitis. Pediatrics 105:25, 2001.
Vernon AN, Georgeson KE: Surgical options for short bowel syndrome. Semin Pediatr Surg 10:91, 2001.
Wilmore DW: Factors correlating with a successful outcome following extensive intestinal resection in newborn infants. J Pediatr 80:88, 1972.

# HEMATOLOGIC SYSTEM AND DISORDERS OF BILIRUBIN METABOLISM

Editor: CHRISTINE A. GLEASON



# PART XV

CHAPTER 75

# Developmental Biology of the Hematologic System

Sandra E. Juul

## OVERVIEW OF EMBRYONIC HEMATOPOIESIS

*Hematopoiesis* is the overall process by which self-renewing stem cells give rise to the multiple lineages of differentiated blood cells (Fig. 75–1). This complex process is the result of the coordinated expression and interaction of many growth factors, some of which act on primitive progenitor cells that can give rise to multiple cell lineages and others of which support lineage-committed multipotential hematopoietic stem cells. Hematopoiesis begins early in embryonic life, with the first hematopoietic cells appearing in the human yolk sac at embryonic day 7.5. By day 10 of gestation, hematopoietic stem cells are present in the aorto-gonado-mesonephron (AGM), and from there activity shifts to the liver and finally to the bone marrow (Huss, 2000). Each cell line undergoes developmental changes that are unique and specific. The developmental peculiarities of each of these systems and the resulting clinical impact of these changes are reviewed individually in the rest of the chapters in Part XV.

## STEM CELL BIOLOGY

Pluripotent stem cells can sustain marrow function throughout a person's lifetime. A unique characteristic of these cells is that their direct offspring include at least one identical daughter cell, thus perpetuating the population. This is in contrast to progenitor cells, which are more differentiated and give rise only to cells more differentiated than themselves. It was long believed that pluripotent stem cells were specific to the bone marrow and gave rise only to hematopoietic tissue and the associated supporting stroma. Recent evidence has demonstrated a more unrestricted potential for these cells. Indeed, progenitor cells have been found in a variety of postnatal tissues with apparently "unorthodox" potential for differentiating into unrelated tissues. For example, bone marrow cells, when placed in a conducive environment, can generate neural cells, and conversely, neural stem cells can reestablish hematopoiesis in irradiated mice (Bjornson et al, 1999; Mezey et al, 2000). This ability of stem cells from one tissue type to differentiate into cells of another tissue type is dependent on the microenvironment.

The developmental changes in the number, function, and location of hematopoietic stem cells are of great interest to transplantation biologists and gene therapists. The cycling potential and proliferative capacity of hematopoietic stem cells vary with the anatomic source of the cells, and with the age at which the cells are harvested. The sensitivity of these cells to recombinant cytokines also changes with age. Thus, improving the understanding of the ontogeny of these cells will be helpful in optimizing their clinical use.

Embryonic and fetal hematopoietic stem cells are capable of repopulating an adult organism (Fleischmann et al, 1984). In contrast, transplanted adult stem cells have a lower capacity for self-renewal, often resulting in late graft failure. This limitation may be because the adult stem cells continue to express the adult differentiation program despite the fetal environment, indicating an irreversible change in gene expression (Fleischmann et al, 1984). Another explanation for the decrease in proliferative potential may have to do with the loss of telomere repeats with each stem cell division, limiting the replicative potential of stem cells (Lansdorp, 1997; Notaro et al, 1997; Vaziri et al, 1994). Mean telomere lengths in donor-recipient pairs have been measured, with a decrease roughly equivalent to 15 years of aging controls noted in the transplant recipients (Wynn et al, 1998). Thus, the increase in cell replication required after engraftment may impose replicative stress on the hematopoietic stem cells, resulting in a pronounced aging effect.

A focus of ongoing research is optimization of techniques by which to harvest stem cells. Cell surface markers, which are dependent on cell maturity and gestational age, are often used to identify and separate hematopoietic stem cells using monoclonal antibodies and fluorescence-activated cell sorter (FACS) analysis. For example, CD34, a cell-surface sialomucin, is a commonly used antigen to select hematopoietic stem cells and early erythropoietic progenitor cells. Combining CD34 positivity with the absence of lineage-specific markers ($lin^-$) allows selection of a cell population highly enriched for the cells desired for transplantation or research purposes. The search is ongoing for still earlier cell populations by a

This chapter is based on work supported by grants RR-00083 and 38782-01A2 from the National Institutes of Health.

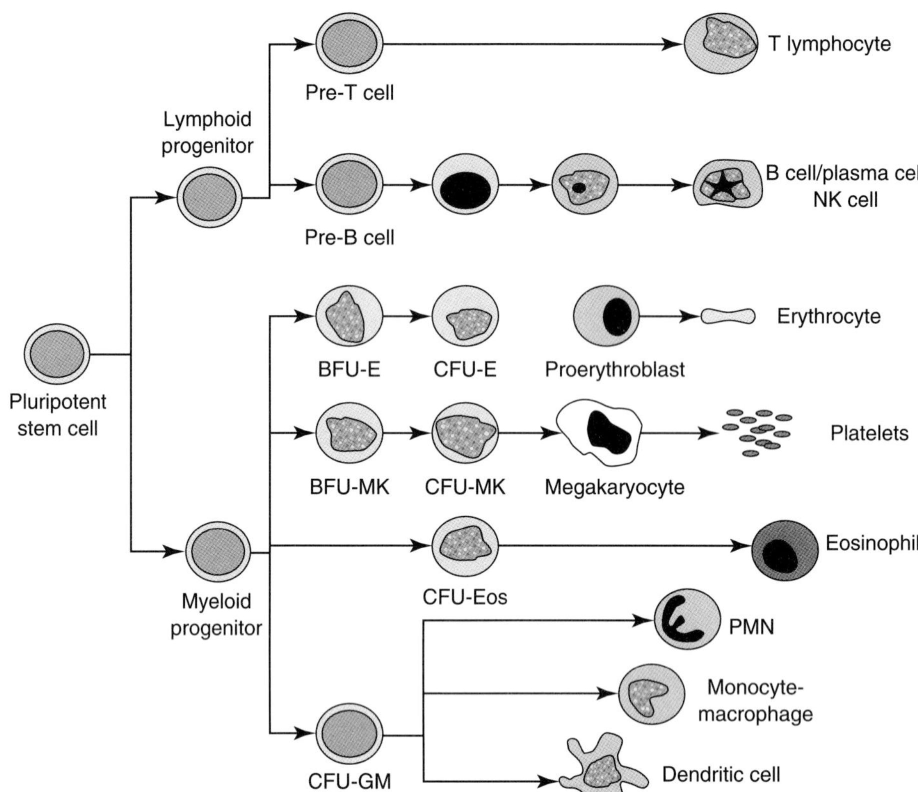


**FIGURE 75–1.** Overview of hematopoiesis. Hematopoietic lineages are outlined in this simplified overview of hematopoiesis. (BFU, burst forming unit; CFU, colony forming unit; E, erythroid; MK, megakaryocyte; GM, granulocyte-macrophage; Eos, eosinophil; NK, non-killer; PMN, polymorphonuclear).

combination of their physical characteristics, growth factor response, and the presence and absence of certain cell markers (Huss, 1997). Similarly, research focused on optimizing various harvest sites is ongoing. Bone marrow and cord blood are rich in stem cells and have long been used as progenitor cell pools. The collection of stem cells from peripheral blood by stimulated apheresis, with ex vivo expansion of select populations, is now also a viable option (Brugger et al, 2000; Pettengell et al, 1994a, 1994b).

This new appreciation for the vast potential of these pluripotent cells has raised political and ethical issues, which are currently being debated. It also has raised interesting new questions about the balance of hematopoiesis in the adult organism. That is, if pluripotent and multipotent cells are common throughout the body, what are the mechanisms by which they are kept in check?

## DEVELOPMENTAL ASPECTS OF ERYTHROPOIESIS

Erythropoiesis is the process of perpetual production of red blood cells. This process undergoes serial adaptations throughout development in order to meet the changing oxygen demands of the embryo, fetus, and neonate. The type of cells produced, the locations in which they are produced, and even the microenvironments present in these locations change as development proceeds. The molecular mechanisms involved in instituting, regulating, and maintaining these adaptations are complex and not yet fully understood. They are still the focus of active investigation.

### Primitive and Definitive Erythropoiesis

The earliest form of erythropoiesis is called *primitive erythropoiesis*. Primitive erythropoiesis takes place at several sites including the yolk sac, the ventral aspect of the aorta, the liver, and bone marrow. It is characterized by large CD34-negative ($CD34^-$) erythroblasts (>20 μm in diameter) that differentiate within blood vessels, remain nucleated, and contain predominantly embryonic hemoglobin. As development proceeds, a transition to definitive erythropoiesis occurs. Definitive erythropoiesis is characterized by smaller (<20 μm) $CD34^+$ erythroblasts, which produce fetal and adult hemoglobins and extrude their nuclei when mature. Unlike primitive erythropoiesis, this process is dependent on Janus kinase (JAK) signal transduction and erythropoietin (Epo) stimulation (Neubauer et al, 1998; Tavassoli, 1991; Wu et al, 1995). Primitive erythroblasts normally undergo apoptosis, becoming extinct during fetal life, whereas definitive erythroblasts are able to self-renew (Dieterlen-Lievre, 1997).

### Switch of the Primary Site of Erythropoiesis

Humans have four main sites of embryonic and fetal erythropoiesis: yolk sac, ventral aspect of the aorta, liver, and bone marrow. In rodents, the spleen also is an important site of hematopoiesis, but there is no evidence for this in healthy humans (Calhoun et al, 1996; Wolf et al, 1983). Studies using an in vitro embryonic stem cell differentiation system have shown that primitive and definitive erythroblasts arise from a common multipotential precursor, which is transiently responsive to specific cytokines such as vascular endothelial growth factor (VEGF) and *c*-kit ligand (Kennedy et al, 1997). Primitive progenitor cells first develop exclusively in the yolk sac, followed by the rise of definitive progenitors, also in the yolk sac (Palis et al, 1999). Another source of the early definitive progenitors is along the ventral aspect of the embryonic aorta (Tavian et al, 1996). Once circulation is established, progenitors from all lineages are detected in the blood, then in the fetal liver, and finally in the marrow (Palis et al, 1999).

### Yolk Sac

The yolk sac is an extraembryonic structure that can be subdivided into the primary and the secondary yolk sac. The primary yolk sac is transient and has no known hematopoietic function. It forms by proliferation and differentiation of primitive endodermal cells 7 to 8 days after conception. These endodermal cells give rise to mesodermal precursors (intermediate cells). The primary yolk sac then collapses into small vesicles, and the secondary yolk sac is formed from its remnants at 12 to 15 days post conception. By 16 to 19 days post conception, primitive erythropoiesis is found in the human yolk sac (Kelemen et al, 1979; Kennedy et al, 1997; Tavassoli, 1991). The secondary yolk sac is an active site of protein synthesis, nutrient transport, and hematopoiesis (Enders and King, 1993). Primitive hematopoietic cells, adherent to surrounding endothelial cells, are first observed at day 16 in the mesodermal layer. These hematopoietic-endothelial cell masses have been described as blood islands (Zon, 1995). As maturation proceeds, these blood islands migrate toward each other, merging to form a network of capillaries. Small clusters of undifferentiated cells, the hemangioblasts, and clusters of primitive erythroblasts are observed in the small vessels present at this developmental stage (Enders and King, 1993). As differentiation proceeds, endothelial and hematopoietic cell lineages emerge. These cell lines share common molecular markers and responsiveness to a cohort of growth factors, and, depending on the microenvironment, can be derived from a common stem cell in culture (Choi, 1998; Choi et al, 1998; Eichmann et al, 1997; Munoz-Chapuli et al, 1999; Robb and Elefanty, 1998; Robertson et al, 1999). Hematopoietic cell antigen is an adhesion molecule that is thought to be a crucial element of the hematopoietic microenvironment present in the yolk sac, essential for both embryonic hematopoiesis and vasculogenesis (Ohneda et al, 2001).

After the sixth week post conception, definitive erythroblasts are found in the yolk sac. A decline in yolk sac hematopoiesis is observed after the eighth week of gestation (Enders and King, 1993). In vivo differences in hematopoietic potential have been observed between yolk sac cells and progenitor cells in the liver. Yolk sac–derived hematopoietic cells have more restricted potential in vivo, as only red cells and macrophages are present in the yolk sac (Enzan, 1986), whereas progenitor cells in the liver develop into the full spectrum of hematopoietic lineages (Palis et al, 1999). However, when yolk sac–derived stem cells are cultured in vitro, or are transplanted, they are multipotent, illustrating the importance of the microenvironment in the development of committed cell lineages (Tavassoli, 1991).

### Aorto-Gonado-Mesonephron

Another site of early erythropoietic activity in the developing human embryo is the ventral aspect of the aorta, in the periumbilical region (Huyhn et al, 1995; Tavian et al, 1996). At around the 23rd postconceptional day in humans, the multipotent hematopoietic progenitor cells in this region are more numerous than in the yolk sac or the liver (Huyhn et al, 1995). It remains unclear whether this is the primary source of definitive hematopoietic stem cells in humans (Zon, 1995) or whether these cells are first derived from the yolk sac and then migrate into this region, the liver, and the bone marrow. By day 40 of gestation, hematopoiesis in the AGM is concluded.

### Liver

A short time after the onset of the circulation (weeks 4 to 5 of gestation), erythropoiesis begins in the liver (Kelemen et al, 1979). As in the yolk sac, primitive erythroblasts predominate in early erythropoiesis. However, over the next 4 weeks, definitive erythrocytes become the predominant red cell form. During this time, the liver mass increases 40-fold, with hematopoietic cells constituting 60% of the liver by weeks 11 to 12 (Thomas and Yoffey, 1964). Meanwhile, other hematopoietic cell lineages also are produced in the liver. Early in this process (5 weeks), the macrophage predominates, with approximately one granulocyte to every nine macrophages (Slayton et al, 1998a). In contrast with the yolk sac, during the period of peak hepatic hematopoiesis (weeks 6 to 18), production of all hematopoietic cell lines—erythrocytes, macrophages, megakaryocytes, granulocytes, and lymphocytes—occurs. Between 18 and 21 weeks of gestation, hematopoiesis in the liver diminishes but the liver continues as an erythropoietic organ until term.

### Bone Marrow

As hepatic hematopoiesis diminishes, the bone marrow becomes the primary site of erythropoiesis and remains so throughout postnatal life. The process of erythropoiesis in marrow begins at about 8 weeks, again, with primitive erythrocytosis (Kelemen et al, 1979). Over the next weeks, a switch to definitive erythropoiesis occurs, and by 14 weeks, only definitive erythroblasts are present. As with the liver, production of all hematopoietic cells occurs in bone marrow. Erythropoietic cells constitute a maximum of 35% of total bone marrow cells at week 12 of gestation, falling to between 20% and 30% thereafter (Charbord et al, 1996; Thomas and Yoffey, 1962).

### Factors Influencing the Sites of Erythropoiesis

The microenvironment at each site of hematopoiesis influences the type and timing of hematopoietic development. The microenvironment includes hematopoietic growth factors and cytokines, as well as the extracellular matrix in which the cells proliferate.

Growth factors are thought to act mainly as permissive and/or selective signals, allowing specific, already committed, cell types to proliferate and differentiate. Growth factors important for definitive erythropoiesis include Epo, stem cell factor (SCF) *c*-kit, interleukin-3 (IL-3), thrombopoietin (TPO), and possibly insulin and insulin-like growth factor I (IGF-1), both of which act as nonessential survival factors for $CD34^+$ cells (Muta et al, 1994; Ratajczak et al, 1998). The foregoing growth factors work in concert to promote erythropoiesis; however, Epo can be considered the primary growth factor in the process of erythropoiesis, as in its absence, definitive erythropoiesis does not occur. Similarly, the absence of the Epo receptor also eliminates definitive erythropoiesis. Null mutations of either Epo or its receptor are therefore lethal at 13 days of gestation in the mouse (Wu et al, 1995).

### Extramedullary Hematopoiesis

After the bone marrow has been established as the primary site of erythropoiesis, extramedullary hematopoiesis occasionally occurs as a pathologic process. This can occur with severe bone marrow failure of any etiology, but common causes include congenital rubella and cytomegalovirus (CMV) or parvovirus B19 infection. Extramedullary hematopoiesis has been documented in many tissues, including the liver, spleen, adrenal glands, pancreas, thyroid gland, endocardium, testes, uterus, skin, and brain. Involvement of the skin results in the classic "blueberry muffin" rash seen in newborns with congenital rubella or CMV infection.

## Ontogeny of Erythrocytes

The earliest precursor cells specific to the erythroid lineage are the burst-forming unit–erythroid (BFU-E) cells. BFU-Es have low numbers of Epo receptors (Sawada et al, 1988, 1990) and respond to Epo, as well as to granulocyte-macrophage colony stimulating factor (GM-CSF) and IL-3. As these cells mature into colony-forming unit–erythroid (CFU-E) cells and proerythroblasts, they become highly dependent on Epo, which is reflected by the high density of Epo receptors on the cell membrane (up to 1000 per cell) (Broudy et al, 1991). Mature erythroblasts have fewer Epo receptors and therefore are less sensitive to Epo stimulation, whereas reticulocytes and erythrocytes have no Epo receptors and are unresponsive to Epo (Fig. 75–2). These mature cells are unique in that they do not have a nucleus, DNA, RNA, ribosomes, or mitochondria. The principal functions of mature erythrocyte metabolism are to maintain adequate adenosine triphosphate (ATP) stores, to produce reducing substances to act as antioxidants, and to produce 2,3-diphosphoglycerate (2,3-DPG), which modifies the oxygen affinity of hemoglobin.

Important developmental changes occur in hematocrit, reticulocyte count, and red cell morphology, membrane content, deformability, life span, and metabolism. Over the course of gestation, there is a rise in expected hematocrit, from 36% ± 3% at 18 to 20 weeks of gestation (fetal samples) to 61% ± 7% expected at term birth. In order to maintain the increase in blood volume and hematocrit associated with fetal growth (up to 7 mL/day during the last trimester), the production of approximately $50 \times 10^9$ erythrocytes per day is required, based on animal experiments (Bell and Wintour, 1985). During this same period of fetal development, erythrocyte size (the mean cell volume) decreases from 134 ± 9 fL to 119 ± 9 fL (Forestier et al, 1986; McIntosh et al, 1988; Zaizov and Matoth, 1976). Mean cell volume continues to drop postnatally, reaching a nadir at 4 to 6 months of life. It then increases until it reaches adult values (88 ± 8 fL) at approximately 1 year of life.

Reticulocytes are erythrocytes that have been recently released from the bone marrow into the circulation. Although the nucleus has been extruded, they retain cytoplasmic organelles such as ribosomes, mitochondria, and Golgi bodies for approximately 24 hours. These newly released cells can be differentiated from mature red blood cells by staining with new methylene blue or brilliant cresyl blue, both of which stain the nucleic acid within the cells. Evaluation of a patient's reticulocyte count can be used to assess the level of erythrocyte production, as high values indicate active erythropoiesis and depressed levels indicate low levels of erythropoiesis. At birth, reticulocyte counts in preterm infants tend to be higher than in term infants (400,000 to 550,000 versus 200,000 to 400,000) (Christensen, 2000). Absolute reticulocyte counts, reticulocyte percentage of total red cells, and corrected reticulocyte counts can be obtained. In general, in evaluating neonates, the corrected reticulocyte count is the most helpful, as this reflects the reticulocyte

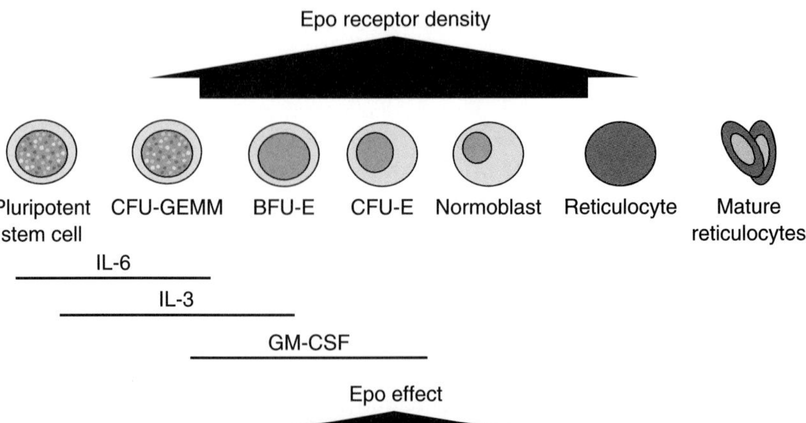


**FIGURE 75–2.** Simplified scheme of erythropoiesis. The timing of cytokine effects during erythropoiesis are delineated. (CFU, colony forming unit; GEMM, granulocyte erythroid monocyte macrophage; BFU, burst forming unit; E, erythroid; IL, interleukin; GM-CSF, granulocyte macrophage-colony stimulating factor; Epo, erythropoietin).

response relative to the hematocrit. This corrected value is obtained as follows: reticulocyte percentage (%) × hematocrit (L/L) ÷ desired or optimal hematocrit (L/L).

Red cell morphology is quite heterogeneous in preterm and term infants as compared with that in adults. Irregularly shaped cells such as poikilocytes, acanthocytes, schizocytes and burr cells are common in the blood smears of neonates. This finding reflects developmental changes in membrane deformability and flexibility. The neonatal red blood cell membrane has decreased deformability, which contributes to its decreased life span of approximately 70 days, compared with 120 days for the adult red blood cell. Membrane characteristics become more adult-like by 4 to 6 weeks of age.

## Developmental Changes in the Regulation of Erythropoiesis

### Erythropoietin

The principal growth factor that regulates erythropoiesis is Epo. This 30.4-kDa glycoprotein contains 165 amino acids and is extensively glycosylated, with a 40% carbohydrate content. Epo maintains red cell production during fetal, neonatal, and adult life by inhibiting apoptosis of erythroid progenitors and by stimulating their proliferation and differentiation into normoblasts (Jelkmann, 1992; Muta et al, 1994; Moritz et al, 1997; Palis and Segel, 1998). Because erythropoietin does not cross the placenta, the Epo concentrations measured in the fetus reflect fetal synthesis (Widness et al, 1989, 1991). Epo production begins early in fetal life, and it has been identified in extraembryonic coelomic fluid and amniotic fluid (Campbell et al, 1992). The primary site of Epo production during fetal life is the liver, but this changes to the kidney postnatally (Koury and Koury, 1993). The liver is less sensitive to hypoxic stimuli than the kidney, so in utero, Epo is thought to work synergistically with other growth factors such as hepatic growth factor, TPO, and IGF-1 (Iguchi et al, 1999; Ikehara, 1996; Kaushansky et al, 1995; Migliaccio and Migliaccio, 1988; Okajima et al, 1998). During human development the kidneys contribute less than 9% of total Epo mRNA expression until the 30th week of gestation, increasing to 27% later in gestation. This increase of renal Epo production after the 30th week of gestation may be a consequence of the growth and maturation of the kidney and the developmental increase in Epo-expressing interstitial cells (Avner, 1992). These data suggest that the switch of Epo production would be complete by several months of life. This switch from liver to kidney as the primary site of Epo production and the relative insensitivity of the liver Epo production to tissue hypoxia may contribute to anemia of prematurity.

During fetal development, circulating Epo concentrations increase from 4 mU/mL at 16 weeks of gestation to 40 mU/mL at term (Fahnenstich et al, 1996; Ireland et al, 1992; Ruth et al, 1988; Widness et al, 1984). After birth in healthy term infants, serum Epo concentrations decrease from between 15 to 40 mU/mL at birth to reach a nadir between weeks 4 to 6 after birth (Brown et al, 1983; Ruth et al, 1990). By 10 to 12 weeks of age they reach adult concentrations (approximately 15 mU/mL) (Kling et al, 1996). These changes in Epo concentrations are consistent with the changes in hemoglobin and hematocrit seen following term birth (physiologic anemia). In premature infants, the anemia is more severe and persists longer, leading to the anemia of prematurity described previously. Epo concentrations in these infants are inappropriately low, forming the rationale for recombinant human Epo therapy.

## Ontogeny of Hemoglobin Chains

### Organization and Structure of the Hemoglobins

Hemoglobin is a tetrameric molecule composed of two pairs of polypeptide subunits. As development proceeds, various hemoglobins are constructed by combining two α-like globins (ζ or α) with two β-like globins (ε, γ, δ, or β) to form a hemoglobin tetramer. These tetramers include the embryonic hemoglobins Hb Gower 1 ($\zeta_2\epsilon_2$), Hb Gower 2 ($\alpha_2\epsilon_2$), and Hb Portland 1 ($\zeta_2\gamma_2$); fetal hemoglobin (HbF) ($\alpha_2\gamma_2$); and the adult hemoglobins HbA ($\alpha_2\beta_2$) and $HbA_2$ ($\alpha_2\delta_2$). Their expression and proportion depend on gestational age but can be modified in part by external mechanisms. The basic function of the various hemoglobins is similar, but their oxygen affinity differs. As the hemoglobins switch from embryonic to fetal to adult forms, oxygen affinity decreases. Thus, the switch from embryonic to fetal to adult hemoglobin synthesis is a major mechanism by which the developing fetus adapts from the intrauterine to the extrauterine environment (Bard, 2000).

### Changes in Hemoglobin Synthesis with Development

The genes within the α-globin as well as the β-globin families are expressed according to a strict ontogenetic schedule, and the quantitative expression of the genes from each of these families is strictly balanced and coordinated (Bard, 2000). Hemoglobin synthesis begins around 14 days post conception, with synthesis of ζ-globin and ε-globin chains. These are replaced by the synthesis of α-globin and γ-globin chains by the fifth to seventh week of gestation (Hb Gower 2, Hb Portland 1, and HbF become predominant) (Gale et al, 1979). By 12 weeks of gestation, HbF ($\alpha_2\gamma_2$) accounts for almost all of the hemoglobin (Cividalli et al, 1974). After the 20th week of gestation, no ε-globin chains are produced, but the production of the ζ-globin chains can persist through the last trimester in pathologic conditions such as homozygous alpha-thalassemia. The expression of the γ-globin gene peaks during midgestation and declines rapidly during the last month of fetal gestation. Beta-globin synthesis, required for HbA, starts at the sixth week of gestation, increasing as γ-globin synthesis declines, a transition that continues to the sixth month of life (Bard, 1975; Kazazian and Woodhead, 1973). Thus, HbA synthesis quantitatively increases first after the 30th week of gestation. At the end of the last trimester, a rapid switch from the synthesis of fetal hemoglobin to adult hemoglobin occurs, falling from 85% at 34 weeks of gestation to 60% to 80% at birth (Peri et al, 1998). The synthesis of δ-globin chains, required for $HbA_2$ ($\alpha_2\delta_2$), begins at weeks 34 to 35 of gestation. After birth, a rapid increase in HbA and $HbA_2$ occurs.

## BILIRUBIN METABOLISM

The primary source of bilirubin in the fetus and newborn is from the breakdown of heme derived from hemoglobin in circulating erythrocytes. Heme is a porphyrin ring surrounding a ferric ion ($Fe^{3+}$). The rate-limiting step in the breakdown of this molecule is the formation of biliverdin, a process controlled by heme oxygenase (Beri and Chandra, 1993; Rodgers and Stevenson, 1990). The iron molecule is recycled, and biliverdin is then reduced to bilirubin IXα by biliverdin reductase. In utero, unconjugated bilirubin is processed by the mother after placental transfer. Thus, under normal circumstances, the fetal liver plays only a minor role in bilirubin excretion. Unconjugated bilirubin is lipophilic and is tightly bound to albumin in the circulation. The conjugation of bilirubin results in a relatively polar, water-soluble molecule, bilirubin diglucuronide, which can be excreted. This process occurs in the liver and is dependent on ligandin, a transfer protein, and uridine diphosphoglucuronyltransferase. The conjugating ability of the fetus and newborn is impaired relative to older cohorts as a result of reduced transferase activity and low levels of uridine diphosphoglucuronic acid (Dennery et al, 2001). Conjugation can be induced in the fetus, however, as during circumstances of increased hemolysis, with its associated increase in bilirubin load, increased conjugated bilirubin can be detected at birth. After birth, the neonate must metabolize the increased load of bilirubin without the assistance of the mother.

## DEVELOPMENTAL ASPECTS OF MEGAKARYOCYTOPOIESIS

Platelets are small (average volume of 7.5 fL), anucleate fragments of megakaryocytes, which circulate as smooth disks when unactivated. The normal circulating lifespan of a platelet is 10 days. Platelets provide the first line of defense in hemostasis. When a breach of the vascular endothelial lining occurs, platelets are activated and adhere to the exposed subendothelium. These activated platelets generate various mediators, including the potent vasoconstrictor thromboxane $A_2$ and adenosine diphosphate (ADP), both of which further contribute to hemostatic plug formation.

### Sites of Megakaryocyte Production

*Megakaryocytopoiesis* is the process by which megakaryocytes and ultimately platelets develop. As with erythropoiesis, the sites of megakaryocytopoiesis change during embryonic and fetal development. In mouse development, megakaryocytes have been identified in the early yolk sac. These cells, when cultured in the presence of SCF, IL-3, IL-6, Epo, TPO, and granulocyte colony-stimulating factor (G-CSF), can produce not only erythroid bursts but also megakaryocyte colonies. The megakaryocyte progenitors share a common progenitor with primitive hematopoietic cells (Xu et al, 2001). In humans, electron micrographic studies have shown megakaryocytes present in the liver and circulatory system as early as 8 weeks post conception (Hesseldahl and Falck Larsen, 1971).

### Megakaryocyte Precursors

Megakaryocytopoiesis begins with the pluripotent hematopoietic stem cells, which give rise to myloid progenitor cells (CFU-S) and then burst-forming unit–megakaryocyte (BFU-MK) cells, followed by colony-forming unit–megakaryocyte (CFU-MK) cells (see Fig. 75–1). Further maturation brings these small mononuclear cells, which are largely indistinguishable from monocytes, to large polyploid cells that are easily recognized on the basis of their phenotype. The process of megakaryocyte differentiation has been separated into four stages. Stage I cells, or megakaryoblasts, are the smallest and most immature. As cells mature through stage II (promegakaryocytes), stage III (granular megakaryocytes), and stage IV (mature megakaryocytes), the nucleus becomes multilobed, the cytoplasm becomes increasingly eosinophilic by Wright-Giemsa staining, and cellular size increases from 6 to 24 μm up to as great as 50 μm. The presence of granules increases steadily until in the mature cells they become organized into "platelet fields." Unlike in other cell lines, as the nucleus of megakaryocytes matures, it undergoes endomitosis or endoreduplication, a process by which cell ploidy is increased in the absence of cell division. Megakaryocytes from adults typically have a modal ploidy of 16N, while comparable samples from preterm or term infants have a significantly lower ploidy of less than 8N (Ma et al, 1996). Megakaryocytes from newborns are also typically smaller than in adults, although they manifest features of mature megakaryocytes. Adult-size megakaryocytes appear by 2 years of age. Typically, smaller cells with lower ploidy produce less platelets than do larger cells with higher ploidy. Nevertheless, the platelet count in fetuses and newborns is within the normal adult range. This is thought to reflect an increased proliferative rate in fetal megakaryocyte progenitors.

### Control of Megakaryocytopoiesis

Multiple cytokines participate in the process of megakaryocytopoiesis; however, TPO is the principal one. IL-3, IL-6, and SCF increase ploidy and size of megakaryocytes. IL-11 also stimulates the proliferation of megakaryocyte progenitors and induces megakaryocyte maturation. Still other growth factors such as Epo, kit ligand, GM-CSF, IL-1, basic fibroblast growth factor, platelet-derived growth factor, and interferon-γ have a less clearly defined role. Some cytokines inhibit thrombopoiesis, including transforming growth factor-β (TGF-β) and platelet factor-4 (Gewirtz et al, 1995). The magnitude of the influence of these growth factors changes with development (Deutsch et al, 1995).

### Thrombopoietin

The presence of a growth factor to regulate platelet formation was first hypothesized in 1958 by Kelemen, but it was not actually realized until 1994, when the protein was isolated by five independent laboratories. TPO is composed of 332 amino acids and contains two domains. The amino terminus is the active domain (153 amino acids) and bears marked homology to Epo. TPO is produced primarily by the liver and kidney, although other tissues express small amounts. TPO acts as a potent stimulator of all stages of megakaryocyte growth and development by binding to its specific cell surface receptor, c-mpl. In TPO and c-mpl knockout models, platelet production is 10% to 15% of controls, confirming that TPO is the primary regulator of platelet production but also indicating that alternative pathways exist for megakaryocytopoiesis. Serum TPO concentrations tend to be lower in preterm infants than in older infants and children, and the TPO response to thrombocytopenia is less robust as gestational age decreases. This diminished response is counterbalanced by an increased sensitivity of megakaryocyte precursors to TPO (Sola et al, 1999, 2000).

### Developmental Changes in Platelet Count

Fetal platelet counts increase linearly with gestation. At 15 weeks of gestation, average platelet counts are 187,000/μL, increasing to 274,000/μL at term (Van den Hof, 1990). Although platelet counts in preterm infants are somewhat lower than those in adults, they remain within the same range (150,000 to 400,000/μL). Thus, a platelet count of less than 150,000/μL is considered abnormal, even in a premature infant.

## DEVELOPMENTAL ASPECTS OF GRANULOCYTOPOIESIS

Early hematopoiesis is characterized almost exclusively by erythropoiesis, although a small number of macrophages are produced in the yolk sac. After circulation begins in the fourth to fifth week of gestation, macrophages appear in the liver, brain, and lungs. During the fifth week, hematopoiesis begins in the liver, and the first hematopoietic cells to appear are macrophages (Kelemen and Janossa, 1980). Whether Kupffer cells originate in the yolk sac and migrate to the liver or rise de novo in the liver is unknown. The marrow space begins to develop around the eighth week after conception, and as is true in the liver, the first hematopoietic cells to appear in the bones are phagocytes (Kelemen et al, 1979; Slayton et al, 1998a). These phagocytic osteoclasts seem to "core out" the marrow space. When hematopoiesis is established in the marrow at 10 to 11 weeks post conception, primarily neutrophils are produced, in contrast to the liver, where primarily macrophages are present (Slayton et al, 1998a, 1998b).

The thymus appears around 8 weeks post conception. T cell progenitors are thought to migrate from the fetal liver to the thymus at 8 to 9 weeks following conception (Haynes et al, 1989), and by the 10th week, lymphoid cells constitute 95% of this organ, with granulocyte precursors and macrophages making up the remainder. B-cell precursors first appear in the omentum and the fetal liver at 8 weeks post conception. B-cell production in the omentum occurs transiently from 8 to 10 weeks, while production continues in the fetal liver.

The spleen is an important secondary lymphatic organ in humans, and lymphocytes begin to appear in the spleen around 11 weeks following conception. By the 22nd week, 70% of the cells are lymphocytes (Kelemen et al, 1979).

The events of erythropoiesis are summarized in Fig. 75–3.

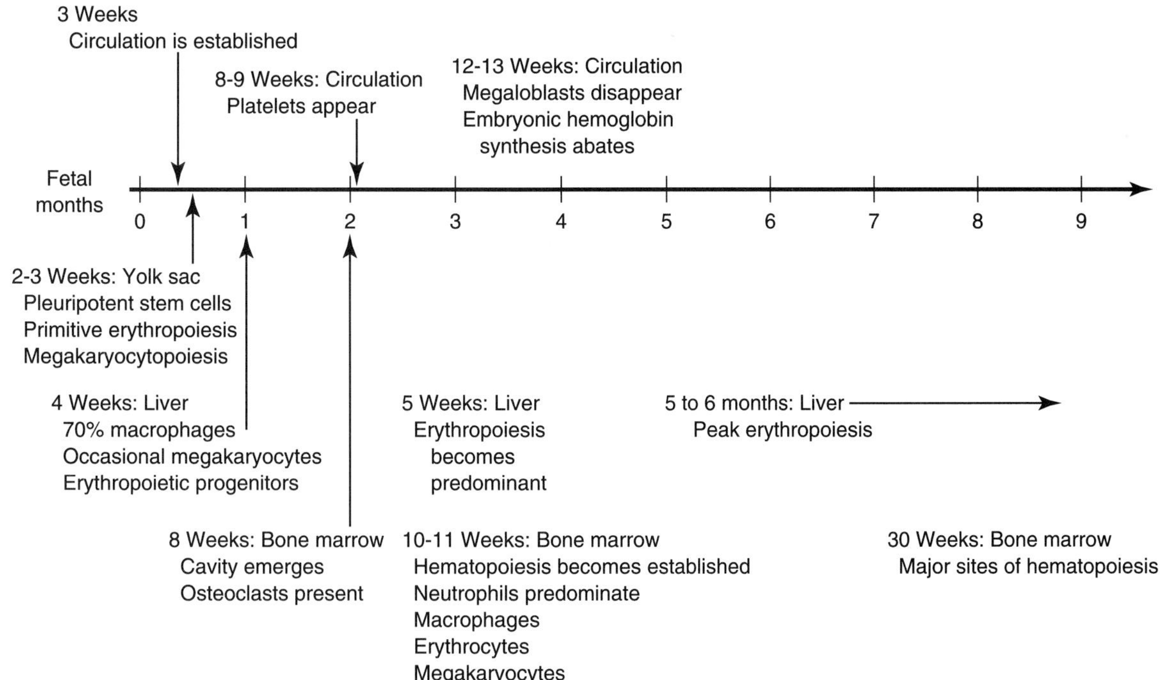


**FIGURE 75–3.** Change sites of hematopoiesis during human gestation. Fetal gestation is shown in months along the central horizontal arrow. The timing of significant events during hematopoiesis are shown from primitive erythropoiesis and megakaryocytopoiess in the yolk sac, to mature hematopoiesis in the bone marrow during late gestation.

## OVERVIEW OF HEMATOPOIETIC CYTOKINES

Hematopoietic growth factors can be classified into two groups: those responsible for the regulation of myeloid and erythroid growth and differentiation, called *colony-stimulating factors* (CSFs), and those concerned with immunity, called *lymphokines*. Once sequenced, lymphokines are assigned interleukin (IL) numbers. There is a great deal of functional overlap between hematopoietic growth factors (redundancy), and each growth factor has a multiplicity of biologic actions (pleiotropy). Thus, more than one cytokine controls cells in any cell lineage, and most factors affect cells in more than one lineage (Metcalf, 1994; Nicola, 1994; Nicola and Metcalf, 1991).

Epo, GM-CSF, and G-CSF belong to a family of hematopoietic cytokines that includes growth hormone, prolactin, and IL-2 through IL-7 (Bazan, 1989). These cytokines share a predicted tertiary structure and function by binding to specific cell surface receptors. Specific ligand binding results in allosteric changes in the receptor molecules, which, depending on the type of receptor, results either in protein kinase activation, as with macrophage colony-stimulating factor (M-CSF) (Nicola et al, 1997), or in a cascade of intracellular signaling via the JAK-2 mechanism, as is characterized by Epo (Watowich et al, 1996).

The receptors for most of these cytokines belong to a receptor superfamily. Family members include receptors for GM-CSF, G-CSF, IL-3 through IL-7, growth hormone, prolactin, neurociliary trophic factor, and TPO. Members of this family share structural similarities and an absence of a tyrosine kinase domain in the cytoplasmic domain (Bazan, 1990; Watowich et al, 1996). These cytokine receptors often are assembled as multisubunit complexes and have been grouped into subfamilies on the basis of the pattern subunit formation. In some cases (e.g., GM-CSF receptor [GM-CSF-R]), an accessory protein contributes to the stability of the receptor complex (Brizzi et al, 1991).

Many of the hematopoietic cytokines were discovered by virtue of their growth-promoting effects on hematopoietic cell lines or their specific immune functions. It initially was assumed that the effects of these cytokines were specific to the hematopoietic system. This view has now been challenged, as evidence has accumulated that many of these growth factors have other important roles that are not hematopoietic (Juul, 2000). Indeed, this is an area of active research, as some of these cytokines have potential as protective agents in the brain, gut, and elsewhere (Cerami, 2001; Juul et al, 2001; Ledbetter and Juul, 2000).

## REFERENCES


Avner ED: Embryogenesis and anatomic development of the kidney. In Polin RA, Fox WW (eds): Fetal and Neonatal Physiology, vol II. Philadelphia, WB Saunders, 1992, pp 1181-1187.

Bard H: Hemoglobin synthesis and metabloism during the neonatal period. In Christensen RD (ed): Hematologic Problems of the Neonate. Philadelphia, WB Saunders, 2000, pp 365-388.

Bard H: The postnatal decline of hemoglobin F synthesis in normal full-term infants. J Clin Invest 55:395-398, 1975.

Bazan JF: Haemopoietic receptors and helical cytokines. Immunol Today 11:350-354, 1990.

Bazan JF: A novel family of growth factor receptors: A common binding domain in the growth hormone, prolactin, erythropoietin and IL-6 receptors, and the p75 IL-2 receptor beta-chain. Biochem Biophys Res Commun 164:788-795, 1989.

Bell RJ, Wintour EM: The effect of maternal water deprivation on ovine fetal blood volume. J Exp Physiol 70:95-99, 1985.

Beri R, Chandra R: Chemistry and biology of heme. Effect of metal salts, organometals, and metalloporphyrins on heme synthesis and catabolism, with special reference to clinical implications and interactions with cytochrome P-450. Drug Metab Rev 25:49-152, 1993.

Bjornson CR, Rietze RL, Reynolds BA, et al: Turning brain into blood: A hematopoietic fate adopted by adult neural stem cells in vivo. Science 283:534-537, 1999.

Brizzi MF, Avanzi GC, Pegoraro L: Hematopoietic growth factor receptors. Int J Cell Cloning 9:274-300, 1991.

Broudy VC, Lin N, Brice M, et al: Erythropoietin receptor characteristics on primary human erythroid cells. Blood 77: 2583-2590, 1991.

Brown MS, Phibbs RH, Garcia JF, Dallman, PR: Postnatal changes in erythropoietin levels in untransfused premature infants. J Pediatr 103:612-617, 1983.

Brugger W, Scheding S, Ziegler B, et al: Ex vivo manipulation of hematopoietic stem and progenitor cells. Semin Hematol 37:42-49, 2000.

Calhoun DA, Li Y, Braylan RC, Christensen RD: Assessment of the contribution of the spleen to granulocytopoiesis and erythropoiesis of the mid-gestation human fetus. Early Hum Dev 46:217-227, 1996.

Campbell J, Wathen N, Lewis M, et al: Erythropoietin levels in amniotic fluid and extraembryonic coelomic fluid in the first trimester of pregnancy. Br J Obstet Gynaecol 99:974-976, 1992.

Cerami A: Beyond erythropoiesis: Novel applications for recombinant human erythropoietin. Semin Hematol 38:33-39, 2001.

Charbord P, Tavian M, Humeau L, Peault B: Early ontogeny of the human marrow from long bones: An immunohistochemical study of hematopoiesis and its microenvironment. Blood 87:4109-4119, 1996.

Choi K: Hemangioblast development and regulation. Biochem Cell Biol 76:947-956, 1998.

Choi K, Kennedy M, Kazarov A, et al: A common precursor for hematopoietic and endothelial cells. Development 125: 725-732, 1998.

Christensen RD: Expected hematologic values for term and preterm neonates. In Christensen RD (ed): Hematologic Problems of the Neonate. Philadelphia, WB Saunders, 2000, pp 117-136.

Cividalli G, Nathan DG, Kan YW, et al: Relation of beta to gamma synthesis during the first trimester: An approach to prenatal diagnosis of thalassemia. Pediatr Res 8:553-560, 1974.

Dennery PA, Seidman DS, Stevenson DK, et al: Neonatal hyperbilirubinemia. N Engl J Med 344:581-590, 2001.

Deutsch VR, Olson TA, Nagler A, et al: The response of cord blood megakaryocyte progenitors to IL-3, IL-6 and aplastic canine serum varies with gestational age. Br J Haematol 89: 8-16, 1995.

Dieterlen-Lievre F: Intraembryonic hematopoietic stem cells. Hematol Oncol Clin North Am 11:1149-1171, 1997.

Eichmann A, Corbel C, Nataf V, et al: Ligand-dependent development of the endothelial and hemopoietic lineages from embryonic mesodermal cells expressing vascular endothelial growth factor receptor 2. Proc Natl Acad Sci USA 94: 5141-5146, 1997.

Enders A, King B: Development of the human yolk sac. In Nogales FF (ed): The Human Yolk Sac and Yolk Sac Tumors. Berlin, Springer, 1993, p 33.

Enzan H: Electron microscopic studies of macrophages in early human yolk sacs. Acta Pathol Jpn 36:49-64, 1986.

Fahnenstich H, Dame C, Allera A, Kowalewski S: Biochemical monitoring of fetal distress with serum-immunoreactive erythropoietin. J Perinat Med 24:85-91, 1996.

Fleischmann WR Jr, Fleischmann CM, Fiers W: Potentiation of interferon action by mixtures of recombinant DNA-derived human interferons. Antiviral Res 4:357-360, 1984.

Forestier F, Daffos F, Galacteros F, et al: Hematological values of 163 normal fetuses between 18 and 30 weeks of gestation. Pediatr Res 20:342-346, 1986.

Gale RE, Clegg JB, Huehns, ER: Human embryonic haemoglobins Gower 1 and Gower 2. Nature 280:162-164, 1979.

Gewirtz AM, Zhang J, Ratajczak J, et al: Chemokine regulation of human megakaryocytopoiesis. Blood 86:2559-2567, 1995.

Haynes BF, Denning SM, Singer KH, Krtzberg J: Ontogeny of T-cell precursors: A model for the initial stages of human T-cell development. Immunol Today 10:87-91, 1989.

Hesseldahl H, Falck Larsen J: Hemopoiesis and blood vessels in human yolk sac. An electron microscopic study. Acta Anat 78:274-294, 1971.

Huss R: New definition and methods for isolation of the earliest peripheral blood-derived hematopoietic stem cells. Beitr Infusionsther Transfusionsmed 34:128-132, 1997.

Huss R: Perspectives on the morphology and biology of CD34-negative stem cells. J Hematother Stem Cell Res 9:783-793, 2000.

Huyhn A, Dommergues M, Izac B, et al: Characterization of hematopoietic progenitors from human yolk sacs and embryos. Blood 86:4474-4485, 1995.

Iguchi T, Sogo S, Hisha H, et al: HGF activates signal transduction from EPO receptor on human cord blood $CD34^{+}CD45^{+}$ cells. Stem Cells 17:82-91, 1999.

Ikehara S: Role of hepatocyte growth factor in hemopoiesis. Leuk Lymphoma 23:297-303, 1996.

Ireland R, Abbas A, Thilaganathan B, et al: Fetal and maternal erythropoietin levels in normal pregnancy. Fetal Diagn Ther 7:21-25, 1992.

Jelkmann W: Erythropoietin: Structure, control of production, and function. Physiol Rev 72:449-489, 1992.

Juul SE: Nonhematopoietic actions of hematopoietic growth factors in the fetus and neonate. In Christensen RD (ed): Hematologic Problems of the Neonate. Philadelphia, WB Saunders, 2000, pp 61-78.

Juul SE, Ledbetter DJ, Joyce AE, et al: Erythropoietin acts as a trophic factor in neonatal rat intestine. Gut 49:182-189, 2001.

Kaushansky K, Broudy VC, Grossman A, et al: Thrombopoietin expands erythroid progenitors, increases red cell production, and enhances erythroid recovery after myelosuppressive therapy. J Clin Invest 96:1683-1687, 1995.

Kazazian HH Jr, Woodhead AP: Hemoglobin A synthesis in the developing fetus. N Engl J Med 289:58-62, 1973.

Kelemen E, Calvo W, Fliedner TM: Atlas of Human Haematopoietic Development. New York, Springer, 1979.

Keleman E, Cserhati I, Tanos B: Demonstration and some properties of human thrombopoietin in thrombocythaemic sera. Acta Haematol. 20:350-355, 1958.

Kelemen E, Janossa M: Macrophages are the first differentiated blood cells formed in human embryonic liver. Exp Hematol 8:996-1000, 1980.

Kennedy M, Firpo M, Choi K, et al: A common precursor for primitive erythropoiesis and definitive haematopoiesis. Nature 386:488-493, 1997.

Kling PJ, Schmidt RL, Roberts RA, Widness JA: Serum erythropoietin levels during infancy: Associations with erythropoiesis. J Pediatr 128:791-796, 1996.

Koury ST, Koury MJ: Erythropoietin production by the kidney. Semin Nephrol 13:78-86, 1993.

Lansdorp PM: Self-renewal of stem cells. Biol Blood Marrow Transplant 3:171-178, 1997.

Ledbetter DJ, Juul SE: Erythropoietin and the incidence of necrotizing enterocolitis in infants with very low birth weight. J Pediatr Surg 35:178-181; discussion 35:182, 2000.

Ma DC, Sun YH, Chang KZ, Zuo W: Developmental change of megakaryocyte maturation and DNA ploidy in human fetus. Eur J Haematol 57:121-127, 1996.

McIntosh N, Kempson C, Tyler RM: Blood counts in extremely low birthweight infants. Arch Dis Child 63:74-76, 1988.

Metcalf D: Implications of the polyfunctionality of hemopoietic regulators. Stem Cells 12:259-275, 1994.

Mezey E, Chandross KJ, Harta G, et al: Turning blood into brain: Cells bearing neuronal antigens generated in vivo from bone marrow. Science 290:1779-1782, 2000.

Migliaccio AR, Migliaccio G: Human embryonic hemopoiesis: Control mechanisms underlying progenitor differentiation in vitro. Dev Biol 125:127-134, 1988.

Moritz KM, Lim GB, Wintour EM: Developmental regulation of erythropoietin and erythropoiesis. Am J Physiol 273: R1829-1844, 1997.

Munoz-Chapuli R, Perez-Pomares JM, Macias D, et al: Differentiation of hemangioblasts from embryonic mesothelial cells? A model on the origin of the vertebrate cardiovascular system. Differentiation 64:133-141, 1999.

Muta K, Krantz SB, Bondurant MC, Wickrema A: Distinct roles of erythropoietin, insulin-like growth factor I, and stem cell factor in the development of erythroid progenitor cells. J Clin Invest 94:34-43, 1994.

Neubauer H, Cumano A, Muller M, et al: Jak2 deficiency defines an essential developmental checkpoint in definitive hematopoiesis. Cell 93:397-409, 1998.

Nicola NA: Cytokine pleiotropy and redundancy: A view from the receptor. Stem Cells 12:3-12, discussion 12-14, 1994.

Nicola NA, Metcalf D: Subunit promiscuity among hemopoietic growth factor receptors. Cell 67:1-4, 1991.

Nicola NA, Smith A, Robb L, et al: The structural basis of the biological actions of the GM-CSF receptor. Ciba Found Symp 204:19-27, 1997.

Notaro R, Cimmino A, Tabarini D, et al: In vivo telomere dynamics of human hematopoietic stem cells. Proc Natl Acad Sci U S A 94:13782-13785, 1997.

Ohneda O, Ohneda K, Arai F, et al: ALCAM (CD166): Its role in hematopoietic and endothelial development. Blood 98: 2134-2142, 2001.

Okajima Y, Matsumura I, Nishiura T, et al: Insulin-like growth factor-I augments erythropoietin-induced proliferation through enhanced tyrosine phosphorylation of STAT5. J Biol Chem 273:22877-22883, 1998.

Palis J, Robertson S, Kennedy M, et al: Development of erythroid and myeloid progenitors in the yolk sac and embryo proper of the mouse. Development 126:5073-5084, 1999.

Palis J, Segel GB: Developmental biology of erythropoiesis. Blood Rev 12:106-114, 1998.

Peri KG, Gagnon C, Bard H: Quantitative correlation between globin mRNAs and synthesis of fetal and adult hemoglobins during hemoglobin switchover in the perinatal period. Pediatr Res 43:504-508, 1998.

Pettengell R, Luft T, Henschler R, et al: Direct comparison by limiting dilution analysis of long-term culture-initiating cells in human bone marrow, umbilical cord blood, and blood stem cells. Blood 84:3653-3659, 1994a.

Pettengell R, Woll PJ, O'Connor DA, et al: Viability of haemopoietic progenitors from whole blood, bone marrow and leukapheresis product: Effects of storage media, temperature and time. Bone Marrow Transplant 14:703-709, 1994b.

Ratajczak J, Zhang Q, Pertusini E, et al: The role of insulin (INS) and insulin-like growth factor-I (IGF-I) in regulating human erythropoiesis. Studies in vitro under serum-free conditions—comparison to other cytokines and growth factors. Leukemia 12:371-381, 1998.

Robb L, Elefanty AG: The hemangioblast—an elusive cell captured in culture. Bioessays 20:611-614, 1998.

Robertson S, Kennedy M, Keller G: Hematopoietic commitment during embryogenesis. Ann N Y Acad Sci 872:9-15; discussion 872:15-16, 1999.

Rodgers PA, Stevenson DK: Developmental biology of heme oxygenase. Clin Perinatol 17:275-291, 1990.

Ruth V, Autti-Ramo I, Granstrom ML, et al: Prediction of perinatal brain damage by cord plasma vasopressin, erythropoietin, and hypoxanthine values. J Pediatr 113:880-885, 1988.

Ruth V, Widness JA, Clemons G, Raivio KO: Postnatal changes in serum immunoreactive erythropoietin in relation to hypoxia before and after birth. J Pediatr 116:950-954, 1990.

Sawada K, Krantz SB, Dai CH, et al: Purification of human blood burst-forming units–erythroid and demonstration of the evolution of erythropoietin receptors. J Cell Physiol 142:219-230, 1990.

Sawada K, Krantz SB, Sawyer ST, Civin CI: Quantitation of specific binding of erythropoietin to human erythroid colony-forming cells. J Cell Physiol 137:337-345, 1988.

Slayton WB, Juul SE, Calhoun DA, et al: Hematopoiesis in the liver and marrow of human fetuses at 5 to 16 weeks postconception: Quantitative assessment of macrophage and neutrophil populations. Pediatr Res 43:774-782, 1998a.

Slayton WB, Li Y, Calhoun DA, et al: The first-appearance of neutrophils in the human fetal bone marrow cavity. Early Hum Dev 53:129-144, 1998b.

Sola MC, Du Y, Hutson AD, et al.: Dose-response relationship of megakaryocyte progenitors from the bone marrow of thrombocytopenic and non-thrombocytopenic neonates to recombinant thrombopoietin. Br J Haematol 110:449-453, 2000.

Tavassoli M: Embryonic and fetal hemopoiesis: An overview. Blood Cells 17:269-281, 1991.

Tavian M, Coulombel L, Luton D, et al: Aorta-associated $CD34^+$ hematopoietic cells in the early human embryo. Blood 87:67-72, 1996.

Thomas D, Yoffey JM: Human foetal haemopoiesis. II. Hepatic haematopoiesis in the human foetus. Br J Haematol 10:193, 1964.

Thomas DB, Yoffey JM: Human foetal haemopoiesis. I. The cellular composition of foetal blood. Br J Haematol 8:290, 1962.

Van den Hof MC, Nicolaides KH: Platelet count in normal, small, and anemic fetuses. Am J Obstet Gynecol 162:735-739, 1990.

Vaziri H, Dragowska W, Allsopp RC, et al: Evidence for a mitotic clock in human hematopoietic stem cells: loss of telomeric DNA with age. Proc Natl Acad Sci U S A 91:9857-9860, 1994.

Watowich SS, Wu H, Socolovsky M, et al: Cytokine receptor signal transduction and the control of hematopoietic cell development. Annu Rev Cell Dev Biol 12:91-128, 1996.

Widness JA, Clemons GK, Garcia JF, et al: Increased immunoreactive erythropoietin in cord serum after labor. Am J Obstet Gynecol 148:194-197, 1984.

Widness JA, Malone TA, Mufson RA: Impermeability of the ovine placenta to 35S-recombinant erythropoietin. Pediatr Res 25:649-651, 1989.

Widness JA, Sawyer ST, Schmidt RL, Chestnut DH: Lack of maternal to fetal transfer of $^{125}$I-labelled erythropoietin in sheep. J Dev Physiol 15:139-143, 1991.

Wolf BC, Luevano E, Neiman RS: Evidence to suggest that the human fetal spleen is not a hematopoietic organ. Am J Clin Pathol 80:140-144, 1983.

Wu H, Liu X, Lodish HF: Generation of committed erythroid BFU-E and CFU-E progenitors does not require erythropoietin or the erythropoietin receptor. Cell 83:59-67, 1995.

Wynn RF, Cross MA, Hatton C, et al: Accelerated telomere shortening in young recipients of allogeneic bone-marrow transplants. Lancet 351:178-181, 1998.

Xu MJ, Matsuoka S, Yang FC, et al: Evidence for the presence of murine primitive megakaryocytopoiesis in the early yolk sac. Blood 97:2016-2022, 2001.

Zaizov R, Matoth Y: Red cell values on the first postnatal day during the last 16 weeks of gestation. Am J Hematol 1:275-278, 1976.

Zon LI: Developmental biology of hematopoiesis. Blood 86:2876-2891, 1995.

CHAPTER

# 76

# Hemostatic Disorders of the Newborn

Stefan Kuhle, Lesley Mitchell, Patricia Massicotte, and Maureen Andrew*

The diagnosis and management of acquired and hereditary hemostatic disorders in newborns differ from those of such disorders in older patients, owing to the presence at birth of a unique hemostatic system and to the age specificity of many pathologic conditions. For example, physiologic levels of many coagulation proteins are decreased compared with those in adults, making the diagnosis of most inherited and acquired hemostatic problems challenging. The hemostatic system is dynamic and age dependent; therefore, multiple reference ranges reflecting both gestational and postnatal ages of infants are necessary (Andrew et al, 1987b, 1988). Because most severe deficiencies manifest in the neonatal period, the index of suspicion for detection of these disorders must be increased.

After confirming the presence of a hemostatic problem, the clinician is faced with the challenge of providing both safe and effective treatment. The efficacy and safety of therapeutic interventions require testing in randomized, controlled trials, whenever feasible. However, in dealing with rare or consistently life-threatening events, alternative study designs can be useful. Guidelines for the classification of study design allowing an estimation of the strength of the findings have been established (Hirsh et al, 2001). Conclusions from studies with strong designs are necessarily given greater weight than that assigned to conclusions from studies with weaker designs.

This chapter provides a brief review of developmental hemostasis and the diagnosis and management of both bleeding and thromboembolic disorders in newborns.

## PHYSIOLOGY OF HEMOSTASIS

### Coagulation System

Physiologically, blood is maintained in a fluid phase. In response to a damaged vessel wall, platelets, plasma coagulation proteins, and the damaged vessel contribute to the formation of a hemostatic plug. Figure 76–1 provides a scheme of the current concepts of the coagulation system as discussed in a recent review (Dahlback, 2000). The central purpose of coagulant proteins is to generate thrombin from prothrombin. Thrombin is a serine protease with potent coagulant functions: (1) it activates factor V (FV), FVIII, and FXI, thereby enhancing its own generation; (2) it cleaves fibrinopeptide A (FPA) and FPB from fibrinogen, resulting in fibrin formation; (3) it promotes fibrin cross-linking by activating FXIII; and (4) it is a potent physiologic activator of platelets.

#### Coagulant Proteins

Components of the coagulation system do not cross the placenta but are synthesized by the fetus, with detectable levels at the end of the first trimester (Heikinheimo, 1964). Plasma concentrations of coagulant proteins in healthy fetuses and preterm and full-term newborns are available (Andrew et al, 1988; Reverdiau-Moalic et al, 1996) and are summarized in Tables 76–1, 76–2, and 76–3. Those fetal reference values may potentially provide a good assessment of the coagulation system of the very premature infant. Plasma concentrations of most coagulant proteins in newborns differ significantly from those in adults (see Tables 76–2 and 76–3). Plasma levels of the vitamin K–dependent coagulant proteins—FII, FVII, FIX, FX—and the contact factors—FXI, FXII, prekallikrein, and high-molecular-weight kininogen—are approximately 50% of adult values at birth. In contrast, plasma concentrations of fibrinogen, FV, and FVIII are not decreased at birth or during infancy (Andrew et al, 1987b, 1988). Plasma concentrations of von Willebrand factor (vWF), vWF high-molecular-weight multimers, and vWF collagen-binding activity are increased during the first weeks of life (Katz et al, 1989; Thomas et al, 1995). By 6 months of age, plasma concentrations of most coagulant proteins are in the lower part of the adult normal range (see Tables 76–2 and 76–3).

#### Inhibitors of Coagulation

Several proteins are involved in regulation of the coagulation system. The direct plasma inhibitors of thrombin include antithrombin (AT), $\alpha_2$-macroglobulin ($\alpha_2$M), and heparin cofactor II (HCII). AT-mediated inhibition of thrombin is potentiated by certain glycosaminoglycans, most important of which is heparin. At birth, plasma concentrations of the direct inhibitors AT and HCII are approximately 50% of adult values, whereas $\alpha_2$M levels are increased, compensating in large part for the decreased plasma concentrations of AT (Schmidt et al, 1989a). By 6 months of age, plasma concentrations of AT and HCII reach adult levels, whereas $\alpha_2$M levels are nearly twice the adult values (see Tables 76–2 and 76–3).

The indirect inhibitors of thrombin include protein C, protein S, and tissue factor pathway inhibitor (TFPI). When thrombin is generated in vivo, it binds to an endothelial cell receptor, thrombomodulin (TM), and can no longer cleave fibrinogen, FV, and FVIII, nor can it activate platelets. However, thrombin can activate protein C to its activated form (aPC). Activated protein C, a VK-dependent serine protease, enzymatically inactivates FVa and FVIIIa by limited proteolytic cleavage. The enzymatic activity of aPC is enhanced by another VK-dependent protein, protein S, which acts as a cofactor. Plasma concentrations of protein C and protein S are reduced at birth by 60% and remain decreased during the first weeks of life

*Deceased.

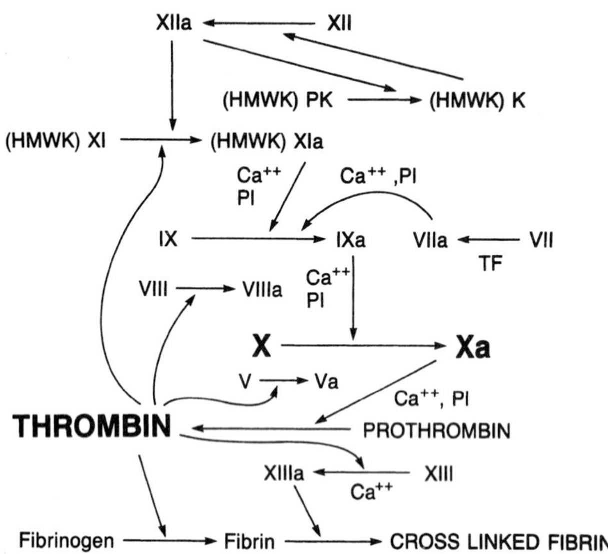


**FIGURE 76–1.** Physiology of normal hemostasis.

(see Tables 76–2 and 76–3). Protein C circulates in a fetal form that differs from the adult form by a twofold increase in single-chain protein C (Greffe et al, 1989). Protein S circulates only in the free, active form in newborn plasma, because C4b-binding protein is absent in newborns (Schwarz et al, 1988). In contrast with proteins C and S, plasma concentrations of TM are increased in fetuses, newborns, and infants (Menashi et al, 1999). Whether this reflects increased endothelial expression of TM in the young is unknown. A second, indirect mechanism for regulating thrombin generation is via TFPI, an inhibitor of the FVIIa/tissue factor pathway. TFPI forms a complex with FXa, and the TFPI/FXa complex inhibits FVIIa, thereby inhibiting the generation of thrombin. Information on the influence of age on TFPI is limited. Plasma concentrations of TFPI in fetuses and neonates at birth are decreased compared with those in adults (Reverdiau-Moalic et al, 1996; Weissbach et al, 1994).

### Thrombin Regulation of Plasma

#### *Thrombin Generation*

Values for the prothrombin time (PT) and the activated partial thromboplastin time (APTT) are prolonged in newborns. More sensitive assays show that thrombin generation is delayed and decreased by approximately 50% in plasmas from newborns compared with adult values (Schmidt et al, 1989b). The plasma concentration of prothrombin is directly related to the amount of thrombin generated in newborn plasma (Andrew et al, 1990c).

#### *Thrombin Inhibition*

The inhibition of iodine-125–labeled thrombin in newborn plasma is slower than in adult plasma, probably reflecting the low plasma concentrations of AT (Schmidt et al, 1989a). However, the total capacity to inhibit thrombin is similar for newborns and for adults owing to the increased binding of thrombin by $\alpha_2$M in newborns (Schmidt et al, 1989a). In addition to the increased binding of thrombin to $\alpha_2$M in newborn plasma, the amount of thrombin complexing to HCII is increased owing to a circulating dermatan sulfate proteoglycan (DSPG) that specifically catalyzes thrombin inhibition by HCII (Andrew et al, 1992b). DSPG also is present in plasmas from pregnant women and probably is released from the placenta (Delorme et al, 1998). The length of time DSPG circulates in newborns is not known, except that it is still present during the first week of life in sick infants with respiratory distress syndrome (RDS) (Shah et al, 1992).

### Conversion of Fibrinogen to Fibrin

#### *Fibrinogen*

At birth, plasma concentrations of fibrinogen are similar to adult levels. Fibrinogen is present in a fetal form that has an increased sialic acid content compared with adult fibrinogen (Francis and Armstrong, 1982). The thrombin clotting time (TCT), if the determination is performed without calcium in the system, is prolonged in newborns, reflecting the presence of fetal fibrinogen. If sialic acid is removed, fetal fibrinogen appears indistinguishable from adult fibrinogen (Francis and Armstrong, 1982). The physiologic significance of fetal fibrinogen is unknown.

#### *Fibrin Clots*

The capacity of newborn fibrin clots to bind thrombin has been assessed by measuring FPA production by fibrin clots prepared from adult and from cord plasma (Patel et al, 1996). Cord plasma clots generate significantly less FPA compared with clots formed in adult plasma, owing to decreased concentrations of prothrombin (Patel et al, 1996). Increasing cord plasma concentrations of prothrombin increase FPA production by cord clots. This observation suggests that thrombi in newborns with low plasma concentrations of prothrombin may have a decreased propensity to propagate.

## Fibrinolysis

Once a fibrin clot has formed in vivo, it is modified by the fibrinolytic system (Fig. 76–2). Activities of the fibrinolytic system are localized to the fibrin clot through specific lysine-binding sites. Plasminogen is converted to plasmin by tissue plasminogen activator (tPA) and urokinase. Analogous to thrombin, plasmin is the critical enzyme in fibrinolysis. Plasmin is a serine proteinase that cleaves fibrin in sequential steps, resulting in fibrin degradation products and the specific fibrin fragment, D-dimer. The fibrinolytic system is regulated by both the direct inhibitors of plasmin and inhibitors of plasminogen activators. Plasmin is inhibited primarily by $\alpha_2$-antiplasmin ($\alpha_2$AP). However, when bound to the fibrin surface, plasmin is relatively protected from

**TABLE 76–1**

**Reference Values for Coagulation Parameters in Fetuses and Full-Term Infants versus Adults**

| Parameter | Fetus: Weeks of Gestation 19-23 (n = 20) | 24-29 (n = 22) | 30-38 (n = 22) | Newborn (n = 60) | Adult (n = 40) |
|---|---|---|---|---|---|
| **A. Coagulation Screening Tests and Coagulation Factors*** | | | | | |
| *Coagulation Tests* | | | | | |
| PT (sec) | 32.5 (19-45) | 32.2 (19-44)† | 22.6 (16-30)† | 16.7 (12.0-23.5)‡ | 13.5 (11.4-14.0) |
| PT (INR) | 6.4 (1.7-11.1) | 6.2 (2.1-10.6)† | 3.0 (1.5-5.0)‡ | 1.7 (0.9-2.7)‡ | 1.1 (0.8-1.2) |
| APTT (sec) | 168.8 (83-250) | 154.0 (87-210)† | 104.8 (76-128)* | 44.3 (35-52)‡ | 33.0 (25-39) |
| TCT (sec) | 34.2 (24-44)‡ | 26.2 (24-28) | 21.4 (17.0-23.3) | 20.4 (15.2-25.0)† | 14.0 (12-16) |
| *Coagulation Factors* | | | | | |
| I (g/L) (Von Clauss) | 0.85 (0.57-1.50) | 1.12 (0.65-1.65) | 1.35 (1.25-1.65) | 1.68 (0.95-2.45)† | 3.0 (1.78-4.50) |
| I Ag (g/L) | 1.08 (0.75-1.50) | 1.93 (1.56-2.40) | 1.94 (1.30-2.40) | 2.65 (1.68-3.60)† | 3.5 (2.50-5.20) |
| IIc (%) | 16.9 (10-24) | 19.9 (11-30)‡ | 27.9 (15-50)† | 43.5 (27-64)† | 98.7 (70-125) |
| VIIc (%) | 27.4 (17-37) | 33.8 (18-48)‡ | 45.9 (31-62) | 52.5 (28-78)† | 101.3 (68-130) |
| IXc (%) | 10.1 (6-14) | 9.9 (5-15) | 12.3 (5-24)† | 31.8 (15-50)† | 104.8 (70-142) |
| Xc (%) | 20.5 (14-29) | 24.9 (16-35) | 28.0 (16-36)† | 39.6 (21-65)† | 99.2 (75-125) |
| Vc (%) | 32.1 (21-44) | 36.8 (25-50) | 48.9 (23-70)† | 89.9 (50-140) | 99.8 (65-140) |
| VIIIc (%) | 34.5 (18-50) | 35.5 (20-52) | 50.1 (27-78)† | 94.3 (38-150) | 101.8 (55-170) |
| XIc (%) | 13.2 (8-19) | 12.1 (6-22) | 14.8 (6-26)† | 37.2 (13-62)† | 100.2 (70-135) |
| XIIc (%) | 14.9 (6-25) | 22.7 (6-40) | 25.8 (11-50)† | 69.8 (25-105)† | 101.4 (65-144) |
| PK (%) | 12.8 (8-19) | 15.4 (8-26) | 18.1 (8-28)† | 35.4 (21-53)† | 99.8 (65-135) |
| HMWK (%) | 15.4 (10-22) | 19.3 (10-26) | 23.6 (12-34)* | 38.9 (28-53)† | 98.8 (68-135) |
| **B. Inhibitors of Coagulation*** | | | | | |
| AT (%) | 20.2 (12-31)‡ | 30.0 (20-39) | 37.1 (24-55)† | 59.4 (42-80)† | 99.8 (65-130) |
| HCII (%) | 10.3 (6-16)‡ | 12.9 (5.5-20) | 21.1 (11-33 )† | 52.1 (19-99)† | 101.4 (70-128) |
| TFPI (%)‡ | 21.0 (16.0-29.2) | 20.6 (13.4-33.2) | 20.7 (10.4-31.5)† | 38.1 (22.7-55.8)† | 73.0 (50.9-90.1) |
| PC Ag (%) | 0.5 (6-14) | 12.1 (8-16) | 15.0 (8-30)† | 32.5 (21-47)† | 100.8 (68-125) |
| PC activity (%) | 9.6 (7-13) | 10.4 (8-13) | 14.1 (8-18)‡ | 28.2 (14-42)† | 98.8 (68-125) |
| Total PS (%) | 15.1 (11-21) | 17.4 (14-25) | 21.0 (15-30)† | 38.5 (22-55)† | 99.6 (72-118) |
| Free PS (%) | 21.7 (13-32) | 27.9 (19-40) | 27.0 (18-40)† | 49.3 (33-67)† | 98.7 (72-128) |
| Free PS/total PS ratio | 0.82 (0.75-0.92) | 0.83 (0.76-0.95) | 0.79 (0.70-0.89)† | 0.64 (0.59-0.98)† | 0.41 (0.38-0.43) |
| C4b-BP (%) | 1.8 (0-6) | 6.1 (0-12.5) | 9.3 (5-14) | 18.6 (3-40)† | 100.3 (70-124) |

*All values are means, followed in parentheses by the lower and upper boundaries including 95% of the population. The significant differences between any two groups are denoted by *P* values, using Dunnett multiple regression.

†$P < .01$.

‡$P < .05$.

§For TFPI, 20 samples were assayed for each group, but only 10 for 19- to 23-week-old fetuses.

Ag, antigen; APTT, activated partial thromboplastin time; AT, antithrombin; BP, binding protein; c, coagulant activity; HCII, heparin cofactor II; HMWK, high-molecular-weight kininogen; INR, international normalized ratio; PC, protein C; PK, prekallikrein; PS, protein S; PT, prothrombin time; TCT, thrombin clotting time; TFPI, tissue factor pathway inhibitor.

Data from Reverdiau-Moalic et al, (1996).

inhibition by $\alpha_2$AP. The activators of plasminogen are inhibited by plasminogen activator inhibitors (PAIs), of which PAI-1 is the most important during infancy and childhood.

## The Fibrinolytic System in Newborns

### *Plasma Concentrations*

Plasma concentrations of components of the fibrinolytic system are age dependent (Table 76–4). At birth, plasminogen levels are about 60% to 70% of adult values; $\alpha_2$AP levels are approximately 85% of adult values (Andrew et al, 1990b). Plasma concentrations of PAI-1 and tPA in cord blood (Astedt and Lindoff, 1997) and neonatal blood (Andrew et al, 1990b) are significantly increased over adult values.

### *Fetal Plasminogen*

At birth, plasminogen is present in a "fetal" form characterized by increased amounts of mannose and sialic acid. Fetal plasminogen may have mildly decreased enzymatic activity as well as decreased binding to cellular receptors for plasminogen (Edelberg et al, 1990). The physiologic significance of fetal plasminogen is unknown.

**TABLE 76–2**

**Reference Values for Coagulation Tests and Inhibitors of Coagulation in Healthy Premature Infants* versus Adults**

| Parameter | Infant | | | | | Adult |
|---|---|---|---|---|---|---|
| | Day 1 | Day 5 | Day 30 | Day 90 | Day 180 | |
| A. Coagulation Tests† | | | | | | |
| PT (sec) | 13.0 (10.6-16.2)‡ | 12.5 (10.0-15.3)‡ | 11.8 (10.0-13.6)‡ | 12.3 (10.0-14.6)‡ | 12.5 (10.0-15.0)‡ | 12.4 (10.8-13.9) |
| INR | 1.0 (0.61-1.70) | 0.91 (0.53-1.48) | 0.79 (0.53-1.11) | 0.88 (0.53-1.32) | 0.91 (0.53-1.48) | 0.89 (0.64-1.17) |
| APTT (sec) | 53.6 (27.5-79.4)§ | 50.5 (26.9-74.1)§ | 44.7 (26.9-62.5) | 39.5 (28.3-50.7) | 37.5 (27.2-53.3)‡ | 33.5 (26.6-40.3) |
| TCT (sec) | 24.8 (19.2-30.4)‡ | 24.1 (18.8-29.4)‡ | 24.4 (18.8-29.9)‡ | 25.1 (19.4-30.8)‡ | 25.2 (18.9-31.5)‡ | 25.0 (19.7-30.3) |
| Fibrinogen (g/L) | 2.43 (1.50-3.73)‡§ | 2.80 (1.60-4.18)‡§ | 2.54 (1.50-4.14)‡ | 2.46 (1.50-3.52)‡ | 2.28 (1.50-3.60) | 2.78 (1.56-4.00) |
| FII (U/mL) | 0.45 (0.20-0.77) | 0.57 (0.29-0.85)§ | 0.57 (0.36-0.95)§ | 0.68 (0.30-1.06) | 0.87 (0.51-1.23) | 1.08 (0.70-1.46) |
| FV (U/mL) | 0.88 (0.41-1.44)‡§ | 1.00 (0.46-1.54) | 1.02 (0.48-1.56)‡ | 0.99 (0.59-1.39) | 1.02 (0.58-1.46)‡ | 1.06 (0.62-1.50) |
| FVII (U/mL) | 0.67 (0.21-1.13) | 0.84 (0.30-1.38) | 0.83 (0.21-1.45) | 0.87 (0.31-1.43) | 0.99 (0.47-1.51)‡ | 1.05 (0.67-1.43) |
| FVIII (U/mL) | 1.11 (0.50-2.13)‡ | 1.15 (0.53-2.05)‡§ | 1.11 (0.50-1.99)‡§ | 1.06 (0.58-1.88)‡§ | 0.99 (0.50-1.87)‡§ | 0.99 (0.50-1.49) |
| vWF (U/mL) | 1.36 (0.78-2.10) | 1.33 (0.72-2.19) | 1.36 (0.66-2.16) | 1.12 (0.75-1.84)‡ | 0.98 (0.54-1.58)‡ | 0.92 (0.50-1.58) |
| FIX (U/mL) | 0.35 (0.19-0.65)§ | 0.42 (0.14-0.74)§ | 0.44 (0.13-0.80) | 0.59 (0.25-0.93) | 0.81 (0.50-1.20) | 1.09 (0.55-1.63) |
| FX (U/mL) | 0.41 (0.11-0.71) | 0.51 (0.19-0.83) | 0.56 (0.20-0.92) | 0.67 (0.35-0.99) | 0.77 (0.35-1.19) | 1.06 (0.70-1.52) |
| FXI (U/mL) | 0.30 (0.08-0.52)§ | 0.41 (0.13-0.69)§ | 0.43 (0.15-0.71)§ | 0.59 (0.25-0.93)§ | 0.78 (0.46-1.10) | 0.97 (0.67-1.27) |
| FXII (U/mL) | 0.38 (0.10-0.66)§ | 0.39 (0.09-0.69)§ | 0.43 (0.11-0.75) | 0.61 (0.15-1.07) | 0.82 (0.22-1.42) | 1.08 (0.52-1.64) |
| PK (U/mL) | 0.33 (0.09-0.57) | 0.45 (0.25-0.75) | 0.59 (0.31-0.87) | 0.79 (0.37-1.21) | 0.78 (0.40-1.16) | 1.12 (0.62-1.62) |
| HK (U/mL) | 0.49 (0.09-0.89) | 0.62 (0.24-1.00)§ | 0.64 (0.16-1.12)§ | 0.78 (0.32-1.24) | 0.83 (0.41-1.25)‡ | 0.92 (0.50-1.36) |
| FXIIIa (U/mL) | 0.70 (0.32-1.08) | 1.01 (0.57-1.45)‡ | 0.99 (0.51-1.47)‡ | 1.13 (0.71-1.55)‡ | 1.13 (0.65-1.61)‡ | 1.05 (0.55-1.55) |
| FXIIIb (U/mL) | 0.81 (0.35-1.27) | 1.10 (0.68-1.58)‡ | 1.07 (0.57-1.57)‡ | 1.21 (0.75-1.67) | 1.15 (0.67-1.63) | 0.97 (0.57-1.37) |
| B. Inhibitors of Coagulation† | | | | | | |
| AT (U/mL) | 0.38 (0.14-0.62)§ | 0.56 (0.30-0.82)‡ | 0.59 (0.37-0.81)§ | 0.83 (0.45-1.21)§ | 0.90 (0.52-1.28)§ | 1.05 (0.79-1.31) |
| $\alpha_2$M (U/mL) | 1.10 (0.56-1.82)§ | 1.25 (0.71-1.77)‡ | 1.38 (0.72-2.04) | 1.80 (1.20-2.66) | 2.09 (1.10-3.21) | 0.86 (0.52-1.20) |
| $C_1$E-INH (U/mL) | 0.65 (0.31-0.99) | 0.83 (0.45-1.21) | 0.74 (0.40-1.24)§ | 1.14 (0.60-1.68)‡ | 1.40 (0.96-2.04) | 1.01 (0.71-1.31) |
| $\alpha_1$AT (U/mL) | 0.90 (0.36-1.44)‡ | 0.94 (0.42-1.46)‡ | 0.76 (0.38-1.12)§ | 0.81 (0.49-1.13)‡§ | 0.82 (0.48-1.16)‡ | 0.93 (0.55-1.31) |
| HCII (U/mL) | 0.32 (0.10-0.60)§ | 0.34 (0.10-0.69) | 0.43 (0.15-0.71) | 0.61 (0.20-1.11) | 0.89 (0.45-1.40)‡§ | 0.96 (0.66-1.26) |
| Protein C (U/mL) | 0.28 (0.12-0.44)§ | 0.31 (0.11-0.51) | 0.37 (0.15-0.59)§ | 0.45 (0.23-0.67)§ | 0.57 (0.31-0.83) | 0.96 (0.64-1.28) |
| Protein S (U/mL) | 0.26 (0.14-0.38)§ | 0.37 (0.13-0.61) | 0.56 (0.22-0.90) | 0.76 (0.40-1.12)§ | 0.82 (0.44-1.20) | 0.92 (0.60-1.24) |

*Born at 30 to 36 weeks of gestation, with measurements at given intervals during first 6 months of life.

†All values except those for fibrinogen are expressed in U/mL, where pooled plasma contains 1.0 U/mL. Values are given as means, followed by the lower and upper boundaries encompassing 95% of the population. Some measurements were skewed owing to a disproportionate number of high values. The lower limit excludes the lower 2.5% of the population. *Coagulation Tests*: Between 40 and 96 samples were assayed for each value for the entire period of time. *Inhibitors of Coagulation*: Between 40 and 75 samples were assayed for each value for the entire period of time.

‡Values not statistically different from adults.

§Values different from those in full-term infant.

APTT, activated partial thromboplastin time; AT, antithrombin; $\alpha_1$AT, $\alpha_1$-antitrypsin; $C_1$E-INH, $C_1$-esterase inhibitor; HCII, heparin cofactor II; HK, high-molecular-weight kininogen; INR, international normalized ratio; $\alpha_2$M, $\alpha_2$-macroglobulin PK, prekallikrein; PT, prothrombin time; TCT, thrombin clotting time; VIII, factor VIII procoagulant; vWF, von Willebrand factor.

Data for **A** from (Andrew et al (1988)) data for **B** from (Andrew et al (1990b)).

**TABLE 76-3**

**Reference Values for Coagulation Tests and Inhibitors of Coagulation in Healthy Full-Term Infants* versus Adults**

| Parameter | Infant | | | | | Adult |
|---|---|---|---|---|---|---|
| | Day 1 | Day 5 | Day 30 | Day 90 | Day 180 | |
| A. Coagulation Tests† | | | | | | |
| PT (s) | 13.0 (10.1-15.9)‡ | 12.4 (10.0-15.3)‡ | 11.8 (10.0-14.3)‡ | 11.9 (10.0-14.2)‡ | 12.3 (10.7-13.9)‡ | 12.4 (10.8-13.9) |
| INR | 1.00 (0.53-1.62) | 0.89 (0.53-1.48) | 0.79 (0.53-1.26) | 0.81 (0.53-1.26) | 0.88 (0.61-1.17) | 0.89 (0.64-1.17) |
| APTT (s) | 42.9 (31.3-54.5) | 42.6 (25.4-59.8) | 40.4 (32.0-55.2) | 37.1 (29.0-50.1)‡ | 35.5 (28.1-42.9)‡ | 33.5 (26.6-40.3) |
| TCT (s) | 23.5 (19.0-28.3)‡ | 23.1 (18.0-29.2) | 24.3 (19.4-29.2)‡ | 25.1 (20.5-29.7)‡ | 25.5 (19.8-31.2)‡ | 25.0 (19.7-30.3) |
| Fibrinogen (g/L) | 2.83 (1.67-3.99)‡ | 3.12 (1.62-4.62)‡ | 2.70 (1.62-3.78)‡ | 2.43 (1.50-3.79)‡ | 2.51 (1.50-3.87)‡ | 2.78 (1.56-4.00) |
| FII (U/mL) | 0.48 (0.26-0.70) | 0.63 (0.33-0.93) | 0.68 (0.34-1.02) | 0.75 (0.45-1.05) | 0.88 (0.60-1.16) | 1.08 (0.70-1.46) |
| FV (U/mL) | 0.72 (0.34-1.08) | 0.95 (0.45-1.45) | 0.98 (0.62-1.34) | 0.90 (0.48-1.32) | 0.91 (0.55-1.27) | 1.06 (0.62-1.50) |
| FVII (U/mL) | 0.66 (0.28-1.04) | 0.89 (0.35-1.43) | 0.90 (0.42-1.38) | 0.91 (0.39-1.43) | 0.87 (0.47-1.27) | 1.05 (0.67-1.43) |
| FVIII (U/mL) | 1.00 (0.50-1.78)‡ | 0.88 (0.50-1.54)‡ | 0.91 (0.50-1.57)‡ | 0.79 (0.50-1.25)‡ | 0.73 (0.50-1.09) | 0.99 (0.50-1.49) |
| vWF (U/mL) | 1.53 (0.50-2.87) | 1.40 (0.50-2.54) | 1.28 (0.50-2.46) | 1.18 (0.50-2.06) | 1.07 (0.50-1.97) | 0.92 (0.50-1.58) |
| FIX (U/mL) | 0.53 (0.15-0.91) | 0.53 (0.15-0.91) | 0.51 (0.21-0.81) | 0.67 (0.21-1.13) | 0.86 (0.36-1.36) | 1.09 (0.55-1.63) |
| FX (U/mL) | 0.40 (0.12-0.68) | 0.49 (0.19-0.79) | 0.59 (0.31-0.87) | 0.71 (0.35-1.07) | 0.78 (0.38-1.18) | 1.06 (0.70-1.52) |
| FXI (U/mL) | 0.38 (0.10-0.66) | 0.55 (0.23-0.87) | 0.53 (0.27-0.79) | 0.69 (0.41-0.97) | 0.86 (0.49-1.34) | 0.97 (0.67-1.27) |
| FXII (U/mL) | 0.53 (0.13-0.93) | 0.47 (0.11-0.83) | 0.49 (0.17-0.81) | 0.67 (0.25-1.09) | 0.77 (0.39-1.15) | 1.08 (0.52-1.64) |
| PK (U/mL) | 0.37 (0.18-0.69) | 0.48 (0.20-0.76) | 0.57 (0.23-0.91) | 0.73 (0.41-1.05) | 0.86 (0.56-1.16) | 1.12 (0.62-1.62) |
| HMWK (U/mL) | 0.54 (0.06-1.02) | 0.74 (0.16-1.32) | 0.77 (0.33-1.21)‡ | 0.82 (0.30-1.46)‡ | 0.82 (0.36-1.28)‡ | 0.92 (0.50-1.36) |
| FXIIIa (U/mL) | 0.79 (0.27-1.31) | 0.94 (0.44-1.44)‡ | 0.93 (0.39-1.47)‡ | 1.04 (0.36-1.72)‡ | 1.04 (0.46-1.62)‡ | 1.05 (0.55-1.55) |
| FXIIIb (U/mL) | 0.76 (0.30-1.22) | 1.06 (0.32-1.80)‡ | 1.11 (0.39-1.73)‡ | 1.16 (0.48-1.84)‡ | 1.10 (0.50-1.70)‡ | 0.97 (0.57-1.37) |
| B. Inhibitors of Coagulation† | | | | | | |
| AT (U/mL) | 0.63 (0.39-0.87) | 0.67 (0.41-0.93) | 0.78 (0.48-1.08) | 0.97 (0.73-1.21)‡ | 1.04 (0.84-1.24)‡ | 1.05 (0.79-1.31) |
| $\alpha_2$M (U/mL) | 1.39 (0.95-1.83) | 1.48 (0.98-1.98) | 1.50 (1.06-1.94) | 1.76 (1.26-2.26) | 1.91 (1.49-2.33) | 0.86 (0.52-1.20) |
| $C_1$E-INH (U/mL) | 0.72 (0.36-1.08) | 0.90 (0.60-1.20)‡ | 0.89 (0.47-1.31) | 1.15 (0.71-1.59) | 1.41 (0.89-1.93) | 1.01 (0.71-1.31) |
| $\alpha_1$AT (U/mL) | 0.93 (0.49-1.37)‡ | 0.89 (0.49-1.29)‡ | 0.62 (0.36-0.88) | 0.72 (0.42-1.02) | 0.77 (0.47-1.07) | 0.93 (0.55-1.31) |
| HCII (U/mL) | 0.43 (0.10-0.93) | 0.48 (0.00-0.96) | 0.47 (0.10-0.87) | 0.72 (0.10-1.46) | 1.20 (0.50-1.90) | 0.96 (0.66-1.26) |
| Protein C (U/mL) | 0.35 (0.17-0.53) | 0.42 (0.20-0.64) | 0.43 (0.21-0.65) | 0.54 (0.28-0.80) | 0.59 (0.37-0.81) | 0.96 (0.64-1.28) |
| Protein S (U/mL) | 0.36 (0.12-0.60) | 0.50 (0.22-0.78) | 0.63 (0.33-0.93) | 0.86 (0.54-1.18)‡ | 0.87 (0.55-1.19)‡ | 0.92 (0.60-1.24) |

*Measurements at intervals during the first 6 months of life.

†All values except those for fibrinogen are expressed in U/mL, where pooled plasma contains 1.0 U/mL. Values are means, followed in parentheses by the lower and upper boundaries encompassing 95% of the population. Some measurements were skewed owing to a disproportionate number of high values. The lower limit excludes the lower 2.5% of the population. *Coagulation Tests*: Between 40 and 77 samples were assayed for each value for newborn. *Inhibitors of Coagulation*: Between 40 and 75 samples were assayed for each value for newborn.

‡Values not statistically different from adults.

APTT, activated partial thromboplastin time; AT, antithrombin; $\alpha_1$AT, $\alpha_1$-antitrypsin; $C_1$E-INH, $C_1$-esterase inhibitor; F, factor; HCII, heparin cofactor II; HMWK, high-molecular-weight kininogen; INR, international normalized ratio; $\alpha_2$M, $\alpha_2$-macroglobulin; PK, prekallikrein; PT, prothrombin time; TCT, thrombin clotting time; von Willebrand factor (vWF).

Data for **A** from Andrew et al, 1987a; data for **B** from Andrew et al (1990b).

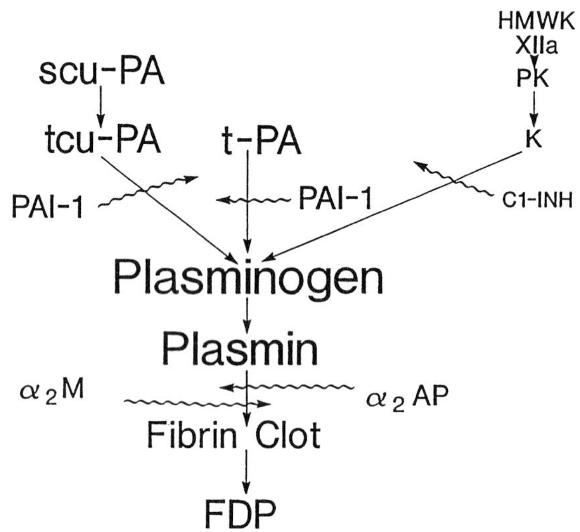


**FIGURE 76–2.** Physiology of fibrinolysis.

### *Activation of the Fibrinolytic System at Birth*

The fibrinolytic system is transiently activated at birth, as evidenced by increased plasma concentrations of plasmin-$\alpha_2$AP, D-dimer, and Bβ15-42–related peptides (Ekelund et al, 1970; Knofler et al, 1998a; Suarez et al, 1985). The clinical significance of an activated fibrinolytic system at birth is uncertain.

### *Regulation of Plasmin*

The capacity to generate plasmin is reduced in cord blood, probably as a result of reduced plasma concentrations of plasminogen (Corrigan et al, 1989). The contribution of "fetal" plasminogen to impaired fibrinolysis is uncertain (Edelberg et al, 1990).

## Platelets

### General Information

Platelets are disk-shaped cells produced by megakaryocytes in the bone marrow and released into the circulation. The plasma membrane of platelets contains several glycoproteins that bind specific adhesive proteins to facilitate platelet-to-surface interactions (adhesion) and platelet-to-platelet interactions (aggregation). Under normal circumstances, platelets circulate without adhering to vessel walls or to other cells. When the endothelial lining of blood vessels is damaged or removed, platelets adhere to subendothelial molecules, are activated, undergo shape change, spread over the surface, and bind to each other. Adhesion initiates the secretion of platelet granule contents. These substances promote adhesion and formation of aggregates. Activated platelets also participate in coagulation by providing a lipoprotein surface on which the soluble coagulation factor complexes can assemble, resulting in the generation of thrombin and the formation of fibrin. As discussed previously, thrombin itself is a potent stimulus of platelet aggregation. Occupation of platelet surface receptors by a variety of extracellular molecules (such as thrombin, collagen, and adenosine diphosphate [ADP]) activates membrane-associated enzymes that, in turn, generate intracellular second messengers that promote platelet activation and secretion. Platelet secretion is a process whereby platelet granules form a cluster and fuse with the membranes of other granules and the surface-connected open canalicular system.The process of platelet adhesion is mediated by glycoprotein Ib/IX/V (GPIb/IX/V), an integral membrane protein specific to the platelet membrane. It serves as a binding site for subendothelial vWF, an adhesive protein. Von Willebrand factor is secreted by endothelial cells and platelets and is present in the subendothelium and in plasma. Both the plasma concentrations of vWF and the proportion of high-molecular-weight multimers of vWF are important for adhesive function. Following activation of platelets, the GPIIb/IIIa complex on the platelet surface exposes a binding site for fibrinogen and, to a lesser extent, vWF, fibronectin, and thrombospondin. Platelet-to-platelet adherence or aggregation is mediated by fibrinogen bound to GPIIb/IIIa. GPIIb/IIIa is the most abundant platelet surface glycoprotein, with approximately 50,000 molecules per platelet.

### Platelets in the Newborn

Platelet counts in newborns are similar to adult values, ranging between 150 and 400 × $10^9$/L, with mean volumes of 7 to 9 fL. Values in fetuses between 18 and 30 weeks of gestation are also within this range, with average values of 250 × $10^9$/L (Forestier et al, 1986). The life span of platelets in healthy infants probably is similar to that in adults at approximately 7 to 10 days, at which time platelets are removed from the circulation by macrophages in the reticuloendothelial system. In a rabbit model, platelet survival times were comparable for rabbit pups and adults (Castle et al, 1988).

### *Platelet Function*

Until recently, little information was available on the function of platelets taken directly from infants because of the volume of blood required and the technical difficulty of obtaining an adequate sample. With the advent of flow cytometry, recent studies using that technique have provided new insights into platelet function of the newborn. However, the limited availability of flow cytometry has hindered its use in routine clinical practice.

Most studies show that cord and newborn platelets function differently from adult platelets. Neonatal platelets have been demonstrated to have fewer pseudopods, smaller glycogen deposits, less visible microtubular structures, and markedly fewer alpha granules (Saving et al, 1994). Flow cytometry studies show that, without added agonists, expression of GPIb or GPIIb/IIIa in newborn platelets does not differ from that in adult platelets.

**Adhesion.** The components required for platelet adhesion, GP Ib and vWF, are present early in fetal life (Gruel et al, 1986). Both plasma concentrations and the proportion of high-molecular-weight multimers of vWF are increased in newborns (Katz et al, 1989) and these changes may be

**TABLE 76–4**

**Reference Values for Components of Fibrinolytic System in Full-Term and Premature Infants* versus Adults**

| Parameter | Infant | | | | | Adult |
|---|---|---|---|---|---|---|
| | Day 1 | Day 5 | Day 30 | Day 90 | Day 180 | |
| A. Healthy Full-Term Infants† | | | | | | |
| Plasminogen (U/mL) | 1.95 (1.25-2.65) | 2.17 (1.41-2.93) | 1.98 (1.26-2.70) | 2.48 (1.74-3.22) | 3.01 (2.21-3.81) | 3.36 (2.48-4.24) |
| TPA (ng/mL) | 9.6 (5.0-18.9) | 5.6 (4.0-10.0)‡ | 4.1 (1.0-6.0)‡ | 2.1 (1.0-5.0)‡ | 2.8 (1.0-6.0)‡ | 4.9 (1.4-8.4) |
| $\alpha_2$AP (U/mL) | 0.85 (0.55-1.15) | 1.00 (0.70-1.30)‡ | 1.00 (0.76-1.24)‡ | 1.08 (0.76-1.40)‡ | 1.11 (0.83-1.39)‡ | 1.02 (0.68-1.36) |
| PAI-1 (U/mL) | 6.4 (2.0-15.1) | 2.3 (0.0-8.1)‡ | 3.4 (0.0-8.8)‡ | 7.2 (1.0-15.3) | 8.1 (6.0-13.0) | 3.6 (0.0-11.0) |
| B. Healthy Premature Infants (30-36 Weeks of Gestation)† | | | | | | |
| Plasminogen (U/mL) | 1.70 (1.12-2.48)§ | 1.91 (1.21-2.61)§ | 1.81 (1.09-2.53) | 2.38 (1.58-3.18) | 2.75 (1.91-3.59)§ | 3.36 (2.48-4.24) |
| tPA (ng/mL) | 8.48 (3.00-16.70) | 3.97 (2.00-6.93)‡ | 4.13 (2.00-7.79)‡ | 3.31 (2.00-5.07)‡ | 3.48 (2.00-5.85)‡ | 4.96 (1.46-8.46) |
| $\alpha_2$AP (U/mL) | 0.78 (0.40-1.16) | 0.81 (0.49-1.13)§ | 0.89 (0.55-1.23)§ | 1.06 (0.64-1.48)‡ | 1.15 (0.77-1.53) | 1.02 (0.68-1.36) |
| PAI-1 (U/mL) | 5.4 (0.0-12.2)‡§ | 2.5 (0.0-7.1)‡ | 4.3 (0.0-10.9)‡ | 4.8 (1.0-11.8)‡§ | 4.9 (1.0-10.2)‡§ | 3.6 (0.0-11.0) |

*Measurements at given intervals during first 6 months of life.

†For $\alpha_2$AP, values are expressed as U/mL, where pooled plasma contains 1.0 U/mL. Plasminogen units are those recommended by the Committee on Thrombolytic Agents. Values for tPA are given as ng/mL. Values for PAI-1 are given as U/mL, where 1 unit of PAI-1 activity is defined as the amount of PAI-1 that inhibits 1 international unit (IU) of human single-chain tPA. All values are means, followed in parentheses by the lower and upper boundaries encompassing 95% of the population.

‡Values not statistically different from adults.

§Values different from those in full-term infant.

$\alpha_2$AP, $\alpha_2$-antiplasmin; PAI-1, plasminogen activator inhibitor-1; tPA, tissue plasminogen activator.

Data from Andrew et al (1990b).

responsible for enhanced cord platelet aggregation by low concentrations of ristocetin (Ts'ao et al, 1976). The multimeric forms of vWF appear similar to those released by endothelial cells, suggesting that mechanisms for processing the multimers may not be fully developed at birth.

**Activation and Secretion.** Recent studies, using whole-blood flow cytometry, show that platelets of preterm and term neonates are hyporeactive to thrombin, a combination of ADP and epinephrine, and a thromboxane $A_2$ analogue (Rajasekhar et al, 1994, 1997). The reason for this hyporeactivity is not completely understood. Agonist receptors, with the exception of the α-adrenergic receptor (Corby and O'Barr, 1981a), do not appear to be decreased in number. Studies of activation pathways showed that inositol phosphate production and protein phosphorylation, as well as production of arachidonic acid and its metabolites, are normal (Israels et al, 1990). A more recent study linked the transient platelet hyporeactivity to a defect in the thromboxane $A_2$ postreceptor signal transduction pathway (Israels et al, 1999).

On the basis of evidence from studies using cord blood, platelets of newborns formerly were thought to be in a state of transient dysfunction secondary to platelet activation during the birth process (Suarez et al, 1988). More recent studies using flow cytometry, however, suggest that hyporeactivity of newborn platelets is not caused by preactivation during birth (Grosshaupt et al, 1997) but is rather a developmental phenomenon that resolves around day 10 of life (Gatti et al, 1996). The clinical significance of these findings remains unknown.

**Aggregation.** Platelet GPIIb/IIIa is present on fetal platelet membranes from early gestation (Gruel et al, 1986). Although the collagen receptor GPIa/IIa is found in adult concentrations on neonatal platelets, the platelet aggregation response to collagen is markedly reduced, probably owing to an impaired intracellular signal transduction (Israels et al, 1999). Collagen-induced aggregation normalizes between the fifth and ninth days of life (Tanindi et al, 1995). Platelet aggregation in response to epinephrine is diminished owing to decreased numbers or occupation of α-adrenergic receptors (Corby and O'Barr, 1981a).

Some studies show that the capacity of cord and neonatal platelets to aggregate following exposure to ADP, thrombin, and arachidonic acid may be similar to that of adult platelets (Corby and O'Barr, 1981b; Israels et al, 1990; Knofler et al, 1998b).

### *Platelet Function Testing*

For many years, the bleeding time has been the most commonly used test of primary hemostasis in infants and children. However, poor reproducibility, operator dependence, and poor predictability of bleeding risk have limited its usefulness. The Platelet Function Analyzer (PFA-100) provides a promising alternative to the bleeding time. The PFA-100 is a high-shear system for the in vitro evaluation of primary hemostasis in anticoagulated whole blood, simulating injury to a small vessel (Kundu et al, 1995). As with the bleeding time (Andrew et al, 1990a), PFA-100 closure times in newborns are shorter than in adults (Carcao et al, 1998). Increased plasma concentrations of vWF and enhanced function of vWF due to increased amounts of high-molecular-weight multimers partly account for this finding in newborns. The contribution of a higher hematocrit to the shortening of PFA-100 closure times in newborns is controversial (Israels et al, 2001; Roschitz et al, 2001). The clinical significance of mild platelet aggregation defects or platelet hyporeactivity in newborns is uncertain when BT and PFA-100 closure time in newborns are shorter than in adults.

## HEMORRHAGIC DISORDERS

All infants with clinically significant bleeding should be evaluated for a hemostatic deficit. Although acquired problems are more frequent, severe forms of hereditary factor deficiencies often first manifest in early infancy and should be seriously considered in otherwise healthy infants. Clinical presentation, diagnosis, and management of hemorrhagic disorders in newborns differ considerably from those in older infants and children.

### Approach to the Newborn with Bleeding

#### History and Physical Examination

Evaluation of any newborn with hemorrhagic complications includes a careful history of familial bleeding problems, maternal illnesses (e.g., infections, immune thrombocytopenia), outcome of previous pregnancies, drug administration (maternal and neonatal), and documentation that vitamin K was given at birth. Simple observations on physical examination, such as localized versus diffuse bleeding and healthy or sick appearance of the newborn, have tremendous importance for the classification of hemorrhagic disorders. Whereas vitamin K deficiency or inherited coagulation defects characteristically manifest with large ecchymoses or localized bleeding in apparently healthy newborns, bleeding due to disseminated intravascular coagulation (DIC) or liver injury generally is seen in sick infants with diffuse bleeding from several sites. Infants with isolated platelet disorders generally appear healthy except for progressive petechiae, ecchymoses, and/or mucosal bleeding. Common bleeding sites in the newborn include the umbilicus, mucous membranes, circumcision wounds, the scalp, and the skin. Hemarthrosis, a common presentation of severe hemophilia in older children, is rarely seen in newborns. In a small but important proportion of infants, intracranial hemorrhage (ICH) is the initial manifestation of a bleeding tendency. In sick newborns, bleeding from the lungs, the gastrointestinal tract, the urinary tract, or peripheral blood sampling sites may be the first sign of a coagulopathy. In otherwise healthy infants, the most common causes of bleeding are thrombocytopenia secondary to transplacental passage of a maternal antiplatelet antibody, vitamin K deficiency, and, less commonly, a hereditary coagulation factor deficiency. Although sick infants may have an underlying hereditary defect, acquired disorders such as DIC and liver failure are more common.

### Laboratory Evaluation

In a majority of newborns with a hemorrhagic disorder, history and physical examination alone will point to the correct diagnosis, with laboratory tests providing confirmation. The initial workup usually includes a PT, APTT, TCT, fibrinogen level, platelet count, and on rare occasion, a bleeding time or PFA-100 assay. Abnormalities in these tests will usually guide the selection of additional tests such as specific factor assays (Fig. 76–3). Deficiencies of FXIII, $\alpha_2$AP, and PAI do not alter the results of the screening tests, and these must be measured directly if deficiencies are suspected.

Ideally, samples should be taken from a peripheral vein. This approach often is not feasible in small preterm infants or in infants with difficult venous access after repeated sampling. If samples are drawn from central lines, even minute contamination with heparin may give erroneous results. In these instances, preanalysis incubation of the sample with protamine or heparinase may be used to eliminate heparin contamination (Ellis, 1993; Keller et al, 1998).

All laboratory results must be considered in the context of age-related reference values. Differentiation of hereditary and acquired deficiencies from physiologic values can be difficult for most coagulation proteins, a problem unique to newborns.

### Management

The appropriate management of an infant with a hemorrhagic disorder is dependent on the current identification of the hemostatic defect. Options for replacement therapy include specific factor concentrates, fresh frozen plasma (FFP), platelet concentrates, and cryoprecipitate. Other therapeutic considerations are related to whether venous access can be maintained, particularly if an exchange

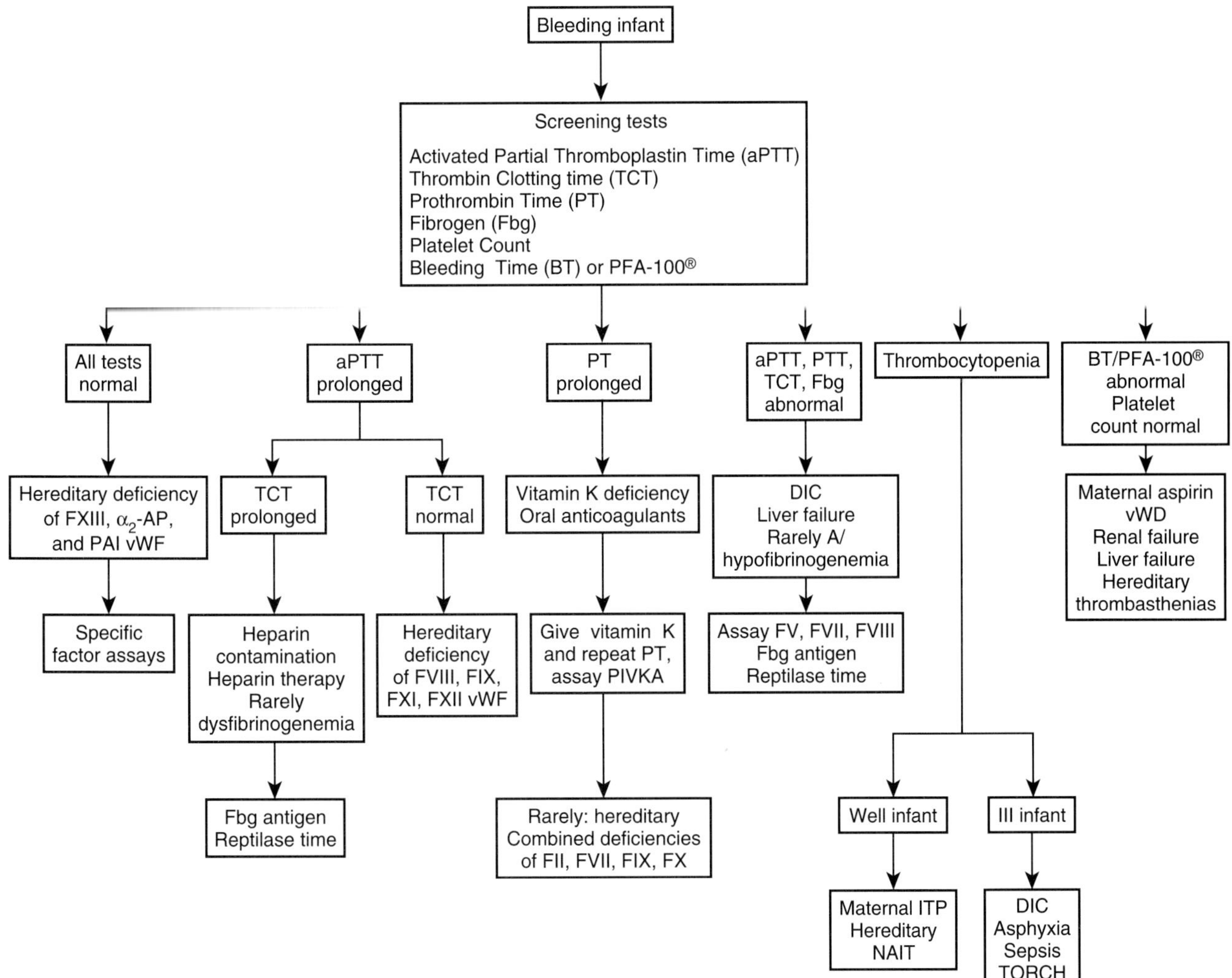


**FIGURE 76–3.** Flow diagram for the evaluation of a bleeding newborn. $\alpha_2$AP, $\alpha_2$-antiplasmin; APTT, activated partial thromboplastin time; BT, bleeding time; DIC, disseminated intravascular coagulation; F, factor; Fbg, fibrinogen; FSPs, fibrin split products; ITP, idiopathic thrombocytopenic purpura; NAIT, neonatal alloimmune thrombocytopenia; PAI, plasminogen activator inhibitor; PIVKA, protein induced in the absence of vitamin K; PT, prothrombin time; TCT, thrombin clotting time; TORCH, *t*oxoplasmosis, *o*ther infections, *r*ubella, *c*ytomegalovirus infection, *h*erpes simplex; vWD, von Willebrand disease; vWF, von Willebrand factor. *(Data from Kisker, 1998.)*

transfusion is planned, and also the risk of viral transmission and graft-versus-host disease.

## Hereditary Hemorrhagic Disorders

### Hemophilia A and B

The terms *hemophilia A* and *hemophilia B* designate hereditary deficiencies of FVIII and FIX, respectively. On the basis of the factor levels, the hemophilias are classified as severe (<1% of the normal level), moderate (1% to 5%), or mild (>5% to <40%). Severe hemophilia is the most common hereditary coagulation defect to manifest in newborns. Hemophilia is inherited as an X-linked recessive trait. About 20% to 30% of cases are from spontaneous mutations. Hemophilia occurs in 1/5000 male births, with approximately 80% to 85% of cases accounting for hemophilia A and 15% to 20% for hemophilia B. Both forms are clinically indistinguishable but differ in laboratory and management aspects. A positive family history is usually present in about two thirds of cases. Very rarely, hemophilia may occur in females and manifest at birth.

#### Pregnancy and Perinatal Management

In affected families, early genetic diagnosis in the fetus can be made by chorionic villus sampling at 11 to 13 weeks of gestation or by amniocentesis around 16 weeks. Cordocentesis for fetal blood sampling for FVIII or FIX is possible after 18 to 20 weeks of gestation (Ljung, 1999). Controversy exists concerning the safest delivery mode of newborns with suspected or proven hemophilia. As yet, no firm evidence-based recommendations can be given. Vaginal delivery appears to be reasonably safe (Ljung et al, 1994) and is used by most centers (Kulkarni et al, 1999). Delivery by cesarean section does not completely eliminate the risk of ICH (Michaud et al, 1991). Vacuum extraction should strictly be avoided as it carries a significant bleeding risk (Ljung et al, 1994). Close communication among hematologist, neonatologist, and obstetrician is of utmost importance. After birth, a cord blood sample for the appropriate clotting factor assay should be taken. Heel sticks or venipunctures in a newborn with hemophilia should be performed only when absolutely necessary. After puncture, local pressure should be applied for 5 to 10 minutes, and the site should be closely observed for 24 hours. Vitamin K may be given intramuscularly, but the same precautions as for venipunctures apply (Kulkarni and Lusher, 2001).

#### Clinical Presentation

Recent studies indicate that 40% to 70% of children with severe hemophilia are diagnosed in the neonatal period (Conway and Hilgartner, 1994; Pollmann et al, 1999), and the vast majority present with bleeding symptoms. The most common presentations are ICH, cephalohematoma, and bleeding from the umbilical stump or following venipuncture, heel prick, or circumcision (Kulkarni and Lusher, 2001).

#### Diagnosis

Severe and moderate hemophilia A as well as severe hemophilia B can be reliably diagnosed in the neonatal period, as factor levels in affected newborns are well below physiologic values. Infants with moderate hemophilia B or with mild forms of hemophilia A or B, however, may have normal PT and APTT values. Therefore, if hemophilia is suspected, specific factor assays should be performed regardless of the PT or APTT value.

#### Treatment

Currently, administration of FVIII and FIX concentrates (highly purified or recombinant) is the treatment of choice for hemophilia. In cases of severe bleeding with pending factor assay results, FFP may be used. Dosage of replacement factor strongly depends on the site and severity of the bleed. Target levels of FVIII/IX range from 40% to 50% in muscular bleeds to 100% in ICH (DiMichele and Neufeld, 1998). In newborns with hemophilia and ICH, treatment with factor concentrates should be continued for at least 2 weeks, and early prophylactic treatment should be considered (Kulkarni and Lusher, 2001). Insufficient data are available to support the benefit of prophylactic doses of FVIII given while the baby is still in the intrauterine environment or shortly after birth to offset the trauma of labor in newborns suspected or confirmed to have hemophilia (Buchanan, 1999). In neonates with severe hemophilia undergoing circumcision, use of local fibrin glue has reduced the need for postoperative factor replacement (Kavakli, 1999).

### Other Hereditary Coagulation Factor Deficiencies

#### Overview

Von Willebrand disease (vWD), the most common hereditary bleeding disorder, found in up to 1% of the general population (Rodeghiero et al, 1987), only rarely manifests during infancy, because of elevated levels of vWF after birth with an increased proportion of high-molecular-weight multimers.

Severe deficiencies of prothrombin, FV, FVII, FX, FXI, fibrinogen, FXIII, $\alpha_2$AP, and PAI all can manifest with bleeding in the first days of life in otherwise healthy infants. However, the severe forms of these disorders are rare, and their prevalence ranges from 1/500,000 to 1/1,000,000 (Peyvandi and Mannucci, 1999). Deficiencies of FXII, high-molecular-weight kallikrein (HMWK), and prekallikrein generally are not associated with bleeding.

Inheritance of vWD usually follows an autosomal dominant pattern, although autosomal recessive cases have been reported. Hereditary deficiencies of prothrombin, FV, FVII, FX, FXI, FXIII, fibrinogen, and $\alpha_2$AP are inherited in an autosomal recessive fashion, and consanguinity often is found in affected families.

#### Clinical Presentation

Von Willebrand disease does not usually present in the neonatal period. However, there are rare reports of ICH, thrombocytopenia, and soft tissue bleeds in newborns with vWD type II or III (Bignell et al, 1990; Donner et al, 1987; Gazengel et al, 1988).

Bleeding symptoms in hereditary deficiencies of prothrombin, FV, FVII, FX, FXI, FXIII, fibrinogen, and $\alpha_2$AP generally appear to be less severe than those of hemophilia A and B. There are no specific bleeding manifestations typical for a single disorder. Bleeding from the umbilical stump, previously thought to be typical of inherited defects of fibrin formation (FXIII deficiency and afibrinogenemia), has recently also been described in deficiencies of prothrombin, FV, and FX (Peyvandi and Mannucci, 1999).

### Diagnosis

Diagnosis of vWD in newborns may be difficult owing to the increased proportion of high-molecular-weight multimers. However, those forms of vWD that may manifest in the neonatal period, such as type IIB or type III, should not pose any diagnostic difficulties, as vWF levels and multimeric structure are clearly departed from normal. In cases with known mutations, DNA analysis may be used to ascertain the diagnosis (Mannhalter et al, 1991).

Homozygous forms of FV, FVII, and FXIII deficiency result in factor levels that are easily distinguishable from normal values for newborns. By contrast, in homozygous deficiencies of prothrombin, FX, and FXI, there may be an overlap between the plasma concentrations of the respective factors and neonatal physiologic values.

### Treatment

Treatment of hereditary hemorrhagic disorders is aimed at increasing plasma concentrations of the deficient coagulation protein to a minimal hemostatic level when a newborn is bleeding or a hemostatic challenge is planned. The minimal hemostatic plasma concentration of a particular coagulation protein varies and is dependent on the protein and the nature of the hemostatic challenge. Specific replacement therapy is available for deficiencies of FVII, FXI, FXIII, and fibrinogen and for vWD. Nonspecific treatment modalities comprise FFP, cryoprecipitate, and antifibrinolytics.

## Acquired Hemorrhagic Disorders

### Vitamin K Deficiency

The discovery of vitamin K and its important role in hemostasis was intertwined with the role of vitamin K in the treatment and subsequent prevention of hemorrhagic disease of the newborn (HDN). This term was coined in 1894 by Townsend, who first described the picture of bleeding from multiple sites in otherwise healthy infants in the absence of trauma, asphyxia, or infection on days 1 to 5 of life. The link between vitamin K deficiency and spontaneous hemorrhage was first reported in 1929. Recognition of the association between vitamin K deficiency and HDN quickly followed, with subsequent treatment of infants with HDN. Replacement of the original term *hemorrhagic disease of the newborn* with *vitamin K deficiency bleeding* (VKDB) has been suggested, because the former entity included many infants with bleeding from other causes (Sutor et al, 1999).

#### Clinical Presentation

Generally, infants are at greater risk for VKDB than are similarly affected adults, because plasma concentrations of vitamin K–dependent factors are physiologically decreased. Breast-fed infants are at higher risk owing to the low vitamin K content of breast milk. The clinical presentation of VKDB can be classified into three patterns—early, classic, late—based on the timing and type of complications.

The *early* form of VKDB manifests in the first 24 hours of life and is almost exclusively linked to maternal use of specific medications that interfere with vitamin K stores or function. These medications include anticonvulsants (carbamazepine, phenytoin, and barbiturates), antibiotics (cephalosporins), tuberculostatic agents (rifampicin, isoniazid), and vitamin K antagonists (Sutor et al, 1999). The *classic* form of VKDB manifests on days 2 to 7 of life in breast-fed, healthy full-term infants. Etiologic factors include poor placental transfer of vitamin K, marginal vitamin K content in breast milk, delayed or inadequate feeding, malabsorption, and a sterile gut. VKDB rarely occurs in formula-fed infants because formula has a higher content of vitamin K (>50 μg/L) than that of breast milk (<5 μg/L) (Greer et al, 1991). In the absence of prophylactic vitamin K, the frequency of classic VKDB ranges from 0.25% to 1.7% (American Academy of Pediatrics, 1993). Common bleeding sites are the gastrointestinal tract, the umbilical stump, venipuncture or heel prick sites, and circumcision wounds. Intracranial hemorrhage is infrequent in classic VKDB but can cause significant morbidity or death. The *late* form of VKDB manifests between weeks 2 and 8 of life and rarely after 3 months of life. It occurs almost exclusively in breast-fed infants, and boys are affected twice as often as girls (Sutor et al, 1995). A clustering of cases in warmer months has been described (McNinch and Tripp, 1991). The incidence ranges between 4.4/100,000 and 10.5/100,000 births (Von Kries and Hanawa, 1993). Late VKDB is mostly secondary to disorders that compromise the supply of vitamin K, such as biliary atresia or other hepatobiliary diseases (Loughnan and McDougall, 1993). Warning signs are rare in the idiopathic forms, but infants with underlying hepatobiliary diseases may show prolonged jaundice, minor bleedings, failure to thrive, and vomiting.

On rare occasions, deficiency of vitamin K–dependent coagulation factors is due to a genetic defect of vitamin K metabolism (Oldenburg et al, 2000). Affected patients may present with bleeding in the intrauterine or early neonatal period.

#### Laboratory Diagnosis

Deficiency of vitamin K leads to decreased activity of vitamin K–dependent coagulation factors (II, VII, IX, X); vitamin K–independent factors are in the normal range. Accordingly, a clearly prolonged PT (international normalized ratio [INR] >3.5) in the presence of normal fibrinogen concentration and platelet count is highly suggestive of vitamin K deficiency. Rapid normalization of these values within 30 to 120 min after parenteral vitamin K administration is diagnostic of vitamin K deficiency (Sutor et al, 1999). Patients with vitamin K deficiency produce decarboxylated forms of the vitamin K–dependent factors (PIVKAs [proteins induced in vitamin K absence]). PIVKA-II has a half-life of up to 70 hours (Shapiro et al, 1986) and thus can be measured even after vitamin K therapy and normalization of the PT. The most common conditions that need to be excluded are liver disease and DIC. Children with liver disease usually also have deficiencies of vitamin K–independent coagulation factors, such as fibrinogen, FV, FVIII, or AT. Infants with DIC generally are severely ill and show deficiencies of all coagulation factors, a low platelet count, and elevated levels of fibrin degradation products. Hereditary coagulation factor deficiencies can be excluded by single factor analysis. Common to all these conditions is the lack of normalization of the PT after vitamin K administration.

### Prophylactic Vitamin K Administration

Several studies have unequivocally demonstrated that prophylactic administration of vitamin K to newborns is effective in reducing the incidence of VKDB. Two major randomized controlled trials that assessed the benefits of vitamin K prophylaxis using clinical bleeding as the outcome measure showed a significantly positive result for prophylactic (intramuscular) vitamin K administration (Sutherland and Glueck, 1967; Vietti et al, 1960). In addition, biochemical evidence of vitamin K deficiency has been found in infants who did not receive vitamin K at birth (Motohara et al, 1985). Population-based studies show that VKDB rarely occurs when vitamin K prophylaxis is used, but it does occur when prophylactic vitamin K is withdrawn (McNinch and Tripp, 1991). Methods for prophylaxis of vitamin K deficiency vary in different parts of the world; regimens consist of either a single intramuscular dose of 1 mg or an oral dose of 2 to 4 mg at birth, with two or multiple subsequent doses during the first 6 to 12 weeks of life. Both routes are effective in preventing classic VKDB (Von Kries and Hanawa, 1993). However, no randomized clinical trial has assessed the efficacy of these regimens for the prevention of late VKDB. Available evidence suggests that a single dose (1.0 mg) of vitamin K given intramuscularly after birth appears to be effective in preventing virtually all cases of late VKDB (Von Kries and Hanawa, 1993). Disadvantages of intramuscular vitamin K prophylaxis are local trauma (such as nerve or vessel injury, osteomyelitis, or abcesses), poor acceptance by parents, and relatively high cost. Other concerns are the high blood levels of vitamin K after intramuscular injection (McNinch et al, 1985) and the potentially elevated risk of cancer (see later on). Use of the oral route of administration of vitamin K is less expensive and less traumatic than use of the intramuscular route. A disadvantage is the unreliable intake due to regurgitation or malabsorption. As oral vitamin K lacks the depot effect of the intramuscular preparation, the duration of effect of a single dose is comparatively short. Accordingly, oral vitamin K is not as effective as intramuscular vitamin K in the prevention of late vitamin K deficiency. Strategies to improve the efficacy of oral vitamin K and to prevent late VKDB include the use of a new mixed-micellar water-soluble vitamin K formulation, repeated administration of oral vitamin K at single doses of 2 mg, and continuous low-dose vitamin K supplementation (1 mg weekly or 25 μg daily) (Cornelissen et al, 1993; Hansen and Ebbesen, 1996; Schubiger et al, 1999; Von Kries et al, 1999). The last regimen seems to be as effective as the intramuscular preparation in the prevention of late VKDB but requires appropriate compliance and may not protect infants with cholestatic liver disease from late VKDB.

In small preterm infants, the first dose of vitamin K often is given as an intravenous bolus. No evidence-based recommendations on the appropriate dose are available. A recent study showed that the intravenous administration of 0.2-0.4 mg/kg vitamin K results in vitamin K plasma levels comparable to those after intramuscular injection (Raith et al, 2000). Vitamin K plasma concentrations remained well above the critical level below which bleeding manifestations can be anticipated (Stoeckel et al, 1996) for at least 1 week. As a single dose of intravenous vitamin K provides no protection from late VKDB (Loughnan et al, 1996), subsequent oral or intravenous doses must be given. In preterm infants who received a single intramuscular injection of vitamin K at birth, plasma concentrations of vitamin K at 2 and 6 weeks of life were higher than those in formula-fed term infants, probably as a result of a high vitamin K intake through parenteral nutrition (Kumar et al, 2001).

Pregnant women receiving oral anticonvulsant therapy should be given about 10 to 20 mg/day of vitamin K orally for 15 to 30 days before delivery to prevent overt vitamin K deficiency in their infants at birth (Cornelissen et al, 1993).

### Vitamin K and Childhood Cancer

In 1990, an unexpected association between childhood cancer and prophylactic vitamin K was reported by Golding and colleagues (1990). A case-control study by the same investigators found a significant association between intramuscular vitamin K and cancer when compared with no vitamin K or oral vitamin K (Golding et al, 1992). Subsequently, several studies have investigated that association. Although taken as a whole these studies failed to establish a significant link between intramuscular vitamin K and childhood cancer (Ross and Davies, 2000), a minimal residual risk cannot be excluded (Parker et al, 1998).

### Treatment of Vitamin K Deficiency

An infant suspected of having VKDB should be treated immediately with vitamin K pending laboratory confirmation. Vitamin K should not be given intramuscularly to infants with VKDB, because large hematomas may form at the site of the injection. The absorption of subcutaneous vitamin K is rapid, and its effect is only slightly slower than systematically administered vitamin K. Intravenous vitamin K should be given slowly because it may induce an anaphylactoid reaction. Infants with major bleeding secondary to vitamin K deficiency also should be treated with plasma products to rapidly increase levels of vitamin K–dependent proteins. Plasma is the product of choice for treatment of a non–life-threatening hemorrhagic event; prothrombin complex concentrate (PCC) at a minimum dose of 50 U/kg should be given for life-threatening bleeding.

## Disseminated Intravascular Coagulation

### Etiology

DIC is not a primary diagnosis but a secondary process related to a variety of primary disease states. Common etiologic disorders in the neonatal period include asphyxia, shock, infection, RDS, necrotizing enterocolitis (NEC), and meconium aspiration syndrome. Rare causes are hypothermia, hemolytic disorders, and hemangiomas. The pathogenic mechanism of DIC is an inappropriate, systemic activation of coagulation with the resultant generation of excess thrombin and decreased generation of anticoagulant factors such as AT, protein C, and protein S. These changes lead to diffuse intravascular thrombus formation (from which the term *disseminated intravascular coagulation* historically originated) and consumption of coagulation factors and platelets. The simultaneous inhibition of the fibrinolytic pathway due to increased concentrations of PAI-1 prevents removal of fibrin from small vessels, leading to extensive thrombosis and organ failure. The consumption of platelets and coagulation factors may in turn cause severe, diffuse hemorrhage (Levi and ten Cate, 1999).

### Clinical Presentation

Unlike bleeding due to vitamin K deficiency or inherited factor deficiencies, DIC occurs in sick infants, most commonly premature infants. Intensity and duration of activation of the hemostatic system, degree of impaired blood flow, and liver function all influence the clinical severity of DIC. Some infants with laboratory evidence of DIC may show little or no clinical signs, whereas those clinically affected usually present with multiorgan failure and/or bleeding from multiple sites. Common bleeding manifestations include oozing from mucous membranes or sites of invasive procedures, hematuria, pulmonary hemorrhage, bruising, and in some cases ICH.

### Laboratory Diagnosis

The diagnosis of DIC is based on compatible clinical features in conjunction with abnormalities of specific coagulation tests. Laboratory findings in severe DIC are characterized by prolonged PT and APTT, depletion of certain coagulation factors (fibrinogen, FV, FVIII), increased fibrin degradation products, thrombocytopenia, and a microangiopathic hemolytic anemia with schistocyte formation. Yet diagnosis of DIC in the newborn is difficult, and no clear-cut diagnostic criteria are available. The diagnostic difficulties are due to an overlap of physiologic and pathologic values for several procoagulant and anticoagulant factors, physiologically elevated markers of thrombin formation and fibrinolysis, and the limited blood volume available for diagnostic workup. In practice, no single laboratory test can be used to confirm or exclude DIC. Although abnormal global coagulation tests strongly support the diagnosis of DIC, normal results do not rule out activation of the coagulation and fibrinolytic system (Schmidt et al, 1993). The availability of sensitive markers for endogenous thrombin and plasmin generation has complicated the diagnosis of DIC in newborns. For example, plasma concentrations of thrombin-AT complexes are increased in the first hours of postnatal life in healthy infants (Knofler et al, 1998a), reflecting activation of the coagulation system during birth. Positive results for these sensitive paracoagulation tests thus do not necessarily indicate the presence of DIC or the need to intervene. On the other hand, D-dimer levels may be normal if fibrinolytic activity is suppressed by elevated PAI-1 levels, a common finding in newborns, even in the absence of sepsis (Andrew et al, 1990b).

### Treatment

The cornerstone of management of DIC remains the successful treatment of the underlying problem. The decision to treat the hemostatic disorder is often difficult to make. In the absence of clinical manifestations, newborns probably do not require therapy for the hemostatic disorder itself. In the presence of clinically significant bleeding, therapeutic intervention with plasma products is indicated and often improves hemostasis. For infants between these two ends of the spectrum, treatment is dictated by the severity of the hemostatic impairment and the underlying problem. In general, the more pronounced the laboratory abnormalities, the greater the risk of bleeding or thrombotic complications. The argument that replacement therapy may "fuel the fire" is theoretical, and this association has not been proved. Therapeutic interventions in neonates with DIC include administration of FFP, cryoprecipitate, factor concentrates, and anticoagulants and exchange transfusions. Unfortunately, no recent clinical studies on replacement therapy in newborns with DIC are available to permit strong recommendations to be made. The following discussion provides a brief overview of the currently used treatment modalities for neonatal DIC.

The most extensively used treatment is administration of FFP, which contains adult concentrations of all the coagulation proteins. The major drawback is that the large volumes of FFP required to achieve sufficient concentrations of coagulation factors may result in fluid overload. Potential adverse effects include viral transmission and graft-versus-host disease. Cryoprecipitate provides high concentrations of fibrinogen and FVIII, two proteins that are frequently depleted in DIC. Prothrombin complex concentrates have been used in newborns but generally are not recommended because of the potential thrombotic and infectious side effects (Roddie et al, 1999). Exchange transfusions occasionally are used in severe DIC, but their effects are transient unless the underlying problem resolves.

The rationale for use of heparin in the treatment of DIC is to reduce the generation of excess thrombin in the early stages of DIC. Heparin treatment has to be initiated prior to microthrombus formation to provide at least a theoretical benefit. Efficacy of heparin treatment also depends on the AT-prothrombin ratio, which may be low in neonatal sepsis, resulting in a reduced heparin sensitivity. To date, no evidence is available to support the use of heparin for infants with DIC.

The observation that plasma concentrations of the coagulation inhibitors AT and protein C are decreased during DIC provides the rationale for the use of AT and protein C concentrates in these patients. So far, only two small uncontrolled studies have investigated the use of AT and/or protein C concentrates in newborns with DIC (Kreuz et al, 1999; Nowak-Gottl et al, 1992). Both studies showed 100% survival, effective treatment of purpura fulminans, and marked improvement in laboratory parameters. However, a carefully designed randomized controlled trial of AT substitution in newborns with RDS reported a trend toward higher bleeding rates and increased mortality in the AT-treated group (Schmidt et al, 1998). On the basis of the data available, treatment with AT and protein C concentrates currently cannot be recommended for routine use. Well-designed controlled trials are required to determine the safety and efficacy of AT and protein C concentrates in neonatal DIC. In the absence of definitive clinical trials, reasonable goals in the treatment of DIC are to maintain platelet counts above $50 \times 10^9$ /L, fibrinogen concentrations over 1.0 g/L, and PT values at normal levels for postnatal and gestational ages.

## Liver Disease

The coagulopathies of liver disease in newborns are similar to those in adults and reflect the failure of hepatic synthetic functions superimposed on a physiologic immaturity, activation of the coagulation and fibrinolytic systems, poor clearance of activated coagulation factors, loss of hemostatic proteins into ascitic fluid, and splenic sequestration of platelets. Some of the common pathologic causes of hepatic dysfunction in newborns are viral hepatitis, hypoxia, total parenteral nutrition, biliary atresia, congenital heart disease with low cardiac output, inherited metabolic disorders, shock, and fetal hydrops. The clinical presentation is variable and usually depends on the underlying disorder. Symptoms include ecchymosis and petechiae, mucous membrane bleeding, hemorrhage from gastrointestinal varices or into the abdomen, and ICH. Laboratory abnormalities in newborns with liver failure include prolongation of PT and APTT, thrombocytopenia, and a prolonged bleeding time. Plasma concentrations of FV, FVII, fibrinogen, AT, and plasminogen are decreased; fibrin degradation products and D-dimer are frequently increased. Normal levels of FVIII, reflecting significant extrahepatic synthesis, can help distinguish severe liver disease from DIC. The etiology of thrombocytopenia and platelet dysfunction is multifactorial and includes impaired platelet production, inappropriate platelet activation and degranulation, splenic sequestration, and accelerated clearance. Patients with clinical bleeding may benefit temporarily from replacement of coagulation proteins with FFP, cryoprecipitate, and platelet transfusion. However, without recovery of hepatic function, replacement therapy is futile. Vitamin K should be administered to infants in whom cholestatic liver disease is suspected. Prothrombin complex concentrate should be avoided in newborns owing to the high risk of transmitting hepatitis and the risk of thrombotic disease, especially in patients with liver disease (Roddie et al, 1999). No data are available to support a role for AT concentrates in treatment of neonatal liver disease.

## Intraventricular Hemorrhage

Intraventricular hemorrhage (IVH) is most commonly seen in premature infants and is characterized by bleeding from the fragile microvasculature of the subependymal germinal matrix, which may extend into the lateral ventricles. Intraventricular hemorrhage is found in about 20% of premature infants with birth weights less than 1500 g and is the major risk factor for long-term neurologic morbidity in this group. A combination of vascular, intravascular, and extravascular factors is operative in the pathogenesis of IVH (Volpe, 2001). The role of hemostasis in this context is controversial. Proposed mechanisms include decreased activities of coagulation factors, thrombocytopenia, platelet dysfunction, and enhanced local fibrinolytic activity (Andrew et al, 1987a; Beverley et al, 1984; Chen and Lorch, 1996; Setzer et al, 1982; Van de Bor et al, 1986). However, lack of uniformity in the results obtained on this topic suggests that its role is merely contributory, if it has any at all. Two studies on the influence of prothrombotic conditions on the incidence of IVH showed conflicting results (Gopel et al, 2001; Petaja et al, 2001).

A number of clinical trials have assessed various hemostatic prevention strategies for IVH and are summarized next.

### Antenatal Vitamin K

Five clinical trials have investigated the effect of antenatal vitamin K (with or without addition of phenobarbital) on plasma activities of vitamin K–dependent coagulation proteins and IVH in premature infants. (Kazzi et al, 1989; Morales et al, 1988; Pomerance et al, 1987; Thorp et al, 1994; Yang et al, 1989). Two reported a benefit, and three did not. The inconsistencies in results and methodologic problems prevent a recommendation for antenatal vitamin K.

### Coagulation Factor/Platelet Replacement

Since 1980, five clinical trials have assessed coagulation factor and platelet replacement in newborns at risk for IVH. Three trials assessed FFP because of the potential contribution to IVH of low plasma concentrations of many coagulation proteins at birth. Two trials failed to show a benefit (Northern Neonatal Nursing Initiative Trial Group, 1996; Wright, 1995), whereas a positive effect was reported in the third but without a placebo control (Beverley et al, 1985). It is possible that the observed beneficial effect was the result not of the increase in plasma concentrations of coagulation proteins but of volume expansion. One trial assessed the effects of FXIII concentrates because of the potential benefit of enhanced fibrin cross-linking (Shirahata et al, 1990). Although this study reported a significant effect, the analysis was performed only on a small subset of infants. In addition, there is no strong biologic rationale for this approach because FXIII levels are well within the adult range at birth. Another trial investigated the effects of platelet concentrates administered to thrombocytopenic premature infants because of the association of thrombocytopenia and IVH (Andrew et al, 1993). No beneficial effect on IVH was shown in this study, which was designed to detect a 25% effect or greater.

### Fibrinolytic or Antifibrinolytic Therapy

One trial assessed the effects of an antifibrinolytic agent, tranexamic acid, because fibrinolytic activity is increased at birth and could contribute to IVH (Hensey et al, 1984). No significant effect was demonstrated.

### Conclusion

At this time, no firm recommendations can be made for any of the intervention modalities discussed because of inconsistent results. Ongoing clinical studies are necessary to test potentially beneficial therapeutic agents within the context of improving clinical care.

## Extracorporeal Membrane Oxygenation

Extracorporeal membrane oxygenation (ECMO) is an increasingly used technique for the treatment of respiratory and/or cardiac failure refractory to conventional forms of therapy. The most common indications for the use of ECMO are meconium aspiration syndrome, congenital diaphragmatic hernia, RDS, pulmonary hypertension, sepsis, and pneumonia. Survival rates depend on the primary diagnosis and range from 55% in congenital heart disease to almost 100% in meconium aspiration syndrome (Bartlett, 1997; Rais-Bahrami and Short, 2000).

During ECMO, gas exchange occurs through a semipermeable membrane in an extracorporeal circuit driven by a servo-regulated pump. To combat the activation and consumption of platelets and clotting factors by the extracorporeal surfaces, the patient must be systemically heparinized during the ECMO session. Therapeutic heparin levels are usually achieved by using a bolus of 100 U/kg of unfractionated heparin (UFH) followed by a continuous infusion of UFH at a rate of about 25 to 50 U/kg/h. Most centers use the activated clotting time (ACT) to monitor anticoagulation, targeting an ACT two to three times the baseline value (180 to 220 seconds) in noncomplicated cases. The correlation between the ACT and heparin levels in children on extracorporeal circuits is poor, probably as a result of concurrent hemodilution of hemostatic factors and activation of the hemostatic system and platelets (Chan et al, 1997).

The most common reported complication of ECMO with major impact on mortality and long-term morbidity is ICH. The increased risk of bleeding is mostly due to the use of heparin in association with contact-induced platelet and clotting factor consumption (Urlesberger et al, 1996) and platelet dysfunction (Cheung et al, 2000). The alteration of physiologic pulsatile blood flow during venoarterial ECMO impairs cerebral autoregulation (Short et al, 1993), which may further contribute to the development of ICH. The overall incidence of ICH in neonatal ECMO patients is reported at 10% to 20%, with an overall mortality rate of 50% (Bulas et al, 1996; Hardart and Fackler, 1999; Upp et al, 1994). The incidence of ICH is increased in neonates less than 35 weeks of gestational age. Other recognized risk factors for ICH include acidosis, sepsis, coagulopathy, and treatment with epinephrine (Hardart and Fackler, 1999).

# THROMBOEMBOLIC DISORDERS

Improvements in pediatric tertiary care during the last decade have led to a significant increase in the incidence of thromboembolic events (TEs) during childhood. Both the rise in survival rates for previously fatal conditions and the increased use of thrombogenic surfaces such as catheters, ECMO circuits, and cardiopulmonary bypass circuits account for this phenomenon. Based on the results of national and international pediatric thrombosis registries, it is estimated that more than 50% of TEs in children occur during the neonatal period (Andrew et al, 1994a; Schmidt and Andrew, 1995; van Ommen et al, 2001). The incidence of TE in newborns is approximately 2.4/1000 admissions to the neonatal intensive care unit (NICU) (Schmidt and Andrew, 1995), which is about the same as the incidence of TE in the general adult population (Heit et al, 2001). The single most common risk factor for TE is the presence of a central catheter—a finding in about 80% of affected neonates (Schmidt and Andrew, 1995; van Ommen et al, 2001). Historically, neonatal hemostasis has focused on bleeding disorders only. Clinicians should now be aware of the increased frequency and importance of neonatal thrombosis.

## Hereditary Prothrombotic Disorders

An ever-growing number of established or candidate hereditary risk factors for venous and/or arterial TE have been described. It cannot be stressed enough, however, that acquired risk factors (e.g., central catheters) are significantly more important in relation to neonatal TE than hereditary prothrombotic disorders alone. Hereditary prothrombotic disorders rarely manifest with TE during the neonatal period unless a significant acquired risk factor is present (Martinelli et al, 2000; Sanson et al, 1999; Schmidt and Andrew, 1995; van Ommen et al, 2001). Furthermore, sufficient evidence currently is available for only a few hereditary prothrombotic disorders to link them to neonatal TE. Assessing the attributable risk of a single prothrombotic abnormality for a specific neonatal thromboembolic disorder requires a large case-control study. To date, most studies assessing prothrombotic risk factors in children did not differentiate between neonates and older children, owing to the low incidence of childhood TE. Sometimes it is difficult to ascertain whether a patient has a true hereditary deficiency of an inhibitor protein and not an acquired transient deficiency due to the underlying disorder or the TE itself. Difficulty in diagnosis of a potential inhibitor deficiency may be further compounded by an overlap of neonatal physiologic values and deficiency states. Therefore, testing for prothrombotic conditions should be delayed until the infant reaches 3 months of age, unless the presentation is unusually severe (e.g., purpura fulminans). If a rare hereditary prothrombotic condition such as AT or protein C deficiency is suspected, familial testing may assist in confirmation of the diagnosis. Routine screening for hereditary prothrombotic conditions is not cost effective and probably is not indicated, as TEs develop in only a small minority of neonates with hereditary prothrombotic disorders. In a majority of cases, the risks of long-term continuous prophylaxis starting in the neonatal period probably outweigh the benefits.

### Activated Protein C Resistance/Factor V Leiden Mutation

Activated protein C is a natural anticoagulant that proteolyzes FVa and FVIIIa, thereby inhibiting conversion of prothrombin to thrombin and of FX to FXa, respectively.

In 95% of cases, aPC resistance (aPCR) is caused by a mutation in the FV gene, the FV Leiden mutation. Activated protein C resistance is the single most common hereditary prothrombotic disorder in Caucasians, found in about 5% of the population (Rees et al, 1995). In heterozygous adult carriers, the relative risk for TE is increased sevenfold (van der Meer et al, 1997). This increases to 80-fold in homozygous persons (Rosendaal et al, 1995). Despite its relative frequency, heterozygous or homozygous FV Leiden mutation rarely manifests in the neonatal period (Simioni et al, 1999). When a TE occurs in newborns with the FV Leiden mutation, another prothrombotic disorder or a significant acquired risk factor usually is present (Nowak-Gottl et al, 1996). An increased frequency of FV Leiden has been reported in children with porencephaly (Debus et al, 1998) and with cerebral palsy (Nelson et al, 1998). Testing for aPCR in newborns and infants is hampered by elevated levels of FV and FVIII and a reduced capacity to generate thrombin (Andrew et al, 1990c), which strongly interferes with the test result (Montaruli et al, 1997; Nowak-Gottl et al, 1996). Diagnosis of the FV Leiden mutation by DNA testing is preferable and necessary for definitive diagnosis.

### Prothrombin Gene Mutation *G20210A*

A mutation of the prothrombin gene at position 20210 was recently found to be associated with an increased risk of venous TE in adults (Poort et al, 1996). To date, there is no evidence that either a homozygous or a heterozygous prothrombin gene mutation is a risk factor for neonatal TE.

### Antithrombin Deficiency

AT is the major inhibitor of thrombin and other serine proteases such as FXa, FIXa, FXIa, and FXIIa. Persons with heterozygous AT deficiency usually present with venous TE in early adulthood, occurring either spontaneously or in association with relatively minor acquired risk factors for TE (Thaler and Lechner, 1981). The prevalence of AT deficiency in the general population is estimated at 1/600 (Tait et al, 1994).

Several publications have reported on newborns with heterozygous AT deficiency and severe TE. The clinical presentation was variable, reflecting the site of the thrombi. In these case reports, the TEs often were spontaneous, occurred in venous or arterial vessels, and included unusual locations like the brain (Brenner et al, 1988), pulmonary artery (Martin Montaner et al, 1987), aorta (Sanchez et al, 1998), and coronary arteries (Jochmans et al, 1994). Larger cohort studies on childhood TE, however, have failed to identify significant numbers of neonates with AT deficiency (Aschka et al, 1996; Heller et al, 2000). Therefore, the attributable risk of AT deficiency in neonatal TE is likely to be small. Homozygous or compound heterozygous AT deficiency type I manifesting with purpura fulminans and extensive thrombosis has been reported in two siblings born to consanguineous parents (Hakten et al, 1989). Both children died in the neonatal period. Homozygous AT deficiency type II has been described in four newborns and infants (Chowdhury et al, 1994; Kuhle et al, 2001), all of whom shared the same mutation. Presentation included deep venous thrombosis (DVT) of the leg, pulmonary artery thrombosis, and arterial ischemic stroke in two children. Treatment of newborns and infants with AT deficiency and TE includes anticoagulation with UFH or low-molecular-weight heparin (LMWH) and transfusion of AT concentrates. In the absence of firm data, recommendations on dose and duration of AT replacement cannot be given at this time.

### Protein C Deficiency

Protein C is a vitamin K–dependent serine protease produced in the liver. Following activation by thrombin and thrombomodulin, aPC proteolyzes FVa and FVIIIa. Heterozygous deficiency of protein C results in a 10-fold increased risk for TE in adults (Allaart et al, 1993). The prevalence of protein C deficiency in the general population is estimated at 1/200 to 1/300 (Miletich et al, 1987).

#### *Heterozygous Protein C Deficiency*

Heterozygous protein C deficiency does not usually manifest with TE during childhood (De Stefano et al, 1994). Some cohort studies, however, suggest that the attributable risk for cerebral TE in children is slightly elevated (Debus et al, 1998; deVeber et al, 1998b; Vielhaber et al, 1998). Two studies in neonates found an elevated attributable risk for abdominal venous thrombosis and arterial ischemic stroke in newborns with protein C deficiency (Gunther et al, 2000; Heller et al, 2000). However, a majority of children had additional, acquired clinical risk factors for TE that unmasked the defect.

#### *Homozygous Protein C Deficiency*

Homozygous deficiency of protein C is a rare and life-threatening disorder that usually manifests within hours after birth, but presentation later in childhood has been described.

##### Clinical Presentation

The classic clinical presentation of homozygous protein C deficiency consists of cerebral and ophthalmic damage that occurred in utero, purpura fulminans within hours or days of birth, and, in rare cases, large-vessel thrombosis. Purpura fulminans is an acute, lethal syndrome of DIC with rapidly progressive hemorrhagic necrosis of the skin due to dermal vascular thrombosis. The skin lesions start as small ecchymotic sites that increase in a radial fashion and become purplish black with bullae and then necrotic and gangrenous. The lesions occur mainly on the extremities but can occur on the buttocks, abdomen, scrotum, and scalp. They also occur at pressure points, at sites of previous punctures, and at previously affected sites (Marlar and Neumann, 1990).

### Diagnosis

The diagnosis of homozygous protein C deficiency usually is unanticipated and is made at the time of the clinical presentation. Prerequisites are the appropriate clinical picture, a protein C level that is usually undetectable, a heterozygous state in the parents, and, ideally, the identification of the molecular defect. The presence of very low levels of protein C in the absence of clinical manifestations and family history cannot be considered diagnostic because physiologic plasma levels can be as low as 0.12 U/mL (Andrew et al, 1988).

### Treatment

Although numerous forms of initial therapy have been used, administration of 10 to 20 mL/kg of FFP every 6 to 12 hours is usually the form of therapy immediately available. Plasma levels of protein C achieved with 10 mL/kg of FFP vary from 15% to 32% at 30 minutes after the infusion and from 4% to 10% at 12 hours (Marlar et al, 1989). If available, protein C concentrates are preferable to FFP, as they are more concentrated and safer in terms of risk of viral transmission. Doses of protein C concentrate have ranged from 20 to 60 U/kg. In one study, a dose of 60 U/kg resulted in peak protein C levels above 0.60 U/mL (Dreyfus et al, 1991). Replacement therapy was continued until all of the clinical lesions resolved, which was usually 6 to 8 weeks. In addition to the clinical course, plasma D-dimer concentrations were useful for monitoring the effectiveness of protein C replacement. Following resolution of skin lesions, long-term oral anticoagulation should be instituted. To avoid skin necrosis when oral anticoagulation therapy is initiated, replacement therapy should be continued until the INR is therapeutic. The therapeutic range for the INR can be individualized to some extent but is usually between 3.0 and 4.5 (Monagle et al, 2001). The risk with oral anticoagulation therapy includes bleeding with high INRs and recurrent purpuric lesions with low INRs. Frequent monitoring of INR values is required to avoid these complications. Recurrence of skin lesions should be treated with FFP or protein C concentrates. Bone development should also be monitored, as long-term warfarin therapy may have a negative effect on bone mineral density (Cheung et al, 2001). Two case reports have described the successful use of subcutaneous protein C administrations at a dose of 250 to 350 U/kg every third day (Minford et al, 1996; Sanz-Rodriguez et al, 1999) in children with homozygous protein C deficiency. Successful prophylactic long-term treatment with LMWH has been described in two sisters with homozygous protein C deficiency and measurable plasma concentrations of protein C (Monagle et al, 1998). Liver transplantation has been performed successfully in one patient with homozygous protein C deficiency (Marlar et al, 1989).

## Protein S Deficiency

Protein S is a vitamin K–dependent protein that functions as a cofactor of aPC by enhancing its proteolytic activity against FVa and FVIIIa. The prevalence of protein S deficiency in the general population is unknown. In persons with heterozygous protein S deficiency, TE usually does not occur before puberty (De Stefano et al, 1994).

To date, there have been no reports of newborns with heterozygous protein S deficiency and TE. Homozygous protein S deficiency and compound heterozygous protein S deficiency have been described in a small number of newborns (Mahasandana et al, 1990b; Marlar and Neumann, 1990; Pegelow et al, 1988). A majority of these presented with purpura fulminans similar to that seen in homozygous protein C deficiency. The plasma concentrations of protein S in those infants who presented with purpura fulminans were less than 1%. Because no protein S concentrates are available, treatment of purpura fulminans secondary to homozygous protein S deficiency requires FFP or cryoprecipitate. A pharmacokinetic study following administration of 10 mL/kg FFP found protein S levels of 23% and 14% at 2 and 24 hours, respectively (Mahasandana et al, 1990a). Long-term treatment strategies are similar to those in homozygous protein C deficiency.

# Acquired Prothrombotic Disorders

## Central Venous Lines

Presence of a central venous line (CVL) is the single most common risk factor associated with TE in newborns (Schmidt and Andrew, 1995; van Ommen et al, 2001). CVLs in newborns are placed either in the upper venous system (jugular or subclavian vein), in the lower venous system (femoral vein), or through peripheral veins into the inferior vena cava ("long lines"). A number of studies have investigated the incidence of CVL-related TE in neonates. The incidence reported ranged from 1% to up to 47% (Abdulla et al, 1990; Hruszkewycz et al, 1991; Mehta et al 1992; Neubauer, 1995; Salonvaara et al, 1999; Tanke et al, 1994), depending on the criterion used for diagnosis (loss of CVL patency versus objective tests), the radiographic test used, the study design, the duration of use, and the patient group studied.

### Clinical Presentation and Diagnosis

Presenting symptoms and signs of CVL-related thrombosis include loss of CVL patency, swelling and discoloration of the affected limb, swelling of the face, pulmonary embolism (PE), chylothorax, and superior vena cava syndrome. In the lower venous system, ultrasound examination is an appropriate first choice for the diagnosis of DVT. In the upper venous system, ultrasound examination has been shown to have poor sensitivity for the diagnosis of DVT because of the lack of compressibility of intrathoracic vessels, obstruction of view by the clavicle, and inability to distinguish flow through large collaterals from the normal venous system (Male et al, 2002). Ultrasound examination may be used to screen for DVT in the upper venous system. However, if findings on the ultrasound study are negative and the infant is symptomatic, venography should be used. Injection of contrast material through the CVL ("lineogram") enables visualization of thrombi only at the tip of the catheter, not on the vessel wall along the course of the CVL (Chait et al, 2001).

### Prophylaxis of Central Venous Line–Related TE

A recent meta-analysis has shown that prophylactic use of heparin (UFH and LMWH) or heparin-bonded catheters significantly reduces catheter-related DVT and may also decrease the rate of bacterial colonization (Randolph et al, 1998). However, studies included in this meta-analysis were done mainly in adults and used varying concentrations of UFH and LMWH. Further studies are needed assess the efficacy in children and to determine the most cost-effective regimen.

#### Therapy

In the absence of sufficient data, the following options exist for treatment of CVL-related DVT in neonates: (1) short-term anticoagulation, (2) conventional anticoagulation therapy, and (3) close monitoring of the thrombus with objective tests. If anticoagulation is used, the current guidelines (Monagle et al, 2001) recommend a short course (10 to 14 days) of therapeutic doses of UFH or LMWH. Depending on the location and extension of the thrombus, longer courses (3 months) of therapy may be required. The decision to remove a CVL associated with a large-vessel DVT should be individualized. Consideration should be given to anticoagulation therapy before CVL removal, especially in patients with right-to-left shunts.

#### Clinical Impact of CVL-Related DVT

Even clinically silent CVL-related DVTs are of clinical importance and require treatment, for a number of reasons. First, evidence suggests that CVL-related DVT is associated with recurrent CVL-related infection (Randolph et al, 1998). Second, CVL-related DVT may cause PE, with potentially fatal results (Monagle et al, 2001). Third, many newborns with CVL have right-to-left shunting, which puts them at risk for embolic stroke. Finally, post-thrombotic syndrome (PTS) is increasingly recognized as a complication of childhood DVT, occurring in about 10% of patients (Monagle et al, 2001).

### Umbilical Venous Catheters

Umbilical venous catheters (UVCs) are placed through the umbilical vein into the inferior vena cava. With appropriate positioning of UVC above the diaphragm, the incidence of portal vein thrombosis was 1.3% in an ultrasound study (Schwartz et al, 1997) and 30% when venography was used (Roy et al, 1997). Comprehensive long-term follow-up data are not available, but case reports have described the development of portal hypertension, splenomegaly, and gastric and esophageal varices following UVC placement (Junker et al, 1976).

### Umbilical Artery Catheters

Umbilical artery catheters (UACs) are used in critically ill newborns for performing arterial blood gas analyses and for continuous monitoring of blood pressure, and to facilitate repeated blood sampling. The tip of the catheter is placed either "high" (between T6 and T10) or "low" (at L3 to L5). A recent meta-analysis found that high positioning of the UAC tip results in longer usability and less complications than with low positioning (Barrington, 2000b). However, there is currently no convincing evidence that the position of the UAC tip influences the incidence of TE. The incidence for UAC-related TE is reported at about 30% when objective radiographic tests are used for the diagnosis (Boo et al, 1999; Seibert et al, 1987). A majority of UAC-related TEs cause minimal or no symptoms, but up to 5% of patients present with major symptoms of ischemia or organ dysfunction (Caeton and Goetzman, 1985). Ultrasound examination and angiography are used for the diagnosis of UAC-related TE. However, the sensitivity of ultrasonography for the diagnosis of aortic TE remains to be proved.

A continuous infusion of low-dose UFH significantly prolongs the patency of the UAC (Barrington, 2000a). However, a reduction in incidence of TE could not be shown. The effective concentration of UFH in the infusate may be as low as 0.25 U/mL. The association of heparin with intraventricular hemorrhage (IVH) has been assessed in four studies. Two randomized trials showed no difference in rate of IVH between patients receiving UFH and those receiving no UFH (Ankola and Atakent, 1993; Chang et al, 1997). However, both studies lacked sufficient power (i.e., did not have adequate patient numbers) to answer the question. The remaining case-control study and retrospective cohort study reported an increased risk of IVH in association with heparin, with an odds ratio of 3.9 (95% confidence interval [CI] 1.4-11) (Lesko et al, 1986) and 1.96 (95% CI 1.32-2.91) (Malloy and Cutter, 1995), respectively. The limitations of the designs of these two studies make it impossible to determine whether heparin is associated with IVH or is simply a marker of disease severity. Therefore, the evidence associating heparin use and IVH is inconclusive.

## Thromboembolic Complications in Specific Organ Sites

### Pulmonary Embolism

Most reported studies on PE group newborns, infants, and older children together, which necessitates a joint analysis and limits the information available specifically on newborns. Given the fact that in the pediatric population DVT is most prevalent among newborns, there is no reason to assume that PE is less common in this age group. Therefore, data on PE in the following section are extrapolated from children. PE represents the major cause of DVT-associated mortality in children (Monagle et al, 2000). A prospective cohort study reported an incidence of PE of 8.6 cases per 100,000 hospital admissions (Andrew et al, 1994a). However, clinical studies probably underestimate the true incidence of PE in children owing to a decreased index of suspicion and absence of standardized diagnostic techniques. CVL-related thrombi in the upper venous system are the major source for PE in children (Monagle et al, 2000). The incidence of PE in children with CVL was found to be as high as 15% to 30% when objective radiographic tests were used for the diagnosis (Dollery et al, 1994; Massicotte et al, 1998a).

PE often is not diagnosed during life in newborns owing to the subtlety of symptoms, the inability to verbalize symptoms, and the presence of underlying cardiorespiratory problems that may mask PE. Respiratory distress, hemoptysis or bloody tracheal aspirate, cyanosis, acute right-sided heart failure, hypotension, increasing oxygen requirements, arrhythmias, and pallor all may be linked to neonatal PE. Any unexplained deterioration in a newborn with a CVL should raise the suspicion of PE.

Performance of pulmonary angiography, the gold standard radiographic test for diagnosis of PE, and the more commonly used ventilation-perfusion scan is not always feasible in critically ill neonates. Pulmonary angiography is difficult to perform in neonates, carries a higher rate of complications in critically ill patients, and requires an experienced radiologist. Ventilation-perfusion scans may be difficult to interpret in neonates with underlying cardiorespiratory disorders because of to imbalances in pulmonary blood flow between the right and left lungs, or even within each lung. Accordingly, both tests have not been validated for the diagnosis of PE in neonates. Echocardiography may be used at the bedside for direct imaging of PE in the central pulmonary arteries. Increased right ventricular volume or pressure may provide an indirect index of more peripheral PE (Pollard et al, 1995). If none of these radiographic tests is feasible, searching for the source of the PE by ultrasound examination and venography may give indirect clues to the diagnosis of PE.

Insufficient data are available to make firm recommendations on the treatment of neonatal PE. Current guidelines recommend intravenous treatment with therapeutic doses of UFH (Monagle et al, 2001). In life-threatening situations or after failure of UFH therapy, thrombolytic therapy or embolectomy might be considered.

## Renal Vein Thrombosis

About 80% of childhood cases of renal vein thrombosis (RVT) occur during the neonatal period (Andrew and Brooker, 1996). RVT accounts for approximately 20% to 40% of neonatal TEs, with about half of the patients being preterm infants (Nowak-Gottl et al, 1997; Schmidt and Andrew, 1995). In up to 20% of cases, RVT is bilateral; in 30%, RVT extends into the inferior vena cava (Bokenkamp et al, 2000). Typically, RVT manifests with hematuria, flank mass, and thrombocytopenia. Occasionally, a transient hypertension is observed. In about 10% of cases, an associated adrenal hemorrhage is found on ultrasound examination. Risk factors for RVT in the newborn include asphyxia, shock, congenital heart disease, dehydration, polycythemia (predominantly infants of diabetic mothers), and sepsis. Diagnosis is usually made by ultrasound studies. Mortality and long-term morbidity associated with RVT are considerable (Bokenkamp et al, 2000). The role of antithrombotic therapy in RVT and its impact on outcome remain uncertain (Nuss et al, 1994). In the absence of clinical trials, one approach is to use supportive therapy for unilateral RVT without uremia or extension into the inferior vena cava (IVC). Anticoagulation should be considered for unilateral RVT extending into the IVC or for bilateral RVT because of the risk of PE and renal failure. Thrombolytic therapy should be considered in cases of bilateral RVT and pending renal failure.

## Arterial Ischemic Stroke

About 25% of cases of arterial ischemic stroke during childhood occur in neonates and young infants (deVeber et al, 2000). The incidence of neonatal arterial ischemic stroke based on clinical data is estimated at 1/4000 live births (Estan and Hope, 1997). However, this figure probably is an underestimate, as the diagnosis of arterial ischemic stroke is frequently delayed owing to the subtlety or lack of symptoms, or may be made only at autopsy (Barmada et al, 1979). Arterial ischemic stroke is most commonly found in full-term newborns but has also been described in preterm infants (de Vries et al, 1997). All three major cerebral arteries and their branches may be affected. However, most lesions are diagnosed in the territory of the middle cerebral artery. Some authors have reported a predominance of left-sided lesions. The vascular anatomy of the aortic arch favoring blood flow to the left common carotid artery or regional differences in cerebral metabolism associated with a higher susceptibility to ischemic injury may explain this predilection (Levy et al, 1985; Trauner et al, 1993).

The typical clinical presentation of neonatal arterial ischemic stroke is focal or generalized seizures. A prospective magnetic resonance imaging (MRI) study in a cohort of term newborns with seizures found an arterial ischemic stroke in 50% of the cases (Mercuri et al, 1995). Abnormalities in muscular tone, lethargy, jitteriness, and feeding problems also have been reported as presenting signs.

Acquired risk factors that have been described in association with neonatal arterial ischemic stroke include asphyxia, sepsis, pulmonary hypertension, congenital heart disease, dehydration, and meningitis (deVeber et al, 1997; Klesh et al, 1987; Ment et al, 1986; Pellicer et al, 1992). However, in a majority of cases, no acquired risk factor can be identified (deVeber et al, 1997). The incidence of hereditary prothrombotic disorders reported in neonates with arterial ischemic stroke varies widely, ranging from 10% to 60% of cases (deVeber et al, 1997; Gunther et al, 2000; Mercuri et al, 2001). The strength of the association and the etiologic role of these conditions in arterial ischemic stroke, however, are not well established.

Cranial ultrasound examination in conjunction with transcranial Doppler techniques may be used for bedside screening for neonatal arterial ischemic stroke. However, the sensitivity of ultrasonography is low, and definitive diagnosis should be made by computed tomography (CT) or MRI with angiography (MRA). MRI is preferred to CT, as it has a higher sensitivity for hypoxic-ischemic brain injury in the neonate (Barkovich, 1997).

The role of anticoagulant therapy in neonatal arterial ischemic stroke is uncertain, as there are no controlled trials assessing the benefits and risks of such treatment. In the absence of studies on neonates with arterial ischemic stroke, treatment guidelines are extrapolated from adult studies. The optimal duration of therapy is unknown. Current guidelines recommend a short course (10 to 14 days) of UFH or LMWH at therapeutic doses (Monagle et al, 2001). Because neonates have a low risk of recurrence of arterial ischemic stroke, subsequent long-term treatment with aspirin usually is not necessary.

Published data on the long-term prognosis with neonatal arterial ischemic stroke show a wide range of outcomes, probably reflecting differences in patient population and study design. Large prospective studies have reported a normal outcome in about 30% to 50% of survivors;

the remaining 50% to 70% develop hemiplegia, cerebral palsy, seizures, visual impairment, and/or mental disability (deVeber et al, 2000; Mercuri et al, 2001; Sreenan et al, 2000).

### Sinovenous Thrombosis

A large population-based study has estimated the incidence of childhood sinovenous thrombosis (SVT) at 0.67 case per 100,000 children, with about 50% cases manifesting during the neonatal period (deVeber and Andrew, 2001).

The clinical presentation is subtle and diffuse, includes seizures, lethargy and jitteriness, and may develop gradually over many hours or days. Physical findings comprise a tense fontanel, dilated scalp veins, and, rarely, swelling of the eyelids. Owing to the frequency of diffuse neurologic signs and seizures, a high index of suspicion for SVT is necessary.

Most neonates have one or two risk factors associated with SVT, among which perinatal asphyxia, dehydration, and sepsis are the most frequently encountered. Hereditary prothrombotic disorders are found in about 20% of affected neonates (deVeber and Andrew, 2001; deVeber et al, 1998b).

Doppler ultrasound examination may be used to screen for abnormalities in sinovenous blood flow (Bezinque et al, 1995). However, MRI and MR venography, if available, are the radiographic methods of choice for the definitive diagnosis of SVT and follow-up evaluation. Alternatively, cranial CT can be used, but sensitivity and specifity in neonates are lower than for MRI (deVeber and Andrew, 2001).

Results from adult studies and a cohort study in children suggest that anticoagulant therapy may be useful in neonates with SVT (deVeber et al, 1998a). However, owing to the lack of clinical studies in neonates with SVT, no firm recommendations on treatment can be made. One approach is to treat neonates for 10 to 14 days with therapeutic doses of UFH or LMWH and then reassess the situation (Monagle et al, 2001).

The long-term prognosis for SVT in neonates is not known. The mortality rate has been reported at about 4%. At the age of 2 years, 77% of survivors were found to be neurologically normal. Among those with neurologic defects, motor impairment was present in 80%. The presence of cortical infarctions was a predictor for adverse neurologic outcome. Recurrence of thrombosis occurs in about 8% of neonates (deVeber and Andrew, 2001).

## Anticoagulant and Thrombolytic Therapy

The lack of consensus regarding prophylaxis and treatment of TE in newborns reflects the lack of controlled trials in this area. Recommendations for adult patients provide useful guidelines but may not reflect optimal therapy for newborns due to marked differences in the coagulation system and the distinct etiology and pathogenesis of neonatal TE. Current therapeutic options for TE in newborns include supportive care alone with close observation of the thrombus, UFH or LMWH, oral anticoagulants (OAs), and thrombolytic therapy.

### Unfractionated Heparin

UFH is the most widely used anticoagulant drug in children. The anticoagulant activities of UFH are mediated by catalysis of AT inhibition of thrombin and FXa. Some observations suggest that heparin requirements in newborns will be decreased compared with those in adults. For example, (1) the capacity of plasma from healthy newborns to generate thrombin is both delayed and decreased compared with adults and is similar to that of plasma from adults receiving therapeutic amounts of UFH (Schmidt et al, 1989b); (2) at UFH concentrations in the therapeutic range, the capacity of plasmas from healthy newborns to generate thrombin is barely measurable (Schmidt et al, 1989b); and (3) the amount of clot-bound thrombin is decreased in newborns owing to low plasma concentrations of prothrombin, which probably decreases heparin requirements (Ansell et al, 1995). Other observations suggest that heparin requirements will be increased compared with adults. For example, (1) the clearance of UFH is accelerated in newborns (McDonald et al, 1981); (2) plasma concentrations of AT are decreased to levels frequently less than 0.40 U/mL in premature infants, which may limit the antithrombotic activities of UFH (Vieira et al, 1991); and (3) studies in a newborn piglet model of venous thrombosis have shown that low AT levels limit the anticoagulant and antithrombotic effectiveness of heparin (Schmidt et al, 1988). These findings suggest that the optimal dosing of UFH therapy in newborns probably will differ from that in adults.

#### Therapeutic Range

Therapeutic ranges reflect the optimal risk-benefit ratio of anticoagulant therapy with regard to recurrent thrombotic events and bleeding complications. In the absence of clinical trials in newborns, these ranges are extrapolated from adult studies. The therapeutic range for adults is an APTT between 60 and 85 seconds. The APTT should reflect a heparin level by protamine titration of 0.2 to 0.4 U/mL or an anti-Xa level of 0.3 to 0.7 U/mL (Hirsh, 1991). The APTT correctly predicts the heparin level in about 70% of pediatric patients (Andrew et al, 1994b). However, recent data show that this relationship has changed, with about 70% of APTT values not corresponding to anti-Xa levels (unpublished data). The reasons for this finding are unclear. Most likely it reflects a change in the patient populations receiving UFH.

#### Dosing

Average doses of heparin required in newborns to achieve adult therapeutic APTT values are bolus doses of 75 to 100 U/kg and maintenance doses of 28 U/kg/hour (Monagle et al, 2001). The duration of heparin therapy required for the treatment of neonatal TE is uncertain. One approach is to treat for 10 to 14 days with UFH alone (Monagle et al, 2001). The thrombus size should be carefully monitored using an objective test to detect any changes. If extension of the thrombus occurs despite anticoagulation therapy, further treatment with heparin (preferably LMWH) or OA should be considered. A nomogram to facilitate appropriate dosing of UFH in newborns is provided in Table 76–5.

**TABLE 76–5**

**Protocol for Systemic Heparin Administration and Adjustment for Pediatric Patients**

I. Loading dose: heparin 75 units/kg given IV over 10 minutes.

II. Initial maintenance dose: 28 units/kg/hour for infants younger than 1 year; 20 units/kg/hour for children older than 1 year.

III. Adjust heparin to maintain APTT at 60-85 seconds (assuming this reflects an anti–factor Xa level of 0.30-0.70 unit/mL):

| APTT (sec) | Bolus (u/kg) | Hold (min) | Rate Change, (%) | Repeat |
|---|---|---|---|---|
| <50 | 50 | 0 | +10% | After 4 hr |
| 50-59 | 0 | 0 | +10% | After 4 hr |
| 60-85 | 0 | 0 | 0 | Next day |
| 86-95 | 0 | 0 | −10% | After 4 hr |
| 96-120 | 0 | 30 | −10% | After 4 hr |
| >120 | 0 | 60 | −15% | After 4 hr |

IV. Obtain blood for APTT 4 hours after administration of the heparin loading dose and 4 hours after every change in the infusion rate.

V. When APTT values are therapeutic, perform a daily CBC and APTT determination.

APTT, activated partial thromboplastin time; CBC, complete blood count.
Data from Monagle et al (2001).

### Adverse Effects

There are three clinically important adverse effects of heparin therapy: major bleeding, osteoporosis, and heparin-induced thrombocytopenia (HIT).

Data from a pediatric cohort study (Andrew et al, 1994b) suggest that major bleeding is an infrequent event in children receiving UFH for the treatment of DVT. However, doses used in this study were lower than those used today and case reports have reported major bleeding events secondary to UFH therapy in children. A recent retrospective study found major bleeding events in 18% of children receiving therapeutic UFH (unpublished data).

Heparin-induced osteoporosis is a known complication of long-term therapy with UFH in adults. There are only three case reports describing heparin-induced osteoporosis in children (Monagle et al, 2001). Long-term data on UFH therapy in a larger group of pediatric patients are not available yet, however. Given the clear association between heparin and osteoporosis in adults, long-term use of heparin in newborns and children should be avoided when possible.

HIT is a serious and relatively common complication of heparin therapy in adults. In the only published case series of newborns with HIT, this complication developed in about 1% of newborns admitted to the NICU during the study period (Spadone, 1996). UFH had been given prophylactically to maintain UAC patency. About 85% of newborns with HIT suffered aortic TE with a mortality rate of 21% (Spadone, 1996). A high index of suspicion is needed for the diagnosis of neonatal HIT in the setting of low-dose prophylactic UFH and multiple coexisting disorders that can cause thrombocytopenia in critically ill neonates. In the absence of an alternative cause for thrombocytopenia, UFH should be discontinued, and the patient should be evaluated for HIT. Danaparoid may be used if anticoagulation is required (Monagle et al, 2001).

## Low-Molecular-Weight Heparin

In adults, LMWH has consistently been shown to be as efficacious and safe as UFH for the prevention and treatment of thrombotic complications. In contrast with UFH, the LMWH-AT complex is too small to inhibit thrombin but does retain its activity against FXa. The advantages of LMWH include predictable pharmacokinetics, minimal monitoring, ease of administration, equivalent or decreased risk of bleeding, equal or increased efficacy, and potentially less risk of osteoporosis with long-term use. Although LMWHs are more expensive than UFH, reduction in laboratory testing, nursing hours, intravenous starts, and phlebotomy time results in lower total costs (Massicotte et al, 1996).

### Therapeutic Range

Therapeutic ranges for LMWH therapy as monitored by the anti-Xa level are extrapolated from adults. The target range is an anti-Xa level of 0.10 to 0.30 U/mL for prophylaxis and 0.50 to 1.0 U/mL for therapy (Monagle et al, 2001). Anti-Xa level determinations are performed 4 hours after a subcutaneous injection.

### Dosing

Two clinical trials have established doses required to achieve adult therapeutic anti-Xa levels for two LMWHs: enoxaparin (Lovenox, Aventis Pharma, Bridgewater, NJ) and reviparin (Clivarin, Knoll Pharmaceuticals, Germany) (Massicotte et al, 1996, 1999). Peak anti-Xa levels for both preparations occur 4 hours after subcutaneous injection. Newborns have increased dose requirements compared with older children, probably owing to altered pharmacokinetics (Andrew et al, 1989). Dosing requirements and a nomogram to facilitate appropriate dosing of LMWH in newborns are provided in Tables 76–6 and 76–7. The optimal duration of LMWH therapy in the treatment of neonatal TE is uncertain. As with UFH, an initial short course (10 to 14 days) may be used; this may be extended to 3 months if the thrombus size increases (Monagle et al, 2001). If LMWH is used for longer than 3 months, bone density should be monitored to detect heparin-induced osteoporosis.

### Adverse Effects

The important adverse effects of LMWH are similar to those of UFH but usually are less frequent and less severe. However, in one large study, major bleeding events occurred in 5% of children receiving therapeutic doses of LMWH (Dix et al, 2000). Other studies did not report major bleeds during LMWH treatment in children (Hofmann et al, 2001; Nohe et al, 1999). In addition, there are no reports of heparin-induced osteoporosis or HIT in newborns and infants who received LMWH therapy.

**TABLE 76-6**

**Dosing for Low-Molecular-Weight Heparins**

| Reviparin: Weight-Dependent Dosing | <5 kg | >5 kg |
|---|---|---|
| Initial treatment dose | 150 u/kg/dose q12h | 100 u/kg/dose q12h |
| Initial prophylactic dose | 50 u/kg/dose q12h | 30 u/kg/dose q12h |
| **Enoxaparin: Age-Dependent Dosing** | **<2 mo** | **>2 mo** |
| Initial treatment dose | 1.5 mg/kg/dose q12h | 1.0 mg/kg/dose q12h |
| Initial prophylactic dose | 0.75 mg/kg/dose q12h | 0.5 mg/kg/dose q12h |

Enoxaparin contains 100 anti–factor Xa units/mg.

Data from Monagle et al (2001).

## Oral Anticoagulation

OAs function by reducing plasma concentrations of the vitamin K–dependent proteins. At birth, levels of the vitamin K–dependent proteins are similar to those found in adults receiving therapeutic amounts of OAs. In keeping with this observation, the pattern of thrombin generation in healthy newborns is similar to that in adults receiving warfarin (Massicotte et al, 1998b). In addition, stores of vitamin K are low, and a small number of newborns have evidence of a functional vitamin K deficiency state (Bovill et al, 1993). Therefore, there is a potential risk of hemorrhage from further anticoagulation. OA therapy in newborns and infants is extremely difficult to perform and should be avoided, when possible, during the first year of life. There are, however, exceptions to this rule, such as homozygous protein C and protein S deficiency and presence of prosthetic heart valves.

### Therapeutic Range and Dose

The optimal therapeutic INR range for newborns is unknown and almost certainly differs from that for adults. Recommendations for OA therapy in adults can be used as a guideline, with the goal of using the lowest effective dose, which can be individualized to some extent. Maintenance doses for therapeutic amounts of OA are age dependent, with infants having the highest requirements per unit of body weight (0.33 mg/kg) (Streif et al, 1999).

### Monitoring

Close monitoring of oral anticoagulation in newborns is required to prevent hemorrhagic and recurrent thrombotic complications. Unfortunately, infants have poor venous access as well as poor venous access and frequently complicated medical problems. Weekly or twice-weekly measurements of the INR are often required with frequent dose adjustments (Streif et al, 1999). Reducing or removing vitamin K supplementation of total parenteral nutrition significantly reduces the dose requirements. Most infants requiring OA also require other medications on an intermittent and long-term basis. The effects of dosage changes and the introduction of new medications must be closely supervised. A whole blood monitor has been used with success in the monitoring of OA in infants (Marzinotto et al, 2000). However, these infants were managed in a pediatric anticoagulation clinic with expert staff available at all times.

### Adverse Effects

The most important adverse effect of OA therapy is bleeding. A large cohort study on warfarin therapy in children found an overall incidence of major bleeding of 0.5% per patient year, which is comparable to that in adults (Streif et al, 1999). The rate of serious bleeding in children who receive OA for prosthetic heart valves is less than 3.2% (Solymar et al, 1991). A recent study suggests that long-term warfarin therapy in young patients may negatively influence bone mineral density (Cheung et al, 2001). Further studies are required to determine the mechanism, impact, and possible prevention of this side effect.

## Thrombolytic Therapy

The action of thrombolytic agents is mediated by converting endogenous plasminogen to plasmin. In the newborn, plasminogen concentrations are reduced to about 50% of adult values (Andrew et al, 1987b). Low plasminogen levels

**TABLE 76-7**

**Nomogram for Monitoring Reviparin/Enoxaparin Therapy in Pediatric Patients**

| Anti–Factor Xa Level | Hold Next Dose? | Dose Change? | Repeat Anti–Factor Xa Level? |
|---|---|---|---|
| <0.35 unit/mL | No | Increase by 25% | 4 hours after next dose |
| 0.35-0.49 unit/mL | No | Increase by 10% | 4 hours after next dose |
| 0.5-1.0 unit/mL | No | No | Next day, then 1 week later and monthly thereafter while receiving Reviparin-Na treatment (at 4 hours after AM dose) |
| 1.1-1.5 units/mL | No | Decrease by 20% | Before next dose |
| 1.6-2.0 units/mL | 3 hours | Decrease by 30% | Before next dose; then 4 hours after next dose |
| >2.0 units/mL | Until anti-Xa 0.5 unit/mL | Decrease by 40% | Before next dose; if not <0.5 unit/mL, repeat every 12 hours |

Data from Monagle et al (2001).

result in an impaired capacity to generate plasmin (Corrigan et al, 1989) and a decreased capacity to lyse fibrin clots in response to thrombolytic drugs (Andrew et al, 1992a). Increasing plasma concentrations of plasminogen with purified plasminogen resulted in fibrin clot lysis that was greater than for adult plasma, probably owing to the decreased levels of $\alpha_2$-antiplasmin in newborns' plasma (Andrew et al, 1992a).

### Indications

There are two classes of thrombolytic agents: (1) the nonselective plasminogen activators such as streptokinase (SK) and urokinase (UK) and (2) the more specific fibrin-bound plasminogen activators such as tissue plasminogen activator (tPA) and its recombinant variants. No studies are available comparing the efficacy and safety of these agents in vivo. SK is not used in neonates and children because of its potential for allergic reactions and its reduced efficacy at low plasminogen concentrations (Andrew et al, 1992b). UK was widely used in pediatric patients until the Food and Drug Administration (FDA) warning about a potential risk for viral transmission issued in 1999 substantially diminished its popularity (Food and experimental evidence of Drug Administration, 1999). Tissue plasminogen activator has become the thrombolytic agent of choice in newborns and infants for its fibrin specificity, low immunogenicity and experimental evidence of improved clot lysis compared with that achieved with SK and UK (Andrew et al, 1992a). However, the costs for tPA are considerably higher, and no controlled clinical trial has proved its superiority to other thrombolytic agents.

Indications for the use of thrombolytic therapy in infants are (1) to restore patency of blocked central venous or arterial lines and (2) to treat serious thrombotic complications, defined by severe organ or limb impairment. The clinical objective in the latter situation is to remove the clot as quickly and safely as possible. The surgical removal of a clot in a major vessel in infants can be curative; however, it is technically difficult owing to the small size of neonatal vessels and poses a considerable life-threatening risk to affected infants, who often are premature. In the absence of contraindications, the use of thrombolytic agents for these infants is a preferred approach. Contraindications to the use of thrombolytic therapy in newborns include general surgery within the previous 10 days, neurosurgery within the previous 3 weeks, recent history of major bleeding (intracranial, gastrointestinal, or pulmonary), perinatal asphyxia, arterial hypertension, and severe thrombocytopenia.

### Therapeutic Range and Monitoring

There is no therapeutic range for thrombolytic agents. However, a variety of coagulation tests are used to monitor the activities of thrombolytic agents to ensure that a fibrinolytic effect is present. These tests include determination of fibrinogen concentrations, thrombin clotting time, and fibrin/fibrinogen degradation products and D-dimer assay. The clinically most useful test is the fibrinogen level. A commonly used lower limit for fibrinogen level below which FFP or cryoprecipitate should be administered is 100 mg/dL. The APTT is not helpful in the setting of low fibrinogen levels, concomitant heparin use, and fibrin split products (Bovill et al, 1992). Measurement of fibrin degradation products is helpful to determine whether a fibrinolytic effect is present. When thrombolytic therapy is used, it is advisable, when possible, to correct other concurrent hemostatic problems such as thrombocytopenia and vitamin K deficiency.

### Low-Dose Therapy for Restoring Catheter Patency

SK should not be used to reestablish CVL patency because of the possibility of allergic reactions with repeated doses. UK is no longer used for restoration of CVL patency following the FDA warning about potential infectious hazards with its use. Alteplase (recombinant tPA) appears to be a safe and effective alternative to UK (Choi et al, 2001). The commonly used low-dose guideline for newborns and infants weighing less than 10 kg is to instill 0.5 mg of alteplase diluted in normal saline to a volume required to fill the line and let it dwell for 2 to 4 hours (Monagle et al, 2001).

### Systemic Thrombolytic Therapy

Although more information is available on the use of SK and UK, this section deals with tPA only, which is currently the treatment of choice for systemic thrombolytic therapy in newborns. The recommended regimen is to administer tPA as a continuous infusion (no bolus) at a rate of 0.1 to 0.6 mg/kg/hour for 6 hours (Monagle et al, 2001). Currently, no evidence exists for an advantage of catheter-directed over systemic lysis in terms of efficacy and safety. During or immediately after completion of thrombolytic therapy, UFH at a rate of 10 to 20 U/kg/hour may be administered to prevent reocclusion of the vessel (Monagle et al, 2001). However, currently no data are available showing a beneficial effect of such adjuvant therapy. If an infant does not respond to thrombolytic therapy, replacement of plasminogen through administration of FFP at a dose of 10 to 20 mL/kg may be considered.

### Adverse Effects

The most important adverse effect of thrombolytic therapy is bleeding. Bleeding from sites of invasive procedures is reported in about 10% of newborns and infants receiving thrombolytic therapy. The incidence of major bleeding in this patient group is about 4% (Nowak-Gottl et al, 1999). The incidence of ICH secondary to thrombolytic therapy is age dependent and is highest in preterm infants during the first week of life (Zenz et al, 1997). However, three recent cohort studies with a total number of 37 newborns (10 of whom were younger than 34 weeks of gestational age) receiving tPA did report one case of ICH in a neonate with severe thrombocytopenia (Farnoux et al, 1998; Hartmann et al, 2001; Weiner et al, 1998). In the absence of controlled trials, these data should be regarded with caution, as different protocols for thrombolysis and adjuvant therapy were used in the different studies.

Treatment of mild bleeding secondary to thrombolytic therapy consists of local measures (pressure, topical thrombin preparations), and transfusion of packed red blood cells when necessary. Treatment of major bleeding consists of stopping the thrombolytic therapy and administration of FFP, with consideration of an antifibrinolytic agent.

## PLATELET DISORDERS

### Thrombocytopenia

Healthy newborns and fetuses have platelet counts in the same range as for adults; therefore, a platelet count less than 150 × $10^9$/L is the accepted definition of thrombocytopenia for all infants. Thrombocytopenia is classified as mild (100 to 150 × $10^9$ platelets/L), moderate (50 to 100 × $10^9$/L), or severe (<50 × $10^9$/L). The clinical significance of mild thrombocytopenia is unclear. However, it may be indicative of an underlying pathologic process and should be investigated. The reported overall incidence of neonatal thrombocytopenia ranges from 0.7% (Uhrynowska et al, 1997) to 4% (Burrows and Kelton, 1988), depending on the population studied, the definition of thrombocytopenia, and the timing of blood sampling (immediately postnatally versus during the first week of life). This relatively low overall frequency contrasts with a high incidence of thrombocytopenia in infants admitted to the NICU. About 20% to 40% of sick neonates develop thrombocytopenia (Castle et al, 1986; Mehta et al, 1980; Murray and Roberts, 1995). In more than 50% of affected neonates, platelet counts fall below 100 × $10^9$/L, and 20% of neonates have platelet counts less than 50 × $10^9$/L (Castle et al, 1986). The natural history of thrombocytopenia in sick newborns is remarkably consistent. It is present by day 2 of life in 75% of affected infants, reaches a nadir by day 4, and resolves with recovery of the platelet count to more than 150 × $10^9$/L by day 10 of life in nearly 90% of infants (Castle et al, 1986).

### Causes of Thrombocytopenia in the Newborn

A large number of conditions have been associated with thrombocytopenia in the newborn (Table 76–8). A detailed description of each disorder is beyond the scope of this discussion. This section focuses on those conditions that are most frequently encountered.

**Infections.** Thrombocytopenia is a common finding in septic neonates. About 60% of newborns with proven infection become thrombocytopenic, with platelet counts of less than 100 × $10^9$/L (Modanlou and Ortiz, 1981). Responsible mechanisms include immune-mediated platelet destruction, decreased production, and DIC (Murray et al, 1994; Tate et al, 1981). Thrombocytopenia may be found in up to 90% of newborns with NEC, with platelet counts of less than 50 × $10^9$/L in about half of the cases (Hutter et al, 1976). Congenital intrauterine infections of the TORCH group (*t*oxoplasmosis, *o*ther infections, *r*ubella, *c*ytomegalovirus infection, *h*erpes simplex) as well as parvovirus B19 infection also may result in neonatal thrombocytopenia (Hohlfeld et al, 1994; Srivastava et al, 1990). The underlying mechanism is probably a mix of diminished production, increased destruction, and sequestration in an enlarged spleen.

**Asphyxia.** Asphyxia has been identified as a major risk factor for neonatal thrombocytopenia (Castle et al, 1986). The most important mechanism responsible is DIC caused by

**TABLE 76–8**

**Causes of Neonatal Thrombocytopenia**

**Decreased Platelet Production**
Congenital thrombocytopenias
- Amegakaryocytic thrombocytopenia
- Thrombocytopenia–absent radius (TAR) syndrome
- Amegakaryocytic thrombocytopenia without limb abnormalities
- Wiskott-Aldrich syndrome
- Chédiak-Higashi syndrome
- May-Hegglin anomaly
- Alport syndrome
- Fechtner syndrome
- Trousseau syndrome
- Mediterranean macrothrombocytopenia
- Bernard-Soulier syndrome

Marrow-infiltrative disorders
- Congenital leukemia
- Congenital neuroblastoma
- Letterer-Siwe disease

Osteopetrosis

**Increased Platelet Destruction**
- Intravascular coagulation
- Disseminated (e.g., DIC associated with severe birth asphyxia)
- Localized (e.g., renal vein thrombosis, necrotizing enterocolitis, maternal eclampsia, HELLP syndrome, Kasabach-Merritt syndrome)

Systemic infections (bacterial, viral, fungal, protozoal)
- Congenital
- Acquired

Immune-mediated
- Neonatal alloimmune thrombocytopenia
- Neonatal autoimmune thrombocytopenia
- Drug-induced thrombocytopenia (e.g., quinine)
- Von Willebrand disease (type IIB)

**Combination of Decreased Production and Increased Destruction**
Infection
- Congenital (e.g., TORCH association)
- Acquired (e.g., bacterial sepsis)

Erythroblastosis fetalis

**Miscellaneous**
Exchange transfusion
Extracorporeal membrane oxygenation
Polycythemia
Chromosomal abnormalities (e.g., Down syndrome)
Neonatal cold injury
Mechanical ventilation
Pulmonary hypertension

DIC, disseminated intravascular coagulation; HELLP, hemolysis, elevated liver enzymes, low platelets; TORCH, toxoplasmosis, other infections, rubella, cytomegalovirus infection, herpes simplex.

Data from Blanchette and Rand ML (1997).

activation of the extrinsic coagulation pathway secondary to the release of tissue factor from damaged tissues.

**Intrauterine Growth Restriction and Pregnancy-Induced Hypertension.** Thrombocytopenia is a common finding in small-for-gestational-age preterm infants and preterm infants born to hypertensive mothers (Burrows and Andrew, 1990; Philip and Tito, 1989). Neutropenia and an increased nucleated red cell count frequently accompany the thrombocytopenia in these patients. The platelet count rarely drops below 50 × $10^9$/L and normalizes by 7 to 10 days of life (Burrows and Andrew, 1990; Murray et al, 1998). The underlying mechanism is not known.

**Hemangiomas.** The presence of giant hemangiomas, or Kasabach-Merritt syndrome, is associated with a local consumptive coagulopathy characterized by hypofibrinogenemia, elevated fibrin degradation products, microangiopathic fragmentation of red blood cells, and thrombocytopenia. The thrombocytopenia is usually severe, with platelet counts less than 50 × $10^9$/L. Treatment options include steroids, surgery, embolization, irradiation, and α-interferon (IFN) therapy. The last treatment option is relatively contraindicated in the first months of life owing to reports of spastic diplegia in infants who had received IFN (Barlow et al, 1998).

**Chromosomal Abnormalities.** Thrombocytopenia may be a feature of chromosomal abnormalities such as trisomies 13, 18, and 21 and monosomy X (Turner syndrome). A retrospective study of fetal blood samples found thrombocytopenia in 54% of fetuses with trisomy 13, in 87% of fetuses with trisomy 18, and in 7% of fetuses with trisomy 21 (Hohlfeld et al, 1994). With trisomy 21, a transient moderate thrombocytopenia lasting 2 to 3 weeks may be found in 5% to 30% of newborns (Hord et al, 1995; Miller and Cosgriff, 1983).

## Diagnostic Approach to the Thrombocytopenic Newborn

In evaluation of a thrombocytopenic newborn, the general clinical condition of the infant, maternal and perinatal history, age at onset of thrombocytopenia, severity of thrombocytopenia, and the presence of abnormal findings on physical examination are important considerations. A cranial ultrasound examination should be performed in every neonate with severe thrombocytopenia to rule out intracranial bleeding.

### *History and Physical Examination*

Simple observation of the clinical appearance of the newborn can have a tremendous impact on further management of thrombocytopenic infants. Whereas infections, asphyxia, and placental insufficiency account for a majority of thrombocytopenias in sick neonates, thrombocytopenia in the apparently healthy neonate is mainly due to transmission of maternal antiplatelet antibodies. An onset during fetal life or in the early neonatal period (i.e., during the first 72 hours) is most often due to maternal factors or perinatal events. A careful history including family bleeding problems, maternal illnesses and medication use, platelet count, outcome of previous pregnancies, and perinatal events may provide clues to enable correct diagnosis. Common conditions causing early thrombocytopenia are immune thrombocytopenia, preeclampsia, placental insufficiency, congenital infections, asphyxia, and maternal medications. Thrombocytopenia beyond the first 3 days of life is most commonly due to sepsis or NEC. On physical examination, particular attention should be given to the presence of conditions associated with neonatal thrombocytopenia such as dysmorphic features and skeletal abnormalities (thrombocytopenia–absent radii or other dysmorphic syndromes), hemangiomas (Kasabach-Merritt syndrome), and hepatosplenomegaly (congenital infections).

### *Laboratory Evaluation*

The first step in the laboratory evaluation of a thrombocytopenic newborn should include a complete blood count with examination of a peripheral blood smear and a coagulation screen. These tests can help to diagnose potentially life-threatening conditions such as infections, DIC, or NEC. The presence of giant platelets, leukocyte inclusions, or very small platelets in the blood smear may indicate the presence of a hereditary hematologic disorder. A platelet count should also be performed on the infant's mother. Other laboratory tests for the evaluation of thrombocytopenic neonates include mean platelet volume determination, reticulated platelet counts, platelet survival study, platelet-associated immunoglobulin G (IgG) assay, and measurement of thrombopoietin levels (Castle et al, 1986; Peterec et al, 1996; Sola et al, 1999a). Although these tests may be helpful in determining the underlying mechanism of the thrombocytopenia (decreased production, increased destruction, or splenic sequestration), they are relatively nonspecific and not readily available and therefore are rarely used in routine clinical practice. Bone marrow biopsies should be performed in cases of persistent thrombocytopenia of unknown origin. A bone marrow biopsy technique suitable for neonates has recently been described (Sola et al, 1999b).

### Treatment

Currently, platelet transfusions remain the only treatment option for most sick thrombocytopenic infants. In the future, megakaryocytopoietic cytokines such as interleukin-11 or thrombopoietin may provide an alternative form of management for some forms of neonatal thrombocytopenia.

Evidence-based recommendations on what platelet count constitutes an indication for intervention are lacking. However, there is general agreement that in sick preterm infants, the platelet count should be maintained well above 50 × $10^9$/L, especially during the first week of life to reduce the risk of intraventricular hemorrhage (IVH) (Andrew et al, 1987a, 1993; Blanchette and Rand, 1997; Calhoun et al, 2000). The importance of moderate thrombocytopenia in sick premature infants is unclear (Andrew et al, 1993). In one study, maintaining a platelet count over 150 × $10^9$/L with platelet concentrates did not have a beneficial effect on incidence of IVH, although it did reduce requirements for red blood cell transfusions and FFP (Andrew et al, 1993).

Platelet concentrates for newborns should be ideally leukocyte depleted and CMV negative (Blanchette et al, 1995). Usually, 10 to 20 mL/kg is administered. The routine use of volume-reducing procedures should be avoided when possible because of the potentially negative effects on the platelets (Hume et al, 1997). However, a recent study failed to show an effect of volume reduction on in vitro platelet function and in vivo platelet recovery (Rand et al, 2001). At 1 hour following transfusion, a platelet count should be performed to assess the response to the platelet concentrate. The life span of transfused platelets varies with the underlying mechanism of thrombocytopenia. Adult studies have shown a mean platelet survival of 5.4 days in patients with decreased platelet production, compared with 2.7 days in patients with increased platelet destruction (Tomer et al, 1991).

## Immune Thrombocytopenia in the Newborn

Immune thrombocytopenia should always be suspected in otherwise healthy infants with isolated severe thrombocytopenia. An IgG antiplatelet autoantibody or alloantibody is produced in mothers and crosses the placenta, causing fetal thrombocytopenia. Because the antibody is not autologous, the thrombocytopenia persists only as long as the maternal IgG antibody remains in the infant's circulation. Normally, this would be several months, because the half-life of IgG is approximately 21 days. Because the antibody binds to platelets, however, its life span is dependent on the life span of the sensitized platelets and therefore may be very short. As a result, neonatal immune thrombocytopenic disorders are usually short-lived but can cause serious bleeding, making the correct diagnosis and management of these disorders all the more important. The differentiation of autoimmune from alloimmune thrombocytopenia is critical, because the management and severity of these disorders are quite different.

### *Neonatal Alloimmune Thrombocytopenia*

Neonatal alloimmune thrombocytopenia (NAIT) is similar to hemolytic disease of the newborn and neonatal alloimmune neutropenia. All three disorders are caused by maternal IgG alloantibodies that cross the placenta into the fetal circulation, bind to specific cell antigens, and accelerate the removal of the cell type in question from the circulation. Unlike hemolytic disease of the newborn, NAIT may occur with the first pregnancy, as fetal platelets may leak into the maternal circulation, causing sensitization and subsequent production and transmission of antibodies directed against fetal platelets. Mothers of infants with NAIT have normal platelet counts and no bleeding history, although they may have previously delivered thrombocytopenic newborns. Maternal IgG alloantibodies are directed against specific paternally derived antigens on the infant's platelets, which are absent from the mother's platelets. The most frequently implicated alloantigen in the white population is the HPA-1a ($Pl^{A1}$) antigen (found in >80% of cases), which is present on the platelets of 98% of the general population. The second most common alloantigen is HPA-5b ($Br^a$) (Mueller-Eckhardt et al, 1989). The frequency of platelet antigens differs between ethnic groups. The HPA-1b ($Pl^{A2}$) antigen usually is not found in African American and Oriental populations (Mueller-Eckhardt et al, 1994; Ramsey and Salamon, 1986). Accordingly, NAIT due to HPA-1b incompatibility is virtually unknown in these populations. ABO and human leukocyte antigen (HLA) alloantibodies are infrequent causes of NAIT (Mueller-Eckhardt et al, 1989). One potential explanation is that maternal HLA alloantibodies do not enter the fetal circulation in sufficient quantities because they are absorbed by foreign HLA antigens on the placenta.

#### Incidence

The pooled incidence of NAIT derived from five large studies including a total of 40,027 newborns is 0.18% (Blanchette et al, 2000). This incidence is considerably lower than the actual risk based on the frequency of the alloantigens, which is estimated to be about 2.5% for the most prevalent maternal antigen (HPA-1b) implicated (Williamson et al, 1998). There is evidence that one or more immune response genes determine the formation of alloantibodies. For example, women possessing the HLA-DR3 alloantigen have a 140-fold increased risk of forming anti–HPA-1a alloantibodies (Williamson et al, 1998). Alloimmunization against HPA-5b antigen is associated with HLA-DRw6 (Mueller-Eckhardt and Kiefel, 1989).

#### Clinical Presentation

The clinical presentation of NAIT is usually severe, isolated thrombocytopenia in a healthy, full-term infant. First-born infants are affected as often as subsequent infants. However, subsequent siblings are invariably as affected as or more affecteds than the previous sibling. Minor bleeding in the form of petechiae, gastrointestinal tract hemorrhage, hematuria, or hemoptysis is a frequent fiding. Of great concern and associated with serious morbidity is the occurrence of ICH in as many as 15% of infants who have symptoms of thrombocytopenia (Mueller-Eckhardt et al, 1989). ICH may occur prenatally as well as postnatally. The severity of bleeding in infants with NAIT may reflect not only the severe thrombocytopenia but also an additional platelet dysfunction caused by antiplatelet alloantibody impairing aggregation through binding to GPIIb/IIIa (van Leeuwen et al, 1984).

#### Diagnosis

The diagnosis of NAIT is based on the clinical presentation and the presence of severe thrombocytopenia with a platelet count frequently less than $10 \times 10^9$/L. Neonatal alloimmune thrombocytopenia should be confirmed by serologic and/or DNA testing; however, specific therapy should be instituted immediately. Testing can be performed in almost all cases on only the parents of the newborn (Bussel et al, 1991). Serologic testing includes typing of the parents' platelet antigens and testing for the presence of antiplatelet alloantibody in the maternal serum. DNA-based platelet typing, although more expensive, offers several advantages over serologic testing (Bussel, 2001). Determining the paternal zygosity for the implicated alloantigen is important for predicting the risk of recurrence in future pregnancies. Not infrequently, alloantibodies are undetectable in the maternal serum (Mueller-Eckhardt et al, 1989). In such cases, the antibodies may be detected a few weeks or months after delivery (Schabel et al, 1996).

### Prevention

In women who have had a previously affected infant, there is a high probability that all subsequent infants will be affected (Bussel et al, 1997). Because of the risk of ICH in utero, it is important that monitoring for the presence of ICH and therapeutic interventions commence prenatally. However, general agreement on the optimal management strategy is lacking (Bussel et al, 1996). In some centers, cordocentesis with regular platelet transfusions is performed (Murphy et al, 1994). This strategy effectively increases the fetal platelet count but entails a significant risk of complications due to repeated cordocenteses. An alternative, less invasive approach is the intravenous administration of IgG with or without corticosteroids to the mother in the latter part of the pregnancy (Bussel et al, 2001). The relative safety and efficacy of these differing approaches require further clarification. Elective delivery is recommended at the time of fetal maturity to facilitate the postnatal management of the infant (Blanchette et al, 2000). The necessity of cesarean section to prevent ICH has not been proved.

### Treatment

The choice of treatment depends on the severity of the thrombocytopenia. In an affected newborn with a platelet count below $30 \times 10^9$/L, transfusion of platelet antigen-negative platelets from the mother or an antigen-negative donor should be given as soon as possible (Blanchette et al, 2000). These platelets can be prepared before delivery if a planned cesarean section is the mode of delivery. Maternal platelets are preferred to matched platelets from an unrelated donor because of their certain compatibility, availability, and safety. Maternal platelets must be washed and centrifuged to remove maternal alloantibody and irradiated to prevent graft-versus-host disease caused by maternal lymphocytes. Random donor platelets should be used in an infant with significant hemorrhage while awaiting maternal platelets. The infusion of random donor platelets may transiently help the bleeding infant, and the lack of a sustained increase in platelet number confirms the diagnosis of NAIT. In those infants with platelet counts between 30 and $50 \times 10^9$/L, intravenous IgG in a dose of 1 g/kg/day on two consecutive days may be used to effectively raise the platelet count (Blanchette et al, 2000). IgG is not as rapidly effective as compatible platelets, however. No convincing evidence is available to support the use of corticosteroids or exchange transfusions. Data on the safety of breast-feeding affected infants are sparse, and thus no recommendations can be made (Reese et al, 1994).

## *Autoimmune Neonatal Thrombocytopenia*

Newborns with thrombocytopenia secondary to maternal autoimmune disorders present with a milder clinical course than that of newborns affected with alloimmune disorders. Usually, the mother has idiopathic thrombocytopenic purpura (ITP), but autoimmune platelet consumption also can be associated with other maternal disorders such as systemic lupus erythematosus, lymphoproliferative disorders, and hyperthyroidism. Serologically, the antibody is directed against antigens common to maternal and neonatal platelets. Maternal ITP must be distinguished from the mild thrombocytopenia that frequently occurs in healthy pregnant women at term. The latter, referred to as gestational thrombocytopenia, appears to have no adverse effect on either the mothers or their infants and does not necessitate any specific treatment or delivery by cesarean section (Burrows and Kelton, 1993). The overall incidence of thrombocytopenia in the offspring of mothers with ITP is about 15% to 45%. Severe thrombocytopenia is found in about 5% to 15% of newborns of affected mothers (al Mofada et al, 1994; Burrows and Kelton, 1990). The varying results are explained by differing definitions of thrombocytopenia and by differential timing of the blood sampling. The platelet count nadir in neonates born to mothers with ITP occurs not at birth but a few days after birth (Burrows and Kelton, 1990). Therefore, the platelet count should be monitored closely for the first week of life. Maternal platelet counts in mothers with ITP do not predict which infants will be thrombocytopenic. Some women who are "cured" of ITP by splenectomy can still deliver thrombocytopenic babies, whereas other women who are severely thrombocytopenic will not necessarily deliver thrombocytopenic infants. There are no reliable clinical or laboratory predictors of severe thrombocytopenia in the infant except for direct determination of the fetal platelet count by cordocentesis. However, this procedure entails risks (Pielet et al, 1988) that outweigh the relatively infrequent risk of significant bleeding complications in this disorder. A review of 474 cases reported in the literature until 1991 found a 3% incidence for ICH in newborns with moderate to severe thrombocytopenia (Cook et al, 1991). More recent cohort studies did not report any cases of significant bleeding—in particular, no ICH—in affected newborns (al Mofada et al, 1994; Burrows and Kelton, 1990; Sainio et al, 1998).

Given the low risk for the newborn, the pregnant mother should be managed according to her own platelet count and not the hemostatic risk to the infant (Cook et al, 1991). If the woman has had previous uncomplicated deliveries and the obstetrician anticipates no problems, spontaneous vaginal delivery is appropriate. Infants for whom a difficult procedure is anticipated can be delivered by cesarean section, but the evidence indicating that this approach is safer for the fetus is lacking.

Clinically, affected infants present as full term and healthy appearing, with at most mild clinical manifestations of thrombocytopenia in the form of petechiae. These infants usually do not have clinical or laboratory evidence of any other neonatal problems, such as DIC, hepatosplenomegaly, and prematurity. The diagnosis of autoimmune thrombocytopenia in newborns is made predominantly by the clinical presentation of mother and infant as well as the exclusion of other known causes of thrombocytopenia.

Possible therapeutic interventions for affected newborns with autoimmune thrombocytopenia include platelet transfusions, high-dose IgG, and corticosteroids. The effect of platelet transfusions can be anticipated to be very short-lived. Intravenous IgG has been used after delivery and is safe and effective, with in an 80% response rate in the infant when it is used alone or in combination with steroids (Ballin et al, 1988). It is unclear whether the addition of steroids to intravenous IgG is beneficial. Clearly, prospective studies are required to confirm the high rate of response to intravenous IgG and the beneficial effects of intravenous IgG over other forms of therapy. If the infant is bleeding, platelet transfusions should also be given at doses of 10 to 20 mL/kg. A poor response in platelet count as well as a rapid fall in platelet number supports the diagnosis of autoimmune thrombocytopenia. If the infant does not respond and has evidence of bleeding, adjunctive steroids should be given and intravenous IgG therapy repeated.

## Qualitative Platelet Disorders

Qualitative platelet disorders may be hereditary or acquired. Hereditary disorders of platelet function such as Glanzmann thrombasthenia or Bernard-Soulier syndrome rarely manifest with bleeding in the neonatal period.

Acquired impairment of platelet function in the newborn has been reported to occur in response to maternal and neonatal drugs. Aspirin crosses the placenta and can be detected in fetuses following maternal ingestion. However, the evidence linking maternal analgesic doses of aspirin to clinically important bleeding in newborns is weak (Corby, 1978). Low-dose aspirin appears to be safe for the fetus (Dasari et al, 1998).

Ex vivo studies from newborns receiving inhaled nitric oxide (NO) for the treatment of pulmonary hypertension show a prolonged bleeding time and inhibition of platelet aggregation (Cheung et al, 1998; George et al, 1998). The clinical significance of these findings is uncertain.

Platelet dysfunction also has been reported in infants undergoing ECMO, as well as in infants with congenital heart disease, hyperbilirubinemia, renal failure, or hepatic failure. The extent to which the platelet function defect contributes to clinical bleeding manifestations in these conditions is not known.

## Acknowledgments

Our friend and colleague Dr. Maureen Andrew, who passed away in 2001, was instrumental in completion of the work reported here, and we respectfully dedicate this chapter to her memory.

We thank Dr. Anthony Chan, Dr. Margaret Rand, and Dr. Manuel Carcao for critical review of the manuscript. We also are indebted to Lu Ann Brooker for editing of the manuscript.

Dr. Kuhle gratefully acknowledges the support of the Austrian Science Foundation (FWF), Vienna, Austria, in the form of an Erwin Schrödinger scholarship for his work contributing to this chapter (Project J–2038/2001).

## SELECTED READINGS

Andrew M, David M, Adams M, et al: Venous thromboembolic complications (VTE) in children: First analysis of the Canadian Registry of VTE. Blood 83:1251-1257, 1994.

Andrew M, Paes B, Johnston M: Development of the hemostatic system in the neonate and young infant. Am J Pediatr Hematol Oncol 12:95-104, 1990.

Andrew M, Paes B, Milner R, et al: Development of the human coagulation system in the full-term infant. Blood 70:165-172, 1987.

Andrew M, Paes B, Milner R, et al: Development of the human coagulation system in the healthy premature infant. Blood 72:1651-1657, 1988.

Blanchette VS, Johnson J, Rand M: The management of alloimmune neonatal thrombocytopenia. Baillieres Best Pract Res Clin Haematol 13:365-390, 2000.

Bokenkamp A, von Kries R, Nowak-Gottl U, et al: Neonatal renal venous thrombosis in Germany between 1992 and 1994: Epidemiology, treatment and outcome. Eur J Pediatr 159: 44-48, 2000.

Bussel JB: Alloimmune thrombocytopenia in the fetus and newborn. Semin Thromb Hemost 27:245-252, 2001.

Carcao MD, Blanchette V, Dean J, et al: The Platelet Function Analyzer (PFA-100): A novel in-vitro system for evaluation of primary haemostasis in children. Br J Haematol 101:70-73, 1998.

Choi M, Massicotte M, Marzinotto V, et al: The use of alteplase to restore patency of central venous lines in pediatric patients: A cohort study. J Pediatr 139:152-156, 2001.

Dahlback B: Blood coagulation. Lancet 355:1627-1632, 2000.

deVeber G, Andrew M: Cerebral sinovenous thrombosis in children. N Engl J Med 345:417-423, 2001.

George D, Bussel J: Neonatal thrombocytopenia. Semin Thromb Hemost 21:276-293, 1995.

Gupta AA, Leaker M, Andrew M, et al: Safety and outcomes of thrombolysis with tissue plasminogen activator for treatment of intravascular thrombosis in children. J Pediatr 139:682-688, 2001.

Kuhne T, Imbach P: Neonatal platelet physiology and pathophysiology. Eur J Pediatr 157:87-94, 1998.

Kulkarni R: Bleeding in the newborn. Pediatr Ann 30:548-556, 2001.

Kulkarni R, Lusher J: Perinatal management of newborns with haemophilia. Br J Haematol 112:264-274, 2001.

Lane DA, Grant P: Role of hemostatic gene polymorphisms in venous and arterial thrombotic disease. Blood 95:1517-1532, 2000.

Massicotte MP: Low-molecular-weight heparin therapy in children. J Pediatr Hematol Oncol 23:189-194, 2001.

Massicotte MP, Dix D, Monagle P, et al: Central venous catheter related thrombosis in children: Analysis of the Canadian Registry of Venous Thromboembolic Complications. J Pediatr 133: 770-776, 1998.

Mercuri E, Cowan F: Cerebral infarction in the newborn infant: Review of the literature and personal experience. Europ J Paediatr Neurol 3:255-263, 1999.

Monagle P, Adams M, Mahoney M, et al: Outcome of pediatric thromboembolic disease: A report from the Canadian Childhood Thrombophilia Registry. Pediatr Res 47:763-766, 2000.

Monagle P, Michelson A, Bovill E, et al: Antithrombotic therapy in children. Chest 119:344S-370S, 2001.

Nowak-Gottl U, Auberger K, Halimeh S, et al: Thrombolysis in newborns and infants. Thromb Haemost 82 Suppl 1:112-116, 1999.

Nowak-Gottl U, von Kries R, Gobel U: Neonatal symptomatic thromboembolism in Germany: Two year survey. Arch Dis Child Fetal Neonatal Ed 76:F163-F167, 1997.

Roberts IA, Murray N: Management of thrombocytopenia in neonates. Br J Haematol 105:864-870, 1999.

Roschitz B, Sudi K, Kostenberger M, et al: Shorter PFA-100 closure times in neonates than in adults: Role of red cells, white cells, platelets and von Willebrand factor. Acta Paediatr 90:664-670, 2001.

Ross JA, Davies S: Vitamin K prophylaxis and childhood cancer. Med Pediatr Oncol 34:434-437, 2000.

Schmidt B, Andrew M: Neonatal thrombosis: Report of a prospective Canadian and international registry. Pediatrics 96:939-943, 1995.

Schmidt B, Gillie P, Mitchell L, et al: A placebo-controlled randomized trial of antithrombin therapy in neonatal respiratory distress syndrome. Am J Respir Crit Care Med 158:470-476, 1998.

Sola MC, Del Vecchio A, Rimsza L: Evaluation and treatment of thrombocytopenia in the neonatal intensive care unit. Clin Perinatol 27:655-679, 2000.

Sutor AH, von Kries R, Cornelissen E, et al: Vitamin K deficiency bleeding (VKDB) in infancy. ISTH Pediatric/Perinatal Subcommittee. International Society on Thrombosis and Haemostasis. Thromb Haemost 81:456-461, 1999.

Van Ommen CH, Heijboer H, Buller HR, et al: Venous thromboembolism in childhood: A prospective two-year registry in the Netherlands. J Pediatr 139:676-681, 2001.

Zipursky A: Prevention of vitamin K deficiency bleeding in newborns. Br J Haematol 104:430-437, 1999.

## REFERENCES

Abdulla F, Dietrich KA, Pramanik AK: Percutaneous femoral venous catheterization in preterm neonates. J Pediatr 117: 788-790, 1990.

al Mofada SM, Osman M, Kides E, et al: Risk of thrombocytopenia in the infants of mothers with idiopathic thrombocytopenia. Am J Perinatol 11:423-426, 1994.

Allaart CF, Poort S, Rosendaal F, et al: Increased risk of venous thrombosis in carriers of hereditary protein C deficiency defect. Lancet 341:134-138, 1993.

American Academy of Pediatrics: Controversies concerning vitamin K and the newborn. Pediatrics 91:1001-1003, 1993.

Andrew M, Brooker L: Hemostatic complications in renal disorders of the young. Pediatr Nephrol 10:88-99, 1996.

Andrew M, Brooker L, Leaker M, et al: Fibrin clot lysis by thrombolytic agents is impaired in newborns due to a low plasminogen concentration. Thromb Haemost 68:325-330, 1992a.

Andrew M, Castle V, Saigal S, et al: Clinical impact of neonatal thrombocytopenia. J Pediatr 110:457-464, 1987a.

Andrew M, David M, Adams M, et al: Venous thromboembolic complications (VTE) in children: first analyses of the Canadian Registry of VTE. Blood 83:1251-1257, 1994a.

Andrew M, Marzinotto V, Massicotte P, et al: Heparin therapy in pediatric patients: A prospective cohort study. Pediatr Res 35:78-83, 1994b.

Andrew M, Mitchell L, Berry L, et al: An anticoagulant dermatan sulfate proteoglycan circulates in the pregnant woman and her fetus. J Clin Invest 89:321-326, 1992b.

Andrew M, Ofosu F, Brooker L, et al: The comparison of the pharmacokinetics of a low molecular weight heparin in the newborn and adult pig. Thromb Res 56:529-539, 1989.

Andrew M, Paes B, Bowker J, et al: Evaluation of an automated bleeding time device in the newborn. Am J Hematol 35:275-277, 1990a.

Andrew M, Paes B, Johnston M: Development of the hemostatic system in the neonate and young infant. Am J Pediatr Hematol Oncol 12:95-104, 1990b.

Andrew M, Paes B, Milner R, et al: Development of the human coagulation system in the full-term infant. Blood 70:165-172, 1987b.

Andrew M, Paes B, Milner R, et al: Development of the human coagulation system in the healthy premature infant. Blood 72:1651-1657, 1988.

Andrew M, Schmidt B, Mitchell L, et al: Thrombin generation in newborn plasma is critically dependent on the concentration of prothrombin. Thromb Haemost 63:27-30, 1990c.

Andrew M, Vegh P, Caco C, et al: A randomized, controlled trial of platelet transfusions in thrombocytopenic premature infants. J Pediatr 123:285-291, 1993.

Ankola PA, Atakent Y: Effect of adding heparin in very low concentration to the infusate to prolong the patency of umbilical artery catheters. Am J Perinatol 10:229-232, 1993.

Ansell JE, Patel N, Ostrovsky D, et al: Long-term patient self-management of oral anticoagulation. Arch Intern Med 155:2185-2189, 1995.

Aschka I, Aumann V, Bergmann F, et al: Prevalence of factor V Leiden in children with thromboembolism. Eur J Pediatr 155:1009-1014, 1996.

Astedt B, Lindoff C: Plasminogen activators and plasminogen activator inhibitors in plasma of premature and term newborns. Acta Paediatr 86:111-113, 1997.

Ballin A, Andrew M, Ling E, et al: High-dose intravenous gammaglobulin therapy for neonatal autoimmune thrombocytopenia. J Pediatr 112:789-792, 1988.

Barkovich AJ: The encephalopathic neonate: choosing the proper imaging technique. Am J Neuroradiol 18:1816-1820, 1997.

Barlow CF, Priebe C, Mulliken J, et al: Spastic diplegia as a complication of interferon alfa-2a treatment of hemangiomas of infancy. J Pediatr 132:527-530, 1998.

Barmada MA, Moossy J, Shuman R: Cerebral infarcts with arterial occlusion in neonates. Ann Neurol 6:495-502, 1979.

Barrington KJ: Umbilical artery catheters in the newborn: effects of heparin. Cochrane Database Syst Rev CD000507, 2000a.

Barrington KJ: Umbilical artery catheters in the newborn: effects of position of the catheter tip. Cochrane Database Syst Rev CD000505, 2000b.

Bartlett RH: Extracorporeal Life Support Registry Report 1995. ASAIO J 43:104-107, 1997.

Beverley DW, Chance G, Inwood M, et al: Intraventricular haemorrhage and haemostasis defects. Arch Dis Child 59: 444-448, 1984.

Beverley DW, Pitts-Tucker T, Congdon P, et al: Prevention of intraventricular haemorrhage by fresh frozen plasma. Arch Dis Child 60:710-713, 1985.

Bezinque SL, Slovis T, Touchette A, et al: Characterization of superior sagittal sinus blood flow velocity using color flow Doppler in neonates and infants. Pediatr Radiol 25:175-179, 1995.

Bignell P, Standen G, Bowen D, et al: Rapid neonatal diagnosis of von Willebrand's disease by use of the polymerase chain reaction. Lancet 336:638-639, 1990.

Blanchette VS, Johnson J, Rand M: The management of alloimmune neonatal thrombocytopenia. Baillieres Best Pract Res Clin Haematol 13:365-390, 2000.

Blanchette VS, Kuhne T, Hume H, et al: Platelet transfusion therapy in newborn infants. Transf Med Rev IX:215-230, 1995.

Blanchette VS, Rand ML: Platelet disorders in newborn infants: Diagnosis and management. Semin Perinatol 21:53-62, 1997.

Bokenkamp A, Von Kries R, Nowak-Gottl U, et al: Neonatal renal venous thrombosis in Germany between 1992 and 1994: Epidemiology, treatment and outcome. Eur J Pediatr 159: 44-48, 2000.

Boo NY, Wong NC, Zulkifli SS, et al: Risk factors associated with umbilical vascular catheter–associated thrombosis in newborn infants. J Paediatr Child Health 35:460-465, 1999.

Bovill EG, Becker R, Tracy RP: Monitoring thrombolytic therapy. Prog Cardiovasc Dis 34:279-294, 1992.

Bovill EG, Soll R, Lynch M, et al: Vitamin $K_1$ metabolism and the production of des-carboxy prothrombin and protein C in the term and premature neonate. Blood 81:77-83, 1993.

Brenner B, Fishman A, Goldsher D, et al: Cerebral thrombosis in a newborn with a congenital deficiency of antithrombin III. Am J Hematol 27:209-211, 1988.

Buchanan GR: Factor concentrate prophylaxis for neonates with hemophilia. J Pediatr Hematol Oncol 21:254-256, 1999.

Bulas DI, Taylor G, O'Donnell R, et al: Intracranial abnormalities in infants treated with extracorporeal membrane oxygenation: update on sonographic and CT findings. Am J Neuroradiol 17:287-294, 1996.

Burrows RF, Andrew M: Neonatal thrombocytopenia in the hypertensive disorders of pregnancy. Obstet Gynecol 76: 234-238, 1990.

Burrows RF, Kelton J: Incidentally detected thrombocytopenia in healthy mothers and their infants. N Engl J Med 319:142-145, 1988.

Burrows RF, Kelton J: Fetal thrombocytopenia and its relation to maternal thrombocytopenia. N Engl J Med 329:1463-1466, 1993.

Burrows RF, Kelton JG: Low fetal risks in pregnancies associated with idiopathic thrombocytopenic purpura do not justify obstetrical interventions. Am J Obstet Gynecol 163:1147-1150, 1990.

Bussel J, Berkowitz RL, MacFarland JG: Multicenter study of antenatal management of fetal alloimmune thrombocytopenia (AIT): Stratification into 4 risk groups prior to randomization [abstract]. Thromb Haemost 86:P1234, 2001.

Bussel J, Kaplan C, McFarland J, et al: Recommendations for the evaluation and treatment of neonatal autoimmune and alloimmune thrombocytopenia. Thromb Haemost 65:631-634, 1991.

Bussel JB: Alloimmune thrombocytopenia in the fetus and newborn. Semin Thromb Hemost 27:245-252, 2001.

Bussel JB, Skupski D, MacFarland J: Fetal alloimmune thrombocytopenia: Consensus and controversy. J Matern Fetal Med 5:281-292, 1996.

Bussel JB, Zabusky MR, Berkowitz R, et al: Fetal alloimmune thrombocytopenia. N Engl J Med 337:22-26, 1997.

Caeton AJ, Goetzman B: Risky business. Umbilical arterial catheterization [editorial]. Am J Dis Child 139:120-121, 1985.

Calhoun DA, Christensen R, Edstrom C, et al: Consistent approaches to procedures and practices in neonatal hematology. Clin Perinatol 27:733-753, 2000.

Carcao MD, Blanchette V, Dean JA, et al: The platelet function analyzer (PFA-100): A novel in vitro system for evaluation of primary haemostasis in children. Br J Haematol 101:70-73, 1998.

Castle V, Andrew M, Kelton J, et al: Frequency and mechanism of neonatal thrombocytopenia. J Pediatr 108:749-755, 1986.

Castle V, Coates G, Mitchell L, et al: The effect of hypoxia on platelet survival and site of sequestration in the newborn rabbit. Thromb Haemost 59:45-48, 1988.

Chait P, Dinyari M, Massicotte MP: The sensitivity and specificity of lineograms and ultrasound compared to venography for the diagnosis of central venous line related thrombosis in symptomatic children: The LUV study [abstract]. Thromb Haemost Suppl:P697, 2001.

Chan AKC, Leaker M, Burrows F, et al: Coagulation and fibrinolytic profile of paediatric patients undergoing cardiopulmonary bypass. Thromb Haemost 77:270-277, 1997.

Chang GY, Lueder F, DiMichele D, et al: Heparin and the risk of intraventricular hemorrhage in premature infants. J Pediatr 131:362-366, 1997.

Chen JP, Lorch V: Intraventricular haemorrhage in preterm infants: Evidence of suppressed fibrinolysis. Blood Coagul Fibrinolysis 7:289-294, 1996.

Cheung AM, Halton J, Dinyari M: Bone mineral density (BMD) in a cohort of children on long term warfarin therapy (>1year). Thromb Haemost 86:OC1729, 2001(Abstract).

Cheung PY, Salas E, Etches P, et al: Inhaled nitric oxide and inhibition of platelet aggregation in critically ill neonates. Lancet 351:1181-1182, 1998.

Cheung PY, Sawicki G, Salas E, et al: The mechanisms of platelet dysfunction during extracorporeal membrane oxygenation in critically ill neonates. Crit Care Med 28:2584-2590, 2000.

Choi M, Massicotte M, Marzinotto V, et al: The use of alteplase to restore patency of central venous lines in pediatric patients: a cohort study. J Pediatr 139:152-156, 2001.

Chowdhury V, Lane D, Mille B, et al: Homozygous antithrombin deficiency: report of two new cases (99 Leu to Phe) associated with arterial and venous thrombosis. Thromb Haemost 72: 198-202, 1994.

Conway JH, Hilgartner M: Initial presentations of pediatric hemophiliacs. Arch Pediatr Adolesc Med 148:589-594, 1994.

Cook RL, Miller R, Katz V, et al: Immune thrombocytopenic purpura in pregnancy: a reappraisal of management. Obstet Gynecol 78:578-583, 1991.

Corby DG: Aspirin in pregnancy: maternal and fetal effects. Pediatrics 62:930-937, 1978.

Corby DG, O'Barr T: Decreased alpha-adrenergic receptors in newborn platelets: cause of abnormal response to epinephrine. Dev Pharmacol Ther 2:215-225, 1981a.

Corby DG, O'Barr T: Neonatal platelet function: a membrane-related phenomenon? Haemostasis 10:177-185, 1981b.

Cornelissen EAM, Steegers-Theunissen R, Kollee LA, et al: Supplementation of vitamin K in pregnant women receiving anticonvulsant therapy prevents neonatal vitamin K deficiency. Am J Obstet Gynecol 168:884-888, 1993.

Cornelissen E, Kollee LAA, De Abreu RA, et al: Prevention of vitamin K deficiency in infancy by weekly administration of vitamin K. Acta Paediatr 82:656-659, 1993.

Corrigan JJ Jr, Sleeth J, Jeter M, et al: Newborn's fibrinolytic mechanism: components and plasmin generation. Am J Hematol 32:273-278, 1989.

Dahlback B: Blood coagulation. Lancet 355:1627-1632, 2000.

Dasari R, Narang A, Vasishta K, et al: Effect of maternal low dose aspirin on neonatal platelet function. Indian Pediatr 35:507-511, 1998.

Debus O, Koch H, Kurlemann G, et al: Factor V Leiden and genetic defects of thrombophilia in childhood porencephaly. Arch Dis Child Fetal Neonatal Ed 78:F121-F124, 1998.

Delorme MA, Xu L, Berry L, et al: Anticoagulant dermatan sulfate proteoglycan (decorin) in the term human placenta. Thromb Res 90:147-153, 1998.

De Stefano V, Leone G, Mastrangelo S, et al: Clinical manifestations and management of inherited thrombophilia: retrospective analysis and follow-up after diagnosis of 238 patients with congenital deficiency of antithrombin III, protein C, protein S. Thromb Haemost 72:352-358, 1994.

deVeber G, Adams M, Andrew M: Cerebral thromboembolism in neonates: Clinical and radiographic features [abstract]. Thromb Haemost 78 (suppl.):725, 1997.

deVeber G, Andrew M, the Canadian Pediatric Stroke Study Group: Cerebral sinovenous thrombosis in children. N Engl J Med 345:417-423, 2001.

deVeber G, Chan A, Monagle P, et al: Anticoagulation therapy in pediatric patients with sinovenous thrombosis: a cohort study. Arch Neurol 55:1533-1537, 1998a.

deVeber G, Monagle P, Chan A, et al: Prothrombotic disorders in infants and children with cerebral thromboembolism. Arch Neurol 55:1539-1543, 1998b.

deVeber GA, MacGregor D, Curtis R, et al: Neurologic outcome in survivors of childhood arterial ischemic stroke and sinovenous thrombosis. J Child Neurol 15:316-324, 2000.

de Vries LS, Groenendaal F, Eken P, et al: Infarcts in the vascular distribution of the middle cerebral artery in preterm and fullterm infants. Neuropediatrics 28:88-96, 1997.

DiMichele D, Neufeld E: Hemophilia. A new approach to an old disease. Hematol Oncol Clin North Am 12:1315-1344, 1998.

Dix D, Andrew M, Marzinotto V, et al: The use of low molecular weight heparin in pediatric patients: a prospective cohort study. J Pediatr 136:439-445, 2000.

Dollery CM, Sullivan I, Bauraind O, et al: Thrombosis and embolism in long-term central venous access for parenteral nutrition. Lancet 344:1043-1045, 1994.

Donner M, Holmberg L, Nilsson I: Type IIB von Willebrand's disease with probable autosomal recessive inheritance and presenting as thrombocytopenia in infancy. Br J Haematol 66:349-354, 1987.

Dreyfus M, Magny J, Bridey F, et al: Treatment of homozygous protein C deficiency and neonatal purpura fulminans with a purified protein C concentrate. N Engl J Med 325:1565-1568, 1991.

Edelberg JM, Enghild J, Pizzo S, et al: Neonatal plasminogen displays altered cell surface binding and activation kinetics. Correlation with increased glycosylation of the protein. J Clin Invest 86:107-112, 1990.

Ekelund H, Hedner U, Nilsson I: Fibrinolysis in newborns. Acta Paediatr Scand 59:33-43, 1970.

Ellis MR III: Coagulopathy screening in children with heparinized central venous catheters. Pediatrics 91:1147-1150, 1993.

Estan J, Hope P: Unilateral neonatal cerebral infarction in full term infants. Arch Dis Child Fetal Neonatal Ed 76:F88-F93, 1997.

Farnoux C, Camard O, Pinquier D, et al: Recombinant tissue-type plasminogen activator therapy of thrombosis in 16 neonates. J Pediatr 133:137-140, 1998.

Food and Drug Administration (FDA): Important drug warning regarding the use of Abbokinase (urokinase). Rockville, Md, Public Health Services, 1999.

Forestier F, Daffos F, Galacteros F, et al: Hematological values of 163 normal fetuses between 18 and 30 weeks of gestation. Pediatr Res 20:342-346, 1986.

Francis JL, Armstrong D: Sialic acid and enzymatic desialation of cord blood fibrinogen. Haemostasis 11:223-228, 1982.

Gatti L, Guarneri D, Caccamo M, et al: Platelet activation in newborns detected by flow-cytometry. Biol Neonate 70: 322-327, 1996.

Gazengel C, Fischer A, Schlegel N, et al: Treatment of type III von Willebrand's disease with solvent/detergent-treated factor VIII concentrates. Nouv Rev Fr Hematol 30:225-227, 1988.

George TN, Johnson K, Bates J, et al: The effect of inhaled nitric oxide therapy on bleeding time and platelet aggregation in neonates. J Pediatr 132:731-734, 1998.

Golding J, Greenwood R, Birmingham K, et al: Childhood cancer, intramuscular vitamin K, and pethidine given during labour. BMJ 305:341-346, 1992.

Golding J, Paterson M, Kinlen LJ: Factors associated with childhood cancer in a national cohort study. Br J Cancer 62:304-308, 1990.

Gopel W, Gortner L, Kohlmann T, et al: Low prevalence of large intraventricular haemorrhage in very low birthweight infants carrying the factor V Leiden or prothrombin G20210A mutation. Acta Paediatr 90:1021-1024, 2001.

Greer FR, Marshall S, Cherry J, et al: Vitamin K status of lactating mothers, human milk, and breast-feeding infants. Pediatrics 88:751-756, 1991.

Greffe BS, Marlar R, Manco-Johnson M: Neonatal protein C: Molecular composition and distribution in normal term infants. Thromb Res 56:91-98, 1989.

Grosshaupt B, Muntean W, Sedlmayr P: Hyporeactivity of neonatal platelets is not caused by preactivation during birth. Eur J Pediatr 156:944-948, 1997.

Gruel Y, Boizard B, Daffos F, et al: Determination of platelet antigens and glycoproteins in the human fetus. Blood 68: 488-492, 1986.

Gunther G, Junker R, Strater R, et al: Symptomatic ischemic stroke in full-term neonates: Role of acquired and genetic prothrombotic risk factors. Stroke 31:2437-2441, 2000.

Hakten M, Deniz U, Ozbay G, et al: Two cases of homozygous antithrombin III deficiency in a family with congenital deficiency of ATIII. In Sinzinger H, Vinazzer H (eds): Thrombosis and Haemorrhagic Disorders. Wurzburg, Schmidt and Meyer Verlag, 1989, pp 177-181.

Hansen KN, Ebbesen F: Neonatal vitamin K prophylaxis in Denmark: Three years' experience with oral administration during the first three months of life compared with one oral administration at birth. Acta Paediatr 85:1137-1139, 1996.

Hardart GE, Fackler J: Predictors of intracranial hemorrhage during neonatal extracorporeal membrane oxygenation. J Pediatr 134:156-159, 1999.

Hartmann J, Hussein A, Trowitzsch E, et al: Treatment of neonatal thrombus formation with recombinant tissue plasminogen activator: six years experience and review of the literature. Arch Dis Child Fetal Neonatal Ed 85:F18-F22, 2001.

Heikinheimo R: Coagulation with fetal blood. Biol Neonate 7:319-327, 1964.

Heit JA, Silverstein M, Mohr D, et al: The epidemiology of venous thromboembolism in the community. Thromb Haemost 86:452-463, 2001.

Heller C, Schobess R, Kurnik K, et al: Abdominal venous thrombosis in neonates and infants: Role of prothrombotic risk factor. Br J Haematol 111:534-539, 2000.

Hensey OJ, Morgan M, Cooke R: Tranexamic acid in the prevention of periventricular haemorrhage. Arch Dis Child 59:719-721, 1984.

Hirsh J: Heparin. N Engl J Med 324:1565-1574, 1991.

Hirsh J, Dalen J, Guyatt G: The sixth (2000) ACCP guidelines for antithrombotic therapy for prevention and treatment of thrombosis. American College of Chest Physicians. Chest 119:1S-2S, 2001.

Hofmann S, Knoefler R, Lorenz N, et al: Clinical experiences with low-molecular weight heparins in pediatric patients. Thromb Res 103:345-353, 2001.

Hohlfeld P, Forestier F, Kaplan C, et al: Fetal thrombocytopenia: A retrospective survey of 5,194 fetal blood samplings. Blood 84:1851-1856, 1994.

Hord JD, Gay J, Whitlock J: Thrombocytopenia in neonates with trisomy 21. Arch Pediatr Adolesc Med 149:824-825, 1995.

Hruszkewycz V, Holtrop PC, Batton D, et al: Complications associated with central venous catheters inserted in critically ill neonates. Inf Control Hosp Epidemiol 12:544-548, 1991.

Hume H, Blanchette V, Strauss R, et al: A survey of Canadian neonatal blood transfusion practices. Transfus Sci 18:71-80, 1997.

Hutter JJ Jr, Hathaway W, Wayne E: Hematologic abnormalities in severe neonatal necrotizing enterocolitis. J Pediatr 88:1026-1031, 1976.

Israels SJ, Cheang T, McMillan-Ward E, et al: Evaluation of primary hemostasis in neonates with a new in vitro platelet function analyzer. J Pediatr 138:116-119, 2001.

Israels SJ, Cheang T, Roberston C, et al: Impaired signal transduction in neonatal platelets. Pediatr Res 45:687-691, 1999.

Israels SJ, Daniels M, McMillan E: Deficient collagen-induced activation in the newborn platelet. Pediatr Res 27:337-343, 1990.

Jochmans K, Lissens W, Vervoort R, et al: Antithrombin-Gly 424 Arg: a novel point mutation responsible for type 1 antithrombin deficiency and neonatal thrombosis. Blood 83:146-151, 1994.

Junker P, Egeblad M, Nielsen O, et al: Umbilical vein catheterization and portal hypertension. Acta Paediatr Scand 65:499-504, 1976.

Katz JA, Moake J, McPherson P, et al: Relationship between human development and disappearance of unusually large von Willebrand factor multimers from plasma. Blood 73:1851-1858, 1989.

Kavakli K: Fibrin glue and clinical impact on haemophilia care. Haemophilia 5:392-396, 1999.

Kazzi NJ, Ilagan N, Liang K, et al: Maternal administration of vitamin K does not improve the coagulation profile of preterm infants. Pediatrics 84:1045-1050, 1989.

Keller FG, DeFazio J, Jencks F, et al: The use of heparinase to neutralize residual heparin in blood samples drawn through pediatric indwelling central venous catheters. J Pediatr 132:165-167, 1998.

Kisker C: Pathophysiology of bleeding disorders in the newborn. In Polin RA, Fox WW (eds): Fetal and Neonatal Physiology. Philadelphia, WB Saunders, 1998, pp 1848-1861.

Klesh KW, Murphy T, Scher M, et al: Cerebral infarction in persistent pulmonary hypertension of the newborn. Am J Dis Child 141:852-857, 1987.

Knofler R, Hofmann S, Weissbach G, et al: Molecular markers of the endothelium, the coagulation and the fibrinolytic systems in healthy newborns. Semin Thromb Hemost 24:453-461, 1998a.

Knofler R, Weissbach G, Kuhlisch E: Platelet function tests in childhood. Measuring aggregation and release reaction in whole blood. Semin Thromb Hemost 24:513-521, 1998b.

Kreuz W, Veldmann A, Fischer D, et al: Neonatal sepsis: A challenge in hemostaseology. Semin Thromb Hemost 25:531-535, 1999.

Kuhle S, Lane D, Jochmanns K, et al: Homozygous antithrombin deficiency type II (99 Leu to Phe mutation) and childhood thromboembolism. Thromb Haemost 86:1007-1011, 2001.

Kulkarni R, Lusher J: Perinatal management of newborns with haemophilia. Br J Haematol 112:264-274, 2001.

Kulkarni R, Lusher J, Henry R, et al: Current practices regarding newborn intracranial haemorrhage and obstetrical care and mode of delivery of pregnant haemophilia carriers: A survey of obstetricians, neonatologists and haematologists in the United States, on behalf of the National Hemophilia Foundation's Medical and Scientific Advisory Council. Haemophilia 5:410-415, 1999.

Kumar D, Greer F, Super D, et al: Vitamin K status of premature infants: Implications for current recommendations. Pediatrics 108:1117-1122, 2001.

Kundu SK, Heilmann E, Sio R, et al: Description of an in vitro platelet function analyzer—PFA-100. Semin Thromb Hemost 219(suppl 2):106-112, 1995.

Lesko SM, Mitchell A, Epstein M, et al: Heparin use as a risk factor for intraventricular hemorrhage in low-birth-weight infants. N Engl J Med 314:1156-1160, 1986.

Levi M, ten Cate H: Disseminated intravascular coagulation. N Engl J Med 341:586-592, 1999.

Levy SR, Abroms I, Marshall P, et al: Seizures and cerebral infarction in the full-term newborn. Ann Neurol 17:366-370, 1985.

Ljung R, Lindgren A, Petrini P, et al: Normal vaginal delivery is to be recommended for haemophilia carrier gravidae. Acta Paediatr 83:609-611, 1994.

Ljung RC: Prenatal diagnosis of haemophilia. Haemophilia 5: 84-87, 1999.

Loughnan PM, McDougall P: Epidemiology of late onset haemorrhagic disease: A pooled data analysis. J Paediatr Child Health 29:177-181, 1993.

Loughnan PM, McDougall P, Balvin H, et al: Late onset haemorrhagic disease in premature infants who received intravenous vitamin $K_1$. J Paediatr Child Health 32:268-269, 1996.

Mahasandana C, Suvatte V, Chuansumrit A, et al: Homozygous protein S deficiency in an infant with purpura fulminans. J Pediatr 117:750-753, 1990a.

Mahasandana C, Suvatte V, Marlar, R, et al: Neonatal purpura fulminans associated with homozygous protein S deficiency. Lancet 335:61-62, 1990b.

Male C, Chait P, Ginsberg J, et al: Comparison of venography and ultrasound for the diagnosis of deep vein thrombosis in the upper body in children: A substudy of the PARKAA trial. Thromb Haemost 87:593-598, 2002.

Malloy MH, Cutter G: The association of heparin exposure with intraventricular hemorrhage among very low birth weight infants. J Perinatol 15:185-191, 1995.

Mannhalter C, Kyrle P, Brenner B, et al: Rapid neonatal diagnosis of type IIB von Willebrand disease using the polymerase chain reaction. Blood 77:2539-2540, 1991.

Marlar RA, Montgomery R, Broekmans A: Report on the diagnosis and treatment of homozygous protein C deficiency. Report of the Working Party on Homozygous Protein C Deficiency of the ICTH—Subcommittee on Protein C and Protein S. Thromb Haemost 61:529-531, 1989.

Marlar RA, Neumann A: Neonatal purpura fulminans due to homozygous protein C or protein S deficiencies. Semin Thromb Hemost 16:299-309, 1990.

Martin Montaner MI, Alzina de V, Aranda Arrufat, et al: [Thrombosis of the pulmonary artery associated with maternal deficiency of antithrombin III]. An Esp Pediatr 26:115-117, 1987.

Martinelli I, Bucciarelli P, Margaglione M, et al: The risk of venous thromboembolism in family members with mutations in the genes of factor V or prothrombin or both. Br J Haematol 111:1223-1229, 2000.

Marzinotto V, Monagle P, Chan A, et al: Capillary whole blood monitoring of oral anticoagulants in children in outpatient clinics and the home setting. Pediatr Cardiol 21:347-352, 2000.

Massicotte MP, Dix D, Monagle P, et al: Central venous catheter related thrombosis in children: Analysis of the Canadian Registry of Venous Thromboembolic Complications. J Pediatr 133: 770-776, 1998a.

Massicotte MP, Marzinotto V, Julian J, et al: Dose finding and pharmacokinetics of prophylactic doses of a low molecular weight heparin (reviparin™) in pediatric patients. Blood 94:pt 1 of 2, 1999(Abstract).

Massicotte P, Adams M, Marzinotto V, et al: Low-molecular-weight heparin in pediatric patients with thrombotic disease: a dose finding study. J Pediatr 128:313-318, 1996.

Massicotte P, Leaker M, Marzinotto V, et al: Enhanced thrombin regulation during warfarin therapy in children compared to adults. Thromb Haemost 80:570-574, 1998b.

McDonald MM, Jacobson L, Hay W Jr, et al: Heparin clearance in the newborn. Pediatr Res 15:1015-1018, 1981.

McNinch A, Tripp JH: Haemorrhagic disease of the newborn in the British Isles: two year prospective study. BMJ 303:1105-1109, 1991.

McNinch AW, Upton C, Samuels M, et al: Plasma concentrations after oral or intramuscular vitamin $K_1$ in neonates. Arch Dis Child 60:814-818, 1985.

Mehta P, Vasa R, Neumann L, et al: Thrombocytopenia in the high-risk infant. J Pediatr 97:791-794, 1980.

Mehta S, Connors A Jr, Danish E, et al: Incidence of thrombosis during central venous catheterization of newborns: A prospective study. J Pediatr Surg 27:18-22, 1992.

Menashi S, Aurousseau M, Gozin D, et al: High levels of circulating thrombomodulin in human foetuses and children. Thromb Haemost 81:906-909, 1999.

Ment LR, Ehrenkranz R, Duncan C: Bacterial meningitis as an etiology of perinatal cerebral infarction. Pediatr Neurol 2: 276-279, 1986.

Mercuri E, Cowan F, Gupte G, et al: Prothrombotic disorders and abnormal neurodevelopmental outcome in infants with neonatal cerebral infarction. Pediatrics 107:1400-1404, 2001.

Mercuri E, Cowan F, Rutherford M, et al: Ischaemic and haemorrhagic brain lesions in newborns with seizures and normal Apgar scores. Arch Dis Child Fetal Neonatal Ed 73:F67-F74, 1995.

Michaud JL, Rivard G, Chessex P: Intracranial hemorrhage in a newborn with hemophilia following elective cesarean section. Am J Pediatr Hematol Oncol 13:473-475, 1991.

Miletich J, Sherman L, Broze G Jr: Absence of thrombosis in subjects with heterozygous protein C deficiency. N Engl J Med 317:991-996, 1987.

Miller M, Cosgriff J: Hematological abnormalities in newborn infants with Down syndrome. Am J Med Genet 16:173-177, 1983.

Minford AM, Parapia L, Stainforth C, et al: Treatment of homozygous protein C deficiency with subcutaneous protein C concentrate. Br J Haematol 93:215-216, 1996.

Modanlou HD, Ortiz O: Thrombocytopenia in neonatal infection. Clin Pediatr (Phila) 20:402-407, 1981.

Monagle P, Adams M, Mahoney M, et al: Outcome of pediatric thromboembolic disease: A report from the Canadian Childhood Thrombophilia Registry. Pediatr Res 47:763-766, 2000.

Monagle P, Andrew M, Halton J, et al: Homozygous protein C deficiency: Description of a new mutation and successful treatment with low molecular weight heparin. Thromb Haemost 79:756-761, 1998.

Monagle P, Michelson A, Bovill E, et al: Antithrombotic therapy in children. Chest 119:344S-370S, 2001.

Montaruli B, Schinco P, Pannocchia A, et al: Use of modified functional assays for activated protein C resistance in patients with basally prolonged aPTT. Thromb Haemost 78:1042-1048, 1997.

Morales WJ, Angel J, O'Brien W, et al: The use of antenatal vitamin K in the prevention of early neonatal intraventricular hemorrhage. Am J Obstet Gynecol 159:774-779, 1988.

Motohara K, Endo F, Matsuda I: Effect of vitamin K administration on acarboxy prothrombin (PIVKA-II) levels in newborns. Lancet 2:242-244, 1985.

Mueller-Eckhardt C, Kiefel V: HLA-DRw6, a new immune response marker for immunization against the platelet alloantigen Br[a]. Vox Sang 57:90, 1989.

Mueller-Eckhardt C, Kiefel V, Grubert A: 348 cases of suspected neonatal alloimmune thrombocytopenia. Lancet 1:363-366, 1989.

Mueller-Eckhardt C, Santoso S, Kiefel V: Platelet alloantigens—molecular, genetic, and clinical aspects. Vox Sang 67(suppl 3):89-93, 1994.

Murphy MF, Waters A, Doughty H, et al: Antenatal management of fetomaternal alloimmune thrombocytopenia—report of 15 affected pregnancies. Transfus Med 4:281-292, 1994.

Murray NA, Roberts I: Circulating megakaryocytes and their progenitors (BFU-MK and CFU-MK) in term and pre-term neonates. Br J Haematol 89:41-46, 1995.

Murray NA, Watts TL, Roberts IA: Inhibition of megakaryocytes and their progenitors in early thrombocytopenia in preterm neonates. Blood 94:450a, 1994(Abstract).

Murray NA, Watts, T, Roberts I: Endogenous thrombopoietin levels and effect of recombinant human thrombopoietin on megakaryocyte precursors in term and preterm babies. Pediatr Res 43:148-151, 1998.

Nelson KB, Dambrosia J, Grether J, et al: Neonatal cytokines and coagulation factors in children with cerebral palsy. Ann Neurol 44:665-675, 1998.

Neubauer AP: Percutaneous central i.v. access in the neonate: Experience with 535 Silastic catheters. Acta Paediatr 84:756-760, 1995.

Nohe N, Flemmer A, Rumler R, et al: The low molecular weight heparin dalteparin for prophylaxis and therapy of thrombosis in childhood: A report on 4 cases. Eur J Pediatr 158:S134-S139, 1999.

The Northern Neonatal Nursing Initiative Trial Group: Randomised trial of prophylactic early fresh-frozen plasma or gelatin or glucose in preterm babies: Outcome at 2 years. Lancet 348:229-232, 1996.

Nowak-Gottl U, Koch H, Aschka I, et al: Resistance to activated protein C (APCR) in children with venous or arterial thromboembolism. Br J Haematol 92:992-998, 1996.

Nowak-Gottl U, Auberger K, Halimeh S, et al: Thrombolysis in newborns and infants. Thromb Haemost 82(suppl 1):112-116, 1999.

Nowak-Gottl U, Groll A, Kreuz WD, et al: Treatment of disseminated intravascular coagulation with antithrombin III concentrate in children with verified infection. Klin Padiatr (Germany) 204(3):134-140, 1992.

Nowak-Gottl U, Kohlhase B, Vielhaber H, et al: APC resistance in neonates and infants: Adjustment of the APTT-based method. Thromb Res 81:665-670, 1996.

Nowak-Gottl U, Von Kries R, Gobel U: Neonatal symptomatic thromboembolism in Germany: Two year survey. Arch Dis Child Fetal Neonatal Ed 76:F163-F167, 1997.

Nuss R, Hays T, Manco-Johnson M: Efficacy and safety of heparin anticoagulation for neonatal renal vein thrombosis. Am J Pediatr Hematol Oncol 16:127-131, 1994.

Oldenburg J, von Brederlow B, Fregin A, et al: Congenital deficiency of vitamin K dependent coagulation factors in two families presents as a genetic defect of the vitamin K-epoxide-reductase-complex. Thromb Haemost 84:937-941, 2000.

Parker L, Cole M, Craft A, et al: Neonatal vitamin K administration and childhood cancer in the north of England: Retrospective case-control study. BMJ 316:189-193, 1998.

Patel P, Weitz J, Brooker L, et al: Decreased thrombin activity of fibrin clots prepared in cord plasma compared with adult plasma. Pediatr Res 39:826-830, 1996.

Pegelow CH, Curless R, Bradford B: Severe protein C deficiency in a newborn. Am J Pediatr Hematol Oncol 10:326-329, 1988.

Pellicer A, Cabanas F, Garcia-Alix A, et al: Stroke in neonates with cardiac right-to-left shunt. Brain Dev 14:381-385, 1992.

Petaja J, Hiltunen L, Fellman V: Increased risk of intraventricular hemorrhage in preterm infants with thrombophilia. Pediatr Res 49:643-646, 2001.

Peterec SM, Brennan S, Rinder H, et al: Reticulated platelet values in normal and thrombocytopenic neonates. J Pediatr 129:269-274, 1996.

Peyvandi F, Mannucci P: Rare coagulation disorders. Thromb Haemost 82:1207-1214, 1999.

Philip AG, Tito A: Increased nucleated red blood cell counts in small for gestational age infants with very low birth weight. Am J Dis Child 143:164-169, 1989.

Pielet BW, Socol M, MacGregor S, et al: Cordocentesis: An appraisal of risks. Am J Obstet Gynecol 159:1497-1500, 1988.

Pollard AJ, Sreeram N, Wright J, et al: ECG and echocardiographic diagnosis of pulmonary thromboembolism associated with central venous lines. Arch Dis Child 73:147-150, 1995.

Pollmann H, Richter H, Ringkamp H, et al: When are children diagnosed as having severe haemophilia and when do they start to bleed? A 10-year single-centre PUP study. Eur J Pediatr 158(suppl 3):S166-S170, 1999.

Pomerance JJ, Teal J, Gogolok J, et al: Maternally administered antenatal vitamin $K_1$: Effect on neonatal prothrombin activity, partial thromboplastin time, and intraventricular hemorrhage. Obstet Gynecol 70:235-241, 1987.

Poort SR, Resendaal FR, Reitsma PH, Bertina RM: A common genetic variation in the 3′-untranslated region of the prothrombin gene is associated with elevated plasma prothrombin levels and an increase in venous thrombosis. Blood 88:3698-3703, 1996.

Rais-Bahrami K, Short B: The current status of neonatal extracorporeal membrane oxygenation. Semin Perinatol 24:406-417, 2000.

Raith W, Fauler G, Pichler G, et al: Plasma concentrations after intravenous administration of phylloquinone (vitamin $K_1$) in preterm and sick neonates. Thromb Res 99:467-472, 2000.

Rajasekhar D, Barnard M, Bednarek F, et al: Platelet hyporeactivity in very low birth weight neonates. Thromb Haemost 77:1002-1007, 1997.

Rajasekhar D, Kestin A, Bednarek F, et al: Neonatal platelets are less reactive than adult platelets to physiological agonists in whole blood. Thromb Haemost 72:957-963, 1994.

Ramsey G, Salamon D: Frequency of *PLA1* in blacks. Transfusion 26:531-532, 1986.

Rand ML, Blanchette VS, Weitzman S: Volume reduction of pre-storage leuko-reduced platelet concentrates does not affect platelet function in vitro or platelet recovery in vivo [abstract]. Blood 98:58a, 2001.

Randolph AG, Cook D, Gonzales C, et al: Benefit of heparin in central venous and pulmonary artery catheters: A meta-analysis of randomized controlled trials. Chest 113:165-171, 1998.

Rees CD, Cox M, Clegg JB: World distribution of factor V Leiden. Lancet 346:1133-1134, 1995.

Reese J, Raghuveer T, Dennington P, et al: Breast feeding in neonatal alloimmune thrombocytopenia. J Paediatr Child Health 30:447-449, 1994.

Reverdiau-Moalic P, Delahousse B, Body G, et al: Evolution of blood coagulation activators and inhibitors in the healthy human fetus. Blood 88:900-906, 1996.

Roddie PH, Stirling C, Mayne E, et al: Thrombosis and disseminated intravascular coagulation following treatment with the prothrombin complex concentrate, DEFIX. Thromb Haemost 81:667, 1999.

Rodeghiero F, Castaman G, Dini E: Epidemiological investigation of the prevalence of von Willebrand's disease. Blood 69:454-459, 1987.

Roschitz B, Sudi K, Kostenberger M, et al: Shorter PFA-100 closure times in neonates than in adults: role of red cells, white cells, platelets and von Willebrand factor. Acta Paediatr 90:664-670, 2001.

Rosendaal FR, Koster T, Vandenbroucke J, et al: High risk of thrombosis in patients homozygous for factor V Leiden (activated protein C resistance). Blood 85:1504-1508, 1995.

Ross JA, Davies S: Vitamin K prophylaxis and childhood cancer. Med Pediatr Oncol 34:434-437, 2000.

Roy M, Turner-Gomes SO, Gill G: Incidence and diagnosis of neonatal thrombosis associated with umbilical venous catheters. Pediatr Res 41:173a, 1997(Abstract).

Sainio S, Joutsi L, Jarvenpaa A, et al: Idiopathic thrombocytopenic purpura in pregnancy. Acta Obstet Gynecol Scand 77:272-277, 1998.

Salonvaara M, Riikonen P, Kekomaki R, et al: Clinically symptomatic central venous catheter–related deep venous thrombosis in newborns. Acta Paediatr 88:642-646, 1999.

Sanchez J, Velasco F, Alvarez R, et al: Aortic thrombosis in a neonate with hereditary antithrombin III deficiency: Successful outcome with thrombolytic and replacement treatment. Acta Paediatr 85:245-247, 1998.

Sanson BJ, Simioni P, Tormene D, et al: The incidence of venous thromboembolism in asymptomatic carriers of a deficiency of antithrombin, protein C, or protein S: a prospective cohort study. Blood 94:3702-3706, 1999.

Sanz-Rodriguez C, Gil-Fernandez J, Zapater P, et al: Long-term management of homozygous protein C deficiency: Replacement therapy with subcutaneous purified protein C concentrate. Thromb Haemost 81:887-890, 1999.

Saving KL, Jennings D, Aldag J, et al: Platelet ultrastructure of high-risk premature infants. Thromb Res 73:371-384, 1994.

Schabel A, Konig A, Brand U, et al: [Severe neonatal alloimmune thrombocytopenia with delayed antibody detection]. Beitr Infusionsther Transfusionsmed 33:156-159, 1996.

Schmidt B, Andrew M: Neonatal thrombosis: Report of a prospective Canadian and international registry. Pediatrics 96:939-943, 1995.

Schmidt B, Andrew M, Weitz J: Do coagulation screening tests detect increased generation of thrombin and plasmin in sick newborn infants? Thromb Haemost 69:418-421, 1993.

Schmidt B, Buchanan M, Ofosu F, et al: Antithrombotic properties of heparin in a neonatal piglet model of thrombin-induced thrombosis. Thromb Haemost 60:289-292, 1988.

Schmidt B, Gillie P, Mitchell L, et al: A placebo-controlled randomized trial of antithrombin therapy in neonatal respiratory distress syndrome. Am J Respir Crit Care Med 158:470-476, 1998.

Schmidt B, Mitchell L, Ofosu F, et al: Alpha-2-macroglobulin is an important progressive inhibitor of thrombin in neonatal and infant plasma. Thromb Haemost 62:1074-1077, 1989a.

Schmidt B, Ofosu F, Mitchell L, et al: Anticoagulant effects of heparin in neonatal plasma. Pediatr Res 25:405-408, 1989b.

Schubiger G, Stocker C, Banziger O, et al: Oral vitamin $K_1$ prophylaxis for newborns with a new mixed-micellar preparation of phylloquinone: 3 years experience in Switzerland. Eur J Pediatr 158:599-602, 1999.

Schwartz DS, Gettner P, Konstantino M, et al: Umbilical venous catheterization and the risk of portal vein thrombosis. J Pediatr 131:760-762, 1997.

Schwarz HP, Muntean W, Watzke H, et al: Low total protein S antigen but high protein S activity due to decreased C4b-binding protein in neonates. Blood 71:562-565, 1988.

Seibert JJ, Taylor B, Williamson S, et al: Sonographic detection of neonatal umbilical-artery thrombosis: clinical correlation. Am J Roentgenol 148:965-968, 1987.

Setzer ES, Webb I, Wassenaar J, et al: Platelet dysfunction and coagulopathy in intraventricular hemorrhage in the premature infant. J Pediatr 100:599-605, 1982.

Shah JK, Mitchell L, Paes B, et al: Thrombin inhibition is impaired in plasma of sick neonates. Pediatr Res 31:391-395, 1992.

Shapiro AD, Jacobson L, Aramon M, et al: Vitamin K deficiency in the newborn infant: Prevalence and perinatal risk factors. J Pediatr 109:675-680, 1986.

Shirahata A, Nakamura T, Shimono M, et al: Blood coagulation findings and the efficacy of factor XIII concentrate in premature infants with intracranial hemorrhages. Thromb Res 57:755-763, 1990.

Short BL, Walker L, Bender K, et al: Impairment of cerebral autoregulation during extracorporeal membrane oxygenation in newborn lambs. Pediatr Res 33:289-294, 1993.

Simioni P, Sanson B, Prandoni P, et al: Incidence of venous thromboembolism in families with inherited thrombophilia. Thromb Haemost 81:198-202, 1999.

Sola MC, Calhoun D, Hutson A, et al: Plasma thrombopoietin concentrations in thrombocytopenic and non-thrombocytopenic patients in a neonatal intensive care unit. Br J Haematol 104: 90-92, 1999a.

Sola MC, Rimsza L, Christensen R: A bone marrow biopsy technique suitable for use in neonates. Br J Haematol 107:458-460, 1999b.

Solymar L, Rao P, Mardini M, et al: Prosthetic valves in children and adolescents. Am Heart J 121:557-568, 1991.

Spadone D: Heparin induced thrombocytopenia in the newborn. J Vasc Surg 15:306-312, 1996.

Sreenan C, Bhargava R, Robertson C: Cerebral infarction in the term newborn: Clinical presentation and long-term outcome. J Pediatr 137:351-355, 2000.

Srivastava A, Bruno E, Briddell R, et al: Parvovirus B19-induced perturbation of human megakaryocytopoiesis in vitro. Blood 76:1997-2004, 1990.

Stoeckel K, Joubert P, Gruter J: Elimination half-life of vitamin $K_1$ in neonates is longer than is generally assumed: Implications for the prophylaxis of haemorrhaghic disease of the newborn. Eur J Clin Pharmacol 49:421-423, 1996.

Streif W, Andrew M, Marzinotto V, et al: Analysis of warfarin therapy in pediatric patients: A prospective cohort study of 319 patients. Blood 94:3007-3014, 1999.

Suarez CR, Gonzalez J, Menendez C, et al: Neonatal and maternal platelets: Activation at time of birth. Am J Hematol 29:18-21, 1988.

Suarez CR, Walenga J, Mangogna L, et al: Neonatal and maternal fibrinolysis: Activation at time of birth. Am J Hematol 19: 365-372, 1985.

Sutherland JM, Glueck H: Hemorrhagic disease of the newborn; breast feeding as a necessary factor in the pathogenesis. Am J Dis Child 113:524-533, 1967.

Sutor AH, Dagres N, Niederhoff H: Late form of vitamin K deficiency bleeding in Germany. Klin Padiatr 207:89-97, 1995.

Sutor AH, Von Kries R, Cornelissen E, et al: Vitamin K deficiency bleeding (VKDB) in infancy. ISTH Pediatric/Perinatal Subcommittee. International Society on Thrombosis and Haemostasis. Thromb Haemost 81:456-461, 1999.

Tait RC, Walker I, Perry D, et al: Prevalence of antithrombin deficiency in the healthy population. Br J Haematol 87:106-112, 1994.

Tanindi S, Kurekci A, Koseoglu V, et al: The normalization period of platelet aggregation in newborns. Thromb Res 80:57-62, 1995.

Tanke RB, van Megen R, Daniels O: Thrombus detection on central venous catheters in the neonatal intensive care unit. Angiology 45:477-480, 1994.

Tate DY, Carlton G, Johnson D, et al: Immune thrombocytopenia in severe neonatal infections. J Pediatr 98:449-453, 1981.

Thaler E, Lechner K: Antithrombin III deficiency and thromboembolism. Clin Haematol 10:369-390, 1981.

Thomas KB, Sutor A, Altinkaya N, et al: Von Willebrand factor-collagen binding activity is increased in newborns and infants. Acta Paediatr 84:697-699, 1995.

Thorp JA, Parriott J, Ferrette-Smith D, et al: Antepartum vitamin K and phenobarbital for preventing intraventricular hemorrhage in the premature newborn: a randomized, double-blind, placebo-controlled trial. Obstet Gynecol 83:70-76, 1994.

Tomer A, Hanson S, Harker L: Autologous platelet kinetics in patients with severe thrombocytopenia: discrimination between disorders of production and destruction. J Lab Clin Med 118: 546-554, 1991.

Trauner DA, Chase C, Walker P, et al: Neurologic profiles of infants and children after perinatal stroke. Pediatr Neurol 9: 383-386, 1993.

Ts'ao CH, Green D, Schultz K: Function and ultrastructure of platelets of neonates: Enhanced ristocetin aggregation of neonatal platelets. Br J Haematol 32:225-233, 1976.

Uhrynowska M, Maslanka K, Zupanska B: Neonatal thrombocytopenia: Incidence, serological and clinical observations. Am J Perinatol 14:415-418, 1997.

Upp JR Jr, Bush P, Zwischenberger J: Complications of neonatal extracorporeal membrane oxygenation. Perfusion 9:241-256, 1994.

Urlesberger B, Zobel G, Zenz W, et al: Activation of the clotting system during extracorporeal membrane oxgenation in term newborn infants. J Pediatr 129:264-268, 1996.

Van de Bor BM, Briet E, Van Bel F, et al: Hemostasis and periventricular-intraventricular hemorrhage of the newborn. Am J Dis Child 140:1131-1134, 1986.

van der Meer FJ, Koster T, Vandenbroucke J, et al: The Leiden Thrombophilia Study (LETS). Thromb Haemost 78:631-635, 1997.

van Leeuwen EF, Leeksma O, van Mourik J, et al: Effect of the binding of anti-Zwa antibodies on platelet function. Vox Sang 47:280-289, 1984.

van Ommen CH, Heijboer H, Buller H, et al: Venous thromboembolism in childhood: A prospective two-year registry in The Netherlands. J Pediatr 139:676-681, 2001.

Vieira A, Berry L, Ofosu F, et al: Heparin sensitivity and resistance in the neonate: An explanation. Thromb Res 63:85-98, 1991.

Vielhaber H, Ehrenforth S, Koch H, et al: Cerebral venous sinus thrombosis in infancy and childhood: Role of genetic and acquired risk factors of thrombophilia. Eur J Pediatr 157: 555-560, 1998.

Vietti TJ, Murphy T, James J, et al: Observation on the prophylactic use of vitamin K in the newborn. J Pediatr 56:343-346, 1960.

Volpe JJ: Neurology of the Newborn, 3rd ed. Philadelphia, WB Saunders, 2001.

Von Kries R, Hanawa Y: Neonatal vitamin K prophylaxis. Report of Scientific and Standardization Committee on Perinatal Hemostasis. Thromb Haemost 69:293-295, 1993.

Von Kries R, Hachmeister A, Gobel U: Can 3 oral 2 mg doses of vitamin K effectively prevent late vitamin K deficiency bleeding? Eur J Pediatr 158(suppl 3):S183-S186, 1999.

Weiner GM, Castle V, DiPietro M, et al: Successful treatment of neonatal arterial thromboses with recombinant tissue plasminogen activator. J Pediatr 133:133-136, 1998.

Weissbach G, Harenberg J, Wendisch J, et al: Tissue factor pathway inhibitor in infants and children. Thromb Res 73:441-446, 1994

Williamson LM, Hackett G, Rennie J, et al: The natural history of fetomaternal alloimmunization to the platelet-specific antigen HPA-1a (Pl[A1], Zwa) as determined by antenatal screening. Blood 92:2280-2287, 1998.

Wright IM: Prevention of intraventricular haemorrhage in preterm infants in Britain and Ireland. Arch Dis Child Fetal Neonatal Ed 72:F79, 1995.

Yang YM, Simon N, Maertens P, et al: Maternal-fetal transport of vitamin $K_1$ and its effect on coagulation in premature infants. J Pediatr 115:1009-1013, 1989.

Zenz W, Arlt F, Sodia S, et al: Intracerebral hemorrhage during fibrinolytic therapy in children: a review of the literature of the last thirty years. Semin Thromb Hemost 23:321-332, 1997.

CHAPTER 77

# Erythrocyte Disorders in Infancy

William C. Mentzer and Bertil E. Glader

## NORMAL ERYTHROCYTE PHYSIOLOGY IN THE FETUS AND NEWBORN

### Fetal Erythropoiesis

Fetal erythropoiesis occurs sequentially during embryonic development in three different sites: yolk sac, liver, and bone marrow. The growth factors and cytokines that regulate embryonic hematopoiesis in humans are not yet defined, but animal work suggests that they are different from those that regulate proliferation and differentiation of stem cells in later life (Zon, 1995). Yolk sac formation of red blood cells (RBCs) is maximal between 2 and 10 weeks of gestation. Myeloid, or bone marrow, production of RBCs begins around week 18, and by the 30th week of fetal life, bone marrow is the major erythropoietic organ. At birth, almost all RBCs are produced in the bone marrow, although a low level of hepatic erythropoiesis persists through the first few days of life. Sites of fetal erythropoiesis occasionally are reactivated in older patients with hematologic disorders such as myelofibrosis, aplastic anemia, and severe hemolytic anemia.

RBC production in extrauterine life is controlled in part by erythropoietin, a humoral erythropoietic-stimulating factor (ESF) produced by the kidney. The role of erythropoietin in the developing fetus has not been completely defined. Current thought is that ESF does not influence yolk sac or hepatic erythropoiesis but may partially regulate myeloid RBC production (Finne and Halvorsen, 1972). ESF is detected in fetal blood and amniotic fluid during the last trimester of pregnancy. The concentration of this hormone increases directly with the period of gestation, and thus, erythropoietin levels in term newborns are significantly higher than in premature infants. This difference may reflect some degree of fetal hypoxia during late intrauterine life. Increased ESF titers also are seen in placental dysfunction, fetal anemia, and maternal hypoxia (Finne, 1966). Fetal RBC formation is not influenced by maternal erythropoietin, because transfusion-induced maternal polycythemia (decreased maternal ESF levels) has no effect on fetal erythropoiesis (Jacobson et al, 1959). Maternal nutritional status also is not a significant factor in the regulation of fetal erythropoiesis, because iron, folate, and vitamin $B_{12}$ are trapped by the fetus irrespective of maternal stores. Most studies have demonstrated that women with severe iron deficiency bear children with normal total body hemoglobin content (Lanzkowsky, 1961).

Hemoglobin, hematocrit, and RBC count increase throughout fetal life (Table 77–1). Extremely large RBCs (mean corpuscular volume [MCV] of 180 fL) with an increased hemoglobin content (mean corpuscular hemoglobin [MCH] of 60 pg/cell) are produced early in fetal life. The size and hemoglobin content of these cells decrease throughout gestation, but the mean corpuscular hemoglobin concentration (MCHC) does not change significantly. Even at birth, the MCV and MCH are greater than those in older children and adults. Many nucleated RBCs and reticulocytes are present early in gestation, and the percentage of these cells also decreases as the fetus ages.

Hemoglobin production increases markedly during the last trimester of pregnancy. The actual hemoglobin concentration increases, but, more important, body weight, blood volume, and total body hemoglobin triple during this period. Fetal iron accumulation parallels the increase in total body hemoglobin content. The neonatal iron endowment at birth, therefore, is directly related to total body hemoglobin content and length of gestation. Term infants have more iron than premature infants.

### RBC Physiology at Birth

In utero, the $Po_2$ in blood delivered to the tissues is only one-third to one-fourth the value in adults. This relative hypoxia may be responsible for the increased content of erythropoietin and signs of active erythropoiesis (nucleated RBCs, increased reticulocytes) seen in newborns at birth. When lungs become the source of oxygen, hemoglobin-oxygen saturation increases to 95% and erythropoiesis decreases. Within 72 hours after birth, erythropoietin is undetectable, nucleated RBCs disappear, and reticulocytes decrease to less than 1%.

The concentration of hemoglobin during the first few hours of life increases to values greater than those in cord blood. This is both a relative increase caused by a reduction in plasma volume (Gairdner et al, 1958) and an absolute increase caused by placental blood transfusion (Usher et al, 1963). The umbilical vein remains patent long after umbilical arteries have constricted, and thus transfusion of placental blood occurs when newborns are placed at a level below the placenta. The placenta contains approximately 100 mL of fetal blood (30% of the infant's blood volume). Approximately 25% of placental blood enters the newborn within 15 seconds of birth, and by 1 minute, 50% is transfused. The time of cord clamping is thus a direct determinant of neonatal blood volume. The blood volume in term infants (mean of 85 mL/kg) varies considerably (50 to 100 mL/kg) because of different degrees of placental transfusion (Usher et al, 1963). These differences are readily apparent when the effects of early versus delayed cord clamping are compared at 72 hours of age: 82.3 mL/kg (early clamping) versus 92.6 mL/kg (delayed clamping). These changes are largely the result of differences in RBC mass (early clamping, 31 mL/kg; delayed clamping, 49 mL/kg). The blood volume in premature infants (89 to 105 mL/kg) is slightly greater than that in term infants, but this difference is due in large part to an increased plasma volume (Usher and Lind, 1965).

**TABLE 77–1**

**Mean Red Blood Cell (RBC) Values During Gestation**

| Age (wk) | Hb (g/dL) | Hematocrit (%) | RBC ($10^6/mm^3$) | Mean Corpuscular Volume (fL) | Mean Corpuscular Hb (pg) | Mean Corpuscular Hb Concentration (g/dL) | Nucleated RBCs (% of RBCs) | Reticulocytes (%) | Diameter (μm) |
|---|---|---|---|---|---|---|---|---|---|
| 12 | 8.0-10.0 | 33 | 1.5 | 180 | 60 | 34 | 5.0-8.0 | 40 | 10.5 |
| 16 | 10.0 | 35 | 2.0 | 140 | 45 | 33 | 2.0-4.0 | 10-25 | 9.5 |
| 20 | 11.0 | 37 | 2.5 | 135 | 44 | 33 | 1.0 | 10-20 | 9.0 |
| 24 | 14.0 | 40 | 3.5 | 123 | 38 | 31 | 1.0 | 5-10 | 8.8 |
| 28 | 14.5 | 45 | 4.0 | 120 | 40 | 31 | 0.5 | 5-10 | 8.7 |
| 34 | 15.0 | 47 | 4.4 | 118 | 38 | 32 | 0.2 | 3-10 | 8.5 |

Hb, hemoglobin.

Data from Oski FA, Naiman JL: Hematologic Problems in the Newborn, 3rd ed. Philadelphia, WB Saunders, 1982.

The RBC mass in premature infants, expressed in milliliters per kilogram, is the same as in term newborns.

## Fetal and Neonatal Hemoglobin Function

A variety of hemoglobins are present during fetal and neonatal life (see Hemolysis Due to Hemoglobin Disorders). Fetal hemoglobin is the major hemoglobin in utero, whereas hemoglobin A is the normal hemoglobin of extrauterine life. A single RBC may contain both hemoglobin F and hemoglobin A in varying proportions, depending on gestational and postnatal age. One major difference between hemoglobins A and F is related to oxygen transport.

The transport of oxygen to peripheral tissues is regulated by several factors, including blood oxygen capacity, cardiac output, and hemoglobin-oxygen affinity. (1) Oxygen capacity is a direct function of hemoglobin concentration (1 g hemoglobin combines with 1.34 mL oxygen). (2) Compensatory changes in cardiac output can maintain normal $O_2$ delivery under conditions in which oxygen capacity is significantly reduced. (3) The oxygen affinity of hemoglobin also influences oxygen delivery to tissues. Hemoglobin A is 95% saturated at arterial oxygen tensions (100 mm Hg), but this decreases to 70% to 75% saturation at a venous $Po_2$ of 40 mm Hg. The difference in $O_2$ content at arterial and venous oxygen tensions reflects the amount of oxygen that can be released. Changes in hemoglobin affinity for oxygen can influence oxygen delivery (Oski and Delivoria-Papadopoulos, 1970) (Fig. 77–1). At any given $Po_2$, more oxygen is bound to hemoglobin when oxygen affinity is increased. Stated in physiologic terms, increased hemoglobin-oxygen affinity reduces oxygen delivery, whereas decreased hemoglobin-oxygen affinity increases oxygen release to peripheral tissues.

The oxygen affinity of hemoglobin A in solution is greater than that of hemoglobin F. Paradoxically, however, whole blood from normal children (hemoglobin A) has a lower oxygen affinity than that of neonatal blood (hemoglobin F) (Allen et al, 1953). This difference is related to an intermediate of RBC metabolism, 2,3-diphosphoglycerate (2,3-DPG). This organic phosphate compound interacts with hemoglobin A to decrease its affinity for oxygen, thereby enhancing $O_2$ release. Fetal hemoglobin does not interact with 2,3-DPG to any significant extent (Bauer et al, 1968); consequently, cells containing hemoglobin F have a higher oxygen affinity than those containing hemoglobin A.

The increased oxygen affinity of fetal RBCs is advantageous for extracting oxygen from maternal blood within the placenta. A few months after birth, however, infant blood acquires the same oxygen affinity as that of older children (Fig. 77–2). The postnatal decrease in oxygen affinity is due to a reduction in hemoglobin F and an increase in hemoglobin A (which interacts with 2,3-DPG). Oxygen delivery (the difference in arterial and venous $O_2$ content) actually increases while oxygen

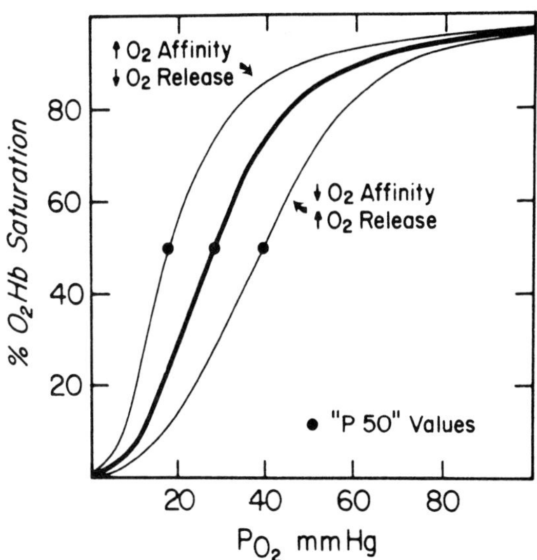


**FIGURE 77–1.** The oxygen dissociation curve for normal adult hemoglobin *(dark line)*. The percent oxygen saturation (ordinate) is plotted for arterial oxygen tensions between 0 and 100 mm Hg (abscissa). As the curve shifts to the right, more oxygen is released at any given $Po_2$. Conversely, as the curve shifts to the left, more oxygen is retained on hemoglobin at any given $Po_2$. The "P 50" refers to that $Po_2$ in which hemoglobin is 50% saturated with oxygen. This term is useful in comparing the oxygen affinities of different hemoglobins. *(From Oski FA, Delivoria-Papadopoulos M: The red cell, 2,3-diphosphoglycerate, and tissue oxygen release. J Pediatr 77:941, 1970.)*

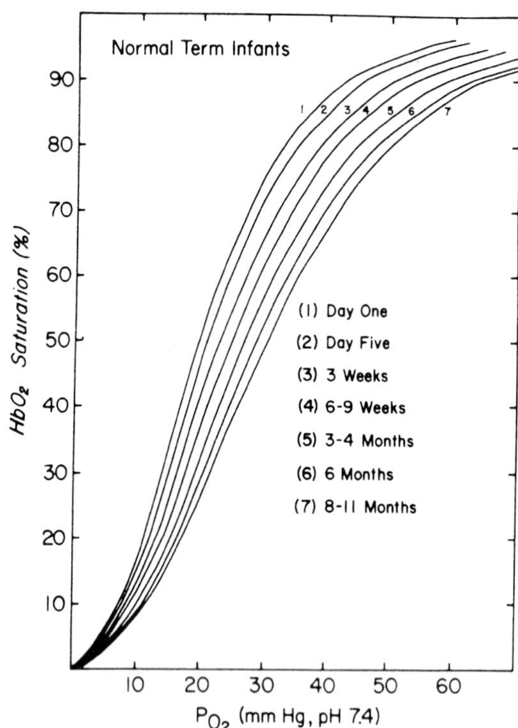


**FIGURE 77–2.** The oxygen affinity of blood from term infants at birth and at different postnatal ages. The gradual rightward shift of the oxygen saturation curve indicates increased oxygen release from hemoglobin as infants get older. This decreased oxygen affinity is due to a decrease in hemoglobin F and an increase in hemoglobin A. *(From Oski FA, Delivoria-Papadopoulos M: The red cell, 2,3-diphosphoglycerate, and tissue oxygen release. J Pediatr 77:941, 1970.)*

capacity (hemoglobin concentration) decreases during the 1st week of life (Fig. 77–3). This enhanced delivery is largely a reflection of the decreased oxygen affinity of infant blood (Delivoria-Papadopoulos et al, 1971). The oxygen affinity of blood from premature infants is higher than that of term infants, and the normal postnatal changes (decrease in oxygen affinity, increase in oxygen delivery) occur much more gradually in premature infants (see Fig. 77–3).

## GENERAL APPROACH TO ANEMIC INFANTS

### Medical History and Physical Examination

The cause of anemia frequently can be ascertained by medical history and physical examination. Particular importance is given to family history (anemia, cholelithiasis, unexplained jaundice, splenomegaly), maternal medical history (especially infections), and obstetric history (previous pregnancies, length of gestation, method and difficulty of delivery). The age at which anemia becomes manifest also is of diagnostic importance. Significant anemia at birth invariably is due to blood loss or alloimmune hemolysis. After 24 hours, internal hemorrhages and other causes of hemolysis become evident. Anemia that appears several weeks after birth can be caused by a variety of conditions, including abnormalities in the synthesis of hemoglobin beta chains, hypoplastic RBC disorders, and the physiologic anemia of infancy or prematurity.

Infants with anemia resulting from chronic blood loss may appear pale, without other evidence of clinical distress. Acute blood loss can produce hypovolemic shock and a clinical state similar to severe neonatal asphyxia. Newborns with hemolytic anemia frequently show a greater-than-expected degree of icterus. In addition, hemolysis often is associated with hepatosplenomegaly, and in cases resulting from congenital infection, other stigmata may be present.

### Laboratory Evaluation of Anemia

A simple classification of neonatal anemia based on physical examination and simple laboratory tests is presented in Table 77–2. More esoteric RBC tests are described elsewhere (Alter, 1989).

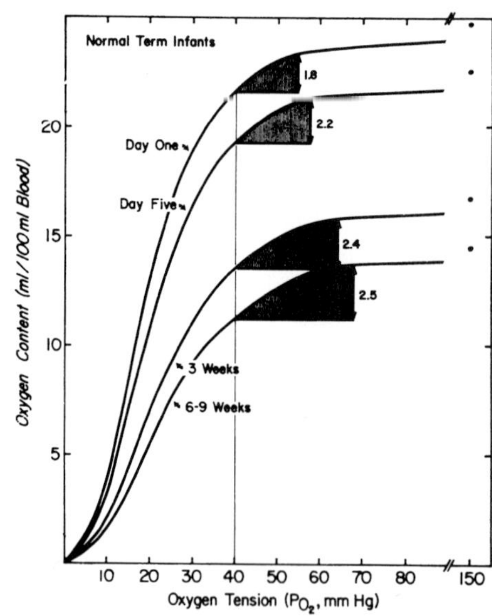


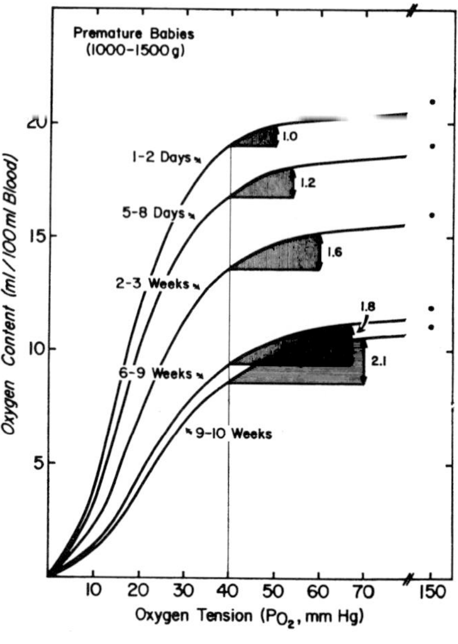


**FIGURE 77–3.** Oxygen delivery in normal term and premature infants. Oxygen content (a function of total hemoglobin) is on the ordinate. Oxygen tension is on the abscissa. Oxygen delivery is measured by the difference in oxygen content at arterial (100 mm Hg) and venous (40 mm Hg) oxygen tensions. For both term and premature infants, oxygen delivery *(shaded areas)* increases with age. This occurs despite a decrease in oxygen content. *(From Delivoria-Papadopoulos M, Roncevic NP, Oski FA: Postnatal changes in oxygen transport of term, premature, and sick infants: The role of red cell 2,3-diphosphoglycerate and adult hemoglobin. Pediatr Res 5:235, 1971.)*

**TABLE 77–2**

**Differential Approach to Anemia in the Newborn Period**

| Hemoglobin | Reticulocytes | Bilirubin | Coombs Test | Clinical Considerations |
|---|---|---|---|---|
| Decreased | Normal/decreased | Normal | Negative | Physiologic anemia of infancy and prematurity<br>Hypoplastic anemia |
| Decreased | Normal/increased | Normal | Negative | Hemorrhagic anemia |
| Decreased | Normal/increased | Increased | Positive | Immune-mediated hemolysis |
| Decreased | Normal/increased | Increased | Negative | Acquired or hereditary red blood cell defects<br>Enclosed hemorrhage with resorption of blood<br>Coombs-negative ABO incompatibility |

### Red Blood Cell Count, Hemoglobin, Hematocrit, and Red Blood Cell Indices

RBC values during the neonatal period are more variable than at any other time of life. The diagnosis of anemia must therefore be made in terms of "normal" values appropriate for gestational and postnatal ages. The mean cord blood hemoglobin of healthy term infants ranges between 14 and 20 g/100 mL (Table 77–3). Shortly after birth, however, hemoglobin concentration increases. This increase is both relative (owing to a reduction of plasma volume) and absolute (owing to placental RBC transfusion). Failure of hemoglobin to increase during the first few hours of life may be the initial sign of hemorrhagic anemia. RBC values at the end of the first week are virtually identical with those seen at birth. Anemia during the first week of life is thus defined as any hemoglobin value less than 14 g/100 mL. A significant hemoglobin decrease during this time, although within the normal range, is suggestive of hemorrhage or hemolysis. For example, 14.5 g hemoglobin at 7 days of age is abnormal for a term infant whose hemoglobin was 18.5 g at birth. A slight hemoglobin reduction normally occurs in premature infants during the first week of life. Beyond the first week, however, the hemoglobin concentration decreases in both term and premature infants (see later section, Physiologic Anemia of Infancy and Prematurity).

The electronic equipment currently used for blood counts also gives statistical information regarding erythrocyte size (MCV) and hemoglobin content (MCH). The normal MCV in older children ranges from 75 to 90 fL. MCV values of less than 75 fL are considered microcytic, whereas those over 100 fL indicate macrocytosis. Normal infant RBCs are large (MCV 105 to 125 fL), and not until 8 to 10 weeks of age does cell size approach that in older children. Neonatal microcytosis is defined as an MCV of less than 95 fL at birth. The RBC hemoglobin content of neonatal cells (MCH 35 to 38 pg/cell) is greater than that seen in older children (MCH 30 to 33 pg/cell). Neonatal hypochromia is defined as an MCH of less than 34 pg/cell. Hypochromia and microcytosis generally occur together, and invariably these abnormalities are due to hemoglobin production defects. Neonatal hypochromic microcytosis is seen with iron deficiency (chronic blood loss) and thalassemia disorders (alpha- and gamma-thalassemias).

The site at which blood is obtained is important, because hemoglobin and hematocrit are higher in capillary blood than in simultaneously obtained central venous samples (up to 20%). This difference can be minimized by warming an extremity to obtain "arterialized capillary blood" (Oh and Lind, 1966). In the face of acute hemorrhage, however, central venous samples must be obtained because of marked peripheral vasoconstriction.

**TABLE 77–3**

**RBC Values in Term and Premature Infants During the First Week of Life**

| | Hb (g/100 mL) | Hct (%) | Reticulocytes (%) | Nucleated RBCs (cells/1000 RBCs) |
|---|---|---|---|---|
| Term | | | | |
| Cord blood | 17.0 (14-20) | 53.0 (45-61) | <7 | <1.00 |
| Day 1 | 18.4 | 58.0 | <7 | <0.40 |
| Day 3 | 17.8 | 55.0 | <3 | <0.01 |
| Day 7 | 17.0 | 54.0 | <1 | 0 |
| Premature (birth weight <1500 g) | | | | |
| Cord blood | 16.0 (13.0-18.5) | 49 | <10 | <3.00 |
| Day 7 | 14.8 | 45 | <3 | <0.01 |

Hct, hematocrit; Hb, hemoglobin; RBCs, red blood cells.

### Reticulocyte Count

The normal reticulocyte count in children and older infants is 1% to 2% of the circulating red cells. The reticulocyte count in term infants ranges between 3% and 7% at birth, but this decreases to 1% to 3% by 4 days and to less than 1% by 7 days of age (see Table 77–3). In premature infants, reticulocyte values at birth are higher (6% to 10%) and may remain elevated for a longer period of time. Nucleated RBCs are seen in newborn infants, but they generally disappear by the third day of life in term infants and in 7 to 10 days in premature infants. The persistence of reticulocytosis or nucleated RBCs suggests the possibility of hemorrhage or hemolysis. Hypoxia, in the absence of anemia, also can be associated with increased release of reticulocytes and nucleated RBCs.

### Peripheral Blood Smear

Examination of the peripheral blood smear is an invaluable aid in the diagnosis of anemia. In particular, the smear is evaluated for alterations in the size and shape of RBCs as well as abnormalities in leukocytes and platelets. Erythrocytes of older children are approximately the size of a small lymphocyte nucleus, whereas those of newborns are slightly larger. RBC hemoglobinization (e.g., hypochromia) is estimated by observing the area of central pallor, which is one-third the diameter of normal RBCs and more than one-half the diameter of hypochromic cells. Spherocytes are detected by the complete absence of central pallor. The degree of reticulocytosis can be estimated, because these cells are larger and have a bluish coloration.

### Direct Antiglobulin Test

Most cases of neonatal hemolytic anemia are due to isoimmunization. The direct antiglobulin test (DAT), also known as the direct Coombs test, detects the presence of antibody on RBCs or in the plasma (indirect Coombs test). The clinician must search diligently to rule out an alloimmune disorder before embarking on a more wide-ranging (and expensive) workup of hemolysis.

## Blood Transfusions in the Treatment of Anemia

A hemoglobin of 14 g/100 mL corresponds to an RBC mass of 31 mL/kg. Thus, an RBC transfusion of 2 mL/kg will increase the hemoglobin concentration by approximately 1 g/100 mL. Packed RBCs (hematocrit approximately 67%) contain 2 mL of RBCs/3 mL of packed RBCs. Whole blood (hematocrit approximately 33%) contains 2 mL of RBCs/6 mL whole blood. Thus, the transfusion of 3 mL of packed RBCs/kg or 6 mL of whole blood/kg increases hemoglobin concentration by approximately 1 g/100 mL.

Packed RBCs are the product of choice when transfusion is necessary for simple anemia, as occurs in hemolysis. If anemia is accompanied by hypovolemia from acute blood loss, volume expansion must be achieved promptly, using either whole blood or packed RBCs and a colloid such as 5% serum albumin or plasma protein fraction (infused separately). Because of the reduced availability of whole blood, owing to the demand for its components, the usual choice is packed RBCs and colloid. The previously common practice of reconstituting RBCs with fresh frozen plasma to make "whole blood" is no longer acceptable, because the increased donor exposure increases the risk of transmitting infectious disease. When packed RBCs need to be diluted to facilitate nonurgent transfusion, isotonic saline is the preferred diluent. If exchange transfusion is needed to treat hyperbilirubinemia, the capability of albumin to improve bilirubin binding and removal is ample reason to request whole blood. Although fresh blood less than 2 days old is ideal because there is a reduced risk of hyperkalemia, this is not usually available. An acceptable substitute is packed RBCs less than 4 to 5 days old. These packed RBCs provide adequate oxygen delivery; hyperkalemia can be prevented by washing the RBCs once in saline and then reconstituting with normal saline. Washing is not required for the usually small, simple transfusions of packed RBCs, because the small volume of plasma minimizes any toxic effect of increased concentration of potassium in the plasma.

Blood currently available in most blood banks is anticoagulated with citrate-phosphate-dextrose (CPD), CPD-adenine (CPDA-1), or adenine-saline (AS-3), with a shelf life of 21, 35, or 42 days, respectively. Hematocrit usually ranges between 65% and 80% for packed RBCs. Near-normal 2,3-DPG levels are maintained for up to 12 to 14 days, which is advantageous in transfusing infants with acute hypoxia or those receiving large volumes of blood. Hematocrits range from 55% to 65%, thus facilitating flow during infusion. The newest of these preparations, AS-3, is well tolerated by newborns even after up to 42 days of storage, so long as only small-volume transfusions are given at any one time (Strauss, 2000). Designation of a single AS-3–preserved red cell donation for use by one neonate is an effective way to limit donor exposures and reduce the risk of transfusion-associated infections (Goldman, 2001).

Preterm infants born weighing less than 1250 g are uniquely susceptible to potentially serious cytomegalovirus (CMV) infection from transfused blood, particularly if they lack immunity because their mothers are seronegative. CMV infection can be prevented by using blood products only from seronegative donors (Yeager et al, 1981). Because approximately 40% to 60% of adults are seropositive, this limits the availability of seronegative donors. Reserving seronegative blood for the minority of infants who are seronegative can reduce the demand for such donors. Alternatively, because CMV resides mainly in leukocytes, removal of such cells also can prevent transmission of the virus. Transfusion of frozen thawed, deglycerolized RBCs (Brady et al, 1984) and use of high-efficiency leukocyte depletion filters (Gilbert et al, 1989) have proved effective. Transfusion of conventional saline-washed RBCs is not adequate for prevention of infection, presumably because they contain greater numbers of residual leukocytes (Demmler et al, 1986). A potential disadvantage of using CMV-seronegative blood in CMV-positive infants receiving large amounts of blood is dilution of infant's antibody level, resulting in increased susceptibility to nursery-acquired CMV infection. Currently, a majority of neonatal services utilize leukocyte-reduced red cell products rather than relying on CMV-negative products to prevent CMV infection (Engelfreit and Reesink, 2001).

Graft-versus-host (GVH) reaction rarely follows transfusion and occurs mainly in certain newborns at risk. For this to occur, viable lymphocytes in cellular blood products must be able to engraft and react against foreign antigens on tissues of the recipient. Infants at risk include those with congenital or acquired defects of cellular immunity, those who as fetuses received intrauterine transfusion of RBCs or platelets, newborns receiving exchange transfusion following intrauterine transfusion (Naiman et al, 1969; Parkman et al, 1974), and infants receiving directed blood donations from first-degree relatives (whose genetic similarity may increase the likelihood of engraftment). Irradiation of RBCs, whole blood, platelets, and granulocytes with a minimum of 1500 rads has proved effective in preventing GVH reaction. Reports of GVH reaction after RBC transfusion in very premature infants without known risk factors (Enoki et al, 1985; Sanders et al, 1989) have prompted most neonatal services to irradiate all RBC blood products (Engelfreit and Reesink, 2001).

## HEMORRHAGIC ANEMIA

Anemia frequently follows fetal blood loss, bleeding from obstetric complications, and internal hemorrhages associated with birth trauma (Table 77–4). Iatrogenic anemia due to repeated removal of blood for laboratory testing is common in premature infants. The clinical presentation of anemia depends on the magnitude and acuteness of blood loss.

Infants with anemia subsequent to moderate hemorrhage or chronic blood loss are generally asymptomatic. The only physical finding is pallor of the skin and mucous membranes. Laboratory studies can range from a mild normochromic normocytic anemia (hemoglobin 9 to 12 g/100 mL) to a more severe hypochromic microcytic anemia (hemoglobin 5 to 7 g/100 mL). The only therapy required for asymptomatic children is iron (2 mg elemental iron/kg three times a day for 3 months). RBC replacement is indicated only if there is evidence of clinical distress (tachycardia, tachypnea, irritability, feeding difficulties). In most cases, increasing the hemoglobin to 10 to 12 g/100 mL removes all signs and symptoms associated with anemia. Because severely anemic infants are frequently in incipient heart failure, however, these children should be transfused very slowly (2 mL/kg/hour). If signs of congestive heart failure appear, a rapid-acting diuretic (furosemide, 1 mg/kg intravenously) should be given before proceeding with the transfusion. An alternative approach is to administer a partial exchange transfusion with packed RBCs to severely anemic infants. This approach increases the hemoglobin concentration without the danger of increasing blood volume and precipitating congestive heart failure.

A simple formula for the volume of RBCs needed in a partial exchange transfusion to correct severe anemia has been described by Nieburg and Stockman (1977):

$$\text{Packed RBC volume needed (mL)} = \text{body weight (kg)} \times 75\ \text{mL/kg} \times \text{desired hemoglobin change} \div [22\ \text{g/dL} - \text{Hb}_w]$$

where 75 mL/kg approximates the average blood volume and 22 g/dL represents the hemoglobin concentration of packed RBCs. The term $\text{Hb}_w$ is a reflection of the hemoglobin removed during the exchange transfusion, approximated by (initial hemoglobin + desired hemoglobin)/2. For each infusion and withdrawal, syringe volumes up to 5% of the blood volume are well tolerated. For example, in the case of a 3-kg newborn with a hemoglobin of 3 g/dL that needs to be raised to a hemoglobin of 10 g/dL, approximately 100 mL of packed RBCs is needed for the procedure; syringe volumes of 15 mL can be used for each cycle of infusion and withdrawal of blood.

Infants who rapidly lose large volumes of blood appear to be in acute distress (pallor, tachycardia, tachypnea, weak pulses, hypotension, and shock). This presentation is distinct from that seen in neonatal respiratory asphyxia (slow respirations with intercostal retractions, bradycardia, and pallor with cyanosis) (Table 77–5). The clinical response to assisted ventilation and oxygen also is different: Infants with respiratory problems demonstrate a marked improvement, whereas there is little change in anemic newborns. Cyanosis is not a feature of severe anemia because the hemoglobin concentration is too low (clinical cyanosis indicates at least 5 g/100 mL of deoxygenated hemoglobin). The hemoglobin concentration immediately after an acute hemorrhage may be normal, because the initial response to acute volume depletion is vasoconstriction. A decreased hemoglobin may not be seen until the plasma volume has reexpanded several hours later. In view of these hemodynamic considerations, it is apparent that the diagnosis of acute hemorrhagic anemia is based largely on physical findings and evidence of blood loss. It is important to recognize these clinical features because immediate therapy is required. Treatment is directed at rapid expansion of the vascular space (20 mL fluid/kg). This is most quickly

**TABLE 77–4**

**Causes of Hemorrhagic Anemia in Newborns**

| |
|---|
| Fetal hemorrhage |
| Spontaneous fetomaternal hemorrhage |
| Hemorrhage following amniocentesis |
| Twin-twin transfusion |
| Nuchal cord |
| Placental hemorrhage |
| Placenta previa |
| Abruptio placentae |
| Multilobed placenta (vasa previa) |
| Velamentous insertion of cord |
| Placental incision during cesarean section |
| Umbilical cord bleeding |
| Rupture of umbilical cord with precipitous delivery |
| Rupture of short or entangled cord |
| Postpartum hemorrhage |
| Bleeding from umbilicus |
| Cephalhematomas, scalp hemorrhages |
| Hepatic rupture, splenic rupture |
| Retroperitoneal hemorrhages |

**TABLE 77-5**

**Comparative Clinical Findings in Neonatal Asphyxia and Acute Hemorrhage**

| | Neonatal Asphyxia | Acute Blood Loss |
|---|---|---|
| Heart rate | Decreased | Increased |
| Respiratory rate | Decreased | Increased |
| Intercostal retractions | Present | Absent |
| Skin color | Pallor with cyanosis | Pallor without cyanosis |
| Response to oxygen and assisted ventilation | Marked improvement | No significant change |

accomplished by rapid infusion of either isotonic saline or 5% albumin, followed by either type-specific, cross-matched whole blood or packed RBCs resuspended with saline, depending on availability. Fresh frozen plasma, formerly used for reconstituting RBCs, is no longer acceptable because of the risk of transfusion-transmissible infection. In infants in whom anemia and hypoxia are severe, non–cross-matched group O, Rh-negative RBCs are an acceptable alternative to cross-matched RBCs. Infants with hypovolemic shock caused by acute external blood loss usually show marked clinical improvement after this treatment. A poor response is seen in newborns with severe internal hemorrhage.

## Fetal Hemorrhage

### Fetomaternal Hemorrhage

Significant bleeding into the maternal circulation occurs in approximately 8% of all pregnancies and thus represents one of the most common forms of fetal bleeding. Small amounts of fetal blood are lost in most cases, but in 1% of pregnancies, fetal blood loss may exceed 40 mL (Cohen et al, 1964). Fetomaternal hemorrhage occasionally follows amniocentesis and placental injury (Zipursky et al, 1963), although anemia is seen only after unsuccessful amniocentesis or when there is evidence of a bloody tap (Woo Wang et al, 1967). For this reason, infants born to mothers who have had amniocentesis should be observed closely for signs of anemia. The effects of anemia resulting from fetomaternal hemorrhage are variable. Large acute hemorrhages can produce hypovolemic shock (Raye et al, 1970), whereas slower, more chronic blood loss results in hypochromic microcytic anemia resulting from iron deficiency (Pearson and Diamond, 1959). Some infants with severe chronic anemia (hemoglobin as low as 4 to 6 g/100 mL) may have minimal symptoms.

An examination of maternal blood for the presence of fetal cells is necessary in any infant with suspected fetomaternal hemorrhage. Two techniques are available. The Kleihauer-Betke preparation involves examination of a stained specimen of maternal blood by microscopy following differential elution of hemoglobin A but not hemoglobin F from the red cells. Alternative, flow cytometry–based techniques are probably more accurate but are less widely available and require blood group antigen incompatibility between fetus and mother (Chapman et al, 1999, Fong et al, 2000).

Approximately 50 mL of fetal blood must be lost to produce significant neonatal anemia. This volume is greater than 1% of the maternal blood volume, and therefore fetal cells within the maternal circulation may be detected readily. Tests that depend on the presence of fetal hemoglobin are not valid when a maternal hemoglobinopathy with increased hemoglobin F levels coexists. In addition, fetomaternal ABO incompatibility may cause rapid removal of fetal RBCs, thus obscuring any significant hemorrhage. For this reason, it is important to examine maternal blood as soon as anemia from fetal hemorrhage is suspected. An unusual form of fetal blood loss is presumed to occur in infants born with a nuchal cord. In these cases, anemia is caused by compression of the umbilical vein, preventing placental blood from returning to the fetus (Shepherd et al, 1985).

### Twin-Twin Transfusion

Transfusion of blood from one monozygous twin to another can result in anemia in the donor twin and polycythemia in the recipient. Significant hemorrhage is seen only in monochorionic monozygous twins (approximately 70% of all monozygous twins). In approximately 15% to 35% of these pregnancies, there is a twin-to-twin transfusion (Rausen et al, 1965; van Gemert et al, 2001). Bleeding occurs because of vascular anastomosis in monochorionic placentas. The anemic donor twin is usually smaller than the polycythemic recipient, with a greater than 20% difference in birth weight. Polyhydramnios is frequently seen in the recipient twin and oligohydramnios is seen in the donor. The high rate of intrauterine mortality (approximately 63% with conservative management) has spurred attempts at fetal therapy, including decompression amniocentesis, laser coagulation of vascular anastamoses, interfetal septal disruptions, and selective feticide (Seng and Rajadurai, 2000; van Gemert et al, 2001). Twin-twin transfusions should be suspected when the hemoglobin concentration of identical twins differs by more than 5 g/100 mL; however, such a difference in hemoglobin concentration does not prove there has been a twin-twin transfusion. Recent studies indicate that this major hemoglobin difference can exist in some dichorionic twins, in whom there are no vascular anastomoses and therefore no possibility for twin-twin transfusion (Danskin and Neilson, 1989).

## Placental Blood Loss

Placental bleeding during pregnancy is common, but in most cases hemorrhage is from the maternal aspect of the placenta. In placenta previa, however, the thinness of the placenta overlying the cervical os frequently results in fetal blood loss. The vascular communications between multilobular placental lobes also are very fragile and are easily subjected to trauma during delivery. *Vasa previa* is the condition in which one of these connecting vessels overlies the cervical os and thus is prone to rupture during delivery. *Abruptio placentae* generally causes fetal anoxia and death, although some infants survive but can be severely anemic. Bleeding also follows inadvertent placental incision during cesarean section (Montague and Krevans, 1966), and thus the placenta should be inspected for injury following all cesarean sections.

### Umbilical Cord Bleeding

The normal umbilical cord is resistant to minor trauma and does not bleed. The umbilical cord of dysmature infants, however, is weak and liable to rupture and hemorrhage (Raye et al, 1970). In cases of precipitous delivery, a rapid increase in cord tension can rupture the fetal aspect of the cord, causing serious acute blood loss. Short or entangled umbilical cords and abnormalities of umbilical blood vessels (velamentous insertions into the placenta) are also liable to rupture and hemorrhage. Bleeding from injured umbilical cords is rapid but generally ceases after a short period of time, owing to arterial constriction. The umbilical cord should always be inspected for abnormalities or signs of injury, particularly after unattended, precipitous deliveries.

### Hemorrhage after Delivery

Hemorrhagic anemia due to internal bleeding is occasionally associated with birth trauma. Characteristically, internal hemorrhages are asymptomatic during the first 24 to 48 hours of life, with signs and symptoms of anemia developing after this time. Cephalhematomas can be sufficiently large to cause anemia and hyperbilirubinemia, secondary to the resorption of blood (Leonard and Anthony, 1961). Subgaleal hemorrhages are seen infrequently, sometimes after vacuum extraction used during delivery. These hemorrhages may be extensive because bleeding is not limited by periosteum. Adrenal and kidney hemorrhages occasionally follow difficult breech deliveries. Splenic rupture and hemorrhage occur most commonly in association with splenomegaly, as in erythroblastosis fetalis. Hepatic hemorrhages are generally subcapsular and may be asymptomatic. Rupture of the hepatic capsule results in hemoperitoneum and hypovolemic shock. Hepatic hemorrhages are suspected when a previously healthy infant goes into shock with clinical manifestations of an increasing right upper quadrant abdominal mass, shifting dullness on percussion, and evidence of free fluid on abdominal radiographs. In contrast with newborns with acute blood loss from fetomaternal or umbilical vessel bleeding, infants with hepatic hemorrhage generally demonstrate a poor clinical response to blood replacement.

## HEMOLYTIC ANEMIA

RBCs from children and adults normally circulate for 100 to 120 days. Erythrocyte survival in newborns is somewhat shorter: 70 to 90 days in term infants, 50 to 80 days in premature infants (Pearson, 1967). Hemolytic anemia, which further shortens RBC survival, may arise for many reasons (Table 77–6). The precise mechanism of cell destruction is not always known, although membrane deformability is thought to be an important determinant (LaCelle, 1970). Erythrocytes are 7 to 8 μm wide, whereas the vascular diameter in some areas of the microcirculation may be less than 3 μm. Consequently, RBCs must deform their membranes and intracellular contents in order to pass through these narrow channels. This requirement is no problem for normal RBCs. Abnormalities in RBC metabolism, hemoglobin, or cell shape, however, all lead to decreased RBC membrane deformability. The consequence of this decreased membrane flexibility is RBC sequestration and removal by reticuloendothelial cells of the spleen and liver.

In older infants and children, the usual response to increased RBC destruction is enhanced erythropoiesis, and there may be little or no anemia if the rate of production matches the accelerated rate of destruction. In these cases of well-compensated hemolysis, the major manifestations are due to increased erythrocyte destruction (hyperbilirubinemia) and augmented erythropoiesis (reticulocytosis). During the early neonatal period, however, the increased oxygen-carrying capacity of blood (see later section, Physiologic Anemia of Infancy and Prematurity) may blunt any compensatory erythropoietic activity in cases of mild hemolysis. Consequently, hyperbilirubinemia in excess of normal neonatal levels may be the only apparent manifestation of hemolysis. In most cases of significant hemolysis, however, some degree of reticulocytosis is usually present. The degree of hyperbilirubinemia and reticulocytosis must be interpreted in terms of values appropriate for gestational and postgestational ages.

**TABLE 77–6**

**Causes of Hemolytic Anemia During the Newborn Period**

**Immune Disorders**
- Isoimmune: Rh and ABO incompatibility
- Maternal immune disease: autoimmune hemolytic anemia, systemic lupus erythematosus
- Drug-induced: penicillin

**Acquired Red Blood Cell (RBC) Disorders**
- Infection: cytomegalovirus toxoplasmosis, syphilis, bacterial sepsis
- Disseminated and localized intravascular coagulation, respiratory distress syndrome

**Hereditary RBC Disorders**
- Membrane defects: hereditary spherocytosis, hereditary elliptocytosis
- Enzyme abnormalities: glucose-6-phosphate dehydrogenase pyruvate kinase
- Hemoglobinopathies: alpha-thalassemia syndromes, gamma/beta-thalassemia

### Immune Hemolysis

Placental transfer of maternal antibodies directed against fetal RBC antigens is the most common cause of neonatal hemolysis. This phenomenon is a consequence of maternal sensitization to fetal RBC antigens inherited from the father. Hemolysis occurs only in the fetus. The spectrum of clinical problems ranges from minimal anemia and hyperbilirubinemia to severe anemia with hydrops fetalis. At one time, before effective prevention of Rh sensitization was available, hemolytic disease of the newborn was responsible for more than 10,000 deaths annually in the United States (Freda et al, 1975). Since the development of immunoprophylaxis against Rh(D) sensitization, the overall incidence of alloimmune hemolysis has decreased dramatically. Nevertheless, a majority of *serious* alloimmune hemolysis cases are still due to Rh(D) incompatibility, although ABO maternal-fetal incompatibility is much more common. A much smaller fraction of neonatal hemolytic disease is due to sensitization to Kell, Duffy, Kidd, and other Rh antigens such as c and E.

### Rh Hemolytic Disease: Erythroblastosis Fetalis

The role of Rh antibody in classic erythroblastosis fetalis was first elucidated by Levine and Katzin in 1941. Several Rh antigens are recognized, each of which is detected by specific antibodies. It is known that Rh blood group antigens are determined by at least two homologous but distinct membrane-associated proteins. Two of these membrane proteins have separate isoforms (C and c; E and e), which are detected by specific antibodies (anti-C and anti-c; anti-E and anti-e). The most important of the membrane Rh proteins is the D antigen. Rh-positive RBCs are those that possess this antigen. A lowercase d is used to denote the absence of D, or Rh-negative status; it is not related to a specific antigen—no "anti-d" serum has been identified. Rh proteins are encoded by two separate genes located on chromosome 1; they are designated *RHCE* and *RHD* (Mouro et al, 1993). The *RHCE* gene encodes both the C/c and E/e proteins. The *RHD* gene encodes the Rh D proteins. The Rh-negative phenotype results from deletion of the *RHD* gene on both chromosomes. In most cases, the Rh-negative phenotype also is associated with Rh c and Rh e (i.e., Rh cde). The frequency of Rh negativity varies in different racial groups. It is high in whites (15%), lower in blacks (5%), and virtually nonexistent in Asians. The Rh-positive phenotype may result from homozygosity (DD) or heterozygosity (Dd) for the D antigen. In Rh-positive whites, approximately 44% are homozygous (DD) and 56% are heterozygous (Dd). Knowledge of differences in *RHD* genotype is important because approximately 25% of fetuses of couples with an Rh(D)-negative mother and an Rh(D)-positive father will be Rh(D)-negative.

Current understanding of the natural history of Rh sensitization is derived largely from clinical experience gained before the immunologic prevention of neonatal hemolysis was readily available. The pathophysiology of alloimmune hemolysis resulting from Rh incompatibility includes the following: an Rh-negative mother, an Rh-positive fetus, leakage of fetal RBCs into maternal circulation, maternal sensitization to D antigen on fetal RBCs, production and transplacental passage of maternal anti-D antibodies into fetal circulation, attachment of maternal antibodies to Rh-positive fetal RBCs, and destruction of antibody-coated fetal RBCs. Historically, Rh hemolytic disease was rare (occurring in 1% of cases) during the first pregnancy involving an Rh-positive fetus but increased significantly with each subsequent pregnancy. Small volumes of fetal RBCs enter the maternal circulation throughout gestation, although the major fetomaternal bleeding responsible for sensitization occurs during delivery (Zipursky et al, 1963). Once sensitization has occurred, reexposure to Rh(D) RBCs in subsequent pregnancies leads to an anamnestic response, with an increase in the maternal anti-D titer. Currently, significant hemolysis occurring in the first pregnancy indicates prior maternal exposure to Rh-positive RBCs, a consequence of fetal bleeding associated with a previous spontaneous or therapeutic abortion, ectopic pregnancy, or a variety of different prenatal procedures. On occasion the sensitization may be a consequence of an earlier transfusion in which Rh-positive RBCs were administered by mistake or in which some other blood component (e.g., platelets) containing Rh(D) RBCs was transfused.

The major factor responsible for the reduced death rate is the development of Rh immune globulin to prevent maternal sensitization. Important early observations were that fetomaternal RBC transfer (and thereby sensitization) occurs primarily during delivery and that the frequency of Rh immune hemolytic disease was much lower in ABO-incompatible pregnancies (maternal RBC type O, fetal RBC type A or B). The apparent beneficial effect of ABO incompatibility is due to the fact that maternal anti-A and anti-B antibodies recognize the corresponding A and B fetal RBCs, leading to their destruction before sensitization can occur. As a result of these early observations, it became standard practice for unsensitized Rh-negative mothers to receive a single intramuscular dose of Rh immune globulin (300 $\mu$g) within 72 hours of delivering of an Rh-positive infant (Freda et al, 1975). The results of this therapy were remarkable, with the virtual elimination of Rh(D) sensitization as a major cause of hemolytic disease in newborns. The few treatment failures seen were attributed to fetomaternal bleeding of greater than 30 mL at delivery or bleeding that occurred antenatally. The current standard of practice is to administer a full dose of Rh immune globulin to all unsensitized Rh-negative women at 28 weeks of gestation, with an additional dose given at birth if the infant is Rh-positive. Moreover, the dose of Rh immune globulin should be increased proportionately when there is evidence of larger-than-normal fetomaternal bleeding at delivery. All newborns should be screened using the rosette test to screen for fetal red cells (Brecher, 2002). Positive results should be followed by a quantitative test such as the Kleihauer-Betke test (Judd, 2001). In suspicious cases (e.g., with placental abruption or neonatal anemia), the volume of fetal hemorrhage can be quantified using the Kleihauer-Betke procedure. Rh immune globulin also should be administered to unsensitized Rh-negative women after any event known to be associated with increased risk of fetomaternal hemorrhage (e.g., spontaneous or therapeutic abortion, amniocentesis, chorionic villus biopsy). The risk of anti-Rh desensitization ranges from 0.6% to 5.4% when nonsensitized Rh-negative women undergo amniocentesis (Spinnato, 1992).

In pregnant Rh-negative women previously sensitized to Rh(D), the transplacental passage of maternal anti-D leads to a positive DAT on Rh(D) fetal RBCs. Depending on the amount of anti-D absorbed, a variable degree of fetal hemolysis occurs, thereby leading to anemia, hepatosplenomegaly, and increased bilirubin formation. In utero, bilirubin is removed by transfer across the placenta into the maternal circulation; therefore, hyperbilirubinemia is not a problem until after delivery, when levels may increase because of immaturity of hepatic conjugating enzymes. The major threat to the fetus is severe anemia leading to hydrops fetalis and intrauterine death. The clinical severity of neonatal hemolytic disease varies.

*Mild hemolytic disease* is most common, manifested by a positive DAT with minimal hemolysis, little or no anemia (cord blood hemoglobin greater than 14 g/dL), and minimal hyperbilirubinemia (cord blood bilirubin less than 4 mg/dL). Aside from early phototherapy, these newborns generally require no therapy unless the postnatal rate of rise in bilirubin is greater than expected. Infants who do not become sufficiently jaundiced to require exchange transfusion are at risk of development of severe late anemia associated with a low reticulocyte count, usually at 3 to 6 weeks of age; thus, it is important to closely monitor hemoglobin levels after hospital discharge.

*Moderate hemolytic disease* is found in a smaller fraction of affected infants. This form is characterized by hemolysis, moderate anemia (cord blood hemoglobin less than 14 g/dL), and increased cord blood bilirubin levels (greater than 4 mg/dL). The peripheral blood may reveal numerous nucleated RBCs, decreased numbers of platelets, and occasionally a leukemoid reaction with large numbers of immature granulocytes. The cause of thrombocytopenia is not understood, but it is unlikely to be an immune reaction, because platelets lack Rh antigens. Similarly, the cause of the leukemoid reaction is not defined, although rarely it may be confused with congenital leukemia. Infants with Rh disease also may exhibit marked hepatosplenomegaly, a consequence of extramedullary hematopoiesis and sequestration of antibody-coated RBCs. The risk of development of bilirubin encephalopathy is high if these neonates do not receive treatment. Thus, early exchange transfusion with type O Rh-negative fresh RBCs (less than 5 days old) is usually necessary, in conjunction with intensive phototherapy. This approach has been responsible for the favorable outcome for most infants with moderate alloimmune hemolysis. It is common for newborns who receive exchange transfusion to demonstrate a lower-than-normal hemoglobin concentration at the nadir of their "physiologic" anemia. Therefore, follow-up evaluation of hemoglobin for at least 2 months is important. The decrease in hemoglobin may be due in part to persistence of some anti-D antibody and destruction of the patient's own Rh(D)-positive RBCs. Also, this low hemoglobin measurement may reflect the decreased oxygen affinity and enhanced oxygen delivery of adult RBCs used for the exchange process, thereby blunting the expected erythropoietic response to hypoxia. Preliminary data suggest that the administration of recombinant human erythropoietin (rHuEPO) may minimize this late anemia of Rh hemolytic disease (Scaradavou et al, 1993; Ovali et al, 1996).

*Severe hemolytic disease* is seen in approximately 25% of affected infants, who are either stillborn or hydropic at birth. Understanding of hydrops fetalis, originally attributed to high-output cardiac failure secondary to severe anemia, is incomplete. Two other consequences of anemia also may contribute to the edema of hydrops. One of these is low colloid osmotic pressure resulting from hypoalbuminemia, a consequence of hepatic dysfunction. The second is a capillary leak syndrome secondary to tissue hypoxia. Management of seriously affected fetuses is directed at the prevention of severe anemia and death. To accomplish this, it first is necessary to identify those fetuses at risk. An increase in the maternal anti-D titer in a previously sensitized Rh-negative woman is a good serologic measure of a fetus in potential jeopardy. Moreover, a previous history of neonatal hemolytic disease resulting from anti-D antibodies suggests that the current fetus also may be at risk. In this regard it may be useful to know the fetal Rh blood type because this identifies those Rh-negative infants who are not at risk. In many cases this can be accomplished by direct Rh typing of fetal RBCs obtained via cordocentesis. Alternatively, molecular biologic techniques can be used to determine the Rh genotype in DNA obtained from amniocytes or chorionic villus samples (Bennett et al, 1993; Fisk et al, 1994). When the fetus is found to be Rh-negative, no further maternal monitoring or fetal blood studies are necessary.

An increase in the maternal titer of immunoglobulin G (IgG) anti-D indicates maternal sensitization but does not accurately predict the potential severity of fetal hemolysis. A better correlation is obtained by spectrophotometric estimation of bile pigment in amniotic fluid as measured by the deviation in optical density (OD) at 450 nm (Fig. 77–4). Amniocentesis should be done when the indirect antiglobulin test exceeds a critical threshold level (1:16 to 1:32). Plotting the "delta OD 450 nm" against fetal age provides a good correlation with the severity of fetal hemolysis during the third trimester, and the trend of two or more values is a more reliable predictor of severity of fetal disease (Liley, 1961). Fetuses with amniotic fluid delta OD values in zone 3 (see Fig. 77–4) or increasing toward zone 3 are at greatest risk of intrauterine death from severe anemia and hydrops fetalis.

In earlier studies, at-risk fetuses greater than 32 weeks of gestation with evidence of mature lung function were delivered early. However, for those fetuses less than 32 weeks of gestation with immature lung function, early delivery was not possible and fetal RBC transfusions were given. Initially, intrauterine RBC transfusions were administered through the peritoneal cavity, and this procedure ameliorated the anemia sufficiently to save many otherwise doomed fetuses (Liley, 1963). However, in some of these cases in which hydrops was already present, the success rate was much lower because RBC absorption from the peritoneal cavity (complicated by ascites) was too slow to reverse the effects of severe anemia and hypoxia.

In severely affected fetuses, hydrops may occur as early as 20 to 22 weeks of gestation. Moreover, in these instances, the Liley amniocentesis curves (which were derived from studies of fetuses after 27 weeks of gestation) do not accurately predict severe disease (Nicolaides et al, 1988). However, the development of high-resolution ultrasound techniques has been a major advance that facilitates detection of early hydrops (ascites and edema)

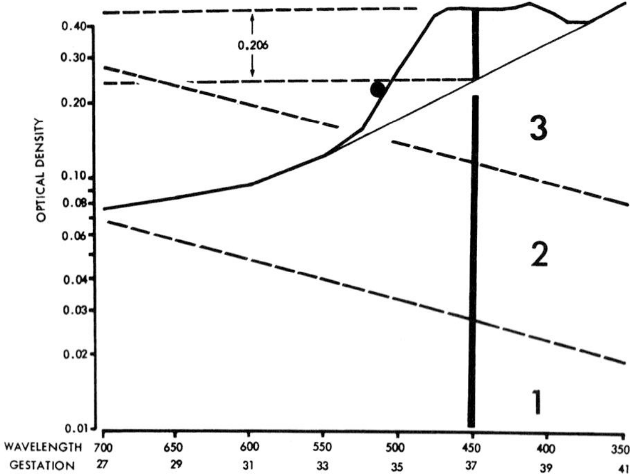


**FIGURE 77–4.** This composite graph depicts how spectrophotometric estimation of amniotic fluid bilirubin levels can be used as an indicator of fetal jeopardy from hemolytic disease. To begin, the optical density of amniotic fluid (ordinate) is measured from 700 to 350 nm (abscissa—top). This absorption curve is depicted as the *heavy solid line*. Next, the contribution of bilirubin to this absorption is calculated by subtracting the optical density of the projected baseline (*fine solid line*) from the measured optical density at 450 nm. In this case, the calculated value is 0.206. This calculated contribution of bilirubin is then plotted as a function of gestational age (abscissa—bottom). In this particular patient, the gestational age of 34.5 weeks and the bilirubin absorption of 0.206 determine the point indicated by the *solid dot*. The *dashed lines* demarcate three zones: Zone 1 indicates an unsensitized infant or one with very mild hemolytic disease. Zone 2 indicates mild to moderate hemolytic disease. Zone 3 represents severe hemolytic disease with impending fetal death. Because the bilirubin concentration of amniotic fluid decreases with gestational age, the absolute optical density that places a fetus in zone 3 decreases as the length of gestation increases. In the case depicted here, an absorption of 0.206 at 34.5 weeks of gestation indicated severe (zone 3) disease, placing the fetus at serious risk. *(From Bowman JM, Pollock JM: Amniotic fluid spectrophotometry and early delivery in the management of erythroblastosis fetalis. Pediatrics 35:815, 1965. Reproduced with permission from Pediatrics.)*

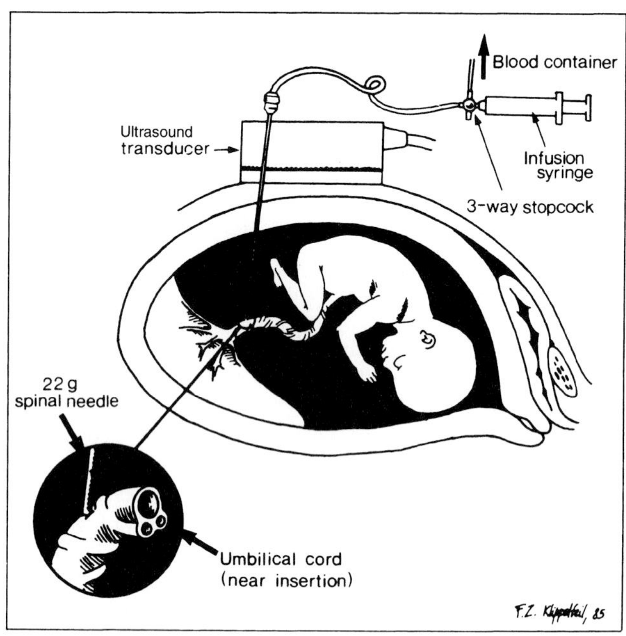


**FIGURE 77–5.** Diagrammatic view of in utero direct intravascular transfusion. U/S, ultrasound. *(From Grannum PA, Copel JA, Plaxe SC, et al: In utero exchange transfusion by direct intravascular injection in severe erythroblastosis fetalis. N Engl J Med 314:1431, 1986. Reprinted by permission of the New England Journal of Medicine.)*

and enables direct percutaneous umbilical blood sampling (PUBS) (cordocentesis) for determination of red cell antigen typing and measurement of fetal hematocrit or hemoglobin levels (Fig. 77–5). Fetal hydrops does not occur until hemoglobin concentration of the fetus decreases below approximately about 4 g/dL (or hematocrit below approximately 15%). However, the hemoglobin concentration of normal fetuses increases gradually during the latter part of pregnancy; thus, hemoglobin values in affected fetuses must be interpreted relative to those in normal subjects for the same stage of gestation (Nicolaides et al, 1988). A reference range for normal fetuses and fetuses with varying degrees of hemolysis is seen in Figure 77–6. Expressing the degree of anemia as "hemoglobin deficit" (grams per deciliter below the normal mean hemoglobin value for age), three zones of severity have been defined:

Zone I (mild): deficit less than 2 g/dL
Zone II (moderate): deficit 2 to 7 g/dL
Zone III (severe, hydropic): deficit 7 to 10 g/dL

The use of ultrasound examination, which allows fetal blood sampling through a 22-gauge spinal needle, has reduced the rate of fetal trauma and morbidity associated with cordocentesis to less than 2% (Parer, 1988). Cordocentesis also has facilitated direct intravascular RBC

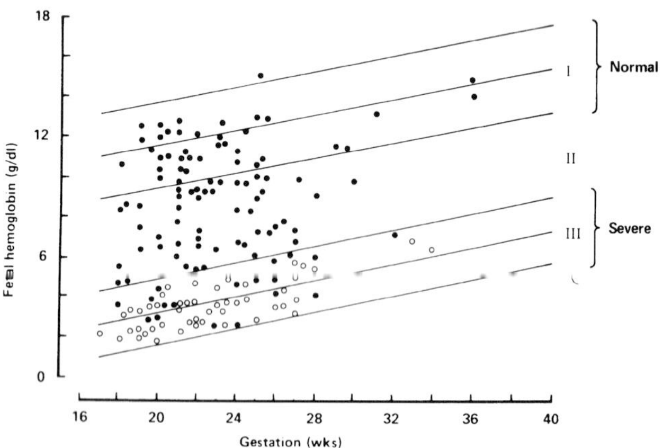


**FIGURE 77–6.** Fetal hemoglobin concentration of 48 hydropic *(open circles)* and 106 nonhydropic *(solid circles)* fetuses from red blood cell isoimmunized pregnancies at time of first fetal blood sampling. Values are plotted on the reference range of fetal hemoglobin for gestation. The individual 95% confidence intervals of the normal hemoglobin for gestation define zone I, and the individual 95% confidence intervals of the hemoglobin for gestation define zone III. Zone II indicates moderate anemia. *(From Nicolaides JH, Soothill PW, Clewell WH, et al: Fetal hemoglobin measurement in the assessment of red cell isoimmunization. Lancet 1:1073, 1988.)*

transfusion to correct severe life-threatening anemia, with the reversal of established hydrops in most cases (Grannum et al, 1988; Rodeck et al, 1984). Depending on the age of the fetus and severity of anemia, the desired volume of RBCs transfused generally is that which will achieve a post-transfusion hematocrit of approximately 35% to 45%. When RBC transfusion induces a reversal of hydrops, the serum albumin also increases; this finding supports the role of anemia in the pathogenesis of the low albumin levels. Both simple transfusions and exchange transfusions have been performed in a number of fetuses (Grannum et al, 1986). Most perinatologists prefer simple RBC transfusion because of its shorter duration, aiming for a post-transfusion hematocrit no greater than 45% to avert circulatory overload (Weiner et al, 1991).

Hyperbilirubinemia (with elevation of the conjugated fraction) often develops in newborns who have received intrauterine RBC transfusions and often predicts the need for exchange transfusions. This hyperbilirubinemia reflects the severity of hemolysis and its effects on the fetal liver. In some cases, anemia may be minimal or absent, and the DAT may be negative if the Rh-negative RBCs transfused prenatally still predominate. In such cases the infant may not require exchange transfusion. Neonatal exchange transfusion, amniocentesis, selective early induction of delivery, and intrauterine fetal blood transfusions all have contributed to the declining neonatal death rate from Rh incompatibility (Fig. 77–7).

### ABO Incompatibility

Hemolysis associated with ABO incompatibility is similar to Rh hemolytic disease in that maternal anti-A or anti-B antibodies enter the fetal circulation and react with A or B antigens on the erythrocyte surface (Table 77–7). In persons with type A and type B blood, naturally occurring anti-B and anti-A isoantibodies largely are IgM molecules that do not cross the placenta. In contrast, the alloantibodies present in persons with type O blood are predominantly IgG molecules (Abelson and Rawson, 1961). For this reason, ABO incompatibility is largely limited to type O mothers with type A or B fetuses. The presence of IgG anti-A or anti-B antibodies in type O mothers also explains why hemolysis caused by ABO incompatibility frequently occurs during the first pregnancy without prior "sensitization." ABO incompatibility is present in approximately 12% of pregnancies, although evidence of fetal RBC sensitization (i.e., positive result on DAT) is found in only 3% of births, and less than 1% of live births are associated with significant hemolysis (Kaplan et al, 1976; Zipursky et al, 1963). The relative mildness of neonatal ABO hemolytic disease contrasts sharply with the findings in Rh incompatibility. In large part, this is because A and B antigens are present in many tissues besides RBCs; consequently, only a small fraction of anti-A or anti-B antibody that crosses the placenta actually binds to erythrocytes, the remainder being absorbed by other tissues and soluble A and B substances in plasma.

Although hemolytic disease resulting from ABO incompatibility is clinically milder than Rh disease, severe hemolysis occasionally occurs, and hydrops fetalis has been reported. In such cases it is essential to exclude other antibodies and nonimmune causes of hemolysis such as glucose-6-phosphate dehydrogenase (G6PD) deficiency or hereditary spherocytosis. In most cases, pallor and jaundice are minimal (see Table 77–7). Hepatosplenomegaly is uncommon. Laboratory features include evidence of minimal to moderate hyperbilirubinemia and, occasionally, some degree of anemia. The DAT frequently is negative,

**TABLE 77-7**

**Clinical and Laboratory Features of Immune Hemolysis Due to Rh Disease and ABO Incompatibility**

| | Rh Disease | ABO Incompatibility |
|---|---|---|
| **Clinical Features** | | |
| Frequency | Unusual | Common |
| Pallor | Marked | Minimal |
| Jaundice | Marked | Minimal to moderate |
| Hydrops | Common | Rare |
| Hepatosplenomegaly | Marked | Minimal |
| **Laboratory Features** | | |
| Blood type | | |
| Mother | Rh(−) | O |
| Infant | Rh(+) | A or B |
| Anemia | Marked | Minimal |
| Direct Coombs test | Positive | Frequently negative |
| Indirect Coombs test | Positive | Usually positive |
| Hyperbilirubinemia | Marked | Variable |
| RBC morphology | Nucleated RBCs | Spherocytes |

RBC, red blood cell.

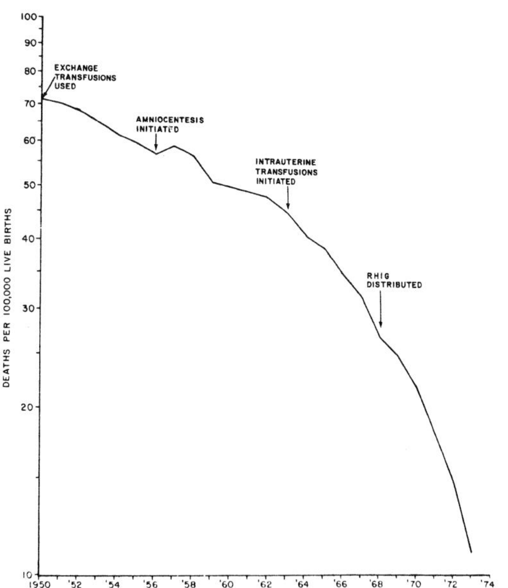


**FIGURE 77–7.** Infant death rates from hemolytic disease of the newborn, United States, 1950 to 1973. *(From Centers for Disease Control: Rh Hemolytic Disease Surveillance Annual Report, Atlanta, GA, June 1975.)*

although the indirect antiglobulin test (neonatal serum plus adult group A or B RBCs) more commonly is positive. This paradox is related to the fact that fetal RBCs, compared with adult erythrocytes, have less type-specific antigen on their surface (Voak and Williams, 1971). Heat elution is the most sensitive test for anti-A or anti-B antibodies on infant red cells, but like the antiglobulin tests, it has poor predictive value for hemolysis. Studies of the subclass of the IgG anti-A and anti-B in maternal serum and on red cells of ABO-incompatible infants point to a possible explanation (Brouwers et al, 1988). The most common subclass is IgG2, which crosses the placenta but does not bind to Fc receptors of phagocytic cells and therefore is incapable of causing cell lysis. This finding accounts for the frequent observation of positive indirect and direct antiglobulin tests with little or no hemolysis. On the other hand, IgG3 antibodies and, to a lesser extent, IgG1 antibodies, although present in lower concentrations on fetal RBCs, do bind to Fc receptors and have strong lytic activity. This seems to account for cases of hemolysis associated with a negative or only weakly positive DAT.

The peripheral blood smear is characterized by marked spherocytosis, which is thought to be due to the reduced RBC surface area that results as antibody and membrane are removed by splenic macrophages. Autoimmune hemolytic anemia in older children is associated with antibodies directed against the Rh locus, and these cases also are characterized by spherocytosis. For unknown reasons, spherocytes are not a prominent feature of neonatal hemolysis resulting from Rh incompatibility.

Hemolysis in ABO incompatibility is usually mild, presenting with some degree of hyperbilirubinemia. Of major concern in the current cost-conscious health care environment is that some infants with ABO incompatibility may be discharged home from medical establishments before significant clinical jaundice is evident. *It is critical that infants with ABO incompatibility be monitored closely for evolving jaundice and hyperbilirubinemia in the first few days of life.* In most cases, hyperbilirubinemia is readily controlled by phototherapy (Osborn et al, 1984). When hyperbilirubinemia is not controlled by phototherapy, exchange transfusion is necessary using group O Rh-compatible RBCs. Tin-protoporphyrin, an inhibitor of heme catabolism to bilirubin, may help prevent hyperbilirubinemia in ABO-incompatible infants (Kappas et al, 1988). Additional follow-up at 2 to 3 weeks of age to check for anemia in these infants is essential.

### Minor Blood Group Incompatibility

With the sharp decline of hemolytic disease caused by Rh incompatibility, the proportion of cases caused by Rh c, Rh E, Kell, Duff, and Kidd incompatibility has increased from the previous estimates of 1% to 3%, to as high as 20% (for Kell sensitization). The pathophysiology of these disorders is similar to that of Rh and ABO incompatibility. The infrequency of minor group incompatibility is primarily a reflection of the lower antigenicity of these RBC antigens. Diagnosis of minor group incompatibility is suggested by hemolytic anemia with a positive DAT in the absence of ABO or Rh incompatibility and with a negative maternal DAT. Definitive diagnosis requires identification of the specific antibody in neonatal serum or an eluate from neonatal RBCs. This is readily accomplished by testing maternal serum against a variety of known RBC antigens. With some antibodies such as Kell, antibody titer and amniocentesis findings may underestimate the severity of fetal hemolysis. Therefore, frequent ultrasound monitoring may be necessary, with performance of fetal blood sampling in worrisome cases. Fetal blood sampling also is useful in determining whether the fetus of a heterozygous father has inherited the offending RBC antigen. This test identifies those fetuses that need further serial evaluations.

### Immune Hemolytic Anemia Due to Maternal Disease

Maternal autoimmune hemolytic anemia or lupus erythrematous during pregnancy may be associated with passive transfer of IgG antibody to the fetus. The diagnosis is suggested by the presence of neonatal hemolytic disease, a positive DAT, absence of Rh or ABO incompatibility, and antiglobulin-positive hemolysis in the mother. Treatment with prednisone in the mother may reduce both maternal hemolysis and the risk of neonatal morbidity. As in other cases of neonatal hemolysis, attempts are made to prevent hyperbilirubinemia and kernicterus.

### Drug-Induced Immune Hemolysis

The classic example of drug-induced immune hemolysis is seen following administration of penicillin and appears when an antibody is directed to a complex of penicillin bound to the RBC membrane. No hemolysis occurs in the absence of penicillin, even though antibody persists in the circulation. This type of drug-mediated immune hemolysis is seen rarely in newborn infants. Cephalosporin drugs also have been implicated to cause immune-mediated hemolysis by a similar mechanism. In all of these cases, the DAT may be positive only when the test is done in the presence of the drug in question. Moreover, hemolysis ceases once the drug is withdrawn.

## Nonimmune Acquired Hemolytic Disease

### Infection

Cytomegalic inclusion disease, toxoplasmosis, syphilis, and bacterial sepsis all can be associated with hemolytic anemia. In most of these conditions, some degree of thrombocytopenia also exists. Generally, hepatosplenomegaly is present. In cases of bacterial sepsis, both the direct and indirect bilirubin levels may be elevated. The mechanism of hemolysis is not clearly defined, but it may be related to RBC sequestration in the presence of marked reticuloendothelial hyperplasia associated with infection. Documentation of infection as the cause of hemolysis is made by the presence of other clinical and laboratory evidence of neonatal infections. Hemolysis caused by infections may be exhibited early in the neonatal period, or it can be delayed for several weeks.

### Schistocytic Anemias

Disseminated intravascular coagulation (DIC) is discussed in Chapter 76. The hemolytic component of this disorder is secondary to the deposition of fibrin within the vascular walls. When erythrocytes interact with fibrin, fragments of RBCs are broken off, producing fragile, deformed RBCs, or schistocytes. These cells are relatively rigid and thus incapable of normal deformation within the microcirculation. The hemolytic-uremic syndrome represents a localized form of intravascular coagulation that is characterized by thrombocytopenia, renal disease, and hemolytic anemia. Hemolysis is characterized by RBC fragmentation, presumably for the aforementioned reasons. Abnormalities of the placental microcirculation or macrovascular anomalies such as an umbilical vein varix are rare causes of congenital schistocytic anemia (Batton et al, 2000).

## Hereditary Red Blood Cell Disorders

### Membrane Defects

The customary findings in RBC membrane disorders are the presence of dominant inheritance, abnormal RBC morphology (Fig. 77–8), and either increased or decreased osmotic fragility. Aside from hereditary spherocytosis, these disorders are uncommon.

### Hereditary Spherocytosis

The hallmark of hereditary spherocytosis is the presence in the circulation of spherocytes, cells that have become spheroid because of a loss of membrane surface with no concomitant loss in volume. Inherited mutations in components of the membrane cytoskeleton (spectrin, ankyrin,

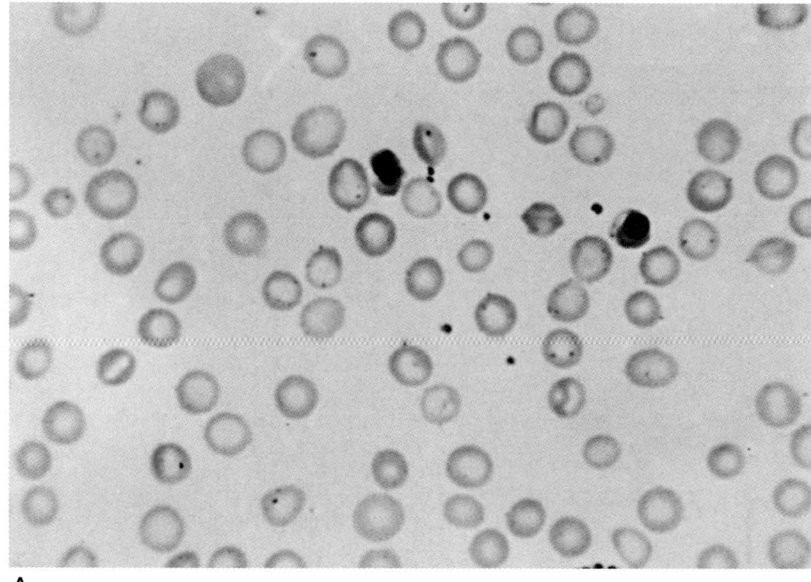


**FIGURE 77–8. A,** Hypochromic-microcytic red blood cells (RBCs) secondary to chronic fetal blood loss. **B,** Fetal RBCs in the maternal blood after a fetomaternal hemorrhage (acid-elution technique).

*Continued*

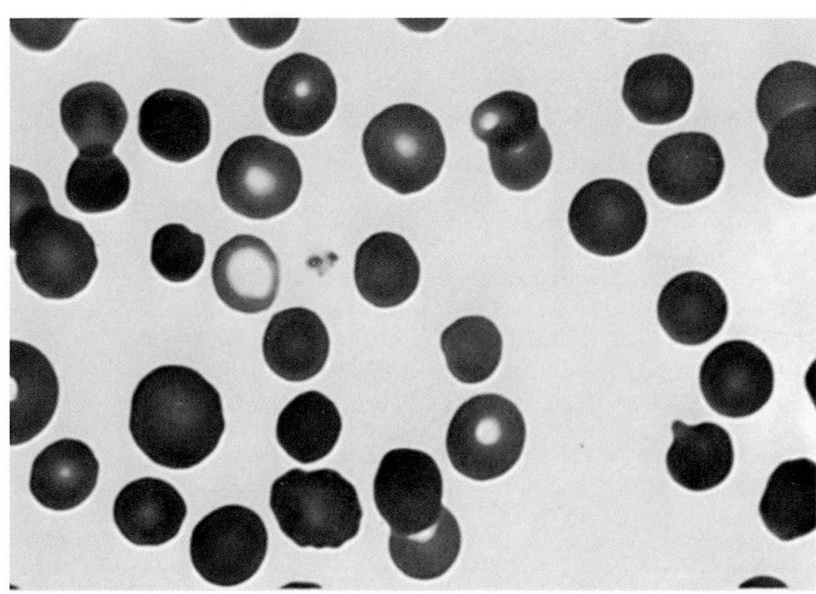

C

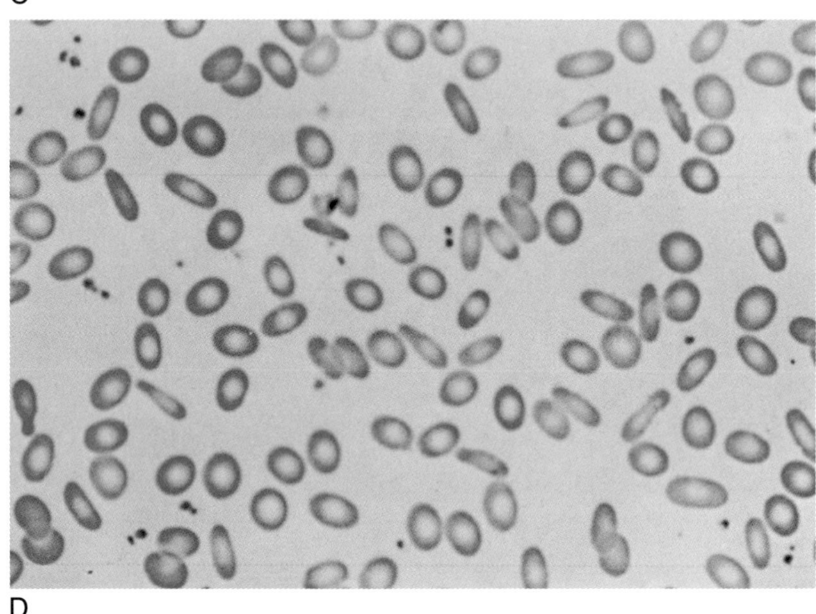

D

**FIGURE 77–8. Cont'd C,** Hereditary spherocytosis. **D,** Hereditary elliptocytosis.

*Continued*

or band 3) weaken the stability of the interactions between the cytoskeleton and the membrane lipid bilayer, promoting vesiculation and loss of bits of the bilayer, thus leading to progressive loss of membrane surface area (Palek and Jarolim, 1993). As the RBC becomes more spherical, it loses flexibility and becomes vulnerable to entrapment in the spleen, where metabolic depletion and attack by the reticuloendothelial system lead to hemolysis. Removal of the spleen allows the spherocytes to have a near-normal life span despite their cytoskeletal defects and abnormal shape.

The clinical manifestations of hereditary spherocytosis range from hydrops fetalis with fetal death (Gallagher et al, 1997) to fully compensated, lifelong hemolysis marked by reticulocytosis but no anemia (Mentzer et al, 2004). Neonatal hemolysis or hyperbilirubinemia appears in approximately half of all affected infants (Stamey and Diamond, 1957). In most cases, other family members are affected in a pattern consistent with autosomal dominant inheritance. In 20% to 30% of cases, recessive inheritance is noted, and only homozygotes express the clinical features of spherocytosis. Occasionally, the appearance of a new case of spherocytosis in a previously unaffected family is due to spontaneous mutation.

The diagnosis of spherocytosis is suspected when spherocytes are seen on the blood smear and the RBC osmotic fragility is increased in a patient with laboratory evidence of hemolysis. In the newborn, morphologic assessment of the RBCs is sometimes difficult because even normal newborns may possess a minor population of spherocytes; conversely, in hereditary spherocytosis, fewer spherocytes may be evident than will be the case later in life. Furthermore, interpretation of the osmotic fragility curve has to take into account the relative osmotic resistance of normal

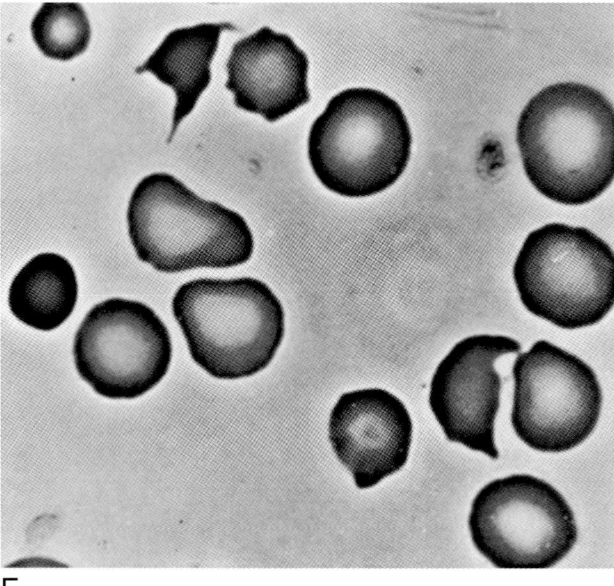


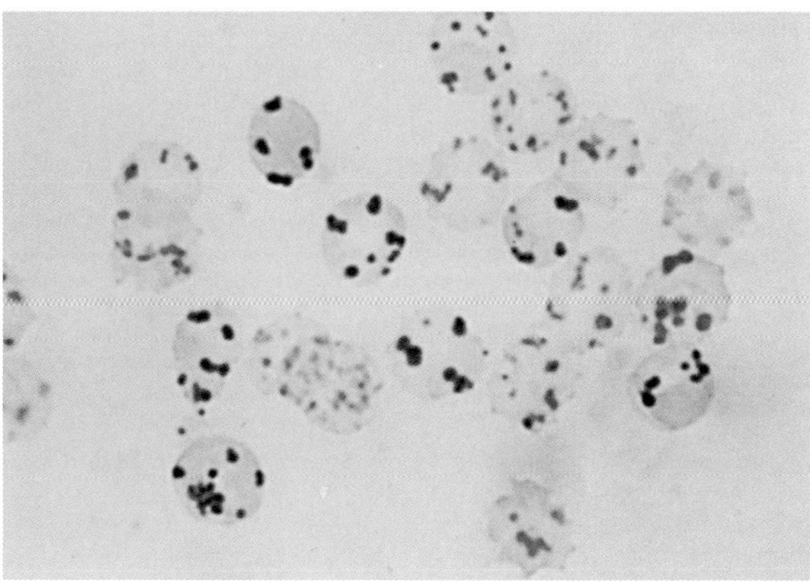


**FIGURE 77–8. Cont'd E,** Glucose-6-phosphate dehydrogenase (G6PD)-deficient RBCs during acute hemolytic episode. **F,** Heinz bodies from a patient with G6PD-deficient hemolysis (stained with supravital dye).

neonatal RBCs. If this is done by using newborns rather than normal adults as controls, the fragile RBCs of infants who have hereditary spherocytosis can easily be identified (Schröter and Kahsnitz, 1983). Immune hemolysis, which also generates spherocytes, must always be ruled out in the workup of a suspected case of hereditary spherocytosis. In the newborn, maternal antibody rather than autoantibody must be suspected if immune hemolysis is present. Spherocytes are commonly observed in ABO incompatibility but not in Rh disease. Blood typing and a Coombs test usually confirm a diagnosis of ABO incompatibility, but the Coombs test result may occasionally be negative and thus misleading. In this situation, evaluation of the family for other persons affected with spherocytosis may point to a hereditary rather than an acquired cause. Sometimes it is necessary to wait until the infant is 3 months of age or so to obtain a definitive laboratory diagnosis of hereditary spherocytosis, because, by this age, the confounding effects of maternal antibody and fetal RBCs are no longer present.

Treatment during the newborn period is directed toward management of hyperbilirubinemia, which often is present. Occasionally, RBC transfusions may be required at birth for management of symptomatic anemia (Gallagher et al, 1997). A common occurrence is the appearance of a transient but severe anemia during the first 20 days of life due to underproduction of erythropoietin in the face of continuing hemolysis (Delhommeau et al, 2000). Careful monitoring of affected infants after discharge from the nursery is warranted. Splenectomy is the definitive treatment for hereditary spherocytosis, but it is best deferred until the child is at least 5 years of age because of the increased risk of overwhelming sepsis with encapsulated organisms such as *Haemophilus influenzae* or *Streptococcus pneumoniae* (Diamond, 1969) that occurs following splenectomy in infants and young children. Partial splenectomy may reduce the rate of hemolysis without increasing the risk of overwhelming infection and is an attractive therapeutic option in young children with severe hemolysis (Bader-Meunier et al, 2001).

## Hereditary Elliptocytosis

Hereditary elliptocytosis is an autosomal dominant, clinically heterogeneous group of disorders that are caused by mutations of the RBC membrane cytoskeletal proteins (usually spectrin or protein 4.1) that weaken skeletal protein interactions and increase RBC mechanical fragility (Mentzer et al, 2004; Palek and Jarolim, 1993). Heterozygotes usually exhibit elliptocytes on the blood smear, but in most instances hemolysis is absent. Homozygotes or compound heterozygotes may have sufficient weakening of the cytoskeleton to cause significant hemolysis accompanied by striking abnormalities in RBC morphology (homozygous hereditary elliptocytosis or hereditary pyropoikilocytosis). Transient poikilocytosis and hemolysis may occur during the newborn period in infants destined ultimately to have asymptomatic elliptocytosis (Austin and Desforges, 1969). RBC membrane mechanical fragility is strikingly abnormal in these infants, probably as a consequence of the destabilizing influence of large amounts of free intraerythrocytic 2,3-DPG, a byproduct of the presence of fetal hemoglobin (Mentzer et al, 1987). As fetal hemoglobin levels decline postnatally in affected infants, membrane mechanical fragility lessens, hemolysis disappears, and RBC morphology undergoes a transition from poikilocytosis to elliptocytosis. Without knowledge of the membrane protein mutations present in the infant and the infant's family, it is difficult to predict at birth who will have transient poikilocytosis with ultimate recovery and who is destined to have lifelong pyropoikilocytosis with hemolysis.

## Red Blood Cell Enzyme Abnormalities

Hyperbilirubinemia, anemia, and even hydrops fetalis can be the result of inherited RBC enzymopathies. Except for G6PD deficiency (sex-linked) and adenosine deaminase excess (autosomal dominant), these disorders are inherited in autosomal recessive fashion, and heterozygotes are clinically normal. RBC morphology is usually normal, and diagnosis requires assay of the activity of the enzyme suspected to be abnormal. It usually is prudent to rule out common causes of hemolysis that are easily diagnosed before embarking on an expensive search for RBC enzymopathies, which, except for G6PD deficiency, are rare. Overviews of this group of disorders are available elsewhere (Luzzato, 1997; Mentzer, 2003), and the special features of RBC enzymopathies in the newborn period have also been summarized (Matthay and Mentzer, 1981).

### Glucose-6-Phosphate Dehydrogenase Deficiency

G6PD deficiency is a sex-linked disorder that affects millions of people throughout the world, particularly in Mediterranean countries, Africa, and China. Like sickle cell trait and thalassemia, G6PD deficiency is thought to have become common because it provides a measure of protection against malaria. In all but a few G6PD-deficient persons, hemolysis and anemia are present only after exposure to medications that are potent oxidants or during infections. Occasionally, hemolytic anemia is chronic rather than episodic and is present even in the absence of obvious exposure to oxidant stress. Rarely, anemia may be so severe as to require regular RBC transfusions. The clinical heterogeneity of G6PD deficiency is due to the very large number of different mutations, usually single amino acid substitutions, that lead to altered enzyme function (Beutler et al, 1996; Miwa and Fujii, 1996). Normal RBCs contain abundant amounts of reduced glutathione (GSH), a sulfhydryl-containing tripeptide that serves as an intracellular antioxidant, neutralizing peroxides that form during metabolism or are introduced directly from the extracellular environment. Because of their enzyme deficiency, G6PD-deficient RBCs have a limited capacity to regenerate GSH from oxidized glutathione (Fig. 77–9). In the absence of GSH, RBCs are vulnerable to oxidant injury. The effects of oxidants on the RBC are multifocal. Denatured globin precipitates termed *Heinz bodies* bind to the cell membrane, unfavorably altering its structure and function. Membrane lipid peroxidation may contribute to altered function. The activity of intracellular enzymes may decline. The ultimate result of these insults is hemolysis.

#### Severity of Clinical Disease

Race and gender are determinants of the severity of hemolysis and neonatal hyperbilirubinemia in G6PD deficiency.

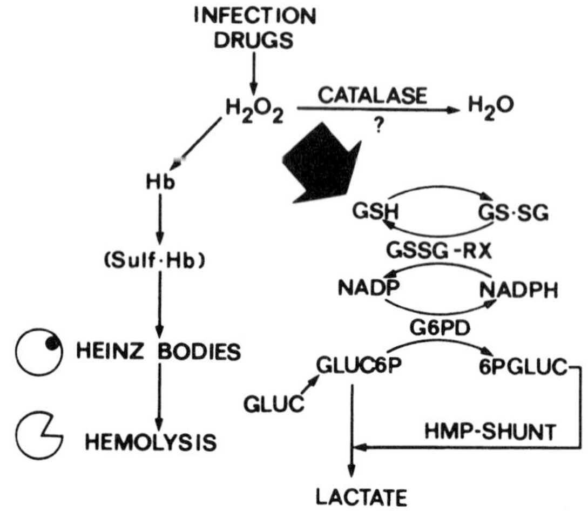


**FIGURE 77–9.** Glucose-6-phosphate hemolysis pathophysiology. GSH, reduced glutathione; GS-SG, oxidized glutathione; GSSG-RX, glutathione reductase; GLUC6P, glucose-6-phosphate; 6PGLUC, 6-phosphogluconate; G6PD, glucose-6-phosphate dehydrogenase; HMP-SHUNT, hexose monophosphate shunt.

***Race.*** The mutation G6PD A– that is responsible for nearly all of the G6PD deficiency seen in Africans (and is present in approximately 10% of American blacks) affects the stability of the enzyme, causing a gradual decline in activity during the life span of the RBC. Only in the oldest RBCs does enzyme activity reach low enough levels to create vulnerability to oxidant hemolysis. For this reason, hemolysis, if it occurs, is usually mild and self-limited. In contrast, in Asians and persons of Mediterranean descent, the common mutations causing G6PD deficiency alter enzyme activity in young and old RBCs alike. Hemolysis is usually more severe and can be fatal. In these ethnic groups, inheritance of an as-yet-unidentified factor renders some G6PD-deficient persons susceptible to severe and even fatal episodes of hemolysis following exposure to fava beans (favism). The hemolytic factor can be transmitted to neonates via breast milk (Kaplan et al, 1998). Favism is not seen in blacks.

***Gender.*** The gene for G6PD is located on the X chromosome. All of the RBCs of hemizygous G6PD-deficient males are affected by the enzyme deficiency. In contrast, a variable proportion of the RBCs of heterozygous G6PD-deficient females are enzyme deficient, depending on whether the process of random inactivation of the X chromosome that occurs early in embryonic development involves the chromosome carrying the normal or the mutant G6PD gene (Lyon, 1961). When a large proportion of their RBCs are enzyme deficient, females exhibit hemolysis, after exposure to oxidants, in similar degree to that seen in their male counterparts. When a smaller proportion of cells are affected, hemolysis is milder or absent. For these reasons, hemolysis is more commonly seen in G6PD-deficient populations of male hemizygotes than those of female heterozygotes. It is worthy of note that both homozygotes and heterozygotes may exhibit hyperbilirubinemia even in the absence of evidence of hemolysis (Kaplan et al, 1999).

### Diagnosis

The diagnosis of G6PD deficiency is suggested by the appearance of a Coombs-negative anemia in association with infection or the administration of drugs. Cells that appear as if a "bite" had been taken from them (as a result of splenic removal of Heinz bodies) are occasionally seen on the peripheral blood smear. Supravital stains of the peripheral blood with crystal violet may reveal Heinz bodies during hemolytic episodes. Although screening tests are available, definitive diagnosis requires assay of RBC G6PD activity or identification of a specific G6PD mutation by DNA analysis (Beutler, 1996; Miwa and Fujii, 1996). Measurement of enzyme activity may not reveal the deficiency in American blacks immediately after a hemolytic episode, because the population of deficient cells has been eliminated, or in transfused patients because of the presence of normal, enzyme-replete RBCs. Repeating the assay after at least 3 months ensures that any transfused cells are gone and that the population of deficient cells has been regenerated so that a more accurate determination of the presence of G6PD deficiency can be made.

### Etiology

Hemolysis and/or hyperbilirubinemia resulting from G6PD deficiency are well documented in the newborn period (Valaes, 1994). In fact, the onset of jaundice may often occur in utero (Kaplan et al, 2001a). Early and continuing monitoring of serum bilirubin levels in infants known to be G6PD deficient is warranted (Kaplan et al, 2000, 2001b). Although the usual factors (drugs and infection) may be implicated, often there is no obvious cause for hemolysis. Premature (Eshaghpour et al, 1967) but not term (O'Flynn and Hsia, 1963) black G6PD-deficient newborns have more hyperbilirubinemia than is seen in normal infants. Severe hemolysis and hyperbilirubinemia can follow exposure to known hemolytic agents in black G6PD-deficient newborns (Brown, 1992) but can be seen even in the absence of exposure to such agents in Asian or white G6PD-deficient infants. These ethnic differences reflect the different G6PD mutations that are present in blacks, Asians, and whites. In one study from Greece (Doxiadis and Valaes, 1964), approximately 30% of all exchange transfusions done in the nursery were in G6PD-deficient infants who had no evidence of isoimmune hemolytic anemia. In Taiwan, the incidence of hyperbilirubinemia requiring phototherapy was higher in G6PD-deficient than in normal infant males, particularly if the nt 1376 mutation was present. Other mutations were associated with lesser degrees of hyperbilirubinemia and responded more favorably to phototherapy (Huang et al, 1996). The degree of hyperbilirubinemia reflects both the increased bilirubin load presented to the liver by hemolysis of G6PD deficient RBCs and the presence or absence of the variant form of uridine-diphosphoglucuronylsyl-transferase responsible for Gilbert syndrome (Kaplan et al, 2001b). The relative importance of the latter is underscored by the observations that most jaundiced G6PD-deficient neonates are not anemic and that often, evidence for increased bilirubin production secondary to hemolysis is lacking (Kaplan et al, 1999).

### Treatment

Therapy for neonatal hemolysis and hyperbilirubinemia resulting from G6PD deficiency includes (1) phototherapy or exchange transfusion to prevent kernicterus, (2) RBC transfusion for symptomatic anemia, (3) removal of potential oxidants that may be contributing to hemolysis, and (4) treatment of infections using agents that do not themselves initiate hemolysis. In infants known to be G6PD deficient, prevention of severe hyperbilirubinemia by administration of a single intramuscular dose of tin-mesoporphyrin, an inhibitor of heme oxygenase, is highly effective and safe (Valaes et al, 1994; Kappas et al, 2001). Neonatal screening for G6PD deficiency has been very effective in reducing the incidence of favism later in life in Sardinia (Meloni et al, 1992) and in other regions where this potentially fatal complication is common (Valaes, 1994). In the United States, where the most common G6PD mutation is the A– variant found in blacks (who are not susceptible to favism and in whom life-threatening hemolytic episodes are rare), neonatal screening has not been thought to be cost-effective.

### Comment

As illustrated by this case, G6PD deficiency should be considered in the differential diagnosis not only for hyperbilirubinemia and hemolytic anemia but also for hydrops fetalis. The reason for the disastrous course in this infant is not known. Infection, ascorbic acid (an intracellular oxidant), or favism could have been responsible.

**CASE STUDY 1**

A male infant weighing 2722 g was born at 38 weeks of gestation to a 30-year-old Chinese, gravida 3, para 1, aborta 1 mother. Apgar score at birth was 1. Despite intensive resuscitative measures, the infant died after 2 hours, never having established spontaneous respirations. Autopsy disclosed hepatosplenomegaly, bile-filled canaliculi within the liver, bone marrow erythroid hyperplasia, and other evidence of severe intrauterine hemolysis. Hemoglobin was 9.8 g/100 mL, and the white blood cell count was 7200/μL. There was marked polychromatophilia (reticulocytosis), and numerous nucleated RBCs were seen in the peripheral smear. The infant's blood type was AB-positive, the mother's blood type was B-positive, and the Coombs test (direct and indirect) was negative. Hemoglobin electrophoresis revealed 52% hemoglobin F, 45% hemoglobin A, and no hemoglobin Barts or hemoglobin H. RBC G6PD activity was decreased in the infant and in his mother. Four weeks before delivery, the mother had an upper respiratory infection and took ascorbic acid (250-500 mg/day) for a period of 2 weeks as treatment. On at least one occasion during the last month of pregnancy, she also ate fava beans (Mentzer and Collier, 1975).

### Pyruvate Kinase Deficiency

Pyruvate kinase (PK) deficiency is an autosomal recessive disorder that occurs in all ethnic groups (Mentzer, 2003). Although the most common of the Embden-Meyerhof glycolytic pathway defects, it is rare in comparison with G6PD deficiency. Over 400 cases, mostly in Northern Europeans, have been described (Zanella and Bianchi, 2000). PK is one of the two enzymes that generate adenosine triphosphate (ATP) in RBCs. Impairment of ATP production is the central pathophysiologic abnormality in PK deficiency. Because nonerythroid tissues have alternative means of generating ATP, clinical abnormalities in PK deficiency are limited to RBCs. More than 130 PK mutations have been defined at the nucleic acid level and many more in terms of abnormalities of the PK protein (Zanella and Bianchi, 2000). Reflecting this genetic diversity, the hemolytic anemia that characterizes PK deficiency varies considerably in severity from family to family. Approximately one third of PK-deficient babies experience hyperbilirubinemia during the newborn period. Jaundice tends to appear early (on the first day of life) and may necessitate exchange transfusion (Matthay and Mentzer, 1981). Death or kernicterus may occur. Severe intrauterine anemia and hydrops fetalis have been reported (Zanella and Bianchi, 2000).

The diagnosis of PK deficiency should be considered in a jaundiced newborn with evidence of nonimmune hemolysis in the absence of infection or exposure to hemolytic agents. Hemoglobinopathies and membrane disorders should be ruled out by examination of the blood smear and other appropriate diagnostic tests before proceding to assay of RBC PK activity, which is the definitive test for the disorder. RBC morphology is basically normal in PK deficiency, although a few dense cells with irregular margins (echinocytes) are occasionally seen. PK heterozygotes are clinically and hematologically normal but usually have roughly half the normal amount of RBC PK activity.

Treatment of hyperbilirubinemia by phototherapy and exchange transfusion if necessary is usually the only therapy necessary in the newborn period. RBC transfusions for anemia may occasionally be required. Splenectomy may reduce the rate of hemolysis but should be avoided in infancy and early childhood owing to the high risk of infection after splenectomy.

## Hemolysis Due to Hemoglobin Disorders

To understand the hemoglobinopathies that are seen in the newborn, it is first necessary to review the normal developmental changes that occur in globin synthesis during fetal and neonatal life. In adults, the predominant hemoglobin tetramer—hemoglobin A—is composed of two alpha globin chains and two beta globin chains. In very young embryos, alpha chains are replaced by zeta chains and beta chains by epsilon chains. The transition from zeta to alpha globin chains is complete by the end of the first trimester. Epsilon chains disappear more slowly and are replaced first by gamma chains and then later by the beta chains of adult hemoglobin. By the time of birth, the transition from gamma to beta globin synthesis is well under way (Fig. 77–10). The various possible combinations of these different globin chains form a number of different hemoglobin tetramers that are characteristically found in embryonic, fetal, or postnatal life (Fig. 77–11). In contrast with globin, the heme moiety is unchanged in structure in embryonic, fetal, and postnatal hemoglobin molecules.

Fetal hemoglobin ($\alpha_2\gamma_2$) is the major hemoglobin found in fetuses after the first trimester. Its replacement by adult hemoglobin (hemoglobin A) begins before birth, so that only approximately 60% to 90% of the hemoglobin found in the normal term infant is fetal hemoglobin (hemoglobin F). After birth, gamma chain synthesis declines rapidly as beta chain synthesis increases (see Fig. 77–10) so that most newly formed hemoglobin is hemoglobin A. As RBCs made before birth are replaced

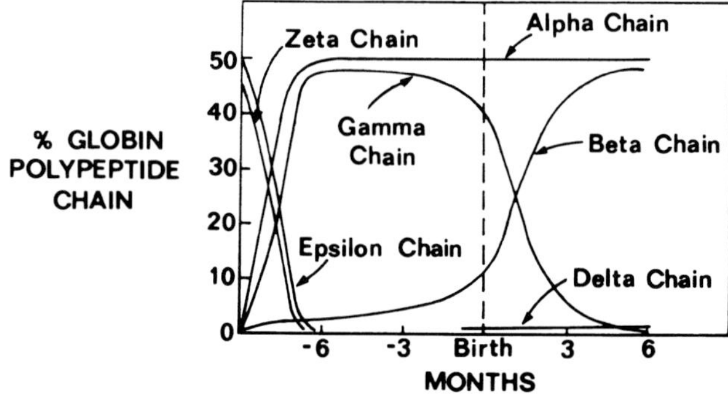


**FIGURE 77–10.** Fetal and neonatal hemoglobin production.

| | HEMOGLOBIN | GLOBIN POLYPEPTIDES | % IN CORD BLOOD |
|---|---|---|---|
| EMBRYONIC | GOWER - 1 | Zeta-2, Epsilon-2 ($\zeta_2\epsilon_2$) | 0 |
| | GOWER - 2 | Alpha-2, Epsilon-2 ($\alpha_2\epsilon_2$) | 0 |
| | PORTLAND | Zeta-2, Gamma-2 ($\zeta_2\gamma_2$) | 0 |
| FETAL | BARTS | Gamma-4 ($\gamma_4$) | <1% |
| | Hgb F | Alpha-2, Gamma-2 ($\alpha_2\gamma_2$) | 60-85% |
| ADULT | Hgb A | Alpha-2, Beta-2 ($\alpha_2\beta_2$) | 15-40% |
| | Hgb $A_2$ | Alpha-2, Delta-2 ($\alpha_2\delta_2$) | <1% |

**FIGURE 77–11.** Hemoglobin composition of cord blood.

by cells made postnatally, the percentage of hemoglobin F declines rapidly, reaching a level of approximately 5% by 6 months of age (Fig. 77–12). Only trace amounts of the minor adult hemoglobin, hemoglobin $A_2$ ($\alpha_2\delta_2$), and of the homotetramer of gamma globin chains, hemoglobin Barts, are present in cord blood. With postnatal maturation, the hemoglobin $A_2$ level increases gradually to the adult level of 2% to 3%, while hemoglobin Barts quickly disappears.

Beta globin disorders such as sickle cell disease or beta-thalassemia major do not become apparent clinically until several months of age, when the switch from hemoglobin F to hemoglobin A synthesis reveals the defect. In contrast, gamma globin mutations are most evident in fetal and neonatal life and then disappear by approximately 3 months of age as gamma globin synthesis is replaced by beta globin synthesis. Structural mutations of gamma globin may be associated with transient cyanosis during the newborn period if they form methemoglobin (see later section, Methemoglobinemia) or are associated with low oxygen affinity (Kohli-Kumar et al, 1995). The alpha globin disorders are evident at all stages of development from fetal to adult.

## Thalassemia Syndromes

The fundamental lesion in the thalassemias is absent or deficient synthesis of one or another of the normal globin chains, leading to a relative excess of the complementary or partner chain. For example, in alpha-thalassemia there is diminished synthesis of alpha globin chains, leading to an excess of beta chains (or, in the fetus, of gamma chains). The opposite is true of beta-thalassemia, in which it is excess alpha globin chains that accumulate. Aggregates of free alpha chains or homotetramers of beta chains (hemoglobin H) or of gamma chains (hemoglobin Barts) form in the absence of more suitable partner globin chains, leading to RBC membrane damage and rapid hemolysis. In addition, the decrease in overall production of hemoglobin produces small RBCs (microcytosis) that are often filled with less than the normal amount of hemoglobin (hypochromia). Although in most instances the globin chains produced by the thalassemic locus are normal in structure, there are mutations, termed *thalassemic hemoglobinopathies*, in which a structurally abnormal globin chain is found. In these cases, the instability of the hemoglobin tetramer formed from abnormal globin chains may also contribute to the hemolytic process.

### Alpha-Thalassemia

Alpha-thalassemia is of particular importance to neonatologists because its clinical manifestations are present in utero and at birth. The more severe forms of alpha-thalassemia are found in Southeast Asians (Glader and Look, 1996) and less commonly in infants of Mediterranean origin. The molecular basis for alpha-thalassemia is usually deletion of one or more of the four alpha globin genes. Nondeletional forms of alpha-thalassemia also are known but are less common. A thalassemic hemoglobinopathy involving the abnormal hemoglobin Constant Spring also may behave functionally as a mild form of alpha-thalassemia. Clinical severity is dictated by how many alpha globin genes are absent or nonfunctional. An infant can inherit no, one, or two alpha-thalassemia genes from each parent, giving rise to the following four clinical syndromes:

1. *Silent carrier state*. Deletion or nonfunction of a single alpha globin gene is not accompanied by any clinical or hematologic abnormalities.

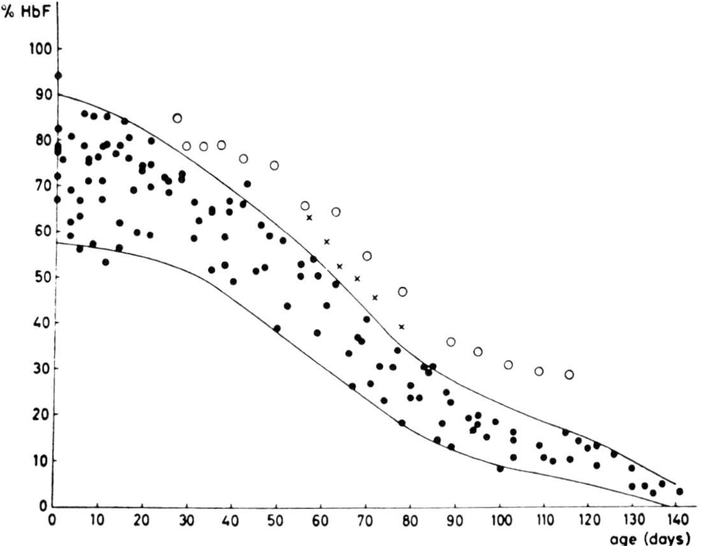


**FIGURE 77–12.** Decreasing concentration of fetal hemoglobin after birth. *(From Garby L, Sjöhn S, Vuille JC: Studies of erythro-kinetics in infancy. II. The relative rates of synthesis of haemoglobin F and haemoglobin A during the first months of life. Acta Paediatr 51:245, 1962.)*

2. *Alpha-thalassemia trait.* Deletion or nonfunction of two alpha globin genes, in *cis* or *trans*, is associated with mild microcytic anemia, without hemolysis or reticulocytosis.
3. *Hemoglobin H disease.* When three of four alpha globin genes are deleted or nonfunctional, a moderate hemolytic anemia is found. The RBCs are hypochromic and microcytic and contain inclusions of hemoglobin Barts or hemoglobin H when appropriate staining is performed. Surprisingly, the clinical severity of deletional hemoglobin H disease is less than that of nondeletional hemoglobin H disease (Chen et al, 2000).
4. *Homozygous alpha-thalassemia.* Lack of all four alpha globin genes is associated with a severe intrauterine hemolytic anemia and hydrops fetalis, with massive hepatosplenomegaly, and, in most instances, fetal demise. The RBCs are very hypochromic, fragmented, and bizarre in shape. Erythroblastosis is present (Chui and Waye, 1998).

The diagnosis of the alpha-thalassemia syndromes is easily made during the newborn period by correlation of the clinical and hematologic appearance of the child with the amount of hemoglobin Barts ($\gamma_4$) present in the RBCs (Lorey et al, 2000) (Table 77–8). Screening of all newborns for hemoglobin H disease is justified in populations with a substantial number of at-risk pregnancies (Lorey et al, 2000). The large amount of hemoglobin Barts found in the RBCs of homozygotes for alpha-thalassemia contributes to the clinical severity of the syndrome, because the markedly increased oxygen affinity of this hemoglobin makes it incapable of delivering oxygen to the tissues. DNA-based diagnostic tests are available for prenatal diagnosis, which is often carried out when a pregnancy at risk for a fetus with homozygous alpha-thalassemia is identified (Chui and Waye, 1998). The increased risk of eclampsia in mothers of such fetuses is an important justification for early identification and termination of the pregnancy.

No treatment is needed for the silent carrier state or for alpha-thalassemia trait, but studies to determine the thalassemia status of other family members, particularly those in their reproductive years, are recommended so that genetic counseling (and prenatal diagnosis if indicated) can be provided. Parents of infants who have hemoglobin H disease should be instructed to avoid oxidant agents that can cause hemolysis (the same list that is given to patients with G6PD deficiency). Although these infants are usually only mildly anemic, they may experience severe episodes of hemolysis during infections or with exposure to oxidant agents. Fetuses with homozygous alpha-thalassemia that are not aborted are usually stillborn, but several affected children have been born alive, resuscitated, and placed on chronic RBC transfusion programs (Beaudry et al, 1986; Bianchi et al, 1986, Singer et al, 2000). If a suitable donor is available, these infants can be considered for curative bone marrow transplantation (Chik et al, 1998). Experimental treatment of homozygous alpha-thalassemia in utero by means of hematopoietic stem cell transplantation is currently under evaluation.

### *Beta-Thalassemia*

Like alpha-thalassemia, beta-thalassemia is found in regions of the world where malaria was formerly endemic: Southeast Asia, India, Africa, and the Mediterranean basin. Although deletion of the beta globin locus is an occasional cause of beta-thalassemia, most cases are caused by point mutations that affect transcription, messenger RNA (mRNA) processing, or translation (Galanello, 1995; McDonagh and Nienhuis, 1993; Olivieri, 1999). Two general types of beta-thalassemia are recognized. In

**TABLE 77–8**

**Alpha-Thalassemia Syndromes**

| | | Anemia | Hemolysis | α:β Chain Synthesis | Abnormal Hemoglobins Cord Blood | Adult Blood |
|---|---|---|---|---|---|---|
| Normal | α/α<br>α/α | None | None | 0.95-1.10 | 0%-1% $\gamma_4$ | — |
| Silent carrier | α/–<br>α/α | None | None | 0.85-0.95 | 1%-2% $\gamma_4$ | — |
| Alpha-thalassemia trait | –/–<br>α/α | Mild<br>Hypochromic<br>Microcytic | None | 0.72-0.82 | 5%-6% $\gamma_4$ | — |
| Hemoglobin "H" disease | –/–<br>α/– | Moderate<br>Hypochromic<br>Microcytic | Moderate | 0.30-0.52 | 20%-40% $\gamma_4$<br>0%-5% $\beta_4$ | 20%-40% $\beta_4$ |
| Homozygous alpha-thalassemia ("hydrops") | –/–<br>–/– | Severe<br>Hypochromic<br>Microcytic | Severe | 0 | 70%-80% $\gamma_4$<br>15%-20% $\beta_4$<br>0%-10% $\zeta_2\gamma_2$ | |

beta$^0$-thalassemia, no beta globin at all is produced by the thalassemic locus, whereas in beta$^+$-thalassemia, there is reduced but measurable output of beta globin. The severity of homozygous beta-thalassemia (or beta-thalassemia major) is greatest when two beta$^0$-thalassemia genes are inherited; clinical disease usually is much milder when two beta$^+$-thalassemia genes are inherited. Severe beta-thalassemia is associated with lifelong hemolytic anemia, dependence on regular RBC transfusions for survival, and the gradual development of transfusion-associated hemosiderosis (Olivieri, 1999). The clinical abnormalities of beta-thalassemia are not evident at birth but first manifest only after 3 months of age, when beta globin normally becomes the dominant form of non-alpha globin synthesized. Although affected newborns appear clinically normal, the diagnosis of beta$^0$-thalassemia can be made at birth by detecting a complete absence of hemoglobin A, using hemoglobin electrophoresis or similar techniques. Definitive diagnosis of beta$^+$-thalassemia by these techniques, however, is not possible in the newborn period, because the reduced amount of hemoglobin A produced overlaps the range for normal babies. Direct identification of beta-thalassemia mutations by DNA diagnostic techniques is increasingly available and allows the identification at birth of all infants with beta-thalassemia major. These techniques, however, are more commonly used for prenatal diagnosis of beta-thalassemia syndromes. DNA can be obtained during midtrimester from fetal amniocytes (15 to 17 weeks) or during the first trimester from chorionic villi (9 to 11 weeks) and the assay completed within a few days, allowing families to make informed decisions regarding termination of pregnancy (Kazazian and Boehm, 1988). The implementation of a strategy of carrier detection, genetic counseling, and prenatal diagnosis in countries where beta-thalassemia is common has led to a striking reduction in the number of births of infants with beta-thalassemia major (Cao et al, 1996).

### Hemoglobin E/Beta-Thalassemia

Hemoglobin E is a structurally abnormal hemoglobin that results from an amino acid substitution (lysine for glutamine) at the number 26 amino acid of beta globin, counting from the N terminus. Because this mutation also adversely affects mRNA processing, there is reduced output of beta globin mRNA. Hemoglobin E trait is therefore an example of a thalassemic hemoglobinopathy. The thalassemic component of the condition is mild (a beta$^+$-thalassemia) so that hemoglobin E carriers are microcytic but not anemic. Even hemoglobin E homozygotes have little or no anemia. However, coinheritance of hemoglobin E trait and beta$^0$-thalassemia trait can give rise to a transfusion-dependent form of beta-thalassemia major (Fucharoen et al, 2000). As with other types of beta-thalassemia major, clinical abnormalities are not seen until the infant is 3 to 6 months of age. However, the presence of hemoglobin E is easily detected at birth by hemoglobin electrophoresis or related techniques. Infants found to have hemoglobin E need careful follow-up evaluation to exclude the possibility of hemoglobin E beta-thalassemia. DNA-based detection of the hemoglobin E mutation is feasible (Embury et al, 1990) and has been applied to both prenatal and neonatal diagnosis.

### Gamma-Thalassemia

Large deletions within the beta globin gene cluster may remove both gamma globin genes ($^A\gamma$ and $^G\gamma$) as well as the delta and beta globin genes. The resulting gamma-delta-beta-thalassemia is lethal in the homozygous state but in the heterozygote produces a transient but moderately severe microcytic anemia in the newborn. Over the first few months of life, the anemia resolves to a variable extent without specific therapy, and eventually the hematologic picture is that of beta-thalassemia trait. At least eight different gamma-delta-beta deletions have been reported, all but one in families of European origin (McDonagh and Nienhuis, 1993).

### Comment

We frequently see newborns with severe hemolytic anemia that resolves or decreases in severity spontaneously over the first few months of life, suggesting that some unique property of the fetal RBC contributes to the severity of hemolysis. The presence of a hypochromic microcytic anemia not related to iron deficiency (which can occur with chronic fetal blood loss) suggests one of the thalassemia disorders. Either alpha- or gamma-thalassemia could produce this degree of anemia. The absence of hemoglobin Barts in the cord blood RBCs rules out alpha-thalassemia. Measurement of reticulocyte globin chain synthesis in vitro showed diminished production of both gamma and beta chains, consistent with a diagnosis of gamma-beta-thalassemia. The severe neonatal hemolytic anemia was due to accumulation of excess alpha globin chains, unable to form normal hemoglobin tetramers because of the lack of partner gamma or beta chains. As the infant matured and began to synthesize more beta chains, the globin chain imbalance lessened and hemolysis diminished. Eventually, the hematologic picture in the infant resembled that in her father, that is, classic beta-thalassemia trait.

**CASE STUDY 2**

A full-term 2300-g girl became jaundiced at 24 hours of age (total bilirubin 13.7 mg/dL). The hemoglobin was 10.4 g/dL, hematocrit 32%, RBC count 3.8 × $10^6$/mL, MCV 84 fl, and MCH 27 pg/cell. The reticulocyte count was 26%, and there were 400 nucleated RBCs/100 WBCs. Rh and ABO incompatibility were absent; the Coombs test was negative. Iron and iron-binding capacity were normal, and there was no detectable RBC enzyme deficiency. The hemoglobin F level was 52% (normal is 60% to 85%). Hemoglobin Barts was not detected. An RBC transfusion was given, and over the next few days, nucleated RBCs disappeared, the reticulocyte count decreased, and the hematocrit remained stable. The mother was hematologically normal, but the father had a mild hypochromic microcytic anemia that resembled beta-thalassemia trait. At several months of age, the infant had improved and had only a mild hypochromic microcytic anemia that clearly resulted from beta-thalassemia trait (Kan et al, 1972).

### Sickle Cell Disease

The sickling hemoglobinopathies are beta globin mutations that, as with beta-thalassemia, do not become clinically evident until the infant reaches several months of age. Sickle cell anemia, the most severe of the disorders, is the result of inheritance of two beta$^S$ mutations (substitution of valine for glutamic acid at the sixth amino acid on the beta globin chain), one from each parent. Sickle-beta$^0$-thalassemia, phenotypically identical to sickle cell anemia, is caused by inheritance of one beta$^S$ and one beta-thalassemia mutation. The third common form of sickle cell disease, hemoglobin S-C disease, is somewhat milder than sickle cell anemia or sickle-beta$^0$-thalassemia. It is the consequence of inheritance of one beta$^S$ mutation and one beta$^C$ mutation (the substitution of lysine for glutamic acid at the sixth amino acid on the beta globin chain). Although no clinical abnormalities are present at birth, early diagnosis is important, because two potentially fatal but largely preventable complications may occur during the first year of life (Lenfant, 2002). The first is the splenic sequestration crisis, an unpredictable pooling of large numbers of RBCs in the spleen, which leads to a rapid decrease in hematocrit and, in the most severe cases, cardiovascular collapse and death. The second is overwhelming septicemia, usually caused by *S. pneumoniae* or *H. influenzae*. The unusually high susceptibility to infection with encapsulated organisms such as *S. pneumoniae* is the consequence of functional asplenia, which commonly appears by 1 year of age in infants with sickle cell anemia or sickle-beta$^0$-thalassemia (but not until later in persons with hemoglobin S-C disease). Prompt treatment of splenic sequestration with RBC transfusions is lifesaving so that parents are taught to recognize early manifestations such as splenic enlargement, lethargy, or pallor. Overwhelming sepsis can be prevented in most instances by early immunization with *H. influenzae* and conjugated pnuemococcal vaccines, beginning at 2 months of age, and by institution of daily prophylactic penicillin at a dose of 125 mg twice daily (Gaston et al, 1986). It is the need to institute these prophylactic measures within the first 1 to 2 months of life that provides a compelling rationale for neonatal diagnosis of the sickling disorders. In many states, all newborns are screened for these disorders, whereas in others, only high-risk ethnic groups are targeted. Usually a dried sample of blood on filter paper, collected at the same time as for other screening tests for inherited metabolic disorders, is used, but cord blood also is satisfactory. Tests that quantitate the amount of hemoglobin S, such as high-performance liquid chromatography, thin-layer isoelectric focusing, or electrophoresis on both cellulose acetate (in an alkaline buffer) and citrate agar (in an acid buffer), are adequate, but sickle solubility tests or the sodium metabisulfate "sickle prep" are not, because sickle cell disease cannot be distinguished from sickle cell trait and the tests are not sensitive enough to detect reliably the small percentage of hemoglobin S present in the RBCs of the newborn.

Prior transfusion with normal adult RBCs may cause a false-negative newborn screening result and delay the diagnosis (Reed et al, 2000). An excellent overview of issues related to newborn screening for sickle cell disease has been published by Wethers and colleagues (1989). Extensive experience with mandatory statewide screening for all infants has been accumulated in New York (Diaz-Barrios, 1989), California (Lorey et al, 1996), and elsewhere (Wethers et al, 1989).

Infants without a hemoglobinopathy born to mothers with sickle cell disease present more of a clinical problem during gestation and the neonatal period than is the case with infants who actually have sickle cell disease. Spontaneous abortion, intrauterine growth restriction (present in approximately 15% of cases), stillbirth (in 6%), preterm labor and delivery, and perinatal mortality (in approximately 15%) all are more frequent in the infants of mothers with sickle cell anemia (Koshy and Burd, 1995). These problems may be traced to abnormalities of the placenta such as small size, infarction, and an increased incidence of placenta previa and abruptio placentae, which appears to be the consequence of sickle vaso-occlusive events within the maternal side of the placental circulation. They are not caused by the presence of the sickle trait, beta-thalassemia trait, or hemoglobin C trait in the infant, because no hematologic disease is associated with the carrier state for these mutations, even in adult life when they are fully expressed, except under conditions of extreme hypoxia.

One caveat regarding sickle trait blood is that blood from an adult donor who has sickle trait should not be used for exchange transfusions in the newborn, particularly if hypoxemia is present, because use of sickle trait RBCs in this setting may contribute to a fatal outcome (Veiga and Vaithianathan, 1963).

## HYPOPLASTIC ANEMIA

The two major causes of pure RBC aplasia in children are Diamond-Blackfan anemia (DBA) and transient erythroblastopenia of childhood (TEC). Approximately 25% of infants with DBA are anemic at birth. In contrast, TEC is a disease that rarely manifests before 1 to 2 months of age (Alter and Young, 1998), and although it can manifest in the first year of life (Miller and Berman, 1994; Ware and Kinney, 1991), most children with this disorder are older infants or young children.

### Diamond-Blackfan Anemia

Also known as *congenital hypoplastic anemia*, DBA is a red cell aplasia characterized by the absence of recognizable erythroid precursor cells in the bone marrow (Alter and Young, 1998). An as-yet-uncharacterized defect in erythroid progenitor cells appears to be responsible for the profound erythroid hypoplasia. Most cases are sporadic, although 10% to 20% clearly are inherited, most commonly following an autosomal dominant pathway. Recent studies have identified that a significant fraction of DBA cases are linked to genes on chromosome 19q (Gustavsson et al, 1997) and chromosome 8p (Gazda et al, 2001). The relationship of these findings to the pathophysiology of DBA currently is being defined. Anemia is lifelong, but the onset of the disease is variable. Approximately 10% of affected infants are severely anemic in the newborn period, and pallor at birth or soon thereafter has been a feature of the disease in most cases (Alter and Young, 1998). Growth retardation, skeletal abnormalities, or other congenital anomalies are seen in almost one third of patients. The diagnosis of DBA is suggested by anemia and reticulocytopenia appearing in the first 6 months of life. Certain unusual features of the RBCs (macrocytosis, elevated fetal hemoglobin, increased adenosine deaminase activity) may assist in diagnosis. Many patients achieve durable remissions from anemia when treated with corticosteroids. Those who do not receive corticosteroids will require chronic RBC transfusions and are at risk of transfusion hemosiderosis. Transfusion-dependent DBA can be cured by allogeneic bone marrow transplantation from tissue-compatible siblings (Vlachos et al, 2001). At present, the use of unrelated donors for bone marrow transplants is not recommended, but this may change in the future. The incidence of leukemia may be increased in older patients with DBA, but the basis for this predisposition is unknown (Alter and Young, 1998; Glader, 1987). An increased incidence of osteosarcoma also is now recognized (Lipton et al, 2001).

### Transient Erythroblastopenia of Childhood

TEC is an acquired hypoplastic anemia that usually appears several weeks after an acute viral infection (Wranne, 1970). Evidence of a humoral or cellular immune response directed against erythroid precursor cells has been obtained in many affected children. As in DBA, the hallmarks of the disorder are anemia and reticulocytopenia, with an absence of erythroid precursors in the bone marrow. The platelet count sometimes is increased, and neutropenia may be present (Rogers et al, 1989). The abnormal RBC features seen in DBA are not seen in TEC. The natural history of TEC is one of spontaneous recovery over a period of several weeks, and because most children are recognized at the nadir of their anemia, evidence of recovery may already be present. RBC transfusion may be required to treat symptomatic anemia, but steroid therapy is unnecessary and not effective. There are no long-term hematologic sequelae of TEC, and recurrences are rare.

## PHYSIOLOGIC ANEMIA OF INFANCY AND PREMATURITY

At birth, the mean hemoglobin of term infants (17 g/100 mL) is slightly greater than in premature infants (16 g/100 mL). The hemoglobin concentration in term infants subsequently decreases to a plateau at which it remains throughout the first year of life (Table 77–9). Termed *physiologic anemia of infancy*, this anemia characterized by low (relative to adult values) hemoglobin is a normal part of development and has no adverse clinical effects. A similar process (*anemia of prematurity*) occurs in premature infants, but the hemoglobin decreases more rapidly and reaches a lower nadir. After 1 year of age, there is little difference between the hemoglobin values of term and premature infants.

### Physiologic Anemia of Infancy

With the onset of respirations at birth, considerably more oxygen is available for binding to hemoglobin, and the hemoglobin-oxygen saturation increases from approximately 50% to 95% or more. Furthermore, the normal developmental switch from fetal to adult hemoglobin synthesis actively replaces high-oxygen-affinity fetal hemoglobin with lower-oxygen-affinity adult hemoglobin, which can deliver a greater fraction of hemoglobin-bound oxygen to the tissues. Therefore, immediately after birth the increase in blood oxygen content and tissue oxygen delivery down-regulates erythropoietin production; as a consequence, erythropoiesis is suppressed. In the absence of erythropoiesis, hemoglobin levels decrease because there is no replacement of aged RBCs as they are normally removed from the circulation. Iron from degraded RBCs is stored for future hemoglobin synthesis. The hemoglobin concentration continues to decrease until tissue oxygen needs are greater than oxygen delivery. Normally, this point is reached between 6 and 12 weeks of age, when the hemoglobin concentration is 9.5 to 11 g/dL. As hypoxia is detected by renal or hepatic oxygen sensors, erythropoietin production increases and erythropoiesis resumes. The iron previously stored in reticuloendothelial tissues can then be used for hemoglobin synthesis. The supply of stored iron is sufficient for hemoglobin synthesis, even in

**TABLE 77–9**

**Hemoglobin Changes During the First Year of Life**

| Week | Term | Premature (1.2-2.5 kg) | Premature (<1.2 kg) |
|---|---|---|---|
| 0 | 17.0 (14.0-20.0) | 16.4 (13.5-19.0) | 16.0 (13.0-18.0) |
| 1 | 18.8 | 16.0 | 14.8 |
| 3 | 15.9 | 13.5 | 13.4 |
| 6 | 12.7 | 10.7 | 9.7 |
| 10 | 11.4 | 9.8 | 8.5 |
| 20 | 12.0 | 10.4 | 9.0 |
| 50 | 12.0 | 11.5 | 11.0 |
| Lowest hemoglobin: mean (range) | 10.3 (9.5-11.0) | 9.0 (8.0-10.0) | 7.1 (6.5-9.0) |
| Time of nadir | 6-12 wk | 5-10 wk | 4-8 wk |

the absence of dietary iron intake, until approximately 20 weeks of age. It is unnecessary to administer iron during this period, because it does not prevent the physiologic decrease in hemoglobin. Any iron administered is added to stores for future use. This physiologic hemoglobin decrease does not represent anemia in the true sense of the term; rather, it is a normal adjustment reflecting the presence of excess capability for oxygen delivery relative to tissue oxygen requirements. There is no hematologic problem, and no therapy is required.

## Anemia of Prematurity

The physiologic anemia seen in preterm infants is more profound and occurs earlier (see Table 77–9). Because symptoms may occur, the anemia of prematurity is considered nonphysiologic. The cause of anemia is multifaceted. The lower hemoglobin may be in part a physiologic response to the lower oxygen consumption in premature infants compared with that in term infants, a consequence of their diminished metabolic oxygen needs (Mestyan et al, 1964). An important component in the first few weeks of life is blood loss due to sampling for the many laboratory tests necessary to stabilize the clinical status of these infants, particularly those with cardiorespiratory problems. The erythropoietic response to anemia also is suboptimal, a significant problem because demands on erthyropoiesis are heightened by the short survival of the RBCs of premature infants (approximately 40 to 60 days instead of 120 days as in adults) and the rapid expansion of the RBC mass that accompanies growth. The basis for suboptimal erythropoiesis in prematurity appears to be inadequate synthesis of erythropoietin in response to hypoxia. Figure 77–13 illustrates the magnitude of the deficiency, which, as shown by Stockman and colleagues (1984), is greatest in the smallest, least mature infants. Because the liver is the predominant source of erythropoietin during fetal life, it has been proposed that relative insensitivity of the hepatic oxygen sensor to hypoxia explains the blunted erythropoietin response seen in premature infants (Dallman, 1993). The spontaneous resolution of the anemia that occurs by approximately 40 weeks of gestational age is in keeping with a developmental switch from the relatively insensitive hepatic oxygen sensor to the renal oxygen sensor, which is exquisitely sensitive to hypoxia, because by this time the predominant site of erythropoietin synthesis has shifted to the kidneys. The problem does not lie with altered sensitivity of erythroid progenitors to erythropoietin because this has been shown to be normal (Shannon et al, 1987).

The anemia of prematurity occurs even in nutritionally replete infants, but it may be heightened by deficiencies of folate, vitamin $B_{12}$, or vitamin E (Worthington-White et al, 1994). Premature infants are endowed at birth with significantly less vitamin E than is present in term infants, and unless supplemental vitamin E is provided, this deficiency state persists for 2 to 3 months. Vitamin E is an antioxidant compound vital to the integrity of erythrocytes, and in its absence, these cells are susceptible to lipid peroxidation and membrane injury. One clinical consequence of vitamin E deficiency is that hemolytic anemia can occur in small premature infants (weighing less than 1500 g) at 6 to 10 weeks of age (Oski and Barness, 1967; Ritchie et al, 1968). This hemolytic anemia, which is characterized by reduced vitamin E levels and increased RBC peroxide hemolysis, rapidly disappears following vitamin E administration. A logical conclusion is that vitamin E deficiency might contribute to the anemia of prematurity in a more general sense. In fact, premature infants given daily vitamin E (15 IU/day) had higher hemoglobin levels and lower reticulocyte levels than a control group not given the vitamin, as shown in Table 77–10 (Oski and Barness, 1967). A more recent study found no hematologic benefit for the administration of 25 IU of vitamin E daily to premature infants (Zipursky et al, 1987). Although it has become standard practice to administer vitamin E to all premature infants, the hemoglobin nadir in these babies is still lower than that in term newborns, indicating that anemia is largely caused by other factors such as erythropoietin deficiency.

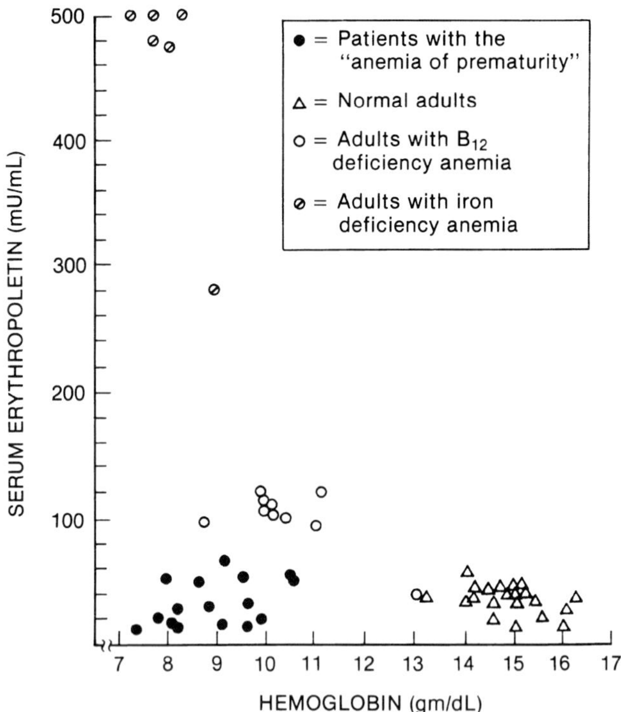


**FIGURE 77–13.** Hemoglobin levels and corresponding serum erythropoietin levels are shown. Values are from infants with the anemia of prematurity, normal adults, adults with vitamin $B_{12}$ deficiency anemia, and adults with iron deficiency anemia. *(From Ross MP, Christensen RD, Rothstein G, et al: A randomized trial to develop criteria for administering erythrocyte transfusions to anemic preterm infants from 1 to 3 months of age. J Perinatol 9:246, 1989. Reprinted by permission of Appleton & Lange, Inc.)*

### Treatment of Anemia of Prematurity with Recombinant Human Erythropoietin

Because a relative deficiency of erythropoietin is present in the anemia of prematurity, a number of studies have evaluated the safety and efficacy of rHuEPO therapy in this setting. If adequate doses of rHuEPO are used,

**TABLE 77-10**

**Effect of Supplemental Vitamin E on Anemia of Prematurity***

| | Control | Vitamin E |
|---|---|---|
| Birth weight | 1176 ± 182 g | 1278 ± 180 g |
| Vitamin E (mg/100 mL) | 0.22 ± 0.10 | 1.00 ± 0.25 |
| $H_2O_2$ hemolysis (%) | 66 ± 21 | 9 ± 9 |
| Lowest hemoglobin (g/100 mL) | 7.7 ± 1.5 | 9.2 ± 1.3 |
| Highest reticulocytes (%) | 6.7 ± 2.5 | 3.1 ± 0.7 |

*Premature infants were given prophylactic vitamin E (15 international units [IU]/day), and the vitamin E level, peroxide hemolysis, hemoglobin concentration, and reticulocyte count were measured after 6 to 8 weeks. These values were compared with those from a group of control infants not given vitamin E supplements.

Data from Oski FA, Barness LA: Vitamin E deficiency: A previously unrecognized cause of hemolytic anemia in the premature infant. J Pediatr 70:211, 1967.

reticulocytosis and a retardation in the development of anemia are regularly achieved (Gallagher and Ehrenkranz, 1993; Mentzer and Shannon, 1995). Several large multicenter trials have documented a modest but statistically significant reduction in the RBC transfusion requirements of treated infants compared with control subjects (Maier et al, 1994; Meyer et al, 1994; Shannon et al, 1995). Erythropoietin treatment may have a particularly important role to play in the management of infants whose parents refuse to allow blood transfusions on religious grounds (Davis et al, 1991). The optimal timing for initiation of rHuEPO therapy and the optimal dose have yet to be determined. To achieve the best results, supplemental oral iron at a dose of at least 6 mg/kg per day needs to be administered. It may be possible to use parenteral iron supplements, particularly in young very-low-birth-weight infants who are not able to take oral iron (Heese et al, 1990). Adequate vitamin E supplementation is of particular importance if intramuscular iron is used (Graeber et al, 1977). Although concern was raised over two rHuEPO-treated infants in one study who subsequently died of sudden infant death syndrome (SIDS) (Emmerson et al, 1993), SIDS has not been a feature of rHuEPO treatment in other studies. Early concerns about rHuEPO-induced neutropenia (Christensen et al, 1991) have, similarly, not been borne out (Shannon et al, 1995). Therefore, the current consensus is that use of this agent appears to be safe in premature infants. Very small premature infants (less than 1300 g birth weight) are those most likely to benefit from therapy (Strauss, 1994). There is disagreement regarding the cost-benefit relation of rHuEPO therapy (Maier et al, 1994; Shireman et al, 1994; Wandstrat and Kaplan, 1995; Zipursky, 2000).

A meta-analysis of 21 prospective controlled trials of rHuEPO treatment of the anemia of prematurity was recently published (Vamvakas and Strauss, 2001). Although there was considerable variation between studies, in general the efficacy of rHuEPO in reducing the need for red cell transfusions was modest. The authors concluded that it was premature to recommend rHuEPO for standard therapy for the anemia of prematurity.

### Red Blood Cell Transfusion Therapy in Premature Infants

It has been estimated that of the approximately 38,000 infants born weighing less than 1500 g in the United States each year, 80% will receive multiple RBC transfusions (Strauss, 1991). Most transfusions given in the first several weeks of life are to replace losses from phlebotomy required for laboratory monitoring during ventilator support and other intensive care measures. The mean blood loss resulting from phlebotomy during the first week of life in one group of 20 successive very ill premature infants admitted to the intensive care nursery was 38.9 mL, an impressive figure considering that the total blood volume of such infants is approximately 80 mL/kg body weight (Shannon, 1990). After the first few weeks of life, most transfusions are given to treat the symptoms of anemia of prematurity. The risks associated with use of allogeneic RBC transfusion in premature infants include exposure to viral infections, graft-versus-host disease, electrolyte and acid-base imbalances, exposure to plasticizers, hemolysis when T antigen activation of RBCs has occurred, and immunosuppression (Strauss, 1991).

Many strategies to reduce the need for allogeneic RBC transfusion in premature infants have been developed. Reducing phlebotomy losses by use of noninvasive monitoring techniques has been of only limited usefulness (Strauss, 1991). Donor exposures can be reduced by assigning a specified bag of adult donor blood to a sick neonate for multiple transfusions (Cook et al, 1993), particularly because it has been shown that blood stored for up to 35 days in CPDA-1 (Liu et al, 1994) or A3-3 (Goldman et al, 2001; Strauss et al, 2000) is safe for use in this setting . Defining strict criteria for RBC transfusions also can reduce the number of donor exposures in routine nursery practice (Batton et al, 1992). Traditionally, RBC transfusions have been given to replace phlebotomy losses or in the presence of symptoms thought to reflect hypoxia (e.g., tachycardia, tachypnea, dyspnea, apneic spells, poor feeding) (Oski and Naiman, 1982; Wardrop et al, 1978). However, studies to validate such practices have yielded conflicting results. Stockman and Clark (1984) showed a beneficial effect of transfusion on weight gain, but no benefit was found by Blank and coworkers (1984). Similarly, apneic spells were reduced in frequency following RBC transfusion in the studies of Joshi and associates (1987) and Ross and coworkers (1989) but not in those of Blank and colleagues (1984), Keyes and coworkers (1989), or Bifano and colleagues (1992). Lachance and colleagues (1994) measured oxygen consumption, myocardial function, resting energy expenditure, and other physiologic variables before and after RBC transfusions. They concluded that in asymptomatic anemic premature infants, oxygenation was well maintained without RBC transfusions when the hemoglobin level was 6.5 g/dL or more. Nelle and coworkers (1994) studied a similar group of asymptomatic anemic premature infants and found that RBC transfusion improved systemic oxygen transport as well as transport in the cerebral and gastrointestinal arteries. When clinical features of hypoxia are absent or findings are equivocal, an elevated blood lactate level may predict a need for transfusion (Izraeli et al, 1993) but in the experience of Frey and Losa (2001) adds little value to the decision-making process in the individual patient. At present, most NICUs have abandoned earlier practices of automatically replacing phlebotomy losses in favor of transfusing for clear-cut symptoms of hypoxia or for significant anemia unaccompanied by evidence of an adequate erythropoietic response (Alagappan et al, 1998; Engelfriet and Reesink, 2001).

## POLYCYTHEMIA

Neonatal polycythemia usually is caused by one of two conditions: increased intrauterine erythropoiesis or fetal hypertransfusion (Table 77–11). Other causes seen in older children, such as arterial hypoxemia (cyanotic heart disease, pulmonary disease), abnormal hemoglobins, or hypersecretion of erythropoietin by tumors, are rare, and primary polycythemia or polycythemia vera is virtually nonexistent. In normal term infants, delayed clamping of the cord leading to an increased transfer of placental blood to the infant is the most common cause of polycythemia. In the setting of acute intrapartum hypoxia, increased placental transfusion also may account for the observed increase in fetal RBC mass, according to animal studies by Oh and coworkers (1975). Placental insufficiency and chronic intrauterine hypoxia, as seen typically in small-for- gestational-age infants, most commonly underlie increased intrauterine erythropoiesis.

As the hematocrit increases, blood viscosity increases exponentially (Fig. 77–14). Blood flow is impaired by hyperviscosity at hematocrits of 60% or more. Oxygen transport, which is determined by both hemoglobin levels (i.e., oxygen-binding capacity) and blood flow, is maximal in the normal hematocrit range. At low hematocrits, oxygen transport is limited by reduced oxygen-binding capacity, whereas at higher hematocrits, reduction in blood flow secondary to hyperviscosity may similarly limit oxygen transport. At any given hematocrit, expansion of the blood volume beyond the normal level (hypervolemia) distends the vasculature, decreases peripheral resistance, and increases blood flow and, ultimately, oxygen transport. These physiologic observations have implications for therapy of polycythemia.

Most polycythemic infants have no symptoms, particularly if the polycythemia becomes apparent only on routine neonatal screening. Symptoms, when present, usually are attributable to hyperviscosity and poor tissue perfusion or to associated metabolic abnormalities such as hypoglycemia and hypocalcemia. Common early signs and symptoms include plethora, cyanosis (resulting from peripheral stasis), lethargy, hypotonia, poor suck and feeding, and tremulousness. Serious complications include cardiorespiratory distress (with or without congestive heart failure), seizures, peripheral gangrene, NEC, renal failure (occasionally resulting from renal vein thrombosis), and priapism. Because the elevated RBC mass increases the catabolism of hemoglobin, hyperbilirubinemia is common and gallstones occasionally occur.

In the symptomatic infant, a venous hematocrit of 65% or more (or a hemoglobin greater than 22 g/dL) confirms the presence of polycythemia. In screening apparently healthy newborns for polycythemia, however, account must be taken of a number of physiologic variables that influence the hematocrit during the first 12 hours of life:

1. Time of cord clamping—immediate clamping (within 30 seconds) minimizes placental transfusion.
2. Age at sampling—values increase from birth to a peak at 2 hours, gradually decreasing to cord levels around 12 to 18 hours (Ramamurthy and Berlanga, 1987; Shohat et al, 1984).
3. Site of sampling—values from blood extracted by the heelstick method exceed those from venous blood (the difference can be minimized by prewarming the heel).
4. Method of hematocrit determination—spun values are higher than those obtained by electronic cell counter and show better correlation with blood viscosity (Villalta et al, 1989)

One way to standardize and simplify screening for polycythemia is as follows: At birth, clamp the cord at about 30 to 45 seconds; at 4 to 6 hours of age, obtain a blood sample from a warmed heelstick and perform a spun hematocrit determination. If the result is greater than 70%, repeat the test on a venous sample. A venous hematocrit of 65% or more indicates polycythemia. By this approach, 1% to 5% of newborns are polycythemic; the range largely reflects differences in altitude at which the study population resides. Because the hematocrit is lower with increasing prematurity, polycythemia is seen less frequently in preterm infants than in term babies.

Following diagnosis, an attempt should be made to determine the cause of polycythemia (see Table 77–11). The condition is particularly common in infants of diabetic mothers or those with Down syndrome (Mentzer,

**TABLE 77–11**

**Etiology of Neonatal Polycythemia**

| Active (Increased Intrauterine Erythropoiesis) | Passive (Secondary to Erythrocyte Transfusions) |
|---|---|
| Intrauterine hypoxia | Delayed cord clamping |
| Placental insufficiency | Intentional |
| Small-for-gestational-age infant | Unassisted delivery |
| Postmaturity | Maternofetal transfusion |
| Toxemia of pregnancy | Twin-twin transfusion |
| Drugs (propranolol) | |
| Severe maternal heart disease | |
| Maternal smoking | |
| Maternal diabetes | |
| Neonatal hyperthyroidism or hypothyroidism | |
| Congenital adrenal hyperplasia | |
| Chromosome abnormalities | |
| Trisomy 13 | |
| Trisomy 18 | |
| Trisomy 21 (Down syndrome) | |
| Hyperplastic visceromegaly (Beckwith syndrome) | |
| Decreased fetal erythrocyte deformability | |

Data from Oski FA, Naiman JL: Hematologic Problems in the Newborn, 3rd ed. Philadelphia, WB Saunders, 1982.

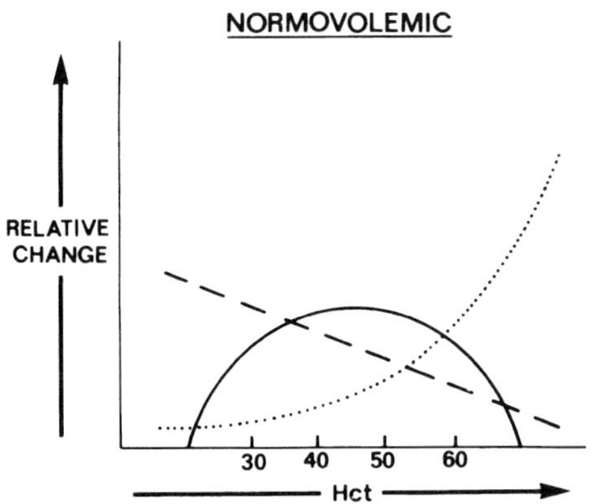


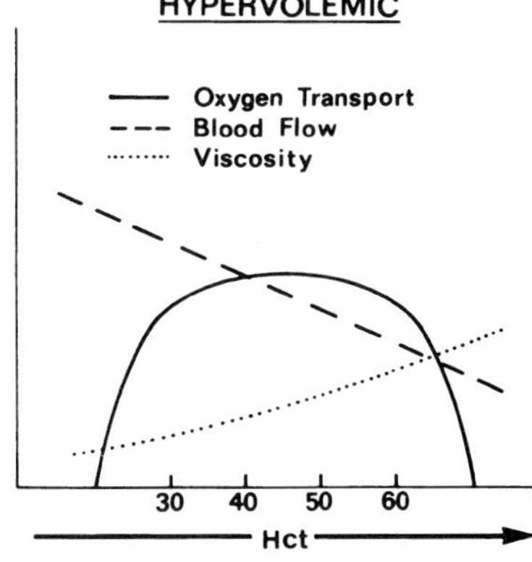


**FIGURE 77–14.** Effect of hematocrit on viscosity, blood flow, and oxygen transport.

1978) and may also occur in the setting of maternal hypertension (Kurlat and Sola, 1992) or, rarely, fumaric aciduria (Kerrigan et al, 2000). However, no apparent cause is found in most cases. Studies to determine the effects of polycythemia are dictated by the clinical findings but should usually include serum bilirubin, glucose, calcium, urea nitrogen, and creatinine levels.

Treatment by isovolumetric partial exchange transfusion is recommended to reduce the RBC mass without inducing hypovolemia. A beneficial effect of isovolumetric hemodilution on skin capillary perfusion (Norman et al, 1992) and on skin vasomotor activity (Norman et al, 1993) has been documented in polycythemic infants. At the University of California at San Francisco, all symptomatic newborns whose venous hematocrit is greater than 60% and asymptomatic newborns whose hematocrit is greater than 65% undergo partial exchange transfusion, using either normal saline or 5% albuminated saline (Levy et al, 1990). Unlike fresh frozen plasma, these products do not carry a risk of transmitting viral infections. Furthermore, partial exchange transfusion with fresh frozen plasma has been associated with the appearance of NEC (Black et al, 1985), whereas purified plasma protein derivatives such as albumin have not (Hein and Lathrop, 1987). Withdrawal of blood for a partial exchange transfusion is most easily done using an umbilical artery catheter. Any vessel may be used for blood withdrawal, and all but arterial lines can be used to infuse volume. An umbilical venous catheter inserted into the right atrium also provides acceptable access, but if correct placement cannot be achieved, the catheter should be inserted just far enough into the vessel to allow blood to be withdrawn. Calculation of the total volume of blood to be exchanged for diluent uses the following formula (Oski and Naiman, 1982):

$$\text{Exchange volume} = \frac{\text{observed Hct} - \text{desired Hct} \times \text{BV (mL/kg)} \times \text{weight (kg)}}{\text{observed Hct}}$$

where blood volume (BV) usually is 100 mL/kg but in infants of diabetic mothers may be lower (80 to 85 mL/kg).

**Example**: A 3-kg dyspneic infant with an 80% hematocrit requires a partial exchange transfusion.

$$\text{Blood volume} = 3\ \text{kg} \times 100\ \text{mL/kg} = 300\ \text{mL}$$

$$\frac{\text{observed Hct} - \text{desired Hct}}{\text{observed Hct}} = \frac{80-55}{80} = 0.31$$

Therefore, volume of exchange = 300 mL × 0.31 = 93 mL.

Some neonatal programs have more stringent hematocrit thresholds (e.g., >70%) (Carmi et al, 1992; Levy et al, 1990) for partial exchange transfusion of asymptomatic polycythemic infants than that cited previously (>65%). Although asymptomatic infants have an increased risk of late, mild neuropsychologic handicaps, prospective studies have failed to demonstrate major benefit from partial exchange transfusion (Delaney-Black et al, 1989). Because coexisting hypoglycemia is an important determinant of adverse neurologic outcome, careful monitoring and maintenance of adequate glucose levels and hydration are essential.

### *Comment*

The clinical findings in this infant were initially suggestive of organic heart disease. Rapid disappearance of the cardiac abnormalities following recognition and treatment of polycythemia indicated that these abnormalities were the result of polycythemia-induced hyperviscosity. In older children with cyanotic heart disease, polycythemia is a physiologic response that allows adequate oxygen transport to occur in the presence of arterial hypoxemia. Phlebotomy in these children may produce an acute hypoxic insult and should be undertaken with caution if at all. In striking contrast, in the newborn period, infants with cyanotic heart disease are not polycythemic (Gatti et al, 1966). Therefore, phlebotomy should improve, not worsen, oxygen transport, as it did in this case.

### CASE STUDY 3

A gravida 2, para 1 white woman delivered a 2950-g male infant after a normal pregnancy, labor, and delivery. At birth, the child had an Apgar score of 6. Physical examination revealed a cyanotic infant with a grade III/VI systolic heart murmur. The liver edge was palpable 2 cm below the right costal margin, and the spleen tip was palpable. Chest radiograph revealed a markedly enlarged heart with increased pulmonary vascular markings. The hemoglobin was 26 g/dL, and the hematocrit was 79%. There were no other hematologic abnormalities. The infant underwent partial exchange transfusion with 5% albumin, and the postexchange hematocrit was 62%. Subsequently, the infant's color improved, the heart murmur disappeared, and there were no remaining signs of congestive heart failure.

## METHEMOGLOBINEMIA

Methemoglobin is an oxidized derivative of hemoglobin in which heme iron is in the ferric ($Fe^{3+}$) or oxidized state rather than the ferrous ($Fe^{2+}$) or reduced state. Because methemoglobin is unable to bind (or release) oxygen, the presence of significant amounts of this respiratory pigment adversely affects blood oxygen-binding capacity and oxygen transport. Normally, small amounts of methemoglobin are formed daily in vivo by the action of endogenous agents, which may include oxygen itself (auto-oxidation). However, any methemoglobin formed is rapidly reduced through the action of RBC NADH-methemoglobin reductase (also known as cytochrome $b_5$ reductase), so that in normal persons, levels of methemoglobin seldom exceed 1%. A second methemoglobin reductase, dependent on NADPH as cofactor, also is present in RBCs. Although this enzyme is not active under normal physiologic conditions, it is greatly activated by the presence of certain redox compounds such as methylene blue, forming the basis for treatment of methemoglobinemia by this agent.

*Acquired methemoglobinemia* occurs when normal persons are exposed to chemicals such as aniline dyes that readily oxidize hemoglobin iron. Newborns are particularly susceptible because fetal hemoglobin is more readily oxidized to the ferric state than is hemoglobin A (Martin and Huisman, 1963) and because RBC NADH-methemoglobin reductase activity is low during the first few months of life (Bartos and Desforges, 1966). Merely marking the diapers of newborns with aniline dyes has caused methemoglobinemia. Drugs such as prilocaine, administered before birth to provide local anesthesia, can produce methemoglobinemia in both mother and infant (Climie et al, 1967). Although in most infants, no increase in methemoglobin levels follows the use of lidocaine-prilocaine cream (Emla Cream) to provide analgesia during circumcision (Taddio et al, 1997), a few case reports of visible cyanosis due to methemoglobinemia in infants treated with this cream have appeared (Couper, 2000; Tse et al, 1995). Perhaps the best-known agent that may cause methemoglobinemia is nitrite, either present de novo in ingested material or generated by administering nitric oxide to term babies in high concentrations for treatment of persistent pulmonary hypertension (Davidson et al, 1998). Nitrates can be converted to nitrite by the action of intestinal bacteria. It is for this reason that well water (Comly, 1945) or foods with a high nitrate content (e.g., cabbage, spinach, beets, carrots) (Keating et al, 1973) can produce methemoglobinemia in infants. Accumulation of nitrate in the intestinal tract of infants with diarrhea and acidosis (Kay et al, 1990; Yano et al, 1982) or symptomatic dietary protein intolerance (Murray and Christie, 1993) is thought to underlie the transient methemoglobinemia that occurs in these conditions.

*Congenital methemoglobinemia* is due to inherited disorders of hemoglobin structure or to a severe deficiency of NADH methemoglobin reductase activity. The seven inherited abnormalities of hemoglobin structure that give rise to methemoglobinemia, known collectively as the hemoglobin M disorders, are rare autosomal dominant defects caused by point mutations that alter a single amino acid in the structure of normal globin. The altered conformation that ensues favors the persistence of the ferric rather than the ferrous form of heme iron. The normal methemoglobin reductive capacity of the RBC cannot compensate for such instability of ferrous heme. Two of the mutations affect the alpha globin chain, three affect the beta globin chain, and two affect the gamma chain. Only the alpha and gamma globin chain mutations are associated with neonatal methemoglobinemia, because these are the globins that form hemoglobin F, the predominant hemoglobin found in neonatal RBCs. Neonatal methemoglobinemia is transient when produced by one of the two gamma chain mutations, hemoglobin FM-Osaka (Hayashi et al, 1980) or hemoglobin FM-Fort Ripley (Priest et al, 1989), because the normal developmental switch from fetal to adult hemoglobin eliminates all but a trace of the mutant hemoglobin. Hemoglobin M heterozygotes inheriting alpha or beta globin mutations appear cyanotic all their lives because of the increased methemoglobin levels present in their RBCs, but they are otherwise asymptomatic. No therapy is needed (and none is possible). The homozygous state is incompatible with life. Diagnosis of the hemoglobin M disorders is by hemoglobin electrophoresis.

*NADH-methemoglobin reductase deficiency* is an uncommon autosomal recessive disorder. Heterozygotes are asymptomatic and do not have methemoglobinemia under normal circumstances. If challenged by drugs or chemicals that cause methemoglobinemia, however, patients become cyanotic and symptomatic at doses that have no effect in normal persons. Homozygotes have lifelong methemoglobin levels of 15% to 40% and are cyanotic but otherwise asymptomatic unless exposed to toxic agents. Diagnosis of NADH-methemoglobin reductase deficiency is by assay of the RBC enzyme activity, a procedure available only in specialized hematology laboratories.

The cardinal clinical manifestation of methemoglobinemia is cyanosis not resulting from cardiac or respiratory disease. Cyanosis present at birth suggests hereditary methemoglobinemia, whereas that appearing suddenly in an otherwise asymptomatic infant is more consistent with acquired methemoglobinemia (Table 77–12). The blood is dark and, unlike deoxygenated venous blood, does not turn red when exposed to air. Rapid screening for methemoglobinemia can be done by placing a drop of blood on filter paper and then waving the filter paper in air to allow the blood to dry. Deoxygenated normal hemoglobin turns red, whereas methemoglobin remains brown. Methemoglobin levels of 10% or more can be detected (Harley and Celermajer, 1970). More accurate determination of methemoglobin levels is accomplished in the blood gas laboratory by co-oximetry or in the clinical laboratory using a spectrophotometer. Cyanosis is first clinically evident when methemoglobin levels reach approximately 10% (1.5 g/dL), but symptoms attributable to hypoxemia and diminished oxygen transport do not appear until levels increase to 30% to 40% of total hemoglobin. Death occurs at levels of 70% or greater. Methemoglobinemia is not associated with anemia, hemolysis, or other hematologic abnormalities.

In newborns, treatment with intravenous methylene blue (1 mg/kg as a 1% solution in normal saline) is indicated when methemoglobin levels are greater than 15% to 20%. Doses greater than 1 mg/kg should be avoided, as they may be toxic (Porat et al, 1996). The response to methylene blue is both therapeutic and diagnostic. Methemoglobin levels decrease rapidly, within 1 to 2 hours, if

**TABLE 77-12**

**Approach to Infants with Cyanosis and Methemoglobinemia**

**Cyanosis with respiratory and cardiac abnormalities:**
- Blood turns red when mixed with air
- Decreased arterial $Po_2$
- Consider pulmonary, cardiac, or central nervous system disease

**Cyanosis with or without respiratory or cardiac abnormalities:**
- Blood turns red when mixed with air
- Normal arterial $Po_2$
- Consider polycythemia syndromes

**Cyanosis without respiratory or cardiac abnormalities:**
- Blood remains dark after mixing with air
- Normal arterial $Po_2$

Consider methemoglobinemia syndromes
1. *With rapid clearing of methemoglobin following methylene blue:*
   a. Consider toxic methemoglobinemia (look for environmental oxidants)
   b. Consider NADH-methemoglobin reductase deficiency (perform enzyme assay)
2. *With reappearance of methemoglobinemia after initial response to methylene blue:*
   a. Consider NADH-methemoglobin reductase deficiency
3. *With no change in methemoglobin following methylene blue:*
   a. Consider hemoglobin M disorders (perform hemoglobin electrophoresis)
   b. Consider associated glucose-6-phosphate dehydrogenase deficiency (perform enzyme assay)

methemoglobinemia is caused by a toxic agent or by a deficiency of NADH-methemoglobin reductase. In contrast, the hemoglobin M disorders do not respond to methylene blue. Reappearance of methemoglobinemia after an initial response to methylene blue suggests a deficiency of NADH-methemoglobin reductase or the persistence of an occult oxidant. A poor response to methylene blue also is seen in G6PD-deficient persons, not because G6PD deficiency is a cause of methemoglobin formation but because there is suboptimal generation of NADPH, a required cofactor in the reduction of methemoglobin by methylene blue in deficient persons. In general, most infants with hereditary methemoglobinemia are asymptomatic and require no therapy. Older children sometimes are given daily administration of oral ascorbic acid or methylene blue to decrease cyanosis for cosmetic reasons. Methylene blue produces blue urine, but this is harmless.

## REFERENCES

### Normal Erythrocyte Physiology in the Fetus and Newborn

Allen DW, Wyman J, Smith GA: The oxygen equilibrium of fetal and adult hemoglobin. J Biol Chem 203:81, 1953.

Bauer C, Ludwig I, Ludwig M: Different effects of 2,3-diphosphoglycerate and adenosine triphosphate on oxygen affinity of adult and fetal hemoglobin. Life Sci 7:1339, 1968.

Delivoria-Papadopoulos M, Roncevic NP, Oski FA: Postnatal changes in oxygen transport of term, premature, and sick infants: The role of red cell 2,3-diphosphoglycerate and adult hemoglobin. Pediatr Res 5:235, 1971.

Finne PH: Erythropoietin levels in cord blood as an indicator of intrauterine hypoxia. Acta Paediatr Scand 55:478, 1966.

Finne PH, Halvorsen S: Regulation of erythropoiesis in the fetus and newborn. Arch Dis Child 47:683, 1972.

Gairdner D, Marks J, Roscoe JD, et al: The fluid shift from the vascular compartment immediately after birth. Arch Dis Child 33:489, 1958.

Jacobson LO, Marks EK, Gaston EO: Studies on erythropoiesis. XII. The effect of transfusion-induced polycythemia in the mother on the fetus. Blood 14:644, 1959.

Lanzkowsky P: The influence of maternal iron deficiency on the haemoglobin of the infant. Arch Dis Child 36:205, 1961.

Oski FA, Delivoria-Papadopoulos M: The red cell, 2,3-diphosphoglycerate, and tissue oxygen release. J Pediatr 77:941, 1970.

Usher R, Lind J: Blood volume of the newborn premature infant. Acta Paediatr Scand 54:419, 1965.

Usher R, Shepard M, Lind J: The blood volume of the newborn infant and placental transfusion. Acta Paediatr Scand 52:497, 1963.

Zon LI: Developmental biology of hematopoiesis. Blood 86:2876, 1995.

### General Approach to Anemic Infants

Alter BE: Methods in Haematology, vol 21: Perinatal Haematology. Edinburgh, Churchill Livingstone, 1989.

Brady MT, Milam JD, Anderson DC, et al: Use of deglycerolized red blood cells to prevent posttransfusion infection with cytomegalovirus in neonates. J Infect Dis 150:334, 1984.

Demmler GJ, Brady MT, Bijou H, et al: Posttransfusion cytomegalovirus infection in neonates: Role of saline washed red blood cells. J Pediatr 108:762, 1986.

Engelfriet CP, Reesink HW: Red cell transfusions in neonatal care. Vox Sang 80:122, 2001.

Enoki M, Goto R, Goto A, et al: Graft-versus-host reaction in an extremely premature infant after repeated blood transfusions. Acta Neonatol Jpn 21:696, 1985.

Gilbert GL, Hayes K, Hudson IL, et al: Prevention of transfusion-acquired cytomegalovirus infection in infants by blood filtration to remove leucocytes. Lancet 1:1228, 1989.

Goldman MJ, Garcia C, Spurll G: Reduction of donor exposures in premature infants by the use of designated adenine-saline preserved split red blood cell packs. J Perinatol 21:363, 2001.

Naiman JL, Punnett HH, Lischner HW, et al: Possible graft-versus-host reaction after intrauterine transfusion for Rh erythroblastosis fetalis. N Engl J Med 281:697, 1969.

Oh W, Lind J: Venous and capillary hematocrit in newborn infants and placental transfusion. Acta Paediatr Scand 55:38, 1966.

Parkman R, Mosier D, Umansky I, et al: Graft-versus-host disease after intrauterine and exchange transfusions for hemolytic disease of the newborn. N Engl J Med 209:359, 1974.

Sanders MR, Graeber JE, Vogelsang G, et al: Post-transfusion graft versus host disease in a premature infant without known risk factors. Pediatr Res 25:272A, 1989.

Strauss RG, Burmeister LF, Johnson K, et al: Feasibility and safety of AS-3 red blood cells for neonatal transfusions. J Pediatr 136:215, 2000.

Yeager AS, Grumet FC, Hafleigh EB, et al: Prevention of transfusion-acquired cytomegalovirus infections in newborn infants. J Pediatr 98:281, 1981.

### Hemorrhagic Anemia

Chapman JF, Bain BJ, Bates SC, et al: The estimation of fetomaternal haemorrhage. Transfusion Medicine 9:87, 1999.

Cohen F, Zuelzer WW, Gustafson DC, Evans MM: Mechanisms of isoimmunization. I. The transplacental passage of fetal erythrocytes in homo-specific pregnancies. Blood 23:621, 1964.

Danskin FH, Neilson JP: Twin-to-twin transfusion syndrome: What are appropriate diagnostic criteria? Am J Obstet Gynecol 161:365, 1989.

Fong EA, Davies JI, Grey DE, et al: Detection of massive transplacental haemorrhage by flow cytometry. Clin Lab Haem 22:325, 2000.

Leonard S, Anthony B: Giant cephalohematoma of newborn. Am J Dis Child 101:170, 1961.

Montague ACW, Krevans JR: Transplacental hemorrhage in cesarean section. Am J Obstet Gynecol 95:1115, 1966.

Nieburg PI, Stockman JA: Rapid correction of anemia with partial exchange transfusion. Am J Dis Child 131:60, 1977.

Oski FA, Naiman JL: Hematologic Problems in the Newborn, 3rd ed. Philadelphia, WB Saunders, 1982.

Pearson HA, Diamond LK: Fetomaternal transfusion. Am J Dis Child 97:267, 1959.

Rausen AR, Seki M, Strauss L: Twin transfusion syndrome. A review of 19 cases studied at one institution. J Pediatr 66:613, 1965.

Raye JR, Gutberlet RL, Stahlman M: Symptomatic posthemorrhagic anemia in the newborn. Pediatr Clin North Am 17:401, 1970.

Seng YC, Rajadurai VS: Twin-twin transfusion syndrome: A five year review. Arch Dis Child Fetal Neonatal Ed 83:F168, 2000.

Shepherd AJ, Richard J, Brown JP: Nuchal cord as a cause of neonatal anemia. Am J Dis Child 139:71, 1985.

Van Gemert MJC, Umur A, Tijssen JGP, Ross MG: Twin-twin transfusion syndrome: Etiology, severity and rational management. Curr Opin Obstet Gynecol 13:193, 2001.

Woo Wang MYF, McCutcheon E, Desforges JF: Fetomaternal hemorrhage from diagnostic transabdominal amniocentesis. Am J Obstet Gynecol 97:1123, 1967.

Zipursky A, Pollock J, Chown B, Israels LG: Transplacental fetal maternal hemorrhage after placental injury during delivery or amniocentesis. Lancet 2:493, 1963.

## Hemolytic Anemia

Abelson NM, Rawson AJ: Studies of blood group antibodies. V. Fractionation of examples of anti-B, anti-A,B, anti-M, anti-P, anti-JK$^{a}$, anti-Le$^{a}$, anti-D, anti-CD, anti-K, anti-Fy$^{a}$, anti-S, and anti-Good. Transfusion 1:116, 1961.

Austin RF, Desforges JF: Hereditary elliptocytosis: An unusual presentation of hemolysis in the newborn associated with transient morphologic abnormalities. Pediatrics 44:196, 1969.

Bader-Meunier B, Gauthier F, Archambaud F, et al. Long-term evaluation of the beneficial effect of subtotal splenectomy for management of hereditary spherocytosis. Blood 97:399, 2001.

Bard H: The postnatal decline of hemoglobin F synthesis in normal full-term infants. J Clin Invest 55:395, 1975.

Batton DG, Amanullah A, Comstock C: Fetal schistocytic hemolytic anemia and umbilical vein varix. J Pediatr Hematol Oncol 22:259, 2000.

Beaudry MA, Ferguson DJ, Pearse K, et al: Survival of a hydropic infant with homozygous alpha-thalassemia-1. J Pediatr 108:713, 1986.

Bennett PR, Le Van Kim C, Colin Y, et al: Prenatal determination of fetal RhD type by DNA amplification. N Engl J Med 329:607, 1993.

Beutler E, Vulliamy T, Luzzatto L: Hematologically important mutations: Glucose-6-phosphate dehydrogenase. Blood Cells, Mol Dis 22:49, 1996.

Bianchi DW, Beyer EC, Stark AR, et al: Normal long-term survival with alpha-thalassemia. J Pediatr 108:716, 1986.

Brecher ME (ed): Technical Manual, 14th ed. Bethesda, Md, American Association of Blood Banks, 2002.

Brouwers HAA, Overbeeke MAM, van Ertbrugeen I, et al: What is the best predictor of the severity of ABO-haemolytic disease of the newborn? Lancet 2:641, 1988.

Brown AK: Hyperbilirubinemia in black infants: Role of glucose-6-phosphate dehydrogenase deficiency. Clin Pediatr 31:712, 1992.

Cao A, Galanello R, Rosatelli MC, et al: Clinical experience of management of thalassemia: The Sardinian experience. Semin Hematol 33:66, 1996.

Chen FE, Ool C, Yin S, et al: Genetic and clinical features of hemoglobin H disease in Chinese patients. N Engl J Med 343:544, 2000.

Chik KW, Shing MM, Leung TF, et al: Treatment of hemoglobin Bart's hydrops with bone marrow transplantation. J Pediatr 132:1039, 1998.

Chui DHK, Waye JS: Hydrops fetalis caused by α-thalassemia: An emerging health care problem. Blood 91:2213, 1998.

Delhommeau F, Cynober T, Schischmanoff PO, et al: Natural history of hereditary spherocytosis during the first year of life. Blood 95:393, 2000.

Diamond LK: Splenectomy in childhood and the hazard of overwhelming infection. Pediatrics 43:886, 1969.

Diaz-Barrios V: New York's experience. Pediatrics (Suppl) 83:2, 1989.

Doxiadis SA, Valaes T: The clinical picture of glucose-6-phosphate dehydrogenase deficiency in early infancy. Arch Dis Child 39:545, 1964.

Embury SH, Kropp GL, Stanton TS: Detection of the hemoglobin E mutation using the color complementation assay: Application to complex genotyping. Blood 78:619, 1990.

Eshaghpour E, Oski FA, Williams M: The relationship of erythrocyte glucose-6-phosphate dehydrogenase deficiency to hyperbilirubinemia in Negro premature infants. J Pediatr 70:595, 1967.

Fisk NM, Bennett P, Warwick RM, et al: Clinical utility of fetal RhD typing in alloimmunized pregnancies by means of polymerase chain reaction on amniocytes or chorionic villi. Am J Obstet Gynecol 171:50, 1994.

Freda VJ, Gorman JG, Pollack W, Bowe E: Prevention of Rh hemolytic disease: 10 years' clinical experience with Rh immune globulin. N Engl J Med 292:1014, 1975.

Fucharoen S, Ketvichit P, Pootrakul P, et al: Clinical manifestation of beta-thalassemia/hemoglobin E disease. J Pediatr Hematol Oncol 22:552, 2000.

Galanello R: Molecular basis of thalassemia major. Int J Pediatr Hematol Oncol 2:383, 1995.

Gallagher PG, Petruzzi MJ, Weed SA, et al: Mutation of a highly conserved residue of β1 spectrin associated with fatal and near-fatal neonatal hemolytic anemia. J Clin Invest 99:267, 1997.

Gaston MH, Vertier JI, Wood G, et al: Prophylaxis with oral penicillin in children with sickle cell anemia. N Engl J Med 314:1593, 1986.

Glader BE, Look K: Hematologic disorders in children in Southeast Asia. Pediatr Clin North Am 43:665, 1996.

Grannum PA, Copel JA, Moya FR, et al: The reversal of hydrops fetalis by intravascular transfusion in severe isoimmune fetal anemia. Am J Obstet Gynecol 158:914, 1988.

Grannum PA, Copel JA, Plaxe SC, et al: In utero exchange transfusion by direct intravascular injection in severe erythroblastosis fetalis. N Engl J Med 314:1431, 1986.

Huang CS, Hung KL, Huang MJ, et al: Neonatal jaundice and molecular mutations in glucose-6-phosphate dehydrogenase deficient newborn infants. Am J Hematol 51:19, 1996.

Judd WJ: Practice guidelines for prenatal and perinatal immunohematology, revisited. Transfusion 41:1445-1452, 2001.

Kan YW, Forget BG, Nathan DG: Gamma-beta thalassemia: A cause of hemolytic disease of the newborn. N Engl J Med 286:129, 1972.

Kaplan M, Algur N, Hammerman C: Onset of jaundice in glucose-6-phosphate dehydrogenase–deficient neonates. Pediatr 108:956, 2001a.

Kaplan M, Beutler E, Vreman HJ, et al: Neonatal hyperbilirubinemia in glucose-6-phosphate dehydrogenase–deficient heterozygotes. Pediatr 104:68, 1999.

Kaplan M, Hammerman C, Beutler E: Hyperbilirubinaemia, glucose-6-phosphate dehydrogenase deficiency and Gilbert syndrome. Eur J Pediatr 160:195, 2001b.

Kaplan M, Hammerman C, Feldman R, et al: Predischarge bilirubin screening in glocose-6-phosphate dehydrogenase–deficient neonates. Pediatr 105:533, 2000.

Kaplan E, Herz F, Scheye E: ABO hemolytic disease of the newborn, without hyperbilirubinemia. Am J Hematol 1:279, 1976.

Kaplan M, Vreman HJ, Hamerman C, et al: Favism by proxy in nursing glucose-6-phosphate dehydrogenase–deficient neonates. J Perinatol 18:477, 1998.

Kappas A, Drummond GS, Manola T, et al: Sn-protoporphyrin use in the management of hyperbilirubinemia in term infants with direct Coombs-positive ABO incompatibility. Pediatrics 81:485, 1988.

Kappas A, Drummond GS, Valaes T: A single dose of Sn-mesoporphyrin prevents development of severe hyperbilirubinemia in glucose-6-phosphate dehydrogenase–deficient newborns. Pediatrics 108:25, 2001.

Kazazian HH, Boehm CD: Molecular basis and prenatal diagnosis of β-thalassemia. Blood 72:1107, 1988.

Kohli-Kumar M, Zwerdling T, Rucknagel DL: Hemoglobin F-Cincinnati, $a_2{}^{G}\gamma_2$41(C7) Phe6Ser in a newborn with cyanosis. Am J Hematol 49:43, 1995.

Koshy M, Burd L: Obstetric and gynecologic issues. In Embury SH, Hebbel RP, Mohandas N, Steinberg MH (eds): Sickle Cell Disease: Basic Principles and Clinical Practice. New York, Raven Press, 1995, p 689.

LaCelle PL: Alteration of membrane deformability in hemolytic anemias. Semin Hematol 7:355, 1970.

Lenfant C: The Management of Sickle Cell Disease, 4th ed. National Institutes of Health Publication No 02–2117. Bethesda, MD. National Heart, Lung, and Blood Institute, 2002. Also available on line: http://www.nhlbi.nih.gov

Levine P, Burnham L, Katzen EM, Vogel P: The role of isoimmunization and the pathogenesis of erythroblastosis fetalis. Am J Obstet Gynecol 42:925, 1941.

Liley AW: Liquor amnii analysis in the management of pregnancy complicated by rhesus sensitization. Am J Obstet Gynecol 82:1359, 1961.

Liley AW: Intrauterine transfusion of fetus in hemolytic disease. BMJ 2:1107, 1963.

Lorey F, Arnopp J, Cunningham GC: Distribution of hemoglobinopathy variants by ethnicity in a multiethnic state. Genet Epidemiol 13:501, 1996.

Lorey F, Cunningham G, Vichinsky EP, et al: Universal newborn screening for Hb H disease in California. Genet Testing 5:93, 2000.

Luzzatto L: Glucose-6-phosphate dehydrogenase deficiency and hemolytic anemia. In Nathan DG, Orkin SH (eds): Nathan and Oski's Hematology of Infancy and Childhood, 5th ed. Philadelphia, WB Saunders, 1998.

Lyon MF: Gene action in the X-chromosome of the mouse. Nature 190:372, 1961.

Matthay KK, Mentzer WC: Erythrocyte enzymopathies in the newborn. Clin Haematol 10:31, 1981.

McDonagh KT, Nienhuis AW: The thalassemias. In Nathan DG, Oski FA (eds): Hematology of Infancy and Childhood, 4th ed. Philadelphia, WB Saunders, 1993, p 783.

Meloni T, Forteleoni G, Meloni GF: Marked decline of favism after neonatal glucose-6-phosphate dehydrogenase screening and health education: The northern Sardinian experience. Acta Haematol 87:29, 1992.

Mentzer WC: Pyruvate kinase deficiency and disorders of glycolysis. In Nathan DG, Orkin SH, Look AT, Ginsburg D (eds): Hematology of Infancy and Childhood, 6th ed. Philadelphia, WB Saunders, 2003, p 685.

Mentzer WC Jr, Collier E: Hydrops fetalis associated with erythrocyte G-6-PD deficiency and maternal ingestion of fava beans and ascorbic acid. J Pediatr 86:565, 1975.

Mentzer WC, Glader BE: Hereditary spherocytosis and other anemias due to abnormalities of the red cell membrane. In Greer JP, Foerster J, Lukens JN, et al (eds): Wintrobe's Clinical Hematology, 11th ed. Philadelphia, Lippincott Williams & Wilkins, 2004, p 1089.

Mentzer WC, Iarocci TA, Mohandas N, et al: Modulation of erythrocyte membrane mechanical stability by 2,3-diphosphoglycerate in the neonatal poikilocytosis/elliptocytosis syndrome. J Clin Invest 79:943, 1987.

Miwa S, Fujii H: Molecular basis of erythroenzymopathies associated with hereditary hemolytic anemia: Tabulation of mutant enzymes. Am J Hematol 51:122, 1996.

Mouro I, Colin Y, Cherif-Zahar B, et al: Molecular genetic basis of the human rhesus blood group system. Nature Genet 5:62, 1993.

Nicolaides JH, Soothill PW, Clewell WH, et al: Fetal hemoglobin measurement in the assessment of red cell isoimmunization. Lancet 1:1073, 1988.

O'Flynn MED, Hsia DY: Serum bilirubin levels and glucose-6-phosphate dehydrogenase deficiency in newborn American Negroes. J Pediatr 63:160, 1963.

Olivieri NF: The β-thalassemias. N Engl J Med 341:99, 1999.

Osborn LM, Lenarsky C, Oakes RC, et al: Phototherapy in full-term infants with hemolytic disease secondary to ABO incompatibility. Pediatrics 74:371, 1984.

Ovali F, Samanci N, Dagoglu T, et al: Management of late anemia in rhesus hemolytic disease: Use of recombinant human erythropoietin (a pilot study). Pediatr Res 39:831, 1996.

Palek J, Jarolim P: Clinical expression and laboratory detection of red blood cell membrane protein mutations. Semin Hematol 30:249, 1993.

Parer JT: Severe Rh isoimmunization: Current methods of in utero diagnosis and treatment. Obstet Gynecol 158:1323, 1988.

Pearson HA: Life-span of the fetal red blood cell. J Pediatr 70:166, 1967.

Reed W, Lane PA, Lorey F, et al: Sickle-cell disease not identified by newborn screening because of prior transfusion. J Pediatr 136:248, 2000.

Rodeck CH, Nicolaides KH, Warsof SL, et al: The management of severe rhesus isoimmunization by fetoscopic intravascular transfusions. Am J Obstet Gynecol 150:769, 1984.

Scaradavou A, Inglis S, Peterson P, et al: Suppression of erythropoiesis by intrauterine transfusions in hemolytic disease of the newborn: Use of erythropoietin to treat the late anemia. J Pediatr 123:279, 1993.

Schröter W, Kahsnitz E: Diagnosis of hereditary spherocytosis in newborn infants. J Pediatr 103:460, 1983.

Singer ST, Styles L, Bojanowski J, et al. Changing outcome of homozygous α-thalassemia: Cautious optimism. J Pediatr Hematol Oncol 22:539, 2000.

Spinnato JA: Hemolytic disease of the fetus: A plea for restraint. Obstet Gynecol 80:873, 1992.

Stamatoyannopoulos G: Gamma-thalassemia. Lancet 2:192, 1971.

Stamey CC, Diamond LK: Congenital hemolytic anemia in the newborn. Am J Dis Child 94:616, 1957.

Tchernia G, Gauthier F, Mielot F, et al: Initial assessment of the beneficial effect of partial splenectomy in hereditary spherocytosis. Blood 81:2014, 1993.

Valaes T: Severe neonatal jaundice associated with glucose-6-phosphate dehydrogenase deficiency: Pathogenesis and global epidemiology. Acta Paediatr Suppl 394:58, 1994.

Valaes T, Petmezaki S, Henschke C, et al: Control of jaundice in preterm newborns by an inhibitor of bilirubin production: Studies with tin-mesoporphyrin. Pediatrics 93:1, 1994.

Veiga S, Vaithianathan T: Massive intravascular sickling after exchange transfusion with sickle cell trait blood. Transfusion 3:387, 1963.

Voak D, Williams MA: An explanation of the failure of the direct antiglobulin test to detect erythrocyte sensitization in ABO hemolytic disease of the newborn and observations on pinocytosis of IgG anti-A antibodies by infant (cord) red cells. Br J Haematol 20:9, 1971.

Weiner CP, Williamson RA, Wenstrom KD, et al: Management of fetal hemolytic disease by cordocentesis. Am J Obstet Gynecol 165:1302, 1991.

Wethers D, Pearson H, Gaston M: Newborn screening for sickle cell disease and other hemoglobinopathies. Pediatrics (Suppl) 83:813, 1989.

Zanella A, Bianchi P: Red cell pyruvate kinase deficiency: From genetics to clinical manifestations. Baillieres Clin Haematol 13:57, 2000.

Zipursky A, Pollock J, Chown B, et al: Transplacental fetal hemorrhage after placental injury during delivery or amniocentesis. Lancet 2:493, 1963.

### Hypoplastic Anemia

Alter BP: The inherited bone marrow failure syndromes. In Nathan DG, Orkin SH (eds): Nathan and Oski's Hematology of Infancy and Childhood, 6th ed. Philadelphia, WB Saunders, 2003, p 280.

Diamond LK, Blackfan KD: Hypoplastic anemia. Am J Dis Child 56:464, 1938.

Gazda H, Lipton JM, Willig TN, et al: Evidence for linkage of familial Diamond-Blackfan anemia to chromosome 8p23.3-p22 and for non-19q non 8p disease. Blood 97:2145, 2000.

Glader BE: Diagnosis and management of red cell aplasia in children. Hematol Oncol Clin North Am 1:431, 1987.

Gustavsson P, Willig TN, van Haeringen A, et al: Diamond-Blackfan anaemia: Genetic homogeneity for a gene on chromosome 19q13 restricted to 1.8 Mb. Nat Genet 16:368, 1997.

Lipton JM, Federman N, Khabbaze Y, et al: Osteogenic sarcoma associated with Diamond-Blackfan anemia: A report from the Diamond Blackfan Anemia Registry. J Pediatr Hematol Oncol 23:377, 2001.

Miller R, Berman B: Transient erythroblastopenia of childhood in infants <6 months of age. Am J Pediatr Hematol Oncol 16:246, 1994.

Rogers ZR, Bergstrom SK, Amylon MD, et al: Reduced neutrophil counts in children with transient erythroblastopenia of childhood. J Pediatr 15:746, 1989.

Vlachos A, Federman N, Reyes-Haley C, et al: Hematopoietic stem cell transplantation for Diamond-Blackfan anemia: A report from the Diamond Blackfan Anemia Registry. Bone Marrow Transplant 27:381, 2001.

Wranne L: Transient erythroblastopenia in infancy and childhood. Scand J Haematol 7:76, 1970.

Ware RE, Kinney TR: Transient erythroblastopenia in the first year of life. Am J Hematol 37:156, 1991.

### Physiologic Anemia of Infancy and Prematurity

Alagappan A, Shattuck KE, Malloy MH: Impact of transfusion guidelines on neonatal transfusions. J Perinatology 18:92, 1998.

Batton DG, Goodrow D, Walker RH: Reducing neonatal transfusions. J Perinatol 12:152, 1992.

Bifano EM, Smith F, Borer J: Relationship between determinants of oxygen delivery and respiratory abnormalities in preterm infants with anemia. J Pediatr 120:292, 1992.

Blank JP, Sheagren TG, Vajara J, et al: The role of RBC transfusion in the premature infant. Am J Dis Child 138:831, 1984.

Brown MS, Berman ER, Luckey D: Prediction of the need for transfusion during anemia of prematurity. J Pediatr 116:773, 1990.

Christensen RD, Liechty KW, Koenig JM, et al: Administration of erythropoietin to newborn rats results in diminished neutrophil production. Blood 78:1241, 1991.

Cook S, Gunter J, Wissel M: Effective use of a strategy using assigned red cell units to limit donor exposure for neonatal patients. Transfusion 33:379, 1993.

Dallman PR: Anemia of prematurity: The prospects for avoiding blood transfusions with recombinant erythropoietin. Adv Pediatr 40:385, 1993.

Davis P, Herbert M, Davies DP, et al: Erythropoietin for anaemia in a preterm Jehovah's Witness baby. Early Hum Dev 1:279, 1991.

Emmerson AJB, Coles HJ, Stern CMM, et al: Double blind trial of recombinant human erythropoietin in preterm infants. Arch Dis Child 63:291, 1993.

Engelfriet CP, Reesink HW, Strauss RG, et al: Red cell transfusions in neonatal care. Vox Sang 80:122, 2001.

Frey B, Losa M: The value of capillary whole blood lactate for blood transfusion requirements in anaemia of prematurity. Intensive Care Med 27:222, 2001.

Gallagher PG, Ehrenkranz RA: Erythropoietin therapy for anemia of prematurity. Clin Perinatol 20:169, 1993.

Goldman MJ, Garcia C, Spurll G: Reduction of donor exposures in premature infants by the use of designated adenine-saline preserved split red blood cell packs. J Perinatol 21:363, 2001.

Graeber JE, Williams ML, Oski FA: The use of intramuscular vitamin E in the premature infant. J Pediatr 90:282, 1977.

Heese H De V, Smith S, Watermeyer S, et al: Prevention of iron deficiency in preterm neonates during infancy. S Afr Med J 77:339, 1990.

Izraeli S, Ben-Sira L, Harell D, et al: Lactic acid as a predictor for erythrocyte transfusion in healthy preterm infants with anemia of prematurity. J Pediatr 122:629, 1993.

Joshi A, Gerhardt T, Schandloff P, et al: Blood transfusion effect on the respiratory pattern of premature infants. Pediatrics 80:79, 1987.

Keyes WG, Donohue PK, Spivak JL, et al: Assessing the need for transfusion of premature infants and role of hematocrit, clinical signs and erythropoietin level. Pediatrics 84:412, 1989.

Lachance C, Chessex P, Fouron JC, et al: Myocardial, erythropoietic, and metabolic adaptations to anemia of prematurity. J Pediatr 125:278, 1994.

Liu EA, Mannino FL, Lane TA: Prospective, randomized trial of the safety and efficacy of a limited donor exposure transfusion program for premature neonates. J Pediatr 125:92, 1994.

Maier RF, Obladen M, Scigalla P, et al: The effect of epoetin beta (recombinant human erythropoietin) on the need for transfusion in very-low-birth-weight infants. N Engl J Med 330:1173, 1994.

Mentzer WC, Shannon KM: The use of recombinant human erythropoietin in preterm infants. Int J Pediatr Hematol Oncol 2:97, 1995.

Mestyan J, Fekete M, Bata G, et al: The basal metabolic rate of premature infants. Biol Neonatol 7:11, 1964.

Meyer MP, Meyer JH, Commerford A, et al: Recombinant human erythropoietin in the treatment of the anemia of prematurity: Results of a double-blind, placebo-controlled study. Pediatrics 93:918, 1994.

Nelle M, Höcker C, Zilow EP, et al: Effects of red cell transfusion on cardiac output and blood flow velocities in cerebral and gastrointestinal arteries in premature infants. Arch Dis Child 71:F45, 1994.

Oski FA, Barness LA: Vitamin E deficiency: A previously unrecognized cause of hemolytic anemia in the premature infant. J Pediatr 70:211, 1967.

Oski FA, Naiman JL: Hematologic Problems in the Newborn, 3rd. Philadelphia, WB Saunders, 1982.

Ritchie JH, Fish MB, McMasters V, et al: Edema and hemolytic anemia in premature infants. N Engl J Med 279:1185, 1968.

Ross MP, Christensen RD, Rothstein G, et al: A randomized trial to develop criteria for administering erythrocyte transfusions to anemic preterm infants 1 to 3 months of age. J Perinatol 9:246, 1989.

Shannon KM: Anemia of prematurity: Progress and prospects. Am J Pediatr Hematol Oncol 12:14, 1990.

Shannon KM, Keith JF III, Mentzer WC, et al: Recombinant human erythropoietin stimulates erythropoiesis and reduces erythrocyte transfusions in very low birth weight preterm infants. Pediatrics 95:1, 1995.

Shannon KM, Naylor GS, Torkildson JC, et al: Circulating erythroid progenitors in the anemia of prematurity. N Engl J Med 317:728, 1987.

Shireman TI, Hilsenrath PE, Strauss RG, et al: Recombinant human erythropoietin vs transfusions in the treatment of anemia of prematurity. Arch Pediatr Adolesc Med 148:582, 1994.

Stockman JA, Clark DA: Weight gain: A response to transfusion in selected preterm infants. Am J Dis Child 138:828, 1984.

Stockman JA III, Graeber JE, Clark DA, et al: Anemia of prematurity: Determinants of the erythropoietin response. J Pediatr 105:786, 1984.

Strauss RG: Erythropoietin and neonatal anemia. N Engl J Med 330:1227, 1994.

Strauss RG: Transfusion therapy in neonates. Am J Dis Child 145:904, 1991.

Strauss RG, Burmeister LF, Johnson K, et al: Feasibility and safety of AS-3 red blood cells for neonatal transfusions. J Pediatr 136:215, 2000.

Vamvakas EC, Strauss RG: Meta-analysis of controlled clinical trials studying the efficacy of rHuEPO in reducing blood transfusions in the anemia of prematurity. Transfusion 41:406, 2001.

Wandstrat TL, Kaplan B: Use of erythropoietin in premature neonates: Controversies and the future. Pediatrics 29:166, 1995.

Wardrop CA, Holland BM, Veale KE, et al: Nonphysiological anaemia of prematurity. Arch Dis Child. 53:855, 1978.

Worthington-White DA, Behnke M, Gross S: Premature infants require additional folate and vitamin $B_{12}$ to reduce the severity of the anemia of prematurity. Am J Clin Nutr 60:930, 1994.

Zipursky A, Brown EJ, Watts J, et al: Oral vitamin E supplementation for the prevention of anemia in premature infants: A controlled trial. Pediatrics 79:61, 1987.

Zipursky A: Erythropoietin therapy for premature infants: Cost without benefit? Pediatr Res 48:136, 2000.


### Polycythemia


Black VD, Rumack CM, Lubchenko LO, et al: Gastrointestinal injury in polychemic term infants. Pediatrics 76:225, 1985.

Carmi D, Wolach B, Dolfin T, et al: Polycythemia of the preterm and full-term newborn infant: Relationship between hematocrit and gestational age, total blood solutes, reticulocyte count, and blood pH. Biol Neonate 61:173, 1992.

Delaney-Black V, Camp BW, Lubchenko LO, et al: Neonatal hyperviscosity association with lower achievement and IQ scores at school age. Pediatrics 83:662, 1989.

Gatti RA, Muster AJ, Cole RB, et al: Neonatal polycythemia with transient cyanosis and cardiorespiratory abnormalities. J Pediatr 69:1063, 1966.

Hein HA, Lathrop SS: Partial exchange transfusion in term, polycythemic neonates: Absence of association with severe gastrointestinal injury. Pediatrics 80:75, 1987.

Kerrigan JF, Aleck KA, Tarby TJ, et al: Fumaric aciduria: Clinical and imaging features. Ann Neurol 47:583, 2000.

Kurlat I, Sola A: Neonatal polycythemia in appropriately grown infants of hypertensive mothers. Acta Paediatr 81:662, 1992.

Levy I, Pmerlob P, Ashkenazi S, et al: Neonatal polycythaemia: Effort of partial dilutional exchange transfusion with human albumin on whole blood viscosity. Eur J Pediatr 149:354, 1990.

Mentzer WC: Polycythaemia and the hyperviscosity syndrome in newborn infants. Clin Haematol 7:63, 1978.

Norman M, Fagrell B, Herin P: Effects of neonatal polycythemia and hemodilution on capillary perfusion. J Pediatr 121:103, 1992.

Norman M, Fagrell B, Herin P: Skin microcirculation in neonatal polycythaemia and effects of haemodilution. Interaction between haematocrit, vasomotor activity and perfusion. Acta Paediatr 82:672, 1993.

Oh W, Omori K, Emmanouilides GC, Phelps DL: Placenta to lamb fetus transfusion in utero during acute hypoxia. Am J Obstet Gynecol 122:316, 1975.

Oski FA, Naiman JL: Hematologic Problems in the Newborn, 3rd. Philadelphia, WB Saunders, 1982.

Ramamurthy RS, Berlanga M: Postnatal alteration in hematocrit and viscosity in normal and polycythemic infants. J Pediatr 110:929, 1987.

Shohat M, Merlob P, Reisner SH: Neonatal polycythemia: Early diagnosis and incidence relating to time of sampling. Pediatrics 73:7, 1984.

Villalta IA, Pramanik AK, Diaz-Blanco J, et al: Diagnostic errors in neonatal polycythemia based on method of hermatocrit determination. J Pediatr 115:460, 1989.


### Methemoglobinemia


Bartos HR, Desforges JF: Erythrocyte DPNH dependent diaphorase levels in infants. Pediatrics 37:991, 1966.

Climie CR, McLean S, Starmer GA, Thomas J: Methaemoglobinaemia in mother and foetus following continuous epidermal analgesia with prilocaine. Br J Anaesthesiol 39:155, 1967.

Comly HR: Cyanosis in infants caused by nitrates in well water. JAMA 129:112, 1945.

Couper R: Methaemoglobinaemia secondary to topical lignocaine/prilocaine in a circumcised neonate. J Paediatr Child Health 36:406, 2000.

Davidson D, Barefield ES, Kattwinkel J, et al: Inhaled nitric oxide for the early treatment of persistent pulmonary hypertension of the term newborn: A randomized, double-masked, placebo-controlled, dose-response, multicenter study. Pediatrics 101:325, 1998.

Harley JD, Celermajer JM: Neonatal methaemoglobinaemia and the "red-brown" screening test. Lancet 2:1223, 1970.

Hayashi A, Fujita T, Fujimura M, et al: A new abnormal fetal hemoglobin, Hb FM-Osaka. Hemoglobin 4:447, 1980.

Kay MA, O'Brien W, Kessler B, et al: Transient organic-aciduria and methemoglobinemia with acute gastroenteritis. Pediatrics 85:589, 1990.

Keating JP, Lell ME, Strauss AW, et al: Infantile methemoglobinemia caused by carrot juice. N Engl J Med 288:824, 1973.

Martin H, Huisman THJ: Formation of ferrihaemoglobin of isolated human haemoglobin types by sodium nitrate. Nature 200:898, 1963.

Murray KF, Christie DL: Dietary protein intolerance in infants with transient methemoglobinemia and diarrhea. J Pediatr 122:90, 1993.

Porat R, Gilbert S, Magilner D: Methylene blue–induced phototoxicity: An unrecognized complication. Pediatr 97:717, 1996.

Priest JR, Watterson J, Jones RT, et al: Mutant fetal hemoglobin causing cyanosis in a newborn. Pediatrics 83:734, 1989.

Taddio A, Stevens B, Craig K, et al: Efficacy and safety of lidocaine-prilocaine cream for pain during circumcision. N Engl J Med 336:1197, 1997.

Tse S, Barrington K, Byrne P: Methemoglobinemia associated with prilocaine use in neonatal circumcision. Am J Perinatol 12:331, 1995.

Yano SS, Danish EH, Hsia YE: Transient methemoglobinemia with acidosis in infants. J Pediatr 100:415, 1982.

CHAPTER 78

# Neonatal Leukocyte Physiology and Disorders

Elvira Parravicini, Carmella van de Ven, and Mitchell S. Cairo

This chapter presents an overview of neonatal leukocyte physiology and quantitative and qualitative disorders of leukocytes. Topics include the normal physiology and defects associated with neonatal hematopoiesis, neutrophils, lymphocytes, monocytes, and dendritic cells. Novel therapeutic approaches also are discussed.

## HEMATOPOIESIS

Hematopoiesis is a complex process that begins with an uncommitted pluripotent hematopoietic stem cell that progresses through a series of steps to development of a single-lineage progenitor cell. The final result of this physiologic process is a mature, lineage-restricted effector cell that circulates either in the bloodstream or within tissue. In 1961 Till and McCulloch demonstrated that when bone marrow cells were transfused into lethally irradiated mice, separate colonies of hematopoietic cells could be identified in the spleen of the recipient. Each colony, containing neutrophils, monocytes, erythrocytes, megakaryocytes, eosinophils, and basophils, was derived from an individual cell, and many of the colonies contained cells that were capable of such colony formation when transplanted into a second irradiated animal. Such cells, which are capable of unlimited self-renewal, have been referred to as *pluripotent stem cells*.

### Fetal and Neonatal Hematopoiesis

In human ontogeny, the process of maturation involves the orderly shift of hematopoiesis from extramedullary organs to the bone marrow (Nathan, 1989). Hematopoiesis is first observed by day 15 in blood islands formed by the yolk sac (Zon, 1995). The erythroid lineage is predominant during yolk sac hematopoiesis. Yolk sac erythrocytes are large nucleated cells, expressing the products of certain genes that are unique to this phase of development. Hematopoietic progenitor cells that migrate to the fetal liver and subsequently to the fetal bone marrow are thought to originate from either the yolk sac or dorsal mesenteric hematopoietic cells (Zon, 1995). The transition of embryonal hematopoiesis from the yolk sac to the liver is associated with development of a differentiating program in proliferating stem cells as shown by their erythroid progeny and therefore parallels changes in multiple parameters (e.g., morphology and globin expression).

Granulocyte-macrophage colony-forming units (CFU-GMs) have been identified in fetal liver as early as 5 weeks of gestation. However, their number is low compared with that of cells of the erythroid lineage. Neutrophils have been identified in the bone marrow of fetuses as early as 14 weeks of gestation, but they are limited in number. Myeloid cells (neutrophil progenitor cells) constitute less than 5% of nucleated marrow cells in the fetus, compared with 31% to 69% in term neonates and 25% to 52% in adults.

### Hematopoietic Growth Factors

The regulation of hematopoiesis is a complex biologic process involving multifactorial mechanisms. As reported by our group (Abu-Ghosh et al, 2000), in vitro culture of hematopoietic progenitor cells has enabled the categorization, functional analysis, and definition of the growth factor requirements of the various committed progenitor cells (Fig. 78–1).

The hematopoietic pluripotent stem cell (PPSC) that expresses CD34 represents an early and primitive hematopoietic stem cell that can be identified by immunophenotyping. This cell can either undergo self-renewal or proliferate and differentiate into any of the hematopoietic blood lineages depending on its exposure to individual and combinations of hematopoietic growth factors (HGFs). Primitive progenitor cells maintain their multipotent potential, whereas more mature progenitor cells become committed as they differentiate into specific lineages. A relatively small and common set of pluripotent stem cells gives rise to large numbers of functionally diverse mature cells.

Cell proliferation and differentiation is regulated and controlled by highly specific protein factors, affecting single- and multiple-lineage hematopoiesis. These growth-promoting factors are named colony-stimulating factors (CSFs). CSFs are a group of glycoproteins with molecular masses of 18 to 90 kD, defined by their abilities to support proliferation and differentiation of hematopoietic cells of various lineages (see Fig. 78–1).

#### Granulocyte Colony-Stimulating Factor

Human granulocyte colony-stimulating factor (G-CSF) was first purified to homogeneity from a medium conditioned by the bladder carcinoma cell line 5637. The molecular mass of this glycoprotein is between 18 and 20 kD and the gene has been localized to chromosome 17q11-21. It has been identified in the 15 to 17 chromosomal translocation commonly found in acute promyelocytic leukemia. G-CSF is produced primarily by mature macrophages, endothelial cells, fibroblasts, and mesothelial cells. Its production can be stimulated in these cells by tumor necrosis factor, lipopolysaccharide (LPS), and the interleukins IL-1, IL-3, and IL-6 and also stem cell factor

This chapter is based on work supported in part by a grant from the Pediatric Cancer Research Foundation.

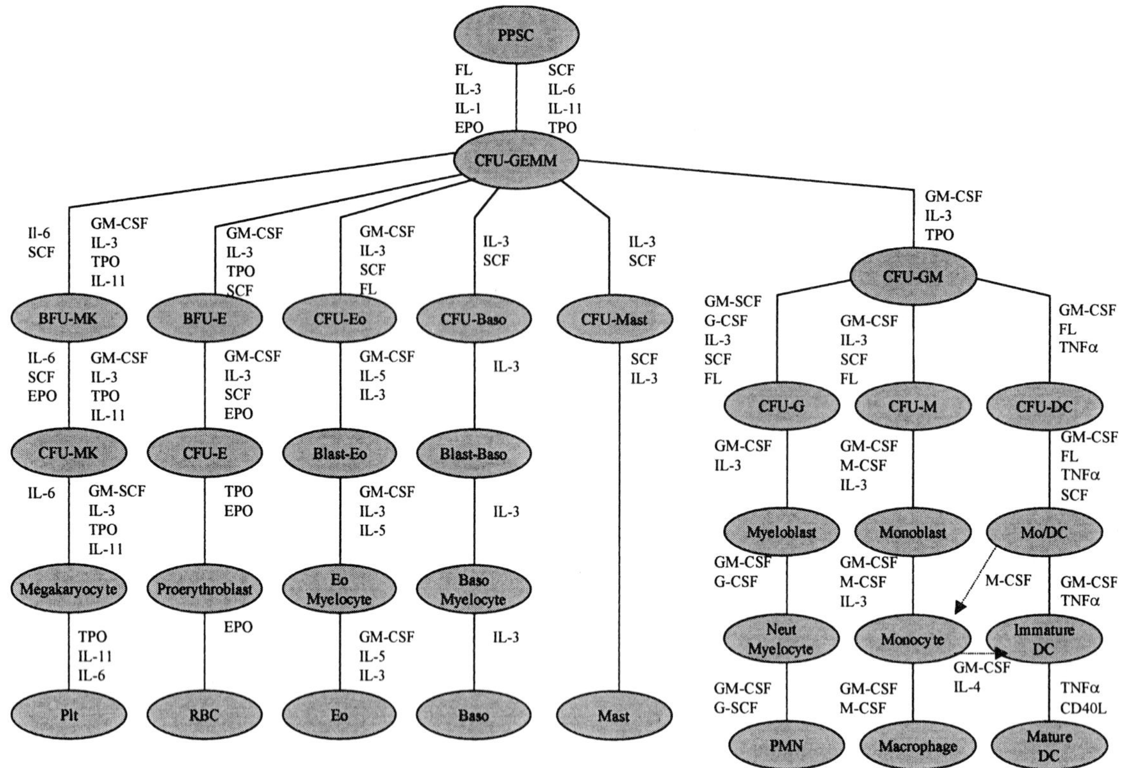


**FIGURE 78–1.** Hematopoiesis and hematopoietic growth factors. Baso, basophil; BFU, burst-forming unit; CFU, colony-forming unit; CSF, colony-stimulating factor; DC, dendritic cell; E, erythroid; Eo, eosinophil; EPO, erythopoietin; FL, Flt 3 ligand; G, granulocyte; GEMM, granulocyte, erythrocyte, macrophage, and megakaryocyte; GM, granulocyte-macrophage; IL, interleukin; M, macrophage; MK, megakaryocyte; Mo, monocyte; Neut, neutrophil; Plt, platelet; PMN, polymorphonuclear neutrophil leukocyte; PPSC, pluripotent stem cell; RBC, red blood cell; SCF, stem cell factor; TNFα, tumor necrosis factor-α; TPO, thrombopoietin.

(SCF) (Lieschke and Burgess, 1992). G-CSF stimulates the proliferation of committed myeloid progenitor cells and has specific activity toward granulocyte colony formation with pure neutrophil colony proliferation. G-CSF affects mature neutrophil effector function in that it primes neutrophils to increase expression of chemotactic receptors and to enhance bactericidal and phagocytic activity, superoxide generation, and antibody-dependent cellular cytotoxicity.

Clinical studies have shown that G-CSF therapy results in a dose-dependent increase in the circulating neutrophil count in children and adults with congenital and acquired neutropenia syndromes as well as chemotherapy-induced neutropenia (Bonilla et al, 1989; Hammond et al, 1989). Significant differences in G-CSF production, G-CSF gene expression, and circulating G-CSF level exist between adults and newborns (Cairo et al, 1993). Gessler and coworkers (1995) reported G-CSF serum levels at birth with respect to neutrophil count, infection, and gestational age. Serum concentrations of G-CSF in term and preterm neonates without infection reached peak levels within the first 7 hours of life (mean values of 261 pg/mL and 126 pg/mL in term and preterm infants, respectively). Levels decreased to normal adult range (<50 pg/mL) between 4 and 7 days of age and were unchanged at 2 to 3 weeks of age.

From neonatal animal model studies it appears that the administration of recombinant human G-CSF (rhG-CSF) has significant effects on neonatal rat hematopoiesis, with a marked increase in the circulating neutrophil count, bone marrow myeloid progenitor pool, and neutrophil storage pool (NSP) (Cairo et al, 1990b). Combining G-CSF with earlier-acting cytokines such as SCF, IL-6, and IL-11 further enhances these effects on neonatal rat hematopoiesis (Cairo et al, 1991a, 1992a, 1993, 1994).

G-CSF acts in synergism with antibiotics in improving survival during neonatal sepsis, but only if given before or at the starting of the development of experimental sepsis (Cairo et al, 1990b, 1992b). Additionally, improved survival during experimental sepsis in neonatal rats has been demonstrated following prophylactic use of G-CSF in combination with antibiotics and either SCF or IL-11 (Cairo et al, 1992a, 1994; Chang et al, 1994).

G-CSF has been used in clinical trials for both prevention and therapy of neonatal sepsis. One study investigated the safety, pharmacokinetics, and biologic efficacy of administration of G-CSF to newborn infants with sepsis (Gillan et al, 1994). Forty-two newborn infants, both term and preterm, with presumed sepsis within the first 3 days of life were randomized to receive either placebo or varying doses of rhG-CSF. The growth factor was given for 3 days at doses of 1, 5, or 10 μg/kg every day or 5 or 10 μg/kg twice a day. The half-life of rhG-CSF was 4.4 ± 0.4 hours. Intravenous rhG-CSF was well tolerated at all gestational ages and was not associated with any recognized acute toxicity. RhG-CSF induced a significant increase in the absolute neutrophil count (ANC) within 24 hours following doses of 5 and 10 μg/kg given either every 24 hours or divided every 12 hours. The increased neutrophil count was maintained for 96 hours, 48 hours after the last rhG-CSF dose. Bone marrow aspirates demonstrated a dose-dependent increase in NSP following treatment with rhG-CSF. In addition, polymorphonuclear neutrophil (PMN) C3bi expression was significantly increased at 24 hours following administration of 10 μg/kg of rhG-CSF every 24 hours. The enhancement of neonatal neutrophil C3bi expression indicates that rhG-CSF may induce functional maturation of neonatal neutrophils. A recent 2-year follow-up analysis in these patients has shown that rhG-CSF therapy for presumed neonatal sepsis was not associated with long-term hematologic, immunologic, or developmental adverse effects (Rosenthal et al, 1995).

A randomized, placebo-controlled trial of G-CSF administration to infants with neutropenia and clinical sign of early-onset sepsis was recently reported (Schibler et al, 1998). Twenty infants, term and preterm, were given G-CSF (10 μg/kg/day) or placebo for 3 days. ANC, ratio of immature to total neutrophils (I/T ratio), bone marrow NSP, bone marrow neutrophil proliferative pool (NPP), and plasma concentration of G-CSF were evaluated and found to be similar in treated and control infants. No significant differences were found in outcome measures such as severity of illness and mortality.

### Granulocyte-Macrophage Colony-Stimulating Factor

Granulocyte-macrophage colony-stimulating factor (GM-CSF) was purified from a medium conditioned by the human T-cell lymphotropic virus-II (HTLV-II)–infected T-lymphoblast cell line MO. Characterization of the purified material showed that GM-CSF is a glycoprotein of 22 kD, and the gene is located on chromosome 5q21-32. Potential physiologic sources for GM-CSF are T and B lymphocytes, macrophages, fibroblasts, mast cells, endothelial cells, mesothelial cells, and osteoblasts.

GM-CSF acts as a potent growth factor both ex vivo and in vivo by stimulating proliferation and maturation of myeloid progenitor cells, subsequently giving rise to neutrophils, eosinophils, and monocytes. GM-CSF has direct and indirect effects on human neutrophils. Direct effects include inhibition of neutrophil migration, enhanced degranulation, induction of adhesion, and changes in cytoskeleton and cell shape. Indirect actions enhance the ability of the neutrophil to respond to triggering stimuli. Among these effects are increased superoxide generation, $Ca^{2+}$ fluxes, and production of inflammatory mediators such as leukotriene $B_4$.

Administration of GM-CSF in clinical trials results in an immediate and transient decrease in circulating neutrophils, eosinophils, and monocytes, followed by a recovery to baseline within 2 hours. A second phase follows in which the number of leukocytes increases, with a marked "shift to the left" as a result of demargination from the bone marrow NSP and increased myeloid production in the marrow.

The effect of GM-CSF on the incidence of sepsis in human neonates also has been evaluated. A phase I/II trial determined the feasibility, safety, and biologic response of GM-CSF in very low-birth-weight (VLBW) (≤1500 g) neonates. Twenty neonates (500 to 1500 g) were randomized in the first 3 days of life to receive GM-CSF at 5 μg/kg/day or 5 μg/kg/twice a day or 10 μg/kg/day or placebo. The study demonstrated that GM-CSF was well tolerated with no toxic acute effects. GM-CSF induced a significant increase in ANC, absolute monocyte count (AMC), bone marrow NSP, and neutrophil C3bi expression (Cairo et al, 1995).

A phase III multicentric, randomized, prospective, double-blind, placebo-controlled trial was performed to determine whether prophylactic administration of GM-CSF would reduce nosocomial infections in VLBW neonates. Two hundred sixty-four infants (500 to 1500 g) were randomized in the first 3 days of life to receive either GM-CSF (8 μg/kg/day) for 7 days and then every other day for 21 days or placebo. No toxicity was recorded. The ANC was significantly elevated in the GM-CSF group on days 7, 14, and 21, and the absolute eosinophil count (AEC) on days 7 and 28. However, there was no difference in the incidence of confirmed nosocomial infections between the two groups (Cairo et al, 1999).

## NEONATAL NEUTROPENIA

Manroe and colleagues (1979) established reference values for ANCs in term and preterm infants during the first 28 days of life for both healthy infants and those with perinatal complications. Mouzinho and associates (1994) studied serial white blood cells counts in healthy preterm VLBW infants to investigate whether this subgroup of patients had different neutrophil counts from those found in previous studies in cohorts consisting mostly of term infants. They found that there was a wider range of the absolute total neutrophil count, mostly resulting from a downward shift of the lower boundary, especially during the first 60 hours of life. However, there was no difference in absolute total immature neutrophil counts or in I/T ratio. Similar findings were noted by Gessler and colleagues (1995), who studied, retrospectively, neutropenia in low-birth-weight infants and its relationship to maternal disease, sepsis, and antibiotic therapy. They noted that neutropenia during the second week of life was most commonly related to antibiotic use.

Neutropenia may be caused by any one or a combination of defects in production or maturation of neutrophils or in release of neutrophils from the bone marrow to the peripheral blood. The pathophysiologic mechanism responsible for neonatal neutropenia may be either exhaustion of myeloid committed progenitor cells or inadequate response of progenitor cells to proliferative or maturational signals. In a series of studies, Christensen and Rothstein (1984) documented significant differences in myeloid progenitor pools and cell kinetics in fetal and neonatal rats compared with adult rats. In the newborn rat, the myeloid progenitor pool, consisting of CFU-GMs in the bone marrow, is only 25% of that of adult animals and requires 4 weeks of maturation to reach adult levels. Additionally, despite a lower number, the CFU-GM of the newborn rat is in a state of near-maximal proliferative capacity, the maximal rate of proliferation being 75% to 80%, whereas that of the adult CFU-GM is only 25% (Christensen and Rothstein, 1984). Concomitantly with reduced numbers of myeloid progenitor cells (lower numbers of CFU-GMs) and lower expansion capacity (already near maximal proliferative rate), the neonatal rat also possesses reduced numbers (25% of adult) of NSP, defined as the percentage of metamyelocytes, bands, and mature neutrophils in the bone marrow. The NSP reach adult levels in the neonate rat at 4 weeks of age. Following experimental sepsis with group B streptococci (GBS), adult rats respond with a transient decrease in circulating neutrophil counts followed by significant neutrophilia associated with a two- to threefold increase in the progenitor pool (CFU-Meg) and an increase in the proliferative rate to 75% of the maximal capacity (Christensen et al, 1982, 1983). In contrast, neonatal rats under the same conditions had a decrease by 50% of their progenitor pool and failed to increase their myeloid proliferative rate, which, as discussed previously, was already at near-maximal levels. Most important, during experimental sepsis, neonatal rats had further depletion of their already reduced NSP reserves by almost 80%, compared with a decline of 33% in adult rats.

## Kostmann Syndrome

Kostmann syndrome is an autosomal recessive disorder that manifests within the first few months of life with severe, persistent neutropenia, with ANCs of less than 500/mm$^3$ and often less than 200/mm$^3$. Bone marrow examination typically demonstrates a maturational arrest at the promyelocyte stage (Kostmann, 1956). Affected children have recurrent infections, especially of the skin and oral mucosa.

Recently, Dale and colleagues (2000) described the occurrence of mutations of the gene encoding neutrophil elastase in 22 patients with severe congenital neutropenia. This is the well-known locus for autosomal dominant cyclic neutropenia. Neutrophil elastase is a protease that is synthesized and packaged in promyelocytes at early stages of neutrophil development. The pathogenic role of elastase mutation in causing neutropenia, in both congenital and cyclic neutropenia, may be linked to the poor survival of early myeloid precursor cells.

G-CSF has been used with success in increasing the ANC and decreasing the number of infections in patients with congenital neutropenia (Bonilla et al, 1989; Welte et al, 1990). Dale and associates (1993) have described the successful use of G-CSF in the treatment of infants, children, and adults with either congenital neutropenia or cyclic neutropenia, with significant laboratory and clinical responses. Bone marrow transplantation also has been used for those patients in whom medical therapy fails and who have a human leukocyte antigen (HLA)-identical unaffected sibling.

## Alloimmune Neonatal Neutropenia

Alloimmune neonatal neutropenia occurs as a result of maternal sensitization to neutrophil antigens present on the infant's neutrophils, paternally acquired, that are not present on the maternal neutrophils, with subsequent production of immnuoglobulin G (IgG). Neutrophil-specific antibodies are found in the maternal and infant sera, but the mother has a normal neutrophil count. It is estimated to occur at a frequency of 3% of live births (Curnette, 1993). The most common antigens involved are NA1 and NA2. Peripheral blood counts show profound neutropenia and often demonstrate a monocytosis and eosinophilia. The condition is self-limiting and typically lasts for 6 to 7 weeks, during which time the neonate is susceptible to infections, mostly cutaneous in nature but occasionally life-threatening, necessitating intensive support. Therapeutic interventions that have been attempted include, in addition to antimicrobials, intravenous immune globulin (IVIG) infusions, with mixed success, as well as granulocyte transfusions that lack the disparate antigen.

## Maternal Hypertension–Associated Neutropenia

One of the most common and well-described causes of transient neonatal neutropenia is maternal hypertension. Infants of hypertensive mothers seem to have decreased production of neutrophils, but the cause is uncertain. Several studies showed a decrease in neutrophil progenitor cells, decreased cycling of these cells, a relatively normal NPP and NSP, and the absence of a "left shift" (Koenig et al, 1989). In fact, many investigators have documented an increased incidence of nosocomial infections if neutropenia is associated with maternal hypertension (Doron et al, 1994). In a prospective study, Mouzinho and colleagues (1994) analyzed the incidence of neonatal neutropenia in relation to birth weight, gestational age, and severity of maternal hypertension. They concluded that the neonatal neutropenia was inversely related to the birth weight and gestational age and directly related to the severity of the preeclampsia. The incidence was nearly 80% among neonates born at less than 30 weeks of gestation and was statistically different from that in similar infants born to normotensive mothers. In most cases, the neutropenia resolved within 72 hours, but in some cases the neutropenia persisted and G-CSF was used to increase the neutrophil count (La Gamma et al, 1995).

## Congenital Disorders Associated with Neonatal Neutropenia

### *Cartilage-Hair Hypoplasia*

Cartilage-hair hypoplasia (CHH), inherited as an autosomal recessive trait common among Amish populations, is characterized by short-limbed dwarfism, fine hair, and increased susceptibility to infections. Immunologic and hematologic investigations in patients with recurrent infections revealed the presence of chronic noncyclic neutropenia and lymphopenia. Neutropenia may be due to an arrest of myeloid maturation, with underproduction of mature neutrophils and diminished bone marrow storage pools. Lymphopenia, decreased delayed hypersensitivity, and impaired in vitro responsiveness of lymphocytes to mitogens suggest functional dysfunction of small lymphocytes (Lux et al, 1970).

### *Schwachman Syndrome*

Schwachman syndrome is a rare multiorgan disease of unknown origin, characterized by metaphyseal chondrodysplasia, dwarfism, pancreatic exocrine insufficiency, and neutropenia. Clinical manifestations begin in neonatal age with diarrhea, weight loss, failure to thrive, eczema, otitis media, and pneumonia. By 2 years of age, dwarfism is evident; later, gait disturbances result from metaphyseal chondrodysplasia. Neutropenia is severe (ANC of 200 to 400/mm$^3$) and causes recurrent infections. Aplastic anemia occurs in about 25% of the cases, and leukemic transformation has been described. In vivo administration of G-CSF has been reported to increase the neutrophil count to normal levels.

### *Reticular Dysgenesis*

Reticular dysgenesis is characterized by extremely severe neutropenia, leukopenia, agammaglobulinemia, and presence of rudimentary thymic, lymphoid, and splenic tissue. In the bone marrow, erythroid and magakaryocyte elements are normal, but myeloid cells are absent or sparse, possibly owing to a maturation defect in a progenitor cell (Roper et al, 1985). Use of GM-CSF or G-CSF has been ineffective. Allogeneic bone marrow transplantation remains the only available curative option.

## QUALITATIVE DEFECTS (DYSFUNCTION) OF NEONATAL PHAGOCYTIC IMMUNITY

The immaturity of the neonatal phagocytic immune system in both humans and animals predisposes the neonate to greatly increased morbidity and mortality during bacterial sepsis. Neutrophils and macrophages play vital roles as effector cells in the phagocytic system. The efficient function of the phagocyte system depends on several factors, including the presence of adequate numbers of phagocytes in the peripheral blood, the ability to respond to signals from the sites of inflammation, the ability to migrate to these sites, and the capability to ingest and kill invading microorganisms. The immaturity of neonatal host defense is characterized by profound deficiencies in quantitative and qualitative phagocytic effector cell function.

Stressed and septic neonates exhibit significant dysfunction of the phagocytic process. Chemotaxis is the initial step in the inflammatory response. Chemotaxis is a process that involves numerous changes in cellular motility and mobility, followed by intracellular biochemical changes. It begins with stimuli from the invading microorganism and continues with the directed migration of neutrophils to the site of invasion, ingestion of the pathogen, and killing by oxygen- dependent and -independent mechanisms. Qualitative abnormalities of neonatal neutrophils include decreased deformability and impaired functions including chemotaxis, phagocytosis, adherence, bacterial killing, aggregation, and oxidative metabolism (Cairo et al, 1990c).

GM-CSF increases adult neutrophil oxidative metabolism by augmenting *N*-formyl-L-methionyl–L-leucyl-phenylalanine (FMLP)-, C5a-, and leukotriene $B_4$–induced superoxide anion production. Additionally, GM-CSF increases FMLP-stimulated chemotaxis, promotes phagocytosis of *Staphylococcus aureus*, and augments neutrophil aggregation by the increased expression of surface adhesion (Gasson et al, 1984; Weisbart et al, 1985) (Table 78–1). Our laboratory investigated the biologic effects of GM-CSF on cord blood (CB) neutrophil oxidative metabolism, bacterial killing, and chemotaxis (Cairo et al, 1989). We determined that GM-CSF is not a direct stimulant of in vitro neonatal neutrophil function; however, when CB was preincubated with GM-CSF and stimulated with FMLP or opsonized zymosan particles, a significant increase in superoxide production was observed. Priming with GM-CSF and subsequent stimulation with phorbolmyristate acetate (PMA) did not evoke a significant difference in superoxide release when CB neutrophils were compared with unprimed controls. Furthermore, when CB was compared with adult neutrophils, an earlier but less maximal superoxide generation was seen in CB.

The diminished inflammatory response of CB neutrophils results in a high incidence of microbial invasion. Significant defects in the up-regulation of surface-active glycoprotein receptors (C3bi) and reduced aggregation also predispose the neonate to impaired response to bacterial infection. C3bi expression has been compared in adult blood and CB neutrophils and found to be significantly less in CB when stimulated by FMLP- or zymosan-activated serum. (Cairo et al, 1990c). However, CB neutrophils incubated with GM-CSF demonstrated a significant induction of C3bi expression. Also, a significant increase of C3bi expression was seen when CB neutrophils were pretreated with GM-CSF and subsequently stimulated with calcium ionophore A23187. The up-regulation of C3bi receptor by GM-CSF also appears to correlate with enhancement of CB neutrophil aggregation. GM-CSF also primes CB neutrophils for increased neutrophil aggregation following agonist (FMLP) stimulation.

G-CSF and tumor necrosis factor-α (TNF-α) also have been reported to modulate the function of adult and CB neutrophils in a manner similar to that for GM-CSF.

**TABLE 78–1**

**Comparison of GM-CSF Effects on Adult and Cord Blood in Vitro Neutrophil Function**

| | Adult | Cord Blood |
|---|---|---|
| Superoxide production | ↑↑↑↑ | ↑↑ |
| Chemotaxis | ↑ | ↑ |
| Bacterial killing | ↑↑ | ↑↑ |
| C3bi receptor expression | ↑↑ | ↑↑ |
| Aggregation | ↑ | ↑ |

GM-CSF, granulocyte-macrophage colony-stimulating factor.

Priming CB neutrophils with G-CSF or TNF-α and subsequent stimulation with FMLP induces the expression of C3bi receptors, enhances bacterial and phagocytic activity, and superoxide generation.

## LYMPHOCYTE PHYSIOLOGY AND DYSFUNCTION

### Granulocyte Colony-Stimulating Factor

Our laboratory has demonstrated a significant reduction in G-CSF messenger RNA (mRNA) transcript expression as well as decreased production of G-CSF protein in stimulated CB versus adult peripheral blood (APB) mononuclear cells (MNCs). (Cairo et al, 1992b). Furthermore, we have determined that circulating serum G-CSF levels, measured by enzyme-linked immunosorbent assay (ELISA), in CB from term infants are low but similar to healthy adult levels (50 pg/mL). However, we found that G-CSF levels are approximately threefold higher in CB from healthy preterm infants than in CB from term infants between days of life 1 and 3. G-CSF production in the first days of life is associated with peak values at 7 hours of life, followed by a peak neutrophil count approximately 6 hours later.

### Granulocyte-Macrophage Colony-Stimulating Factor

On stimulation of mononuclear cells with phytohemagglutinin and phorbol-12-myristate-6-acetate (PMA), we have observed a sevenfold decrease of GM-CSF protein production in CB versus APB. Additionally, a fourfold decrease in the expression of GM-CSF mRNA and a threefold lower GM-CSF half-life were measured in CB versus APB stimulated MNCs. Although no difference in rate of transcriptional activation from activated CB and APB MNCs was noted, actinomycin D transcriptional decay studies demonstrated reduced GM-CSF half-life in activated CB compared with APB mononuclear cells (Cairo et al, 1991a).

We thus established that the decrease in GM-CSF mRNA expression and protein in activated CB versus APB MNCs is due to a decrease in posttranscriptional mRNA stability and not to alterations in GM-CSF gene transcription. The cytoplasmic instability of GM-CSF mRNA is regulated in part by adenosine + uridine–rich elements in the 3′-untranslated region of the cytokine transcript. We have previously investigated the molecular basis for the differential stability of GM-CSF mRNA in CB and APB MNCs using electrophoretic mobility-shift assays. We demonstrated that the destabilization of GM-CSF mRNA in CB MNC is translation dependent and that increased levels of the specific RNA binding protein AUF-1 isoforms in the CB MNC may target transcripts for increased degradation and contribute to the dysregulation of phagocytic immunity (Buzby et al, 1996).

### Macrophage Colony-Stimulating Factor

Macrophage colony-stimulating factor (M-CSF) is a hematopoietic growth factor that regulates the proliferation, differentiation and functional activation of monocytes. Normally detected in human serum, M-CSF plays an important role in enhancing the effector functions of mature monocytes and macrophages. M-CSF serum levels are increased in CB and further increased in the neonate. Our laboratory studied the regulation of the M-CSF gene expression under basal and activated conditions and the transcriptional and post-transcriptional regulation of M-CSF in CB versus APB. Both CB and adult blood MNCs constitutively express M-CSF mRNA on adhesion to tissue culture flasks. However, when GM-CSF was added as a costimulator, CB MNCs produced two- to threefold less M-CSF protein compared with APB MNCs, and a fourfold decrease in M-CSF mRNA expression was shown in both unstimulated and GM-CSF–induced CB versus APB MNCs. Furthermore, we determined that M-CSF mRNA expression peaked between 16 and 24 hours after stimulation and fell to normal levels by 48 hours in both CB and APB (Suen et al, 1994). This study also demonstrated that the transcriptional rates of the M-CSF gene were similar in CB and APB even after stimulation with rhGM-CSF. However, actinomycin D decay studies showed the half-life of M-CSF mRNA in CB MNCs was significantly lower, and the induction of M-CSF mRNA after cycloheximide administration in CB compared with APB MNCs was significantly increased, suggesting that one or more labile proteins may be involved in regulating M-CSF transcript stability (Suen et al, 1994).

## NEGATIVE REGULATORS OF HEMATOPOIESIS

Cytokines also play a predominant role as negative regulators of hematopoiesis. These negative growth factors regulate early hematopoiesis with suppressive effects on the proliferation of early myeloid and lymphoid progenitors. The most notable negative regulators of hematopoiesis are transforming growth factor-β1 (TGF-β1), macrophage inflammatory protein-1α (MIP-1α), and IL-8. TGF-β1 induces a wide range of responses including the inhibition of lymphocyte, thymocyte, and epithelial cell proliferation as well as the suppression and proliferation of early progenitor cells. MIP-1α and IL-8 also have suppressive effects on early progenitors, similar to TGF-β1. Our laboratory measured the protein levels of TGF-β1 and MIP-1α in the conditioned media of phytohemagglutinin and PMA-stimulated CB and APB MNCs. Both TGF-β1 and MIP-1α levels were significantly less in CB supernatants compared with APB supernatants. Furthermore, the mRNA expression of TGF-β1, MIP-1α, and IL-8 in stimulated CB and APB MNCs was found to be significantly less in CB MNCs; yet no significant difference was seen in the transcription rate of either the TGF-β1 or MIP-1α genes in CB compared with APB. These results suggested that the reduced mRNA of the negative regulators, TGF-β1 and MIP-1α, may be secondary to alterations in posttranscriptional regulation, and that the altered expression of both positive and negative regulators may be involved in the immaturity of host defense in the neonate (Chang et al, 1994).

# MONOCYTES AND DENDRITIC CELLS

## Monocytes

### Ontogeny

Embryonic macrophages are found among hematopoietic cells in the yolk sac at 3 to 6 weeks of gestation. After 6 weeks, the fetal liver becomes the primary site of hematopoiesis for the next 6 to 22 weeks of gestation, when the bone marrow becomes the lifelong center of blood cell production (Palis et al, 2001). Monocytes are present in high proportions in the early hematopoietic tissues, with approximately 70% of hematopoietic cells at 4.5 weeks of gestation morphologically identifiable as monocytes. This proportion decreases to 1% to 2% over the next 6 weeks as erythroid cells become predominant. The precursors of monocytes, monoblasts, and promonocytes continue to be present in the fetal liver; however, intravascular monocytes are not observed until the fifth month of gestation. Circulating monocytes do not appear with regularity until hematopoiesis is first established in the bone marrow after the tenth week of gestation.

At birth, the number of circulating granulocyte-monocyte progenitor cells (CFU-GMs), the committed progenitor precursor to monocytes, are increased in cord blood before 32 weeks, but levels fall shortly after birth. The estimated total bone marrow cellularity of the term neonate at birth is approximately $1.36 \times 10^{11}$ cells/L, and the total cell numbers decline over the first 1 to 2 weeks to $3.5 \times 10^{10}$/L. These levels remain low through the neonatal period, in which circulating monocyte counts are highest in the first week of life, ranging from 1340 to 2200 cells/μL, and gradually fall in successive weeks to 700 cells/mm$^3$ at 3 weeks and 450 cells/mm$^3$ by 6 years of age.

### Morphology

Immunophenotyping using fluorescent conjugated monoclonal antibodies also has been used to identify monocyte cell subpopulations and give insight to cell activation and function. During ontogeny, macrophages in the fetal liver express CD11b as early as 12 weeks of gestation. The classic monocyte marker, CD14, does not appear until about 15 to 21 weeks of gestation. CD14 expression on circulating MNCs is equivalent in CB and APB. CD11a, CD11b, and CD11c are expressed in lower densities on CB monocytes than on adult cells. There is also lower expression of class II major histocompatibility complex (MHC) antigens HLA-DR, HLA-DP, and HLA-DQ on neonatal monocytes compared with adult monocytes. HLA-DR expression also is significantly lower in CD14$^+$ populations in CB compared with APB CD14$^+$. The density of these class II MHC antigens has been correlated with antigen-presenting capacity of monocytes in vitro; however, it has not been determined whether this deficiency affects neonatal host defense. Other important monocyte markers are the receptors for the Fc moiety of IgG (FcγR). These receptors are important in the process of monocyte and macrophage phagocytosis of microbes and antibody-dependent cytotoxicity. Monocytes constitutively express the high- affinity receptor FcγRI (CD64) and FcγRII (CD32). FcγR-III$^+$ monocytes in adult blood are significantly higher compared with CB samples. Despite the difference in the FcγR-III$^+$ populations, the intensity of FcγR-III expression is higher in CB than in APB.

### Function

Monocytes exhibit the characteristic properties of phagocytosis—namely, movement, adherence, endocytosis, and microbial activity. Monocytes are capable of directed movement (chemotaxis) in response to substances (chemokines) produced by bacteria or by accessory cells at the site of injury or invasion. Chemotactic capabilities of neonatal and adult peripheral blood monocytes have been compared, and chemotaxis was found to be less pronounced in neonates than in adults.

The cascade of reactions within the immune response to infection involves monocyte up-regulation and adherence via CD11b/CD18 receptors followed by cell activation and the release of cytokines (TNF, IL-1, and IL-6) and bactericidal products—superoxide radicals, nitric oxide, and granule contents released in the process of degranulation. Adherence requires the interaction of monocytes and the endothelium. Activated monocytes migrate from circulation into the tissues by firmly adhering to endothelial surfaces through the interaction of the integrins (CD11a-c and CD18) expressed on the monocyte cell membrane and the intercellular adhesion molecule-1 (ICAM-1) or ICAM-2 on the endothelial surface. Finally, the activated monocyte moves through the endothelium to the site of inflammation or infection. Preliminary studies demonstrate that levels of monocyte adhesion molecule expression are comparable in neonate and adult peripheral blood (Schibler, 2000). The β-2 integrin, CR3, plays a major role in the migration to sites of infection by mediating the binding to ICAM-1 and also is responsible for mediating the recognition of opsonized microbial pathogens. Neonatal monocytes express approximately 85% as much CR3 as that expressed by adult monocytes.

Antimicrobial activity of monocytes includes oxygen-dependent mechanisms such as the respiratory burst, which through a complex series of reactions forms highly reactive hydroxyl radicals that damage host and microbial membranes. The ability of monocytes of fetal and neonatal monocytes to kill pathogens (*Staphylococcus aureus*, *S. epidermidis*, *Escherichia coli*, and *Candida albicans*) is shown to be equivalent to that of APB monocytes. However, a recent study of isolated CB plastic adherent monocytes from preterm and full-term infants revealed a significant decrease in superoxide production and degranulation in preterm compared with full-term monocytes.

Activated monocytes and macrophages produce several cytokines and chemokines contributing to the inflammatory process. IL-1, interferon-α (IFN-α), and TNF-α are synthesized at similar levels in adults and neonates. Kaufman and colleagues (1999) found a significant decrease in the secretion of TNF-α by LPS-stimulated adherent monocytes from preterm infants compared with full-term infants; however, no difference was seen in the production of IL-1β or IL-6. They showed a significant decrease in the expression of CD11b and CD18 adhesion receptor subunits in monocytes collected from preterm infants compared with that in full-term infants.

## Dendritic Cells

Dendritic cells (DCs) are specialized mononuclear cells with highly developed antigen-presenting capabilities that play a pivotal role in humoral and cellular immunity by initiating primary and secondary T cell responses. DCs can be categorized into several types: follicular, lymphoid, and circulating blood DCs. Follicular DCs are located in the paracortical areas of the spleen and lymph nodes and express receptors for immunoglobulin and complement. Their role is to present antigen to B lymphocytes. Lymphoid DCs are highly motile, low density cells found in several locations. These DCs express high levels of costimulatory molecules and class II MHC and function to present antigen to T cells. Circulating blood DCs constitute from 0.1% to 1.0% of peripheral blood mononuclear cells and migrate to the lymph nodes. The function of circulating DCs is similar to that of the lymphoid DCs—stimulating T cells by the presentation of antigen. DCs are derived from pluripotent hematopoietic stem cells (CD34$^+$) that differentiate along myeloid or lymphoid lineages. Recent studies have suggested that DCs derived from a novel population of progenitors (CD34$^+$/CD7$^+$/CD45RA$^+$) in cord blood represent an original lymphoid DC population. These DCs produce two- to fourfold higher levels of IL-6, IL-12, and TNF-α on stimulation with CD40L and demonstrate a higher allogeneic T-lymphocyte reactivity. Two classes of dendritic cells have been characterized on the basis of expression of CD8a. CD8a$^+$ DCs are derived from lymphoid tissue, and CD8a$^-$ DCs are derived from myeloid tissue.

Caux and colleagues (1997) generated DCs in vitro from CB D34$^+$ hematopoietic stem cells stimulated with GM-CSF plus TNF-α. Two subsets of DCs were generated: one expressing CD1a and the other, CD14 surface antigens. These subsets further differentiated along two independent DC pathways, with cells expressing either the CD1a$^+$ or CD14$^+$ membrane antigen. CD1a$^+$ cells differentiated into Langerhans cells, characterized by Birbeck granules, the Lag antigen, and E-cadherin. CD14$^+$ progenitors matured into CD1a$^+$DCs that expressed CD2, CD9, and CD 68 and could be induced to differentiate into circulating blood DCs. CD40 activates CB CD34$^+$ cells to proliferate and differentiate independently of GM-CSF into a cell population with prominent DC characteristics. DCs generated with CD40 are able to prime allogeneic T cells and express high levels of HLA-DR but lack the characteristic CD1a and CD40 surface molecules (Flores-Romo et al, 1997).

Mature DCs express high levels of CD80 and CD83 on the cell membrane. Several agents have been shown to increase CD80 and CD83 expression on DCs, including TNF-α, bacterial LPS, and monocyte-conditioned media. Interactions with other cells also can induce activation and maturation of DCs, as demonstrated by the cross-linking of CD40 that is mediated by T cells.

We have recently demonstrated the ability to generate CB DCs ex vivo in serum-free media with GM-CSF, IL-4, Flt-3 ligand, TGF-β, and TNF-α. We found that the ex vivo–generated CB DCs from plastic adherent MNCs exhibit morphology and immunophenotypic characteristics similar to those of APB DCs; however, CB adherent MNC-derived DCs have differential potency in stimulating allogeneic mixed leukocyte reaction when compared with adult adherent MNC-derived DCs (Bracho et al, 2001).

### *Morphology*

The cardinal properties of DCs include the ability to take in, process, and present antigen and the ability to migrate selectively through tissues and interact with, stimulate, and direct T-cell responses. DCs have a distinct morphology and are noted for their irregular shape with veil-like ruffled cell membranes (lamellipodia) that include many pseudopods and numerous membrane processes. Microscopic examination of DCs reveals prominent mitochondria and endosomes and lysosomes within the cytoplasm, which are necessary for the processing of antigen. The morphology of DCs in CB and APB is identical; however, the mean percentage of DCs is lower in CB (0.5%) than in adult blood (1%).

Immunophenotyping studies have shown that DCs express numerous surface molecules commonly found on mononuclear cells, MHC molecules, CD4, CD45 isoforms, adhesion molecules (ICAM-1, -2, -3 and leukocyte function–associated antigen-1 [LFA-1]), and Fc receptors (FcγI [CD64], FcγII [CD3]). Maturation of DCs is commonly associated with high expression of CD80 and CD83 (Fig. 78–2). On stimulation, DCs up-regulate costimulatory molecules CD40, CD80, and CD86. Flow cytometric studies, however, show levels of ICAM-1 (CD54), MHC class I (HLA-ABC) and II (HLA-DR), CD80, and CD40 antigens to be significantly lower on CB DCs (Goriely et al, 2001; Hunt et al, 1994). Liu and colleagues (2001) compared the phenotypic and functional characteristics of monocyte-derived DCs in CB versus APB. After 7 days of culture with GM-CSF plus IL-4, CB monocytes generated fewer CD1a$^+$ cells than those generated by APB monocytes, and the cultured CB DCs had a reduced intensity of CD1a expression and MHC class II molecules. These investigators further reported that both the endocytotic ability and ability to stimulate CD3$^+$ T cells was reduced in CB DCs compared with APB DCs.

## Function

Functional differences between neonatal and adult DCs have been examined by several investigators. CB DCs have been found to be poor stimulators of T cells in a mixed leukocyte reaction when either adult blood or CB mononuclear cells or T cells were used as responder cells (Bracho et al, 2001). In contrast, CB T cells and mononuclear cells responded normally to allogeneic adult DCs. Furthermore, CB DCs performed poorly as accessory cells for T-cell mitogenic responses (Hunt et al, 1994). Recent studies of the ontogeny of DCs have shown that DCs from 3- and 7-day-old mice were severely defective in presenting tetanus toxoid to antigen-specific T-cell clones. However, the ability of the neonatal DCs to present antigen improved with age, reaching adult levels by 4 weeks of age.

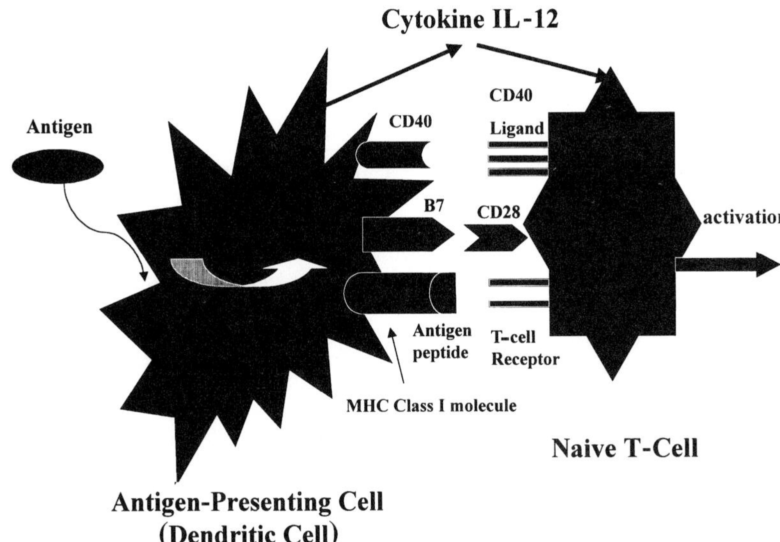


**FIGURE 78–2.** Dendritic cell (DC) (antigen-presenting cell [APC]) stimulation of naive T cell. The DC encounters and takes up an antigen; processes the antigen, subsequently releasing interleukin-12 (IL-12); and expresses CD40 and B7 proteins on its cell membranes. Once the antigen is processed by the DC, it is presented as a major histocompatibility complex (MHC) class I molecule at the cell surface. The naive T cell is stimulated by IL-12 and responds to the DC via CD40 ligand, T-cell receptor, and CD28 cell surface proteins.

Cytokine production by stimulated neonatal DCs can provide insight into the defect of their impaired immune response. IL-12 plays a critical role in the stimulation of T cells by mature DCs. Goriely and colleagues (2001) reported comparable levels of IL-6, IL-8, TNF-α, and IL-10 in newborn and adult DCs after stimulation with LPS or CD40 ligand. However, IL-12 (p40) levels secreted by neonatal DCs were significantly lower on stimulation with LPS but not with CD40 ligand. Also, after either LPS or CD40 ligand stimulation, neonatal DCs produced lower levels of IL-12 (p70) than adult DCs. CB DCs stimulated with LPS, CD40 ligand, or poly(I;C) showed a selective defect in the synthesis of IL-12. Furthermore, when stimulated with poly (I;C), neonatal DCs produced deficient levels of IL-12 (p70) but their production of IL-12 (p40) was similar to that of adult DCs. Neonatal DCs were also placed in mixed leukocyte culture with adult $CD4^+$ T cells, and neonatal DCs induced significantly lower levels of IFN-γ but higher levels of IL-10 than did adult DCs. Analysis of IL-12 (p35) mRNA from LPS stimulated neonatal and adult DCs by real-time polymerase chain reaction (PCR) assay revealed significantly lower levels in neonatal versus adult DCs; however, the addition of rIFN-γ to LPS- stimulated newborn DCs restored the expression of and synthesis of IL-12 to adult levels.

## SUMMARY

Immaturity of neonatal neutrophils, monocytes, lymphocytes, and dendritic cells predisposes the newborn to an increased incidence and/or severity of infectious complications. An increased understanding of the genetic mechanisms responsible for these defects will provide insight regarding future treatment strategies to prevent and/or treat serious or overwhelming infection in the newborn.

## Acknowledgment

The authors would like to thank Linda Rahl for her expert editorial assistance in the preparation of this chapter.

## REFERENCES

Abu-Ghosh AM, Bracho F, Kirov I, et al: Hematopoietic colony-stimulating factors. In Grenvik A, Ayers SM, Holbrook PR, Shoemaker WC (eds): Textbook of Critical Care, 4th ed. Philadelphia, WB Saunders, 2000, pp 542-561.

Bonilla MA, Gillio AP, Ruggeiro M, et al: Effects of recombinant human granulocyte colony-stimulating factor on neutropenia in patients with congenital agranulocytosis. N Engl J Med 320:1574-1580, 1989.

Bracho FA, Bradley MB, Hughes RL, et al: Despite similar morphology and immunophenotypic characteristics, ex-vivo expanded dendritic cells (DC) derived from cord blood (CB) vs. mobilized adult peripheral blood (APB) plastic adherent mononuclear cells are significantly deficient in stimulating allogeneic T-cells [abstract]. Blood 98:659, 2000.

Buzby JS, Lee SM, Van Winkle P, et al: Increased granulocyte-macrophage colony-stimulating factor mRNA instability in cord versus adult mononuclear cells is translation-dependent and associated with increased levels of A + U-rich element–binding factor. Blood 88:2889-2897, 1996.

Cairo MS, Agosti JM, Ellis R, et al: A randomized, double-blind, placebo-controlled trial of prophylactic recombinant human granulocyte-macrophage colony-stimulating factor to reduce nosocomial infaction in very low birthweight neonates. J Pediatr 134:64-70, 1999.

Cairo MS, Christensen R, Sender LS, et al: Results of a phase I/II trial of recombinant human granulocyte-macrophage colony-stimulating factor in very low birthweight neonates: Significant induction of circulatory neutrophils, monocytes, platelets and bone marrow neutrophils. Blood 86:2509-2515, 1995.

Cairo MS, Gillan ER, Buzby JS, et al: Circulating Steel factor (SLF) and G-CSF levels in pretem and term newborn and adult peripheral blood. Am J Pediatr Hematol Oncol 15:311-315, 1993.

Cairo MS, Mauss D, Kommareddy S, et al.: Prophylactic or simultaneous administration of recombinant human granulocyte colony-stimulating factor in the treatment of group B streptococcal sepsis in neonatal rats. Pediatr Res 27:612-616, 1990a.

Cairo MS, Plunkett JM, Mauss D, et al.: Seven-day administration of recombinant human granulocyte colony-stimulating factor to newborn rats: Modulation of neonatal neutrophilia, myelopoiesis, and group B streptococcus sepsis. Blood 76:1788-1794, 1990b.

Cairo MS, Plunkett JM, Nguyen A, et al: Effect of stem cell factor with and without granulocyte colony-stimulating factor on neonatal hematopoiesis: In vivo induction of newborn myelopoiesis and reduction of mortality during experimental group B streptococcal sepsis. Blood 80:96-101, 1992a.

Cairo MS, Plunkett JM, Schendel P, et al: The combined effects of interleukin-11, stem cell factor, and granulocyte colony-stimulating factor on newborn rat hematopoiesis: Significant enhancement of the absolute neutrophil count. Exp Hematol 22:1118-1123, 1994.

Cairo MS, Suen Y, Knoppel E, et al: Decreased G-CSF and IL-3 production and gene expression from mononuclear cells of newborn infants. Pediatr Res 31:574-578, 1992b.

Cairo MS, Suen Y, Knoppel E, et al: Decreased stimulated GM-CSF production and GM-CSF gene expression but normal numbers of GM-CSF receptors in human term newborns compared to adults. Pediatr Res 30:362-367, 1991a.

Cairo MS, van de Ven C, Mauss D, et al: Modulation of neonatal rat myeloid kinetics resulting in peripheral neutrophilia by single pulse administration of Rh granulocyte-macrophage colony-stimulating factor and Rh granulocyte colony-stimulating factor. Biol Neonate 59:13-21, 1991b.

Cairo MS, VandeVen C, Toy C, et al: Lymphokines: Enhancement by granulocyte-macrophage and granulocyte colony-stimulating factors of neonatal myeloid kinetics and functional activation of polymorphonuclear leukocytes. Rev Infect Dis 12:S492-S497, 1990c.

Cairo MS, VandeVen C, Toy C, et al: Recombinant human granulocyte-macrophage colony stimulating factor primes neonatal granulocytes for enhanced oxidative metabolism and chemotaxis. Pediatr Res 26:395-399, 1989.

Caux C, Massacrier C, Vanbervliet B, et al: CD34$^+$ hematopoietic progenitors from human cord blood differentiate along two independent dendritic cell pathways in response to granulocyte-macrophage colony-stimulating factor plus tumor necrosis factor alpha: II. Functional analysis. Blood 90:1458-1470, 1997.

Chang M, Suen Y, Lee S, et al: Transforming growth factor-β1, macrophage inflammatory protein-1α, and interleukin-8 gene expression is lower in stimulated human neonatal compared to adult mononuclear cells. Blood 84:118-124, 1994.

Christensen RD, Macfarlane JL, Taylor NL, et al: Blood and marrow neutrophils during experimental group B streptococcal infection: Quantification of the stem cell, proliferative, storage and circulating pools. Pediatr Res 16:549-553, 1982.

Christensen RD, Hill HR, Rothstein G: Granulocytic stem cell (CFU-C) proliferation in experimental group B streptococcal sepsis. Pediatr Res 17:278-280, 1983.

Christensen RD, Rothstein G: Pre- and post-natal development of granulocyte stem cells (CFUc) in the rat. Pediatr Res 18:599-602, 1984.

Curnette J: Disorders of granulocyte function and granulopoiesis. In Nathan DG, Oski FA (eds): Hematology of Infancy and Childhood, 4th ed. Philadelphia, WB Saunders, 1993, pp 904-961.

Dale DC, Bonilla MA, Davis MW, et al: A randomized controlled phase III trial of recombinant human granulocyte colony-stimulating factor (filgrastim) for treatment of severe chronic neutropenia. Blood 81:2496-2502, 1993.

Dale CD, Person RE, Bolyard AA, et al: Mutations in the gene encoding neutrophil elastase in congenital and cyclic neutropenia. Blood 96:2317-2322, 2000.

Doron MW, Makhluof RA, Katz VL, et al.: Increased incidence of sepsis at birth in neutropenic infants of mother with preeclampsia. J Pediatr 125:452, 1994.

Flores-Romo L, Björck P, Duvert V, et al: CD40 ligation on human cord blood CD34$^+$ hematopoietic progenitors induces their proliferation and differentiation into functional dendritic cells. J Exp Med 185:314-349, 1997.

Gasson JC, Weisbart RH, Kaufman SE, et al: Purified human granulocyte-macrophage colony-stimulating factor: Direct action on neutrophils. Science 226:1339-1342, 1984

Gessler P, Luders R, Konig S, et al: Neonatal neutropenia in low birthweight premature infants. Am J Perinatol 12:34-38, 1995.

Gillan ER, Christensen R, Suen Y, et al.: A randomized, placebo-controlled trial of recombinant human granulocyte-colony stimulating factor administration in newborn infants with presumed sepsis: Significant induction of peripheral and bone marrow neutrophilia. Blood 84:1427-1433, 1994.

Goriely S, Vincart B, Stordeur P, et al: Deficient IL-12 (p35) gene expression by dendritic cells derived from neonatal monocytes. J Immunol 166:2141-2146, 2001.

Hammond WP, Price TH, Souza LM, et al: Treatment of cyclic neutropenia with granulocyte colony-stimulating factor. N Engl J Med 320:1306-1311, 1989.

Hunt DW, Huppertz HI, Jiang HJ, et al: Studies of human cord blood dendritic cells: evidence for functional immaturity. Blood 84:4333-4343, 1994.

Kaufman D, Kilpatrick L, Hudson RG, et al: Decreased superoxide production, degranulation, tumor necrosis factor-alpha secretion and CD11b/CD18 receptor expression by adherent monocytes from preterm infants. Clin Diag Lab Immunol 6:525-529, 1999.

Koenig JM, Christensen RD: Incidence, neutrophil kinetics, and natural history of neonatal neutropenia associated with maternal hypertension. N Engl J Med 321:557-562, 1989.

Kostmann R: Infantile genetic agranulocytosis. Acta Paediatr Scand Suppl 105:1, 1956.

La Gamma E, Alpan O, Kocherlakota P: Effect of granulocyte colony-stimulating factor on preeclampsia-associated neonatal neutropenia. J Pediatr 126:457-459, 1995.

Lieschke GJ, Burgess AW: Granulocyte colony-stimulating factor and granulocyte-macrophage colony-stimulating factor. N Engl J Med 327:28-35, 1992.

Liu E, Tu W, Law HK, et al: Decreased yield, phenotypic expression and function of immature monocyte-derived dendritic cells in cord blood. Br J Haematol 113:240-246, 2001.

Lux SE, Johnston RB, August CS, et al.: Chronic neutropenia and abnormal cellular immunity in cartilage-hair hypoplasia. N Engl J Med 282:231-236, 1970.

Manroe BL, Weinberg AG, Rosenfeld CR, et al: The neonatal blood count in health and disease. J Pediatr 95:89-98, 1979.

Mouzinho A, Rosenfeld C, Sanchez P, et al: Revised reference ranges for circulating neutrophils in very-low-birth-weight neonates. Pediatrics 94:76-82, 1994.

Nathan DG: The beneficence of neonatal hematopoiesis. N Engl J Med 321:1190-1191, 1989.

Palis J, Yoder MC: Yolk-sac hematopoiesis: The first blood cells of mouse and man. Exp Hematol 29:927-936, 2001.

Roper M, Parmley RT, Crist WM, et al: Severe congenital leukopenia (reticular dysgenesis). Immunologic and morphologic characterizations of leukocytes. Am J Dis Child 139:832, 1985.

Rosenthal J, Healey T, Ellis R, et al: A two-year follow-up of neonates with presumed sepsis treated with recombinant human granulocyte colony-stimulating factor during the first week of life. J Pediatr 128:135-137, 1995.

Schibler KR, Osborne KA, Leung LY, et al: A randomized, placebo-controlled trial of granulocyte colony-stimulating factor administration to newborn infants with neutropenia and clinical signs of early-onset sepsis. Pediatrics 102:6-13, 1998.

Schibler K: Leukocyte development and disorders during the neonatal period. In Christensen RD (ed): Hematologic Problems of the Neonate. Philadelphia, WB Saunders, 2000, pp 43-59.

Suen Y, Chang M, Lee S, et al: Regulation of interleukin-11 protein and mRNA expression in neonatal and adult fibroblasts and endothelial cells. Blood 84:4125-4134, 1994.

Till J, McCulloch E: A direct measurement of the radiation sensitivity of normal mouse bone marrow cells. Radiat Res 14:213-222, 1961.

Weisbart RH, Golde DW, Clark SC, et al: Human granulocyte macrophage colony stimulating factor is a neutrophil activator. Nature 314:361-363, 1985.

Welte K, Zeidler C, Reiter A, et al: Differential effects of granulocyte-macrophage colony-stimulating factor and granulocyte colony-stimulating factor in children with severe congenital neutropenia. Blood 75:1056-1063, 1990.

Zon L: Developmental biology of hematopoiesis. Blood 86: 2876-2891, 1995.

CHAPTER 79

# Neonatal Hyperbilirubinemia

**Ashima Madan, James R. MacMahon, and David K. Stevenson**

## PHYSIOLOGIC JAUNDICE

The following terms are relevant to a discussion of jaundice and hyperbilirubinemia. This listing is of interest not only in an etymologic sense but also because it reflects a historical appreciation of these entities:

- Bile—from Latin *bilis* ("bile"), but the Latin probably had Celtic origins (*bistlis*).
- Bilirubin and biliverdin—simply "red bile" and "green bile," latinized.
- Icterus—from Greek *ikteros*, meaning "yellow colored," a word applied to a yellow bird as well.
- Jaundice—from Old French *jaundice*, a word rooted in the Latin *galbinus*, meaning "greenish yellow," from *galbus* ("yellow").

Jaundice is the visible manifestation in skin and sclera of elevated serum concentrations of bilirubin. Most adults are jaundiced when serum total bilirubin (STB) levels exceed 2.0 mg/dL (34 μmol/L). Neonates, however, may not appear jaundiced until the STB concentration exceeds 5.0 to 7.0 mg/dL (86 to 119 μmol/L). Some degree of jaundice develops in 60% to 70% of the approximately 4 million infants born each year in the United States. In those born prematurely, the incidence probably exceeds 80%.

Chemical hyperbilirubinemia, defined as an STB level of 2.0 mg/dL (34 μmol/L) or more, is virtually universal in newborns during the first week of life. STB concentrations in premature infants are even higher, persist longer, and are more likely to be associated with neurologic injury than those in term neonates (Lockitch, 1994). Debate and controversy remain in efforts to define either normal or physiologic ranges of STB concentrations in newborns, because the data are influenced by such variables as length of gestation, birth weight, nutritional status, mode of feeding, race, and even geographic location. At issue is whether the normal range should be defined by the rate of increase in STB concentration, a level for a specific postpartum age, the duration of STB elevation, or the maximal level attained.

Traditionally, a distinction has been made between benign physiologic jaundice and hyperbilirubinemia, which is either pathologic in origin or severe enough to be considered deserving of further evaluation and intervention. This latter entity has been called "nonphysiologic," although frequently no disease is identified as being causative or consequent.

STB concentrations have been defined as nonphysiologic if the concentration exceeds 5 mg/dL (86 μmol/L) on the first day of life in a term neonate, 10 mg/dL (171 μmol/L) on the second day, or 12 to 13 mg/dL (205 to 222 μmol/L) thereafter, based on data from the National Collaborative Perinatal Project (Hardy et al, 1979). In recent years, the significance of these numbers has been questioned. Indeed, data from a mixed population of infants weighing 2500 g or more in San Francisco revealed that, using these parameters, 13.4% of the infants would be classified as having nonphysiologic jaundice (10% of whites, 4.4% of blacks, and 23% of Asians) (Newman et al, 1990). The data of Maisels and Gifford (1986) indicate that the 97th percentile of maximal STB concentration in healthy mature newborns is 12.4 mg/dL (212 μmol/L) for formula-fed infants and 14.8 mg/dL (253 μmol/L) for breast-fed infants. Any STB elevation exceeding 17 mg/dL (291 μmol/L) should be presumed pathologic and warrants investigation for a cause and possible therapeutic intervention, such as phototherapy.

The elevation of STB concentrations in healthy-appearing infants results from the convergence of several developmental factors specific to the neonate. Gartner and coworkers (1977) divided the clinical course of physiologic jaundice into two phases. Phase I includes the first 5 days of life in term infants and is characterized by a rapid increase in STB levels for 3 or 4 days, after which the level begins to decline. Phase II is characterized by stable, but elevated STB levels lasting about 2 weeks. In contrast, in preterm infants, phase I lasts 6 to 7 days, and the STB levels reached are higher than those in term infants. After phase II, STB levels become comparable with adult levels. Data from multiple studies show that physiologic jaundice usually results in peak STB levels between days 3 and 5 of life. Maisels (1981) proposed criteria that can be used to exclude the diagnosis of physiologic jaundice. His original criteria have been amended to accommodate conditions related to breast-feeding, state of hydration, and so on. In addition, it must be remembered that absence of these criteria does not guarantee that the jaundice is physiologic (Table 79–1).

## PHYSIOLOGIC MECHANISMS

Distinctive aspects of normal newborn physiology that contribute to neonatal hyperbilirubinemia include: (1) increased bilirubin synthesis; (2) less effective binding and transportation; (3) less efficient hepatic conjugation and excretion; and (4) enhanced absorption of bilirubin via the enterohepatic circulation.

### Increased Bilirubin Synthesis

Bilirubin is a breakdown product of hemoglobin. The bilirubin load is greater in neonates because in this population, not only does hemoglobin break down at two to three times the adult rate (Maisels et al, 1971), but also there is an increased rate of red blood cell (RBC) degradation in the marrow even before release. In addition, bilirubin synthesis in healthy neonates results from a greater erythrocyte mass

**TABLE 79-1**

**Criteria that Rule Out the Diagnosis of Physiologic Jaundice**

1. Clinical jaundice in the first 24 hours of life
2. STB* concentration increasing by more than 0.2 mg/dL (3.4 μmol/L) per hour or 5 mg/dL (85 μmol/L) per day
3. STB concentration exceeding the 95th percentile for age in hours†
4. Direct serum bilirubin concentration exceeding 1.5-2 mg/dL (26-34 μmol/L)
5. Clinical jaundice persisting for more than 2 weeks in a full-term infant

*STB, serum total bilirubin.

†Based on a nomogram for hour-specific serum total bilirubin values (see Fig. 79–1).

at birth and a shorter half-life of neonatal RBCs. Normal term newborns have a hemoglobin level of approximately 17 to 19 g/dL, and a hematocrit of approximately 50% to 60%. Polycythemia, defined as a hematocrit greater than 65%, occurs in 1.4% to 1.8% of infants born at sea level and in 4% of those born at higher altitudes.

The life span of erythrocytes is less than 70 days for premature infants. It is estimated to be approximately 70 to 90 days in healthy term infants, compared with 120 days in adults.

### Binding and Transport

Circulating bilirubin is bound to plasma albumin. It is believed that the neurotoxicity associated with hyperbilirubinemia is primarily the result of unbound or "free" bilirubin, so the amount of albumin available for binding is important. The full-term newborn infant has a significantly lower plasma albumin level than that for the adult and, correspondingly, fewer bilirubin binding sites. The albumin level is inversely correlated with gestational age, so this lack of binding sites is more pronounced in preterm infants. Plasma albumin level increases rapidly over the first few days after birth, resulting in a mean increase over the first 7 days of almost 30%. Adult levels are reached by about 5 months of age (Notarianni, 1990).

Albumin binding of compounds in neonates is similar to that in adults in that acidic drugs and bilirubin are bound to albumin, but the binding affinity may be altered. In particular, affinity may be altered in the first several days after birth. This may be due to the presence of endogenous displacing agents in newborns, as well as structural differences in the albumin that resolve with maturity, adult characteristics being attained by 10 to 12 months of age (Miyoshi et al, 1966).

### Conjugation and Excretion

During intrauterine life, fetal removal of bilirubin is accomplished by way of the placenta and maternal-fetal circulation, and the bilirubin in cord blood is virtually all unconjugated. At birth, blood supply to the right lobe of the liver changes from the high oxygen content of the umbilical vein to the low oxygen content of the portal vein. Blood flow through the hepatic arteries develops only in the first week of extrauterine life. In addition, the ductus venosus may remain partially patent for several days, allowing blood to bypass the liver completely. All of these factors can contribute to a delay in the plasma clearance of bilirubin.

The conjugating capacity of normal infants varies greatly, with delayed conjugation and excretion, in some cases, related to the immaturity of the liver cell itself. The activity of the uridine diphosphate-glucuronosyltransferase (UGT) system in the newborn liver must be induced. Elevated conjugated bilirubin levels at birth, in cases of severe fetal hemolysis, suggest that elevated STB levels may be necessary to induce the conjugating enzymes. Production of UGT has been shown to be enhanced when certain drugs are administered. Phenobarbital is known to have this effect, and its clinical application is discussed later. Other pharmacologic substances, however, can inhibit UGT activity. Steroids structurally related to estrogen and progesterone have been shown to have this effect in vitro and in vivo, as have phenothiazines and the ester propionate preparation of erythromycin (Hsia et al, 1960).

### Enhanced Enterohepatic Circulation

Intestinal absorption of bilirubin successfully excreted into the intestine is enhanced by several features of newborn physiology, thereby adding to the tendency of newborns to become jaundiced. Conjugated bilirubin, as either the mono or diglucuronide, is unstable and can be spontaneously or enzymatically hydrolyzed back to unconjugated bilirubin, which can be easily reabsorbed through the mucosa. In addition, absorption is enhanced by the sterility of the intestinal contents. Older children and adults have intestinal flora, which can metabolize conjugated bilirubin to the water-soluble and readily excretable breakdown products urobilin and stercobilin. Newborns have no such advantage; instead, the neonatal intestinal mucosa has a greater concentration of β-glucuronidase than is found in the adult. This enzyme can deconjugate bilirubin to form more unconjugated bilirubin, which can be absorbed via the enterohepatic circulation, adding further to the circulating unconjugated bilirubin load. Two other factors accelerating the deconjugation of bilirubin glucuronides in the newborn intestine are the mildly alkaline pH of the proximal intestine, which facilitates nonenzymatic hydrolysis, and the predominance of monoglucuronides as the main excretion form of bilirubin in the first few days of life.

### Clinical Relevance

All of the aforementioned factors have the combined effect of potentially increasing STB levels in the healthy newborn. The premature newborn is even more susceptible to almost all of these influences. Because individual variation in the maturation of any of these systems is great, STB levels in a normal neonatal population vary widely. Slight perturbations in any of these processes could result in increased STB levels. For example, through studies of carbon monoxide (CO) production, it has been determined that infants of diabetic mothers have an increased propensity for jaundice because of enhanced formation and impaired elimination of bilirubin. Any pathologic process that increases the production or impairs the elimination of bilirubin can exacerbate the normally occurring physiologic jaundice in newborns. In the clinical setting, any such pathologic disorder should be identified and treated as appropriate. What remains controversial is the danger posed by increased STB levels encountered in the absence of pathologic disorders, as well as when to pursue investigations to identify or rule out disease.

## EPIDEMIOLOGY

Although all infants experience some degree of (hyper) bilirubinemia in the first few days of life and most have some physiologic jaundice, the extent and duration of the elevation vary among populations of different racial compositions or in different geographic distributions. The pattern of physiologic jaundice described previously in this chapter, with STB reaching maximal levels on the third or fourth day of life, is commonly seen in term infants of European or African ancestry. In the United States, black infants have slightly lower peak STB concentrations than those in other groups. In contrast, infants of Asian or Native American ancestry have a different pattern of neonatal jaundice, which is characterized by a more rapid increase of STB concentrations in the first few days, higher peak STB levels, and relatively prolonged courses, with the peak STB levels reaching their maximum several days later. The subsequent return to more normal levels occurs more slowly in these populations as well (Gartner, 1994).

Investigations involving infants in Japan, Asians born in the United States, Navajo, Sioux, Eskimos in Alaska, and Hispanics in Los Angeles (mostly from families in northern Mexico) have consistently shown higher STB levels in the first few days of life in all these groups. The reasons for such racial or ethnic differences are unclear. Studies assessing CO production suggest that an increased rate of heme catabolism leading to increased synthesis of bilirubin may be an important contributing cause. There is no strong evidence in favor of enhanced intestinal absorption or diminished conjugation or excretion in these populations (Johnson, 1992). However, in larger studies that have assessed the increase in bilirubin synthesis in Asians, it is clear that not all persons in a population are high producers of bilirubin (Fischer et al, 1988). Whether these populations are at higher risk for toxic effects of hyperbilirubinemia has not yet been determined. Italian studies looking for specific genetic markers within racial groups suggest that certain genetic traits involving red cell membrane stability as well as factors involved with bilirubin conjugation may contribute to neonatal jaundice, although environmental as well as genetic factors also may play a role (Lucarini et al, 1991). It has been shown that variations in the UGT 1A1 gene contribute to some of the observed racial differences. For example, polymorphisms due to differences in the number of thymine-adenine (TA) repeats in the promoter region of the gene vary among individuals of Asian, African, and Caucasian ancestry and correlate with variations in UGT enzyme activity and affect bilirubin metabolism (Beutler et al, 1998). Another cause of racial variation is due to a common mutation in the UGT gene (Gly71Arg), which occurs in Asians and results in an increased incidence (approximately 20%) of severe hyperbilirubinemia (Akaba et al, 1998). The knowledge that racial groups differ in the peak STB levels could have important implications for management of these infants.

## BREAST-FEEDING AND JAUNDICE

For several years there has been considerable controversy regarding the influence of breast-feeding on STB levels. Most studies indicate that infants who are breast-fed are several times more likely to have STB levels greater than 12 mg/dL (205 μmol/L) than infants who are formula-fed. In addition, breast-fed infants are believed to have higher STB levels throughout the first several weeks of life. Is physiologic jaundice in the newborn exaggerated in breast-fed babies? Many studies have attempted to answer this question, and the results are conflicting. A meta-analysis of a large series of studies showed that nearly 13% of breast-fed babies versus 4% of those formula-fed had STB levels of 12 mg/dL (205 μmol/L) or higher on days 3 to 6 of life, and 2% of breast-fed infants versus 0.3% of formula-fed infants had STB levels exceeding 15 mg/dL (257 μmol/L) (Schneider, 1986). The consensus of practitioners and investigators in the past decade is that breast-feeding is indeed associated with statistically significant elevations of STB concentrations.

Two separate patterns of jaundice in breast-feeding infants have been described. The first has been termed *breast-feeding–associated jaundice*, or simply *breast-feeding failure jaundice*, a condition that occurs in the first week of life; the second is less common and is called *breast milk jaundice* and manifests as prolonged hyperbilirubinemia lasting into the third week of life or beyond. As the epidemiology of these conditions is better understood, they may no longer be perceived as disease states; rather, they may be related to feeding practices or may simply represent an extension of physiologic jaundice.

### Breast-Feeding Failure Jaundice

Several reports suggest that the cause of breast-feeding failure jaundice may be nutritional and that it can be prevented by frequent (e.g., nine times daily) breast-feeding in the first 3 days of life, and avoidance of supplementation with water or glucose solutions (De Carvalho et al, 1982; Varimo et al, 1986; Yamauchi and Yamanouchi, 1990). Attention has focused on such factors as dehydration, caloric intake, frequency and volume of feedings, and supplementation. Of these, dehydration has been questioned as a major issue because of normal serum osmolalities, an absence of hematocrit changes consistent with the degree of hyperbilirubinemia, and the finding in some studies that water supplementation actually leads to further elevation of STB levels. Breast-fed infants pass fewer stools in the first few days of life, suggesting that increased amounts of bilirubin are absorbed into the enterohepatic circulation. To overcome this, early and frequent feedings may increase evacuation and decrease intestinal transit time. Additional evidence indicates that caloric intake can influence STB levels independently of other factors. In studies with adults and a variety of animals, starvation or general deprivation of calories has been shown to increase STB levels in association with changes in liver function. The mechanisms for this "starvation jaundice" are not known but may involve shifts in bilirubin pools, less efficient hepatic conjugation, enhanced bilirubin absorption from the intestines, or a systemic effect modulating cell transport of bilirubin. Consistent with the concept that the increase in STB concentration is related to conjugation and absorption rather than bilirubin production or heme catabolism are findings from studies showing that there is no difference in CO production (a surrogate for bilirubin production) between breast-fed and formula-fed infants (Stevenson et al, 1994). With improved management of breast-feeding in conjunction with the use of lactation consultants, the incidence of breast-feeding failure jaundice in newborns might be reduced.

Changes in hospital breast-feeding policies and practitioner approaches to breast-feeding may not only prevent toxicity from hyperbilirubinemia but also lead to reductions in unnecessary laboratory testing, hospitalization, and medical intervention. Breast-feeding jaundice is an important issue for the practitioner, especially because the incidence of breast-feeding has increased from 33% of infants in the United States in 1975 (Gartner, 1994) to 50% to 60% in recent years (Martinez and Krieger, 1985; Ryan et al, 1991), and the length of routine newborn hospital length of stay has shortened to about 1 day. Breast-feeding jaundice is a diagnosis of exclusion, and most important, increased bilirubin production must be eliminated as a contributing cause.

### Breast Milk Jaundice

The second identified pattern of jaundice in some otherwise healthy breast-fed infants has been called "breast milk jaundice." Considered by some researchers to be an extension of physiologic hyperbilirubinemia, this entity was first described in 1963 (Arias et al, 1963) and was considered to be a disease that occurred in less than 1% to 2% of the breast-feeding population. More recent epidemiologic studies suggest it is much more frequent, affecting as many as 10% to 30% of the breast-fed infants in the second to sixth weeks of life, with some experiencing hyperbilirubinemia well into the third month (Gartner, 1994; Linn et al, 1985).

One hypothesis addressing this prolonged jaundice associated with breast-feeding suggests that it results from enhanced enterohepatic absorption of unconjugated bilirubin related to the presence of an unidentified factor in human milk. This theory proposes that among breast-fed infants who do not have the prolonged jaundice, either the infants do not respond to this factor in their mother's milk or their mother's milk does not contain it. No specific factor has been identified, and these etiologic theories are still considered speculative.

The cause of breast milk jaundice has been pursued ever since it was first considered a disease state. Several metabolites in breast milk have been considered as etiologic agents, and usually their proposed mechanism of action has been described as inhibiting conjugation or enhancing the intestinal absorption of bilirubin through the enterohepatic circulation. Early studies suggested that the prolonged unconjugated hyperbilirubinemia in otherwise healthy breast-fed infants was due to the inhibition of hepatic UGT. Initially, an unusual steroid metabolite of progesterone, pregnane-3α,20β-diol, was considered as a likely candidate because it was known to inhibit hepatic UGT in vitro. Later studies cast doubt on the relevance of this chemical to breast milk jaundice. Other inhibitors of UGT have been implicated, such as free fatty acids and several lipases (including lipoprotein lipase [serum-stimulated lipase] and bile salt–stimulated lipase). Other studies suggest that yet another factor such as β-glucuronidase might be present that could deconjugate bilirubin in the intestine, allowing for increased intestinal bilirubin reabsorption. However, no clear relationship between the levels of this enzyme in breast milk and the infant's STB level has been demonstrated, and none of the aforementioned theories have been confirmed. Consideration that breast milk jaundice may be a normal event does nothing to explain its cause, so the search for a true link between breast milk composition and breast milk jaundice will continue.

Over the past 40 years, much investigation has been carried out to explain both breast-feeding failure jaundice and breast milk jaundice. No single and exclusive cause for either condition has been identified.

## UNCONJUGATED HYPERBILIRUBINEMIA: OVERVIEW

Overproduction of bilirubin combined with immature mechanisms for conjugation and enhanced intestinal enterohepatic circulation of bilirubin contributes to the development of neonatal jaundice. In most infants, this increase in STB is mild enough to be considered physiologic and nontoxic, and the excess bilirubin is composed almost entirely of the unconjugated form. When excessive production of bilirubin saturates the immature mechanism for bilirubin uptake and conjugation, however, or when the process of bilirubin uptake and conjugation is defective or deficient, the level of unconjugated bilirubin in the serum can accumulate to toxic concentrations. Accordingly, a variety of pathologic conditions may result in severe or prolonged unconjugated hyperbilirubinemia (Table 79–2). Even though the most prevalent of these involve the overproduction of bilirubin, impaired uptake and conjugation and excessive enterohepatic circulation of bilirubin can be responsible for severe clinical disorders. Because most cases of dangerous or extreme hyperbilirubinemia are related to hemolysis, identification of overproduction of bilirubin is useful in the early identification of the increased risk for bilirubin toxicity. Measurements of levels of end-tidal CO, corrected for inhaled CO ($ETCO_c$), or of carboxyhemoglobin, also corrected for inhaled CO ($COHb_c$), can help identify these infants, as there is a one-to-one correlation of CO production with bilirubin production.

In a review of 88,000 liveborn infants in Melbourne, Australia, from 1971 to 1989, it was determined that 12.4%

**TABLE 79–2**

**Causes of Unconjugated Hyperbilirubinemia**

A. Excessive production of bilirubin (hemolytic disease of newborn)
   1. Blood group heterospcificity (incompatibility)
      a. Rh isoimmunization
      b. ABO incompatibility
      c. Minor blood group incompatibility
   2. Red blood cell enzyme abnormalities
      a. Glucose-6-phosphate dehydrogenase deficiency
      b. Pyruvate kinase deficiency
   3. Sepsis
   4. Red blood cell membrane defects
      a. Hereditary spherocytosis
      b. Elliptocytosis
      c. Poikilocytosis
   5. Extravascular blood
   6. Polycythemia

B. Impaired conjugation or excretion
   1. Hormonal deficiency
      a. Hypothyroidism
      b. Hypopituitarism
   2. Disorders of bilirubin metabolism
      a. Crigler-Najjar syndrome type I
      b. Crigler-Najjar syndrome type II (Arias disease)
      c. Gilbert disease
      d. Lucey-Driscoll syndrome
   3. Enhanced enterohepatic circulation
      a. Intestinal obstruction, pyloric stenosis
      b. Ileus, meconium plugging, cystic fibrosis

of all of the infants had hyperbilirubinemia, defined as STB levels greater than 9 mg/dL (154 μmol/L) (Guaran et al, 1992). Correlates of jaundice were determined in 32% of the infants. Most often these were prematurity (20%) followed by isoimmunization (7%), with sepsis, bruising, and glucose-6-phosphate dehydrogenase (G6PD) deficiency accounting for less than 2% each. Of the infants defined as having hyperbilirubinemia, the maximum levels of STB exceeded 20 mg/dL (342 μmol/L) in 2% (212 of 10,944), representing 0.25% of all the births. Nearly 60% of these infants had some determined cause of jaundice, with the hemolysis of isoimmunization (found in 54 of 212) being the most common identifiable cause of the severe hyperbilirubinemia. The largest single group with high STB levels, however, comprised infants with no known cause of jaundice (90 of 212).

## CAUSES OF UNCONJUGATED HYPERBILIRUBINEMIA

In the newborn period, unconjugated hyperbilirubinemia is the manifestation of a large and diverse group of clinical entities. To emphasize the pathophysiologic processes involved, the following discussion considers conditions associated with excess bilirubin production separately from those related to impaired conjugation, excretion, or elimination. This distinction is of clinical relevance in that excessive bilirubin production can be identified from the CO production resulting from heme degradation. In addition, the risk of neurotoxicity in the newborn infant is greater in conditions associated with increased bilirubin production than in those associated primarily with impaired bilirubin excretion or elimination. The former conditions tend to manifest earlier in more unstable infants, and the latter manifest later in otherwise well infants.

The following sections describe the major pathologic conditions responsible for unconjugated hyperbilirubinemia (see Table 79–2).

### Excessive Production of Bilirubin: Hemolytic Disease of the Newborn

#### Blood Group Incompatibility

##### *Rh Isoimmunization*

The most common identified pathologic cause leading to hyperbilirubinemia is hemolytic disease of the newborn. The destruction of RBCs in the fetus and newborn most commonly results from Rh or ABO blood group incompatibility with the maternal blood type.

The first understanding of hemolytic disease in the newborn resulted from studies of erythroblastosis fetalis due to Rh incompatibility. The Rh antibody is produced by an Rh negative mother in response to the presence of Rh antigen on the fetal RBC membrane. The initial maternal response to this antigenic stimulus is to produce immunoglobulin M (IgM) antibodies, which do not cross the placenta in significant amounts. Later, IgG antibodies are formed that cross into the fetus and attach to antigenic sites on the RBC membrane. Although small volumes of fetal RBCs may enter the maternal circulation throughout pregnancy, the major sensitizing event occurs during delivery, when a greater amount of fetal blood may enter the maternal circulation. For this reason, Rh incompatibility is less likely to cause hemolysis or hyperbilirubinemia with the first pregnancy, but repeated pregnancies can result in progressively more severe life-threatening complications. Mothers can be sensitized by the transplacental hemorrhage of as little as 0.5 mL of blood, an amount that can easily pass from fetus to mother during active labor or during obstetric complications or procedures such as amniocentesis or therapeutic abortions. The development of maternal sensitization can be identified by the indirect antiglobulin (Coombs) reaction in the mother, which identifies the presence of IgG antibody in her circulation, or from spectrophotometric examination of amniotic fluid. Because the placenta efficiently transports bilirubin to the mother, affected infants do not appear significantly jaundiced at birth, but the hemolysis can result in severe anemia, hydrops, or intrauterine death. After delivery of the infant, the hemolysis resulting from Rh sensitization may result in rapid development of hyperbilirubinemia, with attainment of bilirubin levels requiring intervention. Presence of the Rh antigen in an infant is identified by blood typing. Isoimmunization, which is the attachment of maternal antibody to fetal RBCs, can be identified with a positive direct antiglobulin (Coombs) reaction in the infant. RBCs coated with maternal antibodies are destroyed in the fetal or newborn liver and spleen, resulting in catabolism of excessive amounts of hemoglobin to bilirubin. The severity of the Rh-induced hemolysis depends on several factors, including the antigenicity of the fetal erythrocytes (e.g., males in general are more antigenic than females), degree of sensitization, the specific Rh antigen involved, and the amount of maternal-fetal transfusion. Fifteen percent to 20% of Rh-positive infants born to Rh-negative sensitized mothers show no clinical signs of illness, whereas 25% have severe disease with fetal death, hydrops, or severe anemia at birth. The administration of blocking antibodies (RhoGAM) to pregnant Rh-negative women has greatly decreased the incidence of hydrops fetalis in the United States.

### *ABO Incompatibility*

Hemolytic disease caused by reaction of maternal anti-A or anti-B antibodies with fetal A or B antigens on the erythrocyte surface, a process similar to that in Rh incompatibility, is more common but generally milder than hemolytic disease caused by Rh incompatibility. This condition occurs almost exclusively in type O mothers, in that the relevant antibodies produced by type A mothers or type B mothers are mostly IgM antibodies that do not cross the placenta. The jaundice of ABO heterospecificity usually appears within the first 24 to 72 hours after birth, later than that of Rh incompatibility. In the circumstances of the ABO heterospecificity, only half of infants with a positive direct Coombs' test have significant hemolysis; and some infants without a positive direct Coombs' test may exhibit hemolysis. Thus, the measurement of an $ETCO_c$ level can identify hemolysis in these infants.

### *Minor Blood Group Incompatibility*

Traditionally, less than 2% of infants with hemolytic disease have isoimmunization caused by minor blood group antibodies, such as Kell, Duffy, and Kidd. However, because the cases resulting from Rh incompatibility have dramatically declined since the use of blocking antibodies (RhoGAM) was instituted, there is a higher percentage of contribution from minor blood group incompatibilities. Maternal antibody titers with some antigen such as Kell are not always predictive of the presence or degree of hemolysis. Only about 50% of infants with a positive direct Coombs test have hemolysis. The presence and severity of hemolysis can be followed using sequential hematocrits, reticulocyte counts, red blood cell smears in combination with STB, and if available, by estimating total CO production as an index of total bilirubin production using a surrogate measure, such as $ETCO_c$. Diagnosis requires identification of the specific antibody in neonatal serum or an eluate from neonatal RBCs.

## Red Blood Cell Enzyme Abnormalities

A group of RBC enzymopathies have been identified which result in chronic spontaneous hemolysis of early onset that persists throughout life. In the newborn period, marked hyperbilirubinemia can occur as a result of the severe hemolysis (Matthay and Mentzer, 1981; Olsen, 1969; Valaes, 1969). The two most studied defects, G6PD deficiency and pyruvate kinase (PK) deficiency, may be associated with hemolytic anemia and jaundice even in the absence of a recognized trigger agent or event in the neonatal period.

### *Glucose-6-Phosphate Dehydrogenase Deficiency*

G6PD deficiency is a heterogeneous sex-linked recessive trait whose occurrence has a geographic distribution, with increased prevalence in African, Mediterranean, and Asian regions. Some of the clinical manifestations of this condition, such as favism and hemolytic reactions to certain drugs, were well recognized long before identification of the enzyme deficiency. Although severe neonatal jaundice is the most common clinical manifestation of G6PD deficiency, the relationship between hyperbilirubinemia and the hemolytic anemia was established only when the enzyme deficiency was identified in the late 1950s (Newton and Frajola, 1958; Zinkham and Lenhard, 1959). Since then, it has become apparent that the situation in the neonatal period is special, because severe jaundice rather than the anemia may predominate in the clinical presentation. Moreover, severe neonatal jaundice can develop in the absence of significant hemolysis in some G6PD-deficient babies. In G6PD deficiency, RBCs cannot activate the pentose phosphate metabolic pathway and therefore are unable to defend adequately against oxidant stresses. Because of this phenomenon, severe hyperbilirubinemia can result from hemolysis associated with sepsis, exposure to chemicals such as naphtha in mothballs, or administration of pharmaceutical agents (Table 79–3). Even though some of these agents and stresses have received public attention, others represent generally unsuspected dangers, such as the intramuscular injection of vitamin K analogues or the inhalation of paradichlorobenzene, which is used in many countries in moth repellents, car and carpet fresheners, and bathroom deodorizers (Siegel and Wason, 1986; Valaes, 1994). Exposure of the newborn to a hemolytic agent can occur transplacentally, via breast milk, or directly by inhalation, ingestion, or injection. RBCs deficient in G6PD also are unable to reduce methylene blue to leukomethylene blue; therefore, exposure to even normally acceptable levels of methylene blue causes hemolytic anemia and hyperbilirubinemia when the dye accumulates and functions as a hemoglobin-oxidizing agent. Thus, severe hyperbilirubinemia and even kernicterus have resulted from the use of methylene blue in patients with unsuspected G6PD deficiency.

Understanding of the processes leading to the clinical manifestations of G6PD deficiency has come from studies examining the intracellular events following exposure of RBCs to naphthoquinones (Harley and Robin, 1962, 1963; Sass-Kortsak et al, 1962). In these studies, oxidation of hemoglobin to methemoglobin, Heinz body formation, and growth-stimulating hormone depletion were described even in normal erythrocytes. All of these phenomena are exaggerated in RBCs deficient in G6PD because the pentose phosphate pathway is essential to the defense against such oxidative stress. The data in these studies suggest that

**TABLE 79-3**

**Agents Producing Hemolysis in Patients with Glucose-6-Phosphate Dehydrogenase Deficiency**

| Antimalarials | Others |
|---|---|
| Pamaquine | Ascorbic acid |
| Pentaquine | Chloramphenicol |
| Plasmoquine | Chloroquine |
| Primaquine | Aniline dyes |
| Quinacrine | Dimercaprol (BAL) |
| Quinine | Fava beans |
| Quinocide | Methylene blue |
| **Sulfonamides** | **Nalidixic acid** |
| Sulfacetamide | Naphthalene* (used in mothballs) |
| Sulfamethoxazole | |
| Sulfanilamide | Naphthoquinones* (used in mothballs) |
| Sulfamethoxypyridazine | |
| Sulfapyridine | Paradichlorbenzenes (moth repellent, car freshener, bathroom deodorizer) |
| Sulfisoxazole | |
| Trisulfapyrimidine | |
| | Phenylhydrazene |
| **Sulfones** | Probenecid |
| Nitrofurans | Quinidine |
| Furaltadone | |
| Furazolidone | **Tolbutamide** |
| Nitrofurantoin | Vitamin K, water-soluble analogues |
| Nitrofurazone | |
| Thiazolesulfone | Menadione diphosphate |
| **Antipyretics and Analgesics** | Menadione sodium disulfate |
| Acetophenetidin | |
| Acetylsalicylic acid | |
| Aminopyrine | |
| Antipyrone | |
| *p*-Aminosalicylic acid | |

*Associated with most severe and numerous hemolytic episodes.

Adapted from Oski FA, Nalman JL: Hematologic Problems in the Newborn, 2nd ed. Philadelphia, WB Saunders, 1972; and from Valaes F: Severe neonatal jaundice associated with glucose-6-phosphate dehydrogenase deficiency: Pathogenesis and global epidemiology. Acta Paediatr Suppl 394:58-76, 1994.

neonates with G6PD deficiency may be particularly susceptible to the hemolytic action of vitamin K analogues. Experts currently recommend that oral vitamin $K_1$ be given for prevention of hemorrhagic disease in newborns in populations with a high incidence of G6PD deficiency (Jørgensen et al, 1991; Valaes, 1994).

Different genetic forms of the enzyme deficiency have characteristic risks, with the form found in the Mediterranean region exhibiting a more severe type of deficiency (Gd$^{\text{Mediterranean}}$) than the form found in West Africa (Gd $A^-$ type). The association between G6PD deficiency and neonatal hyperbilirubinemia and kernicterus initially was reported from Greece (Doxiadis et al, 1961), and in 1969 it was recognized as a serious public health problem there (Valaes et al, 1969). Reports from other Mediterranean countries followed. A similar relationship between G6PD deficiency and hyperbilirubinemia was reported in neonates in China and in ethnic groups of other East Asian countries (Lie-Injo et al, 1977; Phornphutkul et al, 1969), and it appears that the Asian forms of this condition have a severe reduction in enzyme activity similar to that in the Mediterranean forms. Reports from Africa associating G6PD deficiency of the Gd $A^-$ type with neonatal hyperbilirubinemia and kernicterus in infants in Nigeria, Senegal, Ghana, and South Africa were significant because the earlier reports had suggested that only the Gd$^{\text{Mediterranean}}$ form of the enzyme deficiency was severe enough to cause kernicterus. Early reports suggesting that black infants with G6PD deficiency exhibit no increased incidence or severity of hemolysis and jaundice have been shown to be incorrect, although their enzyme deficiency, the Gd $A^-$ type form of the disease, is less severe than the others. The susceptibility to hemolysis is dependent not only on the level of enzyme deficiency but also on the amount of oxidant stress or degree of exposure to an offending agent.

Between 200 million and 400 million people are estimated to carry the G6PD deficiency gene. In Greece, for example, the prevalence is estimated at 2% to 4% (Valaes, 1994). Even though the distribution of this genetic trait has historically been centered in the tropics, where malaria has flourished, several centuries of migration have led to worldwide dissemination of the gene. Therefore, physicians in all countries need to be familiar with the clinical manifestations and risks of G6PD deficiency.

Severe jaundice develops in approximately 5% of white or Asian infants with this disorder, usually after 24 to 48 hours of life and sometimes only after some trigger event. Maximal STB level is reached between the third and fifth days of life. One report of such a case (Penn et al, 1994) is a reminder to practitioners that the cause may be subtle but the consequences devastating. A G6PD screen is recommended in infants of Mediterranean, Nigerian, or Asian descent who have STB levels greater than 17 mg/dL (291 μmol/L) and a Coombs'-negative hemolytic anemia. However, the G6PD screen can sometimes be falsely negative in infants experiencing a hemolytic crisis.

The incidence of hyperbilirubinemia is increased when infants have both the Gilbert polymorphism and G6PD deficiency. Kaplan and coworkers (1997) observed that infants with the normal variant in the Gilbert promoter region had a similar incidence of hyperbilirubinemia (greater than 15 mg/dL [257 μmol/L]) to that in infants with and without G6PD deficiency (9.7% versus 9.9%). However, among G6PD-deficient infants who were homozygous or heterozygous for the Gilbert variant, hyperbilirubinemia was more frequent (50% versus 32%).

### *Pyruvate Kinase Deficiency*

Pyruvate kinase (PK) deficiency is the second most common cause of enzymatic-related hemolytic anemia. It is an autosomal recessive disorder that occurs uncommonly in all ethnic groups. PK is a key enzyme in the production of adenosine triphosphate (ATP) in RBCs. Its deficiency leads to shortened RBC survival, with excess hemolysis. Unexplained jaundice in a newborn with no isoimmunization or no sepsis or drug administration, but with evidence of hemolysis (excessive CO production, anemia, reticulocytosis), raises the possibility of this disorder.

## Septicemia

Sepsis is one of the important treatable problems associated with bilirubin overproduction. From the earliest studies of septicemia in newborns, it was observed that 25% to 30% had clinical jaundice early in the illness, sometimes reaching extreme levels. The hyperbilirubinemia in septic neonates is thought to be a consequence of rapid hemolysis, although there are several theories regarding the mechanism of occurrence. Neonatal erythrocytes are susceptible to cell injury and Heinz body formation in response to oxidative stress. In addition, heme oxygenase (HO) is induced by oxidants, and its induction could lead to increased catabolism of heme to bilirubin. Unstable hemoglobins are known to precipitate to form Heinz bodies when exposed to certain chemicals (e.g., methylene blue), resulting in production of erythrocytes that tend to lyse. It is possible that some aspect of sepsis has similar effects.

Available evidence suggests that bilirubin is a protective antioxidant (Dennery et al, 1995; Stocker et al, 1987) and that initially in infection, STB levels may be decreased as a result of its consumption (Benaron and Bowen, 1991). However, the hemolysis that can occur in association with sepsis probably overwhelms this effect, resulting in hyperbilirubinemia.

## Red Blood Cell Membrane Defects

### *Hereditary Spherocytosis*

Hereditary spherocytosis is characterized by spherocytic erythrocytes that are abnormally fragile under osmotic stress owing to abnormalities of the RBC cytoskeleton. This condition is inherited as a mendelian dominant trait, but in 10% to 25% of cases, neither parent is found to have spherocytes (Robinson, 1957). The incidence of this disorder in the United States is 1:5000 and may be higher in other parts of the world. Many families with hereditary spherocytosis have mutations in the gene encoding spectrin, an essential component of the RBC cytoskeleton. Cells from persons with spherocytosis also contain less lipid than normal.

Jaundice develops in approximately 50% of infants with spherocytes and may be misdiagnosed as physiologic jaundice. Because isoimmunization is not involved as an etiologic factor, the direct Coombs' test in the infant is negative. The diagnosis is made by examination of a peripheral smear of blood and recognition of the abnormal shape of erythrocytes. RBC osmotic fragility tests also are abnormal.

### *Hereditary Elliptocytosis*

Hereditary elliptocytosis is a heterogeneous group of autosomal dominant defects that, as with spherocytosis, result in an abnormal RBC cytoskeleton. The membrane defect is caused by abnormalities of either spectrin or glycophorin C. The incidence of hereditary elliptocytosis is approximately 1:4000; the disorder generally is defined by the presence of more than 25% elliptocytes on the RBC smear. This disorder usually is asymptomatic in the newborn period; however, occasionally there is enough hemolysis resulting from increased osmotic fragility to cause hyperbilirubinemia. The peripheral smear in these cases demonstrates many budding erythrocytic forms similar to those seen in pyropoikilocytosis (Austin and Desforges, 1969).

## Extravascular Blood

Presence of blood that has been swallowed or remains entrapped after a hemorrhagic event, such as with severe bruising, cephalohematoma, or liver, splenic, or adrenal hemorrhages, commonly leads to hyperbilirubinemia because of the excess bilirubin production resulting from the breakdown of extravasated RBCs. The common sites for such substantial collections of blood in term infants are cephalohematomas and the space beneath the galeal aponeurosis; in preterm infants, intraventricular hemorrhages are more frequent.

## Polycythemia

Because neonatal erythrocytes have a shorter life span than that of erythrocytes of older infants and children, an excess in the number of erythrocytes at birth can be associated with increased heme degradation and bilirubin production. For this reason, any infant who is plethoric or polycythemic runs some risk for development of hyperbilirubinemia. Because polycythemia is regularly associated with specific clinical entities in newborns, such as late cord clamping, trisomy 21, or maternal diabetes, these conditions can be associated with increased risk of neonatal jaundice.

Infants of diabetic mothers may be at increased risk for development of hyperbilirubinemia secondary to certain contributory factors, in addition to polycythemia. For example, hypoglycemia can be associated with high levels of unconjugated bilirubin. In this instance, the cause is not only excess bilirubin production but also limitation of conjugation. Glucose is a substrate that participates in the synthesis of the bilirubin conjugate; its absence may reduce the capacity to conjugate bilirubin, accentuating jaundice in young infants.

## Impaired Conjugation or Impaired Excretion of Bilirubin: Nonhemolytic Unconjugated Hyperbilirubinemia

### Hypothyroidism

Congenital hypothyroidism can be accompanied by prolonged hyperbilirubinemia (unconjugated), presumably as a result of a delay in maturation of the bilirubin-conjugating enzymes (MacGillivray et al, 1967). First recognized in 1954, this association has been documented in approximately 10% of all newborns with hypothyroidism. Several mechanisms may be involved in this process, because only some of these hypothyroid patients with jaundice demonstrate rapid resolution of the problem after hormonal therapy. It is unclear whether the protracted jaundice in hypothyroidism is a consequence of delayed maturation of hepatic conjugating capacity, but a similar picture of protracted jaundice, often in association with refractory hypoglycemia, is seen in infants with congenital hypopituitarism.

The exact impact of the thyroid hormones on conjugation, or other role, awaits further study. The prolonged jaundice associated with congenital hypothyroidism may stem from a delayed maturation of the ability of the liver to conjugate bilirubin because of the hormone-dependent variations in UGT activity. Reports also suggest that the thyroid hormones cause changes in protein expression, rather than enzyme latency, although some coordinated regulation of glucuronidation and levels of cytochrome P-450 also has been hypothesized (Goudonnet et al, 1990). Differential actions of thyroid hormones and chemically related compounds on UGT and cytochrome P-450 isozymes in animal studies suggest that the physicochemical characteristics of the hormones are important in determining the impact of these chemicals (Goudonnet et al, 1990). Clinically, a similar picture is seen in infants with congenital hypopituitarism, although this condition is much less common than hypothyroidism.

## Inherited Disorders of Bilirubin Metabolism

The entire group of inherited disorders of bilirubin metabolism (nonhemolytic unconjugated hyperbilirubinemia) can be simplistically divided into three major types according to the degree of bilirubin UGT activity and response to enzyme-inducing agents such as phenobarbital. The pattern of inheritance is different among these groups as well. The principal features of these three forms of the disorder are listed in Table 79–4.

### *Crigler-Najjar Syndrome Type I*

In the 1950s, just when the Rh isoimmunization problems were being clarified and understood as the major cause of kernicterus, a report of congenital familial nonhemolytic jaundice with kernicterus was published by Crigler and Najjar (1952). That report describes a severe, often lethal, unconjugated hyperbilirubinemia afflicting as many as 15 children in one family pedigree with no evidence of blood group incompatibility, hemolysis, or primary biliary obstruction. STB levels were 25 to 35 mg/dL (428 to 599 μmol/L), but other liver function tests were normal. Subsequent reports have documented STB levels as high as 45 mg/dL (770 μmol/L). Crigler-Najjar syndrome has come to be recognized as the most severe form of a group of inherited disorders of bilirubin metabolism that result from reduction or absence of UGT activity. In 1969, Arias and colleagues described a second type of severe nonhemolytic hyperbilirubinemia that is more common. The original condition described by Crigler and Najjar became known as Crigler-Najjar syndrome type I, and the new condition was called Crigler-Najjar syndrome type II, or Arias disease (Arias, 1971). The type I form of this inherited disorder is extremely rare (incidence estimated at 1 case per million). Family studies of type I patients have exposed partial deficiencies in glucuronidation of salicylates and menthol among siblings, parents, and grandparents of affected patients (Childs et al, 1959), supporting the view that this syndrome is inherited as an autosomal recessive characteristic that results in the virtual absence of UGT activity. The parents of these patients are anicteric heterozygotes. The patients with type I disease have pale

**TABLE 79–4**

**Congenital Nonhemolytic Unconjugated Hyperbilirubinemia: Clinical Syndromes**

| | Severity | | |
|---|---|---|---|
| **Characteristic** | **Marked (Crigler-Najjar Syndrome type I)** | **Moderate (Arias disease, Crigler-Najjar Syndrome type II)** | **Mild (Gilbert Disease)** |
| Steady-state serum total bilirubin | >20 mg/dL | <20 mg/dL | <5 mg/dL |
| Range of bilirubin values | 14-50 mg/dL | 5.3-37.6 mg/dL | 0.8-10 mg/dL |
| Total bilirubin in bile | <10 mg/dL (increased with phototherapy) | 50-100 mg/dL | Normal |
| Conjugated bilirubin in bile | Absent | Present (only monoglucuronide) | Present (50% monoglucuronide) |
| Bilirubin clearance | Extremely decreased | Markedly decreased | 20-30% of normal |
| Hepatic bilirubin uptake | Normal | Normal | Reduced |
| Bilirubin UGT activity | None detected | None detected | Decreased |
| Genetics | Autosomal recessive | Heterogeneity of defect distinctly possible | Genetic polymorphisms including additional thymine-adenine (TA) repeats are present in the promoter region of the Ugt gene. Other polymorphisms, such as the Gly71Arg mutation identified in the Asian population, lead to a relative deficiency or decrease in conjugation and decreased elimination of bilirubin |

*UGT, uridine diphosphate glucuronosyltransferase.

Adapted and modified from Valaes T: Bilirubin metabolism: Review and discussion of inborn errors. Clin Perinatol 3:177, 1976.

bile containing no bilirubin. Whereas in the past, kernicterus resulted early in life, patients with this condition can currently be treated with long-term phototherapy and agents that reduce the enterohepatic circulation of bilirubin, allowing the possibility of leading a normal life.

If Crigler-Najjar syndrome type I is left untreated, bilirubin production from the breakdown of hemoglobin in erythrocytes and other heme proteins occurs normally, but the unconjugated bilirubin accumulates in plasma and tissues. A new steady state is eventually attained as bilirubin is degraded by other pathways.

The Gunn rat provides an animal model of Crigler-Najjar type I disease (Gunn, 1938). This animal produces no UGT and experiences severe jaundice. This animal model has served well in the understanding of the biologic processes involving bilirubin metabolism and the genetic defects associated with deficiency of conjugating enzymes.

### Crigler-Najjar Syndrome Type II

Crigler-Najjar syndrome type II, or Arias disease, is more common but more difficult to recognize in the first week of life. Children with type II disease excrete small amounts of bilirubin glucuronide into the bile, which is yellow. The hyperbilirubinemia experienced by these patients is less severe than in type I disease, with levels ranging from 8 to 25 mg/dL (137 to 428 μmol/L), with less risk of kernicterus. Type II disease usually is inherited in an autosomal recessive manner, although autosomal dominant transmission occurs in some cases. Initially the inheritance was thought to be autosomal dominant, because abnormalities of glucuronidation were found in only one parent of each patient. However, subsequent studies identified mild STB elevations and decreased UGT activity in some siblings and other parents (Labrune et al, 1989; Okolicsanyi et al, 1988). Some investigations have suggested that this condition could be a homozygous form of Gilbert disease. Patients with this form of UGT deficiency are clinically cured by the use of phenobarbital or other substances known to induce the enzyme activity.

This characteristic differentiates the two types of Crigler-Najjar syndrome, because type I patients experience no decrease in STB or enhanced conjugation in response to drug therapy (Sinaasappel and Jansen, 1991).

In the more than 50 years since the report by Crigler and Najjar, advances in molecular biology and genetics have led to an understanding of the molecular basis of these defects in glucuronidation. The organizational gene, termed UGT1A1, that expresses bilirubin uridine 5′-diphosphate glucuronosyltransferase (bilirubin UGT) in humans and rats has been identified and described. It consists of five exons, four of which encode the carboxyl-terminal domain of all UGT isoforms; the fifth exon encodes the amino-terminal half of each isoform. Because UGT is the only physiologically significant form of the enzyme, a mutation in any of the five exons can lead to either type I or type II disease, depending on the severity of the impact of the mutation on enzyme activity. Patients with as little as 4% of normal enzyme activity are clinically in the type II category; they have moderate elevations of bilirubin without ill health or neurotoxicity.

Because all of these patients are normal in every regard except for a single-gene defect that happens to code for this one enzyme, therapeutic intervention using gene therapy has been proposed. Several modes of gene therapy have been suggested, including transplantation of normal hepatocytes, retrovirus-mediated gene transfer, adenovirus-mediated gene transfer, and noninvasive receptor-mediated delivery of hepatocytes (Kren et al, 1999; Sauter et al, 2000; Tada et al, 1998). Until these techniques are successfully tested, liver transplantation will be the main mode of treatment for more severely afflicted persons.

### Gilbert Disease

A mild form of UGT deficiency was identified before Crigler and Najjar reported their severe family pedigree. Known as Gilbert disease, this condition initially was described in 1901 (Gilbert and Lereboullet, 1901) and later acquired a variety of names including *physiologic hyperbilirubinemia*, *icterus intermittens juvenilis*, *constitutional hepatic dysfunction*, and *familial nonhemolytic jaundice* (Crigler and Najjar, 1952). Although many patients with this condition have severe neonatal hyperbilirubinemia, the diagnosis most often is made in later adolescence. It is estimated that 5% to 10% of the general population may have this condition, which is characterized by a hereditary, mild chronic or recurrent nonhemolytic jaundice with otherwise normal results on liver function tests and no excess pigment in the urine (Odell and Gourley, 1989). Affected persons have a two-base-pair (TA) addition mutation in the TATAA element of the promoter region of the gene encoding UGT. The variant promoter contains seven TA repeats (Bosma et al, 1995) instead of the usual six. This results in a decreased (one-third normal) production of the UGT enzyme. Although Gilbert disease typically manifests in the older child or adolescent, homozygous newborns have an increased likelihood of developing jaundice during the first 2 days of life compared with heterozygotes. In addition, hyperbilirubinemia has been shown to be more frequent in G6PD-deficient infants who were homozygous (50%) for the Gilbert variant than in those who were heterozygotes (32%) (Beutler et al, 1998; Bosma et al, 1995; Kaplan et al, 1997; Koiwai et al, 1995). Older patients often complain of fatigue and asthenia associated with their jaundice. Because caloric deprivation results in hyperbilirubinemia in the child or adult with this disease, it is possible that many infants with unexplained hyperbilirubinemia are actually demonstrating the earliest manifestations of this disease. Like Crigler-Najjar syndrome type II, Gilbert disease can be treated with phenobarbital, which induces the necessary enzymes, although no specific treatment is usually necessary. This condition represents a heterogeneous group of disorders that result in at least a 50% decrease in UGT activity (Gourley, 1994).

### Lucey-Driscoll Syndrome

The Lucey-Driscoll syndrome originally was described in 24 infants born to eight mothers. Kernicterus developed in four of the infants in the original report as a result of their intense hyperbilirubinemia. The sera from the mothers of these infants contained a substance that markedly inhibited the conjugation in vitro of aglycones such as *O*-aminophenol. This inhibitory material also was detected in the sera of the infants and was postulated to have been transplacentally acquired. The substance eventually disappears from the circulation of both the mother and the infant and is believed to be a gestational hormone. This syndrome should be considered in those circumstances in which siblings experience intense, transient hyperbilirubinemia of unexplained cause.

### Enhanced Enterohepatic Circulation of Bilirubin

In young infants, unconjugated hyperbilirubinemia has been documented with high intestinal obstruction, especially with hypertrophic pyloric stenosis. Jaundice rapidly disappears after operation. It was previously thought that this entity represented a condition in which enhanced enterohepatic circulation of bilirubin resulted in unconjugated hyperbilirubinemia. Studies have now shown that an essential etiologic feature of jaundice with pyloric stenosis is a markedly reduced activity of UGT at the time of corrective surgery. Normal enzyme activity is seen in nonjaundiced infants with pyloric stenosis. Therefore, concerns have been raised that jaundice with pyloric stenosis may represent an early manifestation of Gilbert syndrome exposed by factors related to undernutrition. Other researchers have suggested that this jaundice results from reduced portal and hepatic artery blood flow or simply a delay in maturation of the enzymes needed for conjugation. Until long-term enzyme presence and activity have been assessed after treatment of upper intestinal obstruction, the cause of this jaundice may be unclear.

Other intestinal conditions thought to cause hyperbilirubinemia via increased enterohepatic circulation include lower intestinal obstruction, hypoperistalsis, paralytic ileus regardless of cause (e.g., drug-induced), and meconium plugging. In all of these conditions, there is virtually no removal of bilirubin secreted into the intestines, and reabsorption is enhanced by the stasis and the sterility of the intestinal lumen.

## BILIRUBIN TOXICITY, ENCEPHALOPATHY, AND KERNICTERUS

Neonatal jaundice can be an entirely benign physiologic process, or it can also be the first sign of serious illness with associated toxicity manifested in the nervous system. The terms *bilirubin encephalopathy* and *kernicterus* represent clinical and pathologic abnormalities resulting from bilirubin toxicity in the central nervous system. Often the term *kernicterus* is used to include an entire spectrum of clinical and pathologic manifestations attributed to bilirubin. However, kernicterus, by strict definition, includes only the neuropathologic changes that are characterized by pigment deposition in specific regions of the brain, especially the basal ganglia, pons, and cerebellum. Of all infants in whom kernicterus develops, 50% die, and the survivors may have choreoathetoid cerebral palsy, high-frequency auditory nerve deafness, and mental retardation. The term *bilirubin encephalopathy* is correctly applied to the clinical manifestations of the effects of bilirubin on the central nervous system; a broad spectrum of neurologic signs is attributed to bilirubin, ranging from subtle behavioral changes such as lethargy and irritability to seizures, hearing deficits, mental retardation, and death. Because it is not clear under what conditions neurotoxicity develops or at what STB concentration this damage occurs, little agreement exists about what constitutes a "safe" level of bilirubin. The effect of even moderate increases in STB levels on early development remains a source of controversy, especially because some clinical manifestations are reversible on reduction of the STB concentration.

Before exchange transfusions were used to control STB levels in isoimmune hemolytic disease, kernicterus was a common postmortem finding in infants dying with severe jaundice. Kernicterus has been documented in ill, low-birth-weight (mainly premature) infants whose STB levels remained much lower than the levels formerly associated with kernicterus. Whether this "low-bilirubin kernicterus" is associated with prematurity alone or is necessarily associated with stresses such as hypoxia, acidosis, respiratory distress, and neonatal septicemia is uncertain.

In the following paragraphs, the history of kernicterus is reviewed, clinical findings are described, and the current understanding of the processes leading to bilirubin neurotoxicity is discussed. Finally, new approaches to diagnosis, prediction of risk, and prevention are presented.

### Historical Overview

The relation between the clinical encephalopathy associated with elevated STB concentration and the gross pathologic changes seen as yellow staining of specific areas of the central nervous system was observed and described as early as 1875 (Orth, 1875). Schmorl, in 1904, coined the term *kernikterus* for such focal icteric pigmentation in degenerated zones of the brain (*kern*, "nucleus" or "ganglion," and *ikterus*, "yellow") (Schmorl, 1904). He observed that the staining of the neural tissue occurred in only a minority of infants having severe jaundice; he identified only six instances of kernicterus in 120 cases of jaundice of the newborn that came to autopsy.

Beneke (1907) was the first to suggest that septicemia might play an important role in icterus gravis neonatorum, and he theorized that the pigmentation of brain tissue was caused by: (1) a peculiar attraction of bile pigments to ganglion cells, leading to their necrosis; (2) damage to ganglion cells by bile salts, which then became pigmented; or (3) schemic or traumatic insult that allowed the cells to become pigmented.

As early as 1915, the literature included descriptions of children who survived severe neonatal jaundice with resultant mental retardation and neuromuscular dysfunction, the jaundice being considered the causal agent (Guthrie, 1913; Spiller, 1915). In 1916, an advance in the understanding of this disease was made possible by the observation of Van den Bergh and Muller that serum from patients with hemolytic jaundice could be differentiated from serum of patients with obstructive jaundice on the basis of chemical reactions. They observed that the hemolytic serum did not react promptly with diazotized sulfanilic acid except in the presence of alcohol; the other serum reacted in an aqueous solution. They termed these reactions "indirect" and "direct," which have come to be recognized as unconjugated and conjugated bilirubin, respectively (Van den Bergh and Muller, 1916).

Diamond and colleagues in 1932 recognized that generalized edema of the fetus (hydrops fetalis), icterus gravis, and congenital anemia of the newborn (until that time considered three unrelated syndromes) were in fact all part of a single condition, which they termed *erythroblastosis fetalis* (Diamond et al, 1932). This was followed by the demonstration in 1939 of a serologic basis for maternal-fetal blood group incompatibility and the identification of the Rh system of antigens (Landsteiner and Weiner, 1940; Levine and Stetson, 1939).

By 1950, kernicterus was thought to occur almost entirely as a sequel to erythroblastosis fetalis, and the relationship between the damage and the severity of jaundice was recognized. Even then, only the Rh incompatibility was considered critical. There was debate about whether other blood groups played any role at all; prematurity, sepsis, pulmonary damage, and maternal diabetes were seen as cofactors in the development of clinical or pathologic disease.

With the publication describing congenital familial nonhemolytic jaundice with kernicterus in 1952, Crigler and Najjar not only exposed a new disease or family of diseases (currently understood to be hereditary deficiencies of UGT) but also advanced the understanding of kernicterus as a process related more to elevated unconjugated bilirubin levels than to specific blood group incompatibilities or even hemolysis (Crigler and Najjar, 1952).

In a series of publications between 1950 and 1952, Diamond, Allen, Hsia, and coworkers summarized the contemporary knowledge and state-of-the-art approaches regarding kernicterus, erythroblastosis, and interventions to prevent neurologic damage from high serum concentrations of unconjugated bilirubin (Allen et al, 1950). In concluding the series of articles, they wrote "kernicterus is likely to occur in babies with serum bilirubin above 30 mg per 100 cc and unlikely to occur when serum bilirubin remains below 20 mg per 100 cc" (Hsia et al, 1952). Often taken out of context, this sentence has had an enduring effect on decisions regarding clinical intervention, standards of care, hospitalization policies, and even legal concerns. Controversies about appropriate treatment of hyperbilirubinemia to prevent kernicterus continue.

In a review of the incidence of kernicterus, Johnson and Brown (1999) identified 41 cases occurring in the United States in the last 30 years. Of these, 31 occurred after 1990. This increase has been attributed partly to shorter hospital stays, decreased vigilance in diagnosing jaundice, lack of physician compliance with current guidelines, and an altered physician perception of the toxicity of bilirubin. Indeed, physicians trained after the 1970s have rarely seen classical kernicterus, owing to the successful implementation of the use of RhoGAM to prevent isoimmunization and the treatment of jaundice with phototherapy. Many of the recently reported cases are found in healthy, breast-feeding term male infants with no other obvious cause for jaundice.

The progress in preventing maternal-fetal blood group incompatibility and in reducing STB concentration coincided with the development of neonatology as a specialty and the ability to rescue sick premature infants. Kernicterus was reappearing in the autopsies of sick low-birth-weight infants, particularly in those who had experienced severe respiratory distress, acidosis, or sepsis. It was evident in neonates whose STB level was never elevated to the extremes reported earlier, suggesting that bilirubin toxicity in low-birth-weight infants might be in some way different from that in full-term infants with erythroblastosis fetalis. Again the question arises: Is bilirubin the cause of the damage or is staining of tissue caused by antecedent injury? Are patients dying with kernicterus or of kernicterus? In some cases, bilirubin encephalopathy is observed before death, and the yellow neuronal staining in a classic distribution of kernicterus is the only prominent finding in the central nervous system at autopsy, providing evidence of a real toxicity attributed to bilirubin itself.

## Clinical Manifestations of Bilirubin Toxicity

Bilirubin toxicity usually does not become overt until high STB levels have been established for several hours. Acute bilirubin encephalopathy typically progresses through three stages. Stage 1 occurs during the first few days, with the infant having decreased activity, poor sucking, hypotonia, and a slightly high-pitched cry. If the STB level is rapidly decreased (e.g., by way of exchange transfusion), the abnormalities often can be reversed. Stage 2 develops after a week, with the infant demonstrating the features of stage 1 and also rigid extension of all four extremities, tight-fisted posturing of arms, crossed extension of the legs, and a high-pitched, irritable cry. Sometimes these changes are accompanied with seizure activity, backward arching of the neck (retrocollis) and trunk (opisthotonos), and fever. Stage 3 typically begins after the first week, with the infant demonstrating hypertonia with marked retrocollis and opisthotonos, stupor or coma, and a shrill cry. After several months in patients who survive, chronic bilirubin encephalopathy develops and has three major features: movement disorder (chorea, ballismus, tremor), gaze abnormalities (especially limitation of upward gaze), and auditory abnormalities. The most common findings later in childhood are choreoathetosis, ocular paralysis, and eighth nerve deafness; severe mental retardation and spastic cerebral palsy occur in a minority. In general, the motor findings are the most obvious abnormalities in long-term survivors. In addition to the neurologic abnormalities, some children with bilirubin encephalopathy have dental enamel hypoplasia.

A scoring system developed by Johnson and coworkers (1999) can be used to define the presence and severity of the neurologic sequelae associated with excessive hyperbilirubinemia. Mental state, muscle tone, and cry are characterized and then grouped into three levels of increasing abnormalities: stage IA, minimal signs; stage IB, progressive but reversible with treatment (4 to 6); and stage II, advanced and largely irreversible (7 to 9). Characteristics for each category are weighted as 1, 2, or 3 according to severity and then summed for an overall score; the higher the score, the greater the risk.

The first magnetic resonance imaging (MRI) study showing brain damage associated with hyperbilirubinemia was reported in a full-term infant with G6PD deficiency. MRI at 8 days of life showed abnormally high signal intensity on T1-weighted images in the basal ganglia, thalamus, and internal capsule. Similar but less intense signal was seen on T2-weighted images. Subsequently, there have been several reports of abnormalities seen in the globus pallidus on MRI in infants with bilirubin encephalopathy. A high-intensity signal in the posteromedial aspect of the globus pallidus on MRI is diagnostic of bilirubin injury.

Classic features of kernicterus are not often seen in neonatal follow-up clinics for premature and low-birth-weight infants, because even mild hyperbilirubinemia is usually aggressively treated in this population. However, a spectrum of mild neurologic disabilities and subtle developmental delays has been associated with moderate elevation of serum indirect bilirubin concentration. Because developmental delays related to other factors of prematurity, neonatal illness, or environmental situations are commonly associated with neonatal intensive care, there is controversy regarding the reversibility or long-term implications of the subtle neurologic damage attributed to bilirubin in low-birth-weight babies. Debates about the need for aggressive or conservative treatment for mild to moderate hyperbilirubinemia in infants persist.

Results from the Collaborative Perinatal Project (Hardy et al, 1979) showed that neurodevelopment during the first year of life was correlated with maximal STB concentration soon after birth. Results from a multicenter study from Netherlands reported that, although there was a dose-response relationship between maximum STB concentration and the risk of impaired development at 2 years of age, the effect did not persist at 5 years of age (van de Bor et al, 1989). A 17-year follow-up study revealed an association between severe hyperbilirubinemia and low intelligence quotient (IQ) in boys but not in girls (Seidman et al, 1991). This finding also was noted in a large study of 31,759 untreated infants with an STB of less than 20 mg/dL (342 μmol/L).

**TABLE 79–5**

**Factors that Increase Susceptibility to Neurotoxicity Associated with Hyperbilirubinemia**

| | |
|---|---|
| Asphyxia | Caloric deprivation |
| Hyperthermia | Prolonged hyperbilirubinemia |
| Septicemia | Young gestational age |
| Hypoalbuminemia | Low birth weight |
| Acidosis | Excessive hemolysis |

## Pathophysiology of Bilirubin Toxicity

To understand neonatal bilirubin toxicity more completely, several factors need further exploration, including how bilirubin enters the brain, what it does to the neurons, whether neurotoxicity can be predicted in time to be prevented, and what effects are reversible (Table 79–5).

### Entry of Bilirubin into the Brain

The mechanism by which unconjugated bilirubin enters the brain and damages it is unclear. Several hypotheses regarding entrance of bilirubin into the brain have been advanced and are not yet disproved.

One hypothesis involving free bilirubin (i.e., bilirubin that is not bound to albumin) has been widely accepted although never conclusively proved. Recognizing the lipophilic nature of free bilirubin, this hypothesis presumes that free bilirubin, in equilibrium with bound bilirubin, has access to tissues. Thus, any increase in the amount of free bilirubin or reduction in the amount or binding capacity of albumin could increase the level of unbound bilirubin within the brain tissue, saturating membranes and causing precipitation of bilirubin acid within the nerve cell membrane. This hypothesis arose to explain an outbreak of kernicterus in premature infants given sulfisoxazole (Odell, 1959). The drug was shown to compete with bilirubin for albumin binding sites, thereby increasing plasma free bilirubin levels. Benzoate, a metabolite of benzyl alcohol (a preservative found in intravenous flush solutions), also has been found to compete with these binding sites and, in sufficient quantities, can produce toxic levels of free bilirubin (Ahlfors, 2000b). Consistent with this hypothesis is the knowledge that even during physiologic hyperbilirubinemia, some unbound bilirubin crosses the blood-brain barrier freely.

The clinical significance of this passage of free bilirubin into the brain during physiologic jaundice is unclear. Could this be the cause of transient changes in attention, alertness, and motor performance documented during moderate STB elevations? This theory raises concern about the duration of jaundice as well as the peak STB level attained and suggests that any situation that decreases the affinity or binding capacity of albumin, or increases movement of bilirubin into tissue (e.g., acidosis, hypoalbuminemia, action of competitively bound drugs), would thus exacerbate the entry of bilirubin into brain tissue.

A second hypothesis not only involves the binding of bilirubin to albumin but also focuses on the state of the bilirubin available to cross cell membranes. This hypothesis is based on close examination of the chemical nature of bilirubin in solution and seeks to explain the increased risk to acidotic infants. At alkaline pH, bilirubin forms a water-soluble sodium salt, but the solubility of this substance at neutral or lower pH is extremely low. Bilirubin is therefore found in plasma as a dianion bound to albumin after dissociation of two hydrogen ions. The amount of bilirubin acid (i.e., bilirubin that has not dissociated the hydrogen ions) may be excessive, however, and bilirubin acid tends to precipitate readily from serum only when a lipid membrane is present, suggesting that it is the supersaturated bilirubin acid that precipitates in the tissues of icteric infants (Brodersen and Stern, 1990). In this model, the degree of supersaturation is determined by the concentration of free bilirubin, relative to the solubility at the pH of plasma. However, it is accepted that some bilirubin can pass from albumin to tissues by direct contact of the bilirubin-albumin molecule with a cellular surface. In this theory, the rate of tissue uptake of bilirubin would depend on both the concentration of albumin-bound bilirubin and the pH, with low pH enhancing precipitation and tissue uptake. Any increase in free albumin could reverse the process. This theory provides an explanation for the role that acidosis may play in the development of kernicterus (Gartner et al, 1970; Stern and Denton, 1965). The low albumin levels of premature infants coupled with the acidosis of respiratory distress place these infants at risk for kernicterus in the face of only moderate hyperbilirubinemia. Whether brain bilirubin oxidase can degrade bilirubin rapidly enough to prevent the deposition of bilirubin acid at the cellular level is controversial, and variations of this hypothesis have been suggested (Wennberg, 1988). It is still unclear whether bilirubin acid or bilirubin acid salt (monobasic bilirubin) is the form of bilirubin involved in the crossing of cell membranes or in tissue binding.

A third theory suggests that bound bilirubin enters the brain mainly through a damaged blood-brain barrier. The importance of a mature and intact blood-brain barrier stems from demonstration that the barrier to albumin and bilirubin can be reversibly opened under conditions of vascular injury, abnormal circulation, or abnormal osmolality (Bratlid, 1991). Hyperthermia and septicemia may have similar effects (Levine, 1983). Such loss of integrity of the blood-brain barrier could make entry of bilirubin into the brain possible at any STB concentration. According to this hypothesis, the local toxicity of bilirubin to the central nervous system would still require dissociation of the bilirubin from albumin at the cell membrane or in the cell, because free bilirubin is known to be more toxic than bound bilirubin in in vitro preparations. Even with a damaged blood-brain barrier, however, more bilirubin than albumin enters the brain, suggesting that several mechanisms of bilirubin entry may be operant simultaneously (see Table 79–5).

Recent studies suggest that unconjugated bilirubin is a substrate for P-glycoprotein (P-gp) (Jetté et al, 1995; Watchko et al, 1998) and that the blood-brain barrier P-gp may play a role in limiting the passage of bilirubin into the CNS. P-gp is an ATP-dependent integral plasma membrane transport protein that translocates a wide range of substrates across biologic membranes.

## Bilirubin Toxicity at the Cellular Level

Similar to the controversy regarding the entry of bilirubin into brain tissue is that concerning how bilirubin actually exerts its toxic effect at the cellular level. Four possible mechanisms have been proposed: interruption of normal neurotransmission, mitochondrial dysfunction, cellular and intracellular membrane impairment, and interference with enzyme activity (Palmer and Smith, 1990).

*Neurotransmission* has been theorized as an early target of bilirubin toxicity because reversible changes in brainstem auditory evoked responses (BAERs) have been recorded at moderate levels of hyperbilirubinemia. Bilirubin has been shown in vitro to inhibit phosphorylation of enzymes (e.g., synapsin I) that are critical in neurotransmitter release (Hansen et al, 1988; Morphis et al, 1982). In addition, changes in membrane potential in cells involved in synapse transmission are known to occur in the presence of varying levels of bilirubin. Bilirubin also has been reported to inhibit uptake of tyrosine, a marker for synaptic transmission, as well as the function of *N*-methyl-D-aspartate receptor ion channels.

*Mitochondrial dysfunction* has long been believed to be important in the pathogenesis of irreversible bilirubin encephalopathy. Some researchers have hypothesized that bilirubin acid precipitates in phospholipid membranes, resulting in mitochondrial dysfunction. Others, however, postulate *cellular/intracellular membrane impairment*, suggesting that bilirubin forms reversible complexes with various cellular membranes. This pathomechanism would explain the reversal of some clinical signs of bilirubin toxicity in response to exchange transfusions and rapid reduction of STB levels. Further research is necessary to elucudate the molecular mechanisms more fully. Perhaps the impact of bilirubin on either neurotransmission or on mitochondrial function relates to the effect of bilirubin acid on the ability of ions (e.g., hydrogen, sodium, potassium) to cross the membranes. Bilirubin inhibits ion exchange and water transport in renal cells, which may explain the neuronal swelling that occurs in bilirubin encephalopathy associated with kernicterus. Hydrogen ion gradients across cellular and mitochondrial membranes may be important in controlling mitochondrial function and neurotransmitter release at the synapses. Any changes in the ability of the membranes to maintain hydrogen ion gradients may be critical in bilirubin toxicity, especially because the binding of bilirubin to cells or mitochondria is proportional to the hydrogen concentration in the local environment (Nelson et al, 1974; Odell, 1965; Wennberg, 1988). In addition, increased levels of lactate, decreased levels of cellular glucose and impaired cerebral glucose metabolism have been shown to be associated with hyperbilirubinemia in the neonatal rat.

A fourth hypothesis to explain intracellular bilirubin toxicity is *interference with enzyme activity*. This theory holds that bilirubin acid is capable of binding receptor sites on specific enzymes, rendering the enzymes inoperative or at least severely diminishing their activities.

The pathogenesis of kernicterus, especially the "low-bilirubin" variety, and the exact mechanism of bilirubin toxicity to the central nervous system are still not fully understood. Bilirubin encephalopathy is a multifactorial process that requires a critical level of free bilirubin, access to the brain across the blood-brain barrier, and presence of susceptible nerve cells. The severity and duration of hyperbilirubinemia, the maturity of the structures involved, the binding capability of albumin, the physiologic environment, and the cell membrane composition and metabolic state probably all are critical to the development of neurodysfunction. Decisions based simply on the total or unconjugated serum bilirubin levels seem simplistic; these other factors must be taken into consideration as well.

## Predicting Encephalopathy and Reversibility of Damage

From the aforementioned information, it is understandable that controversy remains regarding the toxicity of low and moderate levels of bilirubin in the premature and the full-term infant. Despite progress made in clinical management, there is no agreement on what constitutes a "safe" level of bilirubin. New assessment tools have been sought to identify factors that could be used to predict impending encephalopathy or to identify subtle findings that could be reversed. Various new techniques are being used in this regard (Vohr, 1990).

### *Brainstem Evoked Auditory Response*

Because the auditory pathway of the neonate is particularly vulnerable to insult from bilirubin, BAER testing has been suggested as a tool that could identify or predict early effects of hyperbilirubinemia on the central nervous system. Studies have regularly correlated increased bilirubin concentrations with changes in amplitude and latency of these responses. BAER testing is accurate and noninvasive and assesses the functional status of the auditory nerve in the brainstem auditory pathway. A sound stimulus is introduced to the infant, and the waveforms that are generated as the electrical impulse passes through the auditory pathway are measured. Recorded parameters include the threshold sensitivity, latency (the conduction time interval from sound stimulus to the appearance of waveforms), the interpeak latency, the amplitude of the waves, and the slope of latency changes with time and magnitude of the stimulus. Wave I reflects peripheral conduction time, wave III reflects the superior olive, and waves IV and V represent the inferior colliculus. Interpeak latencies I to III and I to V are useful in assessing damage from bilirubin. When electrodes are left in place, serial examinations can be made to assess response to therapy or impending brain injury. In a study of 50 full-term infants with moderate hyperbilirubinemia (STB levels of 10 to 20 mg/dL [171 to 342 μmol/L]), the latency of BAER waves IV and V was longer than in those infants with lower STB levels (Shapiro and Nakamura, 2001). These abnormalities in most infants resolve as STB values become normal by 6 months of age. Some of the changes in BAER can also be reversed with an exchange transfusion. Changes in BAER also have been noted with elevated free bilirubin levels. An abnormal BAER and normal otoacoustic emission (OAE) suggest an auditory neuropathy. Auditory neuropathy has been observed in one third to one half of infants reported to have significant hyperbilirubinemia. Recent findings indicate that it is more likely to be reversible than are other types of auditory neuropathy. BAER testing could be used to screen hyperbilirubinemic full-term and premature infants for sensorineural hearing loss and could be incorporated into the assessment of need for exchange transfusions (Nwaesei et al, 1984; Wennberg et al, 1982).

### *Infant Cry Analysis*

Analysis of characteristics of infant crying, or "cry analysis," has progressed so that alterations in cry characteristics have been documented in several perinatal risk situations including hyperbilirubinemia. Early work in this field involved spectrographic methods, but recent advances in high-speed computer technology have improved the ability to measure cry characteristics efficiently and accurately (Lester, 1987). It has been shown that with moderately elevated STB levels, there is interference with neural conduction, as demonstrated by the BAER, and changes in neural function in adjoining pathways, with resultant effects on the vocal cords (increased tension or phonation).

### *Nuclear Magnetic Resonance Techniques*

Nuclear magnetic resonance (NMR) techniques, both imaging and spectroscopy, have been proposed as a rapid, noninvasive measure of impending or actual brain cell injury in the face of hyperbilirubinemia (Palmer and Smith, 1990). NMR spectroscopy is a form of spectroscopy using magnetism and radio-frequency energy. It is a noninvasive method that could be used to characterize anatomic structural changes in variable metabolic states. Compared with ultrasonography or computed tomography (CT), MRI provides superior anatomic detail without exposing the neonate to ionizing radiation. NMR spectroscopy, especially using phosphorus3s1, with its ability to measure phosphorus metabolites, is being used to improve understanding of the interaction of hyperbilirubinemia and asphyxia. Phosphorus3s1 NMR spectroscopy captures the phosphorus metabolites as levels decline, elevate, and shift in relation to each other to maintain cellular homeostasis in the face of oxygen depletion.

Brain biochemical activity and "energy failure" are detectable by these techniques, allowing for identification and study of the progression from initial to irreversible tissue damage. Using phosphorus3s1 NMR spectroscopy, studies involving animal models have demonstrated that the cumulative effect of bilirubin and hypoxia is far more significant than either alone in disrupting brain energy metabolism (Ives et al, 1988). Similarly, hyperosmolar blood-brain barrier opening and hyperbilirubinemia have been shown to disturb cortical energy metabolism only when they coexist (Ives et al, 1989). NMR spectroscopic changes have also been reported in a jaundiced newborn rhesus monkey after displacement of bilirubin with a sulfa drug (Ahlfors et al, 1986).

NMR technology may enable the diagnosis of reversible brain injury in sufficient time to intervene and to determine what changes are irreversible for timely prognostication. Diffusion-weighted NMR imaging (DWI) applies a special gradient on the water signal to measure its diffusivity, which can be used as an early physiologic marker of neuronal injury. In other models of brain injury, such as neonatal hypoxic-ischemic encephalopathy or stroke, DWI shows significant changes quite early while still reversible and before the more permanent injury occurs that is normally shown by conventional NMR imaging (Fisher et al, 1995; Rhine et al, 1994). This capability could have important implications in bilirubin encephalopathy if DWI is shown to demonstrate ongoing, severe neuronal dysfunction in the affected regions of the brain (e.g., basal ganglia), which might prompt intervention such as exchange transfusion. In brain studied after exposure to extreme hyperbilirubinemia, conventional NMR images have been anatomically specific and symmetrical, the observed abnormalities having the distribution characteristic of kernicterus (Martich-Kriss et al, 1995; Penn et al, 1994). Further spectroscopic and imaging studies are needed to better characterize kernicterus and to help determine which changes suggestive of neurotoxicity might be found in more moderate hyperbilirubinemia.

### Practical Considerations

The question of what constitutes a critical threshold of bilirubin for the neonate in terms of long-term or permanent morbidity remains unanswered. A safe level of STB and a safe duration of exposure have not been determined, nor have all the factors (e.g., acidosis, hypoxia) that influence the risk of long-term neurodevelopmental handicaps been fully explained. Until these issues are adequately understood, a cautious approach to clinical management must be pursued.

## MANAGEMENT OF NEONATAL HYPERBILIRUBINEMIA

Hyperbilirubinemia remains a common, important, and sometimes pathologic condition of the newborn. Because the risk of jaundice-associated neurotoxicity continues to be a major concern of physicians caring for newborns, management of neonatal hyperbilirubinemia is a subject of considerable discussion and debate. Issues affecting management decisions and current recommendations are discussed in this section.

The occurrence of bilirubin encephalopathy in newborns has been greatly reduced since the introduction of blood exchange transfusion in the 1950s for the treatment of hyperbilirubinemia associated with hemolytic disease of the newborn, and since Rh-negative mothers have routinely received the anti-Rh globulin as a measure to prevent isoimmunization. A single reliable criterion for instituting treatment of hyperbilirubinemia has not been possible, however, because low STB levels can be associated with bilirubin encephalopathy in small premature infants, and hypoxia, acidosis, and sepsis also may be associated with higher risk. The neurotoxicity of bilirubin is not an all-or-none phenomenon but instead ranges from subtle reversible changes in neural function to permanent structural and functional impairment related to discrete cell death and regional yellow staining of brain tissue. Besides the classic signs of kernicterus, neurologic sequelae (e.g., disturbances of visual-motor function, impaired nonverbal intelligence) have been described in surviving premature infants who had hyperbilirubinemia in the neonatal period. However, whether such nonspecific findings may have been related to either the degree or the duration of hyperbilirubinemia or to some other factors is uncertain and will not be ascertained by further analysis of current data. Thus, predictors of bilirubin encephalopathy, besides STB concentration, have been sought, and guidelines for intervention have been fraught with lively controversy. Criteria based entirely on clinical experience and measurement of STB have weaknesses and may result in overtreatment of term infants. In contrast, more liberal criteria may lead to undertreatment of some infants, inadvertently contributing to permanent damage in susceptible infants. Understanding susceptibility is key to solving this clinical problem. Some researchers have argued for a case-based approach using not only the determination of total unconjugated serum bilirubin concentrations to develop criteria for treatment plans but also measures of albumin binding capacity, determination of the integrity and maturity of the blood-brain barrier, and an assessment of the conjugating power of the liver. Because the basic mechanisms behind the development of bilirubin toxicity are not completely understood, however, such new treatment criteria have not been systematically or successfully implemented (Bratlid, 1995).

### The Term Infant

Because health term neonates are as a group at less risk for bilirubin encephalopathy than premature or sick infants, most authors discussing clinical management of neonatal hyperbilirubinemia frame their discussion in the context of only one of these groups. As medical practice faces increasing economic constraints, decisions regarding the management of hyperbilirubinemia include not only which tests to complete and which clues to follow but also the balance of risks of undertreatment with the cost and consequences of overtreatment.

With regard to management of the jaundiced term neonate who is deemed to be "healthy," controversy has characterized the discussions for several decades. In 1959, Mores and associates evaluated 54 full-term infants without evidence of isoimmunization who had STB levels greater than 20 mg/dL (342 μmol/L) and who received no exchange transfusion. Citing normal development in all 54 subjects after 2 years of follow-up, these investigators concluded that "it is useless to perform an exchange transfusion on full-term infants with intensive jaundice without isoimmunization because these infants are neither in danger, nor ill; they are only icteric" (Mores et al, 1959). Since that time, much has been learned about the processes of bilirubin metabolism but not much more about the mechanisms of neurotoxicity. Although many studies confirm the low risk to term infants who do not have excessive hemolysis or rigid elements in STB levels, any statement suggesting total absence of risk is viewed as overly simplistic and dangerous.

In response to these controversies, the American Academy of Pediatrics (AAP) published guidelines for the management of the jaundiced neonate (AAP, 1994). Intended to apply only to the healthy full-term neonate, these guidelines describe a range of acceptable practices, recognizing that more precise recommendations cannot be formulated from current scientific literature, and acknowledging that: (1) "factors influencing bilirubin toxicity to the brain cells of newborn infants are complex and incompletely understood"; (2) "It is not known at what bilirubin concentration or under what circumstances significant risk of brain damage occurs or when the risk of brain damage exceeds the risk of treatment"; and (3) "Concentrations considered harmful may vary in different ethnic groups, or geographic locations. . . . Reasons for apparent geographic differences in risk for kernicterus are not clear." In addition, these recommendations were presented at a time when the management decisions were increasingly problematic because of mounting pressures for early discharge from the hospital and a greater prevalence of breast-feeding in the American population.

## Evaluation and Diagnostic Procedures

The AAP "practice parameter" lists factors to be considered in assessing a jaundiced infant (Table 79–6). Regarding the evaluation of the jaundiced newborn, the AAP recommendations reinforce the fact that because the determination of specific risk factors and the identification of illnesses early are crucial in the management of these patients, a careful history and physical examination remain the most important diagnostic procedures.

Of particular significance is a family history of severe unexplained jaundice requiring exchange transfusion, suggesting the possibility of G6PD deficiency or some other cause of hemolytic disease. When the family history, ethnic or geographic origin, or timing of jaundice suggests such a diagnosis, appropriate laboratory assessment in the infant should be performed (Table 79–7).

Maternal prenatal testing should routinely include ABO and Rh typing and a serum screen for unusual isoimmune antibodies. When the mother has not had prenatal determination of blood group or is Rh- negative, a direct Coombs' test and Rh typing of the infant's cord blood are recommended to anticipate and closely monitor an infant at risk of severe hemolysis and to determine the need for the mother to receive Rho(D) antibody (anti-Rh globulin).

STB determinations are indicated in all infants who appear jaundiced in the first 24 hours of life, because such an early appearance of jaundice is almost always associated with hemolytic disease or illness. In other infants, STB levels are indicated if estimates from sequential observations show that the jaundice is moderate or worse (estimate of STB in excess of 12 mg/dL [200 μmol/L]).

**TABLE 79–6**

**Factors to Be Considered in Assessment of the Jaundiced Infant**

Factors that suggest the possibility of hemolytic disease
Family history of significant hemolytic disease
Onset of jaundice before age 24 hours
An increase in STB levels of more than 0.5 mg/dL/hour
Pallor, hepatosplenomegaly
Rapid increase in the STB level after 24 to 48 hours (consider G6PD deficiency)
Ethnicity suggestive of inherited disease (e.g., G6P deficiency)
Failure of phototherapy to lower the STB level
Clinical signs suggesting other diseases (e.g., sepsis, galactosemia) in which jaundice may be one manifestation
Vomiting
Lethargy
Poor feeding
Hepatosplenomegaly
Excessive weight loss
Apnea
Temperature instability
Tachypnea
Signs of cholestatic jaundice suggesting the need to rule out biliary atresia or other causes of cholestasis
Dark urine or urine positive for bilirubin
Light-colored stools
Persistent jaundice for more than 3 weeks

*G6PD, glucose-6-phosphate dehydrogenase; STB, serum total bilirubin.

Data from the American Academy of Pediatrics: Practice parameter: Management of hyperbilirubinemia in the healthy term newborn. Pediatrics 94:559, 1994.

## Prediction of the Risk of Hyperbilirubinemia

Visual assessment of STB levels as suggested by Kramer (1969), which relies on the cephalocaudal progression of jaundice with a rising STB level (head and neck, 4 to 8 mg/dL [68 to 292 μmol/L]; upper trunk, 5 to 12 mg/dL [86 to 205 μmol/L]; lower trunk and thighs, 8 to 16 mg/dL [137 to 274 μmol/L]; palms and soles, greater than 15 mg/dL [257 μmol/L], is now known to be fraught with error. There is also considerable interlaboratory variation among STB levels measured at different laboratories (Vreman et al, 1996b). Bhutani and colleagues (1999), in a study of 1997 infants, found the practice of reporting the STB level on the basis of age in days rather than hours to be misleading and ineffective at accurately predicting which infants are at high risk for severe hyperbilirubinemia. Because jaundice is a common occurrence in newborn infants and severe hyperbilirubinemia is a relatively rare event, there has been considerable interest in developing a selective approach to follow-up evaluation and surveillance of these infants. The approaches that are currently suggested include universal bilirubin screening of all infants prior to discharge by either STB level determination or a transcutaneous bilirubin measurement (TcB) and ETCOc to assess rate of bilirubin production and to diagnose hemolysis.

Bhutani and colleagues (1999) generated a percentile-based bilirubin nomogram using hour-specific predischarge STB levels from a racially diverse group of term healthy newborns with no Rh or ABO incompatibility (42% white, 42.4% African American, 8% Hispanic, 4.3% Asian, other 2.8%, and 4.7% undisclosed) who did not need phototherapy before 60 hours of age and of whom 60% were breastfed (Fig. 79–1). Postdischarge STB levels were measured by a hospital-based bilirubin assay within 3 days after discharge. The risk for significant hyperbilirubinemia (STB greater than 17 mg/dL [291 μmol/L]) for infants with a predischarge STB above the 95th percentile (high-risk zone) was 57%, for infants with STB between the 75th and 95th percentiles (high-intermediate risk) it was 13%, for infants with STB between the 40th and 75th percentiles (low-intermediate risk) it was 2.1%, and for infants with STB below the 40th percentile (low risk) it was 0. The applicability of the nomogram was not significantly altered by including near-term infants or those who had hemolysis secondary to blood group incompatibility except for jaundice at less than 24 hours of age. Measurement of a predischarge bilirubin at the time of newborn screening (beyond 24 hours) along with an assessment of individual risk factors for jaundice such as gestational age, race, method of feeding, presence of polycythemia, blood group incompatibility or bruising, can help in the timing of follow-up examination of a select group of infants. Limitations of this approach are the need for blood sampling (although this can be done with the newborn screen) and the cost of STB measurement.

TcB is based on the measurement of light reflected from the skin. Older devices reported a jaundice index that, despite correlation with serum bilirubin levels, was

**TABLE 79-7**

**Data Collection in the Diagnosis of Neonatal Jaundice**

| Information | Significance |
|---|---|
| **Family History** | |
| Parent or sibling with history of jaundice or anemia | Suggests hereditary hemolytic anemia such as hereditary spherocytosis |
| Previous sibling with neonatal jaundice | Suggests hemolytic disease due to ABO or Rh isoimmunization |
| History of liver disease in siblings or disorders such as cystic fibrosis, galactosemia, tyrosinemia, hypermethioninemia, Crigler-Najjar syndrome, or $\alpha_1$-antitrypsin deficiency | All associated with neonatal hyperbilirubinemia |
| **Maternal History** | |
| Unexplained illness during pregnancy | Consider congenital infections such as rubella, cytomegalovirus, toxoplasmosis, herpes, syphilis, hepatitis A or B, Epstein-Barr virus |
| Diabetes mellitus | Increased incidence of jaundice among infants of diabetic mothers |
| Drug ingestion during pregnancy | Ingestion of sulfonamides, nitrofurantoins, antimalarials may initiate hemolysis in G6PD-deficient infant |
| **History of Labor and Delivery** | |
| Vacuum extraction | Increased incidence of cephalhematoma and jaundice |
| Oxytocin-induced labor | Increased incidence of hyperbilirubinemia |
| Delayed cord clamping | Increased incidence of hyperbilirubinemia among polycythemic infants |
| Apgar score | Increased incidence of jaundice in asphyxiated infants |
| **Infant History** | |
| Delayed passage of meconium or infrequent stools | Increased enterohepatic circulation of bilirubin; consider intestinal atresia, annular pancreas, Hirschsprung disease, meconium plug, drug-induced ileus (hexamethonium) |
| Caloric intake | Inadequate caloric intake results in delay in bilirubin conjugation |
| Vomiting | Suspect sepsis, galactosemia, or pyloric stenosis; all associated with hyperbilirubinemia |
| **Infant Physical Examination** | |
| Small for gestational age | Infants frequently polycythemic and jaundiced |
| Head size | Microcephaly seen with intrauterine infections associated with jaundice |
| Cephalhematoma | Entrapped hemorrhage associated with hyperbilirubinemia |
| Plethora | Polycythemia |
| Pallor | Suspect hemolytic anemia |
| Petechiae | Suspect congenital infection, overwhelming sepsis, or severe hemolytic disease as cause of jaundice |
| Appearance of unbilical stump | Omphalitis and sepsis may produce jaundice |
| Hepatosplenomegaly | Suspect hemolytic anemia or congenital infection |
| Optic fundus abnormalities | Chorioretinitis suggests congenital infection as cause of jaundice |
| Umbilical hernia | Consider hypothyroidism |
| Congenital anomalies | Jaundice occurs with increased frequency among infants with trisomic conditions |
| **Laboratory Data** | |
| ***Maternal*** | |
| Blood group and indirect Coombs' test | Necessary for evaluation of possible ABO or Rh incompatibility |
| Serologic studies | Rule out congenital syphilis |
| ***Infant*** | |
| Hemoglobin determination | Anemia suggests hemolytic disease or large entrapped hemorrhage; hemoglobin above 22 g/dL associated with increased incidence of jaundice |
| Reticulocyte count | Elevation suggests hemolytic disease |
| Red blood cell morphology | Spherocytes suggest ABO incompatibility or hereditary spherocytosis; red blood cell fragmentation seen in disseminated intravascular coagulation |
| Platelet count | Thrombocytopenia suggests infection |
| White blood cell count | Total white blood cell count less than 5000/mm$^3$ or band-to-neutrophil ratio >0.2 suggests infection |
| Sedimentation rate determination | Values in excess of 5 during the first 48 hours indicate infection or ABO incompatibility |
| Direct bilirubin assay | Elevation suggests infection or severe Rh incompatibility |
| Immunoglobulin M assay | Elevation indicates infection |
| Blood group studies and direct and indirect Coombs' test | Required to rule out hemolytic disease as a result of isoimmunization |
| Carboxyhemoglobin level determination | Elevated in infants with hemolytic disease or entrapped hemorrhage |
| Urinalysis | Presence of reducing substance suggests diagnosis or galactosemia |

G6PD, glucose-6-phosphate dehydrogenase.

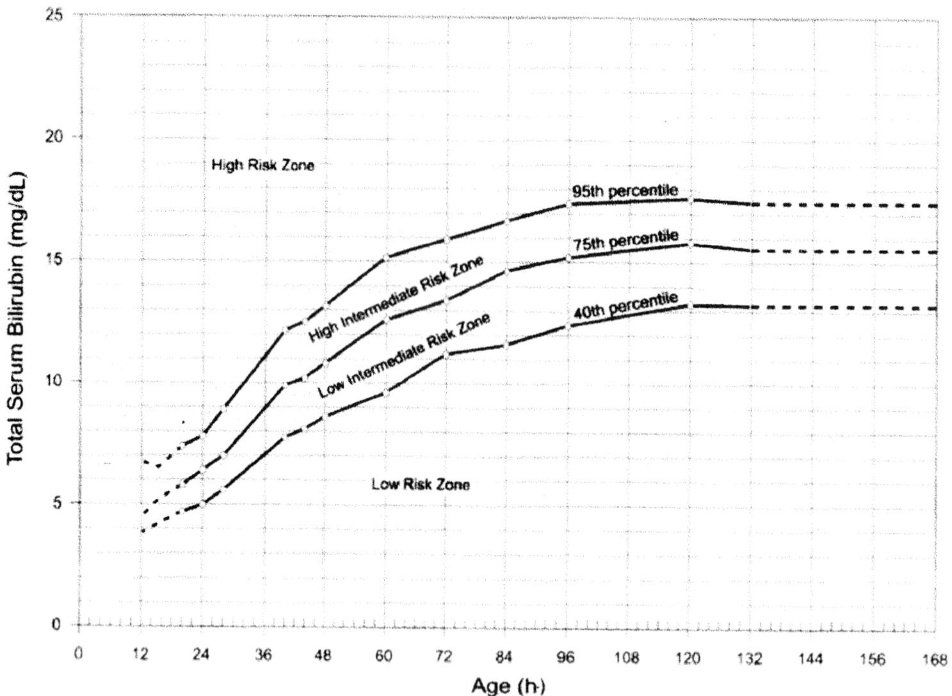


**FIGURE 79–1.** Nomogram displaying risk designation of term and near-term well infants based on hour-specific serum total bilirubin values. The high-risk zone is designated by the 95th percentile track. The intermediate risk zone is subdivided into upper and lower risk zones by the 75th percentile track. The low risk zone is below the 40th percentile. *(From Bhutani VK, Johnson L, Sivieri EM: Predictive ability of a predischarge hour–specific serum bilirubin for subsequent significant hyperbilirubinemia in healthy and near-term newborns. Pediatrics 103:6-14, 1999. Reproduced by permission of Pediatrics, Copyright 1999.)*

affected by skin thickness and skin color. One device also required a baseline skin color measurement, thus limiting its usefulness for widespread use. A newer point-of-care device (BiliCheck, SpectRx Inc., Norcross, Georgia) that measures the entire spectrum of visible light reflected from the skin (380 to 760 nm) has been shown to provide an accurate assessment of STB in term and near-term newborn infants of diverse races and ethnicities. It is important to note that transcutaneous devices measure not serum bilirubin but the amount of bilirubin that has moved into the tissue. The efficacy of this device in preterm infants, infants undergoing phototherapy, and those with STB levels less than 15 mg/dL (257 μmol/L) needs to be tested. Use of TcB for screening may decrease the need for phlebotomy and possibly reduce costs. An alternative approach is measurement of STB in all jaundiced infants and follow-up evaluation within 2 days of all infants discharged prior to 48 hours.

## Measurement of $ETCO_c$

Because the breakdown of heme by the rate-limiting enzyme HO leads to the formation of equimolar amounts of CO and biliverdin, with biliverdin immediately reduced to bilirubin, the measurement of CO in the exhaled breath of the newborn can be used as an index of heme degradation and bilirubin production in vivo. The $ETCO_c$ is an index of the rate of bilirubin production and can aid the practitioner in diagnosing hemolysis. A large multicenter trial conducted at nine centers with the objective of determining whether a measurement of $ETCO_c$ at 30 ± 6 hours of age, alone or in combination with an STB measurement obtained at the same time, could predict the development of severe hyperbilirubinemia showed that addition of the $ETCO_c$ measurement did not improve the predictive ability of the hours of age-specific STB (Stevenson et al, 2001). However, use of the $ETCO_c$ along with the STB level has several benefits. It can help distinguish between cases of increased bilirubin production versus decreased elimination or impaired bilirubin conjugation. In a retrospective study of results of 2443 direct Coombs' tests, 8% were found positive, suggesting Gilbert syndrome or a condition affecting conjugation. Only 17% of infants with a positive Coombs' test subsequently developed hyperbilirubinemia that needed treatment with phototherapy (unpublished observation). Therefore, routine measurement of the Coombs' test is not necessary in infants delivered to O-positive mothers. The Coombs' test is not a good predictor of the risk of hemolysis. In addition, use of the peripheral blood smear and reticulocyte counts has not been useful in diagnosing hemolysis.

Assessment of risk factors for jaundice helps in identification of infants who are most at risk for development of hyperbilirubinemia. It is recommended that depending on the incidence of hyperbilirubinemia and the demographics of the population, each institution develop its own criteria for decision making and timing for follow-up evaluation of infants.

With increasing pressure to discharge babies from the hospital at 24 hours of age or younger, most jaundiced infants will not be diagnosed by nursery personnel. Therefore, 2 to 3 days after discharge (corresponding with the time of the normal transitional peak of hyperbilirubinemia), follow-up evaluation should be provided by a health care professional in an office or clinic or at home for all newborns discharged at less than 48 hours after birth. Because bacterial sepsis is a significant risk factor for bilirubin encephalopathy and may be associated with elevated bilirubin levels caused by hemolysis or inadequate nutrition or hydration, further evaluation of newborns in whom abnormal signs such as feeding difficulty, lethargy, apnea, or temperature instability develop must be initiated to rule out underlying illness or sepsis (see Table 79–6).

Because approximately one third of healthy breast-fed infants have jaundice that persists beyond 2 weeks of age (Linn et al, 1985), breast-feeding need not be routinely interrupted solely for the purpose of establishing a diagnosis of breast milk or breast-feeding jaundice (Gartner, 1994).

Any report of dark urine, light stools, or persistence of jaundice beyond 2 weeks should prompt a measurement of direct (conjugated) serum bilirubin levels. Otherwise, determination of direct bilirubin levels is most often not useful in the healthy neonate. Other data that are useful in evaluating an infant with neonatal jaundice are listed in Table 79–7.

## Susceptibility to Bilirubin Neurotoxicity

An appreciation of the factors that may be associated with increased risk for brain injury associated with increased hyperbilirubinemia is central to determining which patients should be treated and which intervention should be undertaken. Some patients demonstrate a steady and excessive increase in STB levels over the first several days of extrauterine life, enabling clinicians to predict STB levels by extrapolation. Other infants exhibit a more sudden change in STB concentration, making prediction of the course of hyperbilirubinemia impossible (e.g., in G6PD-deficient or septic infants).

Specific clinical situations such as sepsis, isoimmunization, and other causes of hemolysis are known to be associated with elevated risks for neurotoxicity, even at STB levels otherwise considered moderate or mild. The reason for this increased risk is not known with certainty, but increased bilirubin production is a finding common to these situations.

Some experts think that bilirubin production rates may be the critical piece of information distinguishing jaundiced infants at excessive risk of encephalopathy from those who, although equally jaundiced in appearance and having similarly elevated STB concentrations, are at less risk. The saturation of the albumin binding sites and elevated levels of unbound bilirubin may be critical to the neurotoxic effects of bilirubin. In addition to the capacity of albumin to bind bilirubin in the circulation, the total tissue load of bilirubin may be important to consider.

When STB concentrations are lower than the level that saturates the bilirubin-binding sites of albumin, the measured "STB" represents all the unconjugated bilirubin in circulation, whether bound to albumin or not. However, this STB concentration does not reflect the tissue load or total body load of bilirubin. This is a critical difference, because a high bilirubin production rate is thought to result in a more rapid transfer of bilirubin to tissue, causing patients with high rates of production to have substantially higher tissue loads than in patients with low production rates. If the capacity to keep bilirubin in circulation is exceeded more rapidly, a surrogate for this circumstance is the rate of increase of bilirubin in circulation or the postnatal age at which a particular level is reached; for example, a STB concentration of 20 mg/dL (342 μmol/L) at 48 hours of age represents a different risk from that of 20 mg/dL (342 μmol/L) at 7 days of age. When the STB concentration increases enough to "saturate" the albumin binding sites and the body load is particularly heavy, the tissue load is already high, and any further increase in serum bilirubin represents bilirubin with great potential to enter the brain, which may have been spared until that time. If the tissue load is small, however, further deposition of bilirubin in the body may be possible, relieving the brain of immediate risk. It has been hypothesized that this high tissue load in patients with increased bilirubin production may explain why these patients are vulnerable to brain damage at the same STB levels that do not seem to endanger babies with low rates of bilirubin production. This concept of a total body load or tissue load also may explain why infants with increased bilirubin production (e.g., hemolysis) have a more profound rebound in STB levels after treatment with either exchange transfusion or phototherapy. If this hypothesis is sustained, identifying patients with increased bilirubin production will be extremely useful in determining the level of risk for neurotoxicity and scheduling interventions.

## Treatment Guidelines

The AAP guidelines for treatment of and intervention for hyperbilirubinemia in the healthy term newborn are summarized in Table 79–8 and in Figure 79–2. The guidelines are recommended for infants initially seen with elevated STB levels as well as for infants requiring follow-up evaluation for clinical jaundice. Because direct bilirubin measurements vary substantially as a function of differences of individual laboratories and their instrumentation, the direct bilirubin measurement should not be subtracted from the STB level in determining management strategy (Vreman et al, 1996b). Infants less than 24 hours of age who are jaundiced are generally considered to have a "pathologic" process and require further evaluation. Uncertainty remains about what specific STB levels warrant exchange transfusion, and intensive phototherapy is recommended while preparations are being made for exchange transfusion. Implementation of phototherapy is especially relevant for infants who have an STB concentration in the exchange transfusion range when initially seen (see Table 79–8). Intensive phototherapy is expected to cause a decline in STB level of 1 to 2 mg/dL (17 to 34 μmol/L) within 4 to 6 hours (AAP, 1994); if no decline occurs, the presence of hemolytic disease or some other pathologic process is suggested and warrants further investigation, and most experts recommend exchange

**TABLE 79-8**

**American Academy of Pediatrics Guidelines for Management of Hyperbilirubinemia in the Healthy Term Newborn**

| | Serum Total Bilirubin Level (mg/dL [μmol/L]) | | | |
|---|---|---|---|---|
| **Age (h)** | **Consider Phototherapy*** | **Phototherapy** | **Exchange Transfusion if Intensive Phototherapy Fails†** | **Exchange Transfusion and Intensive Phototherapy** |
| 25-48§ | ≥12 [170] | ≥15 [260] | ≥20 [340] | ≥25 [430] |
| 49-72 | ≥15 [260] | ≥18 [310] | ≥25 [430] | ≥30 [510] |
| >72 | ≥17 [290] | ≥20 [340] | ≥25 [430] | ≥30 [510] |

*Phototherapy at these serum total bilirubin (STB) levels is a clinical option, meaning that the intervention is available and may be used on the basis of individual clinical judgment.

†Intensive phototherapy should produce a decline in STB of 1-2 mg/dL within 4-6 hours, and the STB level should continue to decline and remain below the threshold level for exchange transfusion. If this does not occur, phototherapy has failed. Intensive phototherapy includes the use of more than one bank of lamps containing "special blue" bulbs, maximizing the surface area illuminated by using a phototherapy blanket or other means, and providing phototherapy on a continuous, uninterrupted schedule.

§Term infants who are clinically jaundiced at <24 hours old are not considered healthy and require further evaluation.

Used with permission of the American Academy of Pediatrics: Practice parameter: Management of hyperbilirubinemia in the healthy term newborn. Pediatrics 94:560, 1994.

transfusion. Practices vary between ordering sequential individualized laboratory tests and "batching" them in a "hyperbilirubinemia workup." For example, once an STB level is obtained and is seen to be elevated, some clinicians obtain a direct Coombs' test and blood group type and await the results before proceeding to further tests. Others, to minimize patient inconvenience and to gather more complete information initially, study hemoglobin, reticulocyte count, blood group, direct Coombs' test, and blood cell count and differential and inspect a blood film all at once. Consideration of practical and economic issues plays a role in such decisions, and practice variations are expected.

The controversies remaining in the AAP recommendation center on two areas. First, the guidelines are said to apply to infants without signs of illness or apparent hemolytic disease. The bilirubin levels cited by the committee's policy for initiating phototherapy are high enough that increased bilirubin production could well be a contributing cause, and it becomes the responsibility of the physician to determine whether such a contributing cause is likely. Assuming the absence of hemolysis when the Coombs test' result is negative does not suffice, because this test identifies isoimmunization primarily. Obtaining a direct estimate of bilirubin production by measuring the $COHb_c$ level or $ETCO_c$ can be a very useful way to exclude hemolysis. Although the feasibility of both of these techniques has been demonstrated, they have not been available to most physicians until recently.

The second area of controversy involves the levels of STB cited for initiating phototherapy or considering exchange transfusion. Some experts think that the AAP recommendation is overly simplistic because the guidelines do not consider the duration of moderate to severe hyperbilirubinemia and because they belittle the risk of hyperbilirubinemia when the STB level ranges from 25 to 30 mg/dL (425 to 510 μmol/L), especially without knowing the albumin binding capacity or its affinity for bilirubin.

## Management of the Preterm Infant

The increased intensity and duration of hyperbilirubinemia in the preterm infant as well as the assumed immaturity of the blood-brain barrier have lead to concern about greater risks of bilirubin encephalopathy in this patient population. Is the "healthy" preterm infant at greater risk

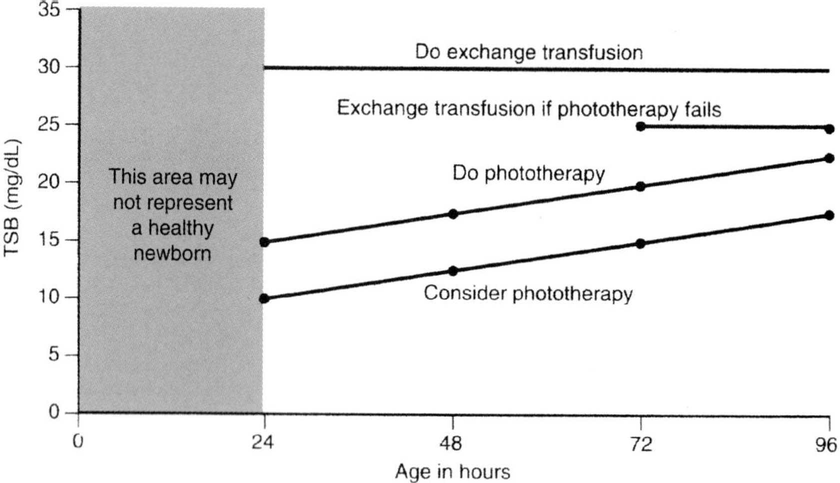


**FIGURE 79-2.** Guidelines for treatment and intervention of hyperbilirubinemia in the healthy term newborn. *(From Gartner LM: Neonatal jaundice. Pediatr Rev 15:429, 1994. Reproduced by permission of Pediatrics in Review, Copyright 1994.)*

of bilirubin encephalopathy at STB concentrations less than 20 mg/dL (340 μmol/L)? Or is the premature infant at greater risk because of the greater frequency of pathologic conditions such as sepsis, acidosis, hypoxia, shock, and intracranial hemorrhage in such patients? Many clinicians use gestational age, birth weight, and health status adjustments to determine the need for phototherapy and exchange transfusion, although controlled trials supporting these policies have not been carried out. The guidelines in Table 79–9 suggest one approach to the implementation of exchange transfusion in premature babies.

Because neurotoxicity has been related to the STB level, this measure has traditionally been the parameter most often used in assessing the severity of hyperbilirubinemia and in decisions regarding management. During the years in which practice guidelines suggested instituting phototherapy to keep the STB level less than 20 mg/dL (340 μmol/L) in term infants, severe bilirubin encephalopathy rarely occurred. In infants weighing less than 1500 g, efforts were usually made to keep the STB concentration less than 12 mg/dL (200 μmol/L) and less than 14 mg/dL (240 μmol/L) in infants weighing 1500 to 2500 g, with similar good results. There is concern, however, that more subtle neurodevelopmental abnormalities may occur at these levels and that prolonged elevations at lower levels also may be damaging, suggesting that the current guidelines for premature or low-birth-weight infants may still not be adequate to eliminate risk.

## Other Management Considerations: Identifying Treatment Criteria

The importance of excess bilirubin production as a risk factor for encephalopathy must be stressed. Excess bilirubin production includes hemolysis resulting from isoimmune reactions, hemolysis from other causes (e.g., G6PD deficiency, erythrocyte membrane disorders), and nonhemolytic processes leading to excess bilirubin production. A Coombs' test is not sufficient to identify all causes of excess bilirubin production and is not a good measure of the degree or intensity of hemolysis.

Researchers continue to work toward identifying parameters to help clinicians evaluate hyperbilirubinemia so that intervention can be instituted appropriately, and in a timely manner. In addition to the factors listed in Table 79–6, the STB concentration has been the critical parameter in developing management guidelines. Other measures are listed in Table 79–10, and some of these hold promise for becoming useful tools in the decision-making process. However, they have not yet been included in standard practice parameters (see Table 79–7).

### Free Plasma Bilirubin

Free plasma bilirubin is the fraction of bilirubin not bound to albumin. This has been considered the critical portion of unconjugated bilirubin because of its ability to cross the blood-brain barrier easily. Although there is a constant dynamic state between bound and unbound bilirubin at the albumin binding sites, free bilirubin levels are known to increase when plasma albumin levels are diminished or when bilirubin is displaced from the albumin by drugs and chemicals that competitively attach to the albumin binding sites. Encephalopathy is virtually nonexistent if the unbound bilirubin levels are maintained at less than 0.8 μg/dL in infants weighing less than 1500 g and at less than 0.1 μg/dL (1.7 μmol/L) in infants weighing 1500 to 2500 g (Bratlid, 1995; Nakamura et al, 1992). Studies using BAER have demonstrated significantly more abnormalities in newborns with unbound bilirubin concentrations of 1.0 μg/dL (17 μmol/L) or greater, suggesting that measuring unbound bilirubin concentrations may be helpful for evaluating bilirubin effects and may predict the risk of bilirubin encephalopathy in full-term newborns with hyperbilirubinemia. Until recently, there has been no simple accurate method of determining free

**TABLE 79–9**

**Guidelines for the Management of Hyperbilirubinemia Based on Birth Weight and Relative Health of the Newborn**

| | Serum Total Bilirubin Level (mg/dL) | | | |
|---|---|---|---|---|
| | Healthy | | Sick | |
| Birth Weight | Phototherapy | Exchange Transfusion | Phototherapy | Exchange Transfusion |
| Premature | | | | |
| <1000 g | 5-7 | Variable | 4-6 | Variable |
| 1001-1500 g | 7-10 | Variable | 6-8 | Variable |
| 1501-2000 g | 10-12 | Variable | 8-10 | Variable |
| 2001-2500 g | 12-15 | Variable | 10-12 | Variable |
| Term | | | | |
| >2500 g | 15-18 | 20-25 | 12-15 | 18-20 |

Data from Halamek LP, Stevenson DK: Neonatal jaundice and liver disease. In Fanaroff AA, Martin RJ (eds): Neonatal-Perinatal Medicine. Diseases of the Fetus and Infant, 7th ed. St. Louis, Mosby–Year Book, 2001, p 1335.

**TABLE 79–10**

**Potential Criteria for Treatment of Neonatal Jaundice**

| |
|---|
| Serum total bilirubin concentration |
| Transcutaneous bilirubin concentration |
| Unconjugated serum bilirubin concentration |
| Free plasma bilirubin (not bound to albumin) |
| Reserve albumin-binding capacity |
| Bilirubin production rates |
| Serum carboxyhemoglobin (COHb) levels |
| End-tidal carbon monoxide ($ETCO_c$) levels |
| Neurophysiologic criteria |
| Visual evoked potentials |
| Somatosensory potentials |
| Auditory evoked potentials |

bilirubin levels, but unbound bilirubin concentrations can now be measured by the peroxidase method using a commercially available device (Nakamura et al, 1992). A recent modification of this method overcomes the limitations, such as inaccuracy due to the presence of bilirubin-binding competitors (e.g., benzoate), rate-limiting dissociation of bilirubin from albumin, or high levels of antioxidants, conjugated bilirubin, or free radical–producing drugs (Ahlfors, 2000a, 2000b).

### Reserve Albumin Binding Capacity

Some authors have suggested the use of the reserve albumin binding capacity to determine how much of a range of safety is available before albumin binding sites become saturated. The conceptual basis for this proposal is the knowledge that unbound bilirubin accumulates in the brain only after the albumin binding sites have been saturated, and the theory that the oversaturation by bilirubin allows unbound bilirubin to gain access to the brain. However, the dynamic process involved in attachment of bilirubin to albumin suggests that this parameter might be an unreliable measure of the amount of unbound bilirubin. Even when the binding sites are not fully occupied with bilirubin, there is some unbound bilirubin that can diffuse across the blood-brain barrier. Using the availability of binding sites, as a proxy for unbound bilirubin levels could therefore be unreliable, underestimating risks of neurotoxicity. Among the tests currently suggested for estimating albumin binding capacity are bilirubin titration tests, dye binding tests, and selective binding of tracer ligands. Some of these tests are semiquantitative, and most are impractical in the neonatal clinical setting (Bratlid, 1995).

### Bilirubin Production Rates

Unconjugated bilirubin production has traditionally been estimated from the rate of increase in STB concentration during the first 24 to 48 hours after birth. However, the rate of increase in STB reflects not only bilirubin production but also distribution and elimination.

Techniques have recently been developed that result in clinically useful measurements of $ETCO_c$ or percutaneous measurement of $COHb_c$. These measures correlate well with bilirubin production rates. Monitoring bilirubin production rates as well as STB concentration has been suggested as a guide to initiation of treatment and management for severe neonatal jaundice. Continuous monitoring of these parameters would be ideal, especially in situations of rapid increase in STB concentration, and instruments capable of such measures are becoming available for clinical application using portable electrochemical sensors (Stevenson et al, 1994; Vreman et al, 1994, 1996a).

## Modes of Intervention to Reduce Serum Bilirubin Concentration

Once the clinician has determined that a neonate's STB concentration is elevated enough to present a risk of encephalopathy or is increasing in a way that predicts significant risk, intervention to reduce the STB concentration becomes imperative. Therapeutic intervention decisions must be tempered by clinical judgment based on the history, course, and physical findings. The currently accepted modes of intervention and others that are still in various stages of investigation are listed in Table 79–11.

### Hydration

There is no evidence that excess fluid administration affects the STB concentration. Some infants however, especially those being breast-fed, may be mildly dehydrated and may need supplemental fluid intake to correct their dehydration. Reduction in STB concentration, which appears to be a response to rehydration, especially with increased oral nutrition, may be related to the correction of dehydration, to more effective intestinal motility (with the increased oral intake leading to elimination of conjugated bilirubin via stool), or to enhanced removal of photoproducts in both urine and stool. Because milk-based formula is less likely to enhance reabsorption of bilirubin by the enterohepatic circulation, it often is recommended for use for oral correction of mild dehydration in hyperbilirubinemic children.

### Phototherapy

Although Native Americans had long been aware of the beneficial effects of the sun in reducing the yellow color

**TABLE 79–11**

**Treatment Modalities to Reduce Serum Bilirubin Concentration**

| |
|---|
| Hydration |
| Phototherapy |
| Exchange transfusion |
| Drugs to increase conjugation |
| Inhibition of reabsorption (binding in the gut) |
| Inhibition of bilirubin production |

of babies exposed to its light, phototherapy for neonatal hyperbilirubinemia was first proposed in 1958 by Cremer and colleagues in England (Cremer et al, 1958). Subsequently, this therapy has been used for the reduction of elevated STB levels and for the "prophylactic" prevention of hyperbilirubinemia in premature infants. With the development of Rh-immune globulins to prevent maternal isoimmunization and the introduction of phototherapy, the need for exchange transfusions in healthy term infants was reduced significantly. Phototherapy has remained the mainstay of treatment for hyperbilirubinemia.

Phototherapy has become the most common treatment used for neonatal hyperbilirubinemia (Costarino et al, 1985). Still, there is no standardized method for delivering phototherapy. The phototherapy units vary widely, the types of lamps used differ, the amount of skin exposed to phototherapy often depends on other clinical issues, and the intensity of the light varies according to the lamp power and the distance from the skin. Usually the dose of phototherapy is based on what is convenient to administer, rather than what is most effective.

The efficacy of phototherapy is influenced by the following factors: (1) the spectrum of light delivered, the blue-green region of the visible spectrum being the most effective; (2) the energy output or irradiance of the phototherapy light, measured in $\mu W/cm^2/nm$; and (3) the surface area of the infant exposed to phototherapy (Landry et al, 1985).

The amount of light to which an infant is exposed during phototherapy is minute compared with exposure later in life, even during the first year of life. With the light sources currently used, it is impossible to overdose the patient with phototherapy. Conventional phototherapy involves exposing a maximal area of skin to an irradiance of 6 to 12 $\mu W/cm^2/nm$ (Dennery et al, 2001; Garg et al, 1995).

High-intensity phototherapy involves increasing the irradiance to more than 25 $\mu W/cm^2/nm$ and was first described in 1977 (Tan, 1977). The rationale for high-intensity phototherapy is the demonstration of a dose-response relationship to bilirubin degradation until a saturation dose is reached at about 40 $\mu W/cm^2/nm$ of appropriate light. The use of high-intensity phototherapy has been advocated by investigators who have documented more effective reduction of STB levels with no long-term complications.

Commonly used phototherapy units contain a number of "daylight," "cool white," or "special blue" fluorescent tubes. Others use tungsten-halogen lamps. These lamps may be part of a radiant warming device, included as a bank of lights shining on the baby, or included in fiberoptic vests or blankets, which are used to increase the surface area exposed or to aid in continuing phototherapy while a baby is held or fed. The special blue fluorescent tubes make the baby appear blue, occasionally causing discomfort to nursery personnel. Recently, high-intensity gallium nitride light-emitting diodes (LEDs) have been proposed as a potential light source for delivering phototherapy (Vreman et al, 1998). LEDs deliver high-intensity narrow-band light with minimal heat generation, are lightweight and portable, and can be used in a variety of applications. In a preliminary clinical trial, blue LED phototherapy was as efficacious as conventional fluorescent phototherapy (Seidman et al, 2000). The potential benefits and versatility of this type of phototherapy are promising.

Recommendations to optimize phototherapy include using the most effective spectrum, using the maximum irradiance available, and exposing as much skin as possible to the therapy. Intermittent skin exposure using one continuous light source and rotating the baby to expose different areas of the skin has not been shown to improve the effect of phototherapy. There is no convincing rationale for using intermittent phototherapy, but interrupting phototherapy for feeding or brief parental visits may be tolerated in less severely affected infants. Therefore, the systems that provide a fiberoptic light source in the mattress under the baby and standard lighting above have been recommended. The administration of high-intensity phototherapy using a transparent waterbed has been shown to be significantly more effective at reducing bilirubin levels than conventional phototherapy (Garg et al, 1995).

Despite its apparent safety and enthusiastic application, the photochemical reactions responsible for the decline in STB levels are incompletely understood. Bilirubin is known to undergo photodegradation in vivo and in vitro, resulting in photoproducts that are more polarized and therefore more water soluble and potentially excretable than native bilirubin. Bilirubin is a yellow pigment with a peak absorption at a wavelength of 450 nm. The initial and most rapid reactions occurring as a result of phototherapy produce configurational isomers, characterized by changes in the shape of the bilirubin molecule but not its structure (McDonagh and Lightner, 1988). These isomers are the most abundant serum photoisomers and may account for up to 20% of STB in infants undergoing phototherapy. The most prominent of these configurational isomers is called 4Z,15E bilirubin (native bilirubin being 4Z,15Z bilirubin). The second most rapid photochemical reaction leads to the formation of structural isomers, the most prominent known as lumirubin. Formation of this compound appears to be irreversible. Although certain phototherapy reactions reach their peak at relatively low levels of irradiance (6 to 9 $\mu W/cm^2/nm$), the production of lumirubin is directly proportional to the energy output on the skin (Garg et al, 1995). High-intensity phototherapy results in greater amounts of lumirubin among the photoisomers.

In summary, it appears that the decrease in STB levels resulting from phototherapy is mainly a result of excretion of photoproducts in the bile and subsequent removal in stool. Configurational isomers are maximally produced at conventional levels of irradiance, but structural isomers are more efficiently produced by high-intensity phototherapy and may account for the increased efficacy of high-intensity phototherapy. Because these photoproducts are not conjugated for excretion but merely rendered more polar, their reabsorption by way of the enterohepatic circulation can diminish the effectiveness of phototherapy.

Phototherapy is relatively a safe and simple method of treatment. The possible side effects of phototherapy have been subject to extensive and controversial debate. Associated side effects that may occur, especially in premature infants, include rashes (erythema), oxidative injury, dehydration (transdermal water loss), and ultraviolet (UV) light irradiation (Aouthmany, 1999; Ente and Klein, 1970; Porat et al, 1996). Although irradiation of cells with light intensities similar to those used in phototherapy can produce DNA damage (Speck and Rosenkranz, 1976), no changes in growth, development, or infant behavior have been reported in long-term follow-up studies of infants who have received phototherapy (Granati et al, 1984; Teberg et al, 1977).

### *Rebounding Bilirubin Levels*

In the absence of hemolytic disease in healthy term infants, the cessation of phototherapy results in a mild rebound in the level of STB concentration. In one small study involving term and preterm infants, the average rebound after cessation of phototherapy was less than 1 mg/dL (17 μmol/L) (Lazar et al, 1993; Maisels and Kring, 2002).

Hospital discharge does not need to be delayed for observation for rebound in such cases. However, in the presence of hemolytic disease or in sick or low-birth-weight infants, such reassurance may not be warranted. Because hemolysis or other processes responsible for increased bilirubin production may continue, the rebound in these cases depends not only on the effectiveness of phototherapy but also on the severity of the bilirubin production.

### Exchange Transfusion

Although the first successful exchange transfusion performed on an infant with familial icterus gravis was reported in 1925 (Hart, 1925), this mode of intervention was not accepted until hemolytic disease of the newborn was conceptually understood in the 1940s. Exchange transfusion decreases the risk of bilirubin encephalopathy by reducing the total bilirubin load, increasing the binding sites of plasma albumin, and shifting bilirubin out of tissue into the plasma as well as providing erythrocytes less apt to hemolyze. Early attempts at exchange transfusion involved removing blood from the sagittal sinus or radial artery and infusing blood into the saphenous vein. With the development of polyethylene tubing, Diamond and coworkers in 1946 introduced the technique of alternate removal and administration of blood for each transfusion via umbilical vein catheterization (Diamond et al, 1951).

Before exchange transfusion came into common usage in the 1950s, kernicterus affected 15% of liveborn infants with erythroblastosis. Seventy percent of patients with kernicterus died within 1 week of birth, and many of the remainder died during the first year of life (Hsia et al, 1952). Survivors had permanent neurologic sequelae, and this entity was thought to account for 10% of all cases of cerebral palsy. Considering the severe morbidity of this condition, the major contribution provided by exchange transfusion can be appreciated, even though the procedure was recognized as having inherent risks of its own. With the initiation of exchange transfusion as an intervention for the hyperbilirubinemia of erythroblastosis fetalis, the history of kernicterus in newborns was forever changed. Despite many advances in the understanding of hemolytic and neonatal physiology, exchange transfusion remains the ultimate treatment to prevent neurotoxic damage from hyperbilirubinemia.

Exchange transfusion should be considered in cases of hemolysis in which intensive phototherapy has failed to decrease the STB levels by 1 to 2 mg/dL (17 to 34 μmol/L) in 4 to 6 hours or when the rate of rise of STB indicates that the level will reach 25 mg/dL (428 μmol/L) within 48 hours. It also should be performed in infants with high STB concentrations and early signs of kernicterus and in cases of hemolysis with anemia and hydrops. Exchange transfusion removes much of the circulating bilirubin and "sensitized" red cells (erythrocytes with maternal antibodies attached), replacing them with red cells compatible with the mother's antibody-rich serum and providing fresh albumin with binding sites for bilirubin. The process is tedious in that 5- to 10-mL aliquots are removed and replaced sequentially until about twice the volume (blood volume is 85 to 90 mL/kg) of the neonate's circulating blood volume has been exchanged. The anticoagulant of choice in the blood being infused is citrate-phosphate-dextrose. Because the citrate chelates calcium ions, there may be a need for calcium gluconate infusion during the course of the exchange. High concentration of glucose in the infusate may stimulate insulin production, increasing the risk of severe hypoglycemia (Rubaltelli and Griffith, 1992).

Blood stored for more than 4 days has excessive potassium levels, and such blood requires erythrocyte washing and resuspension in compatible plasma. All of these issues, as well as the temperature of the infusate and the environment, lead to possible stress and instability in the infant, especially in one who is ill and of low birth weight. The amount of bilirubin removed by each transfusion is a function of the initial STB level and the amount of blood exchanged. After an exchange transfusion, low levels of STB concentration may increase rapidly for several hours as bilirubin in tissues "migrates" back into the circulation. Typically, STB levels fall to one half of the pre-exchange value. In some cases (particularly in infants with hemolytic disease), the procedure may need to be repeated to lower the STB concentration sufficiently. Administration of 1 g/kg of albumin 1 to 2 hours before the procedure helps to shift more extravascular bilirubin into the circulation. Intravenous immune globulin (500 mg/kg) given over 2 hours may reduce the chance for a repeat exchange transfusion. Correction of metabolic acidosis by administration of sodium bicarbonate is recommended.

Exchange transfusions are not free of risk. Some reports estimate a risk of morbidity resulting from the procedure at 5%, with apnea, bradycardia, cyanosis, vasospasm, and hypothermia being the most common problems. Other risks include coagulation disturbances, electrolyte imbalances, thrombocytopenia, necrotizing enterocolitis, portal vein thrombosis, blood-borne infections, cardiac arrhythmias, and sudden death. Monitoring of electrolytes, platelet count, coagulation parameters, and arterial blood gases is recommended during the procedure. The procedure should therefore be instituted only when intensive phototherapy does not control the rapid rate of rise of STB levels and the risk of bilirubin encephalopathy outweighs the risk from the procedure itself. Mortality rate estimates run as high as 0.5%.

### Inducing Enzymes to Increase Conjugation

Increasing the ability of the body to excrete bilirubin by stimulating the ability of the liver to conjugate it has been attempted since Trolle (1961) observed less hyperbilirubinemia in infants of mothers receiving phenobarbital as anticonvulsant therapy.

Several pharmacologic agents have been identified as liver enzyme inducers, and those inducing UGT have been shown to increase the conjugation and excretion of bilirubin. Phenobarbital and nicotinamide were the first agents used for prevention and treatment of hyperbilirubinemia in newborns, and phenobarbital continues to be used in Gilbert disease and Crigler-Najjar syndrome type II (Arias disease). Type I disease does not respond well to this therapy (Rubaltelli and Griffith, 1992).

The effect of phenobarbital (at a dosage of 2.5 mg/kg/ day) on STB levels begins within a few days of its administration. This characteristic has made it less than optimal for use in the usual neonatal hyperbilirubinemia, because the STB is already high or rapidly increasing in the first few days. Phototherapy has been shown to be more effective in this situation, and adding phenobarbital to phototherapy has not been shown to have any advantage. However, postnatal phenobarbital administration may provide a useful approach to later elevation of STB levels, such as that seen in the hyperbilirubinemia in Asians, Native Americans, and other ethnic and genetic subgroups. It has been used with some success in congenital disorders of bilirubin metabolism, in which it lowers STB levels for 15 to 20 days, after which a new steady state is reached that is lower than pretreatment levels.

Prenatal administration of phenobarbital in anticipation of hyperbilirubinemia has been suggested in an effort to "prime the pump" of the conjugation process. One untoward side effect of this approach, however, is a decrease in prothrombin levels in the newborn, but this effect can be remedied by vitamin K administration. In a study involving prenatal administration of phenobarbital during the last week of the pregnancy to mothers whose infants were at risk for jaundice, treated infants had a reduced incidence of STB levels greater than 16 mg/dL (274 μmol/L) (Yaffe and Dorn, 1990).

Several chemicals used in traditional Chinese medicine have an enzyme-inducing effect similar to that of phenobarbital (Yin et al, 1991a). In studies involving rats and rabbits, *yin zhi huang* in a dose of 30 to 60 mg/kg/day has been shown to accelerate the plasma clearance and conjugation of bilirubin to an even greater degree than occurs with phenobarbital at 60 mg/kg/day. Both drugs increase glucuronyltransferase activity, but because they have dissimilar effects on other liver enzymes, it appears that their mechanisms of action may be different. Yin zhi huang, which is widely used in Asia to treat neonatal hyperbilirubinemia, is a decoction of four plants: *Artemisia*, *Gardenia*, *Rheum*, and *Scutellaria baicalensis*. The gardenia portion and phenobarbital have similar inducing effects also on glutathione-*S*-transferase, an enzyme involved in intracellular bilirubin transport in the liver (Yin et al, 1991b).

## Blocking Bilirubin Reabsorption

Neonatal hyperbilirubinemia is exacerbated by, if not caused by, enhanced reabsorption in the enterohepatic circulation. The absence of intestinal flora in neonates prevents the degradation of bilirubin in meconium and stool to products such as urobilinogen, which could be excreted. Bilirubin glucuronide arriving in the intestines is readily deconjugated to bilirubin and reabsorbed. Some of the products of phototherapy, especially the configurational isomers of bilirubin, also return to the native bilirubin form and may be reabsorbed. To counteract this process, various strategies have been used to bind the bilirubin in the intestinal lumen to substances that resist absorption. Seen as an effective low-risk, low-cost therapy, products such as activated charcoal and dried agar (an extract of seaweed) have been used with inconsistent results. A review of the early studies involving agar identified methodologic problems, allowing neither recommendation nor rejection of this approach (Kemper et al, 1988).

More recent studies using doses of 500 mg/kg of agar every 6 hours suggest that agar therapy can be used to augment the efficacy of phototherapy, and perhaps it could be used as therapy by itself (Caglayan et al, 1993). Besides resulting in a more rapid decline in STB levels, the use of agar increased stool frequency, suggesting enhanced clearance of intraluminal bilirubin regardless of binding. Cholestyramine was similarly considered but was found to cause hyperchloremic acidosis (Nicolopoulos et al, 1978).

Bilirubin oxidase derived from the fungus *Myrothecium verrucarea* has been suggested as another oral agent, but its effectiveness in interrupting reabsorption is based on its ability to degrade bilirubin to biliverdin and other nontoxic substances enzymatically, rather than by binding the pigment in the lumen (Murao and Tanaka, 1981). Studies involving the Gunn rat support this approach, but adequate data in humans are not yet available (Johnson et al, 1988).

## *Inhibiting Bilirubin Production*

Whereas other modes of intervention are directed at disposing of excess bilirubin already produced, attempts to decrease the production of bilirubin have met with moderate success. Studies in vitro and in both animals and humans have shown that certain metalloporphyrins can reduce the production of bilirubin, substantially reducing STB levels. These studies suggest that, in cases of hyperbilirubinemia caused by excess bilirubin production (i.e., catabolism of heme), these metalloporphyrins could be used to prevent the accumulation of dangerous STB levels, thus obviating more expensive, time-consuming, or hazardous interventions such as phototherapy and exchange transfusion. The mechanism of action of these compounds is competitive inhibition of the activity of HO, the rate-limiting enzyme in heme catabolism. Tin or zinc protoporphyrin, tin or zinc mesoporphyrin, and other synthetic analogues of the natural metalloporphyrin (ferroporphyrin-heme) are potent competitors of HO, the critical enzyme in the catabolism of heme. Their action is based on the fact that the catalytic site of HO recognizes metalloporphyrins with central metal ions other than iron (Fig. 79–3). HO actually favors some of these metalloporphyrins over heme as a substrate, sometimes by a large factor (Cornelius and Rodgers, 1984; Valaes et al, 1994; Vreman et al, 1990, 1991).

The potency of metalloporphyrins and their side effects are influenced by the central metal cation and the nature of the side chains. Tin porphyrins are more potent than zinc or cobalt porphyrins. With side chains composed

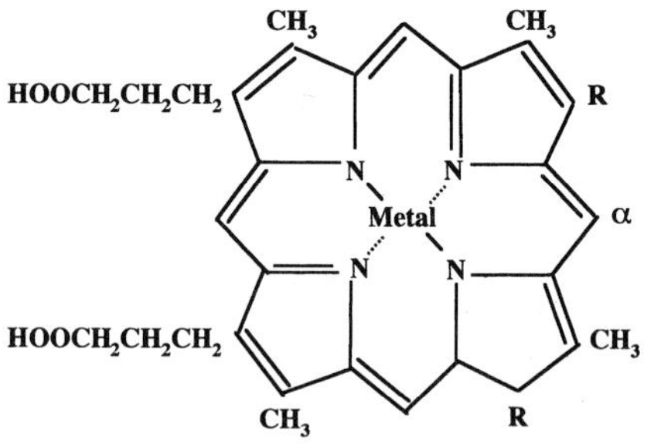

**Porphyrin Type Based on Ring Substituent and Chelated Metal**

| Metal | Deuteroporphyrin (R = —H) | Mesoporphyrin (R = —$CH_2$—$CH_3$) | Protoporphyrin (R = —CH=$CH_2$) | Bis(glycol)porphyrin (R = —CHOH—$CH_2$OH) |
|---|---|---|---|---|
| Metal-Free | MfDP | MfMP | MfPP | MfBG |
| Iron ($Fe^{2+}$) | FeDP | FeMP | **FePP (Hemin)** | FeBG |
| Zinc ($Zn^{2+}$) | ZnDP | ZnMP | ZnPP | ZnBG |
| Tin ($Sn^{4+}$) | SnDP | SnMP | SnPP | SnBG |
| Chromium ($Cr^{2+}$) | CrDP | CrMP | CrPP | CrBG |
| Manganese ($Mn^{2+}$) | MnDP | MnMP | MnPP | MnBG |
| Copper ($Cu^{2+}$) | CuDP | CuMP | CuPP | CuBG |
| Nickel ($Ni^{2+}$) | NiDP | NiMP | NiPP | NiBG |
| Magnesium ($Mg^{2+}$) | MgDP | MgMP | MgPP | MgBG |

**FIGURE 79–3.** Metalloporphyrin complexes and their chemical structures. Substrates and inhibitors of heme oxygenase belong to a large family of metalloporphyrins with varying metal moieties and porphyrin ring substituents. Heme or FePP is indicated in bold. *(From Vreman HJ, Wong RJ, Stevenson DK: Alternative metalloporphyrins for the treatment of neonatal jaundice. J Perinatol 21:S110, 2001. Reproduced by permission of the Journal of Perinatology, Copyright 2001.)*

of ethyl groups, mesoporphyrins are far more potent and stable than the other forms. When these agents were administered intramuscularly in doses from 1 to 6 μmol/kg, a 76% reduction in phototherapy requirements with a lowering of peak STB levels of 41% was observed, with minimal side effects (Valaes et al, 1994). In another randomized trial, the need for phototherapy was completely eliminated in full-term infants treated with 6 μmol of tin mesoporphyrin (SnMP)/kg (Martinez et al, 1999). These infants also had significantly shorter hospital stays and peak STB levels less than 19.6 mg/dL (335 μmol/L). Even with these promising results, metalloporphyrins are not currently approved for use in newborn infants. In another study, term infants with G6PD deficiency given SnMP at approximately 27 hours of age had lower and earlier peak STB values than those seen in control infants with and without G6PD deficiency. No treated infant required phototherapy, compared with 31% and 15% in the controls with and without G6PD deficiency, respectively.

Because these synthetic metalloporphyrins do not bind molecular oxygen, they are not metabolically degraded by ring rupture and do not add to the body pool of bilirubin. The metalloporphyrins also do not affect the metabolic disposition of preformed bilirubin, but they may have some inhibitory effect on the biliary excretion of bilirubin (Beri and Chandra, 1993).

The potential benefits of this chemopreventive approach to the management of hyperbilirubinemia could be substantial, especially in premature infants, in whom threshold levels for the manifestation of bilirubin toxicity are controversial and uncertain. Proponents of metalloporphyrins have demonstrated the effectiveness and apparent innocuousness of these compounds, but research continues in identifying which of the compounds is most effective at reducing bilirubin production without toxic side effects. For example, if phototherapy were to be used in conjunction with metalloporphyrin therapy, the effect of photodegradation on the metalloporphyrin and any ensuing risks would become substantial issues. For example, adults and children with cholestasis have high levels of copper porphyrins that are vulnerable to photo-induced chemical alterations resulting in the formation of brown pigments, made famous by the term *bronze baby syndrome* (Rubaltelli et al, 1983).

Each metalloporphyrin currently being evaluated has its own characteristics related to efficacy and side effects. These compounds are administered intramuscularly in a dose based on body weight, and their effectiveness appears to be dose related (and compound specific) in all gestational age groups tested. Administration of these compounds also produces a dose-dependent decrease in the proportion of newborns requiring phototherapy. When phototherapy is used as an adjunct to metalloporphyrin administration, a decrease in the duration of phototherapy is seen, especially on days 3 to 7 of life, which is related to metalloporphyrin dose. It is not clear which of these metalloporphyrins will eventually prove to be most efficacious and safe, and research in their use continues (Vreman et al, 2001). Although metalloporphyrins hold promise for the future, especially in countries where phototherapy or exchange transfusions are not easily available, they have currently not been approved by the Food and Drug Administration for use in newborns.

### Interruption of Breast-Feeding

Breast-fed babies generally have STB concentrations slightly above those of formula-fed babies. Some babies may experience prolonged jaundice, termed *breast milk jaundice*. Interrupting or continuing breast-feeding is a management decision that clinician and mother must decide on together. Options include continuing breast-feeding with optimal support, supplementing breast-feeding with bottle-feeding to guarantee optimal hydration, and discontinuing breast-feeding and relying on formula or parenteral feeding.

The choice among these options may depend on the strength and condition of the infant, the availability of the parents, the infant's environment, and the intensity of the treatments prescribed. There is no one certain way, but every attempt to accommodate long-term breast-feeding should be encouraged. The 1994 AAP practice parameter "Managing Hyperbilirubinemia in the Healthy Term Newborn" included a statement discouraging the interruption of breast-feeding in healthy term newborns and encouraging continued and frequent breast-feeding (at least 8 to 10 times every 24 hours).

## SUMMARY

The management of hyperbilirubinemia presents a complicated scenario to the clinician. The purpose of treatment is to prevent neurotoxic effects of bilirubin and to identify and treat illnesses that can be associated with excess bilirubin production, impaired conjugation, or inadequate elimination of the pigment. Modes of treatment include interfering with bilirubin production; enhancing the transport, binding, or conjugation of bilirubin; and removing bilirubin in urine, feces, and blood. Controversies remain regarding which treatment or combination of therapies is safest and most effective and which criteria should serve as indicators for instituting therapy.

## Acknowledgments

We acknowledge the contribution of Dr. Frank A. Oski, whose work on the original chapter served as an invaluable template for subsequent revisions. We also thank Ronald J. Wong for his contributions and critical review of this chapter.

## REFERENCES

Academy of Pediatrics: Practice parameter: Management of hyperbilirubinemia in the healthy term newborn. Provisional Committee for Quality Improvement and Subcommittee on Hyperbilirubinemia. Pediatrics 94:558-565, 1994.

Ahlfors CE: Measurement of plasma unbound unconjugated bilirubin. Anal Biochem 279:130-135, 2000a.

Ahlfors CE: Unbound bilirubin associated with kernicterus: A historical approach. J Pediatr 137:540-544, 2000b.

Ahlfors CE, Bennett SH, Shoemaker CT, et al: Changes in the auditory brainstem response associated with intravenous infusion of unconjugated bilirubin into infant rhesus monkeys. Pediatr Res 20:511-515, 1986.

Akaba K, Kimura T, Sasaki A, et al: Neonatal hyperbilirubinemia and mutation of the bilirubin uridine diphosphate-glucuronosyltransferase gene: A common missense mutation among Japanese, Koreans and Chinese. Biochem Mol Biol Int 46:21-26, 1998.

Allen FHJ, Diamond LK, Vaughn VCI: Erythroblastosis fetalis: VI. Prevention of kernicterus. Am J Dis Child 80:779-791, 1950.

Aouthmany MM: Phototherapy increases hemoglobin degradation and bilirubin production in preterm infants. J Perinatol 1999;19:271-274.

Arias IM: Inheritable and congenital hyperbilirubinemia. Models for the study of drug metabolism. N Engl J Med 285:1416-1421, 1971.

Arias IM, Gartner LM, Seifter S, et al: Neonatal unconjugated hyperbilirubinemia associated with breast feeding and a factor in milk that inhibits glucuronide formation *in vitro*. J Clin Invest 42:913, 1963.

Austin RF, Desforges JF: Hereditary elliptocytosis: An unusual presentation of hemolysis in the newborn associated with transient morphologic abnormalities. Pediatrics 44:196-200, 1969.

Benaron DA, Bowen FW: Variation of initial serum bilirubin rise in newborn infants with type of illness. Lancet 338:78-81, 1991.

Beneke R: Uber den kernicterus der neugeborenen. Munch Med Wochnsch 54:2023, 1907.

Beri R, Chandra R: Chemistry and biology of heme. Effect of metal salts, organometals, and metalloporphyrins on heme synthesis and catabolism, with special reference to clinical implications and interactions with cytochrome P-450. Drug Metab Rev 25:49-152, 1993.

Beutler E, Gelbart T, Demina A: Racial variability in the UDP-glucuronosyltransferase 1 (UGT1A1) promoter: A balanced polymorphism for regulation of bilirubin metabolism? Proc Natl Acad Sci USA 95:8170-8174, 1998.

Bhutani VK, Johnson L, Sivieri EM: Predictive ability of a predischarge hour-specific serum bilirubin for subsequent significant hyperbilirubinemia in healthy term and near-term newborns. Pediatrics 103:6-14, 1999.

Bosma PJ, Chowdhury JR, Bakker C, et al: The genetic basis of the reduced expression of bilirubin UDP-glucuronosyltransferase 1 in Gilbert's syndrome. N Engl J Med 333:1171-1175, 1995.

Bratlid D: Bilirubin toxicity: Pathophysiology and assessment of risk factors. NY State J Med 91:489-492, 1991.

Bratlid D: Neonatal and congenital hyperbilirubinemias: Evaluation of neonatal jaundice. Paper presented at the International Bilirubin workshop, Trieste, Italy, 1995.

Brodersen R, Stern L: Deposition of bilirubin acid in the central nervous system—A hypothesis for the development of kernicterus. Acta Paediatr Scand 79:12-19, 1990.

Caglayan S, Candemir H, Aksit S, et al: Superiority of oral agar and phototherapy combination in the treatment of neonatal hyperbilirubinemia. Pediatrics 92:86-89, 1993.

Childs B, Sidbury JB, Migeon CJ: Glucuronic acid conjugation by patients with familial non-hemolytic jaundice and their relatives. Pediatrics 23:903-913, 1959.

Cornelius CE, Rodgers PA: Prevention of neonatal hyperbilirubinemia in rhesus monkeys by tin-protoporphyrin. Pediatr Res 18:728-730, 1984.

Costarino AT, Ennever JF, Baumgart S, et al: Bilirubin photoisomerization in premature neonates under low- and high-dose phototherapy. Pediatrics 75:519-522, 1985.

Cremer RJ, Perryman PW, Richards DH: Influence of light on the hyperbilirubinaemia of infants. Lancet 1:1094-1097, 1958.

Crigler JFJ, Najjar VA: Congenital familial non-hemolytic jaundice with kernicterus. Pediatrics 10:169-180, 1952.

De Carvalho M, Klaus MH, Merkatz RB: Frequency of breast-feeding and serum bilirubin concentration. Am J Dis Child 136:737-738, 1982.

Dennery PA, McDonagh AF, Spitz DR, et al: Hyperbilirubinemia results in reduced oxidative injury in neonatal Gunn rats exposed to hyperoxia. Free Radic Biol Med 19:395-404, 1995.

Dennery PA, Seidman DS, Stevenson DK: Neonatal hyperbilirubinemia. N Engl J Med 344:581-590, 2001.

Diamond LK, Allen FHJ, Thomas WOJ: Erythroblastosis fetalis: VII. Treatment with exchange transfusion. N Engl J Med 244:39, 1951.

Diamond LK, Blackfan KD, Baty JM: Erythroblastosis fetalis and its association with universal edema of the fetus, icterus gravis neonatorum, and anemia of the newborn. J Pediatr 1:269, 1932.

Doxiadis SA, Fessas P, Valaes T: Glucose-6-phosphate dehydrogenase deficiency: A new etiologic factor in severe neonatal jaundice. Lancet 1:297-301, 1961.

Ente G, Klein SW: Hazards of phototherapy. N Engl J Med 283:544-545, 1970.

Fischer AF, Nakamura H, Uetani Y, et al: Comparison of bilirubin production in Japanese and Caucasian infants. J Pediatr Gastroenterol Nutr 7:27-29, 1988.

Fisher M, Prichard JW, Warach S: New magnetic resonance techniques for acute ischemic stroke. JAMA 274:908-911, 1995.

Garg AK, Prasad RS, Hifzi IA: A controlled trial of high-intensity double-surface phototherapy on a fluid bed versus conventional phototherapy in neonatal jaundice. Pediatrics 95:914-916, 1995.

Gartner LM: Neonatal jaundice. Pediatr Rev 15:422-432, 1994.

Gartner LM, Lee KS, Vaisman S, et al: Development of bilirubin transport and metabolism in the newborn rhesus monkey. J Pediatr 90:513-531, 1977.

Gartner LM, Snyder RN, Chabon RS, et al: Kernicterus: High incidence in premature infants with low serum bilirubin concentrations. Pediatrics 45:906-917, 1970.

Gilbert A, Lereboullet P: La cholemie simple familial. Semaine Medicále 21:241-443, 1901.

Goudonnet H, Magdalou J, Mounie J, et al: Differential action of thyroid hormones and chemically related compounds on the activity of UDP-glucuronosyltransferases and cytochrome P-450 isozymes in rat liver. Biochim Biophys Acta 1035:12-19, 1990.

Gourley GR: Disorders of bilirubin metabolism. In Suchy FJ (ed): Liver Disease in Children. St. Louis, Mosby–Year Book, 1994, pp 401-413.

Granati B, Largajolli G, Rubaltelli FF, et al: Efficacy and safety of the "integral" phototherapy for neonatal hyperbilirubinemia. Results of a follow-up at 6 years of age. Clin Pediatr (Phila) 23:483-486, 1984.

Guaran RL, Drew JH, Watkins AM: Jaundice: Clinical practice in 88,000 liveborn infants. Aust N Z J Obstet Gynaecol 32: 186-192, 1992.

Gunn CH: Hereditary acholuric jaundice in new mutant strain of rats. J Hered 29:137-139, 1938.

Guthrie L: Case of kernikterus associated with choreiform movements. Proc Soc Exp Med 7:86-87, 1913.

Hansen TW, Bratlid D, Walaas SI: Bilirubin decreases phosphorylation of synapsin I, a synaptic vesicle-associated neuronal phosphoprotein, in intact synaptosomes from rat cerebral cortex. Pediatr Res 23:219-223, 1988.

Hardy JB, Drage JS, Jackson EC: The First Year of Life: The Collaborative Perinatal Project of the National Institutes of Neurological and Communicative Disorders of Stroke. Baltimore, Johns Hopkins University Press, 1979, p 104.

Harley JD, Robin H: Haemolytic activity of Vitamin $K_3$: Evidence for a direct effect on cellular enzymes. Nature 193:478-480, 1962.

Harley JD, Robin H: Adaptive mechanisms in erythrocytes exposed to naphthoquinones. Aust J Exp Biol 41:281-292, 1963.

Hart AP: Familial icterus gravis of the newborn and its treatment. Can Med Assoc J 15:1008, 1925.

Hsia DYY, Allen FHJ, Diamond LK: Erythroblastosis fetalis: VIII. Studies of serum bilirubin in relation to kernicterus. N Engl J Med 247:668-671, 1952.

Hsia DYY, Dowben RM, Shaw R: Inhibition of glucuronyl transferase by progestational agents from serum of pregnant women. Nature 187:693, 1960.

Ives NK, Bolas NM, Gardiner RM: The effects of bilirubin on brain energy metabolism during hyperosmolar opening of the blood-brain barrier: An *in vivo* study using $^{31}$P nuclear magnetic resonance spectroscopy. Pediatr Res 26:356-361, 1989.

Ives NK, Cox DW, Gardiner RM, et al: The effects of bilirubin on brain energy metabolism during normoxia and hypoxia: An *in vitro* study using $^{31}$P nuclear magnetic resonance spectroscopy. Pediatr Res 23:569-573, 1988.

Jetté L, Murphy GF, Leclerc JM, et al: Interaction of drugs with P-glycoprotein in brain capillaries. Biochem Pharmacol 50: 1701-1709, 1995.

Johnson JD: Jaundice in Navajo neonates. Clin Pediatr (Phila) 31:716-718, 1992.

Johnson L, Brown AK, Bhutani VK: BIND: A clinical score for bilirubin induced neurologic dysfunction in newborns. Pediatrics 104:746-747, 1999.

Johnson LH, Brown AK: A pilot registry for acute and chronic kernicterus in term and near-term infants. Pediatrics 104:736, 1999.

Johnson LH, Dworanczyk R, Abbasi M, et al: Bilirubin oxidase (BOX) feedings significantly decrease serum bilirubin (B) in jaundiced infant Gunn rats. Pediatr Res 22:412A, 1988.

Jørgensen FS, Felding P, Vinther S, et al: Vitamin K to neonates. Peroral versus intramuscular administration. Acta Paediatr Scand 80:304-307, 1991.

Kaplan M, Renbaum P, Levy-Lahad E, et al: Gilbert syndrome and glucose-6-phosphate dehydrogenase deficiency: A dose-dependent genetic interaction crucial to neonatal hyperbilirubinemia. Proc Natl Acad Sci USA 94:12128-12132, 1997.

Kemper K, Horwitz RI, McCarthy P: Decreased neonatal serum bilirubin with plain agar: A meta-analysis. Pediatrics 82:631-638, 1988.

Koiwai O, Nishizawa M, Hasada K, et al: Gilbert's syndrome is caused by a heterozygous missense mutation in the gene for bilirubin UDP-glucuronosyltransferase. Hum Mol Genet 4:1183-1186, 1995.

Kramer LI: Advancement of dermal icterus in the jaundiced newborn. Am J Dis Child 118:454-458, 1969.

Kren BT, Parashar B, Bandyopadhyay P, et al: Correction of the UDP-glucuronosyltransferase gene defect in the Gunn rat model of Crigler-Najjar syndrome type I with a chimeric oligonucleotide. Proc Natl Acad Sci USA 96:10349-10354, 1999.

Labrune P, Myara A, Hennion C, et al: Crigler-Najjar type II disease inheritance: A family study. J Inherit Metab Dis 12:302-306, 1989.

Landry RJ, Scheidt PC, Hammond RW: Ambient light and phototherapy conditions of eight neonatal care units: A summary report. Pediatrics 75:434-436, 1985.

Landsteiner K, Weiner AS: An agglutinable factor in human blood recognizable by immune sera for Rhesus blood. Proc Soc Exp Biol 43:223, 1940.

Lazar L, Litwin A, Merlob P: Phototherapy for neonatal nonhemolytic hyperbilirubinemia. Analysis of rebound and indications for discontinuing therapy. Clin Pediatr (Phila) 32:264-267, 1993.

Lester BM: Developmental outcome prediction from acoustic cry analysis in term and preterm infants. Pediatrics 80:529-534, 1987.

Levine P, Stetson R: An unusual case of intra-group agglutinization. JAMA 113:126, 1939.

Levine RL: Bilirubin and the blood brain barriers. In Levine RL and Maisels MJ (eds): Hyperbilirubinemia in Newborn. Report of the 85th Ross Conference on Pediatric Research. Columbus, Ohio, Ross Laboratories, 1983, pp 125-140.

Lie-Injo LE, Virik HK, Lim PW, et al: Red cell metabolism and severe neonatal jaundice in West Malaysia. Acta Haematol 58:152-160, 1977.

Linn S, Schoenbaum SC, Monson RR, et al: Epidemiology of neonatal hyperbilirubinemia. Pediatrics 75:770-774, 1985.

Lockitch G: Beyond the umbilical cord: Interpreting laboratory tests in the neonate. Clin Biochem 27:1-6, 1994.

Lucarini N, Gloria-Bottini F, Tucciarone L, et al: Role of genetic variability in neonatal jaundice. A prospective study on full-term, blood group-compatible infants. Experientia 47: 1218-1221, 1991.

MacGillivray MH, Crawford JD, Robey JS: Congenital hypothyroidism and prolonged neonatal hyperbilirubinemia. Pediatrics 40:283-286, 1967.

Maisels MJ: Neonatal jaundice. In Avery GB (ed): Neonatology. Philadelphia, JB Lippincott, 1981, pp 484.

Maisels MJ, Gifford K: Normal serum bilirubin levels in the newborn and the effect of breast-feeding. Pediatrics 78:837-843, 1986.

Maisels MJ, Kring E: Rebound in serum bilirubin level following intensive phototherapy. Arch Pediatr Adolesc Med 156: 669-672, 2002.

Maisels MJ, Pathak A, Nelson NM, et al: Endogenous production of carbon monoxide in normal and erythroblastotic newborn infants. J Clin Invest 50:1-8, 1971.

Martich-Kriss V, Kollias SS, Ball WS, Jr.: MR findings in kernicterus. Am J Neuroradiol 16:819-821, 1995.

Martinez GA, Krieger FW: 1984 milk-feeding patterns in the United States. Pediatrics 76:1004-1008, 1985.

Martinez JC, Garcia HO, Otheguy LE, et al: Control of severe hyperbilirubinemia in full-term newborns with the inhibitor of bilirubin production Sn-mesoporphyrin. Pediatrics 103:1-5, 1999.

Matthay KK, Mentzer WC: Erythrocyte enzymopathies in the newborn. Clin Haematol 10:31-55, 1981.

McDonagh AF, Lightner DA: Phototherapy and the photobiology of bilirubin. Semin Liver Dis 8:272-283, 1988.

Miyoshi K, Saijo K, Kotani Y, et al: Characteristic properties of fetal human albumin (Alb F) in isomerization equilibrium. Tokushima J Exp Med 13:121-128, 1966.

Mores A, Fargasova I, Minarikova E: The relation of hyperbilirubinemia in newborns without isoimmunization to kernicterus. Acta Pediatr Scand 48:590, 1959.

Morphis L, Constantopoulos A, Matsaniotis N, et al: Bilirubin-induced modulation of cerebral protein phosphorylation in neonate rabbits *in vivo*. Science 218:156-158, 1982.

Murao S, Tanaka N: A new enzyme "bilirubin oxidase" produced by *Myrothecium verrucarea* MT-1. Agricult Biolog Chem 45:2383-2385, 1981.

Nakamura H, Yonetani M, Uetani Y, et al: Determination of serum unbound bilirubin for prediction of kernicterus in low birthweight infants. Acta Paediatr Jpn 34:642-647, 1992.

Nelson T, Jacobsen J, Wennberg RP: Effect of pH on the interaction of bilirubin with albumin and tissue culture cells. Pediatr Res 8:963-967, 1974.

Newman TB, Easterling MJ, Goldman ES, et al: Laboratory evaluation of jaundice in newborns. Frequency, cost, and yield. Am J Dis Child 144:364-368, 1990.

Newton WAJ, Frajola WJ: Drug-sensitive chronic hemolytic anemia: Family studies. Clin Res 6:392, 1958.

Nicolopoulos D, Hadjigeorgiou E, Malamitsi A, et al: Combined treatment of neonatal jaundice with cholestyramine and phototherapy. J Pediatr 93:684-688, 1978.

Notarianni LJ: Plasma protein binding of drugs in pregnancy and in neonates. Clin Pharmacokinet 18:20-36, 1990.

Nwaesei CG, Van Aerde J, Boyden M, et al: Changes in auditory brainstem responses in hyperbilirubinemic infants before and after exchange transfusion. Pediatrics 74:800-803, 1984.

Odell GB: Studies in kernicterus. I. The protein binding of bilirubin. J Clin Invest 38:823, 1959.

Odell GB: The influence of pH on distribution of bilirubin between albumin and mitochondria. Proc Soc Exp Biol Med 120:352, 1965.

Odell GB, Gourley GR: Hereditary hyperbilirubinemia. In Lebenthal E (ed): The Textbook of Gastroenterology and Nutrition in Infancy, 2nd ed. New York, Raven Press, 1989, pp 949-967.

Okolicsanyi L, Nassuato G, Muraca M, et al: Epidemiology of unconjugated hyperbilirubinemia: Revisited. Semin Liver Dis 8:179-182, 1988.

Olsen JE: Neonatal nonspherocytic hemolytic anemia due to glucose-6-phosphate dehydrogenase deficiency in a Danish infant. Acta Paediatr Scand 58:187-190, 1969.

Orth J: Ueber das vorkomen von bilirubinkrystallen bei neugebornen kindern. Arch F Anat Pathol 63:447, 1875.

Palmer C, Smith MB: Assessing the risk of kernicterus using nuclear magnetic resonance. Clin Perinatol 17:307-329, 1990.

Penn AA, Enzmann DR, Hahn JS, et al: Kernicterus in a full term infant. Pediatrics 93:1003-1006, 1994.

Phornphutkul C, Whitaker JA, Worathumrong N: Severe hyperbilirubinemia in Thai newborns in association with erythrocyte G6PD deficiency. Clin Pediatr (Phila) 8:275-278, 1969.

Porat R, Gilbert S, Magilner D: Methylene blue–induced phototoxicity: An unrecognized complication. Pediatrics 97:717-721, 1996.

Rhine WD, Benitz WE, Dennery PA, et al: Bilirubin measurements and long-term neurologic outcome. Pediatrics 94:246, 1994.

Robinson GC: Hereditary spherocytosis in infancy. J Pediatr 50:447, 1957.

Rubaltelli FF, Griffith PF: Management of neonatal hyperbilirubinaemia and prevention of kernicterus. Drugs 43:864-872, 1992.

Rubaltelli FF, Jori G, Reddi E: Bronze baby syndrome: A new porphyrin-related disorder. Pediatr Res 17:327-330, 1983.

Ryan AS, Rush D, Krieger FW, et al: Recent declines in breast-feeding in the United States, 1984 through 1989. Pediatrics 88:719-727, 1991.

Sass-Kortsak A, Thalme B, Ernster L: Commentary: Haemolytic activity of Vitamin $K_3$. Nature 193:480-481, 1962.

Sauter BV, Parashar B, Chowdhury NR, et al: A replication-deficient rSV40 mediates liver-directed gene transfer and a long-term amelioration of jaundice in Gunn rats. Gastroenterology 119:1348-1357, 2000.

Schmorl G: Zur kenntnis des icterus neonatorum, insbesondere der dabei auftretenden Gehirnveranderungen. Verhandl D Deutsch path Gesellsch 6:109, 1904.

Schneider AP: Breast milk jaundice in the newborn. A real entity. JAMA 255:3270-3274, 1986.

Seidman DS, Moise J, Ergaz Z, et al: A new blue light–emitting phototherapy device: A prospective randomized controlled study. J Pediatr 136:771-774, 2000.

Seidman DS, Paz I, Stevenson DK, et al: Neonatal hyperbilirubinemia and physical and cognitive performance at 17 years of age. Pediatrics 88:828-833, 1991.

Shapiro SM, Nakamura H: Bilirubin and the auditory system. J Perinatol 21:S52-S55, 2001.

Siegel E, Wason S: Mothball toxicity. Pediatr Clin North Am 33:369-374, 1986.

Sinaasappel M, Jansen PL: The differential diagnosis of Crigler-Najjar disease, types 1 and 2, by bile pigment analysis. Gastroenterology 100:783-789, 1991.

Speck WT, Rosenkranz HS: Intracellular deoxyribonucleic acid-modifying activity of phototherapy lights. Pediatr Res 10:553-555, 1976.

Spiller WG: Severe jaundice in the newborn child a cause of spastic cerebral diplegia. Am J Med Sci 149:345, 1915.

Stern L, Denton RL: Kernicterus in small premature infants. Pediatrics 10:483-485, 1965.

Stevenson DK, Fanaroff AA, Maisels MJ, et al: Prediction of hyperbilirubinemia in near-term and term infants. Pediatrics 108:31-39, 2001.

Stevenson DK, Vreman HJ, Oh W, et al: Bilirubin production in healthy term infants as measured by carbon monoxide in breath. Clin Chem 40:1934-1939, 1994.

Stocker R, Yamamoto Y, McDonagh AF, et al: Bilirubin is an antioxidant of possible physiological importance. Science 235:1043-1046, 1987.

Tada K, Chowdhury NR, Neufeld D, et al: Long-term reduction of serum bilirubin levels in Gunn rats by retroviral gene transfer *in vivo*. Liver Transpl Surg 4:78-88, 1998.

Tan KL: The nature of the dose-response relationship of phototherapy for neonatal hyperbilirubinemia. J Pediatr 90: 448-452, 1977.

Teberg AJ, Hodgman JE, Wu PY: Effect of phototherapy on growth of low-birth-weight infants—two-year follow-up. J Pediatr 91:92-95, 1977.

Trolle D: Discussion on the advisability of performing exchange transfusion in neonatal jaundice of unknown etiology. Acta Pediatr Scand 50:392, 1961.

Valaes T: Bilirubin and red cell metabolism in relation to neonatal jaundice. Postgrad Med J 45:86-106, 1969.

Valaes T: Severe neonatal jaundice associated with glucose-6-1phosphate dehydrogenase deficiency: Pathogenesis and global epidemiology. Acta Paediatr Suppl 394:58-76, 1994.

Valaes T, Karaklis A, Stravrakakis D, et al: Incidence and mechanism of neonatal jaundice related to glucose-6-phosphate dehydrogenase deficiency. Pediatr Res 3:448-458, 1969.

Valaes T, Petmezaki S, Henschke C, et al: Control of jaundice in preterm newborns by an inhibitor of bilirubin production: Studies with tin-mesoporphyrin. Pediatrics 93:1-11, 1994.

van de Bor M, van Zeben-van der Aa TM, Verloove-Vanhorick SP, et al: Hyperbilirubinemia in preterm infants and neurodevelopmental outcome at 2 years of age: Results of a National Collaborative Survey. Pediatrics 83:915-920, 1989.

Van den Bergh AAH, Muller P: Uber eine direkte und eine indirekte diazoreaktionen auf bilirubin. Biochem Z 77:90, 1916.

Varimo P, Similä S, Wendt L, et al: Frequency of breast-feeding and hyperbilirubinemia. Clin Pediatr (Phila) 25:112, 1986.

Vohr BR: New approaches to assessing the risks of hyperbilirubinemia. Clin Perinatol 17:293-306, 1990.

Vreman HJ, Baxter LM, Stone RT, et al: Evaluation of a fully automated end-tidal carbon monoxide instrument for breath analysis. Clin Chem 42:50-56, 1996a.

Vreman HJ, Lee OK, Stevenson DK: *In vitro* and *in vivo* characteristics of a heme oxygenase inhibitor: ZnBG. Am J Med Sci 302:335-341, 1991.

Vreman HJ, Rodgers PA, Stevenson DK: Zinc protoporphyrin administration for suppression of increased bilirubin production by iatrogenic hemolysis in rhesus neonates. J Pediatr 117:292-297, 1990.

Vreman HJ, Stevenson DK, Oh W, et al: Semiportable electrochemical instrument for determining carbon monoxide in breath. Clin Chem 40:1927-1933, 1994.

Vreman HJ, Verter J, Oh W, et al: Interlaboratory variability of bilirubin measurements. Clin Chem 42:869-873, 1996b.

Vreman HJ, Wong RJ, Stevenson DK: Alternative metalloporphyrins for the treatment of neonatal jaundice. J Perinatol 21:S108-113, 2001.

Vreman HJ, Wong RJ, Stevenson DK, et al: Light-emitting diodes: A novel light source for phototherapy. Pediatr Res 44:804-809, 1998.

Watchko JF, Daood MJ, Hansen TW: Brain bilirubin content is increased in P-glycoprotein-deficient transgenic null mutant mice. Pediatr Res 44:763-766, 1998.

Wennberg RP: The importance of free bilirubin acid salt in bilirubin uptake by erythrocytes and mitochondria. Pediatr Res 23:443-447, 1988.

Wennberg RP, Ahlfors CE, Bickers R, et al: Abnormal auditory brainstem response in a newborn infant with hyperbilirubinemia: improvement with exchange transfusion. J Pediatr 100:624-626, 1982.

Yaffe SJ, Dorn LD: Effects of prenatal treatment with phenobarbital. Dev Pharmacol Ther 15:215-223, 1990.

Yamauchi Y, Yamanouchi I: Breast-feeding frequency during the first 24 hours after birth in full-term neonates. Pediatrics 86:171-175, 1990.

Yin J, Miller M, Wennberg RP: Induction of hepatic bilirubin-metabolizing enzymes by the traditional Chinese medicine *yin zhi huang*. Dev Pharmacol Ther 16:176-184, 1991a.

Yin J, Wennberg RP, Xia YC, et al: Effect of a traditional Chinese medicine, *yin zhi huang*, on bilirubin clearance and conjugation. Dev Pharmacol Ther 16:59-64, 1991b.

Zimmerman HM, Yannet H: Kernicterus: Jaundice of the nuclear masses of the brain. Am J Dis Child 45:740-753, 1933.

Zinkham WH, Lenhard RE: Metabolic abnormalities of erythrocytes from patients with congenital non-spherocytic hemolytic anemia. J Pediatr 55:319-336, 1959.

# PART XVI

# RENAL AND GENITOURINARY SYSTEMS

Editors: **ROBERTA A. BALLARD** and **ISTVAN SERI**

CHAPTER 80

# Renal Morphogenesis and Development of Renal Function

Jean-Pierre Guignard

## RENAL MORPHOGENESIS

The fetal kidney develops from three successive mesodermic structures: the pronephros, the mesonephros, and the metanephros. The pronephric tubule extends into the intermediate mesoderm of the mesonephros to form the wolffian duct. The metanephros develops from an outbranch of the wolffian duct called the *ureteric bud* that extends into a mass of undifferentiated metanephric mesenchyme. Reciprocal inductive interactions between the ureteric bud epithelium and the metanephric mesenchyme result in the formation of both the collecting duct system and the nephrons of the permanent kidney. Cells of the metanephric mesenchyme adjacent to the tip of the ureteric bud are induced to aggregate and signal the ureteric bud to grow and branch repeatedly (branching morphogenesis), eventually leading to the formation of the renal collecting system. The ureteric bud also induces the mesenchyme to undergo a mesenchymal-epithelial transformation resulting in the formation of the glomeruli and renal tubules. Ureteric bud outgrowth requires inductive signals derived from the metanephric mesenchyme under the control of transcription factors and signaling molecules including Wilms tumor gene 1 (WT1) and glial cell line-derived neurotrophic factor (GDNF). Normal ureteric bud response to these inductive signals is under the control of several transcription factors such as Pax2 and Lim1 and the *Formin* gene.

Differentiation of the metanephros starts around 5 weeks of gestation, and the first nephrons are formed by week 8. Nephrogenesis continues up to weeks 34 to 35, with the deep nephrons being formed first. From the completion of nephrogenesis around week 35 until birth, the nephrons only grow in size. At birth, juxtamedullary nephrons are more mature than superficial nephrons. The total number of nephrons varies widely from 600,000 to 1.2 million per kidney. Fetal growth retardation reduces the number of nephrons, so that a positive correlation exists between birth weight and the final number of nephrons (Merlet-Bénichou et al, 1999). Exposure to drugs and vitamin A deficiency can also impair nephrogenesis, leading to a permanent nephron deficit (Gilbert and Merlet-Bénichou, 2000).

Mutations in any one of the genes controlling renal morphogenesis result in severe renal developmental defects. The angiotensinogen and angiotensin receptor genes, best known for controlling renal hemodynamics, also play a role in the development of calyces and pelvis. Mutational inactivation of the angiotensin receptor 2 (Agtr2), encoded on the X chromosome, results in a range of anomalies including vesicoureteral reflux, duplex kidney, renal ectopia, ureteropelvic junction stenosis, ureterovesical junction stenosis, renal dysplasia, renal hypoplasia, multicystic dysplastic kidney, and renal agenesis (the CAKUT sequence—*c*ongenital *a*nomalies of the *k*idney and *u*rinary *t*ract) (Nishimura et al, 1999).

Major renal malformations resulting from mutations in transcription factors, signaling molecules and gene products have been discussed in recent reviews (Burrow, 2000; Piscione and Rosenblum, 1999).

The glomerular diameter approximates 110 μm at birth (200 μm in the adult), and the average proximal tubular length reaches 2 mm (20 mm in the adult). Postnatal growth is characterized by accelerated growth of the proximal tubular volume compared with the glomerular filtering area. The glomerular basement membrane, which behaves as a filtration barrier, is thinner in neonates (100 nm) than in adults (300 nm). The size of the apertures in this "barrier" limits the passage of compounds through the capillary wall. In addition, an electrostatic barrier, resulting from the presence of negatively charged glycosialoproteins in the glomerular capillary wall, further restricts the filtration of negatively charged molecules. In the adult, the molecular weight cutoff for the filter is about 70,000. Molecules with a radius less than 1.8 nm are filtered freely. Molecules larger than 3.6 nm are not filtered. The permeability of the glomerular basement membrane is greater in newborn animals than in more mature animals (Savin et al, 1985).

During the second half of gestation, kidney weight increases proportionally to gestational age, body weight, and the body surface area. The kidney and bladder can be visualized by ultrasonography from week 15 of gestation; the precise renal architecture is only clearly defined by week 20. Kidney size as measured by ultrasonography increases proportionally to gestational age: $Y$ (kidney size in mm) = 16.19 + 0.61 gestational weeks (Jeanty et al, 1982). The ratio between the renal and the abdominal circumferences at the level of the umbilical vein remains constant during gestation, with values ranging from 0.27 to 0.30 (Grannum et al, 1980). At birth, renal volume approximates 10 mL, and it reaches 23 mL by the third week of life. Each kidney weighs about 12.5 g (~150 g in the adult) and has a length of about 4.5 cm (11.5 cm in the adult) at birth. The surface of the kidney is lobulated and remains so for months after birth. Fetal bladder volume can also be assessed by ultrasonography. With a maximal capacity of 10 mL at 32 weeks, the bladder can contain up to 40 mL near term.

## RENAL FUNCTION IN UTERO

The placenta is the major regulatory organ of the fetus, so that renal growth does not appear to be governed by functional requirements. Urine formation starts around 10 to 12 weeks of gestation. Fetal urine is a major constituent of amniotic fluid, and its production increases with age. Mean hourly urine flow rate is high and approximates 5 mL at 20 weeks, 10 mL at 30 weeks, and 30 mL at 40 weeks of postconceptional age (Rabinovitz et al, 1989). Fetal oliguria with a consequent decrease in amniotic fluid results in the oligohydramnios sequence, which includes facial compression (loose skin folds, flattened or beaked nose, large flat ears), positional deformities (asymmetrical club feet, major contractures, broad flat hands), and pulmonary hypoplasia.

The fetal urine is hypotonic throughout gestation, with sodium as the major osmotic component. The kidney actively reabsorbs electrolytes and solutes from the glomerular ultrafiltrate. Elevated concentrations of sodium (>100 mmol/L), chloride (>90 mmol/L), and osmolality (>210 mOsm/L) in the urine of a dilated kidney have been considered as indicating poor renal postnatal prognosis (see Chapter 81). However, the sensitivity (40% to 80%) and the specificity (<80%) of these parameters are not ideal.

Fetal renal blood flow (RBF), as measured by Doppler ultrasonography, reaches 20 mL/minute at 25 weeks of gestation and 60 mL/minute near term (Veille et al, 1993). The low rate of RBF in the fetus is associated with an elevated renal vascular resistance (RVR). Of interest, the fetus appears to be able to autoregulate RBF within modest limits.

Fetal glomerular filtration rate (GFR) increases rapidly as the number and size of nephrons increase. When the full complement of nephrons is attained, GFR increases in parallel with renal mass, and hence with body weight and body surface area. From 28 to 35 weeks of gestation, GFR (measured by inulin clearance in 1- to 2-day-old neonates) increases proportionally to gestational age (GFR = −28.1 + 1.37 × weeks of gestation) and then levels off up to the time of birth (Fig. 80–1).

Several vasoactive agents and hormones play a major role in modulating the fetal RBF and GFR, including the renin-angiotensin system, the catecholamines, the prostaglandins, the kallikrein-kinin system, endothelin, nitric oxide, and atrial natriuretic peptide (Table 80–1). Interference with these systems can lead to severe renal dysfunction in the fetus. A clinical example is fetal renal failure after administration to the mother of inhibitors of angiotensin-converting enzyme (ACE) or of prostaglandin synthesis (see Chapter 87).

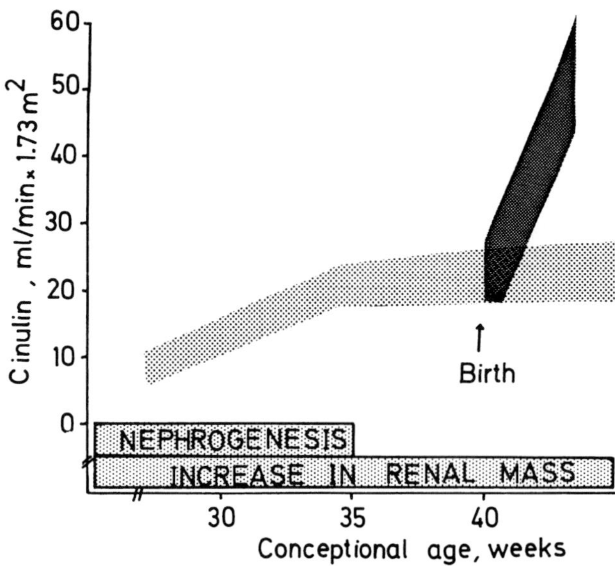


**FIGURE 80–1.** Maturation of GFR ($C_{inulin}$) in relation to conceptional age. *(From Guignard J-P: The Neonatal Stressed Kidney. In Gruskin AB, Norman ME [eds]: Pediatric Nephrology. The Hague, Martinus Nijhoff, 1981.)*

With that due to ACE inhibition, the decrease in the GFR probably results from the attenuated vasoconstriction of the efferent artery by angiotensin II inhibition, whereas reduced prostaglandin-dependent afferent vasodilation and the unopposed vasoconstrictive effects of angiotensin II and catecholamines may explain the drop in GFR observed in fetuses of mothers given nonselective or cyclooxygenase type 2 (COX-2)–selective nonsteroidal anti-inflammatory drugs (NSAIDs) (Guignard, 2002).

## POSTNATAL MATURATION OF RENAL BLOOD FLOW

Renal blood flow is determined primarily by the mean arterial pressure and the resistance at the level of the renal arterioles. In the adult, physiologic intrinsic autoregulation maintains a constant RBF at perfusion pressures varying from 80 to 200 mm Hg. This means that as perfusion pressure increases, the resistance to flow also increases. Both afferent and efferent arterioles participate in the vasoconstriction. In children and adults, RBF approximates 20% to

**TABLE 80–1**

**Vasoactive Factors Modulating Renal Blood Flow and Glomerular Filtration Rate in the Immature Kidney**

| | |
|---|---|
| Adenosine | Nitric oxide |
| Angiotensin II | Norepinephrine |
| Atrial natriuretic peptide | Prostaglandin $E_1$ |
| Bradykinin | Prostaglandin $E_2$ |
| Dopamine | Thromboxane $A_2$ |
| Endothelin | Vasopressin |
| Epinephrine | |

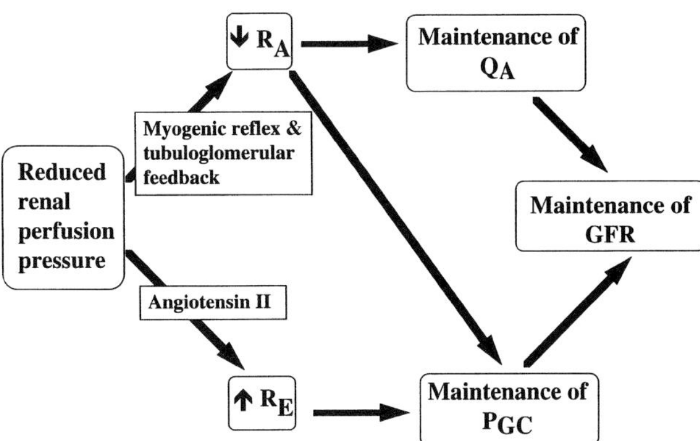


**FIGURE 80–2.** Mechanisms contributing to the autoregulation of renal blood flow and glomerular filtration rate (GFR). $P_{GC}$, glomerular capillary hydraulic pressure; $Q_A$, glomerular plasma flow rate; $R_A$, afferent arteriolar resistance; $R_E$, efferent arteriolar resistance. *(From Badr KF, Ichikawa I: Prerenal failure: A deleterious shift from renal compensation to decompensation. N Engl J Med 319:623, 1988.)*

25% of cardiac output, and it is around 1200 mL/minute × 1.73 $m^2$ of body surface area. The major part of the blood flow supplies the cortex, with medullary blood flow representing only 10% of the total RBF.

During fetal life, RBF is low, representing only 2% to 4% of the total cardiac output. This proportion increases after birth, from a value of 5% in the first 12 hours of life to 10% at the end of the first week. During the first 5 months, RBF increases rapidly from a value of 250 mL/minute × 1.73 $m^2$ at 8 days of age to approximately 770 mL/minute × 1.73 $m^2$ by 5 months of age. The postnatal maturation of RBF is associated with a striking decrease in RVR and a marked increase in systemic blood pressure. The decrease in RVR occurs along with a decrease in the resistance of both the afferent and the efferent arterioles. Animal studies suggest that autoregulation of RBF is present in the immature kidney but is set at a lower range of blood pressure (Chevalier et al, 1987).

Several autocrine, paracrine, and endocrine factors regulate RBF, intrarenal hemodynamics, and GFR (Bailie, 1992; Guignard et al, 1991; Seri, 1995) (Fig. 80–2; see also Table 80–1). Overactivation of the vasoconstrictive forces that regulate renal hemodynamics in the neonatal period may impair the maturation of RBF and induce renal hypoperfusion. Such activation is seen during respiratory distress, hypoxemia, asphyxia, metabolic acidosis, hypercapnia, hyper- and hypothermia, and positive pressure ventilation as well as in response to the administration of various medications. (Guignard and John, 1986; Toth-Heyn et al, 2000)

## POSTNATAL MATURATION OF GLOMERULAR FILTRATION RATE

### Determinants of Glomerular Filtration Rate

The rate of filtration is governed by the rate at which plasma flows through the glomerular capillaries, the balance of Starling forces across the glomerular capillary walls, the permeability of the basement membrane of the glomerular capillary wall to water and small solutes, and the total surface area of the capillaries. The ultrafiltration coefficient ($K_f$) represents the product of the permeability of the glomerular membrane and the glomerular filtering area. GFR is proportional to the Starling forces across the glomerular capillaries times the $K_f$:

$$GFR = K_f \times [P_{GC} - (P_{IT} + \pi_{GC})]$$

where $P_{GC}$ is the hydrostatic pressure in the glomerular capillary, $P_{IT}$ is the proximal intratubular hydrostatic pressure, and $\pi_{GC}$ is the oncotic pressure in the glomerular capillary. In adults, the average value of $P_{GC}$ probably approximates 60 mm Hg, the pressure in Bowman's capsule 15 mm Hg, and the oncotic glomerular capillary pressure 25 mm Hg. Thus, the average net filtration pressure is probably close to 20 mm Hg at the afferent end of the glomerular capillaries. It decreases to 10 mm Hg at the end of the efferent glomerular capillaries. Because of the very low mean arterial pressure present in neonates, the net transglomerular filtration pressure is probably not greater than 3 to 5 mm Hg. The relative state of vasoconstriction of the afferent and efferent arterioles plays a major role in regulating the intracapillary hydrostatic pressure. The factors modulating the state of vascular contraction are listed in Table 80–1.

During the early neonatal period, the factors regulating GFR mature rapidly. Systemic blood pressure and mean transcapillary hydraulic pressure increase, followed by a parallel increase in GFR (Guignard and John, 1986). The plasma oncotic pressure also increases but at a lower rate than for the transcapillary hydraulic pressure, so that the net ultrafiltration pressure increases. The low glomerular plasma flow rate present at birth is due to elevated afferent and efferent arteriolar resistances. A systemic increase in the ultrafiltration coefficient also occurs during maturation and may be attributed to an increase in both the hydraulic permeability and the glomerular capillary area.

In the fetus and neonate, the low systemic blood pressure and hence the low glomerular capillary hydrostatic pressure are the main factors limiting the rate of filtration. Vasoactive factors modulating the intraglomerular filtration pressure thus play a key role in maintaining filtration (Bailie, 1992; Guignard et al, 1991). Vasodilatory prostaglandins, the concentration of which is elevated during fetal and early postnatal life, improve filtration by dilating the afferent arteriole. Angiotensin II also increases filtration by preferentially constricting the efferent arteriole. Minute-to-minute regulation of the contractile tone also depends on endothelium-released vasoactive factors such as nitric oxide and endothelin. Although endogenous endothelin behaves as a potent constrictor in the adult, it may actually vasodilate the afferent artery in the immature kidney (Semama et al, 1993). Atrial natriuretic peptide, the concentration of which also is elevated in the fetus, vasodilates the afferent arteriole (Robillard et al, 1992). Adenosine, a regulator of the tubuloglomerular feedback mechanism, is an efferent vasodilator. When acting in conjunction with elevated levels of angiotensin II, it also vasoconstricts the afferent arteriole (Gouyon and Guignard, 1989). Although the overactivation of adenosine plays a critical role in the pathogenesis of the hypoxemia-induced vasomotor insufficiency, the exact physiologic role of intrarenal adenosine in the fetus and neonate is still ill defined.

## Assessment of Glomerular Filtration Rate

Determination of inulin clearance is the "gold standard" for assessing GFR in both the immature and the mature kidney. Inulin is freely filtered even in the preterm neonate with a gestational age as low as 27 weeks. The postnatal development of GFR has been assessed in premature neonates at different gestational ages and in term neonates. From a value of 20 mL/minute × 1.73 $m^2$ at birth, GFR doubles in the first 2 weeks of life in term neonates (Guignard et al, 1975) (Figs. 80–3 and 80–4). GFR is lower in premature infants and, owing to incomplete nephrogenesis, also develops at a lower velocity.

Creatinine, the most commonly used glomerular marker in mature persons, also is frequently used to assess GFR in neonates. However, the use of creatinine presents several drawbacks. The concentration of creatinine is elevated at birth, reflecting maternal levels. A complete equilibration between the maternal and fetal plasma creatinine levels is achieved throughout pregnancy (Guignard and Drukker, 1999). During the first postnatal week, the highest levels are observed in the most premature neonates (Bueva and Guignard, 1994) (Fig. 80–5). In term neonates, serum creatinine decreases rapidly to reach stable neonatal levels close to 0.40 mg/dL (35 μmol/L) by 1 to 2 weeks postnatally. In very premature infants, there is a transient increase in serum creatinine, peaking on postnatal day 4 (Gallini et al, 2000) (Fig. 80–6), followed by a progressive decline toward normal neonatal levels by 3 to 4 weeks of life. The transient increase in plasma creatinine is caused in part by passive reabsorption (back-diffusion) of creatinine across leaky tubules (Matos et al, 1998). The reabsorption of creatinine by the premature infant accounts for the negative correlation between gestational age and the plasma creatinine during the first postnatal weeks (see Fig. 80–4) as well as for the finding that, in very premature neonates, creatinine clearance underestimates inulin clearance (Coulthard and Ruddock, 1983). In spite of these drawbacks, creatinine clearance correlates with inulin clearance (Stonestreet et al, 1979; Van den Anker et al, 1995), and creatinine clearance studies in neonates have confirmed the rapid development of GFR during the first postnatal weeks and that GFR develops at a lower velocity in premature infants (Bueva and Guignard, 1994; Vanpee et al, 1992). The differences in the GFR among infants with different gestational and postnatal ages explain why the specific dosage recommendations are tailored to the given gestational and postnatal ages for medications eliminated primarily via glomerular filtration (e.g., aminoglycosides, vancomycin, digoxin).

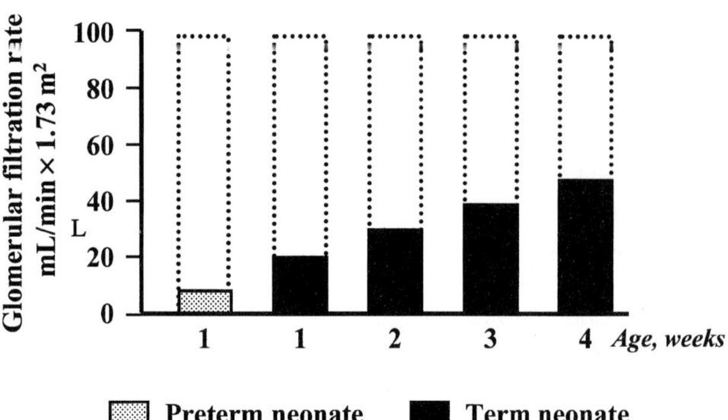


**FIGURE 80–3.** Glomerular filtration rate during the first month of life of preterm and term neonates, compared with adult values *(open columns). (Adapted from Guignard JP, Torrado A, Da Cunha O, et al: Glomerular filtration rate in the first three weeks of life. J Pediatr 87:268, 1975.)*

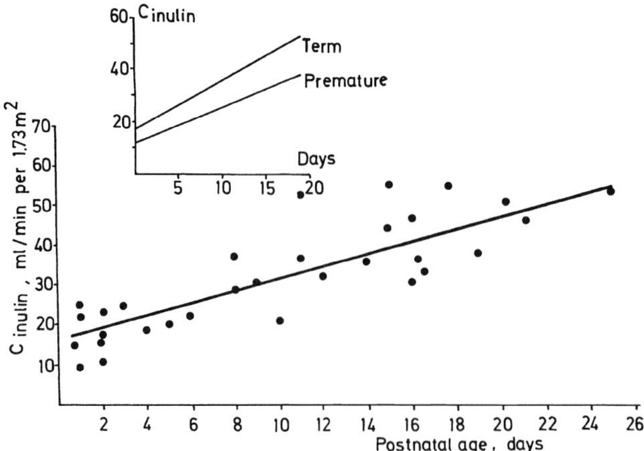


**FIGURE 80–4.** Maturation of GFR ($C_{inulin}$) in relation to postnatal age in term and preterm infants. *(From Guignard J-P: The Neonatal Stressed Kidney. In Gruskin AB, Norman ME [eds]: Pediatric Nephrology. The Hague, Martinus Nijhoff, 1981.)*

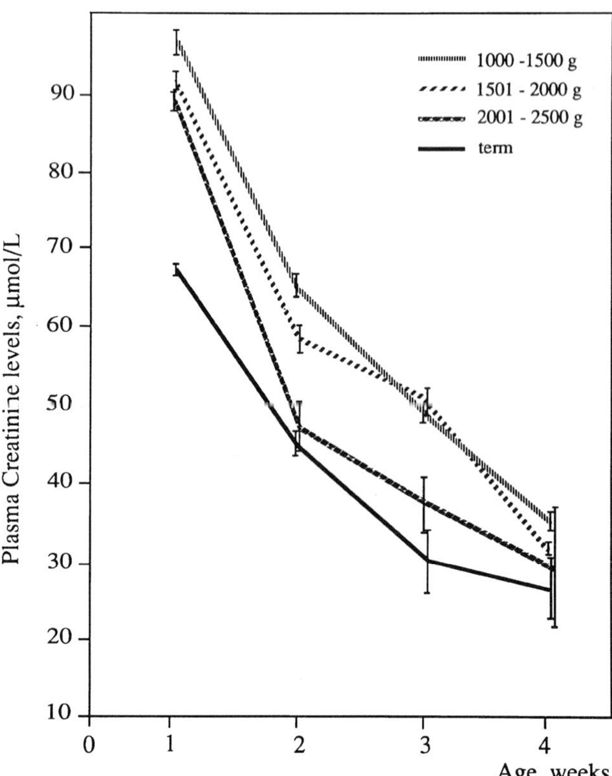


**FIGURE 80–5.** Plasma creatinine in term and low-birth-weight infants during the first 4 weeks of life. *(From Bueva A, Guignard JP: Renal function in preterm neonates. Pediatr Res 36:572, 1994.)*

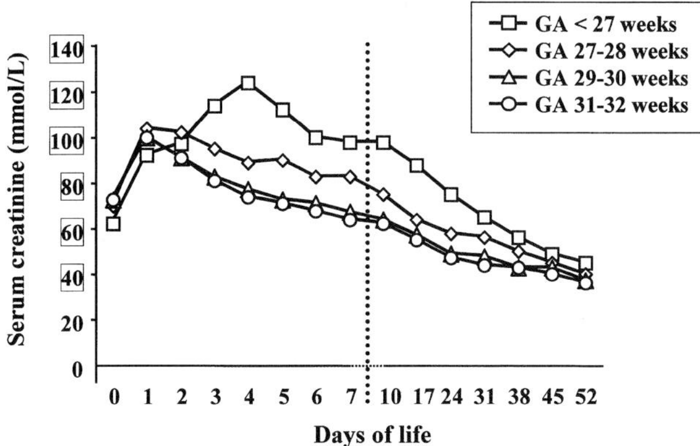


**FIGURE 80–6.** Serum creatinine concentration (μmol/L) in the first 52 days of life of premature infants. *(Adapted from Gallini F, Maggio L, Romagnoli C, et al: Progression of renal function in premature neonates with gestational age ≤ 32 weeks. Pediatr Nephrol 15:119, 2000.)*

## REGULATION OF BODY FLUID TONICITY AND VOLUME

The kidney is responsible for maintaining the extracellular fluid (ECF) volume and osmolality despite large variations in salt and water intake. By modulating the renal conservation of water, the antidiuretic hormone (ADH) system plays a central role in the regulation of body fluid tonicity. Sodium chloride, the major osmotically active solute in ECF, determines its volume. The balance between the intake and the renal excretion of sodium thus regulates ECF volume (see Chapter 30).

### Sodium, Chloride, and Water Reabsorption

Active sodium reabsorption occurs throughout the nephron, driven by the $Na^+,K^+$-ATPase localized at the basolateral membrane. Two thirds of the filtered $Na^+$ load is reabsorbed in the proximal tubule via the $Na^+$-glucose, $Na^+$-amino acid, $Na^+$-$P_i$, and $Na^+$-lactate symporters, and by the $Na^+$-$H^+$ antiporter. Because water passively follows $Na^+$ across the highly water-permeable proximal tubule, the osmolality of the proximal tubule fluid remains isotonic. Twenty percent of the filtered sodium load is reabsorbed in the ascending limb of the loop of Henle, which is relatively impermeable to water. Accumulation of NaCl and recycling of urea into the medullary interstitium lead to the formation of a hyperosmotic medulla. The thick ascending limb also reabsorbs calcium, magnesium, and potassium. The distal tubule and collecting duct reabsorb 10% of the filtered $Na^+$ and $Cl^-$ load. In the distal tubule, the continuing NaCl reabsorption in the absence of water reabsorption further decreases the osmolality of the tubular fluid, allowing the formation of hypotonic urine. Excretion of solute-free water thus is dependent on $Na^+$ delivery to and reabsorption at the distal diluting site. The permeability of the collecting duct to water depends on the presence of ADH or arginine vasopressine (AVP). The release of AVP by the posterior pituitary is regulated by osmoreceptors located in the supraoptic nucleus of the hypothalamus. By binding to its cell membrane receptors and activating adenylate cyclase, AVP increases the intracellular levels of cAMP. This increase ultimately leads to phosphorylation of the aquaporin water channels, which in turn results in insertion of these channels into the luminal membrane of the collecting duct cells, rendering the collecting duct permeable to water. In the absence of AVP, a large volume of hypotonic urine is excreted. In contrast, when elevated levels of AVP are present, water passively diffuses out of the collecting duct into the hyperosmotic interstitium, and a small volume of concentrated urine is excreted.

Water transport depends on the intact function of the aquaporin water channels. Ten aquaporins (AQPs), designated 0-9, have been described in mammals, six of which—AQP1-4, AQP6, AQP7—are expressed in the kidney (Nielsen et al, 2000). AQP2 is the vasopressin-responsive AQP in collecting duct cells. Mutations in the AVP V2 receptor gene located on Xq28 are responsible for *X-linked recessive diabetes insipidus*. When inherited as an autosomal recessive or dominant trait, diabetes insipidus usually is caused by various mutations in the *AQP2* gene located on chromosome 12q13.

#### Sodium

During development, proximal $Na^+$ reabsorption increases three- to fourfold (Celsi et al, 1986). The increase in active $Na^+$ reabsorption is associated with a threefold increase in $Na^+,K^+$-ATPase activity in the corresponding segment (Celsi et al, 1986) and with an increase in the number of cotransporters for glucose and bicarbonate reabsorption (Schwartz and Evan, 1983). The immature proximal tubule has a lower reflection coefficient for mannitol, indicating increased permeability of the proximal tubule to various solutes. The low capacity of the immature thick ascending limb of the loop of Henle to reabsorb $Na^+$ is associated with a low activity of the tubular $Na^+$, $K^+$-ATPase. As a consequence of the reduced $Na^+$ reabsorption in the loop of Henle, immature nephrons deliver a greater fraction of filtered $Na^+$ to the distal nephrons. The activity of the $Na^+,K^+$-ATPase also increases in this segment during development. As a result of the maturational process, the fractional excretion of $Na^+$ (FENa) decreases during development, from a value of 13% in the fetus to 3% in premature neonates less than 30 weeks of gestation, and to 1% in term neonates (Bueva and Guignard, 1994). Very low-birth-weight (VLBW) infants may be at risk for negative sodium balance around postnatal weeks 2 to 3, when $Na^+$ retention is required for growth.

The study of the developmental changes in the various tubular epithelial transport mechanisms and the delineation of the molecular basis of such mechanisms and associated genetic defects have shed new light on a number of rare pediatric renal tubular disorders (Zelikovic, 2001) related to abnormalities of sodium and water homeostasis. Constitutive activation of the amiloride-sensitive epithelial $Na^+$ channel (ENaC) is seen in Liddle syndrome, characterized by salt retention, early-onset hypertension, metabolic alkalosis, and hypokalemia. Autosomal recessive pseudohypoaldosteronism, characterized by renal salt wasting and end-organ unresponsiveness to mineralocorticoids, is due to decreased activity of ENaC. The activity of ENaC is under the tight control of aldosterone and vasopressin (Rossier et al, 2002). ENaC is composed of three subunits: $\alpha$, $\beta$, and $\gamma$. The $\alpha$ subunit of ENaC is the most important and it is also expressed in other organs such as the lungs. Thus, the $\alpha$ subunit of ENaC is required not only for channel function in the collecting duct of the kidney but also for active lung fluid clearance.

### Chloride

A major fraction of chloride reabsorption in the proximal tubular occurs by paracellular diffusion. Active chloride countertransport with organic anions (fumarate, oxalate) also takes place in the proximal tubule. In the ascending limb of Henle, the $Na^+,K^+$-ATPase is the driving force for active NaCl reabsorption and accumulation in the medullary interstitium. Here, $Na^+$-$K^+$-$2Cl^-$ cotransporters and $Cl^-$ channels are involved in the transport of chloride. Renal salt wasting with hypokalemic metabolic alkalosis, hyperreninemic hyperaldesteronism, and normal blood pressure are the features of *Bartter syndrome*. Antenatal Bartter syndrome, called "hyperprostaglandin E syndrome," is the most severe form of the disease. Congenital defects in the genes encoding various chloride transporters, cotransporters, and channels in the thick ascending limb and distal tubule are responsible for the various forms of Bartter syndrome and Gitelman syndrome (Rodriguez-Soriano, 1998; Scheinmann et al, 1989).

## Body Fluid Tonicity

Although the volume of body fluids varies during growth, the tonicity of ECF is maintained constant by the kidneys, which excrete or retain appropriate amounts of water.

### Excretion of Free Water

When plasma osmolality decreases, the release of ADH also diminishes, leading to the excretion of dilute urine. The newborn infant, preterm or term, is able to decrease urine osmolality to values as low as 40 mOsm/kg $H_2O$ (Guignard et al, 1976). Because GFR is low in the newborn infant, ability to excrete large amounts of free water and consequently to cope with a hypotonic fluid load is limited. Excessive hypotonic fluid loading leads to hyponatremia.

Hyponatremia also may occur in the syndrome of inappropriate secretion of antidiuretic hormone (SIADH), when the excretion of free water is impaired. This syndrome can occur in term as well as in preterm infants presenting with various cerebral injuries or pulmonary disorders, in infants undergoing mechanical ventilation, and in response to some drugs. Because the renal response to AVP is maturation dependent, the more immature the neonate, the less severe the clinical presentation of the SIADH.

### Concentration of Urine

By comparison with adults, who can concentrate urine up to 1400 mOsm/kg $H_2O$, the concentrating ability is limited in the neonate. The maximal urine osmolality achieved following dehydration or exogenous vasopressin (DDAVP) administration (10 $\mu$g) remains below 430 mOsm/kg $H_2O$ and 630 mOsm/kg $H_2O$ in 1- to 3-week-old and 4- to 6-week-old term infants, respectively. Osmolalities achieved by preterm neonates are slightly lower (Svenningssen and Aronson, 1974). The relative ineffectiveness of the concentrating ability of the neonate is related to several factors including the low corticomedullary solute gradient associated with a limited accumulation of sodium chloride and urea in the medullary interstitium, the decreased formation of cAMP in response to ADH, the shortness of the loops of Henle, and the interference of prostaglandins with the vasopressin-stimulated cyclic adenosine monophosphate (cAMP) synthesis.

## Extracellular Fluid Volume

The ECF volume is a function of the ECF sodium content. Under normal conditions, plasma volume is closely related to ECF volume. Volume receptors distributed both on the venous (low-pressure receptors) and the arterial (high-pressure receptors) sides of the circulation sense the changes in plasma volume. Arterial sensors perceive the "effective arterial volume." Atrial filling volume is monitored by stretch receptors, which mediate the release of the natriuretic peptide (Semmekrot and Guignard, 1991) promoting diuresis and natriuresis. Effective renal arterial volume also is sensed by baroreceptors located in the juxtamedullary apparatus of the kidney. A decrease in renal perfusion pressure activates the renin-angiotensin-aldosterone system (see Fig. 80–2). Angiotensin II, a potent renal and peripheral vasoconstrictor, promotes sodium reabsorption, stimulates thirst, and favors the renal production of prostaglandins and bradykinin, hormones that play a role in sodium homeostasis. Aldosterone increases sodium reabsorption in the distal tubule, leading to further conservation of ECF volume.

The neonatal period is characterized by the rapid physiologic constriction of the expanded ECF volume, as well as by elevated levels of several hormonal systems participating in the regulation of sodium balance. Although angiotensin II induces sodium retention by a direct action on the proximal tubule and by stimulating aldosterone secretion, the role of atrial natriuretic peptide in defending the plasma volume is still unclear. The elevated levels of plasma renin activity, which are inversely correlated with gestational age, may be of importance in the maintenance and distribution of blood flow to various organs. The integrity of the renin-angiotensin system also appears to be crucial for the maintenance of renal blood flow and GFR at low perfusion pressure in the neonate (Guignard et al, 1991). Other factors that may be involved in regulating sodium excretion include atrial natriuretic peptide, bradykinin, dopamine, nitric oxide, endothelin, and adrenomedullin. Dopamine, synthesized by the proximal tubule cells in the kidneys, reduces sodium reabsorption by inhibiting the $Na^+,K^+$-ATPase and by decreasing $Na^+$-$H^+$ antiporter and sodium–inorganic phosphate ($Na^+$-$P_i$) cotransporter activity (Seri, 1995). Agents such as nitric oxide, endothelin, and adrenomedullin all can increase sodium excretion and may participate in the homeostasis of sodium.

## REGULATION OF ACID-BASE BALANCE

The kidneys maintain the acid-base balance by preventing the loss of bicarbonate in the urine and by excreting the daily production of fixed acids. Bicarbonate reabsorption occurs mainly in the proximal tubule (80%) and to a lesser extent in the thick ascending limb of Henle (15%) and the cortical collecting duct (5%). It is mediated by active secretion of hydrogen ions and is closely linked to the tubular reabsorption of sodium. Hydrogen ion secretion occurs through the $Na^+$-$H^+$ antiporter (NHE-3) but also is mediated in part by $H^+$-ATPase. In the tubular lumen, secreted $H^+$ reacts with filtered $HCO_3^-$ to form $H_2CO_3$, which quickly dissociates under the influence of the brush border carbonic anhydrase enzyme (CA IV). Luminal $CO_2$ diffuses freely back into the tubular cells. $H_2CO_3$ is then formed within the cell by the hydration of $CO_2$, a reaction catalyzed by carbonic anhydrase type 2 (CA II). After crossing the luminal membrane as $CO_2$, most $HCO_3^-$ exits the tubular cells via an $Na^+$-$HCO_3^-$ cotransporter (NBC I, II, and III) which couples the transport of 1 $Na^+$ with 3 $HCO_3^-$, or in exchange for $Cl^-$ via a $Cl^-$-$HCO_3^-$ antiporter.

The excretion of fixed acids occurs mainly in the distal tubule, where secreted $H^+$ is buffered by $NH_3$ and $HPO_4^{2-}$ and is excreted as $NH_4^+$ and $H_2PO_4^-$ (titratable acid). Free $H^+$ concentration determines the urine pH. The ability of the collecting duct to lower the urine pH is critically important for the excretion of urinary buffers and ammonium. $NH_4^+$ is produced by the kidneys; its synthesis and subsequent excretion can be regulated in response to acid-base requirements of the body. To produce $NH_4^+$, the kidneys metabolize glutamine, excrete $NH_4^+$ with the acid salts, and return the generated $HCO_3^-$ to the blood. $NH_3$ synthesis is up-regulated by metabolic acidosis and by hypokalemia.

During fetal life, the placenta is responsible for the excretion of $H^+$. In experimental studies, the fetus responds to acid loading by increasing the excretion of $NH_4^+$ and titratable acid, and by decreasing the urine pH. In early postnatal life, several transporters and enzymes involved in bicarbonate reabsorption are weakly expressed, so that the functioning of the $Na^+$-$H^+$ antiporter is clearly impaired (Rodriguez-Soriano, 2000). The proximal reabsorption of bicarbonate is reduced, resulting in low bicarbonate threshold. This low threshold is responsible for the low "physiologic" plasma bicarbonate concentration in neonates: 16 to 20 mmol/L in extremely immature infants and 19 to 21 mmol/L in term infants (Schwartz et al, 1979). In addition to immature carbonic anhydrase activity, the relative expansion of ECF volume at birth may account for the reduced bicarbonate threshold. Immature carbonic anhydrase (CA II and CA IV) enzyme activities also may play an important role in the low bicarbonate proximal reabsorption rate. Maturation of $HCO_3^-$ reabsorption increases proportionally to the increase in proximal tubular basolateral area and $Na^+$,$K^+$-ATPase activity (Rodriguez-Soriano, 2000). Administration of glucocorticoids stimulates the maturation of both the $Na^+$-$H^+$ antiporter activity and the expression of the $Na^+$-$H^+$ antiporter messenger RNA (mRNA) (Shah et al, 1999).

Distal tubular acidification is more mature than proximal tubular bicarbonate reabsorption. The ability of the neonate to excrete an acid load is well developed. Deficient ammoniagenesis results, however, in low glutamine uptake, decreased $NH_3$ production and excretion, and, ultimately, impaired ability to excrete an acid load.

Mutation in the various genes encoding the $Na^+$-$HCO_3^-$ cotransporter (NBC-1), the $Cl^-$-$HCO_3^-$ exchanger (AE1), the $H^+$-ATPase, and CA II are responsible for the various forms of renal tubular acidosis (Rodriguez-Soriano, 2000, 2002).

Under normal conditions, very little bicarbonate is lost in the urine. The reabsorption of bicarbonate is increased by extracellular volume contraction, hypercapnia, hypokalemia, chloride deficiency, glucocorticoids, angiotensin, aldosterone and alpha-adrenergic stimulation; it is depressed by volume expansion and parathormone (PTH) (Rodriguez-Soriano, 2000, 2002). The postnatal renal compensation for hypercapnia involves increased bicarbonate reabsorption and excretion of fixed acids, in order to blunt a decrease in plasma pH. Animal studies and clinical observations indicate that this compensating mechanism is functional in the neonate (van der Heijden and Guignard, 1989).

## REGULATION OF POTASSIUM HOMEOSTASIS

Ninety-eight percent of the potassium in the body is intracellular, resulting in a high intracellular concentration of potassium. High intracellular concentration of potassium also is required for cell growth and division. Potassium homeostasis depends on an internal balance that maintains a constant potassium concentration in the intracellular and extracellular fluid space, and also on an external balance that requires that the potassium absorbed by the gastrointestinal tract in excess of the amount needed for growth be eventually excreted by the kidneys.

In the proximal tubule, some 70% of filtered potassium is reabsorbed, predominantly passively, although active reabsorption against a concentration gradient also occurs. About 20% of filtered potassium is reabsorbed in the ascending limb of the loop of Henle. The overall rate of potassium excretion is determined by the function of the distal tubule and collecting duct. Plasma potassium concentration and aldosterone are the major physiologic regulators of potassium secretion. Hyperkalemia stimulates the $Na^+$,$K^+$-ATPase activity, increases the permeability of the luminal membrane to potassium, and stimulates the secretion of aldosterone by the adrenal cortex. Aldosterone in turn stimulates sodium reabsorption and enhances potassium secretion by stimulating the basolateral $Na^+$,$K^+$-ATPase, leading to an elevation of the intracellular concentration of potassium, and also by increasing the permeability of the luminal membrane to potassium. Aldosterone probably plays a more important role in determining potassium balance than in regulating sodium excretion. The aldosterone-sensitive transport mechanisms for sodium and potassium are largely independent of each other. Other factors favoring potassium secretion by the distal tubule and collecting duct include a rise in tubular flow rate, alkalosis, and an increase in the tubular fluid sodium concentration.

Potassium excretion remains low throughout gestation, and the fetal potassium concentration is maintained at levels exceeding 5 mmol/l. Postnatal growth is associated with an increase in total body potassium from approximately

8 mmol/cm body height at birth to more than 14 mmol/cm body height by 18 years of age (Butte et al, 2000).

In neonatal tissues, $K^+$ content is significantly higher than in adult tissues. The plasma $K^+$concentration is also more elevated during the first 3 to 4 postnatal months. The intracellular versus extracellular potassium distribution in infancy may be influenced not only by the expression of the $Na^+$,$K^+$-ATPase and potassium transporters and channels but also by the expression of hormone receptors and intracellular messengers.

In healthy preterm infants with a positive potassium balance, potassium excretion remains stable during the first postnatal month, with mean values ranging from 1.29 to 1.48 mmol/kg/day (Guignard and John, 1986). Some 85% to 90% of ingested potassium is eliminated in the intestine, and the remaining in the urine (Aizman et al, 1998). The high urine sodium-to-potassium ratio present at birth decreases significantly with gestational age and postnatal age (Sulyok et al, 1979), and it is thought to indicate the relative unresponsiveness of the distal tubule and collecting duct to aldosterone. The limited potassium excretory capacity of the collecting duct and the increased distal tubular reabsorptive activity of the neonate contribute to the positive potassium balance necessary in early postnatal life. Transient hyperkalemia sometimes occurs in the early neonatal period in VLBW infants. Lower renal $K^+$ excretory and tissue $K^+$-binding capacities and a low tissue $K^+$ uptake due to low $Na^+$,$K^+$-ATPase activity are thought to be responsible for this non-oliguric hyperkalemia (Lorenz et al, 1997). In contrast with healthy premature infants, critically ill and stressed premature neonates may develop a negative potassium balance. In sick neonates, potassium losses can be exaggerated by the use of diuretics, and volume expansion.

## REGULATION OF CALCIUM, PHOSPHATE, AND MAGNESIUM HOMEOSTASIS

The kidney, in conjunction with the gastrointestinal tract and bone, plays a major role in maintaining calcium, phosphate, and magnesium homeostasis.

### Regulation of Calcium Homeostasis

The blood ionic calcium concentration in plasma is maintained within narrow limits at approximately 1.10 to 1.30 mmol/L. The distribution of calcium between the intracellular (bone) and extracellular compartment is regulated mainly by PTH. The parathyroid gland has the ability to determine the level of blood-ionized calcium by a calcium sensor (CaSR) located on the extracellular membrane. The CaSR appears to act via a G protein–coupled signaling system and its gene has been cloned (Brown, 1999). Loss-of-function and gain-of-function mutations in the *CaSR* gene are responsible for the *autosomal dominant familial hypercalcemia with hypocalciuria* and *autosomal dominant hypoparathyroidism with hypocalcemia* (Langman, 2000).

PTH increases plasma calcium concentration by stimulating bone resorption, by activating the synthesis of 1,25-dihydroxyvitamin $D_3$ (1,25$(OH)_2D_3$ or calcitriol), and by increasing calcium reabsorption by the kidney. Normally, 99% of the filtered calcium is reabsorbed by the nephron, mainly by the proximal tubule and the loop of Henle. In the proximal tubule and the thick ascending limb, calcium reabsorption is passive and closely linked to sodium reabsorption. By contrast, in the distal tubule and collecting duct, calcium reabsorption is active and independent of sodium transport, so that net calcium and sodium excretions do not always change in parallel. PTH is the main regulator of the renal excretion of calcium, and it strongly stimulates calcium reabsorption in the distal tubule and collecting duct, resulting in a reduced calcium excretion. Volume expansion depresses both sodium and passive calcium reabsorption in the proximal tubule and thus increases calcium excretion. Calcium excretion is increased by acidosis and decreased by alkalosis. Finally, 1,25$(OH)_2D_3$ stimulates distal calcium reabsorption and thus decreases its excretion. Whereas the single most important action of PTH is on bone, that of vitamin $D_3$ is on the intestine.

During weeks 26 to 36 of gestation, the mean intrauterine accumulation of calcium is about 130 mg/kg/day (Forbes, 1976; Wharton et al, 1987). The calcium levels in fetal plasma are higher than the maternal levels (Delivoria et al, 1967), averaging 1.40 to 1.60 mmol/L. Of interest, the fetal kidney also is able to effectively produce 1,25$(OH)_2D_3$ (Moore et al, 1985). The 25-hydroxyvitamin $D_3$–1α hydroxylase is produced by the renal proximal tubule mitochondria. The 1,25$(OH)_2D_3$ binds to an intracellular receptor to stimulate intestinal calcium reabsorption. During the neonatal period, the urinary calcium-to-creatinine ratio is higher in neonates than later in infancy (2.5 versus 0.7) (Matos et al, 1997). Loop diuretics are potent calciuric agents that may lead to neonatal nephrocalcinosis.

### Regulation of Phosphate Homeostasis

Plasma phosphate concentration is regulated by the kidney. In the urine, phosphate binds $H^+$ ions and is eliminated as acid phosphate (a component of titratable acid). Phosphate release from the intracellular stores (mainly bone) is increased by PTH and 1,25$(OH)_2D_3$. The proximal tubule reabsorbs approximately 80% of the filtered phosphate load; 10% is reabsorbed by the distal tubule; and 10% is excreted in the urine. Factors that increase the excretion of phosphate include PTH, glucocorticoids, volume expansion, dopamine administration, and acidosis. PTH is the main physiologic hormone regulating renal phosphate excretion, and it exerts this effect mainly by the inhibition of the $Na^+$-$P_i$ cotransporter in the proximal tubule. There are three $Na^+$-$P_i$ cotransporters: type I and type IIa and IIb. The type IIa cotransporter plays a key role in determining brush border $Na^+$-$P_i$ cotransport, and thus the overall $P_i$ homeostasis (Mürer et al, 2000). Several genetic defects resulting in isolated renal phosphate wasting are X-linked hypophosphatemic rickets, autosomal dominant hypophosphatemic rickets without hypercalciuria, and hereditary hypophosphatemic rickets with hypercalciuria. The X-linked syndrome is caused by mutation in the Phex gene that indirectly affects the $Na^+$-$P_i$ cotransporter. Calcitonin and glucagon increase the excretion of phosphate. Phosphate renal transport also is modulated by changes in dietary intake.

During weeks 26 to 36 of gestation, the mean intrauterine accumulation of inorganic phosphate is close to 75 mg/kg/day (Wharton et al, 1987). At birth, approximately 80% of the phosphorus is in the bones (Royer, 1981). During early postnatal life, owing to the efficient intestinal absorption and renal retention of phosphate, the neonate is in a positive phosphate balance and presents with elevated plasma concentrations of this anion (Brodehl et al, 1982; Key and Carpenter, 1990). Although fetuses and neonates appear to synthesize PTH in response to hypocalcemia (Garel, 1987), the phosphaturic response to PTH is attenuated. This phenomenon may be due to a decreased sensitivity of the proximal tubule to the hormone and probably reflects homeostatic regulation at a time when phosphate retention is essential for growth. Growth hormone stimulates renal phosphate retention and increases the plasma concentration of phosphate.

### Regulation of Magnesium Homeostasis

Magnesium is the second most abundant intracellular cation. It plays a major role in the regulation of protein synthesis and bone formation and also plays a role in the regulation of potassium and calcium channels in cell membranes. The kidney maintains magnesium balance by excreting in the urine the amount of magnesium that is absorbed by the gastrointestinal tract in excess of the amount retained for growth. In normal conditions, approximately 3% of the filtered magnesium load is excreted in the urine. Magnesium is passively reabsorbed by the proximal tubule and the thick ascending limb. Regulation of magnesium excretion takes place in the thick ascending limb, where approximately 65% of the filtered load is reabsorbed. Factors that increase magnesium excretion include ECF volume expansion, acidosis, hypercalcemia, and hypermagnesemia. PTH decreases the excretion of magnesium. Most diuretics increase magnesium excretion.

During weeks 26 to 36 of gestation, the mean intrauterine accumulation of magnesium approximates 3.5 mg/kg/day (Wharton et al, 1987). At birth, the urinary excretion of magnesium is low (Chan et al, 1984). Magnesium excretion increases 10-fold during the first month of life, reaching values close to 2 mg/kg/day (De Santo et al, 1988). Plasma magnesium levels follow a circadian rhythm, being higher at night (De Santo et al, 1988). Neonatal hypomagnesemia is associated with intrauterine growth restriction, whereas neonatal hypermagnesemia frequently occurs following maternal magnesium administration in the immediate prenatal period. Mutations in the gene encoding the $Na^+,K^+$-ATPase γ subunit, localized on the basolateral membrane of the distal convoluted tubule, lead to magnesium wasting in the so-called *isolated renal magnesium wasting syndrome*, a rare autosomal dominant disorder.

## SUMMARY

Normal renal maturation and adaptive responses at birth play an essential role in the neonate and contribute to the establishment of an intracellular and extracellular milieu necessary for survival and appropriate growth. Renal development and function are regulated by numerous hormones, paracrine factors, and signaling molecules. Recent advances in the understanding of the molecular basis of renal development and function have provided invaluable insights in the pathophysiology of inherited and acquired renal conditions during development. An understanding of the basic principles of renal developmental physiology is essential for the successful clinical management of sick preterm and term neonates.

## SELECTED READINGS


Clark AT, Bertram JF: Advances in renal development. Curr Opin Nephrol Hypertens 9:247, 2000.

Drukker A, Guignard J-P: Renal aspects of the term and preterm infant: A selective update. Curr Opin Pediatr 14:175, 2002.

Guignard J-P: Renal function in the newborn infant. Pediatr Clin North Am 29:777, 1982.

Guillery EN: Fetal and neonatal nephrology. Curr Opin Pediatr 9:148, 1997.

Merlet-Benichou C: Influence of fetal environment on kidney development. Int J Dev Biol 43:453, 1999.

Satlin LM, Guay-Woodford L, Chevalier RL: Proceedings of the Eighth International Workshop on Developmental Nephrology: genes, morphogenesis, and function. The sessions. Pediatr Nephrol 18:174, 2003.

Toth-Heyn P, Guignard J-P: Bradykinin in the newborn kidney. Nephron 91:571, 2002.


## REFERENCES


Aizman R, Grahnquist L, Celsi G: Potassium homeostasis: Ontogenic aspects. Acta Paediatr 87:609, 1998.

Bailie MD: Development of the endocrine function of the kidney. Clin Perinatol 19:59, 1992.

Brodehl J, Gellissen K, Weber HP: Postnatal development of tubular phosphate reabsorption. Clin Nephrol 17:163, 1982.

Brown EM: Physiology and pathophysiology of the extracellular calcium-sensing receptor. Am J Med 106:238, 1999.

Bueva A, Guignard JP: Renal function in preterm neonates. Pediatr Res 36:572, 1994.

Burrow CR: Regulatory molecules in kidney development. Pediatr Nephrol 14:240, 2000.

Butte NF, Hopkinson JM, Wong WW, et al: Body composition during the first 2 years of life: an updated reference. Pediatr Res 47:578, 2000.

Celsi G, Larsson L, Aperia A: Proximal tubular reabsorption and Na,K-ATPase activity on remnant kidney of young rats. Am J Physiol 251:F588, 1986

Chan GM, Nordmeyer FR, Richter BE, et al: Comparison of serum total calcium, dialysable calcium and dialysable magnesium in well and sick neonates. Clin Physiol Biochem 2:154, 1984.

Chevalier RL, Carey RM, Kaiser DC: Endogenous prostaglandins modulate autoregulation of renal blood flow in young rats. Am J Physiol 253:F66, 1987.

Coulthard MG, Ruddock V: Validation of inulin as a marker for glomerular filtration in preterm babies. Kidney Int 23:407, 1983.

Delivoria-Papadopoulos M, Battaglia FC, Bruns PD, et al: Total, protein-bound, and ultrafilterable calcium in maternal and fetal plasma. Am J Physiol 21:363, 1967.

De Santo NG, Dilorio B, Capasso G, et al: Circadian rhythm with acrophase at night for urinary excretion of calcium and magnesium in childhood. Population-based data of the Cimitile study in southern Italy. Miner Electrolyte Metab 14:235, 1988.

Forbes GB: Calcium accumulation by the human fetus. Pediatrics 57:976, 1976.

Gallini F, Maggio L, Romagnoli C, et al: Progression of renal function in premature neonates with gestational age ≤ 32 weeks. Pediatr Nephrol 15:119, 2000.

Garel JM: Hormonal control of calcium metabolism during the reproductive cycle in mammals. Physiol Rev 67:1, 1987.

Gilbert T, Merlet-Bénichou C: Retinoids and nephron mass control. Pediatr Nephrol 14:1137, 2000.

Gouyon JB, Guignard J-P: Adenosine in the immature kidney. Dev Pharmacol Ther 13:113, 1989.

Grannum P, Bracken M, Silverman R, et al: Assessement of kidney size in normal gestation by comparison of ratio of kidney circumference to abdominal circumference. Am J Obstet Gynecol 136:249, 1980.

Guignard JP: The adverse renal effects of prostaglandin-synthesis inhibitors in the newborn rabbit. Semin Perinatol, 26:398, 2002.

Guignard JP, Drukker A: Why do newborn infants have a high plasma creatinine? Pediatric 103:49, 1999.

Guignard JP, Gouyon JB, John EG: Vasoactive factors in the immature kidney. Pediatr Nephrol 5:443, 1991.

Guignard JP, John EG: Renal function in the tiny, premature infant. Clin Perinatol 13:377, 1986.

Guignard JP, Torrado A, Da Cunha O, et al: Glomerular filtration rate in the first three weeks of life. J Pediatr 87:268, 1975.

Guignard JP, Torrado A, Mazouni SM, et al: Renal function in respiratory distress syndrome. J Pediatr 88:845, 1976.

Jeanty P, Dramaix WM, Elkhazen N, et al: Measurement of fetal kidney growth on ultrasound. Radiology 144:159, 1982.

Key LL, Carpenter TO: Metabolism of calcium, phosphorus and other divalent ions. In Ichikawa L (ed): Pediatric Textbook of Fluids and Electrolytes. Baltimore, Lippincott Williams & Wilkins, 1990, p 98.

Langman CB: New developments in calcium and vitamin D metabolism. Curr Opin Pediatr 12:135, 2000.

Lorenz JM, Kleinman LI, Markarian K: Potassium metabolism in extremely low birth weight infants in the first week of life. J Pediatr 131:81, 1997.

Matos V, Van Melle G, Boulat O, et al: Urinary phosphate/creatinine, calcium/creatinine and magnesium/creatinine ratios in a healthy pediatric population. J Pediatr 131:252, 1997.

Matos P, Duarte-Silva M, Drukker A, et al: Creatinine reabsorption by the newborn rabbit kidney. Pediatr Res 44:639, 1998.

Merlet-Bénichou C, Gilbert T, Vilar J, et al: Nephron number: Variability is the rule. Lab Invest 79:512, 1999.

Moore ES, Langmann CB, Favus MJ, et al: Role of fetal 1, 25-dihydroxyvitamin D production in intrauterine phosphorus and calcium homeostasis. Pediatr Res 19:566, 1985.

Mürer H, Hernando N, Forster I, Biber H: Proximal tubular phosphate reabsorption: Molecular mechanisms. Physiol Rev 80:1373, 2000.

Nielsen S, Frokiaer J, Marples D, et al: Aquaporins in the kidney: from molecules to medicine. Physiol Rev 82:205, 2000.

Nishimura H, Yerkes E, Hohenfeller K, et al: Role of the angiotensin type 2 receptor gene in congenital anomalies of the kidney and urinary tract, CAKUT of mice and men. Mol Cell 3:1, 1999.

Piscione TD, Rosenblum ND: The malformed kidney: disruption of the glomerular and tubular development. Clin Genet 13:341, 1999.

Rabinovitz R, Peters MD, Vyas C, et al: Measurement of fetal urine production in normal pregnancy by real-time ultrasonography. Am J Obstet Gynecol 161:1264, 1989.

Robillard JE, Segar JL, Smith FG, et al: Regulation of sodium metabolism and extracellular fluid volume during development. Clin Perinatol 19:15, 1992.

Rodriguez-Soriano J: Bartter and related syndromes: The puzzle is almost solved. Pediatr Nephrol 12:315, 1998.

Rodriguez-Soriano J: New insight in the pathogenesis of renal tubular acidosis—from functional to molecular studies. Pediatr Nephrol 14:1121, 2000.

Rodriguez-Soriano J: Renal tubular acidosis: The clinical entity. J Am Soc Nephrol 13:2160, 2002.

Rossier B, Pradervand S, Schild L, Hummeler E: Epithelial sodium channel and the control of sodium balance: interaction between genetic and environmental factors. Annu Rev Physiol 64:877, 2002.

Royer P: Growth and development of bony tissue. In Davis JA, Dobbing J (eds): Scientific Foundations of Paediatrics. London, William Heinemann Medical Books, 1981, p 565.

Savin VJ, Beason-Griffin C, Richardson WP: Ultrafiltration coefficient of isolated glomeruli of rats aged 4 days to maturation. Kidney Int 28:926, 1985.

Scheinmann SJ, Guay-Woodford LM, Thakker RV, Warnock DG: Genetic disorders of renal electrolyte transport. N Engl J Med 340:1177, 1989.

Schwartz GJ, Haycock JB, Edelmann CM Jr, et al: Late metabolic acidosis: a reassessment of the definition. J Pediatr 95:102, 1979.

Schwartz GJ, Evan AP: Development of solute transport in rabbit proximal tubule. I. HCO-3 and glucose absorption. Am J Physiol 245:F382, 1983.

Semama DS, Thonney M, Guignard JP: Role of endogenous endothelin in renal hemodynamics of newborn rabbits. Pediatr Nephrol 7:886, 1993.

Semmekrot B, Guignard JP: Atrial natriuretic peptide during early human development. Biol Neonate 60:341, 1981.

Seri I: Cardiovascular, renal and endocrine actions of dopamine in neonates and children. J Pediatr 126:333, 1995.

Shah M, Quigley SM, Baum M: Neonatal rabbit proximal tubule baso-lateral membrane $Na^+/H^+$ antiporter and $Cl^-$/base exchange. Am J Physiol 276:R1792, 1999.

Stonestreet BS, Bell EF, Oh W: Validity of endogenous creatinine clearance in low-birth-weight infants. Pediatr Res 13:1012, 1979.

Sulyok E, Nemeth M, Tenyi I, et al: Postnatal development of renin-angiotensin aldosterone system (RAAS) in relation to electrolyte balance in premature infants. Pediatr Res 13:817, 1979.

Svenningsen NW, Aronson AS: Postnatal development of renal concentration capacity as estimated by DDAVP-test in normal and asphyxiated neonates. Biol Neonate 25:230, 1974.

Toth-Heyn P, Drukker A, Guignard J-P: The stressed neonatal kidney: From pathophysiology to clinical management of neonatal vasomotor nephropathy. Pediatr Nephrol 14:227, 2000.

Van den Anker JN, De Groot R, Broerse HM, et al: Assessment of glomerular filtration rate in preterm infants by serum creatinine. Comparison with inulin clearance. Pediatrics 96:1156, 1995.

Van der Heijden AJ, Guignard JP: Bicarbonate reabsorption by the kidney of the newborn rabbit. Am J Physiol 256:F29, 1989.

Vanpee M, Blennow M, Linne T, et al: Renal function in very low birth weight infants: normal maturity reached during early childhood. J Pediatr 121:784, 1992.

Veille JC, Hanson RA, Tatum K, et al: Quantitative assessment of human fetal renal blood flow. Am J Obstet Gynecol 169:1399, 1993.

Wharton BA, et al: Calcium, phosphorus and magnesium. In Nutrition and Feeding of Preterm Infants. Edited by the Committee on Nutrition of the Preterm Infant European Society for Paediatric Gastroenterology and Nutrition. Oxford, Blackwell Scientific Publications, 1987, p 111.

Zelikovic I: Molecular pathophysiology of tubular transport disorders. Pediatr Nephrol 16:919, 2001.

CHAPTER 81

# Clinical Evaluation of Renal and Urinary Tract Disease

Philippe S. Friedlich, Jacquelyn R. Evans, and Istvan Seri

## PRENATAL EVALUATION OF RENAL AND URINARY TRACT DISEASE

### Prenatal Diagnosis

Ultrasound has become the most widely used and effective diagnostic tool in the prenatal evaluation of the fetal kidneys and urinary tract. Since the first report of the in utero ultrasound diagnosis of congenital renal disease in 1970 (Garett et al, 1970), the prenatal diagnosis of most forms of congenital renal and urinary tract malformations has been described. The detection rate of fetal congenital urologic abnormalities by ultrasonography is approximately 0.2% (Arger et al, 1986; Shackelford et al, 1992). Because the incidence of renal and urinary tract malformations in the general population is close to 1%, approximately 1 in 5 cases is diagnosed prenatally by ultrasound.

The most common indication for an ultrasound survey of the fetal genitourinary tract is the presence of oligohydramnios (Bruno et al, 1985). Another important indication is a positive family history of renal disease, because fetal urinary tract abnormalities have been reported in 8% of pregnancies in women with a family history of renal anomalies (Reuss et al, 1987).

The fetal kidneys can be identified by early in the second trimester (Patten et al, 1990). However, a more detailed view of the kidneys is usually appreciated only from weeks 28 to 30 of gestation. The normal ureter cannot be visualized by prenatal ultrasound examination. The normal fetal bladder can be routinely identified by 16 weeks of gestation, although it sometimes can be seen as early as 13 weeks (Patten et al, 1990).

Hydronephrosis is readily identifiable by prenatal ultrasonography and is most frequently due to ureteropelvic obstruction. Other causes of fetal hydronephrosis include bladder outlet or ureteral obstruction, polycystic kidney disease, multicystic dysplastic kidney disease, renal agenesis, congenital megaureter, duplication anomalies, reflux, and prune-belly syndrome. A mildly dilated (1 to 2 mm) renal pelvis has been reported in 41% of routine prenatal ultrasound examinations (Cohen and Haller, 1987). This is often a normal prenatal finding reflecting the functional dilatation of the urinary tract secondary to high fetal urine flow rates.

Although prenatal ultrasonography has become standard for fetal evaluation, there are many potential pitfalls with use of this technique even in experienced hands. Because diagnostic error may occur up to 30% of the cases (Colodny, 1987), appropriate postnatal studies should always confirm the prenatal diagnosis. More recently, ultrafast magnetic resonance imaging (MRI) has been found to be a potentially useful adjunct to ultrasound examination in the evaluation of fetal renal diseases (Hubbard et al, 1999).

Fetal karyotype analysis and, in cases of certain types of obstructive uropathy, serial measurements of urine osmolality and electrolyte and protein excretion assist in the intrauterine diagnostic evaluation of fetuses with suspected renal and urinary tract anomalies (Johnson et al, 1994; Sullivan and Adzick, 1994). Detection of elevated amniotic fluid α-fetoprotein in conjunction with normal acetylcholinesterase activity suggests the intrauterine diagnosis of congenital nephrotic syndrome (Ghidini et al, 1994). Recently, prenatal diagnosis of the autosomal dominant form of polycystic kidney disease using DNA probes also has become available.

### Prenatal Management

In fetuses with severe obstructive uropathy, if the condition is bilateral or if there is a solitary kidney, the decrease in fetal urine output results in severe oligohydramnios or anhydramnios, leading to pulmonary hypoplasia, the Potter sequence, and extremely high neonatal mortality rates. Early obstruction affects normal glomerular and tubular differentiation and, if untreated, leads to the development of irreversible renal dysplasia. Percutaneous vesicoamniotic shunt, bladder stenting, and open bladder marsupialization constitute the choices for fetal intervention (Sullivan and Adzick, 1994). The goal of prenatal management is to relieve the obstruction during the most active period of nephrogenesis—that is, between 20 and 32 weeks of gestation (Crombleholme et al, 1988).

The integrated evaluation of the findings on prenatal ultrasonography, fetal karyotyping, and fetal urine electrolyte, osmolality and protein studies has been used to identify those fetuses with bilateral obstructive uropathies whose have not yet progressed to a stage of irreversible renal damage. Because only the third or fourth urine sample is predictive of long-term prognosis (Evans et al, 1991; Johnson et al, 1994), performance of serial vesicocenteses at 48- to 72-hour intervals is recommended. On the third or fourth urine examination, a sodium level of less than 100 mg/dL, osmolality of less than 200 mOsm/L, total protein of less than 20 mg/dL, and $\beta_2$-microglobulin of less than 4 mg/L are considered to be indications for fetal surgery.

In addition to the predicted long-term renal outcome, other important factors influencing prenatal management of fetuses with obstructive uropathy include gestational age, lung maturity, and presence of associated anomalies. If associated life-threatening anomalies or chromosome abnormalities are detected, the options are expectant management and termination of pregnancy. For the fetus with isolated obstructive uropathy and predicted irreversible renal dysplasia, in utero decompression is not recommended. In fetuses with isolated obstructive uropathy but predicted good long-term renal outcome, treatment depends on gestational age and lung maturity. At less than 32 weeks of gestation, intrauterine decompression is advocated. Indeed, preliminary long-term outcome studies in this group of patients suggest that antenatal vesicoamniotic shunt placement may benefit the fetus suffering from severe obstructive uropathy (Freedman et al, 1999). At 32 weeks of gestation or beyond, maternal steroid treatment and, once lung maturity is achieved, delivery of the infant is recommended. Fetuses with immature lungs and isolated obstructive uropathy with normal or only mildly diminished amniotic fluid volume do not require active intervention in utero (Johnson et al, 1994).

## POSTNATAL EVALUATION OF RENAL AND URINARY TRACT DISEASE

### History

Renal disease in the newborn is more likely when there is a family history of renal disease including urinary tract anomalies, renal agenesis, hereditary nephritis, polycystic kidney disease, medullary cystic disease, vesicoureteral reflux, and renal tubule disorders such as Fanconi syndrome, cystinuria, and nephrogenic diabetes insipidus. Appropriate screening of neonates for renal disease who have a positive family history of inherited diseases associated with renal anomalies also is indicated.

### Prenatal and Perinatal History

A history of oligohydramnios or anhydramnios suggests the presence of bilateral renal agenesis, severe renal dysplasia, or obstructive uropathy. Polyhydramnios, on the other hand, may occur with fetal nephrogenic diabetes insipidus. A difficult delivery secondary to increased abdominal girth may signal the presence of renal masses. A disproportionately large placenta should prompt appropriate studies to rule out congenital nephrotic syndrome in the neonate (Mahan et al, 1984). A history of perinatal asphyxia, acute hemorrhage, sepsis, hyaline membrane disease, antenatal or postnatal indomethacin therapy, and hypernatremic dehydration of the very low-birth-weight (VLBW) neonate are conditions that should alert the clinician to the possibility of the development of postnatal acute renal failure.

### Evaluation of Presenting Signs and Symptoms: Laboratory Tests and Methods of Evaluation of Renal Function

***Urine Collection.*** Urine collection in the newborn is most commonly performed by the use of special collection bags. With the exemption of urine culture studies, this method provides an adequate sample for most of the routine tests. To document urinary tract infection, suprapubic bladder aspiration is recommended as the most reliable method of obtaining a urine specimen. Bladder catheterization is used mainly in infants who fail to pass urine after the first day of life, and in severely ill neonates who are paralyzed or heavily sedated.

***Urinalysis.*** Analysis of the urine in the normal term newborn during the first few days of life shows a specific gravity of 1.001 to 1.021, with a corresponding osmolality of 50 to 800 mOsm/L. Maximum urine osmolality in preterm infants is less than in term neonates. The impaired concentrating capacity of the newborn kidney is the consequence of renal anatomic and functional immaturity, including the decreased hypertonicity of the renal medulla and the relative insensitivity of the immature collecting tubule to vasopressin (Roy et al, 1992).

***Proteinuria.*** During the first few days of life, proteinuria can be detected in 76% of healthy newborns. Conditions affecting renal blood flow and tubular function, such as dehydration or perinatal asphyxia, frequently result in a usually transient but significant proteinuria. However, proteinuria with levels greater than 30 mg/dL in a concentrated urine persisting beyond the first week of life suggests glomerular and/or tubular injury and requires further evaluation (Aviles et al, 1992). Persistent and massive proteinuria may indicate congenital nephrotic syndrome and necessitate renal biopsy.

***Hematuria, Hemoglobinuria, and Myoglobinuria.*** Normal newborns do not have hematuria, hemoglobinuria or myoglobinuria. Hematuria may occur in patients with perinatal asphyxia, acute renal failure, renal vein or artery thrombosis, congenital urinary malformations including autosomal recessive polycystic kidney disease and obstructive uropathies, coagulopathies, urinary tract infections, and trauma. Hematuria in a neonate with an umbilical artery catheter in place should alert the clinician to the possibility of aortic or renal artery thrombosis. Finally, transient hematuria is a common finding in critically ill neonates. Hemoglobinuria and myoglobinuria may manifest in patients with intravascular hemolysis and rhabdomyolysis, respectively.

***Uric Acid, Electrolyte, Glucose, and Amino Acid Excretion.*** Owing to increased uric acid production and fractional excretion, urinary excretion of uric acid is high during the first week in normal preterm and term infants, causing colored diaper stains and false-positive tests for proteinuria. However, because the newborn's urine is dilute and not significantly acidic, uric acid precipitation and acute urate nephropathy are rare in the neonatal period. As a result of the immaturity of their renal tubular transport processes, premature neonates also excrete more sodium, bicarbonate, phosphorus, glucose, and amino acids in the urine than is normal for term neonates (Jones and Chesney, 1992).

***Sediment.*** The urinary sediment of the normal newborn contains fewer than 5 squamous epithelial cells, 0 to 2 red blood cells, and fewer than 5 white blood cells per high-power field. The most common cause of leukocyturia is urinary tract infection. The presence of casts in the sediment usually suggests an involvement of the upper urinary tract in the disease process. Red blood cell casts indicate glomerular injury; white blood cell casts are present with infection or interstitial and/or tubular damage. Epithelial cell casts and granular casts may be seen in newborns with severe dehydration or also may represent interstitial and/or tubular injury. Hyaline casts are detected in cases of severe proteinuria or dehydration.

***Serum Chemistry and Clearance Studies.*** Serum chemistry and clearance studies reflect the status of fluid and electrolyte balance and renal function. Owing mainly to their excessive insensible water losses during the first few days of life (Sedin, 1995), very immature preterm infants cared for under radiant warmers require frequent serum electrolyte studies as well as close monitoring of the changes in their body weight and urine output to guide daily fluid administration (see Chapter 30, Acid-Base, Fluid, and Electrolyte Management).

An ideal endogenous substance that can be utilized to characterize glomerular function must have a constant turnover rate and be freely filtered and must not be reabsorbed, secreted, protein bound, or subject to synthesis, metabolism, or storage by the kidney. Although the turnover rate of creatinine is unknown in sick neonates and creatinine is not only filtered but also secreted and reabsorbed by the immature kidney (Avilles et al, 1992; Bueva and Guignard, 1994), it is the endogenous substance that comes closest to fulfilling these requirements. In clinical practice, sequential determination rather than a single value of serum creatinine gives the most valuable information on glomerular filtration rate (GFR).

In term infants, serum creatinine is approximately 0.8 mg/dL at birth and remains between 0.7 and 0.9 mg/dL during the first 2 days of life (Bueva and Guignard, 1994; Feldman and Guignard, 1982). Thereafter, serum creatinine gradually decreases to approximately 0.5 mg/dL by 1 week of age and to approximately 0.4 mg/dL by the end of the first month (Bueva and Guignard, 1994; Feldman and Guignard, 1982). During the first few days of life, serum creatinine levels are significantly higher in preterm than in term infants (0.8 to 1.8 mg/dL versus 0.7 to 0.9 mg/dL), with the highest levels observed in the most immature neonates (Bueva and Guignard, 1994; Stonestreet and Oh, 1978). This finding supports the notion that GFR is very low in the preterm infant, who immediately after birth is unable to eliminate the excess creatinine transferred in utero from the mother (Avilles et al, 1992; Bueva and Guignard, 1994). However, by the second week of life, serum creatinine begins to fall, and drops below 0.6 mg/dL, even in the 1-month-old VLBW infant (Bueva and Guignard, 1994).

In addition to serum creatinine, blood urea nitrogen (BUN) has been used widely in clinical practice to assess renal function. However, as BUN is also influenced by the state of hydration, protein intake, and urinary flow rate, it is a much less reliable marker of renal function than serum creatinine.

Applying the concept of clearance measurements, the rate of sodium and water reabsorption also may be estimated in the different nephron segments (Aviles et al, 1992). Despite its limitations, this method is the only way to assess sodium and water reabsorption along the nephron in the intact human kidney. The information obtained may then be used to detect changes in proximal and distal tubule sodium and water handling during development and/or disease. For a concise review on this subject, the reader is referred to the article by Avilles and coauthors (1992).

### Evaluation of Presenting Signs and Symptoms: Physical Examination

***Disorders of Micturition.*** Although many healthy newborn infants do not void until 12 to 24 hours of life, 92% to 100% of them will pass urine by the end of the first day (Clark, 1977). The delay in voiding in the healthy newborn is mostly due to labor- and delivery-triggered cardiovascular and hormonal changes and their effects on renal function. Among others, a significant increase in vasopressin (Ramin et al, 1991) and catecholamine release (Lagercrantz and Bistoletti, 1973; Mehandru et al, 1993) occurs during labor and delivery. These hormonal changes contribute to the decrease in the effective circulating plasma volume (Brace, 1992) and also directly cause renal vasoconstriction and an augmentation of sodium and water reabsorption. If a newborn has not passed urine during the first 24 hours of life, the presence of hypovolemia or other causes of compensated shock or severe bilateral renal and/or urinary tract anomalies should be considered.

***Abdominal Masses.*** Deep abdominal palpation can be most easily performed during the first 24 hours of life, when abdominal tone is still somewhat decreased and air does not completely fill the gastrointestinal tract. Thereafter, deep abdominal palpation is best done with the sucking reflex evoked, as this reflex also induces abdominal muscle relaxation. Palpable abdominal masses are present in 0.2% to 0.6% of newborns (Museles et al, 1971; Perlman et al, 1976). Two thirds of these masses are of renal origin; most of the remainder arise from the adrenal gland, the gastrointestinal tract, the female genitalia, or the liver. Hydronephrosis and dysplastic and polycystic kidney disease lead most frequently to palpable renal masses during the neonatal period. In the case of a midline abdominal mass, the presence of posterior urethral valves or a neurogenic bladder should always be considered. The discovered abdominal mass should then be further studied by ultrasonography, computed tomography (CT) scan, and/or MRI and, if appropriate, by renal cystourethrography, radionuclide scan, or intravenous pyelography.

***Edema.*** Accumulation of fluid in the interstitial space is a frequent finding in preterm and term neonates and occurs as a result of an imbalance in Starling forces and/or decreased lymphatic drainage. In the newborn with acute renal failure, *generalized edema* is most frequently due to a relative fluid overload in face of the markedly decreased GFR. In neonatal nephrotic syndrome, edema develops because increased urinary protein losses result in a marked drop in colloid osmotic pressure. In the edematous neonate with renal disease, additional hormonal factors may also contribute to the pathophysiology of edema formation. Such factors include the elevated activity of the renin-angiotensin-aldosterone system, increased bradykinin and prostaglandin production, high neonatal plasma prolactin levels, and the attenuation of the renal effects of atrial natriuretic peptide.

However, generalized edema in the neonatal period occurs most frequently with conditions other than primary renal disease. Otherwise healthy premature neonates and term infants born to diabetic mothers may present with generalized edema due to complex, hormone-regulated alterations in the dynamics of their physiologic fluid shift during early neonatal adaptation. Frequent iatrogenic causes of edema formation include volume overload, aggressive sodium supplementation during the period of early neonatal adaptation, and, in cases of late edema formation in the preterm neonate, maintenance of a high sodium intake after the infant converts from the sodium loosing to the sodium-retaining state (see also Chapter 30, Acid-Base, Fluid and Electrolyte Management). Generalized edema also is a prominent clinical feature of congestive heart failure and of neonatal conditions characterized by generalized capillary leak including hypoxia, sepsis, and shock. Other, less common causes of generalized edema include severe anemia, liver failure, protein-losing enteropathy, congenital infections, syndrome of inappropriate secretion of antidiuretic hormone, congenital analbuminemia, vitamin E deficiency, hyperaldosteronism, and hereditary angioneurotic edema.

Characteristic congenital *localized edema* is present in neonates with gonadal dysgenesis and primary lymphedema (Milroy disease) (Greenlee et al, 1993). Localized edema in the sick neonate also occurs with impairment of venous return and/or lymphatic drainage, as seen in the frequently catheter-related thromboses of major veins including the superior and inferior venae cavae and the femoral and axillary veins. Of iatrogenic origin and mostly of a benign nature is the localized limb edema associated with use of restrictive boards to protect intravenous sites.

***Ascites.*** Renal causes of intraperitoneal accumulation of fluid in the neonate include congenital urinary tract obstruction and nephrotic syndrome. The ascites in congenital urinary tract obstruction represents urine that has entered the peritoneal cavity following the rupture of the renal pelvis or one of the calyces. The ascitic fluid usually undergoes peritoneal dialysis and may lose most of the chemical characteristics of urine. If the abdominal ultrasound examination also demonstrates the presence of a thickened bladder wall, bladder outlet obstruction is the most likely diagnosis. The ascetic fluid in nephrotic syndrome has the character of an exudate. Nonrenal causes of ascites include bacterial or chemical peritonitis, congenital anomalies of the abdominal lymphatic system or biliary tree, malrotation, incomplete volvulus, ruptured ovarian cyst, and, extremely rarely, pancreatitis secondary to congenital pancreatic duct anomaly.

***External Genitalia.*** In general, an association between anomalies of the external genitalia and the upper urinary tract is infrequent. In the male, however, abnormalities of mesonephric development may lead to unilateral or bilateral renal agenesis and lack of testicular development. In the female, such abnormalities may result in unilateral or bilateral renal agenesis and uterine abnormalities. Furthermore, neonates with bilateral cryptorchidism, with unilateral cryptorchidism and hypospadias, or with penoscrotal or perineoscrotal hypospadias, who require thorough clinical and genetic evaluation for appropriate gender assignment, may also benefit from a renal ultrasound study to rule out possible renal and/or upper urinary tract anomalies (Laurance et al, 1976).

***Hypertension*** As discussed in Chapters 82, 83, and 87, renal parenchymal and vascular diseases as well as urinary tract anomalies may lead to the development of systemic hypertension. Therefore, a diagnostic work-up of neonatal hypertension should always include, but not be limited to, the evaluation of renal anatomy, function, and vascular integrity.

### Evaluation of Renal and Urinary Tract Morphology

***Ultrasonography.*** Ultrasonography has become the primary imaging technique in the postnatal evaluation of renal and urinary tract disorders in the newborn. Prenatal findings suggestive of urogenital anomalies require follow-up evaluation with a postnatal sonogram. The most common reasons for postnatal ultrasonographic assessment of the urinary tract are a prenatal finding of fetal hydronephrosis, urinary tract infection, and the detection of an abdominal mass in the newborn. However, oligohydramnios in the absence of signs of placental dysfunction, unexplained tension pneumothorax in a nonventilated infant, failure to void, a poor urinary stream, the presence of a single umbilical artery, abnormal and/or low-set ears, perineal and/or anal anomalies, vertebral anomalies, with or without the VATER (*v*ertebral defects, imperforate *a*nus, *t*racheo*e*sophageal fistula, *r*adial and renal dysplasia) or VACTERL (i.e., VATER plus *c*ardiac abnormalities and *l*imb defects) association, decreased abdominal wall musculature, unexplained elevation of serum creatinine, significant hematuria, proteinuria, renal tubular acidosis, and/or a urinary tract infection also are indications for ultrasonographic evaluation of the urinary tract in the neonatal period. Finally, because prolonged administration of furosemide is associated with an increased incidence of nephrocalcinosis, screening ultrasound examinations are warranted in neonates on chronic diuretic treatment with furosemide in the presence of hematuria.

Doppler ultrasonography, a noninvasive method of detecting renal blood flow, is helpful in the evaluation of suspected renal arterial and venous thrombosis.

***Voiding Cystourethrography.*** Voiding cystourethrography (VCUG), an important complement to ultrasonography, can identify anatomic and/or functional abnormalities in lower urinary tract disorders. It is particularly important in the evaluation of urinary tract infection for the detection and assessment of vesicoureteral reflux.

Radionuclide cystography is associated with significantly decreased radiation exposure to the patient compared to VCUG and has gained acceptance for use in the pediatric population, especially for follow-up evaluation of vesicoureteral reflux in children. However, it has considerable technical limitations in the newborn, and it has not been widely used in this patient population.

***Radionuclide Renal Imaging.*** Renal scintigraphy provides information about renal blood flow and function and is utilized primarily in follow-up evaluation of infants with obstructive uropathy. It has all but replaced intravenous urography in the neonate, especially during the first 2 weeks of life, when renal concentrating ability, essential to visualization of the iodinated agents used in the scan, is limited. Although renal scintigraphy provides less anatomic detail than is shown with intravenous urography, it offers useful physiologic information with reasonable anatomic definition and less radiation exposure. It also is a reliable quantitative method of monitoring renal function before and after surgery for obstructive uropathy.

***Angiography.*** Because of advances in Doppler ultrasonography and radionuclide scintigraphy techniques, renal angiography has been used less frequently in the neonate. It provides accurate anatomic information of the renal arterial and venous circulation but is invasive and poses a significant radiation exposure to the newborn.

***Renal Computed Tomography and Magnetic Resonance Imaging.*** Both renal CT and MRI techniques provide high-resolution cross-sectional imaging. However, with most indications for neonatal renal imaging, CT and MRI do not offer a significant advantage over sonography or renal scintigraphy. CT and MRI also usually require sedation and immobilization. They may play a role in neonatal uroimaging, however, when findings of other techniques are inconclusive.

***Renal Biopsy.*** Ultrasound-guided renal biopsy is performed in neonatal renal diseases if a tissue sample is required for the final diagnosis. Such conditions include, but are not limited to, Finnish-type nephrotic syndrome, nail-patella syndrome, autosomal recessive and autosomal dominant polycystic kidney disease, glomerulocystic kidney disease, and complex tubular functional abnormalities.

## REFERENCES


Arger PH, Coleman BG, Mintz MC, et al: Routine fetal genitourinary tract screening. Radiology 156:485-489, 1986.

Aviles DH, Fildes RD, Jose PA: Evalution of renal function. Clin Perinatol 19:69-84, 1992.

Brace AB: Fluid distribution in the fetus and neonate. In Polin RA, Fox WW (eds): Fetal and Neonatal Physiology. Philadelphia, WB Saunders, 1992, pp 1288-1298.

Bruno AN, Lavin JP, Nasrallah PF: Ultrasound experience with prenatal genitourinary abnormalities. Urology 26:196-201, 1985.

Bueva A, Guignard JP: Renal function in preterm neonates. Pediatr Res 36:572-577, 1994.

Cohen HL, Haller JO: Diagnostic sonography of the fetal genitourinary tract. Urol Radiol 9:88-98, 1987.

Colodny AH: Antenatal diagnosis and management of urinary abnormalities. Pediatr Clin North Am 34:1365-1381, 1987.

Clark DA: Times of first void and first stool in 500 newborns. Pediatrics 60:457-459, 1977.

Crombleholme TM, Harrison MR, Longaker MT, Langer JC: Prenatal diagnosis and management of bilateral hydronephrosis. Pediatr Nephrol 2:334-342, 1988.

Evans MI, Sacks AJ, Johnson MP, et al: Sequential invasive assessment of fetal renal function and intrauterine treatment of fetal obstructive uropathies. Obstet Gynecol 77:545-550, 1991.

Feldman H, Guignard JP: Plasma creatinine in the first month of life. Arch Dis Child 57:123-126, 1982.

Freedman AL, Johnson MP, Smith CA, et al: Long-term outcome in children after antenatal intervention for obstructive uropathies. Lancet 354:374-377, 1999.

Garett WJ, Grunwald G, Robinson DE: Prenatal diagnosis of fetal polycystic kidney disease by ultrasound. Aust N Z J Obstet Gynaecol 10:7-9, 1970.

Ghidini A, Alvarez M, Silverberg G, et al: Congenital nephrosis in low-risk pregnancies. Prenatal Diagn 14:599-602, 1994.

Greenlee R, Hoyme H, Witte M, et al: Developmental disorders of the lymphatic system. Lymphology 26:156-168, 1993.

Hubbard AM, Harty P, States LJ: A new tool for prenatal diagnosis: Ultrafast fetal MRI. Semin Perinatol 23:437-447, 1999.

Johnson MP, Bukowski TP, Reitleman C, et al: In utero surgical treatment of fetal obstructive uropathy: A new comprehensive approach to identify appropriate candidates for vesicoamniotic shunt therapy. Am J Obstet Gynecol 170:1770-1779, 1994.

Jones DP, Chesney RW: Development of tubular function. Clin Perinatol 19:33-57, 1992.

Lagerkrantz H, Bistoletti P; Catecholamine release in the newborn infant at birth. Pediatr Res 11:889-893, 1973.

Laurance BM, Darby CW, Vanderschueren-Lodeweyck M: Two XX males diagnosed in childhood. Endocrine, renal, and laboratory findings. Arch Dis Child 51:144-148, 1976.

Mahan JD, Mauer SM, Sibley RK: Congenital nephrotic syndrome, evolution of medical management and results of renal transplantation. J Pediatr 105:549-557, 1984.

Mehandru PL, Assel BG, Nuamah IF, et al: Catecholamine response at birth in preterm newborns. Biol Neonate 64:82-88, 1993.

Museles M, Gaundry CL, Bason MW: Renal anomalies in the newborn found by deep palpation. Pediatrics 47:97-100, 1971.

Patten RM, Mack LA, Wang KY, Cyr DR: The fetal genitourinary tract. Radiol Clin North Am 28:115-130, 1990.

Perlman M, Williams J: Detection of renal anomalies by abdominal palpation in the newborn infant. BMJ 2:347-349, 1976.

Ramin SM, Porter JC, Gilstrap LC III, Rosenfeld CR: Stress hormones and acid-base status of human fetuses at delivery. J Clin Endocrinol Metab 73:182-186, 1991.

Reuss A, Wladimiroff JW, Niermeijer MF: Antenatal diagnosis of renal tract anomalies by ultrasound. Pediatric Nephrol 1:546-552, 1987.

Roy DR, Layton HE, Jamison RL: Countercurrent mechanism and its regulation. In Seldin DW, Giebisch G (eds): The Kidney: Physiology and Pathophysiology, 2nd ed. New York, Raven Press, 1992, pp 1649-1692.

Sedin G: Fluid management in the extremely preterm infant. In Hansen TN, McIntosh N (eds): Current Topics in Neonatology. London, WB Saunders, 1995, pp 50-66.

Shackelford GD, Kees-Folts D, Cole BR: Imaging the urinary tract. Clin Perinatol 19:85-119, 1992.

Stonestreet BS, Oh W: Plasma creatinine levels in low birth weight infants during the first three months of life. Pediatrics 61:788-789, 1978.

Sullivan KM, Adzick NS: Fetal surgery. Clin Obstet Gynecol 37:355-371, 1994.

CHAPTER

# 82

# Developmental Abnormalities of the Kidneys

Bernard S. Kaplan

The increasing use of prenatal ultrasonography, continuing improvements in ventilator and nutritional support, and progress in dialysis techniques for newborns and renal transplantation for young children have changed the natural history of cystic and dysplastic kidney diseases. Information gathered from many sources must be evaluated carefully for optimal management of a newborn with a genetic or developmental disorder of the kidneys. Clearly, a team approach is needed. Errors occur with insufficient data, inadequate communication, and poor understanding of the natural history of these disorders (Guay-Woodford et al, 1998; Kaplan et al, 1992).

Many newborns who might have died in the past now can be dialyzed from birth and then undergo kidney transplantation when they attain a weight of about 10 kg. A precise diagnosis must be made before starting dialysis because some of these problems impose enormous emotional and financial burdens on families of affected children. The diagnosis depends on the evaluation of the findings on prenatal history, fetal ultrasonography, family history, clinical examination, imaging studies of the infants and parents when indicated, and laboratory studies (including DNA tests if available) and interpretation of pathologic examination findings. Several guiding principles are worth keeping in mind. Few genetic renal disorders are confined to the kidneys, and many syndromes have associated renal involvement. Therefore, ultrasonography of the kidneys and urinary tract should be done in all newborns with multiple defects. Also, ultrasonographic features can change over time. Variable expression of congenital renal defects may occur within and among kindreds; this is particularly true in autosomal recessive polystic kidney disease. Many classifications of cystic and dysplastic kidneys have been devised, but the one shown in Table 82–1 lists the conditions that can be seen in newborns.

## ECTOPIC KIDNEY, HORSESHOE KIDNEY, AND CROSSED FUSED ECTOPIA

Ectopic kidney, horseshoe kidney, and crossed fused ectopia are abnormalities in the position of the kidney(s) that do not have important long-term effects unless these conditions are associated with lower urinary tract anomalies, such as reflux or obstruction. In essence, affected kidneys are at risk for the same problems as those in normal positions. Horseshoe kidney, however, does occur with increased frequency in Turner syndrome and other syndromes. Avoiding cystourethrogram should be done to exclude the possibility of reflux, and a technetium 99m–labeled diethylenetriaminepenta-acetic acid (DTPA) scan also should be performed if there is evidence on ultrasonography of an obstruction.

## MULTICYSTIC KIDNEY

Multicystic kidney is the second most common cause of a flank mass in the newborn, with a prevalence rate of 1/4300. Multicystic kidney is almost always a sporadic, nonsyndromal, congenital anomaly. The diagnosis is made by in utero ultrasonography or by detection of an abdominal mass. Multicystic kidney is rarely the cause of symptoms in the newborn. Pathologic findings are ureteropelvic dysplasia or atresia, enlarged kidney, and cysts of varying size that do not communicate, with no demonstrable pelvis or calyces (Bernstein, 1991) (Fig. 82–1). Multicystic kidney must be differentiated from obstructive cystic renal dysplasia associated with hydronephrosis and other causes of obstructive uropathy by doing a DTPA scan. The multicystic kidney does not function. The contralateral kidney usually is normal, but in up to 50% of the cases it may be hydronephrotic, ectopic, refluxing, or occasionally dysplastic, or it may be absent (Atiyeh et al, 1992). Some investigators have postulated a spectrum, within and among kindreds, of caliceal diverticulum, pyelogenous cyst, ureteropelvic junction stenosis, infundibular stenosis, pelvic stenosis, and multicystic kidney (Kelalis and Malek, 1981). In most patients, follow-up evaluation by ultrasonography is done, and spontaneous involution often occurs without complications of infection, bleeding, or malignancy (Wacksman and Phipps, 1993).

## RENAL ADYSPLASIA AND DYSPLASIA

The term *adysplasia* encompasses a spectrum of renal anomalies that include renal agenesis, hypoplasia, and dysplasia, any of which may occur in an individual patient (such as unilateral agenesis with contralateral dysplasia) or within a kindred (Buchta et al, 1973). Dysplastic kidneys can be unilateral or bilateral, often contain cysts, are disorganized, and may also contain ectopic cartilage and muscle. They may or may not function. The clinical picture depends on the severity of the renal anomaly, whether it is unilateral or bilateral, and the presence of associated anomalies. The newborn may look normal or may have features of the oligohydramnios sequence, prune-belly syndrome, or a malformation syndrome.

Adysplasia and dysplasia can be the result of a single autosomal recessive (Cole et al, 1976) or dominant gene disorder (McPherson et al, 1987). Absent or dysplastic kidneys also can occur by multifactorial inheritance (Holmes, 1989), in chromosomal disorders (Egli and Stalder, 1973), or as a consequence of in utero infections or exposure to toxins. Prenatal diagnosis by ultrasonography is possible, especially if there is oligohydramnios or associated anomalies such as limb defects.

**TABLE 82-1**

**Cystic and Dysplastic Kidneys in Newborns**

Ectopic kidney, horseshoe kidney, crossed fused ectopia
Multicystic kidney
Unilateral renal agenesis
Bilateral renal agenesis
Renal adysplasia/dysplasia
  Isolated adysplasia/dysplasia
 Dysplasia/adysplasia in regional defects
  Prune-belly syndrome (PBS) [McKusick #100100]
  Posterior urethral valves (PUV) [McKusick #100100]
 Adysplasia/dysplasia with multiple-congenital-abnormalities syndromes
  Branchio-otorenal dysplasia (BOR syndrome) [McKusick #113650]
  Mayer-Rokitansky-Küster-Hauser syndrome
  Kallmann syndrome (KAL1) [McKusick #308700]
 Acrorenal syndromes
 Ectodermal dysplasia, ectrodactyly, cleft lip/palate syndrome
  Fanconi pancytopenia syndrome
  Thrombocytopenia–absent radius syndrome
  Townes-Brocks syndrome (TBS) [McKusick #107480]
  Fraser syndrome [McKusick #219000]
  Fryns syndrome
  Pallister-Hall syndrome [McKusick #146510]
Polycystic kidneys
 Autosomal recessive polycystic kidney disease [McKusick #263200]
 Autosomal dominant polycystic kidney disease [McKusick #179300]
 Tuberous sclerosis (TS) [McKusick #191100]
Cystic kidneys with autosomal recessive inheritance
 Meckel syndrome (MKS 1, MKS 2) [McKusick #249000]
 Jeune asphyxiating thoracic dystrophy syndrome [McKusick #208500]
 Renal-hepatic-pancreatic dysplasia (Ivemark syndrome)
Hypoplastic kidneys
Glomerulocystic kidneys
Dysgenetic kidneys
 Congenital hypernephronic nephromegaly with tubular dysgenesis [McKusick #267430]
Overgrowth syndromes
 Beckwith-Wiedemann syndrome [McKusick #130650]
 Perlman syndrome [McKusick #267000]
 Simpson-Golabi-Behmel syndrome type 1 (SGBS1) [McKusick #312870]
In utero exposure to teratogens
 Anticonvulsants; cocaine; indomethacin; lead; phenacetin; salicylate; warfarin; gentamicin
Inborn errors of metabolism
 Glutaric aciduria type II (multiple acyl-CoA dehydrogenase deficiencies)
 Zellweger cerebrohepatorenal syndrome [McKusick #214100]
 Carbohydrate-deficient glycoprotein syndrome

CoA, coenzyme A.

## Unilateral Renal Agenesis

Unilateral renal agenesis usually is an isolated (nonsyndromic), sporadic abnormality that is detected during prenatal ultrasonography. Unilateral renal agenesis is an important finding if the solitary kidney is abnormal, is part of a syndrome, or is an expression of hereditary renal dysplasia (Moerman et al, 1994). The incidence is between 1/500 and 1/800 live births. If the solitary kidney is normal, there is little risk of chronic renal failure in adulthood. The newborn must be examined carefully for additional anomalies: cleft palate, preauricular pits, cardiac and vertebral defects, and müllerian duct aplasia (Tarry et al, 1986). A voiding cystourethrogram should be done to exclude reflux. No further evaluations are needed beyond 1 year of age if at that time renal ultrasonography shows that the kidney is growing normally, with appropriate compensatory hypertrophy.

## Bilateral Renal Agenesis

Bilateral renal agenesis can occur as an isolated (nonsyndromal), sporadic abnormality detected during prenatal ultrasonography. It also can be a component of a syndrome such as the branchio-otorenal dysplasia (BOR) syndrome or can be an expression of hereditary renal adysplasia. Variable expression within a family is possible, with both autosomal recessive and dominant modes of inheritance. The incidence is about 1 in 3000 births. Bilateral renal agenesis is an important cause of the oligohydramnios

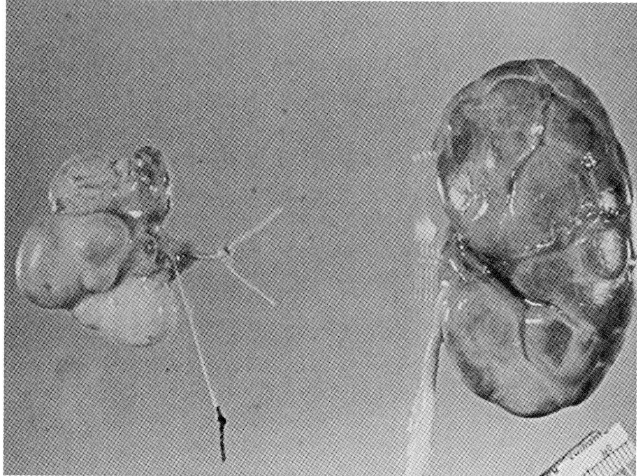

**FIGURE 82–1.** Multicystic kidney with atretic ureter *(right)*. Large cysts with no normal renal tissue.

sequence (Potter syndrome), in which decreased amniotic fluid causes uterine compression of the fetus. This produces the characteristic Potter facies with wide-set eyes, a prominent skin fold that extends from medial canthus to cheek, a parrot-beak nose, pliable low-set ears, and receding chin. Other features are lower limb deformations and, most important, a narrow, small chest with pulmonary hypoplasia. The infant is anuric and dies from pulmonary insufficiency. Bilateral renal agenesis is the most important cause of oligohydramnios, and the diagnosis can be confirmed by prenatal ultrasonography.

## Isolated Dysplasia and Adysplasia

The incidence of isolated (nonsyndromic) bilateral renal dysplasia is about 15 per 100,000 newborns (Holmes, 1989). Modes of transmission are autosomal dominant inheritance with reduced penetrance and multifactorial inheritance. A parent and siblings may be unaffected or have unilateral dysplasia or unilateral agenesis. Sporadic adysplasia may be caused by a new mutation or inheritance of the gene(s) from a nonmanifesting parent. First-degree relatives should be screened by ultrasonography to provide genetic counseling. The empirical risk of bilateral renal adysplasia for future siblings is 3.5% (Carter, 1970). The recurrence risk increases if two siblings are affected.

## Dysplasia and Adysplasia in Regional Defects: Prune-Belly Syndrome and Posterior Urethral Valve

Renal adysplasia occurs in prune-belly syndrome (PBS) [McKusick #100100] and posterior urethral valve (PUV) [McKusick #100100], possibly as a result of obstructive uropathy (Bernstein, 1991). Findings on renal pathologic examination range from minor anomalies to severe dysplasia with and without cysts. The features of PBS are deficient abdominal wall muscles (Fig. 82–2), unilateral or bilateral undescended testes, and urinary tract abnormalities. Females are rarely affected but may have uterine or vaginal anomalies. PBS also is associated with lower intestinal tract malrotation and atresias, lower limb deformations, and cardiovascular defects.

PUV is characterized by presence of a urethral valve (either a flap valve or a diaphragm in the prostatic urethra) and features of obstructive uropathy. A dilated prostatic urethra, megacystis, and megaureters can occur in both PBS and PUV. In both conditions, the most frequent clinical presentation in the newborn is that of the oligohydramnios sequence. The survival of newborns with PBS or PUV depends on the severity of pulmonary hypoplasia and the severity of renal dysplasia. Both

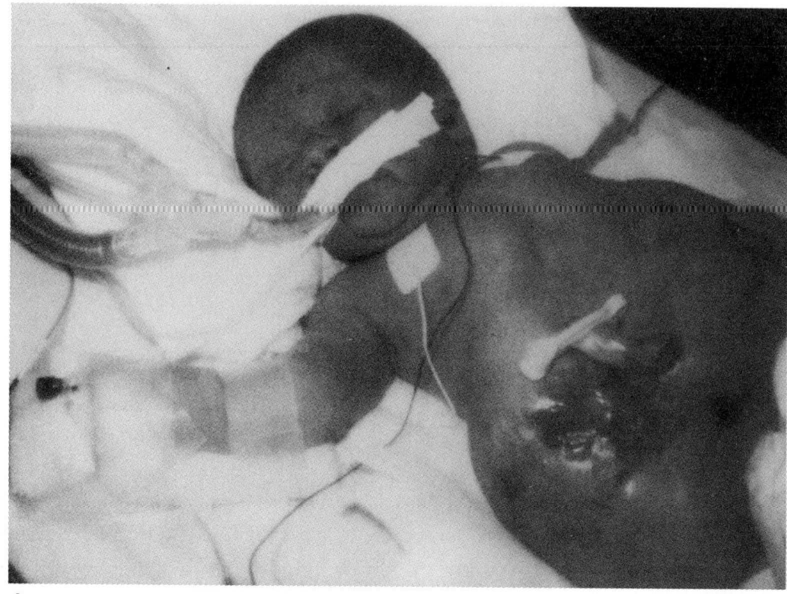

A

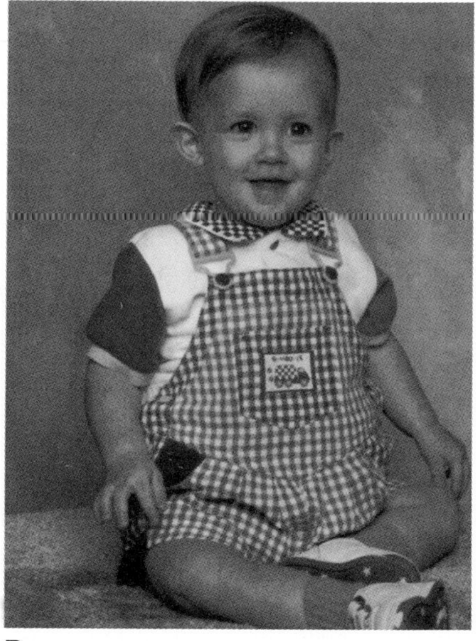

B

**FIGURE 82–2. A,** Newborn with prune-belly syndrome. The abdomen is protuberant, and the outlines of the intestines can be seen. The right ureter ruptured into the amniotic sac, thereby preventing development of the features of oligohydramnios sequence. **B,** The same patient at age 19 months.

conditions are usually isolated occurrences, although PUV may occur in families and in malformation syndromes. Prenatal diagnosis and treatment are discussed in detail in Chapter 81.

## Dysplasia and Adysplasia with Multiple Congenital Anomalies

### Branchio-otorenal Dysplasia (Branchio-otorenal Syndrome)

The spectrum of renal anomalies in BOR syndrome [McKusick #113650] ranges from unilateral dysplasia to bilateral agenesis. The kidneys may be even normal. Renal function ranges from normal to severe reduction in glomerular filtration rate. Extrarenal manifestations are preauricular pits, branchial clefts, sensorineural deafness, and lacrimal duct atresia. The incidence is about 1/40,000. Inheritance is autosomal dominant with high penetrance and variable expression. One mutant gene, *EYA1*, is on chromosome 8q13.3 (Abdelhak et al, 1997; Kumar et al, 1997). The prognosis depends on the severity of the renal disorder.

### Mayer-Rokitansky-Küster-Hauser Syndrome

Females with Mayer-Rokitansky-Küster-Hauser syndrome have renal adysplasia and müllerian anomalies of vaginal atresia and bicornuate or septate uterus (Tarry et al, 1986). The fallopian tubes, ovaries, and broad and round ligaments are normal. There is a normal female karyotype and normal secondary sexual development.

### Kallmann Syndrome (Hypogonadotropic Hypogonadism and Anosmia)

Males with Kallmann syndrome (KAL1) [McKusick #308700] have hypogonadotropic hypogonadism that manifests with delayed puberty and infertility, anosmia caused by agenesis of the olfactory lobes, and renal abnormalities (Colquhoun-Kerr et al, 1999; Deeb et al, 2001; Dissaneevate et al, 1998; Hardelin et al, 1992). Urogenital abnormalities include unilateral renal agenesis, bilateral renal agenesis, multicystic dysplastic kidney, cryptorchidism, testicular atrophy, and micropenis. Males may die at birth as a result of bilateral renal agenesis. Additional features include coloboma of the iris, deafness, midline anomalies, oculomotor apraxia, and congenital facial diplegia (Möbius anomalad). The X-linked form is the result of a mutation in the *KAL1* gene on Xp22.3. Treatment with testosterone or estrogen for induction of puberty induces appropriate pubertal development.

## Acrorenal Syndromes

Radial and renal anomalies occur in many syndromes. In the *ectodermal dysplasia–ectrodactyly–cleft lip and/or palate (EEC 1) syndrome* [McKusick #128930], there are combinations of urogenital defects, ectrodactyly, ectodermal dysplasia, clefting, lacrimal duct anomalies, and conductive hearing loss. Inheritance is autosomal dominant, with variable penetrance and expression. In the *VACTERL/VATER association* [McKusick #192350], there is variable occurrence of vertebral anomalies, anal atresia, congenital cardiac disease, tracheoesophageal fistula, renal abnormalities, and radial-limb dysplasia. Occurrence of VACTERL usually is sporadic. Neonates with features of VACTERL must be tested for Fanconi anemia. Congenital malformations occur in 60% of cases of *Fanconi anemia (pancytopenia) syndrome.* Affected patients may have renal malformations, short stature, café-au-lait spots, radial-ray abnormalities, gastrointestinal, microcephaly, skeletal abnormalities, and, in males, genital anomalies, hypogonadism and infertility (Giampietro et al, 1993). Other features are chromosomal instability and mutagen hypersensitivity in cells. Inheritance is autosomal recessive, with variable expression and mutations in one of at least seven different genes (Joenje and Patel, 2001). Renal anomalies also may occur in *thrombocytopenia–absent radius syndrome* (TAR) [McKusick #274000].

The clinical features of *Townes-Brocks radial-ear-anal-renal syndrome* (TBS) [McKusick #107480] include broad, bifid, or triphalangeal thumb; flat thenar eminences; small, "lop," or "satyr" external ear and preauricular pits or tags; sensorineural hearing loss; and imperforate or stenotic or anteriorly placed anus. Renal and urologic anomalies encompass renal hypoplasia, renal dysplasia, unilateral renal agenesis, horseshoe kidney, posterior urethral valves, uretero-vesical reflux, and meatal stenosis (Salerno et al, 2000). Inheritance is dominant, with a defect in the gene encoding SALL1 on chromosome16q12.1. Renal anomalies can occur in association with numerous other abnormalities in *Fraser syndrome* [McKusick #219000] (Schauer et al, 1990), *Fryns syndrome* [McKusick #229850] (Moerman et al, 1988), and *Pallister-Hall congenital hypothalamic hamartoblastoma syndrome* (PHS) [McKusick #146510] (Killoran et al, 2000).

## POLYCYSTIC KIDNEYS

The term *polycystic kidneys* should be applied only to autosomal recessive polycystic kidneys and autosomal dominant polycystic kidneys. In these conditions, there are many cysts in both kidneys, there is no evidence of renal dysplasia, and there is continuity of the lumen of the nephron from the uriniferous space to the urinary bladder. Patients with tuberous sclerosis can have cystic kidneys that appear identical by ultrasonography to autosomal dominant polycystic kidneys.

### Autosomal Recessive Polycystic Kidney Disease

The incidence of autosomal recessive polycystic kidney disease (ARPKD) [McKusick #263200] is about 1 in 16,000 newborns. Inheritance is autosomal recessive; there may be variable expression within a sibship (Kaplan et al, 1988), and the parents are unaffected. The gene locus is chromosome 6p21.1-p12 (Guay-Woodford et al, 1995; Zerres et al, 1998). In the newborn, the kidneys are much more severely affected than the liver, whereas liver disease is more prominent when the disorder is diagnosed in older children. Features of the oligohydramnios sequence are present if there is severe oliguria or anuria in utero. The abdomen is protuberant, and the kidneys are large and easily palpable. Hypertension often is severe, may be caused by volume expansion, and can be difficult to control. Peripheral renin activity and aldosterone excretion are reduced (Kaplan et al, 1989). Hyponatremia often is induced iatrogenically as a result of inappropriate administration of free water and is not associated with increased urinary losses of sodium (Kaplan et al, 1989). Furosemide or metolazone may correct hyponatremia, but additional sodium chloride also may be needed. The hypertension often responds to treatment with an angiotensin-converting enzyme (ACE) inhibitor and a loop diuretic.

Renal sonography has superseded excretory urography and even histologic studies as the preeminent diagnostic procedure. The sonographic findings in the newborn are large kidneys, increased echogenicity of the parenchyma, loss of corticomedullary differentiation, and loss of central echo complex (Metreweli and Garel, 1980). The cortex is preserved, and the papillae are echogenic. There may be macrocysts that are less than 2 cm in diameter. The liver is echodense, and biliary ducts are dilated. It is important to remember that renal ultrasonography does not always distinguish between autosomal recessive polycystic kidneys and autosomal dominant polycystic kidneys, between autosomal recessive polycystic kidneys and transient nephromegaly (Stapleton et al, 1981), or between autosomal recessive polycystic kidneys and glomerulocystic kidneys (Fitch and Stapleton, 1986). Kidney and liver biopsies are indicated in ambiguous cases.

At postmortem examination, the kidneys are enlarged, are spongy, and maintain their renal contours (Fig. 82–3A). The dilated collecting ducts are neatly arranged perpendicular to the surface of the kidney (see Fig. 82–3B). There are no dysplastic elements. The liver is always involved; portal areas are expanded by increased numbers of dilated bile ductules surrounded by fibrous tissue. The dilated ductules may become cystic. The liver cells are normal.

Autosomal recessive polycystic kidneys can be diagnosed after 24 weeks of gestation by ultrasonographic demonstration of large hyperechogenic kidneys, oligohydramnios, and an empty bladder (Romero et al, 1984). Most infants who are symptomatic at birth die from respiratory or renal causes. Respiratory and renal function can improve in some cases, and a small number of patients who survive the neonatal period may maintain adequate renal function into adolescence. Massively enlarged kidneys may cause respiratory distress by restricting diaphragmatic excursion; therefore, bilateral nephrectomies may improve ventilation. Peritoneal dialysis may then be performed until the infant can have a kidney transplant (Sumfest et al, 1993). Seventy-five percent of infants with ARPKD who survive to 1 year of age can live for more than 15 years (Kaplan et al, 1989).

### Autosomal Dominant Polycystic Kidney Disease

The incidence of autosomal dominant polycystic kidney disease (ADPKD) [McKusick #179300] in liveborn infants is 1/100,000 to 3/100,000. Although the second most common autosomal dominant mutation in humans, with an estimated prevalence in the population of between 1/200 and 1/1000, ADPKD rarely manifests with clinical findings at birth (Fick et al, 1993). The inheritance is autosomal dominant, with variable expression. Negative findings on an ultrasound examination performed after the age of 10 years, and especially past the age of 30, provide reassurance for persons at 50% risk (Bear et al, 1992). Occasionally an infant may have symptoms before the parent does. Prediction by DNA analysis complements ultrasonography for detection, is not age dependent, and may not be informative in every family. Mutations in at least three genes cause ADPKD. Polycystic kidney disease 1 (PKD1), in 85% of families is caused by a mutation on chromosome 16p13.3-p13.12 (Breuning et al, 1987). Patients with PKD2, occurring in about 5% of affected families, have the same phenotype as in PKD1,

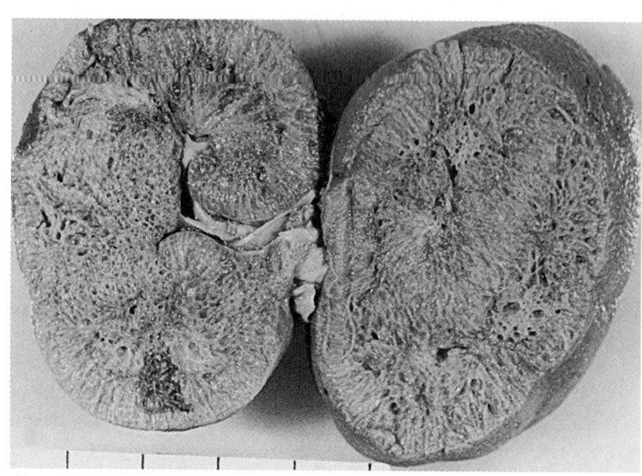
A

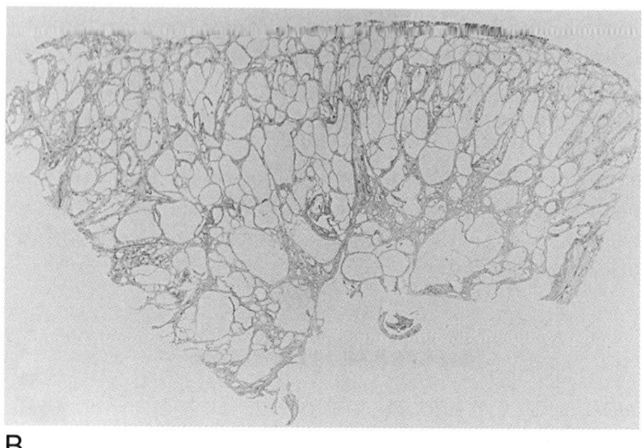
B

**FIGURE 82–3.** **A,** Large spongy kidneys (autosomal recessive kidneys). **B,** Photomicrograph of autosomal recessive kidneys with dilated tubules and paucity of glomeruli.

and the mutation is on chromosome 4q13-q23 (Kimberling et al, 1993; Peters et al, 1993). The location of the third gene, *PKD3*, is unknown. Polycystin-1, the gene product, is a matrix receptor that links the extracellular matrix to the actin cytoskeleton via focal adhesion proteins (Wilson, 2001). The mean age at onset of end-stage renal disease in persons with PKD1 is 56.7 ± 1.9 years, as compared with 69.4 ± 1.7 years in those with PKD2. Hypertension and renal impairment are less frequent and occur later in the families with PKD2. The kidneys are enlarged and lobular, and the calices are stretched and distorted by cysts, which produce smooth or irregular indentations. Numerous cysts of various sizes are seen in the parenchyma in severely affected cases. At postmortem examination, the kidneys are large, with numerous round protuberances on their surfaces (Fig. 82–4). Cysts are irregularly dispersed through the parenchyma and arise from many nephron segments. Ultrasonography and computed tomography (CT) scanning are more sensitive methods for detecting the cysts than intravenous urography (IVU). Cysts may be seen in liver, pancreas, and spleen.

ADPKD may be detected prenatally by ultrasonography (Sedman et al, 1987). Some patients have the oligohydramnios sequence, enlarged kidneys, and hematuria. Associated abnormalities reported in infants with ADPKD are endocardial fibroelastosis, an intracerebral vascular anomaly, pyloric stenosis, and hepatic fibrosis (Cobben et al, 1990). The finding of hepatic fibrosis in some patients can make differentiation between ARPKD and ADPKD difficult. In the past, in about half the reported cases of ADPKD manifesting in utero or in the first few months of life, the patient died before 1 year of age, but recent studies of larger numbers of patients show a much more optimistic prognosis (Fick et al, 1993).

### Tuberous Sclerosis

Tuberous sclerosis (TS) [McKusick #191100] is characterized by hamartomata in numerous organs. Rarely, polycystic or unilateral cystic disease is found in a newborn in whom a diagnosis of TS is made later (Brook-Carter et al, 1994; Sampson et al, 1997). Renal cysts or polycystic disease in TS are identical to simple cysts or ADPKD in their ultrasonographic, IVU, and CT scan appearances. Nonsymptomatic renal lesions (cysts and/or angiomyolipomas) occur in about 60% of persons with TS (Cook, 1996).

Other features include skin lesions (in 96% of patients), epilepsy, learning difficulties, and behavioral problems. "Ash leaf" hypopigmented nevi may be the only skin manifestation of TS in infancy, and babies with polycystic kidneys must be examined for the nevi under ultraviolet light. Shagreen patches and adenoma sebaceum develop before the age of 14 years; nail fibromas appear after 5 years and increase in number and size with age. Ventricular rhabdomyomas and seizures may occur in infancy.

Patients usually survive to adolescence and adulthood, but those with early-onset polycystic kidneys may develop end-stage renal failure. Inheritance is autosomal dominant, with very variable expression within a family, nonpenetrance of the gene, or germinal mosaicism A parent with the gene may appear unaffected, so the parents also must be examined clinically and radiologically for stigmata of TS. TS is linked in half of the cases to a gene *TSC1* ("hamartin") on chromosome 9q34. In other patients, TS is linked to a marker gene, *TSC2* ("tuberin"), near the locus for PKD1 on chromosome 16p13.3 (Kandt et al, 1992; van Slegtenhorst et al, 1998).

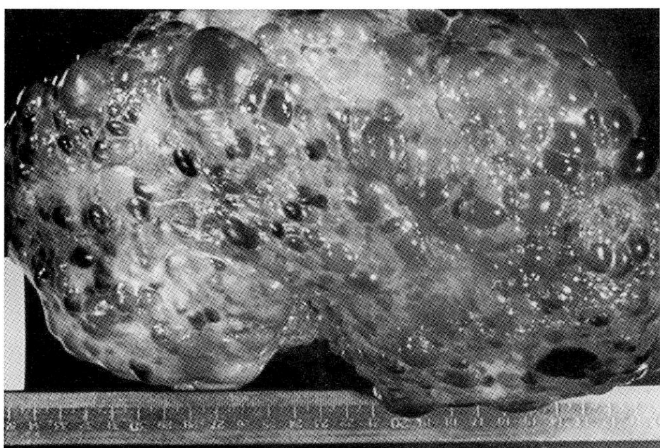

**FIGURE 82–4.** Autosomal dominant polycystic kidney. The kidney is large, and there are numerous cysts on the surface.

## CYSTIC KIDNEYS WITH AUTOSOMAL RECESSIVE INHERITANCE

### Meckel Syndrome

In Meckel syndrome (MKS 1, MKS 2) [McKusick #249000], polycystic kidneys are an invariable finding. A consistent feature is hepatic fibrosis with variable reactive ductule proliferation and dilation and plate fibrosis. Other features include a sloping forehead, posterior encephalocele, microphthalmia, postaxial polydactyly, and ambiguous genitalia. Fifty percent of the patients have oligohydramnios and die in the perinatal period. In Goldston syndrome, there are cystic kidneys, hepatic fibrosis, and Dandy-Walker malformation. This and other syndromes may be either part of the spectrum of MKS or discrete entities (Gloeb et al, 1989). The incidence of MKS is 1/9000. Inheritance is autosomal recessive, with variable expression within and among families (Fraser and Lytwyn, 1981). Gene loci are on chromosomes 17q22-q23 (MKS 1) and 11q13 (MKS 2) (Roume et al, 1998). Prenatal diagnosis is possible by ultrasonography and by detection of increased alpha-fetoprotein levels in amniotic fluid.

### Jeune Asphyxiating Thoracic Dystrophy Syndrome

Jeune asphyxiating thoracic dystrophy syndrome [McKusick #208500] is inherited as an autosomal recessive trait, with variable expression. Respiratory distress, dysostoses, renal cystic disease, and congenital hepatic fibrosis characterize the disorder. Dysostoses include short ribs, small and long thoracic cage, small pelvis, trident acetabular margins, short and thick second and third phalanges, cone-shaped epiphyses, handle-bar clavicle, and mesomelic shortening of the limbs (Donaldson et al, 1985). Three different morphologic lesions of the kidneys have been described: (1) dilated proximal and distal tubules and Bowman capsule with interstitial fibrosis, (2) cystic dysplasia and disorganized renal architecture, and (3) chronic tubulointerstitial disease resembling juvenile nephronophthisis. The differential diagnosis includes Ellis–van Creveld syndrome, Saldino-Noonan short rib–polydactyly syndrome (type II), Majewski short rib–polydactyly syndrome, and Naumoff syndrome (type III). Survivors develop metaphyseal dysplasia with short-limb dwarfism. Treatment of renal failure may require dialysis and transplantation. Prenatal diagnosis by ultrasonography is possible by 18 weeks (Elejade et al, 1985).

### Renal-Hepatic-Pancreatic Dysplasia (Ivemark Syndrome)

Inheritance of renal-hepatic-pancreatic dysplasia (Ivemark syndrome) is autosomal recessive. Patients may have the oligohydramnios sequence. The kidneys may be dysplastic, with peripheral cortical cysts, primitive collecting ducts, glomerular cysts, and metaplastic cartilage (Bernstein et al, 1987). There is fibrosis of the liver and pancreas. Most patients die from respiratory insufficiency in the newborn period. Inheritance is autosomal recessive.

## HYPOPLASTIC KIDNEYS

Hypoplastic kidneys are small, have fewer calices, and may be dysplastic. Simple hypoplasia, oligomeganephronia, and renal dysplasia are the types of kidney hypoplasia that are seen in newborns. In older children, small kidneys also may be the result of chronic pyelonephritis, chronic glomerulonephritis, renovascular accident, or nephronophthisis. In simple hypoplasia, the renal architecture is normal, but there are a decreased number of reniculi and small nephrons. Oligomeganephronic kidneys are small and have a decreased number of enlarged glomeruli. Oligomeganephronia probably is not a specific clinicopathologic entity. Some patients with oligomeganephronic kidneys have chromosome 4 abnormalities (Anderson et al, 1997), and others have heterozygous *PAX2* mutations (Salomon et al, 2001).

## GLOMERULOCYSTIC KIDNEYS

The purest form of glomerulocystic kidney is characterized by dilated Bowman spaces, with few or no cysts in the tubule (Bernstein, 1993). The rest of the renal architecture is normal. The kidneys may be large or small. The liver is normal. Glomerular cysts also are seen in obstructive uropathy, in autosomal dominant polycystic kidneys, in association with malformations of other organs, in dysplastic kidneys, and in the kidneys of infants whose mothers received phenacetin or indomethacin during pregnancy. Glomerular cysts are often subcapsular and may contain more than one glomeruloid structure (Fig. 82–5). Glomerulocystic kidneys may occur sporadically. Autosomal dominant inheritance is found in some kindreds in association with mutations in the gene encoding hepatocyte nuclear factor (HNF)-1β and early-onset diabetes (Bingham et al, 2001).

## DYSGENETIC KIDNEYS

### Renal Tubular Dysgenesis: Congenital Hypernephronic Nephromegaly with Tubular Dysgenesis

Clinical features of congenital hypernephronic nephromegaly with tubular dysgenesis [McKusick #267430], an autosomal recessive condition, include late-onset

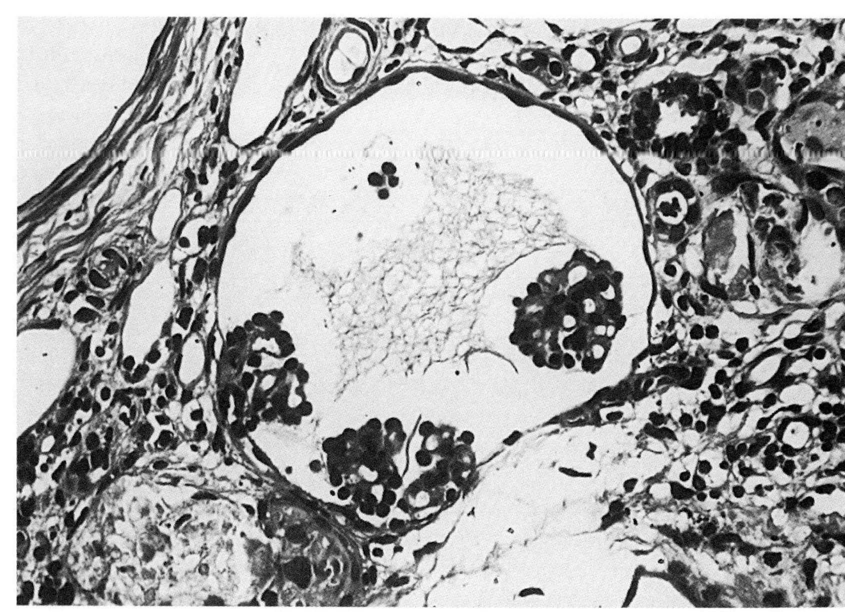

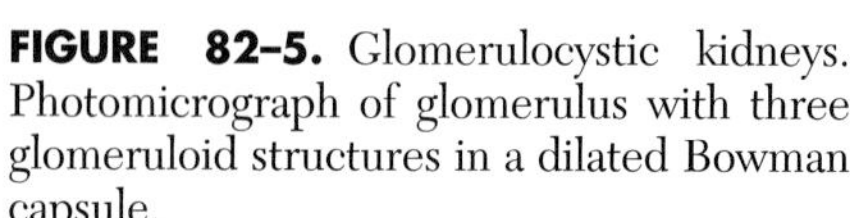

**FIGURE 82–5.** Glomerulocystic kidneys. Photomicrograph of glomerulus with three glomeruloid structures in a dilated Bowman capsule.

oligohydramnios after 24 weeks of gestation and large nonfunctioning kidneys (Allanson et al, 1992). The calvaria may be underdeveloped with wide sutures. Similar calvarial anomalies occur in patients with the Finnish-type congenital nephrotic syndrome and in infants exposed in utero to ACE inhibitors. The kidneys are seen to be enlarged symmetrically on ultrasonography, and the corticomedullary junction is poorly defined. Other features are an apparent increase in the number of glomeruli and immature tubules without proximal convolutions. Prenatal diagnosis is not possible before 20 weeks. All of the patients have died in the neonatal period.

## OVERGROWTH SYNDROMES

Beckwith-Wiedemann syndrome, Simpson-Golabi-Behmel syndrome, and Perlman syndrome are overgrowth syndromes with overlapping features and kidneys that may be abnormal at birth (Coppin et al, 1997).

### Beckwith-Wiedemann Syndrome

Patients with Beckwith-Wiedemann syndrome [McKusick #130650] may have nephromegaly, Wilms tumor, medullary renal cysts, caliceal diverticula, hydronephrosis, and nephrolithiasis (Choyke et al, 1998). The syndrome is caused by a mutation of a gene encoding a human cyclin-dependent kinase inhibitor, p57 (*KIP2*), on chromosome 11p15.5 (Matsuoka et al, 1996). Patients should be screened by renal ultrasound examination for Wilms tumor every 3 months for the first 7 years.

### Perlman Syndrome

In Perlman syndrome [McKusick #267000], characterized by renal hamartomas, nephroblastomatosis, and fetal gigantism, associated features include polyhydramnios, macrosomia, and bilateral nephromegaly with nephroblastomatosis, visceromegaly, cryptorchidism, diaphragmatic hernia, interrupted aortic arch, hypospadias, and polysplenia and renal findings of dysplasia, microcysts, and nephrogenic rests (Greenberg et al, 1988; Schilke et al, 2000). Inheritance is autosomal recessive.

### Simpson-Golabi-Behmel Syndrome

In patients with Simpson-Golabi-Behmel syndrome type 1 (SGBS1) [McKusick #312870], features include pre- and postnatal overgrowth, “coarse” face, hypertelorism, broad nasal root, cleft palate, full lips with a midline groove of the lower lip, grooved tongue with “tongue-tie,” prominent mandible, congenital heart defects, arrhythmias, supernumerary nipples, splenomegaly, large dysplastic kidneys, cryptorchidism, hypospadias, skeletal abnormalities, and postaxial hexadactyly. Inheritance is X-linked. Some cases are caused by a mutation in the gene for glypican-3, which maps to Xq26 (Pilia et al, 1996). The gene responsible for a second SGB syndrome (SGBS2) is located on Xp22 (Brzustowicz et al, 1999).

## IN UTERO EXPOSURE TO TERATOGENS

No convincing proof of a cause-and-effect relationship has been provided for associations of in utero exposure to teratogens. Urogenital anomalies are found occasionally in infants exposed in utero to valproic acid and other anticonvulsant agents (Ardinger et al, 1988). Maternal cocaine (and polydrug) use may produce genitourinary abnormalities (Chasnoff et al, 1988). Indomethacin may cause renal dysgenesis in fetal monkeys and possibly in humans exposed early in utero to prolonged high doses (Kaplan et al, 1994). Prenatal lead exposure is incriminated as a possible cause of the VACTERL association (Levine and Muenke, 1991). Glomerulocystic disease was reported in an infant exposed to phenacetin and salicylate in utero (Krous et al, 1977). Unilateral renal agenesis and abnormalities of position were noted in three infants exposed prenatally to warfarin (Hall, 1989).

## INBORN ERRORS OF METABOLISM

In several inborn errors of energy metabolism that manifest in the newborn period, features include morphologic and functional abnormalities of the kidneys. These are all rare conditions.

### Glutaric Aciduria Type II

The clinical features of glutaric aciduria type IIa, the neonatal-onset form of multiple acyl-coenzyme A (CoA) dehydrogenase deficiencies, include prematurity, hypotonia, hepatomegaly, nephromegaly, craniofacial anomalies, rocker-bottom feet, anterior abdominal wall defects, and external genital anomalies. An odor of sweaty feet may be present. Within 24 hours there is severe hypoglycemia but no ketosis, a metabolic acidosis with an increased undetermined anion gap, lactic acidosis, and mild hyperammonemia. Elevated levels of organic acids are found in body fluids. Renal cystic dysplasia occurs in many cases (Wilson et al, 1989). The deficiencies in electron transfer flavoprotein or electron transfer ubiquinone oxidoreductase are inherited as autosomal recessive traits. Prenatal diagnosis may be possible by assaying enzyme in amniocytes and/or elevated glutaric acid in amniotic fluid. Ultrasonography in utero may show enlarged cystic kidneys. Death occurs within days to months. There is no successful treatment.

### Zellweger Cerebrohepatorenal Syndrome

Clinical features of Zellweger cerebrohepatorenal syndrome [McKusick #214100] are similar to those of glutaric aciduria type II, plus profound hypotonia, nystagmus, cataracts (“oil droplets”), pigmentary retinopathy, optic disc pallor, and stippled epiphyses of patella and acetabulum. Odor is not abnormal. All peroxisomal functions are abnormal: elevated plasma very-long-chain fatty acids, bile acids, pipecolic acid, and phytanic acid and urine dicarboxylic acids, and low cholesterol and triglycerides (Steinberg et al, 1999). Pathologic features are cortical renal cysts, micronodular cirrhosis, brain heterotopias, abnormal brain gyri, and absent corpus callosum. Inheritance is autosomal recessive. Prenatal diagnosis is possible by enzyme assays in amniocytes or chorionic villus cells. Most affected infants die within 6 months but those with a milder form can survive into adolescence with retardation, deafness, and seizures.

### Carbohydrate-Deficient Glycoprotein Syndrome

Multiple renal microcysts are found in the carbohydrate-deficient glycoprotein syndrome (Strom et al, 1993). There is multisystem involvement with olivopontocerebellar atrophy, retinitis pigmentosa, testicular atrophy, hypothyroidism, and immune deficiency. Several glycoproteins are deficient in their carbohydrate moieties. Inheritance is autosomal recessive, and the prognosis is variable.

## REFERENCES


Abdelhak S, Kalatzis V, Heilig R, et al: A human homologue of the *Drosophila* eyes absent gene underlies branchio-oto-renal (BOR) syndrome and identifies a novel gene family. Nat Genet 15:157, 1997.

Allanson JE, Hunter AGW, Mettler GS, Jiminez C: A not uncommon autosomal recessive syndrome: A review. Am J Med Genet 43:811, 1992.

Anderson CE, Wallerstein R, Zamerowski ST, et al: Ring chromosome 4 mosaicism coincidence of oligomeganephronia and signs of Seckel syndrome. Am J Med Genet 72:281, 1997.

Ardinger HH, Atkin JF, Blackston RD, et al: Verification of the fetal valproate syndrome phenotype. Am J Med Genet 29:171, 1988.

Atiyeh B, Husmann D, Baum M: Contralateral renal abnormalities in multicystic-dysplastic kidney disease. J Pediatr 121:65, 1992.

Bear JC, Parfrey PS, Morgan JM, et al; Autosomal dominant polycystic kidney disease: New information for genetic counseling. Am J Med Genet 43:548, 1992.

Bernstein J: The multicystic kidney and hereditary renal adysplasia. Am J Kidney Dis 17:495, 1991.

Bernstein J: Glomerulocystic kidney disease—nosological considerations. Pediatr Nephrol 7:464, 1993.

Bernstein J, Chandra M, Cresswell J, et al: Renal-hepatic-pancreatic dysplasia: A syndrome reconsidered. Am J Med Genet 26:391, 1987.

Bingham C, Bulman MP, Ellard S, et al: Mutations in the hepatocyte nuclear factor-1β gene are associated with familial hypoplastic glomerulocystic kidney disease. Am J Hum Genet 68:219, 2001.

Breuning MH, Reeders ST, Brunner H, et al: Improved early diagnosis of adult polycystic kidney disease with flanking DNA markers. Lancet 2:1359, 1987.

Brook-Carter PT, Peral B, Ward CJ, et al: Deletion of the TSC2 and PKD1 genes associated with severe infantile polycystic kidney disease—a contiguous gene syndrome. Nat Genet 8:328, 1994.

Brzustowicz LM, Farrell S, Khan MB, et al: Mapping of a new SGBS locus to chromosome Xp22 in a family with a severe form of Simpson-Golabi-Behmel syndrome. Am J Hum Genet 65:779, 1999.

Buchta RM, Viseskul C, Gilbert EF, et al: Familial bilateral renal agenesis and hereditary renal adysplasia. Z Kinderheilk 115:111, 1973.

Carter CO: Genetics of polycystic disease of the kidney. Birth Defects 6:11, 1970.

Chasnoff IJ, Chisum CM, Kaplan WE: Maternal cocaine use and genitourinary tract malformations. Teratology 37:201, 1988.

Choyke PL, Siegel MJ, Oz O, et al: Nonmalignant renal disease in pediatric patients with Beckwith-Wiedemann syndrome. AJR Am J Roentgenol 171:733, 1998.

Cobben JM, Breuning MH, Schoots C, et al: Congenital hepatic fibrosis in autosomal-dominant polycystic kidney disease. Kidney Int 38:880, 1990.

Cole BR, Kaufman BL, McAlister WH, et al: Bilateral renal dysplasia in three siblings: Report of a survivor. Clin Nephrol 5:83, 1976.

Colquhoun-Kerr JS, Gu WX, Jameson JL, et al: X-linked Kallmann syndrome and renal agenesis occurring together and independently in a large Australian family. Am J Med Genet 83:23, 1999.

Cook JA, Oliver K, Mueller RF, et al: A cross sectional study of renal involvement in tuberous sclerosis. J Med Genet 33:480, 1996.

Coppin B, Moore I, Hatchwell E: Extending the overlap of three congenital overgrowth syndromes. Clin Genet 51:375, 1997.

Deeb A, Robertson A, MacColl G, et al: Multicystic dysplastic kidney and Kallmann's syndrome: a new association? Nephrol Dial Transplant 16:1170, 2001.

Dissaneevate P, Warne GL, Zacharin MR: Clinical evaluation in isolated hypogonadotrophic hypogonadism (Kallmann syndrome). J Pediatr Endocrinol Metab 11:631,1998.

Donaldson MDC, Warner AA, Trompeter RS, et al: Familial juvenile nephronophthisis, Jeune's syndrome and associated disorders. Arch Dis Child 60:426, 1985.

Egli F, Stalder G: Malformations of kidney and urinary tract in common chromosomal aberrations: I. Clinical studies. Humangenetik 18:1, 1973.

Elejade BR, de Elejade MM, Pansch D: Prenatal diagnosis of Jeune's syndrome. Am J Med Genet 21:433, 1985.

Fick GM, Johnson AM, Strain JD, et al: Characterization of very early onset autosomal dominant polycystic kidney disease. J Am Soc Nephrol 3:1863, 1993.

Fitch SJ, Stapleton FB: Ultrasonographic features of glomerulocystic disease in infancy: Similarity to infantile polycystic kidney disease. Pediatric Radiol 16:400, 1986.

Fivush B, McGrath S, Zinkham W: Thrombocytopenia absent radius syndrome associated with renal insufficiency. Clin Pediatr 29:182, 1990.

Fraser FC, Lytwyn A: Spectrum of anomalies in the Meckel syndrome, or: "May be there is a malformation syndrome with at least one constant anomaly." Am J Med Genet 9:63, 1981.

Giampietro PF, Adler-Brecher B, Verlander PC, et al: The need for more accurate and timely diagnosis in Fanconi anemia: A report from the International Fanconi Anemia Registry. Pediatrics 91:1116, 1993.

Gloeb DJ, Valdes-Dapena M, Saiman F, et al: The Goldston syndrome; report of a case. Pediatr Pathol 9:337, 1989.

Greenberg F, Copeland K, Gresik MV: Expanding the spectrum of the Perlman syndrome. Am J Med Genet 29:773, 1988.

Guay-Woodford LM, Galliani CA, et al: Diffuse renal cystic disease in children: Morphologic and genetic correlations. Pediatr Nephrol 12:173, 1998.

Guay-Woodford LM, Muecher G, Hopkins SD, et al: The severe perinatal form of autosomal recessive polycystic kidney disease maps to chromosome 6p21.1-p12: Implications for genetic counseling. Am J Hum Genet 56:1101, 1995.

Hall BD: Warfarin embryopathy and urinary tract anomalies: Possible new association. Am J Med Genet 34:292, 1989.

Hardelin JP, Levilliers J, del Castillo I, et al: X chromosome-linked Kallmann syndrome: Stop mutations validate the candidate gene. Proc Natl Acad Sci U S A 89:8190, 1992.

Holmes LB: Prevalence, phenotypic heterogeneity and familial aspects of bilateral renal agenesis/dysgenesis. In Liss AR (ed): Genetics of Kidney Disorders. New York, Alan R. Liss, 1989, pp 1-11.

Joenje H, Patel KJ: The emerging genetic and molecular basis of Fanconi anaemia. Nat Rev Genet 2:446, 2001.

Kandt RS, Haines JL, Smith M, et al: Linkage of an important gene locus for tuberous sclerosis to a chromosome 16 marker for polycystic kidney disease. Nat Genet 2:37, 1992.

Kaplan BS, Fay J, Dillon MJ, et al: Autosomal recessive polycystic kidney disease. Pediatr Nephrol 3:43, 1989.

Kaplan BS, Kaplan P, de Chadarevian J-P, et al: Variable expression within a family of autosomal recessive polycystic kidney disease and congenital hepatic fibrosis. Am J Med Genet 29:639, 1988.

Kaplan BS, Kaplan P, Ruchelli E: Hereditary and congenital malformations of the kidneys. Perinat Clin North Am 19:197, 1992.

Kaplan BS, Restaino 1, Raval DS, et al: Renal failure in the newborn associated with in utero exposure to non-steroidal anti-inflammatory agents. Pediatr Nephrol 8:700, 1994.

Kelalis PP, Malek RS: lnfundibular stenosis, J Urol 125:568, 1981.

Killoran CE, Abbott M, McKusick VA, et al: Overlap of PIV syndrome, VACTERL and Pallister-Hall syndrome: Clinical and molecular analysis. Clin Genet 58:28, 2000.

Kimberling WJ, Kumar S, Gabow PA, et al: Autosomal dominant polycystic kidney disease: Localization of the second gene to chromosome 4q13-q23. Genomics 18:467, 1993.

Krous HF, Richie JP, Sellers B: Glomerulocystic kidney: A hypothesis of origin and pathogenesis. Arch Pathol Lab Med 101:462, 1977.

Kumar S, Deffenbacher K, Cremers CW, et al: Branchio-otorenal syndrome: Identification of novel mutations, molecular characterization, mutation distribution, and prospects for genetic testing. Genet Test 1:243, 1997.

Levine F, Muenke M: VACTERL association with high prenatal lead exposure. Pediatrics 87:390, 1991.

Maas SM, de Jong TP, Buss P, et al: EEC syndrome and genitourinary anomalies: An update. Am J Med Genet 63:472, 1996.

Matsuoka S, Thompson JS, Edwards MC: Imprinting of the gene encoding a human cyclin-dependent kinase inhibitor, p57 (*KIP2*), on chromosome 11p15. Proc Nat Acad Sci 93:3026, 1996.

McPherson E, Carey J, Kramer A, et al: Dominantly inherited renal adysplasia. Am J Med Genet 26:863, 1987.

Metreweli C, Garel L: The echographic diagnosis of infantile renal polycystic disease. Ann Radiol 23:103, 1980.

Moerman P, Fryns J-P, Sastrowijoto SH, et al: Hereditary renal adysplasia: New observations and hypotheses. Pediatr Pathol 14:405, 1994.

Moermnan P, Fryns J-P, Vandenberghe K, et al: The syndrome of diaphragmatic hernia, abnormal face and distal limb anomalies (Fryns syndrome): Further delineation of this multiple congenital anomaly (MCA) syndrome. Am J Med Genet 31:80, 1988.

Peters DJM, Spruit L, Saris JJ, et al: Chromosome 4 localization of a second gene for autosomal dominant polycystic kidney disease. Nat Genet 5:359, 1993.

Pilia G, Hughes-Benzie RM, MacKenzie A, et al: Mutations in *GPC3*, a glypican gene, cause the Simpson-Golabi-Behmel overgrowth syndrome. Nat Genet 12:225, 1996.

Romero R, Cullen M, Jeanty P, et al: The diagnosis of congenital renal anomalies with ultrasound: II. Infantile polycystic kidney disease. Am J Obstet Gynecol 150:259, 1984.

Roume J, Genin E, Cormier-Daire V, et al: A gene for Meckel syndrome maps to chromosome 11q13. Am J Hum Genet 63:1095, 1998.

Salerno A, Kohlhase J, Kaplan BS: Townes-Brocks syndrome and renal dysplasia: A novel mutation in the SALL1 gene. Pediatr Nephrol 14:25, 2000.

Salomon R, Tellier AL, Attie-Bitach T, et al: PAX2 mutations in oligomeganephronia. Kidney Int 59:457, 2001.

Sampson JR, Maheshwar MM, Aspinwall R, et al: Renal cystic disease in tuberous sclerosis: role of the polycystic kidney disease 1 gene. Am J Hum Genet 61:843, 1997.

Schauer GM, Dunn LK, Godmilow L, et al: Prenatal diagnosis of Fraser syndrome at 18.5 weeks gestation, with autopsy findings at 19 weeks. Am J Med Genet 37:583, 1990.

Schilke K, Schaefer F, Waldherr R, et al: A case of Perlman syndrome: Fetal gigantism, renal dysplasia, and severe neurological deficits. Am J Med Genet 91:29, 2000.

Sedman A, Bell P, Manco-Johnson M, et al: Autosomal dominant polycystic kidney disease in childhood: A longitudinal study. Kidney Int 31:1000, 1987.

Stapleton FB, Hilton S, Wilcox J: Transient nephromegaly simulating infantile polycystic disease of the kidneys. Pediatrics 67:554, 1981.

Steinberg SJ, Elcioglu N, Slade CM, Peroxisomal disorders: clinical and biochemical studies in 15 children and prenatal diagnosis in 7 families. Am J Med Genet 85:502, 1999.

Strom EH, Stromine P, Westvik J, et al: Renal cysts in the carbohydrate-deficient glycoprotein syndrome. Pediatr Nephrol 7:253, 1993.

Sumfest JM, Burns MW, Mitchell ME: Aggressive surgical and medical management of autosomal recessive polycystic kidney disease. Urology 42:309, 1993.

Tarry WF, Duckett JW, Stephens FD: The Mayer-Rokitansky syndrome: Pathogenesis, classification and management. J Urol 136:648, 1986.

van Slegtenhorst M, Nellist M, Nagelkerken B, et al: Interaction between hamartin and tuberin, the *TSC1* and *TSC2* gene products. Hum Mol Genet 7:1053, 1998.

Wacksman J, Phipps L: Report of the multicystic kidney registry: Preliminary findings. J Urol 150:1870, 1993.

Wilson PD: Polycystin: New aspects of structure, function, and regulation. J Am Soc Nephrol 12:834, 2001.

Wilson GN, de Chadarevian J-P, Kaplan P, et al: Glutaric aciduria type II: Review of the phenotype and report of an unusual glomerulopathy. Am J Med Genet 32:395, 1989.

Zerres K, Mucher G, Becker J: Prenatal diagnosis of autosomal recessive polycystic kidney disease (ARPKD): Molecular genetics, clinical experience, and fetal morphology. Am J Med Genet 76:137, 1998.

CHAPTER

# 83

# Developmental Abnormalities of the Genitourinary System

**Stephen A. Zderic**

This chapter reviews the major presentations that prompt a urologic consultation in the neonatal period. Anomalies of the urinary tract are discussed first, followed by the disorders of the external genitalia. Prenatal ultrasonography allows most urinary tract anomalies and disorders of the external genitalia to be detected prenatally and thus managed early and effectively in the neonatal period. In the past, many neonates with these conditions presented in critical condition with urosepsis weeks or months after birth.

## PRENATAL DIAGNOSIS

Because of the widespread use of ultrasonography in screening for fetal problems, neonatal urology has undergone profound changes in the past two decades or so. Under optimal circumstances, a relationship already has been established between the urologist and members of the family who sought prenatal consultation. These families have a chance to learn about the possible diagnosis, to plan for evaluation and management in the postnatal period. Two decades ago, most children with congenital anomalies of the urinary tract presented with urosepsis. Prenatal ultrasonography identifies the patients at risk; if indicated, in utero decompression of an obstructed urinary tract (i.e., from posterior urethral valves or ureterocele) may be performed or antibiotic prophylaxis may be initiated in the immediate postnatal period. Prenatal diagnosis has also led to a decrease in the incidence of several major uncorrectable congenital urologic anomalies as parents have opted for termination (Cromie, 2001; Ransley, 1996).

Due primarily to the high fetal urine output, most prenatally discovered cases of hydronephrosis will be benign and self-limiting in nature. Therefore, it is important to give realistic advice and also reassurance in cases of functional hydronephrosis. With congenital anatomic obstructions, fetal intervention may be considered in the most severe cases (Crombleholme, 1984). Recent studies suggest that such interventions offer little benefit to renal function (Coplen et al, 1996), however, but may improve pulmonary development. As mentioned earlier, in addition to the obstructive uropathies, intersex states and other disorders of the external genitalia are being detected with prenatal sonography (Rintoul and Crombleholme, 2002).

## HYDRONEPHROSIS

As mentioned earlier, most patients with prenatally diagnosed hydronephrosis have transient dilatations of the urinary tract (Homsy et al, 1986) that may reflect a more distensible fetal urinary tract and large volumes of dilute fetal urine. With the cardiovascular and hormonal changes in the immediate postnatal period, urine output per kilogram of body weight decreases, resulting in the resolution of the prenatally detected "functional" renal and ureteral dilatation. In addition, the ureter may contain small kinks or folds, which normalize over time. The list of explanations for the spontaneous improvement in these systems is seemingly endless. Despite the fact that most dilatations of the fetal urinary tract prove to be of no long-term significance, a subset of these patients will prove to have anatomic obstructions requiring surgical correction (Cendron et al, 1994).

The neonatal evaluation of antenatal hydronephrosis is dictated by the child's gender, whether the hydronephrosis is unilateral or bilateral, and whether a hydroureter is present. Several schools of thought exist regarding how extensive an initial work-up is required (Blyth et al, 1993; Cendron et al, 1994; Woodward and Frank, 2002; Yerkes et al, 1999) (Fig. 83–1). Bilateral hydroureteronephrosis in a boy should lead to a consideration of the presence of a posterior urethral valve (PUV). This condition can be ruled out by performing an ultrasound examination and voiding cystourethrogram (VCUG) within 24 hours of birth. Unilateral hydronephrosis in a male or female can be managed by performing an ultrasound study of the kidneys and bladder at 2 to 5 days of age. Performing an ultrasound study in the first postnatal hours may show minimal to no hydronephrosis, owing to the significant and physiologic decrease in the urine output during the period of transition to extrauterine life. In these cases, a follow-up study should be performed to ensure that, with the ensuing increase in the urine output over the first few days, the collecting system remains unobstructed (Djeter and Gibbons, 1989). For patients with persisting unilateral hydronephrosis, a VCUG and renal diethylenetriaminepenta-acetic acid (DTPA) scan should be performed at about 1 month of age. In the interim, it is absolutely essential that the infant be discharged to home on antimicrobial prophylaxis, usually one dose of amoxicillin (12.5 mg/kg) at bedtime. The algorithm presented in Figure 83–1 is a reasonable approach to the management of neonatal hydronephrosis.

However, ample controversy exists concerning some of the fine points of this management algorithm. Because 20% of children with prenatal hydronephrosis have reflux, should all children get a VCUG irrespective of their first ultrasound findings? Yerkes and colleagues (1999) have suggested that for patients with mild pelviectasis and no caliectasis or hydroureter, the diagnostic yield of the VCUG is low, and the study may be deferred. Other authors argue in favor of a VCUG for all patients with a prenatal diagnosis of hydronephrosis (Herndon et al, 1999). If results on their initial ultrasound examination are negative, should these children then be placed on antimicrobial prophylaxis until their next ultrasound study is done and judged to be normal?

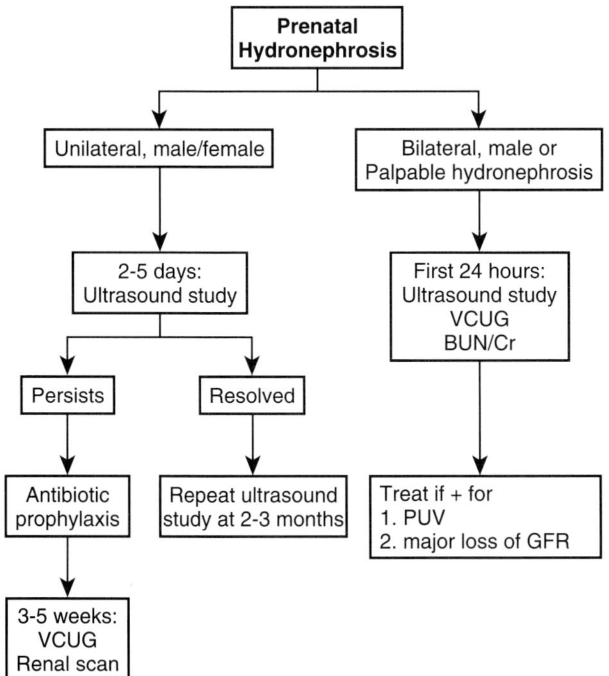


**FIGURE 83–1.** An algorithm for the approach to the work-up of a patient with antenatally diagnosed hydronephrosis. With further experience and clinical outcomes studies, it may be possible to better select which patients require a voiding cystourethrogram (VCUG) and renal MAG3 on DTPA scan. BUN, blood urea nitrogen; Cr, serum creatinine; GFR, glomerular filtration rate; PUV, posterior urethral valve.

With increasing experience and the findings from prospective studies, the algorithm for the postnatal assessment of minimal prenatal hydronephrosis should become more streamlined. It is important to remember that while the uro logic issues are being sorted out, antibiotic prophylaxis is cost effective and protects against urosepsis. Therefore, when the diagnosis is in doubt, the clinician should provide antibiotic prophylaxis.

## OBSTRUCTIVE UROPATHY

### Ureteropelvic Junction Obstruction

The most common obstructive uropathy is seen at the level of the ureteropelvic junction (UPJ). Ultrasonography will reveal a dilated renal pelvis with or without caliectasis, and with no dilatation of the ureter (Fig. 83–2). On the other hand, the presence of a dilated distal ureter is seen with ureterovesical junction obstruction (megaureter). The sonographic appearance of a UPJ obstruction does not always predict its functional significance. Many infants with fairly impressive dilatations of the renal pelvis in the neonatal period show partial or even complete resolution of their hydronephrosis with preservation of renal function (see Fig. 83–2). Functional imaging is obtained before any surgical repair. Although any kidney with an anteroposterior diameter of greater than 2 cm had a greater chance of showing functional compromise in one extensive series (Ransley et al, 1990), many of the patients when evaluated over time may show stable renal function (Koff, 1994). DTPA renal scans allow for careful selection of those patients with a loss of function as defined by a decrease in the glomerular filtration rate. Disagreement remains on how much functional impairment necessitates intervention (Allen, 1992; Koff et al, 1994). Some authorities advocate intervention only if the differential function in the affected kidney falls below 35% (Cartwright et al, 1992), whereas others place the limit at 40%. Still others rely heavily on a "well-tempered" diuretic renogram and the furosemide washout curves to identify those patients whose urinary tract is truly obstructed (Conway and Maizels, 1993).

Many patients will be found to have good function and rapid washout curves despite a significant degree of hydronephrosis (Fig. 83–3). For those patients in whom a UPJ obstruction is diagnosed by sonography, and in whom the renal scan shows diminished function, pyeloplasty is indicated. Placing an infant with a poorly functioning kidney on antimicrobial prophylaxis is not effective because a kidney functioning this poorly will not deliver enough antibiotic into the collecting system, leaving the child at risk for urosepsis. It is important to note that with most severe UPJ obstructions, the kidney does not recover full function following surgical correction. In addition, infection in the presence of a UPJ obstruction makes recovery of function less likely. No preoperative test will predict recovery of renal function following relief of obstructive uropathy; clinicians are left with the option of placing a temporary percutaneous nephrostomy or carrying out a primary repair.

Finally, few prenatally diagnosed cases of UPJ obstruction require immediate repair. These cases rarely result in palpable hydronephrosis, and most affected infants will have good renal function, allowing elective evaluation and repair at 3 to 6 weeks of life. This group of patients may be divided into three subgroups, according to Homsy and colleagues (1990). One third will be obstructed and require immediate intervention, and one third will have a normal postnatal evaluation. The remaining one third may be observed with serial sonograms and renal scans. Of this observed group, up to one third of the patients may ultimately need surgical correction. The postnatal evaluation of prenatally diagnosed hydronephrosis must contain two key elements: (1) antimicrobial prophylaxis until such time as the urinary tract is judged normal, or the patient is less susceptible to infection, and (2) thorough follow-up evaluation. Although expectant management may eliminate surgical procedures that may offer little benefit, this advantage comes at the price of the need for careful follow-up evaluation. This aspect of management must be made clear to the family in no uncertain terms.

### Multicystic Dysplastic Kidney

The diagnosis of multicystic dysplastic kidney (MCDK) is applied to a kidney that on ultrasound examination is seen to consist of multiple cysts of roughly equal size, which gives rise to a fairly classic "bunch of grapes" pattern (Fig. 83–4). The contralateral kidney will show signs of hypertrophy, as manifested by increases in length and width, and the affected kidney will have no function on the DTPA scan. If

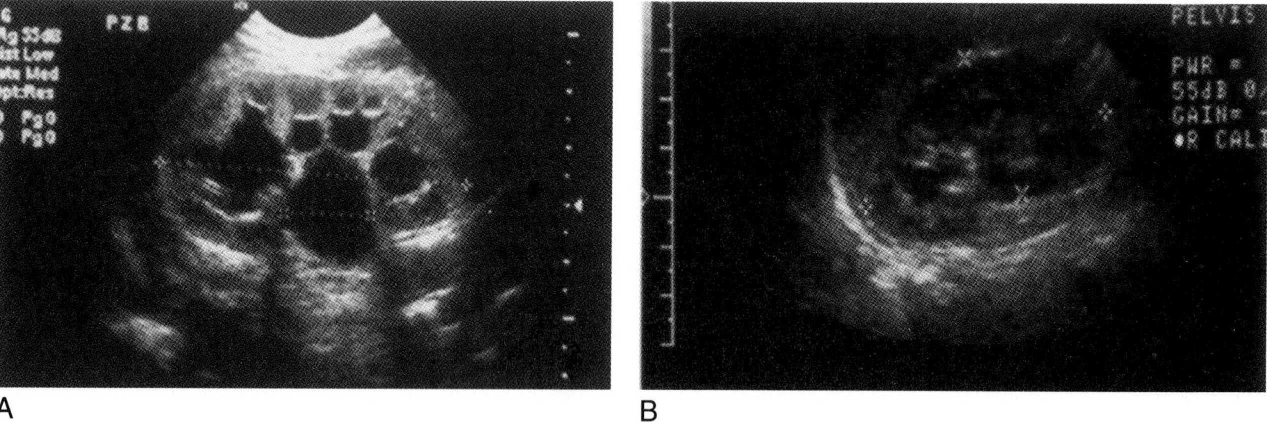

**FIGURE 83–2.** An example of antenatal hydronephosis consistent with a partial ureteropelvic junction obstruction (**A**) that spontaneously resolved over a 6-month interval (**B**).

the MCDK has one large, centrally located cyst, it may not be possible to rule out a severe UPJ obstruction. In these rare instances it may prove necessary to explore the kidney to see if there is any salvageable renal function that might be amenable to relief of the obstruction. In most cases of MCDK, the cysts will involute completely. Should these children have yearly ultrasound examinations to check for involution? It might be argued that no follow-up evaluation is needed. It is reassuring, however, to check on the solitary remaining kidney, as metachronous contralateral obstruction has been reported (Weiser et al, 2002). Concerns have been raised about the occasional case reports of malignancy in MCDK. It has been estimated that 80,000 nephrectomies would have to be performed to save one patient with MCDK from developing a malignancy. In practice, some families opt for nephrectomy if, on yearly sonography, involution fails to occur.

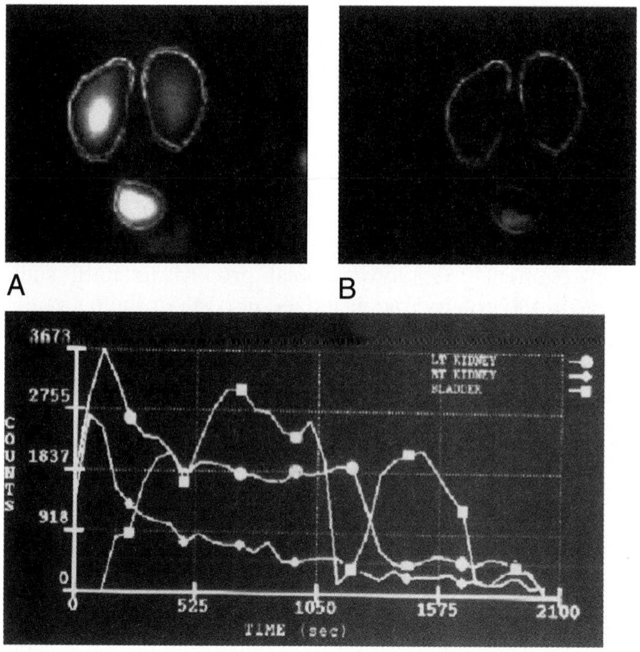

**FIGURE 83–3. A,** This renal MAG3 scan demonstrates equal function in the right and the left kidneys but marked stasis in the left kidney. **B** and **C,** Following administration of furosemide, the stasis in the left renal pelvis clear quickly.

## Ureterovesical Junction Obstruction: Megaureter

Primary megaureters account for 15% of prenatally diagnosed cases of hydronephrosis and are characterized by pelviectasis, caliectasis, and ureteral dilatation. Ureteral dilatation is best seen behind a distended bladder, and a VCUG is indicated to rule out reflux. Reflux into a partially obstructed system can occur, creating the paradoxical refluxing obstructed megaureter. In such cases, the contrast that refluxes into the ureter is quite dilute when compared with that within the bladder. Furthermore, on the post-void views, the contrast will be "held up" within the ureter. Some investigators believe that refluxing primary megaureter should be repaired, because an infection

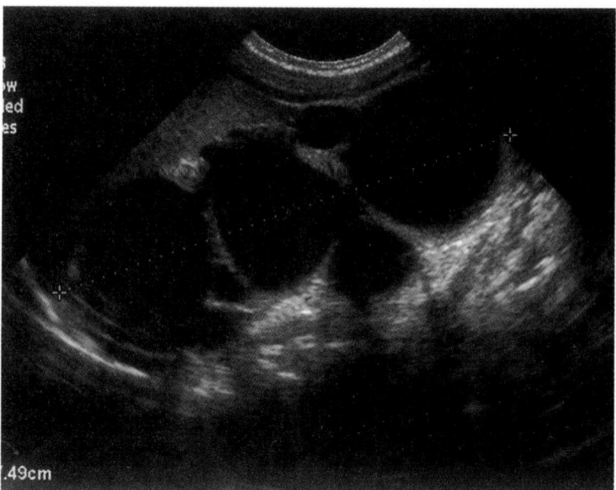

**FIGURE 83–4.** Sonographic view of a multicystic dysplastic kidney in which multiple cysts that do not communicate with another are grouped together, giving the typical "bunch of grapes" appearance. No function was noted on the patient's renal scan, confirming this diagnosis.

developing in a partially obstructed system can be especially severe. The renal DTPA scan is essential to the work-up (Fig. 83–5). If it shows good renal function, these patients may be safely managed on antimicrobial prophylaxis. In a longitudinal study, Baskin and colleagues (1994) showed that renal function is well preserved, and in many instances, the morphologic appearance of the system is substantially improved. Thus, unlike the UPJ obstructions, which are associated with a 20% to 30% risk of renal decompensation with need for subsequent surgery, primary megaureters seem to do better with very few changes in the course of management. The encouraging results achieved by restricting management to thorough follow-up evaluation, with no surgical intervention, in the study by Baskin and colleagues (1994) were obtained in a select group of patients with good renal function at the outset. Good renal function was defined as contribution by the involved kidney of greater than 35% to the overall GFR as determined by scan. On the other hand, for kidneys whose split function fell below 35%, the authors performed surgery to relieve the obstructive uropathy.

### Posterior Urethral Valves

Most cases of posterior urethral valves (PUVs) today will be detected on prenatal sonography; the clinical manifestations vary across a wide spectrum. An extreme example would be the case of a child who was born with chronic renal insufficiency and whose creatinine level is rising, in which prenatal sonography revealed severe oligohydramnios. If the oligohydramnios is severe enough, such infants also may suffer from severe respiratory insufficiency secondary to pulmonary hypoplasia. In highly selected cases, extracorporeal membrane oxygenation (ECMO) has been used to get past the initial period of respiratory failure, and long-term survivors have been reported. Most of these survivors, however, will require renal transplantation at some point (Gibbons et al, 1993). At the other end of the spectrum would be the presence of PUVs of minimal functional significance. If the abnormality is not detected in utero, similar to neonates with other obstructive uropathies, patients with PUVs may present with urosepsis. The prenatal diagnosis by ultrasound examination offers the pediatric urologist an opportunity to intervene before the obstructive uropathy is further compromised by the additional burden of infection.

The postnatal evaluation of a child with suspected PUVs should begin with a renal and bladder ultrasound study. The examination should be performed first without a catheter in the bladder so as to reveal the anatomy of the urinary tract in its distended form. There will usually be severe bilateral hydroureteronephrosis. In severe cases, the renal parenchyma will be of extremely poor quality, comprising a thin rim with a highly echogenic nature. When these findings are associated with a thick-walled bladder in a male infant, the diagnosis is unlikely to be anything other than PUVs. Ultrasound examination of the bladder also may reveal a dilated posterior urethra (Fig. 83–6). A catheter should be passed into the child's bladder and the sonographic examination with the same views repeated to get a sense of whether bladder decompression improves the morphology of the upper urinary tract at all. In some instances, the posterior urethra is so severely distorted that the catheter may curl up within it.

The diagnosis of PUVs is made from a fluoroscopic VCUG. This study will demonstrate a dilated posterior urethra, valve cusps at the distal aspect of the prostatic fossa (see Fig. 83–6), a heavily trabeculated bladder, and an associated high-grade vesicoureteral reflux in many cases. Once the diagnosis is established, endoscopic valve

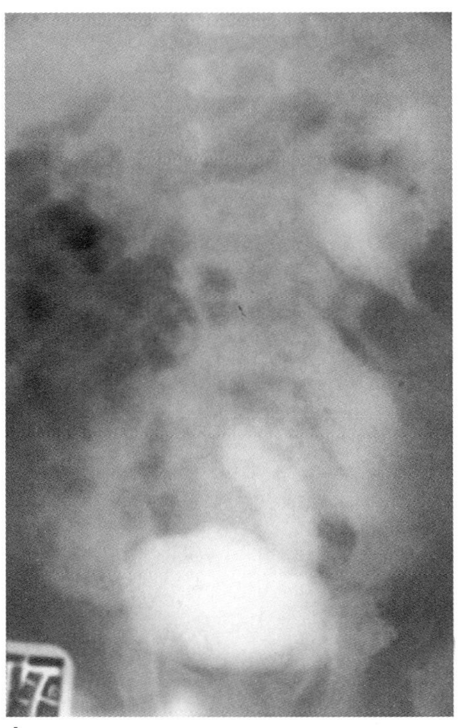

A

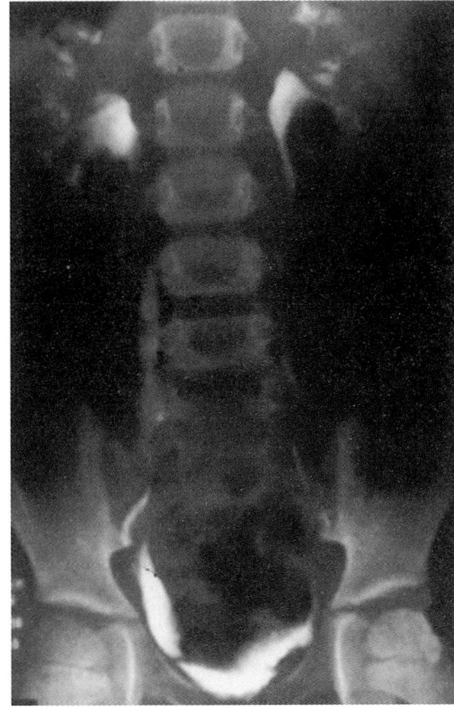

B

**FIGURE 83–5. A,** This radiograph shows significant hydroureteronephrosis that was diagnosed by antenatal sonography and was shown to be consistent with bilateral primary megaureters. Renal function was normal despite the abnormal morphologic appearance. **B,** With time, the radiographic findings showed marked improvement.

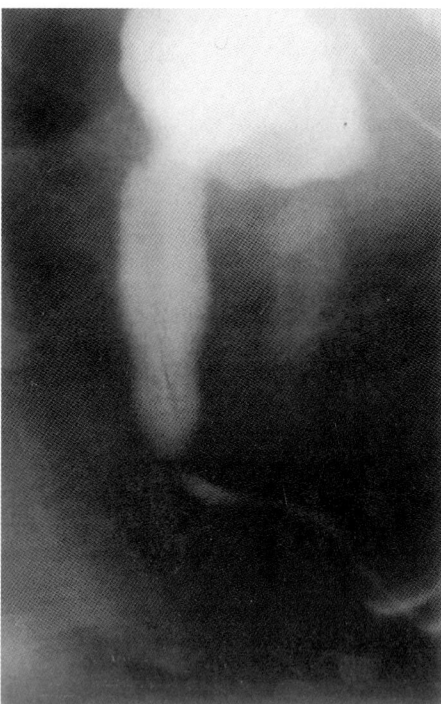

**FIGURE 83–6.** This voiding cystourethrogram shows a classic posterior urethral valve, with narrowing of the urethra at the most distal end of the prostate. This area corresponds to a flap of tissue that serves as an obstructing valve leaflet.

ablation is indicated (Zderic, 1996). In rare instances, the pediatric urologist may opt for a temporizing vesicostomy. A circumcision should be performed at the time of the valve resection, to minimize the chances for development of urinary tract infection (Wiswell and Geschke, 1989) in this patient population at high risk for this complication.

In severe cases of PUV, decompression may result in a postobstructive diuresis. For this reason, neonates with PUVs who undergo decompression with placement of a catheter should remain in the neonatal intensive care unit (NICU) for fluid and electrolyte monitoring. The diuresis can be quite dramatic, necessitating hourly tallies of urine output with appropriate replacement of fluid and electrolyte losses. Failure to keep up with losses can easily produce hypotension, further aggravating the renal insufficiency. Once the child has been catheterized, antibiotics should be started and the child's medical condition should be optimized before any thought is given to operative intervention.

Up to 30% of these patients may require renal replacement therapy during their lifetimes (Smith et al, 1996). In the neonatal period, every effort must be made to optimize renal function and to maintain a sterile urine with the use of antibiotic prophylaxis. In a subset of patients with valves who present with only unilateral reflux and dysplasia, the valve may act as a pop-off valve to lower bladder pressure, sparing the contralateral kidney. A number of these pop-off mechanisms have been described, and all are associated with better long-term renal (Rittenberg et al, 1988) and bladder (Kaefer et al, 1995) function. Families must be cautioned that these infants have poor urinary concentrating ability; their additional fluid requirements make them especially susceptible to dehydration with even mild diarrhea or emesis. The initial follow-up evaluation within 1 month consists of a physical examination, renal-bladder ultrasound study, and serum creatinine measurement. Antibiotic prophylaxis should be maintained for a long period in these patients.

## Ureterocele

The ureterocele is a cystic dilatation of the distal ureter that protrudes into the urinary bladder and may extend past the bladder neck into the urethra. Ureteroceles are found primarily in duplex systems, where they are always associated with the upper pole renal parenchyma. The renal parenchyma seen in the upper pole of the duplex systems usually is of poor quality and may even contain dysplastic elements. The ureterocele is by definition an obstructed system; accordingly, measures must be instituted to prevent the neonate from developing urosepsis. Renal-bladder ultrasound examination of a ureterocele will show three characteristic findings (Fig. 83–7). First, hydronephrosis will always be associated with the upper pole of a duplex system (although single systems also may contain ureteroceles). Second, a significant ureteral dilatation down to the level of the bladder will be seen, and finally a cystic lesion within the lumen of the bladder close to the bladder base will be demonstrated. A VCUG will complete the work-up and aid the urologist in assessing whether any reflux is found into the ipsilateral or contralateral ureter(s). Ureteroceles may prolapse into the urethra; these lesions constititute the most common form of bladder outlet obstruction in female neonates, in whom they manifest as a cystic bulge within the labia.

Several surgical options exist for the management of the newborn with a ureterocele: endoscopic puncture, upper pole partial nephrectomy, and excision of the ureterocele with a combined reimplantation. Finally, an additional surgical approach is to perform a cutaneous ureterostomy and then wait to carry out a definitive lower tract reconstruction in the older child.

## Ectopic Ureters

Most ectopic ureters today will be detected with prenatal sonography that results in a neonatal evaluation. Findings on physical examination in these patients will often be unremarkable. A male will never be incontinent secondary to an ectopic ureter, because the ureter will always enter above the level of the external sphincter. However, in females, the ureter may be ectopic to the urethra or vaginal vault, where it may produce urine on a continuous basis and detected on physical examination. Making this diagnosis early in life prevents urosepsis from developing in an obstructed or partially obstructed system and simplifies the process of toilet training for a young female.

Most ectopic ureters will be found in duplex systems, where they always represent the upper pole moiety. The ultrasound findings in ectopic ureter include the presence of hydronephrosis, usually of an upper pole of a duplex system (although single systems also may be involved), a dilated distal ureter that lies behind the bladder, and an

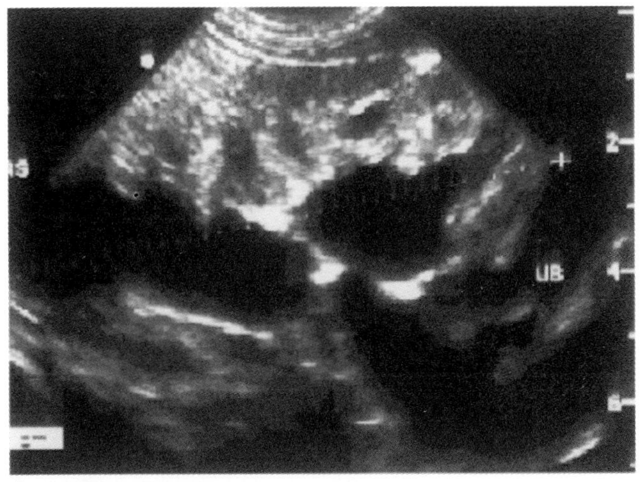
A

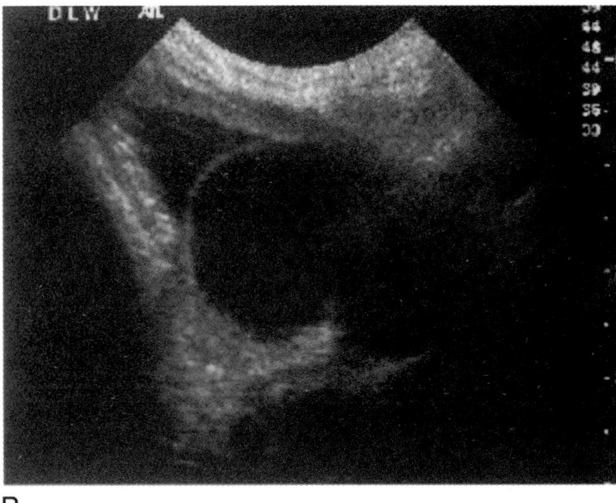
B

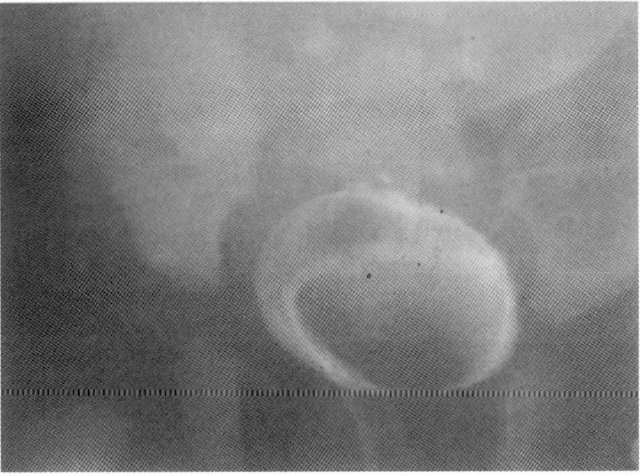
C

**FIGURE 83–7.** These images demonstrate upper pole hydronephosis that is secondary to a dilated ureter (**A**), which empties into a larger ureterocele within the bladder (evident in **B**). There is also secondary dilation of the lower pole renal pelvis. The ureterocele is demonstrated as the cystic filling defect on the bladder views from the ultrasound study (**B**) as well as the voiding cystourethrogram (**C**).

extension of this dilated distal ureter past the bladder neck, with no cystic lesion within the bladder itself, as is seen with a ureterocele. The VCUG is important in the evaluation of these patients, because in 70% of the cases it may demonstrate reflux into the ectopic ureter. However, the reflux may not be apparent on the first void, and it may be necessary to "cycle" the bladder several times before such reflux may be demonstrated.

An endoscopic option does not exist for repairing an ectopic ureter. The open surgical options (Snyder, 1996) include a partial nephrectomy of the upper pole with or without an excision of the distal stump, a complete nephrectomy in a nonfunctioning kidney, a temporizing cutaneous ureterostomy with delayed reimplantation and excision of the distal stump, and an immediate complete reconstruction with reimplantation and excision of the ectopic stump. The urologist's choice among these options will be dictated by the amount of function present within the upper pole segment, which is often 15% or less of total GFR.

### Prune-Belly Syndrome

Patients with prune-belly syndrome present with a lax and floppy abdominal wall that is extremely thin, bilateral undescended testes, a flattened diaphragm with flaring of the ribs, and a massively dilated upper urinary tract and bladder (Fig. 83–8). In severe cases, respiratory insufficiency may mandate temporary mechanical ventilation until the infant is strong enough to be weaned off support. In older series, pulmonary complications were a common source of neonatal demise. Today, with the advent of prenatal sonography, such severe cases are being diagnosed earlier. These neonates are often born with significant renal dysplasia and go on to develop end-stage renal disease. Indeed, if the serum creatinine fails to fall below 1.0 mg/dL by 1 year of age, the infant with prune-belly syndrome is more likely to develop end-stage renal disease (Noh et al, 1999). However, this disease manifests across a wide spectrum; some patients may not develop renal insufficiency until much later in life, if at all, despite their massively dilated urinary tracts.

Prune-belly syndrome is a clinical diagnosis that should lead to the institution of prophylactic antibiotics. An ultrasound study to assess the renal parenchyma also is warranted, but a VCUG is not. Instrumenting a neonate with prune-belly syndrome who is voiding satisfactorily is to be avoided, as such procedures will increase the risk of urosepsis owing to the presence of the huge, floppy, and poorly draining bladder. Furthermore, discovering whether such a child is refluxing or not will add little to neonatal management; these infants will stay on antibiotic

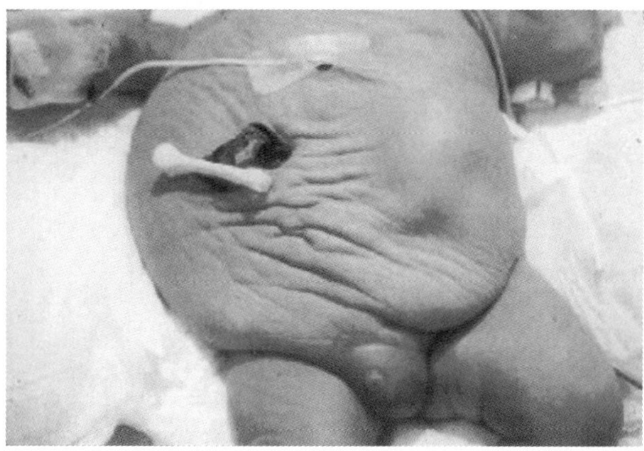

A

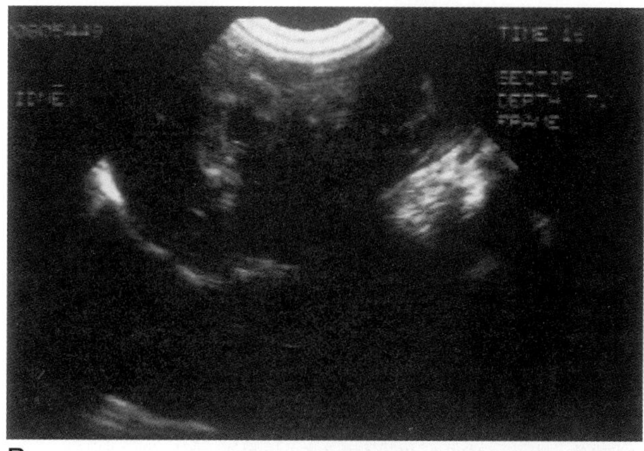

B

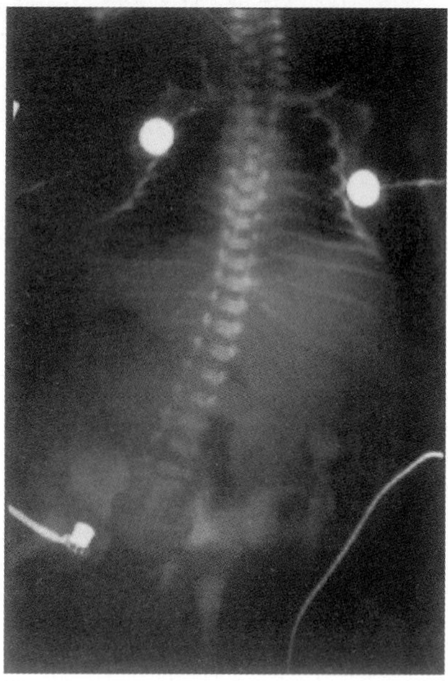

C

**FIGURE 83–8.** (See also Color Plate 83–8.) The classic wrinkled abdominal wall seen in the prune-belly syndrome is accompanied by bilateral undescended testes (**A**). Affected patients will have marked hydronephrosis. In severe cases as illustrated here, these small kidneys may have a markedly dysmorphic sonographic appearance (**B**), and renal insufficiency may be present from the beginning. In cases with severe renal insufficiency, pulmonary development may be compromised, as evident on the radiograph (**C**); the patient required prolonged mechanical ventilation in the neonatal period.

prophylaxis regardless of the VCUG results. The key is to maintain a sterile urine and to institute careful follow-up evaluation (Noh et al, 1999). If, in the neonatal period, the voiding dynamics are significantly altered, a vesicostomy may prove to be an ideal means of decompressing the urinary tract. It can be surprising that despite the tremendous distortions seen within the urinary tract, the bladder may empty quite adequately, and improvement may be seen over time in the quality of the upper tracts. Reconstructive procedures for these children consist of bilateral orchiopexies and an abdominal wall plication

## The Exstrophies

### *Bladder Exstrophy*

The patient with classic bladder exstrophy presents with a bladder plate that is protruding in the suprapubic area and that extends up to just below the umbilicus (Fig. 83–9). In males, there is an associated complete epispadias because the urethra never develops. In both males and females, there is lack of formation of the bladder neck; thus, there is no mechanism for urinary continence. This diagnosis is being increasingly established in utero; failure to image the bladder on several prenatal sonograms should raise suspicion of this diagnosis. Classic exstrophy is not associated with any other associated anomalies, and many families opt to continue with the pregnancy. These children have an excellent prognosis and with proper management can lead nearly normal lives.

The traditional approach to the patient with classic exstrophy used to be a staged reconstruction beginning with a tubularization of the bladder plate within the first 24 hours of life (Canning et al, 1996). These children were left incontinent until the age of 5 to 7 years, when they underwent a second urologic reconstruction to create a competent bladder neck. This took place at a time when the child was capable of self-catheterization, to empty the bladder and to maintain safe storage pressures. In some series, up to 90% of these children required long-term clean intermittent catheterization (CIC) to achieve continence and maintain stable renal function.

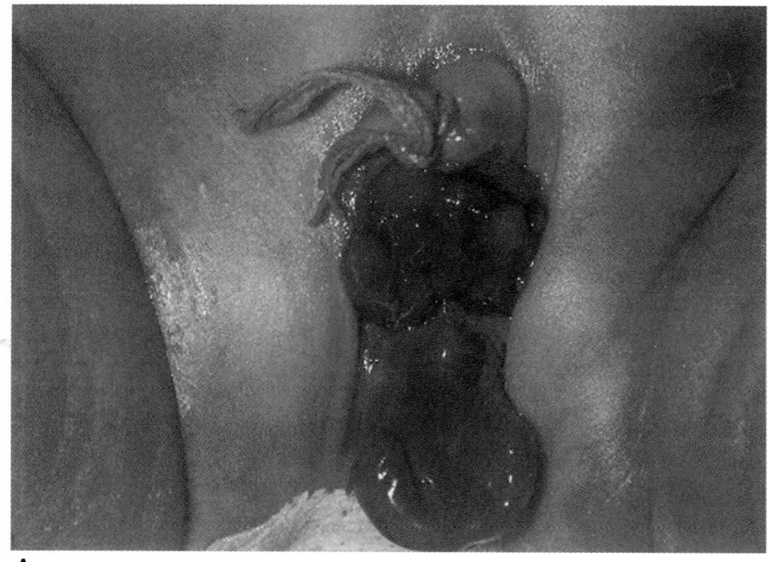


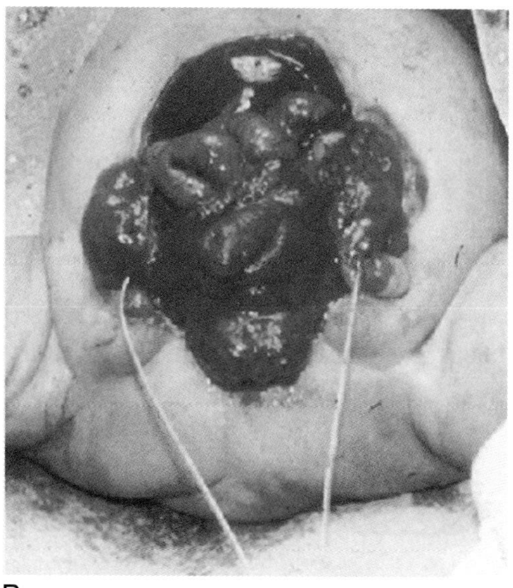


**FIGURE 83–9.** (See also Color Plate 83–9.) The appearance of classic bladder exstrophy (**A**), in contrast with the dramatic appearance of cloacal exstrophy (**B**). In cloacal exstrophy, the bladder halves are separated by the presence of a large cecal plate, and a protruding ileal stump. **B**, In this intraoperative photograph, the omphalocele has been removed to expose the small bowel and liver.

These problems with staged exstrophy reconstruction outcomes led Mitchell and Bagli (1996) to propose a one-stage reconstruction within the first month of life. In males, this procedure includes a splitting of the penis with separation of the corporal bodies and urethral realignment. With this method, the bladder neck is reapproximated in an attempt to provide an anatomic closure offering a resistance that stimulates bladder growth; this approach probably will increase the percentage of patients who are able to void spontaneously while maintaining continence.

### *Cloacal Exstrophy*

The infant with cloacal exstrophy presents with several obvious clinical features (see Fig. 83–9) that include the presence of two bladder halves fully exposed on the abdomen; an abdominal midline that consists of the entire cecal plate that is wide open, allowing for egress of stool; often, a protruding prolapsed distal ileum; and an omphalocele of variable size (Canning et al, 1996; Zderic et al, 2002). In addition to these obvious malformations, 50% of these children will have associated spinal dysraphism of various degrees. From a medical standpoint, the risks of fluid loss, hypothermia, and infection from the exposed viscera mandate covering the exposed viscera with plastic wrap and immediately transferring the patient to the NICU.

The first stage of reconstruction should be undertaken as soon as the child's condition has stabilized. A central line is placed; all of these children will have some element of short bowel syndrome and will require hyperalimentation for varying periods postoperatively. The goals of the initial surgery are to tubularize the cecal plate and create a colostomy, followed by a reapproximation of the two bladder halves. In some instances, only the omphalocele is closed first, and the bladder halves are left in place for a second-stage repair. For most of these children, continence will still come at the expense of intermittent catheterization, because 50% or more have a neural tube deficit.

Male infants with cloacal exstrophy will present with testes and rudimentary corporal bodies. The traditional recommendation for these patients was that they be assigned female gender of rearing, in light of the earlier dismal long-term phalloplasty results. However, today much more is known about the sexual differentiation of the fetal brain. This basic scientific information has been corroborated by several reassigned patients reverting to a male role (Reiner, 2002). Indeed, in view of this information and the newer surgical techniques available (Mitchell and Bagli, 1996), the pendulum is swinging away from reassignment and toward preserving male gender.

### Spina Bifida

The urologist's primary goal in management of the neonatal patient with spina bifida is the preservation of renal function. In these patients, the main threat to renal function may be traced to the abnormal bladder function. The traditional approach to management of patients with spina bifida called for closure of the defect in the neonatal period. However, as spina bifida is frequently diagnosed with prenatal sonography, a randomized clinical trial is being performed at present comparing outcomes of fetal versus neonatal spina bifida repair. Thus, in the next 5 years or so, more will be known about the long-term outcomes for these patients after in utero repair.

At present with postnatal repair, a renal bladder ultrasound study should be obtained within 1 week of closure to look for any evidence of hydronephrosis. If this sonogram is normal, the child is discharged to home and a video-urodynamic assessment is performed at 4 weeks of age. The video-urodynamic studies are then repeated at 6 months of age and thereafter on a yearly basis until age 5. Yearly ultrasound examinations also must be performed to ensure the upper tracts are protected. If the initial ultrasound findings are abnormal, showing dilated upper tracts, the video-urodynamic studies are performed sooner.

The purpose of the urodynamic studies is to identify in advance the "hostile bladder." A "hostile bladder" has poor function, with the potential to compromise renal function. Grading scales have been designed to identify in advance those infants at risk of upper urinary tract damage (Bauer et al, 1984; Bauer, 1992; McGuire et al, 1981; Perez et al, 1992). If there is evidence for the presence of a "hostile bladder," many groups favor the immediate institution of CIC in conjunction with antimicrobial prophylaxis and anticholinergic medications (Kasabian et al, 1992; Sutherland et al, 1995). In addition to the benefits of CIC on preservation of renal function, recent studies suggest that early institution of CIC and anticholinergic therapy may improve bladder compliance in the long run and thus lessen the likelihood of future bladder augmentation surgery (Kaefer et al, 1999).

An additional option is the surgical creation of a vesicostomy. Although CIC offers many benefits, compliance may be difficult with the regimen required to maintain a safe storage pressure. Vesicostomy is a valid option because it is associated with preservation of the upper urinary tract (Snyder et al, 1983) and can dramatically diminish admission rates for urosepsis (Zhylan et al, 1993). This last point is especially a factor in the child with spina bifida who experiences vesicoureteral reflux, because it is impossible to maintain sterile urine with use of CIC. Indeed, a child with spina bifida and vesicoureteral reflux who is maintained on CIC is at greater risk of developing pyelonephritis.

The child without evidence for having a "hostile bladder" may be followed with ultrasound examinations every 6 to 12 months, with the realization that the risk for upper urinary tract decompensation is less than 10%. Such children must, however, be evaluated with at least one examination annually, because the bladder may undergo changes over time, especially within the first 3 years of life. At 3 to 4 years of age, the issues of fecal and urinary continence must be dealt with. These children will require fecal training, and in most cases a daily enema followed by planned timed evacuation. Urinary continence also is rare in this subset of patients. For this reason, these children must master the process of CIC. Once this has been accomplished, further surgical reconstruction of the lower urinary tract may be required in order to achieve urinary continence.

### Imperforate Anus

The diagnosis of imperforate anus will prompt an immediate general surgical consultation and may result in a diverting colostomy. It is worth remembering that affected infants often have associated urologic findings (Rich et al, 1988). Urologic abnormalities are more likely for patients in whom the rectum ends in the supralevator position (30%) as opposed to the infralevator position (15%). Up to 40% of these patients may have an associated lumbosacral lesion such as spina bifida occulta or a tethered cord. This is an important subset of patients to identify, for their bladders are already at risk for voiding dysfunction even before any rectal pull-through is performed. These patients will have a neurogenic bladder and often require intermittent catheterization to achieve continence.

The urologic radiographic work-up for these patients should consist of a renal-bladder ultrasound study and a VCUG. The renal sonogram will identify those patients with renal agenesis, anomalies of renal fusion, or occasional obstructive uropathy. The VCUG will identify those patients with reflux so that antibiotic prophylaxis can be initiated. In addition, the VCUG may identify any signs of a coloprostatic or colovaginal fistula and aid in the subsequent anorectal reconstruction. Finally, a magnetic resonance imaging (MRI) study of the lumbosacral spine will identify that subset of patients with a tethered cord or spinal dysraphism.

### Cloacal Anomalies

Cloacal anomalies of caudal differentiation manifest as a wide spectrum of abnormalities. One common variant in the female neonate is the combination of a completely "normal" although anteriorly placed rectum and a urogenital sinus into which the vagina and urethra merge (Fig. 83–10). Such neonates may present with a pelvic mass that is cystic and posterior to the bladder on pelvic sonography. Close inspection of their genitalia reveals one common sinus, which is narrow and offers high resistance to urinary flow. As a consequence, the bladder empties into a vaginal vault that progressively expands. In severe cases, it may even produce ureteral obstruction and hydronephrosis. The definitive diagnosis is made by a genitogram. Some cases demonstrate complete fusion, so that the urethra, vagina, and rectum empty into the perineum via one common channel. The embryology, anatomy, and complex management of these rare cases have been described in great detail by Hendren (1986) and Pena (1995). These anomalies constitute neonatal surgical emergencies, in which management decisions are highly individualized.

## DISORDERS OF THE GENITALIA

### Undescended Testes

Up to 3% of all term males may have evidence for an undescended testicle, although by 1 year of age, this drops to about 0.8%. Most of these testes that are going to descend do so by 6 to 9 months of life. Up to 30% of patients may present with bilateral undescended testes. The presence of bilateral impalpable undescended testes in a newborn male must be considered to represent an intersex state until proved otherwise. Failure to appreciate the significance of bilateral and impalpable undescended

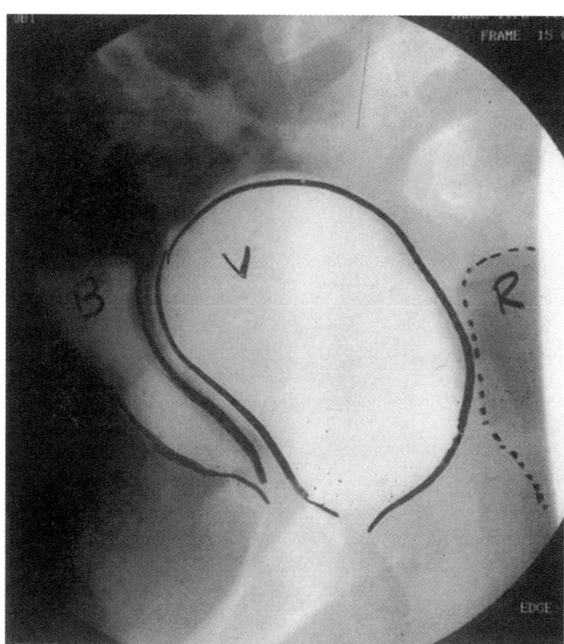


**FIGURE 83–10.** This genitogram, performed by retrograde injection of contrast into a single sinus anterior to the patient's rectum, demonstrates the anteriorly placed bladder (B) and posteriorly placed vagina (V). The vagina and urethra merged into a common sinus, which then traveled a distance of 2 cm prior to emerging on the perineal body. The rectum (R) was normally placed. The vagina distended as a result of urinary entrapment, and the patient presented with a lower abdominal mass.

testes in the NICU means that a diagnosis of congenital adrenal hyperplasia may be missed (Fig. 83–11). Although in most cases of bilateral impalpable testes the infant proves to be a normal male, neonates with congenital adrenal hyperplasia often have inadequate cortisol and mineralocorticoid function, leaving the child susceptible to shock and delaying assignment of gender of rearing. Similar concerns arise if undescended testes are found in the presence of a hypospadias (see later section on ambiguous genitalia).

The neonate with a unilateral undescended testis and a normal phallus may be referred for a urologic follow-up evaluation at 6 months of age. At that time a careful examination will reveal whether the testis is impalpable, in which case surgical intervention should be undertaken. The impalpable testis may be a true intra-abdominal gonad or a testis that is intermittently passing in and out of a large patent processus vaginalis, or the testis may be completely absent secondary to an antenatal torsion. If testicular agenesis is present, the contralateral testis usually has undergone some degree of compensatory hypertrophy, with an increased volume noted on examination or by sonographic measurements (Huff et al, 1992). The measurement of volume alone, however, does not preclude the need for exploration. Parents need to be reminded that in 80% of cases in which exploration is undertaken for an impalpable testis, the testis is found and a successful orchiopexy is performed. The child who presents at 6 months of age with an undescended testis high in the inguinal canal also is a candidate for surgical intervention, because it is unlikely to descend on its own. If, however, the testis is near the scrotum, a repeat examination is prudent. A retractile testis may also present at this point, in which the testis may be pulled into the scrotal sac but will stay down only if there is a gentle overstretch of the cremasteric muscle fibers. Affected infants require close follow-up evaluation.

Long-term issues facing patients with cryptorchidism include a significantly increased risk of infertility and a slightly increased risk of testicular malignancy. Fertility rates vary greatly, depending on whether the cryptorchidism is unilateral or bilateral. Long-term follow-up studies looking at paternity have suggested that 90% of boys with unilateral cryptorchidism report paternity in later years (Cendron et al, 1989; Lee et al, 2001). However, for bilateral undescended testes, the paternity rate dropped to 50% for patients operated on in the first 3 years of life. As the patients' age at bilateral orchiopexy increases, the paternity rates decline (Lee et al, 2001). A number of centers have shown that cryptorchidism results in lower sperm counts despite surgical correction, and that the lowest counts are seen in those patients with bilateral cryptorchidism. Testicular biopsy at the time of orchiopexy may offer a potential to identify those patients at the greatest risk of infertility 20 and 30 years later (Huff et al, 1989). A histologic scoring system allowing for the prediction of a high-risk cohort of patients was recently validated with long-term follow-up semen analyses. The ability to predict low sperm counts using biopsy criteria also may allow for early hormonal treatment to enhance future fertility prospects in this group of patients. Although the timing of orchiopexy has been controversial, Lee and colleagues' (1996) long-term follow-up data suggest that, for bilateral undescended testes, an earlier age of surgery correlates with a better paternity rate.

There is an increased risk of malignancy for a child with an undescended testis, as the relative risk for testicular cancer in patients with an undescended testis increases anywhere from 9- to 40-fold over that in the normal population. This observation must be tempered, however, with the reality that testicular cancer is rare. This means that the overall lifetime risk of developing testicular cancer remains low for the individual patient. Orchiopexy is recommended, to place both testes in their proper scrotal position and to allow for monthly self-examination once the patient enters the pubertal years.

## Testicular Torsion

Torsion of the testes is a rare event in the neonatal period, but there is controversy as to its optimal management. The most important point in arriving at a management decision is a determination of what the scrotum looked like at birth. Was it blue, tense, and painless on initial exam in the delivery room? Was the scrotum normal initially, and then develop swelling accompanied by pain? The newborn that presents in the delivery room with an initially painless, blue, and tense hemiscrotum will be most likely to have an antenatal torsion. In this type of torsion, the entire tunica vaginalis and spermatic vessels

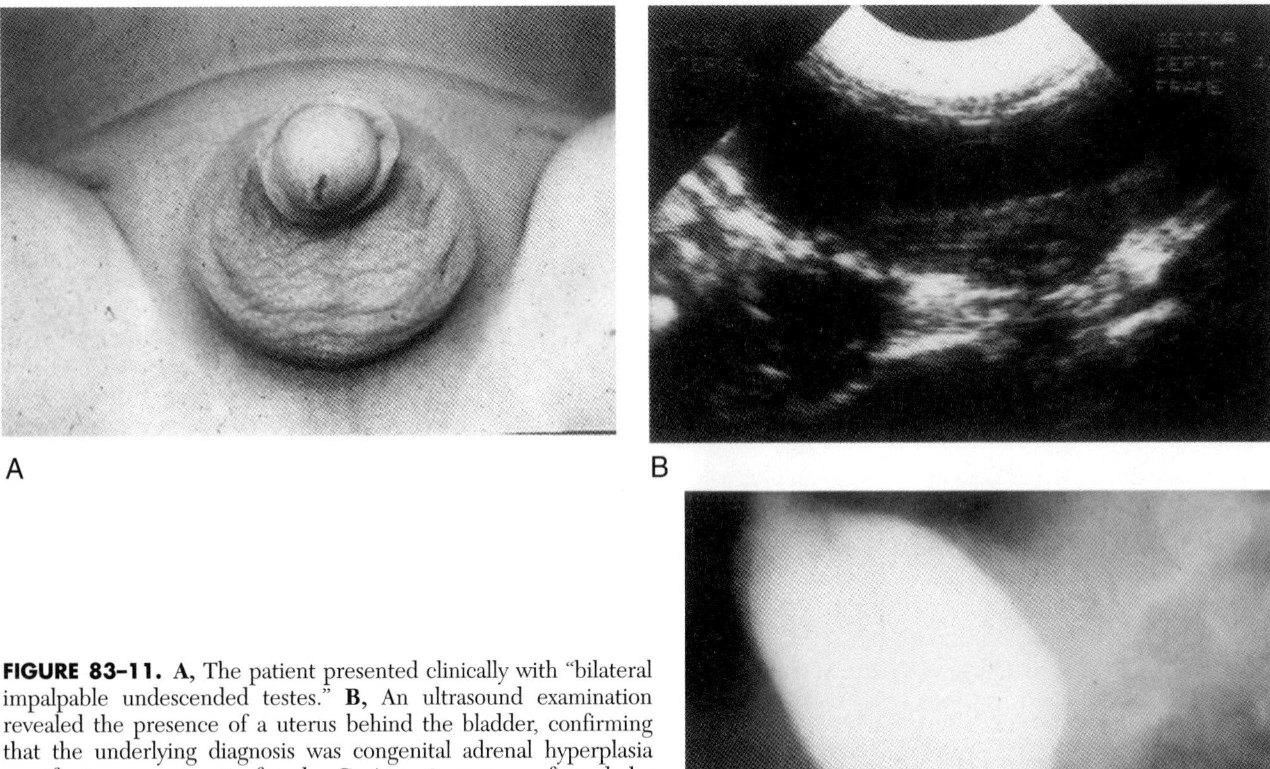


**FIGURE 83–11.** **A,** The patient presented clinically with "bilateral impalpable undescended testes." **B,** An ultrasound examination revealed the presence of a uterus behind the bladder, confirming that the underlying diagnosis was congenital adrenal hyperplasia manifesting in a genetic female. **C,** A genitogram confirmed the presence of a vagina, and a cervical imprint also was noted.

are twisted in such a way as to occlude the vascular pedicle and render the testis ischemic. This may often occur during the last trimester, and thus what one is seeing in the delivery room is a late presentation of a process that has been ongoing for some time. In fact, if the antenatal torsion occurs early enough in gestation all inflammation will have resolved, and the neonate presents with an impalpable testis. Surgical findings include blood vessels and a vas deferens that end blindly at a common point where a small nubbin is occasionally found.

The controversy about management of torsion revolves around what to do for the infant who is born with a clinically apparent torsion. Immediate exploration in the hours after birth does not result in testicular salvage. However, there are several case reports documented in which bilateral metachronous torsions occurred, often with the initially normal testis subsequently undergoing a torsion (Kay et al, 1980). For this reason, some authors have advocated proceeding with an exploration to surgically tack down the normal testis and prevent a torsion in the remaining healthy gonad (Jerkins et al, 1983; Kaplan and Silber, 1989). Testes with antenatal torsion may also present as a firm mass in the neonatal period. The use of Doppler ultrasonography will help differentiate torsion (no flow) from the more rare neonatal yolk sac tumor where testicular blood flow will be seen.

## Hydrocele

A hydrocele is nothing more than a collection of fluid between the tunica vaginalis, the liner of the scrotal sac, and the tunica albuginea, which covers the surface of the testes. In the neonate, this fluid will have its origin within the peritoneal cavity, which communicates with the scrotal sac via an evagination or extension of the peritoneum called a patent processus vaginalis. If the patency is small enough it may actually function as a one-way valve allowing fluid into, but not out of the scrotum. This explains the slow and progressive increases in scrotal size that may be seen in some cases. In other cases with a large patency, the fluid may move in and out of the scrotum with ease such that when the urologist arrives to examine the child, the swelling is gone. It is important to reassure families that these infants will often improve over time. Indeed, as for the frequency of a patent processus vaginalis, in autopsy series of men with no history of hernias or hydroceles, a 20% patency rate was found. Hydroceles may present acutely following the placement of ventriculoperitoneal shunts or peritoneal dialysis catheters. In these instances, both sides should be repaired since there is a 30% chance that the contralateral side will also become symptomatic. Overly aggressive therapy of the neonatal hydrocele is to be avoided because many of these hydroceles will resolve on their own, and because the surgery always carries with it the attendant risk of damage to the vas deferens, and testicular vessels, and may result in testicular atrophy. The likelihood of such an iatrogenic injury is increased in the small neonate (Scherer and Grosfeld, 1993).

### Hernia

In cases where the patency of the processus vaginalis is large enough, it is possible that intestines and other viscera (including the bladder) may migrate into the scrotal sac. This, by definition, is a hernia, which may be easily reducible so that there is no urgency for repair (Scherer and Grosfeld, 1993). In contrast, if a hernia is difficult to reduce or incarcerated, this is cause for alarm and should prompt repair. If the neck of the sac is so tight that the hernia cannot be reduced, the blood supply to the intestine will be compromised and this is classified as a strangulated hernia, and represents a surgical emergency.

### Hypospadias

The diagnosis of hypospadias is established when the urethral meatus is not present in the normal glanular position; it may be present anywhere from the glans to the perineum. In addition, there is an asymmetrical or hooded foreskin, and the penis may be tethered, creating a significant bend (chordee). These infants must not undergo circumcision, because the foreskin is crucial for use in the urethral reconstruction and correction of the chordee. However, up to 10% of patients with a hypospadias may have an intact foreskin, and the diagnosis can be made only after circumcision. These cases constitute the megameatus–intact prepuce (MIP) variants. In such cases, the loss of foreskin does not compromise the hypospadias repair, which is carried out when the infant is 6 months old. It is important to be certain that both testes are descended into their proper scrotal positions; if a hypospadias is seen in conjunction with an undescended testis, the possibility of an intersex state exists (Rajfer and Walsh, 1976). This is particularly true if both testes are undescended and impalpable, in which case a diagnosis of congenital adrenal hyperplasia must be ruled out at once (see later section on ambiguous genitalia).

On making the diagnosis of hypospadias, the examining physician must immediately check to see if both testes are palpable. For an infant with a hypospadias and two testes that are properly placed in the scrotum, an outpatient evaluation with a urologist may be arranged within 1 month, to allay parental concerns, even though the reconstruction is deferred until the infant is 6 months of age. Completely elective outpatient surgery is felt to be safest after 6 months of age

Hypospadias manifests with a wide spectrum of severity. The best results will be obtained in the simpler 90% of cases, in which the meatus is present anywhere along the penile shaft. Snodgrass and Nguyen (2002) have developed a versatile repair that offers success rates of 98% to 99% for hypospadias with the meatus present along the penile shaft. Current hypospadias repairs offer functional improvement in terms of the quality of stream, as well as cosmetic results that are increasingly approaching those seen in normal males. Even the 10% of cases that constitute the most severe penoscrotal hypospadias may be reconstructed with good cosmetic and functional results. The key in all of these cases is the preservation of all genital skin that is to be used in the reconstruction—hence the need to avoid circumcision (Baskin and Duckett, 1996).

### Circumcision

Few topics arouse as much controversy, office visits, phone calls, and annoyance for families, pediatricians, and urologists as the issue of routine circumcision in the newborn male. Circumcision has been practiced for centuries, and despite all-out efforts in the late 1970s and early 1980s to discourage it, families have continued to clamor for this procedure. It is a fact that in the United States, nearly 80% of the male population is circumcised; thus, for many families, the concept that one could forgo this procedure is a surprise. For many families, the need for their children to fit in and look like their siblings or father is a major issue. It is reasonable to assume that the main reason most Americans seek routine circumcision is cosmetic. The other reason that families cite in their decision for circumcision is ease of maintaining hygiene. Superimposed on these notions are a number of other arguments including the "threat" of penile cancer and an "increased risk of sexually transmitted disease." It is true that for patients with poor hygiene, a nonretractile foreskin will mask the onset of carcinoma of the penis. It also is true that this is a rare malignancy in the United States and a common malignancy in underdeveloped nations where circumcision is not practiced. However, this difference fails to explain why in Europe, where the overwhelming majority of men are not circumcised, penile cancer is rare. The reasons relate to access to regular bathing, basic hygiene, and the ability to retract the foreskin when sexual activity begins. The etiology of carcinoma of the penis is polyfactorial, and so long as the foreskin may be retracted to allow for good hygiene, the threat of malignancy is in and of itself a nonindication for circumcision. Likewise, the risk of sexually transmitted diseases is polyfactorial, and circumcision will not eradicate this family of diseases. Educational efforts on behalf of diminished promiscuity, condom use, and basic hygiene will produce a greater benefit for society as a whole than circumcision alone.

All of these rational arguments in favor of noncircumcision tend to fall short of their mark; the vast majority of American parents will request routine circumcision. Parents may cite a significant study reported by Wiswell and Geschke and colleagues, in several stages (Wiswell and Geschke, 1989; Wiswell et al, 1993), that identified a small but very real medical benefit to circumcision. By looking closely at the discharge data from U.S. Army hospitals worldwide, these investigators were able to correlate the status of the foreskin with subsequent outcomes with regard to urinary tract infections. Their findings include that, within the first year of life, although only 20% of the males were not circumcised, this 20% accounted for 80% of all urinary tract infections. In other words, these investigators demonstrated that the presence of foreskin increased the chances of a urinary tract infection by approximately fourfold during the first year of life. It is estimated that 99 children have to undergo circumcision to avoid 1 episode of urinary tract infection in the 100th patient—a small but real medical benefit. Nevertheless, circumcision is to be encouraged for any neonate with an underlying congenital anomaly of the urinary tract such as reflux, posterior urethral valves, or megaureters, where the added burden of a urinary tract infection could have more serious consequences.

The three main techniques for circumcision are use of the Plastibell, the Gomco clamp, and the Mogen clamp. Each has benefits and drawbacks; each physician performing circumcisions will find the method with which he or she feels most comfortable and should use it repetitively. If there is any doubt about a child's particular anatomy, the procedure should be stopped, and urologic consultation obtained. The use of EMLA cream and a circumferential block is highly effective in minimizing the pain associated with the procedure.

The leading contraindication to circumcision is medical fragility of the infant. Circumcision in a premature baby may present a technical challenge related to the infant's smaller size, because a proper fit between child and equipment is essential. In such instances, circumcision should be deferred until just before discharge from the NICU. In the child with a complex medical course, this timing also offers the physician a chance to carry out a circumcision with full cardiovascular and respiratory monitoring, which is not always available in an office-based setting. Circumcision must never be performed in any child with hypospadias or epispadias (Fig. 83–12), because as mentioned earlier, this skin is essential to the urethral reconstruction.

Bleeding after a routine circumcision may be seen in 10% to 20% of the cases, and this minor spotting is no cause for alarm. If the bleeding has passed onto the diaper, and a repositioning of the pressure dressing fails to stop the bleeding, the frenulum should be inspected, because this is where most bleeding vessels are found. If the bleeding persists, the clinician should not hesitate to obtain coagulation studies, because both hemophilia and von Willebrand disease may manifest in this manner. Rarely, there is injury to the glans and urethra. However, the most common problem arising after circumcision is penile adhesions, although this complication may be prevented by teaching parents to pull back on the penile shaft skin and apply petrolatum over the glans. Parents also should be warned that despite a nice skin fit in the neonatal period, the cosmetic appearance of the penis may change as the prepubic fat pad grows. The result may be that a perfect circumcision is obscured as the penis is pulled back into the fat pad; in such cases, reassurance, and not surgical revision, is indicated.

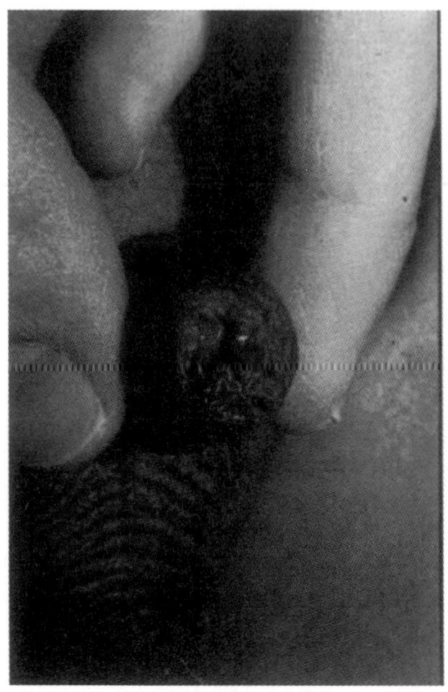
A

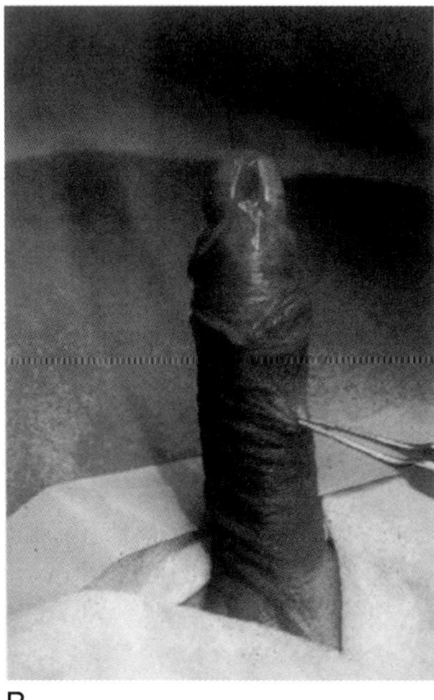
B

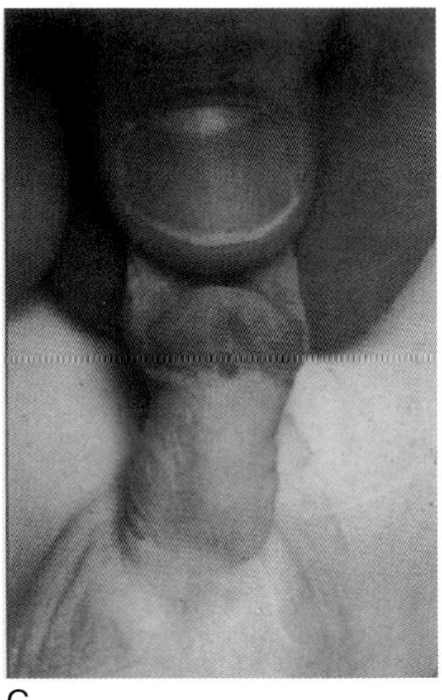
C

**FIGURE 83–12.** Hypospadias may not be discovered until the time of circumcision, because the foreskin has such a normal appearance, as in **A** and **B**. These cases represent the megameatus–intact prepuce variant, in which circumcision is not at all detrimental to future reconstruction. **C,** This photograph shows a more typical hypospadias with an asymmetrical foreskin and a meatus that is present at the glanular margin. In such cases, circumcision should be deferred because the hooded preputial skin may be required for subsequent reconstruction.

### Ambiguous Genitalia

The diagnosis and management of the child with ambiguous genitalia remain a medical and social emergency, and a complete discussion of this topic is beyond the scope of this section. Whereas in the past, this dilemma came as a total surprise in the delivery suite, today prenatal diagnosis has allowed for the discussions about genital ambiguity to begin in advance (Rintoul and Crombleholme, 2002). The widespread use of ultrasonography and increasing use of amniocentesis have allowed for the in utero diagnosis of virilizing congenital adrenal hyperplasia and complete androgen resistance syndromes. Such diagnosis is possible because the sonographic appearance of the genitalia will not match the karyotype obtained at amniocentesis. Still, the clinician must be prepared to deal with the situation in which no amniocentesis data are available and only one maternal sonogram was done in early gestation.

The most common presentation will be the female with congenital adrenal hyperplasia, which varies in its severity of presentation. Findings on physical examination range from severe clitoromegaly to a fully developed phallus with no palpable gonads (see Fig. 83–11). This virilization is caused by enzymatic deficiencies in the pathways of cortisol synthesis, leading to shunting into the androgen biosynthetic pathways (White, 2002). The family history is useful, as an older sibling or relative may have already been diagnosed with this condition. It is also useful to know if a karyotype was done during gestation. If a karyotype was not done or the results are not available, an ultrasound examination of the pelvis may be ordered to look behind the bladder for any müllerian remnants (see Fig. 83–11) and a karyotype should be ordered. Virilizing congenital adrenal hyperplasia is a rare diagnosis, and most males with bilateral impalpable testes will prove to be normal males. However, a delay in establishing this diagnosis is dangerous because replacement therapy with cortisol must be initiated. A delay in diagnosis also has profound implications for gender assignment. A genitogram (see Fig. 83–11) will delineate the extent of surgery required. The timing of surgery and the process of gender assignment are controversial at present, and these issues are addressed in the final paragraph.

Another common presentation is that of the child with androgen insensitivity who presents as a phenotypic female despite an amniocentesis showing an XY karyotype. This situation arises because for virilization to occur, the androgens must first bind to their receptors in the cytosol. Mutations in this receptor or at other points downstream then result in a phenotypic female who at subsequent laparotomy is found to have testes. Furthermore, these testes have continued to produce the müllerian inhibitory substance—hence, the uterus and the upper two thirds of the vaginal vault will be missing. There are no surgical management or gender assignment issues for these patients in the neonatal period.

Mixed gonadal dysgenesis (MGD) is seen in the neonatal unit as patients present with a severe hypospadias and a unilateral undescended testis. However, Rajfer and Walsh (1976) noted that MGD was one of the most common diagnoses made in patients with hypospadias and associated cryptorchidism. These patients may have a normal XY karyotype or a mosaic presentation. At exploratory laparotomy, the gonads are biopsied; a testis will be found on one side and a primitive streak on the opposite side. Rudimentary müllerian structures may be seen on the side of the streak gonad and may include a hypoplastic uterus. Streak gonads are removed because of their malignant potential. Although in past years a female gender assignment was considered, the current trend favors maintaining a male gender of rearing, with subsequent application of now-available advanced hypospadias reconstruction techniques.

The traditional approach to the diagnosis and management of genital ambiguity has undergone a great deal of criticism and increasing scrutiny over the past several years. With the traditional approach, the emphasis was placed on assigning a gender of rearing as soon as possible, and initiating any surgical reconstructions in the neonatal period. In recent years, it has become apparent that there can be problems with such an approach. Physicians, together with the parents, can assign a sex and gender role to a neonate. However, the long-term question arises as to whether a child's own gender identity will be congruent with the assigned gender role. For years it was believed that gender identity was plastic and not fixed until a child was 2 years of age. Given the technical problems encountered in phallic reconstruction, it was believed that if a satisfactory phallus could not be reconstructed, a female sex should be assigned. The recent reports of several patients who, on reaching the teenage years, have reverted back to a male gender after early female gender assignment have challenged this practice (Diamond, 1999; Reiner, 2002). In light of these scientific and clinical concerns, some authors and patients have called for a moratorium on surgery in infancy for patients with genital ambiguity (Diamond, 1999). They propose that all diagnostic tests be performed to allow for a determination of what the best gender assignment will be for the child. However, no irreversible surgery would be performed until it becomes clear what the child's own gender identity is, and a pediatric assent could be obtained. It is important to note that many patients with an XY karyotype assigned to a female gender have compensated to their situation (Schober et al, 2002). However, because the brain is a sexually dimorphic organ, many of the structural differences between the two genders that exist do so on the basis of hormonal imprinting in utero (Gorski, 2002; Swaab et al, 2002).

## REFERENCES

Allen TD: The swing of the pendulum. J Urol 148:534, 1992.

Baskin LS, Zderic SA, Snyder HM, Duckett JW: Primary dilated megaureter: Long term followup. J Urol 152:618, 1994.

Baskin LS, Duckett JW: Hypospadias. In Gillenwater J, Grayhack J, Howards S, Duckett J (eds): Adult and Pediatric Urology, 3rd ed. Chicago, Year Book, 1996, pp 2549-2590.

Bauer SB, Hallett M, Koshboin S, et al: Predictive value of urodynamic evaluation in newborns with myelodysplasia. JAMA 252:650-653, 1984.

Bauer SB: Neurogenic vesical dysfunction in children. In Walsh PC, Retik AB, Stamey TA, Vaughan ED (eds): Campbell's Urology, 6th ed. Philadelphia, WB Saunders, 1992, pp 1634-1637.

Blyth B, Snyder HM, Duckett JW: Antenatal diagnosis and subsequent management of hydronephrosis. J Urol 149:693-8, 1993.

Canning DA, Koo HP, Duckett JW: Anomalies of the bladder and cloaca. In Gillenwater J, Grayhack J, Howards S, Duckett J (eds): Adult and Pediatric Urology, 3rd ed. Chicago, Year Book, 1996, pp 2445-2488.

Cartwright PC, Duckett JW, Keating MA, et al: Managing apparent ureteropelvic junction obstruction in the newborn. J Urol 148:1224, 1992.

Cendron M, Keating MA, Huff DS, et al: Cryptorchidism, orchiopexy and infertility: a critical long-term retrospective analysis. J Urol 142:559-562, 1989.

Cendron M, D'Alton ME, Crombleholme M: Prenatal diagnosis and management of the fetus with hydronephrosis. Semin Perinatol 18:163-181, 1994.

Conway JJ, Maizels M: The "well tempered" diuretic renogram: A standard method to examine the asymptomatic neonate with hydronephrosis or hydroureteronephrosis. J Nucl Med 33:2047-2051, 1993.

Coplen DE., Hare JV, Zderic SA, et al: A 10 year experience with antenatal intervention. J Urol 156:1142-1145, 1996.

Crombleholme TM: Invasive fetal therapy: Current status and future directions. Semin Perinatol 18:385-396, 1984.

Cromie WJ: Implications of antenatal ultrasound screening in the incidence of major genitourinary malformations. Semin Pediatr Surg 10:204-211, 2001.

Diamond M: Pediatric management of ambiguous and traumatized genitalia. J Urol 162:1021-1028, 1999.

Djeter SW, Gibbons MD: The fate of infant kidneys with fetal hydronephrosis but initially normal postnatal sonography. J Urol 142:661-662, 1989.

Gibbons MD, Horan HA, Dejter SW, Keszler M: Extracorporeal membrane oxygenation: An adjunct in the management of the neonate with severe respiratory distress and congenital urinary tract anomalies. J Urol 150:434-437, 1993.

Gorski RA: Hypothalamic imprinting by gonadal steroid hormones. Adv Exp Med Biol 511:57-70, 2002.

Hendren WH: Repair of cloacal anomalies: Current techniques. J Pediatr Surg 21:1159-1176, 1986.

Herndon CD, McKenna PH, Kolon TF, et al: A multicenter outcomes analysis of patients with neonatal reflux presenting with prenatal hydronephrosis. J Urol 162:1203-1208, 1999.

Homsy YL, Williot P, Danais S: Transitional neonatal hydronephrosis: Fact or fantasy? J Urol 136:339-341, 1986.

Homsy YL, Saad F, Laberge I, et al: Transitional hydronephrosis of the newborn and infant. J Urol 144:579-583, 1990.

Huff DS, Snyder HM 3d, Hadziselimovic F, et al: An absent testis is associated with contralateral testicular hypertrophy. J Urol 148:627-628, 1992.

Huff DS, Hadziselimovic F, Synder HM III, et al: Postnatal testicular maldevelopment in unilateral cryptorchidism. J Urol 142:546-548, 1989.

Jerkins GR, Noe HN, Hollabaugh RS, et al: Spermatic cord torsion in the neonate. J Urol 129:543-549, 1983.

Kaefer M, Keating MA, Adams MC, Rink RC: Posterior urethral valves, pressure pop offs, and bladder function. J Urol 154: 708-711, 1995.

Kaefer M, Pabby A, Kelly M, et al: Improved bladder function after prophylactic treatment of the high risk neurogenic bladder in newborns with myelomentingocele. J Urol 162:1068-1071, 1999.

Kaplan GW, Silber I: Neonatal torsion—to pex or not? In King LR (ed): Urologic Surgery in Infants and Children. Philadelphia, WB Saunders, 1989, pp 386-395.

Kasabian NG, Bauer SB, Dyro FM, et al: The prophylactic value of clean intermittent catheterization in the treatment of infants and children with myelomeningocele and neurogenic bladder dysfunction. Am J Dis Child 146:840-844, 1992.

Kay R, Strong DW, Tank ES: Bilateral spermatic cord torsion in the neonate. J Urol 123:293-294, 1980.

Koff SA, Campbell KD: Non-operative management of unilateral neonatal hydronephrosis: Natural history of poorly functioning kidneys. J Urol 152:593-595, 1994.

Lee PA, O'Leary LA, Songer NJ, et al: Paternity after unilateral cryptorchidism: a controlled study. Pediatrics 98:676-679, 1996.

Lee PA, Coughlin MT: Fertility after bilateral cryptorchidism. Evaluation by paternity, hormone, and semen data. Horm Res 55:28-32, 2001.

McGuire EJ, Woodside JR, Borden TA, Weiss RM: The prognostic value of urodynamic testing in myelodysplastic patients. J Urol 126:205-209, 1981.

Mitchell ME, Bagli DJ: Complete penile disassembly for epispadias repair: The Mitchell technique. J Urol 155:300-304, 1996.

Noh PH, Cooper CS, Winkler AC, et al: Prognostic factors for long term renal function in boys with prune belly syndrome. J Urol 162:1399-1401, 1999.

Pena A: Anorectal malformations. Semin Pediatr Surg 4:35-40, 1995.

Perez LM, Khoury J, Webster GD: The value of urodynamic testing in infants less than one year of age with spinal dysraphism. J Urol 148:584-587, 1992.

Rajfer J, Walsh PC: The incidence of intersexuality in patients with hypospadias and cryptorchidism. J Urol 116:769-773, 1976.

Ransley PG, Dhillon HK, Gordon I, et al: The postnatal management of hydronephrosis diagnosed by prenatal ultrasound. J Urol 144:584-589, 1990.

Ransley PG: The Meredith Campbell Lecture. The Impact of Prenatal Diagnosis on the Practice of Pediatric Urology. Presented at the Annual Meeting of the American Urological Association, Orlando, 1996.

Reiner W: Gender identity and sex assignment: A reappraisal for the 21st century. Adv Exp Med Biol 511:175-187, 2002.

Rich MA, Brock WA, Pena A: Spectrum of genitourinary anomalies in patients with imperforate anus. Ped Surg Int 3: 110-113, 1988.

Rintoul N, Crombleholme TM: Prenatal diagnosis and treatment of intersex states. Adv Exp Med Biol 511:225-235, 2002.

Rittenberg MH, Hulbert WC, Snyder HM III, Duckett JW: Protective factors in posterior urethral valves. J Urol 140:993-996, 1988.

Scherer LR 3rd, Grosfeld JL: Inguinal hernia and umbilical anomalies. Pediatr Clin North Am 40:1121-1131, 1993.

Schober JM, Carmichael PA, Hines M., Ransley PG: The ultimate challenge of cloacal exstrophy. J Urol 167:300-304, 2002.

Smith GH, Canning DA, Schulman SL, et al: The long-term outcome of posterior urethral valves treated with primary valve ablation and observation. J Urol 155:1730-1734, 1996.

Snodgrass W, Nguyen M: Tubularized incised plate hypospadias repair. Urology 60:157-162, 2002.

Snyder HM: Anomalies of the ureter. In Gillenwater J, Grayhack J, Howards S, Duckett J (eds): Adult and Pediatric Urology, 3rd ed. Chicago, Year Book, 1996, pp 2197-2232.

Snyder HM, Kalichman MA, Charney E, et al: Vesicostomy for neurogenic bladder with spina bifida: A followup study. J Urol 130:724-727, 1983.

Sutherland RS, Mevorach RA, Baskin LS, Kogan BA: Spinal dysraphism in children: An overview and an approach to prevent complications. Urology 46:294-299, 1995.

Swaab DF, Chung WC, Krujiver F, et al: Sexual differentiation of the human hypothalamus. Adv Exp Med Biol 511:75-95, 2002.

Weiser AC, Amukele SA, Palmer LS: Metachronous presentation of a ureterovesical junction obstruction contralateral to a multicystic dysplastic kidney. J Urol 167:2538-2539, 2002.

White PC: The endocrinologist's approach to the intersex patient. Adv Exp Med Biol 511:107-118, 2002.

Wiswell TE, Geschke DW: Risks from circumcision during the first month of life compared to those for uncircumcised boys. Pediatrics 83:1011-1015, 1989.

Wiswell TE, Hachey WE: Urinary tract infection and the uncircumcised state: An update. Clin Pediatr 32:130, 1993.

Woodward M, Frank D: Postnatal management of antenatal hydronephrosis. Br J Urol Int 89:149-156, 2002.

Yerkes EB, Adams MC, Pope JC, Brock JW: Does every patient with prenatal hydronephrosis need voiding cystourethrography? J Urol 162:1218-1220, 1999.

Zderic SA: The endoscopic management of urethral valves. In Smith AD, Badlani GH, Bagley D, et al (eds): Smith's Textbook of Endourology. St. Louis, Quality Medical Publishing, 1996, pp 1323-1332.

Zderic SA, Canning DA, Carr MC, et al: The CHOP experience with cloacal exstrophy and gender reassignment. Adv Exp Med Biol 511:135-143, 2002.

Zhylan O, Zderic SA, Duckett JW, et al: Vesicostomy in the management of the myelomeningocele patient: An 18 year experience. J Urol 149:259A, 1993.

CHAPTER 84

# Acute and Chronic Renal Failure

Philippe S. Friedlich, Jacquelyn R. Evans, Tivadar Tulassay, and Istvan Seri

## DEFINITION OF NEONATAL ACUTE AND CHRONIC RENAL FAILURE

Neonatal acute renal failure (ARF) is defined as the sudden, severe derangement of glomerular filtration and tubular function and is diagnosed when serum creatinine is greater than 1.5 mg/dL regardless of the rate of urine output. ARF also should be suspected in the newborn if serum creatinine fails to decline below maternal levels by (at least) the fifth to seventh days postnatally or is rising by 0.3 mg/dL/day or faster (Karlowicz and Adelman, 1992).

Neonatal ARF has conventionally been subdivided into prerenal, intrarenal (intrinsic), and postrenal (obstructive) renal failure according to the primary site of the disorder. The overall incidence of neonatal ARF is approximately 20% of all neonatal intensive care unit (NICU) admissions (Karlowicz and Adelman, 1992; Stapleton et al, 1987). Greater than 70% of these cases represent prerenal ARF with the rest being intrinsic or obstructive ARF. It is important to remember that the conventional classification of neonatal *obstructive* renal failure as ARF is incorrect; this disorder rather represents the acute presentation of a chronic renal failure when separation from the placental circulation at birth occurs.

Neonatal chronic renal failure (CRF) develops when derangements of glomerular filtration and/or tubular function continue following the resolution of the acute phase of renal failure.

## PATHOPHYSIOLOGY OF NEONATAL RENAL FAILURE

### Prerenal Acute Renal Failure

Prerenal ARF is the most common form of ARF in the newborn. The cause of prerenal ARF is renal hypoperfusion due to systemic hypotension or to selective decreases in renal blood flow in response to tissue hypoxia without significant systemic hypotension. Under these circumstances, renal autoregulation fails to maintain renal blood flow (RBF) and glomerular filtration rate (GFR) in the physiologic range. Correction of the underlying condition immediately restores normal renal function unless renal hypoperfusion has been so severe or prolonged that renal parenchymal damage has already developed. Once parenchymal damage occurs, prerenal ARF evolves into intrinsic ARF.

In prerenal ARF, despite the decrease in RBF, GFR is initially relatively preserved leading to enhanced tubular reabsorption of solutes and water. The increase in filtration fraction (GFR/RBF × 100) increases peritubular oncotic pressure, resulting in enhanced proximal tubular sodium and water reabsorption (Feld et al, 1986). Furthermore, vasopressin and endothelin secretion as well as the activity of the renin-angiotensin-aldosterone system and the renal sympathetic nerves increases, leading to further enhancement of renal tubular solute and water absorption. The net result of these renal hemodynamic and hormonal changes is oliguria, decreased urinary sodium losses, and increased urinary osmolality. In some newborns, however, oliguria does not develop, because pituitary release of or renal responsiveness to vasopressin is decreased (Dixon and Anderson, 1985), and because in these cases less significant alterations in the renal microcirculation may occur. Thus, the rate of urine output has a somewhat limited diagnostic value in newborns (see later). Urine output is an important prognostic factor, however, because morbidity and mortality in nonoliguric ARF are decreased compared with those in the oliguric form, even if features of intrinsic renal failure develop (Chevalier et al, 1984; Karlowicz and Adelman, 1995).

Severe perinatal blood loss, perinatal asphyxia, respiratory distress syndrome, dehydration in the extremely immature preterm infant due to increased transepidermal free water losses, necrotizing enterocolitis, hydrops, septic shock, other severe illness associated with capillary leak syndrome, and the use of certain pharmacologic agents (see later) are the most frequent conditions associated with absolute or relative decreases of intravascular volume or renal hypoperfusion (or both) resulting in the development of prerenal ARF in the newborn (Table 84–1). In addition, decreases in renal perfusion may occur following primary surgical repair or surgical reduction of omphalocele, gastroschisis, or congenital diaphragmatic hernia. Finally, acute decreases in cardiac output during cardiac surgery or use of extracorporeal membrane oxygenation (ECMO) also may lead to the development of prerenal ARF. In addition, ECMO may result in impaired autoregulation of organ blood flow (Liem et al, 1995), leading to the development of a pressure-passive circulation. Thus, in newborns on ECMO, prerenal failure may develop rapidly unless blood pressure is tightly controlled in the normal range. If blood pressure cannot be appropriately maintained and renal blood flow remains compromised for a prolonged period of time, the prerenal failure may evolve into intrinsic renal failure with potentially permanent damage to the kidneys.

### Intrinsic Acute Renal Failure

Approximately 6% to 8% of newborns admitted to NICUs have intrinsic ARF, with severe perinatal asphyxia being the most common cause (Stapleton et al, 1987). In contrast with prerenal ARF, the renal functional abnormalities in intrinsic ARF are not immediately reversible. The severity of intrinsic ARF ranges from mild tubular dysfunction to acute tubular necrosis, with or without oliguria and anuria, to renal infarction and corticomedullary necrosis with

**TABLE 84–1**

**Causes of Acute Renal Failure in the Newborn***

| Prerenal Acute Renal Failure | Intrinsic Acute Renal Failure | Obstructive Renal Failure |
|---|---|---|
| Loss of effective circulating blood volume | Acute tubular necrosis (long-lasting, severe renal ischemia, nephrotoxins) | Congenital malformations |
| Absolute loss | Congenital malformations | Imperforate prepuce |
| Hemorrhage | Bilateral renal agenesis | Urethral stricture |
| Dehydration | Renal dysplasia | PUV |
| Relative loss | Polycystic kidneys | Urethral diverticulum |
| ↑ Capillary leak (sepsis, NEC, RDS, asphyxia, ECMO) | Infections | Primary VUR |
| Renal hypoperfusion | Congenital infections (syphilis, toxoplasmosis) | Ureterocele |
| All of the above | Pyelonephritis | Megaureter |
| Congestive heart failure | Bacterial endocarditis | UPJ obstruction |
| Cardiac surgery | Renal vascular causes | Extrinsic compression |
| Pharmacologic agents | Renal artery thrombosis | Sacrococcygeal teratoma |
| Indomethacin | Renal vein thrombosis | Hematocolpos |
| Tolazoline | DIC | Intrinsic obstruction |
| ACE inhibitors | Nephrotoxins | Renal calculi |
| | Aminoglycosides | Fungus balls |
| | Indomethacin | Neurogenic bladder |
| | Amphotericin B | |
| | Methicillin | |
| | Radiocontrast dyes | |
| | Intrarenal obstruction | |
| | Uric acid nephropathy | |
| | Myoglobinuria | |
| | Hemoglobinuria | |

*In many cases, a combination of several causative factors contributes to the development of acute renal failure. For instance, absolute hypovolemia, increased capillary leak–induced loss of effective circulating blood volume, and reflex renal vasoconstriction all may contribute to renal hypoperfusion and ensuing renal injury in newborns with severe forms of shock.

ACE, angiotensin-converting enzyme; COX-2, cyclooxygenase type 2; DIC, disseminated intravascular coagulation; ECMO, extracorporeal membrane oxygenation; NEC, necrotizing enterocolitis; PUV, posterior urethral valve; RDS, respiratory distress syndrome; UPJ, ureteropelvic junction; VUR, vesicoureteral reflux.

Data from Karlowicz and Adelman, 1992.

irreversible renal damage. It is of clinical importance that untreated and sustained prerenal or obstructive ARF eventually develops into intrinsic ARF (see earlier). Conditions most commonly associated with the development of intrinsic ARF in the newborn are listed in Table 84–1.

The term *acute tubular necrosis* has been used interchangeably with *acute renal failure*. Although extensive tubule injury is a frequent pathologic finding in ARF, acute tubular necrosis should be used only to refer to cases of intrinsic ARF secondary to renal ischemia or nephrotoxic substances, in which tubular necrosis is always one of the main mechanisms causing renal failure (Kon and Ichikawa, 1984).

The course of intrinsic ARF may be subdivided into initiation, maintenance, and recovery phases. The initiation phase includes the original insult and the associated events. The sustained low GFR, tubular dysfunction, and azotemia represent the maintenance phase. The duration of the maintenance phase depends, at least in part, on the severity and duration of the initial insult. The recovery phase is characterized by the gradual restoration of GFR and tubular functions. Recognition of the different phases of neonatal intrinsic ARF is helpful in the diagnosis, clinical management, and prognostication of the disorder.

Changes in renal hemodynamics brought about by the excessive production and release of vasoconstrictive hormones, including the renin-anigiotensin system, epinephrine, norepinephrine, endothelin, adenosine, vasoconstrictive prostaglandins, and vasopressin, play an important role in the development and maintenance of intrinsic renal failure (Karlowicz and Adelman, 1992; Toth-Heyn et al, 2000). In addition, alterations in the function and ultrastructure of the nephron, including the decrease in the permeability and surface area of the glomerular capillary, intratubular obstruction to tubular flow by cellular debris, and tubular back-leak, contribute to the impairment of renal function in intrinsic ARF. Finally, the deterioration of hemodynamic and tubular functions is associated with intracellular events, such as enhanced free radical injury with reperfusion of the kidneys and accumulation and sequestration of intracellular calcium in mitochondria, resulting in phospholipase activation and the ensuing deterioration of mitochondrial structure and function. If the initiating insult is severe, sustained, or repeated, the intracellular events may lead to widespread epithelial cell death and irreversible tissue damage, resulting in the development of CRF.

### Ischemic-Hypoxic Injury

Despite being the best-oxygenated organ, the kidney is susceptible to ischemic-hypoxic injury because of the redistribution of its blood flow under pathologic circumstances to the "vital" organs and also because of the unique vascular supply of the renal medulla. The presentation and course of the renal damage depend on the severity and duration of the insult. Mild ischemia results in transient loss of renal concentrating capacity, owing to the extreme sensitivity of the medullary thick ascending limb to tissue hypoxia (Brezis et al, 1984). The loss of concentrating capacity may be difficult to detect in immature preterm newborns with the developmentally regulated maturity of their renal concentrating capacity (see Chapter 80). More prolonged injury produces widespread tubular dysfunction, with significant impairments in sodium and water reabsorption and decreases in GFR. This degree of severity of intrinsic ARF is most frequently seen in full-term newborns with severe perinatal asphyxia, who present most commonly with the nonoliguric form of ARF (Karlowicz and Adelman, 1995). Finally, prolonged or repeated insults may result in the irreversible form of intrinsic ARF, with oliguria and anuria and persistent tubular and glomerular damage leading to the development of CRF.

The primary pathomechanism of ischemic-hypoxic intrinsic ARF is the damage to the renal tubular epithelium, resulting in back-leak of the glomerular filtrate and intraluminal obstruction with necrotic cellular debris (Kon and Ichikawa, 1984). The latter results in an elevation of the pericapillary hydrostatic pressure in the Bowman space, leading to further decreases in GFR. The tubuloglomerular feedback mechanism also may be activated by the compensatory increases in the delivery of sodium and water to the distal parts of the nephron in the unobstructed tubules, resulting in a further loss in GFR (Myers and Moran, 1986). In addition, abnormalities in the ultrastructure of the glomerulus and decreases in the total filtering surface area occur (Feld et al, 1986; Kon and Ichikawa, 1984). The cumulative effect of these changes in the most severe cases of intrinsic ARF is the complete cessation of glomerular filtration.

The use of some medications, including captopril or enalapril (Rasoulpour and Marinelli, 1992) (see Chapter 87) and tolazoline (Guignard and Gouyon, 1988), may also lead to the development of ischemic intrinsic ARF in the sick newborn. The angiotensin-converting enzyme (ACE) inhibitors (captopril and enalapril) may induce unpredictable decreases in systemic blood pressure so that renal perfusion pressure drops below the autoregulatory range, leading to tissue hypoperfusion with subsequent hypoxic-ischemic damage to the renal epithelium. Although tolazoline is not available in the United States any more, it is worth mentioning that, in addition to causing systemic hypotension, this drug also may induce severe renal vasoconstriction, further compromising renal perfusion (Guignard and Gouyon, 1988).

## Nephrotoxic Injury

The predominant lesion in nephrotoxic ARF is the damage to the proximal tubule cells (Feld et al, 1986). In clinical practice, aminoglycoside administration to the newborn is one of the most common conditions in which such damage can occur. Aminoglycosides inhibit lysosomal phospholipases, leading to tubule cell phospholipidosis and subsequent necrosis (Giuliano et al, 1984). Changes in the ultrastructure of the glomerulus also occur (Kon and Ichikawa, 1984). The immature kidney appears to be less susceptible to aminoglycoside toxicity than that of the adult (Pelayo et al, 1983). The clinician must also remember that aminoglycoside toxicity is usually *nonoliguri*; therefore, serial monitoring of serum creatinine values is necessary, especially during prolonged administration of these antibiotics, to detect their potential nephrotoxicity in the newborn. The mechanisms of aminoglycoside toxicity may be activated even when serum levels are in the accepted range for toxicity in the newborn (Adelman et al, 1987). The potential long-term consequences of this effect on neonatal renal function are unknown.

Finally, neonates and infants with mitochondrial cytopathies may present with renal dysfunction resembling nephrotoxic injury before the neurologic and neuromuscular symptoms become evident (Buemi et al, 1997). Renal tubulopathy (Fanconi syndrome) is frequently a leading presentation in newborns with mitochondrial cytopathies; affected infants may first present with tubulointerstitial nephropathy developing into terminal uremia.

## Combined Ischemic and Nephrotoxic Injury

Other medications, including amphotericin B and indomethacin, exert their renal side effects by causing both ischemic and direct nephrotoxic renal injury. Amphotericin B alters renal function by reducing RBF and GFR and by directly affecting tubular function, resulting in renal tubular acidosis and increased urinary potassium excretion. Although these nephrotoxic effects are most often reversible, cases of fatal neonatal renal failure due to amphotericin B toxicity have been reported (Baley et al, 1984). Serum creatinine and electrolytes should be closely monitored; the dosing interval should be prolonged if serum creatinine rises, and replacement therapy with potassium and bicarbonate should be provided if indicated. Finally, because liposomal or lipid complex amphotericin B–based products appear to be less nephrotoxic, their use should be considered in neonates at risk for renal insufficiency (Adler-Shobert et al, 2001; Friedlich et al, 1997).

Severe, although usually transient, nephrotoxicity can occur with indomethacin administration. The potentiation of the vasoconstrictive and sodium- and water-retaining effects of angiotensin II, norepinephrine, and vasopressin by the indomethacin-induced inhibition of renal prostaglandin production is the primary mechanism of the renal actions of the drug. Because neonatal renal function is more dependent on local prostaglandin production than that of the euvolemic adult (especially when intravascular volume is decreased as a result of fluid restriction, increased capillary leak, and transepidermal water losses in the preterm infant with patent ductus arteriosus), indomethacin administration is almost always associated with elevated serum creatinine concentrations, decreased urine output, and hyponatremia (Cifuentes et al, 1979). In addition, indomethacin may also exert a direct aldosterone-like effect on the distal tubule. Because the renal side effects of indomethacin are mostly transient, some clinicians prefer to wait until spontaneous recovery of renal function occurs while maintaining a restricted fluid intake without additional sodium supplementation. Whether concomitant low-dose dopamine infusion aids in the recovery from the renal tubular side effects of indomethacin treatment remains to be determined (Baenzinger et al, 1999; Fajardo et al, 1992; Seri, 1995; Seri et al, 2002). If severe oliguria or anuria develops in the preterm infant, however, furosemide administration may become necessary to prevent the persistence of the ARF caused by indomethacin (Yeh et al, 1982). Serum creatinine and electrolytes as well as urine output should be closely monitored in these newborns. If gentamicin or other nephrotoxic medications are being concomitantly administered, the dosing interval for these medications should be prolonged in anticipation of the increases in serum creatinine.

A less common form of neonatal intrinsic ARF associated with hypoxia, perinatal asphyxia, or polycythemia is uric acid nephropathy (Karlowicz and Adelman, 1992; Stapleton et al, 1987). In such cases, precipitation of uric acid or monosodium urate crystals results in obstruction of the renal tubules, causing intrinsic ARF. Because newborns normally excrete more uric acid, they may be prone to the development of uric acid nephropathy if severe and prolonged hyperuricemia develops (Stapleton et al, 1987). In addition, intrinsic ARF, partly as a result of intratubular obstruction, may develop with cases of rhabdomyolysis in severe perinatal asphyxia (Kojima et al, 1985) or with massive hemoglobinuria resulting from intravascular hemolysis. Radiopaque contrast agents also may cause intrinsic ARF, especially in newborns who already have compromised renal function, such as those with congenital heart disease undergoing cardiac catheterization (Karlowicz and Adelman, 1992).

Finally, medications given to pregnant women may cause combined ischemic and nephrotoxic renal injury in the fetus, resulting in the clinical presentation of ARF after birth. A frequently used class of medications that fall into this category are the nonsteroidal anti-inflammatory drugs (NSAIDs) prescribed for tocolysis—both nonselective cyclooxygenase inhibitors such as indomethacin or ketoprofen (Bannwarth et al, 1999) and selective cyclooxygenase type 2 (COX-2) inhibitors such as nimesulide (Peruzzi et al, 1999). Because intrauterine nimesulide exposure may also lead to end-stage intrinsic ARF necessitating dialysis of the newborn (Balasubramanian, 2000; Peruzzi et al, 1999), COX-2 inhibitors must be used with caution in pregnant women.

### Obstructive Renal Failure: Acute Presentation of Chronic Renal Failure

Obstructive renal failure can be caused by a variety of congenital malformations of the kidneys and the urinary collecting system (see Table 84–1) (see also Chapters 82 and 83). Some of these newborns have reversible renal failure, whereas others have renal dysplasia with irreversible intrinsic renal failure at the time of diagnosis. Although prognostication of long-term outcome of renal function in obstructive renal failure is extremely difficult, in newborns with prune-belly syndrome, a nadir serum creatinine greater than 0.7 mg/dL, bilateral renal abnormalities on renal ultrasound scan, and clinical pyelonephritis are prognostic for development of CRF (Noh et al, 1999).

## DIAGNOSIS OF NEONATAL ACUTE AND CHRONIC RENAL FAILURE

Despite its limitations, serum creatinine is the most widely used measure to evaluate glomerular filtration in the clinical setting and is more specific than blood urea nitrogen (BUN) (see Chapter 81, on clinical evaluation in renal/kidney disease). Because the production of BUN is increased by a high dietary protein intake, gastrointestinal bleeding, and hypercatabolic states, BUN levels are elevated out of proportion to changes in GFR under these conditions. Moreover, the renal excretion of urea also is influenced by tubular function, especially under conditions associated with alterations in tubular water reabsorption. Therefore, as a general rule, if the BUN–to–serum creatinine ratio exceeds 20, increased urea production or increased renal urea reabsorption (or both) should be suspected (Feld et al, 1986).

The major goal in the initial evaluation of neonatal ARF is to diagnose prerenal ARF and obstructive renal failure promptly to prevent their transition to intrinsic ARF and then CRF. The medical history of the pregnancy, the findings on prenatal tests and ultrasound studies, and the physical examination usually provide important clues in the newborn presenting with oliguria and anuria in the immediate postnatal period. If obstruction is suspected, a renal and bladder ultrasound study should be performed without delay (see Chapter 83). In cases in which oliguria and elevated serum creatinine values are associated with hematuria or hypertension (or both), the possibility of renal vascular disease should also be considered (see Chapter 87).

The clinically most reliable diagnostic tool to differentiate prerenal ARF from intrinsic ARF is the provision of an appropriate fluid challenge, unless the newborn is suspected of having a urinary outlet obstruction or renal hypoperfusion secondary to congestive heart failure. Isotonic solution (usually normal saline) should be given in a dose of 20 mL/kg or more over a period of 30 minutes to 2 hours. If urine output remains less than 1 mL/kg per hour after 2 hours and there are no clinical signs of intravascular volume deficit, 1 to 2 mg/kg of furosemide should be administered. Low-dose dopamine infusion may be used in addition to the volume challenge, especially if systemic blood pressure is labile or remains low after the volume challenge is completed. Low-dose dopamine improves renal perfusion, increases GFR, and increases renal sodium and free water excretion in the preterm and term infant (Seri, 1995; Seri et al, 1998). In addition, primarily along the proximal parts of the nephron, dopamine inhibits renal tubular $Na^+,K^+$-ATPase activity and decreases renal oxygen consumption when oxygen delivery is limited (Seri, 1995). However, the clinical importance of this effect of the drug remains to be demonstrated, and because dopamine blunts the tubuloglomerular feedback and increases solute delivery to the distal parts of the nephron, oxygen consumption in the outer medulla may increase rather than decrease (Heyman et al, 1995). On the other hand, at least under pathologic conditions, dopamine restores the diminished outer medullary blood flow and ameliorates outer medullary hypoxia caused by indomethacin or by the inhibition of nitric oxide synthesis (Heyman et al, 1995). Therefore, the use of dopamine may be beneficial in the sick preterm and term infant with *prerenal ARF* caused by hypoxemia, acidosis, or indomethacin administration (Seri, 1995; Seri et al, 1998, 2002). Finally, although widely used in children and adults to diagnose prerenal ARF, the mannitol test is contraindicated in newborns with a predisposition to the development of intraventricular hemorrhage or periventricular leukomalacia because of the drug-induced sudden increase in serum osmolality.

Compared with intrinsic ARF, prerenal ARF is associated with a low urinary sodium excretion, fractional excretion of sodium (FENa), and renal failure index and with high urine-to-plasma osmolar and creatinine ratios (Table 84–2). Although these diagnostic indices are helpful in differentiating prerenal ARF from intrinsic ARF in older children and adults, there are important limitations to their use in the sick preterm and term newborn. Some newborns, especially immature preterm infants, with prerenal ARF have values overlapping those attributed to intrinsic ARF (Ellis and Arnold, 1982). Furthermore, FENa in preterm infants born at less than 32 weeks of gestation with normal renal function is usually higher than 3%, and there are no data of FENa in these infants with intrinsic ARF. Finally, because of the developmentally regulated limitation of their concentrating capacity and the effects of low protein intake and urea excretion on urine osmolality (Feld et al, 1986), the urine-to-plasma creatinine ratio instead of the urine-to-plasma osmolal ratio should be used in newborns to evaluate their renal tubular reabsorptive capacity.

Laboratory values to be monitored in ARF include serum sodium, potassium, chloride, bicarbonate, calcium, phosphorus, magnesium, creatinine, uric acid, and glucose as well as BUN and blood gases; a complete blood count with platelets should also be included. If urine is available, a urinalysis, urine culture, and a spot urine sample for sodium, creatinine, and osmolality should be obtained. Findings in a given spot urine sample may significantly differ from those in another one, and repeat analyses or a timed urine collection may become necessary in selected cases to aid in the differential diagnosis.

Neonatal CRF is diagnosed when sustained derangements of glomerular filtration and/or tubular function occur with minimal to no resolution over time. In some cases, the acute phase of the renal compromise has not been detected or has occurred in utero, and the diagnosis of CRF is established without documented evidence of preexisting ARF.

## TREATMENT OF NEONATAL ACUTE AND CHRONIC RENAL FAILURE

### Prerenal Acute Renal Failure

The approach of diagnosing prerenal ARF with the provision of fluid boluses and diuretic treatment (if appropriate) also serves as the initial management of this condition. Most newborns admitted to NICUs with ARF have the prerenal form of ARF and respond to fluid therapy. If systemic hypotension develops despite adequate volume administration, early initiation of dopamine with the subsequent normalization of blood pressure often establishes appropriate renal perfusion (Seri et al, 1993, 1998). In cases of pressor/inotrope-resistant hypotension and shock, a brief course of low-dose hydrocortisone administration has been demonstrated to be effective in restoring systemic perfusion and renal function in preterm neonates (Seri et al, 2001). Other management goals include the maintenance of normoxemia and normal pH to avoid the recurrence of renal vasoconstriction and to improve capillary integrity as well as the replacement of blood and free water losses as needed.

**TABLE 84–2**

**Diagnostic Indices Suggestive of Prerenal or Intrinsic Renal Failure in the Newborn**

| | Prerenal Acute Renal Failure | Intrinsic Acute Renal Failure |
|---|---|---|
| Urine flow rate (mL/kg/hr) | Variable | Variable |
| Urine osmolality (mOsm/L) | >400 | ≤400 |
| Urine-to-plasma osmolal ratio | >1.3 | ≤1.0 |
| Urine-to-plasma creatinine ratio | 29.2 ± 1.6‡ | 9.7 ± 3.6‡ |
| Urine [Na+] (mEq/L) | 10-50 | 30-90 |
| FENa* (%) | <0.3 (0.9 ± 0.6)‡ | >3.0 (4.3 ± 2.2)‡ |
| Renal failure index*† | <3.0 (1.3 ± 0.8)‡ | >3.0 (11.6 ± 9.5)‡ |
| Response to fluid challenge (± furosemide) | Increased urine output | No effect on urine output |

*Fractional excretion of sodium (FENa) = (urine [Na+]/serum [Na+])/(urine [Cr]/serum [Cr]) × 100.

†Renal failure index (RFI) = urine [Na+]/(urine [Cr]/serum [Cr]).

‡Mean ± SD.

Data from Feld at al, 1986; Karlowicz and Adelman, 1992; and Mathew et al, 1980. See text for details.

## Intrinsic Acute Renal Failure and Chronic Renal Failure

Whenever possible, newborns presenting with conditions potentially associated with the development of intrinsic ARF should be monitored closely and, if available, preventive measures applied before the onset of renal injury. In established intrinsic ARF of the newborn, management centers on providing appropriate *supportive care* until renal function recovers (see later). Additional *nonspecific therapy* includes the use of furosemide (Fildes et al, 1986) and dopamine (Karlowicz and Adelman, 1992; Seri et al, 1993, 1998; Tulassay et al, 1983). Although there is no conclusive evidence that the attempt to provide selective renal vasodilatation and diuresis improves prognosis in intrinsic ARF, patients who respond to diuretic management with an increase in urine output early in the course of renal failure are more likely to survive (Fildes et al, 1986). In addition, the use of these medications may aid in ensuring an appropriate fluid and electrolyte balance. If dopamine is used, it should be started early in the course of the disease and at low doses (1 to 4 μg/kg/minute) to avoid unnecessary increases in systemic blood pressure and possible renal vasoconstriction (Karlowicz and Adelman, 1992; Seri, 1995; Seri et al, 1993, 1998; Tulassay et al, 1983). The combined use of dopamine and furosemide may have a synergistic effect on inducing diuresis even in the preterm newborn (Tulassay and Seri, 1986). The potential toxicity of long-term and aggressive furosemide therapy, including ototoxicity, interstitial nephritis, osteopenia, nephrocalcinosis, hypotension, and persistence of patent ductus arteriosus, should be taken into consideration, especially in the preterm newborn (Karlowicz and Adelman, 1992). Because continuous infusion of furosemide is less toxic and more effective than its bolus administration, continuous infusion of the drug should be used in neonates with intrinsic ARF.

There is no accepted *specific therapy* in clinical practice for intrinsic ARF. Experimental findings suggest that early administration of adenosine triphosphate–magnesium chloride (ATP-$MgCl_2$) or thyroxine may decrease the extent of cellular damage in experimental intrinsic ARF (Karlowicz and Adelman, 1992). Both agents exert their protective effects mainly by improving the recovery of renal cellular ATP (Boydstun et al, 1995; Karlowicz and Adelman, 1992). Because of its serious hemodynamic side effects, however, ATP-$MgCl_2$ is probably contraindicated in sick newborns. With regard to thyroxine, there is only one noncontrolled clinical study, in which the hormone was implicated in the recovery of renal function in eight children with ARF (Straub, 1976). The potential of thyroxine as well as adenine nucleotides and several growth factors to facilitate recovery in experimental ARF probably will be used in future clinical trials in an attempt to improve further recovery and survival of patients with intrinsic ARF (Wagener et al, 1995).

*Supportive care* includes prevention, early recognition, and aggressive management of complications of neonatal intrinsic ARF, including fluid overload, hypertension, electrolyte disturbances, nutritional deficiency, metabolic acidosis, and sepsis. Severe fluid restriction limiting intake to insensible and gastrointestinal and renal losses is required to avoid fluid overload with the development of pulmonary edema, congestive heart failure, hypertension, and hyponatremia. Fluid restriction also mandates the placement of a central venous line and the use of high glucose concentrations with little or no sodium and no potassium in the infusate.

Hypertension usually develops as a consequence of fluid overload or hyperreninemia resulting from the renal damage. The evaluation, diagnosis, and treatment of neonatal hypertension are described in Chapter 87.

Hyponatremia, hyperkalemia, hyperphosphatemia, and hypocalcemia frequently develop and necessitate close monitoring and aggressive treatment when indicated. In cases of nonsymptomatic hyponatremia (serum sodium concentrations usually between 120 and 130 mEq/L), further restriction of free water intake is recommended. If hyponatremia at this level results in clinical signs and symptoms (lethargy, seizures) or serum sodium concentration falls below 120 mEq/L, 3% sodium chloride should be administered over 2 hours according to the following formula:

$$Na^+_{required}\,(mEq) = ([Na^+]_{desired} - [Na^+]_{actual}) \times \text{body weight (Kg)} \times 0.8$$

Possible complications of hypertonic saline administration, especially if infused over less than 1 to 2 hours, include congestive heart failure, pulmonary edema, hypertension, intraventricular hemorrhage, and periventricular leukomalacia. Care should be taken not to increase serum sodium concentration more rapidly than 0.5 mEq/hour.

Signs of progressive hyperkalemia on the electrocardiogram, in order of severity, consist of tall peaked T waves, heart block with widened QRS complexes, arrhythmia, the development of sine waves, and finally cardiac arrest. If diuretics are ineffective and all potassium intake has been abolished (including that in medications), with serum potassium levels between 6 and 7 mEq/L and associated electrocardiogram changes or with serum potassium greater than 7 mEq/L in the absence of characteristic electrocardiogram changes, additional treatment is necessary. Under these conditions, management of hyperkalemia includes the administration of calcium gluconate, sodium bicarbonate, and insulin with glucose (Table 84–3). Although sodium polystyrene may also be administered, it must be remembered that up to 6 hours may be required before any effect is seen, and the exchange resin may be ineffective in preterm infants born at less than 29 weeks of gestation (Malone, 1991). Hyperkalemia unresponsive to medical management is one of the most common indications for peritoneal and hemodialysis in the newborn with intrinsic ARF (Coulthard and Vernon, 1995; Karlowicz and Adelman, 1992).

Hyperphosphatemia is common in ARF and should be treated with low phosphorus intake. Significant elevations in serum phosphate represent a risk of development of extraskeletal calcifications of the heart, blood vessels, and kidneys in the newborn, especially when the calcium-phosphorus product exceeds 70 (Lerner and Gruskin, 1990). Low-phosphorus formulas should be provided for those newborns who tolerate feeding. Soy formulas should be avoided because of their high aluminum content. Although calcium carbonate may be used as a phosphate-binding agent, severe hyperphosphatemia is best treated with dialysis.

TABLE 84-3

**Medical Management of Hyperkalemia in the Newborn**

| Drug | Dose | Onset of Action | Duration of Action |
|---|---|---|---|
| Calcium gluconate (10%) | 0.5-1.0 mL/kg (IV over 10 min) | 1-5 min | 15-60 min |
| Sodium bicarbonate (3.75% solution) | 1.0-2.0 mEq/kg (IV over 10 min) | 5-10 min | 2-6 hr |
| Insulin | 1 IU/5 g glucose (IV bolus or continuous infusion) | 15-30 min | 4-6 hr |
| Glucose | ≤14 mg/kg/min (IV bolus or continuous infusion) | 15-30 min | 4-6 hr |
| Sodium polystyrene sulfonate | 1 g/kg dose q6h as needed (orally/rectally) | 1-2 hr* | 4-6 hr |

*Onset of action may take up to 6 hours, and the drug may be ineffective in preterm infants born at less than 29 weeks of gestation (Malone, 1991). See text for details.

Although total calcium levels are frequently low in newborns with intrinsic ARF, ionized calcium is less commonly decreased, because of concurrent hypoalbuminemia and metabolic acidosis. If ionized calcium is decreased and the newborn is symptomatic, 100 to 200 mg/kg of calcium gluconate should be infused over 10 to 20 minutes and repeated every 4 to 8 hours as necessary. The usual maintenance doses of elemental calcium (50 to 100 mg/kg/day) also should be provided, in the form of calcium gluconate or calcium carbonate. If the newborn is being fed, dihydrotachysterol or calciferol may be administered to increase intestinal reabsorption of calcium.

Nutritional deficiency almost always develops in newborns with intrinsic ARF. The goal is to provide 100 kcal/kg/day with carbohydrates and fat, and 1 to 2 g/kg/day of high-biologic-value protein or an amino acid equivalent. Metabolic acidosis usually should be treated only when pH is less than 7.20, unless the newborn presents with associated pulmonary vascular reactivity and persistent pulmonary hypertension. The latter clinical scenario represents an extreme clinical challenge and may require the initiation of ECMO and hemofiltration to treat both the pulmonary vascular disease and the renal disease. Finally, because sepsis is a common cause of death in newborns with intrinsic ARF, infection control must be rigorously observed, and when sepsis is suspected appropriate diagnostic steps should be taken and non-nephrotoxic antibiotic therapy initiated. Because ARF alters the volume of distribution, protein binding, and renal excretion of many antibiotics, drug doses and dosing intervals should frequently be adjusted. Furthermore, many hepatically metabolized antibiotics still require renal excretion of their potentially toxic metabolites.

### Obstructive Renal Failure: Acute-Onset Chronic Renal Failure

Management of obstructive renal failure centers on the immediate relief of the obstruction, supportive medical care, and surgical correction of the underlying congenital malformation. Polyuria with electrolyte losses may occur following the relief of the obstruction, and close monitoring of serum electrolytes and appropriate fluid and electrolyte replacement therapy are necessary in the clinical care of such newborns.

## Management of More Advanced Renal Failure

### Dialysis

When renal failure is prolonged beyond 1 to 2 weeks, supportive therapy becomes unsuccessful and serious complications of intrinsic ARF develop. These complications may also develop in patients with worsening CRF and include severe fluid overload, electrolyte abnormalities (especially hyperkalemia or severe hyponatremia refractory to medical management), symptomatic uremia (tremors, vomiting, irritability), rising serum creatinine and BUN, and hypertension. When complications develop, dialysis should be initiated. However, dialysis should be started when the newborn is *still hemodynamically stable* so that this treatment modality can limit morbidity and mortality from ARF or CRF.

### Peritoneal Dialysis

Peritoneal dialysis has traditionally been preferred over hemodialysis in the newborn, but this may change with the use of cycling hemodialysis (see later). With peritoneal dialysis, the peritoneal catheter may be placed either percutaneously or surgically. One of the major problems with percutaneous catheters is the possibility of leakage around the catheter, rendering the dialysis virtually impossible. In patients with liver immaturity or dysfunction, bicarbonate dialysis may become necessary, because using the standard lactate-containing solution may result in significant metabolic acidosis owing to the inability of the liver to metabolize lactate adequately. Other, immaturity- and size-related technical problems with peritoneal dialysis include the need to deliver very small volumes, the high risk of infection (peritonitis) and bleeding complications, and the obstruction of the catheter by the sometimes very active omentum of the preterm infant (Coulthard and Vernon, 1995). Absolute or relative contraindications to peritoneal dialysis include necrotizing enterocolitis, abdominal wall defects, coagulopathy, hemodynamic instability, and the presence of an intra-abdominal foreign body, such as a ventriculoperitoneal shunt or diaphragmatic patch.

### Hemodialysis

Peritoneal dialysis is unlikely to be successful in cases with the foregoing contraindications. However, the small size of the neonatal arteries and veins restricts the use of hemodialysis because, as described by Poiseuille's law, at any pressure, the rate of flow of a liquid through a tube varies with the fourth power of the radius. Thus, if the catheter that can be used for hemodialysis is half the size of the peritoneal catheter for the same patient, only $^1/_{16}$ of the flow can be achieved at the same pressure. As for the type of catheters, use of a double-lumen catheter is preferred over use of two catheters for sampling and return, but the patient's size may again become a limiting factor. Hemodialysis is controlled by three factors: the membrane surface area, blood flow through the catheter, and dialysate fluid flow rate. Three different types of hemodialysis have been used in neonates and infants: continuous arteriovenous hemofiltration, continuous pumped hemodialysis, and cycling hemodialysis with a reservoir. *Continuous arteriovenous hemofiltration* uses the patient's cardiac output as the driving force for the hemofilter, which has a high ultrafiltration coefficient. The advantage of this technique is that it avoids rapid fluid shifts and the occurrence of hypotension by providing slow, continuous removal of an isotonic solute. *Continuous pumped hemodialysis* has all the limitations inherent to patient size and cannot be used in small or preterm neonates. Recently, *cycling hemodialysis with a reservoir* has been introduced (Coulthard and Sharp, 1995, 2001), allowing for the hemodialysis of preterm neonates weighing as little as 600 g using a manual syringe-driven circuit and a reservoir. This technique does not require priming of the circuit with blood and uses very small volumes. Effective hemodialysis is ensured by pushing the blood several times across the dialyzer in the reservoir before returning it to the neonate. However, more data are needed to assess safety and efficacy of this approach. It is important to note that these techniques require systemic heparinization, with activated clotting time usually kept at 180 to 200 seconds, rendering the technique relatively contraindicated in preterm newborns and others at high risk for intracranial bleeding. Furthermore, clotting of the catheters may occur, especially after prolonged use (Ronco et al, 1986).

### Transplantation

Renal transplantation is the definitive therapy for children with end-stage renal disease. Data on renal transplantation before 6 months of age or below a recipient weight of 6 kg are limited. However, recent data indicate that kidney transplantation results in young infants (<1 year of age) may be comparable to those in older pediatric age groups; the 5-year patient and/or graft survival rate is well over 80% (Humar et al, 2001). It also has been suggested that there is no need to set a minimum age for performing renal transplantation in very young infants (Humar et al, 2001). The patient's potential for growth and development, the primary renal disease, associated anomalies, urologic conditions, and family psychosocial status all are considered in determining eligibility for and the optimal time of transplantation. Although the overall postoperative complication rate is similar to that in older age groups, young infants may present with more vascular thrombotic complications. Long-term neurodevelopmental outcome in high-risk patients appears to be related to prematurity at birth and the presence of brain infarcts, probably secondary to the higher rate of the early post-transplantation thrombotic complications in the young infant (Qvist et al, 2002). Outcome is more favorable if the neonatal and young infant recipients receive their primary transplants from living donors (Humar et al, 2001).

## CLINICAL COURSE OF NEONATAL ACUTE AND CHRONIC RENAL FAILURE

Derangement of glomerular and tubular function may last for up to 3 to 6 weeks in newborns with ARF. In the case of oliguric ARF, if recovery occurs, it is usually heralded by a gradual increase in the urine output over the course of several days and, in some cases, by the appearance of a polyuric phase. The free water and electrolyte losses associated with the polyuric phase of recovery mandate close monitoring of serum electrolytes and appropriate replacement therapy with sodium, potassium, and free water if indicated. Serum creatinine and BUN usually start decreasing later in the course of polyuria.

CRF is characterized by reduced GFR in cases with excessive nephron losses and tubular dysfunction. CRF with reduced GFR develops in approximately 40% of newborns in both acquired oliguric (Stapleton et al, 1987) and nonoliguric (Chevalier et al, 1984) ARF. Newborns with the history of ARF secondary to congenital malformation have the worst long-term prognosis; close to 80% of such infants later develop CRF (Reinold et al, 1977).

In cases of CRF in which renal tubular dysfunction is the dominating pathophysiologic abnormality, a permanent decrease in the concentrating capacity due to injury to the epithelium of the thick ascending limb (see earlier) is the most frequent finding. Other abnormalities include chronic hypertension, renal tubular acidosis, impaired renal growth, and, mostly in cases of renal cortical necrosis, nephrocalcinosis (Karlowicz and Adelman, 1992).

## OUTCOME OF NEONATAL RENAL FAILURE

Overall long-term outcome for neonates with renal failure depends on the primary etiology, the extent of the insult in the acute phase of the renal failure, and associated anomalies. The mortality rate in newborns with ARF caused by congenital malformation or by acquired diseases is around 50% (Karlowicz and Adelman, 1992; Stapleton et al, 1987), whereas newborns with nonoliguric ARF have a much better prognosis (Chevalier et al, 1984; Karlowicz and Adelman, 1992). Although preliminary results appear encouraging, at present only limited data are available on long-term outcome of infants with CRF and renal transplantation.

## REFERENCES

Adelman RD, Wirth F, Rubio T: A controlled study of the nephrotoxicity of mezlocillin and gentamycin plus ampicillin in the newborn. J Pediatr 111:888, 1987.

Adler-Shohet F, Waskin HF, Lieberman JM: Amphotericin B lipid complex for neonatal invasive candidiasis. Arch Dis Child Fetal Neonatal Ed 84:F131, 2001.

Baenzinger O, Waldvogel K, Ghelfi D, et al: Can dopamine prevent the renal side effects of indomethacin? Klin Padiatr 211:438, 1999.

Balasubramanian J: Nimesulide and neonatal renal failure. Lancet 355:575, 2000.

Baley JE, Kliegman RM, Fanaroff AA: Disseminated fungal infections in very low birth weight infants: Therapeutic toxicity. Pediatrics 73:153, 1984.

Bannwarth B, Lagrange F, Pehourcq F, et al: (S)-ketoprofen accumulation in premature neonates with renal failure who were exposed to the racemate during pregnancy. Br J Clin Pharmacol 47:459, 1999.

Boydstun I, Najjar S, Kashgarian M, et al: Postischemic thyroxin stimulates renal mitochondrial adenine nucleotide translocator activity. Am J Physiol 268:E651, 1995.

Brezis M Rosen S, Silva P, Epstein FH: Selective vulnerability of the medullary thick ascending limb to anoxia in the isolated perfused rat kidney. J Clin Invest 73:182, 1984.

Buemi M, Allegra A, Rotig A, et al: Renal failure from mitochondrial cytopathies. Nephron 76:249, 1997.

Chevalier RL, Campbell F, Brenbridge AN: Prognostic factors in neonatal acute renal failure. Pediatrics 74:265, 1984.

Cifuentes RF, Olley PM, Balfe JW, et al: Indomethacin and renal function in premature infants with persistent patent ductus arteriosus. J Pediatr 95:583, 1979.

Coulthard MG and Vernon B. Managing acute renal failure in very low birth weight infants. Arch Dis Child 73:F187, 1995.

Coulthard MG, Sharp J: Hemodialysis and ultrafiltration in babies weighing under 1000 g. Arch Dis Child 73:F162, 1995.

Coulthard MG, Sharp J: Hemodialysing infants: Theoretical limitations, and single versus double lumen lines. Pediatr Nephrol 16:322, 2001.

Dixon BS, Anderson RJ: Nonoliguric acute renal failure. Am J Kidney Dis 6:71, 1985.

Ellis EN, Arnold WC: Use of urinary indices in renal failure in the newborn. Am J Dis Child 136:615, 1982.

Fajardo CA, Whyte RK, Steele BT: Effect of dopamine on failure of indomethacin to close the patent ductus arteriosus. J Pediatr 121:771-5, 1992.

Feld LG, Springate JE, Fildes RD: Acute renal failure: I. Pathophysiology and diagnosis. J. Pediatr 109:401, 1986.

Fildes RD, Springate JE, Feld LG: Acute renal failure: II. Management of suspected and established disease. J Pediatr 109:567, 1986.

Friedlich PS, Steinberg I, Fujitani A, deLemos R: Renal tolerance with the use of intralipid amphotericin B in low birth weight neonates. Am J Perinatol 14:377-382, 1997.

Giuliano RA Paulus GJ, Verpooten GA, et al: Recovery of cortical phospholipidosis and necrosis after acute gentamicin loading in rats. Kidney Int 26:838, 1984.

Guignard JP, Gouyon JB: Adverse effects of drugs on the immature kidney. Biol Neonate 53:243, 1988.

Heyman SN, Kaminski N, Brezis M: Dopamine increases renal medullary blood flow without improving regional hypoxia. Exp Nephrol 3:331, 1995.

Humar A, Arrazola L, Mauer M et al: Kidney transplantation in young children: Should there be a minimum age? Pediatr Nephrol 16:941, 2001.

Karlowicz MG, Adelman RD: Acute renal failure in the newborn. Clin Perinatol 19:139, 1992.

Karlowicz MG, Adelman RD: Nonoliguric and oliguric acute renal failure in asphyxiated term newborns. Pediatr Nephrol 9:718, 1995.

Kojima R, Kobayashi T, Matsuzaki S, et al: Effects of perinatal asphyxia and myoglobinuria on development of acute, neonatal renal failure. Arch Dis Child 60:908, 1985.

Kon V, Ichikawa I: Research seminar: Physiology of acute renal failure. J Pediatr 105:351, 1984.

Lerner GR, Gruskin AB: Acute renal failure. In Nelson NM (ed): Current Therapy in Neonatal-Perinatal Medicine, 2nd ed. Toronto, BC Decker, 1990, pp 173-177.

Liem KD, Hopman JCW, Oeseburg B, et al: Cerebral oxygenation and hemodynamics during induction of extracorporeal membrane oxygenation as investigated by near infrared spectroscopy. Pediatrics 95:555, 1995.

Malone T: Glucose and insulin versus cation-exchange resin for the treatment of hyperkalemia in very low birth weight infants. J Pediatr 118:121, 1991.

Mathew OP, Jones AS, James E, et al: Neonatal renal failure: Usefulness of diagnostic indices. Pediatrics 65:57, 1980.

Myers BD, Moran SM: Hemodynamically mediated acute renal failure. N. Engl J Med 314:97, 1986.

Noh PH, Cooper CS, Winkler AC et al: Prognostic factors for long-term renal function in boys with the prune-belly syndrome. J Urol 162:1399, 1999.

Pelayo JC, Andrews PM, Coffey AK, et al: The influence of age on acute renal toxicity of uranyl nitrate in the dog. Pediatr Res 17:985, 1983.

Peruzzi L, Gianoglio B et al: Neonatal end-stage renal failure associated with maternal ingestion of cyclo-oxygenase-type-2 selective inhibitor nimesulide as tocolytic. Lancet 354:919, 1999.

Qvist E, Pihko H, Fagerrud P, et al: Neurodevelopmental outcome in high-risk patients after renal transplantation in early childhood. Pediatr Transplant 6:53, 2002.

Rasoulpour M, Marinelli KA: Systemic hypertension. Clin Perinatol 19:121, 1992.

Reinold EW, Don TD, Worthen HG: Renal failure during the first year of life. Pediatrics 59:987, 1977.

Ronco C, Brendolan A, Bragantini L, et al: Treatment of acute renal failure in newborns by continuous arteriovenous hemofiltration. Kidney Int 29:9008, 1986.

Seri I: Cardiovascular, renal, and endocrine actions of dopamine in newborns and children. J Pediatr 126:333, 1995.

Seri I, Abbasi S, Wood DC, Gerdes JS: Regional hemodynamic effects of dopamine in the indomethacin-treated preterm infant. J Perinatol 22:300, 2002.

Seri I, Abbasi S, Wood DC, Gerdes JS: Regional hemodynamic effects of dopamine in the sick preterm infant. J Pediatr, 133:728, 1998.

Seri I, Rudas G, Bors ZS, et al: The effect of dopamine on renal function, cerebral blood flow and plasma catecholamine levels in sick preterm newborns. Pediatr Res 34:742, 1993.

Seri I, Tan, R, Evans J: The effect of hydrocortisone on blood pressure in preterm neonates with pressor-resistant hypotension Pediatrics 107:1070, 2001.

Stapleton FB, Jones DP, Green RS: Acute renal failure in newborns: Incidence, etiology and outcome. Pediatr Nephrol 1:314, 1987.

Straub E: Effects of L-thyroxine in acute renal failure. Res Exp Med 168:81, 1976.

Toth-Heyn P, Druckker A, Guignard JP: The stressed neonatal kidney: from physiology to clinical management of vasomotor nephropathy. Pediatr Nephrol 14:227, 2000.

Tulassay T, Seri I: Interaction of dopamine and furosemide in acute oliguria of preterm infants with hyaline membrane disease. Acta Pediatr Scand 75:420, 1986.

Tulassay T, Seri I, Machay T, et al: Effects of dopamine on renal function in premature infants with respiratory distress syndrome. Int J Pediatr Nephrol 4:199, 1983.

Wagener OE, Lieske JC, Toback FG: Molecular and cell biology of acute renal failure: New therapeutic strategies. New Horiz 3:634, 1995.

Yeh TF, Wilks A, Singh J, et al: Furosemide prevents the renal side effects of indomethacin therapy in premature infants with patent ductus arteriosus. J Pediatr 101:433, 1982.

CHAPTER

# 85

# Glomerulonephropathies and Disorders of Tubular Function

Bernard S. Kaplan

## GLOMERULONEPHROPATHIES

Glomerulonephropathies generally manifest with features of the nephrotic syndrome and less often with those of the nephritic syndrome. Massive proteinuria, hypoalbuminemia, hyperlipidemia, and edema characterize the nephrotic syndrome. Newborns may have transient proteinuria without apparent glomerular injury, and serum albumin levels can be in the nephrotic range in normal premature infants. Therefore, the diagnosis of nephrotic syndrome should be made only in patients with persistent, massive proteinuria, severe hypoalbuminemia, hyperlipidemia not caused by hyperalimentation, and edema that is not the result of fluid overload or capillary leak, or both. Nephritis (hematuria, red blood cell casts, oliguria or anuria, hypertension, and azotemia) is uncommon in newborns.

The nephrotic syndrome can be inherited as an entity isolated to the kidneys (congenital nephrotic syndrome of the Finnish type [CNF]) or as part of a defined malformation syndrome (Denys-Drash syndrome, Galloway-Mowat syndrome, or nail-patella syndrome). Glomerulopathies that occur in newborns and infants also can be divided into primary glomerular conditions with nephrotic syndrome (e.g., CNF) and secondary glomerular conditions (e.g., congenital syphilis). Only CNF and congenital syphilis *typically* manifest with nephrotic syndrome at birth. Diffuse mesangial sclerosis (DMS), Denys-Drash syndrome, and Galloway-Mowat syndrome rarely manifest in the neonatal period. Minimal-change nephrotic syndrome, focal segmental glomerulosclerosis, membranous glomerulonephritis, collagen type III glomerulopathy and mercury toxicity do not occur in newborns but occasionally present in infants. However, lupus nephritis and congenital toxoplasmosis have been reported in a neonate (Lam et al, 1999). Renal vein thrombosis can be a consequence of the nephrotic syndrome but is not a cause of the syndrome. There is no convincing evidence that intrauterine infections with cytomegalovirus (Batisky et al, 1993), rubella virus (Beale et al, 1979), or *Toxoplasma* (Shahin et al, 1974) are causes of neonatal nephrotic syndrome. In reports of *unique* family syndromes, congenital nephrotic syndrome occurred in association with congenital anomalies, such as buphthalmos. Finally, there are reports of congenital glomerular injury that elude classification and reports of spontaneous remission of apparent congenital nephrotic syndrome (Haws et al, 1992).

### Congenital Nephrotic Syndrome (CNS) of the Finnish Type

In CNF (NPHS1) [McKusick #256300], inheritance is autosomal recessive and the locus is assigned to 19q12-q13.1 (Kestila et al, 1994). The *NPHS1* gene that is mutated in NPHS1 codes for nephrin, a cell-surface podocyte protein. Two mutations, Fin-major and Fin-minor, are found in over 90% of Finnish patients (Patrakka et al, 2000). CNF occurs in all population groups, but the highest prevalence is in Finland, with an incidence of 12.2 per 100,000 newborns (Huttunen, 1976). There is minor intrafamilial and interfamilial variability in the severity and age at onset of the nephrotic syndrome. Absence of a history of Finnish ancestry does not exclude the diagnosis. Proteinuria is detected within the first week of life in 71% of cases and by 2 months in all affected infants (Huttunen, 1976). Early onset of hypertension and renal failure are uncommon. Infants are often premature and small for gestational age. Although there are no typical dysmorphic features, large anterior fontanels, limb deformations, and pyloric stenosis do occur (Sibley et al, 1986). Maternal serum and amniotic fluid alpha-fetoprotein levels are elevated (Seppala et al, 1976), and increased concentrations of albumin are detected in the amniotic fluid in some cases. The diagnosis may be made coincidentally by the finding of a low thyroxine level during screening for hypothyroidism (Finnegan et al, 1980). Most of these patients have a primary form of hypothyroidism characterized by low thyroxine and high thyroid-stimulating hormone (TSH) levels caused by urinary losses of thyroxine and iodine (McLean et al, 1982). The placenta is large, with a mean placenta-to-neonate weight ratio of 0.43 (normal ratio is around 0.18).

Echodense kidneys are symmetrically enlarged on ultrasonography. Proximal tubules are dilated in 74% of cases, and glomeruli initially appear normal. Ultrastructural studies show the effacement *(fusion)* of epithelial cell foot processes and, later in the course, interstitial fibrosis, lymphocytic and plasma cell infiltration, periglomerular fibrosis, and glomerular sclerosis (Habib, 1993).

The course is characterized by nephrotic syndrome complicated by failure to thrive, recurrent infections, and eventual chronic renal failure. Renal vein thrombosis may occur in utero or post partum. The nephrotic syndrome is resistant to treatment. Aggressive feeding by nasogastric or gastrostomy tube can ensure weight gain. Massive edema is treated with intravenous albumin. Furosemide is added if the patient is not volume depleted. Hypothyroidism is treated with thyroxine. Bilateral nephrectomies and dialysis are indicated if edema, volume depletion, and inanition cannot be controlled. Long-term peritoneal dialysis is difficult but feasible in small infants. The results with living-related-donor renal transplantation are encouraging, and CNF does not recur after transplantation (Mahan et al, 1984). Unfortunately, a unique post-transplantation glomerular lesion resembling transplant glomerulopathy occurs in a quarter of the patients and is resistant to treatment (Laine et al, 1993).

### Diffuse Mesangial Sclerosis

DMS can be inherited as an autosomal recessive condition or occur sporadically, and it is a component of the Denys-Drash syndrome (see later) (Habib, 1993). DMS has been reported in an 18-week fetus (Spear et al, 1991) and occasionally can manifest in the neonatal period (Scott and Rochefort, 1992). Maternal and fetal alpha-fetoprotein concentrations and placental size are usually normal (Scott and Rochefort, 1992). Most patients present with nephrotic syndrome and chronic renal failure between 3 and 6 months and are hypertensive. There are no dysmorphic features. The kidneys are seen to be enlarged and echodense by ultrasound examination. The fully developed renal lesion consists of mesangial sclerosis, collapsed tufts, embedded mesangial cells, thick glomerular basement membranes, and tubulointerstitial lesions (Habib, 1993).

There is no specific treatment. Hypertension is treated with angiotensin-converting enzyme (ACE) inhibitors, but several additional agents often are required. Treatment of DMS includes optimization of caloric intake, peritoneal dialysis, and transplantation. DMS does not recur after transplantation. It is important to determine whether there is a mutation in the *WT1* gene on chromosome 11p to rule out Denys-Drash syndrome. If that cannot be done, renal ultrasound examinations may be warranted every few months to monitor for Wilms tumor.

### Denys-Drash Syndrome

Early onset of nephrotic syndrome with DMS can also occur in the Denys-Drash syndrome. The syndrome consists of overlapping features of ambiguous genitalia, nephrotic syndrome with DMS (Habib, 1993), Wilms tumor, and a zinc finger mutation on chromosome 11p (Schumacher et al, 1998). Occasionally, patients present with nephrotic syndrome in the neonatal period (Maalouf et al, 1998). Siblings are not affected. Most patients die by 4 years of age unless they receive a kidney transplant.

### Galloway-Mowat Syndrome

Galloway-Mowat syndrome is a rare condition that consists of abnormal central nervous system development and nephrotic syndrome (Cooperstone et al, 1993). Inheritance is autosomal recessive, and there may be variable expression in a family (Cohen et al, 1994). Patients may be small for gestational age. The nephrotic syndrome usually manifests before the age of 3 years and often develops before 3 months. There are no consistent glomerular histopathologic changes. The pathogenesis has not been determined. Neurologic findings are microcephaly, wide sulci, abnormal gyral patterns, developmental retardation, and seizures (Kucharczuk et al, 2000). Large floppy ears, a receding forehead, and hiatal hernia are features in some cases (Cooperstone et al, 1993). Death usually occurs before 6 months of age. The nephrotic syndrome does not respond to treatment. Renal transplantation is not encouraged because of the progressive nature of the severe neurologic disorder. Increased values on maternal serum and amniotic fluid alpha-fetoprotein assays and abnormal renal ultrasonographic findings may prove useful for prenatal diagnosis (Palm et al, 1986).

### Congenital Syphilis

Clinical features of nephrotic syndrome predominate over those of nephritis. The diagnosis must be suspected in an infant who has edema, proteinuria, and signs of congenital syphilis (McDonald et al, 1971). The glomerular findings implicate an immune pathogenesis with subepithelial deposits that contain immunoglobulin G (IgG) and treponema antigen (O'Regan et al, 1976). Treatment with penicillin results in permanent remission of the glomerulopathy.

## DISORDERS OF RENAL TUBULAR FUNCTION

The diagnosis of a renal tubular disorder cannot be made without an appreciation of normal renal maturation. Premature newborns (and even full-term newborns) can exhibit sodium and chloride wasting and have variable combinations of aminoaciduria, glucosuria, phosphaturia, impaired potassium excretion, reduced reabsorptive capacity for sodium bicarbonate, and inability to concentrate the urine maximally. In healthy newborns, these are transient aberrations that tend to be isolated and that do not cause problems except for the low bicarbonate threshold in preterm infants. This derangement can lead to mild metabolic acidosis during the first few months of life. Very low-birth-weight newborns may have nonoliguric hyperkalemia, in part secondary to decreased $Na^+,K^+$-ATPase activity, which increases with maturation. Therefore, except in specific circumstances, it is not necessary to embark on a full-scale evaluation.

Some renal tubular disorders may be suspected and confirmed in utero. A prenatal diagnosis, however, requiring chorionic villus sampling or amniocentesis can be made only after the diagnosis of the condition in an older sibling. Postnatally, the possibility of a tubular disorder may arise when abnormal blood gas and electrolyte results are obtained. The initial manifestations of a renal tubular disorder may not include all of the findings associated with the disorder.

Three constellations of fluid and electrolyte imbalances should alert the neonatologist to the possibility of a disorder of renal tubular function. (1) The combination of *metabolic acidosis, hyperkalemia*, and *hyponatremia* is seen in renal dysplasias, obstructive uropathy (especially if complicated by a urinary tract infection), and pseudohypoaldosteronism. Furthermore, congenital adrenal hyperplasia can manifest with these abnormalities. (2) *Metabolic acidosis, hypokalemia*, and *hypophosphatemia* are the characteristic findings seen in patients with the renal tubular Fanconi syndrome. (3) *Metabolic alkalosis, hypokalemia*, and *hyponatremia* occur in the Bartter syndromes.

Important clinical clues to the presence of a renal tubular disorder are poor feeding, unexplained vomiting, dehydration, failure to thrive, drowsiness, irritability, tetany, seizures, and unexplained icterus. Isolated proximal renal tubular acidosis (RTA) is uncommon, and the need for large quantities of bicarbonate to correct a hyperchloremic metabolic acidosis is a clue to the diagnosis. Fructose intolerance and galactosemia must be considered in a jaundiced newborn who has Fanconi syndrome. Hypophosphatemia and renal phosphate wasting are manifestations of X-linked hypophosphatemic rickets, but it is uncommon for this disorder to be diagnosed in a newborn. Hyperchloremic metabolic acidosis with a decrease in the unmeasured anion gap and in the absence of diarrhea raises the possibility of distal RTA. Distal RTA rarely manifests in the neonatal period, however. Pseudohypoaldosteronism, Bartter syndromes, and renal adysplasias must be considered in newborns with severe hyponatremia and renal salt wasting. Infants with Bartter syndrome are hypokalemic, whereas those with renal adysplasia, pseudohypoaldosteronism, and the renal tubular hyperkalemia syndromes are hyperkalemic. Hematuria, renal calculi, and nephrocalcinosis with hypercalciuria can occur in newborns with and without prolonged use of furosemide. Primary hyperoxaluria type 1 may manifest in the newborn period with acute renal failure and nephrocalcinosis (Ellis et al, 2001).

## Renal Fanconi Syndrome of Proximal Tubular Dysfunction

The renal Fanconi syndrome is characterized by generalized proximal renal tubular dysfunction with impaired net reabsorption of amino acids, bicarbonate, glucose, phosphate, urate, sodium, potassium, magnesium, calcium, and low-molecular-weight proteins. Renal excretion of these solutes and water is increased, and the serum concentrations of some are variably reduced. Hypophosphatemia results in vitamin D–resistant rickets, and bicarbonaturia causes a hyperchloremic metabolic acidosis. In newborns, the clinical manifestations of renal Fanconi syndrome may include polyuria, dehydration, metabolic acidosis, and glycosuria. These features are often asynchronous. Growth retardation and rickets mostly occur later in infancy.

### *Hereditary Fructose Intolerance*

Hereditary fructose intolerance (HFI) [McKusick #229600] manifests only in newborns fed sucrose or fructose in formula, antibiotics, fruit juices, or honey. The symptoms are poor feeding, vomiting, and failure to thrive (Gitzelman et al, 1989). The diagnosis can be made by molecular analysis of the aldolase-B gene in blood (Brooks and Tolan, 1993). Inheritance is autosomal recessive. Fructose-containing foods must be withdrawn from the diet as soon as the condition is suspected.

### *Galactosemia*

Classic galactosemia [McKusick #230400] can manifest in neonates with vomiting, diarrhea, hyperbilirubinemia with jaundice, hepatomegaly, ascites, and *Escherichia coli* sepsis a few days after starting milk ingestion. Cataracts are occasionally detectable by slit-lamp examination in neonates. This autosomal recessive disease is caused by deficient activity of galactose-1-phosphate uridyltransferase (GALT) as a result of mutations at the *GALT* gene on chromosome 17q (Tyfield et al, 1999). Two other autosomal recessively inherited disorders of galactose metabolism—transferase and epimerase deficiency—occur more rarely. Newborn screening programs include tests for detection of galactosemia. The diagnosis is suggested by demonstrating increased concentrations of galactose in blood and urine and confirmed by demonstrating deficient red blood cell GALT (or galactokinase). Milk and milk-containing products must be withdrawn from the diet.

### *Cytochrome-c Oxidase Deficiency*

Cytochrome-*c* oxidase deficiency (Biervliet et al, 1977), a fatal infantile cytopathy with variable manifestations in brain, skeletal and cardiac muscle, and liver, and occasionally also manifesting with renal Fanconi syndrome, is one of the "mitochondrial cytopathy" syndromes associated with defects in complex IV of the respiratory chain (cytochrome-*c* oxidase; EC 1.9.3.1). Inheritance appears to be autosomal recessive. Clinical features include neonatal onset of hypotonia; hyporeflexia; respiratory failure; elevated levels of lactic and pyruvic acids in blood, cerebrospinal fluid, or urine; and renal Fanconi syndrome (Lombes et al, 1996). There is no treatment; prognosis is dismal, and most patients die in infancy.

### Cystinosis

Infants affected with cystinosis [McKusick #219800] appear normal at birth and develop manifestations of the renal Fanconi syndrome between 6 and 12 months. The diagnosis should be considered if there are features of the renal Fanconi syndrome in a neonate. Inheritance is autosomal recessive, and there is defective lysosomal transport of cystine. The cystinosis gene, *CTNS*, maps to chromosome 17p13 and encodes an integral membrane protein, cystinosin (Town et al, 1998). Cystinosis can be diagnosed in utero using cystine measurements in chorionic villi by 9 weeks (Smith et al, 1987). Early and adequate treatment with oral cysteamine retards progression to end-stage renal failure (Markello et al, 1993), and administration of 0.55% cysteamine eyedrops from 1 year of age dissolves the corneal cystine crystals (Gahl et al, 2000).

### *Tyrosinemia Type 1*

Type 1 tyrosinemia [McKusick #276700] is caused by deficiency in the gene for fumarylacetoacetate hydrolase on chromosome 15q23-q25. Although type 1 tyrosinemia is an important cause of renal Fanconi syndrome and hepatocellular carcinoma, this condition rarely manifests in the neonate (Vanden Eijnden et al, 2000).

### Renal Glycosuria

Isolated forms of renal glycosuria rarely manifest in the newborn and are benign. Intermittent or constant renal glycosuria can be detected in newborns who have the rare and possibly autosomal recessive condition of glucose and galactose malabsorption (Markello et al, 1993).

### Renal Tubular Acidosis

Primary RTA is characterized by chronic hyperchloremic metabolic acidosis associated with an inability to acidify the urine. It may be a primary disorder or secondary to acquired renal injury. Primary RTA is not associated with the renal Fanconi syndrome. Primary RTA is separated into three main types: proximal RTA (pRTA) (type 2); distal RTA (dRTA) or "classic" RTA (type 1), and hyperkalemic RTA (type 4) (Rodriguez-Soriano, 2002).

#### *Primary Proximal Renal Tubular Acidosis*

Proximal RTA is an integral feature of the renal Fanconi syndrome, and primary pRTA is extremely uncommon. Proximal RTA is the result of an inability to reabsorb filtered bicarbonate in the proximal tubule, with bicarbonate wasting and hyperchloremic metabolic acidosis and normal distal tubular acidification. Therefore, when the filtered bicarbonate is reclaimed up to the maximal renal tubular reabsorptive capacity for a patient with pRTA, the urine pH is appropriate for the severity of the metabolic acidosis, with values below 5.3. When pRTA occurs as an isolated defect, it is usually transient (Nash et al, 1972).

#### *Distal Renal Tubular Acidosis*

Clinical manifestations of dRTA are anorexia, failure to thrive, hypotonia, a persistently low serum bicarbonate, elevated serum chloride, inappropriately high urine pH, and, in some cases, nephrocalcinosis. Additional findings are decreased urinary excretion of titratable acid, ammonium ($NH_4^+$), and citrate. Some patients have congenital high-frequency nerve deafness. Untreated patients develop rickets (Caldas et al, 1992). Distal RTA is often considered in the differential diagnosis of a neonate with a non–anion gap acidosis, but there are few reports of dRTA in neonates (Caldas et al, 1992; McSherry et al, 1978). The possibility of dRTA can be inferred from calculating the rate of excretion of ($NH_4^+$). This can be determined indirectly by calculating the urinary net charge or urine anion gap (Goldstein et al, 1986):

$$Na^+ + K^+ + NH_4^+ = Cl^- + 80$$

The kidney is not the cause of the acidosis if the chloride ($Cl^-$) is greater than the sum of the $Na^+$ (sodium) + $K^+$ (potassium). If the sum of $Na^+ + K^+$ is greater than $Cl^-$, then the urinary ($NH_4^+$) may be less than 80 mmol per day, in keeping with dRTA (Carlisle et al, 1991). The diagnosis of dRTA is often made erroneously in patients with a hyperchloremic metabolic acidosis who have an "inappropriate" urine pH over 6 but who have diarrhea (Izraeli et al, 1990).

Regardless of whether a transient or permanent form of dRTA is suspected, adequate amounts of alkali, as either bicarbonate or citrate, in doses of 2 to 3 mEq/kg/day are required to maintain a normal serum bicarbonate concentration (Igarashi et al, 1992). This can be withdrawn after several months to challenge the diagnosis, or the infant can be allowed to outgrow the dose. Challenge with an ammonium chloride loading test is not necessary because the diagnosis can be inferred from indirect tests such as the urine anion gap.

At least two autosomal recessively inherited forms of dRTA exist. In dRTA *without* nerve deafness, the mutated gene is located on chromosome 7q33-34; the gene product is the 116-kD β subunit of the apical pump (ATP6β1) (Smith et al, 2000). Distal RTA *with* nerve deafness (Karet et al, 1999) is caused by mutations in ATP6β1, located on chromosome 2p13, encoding the β subunit of the apical proton pump, which mediates distal nephron acid secretion.

#### *Renal Tubular Acidosis Caused by Maternal Sniffing of Toluene*

Maternal toluene abuse from paint or glue sniffing during pregnancy causes severe RTA in mother and neonate (Lindemann, 1991).

### Bartter Syndromes: Inherited Hypokalemic Renal Tubular Disorders

The Bartter syndromes are a group of congenital chronic tubular disorders characterized by hypokalemic metabolic alkalosis, polyuria, salt wasting, hyperkaliuria, hyperaldosteronism, resistance to the pressor effect of angiotensin, juxtaglomerular apparatus hyperplasia, increased renal renin production, and, in some patients, hypercalciuria and nephrocalcinosis. Similar features occur with loop diuretic treatment and congenital chloride diarrhea. At least three clinical subtypes of the Bartter syndromes, with marked phenotypic variations within each subtype, are known: the *antenatal hypercalciuric variant*, or hyperprostaglandin E syndrome (HPS/aBS); *classic Bartter syndrome* (cBS); and the *Gitelman variant of Bartter syndrome* (GS). The common characteristics of each subtype are hypokalemic metabolic alkalosis and renal salt wasting.

#### *Antenatal Hypercalciuric Variant*

Antenatal hypercalciuric variant (hyperprostaglandin E syndrome) (HPS/aBS) is a life-threatening neonatal disorder. Features include polyhydramnios, premature delivery, hypokalemia, hypercalciuria, metabolic alkalosis, fever, vomiting, diarrhea and failure to thrive, hyposthenuria, and nephrocalcinosis. The inheritance is autosomal recessive with mutations in the gene for either the furosemide-sensitive Na-K-2Cl cotransporter, NKCC2 (*SLC12A1*), or the inwardly rectifying potassium channel, subfamily J, member 1, ROMK (*KCNJ1*) on chromosome 11q24 (Jeck et al, 2001a). Classic Bartter syndrome also may be caused by a mutation in either of these genes, suggesting that the antenatal and classic forms are different manifestations of severity of the same disorder. In addition, neonates have been identified who have homozygous gene mutations linked to chromosome 1p31, who do not respond to indomethacin treatment, and who have a more severe variant with marked delays in growth and motor development, chronic renal failure, and congenital deafness (Jeck et al, 2001b). There is no cure for Bartter syndrome, but treatment with inhibitors of prostaglandin synthesis improves the polyuria, corrects the biochemical abnormalities, and permits satisfactory growth and development. However, the nephrocalcinosis may not improve (Mourani et al, 2000).

### *Classic Bartter Syndrome*

In classic Bartter syndrome (cBS) [McKusick #241200], the clinical phenotype varies from episodes of neonatal severe volume depletion with hypotension and hypokalemia to mild symptoms in a patient diagnosed in adolescence. Serum magnesium levels are normal. Several reported cases involved mutations in one of three genes encoding ascending limb of Henle transporters: (1) Na-K-2Cl cotransporter (basolateral chloride channel), CLCNKB, on chromosome 1p36; (2) Na-K-2Cl cotransporter gene, *NKCC2* (*SLC12A1*), on chromosome 15q13; or (3) the gene encoding the inwardly rectifying $K^+$ channel, subfamily J, member 1, *ROMK* (*ROMK1/KCNJ1*) on chromosome 11q24. *CLCNKB* mutations also may cause congenital Bartter (HPS/aBS) or a Gitelman-like phenotype.

### *Gitelman Variant of Bartter Syndrome*

The Gitelman variant of Bartter syndrome (GS) [McKusick #263800] usually does not manifest in neonates (Bettinelli et al, 2000). Hypocalciuria and hypomagnesemia are specific clinical features of Gitelman syndrome. The Gitelman variant is caused by mutations in the gene for the thiazide-sensitive Na-Cl cotransporter NCCT (*SLC12A3*) of the distal tubule, on chromosome 16q13.

### Renal Tubular Hyperkalemia

The causes of neonatal renal tubular hyperkalemia (RTH) are marked prematurity, renal adysplasia, urinary tract obstruction, urinary tract infection, pseudohypoaldosteronism, and congenital adrenal hyperplasia (Rodriguez-Soriano et al, 1995). Features of RTH include an inappropriately low urine potassium concentration, renal salt wasting, and metabolic acidosis. The serum creatinine concentration is often increased because of volume depletion (pseudohypoaldosteronism, congenital adrenal hyperplasia), reduced nephron mass (renal adysplasia), or obstruction (posterior urethral valves).

### *Pseudohypoaldosteronism*

Two syndromes of aldosterone resistance exist: pseudohypoaldosteronism type I and pseudohypoaldosteronism type II (Hanukoglu, 1991). Furthermore, there are two clinically and genetically distinct types of type I pseudohypoaldosteronism: the renal pseudohypoaldosteronism and the multiple-organ pseudohypoaldosteronism. Pseudohypoaldosteronism may be inherited as an autosomal dominant or as an autosomal recessive trait. In the dominant form of pseudohypoaldosteronism type I, mutations in the gene *MLR* encoding the mineralocorticoid receptor have been recognized. In the recessive form of pseudohypoaldosteronism type I there are mutations in the genes *SNCC1A*, *SNCC1B*, and *SCNN1G*, which encode subunits of the epithelial $Na^+$ channel (Rodriguez-Soriano, 2000).

#### Renal Pseudohypoaldosteronism Type I

Renal pseudohypoaldosteronism type I usually starts in early infancy and is characterized by diminished renal tubular responsiveness to aldosterone, with hyponatremia, hyperkalemia, markedly elevated plasma aldosterone, and hypereninemia. The clinical expression ranges from that in severely affected patients who die in infancy to an asymptomatic state. Symptomatic patients are treated with sodium supplementation, which usually is no longer necessary by 2 years of age.

#### Multiple Organ Pseudohypoaldosteronism Type I

With multiple organ pseudohypoaldosteronism type I, there is impaired responsiveness to aldosterone in salivary and sweat glands, renal tubules, and colonic mucosal cells. The course is protracted, with life-threatening episodes of salt wasting.

#### Pseudohypoaldosteronism Type II (Gordon Hyperkalemia-Hypertension Syndrome)

Features of pseudohypoaldosteronism type II (Gordon hyperkalemia-hypertension syndrome) are hyperkalemia despite a normal glomerular filtration rate, hypertension, variable mild hyperchloremia, metabolic acidosis, and suppressed plasma renin activity (Schambelan et al, 1981). The metabolic abnormalities are corrected by treatment with thiazide diuretics. There are no reports of neonatal presentation.

### Congenital Nephrogenic Diabetes Insipidus

Nephrogenic diabetes insipidus (NDI) can result from congenital or acquired insults to the kidneys including electrolyte abnormalities (hypokalemia, hypocalcemia), drugs (aminoglycosides), tubular interstitial inflammation, obstruction, and dysplasia. In the congenital or inherited forms of NDI, insensitivity of the distal nephron to the antidiuretic effect of vasopressin results in an inability to concentrate urine, resulting in the excretion of large quantities of hypotonic urine (Bichet et al, 1997; van Lieburg et al, 1999). Affected neonates may be irritable, feed poorly, fail to gain weight, and have unexplained dehydration and fevers. Serum concentrations of sodium, chloride, creatinine, and blood urea nitrogen (BUN) are elevated, and serum levels of vasopressin are normal or increased. There is a blunted response of plasma factor VIII, von Willebrand factor, and plasminogen activator after administration of 1-desamino-8-D-arginine vasopressin (DDAVP). Treatment with hydrochlorothiazide (3 mg/kg/day) and amiloride (0.3 mg/kg/day three times a day) may be preferable to hydrochlorothiazide and indomethacin because indomethacin can cause bleeding. Treatment can prevent dehydration, electrolyte imbalances, cerebral calcification and seizures, and result in normal growth but patients continue to have polydipsia and polyuria.

About 90% of patients with inherited NDI are males with the X-linked form caused by mutations in the arginine vasopressin receptor 2 gene (*AVPR2*) located in chromosomal region Xq28 (Morello and Bichet, 2001) that codes for the V2 receptor. In less than 10% of the families, the inheritance of NDI is autosomal recessive or autosomal dominant. In these cases, mutations have been identified in the aquaporin-2 gene (*AQP2*) on chromosome 12q13 that codes for the vasopressin-sensitive water channel (Goji et al, 1998). The reliability of prenatal diagnosis of the X-linked form of NDI is about 96%.

## REFERENCES


Batisky DL, Roy S III, Gaber LW: Congenital nephrosis and neonatal cytomegalovirus infection: A clinical association. Pediatr Nephrol 7:741, 1993.

Beale MG, Strayer DS, Kissane JM, Robson AM: Congenital glomerulosclerosis and nephrotic syndrome in two infants. Am J Dis Child 133:842, 1979.

Bettinelli A, Ciarmatori S, Cesareo L, et al: Phenotypic variability in Bartter syndrome type I. Pediatr Nephrol 14:940, 2000.

Bichet DG, Oksche A, Rosenthal W: Congenital nephrogenic diabetes insipidus. J Am Soc Nephrol 8:1951, 1997.

Biervliet JPAM, Bruinvis L, Ketting D, et al: Hereditary mitochondrial myopathy with lactic acidemia, a De Toni-Fanconi-Debre syndrome, and a defective respiratory chain in voluntary striated muscle. Pediatr Res 11:1088, 1977.

Brooks CC, Tolan DR: Association of the widespread A 149 P hereditary fructose intolerance mutation with newly identified sequence polymorphisms in the aldolase gene. Am J Med Genet 52:835, 1993.

Caldas A, Broyer M, Dechaux M, et al: Primary distal tubular acidosis in childhood: Clinical study and long-term follow-up of 28 patients. J Pediatr 121:233, 1992.

Carlisle EJF, Donnelly SM, Halperin ML: Renal tubular acidosis (RTA): Recognize the ammonium defect and pHorget the urine pH. Pediatr Nephrol 5:242, 1991.

Cohen AH, Turner MC: Kidney in Galloway-Mowat syndrome: Clinical spectrum with description of pathology. Kidney Int 45:1407, 1994.

Cooperstone B, Friedman A, Kaplan BS: The Galloway-Mowat syndrome of abnormal gyral pattern and glomerulopathy. Am J Med Genet 47:250, 1993.

Ellis SR, Hulton SA, McKiernan PJ, et al: Combined liver-kidney transplantation for primary hyperoxaluria type 1 in young children. Nephrol Dial Transplant 16:348, 2001.

Finnegan JT, Slosberg EJ, Postellon DC, Primack WA: Congenital nephrotic syndrome detected by hypothyroid screening. Acta Paediatr Scand 69:705, 1980.

Gahl WA, Kuehl EM, Iwata F, et al: Corneal crystals in nephropathic cystinosis: Natural history and treatment with cysteamine eyedrops. Mol Genet Metab 71:100, 2000.

Gitzelman R, Steinmann B, van den Berghe G: Disorders of fructose metabolism. In Scriver C, Beaudet AL, Sly WS, Valle D (eds): The Metabolic Basis of Inherited Disease, 6th ed. New York, McGraw-Hill, 1989, pp 399-424.

Goji K, Kuwahara M, Gu Y, et al: Novel mutations in aquaporin-2 gene in female siblings with nephrogenic diabetes insipidus: Evidence of disrupted water channel function. J Clin Endocrinol Metab 83:3205, 1998.

Goldstein MB, Bear R, Richardson RM, et al: The urine anion gap: A clinically useful index of ammonium excretion. Am J Med Sci 282:198, 1986.

Habib R: Nephrotic syndrome in the 1st year of life. Pediatr Nephrol 7:347, 1993.

Hanukoglu A: Type I pseudohypoaldosteronism includes two clinically and genetically distinct entities with either renal or multiple organ defects. J Clin Endocrinol Metab 73:936, 1991.

Haws RM, Weinberg AG, Baum M: Spontaneous remission of congenital nephrotic syndrome: A case report and review of the literature. Pediatr Nephrol 6:82, 1992.

Huttunen N-P: Congenital nephrotic syndrome of Finnish type: Study of 75 patients. Arch Dis Child 51:344, 1976.

Igarashi T, Sekine Y, Kawato H, et al: Transient distal renal tubular acidosis with secondary hyperparathyroidism. Pediatr Nephrol 6:267, 1992.

Izraeli S, Rachmel A, Frishberg Y, et al: Transient renal acidification defect during acute infantile diarrhea: The role of urinary sodium. J Pediatr 117:711, 1990.

Jeck N, Derst C, Wischmeyer E, et al.: Functional heterogeneity of ROMK mutations linked to hyperprostaglandin E syndrome. Kidney Int 59:1803, 2001a.

Jeck N, Reinalter SC, Henne T, et al: Hypokalemic salt-losing tubulopathy with chronic renal failure and sensorineural deafness. Pediatrics 108:E5, 2001b.

Karet FE, Finberg KE, Nelson RD, et al: Mutations in the gene encoding B1 subunit of $H^+$-ATPase cause renal tubular acidosis with sensorineural deafness. Nat Genet 21:84, 1999.

Kestila M, Mannikko C, Gyapay G, et al: Congenital nephrotic syndrome of the Finnish type maps to the long arm of chromosome 19. Am J Hum Genet 54:757, 1994.

Kucharczuk K, de Giorgi AM, Golden J, et al: Additional findings in Galloway-Mowat syndrome. Pediatr Nephrol 14: 406, 2000.

Laine J, Jalanko H, Holthofer H, et al: Post-transplantation nephrosis in congenital nephrotic syndrome of the Finnish type. Kidney Int 44:867, 1993.

Lam C, Imundo L, Hirsch D, et al: Glomerulonephritis in a neonate with atypical congenital lupus and toxoplasmosis. Pediatr Nephrol 13:850, 1999.

Lindemann R: Congenital renal tubular dysfunction associated with maternal sniffing of organic solvents. Acta Paediatr Scand 80:882, 1991.

Lombes A, Romero NB, Touati G, et al: Clinical and molecular heterogeneity of cytochrome *c* oxidase deficiency in the newborn. J Inherit Metab Dis 19:286, 1996.

Mahan JD, Mauer SM, Sibley RK, et al: Congenital nephrotic syndrome: Evolution of medical management and results of renal transplantation. J Pediatr 105:549, 1984.

Maalouf EF, Ferguson J, van Heyningen V, et al: In utero nephropathy, Denys-Drash syndrome and Potter phenotype. Pediatr Nephrol 12:449, 1998.

Markello TC, Bernardini IM, Gahl WA: Improved renal function with cystinosis treated with cysteamine. N Engl J Med 328:1157, 1993.

McLean RH, Kennedy TL, Ratzan SK, et al: Hypothyroidism in congenital nephrotic syndrome. J Pediatr 101:72, 1982.

McDonald R, Wiggelinkhuizen J, Kaschula ROC: The nephrotic syndrome in very young infants. Am J Dis Child 122:507, 1971.

McSherry E, Morris RC Jr: Attainment of normal stature with alkali therapy in infants and children with classic renal tubular acidosis. J Clin Invest 61:509, 1978.

Morello JP, Bichet DG.: Nephrogenic diabetes insipidus. Annu Rev Physiol 63:607, 2001.

Mourani CC, Sanjad SA, Akatcherian CY: Bartter syndrome in a neonate: Early treatment with indomethacin. Pediatr Nephrol 14:143, 2000.

Nash MA, Torrado AD, Griefer I, et al: Renal tubular acidosis in infants and children. J Pediatr 80:738, 1972.

O'Regan S, Fong JSC, de Chadarevian JP, et al: Treponemal antigens in congenital and acquired syphilitic nephritis. Ann Intern Med 85:325, 1976.

Palm L, Hagerstrand I, Kristoffersson U, et al: Nephrosis and disturbances of neuronal migration in male siblings—a new hereditary disorder? Arch Dis Child 61:545, 1986.

Patrakka J, Kestila M, Wartiovaara J, et al: Congenital nephrotic syndrome (NPHS1): Features resulting from different mutations in Finnish patients. Kidney Int 58:972, 2000.

Rodriguez-Soriano J: Potassium homeostasis and its disturbances in children. Pediatr Nephrol 9:364, 1995.

Rodriguez-Soriano J: New insights into the pathogenesis of renal tubular acidosis—from functional to molecular studies. Pediatr Nephrol 14:1121, 2000.

Schambelan M, Sebastian A, Rector FC Jr: Mineralocorticoid-resistant renal hyperkalemia without salt wasting (type II pseudohypoaldosteronism): Role of increased renal chloride reabsorption. Kidney Int 19:716, 1981.

Schumacher V, Scharer K, Wuhl E: Spectrum of early onset nephrotic syndrome associated with WT1 missense mutations. Kidney Int 53:1594, 1998.

Scott RJ, Rochefort M: Fatal perinatal nephropathy with onset in intrauterine life. Arch Dis Child 67:1212, 1992.

Seppala M, Rapola J, Huttunen N-P, et al: Congenital nephrotic syndrome: Prenatal diagnosis and genetic counselling by estimation of amniotic-fluid and maternal serum alpha-fetoprotein. Lancet 11:123, 1976.

Shahin B, Papadopoulou ZL, Jenis EH: Congenital nephrotic syndrome associated with congenital toxoplasmosis. J Pediatr 85:366, 1974.

Sibley RK, Mahan JD, Vernier RL: Congenital and infantile nephrotic syndrome: A clinicopathologic study of 46 cases. Kidney Int 27:544, 1986.

Smith ML, Pellett OL, Cass MM, et al: Prenatal diagnosis of cystinosis utilizing chorionic villus sampling. Prenat Diagn 7:23, 1987.

Smith AN, Skaug J, Choate KA: Mutations in *ATP6N1B*, encoding a new kidney vacuolar proton pump 116-kD subunit, cause recessive distal renal tubular acidosis with preserved hearing. Nat Genet 26:71, 2000.

Spear GS, Steinhaus KA, Quddusi A: Diffuse mesangial sclerosis in a fetus. Clin Nephrol 36:46, 1991.

Town M, Jean G, Cherqui S, et al: A novel gene encoding an integral membrane protein is mutated in nephropathic cystinosis. Nat Genet 18:319, 1998.

Tyfield L, Reichardt J, Fridovich-Keil J, et al: Classical galactosemia and mutations at the galactose-1-phosphate uridyl transferase (GALT) gene. Hum Mutat 13:417, 1999.

Vanden Eijnden S, Blum D, Clercx A, et al: Cutaneous porphyria in a neonate with tyrosinaemia type 1. Eur J Pediatr 159:503, 2000.

van Lieburg AF, Knoers NV, Monnens LA: Clinical presentation and follow-up of 30 patients with congenital nephrogenic diabetes insipidus. J Am Soc Nephrol 10:1958, 1999.

CHAPTER

# 86

# Urinary Tract Infections and Vesicoureteral Reflux

Stephen A. Zderic

This chapter provides an overview of the epidemiology, pathophysiology, radiographic evaluation, and management of urinary tract infections in the neonate. Although the focus here is on the management of vesicoureteral reflux as one of the congenital conditions frequently associated with urinary tract infection, other congenital urologic anomalies also may manifest with urinary tract infection. Of several key points emphasized in this chapter, one of the most important is that reflux itself does not cause urinary tract infection. Therefore, many children may have reflux without any symptoms, and the neonates who develop bladder infections and have reflux will be the ones who present clinically. It also is important to remember that biologic susceptibility plays a major role in the etiology of neonatal urinary tract infections. Finally, it has been recognized that not all damage to the kidneys associated with reflux reflects scarring from infection. Indeed, some kidneys with high-grade reflux have elements of dysplasia and scarring at the time of initial presentation and in the absence of infection.

## URINARY TRACT INFECTIONS

### Epidemiology

Within the first several months of postnatal life, urinary tract infections are more common in boys. After the first 6 months, the incidence in girls increases steadily as that in boys declines (Shortliffe, 1992). Some studies have suggested that the incidence of urinary tract infections is anywhere from 10- to 15-fold higher in girls than in boys between 1 and 3 years of age. A major risk factor for urinary tract infection was delineated by Wiswell reporting alone (1992) and with Geschke (1989), who noted that although only 20% of males were uncircumcised, this group accounted for 80% of all urinary tract infections in boys. These data suggests that circumcision offers protection against urinary tract infections in the first year of life. Wiswell and Geschke's findings offer support for encouraging circumcision in males with congenital structural or functional abnormalities placing them at high risk for pyelonephritis and sepsis, such as patients with posterior urethral valves or reflux.

### Diagnosis

The diagnosis of a urinary tract infection in a young infant is not always straightforward, and a high index of suspicion is required because the symptoms are so generalized. In one series of 100 infants, all infants were febrile with temperatures above 38° C (70% had temperatures above 39° C), 60% were irritable, 50% were feeding poorly, and 40% had vomiting or diarrhea (Ginsburg and McCracken, 1982). The index of suspicion must rise when these aforementioned symptoms are present with no localizing source. In such instances, obtaining a urine specimen for analysis and culture must be included in the evaluation.

Much has been said and written about the procurement of specimens by the techniques of clean catch (not applicable in neonates), use of a bag, catheterization, or suprapubic puncture. Results of studies on bag or clean-catch specimens are valid only if cultures are truly negative. It is intuitively obvious why these collection methods are susceptible to contamination in girls and, especially, in the uncircumcised male (Fig. 86–1). Knowledge of the composition of the preputial or vaginal flora is of little use in managing the febrile child; what matters most is the composition of the urine within the bladder itself. This problem is compounded when bagged specimens are obtained at home and arrive "fresh" at the office only to be sent to a central laboratory before plating. Another problem arises with the definition of what a negative urine culture means. In many instances the reports say the results are negative but only because the presence of 100,000 colony-forming units (CFUs) is used as a cutoff point to define a positive culture. Hoberman and colleagues (1994) have looked at the frequency distribution of the voided or bag specimens and compared the findings with those in post-void specimens obtained by catheterization of febrile infants. The authors found that 10,000 to 49,000 CFUs/mL usually represented contamination, whereas counts in excess of 50,000 CFUs/mL were more characteristic of a true positive. Still, there were overlaps between these groups, and numeric quantitation remains an inexact tool.

The gold standard for specimen collection remains suprapubic aspiration, which is accurate and can be safely performed in a neonate because the bladder is a pelvic organ. A 21-gauge needle may be inserted into the palpable bladder just above the pubic symphysis in the midline to collect an aspirate. However, even urologists rarely use this method of collection; a catheterized specimen is easy to obtain and provides accurate results, especially if the first 2 to 3 mL of urine, which may contain urethral contaminants, is discarded. For a febrile child presenting to an emergency room with possible urosepsis, or requiring hospital admission, documentation of a urinary tract infection should be established on the basis of a catheterized specimen (or a suprapubic aspirate). *Voided clean-catch or bag methods may be used early on in an evaluation before the urinary tract is considered a source.* However, the increased incidence of false-positive findings seen with these collection methods means that more patients will undergo antibiotic therapy and a costly and invasive radiographic work-up. The greatest diagnostic yield from doing these expensive and invasive studies will be in the population of patients whose urinary tract infection was most accurately diagnosed by using catheterized or suprapubic specimens.

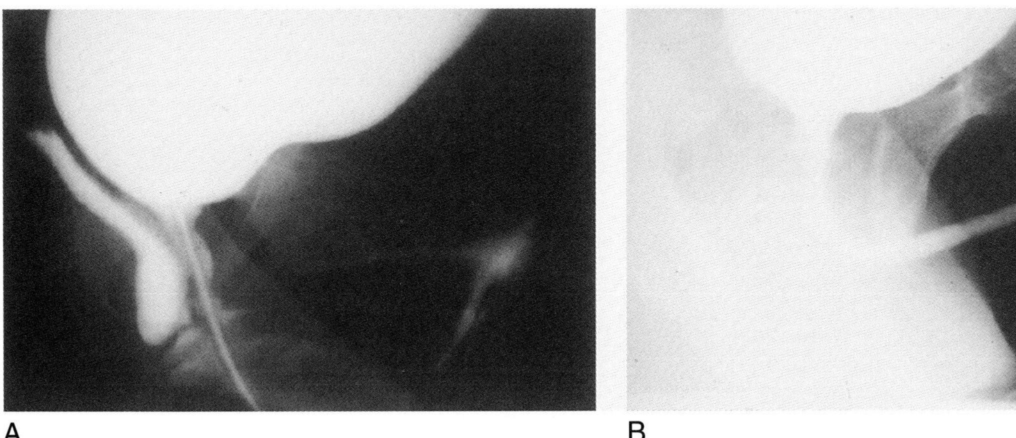

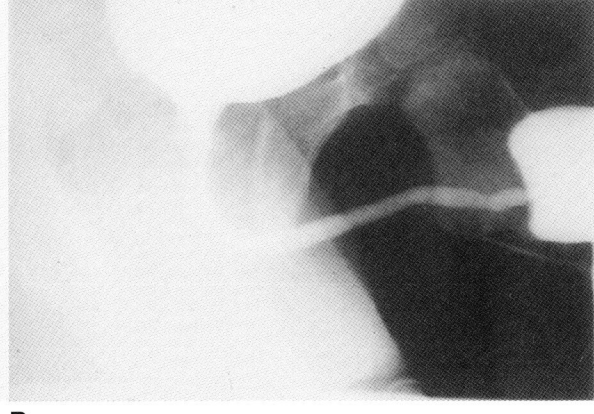

**FIGURE 86–1.** These VCUG findings demonstrate how bagged specimens may lead to false-positive results in infant females or uncircumcised males. Vaginal reflux allows for contaminants in the bagged specimen from an infant female (**A**). In the uncircumcised male, urine may pool underneath the foreskin and acquire contaminating flora (**B**).

### Treatment

The neonate with suspected urosepsis should receive broad-spectrum antibiotic coverage until results of sensitivity testing dictate a shift to single-antibiotic coverage. Ampicillin and gentamicin provide excellent coverage for the most common pathogens that are likely to be present. The most likely pathogen is *Escherichia coli*, but there is always a possibility of *Pseudomonas*, especially in an infant who was just discharged to home following a stay in the neonatal intensive care unit (NICU). The duration of intravenous antibiotic therapy for pyelonephritis can be debated, but parenteral therapy at least avoids the concern of compliance issues. Experimental evidence demonstrates that reflux-associated pyelonephritis in piglet confirmed by technetium 99m dimercaptosuccinic acid (DMSA) scan can be successfully treated with only oral macrodantin (Risdon et al, 1995). Given the expense of hospitalization or home-based intravenous antibiotic therapy, the mandatory duration of parenteral therapy will continue to be debated, especially in the older child (Hoberman et al, 1999). However, in the more susceptible neonate, parenteral therapy should be instituted in a hospital setting and continued until results of a follow-up urine culture become negative (AAP Committee, 1999). At that point, oral antibiotic therapy may be started for a total course of 10 to 14 days.

Once the acute infection has been treated, antibiotic prophylaxis should be instituted until the child is ready for radiographic imaging studies. The use of amoxicillin (12.5 mg/kg) in neonates, or trimethoprim-sulfamethoxazole in infants, is accepted for prophylaxis. The use of trimethoprim-sulfamethoxazole in urology patients for suppression is based on the classic work of Stamey (1980), who demonstrated that low-dose antibiotic treatment does not produce shifts in the fecal flora. In contrast, high doses of trimethoprim-sulfamethoxazole and especially of broad-spectrum antibiotics have been shown to produce greater and more concerning shifts in the fecal flora. This finding is especially significant because the feces serve as the origin for most (>90%) of the bacteria that colonize the perineum and vagina and thus ultimately produce a urinary tract infection.

### The Radiographic Work-up

Once a diagnosis of urinary tract infection has been established and treated, it is important to initiate a radiographic work-up to look for any underlying structural anomalies (AAP Committee, 1999). It has been stated that up to 30% of children with a urinary tract infection have aberrant urinary tract anatomy or function. The radiographic evaluation should consist of an ultrasound study of the *kidneys and bladder*, followed by a carefully done voiding cystourethrogram (VCUG) (Lebowitz and Mandell, 1987). Most often, a 2- to 4-week period is allowed between infection and the radiographic imaging, but this interval is arbitrary. It is more important is to ensure that the urine is sterile before performance of the VCUG. A patient should be maintained on antimicrobial prophylaxis until imaging rules out any urinary tract pathology. On sonography, obtaining both kidney and bladder views is stressed because sometimes the kidneys alone are imaged and shown to be normal, and the work-up is terminated. Then, several infections later, a bladder ultrasound study shows a stone, ureterocele, or diverticulum. Even if a VCUG is being done on the same day of the renal ultrasound examination, a small ureterocele may be missed at the fluoroscopy that would have been seen on the bladder sonogram.

The VCUG must be done carefully and requires patience on the part of all concerned. Because the act of voiding is required to demonstrate reflux in 20% to 30% of reflux cases, such cases would be missed if the child were anesthetized for a static cystogram. The policy at the author's institution is to obtain a classic fluoroscopic study first, to define the anatomy and accurately grade the reflux if it is present. Some groups have advocated that radionuclide VCUG be used as the initial screening study.

However, to appropriately define the anatomy, the contrast VCUG remains the gold standard. As discussed later in the section on reflux, the cornerstone of accurate management is grading of the reflux, which can be provided only by a well-executed VCUG study.

In recent years there has been a growing support in the literature for the use of DMSA scanning to identify patients with acute pyelonephritis. However, it is this author's bias that an *accurately collected* urine specimen showing signs of infection in a febrile patient is adequate. The DMSA scan is very helpful in assessing the patient with abnormal anatomy secondary to exstrophy or spina bifida, whose chronic catheterization regimens result in chronic urinary colonization and a urine culture that will always be positive.

### Pathophysiology

Urinary tract infections are multifactorial in their etiology and clearly represent an altered balance between host and pathogen. Abnormal anatomy serves to exacerbate the effects of a urinary tract infection. The reader is referred to several excellent reviews regarding this issue (Lebowitz and Mandell, 1987; Shortliffe, 1992; Stamey, 1980). Hematogenous spread of bacteria to the urinary tract may occur but is very rare. Most urinary tract infections will start in the bladder and then *ascend* to produce pyelonephritis. This ascent of infected urine from the bladder to the kidney may take place via two major mechanisms: (1) the bacteria may be extremely virulent and produce pili that allow the bacteria to attach themselves to the ureter and migrate upstream, or (2) the patient may have reflux that showers the renal pelvis, allowing for intrarenal reflux and seeding of the renal parenchyma (Fig. 86–2). Once bacteria are injected into the renal parenchyma under high pressures, areas of focal infection and inflammation develop (Fig. 86–3), and a series of complex steps in the inflammatory cascade take place (Roberts, 1992). If this process is not interrupted by treatment, it can produce severe renal injury or scarring. Furthermore, if repeated infectious insults such as these continue without adequate therapy, the long-term result is significant renal scarring, which in its extreme produces reflux nephropathy, leading to end-stage renal disease.

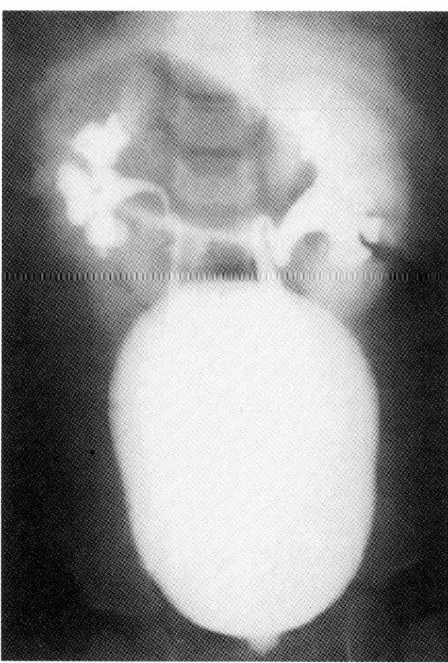

**FIGURE 86–2.** High-grade bilateral vesicoureteral reflux with evidence of pyelotubular backflow within the left kidney is demonstrated on this VCUG in a neonate.

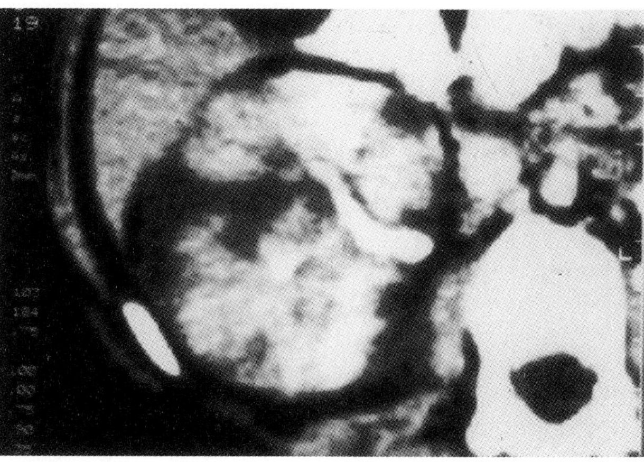

**FIGURE 86–3.** This CT scan of an infant with right pyelonephritis and associated grade II reflux shows the signs of lobar nephronia. Areas within the right kidney function well and excrete contrast—others show signs of poor perfusion.

Equally important in the pathogenesis of urinary tract infections is the biology of the patient (or host). It is accepted that many patients are more susceptible to bacterial urinary tract infections because their bladder mucosa expresses cell surface proteins that have a high affinity for the cell surface antigens on the bacterial cell wall. A great deal is known about the bladder mucosal expression of these complex glycoproteins, with some being mannose sensitive. In these cases, the receptor-ligand interaction between pathogen and host is based on the molecular recognition of mannose-6-phosphate (Schaeffer et al, 1984).

## Urinary Tract Infections Complicated by Obstructive Uropathy

An important consideration is what happens when urinary tract infections develop in a newborn with an abnormal urinary tract. It used to be extremely common for obstructive uropathies to present after urosepsis had developed. With the widespread use of prenatal sonography, however, most neonates with an obstructive uropathy are identified at birth, and antibiotic prophylaxis is initiated. However, on occasion even today, a neonate may still present with urosepsis secondary to an obstructive uropathy. In such cases, the obstructive uropathy may have developed after the initial early normal prenatal ultrasound examination, or the problem went undiscovered because of a lack of access to prenatal care.

The most common pathologic factor associated with a febrile urinary tract infection in a neonate or infant is vesicoureteral reflux. However, on occasion, an obstructed system will be discovered during the work-up. The presence of obstruction produces a dangerous combination of bacteria, urinary stasis, and a warm environment with a near-ideal culture broth. Thus, one must always consider the possibility of an infection developing in an obstructed system. Keeping this possibility in mind is important because the management may be altered by the use of surgical drainage (by either ureterostomy or percutaneous nephrostomy). During treatment for acute pyelonephritis, the patient may not defervesce for 48 to 72 hours. *However, beyond 72 hours, underlying obstruction must be suspected if fever persists or the neonate's condition worsens.* Under these circumstances, an ultrasound study to rule out obstruction is warranted. Infections may become established in primary megaureters, ureteroceles, or ectopic ureters (Fig. 86–4) and, on rare occasions, in ureteropelvic junction (UPJ) obstructions. Urine production allows for some antibiotic to reach these bacteria, and a good response may be seen if the patient receives treatment early in the course of the infection. In advanced cases, especially in those associated with poor renal function, temporary drainage procedures such as percutaneous nephrostomy will allow for eradication of the infection and for the patient's condition to stabilize before definitive repair.

## VESICOURETERAL REFLUX

Vesicoureteral reflux exists when urine flows from the bladder back toward the kidney; this reverse flow may occur during bladder filling or emptying (voiding). Using the contrast VCUG, it is possible to grade reflux from I through V (Fig. 86–5). Grading reflux allows physicians to communicate findings quickly and to understand what the chances of spontaneous resolution are. Many additional findings appear on the VCUG images besides just the grade. Was there reflux on filling, and did it start at the beginning or at the end of the filling phase? How much contrast was added to the bladder prior to the initiation of voiding? Was there evidence of a pyelotubular backflow? (See Fig. 86–2.) By evaluating the findings in detail, a better understanding of the severity, potential treatment modalities, and outcome can be achieved and utilized for the benefit of the patient.

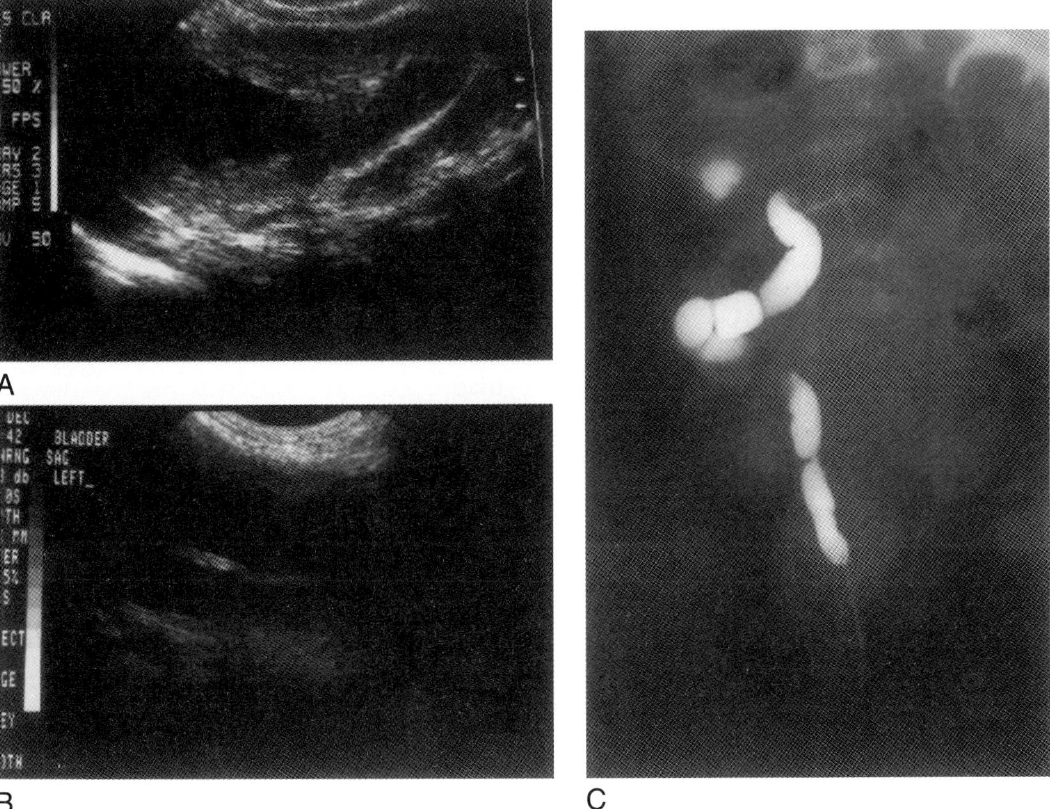


**FIGURE 86–4.** Ectopic ureter and urosepsis. This 3-month-old infant presented with a high fever and a positive urine culture that failed to respond to parenteral antibiotic therapy. **A** and **B,** The ultrasound showed signs of right hydronephrosis and hydroureter; **C,** a retrograde pyelogram confirmed a diagnosis of ectopic ureter. Most such cases are identified by fetal sonography. However, in this instance, the young parents did not seek prenatal care. Following a cutaneous diversion of this ectopic ureter, the infant became afebrile, and ureteral reimplantation was successfully performed 6 months later.

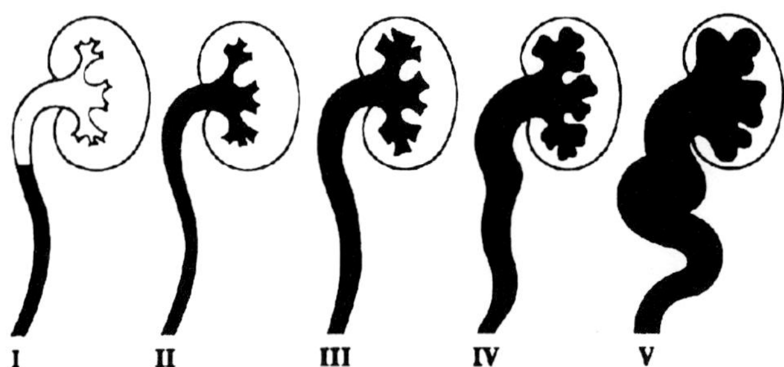


**FIGURE 86–5.** Grading scale for reflux. The International Reflux Study used this grading scale, which is based on the findings on a conventional fluoroscopic voiding cystourethrogram.

The etiology of reflux remains debated, but there is growing agreement that reflux constitutes a syndrome. Some patients with reflux have a congenital anatomic basis for the reflux. The normal course of the ureter travels through the bladder wall and underneath the mucosal layer to create a flap valve mechanism, which prevents vesicoureteral reflux. Reflux due to anatomic abnormalities in bladder insertion of the ureter is referred to as *primary reflux*. In other patients, reflux occurs secondary to increases in bladder pressure, a condition referred to as *secondary reflux*. For example, many patients with posterior urethral valves may have reflux, which disappears once the valves are resected. This distinction is important because the rules for primary reflux resolution do *not* apply to cases of reflux secondary to obstructing lesions such as posterior urethral valves or the neurogenic bladder seen with spina bifida.

Growing clinical (Sillen et al, 1992, 1996a, b) evidence suggests that voiding pressures are dramatically increased in infants with reflux, especially in boys. Sillen (2001) has shown that, even in normal males, voiding pressures are elevated in the neonatal period and decline dramatically during the first 2 years of life. Sillen's data demonstrate that voiding pressures in boys with high-grade reflux are often three- to fourfold higher than those seen in older children. In these boys, the reflux often resolves in a surprisingly short period of time, implying that with maturation of bladder function, the pressures drop. Of interest, female newborns do not fare as well with regard to the resolution of neonatal reflux on a grade-for-grade basis, nor are their voiding pressures as elevated. These clinical observations are supported by experimental findings suggesting that there are gender-related differences in bladder neck function. The key concept is that voiding pressures are elevated, especially in the male neonate with reflux, and that these pressures diminish over time. These observations have a great bearing on how reflux resolution rates should be interpreted in the newborn.

However, outcomes for reflux resolution in neonates must be studied further (Sillen, 1999a, b). This should be made easier by the increased number of cases detected by prenatal ultrasonography. Evidence from a multicenter study suggests that reflux detected in the first months of life as part of a work-up for prenatal hydronephrosis has a better chance for spontaneous resolution, grade for grade, than that diagnosed in the child presenting at 2 to 4 years of age (Herndon et al, 1999). Given this information, recommendations that can be made about neonatal reflux management will be altered by the mode of presentation and social circumstances (compliance issues). For a newborn with prenatally diagnosed grade IV or V reflux, expectant observation with antibiotic prophylaxis seems most reasonable. However, this course of action demands that parents comply with antibiotic prophylaxis and understand that a breakthrough infection rate as high as 20% is possible (Herndon et al, 1999). This series also pointed out the benefit for circumcision in males with known reflux (Herndon et al, 1999). The case can be made for a more aggressive surgical approach if a neonate presents with *urosepsis and high-grade* (*IV or V*) *reflux*. It is absolutely crucial for any parent and referring physician to understand that successful reimplantation surgery diminishes but does not eradicate the likelihood of pyelonephritis. A child with innate susceptibility will still experience bladder infections despite the absence of reflux.

Several studies have shown that siblings of patients with reflux also have a higher likelihood of having reflux (Jerkins and Noe, 1982; Noe, 1995). Sibling screening studies in the first year of life have shown that anywhere from 20% to 50% of the siblings will have a VCUG that is positive for reflux (Noe, 1995; Parekh et al, 2002). It can be argued that all siblings should be screened, perhaps even up to the age of 9 years. Several studies have shown an increased incidence of renal scarring in siblings whose reflux was discovered by screening (Sweeney et al, 2001; Wan et al, 1996). Parekh and colleagues (2002) suggest that sibling reflux follows a more benign course and noted no renal scarring following antibiotic prophylaxis. On the other hand, would the cohort of patients in their study have done just as well if undiagnosed and left off antibiotic prophylaxis? It behooves us to remember that many asymptomatic infants have undiagnosed reflux, never develop urinary tract infections, resolve their reflux, and live normal lives. The extent to which screening averts renal complications will be best answered by prospective trials.

It is clear that identifying neonates with reflux and starting antibiotic prophylaxis offer benefit in terms of reducing the number of episodes of pyelonephritis. Clearly, episodes of pyelonephritis and the associated renal inflammation that results (see Fig. 86–3) can do harm if left untreated. It is estimated that each episode of febrile urinary tract infection may lead to a 5% risk of formation of a new renal scar per episode. All authorities agree that repeated and untreated infection does harm to the kidney. It is, however, very important to note that not all of the renal insufficiency in patients with reflux reflects damage by infection. This case is demonstrated in Figure 86–6, in which a VCUG was done for antenatal reflux and demonstrated massive grade V reflux. In the patient, a newborn child, urinary tract infection had never been noted, yet the creatinine was already abnormal and the ultrasound findings demonstrated increased echogenicity and a loss of corticomedullary differentiation. In this setting, the high-grade reflux is associated with renal dysplasia at the onset, and renal failure will be progressive.

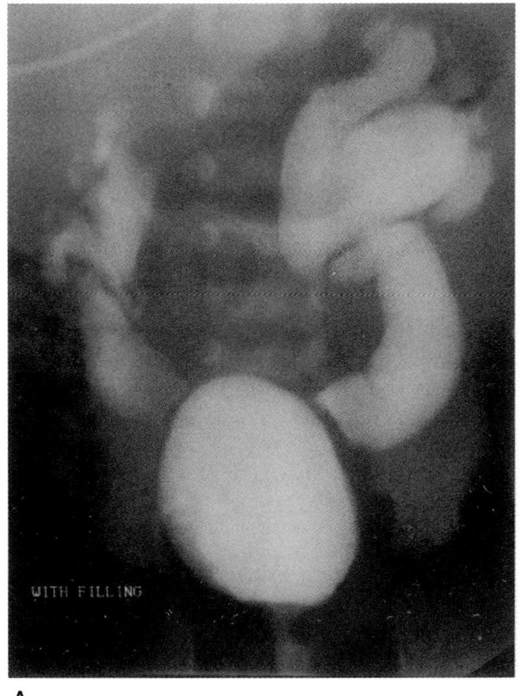


A

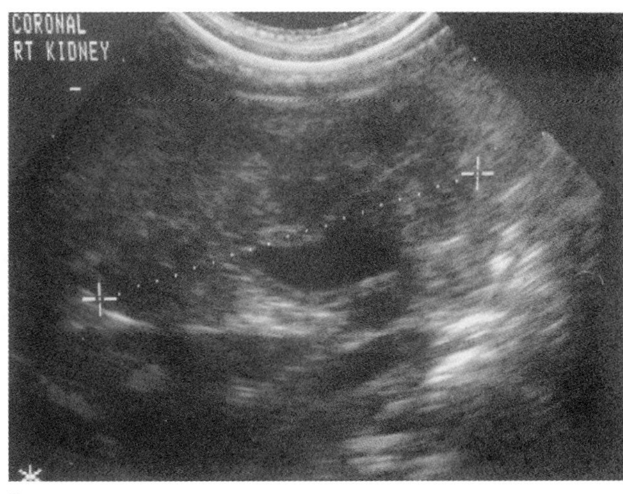


B

**FIGURE 86–6.** Dysplasia and high-grade reflux. This case demonstrates the association of bilateral grade V reflux with renal dysplasia. The voiding cystourethrogram (**A**) and ultrasound scan (**B**) shown here were performed within the first 2 weeks of life, and the child had never had a diagnosed urinary tract infection during this interval. Despite sterile urine, the creatinine was elevated, and the renal sonogram showed increased echogenicity and poor corticomedullary differentiation. This case points out that renal insufficiency associated with reflux often is present at the outset and is not always secondary to infection.

## REFERENCES


AAP Committee on Quality Improvement and Subcommittee on Urinary Tract Infection: Practice parameter: The diagnosis, treatment, and evaluation of the initial urinary tract infection in febrile infants and young children. Pediatrics 103:843-852, 1999.

Ginsberg CM, McCracken GH Jr: Urinary tract infections in young infants. Pediatrics 69:409-412, 1982.

Herndon CD, McKenna PH, Kolon TF, et al: A multicenter outcomes analysis of patients with neonatal reflux presenting with prenatal hydronephrosis. J Urol 162:1203-1208, 1999.

Hoberman A, Wald ER, Reynolds EA, et al: Pyuria and bacteruria in catheterized urine specimens obtained from young children with fever. J Pediatr 124:513-519, 1994.

Hoberman A, Wald ER, Hickey RR, et al: Oral versus initial intravenous therapy for urinary tract infections in young febrile children. Pediatrics 104:79-86, 1999.

Jerkins GR, Noe HN: Familial vesicoureteral reflux: A prospective study. J Urol 128:774-775, 1982.

Lebowitz RL, Mandell J: Urinary tract infections in children: Putting radiology in its place. Radiology 165:1-9, 1987.

Noe HN: The current status of screening for vesicoureteral reflux. Pediatr Nephrol 9:638, 1995.

Parekh DJ, Pope JC, Adams MC, Brock JW: Outcome of sibling vesicoureteral reflux. J Urol 167:283-284, 2002.

Risdon RA, Godley ML, Parkhouse HF, et al: Renal pathology and the $^{99m}$Tc-DMSA image during the evolution of the early pyelonephritic scar: An experimental study. J Urol 151:767-773, 1994

Roberts JA: Vesicoureteral reflux and pyelonephritis in the monkey: A review. J Urol 148:1721-1724, 1992.

Schaeffer AW, Chmiel JS, Duncan JL, et al: Manose sensitive adherents of *E. coli* to epithelial cells from women with recurrent urinary tract infections. J Urol 131:906-910, 1984.

Shortliffe LM: Urinary tract infections in infants and children. In Walsh PC, Retik AB, Stamey TA, Vaughan ED (eds): Campbell's Urology, 6th ed. Philadelphia, WB Saunders, 1992, pp 1669-1686.

Sillen U: Bladder function in healthy neonates and its development during infancy. J Urol 166:2376-2381, 2001.

Sillen U, Bachelard M, Hansson S, et al: Video cystometric recording of dilating reflux in infancy. J Urol 155:1711-1715, 1996a.

Sillen U, Bachelard M, Hermanson G, Hjalmas K: Gross bilateral reflux in infants: Gradual decrease of initial detrusor hypercontractility. J Urol 155:668-672, 1996b.

Sillen U, Hjalmas K, Aili M, et al: Pronounced detrusor hypercontractility in infants with gross bilateral reflux. J Urol 148:598-599, 1992.

Stamey TA: Pathogenesis and Treatment of Urinary Tract Infections. Baltimore, Williams & Wilkins, 1980.

Sweeney B, Cascio S, Veldayudham M, Puri P: Reflux nephropathy in infants presenting with and without urinary tract infection. J Urol 166:648-650, 2001.

Wan J, Greenfield SP, Ng M, et al: Sibling reflux: A dual center retrospective study. J Urol 156:677-679, 1996.

Wiswell TE: John K. Lattimer lecture. Prepuce presence portends prevalence of potentially perilous periurethral pathogens. J Urol 148:739-742, 1992.

Wiswell TE, Geschke DW: Risks from circumcision during the first month of life compared to those for uncircumcised boys. Pediatrics 83:1011-1015, 1989.

CHAPTER

# 87

# Renal Vascular Disease in the Newborn

**Tivadar Tulassay, Rangasamy Ramanathan, Jacquelyn R. Evans, and Istvan Seri**

For the pediatric patient population, the neonatal period represents the time of greatest risk for thromboembolic complications, with neonates presenting with 5.1 symptomatic thromboses per 100,000 live births (Nowak-Göttl et al, 1997). This high incidence decreases significantly after the first year of life. Neonatal hemostasis is characterized by a decrease in both the concentration and the function of the procoagulant and anticoagulant proteins. In addition, there is a decreased response of neonatal platelets to physiologic agonists, although, by affecting blood rheology and offering an additional source for adenosine diphosphate (ADP) release, the higher hematocrit may partially compensate for the immaturity of platelet function (Israels et al, 2001). However, under pathologic conditions, such as hypoxia, hypovolemia, hypotension, maternal diabetes, infection, and polycythemia, this delicate balance is easily disrupted, leading to an increased incidence of bleeding or thrombosis in the sick newborn. Among the recently recognized genetic conditions, hereditary thrombophilia with the G1691A mutation in the factor V gene (factor V Leiden) is the most commonly found prothrombotic risk factor for early spontaneous thrombosis during infancy (Nowak-Göttl et al, 2001; Schobess et al, 1999). In addition to the pathologic conditions, the placement of an indwelling arterial or venous catheter resulting in endothelial injury plays a major role in thrombus formation in neonates. This notion is supported by the observation that 44% to 89% of all major vessel thromboses in the newborn are associated with catheter placement (Nowak-Göttl et al, 1997; Schmidt and Andrew, 1995). Symptomatic thromboembolic complications with umbilical artery catheters alone are estimated at 1% to 9% (Weiner et al, 1998); placement of an umbilical vein catheter in sick neonates is associated with portal vein thrombosis in 1.3% of the cases (Schwartz et al, 1997). The incidence of asymptomatic aortic and ductus venosus, inferior vena cava, and right atrial thrombosis associated with umbilical catheters is in the 17% to 31% range (Horgan et al, 1987; Oppenheimer et al, 1982, Roy et al, 2002). It has recently been found that Doppler echocardiography is less sensitive than contrast venography in detecting asymptomatic thrombosis associated with umbilical vein catheter placement (Roy et al, 2002). Finally, although relatively rarely reported, neonatal thromboembolism may result in death or severe organ failure as a consequence of irreversible tissue damage.

The neonatal kidney is especially at high risk for thrombus formation. In addition to the use of umbilical artery catheters (see later), the low renal blood flow, the relatively small caliber of the renal vessels, high catecholamine levels, and the enhanced renal vasoconstrictive and angioproliferative effects of endothelin and angiotensin II contribute to the increased risk of thrombogenesis in the neonatal kidney. The incidence of renovascular thrombosis in the newborn is unknown. In the past, renal venous thrombosis was more common. Since the introduction of umbilical arterial catheters in the routine care of the sick newborn, however, aortic and associated renal arterial thrombosis has become more frequent. Although renal vascular events usually manifest with the development of renal dysfunction, the function of other organs also may be affected, leading to the development of adrenal hemorrhage, necrotizing enterocolitis, congestive heart failure, systemic hypertension, inadequate perfusion of the lower extremities, and multiorgan failure.

## RENAL ARTERIAL OBSTRUCTION

### Etiology and Incidence

In the vast majority of the cases, renal arterial obstruction is the consequence of intra-arterial thrombus formation. Before the introduction of umbilical artery catheterization, only a few cases of renal artery thrombosis were reported, with shock, coagulopathy, and congestive heart failure being the principal causative factors (Adelman, 1988). The introduction of umbilical artery catheterization in the early 1970s resulted in a significant increase in the incidence of neonatal aortic thrombosis. Because the presence of a catheter-related aortic thrombus is associated with involvement of one or both of the renal arteries in 30% to 50% of affected newborns, umbilical artery catheter placement also increases the incidence of renal artery thrombosis (Schmidt and Andrew, 1995; Seibert et al, 1987). Ultrasonographic findings suggest that catheter-related asymptomatic aortic thrombi are present in 17% to 31% of newborns (Horgan et al, 1987; Oppenheimer et al, 1982), although the Doppler ultrasound technique may underestimate the real incidence (Roy et al, 2002; Schmidt and Andrew, 1995). The incidence of *severe symptomatic thrombosis* after umbilical artery catheter placement is much lower and is reported to be around 1% (O'Neill et al, 1981). Because the trauma to the vessel wall inflicted at the time of the placement of the catheter appears to play the most important role in aortic thrombus formation (Goetzman et al, 1975; Rasoulpour and Marinelli, 1992), the procedure should be done carefully to minimize endothelial injury and the attendant risk of thrombus formation. Because continuous infusion of low-dose heparin prolongs the patency of umbilical artery lines (Rajani et al, 1979), its use has been recommended and practiced in most intensive care units. However, the reports are conflicting regarding the effect of low-dose heparin infusion on the incidence of thrombotic sequelae (Ankola and Atakent, 1993; Horgan et al, 1987). On the other hand, heparin bonding of catheters has been shown to be clearly associated with significantly fewer thrombotic complications (Krafte-Jacobs et al, 1995). Owing to the possible relationship between heparin use and systemic fungal infections in extremely low-birth-weight (ELBW) neonates, however, the routine use of heparin may have to be reassessed, at least for this patient population (Stephenson, 2001).

In addition to the endothelial injury caused by catheter placement, several other risk factors for aortic and renal arterial thrombosis have been identified. Systemic infection, birth weight less than 1500 g, perinatal asphyxia, polycythemia, intrauterine cocaine exposure, maternal diabetes mellitus, maternal lupus, congenital heart disease, hypercoagulability, dehydration (especially hypernatremic dehydration), and infusion of calcium salts, hyperalimentation solutions, or intravenous fat preparations through the umbilical arterial catheter are the most important additional risk factors for aortic and renal artery thrombosis in the newborn (Schmidt and Andrew, 1995; Seibert et al, 1987; Vailas et al, 1986).

Finally, resistance to activated protein C has been identified as a risk factor for thrombotic disease, even in the absence of umbilical catheter placement (Manco-Johnson et al, 1988). In over 90% of cases, the basis for the activated protein C resistance is a mutation in the coagulation factor V gene (factor V Leiden) that renders factor V Leiden more resistant to inactivation by activated protein C. The prevalence of factor V Leiden mutation in neonates with arterial thrombosis reaches 23% (Hagstrom et al, 1998). In cases of homozygous congenital protein C deficiency with associated thrombosis, in addition to anticoagulant therapy, the administration of supplemental protein C is necessary to correct the hypercoagulable prothrombotic condition (Dreyfus et al, 1991).

## Thromboembolic Complications of Umbilical Artery Catheters in Neonates

Umbilical artery catheters are extensively used for blood pressure monitoring, blood gas sampling, and fluid administration in critically ill newborn infants. As mentioned earlier, however, there are significant variations in the type and size of catheter used, catheter tip position, presence of end or side holes in the catheter, type of fluids or drugs infused, duration of catheterization, and heparinization of the infusate.

Catheter materials used include polyvinyl chloride, polyurethane, Silastic or silicone-based polymer, and heparin-coated or heparin-bonded catheters. The soft Silastic catheters may cause less intimal tear at the time of insertion, and Silastic or heparin-coated catheters may be less thrombogenic. However, a randomized study comparing polyvinyl chloride and heparin-bonded polyurethane catheters in 125 infants without additional heparin in the infusate showed no difference in the incidence of aortic thrombosis (Jackson et al, 1987). Of interest, heparin-coated catheters may reduce infections by inhibiting bacterial adherence to the catheter (Applegren et al, 1996; Mermel et al, 1993). Finally, although the use of antiseptic-impregnated catheters has not yet been studied extensively in newborns, silver-impregnated catheters have been shown to reduce catheter-related sepsis in adults.

Umbilical artery catheter tip positioning may also influence the risk of aortic and/or renal artery thrombosis, ischemic events, intraventricular hemorrhage, and necrotizing enterocolitis. However, there are conflicting data on clinically significant complications associated with high versus low umbilical artery lines. In an earlier study, high umbilical artery catheters placed at a T6 to T10 vertebral level have been reported to be associated with a lower incidence of clinically significant vascular complications, without an increase in hypertension, intraventricular hemorrhage, or necrotizing enterocolitis (Harris and Little, 1978). However, another study found that newborns with a high umbilical artery catheter in place more frequently develop aortic and renal thrombosis (Seibert et al, 1987). Finally, a recent meta-analysis comparing the complications associated with high versus low positioning of the umbilical artery line suggests a probable reduction in aortic thrombosis and a longer catheter life with high line positioning (Barrington, 2002).

Position of the hole at the tip of the catheter also may influence the incidence of aortic thrombosis, because the use of side-hole catheters has been associated with a higher incidence of this complication than is seen with end-hole catheters (Wesstrom et al, 1979). No data regarding about the optimal size of the catheter are available. The authors' preference is to use a 3.5 French catheter in infants weighing less than 1000 g and a 5.0 French catheter in infants weighing greater than 1000 g. In addition to the short-term side effects, long-term complications have been reported following neonatal umbilical catheterization including acquired coarctation of abdominal aorta and renal artery stenosis (Adelman and Morrell, 2000).

### Clinical Presentation and Laboratory Findings

The symptoms of aortic and renal artery thrombosis depend on the severity and extension of thrombus formation. Some infants may remain asymptomatic for a longer period of time, whereas others may show severe symptoms immediately after thrombus formation. Thrombosis of the abdominal aorta and the renal arteries should be suspected in newborns with a history of umbilical artery catheterization who exhibit signs of congestive heart failure, hypertension, oliguria, renal failure, bowel ischemia or frank necrotizing enterocolitis (secondary to obstruction of the superior or inferior mesenteric artery), or decreased femoral pulses with lower limb ischemia (Schmidt and Andrew, 1995; Vailas et al, 1986). The finding that symptoms of arterial or renal vein thrombosis occur sooner in term (within the first few postnatal days) than in preterm neonates (at a median postnatal age of 8 days) implies that increased vigilance of monitoring for potential signs of thromboembolic complications, for a longer time period, is indicated in the preterm patient population (Nowak-Göttl et al, 1997). Aortic and renal artery thrombosis may be classified according to the severity of the clinical findings. *Minor thrombosis* manifests with mildly decreased limb perfusion, hypertension, and hematuria; *moderate thrombosis* is present when decreased limb perfusion, hypertension, oliguria, and congestive heart failure occur; and *major thrombosis* is characterized by hypertension and signs of multiorgan failure. Laboratory abnormalities most commonly associated with aortic thrombosis are thrombocytopenia, hypofibrinogenemia, elevated fibrin split products, variable prothrombin and thromboplastin times, conjugated hyperbilirubinemia, elevated blood urea nitrogen and serum creatinine, hyperreninemia, and hematuria.

### Diagnosis

Because ultrasonography fails to detect small intra-arterial renal thrombi (Roy et al, 2002, Schmidt and Andrew, 1995; Seibert et al, 1987; Vailas et al, 1986) and, in some cases, even larger asymptomatic venous thrombosis (Roy et al, 2002), the "gold standard" imaging technique for the diagnosis of neonatal thrombosis remains angiography. However, in clinical practice, the diagnosis of aortic and main renal artery thrombosis is most frequently made by real-time and Doppler ultrasonography (Schmidt and Andrew, 1995). Radionuclide imaging also may be useful in cases of suspected catheter-related renal artery thrombosis if the ultrasonographic findings are inconclusive (Molteni et al, 1993; Schmidt and Andrew, 1995). In cases in which intrathrombic fibrinolytic therapy or surgical intervention is considered, aortography performed through the umbilical artery line should confirm the diagnosis (Richardson et al, 1988; Schmidt and Andrew, 1995).

### Treatment

Prospective studies have shown that a large number of newborns with umbilical artery catheters may develop asymptomatic aortic thrombosis (Oppenheimer et al, 1982; Seibert et al, 1987, 1991; Vailas et al, 1986). Because most of these thrombi resolve spontaneously, only supportive care, removal of the umbilical artery catheter, and close ultrasonographic follow-up evaluation are recommended for management of the asymptomatic or the minimally symptomatic newborn (Schmidt and Andrew, 1995; Vailas et al, 1986). In more severe cases, when fibrinolytic therapy is considered, the umbilical artery line may be left in place (see later).

In the symptomatic patient with stable thrombosis of the aorta and renal arteries and only mild signs of organ dysfunction, supportive medical management consists of treatment of systemic hypertension and of the usually transient renal insufficiency and mild congestive heart failure. At present, heparin is the anticoagulant of choice in these newborns (Payne et al, 1989; Richardson et al, 1988; Schmidt and Andrew, 1995). The initial loading dose is 75 to 100 IU/kg followed by 28 IU/kg/hour continuous infusion (Andrew et al, 1994). Laboratory monitoring to avoid excessive heparinization and close follow-up of the clinical response by Doppler flow measurements and real-time ultrasonography are obligatory. Heparin has a large volume of distribution in newborns, resulting in faster drug clearance (Schmidt and Andrew, 1995). Newborns at high risk for intracranial bleeding and those with established intracranial bleeding or with active bleeding elsewhere may not be candidates for systemic heparinization. The duration of heparin therapy depends on the clinical response measured by the improvement in organ function and should be at least 7 days (Schmidt and Andrew, 1995). It is important to note that in some newborns, a resistance to heparin therapy secondary to inherited or acquired antithrombin III deficiency may occur. In such cases, the administration of supplemental antithrombin III may be necessary to restore the effectiveness of heparin treatment. Recently, the use of low-molecular-weight heparins (LMWHs) has been advocated in the management of neonatal thrombosis because of the potential advantages LMWHs offer over unfractionated heparin. These advantages include a longer half-life with predictable pharmacokinetics, better bioavailability, ease of subcutaneous administration, decreased risk of osteopenia and heparin-induced thrombocytopenia, lack of interference by concurrent medications, and decreased risk for hemorrhagic complications. LMWHs also have a greater activity against factor Xa when compared with heparin. In adults and in children, LMWHs have been proved to be safe and effective in the treatment of venous and arterial thrombosis (Weitz, 1997), and in a recent prospective cohort study, 48 neonates also were successfully treated with the LMWH enoxaparin (Dix et al, 2000). Finally, there is no evidence that long-term oral anticoagulation therapy is necessary after the resolution of neonatal aortic and renal thrombosis.

Medical management of cases with potential life-threatening complications of aortic or renal thrombosis includes systemic (Schmidt and Andrew, 1995) or intrathrombic (Schmidt and Andrew, 1995; Strife et al, 1988) application of fibrinolytic therapy and aggressive supportive care directed at organ dysfunction. The intrathrombic infusion of the fibrinolytic agent reduces cumulative dose requirements and possibly the untoward systemic effects of fibrinolytic therapy. Close ultrasonographic or angiographic follow-up is considered mandatory to evaluate the thrombolytic response to these agents. The fibrinolytic agents used in the clinical management of newborns with major thrombosis have been streptokinase, urokinase, and tissue plasminogen activator (Schmidt and Andrew, 1995). These fibrinolytic agents act by directly or indirectly converting plasminogen to plasmin, thus activating fibrinolysis. Streptokinase forms a protein complex with plasminogen, which in turn converts other plasminogen molecules to plasmin (Holden, 1990). The theoretical drawbacks of streptokinase use are depletion of the substrate and possible toxic reactions. However, it is primarily because of the antigenicity and systemic side effects of streptokinase that its use has been abandoned (Hartmann et al, 2001). Urokinase, a nonantigenic protein, directly converts plasminogen to plasmin in both the systemic circulation and the thrombus (Holden, 1990). Laboratory responses to urokinase include a decrease in fibrinogen concentration and an increase in fibrin split products. In cases with poor laboratory and clinical responses, supplementation of plasminogen by the administration of fresh frozen plasma has been recommended. Although urokinase has been the most frequently used fibrinolytic agent in newborns (Schmidt and Andrew, 1995), owing to its potential contamination with reovirus, the Food and Drug Administration (FDA) has recently recommended to consider other treatment options before urokinase is administered until the problem with the viral contamination has been solved. The third fibrinolytic agent, tissue plasminogen activator (tPA), is a fibrin-specific plasminogen activator that binds poorly to circulating plasminogen or fibrinogen (Haire, 1992). This agent offers several theoretical advantages in the newborn, including a short half-life, minimal antigenicity, direct activation of plasminogen, lack of inhibition by $\alpha_2$-antiplasmin, and localization of fibrinolytic activity (Kennedy et al, 1990). Thus, at least in theory, the use of this agent minimizes systemic proteolysis, with maximal fibrinolytic activity on the surface of the thrombus. Indeed, several investigators have recently reported the use of recombinant tissue plasminogen activator (r-tPA) in neonates to treat life- or limb-threatening neonatal arterial thrombosis (Dillon et al, 1993; Weiner et al, 1998, Hartmann et al, 2001). The published data indicate that successful lysis with r-tPA occurs in most patients and that hemorrhagic complications are unusual although may happen. An absolute contraindication to the use of r-tPA in neonates is the presence of intraventricular hemorrhage and/or significant cerebral ischemic changes. The protocol for r-tPA therapy in neonates should include monitoring for the presence of intraventricular hemorrhage and/or cerebral ischemic changes before and during therapy, normalizing blood pressure prior to r-tPA administration, limiting its dose to 0.4 mg/kg/hour, maintaining the fibrinogen level at greater than 150 mg/dL, and performing sonographic evaluations of thrombus during and after r-tPA administration to assess lysis and long-term outcome (Weiner et al, 1998). Recently, r-tPA at 0.7 mg/kg given as an initial bolus over 30 to 60 minutes followed by 0.2 mg/kg/hour along with low-dose heparin at 4 to 10 IU/kg/hour was used successfully in treatment of catheter-related thrombosis in neonates (Hartmann et al, 2001). This protocol appears to be effective and safe without apparent increases in the risk of intracranial bleeding. According to the available and limited information comparing the use of urokinase and r-tPA in neonates, there is probably no real difference between them in effectiveness and toxicity (Nowak-Göttl et al, 1999). However, more information is needed to appropriately address this question. Finally, it is unclear at present if concomitant systemic heparinization offers any benefit without increasing the risk of bleeding complications.

The major complication of fibrinolytic therapy is the occurrence of intracranial hemorrhage, especially in the sick preterm infant (Strife et al, 1988). Therefore, intrathrombic rather than systemic fibrinolytic therapy with radiologic imaging studies including serial head ultrasound examinations and laboratory monitoring of the appropriate coagulation parameters before, during, and after treatment constitute the suggested specific management of the newborn at high risk for intracranial bleeding who presents with a life-threatening aortic or renal arterial thrombosis. Although surgical thrombectomy has been successfully performed in newborns (Payne et al, 1989; Schmidt and Andrew, 1995), guidelines for the indication and timing of surgical management of neonatal aortic and renal thrombosis are not well established. Moreover, it must be emphasized that there is also no validated approach at present for the use of anticoagulant or fibrinolytic agents in newborns with aortic and renal thrombosis owing to the lack of scientific evidence concerning optimal management strategies. The above-described empiric approach to medical management has summarized, in the absence of well-designed controlled clinical studies, the most recent recommendations based on the results of case reports.

### Prognosis

Gestational and postnatal age, underlying pathologic conditions of the newborn, and the age, size, and location of the thrombus all have an impact on the outcome of neonatal aortic and renal arterial thrombosis. The overall mortality rate lies between 9% and 20% (Nowak-Göttl et al, 1997; Schmidt and Andrew, 1995). Mortality rates with major aortic and renal arterial thrombosis, however, are higher (Vailas et al, 1986), whereas most newborns with minor or moderate thrombi recover. Concerning the recovery of blood flow through the affected vessel, a complete resolution or partial vessel patency occurs in approximately 60% of the cases following neonatal thromboembolism (Nowak-Göttl et al, 1997).

The most frequent long-term morbidity in the affected newborn is renovascular hypertension. Although hypertension may persist for months or sometimes years, blood pressure eventually becomes normal, and the majority of the patients remain normotensive even after the antihypertensive treatment has been discontinued. It is not known, however, whether these children will have a higher incidence of hypertension or renal failure in adulthood. Chronic renal insufficiency develops less frequently during infancy and early childhood and is always the consequence of severe aortic and bilateral renal arterial thrombosis causing irreversible renal parenchymal damage.

## RENAL VEIN OBSTRUCTION

Although renal vein thrombosis may occur at any age, newborns are particularly at risk for the development of this vascular event, because 60% to 75% of the patients with renal vein thrombosis are younger than 1 month of age. Prenatally demonstrated renal vein thrombosis has also been reported, mainly in fetuses of diabetic mothers (Duncan et al, 1991; Sanders and Jaquier, 1989).

### Incidence

Earlier autopsy findings indicate that the incidence of renal vein thrombosis is 1/40 to 1/300 in newborns who died (Arneil et al, 1973). A more recent estimate of the minimal incidence of renal vein thrombosis in term neonates is 2.2 cases per 100,000 live births, with a sixfold higher rate in preterm neonates (Böbenkamp et al, 2000).

### Etiology

The anatomy of the renal vasculature and the differences between the left and the right renal venous drainage determine the response of the renal venous system to injury. The drainage of the left adrenal vein into the left main renal vein explains why ipsilateral adrenal hemorrhage more frequently accompanies left-sided than it does right-sided renal vein thrombosis. The lack of venous collaterals in the right kidney is responsible for the more rapid and severe occurrence of clinical symptoms of venous thrombosis on this side. In the primary and most frequent form of renal vein thrombosis in the newborn, clotting starts in the small intrarenal veins when venous stasis occurs. As a result of the free anastomoses within the renal venous system, microthrombi spread distally and involve the renal cortex and medulla extending into larger veins (Arneil et al, 1973). In the secondary form of renal vein thrombosis, a thrombus in the inferior vena cava extends into the renal vein.

Renal vein thrombosis in the newborn has been frequently associated with known risks—catheters, surgery, trauma, and infection. Genetic factors also may predispose the infant to develop thrombosis, and the pathogenic role of inherited prothrombotic states (i.e., activated protein C resistance, factor V Leiden) has now been well demonstrated (Hangstrom et al, 1998). Association of factor V Leiden with methyltetrahydrofolate reductase and platelet glycoprotein IIIa (GPIIIa) polymorphisms also may result in renal vein thrombosis (Giordano et al, 2001). In addition to prethrombotic or hypercoagulable prothrombotic states, conditions associated with decreases in renal blood flow are important factors frequently involved in the pathogenesis of renal vein thrombosis in the newborn. The normally low venous blood flow in the newborn may be further reduced by intravascular volume loss (from bleeding or dehydration), hypoxia, infection, polycythemia, or cyanotic congenital heart disease. The ensuing venous stasis and hemoconcentration, especially when accompanied by disturbances in fluid and electrolyte homeostasis and acid-base balance, result in sludging and thrombosis in the small interlobular veins. The microthrombi in the small veins then spread distally to involve the larger vessels. In thromboembolic states, subsequent renal vein involvement occurs with the proximal extension of the thrombus from the pelvicaliceal veins and from the inferior vena cava. In the newborn, renal vein thrombosis most frequently occurs after a central line placement through the femoral vein or if hemorrhagic shock develops. Finally, infants of diabetic mothers are at an especially high risk for renal vein thrombosis as a result of a combination of several risk factors, including their hypercoagulable state and relatively low extracellular water content as well as the often associated polycythemia, perinatal asphyxia, and respiratory distress.

### Thromboembolic Complications of Umbilical Venous Catheters In Neonates

Umbilical venous catheterization is an alternative initial option for central venous access, especially in infants weighing less than 1000 g. As mentioned earlier, this route allows for administration of hypertonic nutrient fluids, drugs, and pressors, and for continuous infusion of medications. Verification of catheter tip position by radiography is extremely important and should be done before using the line. The tip should lie in the inferior vena cava, 0.5 to 1.0 cm above the diaphragm, avoiding hepatic and portal veins. Placing the catheter tip in the right atrium increases the risk for cardiac tamponade via perforation of the atrial wall by the catheter or transudation of the infusate through the thin atrial wall into the pericardial space. Potential complications of umbilical venous catheter placement include portal vein, hepatic vein, or inferior vena cava thrombosis; thrombotic endocarditis; obstruction of pulmonary venous return in infants with infradiaphragmatic total anomalous pulmonary venous return; air embolism; and infection.

### Clinical Presentation and Laboratory Findings

The classic diagnostic triad of a palpable abdominal mass, gross hematuria, and thrombocytopenia is infrequently seen in the neonate. The development of a unilateral or bilateral flank mass in association with a sudden deterioration of clinical status, however, should raise the possibility of renal vein thrombosis in the newborn. Other clinical signs and laboratory findings consistent with renal vein thrombosis include oliguria or anuria, gross hematuria, thrombocytopenia, hemolytic anemia, metabolic acidosis, and azotemia. Prothrombin time and partial thromboplastin time may be prolonged because of consumption of coagulation factors. At the beginning of the clinical course, blood pressure often is low. Although hypertension may develop later in the course, the increase in blood pressure usually does not reach the level seen in cases of renal artery thrombosis. Some newborns, however, whose early clinical symptoms are mild or overlooked, may present with hypertension days or weeks after the development of the renal vein thrombosis.

### Diagnosis

The diagnosis of renal vein thrombosis in the newborn is suspected based on the clinical presentation and laboratory findings, as just described, and confirmed by the results of real-time and Doppler ultrasonography (Nowak-Göttl et al, 1997; Schmidt and Andrew, 1995; Slovis et al, 1993; Weiner et al, 1998). Sonography confirms the diagnosis with approximately 92% accuracy (Ricci and Lloyd, 1990), and performance of additional studies such as angiography is infrequently needed. The real-time ultrasonographic features are nonspecific and include renal enlargement and evidence of edema causing distortion of the renal architecture with an inhomogeneous appearance of the parenchyma and loss of corticomedullary differentiation. The findings on color Doppler sonography are more specific, making the diagnosis relatively easy once the thrombus has reached the larger renal veins. Using high-frequency transducers (7.0 to 10 MHz), a hypoechoic apex and renal papilla can be identified, with a ring of reduced echogenicity seen around the affected pyramids 1 to 2 weeks after the acute phase (Wright et al, 1996). Among the survivors, characteristic calcification of intrarenal veins is detected in 60% of the cases (Slovis et al, 1993).

Renal vein thrombosis should always be differentiated from renal artery thrombosis. The latter occurs mostly in newborns with catheterization of the umbilical artery, it does not present with renal enlargement, and the subsequent systemic hypertension is usually more severe than that in renal vein thrombosis.

### Treatment

Initial treatment is directed at correcting the abnormalities in the fluid, electrolyte, and acid-base balance. The use of hypertonic infusions, nephrotoxic medications, and hyperosmolar radiographic contrast agents should be avoided. Diuretics are of limited value, and their use may further perpetuate hemoconcentration. If hemoconcentration cannot be corrected by infusion therapy, peritoneal dialysis may be indicated.

Although the correction of hemoconcentration and hyperviscosity in most patients prevents further propagation of the thrombus, intravenous heparin may be of value in preventing extension of the thrombus (Ricci and Lloyd, 1990). According to findings in earlier studies, heparin treatment does not prevent the development of renal dysfunction (Mocan et al, 1991; Nuss et al, 1994). More recently, however, anticoagulation with heparin and/or LMWH in neonates with renal vein thrombosis showed significant improvement in long-term renal outcome (Zigman et al, 2000). Successful thrombolytic therapy with urokinase infused through a lower extremity vein also has been reported (Duncan et al, 1991). It is important to note that the combined use of thrombolytic and anticoagulation therapy in preterm neonates may be complicated by severe intracranial bleeding and without the resolution of the renal vein thrombosis (Weinschenk et al, 2001). Because active bleeding and the risk for intraventricular hemorrhage are the main contraindications to anticoagulant and thrombolytic therapy, their use is recommended mostly in the full-term newborn with life-threatening thromboembolic complications (see earlier).

The role of surgical intervention in the treatment of renal vein thrombosis has been extensively debated. Theoretically, in the primary form of renal vein thrombosis, thrombectomy precludes extension of the thrombus into the vena cava or opposite kidney and prevents infections and the development of hypertension caused by renal ischemia. Because the smaller intrarenal veins are almost always occluded, however, extraction of thrombus from the main renal vein does not alleviate renal infarction in most cases of renal vein thrombosis. Moreover, an advantage of early thrombectomy or nephrectomy has not been demonstrated, even with bilateral involvement (Ricci and Lloyd, 1990).

### Prognosis

The survival rate for newborns with renal vein thrombosis has improved during the past decade and is around 80% to 95% (Ricci and Lloyd, 1990; Schmidt and Andrew, 1995). Most deaths are due to the underlying disease and not the renal vein thrombosis or the ensuing renal dysfunction. The extent of recovery of the involved kidney after renal vein thrombosis varies, ranging from complete restoration of renal function to the development of a nonfunctioning shrunken kidney, partially fibrous kidney, renal hypertension, nephrotic syndrome, or chronic renal tubular dysfunction. Kidney atrophy is already present at 1 year of age in two thirds of the patients with a sonographic diagnosis of neonatal renal vein obstruction (Böbenkamp et al, 2000). Although long-term follow-up data on survivors of neonatal renal vein thrombosis are limited, at a follow-up period of 5 to 12 years, blood pressure, glomerular filtration rate, and urinary concentration ability remained within normal limits in a majority of affected children (Keidan et al, 1994; Mocan et al, 1991). Because persistent renal imaging abnormalities were present in more than 80% of these patients (Mocan et al, 1991), however, the long-term outcome of renal function in patients with neonatal renal vein thrombosis remains uncertain, and continuing follow-up is absolutely necessary.

## RENAL CORTICAL AND MEDULLARY NECROSIS

Renal cortical necrosis, renal medullary necrosis, and combined cortical and medullary necrosis are uncommon disorders in the newborn. They occur only in critically ill newborns who, in most of the cases, present with irreversible shock. Therefore, renal cortical and medullary necrosis is the manifestation of an end-organ insult to the kidney caused most frequently by extreme perinatal or postnatal stress, and it is seldom recognized while the newborn is alive.

### Incidence and Etiology

Autopsy findings indicate that the incidence of renal cortical and medullary necrosis is around 5% in infants who die at less than 3 months of age (Lerner et al, 1992). Risk factors for the development of renal cortical and medullary necrosis include prematurity, congenital heart disease associated with low renal perfusion or poor tissue oxygenation, perinatal asphyxia, sepsis, bleeding diathesis or coagulopathy, and respiratory distress resulting in cardiovascular compromise. In addition, the use of contrast agents during cardiac catheterization also appears to be a risk factor.

### Pathomechanism and Clinical Presentation

The clinical manifestations of renal cortical and medullary necrosis (hematuria, oliguria or anuria, and renal enlargement) are nonspecific and are present in several more common neonatal renal abnormalities. Because renal cortical and medullary necrosis occurs only in newborns with shock caused by a life-threatening condition, its recognition is often delayed or the diagnosis is never even considered. It is unclear why some affected newborns preferentially develop medullary necrosis, whereas others present with cortical necrosis of the kidney. The severity of the intrarenal arteriolar vasoconstriction and the magnitude of the underlying resistance of the capillary bed in the renal cortex and medulla may have a major impact on the primary localization of the necrotic process.

Increased local production of vasodilator prostaglandins attenuates renal vasoconstriction occurring with acute circulatory collapse (Gleason, 1987). Because inhibition of prostaglandin synthesis by indomethacin enhances renal ischemia under these circumstances, administration of the drug may contribute to the development of renal cortical and medullary necrosis in premature newborns with severely compromised cardiovascular status.

Hyperosmotic radiocontrast agents also may produce marked and protracted medullary vasoconstriction and hypoxia, probably by affecting renal medullary prostaglandin synthesis (Gruskin et al, 1974; Nygren et al, 1988). Their use in newborns with congenital heart disease during cardiac catheterization may contribute to the development of renal cortical and medullary necrosis in this patient population. Whether the use of isosmotic contrast agents results in similar renal response is unknown.

### Diagnosis, Management, and Prognosis

There are no specific clinical, laboratory, or imaging findings to aid in the diagnosis of neonatal renal cortical and medullary necrosis, and no specific therapy is available. In all critically ill newborns with shock or thrombosis of the renal vessels, or after the administration of a hyperosmolar contrast agent during cardiac catheterization, the clinician should maintain a high degree of suspicion until the presence of a major renal insult can safely be ruled out. Considerations in the differential diagnosis include all causes of neonatal acute renal failure, including bilateral renal artery or renal vein thrombosis, autosomal recessive polycystic kidney disease, and bilaterally multicystic or hydronephrotic kidneys. During the acute phase, renal scintigraphy and magnetic resonance imaging (MRI) may be of value in the diagnosis. The decreased ability of the critically ill newborn to tolerate transport in the acute phase of the disease, however, renders these studies impractical.

The prognosis for neonatal renal cortical and medullary necrosis depends on the underlying disease. Excretory urography in survivors shows characteristic bizarre-appearing dilated calices with a variable amount of scarring. These morphologic changes are most frequently associated with reduced glomerular filtration rate, renal concentrating defect, hypertension, and segmental hypoplasia. As in the cases of renal artery and vein thrombosis, the long-term effects of neonatal cortical and medullary necrosis on renal function remain to be determined.

## ADRENAL HEMORRHAGE

### Incidence

The incidence of detected neonatal adrenal hemorrhage ranges from 1.7 to 2.1 per 1000 births (Marino et al, 1990). Because adrenal bleeding may remain asymptomatic, the real occurrence is probably higher. Among newborns who die, the incidence of adrenal hemorrhage is around 10%. In a majority of the cases, the bleeding locates to one side, and only 5% to 8% of adrenal hemorrhages are bilateral (Marino et al, 1990).

### Pathomechanism

The fetal and neonatal adrenal glands are relatively large and are more vascularized than later in life, which may predispose them to bleeding. Risk factors associated with adrenal hemorrhage in the newborn include birth trauma, perinatal asphyxia, shock, infection, thrombosis of the inferior vena cava and left renal vein, and hemorrhagic disorders.

### Clinical Presentation

Clinical symptoms are nonspecific and most frequently include unexplained and persistent jaundice, mild anemia, and abdominal distention associated with an abdominal mass. In the case of bilateral adrenal hemorrhage, hypoglycemia and hypotension may be the presenting findings. In boys, neonatal adrenal hemorrhage may present with the clinical manifestation of a scrotal hematoma (Miele et al, 1997; Putnam, 1989). The simultaneous occurrence of adrenal bleeding and incomplete rotation of the colon leading to early duodenal obstruction also has been reported (Cheves et al, 1989). Finally, some infants remain completely asymptomatic, and the diagnosis is made only incidentally.

### Diagnosis

Suprarenal masses in the newborn that should be considered in the differential diagnosis of neonatal adrenal hemorrhage include abscesses; neuroblastoma; renal duplication; hydronephrosis; Wilms tumor; enteric duplications; and renal, pancreatic, hepatic, ovarian, and choledochal cysts. If adrenal hemorrhage is suspected, laboratory tests including a complete blood cell count, serum bilirubin, serum glucose, and urinary excretion of catecholamines and their metabolites aid in establishing the diagnosis. In typical cases, the diagnosis is confirmed by ultrasonography. Usually the whole gland is affected, but occasionally an uninvolved adrenal limb may be detected adjacent to the suprarenal mass. Because hemorrhage into the adrenal gland usually is followed by necrosis and later resolution with fibrosis and calcification, the evolution of these signs is characteristic on the sonographic follow-up examinations. Calcification of the adrenal gland is usually noted about 2 weeks after the hemorrhage. Despite the high resolution of ultrasound imaging, the use of MRI, computed tomography, or radionuclide renal scan sometimes is necessary to differentiate between an atypical adrenal hemorrhage and neuroblastoma or a renal mass. Surgical exploration is seldom needed.

In utero adrenal bleeding of the fetus should be considered if a cystic mass in the suprarenal area is detected on prenatal ultrasonography (Marino et al, 1990). It is extremely difficult, however, to distinguish between fetal adrenal hemorrhage and cystic neuroblastoma without histologic examination. Because adrenal hemorrhage shows progressive changes within 2 weeks, whereas neuroblastoma usually remains unchanged during this time, a repeat prenatal ultrasound study may be helpful in establishing the diagnosis. A hemorrhage into an adrenal neuroblastoma may also cause progressive cystic changes on repeat ultrasonographic examinations, making the prenatal differential diagnosis extremely difficult. In such cases, intrauterine evaluation of the suprarenal mass by MRI may be informative.

The occurrence of benign hemorrhagic adrenocortical cysts also has been reported in Beckwith-Wiedemann syndrome, a condition also associated with a high incidence of adrenocortical carcinoma (McCauley et al, 1991). The differentiation of these benign hemorrhagic lesions of the adrenals from common adrenal hemorrhage may be difficult by imaging studies alone.

### Outcome

In a majority of cases, the prognosis for neonatal adrenal hemorrhage is excellent. The disease is self-limiting and except for the rare bilateral cases requires no specific treatment.

## HYPERTENSION IN THE NEWBORN

The first reported blood pressure measurement in the newborn was performed in the late 19th century by the direct determination of the pressure in the umbilical artery (Ribemont, 1879). Since then, the ever-increasing body of information on arterial blood pressure in the newborn has generated many new and as-yet unanswered questions. For example, because the physiologic blood pressure range in the neonatal period, especially in the immature preterm infant, remains unknown, hypotension and hypertension cannot be adequately defined in this patient population.

### Blood Pressure Measurement Techniques

The requirements for the techniques of blood pressure measurement include that the method should be simple, painless, and reliable with an acceptable risk-to-benefit ratio, and it should give information continuously or at least in frequent intervals without disturbing the newborn.

#### *Invasive Measurement*

The most widely used method of blood pressure measurement in the critically ill newborn is by means of an indwelling umbilical or peripheral artery catheter connected to a transducer. Three sources of error are of importance when this method is used. First, if the catheter is too small in diameter, it underestimates the systolic pressure because of loss of higher frequencies. Second, the position of the catheter tip too close to the wall of the vessel or the presence of a clot at the tip of the catheter may result in damping of the pressure waves, leading to an underestimation of the blood pressure. Finally, the presence of even small air bubbles in the system generates a resonant frequency, which then alters the measured systolic, diastolic, and, to a lesser extent, mean blood pressure values (Weindling, 1989). The position of the umbilical arterial catheter tip in the aorta (high versus low) does not influence the measured value. Occasionally, both peripheral and umbilical artery lines are placed and transduced in extremely labile, critically ill full-term newborns. In these cases, the peripheral artery catheter may read higher systolic pressures than the umbilical line (Adelman, 1988).

#### *Noninvasive Measurement*

Three noninvasive methods are used in clinical practice. The traditional methods using auscultation, palpation, or the flush technique are insensitive, especially when the stroke volume is low. The Doppler ultrasound method is reliable for the measurement of systolic values, but it cannot accurately detect the diastolic pressure (Emery and Greenough, 1992). Automatic oscillometry is the most commonly used noninvasive technique that provides an accurate, reproducible, and convenient estimate of blood pressure (including the mean blood pressure) in most newborns, provided that the appropriate size cuff is used with a cuff width–to–arm circumference ratio of 0.44 to 0.55 (Low et al, 1995; Sonesson and Broberger, 1987). Oscillometry is the only noninvasive method that actually measures mean blood pressure instead of calculating it. In very low-birth-weight (VLBW) newborns, however, as well as in cases of extreme hypotension, some inaccuracy is possible (Rasoulpour and Marinelli, 1992).

### Definition and Incidence

Despite the large body of information on blood pressure values in the neonatal period, there is no accurate definition of pathologic blood pressure values for the newborn and, in particular, for the VLBW infant (see earlier). In the clinical practice, the infant's blood pressure and tissue perfusion generally are considered to be adequate as long as urine output and capillary refill are within normal limits in the absence of metabolic acidosis. Although this approach may be an appropriate clinical approximation for hypotension, it does not allow for prompt detection of mild systemic hypoperfusion. In addition, the indirect clinical assessment is not at all useful to determine the blood pressure values representing hypertension because there are no specific clinical or laboratory signs to indicate the level of systemic blood pressure elevation that has the potential of causing end-organ damage in the given newborn. In the pediatric population, hypertension is defined as the average systolic or diastolic blood pressure (or both) at the 95th percentile or greater for age and gender when measured on at least three occasions. This definition, however, cannot be applied to neonatal hypertension because it presupposes an accurate definition of normal neonatal blood pressure (see earlier). Therefore, neonatal hypertension remains arbitrarily defined as systolic blood pressure greater than 90 mm Hg and diastolic blood pressure greater than 60 mm Hg in the full-term newborn and systolic blood pressure greater than 80 mm Hg and diastolic blood pressure greater than 50 mm Hg in the preterm infant (Adelman, 1988). At present, this arbitrary definition is widely accepted and referred to in the literature. On the basis of these criteria, the reported incidence of neonatal hypertension ranges from 0.7% to 3.2% (Adelman, 1988; Rasoulpour and Marinelli, 1992, Singh et al, 1992, Nuntnarumit et al, 1999). In the ELBW infant (weighing less than 1000 g), however, even the arbitrary limits of hypertension are not agreed on (Spinazzola et al, 1991). Obviously, additional well-designed studies are needed to follow the normal changes in neonatal blood pressure with time, to provide more appropriate 95% confidence limits for use in the diagnosis of neonatal hypertension.

Factors directly associated with increases in blood pressure in the newborn include maternal smoking during pregnancy (Beratis et al, 1996); maternal age (Gillman et al, 2001); gestational and postnatal age (Georgieff et al, 1996; Rasoulpour and Marinelli, 1992; Spinazzola et al, 1991; Versmold et al, 1981; Zubrow et al, 1995); route of delivery (Engle, 2001); stress; agitation; application of topical mydriatics; crying; upright position; and, provided that the newborn is euvolemic, abdominal compression. Endotracheal suctioning results in a biphasic blood pressure response, with an initial brief drop followed by a greater rise of longer duration (Perry et al, 1990). It has been suggested that neonatal blood pressure is higher in preterm infants whose mother received antenatal steroids (Demarani et al, 1999; Moise et al, 1995). Conversely, some investigators reported no increases in blood pressure in neonates whose mothers received steroids antenatally (LeFlore et al, 2000; Omar et al, 1999).

### Blood Pressure Standards

The determination of normal values for blood pressure in newborn infants has been attempted by numerous investigations, and there is good agreement on several principles. Mean blood pressure increases with postnatal age by 1 to 2 mm Hg per day during the first week and by approximately 1 mm Hg per week during the first 6 weeks of life. Because blood pressure is affected by gestational age and birth weight, it is lower in premature infants than in full-term newborns (Emery and Greenough, 1992; Hegyi et al, 1994; Nuntnarumit et al, 1999; Versmold et al, 1981; Weindling, 1989). Small-for-gestational age infants may have lower blood pressure than that in larger babies with comparable gestational age. Among premature infants, however, the limits of systolic and diastolic blood pressure appear to be less dependent on weight and gestational age if they do not require mechanical ventilation and have a stable cardiovascular status (Hegyi et al, 1994). Systolic blood pressure in newborn infants usually stabilizes at a mean of 92 mm Hg (95% confidence interval [CI] 72 to112) at a postconceptional age of 44 to 48 weeks, irrespective of gestation at birth (Northern Neonatal Nursing Initiative, 1999).

As mentioned earlier, there is a paucity of data on the reference values for arterial blood pressure in the newborn period. Normative data for blood pressure in the newborns, including VLBW neonates, may be influenced by management protocols used in the given institution (Al-Aweel et al, 2001; Nuntnarumit et al, 1999; Nwankwo et al, 1997). The Joint Working Group of the British Association of Perinatal Medicine has recommended that mean arterial blood pressure be maintained at or above the gestational age of the infants in weeks during the first day of life (Report of the Joint Working Group, 1992). Although this approach seems to be practical, its safety requires further investigation. Moreover, recent data suggest that 90% of extremely preterm neonates not receiving pressor or inotrope support will have a mean arterial blood pressure higher than 30 mm Hg by the end of the third postnatal day (Nuntnarumit et al, 1999) (Fig. 87–1). Table 87–1 describes the normal blood pressure values in healthy term newborns during the first year of life, and Table 87–2 depicts the increase in systolic blood pressure in preterm infants during the first postnatal week.

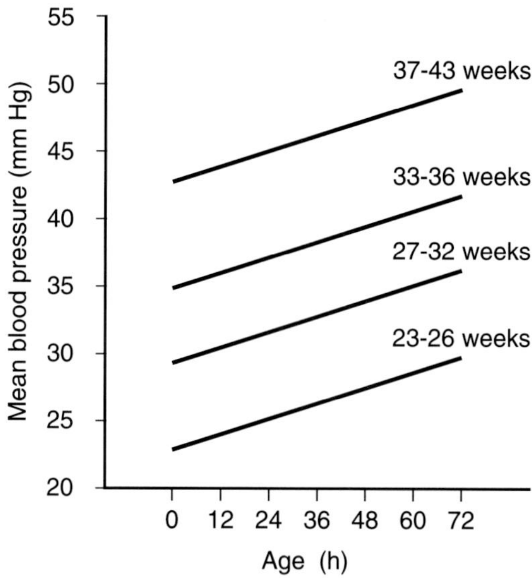


**FIGURE 87–1.** Gestational age– and postnatal age–dependent nomogram for mean blood pressure values in neonates during the first 3 days of life. The nomogram is derived from continuous arterial blood pressure measurements obtained from 103 neonates with gestational ages between 23 and 43 weeks. Each line represents the lower limit of 80% confidence interval of mean blood pressure for each gestational age group. Thus, 90% of infants for each gestational age group are expected to have a mean blood pressure equal to or greater than the value indicated by the corresponding line (the lower limit of confidence interval). *(From Nuntnarumit P, Yang W, Bada-Ellzey HS: Blood pressure measurements in the newborn. Clin Perinatol 26:981-996, 1999.)*

### Etiology

Neonatal hypertension is associated with certain congenital malformations and acquired diseases (Table 87–3). The most common causes of hypertension seen in neonatal intensive care units are thrombosis of the renal artery due to umbilical arterial catheterization, bronchopulmonary dysplasia, extracorporeal membrane oxygenation, and coarctation of the aorta (Flynn, 2000; Rasoulpour and Marinelli, 1992; Seibert et al, 1991).

### Clinical Signs

Approximately one third of patients with neonatal hypertension remain asymptomatic (Adelman, 1987). In those who develop clinical signs, the findings are rather nonspecific, and the presence or severity of the signs and symptoms is not related to the magnitude of the blood pressure elevation. The clinical manifestations of neonatal hypertension include signs of dysfunction of the cardiovascular system (congestive heart failure, decreased or unequal pulses, cardiomegaly, hepatomegaly, vasomotor instability), the respiratory system (tachypnea, cyanosis), the central nervous system (tremors, seizures, lethargy, coma, apnea, abnormal muscle tone, opisthotonos, asymmetrical reflexes, facial palsy, hypertensive retinopathy, cerebral edema and hemorrhage), and the kidneys (dehydration, sodium wasting, oliguria or anuria, renal enlargement). In addition, nonspecific general symptoms of hypertension (abdominal distention, edema, fever, and failure to thrive) also may be encountered. Most infants develop hypertension during the first 2 weeks of life, with a range of 1 to 45 days (Adelman, 1988). Approximately 50% of newborns with hypertension exhibit signs of hypertensive retinopathy, including a decreased ratio of the arterial to venous caliber, vascular tortuosity, and exudate formation (Skalina et al, 1983).

### Evaluation of Neonatal Hypertension

After the thorough review of the history and the findings on physical examination, appropriate laboratory and imaging studies should be performed according to the suspected cause. In the hypertensive newborn with an indwelling umbilical artery catheter, a urinalysis and the evaluation of serum electrolytes, creatinine, and blood urea nitrogen should be immediately followed by real-time and Doppler ultrasonographic studies of the kidneys, perirenal regions, renal arteries and veins, aorta, and inferior vena cava. Dynamic (technetium 99 m diethylenetriaminepenta-acetic acid) and static (technetium 99 m dimercaptosuccinic acid) renal radionuclide scans are additional valuable tests in

**TABLE 87–1**

**Blood Pressure in Healthy Term Newborns and Infants During the First Year of Life**

| Age | n | State | Measured Pressures (mm Hg) | | |
|---|---|---|---|---|---|
| | | | Systolic | Diastolic | Mean |
| 1 hour[a] | 17 | | 70 | 44 | 53 |
| 12 hours[a] | 17 | | 66 | 41 | 50 |
| 1 day[b] | 46 | Asleep | 70 ± 9 | 42 ± 12 | 55 ± 11 |
| | | Awake | 71 ± 9 | 43 ± 10 | 55 ± 9 |
| 3 days[b] | 46 | Asleep | 75 ± 11 | 48 ± 10 | 59 ± 9 |
| | | Awake | 77 ± 12 | 49 ± 10 | 63 ± 13 |
| 6 days[b] | 46 | Asleep | 76 ± 10 | 46 ± 12 | 58 ± 12 |
| | | Awake | 76 ± 10 | 49 ± 11 | 62 ± 12 |
| 2 weeks[c] | 566 | | 78 ± 10 | 50 ± 9 | |
| 3 weeks[c] | 77 | | 79 ± 8 | 49 ± 8 | |
| 4 weeks[c] | 642 | | 85 ± 10 | 46 ± 9 | |
| 6 weeks[d] | 131 | Asleep | 89 ± 11 | | |
| | | Awake | 96 ± 11 | | |
| 6 months[c] | 525 | | 92 ± 9 | 55 ± 9 | |
| 6 months[d] | 858 | | 93 ± 14 | | |
| 12 months[c] | 427 | | 95 ± 8 | 56 ± 8 | |
| 12 months[d] | 1338 | | 94 ± 11 | | |

Data from:
[a]Kitterman et al, 1969 (average values)
[b]Tan, 1987
[c]Zinner et al, 1985
[d]de Swiet et al, 1980

newborns with suspected renovascular hypertension, providing information about renal blood flow and its intrarenal distribution as well as about renal function. Aortography performed through the umbilical artery catheter is seldom indicated. Evaluation of the role of pain sensation or agitation in the cause of hypertension and four-extremity blood pressure measurements also should be part of the initial work-up. A more detailed cardiac evaluation, including an electrocardiogram, a chest radiograph, and an echocardiographic study, is necessary in cases in which a cardiac cause of the hypertension is suspected. In most newborns, the usual work-up as described previously is sufficient for the diagnosis. If the clinical or laboratory findings so indicate, however, further studies may be warranted to rule out other, less frequent conditions associated with neonatal hypertension, including endocrine disorders and pheochromocytoma.

**TABLE 87–2**

**Systolic Blood Pressure in Preterm Infants with Birth Weight <1500 g During the First Week of Life**

| Age (days) | n | Systolic Blood Pressure (mm Hg) | +2 SD* (mm Hg) |
|---|---|---|---|
| 1 | 44 | 39.2 ± 7.6 | 54.4 |
| 2 | 37 | 45.3 ± 7.8 | 60.9 |
| 3 | 33 | 45.2 ± 7.8 | 60.8 |
| 4 | 27 | 46.0 ± 8.9 | 63.8 |
| 5 | 23 | 46.0 ± 8.7 | 63.4 |
| 6 | 22 | 47.5 ± 9.9 | 67.3 |
| 7 | 19 | 51.1 ± 9.9 | 70.9 |

*In children, mean pressure plus 2 standard deviations is considered as the upper limit of normal (see text for details).

From Emery EF, Greenough A: Non-invasive blood pressure monitoring in preterm infants receiving intensive care. Eur J Pediatr 151:136, 1992. © 1992 Springer-Verlag.

### Treatment

As a result of inability to define neonatal hypertension accurately and the lack of information about the short-term and long-term side effects of antihypertensive medications in the newborn, firm clinical guidelines regarding the treatment of neonatal hypertension cannot be postulated. In asymptomatic newborns, with only mild to moderate elevation of blood pressure and without an identified cause, close observation, with no aggressive antihypertensive treatment, is recommended, unless clinical or echocardiographic evidence of hypertension develops. The definitive therapy of neonatal hypertension is to treat the primary cause whenever possible (e.g., removal of the umbilical catheter, discontinuation of an offending medication). In asymptomatic newborns with severe hypertension and in all symptomatic newborns even with only mild to moderate blood pressure elevation, treatment of the hypertension with antihypertensive agents is the presently accepted clinical practice (Table 87–4).

For mild hypertension with a component of fluid retention, diuretic therapy using furosemide or a thiazide diuretic with or without spironolactone is recommended. In the long-term diuretic treatment of neonatal hypertension, thiazide diuretics are preferred over furosemide because long-term furosemide treatment is associated with potentially detrimental side effects, including severe electrolyte imbalance resulting in failure to thrive, calciuria, nephrocalcinosis, and osteopenia.

**TABLE 87–3**

**Causes of Neonatal Hypertension**

**Vascular**
Renal artery thrombosis
Aortic thrombosis
Coarctation of the aorta
Hypoplastic aorta
Renal vein thrombosis
Thrombosis of the ductus arteriosus
Renal artery stenosis/intimal hyperplasia
Idiopathic arterial calcification

**Renoparenchymal**
Acute renal failure
Polycystic kidney disease
Renal cortical and medullary necrosis
Hypoplastic, dysplastic kidney
Acute renal infection
Pyelonephritis with scarring
Obstructive uropathy
Constrictive perirenal hematoma or urinoma
Congenital mesoblastic nephroma
Nephrolithiasis
Following pyeloplasty of a hydronephrotic kidney
Multicystic kidney

**Endocrine**
Pheochromocytoma
Neuroblastoma
Adrenal disorders (hyperplasia, hyperaldosteronism, carcinoma, hematoma)
Hyperthyroidism

**Other**
Drugs (corticosteroids, theophylline, pancuronium, intrauterine cocaine exposure, phenylephrine eye drops)
Extracorporeal membrane oxygenation
Bronchopulmonary dysplasia
Increased intracranial pressure/seizures
Fluid and electrolyte overload
Following closure of an abdominal wall defect

For the initial treatment of moderate to severe hypertension, the direct-acting vascular smooth muscle relaxant hydralazine is used frequently. Hydralazine also may decrease pulmonary vascular resistance in infants with bronchopulmonary dysplasia. Hydralazine may be given alone or in combination with a beta blocker. Among the beta blockers, the nonselective agent propranolol has been used most widely because it appears to increase the efficacy of hydralazine while decreasing thiazide-induced tachycardia. Propranolol may precipitate heart failure, however, and cause hypoglycemia and bronchospasm.

The use of an angiotensin-converting enzyme (ACE) inhibitor, primarily captopril, has become the treatment of choice in severe neonatal renovascular hypertension not responding to other medications. Mostly because of the higher postnatal renin levels and the immaturity of their renal function, newborns are extremely sensitive to the antihypertensive effects of captopril. When it was given at the originally recommended higher doses (0.3 mg/kg), unpredictable decreases in the systemic blood pressure occurred in some of the newborns, resulting in renal failure (Rasoulpour and Marinelli, 1992) and neurologic complications (Perlman and Volpe, 1989). Therefore, captopril should be started at lower doses, and the dose should be titrated so that the lowest effective dose is administered long-term (see Table 87–4). The intravenous ACE inhibitor enalaprilat also has been used successfully for the treatment of severe neonatal renovascular hypertension (Mason et al, 1992).

Hypertensive emergencies in the newborn are usually managed with hydralazine, diazoxide, sodium nitroprusside, or nicardipine. To avoid a rapid and substantial drop in blood pressure and thus tissue perfusion, stepwise dose increases are recommended. Diazoxide, a direct arteriolar smooth muscle relaxant, must be given rapidly because it avidly binds to protein. Side effects with repeated use include sodium and water retention and hyperglycemia. Sodium nitroprusside acts via the generation of nitric oxide, and thus its effect is dependent on the intact function of the endothelium. This photosensitive agent is an extremely potent vasodilator and must be administered in titrated continuous infusion while being shielded from light. Owing to its mechanism of action and metabolism, it may cause methemoglobinemia and cyanide toxicity. Because its administration to newborns in doses of 0.2 to 6 μg/kg/minute for up to 4 days has been found safe, routine monitoring of thiocyanate levels may not be necessary if the drug is administered in the aforementioned dose range and for a short period only (Benitz et al, 1985). The development of an unexplained metabolic acidosis with increased mixed venous oxygen content must prompt the discontinuation of the drug infusion and the measurement of plasma cyanide levels. Nicardipine is a dihydropyridine calcium channel–blocking agent that, when administered by intravenous infusion, has a powerful, titratable antihypertensive effect. In a dose of 0.8 to 1.8 μg/kg/minute, nicardipine effectively lowers blood pressure also in the neonatal period (Flynn et al, 2001). However, since the immature myocardium is more dependent on the transport of extracellular calcium for its function, more data are needed to establish the safety and long-term efficacy of calcium channel blockers in the neonatal patient population.

In hypertensive infants with stenosis of the renal artery, a balloon angioplasty or surgical reconstruction of the renal artery may be attempted. Only the poorly functioning, sclerotic, and shrunken kidney with established hypertension represents an indication for nephrectomy.

### Prognosis

In a majority of the cases of neonatal hypertension, systemic blood pressure can be adequately controlled by pharmacologic management, and the hypertension eventually resolves (Adelman, 1987; Rasoulpour and Marinelli, 1992). The long-term outcome, however, remains unclear. Newborns with hypertension of renovascular or renoparenchymal origin and those with persistent abnormalities of renal size and function, especially with concurrent bronchopulmonary dysplasia, require close and long-term follow-up,

**TABLE 87-4**

**Antihypertensive Agents Used in the Treatment of Hypertension in Newborns**

| Medication | Route | Dose | Comments |
|---|---|---|---|
| **Diuretics** | | | |
| Furosemide | IV, oral (q8h, q12h, q24h) | 1-2 mg/kg/dose | Hyponatremia, hypokalemia, hypochloremia, hypercalciuria, nephrocalcinosis, osteopenia, ototoxicity, growth retardation |
| Chlorothiazide | IV, oral | 5-50 mg/kg/day (q12h) | Hyponatremia, hypokalemia, hypochloremia, calcium sparing |
| Spironolactone | Oral | 1-3 mg/kg/day | Weak diuretic, hyperkalemia |
| **Adrenergic blockers** | | | |
| Beta-adrenergic blockers | | | |
| Propranolol | Oral | 0.5-2 mg/kg/day | Precipitation of heart failure, bronchospasm, hypoglycemia, decreased renin release, recommended in combination with hydralazine |
| Alpha$_1$/beta-adrenergic blockers | | | |
| Labetalol | IV | 0.25-1 mg/kg/hr | Limited experience in neonatal hypertensive emergencies |
| **Vasodilators** | | | |
| Hydralazine* | IV | 0.1-2 mg/kg/dose (q6-12h) | Reflex tachycardia, paroxysmal atrial tachycardia, emesis, diarrhea, positive ANA assay (SLE-like syndrome) |
| | Oral | 0.25-1 mg/kg/dose (q6-12h) | |
| Diazoxide* | IV | 1-3 mg/kg/dose | Hypotension, hyperglycemia, sodium and water retention |
| Nitroprusside* | IV | 0.2-10 μg/kg/min | Thiocyanate and cyanide toxicity, methemoglobinemia; drug must be protected from light due to increased photochemical degradation |
| **Angiotensin-Converting Enzyme Inhibitors** | | | |
| Captopril | Oral | 10-50 μg/kg/dose (q8-24h) May titrate to 0.5 mg/kg/dose | Oliguria, renal failure, hyperkalemia, apnea, seizures, cough |
| Enalaprilat | IV | 5-15 μg/kg/dose (q8-24h) | Oliguria, renal failure, hyperkalemia, cough |

*Recommended in neonatal hypertensive emergencies.

ANA, antinuclear antibody; SLE, systemic lupus erythematosus.

because the scars and atrophic regions in the kidney carry the possibility of recurrence of hypertension as well as that of the development of renal insufficiency at a later age.

## REFERENCES


Adelman RD: Long-term follow up of neonatal renovascular hypertension in the newborn. Pediatr Nephrol 1:35-41, 1987.

Adelman RD: The hypertensive newborn. Clin Perinatol 15: 567-585, 1988.

Adelman RD, Morrell RE: Coarctation of the abdominal aorta and renal artery stenosis related to an umbilical artery catheter placement in a neonate. Pediatrics 106:E36, 2000.

Al-Aweel I, Pursley DM, Rubin LP, et al: Variations in prevalence of hypotension, hypertension, and vasopressor use in NICUs. J Perinatol 21:272-278, 2001.

Andrew M, Marzinotto V, Massicotte P, et al: Heparin therapy in pediatric patients: A prospective cohort study. Pediatr Res 35:78-83, 1994.

Ankola PA, Atakent YS: Effect of adding heparin in very low concentration to the infusate to prolong the patency of umbilical artery catheters. Am J Perinatol 10:229-232, 1993.

Applegren P, Ransjo I, Bindslev L, et al: Surface heparinization of central venous catheters reduces microbial colonization in vitro and in vivo: Results from a prospective, randomized trial. Crit Care Med 24:1482-1489, 1996.

Arneil GC, MacDonald AM, Sweet EM: Renal venous thrombosis. Clin Nephrol 1:119-131, 1973.

Barrington KJ: Umbilical artery catheters in the newborn: Effects of catheter materials. Cochrane Syst Rev 1, CD000949, 2002.

Benitz WE, Malachowski N, Cohen RS, et al: Use of sodium nitroprusside in newborns: Efficacy and safety. J Pediatr 106:102-110, 1985.

Beratis NG, Panagoulias D, Varvarigou A: Increased blood pressure in newborns and infants whose mothers smoked during pregnancy. J Pediatr 128:806-812, 1996.

Böbenkamp A, vonKries R, Nowak-Göttl U, et al: Neonatal renal venous thrombosis in Germany between 1992 and 1994: Epidemiology, treatment and outcome. Eur J Pediatr 159: 44-48, 2000.

Cheves H, Bledsoe F, Rhea WG, Bomar W: Adrenal hemorrhage with incomplete rotation of the colon leading to early duodenal obstruction: Case report and review of the literature. J Pediatr Surg 24:300-302, 1989.

de Swiet M, Fayers P, Shinebourne EA: Systolic blood pressure in a population of infants in the first year of life: The Brompton study. Pediatrics 65:1028-1035, 1980.

Dillon PW, Fox PS, Berg CJ, et al: Recombinant tissue plasminogen activator for neonatal and pediatric vascular thrombolytic therapy. J Pediatr Surg 28:1264-1268, 1993.

Demarani S, Dollberg S, Hoath SB, et al: Effects of antenatal corticosteroids on blood pressure in very low birth weight infants during the first 24 hours of life. J Perinatol 19:419-425, 1999.

Dreyfus M, Magny JF, Brifey F, et al: Treatment of homozygous protein C deficiency and neonatal purpura fulminans with purified protein C concentrate. N Engl J Med 325:1565-1568, 1991.

Dix D, Andrew M, Marzinotto V, et al: The use of low molecular weight heparin in pediatric patients: A prospective cohort study. J Pediatr 136:439-445, 2000.

Duncan BW, Adzick NS, Longaker MT, et al: In utero arterial embolism from renal vein thrombosis with successful postnatal thrombolytic therapy. J Pediatr Surg 26:741-743, 1991.

Emery EF, Greenough A: Non-invasive blood pressure monitoring in preterm infants receiving intensive care. Eur J Pediatr 151:136-139, 1992.

Engle WD: Blood pressure in the very low birth weight neonates. Early Hum Dev 62:97-130, 2001.

Flynn JT: Neonatal hypertension: Diagnosis and management. Pediatr Nephrol 14:332-341, 2000.

Flynn JT, Mottes TA, Brophy PD, et al: Intravenous nicardipine for treatment of severe hypertension in children. J Pediatr 139:38-43, 2001.

Georgieff MK, Mills MM, Gomez-Marin O, Sinaiko AR: Rate of change of blood pressure in premature and full term infants from birth to 4 months. Pediatr Nephrol 10:152-155, 1996.

Gillman MW, Link CL, Rich-Edwards JW, et al: Maternal age and newborn blood pressure [abstract]. Circulation 103:1347, 2001.

Giordano P, Laforgia N, Di Giulio G, et al: Renal vein thrombosis in a newborn with prothrombotic genetic risk factors. J Perinat Med 29:163-166, 2001.

Gleason CA: Prostaglandins and the developing kidney. Semin Perinatol 11:12-21, 1987.

Goetzman BW, Stadalnik RC, Bogren HG, et al: Thrombotic complications of umbilical artery catheters: A clinical and radiographic study. Pediatrics 56:374-379, 1975.

Gruskin AB, Auerbach VH, Black IF: Intrarenal blood flow in children with normal kidneys and congenital heart disease: Changes attributable to angiography. Pediatr Res 8:561-572, 1974.

Hagstrom JN, Walter J, Bluebond-Langner R et al: Prevalence of the factor V Leiden mutation in children and neonates with thromboembolic disease. J Pediatr 133:777-781, 1998.

Haire WD: Pharmacology of fibrinolysis. Chest 101:91S-97S, 1992.

Harris MS, Little GA: Umbilical artery catheters: High, low or no. J Perinat Med 6:15, 1978.

Hartmann J, Becker J, Hussein A, et al: Treatment of neonatal thrombus formation with recombinant tissue plasminogen activator: Six years experience and review of literature. Arch Dis Child Fetal Neonatal Ed 85:F18-F22, 2001.

Hegyi T, Carbone MT, Anwar M, et al: Blood pressure ranges in premature infants: I. The first hours of life. J Pediatr 124: 627-633, 1994.

Holden RW: Plasminogen activators: Pharmacology and therapy. Radiology 174:993-1001, 1990.

Horgan MJ, Bartoletti A, Polansky S, et al: Effect of heparin infusates in umbilical arterial catheters on frequency of thrombotic complications. J Pediatr 111:774-778, 1987.

Israels SJ, Cheang T, McMillan-Ward EM, Cheang M: Evaluation of primary hemostasis in neonates with a new in vitro platelet function analyzer. J Pediatr 138:116-119, 2001.

Jackson JC, Truog WE, Watchko JF, et al: Efficacy of thromboresistant umbilical artery catheters in reducing aortic thrombosis and related complications. J Pediatr 110:102-105, 1987.

Keidan I, Lotan D, Gazit G, et al: Early neonatal renal venous thrombosis: Long-term outcome. Acta Paediatr 83:1225-1227, 1994.

Kennedy LA, Drummond WH, Knight ME, et al: Successful treatment of neonatal aortic thrombosis with tissue plasminogen activator. J Pediatr 116:798-801, 1990.

Kitterman JA, Phibbs RH, Tooley WH: Aortic blood pressure in normal newborn infants during the first 12 hours of life. Pediatrics 44:959-968, 1969.

Krafte-Jacobs B, Sivit CJ, Mejia R, Pollack MM: Catheter-related thrombosis in critically ill children: Comparison of catheters with and without heparin bonding. J Pediatr 126: 50-54, 1995.

LeFlore JL, Engle WD, Rosenfeld CR: Determinants of blood pressure in very low birth weight neonates: Lack of effect of antenatal steroids. Early Hum Dev 59:37-50, 2000.

Lerner GR, Kurnetz R, Bernstein J, et al: Renal cortical and renal medullary necrosis in the first 3 months of life. Pediatr Nephrol 6:516-518, 1992.

Low JA, Panagiotopoulos C, Smith JT, et al: Validity of newborn oscillometric blood pressure. Clin Invest Med 18:163-167, 1995.

Manco-Johnson MJ, Marlar RA, Jacobson LJ, et al: Severe protein C deficiency in newborn infants. J Pediatr 113:359-363, 1988.

Marino J, Martinez-Urrutia MJ, Hawkins F, et al: Encysted adrenal hemorrhage: Prenatal diagnosis. Acta Paediatr Scand 79:230-231, 1990.

Mason T, Polak MJ, Pyles L, et al: Treatment of neonatal renovascular hypertension with intravenous enalapril. Am J Perinatol 9:254-257, 1992.

McCauley RG, Beckwith JB, Elias ER, et al: Benign hemorrhagic adrenocortical macrocysts in Beckwith-Wiedemann syndrome. AJR Am J Roentgenol 157:549-552, 1991.

Mermel LA, Stolz SM, Maki DG: Surface antimicrobial activity of heparin-bonded and antiseptic-impregnated vascular catheters. J Infect Dis 167:920-924, 1993.

Miele V, Galuzzo M, Patti G, et al: Scrotal hematoma due to neonatal adrenal hemorrhage: The value of ultrasonography in avoiding unnecessary surgery. Pediatr Radiol 27:672-674, 1997.

Mocan H, Beattie TJ, Murphy AV: Renal venous thrombosis in infancy: Long-term follow-up. Pediatr Nephrol 5:45-49, 1991.

Moise AA, Wearden CA, Kozinetz CA, et al: Antenatal steroids are associated with less need for blood pressure support in extremely premature infants. Pediatrics 95:845-850, 1995.

Molteni KH, George J, Messersmith R, et al: Intra-thrombic urokinase reverses neonatal renal artery thrombosis. Pediatr Nephrol 7:413-415, 1993.

Northern Neonatal Nursing Initiative: Systolic blood pressure in babies of less than 32 weeks gestation in the first year of life. Arch Dis Child 80:F38-F42, 1999.

Nowak-Göttl U, von Kreis R, Göbel U: Neonatal symptomatic thromboembolism in Germany: Two year survey. Arch Dis Child 76:F163-F167, 1997.

Nowak-Göttl U, Auberger K, Halimeh S, et al: Thrombolysis in the newborns and infants. Thromb Haemost 82(Suppl 1):112-116, 1999.

Nowak-Göttl U, Kosch A, Schlegel N: Thromboembolism in newborns, infants and children. Thromb Haemost 86:464-474, 2001.

Nuntnarumit P, Yang W, Bada-Ellzey HS: Blood pressure measurements in the newborn. Clin Perinatol 26:981-96, 1999.

Nuss R, Hays T, Manco-Johnson M: Efficacy and safety of heparin anticoagulation for neonatal renal vein thrombosis. Am J Pediatr Hematol Oncol 16:127-131, 1994.

Nygren A, Ulfendahl HR, Hansell P, Erikson U: Effects of intravenous contrast media on cortical and medullary blood flow in the rat kidney. Invest Radiol 23:753-761, 1988.

Nwankwo MU, Lorenz JM, Gardiner JC: A standard protocol for blood pressure measurement in the newborn. Pediatrics 99:E10, 1997.

Omar SA, De Cristofaro JD, Agarwal BI, LaGamma EF: Effects of prenatal steroids on water and sodium homeostasis in extremely low birth weight neonates. Pediatrics 104:482-488, 1999.

O'Neill JA Jr, Neblett WW III, Born ML: Management of major thromboembolic complications of umbilical artery catheters. J Pediatr Surg 16:972-978, 1981.

Oppenheimer DA, Carroll BA, Garth KE: Ultrasonic detection of complications following umbilical arterial catheterization in the newborn. Radiology 145:667-672, 1982.

Payne RM, Martin TC, Bower RJ, Canter CE: Management and follow-up of arterial thrombosis in the neonatal period. J Pediatr 114:853-858, 1989.

Perlman JM, Volpe JJ: Neurologic complications of captopril treatment of neonatal hypertension. Pediatrics 83:47-52, 1989.

Perry EH, Bada HS, Ray JD, et al: Blood pressure increases, birth weight-dependent stability boundary, and intraventricular hemorrhage. Pediatrics 85:727-732, 1990.

Putnam MH: Neonatal adrenal hemorrhage presenting as a right scrotal mass. JAMA 261:2958, 1989.

Rajani K, Goetzman BW, Wennberg RP, et al: Effect of heparinization of fluids infused through an umbilical artery catheter on catheter patency and frequency of complications. Pediatrics 63:552-556, 1979.

Rasoulpour M, Marinelli KA: Systemic hypertension. Clin Perinatol 19:121-137, 1992.

Report of a Joint Working Group of the British Association of Perinatal Medicine and the Research Unit of the Royal College of Physicians: Development of audit measures and guidelines for good practice in the management of neonatal respiratory syndrome. Arch Dis Child 67:1220-1227, 1992.

Ribemont A: Recherches sur la tension du sang dan les vaisseaux du foetus et du nouveau-n propos du moment on lon doit lier le cordon ombilical. Arch Tocol 6:577, 1879.

Ricci MA, Lloyd DA: Renal venous thrombosis in infants and children. Arch Surg 125:1195-1199, 1990.

Richardson R, Applebaum H, Touran T, et al: Effective thrombolytic therapy of aortic thrombosis in the small premature infant. J Pediatr Surg 23:1198-1200, 1988.

Roy M, Turner-Gomes S, Gill G, et al: Accuracy of Doppler echocardiography for the diagnosis of thrombosis associated with umbilical venous catheters. J Pediatr 140:131-134, 2002.

Sanders LD, Jaquier S: Ultrasound demonstration of prenatal renal vein thrombosis. Pediatr Radiol 19:133-135, 1989.

Schmidt B, Andrew M: Neonatal thrombosis: Report of a prospective Canadian and international registry. Pediatrics 96:939-941, 1995.

Schobess R, Junker R, Auberger K, et al: Factor V G1691A and prothrombin G20210A in childhood spontaneous venous thrombosis: Evidence of an age-dependent thrombotic onset in carriers of factor V G1691A and prothrombin G20210A mutation. Eur J Pediatr 158(suppl 3):S105-S108, 1999.

Schwartz DS, Gettner P, Konstantino M, et al: Umbilical venous catheterization and the risk of portal vein thrombosis. J Pediatr 131:760-762, 1997.

Seibert JJ, Taylor BJ, Williamson SL, et al: Sonographic detection of neonatal umbilical-artery thrombosis: Clinical correlation. AJR Am J Roentgenol 148:965-968, 1987.

Seibert JJ, Northington FJ, Miers JF, Taylor BJ: Aortic thrombosis after umbilical artery catheterization in newborns: Prevalence of complications on long-term follow-up. AJR Am J Roentgenol 156:567-569, 1991.

Singh HP, Hurley RM, Myers TF: Neonatal hypertension: incidence and risk factors. Am J Hypertens 5:51-55, 1992.

Skalina ME, Annable WL, Kliegman RM, Fanaroff AA: Hypertensive retinopathy in the newborn infant. J Pediatr 103:781-786, 1983.

Slovis TL, Bernstein J, Gruskin A: Hyperechoic kidneys in the newborn and young infant. Pediatr Nephrol 7:294-302, 1993.

Sonesson SE, Broberger U: Arterial blood pressure in the very low birthweight newborn: Evaluation of an automatic oscillometric technique. Acta Paediatr Scand 76:338-341, 1987.

Spinazzola RM, Harper RG, de Soler M, Lesser M: Blood pressure values in 500- to 750-gram birthweight infants in the first week of life. J Perinatol 11:147-151, 1991.

Stephenson J: Can a common medical practice transform *Candida* infections from benign to deadly? JAMA 286:2531-2, 2001.

Strife JL, Ball WS Jr, Towbin R, et al: Arterial occlusions in newborns: Use of fibrinolytic therapy. Radiology 166:395-400, 1988.

Tan KL: Blood pressure in full-term healthy newborns. Clin Pediatr 26:21-24, 1987.

Vailas GN, Brouillette RT, Scott JP, et al: Neonatal aortic thrombosis: Recent experience. J Pediatr 109:101-108, 1986.

Versmold HT, Kitterman JA, Phibbs RH, et al: Aortic blood pressure during the first 12 hours of life in infants with birth weight 610 to 4,220 grams. Pediatrics 67:607-613, 1981.

Weindling AM: Blood pressure monitoring in the newborn. Arch Dis Child 64:444-447, 1989.

Weiner G, Castle V, DiPietro M, Faix R: Successful treatment of neonatal arterial thromboses with recombinant tissue plasminogen activator. J Pediatr 133:133-136, 1998.

Weinschenk N, Pelidis M, Fiascone J: Combination thrombolytic and anticoagulant therapy for bilateral renal vein thrombosis in premature infants. Am J Perinatol 18:293-297, 2001.

Weitz JI: Drug therapy: Low-molecular weight heparins. N Engl J Med 337:688-698, 1997.

Wesstrom G, Finnstrom O, Stenport G: Umbilical artery catheterization in newborns. I. Thrombosis in relation to catheter type and position. Acta Pediatr Scand 68:575-581, 1979.

Wright NB, Blanch G, Walkinshaw S, Pilling DW: Antenatal and neonatal renal vein thrombosis: new ultrasonic features with high frequency transducers. Pediatr Radiol 26:686-689, 1996.

Zigman A, Yazbeck S, Emil S, Nguyen L: Renal vein thrombosis: A 10-year review. J Pediatr Surg 35:1540-1542, 2000.

Zinner SH, Rosner B, Oh W, Kass EH: Significance of blood pressure in infancy: Familial aggregation and predictive effect on later blood pressure. Hypertension 7:411-416, 1985.

Zubrow AB, Hulman S, Kushner H, Falkner B: Determinants of blood pressure in infants admitted to neonatal intensive care units: a prospective multicenter study. J Perinatol 15:470-479, 1995.

# PART XVII

# ENDOCRINE DISORDERS

Editor: H. WILLIAM TAEUSCH

CHAPTER 88

## Embryology, Developmental Biology, and Anatomy of the Endocrine System

Lewis P. Rubin

### ENDOCRINE AND NEUROENDOCRINE DEVELOPMENT IN THE FETUS AND PERINATAL TRANSITION

The endocrine system consists of a number of interacting effector–target organ feedback pathways. The placental-fetal endocrine tissues sustain the intrauterine milieu and promote adaptation for postnatal life. During this perinatal transition, the organism shifts from dependence on the placenta to independent homeostatic regulation (Gluckman et al, 1999). The functional development of the endocrine glands and hormonal responsiveness of target tissues are influenced by fetal genotype, maternal genotype, maternal prepregnancy and pregnancy health and nutrition, and pregnancy-associated and other maternal stresses.

Much of the understanding about the developmental biology of the endocrine system is derived from large-animal fetal physiology models and gene manipulation in mice. An important caveat in comparing ontogenic studies in different species, however, is to consider the similarities with and differences from human fetuses and newborns. A critical point for interspecies comparisons is the relationship between birth and the maturational state of the neonate. Different species (and different organ systems of a single species) may be classified either as immature (altricial) or more developed (precocial). The human newborn has a relatively mature (precocial) brain and lung and mature neuroendocrine and parathyroid-renal pathways but is relatively clumsy—that is, motorically immature (altricial).

The human fetal endocrine system develops more or less independently of maternal endocrine influences. This separation is possible because the placenta is an efficient barrier to fetal access to most maternal hormones including steroids, sterols, peptides, glycoproteins, and catechols. Nevertheless, transplacental passage of even minute amounts of several maternal hormones can be essential for normal fetal development. For example, in human fetuses with congenital hypothyroidism (Chapter 92, on thyroid disorders), maternal-fetal transfer of thyroid hormone ($T_4$) may result in neonatal plasma levels 25% to 50% of those in normal newborns (Vulsma et al, 1989). Therefore, the outcome in congenital hypothyroidism is generally good when $T_4$ replacement is initiated within the first 2 weeks after birth. In contrast, maternal hypothyroidism during pregnancy adversely affects neurodevelopmental outcome in the offspring (Haddow et al, 1999), and the combination of severe maternal and fetal hypothyroxinemia results in profound neurodevelopmental disability (Yasuda et al, 1999).

Disturbances in transplacental substrate transfer, such as that of calcium (Chapter 89) and glucose (Chapter 93), also may modify the development of fetal and neonatal hormonal pathways. Maternal immunoglobins and certain therapeutic agents also are transported to the fetus. In the example of Graves disease, transplacental transfer of maternal thyroid-stimulating antibodies may cause fetal hyperthyroidism, and maternal antithyroid medications (propylthiouracil, methimazole) in sufficient doses suppress fetal thyroid function (Chapter 92).

### MOLECULAR DETERMINANTS OF ENDOCRINE DEVELOPMENT

Genotyping studies have shown that functional mutations in a single gene, usually encoding a transcription factor, can produce endocrine organ hypoplasia or aplasia. Important clinical examples include mutations in *HESX1* in septo-optic dysplasia with pituitary hypoplasia (Dattani et al, 1998), *IPF1* in pancreatic agenesis (Stoffers et al, 1997), *PAX8* in congenital hypothyroidism associated with thyroid hypoplasia (Congdon et al, 2001), or *DAX-1* in X-linked adrenal hypoplasia congenita and hypogonadotropic hypogonadism (Achermann et al, 2001).

Congenital (non-neoplastic) endocrine hyperfunction also is often caused by single-gene mutations that in this case lead to gene inactivation (*CaR, SUR1, Kir6.2*) or activation (*TSHR, LHR, GK, GLUD1*) (Table 88–1). All proteins currently known to cause fetal and neonatal non-neoplastic endocrine hyperfunction disrupt hormone exocytosis or cell sensing of an extracellular regulator of hormone exocytosis (Marx, 1999).

A second important genetic mechanism for developmental endocrinopathies involves genomic imprinting. In mammals, some (imprinted) genes are expressed solely from either the paternally or the maternally inherited allele.

**TABLE 88-1**

**Features of Nonneoplastic Endocrine Hyperfunction Disorders**

| Tissue Expressing Hyperfunction | Syndrome | Gene Mutated | Typical Age at Onset (yr) | Treatment |
|---|---|---|---|---|
| Parathyroid cells | FHH | *CaR* | 0 | None |
| | NSHPT | *CaR* | 0 | Excision* |
| Pancreatic islet beta cells | PHHI-1 | *SUR1* | 0 | Excision† |
| | PHHI-2 | *Kir6.2* | 0 | Excision† |
| | PHHI-3 | *GK* | 15 | Diazoxide |
| | PHHI-4 | *GLUD1* | 0 | Diazoxide |
| Thyrocytes | Congenital thyrotoxicosis | *TSHR* | 0-10 | Medical or ablative |
| Leydig cells | Testotoxicosis | *LHR* | 3 | Medical |

*Total excision of all tissue.

†Near-total excision.

*CaR*, calcium receptor gene; FHH, familial hypocalciuric hypercalcemia; *GK*, glucokinase gene; *GLUD1*, glutamate dehydrogenase type 1 gene; *Kir6.2*, beta cell ATP-binding subunit of inward-rectifying potassium channel gene; *LHR*, luteinizing hormone receptor gene; NSPHT, neonatal severe hyperparathyroidism; PHHI, persistent hyperinsulinemic hypoglycemia of infancy (types 1 to 4); *SUR1*, beta cell–specific sulfonylurea receptor (component of potassium channel) gene; *TSHR*, thyroid-stimulating hormone receptor gene.

Data from Marx, 1999.

Maternal and paternal imprints are established, respectively, in dividing diplotene oocytes and prospermatogonia. Lack of imprinting of specific chromosomes or chromosome segments occurs as a result of uniparental disomy or deletions of imprinted centers. Imprinting defects can cause distinct developmental abnormalities according to the chromosome involved (Tilghman, 1999). The chief mechanism involves differential methylation of specific sites in or near imprinted genes. These methylation marks are maintained throughout development and are only erased and reestablished in the germ line. Human endocrinopathies caused by imprinting defects include transient neonatal diabetes mellitus (Chapter 93) and Albright hereditary osteodystrophy (*GNAS1* imprinting defect) (Chapter 89). The single-copy *GNAS1* gene coding for the $G_s$ $\alpha$ subunit is the only G protein $\alpha$ subunit yet shown to produce human disease.

## STEROIDOGENESIS AND THE MATERNAL-PLACENTAL-FETAL UNIT

During pregnancy, the mother, fetus, and placenta function in concert as a steroidogenic unit for estrogen and progesterone production. Maternal cholesterol is the principal substrate for placental synthesis of progesterone precursors for fetal androgen production. Although the placenta lacks 17-hydroxylase and 17,20-desmolase (CYP17) activities for estrogen synthesis, the human fetal adrenal compensates with a considerable output of Δ5-steroids (17-hydroxylated precursors), particularly dihydroepiandrosterone sulfate (DHEAS) (Fig. 88–1). In primates, estrogen plays an integrative role in modulating placental-fetal communication and intrauterine development (Albrecht and Pepe, 1999). Estrogen promotes placental trophoblast differentiation into syncytiotrophoblast and up-regulates key enzymes in progesterone biosynthesis and cortisol-cortisone conversion.

Throughout most of gestation, protection from hypercortisolism is crucial for normal neuroendocrine development. Late in gestation, with activation of the fetal hypothalamic-pituitary-adrenal (HPA) axis, fetal cortisol acts as a trigger for parturition; lung, gastrointestinal, brain, and adrenal medullary maturation; induction of numerous metabolic pathways; and increased beta-adrenergic receptor density in heart, lung, and brown fat. In fact, studies on the role of glucocorticoids in preterm labor and fetal maturation have led to the successful, widespread use of antenatal glucocorticoids to accelerate fetal, especially lung, maturation (Liggins and Howie, 1972) (see also Chapter 6). On the other hand, chronic or repetitive fetal

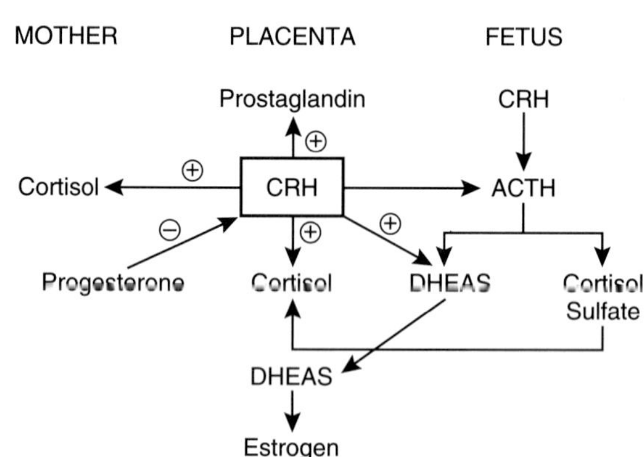


**FIGURE 88–1.** Schematic representation of the interrelationships among the mother, placenta and fetus in the upregulation of placental CRH production in response to stress. Maternal and/or fetal cortisol stimulates placental CRH expression. Placental CRH, in turn, stimulates the fetal HPA axis and secretion of DHEAS from the fetal zone of adrenal cortex. ACTH, adrenocorticotropic hormone; CRH, cortisol-releasing hormone; DHEAS, dehydroepiandrosterone sulfate; HPA, hypothalamic-pituitary-adrenal. *(Adapted from Challis JRG, Sloboda D, Matthews SG, et al: The fetal placental hypothalamic-pituitary-adrenal [HPA] axis, parturition and postnatal health. Mol Cell Endocrinol 185:135, 2001.)*

exposure to antenatal glucocorticoid has a profound, sometimes deleterious influence on postnatal adaptation and activity of the endocrine pancreas, pituitary-adrenal axis, and cardiovascular activity (Challis et al, 2001) (see later section,"The 'Fetal Origins of Adult Disease' Hypothesis").

Therefore, it is not surprising that in all species studied, including humans (Beitins et al, 1973), fetal access to maternal glucocorticoid is restricted and fetal glucocorticoid levels (cortisol or corticosterone) are low. This maternal-to-fetal gradient is maintained by the enzyme 11β-hydroxysteroid dehydrogenase (11βHSD). The type 1 enzyme isoform is bidirectional. The type 2 isoform (11βHSD2) unidirectionally converts cortisol and corticosterone to inactive cortisone and 11-dehydrocorticosterone, respectively. The low cortisol-to-cortisone ratio (approximately 0.3) in the fetal circulation reflects a low fetal cortisol production and high placental 11βHSD2 activity. The cortisol-to-cortisone ratio rises after birth.

As pregnancy progresses, the maternal-placental-fetal steroidogenic unit activates the fetal HPA axis. This is a central mechanism for the fetus to exert an influence on gestation. For example, placental production of corticotropin-releasing hormone (CRH) is correlated with the length of gestation. A CRH/adrenocorticotropic hormone (ACTH)/cortisol surge occurs near term that induces involution of the fetal adrenal cortex, increased adrenal 3β-hydroxysteroid dehydrogenase (3βHSD) activity, and a relative reduction in the placental 11βHSD2-to-11βHSD1 ratio. In humans, the fall in placental 11βHSD2 mRNA expression and rise in fetoplacental cortisol levels lead to a rise in placental prostaglandin ($PGE_2$ and $PGF_{2\alpha}$) synthesis that, in turn, stimulates uterine contractility and further CRH expression (see Fig. 88–1). The increased fetal adrenal cortisol production and decreased placental cortisol clearance in preparation for parturition synchronize the maturation of critical organs (lung, liver, intestine, adrenal, brain). In effect, term birth may be viewed as an escape mechanism from this intrauterine environment of increasing hypercortisolemia. In primates, the postnatal transition is promoted by disconnection from this robust placental steroid production.

A critical aspect of intrauterine endocrinology is the opposite effects of the increase in late fetal cortisol levels on hypothalamic and placental CRH expression. Specifically, cortisol inhibits hypothalamic CRH production via the HPA-negative feedback loop but stimulates placental CRH production, an effect mediated via the cAMP response element in the CRH promoter (Cheng et al, 2000). Positive feedback loops are intrinsically unstable and, in this instance, terminate in birth.

It is possible that placental CRH in humans may have evolved to meet the need for high fetal adrenal production of estrogen precursors such as DHEAS (Majzoub et al, 1999). Fetoplacental 17β-estradiol ($E_2$) and progesterone plasma levels are quite high and fall approximately 100-fold during the first day after birth. From this perspective, birth may have adverse endocrine consequences for the preterm newborn. In extremely preterm infants, the consequences of $E_2$ and progesterone withdrawal so early in development are largely unknown. Extremely preterm infants have different steroid hormone profiles from the norms for infants born at term. Whether these "abnormal" hormone levels are maladaptive and related to morbidity is controversial. One pilot study of $E_2$ and progesterone supplementation in extremely low-birth-weight (ELBW) infants showed trends toward increased bone mineral accretion and a decreased incidence of chronic lung disease (Trotter et al, 1999). Randomized clinical trials of "physiologic replacement" in extremely preterm newborns may answer these important clinical questions.

## HYPOTHALAMIC-PITUITARY-ADRENAL AXIS

The HPA system maintains homeostasis in a stable environment, facilitates adaptation to environmental stresses, and regulates somatic growth, reproduction, and lactation. Advancing pregnancy is associated with HPA axis maturation.

The hypothalamus forms an interface between the endocrine and autonomic systems and regulates thermoregulation, blood pressure, energy balance, and behavioral responses. Early specification signals are required before or during gastrulation for forebrain induction. Later in embryogenesis, ventralizing and rostralizing signals from the axial mesoderm (e.g., Sonic Hedgehog [Shh]) are required to induce the cell types of the presumptive hypothalamus (Michaud, 2001). The fetal hypothalamus begins to form soon after the appearance of the hypothalamic sulcus in the 32-day embryo. Between 6 and 12 weeks, the basal hypothalamus differentiates into distinct nuclei and fiber tracts and produces hormones detectable by immunohistochemistry or immunoassay. Portal vascular connections to the anterior pituitary are established by about 12 weeks (Thliveris and Currie, 1980), although the definitive hypothalamo-hypophyseal portal system develops primarily in the third trimester. Failure of ventral forebrain induction causes holoprosencephaly (see Chapter 63). Endocrine deficiencies caused by hypothalamic and/or pituitary dysfunction may be the only clinical sign in milder forms of (lobar) holoprosencephaly.

Neuropeptide secretion from hypothalamic neurons and negative and positive feedback loops from target organs regulate the synthesis and secretion of distinct pituitary hormones. The anterior pituitary gland (adenohypophysis) derives from ectodermal thickening of the diencephalon and roof of the oral pit. The pituitary diverticulum (Rathke's pouch) bulges into the floor of the prosencephalon by week 4. In week 6, sphenoidal mesenchyme pinches off the pituitary diverticulum from the oral pit. The precursor cells of the anterior pituitary begin to differentiate by week 8. These distinct pituitary cell types arise in a temporally and spatially specific pattern and in tandem with their inputs from hypothalamic nuclei. Development of the hypothalamo-hypophyseal portal veins permits the local circulation of releasing hormones, including thyrotropin-releasing hormone (TRH), growth hormone–releasing hormone (GHRH), CRH, and somatostatin (SS).

During the second trimester, the anterior pituitary differentiates into the five endocrine cell types that secrete six hormones: (1) pro-opiomelanocortin (POMC), which is proteolytically cleaved to ACTH in corticotropes and melanocyte-stimulating hormone (MSHα) in melanotropes;

(2) thyroid-stimulating hormone (TSH) in thyrotropes; (3) growth hormone (GH) in somatotropes; (4) prolactin (PRL) in lactotropes; and (5) follicle-stimulating hormone (FSH) and (6) luteinizing hormone (LH) in gonadotropes (Fig. 88–2). Serum GH concentrations peak at 20 to 24 weeks (Suganuma et al, 1989) and decline steadily thereafter, perhaps as a result of hypothalamic-pituitary maturation and increased interaction between GHRH and somatotropin release–inhibiting hormone (SRIH).

Anterior pituitary organogenesis illuminates how mutation of a single regulatory gene can cause multiple hormone deficiencies—in this case, multiple pituitary hormone deficiencies (MPHD), or panhypopituitarism—even though the genes encoding those hormones are dispersed throughout the genome. Transient embryonic morphogenetic signaling gradients induce overlapping expression patterns of transcription factors (repressors, activators) and coregulators and direct the positional fates of specific cell types. These pituitary and hypothalamic transcription factors coordinate gland formation, differentiation, expansion, and definitive function of the distinct pituitary cell types (Parks et al, 1999). Pituitary development and hormone expression require Pit-1, a pituitary-specific transcription factor. *PIT1* gene expression directs differentiation and proliferation of somatotrophs, lactotrophs, and thyrotrophs and transactivation of the genes encoding GH, PRL, and TSH. Several *PIT1* mutations have been shown to be responsible for a phenotype of multiple congenital pituitary hormone deficiencies involving GH, PRL, and TSH (Vallette-Kasic et al, 2001). The repressor *HESX1* ("homeobox gene expressed in embryonic stem cells," or Rpx for "Rathke pouch homeobox") is expressed early in the anterior region of the embryo and is involved in the initial determination of the optic nerves and anterior pituitary (see Fig. 88–2). *HESX1* mutations cause some recessive and autosomal forms of hypopituitarism and septo-optic dysplasia.

The neural component of the pituitary, the posterior pituitary gland or neurohypophysis, grows from an infundibular sac projecting from the floor of the diencephalon (at 5 to 8 weeks). Magnocellular neurons from the hypothalamus synapse with posterior lobe neurosecretory cells. Two hormones, oxytocin and vasopressin, are secreted directly into the general circulation.

The mammalian adrenal (or suprarenal) glands develop as a fusion of two distinct embryologic tissues, the cortex and the medulla (Fig. 88–3). The adrenal cortex arises bilaterally from coelomic mesothelium between the base of the mesentery (mesogastrium) medially and the mesonephros and undifferentiated gonad (urogenital ridge) laterally. The close proximity of these embryonic structures explains why ectopic cortical tissue may be located below the kidneys and sometimes is associated with the ovaries or testes. In week 6, coelomic cells become embedded in the underlying mesoderm, where they meet and envelop neural crest cells migrating from the sympathetic chain.

This migration of neuroblasts (neuroectoderm) forms the ganglia of the sympathetic trunk and sympathetic plexuses as well as the catecholamine-secreting paraganglia (chromaffin tissue). In the human embryo, the sympathetic trunk arises by about week 7. After weeks 10 to 12, chromaffin tissue develops along the aorta and subsequently differentiates into paraganglia and the adrenal medulla. Most of the paraganglia reach a maximal size by about 28 weeks; however, the organ of Zuckerkandl ventral to the aortic bifurcation continues to enlarge until term (Lagerkrantz, 1998). Usually, paraganglionic sites of chromaffin tissue involute with age, but they may develop into extra-adrenal pheochromocytomas.

The adrenal medulla functions as a classic endocrine tissue; that is, it secretes hormones directly into the blood stream. The medulla also participates in sympathetic control via preganglionic sympathetic nerve fibers. Pheochromocytoblasts give rise to the medullary pheochromocytes, which are epinephrine- and norepinephrine-secreting homologues of sympathetic postganglionic cells. Medullary cells are chromaffin (stain brown with chromium salts) and argyrophilic (stain with silver salts). By 3 months, adrenal pheochromocytes secrete epinephrine and norepinephrine into the medullary sinusoids and then into the systemic circulation. In the human fetus, the hypothalamic-pituitary-medullary adrenal axis becomes sufficiently functional by midgestation so that fetal stress responses can be independent of those of the mother (Gitau et al, 2001). This fetal stress response contrasts to fetal cortisol output. The fetal adrenal cortex minimally secretes cortisol before midgestation and fetal cortisol surges are determined by placental transfer from the mother.

From the third month, the superficial shell of adrenal cortical cells forms the precursor of the postnatal zona glomerulosa and zona fasciculata, that is, the definitive or adult cortex. The more superficial zona glomerulosa has a pseudoglomerular histologic appearance and secretes the mineralocorticoid aldosterone. The zona fasciculata contains large cells packed in radiate columns alternating with sinusoids and arterioles and secretes cortisol. The third definitive cortical layer, a network of cell cords called the zona reticularis, is absent at birth and develops from 3 years onward. It is an extragonadal source of sex steroids.

Deep to the presumptive definitive layer, cells proliferate inward, forming the impermanent fetal cortex. The outer (transitional) zone of the fetal cortex contains smaller (10- to 20-μm-diameter) basophilic cells. This transitional zone, between the inner (fetal) and outer (definitive) zones, expresses CYP17 and 3βHSD only relatively late in gestation, so that adrenal cortisol production also increases only relatively late in normal gestation. Most of the inner fetal zone consists of large (20- to 50-μm) eosinophilic cells that are the primary site for steroidogenesis, including abundant secretion of Δ5-steroid substrates for placental estrogen production (see earlier section, "Steroidogenesis and the Maternal-Placental-Fetal Unit"). The fetal zone accounts for about 80% of fetal adrenal mass, or about 8 g at birth. During the first year, the fetal cortex regresses, and the adrenal mass diminishes to 2 to 3 g.

Evaluation of the HPA axis in infants is used to test for primary adrenal suppression as well as for secondary adrenal insufficiency, either in preterm neonates who are thought to be cortisol deficient (Watterberg et al, 2001) or following dexamethasone treatment. In the latter case, a CRH test may more reliably indicate suppressed cortisol secretion than the short ACTH(1-24) test (Karlsson et al,

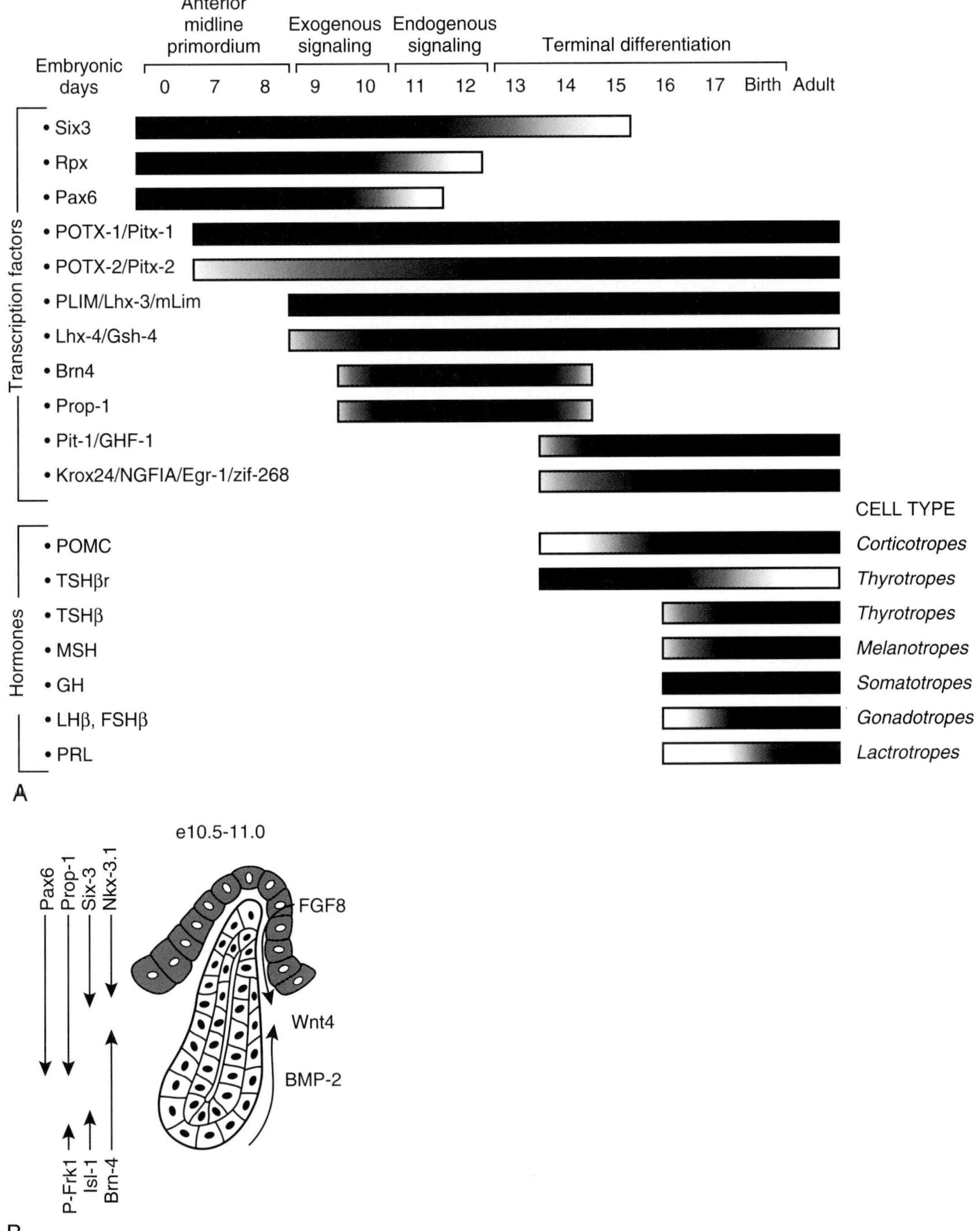


**FIGURE 88–2.** Expression of transcription factors and hormones during pituitary gland development in the mouse. **A,** Pituitary gland commitment has been divided into three phases. Phase 1, encompassing embryonic days 6 to 8.5 (e6-e8.5), is characterized by development and differentiation of stomodeum and oral ectoderm and the expression of *Rpx, Six-3, Pax6, Pitx-1,* and *Pitx-2.* Phase 2 (e8.5-e10.5), induction from exogenous signals, and phase 3 (e10.5-e12.5), induction from endogenous signals, are characterized by appearance of Rathke's pouch and expression of *PLIM* and *Lhx-4.* The pituitary gland cell lineage determination involves phase 3 (e12.5-adult) and the expression of *Pit-1.* POMC in corticotropes is the first hormone to appear (e12.5); TSHβ appears on e13.5, MSH on e14.5, GH on e15.5 and LHβ, FSHβ, and PRL before birth. **B,** Ventral-dorsal gradient of expression of transcription factors and signaling molecules in e10.5-e11 pituitary gland. FSHβ, follicle-stimulating hormone-β; GH, growth hormone; LHβ, luteinizing hormone-β; MSH, melanocyte-stimulating hormone; POMC, pro-opiomelanocortin; PRL, prolactin-releasing hormone; TSHβ, thyroid-stimulating hormone-β. *(From Kioussi C, Carriere C, Rosenfeld MG: A model for the development of the hypothalamic-pituitary axis: Transcribing the hypophysis. Mech Dev 81:23, 1999.)*

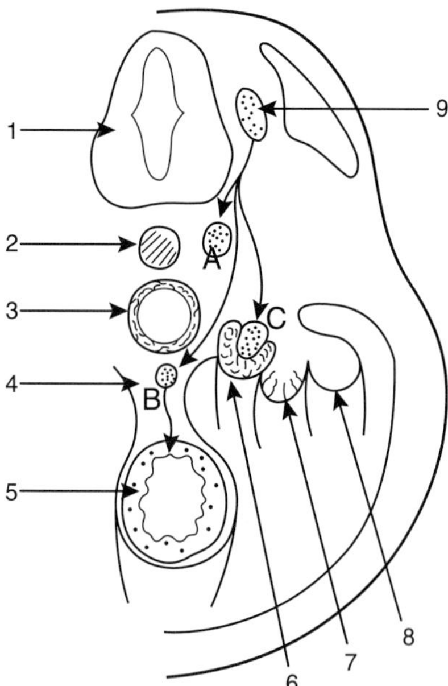


**FIGURE 88–3.** Transverse cross section of human adrenal development: neural tube (1), chorda (2), aorta (3), base of the mesentery (4), digestive tube (5), adrenal cortex (6), undifferentiated gonad (7), mesonephros (8). Migration of neuronal cells *(arrows)* from the neural crest (9) forms the sympathetic trunk ganglia (A), sympathetic plexuses (B), and the medulla and paraganglia (C). *(From Avisse C, Marcus C, Patey M, et al: Surgical anatomy and embryology of the adrenal glands. Surg Clin North Am 80:403, 2000.)*

2000). It is not yet clear whether the low circulating cortisol levels in ELBW infants reflect clinically relevant glucocorticoid deficiency (Chrousos, 2001).

## HYPOTHALAMIC-PITUITARY-THYROID AXIS

Maturation of the thyroid axis occurs in three phases: hypothalamic, pituitary, and thyroidal. At 10 to 20 weeks of gestation, secretory granules can be identified in differentiating pituitary thyrotropes, and TSH is detectable by bioassay and immunoassay.

The thyroid is the first endocrine gland to develop in the embryo. It forms at about 24 days from a pharyngeal outpouching, the thyroid diverticulum; as the anterior embryo grows, it migrates ventrally to the developing hyoid bone and laryngeal cartilages. By 7 weeks, the thyroid gland has assumed its definitive lobar shape and reached its final location in the neck. By 10 to 11 weeks, clusters of endodermal epithelial cells form single layers around lumens, the thyroid follicles, in which colloid begins to appear. Umbilical blood sampling has demonstrated that fetal TSH and $T_4$ are already detectable by 12 weeks and increase gradually through pregnancy to about 7 mU/L for TSH and 19.9 pmol/L for $T_4$ by term (Thorpe-Beeston et al, 1991). The fetal pituitary-thyroid feedback mechanism appears to be fully responsive by 18 to 20 weeks (Fisher, 1997). By that time, in pregnant women with Graves disease, transplacental passage of maternal thyroid-stimulating autoantibodies can induce fetal hyperthyroidism (Rakover et al, 1999).

Because pituitary and thyroid differentiation are contemporaneous, it has been suggested that the controlling events are independent. During the second half of gestation, fetal thyroid gland function is believed to mature under the influence of increased hypothalamic TRH secretion, pituitary TSH secretion, thyroid cell sensitivity to TSH, and pituitary sensitivity to negative feedback by $T_4$ (Chapter 92). However, as described previously (under "Endocrine and Neuroendocrine Development in the Fetus and Perinatal Transition"), small amounts of maternal thyroid hormones cross the placenta; adequate functioning of both maternal and fetal thyroid glands is important for normal fetal development. In congenital hypothyroidism due to defects in glandular ontogenesis (athyreosis), maternal thyroid hormones lessen the impact on fetal neurological development. Early neonatal diagnosis and $T_4$ treatment permit normalized growth and development. In contrast, when the mother is hypothyroid throughout gestation, the fetal consequences are more severe (Glinoer and Delange, 2000).

## ENDOCRINE PANCREAS

During the first 4 weeks of gestation, the ventral and dorsal pancreatic anlage arises from evaginations of the embryonic foregut. After rotation of the stomach and duodenum, the ventral pancreatic bud migrates and fuses with the dorsal bud. By branching morphogenesis, the ductal pluripotential epithelial cells give rise to endocrine and acinar cells under the influence of locally acting signals and activation of lineage-specific transcription factors (Hill and Duvillie, 2000; Peters et al, 2000). Beginning by week 7, scattered endocrine cells produce somatostatin, pancreatic polypeptide (PP), glucagons, and, by week 9, insulin. Pax and Ndx family transcription factors control the further fate determination of alpha, beta, delta, and PP endocrine cells (Fig. 88–4). Ongoing beta cell proliferation and differentiation are dependent on insulin-like growth factor-I (IGF-II) gene expression in the islets.

In the human, islet formation begins by week 12. Polyclonal clusters of endocrine cells aggregate in response to developmental expression of cell adhesion molecules (e.g., N-CAM and cadherins). In 24-week fetuses, islets generally remain in direct contact with the ducts, whereas by term, the islets have separated from the ducts; in adults, the islets are dispersed throughout the lobule (Watanabe et al, 1999). Islet volume also increases from about 4% to 13% of total pancreatic tissue by term (Peters et al, 2000). Endodermal differentiation into pancreatic endocrine cells, like other epithelial differentiation, depends on inductive signals derived from surrounding mesenchyme. Targeted gene deletion studies in mice have demonstrated critical roles for several transcription factors in pancreatic endocrine development (Sander and German, 1997) (see Fig. 88–4).

Human postnatal insulin kinetics and end-organ sensitivity to insulin appear to be established during the third trimester in preparation for extrauterine fuel metabolism. Recent observations indicate that both the

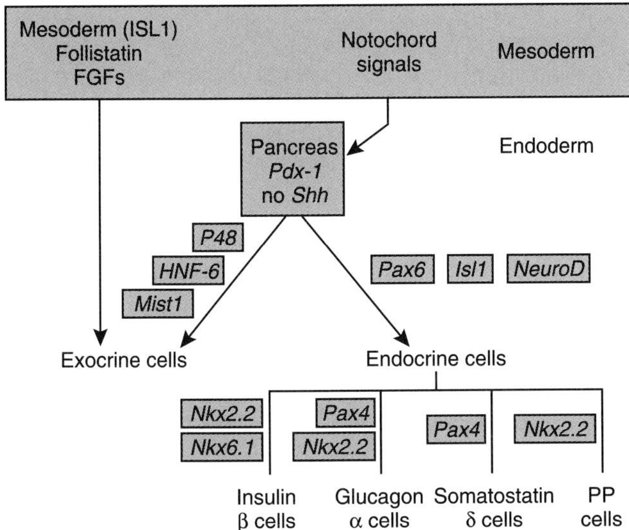


**FIGURE 88–4.** Molecular control of cell fate choices in the pancreas. *Pax6* and *Isl1* are expressed early, and their disruption leads to the reduction or absence of endocrine differentiation, which suggests that they could be expressed in endocrine progenitors able to give rise to all cell types. In *Isl1* mutant mice, *Pax6* is not expressed, which suggests *Pax6* is downstream of *Isl1*. Although *Pax4, NeuroD, Ndx2.2* and *Ndx6.1* are expressed as early as *Pax6* and *Isl1*, they affect the differentiation of only a subset of lineages. *Pax4* is required for glucagon- and somatostatin-producing cell differentiation. *Ndx2.2* is expressed in all islet cells, except somatostatin-producing cells, and its inactivation leads to the absence of the cell types where it is expressed. *Ndx6.1* is itself required for insulin cell differentiation. Although *Mist1* and *HNF-6* are expressed in endocrine cell lineages, their function has not yet been assessed by inactivation experiments. FGFs, fibroblast growth factors; PP, pancreatic peptide. *(From Grapin-Botton A, Melton DA: Endoderm development: From patterning to organogenesis. Trends Genet 16: 124, 2000.)*

maternal environment and the fetal genome influence the number and/or function of pancreatic beta cells in early life, with lifelong implications for postnatal diabetes (Hill and Duvillie, 2000; Hoet and Hanson, 1999). In contrast, insulin gene knockout mice (Duvillie et al, 1997) and human newborns with pancreatic agenesis (Stoffers et al, 1997) show severe intrauterine growth restriction/retardation (IUGR), which is consistent with insulin's role in mitogenesis and growth.

## PARATHYROID-RENAL AXIS

The parathyroid-renal (parathyroid hormone [PTH]–vitamin D) axis is the principal regulatory pathway in mammalian mineral and bone homeostasis (Chapter 89). The parathyroid glands arise from the dorsal parts of pharyngeal or branchial ("gill") pouches 3 and 4. These paired endodermal cell masses migrate ventrally and come to rest and differentiate in the back of the thyroid lobes as the superior (fourth pouch) and inferior (third pouch) parathyroid glands. The presence of immunoreactive PTH-containing cells can be detected in the human fetal parathyroids at 10 weeks. Defects in neural crest cell migration, such as DiGeorge syndrome (Chapter 89), result in embryonic field defects including parathyroid aplasia or hypoplasia. The caudal pharyngeal complex (pouches 4 and 5) develops into the calcitonin-secreting C cells in the thyroid gland. Calcitonin is detectable in fetal thyroidal C cells as early as 14 weeks. The fetal renal tubules can synthesize the active hormonal form of vitamin D, 1,25-dihydroxyvitamin D [$1,25(OH)_2D$], at least as early as the second half of gestation. Fetal plasma $1,25(OH)_2D$ levels remain low, however, as a result of high placental clearance.

## GONADAL AXES

Human reproductive system development is regulated by complex genetic, endocrine, and environmental signals. Gender-specific organogenesis begins in the early embryo, and sexual dimorphism results in the development of either ovaries or testes by birth. Further sexual maturation occurs in the perinatal period and at puberty (Chapter 91).

In mammals, genetic sex is determined by inheritance of either an X or a Y chromosome from the male gamete. The initial stages of gonadal and genital development in male and female embryos are morphologically indistinguishable. The gonads arise from thickening of the ventrolateral surface of the embryonic mesonephros (the genital ridge). At least four genes are required for testicular induction of the bipotential gonads: the orphan nuclear receptor steroidogenic factor-1 gene (*SF-1*), the Wilms tumor–associated gene (*WT1*), and the homeobox genes *Lhx1* (*Lim1*) and *Lhx9*. The two pituitary gonadotropins, LH and FSH, play a key role in cell fate determination and maturation of the sexual organs. Mutations in gonadotropin subunit or gonadotropin receptor genes have been associated with various types of hypogonadism in males and females.

In females, the müllerian ducts give rise to the uterus, fallopian tubes, and proximal vagina. The fetal ovarian germ cells are maintained in early meiotic arrest. The fetal ovary is characterized by late expression of the LH receptor (compared with that in the testis), late onset of aromatase activity, and low $E_2$ content. The postnatal ovarian follicles are prominent, and serum $E_2$ levels in female neonates remain low.

In males, wolffian ducts develop into epididymis, vas deferens, seminal vesicles, and prostate. Divergence from the female developmental pathway toward male sexual differentiation requires secretion of several testicular hormones. After gonad formation, expression of the *SRY* ("sex-determining region of the Y chromosome") gene initiates the male developmental cascade. *SRY* contains a high-mobility group (HMG) box, a conserved transcription factor motif that, in this instance, targets testicular Sertoli cell differentiation. Mutations in the HMG box are associated with 46,XY pure gonadal dysgenesis and sex reversal. Early events in testis development are differentiation of Sertoli cells and androgen-producing Leydig cells, LH receptor and steroid enzyme expression, autonomous steroid secretion, and high testosterone content. In contrast, germ cell maturation occurs later in gestation. Postnatally, testicular Leydig and Sertoli cells are prominent, and serum testosterone levels are high.

Müllerian-inhibiting substance (MIS) produced by Sertoli cells induces müllerian duct regression. LH and placental human chorionic gonadotropin induce Leydig cell androgen synthesis. In turn, testosterone and dihydrotestosterone promote development of the wolffian duct derivatives (male internal reproductive tract) and the virilization of the external genitalia. Therefore, inadequate fetal and neonatal testosterone secretion (e.g., due to hypogonadotropic hypogonadism or panhypopituitarism) impairs normal phallus and scrotum development. Leydig insulin-like 3 hormone (INSL3) may mediate transabdominal testicular descent into the scrotum (Nef and Parada, 2000). Female embryonic differentiation continues when the absence of MIS permits persistence of the müllerian structures, a lack of androgens permits wolffian duct degeneration, and the absence of INSL3 maintains the gonads in the abdomen.

## FETAL AND NEONATAL CIRCADIAN RHYTHMS

Neuroendocrine rhythmicity is an essential aspect of normal physiology and behavior. Certain rhythms occur in response to light-dark cycles. *Ultradian rhythms* have a periodicity shorter than 1 day but longer than 1 hour. Others, termed *circadian rhythms*, occur with a periodicity roughly matching the earth's rotation (24 hours) and persist even in the absence of environmental stimuli. Currently, little is known about either the maturational onset of ultradian or circadian hormonal secretion or the effects of perturbing factors such as prematurity or intrauterine and neonatal hormone treatment on endocrine periodicity.

In mammals, the master clock or pacemaker that controls circadian rhythms is located in oscillating neurons of the hypothalamic suprachiasmatic nuclei (SCN). The molecular mechanisms of rhythmogenic SCN function involve pulsed expression of specific transcription factors that induce the oscillatory secretion of neuropeptides including somatostatin, vasoactive intestinal peptide (VIP), arginine vasopressin (AVP), and neurotensin. Efferent pathways project from the SCN to other nuclei, such as the paraventricular nucleus (PVN). SCN efferents to the PVN stimulate secretion of CRH, which results in circadian adrenal cortisol secretion (see earlier section, "Hypothalamic-Pituitary-Adrenal Axis"), and pineal gland expression of melatonin.

Regulation and entrainment of the circadian clock(s) occur by transcriptional negative feedback loops and post-transcriptional controls. In the human fetus, heart rate, fetal movements, and some other outputs may be entrained to maternal rhythms. However, by late pregnancy the fetus establishes a circadian rhythm of cortisol secretion, presumably controlled by the fetal hypothalamic pacemaker (Seron-Ferre et al, 2001). ELBW infants (birth weight less than 1000 g and gestational age less than 28 weeks) show little short-term pulsatility in circulating cortisol levels over time (Jett et al, 1997). Nevertheless, available data suggest that the adult pattern of circadian cortisol secretion is established by 2 to 4 months after birth, irrespective of gestational age. In contrast, the onset of circadian melatonin secretion is related to post-conceptional age, not postnatal age.

The influence of the neonatal intensive care unit (NICU) environment on biologic rhythms of preterm infants is, as yet, poorly understood. Gene profiling experiments and clinical trials in newborns probably will yield a more detailed perspective on the developmental regulation and entrainment of circadian clocks.

## THE "FETAL ORIGINS OF ADULT DISEASE" HYPOTHESIS

Research from a wide range of disciplines has shown that endocrine function in adult life is determined, in part, by environmental influences acting at different stages of development spanning conception into infancy. Programming is a process by which environmental stimuli during critical periods of growth and development have lasting effects on the structure or function of tissues and physiologic systems. Intrauterine stresses can have an impact on HPA axis development and can program distinct autonomic, neuroendocrine, and behavioral responses into adulthood.

The "fetal origins" or so-called thrifty phenotype hypothesis proposes that the fetus adapts to a limited supply of nutrients in a manner that permanently alters its physiology and metabolism, with increased risk of disease in later life (Hales and Barker, 1992). The Dutch famine of 1944 to 1945 provided a unique opportunity to examine the long-term effects of intrauterine malnutrition in humans. The famine was imposed for a defined period on a previously well-nourished population. Extensive and reliable records have permitted unprecedented analysis of a birth cohort exposed to this discrete intrauterine insult. Additionally, David Barker and colleagues in Southampton, United Kingdom, have exploited detailed obstetric records in British hospitals to establish that IUGR is a strong predictor of adult metabolic and cardiovascular disease (e.g., Barker, 1998). For example, the relative risk for insulin resistance and "syndrome X" (the metabolic syndrome), consisting of type 2 diabetes, hypertension, and hyperlipidemia, is significantly higher in persons who were thin at birth with a low ponderal index. Clinical studies also uphold the association of maternal psychosocial or other stress in pregnancy with qualitative and quantitative changes in birth outcome and fetal and neonatal neuroendocrine activity (Wadhwa et al, 1996).

Increased fetal access to glucocorticoids during critical developmental periods may be a common mechanism explaining how these diverse maternal and uteroplacental stresses, including maternal undernutrition, psychosocial stress, and uteroplacental hypoxemia, induce fetal programming. Increased fetal glucocorticoids and stress both program specific effects in the brain, notably the HPA axis and dopaminergic-motor systems (Matthews, 2000; Welberg and Seckl, 2001), and can induce IUGR. The principal stress-mediated catecholamines (norepinephrine, epinephrine) transcriptionally repress placental trophoblast 11βHSD2 expression via alpha-adrenergic pathways (Sarkar et al, 2001), thereby increasing transplacental transfer of maternal cortisol to the developing fetus.

IUGR and metabolic programming interact with the genotype to influence the onset of endocrine, metabolic and cardiovascular disease in later life (e.g., Ibanez et al, 2001). Intrauterine stress producing low birth weight is associated with altered basal and stimulated cortisol levels as an early marker of HPA responsiveness, followed by glucose intolerance (insulin resistance) and hypertension (Levitt et al, 2000).

IUGR also results in a reduced beta cell population at birth (Van Assche et al, 1977). Fetal beta cell growth and development may be more sensitive to ambient amino acid than to glucose concentrations, suggesting a role for intrauterine protein availability for normal insulin homeostasis. In IUGR due to fetal malnutrition, altered expression of IGF-II (an islet cell survival factor) or IGF-binding proteins may severely alter beta cell ontogeny, resulting in a population of beta cells poorly suited for responding to subsequent metabolic stress (Hill and Duvillie, 2000). Fetal hypercortisolism also can decrease expression of IGFs and IGF receptors in late gestation (Price et al, 1992).

## THE ENVIRONMENTAL ENDOCRINE HYPOTHESIS

Recent environmental changes appear to have potentially important effects on the development of the endocrine system. Specifically, industrial and agricultural chemicals, through their actions on endocrine function, may be responsible for a number of reproductive and developmental abnormalities in a wide range of species, including humans (Cooper and Kavlock, 1997; Krimsky, 2000). These exogenous agents, or "endocrine disruptors," can interfere with the synthesis, storage and release, transport, metabolism, binding, action, or elimination of natural hormones. This importance of environmental endocrine-disrupting chemicals for public health and ecology, first stressed by Theo Colborn in the late 1980s, prompted passage in the United States of the Food Quality Protection Act and the Safe Drinking Water Estrogenic Substances Screening Act of 1996.

Three independent lines of research have provided the initial evidence for the importance of environmental agents on human endocrine development: recognition of the adverse effects of the potent synthetic estrogens—specifically, diethylstilbestrol (DES) and related compounds—on female and male reproductive tract development; field and laboratory studies associating wildlife reproductive malformations with chemical pollutants; and research linking xenoestrogens to declines in human sperm counts (Krimsky, 2000). Structural abnormalities of the reproductive tract including hypospadias and cryptorchidism, which have potential hormone-mediated origin and a critical developmental component, show upward secular trending.

During development, reproductive tract tissues are especially sensitive to low concentrations of sex steroids. Androgens secreted by a maternal adrenal tumor can virilize a female fetus (Kirk et al, 1992). Increased placental estradiol production has been associated with cryptorchidism in male newborns (Hadziselimovic et al, 2000). One mechanism is estrogenic down-regulation of insulin-3 (Insl3) expression by embryonic Leydig cells (Nef et al, 2000). Similarly, endocrine disruptors with antiandrogenic or estrogenic activity can have feminizing effects in the developing male fetus. Estrogens may induce adverse reproductive changes in female fetuses, but antiandrogens have little effect (Toppari and Skakkebaek, 1998). Changes induced by intrauterine exposure to endocrine disruptors may be irreversible, in contrast with the reversible changes induced by transient hormone exposure in the adult (Bigsby et al, 1999).

Endocrine disruptors such as organochlorines (e.g., the pesticide DDT) can alter normal gonadal ontogeny. In female fetuses, the onset of meiosis is delayed, and in male fetuses, testosterone synthesis is increased (Rhind et al, 2001). Prenatal exposure to the estrogenic agent DES increases risk of reproductive teratogenicity in female and male offspring. Exposure of the conceptus to antiandrogenic pharmaceuticals such as the androgen receptor antagonist flutamide and the 5α-reductase inhibitor finasteride generally affects males, causing hypospadias, cryptorchidism, reduced testicular mass, or decreased sperm production. Exposure to polychlorinated biphenyl (PCB) congeners, either in utero or via breast-feeding, has structural, functional, and behavioral influences, particularly on thyroidal axis development and differentiation of the male reproductive tract (Brouwer et al, 1998). It is evident that the endocrine system presents a number of target sites for adverse effects of environmental agents. Much more information is needed about the specific ecologic and public health risks.

## SELECTED READINGS


Avisse C, Marcus C, Patey M, et al: Surgical anatomy and embryology of the adrenal glands. Surg Clin North Am 80:403, 2000.

Barker DJP (ed): Mothers, Babies and Health in Later Life, 2nd ed. Edinburgh, Churchill Livingstone, 1998.

Brivanlou AH, Darnell JE Jr: Signal transduction and the control of gene expression. Science 295:813, 2002.

Brookes M, Zietman AL (eds): Clinical Embryology: A Color Atlas and Text. Boca Raton, Fla, CRC Press, 1998.

Challis JRG, Matthews SG, Gibb W, Lye SJ: Endocrine and paracrine regulation of birth at term and preterm. Endocr Rev 21:514, 2000.

Dasen JS, Rosenfeld MG: Signaling and transcriptional mechanisms in pituitary development. Annu Rev Neurosci 24:327, 2001.

Endocrine Disruptors Research Initiative: http://www.epa.gov/endocrine

Fisher DA: The unique endocrine milieu of the fetus. J Clin Invest 78:603, 1986.

Hoet JJ, Hanson MA: Intrauterine nutrition: Its importance during critical periods for cardiovascular and endocrine development. J Physiol 514:617, 1999.

Krimsky S: Hormonal Chaos: The Scientific and Social Origins of the Environmental Endocrine Hypothesis. Baltimore, Johns Hopkins University Press, 2000.

Lockitch G, Halstead AC, Dimmick JE: Endocrine system. In Dimmick JE, Kalousek DK (eds): Developmental Pathology of the Embryo and Fetus. Philadelphia, JB Lippincott, 1992, p 707.

Nef S, Parada LF: Hormones in male sexual development. Genes Dev 14:3075, 2000.

O'Regan D, Welberg LLAM, Holmes MC, Seckl JR: Glucocorticoid programming of pituitary-adrenal function: mechanisms and physiological consequences. Semin Neonatol 6:319, 2001.

Tilghman SM: The sins of the fathers and mothers: Genomic imprinting in mammalian development. Cell 96:185, 1999.

## REFERENCES


Achermann JC, Ito M, Silverman BL, et al: Missense mutations cluster within the carboxyl-terminal region of DAX-1 and impair transcriptional repression. J Clin Endocrinol Metab 86:3171, 2001.

Albrecht ED, Pepe GJ: Central integrative role of oestrogen in modulating the communication between the placenta and fetus that results in primate fetal-placental development. Placenta 20:129, 1999.

Barker DJP (ed): Mothers, Babies and Health in Later Life, 2nd ed. Edinburgh, Churchill Livingstone, 1998.

Beitins IZ, Bayard F, Ances IG, et al: The metabolic clearance rate, blood production, interconversion and transplacental passage of cortisol and cortisone in pregnancy near term. Pediatr Res 7:509, 1973.

Bigsby R, Chapin RE, Daston GP, et al: Evaluating the effects of endocrine disruptors on endocrine function during development. Environ Health Perspect 107(suppl 4):613, 1999.

Brouwer A, Ahlborg UG, van Leeuwen FXR, Feeley MM: Report of the WHO Working Group on the Assessment of Health Risks for Human Infants from Exposure to PCDDs, PCDFs and PCBs. Chemosphere 37:1627, 1998.

Challis JRG, Sloboda D, Matthews SG, et al: The fetal placental hypothalamic-pituitary-adrenal (HPA) axis, parturition and post natal health. Mol Cell Endocrinol 185:135, 2001.

Cheng YH, Nicholson RC, King B, et al: Glucocorticoid stimulation of corticotropin-releasing hormone gene expression requires a cyclic adenosine 3',5'-monophosphate regulatory element in human primary placental cytotrophoblast cells. J Clin Endocrinol Metab 85:1937, 2000.

Chrousos CP: Adrenal suppression versus clinical glucocorticoid deficiency in the premature infant: no simple answers. J Clin Endocrinol Metab 86:473, 2001.

Congdon T, Nguyen LQ, Nogueira CR, et al: A novel mutation (*Q40P*) in *PAX8* associated with congenital hypothyroidism and thyroid hypoplasia: Evidence for phenotypic variability in mother and child. J Clin Endocrinol Metab 86:3962, 2001.

Cooper RL, Kavlock RJ: Endocrine disruptors and reproductive development: A weight-of evidence overview. J Endocrinol 152:159, 1997.

Dattani MT, Martinez-Barbera JP, Thomas PQ, et al: Mutations in the homeobox gene *HESX1/Hesx1* associated with septo-optic dysplasia in human and mouse. Nat Genet 19:125, 1998.

Duvillie B, Cordonnier C, Deltour L, et al: Phenotypic alterations in insulin deficient mutant mice. Proc Natl Acad Sci U S A 94:5137, 1997.

Fisher DA: Fetal thyroid function: Diagnosis and management of fetal thyroid disorders. Clin Obstet Gynecol 40:16, 1997.

Gitau R, Fisk NM, Teixeira MA, et al: Fetal hypothalamic-pituitary-adrenal stress responses to invasive procedures are independent of maternal responses. J Clin Endocrinol Metab 86:104, 2001.

Glinoer D, Delange F: The potential repercussions of maternal, fetal, and neonatal hypothyroxinemia on the progeny. Thyroid 19:871, 2000.

Gluckman PD, Sizonenko SV, Bassett NS: The transition from fetus to neonate—an endocrine perspective. Acta Paediatr Suppl 88:7, 1999.

Grapin-Botton A, Melton DA: Endoderm development: From patterning to organogenesis. Trends Genet 16:124, 2000.

Haddow JE, Palomaki GE, Allan WC, et al: Maternal thyroid deficiency during pregnancy and subsequent neuropsychological development of the child. N Engl J Med 341:549, 1999.

Hadziselimovic F, Geneto R, Emmons LR: Elevated placental estradiol: A possible etiological factor of human cryptorchidism. J Urol 164:1696, 2000.

Hales C, Barker D: Type 2 diabetes mellitus: The thrifty phenotype hypothesis. Diabetologia 35:595, 1992.

Hill DJ, Duvillie B: Pancreatic development and adult diabetes. Pediatr Res 48:269, 2000.

Hoet JJ, Hanson MA: Intrauterine nutrition: Its importance during critical periods for cardiovascular and endocrine development. J Physiol 514:617, 1999.

Ibanez L, Ong K, Potau N, et al: Insulin gene variable number of tandem repeat genotype and the low birth weight, precocious pubarche, and hyperinsulinism sequence. J Clin Endocrinol Metab 86:5788, 2001.

Jett PL, Samuels MH, McDaniel PA, et al: Variability of plasma cortisol levels in extremely low birth weight infants. J Clin Endocrinol Metab 82:2921, 1997.

Karlsson R, Kallio J, Irjala K, et al: Adrenocorticotropin and corticotrophin-releasing hormone tests in preterm infants. J Clin Endocrinol Metab 85:4592, 2000.

Kioussi C, Carriere C, Rosenfeld MG: A model for the development of the hypothalamic-pituitary axis: Transcribing the hypophysis. Mech Dev 81:23, 1999.

Kirk JM, Perry LA, Shand WS, et al: Female pseudohermaphroditism due to a maternal adrenocortical tumor. J Clin Endocrinol Metab 75:646, 1992.

Krimsky S: Hormonal Chaos: The Scientific and Social Origins of the Environmental Endocrine Hypothesis. Baltimore, Johns Hopkins University Press, 2000.

Lagerkrantz H: Sympathoadrenal mechanisms during development. In Polin RA, Fox WW (eds): Fetal and Neonatal Physiology, 2nd ed. Philadelphia, WB Saunders, 1998, p 220.

Levitt NS, Lambert EV, Woods D, et al: Impaired glucose tolerance and elevated blood pressure in low birth weight, nonobese, young South African adults: Early programming of cortisol axis. J Clin Endocrinol Metab 85:4611, 2000.

Liggins GC, Howie RN: A controlled trial of antepartum glucocorticoid treatment for prevention of the respiratory distress syndrome in premature infants. Pediatrics 50:515, 1972.

Majzoub JA, McGregor JA, Lockwood CJ, et al: A central theory of preterm and term labor: Putative role for corticotropin-releasing hormone. Am J Obstet Gynecol 180:S232, 1999.

Marx SJ: Contrasting paradigms for hereditary hyperfunction of endocrine cells. J Clin Endocrinol Metab 84:3001, 1999.

Matthews SG: Antenatal glucocorticoids and programming of the developing CNS. Pediatr Res 41:291, 2000.

Messiano S, Jaffe RB: Developmental and functional biology of the primate fetal adrenal cortex. Endocr Rev 18:378, 1997.

Michaud JL: The developmental program of the hypothalamus and its disorders. Clin Genet 60:255, 2001.

Nef S, Parada LF: Hormones in male sexual development. Genes Dev 14:3075, 2000.

Nef S, Shipman T, Parada LF: A molecular basis for estrogen-induced cryptorchidism. Dev Biol 224:354, 2000.

Ong KKL, Dunger DB: Developmental aspects in the pathogenesis of type 2 diabetes. Mol Cell Endocrinol 185:145, 2001.

Parks JS, Brown MR, Hurley DL, et al: Heritable disorders of pituitary development. J Clin Endocrinol Metab 84:4362, 1999.

Peters J, Jurgensen A, Kloppel G: Ontogeny, differentiation and growth of the endocrine pancreas. Virchows Arch 436:527, 2000.

Petry CJ, Ozanne SE, Hales CN: Programming of intermediary metabolism. Mol Cell Endocrinol 185:81, 2001.

Price WA, Stiles AD, Moats-Staats BM, D'Ercole AJ: Gene expression of the insulin-like growth factors (IGFs), the type 1 IGF receptor, and IGF binding proteins in dexamethasone-induced fetal growth retardation. Endocrinology 130:1424, 1992.

Rakover Y, Weiner E, Mosh N, Shalev E: Fetal pituitary negative feedback at early gestational age. Clin Endocrinol 50:809, 1999.

Rhind SM, Rae MT, Brooks AN: Effects of nutrition and environmental factors on the fetal programming of the reproductive axis. Reproduction 122:205, 2001.

Sander M, German MS: The beta cell transcription factors and development of the pancreas. J Mol Med 75:327, 1997.

Sarkar S, Tsai SW, Nguyen TT, et al: Inhibition of placental 11β-hydroxysteroid dehydrogenase type 2 by catecholamines via α-adrenergic signaling. Am J Physiol Reg Integ Com Physiol 281:R1966, 2001.

Seron-Ferre M, Riffo, Valenzuela GJ, Germain AM: Twenty-four-hour pattern of cortisol in the human fetus at term. Am J Obstet Gynecol 184:1278, 2001.

Stoffers DA, Zinkin NT, Stanojevic V, et al: Pancreatic aganesis attributable to a single nucleotide deletion in the human *IPF1* gene coding sequence. Nat Genet 15:106, 1997.

Suganuma N, Seo H, Yamamoto N, et al: The ontogeny of growth hormone in the human fetal pituitary. Am J Obstet Gynecol 160:729, 1989.

Thliveris JA, Currie RW: Observations on the hypothalamohypophyseal portal vasculature in the developing human fetus. Am J Anat 157:441, 1980.

Thorpe-Beeston JG, Nicoliades KH, Felton CV, et al: Maturation of the secretion of thyroid hormone and thyroid-stimulating hormone in the fetus. N Engl J Med 324:532, 1991.

Tilghman SM: The sins of the fathers and mothers: Genomic imprinting in mammalian development. Cell 96:185, 1999.

Tobet SA, Bless EP, Schwarting GA: Developmental aspect of the gonadotropin-releasing hormone system. Mol Cell Endocrinol 185:173, 2001.

Toppari J, Skakkebaek NE: Sexual differentiation and environmental endocrine disrupters. Ballieres Clin Endocrinol Metab 12:143, 1998.

Trotter A, Maier L, Grill HJ, et al: Effects of postnatal estradiol and progesterone replacement in extremely preterm infants. J Clin Endocrinol Metab 84:4531, 1999.

Valette-Kasic S, Pellegrini-Bouiller I, Sampieri F, et al: Combined pituitary hormone deficiency due to the F135C human Pit-1 (Pituitary-specific factor-1) gene mutation: Functional and structural correlates. Mol Endocrinol 15:411, 2001.

Van Assche FA, De Prins F, Aerts L, Verjans M: The endocrine pancreas in small-for-dates infants. Br J Obstet Gynaecol 84:751, 1977.

Vulsma T, Gons MH, de Vijlder JJM: Maternal-fetal transfer of thyroxine in congenital hypothyroidism due to a total organification defect or thyroid aganesis. N Engl J Med 321:13, 1989.

Wadhwa PD, Dunkel-Schetter C, Chicz-DeMet A, et al: Prenatal psychosocial factors and the neuroendocrine axis in human pregnancy. Psychosom Med 58:432, 1996.

Watanabe T, Yaegashi H, Koizumi M, et al: Changing distribution of islets in the developing human pancreas: a computer-assisted three-dimensional reconstruction study. Pancreas 18:349, 1999.

Welberg LAM, Seckl JR: Prenatal stress, glucocorticoids and the programming of the brain. J Neuroendocrinol 13:113, 2001.

Watterberg KL, Gerdes JS, Cook KL: Impaired glucocorticoid synthesis in premature infants developing chronic lung disease. Pediatr Res 50:190, 2001.

Yasuda T, Ohnishi H, Wataki K, et al: Outcome of a baby born from a mother with acquired juvenile hypothyroidism having undetectable thyroid hormone concentrations. J Clin Endocrinol Metab 84:2630, 1999.

CHAPTER 89

# Disorders of Calcium and Phosphorus Metabolism

Lewis P. Rubin

## HOMEOSTATIC CONTROL OF CALCIUM AND MAGNESIUM

Calcium plays two important physiologic roles. Calcium salts in bone provide structural integrity. Regulation of calcium ions present in the cytosol and extracellular fluid (ECF) is essential for maintenance and control of many biologic processes, including cell-cell communication, cell aggregation and division, coagulation, neuromuscular excitability, membrane integrity and permeability, enzyme activity, and secretion. This diversity of functions is made possible by the maintenance of a large electrochemical gradient between the ECF $Ca^{2+}$ concentration, which is in the 1 mmol/L range, and resting intracellular (cytosolic) $Ca^{2+}$concentration, which is about 0.1 μmol/L.

Significant alterations in serum calcium concentration occur frequently in the neonatal period. It is important to evaluate these alterations in light of the normal dynamic changes that take place during the perinatal transition. After the first 2 to 3 extrauterine days, normal serum calcium concentrations vary only slightly with age, range between 8.8 and 10.6 mg/dL, and average about 10 mg/dL. In the United States, serum or plasma calcium levels usually are reported as mg/dL, which may be converted to molar units by dividing by 4 (e.g., 10 mg/dL is equivalent to 2.5 mmol/L).

Approximately 55% to 60% of the total plasma calcium is diffusible (or ultrafilterable), and the rest is protein bound. Most diffusible calcium is ionized, but about 5% of total circulating calcium is complexed to plasma anions, such as phosphates, citrate, and bicarbonate. Ionized calcium ($Ca^{2+}$) is the only biologically available fraction of ECF calcium. It is subject to precise metabolic control.

Hypoalbuminemia leads to a decline in total serum calcium, but proportionate increases in the ionized fraction usually maintain serum $Ca^{2+}$ within the normal range. Acute alkalosis (e.g., hyperventilation or bicarbonate infusion) or rapid administration of citrate-buffered blood (e.g., during exchange transfusion, initiation of extracorporeal membrane oxygenation [ECMO], cardioplegia, or organ transplantation) may acutely lower serum $Ca^{2+}$ by increasing albumin binding or citrate chelation, respectively. These conditions can produce transient clinical manifestations of hypocalcemia but do not lower the total serum calcium concentration. Electrocardiogram Q-Tc intervals and algorithms for correcting serum total calcium for alterations in serum albumin concentration and/or pH or for calculating "free" calcium concentration have not proved to be reliable compared with actual measurement of $Ca^{2+}$ using ion-selective electrodes (Clase et al, 2000). For routine clinical purposes, measuring total serum calcium often suffices.

Although the intestine has considerable absorptive capacity for calcium, renal tubular calcium reabsorption usually exceeds intestinal absorption by at least 40-fold. Most of the tubular $Ca^{2+}$ load is reabsorbed in the proximal tubule and thick ascending limb of the loop of Henle via paracellular, passive flux (coupled with sodium reabsorption) driven by the existing electrochemical gradient. A transcellular pathway in the distal nephron tightly regulates the rest of urinary $Ca^{2+}$ reabsorption. Calcitropic hormones regulate the distal $Ca^{2+}$-selective, $Na^+$-independent channels.

More than 98% of total body calcium is deposited in the skeleton as hydroxyapatite [$Ca_5(OH)(PO_4)_3$]; the ECF and soft tissues contain the remainder. A small fraction of skeletal calcium freely exchanges with the ECF and serves as an important buffer of circulating calcium. Consequently, decreased skeletal calcium is a hallmark of most chronic metabolic bone diseases.

Magnesium homeostasis also is largely renally mediated. Approximately 80% of total plasma magnesium is filtered through the glomerulus and is reabsorbed mainly in cortical segments of the thick ascending limb of the loop of Henle. Once the maximal tubular reabsorption is exceeded, filtered magnesium is excreted into the urine. Hormones regulate magnesium reabsorption by changing the transepithelial voltage and paracellular permeability of tubular cells.

## HOMEOSTATIC CONTROL OF PHOSPHORUS

Blood inorganic phosphate ($P_i$) concentration varies with age. It is highest during infancy and gradually declines to adulthood. Approximately 10% of plasma $P_i$ is noncovalently bound to protein, whereas 90% circulates as $HPO_4^{2-}$ and $HPO_4^-$ ions or as complexes with sodium, calcium, or magnesium. About 80% to 85% of total body phosphorus is contained in the hydroxyapatite lattice of bone, where it contributes to mechanical support. The remainder is distributed in the ECF, largely as inorganic ions or complexes, and in soft tissues as phosphate esters. Intracellular phosphate esters and phosphorylated intermediates regulate cell metabolism and gene expression (via phosphorylase, kinase, and phosphatase activities) and generate and transfer cellular energy (e.g., via adenosine triphosphate [ATP]). Cytosolic and ECF phosphorus levels (approximately 0.1 mmol/L and 0.2 mmol/L, respectively) are less stringently regulated than are levels of $Ca^{2+}$ and $Mg^{2+}$.

Dietary phosphate generally is absorbed in proportion to its content in food. Although phosphorus and calcium can be absorbed along the entire length of the small intestine, most phosphate transport takes place in the jejunum and ileum, whereas most calcium absorption occurs in the duodenum. The renal proximal tubule is the principal regulatory site for phosphorus homeostasis. Renal regulation is accomplished primarily by varying the threshold for phosphate reabsorption (the tubular maximum for $P_i$/glomerular filtration rate, or TmP/GFR). Hormones (parathyroid hormone [PTH], parathyroid hormone–related protein [PTHrP], growth hormone) and dietary phosphate reset this theoretical threshold by regulating apical tubular $Na^+$-$P_i$ cotransporters (Murer and Biber, 1995). Essentially, the TmP/GFR is the "set point" that defines the fasting serum phosphorus concentration. At lower serum phosphorus levels, most filtered phosphorus is reabsorbed; at higher levels, most filtered phosphorus is excreted. To assess the TmP/GFR, a fasting urine specimen is obtained for measurement of phosphorus and creatinine along with simultaneous determination of serum phosphorus and creatinine. A nomogram has been constructed so that TmP/GFR can easily be derived from these values (Walton and Bijvoet, 1975).

The higher serum phosphate levels in infants (e.g., 4.5 to 9.3 mg/dL) compared with those in adults (3.0 to 4.5 mg/dL) reflect infants' greater tubular phosphate resorption. This adaptation permits avid tubular phosphate conservation despite high ambient serum phosphate levels. For this reason, neonatal disorders of chronic hypophosphatemia and/or phosphorus depletion usually result from inadequate dietary supply (as in preterm infants) or intrinsic (e.g., familial hypophosphatemic rickets) or extrinsic (e.g., hyperparathyroidism) alterations in TmP/GFR. Similarly, chronic hyperphosphatemia usually implies either intrinsic (e.g., renal insufficiency) or extrinsic (e.g., hypoparathyroidism) abnormalities in TmP/GFR.

## THE PARATHYROID-RENAL HORMONAL AXIS

In mammals, calcium and phosphate homeostasis is controlled by a parathyroid-renal hormonal axis involving PTH and 1,25-dihydroxyvitamin D [$1,25(OH)_2D$]. The influence of these two hormones on bone deposition, mobilization of mineral, and regulation of intestinal and renal absorption is depicted in Figure 89–1. Deficiency or excess of either hormone causes hypocalcemia or hypercalcemia, respectively.

### Parathyroid Hormones

PTH is a 9500-dalton, single-chain polypeptide. PTH is synthesized by the four parathyroid glands, which are derived from the embryonic third and fourth pharyngeal pouches. The messenger RNA (mRNA) for PTH (pre-proPTH) encodes the 84 amino acids of the mature peptide, an N-terminal "pre" sequence of 25 amino acids, and a basic "pro" hexapeptide, which is clipped intracellularly. Following secretion, the intact PTH molecule [PTH (1-84)] is further metabolized and rapidly cleared from the circulation, with a half-life of less than 4 minutes. The N-terminal region of the PTH molecule [PTH(1-34)] binds the PTH receptor and shows full biologic activity, whereas the C terminus has specific, albeit poorly understood activities in osteoclasts and osteoclastic precursors.

Secretion of PTH fragments by the parathyroid glands and prolonged clearance of C-terminal PTH metabolites add considerable immunoheterogeneity to circulating PTH. The numerous inconsistencies found in reports on PTH pathophysiology until the late 1980s are due to use of earlier-generation "C-terminal" and "mid-molecule" PTH assays. In contrast, current two-site "intact PTH" assays are sufficiently sensitive and specific to detect physiologic levels of biologically active PTH(1-84) and to distinguish hypoparathyroid from euparathyroid states. The normal circulating levels of intact PTH range from approximately 10 to 60 pg/mL; the maximally stimulated

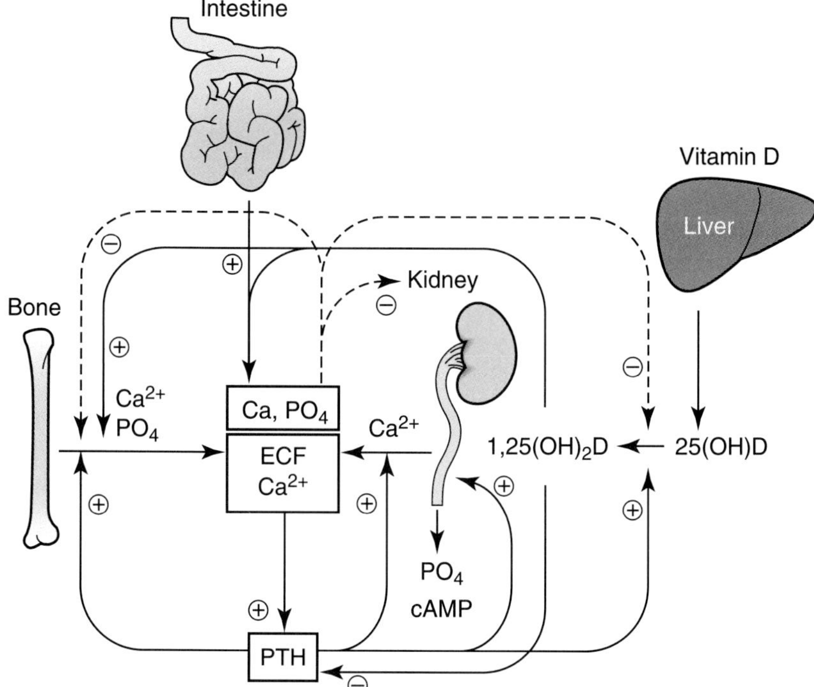


**FIGURE 89–1.** Hormonal regulation of calcium and phosphate by PTH and $1,25(OH)_2D$. Decreased $Ca^{2+}$ stimulates PTH and $1,25(OH)_2D$ secretion. Renal, gastrointestinal, and skeletal mechanisms increase $Ca^{2+}$, inhibiting PTH secretion and closing the negative feedback loop. $Ca^{2+}$, ionized calcium; cAMP, cyclic adenosine monophosphate; ECF, extracellular fluid; 25(OH)D, 25-hydroxyvitamin D; $1,25(OH)_2D$, 1,25-dihydroxyvitamin D; $PO_4$, inorganic phosphate; PTH, parathyroid hormone; *(From Brown EM, MacLeod RJ: Extracellular calcium sensing and extracellular calcium signaling. Physiol Rev 81:239, 2001.)*

(hypocalcemic) and maximally suppressed (hypercalcemic) levels for normal parathyroid function are about 100 to 150 pg/mL and 2 to 5 pg/mL, respectively.

Parathyroid cells are exquisitely responsive to changes in ambient $Ca^{2+}$. PTH secretory dynamics may be described as an inverse sigmoid hysteretic relationship between serum PTH and $Ca^{2+}$ with a parathyroid cell "set point" (the $Ca^{2+}$ at which PTH secretion is half-maximal) of 1.2 to 1.25 mmol/L. The parathyroid "calcistat" detects perturbations of blood $Ca^{2+}$ of as small as 0.025 to 0.05 mmol/L and promptly adjusts PTH secretion. The molecular mechanism that enables certain cells (e.g., parathyroid cells, thyroidal C cells, renal tubular cells, osteoblasts) to sense these minute changes in ECF $Ca^{2+}$ involves a heptahelical G protein–coupled receptor (GPCR), the $Ca^{2+}$-sensing receptor (CaR). ECF $Ca^{2+}$ (and, at lower potency, $Mg^{2+}$) binds the CaR, activates several intracellular effector pathways, and ultimately leads to oppositely directed changes in PTH secretion and altered renal cation handling (Brown and MacLeod, 2001). As described later, loss-of-function (or inactivating) mutations in the *CaR* gene are responsible for neonatal hyperparathyroidism and familial hypocalciuric hypercalcemia, whereas gain-of-function *CaR* mutations result in autosomal dominant neonatal hypocalcemia.

PTH mobilizes calcium and phosphorus from bone, stimulates calcium reabsorption, inhibits phosphorus reabsorption by reducing TmP/GFR, and stimulates the renal synthesis of $1,25(OH)_2D$, which participates with PTH in reabsorbing bone mineral and also increases efficiency of intestinal absorption of calcium and phosphorus. Therefore, PTH secretion causes the serum calcium concentration to rise and the serum phosphorus concentration to be maintained or decline.

PTH-related protein (PTHrP) is a second member of the PTH family, first identified as the cause of humoral hypercalcemia of malignancy. The amino acid sequences of PTHrP and PTH are homologous at the N terminus, and 8 of the first 13 amino acids are identical. Beyond this region, the sequences have little in common. PTHrP is a multifunctional molecule, like neuropeptides such as pro-opiomelanocortin (the precursor of corticotropin, endorphins, and melanocyte-simulating hormones). The three PTHrP isoforms (139, 141 and 173 amino acids) give rise to several secreted peptide fragments. PTHrP is widely expressed, especially in fetal tissues, and has important local functions in morphogenesis and differentiation. The normal circulating levels of PTHrP are considerably lower than the levels of PTH, and it is doubtful that PTHrP has a major role in calcium homeostasis. Two important exceptions are in the fetus and lactating woman, for whom PTHrP appears to be an important calcitropic hormone.

The principal PTH receptor (type 1 PTH/PTHrP receptor) is a GPCR belonging to a newly recognized receptor subfamily that includes receptors for calcitonin, secretin, and corticotropin-releasing hormone. This versatile PTH/PTHrP receptor mediates actions of its two physiologic ligands in multiple tissues and signals through several second messenger pathways. The best-characterized effector of PTH action is cyclic adenosine monophosphate (cAMP).

## Vitamin D

Vitamin D is a secosteroid synthesized in the skin or absorbed from the diet. Exposure to sunlight (wavelength of 290 to 320 nm) cleaves the B ring of 7-dehydrocholesterol (7-DHC), or provitamin D, the immediate precursor of cholesterol, to form a sterol, previtamin D. Previtamin D in the skin undergoes isomerization to the biologically inert vitamin D. Vitamin D enters the circulation bound to vitamin D–binding protein and is transported to the liver, where a mitochondrial cytochrome P450 vitamin D–25-hydroxylase produces 25-hydroxyvitamin D [25(OH)D]. 25(OH)D (provitamin D) is the major circulating vitamin D metabolite. Because activity of hepatic 25-hydroxylase is not tightly regulated, measurement of serum 25(OH)D is a useful assessment of vitamin D stores. In renal proximal tubule cells, mitochondrial cytochrome P450 25 (OH)D–1α-hydroxylase metabolizes 25(OH)D to the biologically active hormone, $1,25(OH)_2D$. The normal circulating level of 25(OH)D is approximately 10 to 50 ng/mL. The normal circulating concentration of $1,25(OH)_2D$ ranges from 30 to 75 pg/mL, or about 1/1000 that of 25(OH)D.

Serum 25(OH)D levels are increased by sunlight exposure and by vitamin D ingestion and are decreased in vitamin D deficiency and in hepatobiliary disorders. Circulating $1,25(OH)_2D$ levels are increased by hyperparathyroidism and phosphate depletion and are reduced in hypoparathyroidism. $1,25(OH)_2D$ is biologically inactivated through a series of reactions beginning with 24-hydroxylation. $1,25(OH)_2D$ induces the 24-hydroxylase in vitamin D target cells, whereas hypocalcemia, by increasing PTH levels, suppresses this enzyme. 24-Hydroxylase metabolizes 25(OH)D as well as $1,25(OH)_2D$. In vitamin D–sufficient states, the kidney preferentially 24-hydroxylates the prohormone, 25(OH)D, to $24,25(OH)_2D$. In contrast, when vitamin D action is required, 25(OH)D–1α-hydroxylase is preferentially activated for $1,25(OH)_2D$ synthesis.

A chief biologic function of $1,25(OH)_2D$ is to increase intestinal absorption of calcium and phosphorus. During low calcium intake, PTH levels increase and stimulate the renal conversion of 25(OH)D to $1,25(OH)_2D$, which in turn stimulates osteoclast differentiation and bone resorption. Most of the identified biologic actions of $1,25(OH)_2D$ are mediated via binding to the vitamin D receptor (VDR), a member of the intracellular receptor superfamily, and via VDR interaction with specific response elements (VDREs) in promoters of vitamin D–responsive genes.

The parathyroid-renal [PTH-$1,25(OH)_2D$] axis, reminiscent of the hypothalamic-pituitary-adrenal axis, is the principal means for systemic response to a prolonged or major hypocalcemic challenge. In this long-loop feedback system, $1,25(OH)_2D$-mediated calcium absorption provides the ultimate feedback on PTH secretion. PTH secreted in response to hypocalcemia is the principal regulator of renal production of $1,25(OH)_2D$ that, in turn, feeds back to suppress PTH gene expression (see Fig. 89–1). Maximal adjustments of intestinal calcium absorption via the PTH-$1,25(OH)_2D$ axis require 1 to 2 days to become fully operative, so $1,25(OH)_2D$ effects come into play only when a hypocalcemic stress persists. In contrast, PTH regulates the minute-to-minute perturbations of ECF [$Ca^{2+}$].

### Calcitonin

Calcitonin, a peptide hormone synthesized by thyroid parafollicular C cells, has an antihypercalcemic effect, that is, an effect opposite that of the actions of PTH. Human calcitonin is a 32-amino-acid chain with a 1,7-disulfide bridge and a C-terminal prolinamide. Alternative splicing of several transcripts from the single calcitonin gene produces several polypeptide products. These peptides have uncertain calcitropic importance. The primary stimulus for calcitonin secretion is a rise in circulating calcium concentration. Calcitonin lowers serum calcium and phosphorus chiefly by inhibiting bone resorption.

Currently, there is no compelling evidence that the calcitonin-like calcium-lowering hormones are critical regulators of calcium homeostasis in nonpregnant adult humans, perhaps because the low prevailing rates of bone turnover blunt the impact of the antiresorptive actions. However, calcitonin may have important calcitropic functions in pregnant and lactating women and in the fetus and neonate, and in other mammals, particularly rodents, whose bones are constantly growing. In human newborns, the C cell population and serum calcitonin concentrations are much greater than in adults.

## PERINATAL MINERAL METABOLISM

During human pregnancy, approximately 30 g of calcium and more than 16 g of phosphorus are transferred transplacentally from the maternal circulation to the growing fetus, the bulk during the third trimester when fetal calcium accretion is approximately 140 to 150 mg/kg per day. A mid-molecule PTHrP hormone (Kovacs et al, 1996) that is expressed principally by placenta regulates this transplacental calcium pump. In humans, a doubling of maternal intestinal calcium absorption and a net increase of calcium accretion into bone compensate for the formidable demand on maternal calcium.

### Pregnancy

Pregnancy constitutes a unique hormonal milieu that promotes a state of "physiologic absorptive hypercalciuria" (Gertner et al, 1986). Maternal total serum calcium declines slightly during pregnancy, reaches a nadir in the mid-third trimester, and then increases slightly toward term. The maternal serum phosphorus and magnesium profiles are similar to that of calcium. Maternal serum 25(OH)D varies with the season and with vitamin D intake, but the vitamin D transport protein (DBP) increases during pregnancy. Serum $1,25(OH)_2D$ concentrations increase early in pregnancy and continue to rise through gestation (Seely et al, 1997). The calculated concentration of free $1,25(OH)_2D$ also rises. For many years, it was believed that PTH levels also increased steadily through pregnancy. However, use of newer immunometric "sandwich" assays indicates that PTH actually declines during the course of pregnancy (Davis et al, 1988; Saggese et al, 1991; Seely et al, 1997). PTHrP levels, in contrast, may be higher in pregnant than in nonpregnant women (Bertelloni et al, 1994). The role of circulating calcitonin in pregnancy is uncertain.

$1,25(OH)_2D$ drives the maternal enhanced intestinal mineral absorption. Following parturition, $1,25(OH)_2D$ concentrations and calcium absorption rates (Kent et al, 1991) fall to prepregnancy levels. The interplay of calcitropic and progestational hormones in pregnancy protects the maternal skeleton from demineralization. In contrast, during the relatively low estrogen state of lactation, calcium is mobilized from bone stores, possibly under the influence of PTHrP (Dobnig et al, 1995).

In the third trimester, total and ionized calcium and phosphorus levels in fetal plasma are higher than maternal levels, and there is a state of "physiologic fetal hypercalcemia" (Rubin et al, 1991). Fetal plasma PTH is low, and calcitonin and PTHrP levels are relatively high. Even these low circulating PTH levels may be functionally important in fetal calcium and magnesium metabolism (Kovacs et al, 2001). There also is a close correlation between maternal and fetal serum 25(OH)D levels, consistent with transplacental transfer of this metabolite. Low levels may be found in infants born to women with low circulating 25(OH)D resulting from poor dietary intake of vitamin D and lack of sunlight exposure. Fetal plasma $1,25(OH)_2D$ also is relatively low, despite robust renal 25(OH)D–1α-hydroxylase activity, whereas concentrations of $24,25(OH)_2D$ are high. In fact, the major function of the fetal kidneys in calcium homeostasis may be production of $1,25(OH)_2D$, rather than renal tubular regulation of calcium excretion. The high circulating concentrations of calcitonin may support this stimulated fetal 25(OH)D–1α-hydroxylase activity. In contrast, the relatively low circulating fetal $1,25(OH)_2D$ concentrations are a consequence of enhanced placental clearance (Ross et al, 1989). Constitutively activated placental 24-hydroxylase activity (Rubin et al, 1993) also preferentially hydroxylates maternally derived 25(OH)D to $24,25(OH)_2D$. This placental capacity to metabolize 25(OH)D and $1,25(OH)_2D$ probably accounts for the enhanced clearance of fetal $1,25(OH)_2D$, limits access of placentally synthesized $1,25(OH)_2D$ to the fetal and maternal circulations, and, in effect, partitions the maternal and fetal vitamin D pools.

### The Neonate

Placental transfer of calcium ceases abruptly at birth. In healthy term newborns, total calcium concentration and $[Ca^{2+}]$ decline from nearly 11 mg/dL and 6 mg/dL, respectively, in umbilical cord blood to serum levels of 8 to 9 mg/dL and 5 mg/dL by 24 to 48 hours. The nadir of $[Ca^{2+}]$ may range from 4.4 to 5.4 mg/dL. Concomitant rises in PTH and $1,25(OH)_2D$ stabilize serum calcium as the newborn adapts to extrauterine mineral homeostasis and dietary calcium intake. In preterm infants, calcium absorption from the intestine is nonsaturable and may be vitamin D independent (Bronner et al, 1992). Serum calcitonin levels increase sharply during the first day and remain elevated compared with those in adults. In the mother, prolactin helps stimulate PTHrP expression in lactating breast tissue. PTHrP is secreted into milk at concentrations 10,000-fold higher than its serum concentration. It is likely that the abundant milk PTHrP content ingested by the neonate also is important for mineral regulation. By 2 weeks of life, serum calcium rises to the mean values observed in older children and adults.

During the first week of life, urinary phosphate excretion is significantly higher in preterm than in term infants but then approximates that of term infants, possibly owing to accelerated postnatal renal maturation. Calcium excretion is low during the first week, when the newborn must compensate for the postpartum fall in serum calcium. After the first several days, calcium excretion increases with a magnitude inversely proportional to gestation. The high urinary calcium-to-creatinine ratio (UCa/Cr) of young infants then steadily declines with age (Sargent et al, 1993). However, in preterm breast-fed infants who are more than 2 weeks old, the UCa/Cr can exceed 2.0 (Karlen et al, 1985). These changes may reflect the relative phosphate deficiency in many preterm infants, which results in an adaptively low urinary phosphate excretion, decreased bone mineralization, and, consequently, relatively high urinary calcium excretion.

## CALCIUM METABOLISM IN THE NEWBORN

### Neonatal Hypocalcemia

*Neonatal hypocalcemia* has been variously defined as a serum calcium level of less than 8 mg/dL, less than 7.5 mg/dL, or less than 7.0 mg/dL and as a $Ca^{2+}$ level of less than 4.0 mg/dL. Under conditions of normal acid-base status and normal serum albumin, serum total calcium and $Ca^{2+}$ levels are linearly correlated, so total serum calcium measurements remain useful as a screening test. However, because $Ca^{2+}$ is the physiologically relevant fraction, in sick infants it may be preferable to assay $[Ca^{2+}]$ directly in freshly obtained blood samples. A precise definition of hypocalcemia, like hypoglycemia, in preterm infants is particularly difficult to formulate. Preterm hypocalcemia is probably best defined with reference to $[Ca^{2+}]$.

A useful approach to the classification of neonatal hypocalcemia is by time of onset. "Early"- and "late"-occurring hypocalcemia (Table 89–1) have different causes, usually occur in different clinical settings, and should prompt different approaches to evaluation and management.

#### Clinical Findings

Because $Ca^{2+}$ couples excitation and contraction in skeletal and cardiac muscle, increased neuromuscular excitability (tetany) is a cardinal feature of hypocalcemia. However, hypocalcemic signs in neonates are variable and may not correlate with the magnitude of the decline in $[Ca^{2+}]$. Although some infants are severely affected, others having equally depressed serum calcium levels may be asymptomatic.

Tetanic infants are jittery and hyperactive and frequently exhibit muscle jerking and twitching. Generalized or focal clonic seizures may occur at any time during the calcium derangement. Hyperacusis may be detected as an exaggerated response to environmental noises (e.g., a "spontaneous" Moro reflex). Occasionally, respiratory or gastrointestinal signs, rather than neurologic findings, predominate. Laryngospasm with inspiratory stridor, sometimes severe enough to cause cyanosis or anoxia, or wheezing due to bronchospasm may be a presenting manifestation. Vomiting, possibly related to pylorospasm, sometimes causes hematemesis or melena. At times, the gastrointestinal signs are severe enough to mimic those of intestinal obstruction. Other signs of neonatal tetany include extensor hypertonia, apnea, tachycardia, tachypnea, and edema. Carpopedal spasm and Chvostek sign are not as reliably elicited in hypocalcemic newborns as in older children or adults.

### Early Neonatal Hypocalcemia

Hypocalcemia occurring during the first 3 days of life, usually between 24 and 48 hours postpartum, is termed *early neonatal hypocalcemia*. It is a pathologic exaggeration of the normal decline in circulating calcium. Early neonatal hypocalcemia is characteristically seen in any of four circumstances: prematurity, severe stress or asphyxia, maternal diabetes, and significant intrauterine growth restriction (IUGR). Typically, in preterm infants, there is a steeper and more rapid postnatal decline in serum calcium than in term newborns; the magnitude of the depression is inversely proportional to gestational age. Untreated, many low-birth-weight (LBW) infants and essentially all extremely low-birth-weight (ELBW) infants exhibit total calcium levels of less than 7.0 mg/dL by day 2. However, the fall in $[Ca^{2+}]$ is not proportional to the fall in total calcium concentration, and the ratio of ionized to total calcium in these newborns is higher. This "sparing" of $Ca^{2+}$ may be related to the lower serum protein concentration and pH in prematurity. The sparing effect on $[Ca^{2+}]$ also, in part, explains the frequent absence of hypocalcemic signs in preterm infants.

The neonatal parathyroid glands, regardless of degree of prematurity, can mount an appropriate PTH response to hypocalcemia. In fact, hypocalcemia in extremely preterm newborns (Rubin et al, 1991) or infants undergoing cardiac bypass (Robertie et al, 1992) stimulates increases in serum PTH at least as great as those seen in adults during citrate-induced hypocalcemia (Grant et al, 1990). Resistance to PTH action plays an uncertain role in early neonatal hypocalcemia. A several day delay in the phosphaturic and renal cAMP responses to PTH has inconsistently been reported, suggesting that there might be a maturational delay in renal responses to PTH. High renal sodium excretion in preterm infants also probably aggravates calciuric losses. In addition, the preterm infant's exaggerated rise in calcitonin may promote hypocalcemia. Currently, there is no convincing evidence that abnormalities in vitamin D metabolism are involved in the etiopathogenesis of hypocalcemia in preterm infants. Like fetuses, even ELBW newborns efficiently synthesize 1,25$(OH)_2$D when vitamin D stores are adequate.

Early neonatal hypocalcemia with hyperphosphatemia is frequently observed in severely stressed or asphyxiated infants. The causes are probably multifactorial and may include, to varying degrees, renal insufficiency, tissue catabolism, and acidosis. There is an exaggerated serum calcitonin response and elevated PTH levels. Low serum $Ca^{2+}$ and elevated serum magnesium levels have been correlated with severity of hypoxic-ischemic encephalopathy and poor outcome (Ilves et al, 2000).

Infants of diabetic mothers (IDMs) show an exaggerated postnatal drop in circulating calcium levels compared to

**TABLE 89–1**

**Causes of Neonatal Hypocalcemia**

| | |
|---|---|
| Early-onset hypocalcemia (<48 hr of age) | Abnormal vitamin D [1,25(OH)$_2$D] production or action ("hypocalcemic rickets") |
| Prematurity | Vitamin D deficiency (secondary to maternal vitamin D deficiency) |
| Perinatal distress/asphyxia | Acquired or inherited disorders of vitamin D metabolism |
| Infants of diabetic mothers | Resistance to the actions of vitamin D |
| Intrauterine growth restriction | Hyperphosphatemia |
| Late-onset hypocalcemia (1st week of life) | Excessive dietary phosphate |
| High phosphate load ± hypoparathyroidism or vitamin D deficiency | Phosphate-containing enemas |
| Neonatal hypoparathyroid syndromes | Rhabdomyolysis-induced acute renal failure |
| Parathyroid agenesis | Hyperphosphatemic renal insufficiency |
| DiGeorge syndrome (22q11.2 deletions) | "Hungry bones syndrome" (mineralization outpacing osteoclastic bone resorption) |
| Familial isolated hypoparathyroidism | Other causes |
| PTH gene mutations | Metabolic or respiratory alkalosis |
| Autosomal dominant hypocalcalcemic hypocalciuria (ADHH) | Phototherapy |
| Activating mutations of the $Ca^{2+}$-sensing receptor | Long chain 3-hydroxyacyl-CoA dehydrogenase deficiency (LCHAD) |
| Neonatal hypoparathyroidism secondary to maternal hyperparathyroidism | Pancreatitis |
| Autoimmune–candidiasis–ectodermal dystrophy (APECED or APS1) | Sepsis, septic shock |
| Hypoparathyroidism associated with skeletal dysplasias | Rotavirus gastroenteritis |
| Kenny-Caffey syndrome | Osteopetrosis and other skeletal dysplasias |
| Sanjad-Sakati (hypoparathyroidism-retardation-dysmorphism [HRD]) syndrome | Pseudohypocalcemia (hypoalbuminemia) |
| Osteogenesis imperfecta type II | Medications |
| PTH resistance (transient neonatal pseudohypoparathyroidism) | Bicarbonate |
| Hypomagnesemia ± distal renal tubular acidosis | Rapid transfusion or plasmapheresis with citrated blood |
| Primary hypomagnesemia | Furosemide-induced |
| Renal tubular acidosis type 1 | Lipid infusions |

CoA, coenzyme A; 1,25(OH)$_2$D, 1,25-dihydroxyvitamin D.

gestational age controls. The course usually is similar to that of early neonatal hypocalcemia in preterm infants, although hypocalcemia sometimes persists for several additional days. Maternal and neonatal hypomagnesemia (Mimouni et al, 1986) and low fetal PTH/PTHrP biologic activity (Rubin et al, 1991) may be causative factors. The greater bone mass and relative undermineralization typical of macrosomic IDMs also may increase the neonatal demand for calcium, producing a more profound and prolonged decline in postnatal serum calcium levels. Similar mechanisms may come into play in the transient hypocalcemia often observed in small-for-gestational-age (SGA) infants. Hypercalcitonemia, hypoparathyroidism, abnormalities in vitamin D metabolism, and hyperphosphatemia all have been implicated, but none has been consistently found.

Historically, symptomatic neonatal hypocalcemia in IDMs has been associated with the severity of maternal diabetes (e.g., White classification) and inadequate glycemic control. Not surprisingly, preterm IDMs who have sustained IUGR and asphyxia as a result of uteroplacental insufficiency invariably become quite hypocalcemic. In recent years, improved metabolic control for pregnant diabetic women has markedly diminished the occurrence and severity of early neonatal hypocalcemia in IDMs (Demarini et al, 1994). Healthy IDMs who are able to begin milk feedings on the first day do not require serum calcium monitoring unless suspicious signs (e.g., jitteriness, stridor) are noted.

### Late Neonatal Hypocalcemia

Late neonatal hypocalcemia, or hypocalcemia developing after 3 to 5 days of life, occurs more frequently in term than in preterm newborns and is not correlated with maternal diabetes, birth trauma, or asphyxia. Historically associated with cow milk or cow milk formula feedings, it also occasionally occurs in breast-fed infants. The entity of "late infantile tetany" seen in infants fed whole cow's milk has become a rarity with adjustment of phosphorus content in humanized cow milk and soy infant formulas.

The hyperphosphatemia that is a prominent feature of late neonatal hypocalcemia may result from varying combinations of dietary phosphate load, immature renal tubular phosphate excretion, transiently low levels of circulating PTH, hypomagnesemia, and marginal maternal vitamin D intake. A relatively high dietary phosphate load coupled with a low GFR leads to an increase in serum phosphate levels and a reciprocal decline in serum calcium levels. The normal response to hypocalcemia is an increase in PTH secretion, leading to increased urinary phosphate excretion and tubular calcium resorption. It is relevant, therefore, that low circulating PTH levels have sometimes been observed in infants with late neonatal hypocalcemia. Serum calcium levels frequently increase when these infants are placed on a low-phosphate formula and calcium supplements. After several days to weeks, serum PTH usually increases, and the infants then can tolerate more dietary phosphate. The pathogenesis of this "transient hypoparathyroidism" in late neonatal hypocalcemia is not readily apparent. Some of these infants show a persistent or recurrent inability to mount an adequate PTH response to a hypocalcemic challenge, indicating partial hypoparathyroidism (see later).

In other infants, maternal vitamin D deficiency can cause late (or occasionally an "early") neonatal hypocalcemia. This possibility is investigated by assaying maternal and neonatal serum 25(OH)D levels. A role for maternal vitamin D deficiency also is implicated by the increased incidence of late neonatal hypocalcemia in winter. The high prevalence of enamel hypoplasia of incisor teeth reported in affected infants indicates a defect in mineralization during the third trimester of pregnancy.

Hypocalcemia and hyperphosphatemia after the first 2 to 3 days always should prompt a thorough investigation for underlying cause(s) (see Table 89–1). Hypocalcemia in this setting usually implies primary or secondary dysregulation of the parathyroid-renal [PTH-1,25$(OH)_2$D] axis, hypomagnesemia, or renal insufficiency. The primary hormonal and end-organ disturbances that cause neonatal hypoglycemic syndromes are described in a later section. As a cautionary note, earlier observations of generally favorable neurologic outcomes in newborns with hypocalcemic or hypomagnesemic seizures (which may have been related to a nutritional metabolic disturbance) may be less relevant to the current neonatal population, in which hypocalcemia or hypomagnesemia due to dietary phosphate overload seldom is observed. In this group, neurologic prognosis may be more closely related to the causative disorder (Lynch and Rust, 1994).

## Hypocalcemia Caused by Hypoparathyroid Syndromes

Improved clinical assays have increased recognition of PTH deficiency manifesting during the first weeks of life. Cytogenetic and molecular genetic diagnosis also permits characterization of several types of congenital hypoparathyroidism. The biochemical hallmarks of hypoparathyroidism are hypocalcemia and hyperphosphatemia in the presence of normal renal function. Serum PTH concentrations are inappropriately low or undetectable.

Isolated hypoparathyroidism is usually sporadic but may show X-linked, autosomal recessive or autosomal dominant inheritance. Congenital hypoparathyroidism may be part of the DiGeorge syndrome (DGS), which comprises hypoparathyroid hypocalcemia, thymic hypoplasia with T-cell incompetence, conotruncal cardiac defects, and dysmorphic facies. The DGS phenotype results from defects in cervical neural crest cell migration into the derivatives of the third and fourth pharyngeal (branchial) pouches. More than 90% of persons with a clinical diagnosis of DGS have deletions (monosomy or partial monosomy) of chromosome region 22q11.2 detectable by fluorescence in situ hybridization (FISH) using 22q11 probes or by high-resolution G band karyotyping. Recent studies suggest that haploinsufficiency of the *UFD1* gene within the 22q11.2 region results in the DGS phenotype (Yamagishi et al, 1999). However, the rare identification of other cytogenetic abnormalities suggests that several distinct molecular defects can lead to disturbed cranial neural crest cell migration.

DGS is sporadic in about 90% of cases. In many familial clusters the variable phenotype behaves as an autosomal dominant trait. In familial transmission, there appears to be a strong tendency for 22q11.2 deletions to be maternal in origin (Demczuk et al, 1996). In members of the same family, the 22q11 deletion may be associated with different phenotypic features, depending on whether endocrinologic, cardiac, craniofacial, or palatal abnormalities are the focus of attention. The clinical spectrum in DGS encompasses features previously categorized as Shprintzen (velocardiofacial) syndrome, conotruncal anomaly face (Takao) syndrome, and isolated cardiac outflow tract defects. Even transient congenital hypoparathyroidism in the absence of a DGS phenotype can be associated with a 22q11 deletion, so these infants should be evaluated and monitored for recurrence of hypocalcemia. The incidence of DGS may be at least 1 case per 5000 live births (Ryan et al, 1997).

DGS often manifests in the first week of life with hypocalcemic tetany or seizures. Craniofacial features include microretrognathia, submucous cleft palate, low-set and abnormal pinnae, telecanthus with short palpebral fissures, short philtrum, and a relatively small mouth. The presence of cardiac outflow tract or aortic arch abnormalities (especially pulmonary atresia/tetralogy of Fallot, type B interrupted aortic arch, truncus arteriosus, anomalies of aortic arch laterality, or abnormal branching of the brachiocephalic vessels), even in the absence of other DGS features, should prompt investigation with a standard karyotype to exclude major rearrangements and with FISH using DGS probes to detect microdeletions. Parents of an infant with DGS should be screened for carrier status. These infants require close anticipatory monitoring for the onset of hypocalcemia. Absence of a thymic shadow on chest radiograph is not a reliable indicator. A variety of T-cell and B-cell disorders is relatively common in DGS but severe T-cell immunodeficiency is rare. Nevertheless, because of the potential for inducing graft-versus-host disease, until T-cell immunocompetence has been demonstrated, irradiated red blood cell transfusions may be preferred.

A normal serum PTH obtained when an infant is relatively normocalcemic also does not exclude the diagnosis of DGS. Infants with DGS may show resolution of hypoparathyroidism by early childhood, although PTH reserves may remain inadequate for defense against hypocalcemic stresses.

Hypoparathyroidism is a prominent feature of several rare skeletal dysplasias. Kenny-Caffey syndrome is an autosomal recessive (sometimes dominant) skeletal dysplasia featuring transient neonatal hypoparathyroidism and dwarfism, macrocephaly, delayed fontanel closure, dysmorphic facies, and cortical thickening of tubular bones (Fanconi et al, 1992). In Sanjad-Sakati syndrome (Sanjad et al, 1991), or hypoparathyroidism-retardation-dysmorphism (HRD) syndrome, hypoparathyroidism is associated with IUGR and poor postnatal growth, characteristic facies (deep-set eyes, depressed nasal bridge, beaked nose, long philtrum, thin upper lip, micrognathia, large and floppy earlobes), small hands and feet, skeletal defects, and developmental delay. This autosomal recessive disorder has been described in persons of Gulf Arab and Bedouin ancestry. The gene for Sanjad-Sakati syndrome (*hrd* locus) maps to chromosome 1q42-q43, which also is the autosomal recessive Kenny-Caffey locus, suggesting that these are allelic disorders (Diaz et al, 1999).

Although osteogenesis imperfecta (OI) type II usually is perinatally lethal, some infants have prolonged survival. Knisely and colleagues (1988) showed that acute parathyroid hemorrhage ("parathyroid apoplexy") is a common event in OI II and may contribute to early death. Autoimmune–candidiasis–ectodermal dystrophy (APECED), also known as autoimmune polyglandular syndrome type I (APS 1), is a rare autosomal recessive disorder characterized by hypoparathyroidism, adrenal insufficiency, and chronic mucocutaneous candidiasis. In afflicted persons, the development of chronic active hepatitis, malabsorption, juvenile-onset pernicious anemia, alopecia, and primary hypogonadism is frequent. APECED results from inheritance of mutations in an autoimmune regulator gene (*AIRE*). When APECED is diagnosed in early infancy, which is rare, hypocalcemia (with or without candidiasis) typically is the presenting sign.

A major breakthrough in the last decade has been the association of several forms of autosomal dominant and autosomal recessive congenital hypoparathyroidism, with allelic variants of the *preproPTH* and calcium-sensing receptor (*CaR*) genes. Affected infants have subnormal or undetectable serum PTH levels but do not have congenital anomalies or developmental field defects, DGS locus deletions, candidiasis or autoimmune polyglandular failure, or antiendocrine antibodies. Autosomal dominant and autosomal recessive forms of familial isolated hypoparathyroidism have been related to mutations in the *preproPTH* gene (Sunthornthevarakul et al, 1999). Activating *CaR* gene mutations cause autosomal dominant hypocalcemic hypocalciuria (ADHH) or "CaR hyperfunction." The parathyroid and renal calcistat is reset downward, so that hypocalcemia does not elicit normal compensatory PTH secretion or renal calcium reabsorption. Because de novo *CaR* mutations producing CaR hyperfunction may account for many cases of so-called sporadic idiopathic hypoparathyroidism (D'Souza-Li et al, 2002; Lienhardt et al, 2001), mutational analysis of the *CaR* gene should be considered in the work-up of isolated hypoparathyroidism in infants, especially when hypocalcemia manifests with inappropriately normal urinary calcium excretion (relative hypercalciuria). In fact, hypercalciuria and nephrocalcinosis can develop even when serum calcium remains below the normal range. Therefore, these patients require close monitoring of urinary calcium excretion for adjusting therapy with $1,25(OH)_2D$ analogues (Lienhardt et al, 2001).

Resistance to PTH comes in three forms. Deletion of the PTH/PTHrP receptor is embryologically or perinatally lethal. Loss of one allele for *GNAS1*, which encodes $G_s\alpha$, the G protein $\alpha$ subunit required for receptor-stimulated cAMP generation, produces pseudohypoparathyroidism type 1a (PHP1a). PHP1a is characterized by PTH-resistant (pseudo)hypoparathyroidism and characteristic somatic features (short stature, brachydactyly, and subcutaneous ossification), which collectively are known as Albright hereditary osteodystrophy. Isolated PTH resistance in the absence of this somatic phenotype is called pseudohypoparathyroidism type 1b (PHP1b). This disorder was recently shown to be an imprinting defect in which both *GNAS1* alleles have an unmethylated (paternal) pattern (Liu et al, 2000). Although persons eventually diagnosed with a PTH resistance syndrome usually do not show hypocalcemia during the first month of life, transient neonatal pseudohypoparathyroidism has occasionally been reported (Minagawa et al, 1995). Neonatal PTH resistance, which has an unknown frequency, manifests as hypocalcemic seizures with hyperphosphatemia and an elevated PTH. Molecular characterizations have not been performed.

### Neonatal Hypocalcemia Associated with Maternal Hyperparathyroidism

Hypocalcemia is commonly observed in newborns of hyperparathyroid mothers. These infants frequently show increased neuromuscular irritability during the first 3 weeks of life but occasionally may do so much later as limited PTH reserve and latent hypoparathyroidism emerge under stress or with time (Cuneo et al, 1996). The serum calcium levels usually range from 5.0 to 7.5 mg/dL, and the serum phosphate levels are often greater than 8.0 mg/dL. Hypocalcemic signs may be exacerbated by high-phosphate diets. In some instances, the signs of hypocalcemia can be quite severe and resistant to therapy. Calcium supplementation, which in some instances must be continued for several weeks, produces eventual improvement.

In maternal hyperparathyroidism, the increased maternal serum calcium facilitates transplacental calcium transport, producing fetal hypercalcemia greater than the moderate elevations of serum calcium normally observed in the third trimester. As a result, fetal PTH secretion is suppressed more than it is in normal pregnancy. The suppressed parathyroids are unable to maintain normal serum calcium levels post partum. The reason for the hypomagnesemia observed in some infants born to hyperparathyroid mothers is uncertain, but this derangement may be due to (1) maternal magnesium depletion as a complication of hyperparathyroidism; (2) transient neonatal hypoparathyroidism; or (3) hyperphosphatemia, which may result from transient hypoparathyroidism or high dietary phosphate intake, or both.

Maternal serum calcium and phosphorus should be assayed whenever this diagnosis is suspected. Hypocalcemic tetany occurring in the infant may lead to diagnosis of hyperparathyroidism in an asymptomatic mother. Maternal serum calcium values in the upper normal range can be falsely reassuring if the samples were obtained during pregnancy, a time when serum calcium levels normally decline.

## Neonatal Hypocalcemia Associated with Hypomagnesemia or Renal Tubular Acidosis

Hypomagnesemia causes hypocalcemia by interfering with the parathyroid cell CaR-mediated release of PTH and blunting end-organ PTH response. Depression of serum magnesium levels in newborns may be chronic, sometimes as primary hypomagnesemia with secondary hypocalcemia, or transient.

Hypomagnesemia with secondary hypocalcemia (HSH) can manifest within the first weeks of life with persistent hypocalcemia, tetany, and seizures uncontrollable by anticonvulsants or calcium gluconate. Delay in establishing the diagnosis may lead to permanent neurologic impairment. This rare autosomal recessive disorder results from defective intestinal magnesium absorption and renal magnesium leak. HSH is caused by mutations in the gene encoding TRPM6, a member of the transient receptor potential (TRP) channel family that is expressed in intestinal epithelia and renal tubules (Schlingmann et al, 2002; Walder et al, 2002). In contrast, in the intestinal defect of primary familial hypomagnesemia, serum magnesium is low despite a normal renal fractional excretion of magnesium (<5%) (Shalev et al, 1998).

Several forms of primary renal hypomagnesemia have been described, including autosomal recessive familial hypomagnesemia with hypercalciuria and nephrocalcinosis caused by mutations in the claudin-like paracellin-1 gene (*PCLN1, CLDN16*) (Simon et al, 1999) and a genetically heterogeneous autosomal dominant "isolated renal magnesium wasting" (Kantorovich et al, 2002). The clinical spectrum includes polyuria, hyposthenuria, moderate metabolic acidosis with an inappropriately high urine pH and a positive urine anion gap, low citrate excretion, renal magnesium and calcium wasting, secondary renal potassium wasting, nephrocalcinosis, muscle weakness, persistent tetany, seizures, and sometimes abnormal facies and sensorineural hearing loss. The partial distal acidification defect, which is probably secondary to a medullary interstitial nephropathy, can be functionally distinguished from primary distal renal tubular acidosis (RTA1) (Rodriguez-Soriano and Vallo, 1994). In primary hypomagnesemia, the serum magnesium is frequently less than 0.8 mg/dL (normal 1.6 to 2.8 mg/dL), and the magnesium deficiency leads to parathyroid failure and peripheral PTH resistance, despite hypocalcemia. High-dose enteral magnesium leads to spontaneous parallel increases in serum PTH and calcium levels and renal phosphate clearance. Renal transplantation normalizes serum magnesium and urinary calcium.

A transient hypomagnesemia in newborns often occurs in association with hypocalcemia. Less commonly, the serum calcium level may be normal. In transient hypomagnesemia, the decrease in serum magnesium level typically is less severe (0.8 to 1.4 mg/dL) than in magnesium transport defects. In many infants with transient hypomagnesemia, the serum magnesium level increases spontaneously as the serum calcium level returns to normal following the administration of calcium supplements. However, in other cases, the hypocalcemia responds poorly to calcium therapy, but when magnesium salts are given, both serum calcium and magnesium levels rise.

Secondary hypomagnesemia from renal magnesium wasting can be caused by administration of loop diuretics, aminoglycosides, or amphotericin B or by urinary tract obstruction, or may occur in the diuretic phase of acute renal failure. The disorder also may be mistaken for neonatal hypoparathyroidism because of the tetany and hypocalcemia, or as Bartter syndrome (hypokalemic alkalosis with hypercalciuria) because of secondary potassium wasting. The clinician's index of suspicion should be raised whenever hypomagnesemia occurs in one of these situations. Finding low serum magnesium levels with inappropriately high urinary magnesium excretion confirms the diagnosis of renal magnesium wasting. A common laboratory feature of magnesium depletion, regardless of cause, is hypokalemia. Attempts to replete the potassium deficit with potassium therapy alone usually is not successful without concurrent magnesium therapy.

The distal type of renal tubular acidosis, RTA1, is characterized by hypocalcemia, hypercalciuria, varying degrees of hypomagnesemia, hyperchloremia, low serum bicarbonate, and a fixed urinary specific gravity and urinary pH (about 5.0). The mineral excretion defect leads to nephrocalcinosis and metabolic bone disease. RTA1 sometimes manifests during early infancy, when the hypocalcemia may precede the RTA. Lewis (1992) proposed that Tiny Tim in Dickens' *A Christmas Carol* had RTA1, which would account for Tim's growth failure, osteomalacia, fractures, and neuromuscular weakness.

## Hypocalcemia Resulting from Vitamin D Disorders

In older children and adults, hypocalcemia rarely occurs as an isolated finding that results from disorders of vitamin D intake or metabolism. Most persons with abnormalities in either the production or the action of $1,25(OH)_2D$ present with rickets or osteomalacia. In contrast, young infants may exhibit hypocalcemic tetany before rachitic features become very conspicuous. Abnormalities in vitamin D metabolism can be divided into three broad categories: vitamin D deficiency, acquired or inherited disorders of vitamin D metabolism, and resistance to the actions of vitamin D.

Maternal vitamin D deficiency is the major risk factor for neonatal vitamin D deficiency presenting as hypocalcemia. Maternal vitamin D deficiency has become unusual in countries where vitamin D supplementation of dairy products and other foods is common. It does occur, however, when both sunlight exposure and dietary intake of vitamin D are inadequate. Female immigrants from the Middle East or South Asia who continue to wear traditional dress *and* have inadequate dietary vitamin D intake are particularly at high risk (Shaw and Pal, 2002), especially during pregnancy. Breast-fed infants of lactovegetarian mothers also are susceptible to early-onset hypocalcemic rickets. Nutritional rickets in newborns can be prevented by daily supplementation of 400 IU for infants and 400 IU daily for mothers during pregnancy and lactation or 1000 IU daily if begun in the third trimester.

Intestinal absorption of fat-soluble vitamin D requires a functioning exocrine pancreas, biliary tract, and bowel mucosa. Consequently, pregnant women with malabsorption syndromes may be vitamin D deficient. Anticonvulsant therapy (e.g., with phenobarbital or diphenylhydantoin) during pregnancy, which increases hepatic catabolism of 25(OH)D, also can induce maternal and fetal vitamin D deficiency. Pregnant women who take anticonvulsants should receive vitamin D supplementation (800 to 1000 IU/day).

## Phosphate-Induced Hypocalcemia

Hypocalcemia is the systemic response to hyperphosphatemia. Conditions conducive to phosphate-induced neonatal hypocalcemia are excessive dietary phosphate, rhabdomyolysis-induced acute renal failure, and hyperphosphatemic renal insufficiency. Phosphate-containing enemas can produce significant phosphate absorption. Their use is hazardous and contraindicated for infants.

## Other Causes of Neonatal Hypocalcemia

It is important to recognize that hypocalcemia may be precipitated whenever skeletal mineralization significantly outpaces the rate of osteoclastic bone resorption. Examples of this type of hypocalcemia occur with overzealous vitamin D replacement in infants with rickets or hypoparathyroidism. Pancreatitis can cause hypocalcemia and tetany through the action of pancreatic lipase on retroperitoneal and omental fat to release free fatty acids (FFAs). FFAs avidly chelate calcium and remove it from the ECF. Pancreatitis also may release pancreatic calcium-lowering factors (Tomomura et al, 1995). Sepsis and septic shock cause hypocalcemia by unknown mechanisms. Neonatal or infantile hypocalcemia and hypocalcemic seizures may accompany long-chain 3-hydroxyacyl-coenzyme A (CoA) dehydrogenase deficiency (LCHAD) (Ibdah et al, 1999) and severe cases of rotavirus gastroenteritis (Foldenauer et al, 1998). Hypocalcemic jitteriness or seizures can be the presenting sign of infantile osteopetrosis (Srinivasan et al, 2000). Prompt recognition permits early evaluation for bone marrow or hematopoietic stem cell transplantation. Certain other skeletal dysplasia syndromes are associated with neonatal hypocalcemia, which may be severe.

Several common therapeutic interventions can induce hypocalcemia. Bicarbonate therapy, as well as any form of metabolic or respiratory alkalinization, decreases both ionized calcium levels and bone resorption of calcium. Blood transfusion or plasmapheresis can promote calcium complexes with the infused citrate, decreasing $Ca^{2+}$. Hypocalcemia after initiation of ECMO is related to composition of the circuit-priming solution and to acute citrate loading and may lead to hemodynamic instability (Meliones et al, 1995). Furosemide therapy promotes calciuresis and nephrolithiasis. Phototherapy for hyperbilirubinemia may be associated with mild hypocalcemia. This effect has been attributed to decreased melatonin secretion, which potentiates glucocorticoid actions on bone metabolism. Lipid infusions may elevate serum FFAs, which form insoluble complexes with calcium. Most of these effects are transient, and cessation of therapy is followed by a return to normal serum calcium levels. The major exception is aggressive furosemide therapy, which when prolonged may lead to bone demineralization and renal dysfunction (Downing et al, 1992).

### Treatment

The decision to treat hypocalcemia in an infant depends on the severity of the hypocalcemia and the presence of clinical signs and symptoms. The morbidity associated with calcium treatment must be weighed against the potential benefits. Hypocalcemic preterm infants who have no symptoms and are not ill from any other cause probably do not need specific treatment. Early neonatal hypocalcemia should resolve by day 3. Some clinicians begin treatment in preterm newborns once serum calcium levels have dropped to 6.0 to 6.5 mg/dL or after $[Ca^{2+}]$ has decreased to 2.5 to 3.0 mg/dL. Another reasonable approach is to initiate prophylactic calcium infusions (or calcium-containing parenteral nutrition) for all ELBW infants within the first 24 hours. There is no role for prophylaxis or treatment with pharmacologic doses of vitamin D. For newborns who exhibit cardiovascular compromise (e.g., severe respiratory distress, pulmonary hypertension, asphyxia, sepsis) or who require cardiotonic drugs or blood pressure support, monitoring blood $[Ca^{2+}]$ is particularly helpful, with the aim of preventing the onset of significant hypocalcemia.

The mainstay of treatment for neonatal hypocalcemia is intravenous administration of calcium salts. Calcium gluconate is preferred over calcium chloride (which, in sufficient doses, produces hyperchloremic acidosis) or calcium lactate. A 10% solution of calcium gluconate contains 9.4 mg Ca/mL. A constant infusion of approximately 45 to 75 mg/kg/day usually produces a sustained increase in serum calcium level (7 to 8 mg/dL). Bolus infusions are hazardous and only transiently effective.

The risks associated with calcium infusions can be minimized by attention to detail. Rapid intravenous infusion of calcium can cause sudden elevation in serum calcium, leading to bradyarrhythmias. Bolus infusion of calcium should be reserved for treating hypocalcemic tetany and seizures. Extravasation of calcium solutions into subcutaneous tissues may cause necrosis and subcutaneous calcification. Therefore, meticulous care of peripheral intravenous catheter sites is particularly important when calcium-containing solutions are infused. Inadvertent intrahepatic infusion of calcium through an umbilical vein catheter (due to failure to reach the inferior vena cava) can cause hepatic necrosis. Rapid intra-aortic infusion via an umbilical artery can cause arterial spasm and, at least experimentally, intestinal necrosis.

***Hypocalcemic Crisis.*** For emergency treatment of hypocalcemic crisis with seizures, tetany, or apnea, 1 to 2 mL/kg of a 10% solution of calcium gluconate should be administered over 5 to 10 min. The initial serum calcium level may be less than 5.0 mg/dL. Careful observation of the infant and of the infusion site is essential, and the infusion should be discontinued if there is bradycardia or when the desired clinical result is obtained. The intravenous dose of calcium gluconate necessary to stop convulsions is usually 1 to 3 mL/kg. Toxic reactions are avoided if the maximum intravenous dose of calcium gluconate given at any one time does not exceed 2 mL/kg; doses above 3 mL/kg should be administered with caution. If necessary, intravenous calcium therapy may be repeated 3 or 4 times in 24 hours to help control acute symptoms.

***Nonemergency Treatment.*** After acute symptoms have been controlled, calcium therapy should be continued as needed to maintain serum calcium above 7.0 mg/dL. In part, the level of serum calcium to be achieved depends on serum total protein, particularly albumin. In hypoalbuminemic infants, lower levels of total serum calcium are normally present. In preterm and sick infants for whom oral intake is limited, 5 to 8 mL/kg of 10% calcium gluconate (45 to 75 mg Ca/kg) may be infused with intravenous fluids over a 24-hour period. The lower dose range is preferred whenever there is hyperphosphatemia. If oral feedings are tolerated, 10% calcium gluconate may be given in the same daily dose divided into 4 to 6 feedings. Alternatively, calcium glubionate (Neo-Calglucon), which contains 23.6 mg Ca/mL, may be given in a dose of 2 mL/kg/day divided into feedings. Oral calcium gluconate is better tolerated by young infants because the high sugar content and osmolality of calcium glubionate may cause gastrointestinal irritation or diarrhea. Intravenous or oral calcium supplements should be continued until the serum calcium level stabilizes.

Dietary factors and hypoparathyroidism are important in the pathogenesis of late neonatal hypocalcemia. Therefore, therapy is often directed at reducing the phosphate load and increasing the calcium-to-phosphorus ratio of feedings to 4:1. This can be accomplished by the use of low-phosphorus feedings such as human milk or Similac PM 60/40 Low Iron in conjunction with calcium supplements. These measures inhibit intestinal absorption of phosphorus. Phosphate binders generally are not necessary. Serum calcium and phosphorus levels should be monitored at least once to twice weekly and the calcium supplements discontinued in a stepwise fashion after several weeks.

***Magnesium Administration.*** When hypomagnesemia contributes to (or causes) hypocalcemia, administration of magnesium salts is indicated. Magnesium may be given intramuscularly as a 50% solution of magnesium sulfate (50% $MgSO_4 \cdot 7H_2O$ contains 4 mEq/mL of magnesium). The suggested intramuscular or intravenous dose of 50% magnesium sulfate is 0.1 to 0.2 mL/kg. Intravenous infusions should be administered slowly using electrocardiographic monitoring to detect acute rhythm disturbances, which may include prolonged atrioventricular conduction time and sinoatrial or atrioventricular block. The magnesium dose may be repeated every 12 to 24 hours, depending on the clinical and serum magnesium response. Serum magnesium levels should be carefully monitored to guard against hypermagnesemia. Many infants with transient hypomagnesemia will respond sufficiently to one or two magnesium injections. Infants with primary hypomagnesemia have permanent magnesium wasting and low serum magnesium levels and require lifelong treatment with magnesium supplements.

***Vitamin D Treatment.*** Infants with normal intestinal absorption who develop late hypocalcemia with vitamin D deficiency rickets usually respond within 4 weeks to 1000 to 2000 IU/day of oral vitamin D. These infants should receive at least 40 mg/kg/day of elemental calcium in order to prevent hypocalcemia because the unmineralized osteoid may avidly incorporate calcium once vitamin D is provided ("hungry bones" syndrome). The PTH-dependent renal production of $1,25(OH)_2D$ is deficient in all hypoparathyroid states. Therefore, in persistent congenital hypoparathyroidism, long-term treatment with vitamin D or a shorter-acting vitamin D analogue is indicated.

## Neonatal Hypercalcemia

Hypercalcemia usually is defined as total serum calcium concentration greater than 11.0 mg/dL and $[Ca^{2+}]$ greater than 5.0 mg/dL. Neonatal hypercalcemia is found in association with several clinical entities (Table 89–2). It may be asymptomatic and discovered incidentally or may manifest dramatically (especially if serum calcium is 14.0 mg/dL or greater) and be life-threatening, requiring immediate intervention. The clinical findings may include poor feeding, vomiting, constipation, polyuria, hypertension, tachypnea, dyspnea, hypotonia, lethargy, and seizures. Polyuria is due to an impaired renal response to vasopressin (nephrogenic diabetes insipidus) and may lead to dehydration. The hypertension is probably due to a direct vasoconstrictive effect of the elevated ECF calcium as well as to increased activity of the renin-angiotensin system resulting from renal arteriolar constriction. The central nervous manifestations result from

**TABLE 89–2**

**Causes of Neonatal Hypercalcemia**

Iatrogenic (calcium salts)
Parathyroid hyperfunction
- Neonatal severe primary hyperparathyroidism (NSPHP)
  - $Ca^{2+}$-sensing receptor mutation homozygosity
- Familial (benign) hypercalcemic hypocalciuria (FBHH)
  - $Ca^{2+}$-sensing receptor mutation heterozygosity
- Neonatal hyperparathyroidism associated with multiple endocrine adenomatosis
- Renal tubular acidosis with secondary hyperparathyroidism
- Neonatal hyperparathyroidism secondary to maternal hypoparathyroidism

Williams syndrome (elastin gene locus deletions)
Idiopathic infantile hypercalcemia ("Lightwood-type")
Phosphate depletion
Hypervitaminosis D
- Vitamin D intoxication
- Subcutaneous fat necrosis

Blue diaper syndrome
Hypercalcemia associated with skeletal dysplasias
- Infantile hypophosphatasia
- Jansen metaphyseal chondrodysplasia (activating mutations of the PTH/PTHrP receptor)

Other causes
- Tumor-associated hypercalcemia
- Congenital lactase deficiency
- Acute adrenal insufficiency
- Hypervitaminosis A
- Thyrotoxicosis
- Prolonged ECMO

ECMO, extracorporeal membrane oxygenation; PTH, parathyroid hormone; PTHrP, parathyroid hormone–related protein.

direct neuronal effects of calcium, hypertensive encephalopathy, and cerebral ischemia. Persistent hypercalcemia may produce extraskeletal calcification in the kidney, skin, subcutaneous tissue, falx cerebri, arteries, myocardium, lung, or gastric mucosa. Nephrocalcinosis, nephrolithiasis, diffuse bone undermineralization (and occasionally osteitis fibrosa) are well-recognized hypercalcemic complications. In infants, the predominant manifestation of chronic, moderate elevations of serum calcium may be failure to thrive. The physical examination usually is otherwise normal, except in those infants with subcutaneous fat necrosis, Williams syndrome, or skeletal dysplasias.

Normally, the parathyroid-renal axis prevents hypercalcemia via inhibition of PTH secretion and $1,25(OH)_2D$ synthesis, which reduces calcium absorption from the intestine, mobilization from bone, and reabsorption from the kidney. (The physiologic role of calcitonin is uncertain.) An elevated serum calcium, therefore, indicates that there is inappropriate calcium influx to the ECF from one or more of these pools. Because the kidney is the principal organ for stoichiometric calcium balance, hypercalcemia usually means the renal capacity to excrete calcium has been exceeded. In fact, abnormalities in distal tubular resorption are involved in the pathogenesis of many hypercalcemic conditions (e.g., hyperparathyroidism) and renal impairment frequently accompanies many hypercalcemic syndromes.

### Neonatal Hyperparathyroid Syndromes and Familial Hypocalciuric Hypercalcemia

Neonatal severe primary hyperparathyroidism (NSPHP) is a rare, life-threatening disorder. The enlarged parathyroid glands are resistant to regulation by $Ca^{2+}$, resulting in marked hypercalcemia, although milder clinical expression also occurs. These infants usually appear normal at birth but may have a narrow thorax, depressed sternum, or thoracolumbar kyphosis. Signs of hypercalcemia usually develop during the first days of life. Serum calcium levels may range between 15 and 30 mg/dL, serum phosphorus concentration is frequently less than 3.5 mg/dL with significant hyperphosphaturia, and PTH levels are very elevated. Anemia, hepatomegaly, and splenomegaly have been reported. Skeletal radiographs may show generalized undermineralization, irregular metaphyses (subperiosteal erosions), and multiple pathologic fractures of the long bones and ribs. Nephrocalcinosis is common. The bone findings initially may be mistaken for osteogenesis imperfecta (Bai et al, 1997).

Inheritance studies have long suggested a connection between NSPHP and a milder disease, familial (benign) hypocalciuric hypercalcemia (FBHH) as well as a relationship of both to PTH-independent "resetting" of parathyroid $Ca^{2+}$ sensing and renal calcium handling. Sequencing of the parathyroid and renal CaR has clarified these relationships. Partial or total inactivating *CaR* mutations cause increased renal tubular calcium reabsorption (hypercalciuria) and persistent PTH secretion despite hypercalcemia. Homozygosity for inactivating *CaR* mutations causes NSPHP, whereas heterozygosity results in the autosomal dominant FBHH. Additionally, certain de novo or inherited heterozygous *CaR* mutations account for some cases of NSPHP.

Newborns (and older children and adults) with FBHH have mild (often asymptomatic) and intermittent hypercalcemia without hypercalciuria. In distinction to neonatal hyperparathyroidism, circulating levels of PTH, phosphorus, and $1,25(OH)_2D$ tend to be normal. Persons who have FBHH are at risk for having a child with NSPHP. Conversely, parents of an infant with hyperparathyroidism should be screened with serum calcium and phosphorus levels and a urinary UCa/Cr. A UCa/Cr below 0.01 supports the diagnosis. Early diagnosis and parathyroidectomy have been necessary for survival in fulminant NSHPT. However, conservative management may be warranted in less severe cases, which can be self-limiting and are often due to heterozygous *CaR* mutations.

Neonatal hyperparathyroidism occasionally occurs as part of the syndrome of multiple endocrine adenomatosis. There also have been reports of sporadic and familial forms of renal tubular acidosis with secondary hyperparathyroidism manifesting as hyperchloremia, hypercalcemia, elevated serum PTH, and severe metabolic acidosis (Nishiyama et al, 1990; Savani et al, 1993). Serum calcium and PTH may promptly revert to normal values after initiation of alkali therapy. Often, the acidification defect is transient (Igarashi, 1992). As the hyperparathyroidism and ECF volume contraction are corrected, serum calcium normalizes.

### Neonatal Hyperparathyroidism Associated with Maternal Hypoparathyroidism

Fetal and neonatal hyperparathyroidism may occur in infants born to mothers with poorly controlled (hypocalcemic) hypoparathyroidism. Maternal hypocalcemia leads to impaired transplacental calcium transfer and causes chronic stimulation of the fetal parathyroid glands. In contrast with infants with NSPHP, these newborns are frequently of low birth weight and have depressed or normal (rather than elevated) serum calcium levels and normal to mildly elevated (rather than depressed) serum phosphorus levels. The reasons for these differences between the two groups are unknown.

Mortality rates are high in infants born to poorly or untreated hyperparathyroid mothers, especially if there is significant IUGR. In survivors, the skeletal abnormalities usually regress and bone radiographs normalize by 4 to 7 months. Correction of hypocalcemia in hypoparathyroid women during pregnancy using calcium and vitamin D supplements prevents the development of fetal hyperparathyroidism.

### Williams Syndrome and Idiopathic Infantile Hypercalcemia

Williams syndrome (WS) (or Williams-Beuren syndrome) is an autosomal dominant disorder that, in fully expressed form, includes transient hypercalcemia in infancy, supravalvular aortic stenosis, multiple peripheral pulmonary arterial stenoses, "elfin" facies, mental and height deficiency, and dental malformations. The typical facial features include supraorbital fullness with a broad forehead, short palpebral fissures with a medial flare to the eyebrows, a flat nasal bridge with a full tip and anteverted nostrils, ocular hypertelorism, strabismus, stellate iris, malar hypoplasia with a wide mouth and a full lower lip, and hypoplastic teeth with malocclusion. Hallux valgus with a small curved fifth digit is common. Pectus excavatum and umbilical or inguinal hernia are less commonly noted.

Two thirds of newborns with WS are small for gestational age, and many are born post-dates. The frequency of WS is estimated to be about 1/10,000 to 1/20,000. Hemizygosity for elastin gene mutations and deletions are responsible, at least in part, for the manifestations. WS often results from a contiguous gene deletion in which up to 2.5 Mb of genomic DNA distal to the elastin gene locus may be missing (Urban et al, 1996). Deletion of several specific genes in the *WS* region (7q11.23) appears to account for the distinct physiognomic and cognitive features. Expression of the full WS phenotype may be related to the size of the deletion. FISH for the detection of elastin locus deletions is the appropriate initial diagnostic assay.

Although the hypercalcemia is often diagnosed after the first month, the child with WS sometimes comes to clinical attention in the neonatal period (Shimizu et al, 1994). Heightened awareness of the syndrome should increase the frequency of neonatal diagnosis. The hypercalcemia rarely persists beyond several months and generally resolves spontaneously, but hypercalciuria may persist. The pathogenesis of hypercalcemia in WS remains unknown. Elevated serum calcium associated with normal or increased serum phosphorus levels and characteristic radiographic findings differentiate WS from primary hyperparathyroidism. In some older infants, the serum calcium level is normal, but the presence of nephrocalcinosis and other soft tissue calcifications suggests that hypercalcemia occurred earlier. Increased calcium absorption has been demonstrated, but enhanced vitamin D sensitivity or other disorders of specific calcitropic hormones have not been consistently found. A cautionary note is that many of these children were studied after their hypercalcemia had resolved. A low-calcium diet usually controls the hypercalcemia.

In the early 1950s in England, Lightwood (1952) reported a series of infants with severe hypercalcemia. Hypervitaminosis D was suggested by the findings of osteoporosis and dense bands of mineralization at the metaphyseal ends of long bones. Epidemiologic investigations revealed that a majority of these infants were born to mothers who ingested foods heavily fortified with vitamin D. Some infants also had received 3000 to 4000 IU of vitamin D daily in an effort to prevent nutritional deficiencies. With reduction of vitamin D supplementation, the incidence of infantile hypercalcemia has declined dramatically. However, in other instances, no known previous exposure to excessive maternal vitamin D intake has occurred. The incidence of this milder (Lightwood-type) "idiopathic" infantile hypercalcemia (IIH) without WS phenotypic features has remained relatively fixed over time. Further distinction between these conditions probably awaits more extensive genetic analysis and definition of the mineral metabolic derangement(s). In contrast with those in WS, serum calcium levels remain elevated for a prolonged period in severely affected infants with IIH. There may be an exaggerated increase in serum $1,25(OH)_2D$ in response to exogenous PTH administration (Pronicka et al, 1988). Therefore, in addition to dietary calcium restriction and avoidance of vitamin D, glucocorticoid therapy to reduce gastrointestinal calcium absorption is sometimes warranted.

## Neonatal Hypercalcemia Associated with Subcutaneous Fat Necrosis

Hypercalcemia is an occasional, severe complication of subcutaneous fat necrosis in newborns. The erythematous to violaceous, indurated subcutaneous nodules and plaques often overlie bony prominences on the buttocks, thighs, trunk, cheeks, or arms and may appear up to several weeks after delivery. The lesions may resemble those of sclerema neonatorum. Frequently, there is a history of difficult delivery, trauma, hypothermia, or asphyxia. Hypercalcemic infants may present with poor weight gain despite adequate energy intake or with nephrocalcinosis. Hypercalcemia should be sought for in all infants with subcutaneous fat necrosis. Laboratory evaluation shows high blood $1,25(OH)_2D$ levels and usually normal phosphorus and alkaline phosphatase. Radiographs of the long bones also are usually normal, although periosteal elevation, features similar to those of WS, or ectopic calcification may be present. Skin and subcutaneous tissue punch biopsy specimens show lobular panniculitis with necrotic adipocytes, abundant histiocytes, and giant cells with radial crystals. Distinctive, needle-shaped clefts in the fat lobules are pathognomonic findings (Hicks et al, 1993). Magnetic resonance imaging (MRI) may point to the correct diagnosis without biopsy.

Unregulated production of $1,25(OH)_2D$ by activated macrophages induces hypercalcemia (Kruse et al, 1993) similar to the hypercalcemia encountered in sarcoidosis and other granulomatous diseases. Lesion prostaglandin E release also may contribute to hypercalcemia and osteoclastic bone resorption. Hypercalcemia associated with subcutaneous fat necrosis may persist for days to weeks. Prognosis depends on its duration. Treatment consists of glucocorticoids, intravascular volume expansion, furosemide diuresis, and a low-calcium, low-vitamin D diet.

## Blue Diaper Syndrome

Blue diaper syndrome is a rare familial disease in which hypercalcemia and nephrocalcinosis are associated with a defect in the intestinal transport of tryptophan (Drummond et al, 1964). Bacterial degradation of tryptophan in the intestine leads to excessive indole production, which is converted to indican in the liver. Oxidative conjugation of indican in the urine forms the water-insoluble dye indigo blue (indigotin), with a consequent peculiar bluish discoloration of the diaper. The clinical course is characterized by failure to thrive, recurrent unexplained fever, infections, marked irritability, and constipation. The mechanism of the hypercalcemia is uncertain, although oral tryptophan loading in human subjects and experimental animals also elevates serum calcium. Treatment consists of glucocorticoids and a low-calcium, low–vitamin D diet.

## Hypercalcemia Associated with Skeletal Dysplasias

Several skeletal dysplasia syndromes are associated with hypercalcemia. Their distinctive phenotypes suggest appropriate diagnosis.

Hypophosphatasia is a rare autosomal recessive condition caused by deficiency of tissue-nonspecific alkaline phosphatase. The perinatal and early infantile onsets are characterized by defective bone mineralization. Prominent features are craniosynostosis, severe rickets, and hypercalcemia. More than 50% of patients with the infantile form have not survived the first year. Attempts to control the hypercalcemia, hypercalciuria, and chronic bone demineralization using chlorothiazide, calcitonin, and bisphosphonates have been disappointing (Deeb et al, 2000).

Jansen metaphyseal chrondrodysplasia manifests in newborns with hypercalcemia and skeletal radiographs that mimic rachitic changes. This severe autosomal recessive disorder results from gain-of-function mutations in the PTH/PTHrP receptor leading to ligand-independent receptor activation (Schipani et al, 1996). PTH and PTHrP levels are low or undetectable. The functional consequences are premature chrondrocyte maturation, accelerated endochondral bone formation, and hypercalcemia.

## Hypercalcemia Associated with Phosphate Depletion

Neonatal hypercalcemia due to phosphate depletion is most often seen in very-low-birth-weight (VLBW) infants who are fed unsupplemented human milk. The low phosphate content of human milk leads to hypophosphatemia, which stimulates renal $1,25(OH)_2D$ synthesis, leading to increased intestinal calcium absorption. When phosphate is limited, little calcium can be deposited in bone, leading to rickets, hypercalcemia, and hypercalciuria. Extremely high serum calcium levels (greater than 15 mg/dL, with serum phosphorus less than 2 mg/dL and suppressed PTH) may be observed in VLBW infants in this setting. These infants respond to cautious phosphate replenishment. The condition is preventable by anticipatory monitoring of serum calcium and phosphorus levels in high-risk infants. Hypophosphatemic bone disease in VLBW infants is discussed later (see section "Osteopathy of Prematurity").

## Vitamin D Toxicity

Excessive supplementation with vitamin D will cause hypercalcemia in newborns and infants. In preterm infants, prolonged feeding with premature formula (Nako et al, 1993) or mineral- and vitamin D–supplemented human milk fortifiers also has led to mild to significant hypercalcemia. Infants respond to discontinuation of vitamin D supplements. These occurrences have prompted vitamin reformulation of premature nutritional products. Laboratory studies of hypervitaminosis D typically show elevation of 25(OH)D but not of $1,25(OH)_2D$. Serum PTH usually is suppressed by the hypercalcemia. Biochemical resolution may be protracted because vitamin D accumulates in body fat.

## Other Causes of Neonatal Hypercalcemia

Hypervitaminosis A and thyrotoxicosis also accelerate bone turnover and can induce hypercalcemia. Tumor-associated hypercalcemia in neonates is extremely rare. Most cases have been associated with congenital mesoblastic nephroma, the most common renal tumor of early infancy. Congenital lactase deficiency is associated with rapid onset of hypercalcemia, hypercalciuria, and medullary nephrocalcinosis (Saarela et al, 1995). The calcium derangements are well managed by a lactose-free diet. Modest hypercalcemia may occur in acute adrenal insufficiency. The pathogenesis is uncertain. Iatrogenic hypercalcemia may be induced, especially in VLBW infants, by administration of parenteral calcium supplementation in association with indomethacin treatment for patent ductus arteriosus (Rodd and Goodyer, 1999). Prolonged ECMO support has been associated with hypercalcemia (greater than 11 mg/dL) in some infants (Fridriksson et al, 2001). The cause is not known.

### Treatment

The first principle in the medical management of hypercalcemia is to increase the urinary calcium excretion by maximizing glomerular filtration rate (GFR) and urinary sodium excretion. In the normal kidney, sodium and calcium clearances are very closely linked during water or osmotic diuresis. Two-thirds normal to isotonic saline containing 20 to 30 mEq of potassium chloride per liter may be infused intravenously at a rate to correct dehydration and maximize GFR. After rehydration, furosemide (1 mg/kg) may be given intravenously at 6- to 8-hour intervals to inhibit tubular reabsorption of calcium.

When severe hypercalcemia is associated with hypophosphatemia, 30 to 50 mg/kg/day of oral or intravenous phosphorus as a phosphate salt may be given. Unlike sodium, phosphate does not remove calcium from the body but causes a redistribution of calcium. The goal of phosphate therapy is to maintain serum phosphorus levels in a range of 3 to 5 mg/dL. The oral route is preferable because of the potential for serious complications with intravenous phosphate treatment. Therapy usually results in a significant reduction in serum calcium concentration over 1 to 2 days. In more severe and resistant cases, glucocorticoids (e.g., prednisone, 2 mg/kg per day) may be added. Glucocorticoids suppress intestinal calcium absorption and increase renal excretion. Although glucocorticoids are effective in several types of hypercalcemia, they are relatively ineffective for the treatment of hypercalcemia associated with primary hyperparathyroidism. Experience with use of other antihypercalcemic agents (e.g., calcitonin or bisphosphonates) is limited in newborns.

The mainstays of the nonacute treatment of milder neonatal hypercalcemia are restriction of dietary calcium, elimination of vitamin D supplements, and limiting sunlight exposure.

### Neonatal Disorders of Serum Magnesium

Neonatal hypomagnesemia is discussed in a preceding section, "Neonatal Hypocalcemia Associated with Hypomagnesemia or Renal Tubular Necrosis."

Neonatal hypermagnesemia usually is due to maternal magnesium sulfate administration for preeclamptic seizure prophylaxis or for tocolysis of premature uterine contractions. Later-onset neonatal hypermagnesemia can result from use of magnesium hydroxide–containing antacids ("milk of magnesia"). The hypermagnesemic newborn may exhibit varying degrees of flaccidity, unresponsiveness, respiratory insufficiency and apnea, ileus, or delayed passage of meconium. The signs may be mistaken for those of perinatal asphyxia. Occasionally, temporizing endotracheal intubation and mechanical ventilation are required. Feedings should be deferred until normalization of bowel function occurs. Prolonged fetal hypermagnesemia also increases the risk of meconium obstruction. Aside from this latter possibility, the neonatal effects of hypermagnesemia appear to be transient and usually disappear within several hours. Generally, newborns effectively excrete a magnesium load, and serial monitoring of serum levels usually is not necessary. However, in preterm newborns, who have limited renal excretory capacity for magnesium, hypermagnesemia may persist for more than 48 hours. No magnesium should be added to parenteral nutrition solutions until serum magnesium falls. Early hypermagnesemia in preterm infants also may suppress PTH secretion (Rantonen et al, 2001). Infusion of calcium salts may antagonize some of the adverse effects of excess magnesium.

**TABLE 89–3**

**Forms of Metabolic Bone Disease Manifesting in Newborns and Infants**

| |
|---|
| Vitamin D deficiency |
| Maternal vitamin D deficiency (congenital rickets) |
| Inadequate intake of dietary vitamin D |
| Lack of adequate sunlight exposure + dietary inadequacy |
| Vitamin D malabsorption |
| Hepatic disease (steatorrhea) |
| Short gut syndrome |
| Pancreatic insufficiency |
| Vitamin D metabolic defects |
| Hepatic rickets (inadequate vitamin D 25-hydroxylation) |
| Vitamin D–dependent rickets (VDDRI)—defects in 1α-hydroxylation |
| Renal insufficiency (renal osteodystrophy) |
| Antoconvulsants (increased 25(OH)D metabolism) |
| Vitamin D receptor defects |
| Vitamin D–resistant rickets (VDRRII) |
| Phosphate deficiency rickets |
| Osteopathy of prematurity |
| X-linked hypophosphatemic rickets |
| Fanconi syndrome |
| Antacid-induced osteopathy (aluminum hydroxide) |
| Tumor (including hemangioma)-associated rickets |
| Calcium deficiency rickets |
| Osteopathy of prematurity |
| Inadequate intake of dietary calcium after weaning |
| Inadequate calcium in TPN solution |

25(OH)D, 25-hydroxyvitamin D; TPN, total parenteral nutrition.

## METABOLIC BONE DISEASE IN NEWBORNS AND INFANTS

Forms of metabolic bone disease manifesting in infants and children are listed in Table 89–3. The following definitions are presented as a background for the discussions of specific entities in this section.

*Osteopenia* is defined as radiographic evidence of diminished bone density. Osteopenia is present in rickets, osteomalacia, and osteoporosis.

*Rickets* is a disorder of the bone matrix, or osteoid, in growing bone resulting from undermineralization of cartilage; it involves both the growth plate (physis) and newly formed trabecular and cortical bone. In infancy, the most rapidly growing bones are the skull, upper limbs, and ribs. Early development of rickets, therefore, leads to craniotabes ("Ping-Pong ball" sign), widened cranial sutures, frontal bossing, swollen epiphyses of the wrists, costochondral beading ("rachitic rosary"), and Harrison's sulcus (caused by diaphragmatic depression of the lower thorax on inspiration). There is an increased risk of pneumonia. Manifestations of muscle weakness (myopathy) may include dilated cardiomyopathy and ventricular dysfunction, which respond to vitamin D therapy (Mustafa et al, 1999). The radiographic features in rickets reflect expansion of the cartilaginous growth plate and delayed mineralization and include lucency and widening of the gap between metaphysis and epiphysis (the zone of provisional calcification); irregularity, cupping, or fraying of the metaphyseal margin; and osteopenia. Serum phosphorus or serum calcium or both characteristically are depressed, and serum alkaline phosphatase is elevated. An exception is the hyperphosphatemia of renal osteodystrophy.

*Osteomalacia* is rickets that occurs in the absence of linear growth. This is the typical pattern in adults, but it also can occur in poorly nourished preterm infants. In osteomalacia, the radiographic features of rickets at the cartilage-shaft junction are generally absent.

*Osteoporosis* in adults is defined as a state of reduced bone mass per unit volume with a normal ratio of mineral to matrix. Unlike in rickets and osteomalacia, where mineralization defects predominate, the primary abnormality in osteoporosis is either a decrease in matrix formation or an increase in matrix and mineral resorption. There is no generally accepted pediatric definition for osteoporosis (Rauch and Schoenau, 2002).

### Osteopathy of Prematurity

In preterm infants, osteopenia with or without rachitic changes at the cartilage-shaft junction may be observed between 3 and 12 weeks of age. This metabolic bone disorder has also been called "rickets of prematurity" and "osteopenia of prematurity." Its incidence and severity increase with decreasing gestation and birth weight and it is more common in preterm infants with a complicated medical course and delayed nutrition. On the other hand, osteopathy usually is not a problem for healthier, larger preterm infants. In osteopathic VLBW babies, postnatal bone mineralization lags significantly behind the expected intrauterine bone mineralization rate. The pathogenesis of this disorder is increased endosteal resorption rather than decreased bone formation; that is, it is a high-turnover osteopathy (Beyers et al, 1994).

The clinical findings in VLBW infants with severe osteopathy, as in older, term infants with rickets, include a widened anterior fontanel, craniotabes, bony expansion of the wrists, costochondral beading, and rib or long bone fractures. Undermineralization, softening, or fractures of the ribs can lead to respiratory distress (especially tachypnea), atelectasis, or pneumonia. In most premature infants, osteopathy is self-limiting. However, long-term effects of osteopathy of prematurity may include delayed dental maturation (Seow, 1996) and reduced stature into school age (Fewtrell et al, 2000). Bone mineral content later in childhood for these preterm newborns also is influenced by polymorphisms in multiple bone regulatory genes (Backstrom et al, 2001).

Although the clinical features of nutritional rickets in term infants and osteopathy of prematurity are similar, the latter has a distinctive pathogenesis. Preterm osteopathy is caused chiefly by deficiencies in dietary phosphate and calcium, rather than by vitamin D deficiency. Eighty percent of bone mineralization in the fetus occurs during the third trimester, when fetal calcium and phosphorus requirements are at least 100 to 120 mg/kg/day and 60 to 75 mg/kg/day, respectively. Diets particularly low in mineral (and especially phosphorus) content predispose preterm infants to osteopathy. The greatest risks for phosphate deficiency result from feeding unsupplemented human milk or milk formulas not designed for use in preterm infants and from prolonged parenteral nutrition.

Typically, neither hyperparathyroidism nor vitamin D deficiency is present in phosphate-deficient osteopathy of prematurity. In contrast, the pathogenesis of calcium deficiency rickets and that of vitamin D deficiency are similar in that hypocalcemia causes hyperparathyroidism. The elevated PTH increases bone resorption and enhances renal $1,25(OH)_2D$ synthesis, which in turn increases intestinal calcium and phosphorus absorption. Individual preterm babies may exhibit predominantly phosphate depletion, but mixed phosphate and calcium deficiency is more common; isolated calcium deficiency is rare. In dual mineral deficiency, laboratory values may show low, normal, or slightly elevated serum calcium and low to low-normal phosphorus. In severe or complicated bone disease, serum 25(OH)D is a useful screen for evaluating the sufficiency of vitamin D stores; levels less than 6 ng/mL indicate severe vitamin D deficiency. For evaluating bone mineral status in preterm neonates, measurement of cortical thickness and visual inspection of the humerus on a chest radiograph probably constitute the simplest and best method (Fig. 89–2).

Serum alkaline phosphatase, a marker of osteoblastic bone formation, is frequently used to monitor skeletal metabolism in preterm infants. However, the magnitude of elevations in alkaline phosphatase (or osteocalcin) concentrations is not a good predictor of the extent of the bone mineral deficits (Ryan et al, 1993; Pittard et al, 1992). Serial urinary biochemical markers of bone metabolism (e.g., pyridinoline, deoxypyridinoline) have not yet been useful in predicting severe osteopathy, because levels are related to bone volume and normative data for growing preterm infants are lacking. Longitudinal assessment of bone mineral content by dual x-ray absorptiometry (DXA) or quantitative ultrasonography is not widely available.

Phosphate depletion and rickets occur in rapidly growing preterm infants fed unsupplemented human milk, which has low phosphate content. Characteristically, these infants develop hypophosphatemia, hypophosphaturia, hypercalcemia, and hypercalciuria. Serum PTH may be low or normal, 25(OH)D is normal, and $1,25(OH)_2D$ is elevated. The hypophosphatemia stimulates the production of $1,25(OH)_2D$, which in turn increases intestinal calcium

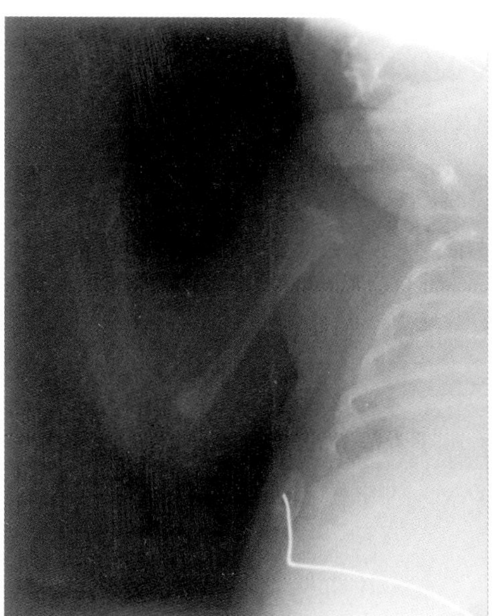

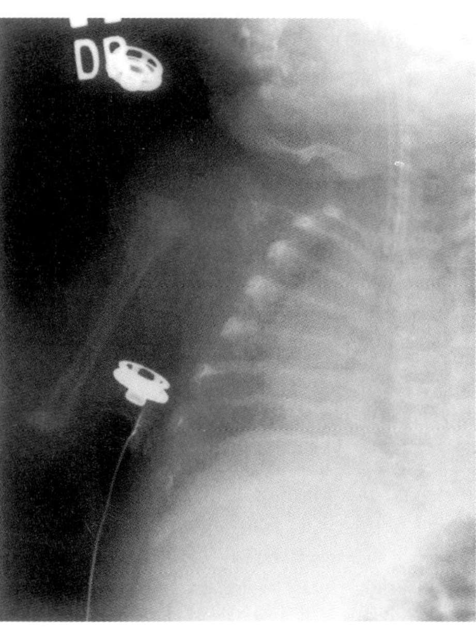

**FIGURE 89–2.** Chest radiographs from a 700-g-birth-weight, 25-week-gestation infant with bronchopulmonary dysplasia and osteopathy of prematurity. **Left panel,** At 34 weeks of postconceptional age, mild osteopenia and metaphyseal changes (especially in right arm and wrist) are evident. **Right panel,** Two weeks later, signs of rachitic healing can be seen in ribs and long bones.

absorption. However, in the presence of hypophosphatemia, only limited amounts of calcium can be deposited in bone, leading to hypercalcemia and hypercalciuria. The hypercalcemia inhibits PTH secretion.

This form of rickets does not respond to vitamin D therapy. In fact, vitamin D supplementation without prior correction of the underlying dietary phosphate deficiency may aggravate the hypercalcemia and hypercalciuria by enhancing intestinal calcium absorption. The bone disease in these infants does respond to increased dietary phosphate, accomplished by adding a human milk supplement designed for preterm infants or switching to a preterm milk formula; both diets provide additional calcium as well as phosphorus. Addition of 20 to 25 mg/kg/day of potassium phosphate also will increase serum phosphorus levels. However, because phosphate repletion promotes bone mineralization, serum calcium may fall to subnormal levels ("hungry bones" syndrome) unless supplemental calcium (e.g., 30 mg/kg/day) also is provided. Recommended intakes of calcium and phosphorus (Atkinson, 1994; Schanler and Rifka, 1994) allow normalized bone growth and mineralization in preterm infants. For VLBW infants, it is important to maintain a mineral-enriched diet and to perform serial laboratory monitoring for several weeks to months after hospital discharge.

Human milk has a total antirachitic sterol activity of only 25 to 50 IU/L (Reeve et al, 1982), which may be insufficient for maintaining normal 25(OH)D levels in preterm infants. Therefore, preterm infants fed unsupplemented human milk also should receive 400 to 600 IU daily of vitamin D. There is no apparent benefit for additional vitamin D intake for VLBW infants who are receiving standard high-calcium, high-phosphorus preterm infant formulas.

Additional, non-nutritional risk factors for osteopathy in ill preterm infants are the early withdrawal of placental estradiol and progesterone (Trotter et al, 1999), lack of mobility (Moyer-Mileur et al, 2000), and therapy with dexamethasone (Kamitsuka et al, 1995), methylxanthines (Zanardo et al, 1995), or aminoglycosides (Giapros et al, 1995), any of which can increase urinary calcium excretion and contribute to serum mineral imbalance, nephrocalcinosis, and osteopenia. The importance of mechanical stimulation in preterm infants and term newborns with muscle weakness or paralysis is gaining better appreciation in neonatology. Glucocorticoids decrease bone formation by inhibiting osteoblast growth and increasing cell death of osteoblasts and osteocytes (Ng et al, 2002; Weinstein et al, 1998) and, at least over several months, increase osteoclastogenesis and bone resorption. Copper deficiency is a rare contributor to osteopenia in preterm infants (Tanaka et al, 1980).

## Nutritional (Vitamin D Deficiency) Rickets

In North America, Europe, and northern Asia, rickets most often occurs in exclusively breast-fed infants who also have little exposure to sunlight. Historically, a marked rise in prevalence in nutritional rickets has accompanied industrialization and urban crowding. Clinical rickets often manifests at 4 months of age or later, but onset in early infancy is not uncommon. In the United States, there has been a recent apparent increase in the incidence of nutritional rickets. Because deeply dark-skinned infants who are breast-fed or are not exposed much to sunlight are at greatest risk, vitamin D supplementation for these babies is warranted (Kreiter et al, 2000; Shaw and Pal, 2002). Recent data also suggest vitamin D supplementation of breast-fed infant girls during the first year of life increases bone mineral mass in later childhood (Zamora et al, 1999). This author and others (Welch et al, 2000) advocate a simple approach of universal vitamin D supplementation for all breast-fed babies. Stoss therapy, which occasionally is used to treat rickets, consists of a single intramuscular large dose (150,000 to 500,000 IU) of vitamin D.

In tropical areas, the daily requirements for vitamin D usually are met by skin exposure to sunlight, and vitamin D deficiency rickets is less common. Instead, recent reports suggest dietary insufficiency of calcium contributes to the development of rickets in Africa and Asia. As a consequence, in tropical populations, rickets usually occurs later than at higher latitudes, between 1 and 2 years of age, after weaning and with introduction of a low-calcium diet.

Congenital rickets should always prompt an investigation for maternal vitamin D deficiency. Rickets, hypercalciuria, and hypophosphatemia also occur in Fanconi renotubular syndrome. Prolonged treatment with aluminum-containing antacids can induce hypophosphatemia and rickets (Pattaragarn and Alon, 2001). These antacids should be avoided or used with caution during infancy.

## Renal Osteodystrophy

Because normal renal function is essential for physiologic mineral and bone metabolism, renal insufficiency induces hyperphosphatemia and bone disease. Renal osteodystrophy can be predominantly a high- or low-bone-turnover form, or the two forms may alternate predominance during the clinical course in an individual infant. High bone turnover or osteitis fibrosa is a manifestation of secondary hyperparathyroidism. Parathyroid hyperfunction often occurs early in the course of renal failure. Contributing factors include phosphate retention, impaired renal $1,25(OH)_2D$ synthesis, hypocalcemia, parathyroid gland hyperplasia, and skeletal resistance to PTH actions. Low-turnover osteodystrophy (adynamic bone or osteomalacia) results from suppressed bone formation; in older children and adults, it is more common among dialyzed patients. The relative incidences of these forms of renal osteodystrophy in newborns are not known.

A principal goal of therapy is to lower serum phosphate, in order to prevent hypocalcemia and severe hyperparathyroidism. Phosphate restriction is accomplished with feeding breast milk or Similac PM 60/40. Hypocalcemia and metabolic acidosis should be treated with appropriate supplements. If serum $1,25(OH)_2D$ is low, $1,25(OH)_2D$ therapy will increase intestinal calcium absorption, transcriptionally suppress *PTH* gene expression, and decrease parathyroid hyperplasia. Serum calcium, phosphorus, and PTH levels, as well as linear growth and bone radiographs, should be serially monitored. Management of severe renal osteodystrophy in neonates is particularly complicated by the increased phosphate requirements for growth. Calcium supplementation and use of potent vitamin D metabolites also may produce an "oversuppression" of PTH. As with any complex disorder, effective clinical management requires close monitoring and an integrated team approach.

## Inherited Metabolic Bone Disease in Infancy

Three major forms of metabolic bone disease or rickets have been described that can present in newborns and infants. Vitamin D–dependent rickets (VDDRI), also called vitamin D pseudodeficiency or Prader-type rickets, is caused by mutations in the vitamin D 1α-hydroxylase gene. This autosomal recessive disorder is most common in French Canadian kindreds. Muscle weakness and rickets appear shortly after birth. Treatment with 1α-hydroxylated vitamin D analogues induces remission.

The autosomal recessive form of $1,25(OH)_2D$-resistant rickets (VDRRII) is caused by a wide range of mutations in the vitamin D receptor (VDR). Affected infants show early-onset rickets, hypocalcemia, elevated serum $1,25(OH)_2D$ levels, secondary hyperparathyroidism, and often alopecia. Depending on the genotype, there is a variable response to supraphysiologic doses of $1,25(OH)_2D$ analogues.

X-linked dominant hypophosphatemia (XLH), also known as familial hypophosphatemic rickets or vitamin D–resistant rickets, is a disorder of phosphate homeostasis. Its prevalence is 1/20,000. XLH is characterized by poor linear growth, rickets, and hypophosphatemia associated with a low TmP and renal tubular phosphate leak. Defective regulation of vitamin D metabolism results in inappropriately normal $1,25(OH)_2D$ concentrations in the face of hypophosphatemia. The responsible gene is designated *PHEX* ("phosphate-regulating gene with homology to endopeptidases on the X chromosome"). The role that *PHEX* plays in the pathophysiology of XLH and renal phosphate transport currently is unresolved.

Neonatal rickets with increased bone density rather than osteopenia can occur in infantile osteopetrosis, a rare autosomal recessive disorder of osteoclast formation. Diagnosis may be obscured by concurrent maternal vitamin D deficiency (Popp et al, 2000).

## SELECTED READINGS


Ariceta G, Rodriguez-Soriano J, Vallo A: Magnesium homeostasis in premature and full-term neonates. Pediatr Nephrol 9:423, 1995.

Baker SS, Cochran WJ, Flores CA, et al: American Academy of Pediatrics Committee on Nutrition. Calcium requirements of infants, children, and adolescents. Pediatrics 104:1152, 1999.

Chesney RW: Vitamin D deficiency and rickets. Rev Endocr Metab Disord 2:145, 2001.

DiMeglio LA and Econs MJ: Hypophosphatemic rickets. Rev Endocr Metab Disord 2:165, 2001.

Ernst JA, Cruse WK, Lemons JA: Metabolic balance studies in premature infants. Clin Perinatol 22:177, 1995.

Marx SJ: Hyperparathyroid and hypoparathyroid disorders. N Engl J Med 343:1863, 2000.

Pearce S, Steinmann B: Casting new light on the clinical spectrum of neonatal severe hyperparathyroidism. Clin Endocrinol 50:691, 1999.

Prentice A: Calcium in pregnancy and lactation. Annu Rev Nutr 20:249, 2000.

Schanler RJ: The use of human milk for premature infants. Pediatr Clin North Am 48:207, 2001.

Vieth R: Vitamin D supplementation, 25-hydroxyvitamin D concentrations, and safety. Am J Clin Nutr 69:842, 1999.


## REFERENCES


Atkinson SA: Calcium and phosphorus needs of premature infants. Nutrition 10:66, 1994.

Backstrom MC, Mahonen A, Ala-Houlala M, et al: Genetic determinants of bone mineral content in premature infants. Arch Dis Child 85:F214, 2001.

Bai M, Pearce SHS, Kifor O, et al: In vivo and in vitro characterization of neonatal hyperparathyroidism resulting from a de novo, heterozygous mutation in the $Ca^{2+}$-sensing receptor gene: Normal maternal calcium homeostasis as a cause of secondary hyperparathyroidism in familial benign hypocalciuric hypercalcemia. J Clin Invest 99:88, 1997.

Bertelloni S, Baroncelli GI, Pelletti A, et al: Parathyroid hormone–related protein in healthy pregnant women. Calcif Tissue Int 54:195, 1994.

Beyers N, Alheit B, Taljaard JF, et al: High turnover osteopenia in preterm babies. Bone 15:5, 1994.

Bronner F, Salle BL, Putet G, et al: Net calcium absorption in premature infants: Results of 103 metabolic balance studies [published erratum appears in Am J Clin Nutr 57:451, 1993]. Am J Clin Nutr 56:1037, 1992.

Brown EM, MacLeod RJ: Extracellular calcium sensing and extracellular calcium signaling. Physiol Rev 81:239, 2001.

Clase CM, Norman GL, Beecroft ML, Churchill DN: Albumin-corrected calcium and ionized calcium in stable haemodialysis patients. Nephrol Dial Transpl 15:1841, 2000.

Cuneo BF, Langman CB, Ilbawi MN, et al: Latent hypoparathyroidism in children with conotruncal cardiac defects. Circulation 93:1702, 1996.

Davis OK, Hawkins DS, Rubin LP, et al: Serum parathyroid hormone (PTH) in pregnant women determined by an immunoradiometric assay for intact PTH. J Clin Endocrinol Metab 67:850, 1988.

Deeb AA, Bruce SN, Morris AAM, Cheetham TD: Infantile hypophosphatasia: Disappointing results of treatment. Acta Paediatr 89:740, 2000.

Demarini S, Mimouni F, Tsang RC, et al: Impact of metabolic control of diabetes during pregnancy on neonatal hypocalcemia: A randomized study. Obstet Gynecol 83:918, 1994.

Demczuk S, Levy A, Aubry M, et al: Excess of deletions of maternal origin in the DiGeorge/velo-cardio-facial syndromes: A study of 22 new patients and a review of the literature. Hum Genet 96:9, 1996.

Diaz GA, Gelb BD, Ali F, et al: Sanjad-Sakati and autosomal recessive Kenny-Caffey syndromes are allelic: Evidence for an ancestral founder mutation and locus refinement. Am J Med Genet 85:48, 1999.

Dobnig H, Kainer F, Stepan V, et al: Elevated parathyroid hormone-related peptide levels after human gestation: Relationship to changes in bone and mineral metabolism. J Clin Endocrinol Metab 80:3699, 1995.

Downing GJ, Egelhoff JC, Daily DK, et al: Kidney function in very low-birth-weight infants with furosemide-related renal calcifications at ages 1 to 2 years. J Pediatr 120:599, 1992.

Drummond KN, Michael AF, Ulstrom RA, Good RA: The blue diaper syndrome: Familial hypercalcemia with nephrocalcinosis and indicanuria: A new familial disease, with definition of the metabolic abnormality. Am J Med 37:928, 1964.

D'Souza-Li L, Yang B, Canaff L, et al: Identification and functional characterization of novel calcium-sensing receptor mutations in familial hypocalciuric hypercalcemia and autosomal dominant hypocalcemia. J Clin Endocrinol Metab 87:1309, 2002.

Fanconi S, Fischer JA, Wieland P, et al: Kenny syndrome: Evidence for idiopathic hypoparathyroidism in two patients and for abnormal parathyroid hormone in one. J Pediatr 109:469, 1992.

Fewtrell MS, Cole TJ, Bishop NJ, Lucas A: Neonatal factors predicting childhood height in preterm infants: Evidence for a persisting effect of early metabolic bone disease? J Pediatr 137:668, 2000.

Foldenauer A, Vossbeck S, Pohlandt F: Neonatal hypocalcaemia associated with rotavirus diarrhoea. Eur J Pediatr 157:838, 1998.

Fridriksson JH, Helmrath MA, Wessel JJ, Warner BW: Hypercalcemia associated with extracorporeal life support in neonates. J Pediatr Surg 36:493, 2001.

Gertner JM, Coustan DR, Kliger AS, et al: Pregnancy as a state of physiologic absorptive hypercalciuria. Am J Med 81:451, 1986.

Giapros VI, Andronikou S, Cholevas VI, Papadopoulou ZL: Renal function in premature infants during aminoglycoside therapy. Pediatr Nephrol 9:163, 1995.

Grant FD, Conlin PR, Brown EM: Rate and concentration dependence of parathyroid hormone dynamics during stepwise changes in serum ionized calcium in normal humans. J Clin Endocrinol Metab 71:370, 1990.

Hicks MJ, Levy ML, Alexander J, Flaitz CM: Subcutaneous fat necrosis of the newborn and hypercalcemia: Case report and review of the literature. Pediatr Dermatol 10:271, 1993.

Ibdah JA, Dasouki MJ, Strauss AW: Long-chain 3-hydroxylacyl-CoA dehydrogenase deficiency: Variable expressivity of maternal illness during pregnancy and unusual presentation with infantile cholestasis and hypocalcaemia. J Inher Metab Dis 22:811, 1999.

Igarashi T, Sekine Y, Kawato H, et al: Transient neonatal distal renal tubular acidosis with secondary hyperparathyroidism. Pediatr Nephrol 6:267, 1992.

Ilves P, Kiisk M, Soopold T, Talvik T: Serum total magnesium and ionized calcium concentrations in asphyxiated term newborn infants with hypoxic-ischaemic encephalopathy. Acta Paediatr 89:680, 2000.

Kamitsuka MD, Williams MA, Nyberg DA, et al: Renal calcification: A complication of dexamethasone therapy in preterm infants with bronchopulmonary dysplasia. J Perinatol 15:359, 1995.

Kantorovich V, Adams JS, Gaines JE, et al: Genetic heterogeneity in familial renal magnesium wasting. J Clin Endocrinol Metab 87:612, 2002.

Karlen J, Aperia A, Zetterstrom R: Renal excretion of calcium and phosphate in preterm and term infants. J Pediatr 106:814, 1985.

Kent GN, Price RI, Gutteridge DH, et al: The efficiency of intestinal calcium absorption is increased in late pregnancy but not in established lactation. Calcif Tissue Int 48:293, 1991.

Knisely AS, Magid MS, Felix JC, Singer DB: Parathyroid gland hemorrhage in perinatally lethal osteogenesis imperfects. J Pediatr 112:720, 1988.

Kovacs CS, Lanske B, Hunzelman JL, et al: Parathyroid hormone–related peptide (PTHrP) regulates fetal-placental calcium transport through a receptor distinct from the PTH/PTHrP receptor. Proc Natl Acad Sci U S A 93:15233, 1996.

Kovacs CS, Manley NR, Moseley JM, et al: Fetal parathyroids are not required to maintain placental calcium transport. J Clin Invest 107:1007, 2001.

Kreiter SR, Schwartz RP, Kirkman HN Jr, et al: Nutritional rickets in African American breast-fed infants. J Pediatr 137:153, 2000.

Kruse K, Irle U, Uhlig R: Elevated 1,25-dihydroxyvitamin D serum concentrations in infants with subcutaneous fat necrosis. J Pediatr 122:460, 1993.

Lewis DW: What was wrong with Tiny Tim? Am J Dis Child 146:1403, 1992.

Lienhardt A, Bai M, Lagarde J-P, et al: Activating mutations of the calcium-sensing receptor: management of hypocalcemia. J Clin Endocrinol Metab 86:5323, 2001.

Lightwood RL: Idiopathic hypercalcemia with failure to thrive. Arch Dis Child 27:302, 1952.

Liu J, Litman D, Rosenberg MJ, et al: A *GNAS1* imprinting defect in pseudohypoparathyroidism type 1B. J Clin Invest 106:1167, 2000.

Lynch BJ, Rust RS: Natural history and outcome of neonatal hypocalcemic and hypomagnesemic seizures. Pediatr Neurol 11:23, 1994.

Meliones JN, Moler FW, Custer JR, et al: Normalization of priming solution ionized calcium concentration improves hemodynamic stability of neonates receiving venovenous ECMO. ASAIO J 41:884, 1995.

Mimouni F, Tsang RC, Hertzberg VS, Miodovnik M: Polycythemia, hypomagnesemia and hypocalcemia in infants of diabetic mothers. Am J Dis Child 140:798, 1986.

Minagawa M, Yasuda T, Kobayashi Y, Niimi H: Transient pseudohypoparathyroidism of the neonate. Eur J Endocrinol 133:151, 1995.

Moyer-Mileur L, Brunstetter V, McNaught TP, et al: Daily physical activity program increases bone mineralization and growth in preterm very low birth weight infants. Pediatrics 106:1088, 2000.

Murer H, Biber J: Molecular mechanisms in renal phosphate reabsorption. Nephrol Dial Transplant 10:1501, 1995.

Mustafa A, Bigras JL, McCrindle BW: Dilated cardiomyopathy as a first sign of nutritional vitamin D deficiency in infancy. Can J Cardiol 16:699, 1999.

Nako Y, Fukushima N, Tomomasa T, et al: Hypervitaminosis D after prolonged feeding with a premature formula. Pediatrics 92:862, 1993.

Nishiyama S, Tomoeda S, Inoue F, et al: Self-limited neonatal familial hyperparathyroidism associated with hypercalciuria and renal tubular acidosis in three siblings. Pediatrics 86:421, 1990.

Ng PC, Lam CWK, Wong GWK, et al: Changes in markers of bone metabolism during dexamethasone treatment for chronic lung disease I preterm infants. Arch Dis Child 86:F49, 2002.

Pattaragarn A, Alon US: Antacid-induced rickets in infancy. Clin Pediatr 40:389, 2001.

Pittard WB 3rd, Geddes KM, Hulsey TC, Hollis BW: Osteocalcin, skeletal alkaline phosphatase, and bone mineral content in very low-birth-weight infants: A longitudinal assessment. Pediatr Res 31:181, 1992.

Popp D, Zieger B, Schmitt-Graff A, et al: Malignant osteopetrosis obscured by maternal vitamin D deficiency in a neonate. Eur J Pediatr 158:412, 2000.

Pronicka E, Kulczyka H, Lorenc R, et al: Increased serum level of 1,25-dihydroxy-vitamin $D_3$ after parathyroid hormone in the normocalcemic phase of idiopathic hypercalcemia. J Pediatr 112:930, 1988.

Rantonen T, Kaapa P, Jalonen J, et al: Antenatal magnesium sulphate exposure is associated with prolonged parathyroid hormone suppression in preterm neonates. Acta Paediatr 90:278, 2001.

Rauch F, Schoenau E: Skeletal development in premature infants: A review of bone physiology beyond nutritional aspects. Arch Dis Child 86:F82, 2002.

Reeve LE, Chesney RW, DeLuca HF: Vitamin D of human milk: Identification of biologically active forms. Am J Clin Nutr 36:122,1982.

Robertie PG, Butterworth JF 4th, Prielipp RC, et al: Parathyroid hormone in marked hypocalcemia in infants and young children undergoing repair of congenital heart disease. J Am Coll Cardiol 20:672, 1992.

Rodd C, Goodyer P: Hypercalcemia of the newborn: Etiology, evaluation, and management. Pediatr Nephrol 13:542, 1999.

Rodriguez-Soriano J, Vallo A: Pathophysiology of the renal acidification defect present in the syndrome of familial hypomagnesaemia-hypercalciuria. Pediatr Nephrol 8:431, 1994.

Ross R, Halbert K, Tsang RC: Determination of the production and metabolic clearance rates of 1,25-dihydroxyvitamin $D_3$ in the pregnant sheep and its chronically catheterized fetus by primed infusion technique. Pediatr Res 26:633, 1989.

Rubin LP, Posillico JT, Anast CS, Brown EM: Circulating levels of biologically active and immunoreactive intact parathyroid hormone in human newborns. Pediatr Res 29:201, 1991.

Rubin LP, Yeung B, Vouros P, et al: Evidence for human placental synthesis of 24,25-dihydroxyvitamin $D_3$ and 23,25-dihydroxy vitamin $D_3$. Pediatr Res 34:98, 1993.

Ryan AK, Goodship JA, Wilson DI, et al: Spectrum of clinical features associated with interstitial chromosome 22 q 11 deletions: A European collaborative study. J Med Genet 34:798, 1997.

Ryan SW, Truscott J, Simpson M, James J: Phosphate, alkaline phosphatase and bone mineralization in preterm infants. Acta Paediatr 82:516, 1993.

Saarela T, Simila S, Koivisto M: Hypercalcemia and nephrocalcinosis in patients with congenital lactase deficiency. J Pediatr 127:920, 1995.

Saggese G, Baroncelli GI, Bertelloni S, et al: Intact parathyroid hormone levels during pregnancy, in healthy term neonates and in hypocalcemic preterm infants. Acta Paediatr Scand 80:36, 1991.

Sanjad SA, Sakati NA, Abu Osba YK, et al: A new syndrome of congenital hypoparathyroidism, seizure, growth failure and dysmorphic features. Arch Dis Child 66:193, 1991.

Sargent JD, Stukel TA, Kresel J, Klein RZ: Normal values for random urinary calcium to creatinine ratios in infancy. J Pediatr 123:393, 1993.

Savani RC, Mimouni F, Tsang RC: Maternal and neonatal hyperparathyroidism as a consequence of maternal renal tabular acidosis. Pediatrics 91:661, 1993.

Schanler RJ, Rifka M: Calcium, phosphorus and magnesium needs for the low-birth-weight infant. Acta Paediatr Suppl 405:111, 1994.

Schipani E, Langman CB, Parfitt AM, et al: Constitutively activated receptors for parathyroid hormone and parathyroid hormoneBrelated peptide in Jansen's metaphyseal chondrodysplasia. N Engl J Med 335:736, 1996.

Schlingmann KP, Weber S, Peters M, et al: Hypomagnesemia with secondary hypocalcemia is caused by mutations in *TRPM6*, a new member of the *TRPM* gene family. Nat Genet 31:166, 2002.

Seely EW, Brown EM, DeMaggio DM, et al: A prospective study of calciotropic hormones in pregnancy and postpartum: Reciprocal changes in serum intact parathyroid hormone and 1,25-dihydroxyvitamin D. Am J Obstet Gynecol 176:214, 1997.

Seow WK: A study of the development of the permanent dentition in very-low-birth weight children. Pediatr Dent 18:379, 1996.

Shalev H, Phillip M, Galil A, et al: Clinical presentation and outcome in primary familial hypomagnesaemia. Arch Dis Child 78:127, 1998.

Shaw NJ, Pal BR: Vitamin D deficiency in UK Asian families: Activating a new concern. Arch Dis Child 86:147, 2002.

Shimizu H, Kodama S, Takeuchi A, et al: Idiopathic infantile hypercalcemia discovered in the newborn period. Acta Paediatr Jpn 36:720, 1994.

Simon DB, Lu Y, Choate KA, et al: Paracellin-1, a renal tight junction protein required for paracellular $Mg^{2+}$ resorption. Science 285:103, 1999.

Srinivasan M, Abinun M, Cant AJ, et al: Malignant infantile osteopetrosis presenting with neonatal hypocalcaemia. Arch Dis Child Fetal Neonatal Ed 83:F21, 2000.

Sunthornthevarakul T, Churesigaew S, Ngowngarmratana S: A novel mutation of the signal peptide of the preproparathyroid hormone gene associated with autosomal recessive familial isolated hypoparathyroidism. J Clin Endocrinol Metab 84:3792, 1999.

Tanaka Y, Hatano S, Nishi Y, Usui T: Nutritional copper deficiency in a Japanese infant on formula. J Pediatr 96:255, 1980.

Tomomura A, Tomomura M, Fukushige T, et al: Molecular cloning and expression of serum calcium-decreasing factor (caldecrin). J Biol Chem 270:30315, 1995.

Trotter A, Maier L, Grill HJ, et al: Effects of postnatal estradiol and progesterone replacement in extremely preterm infants. J Clin Endocrinol Metab 84:4525, 1999.

Urban Z, Helms C, Gerardo A, et al: 7q11.23 deletions in Williams syndrome arise as a consequence of unequal meiotic crossover [letter]. Am J Hum Genet 59:958, 1996.

Walder RY, Landau D, Meyer P, et al: Mutation of *TRPM6* causes familial hypomagnesemia with secondary hypocalcemia. Nat Genet 31:171, 2002.

Walton R, Bijvoet O: Nomogram for the derivation of renal threshold phosphate concentration. Lancet 2:309, 1975.

Weinstein RS, Jilka RL, Parfitt AM, Manolagas SC: Inhibition of osteoblastogenesis and promotion of apoptosis of osteoblasts and osteocytes by glucocorticoids. Potential mechanisms of their deleterious effects on bone. J Clin Invest 102:274, 1998.

Welch TR, Bergstrom WH, Tsang RC: Vitamin D-deficient rickets: The reemergence of a once-conquered disease. J Pediatr 137:143, 2000.

Yamagishi H, Garg V, Matsuoka R, et al: A molecular pathway revealing a genetic basis for human cardiac and craniofacial defects. Science 283:1158, 1999.

Zamora SA, Rizzoli R, Belli DC, et al: Vitamin D supplementation during infancy is associated with higher bone mineral mass in prepubertal girls. J Clin Metab Endocrinol 84:4541, 1999.

Zanardo V, Dani C, Trevisanuto D, et al: Methylxanthines increase renal calcium excretion in preterm infants. Biol Neonate 68:169, 1995.

CHAPTER

# 90

# Disorders of the Adrenal Gland

Kathleen E. Bethin and Louis J. Muglia

Normal adrenal function is critically important for maintenance of intrauterine homeostasis, promotion of organ maturation, and adaptation to extrauterine life. As further testimony to the importance of the adrenal in perinatal adaptation, in some species, fetal glucocorticoid production serves as the trigger for parturition (Challis and Lye, 1994; Gross et al, 2000). Failure to recognize adrenal disease in the newborn, analogous to adrenal insufficiency in adults, has dire, often life-threatening consequences.

The mature adrenal consists of cortical steroidogenic cells and medullary chromaffin catecholamine-producing cells. The catecholamine-producing cells of the adrenal medulla arise from neural crest cells that migrate during intrauterine development from their paraspinal site of origin into the primitive adrenocortical condensation and serve as an endocrine arm of the sympathetic nervous system. This chapter focuses on the development, function, and pathophysiology of the steroidogenic adrenal cortex.

In the neonate, as in the adult, the adrenal cortex produces glucocorticoids and mineralocorticoids as its primary functional products. The fetal adrenal additionally must generate copious amounts of dehydroepiandrosterone sulfate (DHEAS) to serve as a substrate for placental estradiol and estriol production during pregnancy (Mesiano and Jaffe, 1997). The mammalian adrenal has accomplished the ability to preferentially produce a given steroid as its main product by the presence or absence of steroidogenic enzymes in discrete compartments. The DHEAS-producing fetal cortex lacks 3β-hydroxysteroid dehydrogenase (Mesiano and Jaffe, 1997); the aldosterone-producing zona glomerulosa of the adult cortex lacks 17-hydroxylase but produces a unique form of 11-hydroxylase that also possesses aldosterone synthase activity (White et al, 1994); and the glucocorticoid-producing zona fasciculata of the adult cortex lacks aldosterone synthase activity but produces 17-hydroxylase/17,20-lyase for generation of glucocorticoids and androgens, respectively (Fig. 90–1). The zona reticularis does not appear as a discrete histologic region of the adrenal until the middle of the first decade of life and is associated with increased adrenal androgen production (adrenarche).

Cortisol and aldosterone, the primary glucocorticoid and mineralocorticoid, respectively, in humans, modulate cellular function by interaction with high affinity receptors located in the cytoplasm in the non–ligand-bound state (Truss and Beato, 1993). Products of two different genes exhibit high-affinity glucocorticoid binding: the mineralocorticoid (type I) receptor and the glucocorticoid (type II) receptor. When ligand is bound, the receptor undergoes a conformational change such that the chaperone proteins that normally mask the receptor's nuclear translocation sequence are exposed, allowing dimerization and subsequent entry into the nucleus, where specific genes are either activated or repressed by a variety of recently elucidated mechanisms (Collingwood et al, 1999). Primary adrenal insufficiency often combines defects in mineralocorticoid and glucocorticoid production and subsequent actions through their receptors in target tissues. Defects in mineralocorticoid action may result in dramatic salt-wasting crises in the first week of life; isolated glucocorticoid deficiency as occurs in secondary and tertiary hypoadrenalism (defects of the pituitary and hypothalamus, respectively) causes substantial morbidity as well. Glucocorticoids regulate carbohydrate metabolism (Van Cauter et al, 1992), free water excretion (Green et al, 1970), vascular tone (Munck and Guyre, 1984), and the inflammatory response (Chrousos, 1995), although the essential actions of glucocorticoids remain uncertain. Recent studies in mice deficient in the glucocorticoid receptor (Cole et al, 1995) or corticotropin-releasing hormone (CRH) (Muglia et al, 1995; Muglia et al, 1999) have demonstrated an essential role for glucocorticoids in promoting lung maturation. Of interest, CRH-deficient offspring of heterozygous parents survive normally, but CRH-deficient offspring of CRH-deficient parents die on the first day of life due to abnormal lung development. The placenta possesses a significant amount of 11β-hydroxysteroid dehydrogenase and is capable of metabolizing glucocorticoid to inactive products (Pepe and Albrecht, 1990). The findings in CRH-deficient mice, however, implicate the ability of maternal glucocorticoid to cross the placenta and maintain appropriate tissue maturation if the fetus is glucocorticoid deficient and may explain why infants with congenital adrenal hyperplasia (CAH) or other states of inadequate glucocorticoid production do not exhibit overt pulmonary insufficiency.

## CONTROL OF GLUCOCORTICOID AND MINERALOCORTICOID PRODUCTION

Two distinct regulatory circuits control adrenal glucocorticoid and mineralocorticoid secretion. The hypothalamic-pituitary-adrenal (HPA) axis determines the set point for circulating glucocorticoid (cortisol) concentration. The neuropeptide corticotropin-releasing hormone (CRH) and arginine vasopressin are synthesized in the hypothalamic paraventricular nucleus and released into the hypophysial portal circulation at the median eminence in response to stress (Aguilera, 1994) and, beginning at approximately 6 months of age (Onishi et al, 1983), to circadian cues. These neuropeptides stimulate release of adrenocorticotropin—adrenocorticotropic hormone (ACTH)—from anterior pituitary corticotrophs. ACTH released into the systemic circulation augments adrenocortical secretion of DHEAS and cortisol by acting on the ACTH receptor (Clark and Cammas, 1996), a member of the melanocortin receptor family. The ACTH receptor is present on

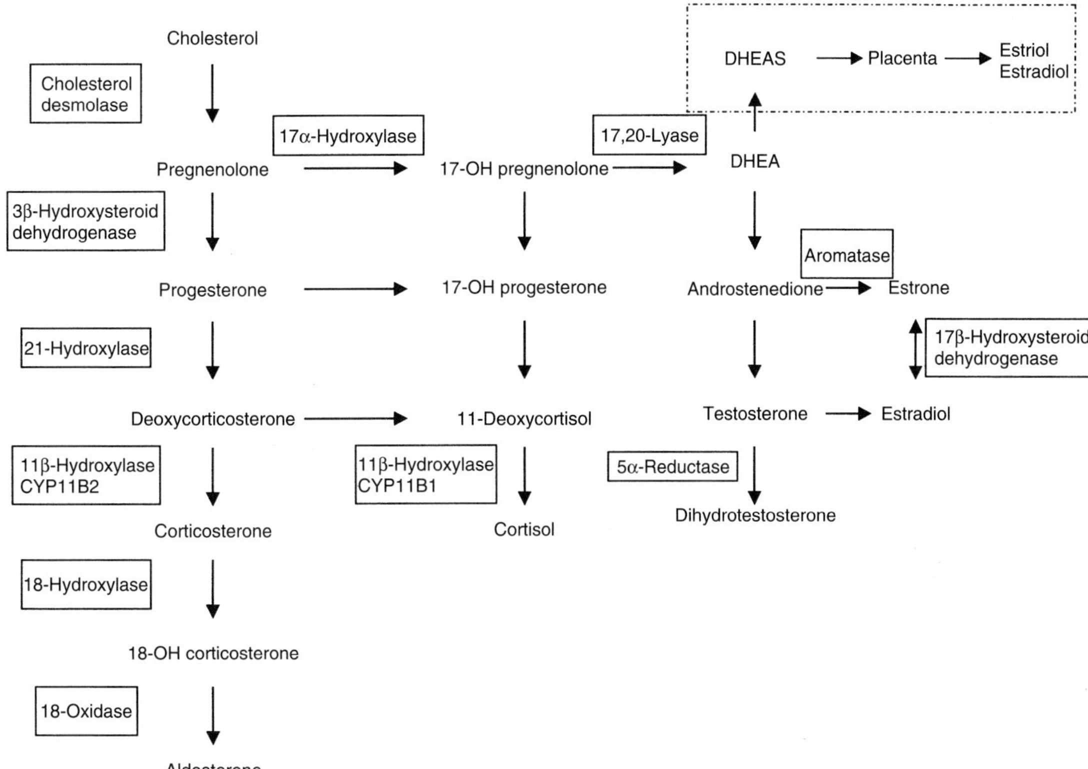


**FIGURE 90–1.** Steroid biosynthetic pathways. The synthesis of cortisol, aldosterone, testosterone, and estrogen from cholesterol is shown. The enzymes that catalyze the reactions are indicated in *boxes*. The *dashed box* outlines the pathway of estriol and estradiol synthesis by the placenta from dehydroepiandrosterone sulfate (DHEAS) produced by the fetal adrenal. DHEA, dehydroepiandrosterone.

steroidogenic cells of the fetal zone and transitional zone of the fetal adrenal as well as the adult cortex. The resulting increase in plasma cortisol concentration limits further release of hypothalamic neuropeptides and ACTH by negative feedback through glucocorticoid receptors at central nervous system and pituitary sites. As a corollary, if glucocorticoid production is impaired by intrinsic adrenal dysfunction, neuropeptide and ACTH release are augmented.

The components of the HPA axis are present early in human development (Mesiano and Jaffe, 1997). As detailed later on, the fetal adrenal begins to develop at the fourth week of gestation, a time similar to that for initial evagination of the pituitary primordium (Conklin, 1968). ACTH-producing pituitary cells can be detected at 7 weeks of gestation, and an intact hypophysial portal vascular system by 12 weeks (Baker and Jaffe, 1975; Thliveris and Currie, 1980). Nerve terminals containing CRH can be detected in the hypothalamus by approximately 16 weeks of gestation. Because virilization due to increased production of adrenal androgens in females with congenital adrenal hyperplasia occurs before 12 weeks of gestation, the ACTH-producing corticotrophs probably undergo cortisol-mediated feedback modulation at the initial stages of hypothalamic-pituitary development.

Mineralocorticoid (aldosterone) release by the zona glomerulosa of the adrenal is determined by the renin-angiotensin system, with acute modulation of lower magnitude also by ACTH (Dzau, 1988). Decreases in vascular volume result in increased secretion of renin by the renal juxtaglomerular apparatus. Renin, a proteolytic enzyme, cleaves angiotensinogen to angiotensin I. Angiotensin I is then cleaved and activated by angiotensin-converting enzyme (ACE) in the lung and other peripheral sites to angiotensin II. Angiotensin II and its metabolite angiotensin III possess vasopressor and potent aldosterone secretory activity. Although angiotensin II receptors are present on cells of the definitive zone at 16 weeks of gestation, significant aldosterone production by the fetal adrenal does not occur until the third trimester of pregnancy (Mesiano and Jaffe, 1997).

## ADRENAL DEVELOPMENT

The development of the human adrenal gland begins at approximately the fourth week of gestation and continues through adolescence and young adulthood, as recently reviewed in detail (Mesiano and Jaffe, 1997). The developing adrenal cortex can first be identified as a thickening of coelomic epithelium between the primitive urogenital ridge and the dorsal mesentery. By the eighth week of gestation, the rudimentary adrenal cortex, or adrenal blastema, consists of functionally distinct zones: the fetal zone, definitive zone, and transitional zone (Fig. 90–2) (Mesiano and Jaffe, 1997). It is unclear whether these zones arise from a single progenitor population. During most of embryogenesis, 80% to 90% of the adrenal cortex is made up of the fetal zone, with the remainder consisting of the definitive and transitional zones, destined to become the adult cortex. The fetal zone produces mainly DHEAS due to limited 3β-hydroxysteroid dehydrogenase activity, and the definitive and transitional zones primarily produce corticoids in response to ACTH (Mesiano and Jaffe, 1997). A distinct adrenal medulla does not start to form until the first week of postnatal life and an adult-like medulla is not apparent until 12 to 18 months of life.

Beginning at 8 to 10 weeks of gestation, the fetal adrenal cortex produces significant levels of DHEAS. Production of DHEAS by the fetal adrenal increases throughout pregnancy to very high levels at term. The adrenal-derived DHEAS serves as the critical substrate for placenta estradiol and estriol synthesis. The measurement of these estrogens in maternal serum thus provides a valuable index of steroid-producing function of the fetoplacental unit (Yen, 1991). Cortisol, corticosterone and aldosterone

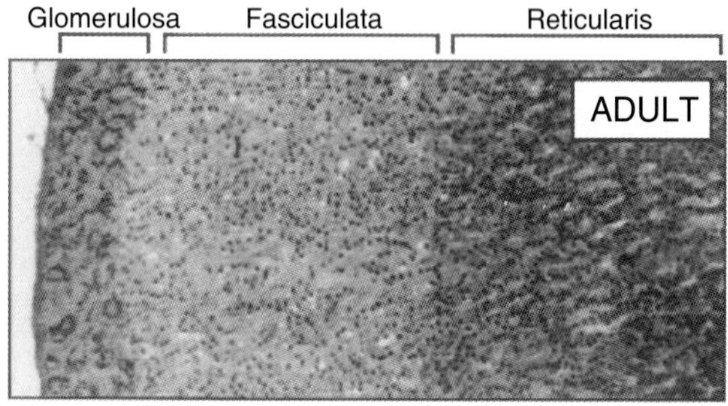


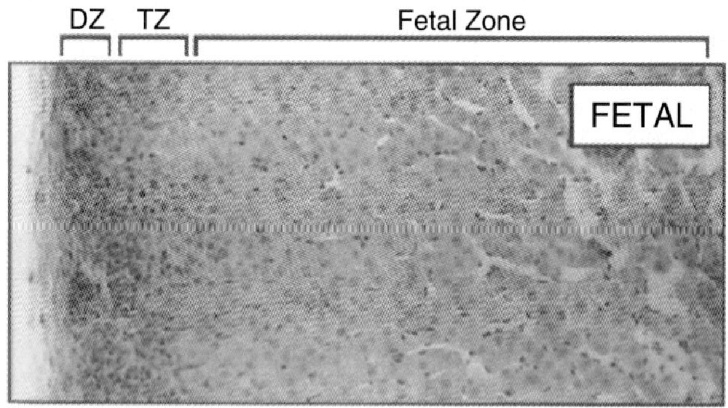


**FIGURE 90–2. Upper panel,** Morphology of the human adult adrenal cortex. The cortex is composed of the zona glomerulosa, zonal fasciculata, and zona reticularis. The adrenal medulla (not shown) is medial to the zona reticularis. **Lower panel,** Morphology of the fetal (midgestation) adrenal cortex. The fetal adrenal cortex is composed primarily of the inner large fetal zone (FZ) and the smaller outer definitive zone (DZ). The transitional zone (TZ) is at the outer edge of the fetal zone. *(Reproduced with permission from Mesiano S, Jaffe RB: Developmental and functional biology of the primate fetal adrenal cortex. Endocr Rev 18:378-403, 1997. Copyright 1997 by The Endocrine Society.)*

production can be detected by 10 to 20 weeks from the fetal adrenal (Partsch et al, 1991).

By 16 to 20 weeks of gestation, the fetal adrenal is dominated by the large steroid-secreting cells of the fetal zone and a narrow band of proliferative cells that represent the definitive zone. By late gestation, the definitive zone resembles the adult zona glomerulosa. A third zone called the transitional zone exists between the fetal and definitive zones. These cells are thought to produce cortisol and, by 30 weeks of gestation, resemble the zona fasciculata (Mesiano and Jaffe, 1997). Postnatally, the adrenal gland undergoes extensive remodeling with the expansion of the preexisting zona glomerulosa and zona fasciculata and apoptosis of the fetal zone.

By 20 weeks of gestation, the adrenal is the size of the fetal kidney, and between 20 and 30 weeks, its size doubles to 10 to 20 times the relative size of the adult adrenal (Mesiano and Jaffe, 1997). This growth is dependent on ACTH, as evidenced by failure of the fetal zone to increase beyond the size of a 15-week embryo in infants with anencephaly and the markedly enlarged fetal zone in infants with CAH. Furthermore, mice and humans with pro-opiomelanocortin (POMC) deficiency demonstrate severe adrenocortical atrophy. Despite this dependence on ACTH for growth of the fetal adrenal gland, plasma ACTH levels fall by almost 50% during the period of most rapid adrenal growth. The explanation for this apparent discrepancy is that the fetal adrenal gland becomes more responsive to ACTH during the second and third trimesters as a result of increased expression of the ACTH receptor. Although ACTH is the principal regulator of fetal adrenal growth, several other factors must be involved in adrenal growth (Mesiano and Jaffe, 1997). In anencephalic infants, the definitive zone is normal and development of the fetal zone is normal until 10 to 15 weeks of gestation (Gray and Abramovich, 1980). Additionally, the fetal zone rapidly involutes once the newborn is delivered and the uterine cord clamped, despite continued ACTH exposure (Gray and Abramovich, 1980).

The molecular basis of adrenal development has recently begun to be elucidated. Several transcription factors are critically important for normal adrenal development. Steroidogenic factor-1 (SF-1), or adrenal 4-binding protein, is a member of the nuclear receptor superfamily (Parker, 1998). SF-1 knockout mice lack adrenals and gonads, and subsequent identification of SF-1 mutations in humans with adrenal insufficiency confirms the essential role of SF-1 in development (Parker, 1998). SF-1 expression is found in the early urogenital ridge of the mouse in cells that give rise to both the bipotential gonad and adrenal cortex. Expression of SF-1 remains high throughout embryogenesis and postnatal and adult life (Parker, 1998).

DAX1 (dosage-sensitive sex reversal–adrenal hypoplasia congenita critical region on the X chromosome) is an orphan nuclear receptor that co-localizes with SF-1 in the cells of the adrenals, gonads, gonadotropes, and ventral-medial lateral nucleus of the hypothalamus. Deletion of DAX1 results in adrenal hypoplasia congenita. Although the exact role of DAX1 in adrenal development is not known, it has been shown to interact with SF-1 (Ikeda et al, 2001). Normally, DAX1 recruits the nuclear corepressor N-CoR to SF-1 and represses SF-1 (Crawford et al, 1998).

Similarly, the *WT1* (Wilms tumor gene) protein has been shown to interact with SF-1. *WT1* encodes 24 different protein isoforms that act as transcription factors. *WT1* is detected in the urogenital ridge of the mouse embryo but is not detected in adult or fetal adrenals. Mutations in *WT1* have resulted in abnormal development of the adrenal in the mouse but have not been clearly correlated with abnormal human adrenal development (Vidal and Schedl, 2000).

## ASSESSING ADRENAL FUNCTION IN THE NEWBORN

The spectrum of adrenal steroid production changes significantly over the first days and months of life. In determining whether steroidogenic function in the newborn adrenal is "normal," special attention must be given to the age-related changes in adrenal steroid intermediates and circulating cortisol and aldosterone concentrations that reflect ongoing adrenal maturation. The third-trimester fetal zone, the predominant component of the adrenal cortex in the fetus, preferentially produces DHEA and DHEAS as a result of absent 3β-hydroxysteroid dehydrogenase activity. Rapid loss of the fetal zone in the days following birth results in a dramatic fall in circulating DHEA concentration over the first week to 1 month postnatally. DHEA concentrations above 1000 ng/dL are common in healthy newborn males and females on day 1 of life (de Peretti and Forest, 1976; Lee et al, 1989). The variable pattern of decline in the ensuing weeks probably reflects variation in remodeling of the fetal zone and emergence of the zona fasciculata of the adult cortex. In addition to impaired 3β-hydroxysteroid dehydrogenase activity, preterm infants have sustained elevations in 17-hydroxyprogesterone and the 17-hydroxyprogesterone-to-cortisol ratio, suggesting a reduction in 21-hydroxylase activity (Al Saedi et al, 1995; Lee et al, 1989). Because blood-spot 17-hydroxyprogesterone concentration is used as a newborn screen for CAH in many states (Mitchell et al, 1990), many preterm infants initially test abnormal. Subsequent follow-up testing is then required to determine whether CAH is present. Plasma aldosterone concentrations tend to be higher in preterm infants than in term infants also, both of which are higher than in older children and adults (Doerr et al, 1988; Kotchen et al, 1972).

In the ill newborn with hypotension or other evidence of cardiovascular instability, the question often arises as to whether these manifestations reflect underlying glucocorticoid insufficiency. Random plasma cortisol measurement is often inadequate to answer this question, as up to 10% of stressed newborns have low or undetectable cortisol levels but subsequently are capable of mounting an adequate cortisol response to exogenous ACTH administration (Thomas et al, 1986). In these infants, cosyntropin [(1-24)ACTH] testing should be performed for establishing adrenal function. The standard 0.25-mg cosyntropin dose with sampling at 30 or 60 minutes after administration has been widely employed for this purpose, although lower dose cosyntropin testing has been favored in some studies to reveal more subtle deficits in adrenal responsiveness (Korte et al, 1996). In a study by Hingre and colleagues, all prematurely born infants (less than 30 weeks of gestation) that were sick had plasma cortisol levels that were comparable with healthy term infants (Hingre et al, 1994). The failure of stressed newborns, particularly those born prematurely, to mount a cortisol response of the same magnitude as older children and adults may reflect inadequate maturation of steroidogenic enzymes, or could represent the human counterpart of the stress-hyporesponsive period that has been extensively documented in studies of newborn animals (Dent et al, 2000; Sapolsky and Meaney, 1986). In the stress hyporesponsive period, the pituitary releases minimal ACTH in response to stress resulting in little adrenocortical activity.

## DISORDERS OF ADRENAL INSUFFICIENCY

### Neonatal Primary Adrenal Insufficiency

#### Biosynthetic Defects

##### *Congenital Adrenal Hyperplasia*

Enzymatic defects of steroid metabolism are one of the most common causes of neonatal adrenal insufficiency. The most frequent of these are the enzyme defects that cause CAH. This disorder occurs with any enzyme defect involved in the biosynthesis of cortisol from cholesterol that results in impaired production of cortisol. Loss of negative feedback by cortisol leads to increased secretion of ACTH from the pituitary and hyperplasia of the adrenal cortex. Females with CAH often are recognized at birth because of ambiguous genitalia due to virilization from adrenal androgens produced in excess. The phenotypic features of affected females range from mild clitoromegaly and posterior labial fusion to male-appearing genitalia without palpable testes in the scrotum. Genitalia of males with CAH are not affected unless the enzyme defect leads to decreased testosterone production, as seen with 3β-hydroxysteroid dehydrogenase deficiency. In this case, inadequate virilization occurs. Newborns with CAH may also present with hyperpigmentation, hypoglycemia, or acidosis. Depending on the degree of enzyme activity, patients with CAH may have either simple virilizing CAH or salt-wasting CAH. Infants with salt-wasting CAH do not exhibit salt-wasting until 5 to 15 days of life. Accordingly, males with undiagnosed salt-wasting CAH often present in adrenal crisis 1 to 2 weeks after birth (New, 1995; White and Speiser, 2000).

The most common form of CAH is 21-hydroxylase deficiency, inherited as an autosomal recessive trait, with an incidence of approximately 1/15,000 worldwide. The incidence may be as high as 1/300 in certain ethnic populations, such as the Yupik Eskimos of Alaska. A defect in 21-hydroxylase results in abnormally high levels of its substrate, 17-hydroxyprogesterone, and the androgens androstenedione and DHEA. These excess androgens result in virilization of affected female infants (Miller, 1991; New, 1995; White, 2001; White and Speiser, 2000).

The molecular biology of the 21-hydroxylase locus has been extensively characterized. There are two homologous genes within the class III region of the major histocompatibility locus on chromosome 6p21.3 that encode

21-hydroxylase and a related pseudogene. *P450c21B*, or *CYP21*, is the active gene; the pseudogene *P450c21A*, or *CYP21P*, contains at least nine different mutations. *CYP21P* and *CYP21* are 98% identical and therefore frequently recombine, resulting in most of the known mutations that cause CAH. Gene deletions and gene conversions in the homozygous form all cause the salt-losing form of CAH, although many point mutations also cause salt-losing CAH. Approximately 20% of mutations are a deletion of the 3′ end of *CYP21P*, *C4B*, which encodes the fourth component of complement, and the first 3 to 7 exons of *CYP21*, resulting in a nonfunctional hybrid gene composed of the 5′ end of *CYP21P* and the 3′ end of *CYP21*. Another 20% to 25% of mutations are a point mutation in intron 2 of *CYP21*, resulting in an abnormally spliced product (Miller, 1991; White, 2001; White and Speiser, 2000). If there is an affected proband, defects in *CYP21* can be detected by polymerase chain reaction (PCR) analysis of polymorphic microsatellite markers based on linkage analysis (New et al, 2001; White and Speiser, 2000). Postnatally, a defect in 21-hydroxylase activity can be detected by measuring elevated 17-hydroxyprogesterone and adrenal androgens after day 2 of life. Many states measure 17-hydroxyprogesterone levels on the standard newborn screen.

Although biochemical evaluation is required for diagnosis of CAH, imaging methods can be useful in the evaluation of suspected adrenal disorders. In an infant with genital ambiguity, a pelvic ultrasound examination to look for the presence of a uterus is helpful in identifying a virilized female. Ultrasonography also is the preferred imaging modality for evaluation of the adrenals in the neonate. The adrenals of the neonate are easier to visualize by ultrasound examination than the adult glands, because the adrenals relative to the kidneys are much larger, there is decreased perirenal fat, and the adrenals are more superficially located (Ghiacy et al, 1985). Neonates with CAH tend to have longer and wider adrenals than those in normal infants (Sivit et al, 1991). In addition, neonates with CAH tend to have abnormal surface characteristics and echogeneicity of their adrenals when compared with neonates with ambiguous genitalia of other causes. When all three characteristics are studied, adrenal ultrasound examination has a specificity of 92% and sensitivity of 100% in detecting CAH (Al-Alwan et al, 1999).

Although far less common than 21-hydroxylase deficiency, 11β-hydroxylase or 3β-hydroxysteroid dehydrogenase deficiency also needs to be considered in an infant suspected of having CAH. Mutations in *CYP11B1* (*P450c11*) cause 11β-hydroxylase deficiency. *CYP11B1* is a mitochondrial enzyme that catalyzes the 11β-hydroxylation of 11-deoxycortisol to cortisol. *CYP11B2* encodes aldosterone synthase, which 11-hydroxylates 11-deoxycorticosterone (DOC) to corticosterone and 18-hydroxylates and then 18-oxidizes corticosterone to aldosterone. *CYP11B1* and *CYP11B2* are 40 kilobases apart on chromosome 8q24 and are 95% identical within the coding region. Affected females are virilized because of high DHEA and androstenedione levels. Diagnosis is made by measuring high levels of 11-deoxycortisol. Because DOC has mineralocorticoid activity and also is elevated in 11β-hydroxylase deficiency, affected patients usually maintain normal sodium levels, have suppressed plasma renin activity, and may be hypertensive or hypokalemic. However, newborns may have mild transient salt loss. Mutations in *CYP11B2* result in deficiencies of 18-hydroxylase or 18-methyl oxidase activity with normal 11-hydroxylase activity. Because aldosterone does not "feed back" to ACTH, affected patients have salt loss and hyperreninemia without virilization or hyperpigmentation. In addition, these newborns are not deficient in cortisol, so hypoglycemia is not a problem (White et al, 1994).

3β-hydroxysteroid dehydrogenase deficiency is rare. Affected females show mild virilization because of the androgenic effects of large amounts of DHEA caused by this enzyme deficiency. Affected males are undervirilized because 3β-hydroxysteroid dehydrogenase is necessary for testosterone production. These patients also tend to have severe mineralocorticoid deficiencies. There are two isoenzymes for 3β-hydroxysteroid dehydrogenase (HSD). The type I enzyme is expressed in the placenta, skin, and adipose tissue; the type II enzyme is expressed in the adrenals and gonads. *HSD3B1* and *HSD3B2* encode active enzymes and are located on chromosome 1p11-13. The classic form of 3β-hydroxysteroid dehydrogenase deficiency is caused by mutations in *HSD3B2*. Because the *HSD3B1* is unaffected, steroid biosynthesis in the placenta is normal (White, 2001).

Other enzymatic defects in the cortisol synthesis pathway also may cause adrenal insufficiency but are exceedingly rare. 17α-hydroxylase/17,20-lyase deficiency (P450c17) has been reported in 120 persons. These patients overproduce deoxycorticosterone and cannot produce testosterone. Therefore, affected patients retain sodium and are hypertensive. Affected male patients have incomplete sexual development, and affected females are phenotypically normal but fail to undergo adrenarche and puberty (Miller, 1991).

Another rare recessive condition that also causes adrenal insufficiency and 46,XY sex reversal is congenital lipoid adrenal hyperplasia (StAR [*st*eroidogenic *a*cute *r*egulatory] protein deficiency). The defective gene is on chromosome 8 and encodes the StAR protein, which transports cholesterol from the outer to the inner mitochondrial membrane (Lin et al, 1995).

### Familial Glucocorticoid Deficiency and Adrenoleukodystrophy

Familial isolated glucocorticoid deficiency is a rare autosomal recessive disorder. Affected infants demonstrate adrenal unresponsiveness to ACTH and severe glucocorticoid deficiency without mineralocorticoid deficiency. Affected patients may present in the neonatal period with hypoglycemia, hyperpigmentation, muscle weakness, or seizures. Several affected families have defects in the coding region of the ACTH receptor (MC2R) gene. However, many other affected families have no detectable mutation and may have a postreceptor defect. Allgrove or triple A syndrome is a similar disorder that combines alacrima and achalasia with adrenal insufficiency. Some of these families have a defect in the *AAAS* (*a*lacrima–*a*chalasia–*a*drenal insufficiency *s*yndrome) gene, which is postulated to be involved in either cytoplasmic trafficking or peroxisomal activities (Allolio and Reincke, 1997; Stratakis et al, 1994; Weber and Clark, 1994; Weber et al, 1995; Yamaoka et al, 1992).

Neonatal adrenoleukodystrophy (NALD) is a fatal autosomal recessive disease of impaired peroxisome biogenesis. NALD belongs to a class of disorders involving peroxisomal biogenesis, including Zellweger syndrome and infantile Refsum disease. NALD is the only one of the three diseases that often involves adrenal insufficiency. NALD is a result of a defect in peroxisome biogenesis. Mutations in seven different peroxisome biogenesis factors have been shown to cause NALD (Moser, 1999). Mutations in PEX1 (peroxisome biogenesis factor 1), a member of the AAA ATPase family, are the most common cause of NALD (Tamura et al, 2001). As in X-linked adrenoleukodystrophy, patients with NALD accumulate very long-chain fatty acids and develop degenerative changes of the white matter of the nervous system and adrenal atrophy. Infants with NALD characteristically demonstrate dolichocephaly, prominent and high forehead, esotropia, epicanthic folds, broad nasal bridge, high-arched palate, low-set ears, and anteverted nostrils. Affected patients usually die in early childhood (Moser, 1999; Tamura et al, 2001; Walter et al, 2001). X-linked adrenoleukodystrophy (X-ALD) is a recessively inherited X-linked defect of the adrenoleukodystrophy protein. It is also a peroxisomal defect that usually results in adrenal insufficiency and CNS deterioration. However, X-ALD does not usually manifest before early childhood and often manifests later (Laureti et al, 1996; Moser et al, 1984).

### *Other Adrenal Diseases*

The clinical picture of adrenal insufficiency and 46,XY gonadal dysgenesis may be caused by a deficiency of 7-dehydrocholesterol C-7 reductase, or Smith-Lemli-Opitz syndrome. The biochemical abnormalities of this syndrome include low cholesterol and high 7-dehydrocholesterol (Bialer et al, 1987; Tint et al, 1995). Other symptoms that may be exhibited include failure to thrive, altered muscle tone, microcephaly, dysmorphic facies, moderate to severe mental retardation, genitourinary anomalies, and limb anomalies. The incidence of Smith-Lemli-Opitz syndrome in persons of Northern and Central European ancestries is 1/20,000 to 1/30,000 (Jones, 1997).

Complete deficiency of lysosomal esterase also may result in adrenal insufficiency in Wolman disease, a rare autosomal recessive disease. Wolman disease usually is fatal in the first year of life. Affected infants exhibit mild mental retardation, hepatosplenomegaly, vomiting, diarrhea, growth failure, and adrenal calcifications. Calcifications that delineate the outline of both adrenals are pathognomonic for this condition (Anderson et al, 1994; Wolman, 1995).

## Acquired Adrenal Insufficiency

The incidence of adrenal hemorrhage in the neonate is reported to be 1.7 cases per 1000 autopsied infants and as high as 3% of infants screened by abdominal ultrasound examination. The etiology of neonatal adrenal hemorrhage is unknown, but it has been associated with birth trauma related to difficult deliveries, sepsis, coagulopathies, traumatic shock, and ischemic disorders. Infants with minimal hemorrhage may be asymptomatic and discovered incidentally to have adrenal calcifications, indicating an earlier hemorrhage. Major adrenal hemorrhage may manifest as an abdominal mass, anemia from blood loss, or jaundice from reabsorption of the hematoma. Hemorrhage also may lead to adrenal insufficiency, which may manifest as neonatal hypoglycemia, hypotension, hypothermia, apnea, or shock. Because of the location of the right adrenal between the liver and spine, it is the adrenal most often affected by hemorrhage (Velaphi and Perlman, 2001).

*Neisseria meningitidis* is a well-known cause of the Waterhouse-Friderichsen syndrome, or adrenal hemorrhage in association with fulminant septicemia (Enriquez et al, 1990). Other infections in the neonate that have been associated with adrenal hemorrhage and insufficiency include those due to herpesvirus (HSV), *Bacteroides*, herpes simplex virus type 6 (HSV-6), echovirus types 11 and 6 (Bekdash and Slim, 1981; Jain et al, 1996; Morrison et al, 1988; Nakamura et al, 1985; Ohta et al, 1978; Phinney et al, 1982; Schmitt et al, 1996; Ventura et al, 2001).

## Abnormalities of Development: DAX1 and SF-1 Deficiency

Mutations in DAX1 are associated with adrenal hypoplasia congenita (AHC) and have been reported in approximately 70 patients (Achermann et al, 2001). These infants exhibit primary adrenal insufficiency associated with hypogonadotropic, hypogonadism. Approximately 60% of boys with DAX1 mutation present with the typical signs and symptoms of adrenal insufficiency, including failure to thrive, poor weight gain, vomiting, prolonged jaundice, hyperpigmentation, and shock. The remaining patients present during childhood and have a more insidious onset of symptoms, including nausea, weight loss, and hyperpigmentation (Achermann, 2001; Habiby et al, 1996). Correlation between specific DAX1 mutations and age at presentation is lacking. Although DAX1 mutations are rare, 70% of boys with adrenal insufficiency and hypogonadotropic hypogonadism have been shown to have a mutation in DAX1 (Achermann, 2001).

Mutations in SF-1 are even rarer, and only two such patients have been reported (Achermann et al, 2001; Achermann et al, 1999; Biason-Lauber and Schoenle, 2000). The first patient had primary adrenal insufficiency and XY sex reversal (Achermann et al, 1999). The second patient had adrenal insufficiency but normal ovarian function at 27 months of age (Biason-Lauber and Schoenle, 2000). Both patients were heterozygotes for different point mutations in SF-1. The first patient described with an SF-1 mutation with adrenal insufficiency and XY sex reversal exhibited signs of adrenal insufficiency within the first 2 weeks of life and presented with vascular collapse at 17 days of life. In the second case, the patient presented at 14 months of age in adrenal crisis 1 week after the onset of otitis media and tonsillitis.

## Secondary and Tertiary Adrenal Insufficiency

Secondary and tertiary forms of adrenal insufficiency result from defects in pituitary corticotroph and hypothalamic function, respectively. Supraphysiologic doses of glucocorticoids often are used for the treatment of hyaline membrane disease. With prolonged (more than 7 to 10 days) use of supraphysiologic doses of glucocorticoids, these neonates are at risk for iatrogenic suppression of corticotroph ACTH release, with secondary adrenocortical atrophy and adrenal insufficiency (Axelrod, 1976). The duration of recovery of corticotroph function from adrenal suppression, once administration of glucocorticoids is discontinued, is quite variable, with evidence of suppression of the HPA axis evident in some patients for more than 1 year (Livanou et al, 1967). In addition to prolonged use of steroids placing these infants at risk for adrenal suppression, there has recently been a concern that dexamethasone use in preterm infants may adversely affect brain development (Tarnow-Mordi and Mitra, 1999; Thebaud et al, 2001).

Secondary or tertiary adrenal insufficiency in the neonate often is a consequence of abnormalities in development of the hypothalamus and pituitary associated with adrenal insufficiency, including de Morsier syndrome (septo-optic dysplasia) (de Morsier, 1956; Willnow et al, 1996), hydranencephaly or anencephaly, and pituitary hypoplasia or aplasia. If these infants have concomitant diabetes insipidus, they have an increased risk of sudden death during childhood (Brodsky et al, 1997). Patients with developmental abnormalities of the pituitary or hypothalamus often have deficiencies of other hormones. Signs of hypopituitarism in a neonate include hypoglycemia, prolonged jaundice, shock, and microphallus in males. Homozygous inactivating mutations of the pituitary homeobox gene, *HESX1*, have recently been associated with septo-optic dysplasia (Parks et al, 1999; Thomas et al, 2001). Trauma to the hypothalamus, pituitary, or hypophysial portal circulation from significant head injury, cerebrovascular accident, Sheehan syndrome, or hydrocephalus also may be a cause of central adrenal insufficiency. Historic factors associated with increased risk for central adrenal insufficiency include maternal drug use and traumatic delivery.

Least commonly, there have been case reports of families with inherited abnormalities of neuropeptides involved in HPA axis regulation. Adrenal insufficiency, pigmentary abnormalities, and obesity have been described in families with a defect in POMC (Krude et al, 1998; Pernasetti et al, 2000). One kindred has been reported with Arnold-Chiari type I malformation and suspected *CRH* deficiency. The mutation in this kindred is linked to the *CRH* locus; however, a specific mutation in the *CRH* gene has not yet been defined (Kyllo et al, 1996).

## Therapy of Adrenal Insufficiency Disorders

### Primary Adrenal Insufficiency

#### *Chronic Replacement*

Studies in adults and adolescents have determined that the daily production rate of cortisol is 5.7 to 7 mg/m²/day. Because of variable oral absorption, replacement hydrocortisone should be initiated at 10 to 15 mg/m²/day divided three times per day (Esteban et al, 1991; Kerrigan et al, 1993; Linder et al, 1990). Because the bioavailability of oral steroids varies from person to person, infants need to be monitored closely for signs of either inadequate cortisol replacement or cortisol excess (Heazelwood et al, 1984). Although adults and older children may be able to take hydrocortisone twice daily, most infants should be dosed three times daily to avoid hypoglycemia associated with low cortisol on a twice-daily regimen (DeVile and Stanhope, 1997; Groves et al, 1988). Although other steroids may be used, hydrocortisone is preferred in infants because it has less growth suppressive effects than those associated with use of synthetic steroids (Stempfel et al, 1968; Van Metre et al, 1960). In primary adrenal insufficiency, aldosterone production is usually diminished. Physiologic doses of hydrocortisone do not provide enough mineralocorticoid activity to prevent salt wasting, so these infants often require 0.05 to 0.2 mg/day of fludrocortisone acetate (Florinef). Because after the first month of life aldosterone production does not vary, the dose of fludrocortisone does not change with growth and aging (Doerr et al, 1987; Sippel et al, 1978; Weldon et al, 1967). Infants with mineralocorticoid deficiency require 1 to 4 g of NaCl added to their diet, because formula and breast milk are low in salt (Mullis et al, 1990).

#### *Stress Replacement*

The normal response to surgery, trauma, or critical illness is to increase plasma ACTH and cortisol levels. The daily secretion rate of cortisol has been found to be proportional to the degree of stress and ranges from 60 to 167 mg/day in adults after surgery (Chernow et al, 1987; Espiner, 1966; Hume et al, 1962; Ichikawa, 1966; Kehlet and Binder, 1973; Wise et al, 1972). Based on data from adults, it is recommended that infants with adrenal insufficiency receive 30 to 100 mg/m²/day divided every 6 to 8 hours of hydrocortisone when stressed. Stress doses of hydrocortisone should be given with the onset of fever, gastrointestinal or other significant illness, and continued for 24 hours after the symptoms resolve (Miller, 1991; New, 1995; Nickels and Moore, 1989). If oral steroids are not tolerated, an intramuscular or intravenous dose should be given. For surgery, infants should be given 30 to 100 mg/m² of intravenous hydrocortisone on call to the operating room before the administration of anesthesia. Stress dosing for hydrocortisone (30 to 100 mg/m²/day divided every 6 to 8 hours) should be continued postoperatively for the next 24 to 48 hours. Electrolytes should be closely monitored, but changes in the dose of fludrocortisone are not needed.

In the event of a suspected adrenal crisis, blood for determination of electrolytes, aldosterone, plasma renin activity, cortisol, and ACTH should be drawn and treatment started before the results are obtained. Fluid resuscitation with normal saline containing 5% dextrose should be given as a bolus to restore cardiovascular stability. Plasma sodium should be monitored closely, as rapid correction of hyponatremia with sodium repletion of more than 0.5 to 1 mEq/L/hour increases the risk of central pontine myelinolysis. The sodium deficit may be calculated by subtracting the infant's sodium from a "normal" sodium of 140 mEq/L and then multiplying this value by 0.6 × (weight in kg). The rate of replacement should occur over an initial rate such that the sodium increase does not exceed 0.5 mEq/L/hour. Intravenous hydrocortisone should be given initially at 100 mg/m$^2$ and then continued at 100 mg/m$^2$/day divided, every 6 to 8 hours, until the infant is stable. If the diagnosis of adrenal insufficiency is unclear, then an equivalent dose of dexamethasone (2.5 mg/m$^2$/day) should be given in place of the hydrocortisone. Because dexamethasone does not cross-react in standard cortisol assays, it allows a cosyntropin stimulation test to be performed shortly after the initiation of therapy. Long-term dexamethasone therapy is not recommended, as it may be more growth-suppressing than hydrocortisone (Laron and Pertzelan, 1968; Stempfel et al, 1968; Van Metre et al, 1960; White and Speiser, 2000).

### *Special Considerations in Virilizing Forms of Congenital Adrenal Hyperplasia*

Treatment of CAH consists of sufficient cortisol to suppress ACTH production to prevent further virilization and rapid fusion of the growth plates. The dose of cortisol required is usually 10 to 20 mg/m$^2$/day divided, three times per day (New, 1995; White, 2001; White and Speiser, 2000). Thrice-daily therapy is preferable, to adequately suppress adrenal androgen production. Although hydrocortisone is the usual form of therapy because it is less growth suppressing than synthetic steroids (Brook et al, 1974; DiMartino-Nardi et al, 1986; Jaaskelainen and Voutilainen, 1997; New et al, 1989; Silva et al, 1997; Urban et al, 1978), a recent study has shown that some children with CAH may have adequate growth with daily dexamethasone therapy (Rivkees and Crawford, 2000). Patients with salt-losing CAH have elevated plasma renin activity and require mineralocorticoid replacement with 0.05 to 0.2 mg per day of fludrocortisone. Angiotensin II, which is increased by elevations in plasma renin, is a mild stimulator of ACTH secretion (Ames et al, 1965; Rayyis and Horton, 1971; Rosler et al, 1977). Therefore, patients without salt loss but with mildly elevated plasma renin activity may require less hydrocortisone for androgen suppression if fludrocortisone is added to their regimen.

Females born with virilizing forms of CAH often are born with ambiguous genitalia. Recent clinical trials have demonstrated that severity of virilization may be reduced by prenatal treatment of the affected female fetus and mother with dexamethasone. Once a child is born with CAH, there is a 1 in 4 chance that the parents will have another affected child and a 1 in 8 chance that it will be an affected female. In subsequent pregnancies, as soon as the mother knows that she is pregnant, dexamethasone therapy is begun. After diagnosis is made by DNA analysis from chorionic villus sampling at 8 to 12 weeks, therapy in unaffected or male patients is discontinued (Carlson et al, 1999; Miller, 1999; New et al, 2001; Speiser, 1999; White and Speiser, 2000). To date, there have been no congenital abnormalities attributed to dexamethasone therapy (New et al, 2001).

For patients with ambiguous genitalia, corrective surgery is usually performed in stages after birth. Most virilized female infants undergo clitoroplasty during the first year of life (Gonzalez and Fernandes, 1990; Newman et al, 1992), although the timing of gender assignment and surgical correction remains controversial (Schober, 1998; Wilson and Reiner, 1998). As management of CAH has improved, many women with CAH have been able to spontaneously conceive and give birth (Premawardhana et al, 1997).

### Secondary or Tertiary Adrenal Insufficiency

Cortisol replacement for patients with secondary or tertiary adrenal insufficiency is the same as described for patients with primary adrenal insufficiency. To minimize growth suppression, these children may be treated with doses of hydrocortisone that are slightly less than physiologic replacement doses. Furthermore, because mineralocorticoid production is under the control of the renin-angiotensin system, patients with secondary or tertiary adrenal insufficiency do not require mineralocorticoid replacement. However, these infants do require evaluation for deficiencies of other pituitary hormones.

## DISORDERS OF ADRENAL EXCESS

Diseases of adrenal excess are rare in infancy. Adrenocortical tumors are the most common cause of noniatrogenic adrenal excess in infants. The annual incidence of adrenocortical tumors for children below the age of 15 is 0.3 to 0.38 per million children. Presenting signs of an adrenocortical tumor include an abdominal mass, pubic hair, clitoromegaly, hypertrophy of the phallus, hypertension, acne, hirsutism, "moon face," acne, facial hair, weight gain, centripetal fat distribution, accelerated growth velocity, "buffalo hump," and seizures (Mendonca et al, 1995; Sandrini et al, 1997). In one study of 73 children from southern Brazil with adrenocortical tumors, 40% of the children presented with only signs of virilization, 50% presented with signs of virilization and Cushing syndrome, and 3% presented with only signs of Cushing syndrome (Sandrini et al, 1997).

The most important treatment is surgical resection. It is critical to remember that the normal adrenal has been suppressed by dysregulated steroid production by the tumor and that stress doses of hydrocortisone are necessary perioperatively and replacement doses required postoperatively. Chemotherapy has been used on a case-by-case basis but has not been proved as a first-line therapy for adrenocortical tumors in children (Sandrini et al, 1997). Pituitary adenomas or carcinomas are very rare but also may cause Cushing disease or virilization from overproduction of ACTH.

**CASE STUDY 1**

A 20-day-old infant with apparently male phenotype presented to the emergency department with lethargy after refusing to eat for the previous 7 hours. The infant was the 3.235-kg, full-term product of an uncomplicated pregnancy. The newborn examination performed in the nursery identified perineal hypospadias, but the infant was discharged home on day 2 of life. Over the first 2 weeks of life, weight gain was poor, and appetite was markedly decreased over the 1 to 2 days before evaluation in the emergency department. In the emergency department on presentation, the infant was limp and poorly responsive. Initial blood glucose was 30 mg/dL. The infant's mental status was improved after administration of 25% dextrose via an intraosseous line. Resuscitation was continued with dextrose containing normal saline. Initial laboratory values were significant for Na (105 mEq/L), K (8.7 mEq/L), Cl (75 mEq/L), total $CO_2$ (15.8 mEq/L), BUN (40.5 mg/dL), and creatinine (0.6 mg/dL). After the laboratory results were obtained, the infant was given 100 mg/$m^2$ of intravenous hydrocortisone. The physical examination was notable for a weight of 3.1 kg and a phallus with a length of 2.5 cm, a midshaft diameter of 1.5 cm with hypospadias near the perineum, a hyperpigmented and rugated shawl scrotum, and no palpable testes. Family history was significant for a male sibling who died at age 1 week. Additional evaluation revealed 46,XX chromosomes and enlarged adrenals and a small uterus on ultrasound examination. The 17-hydroxyprogesterone concentration was 20,700 ng/dL before hydrocortisone administration. These laboratory results all were consistent with classic salt-wasting 21-hydroxylase deficiency. The infant's electrolytes were normalized over several days, and the infant was discharged home on hydrocortisone, fludrocortisone, and salt supplementation.

### *Comment*

An important point in this case is that the presence of bilateral undescended testes, with or without other evidence of genitourinary anomalies, should be considered ambiguous genitalia and merits further work-up in the immediate perinatal period. Additionally, the institution of state newborn screening for elevated 17-hydroxyprogesterone may allow earlier detection of salt-wasting 21-hydroxylase deficiency, before occurrence of a life-threatening event.

## REFERENCES


Achermann JC, Ito M, Hindmarsh PC, Jameson JL: A mutation in the gene encoding steroidogenic factor-1 causes XY sex reversal and adrenal failure in humans. Nat Genet 22:125-126, 1999.

Achermann JC, Meeks, JJ, Jameson JL: Phenotypic spectrum of mutations in DAX-1 and SF-1. Mol Cell Endocrinol 185:17-25, 2001.

Aguilera G: Regulation of pituitary ACTH secretion during chronic stress. Front Neuroendocrinol 15:312-350, 1994.

Al-Alwan I, Navarro O, Daneman D, Daneman A: Clinical utility of adrenal ultrasonography in the diagnosis of congenital adrenal hyperplasia. J Pediatr 135:71-75, 1999.

Allolio B, Reincke M: Adrenocorticotropin receptor and adrenal disorders. Horm Res 47:273-278, 1997.

Al Saedi S, Dean H, Dent W, Cronin C: Reference values for serum cortisol and 17-hydroxyprogesterone in preterm infants. J Pediatr 126:985-987, 1995.

Ames RP, Borkowski AJ, Sicinski AM, Laragh JH: Prolonged infusions of angiotensin II and norepinephrine and blood pressure, electrolyte balance, and aldosterone and cortisol secretion in normal man and in cirrhosis with ascites. J Clin Invest 44:1171-1186, 1965.

Anderson RA, Byrum RS, Coates PM, Sando GN: Mutations at the lysosomal acid cholesteryl ester hydrolase gene locus in Wolman disease. Proc Natl Acad Sci U S A 91:2718-2722, 1994.

Axelrod L: Glucocorticoid therapy. Medicine 55:39-65, 1976.

Baker BL, Jaffe RB: The genesis of cell types in the adenohypophysis of the human fetus as observed with immunocytochemistry. Am J Anat 143:137-161, 1975.

Bekdash BA, Slim MS: Adrenal abscess in a neonate due to gas-forming organisms: A diagnostic dilemma. Z Kinderchir 32:184-187, 1981.

Bialer MG, Penchaszadeh VB, Kahn E, et al: Female external genitalia and müllerian duct derivatives in a 46,XY infant with the Smith-Lemli-Opitz syndrome. Am J Med Genet 28:723-731, 1987.

Biason-Lauber A, Schoenle EJ: Apparently normal ovarian differentiation in a prepubertal girl with transcriptionally inactive steroidogenic factor 1 (NR5A1/SF-1) and adrenocortical insufficiency. Am J Hum Genet 67:1563-1568, 2000.

Brodsky MC, Conte FA, Taylor D, et al: Sudden death in septo-optic dysplasia: Report of 5 cases. Arch Ophthalmol 115:66-70, 1997.

Brook CG, Zachmann M, Prader A, Murset G: Experience with long-term therapy in congenital adrenal hyperplasia. J Pediatr 85:12-19, 1974.

Carlson AD, Obeid JS, Kanellopoulou N, et al: Congenital adrenal hyperplasia: Update on prenatal diagnosis and treatment. J Steroid Biochem Mol Biol 69:19-29, 1999.

Challis JRG, Lye SJ:Parturition. In Knobil E, Neill JD (eds): The Physiology of Reproduction. New York, Raven Press, 1994, pp 985-1031.

Chernow B, Alexander HR, Smallridge RC, et al: Hormonal responses to graded surgical stress. Arch Intern Med 147:1273-1238, 1987.

Chrousos GP: The hypothalamic-pituitary-adrenal axis and immune-mediated inflammation. N Engl J Med 332:1351-1362, 1995.

Clark AJ, Cammas FM: The ACTH receptor. Baillieres Clin Endocrinol Metab 10:29-47, 1996.

Cole TJ, Blendy JA, Monaghan AP, et al: Targeted disruption of the glucocorticoid receptor gene blocks adrenergic chromaffin cell development and severely retards lung maturation. Genes Dev 9:1608-1621, 1995.

Collingwood TN, Urnov FD, Wolffe AP: Nuclear receptors: Coactivators, corepressors and chromatin remodeling in the control of transcription. J Mol Endocrinol 23:255-275, 1999.

Conklin JL: The development of the human fetal adenohypophysis. Anat Rec 160:79-91, 1968.

Crawford PA, Dorn C, Sadovsky Y, Milbrandt J: Nuclear receptor DAX-1 recruits nuclear receptor corepressor N-Cor to steroidogenic factor 1. Mol Cell Biol 18:2949-2956, 1998.

de Morsier G: Etudes sur les dysraphies cranioencephaliques. III. Agenesie du septum lucidum avec malformation du tractus optique. La dysplasie septo-optique. Schweiz Arch Neurol Neurochir Psychiatr 77:267-292, 1956.

Dent GW, Okimoto DK, Smith MA, Levine S: Stress-induced alterations in corticotropin-releasing hormone and vasopressin gene expression in the paraventricular nucleus during ontogeny. Neuroendocrinology 71:333-342, 2000.

de Peretti E, Forest, MG: Unconjugated dehydroepiandrosterone plasma levels in normal subjects from birth to adolescence in human: The use of a sensitive radioimmunoassay. J Clin Endocrinol Metab 43:982-991, 1976.

DeVile CJ, Stanhope R: Hydrocortisone replacement therapy in children and adolescents with hypopituitarism. Clin Endocrinol 47:37-41, 1997.

DiMartino-Nardi J, Stoner E, O'Connell A, New MI: The effect of treatment of final height in classical congenital adrenal hyperplasia (CAH). Acta Endocrinol Suppl 279:305-314, 1986.

Doerr HG, Sippell WG, Versmold HT, et al: Plasma mineralocorticoids, glucocorticoids, and progestins in premature infants: Longitudinal study during the first week of life. Pediatr Res 23:525-529, 1988.

Doerr HG, Sippell WG, Versmold HT, et al: Plasma aldosterone and 11-deoxycortisol in newborn infants: A reevaluation. J Clin Endocrinol Metab 65:208-210, 1987.

Dzau VJ: Molecular and physiological aspects of tissue renin-angiotensin system: Emphasis on cardiovascular control. J Hypertens Suppl 6:S7-S12, 1988.

Enriquez G, Lucaya J, Dominguez P, Aso C: Sonographic diagnosis of adrenal hemorrhage in patients with fulminant meningococcal septicemia. Acta Paediatr Scand 79:1255-1258, 1990.

Espiner E: Urinary cortisol excretion in stress situations and in patients with Cushing's syndrome. J Endocrinol 35:29-44, 1966.

Esteban NV, Loughlin T, Yergey AL, et al: Daily cortisol production rate in man determined by stable isotope dilution/mass spectrometry. J Clin Endocrinol Metab 72:39-45, 1991.

Ghiacy S, Dubbins PA, Baumer H: Ultrasound demonstration of congenital adrenal hyperplasia. J Clin Ultrasound 13:419-420, 1985.

Gonzalez R, Fernandes ET: Single-stage feminization genitoplasty. J Urol 143:776-778, 1990.

Gray ES, Abramovich DR: Morphologic features of the anencephalic adrenal gland in early pregnancy. Am J Obstet Gynecol 137:491-495, 1980.

Green HH, Harrington AR, Valtin H: On the role of antidiuretic hormone in the inhibition of acute water diuresis in adrenal insufficiency and the effects of gluco- and mineralocorticoids in reversing inhibition. J Clin Invest 49:1724-1736, 1970.

Gross G, Imamura T, Muglia LJ: Gene knockout mice in the study of parturition. J Soc Gynecol Invest 7:88-95, 2000.

Groves RW, Toms GC, Houghton BJ, Monson JP: Corticosteroid replacement therapy: Twice or thrice daily? J R Soc Med 81:514-516, 1988.

Habiby RL, Boepple P, Nachtigall L, et al: Adrenal hypoplasia congenita with hypogonadotropic hypogonadism: Evidence that DAX-1 mutations lead to combined hypothalamic and pituitary defects in gonadotropin production. J Clin Invest 98:1055-1062, 1996.

Heazelwood VJ, Galligan JP, Cannell GR, et al: Plasma cortisol delivery from oral cortisol and cortisone acetate: Relative bioavailability. Br J Clin Pharmacol 17:55-59, 1984.

Hingre RV, Gross SJ, Hingre KS, et al: Adrenal steroidogenesis in very low birth weight preterm infants. J Clin Endocrinol Metab 78:266-270, 1994.

Hume DM, Bell CC, Bartter F: Direct measurement of adrenal secretion during operative trauma and convalescence. Surgery 52:174-187, 1962.

Ichikawa Y: Metabolism of cortisol-4-C14 in patients with infections and collagen diseases. Metabolism 15:613-625, 1966.

Ikeda Y, Takeda Y, Shikayama T, et al: Comparative localization of Dax-1 and Ad4BP/SF-1 during development of the hypothalamic-pituitary-gonadal axis suggests their closely related and distinct functions. Dev Dyn 220:363-376, 2001.

Jaaskelainen J, Voutilainen R: Growth of patients with 21-hydroxylase deficiency: An analysis of the factors influencing adult height. Pediatr Res 41:30-33, 1997.

Jain R, Shareef M, Rowley A, et al: Disseminated herpes simplex virus infection presenting as fever in the newborn—a lethal outcome. J Infect 32:239-241, 1996.

Jones KL: Smith-Lemli-Opitz syndrome. In Jones KL (ed): Smith's Recognizable Patterns of Human Malformation, 5th ed. Philadelphia, WB Saunders, 1997, pp 112-115.

Kehlet H, Binder C: Adrenocortical function and clinical course during and after surgery in unsupplemented glucocorticoid-treated patients. Br J Anaesth 45:1043-1048, 1973.

Kerrigan JR, Veldhuis JD, Leyo SA, et al: Estimation of daily cortisol production and clearance rates in normal pubertal males by deconvolution analysis. J Clin Endocrinol Metab 76:1505-1510, 1993.

Korte C, Styne D, Merritt TA, et al: Adrenocortical function in the very low birth weight infant: Improved testing sensitivity and association with neonatal outcome. J Pediatr 128:257-263, 1996.

Kotchen TA, Strickland AL, Rice TW, Walters DR: A study of the renin-angiotensin system in newborn infants. J Pediatr 80:938-946, 1972.

Krude H, Biebermann H, Luck W, et al: Severe early-onset obesity, adrenal insufficiency and red hair pigmentation caused by POMC mutations in humans. Nat Genet 19:155-157, 1998.

Kyllo JH, Collins MM, Vetter KL, et al: Linkage of congenital isolated adrenocorticotropic hormone deficiency to the corticotropin releasing hormone locus using simple sequence repeat polymorphisms. Am J Med Genet 62:262-267, 1996.

Laron Z, Pertzelan A: The comparative effect of 6 alpha-fluoroprednisolone, 6 alpha-methylprednisolone, and hydrocortisone on linear growth of children with congenital adrenal virilism and Addison's disease. J Pediatr 73:774-782, 1968.

Laureti S, Casucci G, Santeusanio F, et al: X-linked adrenoleukodystrophy is a frequent cause of idiopathic Addison's disease in young adult male patients. J Clin Endocrinol Metab 81:470-474, 1996.

Lee MM, Rajagopalan L, Berg GJ, Moshang TJ: Serum adrenal steroid concentrations in premature infants. J Clin Endocrinol Metab 69:1133-1136, 1989.

Lin D, Sugawara T, Strauss JF 3rd, et al: Role of steroidogenic acute regulatory protein in adrenal and gonadal steroidogenesis. Science 267:1828-18231, 1995.

Linder BL, Esteban NV, Yergey AL, et al: Cortisol production rate in childhood and adolescence. J Pediatr 117:892-896, 1990.

Livanou T, Ferriman D, James VHT: Recovery of hypothalamo-pituitary-adrenal function after corticosteroid therapy. Lancet 2:856-859, 1967.

Mendonca BB, Lucon AM, Menezes CAV, et al: Clinical, hormonal and pathological findings in a comparative study of adrenocortical neoplasms in childhood and adulthood. J Urol 154:2004-2009, 1995.

Mesiano S, Jaffe RB: Developmental and functional biology of the primate fetal adrenal cortex. Endocr Rev 18:378-403, 1997.

Miller WL: Congenital adrenal hyperplasias. Endocrinol Metab Clin North Am 20:721-749,1991.

Miller WL: Dexamethasone treatment of congenital adrenal hyperplasia in utero: An experimental therapy of unproven safety. J Urol 162:537-540, 1999.

Mitchell ML, Lawler M, Walraven C, Hermos R: To screen or not to screen for congenital adrenal hyperplasia: Is that the question? In Knoppers BM, Laberge CM (eds): Genetic Screening. From Newborns to DNA Typing. Amsterdam, Elsevier Science Publishers, 1990, pp 11-18.

Morrison SC, Comisky E, Fletcher BD: Calcification in the adrenal glands associated with disseminated herpes simplex infection. Pediatr Radiol 18:240-241, 1988.

Moser HW: Genotype-phenotype correlations in disorders of peroxisome biogenesis. Mol Genet Metab 68:316-327, 1999.

Moser HW, Moser AE, Singh I, O'Neill BP: Adrenoleukodystrophy: Survey of 303 cases: Biochemistry, diagnosis, and therapy. Ann Neurol 16:628-641, 1984.

Muglia L, Jacobson L, Dikkes P, Majzoub JA: Corticotropin-releasing hormone deficiency reveals major fetal but not adult glucocorticoid need. Nature 373:427-432, 1995.

Muglia LJ, Bae DS, Brown TT, et al: Proliferation and differentiation defects during lung development in corticotropin-releasing hormone-deficient mice. Am J Respir Cell Mol Biol 20:181-188, 1999.

Mullis PE, Hindmarsh PC, Brook CG: Sodium chloride supplement at diagnosis and during infancy in children with salt-losing 21-hydroxylase deficiency. Eur J Pediatr 150:22-25, 1990.

Munck A, Guyre PM: Glucocorticoid physiology, pharmacology, stress. Adv Exp Med Biol 196:81-96, 1984.

Nakamura Y, Yamamoto S, Tanaka S, et al: Herpes simplex viral infection in human neonates: An immunohistochemical and electron microscopic study. Hum Pathol 16:1091-1097, 1985.

New MI: Congenital adrenal hyperplasia. In DeGroot LJ (ed): Endocrinology, 3rd ed. Philadelphia, WB Saunders, 1995, pp 1813-1835.

New MI, Carlson A, Obeid J, et al: Extensive personal experience: Prenatal diagnosis for congenital adrenal hyperplasia in 532 pregnancies. J Clin Endocrinol Metab 86:5651-5657, 2001.

New MI, Gertner JM, Speiser PW, Del Balzo P: Growth and final height in classical and nonclassical 21-hydroxylase deficiency. J Endocrinol Invest 12:91-95, 1989.

Newman K, Randolph J, Parson S: Functional results in young women having clitoral reconstruction as infants. J Pediatr Surg 27:180-183, discussion 183-184, 1992.

Nickels DA, Moore DC: Serum cortisol responses in febrile children. Pediatr Infect Dis J 8:16-20, 1989.

Ohta S, Shimizu S, Fujisawa S, Tsurusawa M: Neonatal adrenal abscess due to *Bacteroides*. J Pediatr 93:1063-1064, 1978.

Onishi S, Miyazawa G, Nishimura Y, et al: Postnatal development of circadian rhythm in serum cortisol levels in children. Pediatrics 72:399-404, 1983.

Parker KL: The roles of steroidogenic factor 1 in endocrine development and function. Mol Cell Endocrinol 145:15-20, 1998.

Parks JS, Brown MR, Hurley DL, et al: Heritable disorders of pituitary development. J Clin Endocrinol Metab 84:4362-4370, 1999.

Partsch C, Sippell W, MacKenzie I, Aynsley-Green A: The steroid hormonal milieu of the undisturbed human fetus and mother at 16-20 weeks gestation. J Clin Endocrinol Metab 73:969-974, 1991.

Pepe GJ, Albrecht ED: Regulation of the primate fetal adrenal cortex. Endocr Rev 11:151-176, 1990.

Pernasetti F, Toledo SP, Vasilyev VV, et al: Impaired adrenocorticotropin-adrenal axis in combined pituitary hormone deficiency caused by a two-base pair deletion (301-302delAG) in the prophet of Pit-1 gene. J Clin Endocrinol Metab 85:390-397, 2000.

Phinney PR, Fligiel S, Bryson YJ, Porter DD: Necrotizing vasculitis in a case of disseminated neonatal herpes simplex infection. Arch Pathol Lab Med 106:64-67, 1982.

Premawardhana LD, Hughes IA, Read GF, Scanlon MF: Longer term outcome in females with congenital adrenal hyperplasia (CAH): The Cardiff experience. Clin Endocrinol 46:327-332, 1997.

Rayyis SS, Horton R: Effect of angiotensin II on adrenal and pituitary function in man. J Clin Endocrinol Metab 32:539, 1971.

Rivkees SA, Crawford JD: Dexamethasone treatment of virilizing congenital adrenal hyperplasia: The ability to achieve normal growth. Pediatrics 106:767-773, 2000.

Rosler A, Levine LS, Schneider B, et al: The interrelationship of sodium balance, plasma renin activity, and ACTH in congenital adrenal hyperplasia. J Clin Endocrinol Metab 45:500, 1977.

Sandrini R, Ribeiro RC, DeLacerda L: Childhood adrenocortical tumors. J Clin Endocrinol Metab 82:2027-2031, 1997.

Sapolsky RM, Meaney MJ: Maturation of the adrenocortical stress response: Neuroendocrine control mechanisms and the stress hyporesponsive period. Brain Res 396:64-76, 1986.

Schmitt K, Deutsch J, Tulzer G, et al: Autoimmune hepatitis and adrenal insufficiency in an infant with human herpesvirus-6 infection. Lancet 348:966, 1996.

Schober JM: A surgeon's response to the intersex controversy. J Clin Ethics 9:393-397, 1998.

Silva IN, Kater CE, Cunha CF, Viana, MB: Randomised controlled trial of growth effect of hydrocortisone in congenital adrenal hyperplasia. Arch Dis Child 77:214-218, 1997.

Sippel WG, Becker H, Versmold HT, et al: Longitudinal studies of plasma aldosterone, corticosterone, deoxycorticosterone, progesterone, 17-hydroxyprogesterone, cortisol, and cortisone determined simultaneously in mother and child at birth and during the early neonatal period. I. Spontaneous delivery. J Clin Endocrinol Metab 46:971-985, 1978.

Sivit CJ, Hung W, Taylor GA, et al: Sonography in neonatal congenital adrenal hyperplasia. AJR Am J Roentgenol 156:141-143, 1991.

Speiser PW: Prenatal treatment of congenital adrenal hyperplasia. J Urol 162:534-536, 1999.

Stempfel RS Jr, Sheikholislam BM, Lebovitz HE, et al: Pituitary growth hormone suppression with low-dosage, long-acting corticoid administration. J Pediatr 73:767-773, 1968.

Stratakis CA, Karl M, Schulte HM, Chrousos GP: Glucocorticosteroid resistance in humans: Elucidation of the molecular mechanisms and implications for pathophysiology. Ann N Y Acad Sci 746:362-374, discussion 374-376, 1994.

Tamura S, Matsumoto N, Imamura A, et al: Phenotype-genotype relationships in peroxisome biogenesis disorders of PEX1-defective complementation group 1 are defined by Pex1p-Pex6p interaction. Biochem J 357:417-426, 2001.

Tarnow-Mordi W, Mitra A: Postnatal dexamethasone in preterm infants. BMJ 319:1385-1386, 1999.

Thebaud B, Lacaze-Masmonteil T, Watterberg K: Postnatal glucocorticoids in very preterm infants: "The good, the bad, and the ugly"? Pediatrics 107:413-415, 2001.

Thliveris JA, Currie RW: Observations on the hypophyseal portal vasculature in the developing human fetus. Am J Anat 157:441-444, 1980.

Thomas PQ, Dattani MT, Brickman JM, et al: Heterozygous HESX1 mutations associated with isolated congenital pituitary hypoplasia and septo-optic dysplasia. Hum Mol Genet 10:39-45, 2001.

Thomas S, Murphy JF, Dyas J, et al: Response to ACTH in the newborn. Arch Dis Child 61:57-60, 1986.

Tint GS, Salen G, Batta AK, et al: Correlation of severity and outcome with plasma sterol levels in variants of the Smith-Lemli-Opitz syndrome. J Pediatr 127:82-87, 1995.

Truss M, Beato M: Steroid hormone receptors: Interaction with deoxyribonucleic acid and transcription factors. Endocr Rev 14:459-479, 1993.

Urban MD, Lee PA, Migeon CJ: Adult height and fertility in men with congenital virilizing adrenal hyperplasia. N Engl J Med 299:1392-1396, 1978.

Van Cauter E, Shapiro ET, Tillil H, Polonsky KS: Circadian modulation of glucose and insulin responses to meals: Relationship to cortisol rhythm. Am J Physiol 262:E467-E475, 1992.

Van Metre TEJ, Niemann WA, Rosen LJ: A comparison of the growth suppressive effect of cortisone, prednisone and other adrenal cortical hormones. J Allergy 31:531, 1960.

Velaphi S, Perlman JM: Neonatal adrenal hemorrhage: Clinical and abdominal sonographic findings. Clin Pediatr 40:545-548, 2001.

Ventura KC, Hawkins H, Smith MB, Walker DH: Fatal neonatal echovirus 6 infection: Autopsy case report and review of the literature. Mod Pathol 14:85-90, 2001.

Vidal V, Schedl A: Requirement of WT1 for gonad and adrenal development: Insights from transgenic animals. Endocr Res 26:1075-1082, 2000.

Walter C, Gootjes J, Mooijer PA, et al: Disorders of peroxisome biogenesis due to mutations in PEX1: Phenotypes and PEX1 protein levels. Am J Hum Genet 69:35-48, 2001.

Weber A, Clark AJ: Mutations of the ACTH receptor gene are only one cause of familial glucocorticoid deficiency. Hum Mol Genet 3:585-588, 1994.

Weber A, Toppari J, Harvey RD, et al: Adrenocorticotropin receptor gene mutations in familial glucocorticoid deficiency: Relationships with clinical features in four families. J Clin Endocrinol Metab 80:65-71, 1995.

Weldon VV, Kowarski A, Migeon CJ: Aldosterone secretion rates in normal subjects from infancy to adulthood. Pediatrics 39: 713-723, 1967.

White PC: Congenital adrenal hyperplasias. Best Pract Res Clin Endocrinol Metab 15:17-41, 2001.

White PC, Curnow KM, Pascoe L: Disorders of the 11 beta-hydroxylase isozymes. Endocr Rev 15:421-438, 1994.

White PC, Speiser PW: Congenital adrenal hyperplasia due to 21-hydroxylase deficiency. Endocr Rev 21:245-291, 2000.

Willnow S, Kiess W, Butenandt O, et al: Endocrine disorders in septo-optic dysplasia (De Morsier syndrome)—evaluation and follow up of 18 patients. Eur J Pediatr 155:179-284, 1996.

Wilson BE, Reiner WG: Management of intersex: A shifting paradigm. J Clin Ethics 9:360-369, 1998.

Wise L, Margraf HW, Ballinger WF: A new concept on the pre-and postoperative regulation of cortisol secretion. Surgery 72:290-299, 1972.

Wolman M: Wolman disease and its treatment. Clin Pediatr 34:207-212, 1995.

Yamaoka T, Kudo T, Takuwa Y, et al: Hereditary adrenocortical unresponsiveness to adrenocorticotropin with a postreceptor defect. J Clin Endocrinol Metabol 75:270-274, 1992.

Yen S: Endocrine-metabolic adaptations in pregnancy. In Yen SSC, Jaffe RB (eds): Reproductive Endocrinology: Physiology, Pathophysiology, and Clinical Management, 3rd ed. Philadelphia, WB Saunders, 1991.

CHAPTER 91

# Ambiguous Genitalia in the Newborn

Gregory Goodwin and Anthony Caldamone

Disorders of sex differentiation can be generally classified as (1) masculinization of the 46,XX female, (2) incomplete masculinization of the 46,XY male, (3) gonadal differentiation and chromosomal disorders, including true hermaphroditism, or (4) syndromes associated with incomplete genital development (Table 91–1). The first two categories comprise the majority of definable cases of ambiguous genitalia.

This chapter presents an overview of the pathophysiology of intersex disorders, including a discussion of the practical aspects of diagnosis and management. An overview of the traditional surgical methods used in the management of infants with intersex disorders, including the risks and benefits of these procedures, is included at the end of the chapter.

## GENERAL CONSIDERATIONS IN THE APPROACH TO THE CHILD WITH AMBIGUOUS GENITALIA

The medical evaluation of ambiguous genitalia is necessarily time consuming. Open and honest discussions with the parents are invaluable in allaying anxiety and establishing a trusting relationship. Full disclosure of available information is essential in this regard.

Care must be taken to avoid premature gender assignment for the infant. Proper evaluation of the infant with ambiguous genitalia requires a multidisciplinary team that should include the primary care physician, neonatologist, pediatric endocrinologist, pediatric urologist, and pediatric geneticist. Psychological assessment and support of the family are essential in the newborn period, along with long-term psychological follow-up evaluation (Slijper et al, 1998). Decisions regarding the gender of rearing should be made collaboratively between the multidisciplinary team and the parents, with the recognition that cultural and psychosocial factors are likely to be influential (Grumbach and Conte, 1998; Kuhnle and Krahl, 2002).

In the past, gender assignment was based largely on phallic size, relative ease of surgical reconstruction, or the potential for fertility. This approach has come under criticism, however, as dissatisfaction with gender assignment based on these criteria has been reported in several case studies (Diamond and Sigmundson, 1997b; Phornphukutul et al, 2000; Reiner, 1996). The importance of prenatal androgen imprinting has been implicated as an important variable in some of these cases (Reiner, 1997). Furthermore, more recent studies in undervirilized 46,XY males indicate that a small phallus can be associated with a satisfying adult sex life (Reilly and Woodhouse, 1989). Thus, female gender assignment may not be warranted for intermediately undervirilized 46,XY males.

The degree of genital virilization is still an important determinant of gender assignment in the infant with ambiguous genitalia; however, other, incompletely understood factors appear to be involved. The formation of a healthy gender identity seems to involve a complex interplay between psychobiologic and environmental factors (Meyer-Bahlburg et al, 1996; Money et al, 1972; Slijper et al, 1998).

## THE EMBRYOLOGY OF SEXUAL DIFFERENTIATION

Normal and abnormal sexual differentiation constitute superb examples of how an understanding of embryology is critical to the approach to and management of a group of complex and intriguing clinical disorders.

Sexual differentiation is a sequential process that can be divided into three stages. Jost established the sequence as follows: Chromosomal sex is determined at fertilization and dictates the differentiation of the gonad, which in turn dictates the phenotypic sex, or the differentiation of the internal ductal system and external genitalia (Grumbach and Conte, 1998).

Chromosomal sex is determined at the moment of conception by the sex chromosome complement of the fertilizing sperm. If this sperm carries an X chromosome, a 46,XX (normal female) complement results; if the sex chromosome is Y, a 46,XY (normal male) genotype results. The *SRY* (for "sex-determining region of the Y chromosome") gene is necessary but not sufficient for testicular differentiation. *SRY* causes the medullary region of the gonad to develop into Sertoli cells and later into testis cords and seminiferous tubules.

In addition to X chromosome genes, autosomal genes also may influence sexual differentiation, insofar as mutations to these genes result in disorders of sexual differentiation. Some of these genes include *WT1* (Wilms tumor gene 1), associated with Denys-Drash syndrome and WAGR (*W*ilms tumor, *a*niridia, *g*enitourinary abnormalities, mental *r*etardation) syndrome; the sex reversal or adrenal hypoplasia gene (*DAX1*); the steroidogenic factor 1 gene (SF-1); and *SOX9*, which has been associated with camptomelic dysplasia (Grumbach and Conte, 1998).

The gonad develops from both somatic and germ cells. The somatic cells are located at the ventral region of the mesonephros and arise from the mesonephric cells and the coelomic epithelium. Somatic cells become the Sertoli cells of the testis and the granulosa cells of the ovary. The germ cells migrate from a more inferior position on the yolk sac to the genital ridge, just medial to the mesonephros on each side (Fig. 91–1, upper left). This occurs between the fourth and sixth weeks of gestation. Once the germ cells reach the gonadal ridge, they become surrounded by the somatic cells, which appear to regulate germ cell differentiation.

Gonadal sex is established by the seventh week of gestation. At this stage, the fetus contains two internal ductal systems—wolffian and müllerian—and undifferentiated external genital primordia. The wolffian or mesonephric duct is a tubular structure that connects the capillary

**TABLE 91–1**

**Differential Diagnosis of Ambiguous Genitalia**

| |
|---|
| **46,XX Virilized Female** |
| Congenital adrenal hyperplasia |
| 21-Hydroxylase deficiency |
| 11-Hydroxylase deficiency |
| 3β-Hydroxysteroid dehydrogenase deficiency |
| Aromatase deficiency (fetal and maternal virilization) |
| Virilizing maternal conditions |
| Congenital adrenal hyperplasia |
| Adrenal/ovarian tumors/luteoma of pregnancy |
| Maternal ingestion of progestins, androgens |
| **46,XY Undervirilized Male** |
| Androgen insensitivity |
| Partial (PAIS) |
| Complete (CAIS) |
| 5α-Reductase-2 deficiency |
| Testosterone biosynthetic defects |
| 17β-Hydroxysteroid hydrogenase 3 deficiency |
| 3β-Hydroxysteroid dehydrogenase deficiency |
| 17α-Hydroxylase/17,20-lyase deficiency |
| Congenital lipoid adrenal hyperplasia |
| Leydig cell hypoplasia |
| Idiopathic/undetermined |
| Drug ingestion: progestins, spironolactone, cimetidine, phenytoin |
| Persistent müllerian duct syndrome |
| **Gonadal Differentiation/Chromosomal Disorders** |
| 46,XY gonadal dysgenesis |
| Complete (Swyer syndrome) |
| Partial |
| Mixed (45,X/46,XY) |
| True hermaphroditism |
| 46,XX, 46,XY, 46,XX/46,XY |
| **Syndromes Associated with Ambiguous Genitalia** |
| Gonadal dysgenesis |
| 46,XY partial gonadal dysgenesis (Turner syndrome features) |
| Camptomelic dysplasia |
| Renal degenerative diseases and gonadal dysgenesis |
| Denys-Drash syndrome |
| Frasier syndrome |
| WAGR (*W*ilms tumor, *a*niridia, *g*enitourinary abnormalities, mental *r*etardation) syndrome |
| Smith-Lemli-Opitz syndrome (7-dehydrocholesterol reductase deficiency) |
| Robinow syndrome |

network of the mesonephros to the urogenital sinus. Evagination of the coelomic epithelium leads to formation of a second tubular structure adjacent to the mesonephric duct, the paramesonephric, or müllerian, duct. The distal ends of these two ducts are joined. That portion of the urogenital sinus distal to the termination of these ducts contributes to external genital development, whereas the proximal portion develops into the bladder, trigone, and posterior urethra.

Phenotypic sexual differentiation is predicated on establishment of gonadal sex. If an ovary develops, the wolffian ducts involute due to lack of testosterone, and only its terminal portion persists as Gartner's duct. The müllerian ducts develop into the proximal vagina, uterus, and fallopian tubes (see Fig. 91–1). The unfused cephalic portions of the müllerian ducts form the fallopian tubes, while the caudal ends fuse to form the ureterovaginal canal (see Fig. 91–1). The union of the fused caudal ends of the müllerian ducts and urogenital sinus forms the vagina. The proximal two thirds of the vagina is of müllerian duct origin, and the distal third is of urogenital sinus origin.

Male phenotypic differentiation is the result of the elaboration of two distinct testicular hormones: testosterone and müllerian-inhibiting factor (MIF). These factors are produced and secreted by the 8-week stage of development, and they are essential for normal male differentiation. Involution of the müllerian ducts is caused by MIF, which is a glycoprotein secreted by the fetal Sertoli cells. The remnants of the müllerian ducts persist caudally as the prostatic utricle and cephalically as the appendix testis. MIF exerts its action unilaterally and locally (exocrine secretion) rather than bilaterally via the systemic circulation.

Immediately after müllerian duct regression, the wolffian ducts develop under the influence of testosterone secreted by the fetal Leydig cells. The Leydig cells, like the Sertoli cells, differentiate from the mesenchymal cells within the gonadal ridges. This occurs at 9 to 10 weeks of gestation. Under the influence of testosterone, the wolffian ducts evolve into the epididymis, vas deferens, and seminal vesicles (see Fig. 91–1). The mesonephric tubules develop into the ductuli efferentes, which will provide continuity between the seminiferous tubules and rete testis to the vas deferens. This process occurs as a direct action of testosterone on the ductal structures.

Virilization of the male external genitalia, starting at about 8 weeks of gestation (see Fig. 91–1), relies on the ability of the tissues involved to convert testosterone into a more potent androgen, dihydrotestosterone. The target cells possess the enzyme 5α-reductase, which is necessary for this conversion. By 12 to 14 weeks of gestation, formation of the male external genitalia is nearly complete. Androgen exposure after this time results in further phallic enlargement.

## CLINICAL ASSESSMENT OF DISORDERS OF SEX DIFFERENTIATION

### History

A detailed *family history* is important in the evaluation of ambiguous genitalia and information on early neonatal deaths, consanguinity, or urogenital anomalies should be obtained. A family history of female infertility or amenorrhea may be suggestive of an intersex disorder. In one study of androgen insensitivity disorders, a positive family history of a sex differentiation disorder was often overlooked (Viner et al, 1997).

The presence of *maternal virilization* may be suggestive of a variety of disorders that may effect fetal masculinization. Features of maternal virilization include hirsutism, severe acne, deepening of the voice, and clitoromegaly on examination.

The ingestion of any recreational drugs, alcohol, or medications by the mother during pregnancy should be noted. Particular attention to medications with androgenic

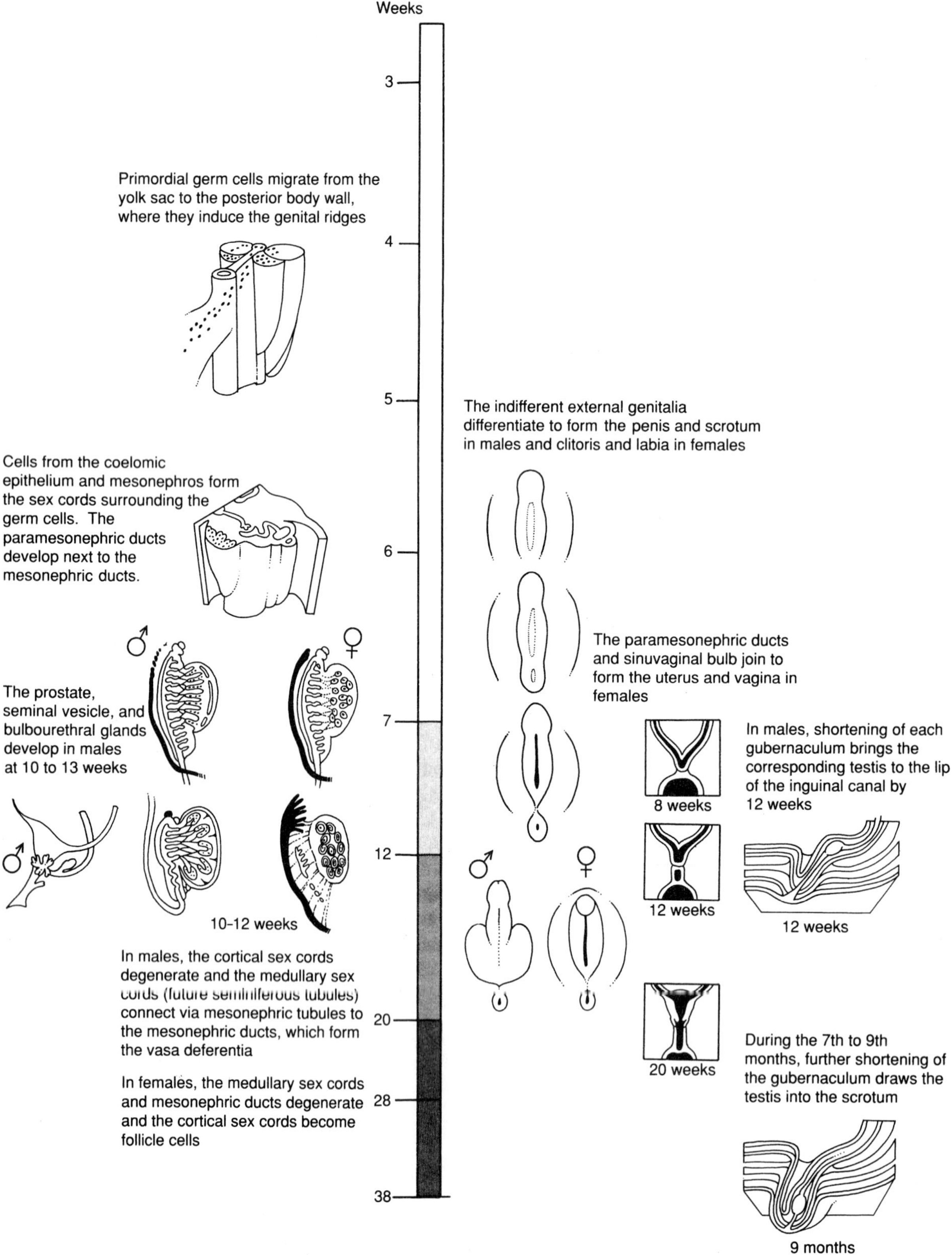

Weeks
3
4
5
6
7
12
20
28
38
Primordial germ cells migrate from the yolk sac to the posterior body wall, where they induce the genital ridges
Cells from the coelomic epithelium and mesonephros form the sex cords surrounding the germ cells. The paramesonephric ducts develop next to the mesonephric ducts.
The prostate, seminal vesicle, and bulbourethral glands develop in males at 10 to 13 weeks
10-12 weeks
In males, the cortical sex cords degenerate and the medullary sex cords (future seminiferous tubules) connect via mesonephric tubules to the mesonephric ducts, which form the vasa deferentia
In females, the medullary sex cords and mesonephric ducts degenerate and the cortical sex cords become follicle cells
The indifferent external genitalia differentiate to form the penis and scrotum in males and clitoris and labia in females
The paramesonephric ducts and sinuvaginal bulb join to form the uterus and vagina in females
8 weeks
12 weeks
20 weeks
In males, shortening of each gubernaculum brings the corresponding testis to the lip of the inguinal canal by 12 weeks
12 weeks
During the 7th to 9th months, further shortening of the gubernaculum draws the testis into the scrotum
9 months


**FIGURE 91–1.** Embryologic time line for gonadal and internal and external genitalia development. *(From Larsen WJ: Human Embryology. New York, Churchill Livingstone, 1993, p. 237.)*

or progestational activity is indicated. Medications that affect fetal genital development include cimetidine, spironolactone, hydantoin, and progestational agents (Grumbach and Conte, 1998).

### Physical Examination

There is significant overlap of the genital anatomy among the various sex differentiation disorders. The physical examination, however, may provide the first clues to the underlying pathology. In addition, the physical examination will provide important information about the degree of virilization of the external genitalia and the presence or absence of palpable gonads.

***Clitoris.*** Significant clitoral enlargement deserves a careful evaluation. Keep in mind that premature infants have relatively underdeveloped labia majora, so that the clitoris may appear enlarged. A truly enlarged clitoris can be distinguished from a generous clitoral hood by the presence of palpable corporal or erectile tissue.

***Penis/Phallus.*** Measurements of the phallic stretch length and mid-shaft diameter are important in determining the degree of virilization. The phallus should be stretched and measured from the pubic ramus to the tip of the glans. Gestational age–corrected phallic stretch lengths are shown in Figure 91–2. The presence of a chordee structure on the ventral surface of the phallus may impair measurement of the true phallic length (Feldman and Smith, 1975) (Fig. 91–3). A chordee is residual urethral tissue that tethers the phallus to the perineum. Measurement of the mid-shaft diameter is particularly useful in this circumstance. For term male infants, a normal mid-shaft diameter is approximately 1 cm (Feldman and Smith, 1975).

A microphallus deserves careful evaluation for the presence of hypopituitarism or growth hormone deficiency, particularly in the presence of hypoglycemia or unexplained jaundice. Microphallus and undescended testes may occasionally be the presenting phenotype for an intersex disorder.

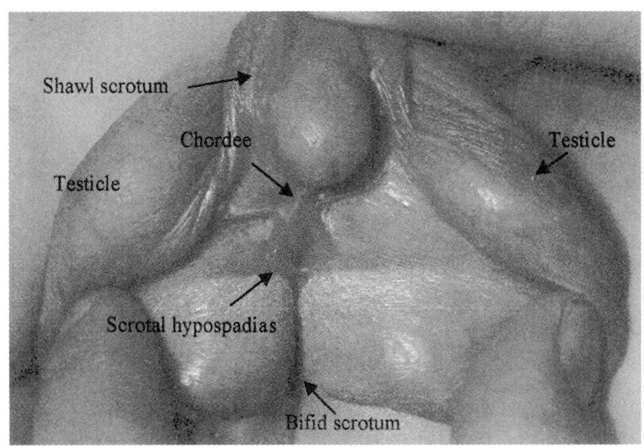


**FIGURE 91–3.** Undervirilized male demonstrating bifid scrotum, scrotal hypospadias, chordee, and bilateral descended testes.

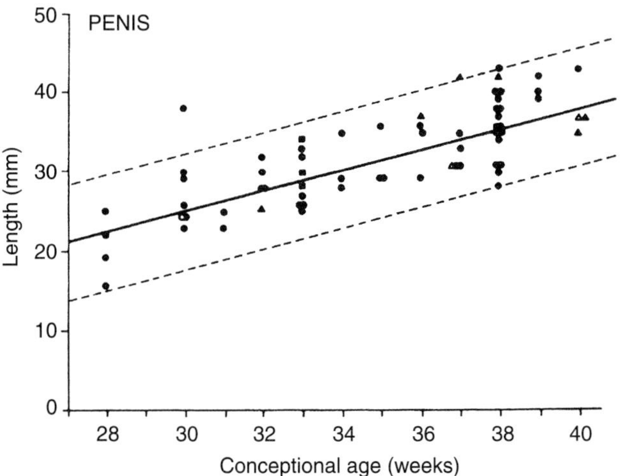


**FIGURE 91–2.** Penis stretch length in 63 normal premature and full-term male infants (●), showing lines of mean ±2 SD. Superimposed are data for two small-for-gestational age infants (△), seven large-for-gestational age infants (▲), and twins (■). *(Reproduced with permission from J Pediatr 86:395, 1975.)*

***Labioscrotal Folds.*** Assessment of the degree of fusion of the labioscrotal folds should be performed. When the infant is exposed to androgens during embryogenesis, fusion of the labioscrotal folds progresses from a posterior to an anterior direction. The spectrum of labial fusion can vary from mild posterior fusion to complete labial fusion (Fig. 91–4). Note whether the folds are rugate or hyperpigmented. Is the phallus positioned in the normal superior position relative to the scrotum or is there a shawl scrotum? (See Fig. 91–3.) Is the scrotum fused normally in the midline or is the scrotum bifid? (See Fig. 91–3.)

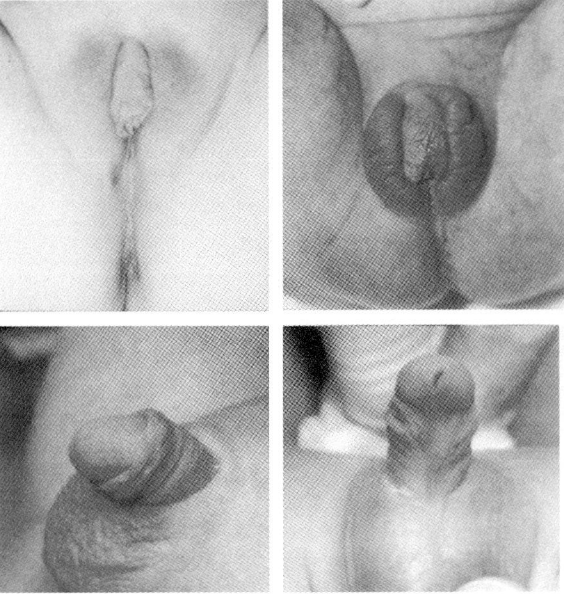

**FIGURE 91–4.** Virilization of external genitalia in 46,XX congenital adrenal hyplasia (21-hydroxylase deficiency). **Upper left panel,** There is a mild to moderate degree of virilization, with primarily clitoral hypertrophy and significant fusion of the labia. **Upper right panel,** Virilization is moderate, with clitoromegaly, labial fusion, and rugation of labial folds. **Lower panels,** Complete masculinization is evident.

***Gonads.*** Careful examination for the presence of gonads should be performed in all infants with ambiguous genitalia. The presence of bilateral gonads in the labial folds is highly suggestive of an undermasculinized genetic male (see Fig. 91–3). A unilaterally palpable gonad is often seen in infants with mixed gonad dysgenesis or hermaphroditism (Fig. 91–5), although other disorders such as androgen insensitivity can manifest similarly. When cryptorchidism and hypospadias occur simultaneously, there is a greater than 25% chance of an intersex problem (Albers et al, 1997; Rajfer and Walsh, 1976).

***Hypospadias/Perineum.*** The severity of hypospadias can vary, with the condition ranging from mild glandular to penoscrotal, although most disorders of sexual differentiation manifest with severe penoscrotal or scrotal hypospadias (see Figs. 91–3 and 91–5). Examination for the presence of separate urethral and vaginal openings versus a single perineal opening (urogenital sinus) conveys important anatomic information. The vagina may be blind ending or completely formed. A urogenital sinus results from failure of the urologic and genital tracts to completely differentiate. In virilized females, the level at which the vagina enters the sinus (low- versus high-level vaginal entry) has important implications for determining the ease of subsequent surgical exterioration of the vagina (Fig. 91–6). Also, when the urethra enters a urogenital sinus, there is potential for urinary stasis and hence urinary tract infections

Excessive pigmentation of the genitals or signs of dehydration should alert the examiner to the possibility of congenital adrenal hyperplasia (CAH).

*Dysmorphic features* suggestive of Turner syndrome point to the possibility of gonadal dysgenesis or mixed gonadal dysgenesis. Such abnormalities or multiple congenital anomalies may indicate any of a variety of syndromes associated with ambiguous genitalia (see Table 91–1).

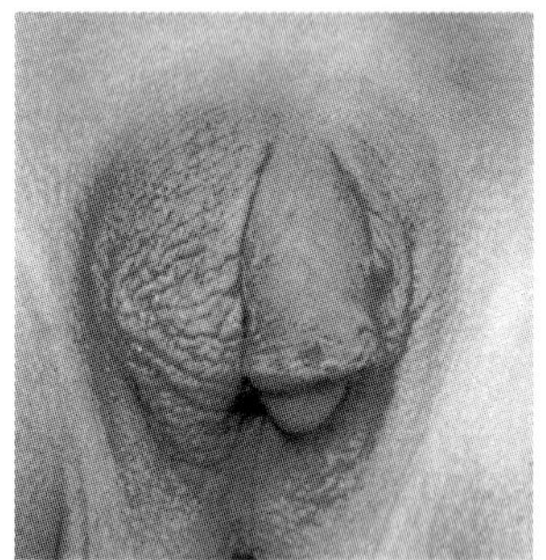

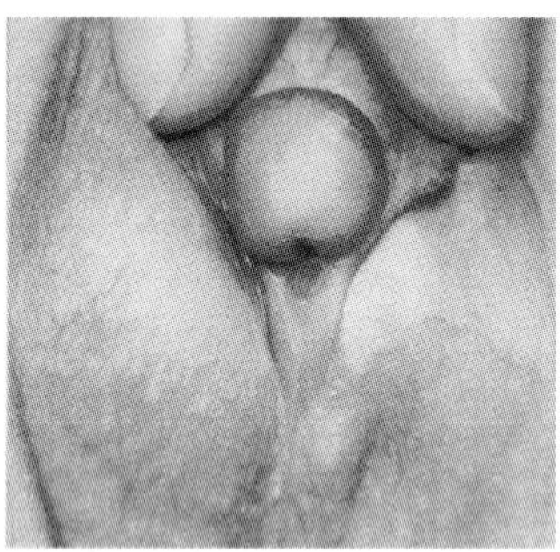

**FIGURE 91–5.** Asymmetric external genitals with left unilateral descended testis (**left**), penoscrotal hypospadias and chordee (**right**). Asymmetrical external genital development or gonadal descent would be characteristic of mixed gonadal dysgenesis or hermaphroditism.

### Radiologic Investigations

***Pelvic Ultrasonography.*** Pelvic ultrasonography reveals vital information in the evaluation of intersex disorders. The presence or absence of a uterus is a critically important determinant in the initial evaluation (Figs. 91–7, 91–8, and 91–9). The newborn period is a time when the uterus, ovaries, and adrenals are optimally visualized (Wright et al, 1995). The presence of a well-developed uterus will direct the differential diagnosis toward virilization of the female, true hermaphroditism, or persistent müllerian duct syndrome (PMDS). A rudimentary uterus may be seen in gonadal dysgenesis or hermaphroditism, however. Ultrasonography can locate undescended testes and determine gonadal size or irregularity, such as an oblong ovotestis. In hermaphroditism, loss of the uniform testicular echotexture may suggest the presence of an ovotestis. Ultrasound examination can determine if the adrenal glands appear enlarged, as in CAH. Note that normal adrenal size does not rule out CAH, however.

***Genitourethrogram.*** A genitourethrogram is a fluoroscopy-guided genital dye study that can provide important information on the urethra and internal genital ducts (Wright et al, 1995). An experienced radiologist should perform this study. It is important to ensure that all perineal orifices are

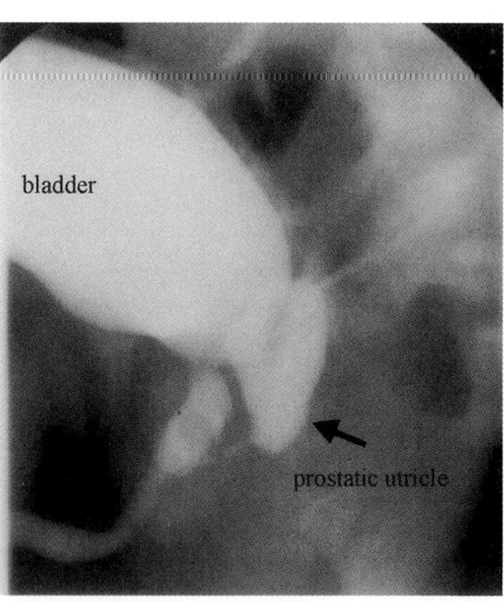


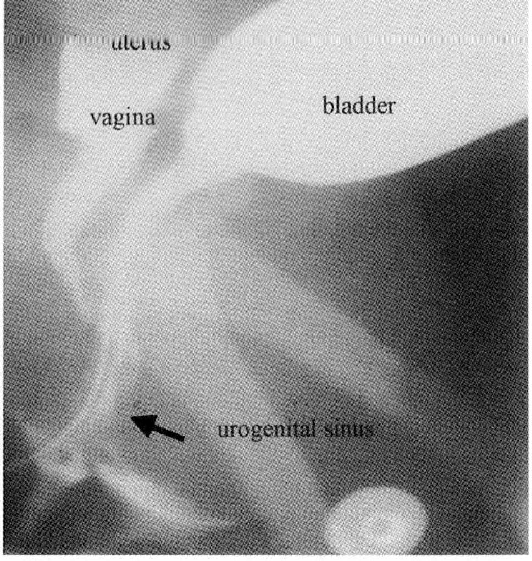


**FIGURE 91–6.** Genitourethrograms. **Left,** Genitogram from a 46,XY infant with microphallus and undescended testes with a clearly delineated prostatic utricle (see Case Study 2). **Right,** Genitogram from a 46,XX infant with congenital adrenal hyperplasia and severe masculinization of external genitals. The confluence of the vagina with the urogenital sinus is of intermediate severity.

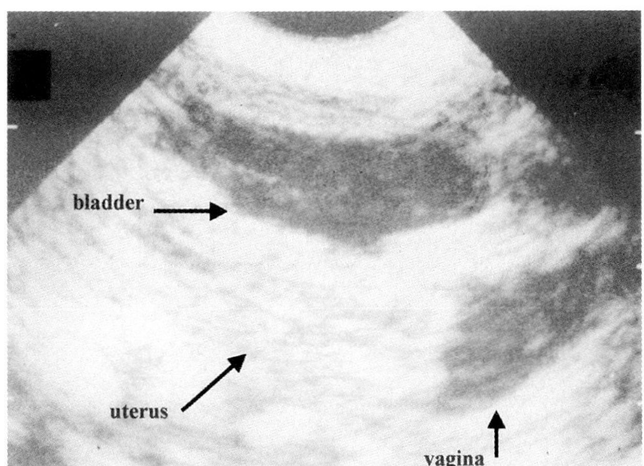


**FIGURE 91–7.** Ultrasound image from a 46,XX infant with ambiguous genitalia. Note the presence of a well-developed uterus with an endometrial stripe.

examined. The main features to be noted are the presence or absence of a vagina (or prostatic utricle) and the relationship between the vagina and the urethra (see Fig. 91–6). Demonstration of the level at which the vagina opens into the urogenital sinus and its relationship to the external sphincter has important surgical implications. Recognition of male or female urethral configurations also may be possible during genitourethrography.

***Magnetic Resonance Imaging.*** Magnetic resonance imaging (MRI) has been used to assess the internal genitalia of a limited number of infants and children with genital differentiation disorders. The strength of MRI lies in its ability to image large areas in multiple planes and characterize soft tissues. Detailed information about müllerian and wolffian structures and the position of the gonads may be obtained; however, thin sections (3 to 5 mm) are required for an adequate study. Streak gonads remain difficult to visualize. MRI has the capability to differentiate between an enlarged clitoris and a penis, as the bulbospongiosus muscle and transverse perineal muscle are absent or poorly visualized in the virilized female (Wright et al, 1995). MRI is a promising modality for the evaluation of ambiguous genitalia; however, further studies are needed to demonstrate efficacy over other imaging modalities.

### Laboratory Investigations

Endocrine and genetic laboratory studies are germane in the evaluation of ambiguous genitalia in the newborn. Day 1 of life is an ideal time to obtain serum testosterone and dihydrotestosterone (DHT) levels, as testosterone levels fall rapidly in the first several days of life (Forest et al, 1980). *Chromosomal* studies should optimally be obtained on day 1, as at least 48 to 72 hours are required to complete the study. On day 2 or 3 of life, determinations of serum *17-hydroxyprogesterone*, 17-hydroxypregnenolone, 11-deoxycortisol, dehydroepiandrosterone (DHEA), androstenedione, and plasma renin activity are performed if CAH is suspected.

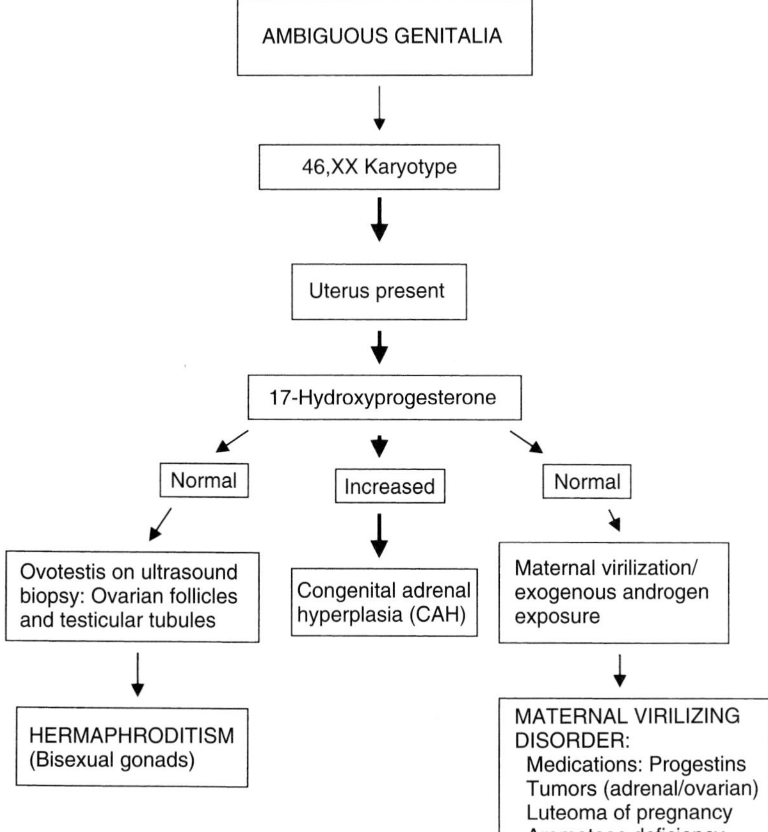


**FIGURE 91–8.** Algorithm for evaluation of the 46,XX infant with ambiguous genitalia. The presence of a uterus would be determined radiographically by ultrasound examination, genitourethrogram, or magnetic resonance imaging.

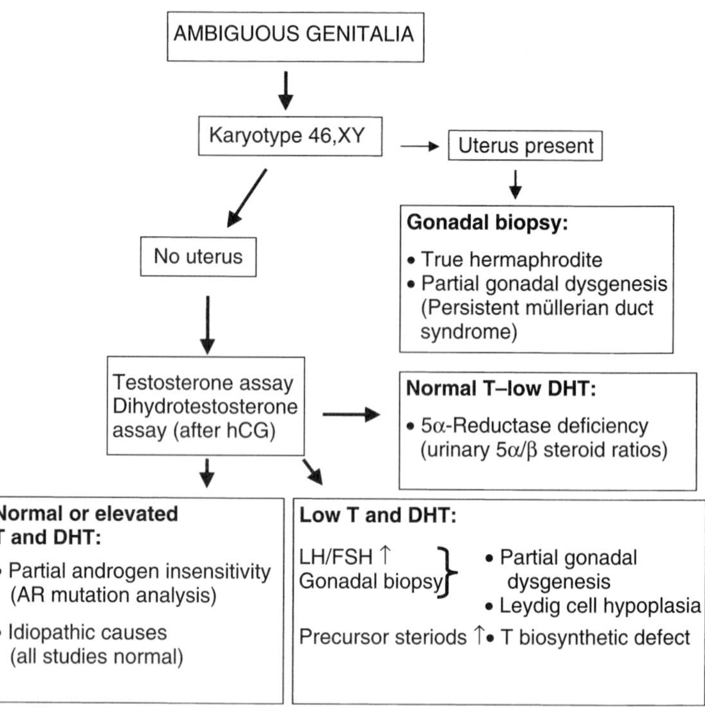


**FIGURE 91–9.** Algorithm for evaluation of the infant with ambiguous genitalia and 46,XY karyotype. The presence or absence of a uterus would be determined by radiographic imaging including ultrasound examination, genitourethrogram, or magnetic resonance imaging, as appropriate. Testosterone (T) and dihydrotestosterone (DHT) levels ideally should be obtained after human chorionic gonadotropin (hCG) stimulation. AR, androgen receptor; FSH, follicle-stimulating hormone; LH, luteinizing hormone.

Some clinicians perform an adrenocorticotropic hormone (ACTH) stimulation test at this time to more clearly demonstrate a block in steroid biosynthesis. Results of these studies should be sent immediately to the appropriate reference laboratory for analysis. Alerting the reference laboratory to the urgent nature of the studies performed will facilitate rapid processing. 17-Hydroxyprogesterone levels are physiologically elevated in the first day of life, and screening for congenital adrenal hyperplasia should preferably not be done at this time. Serum gonadotropins are often suppressed in the immediate newborn period, so they should be measured after 1 week of life. Luteinizing hormone (LH) and follicle-stimulating hormone (FSH) levels are helpful in assessing for androgen insensitivity, gonadal dysgenesis, and LH receptor abnormalities. Repeat LH, FSH, testosterone, and DHT should be done between 2 and 8 weeks of life in the evaluation of undervirilized males. This time period coincides with the physiologic testosterone surge seen in normal male infants (Forest et al, 1980). When congenital adrenal hyperplasia is suspected, daily electrolytes are important to determine.

A *human chorionic gonadotropin* (hCG) *test* will be useful in the evaluation of suspected incomplete masculinization of the genetic male. Human chorionic gonadotropin binds the LH receptor and stimulates the testes to synthesize sex steroids. An adequate testosterone response rules out a testosterone biosynthetic defect, and a normal testosterone-to-DHT ratio argues against 5α-reductase-2 deficiency. In addition, the test may result in phallic enlargement. Almaguer and colleagues (1993) reported an increase in phallic length of 0.25 to 0.75 cm in six 46,XY males with idiopathic microphallus within 5 days of beginning injections. A bolus of 1500 IU of hCG was given intramuscularly on 3 consecutive days, with steroids and phallic length measured on the fifth day. Growth of the phallus in response to hCG suggests that the phallus will further virilize at puberty, although no longitudinal study has documented this assumption. A testosterone level greater than 200 ng/dL with a testosterone-to-DHT ratio of less than 8:1 is considered a normal response to hCG.

Fluorescence in situ hybridization (FISH) can rapidly determine the sex chromosome complement of the newborn by using X chromosome– and Y chromosome–specific centromeric probes (Schwartz et al, 1997) (Fig. 91–10). In addition, this methodology allows for the detection of low levels of chromosomal mosaicism because hundreds of cells can be analyzed rapidly. FISH analysis for determination of sex chromosome constitution has been shown to be

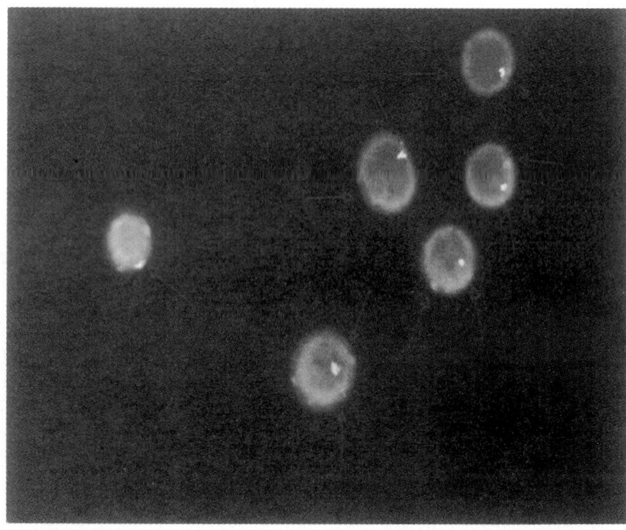

**FIGURE 91–10.** (See also Color Plate 91–10.) Fluorescence in situ hybridization (FISH) technique demonstrating the sex chromosome constitution of peripheral blood leukocytes. Centromeric probes to the X and Y chromosomes are represented by green (X) and orange (Y) markers.

highly reliable, although this methodology has not been used extensively in the evaluation of ambiguous genitalia of the newborn. Therefore, results should be interpreted with some degree of caution until confirmation by karyotypic analysis is available.

In a small percentage of ambiguous genitalia cases, laparoscopy with *gonadal biopsy* is necessary to confirm the diagnosis of true hermaphroditism, gonadal dysgenesis, or Leydig cell aplasia. Obtaining a karyotype from gonadal tissue may be helpful when sex chromosome mosaicism is suspected.

## DISORDERS RESULTING IN AMBIGUOUS GENITALIA

### Virilization of the Female

Virilization of the female infant is most commonly caused by *congenital adrenal hyperplasia* (CAH), although other virilizing conditions can be involved (see Fig. 91–8). CAH encompasses a group of disorders of adrenal steroid hormone biosynthesis, of which over 95% are due to *21-hydroxylase deficiency* (New, 1992) (Fig. 91–11).

Occasionally, the presence of excess androgens of maternal origin can result in virilization of the female infant. Progestational agents used to prevent miscarriages have caused fetal masculinization (Grumbach and Conte, 1998). A unique cause of both maternal and fetal masculinization is placental aromatase deficiency (Conte et al, 1994).

#### Congenital Adrenal Hyperplasia

21-Hydroxylase deficiency is the most common cause of ambiguous genitalia in the newborn female (New, 1992). 21-Hydroxylase deficiency has a population frequency of approximately 1/15,000, and the disorder is inherited in an autosomal recessive fashion. Males and females are equally affected; however, in classic cases, females usually are virilized at birth, resulting in the clinical presentation of ambiguous genitalia.

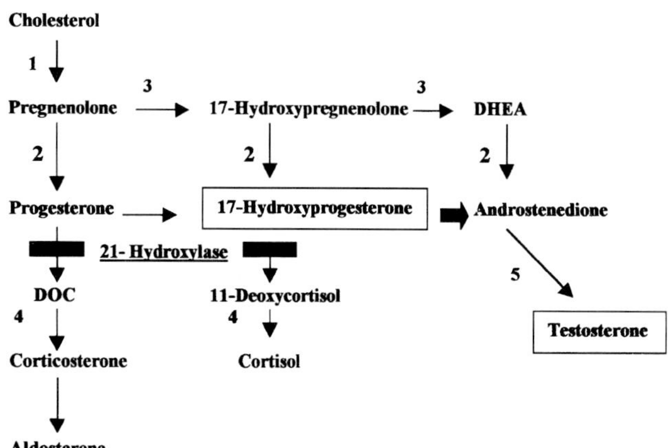


**FIGURE 91–11.** Steroid biosynthetic pathway demonstrating the defect in 21-hydroxylase deficiency (*solid bars*) and accumulated precursor 17-hydroxyprogesterone. Note increased shunting into androgen-producing pathways. Steroidogenic enzymes are indicated as follows: (1) steroidogenic acute regulatory protein (StAR) and side chain cleavage, (2) 3β-hydroxysteroid dehydrogenase, (3) 17α-hydroxylase/17,20-lyase, (4) 11β-hydroxylase, and (5) 17β-hydroxysteroid dehydrogenase. DHEA, dehydroxyepiandrosterone; DOC, deoxycorticosterone.

Deficiency of the 21-hydroxylase enzyme results in excess accumulation of the substrate17-hydroxyprogesterone, which is shunted into the androgen synthesizing pathway resulting in excess levels of androstenedione (see Fig. 91–11). Androstenedione is then converted peripherally to testosterone. The excess production of androgens results in masculinization of the external genitalia of the female fetus, while the male infant with 21-hydroxylase deficiency is phenotypically normal. The degree of masculinization in the female is variable, and may range from mild enlargement of the clitoris to complete closure of the urethra at the tip of the phallus (see Fig. 91–4). The degree of virilization can be classified by Prader stages ranging from I to V (Fig. 91–12). Stage I represents mild enlargement of the clitoris only, and stage V, complete masculinization of the external genitalia,

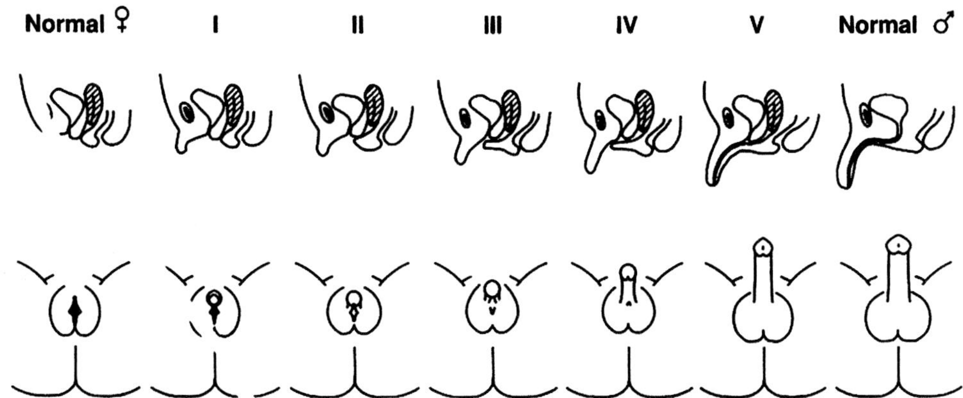


**FIGURE 91–12.** The stages of virilization of the female with congenital adrenal hyperplasia as developed by Prader. Stage I indicates mild clitoromegaly only; stage V indicates complete masculinization. *(Reproduced with permission from Migeon CJ, Berkovitz G, Brown T: Sexual differentiation and ambiguity. In Kappy MS, Blizzard RM, Migeon CJ [eds]: Wilkens' The Diagnosis and Treatment of Endocrine Disorders in Childhood and Adolescence, 4th ed. Springfield, IL, Charles C Thomas, 1994, p 573.)*

with intermediate stages designating lesser degrees of involvement. The internal genitalia (ovaries, uterus, fallopian tubes) of virilized females are normal, however, and wolffian duct–derived structures are absent.

The degree of masculinization of the external genitalia of 46,XX fetuses is dependent on the timing and magnitude of androgen exposure of the fetus. Exposure of the female fetus to high androgen levels earlier then 12 weeks of gestation results in fusion of the labial folds with formation of a urogenital sinus. In severely masculinized cases, the external genitalia may appear completely male (see Fig. 91–4, lower panels). High-level androgen exposure after 12 weeks of gestation will result in mainly clitoral hypertrophy (see Fig. 91–4, upper left panel).

21-Hydroxylase deficiency will result in mineralocorticoid deficiency and salt loss in up to 75% of cases (New, 1992; Therrell et al, 1998). However, clinical manifestations of salt loss typically will not become apparent until several days or weeks after birth. Therefore, all infants with suspected salt-losing CAH need to be followed carefully during this time. Note that the male infant with salt-losing CAH will be phenotypically normal, and he is at great risk for salt-losing crisis after discharge from the newborn nursery. Fortunately, many (approximately 18) state newborn screening programs now screen for CAH to prevent males from developing salt-losing crisis, and also to prevent incorrect gender assignment of profoundly virilized female infants (Therrell et al, 1998) (Case Study 1).

**CASE STUDY 1**

**History**

- A 3.5-kg term infant born after uncomplicated pregnancy
- Cryptorchidism and hypospadias noted, so infant discharged home as a male with plan for outpatient surgical evaluation
- Infant fed poorly at home, with intake of approximately 4 oz/day, no vomiting
- *Day 5 of life*: notification of abnormal newborn screen for congenital adrenal hyperplasia by health department. Referred to emergency room.

**Evaluation**

- On presentation to emergency department: infant was well appearing, weight 2.9 kg (representing a loss of 0.6 kg)
- Genital examination: 2.3 × 1.1 cm phallus, severe hypospadias, marked labial fusion, no palpable gonads, marked hyperpigmentation of genitalia
- Electrolytes: sodium 140 mEq/L, potassium 5.8 mEq/L, chloride 107 mEq/L, $CO_2$ 19 mEq/L, BUN 15 mg/dL, Cr 1.0 mg/dL
- Glucose 94 mg/dL
- Ultrasound examination: uterus present, enlarged adrenals, no gonads seen
- Karyotype 46,XX
- 17-Hydroxyprogesterone 20,000 ng/dL (normal: less than 200) (unstimulated)
- Plasma renin activity 201 ng/mL/hour (normal: less than 26)

**Management and Outcome**

- Gender was reassigned female
- Hydrocortisone (Cortef) and fludrocortisone acetate (Florinef) started along with NaCl supplements
- *Day 10 of life*: weight 3.2 kg, feeding 4 oz/4 hours
- *By 4 months of age*: significant reduction in clitoral and labial enlargement as well as resolution of hyperpigmentation.
- *By 3 years of age*: the clitoral size had not normalized and the mother became very concerned about the child showing signs of gender "confusion," and hence clitoral reduction surgery was performed.

The diagnosis of 21-hydroxylase deficiency should be suspected in all newborns with ambiguous genitalia (or clitoral hypertrophy) and absent gonads in the labial/scrotal folds. A serum 17-hydroxyprogesterone level obtained after the first day of life will often be diagnostic. 17-hydroxyprogesterone levels are usually 50- to 100-fold above the normal range in classic cases, with typical random levels of 10,000 ng/dL or higher (New, 1992). In some cases of 21-hydroxylase deficiency, ACTH stimulation testing may be necessary to establish the diagnosis.

Levels of androstenedione, testosterone, electrolytes, and plasma renin activity should also be determined. Plasma renin activity is a very sensitive indicator of the intravascular volume status of the infant. Impaired sodium-potassium and sodium-hydrogen exchange due to aldosterone deficiency in the distal tubule of the kidney results in hyponatremic dehydration, hyperkalemia, and metabolic acidosis.

Assessment for the less common forms of CAH resulting in ambiguous genitalia—11β-hydroxylase deficiency and 3β-hydroxysteroid dehydrogenase deficiency (3β-HSD)—include measuring 11-deoxycortisol, DOC, and 17-hydroxypregnenolone. (Use of a comprehensive steroid panel from a reliable reference laboratory will limit the amount of required blood to 3 to 5 mL.)

11β-Hydroxylase deficiency accounts for approximately 5% of CAH cases worldwide, and this disorder will result in masculinization of the female fetus (see Fig. 91–11). However, presence of volume overload and hypertension distinguishes this disorder from 21-hydroxylase deficiency (New, 1992). Presumably, the hypertension is due to the excess mineralocorticoid activity of the DOC metabolite. Typically, 11-deoxycortisol (compound S) is elevated and plasma rennin activity is suppressed in this disorder.

3β-HSD may result in ambiguous genitalia in the newborn period (see Fig. 91–11). Unlike 21-hydroxylase deficiency, this enzyme is present in the gonads as well as the adrenals, and deficiency of 3β-HSD may result in undermasculinization of the male infant as well as mild masculinization of the female infant. The 3β-HSD enzyme is needed for testosterone biosynthesis; hence the male fetus may be inadequately masculinized. This enzyme deficiency results in excess production of the steroid DHEA, which can be converted to more potent androgens peripherally. The female infant with this disorder can have clitoromegaly, although such children often are phenotypically normal.

A marked increase in the ratios of 17-hydroxyprogesterone to 17-hydroxypregnenolone and of androstenedione to DHEA is diagnostic in mutation-positive forms of this disorder (Sakkal-Alkaddour et al, 1996).

Treatment of CAH in the newborn period consists of glucocorticoid and mineralocorticoid replacement. Hydrocortisone is the most physiologic form of synthetic glucocorticoids and is less likely to result in unwanted side effects. Hydrocortisone is administered orally at a dose of approximately 25 mg/m$^2$/day in the newborn period (divided into three doses). No liquid preparation of hydrocortisone is currently available, so tablets must be crushed and administered carefully with formula or food. Mineralocorticoid replacement (fludrocortisone acetate [Florinef]) at a starting dose of 0.1 mg/day in the newborn is recommended. Sodium chloride supplements (approximately 1-2 g/day) may be a useful adjunctive therapy in salt-losing CAH, as formula and human milk have low salt contents. Once therapy is initiated, careful monitoring of the infant's growth as well as determination of serum 17-hydroxyprogesterone, androstenedione, testosterone, and plasma renin activity is recommended.

Salt-losing crisis and acute adrenal insufficiency should be treated with stress doses of hydrocortisone (100 mg/m$^2$/day), which can be given either continuously as a drip or divided into equal doses every 6 hours. Intravenous fluids with ample sodium chloride (normal saline for boluses and one-half normal saline for maintenance fluids) are an essential component of treating salt-losing crisis. Care should be taken not to over- or underhydrate the infant. Hyperkalemia often improves after sodium chloride and hydrocortisone are provided intravenously, although severe cases of hyperkalemia may require additional therapies.

Gender assignment in 46,XX infants with 21-hydroxylase deficiency has traditionally been female (American Academy of Pediatrics Committee, 2000; Forest, 2001; Donahoe, 1991; Migeon et al, 1994; New, 1992). Gender identity of 46,XX adults with CAH typically is female, with varying degrees of masculinized behavior (Money and Ehrhardt, 1972; Reiner, 1997). Cases of gender identity disorder have been reported in treated CAH females, however (Slijper et al, 1998), and cases of gender reassignment from female to male have been reported (Meyer-Bahlburg et al, 1996). Persons with undiagnosed 46,XX CAH who are profoundly virilized have functioned successfully as males (Blizzard, 1999). Diamond and Sigmundson (1997a) have suggested male gender assignment in profoundly virilized 46,XX individuals, although female gender assignment is likely to prevail in current practice until evidence is obtained to indicate otherwise (Lee, 2001).

In addition to medical therapies for CAH, efforts to normalize the appearance of the external genitalia may be pursued. It should be kept in mind that hypertrophy of the clitoris will gradually lessen after medical therapy is instituted; however, complete normalization in the more virilized cases is not likely to occur. In severe cases of clitoral enlargement, clitoral reduction surgery is a treatment option, although suboptimal cosmetic results have been reported in long-term outcome studies. Atrophy or loss of the clitoris or excessive regrowth of clitoral tissue has been described in examinations of adolescent and adult patients who underwent genital surgery in early childhood (Alizai et al, 1999; Creighton et al, 2001). The risk of surgery needs to be balanced against the potential detrimental effects of masculinized genitalia on the development of a poor body image (Meyer-Bahlburg et al, 1996) and of social stigmatization by family or community members (Money et al, 1986).

Surgical correction of the vagina in CAH is performed to exteriorize the vagina and also to enlarge the vaginal opening so that successful intercourse may occur later in life (see later section on surgery). Considerable debate exists about when to perform vaginal exteriorization surgery. A number of studies have demonstrated the development of vaginal stenosis when vaginoplasties are performed in the prepubertal period (Alizai et al, 1999; Creighton et al, 2001; Krege et al, 2000). The investigators advocate delaying vaginoplasty until puberty or later, when manual dilation can be undertaken by the patient and estrogenization of the vaginal mucosa may help prevent stricture formation. Others recommend that vaginoplasties be undertaken early in life, as the procedure is technically easier in the first several years of life and the emotional trauma of a major surgery at adolescence is avoided (Donahoe, 1991; Schnitzer and Donahoe, 2001).

Patient advocate groups such as the Intersex Society of North America (ISNA) and others have called for a general moratorium on all nonessential genital surgery in infancy, until affected persons are old enough to express their wishes and give consent (Diamond and Sigmundson, 1997a). Problems with loss of sexual sensation and pleasure have been reported in adult patients as a consequence of genital surgery in early life. However, in cases of severe discordance between assigned sex and genital appearance, the psychosocial consequences of uncorrected genital anomalies may be damaging (Money and Ehrhardt, 1972; Money et al, 1986). Participation of the parents in the decision to pursue genital surgery after they have been fully informed of the benefits and risks is perhaps the most judicious approach at this time (Daaboul and Frader, 2001; Lee, 2001; Reiner, 1997).

Significant reductions in fertility have been reported in women with salt-losing CAH (Kuhnle et al, 1995; Mulaikal et al, 1987). Suggested explanations for reduced fertility included increased anovulatory cycles, low rates of heterosexual activity, inadequate vaginal introitus, and poor compliance with medical treatment (Mulaikal et al, 1987). Problems with a disturbed body image and feeling less feminine were associated with a lower rate of success among women with CAH in terms of the ability to establish a partnership or marry (Kuhnle et al, 1995). Overall quality of life for female patients with CAH was comparable with that for controls, however, suggesting that affected women may develop coping strategies and cognitive appraisals that enable them to accept their life and view it as satisfying (Kuhnle et al, 1995).

### Increased Maternal Androgens and Progestins

Masculinization of the female fetus has been reported in pregnant mothers taking various *progestational agents* to prevent miscarriage. These agents include norethindrone, ethisterone, and medroxyprogesterone. Danazol, which has been used in the treatment of endometriosis, has been associated with fetal masculinization (Grumbach and Conte, 1998). Masculinization of the female fetus due to *maternal virilizing ovarian* or *adrenal tumors* or *luteomas* of pregnancy have been reported. In such cases, virilization beyond the time of birth does not occur, and the prognosis is good (Grumbach and Conte, 1998).

### Placental Aromatase Deficiency

Placental aromatase deficiency has been associated with masculinization of the female fetus. Aromatase is a cytochrome P-450 enzyme that is responsible for the conversion of testosterone to estradiol and of androstenedione to estrone. Autosomal recessive inheritance of aromatase deficiency causes virilization of the female due to failure to metabolize the large amounts of androstenedione and testosterone produced by the placenta. This disorder also will cause significant virilization of the mother. The affected infant will be virilized with normal müllerian structures. Gonadotropins are elevated in infancy, and ovarian cysts may develop. At puberty, females have hypergonadotropic hypogonadism with failure to feminize and progessive virilization. Plasma androstenedione and testosterone are elevated, while estrone and estradiol levels are low. Postpubertal patients have delayed bone maturation, tall stature, and osteopenia (Conte et al, 1994).

## The Incompletely Masculinized Male

Incomplete masculinization refers to absence of or incomplete masculinization of the external and internal genitalia in a person with a 46,XY karyotype and normal testes. Disorders leading to incomplete masculinization of the male include (1) androgen receptor defects, (2) testosterone biosynthetic defects, (3) 5α-reductase deficiency, (4) Leydig cell hypoplasia, and (5) effects of maternal medications (see Fig. 91–9).

It should be noted that in 25% to 50% of undermasculinized males, a specific etiology cannot be found (Al-Agha et al, 2001; Eil et al, 1984). Other factors such as medications and placental insufficiency may potentially interfere with genital masculinization. Placental insufficiency may be related to genital underdevelopment through the presumed mechanism of inadequate human chorionic gonadotropin (hCG) production. Placental hCG is required for early fetal testosterone production and hence early fetal genital development.

Medications such as cimetidine, spironolactone, phenytoin (Dilantin), phenobarbital, medroxyprogesterone, and cyproterone acetate have been associated with altered androgen action or metabolism. Their use during pregnancy may therefore be detrimental to male genital development (Donahoe, 1991; Grumbach and Conte, 1998). Furthermore, various xenobiotics can bind the androgen receptor, and thus speculations on the role of environmental factors in abnormal sex differentiation have been made (Danzol, 1998).

### Androgen Receptor Defects (Androgen Insensitivity)

Disorders of the androgen receptor are the most common definable cause of incomplete masculinization of the genetic male (Quigley et al, 1995). Disorders of the androgen receptor can be divided into complete androgen insensitivity (CAIS) and partial androgen insensitivity (PAIS) syndromes. The gene for the androgen receptor (*AR*) is located on the X chromosome, and over 300 mutations have been found (Griffin et al, 2001). Mutations have been found throughout the *AR* gene, with most mutations occurring in the DNA or steroid-binding domains. Despite extensive characterization of the molecular genetics of *AR* mutations, no genotype-phenotype correlation has been found (Quigley et al, 1995).

The sex-differentiating actions of testosterone and DHT are mediated by the androgen receptor. Dihydrotestosterone is important in the differentiation of the male external genitalia and prostate, whereas testosterone is important in the differentiation of internal wolffian ducts to epididymis, vas deferens, and seminal vesicles.

#### *Complete Androgen Insensitivity*

Complete androgen insensitivity syndrome (CAIS) in a 46,XY individual is characterized by phenotypically normal female external genitalia (Fig. 91–13). Affected children will present with an inguinal hernia prepubertally or because of primary amenorrhea postpubertally. Robust breast development occurs at puberty that is due to peripheral aromatization of testosterone to estrogen. There is usually scant or absent pubic and axillary hair with some vulvar hair. The vagina is short and blind ending, and müllerian structures (cervix, uterus, fallopian tubes) are absent. There are only vestigial or no wolffian duct–derived internal structures. The testes are located in the abdomen or inguinal canal or in the labia majora. Gender identity and role behaviors are typically female. Removal of the testes is recommended because of risk for development of gonadoblastoma, although there is no consensus on the timing of orchidectomy (Forest, 2001; Migeon et al, 1994).

#### *Partial Androgen Insensitivity*

Partial androgen insensitivity syndrome (PAIS) is characterized by varying degrees of ambiguity of the external genitalia. The term *Reifenstein syndrome* formerly was

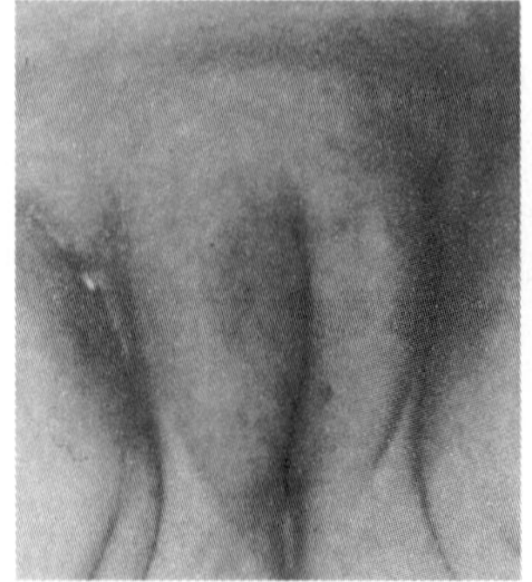

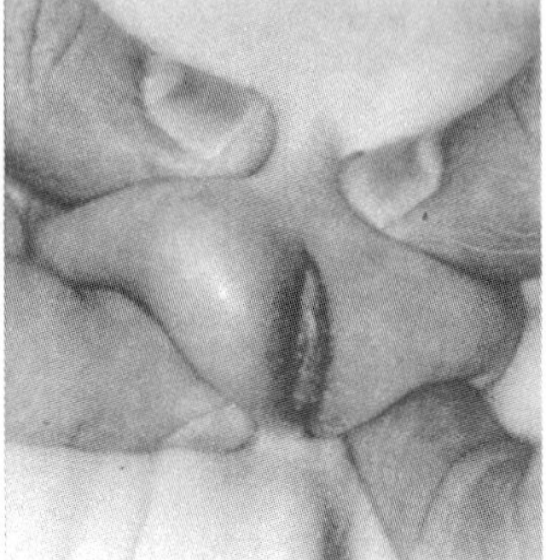

**FIGURE 91–13. Left panel,** Appearance of external genitalia of a 46,XY infant with complete androgen insensitivity syndrome (CAIS). **Right panel,** Note presence of bilateral palpable gonads.

used to describe partial androgen insensitivity with intermediate degrees of masculinization. Affected infants present with a small phallus and a ventral chordee that "tethers" the phallus to the perineum. There is often a penoscrotal hypospadias and a bifid scrotum, which may or may not contain gonads (see Fig. 91–3). Cryptorchidism is not uncommon. Müllerian structures are absent, and the wolffian duct–derived structures are absent or poorly developed. A genitourethrogram may demonstrate a urogenital sinus.

The diagnosis of partial androgen insensitivity is complex. A family history of ambiguous genitalia in male relatives would be suggestive of this diagnosis. However, Viner and colleagues (1997) reported a positive family history in only 25% of patients with PAIS. 5α-Reductase deficiency and testosterone biosynthetic defects should be ruled out by appropriate steroid analysis. This can be accomplished by measuring intermediates in testosterone biosynthesis as well as measuring the ratio of testosterone to DHT. It should be noted that abnormal testosterone-DHT ratios can be seen in PAIS (Ahmed et al, 1999). This may be due to poor development of tissues, which express 5α-reductase-2 in PAIS (Griffin et al, 2001).

Androgen levels in normal newborns are highest at birth and then decline rapidly during the first week. A second testosterone surge occurs between 15 and 60 days of life (Forest et al, 1980). Androgen and LH levels should be obtained at these peak production times. Alternatively, an hCG stimulation test may be performed as follows: a dose of 1500 IU of hCG is given intramuscularly (IM) once daily for 3 days; androgen and gonadotropin levels are measured at baseline and then 24 hours after the third dose. Abnormally elevated levels of LH and/or testosterone in the first several months of life are suggestive of androgen insensitivity. However, a recent report of five neonatal cases of PAIS showed testosterone values in the high-normal range on days 2 to 7 of life (mean, 107 ± 27 ng/dL) and on day 30 (mean, 411 ± 154 ng/dL) (Bouvattier et al, 2002). LH levels were elevated in comparison with historic controls (mean LH levels on days 7 to 15 of life were 5.2 IU/L ± 4.0 ng/dL; on day 30 of life mean levels were 8.7 IU/L ± 2.5 ng/dL). Testosterone response to hCG and LH response to gonadotropin-releasing hormone (GnRH) were exaggerated (Bouvattier et al, 2002).

Androgen receptor binding assay was considered the gold standard for defining this disorder in the past. However, normal ligand binding does not rule out androgen insensitivity, as there may be mutations in domains of the androgen receptor not involved in ligand binding. Direct sequencing of the androgen receptor for mutation analysis is commercially available (GeneTest) and can detect up to 95% of mutations associated with androgen insensitivity. Androgen receptor mutations, however, are not always found in cases of suspected androgen insensitivity, and it is speculated that defects in androgen receptor–interacting proteins may then be involved.

Determining the gender of rearing in partial androgen insensitivity is a difficult task, and multiple factors must be considered. If there is a significant degree of virilization (Prader stages IV and V) (see Fig. 91–12), then male sex assignment is made (Reiner, 1997; Diamond and Sigmundson, 1997a). If masculinization is severely limited (Prader stages 1 and 2), then female sex assignment is recommended. In intermediate forms (Prader stage 3), responsiveness to exogenously administered hCG or testosterone may be of help in the decision-making process (Daaboul and Frader, 2001; Grumbach and Conte, 1998). However, adult males with a small phallus have reported satisfactory sex lives (Reilly and Woodhouse, 1989). These cases perhaps de-emphasize the importance of phallic size in male sex assignment. Slijper and colleagues (1998) report the absence of serious gender identity disorder in five undervirilized 46,XY males, although these boys were "more fearful and bothered about the smallness of their penises." Money and colleagues (1972) caution about the devastating psychosocial effects of male sex assignment when the phallus is only slightly larger than a clitoris and does not respond to testosterone, however.

In a study of 32 undervirilized males assigned female gender of rearing, significant gender transposition (a term meaning gender change as well as homosexual orientation) correlated with the presence of childhood stigmatization and a relatively late age of feminizing surgery (Money et al, 1986). Stigmatization in the home was reflected by treating the child differently from other children, including elaborate efforts at maintaining the privacy of the genital anomaly, keeping the child at home and forbidding play with neighborhood children, and refusal of open communication within the family about the medical condition. Stigmatization in the community was reflected by teasing about the genital anomaly, body habitus, mannerisms, and so on.

Stigmatization by parents or the community also was found to be associated with gender transposition in undervirilized males assigned male gender of rearing; cosmetic inadequacy of the external genitalia was less important (Money and Norman, 1987).

These studies point to the importance of a nurturing, supportive environment to a successful long-term outcome for these children. More comprehensive long-term outcome studies of partial androgen insensitivity are greatly needed, however.

### 5α-Reductase-2 Deficiency

5α-Reductase-2 deficiency is an autosomal recessive disorder that results in an inability to convert testosterone to DHT. DHT is required for the development of the male external genitalia.

At birth, these 46,XY infants typically have a very small phallus that appears to be a normal or slightly enlarged clitoris. However, more significant virilization of the phallus may occur, and the affected child will then be identified as a male with hypospadias. There is usually severe penoscrotal hypospadias. The scrotum is bifid, with slight posterior fusion. The testes are usually in the inguinal canals or labial folds. Approximately half of these patients have a penoscrotal urethra with a separate blind-ending vagina; a smaller percentage have a single urogenital sinus opening on the perineum (Griffin et al, 2001).

Müllerian structures are absent, and wolffian duct–derived structures (vas deferens, epididymis, seminal vesicles) are well developed. The prostate is poorly developed.

At the time of puberty, individuals with this disorder will characteristically virilize. The phallus will typically increase to a length of 4 to 8 cm (Migeon et al, 1994). In affected persons who were raised as females, a change to the male gender role after puberty is commonly seen (Griffin et al, 2001; Imperato-McGinley, 1997). Unlike in partial androgen insensitivity, gynecomastia does not occur in the pubertal period.

5α-Reductase-2 deficiency has been diagnosed in the postpubertal period in most cases, although diagnosis in the newborn period has been reported (Imperato-McGinly et al, 1986; Odame et al, 1992). The disorder is diagnosed by assessing the ratio of testosterone to DHT in blood (Peterson et al, 1977). The normal testosterone-DHT ratio in the newborn period is 4:1, whereas the ratio in infants and children with this disorder is often greater than 14:1. An hCG stimulation test usually is needed to obtain a more definitive diagnosis in the prepubertal period. A positive response to hCG rules out Leydig cell aplasia or a testosterone biosynthetic defect. Measurement of normal androstenedione levels will rule out the testosterone biosynthetic defect: 17β-HSD dehydrogenase deficiency. This enzyme is responsible for the conversion of androstenedione to testosterone, and the clinical presentation in infancy can be similar to that of 5α-reductase deficiency.

In addition, abnormal ratios of 5β- to 5α-urinary steroids can establish a definitive diagnosis of 5α-reductase deficiency-2 (Imperato-McGinley et al, 1986). Distinguishing 5α-reductase deficiency from partial androgen insensitivity is important, as androgen insensitivity can cause a secondary DHT deficiency due to the incomplete development of tissues that express 5α-reductase activity (Griffin et al, 2001). Measurement of urinary 5β- to 5α-glucocorticoids will help make this distinction, as only 5α-reductase deficiency will also affect glucocorticoid metabolism. Analysis of 5α-reductase-2 activity in genital fibroblasts also can be determined. Finally, analysis for mutations in *SRD5A2* gene is diagnostic; however, this test is not currently commercially available.

Sex assignment in cases of 5α-reductase deficiency is a complicated issue, but there is long-term outcome information available. As in androgen insensitivity disorders, sex assignment is often significantly influenced by the degree of masculinization at birth, and because infants with this disorder usually are markedly undervirilized, female sex assignment has been advocated (Grumbach and Conte, 1998; Migeon et al, 1994). However, if the disorder is diagnosed early, topical DHT treatment has been shown to enlarge the phallus (Odame et al, 1992). In addition, the natural history of the disorder is for masculinization of the phallus to occur at puberty. There are frequent reports of reversal from female to male gender behavior after puberty (Wilson, 2001; Wilson et al, 1993). The accumulated evidence would support male sex assignment in this disorder (Imperato-McGinley, 1997), although female sex assignment is likely in the newborn period if the diagnosis is overlooked.

## Testosterone Biosynthetic Defects

Five enzymes are necessary for the synthesis of testosterone. A defect at any step will result in inadequate testosterone synthesis (see Fig. 91–11). Defects in the first three enzymes of the testosterone synthesis pathway will also affect adrenal steroid production, resulting in both an undervirilized male and CAH. Because testosterone production is impaired in these disorders, wolffian duct structures are likely to be underdeveloped, whereas müllerian structures are absent due to normal testicular MIF production. These enzyme deficiencies are quite rare, however, so these disorders are discussed only briefly here.

### *17β-Hydroxysteroid Dehydrogenase-3 Deficiency (17-Ketosteroid Reductase Deficiency)*

The final step in testosterone biosynthesis involves the conversion of androstenedione to testosterone by the enzyme 17β-HSD in the testicle. Mutations that impair the function of 17β-HSD are the cause of this relatively rare autosomal recessive disorder (Wilson, 2001).

The clinical presentation is that of an external female at birth with perhaps a mild degree of clitoral enlargement. The phenotype is female; therefore, these infants typically are raised as females. At puberty, there is progressive masculinization, with enlargement of the phallus to 4 to 6 cm with labial enlargement and rugation. By late puberty, the testes are found at the lower ring of the inguinal canal, and they are of normal size and consistency. Internal wolffian duct–derived structures are found. In addition, a male body habitus develops, and deepening of the voice and male body hair, including mustache and beard are found (Migeon et al, 1994).

Most patients are diagnosed at puberty or as adults. Endocrine studies reveal markedly elevated androstenedione levels, whereas testosterone levels are in the low-normal range (Mendonca et al, 2000). Plasma LH levels are consistently high. In infancy or childhood, the presence of inguinal hernias may bring the child to medical attention. Androstenedione levels in the prepubertal patient may be normal, and the hCG stimulation test is required to elucidate the defect.

Gender of rearing often is influenced by the cultural context. In societies in which a high priority is given to the male gender, gender reassignment at puberty has been successful (Forest, 2001). Mendonca and colleagues (2000) have observed changes in gender role (female to male) in 3 of 10 affected individuals. Despite virilization in some affected persons, however, the female gender role was maintained.

### *Congenital Lipoid Adrenal Hyperplasia*

Lipid accumulation in both the adrenals and gonads is characteristic of this disorder pathologically—hence the name *congenital lipoid adrenal hyperplasia*. Because all adrenal and gonadal steroid synthesis is affected by this disorder, infants are likely to present with complete adrenal insufficiency, characterized by vomiting, weight loss, and hypotension. The phenotype is likely to be female, although there is clinical variability. In the 35 cases reported in the medical literature, only 11 patients have survived beyond infancy (Forest, 2001).

Endocrinologic findings include elevation of ACTH and plasma renin activity but low or unmeasurable levels of all steroid hormones. The main consideration in the differential diagnosis is CAH. The presence of markedly enlarged lipid-laden adrenals on ultrasound, CT, or MRI studies is highly suggestive of the disorder. Successful treatment has occurred and requires replacement of both glucocorticoids and mineralocorticoids. All persons diagnosed with this disorder have been raised as females (Grumbach and Conte, 1998).

In vitro studies performed on either adrenal or testicular tissue demonstrated an inability to convert cholesterol to pregnenolone in these patients. A defect in the first step of adrenal and gonadal steroid biosynthesis mediated by the cytochrome P-450 side chain cleavage (P450scc) enzyme was suspected. However, subsequent molecular studies demonstrated mutations in the steroidogenic acute regulatory protein (StAR) (Grumbach and Conte, 1998). StAR acts to promote sterol translocation to the P450scc enzyme in mitochondria (see Fig. 91–11).

### *3β-Hydroxysteroid Dehydrogenase Deficiency II*

3β-HSD deficiency was first reported by Bongiovanni (1962). 3β-HSD is an important enzyme required for the conversion of Δ-5 to Δ-4 steroids in the adrenals and gonads (see Fig. 91–11). There is marked heterogeneity in clinical presentation, and both genders are affected (Forest, 2001). With severe deficiency of 3β-HSD, salt-losing crisis may occur. Male infants may have ambiguous or completely feminine external genitalia, whereas female infants may be mildly virilized. Severely undervirilized males may have normal mineralocorticoid activity; fully masculinized males may display salt loss.

Diagnosis of this disorder in the newborn period may be difficult because of relatively high levels of Δ-5 steroids physiologically. The diagnosis is based on the ratio of 17-hydroxyprogesterone to 17-hydroxypregnenolone and of DHEA to androstenedione in the basal and stimulated states (Sakkal-Alkaddour et al, 1996).

### *17α-Hydroxylase/17,20-Lyase Deficiency*

A single enzyme encoded on the P450c17 gene mediates the 17-hydroxylation of pregnenolone and progesterone and the conversion of 17-hydroxypregnenolone and 17-hydroxyprogesterone to DHEA and androstenedione. Clinical disorders of this enzyme affect primarily either the hydroxylation or the lyase reaction. Cases of primarily 17-hydroxylase deficiency should be considered in undervirilized males or females with hyporeninemic hypertension and hypokalemic alkalosis. The hypertension is due to elevated levels of DOC and corticosterone (see Fig. 91–11). Most cases are diagnosed in the pubertal period because the 46,XY phenotype is largely female. Of interest, although cortisol synthesis is blocked, the overproduction of DOC and corticosterone is protective against adrenal insufficiency. This disorder is treated with glucocorticoid, which suppresses ACTH overproduction and subsequently suppresses DOC and corticosterone overproduction (Grumbach and Conte, 1998). Sex steroid replacement is needed at puberty.

17,20-Lyase deficiency results in varying degrees of undermasculinization of the 46,XY infant. The phenotype ranges from complete female external genitalia to ambiguous genitalia to a mildly undervirilized male. 46,XX females will present with failure to enter puberty. Gonadotropins will be elevated, along with impaired formation of DHEA and androstenedione (see Fig. 91–11). DOC and corticosterone are normal in this form of the disorder. Human chorionic gonadotropin and ACTH stimulation tests may be helpful to more fully reveal the steroid biosynthetic block.

### Leydig Cell Hypoplasia

Failure of testicles to produce testosterone in response to hCG is characteristic of this disorder. Histologic examination of the testes reveals absent or low numbers of Leydig cells, normal-appearing Sertoli cells, and seminiferous tubules with spermatogenic arrest (Grumbach and Conte, 1998). LH receptor mutations have been described in this disorder. Phenotypically, the external genitalia vary from those of a normal female to those of a male with microphallus. Müllerian-derived structures are absent in all patients, whereas wolffian structures may be present. LH and FSH levels are elevated in postpubertal patients and LH levels decrease after testosterone administration. In less severe forms of the disorder, testosterone therapy augments phallic growth. In severe forms of testicular unresponsiveness to hCG/LH, gender assignment has been female. The gonads are removed, and estrogen replacement therapy is instituted at the time of expected puberty (Grumbach and Conte, 1998).

### Persistent Müllerian Duct Syndrome

The diagnosis of PMDS often is made in otherwise phenotypically normal 46,XY males at the time of surgery for an inguinal hernia or orchidopexy. In the case of hernia repair, a fallopian tube and uterus are often found along with a partially descended testis. In other cases, testes, uterus, and fallopian tubes are found in the pelvis. PMDS is inherited autosomally recessively, although the female phenotype is completely normal. The disorder has been found to be due to a mutation in the antimüllerian hormone or receptor (Grumbach and Conte, 1998). Therapy involves orchidopexy and partial hysterectomy, with care taken to avoid injuring the vas deferens that is embedded in the uterine wall.

## Gonadal Differentiation and Chromosomal Disorders

### 46,XY Complete Gonadal Dysgenesis

46,XY complete gonadal dysgenesis was first described by Swyer in 1955 (Grumbach and Conte, 1998). The phenotype of the external genitalia was female with normal development of müllerian–derived internal structures. Streak gonads are found that are completely

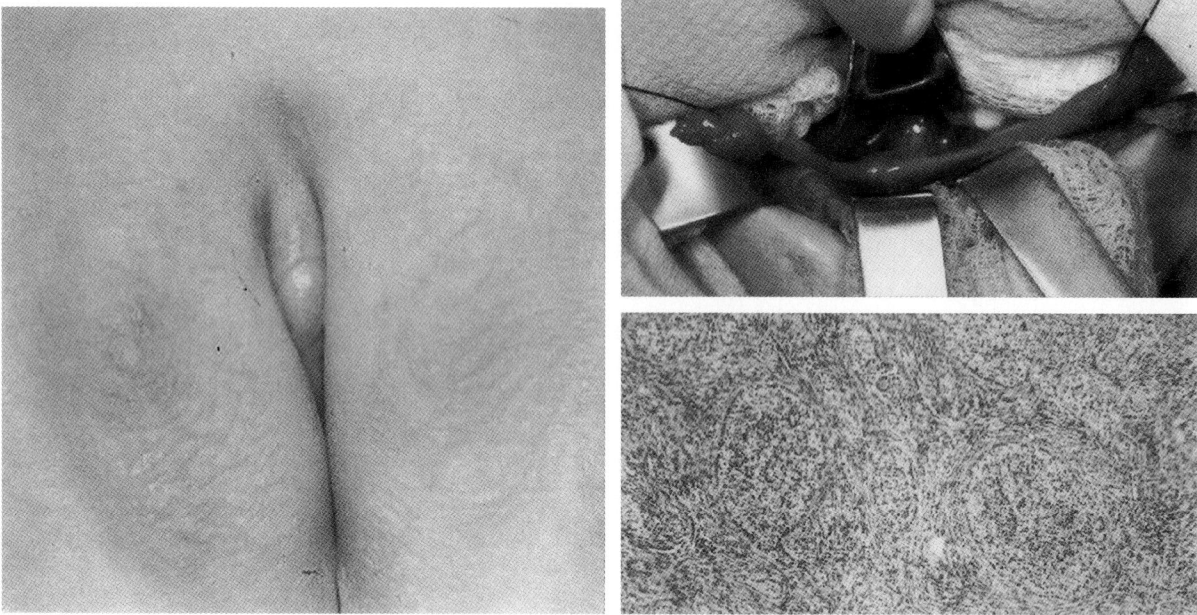

**FIGURE 91–14. Left panel,** Appearance of external genitalia in complete gonadal dysgenesis in a 46,XY infant with features of Turner syndrome. **Upper right panel,** Uterus and fallopian tubes were found at surgery, along with a gonadoblastoma, at 1 year of age. **Lower right panel,** Micrograph of tumor cells.

nonfunctional; therefore, müllerian structures do not regress, and wolffian structures are poorly developed or absent (Fig. 91–14). Most affected persons present in the teenage years with lack of pubertal development. Serum gonadotropin levels are elevated. Mutations in the *SRY* gene account for only a small proportion of these cases (Forest, 2001). Familial cases have been reported. In up to 30% of affected persons, gonadoblastomas will develop in the streak gonad; therefore, removal of the streak gonad is recommended (Migeon et al, 1994) (see Fig. 91–14). Estrogen replacement therapy will provide appropriate feminization.

### 46,XY Partial Gonadal Dygenesis

Patients with 46,XY partial gonadal dygenesis will typically present in the newborn period for evaluation of ambiguous genitalia (Berkovitz et al, 1991). The extent of masculinization of the external genitalia depends on the extent of testicular differentiation. Gonadal tissue is usually intra-abdominal, but testes can be found in the scrotum. One quarter of these patients will have phenotypic features of Turner syndrome (Migeon et al, 1994). Testosterone response to hCG is variable but usually low. In most cases, there is a mix of müllerian and wolffian structures. The presence of müllerian structures on genitourethrogram or ultrasound increases the index of suspicion for this disorder. The diagnosis is confirmed by gonadal biopsy. Some affected children are found to have one dysgenetic gonad on one side and a streak gonad on the other; others have bilateral dysgenetic gonads. Dysgenetic gonads are histologically defined by poorly formed and disorganized seminiferous tubules surrounded by wavy ovarian stroma. In many cases, the dysgenetic gonads resemble ovotestes, except that primordial ovarian follicles are lacking (Berkovitz et al, 1991) (Case Study 2).

**CASE STUDY 2**

#### History

- Infant born at 35 weeks of gestation, weight 2.49 kg (50% percentile for gestational age)
- Pregnancy complicated by maternal hypertension treated with propranolol
- Cesarean section performed for breech position, oligohydramnios, and poor growth.

#### Physical Examination and Laboratory Studies

- Genital examination: phallus 1.4 cm in length with poorly formed glans, no palpable testes; no hypospadias
- Ultrasound examination: presence of uterus, no gonads seen
- Genitogram: large prostatic utricle, no uterus (see Fig. 91–6, left panel)
- Karyotype and FISH: 46,XY, no mosaicism
- Endocrine studies

  *Day 3 of life*:
  17-Hydroxyprogesterone 107 ng/dL (normal: less than 570)
  Testosterone 4 ng/dL (37 to 198)
  DHT less than 2.0 ng/dL (10 to 53)
  Androstenedione 58 ng/dL (80 to 446)

  *Day 11 of life*:
  Müllerian inhibitory factor 3.0 ng/mL (mean 30)
  hCG stimulation test (1500 units IM every other day × 3): testosterone increased from 18 to 65 ng/dL (normal response is greater than 150)
- Gonadal biopsies: dysgenetic testes identified and removed.

### Diagnosis

- 46,XY partial gonadal dysgenesis

### Management and Outcome

- Testosterone enanthate 25 mg IM given × 1; phallic growth increased from 1.6 to 2.1 cm
- Male gender assignment made

---

## Mixed Gonadal Dysgenesis

Mixed gonadal dysgenesis (MGD) refers to asymmetrical gonadal dysgenesis with ambiguous genitalia (see Fig. 91–5) and a mosaic karyotype with an XY cell line. The most common karyotype is 45,XO/46,XY. There is a wide spectrum of phenotypes, ranging from a female with clitoral enlargement to a male with hypospadias. Asymmetrical external and internal genital development has been classically described in this syndrome (Forest, 2001). Considerable phallic development was described in a majority of patients in one study, and there was often penoscrotal hypospadias (Davidoff and Federman, 1973). The phenotypic features of Turner syndrome are described in a significant percentage of patients, although these features may not be readily apparent in the newborn period. An incompletely formed uterus is found in almost all patients. Fallopian tubes are always found on the side of the streak gonad and often found on the side with the dysgenetic gonad. Wolffian structures may be developed on the side with the dysgenetic gonad.

A genitourethrogram is likely to demonstrate internal müllerian structures which can be confirmed at laparoscopy. Demonstration of abnormal gonadal histopathology will confirm the diagnosis. It should be noted that MGD shares many features with partial gonadal dysgenesis, and some authors view these disorders as representing a continuum of gonadal dysgenesis (Berkovitz et al, 1991). Histologic analysis will also differentiate this disorder from true hermaphroditism.

Although the characteristic karyotype is 45,XO/46,XY, it should be pointed out that this genotype has been associated with normal male differentiation in the majority of cases diagnosed by prenatal amniocentesis (Wheeler et al, 1988).

Some authors advocate female sex assignment in MGD, because surgical repair of the vagina is usually easy and a uterus or hemiuterus is present. In addition, the dysgenetic gonad is at risk for development of a tumor and should be removed, particularly if the gonad cannot be brought down into the scrotum (Forest, 2001). However, sex assignment is likely to be guided by the degree of virilization, with the more virilized cases being assigned as males. The capacity for near normal androgen production in this disorder has been described (Davidoff and Federman, 1973). In all cases, the streak gonads should be removed because of the risk for malignancy.

## *Testicular Regression Syndrome*

Testicular regression syndrome refers to the spectrum of disorders affecting persons with 46,XY karyotype who demonstrate evidence of prior testicular function, followed by usually symmetrical gonadal regression. Loss of testicular function between weeks 8 and 10 of gestation would result in ambiguous genitalia and variable internal genitalia. Loss of testicular function after 12 to 14 weeks of gestation would result in normal male genital differentiation with a small phallus. When the male external and internal ducts are completely normal, the term *vanishing testis syndrome* is used by some authors. Presumably the testes were lost during the second half of pregnancy. Testicular torsion has been invoked as a possible explanation in this syndrome.

FSH levels are elevated in infancy, and an exaggerated response to gonadotropin-releasing hormone (GnRH) in the prepubertal period typically is seen (Grumbach and Conte, 1998) Antimüllerian hormone (AMH) levels in infancy and childhood are very low in anorchia and intermediately low with abnormal testes (Lee et al, 1997).

## True Hermaphroditism

True hermaphroditism is defined as the presence of both testicular tissue with distinct seminiferous tubules and ovarian tissue containing mature graafian follicles in a single individual. Both testicular and ovarian elements may be found in the same gonad, or one testicle and one ovary may be found in the same individual. In the majority of cases the karyotype is 46,XX; 46,XX/46,XY chimerism and 46,XY karyotypes also can be found. Clinically, the external genitalia are often ambiguous, but predominantly male or female phenotypes have been described (Grumbach and Conte, 1998; Hadjiathanasiou et al, 1994). In ambiguous cases, a relatively marked degree of virilization can be found. Almost all have some degree of hypospadias and incomplete labioscrotal fold fusion. The labioscrotal folds are asymmetrical, with an appearance of a hemiscrotum on one side and labium majora on the other was seen in 10 of 22 cases (Hadjiathanasiou et al, 1994). At least one gonad is usually palpable. A vagina and uterus are present in most patients, and a genitourethrogram may be required for elucidation. Internal duct development is consistent with the associated gonad, although müllerian ducts predominate with an ovotestis. Breast development is common during puberty and menses can occur in up to 50%.

The diagnosis should be suspected in 46,XX/46,XY individuals with ambiguous genitalia. Palpation of a polarized gonad should also lead the clinician to suspect the diagnosis. In one study, 11 of 12 46,XX true hermaphrodites examined before 6 months of age had baseline testosterone levels greater than 40 ng/dL; normal levels for females of this age would be less than 15 ng/dL (Hadjiathanasiou et al, 1994).

Gender assignment depends on the degree of masculinization, capacity of testicular tissue to secrete testosterone, and the presence or absence of a uterus and tubes. In general, a female gender assignment is favored because of the presence of ovarian tissue and external genitalia that can more easily be reconstructed as female. Male gender assignment is more likely if there is significant virilization. Removal of ductal or gonadal structures not consonant with the gender of rearing is recommended. Testes are usually dysgenetic, which carries an increased risk of gonadoblastoma formation; therefore, careful follow-up evaluation is indicated. As in all cases of intersex, gender identity/behavior issues, along with general psychological well-being, should be longitudinally evaluated.

### Syndromes Associated with Ambiguous Genitalia

*Denys-Drash syndrome* is a rare syndrome consisting of the classic triad of congenital nephrotic syndrome leading to end-stage renal failure, XY ambiguous genitalia, and Wilms tumor. The external genitalia of 46,XY individuals are either ambiguous or female. Gonadal development encompasses a spectrum from streak gonads to dysgenetic testes. Nephropathy and proteinuria are noted at an early age, and renal biopsy will demonstrate mesangial sclerosis. Greater than 90% of cases will have a mutation in the *WT1* gene. *WT1* is a gene critical for the development of the normal genital tract. *WT1* also is associated with the WAGR syndrome. Large deletions of chromosome 11p13 that encompass the *WT1* gene are responsible for this disorder. *Frasier syndrome* also involves the *WT1* gene. This syndrome manifests in 46,XY females with gonadal dysgenesis and progressive glomerulopathy.

*Camptomelic dysplasia* is a rare autosomal dominant disorder associated with often lethal skeletal dysplasia, in which 75% of affected 46,XY males have dysgenetic testes associated with undervirilization (Grumbach and Conte, 1998). Manifestations of this disorder include bowing of the femora and tibiae, hypoplastic scapulae, 11 rib pairs, pelvic malformations, bilateral clubfoot, cleft palate, macrocephaly, micrognathia, hypertelorism, and a variety of cardiac and renal defects. The disorder is caused by heterozygous mutations in the *SOX9* gene (Grumbach and Conte, 1998). Most patients die in the neonatal period from respiratory distress.

*Smith-Lemli-Opitz syndrome* is an autosomal recessive disorder with an estimated frequency of 1/20,000 to 1/40,000. The disorder is caused by 7-dehydrocholesterol reductase deficiency (Forest, 2001). This enzyme catalyzes the final step in cholesterol biosynthesis; thus, the combination of low serum cholesterol and a high serum 7-dehydrocholesterol is suggestive of the diagnosis. Growth and developmental delay and multiple congenital anomalies characterize this disorder. Genital anomalies include hypospadias, crytorchidism, micropenis, and hypoplastic scrotum. Craniofacial abnormalities include microcephaly, narrow bifrontal diameter, broad maxillary ridges, ptosis of the eyelids, micrognathia, and anteverted nostrils (Jones, 1997). Syndactyly of the second or third toes is a common feature. Adrenal insufficiency has been reported in this condition. Treatment with cholesterol improves growth and neurodevelopmental status.

*Robinow syndrome* is an autosomal dominant disorder characterized by a flat facial profile, short forearms, and hypoplastic genitals (Jones, 1997). Sporadic cases have been reported. In males, microphallus may be severe, although normal virilization at the time of puberty has been reported (Jones, 1997). Undescended testes have been reported in 65% of affected boys. Females have characteristic hypoplastic labia and clitoris. Other features include small size at birth, macrocephaly, frontal bossing, hypertelorism, prominent eyes, small upturned nose, micrognathia, and posteriorly rotated ears. Short forearms are seen in 100% of described cases. Other skeletal abnormalities include thoracic hemivertebrae, fusion or absence of ribs, and scoliosis. The abnormal facial features become less pronounced as the child grows, and cognitive performance has been normal in most affected persons.

### Other Disorders of Genital Differentiation

*Hypospadias* is one of the most common anomalies of male genital development, with an estimated incidence of 4 to 8 cases per 1000 male births (Grumbach and Conte, 1998). Hypospadias can be classified as glandular, penile, penoscrotal, scrotal, and perineal. Typically, the more severe forms of hypospadias have been associated with intersex disorders, although the phenotypic spectrum of intersex disorders is wide. In a study of 33 patients with severe (scrotal or penoscrotal) hypospadias, 12 were found to have an intersex disorder, which included Denys-Drash syndrome (in 3 of the 12), partial androgen insensitivity (in 2), true hermaphroditism (in 2), chromosomal abnormality (in 1), MIF abnormality (in 1), gonadal dysgenesis (in 1), 5α-reductase deficiency (in 1), and 46,XX male karyotype (in 1, *SRY* positive) (Albers et al, 1997). It should be noted that in 11 of the 12 patients, the testes were undescended. Aarskog (1970) found an approximately 15% prevalence of intersex disorders in association with hypospadias, and a significant role for maternal progestins was found.

Thus, severe cases of hypospadias require a thorough evaluation including karyotype and hCG stimulation testing, along with examination of the genitourinary tract, particularly if accompanied by undescended testes.

## OVERVIEW OF THE SURGICAL MANAGEMENT OF INTERSEX DISORDERS

Surgery for intersex conditions has recently come under criticism. The criticism has focused not only on the timing of surgery but on whether reconstructive surgery should be done at all. Some authorities have advised that surgery be postponed until the affected person is of an age to make his or her own decision regarding the advisability of surgical correction (Diamond and Sigmundson, 1997a). Others have found that delay in surgery may be associated with problematic outcomes (Meyer-Bahlburg et al, 1996; Money et al, 1986; Reiner, 1997). It is imperative that these divergent viewpoints be discussed with the parents of an infant with an intersex condition.

These issues must be kept in mind in any decision regarding surgery for management of intersex conditions. Current surgical techniques that are available for correction of ambiguous genitalia and intersex conditions are presented next.

### Feminizing Genitoplasty

Feminizing genitoplasty is one of the more common procedures done for correction of ambiguous genitalia. Feminizing genitoplasty is indicated in the genetic female who is externally virilized, most commonly as the result of CAH. The degree of virilization can be quite variable (see Fig. 91–4). The degree of virilization will have a significant influence on the type of procedure done, especially the vaginoplasty portion of this operation. Reconstruction in this group of patients has three components: (1) clitoral reduction, (2) vaginoplasty, and (3) labial reconstruction. The timing of surgical correction also has undergone some changes over the years. The current thinking is that once a decision is made to proceed with genital reconstruction, performing this type of surgery at a younger age will have distinct advantages, including easier mobilization of the urogenital sinus and a more benign postoperative course.

### Clitoral Reduction

Attempts at managing the enlarged clitoris in genetic females with clitoral hypertrophy started with total clitorectomy. Young (1937) originally advocated this procedure. Later, Lattimer (1961) suggested a recession rather than a resection of the clitoris, and he hoped to be able to preserve the arousal function of the clitoris. This led to cases in which painful clitoral erections occurred later in life; therefore, further modification was needed. In 1973, Spence and Allen (1973) advocated the preservation of the glands with reduction in the size of the clitoris. Since then, several reports have looked at preservation of the neurovascular bundle using a clitoral reduction/recession type of approach. Kogan (1987) and Snyder (1983) and their colleagues separately described a similar approach in which the erectile tissue of the clitoris is removed but preservation of the neurovascular bundle and the glands is afforded to preserve the neurologic and arousal functions of the clitoris. If, however, the gland is unusually large in size, then a reduction of the gland size may be indicated as well.

### Vaginoplasty

Reconstruction of the vagina in cases of virilization in females requires an understanding of the anatomy. One may consider the anatomic abnormality an embryologic arrest of maturation with a persistence of an early embryologic stage. The anatomic issue that is important to the surgical management of the common urogenital sinus is the site of the confluence of the genital tract and the urethra. This varies considerably but is somewhat predictable by the appearance of the degree of external virilization. Those children with severe degrees of external virilization are more likely to have a higher confluence of the urethral and vaginal channels, leading to a longer urogenital sinus or a more masculinized urogenital sinus. In the classic article on urogenital sinus abnormalities, Hendron and Crawford (1969) described the variable anatomy that can be seen in these children and noted that the operative procedures needed to be tailored toward the location of the confluence of the urinary and genital tracts. One may describe the confluence anatomically as it relates to the external sphincter, with confluences distal to the external sphincter being considered low and those proximal to the external sphincter referred to as high. One also may describe the variable anatomy according to the length of the urethra from the bladder neck to the point of the confluence. If that length of urethra was long, then one would consider this a low confluence, whereas if the length of the urethra was short and therefore close to the bladder neck, then a high confluence would be present (see Fig. 91–6, right).

The low-confluence cases can generally be repaired either by a cutback procedure on the fused labial scrotal folds or by a flap vaginoplasty. A cutback procedure would be indicated in cases with a minor degree of fusion of the labioscrotal folds. The mid- to high vaginal confluence, however, generally requires either a pull-through vaginoplasty or a total urogenital mobilization, to bring the vagina down to the perineum.

### Flap Vaginoplasty

The flap vaginoplasty should be used for a low confluence of the urogenital sinus. The procedure entails mobilization of a perineum-based flap with its apex at the meatus of the urogenital sinus. Dissection then proceeds along the posterior wall of the urogenital sinus until the vaginal opening is identified. The perineum-based flap is then inserted into the posterior wall of the vagina, therefore, exteriorizing the vagina to the perineum.

### Total Urethral Mobilization

Total urogenital mobilization can be used for the high urogenital sinus. This has been advocated by Pena (1997) and subsequently was substantiated by reports from Rink and colleagues (1997). This approach has been shown to have a superior cosmetic result, compared with that obtained with a flap vaginoplasty, for a mid to high confluence. In addition, there has been a reduced incidence of urethral vaginal fistula and vaginal stenosis. The mobilization occurs in a plane both anterior to the urogenital sinus and up to the bladder neck under the pubic symphysis and posteriorly along the urogenital sinus, and then along the posterior wall of the vagina.

### Pull-Through Vaginoplasty

The pull-through vaginoplasty is reserved for use in severely masculinized genetic females, whose surgical management continues to present a major challenge. Initially, the approach was a combined perineal and abdominal approach with complete mobilization of the vagina and uterus and separation of the vagina from the urethra at the confluence. The abdominal mobilization will then allow the vagina to be brought down to the perineum. A modification of this approach was described by Passerini-Glazel (1989) in which the more distal urogenital sinus tissue was used to provide an anterior vaginal wall flap, which will then connect to the true vagina. This will allow for a complete perineal approach to the procedure as well.

## Vaginal Agenesis

Vaginal replacement has a role in certain intersex conditions or structural abnormalities of the genital urinary tract. The intersex conditions in which vaginal replacement may be indicated are 46,XX vaginal agenesis, 46,XY male karyotype with severely inadequate virilization or complete androgen insensitivity syndrome, and structural urogenital defects such as cloacal exstrophy or persistent cloaca, or following a pelvic exenteration for malignancy. There are a variety of tissues and techniques used for vaginal reconstruction; skin grafting, progressive perineal indentation, split-thickness or fold thickness tissue grafts with expanders, myocutaneous flaps, and bowel. The critical point in creating a vagina is to maintain an adequate perineal opening, an adequate-length tunnel, and good fixation to pelvic structures. This area is highly controversial in terms of the best management. Overall, the most popular tissue for vaginal plate replacement has been the split-thickness skin graft as described by McIndoe (1950). The major disadvantage of this technique has proved to be the need for long-term dilatation to maintain patency and to avoid vaginal stenosis. The use of bowel segments for vaginal replacement was first described by Baldwin (1904). Due to an extraordinarily high mortality rate associated with this approach, earlier attempts using this technique were abandoned. Since then, this approach has been taken up by many groups and has been shown to be highly successful, with minimal complication rates. A major advantage of a bowel-segment vagina over a skin graft is the minimal risk of "poor take" due to the vascularized pedicle to the segment of bowel that is used. Length and patency of the bowel are not issues for similar reasons, because it maintains its blood supply. No dilatation is needed. Early on, intestinal mucus production can be a problem, but this lessens over time, and mucus may act as a natural lubricant. Minimal perineal scarring is associated with this approach as well, and it can be done at a very young age (Hensle and Dean, 1992).

### Male Pseudohermaphroditism

Inadequate virilization results in hypospadias, with or without cryptorchidism. In more severe cases, such as a complete form of androgen insensitivity, these children may appear as phenotypic normal females and present at the time of puberty with primary amenorrhea. Vaginoplasty is frequently needed after puberty in that population. Those children presenting with varying degrees of hypospadias, with or without cryptorchidism, will usually require a repair following the usual principles of hypospadias and cryptorchidism repair. These are generally done at 6 months of age and are tolerated well as outpatient procedures.

### Gonadectomy

Gonadectomy is required under two circumstances in intersex conditions. Gonadectomy would be recommended when the gonads are inconsistent with the sex of rearing. This is most commonly seen in androgen insensitivity syndrome (46,XY karyotype) in which normal testes are present but a female gender assignment has been made. The timing of the gonadectomy is controversial; however, it is currently thought to be best managed once the diagnosis has been made, because the role of postnatal testosterone imprinting in a child's psychosocial development is uncertain.

The other circumstance in which gonadectomy is recommended is in intersex states in which gonadal malignancy is a significant risk. This is most likely to occur in cases in which dysgenetic gonads and a Y chromosome are present. An example is shown in Figure 91–14, in which a 1-year-old infant with pure XY gonadal dysgenesis was found to have a gonadoblastoma on gonadectomy. Other syndromes in which gonadal malignancy is a concern include mixed gonadal dysgenesis and the presence of a dysplastic testis in a dysgenetic XY male.

## CONCLUSIONS

Significant advances have been made in our understanding of the pathophysiology and molecular genetics of intersex disorders. A systematic diagnostic approach to the infant with ambiguous genitalia should be undertaken to identify the underlying disorder. Establishing the diagnosis will often provide a better understanding of the natural history of the disorder.

The need for surgical intervention in intersex disorders should be assessed on a case-by-case basis. The parents need to be informed about the risks and benefits of surgery. Surgery on the external genitalia should perhaps be reserved for those individuals with significant discord between the sex of rearing and the appearance of the external genitalia.

The infant and the family of a child with an intersex condition often may have to cope with difficult psychosocial challenges throughout life. Physicians caring for these patients should try and ensure the integration of well-trained mental health professionals into the longitudinal care of these complex infants and children.

## REFERENCES


Aarskog D: Clinical and cytogenetic studies in hypospadias. Acta Paediatr Scand 203(suppl):1-62, 1970.

Ahmed SF, Cheng A, Hughes IA: Assessment of the gonadotropin-gonadal axis in androgen insensitivity syndrome. Arch Dis Child 80:324-329, 1999.

Al-Agha AE, Thomsett MJ, Batch JA: The child of uncertain sex: 17 years of experience. J Paediatr Child Health 37:348-351, 2001.

Albers N, Ulrichs C, Gluer S, et al: Etiologic classification of severe hypospadias: Implications for prognosis and management. J Pediatr 131:386-392, 1997.

Alizai NK, Thomas DFM, Lilford RJ, et al: Feminizing genitoplasty for congenital adrenal hyperplasia: What happens at puberty? J Urol 161:1588-1591, 1999.

Almaguer MC, Saenger P, Linder BL: Phallic growth after hCG. Clin Pediatr 32:329-333, 1993.

American Academy of Pediatrics Committee on Genetics, Section on Endocrinology/Section on Urology: Evaluation of the newborn with developmental anomalies of the external genitalia. Pediatrics 106:138-142, 2000.

Azziz R, Mulaikal RM, Migeon CJ, et al: Congenital adrenal hyperplasia: Long-term results following vaginal reconstruction. Fertil Steril 46:1011-1014, 1986.

Baldwin J: The formation of an artificial vagina by intestinal transplantation. Ann Surg 40:398, 1904.

Berkovitz GD, Fechner PY, Zacur HW, et al: Clinical and pathological spectrum of 46,XY gonadal dysgenesis: Its relevance to the understanding of sex differentiation. Medicine 70:375-383, 1991.

Blizzard RM: Adult consequences of pediatric endocrine disease. I: Congenital adrenal hyperplasia. Growth Genet Horm 15:33-41, 1999.

Bongiovanni AM: Adreno-genital syndrome with deficiency of 3β-hydroxysteroid dehydrogenase J Clin Invest 41:2086-2092, 1962.

Bouvattier C, Carel J, Lecointre C, et al: Postnatal changes of T, LH, and FSH in 46,XY infants with mutations in the *AR* gene. J Clin Endocrinol Metab 87:29-32, 2002.

Conte FA, Grumbach MM, Ito Y, et al: A syndrome of female pseudohermaphroditism, hypergonadotropic hypergonadism, and multicystic ovaries associated with missense mutations in the gene encoding aromatase (P450arom). J Clin Endocrinol Metab 78:1287-1292,1994.

Creighton SM, Minto CL, Steele SJ: Objective cosmetic and anatomical outcomes at adolescence of feminizing surgery for ambiguous genitalia done in childhood. Lancet 358:124-125, 2001.

Daaboul J, Frader J: Ethics and the management of patients with intersex: A middle way. J Pediatr Endocrinol Metab 14:1575-1583, 2001.

Danzol BJ: The effects of environmental hormones on reproduction. Cell Mol Life Sci 54:1249-1264, 1998.

Davidoff F, Federman DD: Mixed gonadal dysgenesis. Pediatrics 52:725-742, 1973.

Diamond M, Sigmundson K: Management of intersexuality. Arch Pediatr Adolesc Med 151:1046-1050, 1997a.

Diamond M, Sigmundson K: Sex reassignment at birth. Arch Pediatr Adolesc Med 151:298-304, 1997b.

Donahoe P: Clinical management of intersex abnormalities. Curr Probl Surg 28:519-579, 1991.

Eil C, Crawford JD, Donahoe PK, et al: Fibroblast androgen receptors in patients with genitourinary anomalies. J Androl 5:313-320, 1984.

Feldman KW, Smith DW: Fetal phallic growth and penile standards for newborn male infants. J Pediatr 86:395-398, 1975.

Forest MG, de Peretti E, Bertrand J: Testicular and andrenal androgens and their binding to plasma proteins in the perinatal blood: Developmental patterns of plasma testosterone, androstenedione and its sulfate in premature and small for date infants as compared with that of full term infants. J Steroid Biochem 12:25-36, 1980.

Forest MG: Diagnosis and treatment of disorders of sexual development. In Degroot LJ, Jameson JL (eds): Endocrinology, 4th ed. Philadelphia, WB Saunders, 2001.

GeneTests: www.genetests.org

Griffin JE, McPhaul MJ, Russell DW, Wilson JD: The androgen resistance syndromes: Steroid 5α-reductase-2 deficiency, testicular feminization, and related disorders. In Scriver CR, Beaudet AL, Sly WS, Valle D (eds): The Metabolic and Molecular Basis of Inherited Diseases, 8th ed. New York, McGraw-Hill, 2001, p 4117.

Grumbach MM, Conte FA: Disorders of sex differentiation. In Wilson JD, Foster DW, Kronenberg HM, Larsen PR (eds): Williams Textbook of Endocrinology, 9th edition. Philadelphia, WB Saunders, 1998, pp 1303-1426.

Hadjiathanasiou CG, Brauner R, Lortat-Jacob S, et al: True hermaphroditism: Genetic variants and clinical management. J Pediatr 125:738-744, 1994.

Hendren WH, Crawford JD: Adrenogenital syndrome: The anatomy of the anomaly and its repair. J Pediatr Surg 4:49-58, 1969

Hensle TW, Dean GE: Vaginal replacement in children. J Urol 148:677-679, 1992

Imperato-McGinley J, Gautier T, Pichardo M, Shackleton C: The diagnosis of 5α-reductase deficiency in infancy. J Clin Endocr Metab 63:1313-1318, 1986.

Imperato-McGinley J: 5α-Reductase-2 deficiency. In Bardin CW (ed): Current Therapy in Endocrinology and Metabolism, 6th ed. St. Louis, Mosby, 1997, pp 384-386.

ISNA: Intersex Society of North America: www.isna.org

Jones KL (ed): Smith's Recognizable Patterns of Human Malformation, 5th ed. Philadelphia, WB Saunders, 1997, p 112.

Kogan SJ, Smey P, Levitt SB: Subtunical total reduction clitoroplasty: A safe modification of existing techniques. J Urol 130:1079, 1987.

Koplen DE, Manley CB: Timing of general surgery. Chapter 4 in Ehrlich MR, Deiter GJ (eds): Reconstructive and Plastic Surgery of the External Genitalia. Philadelphia, WB Saunders, 1999.

Krege S, Walz KH, Hauffa BP, et al: Long-term follow-up of female patients with congenital adrenal hyperplasia from 21-hydroxylase deficiency, with special emphasis on the results of vaginoplasties. BJU Int 86:253-259, 2000.

Kuhnle U, Bullinger M, Schwarz HP: The quality of life in adult female patients with congenital adrenal hyperplasia: A comprehensive study of the impact of genital malformations and chronic disease on female patients' life. Eur J Pediatr 154:708-716, 1995.

Kuhnle U, Krahl W: The impact of culture on sex assignment and gender development in intersex patients. Persp Bio Med 45:85-103, 2002.

Lattimer JK: Relocation and recession of the enlarged clitoris with preservation of the glans: An alternative to amputation. J Urol 86:113-116, 1961.

Lee MM, Donahoe PK, Silverman BL, et al: Measurement of serum müllerian inhibiting substance in the evaluation of children with nonpalpable gonads. N Engl J Med 336:1480-1486, 1997.

Lee PA: Should we change our approach to ambiguous genitalia? Endocrinologist 11:118-123, 2001.

McIndoe A: Treatment of congenital absence and obliterative conditions of the vagina. Br J Plast Surg 2:254-267, 1950.

Mendonca BB, Inacio M, Arnhold IJP, et al: Male pseudohermaphroditism due to 17β-hydroxysteroid dehydrogenase 3 deficiency. Medicine 79:299-309, 2000.

Meyer-Bahlburg HFL, Gruen RS, New M, et al: Gender change from female to male in classical congenital adrenal hyperplasia. HormBehav 30:319-332, 1996.

Migeon CJ, Berkovitz G, Brown T: Sexual differentiation and ambiguity. In Kappy MS, Blizzard RM, Migeon CJ (eds): Wilkens' The Diagnosis and Treatment of Endocrine Disorders in Childhood and Adolescence, 4th ed. Springfield, IL, Charles C Thomas, 1994, p 573.

Money J, Ehrhardt AA: Man & Woman, Boy & Girl. Baltimore, Johns Hopkins University Press, 1972.

Money J, Norman BF: Gender identity and gender transposition: Longitudinal outcome study of 24 male hermaphrodites assigned as boys. J Sex Marital Ther 13:75-92, 1987.

Money J, Devore H, Norman BF: Gender identity and gender transposition: Longitudinal outcome study of 32 male hermaphrodites assigned as girls. J Sex Marital Ther 12:165-181, 1986.

Mulaikal RM, Migeon CJ, Rock JA: Fertility rates in female patients with congenital adrenal hyperplasia due to 21-hydroxylase deficiency. N Engl J Med 316:178-182, 1987.

New MI: Female pseudohermaphroditism. Semin Perinatol 16:299-318, 1992.

Odame I, Donaldson MDC, Wallace AM, et al: Early diagnosis and management of 5α-reductase deficiency. Arch Dis Child 67:720, 1992.

Passerini-Glazel G: A new one stage procedure for a clitoral vaginoplasty in severely masculinized females with female pseudo hermaphroditism, J Urol 142:565, 1989.

Pena A: Total urogenesis sinus mobilization: An easier way to repair cloacus. J Pediatr Surg 30:2, 1997.

Peterson RE, Imperato-McGinley J, Gautier T, Sturla E: Male pseudohermaphroditism due to steroid 5α-reductase deficiency. Am J Med 62:170-191, 1977.

Phornphutkul C, Fausto-Sterling A, Gruppuso P: Gender self-reassignment in an XY adolescent female born with ambiguous genitalia. Pediatrics 106:135-137, 2000.

Quigley CA, DeBellis A, Marschke KB, et al: Androgen receptor defects: Historical, clinical, and molecular perspectives. Endocr Rev 16:271-321, 1995.

Rajfer J, Walsh PC: The incidence of intersexuality in patients with hypospadias and cryptorchidism. J Urol 116:769, 1976.

Reilly JM, Woodhouse CRJ. Small penis and the male sexual role. J Urol 142:569-571, 1989.

Reiner WG: Case study: Sex reassignment in a teenage girl. J Am Acad Child Adolesc Psychiatry 35:799-803, 1996.

Reiner WG: Sex assignment in the neonate with intersex or inadequate genitalia. Arch Pediatr Adolesc Med 151:1044-1045, 1997.

Rink RC, Pope JC, Kropp BP, et al: Reconstruction of the high urogenital sinus: Early perineal prone approach without division of the rectum. J Urol 158:1293-1297, 1997.

Sakkal-Alkaddour H, Zhang L, Xiaojiang Y, et al: Studies of 3β-hydroxysteroid dehydrogenase genes in infants and children manisfesting premature pubarche and increased adrenocorticotropin-stimulated steroid levels. J Clin Endocrinol Metab 81:3961-3965, 1996.

Schnitzer JJ, Donahoe PK: Surgical treatment of congenital adrenal hyperplasia. Endocrinol Clin North Am 30:137-154, 2001.

Schwartz S, Depinet TW, Leana-Cox J, et al: Sex chromosome markers: Characterization using fluorescence in situ hybridization and review of the literature. Am J Med Genet 71:1-7, 1997.

Slijper FME, Drop SLS, Molenaar JC, et al: Long-term psychological evaluation of intersex children. Arch Sex Behav 27:125-144, 1998.

Snyder HMC, Rettick AB, Bauer SB, et al: Feminizing genitoplasty: A synthesis. J Urol 129:1024-1026, 1983.

Spence HM, Allen TD: Genital reconstruction in the female with the adrenogenital syndrome. Br J Urol 45:126-130, 1973.

Therrell BL, Berenbaum SA, Manter-Kapanke V, et al: Results of screening 1.9 million Texas newborns for 21-hydroxylase-deficient congenital adrenal hyperplasia. Pediatrics 101:583-590, 1998.

Viner RM, Teoh Y, Williams DM, et al: Androgen insensitivity syndrome: A survey of diagnostic procedures and management in the UK. Arch Dis Child 77:305-309, 1977.

Wheeler M, Peakman D, Robinson A, Henry G: 45,X/XY mosaicism: Contrast of prenatal and postnatal diagnosis. Am J Med Genet 29:565-571, 1988.

Wilson JD: Androgens, androgen receptors, and male gender role behavior. Horm Behav 40:358-366, 2001.

Wilson JD, Griffin JE, Russell DW: Steroid 5α-reductase 2 deficiency. Endocr Rev 14:577-593, 1993.

Wright NB, Smith C, Rickwood AMK, Carty HML: Imaging children with ambiguous genitalia and intersex states. Clin Radiol 50:823-829, 1995.

Young HH: Genital abnormalities. In Young HH (eds): Genital Abnormalities, Hermaphroditism and Related Adrenal Diseases. Baltimore, Williams & Wilkins, 1937, p 119.

CHAPTER 92

# Disorders of the Thyroid Gland

Daniel H. Polk and Delbert A. Fisher

## BASIC SCIENCE OF THYROID FUNCTION

### Embryogenesis and Histologic Development of the Thyroid Gland

The human thyroid gland is a derivative of the primitive buccopharyngeal cavity. It develops from contributions of two anlagen: (1) a midline thickening of the pharyngeal floor (median anlage) and (2) paired caudal extensions of the fourth pharyngobranchial pouch (lateral anlagen). All of these structures are discernible by day 16 or 17 of gestation; by day 24, the median anlage has developed a thin flask–like diverticulum extending from the floor of the buccal cavity down to the fourth branchial arch. At 40 days of gestation, the median and lateral anlagen have fused, and by 50 days of gestation, the buccal stalk has ruptured. During this period, the thyroid gland migrates caudally to its definitive location in the anterior neck, helped in part by its relationship with developing cardiac structures.

Developmental abnormalities of the thyroid gland usually represent defects in early morphogenesis resulting from aberrant thyroid tissue migration. The most common anomaly is persistence of the thyroglossal duct. This is not usually associated with altered thyroid status in the newborn but may manifest in later life as an infected fistulous tract. Abnormalities of thyroid embryogenesis (thyroid dysgenesis) include agenesis and presence of ectopic tissue in sublingual, cervical, mediastinal, or even intracardiac locations. Although ectopic thyroid tissue may manifest some function, affected infants usually exhibit some degree of hypothyroidism. In addition, calcitonin deficiency is present in children with congenital hypothyroidism. However, hypoparathyroidism is not associated with thyroid dysgenesis, although the parathyroid glands may be ectopic in these children.

### Thyroid Hormone Synthesis

Circulating plasma iodide enters the thyroid follicular cells and is combined with tyrosine through a series of enzymatically mediated reactions to form the active thyroid hormones 3,5,3′-triiodothyronine ($T_3$) and thyroxine ($T_4$). The steps in the synthesis and release of thyroid hormones include (1) active transport of inorganic iodide from plasma to thyroid cell; (2) synthesis of tyrosine-rich thyroglobulin, which acts as the intermediate iodine acceptor; (3) organification of trapped iodide as iodotyrosines; (4) coupling of monoiodotyrosines (MITs) and diiodotyrosines (DITs) to form the iodothyronines, $T_3$ and $T_4$, with storage of iodotyrosines and iodothyronines in follicular colloid; (5) endocytosis and proteolysis of colloid thyroglobulin to release MIT, DIT, $T_3$, and $T_4$; and, (6) deiodination of released iodotyrosines within the thyroid cell with reutilization of the iodine. These steps and their inhibitors are outlined in Table 92–1. Certain defects in these biochemical processes have been identified, leading in most cases to clinical hypothyroidism. These are discussed later under "Congenital Hypothyroidism."

### Fetal-Placental-Maternal Thyroid Interaction

The relative independence of the maternal and fetal hypothalamic-pituitary-thyroid hormone systems is suggested by several clinical observations. The placenta is impermeable to thyroid-stimulating hormone (TSH) and largely impermeable to the thyroid hormones. These data were reviewed by Roti (1988) and are summarized in Table 92–2. Direct evidence of placental transfer of thyroid hormones is provided by studies using various thyroid hormone analogues and tracers. Human studies have shown limited transfer from mother to fetus. Large doses of $T_4$ given to women produced only minor changes in cord serum concentrations of hormonal iodine. Supraphysiologic doses of $T_3$ chronically administered to pregnant women several weeks before delivery significantly increased maternal serum $T_3$ levels but only minimally lowered fetal $T_4$ values. Thus, it is clear that under physiologic conditions, placental transfer of thyroid hormones is limited. This limitation is due, at least in part, to the presence in placental tissue of an inner-ring (tyrosyl) iodothyronine deiodinase, which converts $T_4$ to inactive reverse $T_3$ ($rT_3$) and converts $T_3$ to inactive diiodothyronine, or $T_2$. Of interest are data suggesting that the maternal compartment may contribute significantly to fetal thyroid hormone levels in the hypothyroid fetus (Vulsma et al, 1989). The physiologic significance of this observation is uncertain.

Maternal immunoglobulins of the IgG subclass are selectively transported across the placenta, particularly late in gestation. Hyperthyroidism or hypothyroidism has been reported in response to maternally derived TSH receptor–stimulating or TSH receptor–blocking antibodies. Usually, these syndromes either are detected by newborn screening or are manifested as neonatal symptoms and signs (Matsurra et al, 1980; Zakarija and McKenzie, 1983). Thyroid scanning in affected infants reveals the presence of a normally situated thyroid gland; the clinical abnormalities wane with degradation of the maternal antibodies. The half-life in newborn blood for the maternally derived IgG antibodies is approximately 20 days.

The placenta is freely permeable to iodide, and the fetal thyroid is particularly sensitive to the inhibitory effects of iodine on thyroid function (Theodoropoulos et al, 1979). Relatively small amounts of maternal iodine exposure have been associated with transient neonatal hypothyroidism. The iodine source may be radiopaque dyes used for radiographic procedures as well as maternal medications, including topically applied iodine washes, which may be absorbed across mucous membrane surfaces.

**TABLE 92–1**

**Biochemical Steps to Thyroid Hormone Synthesis**

| Step | Inhibitor(s) |
|---|---|
| Iodide transport | $ClO_4^-$ and $SCN^-$ |
| Thyroglobulin synthesis | Protein synthesis inhibitors |
| Organification of iodide | PTU, MMI |
| MIT, DIT coupling | PTU, MMI |
| Thyroglobulin endocytosis and proteolysis | $I^-$, $Li^-$, colchicine, cytochalasin B |
| Deiodination | Dinitrotyrosine |

DIT, diiodotyrosine; MIT, monoiodotyrosine; MMI, methimazole; PTU, propylthiouracil.

This effect is described more fully in the section on congenital hypothyroidism.

The thiourylene antithyroid drugs cross the placenta and may compromise fetal and neonatal thyroid function (Marchant et al, 1977). The placenta also is permeable to selected synthetic thyroid hormone analogues such as 3′,5′-dimethyl-5-isopropyl thyronine (DIMIT). There is no current rationale, however, for use of these analogues, because of their low biologic activity. Finally, the placenta is permeable to the hypothalamic peptide thyrotropin-releasing hormone (TRH). Both primate and human fetuses early in the third trimester respond to pharmacologic doses of exogenous TRH with an increase in serum TSH. However, little endogenous TRH is normally detected in adult humans because of the presence of TRH-degrading enzyme systems in the blood. Although the sera of pregnant women contain somewhat lower levels of these enzymes than nonpregnant sera, the nearly unmeasurable levels of TRH in the maternal circulation have little effect on fetal thyroid function.

In addition to producing TRH, the placenta produces thyrotropin-like activity. The alpha subunit of TSH is identical to that of human chorionic gonadotropin (hCG), and the beta subunit of hCG has structural homology with the beta subunit of TSH; thus, hCG has some TSH-like bioactivity. However, the biologic potency of hCG is only about 0.01% that of TSH, and hCG normally has little influence on fetal thyroid system development or function. Because of the hyperthyroidism sometimes seen in patients with choriocarcinoma, a unique chorionic thyrotropin has been proposed, and a glycoprotein with thyrotropic activity has been isolated from human placenta. A structure has never been characterized, however, and it seems likely that this chorionic thyrotropin represents a variant form of hCG (Harada and Hershman, 1978).

In summary, placental permeability to maternal molecules might be a factor affecting fetal thyroid function as a result of maternal pathophysiologic states (acute iodide administration, autoimmune thyroid disease, or pharmacotherapy of thyrotoxicosis). However, the fetal pituitary-thyroid axis normally develops independently of the maternal thyroid axis influence. The placenta and selected fetal tissues may serve as sources of TRH or TSH, but the extent of this influence on fetal thyroid function is uncertain.

**TABLE 92–2**

**Placental Permeability for Substances Affecting Thyroid Function**

| Substance | Placental Permeability |
|---|---|
| $I^-$ | ++++ |
| TRH | +++ |
| Thiourylenes | +++ |
| IgG antibodies | +++ |
| $T_3$ | 0 |
| $T_4$ | + |
| TSH | 0 |

IgG, immunoglobulin G; $T_3$, triiodothyronine; $T_4$, thyroxine; TRH, thyrotropin-releasing hormone; TSH, thyroid-stimulating hormone.

Data from Roti E: Regulation of thyroid-stimulating hormone (TSH) secretion in the fetus and neonate. J Endocrinol Invest 11:145-150, 1988.

## Control of Thyroid Hormone Production

The pattern of perinatal thyroid hormone secretion in the human is shown in Figure 92–1. Maturation of thyroid system control can be considered in three phases: hypothalamic, pituitary, and thyroidal. Changes in these systems are complex and superimposed on the increasing production and increasing serum concentration of serum thyroid hormone–binding globulin (TBG) as well as the changing pattern of fetal tissue iodothyronine deiodination during gestation. Maturation of these latter systems is described in the following section.

Although the fetal thyroid gland is able to concentrate iodide and synthesize thyroglobulin at 70 to 80 days of gestation, little thyroid hormone synthesis occurs until about 18 weeks of gestation. At this time, thyroid follicular cell iodine uptake increases, and $T_4$ becomes measurable in the serum. Both total and free $T_4$ concentrations

**Maturation of Thyroid Hormone Secretion in the Human Fetus**

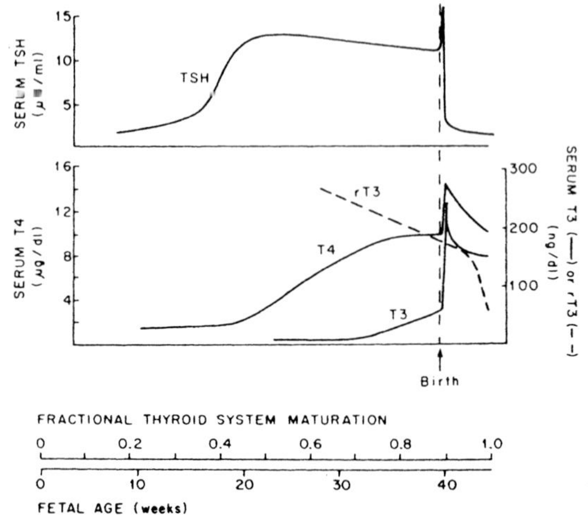


**FIGURE 92–1.** Patterns of circulating levels of thyroid-stimulating hormone (TSH), reverse triiodothyronine ($rT_3$), thyroxine ($T_4$), and $T_3$ in the fetus and newborn.

then increase steadily until the final weeks of pregnancy (Fisher, 1985). This pattern differs from the development of serum $T_3$ levels in the fetus. The fetal serum $T_3$ concentration is low (less than 15 μg/dL) until 30 weeks of gestation and then increases slowly in two distinct phases, a prenatal and a postnatal phase. Prenatally, serum $T_3$ increases slowly after 30 weeks of gestation to reach a level of approximately 50 μg/dL in term cord serum (Fisher and Klein, 1981). Postnatally, both $T_3$ and $T_4$ serum concentrations increase fourfold to sixfold within the first few hours of life, peaking at 24 to 36 hours after birth. These levels then gradually decline to adult values over the first 4 to 5 weeks of life. The prenatal increase in serum $T_3$ seems to be due largely to progressive maturation of hepatic type I (phenolic) outer-ring iodothyronine deiodinase activity and increasing hepatic conversion of $T_4$ to $T_3$, although other tissue sources of deiodinase, such as brown fat and kidney, may be involved.

Fetal serum TSH increases rapidly from a low level at 18 weeks of gestation to a peak value at 24 to 28 weeks and then gradually declines until term. At the time of parturition, partly in response to cold stress, an acute release of TSH occurs, resulting in an elevated level by 30 minutes of life. The level of circulating TSH remains modestly elevated for 2 to 3 days after birth. The increases in thyroid hormone that occur immediately after birth are not totally dependent on TSH and may represent other influences in the thyroid gland at the time of parturition. The high postnatal $T_3$ levels in the days following birth are due to both TSH stimulation of thyroidal $T_3$ secretion and further rapid maturation of tissue outer ring monodeiodinase activity.

Fetal thyroid gland function develops under the influence of a moderately elevated TSH level during the last half of gestation. The increase in serum $T_4$ that occurs during the last trimester is accompanied by a progressive decrease in serum TSH, suggesting that changes in both thyroid follicular cell sensitivity to TSH and pituitary thyrotroph sensitivity to the negative feedback effect of thyroid hormones occur during this period. The pituitary gland contains a type II outer-ring iodothyronine deiodinase, which converts $T_4$ to active $T_3$, which in turn modulates TSH production. In most circumstances, it is circulating $T_4$ that is most important in TSH control. Thus, even when the circulating $T_3$ level is low (as in midgestation), there may be significant negative feedback control (by $T_4$) of pituitary TSH secretion.

The ontogeny of TRH secretion and function in the fetus remains somewhat obscure. TRH immunoactivity is detectable in the hypothalamus by midgestation, increasing markedly in the third trimester after the peak in serum TSH activity is noted. The premature infant (born before 30 to 32 weeks) is characterized by low levels of $T_4$ and free $T_4$, a normal or low level of TSH, and a normal or prolonged TSH response to TRH indicating a state of physiologic TRH deficiency. The full-term human fetus responds to pharmacologic maternal doses of TRH with a somewhat prolonged increase in TSH, suggesting a degree of relative hypothalamic (tertiary) hypothyroidism (Roti et al, 1981). Fetal sources of nonhypothalamic TRH (placenta and pancreas) probably contribute to the elevated circulating levels of fetal and cord blood TRH and presumably account for the high circulating TSH level characteristic of the midgestation fetus. However, the significance of ectopic TRH to the development of thyroid system control remains to be investigated.

In summary, the control of fetal thyroid hormone secretion can be characterized as a balance among increasing hypothalamic TRH secretion, increasing thyroid follicular cell sensitivity to TSH, and increasing pituitary sensitivity to thyroid hormone inhibition of TSH release. The fetus progresses from a state of both primary (thyroidal) and tertiary (hypothalamic) hypothyroidism in midgestation through a state of mild tertiary hypothyroidism during the final weeks of pregnancy and to fully mature thyroid function in the perinatal period.

## Fetal Thyroid Hormone Metabolism

Although the thyroid gland is the sole source of $T_4$, most of the $T_3$ that circulates in the adult is derived from conversion of $T_4$ to $T_3$ via monodeiodination in peripheral tissues. Deiodination of the iodothyronines is the major route of metabolism, and monodeiodination may occur at either the outer (phenolic) ring or the inner (tyrosyl) ring of the iodothyronine molecule. Outer-ring monodeiodination of $T_4$ produces $T_3$, the active form of thyroid hormone with the greatest affinity for the nuclear thyroid hormone receptor. Inner-ring monodeiodination of $T_4$ produces $rT_3$, an inactive metabolite. In mature humans, between 70% and 90% of circulating $T_3$ is derived from peripheral conversion of $T_4$, and 10% to 30%, from direct glandular secretion. Nearly all of the circulating $rT_3$ derives from peripheral conversion, with only 2% to 3% coming directly from the thyroid gland. $T_3$ and $rT_3$ are progressively metabolized to diiodo-, monoiodo-, and noniodinated forms of thyronine, none of which possesses biologic activity.

Two types of outer-ring iodothyronine monodeiodinases (5′-MDIs) have been described. Type I 5′-MDI, expressed predominantly in liver and kidney, is an enzyme inhibited by propylthiouracil, and its activity is stimulated by thyroid hormone. Type II 5′-MDI, located predominantly in brain, pituitary, and brown adipose tissue, is insensitive to propylthiouracil, and its activity is inhibited by thyroid hormone (Refetoff and Larsen, 1989). Type I 5′-MDI activity in the liver, and perhaps the kidney and muscles, probably accounts for most of the peripheral deiodination of $T_4$; type II 5′-MDI acts primarily to increase local intracellular levels of $T_3$ in the brain and pituitary and is important to brown adipose tissue function during the immediate postnatal period. The outer-ring iodothyronine deiodinase also deiodinates $rT_3$ to diiodothyronine.

Both type I 5′-MDI and type II 5′-MDI are present in third-trimester fetuses (Polk et al, 1988b). Both deiodinase species are thyroid hormone responsive. However, hepatic type I 5′-MDI activity becomes thyroid hormone responsive (e.g., activity decreases with hypothyroidism) only during the final weeks of gestation. Brain type II activity, in contrast, is responsive (increases with hypothyroidism) throughout the final trimester of gestation. Thus, type II deiodinase probably plays an important role in providing a source of intracellular $T_3$ to those tissues (such as pituitary and, in some species, brown fat and brain) dependent on $T_3$ during fetal life, whereas the ontogeny of the type I enzyme (to provide increased serum $T_3$ levels) increases only during the final weeks of gestation and during postnatal life.

An inner-ring (tyrosyl) iodothyronine monodeiodinase (type III 5-MDI) has been characterized in most fetal tissues, including the placenta. This enzyme system catalyzes the conversion of $T_4$ to $rT_3$ and $T_3$ to diiodothyronine. Fetal thyroid hormone metabolism is characterized by a predominance of type III enzyme activity, particularly in the liver, kidney, and placenta, and this accounts in part for the increased circulating levels of $rT_3$ observed in the fetus. Placental type III deiodinase contributes to amniotic fluid $rT_3$ levels and presumably also contributes to circulating fetal $rT_3$. However, the persistence of high circulating $rT_3$ levels for several weeks in the newborn indicates that type III 5-MDI activities expressed in nonplacental tissues also are important to the maintenance of high circulating $rT_3$ levels.

Both $T_3$ and $T_4$ in blood are associated with various plasma proteins including TBG, thyroxine-binding prealbumin (TBPA), and albumin. TBG serves as the primary transport protein for both $T_3$ and $T_4$; 70% of the total $T_4$ and 40% to 60% of total $T_3$ are bound to TBG. The rest of the thyroid hormones are distributed almost equally between TBPA and albumin. The binding affinities of these proteins are such that adult-free $T_4$ and $T_3$ concentrations are about 0.03% and 0.3%, respectively, of the total hormone concentrations. TBG, TBPA, and albumin are produced by the liver, and production of these proteins increases progressively during the final half of gestation. Hepatic TBG production is stimulated by estrogen, and the increasing levels of estrogens during pregnancy account, at least in part, for the total plasma $T_4$ concentration, which increases progressively from midgestation until 34 to 35 weeks of gestation.

## Thyroid System Effects and Adaptation to Extrauterine Life

In general, much of the fetal thyroid development is preparatory, providing for the relatively large amounts of thyroid hormones required for normal postnatal development. The production of active thyroid hormones is markedly increased in association with the events of parturition (see Fig. 92–1). During the first hours after birth, there are abrupt threefold to sixfold increases in circulating $T_4$ and $T_3$ levels, coincident with an increase in serum TSH concentrations. The initial increases in circulating thyroid hormone levels are due largely to increased hormone secretion from the thyroid gland. Substances other than TSH also may modulate the acute increases in circulating thyroid hormones at birth. A postnatal increase in serum catecholamine concentrations occurs at the time of parturition (Padbury et al, 1985), and the thyroid gland is adrenergically innervated. The cold-stimulated TSH surge is short-lived, and the decrease in TSH that follows during the 72 to 96 hours after birth is due to feedback inhibition by $T_4$ at either the hypothalamic or the pituitary level (or both). The serum TRH concentration is elevated in cord blood and declines in the days following birth. A clear increase in the serum TRH value coincident with the increase in TSH after parturition has not been reported, but the parallel increases in both TSH and prolactin levels in the early hours after birth support the view that the TSH surge is mediated by TRH (Roti, 1988). Thyroid hormone levels in the newborn gradually return to adult levels by about 1 month of age. The high level of circulating $rT_3$ characteristic of the fetus persists following birth, gradually declining to the adult range by 4 to 6 weeks of age.

The metabolic significance of the neonatal thyroid hormone surge is not entirely clear. Physiologic processes known to be modulated by thyroid hormone in adults, such as thermogenesis and cardiovascular responses, clearly are important in the transition from intrauterine to extrauterine life, and it is tempting to link these transitional events with changes in thyroid hormone metabolism. Several studies using animal models have attempted to establish such a link and support the view that the level of thyroid function during the final weeks of gestation is more important than the neonatal increases in $T_3$ and $T_4$ for successful neonatal transition (Polk et al, 1988a). The situation in the human newborn may be somewhat different. Newborns with congenital thyroid agenesis have few if any signs or symptoms of thyroid hormone deficiency, and their postnatal environmental adaptation usually is not impaired. The precise timing of maturation of thyroid hormone effects on thermogenesis and cardiovascular function in the human newborn has not been defined.

In humans, thyroid hormone nuclear receptors have been reported in fetal lung, brain, heart, and liver at 13 to 19 weeks of gestation by Gonzales and Ballard (1981) and Bernal and Pekonen (1984). The only thyroid hormone actions that have been characterized in the fetus are the effects of hypothyroidism on serum TSH and bone maturation. Most effects of thyroid hormone on perinatal developmental processes occur postnatally (Fig. 92–2).

In summary, thyroid hormones affect important postnatal processes including growth, thermogenesis, and development. The largely successful transition of athyrotic infants to extrauterine life speaks to the limited impor-

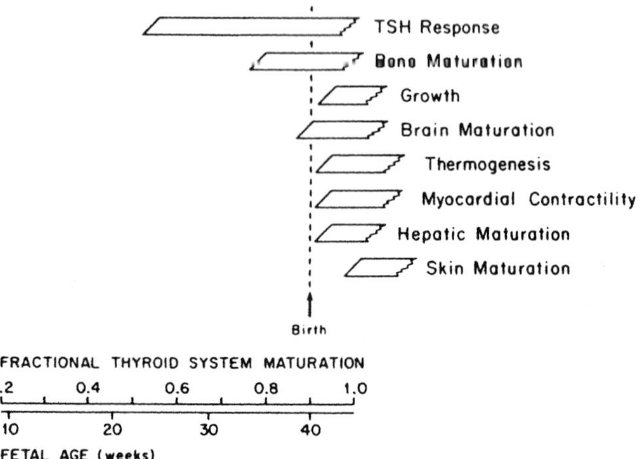


**FIGURE 92–2.** Onset of actions of thyroid hormone in the developing human. The left edge of the bar indicates the initiation of thyroid hormone responsiveness of the indicated parameter.

tance of fetal thyroid hormones in all but the final weeks of gestation. An exception to this may be the fetal brain, a major site of type II iodothyronine monodeiodinase activity in the fetus. The presence of this enzyme system in the brain early in development as well as its demonstrated response to fetal hypothyroidism in the rat and sheep suggests that intracellular conversion of $T_4$ to $T_3$ in the brain is important in these species for normal development and differentiation of the central nervous system. The critical period for this effect is not known for the human fetus, but early treatment of congenital hypothyroidism in the newborn prevents mental retardation, suggesting that the period of thyroid dependency of the human brain extends into the postnatal period.

## CONGENITAL HYPOTHYROIDISM

Congenital hypothyroidism has been recognized for centuries and its treatment known for decades, but only recently has a link between early treatment and the prevention of sequelae been proposed. With today's emphasis on early screening, many conditions that lead to the syndrome of congenital hypothyroidism have been recognized (Table 92–3). The importance of adequate neonatal screening in the management of newborn thyroid diseases must be emphasized. Before the advent of screening, less than one third of the infants found ultimately to have congenital hypothyroidism were given the diagnosis before 3 months of age, and only half by 6 months of age; irreversible brain damage developed in most of these infants (Jacobsen and Brandt, 1981).

**TABLE 92–3**

**Thyroid Disorders and Their Approximate Incidences in the Neonatal Period**

| Disorder | Incidence |
|---|---|
| Thyroid dysgenesis | 1/4,000 |
| Agenesis | |
| Hypogenesis | |
| Ectopia | |
| Thyroid dyshormonogenesis | 1/30,000 |
| TSH receptor defect | |
| Iodide-trapping defect | |
| Organification defect | |
| Iodotyrosine deiodinase deficiency | |
| Defect in thyroglobulin | |
| Transient hypothyroidism | 1/40,000 |
| Drug-induced | |
| Maternal antibody–induced | |
| Idiopathic | |
| Hypothalamic-pituitary hypothyroidism | 1/100,000 |
| Hypothalamic-pituitary anomaly | |
| Panhypopituitarism | |
| Isolated TSH deficiency | |

TSH, thyroid-stimulating hormone.

Newborn screening programs for congenital hypothyroidism are designed to detect elevated serum TSH levels in blood samples collected on filter paper. Some programs measure TSH directly, and others measure TSH in samples with low or low-normal $T_4$ concentrations. In most programs in the United States, an initial $T_4$ measurement is conducted, and TSH is measured in the 10% of samples with the lowest $T_4$ values. An elevated TSH level (greater than 20 μIU/mL) suggests primary hypothyroidism. Most screening programs are just that, and some infants with hypothyroidism are missed in the screening process. Thus, no infant who presents with signs or symptoms suggestive of thyroid dysfunction (Table 92–4) should be excluded from investigation on the basis of previous screening results. A determination of serum $T_4$ and TSH values is necessary in any infant with suspicious clinical or laboratory findings.

### Causative Disorders

The following are the major pathophysiologic states that may lead to congenital thyroid dysfunction (see Table 92–3).

#### Thyroid Dysgenesis

The term *thyroid dysgenesis* describes infants with ectopic or hypoplastic thyroid glands (or both) as well as those with total thyroid agenesis. Thyroid dysgenesis is the etiologic factor in most infants with permanent congenital hypothyroidism detected in newborn screening programs. Some thyroid tissue probably is present in two thirds of these infants, so that the thyroid deficiency in these infants occurs across a spectrum of severity. A normal or near-normal circulating level of $T_3$ in the face of a low $T_4$ value suggests the presence of residual thyroid tissue,

**TABLE 92–4**

**Clinical Signs and Symptoms of Congenital Hypothyroidism in Infancy**

| Age/Manifestation | Frequency (%) |
|---|---|
| **0 to 7 Days** | |
| Prolonged jaundice >3 days | 73 |
| Birth weight >4 kg | 40 |
| Poor feeding | 40 |
| Transient hypothermia | 38 |
| Large posterior fontanel (>5 mm) | 32 |
| **1 to 4 Weeks** | |
| Failure to gain weight | 45 |
| Constipation | 35 |
| Hypoactivity | 33 |
| **1 to 3 Months** | |
| Failure to thrive | 90 |
| Umbilical hernia | 49 |
| Macroglossia | 43 |
| Myxedema | 40 |
| Hoarse cry | 30 |

and this can be confirmed by a thyroid scan. A measurable level of serum thyroglobulin also indicates the presence of some thyroid tissue; athyrotic infants have no circulating thyroglobulin (Dammacco et al, 1985).

Thyroid dysgenesis occurs in 1/4000 liveborn infants and is more prevalent in female than in male infants by a ratio of almost 2:1. Studies by Frasier and colleagues (1982) and Brown and coworkers (1981) suggest the disorder may be less common in African-American (1/32,000) than in white infants and may be more frequent (1/2000) in Hispanic infants. Although thyroid dysgenesis usually is sporadic, rare familial cases have been described, and the incidence is increased in infants with Down syndrome (Fort et al, 1984). Seasonal variations in incidence have been observed in Japan, Australia, and Canada. In isolated instances, thyroid dysgenesis has occurred in association with maternal autoimmune thyroiditis. However, this apparent association may be coincidental; there usually is no correlation between thyroid dysgenesis and the presence of maternal autoimmune thyroiditis or circulating thyroid antimicrosomal or antithyroglobulin autoantibodies (Dussault et al, 1980). Immunoglobulins blocking TSH-stimulated thyroid cell growth in tissue culture have been reported in both maternal and newborn blood in about half of the cases of sporadic congenital hypothyroidism, but a role for such growth-blocking immune globulins in the pathogenesis of congenital hypothyroidism in vivo has not been established.

As discussed, most newborns with thyroid dysgenesis are asymptomatic, and few infants have signs of hypothyroidism during the early weeks of life. Most affected infants have low serum $T_4$ and high TSH concentrations in cord blood or in filter-paper blood spots collected at 2 to 5 days of age. Ten percent to 20% of hypothyroid infants have $T_4$ levels in the low-normal range, with increased TSH values. These infants usually have ectopic functional thyroid tissue on scanning and significant levels of circulating thyroglobulin. Another 5% have a delayed elevation of serum TSH and are missed in the screening process unless a second screening test is done (LaFranchi et al, 1985). Again, thyroid function should be determined in any infant presenting with suspicious clinical signs or symptoms (see Table 92–4). Persons with thyroid dysgenesis also show abnormalities of thyroidal C cells; calcitonin levels and responsiveness are reduced throughout infancy and childhood. Urinary calcium and hydroxyproline levels are increased, and there is a tendency toward osteopenia, but this latter finding seems of limited clinical significance (Kruse et al, 1987).

## Hypothalamic-Pituitary Defects

Congenital hypothyroidism resulting from ineffective TSH stimulation of thyroid hormone secretion can result from a variety of abnormalities in TSH synthesis and metabolism. These include anomalous hypothalamic or pituitary development, isolated or familial deficiencies in TRH or TSH secretion, or TSH deficiency in association with other pituitary hormone deficiencies. Several TSH deficiency syndromes have been described: hypothalamic (tertiary) hypothyroidism with TRH deficiency or pituitary insensitivity (or both), isolated TSH deficiency, familial panhypopituitarism, congenital absence of the pituitary, and panhypopituitarism with absence of the sella turcica. The combined prevalence of these abnormalities associated with congenital hypothyroidism approximates 1/60,000 to 1/140,000 of live births (Stanbury and Dumont, 1983).

## Inborn Defects of Thyroid Hormone Production

Infants with inborn defects in thyroid metabolism account for nearly 10% of newborns with congenital nonendemic hypothyroidism (see Table 92–3). The defects in such patients include (1) a decreased thyroid response to TSH, (2) decreased thyroid iodide trapping, (3) defective organification of trapped iodide, (4) decreased capacity for deiodinating iodotyrosines, and (5) abnormalities in thyroglobulin synthesis, storage, or release. These disorders usually are transmitted as autosomal recessive traits (Lever et al, 1983). Except for the familial incidence and tendency for goiter to develop in affected persons, the clinical manifestations of congenital hypothyroidism resulting from a biochemical defect are similar to those in infants with thyroid dysgenesis. Thyroid enlargement may be present at birth, but in many patients, development of the goiter is delayed.

## Transient Congenital Hypothyroidism

Congenital hypothyroidism may present as a transient defect persisting for a variable period after birth. Usually, transient neonatal hypothyroidism is caused by maternal ingestion of goitrogenic substances that reach the fetus via placental transfer. One frequently ingested goitrogenic drug is iodide prescribed in expectorants for the treatment of asthma or as treatment for maternal thyrotoxicosis. The mothers of affected infants often have taken large doses of iodide for many years without development of large goiters and have been euthyroid during pregnancy. The fetal thyroid gland is unusually sensitive to iodide-induced hypothyroidism because of immaturity of the mechanisms that decrease thyroid iodide uptake in response to high plasma iodide levels. Urine iodine concentrations in affected infants usually exceed 1 mg/L.

Other substances that have been associated with neonatal goiter include thiourylene (antithyroid) drugs, sulfonamides, and hematinic preparations containing cobalt. Neonatal goiters resulting from antithyroid drug administration are uncommon unless large doses of the drugs are given to the mother (more than 150 mg/day of propylthiouracil or equivalent near term). Amniotic injection of radiographic contrast agents used during amniofetography also can lead to transient congenital hypothyroidism.

Maternal-to-fetal transfer of TSH receptor–blocking antibodies also can lead to transient perinatal hypothyroidism (Drexhage and Bottazzo, 1985). This condition is rare but has been reported in the newborns of women with either euthyroid or hypothyroid autoimmune thyroid disease. In these infants, TSH receptor autoantibodies are detectable in maternal and cord blood. These antibodies can be measured either as TSH binding–inhibiting immune globulins (TBIIs) or as TSH (cyclic AMP [cAMP])–blocking antibodies (TBAs). The duration of the hypothyroid state in these newborns is correlated with the initial titer of blocking antibody and the duration of its presence in newborn blood. Transient congenital hypothyroidism must be differentiated from transient hyperthyrotropinemia (see later section, "Thyroid Dysfunction Syndromes in the Premature Infant").

## Diagnosis and Management

### Diagnosis

Infants with congenital hypothyroidism are born with little or no clinical evidence of thyroid hormone deficiency. Thus, detection based on signs and symptoms usually is delayed 6 to 12 weeks or longer. Even though the emphasis in the diagnosis of congenital hypothyroidism currently is on newborn screening, not all infants with congenital hypothyroidism are detected by these systems. Early clinical diagnosis must be based on a high index of suspicion regarding nonspecific symptoms and signs. These are outlined in Table 92–4, along with their relative frequency. The diagnosis should be considered in any infant with prolonged jaundice, transient hypothermia, an enlarged (greater than 1 cm) posterior fontanel, failure to feed properly, or respiratory distress with feeding.

The classic signs evolve during the first weeks after birth. There is a rapid reduction in growth rate after birth, with progressively worsening myxedema in the subcutaneous tissues and in the tongue. The thickened tongue becomes protuberant, and increasing difficulty in nursing and handling salivary secretions is noted. The cry is hoarse because of myxedema of the vocal cords. There is marked muscular hypotonia, with an umbilical hernia, constipation, and bradycardia; extremities are cool to the touch and may exhibit pallor and circulatory mottling. The cardiac silhouette may be enlarged; the electrocardiogram shows low voltage and a prolonged conduction time. Some of the signs and symptoms are present by 6 to 12 weeks, especially lethargy, constipation, and the umbilical hernia. The cretinoid facies and growth retardation become increasingly obvious during the first several months of life.

As discussed previously, infants can escape detection by screening because of a delayed elevation in serum TSH or because of errors in sample collection or laboratory routine; it is estimated that 5% to 8% of affected infants may be missed. Infants with TSH deficiency are not detected, because most newborn screening programs report only those infants with elevated TSH levels. Congenital primary hypothyroidism is associated with a low serum $T_4$ and a high TSH concentration in individual cord blood or neonatal blood samples. A cord serum $T_4$ of 6.0 μg/dL or less with a TSH in excess of 80 μIU/mL suggests hypothyroidism. At 3 to 5 days of age, a serum $T_4$ of less than 7 μg/dL with a serum TSH in excess of 20 μIU/mL suggests hypothyroidism. Up to 10% to 20% of infants with congenital hypothyroidism, however, have $T_4$ values in the low-normal range (7 to 11 μg/dL). During the first 24 to 48 hours of life, serum TSH levels normally are elevated because of the neonatal TSH surge. Obtaining TSH blood samples during this time increases the number of false-positive results, but infants with congenital hypothyroidism usually are not missed.

The diagnosis of congenital hypothyroidism must be confirmed by measurement of serum $T_4$ and TSH concentrations in any infant with suspicious screening or neonatal sampling results. After 7 days of age, a serum $T_4$ of less than 6 μg/dL with a TSH of more than 50 μIU/mL indicates primary hypothyroidism. A serum $T_4$ in the range of 6 to 11 μg/dL with a TSH level of 20 to 50 μIU/mL is suggestive, and repeat testing is necessary. Eight percent to 10% of infants with congenital hypothyroidism have screening TSH values of less than 50 μIU/mL, and 1 in 12 to 24 hypothyroid infants (1/50,000 to 1/100,000 newborns) will have a screening TSH level of less than 20 μIU/mL, with a delayed postnatal increase to hypothyroid levels.

Hypothalamic-pituitary hypothyroidism is more difficult to diagnose. The disorder is characterized by a low serum $T_4$ concentration with a normal TSH value. In contrast, a low $T_4$ and TSH pattern most commonly reflects prematurity or a low TBG concentration. Measurement of a low serum TBG concentration or a normal free $T_4$ level identifies the patients with low TBG. An infant with a low free $T_4$ concentration should be carefully examined for evidence of hypothyroidism, and other tests of pituitary function should be conducted. A subnormal TSH response to TRH confirms a diagnosis of pituitary TSH deficiency. The TSH deficiency may be isolated or associated with other pituitary hormone deficiencies. If the peak level of TSH after TRH stimulation is normal or prolonged, hypothalamic TRH deficiency is likely.

### Treatment

The treatment of hypothyroidism relies on replacement with exogenous thyroid hormone. Sodium L-thyroxine (Na $T_4$) is the drug of choice because of its uniform potency and reliable absorption. Appropriate doses of synthetic $T_4$ produce normal serum levels of $T_3$ via peripheral conversion. The best guide to adequacy of therapy is periodic measurement of circulating levels of $T_4$ and TSH; during the initial stages of treatment, a $T_3$ determination also may be of value. The history and physical examination are important in the follow-up evaluation, but mild hypothyroidism or hyperthyroidism cannot always be excluded on clinical grounds. The usual starting dose of Na $T_4$ for hypothyroid infants is 10 to 15 μg/kg/day; we routinely begin treatment in term infants with a 50-μg $T_4$ tablet daily, crushed and given orally in a small amount of liquid. Using Na $T_4$ for treatment, the goal of therapy is to maintain the serum $T_4$ in the upper normal range (10 to 16 μg/dL), which should result in normal serum $T_3$ levels (70 to 220 ng/dL).

Serum TSH levels may remain elevated in adequately treated patients. The thyroid hormone–pituitary feedback set point seems to be altered in some infants with congenital hypothyroidism, and in such infants the serum TSH concentration remains elevated in the face of a normal or even elevated serum $T_4$ level (McCrossin et al, 1980).

Infants with presumably transient hypothyroidism resulting from maternal goitrogenic drugs need not be treated unless the low serum $T_4$ and elevated TSH levels persist beyond 2 weeks. Hyperthyroid mothers on antithyroid drugs may breast-feed their infants, because the concentration of drug in breast milk is very low. Infants with TSH receptor–blocking antibody–induced hypothyroidism may require treatment for as long as 2 to 5 months.

Adequate dosage of thyroxine in the first year usually ranges between 25 and 50 μg daily. The growth rate should accelerate after initiation of therapy, and any growth deficit is commonly restored within a few months. Bone age is a sensitive index of thyroid deficiency, and delayed bone maturation suggests inadequate treatment even when other signs of hypothyroidism have ameliorated. Overtreatment can induce tachycardia, excessive nervousness, disturbed sleep patterns, and other problems suggesting thyrotoxicosis. Excessive thyroxine administered over a long period can produce premature synostosis of cranial sutures and undue advancement of bone age.

## THYROID DYSFUNCTION SYNDROMES IN THE PREMATURE INFANT

Although the preterm infant is subject to the same pathophysiologic processes affecting the term infant, certain disorders of thyroid function are more common as a result of prematurity and are discussed in the following sections.

### Transient Hypothyroxinemia

Serum $T_4$ concentrations increase progressively with gestational age (see Fig. 92–2). Most term infants have serum $T_4$ concentrations above 6.5 μg/dL; only 2% to 3% have serum $T_4$ levels below this level. In contrast, some 50% of premature infants delivered before 30 weeks of gestation have serum $T_4$ values below 6.5 μg/dL (Hadeed et al, 1981). These preterm infants with hypothyroxinemia also have relatively low levels of free $T_4$. These levels are not as low as those in newborns with congenital hypothyroidism; rather, they are similar to the levels in adults. These relatively low free $T_4$ levels in premature infants are associated with normal or even low serum TSH values and normal TSH and $T_4$ responses to TRH, indicating responsive pituitary and thyroid glands. The hypothyroxinemia is transient, correcting spontaneously (in 4 to 8 weeks) with progressive maturation.

The physiologic significance of these changes remains controversial. Previous studies have suggested that replacement therapy does not improve postnatal growth or subsequent development (Chowdrey et al, 1984). More recent studies, however, have suggested that low $T_4$ values are associated with poorer neurologic outcomes in preterm infants after attempts to adjust for other confounding variables (den Ouden et al, 1996; Reuss et al, 1996). These observations have led to studies examining the influence of thyroxine supplementation on these outcomes. In infants born before 30 weeks of gestation, exogenous thyroxine administration did not improve developmental outcome determined at 2, 5, and 7 years of age (Briet et al, 2001; Van Wassenaer et al, 1997). Moreover, detrimental effects of $T_4$ treatment on cognitive function were noted in preterm infants treated after 29 weeks of gestation. Further studies involving more targeted populations of infants or relying on other dosing strategies are in progress. Currently, it would seem prudent to carefully evaluate preterm infants presenting with elevated TSH levels in the face of low $T_3$ or $T_4$ values for hypothyroidism; a course of replacement therapy may be warranted in these infants. However, the routine treatment of preterm infants with supplemental thyroid hormones should take place under the guidance of approved research protocols.

### Transient Primary Hypothyroidism

Transient hypothyroidism in the newborn, characterized by low serum $T_4$ and high TSH concentrations, is more common in Europe than in the United States; its prevalence varies geographically relative to iodine intake. In Belgium, it occurs in 20% of premature infants, with the incidence increasing as gestational age decreases (Delange et al, 1985). Cord blood $T_4$ and TSH values in these infants usually are in the normal range for premature infants. Premature infants require higher iodine intake levels than those needed in term infants to maintain a positive iodine balance in the extrauterine environment, however, so in iodine-deficient geographic areas, neonatal iodine deficiency may develop in preterm infants. The primary hypothyroid state develops during the first weeks of extrauterine life and often is superimposed on the transient hypothyroxinemia characteristic of prematurity. Urinary iodine excretion and thyroid iodine content are low. The hypothyroidism is transient but may persist for 2 to 3 months; therefore, treatment is recommended. Iodine treatment also corrects this transient primary hypothyroid state. The average time to recovery of function and discontinuation of treatment in Belgium was 50 days.

Premature infants also are particularly susceptible to transient, iodine-induced hypothyroidism (Delange et al, 1985). The mechanism by which the thyroid cell inhibits iodide transport in response to increased plasma iodide levels matures near term. Thus, either in utero or in the postnatal period, administration of iodine-containing drugs to the mother or amniotic injection of radiographic contrast agents for amniofetography has induced hypothyroidism. Premature infants are more susceptible, but iodide-induced hypothyroidism also can develop in term infants. The dose of iodine required is approximately 50 to 100 μg/kg/day. Urine iodine levels in iodine-induced hypothyroid infants usually exceed 1 mg/L. The hypothyroidism, with or without goiter, is characterized by low serum total $T_4$ and free $T_4$ concentrations and high levels of TSH and urinary iodide. Treatment is indicated for these infants.

### Transient Hyperthyrotropinemia

Idiopathic hyperthyrotropinemia is a rare disorder. The serum TSH concentration is increased, often markedly, but other thyroid function parameters are normal, and the infants are euthyroid. In Japan, Miyai and coworkers (1979) have reported an incidence of 1/15,000 to 1/20,000 newborns; the prevalence in Europe and the United States is not precisely known but is much lower. The serum TSH concentration may remain elevated for as long as 9 months before spontaneously normalizing. Affected infants do not require treatment, but prolonged follow-up evaluation is necessary to exclude the possibility of a permanent disorder, such as an ectopic thyroid gland, an inborn defect in thyroid hormonogenesis, or a thyroid hormone resistance syndrome. Transient hyperthyrotropinemia without hypothyroxinemia in the newborn also may occur in response to intrauterine antithyroid drug exposure, intrauterine iodine excess or deficiency, or a maternal TSH receptor–blocking antibody and has been recorded as a TSH assay artifact. The mechanism of transient idiopathic hyperthyrotropinemia is not clear. Delayed maturation of thyroid responsiveness to TSH or of the iodothyronine feedback control of pituitary TSH secretion has been suggested.

### Low Triiodothyronine Syndrome in Premature Infants

In the preterm infant, the changes in thyroid function parameters during neonatal adaptation are qualitatively similar to those in term infants but are quantitatively obtunded (Fisher and Klein, 1981). The neonatal TSH surge and the neonatal $T_4$ and $T_3$ peak responses decrease with decreasing gestational age, and the transient low $T_3$ state that follows probably is related to the state of relative undernutrition in the neonatal period. Premature infants have an increased susceptibility to neonatal morbidity including birth trauma, acidosis, hypoxia, hypoglycemia, hypocalcemia, and infection, all superimposed on feeding disorders and relative malnutrition. All of these factors tend to inhibit peripheral $T_4$-to-$T_3$ conversion, thereby aggravating the extent of the low $T_3$ state characteristic of prematurity. Serum $T_3$ values may remain low in these infants for 1 to 2 months.

Features of the low $T_3$ syndrome in premature infants include a low serum $T_3$ concentration secondary to a decreased rate of conversion of $T_4$ to $T_3$, variable but usually elevated serum $rT_3$ levels, and normal or low total serum $T_4$ concentrations. Free $T_4$ levels usually are in the range of values for healthy premature infants of matched gestational age and weight. TSH values are low in these infants. Treatment is not warranted (Valero et al, 2004).

## DISORDERS OF THYROID HORMONE CARRIER PROTEINS

The wide application of neonatal screening programs for congenital hypothyroidism has resulted in the identification of other causes of low values of $T_3$ and $T_4$ in the newborn. Although physiologically these children are euthyroid, a discussion of these syndromes is warranted due to their impact on reported values of $T_3$ and $T_4$ in the perinatal period.

The major determinants of the levels of circulating thyroid hormones are the concentrations of thyroid hormone–binding proteins. As discussed, TBG, TBPA, and albumin all participate as thyroid hormone carrier proteins. Abnormalities of serum albumin concentration have been described; the major categories are dysalbuminemia and analbuminemia. However, albumin usually binds only about 10% of the circulating $T_4$ and 30% to 50% of $T_3$, and the concentrations of TBG and TBPA are normal or increased in these disorders. Consequently, the levels of thyroid hormones in these patients usually are in the normal range (Hollander et al, 1985). No confirmed primary disorder of TBPA resulting in abnormal thyroid hormone levels has been described to date. Thus, the plasma protein disorders associated with abnormal serum $T_4$ levels include only the variations in TBG and the recently described hyperthyroxinemic state "familial dysalbuminemic hyperthyroxinemia."

### Thyroxine-Binding Globulin Deficiency

The prevalence of TBG deficiency varies from 1/5000 to 1/12,000 newborns and is transmitted as an X-linked trait. Serum TBG levels are very low in affected males and approximately half of normal in carrier females. In about half of the families with this trait, the TBG level shown by radioimmunoassay (RIA) is very low, and in the other half, the defect is partial; serum $T_4$ levels vary similarly. Affected persons are euthyroid, with normal serum TSH responses to exogenous TRH. Treatment is not indicated.

There are many structural defects of the TBG molecule accounting for defective TBG $T_4$ binding. Variants have been reported in Australian aborigines and African-Americans as well as in other populations. These inherited defects seem not to be due to large fragment deletions, insertions, or rearrangements of DNA; consequently, polymorphism studies have not been helpful in detection or screening. A single amino acid substitution (asparagine for isoleucine) at position 96 of the TBG molecule accounts for the marked reduction of $T_4$-binding capacity of TBG-Gary (Takamatsu et al, 1987). Table 92–5 summarizes the reported properties of several variant TBG molecules investigated. Most patients with partial TBG deficiency demonstrated elevated levels of denatured TBG measured by RIA, and each manifested a defective molecule with reduced stability and decreased binding capacity. Patients with severe TBG deficiency have been postulated to have a defect in hepatic TBG synthesis, but the molecular mechanism remains obscure.

### Thyroxine-Binding Globulin Excess

Persons with increased levels of TBG have increased total serum $T_4$ concentrations with normal TSH levels. Serum $T_3$ concentrations are modestly increased. In these persons, as in those with low TBG concentrations, TBG production rates and serum levels are correlated, suggesting that the mechanism for the high TBG concentrations is increased production, presumably by the liver. TBG levels are increased fourfold to fivefold in affected persons. Early reports suggested a dominant mode of inheritance, but subsequent studies are compatible with an X-linked mode of inheritance.

### Familial Dysalbuminemic Hyperthyroxinemia

Several groups of investigators have described euthyroid persons with increased serum $T_4$ concentrations but normal free $T_4$, total serum $T_3$, and TSH levels (Ruiz et al, 1982). Binding of $T_4$ to albumin is increased, and the albumin in these patients has an affinity for $T_4$ binding intermediate between TBG and TBPA. $T_3$ is less avidly bound, accounting for the preferential increase in serum $T_4$ concentration.

TABLE 92-5

**Properties of Reported Abnormal Thyroxine-Binding Globulin Molecules***

| | TBG Concentration | | | |
|---|---|---|---|---|
| | **Normal** | **Denatured** | **$T_4$ Concentration** | **TBG Affinity** |
| Normal TBG | 100 | 100 | 100 | 100 |
| TBG-S | 88 | 100 | 84 | 100 |
| TBG-A | 74 | 100 | 58 | 54 |
| TBG-Quebec | 16 | 260 | 41 | 70 |
| TBG-Montreal | 14 | 390 | 38 | <3 |
| TBG-Gary | 1 | 1000 | 24 | <5 |

*Values listed as percentage of values in normal subjects. Normal absolute values for the measured parameters are TBG RIA, 1.1 to 2.1 mg/dL; TBG-denatured, <2 to 8 μg/dL; $T_4$, 5 to 12 μg/dL; TBG affinity constant for $T_4$, 0.7 to $1.35 \times 10^{-10}$ M.

RIA, radioimmunoassay; $T_4$, thyroxine; TBG, thyroxine-binding globulin.

Data from Takamatsu J, Refetoff S, Charbonneau M, et al: Two new inherited defects of the thyroxine-binding globulin (TBG) molecule presenting as partial TBG deficiency. J Clin Invest 79:833-840, 1987.

Patients with the disorder are euthyroid, with normal thyroid hormone production rates. The abnormal albumin seems to be transmitted as an autosomal dominant trait.

Diagnosis in these patients is confirmed by protein electrophoresis of serum containing labeled $T_4$. The fraction of $T_4$ label associated with TBG, TBPA, or albumin is measured, and the albumin-bound $T_4$ can be calculated and related to normal values. Measurements of TBG and TBPA concentrations also are useful. Antithyroid therapy is not necessary in these patients, but it is important to make the diagnosis to avoid a misdiagnosis of hyperthyroidism.

Finally, although the emphasis of neonatal thyroidology is on early detection and appropriate therapy of the hypothyroid state, hyperthyroid states do occur and are associated with significant morbidity.

### Neonatal Thyrotoxicosis

Neonatal Graves disease is rare, probably because of the low incidence of thyrotoxicosis in pregnancy (1 to 2 cases per 1000 pregnancies) and the fact that the neonatal disease occurs only in about one of 70 cases of thyrotoxic pregnancies (Burrow, 1974). In most cases, the disease is due to transplacental passage of thyroid-stimulating antibody (TSA) from a mother with active or inactive Graves disease or Hashimoto thyroiditis. Thus, prediction of neonatal Graves disease from the maternal clinical status is not always possible. It is possible, however, to predict the occurrence of Graves disease in newborns on the basis of maternal TSA titers. In a report by Zakarija and coworkers (1986), all women with TSA titers exceeding 500% of control values (measured by stimulation of cAMP in human thyroid slices) were delivered of thyrotoxic infants, whereas those with lower titers were delivered of euthyroid infants. In some infants, both TSH receptor–stimulating and TSH receptor–blocking antibodies are acquired from the mother, and the blocking antibodies have been reported to block the effects of the stimulating antibodies for 4 to 6 weeks so that late-onset neonatal Graves disease develops in a previously undiagnosed infant (McKenzie and Zakarija, 1978).

Graves disease in the newborn is manifested by irritability, flushing, tachycardia, hypertension, poor weight gain, thyroid enlargement, and exophthalmos. Thrombocytopenia, hepatosplenomegaly, jaundice, and hypoprothrombinemia also have been observed. Arrhythmias, cardiac failure, and death may occur if the thyrotoxicity is severe and the treatment is inadequate. The mortality rate approaches 25% in disease severe enough to be diagnosed. In some infants, the onset of symptoms and signs may be delayed as long as 8 or 9 days. This delayed onset is due to the postnatal depletion of transplacentally acquired blocking doses of maternal antithyroid drugs and to the abrupt increase in conversion of $T_4$ to active $T_3$ shortly after birth in the newborn. The diagnosis is confirmed by measuring high levels of $T_4$, free $T_4$, and $T_3$ in postnatal blood. Cord blood values may be normal or near normal, whereas levels at 2 to 5 days may be markedly increased; the serum TSH is low. Neonatal Graves disease resolves spontaneously as maternal TSA in the newborn is degraded. The usual clinical course of neonatal Graves disease is 3 to 12 weeks.

The treatment of hyperthyroidism in the newborn includes sedatives and digitalis as necessary. Iodide or antithyroid drugs are administered to decrease thyroid hormone secretion. These drugs have additive effects with regard to inhibition of hormone synthesis; in addition, iodide rapidly inhibits hormone release. Lugol solution (5% iodine and 10% potassium iodide, containing 126 mg/mL of iodine) is given in doses of 1 drop (about 8 mg) three times daily. Methimazole, carbimazole, or propylthiouracil is administered in doses of 0.5 to 1 mg/kg/day, 0.5 to 1 mg/kg/day, or 5 to 10 mg/kg/day, respectively, divided, at 8-hour intervals. A therapeutic response should be observed within 24 to 36 hours. If a satisfactory response is not observed, the dose of antithyroid drug and iodide can be increased by 50%. Corticosteroids in anti-inflammatory doses and propranolol (1 to 2 mg/kg/day) also may be helpful. Radiographic contrast agents (ipodate, 200 mg/kg per day) also may be useful in treatment, either alone or in conjunction with antithyroid drug treatment.

## REFERENCES


Bernal J, Pekonen F: Ontogenesis of nuclear 3,5,3′-triiodothyronine receptors in human fetal brain. Endocrinology 114:667-679, 1984.

Briet J, van Wassenaer A, Dekker F, et al: Neonatal thyroxine supplementation in very preterm children: Developmental outcome evaluated at early school age. Pediatrics 107:712-718, 2001.

Brown A, Fernhoff PM, Milner J, et al: Racial differences in the incidence of congenital hypothyroidism. J Pediatr 99:934-937, 1981.

Burrow GN: The Thyroid Gland in Pregnancy. Philadelphia, WB Saunders, 1974, pp 83-100.

Chowdry P, Scanlon JW, Auerbach R, et al: Results of a controlled double-blind study of thyroid replacement in very low birth weight premature infants with hypothyroxinemia. Pediatrics 73:301-304, 1984.

Dammacco F, Dammacco A, Cavallo T, et al: Serum thyroglobulin and thyroid ultrasound studies in infants with congenital hypothyroidism. J Pediatr 106:451-453, 1985.

Delange F, Bourdoux P, Ermans AM: Transient disorders of thyroid function and regulation in preterm infants. In Delange F, Fisher DA, Malvaux P (eds): Pediatric Thyroidology. Basel, Karger, 1985, pp 369-393.

den Ouden AL, Kok JH, Verkerk RH, et al: The relation between neonatal thyroxine levels and neurodevelopmental outcome at age 5 and 9 years in a national cohort of very preterm and/or very low birth weight infant. Pediatr Res 39:142-145, 1996.

Drexhage HA, Bottazzo GF: The thyroid and autoimmunity. In Delange F, Fisher DA, Malvaux P (eds): Pediatric Thyroidology. Basel, Karger, 1985, pp 90-105.

Dussault JH, Letarte J, Guyda H, et al: Lack of influence of thyroid antibodies on thyroid function in the newborn infant and on a mass screening program for congenital hypothyroidism. J Pediatr 96:385-387, 1980.

Fisher DA: Thyroid hormone and thyroglobulin synthesis and secretion. In Delange F, Fisher DA, Malvaux P (eds): Pediatric Thyroidology. Basel, Karger, 1985, pp 44-56.

Fisher DA, Klein AH: Thyroid development and disorders of thyroid function in the newborn. N Engl J Med 304:702-708, 1981.

Fort P, Lifschitz F, Bellisario R, et al: Abnormalities of thyroid function in infants with Down syndrome. J Pediatr 104:545-549, 1984.

Frasier SD, Penny R, Synder R: Primary congenital hypothyroidism in Spanish-surnamed infants in southern California. J Pediatr 101:315-317, 1982.

Gonzales LA, Ballard PL: Identification and characterization of nuclear 3,5,3'-triiodothyronine binding sites in fetal human lung. J Clin Endocrinol Metab 53:21-28, 1981.

Hadeed AJ, Asay LD, Klein AH, et al: Significance of transient hypothyroxinemia in premature infants with and without respiratory distress syndrome. Pediatr Res 68:494-497, 1981.

Harada A, Hershman JM: Extraction of human chorionic thyrotropin (hCT) from term placentas: Failure to recover thyrotropic activity. J Clin Endocrinol Metab 47:681-685, 1978.

Hollander CS, Bernstein G, Oppenheimer JH: Anomalies in thyroid hormone transport proteins. In Delange F, Fisher DA, Malvaux P (eds): Pediatric Thyroidology. Basel, Karger, 1985, pp 394-406.

Jacobsen BB, Brandt NJ: Congenital hypothyroidism in Denmark. Arch Dis Child 56:131-136, 1981.

Kruse K, Suss A, Busse M, et al: Monomeric serum calcitonin and bone turnover during anticonvulsant treatment and in congenital hypothyroidism. J Pediatr 111:57-63, 1987.

LaFranchi SH, Hanna CE, Krainz PL, et al: Screening for congenital hypothyroidism with specimen collection at two time periods: Results of the Northwest Regional Screening Program. Pediatrics 76:734-740, 1985.

Lever EG, Medeiros-Neto GA, DeGroot LJ: Inherited disorders of thyroid metabolism. Endocr Rev 4:213-247, 1983.

Marchant B, Brownlie BEW, Hant DM, et al: The placental transfer of propylthiouracil, methimazole and carbimazole. J Clin Endocrinol Metab 45:1187-1193, 1977.

Matsurra N, Yamamoto Y, Nohara Y, et al: Familial neonatal transient hypothyroidism due to maternal TSH-binding inhibitor immunoglobulins. N Engl J Med 303:733-741, 1980.

McCrossin RB, Sheffield LJ, Robertson EF: Persisting abnormality in the pituitary-thyroid axis in congenital hypothyroidism. In Nagetaki S, Stockgit JHR (eds): Thyroid Research VIII. Canberra, Australian Academy of Science, 1980, pp 37-40.

McKenzie JM, Zakarija M: Pathogenesis of neonatal Graves' disease. J Endocrinol Invest 2:183-187, 1978.

Miyai K, Amino N, Nishi K, et al: Transient infantile hyperthyrotropinemia. Arch Dis Child 54:965-967, 1979.

Padbury JF, Polk DH, Newnham JP, et al: Neonatal adaptation: Greater sympathoadrenal response in preterm than full-term fetal sheep at birth. Am J Physiol Endocrinol Metab 11:E443-E447, 1985.

Polk DH, Callegari CC, Newnham JP, et al: Effect of fetal thyroidectomy on newborn thermogenesis in lambs. Pediatr Res 21:453-457, 1988a.

Polk DH, Wu SY, Wright C, et al: Ontogeny of thyroid hormone effect on tissue 5'-monodeiodinase activity in fetal sheep. Am J Physiol Endocrinol Metab 17:E337-E341, 1988b.

Refetoff S, Larsen PR: Transport, cellular uptake and metabolism of thyroid hormone. In DeGroot LJ, Jameson JL (eds): Endocrinology. Philadelphia. WB Saunders, 1989, pp 541-561.

Reuss ML, Paneth N, Pihto-Martin JA, et al: The relation of transient hypothyroxinemia in preterm infants to neurological development at two years of age. N Engl J Med 39:142-145, 1996.

Roti E, Gnudi A, Braverman LE, et al: Human cord blood concentrations of thyrotropin, thyroglobulin and iodothyronines after maternal administration of thyrotropin-releasing hormone. J Clin Endocrinol Metab 53:813-817, 1981.

Roti E: Regulation of thyroid-stimulating hormone (TSH) secretion in the fetus and neonate. J Endocrinol Invest 11:145-150, 1988.

Ruiz M, Rajatanavin R, Young RA, et al: Familial dysalbuminemic hyperthyroxinemia. N Engl J Med 306:635-639, 1982.

Stanbury JB, Dumont JE: Familial goiter and related disorders. In Stanbury JB, Wyngaarden JB, Fredrickson, DS (eds): The Metabolic Basis of Inherited Disease. New York, McGraw-Hill, 1983, pp 231-269.

Takamatsu J, Refetoff S, Charbonneau M, et al: Two new inherited defects of the thyroxine-binding globulin (TBG) molecule presenting as partial TBG deficiency. J Clin Invest 79:833-840, 1987.

Theodoropoulos T, Bravermann LE, Vagenakis AG: Iodide-induced hypothyroidism: A potential hazard during perinatal life. Science 205:502-503, 1979.

Valero P, Van Wassenaer AG, de Vijlder JJM, Kok JH: A randomized masked study of T3 plus T4 administration in preterm infants. Ped Res 55:248-253, 2004.

Van Wassenaer AG, Kok JH, de Vijlder JJM, et al: Effects of thyroxine supplementation on neurologic development in infants born at less than 30 weeks gestation. N Engl J Med 336:21-26, 1997.

Vulsma T, Gons MN, de Vijlder JJM: Maternal-fetal transfer of thyroxine in congenital hypothyroidism due to a total organification defect or thyroid agenesis. N Engl J Med 321:13-16, 1989.

Zakarija M, McKenzie JM: Pregnancy-associated changes in the thyroid stimulating antibody of Graves' disease and the relationship to neonatal hyperthyroidism. J Clin Endocrinol Metab 57:1036-1039, 1983.

Zakarija M, McKenzie JM, Hoffman WH: Prediction and therapy of intrauterine and late onset neonatal hyperthyroidism. J Clin Endocrinol Metab 62:368-374, 1986.

CHAPTER

# 93

# Disorders of Carbohydrate Metabolism

Charles A. Stanley and Eugenia K. Pallotto

At the time of birth, the neonate must abruptly switch from having a continuous supply of glucose from the maternal blood in fetal life to maintaining its own supply of glucose during periods of fasting, and when feedings are interspersed intermittently. Glucose homeostasis requires a complex balance between glucose utilization by various organs and production by the liver. This balance is controlled by insulin and an array of counterregulatory hormones that regulate the key metabolic pathways of fuel production during fasting: glycogenolysis, gluconeogenesis, lipolysis, and ketogenesis. Disturbances of these metabolic and endocrine systems may frequently occur in neonates, because of developmental immaturity. Congenital disorders causing hypoglycemia or genetic disorders that result in impairment in carbohydrate metabolism may also present in the neonatal period. Hypoglycemia in a newborn infant represents an urgent diagnostic and therapeutic challenge that must be answered promptly to avoid the adverse consequences of hypoglycemia—most important, damage to the central nervous system (CNS).

This chapter discusses the mechanisms, etiologic factors, and therapeutic strategies for disorders of glucose homeostasis in newborn infants, with special emphasis on neonatal hypoglycemia and a smaller section devoted to hyperglycemia. Disorders of carbohydrate homeostasis caused by inborn errors of metabolism are addressed in detail in Chapter 22.

## HYPOGLYCEMIA

Five systems are involved in maintaining adequate glucose levels for brain metabolism during fasting. Four of these are the major metabolic pathways of fasting adaptation, as shown in Figure 93–1 (Cahill, 1970): (1) hepatic glycogenolysis, (2) hepatic gluconeogenesis, (3) lipolysis, and (4) fatty acid oxidation and ketogenesis. Endocrine control of these four metabolic systems is (5) the important fifth system required for maintaining normal fasting adaptation.

- *Hepatic glycogenolysis*: Once intestinal absorption of a meal is complete and fasting begins, the majority of glucose needed by the body is provided from hepatic glycogen stores. Because the liver contains only 50 to 75 g of glycogen (200 to 300 calories) per kilogram of liver, the supply of glucose from liver stores is sufficient to meet energy requirements for only a few hours.
- *Hepatic gluconeogenesis*: Gluconeogenesis becomes the sole source of glucose as hepatic glycogen stores are depleted. Primary precursors for hepatic gluconeogenesis include amino acids, glycerol from adipose tissue lipolysis and lactate recycled from glycolysis. These precursors are depleted in cases of prolonged demands for glucose. Because there is no reserve of surplus protein in the body and muscle proteolysis is the primary source of amino acids for hepatic gluconeogenesis, the body attempts to limit protein degradation during long-term fasting by switching to fatty acid oxidation.
- *Adipose tissue lipolysis*: Lipolysis releases free fatty acids from adipose tissue stores of triglycerides. Organs such as the heart and kidneys, as well as skeletal muscle, can directly oxidize free fatty acids in place of glucose, thus limiting the need for hepatic gluconeogenesis. Long-chain free fatty acids do not cross the blood-brain barrier; therefore, the brain cannot use them directly. Fatty acids cannot be converted to glucose; however, the glycerol released by lipolysis is used as an important gluconeogenic substrate by liver.
- *Hepatic ketogenesis*: Fatty acids undergo partial oxidation in the liver to produce ketones, β-hydroxybutyrate, and acetoacetate. The brain uses these products of fatty acid oxidation in order to reduce glucose utilization and further reduce the need for protein degradation to support glucose production. Thus, hepatic ketogenesis provides an indirect mechanism for the brain to utilize adipose tissue triglyceride stores during long-term fasting.
- *Hormonal control*: Insulin is the most important hormone involved in the control of fasting adaptation because it acts to inhibit all four of the metabolic fasting systems (Table 93–1). Several counterregulatory hormones oppose the effects of insulin on specific fasting systems (cortisol, growth hormone). Fasting hypoglycemia can result if there is excessive secretion of insulin or a deficiency of one or more counterregulatory hormones.

In infants and children, the pattern of the fasting response is the same as in adults, but the time course is more rapid (Chaussain et al, 1977; Haymond et al, 1982). The accelerated fasting response is due to a greater brain weight relative to body mass. Glucose utilization rates are linearly related to brain size (Zeller and Bougneres, 1992). Therefore, basal glucose consumption in infants is two to three times that in the adult, with preterm infants having higher requirements than those of infants born at term (5 to 8 mg/kg/minute versus 4 to 6 mg/kg/minute, respectively) (Bier et al, 1977; Kalhan and Raghavan, 1998; Ogata, 1986). Infants also have relatively lower muscle mass and less substrate for gluconeogenesis. Thus, fasting hyperketonemia develops within 24 hours in infants and children, compared with 36 to 48 hours in adults.

The fuel and hormonal responses at the time of fasting hypoglycemia provide important information on which of the fasting systems is likely to be involved in the etiology of the hypoglycemia. Specimens of blood and urine obtained at the time of hypoglycemia are termed the "critical" or "Didja" samples (as in "Didja remember to do a glucose [or other] test?"). Plasma samples should be obtained to measure glucose, bicarbonate, lactate, free fatty acids,

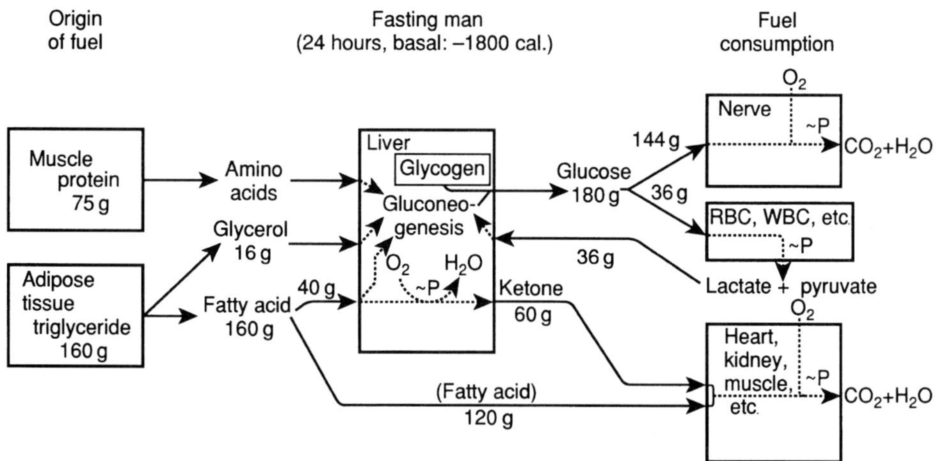


**FIGURE 93–1.** General scheme of fuel metabolism in a normal fasted man, showing the two primary sources, muscle and adipose tissue, and the three types of fuel consumers—nerve, pure glycolyzers (such as the red blood cells [RBC] and white blood cells [WBC]), and the remainder of the body (composed of heart, kidney, and skeletal muscle)—that use fatty acids and ketones. ~P represents energy production. *(Redrawn from Cahill GF: Starvation in man. N Engl J Med 282:668-675, 1970.)*

β-hydroxybutyrate, insulin, cortisol, and growth hormone. Urine should be tested for ketones. Abnormalities in one or more of these levels will direct the clinician toward the mechanism behind the hypoglycemia. Extra plasma and urine specimens should be retained for additional tests that may be required to establish the diagnosis (e.g., acylcarnitine profile for defects in fatty acid oxidation).

## Etiology of Hypoglycemia in Neonates

The etiology of hypoglycemia can be identified by the clinical features and the timing of the episode, along with the response of circulating fuels and hormones during the period of fasting hypoglycemia. Table 93–2 classifies the major causes of disorders in fasting adaptation in infants. Table 93–3 lists the risk factors for the development of hypoglycemia in the newborn period and the fasting system involved.

## Development of Fasting Systems

During fetal life, there is a continuous supply of glucose from the mother through placental transfer. The glucose level of the fetus and that of the mother are highly correlated. Fetal blood glucose is dependent on the maternal-fetal glucose gradient, not on the maternal insulin concentration, as the placenta is impermeable to insulin. Glucose is transported across the placenta by carrier-mediated facilitated diffusion involving non–insulin-dependent glucose transporters. Glut1 and Glut3 both are expressed in the placenta. Glut3 is a high-affinity transporter that is saturated under normal conditions (Simmons, 1998). Glut1 is abundant in both the basal and apical sides of the syncytiotrophoblast, facilitating entry into the cytoplasm from the maternal blood and exit from the cytoplasm to the pericapillary space of the fetus (Arnott et al, 1994; Reid and Boyd, 1994; Sakata et al, 1995; Takata et al, 1992). Glut1 is the predominant isoform in the fetus; its affinity for glucose is very high. Almost all fetal tissues express Glut1, even tissues that do not express it in the adult (Devaskar and Mueckler, 1991). One of its specialized roles is to shuttle glucose between blood and organs that have limited access to small solutes, including brain and red blood cells, in addition to placenta. This transport is acomplished via passive diffusion (Simmons, 1998). After birth, expression of Glut1 decreases, and other isoforms (e.g., Glut2 in liver, Glut4 in muscle) increase (Wang and Brennan, 1988; Werner et al, 1989). Table 93–4 lists the glucose transporters (Devaskar and Mueckler, 1991; Kahn, 1992). The fetus oxidizes glucose for its energy needs, and the remainder is incorporated in glycogen and used for fat biosynthesis. Glucose provides nearly 100% of the energy needs of the fetus.

After the umbilical cord is cut, the formerly continuous maternal glucose supply to the fetus ceases abruptly. Many of the components of the fasting system the neonate needs to maintain normoglycemia are fully functional, but some remain incompletely developed at delivery. Liver glycogen (system 1) and adipose tissue fat stores (system 3) become filled late in the third trimester but may be limited in preterm and small-for-gestational-age (SGA) infants. Hepatic

**TABLE 93–1**

**Hormonal Control of Fasting Adaptation**

| Hormone | Hepatic Glycogenolysis | Hepatic Gluconeogenesis | Adipose Tissue Lipolysis | Hepatic Ketogenesis |
|---|---|---|---|---|
| Insulin | Inhibits | Inhibits | Inhibits | Inhibits |
| Glucagon | Stimulates | | | |
| Cortisol | | Stimulates | | |
| Growth hormone | | | Stimulates | |
| Epinephrine | Stimulates | Stimulates | Stimulates | Stimulates |

**TABLE 93–2**

**Classification of Disorders of Fasting Adaptation in Infants**

**System 1: Glycogenolysis**
Amylo-1,6-glycosidase (debranching enzyme) deficiency (GSD III)
Liver phosphorylase deficiency (GSD VI)
Phosphorylase kinase deficiency (GSD IX)

**System 2: Gluconeogenesis**
Glucose-6-phosphatase deficiency (GSD I)
Fructose-1,6-diphosphatase deficiency
Pyruvate carboxylase deficiency

**System 3: Adipose Tissue Lipolysis**
Congenital lipodystrophy
$Beta_2$ blockers

**System 4: Ketogenesis**
Medium-chain acyl CoA dehydrogenase (MCAD) deficiency
Very long-chain acyl CoA dehydrogenase (vLCAD) deficiency
Long-chain 3-hydroxy-acyl CoA dehydrogenase (LCHAD) deficiency
Carnitine transporter deficiency
Carnitine palmitoyl-transferase 1 deficiency
Carnitine palmitoyl-transferase 2 deficiency
Gluctaric aciduria type 2
Others (there are 12 known disorders in this system)

**System 5: Hormonal Regulation**
Insulin excess
- Congenital hyperinsulinism
- Infant of diabetic mother
- Exogenous insulin
- Beckwith-Wiedemann syndrome
- Sulfonylureas
- Islet cell adenoma

Counterregulatory hormone deficiency
- Panhypopituitarism
- Isolated growth hormone deficiency
- Adrenal insufficiency

Acyl CoA, acyl coenzyme A; GSD, glycogen storage disease.

**TABLE 93–3**

**Risk Factors for Neonatal Hypoglycemia**

| Factor | Affected Fasting System* |
|---|---|
| **Maternal Factors** | |
| Diabetes | 5 |
| Hypertension/eclampsia | 2, 4, and/or 5 |
| Dextrose infusion | 5 |
| Beta agonists | 5 |
| Sulfonylureas | 5 |
| **Fetal Factors** | |
| Prematurity | 2, 4 plus 1 |
| Small for gestational age | 2, 4 plus 1 (?5) |
| Large for gestational age | 5 |
| Congenital heart disease | 1, 2 |
| Microphallus | 5 |
| Midline defects | 5 |
| **Perinatal/Postnatal Factors** | |
| Prolonged fasting | 2, 4 |
| Cold stress | (?1, 2) |
| Sepsis | (?1, 2) |
| Asphyxia | 1, 6 |
| Polycythemia | (1) |

*See Table 93–2.

glycogenolysis (system 1) is functional before term, but several enzymes required for gluconeogenesis (system 2) and, especially, ketogenesis (system 4) are not expressed until after birth.

The immaturity of fasting adaptation in the normal newborn is illustrated in Table 93–5 comparing the circulating fuel concentrations immediately after delivery with those in older children during fasting. When the fasting plasma glucose level falls below 50 mg/dL, normal term neonates have higher lactate and lower ketone concentrations, despite adequate free fatty acid concentrations, than those in older infants (Stanley et al, 1979). This indicates that ketogenesis and gluconeogenesis (systems 2 and 5) are not completely mature. The exact timing of complete maturation of these fasting systems is not known, but maturation probably is accomplished before 1 week of age and possibly as early as 24 hours of life in the normal neonate.

This maturation of the fasting systems after delivery is supported by observations in animal models documenting changes in the enzyme activities involved in ketogenesis and gluconeognensis after birth. Carnitine palmitoyltransferase-1 (CPT-1) and 3-hydroxy-3-methylglutaryl–coenzyme A synthase (HMG-CoA synthase) are two important enzymes involved in ketogenesis. CPT-1 and HMG-CoA synthase are important rate-limiting steps in the conversion of long-chain fatty acids into ketones (Pegorier et al, 1998). In rat liver, neither of these critical enzymes is expressed until after delivery. Increased expression of the CPT-1 and HMG-CoA synthase genes to levels equal to or greater than those in adult rats occurs by 12 to 24 hours following birth. Long-chain fatty acids provided in colostrum appear to be

**TABLE 93–4**

**Characterization of Glucose Transporters**

| Numeric Identification | Tissue Distribution |
|---|---|
| Glut1 | Many adult and fetal tissues; red blood cells, placenta, brain microvessels |
| Glut2 | Liver, pancreatic beta cells, kidney, intestine |
| Glut3 | Many adult and fetal tissues; placenta, brain, kidney |
| Glut4 | White and brown fat, skeletal muscle, heart |
| Glut5 | Jejunum, fat, kidney |
| Glut6 (Glut3P1) | Brain, jejunum, placenta, fat, kidney |
| Glut7 | Liver microsomes |

**TABLE 93–5**

**Comparison of Circulating Fuels in Hypoglycemia in Newborn Infants with Older Children**

| | Glucose (mg/dL) | Lactate (mmol/L) | Free Fatty Acids (mmol/L) | Total Ketones (mmol/L) |
|---|---|---|---|---|
| Term newborns* | 38 | 3 | 1.3 | 0.5 |
| Older children | | | | |
| Basal | 70-90 | 1-2 | 0.5 | 0.1 |
| Hypoglycemia | <40 | 1-2 | 1.5-2.5 | 3-4 |

*Appropriate for gestational age.

Data from Stanley and Baker, 1976; Stanley et al, 1979.

important transcription-activating factors for expression of both genes (Asins et al, 1995; Foster and Bailey, 1976; Pegorier et al, 1998; Serra et al, 1993; Stanley et al, 1983; Thumelin et al, 1993, 1994). Phosphoenolpyruvate carboxykinase (PEP-CK), the rate-limiting step in gluconeogenesis, remains low until after delivery (Kalhan and Raghavan, 1998). Levels of PEP-CK increase in part due to an inhibition of insulin secretion and a surge of glucagon occurring in the time period surrounding delivery (Girard et al, 1973; Granner et al, 1983). Catecholamine release during delivery probably plays a role in the increase in glucagon and decrease in insulin concentrations (Sperling et al, 1984).

Dysregulation of carbohydrate metabolism after birth is evident clinically, as lower glucose measurements have been documented within the first day of life since the first studies in the 1950s. For example, Lubencho and Bard (1971) reported on a group of infants with glucose measurements prior to the first feed on the first day of life. Ten percent of full-term infants with appropriate growth for gestational age had glucose levels of less than 30 mg/dL prior to the first feeding at 6 to 8 hours of age. In contrast, preprandial glucose levels by days 3 to 4 of life were invariably greater than 50 mg/dL in this group. Srinivansan and colleagues (1986) reported glucose measurements in full-term infants with appropriate-for-gestational age (AGA) birth weights. The range of glucose values at 1 hour of life was 17 to 119 mg/dL, with a mean level of 56 mg/dL. On day 3 of life, the mean fasting glucose had increased to 73 mg/dL, with all glucose values greater than 50 mg/dL. A study by Heck and Erenberg (1987) also demonstrated improved ability to maintain glucose levels after the first day of life. The fifth percentile of glucose values, in a group of infants that included more breast-fed babies than in the study by Srinivansan and colleagues, increased from approximately 35 to 45 mg/dL beyond the first 24 hours of life.

## Causes of Neonatal Hypoglycemia

### Self-Limited Disorders

#### *Hypoglycemia during Postnatal Fasting in Normal Neonates*

All neonates are at risk for developing hypoglycemia when exposed to fasting during the first day of life. As shown in Figure 93–2, if the first feeding is withheld until 6 to 8 hours after birth, the frequency of plasma glucose levels falling below 30 mg/dL in term AGA infants is 10%. Thirty percent of these normal neonates were unable to maintain plasma glucose above 50 mg/dL. This marked susceptibility to hypoglycemia disappears rapidly after the first day as the systems of fasting adaptation mature. In a study by Lubchenko and Bard (1971), the frequency of plasma glucose below 50 mg/dL was zero in term AGA infants tested before feedings on the second and third days of life. Similarly, in other groups of infants, including preterm, post-term, large-for-gestational age (LGA), and SGA infants, less than 1% developed a plasma glucose level of less than 50 mg/dL after the first day of life. Hypoglycemia due to immature development of gluconeogenesis and ketogenesis can be avoided easily by feeding earlier than 6 to 8 hours postnatally, preferably within 1 to 2 hours of delivery. Because maturation of these two fasting systems appears to occur during the first 12 to 24 hours

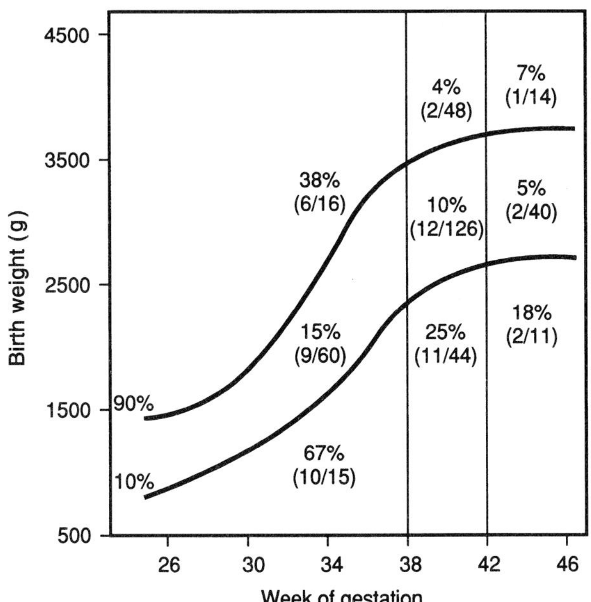


**FIGURE 93–2.** Frequency of hypoglycemia prior to feedings at 6 hours of age in newborn infants grouped by gestational age and birth weight. *(Redrawn from Lubchenco LO, Bard H: Incidence of hypoglycemia in newborn infants classified by birth weight and gestational age. Pediatrics 47:831-838, 1971.)*

of life, the occurrence of hypoglycemia in neonates beyond the first 24 hours of life requires that other possible disorders be considered (Stanley et al, 1979).

### *Postnatal Fasting Hypoglycemia in Preterm or Small-for-Gestational-Age Infants*

Infants who were born prematurely and/or were small for gestational age are at increased risk for hypoglycemia (see Fig. 93–2) (Lubchenko and Bard, 1971). This group of infants with delayed growth in utero has the same impaired gluconeogenesis and ketogenesis as in the AGA infants (Cowett and Schwartz, 1979). These infants have increased glucagon and insulin levels when hypoglycemic. The response to the increased glucagon levels is impaired, suggesting decreased gluconeogenic ability in these infants (Hawdon and Ward Platt, 1993; Hawdon et al, 1993). This hormonal-enzymatic imbalance (high insulin-to-glucagon ratio) probably results in the failure of appropriate gluconeogenesis by delaying PEP-CK induction (the rate-limiting step in gluconeogenesis), because the fall in insulin is one of the main determinants in liver PEP-CK induction, as shown in animal studies (Girard, 1986). Protein, fat, and glycogen stores also may be diminished in these undernourished infants, and they may have an increased glucose utilization rate because of a disproportionately high brain-to-body weight ratio (Hay, 1984; Jones and Roberton, 1984). Management in these high-risk infants includes early institution of oral feedings or intravenous (IV) glucose (Wright et al, 1983). Frequent blood glucose monitoring until oral feedings are tolerated is required to identify those infants who are unable to maintain appropriate fasting blood glucose levels.

## Neonatal Hypoglycemia Due to Transient Forms of Hyperinsulinism

### *Transient Excessive Glucose Utilization (Perinatal Stress-Induced Hyperinsulinism)*

Severe hypoglycemia with excessive glucose utilization is frequently observed in infants with birth asphyxia or other perinatal stresses. This hypoglycemia may last for several days to weeks and may be difficult to manage. A subset of SGA infants probably also fits into this category. Hyperinsulinism has been suggested as the underlying etiology in this group because of several reports documenting high insulin levels as well as good responses to treatment with diazoxide, a drug that acts to suppress beta cell insulin release (Collins and Leonard, 1984, 1990; LeDune, 1972). Glucagon deficiency also has been postulated as playing a role in the etiology of this hypoglycemia (Mehta et al, 1987). Affected infants have excessive glucose requirements, often needing glucose infusion rates greater than 10 to 20 mg/kg/minute. Although very little is known about this form of hyperinsulinism, it may be the most common cause of hypoglycemia beyond the first few days of life. Treatment includes providing adequate dextrose infusions to maintain a plasma glucose level of greater than 60 mg/dL. If high dextrose requirements persist, treatment with oral diazoxide should be considered. Diazoxide treatment may effectively inhibit insulin secretion until the excessive insulin secretion resolves by a few months of age (Collins and Leonard, 1984, 1990). Glucocorticoids have no role in this disorder, as they are not effective in controlling hyperinsulinism. The use of glucocorticoids as a nonspecific therapy, when the underlying etiology of the hypoglycemia has not been identified, should be avoided. Glucagon infusions may help transiently control the hypoglycemia, by mobilizing glycogen stores, and may be useful in providing further diagnostic information. However, use of glucagon is not a practical long-term therapy.

### *Hyperinsulinism in Infants of Diabetic Mothers*

Infants born to mothers with diabetes mellitus may be chronically exposed to hyperglycemia in utero if maternal glucose control is poor. These infants can develop hyperinsulinism in response to the excess glucose exposure (Adam et al, 1969; Schwartz et al, 1994). Because fetal growth is stimulated by high insulin and other metabolic fuels these infants may be markedly obese with excess stores of glycogen, protein, and fat. Increased fetal growth is evident as increased body fat, muscle mass, and organomegaly without increased brain size. The hyperinsulinism may not immediately resolve at birth and therefore these infants are at increased risk of hypoglycemia. These infants have hypertrophy and hyperplasia of the pancreatic islets, as well as an inappropriate preservation of liver glycogen. This is demonstrated by a rise in blood glucose in response to glucagon given during a hypoglycemic episode. Markers of excess insulin include high glucose demands (greater than 6 to 8 mg/kg/minute) as well as suppression of lipolysis and ketogenesis.

Infants of diabetic mothers are at increased risk of additional medical problems including hypocalcemia, hyperbilirubinemia, polycythemia, respiratory distress syndrome, as well as fetal asphyxia and distress. They are at risk for congenital anomalies when maternal glucose is poorly controlled during the critical period of organogenesis between 4 and 10 weeks of gestation. Anomalies include cardiac defects, vertebral abnormalities, and caudal regression syndrome. Meticulous glucose regulation during and prior to pregnancy is critical for decreasing infant morbidity.

All LGA infants should be suspected of having hyperinsulinism. These infants should be given early feedings and have close monitoring of glucose levels. If hypoglycemia develops, IV glucose should be given according to the individual infant's needs. Keeping plasma glucose values within a range of 60 to 80 mg/dL and avoidance of hyperglycemia to prevent further insulin stimulation and possible rebound hypoglycemia will allow for efficient treatment in these infants. Weaning from glucose infusions should be done gradually. If control of glucose levels cannot be achieved beyond the first few days of life, other disorders should be suspected, specifically congenital hyperinsulinism.

### *Miscellaneous Disorders*

Maternal therapy with beta$_2$ agonists or use of high-dextrose IV infusions in the period leading up to delivery has been associated with an increase in neonatal hypoglycemia. The mechanism in both cases probably is related to neonatal hyperinsulinism. The hypoglycemia typically is self-limited and resolves within the first few days of life. Infants with Beckwith-Weidemann syndrome or erythroblastosis fetalis also may display varying degrees of hyperinsulinism. They will often resemble infants with congenital hyperinsulinism, described in the next section.

## Neonatal Hypoglycemia Due to Persistent (Congenital) Forms of Hyperinsulinism

### *Congenital Hyperinsulinism*

Congenital hyperinsulinism is the most common and difficult-to-manage form of persistent hypoglycemia in neonates and infants (Stanley, 1997). Severely affected infants usually present with an abnormally high birth weight but otherwise normal findings on physical examination. In the past, congenital hyperinsulinism had been called "nesidioblastosis," implying a developmental disorder of pancreatic islet formation. However, it is now known that nesidioblastosis is a normal feature of the newborn pancreas and that hyperinsulinism is due to genetic defects in the regulation of insulin secretion.

The pathways involved in insulin release are shown in Figure 93–3. Glucose-stimulated insulin secretion involves increased glucose metabolism via the Glut2 glucose transporter and glucokinase (GK). This leads to an increased ATP/ADP ratio, resulting in inhibition of a plasma membrane ATP-dependent potassium channel. This $K_{ATP}$ channel is composed of a sulfonylurea receptor regulatory subunit (SUR1) complexed with its ion pore (Kir6.2). Closure of the $K_{ATP}$ channel results in membrane depolarization and activation of a voltage-sensitive calcium channel; the resulting increase in cytosolic calcium triggers exocytosis of insulin granules. Insulin secretion also may be stimulated by amino acids through allosteric activation of glutamate dehydrogenase (GDH) by leucine. This results in increased oxidation of glutamate, leading to an increased ATP/ADP ratio, inhibition of the ATP-dependent potassium channel activity, and membrane depolarization.

#### Etiology

Several described defects in the regulation of insulin secretion result in congenital hyperinsulinism. Both recessive and dominant forms of congenital hyperinsulinism have been described and include mutations involving SUR1, Kir6.2, GDH, and GK. Pathologic findings include diffuse involvement of the entire pancreas or focal pancreatic lesions (Delonlay et al, 1997; Glaser et al, 2000; Huopio et al, 2000; Stanley, 1997; Stanley et al, 1998).

#### *Recessive (Diffuse) $K_{ATP}$ Channel Hyperinsulinism*

The genetic defects in this type of hyperinsulinism are recessive, loss-of-function mutations of the genes encoding the SUR1 and Kir6.2 components of the ATP-sensitive potassium channel complex. These two genes are located adjacent to one another on chromosome 11p (Glaser et al, 2000).

#### *Focal $K_{ATP}$ Channel Hyperinsulinism*

In the focal form of the disease, a clone of beta cells expresses a paternally derived mutation of SUR1 or Kir6.2 as a result of the loss of heterozygosity for the maternal allele. Infants with mutations of SUR1 or Kir6.2 (either focal or diffuse disease) are the most severely affected and often present with hypoglycemia on the first day of life. Because diazoxide suppression of insulin secretion depends on a functional $K_{ATP}$ channel (see Fig. 93–3), neonates with diffuse or focal $K_{ATP}$ hyperinsulinism often cannot be managed medically, necessitating surgical pancreatectomy. Infants with focal and with diffuse disease are indistinguishable clinically, however, infants with focal disease (approximately 40% of cases) are potentially curable by surgery, but those with diffuse disease are not (De Lonlay-Debeney et al, 1999).

#### *Dominant $K_{ATP}$ Channel Hyperinsulinism*

A recent report describes a family with a dominantly inherited mutation of SUR1 (Huopio et al, 2000). Clinical disease was less severe than with the typical $K_{ATP}$ channel hyperinsulinism mutation described earlier. Onset of symptoms was

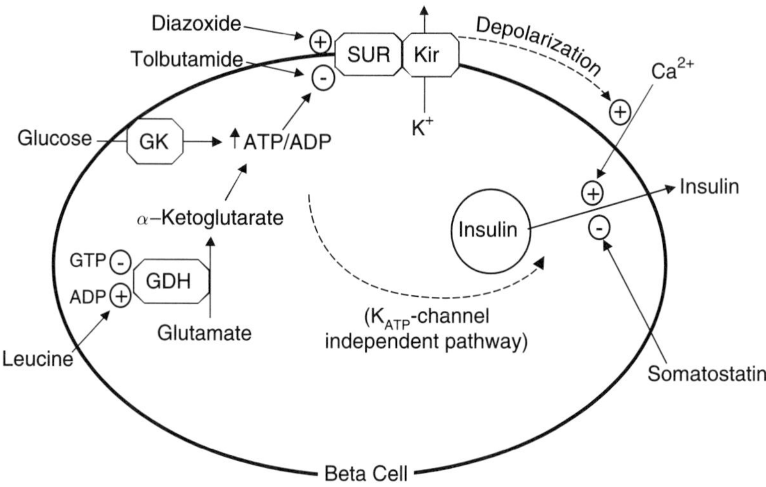


**FIGURE 93–3.** Mechanism of insulin secretion by the beta cell of the pancreas. Glucose is transported into the cell by the insulin-independent glucose transporter (GLUT2). The glucose undergoes phosphorylation by glucokinase (GK). It is then metabolized, with a resultant increase in the ATP/ADP ratio. With this increase in the ATP/ADP ratio, the $K_{ATP}$ channel closes, initiating a cascade of events including membrane depolarization, calcium influx, and release of insulin from storage granules. Leucine stimulates insulin secretion by activating glutamate dehydrogenase (GDH), which increases the oxidation of glutamate, thereby increasing the ATP/ADP ratio. ADP, adenosine diphosphate; ATP, adenosine triphosphate; GTP, guanosine triphosphate; Kir, potassium channel ion pore; SUR, sulfonylurea receptor regulatory subunit.

later in infancy and responded to diazoxide therapy, indicating that complete loss of channel function did not occur. This report suggests that additional phenotypes of $K_{ATP}$ hyperinsulinism are likely to be discovered in the future.

### *Dominant Glucokinase Hyperinsulinism*

Dominant GK hyperinsulinism is associated with a regulatory mutation of GK. Presentation in this form occurs beyond the neonatal period (Glaser et al, 1998).

### Dominant Glutamate Dehydrogenase Hyperinsulinism (Hyperinsulinism/Hyperammonemia Syndrome)

Dominant GDH hyperinsulinism is the result of a gain-of-function mutation of GDH (Huijmans et al, 2000; MacMullen et al, 2001; Miki et al, 2000; Stanley et al, 1998; Yorifuji et al, 1999). Patients present with symptomatic hypoglycemia along with persistent asymptomatic elevation of plasma ammonia. Infants are of normal size at birth, and episodes of hypoglycemia frequently are not detected until beyond the first year of life. Medical therapy with diazoxide is effective. Most cases are sporadic, but familial autosomal dominant inheritance is reported in approximately 20% of cases. Plasma ammonia levels are constant and do not increase with protein feeding, usually in the range of 60 to 105 μmol/L. Treatment is not needed for elevated ammonia levels.

### Clinical Presentation

The infant with congenital hyperinsulinism may present with difficult-to-manage hypoglycemia on the first day of life, requiring glucose infusion rates of greater than 10 to 20 mg/kg/minute (Landau et al, 1982; Stanley and Baker, 1976). Severe forms are associated with $K_{ATP}$ channel defects and usually manifest in the first hours or days after birth. Less severe forms are associated with GDH or GK mutations. Infants with the less severe forms may have normal birth weights, and episodes of hypoglycemia may not be recognized until beyond the neonatal period. Hyperinsulinism can be devastating to the developing brain. The brain is deprived of glucose as well as alternative fuels, because insulin suppresses lipolysis and ketogenesis by inhibiting adipose tissue lipolysis and preventing transport of free fatty acids into the mitochondria for oxidation and ketogenesis (Stanley and Baker, 1976).

### Diagnosis

Using the fasting systems approach, congenital hyperinsulinism can be reliably diagnosed by the pattern of metabolic fuels and hormones at the time of hypoglycemia (glucose less than 50 mg/dL). Plasma insulin levels greater than 2 mU/mL, plasma β-hydroxybutyrate less than 2.0 mmol/L, plasma free fatty acids less than 1.5 mmol/L, and a glycemic response to glucagon greater than 30 mg/dL serve to establish the diagnosis (Finegold et al, 1980; Stanley and Baker, 1976). The glycemic response to glucagon demonstrates inappropriate glycogen conservation during the episode of hypoglycemia and is useful in making the presumptive diagnosis of hyperinsulinism. The lack of an elevated insulin level at the time of hypoglycemia alone does not exclude hyperinsulinism. The hypersecretion of insulin may be episodic, or increased portal vein insulin may not be reflected in peripheral insulin concentrations. Caution must be taken in ruling out pituitary deficiencies if insulin levels are not diagnostically elevated.

### Treatment

The first line of treatment for congenital hyperinsulinism is diazoxide, which acts at the $K_{ATP}$ channel to suppress insulin secretion. If diazoxide fails to control the hypoglycemia, then octreotide, a long-acting somatostatin analogue, may be effective inhibiting insulin secretion (Hirsch et al, 1977). Patients with severe hyperinsulinism often fail to respond to medical management. Surgery may be required to control the hypoglycemia. This may involve resection of a focal lesion, if identified. If a focal lesion is not found, a 95% pancreatectomy is done with the hope that sufficient pancreatic tissue will be removed to control the hypoglycemia. The remaining beta cells still are not normally regulated, so further therapy with diazoxide and/or octreotide or further surgery often is required.

## *Neonatal Hypoglycemia Due to Counterregulatory Hormone Deficiency*

### *Pituitary Deficiency*

Pituitary deficiency is the second most frequent cause of persistent neonatal hypoglycemia. It is often associated with physical features such as midline cleft lip or palate, single central incisor, or optic nerve hypoplasia. Male infants may have micropenis due to gonadotropin deficiency. Caution is advised, because findings on the physical examination also may be normal. Low levels of growth hormone and cortisol, at the time of hypoglycemia, suggest the diagnosis of pituitary deficiency. Provocative testing may be required to confirm the diagnosis. Clinical features in these infants may mimic those of hyperinsulinism, as growth hormone and adrenocorticotropic hormone (ACTH) deficiency permit unopposed insulin action. Thyroid function tests in these infants show low or low-normal levels of thyroxine ($T_4$) and thyroid-stimulating hormone (TSH). Hypoglycemia is correctable with appropriate hormone replacement. A magnetic resonance imaging (MRI) scan should be obtained to identify the presence of other midline defects.

### *Adrenal Insufficiency*

Hypoglycemia is rare in cases of congenital adrenal hyperplasia. It may be present in cases of adrenal hemorrhage, a rare event, or congenital adrenal hypoplasia/aplasia, also rare (Artavia-Loria et al, 1986; Reiner et al, 1983; Toyofuku et al, 1986). Early recognition in these rare cases is crucial, as cortisol deficiency can be life-threatening. Normoglycemia is restored with cortisol replacement.

## *Neonatal Hypoglycemia Due to Defects of Fasting Metabolic Systems*

### *Genetic Metabolic Defects*

Defects in glycogenolysis, gluconeogenesis, and ketogenesis that manifest with hypoglycemia are listed in Table 93–2. They are discussed in greater detail in a separate chapter. Hypoglycemia associated with genetic metabolic defects often is masked by frequent infant feedings in the newborn period. Thus, such defects often are not recognized until after several months of age. The exception to this rule is in affected neonates who are breast-fed, as the delay in establishing lactation can expose infants to prolonged fasting stress. Growth failure, hepatomegaly, and acidosis are often presenting features.

*Persistent hypoglycorrhachia* (glucose transporter 1 [Glut1] deficiency) has been reported (De Vivo et al, 1991). Affected infants have a genetic defect of the glucose transporter required to transfer glucose across the blood-brain barrier. Patients have low cerebrospinal fluid glucose levels (20 to 30 mg/dL) without evidence of meningitis. Cases have been described in which the presenting manifestations were recurrent seizures, progressive microcephaly, and retardation. A ketogenic diet has been used successfully to provide alternative substrate for the brain, permitting normal brain development in some patients.

## Diagnosis and Treatment of Hypoglycemia

### Plasma Glucose Thresholds

Controversy about appropriate glucose thresholds for neonates has continued over the past decades. The uncertainty in this area derives from the perception from 50 or 60 years ago that glucose levels in newborn infants were often lower than the ranges found in infants, children, and adults. Pediatricians were therefore reluctant to apply the same glucose standards to neonates as those used in older children. This reluctance has recently been compounded by concern about medicolegal implications of neonatal hypoglycemia. The fact that hypoglycemia was not purely benign in neonates was first appreciated in the early 1960s, when Cornblath and colleagues (1959) described symptomatic neonatal hypoglycemia. Dr. Cornblath (Cornblath and Schwartz, 1966) proposed that hypoglycemia could be "defined" in neonates as the presence of glucose levels 2 standard deviations below the mean values found in surveys of glucose levels on the first day of life. They also proposed that a different glucose value be used to define hypoglycemia for low-birth-weight infants, because lower glucose levels were more frequent in this group. The problems with this approach are obvious and include the fact that statistical definitions of hypoglycemia only describe what ranges of glucose levels are common, not what is physiologically normal or optimal for newborns. In addition, it is clear that the distribution of glucose values in neonates reflects feeding practices on the first day of life. This effect of changes in nursery practices is apparent in a comparison of mean glucose levels in term infants from 1961 to 1986. The mean glucose level during the first 3 hours after birth increased from 48 mg/dL to 70 mg/dL (Aynsley-Green, 1991).

Despite the perceptions from over 50 years ago, there is no evidence that newborn infants have a lower requirement for plasma glucose concentrations than those in older infants or adults. Before birth, fetal levels of plasma glucose are nearly identical to maternal values, and the fetus is known to be dependent on glucose as its major source of energy. There is also no evidence that the neonatal brain is specially protected to tolerate hypoglycemia better than the brains of older infants and children.

Pathophysiologic responses to hypoglycemia in neonates, older children, and adults occur at similar thresholds of glucose (Koh et al, 1988; Pryds and Christensen, 1990). In adults, visual evoked potentials were abnormal when blood glucose dropped below 47 mg/dL, and a modest decrease in plasma glucose (below 70 mg/dL) caused early impairment in cognitive function without clinical symptoms (DeFeo et al, 1988; Harrad et al, 1985). A compensatory increase in cerebral blood flow was found in preterm infants during hypoglycemia (Pryds and Christensen, 1990). CNS dysfunction has been reported in neonates with asymptomatic hypoglycemia, as noted by abnormalities in sensory evoked potentials (Koh et al, 1988). Studies of preterm infants associated repetitive decreases in glucose (less than 47 mg/dL), with reduced mental and motor developmental scores and increased neurodevelopmental impairment (Lucas et al, 1988).

Because of the aforementioned concerns, the authors do not recommend using different glucose thresholds for diagnosing and treating hypoglycemia in neonates than in older infants and adults. In the neonate, as in older children and adults, hypoglycemia should be considered the result of a failure in one or more of the metabolic and hormonal systems involved in fasting homeostasis. The physiologically optimal range for plasma glucose levels should be considered to be 70 to 100 mg/dL. The goal of therapy in neonates should be identical to that in older children—that is, to maintain plasma glucose at greater than 60 mg/dL, preferably within the optimal range of 75 to 100 mg/dL. A plasma glucose value of 50 mg/dL is the threshold for terminating provocative tests, such as diagnostic fasting tests. This usually provides an adequate margin of safety to obtain necessary information about fasting adaptation without risking severe symptoms, such as seizures. This threshold level of hypoglycemia is influenced by alternative fuel availability. In some disorders, such as fatty acid oxidation defects, infants can have severe symptoms and be dangerously ill with plasma glucose levels in the range of 45 to 60 mg/dL. In other disorders, such as glucose-6-phosphatase deficiency, CNS symptoms are infrequent when glucose levels fall below 40 mg/dL, because high levels of plasma lactate provide alternative fuel for the brain. Plasma glucose levels above 40 mg/dL are not likely to be responsible for severe symptoms such as seizures, but may be suggestive of an underlying abnormality. It should be emphasized that the need for diagnostic work-up is determined not by the level of plasma glucose but rather by clinical factors such as postnatal age, birth history, feeding intervals, and findings on physical examination. This conservative approach to hypoglycemia emphasizes that glucose values of 40 to 60 mg/dL should be considered suboptimal. In neonates on the first day of life who have no other risk factors, hypoglycemia can be assumed to be due to immaturity of fasting that will not persist. In these otherwise normal infants, appropriate early feeding leads to an appropriate elevation in glucose. If adequate response is not obtained, and especially if difficulties persist beyond the first day of life, the possibility of a disorder in one of the fasting systems should be considered.

Several factors may influence the accuracy of glucose measurements. Glucose meters are useful for rapid bedside screening; however, their range of precision is only

±10% to 20% (e.g., at a meter reading of 50 mg/dL, the true value may be as low as 40 mg/dL or as high as 60 mg/dL). Operator technique also may affect results if too much or too little blood is placed on test strips. Corroboration with true laboratory values is required (Perelman et al, 1982). The use of test trips to estimate plasma glucose visually without a meter should be avoided, because this method is grossly inaccurate and outdated. When using whole blood values, one must remember they are 10% to 15% lower than plasma values (Sacks, 1996). When whole blood measurements are performed, falsely low measurements may occur as a result of red cell glycolysis if there is a delay in analyzing specimens or in the presence of polycythemia (hematocrit greater than 70%) (Kaplan et al, 1989). Finally, the site from which the blood was drawn is an important consideration, as arterial glucose values are greater than capillary values, which in turn are greater than venous values (Larsson-Cohn, 1976).

### Clinical Presentation

The classic signs of hypoglycemia relate to adrenergic activation (tachycardia, sweating, jitteriness, etc.) and to CNS impairment (e.g., confusion, lethargy) (Table 93–6). The signs of hypoglycemia in the neonate are more nonspecific, resulting from disturbances in one or more aspects of CNS function. As the signs are often minimal and difficult to appreciate, hypoglycemia should be suspected in any infant who does not appear normal, who has inadequate oral intake, or in any infant known to be at increased risk (see Table 93–3).

### Treatment

Any infant known to be at risk for hypoglycemia should be monitored closely, and either IV glucose or enteral nutrition should be initiated as soon as possible. These include large-for-dates and small-for-dates neonates, neonates with perinatal asphyxia, and infants of diabetic mothers or mothers with toxemia or preeclampsia. In cases of mild or asymptomatic hypoglycemia, enteral feeds should be given if the infant is able to tolerate them. This recommendation applies to otherwise normal infants who have hypoglycemia during the first 24 hours after birth when the problem is believed to be transient and due to a delay in initiation of feedings (e.g., breast-feeding). Beyond the first day, if plasma glucose values below 60 mg/dL continue, further evaluation for the etiology of the hypoglycemia based on the fasting systems approach should be initiated. Breast milk is beneficial when enteral feeds are initiated in that it may be more ketogenic than formula, but it often is not available within the first 24 hours of life. Standard infant formula should be used if breast milk is not available. Breast milk and formula provide carbohydrates, protein, and fat. They are metabolized more slowly than dextrose in water and provide more energy per milliliter despite having less glucose. Fat intake may be beneficial, as it decreases demand for glucose utilization, stimulates gluconeogenesis, and may play important roles in initiating transcription of enzymes of ketogenesis. If clinically tolerated, enteral feeds should be continued even if IV therapy is required for low glucose values (Hawdon et al, 1992; Lucas et al, 1978).

Severe or symptomatic hypoglycemia should be treated with IV glucose. A bolus of 200 mg/kg of glucose (10% dextrose in water [$D_{10}W$], 2 mL/kg) should be used, along with initiation of or increase in the glucose infusion rate (Lilien et al, 1980). A larger bolus of glucose may be harmful to neurologic function and may be followed by rebound hypoglycemia. Dextrose infusion should be started at 5 to 8 mg/kg/minute to maintain plasma glucose above 60 mg/dL. Rates as high as 20 to 30 mg/kg/minute may be required in disorders such as hyperinsulinism or pituitary deficiency or for infants of diabetic mothers. The infusion rate is calculated as follows:

$$\text{rate (mg/kg/minute)} = (\%\ \text{glucose in IV solution} \times \text{IV rate in mL/hr} \times 0.167) \div \text{weight (kg)}$$

Specific therapies such as diazoxide, or somatostatin (octreotide) may be indicated after appropriate diagnostic evaluation to ensure appropriate therapy based on the physiologic mechanism of the hypoglycemia. Glucocorticoids should not be used for nonspecific treatment of hypoglycemia in neonates or older children.

### Diagnosis of Underlying Disorder

In order to appropriately treat infants with evidence of persistent hypoglycemia, the cause of the hypoglycemia must be determined. If the cause of hypoglycemia is clearly a self-limited disorder (such as in the infant of the diabetic mother) then complete diagnostic testing may not be needed. If the etiology is not clear, the history, physical examination, and laboratory findings should be used together to make a diagnosis.

The history should include the duration of fasting prior to the hypoglycemic episode as well as the frequency of episodes. Shorter duration and frequent episodes are consistent with hyperinsulinism. Onset soon after a meal would be consistent with hyperinsulinism or glycogen storage disease. Onset after more prolonged fasting is more consistent with a fatty acid oxidation or gluconeogenic defect. If a midline facial malformation, micropthalmia, or microphallus is present, pituitary deficiency should be suspected. In an LGA infant, congenital hyperinsulinism should be suspected. Growth failure with massive hepatomegaly frequently is associated with glucose-6-phosphatase deficiency or debrancher deficiency glycogen storage disease. A fatty acid oxidation defect may be associated with abnormal liver function tests and hyperammonemia.

An important part of the laboratory evaluation includes the hormonal and fuel responses at the time of fasting

**TABLE 93–6**

**Signs of Neonatal Hypoglycemia**

| | |
|---|---|
| Tremors | Lethargy |
| Irritability | Diaphoresis |
| Poor feeding | Abnormal cry |
| Apnea | Cyanosis |
| Seizures | Limpness |
| Jitteriness | Twitching |
| Hypothermia | Tachycardia |
| Tachypnea | |

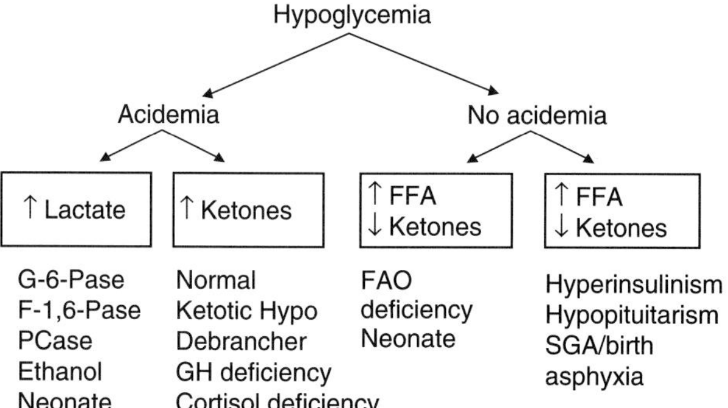


**FIGURE 93–4.** Algorithm for the diagnosis of hypoglycemia based on results of "critical" blood tests at the time of hypoglycemia. FAO, fatty acid oxidation; FFA, free fatty acids; F-1, 6-Pase, fructose-1,6-diphosphatase; GH, growth hormone; G-6-Pase, glucose-6-phosphatase; hypo, hypoglycemia; PCase, pyruvate carboxylase; SGA, small for gestational age.

hypoglycemia. Plasma should be obtained for the "critical" blood measurements at the time of hypoglycemia including levels of lactate, free fatty acids, ketones, insulin, cortisol, and growth hormone (2 to 3 mL). Obtaining an adequate urine sample for the measurement of urinary organic acids is needed (5 to 10 mL). The algorithm presented in Figure 93–4 outlines the differential diagnosis of hypoglycemia based on results of these blood tests. A glucagon stimulation test also provides useful diagnostic information. At the time of hypoglycemia, 0.5 to 1 mg of IV glucagon is given. A rise in glucose greater than 30 mg/dL suggests inappropriate preservation of liver glycogen stores. This may be seen in hyperinsulinism as well as in neonatal panhypopituitarism. Additional tests of pituitary function should be included if pituitary deficiency is suspected.

## HYPERGLYCEMIA

Neonatal hyperglycemia may be seen in the neonatal intensive care unit. It is most commonly a problem encountered in sick neonates, particularly very low-birth-weight (VLBW) infants. This is most commonly seen within 24 hours after birth in the VLBW infant in association with increased glucose infusion rates (greater than 6 mg/kg/minute) but also may be noted at lower glucose infusion rates (Dweck and Cassady, 1974; Zarif et al, 1976). The risk for hyperglycemia is 18 times greater in infants weighing less than 1000 g than in those weighing more than 2000 g (Louik et al, 1985). This risk also is increased in those infants with serious illnesses or stresses such as anesthesia or surgery (Lilien et al, 1979; Ward Platt et al, 1990). Hyperglycemia beyond the initial few days of life in the VLBW infant has been associated with bacterial and fungal infections as well as drugs such as postnatal dexamethasone and methylxanthines (Fanaroff et al, 1998; Farrag and Cowett, 2000; Rowen et al, 1995; Vermont Oxford Network Steroid Study Group, 2001).

Studies of the mechanism of hyperglycemia in the VLBW infant suggest that the neonate has a decreased insulin response to a glucose load, representing a lag in the beta cell response to the hyperglycemia. Other studies suggest that newborns with hyperglycemia have a relative insulin resistance, resulting in decreased suppression of hepatic glucose production throughout a wide range of glucose and insulin infusions and concentrations (Cowett and colleagues, 1983; Hay, 1998). Elevated levels of circulating cortisol, glucagon and catecholamines are implicated when the hyperglycemia is present in association with "stress" conditions such as postsurgery and sepsis (Farrag and Cowett, 2000).

Plasma glucose levels greater than 150 mg/dL generally are considered to indicate hyperglycemia. This level of hyperglycemia is based on statistical studies and does not take into account the underlying events and biologic variations that may be altering the infant's response to exogenous glucose. The long-term effects of mild elevations in glucose are not well studied. In clinical practice, VLBW infants demonstrating glucose intolerance frequently have glucose levels exceeding 200 mg/dL. Physiologic concerns with high glucose levels include osmotic diuresis, dehydration, and weight loss. In severe hyperglycemia (glucose levels greater than 500 mg/dL), cerebral hemorrhage may result from the increased serum osmolarity, causing water to shift from the intracellular to the extracellular compartment (Miranda and Dweck, 1977). Some clinical studies suggest increased mortality, intraventricular hemorrhage, and major handicaps in infants with hyperglycemia (Dweck and Cassady, 1974; Zarif et al, 1976), although it has been difficult to fully evaluate hyperglycemia as an independent risk without other confounding factors. Adult animal and human studies have linked hyperglycemia with increased brain damage when associated with hypoxic brain injury (Binder et al, 1989; Myers and Yamaguchi, 1977; Pulsinelli et al, 1982, 1983).

Therapy for hyperglycemia in the neonate is linked to the severity of glucose elevation. If hyperglycemia is mild and brief (duration less than 24 to 48 hours), a decrease in the glucose infusion rate is frequently successful in treating the hyperglycemia. Use of hypotonic IV solutions should be avoided. In prolonged cases of hyperglycemia, the nutritional needs of the infant may be significantly compromised. Low-dose insulin therapy may be useful in increasing the availability of calories needed for growth from parenteral nutrition when the glucose concentration is consistently greater than 200 to 250 mg/dL (Binder et al, 1989; Collins et al, 1991). Continuous insulin infusions starting at 0.01 unit/kg/hour and increasing gradually up to 0.05 to 0.1 unit/kg/hour will control the hyperglycemia. Caution is indicated regarding use of continuous insulin infusions, as the insulin frequently adsorbs to glass and plastic surfaces and can be degraded by light.

Neonatal onset of diabetes mellitus is rare, with an incidence estimated at about 1/500,000 (Von Muhlendah and Herkenhoff, 1995). Affected infants are usually born small for gestational age. They present within the first 1 to 3 months of life with elevated blood glucose levels and glycosuria. Ketosis may be present but is frequently mild. Infants invariably present with dehydration. They have low insulin levels during the hyperglycemia and decreased insulin response to secretagogues. Insulin therapy usually is required, but the prognosis is excellent, with frequent spontaneous resolution. Three forms have been reported: transient, permanent, and transient with later recurrence (Von Muhlendah and Herkenhoff, 1995). The clinical features of the transient and the permanent forms are similar, but the underlying genetics are different. Paternal uniparental isodisomy of chromosome 6 has been reported in cases of the transient disease form, with linkage to 6q23-q24 (Hermann et al, 2000; Temple et al, 2000). The permanent form of the disease is less understood. It has been associated with abnormalities in pancreatic development including aplasia and hypoplasia (Lemons et al, 1979; Winter et al, 1986). A mutation in the insulin promoter factor-1 (*IFP1*) gene has been identified in a patient with pancreatic agenesis (Stoffers et al, 1977). The *IPF1* locus has been mapped to 13q12.1 (Stoffel et al, 1995). Cases of permanent diabetes mellitus due to complete deficiency of the glycolytic enzyme glucokinase also have been reported (Njolstad et al, 2001).

## REFERENCES


Adam PA, Teramo K, Raiha N, et al: Human fetal insulin metabolism early in gestation: Response to acute elevation of the fetal glucose concentration and placental transfer of human insulin-I-131. Diabetes 18:409-416, 1969.

Arnott G, Coghill G, McArdle HJ, et al: Immunolocalization of Glut1 and Glut3 glucose transporters in human placenta. Biochem Soc Trans 22:272S, 1994.

Artavia-Loria E, Chaussain J, Bougneres PF, et al: Frequency of hypoglycemia in children with adrenal insufficiency. Acta Endocrinol (Suppl) 279:275-278, 1986.

Asins G, Serra D, Arias G, et al: Developmental changes in carnitine palmitoyltransferases I and II gene expression in intestine and liver of suckling rats. Biochem J 306:379-384, 1995.

Aynsley-Green A: Glucose: A fuel for thought! J Pediatr Child Health 27:21-30, 1991.

Bier DM, Leake RS, Haymond MW, et al: Measurement of "true" glucose production rates in infancy and childhood with 6,6 dideuteroglucose. Diabetes 26:1016-1023, 1977.

Binder ND, Raschko PK, Benda GI, et al: Insulin infusion with parenteral nutrition in extremely low birth weight infants with hyperglycemia. J Pediatr. 114:273-280, 1989.

Cahill GF: Starvation in man. N Engl J Med 282:668-675, 1970.

Chaussain JL, Georges P, Calzada L, et al: Glycemic response to 24-hour fast in normal children. III. Influence of age. J Pediatr 91:711-714, 1977.

Collins JE, Leonard JV, Teale D, Marks V: Hyperinsulinemic hypoglycemia in small for dates infants. Arch Dis Child 65:1118-1120, 1990.

Collins JE, Leonard JV: Hyperinsulinism in asphyxiated and small for dates infants with hypoglycemia. Lancet 2:311-313, 1984.

Collins JW, Hoppe M, Brown K, et al: A controlled trial of insulin infusion and parenteral nutrition in extremely low birth weight infants with glucose intolerance. J Pediatr 118:921-927, 1991.

Cornblath M, Odell GB, Levin EY: Symptomatic neonatal hypoglycemia associated with toxemia of pregnancy. J Pediatr 55:545-562, 1959.

Cornblath M, Schwartz R: Disorders of Carbohydrate Metabolism in Infancy. Philadelphia, WB Saunders, 1966, p 82.

Cowett M, Schwartz R: The role of hepatic control of glucose homeostasis in the etiology of neonatal hypo- and hyperglycemia. Semin Perinatol 3:327-340, 1979.

Cowett R, Oh W, Schwartz R: Persistent glucose production during glucose infusion in the neonate. J Clin Invest 71: 467-475, 1983.

DeFeo P, Gallai V, Mazzotta G, et al: Modest decrements in plasma glucose concentration cause early impairment in cognitive function and later activation of glucose counter-regulation in the absence of hypoglycemic symptoms in normal man. J Clin Invest. 82:436-444, 1988.

Delonlay P, Fournet J, Rahier J, Gross-Morand MS: Somatic deletion of the imprinted 11p15 region in sporadic persistent hyperinsulinemic hypoglycemia of infancy is specific of focal adenomatous hyperplasia and endorses partial pancreatectomy. J Clin Invest 100:802-807, 1997.

De Lonlay-Debeney P, Poggi-Travert F, Fournet JC, et al: Clinical features of 52 neonates with hyperinsulinism. N Engl J Med 340:1169-1175, 1999.

Devaskar SU, Mueckler MM: The mammalian glucose transporters. Pediatr Res 31:1-13, 1991.

De Vivo DC, Trifiletti RR, Jacobson RI, et al: Defective glucose transport across the blood-brain barrier as a cause of persistent hypoglycorrhachia, seizures and developmental delay. N Engl J Med 325:703-709, 1991.

Dweck HS, Cassady G: Glucose intolerance in infants of very low birth weight: Incidence of hyperglycemia in birth weights 1100 gm or less. Pediatrics 53:189-195, 1974.

Fanaroff AA, Korones SB, Wright LL, et al: Incidence, presenting features, risk factors and significance of late onset septicemia in very low birth weight infants. Pediatr Infect Dis J 17:593-598, 1998.

Farrag HM, Cowett RM: Glucose homeostasis in the micropremie. Clin Perinatol 27:1-22, 2000.

Finegold DN, Stanley CA, Baker L: Glycemic response to glucagon during fasting hypoglycemia: An aid in the diagnosis of hyperinsulinism. J Pediatr 96:257-259, 1980.

Foster PC, Bailey E: Changes in the activities of the enzymes of hepatic fatty acid oxidation during development of the rat. Biochem J 154:49-56, 1976.

Girard J: Gluconeogenesis in the late fetal and early neonatal life. Biol Neonate 50:237-258, 1986.

Girard J, Caquet D, Bal D, et al: Control of rat liver phosphorylase, glucose-6-phosphatase and phosphoenolpyruvate carboxykinase activities by insulin and glucagon during the perinatal period. Enzyme 15:272-285, 1973.

Glaser B, Kesavan P, Heyman M, et al: Familial hyperinsulinism caused by an activating glucokinase mutation. N Engl J Med 338:226-230, 1998.

Glaser B, Thornton T, Otonski T, et al: Genetics of hyperinsulinism. Arch Dis Child Fetal Neonatal Ed 82:F70-F82, 2000.

Granner D, Andreone T, Sazak K, et al: Inhibition of transcription of the phosphoenol pyruvate carboxykinase gene by insulin. Nature 305:549-541, 1983.

Harrad RA, Cockram CS, Plumb AP, et al: The effect of hypoglycemia on visual function: A clinical and electrophysiological study. Clin Soc (Lond) 69:673-679, 1985.

Hawden HM, Ward Platt MP: Metabolic adaptation in small for gestational age infants. Arch Dis Child. 68:262-268, 1993.

Hawden JM, Weddell A, et al: Hormonal and metabolic response to hypoglycemia in small for gestational age infants. Arch Dis Child 68:269-273, 1993.

Hawdon JM, Ward Platt MP, Aynsley-Green A: Patterns of metabolic adaptation for preterm and term infants in the first neonatal week. Arch Dis Child 67:357-365, 1992.

Hay WW: Nutrient and metabolic needs of the fetus and very small infant: A comparative approach. Biochem Soc Trans 26:75-78, 1998.

Hay WW: Fetal and neonatal glucose homeostasis and their relation to the small for gestational age infant. Semin Perinatol 8:101-116, 1984.

Haymond MW, Karl IE, Clarke WL, et al: Differences in circulating gluconeogenetic substrates during short term fasting in men, women, and children. Metabolism 31:33-42, 1982.

Heck LJ, Erenberg A: Serum glucose levels in term neonates during the first 48 hours of life. J Pediatr 110:119-122, 1987.

Hermann R, Laine A, Johansson C, et al: Transient but not permanent neonatal diabetes mellitus is associated with paternal uniparental isodisomy of chromosome 6. Pediatrics 105:49-52, 2000.

Hirsch HJ, Loo S, Evans N, et al: Hypoglycemia of infancy and nesidioblastosis: Studies with somatostatin. N Engl J Med 296:1323-1326, 1977.

Huijmans JG, Duran M, deKlerk JB, et al: Functional hyperactivity of hepatic gluatamte dehydrogenase as a cause of the hyperinsulinism/hyperammonemia syndrome: Effect of treatment. Pediatrics 106:596-600, 2000.

Huopio H, Reimann F, Ashfield R, et al: Dominantly inherited hyperinsulinism caused by a mutation in the sulfonylurea receptor type 1. J Clin Invest 106:897-906, 2000.

Jones RA, Roberton NR: Problems of the small for dates baby. Clin Obstet Gynecol 11:499-524, 1984.

Kahn BB: Facilitative glucose transporters: Regulatory mechanisms and dysregulation in diabetes. J Clin Invest 89:1367-1374, 1992.

Kalhan SC, Raghavan CV: Metabolism of glucose in the fetus and newborn. In Polin RA, Fox WW (eds): Fetal and Neonatal Physiology, 2nd ed. Philadelphia, WB Saunders, 1998, pp 543-558.

Kaplan M, Blondheim O, Alon I, et al: Screening for hypoglycemia with plasma in neonatal blood of high hematocrit value. Crit Care Med 17:279-282, 1989.

Koh T, Aynsley-Green A, Tarbit M, et al: Neural dysfunction during hypoglycemia. Arch Dis Child 63:1353-1358, 1988.

Landau H, Perlman M, Meyer S, et al: Persistent neonatal hypoglycemia due to hyperinsulinism: Medical aspects. Pediatrics 70:440-446, 1982.

Larsson-Cohn U: Differences between capillary and venous blood glucose during oral glucose tolerance tests. Scan J Clin Lab Invest 36:805-808, 1976.

LeDune MA: Intravenous glucose tolerance and plasma insulin studies in small for dates infants. Arch Dis Child 47:111-114, 1972.

Lemons JA, Ridenour R, Orsini EN, et al: Congenital absence of the pancreas and intrauterine growth retardation. Pediatrics 64:255-256, 1979.

Lilien LD, Pildes RS, Srinivasan G, et al: Treatment of neonatal hypoglycemia with minibolus and intravenous glucose infusion. J Pediatr 97:295-298, 1980.

Lilien L, Rosenfield RL, Baccaro MM, et al: Hyperglycemia in stressed small premature neonates. J Pediatr 94:454-459, 1979.

Louik C, Mitchell AA, Epstein MF, et al: Risk factors for neonatal hyperglycemia associated with 10% dextrose infusion. Am J Dis Child 139:783-786, 1985.

Lubchenco LO, Bard H: Incidence of hypoglycemia in newborn infants classified by birth weight and gestational age. Pediatrics 47:831-838, 1971.

Lucas A, Bloom SR, Aynsley-Green A: Metabolic and endocrine consequences of depriving preterm infants of enteral nutrition. Acta Pediatr Scand 72:245-249, 1983.

Lucas A, Morley R, Coler TJ: Adverse neurodevelopmental outcome of moderate neonatal hypoglycemia. BMJ 297:1304-1308, 1988.

MacMullen C, Fang J, Hsu BY, et al: Hyperinsulinism/hyperammonemia syndrome in children with regulatory mutations in the inhibitory GTP binding domain of glutamate dehydrogenase. J Clin Endocrinol Metab 86:1782-1787, 2001.

Mehta A, Wooten R, Cheng KN, et al: Effect of diazoxide or glucagon on hepatic glucose production during extreme neonatal hypoglycemia. Arch Dis Child 62:924-930, 1987.

Miki Y, Tomohiko T, Obura T, et al: Novel missense mutations in the glutamate dehydrogenase gene in congenital hyperinsulinism-hyperammonemia syndrome. J Pediatr 136:69-72, 2000.

Miranda LE, Dweck HS: Perinatal glucose homeostasis: The unique character of hyperglycemia and hypoglycemia in infants of very low birth weight. Clin Perinatol 4:351-365, 1977.

Myers RE, Yamaguchi S: Nervous system effects of cardiac arrest in monkeys. Arch Neurol 34:65-74, 1977.

Njolstad PR, Oddmund S, Cuesta-Munoz A, et al: Neonatal diabetes mellitus due to complete glucokinase deficiency. N Engl J Med 344:1588-1592, 2001.

Ogata ES: Carbohydrate metabolism in the fetus and neonate and altered neonatal glucoregulation. Pediatr Clin North Am 33:25-45, 1986.

Pegorier JP, Chatelain F, Thumelin S, et al: Role of long-chain fatty acids in the postnatal induction of genes coding for liver mitochondrial beta-oxidative enzymes. Biochem Soc Trans 26:113-120, 1998.

Perelman RH, Gutcher GR, Engle MJ, et al: Comparative analysis of four methods of rapid glucose determination in neonates. Am J Dis Child 136:1051-1053, 1982.

Pryds O, Christensen NJ: Increased cerebral blood flow and plasma epinephrine in hypoglycemic preterm neonates. Pediatrics 85:1172-1176, 1990.

Pulsinelli WA, Levy DE, Sigsbee B, et al: Increased damage after ischemic stroke in patients with hyperglycemia with or without established diabetes mellitus. Am J Med 74:540-544, 1983.

Pulsinelli WA, Waldman S, Rawlinson D, et al: Moderate hyperglycemia augments ischemic brain damage: A neuropathologic study in the rat. Neurology 32:1239-1246, 1982.

Reid NA, Boyd R: Further evidence for the presence of two facilitative glucose isoforms in the brush border membrane of the syncytiotrophoblast of the human full term placenta. Biochem Soc Trans 22:267S, 1994

Reiner WO, Nabben RE, Hustinx TW, et al: Congenital adrenal hypoplasia, progressive muscular dystrophy and severe mental retardation in association with glycerol kinase deficiency in male sibs. Clin Genet 24:243-251, 1983.

Rowen JL, Atkins JT, Levy ML, et al: Invasive fungal dermatitis in the <1000-gram neonate. Pediatrics. 95(5):682-687, 1995.

Sacks DB: Carbohydrates. In Burtis CA, Ashwood ET (eds): Tietz Textbook of Clinical Chemistry. Philadelphia, WB Saunders, 1996, pp 928-1001.

Sakata M, Kurachi H, Imai T, et al: Increase in human placental glucose transporter-1 during pregnancy. Eur J Endocrinol 132:206-212, 1995.

Schwartz R, Gruppuso RA, Petzkold K, et al: Hyperinsulinemia and macrosomia in the fetus of the diabetic mother. Diabetes Care 17:640-648, 1994.

Serra D, Asins G, Hegardt FG: Ketogenic mitochondrial 3-hydroxy 3-methylglutaryl-CoA synthase gene expression in intestine and liver of suckling rats. Arch Biochem Biophys 301:445-448, 1993.

Simmons RA: Cell glucose transport and glucose handling during fetal and neonatal development. In Polin RA, Fox WW (eds): Fetal and Neonatal Physiology, 2nd ed. Philadephia, WB Saunders, 1998, pp 585-592.

Sperling MA, Ganguli S, Leslie N, et al: Fetal-perinatal catecholamine secretion: Role in perinatal glucose homeostasis. Am J Physiol 247:E69-E74, 1984.

Srinivasan G, Pildes RS, et al: Plasma glucose values in normal neonates: A new look. J Pediatr 109:114-117, 1986.

Stanley CA: Hyperinsulinism in infants and children. Pediatr Clin North Am 44:363-374, 1997.

Stanley CA, Anday A, Baker L, et al: Metabolic fuel and hormone responses to fasting in newborn infant. Pediatrics 64:613-619, 1979.

Stanley CA, Gonzalez E, Baker L: Development of hepatic fatty acid oxidation and ketogenesis in the newborn guinea pig. Pediatr Res 17:224-229, 1983.

Stanley CA, Lieu YK, Hsu BY, et al: Hyperinsulinism and hyperammoniemia in infants with regulatory mutations of the glutamate dehydrogenase gene. N Engl J Med 338:1352-1357, 1998.

Stoffel M, Stein R, Wright CVE, et al: Localization of human homeodomain transcription factor insulin promoter factor 1 (IPF1) to chromosome band 13q12.1 Genomics 28:125-126, 1995.

Stoffers DA, Zinkin NT, Stanojevic V, et al: Pancreatic agenesis attributable to a single nucleotide deletion in the human IPF1 gene coding sequence. Nat Genet 15:106-110, 1997.

Takata K, Kasahara T, Kasahara M, et al: Localization of erythrocyte/HepG2-type glucose transporter (Glut 1) in human placental villi. Cell Tissue Res 267:407-412, 1992.

Temple IK, Gardner RJ, MacKay JG, et al: Transient neonatal diabetes: Widening the understanding of the etiopathogenesis of diabetes. Diabetes 49:1359-1366, 2000.

Thumelin S, Esser V, Charvy S, et al: Expression of liver carnitine palmitoyltransferase I and II genes during rat development. Biochem J 300:583-587, 1994.

Thumelin S, Forestier M, Girard J, et al: Developmental changes in mitochondrial 3-hydroxy-3-methylglutaryl-CoA synthase gene expression in rat liver, intestines and kidney. Biochem J 292:493-496, 1993.

Toyofuku T, Takashima S, Takeshita K, et al: Progressive muscular dystrophy with congenital adrenal hypoplasia: An unusual autopsy case. Brain Dev 8:285-289, 1986.

Vermont Oxford Network Steroid Study Group: Early postnatal dexamethasone therapy for the prevention of chronic lung disease. Pediatrics 108:741-748, 2001.

Von Muhlendah KE, Herkenhoff H: Long-term course of neonatal diabetes. N Engl J Med 333:704-708, 1995.

Wang C, Brennan WA Jr: Rat skeletal muscle, liver and brain have different fetal and adult forms of the glucose transporter. Biochim Biophy Acta 946:11-18, 1988.

Ward Platt MP, Tarbit MJ, Aynsley-Green A: The effects of anesthesia and surgery on metabolic homeostasis in infancy and childhoo. J Pediatr Surg 25:472-478, 1990.

Werner H, Adamo H, Lowe WL Jr, et al: Developmental regulation of rat brain/HepG2 glucose transporter gene expression. Mol Endocrinol 3:273-279, 1989.

Winter WE, Maclaren NK, Riley WJ, et al: Congenital pancreatic hypoplasia: A syndrome of exocrine and endocrine pancreatic insufficiency. J Pediatr 109:465-468, 1986.

Wright LL, Stanley CA, Anday EK, Baker L: The effect of early feeding on plasma glucose levels in SGA infants. Clin Pediatr 22:539-541, 1983.

Yorifuji T, Muroi H, Uematsu A, et al: Hyperinsulinism-hyperammonemia syndrome caused by mutant glutamate dehydrogenase accompanied by novel enzyme kinetics. Hum Genet 104:476-479, 1999.

Zarif M, Pildes RS, Vidyasagar D: Insulin and growth hormone responses in neonatal hyperglycemia. Diabetes 25:428-433, 1976.

Zeller J, Bougneres P: Hypoglycemia in infants. Trends Endocr Metab 3:366-370, 1992.

# PART XVIII

# ORTHOPEDIC CONDITIONS

Editor: H. WILLIAM TAEUSCH

CHAPTER 94

## Common Neonatal Orthopedic Ailments

Brian E. Grottkau and Michael J. Goldberg

Although orthopedic afflictions of the newborn generally are not life-threatening, they do have the potential to significantly impair functional performance, even when diagnosed and treated early. A few are also the basis for a disproportionate number of medicolegal proceedings. This chapter discusses the most commonly encountered of these orthopedic problems.

### DEVELOPMENTAL DYSPLASIA OF THE HIP

The term *developmental dysplasia of the hip* (DDH) encompasses a spectrum of pathology from "located" hips that are unstable (femoral head can be moved within or outside the confines of the acetabulum) to frankly dislocated hips in which there is a complete loss of contact between the femoral head and acetabulum. DDH occurs in 11.5 in 1000 infants, with frank dislocations occurring in 1-2/1000 (American Academy of Pediatrics [AAP], 2000; Guille et al, 2000). Risk factors for a positive newborn screening examination include female gender (19/1000 risk), positive family history (boys, 9.4/1000; girls, 44/1000) and breech presentation (boys, 26/1000; girls, 120/1000) (AAP, 2000). The left hip alone is affected in 60%, the right hip in 20%, and both hips in 20% of infants (Guille et al, 2000).

Dislocations can be divided into two groups: teratologic and typical. *Teratologic* dislocations are most frequently associated with neuromuscular conditions such as myelodysplasia and arthrogryposis or with dysmorphic syndromes such as Larsen syndrome. These abnormalities probably occur in either week 12 or 18 of gestation (AAP, 2000). *Typical* dislocations occur in otherwise healthy infants in the prenatal or postnatal period.

Congruent reduction and stability of the femoral head are necessary for normal growth and development of the hip joint. The natural history of untreated DDH is controversial, as newborn instability may resolve or progress to subluxation or dislocation. In cases that progress, infants have significantly increased risk of developing precocious arthritis with moderate to severe hip pain as young adults (Cooperman et al, 1983; Wedge and Wasylenko, 1979). This pain can be debilitating. Early detection and treatment of DDH are therefore important in avoiding the devastating sequelae of a late diagnosis.

There are no pathognomonic signs of a dislocated hip. The physical examination requires patience on the part of the examiner and may be facilitated by having the baby feed from a bottle. Evaluation for asymmetry is perhaps the most important key to the evaluation for DDH, although asymmetry may not be evident in bilateral dislocations. Presence of asymmetrical thigh and/or buttock folds is suggestive of a dislocation, as is a Galeazzi sign. The Galeazzi sign is elicited with the baby placed supine on an examining table so that the pelvis is level, with the hips and knees flexed to 90 degrees. With the baby's hips in neutral abduction, the examiner determines if the knees are at the same height. If one femur appears shorter, the hip may be dislocated posteriorly (Fig. 94–1). Limitations in hip abduction can also herald a dislocated hip. In babies older than 12 weeks, it is the most reliable examination finding suggestive of DDH. Adduction of 30 degrees and abduction of 75 degrees should be possible in most newborns. Variations side to side should be noted. Each of these signs, individually or in combination, may serve to increase the index of suspicion of the examiner and lower the threshold for further diagnostic studies or referral to an orthopedist.

There are two common ways of assessing hip stability in the newborn. The Ortolani test is performed with the calm newborn supine on the examining table. The index and middle fingers of the examiner are placed along the greater trochanter, while the thumb is placed on the medial aspect of the thigh over the lesser trochanter. The pelvis is stabilized by placing the thumb and ring or long finger of the opposite hand on top of both anterior iliac crests simultaneously. Alternatively, the opposite thigh may be held in the same manner as the examined side while the hip is held in abduction. The hip is flexed to 90 degrees and gently abducted while the leg is lifted with the hip in neutral external/internal rotation. A palpable "clunk" is felt as the dislocated femoral head reduces into the acetabulum. This finding is reported as the Ortolani sign (positive result on the Ortolani test). The Barlow test is an attempt to dislocate or subluxate a reduced but unstable hip. The thigh is held and the pelvis stabilized in the same manner as for the Ortolani test. With the hip in neutral external/internal rotation and at 90 degrees of flexion, the leg is then gently adducted with a mild posteriorly

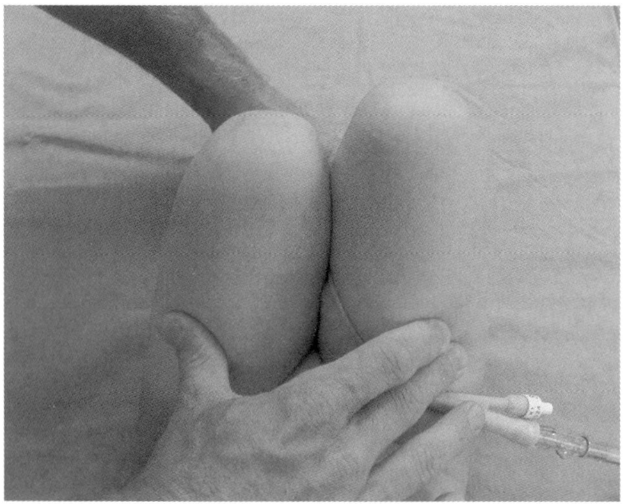

**FIGURE 94–1.** Presence of Galeazzi sign.

directed pressure applied to the knee. A palpable "clunk" or sensation of posterior movement constitutes a positive result (i.e., the Barlow sign). Each hip should be examined separately. High-pitched "clicks" are frequently elicited with hip range of motion. These sounds are most frequently attributed to snapping of the iliotibial band over the greater trochanter and are not associated with dysplasia (Bond et al, 1997). With progressive soft tissue contractures, both the Ortolani and Barlow tests become unreliable after 3 months of age.

Radiologic imaging of the immature hip can be a valuable adjunct to the physical examination. An anteroposterior (AP) roentgenogram of the pelvis is difficult to interpret before age 4 to 5 months. The femoral head is composed entirely of cartilage until the secondary center of ossification appears. Before the appearance of the secondary center, ultrasound examination is the method of choice for visualizing the cartilaginous femoral head and acetabulum. Static ultrasound images allow visualization of acetabular and femoral head anatomy, while the complementary dynamic images give information on the stability of the hip joint (Clarke et al, 1985; Graf, 1984). The primary limitation of hip ultrasonography is that results are dependent on the experience and skill of the operator, especially when performed within the first 3 weeks of life (Marks et al, 1994). For these reasons ultrasonography is recommended as an adjunct to clinical evaluation rather than as a screening tool (AAP, 2000). Studies conducted before 4 weeks of life too often reveal minor degrees of dysplasia that resolve spontaneously. It is the technique of choice for assessing infants at high risk for DDH after 4 to 6 weeks of age and is useful in following the results of intervention. Beginning at 4 to 6 months, the gold standard remains the AP pelvic radiograph.

Recently, the American Academy of Pediatrics published clinical practice guidelines to aid in the early diagnosis and initiation of appropriate intervention of DDH (AAP, 2000). The proposed clinical algorithm is presented in Figure 94–2 and summarized here: All newborns should be examined for DDH by a properly trained health care provider. If an Ortolani or a Barlow sign is noted, the newborn should be referred to an orthopedist. Neither an ultrasound study nor a radiograph is recommended, as treatment decisions will be based on physical examination findings. If findings on the newborn examination are equivocal, a follow-up examination in 2 weeks by the health care provider is recommended. Triple diapering is not recommended, but communication between providers is encouraged if the practitioner examining the newborn in the hospital is different from the 2-week follow-up examiner. If the follow-up examination yields an Ortolani or a Barlow sign or other convincing evidence of DDH, a referral to an orthopedist is necessary. If findings on examination are again equivocal, consideration should be given to referring the baby to an orthopedist for evaluation or obtaining an ultrasound study at age 3 to 4 weeks. If the 2-week follow-up assessment yields normal findings, a follow-up examination is recommended at the next scheduled well-baby visit. Periodically, the hip examination should be repeated in all babies at each of the well-baby visits scheduled throughout the first year of life. At any time during this period, if DDH is suspected, referral to an orthopedist or evaluation by ultrasound examination for an infant younger than 5 months of age or by radiograph if the infant is older than 4 months should be considered. Risk factors for DDH need to be considered in newborns with negative and equivocal examinations. As noted previously, females, infants with a positive family history of DDH, and babies who were born breech are at increased risk for DDH. Newborn girls should be reexamined at 2 weeks in the event of a normal newborn examination and at scheduled well-baby visits subsequently. If examination findings are positive, referral is in order. In infant boys with a positive family history, management should follow the same protocol outlined for girls. Because newborn girls with a positive family history have a 44/1000 risk for DDH, an ultrasound examination at 6 weeks of age or a radiograph of the pelvis at 4 months of age is recommended despite normal findings on the physical examination. Because the risk of DDH is so high in girls (120/1000) born breech, imaging with ultrasound at 4 weeks and/or radiograph at 4 to 6 months of age is recommended in the face of normal findings on the physical examination. Despite newborn screening programs, 1 in 5000 will have a dislocated hip detected at 18 months of age or older (Dezateux and Godward, 1995). It is important to appreciate that not all dislocated hips are present at birth, and not all hips dislocated at birth are detectable in the newborn period.

Treatment of DDH is dependent on the age at presentation. For children 0 to 6 months of age, a reducible hip is treated in a Pavlik harness. The Pavlik is a dynamic splint that allows the infant to actively move the hips through a sphere of motion that encourages deepening and stabilization of the acetabulum (Fig. 94–3). The harness is applied as soon as possible after the diagnosis of DDH is made. The length of treatment is dependent on age at presentation. Progress is judged by serial physical examinations and static and dynamic ultrasonography. If no improvement is noted within 2 to 3 weeks of splint application, this treatment is abandoned, and a closed reduction, usually with arthrographic evaluation and subsequent spica casting, is

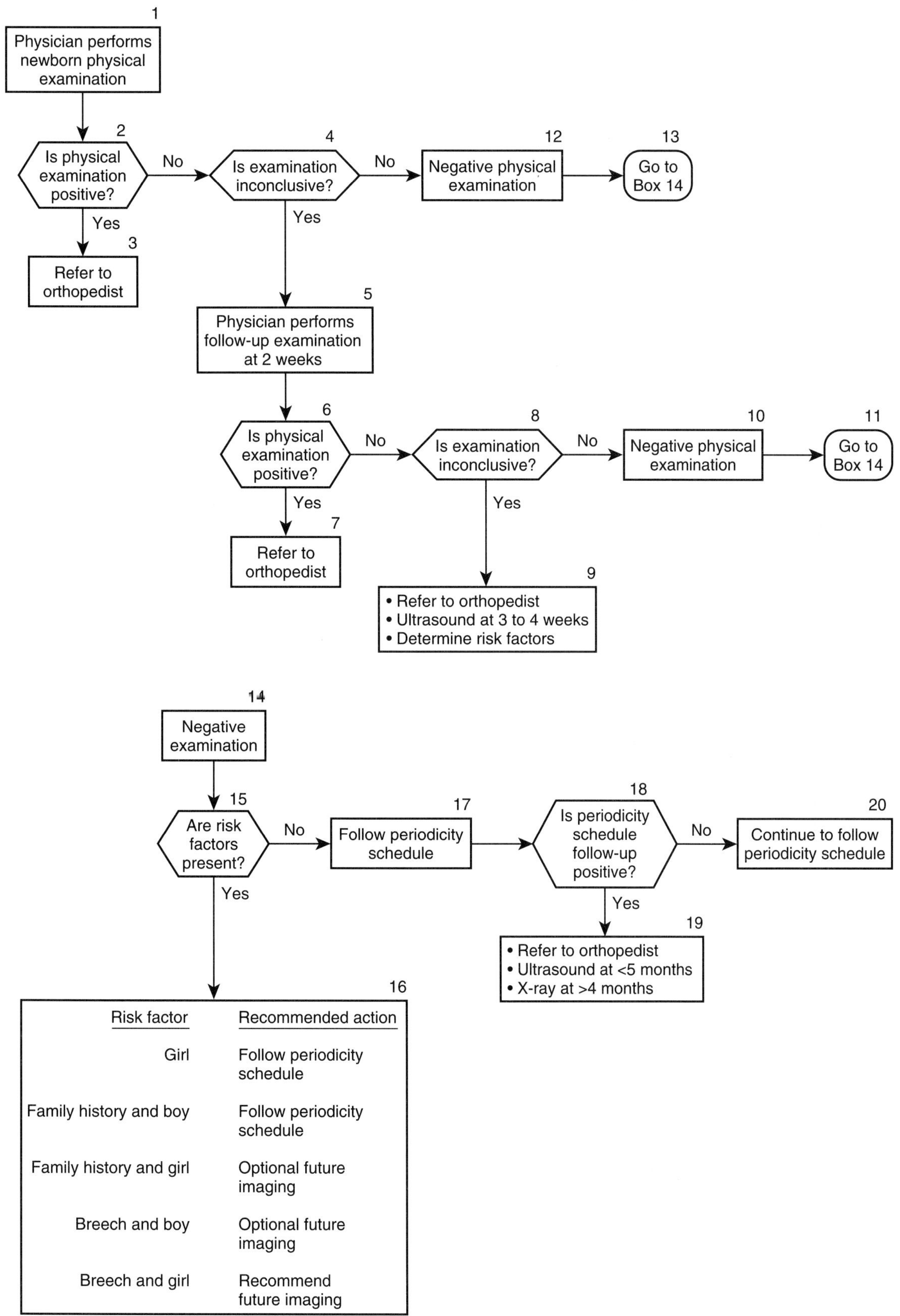


**FIGURE 94–2.** American Academy of Pediatrics clinical algorithm: Screening for developmental hip dysplasia. *(Data from Clinical practice guideline: Early detection of developmental dysplasia of the hip. Committee on Quality Improvement, Subcommitte on Developmental Dysplasia of the Hip. American Academy of Pediatrics. Pediatrics 105:896-905, 2000.)*

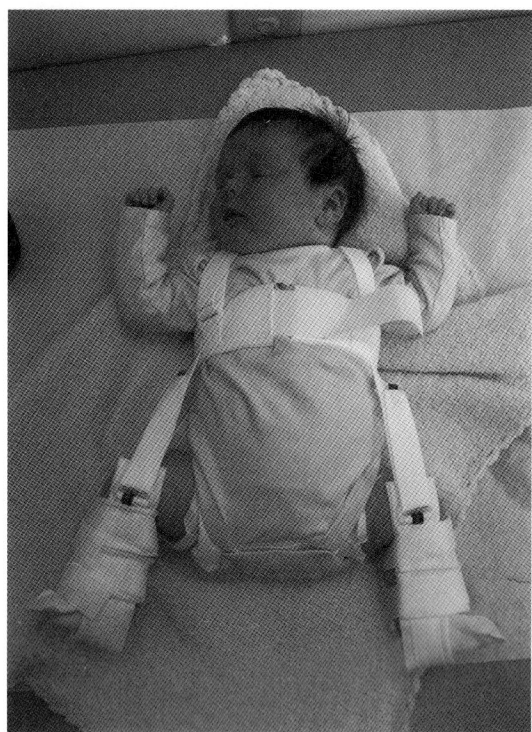

**FIGURE 94–3.** The Pavlik harness.

employed. For an irreducible dislocation, which is unusual in the 0- to 6-month age group, open operative reduction of the hip with subsequent spica casting is undertaken. Pavlik harness treatment is successful more than 90% of the time, however (Guille et al, 1999).

## TORTICOLLIS

Congenital muscular torticollis (CMT) manifests at birth or soon thereafter and is the most frequent cause of "wryneck." However, other conditions, some more serious, may cause torticollis. These include congenital anomalies of the vertebra and skull (Klippel-Feil syndrome, hemivertebrae, basilar invagination, craniosynostosis) (Dubousset, 1986; Hensinger et al, 1974; Raco et al, 1999); abnormalities of the central nervous system (CNS) (syringomyelia, tumors) (Kiwak et al, 1983); Chiari malformations (Dure et al, 1989); ocular abnormalities (Bixenman, 1981); pharyngeal abscess; and gastroesophageal reflux (Sandifer syndrome) (Ramenofsky et al, 1978). Patients with CMT can be divided into those who demonstrate a sternocleidomastoid muscle (SCM) "pseudotumor," those with tightness or fibrosis of the SCM without pseudotumor (termed *muscular torticollis*), and those with all of the characteristic features of congenital torticollis without evidence of contracture or fibrosis of muscle (termed *postural torticollis*) (Cheng et al, 2001). CMT has been estimated to occur in 3/1000 to 20/100,000 live births (Cheng et al, 2001). It is usually discovered between 6 and 8 weeks of life. The infant presents with a "cock robin" appearance, with the head tilted toward and chin rotated away from the affected SCM. Twenty percent to 30% of patients will have a palpable pseudotumor present in the middle to inferior aspect of the affected SCM, which spontaneously regresses with time, leaving a fibrous band (Herring, 2002). More than half will have facial asymmetry. The left and right SCMs are affected in equal proportions. CMT probably results from ischemia within the SCM, leading to fibrosis (Davids et al, 1993). The cause of the ischemia is unknown, but intrauterine crowding may play a role, as there appears to be a 10% to 20% association with DDH and an increased association with metatarsus adductus (Morrison and MacEwen, 1982; Tien et al, 2001).

Excellent results with a manual stretching program can be attained in children first seen before 1 year of age (Morrison and MacEwen, 1982). Initially, the parents are instructed in the technique of stretching the contracted SCM by rotating the infant's chin toward the affected SCM while simultaneously tilting the head away from it. This is completed 10 times each session and held for a count of 10 at least 10 times per day. Unfortunately, compliance may be an issue. If the child fails to improve substantially within 3 to 4 weeks, a physical therapist is enlisted to see the child 2 or 3 times weekly to supervise the program and reinforce the home therapy. Additionally, the parents are instructed to configure the infant's crib and toys in such a manner as to encourage active rotation toward the involved side. There is no justification to undertake surgery in any child less than 1 year of age or in any child who has not completed a minimum of 6 months of therapy (Cheng et al, 2001; Morrison and MacEwen, 1982). In a recent prospective study of 821 children with muscular torticollis, only 8% of patients with the history of a pseudotumor and 3% of those without required surgical intervention following a well-structured stretching program (Cheng et al, 2001). No patients with postural torticollis required surgery. Risk factors for surgery included late initial presentation, presence of a pseudotumor, and rotation deficit of greater than 15 degrees.

The timing of surgical intervention remains controversial. In patients with significant plagiocephaly and facial asymmetry, surgery should be considered just before 2 years of age in order to maximize the chance for complete remodeling. For those with either no or mild facial asymmetry, good to excellent results can be expected with surgery up to 6 years of age (Ling, 1976). Beyond 6 years of age, acceptable results are reported, but the ability to remodel facial asymmetry appears diminished. Surgery entails either release or lengthening of the SCM through cosmetically pleasing incisions.

A less frequent cause of congenital torticollis is osseous fusion between bones in the cervical spine. These fusions may be between the skull and C1 and/or C2 or in the lower cervical spine. They result from failure of the bones to properly segment during embryogenesis. These abnormalities, in combination with a low posterior hairline and a short webbed neck with limited range of motion and head tilt, constitute the triad referred to as *Klippel-Feil syndrome* (Copley and Dormans, 1998). These congenital bone fusions can range from involvement of two segments to involvement of the entire cervical spine. Colloquially, Klippel-Feil syndrome has come to refer to any failure of segmentation in the cervical spine with or without other elements of the triad. In infants and young children, the neck may remain quite flexible despite the bone abnormalities. In a newborn with torticollis who does not improve with passive stretching exercises, radiologic evaluation is mandatory. Cervical spine films are not recommended in all patients initially presenting with neonatal torticollis, as these films are quite difficult to interpret in this age group due to the predominance of cartilage in the bones of the neck. Furthermore, many neonates would be subjected to unnecessary ionizing radiation.

The natural history of Klippel-Feil in most cases is quite favorable, requiring nothing more than periodic observation. In patients with severe involvement, however, the consequences of this disorder can include early spondylosis with the development of pain or stenosis, the development of progressive torticollis and scoliosis, and the occurrence of neurologic compromise and sudden death secondary to even minimal trauma (Herring, 2002). Despite these potentially devastating sequelae, the greatest advantage to early detection of Klippel-Feil syndrome is in being alerted to commonly associated disorders including congenital heart disease (14% to 29%), renal anomalies (25% to 35%), scoliosis (60%), audiologic anomalies (80%), deafness (15% to 35%), synkinesis (15% to 20%), and, less commonly, posterior fossa desmoid tumors (Herring, 2002; Muzumdar and Goel, 2001). The recognition of a Klippel-Feil anomaly should prompt a thorough evaluation for these associations. Treatment for Klippel-Feil most often involves a therapy program of neck flexibility and intermittent observation with activity modification. In the face of progression of deformity or severe deformity, spinal fusion may be warranted.

Sandifer syndrome (gastroesophageal reflux) also can cause a torticollis. With this syndrome, the torticollis is intermittent and may alternate directions, and there is no tightness of the SCM, with normal findings on radiographs (Ramenofsky et al, 1978).

Hemiatlas, or the failure of formation of a portion of the first cervical vertebra, is also a rare cause of torticollis (Dubousset, 1986). In the infant, the neck may be quite flexible and the torticollis passively correctable. An open-mouth (odontoid view) cervical spine radiograph reveals this deformity. If the torticollis is progressive or severe, gradual correction of the deformity with a halo vest followed by posterior occiput–to–cervical spine fusion is necessary. Other potential causes of torticollis in the neonate include CNS tumors and syringomyelia. If radiographs appear normal, a thorough neurologic examination and referral to a neurologist are recommended.

## FOOT DEFORMITIES

Congenital deformities of the foot are relatively common but frequently overlooked in newborns. Consequently, the true incidence of the milder, self-limited deformities is unknown. For identification purposes, congenital foot abnormalities can be divided into those that result in the toes pointing upward (calcaneovalgus) and those that result in the toes pointing inward (metatarsus adductus, clubfoot).

*Calcaneovalgus* is thought to be a postural deformity secondary to intrauterine positioning in which the dorsum of the foot is, or can be, directly apposed to the anterior aspect of the leg. The estimated incidence of calcaneovalgus is 0.4/1000 to 1/1000 live births (Nunes and Dutra, 1986; Wynne-Davies, 1964). It appears to be more common in girls and following breech deliveries (Nunes and Dutra, 1986). There may be an increased association with hip dysplasia, so a thorough hip examination is warranted, as outlined in the previous section on DDH. Calcaneovalgus may be seen in conjunction with external rotation of the tibia, so that the toes appear to be rotated upward and outward. Additionally, a common association occurs with posteromedial bowing of the tibia, a unilateral deformity. This is likely to slowly resolve but eventually leads to a leg length inequality necessitating limb equalization surgery. Early referral to an orthopedist is suggested. Calcaneovalgus needs to be differentiated from congenital vertical talus, a rare condition that frequently is associated with neuromuscular conditions and syndromes. Congenital vertical talus can be differentiated from calcaneovalgus by viewing the hindfoot. If the hindfoot is fixed in equinus (plantar flexion), the foot demonstrates a "rocker bottom" appearance characteristic of congenital vertical talus. This finding mandates referral to an orthopedist. In the calcaneovalgus foot, the hindfoot is in the dorsiflexed position (calcaneus position) so that the plantar aspect of the forefoot is collinear with it. Plantar flexion of the foot is often limited from contracture of the anterior ankle soft tissues. The prognosis for complete resolution with gentle stretching exercises conducted by the parents with diaper changes is excellent in the vast majority of cases. Complete resolution generally occurs by 3 to 6 months of age. Occasionally, in the most severe cases, serial casting is employed to facilitate correction.

The two common neonatal foot deformities resulting in medial deviation of the toes are metatarsus adductus and talipes equinovarus (clubfoot). *Metatarsus adductus* is present at birth but frequently diagnosed later during the first year of life. It has been estimated to occur in 1 in 100 births (Widhe et al, 1988). The pathogenesis is unproved, but the condition is thought to result from intrauterine crowding. Characteristic features include a concave medial border of the foot with a curved lateral border, a "bean-shaped" sole of the foot, a higher-than-normal-appearing arch, fixed adductus of the forefoot when the hindfoot is held in neutral position, separation of the first and second toes, and spontaneous medial deviation of the foot with active movement by the infant (Kite, 1967) (Fig. 94–4). Metatarsus adductus can be classified into cases that passively correct and those that do not. Feet in which passive correction is possible are best left alone and will improve spontaneously. Feet in which passive correction cannot be obtained should be treated with manipulation and serial casting. The corrections can then be maintained with straight-last shoes if necessary or with nighttime bivalved casts. Operative treatment should be considered only in children older than 3 years of age who have a rigid deformity and have failed to respond to a manipulation and serial casting program (Weinstein, 2000). Farsetti and colleagues (1994) reported on 45 feet demonstrating metatarsus adductus, with an average follow-up period of

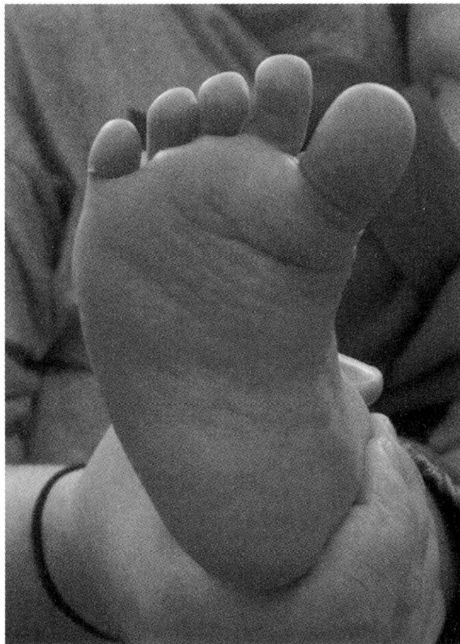

**FIGURE 94–4.** The appearance of the foot with metatarsus adductus.

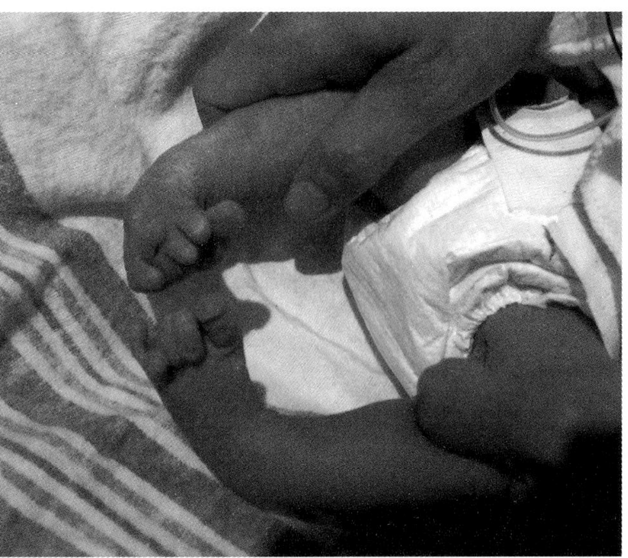

**FIGURE 94–5.** The appearance of an untreated newborn clubfoot.

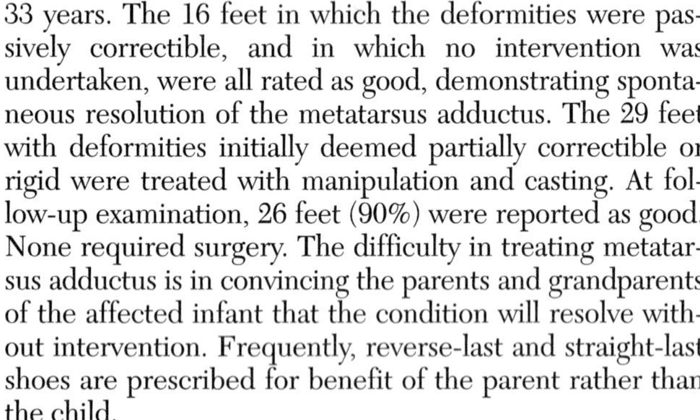

33 years. The 16 feet in which the deformities were passively correctible, and in which no intervention was undertaken, were all rated as good, demonstrating spontaneous resolution of the metatarsus adductus. The 29 feet with deformities initially deemed partially correctible or rigid were treated with manipulation and casting. At follow-up examination, 26 feet (90%) were reported as good. None required surgery. The difficulty in treating metatarsus adductus is in convincing the parents and grandparents of the affected infant that the condition will resolve without intervention. Frequently, reverse-last and straight-last shoes are prescribed for benefit of the parent rather than the child.

The term *clubfoot* describes a foot demonstrating hindfoot equinus (plantar flexion) with adduction and supination of the forefoot (Fig. 94–5). Clubfoot represents a spectrum of congenital deformity that ranges from the mild "postural" clubfoot to the severe arthrogrypotic clubfoot. It occurs in 1/1000 to 2/1000 live births (Herring, 2002). Three prominent theories for the etiology of clubfoot have emerged. An arrest in embryonic development in the 6- to 8-week fetus (Bohm, 1929) secondary to connective tissue abnormalities, a primary germ plasm defect, (Brockman, 1930), and a neuromuscular defect (Handelsman and Badalamente, 1982) each have been proposed. A recently documented risk factor for clubfoot is early amniocentesis (11- to 13-weeks of gestation), which is hypothesized to cause decreased fetal movement during a critical phase of foot development (Tredwell et al, 2001). Although the etiology of clubfoot remains unproved, there appears to be dysplasia of all osseous, muscular, tendinous, cartilaginous, skin, and neurovascular tissues distal to the knee in the affected limb. On the mild end of the spectrum, postural clubfoot appears to represent a packaging problem due to intrauterine positioning. Postural clubfoot is passively correctible, lacks deep medial creasing, demonstrates minimal or no calf atrophy, and responds quickly to a stretching and casting regimen. At the opposite end of the spectrum is the arthrogrypotic or neuromuscular clubfoot that demonstrates severe rigidity; absence of skin creases, suggesting early in utero affliction; and failure to respond to nonoperative therapies. Between these two extremes lies the classic clubfoot deformity. The anatomic deformities in clubfoot are numerous, complex, and somewhat controversial. Although the specific anatomic abnormalities are well beyond the scope of this chapter, the most notable abnormalities include a small, contracted heel cord complex; medial subluxation of the navicular bone on the talar head so that it abuts or nearly abuts the medial malleolus; and parallelism between the calcaneus and talus bones when these are viewed radiographically from the lateral aspect and from an anterior-to-posterior perspective. Clinically, the foot demonstrates a medial crease, with the toes pointed toward the midline, the sole of the foot angulated medially, the hindfoot plantar flexed, and a smaller foot and calf than on the contralateral side (see Fig. 94–5).

All clubfoot deformities should be referred to an orthopedist for treatment. Initial treatment for all cases of congenital clubfoot is nonoperative. The earlier treatment is commenced, the more successful nonoperative treatment is likely to be, owing to improved pliability of the tissues and resilience to immobilization, which can be prolonged over the course of therapy. We prefer to initiate treatment in the newborn nursery within the first 48 hours of delivery. Initial treatment usually consists of a manipulation and serial casting or taping program. Manipulation of the foot is carried out, and the correction is maintained with a long-leg cast. The casts are removed at weekly intervals, with repeated manipulation and casting over 3 to 4 months. By that time, the treating surgeon usually will be able to determine if surgery is warranted as a result of failure or plateauing of the correction. Surgery, if necessary, is generally undertaken at between 9 and 12 months of age, to allow treatment to be completed by the time the child is starting to walk. Attempts at early surgical correction have yielded poor results and high recurrence, and this approach has been abandoned. Despite adept surgical correction, approximately 15% of cases of clubfoot will demonstrate recurrence necessitating further surgical intervention. Some surgeons have advocated a completely nonoperative approach to clubfoot correction (Kite, 1964; Ponsetti, 1996; Seringe and Atia, 1990) based on observations that in operated cases of clubfoot, the feet often appear stiff and gradually develop scarring, which diminishes the result. These programs vary in the specifics of treatment but share a labor-intensive approach. One method necessitates daily manipulations by a trained physical therapist for 8 weeks, with the addition of continuous passive motion during the first 4 weeks. This is followed by strapping and continued bracing. The method has been successfully duplicated at one U.S. hospital (Herring, 2002), with good short-term results. Even these "nonoperative" methods frequently employ heel cord– lengthening surgery or tendon transfers to attain the desired result. Unfortunately, with the economics of the U.S. health care system, this approach is presently impractical for most physicians and hospitals. Untreated clubfoot has a poor natural history, with development of early degenerative changes in the foot joints. With treatment, good results can be expected with both the standard and nonoperative methods in 85% of cases (Weinstein, 2000).

## TORSIONAL DEFORMITIES OF THE LOWER EXTREMITIES

Torsional and angular deformities of the legs constitute the most frequent nontraumatic reason for referral to a children's orthopedist. Torsional deformities of the lower extremities rarely come to the attention of the physician before the child reaches walking age. Occasionally a neonate demonstrates bowing of the legs, or *genu varum*, of a sufficient degree to concern parents or grandparents. The true incidence of genu varum is unknown, but based on our experience, it is extremely common. The overwhelming majority of cases of genu varum resolve spontaneously, with a small minority of affected children manifesting a pathologic condition.

The legs of most neonates are bowed. This results from a combination of an external rotation contracture of the hips and internal tibial torsion. The apex anterior bowing of the femora in conjunction with the external rotation contractures of both hips allow the femoral bowing to be seen tangentially when the baby is viewed from the front. These contractures may not resolve until after walking age. Internal tibial torsion is nearly universal in neonates and spontaneously resolves between 2 and 3 years of age. Internal tibial torsion imparts an appearance of bowing to the tibia. When tibial bowing is viewed in combination with the apparent femoral bowing, a striking amount of leg bowing may be present. This is often concerning to both parent and physician.

Genu varum is physiologic up to the age of 2 years. Salenius and Vankka (1975) documented the tibiofemoral angles both clinically and roentgenographically in 979 children on the basis of 1408 examinations between birth and 16 years of age. They noted that newborns demonstrate a mean varus alignment of 15 degrees, which increases and becomes maximal at 6 months of age and then decreases to neutral at approximately 18 months. The maximum valgus of 12 degrees is then achieved by 3 to 4 years. By age 7, normal adult valgus alignment is achieved (Fig. 94–6). Natural history studies have demonstrated that physiologic genu varum is a self-limited process. Genu varum with angulation greater than 30 degrees has been shown to correct spontaneously with growth (Heath and Staheli, 1993).

Physical examination should include evaluation of the torsional profile (Staheli, 1977), which includes measurements of internal and external rotation of the hips and the thigh-foot angle. Measurement of the thigh-foot angle is performed with the child in the prone position and is an indicator of tibial torsion. The examiner should look for evidence of rhizomelic shortening, which may herald a diagnosis of achondroplasia. Although genu varum progressively worsens with growth in achondroplasia, rather than ameliorating, newborns generally do not demonstrate this disorder. Finally, note is made of whether onset of the varus of the lower extremities is gradual or abrupt. If it was abrupt, can the deformity be localized to the distal femur, the proximal tibia, or the midportion of the tibia? Considerations in the differential diagnosis of genu varum include focal fibrocartilage dysplasia, achondroplasia, osteogenesis imperfecta, vitamin D–resistant rickets, renal osteodystrophy, and tibia vara, or Blount disease. Blount disease does not occur before walking age, and most clinicians agree that this diagnosis cannot be made before 2 years of age.

Radiographs are indicated only with asymmetrical deformities, with short stature, or in infants with progressive deformities. Photographs are the preferred method of follow-up evaluation for progression. Management of physiologic genu varum and tibial torsion consists of serial observation, reassurance, and parental education. Treatment with orthotics such as the Denis Browne splint is not indicated and in fact may be harmful to the ligaments of the knee.

Focal fibrocartilaginous dysplasia (FFD) involving the medial aspect of the proximal tibial metaphysis is a relatively rare cause of tibia vara in the newborn and infant. It was first reported in 1985 (Bell et al, 1985) and continues to be recognized in scattered case reports. The pathophysiologic basis for the disease may be abnormal development of fibrocartilage at the insertion of the pes anserinus (sartorius, gracilis, and semitendinosus tendons). Children with FFD present before 1 year of age with unilateral bowing of the tibia that has prompted radiologic evaluation. The radiographs demonstrate a lytic defect in the proximal medial metaphysic of the tibia with surrounding sclerosis. The natural history of the deformity is that of progression until 2 years of age, with subsequent resolution by 4 years of age. During the progression, the deformity can become quite pronounced and unsettling. Up to 1 cm of tibial length discrepancy is likely. Use of orthotics is not indicated. Surgery is indicated only in patients older than 4 years without evidence of spontaneous resolution (Zayer, 1980).

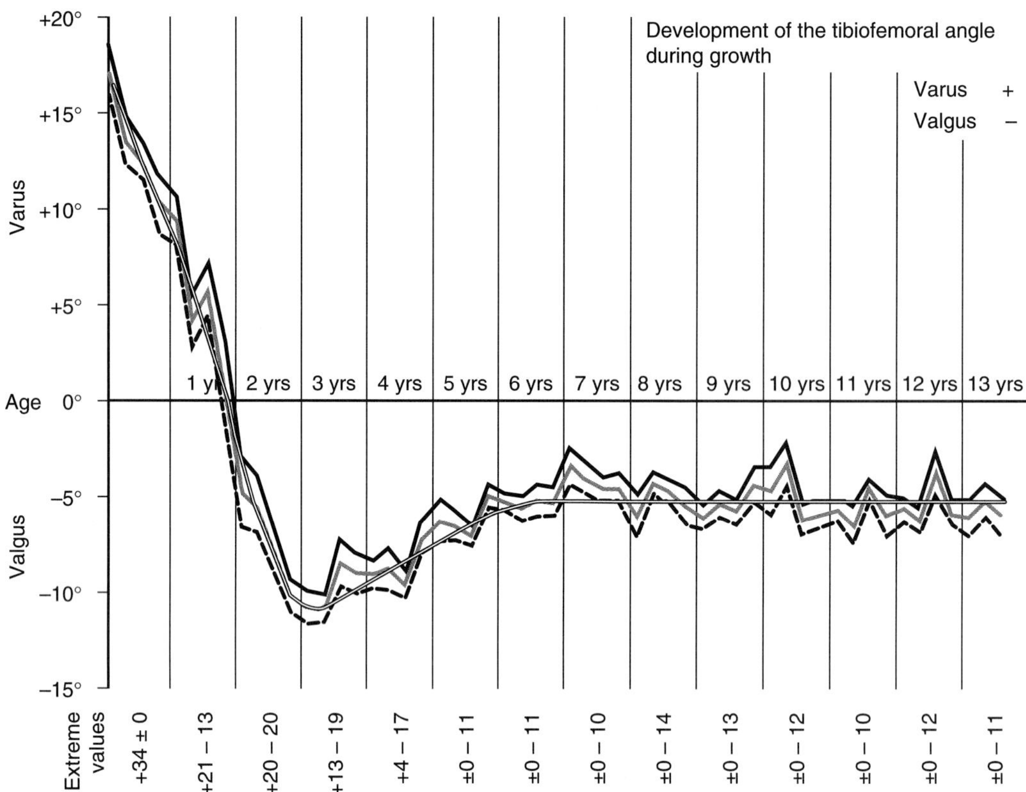


**FIGURE 94–6.** Development of the tibiofemoral angle during growth. *(Data from Salenius P, Vankka GK: The development of the tibiofemoral angle in children. J Bone Joint Surg Am 57:259-261, 1975.)*

Tibial bowing can be the cause of angular deformities in the shaft of the tibia. Two major types of bowing can be identified according to the direction of the apex of the bow. Posteromedial bowing has been previously described in conjunction with calcaneovalgus foot position in the neonate. Its etiology is unknown, but numerous hypotheses have been proffered, including intrauterine fracture with malunion and in utero malpositioning with subsequent growth retardation and soft tissue contractures (Thompson, 2001).

The deformity is unilateral and evident at birth. There is an associated calcaneovalgus foot deformity. Other features include shortening of the tibia and a smaller calf circumference and a smaller foot relative to the contralateral side. Frequently there is a dimple at the apex of the deformity. Radiographic examination of the entire extremity from hip to ankle should be performed. Radiographs demonstrate the degree of bowing well. Other radiographic findings include a normal proximal tibia with thickening and sclerosis of the diaphyseal cortices on the compression side of the deformity with obliteration of the intramedullary canal. There is no increased fracture risk associated with the deformity. Posteromedial bowing tends to resolve with growth, so that much of the deformity resolves by 2 years of age, with continued gradual correction beyond that. The shortening of the tibia and fibula persists, however, and progressively worsens during growth. Leg length inequality at skeletal maturity averages 4.1 cm (Hofmann and Wenger, 1981). Early referral to and serial follow-up assesssments by an orthopedist are necessary to appropriately time epiphysiodesis surgery of the normal leg to allow for equal leg lengths at skeletal maturity. The foot deformity generally resolves by 9 to 12 months with stretching.

The second and most serious type of tibial bowing is anterolateral. It is usually identified at the newborn examination. It most frequently is associated with congenital pseudoarthrosis of the tibia but also can be associated with congenital longitudinal deficiency of the tibia or the fibula. Although its etiology is unknown, congenital pseudoarthrosis of the tibia is associated with neurofibromatosis (NF) in 40% to 80% of the cases (Masserman et al, 1974; Paterson, 1989; Thompson, 2001). It is arguably the most challenging congenital malformation to treat in orthopedics. It is estimated to occur in 1 in 140,000 live births (Crawford and Schorry, 1999). "Congenital pseudoarthrosis" implies that there is a nonunited fracture, which usually is not the case, so the term *congenital tibial dysplasia* (CTD) has been suggested (Crawford and Schorry, 1999). The newborn examination is notable for anterolateral bowing, which is unilateral. Other, cutaneous signs of NF may be evident. If they are not, NF should be considered, and the child serially followed expectantly. If fracture has occurred, motion at the pseudoarthrosis site will be apparent. The foot may be normal or slightly small. The ankle may be in slight valgus to compensate for the bowing.

The natural history of congenital pseudoarthrosis of the tibia is that of fracture with nonunion and repeated surgical attempts at obtaining union. Most of these attempts fail; if one such procedure succeeds, however, repeat fracture is likely, and the cycle begins again. Frequently, amputation is the end result. Because of this possibility, efforts are best directed at prevention of initial fracture. Orthopedic consultation is imperative. In the preambulatory child, a total-contact ankle-foot orthosis should be fabricated and worn at all times except for bathing, to diminish the chance of fracture. When the child begins to walk, the orthosis should be extended above the knee with a drop-lock hinge to allow sitting. Bracing is continued until skeletal maturity is attained. Although no definite proof that long-term bracing affects the natural history of this condition exists, most orthopedists consider that it is warranted. Under no circumstances should an osteotomy be undertaken in a nonfractured tibia to correct the bowing, as pseudoarthrosis is likely to result.

Many treatment options exist once a documented pseudoarthrosis occurs. Long-term immobilization, external fixation, internal fixation, bone transport, bone grafting, microvascular bone transfer, and electrical stimulation each have been attempted, all with less than stellar results (Crawford and Schorry, 1999). When union is achieved, there is concern over its quality and longevity. Amputation has been advocated as a salvage procedure after failed attempts at union and as primary treatment for the initial pseudoarthrosis (Jacobsen et al, 1983). Herring and colleagues (1986) reported that children who underwent Symes amputation (none of whom had CTD as the surgical indication, however) had better psychological and orthopedic functioning than that described in children who underwent numerous corrective surgical procedures. Similar results were reported by other authors (Davidson and Bohne, 1975).

## OBSTETRIC TRAUMA

Birth trauma can be divided into two categories: fractures and neurologic injuries. *Birth fractures* most commonly involve the clavicle, with clavicular fractures occurring in 2/1000 to 35/1000 vaginal births (Cohen and Otto, 1980; Farkas and Levine, 1950; Kaplan et al, 1998; Sanford, 1931). Birth fractures also occur in the proximal humerus (Broker and Burbach, 1990; Fisher et al, 1995), the femur (0.13/1000 births) (Morris et al, 2002), and even the thoracic spine. It is important to note that clavicular fracture can be seen in combination with a proximal humeral physeal separation or in combination with a brachial plexus injury. Risk factors for upper extremity birth fractures in one study included large size of the baby, limited experience of the obstetrician, and a midforceps delivery (Cohen and Otto, 1980). Risk factors for femoral fracture included twin gestation, breech presentation, prematurity, and osteoporosis (Morris et al, 2002). The natural history of isolated birth fractures to the extremities is that of uneventful rapid healing without untoward sequelae. Clavicle fractures may be difficult to diagnose, as the neonate may be asymptomatic. In a study of 300 newborns, radiographs revealed five unsuspected clavicle fractures (Farkas and Levine, 1950). Newborns with either a clavicle fracture or a proximal humeral physeal separation often present with pseudoparalysis of the upper extremity. Considerations in the differential diagnosis include an obstetric brachial plexus palsy and hematogenous metaphyseal osteomyelitis of the humerus with septic glenohumeral arthritis. Pain with direct palpation of the clavicle may be present with obvious deformity. Pain with motion of the shoulder joint and with palpation of the proximal humerus may be caused by either fracture or infection. Eliciting neonatal reflexes such as the Moro reflex and asymmetrical tonic neck reflex (ATNR) may be helpful in evaluating active upper extremity muscle function (Sanford, 1931). Radiographs should be obtained. Ultrasound evaluation of the proximal humerus may be helpful because the proximal humeral epiphysis is entirely cartilaginous at birth and is radiolucent. Ultrasound examination can detect proximal physeal separation, metaphyseal osteomyelitis, and septic shoulder arthritis (Broker and Burbach, 1990; Fisher et al, 1995).

Asymptomatic birth fractures of the clavicle and humerus in neonates can be observed. The fracture will unite in short order, with remodeling of bone with growth. Symptomatic fractures in which the child exhibits pseudoparalysis of the upper extremity should be treated with 2 weeks of immobilization in a soft dressing until symptoms subside. Femoral birth fractures can be treated with a Pavlik harness with good results (Morris et al, 2002). This device provides a simple means of immobilization that is accepted well by new parents. Excellent outcomes with no residual deformities or limb length inequalities can be expected.

*Brachial plexus injuries* represent the second category of birth trauma afflicting newborns. The brachial plexus receives contributions from the anterior spinal nerve roots of C5 through T1. The various nerve roots combine to form trunks, which combine in turn to form divisions, which combine to form cords, which combine and divide to form the peripheral nerves that supply the motor innervation to the upper extremity. The mechanism of injury to the plexus is a forceful separation of the head from the shoulder by lateral bending of the neck with simultaneous shoulder depression during vaginal delivery. These injuries occur in 1/1000 to 4/1000 live births (Greenwald et al, 1984; Hardy, 1981). Obstetric brachial plexus palsies are most common in vertex deliveries with shoulder dystocia, in large-birth-weight babies (in whom the increased size usually is secondary to maternal diabetes), and in multiparous pregnancies (Waters, 1997). It is rarely seen in cesarean section deliveries. Not all cases can be reliably predicted prepartum, nor prevented. Three major injuries are encountered. The most frequent injury is to the upper trunk that involves the C5 and C6 nerve roots primarily and is termed *Erb's palsy*. Affected infants lack external rotation and abduction of the shoulder. Hand function is preserved. The next most frequently occurring injury is a *global plexus palsy* involving the C5 through T1 nerve roots. This results in flaccid paralysis of the involved upper extremity including the hand. Finally, an isolated lower plexus injury involving the C8 and T1 nerve roots is termed *Klumpke's palsy*. This injury is the least common and may be a manifestation of a recovered global plexus injury (Waters, 1997).

The physical examination has proved to be the most reliable method of assessing the level and severity of the neural injury and thereby predicting the potential for spontaneous recovery (Noetzel et al, 2001; Waters, 1997). Myelography, computed tomographic myelography, magnetic resonance imaging, and electrodiagnostic studies have not proved useful in predicting recovery (Waters, 1997). Active shoulder, elbow, wrist, and finger motion need to be assessed. Frequently, such assessment can be facilitated by eliciting some primitive reflexes that are transiently present in normal newborns. The *hand grasp reflex* is normal in all newborns and disappears between 2 and 4 months. The examiner's little finger is placed on the ulnar aspect of the infant's palm, and the infant's fingers reflexively flex and grasp the examiner's finger. The *Moro reflex* begins to fade at 3 months of age. It is elicited by holding the newborn's hands while raising the baby off the table and then suddenly releasing them. In response, the newborn extends the spine, abducts and extends all four limbs and digits, and then subsequently adducts and flexes the limbs and digits. Last, the ATNR, or *fencing reflex*, can be elicited in a normal newborn until the age of 4 months. With the infant lying supine on an examining table, the head is rotated to one side by the examiner. The infant should respond by extending the elbow on the side toward which the face is looking and by flexing the opposite elbow. In newborns with a brachial plexus injury, some of these reflexes will be abnormal due to lack of motor control. For instance, the newborn with an Erb's palsy will, most notably, not be able to actively flex at the elbow during the ATNR or the Moro. The presence or absence of Horner syndrome also must be noted. The infant needs repeat serial examinations until 6 months of age.

Return of biceps function by 3 months is the most important indicator of brachial plexus recovery (Michelow et al, 1994). When biceps recovery is combined with the return of shoulder abduction, wrist extension, and finger extension, there is a 95% chance of normal function (Michelow et al, 1994). When biceps function recovers later than 3 months, it is rare for the child to have complete recovery of normal function (Waters, 1999). A total plexus palsy or the presence of Horner syndrome also heralds a poor prognosis (Michelow et al, 1994; Waters, 1997). In one study of 142 patients with obstetric brachial plexus palsies, 50% demonstrated biceps recovery by 6 weeks, with the remainder demonstrating recovery at varying intervals beyond 6 weeks. At final follow-up evaluation, 67% had excellent shoulder function, 12% good, 5% fair, and 10% poor (Benson et al, 1996). In a similar prospective study, Waters (1999) found that 22 patients out of 66 studied had return of biceps function by 3 months. Each of these went on to have normal function. Infants in whom recovery was delayed until the fourth to the sixth month had significantly worse function.

The initial treatment for obstetric brachial plexus injury is aimed at avoiding contractures of the shoulder, elbow, forearm, and hand during the observation-for-recovery phase. Secondary treatment involves the restoration of neurologic function that will not recover. Finally, augmenting weak muscles, improving functional ranges of motion, and improving the appearance of residual deformities should be undertaken in children without full neurologic recovery.

Each neonate with an obstetric brachial plexus birth palsy must be referred to an orthopedist for early evaluation. Referral to a qualified therapist for passive range of motion exercises also is suggested. Monthly examinations by the orthopedist are undertaken. Brachial plexus exploration with subsequent reconstruction is indicated for infants with total plexus involvement, Horner syndrome, and no return of biceps function at 3 months, and for infants with a C5 to C6 (Erb's) plexopathy and no return of biceps function at 3 to 6 months (Waters, 1997). Surgery is undertaken between 3 and 6 months of age. Utilizing this algorithm prospectively, Waters (1999) operated on 6 infants at 6 months and found that their results were better than those for the 15 patients with biceps recovery at 5 months but worse than those for the 11 patients with biceps recovery at 4 months. Despite treatment as outlined, some children will have residual deficits. Secondary reconstruction for chronic brachial plexopathy resulting in a dysfunctional shoulder can be achieved with a tendon transfer of the latissimus dorsi and teres major to the rotator cuff or by derotational osteotomy of the humerus. These procedures and others designed to correct limitations in hand and forearm function are undertaken after the true scope of the disability has been assessed.

## NEONATAL OSTEOMYELITIS AND SEPTIC ARTHRITIS

*Osteomyelitis* refers to a bacterial infection of bone, and *septic arthritis* is a pyogenic infection of a diarthrodial joint. Incidence rates of 0.12 per 1000 live births and 0.67 per 1000 neonatal intensive care unit (NICU) admissions (Ho et al, 1989) have been reported for septic arthritis. The mortality rate is reported to be 7.3% (Caksen et al, 2000). The hip, knee, and shoulder joints are involved most frequently. Neonates are particularly susceptible to osteomyelitis and septic arthritis, due to an immature immune response resulting in vulnerability to organisms that are not ordinarily virulent in infants and children and a delay in expressing the classic physical findings associated with these conditions (Morrissy, 2001). Two subgroups of neonates are affected: premature neonates requiring prolonged hospitalization and otherwise healthy newborns who present within 2 to 4 weeks of discharge (Morrissy, 2001).

Most cases of neonatal osteomyelitis and septic arthritis result from hematogenous spread, but some occur from direct inoculation during femoral arterial blood sampling. Acute hematogenous osteomyelitis (AHO) and septic arthritis in hospitalized neonates usually occur in premature infants undergoing blood drawing, invasive monitoring, intravenous feedings, and intravenous drug administration, especially in those with indwelling umbilical vessel catheters (Lim et al, 1977). These infections are frequently caused by *S. aureus* or gram-negative organisms (10% to 15%). Up to 40% of these patients may demonstrate multiple areas of involvement characterized by swelling and tenderness and are systemically ill (Bergdahl et al, 1985; Fox and Sprunt, 1978). This contrasts with the typical out-of-hospital newborn with AHO and septic arthritis, who presents in weeks 2 to 4 of life with swelling, pseudoparalysis, and tenderness of the extremity and who feeds well and is not systemically ill (Morrissy, 2001). *S. aureus* and group B streptococci are the most common organisms encountered in this population.

Due to the immature immune response, neonates with AHO and septic arthritis frequently do not necessarily demonstrate fever, leukocytosis, or elevation in their erythrocyte sedimentation rates (Scott et al, 1990). However, C-reactive protein appears to be a reasonable indicator of AHO and septic arthritis (Pulliam et al, 2001; Unkila-Kallio et al, 1994). Blood cultures are positive in only 50% of patients; cultures of synovial aspirates identify an organism in only 30% (Lyon and Evanich, 1999). Plain radiographs demonstrate soft tissue swelling by 3 days, but bone changes are not present for a week after the onset of symptoms (Dormans and Drummond, 1994; Jackson and Nelson, 1982). Bone scan is positive in only 32% of foci of osteomyelitis in neonates due to the usual location of infection near the growth plate (Ash and Gilday, 1980). Ultrasound examination has been advocated as a useful method for the diagnosis and assessment of osteomyelitis (Mah et al, 1994) and is our preferred radiologic method for evaluating the neonate with suspected AHO and/or septic arthritis.

AHO and septic arthritis coexist in up to 76% of neonates as a result of the unique blood supply of the chondroepiphysis (Bergdahl et al, 1985; Fox and Sprunt, 1978), which changes with growth. Infection begins in the metaphyseal veins. Vascular canals traverse the growth plate in the neonate, allowing for rapid spreading of the infection to the cartilaginous chondroepiphysis with subsequent abscess formation. These abscesses frequently rupture into the joint (Ogden, 1979). The growth plate becomes a barrier to the spread of infection in the older child. Additionally, the hip and shoulder, two of the more common sites of neonatal septic arthritis, have intraarticular metaphyses, allowing for a subperiosteal route of decompression for pus into the joint. Due to this unique ability to spread from the metaphysis through the growth plate into the joint, early detection and treatment are necessary to avoid permanent damage to each of these structures. The proteolytic enzymes released by the host response to infection can result in destruction of the growth cartilage and articular cartilage in short order, resulting in growth disturbances and precocious arthritis. When an area of involvement is suspected, aspiration should be undertaken (Morrissy, 2001). This may confirm the diagnosis and provide fluid for Gram stain and culture in order to better direct treatment. If pus is discovered in the neonate, surgical débridement in the operating room is required.

## REFERENCES

### Developmental Dysplasia of the Hip


American Academy of Pediatrics: Clinical practice guideline: Early detection of developmental dysplasia of the hip. Committee on Quality Improvement, Subcommittee on Developmental Dysplasia of the Hip. Pediatrics 105:896-905, 2000.

Bond CD, Hennrikus WL, DellaMaggiore ED: Prospective evaluation of newborn soft-tissue "clicks" with ultrasound. J Pediatr Orthop 17:199-201, 1997.

Clarke NM, Harcke HT, McHugh P, et al: Real-time ultrasound in the diagnosis of congenital dislocation and dysplasia of the hip. J Bone Joint Surg Br 67:406-412, 1985.

Cooperman DR, Wallensten R, Stulberg SD: Acetabular dysplasia in the adult. Clin Orthop 175:79-85, 1983.

Dezateux C, Godward S: Evaluating the national screening programme for congenital dislocation of the hip. J Med Screen 2:200-202, 1995.

Graf R: Fundamentals of sonographic diagnosis of infant hip dysplasia. J Pediatr Orthop 4:735-740, 1984.

Guille JT, Pizzutillo PD, MacEwen GD: Developmental dysplasia of the hip from birth to six months. J Am Acad Orthop Surg 8:232-242, 2000.

Marks DS, Clegg J, al-Chalabi AN: Routine ultrasound screening for neonatal hip instability. Can it abolish late-presenting congenital dislocation of the hip? J Bone Joint Surg Br 76:534-538, 1994.

Wedge JH, Wasylenko MJ: The natural history of congenital disease of the hip. J Bone Joint Surg Br 61:334-338, 1979.


### Torticollis


Bixenman WW: Diagnosis of superior oblique palsy. J Clin Neuroophthalmol 1:199-208, 1981.

Cheng JC, Wong MW, Tang SP, et al: Clinical determinants in the outcome of manual stretching in the treatment of congenital muscular torticollis in infants: A prospective study of 821 cases. J Bone Joint Surg Am 83:679-687, 2001.

Copley LA and Dormans JP: Cervical spine disorders in infants and children. J Am Acad Orthop Surg 6:204-214, 1998.

Davids JR, Wenger DR, Mubarak SJ: Congenital muscular torticollis: Sequela of intrauterine or perinatal compartment syndrome. J Pediatr Orthop 13:141-147, 1993.

Dubousset J: Torticollis in children caused by congenital anomalies of the atlas. J Bone Joint Surg Am 1986;68:178-188.

Dure LS, Percy AK, Cheek WR, et al. Chiari type I malformation in children. J Pediatr 115:573-576, 1989.

Hensinger RN, Lang JE, MacEwen GD: Klippel-Feil syndrome: A constellation of associated anomalies. J Bone Surg Am 56:1246-1253, 1974.

Herring JA: Disorders of the neck. In Herring JA (ed): Tachdjian's Pediatric Orthopaedics, 3rd ed. Philadelphia, WB Saunders, 2002, pp 171-209.

Kiwak KJ, Deray MJ, Shields WD: Torticollis in three children with syringomyelia and spinal cord tumor. Neurology 33:946-948, 1983.

Ling CM: The influence of age on the results of open sternomastoid tenotomy in muscular torticollis. Clin Orthop 116:142-148, 1976.

Morrison DL, MacEwen GD: Congenital muscular torticollis: Observations regarding clinical findings, associated conditions, and results of treatment. J Pediatr Orthop 2:500-505, 1982.

Muzumdar D, Goel A: Posterior cranial fossa dermoid in association with craniovertebral and cervical spinal anomaly: A report of two cases. Pediatr Neurosurg 35:158-161, 2001.

Raco A, Raimondi AJ, De Ponte FS, et al: Congenital torticollis in association with craniosynostosis. Childs Nerv Syst 15:163-168, 1999.

Ramenofsky ML, Buyse M, Goldberg MJ, et al: Gastroesophageal reflux and torticollis. J Bone Joint Surg Am 60:1140-1141, 1978.

Tien YC, Su JY, Lin GT, et al: Ultrasonographic study of the coexistence of muscular torticollis and dysplasia of the hip. J Pediatr Orthop 21:343-347, 2001.


### Foot Deformities


Bohm M: The embryologic origins of clubfoot. J Bone Joint Surg 11:229, 1929.

Brockman EP: Congenital Clubfoot (Talipes Equinovarus). Bristol, England, John Wright & Sons, 1930.

Farsetti P, Weinstein SL, Ponsetti IV: The long-term functional and radiographic outcomes of untreated and non-operatively treated metatarsus adductus. J Bone Joint Surg Am 76: 257-265, 1994.

Handelsman JE, Badalamente MA: Club foot: A neuromuscular disease. Dev Med Child Neurol 24:3-12, 1982.

Herring JA: Disorders of the foot. In Herring JA (ed): Tachdjian's Pediatric Orthopaedics, 3rd ed. Philadelphia, WB Saunders, 2002, pp 891-1037.

Kite JH: The Clubfoot. New York, Grune & Stratton, 1964.

Kite JH: Congenital metatarsus varus. J Bone Joint Surg Am 49:388-397, 1967.

Nunes D, Dutra MG: Epidemiological study of congenital talipes calcaneovalgus. Braz J Med Biol Res 19:59-62, 1986.

Ponsetti IV: Congenital Clubfoot: Fundamentals of Treatment. Oxford, Oxford University Press, 1996.

Seringe R, Atia R: Idiopathic congenital clubfoot: Results of functional treatment (269 feet). Rev Chir Orthop Reparatrice Appar Mot 76:490-501, 1990.

Tredwell SJ, Wilson D, Wilmink MA: Review of the effect of early amniocentesis on foot deformity in the neonate. J Pediatr Orthop 21:636-641, 2001.

Weinstein SL: Long-term follow-up of pediatric orthopaedic conditions: Natural history and outcomes of treatment. J Bone Joint Surg Am 82:980-990, 2000.

Widhe T, Aaro S, Elmstedt E: Foot deformities in the newborn-incidence and prognosis. Acta Orthop Scand 59:176-179, 1988.

Wynne-Davies R: Familial studies of the cause of congenital clubfoot-talipes equinovarus, talipes calcaneovalgus and metatarsus varus. J Bone Joint Surg Br 46:445, 1964.


### Torsional Deformities of the Lower Extremities


Bell SN, Campbell PE, Cole WG, et al: Tibia vara caused by focal fibrocartilaginous dysplasia: Three case reports. J Bone Joint Surg Br 67:780-784, 1985.

Crawford AH, Schorry EK: Neurofibromatosis in children: The role of the orthopaedist. J Am Acad Orthop Surg 7:217-230, 1999.

Davidson WH, Bohne WH: The Syme amputation in children. J Bone Joint Surg Am 57:905-909, 1975.

Heath CH, Staheli LT: Normal limits of knee angle in white children—genu varum and genu valgum. J Pediatr Orthop 13:259-262, 1993.

Herring JA, Barnhill B, Gafffney C: Syme amputation: An evaluation of the physical and psychological function in young patients. J Bone Joint Surg Am 68:573-578, 1986.

Hofmann A, Wenger DR: Posteromedial bowing of the tibia: Progression of discrepancy in leg lengths. J Bone Joint Surg Am 63:384-388, 1981.

Jacobsen ST, Crawford AH, Millar EA, et al: The Syme amputation in patients with congenital pseudoarthrosis of the tibia. J Bone Joint Surg Am 65:533-537, 1983.

Masserman RL, Peterson HA, Bianco AJ Jr: Congenital pseudoarthrosis of the tibia: A review of the literature and 52 cases from the Mayo Clinic. Clin Orthop 99:140-145, 1974.

Paterson D: Congenital pseudoarthrosis of the tibia: An overview. Clin Orthop 247:44, 1989.

Salenius P, Vankka GK: The development of the tibio-femoral angle in children. J Bone Joint Surg Am 57:259-261, 1975.

Staheli LT: Torsional deformity. Pediatr Clin North Am 24:799-811, 1977.

Thompson GH: Angular deformities of the lower extremities in children. In Chapman MW (ed): Chapman's Orthopaedic Surgery. Philadelphia, Lippincott, Williams & Wilkins, 2001, pp 4287-4335.

Zayer M: Osteoarthritis following Blount's disease. Int Orthop 4:63-66, 1980.


### Obstetric Trauma


Benson LJ, Ezaki M, Carter P, et al: Brachial plexus birth palsy: A prospective natural history study. Orthop Trans 20:311, 1996.

Broker FH, Burbach T: Ultrasonic diagnosis of separation of the proximal humeral epiphysis in the newborn. J Bone Joint Surg Am 72:187, 1990.

Cohen AW, Otto SR: Obstetric clavicular fractures: A 3 year analysis. J Reprod Med 25:119, 1980.

Farkas R, Levine S: X-ray incidence of fractured clavicle in vertex presentation. Am J Obstet Gynecol 59:204, 1950.

Fisher NA, Newman B, Lloyd J, et al: Ultrasonic evaluation of birth injury to the shoulder. J Perinatol 15:398, 1995.

Greenwald AG, Schute PC, Shiveley JL: Brachial plexus birth palsy: A 10-year report on the incidence and prognosis. J Pediatr Orthop 4:689-692, 1984.

Hardy AE: Birth injuries of the brachial plexus: Incidence and prognosis. J Bone Joint Surg Br 63:98-101, 1981.

Kaplan B, Rabinerson D, Avrech OM, et al: Fractures of the clavicle in newborns following normal labor and delivery. Int J Gynaecol Obstet 63:15-20, 1998.

Michelow BJ, Clarke HM, Curtis CG, et al: The natural history of obstetrical brachial plexus palsy. Plast Reconstr Surg 93:675-681, 1994.

Morris et al: Birth associated femoral fractures: Incidence and outcome. J Pediatr Orthop 22:27-30, 2002.

Noetzel MJ, Park TS, Robinson, S, et al: Prospective study of recovery following neonatal brachial plexus injury. J Child Neurol 16:488-492, 2001.

Sanford HN: The Moro reflex as a diagnostic aid in fractures of the clavicle in newborn infants. J Dis Child 41:1304, 1931.

Waters PM: Comparison of the natural history, the outcome of microsurgical repair, and the outcome of operative reconstruction in brachial plexus birth palsy. J Bone Joint Surg Am 81:649-659, 1999.

Waters PM: Obstetric brachial plexus injuries: Evaluation and management. J Am Acad Orthop Surg 5:205-214, 1997.


### Neonatal Osteomyelitis and Septic Arthritis


Ash JM, Gilday DL: The futility of bone scanning in neonatal osteomyelitis: Concise communication. J Nucl Med 21:417, 1980.

Bergdahl S, Ekengren K, Eriksson M: Neonatal hematogenous osteomyelitis: Risk factors for long-term sequelae. J Pediatr Orthop 5:564, 1985.

Caksen H, Ozturk MK, Uzum K, et al: Septic arthritis in childhood. Pediatr Int 42:534-540, 2000.

Dormans JP, Drummond DS: Pediatric hematogenous osteomyelitis: New trends in presentation, diagnosis and treatment. J Am Acad Orthop Surg 2:333-341, 1994.

Fox L, Sprunt K: Neonatal osteomyelitis. Pediatrics 62:535, 1978.

Ho NK, Low YP, See HF: Septic arthritis in the newborn—17 years' experience. Singapore Med J 30:356-358, 1989.

Jackson MA, Nelson JD: Etiology and medical management of acute suppurative bone and joint infections in pediatric patients. J Pediatr Orthop 2:313-323, 1982.

Lim MO, Gresham EL, Franken EAJ, et al: Osteomyelitis as a complication of umbilical artery catheterization. Am J Dis Child 131:142, 1977.

Lyon RM, Evanich JD: Culture negative septic arthritis in children. J Pediatr Orthop 19:655-659, 1999.

Mah ET, LeQuesne GW, Gent RJ, et al: Ultrasonic features of acute osteomyelitis in children. J Bone Joint Surg Br 76:969-974, 1994.

Morrissy RT: Bone and joint sepsis. In Morrissy RT and Weinstein SL(eds): Lovell and Winter's Pediatric Orthopaedics, 5th ed. Philadelphia, Lippincott, Williams & Wilkins, 2001, pp 459-505.

Ogden JA: Pediatric osteomyelitis and septic arthritis: The pathology of neonatal disease. Yale J Biol Med 52:423, 1979.

Pulliam PN, Attia MW, Cronan KM: C-reactive protein in febrile children 1 to 36 months of age with clinically undetectable serious bacterial infection. Pediatrics 108:1275-1279, 2001.

Scott RJ, Christofersen MR, Robertson WW Jr, et al: Acute osteomyelitis in children: A review of 116 cases. J Pediatr Orthop 10:649-652, 1990.

Unkila-Kallio L, Kallio MJ, Eskola J, et al: Serum C-reactive protein, erythrocyte sedimentation rate, and white blood cell count in acute hematogenous osteomyelitis of children. Pediatrics 93:59-62, 1994.

# PART XIX

# NEOPLASIA

Editor: H. WILLIAM TAEUSCH

CHAPTER 95

## Congenital Malignant Disorders

Mignon L. Loh and Katherine K. Matthay

Neonatal malignancies differ in incidence, clinical behavior, and heritable features from the cancers seen in older children. Syndromes associated with an inherited predisposition to develop malignancies can manifest in the newborn period. Exposure to potential carcinogens or teratogens during the prenatal period also may be related etiologically. Special consideration must be given to treatment problems unique to the newborn age group, including differences in drug metabolism from older children and the possible intolerance of rapidly growing and developing normal tissues to the inhibitory effects of antineoplastic chemotherapeutic agents and radiation. In addition, special consideration also must be given to the postsurgical management of infants with respect to fluid management, pain control, and nutrition. Late effects on reproductive capacity and intellectual development and the potential for induction of secondary malignancy also are of heightened concerns in the treatment of malignant disorders in the newborn. The epidemiology, etiology, and the diagnosis of neonatal malignancy are reviewed here, followed by discussion of the most commonly encountered malignancies in the newborn.

### EPIDEMIOLOGY, ETIOLOGY, AND DIAGNOSIS OF NEONATAL MALIGNANCY

#### Epidemiology: Incidence and Mortality

A study of U.S. population-based data from the Surveillance, Epidemiology, and End Results (SEER) program gathered between 1976 and 1984 and between 1984 and 1996 reveals an average yearly incidence of malignancy in children in the first year of life of 233/1,000,000 (Ries et al, 1999). Most striking, the peak cancer incidence among all children was during the first year of life, and 13% of these cases were diagnosed in the first month (Ries et al, 1999). Although trend analyses indicate that the incidence of malignancy in the infant population appears to be increasing, these data should be interpreted with caution, due to potential changes in population characteristics, screening fetal ultrasound practices, case ascertainment, and other factors (Gurney et al, 1997; Ries et al, 1999).

The most common malignancy in neonates is neuroblastoma, followed by leukemia and germ cell tumors. In fact, a majority of germ cell tumors occurring in infancy were diagnosed in the first 2 months of life (Ries et al, 1999). In the seventh month of life there is an additional peak of diagnosed cases of leukemia, exceeding that in the first month of life. Female and male infants have similar cancer incidence rates, but white infants have significantly higher rates than those reported in African-American infants for all histologic types. The distribution of the major types of cancers in newborns, infants, and children is depicted in Table 95–1.

The mortality rates for infants with cancer exceed those for older children, even among similar histologic groups (Ries et al, 1999). Despite cure rates exceeding 75% for children older than 1 year diagnosed with acute lymphoblastic leukemia (ALL), infants with ALL continue to experience cure rates of only 40% to 50%. These lower rates probably are due to biologic differences in the leukemias afflicting infants versus older children, as it is well established that infants with leukemia often harbor rearrangements of the *MLL* ("mixed lineage leukemia") gene, whereas older children do not. The poorer survival patterns for infants also are seen in rhabdomyosarcoma and central nervous system (CNS) tumors including primitive neuroectodermal tumor (PNET) and ependymomas, but the reasons for this association are less clear (Ries et al, 1999). Two exceptions are neuroblastoma, for which the incidence in newborns is more than 10 times higher than the mortality rate, and infantile fibrosarcoma, for which cure rates often exceed those achieved in older children or adults (Table 95–2). A study of mortality rates differs markedly from one of incidence, because certain malignancies are rapidly fatal, others lead to death beyond the neonatal period, and a large number are cured or undergo spontaneous regression. The relative frequencies of most types of malignancy in infants are unchanged from those reported earlier (Table 95–3).

#### Etiology

##### *Genetic Predisposition Syndromes and Congenital Defects*

Certain host factors can predispose a person to the development of neoplastic disease. Some of the genes responsible for such predispositions are known, whereas others are not. For instance, an increased incidence of leukemia

**TABLE 95–1**

**Percent Distribution of the Major Types of Cancer in Children, Newborns, and Infants**

| Histologic Type | Children <15 yr (%) | Newborns <30 d (%) | Infants <1 yr (%) |
|---|---|---|---|
| Leukemia | 31 | 13 | 14 |
| Central nervous system tumors | 18 | 3 | 15 |
| Neuroblastoma | 8 | 54 | 27 |
| Lymphoma | 14 | 0.3 | 1 |
| Renal tumors | 6 | 13 | 11 |
| Sarcoma | 11 | 11 | 5 |
| Hepatic tumors | 1.3 | 0 | 3 |
| Teratoma | 0.4 | 0 | 6 |
| Retinoblastoma | 4 | 0 | 13 |
| Other | 6.3 | 5.7 | 5 |

has been noted in persons with trisomy 21, Fanconi anemia, and Bloom syndrome. In addition, children born with immunodeficiency disorders such as ataxia-telangiectasia, Wiskott-Aldrich syndrome, and severe combined immunodeficiency are at higher risk of developing lymphoma later in life.

A small number of well-defined hereditary conditions are associated with an increased incidence of specific neoplasms and are listed in Table 95–4. Except for retinoblastoma, hepatoblastoma, and Wilms tumor, the neoplasms associated with these syndromes seldom manifest in the neonatal period, but the associated abnormalities may be recognized early. The early recognition, in combination with the family history, alerts the clinician to the need for screening. The lack of family history, however, should not dissuade the clinician from investigating these syndromes, as both spontaneous germline mutations and parental mosaicism occur. In many of these neoplasms, the genetic defect has been identified. For example, the *NF1* gene is located at 17q11.2 and encodes a protein, neurofibromin, that normally acts as a guanosine tri-phosphatase activating protein that down regulates the *ras* pathway. Dysregulation of cell growth results when a mutation is present because there is no functional "off" switch, accounting for the increase in malignancies in patients with neurofibromatosis. In Li-Fraumeni syndrome, germline mutations in the tumor suppressor gene *TP53* have been demonstrated in some of the families in which members had sarcomas, breast cancer, brain tumors, and leukemia (Malkin et al, 1990).

An unexpectedly large number of childhood tumors occurs in association with certain congenital defects. For instance, children with congenital aniridia have an increased incidence of Wilms tumors. Aniridia is a rare anomaly found in only 1 of 75,000 persons. It is about 1000 times more likely to occur in children with Wilms tumor (1 in 75). The association with a deletion in the *WT1* gene on chromosome 11p13 has been described in at least 20 patients (Yunis and Ramsay, 1980). Most of these patients also have genitourinary abnormalities and mental retardation; other problems that can be associated with aniridia and Wilms tumor include cardiac septal defects. Collectively, the associated abnormalities are known as the WAGR (*W*ilms tumor, *a*niridia, *g*enitourinary abnormalities, mental *r*etardation) syndrome. From a clinical perspective, if an infant has

**TABLE 95–2**

**Incidence and Mortality Rates of Malignant Tumors in U.S. Newborns and Infants**

| | Incidence | | | | Morality Rate | | | | |
|---|---|---|---|---|---|---|---|---|---|
| | <29 days | | 12 months | | <29 Days | | 12 months | | |
| Tumor Type | No. | Rate | No. | Rate* (A) | No. | Rate | No. | Rate* (B) | Ratio (A/B) |
| Leukemia | 5 | 4.7 | 34 | 31.8 | 101 | 2.6 | 807 | 20.8 | 1.5 |
| Neuroblastoma | 21 | 19.7 | 67 | 62.7 | 70 | 1.8 | 302 | 7.8 | 8 |
| Central nervous system | 1 | 0.9 | 15 | 14 | 12 | 0.3 | 257 | 6.6 | 2.1 |
| Kidney tumors | 5 | 4.7 | 21 | 19.7 | 21 | 0.5 | 141 | 3.6 | 5.4 |
| Reticuloendotheliosis | 0 | 0 | 3 | 2.8 | 7 | 0.2 | 131 | 3.4 | — |
| Sarcoma | 4 | 3.7 | 19 | 17.8 | 29 | 0.7 | 129 | 3.3 | 5.4 |
| Liver tumors | 0 | 0 | 8 | 7.5 | 15 | 0.4 | 99 | 2.6 | 2.9 |
| Lymphoma | 1 | 0.9 | 2 | 1.9 | 2 | <0.1 | 60 | 1.5 | 1.3 |
| Teratoma | 0 | 0 | 3 | 2.8 | 11 | 0.3 | 28 | 0.7 | 4 |
| Carcinona | 1 | 0.9 | 6 | 5.6 | 6 | 0.2 | 18 | 0.5 | 11.2 |
| Germ cell tumors, excluding teratoma | 0 | 0 | 0 | 0 | 0 | 0 | 6 | 0.2 | |
| Retinoblastoma | 0 | 0 | 17 | 15.9 | 1 | <0.1 | 4 | 0.1 | 159 |
| Other | 1 | 0.9 | 1 | 0.9 | 20 | 0.5 | 62 | 1.6 | |
| Total/mean | 39 | 36.4 | 196 | 183.4 | 295 | 7.6 | 2044 | 52.7 | 3.5 |

*Per 1 million live births per year.

Data from Bader JI, Miller RW: U.S. cancer incidence and mortality in the first year of life. Am J Dis Child 133:157, 1979.

**TABLE 95–3**

**Tumor Types in 11 Surveys Consisting of 795 Fetal and Newborn Tumors**

| | Number of Cases (Percent) | | | | | | | | | | | |
|---|---|---|---|---|---|---|---|---|---|---|---|---|
| **Tumor** | **RWHM** | **SJCRH** | **MDA** | **CHB** | **CHSD (1983-1994)** | **CCRG** | **HSC** | **CHOP** | **CHLA (1960-1991)** | **DCR** | **RHSC** | **Total Tumors** |
| Neuroblastoma | 6 (13.0) | 19 (55.9) | 6 (25) | 31 (18) | 8 (10.8) | 27 (26.7) | 48 (47.0) | 11 (50) | 36 (21.6) | 20 (26) | 7 (13.7) | 219 (27.5) |
| Teratoma | 24 (52.2) | 2 (5.9) | — | 49 (29) | 15 (20.3) | 16 (15.8) | — | 3 (13.6) | 62 (37.1)† | 6 (8) | 19 (37.2) | 196 (24.7) |
| Leukemia | — | 6 (17.6) | 3 (12.5) | 21 (12) | 5 (6.8) | 17 (16.8) | 8 (7.8) | 3 (13.6) | 18 (10.8) | 12 (16) | — | 93 (11.7) |
| Sarcoma | — | — | 8 (33) | 17 (10) | 5 (6.8) | 13 (12.9) | 12 (11.8) | 3 (13.6) | 8 (4.8) | 11 (14) | 8 (15.7) | 82 (10.3) |
| Brain tumor | 5 (10.9) | — | 3 (12.5) | 14 (8) | 11 (14.9) | 12 (11.9) | 9 (8.8) | — | 15 (9.0) | 8 (11) | — | 74 (9.3) |
| Renal tumor | 2 (4.3) | 2 (5.9) | — | 8 (5) | 1 (1.3) | 8 (7.9) | 4 (3.9) | 1 (4.6) | 6 (3.6) | 4 (5) | 9 (17.6) | 45 (5.7) |
| Liver tumor | 1 (2.2) | — | — | 8 (50) | 5 (6.8) | 3 (3.0) | 1 (1) | — | 18 (10.8) | 2 (3) | 3 (5.9) | 41 (5.1) |
| Retinoblastoma | — | 3 (8.9) | 2 (8) | 14 (8) | — | — | 17 (16.7) | — | 4 (2.40) | 2 (3) | 3 (5.9) | 45 (5.7) |
| Total in Study‡ | 46 | 34 | 24 | 170 | 74 | 101 | 102 | 22 | 167 | 65 | 51 | 795 (100) |

CCRG, Childhood Cancer Research Group, Oxford[26]; CHB, Children's Hospital, Birmingham, UK[101]; CHLA, Children's Hospital, Los Angeles; CHOP, Children's Hospital of Philadelphia[53]; CHSD, Children's Hospital, San Diego; DCR, Danish Cancer Registry[24]; HSC, The Hospital for Sick Children, Toronto, Canada[30]; MDA, M.D. Anderson Hospital[31]; RHSC, Royal Hospital for Sick Children, Glasgow, Scotland[38]; RWHM, The Royal Women's Hospital and the Mercy Hospital for Women, Melbourne, Victoria, Australia[145];SJCRH, St. Jude Children's Research Hospital.[35]

*The number in parentheses represents the percent of total cases included in that institution's survey.

†2 of 62 were malignant.

‡This figure is the total number of cases recorded for that particular institution's study, not the total number included in the columns in the table.

**TABLE 95–4**

**Hereditary Conditions with Associated Tumors**

| Syndrome | Gene | Locus | Inheritance Pattern | Most Common Tumors |
|---|---|---|---|---|
| Ataxia-telangiectasia | *ATM* | 11q22-q23 | Recessive | Leukemias<br>Lymphomas |
| Beckwith-Wiedemann syndrome | *IGF2* | 11p15 | Some auto dominant imprinting | Wilms tumor<br>Hepatoblastoma<br>Rhabdomyosarcoma |
| Bloom syndrome | *BLM* | 15q26 | Auto recessive | Leukemias |
| Denys-Drash syndrome | *WT1* | 11p13 | Auto dominant | Familial Wilms tumor |
| Down syndrome | | Trisomy 21 | Sporadic | — |
| Fanconi anemia | | Many | Auto recessive | Leukemias |
| Gonadal dysgenesis | | 45X/46XY | ?X-linked | Gonadoblastoma<br>Germinoma |
| Gorlins syndrome | *PTCH2* | 1p33 | Auto dominant | Medulloblastoma<br>Basal cell carcinoma |
| Klinefelter syndrome | ? | XXY | Sporadic | Teratoma<br>Leukemia<br>Breast cancers |
| Li-Fraumeni syndrome | *TP53* | | Auto dominant | Sarcoma, CNS, Breast tumors |
| Neurofibromatosis | *NF1* | 17q11.2 | Auto dominant | Glioma<br>Leukemia (JMML)<br>Sarcoma |
| Retinoblastoma | *RB* | 13q14 | Auto dominant | Retinoblastoma<br>Osteosarcoma<br>Rhabdomyosarcoma |
| Trisomy 18 | ? | Trisomy 18 | Sporadic | Wilms tumor |
| Turner syndrome | | XO | Sporadic | — |
| Von Hippel-Lindau syndrome | *VHL* | 3p26 | Auto dominant | Hemangioblastoma |
| WAGR syndrome | *WT1* | 11p13 | | Wilms tumor |
| Wiskott Aldrich syndrome | *WAS* | Xp11.23 | X-linked | Non-Hodgkin lymphoma |
| X-linked lymphoproliferative disorders | *SAP* | Xq25 | X-linked | EBV lymphomas |

Auto, autosomal; CNS, Central nervous system; EBV, Epstein-Barr virus; JMML, juvenile myelomonocytic leukemia; WAGR, *W*ilms tumors, *a*niridia, *g*enitourinary abnormalities, mental *r*etardation.

aniridia, chromosome analysis should be undertaken. If a deletion of chromosome 11p13 is found, the child should be monitored for the development of Wilms tumor with serial ultrasonographic studies of the kidneys. Wilms tumor develops in approximately half of these patients.

Wilms tumor and several other childhood neoplasms also are associated with the Beckwith-Wiedemann syndrome (BWS) and/or hemihypertrophy syndromes, typified by macroglossia, gigantism, and abdominal wall defects, but also including visceromegaly, flame nevus, neonatal hypoglycemia, microcephaly, and retardation (Sotelo-Avila et al, 1980a, 1980b). The associated neoplasms are seen in approximately 8% of infants with either the complete or partial syndrome and include Wilms tumor, adrenal cortical carcinoma, and hepatoblastoma—tumors of the same organs in which visceromegaly develops. Also reported are rhabdomyosarcoma, neuroblastoma, ganglioneuroma, and adenomas and hamartomas.

BWS is linked with abnormalities of 11p15, where the insulin-like growth factor II gene (*IGF2*) and tumor suppressor gene *H19* are located (Kubota et al, 1994). These two genes are examples of genes that are normally imprinted, or expressed from one parent. The paternal copy of the *IGF2* gene is normally expressed, while the maternal copy is silenced. The maternal copy of *H19* is normally expressed, while the paternal copy is silenced. However, in BWS, uniparental disomy (in which two copies of a chromosomal region come from one parent and none from the other) of the paternal *IGF2* and *H19* locus occurs, which causes a loss of the maternal genes balanced by a gain of the paternal genes (Fig. 95–1). The result is biallelic expression of paternal *IGF2* and no expression of *H19*, leading to the multiorgan hyperplasia (due to increased *IGF2*) and a predisposition to development of neoplasia (due to lack of *H19*).

### *Transplacental Tumor Passage*

Malignancies diagnosed during pregnancy are estimated to occur in 1 out of every 1000 pregnancies (Greenlund et al, 2001; Pavlidis, 2002). The choice to terminate a pregnancy is a painful and individual decision best made in consultation with the family, obstetrician, oncologist, and spiritual counsel (Eisinger and Noizet, 2002; Mathieu et al, 2002;

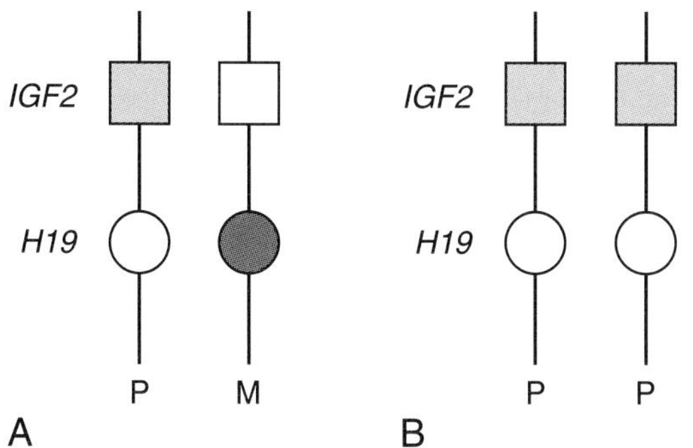


**FIGURE 95-1.** A schematic of uniparental disomy causing Beckwith-Weidemann syndrome. **A,** In the normal pattern of inheritance, there is expression of paternally inherited *IGF-2* and no expression of *H19*. Conversely, there is expression of *H19* from the maternal allele but no expression of *IGF-2*. **B,** Two copies of the paternal allele have been inherited, leading to overexpression of *IGF-2* and no expression of *H19*. M, maternal; P, paternal.

Pautier et al, 2002). Some important factors to consider include the gestational age of the fetus at the time of maternal diagnosis, the stage of the disease and the risks of waiting to treat, and the treatment required. Unfortunately, the most common malignancy among women of childbearing age is leukemia, a disease that is generally fatal if not promptly treated. Most chemotherapy agents are known to be teratogenic in animal models, and some—in particular, all-*trans*-retinoic acid—are known to be potent teratogens in humans. However, there is a dearth of information regarding the pharmacokinetics and transplacental concentrations of many of the chemotherapy agents used. That being said, in numerous case reports in the literature, healthy infants have been born to women diagnosed and treated during pregnancy for leukemia, lymphoma, and breast cancer, among others (Aviles and Neri, 2001; Breccia et al, 2002; Fadilah et al, 2002; Ikeda et al, 2002; McNally et al, 2002; Safdar et al, 2002; Ward and Bristow, 2002).

The transmission of cancer across the placenta is an uncommon but recognized phenomenon. The development of choriocarcinoma in an infant as a complication of placental choriocarcinoma is one example of this rare disease. In addition, both mother and infant have been reported to be affected in some instances (Kishkurno et al, 1997). Chemotherapy has been used successfully in both the mother and infant (McNally et al, 2002). This represents tumor transmission from the fetus to the mother, because the trophoblast, the site of origin, is composed of fetal rather than maternal tissue. In most of the recorded cases, there was either a recognized placental choriocarcinoma or absence of a primary site in the infants with disseminated malignancy. The characteristic presentation is one of hematemesis or hemoptysis, anemia, hepatomegaly, and pulmonary metastases in the infant. The diagnosis is established by the demonstration of an elevated urinary or plasma β-human chorionic gonadotropin (hCG) in the infant (Belchis et al, 1993). The mother is screened for the disease by pathologic examination of the placenta, obtaining a chest radiograph, and following serial hCG levels. The half-life of hCG is on the order of hours, and an assay showing appropriate decay of this marker effectively rules out disease in the mother.

Transmission of maternal leukemia to the infant, either at or shortly after birth, has not been documented (Dildy et al, 1989). A few cases of malignant melanoma of the mother with spread to the fetus have been reported and reviewed (Anderson et al, 1989). Factors suggestive of an unfavorable fetal or infant outcome are maternal age of less than 30 years, primiparity, primary lesion on the leg, onset of disease more than 3 years before pregnancy, metastatic status before pregnancy, birth at greater than 36 weeks of gestation, and male gender. Maternal virilizing tumors have resulted in in utero virilization of the infant as the result of transplacental passage of androgens secreted by the neoplasm, but the tumors have not spread to the fetus (Haymond and Weldon, 1973). Multiple myeloma has been reported in a small number of pregnant women (Lergier et al, 1974). In two instances, no abnormal myeloma protein was found in the infants, but a transient abnormal protein believed to have been passively transferred from the mother was demonstrated in two others. None of the infants had evidence of disease. Recently, transplacental transmission of small cell lung cancer has been reported after the mother presented with advanced-stage disease at the time of delivery (Tolar et al, 2002).

### *Twin-to-Twin Transmission*

Although the risk of development of leukemia is increased slightly in a dizygotic twin or other sibling of a child who has the disease, the chance of developing leukemia is greatest in a monozygotic twin. If one monozygotic twin has leukemia, the co-twin has an approximately 25% chance of developing leukemia, usually within weeks or months of the diagnosis of the sibling. Growing evidence suggests that this increased incidence is likely due to twin-to-twin transmission of a preleukemic clone rather than to the simultaneous development of a shared germline mutation facilitating the later development of leukemia (Ford et al, 1993, 1998).

### *Environmental Factors*

One of the most compelling connections between the environment and an increased risk of developing cancer was demonstrated in 1971 by studies linking maternal exposure to diethylstilbestrol (DES) with clear cell adenocarcinoma of the vagina and cervix in daughters born from those pregnancies (Herbst et al, 1971). According to the calculations of Herbst and colleagues (1977), the risk of development of such tumors is 0.14 to 1.4 per 1000 DES-exposed females up until the age of 24 years. Melnick and coworkers (1987) reported the risk up to age 34 as 1 case per 1000. The tumors are rare in females younger than 14 years of age, but the frequency increases rapidly to a peak at age 17 to 22 years, after which there is a precipitous drop. In addition to neoplastic changes, several nonmalignant epithelial and structural alterations of the lower genital tract have been noted, as have deformities of the endometrial cavity (Cunha et al, 1987; Hatch et al, 2001). Other authors have reported an increased risk of unfavorable outcome of pregnancy in daughters exposed in utero to DES. Detailed studies of males exposed in utero to DES show increased frequencies of testicular hypoplasia, cryptorchidism, epididymal cysts, microphallus, increased abnormal spermatozoal forms, and lowered sperm counts but no increased risk of cancer (Strohsnitter et al, 2001). An estimated 30% of the males studied are probably infertile (Bibbo et al, 1977; Gill et al, 1977).

Other causal relationships between the environment and an increased risk of developing cancer are known. In particular, exposure to ionizing radiation during pregnancy is known to increase the risk of acute leukemias in exposed offspring. Stewart and Draper (1968) examined the risk for development of cancer in children exposed prenatally to diagnostic x-rays when radiography was used routinely to screen mothers for cephalopelvic disproportion and found it to be in excess of what was expected. Since then, other investigators have validated this association (Monson, 1997). A report by Yoshimoto and colleagues (1991) involving longer follow-up suggests that the relative risk of cancer in adult life after intrauterine exposure to radiation from the Hiroshima and Nagasaki atomic bombs was significantly increased.

A comprehensive review summarizes data on the studies of preconceptual and postconceptual parental exposures to chemicals, solvents, radiation, and electromagnetic field exposure as they relate to cancer incidence in offspring (Gold and Sever, 1994). Although many moderately significant correlations have been reported for prenatal exposures and various childhood cancers, the findings are often contradictory. Many possible mechanisms and factors must be considered in studies of the relationship of environmental factors to cancer pathogenesis in children. For example, preconception exposures could lead to genetic alterations transmitted to offspring by either parent. Also, a link to a particular exposure might really be a surrogate for another; thus, occupations in the lumber and paper industries might reflect hydrocarbon exposure as well as wood dust.

The use of fertility drugs may increase the risk of developing cancer in the exposed offspring, but this association is controversial. A case-control study in patients with neuroblastoma showed no association with contraceptive exposure but did suggest a modest increase in risk for children of women exposed to fertility drugs (Olshan et al, 1999). However, in a recent study published by Bruinsma and colleagues (2000), there does not appear to be an increased incidence of cancer among 5249 children born after the use of preconception fertility drugs and in vitro fertilization.

A number of other agents known to be teratogenic also may be carcinogenic to offspring. In utero exposure to phenytoin or other antiepileptic drugs is associated with a well-recognized syndrome in the newborn that includes hypoplasia of the midface, tapering of the fingers and toes, and hypoplasia or aplasia of the nails. At least five children with this syndrome were reported to have neuroblastomas (Ehrenbard and Chaganti, 1981), and one child was found to have an extrarenal Wilms tumor (Taylor et al, 1980). One young adult with a history of exposure in utero to phenytoin had a malignant mesenchymoma (Blattner et al, 1977). Excessive maternal alcohol consumption does appear to be strongly linked with an increased risk of developing cancer in the newborn period, particularly acute myeloid leukemia (Severson et al, 1993; Shu et al, 1996). The fetal alcohol syndrome, a disorder occurring in the children of mothers who consume excessive amounts of alcohol, is characterized by developmental delay, growth deficiency, and multiple minor anomalies. One child with this syndrome has been reported with neuroblastoma (Kinney et al, 1980), a second with hepatoblastoma, and a third with adrenocortical carcinoma, but these are case reports in the literature.

The association of neoplasms with other environmental factors, such as maternal use of tobacco, has not been conclusively proven (Shu et al, 1996). Jick and associates (1981) noted an increase in pregnancies ending in spontaneous abortions and an increased incidence of congenital anomalies in live infants born to women presumed to have used vaginal spermicides near the time of conception. Two of the children were found to have neoplasms shortly after birth. A case-control study from the Children's Cancer Group and the Pediatric Oncology Group of 504 newly diagnosed cases of neuroblastoma reinforced some prior evidence of increased risks in parental electrical, farming and gardening, and painting occupations but failed to confirm other previously reported associations (Olshan et al, 1999).

### Diagnosis and Evaluation

The diagnostic evaluation of a newborn infant suspected to have cancer is obviously guided by the signs and symptoms of the disease. Table 95–5 lists some of the most common signs and symptoms associated with the more common malignancies found in the neonatal period. Prenatal ultrasonography can detect some tumors; however, not all women undergo screening at 18 to 20 weeks. In addition, not all tumors are large enough to be detected at 18 weeks, as the fetus experiences most in utero growth after this point in gestation. However, certain conditions may be associated with malignancies, such as polyhydramnios, hydrops fetalis, or intrauterine growth restriction/retardation.

The laboratory and pathologic evaluations should be directed at making the diagnosis most efficiently, to spare the newborn unnecessary procedures that may lead to significant acute and chronic morbidity. Consultation with a pediatric oncologist should be obtained for help in making the initial diagnosis, as the eventual recommendations for therapy may help to spare the infant the sequelae of major surgery. In particular, surgeons and pathologists should be encouraged to submit any diagnostic tissue for routine histologic examination and immunoperoxidase staining as well as cytogenetic analysis. In addition, samples for tumor banking should be set aside for cryopreservation in compliance with parental consent and adherence to the local institution's guidelines for handling of these rare but potentially precious and informative tumors.

## SPECIFIC NEOPLASMS

### Neuroblastoma

Neuroblastoma is the most common malignant tumor in infants, with approximately 20% of all cases occurring before age 6 months (Huddart et al, 1993). The small round blue cell neoplasm originates from neural crest cells that normally gives rise to the adrenal medulla and sympathetic ganglia (Fig. 95–2). In infants, the first clinical manifestations in more than half the cases usually result from the presence of metastatic disease rather than the primary

**TABLE 95-5**

**Differential Diagnosis of Malignant and Nonmalignant Conditions in Infancy**

| Feature | Malignancy | Nonmalignant Condition |
|---|---|---|
| Skin nodules | Neuroblastoma<br>Acute leukemia<br>Reticuloendothelioses | Congenital viral infections<br>Vasculitis<br>Fibromatosis<br>Neurofibromatososis<br>Xanthoma |
| Head and neck masses | Rhabdomyosarcoma<br>Orbital tumors<br>Cervical tumors<br>Nasopharyngeal<br>Neuroblastoma<br>Lymphoma | Brachial cleft cyst<br>Thyroglossal duct cyst<br>Cystic hygroma<br>Fibromatosis<br>Hemangioma<br>Abscess<br>Cellulitis<br>Reactive hyperplasis of cervical nodes<br>Granulomatous lesions (e.g., atypical tuberculosis) |
| Abdominal or pelvic masses | Neuroblastoma<br>Wilms tumor<br>Sarcoma<br>Malignant teratoma<br>Lymphoma<br>Germ cell tumor | Polycystic kidneys<br>Hydronephrosis<br>Benign teratoma<br>Urinary retention<br>Gastrointestinal duplication<br>Intussusception<br>Chordoma<br>Meningomyelocele<br>Horseshoe kidney<br>Splenomegaly<br>Hepatomegaly |
| Hepatomegaly | Neuroblastoma<br>Acute leukemia<br>Hepatoblastoma | Congenital viral infections<br>Storage diseases<br>Cavernous hemangioma<br>Hemangioendothelioma |
| Signs/symptoms of increased intracranial pressure | Brain tumors<br>Acute leukemia<br>Retinoblastoma | Intracranial hemorrhage<br>Communicating hydrocephalus<br>Dandy-Walker malformation<br>Vascular malformations |
| Anemia | Acute leukemia<br>Neuroblastoma | Acute or chronic blood loss<br>Hypoproliferative anemia (nutritional, congenital)<br>Dyserythropoietic anemias<br>Transient erythroblastopenia |
| Pancytopenia | Acute leukemia<br>Neuroblastoma<br>Retinoblastoma (disseminated) | Congenital viral infections<br>Immune-mediated neutropenia and thrombocytopenia<br>Congenital and acquired aplastic anemias |

tumor. Yet despite the occurrence of widespread disease, the tumors seen in newborn infants are almost always biologically favorable, and carry a remarkably good prognosis.

### Clinical Manifestations

Neuroblastoma may manifest as a tumor mass anywhere sympathetic neural tissue normally occurs. In more than half of affected children, the primary tumor is located within the abdomen, arising in the adrenal medulla or a sympathetic ganglion. The tumor also may arise in the posterior mediastinum with resultant bronchial obstruction. Increasing dyspnea, cough, wheezing, or pulmonary infection may be the presenting sign or symptom. The neoplasm also may arise in the neck or pelvis. Involvement of the stellate ganglion may result in Horner syndrome, which includes sinking in of the eyeball, ptosis of the upper eyelid, slight elevation of the lower lid, miosis, narrowing of the palpebral fissure, and anhidrosis (Fig. 95–3). The neoplasm arising from a paravertebral sympathetic

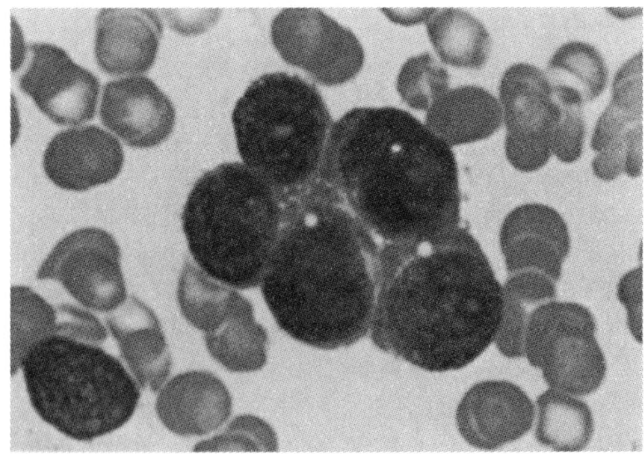

**FIGURE 95–2.** Clump of neuroblastoma cells found in bone marrow aspirate.

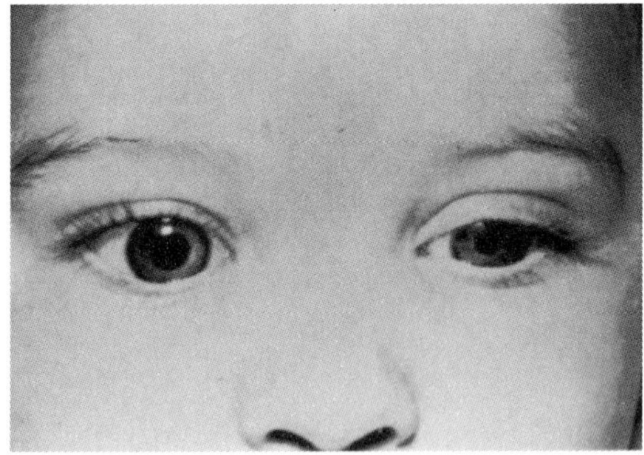

**FIGURE 95–3.** Horner syndrome in an infant with neuroblastoma arising from the left cervical sympathetic ganglion.

ganglion has a tendency to grow into the intervertebral foramina, causing spinal cord compression and resultant paralysis. Careful periodic neurologic evaluation should be performed on the child with a neuroblastoma arising in this location, because the onset of cord compression may necessitate emergency intervention with chemotherapy, surgery, or irradiation.

Metastatic lesions, especially of the skin and liver, are common presenting features during the neonatal period. Often the primary site cannot be discovered. The skin nodules may first become erythematous for 2 or 3 minutes after palpation and then blanch, presumably due to vasoconstriction from release of catecholamines from the tumor cells. This may be a diagnostic sign of subcutaneous neuroblastoma (Fig. 95–4).

The liver often bears the brunt of metastatic dissemination, becoming studded with innumerable foci of tumor growth. The infant has a distended abdomen and respiratory distress (Fig. 95–5) from the rapidly growing hepatic neoplasm. Rarely, stippled calcifications occur in the liver

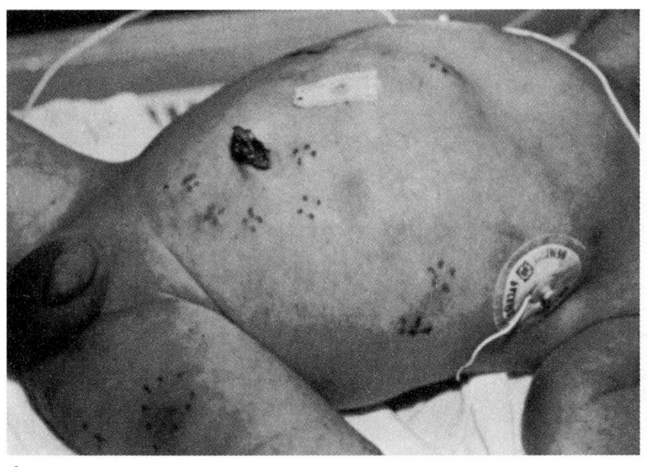

A

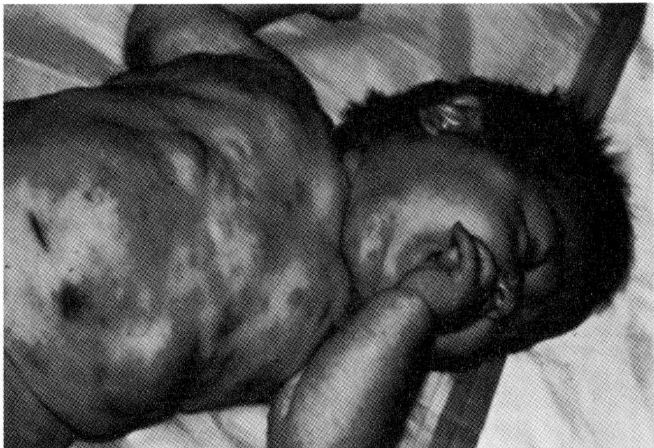

B

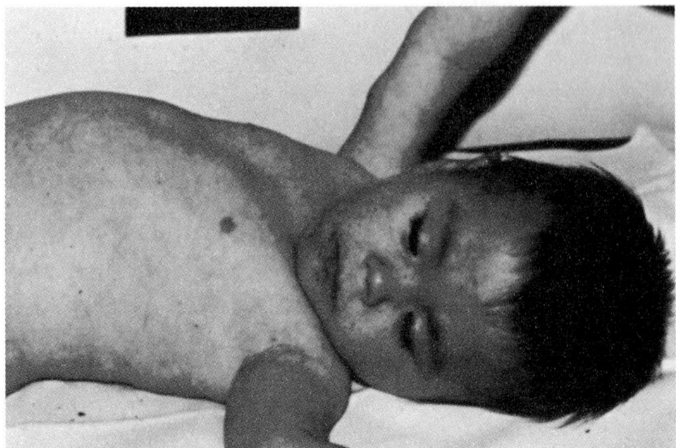

C

**FIGURE 95–4.** A newborn with stage 4S neuroblastoma in whom progression was followed by spontaneous maturation and regression.

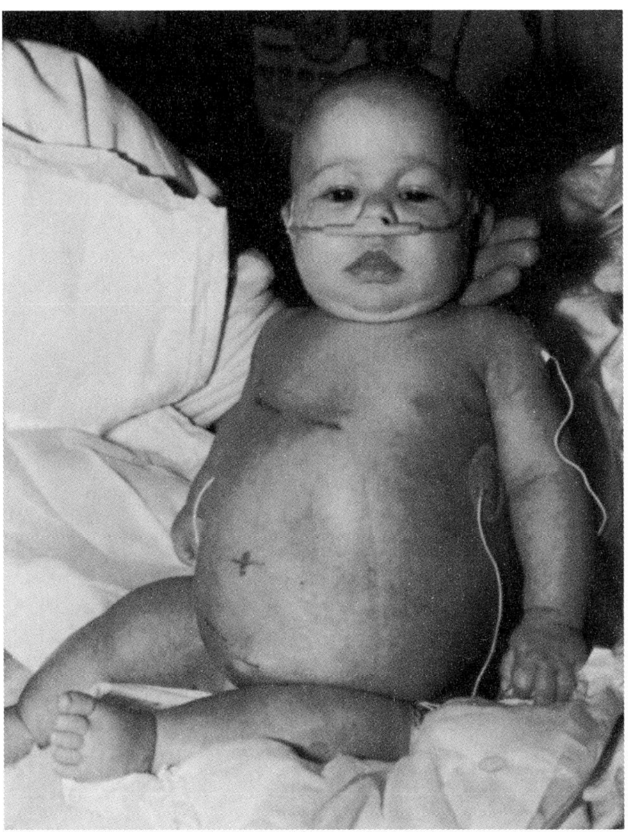

**FIGURE 95–5.** Stage 4S neuroblastoma causing abdominal distention and respiratory distress secondary to hepatic infiltration.

metastases. The liver may be large enough at the time of birth to cause dystocia. The massive liver involvement common in newborns with disseminated neuroblastoma causing respiratory distress and coagulopathy is responsible for the higher mortality rate in newborns than in older infants (Nickerson et al, 2000).

### Unusual Presentations

Several children with neuroblastoma have been reported whose sole presenting manifestation was persistent, intractable diarrhea. The children had been believed to have either cystic fibrosis or celiac syndrome before roentgenographic discoveries of calcified masses were made. Their symptoms dramatically abated following surgical removal of the tumors. It is thought that such symptoms are due to excessive excretion by the tumor of a vasoactive intestinal peptide (Swift et al, 1975).

The association of opsoclonus and myoclonus ("dancing eyes, dancing feet") and neuroblastoma has been described by numerous authors. The usual findings are rapid multidirectional eye movements (opsoclonus), myoclonus, and truncal ataxia (OMA) in the absence of increased intracranial pressure. The condition may be due to an autoimmune reaction, as the presence of antineuronal antibodies has been shown to be significantly more common in children with neuroblastoma and OMA than in case-control neuroblastoma patients (Antunes et al, 2000). This presentation of neuroblastoma is very rarely seen in the newborn, as most patients do not come to medical attention until they are 1 to 3 years of age (Rudnick et al, 2001). Removal of the tumor usually results in a decrease in neurologic signs and symptoms, but the use of steroids is frequently required for complete resolution of the acute condition. In general, the prognosis for survival of children with opsomyoclonus is excellent, although long-term neurologic deficits and learning delays are common and can be quite debilitating. A report from the Netherlands suggests that signs and symptoms may develop in mothers whose fetuses have neuroblastoma. Six women had sweating, pallor, headaches, palpitations, hypertension, and tingling in the feet and hands during the eighth and ninth months of pregnancy (Voute et al, 1970). All of the children delivered were given the diagnosis of neuroblastoma shortly after birth or during the first few months of life. Because the mothers' symptoms disappeared post partum, the authors propose that they were caused by fetal catecholamines entering the maternal circulation.

Neuroblastomas arising from sympathetic ganglia lower in the abdomen give rise to a clinical picture consistent with their location. Thus, presacral neuroblastomas, which arise from the organ of Zuckerkandl, may mimic presacral teratomas and be distinguished from them only by biopsy.

Occasionally, a newborn with congenital neuroblastoma may be thought to have erythroblastosis. Severe jaundice with hepatosplenomegaly and an increase in nucleated red blood cells has been noted. Two newborns with congenital neuroblastoma that metastasized to the liver and placenta initially were thought to have hydrops fetalis (Anders et al, 1970). In one of these infants, the diagnosis was established by histologic examination of the placenta.

Although neuroblastoma usually occurs sporadically, 1% to 2% of patients have a family history of the disease. This frequency is similar to that reported for the other embryonal cancers of childhood in which a familial predisposition is observed. Familial neuroblastoma is inherited in an autosomal dominant mendelian fashion with incomplete penetrance. Affected children from these families differ from those with sporadic disease in that they are often diagnosed at an earlier age (usually infancy) and/or they have multiple primary tumors. These clinical characteristics are hallmarks of the "two-hit" cancer predisposition model first proposed for retinoblastoma. It therefore seems likely that familial neuroblastoma occurs as a result of a germline mutation in one allele of a tumor suppressor gene. In addition, Knudson and Strong proposed that a new germinal mutation in a predisposition gene may account for the initiation of tumorigenesis in up to 22% of cases of nonfamilial neuroblastomas as well. Some recent reports suggest that such cases may involve a constitutional deletion of chromosome 1p36, the same site showing deletion or loss of heterozygosity in many neuroblastoma tumors (Biegel et al, 1993; Fong et al, 1989). At least 14 other cases of constitutional chromosomal rearrangements in neuroblastoma patients have been identified, but the lack of a consistent pattern indicates that many of these rearrangements may be coincidental rather than causal (Maris and Matthay, 1999; Maris et al, 1996). Neuroblastoma also has been reported in families in conjunction with other neurocristopathies, such as Hirschsprung disease and central hypoventilation ("Ondine's curse"). There is remarkable heterogeneity among patients with familial neuroblastoma. Within individual families, the disease can range in severity from an asymptomatic and spontaneously regressing neuroblastoma to a rapidly progressive and fatal disease. The clinical heterogeneity of familial neuroblastoma may partially explain its rarity, because some tumors remain occult or regress and are never detected, whereas others result in death before reproductive age.

### Biochemical Features

Due to the derivation of these cells from neural crest, a hallmark of neuroblastoma cells is the ability to store and secrete catecholamines. Patients with neuroblastoma usually have elevated urinary levels of norepinephrine as well as its biochemical precursors and their metabolites, including dopa, dopamine, normetanephrine, homovanillic acid (HVA), and vanillylmandelic acid (VMA). Ninety percent to 95% of patients have an elevated urinary excretion of VMA or HVA or both. Currently, accurate VMA and HVA determinations can be made on random urine samples when values are normalized for creatinine concentration. In occasional cases, however, there is no elevation of catecholamines, necessitating a 24-hour urine collection. It is therefore important to measure urinary catecholamines in a child before surgical removal of a neuroblastoma or initiation of therapy, to determine whether it is a catecholamine-producing tumor. This unique property of the neoplasm can be used not only as a diagnostic aid but also as a means of assessing the response to therapy or detecting the recurrence of tumor.

### Newborn Screening

Urinary catecholamine screening for neuroblastoma was initially proposed by Woods and Tuchman. The incidence of 8.7 per 1 million children per year is comparable with or higher than that for other congenital diseases for which screening is already in place, such as hypothyroidism, galactosemia, and phenylketonuria (Woods and Tuchman, 1987). The poor prognosis for advanced neuroblastoma in children older than 12 months of age at diagnosis, compared with the favorable outcome for those diagnosed in infancy, raised the expectation that diagnosis at an earlier age might improve overall outcome. Rapid quantitative screening methods have been developed that have high degrees of sensitivity and specificity. However, the cumulative data from 30 years of screening in Japan, the Quebec Neuroblastoma Screening (QNS) Project, and screening projects in Europe have shown that screening infants at 6 months of age or earlier results in a significant apparent increase in the overall incidence of neuroblastoma but fails to reduce the frequency of cases with poor prognosis from advanced-stage disease (Suita et al, 1996; Woods et al, 1996, 2002; Yamamoto et al, 1995). Neuroblastomas detected by screening have almost exclusively favorable biologic features (*MYCN* nonamplified, triploid, favorable Shimada histologic features) (Nakagawara et al, 1991; Takeuchi et al, 1995). Thus, screening practices result in the overdiagnosis of tumors that would otherwise have spontaneously regressed. A recent publication from the Quebec project conclusively showed that screening at 3 weeks and then 6 months in a cohort of 476,654 infants born over a 5-year period did not have any impact on overall mortality rate for the screened cohort compared with multiple control populations from Minnesota, the Delaware Valley, Florida, and the rest of Canada, verifying the earlier studies (Woods et al, 2002). Nor did a second study done to screen children at 1 year of age reveal a favorable impact on outcome (Schilling et al, 2002). Urine screening was done in 1-year-olds in 6 of 16 German states from 1995 to 2000. Children in the remaining states served as controls. A total of 1,475,773 children (61.2% of those who were born between July 1, 1994, and October 31, 1999) underwent screening. In this group, neuroblastoma was detected by screening in 149 children, of whom 3 died. Fifty-five children who had negative results on screening tests were subsequently given a diagnosis of neuroblastoma; 14 of these children died. The screened group and children in the control area had a similar incidence of stage 4 neuroblastoma (3.7 cases per 100,000 screened children and 3.8 per 100,000 controls) and a similar rate of death among children with neuroblastoma (1.3 deaths per 100,000 screened children and 1.2 per 100,000 controls). Comparison of the screened group with the children in the control area revealed substantial overdiagnosis in the former group (an estimated rate of 7 cases per 100,000 children; 95% confidence interval, 4.6 to 9.2); the overdiagnosis rate represents children who had neuroblastoma that was diagnosed by screening but who would not benefit from earlier diagnosis and treatment (Schilling et al, 2002).

### Diagnosis

Neuroblastoma of the newborn most commonly manifests by enlargement of the liver alone, seen in 65% of the cases, followed by subcutaneous metastases, seen in 32%. These percentages differ strikingly from those for older infants and children (Table 95–6). Metastases to lungs, bones, skull, and orbit are rare in the newborn, although clumps of tumor cells often are found if bone marrow aspiration specimens are carefully examined (see Fig. 95–2). Otherwise, a localized primary tumor may be palpable or cause symptoms from spinal cord compression or Horner syndrome. Metastatic evaluation should include computed tomography (CT) or magnetic resonance imaging (MRI) of the primary lesion, MRI of the spine for paraspinal and posterior mediastinal lesions, bone scan, bone marrow aspiration and biopsy, and an [$^{123}$I]- or [$^{131}$I]metaiodobenzylguanidine (MIBG) scan. MIBG is a norepinephrine analogue specifically taken up by neuroblastoma in both bone and soft tissue; thus, MIBG scanning is a sensitive modality for disease localization (Feine et al, 1987; Geatti et al, 1985). Immunocytologic staining of bone marrow with monoclonal antibodies such as neuron-specific enolase (NSE) can increase sensitivity of the detection of bone marrow disease (Moss et al, 1985). The current staging system utilizes the International Neuroblastoma Staging System (INSS) summarized in Table 95–7 (Shimada et al, 1999a; Brodeur et al, 1993).

### Pathologic Classification

The histopathologic appearance of neuroblastoma ranges from undifferentiated neuroblasts, to more mature ganglioneuroblastoma, to fully differentiated and benign ganglioneuroma. The most widely used morphologic classification

**TABLE 95–6**

**Sites of Metastatic Disease at Diagnosis for the 81 Patients with Stage IVS, the 133 Patients with Stage IV <1 Year, and the 434 Patients with Stage IV ≥1 Year.**

| | Stage IVS | Stage IV <1 year | Stage IV ≥1 year | Total (%) |
|---|---|---|---|---|
| ***Sites of Metastases:*** | | | | |
| Bone marrow*, ** | 28 (34.6) | 76 (57.1) | 353 (81.3) | 70.5 |
| Bone** | 0 (0.0) | 65 (48.9) | 296 (68.2) | 55.7 |
| Lymph node | 7 (8.6) | 38 (28.6) | 155 (35.7) | 30.9 |
| Liver*, ** | 65 (80.2) | 71 (53.4) | 56 (12.9) | 29.6 |
| Intracranial/Orbit | 0 (0.0) | 34 (25.6) | 84 (19.6) | 18.2 |
| Adrenal** | 5 (6.2) | 18 (13.5) | 26 (6.0) | 7.6 |
| Skin** | 11 (13.6) | 11 (8.3) | 4 (0.9) | 4.0 |
| Pleura | 0 (0.0) | 6 (4.5) | 16 (3.7) | 3.4 |
| Lung | 0 (0.0) | 3 (2.3) | 18 (4.1) | 3.2 |
| Peritoneum | 0 (0.0) | 5 (3.8) | 9 (2.1) | 2.2 |
| Other | 0 (0.0) | 5 (3.8) | 7 (1.6) | 1.9 |
| CNS | 0 (0.0) | 0 (0.0) | 4 (0.9) | 0.6 |

The * symbol indicates a significant difference between the proportion of patients with stage IVS with the site and the proportion of patients with stage IV <1 year with the site ($p < 0.01$), only for those sites which are included in the definition of stage IVS. The ** symbol indicates a significant difference between the proportion of patients with stage IV <1 year with the site and the proportion of patients with stage IV ≥1 year with the site ($p < 0.02$).

Taken from Dubois S, Kalika Y, Lukens J, et al: Metastatic Sites in Stage IV and IVA neuroblastoma correlate with age, tumor biology, and survival. J Pediatr Hematol Oncol 21:181-189, 1999.

system is based on the system proposed by Shimada and now recommended by the International Neuroblastoma Pathology Committee (INPC) (Brodeur et al, 1993; Shimada et al, 1999a, 1999b). The INPC classification is dependent on age, the degree of differentiation of the neuroblasts, the cellular turnover index, and the presence or absence of Schwannian stromal development. Table 95–8 summarizes the INPC classifications.

**TABLE 95–7**

**International Staging System for Neuroblastoma**

| Stage | Definition |
|---|---|
| Stage 1 | Localized tumor confined to the area of origin; complete gross excision, with or without microscopic residual disease; identifiable ipsilateral and contralateral lymph nodes negative microscopically (adherent nodes may be positive) |
| Stage 2A | Localized tumor with incomplete gross excision; identifiable ipsilateral and contralateral lymph nodes negative microscopically |
| Stage 2B | Localized tumor with complete or incomplete gross excision, with positive ipsilateral nonadherent regional lymph nodes; identifiable contralateral lymph nodes negative microscopically |
| Stage 3 | Unresectable tumor initiating across the midline with or without regional lymph node involvement; or unilateral tumor with contralateral regional lymph node involvement; or, midline tumor with bilateral regional lymph node involvement; bilateral extension by infiltration |
| Stage 4 | Dissemination of tumor to distant lymph nodes, bone, bone marrow, and liver and/or other organs (except as defined in stage 4S) |
| Stage 4S | Localized primary tumor as defined for stage 1 or 2 with dissemination limited to liver, skin, and bone marrow in infant <1 year of age |

Data from Brodeur GM, Pritchard J, Berthold F, et al; Revisions of the international criteria for neuroblastoma diagnosis, staging and response to treatment. J Clin Oncol 11:1466, 1993.

### Genetic Prognostic Factors

The outcome for patients with neuroblastoma has long been known to depend on the age at diagnosis and the stage of disease. However, these two variables alone do not define

**TABLE 95–8**

**International Neuroblastoma Pathology Classifications**

| Age | Neuroblast Differentiation | MKI |
|---|---|---|
| *Favorable* | | |
| <1.5 years | Poor or differentiating | Low or intermediate |
| 1.5-5 years | Differentiating | Low |
| *Unfavorable* | | |
| <1.5 years | Undifferentiated | High |
| 1.5-5 years | Undifferentiated or poorly differentiated | Intermediate or high |
| >5 years | Any | Any |

1. **Ganglioneuroblastoma**
   Composite of schwannian stroma-rich and stroma-poor, or schwannian stroma-rich
2. **Ganglioneuroma**
   Schwannian stroma-dominant
3. **Neuroblastoma**
   Schwannian stroma-poor

a homogeneous group with respect to outcome. Additional molecular characteristics that have been correlated with unfavorable prognosis include N-*myc* oncogene amplification (Seeger et al, 1985); diploid cellular DNA content (Bowman et al, 1997); chromosomal 1p deletions, 11q deletions, and 17q gains (Bown et al, 1999); and low expression of the nerve growth factor receptor TrkA (Nakagawara et al, 1993; Suzuki et al, 1993). Patients with stage 1 and stage 2 neuroblastomas have a 96% to 100% survival rate with surgery alone (Perez et al, 2000). Infants with stage 3 and stage 4 disease have a poorer survival, even with aggressive chemotherapy, although the outcome, with better than 70% surviving overall, is far better than the 10% to 20% reported for older children (Schmidt et al, 2000).

Stage 4S comprises a unique group of patients with disseminated disease but a good prognosis, a combination that occurs exclusively in infants younger than 1 year of age. In this special group of children, typical findings include a small primary tumor that does not cross the midline and remote spread involving the liver, skin, or bone marrow (with less than 15% of marrow replacement with tumor), without roentgenographic evidence of skeletal metastases. The primary tumor may be unidentifiable. Eighteen of 20 infants younger than 1 year of age with stage 4S disease, in the original observation by D'Angio and associates (1971), were cured of their disease. The 5-year survival rate of all those with stage 4S disease is 92% (Nickerson et al, 2000), compared with 30% of all children with stage 4 disease or 70% of infants younger than 1 year with stage 4 disease (D'Angio et al, 1971; Matthay et al, 1999; Schmidt et al, 2000). Haas and colleagues (1988) reviewed outcomes in 212 infants with stage 4S neuroblastoma and found that only 13% died of disease progression, whereas 12% died of therapy-related causes. Biologic differences have been demonstrated between stage 4S and stage 4 neuroblastoma, with lack of elevated serum ferritin levels in stage 4S disease compared with stage 4 disease (Hann et al, 1981). There is usually lack of N-*myc* oncogene amplification in stage 4S tumors, in contrast to stage 4 tumors (Seeger et al, 1985). In general, infants with stage 4S disease can be observed without chemotherapy unless they experience symptoms secondary to local disease progression, such as respiratory distress from increasing hepatomegaly.

Amplification of the N-*myc* oncogene in primary neuroblastoma also has been shown to correlate with advanced-stage disease and with rapid tumor progression regardless of stage (Brodeur et al, 1984; Seeger et al, 1985). Estimated progression-free survival rates were 68%, 30%, and 0%, respectively, for patients whose tumors had 1, 3 to 10, or more than 10 copies of the N-*myc* oncogene. Patients with stage 1, 2, or 4S disease demonstrate N-*myc* amplification only rarely; when present, it has been associated with rapid disease progression in these usually favorable stages (Bourhis et al, 1991; Perez et al, 2000). Approximately 10% of patients with stage 2 disease exhibit amplification; a majority of such patients to date has development of rapid disease progression and death within 2 years of diagnosis. Thus, N-*myc* amplification is a significant prognostic factor that is independent of stage. It is most helpful in identifying newborns with high-risk disease. In the most recent Children's Cancer Group study of stage 4 neuroblastoma in infants, the progression-free survival rate after 3 years was less than 10% in children with tumors that demonstrate N-*myc* amplification, compared with 93% for those with single-copy tumors (Schmidt et al, 2000).

Total cellular DNA content also may predict response to therapy in infants with neuroblastoma (Bowman et al, 1997; Look et al, 1991). Infants with hyperdiploid tumors had a significantly better response to therapy than was noted in those with diploid tumors. Furthermore, hyperdiploidy correlated with stage 4S. Diploidy often correlates with tumor N-*myc* amplification, although in rare cases of hyperdiploidy with N-*myc* amplification, the N-*myc* amplification portends an unfavorable outcome. Other researchers confirmed the poor prognosis of patients with diploid (euploid) tumors and correlated tumor DNA with histologic grading and clinical stage (Gansler et al, 1986; Hayashi et al, 1989).

Tumor karyotype also may influence outcome in neuroblastoma: Abnormalities of the short arm of chromosome 1 are more common in patients with metastatic disease but are rare in patients with stage 1, 2, and 4S disease (Christiansen and Lampert, 1988; Fong et al, 1989). Both allelic losses on chromosome 1 and gains on chromosome 17q are unfavorable prognostic factors in neuroblastoma (Bown et al, 1999; Caron, 1995). It has been shown by multiple groups of investigators that expression of high-affinity nerve growth factor receptors (e.g., glycoprotein [gp] $140^{trk\text{-}A}$) is a favorable prognostic factor, highly predictive of a good outcome regardless of age. Infants whose tumor has high gp $140^{trk\text{-}A}$ expression have an 87% survival rate, compared with those with low expression, who have a 26% survival rate (Nakagawara et al, 1993; Suzuki et al, 1993).

### Treatment

A number of children—most commonly, infants with stage 4S disease—have experienced spontaneous tumor regression despite the presence of metastases. In other instances, malignant neuroblastomas have apparently undergone maturation into benign ganglioneuromas. The case shown in Figure 95–4 is an example of spontaneous maturation and regression (Haas et al, 1988). The diagnosis of neuroblastoma was made before the age of 6 months in 21 of 29 collected case reports in which spontaneous regression occurred (Everson, 1967). The remainder of the cases were diagnosed in patients between 6 and 24 months of age.

The relationship of spontaneous regression to age also has been noted (Evans et al, 1971). In one study, a majority of patients who experienced tumor regression were younger than 6 months of age and were usually those with stage 2 or stage 4S disease (Evans et al, 1971). Some patients with spontaneous regression of stage 4 disease have been reported (Sitarz et al, 1975). The mechanism of the spontaneous regression is uncertain, although in at least three cases, pathologic differentiation and maturation to ganglioneuroma have been documented. Regression has now also been documented in patients with neuroblastomas that are localized and detected either on prenatal ultrasound examination or by urine screening. Such patients have sometimes been observed rather than undergoing surgical resection, with documented regression in 11 patients (Yamamoto et al, 1998).

The unpredictable course of neuroblastoma, with its occasional spontaneous maturation or regression, not only makes the tumor unusual but also causes difficulty in planning therapy. The type and intensity of treatment can be based on the ability to define infants with relatively good, intermediate, and poor prognoses based on stage, Shimada histology, ploidy, and N-*myc* amplification. Patients who have localized disease (stage 1 or 2) without amplification of N-*myc* have a 90% to 100% survival with surgery alone, even if the tumor is not completely resected. Such patients should undergo surgical resection or partial resection, but they probably will not derive any additional benefits from postoperative radiation therapy or chemotherapy. An exception to this rule is in the case of spinal cord compression, in which prompt decompression either with chemotherapy, local irradiation, or laminoplasty may be used to preserve function. There is an increasing trend to use chemotherapy first, given the exquisite sensitivity of the tumor to chemotherapeutic agents, but a rapid deterioration in neurologic function should prompt alternative interventions. A neurosurgeon should always be consulted early in the diagnosis (De Bernardi et al, 2001; Katzenstein et al, 2001). The combination of extensive laminectomy with postoperative irradiation should be avoided, because later spinal deformity is almost inevitable. If a recurrence develops after local therapy for stage 2 neuroblastoma, the patient almost always has a good response and outcome with further treatment (Matthay et al, 1989; Perez et al, 2000).

Patients with stage 4S disease have a highly favorable prognosis and may require minimal therapy. Because many patients undergo spontaneous regression without chemotherapy and the overall disease-free survival rate is 85% to 90%, therapy should be directed toward supportive care, with use of chemotherapy and surgery restricted to relieving symptoms. The main cause of death is massive hepatic involvement resulting in respiratory insufficiency or compromise of renal or gastrointestinal function. In a review of 212 cases in the literature (Haas, 1988), 21 patients died of local disease progression, 20 died of therapy-related causes, and only 7 died of progression to a stage 4 tumor. The hepatic tumor often regresses with low-dose radiation therapy at a dose of 450 cGy given in three fractions through across-table, opposed ports angled to avoid the kidneys, spine, and ovaries. Concomitant low-dose cyclophosphamide often hastens tumor regression. No benefit has been shown to result from resection of the primary tumor, despite anecdotal case reports. Nutritional and blood product support also may be necessary until the lesions begin to resolve. Only in the rare 3% of cases in which progression to a stage 4 lesion occurs is intensive antineoplastic treatment required.

Infants with stage 3 and stage 4 disease usually are treated with combination chemotherapy and local surgery, with radiation therapy given only as necessary to eradicate residual disease. Current Children's Oncology Group protocols assign infants with stage 3 or 4 disease to the intermediate-risk group if the tumors lack N-*myc* amplification. Active drugs that are most commonly used in treatment programs for neuroblastoma include cisplatin, etoposide, doxorubicin, cyclophosphamide, vincristine, and ifosfamide. A small group of infants with a very unfavorable prognosis is comprised of patients with stage 4 disease with amplification of the N-*myc* oncogene; it is possible that for such patients, as in older children with neuroblastoma, standard chemotherapy regimens will be insufficient for cure. In these high-risk patients, intensive chemotherapy with higher doses of the aforementioned agents, in combination with myeloablative therapy followed by bone marrow infusion, may offer additional benefit (Matthay et al, 1999; Valteau-Couanet et al, 2000). In addition, the use of the differentiation agent *cis*-retinoic acid has been shown to improve survival in patients with advanced-stage, high-risk neuroblastoma (Matthay et al, 1999).

## Congenital Leukemia

### Epidemiology

Despite the fact that leukemia is the second most common malignancy diagnosed in infants before the age of 1 year, this disease rarely occurs during the first month of life. Most of the neonatal cases of congenital leukemia are reported to arise from the myeloid lineage, in contrast with the predominance of acute lymphoblastic leukemia (ALL) found in later childhood. In particular, constitutional chromosomal disorders such as trisomy 21 are associated with acute myelogenous leukemia (AML) in the newborn period and, perhaps more intriguingly, with transient myeloproliferative disorder (TMD). However, despite the relative infrequency of congenital leukemia in the newborn period, both myeloid and lymphoid diseases are associated with a high mortality rate secondary to the aggressive biology of the diseases and the complications of the required treatment.

The etiology of infant leukemia is unclear; however genetic epidemiologic studies indicate that many cases, if not all, are initiated in utero. Several studies have demonstrated the presence of leukemia-associated gene rearrangements in the newborn Guthrie "blood spots" of children who subsequently developed leukemia (Ford et al, 1993, 1998).

### Clinical Manifestations

The clinical signs of leukemia may be evident at birth: hepatosplenomegaly, petechiae, and ecchymoses. In addition, myeloid leukemic cell infiltration into the skin (leukemia cutis) results in nodular fibroma-like masses. These tumors are freely movable over the subcutaneous tissue, with a greenish-blue discoloration of the overlying skin (Fig. 95–6). These solid masses of myeloid leukemia are called *chloromas* because of the abundance of myeloperoxidase causing the greenish discoloration. Such cutaneous lesions are commonly found when the disease appears at birth and have been noted in stillborn premature infants with leukemia. They may be the first clinical sign of the disease. If chloromas are present on the head or neck of young infants, further imaging of the head and neck area should be done to assess for the presence of intracranial or skull involvement. At birth, many of the infants have respiratory distress from leukemic infiltration in the lungs. Severe respiratory difficulty may develop soon after birth from pulmonary hemorrhage secondary to thrombocytopenia. In addition, some infants may appear somnolent or have periodic apnea as a result of CNS leukostasis, caused by sludging of the increased white blood cells in the vessels.

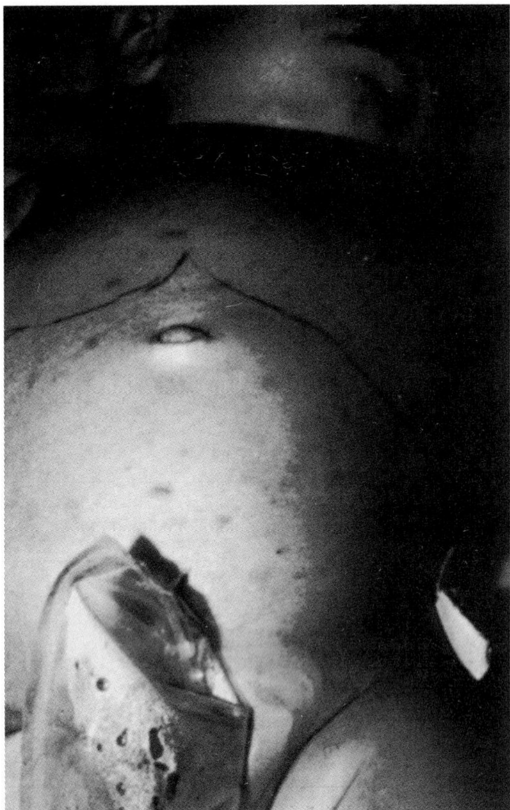

**FIGURE 95–6.** Leukemia cutis in a newborn infant.

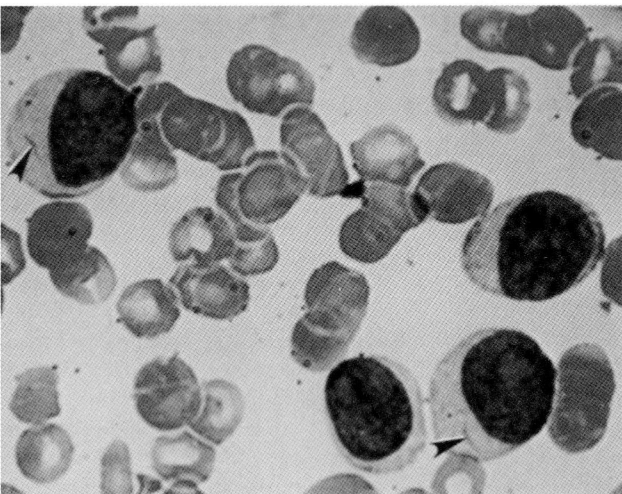

**FIGURE 95–7.** Malignant blast cells with Auer rods *(arrowheads)* present in cytoplasm. This finding is diagnostic of acute myelogenous leukemia.

In those infants in whom signs of the disease develop within the first month but in whom no detectable signs of leukemia were noted at birth, the symptoms often are ill defined, with lethargy, diarrhea, hepatomegaly, and poor feeding with failure to gain weight. In addition, affected infants can present with fever due to bacterial infections. Hemorrhagic manifestations also can be the first signs of the disease, and leukemia cutis is less common.

### Laboratory Manifestations

Hemoglobin levels often appear normal at first, but they soon decline to low levels as the normal decrease in red cell production after birth is combined with the expansion of the leukemia. Total white blood cell counts may be within normal limits or diminished, but leukocytosis is more often present. White blood cell counts of 150,000 to 250,000/mm$^3$ or more are common, and counts as high as 1.3 million/mm$^3$ have been recorded. There is usually a predominance of blast cells and immature granulocytes. Auer rods, pathognomonic of AML, may be present in the blast cells (Fig. 95–7). These intracellular inclusions are composed of lysosomes.

### Differential Diagnosis

A number of newborns described in the earlier literature who were originally believed to have leukemia were later found to have other diseases. Confusion with infections such as congenital syphilis, cytomegalovirus (CMV) infection, toxoplasmosis, and bacterial infections may occur because of the leukocytosis, organomegaly, and thrombocytopenia that can accompany these diseases. The low platelet counts and leukemoid reactions reported in infants with congenital amegakaryocytic thrombocytopenia may also lead to an incorrect diagnosis of leukemia, but the absence of radii commonly seen in these children is a major clue to the correct diagnosis. In addition, infants with trisomy 21 are at higher risk for TMDs and leukemia. These topics are discussed in a section on Down syndrome.

Severe erythroblastosis fetalis can mimic leukemia. Affected infants usually have hepatosplenomegaly, large numbers of nucleated erythroblasts in the peripheral blood, and occasionally, thrombocytopenia. Small infiltrates of extramedullary erythropoiesis may appear in the skin, superficially resembling leukemia cutis. Infants with neonatal neuroblastoma often have hepatomegaly and may also have discolored tumor nodules in the subcutaneous tissue (see Figs. 95–4 and Fig. 95–5). Their blood cell counts are usually normal without circulating blasts, and specimens of bone marrow, if involved, reveal small clusters of neuroblastoma cells (see Fig. 95–2). Although these cells may resemble leukemia blast cells, their tendency to occur in clumps in an otherwise normal bone marrow distinguishes them from leukemic blasts, which usually completely replace the normal bone marrow. In rare cases of complete bone marrow replacement, increased excretion of catecholamine metabolites and the presence of an abdominal mass or other primary lesion are clues to the diagnosis of neuroblastoma. In addition, histochemical stains also can differentiate neuroblastoma from leukemia.

Congenital human immunodeficiency virus (HIV) infection also may rarely be confused with leukemia. Clonal B-cell expansions in such patients may cause lymphadenopathy. One newborn infected with HIV reported by Voelkerding presented with thrombocytopenia and had lymphocyte clusters in the bone marrow that were of B-cell lineage, clonal as defined by immune globulin gene arrangement, and positive for the common acute lymphoblastic leukemia antigen (CD10) (Voelkerding et al, 1988).

However, the patient was well and without evidence of lymphoproliferative disease one year later.

A marked but transient leukemoid reaction may occur in the newborn following in utero exposure to betamethasone (Barak et al, 1992; Calhoun et al, 1996). Lack of the usual clinical and laboratory findings of leukemia and of the appropriate clinical history usually excludes the diagnosis of leukemia.

### Cellular Morphology and Immunophenotype

The bone marrow of a normal newborn is normally hypercellular, so a bone marrow aspirate from an afflicted newborn with leukemia shows extreme hypercellularity in combination with a marked predominance of the immature cells of the cell series affected, either myeloid or lymphoid. ALL and AML are differentiated on the basis of typical morphologic characteristics, such as the presence of granules or Auer rods (in AML) and nuclear and cytoplasmic morphology, cytochemical stains, immunophenotyping, and chromosome analysis. Periodic acid–Schiff stain shows large aggregates of pink glycogen in the cytoplasm of the blast cells in ALL, whereas the pattern in AML is finely granular and diffuse. Most ALL cells stain positively for terminal deoxynucleotidyl transferase, a DNA polymerase that catalyzes the polymerization of deoxynucleotides in thymocytes. This enzyme is present in 90% of cases of ALL but in less than 5% of cases of AML. In addition, the blasts in AML are generally positive for myeloperoxidase, whereas lymphoblasts are not. Both types of leukemia are subclassified according to an international French-American-British (FAB) classification based on morphology and histochemistry (Pui et al, 1995) (see Table 95–8). The most common FAB morphology in infantile and neonatal AML is monocytic (FAB M5) or myelomonocytic (FAB M4) (Odom and Gordon, 1984; van Wering and Kamps, 1986), whereas the most common subtype in ALL is the FAB L1 variety (Sande et al, 1999).

The immunophenotype of the leukemia is determined using a panel of fluorescently labeled monoclonal antibodies against a variety of cluster of differentiation (CD) antigens and is critical for differentiating lymphoid from myeloid leukemias (Pui et al, 1993). The myeloid leukemias react with antibodies to the CD13/CD33 antigens, present on cells of myeloid and monocytic lineage. The only exception is the FAB M7 category, also known as acute megakaryoblastic leukemia, which expresses the CD41/CD42 platelet glycoprotein and CD61. Acute megakaryoblastic leukemia is most commonly seen in patients with trisomy 21. Most of the neonatal and infant acute lymphoblastic leukemia cells exhibit an early precursor B-cell phenotype and often are CD1a, CD19, CD24, and CD15 positive and CD10 negative (Crist et al, 1986; Katz et al, 1988; Pui et al, 1987, 1995). In addition, coexpression of myeloid antigens is frequently present. The frequent rearrangements of the immune globulin heavy-chain gene and occasionally the light-chain gene, but almost never the T-cell receptor gene, also may be helpful in the subclassification and elucidation of the biology of neonatal ALL (Felix et al, 1987; Ludwig et al, 1989). The acute leukemia surface antigen expression is summarized in Table 95–8.

### Genetics and Prognosis

The discovery of chromosomal abnormalities in leukemic cells has contributed greatly to the classification and understanding of the biology of acute leukemias. In addition, certain translocations have prognostic significance for both ALL and AML. The most common chromosome locus involved in infantile ALL and AML is found on 11q23. Abnormalities of 11q23 are found in at least 50% of infant leukemias and in a predominance of neonatal cases (Kaneko et al, 1988). The gene that is disrupted by 11q23 translocations, designated *MLL*, *HRX*, *ALL-1*, or *HTRX-1*, is the human homologue of the trithorax gene in *Drosophila melanogaster* (Ziemin-van der Poel et al, 1991). The trithorax gene is critical for the exoskeletal development of the fly. In mice and in humans, the MLL protein positively regulates *HOX* genes, which are critical for hematopoietic development (Armstrong et al, 2002).

Rearrangements involving 11q23 are the most common clonal chromosomal abnormalities found in infant leukemias (Pui and Evans, 1999; Pui et al, 2000). In older children and adults, this gene is frequently disrupted in secondary (therapy-related) AML induced by epipodophyllotoxin therapy. Epipodophyllotoxins (e.g., etoposide) act by inhibiting topoisomerase 2, a DNA repair enzyme. Accordingly, intrauterine exposure to topoisomerase 2 inhibitors may be responsible for some cases of leukemia in infants (Pui and Evans, 1999; Ross, 2000; Ross et al, 1996). In addition, it has been shown that the nucleotides involved in the breakpoint of the 11q23 locus may be more susceptible to topoisomerase 2–induced breaks (Strick et al, 2000). The Children's Cancer Group has reported a higher incidence of acute myeloid, but not lymphoid, leukemia in the infants of mothers who consumed larger amounts of naturally occurring topoisomerase 2 inhibitors, such as those in foods high in flavonoids and phytates (Ross, 2000; Ross et al, 1996).

The t(4;11)(q21;q23) gene rearrangement is detected in up to 40% of infants with acute lymphoblastic leukemia by molecular analysis. It generally is associated with a poor prognosis when it is accompanied by coexpression of myeloid antigens in infants younger than 6 months of age (Chen et al, 1993; Heerema et al, 1994; Rubnitz et al, 1994). Additional rearrangements can be detected in the remainder of the infant population with other fusion partners, raising the incidence of 11q23 abnormalities up to 80%. The t(4;11)(q21;q23) is the best characterized of the rearrangements involving the *MLL* gene. It generally is associated with hyperleukocytosis, CNS leukemia, and a precursor B-cell immunophenotype with $CD19^+$, $CD15^+$, $CD10^-$. Curiously, older children harboring this same rearrangement do not have the same dismal prognosis as that identified for infants younger than 1 year; reasons for this are still unclear. Recent work in gene expression analysis demonstrates unique genetic signatures that separate infant ALL with *MLL* rearrangements from ALL and AML in older children (Armstrong et al, 2002). These studies may provide the basis for novel drug discovery focusing on genes overexpressed in *MLL*-rearranged leukemias, given the poor prognosis of many of these infants with current therapies.

The t(9;11)(p22;q23), t(1;22)(p13;q13), and t(11;19)(p21;q23) are three of the more frequent cytogenetic abnormalities found in infants with acute myeloid leukemia and 11q23 rearrangements (Sande et al, 1999). Hyperleukocytosis and extramedullary involvement are common in infants with AML. In case reports of leukemia cutis and even leukemia occurring in infants without bone marrow involvement, spontaneous resolution has occurred without chemotherapy (Mora et al, 2000). In general, these leukemias lack 11q23 rearrangements. When 11q23 rearrangements are present, they generally progress to systemic disease; therefore, systemic therapy is advised for those patients with cutaneous disease only who harbor such rearrangements.

### Treatment

The course of congenital leukemia usually has been one of rapid deterioration and death from hemorrhage or infection. Although the length of survival has been significantly prolonged in children with leukemia, success has been limited in newborns. The infant with leukemia frequently presents with hyperleukocytosis (blast cell count in excess of 100,000/mm$^3$). Hyperleukocytosis may result in sludging of blast cells in capillaries with resultant intracranial hemorrhage, respiratory distress, or problems from tumor lysis with hyperkalemia, hyperphosphatemia, hypocalcemia, hyperuricemia, and renal failure. These metabolic problems should be corrected before initiation of chemotherapy. In the infant, exchange transfusion is the easiest way to accomplish this and simultaneously lower the white blood cell count, which further decreases tumor lysis problems once chemotherapy is begun.

Disseminated intravascular coagulation is another common complication seen in hyperleukocytosis and infantile leukemia, especially when monocytic subtypes are suspected. The monoblasts release procoagulants, causing a consumptive coagulopathy, which initially may be exacerbated with further cell lysis from chemotherapy, necessitating support with transfusion of platelets and fresh frozen plasma. In addition, CNS involvement is common in infants with ALL and AML. Evaluation of cerebrospinal fluid and intrathecal prophylactic chemotherapy is a routine part of treatment. Radiation therapy, which is indicated in older children with CNS leukemia, is deferred in most instances until 1 year after diagnosis, to limit potential late effects in neonates.

The current improved success of remission induction with treatment of AML in infants younger than 1 year is similar to that obtained in older children using intensive combination chemotherapy regimens (Bresters et al, 2002; Chessells et al, 2002). The chemotherapy regimens used in infants with myeloid leukemia are identical to those used in older children. The experience with newborns is limited, but between 1984 and 1989, 5 of 12 newborns with AML sustained complete remissions with chemotherapy; all were in the myelomonocytic or monocytic category (Kaneko et al, 1988; Odom and Gordon, 1984).

Up until recently, the treatment outcome in ALL was significantly poorer in infants younger than 1 year at diagnosis (20% to 50% disease-free survival, compared with 80% for older children). Several studies of infant leukemia reported only 10% to 20% survival for infants younger than 6 months of age at diagnosis, compared with 40% for those older than 6 months (Chessells et al, 1994; Heerema et al, 1994). Less than 15% of newborns with acute lymphoblastic leukemia had remissions lasting more than a few months with use of protocols similar to those used in older children. However, recent outcomes for infants have improved slightly with the addition of high-dose cytarabine and high-dose methotrexate. The addition of these two agents has improved the 4-year event-free survival (EFS) rate in some small series to approximately 50% (Silverman et al, 1997). The use of cytarabine, which generally is used in the treatment of AML, may address the more primitive nature of the *MLL*-rearranged ALL cell, with its frequent coexpression of myeloid antigens and lack of CD10 positivity. An international protocol, Interfant 99, currently being used to treat infants in the United States and Europe incorporates these agents; data from this trial are expected to verify their importance in a larger population. In general, the use of bone marrow transplantation has not been shown to be of benefit (Pui et al, 2002). The use of bone marrow transplantation is restricted in the Interfant 99 protocol to those patients who have had poor responses to systemic steroids. These patients tend to relapse within the first year of diagnosis, so that lack of disease beyond the first year is an important landmark in caring for them.

## *Transient Myeloproliferative Disorders and Leukemia in Patients with Down Syndrome*

An increased incidence of acute leukemia in children with Down syndrome (10- to 30-fold increased risk) is well recognized (Fong and Brodeur, 1987). A review of the world literature by Rosner and Lee (1972) revealed 227 children with both disorders; 31% had acute myelogenous leukemia, and 69% had ALL. Among the 47 infants with leukemia, 58% had myeloblastic leukemia and 42% had lymphoblastic leukemia. In infants younger than 3 years of age with Down syndrome and leukemia, the rare megakaryoblastic subtype (M7) predominates and carries a favorable prognosis (Pui, 1995). In addition, neonates with Down syndrome can present with a TMD that usually resolves without treatment. Approximately 30% of these affected children are at risk for developing leukemia later in life. A comprehensive review on the hematopoietic disorders affecting children with Down syndrome summarizes their management (Lange, 2000).

## *Transient Myeloproliferative Disorder*

Patients with Down syndrome can manifest a myeloproliferative disorder in the newborn period indistinguishable from leukemia. Various terms (in addition to "transient myeloproliferative disorder") have been used to describe this phenomenon, including transient leukemia and transient congenital leukemia. TMD also may be seen in trisomy 21 mosaicism (Seibel et al, 1984) and has been reported in two normal infants in whom the trisomy was detected only in the leukemic cells (Ridgway et al, 1990). Some infants with the TMD without Down syndrome also have been described, and true leukemia has subsequently recurred (Brissette et al, 1994). Patients with Down syndrome and

TMD have a 30% chance of developing leukemia later in life, either by developing a recurrence of TMD that progresses to leukemia or by developing a new leukemia unrelated to the TMD.

TMD is a clonal disorder typically manifested by hepatomegaly, splenomegaly, and circulating myeloblasts. There may or may not be associated anemia and thrombocytopenia. The morphology of the blasts often appears to be megakaryoblastic. In general, the blast count of the peripheral blood exceeds that of the marrow. Cytogenetic analysis may or may not reveal abnormalities, but findings often are normal, with the exception of the trisomy 21. Eighteen Down syndrome infants who had a TMD initially indistinguishable from AML experienced complete clinical and hematologic recovery without systemic therapy. Recently, somatic mutations in the *GATA1* transcription factor have been detected in 100% of patients with trisomy 21 and TMD (Mundschau et al, 2003).

In a majority of infants, the blast count slowly decreases over 2 to 3 weeks, and the hemoglobin and platelet counts normalize. However, less commonly, spontaneous resolution does not occur, and the neonate may experience clinical deterioration manifested by progressive hepatosplenomegaly and hepatic dysfunction, formation of pleural or pericardial effusions, and marrow failure. In these cases, treatment with low-dose cytarabine can be life-saving. In some instances, these complications can occur in utero, and varying degrees of hydrops fetalis can result. CNS involvement is rare in these neonates with clinically symptomatic TMD. In addition, 25% of infants with resolved TMD have later experienced recurrence of their disease with progression to AML (Isaacs, 1997). These patients, as well as other patients with Down syndrome and de novo AML, are treated with a less intensive regimen of chemotherapy, with excellent outcomes (Lange et al, 1998).

## *Leukemia and Down Syndrome*

As stated earlier, patients with Down syndrome are at a higher risk of developing leukemia, but the reasons for this increased risk remain unclear. The most popular hypothesis is that there is a leukemia predisposition gene on chromosome 21 which is over-expressed as a result of the constitutional trisomy 21. Acute megakaryoblastic leukemia (AMKL) predominates in infants, while the incidence of ALL increases with age. Similar to what has been described in TMD, mutations in *GATA1* have been reported in all cases of AMKL-DS analyzed to date. Specifically, mutations in *GATA1* have not been detected in non-DS-AMKL (Wechsler et al, 2002).

Patients with Down syndrome and AML have excellent outcomes compared with persons without Down syndrome and AML. In particular, megakaryoblastic AML in normal hosts often carries a dire prognosis, while the same disease in patients with Down syndrome is usually curable (Lange et al, 1998). Reasons for this are unclear but it is well known that patients with Down syndrome also experience greater toxicity from all of the chemotherapy agents used. Some investigators have hypothesized three possible mechanisms to explain simultaneous enhanced efficacy and host toxicity in this population: reduced folate pools, increased free radical generation, and increased generation of the active daunorubicin metabolite (Taub et al, 1996, 1997). Thus, patients with Down syndrome and AML receive treatment protocols involving less intensive chemotherapy regimens, with excellent outcomes. Current treatment protocols sponsored by the Children's Oncology Group are enrolling patients with Down syndrome and TMD or AML in order to capture data on the natural history of TMD, the progression to AML, and secondary biologic factors that may affect the disease.

Older patients with Down syndrome also develop ALL at a higher frequency. Outcomes are similar to those for non–Down syndrome patients and do not appear to be related to tolerance of therapy (Dordelmann et al, 1998). Delays in therapy secondary to excess toxicity, however, can pose unique challenges in the treatment for these patients (Levitt et al, 1990).

## Germ Cell Tumors

Germ cell tumors are neoplasms that contain derivatives of more than one of the three primary germ layers of the embryo. Although these tumors most often are benign in the newborn, one or more of the germ layer derivatives may develop malignant characteristics. A mature teratoma, a term used for a benign germ cell tumor, may arise in a wide variety of locations of the body but usually occurs along the axial midline during early childhood, such as the pineal gland, neck, mediastinum, retroperitoneum, and sacrococcygeal region. In the neonatal period, a majority of teratomas occurs in the sacrococcygeal region, followed next by tumors in the neck. After puberty, teratomas most frequently occur in the gonads, particularly the ovary.

### Staging

Appropriate imaging of the primary tumor using MRI or CT is indicated to best visualize the extent of the disease. In particular, sacrococcygeal tumors should be visualized by MRI to exclude involvement of the spinal cord (Gobel et al, 1998, 2001). In addition, the remainder of the abdomen should be visualized to assess for the extent of local invasion—in particular, involvement of the rectal wall. All patients with germ cell tumors and elevated age-adjusted hormonal markers, such as alpha-fetoprotein (AFP) or hCG, also should have a diagnostic chest CT scan to rule out metastasis. Baseline levels of AFP and hCG are elevated in healthy neonates. The half-life of AFP is 5 to 7 days; that of hCG is 24 to 36 hours. The normal range of serum AFP is discussed in Chapter 18.

### Pathology

Teratomas are composed of tissues arising from all three layers of the embryonic disk. Ectodermal components, including glial tissue, are a major component of teratomas presenting at birth, in particular, sacrococcygeal tumors (Isaacs, 1997). There are often skin, hair, and teeth elements as well. Mesodermal components, including fat, bone, and muscle, also are present. Less commonly seen are endodermal components such as digestive tract tissue.

Occasionally, less mature elements coexist within the teratoma and are typified by higher grade histologic features including nuclear atypia, mitotic activity, and hypercellularity. Hormonal markers, including serum AFP and hCG, often are elevated in the presence of malignant tissue within the teratoma and are useful to follow as therapy progresses. Elevated serum AFP indicates the presence of immature endodermal sinus tissue or yolk sac elements, while elevated hCG indicates the presence of embryonal carcinoma. Choriocarcinoma also manifests with an elevated hCG and clinical bleeding but is rarely found in teratomas of the newborn (Isaacs, 1997). More often, it represents a placental disease or, rarely, a primary intracranial, liver, or kidney tumor.

### *Sacrococcygeal Teratomas*

The sacrococcygeal teratoma is the most common solid tumor in the newborn, although it is rarely malignant. The estimated incidence is 1/20,000 to 1/40,000 births (Isaacs, 1997). Females are affected two to four times more frequently than males. The earliest detection of a teratoma may occur prenatally or at birth. Polyhydramnios, nonimmune fetal hydrops, and dystocia all have been described in association with germ cell tumors. Congenital anomalies are often present in association with sacrococcygeal teratomas, including genitourinary, hindgut, and lower vertebral malformations. In most cases, the tumor manifests as a mass protruding between the coccyx and rectum; the mass may be quite large (Fig. 95–8). About 10% of these tumors are found by rectal examination. Nearly all arise at the tip or inner surface of the coccyx and can be diagnosed early in life by the pediatrician who makes the rectal examination a routine part of the physical examination. An estimated 30 children per year are diagnosed in North America with sacrococcygeal teratomas before the age of 2 to 3 months.

#### Differential Diagnosis

Sacrococcygeal teratomas may be confused with meningomyeloceles, rectal abscesses, pelvic neuroblastomas, pilonidal cysts, and a variety of very rare neoplasms that may occur in that region. Most benign teratomas in this area produce no functional difficulties, even when marked intrapelvic extension is present. Thus, bowel or bladder dysfunction, painful defecation, and vascular or lymphatic obstruction suggest that the lesion is malignant.

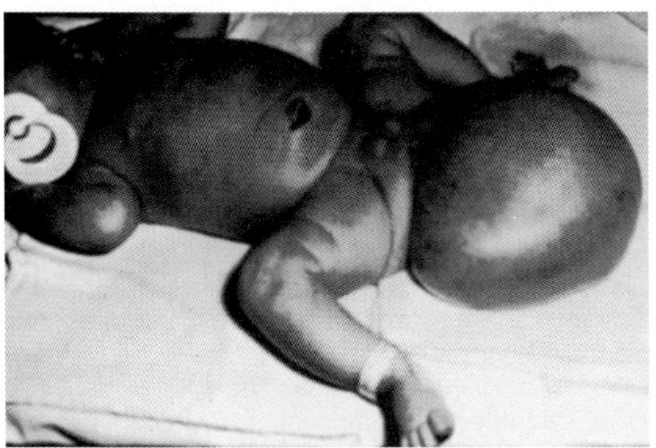

**FIGURE 95–8.** Large sacrococcygeal teratoma in a newborn girl.

#### Treatment

Treatment of sacrococcygeal tumors is primarily surgical if age-adjusted AFP and hCG levels are normal (Gobel et al, 1998). They should be radically excised as soon as possible because small, undifferentiated foci may proliferate and become aggressive. They are attached to the coccyx; therefore, removal of the entire coccyx is an absolutely necessary part of the surgical procedure. Failure to remove the coccyx carries a 30% to 40% risk of local recurrence, and such recurrences may be accompanied by malignant elements. Fetal surgery has been used successfully with long-term survival in at least one report, but the co-morbidities that accompany this high risk procedure preclude its routine use (Graf et al, 2000). Sixty percent to 70% of sacrococcygeal teratomas in newborns are unequivocally benign, as determined by the presence of mature tissues. In general, the risk for malignancy is present only in the sacrococcygeal tumors, whereas those in the nasopharynx, neck, mediastinum, or retroperitoneum do not usually contain malignant germ cell elements. Local recurrence or metastasis of teratoma is rare but may occur when immature elements are present or when surgical resection is incomplete. In the series of 398 cases reported by Altman and associates (1974), 60% of the patients with malignant tumors died within 10 months of surgery, 21% were alive with residual disease, 11% were alive without apparent disease, and 9% were lost to follow-up. These findings contrast markedly with the mortality rate reported for children with benign lesions, which was approximately 5%.

Chemotherapy regimens including cisplatin and/or bleomycin have markedly improved the survival of patients with malignant germ cell tumors. In a nonrandomized trial between 1983 and 1995, 71 patients with malignant sacrococcygeal tumors received a combination of surgery and chemotherapy (Gobel et al, 2001). Treatment decisions were made on the basis of the diagnostic scan and the surgical resection. The 5-year EFS rate was 76%, and the overall survival rate was 81%. Current recommendations for patients presenting with elevated age-adjusted AFP and sacrococcygeal tumors are for complete surgical resection only if the primary tumor is small and focal. Patients who have tumors containing immature elements are followed with serial AFP measurements. They are treated with chemotherapy if the serum AFP remains elevated or begins to increase. In all other cases, chemotherapy regimens containing cisplatin for four cycles is recommended, followed by surgical resection. This approach maximizes the possibility of achieving a complete resection, a goal worth attaining in these tumors. The addition of regimens containing cisplatin, carboplatin, etoposide, and bleomycin to the therapy for disseminated germ cell tumors has improved the disease-free survival rate to more than 50% (Ablin et al, 1991; Marina et al, 1992; Nair et al, 1994). Some infants have died of the complications of the intensive therapy (Raney et al, 1981), and it is important to make appropriate dose modifications.

## Renal Neoplasms

Approximately two thirds of intra-abdominal masses in the neonatal period arise from the kidney. The vast majority of these neoplasms are nonmalignant and are generally due to congenital defects such as polycystic or dysplastic kidneys or other conditions causing hydronephrosis. The most common intrarenal neoplasm manifesting at birth is congenital mesoblastic nephroma, followed by Wilms tumor. In addition, it may be difficult to differentiate an intra-abdominal neuroblastoma from an intrarenal tumor, although this distinction is more easily made with current imaging modalities, such as CT or MRI. Wilms tumor distorts the kidney, whereas neuroblastoma displaces it; this preoperative distinction may be difficult to make when neuroblastoma arises within kidney substance. Less common intrarenal neoplasms also seen in the newborn period are rhabdoid tumor, nephroblastomatosis, cystic renal tumors, renal cell carcinoma, rhabdomyosarcoma, hemangiopericytoma, and lymphoma.

### *Congenital Mesoblastic Nephroma*

The congenital mesoblastic nephroma (CMN), or fetal mesenchymal hamartoma, is clearly distinguishable from Wilms tumor by its benign nature. It is the most common intrarenal neoplasm in the neonate. The involved kidney is usually greatly enlarged and distorted by the tumor, but, contrary to the findings with Wilms tumor, there is usually no lobulation, necrosis, hemorrhage, or discrete capsule between the neoplasm and compressed kidney (Fig. 95–9). Although in most cases the tumor manifests as an asymptomatic abdominal mass, the large size may cause problems. Polyhydramnios and premature labor occur with increased frequency in women whose infants have mesoblastic nephroma. Polyhydramnios occurs in approximately 71% of pregnancies complicated by CMN. The tumor may be diagnosed prenatally with ultrasonography, which helps to differentiate it from Wilms tumor because of its typical sonographic appearance of concentric echogenic ring–echo-poor ring pattern (Chan et al, 1987). Prenatal diagnosis may allow earlier treatment in symptomatic cases; in one such case, compression of the aorta caused severe congestive heart failure in the fetus, necessitating emergency surgery (Matsumura et al, 1993).

Two histologic subtypes of CMN have been identified: the "classic" histologic subtype and the "cellular" variant. The classic histologic subtype has a preponderance of interlacing bundles of spindle-shaped cells, within which dysplastic tubules and glomeruli are irregularly scattered. Extrarenal infiltration is common, especially into the perihilar connective tissues. Since the initial description, a cellular or atypical variant of congenital mesoblastic nephroma with increased cellularity, focal hemorrhage, necrosis, hypercellularity, and a high mitotic index was described. The cellular variants usually manifest at an older age (mean 5.3 months later) than the classic type (mean age at presentation 16 days) (Pettinato et al, 1989). Cytogenetic analysis of the more cellular tumors often reveals trisomy of chromosomes 8, 11, 17, and 20 (Schofield et al, 1993). Recently, a genetic link between CMN and another infantile tumor, congenital infantile fibrosarcoma, has been established, in part due to the characteristic polysomic and histologic features that these tumors share. Both the cellular variant of CMN and infantile fibrosarcoma harbor a cryptic translocation, the t(12;15) (p13q25), which fuses the *TEL* gene on chromosome 12 with the *TRKC* gene on chromosome 15 (Knezevich et al, 1998; Rubin et al, 1998). Of interest, because the classic form of CMN has not been shown to harbor this rearrangement, some investigators speculate that the classic and cellular forms of CMN are genetically distinct (Knezevich et al, 1998). However, mixed lesions also have been observed, and these generally express the t(12;15) rearrangement. Investigations into the biologic events responsible for neoplasia are ongoing (Wai et al, 2000).

Most patients with CMN have been cured by nephrectomy alone, even in the presence of localized extrarenal extension (Pettinato et al, 1989). Radical nephrectomy with complete excision of the tumor is the treatment of choice; however, in rare instances the tumor is unusually aggressive (Isaacs, 1997). In such instances, metastases have been reported to occur in the lungs and the brain. In cases of advanced disease or surgically unresectable disease, chemotherapy has been used with success (Isaacs, 1997; Loeb et al, 2002).

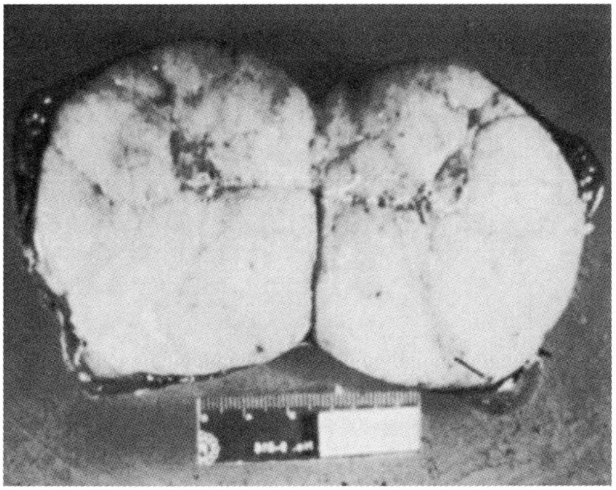

**FIGURE 95–9.** Congenital mesoblastic nephroma compressing and nearly totally replacing the kidney.

## Wilms Tumor

Wilms tumor, or nephroblastoma, is the most common intra-abdominal tumor of childhood but is relatively rare in the neonatal period; it affects 1 in 8000 children. In subsets of children with aniridia, the incidence is much higher. With optimal treatment, cure rates for this neoplasm have increased dramatically, and the overall favorable prognosis for Wilms tumor represents one of the dramatic success stories in the field of cancer therapy. The National Wilms Tumor Study (NWTS), established in 1969, has helped in the rapid accumulation of information regarding the prognosis and treatment of this tumor.

### Clinical Manifestations

Most children with Wilms tumor have either an abdominal or flank mass or an increase in abdominal size noted as the first clinical evidence of disease. This is often first discovered by a parent and brought to the attention of the physician. The tumor lies deep in the flank, is attached to the kidney or is part of it, and usually is firm and smooth. It seldom extends beyond the midline, even though it may grow downward beyond the iliac crest. In 5% to 10% of all cases, tumors involve both kidneys. Gross hematuria is a rare presenting symptom, but microscopic hematuria is found in approximately one fourth of cases. Hematuria in Wilms tumor is not a poor prognostic sign. Hypertension, occasionally noted in older infants and children, has not been observed in the newborn. The tumor may sometimes manifest with abdominal pain and be discovered at laparotomy, and occasionally acute hemorrhage into the tumor may result in a rapidly enlarging mass, usually associated with anemia and fever.

Wilms tumor is seldom diagnosed at birth or during the neonatal period, although several renal tumors have been so large as to have caused dystocia during delivery. Characteristics associated with an earlier presentation include bilaterality and associated aniridia or hypospadias (Pastore et al, 1988) and a positive family history. Rare cases of Wilms tumor associated with polycythemia have been reported; this finding is secondary to an increased production of erythropoietin by the neoplasm. The demonstration of elevated plasma erythropoietin levels in nonpolycythemic children with Wilms tumor studied preoperatively led to the suggestion that this test may be useful in the diagnosis and evaluation of response to therapy.

### Hereditary Associations and Congenital Anomalies

The association among Wilms tumor, hemihypertrophy, cardiac anomalies, congenital aniridia, hamartomas, and genitourinary defects and associated chromosomal changes is discussed earlier in this chapter (under "Genetic Predisposition Syndromes and Congenital Defects"). The finding of hemihypertrophy should alert the physician to observe the child for the possible development of Wilms tumor, adrenal cortical tumor, or hepatoma. Some affected patients may have incomplete forms of BWS (Sotelo-Avila et al, 1980a, 1980b). Occasionally, certain members of a family may have the congenital anomaly and others may have the neoplasm. Meadows and coworkers (1974) described one family in which the mother had congenital hemihypertrophy, three of the children had Wilms tumor, and a fourth had a urinary tract anomaly (Meadows et al, 1974).

The Wilms tumor-aniridia syndrome, a combination of mental retardation, microcephaly, bilateral aniridia, anomalies of the pinna, Wilms tumor, and ambiguous genitalia, is associated with a small deletion of chromosome 11 (11p13-14.1). In some tumor tissues, the same section of DNA deleted from one chromosome may be duplicated on another. Although usually sporadic, this syndrome may occasionally be familial (Yunis and Ramsay, 1980). Rarely, affected persons may demonstrate all of the listed features except the Wilms tumor (Riccardi et al, 1978). In two reports of aniridia in monozygous twins, Wilms tumor developed in only one member of each pair (Maurer et al, 1979). Other congenital conditions that may predispose the patient to Wilms tumor include Turner syndrome and trisomy 18. A variant mutation at 11p13 results in Denys-Drash syndrome: Wilms tumor, genital anomalies, and nephropathy (Coppes and Clericuzio, 1994). Some familial and sporadic cases of Wilms tumor also have been shown to involve loss of heterozygosity at 16q (Newsham et al, 1995) and, in rare cases, changes in chromosome 7 (Wilmore et al, 1994). Bloom syndrome, a rare autosomal recessive disease already known to be associated with a high risk of cancer, has been reported to predispose patients to Wilms tumor (Cairney et al, 1987). Pedigrees showing a predisposition to Wilms tumor are rare, with only 1% of patients having affected siblings or parents; however, such cases tend to occur earlier in infancy. The specific germline abnormality has not yet been successfully localized, although a number of such cases has been examined for the candidate loci on 11p and 16q (Baird et al, 1994). However, the heritability of the unilateral sporadic form of Wilms tumor was examined in 96 long-term survivors (Li, 1988). No Wilms tumor developed in 179 offspring of these patients, confirming the low likelihood of heritability in the sporadic form.

### Prognostic Factors

Several factors seem to influence the response to therapy and ultimate prognosis of the child with Wilms tumor: the histologic pattern, the age of the patient at the time of diagnosis, and the extent of disease. Tumors with better differentiation, showing glomeruloid and tubular formation, indicate a better chance for survival than do those with anaplastic and sarcomatous patterns. Patients younger than 2 years of age at diagnosis have fewer relapses, especially to distant sites, than are seen in older children. Age, however, seems to be of little prognostic significance regarding mortality rate. Specimens weighing more than 250 grams and positive regional lymph nodes, however, are often important predictors of both relapse and death.

### Staging

The most common staging system in use is that devised by the NWTS (Table 95–9). The clinical staging is an important factor in predicting survival; tumors with more extensive spread carry a poorer prognosis. Therefore, adequate evaluation of the extent of tumor involvement is essential and should include CT scans of the abdomen and chest to fully evaluate both kidneys, the inferior vena cava for tumor thrombus, and the liver and lungs, which are the most commonly involved areas of hematogenous spread (Fig. 95–10). Other commonly involved sites of metastatic spread are the retroperitoneum, peritoneum, mediastinum, and pleurae. If histologic studies show a clear cell sarcoma, bone metastases may occur, so a bone scan should be included in the evaluation; rhabdoid tumors, which frequently metastasize to brain, necessitate CT or MRI of the brain.

### Treatment

Before 1950, the two major modalities of therapy for Wilms tumor, surgical removal and radiation therapy, resulted in cure rates approaching 50%. The advantage of treatment with the chemotherapeutic agent dactinomycin was demonstrated in 1966 by Farber, who reported an 89% survival rate in children who had no evidence of metastatic disease at the time of diagnosis and who were followed up

**TABLE 95–9**

**Morphologic and Immunophenotypic Classification of Childhood Acute Leukemia**

| FAB | Morphology | Antigen Expression* |
|---|---|---|
| ALL† | | |
| $L_1$ | Small cells, homogeneous<br>Regular nuclei, scant cytoplasm<br>Inconspicuous nucleoli | Pre=B: HLA-DR, CD10, CD19, CD20, CD24 |
| OR | | OR |
| $L_2$ | Large cells, heterogeneous, irregular or cleft nuclei<br>May be multiple large nucleoli<br>Moderate cytoplasm | T: CD2, CD5, CD7 |
| $L_3$ | Large cells, homogeneous<br>Regular nuclear shape<br>Prominent nucleoli<br>Moderately abundant, deeply basophilic cytoplasm with vacuolation | B: HLA-DR, CD10, CD19, CD20, CD24, Slg* |
| ANLL | | |
| M0 | Minimal myeloid differentiation ($MPO^-$) | CD13, CD33, CD34 |
| M1 | Poorly differentiated myeloblasts ($MPO^+$) | CD13, CD33, CD34 |
| M2 | Myeloblastic with differentiation ($MPO^+$) | CD13, CD33, CD34 |
| M3 | Promyelocytic ($MPO^+$) | CD11b, CD13, CD33, CD34 |
| M4 | Myelomonoblastic ($MPO^+$, $NSE^+$) | CD11b, CD13, CD14, CD15, CD33, CD34 |
| M5 | Monoblastic ($NSE^+$) | CD11b, CD13, CD14, CD15, CD33, CD34 |
| M6 | Erythroleukemic ($MPO^+$, $PAS^+$) | Glycophorin CD34 |
| M7 | Megakaryoblastic ($PPO^+$) | CD41, CD42, CD34, CD61 |

$L_1$ or $L_2$ may show either pre-B or T antigens.

*The indicated FAB type may express some or all of the indicated antigens.

†ALL, acute lymphocytic leukemia; ANLL, acute nonlymphocytic leukemia; FAB, French-American-British; MPO, myeloperoxidase; NSE, nonspecific esterase; PPO, platelet peroxidase; Slg, surface immune globulin.

for at least 2 years, and a 53% survival rate in patients presenting with evidence of metastatic disease. The drug therapy appeared to prevent clinical hematogenous metastases following surgical removal and radiation to the tumor bed, presumably by destroying nondetectable, microscopic tumor foci, especially in the lungs. Vincristine also has striking activity against Wilms tumor and appears to be at least as effective as dactinomycin. Other single agents shown to have activity against this tumor include doxorubicin, cyclophosphamide, ifosfamide, and bleomycin.

Infants younger than 12 months of age have experienced undue toxicities to the liver, hematopoietic system, and lungs from the prescribed doses of dactinomycin, vincristine, and doxorubicin. In the earlier NWTS trials, 47% of infants had severe hematologic toxicity, and toxicity-related deaths occurred in 6%. Dosages were subsequently reduced to 50% of the usual per kilogram dose given to older children, with a decrease in rate of hematologic toxicity to 13% and elimination of toxic deaths. Of importance, dosage reduction did not compromise therapeutic effect as judged by the 2-year relapse-free survival figures (Morgan et al, 1988).

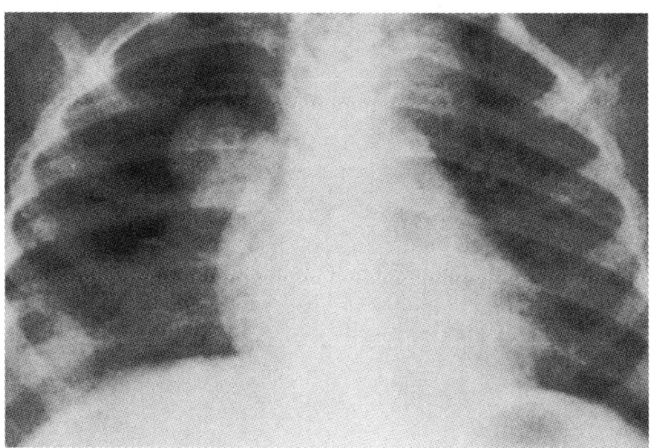

**FIGURE 95–10.** Pulmonary metastases from Wilms tumor.

Results of the first two NWTS trials showed that treatment with vincristine plus dactinomycin is superior to treatment with either drug alone. Postoperative radiation therapy adds little benefit to children with completely excised tumors, and 6 months of therapy with two drugs appears to be as effective as 15 months of therapy in these patients. Patients with more advanced disease fared better following treatment with three drugs (dactinomycin, vincristine, doxorubicin) than with two (dactinomycin, vincristine). Patients with tumors of unfavorable histologic subtype had a significantly poorer prognosis than that for patients whose tumors had favorable histologic features; prognosis also was poorer in those patients with positive nodes (D'Angio et al, 1981). Treatment results from the NTWTS 3 are shown in Table 95–10 (D'Angio et al, 1989). NTWTS 4 demonstrated that children could receive pulse-intensive chemotherapy safely at less cost without sacrificing efficacy (Green et al, 1998). Thus, Wilms tumor, a neoplasm that is fatal if untreated, presently has an overall cure rate approaching 90%.

**TABLE 95–10**

**Treatment Results of the Third National Wilms Tumor Study According to Stage and Histology**

| | | | % Relapse-Free | | % Alive |
|---|---|---|---|---|---|
| **Stage** | **Histology** | **No.** | **2 yr** | **4 Yr** | **4 Yr** |
| I | Favorable | 607 | 91.6 | 90.4 | 96.5 |
| II | Favorable | 278 | 90.4 | 88.1 | 92.3 |
| III | Favorable | 275 | 79.8 | 79.0 | 87.0 |
| IV | Favorable | 120 | 76.0 | 74.9 | 82.5 |
| I-III | Unfavorable | 130 | 69.7 | 64.8 | 68.4 |
| IV | Unfavorable | 29 | 55.6 | 55.6 | 55.3 |
| All patients | | 1439 | 85.0 | 83.3 | 89.1 |

Data from D'Angio GI, Breslow N, Beckwith B. et al. Treatment of Wilms' tumor: Results of the Third National Wilms' Tumor Study. Cancer 64:349, 1989.

### *Persistent Renal Blastema and Nephroblastomatosis*

Accumulations of immature renal tissue are not normally found beyond 36 weeks of gestation, the time at which nephrogenesis normally ceases. Nodular renal blastema is characterized by microscopic nests of primitive cells in the subcapsular renal cortex resembling the blastemal cells of Wilms tumor but lacking mitoses. Although benign, these nodules are believed to have the potential for neoplastic transformation. They are found in 1 of every 200 to 400 postmortem examinations of infants dying from other causes prior to 4 months of age. When nodular renal blastema becomes massive and confluent and replaces the cortex, it is referred to as *nephroblastomatosis* (Bove and McAdams, 1976). Kumar and associates (1978) reported the nodular renal blastema–nephroblastomatosis complex in 8 of 118 patients (6.8%) with Wilms tumor. Five of these eight patients had bilateral tumors. Children with this disorder also may have the congenital anomalies associated with Wilms tumor (Fig. 95–11). The fact that nodular renal blastema is rarely found in older children suggests that a majority of these lesions regresses, a situation analogous to the course of neuroblastoma in situ. It is believed that those that persist give rise to Wilms tumor, whereas a small number progresses to diffuse nephroblastomatosis. Complete progression of nodular renal blastema to nephroblastomatosis to Wilms tumor has been documented (Kulkarni et al, 2002). Children with massive bilateral involvement often respond to therapies used for Wilms tumor. Although persistent renal blastema is not a true malignancy, it probably has been confused with Wilms tumor in the past, and it appears in many instances to be a precursor of this malignancy.

### *Cystic Partially Differentiated Nephroblastoma*

One renal neoplasm in infants is known by a variety of names: polycystic nephroblastoma, benign multilocular cystic nephroma, well-differentiated polycystic Wilms tumor, and cystic partially differentiated nephroblastoma. It is a cystic encapsulated tumor occurring before 2 years of age.

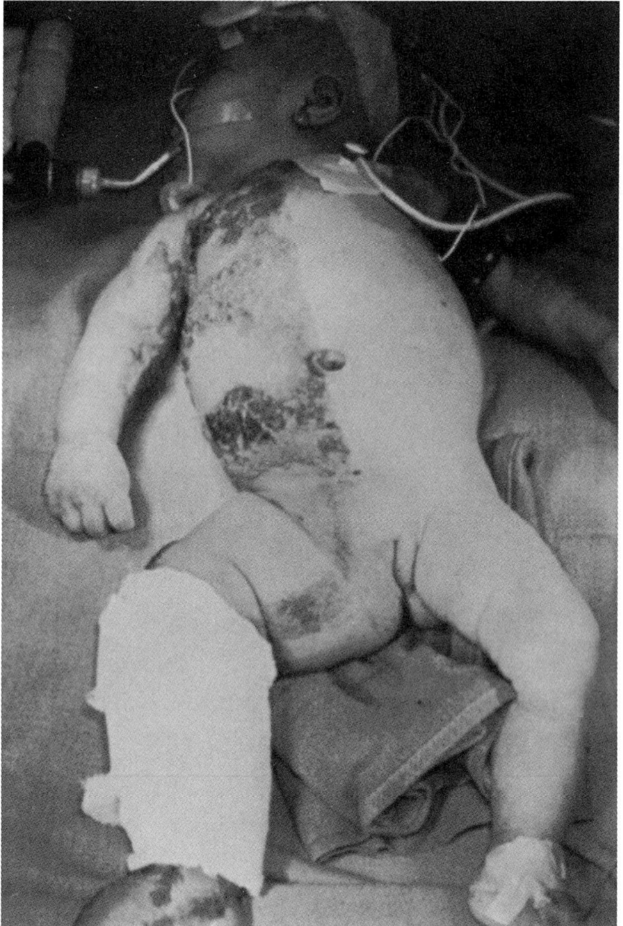

**FIGURE 95–11.** Congenital epidermal nevus in association with hemihypertrophy and nephroblastomatosis.

The cysts are lined by epithelium and show a mixture of partially differentiated and undifferentiated metanephrogenic blastemas, a finding that differentiates this lesion from multilocular cysts of the kidney. The tumor appears to have a benign course, and nephrectomy is the treatment of choice (Joshi et al, 1977). These neoplasms probably represent a differentiated form of nephroblastoma. A number of neonatal renal tumors have been confused with the typical Wilms tumor in the past. Because these neoplasms have been recognized as separate entities, they are more commonly diagnosed during the neonatal period than is the classic nephroblastoma, which rarely occurs during the first month of life.

### *Rhabdoid Tumor of Kidney*

Rhabdoid tumor of the kidney is an uncommon renal tumor of children that is one of the most lethal neoplasms of early neonatal life, with a mortality rate exceeding 80%. It has a predilection for males, with a male-to-female ratio of 1.5:1, and for infants, with median age at diagnosis of 11 months. Overall, rhabdoid tumors comprised 1.8% of all malignant childhood renal tumors entered in the NWTS. Rhabdoid tumors frequently manifest simultaneously with embryonal primary tumors of the CNS, such as medulloblastoma (Bonnin et al, 1984). Originally believed to represent a "rhabdomyosarcomatoid" pattern of Wilms tumor, this lesion subsequently was shown to lack any evidence of myoblastic differentiation or any morphologic or clinical linkage to Wilms tumor. Review of 111 cases by Weeks and coworkers and the NWTS showed several findings suggesting that rhabdoid tumors may arise from cells involved in formation of the renal medulla but that they have no histogenic relationship to Wilms tumor (Weeks et al, 1989). The prognosis is extremely poor, particularly for infants with evidence of dissemination. The only patients who survived were those with completely resected disease and negative lymph nodes (50%), whereas all those with metastases died. A consistently detected cytogenetic abnormality is the deletion of 22q11-12, which has been mapped to the *INI1* or *hSNF5* gene (Versteege et al, 1988). This deletion also is detected in the rhabdoid tumors of the CNS. *INI1* is essential for normal development and has been reported to act as a tumor suppressor gene (Roberts et al, 2000). Mice that are *INI1* heterozygotes develop rhabdoid tumors as early as 5 weeks of age (Roberts et al, 2000).

## Retinoblastoma

Retinoblastoma is a malignant ocular tumor that arises in embryonic retinal cells. The incidence of retinoblastoma in the United States is approximately 1/18,000 live births. Bilateral involvement is observed in 20% to 35% of retinoblastomas; the tumor is detected in only one eye in as many as one fourth of these patients.

### Genetics

The gene for retinoblastoma, located on chromosome 13q14, has been cloned and belongs to a class of tumor suppressor genes whose function is to control cellular growth. When the retinoblastoma gene (*RB*) is inactivated, by either a mutation or a deletion, the block to cellular proliferation is removed, leading to tumor formation. Mutations at the *RB* locus can be inherited in an autosomal dominant pattern or arise spontaneously. The Knudson "two-hit" hypothesis postulates that the first genetic mutation can occur in a germ cell (inherited cases) or in a retinoblast (in sporadic cases); only with the second mutation in a somatic target cell (retinoblast) already carrying a first "hit" will that cell be transformed.

All patients with bilateral retinoblastoma have either a new *RB* germline mutation or an inherited one. Approximately 80% of unilateral retinoblastomas occur as a result of a somatic nonheritable mutation (Cowell and Pritchard, 1987). The germinal trait responsible for retinoblastoma is a dominant one with 80% to 96% penetrance. There is also a small number of patients (5% of retinoblastoma) born with a constitutional deletion of chromosome 13, 13q−, who have the associated anomalies of microencephaly, macrognathia, malformed ears and thumbs, hypertelorism, microphthalmia, ptosis, protruding upper incisors, short stature, cleft palate, developmental delay, and psychomotor retardation (Knudson et al, 1976). Children with the bilateral and hereditary form often are diagnosed at an earlier age, in part because the family history alerts the pediatrician to the need for early screening and in part because the chromosomal abnormality is present at birth, providing a greater susceptibility to tumorigenesis. In rare instances, family history of the disorder may be lacking; hereditary bilateral retinoblastoma may be the result of germline mosaicism in the parent. It is possible using DNA restriction fragment length polymorphisms to predict susceptibility to retinoblastoma (Cavenee et al, 1986; Wiggs et al, 1988).

### Clinical Manifestations

Patients with retinoblastoma commonly present either with leukocoria or "cat's eye" on ocular examination or with strabismus caused by loss of vision in the affected eye. Multifocal retinal involvement is common, occurring in 84% of the cases. Intraocular spread may fill the vitreous body by extension or seeding, whereas exophytic tumors arise from the outer retinal layer and cause retinal detachment. Extraocular spread is seen in less than 15% of patients, usually occurring by direct invasion of the optic nerve and eventually leading to subarachnoid involvement and intracranial spread. In such cases the cerebrospinal fluid may contain tumor cells. Rarely, tumors may spread by invasion of the orbit or by hematogenous dissemination to bones and bone marrow. Children with bilateral retinoblastoma are at risk for dissemination to the pineal gland and should undergo periodic brain MRI for evaluation; this syndrome is known as *trilateral retinoblastoma*.

The diagnosis is made by ophthalmoscopic examination performed with the patient under general anesthesia. CT or MRI of the eye is useful to determine tumor extent and optic nerve involvement. A lumbar puncture for cerebrospinal fluid cytology should be performed if there is optic nerve invasion; bone scan and bone marrow biopsy detect hematogenous spread. In general, repeated metastatic evaluations are not indicated for follow-up study of this tumor because of the extreme rarity of extraocular dissemination. Only cases with extraocular involvement initially or with clinical findings compatible with spread require such evaluations. Tumors are then staged according to the Reese-Ellsworth classification on the basis of the number and size of the lesions and whether they extend anterior to the ora serrata. In addition, any extraocular extension must be characterized.

### Treatment

Because extraocular spread and death from dissemination are rare, the main goal of treatment is local control and preservation of vision. Surgical enucleation is used only when there is no chance for useful vision, if glaucoma is present, or if conservative measures fail to control the tumor. External beam radiation therapy, administered by experienced clinicians using careful positioning and general anesthesia, is known to cure the disease. Doses range from 3500 to 5000 cGy given in three fractions per week. However, patients with hereditary retinoblastoma are at increased risk for radiation-induced sarcomas. Thus, current therapies are focused on avoiding external beam irradiation when possible. If local extension has occurred, the field must be enlarged to include the orbit or a craniospinal field for meningeal or brain involvement (Donaldson and Smith, 1989). In addition, systemic chemotherapy may be used, as there have been some reports of success with this modality (Schouten-van Meeteren et al, 2002).

Small tumors confined to the retina often can be controlled with cryotherapy and photocoagulation. Because of the late effects of radiation on bone growth and the potential for second tumor induction, aggressive cryotherapy and laser therapy are preferable when possible. Use of chemotherapeutic regimens including agents such as vincristine, doxorubicin, cyclophosphamide, cisplatin, and etoposide have achieved responses and may be indicated in patients with advanced local disease before enucleation or disseminated disease. Thus far, no advantage has been demonstrated for the use of chemotherapy as adjuvant treatment given in addition to radiation therapy or enucleation.

### Prognosis

The prognosis for children with unilateral retinoblastoma is excellent, with cure rates of 85% to 90% obtained using conservative local treatment. However, patients with bilateral disease have a much lower long-term survival rate, not because of the retinoblastoma but because of a high predisposition to second malignancy, which may occur at any point in the lifespan. Although patients with hereditary disease are most susceptible to sarcomas in the radiation field, they are at increased risk of sarcomas in other regions. Local extension also confers a poor prognosis, with survival rates of less than 10% with orbital extension or distant dissemination.

## Central Nervous System Tumors

### Incidence and Epidemiology

CNS malignancies are rare in newborns and comprise approximately 13% of infant cancers overall (Gurney et al, 1997). Most of the brain tumors that occur in infants are supratentorial. Half of the CNS malignancies are gliomas, including astrocytomas, which occur at an incidence rate of 15 cases per 1 million infants. Primitive neuroectodermal tumors (PNETs) and medulloblastomas occur at an incidence rate of 9 cases per 1 million infants, followed by ependymomas, which occur at a rate of 5/1 million. In general, infants with CNS malignancies tend to do more poorly than older children. Infants with PNET or ependymoma have particularly poor prognoses. Atypical teratoid or rhabdoid tumor of the CNS occurs rarely but is associated with a high mortality rate (Packer et al, 2002). Although reasons for the poorer outcome are not completely clear, it probably is due to a combination of tumor biology and treatment delivered. Infants are much more susceptible to the side effects of radiation therapy, and the lower radiation doses used to avoid devastating late effects may result in inferior cure rates.

### Clinical Manifestations

Infants who have CNS malignancies often present with signs and symptoms of increased intracranial pressure (ICP) not apparent in older children or adults, such as a bulging fontanelle, split sutures, or rapidly enlarging head size. Poor feeding, vomiting, lethargy, and irritability also can be symptoms of increased ICP. Funduscopic examination may or may not show papilledema. Loss of developmental milestones also can be seen. Specific neurologic abnormalities include Parinaud syndrome (in infants, manifested by impaired upward gaze secondary to increased pressure in the dorsal midbrain), abnormalities related to cranial nerve palsies (i.e., esotropia/exotropia, cranial nerve VI palsy resulting in the inability to abduct the affect eye, or a cranial nerve IV palsy resulting in deviation of the affected eye upward and laterally), and nystagmus. Another common manifestation of CNS malignancies is head tilting secondary to cervical root irritation from posterior cerebellar masses. The *diencephalic syndrome*, which consists of the clinical triad of emesis, emaciation, and euphoria, describes the rare presentation of a hypothalamic lesion that can be seen in older infants. Such infants often present with chronic vomiting and failure to thrive but on clinical examination appear curiously well muscled despite the lack of subcutaneous fat and are extraordinarily good-natured.

### Treatment

The optimal therapy continues to be surgical resection of the tumor, when possible. However, several factors must be taken into consideration in the approach to an infant with a CNS lesion. First, these tumors tend to be highly malignant and invasive, leading to difficulties with resection. Second, these tumors also tend to be highly vascular, making it challenging to remove the tissue with minimal morbidity. Finally, infants tend to present with large tumors, which can also interfere with the resection.

Radiation therapy is a backbone of the treatment given to older children with malignant brain tumors. Infants are highly susceptible to the late effects of radiation therapy, however. They can sustain severe cognitive deficits in addition to growth impairment as a result of craniospinal irradiation. Recent treatment protocols have focused on minimizing the early exposure to high doses of radiation therapy by maximizing effective chemotherapy, when possible. Developments in the subspecialty of radiation oncology have made it possible to deliver more focused radiation, which may help minimize the morbidity that infants may experience. Taken together, all of these factors should alert the clinician to the need for referral of such patients to a center specializing in pediatric care, including a team composed of a pediatric radiation oncologist, a neuro-oncologist, and a pediatric neurosurgeon.

## Sarcomas

Soft tissue sarcomas are rarely seen in newborns; only 13 of 3217 infants and children diagnosed with rhabdomyosarcoma (RMS) were younger than 30 days of age at diagnosis (Lobe et al, 1994). The most commonly diagnosed soft tissue sarcoma in the neonatal age group is infantile or congenital fibrosarcoma, which is diagnosed in all infants between 1 and 12 months at a rate of 5/1 million (Ries et al, 1999). In general, the standard of care for treating infantile fibrosarcoma is complete surgical excision, although neoadjuvant chemotherapy with a variety of agents has been successfully used for tumor shrinkage, with subsequent reduction in the morbidity related to radical surgical procedures. The cure rates for infantile fibrosarcoma, with surgery alone or with chemotherapy and surgery, approach 100% (Kurkchubasche et al, 2000; Loh et al, 2002; Singh et al, 1995).

The initial evaluation of a patient with a congenital fibrosarcoma includes imaging of the primary tumor with either an MRI or a CT study and a chest CT scan. Chemotherapy regimens used successfully for treatment of this tumor include vincristine, actinomycin D, and lower dose cyclophosphamide, as well as etoposide (VP-16) and ifosfamide (Kurkchubasche et al, 2000; Kynaston et al, 1993; Loh et al, 2002; Ninane et al, 1991; Sheng et al, 2001). Doxorubicin, while efficacious, is generally avoided because of the late cardiotoxicity risk. Duration of therapy depends on the size, location, and response of the tumor, but the general goal is to reduce the tumor size to maximize chances of surgical local control. Radiation therapy has been traditionally avoided to spare the infant the associated late effects of poor growth and secondary cancers.

## Histiocytosis

*Histiocytosis* refers to any of a diverse group of poorly understood disorders of abnormal histiocytes in which the cells are derived from the monophagocytic pathway. They occur rarely in neonates. They have been categorized by the Histiocyte Society, an international group, into three classes (Table 95–11). Class I disorders include Langerhans cell histiocytosis (LCH) (formerly known variously as histiocytosis X, Letterer-Siwe disease, Hand-Schüller-Christian disease, and eosinophilic granuloma), and pure cutaneous histiocytosis. The class II disorders include familial erythrophagocytic lymphohistiocytosis and infection-associated hemophagocytic syndrome. The class III disorders are truly malignant disorders of mononuclear phagocytes, including acute monocytic leukemia, malignant histiocytosis, and histiocytic lymphoma. In addition to these three classes, other rare, noncategorized histiocytoses can occur in newborns, in particular, juvenile xanthogranuloma and Omenn disease.

It is postulated that an immunologic stimulus to a normal antigen-processing cell, the Langerhans cell, results in uncontrolled proliferation in class I disorders. The lesions are granulomatous in nature, with infiltration of Langerhans cells with cleaved nuclei and eosinophils. Birbeck granules are seen by electron microscopy, and cell surface antigens include S-100 and CD1a. Multinucleate giant cells are sometimes seen. Class II disorders are believed to represent a secondary histiocytic reaction to an unknown antigenic stimulation or infectious agent, with erythrophagocytosis possibly reflecting foreign antigens adsorbed on erthrocytes or activation of macrophages by excess lymphokine production because of abnormal immunoregulation. The class II lesions are characterized by morphologically normal reactive macrophages without Birbeck granules and with prominent erythophagocytes, and the process involves the entire reticuloendothelial system. The infiltrates are mixed lymphohistiocytic, unlike in class I disease, in which either mixed histiocytic-eosinophilic or pure histiocytic infiltrates are seen.

### *Class I Disorders*

The class I disorders are often classified by the site and/or number of organs involved. In particular, LCH confined to bone is called *eosinophilic granuloma*. This lesion often can be completely ablated with surgical curettage alone or with low-dose radiation (Titgemeyer et al, 2001). However, mono-ostotic LCH in young infants frequently is associated with the appearance of subsequent bone lesions that require chemotherapy with vinblastine and prednisone (Ladisch and Gadner, 1994). Polyostotic LCH can become a chronic disease requiring years of low-dose therapy until it "burns" itself out. In particular, LCH manifesting with diabetes insipidus secondary to pituitary involvement, bone lesions, and exophthalmos (retro-orbital granulomas) formerly was called *Hand-Schüller-Christian disease*.

Disseminated LCH involving skin, hepatosplenomegaly, and lymphadenopathy formerly was called *Letterer-Siwe disease*. The peak incidence is at 6 months of life (Isaacs, 1997), and additional organs, including the bone marrow, lung, and gastrointestinal tract, may be involved. Prognosis is poor for infants who present with disseminated disease (Gadner et al, 1994). The skin involvement of infants with histiocytosis can be mistaken for common conditions such as seborrhea or eczema, particularly in the groin, on the scalp, or over posterior auricles. In addition, chronically draining ears and/or swollen gums with overlying whitish nodules can indicate disease. CNS involvement, while rare, also can occur, either in the sella turcica, causing diabetes insipidus, or in the cerebellar vermis, causing ataxia.

Although LCH appears to respond to low-dose radiation and to many chemotherapeutic agents including vincristine, vinblastine, prednisone, 6-mercaptopurine, chlorambucil, methotrexate, and cyclophophamide, investigators have been unable to show any definitive improvement in cure rates using these modalities. Other agents reported to show efficacy include cladribine and cyclosporine. To optimize therapy, the Histiocyte Society has conducted international randomized trials of therapies for LCH since 1994 (Henter et al, 1997). However, novel approaches are still needed to improve the outcomes in the very young infants with widely disseminated disease.

### *Class II Disorders*

The class II disorders are non–Langerhans cell histiocytoses in which the histiocytic proliferation is stimulated by different pathogenetic mechanisms. Familial erythrophagocytic lymphohistiocytosis (FHL) is a rare and almost always fatal disease of infants and young children. Definitive diagnosis may be preceded by a positive family history, but the inheritance pattern is autosomal recessive, making this an unreliable marker. Patients present with fever, wasting, hepatosplenomegaly, and progressive pancytopenia (Table 95–12). CNS symptoms with seizures, disorientation, and coma with elevated cerebrospinal fluid protein levels and pleocytosis are common. Biopsy specimens of lesions found in the liver, spleen, lymph nodes, lungs, or bone marrow can show erythrophagocytosis and a lymphohistiocytic infiltrate. The disease usually has a fulminant downhill course, but the advent of bone marrow transplantation in recent years has resulted in an estimated 5-year survival rate of 66%, compared with 10% with chemotherapy alone (Arico et al, 1996). Thirty percent of patients with FHL have been reported to harbor mutations in the perforin gene, which encodes an essential protein for cellular immune activation (Stepp et al, 1999).

**TABLE 95–11**

**Classification of Childhood Histiocytoses**

| Feature | Class I | Class II | Class III |
|---|---|---|---|
| Diseases included | Langerhans cell histiocytosis | IAHS; FEL; grouped together as the hemophagocytic lymphohistiocytoses (HLHs) | Malignant histiocytosis; acute monocytic leukemia; true histiocytic lymphoma |
| Cellular characteristics | Langerhans cells with cleaved nuclei and Birbeck granules seen by electron microscopy; cell surface antigens include S100 and CD1a; cells mixed with varying proportions of eosinophils; multinucleated giant cells sometimes seen | Morphologically normal, reactive macrophages with prominent erythrophagocytosis; process involves entire reticuloendothelial system | Neoplastic cellular proliferation of cells exhibiting characteristics of macrophages or dendritic cells or their precursors; localized or systemic |
| Proposed pathophysiologic mechanisms | Iummunologic stimulation of a normal antigen-presenting cell—the Langerhans cell—in an uncontrolled manner | Histiocytic reaction secondary to an unknown antigenic stimulation (FEL) or to an infectious agent (IAHS), with erythrophagocytosis possibly reflecting foreign antigens absorbed on erythrocytes or activation of macrophages by excess lymphokine production due to abnormal immunoregulation | Neoplasm; clonal autonomous uncontrolled proliferative process |

FEL, familial erythrophagocytic lymphohistiocytosis; IAHS, infection-associated hemophagocytic syndrome.

Note: Previously known as histiocytosis X and its related syndromes of eosinophilic granuloma, Hand-Schüller-Christian disease, and Letterer-Siwe disease.

**TABLE 95–12**

**Clinical and Laboratory Findings in the Hemophagocytic Lymphohistiocytoses**

| Required for Diagnosis* | Consistent with Diagnosis |
|---|---|
| Clinical | Clinical |
| Fever | Jaundice |
| Splenomegaly | Edema |
| | Lymphadenopathy |
| Laboratory | Laboratory |
| Cytopenias (affecting ≥2 of 3 lineages in the peripheral blood and not caused by a hypocellular or dysplastic bone marrow): | ↑ Circulating soluble interleukin-2 receptors |
| Hemoglobin (<9.0 g/dL) | |
| Neutrophils (<1.0 × $10^9$/L) | |
| Hypertriglyceridemia or hypofibrinogenemia (fasting triglycerides ≥2.0 mmol/L or ≥3SD of the normal value for age, fibrinogen ≤1.5 g/L or ≤3 SD) | Hepatic enzyme abnormalities<br>↑ Very-low-density lipoprotein<br>↓ High-density lipoprotein<br>↓ Natural killer cell activity |
| Histopathologic criteria: Hemophagocytosis in bone marrow or spleen or lymph nodes; no evidence of malignancy | |

*All are required for the diagnosis of hemophagocytic lymphohistiocytosis [infection-associated hemophagocytic syndrome or familial erthrophagocytic lymphohistiocytosis (FEL)]; in addition, the diagnosis of FEL is justified by a positive family history, and parental consanguinity is suggestive.

Data from Henter J-I, Elinder G, Ost A: Diagnostic guidelines for hemophagocytic lymphohistiocytosis. Semin Oncol 18:29, 1991.

Patients with infection-associated hemophagocytic syndrome (IAHS) can present with clinical features similar to those of FHL. Involvement of the bone marrow is typical, with marked erythrophagocytosis involving normal-appearing histiocytes engulfing red blood cells and platelets. The condition usually is activated in the setting of an immunodeficiency, whether it is secondary to an infection (viral, bacterial, fungal, and parasitic infections all have been reported), malignancy, or immunosuppressive medications. In general, treatment centers on reducing the immunosuppression, through either stopping immunosuppressive drugs or treating the inciting infection. Low-dose etoposide has been used with some success, but many investigators advocate watchful waiting and supportive care.

### *Class III Disorders*

True malignant histiocytosis has been reported occasionally in newborns (Ishii et al, 1998). Acute monocytic leukemia has been classified as a class III histiocytosis but is discussed elsewhere in this chapter. True malignant histiocytosis is characterized clinically by symptoms similar to those of FEL, with fever, hepatosplenomegaly, lymphadenopathy, and pancytopenia. However, the family history is negative, and pathologic examination shows malignant cells with large nuclei and prominent nucleoli that have histochemical features of histiocytes. Erythrophagocytosis may be present but less prominent than in FEL. The disease is more responsive to chemotherapy regimens containing cyclophosphamide, prednisone, doxorubicin, vincristine, etoposide, and cytarabine.

## Hepatoblastoma

Primary malignant tumors of the liver are uncommon in infants and children. The most common malignant neoplasm involving the liver in infancy is metastatic neuroblastoma. Although rare, the most common benign hepatic neoplasms in the neonate are mesenchmymal hamartomas and hemangiomas. The two major histologic types of primary malignant hepatic tumors are hepatoblastoma and hepatocellular carcinoma. Hepatoblastomas usually occur in infants and are rarely seen after 3 years of age. In an older series of 129 infants and children with hepatoblastoma, only 11 were younger than 6 weeks of age (Exelby et al, 1975). Hepatocellular carcinomas appear to have a bimodal age distribution, occurring either in children younger than 4 years or in patients between the ages of 12 and 15 years. Both types of tumors occur more commonly in males. Hepatoblastoma occurs in association with BWS and its variants. Hemihypertrophy occurs in 2% of hepatoblastoma patients. In addition, there is a strong association between prematurity and the development of hepatoblastoma (Ross and Gurney, 1998). Recent analysis of data for 105 children with hepatoblastoma reveals a 15-fold increase in the expected rate for the development of this tumor in patients with birth weights of less than 1000 g (Feusner and Plaschkes, 2002).

Chromosome abnormalities in tumor tissue include loss of heterozygosity at 11p15.5, the Beckwith-Wiedemann locus, and, in non-BWS patients, I(8q) and trisomy 20. There is also an increased risk of hepatoblastoma in familial adenomatosis polyposis coli; the genetic abnormality in this disorder maps to chromosome 5q (Phillips et al, 1989).

The most common presenting manifestations of hepatic tumors are an upper abdominal mass and an enlarging abdomen. Anorexia, weight loss, and pain also are frequent findings. Laboratory studies of liver function are rarely helpful in establishing the diagnosis, and results of such tests usually are normal. AFP often is present in the serum of children with hepatic malignancy.

Hepatic calcification is demonstrated in 10% of cases on plain abdominal roentgenogram. Ultrasonography is useful to distinguish cystic and solid masses from a diffusely enlarged liver. CT shows the extent of tumor involvement, anatomic landmarks, and operability, whereas MRI most accurately shows adenopathy, tumor margins, and vessel involvement. The goal of therapy is to surgically resect the tumor. If one lobe is free of malignancy and there is no evidence of distant metastases, a lobectomy of the involved portion of the liver should be performed. Even though 60% of children with stage I, fully resected tumors are cured of their disease with surgery alone, chemotherapy after complete resection has resulted in an increase in long-term survival rates (96%) in one series (Fuchs et al, 2002). For those children who present with unresectable but nonmetastatic tumors, initial chemotherapy is used to shrink the tumor for resection. Orthotopic liver transplant is curative in those patients with unresectable, nonmetastatic hepatoblastomas.

## TREATMENT CONSIDERATIONS IN INFANTS

### Chemotherapy Dosing

Age-related differences in body composition, drug bioavailability, and drug metabolism have been identified for neonates, infants, children, and adults. Total body water content is higher in neonates (75%) than in adults (55%) (Friis-Hansen, 1971). Extracellular water decreases from 45% in the newborn to 20% in the adult. In addition, many drugs bind less well to circulating serum proteins in the neonate, leading to potentially greater amounts of active drug (Stewart and Hampton, 1987). Also, there is decreased activity of drug-metabolizing enzymes in the newborn period, particularly of the P-450 enzymes (Pelkonen et al, 1973). Finally, kidney function in newborns is less efficient. Taken together, it is plausible that standard doses of chemotherapy tolerated by older children and adults would be toxic to young infants. Unfortunately, available pharmacokinetic data are very limited for educated dosing in infants. Various formulas for dosing infants have been used; most commonly, in infants with body surface areas of less than 0.6 m$^2$, doses per kg are used. However, no one dosing rule is universally applicable in view of the aforementioned variations, juxtaposed against the background of rapid growth and development in this age group (McLeod et al, 1992).

Infants have been shown to experience excessive neurotoxicity from vincristine, with the development of hypotonia, a poor cry, inability to feed, and flaccid paralysis (Reaman et al, 1985). As discussed earlier, infants who received standard doses of actinomycin D, vincristine, and cyclophosphamide (Cytoxan) in early clinical trials for Wilms tumor had a higher rate of hepatotoxicity until the doses were lowered, with no decrease in efficacy observed (Morgan et al, 1988). However, an interesting observation made by Bleyer and colleagues (1977) was that the volume of the CNS in relation to body surface area is much greater in young children than in adults. In fact, current dosing of intrathecal chemotherapy is based on age rather than size, in order to avoid the underdosage of young children with ALL or AML.

### Radiation Effects

The use of radiation therapy in newborn infants is reserved for acute life-threatening situations in which the potential for adverse late effects of radiation, including growth impairment, cognitive impairment, and risk of secondary malignancies, is clearly outweighed by the benefits. The general principle is to use as little radiation as possible to spare the infant potentially morbid side effects.

### Supportive Care

Appropriate supportive care for infants with cancer is paramount. The most important principle in the treatment of cancer in infants is to anticipate problems, so as to prevent rather than treat complications.

#### *Pain Management*

Recent literature demonstrates that infants can experience pain and should be treated appropriately with adequate pain medication (Rouzan, 2001). Signs of pain in the neonate can be subtle and include crying, grimacing, tachycardia, high blood pressure, and poor feeding. Nonsteroidal anti-inflammatory medications are traditionally avoided in patients with cancer because of the risks of interfering with platelet function. In addition, acetaminophen (Tylenol) must be used judiciously in immunocompromised patients to prevent masking a fever that could signify an infection, particularly if a central line is in place or if the white blood cell count is low. Narcotics should be used as needed, with appreciation of the possibility of oversedation or respiratory depression. Parents may express apprehension at the use of narcotics for fear of later addiction, but they should be reassured that addiction is a psychological dependence and unlikely to occur. Patients receiving narcotics for more than 1 week are known to become physically dependent on these drugs, which should be tapered slowly to avoid symptoms of withdrawal.

#### *Nutrition*

Adequate nutrition should be provided to patients, either with oral feedings or via parenteral nutrition by intravenous line. It is easy to lose track of the time during which the infant is without adequate nutrition in the diagnostic workup for the cancer, given the tests, scans, and procedures that must be done with anesthesia. Breast-feeding generally provides optimal nutrition; however, cases of CMV infection have been transmitted from CMV-positive mothers through breast milk to preterm infants and should be recommended for infants with cancer on an individual basis (Hamprecht et al, 2001).

### Intravenous Access

In most cases, it is prudent to place a central venous catheter in a young infant who will need frequent chemotherapy, blood or platelet transfusions, or parenteral nutrition. Some of the chemotherapy drugs used are vesicants and can cause severe burns if infiltrated underneath the skin. Central lines can have single or double lumens, although the size of the baby may affect the type of line placed. In general, it is best to discuss placing a central line with the oncologist, who can better predict the course of therapy. For older infants with more subcutaneous chest wall fat, implantable devices can be placed, which will minimize daily care.

### Transfusions

Any infant suspected of having a malignancy that may require chemotherapy should receive only CMV-negative and irradiated blood products. In addition, the use of leukocyte-depleted products is recommended to minimize future febrile or allergic reactions. A primary CMV infection in an immunocompromised host can be life-threatening. Most blood banks have a policy of transfusing all neonates with CMV-negative blood. Irradiation is also critical to inactivate the donor white blood cells, which, if given unirradiated, could result in an overwhelming graft-versus-host reaction. Donor-designated blood generally is discouraged in infants with congenital leukemia, given the possibility of future bone marrow transplantation.

### Immunizations

Immunizations generally are avoided until the patient has been off chemotherapy for at least 6 months. In addition, all close contacts of the patient should receive the inactivated polio vaccine rather than the live oral polio vaccine. There is no contraindication to immunizing first-degree relatives with the varicella vaccine. However, any person in whom a rash develops after the vaccination should be sequestered from the patient.

### Psychosocial Considerations

Adequate social services and psychological support are critical for families with a sick neonate. In particular, special services are available for families of children with cancer and should be made available as soon as a diagnosis is made. Management of an infant with cancer is best achieved through the efforts of a multidisciplinary team composed of special nurses and social workers in addition to the pediatric oncologist.

### Late Effects

Infants who receive treatment for cancer during the first year of life are at risk for many late effects directly related to chemotherapy, surgery, and radiation therapy, in addition to the psychosocial late effects stemming from their diagnosis. These infants require follow-up evaluations at routine intervals by a pediatric oncologist, who can help identify appropriate screening tests.

## REFERENCES


Ablin AR, Krailo MD, Ramsay NK, et al: Results of treatment of malignant germ cell tumors in 93 children: A report from the Children's Cancer Study Group. J Clin Oncol 9:1782-1792, 1991.

Anders D, Frick R, Kindermann G: [Metastasizing neuroblastoma of the fetus with seeding in the placenta]. Geburtshilfe Frauenheilkd 30:969-975, 1970.

Anderson JF, Kent S, Machin GA: Maternal malignant melanoma with placental metastasis: A case report with literature review. Pediatr Pathol 9:35-42, 1989.

Antunes NL, Khakoo Y, Matthay KK, et al: Antineuronal antibodies in patients with neuroblastoma and paraneoplastic opsoclonus-myoclonus. J Pediatr Hematol Oncol 22:315-320, 2000.

Arico M, Janka G, Fischer A, et al: Hemophagocytic lymphohistiocytosis. Report of 122 children from the International Registry. FHL Study Group of the Histiocyte Society. Leukemia 10:197-203, 1996.

Armstrong SA, Staunton JE, Silverman LB, et al: MLL translocations specify a distinct gene expression profile that distinguishes a unique leukemia. Nat Genet 30:41-47, 2002.

Aviles A, Neri N: Hematological malignancies and pregnancy: A final report of 84 children who received chemotherapy in utero. Clin Lymphoma 2:173-177, 2001.

Baird PN, Pritchard J, Cowell JK: Molecular genetic analysis of chromosome 11p in familial Wilms tumour. Br J Cancer 69: 1072-1077, 1994.

Barak M, Cohen A, Herschkowitz S: Total leukocyte and neutrophil count changes associated with antenatal betamethasone administration in premature infants. Acta Paediatr 81:760-763, 1992.

Belchis DA, Mowry J, Davis JH: Infantile choriocarcinoma: Re-examination of a potentially curable entity. Cancer 72: 2028-2032, 1993.

Bibbo M, Gill WB, Azizi F, et al: Follow-up study of male and female offspring of DES-exposed mothers. Obstet Gynecol 49:1-18, 1977.

Biegel JA, White PS, Marshall HN, et al: Constitutional 1p36 deletion in a child with neuroblastoma. Am J Hum Genet 52: 176-182, 1993.

Blattner WA, Henson DE, Young RC, et al: Malignant mesenchymoma and birth defects: Prenatal exposure to phenytoin. Jama 238:334-335, 1977.

Bleyer AW: Clinical pharmacology of intrathecal methotrexate. II. An improved dosage regimen derived from age-related pharmacokinetics. Cancer Treat Rep 61:1419-1425, 1977.

Bonnin JM, Rubinstein LJ, Palmer NF, et al: The association of embryonal tumors originating in the kidney and in the brain: A report of seven cases. Cancer 54:2137-2146, 1984.

Bourhis J, Dominici C, McDowell H, et al: N-*myc* genomic content and DNA ploidy in stage IVS neuroblastoma. J Clin Oncol 9:1371-1375, 1991.

Bove KE, McAdams AJ: The nephroblastomatosis complex and its relationship to Wilms' tumor: A clinicopathologic treatise. Perspect Pediatr Pathol 3:185-223, 1976.

Bowman LC, Castleberry RP, Cantor A, et al: Genetic staging of unresectable or metastatic neuroblastoma in infants: A Pediatric Oncology Group study. J Natl Cancer Inst 89:373-380, 1997.

Bown N, Cotterill S, Lastowska M, et al: Gain of chromosome arm 17q and adverse outcome in patients with neuroblastoma. N Engl J Med 340:1954-1961, 1999.

Breccia M, Cimino G, Alimena G, et al: AIDA treatment for high-risk acute promyelocytic leukemia in a pregnant woman at 21 weeks of gestation. Haematologica 87:ELT12, 2002.

Bresters D, Reus AC, Veerman AJ, et al: Congenital leukaemia: The Dutch experience and review of the literature. Br J Haematol 117:513-524, 2002.

Brissette MD, Duval-Arnould BJ, Gordon BG, et al: Acute megakaryoblastic leukemia following transient myeloproliferative disorder in a patient without Down syndrome. Am J Hematol 47:316-319, 1994.

Brodeur GM, Pritchard J, Berthold F, et al: Revisions of the international criteria for neuroblastoma diagnosis, staging, and response to treatment. J Clin Oncol 11:1466-1477, 1993.

Brodeur GM, Seeger RC, Schwab M, et al: Amplification of N-myc in untreated human neuroblastomas correlates with advanced disease stage. Science 224:1121-1124, 1984.

Bruinsma F, Venn A, Lancaster P, et al: Incidence of cancer in children born after in-vitro fertilization. Hum Reprod 15: 604-607, 2000. Also available at http://humrep.oupjournals.org/cgi/content/full/15/3/604; http://humrep.oupjournals.org/cgi/content/abstract/15/3/604

Cairney AE, Andrews M, Greenberg M, et al: Wilms tumor in three patients with Bloom syndrome. J Pediatr 111:414-416, 1987.

Calhoun DA, Kirk JF, Christensen RD: Incidence, significance, and kinetic mechanism responsible for leukemoid reactions in patients in the neonatal intensive care unit: A prospective evaluation. J Pediatr 129:403-409, 1996.

Caron H: Allelic loss of chromosome 1 and additional chromosome 17 material are both unfavourable prognostic markers in neuroblastoma. Med Pediatr Oncol 24:215-221, 1995.

Cavenee WK, Murphree AL, Shull MM, et al: Prediction of familial predisposition to retinoblastoma. N Engl J Med 314:1201-1207, 1986.

Chan HS, Cheng MY, Mancer K, et al: Congenital mesoblastic nephroma: A clinicoradiologic study of 17 cases representing the pathologic spectrum of the disease. J Pediatr 111:64-70, 1987.

Chen CS, Sorensen PH, Domer PH, et al: Molecular rearrangements on chromosome 11q23 predominate in infant acute lymphoblastic leukemia and are associated with specific biologic variables and poor outcome. Blood 81:2386-2393, 1993.

Chessells JM, Eden OB, Bailey CC, et al: Acute lymphoblastic leukaemia in infancy: Experience in MRC UKALL trials. Report from the Medical Research Council Working Party on Childhood Leukaemia. Leukemia 8:1275-1279, 1994.

Chessells JM, Harrison CJ, Kempski H, et al: Clinical features, cytogenetics and outcome in acute lymphoblastic and myeloid leukaemia of infancy: Report from the MRC Childhood Leukaemia working party. Leukemia 16:776-784, 2002.

Christiansen H, Lampert F: Tumour karyotype discriminates between good and bad prognostic outcome in neuroblastoma. Br J Cancer 57:121-126, 1988.

Coppes MJ, Clericuzio CL: Molecular genetic analysis of the *WT1* gene in patients suspected to have the Denys-Drash syndrome. Med Pediatr Oncol 23:390, 1994.

Cowell J, Pritchard J: The molecular genetics of retinoblastoma and Wilms' tumor. Crit Rev Oncol Hematol 7:153-168, 1987.

Crist W, Pullen J, Boyett J, et al: Clinical and biologic features predict a poor prognosis in acute lymphoid leukemias in infants: A Pediatric Oncology Group Study. Blood 67:135-140, 1986.

Cunha GR, Taguchi O, Namikawa R, et al: Teratogenic effects of clomiphene, tamoxifen, and diethylstilbestrol on the developing human female genital tract. Hum Pathol 18:1132-1143, 1987.

D'Angio GJ, Breslow N, Beckwith JB, et al: Treatment of Wilms' tumor: Results of the Third National Wilms' Tumor Study. Cancer 64:349-360, 1989.

D'Angio GJ, Evans AE, Breslow N, et al: The treatment of Wilms' tumor: Results of the Second National Wilms' Tumor Study. Cancer 47:2302-2311, 1981.

D'Angio GJ, Evans AE, Koop CE: Special pattern of widespread neuroblastoma with a favourable prognosis. Lancet 1:1046-1049, 1971.

De Bernardi B, Pianca C, Pistamiglio P, et al: Neuroblastoma with symptomatic spinal cord compression at diagnosis: Treatment and results with 76 cases. J Clin Oncol 19:183-190, 2001.

Dildy GA 3rd, Moise KJ Jr, Carpenter RJ Jr, et al: Maternal malignancy metastatic to the products of conception: A review. Obstet Gynecol Surv 44:535-540, 1989.

Donaldson SS, Smith LM: Retinoblastoma: Biology, presentation, and current management. Oncology (Huntingt) 3:45-51; discussion 51-52, 1989.

Dordelmann M, Schrappe M, Reiter A, et al: Down's syndrome in childhood acute lymphoblastic leukemia: Clinical characteristics and treatment outcome in four consecutive BFM trials. Berlin-Frankfurt-Munster Group. Leukemia 12:645-651, 1998.

Ehrenbard LT, Chaganti RS: Cancer in the fetal hydantoin syndrome. Lancet 2:97, 1981.

Eisinger F, Noizet A: [Pregnancy and breast cancer: Decisions and mother's perspectives]. Bull Cancer 89:755-757, 2002.

Evans AE, D'Angio GJ, Randolph J: A proposed staging for children with neuroblastoma. Children's Cancer Study Group A. Cancer 27:374-378, 1971.

Everson TC: Spontaneous regression of cancer. Prog Clin Cancer 3:79-95, 1967.

Exelby PR, Filler RM, Grosfeld JL: Liver tumors in children in the particular reference to hepatoblastoma and hepatocellular carcinoma: American Academy of Pediatrics Surgical Section Survey—1974. J Pediatr Surg 10:329-337, 1975.

Fadilah SA, Ahmad-Zailani H, Soon-Keng C, et al: Successful treatment of chronic myeloid leukemia during pregnancy with hydroxyurea. Leukemia 16:1202-1203, 2002.

Feine U, Muller-Schauenburg W, Treuner J, et al: Metaiodobenzylguanidine (MIBG) labeled with $^{123}I/^{131}I$ in neuroblastoma diagnosis and follow-up treatment with a review of the diagnostic results of the International Workshop of Pediatric Oncology held in Rome, September 1986. Med Pediatr Oncol 15:181-187, 1987.

Felix CA, Reaman GH, Korsmeyer SJ, et al: Immunoglobulin and T cell receptor gene configuration in acute lymphoblastic leukemia of infancy. Blood 70:536-541, 1987.

Feusner J, Plaschkes J: Hepatoblastoma and low birth weight: A trend or chance observation? Med Pediatr Oncol 39:508-509, 2002.

Fong CT, Brodeur GM: Down's syndrome and leukemia: Epidemiology, genetics, cytogenetics and mechanisms of leukemogenesis. Cancer Genet Cytogenet 28:55-76, 1987.

Fong CT, Dracopoli NC, White PS, et al: Loss of heterozygosity for the short arm of chromosome 1 in human neuroblastomas: Correlation with N-*myc* amplification. Proc Natl Acad Sci U S A 86:3753-3757, 1989.

Ford AM, Bennett CA, Price CM, et al: Fetal origins of the *TEL-AML1* fusion gene in identical twins with leukemia. Proc Natl Acad Sci U S A 95:4584-4588, 1998.

Ford AM, Ridge SA, Cabrera ME, et al: In utero rearrangements in the trithorax-related oncogene in infant leukaemias. Nature 363:358-360, 1993.

Friis-Hansen B: Body composition during growth: In vivo measurements and biochemical data correlated to differential anatomical growth. Pediatrics 47 (Suppl 2):264, 1971.

Fuchs J, Rydzynski J, Von Schweinitz D, et al: Pretreatment prognostic factors and treatment results in children with hepatoblastoma: A report from the German Cooperative Pediatric Liver Tumor Study HB 94. Cancer 95:172-182, 2002.

Gadner H, Heitger A, Grois N, et al: Treatment strategy for disseminated Langerhans cell histiocytosis. DAL HX-83 Study Group. Med Pediatr Oncol 23:72-80, 1994.

Gallo GE, Chemes HE: The association of Wilms' tumor, male pseudohermaphroditism and diffuse glomerular disease (Drash syndrome): Report of eight cases with clinical and morphologic findings and review of the literature. Pediatr Pathol 7:175-189, 1987.

Gansler T, Chatten J, Varello M, et al: Flow cytometric DNA analysis of neuroblastoma: Correlation with histology and clinical outcome. Cancer 58:2453-2458, 1986.

Geatti O, Shapiro B, Sisson JC, et al: Iodine-131 metaiodobenzylguanidine scintigraphy for the location of neuroblastoma: Preliminary experience in ten cases. J Nucl Med 26:736-742, 1985.

Gill WB, Schumacher GF, Bibbo M: Pathological semen and anatomical abnormalities of the genital tract in human male subjects exposed to diethylstilbestrol in utero. J Urol 117: 477-480, 1977.

Gobel U, Calaminus G, Engert J, et al: Teratomas in infancy and childhood. Med Pediatr Oncol 31:8-15, 1998.

Gobel U, Schneider DT, Calaminus G, et al: Multimodal treatment of malignant sacrococcygeal germ cell tumors: A prospective analysis of 66 patients of the German cooperative protocols MAKEI 83/86 and 89. J Clin Oncol 19:1943-1950, 2001. Also available at http://www.jco.org/cgi/content/full/19/7/1943; http://www.jco.org/cgi/content/abstract/19/7/1943

Gold EB, Sever LE: Childhood cancers associated with parental occupational exposures. Occup Med 9:495-539, 1994.

Graf JL, Albanese CT, Jennings RW, et al: Successful fetal sacrococcygeal teratoma resection in a hydropic fetus. J Pediatr Surg 35:1489-1491, 2000.

Green DM, Breslow NE, Beckwith JB, et al: Comparison between single-dose and divided-dose administration of dactinomycin and doxorubicin for patients with Wilms' tumor: A report from the National Wilms' Tumor Study Group. J Clin Oncol 16:237-245, 1998.

Greenlund LJ, Letendre L, Tefferi A: Acute leukemia during pregnancy: A single institutional experience with 17 cases. Leuk Lymphoma 41:571-577, 2001.

Gurney JG, Ross JA, Wall DA, et al: Infant cancer in the U.S.: Histology-specific incidence and trends, 1973 to 1992. J Pediatr Hematol Oncol 19:428-432, 1997.

Haas D, Ablin AR, Miller C, et al: Complete pathologic maturation and regression of stage IVS neuroblastoma without treatment. Cancer 62:818-825, 1988.

Hamprecht K, Maschmann J, Vochem M, et al: Epidemiology of transmission of cytomegalovirus from mother to preterm infant by breastfeeding. Lancet 357:513-518, 2001.

Hann HW, Evans AE, Cohen IJ, et al: Biologic differences between neuroblastoma stages IV-S and IV. Measurement of serum ferritin and E-rosette inhibition in 30 children. N Engl J Med 305:425-429, 1981.

Hann HW, Evans AE, Siegel SE, et al: Prognostic importance of serum ferritin in patients with Stages III and IV neuroblastoma: the Childrens Cancer Study Group experience. Cancer Res 45:2843-2848, 1985.

Hatch EE, Herbst AL, Hoover RN, et al: Incidence of squamous neoplasia of the cervix and vagina in women exposed prenatally to diethylstilbestrol (United States). Cancer Causes Control 12:837-845, 2001.

Hayashi Y, Kanda N, Inaba T, et al: Cytogenetic findings and prognosis in neuroblastoma with emphasis on marker chromosome 1. Cancer 63:126-132, 1989.

Haymond MW, Weldon VV: Female pseudohermaphroditism secondary to a maternal virilizing tumor: Case report and review of the literature. J Pediatr 82:682-686, 1973.

Heerema NA, Arthur DC, Sather H, et al: Cytogenetic features of infants less than 12 months of age at diagnosis of acute lymphoblastic leukemia: Impact of the 11q23 breakpoint on outcome: A report of the Children's Cancer Group. Blood 83:2274-2284, 1994.

Henter JI, Arico M, Egeler RM, et al: HLH-94: A treatment protocol for hemophagocytic lymphohistiocytosis. Med Pediatr Oncol 28:342-347, 1997.

Herbst AL, Cole P, Colton T, et al: Age-incidence and risk of diethylstilbestrol-related clear cell adenocarcinoma of the vagina and cervix. Am J Obstet Gynecol 128:43-50, 1977.

Herbst AL, Ulfelder H, Poskanzer DC: Adenocarcinoma of the vagina: Association of maternal stilbestrol therapy with tumor appearance in young women. N Engl J Med 284:878-881, 1971.

Holt SE, Brown EJ, Zipursky A: Telomerase and the benign and malignant megakaryoblastic leukemias of Down syndrome. J Pediatr Hematol Oncol 24:14-17, 2002.

Huddart SN, Muir KR, Parkes S, et al: Neuroblastoma: A 32-year population-based study—implications for screening. Med Pediatr Oncol 21:96-102, 1993.

Ikeda Y, Masuzaki H, Nakayama D, et al: Successful management and perinatal outcome of pregnancy complicated with myelodysplastic syndrome. Leuk Res 26:255-260, 2002.

Isaacs HJ: Tumors of the Fetus and Newborn. Philadelphia, W.B. Saunders Company, 1997.

Ishii E, Ohga S, Tanimura M, et al: Clinical and epidemiologic studies of familial hemophagocytic lymphohistiocytosis in Japan. Japan LCH Study Group. Med Pediatr Oncol 30:276-283, 1998.

Jick H, Walker AM, Rothman KJ, et al: Vaginal spermicides and congenital disorders. JAMA 245:1329-1332, 1981.

Joshi VV, Banerjee AK, Yadav K, et al: Cystic partially differentiated nephroblastoma: A clinicopathologic entity in the spectrum of infantile renal neoplasia. Cancer 40:789-795, 1977.

Kaneko Y, Shikano T, Maseki N, et al: Clinical characteristics of infant acute leukemia with or without 11q23 translocations. Leukemia 2:672-676, 1988.

Katz F, Malcolm S, Gibbons B, et al: Cellular and molecular studies on infant null acute lymphoblastic leukemia. Blood 71:1438-1447, 1988.

Katzenstein HM, Kent PM, London WB, et al: Treatment and outcome of 83 children with intraspinal neuroblastoma: The Pediatric Oncology Group experience. J Clin Oncol 19: 1047-1055, 2001.

Kinney H, Faix R, Brazy J: The fetal alcohol syndrome and neuroblastoma. Pediatrics 66:130-132, 1980.

Kishkurno S, Ishida A, Takahashi Y, et al: A case of neonatal choriocarcinoma. Am J Perinatol 14:79-82, 1997.

Knezevich SR, Garnett MJ, Pysher TJ, et al: *ETV6-NTRK3* gene fusions and trisomy 11 establish a histogenetic link between mesoblastic nephroma and congenital fibrosarcoma. Cancer Res 58:5046-5048, 1998.

Knudson AG, Jr, Meadows AT, Nichols WW, et al: Chromosomal deletion and retinoblastoma. N Engl J Med 295:1120-1123, 1976.

Kubota T, Saitoh S, Matsumoto T, et al: Excess functional copy of allele at chromosomal region 11p15 may cause Wiedemann-Beckwith (EMG) syndrome. Am J Med Genet 49:378-383, 1994.

Kulkarni R, Wolf JS Jr, Padiyar N, et al: Severe intrarenal fibrosis, infundibular stenosis, renal cysts, and persistent perilobar nephrogenic rests in a patient with Beckwith-Wiedemann syndrome 27 years after diffuse nephroblastomatosis and Wilms tumor: Natural progression or a consequence of treatment? J Pediatr Hematol Oncol 24:389-393, 2002.

Kumar AP, Pratt CB, Coburn TP, et al: Treatment strategy for nodular renal blastema and nephroblastomatosis associated with Wilms' tumor. J Pediatr Surg 13:281-285, 1978.

Kurkchubasche AG, Halvorson EG, Forman EN, et al: The role of preoperative chemotherapy in the treatment of infantile fibrosarcoma. J Pediatr Surg 35:880-883, 2000.

Kynaston JA, Malcolm AJ, Craft AW, et al: Chemotherapy in the management of infantile fibrosarcoma. Med Pediatr Oncol 21:488-493, 1993.

Ladisch S, Gadner H: Treatment of Langerhans cell histiocytosis—evolution and current approaches. Br J Cancer Suppl 23:S41-S46, 1994.

Lange B: The management of neoplastic disorders of haematopoiesis in children with Down's syndrome. Br J Haematol 110:512-524, 2000.

Lange BJ, Kobrinsky N, Barnard DR, et al: Distinctive demography, biology, and outcome of acute myeloid leukemia and myelodysplastic syndrome in children with Down syndrome: Children's Cancer Group Studies 2861 and 2891. Blood 91:608-615, 1998.

Lergier JE, Jimenez E, Maldonado N, et al: Normal pregnancy in multiple myeloma treated with cyclophosphamide. Cancer 34:1018-1022, 1974.

Levitt GA, Stiller CA, Chessells JM: Prognosis of Down's syndrome with acute leukaemia. Arch Dis Child 65:212-216, 1990.

Li FP: Heritable fraction of unilateral Wilms tumor. Pediatrics 81:147, 1988.

Lobe TE, Wiener ES, Hays DM, et al: Neonatal rhabdomyosarcoma: The IRS experience. J Pediatr Surg 29:1167-1170, 1994.

Loeb DM, Hill DA, Dome JS: Complete response of recurrent cellular congenital mesoblastic nephroma to chemotherapy. J Pediatr Hematol Oncol 24:478-481, 2002.

Loh ML, Ahn P, Perez-Atayde AR, et al: Treatment of infantile fibrosarcoma with chemotherapy and surgery: Results from the Dana-Farber Cancer Institute and Children's Hospital, Boston. J Pediatr Hematol Oncol 24:722-726, 2002.

Look AT, Hayes FA, Shuster JJ, et al: Clinical relevance of tumor cell ploidy and N-*myc* gene amplification in childhood neuroblastoma: A Pediatric Oncology Group study. J Clin Oncol 9:581-591, 1991.

Ludwig WD, Bartram CR, Harbott J, et al: Phenotypic and genotypic heterogeneity in infant acute leukemia. I. Acute lymphoblastic leukemia. Leukemia 3:431-439, 1989.

Malkin D, Li FP, Strong LC, et al: Germ line p53 mutations in a familial syndrome of breast cancer, sarcomas, and other neoplasms. Science 250:1233-1238, 1990.

Marina N, Fontanesi J, Kun L, et al: Treatment of childhood germ cell tumors: Review of the St. Jude experience from 1979 to 1988. Cancer 70:2568-2575, 1992.

Maris JM, Kyemba SM, Rebbeck TR, et al: Familial predisposition to neuroblastoma does not map to chromosome band 1p36. Cancer Res 56:3421-3425, 1996.

Maris JM, Matthay KK: Molecular biology of neuroblastoma. J Clin Oncol 17:2264-2279, 1999. Also available at http://www.jco.org/cgi/content/full/17/7/2264; http://www.jco.org/cgi/content/abstract/17/7/2264

Mathieu E, Merviel P, Antoine JM, et al: [Cancer and pregnancy: the obstetrician's standpoint]. Bull Cancer 89:758-764, 2002.

Matsumura M, Nishi T, Sasaki Y, et al: Prenatal diagnosis and treatment strategy for congenital mesoblastic nephroma. J Pediatr Surg 28:1607-1609, 1993.

Matthay KK, Sather HN, Seeger RC, et al: Excellent outcome of stage II neuroblastoma is independent of residual disease and radiation therapy. J Clin Oncol 7:236-244, 1989.

Matthay KK, Villablanca JG, Seeger RC, et al: Treatment of high-risk neuroblastoma with intensive chemotherapy, radiotherapy, autologous bone marrow transplantation, and 13-*cis*-retinoic acid. Children's Cancer Group. N Engl J Med 341: 1165-1173, 1999.

Maurer HS, Pendergrass TW, Borges W, et al: The role of genetic factors in the etiology of Wilms' tumor: Two pairs of monozygous twins with congenital abnormalities (aniridia; hemihypertrophy) and discordance for Wilms' tumor. Cancer 43:205-208, 1979.

McLeod HL, Relling MV, Crom WR, et al: Disposition of antineoplastic agents in the very young child. Br J Cancer Suppl 18:S23-S29, 1992.

McNally OM, Tran M, Fortune D, et al: Successful treatment of mother and baby with metastatic choriocarcinoma. Int J Gynecol Cancer 12:394-398, 2002.

Meadows AT, Lichtenfeld JL, Koop CE: Wilms's tumor in three children of a woman with congenital hemihypertrophy. N Engl J Med 291:23-24, 1974.

Melnick S, Cole P, Anderson D, et al: Rates and risks of diethylstilbestrol-related clear-cell adenocarcinoma of the vagina and cervix: An update. N Engl J Med 316:514-516, 1987.

Monson RR: Prenatal X-Ray exposure and cancer in children. In Boice JD, Fraumeni JF Jr (eds): Radiation Carcinogenesis: Epidemiology and Biological Significance. New York, Raven Press, 1997.

Mora J, Dobrenis AM, Bussel JB, et al: Spontaneous remission of congenital acute nonlymphoblastic leukemia with normal karyotype in twins. Med Pediatr Oncol 35:110-113, 2000.

Morgan E, Baum E, Breslow N, et al: Chemotherapy-related toxicity in infants treated according to the Second National Wilms' Tumor Study. J Clin Oncol 6:51-55, 1988.

Moss TJ, Seeger RC, Kindler-Rohrborn A: Immunohistologic detection and phenotyping of neuroblastoma cells in bone marrow using cytoplasmic neuron-specific enolase and cell surface antigens. In Evans A, D'Angio G, Seeger RC (eds): Advances in Neuroblastoma Research. New York, Alan R. Liss, 1985.

Mundschau G, Gurbuxani S, Gamis AS, et al: Mutagenesis of GATA1 is an initiating event in Down syndrome leukemogenesis. Blood 101:4298-4300, 2003.

Nair R, Pai SK, Saikia TK, et al: Malignant germ cell tumors in childhood. J Surg Oncol 56:186-190, 1994.

Nakagawara A, Arima-Nakagawara M, Scavarda NJ, et al: Association between high levels of expression of the *TRK* gene and favorable outcome in human neuroblastoma. N Engl J Med 328:847-854, 1993.

Nakagawara A, Zaizen Y, Ikeda K, et al: Different genomic and metabolic patterns between mass screening-positive and mass screening-negative later-presenting neuroblastomas. Cancer 68:2037-2044, 1991.

Newsham I, Kindler-Rohrborn A, Daub D, et al: A constitutional BWS-related t(11;16) chromosome translocation occurring in the same region of chromosome 16 implicated in Wilms' tumors. Genes Chromosomes Cancer 12:1-7, 1995.

Nickerson HJ, Matthay KK, Seeger RC, et al: Favorable biology and outcome of stage IV-S neuroblastoma with supportive care or minimal therapy: A Children's Cancer Group study. J Clin Oncol 18:477-486, 2000. Also available at http://www.jco.org/cgi/content/full/18/3/477; http://www.jco.org/cgi/content/abstract/18/3/477

Ninane J, Rombouts JJ, Cornu G: Chemotherapy for infantile fibrosarcoma [letter; comments] [see comments]. Med Pediatr Oncol 19:209, 1991.

Odom LF, Gordon EM: Acute monoblastic leukemia in infancy and early childhood: successful treatment with an epipodophyllotoxin. Blood 64:875-882, 1984.

Olshan AF, De Roos AJ, Teschke K, et al: Neuroblastoma and parental occupation. Cancer Causes Control 10:539-549, 1999.

Olshan AF, Smith J, Cook MN, et al: Hormone and fertility drug use and the risk of neuroblastoma: A report from the Children's Cancer Group and the Pediatric Oncology Group. Am J Epidemiol 150:930-938, 1999.

Packer RJ, Biegel JA, Blaney S, et al: Atypical teratoid/rhabdoid tumor of the central nervous system: Report on workshop. J Pediatr Hematol Oncol 24:337-342, 2002.

Pastore G, Carli M, Lemerle J, et al: Epidemiological features of Wilms' tumor: Results of studies by the International Society of Paediatric Oncology (SIOP). Med Pediatr Oncol 16:7-11, 1988.

Pautier P, Lhomme C, Morice P: [Cancer and pregnancy: The medical oncologist's point of view]. Bull Cancer 89:779-785, 2002.

Pavlidis NA: Coexistence of pregnancy and malignancy. Oncologist 7:279-287, 2002.

Pelkonen O, Kaltiala EH, Larmi TK, et al: Comparison of activities of drug-metabolizing enzymes in human fetal and adult livers. Clin Pharmacol Ther 14:840-846, 1973.

Perez CA, Matthay KK, Atkinson JB, et al: Biologic variables in the outcome of stages I and II neuroblastoma treated with surgery as primary therapy: A children's cancer group study. J Clin Oncol 18:18-26, 2000. Also available at http://www.jco.org/cgi/content/full/18/1/18; http://www.jco.org/cgi/content/ abstract/18/1/18

Pettinato G, Manivel JC, Wick MR, et al: Classical and cellular (atypical) congenital mesoblastic nephroma: A clinicopathologic, ultrastructural, immunohistochemical, and flow cytometric study. Hum Pathol 20:682-690, 1989.

Phillips M, Dicks-Mireaux C, Kingston J, et al: Hepatoblastoma and polyposis coli (familial adenomatous polyposis). Med Pediatr Oncol 17:441-447, 1989.

Pilling GP: Wilms' tumor in seven children with congenital aniridia. J Pediatr Surg 10:87-96, 1975.

Pui CH, Behm FG, Crist WM: Clinical and biologic relevance of immunologic marker studies in childhood acute lymphoblastic leukemia. Blood 82:343-362, 1993.

Pui CH, Evans WE: Acute lymphoblastic leukemia in infants. J Clin Oncol 17:438-440, 1999.

Pui CH, Gaynon PS, Boyett JM, et al: Outcome of treatment in childhood acute lymphoblastic leukaemia with rearrangements of the 11q23 chromosomal region. Lancet 359:1909-1915, 2002.

Pui CH, Kane JR, Crist WM: Biology and treatment of infant leukemias. Leukemia 9:762-769, 1995.

Pui CH, Raimondi SC, Murphy SB, et al: An analysis of leukemic cell chromosomal features in infants. Blood 69: 1289-1293, 1987.

Pui CH, Raimondi SC, Srivastava DK, et al: Prognostic factors in infants with acute myeloid leukemia. Leukemia 14:684-687, 2000.

Pui CH: Childhood leukemias. N Engl J Med 332:1618-1630, 1995.

Raney RB Jr, Chatten J, Littman P, et al: Treatment strategies for infants with malignant sacrococcygeal teratoma. J Pediatr Surg 16:573-577, 1981.

Reaman G, Zeltzer P, Bleyer WA, et al: Acute lymphoblastic leukemia in infants less than one year of age: A cumulative experience of the Children's Cancer Study Group. J Clin Oncol 3:1513-1521, 1985.

Riccardi VM, Sujansky E, Smith AC, et al: Chromosomal imbalance in the aniridia-Wilms' tumor association: 11p interstitial deletion. Pediatrics 61:604-610, 1978.

Ridgway D, Benda GI, Magenis E, et al: Transient myeloproliferative disorder of the Down type in the normal newborn. Am J Dis Child 144:1117-1119, 1990.

Ries LAG, Smith MA, Gurney JG, et al: Cancer Incidence and Survival among Children and Adolescents: United States SEER Program 1975-1995. Bethesda, Md, Cancer Statistics Branch, National Cancer Institute, 1999.

Roberts CW, Galusha SA, McMenamin ME, et al: Haploinsufficiency of Snf5 (integrase interactor 1) predisposes to malignant rhabdoid tumors in mice. Proc Natl Acad Sci U S A 97: 13796-13800, 2000.

Rosner F, Lee SL: Down's syndrome and acute leukemia: Myeloblastic or lymphoblastic? Report of forty-three cases and review of the literature. Am J Med 53:203-218, 1972.

Ross JA, Gurney JG: Hepatoblastoma incidence in the United States from 1973 to 1992. Med Pediatr Oncol 30:141-142, 1998.

Ross JA, Potter JD, Reaman GH, et al: Maternal exposure to potential inhibitors of DNA topoisomerase II and infant leukemia (United States): A report from the Children's Cancer Group. Cancer Causes Control 7:581-590, 1996.

Ross JA: Dietary flavonoids and the *MLL* gene: A pathway to infant leukemia? Proc Natl Acad Sci U S A 97:4411-4413, 2000.

Rouzan IA: An analysis of research and clinical practice in neonatal pain management. J Am Acad Nurse Pract 13:57-60, 2001.

Rubin BP, Chen CJ, Morgan TW, et al: Congenital mesoblastic nephroma t(12;15) is associated with ETV6-NTRK3 gene fusion: Cytogenetic and molecular relationship to congenital (infantile) fibrosarcoma. Am J Pathol 153:1451-1458, 1998.

Rubnitz JE, Link MP, Shuster JJ, et al: Frequency and prognostic significance of HRX rearrangements in infant acute lymphoblastic leukemia: A Pediatric Oncology Group study. Blood 84:570-573, 1994.

Rudnick E, Khakoo Y, Antunes NL, et al: Opsoclonus-myoclonus-ataxia syndrome in neuroblastoma: Clinical outcome and antineuronal antibodies—a report from the Children's Cancer Group Study. Med Pediatr Oncol 36:612-622, 2001.

Safdar A, Johnson N, Gonzalez F, et al: Adult T-cell leukemia-lymphoma during pregnancy. N Engl J Med 346:2014-2015, 2002.

Sande JE, Arceci RJ, Lampkin BC: Congenital and neonatal leukemia. Semin Perinatol 23:274-285, 1999.

Schilling FH, Spix C, Berthold F, et al: Neuroblastoma screening at one year of age. N Engl J Med 346:1047-1053, 2002. Also available at http://content.nejm.org/cgi/content/full/346/14/1047; http://content.nejm.org/cgi/content/abstract/346/14/ 1047

Schmidt ML, Lukens JN, Seeger RC, et al: Biologic factors determine prognosis in infants with stage IV neuroblastoma: A prospective Children's Cancer Group study. J Clin Oncol 18: 1260-1268, 2000. Also available at http://www.jco.org/cgi/content/full/18/6/1260; http://www.jco.org/cgi/content/abstract/18/6/1260

Schofield DE, Yunis EJ, Fletcher JA: Chromosome aberrations in mesoblastic nephroma. Am J Pathol 143:714-724, 1993.

Schouten-Van Meeteren AY, Moll AC, Imhof SM, Veerman AJ: Overview: Chemotherapy for retinoblastoma: An expanding area of clinical research. Med Pediatr Oncol 38:428-438, 2002.

Seeger RC, Brodeur GM, Sather H, et al: Association of multiple copies of the N-*myc* oncogene with rapid progression of neuroblastomas. N Engl J Med 313:1111-1116, 1985.

Seibel NL, Sommer A, Miser J: Transient neonatal leukemoid reactions in mosaic trisomy 21. J Pediatr 104:251-254, 1984.

Severson RK, Buckley JD, Woods WG, et al: Cigarette smoking and alcohol consumption by parents of children with acute myeloid leukemia: An analysis within morphological subgroups—a report from the Children's Cancer Group. Cancer Epidemiol Biomarkers Prev 2:433-439, 1993.

Sheng WQ, Hisaoka M, Okamoto S, et al: Congenital-infantile fibrosarcoma. A clinicopathologic study of 10 cases and molecular detection of the *ETV6-NTRK3* fusion transcripts using paraffin-embedded tissues. Am J Clin Pathol 115:348-355, 2001.

Shimada H, Ambros IM, Dehner LP, et al: The International Neuroblastoma Pathology Classification (the Shimada system). Cancer 86:364-372, 1999a.

Shimada H, Ambros IM, Dehner LP, et al: Terminology and morphologic criteria of neuroblastic tumors: recommendations by the International Neuroblastoma Pathology Committee. Cancer 86:349-363, 1999b.

Shu XO, Ross JA, Pendergrass TW, et al: Parental alcohol consumption, cigarette smoking, and risk of infant leukemia: A Childrens Cancer Group study. J Natl Cancer Inst 88:24-31, 1996.

Silverman LB, McLean TW, Gelber RD, et al: Intensified therapy for infants with acute lymphoblastic leukemia: results from the Dana-Farber Cancer Institute Consortium. Cancer 80:2285-2295, 1997.

Singh VP, Kannan N, Rajagopal G, et al: Congenital fibrosarcoma. Report of three cases. Indian J Cancer 32:179-182, 1995.

Sitarz AL, Santulli TV, Wigger HJ, et al: Complete maturation of neuroblastoma with bone metastases in documented stages. J Pediatr Surg 10:533-536, 1975.

Sotelo-Avila C, Gonzalez-Crussi F, Fowler JW: Complete and incomplete forms of Beckwith-Wiedemann syndrome: Their oncogenic potential. J Pediatr 96:47-50, 1980a.

Sotelo-Avila C, Gonzalez-Crussi F, Starling KA: Wilms' tumor in a patient with an incomplete form of Beckwith-Wiedemann syndrome. Pediatrics 66:121-123, 1980b.

Stewart AM, Draper GJ: X-rays and childhood cancer. Lancet 2:828-829, 1968.

Stewart CF, Hampton EM: Effect of maturation on drug disposition in pediatric patients. Clin Pharm 6:548-564, 1987.

Strick R, Strissel PL, Borgers S, et al: Dietary bioflavonoids induce cleavage in the *MLL* gene and may contribute to infant leukemia. Proc Natl Acad Sci U S A 97:4790-4795, 2000.

Strohsnitter WC, Noller KL, Hoover RN, et al: Cancer risk in men exposed in utero to diethylstilbestrol. J Natl Cancer Inst 93:545-551, 2001. Also available at http://jnci.oupjournals.org/cgi/content/full/93/7/545; http://jnci.oupjournals.org/cgi/content/abstract/93/7/545.

Suda J, Eguchi M, Akiyama Y, et al: Differentiation of blast cells from a Down's syndrome patient with transient myeloproliferative disorder. Blood 69:508-512, 1987.

Suita S, Zaizen Y, Sera Y, et al: Mass screening for neuroblastoma: Quo vadis? A 9-year experience from the Pediatric Oncology Study Group of the Kyushu area in Japan. J Pediatr Surg 31:555-558, 1996.

Suzuki T, Bogenmann E, Shimada H, et al: Lack of high-affinity nerve growth factor receptors in aggressive neuroblastomas. J Natl Cancer Inst 85:377-384, 1993.

Swift PG, Bloom SR, Harris F: Watery diarrhoea and ganglioneuroma with secretion of vasoactive intestinal peptide. Arch Dis Child 50:896-899, 1975.

Takeuchi LA, Hachitanda Y, Woods WG, et al: Screening for neuroblastoma in North America: Preliminary results of a pathology review from the Quebec Project. Cancer 76: 2363-2371, 1995.

Taub JW, Matherly LH, Stout ML, et al: Enhanced metabolism of 1-beta-D-arabinofuranosylcytosine in Down syndrome cells: A contributing factor to the superior event free survival of Down syndrome children with acute myeloid leukemia. Blood 87:3395-3403, 1996.

Taub JW, Stout ML, Buck SA, et al: Myeloblasts from Down syndrome children with acute myeloid leukemia have increased in vitro sensitivity to cytosine arabinoside and daunorubicin. Leukemia 11:1594-1595, 1997.

Taylor WF, Myers M, Taylor WR: Extrarenal Wilms' tumour in an infant exposed to intrauterine phenytoin. Lancet 2:481-482, 1980.

Titgemeyer C, Grois N, Minkov M, et al: Pattern and course of single-system disease in Langerhans cell histiocytosis data from the DAL-HX 83- and 90-study. Med Pediatr Oncol 37: 108-114, 2001.

Tolar J, Coad JE, Neglia JP: Transplacental transfer of small-cell carcinoma of the lung. N Engl J Med 346:1501-1502, 2002.

Valteau-Couanet D, Benhamou E, Vassal G, et al: Consolidation with a busulfan-containing regimen followed by stem cell transplantation in infants with poor prognosis stage 4 neuroblastoma. Bone Marrow Transplant 25:937-942, 2000.

van Wering ER, Kamps WA: Acute leukemia in infants: A unique pattern of acute nonlymphocytic leukemia. Am J Pediatr Hematol Oncol 8:220-224, 1986.

Versteege I, Sevenet N, Lange J, et al: Truncating mutations of *hSNF5/INI1* in aggressive paediatric cancer. Nature 394: 203-206, 1998.

Voelkerding KV, Sandhaus LM, Belov L, et al: Clonal B-cell proliferation in an infant with congenital HIV infection and immune thrombocytopenia. Am J Clin Pathol 90:470-474, 1988.

Voute PA, Jr, Wadman SK, van Putten WJ: Congenital neuroblastoma: Symptoms in the mother during pregnancy. Clin Pediatr (Phila) 9:206-207, 1970.

Wai DH, Knezevich SR, Lucas T, et al: The *ETV6-NTRK3* gene fusion encodes a chimeric protein tyrosine kinase that transforms NIH3T3 cells. Oncogene 19:906-915, 2000.

Ward RM, Bristow RE: Cancer and pregnancy: Recent developments. Curr Opin Obstet Gynecol 14:613-617, 2002.

Wechsler J, Greene M, McDevitt MA: Acquired mutations in GATA1 in the megakaryoblastic leukemia of Down syndrome. Nat Genet 32:148-152, 2002.

Weeks DA, Beckwith JB, Mierau GW, et al: Rhabdoid tumor of kidney: A report of 111 cases from the National Wilms' Tumor Study Pathology Center. Am J Surg Pathol 13:439-458, 1989.

Wiggs J, Nordenskjold M, Yandell D, et al: Prediction of the risk of hereditary retinoblastoma, using DNA polymorphisms within the retinoblastoma gene. N Engl J Med 318:151-157, 1988.

Wilmore HP, White GF, Howell RT, et al: Germline and somatic abnormalities of chromosome 7 in Wilms' tumor. Cancer Genet Cytogenet 77:93-98, 1994.

Woods WG, Gao RN, Shuster JJ, et al: Screening of infants and mortality due to neuroblastoma. N Engl J Med 346: 1041-1046, 2002. Also available at http://content.nejm.org/cgi/content/full/346/14/1041; http://content.nejm.org/cgi/content/abstract/346/14/1041

Woods WG, Tuchman M, Robison LL, et al: A population-based study of the usefulness of screening for neuroblastoma. Lancet 348:1682-1687, 1996.

Woods WG, Tuchman M: Neuroblastoma: The case for screening infants in North America. Pediatrics 79:869-873, 1987.

Yamamoto K, Hanada R, Kikuchi A, et al: Spontaneous regression of localized neuroblastoma detected by mass screening. J Clin Oncol 16:1265-1269, 1998.

Yamamoto K, Hayashi Y, Hanada R, et al: Mass screening and age-specific incidence of neuroblastoma in Saitama Prefecture, Japan. J Clin Oncol 13:2033-2038, 1995.

Yoshimoto Y, Kato H, Schull WJ: A review of forty-five years study of Hiroshima and Nagasaki atomic bomb survivors: Cancer risk among in utero-exposed survivors. J Radiat Res (Tokyo) 32:231-238, 1991.

Yunis JJ, Ramsay NK: Familial occurrence of the aniridia-Wilms tumor syndrome with deletion 11p13-14.1. J Pediatr 96: 1027-1030, 1980.

Ziemin-van der Poel S, McCabe NR, Gill HJ, et al: Identification of a gene, *MLL*, that spans the breakpoint in 11q23 translocations associated with human leukemias. Proc Natl Acad Sci U S A 88:10735-10739, 1991.

# DERMATOLOGIC CONDITIONS

Editor: CHRISTINE A. GLEASON

CHAPTER 96

## Newborn Skin: Development and Basic Concepts*

Bernard A. Cohen and Elaine C. Siegfried

### SKIN DEVELOPMENT

Skin is the interface between an organism and its environment. It plays an important role in fluid balance and temperature regulation and provides a barrier against invading microbes and systemic absorption of topically applied agents. This chapter provides an overview of skin development. Emphasis has been placed on factors that influence the clinical management of premature infants and the prenatal diagnosis of heritable skin diseases.

The study of skin ontogenesis has been organized primarily on the basis of the development of individual components: epidermis, basement membrane zone, dermis, immigrant cells, and appendageal structures. However, the initiation, differentiation, and growth of all of its components are intimately related. Prenatal skin biopsy for early diagnosis of severe genodermatoses is a useful procedure that depends on precise knowledge of the details of skin development. Disorders of keratinization, basement membrane integrity, melanocytes, and epidermal appendages have been detected as early as 16 weeks of gestation using this technique. In turn, fetal skin biopsy has helped to further clarify the details of epidermal development (Holbrook, 1991; Holbrook et al, 1993). Recent discoveries of genetic markers for a number of genodermatoses have also allowed for rapid precise prenatal and neonatal diagnoses and added to the understanding of molecular mechanisms of disease.

#### Epidermis

The epidermis consists of ectodermally derived, stratified squamous cells with localized proliferations that form the appendages: hair follicles, sebaceous glands, eccrine sweat glands, apocrine glands, and the nail matrix. Melanocytes immigrate into the epidermis from the neural crest, and Langerhans cells immigrate from mesoderm. The epidermis forms initially as a single layer of "indifferent ectoderm" and then differentiates into two layers of epidermal cells by 6 weeks. The outermost layer, called periderm, covers the basal layer stem cells. During the next 2 weeks, the basal cells give rise to an intermediate layer beneath the periderm. By 8 weeks, epithelial cells are capable of expressing keratins, the major cytoskeletal proteins of the epidermis. K5 and K14 are the high-molecular-weight keratins expressed primarily by basal-layer cells, whereas intermediate-layer cells express K1 and K10 (Smack et al, 1994). Genetic abnormalities of these cytoskeletal components give rise to a spectrum of inherited scaling skin diseases that can now be diagnosed by detection of specific genetic mutations and characteristic features on histologic examination and electron microscopy of skin specimens obtained by fetal skin biopsy, amniocentesis, and chorionic villus biopsy. The third month of gestation is an important period in skin development. Differentiation of the epidermis begins as two or three more layers of "intermediate cells" are added between the basal cells and periderm, while coordinated maturation progresses within other strata of the skin. By 22 to 24 weeks, granular cells have formed beneath the periderm. Granular cells are named for their prominent organelles, the keratohyalin granules. These granules contain a high-molecular-weight protein called profillagrin, which plays a crucial role in terminal differentiation of keratinocytes in the stratum corneum. Cornified cells first appear within the pilosebaceous follicle as early as 15 weeks. Interfollicular keratinization follows at 24 to 26 weeks of gestation. At 28 weeks the stratum corneum consists of two or three cell layers. By 32 weeks there are more than 15 layers of corneocytes, equivalent to those in adult skin (Holbrook, 1991).

#### Basement Membrane Zone

Components of the basement membrane zone appear with the first epidermal cells at 35 days of gestation. Important components of the dermoepidermal junction, such as hemidesmosomes, anchoring filaments, and anchoring fibrils, are completely formed by 8 to 10 weeks. The epidermis and basement membrane generally are flat during fetal development. The undulating rete ridges that expand the surface area of the dermoepidermal junction do not appear until the third trimester and are not fully

*This chapter includes material from the previous edition, to which Nancy B. Esterly, MD, contributed.

developed until 6 months after birth, coincident with accumulation of dermal matrix (Holbrook, 1991).

## Dermis

A network of stellate mesodermal cells is present beneath the epidermis of a 1- to 2-month embryo. The primary matrix secreted by these cells is composed of glycosaminoglycans (GAGs). Hyaluronic acid is the predominant GAG during the first trimester. Matrix proteins also are synthesized in the first trimester, including immature fibers resembling elastin and collagen types I, III, V, and VI. Type III and type V collagen are increased in quantity compared with adult dermis. In the third month, the dermis is transformed from a cellular to a fibrous tissue, coincident with epidermal differentiation. During months 3 to 5, the size and quantity of the matrix proteins increase, and the composition of GAGs changes. Immigrant cells, including Schwann cells, Merkel cells, melanoblasts, pericytes, and mast cells, are found in the dermis by the fifth month. The dermis continues to mature for approximately 6 months postnatally (Holbrook, 1991).

Human fetal skin wounds reportedly heal without scarring. This clinical observation, first made by surgeons pioneering antenatal diagnosis and treatment, has been followed by an explosion of experimental data elucidating the unique aspects of fetal wound healing (Dostal and Gamelli, 1993; Longaker and Adzick, 1991; Mast et al, 1992). Wound healing in the fetus differs from that in the adult in several ways, including nature of tissue environment, inflammatory response, and components of the dermal extracellular matrix (Table 96–1). Wounds can cause scars in some human infants (Cartlidge et al, 1990; Den Ouden et al, 1986), but prospective examination of sternotomy scars (Lista and Thompson, 1988) and bacille Calmette-Guérin (BCG) vaccination sites (Sivarajah et al, 1990) in children found a direct correlation between increasing age and more prominent scarring.

**TABLE 96–1**

**Comparison of Fetal and Adult Wound Repair**

| Variable | Fetus (<24 wk) | Adult |
|---|---|---|
| Tissue environment | Amniotic fluid rich in growth factors and hyaluronic acid<br>Relative hypoxemia<br>Sterile | Air |
| Inflammatory infiltrate | Limited neutrophils and lymphocytes predominate | Macrophages predominate |
| Extracellular matrix | Nonexcessive deposition of Types III and V collagen organized into a reticular pattern<br>Increased amount of hyaluronic acid | Abundant Type I collagen deposited into disorganized bundles |

## Immigrant Cells

Melanocytes from the neural crest and mesenchymally derived Langerhans cells migrate to the epidermis by week 8 but do not develop their characteristic organelles until after 65 days of estimated gestational age (EGA). Melanin production and transfer to adjacent keratinocytes occur during the fourth to the fifth month, but melanin production is relatively low, even at birth. The antigen-presenting function of Langerhans cells has not been documented in utero (Holbrook, 1991).

## Epidermal Appendages

Primordia of hair follicles, apocrine glands, eccrine sweat glands, and nails first appear at 10 to 12 weeks of estimated gestational age (EGA). The pilosebaceous unit is formed, hair is keratinized, and sebum is synthesized as early as 16 to 18 weeks. Sebum production and secretion are greatly increased in the third trimester under the influence of fetal and maternal androgens. The number of lipid-filled sebocytes in amniotic fluid has been used to assess fetal maturity. Sebaceous lipids, squalane, and wax esters constitute most of the vernix caseosa, especially in male infants. The vernix of female infants has a slightly higher proportion of cholesterol and cholesterol esters, lipids derived from keratinocytes (Holbrook, 1991; Nazzaro-Porro et al, 1979). Apocrine gland formation follows that of the sebaceous glands by 8 weeks. Apocrine secretion has been detected during the third trimester but not in the neonatal period. The palmoplantar eccrine sweat ducts are the first portion of the apparatus to develop. By 22 weeks of EGA, they open to the skin surface and join the differentiated secretory cells of the eccrine sweat gland. Maturation of the eccrine apparatus elsewhere on the body follows at 24 to 26 weeks. Neither the morphology of the glandular coil cells nor eccrine gland function is fully developed in the premature infant, but the full complement of the sweat glands and hair follicles is completely formed in utero, making them more densely distributed in infant than in adult skin. However, even in the full-term infant, thermal stress–induced sweating requires a greater stimulus than is needed to induce sweating in older children and adults. This functional response to heat improves with postnatal age (Green and Behrendt, 1973; Harpin and Rutter, 1982). Nail primordia begin to form at 8 to 10 weeks. Nail plate formation is initiated at 17 weeks and is complete by the fifth month (Holbrook, 1991).

# NEWBORN SKIN

The most clinically significant difference between the skin of premature and term infants is in the structure of the stratum corneum. Infants born before 32 weeks of gestation have a very thin stratum corneum, which gives rise to a variety of problems (Rutter, 1988). The primary functions of the stratum corneum are conservation of body water and barrier protection. A premature stratum corneum does not effectively prevent transepidermal water loss, percutaneous absorption of exogenously applied compounds, or invasion of microbes. In the dry postnatal environment, the premature infant experiences excessive losses of body fluid and heat (Baumgart, 1982; Rutter and Hull, 1979). A variety of seemingly benign clinical interventions can dramatically increase these losses. Desiccated skin is even more easily injured, providing a portal of entry for invading microbes and increasing the risk of disseminated infection (Baumgart, 1982; Gunnar et al, 1985; Harper and Rutter, 1983; Rosen et al, 1995; Rutter, 1988). A premature infant's increased ratio of body surface area to body weight, diminished metabolic capacity, and decreased immune responses compound these problems.

Rates of transepidermal water loss (TEWL) are objective measures of stratum corneum integrity. TEWL has been well studied in premature infants, using the evaporimeter, a device that provides direct measurements (Gunnar et al, 1985). During the first 4 weeks after birth, there is an exponential relationship between TEWL and gestational age in appropriate-for-gestational-age (AGA) infants. TEWL is up to 15 times higher in 1-day-old infants born at 25 weeks of gestation than in term neonates. In very low-birth-weight (VLBW) infants, this can translate into a fluid loss of up to 30% of total body weight in 24 hours. As the stratum corneum develops, TEWL gradually decreases, but at 4 weeks postgestation, TEWL from an infant born at 26 weeks is still twice that of a term infant (Fig. 96–1).

Loss of body water is accompanied by evaporative heat loss at a rate of $2.4 \times 10^3$ J/g (or 576 calories of body heat for every milliliter of water) (Hammarlund and Sedin, 1982; Smack et al, 1994). Evaporative losses are greatest in younger, more premature infants. Routine clinical interventions can exacerbate TEWL. Maintenance on an open radiant warmer bed in a nursery with low ambient humidity results in high evaporative loss of body water and heat (LeBlanc, 1991). Higher ambient temperatures are required to maintain normal body temperature under these conditions (Hammarlund and Sedin, 1982).

Traditional efforts to minimize these losses have centered on intravascular fluid replacement and modification of the infant's hospital bed. These approaches have inherent problems. Evaporative losses originate as free water from the extracellular compartment. Replacement has been conventionally determined by calculation based on standardized maintenance fluid requirements and measured changes of body weight and extracellular electrolytes, which have a typical lag time of several hours. Replacement fluids given in the form of isotonic intravenous solutions may result in sodium and glucose overload. Enclosed isolettes with high ambient humidity carry a risk of colonization with pathogenic bacteria, although an increased incidence of infection has not been documented (LeBlanc, 1991). Shielding devices used on open radiant warmer beds limit access to infants. Furthermore, some materials used for shielding (glass, Plexiglas, Lucite, Perspex) absorb infrared energy, blocking overhead transmission of heat to the infant (Baumgart, 1990; LeBlanc, 1991). Pure polyethylene plastic wraps (e.g., Glad Wrap) are transparent to infrared heat, but plastic wrap made of more complex polymers may retain heat and have the potential to burn contacted skin (LeBlanc, 1991). More recent data have focused on limiting skin injury and developing methods to improve the cutaneous barrier.

Clinically occult skin injury accompanies routine care. Skin stripping by removal of adhesive-backed products causes acute injury as well as the potential for secondary infection and significant scarring (Cartlidge et al, 1990). Removal of a piece of tape or an adhesive-backed electrode will markedly compromise the stratum corneum (Cartlidge and Rutter, 1987; Harper and Rutter, 1983), an observation that has been used in a positive way to facilitate transcutaneous monitoring of serum glucose in newborns (De Boer et al, 1994). We have observed several cases of full-thickness skin injuries from presumed innocuous local application of pressure or thermal heat (Fig. 96–2). The precise causes of this type of wound are often difficult

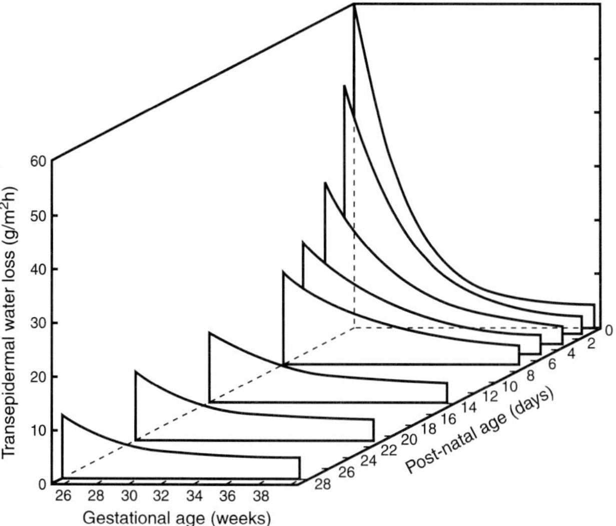


**FIGURE 96–1.** Transepidermal water loss in relation to gestational age at different postnatal ages in appropriate-for-gestational-age infants. *(From Hammarlund K, Sedin G, Stromberg B: Transepidermal water loss in newborn infants: VIII. Relation to gestational age and postnatal age in appropriate and small for gestational age infants. Acta Paediatr Scand 72:721, 1983.)*

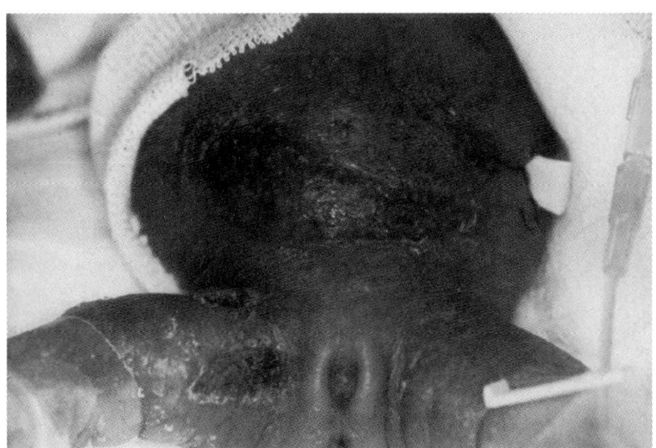

**FIGURE 96-2.** The cause of this full-thickness skin injury in a 26-week-old infant was innocuous enough to elude identification.

to identify and remain unreported. Ultraviolet light burns have occurred in association with white light phototherapy for jaundice, from relatively limited inadvertent exposure to near-ultraviolet A (UVA) light, which is 1000 times less erythemogenic than ultraviolet B (UVB) light (Siegfried et al, 1992). A Plexiglas safety shield, placed in front of daylight fluorescent bulbs, will filter out the UVA. However, white light phototherapy also is a source of infrared heat, and heat stress will exacerbate TEWL. In contrast, phototherapy delivered with blue light alone does not increase TEWL (Kjartansson et al, 1992).

Increased percutaneous absorption of topically applied compounds through an immature stratum corneum has been both advantageous and hazardous to neonates. A finding described in 1971 as "racoon facies" is a visible periorbital ring of pallor from cutaneous vasoconstriction after the application of phenylephrine eyedrops (Rutter, 1987). This effect can be quantified and is directly proportional to measurements of TEWL. Both methods have been established as useful markers of stratum corneum integrity in infants (Plantin et al, 1992; Rutter, 1987). Transdermal delivery may be the optimal route of administration for theophylline (Cartwright et al, 1990; Rutter, 1987) and diamorphine (Barrett et al, 1993) in premature infants. Lidocaine applied topically to premature skin probably is much more effective than after application to mature skin (Barrett and Rutter, 1994). Even supplemental oxygen has been administered percutaneously to very small preterm infants with poor pulmonary function (Cartlidge and Rutter, 1988a, 1988b).

In contradistinction, numerous reports have described percutaneous toxicity in infants caused by absorption of topically applied agents (Lane, 1987; Rutter, 1987). Published accounts serve to document the most severe cases of toxicity, often manifested as nursery epidemics of obvious clinical signs or deaths (Table 96–2). The potential for subclinical toxicities must be considered by everyone caring for small newborns (Table 96–3). When several topical therapeutic options are available, the one with the least potential for toxicity should be used. *Poisindex* is an extensive, frequently updated, computer-based reference source for the identification of potentially toxic compounds (Micromedex, 2002). The information from this database and current published literature indicates a lower risk of percutaneous or systemic toxicity from chlorhexidine skin antisepsis than from povidone-iodine.

The important role of nutrition in skin maturation and wound healing can be overlooked in small, sick infants, who are maintained on varying amounts of complex parenteral fluids. Acquired deficiencies as well as those resulting from inborn errors of metabolism (Table 96–4) are associated with classic cutaneous findings. Deficiencies of

**TABLE 96–2**

**Reported Hazards of Percutaneous Absorption in the Newborn**

| Compound | Reference | Product | Toxicity |
|---|---|---|---|
| Aniline | Rutter, 1987 | Dye used as a laundry marker | Methemoglobinemia,* death |
| Mercury | Dinehart et al, 1988 | Diaper rinses; teething powders | Rash, hypotonia |
| Phenolic compounds: | | | |
| Pentachlorophenol | West et al, 1981 | Laundry disinfectant | Tachycardia, sweating, hepatomegaly, metabolic acidosis, death |
| Hexachlorophene | | Topical antiseptic (pHisoHex) | Vacuolar encephalopathy, death |
| Resorcinol | West et al, 1981 | Topical antiseptic | Methemoglobinemia* |
| Boric acid | Goldbloom and Goldbloom, 1953 | Baby powder | Vomiting, diarrhea, erythroderma, seizures, death |
| Lindane | Rutter, 1987; West et al, 1981 | Scabicide | Neurotoxicity |
| Salicylic acid | Abidel-Magid and El Awad Ahmed, 1994; West et al, 1981 | Keratolytic emollient | Metabolic acidosis, salicylism |
| Isopropyl alcohol (under occlusion) | Rutter, 1987 | Topical antiseptic | Cutaneous hemorrhagic necrosis |
| Silver sulfadiazine | Payne et al, 1992 | Topical antibiotic (Silvadene) | Kernicterus (sulfa component), argyria (silver component) |
| Urea | Anonymous, 1987 | Keratolytic emollient (Carmol) | Uremia |
| Povidine-iodine | Rutter, 1987; West et al, 1981 | Topical antiseptic (Betadine) | Hypothyroidism, goiter |
| Neomycin | Rutter, 1987 | Topical antibiotic | Neural deafness |
| Corticosteroids | Rutter, 1987; West et al, 1981 | Topical anti-inflammatory (Lotrisone) | Skin atrophy, adrenal suppression |
| Benzocaine | Gelman et al, 1996 | Mucosal anesthetic (teething products) | Methemoglobinemia* |
| Prilocaine | Frayling et al, 1990; Reynolds, 1996 | Epidermal anesthetic (Emla) | Methemoglobinemia* |

*Heritable glucose-6-phosphate deficiencies are associated with an increased susceptibility to methemoglobinemia, as is coadministration of several drugs, including sulfonamides, acetaminophen, nitroprusside, phenobarbital, and phenytoin.

TABLE 96–3

**Topically Applied Products that Should Be Used with Caution in the Newborn**

| Compound | Product | Concern |
|---|---|---|
| Triclosan | Lever 2000, liquid deodorant soaps | Risk of toxicities seen with other phenolic compounds |
| Propylene glycol (MacDonald et al, 1987) | Emollients, cleansing agents (Cetaphil lotion) | Excessive enteral and parenteral administration has caused hyperosmolality and seizures in infants |
| Benzethonium chloride | Skin cleansers | Poisoning by ingestion, carcinogenesis |
| Glycerin | Emollients, cleansing agents (Aquanil lotion) | Hyperosmolality, seizures |
| Ammonium lactate | Keratolytic emollient (Lac-Hydrin) | Possible lactic acidosis |
| Coal tar (van Shooten et al, 1994) | Shampoos, topical anti-inflammatory ointments | Excessive use of polycyclic aromatic hydrocarbons is associated with an increased risk of cancer |

TABLE 96–4

**Metabolic and Nutritional Disorders Presenting with Dermatitis**

| Disorder | Reference |
|---|---|
| Acrodermatitis enteropathica | Goskowics and Eichenfield, 1993 |
| Biotin-dependent multiple carboxylase deficiency | Wolf and Heard, 1991 |
| Prolidase deficiency | Bissonnette et al, 1993 |
| Methylmalonic acidemia | Bodemer et al, 1994; de Raeve et al, 1994 |
| Maple syrup urine disease | Giacoia and Berry, 1994 |
| Propionic acidemia | Bodemar et al, 1994; de Raeve et al, 1994 |
| Citrullinemia | Goldblum et al, 1986 |
| Cystic fibrosis | Darmstadt et al, 1992 |
| Gaucher's disease | Sherer et al 1993; Sidransky et al, 1992 |
| Kwashiorkor | Goskowics and Eichenfield, 1993 |

protein, essential fatty acids, zinc, biotin, vitamins A and C, and several B vitamins are possible. Daily requirements for most of these nutrients are higher in premature than in term infants (Table 96–5).

Attention to skin integrity will help control translocation of water through the skin of premature neonates. Appropriate hydration of keratinocytes is essential for normal skin maturation (Rawlings et al, 1994), an optimized barrier against exogenous assault, and maintenance of thermal, fluid, and electrolyte balance. A successful basic skin care regimen should also allow easy access to and handling of infants. Therapeutic goals include minimizing postnatal trauma and providing an artificial barrier until the stratum corneum matures. Currently, there is no uniformly defined or accepted standard of care for the skin of premature infants. Formal clinical investigation has been limited. A few studies have verified the safety and efficacy of semiocclusive, adhesive-backed polyurethane membrane barriers in preventing fluid losses (Barak et al, 1989; Knauth et al, 1989; Mancini et al, 1994; Vernon et al, 1990). However, these dressings are not widely used because they are difficult to apply and thought to limit available area for surface monitors. Neonatal intensive care unit (NICU) staff members often provide topical emollient therapy to infants in a random way. The risks and benefits of the use of commercially available topical emollients have not been well defined. Concerns include the risk of systemic absorption and resulting toxicity, overgrowth of microbes, and secondary heat accumulation that could increase surface and core temperature.

There have been many studies of the mechanism of action and benefits of emollients on injured and diseased skin in adults. Petroleum wax–based ointment emollients (e.g., Vaseline petroleum jelly) act primarily by decreasing TEWL and accelerating barrier recovery (Ghadially and Elias, 1992). Some oils, such as safflower oil, contain essential fatty acids, which greatly influence cutaneous structure and function (Schurer et al, 1991; Ziboh and Chapkin, 1987). However, topical application of safflower oil does not prevent essential fatty acid deficiencies in preterm infants (Lee et al, 1993). Oils, oil- and water-based creams, and lotion emollients have greater tactile acceptance than has been identified for greasy ointments. However, these preparations provide a less effective moisture barrier than is conferred by ointment emollients (Lane and Drost, 1993). In addition, formulation of a cream or lotion emulsion requires the addition of several potentially irritating or toxic ingredients. Eucerin Creme is an emollient that has been studied for use in the nursery (Lane and Drost, 1993). It contains water, petrolatum, mineral oil, ceresin, lanolin alcohol, and methylchloroisothiazolinone/methylisothiazolinone (CMI/MI). Although susceptibility of premature infants to allergic contact sensitization is unknown, CMI/MI has been associated with allergic contact sensitization in up to 10% of exposed adults (Frosch et al, 1994). Aquaphor ointment contains essentially two ingredients: petrolatum in ointment—liquid (mineral oil) and solid (mineral wax) phases—and wool wax alcohol. A recent study documented that application of Aquaphor every 12 hours reduced TEWL, improved skin integrity, did not alter skin flora, and was associated with a significant reduction of

**TABLE 96–5**

**Nutritional Requirements and Cutaneous Signs of Deficiency**

| Nutrient | Infant's Daily Requirement: Premature | Term | Cutaneous Signs |
|---|---|---|---|
| Protein (g/kg/day) | 2.7-3.0 | 2.5-2.7 | "Flaky paint" scaling, hypopigmentation, peripheral edema |
| Linoleic acid (g/kg/day) | 1.2 | 0.3-0.8 | Alopecia, erythema with coarse scaling, erosive intertriginous dermatitis, poor wound healing |
| Zinc (μg/kg/day) | 400 | 100 | Alopecia, acral and periorificial erosive, pustular dermatitis, poor wound healing |
| Biotin (μg/kg/day) | 6.0 | 5.0 (not >20) | Alopecia, intertriginous and periorificial dermatitis, generalized scaling |
| Vitamin C (mg/kg/day) | 25 | 20 (not >80) | Perifollicular hermorrhages, poor wound healing, friable gums |
| Vitamin A (μg/kg/day) | 500 | 175 (not >700) | Generalized scaling |
| Riboflavin (mg/kg/day) | 0.15 | 0.35* (not >1.4) | Intertriginous and periorificial dermatitis, mucositis |
| Pyridoxine (mg/kg/day) | 0.18 | 0.25* (not >1.0) | Intertriginous and periorificial dermatitis, mucositis |
| Niacin (mg/kg/day) | 6.8 | 4.25* (not >17) | Mucositis, symmetrical hyperpigmented plaques at sun-exposed sites |

*For full-term infants, the recommended doses of some water-soluble vitamins are probably high because toxicity has not been reported.

Adapted from Greene HL, Hambridge KM, Schanler R, Tsang RC: Guidelines for the use of vitamins, trace elements, calcium, magnesium, and phosphorus in infants and children receiving total parenteral nutrition: Report of the Subcommittee on Pediatric Parenteral Nutrient Requirements from the Committee on Clinical Practice Issues of the American Society for Clinical Nutrition 1-3. Am J Clin Nutr 48:1324, 1988; © Am J Clin Nutr American Society for Clinical Nutrition; and (2) Miler SJ: Nutritional deficiency and the skin. J Am Acad Dermatol 21:1, 1989. Used with permission.

the incidence of sepsis. No adverse effects were reported (Nopper et al, 1994). Skin surface temperature was stable, and there was no evidence of hyperthermia or burns after application of the petroleum-based emollient used under infrared warmers, even in infants receiving concomitant white light phototherapy, confirming the results of a previous pilot study (Schwayder and Hetzel, 1989). These findings were also corroborated by Pabst and colleagues (1999) in their study of 19 infants between 26 and 30 weeks of gestational age.

Increased understanding of the mechanisms contributing to skin development may one day provide therapy to accelerate barrier maturation in very premature infants. Until that time, therapy should be directed toward providing a safe, temporary barrier and minimizing additional skin injury. Proposed recommendations for the care of premature skin are outlined in Table 96–6. A summary of dressing materials is outlined in Table 96–7.

## DIFFERENTIAL DIAGNOSIS BY CUTANEOUS MORPHOLOGY

Diagnosis of skin disease is based on recognition of definitive morphology of the cutaneous examination. Dermatologists are trained to interpret the important features, including color, shape, texture, and distribution, while ignoring unimportant or misleading features. Skin disease is often categorized into morphologic groups based on the most prominent primary lesion. Use of this classification scheme helps in formulating a differential diagnosis and in directing further investigation. Important morphologic groups in neonatal dermatology are vesicles and pustules, erythroderma, collodion baby, nonblanching violaceous papules and plaques, vascular defects, pigmented lesions, and midline anomalies. Subsequent chapters in this section present more detailed information on specific disorders.

### Vesicles and Pustules

Many conditions cause blisters and pustules in the newborn. Vesicles are, by definition, small intra- or subepidermal pockets of clear fluid. If the lesions are large (greater than 1 cm in diameter), they are referred to as bullae. Pustules are filled with purulent fluid. Diseases in this category range from the totally innocuous and self-limited to the severe and life-threatening.

A directed history, including family history of blistering diseases, and physical examination, including examination of the placenta, can focus the differential diagnosis. Small lesions in an otherwise healthy infant usually suggest a purely cutaneous process. Bullae and widespread involvement should prompt a more aggressive workup.

The initial diagnostic workup should include the following:

- Fluid aspirate taken from an intact pustule for Gram stain, Wright stain, and fungal, viral, and bacterial cultures
- Potassium hydroxide (KOH) preparation (or calcofluor white immunofluorescence), of the blister roof

**TABLE 96-6**

**Proposed Guidelines for Basic Skin Care of the Newborn**

1. *Use adhesives sparingly.*
   Place protective dressing (e.g., DuoDerm or Tegaderm) at sites of frequent taping (endotracheal tube and nasogastric tube placement).
   Use nonadhesive electrodes, and change them only when they become nonfunctional (Cartlidge and Rutter, 1987).
2. *Limit bathing.*
   Defer initial cleansing until body temperature has stabilized.
   Avoid cleansing agents for the first 2 weeks.
   Use warm water and moistened cotton pledgets in a humid environment.
   Surface cleansing is required no more than twice a week.
   If antimicrobial skin preparation is required, use short-contact chlorhexidine (except on the face).
3. *Be aware of the composition and quantity of all topically applied agents.*
   This includes antimicrobial cleansers, diaper wipes, adhesive removers, and perineal products.
   Dispense from single-use containers, if possible.
4. *Ensure adequate intake of protein, essential fatty acids, zinc, biotin, and vitamins A, D, and Bs.*
   Erosive periorifical dermatitis is a sign of nutritional deficiency.
5. *Apply a simple cream or ointment emollient every 8 hours* (Nopper et al, 1994).
6. *Guard against excessive thermal and ultraviolet exposure.*
   Use thermally controlled water for bathing.
   Avoid surface monitors with metal contacts.
   Use Plexiglas shielding over daylight fluorescent phototherapy.
7. *Protect sites of cutaneous injury with the appropriate occlusive dressing.*
   Use a film dressing on nonexudative sites (Barak et al, 1989; Knauth et al, 1989; Vernon et al, 1990).
   Use a hydrogel dressing on exudative wounds.
   Maintain appropriate hydration at the skin-dressing interface.
   Remove necrotic debris with each dressing change.

- Scraping from the base of the blister for Tzanck smear
- Scraping from a carefully selected intact lesion, mounted in mineral oil, for scabies preparation
- Skin biopsy as indicated, depending on the morphology and extent of the lesions, and results of other evaluations

**TABLE 96-7**

**Occlusive Dressing Materials**

| Class | Examples | Indications |
|---|---|---|
| **Films** | | |
| Polyurethane ± adhesive backing | Tegaderm, Op-Site, Bioclusive, Omniderm | Superficial, nonexudative wounds, sites of friction |
| Microporous Teflon/silicone | Silon | |
| **Hydrocolloids** | | |
| Hydrophilic colloidal particles in polyurethane foam | DuoDerm, Cutinova hydro, Restore | Exudative wounds, sites of friction |
| **Hydrogels** | | |
| Cross-linked polyvinyl or other polymer; 80%-99% water | Vigilon, Cutinova gel, Biofilm | Exudative wounds, fragile skin, sites of friction |

Reprinted from Dermatologic Surgery, Kannon GA, Garrett AB: Moist wound healing with occlusive dressings, p 583. Copyright 1995, with permission from Elsevier Science, Inc.

## Differential Diagnosis

### *Infections Localized to Skin*

Candidiasis: KOH (or calcofluor white) preparation of the blister roof reveals pseudohyphae.

Bullous impetigo: Wright stain reveals polymorphonuclear neutrophil leukocytes (PMNs); Gram stain shows gram-positive cocci.

Gram-positive folliculitis: Wright stain reveals PMNs; Gram stain shows gram-positive cocci.

Pityrosporum folliculitis: KOH preparation reveals short hyphae and spores.

Neonatal herpes: Tzanck smear reveals viral cytopathic changes; polymerase chain reaction and immunohistochemical marker assays are highly sensitive studies and can be performed using a smear on glass slides submitted to the laboratory.

Scabies: Mineral oil preparation reveals mites, ova, and feces.

### *Transient Noninfectious Causes*

Erythema toxicum neonatorum: Wright stain shows eosinophils.

Neonatal pustular melanosis: Wright stain shows keratinous debris with PMNs; the Gram stain is negative.

Neonatal acne: Close inspection reveals comedones.

Milia: Wright stain shows keratinocytes only.

Miliaria crystallina: These tiny, superficial noninflammatory vesicles represent obstruction of the sweat duct.

Infantile acropustulosis: This pruritic condition mimics infantile scabies.

Eosinophilic pustular folliculitis

### Bullae and Extensive Blistering

The bullous diseases may be life-threatening and may be impossible to distinguish from one another without skin biopsy. Appropriate therapy depends on correct diagnosis.

Staphylococcal scalded skin syndrome: Skin biopsy reveals a split in the superficial epidermis. Culture of blister contents is negative; the locus of infection is nasopharyngeal, perianal, focus of impetigo, or abcess; mucous membranes may be red but not blistered or eroded.

Congenital herpes simplex infection: Skin, eye, or mouth lesions are presenting signs in one third of infants.

Toxic epidermal necrolysis: Skin biopsy reveals a split at the dermoepidermal junction; mucous membranes are diffusely eroded.

Bullous mastocytosis: Stroking will produce a wheal and flare (Darier sign), and a Tzanck smear may show mast cells.

Genetic disorders: These disorders vary in severity and probability of long-term sequelae. Early diagnosis and genetic counseling are important aspects of management.

Epidermolysis bullosa: Blisters are most prominent at sites of friction. Familial forms are classified as simplex, junctional, and dystrophic, based on the skin cleavage plane. Electron microscopic analysis or immunofluorescence mapping or both are required for precise diagnosis.

Epidermolytic hyperkeratosis: Widespread erythema and blistering may be present at birth, causing confusion with epidermolysis bullosa and other blistering dermatoses. Thick, greasy, foul-smelling scale accentuated in skin creases may not become apparent until later in the first year of life.

Incontinentia pigmenti: Vesicular skin lesions have a characteristic distribution along the lines of Blaschko. This striking pattern is seen with a variety of cutaneous abnormalities as a result of genetic mosaicism. Tzanck smear may show eosinophils but no multinucleate giant cells.

## Erythroderma

Generalized redness and scaling in infancy have an alarming appearance and are often clinically and histologically nonspecific. An infant's general state of well-being is an important clue to the extent of the disease. Definitive diagnosis may be possible only after a period of observation. The erythrodermic newborn will have increased insensible heat and water loss requiring careful monitoring of weight, fluid and electrolytes, and temperature. A neutrothermal and humidified environment may be necessary for the first few days of life.

Careful history, family history, physical examination, and directed laboratory evaluation may help clarify the cause. The spectrum of disease includes common conditions limited to skin, infections, nutritional deficiencies, and immunologic disorders.

Infectious causes of erythroderma should always be considered first. The infant's skin should be carefully examined for more specific primary skin lesions. Laboratory evaluation should include complete blood count, KOH preparation (or calcofluor white immunofluorescence technique), Tzanck smear, and surveillance cultures of the nasopharynx, rectum, umbilicus, conjunctivae, urine, and blood. Consider syphilis serologic studies and human immunodeficiency virus (HIV) assay in epidemiologically relevant locales. Begin empiric therapy, as needed.

The diagnostic evaluation should be more aggressive in any infant who is not thriving, to search for metabolic or immunologic abnormalities. Components of the investigation should include dietary history, electrolytes, protein, albumin, alkaline phosphatase, microscopic examination of hair, and a sweat test. The results of these screening tests can suggest the need for further laboratory evaluation.

More directed laboratory evaluation includes blood smear to look for leukocyte vacuoles, HIV screen, plasma zinc determination, measurement of serum linoleic and arachidonic acids, amino acid profile, specific assays for biotinidase activity, antinuclear antibody (SS-A and SS-B) titers, quantitative immunoglobulins, tests of cell-mediated immunity, skeletal survey, hair examination, and skin biopsy.

### Differential Diagnosis

#### *Systemic Infections Associated with Erythroderma*

Candidiasis
Staphylococcal scalded skin syndrome
Syphilis
Acquired immunodeficiency syndrome (AIDS)

#### *Primary Cutaneous Conditions*

Atopic dermatitis: Pruritus and involvement of the face and extensor extremities with marked sparing of the diaper area are helpful diagnostic clues.

Seborrheic dermatitis: The diaper area and skinfolds are often prominently involved.

Psoriasis: Skin lesions are often sharply circumscribed, but scale may not be prominent.

#### *Genodermatoses*

Skin biopsy helps to distinguish among the ichthyosis-associated abnormalities disorders: lamellar ichthyosis, congenital nonbullous ichthyosiform erythroderma, epidermolytic hyperkeratosis, X-linked ichthyosis, multiple sulfatase deficiency, neutral lipid storage disease, Sjögren-Larsson syndrome, trichothiodystrophy, Netherton syndrome, and X-linked dominant chondrodysplasia punctata. The Foundation for Ichthyosis and Related Skin Types (info@scalyskin.org) is a useful source of information and will assist in the genetic evaluation of patients.

#### *Ectodermal Dysplasias*

Ectodermal dysplasias are a group of disorders involving abnormalities of the skin and its appendages. Excessive desquamation resembling that seen with postmaturity is a characteristic finding. The most well-recognized form is

X-linked recessive hypohidrotic ectodermal dysplasia. Infants with this disorder have a decreased ability to sweat and a tendency toward hyperthermia.

#### *Immunologic Disorders Associated with Erythroderma*

A clinical syndrome of erythroderma, diarrhea, and failure to thrive in infancy was first described in 1908 by Leiner, in association with unsupplemented breast-feeding. Subsequently, similar signs have been reported in infants with increased susceptibility to infection. A defect in yeast opsonization was found in two infants with "Leiner's disease" in 1972. However, this defect, present in 5% of the general population, does not define the disease. Other patients experienced dramatic clinical improvement after infusion of fresh plasma or a purified preparation containing the fifth component of complement, C5. Consequently, "Leiner's disease" has been associated with C5 dysfunction. More recently, a variety of immunologic abnormalities has been reported in infants with similar clinical presentation; this condition has been called *syndrome of erythroderma, failure to thrive,* and *diarrhea in infancy* to avoid confusion (Glover et al, 1988). Other defined disorders in this category include the following:

- Primary immunodeficiencies (severe combined immunodeficiency [SCID], Wiskott-Aldrich syndrome, hyperimmunoglobulin E syndrome, Omenn syndrome)
- Secondary immunodeficiencies (AIDS, graft-versus-host disease)
- Langerhans cell histiocytosis
- Neonatal lupus
- Diffuse cutaneous mastocytosis

#### *Metabolic and Nutritional Disorders Associated with Erythroderma*

Patients with metabolic and nutritional disorders associated with erythroderma often present with erosive, periorificial dermatitis (see Table 96–5).

#### *Other Disorders*

Boric acid poisoning: This condition was reported with the use of boric acid baby powders. It can be clinically indistinguishable from staphylococcal scalded skin syndrome (Goldbloom and Goldbloom, 1953).

## Collodion Baby

Collodion baby represents a distinct subset of neonatal erythroderma that can be a clinical marker of a variety of underlying abnormalities. The phenotype includes parchment-like hyperkeratosis, pseudocontractures, ectropion, eclabium, absence of eyebrows, and sparse hair. These infants have defective cutaneous barrier function, with resultant losses of free water and thermal energy. They are extremely susceptible to hypothermia, hypernatremic dehydration, and percutaneous infection.

## Nonblanching Violaceous Papules and Plaques

Nonblanching violaceous papules and plaques may be localized or disseminated. Infants with widespread lesions have been described as "blueberry muffin babies." The diseases in this category represent a variety of processes; most require aggressive evaluation and treatment.

Initial evaluation of a blueberry muffin infant should include complete blood count with white blood cell differential; platelet count; reticulocyte count; liver function tests; maternal and neonatal TORCH (*t*oxoplasmosis, *o*ther infections, *r*ubella, *c*ytomegalovirus infection, and *h*erpes simplex) infectious agent titers; rapid plasma reagin (RPR) assay; blood cultures for bacteria; urine, nasopharyngeal swab, and rectal swab samples for viral cultures; and ophthalmologic examination.

Skin biopsy is necessary to distinguish between simple hemorrhage into the dermis (purpura) and other infiltrative conditions (e.g., dermal hematopoiesis, tumor) manifesting in the neonatal period.

### Differential Diagnosis

#### *Purpura*

- Ecchymoses: These lesions constitute traumatic purpura, usually secondary to labor and delivery.
- Bland thrombosis: Conditions in this category that can occur in the neonatal period include the following:
  - Embolization of foreign material: This has been reported in infants receiving extracorporeal membrane oxygenation (ECMO).
  - Purpura fulminans: Neonatal purpura fulminans is most often associated with homozygous protein C or protein S deficiency (Marlar et al, 1989).
  - Cryoglobulinemia
- Infectious vasculitis: Purpuric lesions represent infectious, inflammatory microemboli, most commonly associated with the following:
  - Gram-negative bacterial sepsis, including that due to *E. coli* or meningococci, and ecthyma gangrenosum (*Pseudomonas*)
  - Listeriosis
  - Aspergillosis
- Thrombocytopenia, usually manifesting with widely scattered petechiae
- Isoimmune thrombocytopenic purpura (ITP)
- Maternal ITP
- Disseminated intravascular coagulopathy

#### *Dermal Hematopoiesis*

Dermal hematopoiesis is the histologic basis for the blueberry muffin skin lesions. Before 34 weeks of gestation, the skin serves as a hematopoietic center. It has yet to be shown whether blueberry muffin lesions are due to persistence or recurrence of the fetal potential.

- Rubella
- Cytomegalovirus infection
- Syphilis

Other viral infections (e.g., coxsackievirus B2 infection)
Twin-to-twin transfusion syndrome
Rh hemolytic disease of the newborn

#### *Malignancy*

Congenital leukemia
Langerhans cell histiocytosis
Neuroblastoma

### Vascular Defects

It can be difficult to distinguish among the different forms of cutaneous vascular lesions manifesting in the neonatal period. Nonvascular look-alikes also fall into this category but can be differentiated by skin biopsy.

#### *Differential Diagnosis*

#### *Hemangioma*

The most common tumor of infancy, hemangioma usually becomes apparent during the first 2 to 4 weeks after birth and exhibits a characteristic rapid growth phase, peaking at 4 to 6 months in most infants, with stabilization between 6 and 12 months followed by slow involution over the next 5 to 10 years. Although these lesions usually are not associated with extracutaneous findings, hemangiomas in special locations require further evaluation:

Lumbosacral and anogenital: Exclude lumbosacral spine anomalies.
Large facial, scalp, neck, thoracic (PHACES syndrome): Exclude cardiac and posterior fossa anomalies.
"Beard" distribution: Monitor airway.
Large segmental: Evaluate for vascular and soft tissue anomalies of the involved area.

#### *Vascular Malformations*

Vascular malformations are a group of lesions, usually apparent at birth, that do not generally grow or involute. Some vascular malformations are associated with characteristic extracutaneous abnormalities:

Salmon patch
Nevus flammeus (port-wine stain)
Klippel-Trénaunay syndrome
Cobb syndrome
Arterial, lymph, venous, or mixed malformations
Cutis marmorata telangiectatica congenita

#### *Lesions that Mimic Vascular Birthmarks*

Pilomatrixoma
Giant juvenile xanthogranuloma
Langerhans cell histiocytosis
Congenital myofibromatosis

### Pigmented Lesions

It can be difficult to distinguish among the lesions in the pigmented lesion category without histopathologic examination. The majority of congenital pigmented lesions are isolated and benign, but it is important to recognize those that are syndrome-associated or potentially life-threatening. Both melanocytic and nonmelanocytic lesions are included in this category.

In general, skin biopsy of a congenital pigmented lesion can be postponed until after the neonatal period. The one exception is a nodular lesion suggestive of melanoma. (See Chapter 100 for additional details.)

#### **Differential Diagnosis**

Congenital nevocellular nevus
Café au lait macule
Nevus spilus (speckled lentiginous nevus)
Mongolian spot
Smooth muscle hamartoma
Plexiform neurofibroma
Nevus of Ota
Epidermal nevus
Urticaria pigmentosa, solitary mastocytoma
Lentigines

### Midline Facial Lesions

See Chapter 100 for a more detailed discussion of midline facial lesions. The main types are as follows:

Dermoid
Nasal glioma
Encephalocele

### REFERENCES

Abidel-Magid EHM, El Awad Ahmed FR: Salicylate intoxication in an infant with ichthyosis transmitted through skin ointment. Pediatrics 94:939, 1994.

Barak M, Hershkowitz S, Rod R, Dror S: The use of a synthetic skin covering as a protective layer in the daily care of low birth weight infants. Eur J Pediatr 148:665, 1989.

Barrett DA, Rutter N: Percutaneous lignocaine absorption in newborn infants. Arch Dis Child 71:F122, 1994.

Barrett DA, Rutter N, Davis SS: An in vitro study of diamorphine permeation through premature human neonatal skin. Pharm Res 10:583, 1993.

Baumgart S: Radiant energy and insensible water loss in the premature newborn infant nursed under a radiant warmer. Clin Perinatol 9:483, 1982.

Baumgart S: Radiant heat loss versus radiant heat gain in premature neonates under radiant warmers. Biol Neonate 57:10, 1990.

Bissonnette R, Friedmann D, Giroux JM, et al: Prolidase deficiency: A multisystemic hereditary disorder. J Am Acad Dermatol 29:818, 1993.

Bleacher J, Adolph V, Dillon P, Krummel T: Fetal tissue repair and wound healing. Dermatol Clin 11:677, 1993.

Bodemer C, de Prost Y, Bachollet B, et al: Cutaneous manifestations of methylmalonic and propionic acidaemia: A description based on 38 cases. Br J Dermatol 131:93, 1994.

Cartlidge PHT, Fox PE, Rutter N: The scars of newborn intensive care. In Early Human Development. Nottingham, Ireland, Elsevier Scientific, 1990, pp 1-10.

Cartlidge PH, Rutter N: Karaya gum electrocardiographic electrodes for preterm infants. Arch Dis Child 62:1281, 1987.

Cartlidge PH, Rutter N: Percutaneous oxygen delivery to the preterm infant. Lancet 1:315, 1988a.

Cartlidge PH, Rutter N: Percutaneous respiration in the newborn infant: Effect of ambient oxygen concentration on pulmonary oxygen uptake. Biol Neonate 54:68, 1988b.

Cartwright RG, Cartlidge PH, Rutter N, et al: Transdermal delivery of theophylline to premature infants using a hydrogel disc system. Br J Clin Pharmacol 29:533, 1990.

Darmstadt GL, Schmidt CP, Wechsler DS, et al: Dermatitis as a presenting sign of cystic fibrosis. Arch Dermatol 128:1358, 1992.

De Boer J, Baarsma R, Okken A, et al: Application of transcutaneous microdialysis and continuous flow analysis for on-line glucose monitoring in the newborn infants. J Lab Clin Med 124:210, 1994.

De Raeve L, De Meirleir L, Ramet J, et al: Acrodermatitis enteropathica-like cutaneous lesions in organic aciduria. J Pediatr 124:416, 1994.

Den Ouden AL, Berger HM, Ruys JH: Scarring of the hands resulting from venipunctures in babies. Eur J Pediatr 145:58, 1986.

Dinehart SM, Dillard R, Raimer SS, et al: Cutaneous manifestations of acrodynia (pink disease). Arch Dermatol 124:107, 1988.

Dostal G, Gamelli R: Fetal wound healing. Surg Gynecol Obstet 176:299, 1993.

Frayling IM, Addison GM, Chattergee K, Meaklin G: Methaemoglobinaemia in children treated with prilocainelignocaine cream. BMJ 301:153, 1990.

Frieden I: Blisters and pustules in the newborn. Curr Probl Pediatr Nov:555, 1989.

Frosch PJ, Lahti A, Hannuksela M, et al: Chloromethylisothiazolone/methylisothiazolone (CMI/MI) use test with a shampoo on patch-test-positive subjects. Contact Derm 32:210, 1994.

Gelman CR, Rumack BH, Hess AJ: Benzocaine [abstract]. Englewood, Colo, Micromedex (electronic version), 1996.

Ghadially R, Elias P: Effects of petrolatum on stratum corneum structure and function. J Am Acad Dermatol 26:387, 1992.

Giacoia GP, Berry GT: Acrodermatitis enteropathica-like syndrome secondary to isoleucine deficiency during treatment of maple syrup urine disease. Am J Dis Child 147:954, 1994.

Glover MT, Atherton DJ, Levinsky RJ: Syndrome of erythroderma, failure to thrive, and diarrhea in infancy: A manifestation of immunodeficiency. Pediatrics 81:66, 1988.

Goldbloom RB, Goldbloom A: Boric acid poisoning. J Pediatr 43:631, 1953.

Goldblum OM, Brusilow SW, Maldonado YA, Farmer ER: Neonatal citrullinemia associated with cutaneous manifestations and arginine deficiency. J Am Acad Dermatol 14:321, 1986.

Goskowics M, Eichenfield LF: Cutaneous findings of nutritional deficiencies in children. Curr Opin Pediatr 5:441, 1993.

Green M, Behrendt H: Sweating responses of neonates to local thermal stimulation. Am J Dis Child 125:20-25, 1973.

Greene HL, Hambridge KM, Schanler R, Tsang RC: Guidelines for the use of vitamins, trace elements, calcium, magnesium, and phosphorus in infants and children receiving total parenteral nutrition: Report of the Subcommittee on Pediatric Parenteral Nutrient Requirements from the Committee on Clinical Practice Issues of the American Society for Clinical Nutrition 1-3. Am J Clin Nutr 48:1324, 1988.

Gunnar S, Hammarlund K, Nilsson GE, et al: Measurements of transepidermal water loss in newborn infants. Clin Perinatol 12:79, 1985.

Hammarlund K, Sedin G: Transepidermal water loss in newborn infants. Acta Pediatr Scand 71:191, 1982.

Harper VA, Rutter N: Barrier properties of the newborn infant's skin. J Pediatr 102:419, 1983.

Harpin VA, Rutter N: Sweating in preterm babies. J Pediatr 100:614, 1982.

High plasma urea concentrations in collodion babies. Arch Dis Child 62:212, 1987.

Holbrook KA: Structure and function of the developing human skin. In Goldsmith LA (ed): Physiology, Biochemistry and Molecular Biology of the Skin. New York, 1991, pp 63-110.

Holbrook KA, Smith LT, Elias S: Prenatal diagnosis of genetic skin disease using fetal skin biopsy samples. Arch Dermatol 129:1437, 1993.

Kannon GA, Garrett AB: Moist wound healing with occlusive dressings. Dermatol Surg 21:583, 1995.

Kjartansson SK, Hammarlund K, Sedin G: Insensible water loss from the skin during phototherapy in term and preterm infants. Acta Pediatr 81:764, 1992.

Knauth A, Gordin M, McNeils W, Baumgart S: Semipermeable polyurethane membrane as an artificial skin for the premature neonate. J Pediatr 83:945, 1989.

Lane AT: Development and care of the premature infant's skin. Pediatr Dermatol 4:1, 1987.

Lane AT, Drost SS: Effects of repeated application of emollient cream to premature neonate's skin. Pediatrics 92:415, 1993.

LeBlanc MH: Thermoregulation: Incubators, radiant warmers, artificial skins, and body hoods. Clin Perinatol 18:403, 1991.

Lee EJ, Gibson RA, Simmer K: Transcutaneous application of oil and prevention of essential fatty acid deficiency in preterm infants. Arch Dis Child 68:27, 1993.

Lista FR, Thomson HG: The fate of sternotomy scars in children. Plast Reconstr Surg 81:35, 1988.

Longaker MT, Adzick NS: The biology of fetal wound healing: A review. Plast Reconstr Surg 87:788, 1991.

MacDonald MG, Getson PR, Glasgow AM, et al: Propylene glycol: Increased incidence of seizures in low birth weight infants. Pediatrics 79:622, 1987.

Mancini AJ, Sookdeo-Drost S, Madison KC, et al: Semipermeable dressings improve epidermal barrier function in premature infants. Pediatr Res 36:306, 1994.

Mast B, Diegelmann R, Krummel T, Cohen I: Scarless wound healing in the mammalian fetus. Surg Gynecol Obstet 174:441, 1992.

Micromedex: Poisindex System. Englewood, Colo, Micromedex, 1995.

Miller SJ: Nutritional deficiency and the skin. J Am Acad Dermatol 21:1, 1989.

Nazzaro-Porro M, Passi S, Bonifort L, Belsito F: Effects of aging on fatty acids in skin surface lipids. J Invest Dermatol 73:112, 1979.

Nopper AJ, Horli K, Sookdeo-Drost S, et al: Topical ointment therapy reduces the risk of nosocomial infection in premature infants. Paper presented at the Annual Meeting of the Society for Pediatric Dermatology at Hilton Head, SC, June 1994.

Pabst RC, Starr KP, Auiyami S, Schwalbe RS, Gewolb IH: The effect of application of aquaphor on skin condition, fluid requirements, and bacterial colonization in very low birth weight infants. J Perinatol 19:278, 1999.

Payne CM, Bladin C, Colchester AC, et al: Argyria from excessive use of topical silver sulphadiazine. Lancet 340:126, 1992.

Plantin P, Jouan N, Karangwa A, et al: Variations of the skin permeability in premature newborn infants: Value of the skin vasoconstriction test with neosynephrine. Arch Franc Pediatr 49:623, 1992.

Rawlings AV, Scott IR, Harding CR, Bowser PA: Stratum corneum moisturization at the molecular level. In Moshell AN (ed): Progress in Dermatology. Evanston, Ill, 1994, pp 1-12.

Report of the Working Party: Diagnosis and treatment of homozygous protein C deficiency. J Pediatr 114:528, 1989.
Reynolds JEF: Prilocaine hydrochloride [abstract]. Englewood, Colo, Micromedex (electronic version), 1996.
Rosen JL, Atkins JT, Levy ML, et al: Invasive fungal dermatitis in the 1000-gram neonate. Pediatrics 95:682, 1995.
Rutter N: The immature skin. Br Med Bull 44:957, 1988.
Rutter N: Percutaneous drug absorption in the newborn: Hazards and uses. Clin Perinatol 14:911, 1987.
Rutter N, Hull D: Water loss from the skin of term and preterm babies. Arch Dis Child 54:858, 1979.
Schurer NY, Plewig G, Elias PM: Stratum corneum lipid function. Dermatologica 183:77, 1991.
Schwayder T, Hetzel F: Effects of emollients on skin temperature under infrared warmers. Paper presented at the 5th International Congress of Pediatric Dermatology, Milan, Italy, July 1989.
Sherer DM, Metlay LA, Sinkin RA, et al: Congenital ichthyosis with restrictive dermopathy and Gaucher disease: A new syndrome with associated prenatal diagnostic and pathology findings. Obstet Gynecol 81:842, 1993.
Sidransky E, Sherer DM, Ginns EI: Gaucher disease in the neonate: A distinct Gaucher phenotype is analogous to a model created by targeted disruption of the glucocerebrosidase gene. Pediatr Res 32:494, 1992.
Siegfried EC, Stone MS, Madison KC: Ultraviolet light burn: A cutaneous complication of visible light therapy for neonatal jaundice. Pediatr Dermatol 9:278, 1992.
Sivarajah N, Jegatheesan J, Gnananathan V: BCG vaccinations and development of a scar. Ceylon Med J 36:75, 1990.
Smack DP, Korge BP, James WD: Keratin and keratinization. J Am Acad Dermatol 30:85, 1994.
Van Shooten FJ, et al: Are coal-tar shampoos safe? Lancet 344:1505, 1994.
Vernon HJ, Lane AT, Wischerath LJ, et al: Semipermeable dressing and transepidermal water loss in premature infants. J Pediatr 86:357, 1990.
West DP, Worobec S, Solomon LM: Pharmacology and toxicology of infant skin. J Invest Dermatol 76:147, 1981.
Wolf B, Heard GS: Biotinidase deficiency. Adv Pediatr 38:1, 1991.
Ziboh VA, Chapkin RS: Biologic significance of polyunsaturated fatty acids in the skin. Arch Dermatol 123:1686, 1987.

CHAPTER

# 97

# Congenital and Hereditary Disorders of the Skin*

**Timothy P. Monahan, Bernard A. Cohen, and Elaine C. Siegfried**

The heritable disorders of skin—the genodermatoses—feature diverse aberrations of color, texture, and structural integrity of the epidermis, epidermal appendages, and connective tissue. Some of these diseases are cutaneous only; others are associated with anomalies of multiple organ systems. Many genodermatoses can be diagnosed prenatally, by skin biopsy (Holbrook et al, 1993) (Table 97–1). This technique is being replaced, however, by molecular diagnostic methods, as the genetic nature of most of these disorders is identified. Enormous progress has been made in the last few years in elucidating the molecular genetics responsible for many of the dermatoses in this chapter. With these exciting new discoveries comes the hope for novel and more efficacious therapies.

## GENODERMATOSES AND MOSAICISM

A *genetic mosaic* is an organism composed of two or more genetically different populations of cells that originate from one zygote. When the skin is involved, unique patterning is seen, reflecting the cellular heterogeneity. Variations of this striking pattern were clinically described and mapped in 1901 by Alfred Blaschko. The distribution is known as *Blaschko's lines*. Blaschko's lines are distinct from dermatomes, skin tension lines, and lines of lymphatic drainage. The pattern is linear and whorled and may be bilaterally symmetrical, with a midline demarcation (Fig. 97–1). An anatomic equivalent has been described in the eyes and teeth (Bolognia et al, 1994).

Several diseases are expressed in this fashion. The first to be recognized were X-linked disorders. Affected females are obligate heterozygotes, due to the Lyon effect of X-inactivation. Examples include female carriers of the X-linked recessive disorder hypohidrotic ectodermal dysplasia and females with the X-linked dominant disorders, incontinentia pigmenti, chondrodysplasia punctata, CHILD syndrome (see later), and focal dermal hypoplasia. These conditions are seen almost exclusively in females, presumably because they are lethal in males. Autosomal mosaicism is not heritable unless the germ cells are affected (Happle, 1993).

*This chapter includes material from a chapter in the previous edition, to which Elaine C. Siegfried, MD, and Nancy B. Esterly, MD, contributed.

## SPECIFIC GENODERMATOSES

### The Ichthyoses

The *ichthyoses* are a diverse group of heritable and acquired skin disorders that share the primary problem of widespread scaly, dry skin. Several distinct types of ichthyosis have been described on the basis of their clinical and histologic features and by their patterns of genetic transmission (Williams, 1983, 1986); however, nosology is constantly evolving. Several types of ichthyoses are primary disorders of cornification, with manifestations confined to the skin. Ichthyosiform syndromes have characteristic extracutaneous manifestations. More precise diagnostic criteria and better treatments are being recognized through collaborative research efforts, including genetic analysis. The National Registry for Ichthyosis and Related Disorders was created in 1995 to aid in this effort and can be contacted by telephone at (800) 595-1265. The Foundation for Ichthyosis and Related Skin Types (FIRST) is a privately funded national organization providing information and support for families with these disorders (for contact information, see Resources section at the end of the chapter).

#### Ichthyoses That Manifest in the Neonatal Period

Three ichthyosiform conditions have alarming presentations at birth. Two of these, the collodion baby and harlequin ichthyosis, have been historically described as distinct entities based on the associated striking and unique clinical appearance. Long-term survival of affected infants and more refined diagnostic studies have permitted identification of these conditions as phenotypically distinct but genotypically heterogeneous. A third condition, epidermolytic hyperkeratosis (autosomal dominant bullous congenital ichthyosiform erythroderma), has an equally striking neonatal appearance. Another severe category of infantile ichthyosis, congenital nonbullous ichthyosiform erythrodermal/lamellar ichthyosis, presents a difficult diagnostic and management problem. Recognition of these conditions and appropriate management are vital to the survival of these infants.

#### *Collodion Baby*

Neonates affected with the uncommon condition termed *collodion baby* have a pathognomonic appearance. With time, they usually manifest more specific features of one of the ichthyoses.

##### Clinical Findings

Collodion babies are often premature and small for gestational age. Their skin is parchment-like, shiny, and thickened at birth, distorting their facial features with ectropion and eclabium, flattening the ears, and resulting in pseudocontractures of the digits (Fig. 97–2). Histologic examination of the skin at this stage has been nonspecific, revealing a markedly thickened, compact stratum

**TABLE 97–1**

**Genodermatoses Diagnosed Prenatally Using Fetal Skin Samples**

| |
|---|
| Epidermolysis bullosa |
| Junctional |
| Recessive dystrophic |
| Dominant dystrophic |
| Epidermolysis bullosa simplex (general) |
| Epidermolysis bullosa simplex Dowling-Meara |
| Unidentified forms |
| Keratinization disorders |
| Bullous congenital ichthyosiform erythroderma |
| Nonbullous congenital ichthyosiform erythroderma/ lamellar ichthyosis |
| Harlequin ichthyosis |
| Sjögren-Larsson syndrome |
| Pigment disorders |
| Tyrosinase-negative oculocutaneous albinism |
| Congenital nevus |
| Incontinentia pigmenti |
| Disorders of epidermal appendages |
| X-linked hypohidrotic ectodermal dysplasia |
| Autosomal-recessive anhidrotic ectodermal dysplasia |
| Other disorders |
| Tay syndrome |
| Chédiak-Higashi syndrome |
| Griscelli disease |
| Restrictive dermopathy |

Adapted from Holbrook et al, 1993.

corneum. Nonetheless, these infants have a very ineffective barrier against transepidermal water loss and invasion of pathogenic microbes, with accompanying temperature instability.

### Causes

Several genetically distinct outcomes have been reported for the collodion baby phenotype (see Table 97–1). Two thirds of these infants have nonbullous ichthyosiform erythroderma. Fifty percent of affected infants have no family history suggestive of ichthyosis (Pongprasit, 1993).

### Diagnosis

Skin biopsy can be helpful, but is not likely to be specific until after the collodion appearance has resolved. Diagnostic studies should be carefully selected, based on the evolution of the cutaneous findings, associated abnormalities, and family history (Table 97–2). Several outcomes have been reported, including complete healing without sequelae (Frenk and de Techtermann, 1992; Shwayder and Ott, 1991). A prolonged period of observation may be required to determine the precise diagnosis and prognosis. As soon as a definite diagnosis has been made, genetic counseling should be provided.

### Treatment

Complications include marked temperature instability, defective barrier function, increased insensible water loss predisposing to hypernatremic dehydration (Buyse et al, 1993), pneumonia secondary to aspiration of squamous material in the amniotic fluid, and cutaneous infections from gram-positive organisms and *Candida albicans*.

Treatment consists of aggressive supportive care. Infants must be placed in a highly humidified isolette. Fluid and electrolyte balance must be closely monitored. A high index of suspicion must be maintained for signs of cutaneous or systemic infection. Overzealous administration of antibiotics, however, may lead to gram-negative infections and subsequent septicemia. Topical skin care should include application of a bland occlusive ointment emollient every 6 to 8 hours until the hyperkeratosis has resolved. Potentially toxic topical agents should be avoided because of the increased risk of percutaneous absorption. Manual débridement is not indicated. The eyes should be protected with a bland lubricating ointment; aggressive surgical management of ectropion is almost never necessary. Systemic retinoids have not been useful (Waisman et al, 1989). With

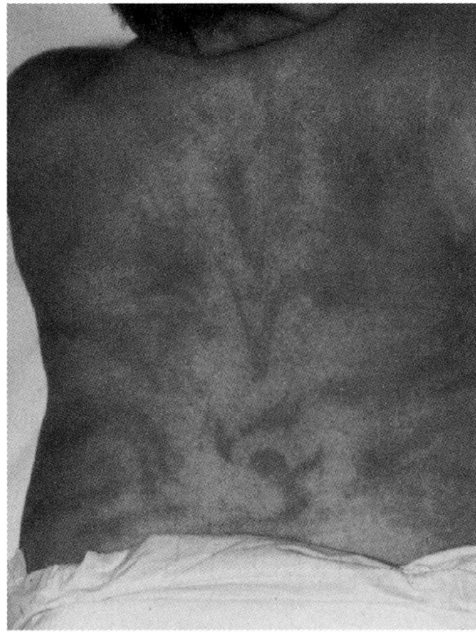

**FIGURE 97–1.** Blashchko's lines are a distinct linear and whorled pattern, to be distinguished from dermatomes or skin tension lines, characterized by midline demarcation with a central V. This pattern is the cutaneous clinical manifestation of a variety of mosaic genetic conditions.

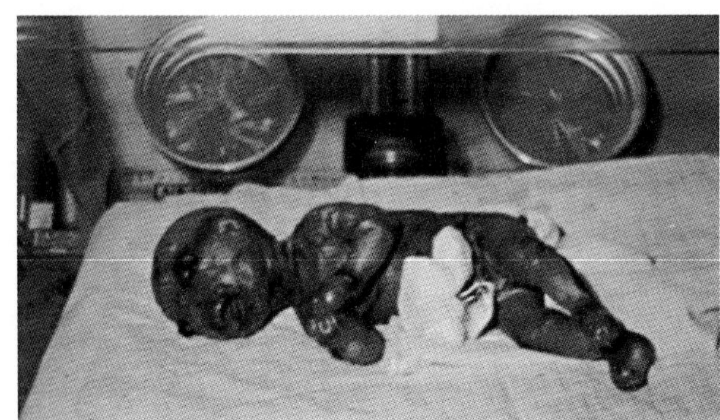

**FIGURE 97–2.** Harlequin fetus. *(Courtesy of Dr. Marvin Cornblath.)*

TABLE 97–2

**Collodion Baby: Differential Diagnosis and Laboratory Evaluation**

| Diagnosis | Inheritance | Associated Abnormalities | Diagnostic Tests* |
|---|---|---|---|
| Nonbullous ichthyosiform erythroderma (>60%) | AR, AD | | Histology is nonspecific; fetal skin biopsy is unreliable; the gene defect has not been identified |
| Lamellar ichthyosis | AR, AD | Persistent ectropion | Histology is nonspecific; fetal skin biopsy is unreliable; the gene defect has been identified |
| X-linked ichthyosis | X-linked recessive | Maternal failure to initiate labor; hypogonadism, undescended testes; corneal opacities (carrier females and affected males) | Histology is nonspecific; decreased serum cholesterol sulfate and steroid sulfatase activity; the gene defect has been mapped to Xp22.3 |
| Netherton syndrome | Sporadic | Ichthyosis linearis circumflexa, atopic diathesis, impaired cellular immunity | Histology is nonspecific; microscopic examination of hair shaft reveals pathognomonic trichorrhexis invagina |
| Gaucher disease | AR | Hepatosplenomegaly, thrombocytopenia, neurologic abnormalities | Liver biopsy; beta-glucocerebroside activity; the gene defect has been mapped to 1q21 and sequenced |
| Trichothiodystrophy (Tay syndrome) | AR | Progeric facies, neurologic abnormalities, hypogonadism, cataracts, dental problems | Hair analyses: polarizing light microscopic examination reveals characteristic banding; there is decreased content of sulfur-rich matrix proteins |
| Sjögren-Larsson syndrome | AR | Spasticity, retardation, seizures | Pathognomonic retinal changes; fibroblast culture for fatty alcohol oxidoreductase activity |
| No detectable abnormality (lamellar exfoliation of the newborn) | AR, sporadic | | Watchful waiting |

*In the immediate neonatal period, skin biopsy may be nonspecific. Histologic evaluation may be postponed until after age 3 to 6 months.

AD, autosomal dominant; AR, autosomal recessive.

Data on diagnostic tests from Paller AS: Laboratory tests for ichthyosis. Derm Clinics 12:99-107, 1994.

optimal supportive care, the thickened stratum corneum usually resolves in 2 to 4 weeks but can persist, especially in infants with lamellar ichthyosis.

### *Harlequin Ichthyosis*

This rare congenital abnormality has a more striking appearance and a graver prognosis than those reported for collodion baby. Most infants have been stillborn or died in infancy. Survival beyond infancy has only recently been possible. The harlequin phenotype is inherited as an autosomal recessive trait; several biochemical defects probably underlie the clinical condition.

#### Clinical Findings

The clinical features are unforgettable. The cutaneous scale is firm and plate-like, distorting and flattening the nose and ears. Skin rigidity also causes deep fissures, marked ectropion, eclabium, and pseudocontractures of all joints. Chemosis of the conjunctivae obscures the globes. The nails and hair are hypoplastic or absent (Fig. 97–3). Primary extracutaneous abnormalities are not prominent.

#### Diagnosis

The diagnosis is made by the pathognomonic appearance. The light microscopic examination always demonstrates compact hyperkeratosis. Additional light and electron microscopic abnormalities of the stratum corneum have not been identified consistently, supporting the theory that harlequin ichthyosis may represent a common phenotype for several different genetic errors of cornification (Hashimoto et al, 1993).

#### Causes

The cause of harlequin ichthyosis is unknown. Although abnormalities of keratinization and epidermal lipid metabolism have been reported, few affected infants have been studied, and no single defect has been identified consistently (Dale and Kam, 1993).

#### Prognosis and Treatment

Treatment consists of supportive care in a humid, temperature-controlled environment and frequent application of topical emollients to the skin and mucosal surfaces, as for collodion baby (Prasad et al, 1994). Nevertheless, infants given these therapies almost invariably succumb to their

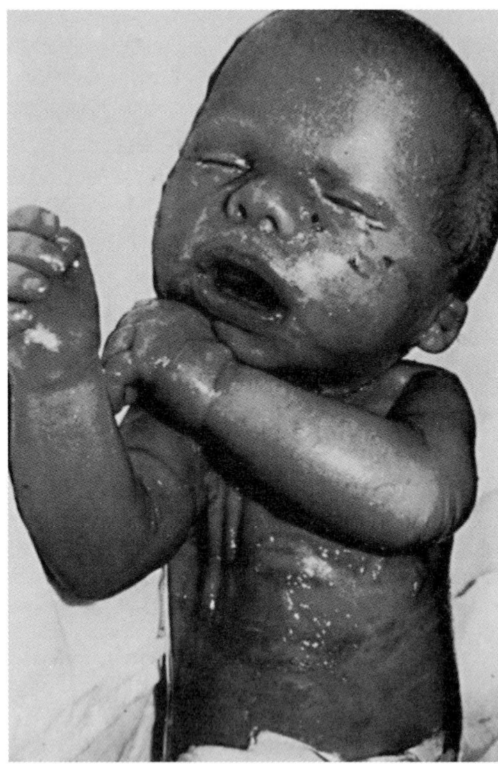

**FIGURE 97–3.** Collodion baby. Note the ectropion, eclabium, and areas of rupture in the membrane over the anterior thorax.

disease from sepsis, inability to feed, and inadequate ventilation. Survival beyond 6 weeks was extremely unusual prior to the use of oral retinoids. Recent reports have documented successful therapy of several affected infants using oral retinoids, with improved quality of life and survival well into childhood. Etretinate has been used most often in the past, at doses of 1 mg/kg/day. Although FDA approval of this drug has been withdrawn, Isotretinoin has been used at a dose of 0.5 mg/kg. Infants receiving retinoids must be monitored for toxic effects. All survivors have had severe ichthyosis as an outcome; some have intellectual impairment. Genetic counseling for the families of these infants is mandatory. Prenatal diagnosis may be made by fetal skin biopsy (Holbrook et al, 1993).

### *Epidermolytic Hyperkeratosis (Congenital Bullous Ichthyosiform Erythroderma)*

Epidermolytic hyperkeratosis (EHK) is rare, with an estimated incidence of 1/250,000. Neonates with EHK are born with generalized erythroderma and blistering. Their clinical appearance shares cutaneous features of other infantile bullous disorders, especially epidermolysis bullosa (EB). Molecular defects responsible for EHK have recently been identified, proving biochemical similarities between EHK, EB simplex, and other disorders of keratinization.

#### Clinical Findings

Infants may be born with generalized erythroderma and blistering. Hyperkeratosis may not be readily apparent. The neonatal course is complicated by temperature instability, susceptibility to hypernatremia, and sepsis, as in the other severe neonatal ichthyoses. With time, the skin changes evolve to include characteristic ridged scales, accentuated in the flexural areas. Palms and soles usually are involved. Excessive bacterial colonization often causes a distressingly foul odor. There are no extracutaneous manifestations.

#### Diagnosis

There is significant clinical similarity to other bullous disorders of infancy, including EB, staphylococcal scalded skin syndrome (SSSS), and toxic epidermal necrosis (TEN). Precise diagnosis can be lifesaving. Skin biopsy should be performed emergently, with examination of frozen sections. The histologic features of EHK are distinctive, showing intercellular edema and coarse, clumped material in the upper granular layers of the epidermis. Prenatal diagnosis is possible by means of fetal skin biopsy (Holbrook et al, 1993).

#### Causes

EHK is transmitted in an autosomal dominant fashion, with a high rate of spontaneous mutation. Ultrastructural analysis of skin from affected patients suggests an abnormality of keratin filaments in the suprabasal cells. Molecular analysis of affected families has identified genetic mutations in the genes encoding the synthesis of the keratin filaments that are preferentially expressed in the superficial epidermis, *K1* (located within the type I keratin gene cluster at chromosome 17q) and *K10* (located within the type II keratin gene cluster at chromosome 12q) (Francis, 1994; Nirunsuksiri et al, 1995; Smack et al, 1994; Steijlen et al, 1994a). The disorder also can be expressed in mosaic fashion as an epidermal nevus oriented along the lines of Blaschko (Paller et al, 1994). Prenatal studies for EHK may be indicated for the offspring of parents with extensive epidermal nevi.

#### Prognosis and Treatment

Infants with widespread blistering should be managed according to the same principles and techniques used for collodion babies. Attention to gentle handling will minimize further trauma. Application of a nonadhesive bioocclusive dressing (e.g., hydrogel, foam) will promote healing of denuded areas. Infants should be closely monitored for the development of secondary infection.

### *Nonbullous Congenital Ichthyosiform Erythroderma/Lamellar Ichthyosis*

The nonbullous form of infantile ichthyosiform skin disease, as distinct from the bullous variety (EHK), initially was characterized by its severity and autosomal recessive inheritance pattern. The term *nonbullous congenital ichthyosiform erythroderma* (NCIE) generally refers to a milder clinical variant. Ultrastructural differences have been described in skin biopsy specimens. The phenotypically more severe lamellar ichthyosis has proved to be genetically distinct as well (Russell et al, 1995).

### Clinical Findings

These conditions are characterized by congenital erythroderma and a varying degree of generalized scaling. Face, flexural sites, palms, and soles are also involved. A majority of collodion babies have these types of ichthyosis. In lamellar ichthyosis, the scales evolve to be thick, dark, and plate-like (Fig. 97–4). Facial involvement causes chronic ectropion. Hair growth may be sparse, and nails may be dystrophic. Children with NCIE have generalized erythema with finer, white scales. There is no associated ectropion. Secondary cutaneous infections with bacteria, yeasts, and dermatophytes are common complications.

### Diagnosis

Before genetic advances, the diagnosis of these forms of ichthyosis had been based on clinical features alone. Skin biopsy is nonspecific; a normal granular layer is present. The differential diagnosis includes other causes of erythroderma and collodion baby (see Chapter 96). Prenatal diagnosis is possible for affected families (Holbrook et al, 1993). For patients without a previously defined family history, the appropriate laboratory assessment can be arranged through the National Registry for Ichthyosis and Related Disorders (see earlier).

### Causes

A majority of cases are inherited in an autosomal recessive fashion, but an autosomal dominant form of lamellar ichthyosis also has been described. In 1995, a common locus of genetic mutations was identified in several families with recessive lamellar ichthyosis (Russell et al, 1995). The linked defects, located on chromosome 14, result in production of abnormal transglutaminase-1. This enzyme normally promotes cross-linking of intracellular proteins in the stratum corneum during terminal differentiation (Huber et al, 1995; Russell et al, 1995). New research has revealed genetic heterogeneity with two other loci on chromosomes 2 and 19. Additionally, a locus on chromosome 3 was identified that was clinically consistent with NCIE (Fischer et al, 2000).

### Prognosis and Treatment

The same management principles recommended for neonates presenting with the collodion baby phenotype can be applied to infants with erythroderma, although their neonatal course is marked by fewer complications. The mainstay of therapy for children with lamellar ichthyosis is the use of topical emollients and keratolytic agents. Successful treatment with topical calcipotriol has been described (Delfino et al, 1994; Russell and Young, 1994). Any topically applied agent will be transcutaneously absorbed to a much higher degree than through normal skin; dosing must be carefully monitored (Abdel-Magid and el-Awad, 1994; Lucker, 1994). Treatment with systemic retinoids has had variable success (Steijlen et al, 1994b; Waisman et al, 1989).

## Ichthyosiform Syndromes

Several syndromes manifesting in the neonatal period have ichthyosis as a major feature.

### *Recessive X-linked Ichthyosis*

Recessive X-linked ichthyosis (RXLI) is an uncommon condition, affecting 1 in 6000 males. Signs of the disorder are present at birth in one fifth of affected infants; 85% develop skin changes by 3 months of age. The characteristic cutaneous finding is coarse brownish scaling, most prominent on the neck and extensor extremities. The palms and soles are spared. Extracutaneous manifestations include hypogonadism and cryptorchidism, present in up to 25% of affected males. Severely affected males may have short stature and mental retardation, a variant that has been referred to as Rud syndrome. Characteristic corneal opacities are seen in affected males and heterozygote females but usually not until late childhood or adolescence. Carrier females experience failure to initiate labor or prolonged labor. Light microscopic and ultrastructural findings in skin biopsy specimens are unremarkable. The

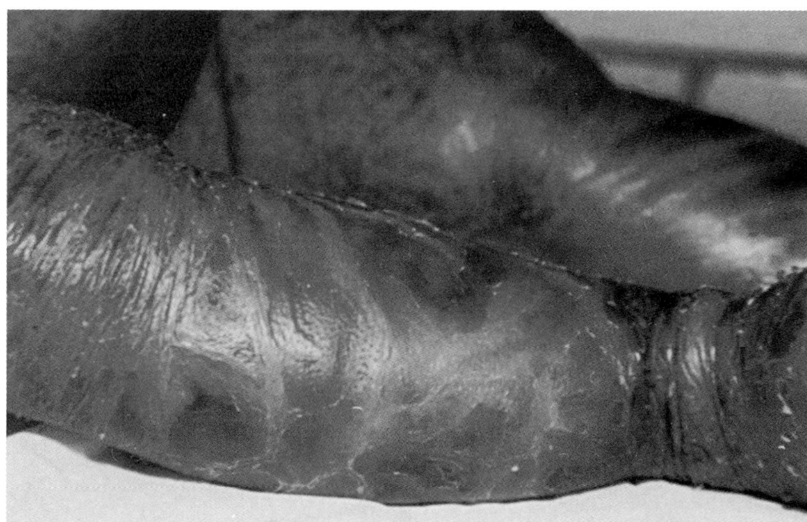

**FIGURE 97–4.** Large dark scales characteristic of lamellar ichthyosis on the leg of an affected infant.

pathogenesis of RXLI is aberrant production of the enzyme steroid sulfatase (a form of arylsulfatase C), with accumulation of cholesterol sulfate (Williams, 1986). The genetic abnormality has been localized to the distal short arm of the X chromosome (Xp22.3).

### *Netherton Syndrome/Ichthyosis Linearis Circumflexa*

Netherton syndrome is a rare, autosomal recessive condition. It often manifests at birth as ichthyosiform erythroderma, with flexural accentuation. The characteristic migratory, polycyclic lesions with a peripheral double-edged scale, referred to as *ichthyosis linearis circumflexa*, do not appear until after age 2 years. The syndrome is characterized by congenital ichthyosis, hair shaft defects (principally trichorrhexis invaginata), and atopic features (pruritus, hay fever, facial angioedema, and elevated immunoglobulin E [IgE]), but until the advent of genetic testing, diagnosis in affected children often was not possible for the first several years of life (Judge et al, 1994b). Generalized aminoaciduria and impaired cellular immunity also have been reported. This distinctive pattern of ichthyosis linearis circumflexa can also manifest as an isolated cutaneous condition. Recently, pathogenic mutations in Netherton syndrome were localized to the *SPINK5* gene on chromosome 5q32, which encodes the serine protease inhibitor LEKTI (Chavanas et al, 2000). Subsequently, prenatal testing for the disorder was successfully attempted (Müller et al, 2002; Sprecher et al, 2001).

### *Sjögren-Larsson Syndrome*

Sjögren-Larsson syndrome, inherited as an autosomal recessive disorder, usually manifests at birth with ichthyosiform erythroderma. The syndrome includes features that become evident only after the neonatal period: spastic diplegia, characteristic retinal lesions ("glistening dots"), and mental retardation. The diagnosis is supported by finding reduced or absent enzymatic activity of fatty aldehyde dehydrogenase from cultured skin fibroblasts, amniocytes, or chorionic cells. The genetic disorder that causes Sjögren-Larsson syndrome has been mapped to a locus on chromosome 17p11.2 that codes for a fatty aldehyde dehydrogenase (De Laurenzi et al, 1996).

### *Chondroplasia Punctata Syndromes (Conradi and Conradi-Hünermann Syndromes)*

The chondroplasia punctata syndromes are a loosely defined group of syndromes sharing distinctive skin and bone abnormalities that are present at birth but may disappear with time. The skin lesions consist of patterned hyperkeratosis along the lines of Blaschko. Orthopedic abnormalities (including asymmetrical shortening of the long bones) prompt radiologic evaluation that reveals chondrodysplasia punctata, characterized by punctate calcifications of the epiphyses and cartilage. Abnormal facies and cataracts are associated features. Autosomal dominant, autosomal recessive, and X-linked dominant forms have been reported. The genetic abnormality associated with X-linked dominant Conradi syndrome has now been mapped to the *EBP* gene locus at Xp11.22-p11.23, which codes for a sterol isomerase (Braverman et al, 1999; Derry et al, 1999).

### *CHILD Syndrome*

CHILD syndrome is characterized by a striking phenotype consisting of *c*ongenital *h*emidysplasia, unilateral *i*chthyosiform erythroderma, and *l*imb *d*efects and also is known as *unilateral congenital ichthyosiform erythroderma*. CHILD syndrome is an X-linked disorder that shares some features with the X-linked dominant Conradi syndrome. Most cases of CHILD syndrome probably are caused by a mutation of the NAD(P)H steroid dehydrogenase–like (NSDHL) protein gene, which has been mapped to Xq28 (Grange et al, 2000). This steroid dehydrogenase functions upstream of the sterol isomerase, which is defective in X-linked dominant Conradi syndrome in the cholesterol biosynthesis pathway. There have also been cases of mutations in the same *EBP* gene of X-linked Conradi syndrome that also included CHILD syndrome (Traupe and Has, 2000).

### *Keratitis-Ichthyosis-Deafness Syndrome*

Keratitis-ichthyosis-deafness (KID) syndrome is a rare disorder of autosomal dominant inheritance that consists of congenital ichthyosiform erythroderma with characteristic pebbly palmoplantar thickening; abnormalities of the nails, hair, and teeth; vascularizing keratitis; and sensorineural deafness. A few affected patients have died in infancy from overwhelming sepsis (Caceres-Rios et al, 1996). Recent evidence points to a mutation in connexin 26 as the pathogenesis of this disorder (van Steensel et al, 2002).

### *Neutral Lipid Storage Disease*

Neutral lipid storage disease, or Chanarin-Dorfman disease, consists of congenital ichthyosiform erythroderma, myopathy, neurosensory deafness, and cataracts. Inheritance is autosomal recessive. Vacuolated leukocytes from lipid droplets, seen on peripheral smear, help establish the diagnosis (Judge et al, 1994a). This disease is characterized by an intracellular accumulation of triacylglycerol droplets. Mutations in a newly discovered protein of the esterase/lipase/thioesterase subfamily, CGI-58, encoded by the *CDS* locus on chromosome 3p21 appear to be the cause of this disease (Lefèvre et al, 2001).

### *Trichothiodystrophy*

Trichothiodystrophy (TTD) is a disorder of autosomal recessive inheritance that includes a spectrum of ectodermal abnormalities: congenital ichthyosis (sometimes manifesting initially as collodion baby), brittle hair, and short stature (Kousseff, 1991). More severely affected patients have a constellation of features that has been referred to as *Tay syndrome*. These features include abnormal dentition, cataracts, nail dystrophy, progeric facies, and photosensitivity, with an increased incidence of skin cancers and a wide variety of central nervous system (CNS) abnormalities. Diagnosis is supported by detection of characteristic alternating light and dark bands within the hair shaft on examination under polarizing microscopy. Further analyses of hair and nails reveal a decrease in the sulfur-rich proteins (Itin and Pittelkow, 1990).

The genetic mutations that cause TTD are the subject of active research. Two genes implicated in TTD, *XPB* and *XPD*, have been found to encode DNA helicase subunits. Other mutations in these two genes can result in xeroderma pigmentosum, or Cockayne syndrome. *XPB* has been localized to chromosome 2q21, and *XPD* has been localized to 19q13.2-q13.3. There is also evidence that a mutation in an unlocalized third gene, *TTDA*, also may cause TTD (van Brabant et al, 2000).

## Primary Cutaneous Ichthyoses

Primary cutaneous ichthyoses are a group of familial disorders that have no prominent extracutaneous manifestations. Lamellar ichthyosis, congenital nonbullous icthyosiform erythroderma, and EHK also are primary cutaneous ichthyoses.

### *Ichthyosis Vulgaris*

Ichthyosis vulgaris is the most common form of ichthyosis, with an estimated incidence of 1/250. It is inherited as an autosomal dominant trait. Onset is usually after the first 3 months of life. Scaling is most prominent on the extensor surfaces of the limbs. The palms and soles also are affected. Affected persons often have coexisting keratosis pilaris and atopic dermatitis (Rabinowitz and Esterly, 1994). Skin biopsy distinguishes ichthyosis vulgaris from the other forms of ichthyosis by revealing small or absent keratohyalin granules. A major component of these granules, profilaggrin, is reduced or undetectable in the skin of affected persons (Nirunsuksiri et al, 1995).

### *Erythrokeratodermia Variabilis*

Erythrokeratodermia variabilis also is a very rare type of ichthyosis that can present in infancy; it usually is inherited in an autosomal dominant fashion, although a probable case of autosomal recessive inheritance has been reported (Armstrong et al, 1997). Affected persons have transient migratory areas of discrete macular erythema as well as fixed hyperkeratotic plaques. A mutation in the connexin 31 gene, which codes for the gap junction protein β3, was reported as the cause of erythrokeratodermia variabilis, but a subsequent case was shown to not have a mutated connexin 31 gene (Wilgoss et al, 1999).

#### Prognosis and Treatment for the Ichthyoses

It is important to distinguish among the various forms of ichthyosis so that the physician can offer a prognosis and appropriate genetic counseling to the family. The prognosis is related to the severity of the condition and the type of ichthyosis. The clinical signs and pedigree data sometimes provide sufficient information to make a diagnosis. Skin biopsy for light microscopy is diagnostic only for EHK and ichthyosis vulgaris. Other general screening laboratory tests are equally nonspecific. Unfortunately, a period of observation beyond the first 4 weeks of life is frequently needed, and laboratory confirmation of the correct diagnosis requires specialized studies (Holbrook et al, 1993).

Standard therapy begins with topical care designed to hydrate the stratum corneum. Frequent, brief tepid water baths should be followed immediately by liberal application of a bland ointment or cream emollient, such as petrolatum, Aquaphor, or Eucerin. Emollients containing keratolytics such as urea (10% to 25%), salicylic acid, propylene glycol, and alpha-hydroxy acids also are effective but are recommended only after infancy because of the risk of toxicity associated with increased percutaneous absorption. Irritating soaps and detergents should be avoided. Topical calcipotriol has been safe and effective as an agent for short-term therapy in adults with a variety of ichthyoses (Kragballe et al, 1995).

## Oculocutaneous Albinism

The term *oculocutaneous albinism* (OCA) refers to a group of congenital disorders that are clinically manifested by an absence of pigment of the skin, hair, and eyes, with associated photophobia and nystagmus. All races are affected; estimates of gene frequency vary depending on the population under consideration. As with many genetic disorders, the incidence of affected persons is increased in certain racial isolates in which there is a high percentage of consanguineous marriages (Witkop et al, 1989).

#### Causes

All forms of OCA but one are inherited in an autosomal recessive fashion. The characteristic pigmentary changes are due to a spectrum of biochemical defects that interfere with melanin synthesis or transport. Three types of oculocutaneous albinism have been mapped to specific chromosomal regions that code for regulatory proteins in the transport and synthesis of tyrosine, a precursor in the melanin synthesis pathway (Oetting and King, 1994). OCA type 1 results from mutations in the gene that codes for tyrosinase (locus 11q14-q21). Tyrosinase is a copper-containing enzyme that catalyzes the two rate-limiting steps in the melanin biosynthetic pathway, and patients with homozygous mutations have a lifelong inability to produce melanin in the eyes, hair, and skin. Over 90 different mutations have been identified (Nakamura et al, 2002). OCA type 2, the most common form of OCA, results from mutations in the *P* gene. Recent findings suggest that the p protein plays a major role in modulating the intracellular transport of tyrosinase (Toyofuku et al,

2002). OCA type 3 is caused by mutations in the tyrosinase-related protein 1 gene (*Tyrp1*). The encoded protein functions to maintain stability of tyrosinase (Sarangarajan and Boissy, 2001). Recent research suggests other genetic mutations may cause a fourth form of OCA (Newton et al, 2001).

### Diagnosis

OCA type 1 can be distinguished from OCA types 2 and 3 on the basis of subtle clinical differences and the presence or absence of tyrosinase activity. OCA type 1 is the tyrosinase-negative variant and can be diagnosed prenatally by fetal skin biopsy (Holbrook et al, 1993). It results from any of several defects in the tyrosinase gene (Tomita, 1994). In type 2 and type 3 OCA, tyrosinase activity is positive. Genetic testing may be necessary to distinguish OCA type 2 from type 3. Oculocutaneous albinism should be distinguished from simple ocular albinism, which has sex-linked, autosomal dominant, and autosomal recessive forms.

### Clinical Findings

Affected infants, regardless of their familial skin type, have a decrease in skin pigment. Hair and iris pigmentation can vary, depending on the genotype. Photophobia and nystagmus of varying degrees are also type specific. Visual acuity is almost always impaired. Patients with tyrosine-negative OCA have the most severe form of visual impairment. Associated abnormalities may include hemorrhagic diathesis (Hermansky-Pudlak syndrome), small stature, and defective mentation. Deafness can occur in association with oculocutaneous albinism as well as with a number of other pigmentary disorders (Konigsmark, 1972).

### Prognosis and Treatment

The most significant associated problems are visual impairment and the increased risk of sun-induced carcinogenesis. Treatment is supportive. Religious use of broad-spectrum sunblock with the highest available sun protection factor (SPF) is mandatory to protect against excessive exposure to sunlight. The safest approach for infants is zinc oxide ointment, sun-protective clothing [Sun Precautions, Seattle, WA; telephone: (800) 882-7860; Web site: www.sunprecautions.com], and sun avoidance. Persons with tyrosinase-positive albinism accumulate pigment with increasing age, decreasing the risk of sun-induced complications. The National Organization for Albinism and Hypopigmentation (NOAH) can provide additional information and support for affected families (see Resources section at the end of the chapter).

## Piebaldism

Piebaldism is an autosomal dominant congenital leukoderma, characterized by a white forelock. Histologic studies show an absence of melanocytes in the depigmented areas of skin and normal melanocytes in the uninvolved skin (Jimbow et al, 1975). The molecular basis of the disease has been identified as a defect of the c-*kit* protooncogene. This gene encodes the cell surface receptor transmembrane tyrosine kinase for an embryonic growth factor. When c-*kit* function is reduced, the migration of melanocytes is curtailed during embryogenesis (Tomita, 1994).

### Clinical Findings

A white forelock is present in 90% of cases. Other areas of the ventral skin may also be devoid of pigment, including the central forehead, chin, and trunk, with relative sparing of the dorsal surface. Eyebrows and midarm and midleg skin may also be depigmented. Within these areas, smaller, normally pigmented or hyperpigmented patches may be evident (Fig. 97–5).

### Diagnosis

Piebaldism is readily differentiated from albinism, in which the absence of pigment is uniform. Vitiligo may have a similar appearance, but it is not congenital and usually does not remain fixed. Occasional families may have associated defects such as sensorineural deafness and mental retardation (Telfer et al, 1971). Piebaldism is unrelated to Waardenburg syndrome, an autosomal dominant condition that features a white forelock, widened nasal bridge, and cochlear deafness.

### Prognosis and Treatment

The leukoderma and white forelock remain constant throughout life. Cosmetic camouflage is a treatment option suitable for infants and children. Surgical options are evolving.

## Aplasia Cutis Congenita

The congenital absence of skin is a cutaneous anomaly most often affecting the scalp but occasionally involving the trunk and extremities.

### Causes

Several distinct subtypes of aplasia cutis have been described based on the distribution, mode of inheritance, and associated abnormalities (Frieden, 1986). Most cases of aplasia cutis congenita occur sporadically; autosomal dominant and autosomal recessive modes of transmission also have been well documented (Sybert, 1985). Associated abnormalities include cleft lip and palate, limb anomalies, cutaneous organoid nevi, and EB. Aplasia cutis may overlie embryologic malformations such as meningomyelocele and spinal dysraphia, omphalocele, and gastroschesis (Frieden, 1986; Sybert, 1985). In addition, scalp defects are associated with specific teratogens (methimazole, intrauterine varicella, herpes simplex) and malformation syndromes (trisomy 13, Johanson-Blizzard syndrome, amniotic band disruption complex, and the ectodermal dysplasias). Extensive aplasia cutis has been associated with elevated alphafetoprotein in maternal serum and amniotic fluid (Gerber et al, 1993).

The cause of aplasia cutis congenita is unknown. Basically, it is a phenotypic physical finding signifying disruption of the skin in utero attributable to any of numerous causes. Findings of a twin fetus papyraceus or a placental

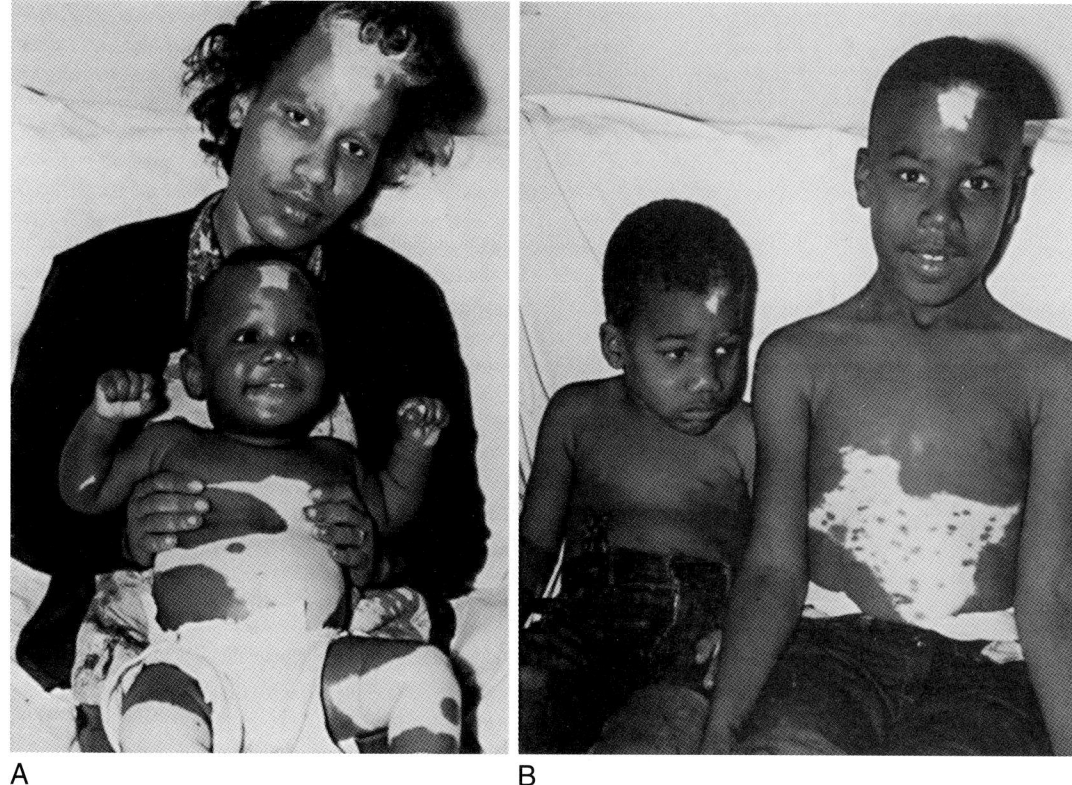


**FIGURE 97–5.** **A,** Mother and child with piebaldism. Both have patches on the forehead, although of different sizes and shapes. The areas of nonpigmentation on the infant's trunk and extremities are unusually extensive. **B,** Siblings with different degrees of piebaldism. *(From Jahn HM, McIntire MS: Am J Dis Child 88:481, 1954. © American Medical Association.)*

infarct have suggested vascular thrombosis as a cause in infants with lesions on the trunk and limbs (Levin et al, 1980).

### Clinical Findings

The defect is usually along the midline of the scalp in the parietal or occipital area. Lesions are sharply marginated and may manifest as ulcers, bullae, or scars. Lesions may be solitary or multiple, measuring up to several centimeters in diameter (Fig. 97–6). Up to 30% of affected infants have underlying defects of the calvaria. Multiple defects, particularly those on the trunk and extremities, may be strikingly symmetrical in distribution (Levin et al, 1980). Larger defects are often deeper and may extend to the dura or meninges. These may be complicated by meningitis, hemorrhage (which can be fatal), or venous thrombosis.

Histologic examination of tissue from the defect demonstrates an absence of epidermis and a diminished number of appendageal structures and dermal elastic fibers or, in deeper lesions, the absence of all layers of the integument. There is no evidence of inflammation or pathogenic organisms.

### Prognosis and Treatment

Cutaneous and bony lesions can heal spontaneously over a period of weeks to months. A hypertrophic or atrophic patch of alopecia remains. Patients with larger and deeper lesions must be observed for the possibility of a complicating meningitis. Prophylactic excision with repair should be considered in these cases. Lesions that fail to heal or produce cosmetically unacceptable scars can be excised with primary closure (Kosnik and Sayers, 1975).

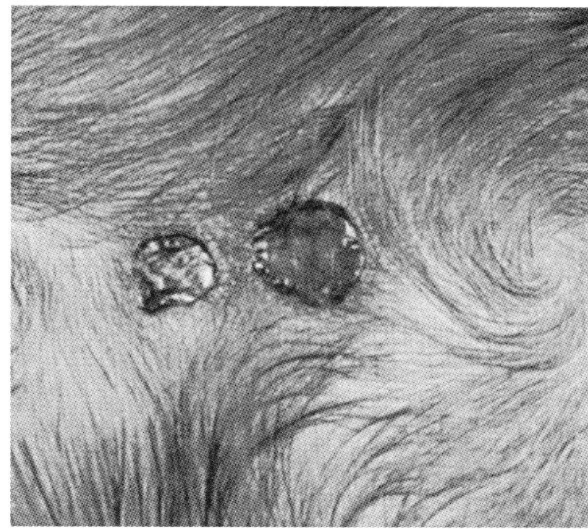

**FIGURE 97–6.** Skin is absent in two sharply marginated areas on the scalp of a normal newborn male infant whose mother's labor and delivery were normal. The defects extended to the subcutaneous tissue and healed in 3 weeks with the formation of thin, white atrophic scars.

## Incontinentia Pigmenti

Incontinentia pigmenti (IP), also known as the Bloch-Sulzberger syndrome, is a disorder of the developing neuroectoderm, characterized by three distinctive, transient stages of cutaneous lesions and variable persistent abnormalities of the CNS, eyes, teeth, hair, and nails.

### Causes

IP is inherited in an X-linked dominant fashion. Surviving females are mosaics, whereas most hemizygous males do not survive embryogenesis. Molecular research points to mutations at one genetic locus at Xq28 as the cause of all true cases of IP. The nuclear factor *k*B essential modulator gene (*NEMO*) codes for a transcription factor. Eighty percent of IP cases were found to result from a single mutation (Berlin et al, 2002).

### Clinical Findings

The diagnosis of IP is made by cutaneous examination. Most patients exhibit three stages of skin lesions that persist for varying periods (O'Brien and Feingold, 1985). The *vesiculobullous* phase presents at birth and generally lasts for several months. It is characterized by widespread inflammatory vesicular lesions on the scalp, trunk, and extremities in a whorled and linear distribution along the lines of Blaschko (Fig. 97–7A). The infant is otherwise well, although markedly elevated leukocyte counts and peripheral eosinophilia with as much as 79% eosinophils may be associated (Berlin et al, 2002). The vesicular phase evolves into a *verrucous* phase, in which warty lesions appear in roughly the same distribution as the blisters but are most pronounced on the hands and feet. The third stage is characterized by macular gray or brown pigmentation distributed along Blashchko's lines, independent of the sites of previous lesions (see Fig. 97–7B). The pigmentary lesions usually fade in later years and may disappear by adulthood. Rarely, the stage three pigmentary changes are present at birth, and the first two stages are never evident (Lerer et al, 1973). Fourth-stage lesions, seen in some affected women, consist of hypopigmented, atrophic, anhidrotic streaks, usually localized to the legs (Moss and Ince, 1987).

Eighty percent of affected persons have extracutaneous involvement, including CNS aberrations (seizures, microcephaly, retardation, and spastic paralysis), patchy alopecia, defective dentition, ocular abnormalities, and less commonly, bone defects (Carney, 1976).

### Diagnosis

Infants with IP usually present with blisters. The linear distribution of blisters is often so characteristic that it permits instant recognition of the disorder. But other causes of blisters must be considered in the differential diagnosis (see Chapter 96). Skin biopsy during the bullous phase will show intraepidermal vesicles filled with eosinophils.

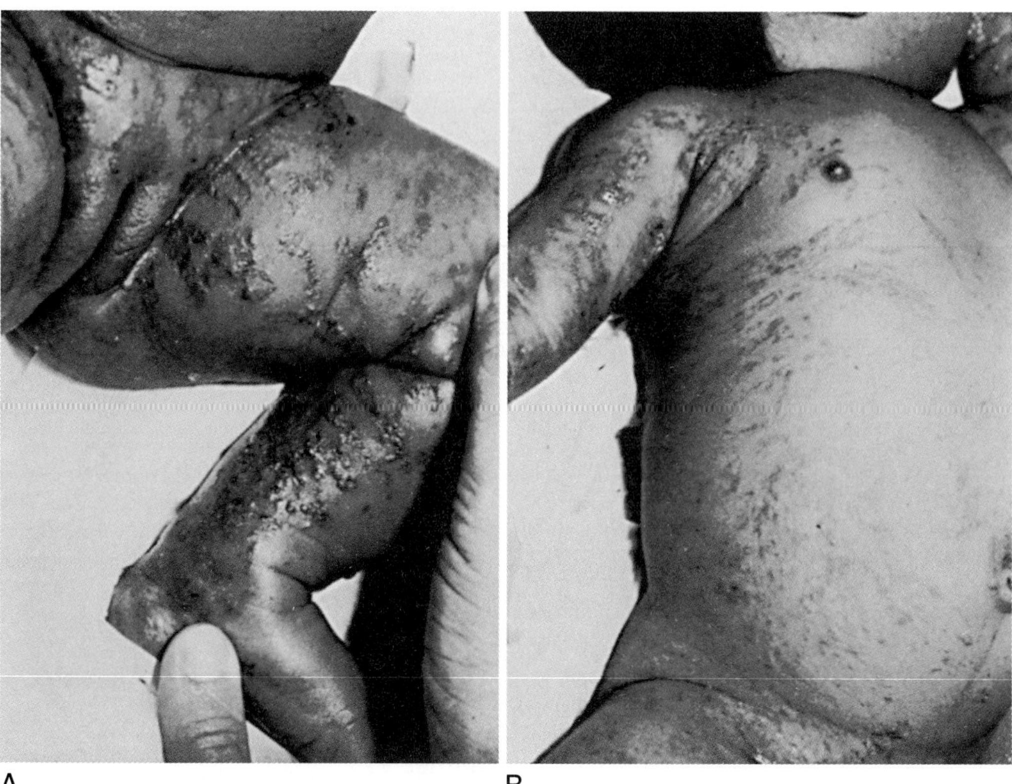

**FIGURE 97–7.** Incontinentia pigmenti. **A,** Inflammatory vesicular and crusted lesions on the legs. **B,** Whorled pigmentation developing on the trunk of a 1-month-old infant, who still has inflammatory lesions on the limbs.

These features are not pathognomonic but help exclude more ominous causes of neonatal blistering. Clinicians should refer patients for genetic testing to the DNA Diagnostic Laboratory at Baylor College of Medicine (see under "Incontinentia Pigmenti" in Resources section).

### Prognosis and Treatment

Treatment of the skin lesions is not necessary. Occasionally, vesicular lesions become extremely inflamed or secondarily infected. Patients should be monitored for the development of other anomalies, especially of the eyes, teeth, and CNS. Genetic counseling is indicated. Two IP support groups for patients and their families are the Incontinentia Pigmenti International Foundation and the Incontinentia Pigmenti Support Network (see Resources section).

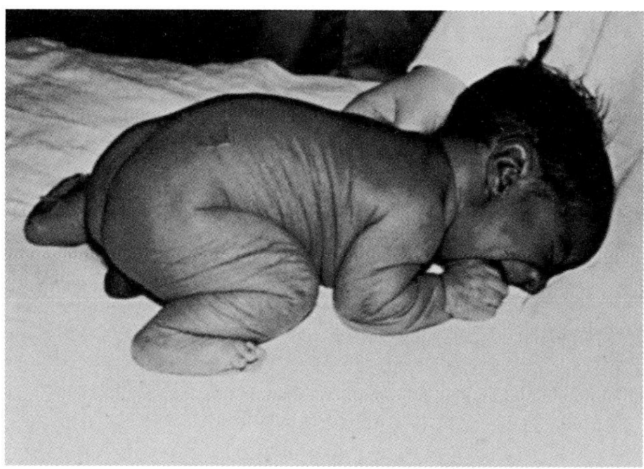

**FIGURE 97–8.** Newborn infant with clinical features of Menkes syndrome and cutis laxa.

## Cutis Laxa

Cutis laxa is a rare, heterogeneous group of genetic abnormalities of connective tissue with striking cutaneous features. Autosomal dominant, autosomal recessive, and X-linked forms have been described (Beighton, 1972; Byers et al, 1980). Cutis laxa–like skin changes can also be found in other disorders (e.g., combined immunodeficiency disease, the Prader-Willi and Langer-Giedion syndromes).

### Clinical Features

Cutis laxa-like skin hangs in pendulous folds, producing a facies with a hooked nose, everted nostrils, a long upper lip, sagging cheeks, and a prematurely aged appearance (Fig. 97–8). The infant may have a hoarse cry due to redundant laryngeal tissue. Persons with the autosomal dominant form of cutis laxa suffer few ill effects, apart from their altered appearance, and enjoy good health and a normal life span. Pulmonary and cardiovascular manifestations are absent or minimal. In contrast, patients with the recessive form of the disorder are often seriously compromised and may die in childhood of pulmonary or cardiovascular complications. Systemic manifestations include diverticula of the gastrointestinal and urogenital tracts, rectal prolapse, multiple hernias, pulmonary emphysema, and cardiac disease (Mehregan et al, 1978). A few infants have been reported who manifested additional defects, such as skeletal anomalies, dislocation of the hips, and intrauterine growth retardation (Sakati et al, 1983).

### Diagnosis

The clinical manifestations of cutis laxa can be attributed to abnormalities of elastin. Elastic fibers are diminished in the papillary and upper dermis, whereas those in the lower dermis undergo fragmentation and granular degeneration (Mehregan et al, 1978). Similar changes occur in the elastic tissue of affected viscera. Autosomal recessive cutis laxa has been associated with a deficiency of lysyl oxidase, a copper-dependent enzyme mapped to chromosome 5 (Khakoo et al, 1997). The X-linked form has been associated with abnormal intracellular copper metabolism, with a decrease in the activity of lysyl oxidase. This form of cutis laxa, once classified as type IX Ehlers-Danlos syndrome, was redefined as occipital horn syndrome, an X-linked recessive condition allelic to Menkes syndrome (Beighton et al, 1988; Byers, 1994; Goldsmith, 1990) (see Fig. 97–8).

### Treatment

Plastic surgery can improve the physical appearance of patients with cutis laxa (Thomas et al, 1993). The internal manifestations are not amenable to therapy.

## Ehlers-Danlos Syndrome

The Ehlers-Danlos syndrome (EDS) is another heterogeneous group of inherited connective tissue disorders. In contrast to patients with cutis laxa, those with EDS have skin that is hyperextensible rather than loose; when stretched, the skin readily snaps back into place. Skin fragility is another feature, leading to easy bruising and bleeding, gaping wounds, and numerous cigarette paper–like scars. Joint hypermobility is another major manifestation. The classification of EDS is evolving, and the latest classification scheme now identifies six major types: the classic type, the hypermobility type, the vascular type, the kyphoscoliosis type, the arthrochalasia type, and the dermatosparaxis type. The kyphoscoliosis and dermatosparaxis types are inherited in an autosomal recessive fashion, whereas inheritance for the other four types is autosomal dominant. In addition, there are other known cases of EDS that do not fit into one of these types and await further characterization (Beighton et al, 1998). Persons with the vascular type of EDS (type IV by previous classification) can be easily distinguished from those with the other forms by their thin, translucent skin, marked bruising, and normal range of motion. It is especially important to identify this group because of its life-threatening complications (Byers, 1994).

### Causes

All forms of EDS are believed to be due to defects in the biogenesis of collagen. The vascular type is characterized by a variety of defects in the synthesis of type III collagen, the kyphoscoliosis type by lysyl hydroxylase deficiency, the arthrochalasia type by defective processing of type I collagen, and the dermatosparaxis type by procollagen *N*-proteinase deficiency. These specific defects can be identified by culture of dermal fibroblasts from a skin biopsy.

### Treatment

Recognition of the correct subtype is important for prognosis. The vascular type of EDS is particularly important to identify because of the life-threatening association with arterial, bowel, and uterine ruptures. There is no effective treatment for the various forms of EDS. Affected patients tolerate surgical procedures poorly because of difficulty in healing and frequent dehiscence of surgical wounds. Repair of cutaneous wounds may require the services of a plastic surgeon, and progressive joint disease will require ongoing orthopedic care. The Ehlers-Danlos National Foundation can provide additional information and support for affected families (see Resources section at the end of the chapter).

## Epidermolysis Bullosa

Epidermolysis bullosa (EB) is a diverse group of diseases that is characterized by skin blistering. Classification is based on clinical characteristics, inheritance pattern, and the level of cleavage within the skin, as determined by skin biopsy. This prominent histologic feature defines three main groups: simplex (cleavage within the basal cells of the epidermis), junctional (within the lamina lucida of the basement membrane zone), and dystrophic (beneath the lamina densa of the basement membrane). At each level, there are several protein components that contribute to skin integrity. These molecules all are expressed in utero during the first trimester, allowing prenatal diagnosis by skin biopsy (Holbrook et al, 1993). Further progress in the field has led to a simplified classification system that recognizes 10 major subtypes; three major EB types, epidermolysis bullosa simplex (EBS), junctional epidermolysis bullosa (JEB), and dystrophic epidermolysis bullosa (DEB); and 11 minor subtypes. (Fine et al, 2000). Research efforts have been greatly enhanced by the Dystrophic Epidermolysis Bullosa Research Association of America (DEBRA) (see Resources section) and the National Epidermolysis Bullosa Registry (see Resources section) (Fine et al, 1994). Identification of the molecular basis of a number of EB genotypes has not only facilitated prenatal and postnatal diagnoses but has also provided insight into the pathogenesis of blistering diseases, as well as the basic mechanisms of epithelial and basement membrane integrity.

### Epidermolysis Bullosa Simplex

EB simplex features blisters that arise within the basal layer of the epidermis. For this reason, the lesions of EB simplex do not scar. Four major subtypes and several minor subtypes have been recognized (Fine et al, 2000). The molecular defects of EB simplex have been localized to the genes encoding specific keratins, *K14* (located on chromosome 17) and *K5* (located on chromosome 12), except for EB with muscular dystrophy, which is due to a defect in plectin. Keratins K5 and K14 are expressed predominantly in the basal cells of the epidermis, and these disorders are closely related to epidermolytic hyperkeratosis (Francis, 1994) (see earlier section on ichthyoses). The four major subtypes are described next.

#### *Epidermolysis Bullosa Simplex, Koebner Subtype*

ES simplex, Koebner subtype (EBS-K), inherited as an autosomal dominant trait, is present at birth or early in infancy. Bullae arise most frequently over pressure points, such as the elbows and knees, as well as on the legs, feet, and hands. Mucous membrane involvement occurs primarily during infancy. The extensive erosions that sometimes result from the trauma of birth may be mistaken for aplasia cutis. Nails may be lost but almost always regrow. The prognosis is relatively good, and the propensity to blister may decrease with age.

#### *Epidermolysis Bullosa Simplex, Dowling-Meara Subtype*

EB simplex, Dowling-Meara subtype (EBS-DM), is inherited as an autosomal dominant trait and causes generalized, often extensive blistering in the neonatal period and early years of life. Herpetiform grouping of the blisters is characteristic. Additional findings include nail dystrophy, palmoplantar keratoderma as a late feature, and improvement with age.

#### *Epidermolysis Bullosa Simplex, Weber-Cockayne Subtype*

EB simplex, Weber-Cockayne subtype (EBS-WC), is inherited in autosomal dominant fashion and usually does not manifest during the neonatal period. The blisters in this disease usually are limited to the hands and feet, although they occasionally occur elsewhere on the body.

#### *Epidermolysis Bullosa Simplex with Muscular Dystrophy*

EB simplex with muscular dystrophy (EBS-MD) is a rare variant that is inherited in an autosomal recessive fashion. Affected persons usually demonstrate blisters on the skin and mucous membranes at birth or shortly thereafter. EBS-MD is associated with tooth enamel hypoplasia and nail dystrophy. Progressive muscular dystrophy usually occurs later in life (Shimizu et al, 1999).

### Junctional Epidermolysis Bullosa

Junctional EB (JEB) is characterized by cleavage within the lamina lucida of the basement membrane zone. Three major subtypes are now recognized: JEB, Herlitz subtype; JEB, non-Herlitz subtype; and JEB with pyloric atresia. Molecular defects have been recognized within several proteins found in the basement membrane zone, including laminin-5, type XVII collagen, and the $\alpha_6,\beta_4$-integrin complex. Several subtypes of JEB are relatively localized and benign (Fine et al, 2000). The major subtypes are described next.

### *Junctional Epidermolysis Bullosa, Herlitz Subtype*

JEB, Herlitz type (JEB-H), was formerly known as EB gravis or letalis because many affected patients die in infancy. Generalized blistering is noted at birth. Persons with this form of JEB can, however, exhibit a spectrum of severity. Bullae and moist erosions occur on the scalp, in the perioral area, and over pressure points elsewhere on the body (Fig. 97–9A). Some of these erosions become the sites of vegetating granulomas, a pathognomonic finding. The hands and feet are relatively spared, and digital fusion, inevitable in the recessive dystrophic type of EB, does not occur. Nails are affected and may be lost permanently. Defective dentition is the rule, but mucous membrane erosions are inconspicuous and rarely cause problems. Laryngeal involvement can occur in childhood, manifested as hoarseness or stridor. These patients grow poorly, appear malnourished, and have chronic recalcitrant anemia

### *Junctional Epidermolysis Bullosa, Non-Herlitz Subtype*

JEB, non-Herlitz subtype (JEB-nH), is a disorder of autosomal recessive inheritance that carries the best prognosis of the major subtypes, with affected persons often surviving into adulthood. Onset is usually at birth, with generalized blistering; dystrophic nails or absence of nails is common (Fine et al, 2000).

### *Junctional Epidermolysis Bullosa with Pyloric Atresia*

JEB with pyloric atresia (JEB-PA) is a rare, autosomal recessively inherited disease characterized by mucocutaneous fragility. JEB-PA is usually fatal in the first few weeks of life, although mild cases have been reported. Polyhydramnios seen at ultrasound examination may be the first clue to gastric outlet obstruction. Generalized blistering and ulcerations of skin and mucous membranes usually are evident at birth. The urinary tract frequently is involved, stenosis being a common complication for survivors (Mellerio et al, 1998).

## Dystrophic Epidermolysis Bullosa

Dystrophic EB is characterized by subepidermal blistering, below the level of the lamina densa of the basement membrane. The anchoring fibrils that link the lower part of the basement membrane to the papillary dermis are composed of type VII collagen. Mutations of the gene that codes for type VII collagen have been identified in most forms of dystrophic EB. This group of diseases is characterized clinically by milia and scarring at the sites of healed blisters. There are three major subtypes and several minor subtypes. All are present at birth (Fine et al, 1991b). Prenatal diagnosis as early as 8 to 10 weeks is possible by molecular techniques for some families. The three major subtypes are described next, as well as one of the more distinctive minor subtypes.

### Dominant Dystrophic Epidermolysis Bullosa

Dominant dystrophic EB (DDEB) is a relatively mild form, inherited as an autosomal dominant trait. Generalized blistering usually is noted at birth. In some cases, blistering may appear only on the hands, feet, elbows, or knees; this pattern is usually due to mechanical trauma. Rarely does scarring cause immobility and deformity of the hands and feet. Small cysts or milia are seen at sites of scarring. There may be mild involvement of the mucous

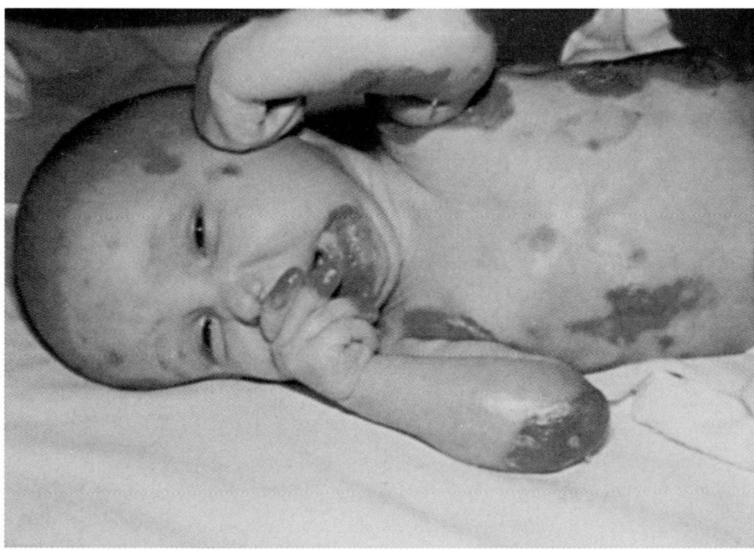

A

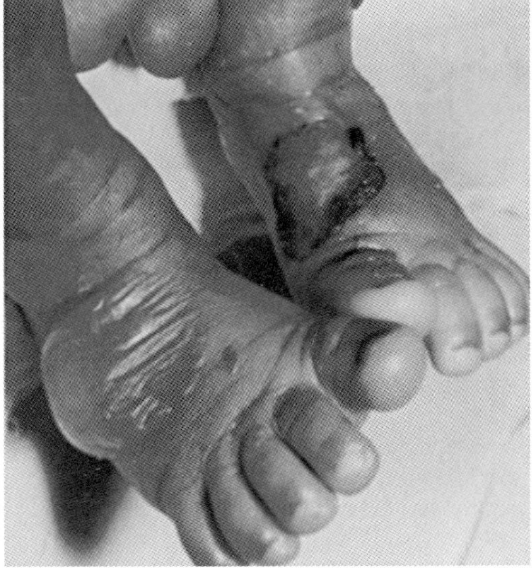

B

**FIGURE 97–9.** **A,** Multiple moist erosions characteristic of junctional epidermolysis bullosa. Note involvement of fingers and perioral skin. **B,** Large bullae on the feet of an infant with a scarring form of epidermolysis bullosa.

membranes; nails may be thick, dystrophic, or destroyed. Some persons affected by this form of EB may note the presence of small, firm, flesh-colored or white skin elevations that appear spontaneously on the trunk and extremities, called *albopapuloid lesions*.

The Cockayne-Touraine and Pasini types of EB formerly were considered to represent two generalized forms of dominant dystrophic EB but are now included within DDEB in the new classification system. The bullae are subepidermal and heal with scarring, but the process may be relatively limited, involving mainly hands, feet (see Fig. 97–9B), and skin over bony protuberances, or may be generalized, particularly in the Pasini variant. Nails may be lost. Milia are common and may appear in profusion in the soft, wrinkled scars; pigmentary changes also are usual. Mucous membrane lesions, if present, are mild, and general health may be unimpaired. The appearance of albopapuloid lesions on the trunk during adolescence is a unique feature of the Pasini variant.

#### *Transient Bullous Dermolysis of the Newborn*

The rare variant transient bullous dermolysis of the newborn was first reported in 1985. Autosomal dominant and recessive forms have been described. The dominant form is now thought to be a form of DDEB. Affected neonates present with alarming acral or generalized blistering that heals with scars. Histologic analyses have localized the abnormality to the precursors of the anchoring fibrils, and genetic studies have shown mutations in a gene that codes for type VII collagen in some cases (Hammami-Hauasli et al, 1998). This condition is unique among the subsets of EB because it spontaneously resolves within the first years of life.

#### *Recessive Dystrophic Epidermolysis Bullosa, Hallopeau-Siemens Subtype*

Recessive dystrophic EB, Hallopeau-Siemens subtype, is the more severe form of recessive dystrophic EB. Infants with Hallopeau-Siemens EB often have extensive denuded lesions at birth and during the neonatal period. Bullae may be hemorrhagic and occur on all surfaces, including the hands and feet; loss of the nails is usual. Over subsequent years the mobility of the fingers and toes becomes severely impaired as fusion of digits, bone resorption, and the inevitable mitten-like deformity of the hands and feet ensue. Mucous membrane involvement may be severe, resulting in esophageal strictures and serious impairment of nutrition due to the restriction of oral intake. These bullae are subepidermal and always eventuate in scarring. Affected persons have a markedly increased risk of skin cancer, with a 39.6% cumulative risk of developing squamous cell carcinoma and a 2.5% cumulative risk of developing malignant melanoma by age 30 (Fine et al, 2000). Electron microscopy reveals diminished or absent anchoring fibrils associated with marked degeneration of type VII collagen in the papillary portion of the dermis. Also evident is excess abnormal collagenase in fibroblast cultures.

#### *Recessive Dystrophic Epidermolysis Bullosa, Non–Hallopeau-Siemens Subtype*

Recessive dystrophic EB, non–Hallopeau-Siemens subtype, is the less severe form of recessive dystrophic EB. It is characterized by onset at birth, generalized blisters to include the mucosal surfaces, atrophic scarring over bony prominences and either nail loss or nail dystrophy. Milia, mild finger flexion contractures, albopapuloid lesions, dental disease, and external ear involvement also are often seen. According to one report, affected patients also have an increased risk of squamous cell carcinoma of about 14% by age 30 (Fine et al, 2000).

## Diagnosis and Treatment of Epidermolysis Bullosa

### Diagnosis

Arriving at the correct diagnosis can be difficult, especially in the neonatal period. The differential diagnosis includes the spectrum of blisters and bullae outlined in Chapter 96. The distribution of blisters can be a clue. In EB, the earliest lesions occur on points of friction, such as the heels, wrists, knees, and sacrum. The fluid within the bullae is likely to be clear or hemorrhagic, rather than purulent. A careful family history for blistering diseases should be obtained. The most precise diagnostic tool is a carefully performed skin biopsy to obtain specimens for immunofluorescence mapping and ultrastructural study. The sample for immunofluorescence should be obtained from normal or perilesional skin, excluding the palms or soles, and placed in Zeus or Michel transport medium. The ideal specimen for electron microscopy is a new spontaneous or induced blister preserved in glutaraldehyde (Fine et al, 1994). After the diagnosis of simplex, junctional, or dystrophic EB is made, further subclassification can be difficult during infancy for subsets without a defined genotype. In these patients without relevant family history, distinguishing clinical features may take months or years to develop.

### Treatment

To date, the mainstay of therapy for this group of disorders is supportive. The infant should be protected from frictional trauma; direct pressure is tolerated. Latex gloves can stick to the skin and should be lubricated with petrolatum. Bedding should be of a soft material. Dressing changes should be performed daily. Adequate premedication for pain control should be given. Bathing may have to be restricted to avoid excessive handling. Compresses with normal saline or Burow solution for eroded areas may be helpful in some instances. Tepid compresses should be used, because warm temperatures increase the tendency to blister. Intact blisters should be lanced with an adequate incision to drain the fluid, while the roof is maintained as a "biologic dressing." Wounds should be covered with petrolatum-impregnated gauze. Topical antibiotics may promote healing, but content and quantity should be carefully monitored in young infants (see Chapter 98). Topical mupirocin is the antibiotic of choice at several EB centers; bacterial resistance has been reported in chronic users with EB. Commercially available nonadhesive dressings are simpler to use and more effective than plain gauze wraps. Exudry pads, secured with Surginet or conforming gauze, are recommended for draining wounds on the body. Omiderm (Doak Pharmaceuticals) is a nonadhesive polyurethane dressing that provides an excellent barrier for moist wounds on the face and hands. Adhesive tape should never be applied, because large areas of epidermis may be torn off with its removal. Dressing should be applied to blistered areas only to maximize the infant's tactile stimulation. For the newborn, environmental temperature must be carefully monitored; overheating may result in extensive blistering. For patients with mucous membrane involvement, soft nipples, bulb syringes, and devices used for feeding infants with cleft palates should be used. Chronic serosanguineous drainage and gastrointestinal involvement often result in poor nutritional status. Iron deficiency anemia is another common complication in infants with severe disease. Routine use of aggressive nutritional supplementation is recommended. After discharge, cribs, high chairs, and infant seats should be well padded, and only soft toys offered for play (Gibbons, 1990).

Caregivers should be given anticipatory guidance about protective measures, wound care, and nutrition. The practitioner should encourage contact with DEBRA, a privately funded organization that is an excellent resource for affected families. DEBRA can provide practical information for day-to-day care and direct families to the appropriate regional center for specialized care (see Resources section). To register newly diagnosed patients, clinicians should contact the National Epidermolysis Bullosa Registry (see Resources section).

## Neonatal Lupus Erythematosus

Neonatal lupus erythematosus (NLE) is an uncommon immune-mediated disease that results from transplacental transfer of maternal immunoglobulin G (IgG) antinuclear antibodies. It manifests within the first 2 months of life. Infants present with a spectrum of signs, including transient cutaneous lesions, thrombocytopenia, hepatitis, and/or congenital heart blocks; all affected infants have serologic evidence of lupus erythematosus during the first few months of life (Lee, 1993; Lee and Weston, 1984; Provost et al, 1987).

### Causes

NLE is always marked by the presence of anti-Ro (SS-A), anti-La (SS-B), and/or anti-$U_1$RNP autoantibodies in the mother and infant. With the exception of congenital heart block, most of the manifestations of neonatal lupus resolve with the disappearance of maternal antibodies, suggesting an important role for these antibodies in pathogenesis. An association with HLA-DR3 in the mother but not the infant also has been documented (Lee and Weston, 1984). Ro-positive HLA-DR2 mothers, in contrast, produce unaffected infants (Provost et al, 1987).

### Clinical Findings

Half of the affected infants have skin lesions. These may be present with or without evidence of systemic disease (Hardy et al, 1979). Skin lesions are typically annular erythematous scaling plaques (Fig. 97–10), with a predilection for sun-exposed areas. These begin to resolve at about 6 months, concurrent with the disappearance of maternal antibodies. Persistent telangiectatic matting in a characteristic distribution, involving the scalp, lips, and vulva, also has been described (Fig. 97–11) (Thornton et al, 1995).

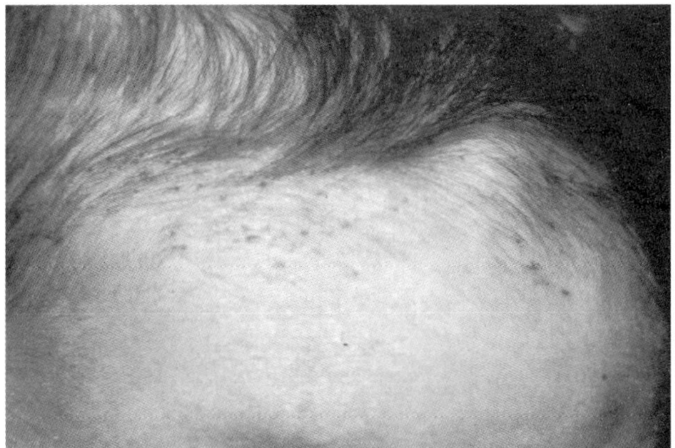

**FIGURE 97–10.** Newborn with cutaneous lesions of neonatal lupus erythematosus.

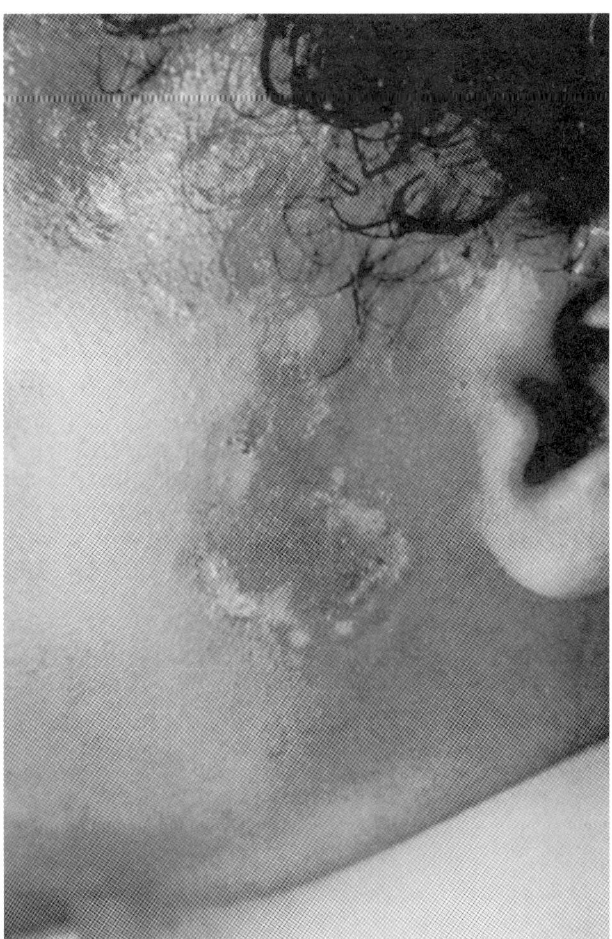

**FIGURE 97–11.** Telangiectatic matting of the scalp, lips, and groin is a recently recognized cutaneous marker of neonatal lupus.

### Diagnosis

The skin lesions of NLE can be mistaken for several cutaneous disorders including syphilis, seborrheic dermatitis, dermatophytosis, atopic dermatitis, and psoriasis. Skin biopsy may demonstrate the histopathologic features of lupus. More reliable, however, is the detection of Ro (SS-A) and/or La (SS-B) antibody in serum from the infant and the mother.

The North American Collaborative Study of NLE is an ongoing prospective study of all aspects of the disease. To arrange for enrollment and serologic testing of patients, clinicians should contact study investigators (see under "Neonatal Lupus Erythematosus" in Resources section).

### Prognosis and Treatment

Affected infants should be protected from sources of ultraviolet light (sunlight and daylight fluorescent bulbs) by application of a broad-spectrum sunscreen such as titanium dioxide, zinc oxide, and sun-protective clothing [Sun Precautions, Seattle, Washington; telephone: (800) 882-7860]. Active skin lesions may be treated with a topical corticosteroid.

The prognosis is excellent, except in affected infants who develop congenital heart block. Most infants with congenital heart block will require a pacemaker, and death will occur in about 20% (Tseng and Buyon, 1997).

It is important to recognize that asymptomatic mothers are at risk for development of disorders associated with their serologic abnormalities (e.g., Sjögren syndrome, subacute cutaneous lupus, systemic lupus erythematosus). There is a 25% risk of involvement for each subsequent pregnancy (Gawkrodger and Beveridge, 1984; McCune et al, 1987).

## Ectodermal Dysplasias

The ectodermal dysplasias (EDs) are a heterogeneous group of inherited disorders characterized by defects in the development of two or more structures of ectodermal origin. The major structures involved are hair follicles, nails, teeth, and sweat glands; sebaceous glands, conjunctivae, and/or the lens also may be affected. A formal classification system has been created for the EDs, based on the specific structures affected (Pinheiro and Freire-Maia, 1994). One hundred fifty-four syndromes have been included in this grouping. Several of these, such as incontinentia pigmenti and syndromes associated with ichthyosis, have not been traditionally regarded as ED. Many others have been reported rarely. The National Foundation for Ectodermal Dysplasias (NFED) is a privately funded organization committed to locating affected families and providing them with information and support (see Resources section). The NFED also coordinates and funds research efforts.

Three of the more well-characterized types of ED are described next.

### Hypohidrotic Ectodermal Dysplasia

Hypohidrotic ED, inherited as an X-linked recessive disorder, was the first type of ED described, as Christ-Siemens-Touraine syndrome. It was previously referred to as "anhidrotic," but affected persons may have a limited capacity to sweat, and the preferred descriptor is *hypohidrotic*. This type of ED occurs in 1 in 100,000 male births and manifests during the first year of life. The most serious problem is diminution of the sweating response due to rudimentary or absent eccrine sweat glands, which results in marked heat intolerance and episodes of hyperpyrexia, frequently misinterpreted as fever of unknown origin (Richards and Kaplan, 1969). If ED is not considered in the differential diagnosis, these infants may be subjected to numerous unnecessary hospitalizations and tests.

#### Clinical Features

Patients with hypohidrotic ED have several characteristic features that may be subtle in the newborn. One common neonatal sign is severe peeling or scaling skin. This skin change, which can be misconstrued as an indication of postmaturity, may provide a valuable clue to the diagnosis (Executive and Scientific Advisory Boards of the NFED, 1989). Thereafter, the skin may appear relatively pale and dry, with a prominent venous pattern over most of the body, but hyperpigmented and wrinkled in the periorbital area (Fig. 97–12).

The craniofacial characteristics of frontal bossing, depression of the midface, flattened nasal bridge, thick protruding lips, and prominent chin may not be readily apparent in the newborn. Likewise, the sparse, unruly, light-colored hair and scanty brows and lashes also are difficult to appreciate in the first few months. The changes in dentition cannot, of course, be detected until late infancy. Hypodontia with conical, poorly formed teeth is the rule; these changes can be identified on dental panoramic radiographs prior to eruption of the teeth. Atrophic rhinitis, diminished lacrimation, hoarseness, and hypoplasia or absence of mucous glands in nasotracheobronchial passages are also frequent findings in these patients (Reed et al, 1970). If the diagnosis is in doubt, palmar skin biopsy may demonstrate absent or hypoplastic eccrine sweat glands. Techniques used to elicit sweating, such as pilocarpine iontophoresis or examination of the

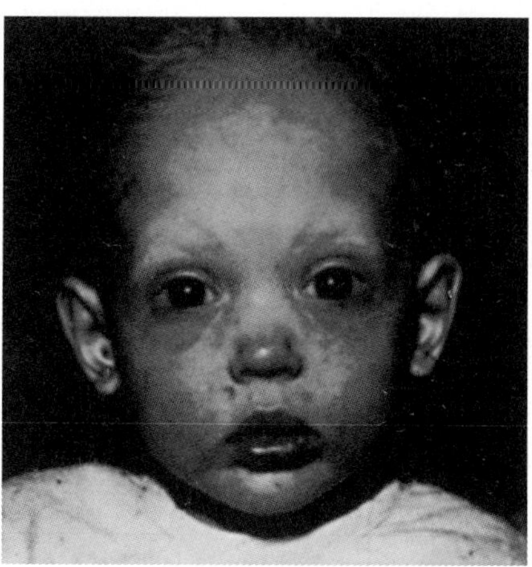

**FIGURE 97–12.** Girl with fully expressed anhidrotic ectodermal dysplasia. Note the sparse wispy hair, hyperpigmentation around the eyes, depressed nasal bridge, and protruding lips and ears.

sweat pores on the palm with *O*-phthalaldehyde, also can be utilized to demonstrate the defect (Esterly et al, 1973). Atopic dermatitis occurs frequently in these children (Reed et al, 1970), as well as a decrease in T-cell function (Davis and Solomon, 1976).

Hypohidrotic ED is transmitted as an X-linked recessive trait. The gene has been localized to Xq11.21.1. First-trimester prenatal diagnosis is possible (Zonana et al, 1990). All affected males fully express the disease, whereas carrier females have variable expression of the clinical signs. This expression can be explained by the inactivation of a random percentage of abnormal X chromosomes. In these females, hypohidrosis can be demonstrated in areas of skin marking the lines of Blaschko (see the section on mosaicism) (Bolognia et al, 1994; Crump and Danks, 1971; Esterly et al, 1973; Gorlin et al, 1970).

Once the diagnosis is made, it is important to educate parents so that these children are protected from overheating. Defective lacrimation can be palliated by the use of artificial tears. The nasal mucosa should be treated with saline drops or irrigation followed by application of petrolatum. Regular dental evaluations should be started early in life and dentures fitted to promote good nutrition, articulation, and normal appearance before the child starts school. Some of these children also choose a wig and reconstructive procedures later in life to improve facial configuration.

### Hidrotic Ectodermal Dysplasia

Hidrotic ED, also known as Clouston syndrome, is an autosomal dominant condition. Affected individuals have characteristic abnormalities of skin, hair, and nails, whereas eccrine and sebaceous functions and dentition are normal. The phenotype is easily recognizable in early childhood, with features including thickened, conical nails and widening of the distal periungual area with cerebriform furrowing. The skin over the joints often is hyperpigmented. The degree of alopecia is variable. The genetic abnormality in hidrotic ED has been mapped to the *GJB6* gene at 13q11-q12.1 encoding connexin 30 (Lamartine et al, 2000).

### Ectodermal Dysplasia–Ectrodactyly–Cleft Lip/Palate Syndrome

The ectodermal dysplasia–ectrodactyly–cleft lip/palate (EEC) syndrome is an autosomal dominant condition featuring ectodermal dysplasia (including dental, ocular, nail, and hair defects), ectrodactyly (lobster-claw deformity of the hand), and cleft lip/palate. The cutaneous and appendageal anomalies include diffuse hypopigmentation affecting both skin and hair, scanty scalp hair and eyebrows, dystrophic nails, and small teeth with enamel hypoplasia. Sweating appears to be intact, and sweat glands are present on skin biopsy. The clefting of the lip is usually complete and bilateral, and the palate has a median cleft. Dry granulomatous lesions in the corners of the mouth often are secondarily infected with *Candida albicans*. Other findings include lacrimal duct scarring, blepharitis and conjunctivitis, xerostomia, conductive hearing loss, and mental retardation. EEC syndrome is caused by a mutation in the p63 gene located at 3q27. The p63 gene, a homologue of the tumor suppressor p53 gene, is highly expressed in the basal layer of many epithelial tissues (Celli et al, 1999).

## REFERENCES


Abdel-Magid EH, el-Awad FR: Salicylate intoxication in an infant with ichthyosis transmitted through skin ointment: A case report. Pediatrics 94:939-940, 1994.

Armstrong DK, Hutchinson TH, Walsh MY, et al: Autosomal recessive inheritance of erythrokeratoderma variabilis. Pediatr Dermatol 14:355-358, 1997.

Beighton P: The dominant and recessive forms of cutis laxa. J Med Genet 9:216, 1972.

Beighton P, de Paepe A, Danks D, et al: International Nosology of Heritable Disorders of Connective Tissue, Berlin, 1986. Am J Med Genet 29:581-585, 1988.

Beighton P, de Paepe A, Steinmann B, et al: Ehlers-Danlos syndromes: Revised nosology, Villefranche, 1997. Am J Med Genet 77:31-37, 1998.

Berlin AI, Paller AS, Chan LS: Incontinentia pigmenti: A review and update on the molecular basis of pathophysiology. J Am Acad Dermatol 47:169-187, 2002.

Bolognia JL, Orlow SJ, Glick SA: Lines of Blaschko. J Am Acad Dermatol 31:157-190, 1994.

Braverman N, Lin P, Moebius FF, et al: Mutations in the gene encoding 3β-hydroxysteroid-$\Delta^8$, $\Delta^7$-isomerase cause X-linked dominant Conradi-Hünermann syndrome. Nat Genet 22: 291-294, 1999.

Buyse L, Marks R, Wijeyesekera K, et al: Collodion baby dehydration: The danger of high transepidermal water loss. Br J Dermatol 120:86-88, 1993.

Byers PH: Ehlers-Danlos syndrome: Recent advances and current understanding of the clinical and genetic heterogeneity. J Invest Dermatol 103:47S-49S, 1994.

Byers PH, Siegel RC, Holbrook KA, et al: X-linked cutis laxa. N Engl J Med 303:61, 1980.

Caceres-Rios H, Tamayo-Sanchez L, Duran-McKinster C, Ruiz-Maldonado R: Keratitis, ichthyosis, and deafness (KID syndrome): Review of the literature and proposal of a new terminology. Pediatr Dermatol 13:105-113, 1996.

Carney RG Jr: Incontinentia pigmenti: A world statistical analysis. Arch Dermatol 112:535, 1976.

Celli J, Duijf P, Hamel BC, et al: Heterozygous germline mutations in the p53 homolog p63 are the cause of EEC syndrome. Cell 99:143-145, 1999.

Chavanas S, Bodemer C, Rochat A, et al: Mutations in SPINK5, encoding a serine protease inhibitor, cause Netherton syndrome. Nat Genet 25:141-142, 2000.

Crump JA, Danks DM: Hypohidrotic ectodermal dysplasia. J Pediatr 78:466, 1971.

Dale BA, Kam E: Harlequin ichthyosis. Arch Dermatol 129: 1471-1477, 1993.

Davis JR, Solomon LM: Cellular immunodeficiency in anhidrotic ectodermal dysplasia. Acta Derm Venereol 56:115, 1976.

De Laurenzi V, Rogers GR, Hamrock DJ: Sjögren-Larsson syndrome is caused by mutations in the fatty aldehyde dehydrogenase gene. Nat Genet 12:52-57, 1996.

Delfino M, Fabbrocini G, Sammarco EM, Santoianni P: Efficacy of calcipotriol versus lactic acid cream in the treatment of lamellar and x-linked ichthyoses. J Dermatol Treat 5:151-152, 1994.

Derry JM, Gormally E, Means GD, et al: Mutations in a $\Delta^8$, $\Delta^7$ sterol isomerase in the tattered mouse and X-linked dominant chondrodysplasia punctata. Nat Genet 22:286-290, 1999.

Emery MM, Siegfried EC, Stone MS, et al: Incontinentia pigmenti: Transmission from father to daughter. J Am Acad Dermatol 29:368-372, 1993.

Esterly NB, Pashayan HM, West CE: Concurrent hypohidrotic ectodermal dysplasia and X-linked ichthyosis. Am J Dis Child 126:539, 1973.

Executive and Scientific Advisory Boards of the National Foundation for Ectodermal Dysplasia: Scaling skin in the newborn: A clue to the early diagnosis of X-linked hypohidrotic ectodermal dysplasia (Christ-Siemens-Touraine syndrome). J Pediatr 114:600, 1989.

Fine JD: Changing clinical and laboratory concepts in inherited epidermolysis bullosa. Arch Dermatol 124:523, 1988.

Fine JD: Epidermolysis bullosa: Clinical aspects, pathology, and recent advances in research. Internat J Dermatol 25:143, 1986.

Fine JD: Laboratory tests for epidermolysis bullosa. Dermatol Clin 12:123-132, 1994.

Fine JD, Bauer EA, Briggaman RA, et al: Revised clinical and laboratory criteria for subtypes of inherited epidermolysis bullosa. J Am Acad Dermatol 24:119-135, 1991a.

Fine JD, Eady RA, Bauer EA, et al: Revised classification system for inherited epidermolysis bullosa: Report of the Second International Consensus Meeting on Diagnosis and Classification of Epidermolysis Bullosa. J Am Acad Dermatol 42:1051-1066, 2000.

Fine JD, Johnson LB, Suchindran CM: The National Epidermolysis Bullosa Registry. J Invest Dermatol 102:54S-56S, 1994.

Fine JD, Johnson LB, Wright JT: Inherited blistering diseases of the skin. Pediatrician 18:175-187, 1991b.

Fischer, J, Faure A, Bouadjar B, et al: Two new loci for autosomal recessive ichthyosis on chromosomes 3p21 and 19p12-q12 and evidence for further genetic heterogenicity. Am J Hum Genet 66:904-913, 2000.

Francis JS: Genetic skin diseases. Curr Opin Pediatr 6:447-453, 1994.

Franco HL, Weston WL, Peebles C, et al: Autoantibodies directed against sicca syndrome antigens in the neonatal lupus syndrome. J Am Acad Dermatol 4:67, 1981.

Freire-Maia N, Pinheiro M: Ectodermal Dysplasias: A Clinical and Genetic Study. New York, Alan R. Liss, 1984.

Frenk E, de Techtermann F: Self-healing collodion baby: Evidence for autosomal recessive inheritance. Pediatr Dermatol 9:95-97, 1992.

Frieden IJ: Aplasia cutis congenita: A clinical review and proposal for classification. J Am Acad Dermatol 14:646, 1986.

Gawkrodger DJ, Beveridge GW: Neonatal lupus erythematosus in four successive siblings born to a mother with discoid lupus erythematosus. Br J Dermatol 111:683, 1984.

Gerber M, de Veciana M, Towers CV, Devore GR: Aplasia cutis congenita: A rare cause of elevated alpha-fetoprotein levels. Am J Obstet Gynecol 172:1040-1041, 1993.

Gibbons S: Care of epidermolysis bullosa patients: A nursing challenge. Dermatol Nursing 2:195-214, 1990.

Goldsmith LA: Look at the genes, see what's in the jeans. Arch Dermatol 126:585-586, 1990.

Gorlin RJ, Old T, Anderson VE: Hypohidrotic ectodermal dysplasia in females: A critical analysis and argument for genetic heterogeneity. Z Kinderheilkd 108:1, 1970.

Grange DK, Kratz LE, Braverman NE, et al: CHILD syndrome caused by deficiency of 3γβ-hydroxysteroid-$\Delta^8$, $\Delta^7$-isomerase. Am J Med Genet 90:328-335, 2000.

Haber RM, Hanna W, Ramsay CA, et al: Hereditary epidermolysis bullosa. J Am Acad Dermatol 13:252, 1985.

Hammami-Hauasli N, Raghunath M, Küster W, et al: Transient bullous dermolysis of the newborn associated with compound heterozygosity for recessive and dominant *COL7A1* mutations. J Invest Dermatol 111:1214-1219, 1998.

Happle R: Mosaicism in human skin. Arch Dermatol 129:1460-1470, 1993.

Hardy JD, Solomon S, Barwell GS, et al: Congenital complete heart block in the newborn associated with maternal systemic lupus erythematosus and other connective tissue disorders. Arch Dis Child 54:7, 1979.

Hashimoto K, De Dobbeleer G, Kanzaki T: Electron microscopic studies of harlequin fetuses. Pediatr Dermatol 10:214-223, 1993.

Hashimoto K, Eng AM: Transient bullous dermolysis of the newborn. J Cutan Pathol 19:49-501, 1992.

Holbrook KA, Smith LT, Elias S: Prenatal diagnosis of genetic skin disease using fetal skin biopsy samples. Arch Dermatol 129:1437-1454, 1993.

Huber N, Rettler I, Bernasconi K, et al: Mutations of keratinocyte transglutaminase in lamellar ichthyosis. Science 267:525-528, 1995.

Itin PH, Pittelkow MR: Trichothiodystrophy: Review of sulfur-deficient brittle hair syndromes and association with the ectodermal dysplasias. J Am Acad Dermatol 22:705-717, 1990.

Jimbow K, Fitzpatrick TB, Szabo G, et al: Congenital circumscribed hypomelanosis: A characterization based on electron microscopic study of tuberous sclerosis, nevus depigmentosus and piebaldism. J Invest Dermatol 64:50, 1975.

Judge MR, Atherton DJ, Salvayre R, et al: Neutral lipid storage disease: Case report and lipid studies. Br J Dermatol 130: 507-510, 1994a.

Judge MR, Morgan G, Harper JI: A clinical and immunological study of Netherton's syndrome. Br J Dermatol 131:615-621, 1994b.

Khakoo A, Thomas R, Trompeter R, et al: Congenital cutis laxa and lysyl oxidase deficiency. Clin Genet 51:109-114, 1997.

King RA, Olds DP: Hairbulb tyrosinase activity in oculocutaneous albinism: Suggestions for pathway control and block location. Am J Med Genet 20:49, 1985.

Konigsmark B: Hereditary childhood hearing loss and integumentary system disease. J Pediatr 80:909, 1972.

Kosnik EJ, Sayers MP: Congenital scalp defects: Aplasia cutis congenita. J Neurosurg 42:32, 1975.

Kousseff BG: Collodion baby: Sign of Tay syndrome. Pediatrics 87:571-574, 1991.

Kragballe K, Steijlen PM, Ibsen HH, et al: Efficacy, tolerability and safety of calcipotriol ointment in disorders of keratinization: Results of a randomized double-blind, vehicle-controlled, right/left comparative study. Arch Dermatol 31:556-560, 1995.

Lamartine J, Munhox Essenfelder G, Kibar Z, et al: Mutations in *GJB6* cause hidrotic ectodermal dysplasia. Nat Genet 26:142-144, 2000.

Lawlor F: Harlequin fetus progression to nonbullous ichthyosiform erythroderma. Pediatrics 82:870, 1988.

Lee LA: Neonatal lupus erythematosus. J Invest Dermatol 100:9-13, 1993.

Lee LA, Weston WL: New findings in neonatal lupus syndrome. Am J Dis Child 138:233, 1984.

Lefèvre C, Jobard F, Caux F, et al: Mutations in *CGI-58*, the gene encoding a new protein of the esterase/lipase/thioesterase subfamily, in Chanarin-Dorfman syndrome. Am J Hum Genet 69:1002-1012, 2001.

Lerer RJ, Ehrenhranz RA, Campbell AGM: Pigmented lesions of incontinentia pigmenti in a neonate. J Pediatr 83:503, 1973.

Levin DL, Nolan KS, Esterly NB: Congenital absence of skin. J Am Acad Dermatol 2:203, 1980.

Lipson AH, Rogers M, Berry A: Collodion babies with Gaucher's disease—a further case. Arch Dis Child 66:667, 1991.

Lucker GPH: Effect of topical calcipotriol on congenital ichthyoses. Br J Dermatol 131:546-550, 1994.

McCune AB, Weston WL, Lee AA: Maternal and fetal outcome in neonatal lupus erythematosus. Ann Intern Med 106:518, 1987.

McKusick VA: Heritable Disorders of Connective Tissue. St. Louis, CV Mosby, 1972.
Mehregan AH, Lee SC, Nabai H: Cutis laxa (generalized elastolysis): A report of four cases with autopsy findings. J Cutan Pathol 5:116, 1978.
Mellerio JE, Pulkkinen L, McMillan JR, et al: Pyloric atresia-junctional epidermolysis bullosa syndrome: Mutations in the integrin beta-4 gene (*ITGB4*) in two unrelated patients with mild disease. Br J Dermatol 139:862-871, 1998.
Moss C, Ince P: Anhidrotic and achromians lesions in incontinentia pigmenti. Br J Dermatol 116:839, 1987.
Müller FB, Hausser I, Berg D, et al: Genetic analysis of a severe case of Netherton syndrome for prenatal testing. Br J Dermatol 146:495-499, 2002.
Nakamura E, Miyamura Y, Matsunaga J, et al: A novel mutation of the tyrosinase gene causing oculocutaneous albinism type 1 (OCA1). J Dermatol Sci 28:102-105, 2002.
Newton JM, Cohen-Barak O, Hagiwara N, et al: Mutations in the human orthologue of the mouse underwhite gene (*uw*) underlie a new form of oculocutaneous albinism, OCA4. Am J Hum Genet 69:981-989, 2001.
Nirunsuksiri W, Presland RB, Brumbaugh SG, et al: Decreased profilaggrin expression in ichthyosis vulgaris is a result of selectively impaired posttranscriptional control. J Biol Chem 270:871-876, 1995.
O'Brien JE, Feingold M: Incontinentia pigmenti: A longitudinal study. Am J Dis Child 139:712, 1985.
Oetting WS, King RA: Molecular basis of oculocutaneous albinism. J Invest Dermatol 103 (suppl 5):131S-136S, 1994.
Paller AS: Laboratory test for ichthyosis. Dermatol Clin 12: 99-107, 1994.
Paller AS, Syder AJ, Yiu-Mo Chan BS, et al: Genetic and clinical mosaicism in a type of epidermal nevus. N Engl J Med 331:1408-1415, 1994.
Pinheiro M, Freire-Maia N: Ectodermal dysplasia: A clinical classification and a casual review. Am J Med Genet 53:153-162, 1994.
Pinnel SR, Krane SM, Kenzora J, et al: A new heritable disorder of connective tissue with hydroxylysine-deficient collagen. N Engl J Med 286:1013, 1972.
Pongprasit P: Collodion baby: The outcome of long-term follow-up. J Med Assoc Thail 76:17-22, 1993.
Prasad RS, Pejaver RK, Hassan A, et al: Management and follow-up of harlequin siblings. Br J Dermatol 130:650-653, 1994.
Pries C, Mittleman D, Miller M, et al: The EEC syndrome. Am J Dis Child 127:840, 1974.
Provost TT, Watson R, Gaither KK, et al: The neonatal lupus erythematosus syndrome. J Rheumatol 14 (suppl 13):199, 1987.
Rabinowitz LG, Esterly NB: Atopic dermatitis and ichthyosis vulgaris. Pediatr Rev 15:220-226, 1994.
Reed WB, Lopez DA, Landing B: Clinical spectrum of anhidrotic ectodermal dysplasia. Arch Dermatol 102:134, 1970.
Richards W, Kaplan M: Anhidrotic ectodermal dysplasia: An unusual cause of hyperpyrexia in the newborn. Am J Dis Child 117:597, 1969.
Roberts LJ: Long-term survival of a harlequin fetus. J Am Acad Dermatol 21:335, 1989.
Rogers M, Scarf C: Harlequin baby treated with etretinate. Pediatr Dermatol 6:216, 1989.
Rosenfeld S, Smith ME: Ocular findings in incontinentia pigmenti. Ophthalmology 92:543, 1985.
Russell LJ, DiGiovanna JJ, Rogers R, et al: Mutations of the gene for transglutaminase 1 in autosomal recessive lamellar ichthyosis. Nat Genet 9:279-283, 1995.
Russell S, Young MJ: Hypercalcemia during treatment of psoriasis with calcipotriol. Br J Dermatol 130:795-796, 1994.
Sakati NO, Nyhan WL, Shear CS, et al: Syndrome of cutis laxa, ligamentous laxity, and delayed development. Pediatrics 72:850, 1983.
Sarangarajan R, Boissy RE: *Tryp 1* and oculocutaneous albinism type 3. Pigment Cell Res 14:437, 2001.
Schachner LA, Hansen RC (eds): Pediatric Dermatology. New York, Churchill Livingstone, 1988.
Shimizu H, Takizawa Y, Pulkkinen L, et al: Epidermolysis bullosa simplex associated with muscular dystrophy: Phenotype-genotype correlations and review of the literature. J Am Acad Dermatol 4141:950-956, 1999.
Shwayder T, Ott F: All about ichthyosis. Pediatr Clin North Am 38:835-857, 1991.
Smack DP, Korge BP, James WD: Keratin and keratinization. J Am Acad Dermatol 30:85-102, 1994.
Solomon LM, Esterly NB: Neonatal Dermatology. Philadelphia, WB Saunders, 1973.
Solomon LM, Keuer EJ: The ectodermal dysplasias. Arch Dermatol 116:1295, 1980.
Sprecher E, Chavanas S, DiGiovanna JJ, et al: The spectrum of pathogenic mutations in *SPINK5* in 19 families with Netherton syndrome: Implications for mutation detection and first case of prenatal diagnosis. J Invest Dermatol 117:179-187, 2001.
Steijlen PM, Kremer H, Fereydoun V, et al: Genetic linkage of the keratin type II gene cluster with ichthyosis bullosa of Siemens and with autosomal dominant ichthyosis exfoliativa. J Invest Dermatol 103:282-285, 1994a.
Steijlen PM, Van Dooren-Greebe RJ, Van de Kerkhof PC: Acitretin in the treatment of lamellar ichthyosis. Br J Dermatol 130:211-214, 1994b.
Sybert VP: Aplasia cutis congenita: A report of 12 new families and a review of the literature. Pediatr Dermatol 3:1, 1985.
Telfer MA, Sugar A, Jaeger EA, et al: Dominant piebald trait (white forehead and leukoderma) with neurological impairment. Am J Hum Genet 23:383, 1971.
Thomas WO, Moses MH, Craver RD, Galen WK: Congenital cutis laxa: A case report and review of loose skin syndromes. Ann Plast Surg 30:252-256, 1993.
Thornton CM, Eichenfield LF, Shinall EA, et al: Cutaneous telangiectases in neonatal lupus erythematosus. J Am Acad Dermatol 33:19-25, 1995.
Tomita Y: The molecular genetics of albinism and piebaldism. Arch Dermatol 130:355-358, 1994.
Toyofuku K, Valencia JC, Kushimoto T, et al: The etiology of oculocutaneous albinism (OCA) type II: The pink protein modulates the processing and transport of tyrosinase. Pigment Cell Res 15:217-224, 2002.
Traupe H, Has CL: The Conradi-Hünermann-Happle syndrome is caused by mutations in the gene that encodes a $\Delta^8$, $\Delta^7$-sterol isomerase and is biochemically related to the CHILD syndrome. Eur J Dermatol 10:425-428, 2000.
Tseng CE, Buyon JP: Neonatal lupus syndromes. Rheum Dis Clin North Am 23:31-54, 1997.
van Brabant AJ, Stan R, Ellis NA: DNA helicases, genomic instability, and human genetic disease. Annu Rev Genomics Hum Genet 1:409-459, 2000.
van Steensel MA, van Geel M, Nahuys M, et al: A novel connexin 26 mutations in a patient diagnosed with keratitis-ichthyosis-deafness syndrome. J Invest Dermatol 118:724-727, 2002.
Waisman Y, Rachmel A, Metzker A, et al: Failure of etretinate therapy in twins with severe congenital lamellar ichthyosis. Pediatr Dermatol 6:226-228, 1989.
Wilgoss A, Leigh IM, Barnes MR, et al: Identification of a novel mutation *R 42 P* in the gap junction protein beta-3 associated with autosomal dominant erythrokeratoderma variabilis. J Invest Dermatol 112:1119-1122, 1999.
Williams ML: A new look at the ichthyoses: Disorders of lipid metabolism. Pediatr Dermatol 3:476, 1986.
Williams ML: The ichthyoses: Pathogenesis and prenatal diagnosis: A review of recent advances. Pediatr Dermatol 1:1, 1983.

Witkop CJ Jr, Quevedo WC Jr, Fitzpatrick TB, King RA: In Albinism: Scriver CR, Beaudet AL, Sly WS, Volle D (eds): The Metabolic Basis of Inherited Disease, 6th ed. New York, McGraw-Hill, 1989, p 2905.
Workshop Proceedings: Pathogenesis, clinical features and management of the non-dermatological complications of epidermolysis. Arch Dermatol 124:705-767, 1988.
Zonana J, Schinzel A, Upadhyaya M, et al: Prenatal diagnosis of X-linked hypohidrotic ectodermal dysplasia by linkage analysis. Am J Med Genet 35:132-135, 1990.

## RESOURCES

### Ichthyosis

Foundation for Ichthyosis and Related Skin Types
650 N. Cannon Ave., Suite 17
Lansdale, PA 19446
Telephone: (215) 631-1413
E-mail: info@scalyskin.org

### Oculocutaneous Albinism

National Organization for Albinism and Hypopigmentation
Telephone: (800) 473-2310
Web site: www.albinism.org

### Incontinentia Pigmenti

Incontinentia Pigmenti International Foundation
30 East 72nd St.
New York, NY 10021
Telephone: (212) 452-1231
Web site: http://imgen.bcm.tmc.edu/ipif/

Incontinentia Pigmenti Support Network
34929 Elm
Wayne, MI 48184
Telephone: (313) 729-7912

Genetic testing:
Baylor College of Medicine
Medical Genetics Laboratory
Houston, TX 77021
Telephone: (800) 411-4363
Web site: www.bcmgeneticlabs.org

### Ehlers-Danlos Syndrome

Ehlers-Danlos National Foundation
6399 Wilshire Boulevard, Suite 2000
Los Angeles, CA 90048
Telephone: (213) 651-3038
Web site: www.ednf.org

### Epidermolysis Bullosa

National Epidermolysis Bullosa Registry
c/o Jo-David Fine, MD, Principal Investigator
OR
c/o Lorraine B. Johnson, ScD, Coordinator
School of Medicine
Department of Dermatology
University of North Carolina at Chapel Hill
Suite 3100, Thurston Building CB #7287
Chapel Hill, NC 27599
Telephone: (919) 966-6383

West Coast registry:
Dr. Lexie Nall, MD
Stanford University Medical Center
Telephone: (415) 725-8839

Dystrophic Epidermolysis Bullosa Research Association of America
5 West 36th St., Room 404
New York, NY 10018
Telephone: (212) 868-1573
Web site: www.debra.org

### Neonatal Lupus Erythematosus

North American Collaborative Study of NLE
c/o Earl Silverman, MD
The Hospital for Sick Children
555 University Ave.
Toronto, Ontario, Canada M5G 1X8
Telephone: (416) 813-6249

### Ectodermal Dysplasia

National Foundation for Ectodermal Dysplasias
410 E. Main St.
Mascoutah, IL 62258
Telephone: (618) 566-2020
Web site: www.nfed.org

CHAPTER

# 98

# Infections of the Skin*

**Elisabeth G. Richard, Bernard A. Cohen, and Elaine C. Siegfried**

As a group of potentially life-threatening and often easily treatable diseases, infections are often suspected first in a neonate with skin lesions. Recognition of characteristic morphologic features, aided by a few easily performed tests, will greatly enhance correct diagnosis and early initiation of appropriate therapy of the most common cutaneous infections. In this chapter, we confine our discussion to disease caused by the most common pathogens responsible for neonatal infections that manifest with skin lesions: *Staphylococcus aureus*, *Streptococcus* species, *Candida albicans*, and herpes simplex virus (HSV).

## *STAPHYLOCOCCUS AUREUS* INFECTIONS

*S. aureus* is a ubiquitous organism, harbored as a commensal organism by greater than 30% of the general population (Ladhani, 2000). Colonization of the anterior nares and perineum is common, with frequent hand carriage (Dancer and Noble, 1991). This bacterial species is responsible for a variety of skin lesions. Infants become colonized with *S. aureus* during the first few weeks of life, following inoculation at the perineum or from handling. Cutaneous signs of *S. aureus* infection are mediated by local or circulating bacterial toxins that act directly on components of the epidermal keratinocytes, or as "superantigens" to stimulate exuberant immunologic responses (Tokura et al, 1994).

### Bullous Impetigo

Impetigo is a group of superficial skin infections caused by group A streptococci or *S. aureus*, or both. Lesions caused by *S. aureus* can be primarily vesicular and thus are referred to as bullous impetigo. This form of impetigo can occur in nursery-based, epidemic patterns, often attributed to nasal carriage of *S. aureus*.

#### Clinical Findings

Impetigo is one of the most common neonatal skin infections. It occurs during the latter part of the first week or as late as the second week of life, manifested as vesicles or pustules on an erythematous base, most often seen in the periumbilical area, diaper area, or skin folds. Because the blisters are superficial, intact lesions are usually less than 1 cm in diameter. Larger lesions are flaccid and rupture so easily that they are usually seen as erosions, with a red moist base that develops a thin, varnish-like crust (Fig. 98–1). These lesions heal rapidly without scarring. Lesions are usually not closely grouped, differentiating them from the vesicles of herpes simplex infection.

#### Etiology

*S. aureus* is the primary cause of both bullous and nonbullous impetigo. Group A streptococci usually are associated with the nonbullous form, especially affecting patients with atopic dermatitis. Bullous impetigo is caused by toxigenic strains of coagulase-positive hemolytic *S. aureus*. Most often, the organism can be classified as one of the group II phage types. The incubation period is 1 to 10 days. Skin lesions are the result of local production of an epidermolytic exotoxin that cleaves a desmosomal protein connecting cells in the granular layer of the epidermis, producing superficial blisters. This is the same toxin produced in staphylococcal scalded skin syndrome (Amagi et al, 2000; Yamaguchi et al, 2002).

#### Epidemiology

Persons with skin lesions are highly contagious, but the disease also can be transmitted by asymptomatic carriers. The anterior nares of 30% of the general population are colonized with *S. aureus*, providing a reservoir for hand carriage and nosocomial spread (Doebbeling, 1994; Kragballe et al, 1995). Colonization of health care workers by methicillin-resistant strains poses a potentially serious problem, and outpatient studies now demonstrate methicillin-resistant strains collected in the community (Yamaguchi et al, 2002).

Sporadic cases of impetigo are common, but many nursery epidemics have been reported and should be treated aggressively (Dave et al, 1994). Infected infants may not develop skin lesions until after discharge, so infection control surveillance should include all exposed patients. Overcrowding, insufficient nursery personnel, and inadequate hand washing contribute to nosocomial spread. Treatment of the umbilical cord with an antimicrobial agent has been shown to control epidemic *S. aureus* infections in the neonatal intensive care unit (NICU) (Haley et al, 1995). In the setting of an outbreak, nursery personnel should be surveyed for colonization of the hands and nares. Application of mupirocin ointment to the anterior nares twice daily for 5 days will eliminate nasal carriage for up to 1 year (Doebbeling et al, 1994). Effective hand washing can prevent nosocomial spread; chlorhexidine is among the safest and most effective antimicrobial cleansers for hospital use (Doebbeling et al, 1992).

#### Diagnosis

The diagnosis is supported by the presence of gram-positive cocci in clusters on Gram stain of the contents from an intact pustule and confirmed by bacterial culture.

*This chapter includes material from the previous edition, to which Nancy B. Esterly, MD, contributed.

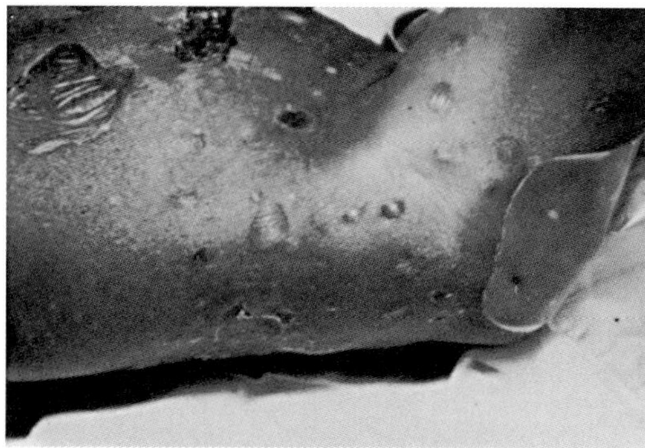

**FIGURE 98–1.** Bullous impetigo. Multiple intact and ruptured bullae on the abdomen, hip, and thigh of a newborn infant. No underlying erythema is present.

### Treatment

Bullous impetigo is benign if treated early, but local proliferation with exotoxin production or dissemination can be life-threatening. Treatment should be instituted promptly, and strict isolation maintained until the lesions have resolved. Infants should be closely monitored, and a high index of suspicion maintained for evidence of systemic disease. Infants with periumbilical lesions are at risk for bacterial omphalitis. Extremely limited infections may be treated with topical mupirocin, but this form of therapy should be used with caution in neonates. Application of compresses with sterile water, normal saline, or Burow solution every few hours helps desiccate blisters. More extensive lesions require a systemically administered penicillinase-resistant antibiotic for 7 to 10 days. Sensitivities of the organism cultured should ultimately determine the choice of antibiotics, especially with the rising incidence of methicillin-resistant strains.

## Staphylococcal Scalded Skin Syndrome

Staphylococcal scalded skin syndrome (SSSS) occurs as a generalized manifestation of a circulating toxin produced by *S. aureus* that specifically cleaves cell-to-cell adhesion proteins in the epidermis. Affected infants are erythrodermic, a striking cutaneous finding that suggests a long list of differential diagnostic possibilities. Early diagnosis and treatment of SSSS can be lifesaving.

### Clinical Findings

Affected infants demonstrate abrupt onset of temperature instability and irritability with generalized skin tenderness and erythema that most often starts on the face and spreads rapidly. Erythema often is accentuated in skin folds. Facial edema, conjunctivitis, and crusting around the eyes, nose, and mouth give the infant a characteristic "sad mask" appearance. Flaccid bullae may develop, followed by widespread exfoliation (Fig. 98–2) involving the entire skin surface within hours to days. Blistering is easily elicited by light stroking of intact skin, a diagnostic feature referred to as a Nikolsky sign. When blisters rupture, the skin peels off in sheets, leaving a painful moist, red base. Widespread skin involvement can exacerbate fluid and electrolyte problems (Frieden, 1989). Whereas in bullous impetigo *S. aureus* is identifiable in the blisters, in SSSS *S. aureus* is present at a primary distant site such as the nose, mouth, or conjunctiva.

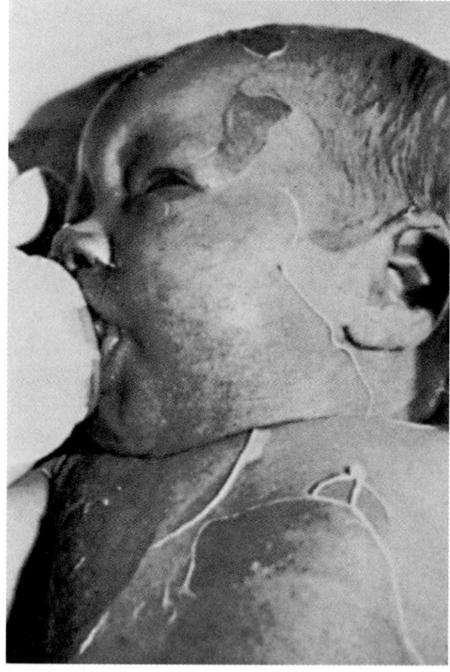

**FIGURE 98–2.** Staphylococcal scalded skin syndrome (Ritter disease). Intense erythema and peeling of large areas of epidermis are seen.

SSSS must be distinguished from toxic epidermal necrolysis, a life-threatening condition involving full-thickness epidermal necrosis, most commonly due to a drug reaction. Intraoral mucosal involvement is rare in SSSS but can be striking in toxic epidermal necrolysis.

### Etiology

The signs and symptoms of SSSS are the result of circulating epidermolytic toxin, produced from an often subclinical focus of *S. aureus* infection. Fresh skin lesions do not contain bacteria, and the blisters are culture negative. Two distinct epidermolytic toxins have been identified in SSSS, produced by toxigenic strains of *S. aureus*, phage group I, II, or III. Approximately 5% of *S. aureus* isolates produce the toxins (Farrell, 1999). The exotoxin cleaves desmosomal proteins within the epidermal granular layer, resulting in blisters (Amagi et al, 2002; Resnick, 1992). Superantigenic stimulation of cytokine production also has been demonstrated (Dave et al, 1994).

### Diagnosis

If the diagnosis is in doubt, skin biopsy prepared for frozen section can be examined emergently. The presence of an intraepidermal rather than full-thickness blister will distinguish SSSS from toxic epidermal necrolysis, allowing rapid initiation of appropriate therapy. Other conditions can be ruled out by examination of formalin-fixed sections. If the clinical impression is strong, surveillance samples will define the primary focus of infection. Gram staining may be performed emergently; cultures will confirm the diagnosis. Common sites of primary infection are the nasopharynx, umbilicus, and ocular conjunctivae; the urine also may demonstrate organisms. Bullous lesions do not contain organisms. Blood culture specimens should be obtained because sepsis, although uncommon, may occur. Phage typing may be of interest in epidemics.

### Treatment

Systemic administration of a penicillinase-resistant penicillin is the therapy of choice. Fluid and electrolyte replacement and measures for maintenance of normal body temperature may be required. Approximately 2 to 3 days after initiation of therapy, the denuded areas become dry, and a flaky desquamation ensues. Crusted and denuded areas may be treated with compresses of Burow or normal saline solution. Application of a bland ointment emollient may accelerate the return of the skin to normal during the flaky desquamative phase. Resolution occurs in another 3 to 5 days. Because the intraepidermal cleavage plane is at the level of the granular layer, scarring occurs only in instances of secondary complications (Frieden, 1989).

## *STREPTOCOCCUS* SPECIES INFECTIONS

Cutaneous streptococcal infections occur in the newborn but are less common than staphylococcal infections. Group A streptococci have been reported to cause disease of epidemic proportions (Dillon, 1966; Peter and Hazard, 1975) following the introduction of the organism into the nursery by maternal carriers or nursery personnel. The umbilicus is a frequent site of infection. Conjunctivitis, paronychia, vaginitis, and an erysipelas-like eruption also have been described (Dillon, 1966; Geil et al, 1970; Isenberg et al, 1984). Because sepsis and meningitis may result, infected infants should be treated promptly, and strict isolation should be instituted. As with staphylococcal infection, serious efforts should be made to identify the source of the organism. Several nursery outbreaks have been difficult to terminate because colonized infants may show little evidence of disease (Lehtonen et al, 1984). Isolation and treatment of infected infants, disinfection of the umbilical stump as the most likely reservoir of the organism, and penicillin prophylaxis for carriers and exposed infants have been the most effective measures. The infections respond readily to penicillin, which should be administered over a 10-day course.

Group B streptococci are now one of the most frequently encountered pathogens in the newborn nursery. Early-onset disease (during the first week of life), probably acquired in utero or during delivery, most commonly becomes manifest as septicemia with respiratory distress and shock. Late-onset disease (after the first week of life) is acquired post partum and more often takes on the form of meningitis. Patients with early-onset disease may harbor the organism on the skin; however, the presence of this agent on the skin is short-lived compared with other sites (Baker, 1977).

Skin infections caused by group B streptococci are uncommon but have been documented (Belgaumkar, 1975; Hebert and Esterly, 1986; Howard and McCrackin, 1974). Vesiculopustular lesions, cellulitis, and small abscesses all have been noted. A 10-day course of procaine penicillin is considered the treatment of choice.

## *CANDIDA ALBICANS* INFECTIONS

*C. albicans* is a frequent pathogen of the female genital tract, especially during pregnancy. Infantile infection may be acquired in utero, during delivery, or postnatally.

### Thrush

#### Clinical Findings

*C. albicans* colonizes the oral cavity and gastrointestinal tract of most neonates, with peak incidence of thrush occurring at 4 weeks of age (Russell and Lay, 1973). The lesions are readily recognized as asymptomatic to moderately painful plaques of white, friable material on an erythematous base over the tongue, palate, buccal mucosa, and gingivae. Candidal infection in the breast-feeding mother–infant dyad is a significant problem, as it can cause considerable pain in the mother and subsequently may lead to premature weaning. Infection frequently recurs and may become chronic (Brent, 2001).

#### Diagnosis

Presumptive diagnosis often is made by physical examination and history, but microscopic examination of scrapings suspended in 10% potassium hydroxide for yeast and pseudohyphal forms is useful. The diagnosis may be confirmed by identification of the organism on culture.

#### Treatment

Nystatin is an antibiotic derived from *Streptomyces noursei* with activity against *Candida* but not dermatophytes. Oral lesions usually respond promptly to a course of nystatin suspension, 100,000 to 200,000 units, administered by mouth four times daily for 14 to 21 days. In refractory cases, an increased dosage of nystatin or systemic therapy may have to be instituted (Hebert and Esterly, 1986). If the breast-feeding mother is affected, treatment of the mother with nystatin cream or oral fluconazole may be indicated. Gentian (crystal) violet is a triphenylmethane antiseptic dye effective against *Candida* species. In a 0.5% or 1% aqueous solution it has been a time-honored, safe, and effective treatment for thrush. Gentian violet is infamous for deep purple staining of the skin, which is transient. Prolonged use of gentian violet has been associated with nausea, vomiting, diarrhea, and mucosal ulceration. Carcinogenicity in mice has been reported (Rosenkranz and Carr, 1971).

### Neonatal and Cutaneous Candidiasis

Neonatal candidiasis manifests 3 to 7 days after birth with mucocutaneous lesions. Infection can be localized or generalized and is usually acquired during birth through an infected birth canal. The disease is rarely invasive in healthy full-term infants.

### Clinical Findings

Localized cutaneous candidal infections are common in infants. Intertriginous areas, particularly the neck folds, axillae, and diaper area (Fig. 98–3A), are most frequently affected. Nails and periungual areas also are sites of predilection. Characteristic primary lesions are tiny vesicopustules that erode and merge, forming bright, erythematous, scaly plaques, often with a scalloped edge. "Satellite" pustules are commonly seen, but by no means are they pathognomonic for this condition. *Oral infection* (thrush) often is seen in neonatal candidiasis following swallowing of infected fluids (Waguespack-LaBiche et al, 1999).

Disseminated neonatal candidiasis can occur as a result of spread from an untreated localized site or by widespread inoculation during the process of birth via passage through an infected birth canal (see Fig. 98–3B). Generalized scaling is the dominant feature, but a careful search may reveal primary vesicopustules and periungual or nail involvement as helpful diagnostic clues (Gibney and Siegfried, 1996). Skin lesions usually resolve with desquamation within 1 to 2 weeks (Darmstadt et al, 2000).

### Diagnosis

The differential diagnosis includes conditions that cause blisters and pustules. A potassium hydroxide preparation that reveals budding yeasts and pseudohyphal forms is the easiest and most cost-effective initial step in establishing the diagnosis. Calcofluor white stain and immunofluorescence microscopy is a more sensitive rapid technique. Positive results on cultures from an intact pustule, skin scrapings, or skin biopsy tissue also support the diagnosis. Cultures of blood, urine, and cerebrospinal fluid are usually negative; however, they are indicated when systemic disease is suspected and in all preterm infants.

### Treatment

The eruption may resolve spontaneously or may become more widespread if left untreated. Localized cutaneous candidiasis in an otherwise healthy infant is most easily treated with a topical candidicidal agent, such as nystatin, one of the imidazoles (e.g., miconazole, clotrimazole, ketoconazole), or ciclopirox olamine. Nystatin in an ointment vehicle may be the least irritating.

## Congenital and Disseminated Candidiasis

Congenital candidiasis is assumed to result from ascending intrauterine infection and usually is noted at birth. This form typically is seen in compromised, premature infants. Disseminated candidiasis also can be acquired during the neonatal period, with 10% of NICU infants becoming colonized in the first week of life. *Candida* septicemia represents 10% to 16% of all cases of sepsis in the NICU, and early recognition and appropriate therapy are lifesaving (Gibney and Siegfried, 1996; Leibovitz, 2002). The estimated crude mortality rate for candidemia is 38% to 75% (Lupetti et al, 2002).

### Clinical Findings

Lesions of congenital candidiasis can be seen on the placenta and fetal membranes, including characteristic granulomas of the umbilical cord (Hebert and Esterly, 1986; Schirar et al, 1974). The cord lesions are multiple yellow-white papules, usually measuring 1 to 3 mm in diameter. The cutaneous eruption of congenital cutaneous candidiasis may be sparse or widespread and consists of papules and vesicopustules on an erythematous base. The face is relatively spared, as are the oral mucous membranes, and there is no predilection for the diaper area. Palmar and plantar pustules, paronychia, and nail dystrophy help distinguish this condition from more common, benign neonatal dermatoses (Fig. 98–4). Bullae and desquamation usually are late features (Fig. 98–5). Very low-birth-weight infants may present with a less specific, scalded skin–like dermatitis due to the organism's penetration of the immature, compromised epidermal barrier, leading to invasive disease.

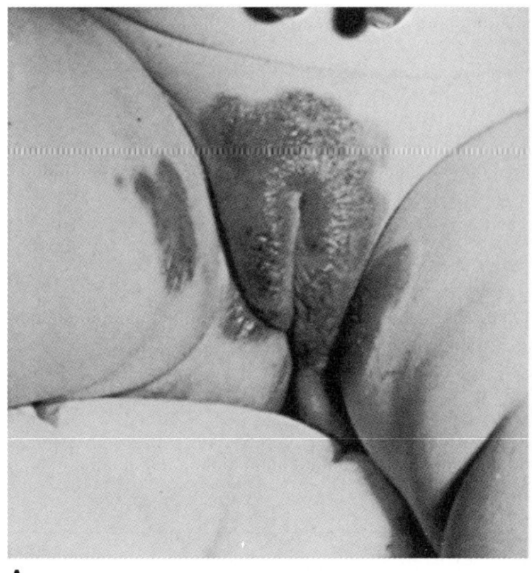
A

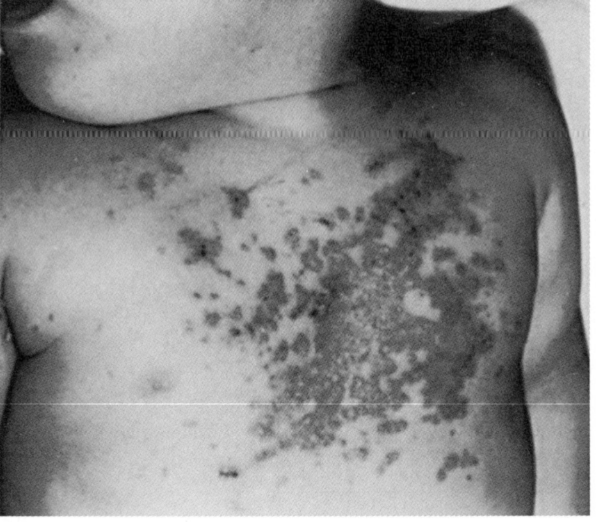
B

**FIGURE 98–3. A,** Sharply demarcated erythematous, scaly candidal rash in the groin. **B,** Candidal eruption on the central chest of an infant.

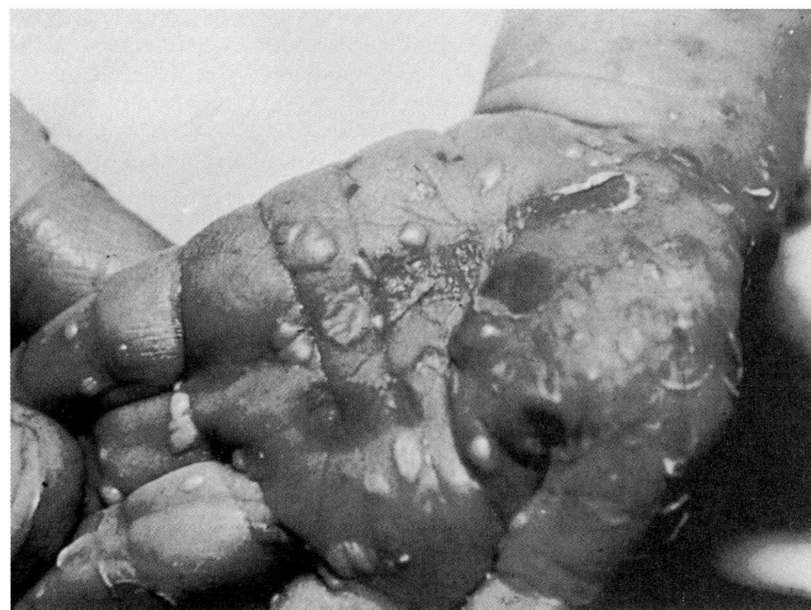

**FIGURE 98–4.** Congenital cutaneous candidiasis, pustular stage, in a 6-day-old infant. A maculopapular rash was present at birth. *(Courtesy of P. J. Kozinn, N. Rudolf, A. A. Tariq, M. R. Reale, and P. K. Goldberg.)*

Systemic involvement occurs via hematogenous or lymphatic spread, most frequently involving the kidney, central nervous system (CNS), and skeletal system. Pneumonia may result from aspiration of infected amniotic fluid and manifests with respiratory distress. Laboratory features include an elevated white blood cell count with a left shift reaching the level of a leukemoid reaction (e.g., 120,000/mm$^3$). In addition, persistent hyperglycemia and glycosuria may be present (Darmstadt et al, 2000).

Risk factors for congenital systemic infection include birth weight of less than 1500 g, indwelling catheters, antibiotic therapy, steroid administration, and hyperalimentation. The indication for parenteral therapy may be stronger in infants with these risk factors (Botas et al, 1995; Johnson et al, 1984).

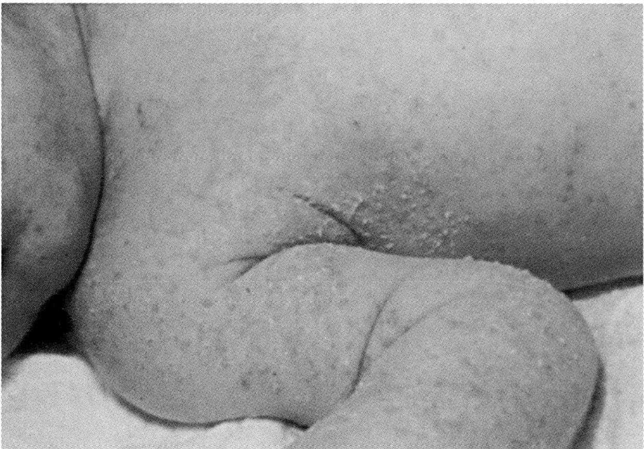

**FIGURE 98–5.** An 8-day-old infant with a generalized erythematous, scaly eruption sparing only the face and scalp. Oral mucosa was not involved. Hyphae and budding yeasts were seen on potassium hydroxide preparation, and *Candida albicans* was cultured from the lesions. The infant's mother had candidal vaginitis during the pregnancy.

### Etiology

Congenital candidiasis is presumed to invade as an ascending infection, crossing the fetal membrane and infecting surfaces that come in contact with amniotic fluid. Disease may be limited to chorioamnionitis and funisitis. Infection also may occur in neonates born to mothers with an intrauterine foreign body such as an intrauterine device (IUD) or a cervical cerclage ring (Darmstadt et al, 2000). Symptomatic vaginitis, chorioamnionitis, and ruptured membranes have no prognostic value for congenital disease (Gibney and Siegfried, 1996; Johnson et al, 1984). Nosocomial acquisition of disseminated disease may be attributed to cluster outbreaks with patient-to-patient spread or caused by horizontal transmission via hospital personnel. Most neonatal fungal infections are caused by *C. albicans* and *Candida parapsilosis*. In recent years, trends indicate a shift toward infection with *C. parapsilosis*, which has a lower associated mortality rate than that for candidemia due to *C. albicans*.

### Diagnosis

The differential diagnosis includes several other neonatal vesiculopustular eruptions that range from benign, self-limited cutaneous processes to rapidly progressive, life-threatening disease. Early and correct diagnosis is essential. Organisms from skin usually are demonstrable on potassium hydroxide or calcofluor white preparations and cultures of scrapings from involved skin. Disseminated disease can be difficult to diagnose. Respiratory distress and infiltrates on chest radiograph will obscure evidence of *Candida* pneumonia because hyaline membrane disease often occurs in the same patient population. Ophthalmologic examination, chest radiograph, and blood, urine, and cerebrospinal fluid cultures may be helpful, but negative findings are not uncommon in disseminated candidiasis (Johnson et al, 1984). Histologic examination of specimens from the placenta and umbilical cord prepared with the appropriate stains may demonstrate fungal elements. Urinalysis positive for budding yeast or urine culture positive for *C. albicans* may be quickly dismissed as being due to contaminants, but such findings are strongly associated with systemic disease in infants at risk. The diagnosis of disseminated candidiasis can be expedited by a positive touch preparation of a punch biopsy specimen. Using this technique, the practitioner firmly imprints the dermal side of the specimen on a microscope slide and then looks for yeast after potassium hydroxide preparation or Gram staining (Held et al, 1988).

### Prognosis and Treatment

Systemic infection with *C. albicans* in premature infants is a serious infection with high morbidity and mortality rates (Johnson et al, 1984). Congenital or acquired candidiasis warrants parenteral antifungal therapy (e.g., with amphotericin B) for infants with any of the following risk factors for disseminated disease: (1) evidence of respiratory distress or sepsis in the immediate neonatal period; (2) birth weight of less than 1500 g; (3) treatment with broad-spectrum antibiotics or corticosteroids; (4) extensive instrumentation during delivery or invasive procedures in the neonatal period; (5) positive systemic cultures; (6) evidence of altered immune response; and (7) birth at less than 27 weeks of gestational age. A critical factor for survival in systemic candidiasis is not limited extent of infection but the early initiation of antifungal therapy (Botas et al, 1995; Johnson et al, 1984). Healthy infants without visceral involvement respond rapidly to topical anticandidal agents (Gibney and Siegfried, 1996).

## HERPES SIMPLEX VIRUS INFECTION

Early recognition and prompt initiation of therapy for neonatal herpes are critical. The consequences of delaying antiviral therapy can be devastating.

### Clinical Findings

Onset of symptoms usually occurs at 1 to 2 weeks for most neonates, but congenital lesions have been reported (Salvador et al, 1994). Infection is categorized by extent of disease, as follows: skin-eye-mucosae (SEM) disease, CNS disease, and disseminated disease. Only one third of infants present with cutaneous involvement (Frieden, 1989), although more than 80% develop typical skin lesions during the course of their disease (Overall, 1994). Characteristic skin lesions begin as isolated or grouped, tense vesicles on an erythematous base and evolve into pustules, crusts, or small erosions over several days. Forty percent of infected infants have SEM disease. With early treatment, these infants have an excellent prognosis; if the infection is left untreated, it will progress in 75% of cases (Arvin and Prober, 1992). Thirty-five percent of infected infants have CNS disease, with a high incidence of developmental abnormalities. One fourth of the infants present with evidence of disseminated disease (e.g., sepsis, liver dysfunction, coagulopathy, respiratory distress). For this group, the prognosis is poor, with a 60% mortality rate and a 40% risk of long-term neurologic impairment in survivors (Arvin and Prober, 1992; Whitley, 1994).

Infants infected in utero have a distinctive clinical presentation. Skin lesions are almost always present at birth and include widespread erosions and bullae, scars, and scalp lesions that resemble those of aplasia cutis. Other frequent findings include chorioretinitis, microcephaly, hydranencephaly, and microphthalmia (Arvin and Prober, 1992).

### Etiology

A majority of cases of neonatal herpes simplex are the result of vertical transmission. Two thirds of cases are caused by HSV-2 and one third by HSV-1. The usual route of infection is via intrapartum contact with genital mucosa, but ascending infection accounts for 5% of cases of neonatal herpes. Infants who become infected in utero are more often premature or small for gestational age, with more widespread and severe disease (Arvin and Prober, 1992).

### Epidemiology

The incidence of neonatal HSV infection is 1/500 to 1/7500 live births. One half of infected infants are born to mothers with primary infections. These women, who are usually without active lesions, have a 50% risk of transmitting disease to their newborns. One half of infants with neonatal herpes are born to mothers with recurrent genital herpes, generally from HSV-2. Most of these women also are asymptomatic at the time of delivery and may have no known history of genital herpes. In this group, the risk of transmitting infection is only 2.5%.

### Diagnosis

A high index of suspicion is required. The differential diagnosis includes the causes of vesicles and pustules in the newborn outlined in Chapter 96. Tzanck smears, viral cultures, and direct fluorescent antibody detection are the most widely used tests to detect herpes infection. The diagnostic yield for each is variable, largely influenced by the age, quality, and handling of the specimen. Optimally, skin scrapings should be obtained from the base of a fresh vesicle. Other sites should be sampled as well, especially in infants suspected of having CNS or disseminated disease. Tzanck smear analysis is rapid and readily available but will reveal characteristic multinucleated giant cells in only 50% of HSV infections (Nahass et al, 1995). Immunofluorescence is 90% to 95% sensitive and specific but requires a specialized laboratory. Viral culture yields positive results for 80% of specimens by 24 hours and for 90% by 48 hours, under optimal conditions of handling and transport. Molecular diagnosis by polymerase chain reaction assay can detect HSV from specimens that would be suboptimal for the other methods (e.g., Tzanck smears, crusts, paraffin-fixed biopsy specimens). Diagnostic polymerase chain reaction assay may be the easiest means of diagnosing HSV infection in the future; however, limitations include the lack of standardization of methodologies, adversely affecting the clinician's ability to interpret results (Kimberlin, 2001; Nahass et al, 1992, 1995).

### Treatment

Early treatment with antiviral agents is critical to decrease the risk of serious complications and death. When diagnostic confirmation is delayed in suspected cases, presumptive therapy should be started. This therapy includes strict isolation and prompt administration of parenteral antiviral therapy. Recent studies indicate that a 21-day course with high-dose (60 mg/kg/day) intravenous acyclovir is more effective at decreasing morbidity and mortality than standard doses (30 mg/kg/day). Adverse effects of high-dose therapy have included temporary neutropenia (Kimberlin et al, 2001). Vidarabine also is effective in preventing severe disease in infants with SEM disease. Treatment is much less effective for infants with more widespread herpes infection (Arvin and Prober, 1992). Morbidity in CNS disease and disseminated disease remains high, with corresponding mortality rates of 15% and 57%, respectively (Jacobs, 1998). Concomitant administration of immunoglobulin products may improve disease outcome for these infants (Whitley, 1994).

Strategies to prevent vertical transmission include cesarean delivery, serologic screening of pregnant women, prophylactic antiviral therapy, and maternal vaccination. Delivery via cesarean section for women with active lesions or prodromal symptoms and prophylactic antiviral treatment for women with gestational HSV are the currently accepted approaches (Enright and Prober, 2002). Because a direct correlation exists between the development of neurologic deficits and the frequency of recurrent cutaneous HSV, the use of suppressive oral acyclovir therapy following acute neonatal SEM disease is under way with the hope that such treatment will limit long-term morbidity (Kimberlin et al, 1996).

## SELECTED READINGS


Adachi J, Endo K, Fukuzumi T, Tanigawa N, Aoki T: Increasing incidence of streptococcal impetigo in atopic dermatitis. J Dermatol Sci 17:45-53, 1998.

Albert S, Baldwin R, Czekajewski S, et al: Bullous impetigo due to group II *Staphylococcus aureus*. Am J Dis Child 120:10, 1970.

Anthony BF, Giuliano DM, Oh W: Nursery outbreak of staphylococcal scalded skin syndrome. Am J Dis Child 124:41, 1972.

Curran JP, Al-Salihi FL: Neonatal staphylococcal scalded skin syndrome: Massive outbreak due to an unusual phage type. Pediatrics 66:285, 1980.

Elias PM, Fritsch P, Epstein EH Jr: Staphylococcal scalded skin syndrome: Clinical features, pathogenesis, and recent microbiological and biochemical developments. Arch Dermatol 113:207, 1977.

Elias PM, Mittermayer H, Tappeiner G, et al: Staphylococcal toxic epidermal necrolysis (TEN): The expanded mouse model. J Invest Dermatol 63:467, 1974.

Gehlbach SH, Gutman LT, Wilfert CM, et al: Recurrence of skin disease in a nursery: Ineffectuality of hexachlorophene bathing. Pediatrics 55:422, 1975.

Guidelines for Perinatal Care: AAP Committee on the Fetus and Newborn. In ACOG Committee on Obstetrics: Maternal and Fetal Medicine, 2nd ed. American Academy of Pediatrics, Elk Grove Village, Ill, 1988.

Johnson DE, Thompson TR, Ferrieri P: Congenital candidiasis. Am J Dis Child 135:273, 1981.

Kam LA, Giacoia GP: Congenital cutaneous candidiasis. Am J Dis Child 129:1215, 1975.

Melish ME, Glasgow LA: Staphylococcal scalded skin syndrome: The expanded clinical syndrome. J Pediatr 78:958, 1971.

Melish ME, Glasgow LA: Staphylococcal scalded skin syndrome—development of an experimental model. N Engl J Med 282:1114, 1970.

Overturf BD, Balfour G: Osteomyelitis and sepsis: Severe complications of fetal monitoring. Pediatrics 55:244, 1975.

Rubenstein AD, Mesher DM: Epidemic boric acid poisoning simulating staphylococcal toxic epidermal necrolysis of the newborn infant: Ritter's disease. J Pediatr 77:884, 1970.

Rudolph N, Tariq AA, Reale MR, et al: Congenital cutaneous candidiasis. Arch Dermatol 113:1101, 1977.

Rudolph RI, Schwartz W, Leyden JJ: Treatment of staphylococcal toxic epidermal necrolysis. Arch Dermatol 110:559, 1974.

Sheagren JN: *Staphylococcus aureus*: The persistent pathogen (Parts I and II). N Engl J Med 310:1368, 1437, 1984.

Stulberg DL: Common bacterial skin infections. Am Fam Physician 66:119-124, 2002.

Wagner MM, Rycheck RR, Yee RB, et al: Septic dermatitis of the neonatal scalp and maternal endomyometritis with intrapartum internal fetal monitoring. Pediatrics 74:81, 1984.


## REFERENCES


Amagi M, Matsuyoshi N, Wang ZH, et al: Toxin in bullous impetigo and staphylococcal scalded-skin syndrome targets desmoglein 1. Nat Med 6:1275-1277, 2000.

Amagi M, Takayuki Y, Hanakawa Y, et al: Staphylococcal exfoliative toxin B specifically cleaves desmoglein 1. J Invest Dermatol 118:845-850, 2002.

Arvin AM, Prober CG: Herpes simplex virus infections: The genital tract and the newborn. Pediatr Rev special edition:11-16, 1992.

Baker CJ: Summary of workshop on infections due to group B streptococcus. J Infect Dis 136:137, 1977.

Belgaumkar TK: Impetigo neonatorum congenita due to group B beta-hemolytic streptococcus infection. J Pediatr 86:982, 1975.

Botas CM, Kurlat I, Young SM, Sola A: Disseminated candidal infections and intravenous hydrocortisone in preterm infants. Pediatrics 95:883-887, 1995.

Brent NB: Thrush in the breastfeeding dyad: Results of a survey on diagnosis and treatment. Clin Pediatr 40:503-506, 2001.

Dancer SJ, Noble WC: Nasal, axillary, and perineal carriage of *Staphylococcus aureus* among women: Identification of strains producing epidermolytic toxin. J Clin Pathol 44:681-684, 1991.

Darmstadt GL, Dinulos JG, Miller Z: Congenital cutaneous candidiasis: Clinical presentation, pathogenesis, and management guidelines. Pediatrics 105:438-444, 2000.

Dave J, Reith S, Nash JQ, et al: A double outbreak of exfoliative toxin-producing strains of staphylococcus aureus in a maternity unit. Epidemiol Infect 112:103-114, 1994.

Dillon HC Jr: Group A Type 12 streptococcal infection in a newborn nursery. Am J Dis Child 112:177, 1966.

Doebbeling BN: Nasal and hand carriage of *Staphylococcus aureus* in healthcare workers. J Chemother 6:11-17, 1994.

Doebbeling BN, Reagan DR, Pfaller MA, et al: Long-term efficacy of intranasal ointment: A prospective cohort study of staphylococcus aureus carriage. Arch Intern Med 154:1505-1508, 1994.

Doebbeling BN, Stanley GL, Sheetz CT, et al: Comparative efficacy of alternative hand-washing agents in reducing nosocomial infections in intensive care units. New Engl J Med 327:88-93, 1992.

Enright AM, Prober CG: Neonatal herpes infection: Diagnosis, treatment and prevention. Semin Neonatol 7:283-291, 2002.

Farrell AM: Staphylococcal scalded-skin syndrome. Lancet 354:880-881, 1999.

Frieden I: Blisters and pustules in the newborn. Curr Probl Pediatr 555-615, 1989.

Geil CC, Castle WK, Mortimer EA Jr: Group A streptococcal infections in newborn nurseries. Pediatrics 46:489, 1970.

Gibney MD, Siegfried EC: Cutaneous congenital candidiasis: A case report. Pediatr Dermatol 2:359-363, 1996.

Haley RW, Cushion NB, Tenover FC, et al: Eradication of endemic methicillin-resistant *Staphyloccus aureus* indications from a neonatal intensive care unit. J Infect Dis 171:614-624, 1995.

Hebert AA, Esterly NB: Bacterial and candidal cutaneous infections in the neonate. Dermatol Clin 4:3, 1986.

Held JL, Berkowitz RK, Grossman ME: Use of touch preparation for rapid diagnosis of disseminated candidiasis. J Am Acad Dermatol 19:1063-1066, 1988.

Howard JB, McCrackin GH Jr: The spectrum of group B streptococcal infections in infancy. Am J Dis Child 128:815, 1974.

Isenberg HD, Tucci V, Lipsitz P, et al: Clinical laboratory and epidemiological investigations of a *Streptococcus pyogenes* cluster epidemic in a newborn nursery. J Clin Microbiol 19:366, 1984.

Jacobs RF: Neonatal herpes simplex virus infections. Semin Perinatol 22:64-71, 1998.

Johnson DE, Thompson TR, Green TP, Ferrieri P: Systemic candidiasis in very low-birth-weight infants (<1,500 grams). Pediatrics 73:138-143, 1984.

Kimberlin D, Powell D, Gruber W, et al: Administration of oral acyclovir suppressive therapy after neonatal herpes simplex virus disease limited to the skin, eyes and mouth: Results of a phase I/II trial. Pediatr Infect Dis J 15:247-254, 1996.

Kimberlin DW: Advances in the treatment of neonatal herpes simplex infections. Rev Med Virol 11:157-163, 2001.

Kimberlin DW, Lin CY, Jacobs RF, et al: Safety and efficacy of high-dose intravenous acyclovir in the management of neonatal herpes simplex virus infections. Pediatrics 108:230-238, 2001.

Kragballe K, Steijlen PM, Ibsen HH, et al: Efficacy, tolerability and safety of calcipotriol ointment in disorders of keratinization: Results of a randomized double-blind, vehicle-controlled, right/left comparative study. Arch Dermatol 131:556-560, 1995.

Ladhani S: Staphylococcal toxins and the scalded skin syndrome. Br J Dermatol 142:195-196, 2000.

Lehtonen OP, Ruuskanen O, Karo P, et al: Group-A streptococcal infection in the newborn. Lancet 2:1473, 1984.

Leibovitz E: Neonatal candidosis: Clinical picture, management controversies and consensus, and new therapeutic options. J Antimicrob Chemother 49 (suppl 1):69-73, 2002.

Lupetti A, Tavanti A, Davini P, et al: Horizontal transmission of *Candida parapsilosis* candidemia in a neonatal intensive care unit. J Clin Microbiol 40:2363-2369, 2002.

Nahass GT, Goldstein BA, Zhu W, et al: Comparison of Tzanck smear, viral culture, and DNA diagnostic methods in detection of herpes simplex and varicella-zoster infection. JAMA 268:2541-2544, 1992.

Nahass GT, Mandel MJ, Cook S, et al: Detection of herpes simplex and varicella-zoster infection from cutaneous lesions in different clinical stages with the polymerase chain reaction. J Am Acad Dermatol 32:730-733, 1995.

Overall JC Jr: Herpes simplex virus infection of the fetus and the newborn. Pediatr Ann 23:131-136, 1994.

Peter G, Hazard J: Neonatal group A streptococcal disease. J Pediatr 87:454, 1975.

Resnick SD: Staphylococcal toxin-mediated syndromes in childhood. Semin Dermatol 11:11-18, 1992.

Rosenkranz HS, Carr HS: Possible hazard in use of gentian violet. BMJ 3:702-703, 1971.

Russell C, Lay KM: Natural history of *Candida* species and yeasts in the oral cavities of infants. Arch Oral Biol 18:957, 1973.

Salvador A, Meislich D, Tunnessen WW Jr: Picture of the month: Intrauterine herpes simplex virus infection. Arch Pediatr Adoles Med 148:1311-1312, 1994.

Schirar A, Rendu C, Vielh JP, Gautray JP: Congenital mycosis (*Candida albicans*). Biol Neonate 24:273, 1974.

Tokura Y, Yagi J, O'Malley M, et al: Superantigenic staphylococcal exotoxins induce T-cell proliferation in the presence of Langerhans cells or class II-bearing keratinocytes to produce T-cell activating cytokines. J Invest Dermatol 112:103-114, 1994.

Waguespack-LaBiche J, Chen SH, Yen A: Disseminated congenital candidiasis in a premature infant. Arch Dermatol 135:510-512, 1999.

Whitley RJ: Neonatal herpes simplex virus infections: Is there a role for immunoglobulin in disease prevention and therapy? Pediatr Infect Dis 13:432-438, 1994.

Yamaguchi T, Yokota Y, Terajima J, et al: Clonal association of *Staphylococcus aureus* causing bullous impetigo and the emergence of new methicillin-resistant clonal groups in Kansai District in Japan. J Infect Dis 15:1511-1516, 2002.

CHAPTER

# 99

# Common Newborn Dermatoses*

**Rebecca A. Kazin, Bernard A. Cohen, and Elaine C. Siegfried**

This chapter describes a group of cutaneous disorders that are unique to neonates. All of these disorders have well-recognized clinical and/or histologic features. Most are asymptomatic and self-limited, so rigorous searches have not been made for precise pathogeneses or definitive therapies. These common neonatal dermatoses may be mistaken for more serious diseases, and serious diseases may be mistaken for common neonatal dermatoses. For this reason, verification of the correct diagnosis can obviate the initiation of aggressive workup and treatment. In other cases, it can be lifesaving. Important considerations in the differential diagnosis based on clinical morphology are outlined in Chapter 96.

## ERYTHEMA TOXICUM NEONATORUM

### Clinical Findings

Erythema toxicum is an inflammatory cutaneous disease of unknown origin that affects about half of all full-term newborns (Berg and Solomon, 1987). It occurs less frequently among preterm infants (Carr et al, 1966; Taylor and Bondurant, 1957). In a majority of infants, the lesions develop between 1 and 3 days of age, but they may appear as late as 3 weeks. No predilection of the disorder for race, gender, season, or geographic location has been reported.

Affected infants appear healthy. The basic skin lesion is a small (1 to 3 mm in diameter) papule that evolves into a pustule, with a prominent halo of erythema, that has been likened to a flea bite. Individual lesions may persist only a few hours, but the eruption lasts for several days or, rarely, for several weeks. The number of lesions present may vary from a few to dozens. The trunk is the most frequent site of predilection, but the face and extremities also may be involved. Palms and soles are almost always spared. Several lesions may coalesce into plaques measuring several centimeters in diameter (Fig. 99–1).

### Diagnosis

A Wright-stained smear of pustule contents reveals large numbers of eosinophils, which supports the diagnosis. Skin biopsy may be necessary in clinically atypical cases. Histologic features consist of eosinophil-filled intraepidermal vesicles and a mixed intradermal inflammatory infiltrate that tends to localize around the superficial portion of the pilosebaceous follicle.

Considerations in the differential diagnosis include other benign, self-limited disorders such as transient neonatal pustular melanosis, miliaria, infantile acropustulosis, and eosinophilic pustular folliculitis, as well as infections such as bacterial folliculitis, bullous impetigo, candidiasis, herpes, and scabies. Urticaria pigmentosa and incontinentia pigmenti are more serious disorders that can be mistaken for erythema toxicum. The diagnostic workup outlined in Chapter 96 can differentiate among these conditions.

### Etiology

Erythema toxicum is a benign inflammatory disease of unknown cause. The eosinophilic infiltrate suggests that erythema toxicum is a hypersensitivity response, but studies attempting to incriminate chemical or microbiologic substances, acquired either transplacentally or vaginally from the mother, such as drugs, topical irritants, sebum, and milk, have failed to provide support for this hypothesis (Bassukas, 1992). At a molecular level, there appears to be an accumulation and activation of immune cells in these lesions as seen by immunohistochemical staining of punch biopsies from cutaneous lesions. Monoclonal antibodies placed in lesional skin detected E-selectin in the vessel wall as well as dendritic cells, eosinophils, macrophages, and E-selectin–expressing cells in these affected areas, whereas uninvolved skin demonstrated reduced or absent immunologic activity (Marchini et al, 2001).

### Treatment and Prognosis

Erythema toxicum is asymptomatic, resolves spontaneously, and requires no treatment. A prolonged course and recurrence are rare. Once the diagnosis is confirmed, anticipatory guidance and reassurance should be provided to parents.

## TRANSIENT NEONATAL PUSTULAR MELANOSIS

### Clinical Findings

This benign disorder is present at birth in 5% of African-American and in 1% of white infants (Ramamurthy et al, 1976). Characteristic lesions are small, superficial pustules that rupture easily, leaving a collarette of fine scale and hyperpigmented macules (Fig. 99–2). The lesions may be profuse or sparse and can involve all body surfaces, including the palms, soles, and scalp (Fig. 99–3). The pustules last about 48 hours; the macules may persist for several months.

### Diagnosis

Affected infants are otherwise well. A Wright-stained smear of pustule contents revealing keratinous debris and variable numbers of polymorphonuclear neutrophils with few or no eosinophils supports the diagnosis. Gram stain and bacterial cultures obtained from intact pustules uniformly fail to disclose the presence of organisms. The differential diagnosis includes the conditions listed for erythema toxicum.

*This chapter includes material from the previous edition, to which Nancy B. Esterly, MD, contributed.

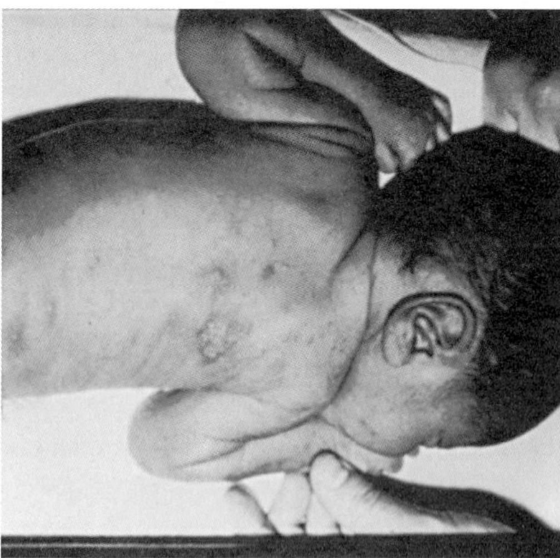

**FIGURE 99–1.** Florid lesions of erythema toxicum on the back of a newborn infant. The pustules are large and surrounded by an erythematous halo. Smears of the pustular contents showed only eosinophils.

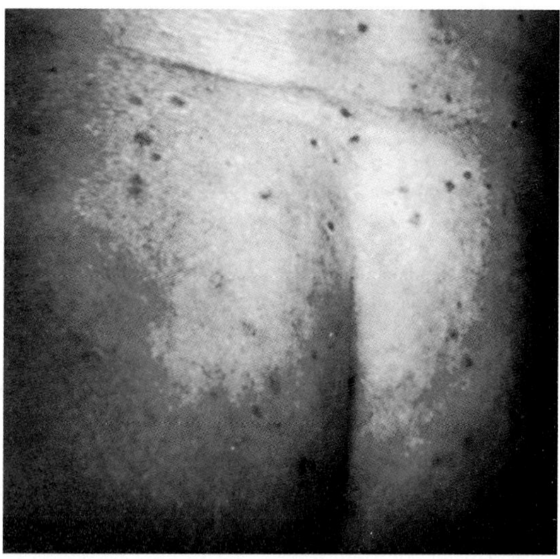

**FIGURE 99–3.** Transient neonatal pustular melanosis. Hyperpigmented macules on the lower back and buttocks, some of which are encircled by scales. *(From Ramamurthy RS, Reveri M, Esterly NB, et al: Transient neonatal pustular melanosis. J Pediatr 88:831, 1976.)*

### Etiology

The cause of transient neonatal pustular melanosis is unknown. A prospective study reported that 17 infants with typical congenital lesions subsequently developed lesions of erythema toxicum, linking the two conditions (Ferrandiz et al, 1992).

### Treatment

The disorder is asymptomatic and self-limited. Once the diagnosis is confirmed, further therapy is not required.

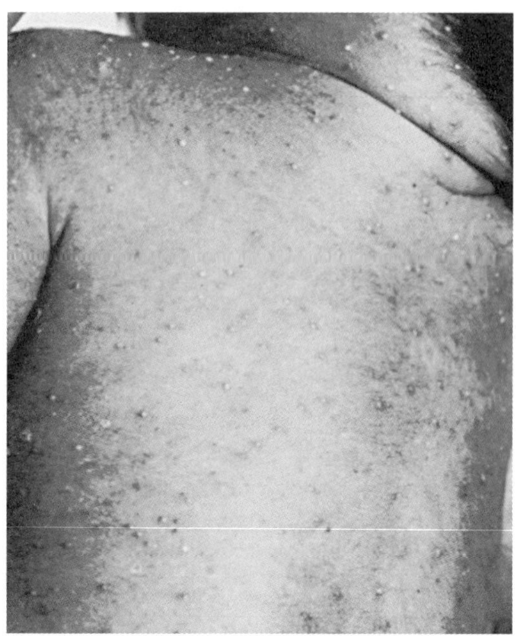

**FIGURE 99–2.** Numerous superficial pustules on the neck and back of a 1-day-old infant. A few pustules have ruptured, leaving a collarette of scales.

## MILIA, EPSTEIN PEARLS, AND SEBACEOUS HYPERPLASIA

### Clinical Findings

*Milia* (a single lesion is a *milium*) are found in 40% of full-term infants (Gordon, 1959). They are single or sparsely scattered 1- to 2-mm pearly lesions that occur on the face. The sites of predilection are the cheeks, forehead, and chin (Fig. 99–4). Large milia (greater than 2 mm in diameter) are found in infants with type I oral-facial-digital syndrome (Solomon et al, 1970). Rarely, milia may occur in unusual sites, such as on the arms, legs, or foreskin.

*Epstein pearls* are milia that occur in the oral mucosa. These tiny cystic lesions occur in about 85% of newborn infants and usually are found on the palate, particularly along the midpalatine raphe and at the junction of the hard and soft palates. They usually are grouped, firm, and movable and appear opaque and white.

### Diagnosis

Histologically, a milium is an invagination of epidermal tissue, arising from the pilosebaceous apparatus of vellus

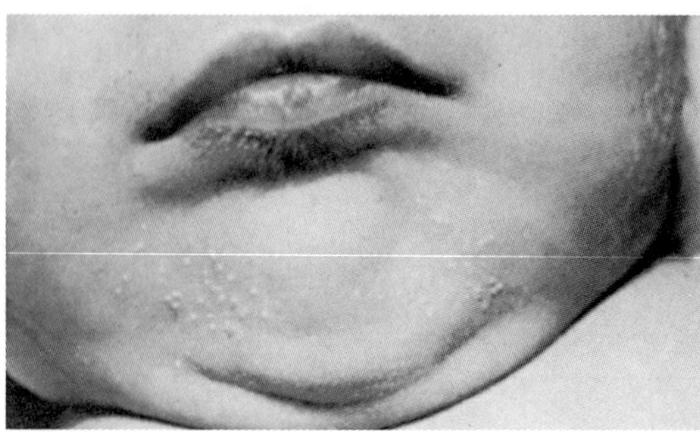

**FIGURE 99–4.** Numerous grouped milia on the chin of a newborn infant.

hair, which forms a cyst filled with several layers of keratin-producing cells. The expressed contents of milial cysts resemble tiny white pearls and consist mostly of keratinocyte debris, a useful diagnostic feature.

Milia may be mistaken for *sebaceous gland hyperplasia*, which occur in the same distribution. The papules of sebaceous gland hyperplasia are smaller (pinpoint) and more yellow and contain sebaceous lipids. Milia usually exfoliate spontaneously within 1 month. Epstein pearls are self-limited but may take several months to resolve. Sebaceous hyperplasia also resolves spontaneously within the first few weeks of life.

## MILIARIA

### Clinical Findings

Miliaria neonatorum is a vesicular or pustular dermatitis arising from the eccrine duct. Four clinical variants have been described, their appearances influenced by the site of obstruction within the duct. *Miliaria crystallina* (sudamina) consists of very superficial, clear, thin-walled, noninflammatory vesicles that rupture easily. The vesicle is localized within the stratum corneum. *Miliaria rubra* (prickly heat) consists of small, erythematous, grouped papules often localized to skin folds and areas covered by clothing. These lesions arise within the deeper levels of the epidermis and are accompanied by inflammation. The papules may become pustular if there is a prominent inflammatory component or secondary bacterial infection, a condition sometimes referred to as *miliaria pustulosa. Miliaria profunda* is a mildly inflammatory papular eruption that arises within the dermal portion of the eccrine duct.

### Etiology

Miliaria is believed to be caused by sweat accumulation into obstructed eccrine ducts. Obstruction of the eccrine duct in adults has been reported to result from a variety of triggers such as cutaneous injury, excessive hydration of the stratum corneum, or overgrowth of microbes (Fitzpatrick, 1990). Premature and even full-term neonates have a full complement of eccrine glands, distributed in greater density than after growth with concomitant increase in skin surface area (Jordan and Blaney, 1982). Immature, incompletely canalized eccrine ducts could predispose the newborn to miliaria (Straka et al, 1991). Overheating from excessive bundling and phototherapy probably contribute to its pathogenesis. The widespread availability of environmental temperature control probably has decreased the incidence of this condition.

Recurrent episodes of pustular miliaria rubra could signal the rare condition type I pseudohypoaldosteronism. This potentially fatal condition of autosomal recessive inheritance is a disorder of mineralocorticoid resistence that leads to salt-wasting crises through the eccrine ducts. If this condition is suspected, an appropriate serologic workup should be initiated. (Urbatsch and Paller, 2002)

### Diagnosis

The differential diagnosis of miliaria includes the conditions listed previously for erythema toxicum. Wright stain of vesicle contents from miliaria crystallina will show few cells; that of miliaria rubra will usually reveal a majority of lymphocytes. If screening studies are nondiagnostic, a skin biopsy will be confirmatory (Fitzpatrick, 1990).

### Treatment

Lesions rapidly resolve after the infant's environmental temperature is reduced. Application of occlusive emollients may exacerbate the eruption.

## ACNE

### Clinical Findings

The appearance of acne in infancy is similar to that of typical acne vulgaris of adolescence. The spectrum of lesions includes comedones, inflammatory papules, pustules, and rarely, cysts, generally limited to the face (Fig. 99–5). Comedones are an easily recognized, pathognomonic feature of acne.

The condition occurs in up to 20% of infants and is more common in boys. Acne occurs in a bimodal distribution during infancy. Early-onset *neonatal acne* occurs after 1 to 2 weeks of age and usually resolves spontaneously by 3 months. *Infantile acne* appears after 3 to 6 months and may persist for years.

### Etiology

The pathophysiologic features of acne are similar at all ages. Important components are the increased size and activity of sebaceous glands, which are influenced by circulating levels of adrenal and gonadal androgens, of both endogenous and maternal origins. The role of *Propionibacterium acnes* in the pathogenesis of infantile acne has not been studied. This lipophilic, anaerobic gram-positive rod plays an important role in the pathogenesis of inflammatory lesions in adolescent acne. A family history of acne is common, and affected infants have a higher risk of developing severe acne later in life (Hellier, 1954), suggesting a genetic predisposition (Forest et al, 1973).

In the past few years, a potential etiologic factor of noncomedonal neonatal acne, or cephalic pustulosis, has been identified. *Malassezia* is a lipophilic yeast that is part of the normal flora of adult skin; a variety of factors,

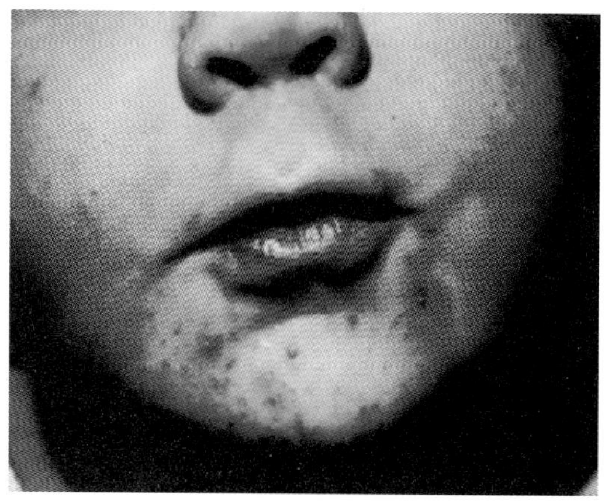

**FIGURE 99–5.** Papules, pustules, and comedones (diagnostic of acne) on the chin and cheeks of a male infant.

including sebaceous gland activity, humidity, heredity, and corticosteroid treatment, may be influential in allowing it to become an opportunistic pathogen. Recently, several investigators have examined the connection between *Malassezia* and neonatal acne. Findings include the rapid progressive skin colonization of neonates by *Malassezia* species as seen on smear and culture examination, specifically *Malassezia sympodialis* and *Malassezia globosa*; higher rates of skin colonization by *Malassezia* in more severe cases of cephalic pustulosis; and isolation of *M. sympodalis* in the neonatal pustules (Bernier et al, 2002; Niamba et al, 1998). In a study conducted to explore this association, 8 of 13 patients (61%) with pustules positive for *Malassezia* showed a favorable response to treatment with 2% ketoconazole (Rapelanoro et al, 1996.)

However, contrary evidence exists, including lack of complete correlation between *Malassezia* and neonatal acne. Other studies have identified patients with neonatal acne in whom *Malassezia* was not found, as well as patients without acne whose pustule cultures were positive for *Malassezia* (Katsambas et al, 1999). Therefore, further investigation is needed to clarify cephalic pustulosis and neonatal acne and to specifically address the possibility that these inconsistencies could be explained by methodologic or pathologic variation, or that *Malassezia* may be one part of a multifactorial process, or that some cases of neonatal acne are not cephalic pustulosis but true comedonal disease (Bergman and Eichenfield, 2002.)

### Diagnosis

Considerations in the differential diagnosis include the papular and pustular disorders listed previously, but the diagnosis of acne can almost always be made by clinical inspection. No other disorder features comedones. Infants with severe or persistent acne should be evaluated for androgenic endocrinopathy.

### Treatment

Aggressive treatment of neonatal acne is rarely required. For initial therapy, topical 2% erythromycin or 2.5% or 5% benzoyl peroxide may be applied daily. Tretinoin and more potent formulations of benzoyl peroxide may be irritating. In more severe cases, a course of enteral erythromycin may be added, in divided doses of 30 to 50 mg/kg/day. Creams, ointments, and topical steroids may exacerbate the condition. If *Malassezia* is isolated or suspected, an antifungal agent may be efficacious (Rapelanoro et al, 1996.)

## INFANTILE ECZEMA

The term *eczema* is derived from a Greek term meaning "to boil over." It refers to a clinical and histologic cutaneous phenotype characterized by erythema, edema, and scaling, often accompanied by crusting and, in severe cases, blistering. The histologic hallmark of acute eczema is epidermal intercellular edema (i.e., spongiosis). Epidermal thickening is present in chronic eczema. A mixed perivascular inflammatory infiltrate usually is seen within the papillary dermis.

Different types of eczema can be defined by a spectrum of unifying clinical features. When a patient presents in infancy with widespread eczema, a precise diagnosis sometimes requires a period of observation. Two common eczematous conditions manifest in otherwise healthy infants: seborrheic dermatitis and atopic dermatitis (AD). These diseases differ in pathogenesis, distribution of skin involvement, prognosis, and range of therapeutic options. Infants with widespread eczema who are not otherwise healthy and those with prominent, erosive periorificial involvement should be evaluated for associated nutritional, metabolic, or immunologic abnormalities. A more extensive differential diagnosis is detailed under "Erythroderma" in Chapter 96.

### Seborrheic Dermatitis

#### Clinical Findings

Infantile seborrheic dermatitis is characterized by greasy yellow scales on an erythematous base and minimal pruritus. Onset usually is within the first 2 months of life. The most common sites of involvement are the face, scalp, and diaper area. The condition may be localized or disseminated. Flexural areas such as the posterior auricular sulcus, neck, axillae, and inguinal folds also can be affected. Hypopigmentation is often striking in dark-skinned infants (Fig. 99–6). In severe cases, fissures may develop and become secondarily infected.

#### Causes

*Pityrosporum ovale* is a lipophilic yeast that is commonly present on normal skin, increasing in density during and after puberty. The mycelial form has been identified as a causative agent in tinea versicolor. For a century, the yeast form has been linked to adult seborrheic dermatitis. Therapeutic trials with yeast-inhibiting agents have supported a causal role (Straka et al, 1991). There is a higher incidence of seborrheic dermatitis in immunocompromised patients, especially those with acquired immunodeficiency syndrome (AIDS) (Prose, 1991). The association between *P. ovale* and infantile seborrheic dermatitis also has been confirmed (Broberg and Faergemann, 1989; Ruiz-Maldonado et al, 1989). The pathogenesis of the disorder, and the reasons carriers remain asymptomatic and immunocompromised persons can be more severely affected, remain unclear.

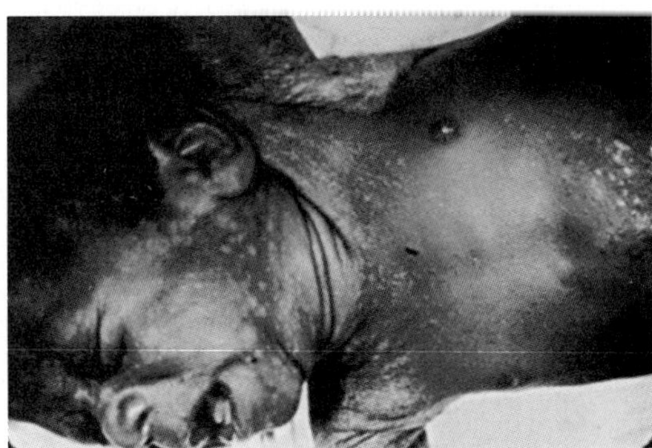

**FIGURE 99–6.** Infant with seborrheic eczema on the face and neck and in the axillae. Note the scaling and hypopigmentation. Temporary hypopigmentation is common in African-American infants with this disorder.

### Treatment

Infantile seborrheic dermatitis spontaneously resolves by the end of the first year of life. For infants with disfiguring or symptomatic disease, there are several therapeutic alternatives. Topical agents effective against *P. ovale* include topical ketoconazole, in a cream or shampoo base (Cutsem et al, 1990), shampoos containing 1% zinc pyrithione or 1% to 2.5% selenium sulfide, and propylene glycol (Faergemann, 1988). Propylene glycol is a hygroscopic preservative, with antimycotic activity against *P. ovale*, that has been widely used for more than a century in foods and cosmetics. It is commercially available as a 1.5% soapless cleanser (Cetaphil lotion, Galderma Laboratories, Inc., Fort Worth, Texas). The safety and efficacy for none of these products have been established in infants. Nevertheless, widespread availability and popular use have not produced reports of toxicity. Brief application with daily bathing usually is effective and limits excessive percutaneous absorption. Daily application of 0.5% to 1% hydrocortisone cream is another short-term alternative.

## Atopic Dermatitis

### Clinical Findings

AD is a chronic, severely pruritic, familial disorder defined by a spectrum of defined cutaneous and extracutaneous manifestations (Hanifin, 1991; Paller, 1991). In 60% of cases, signs and symptoms begin in infancy; up to 10% of 1-year-old children are affected (Kay et al, 1994). The most easily recognized of the diagnostic criteria for AD may not be present until early childhood. These criteria include onset of rash before the age of 2 years, flexural skin lesions, asthma or hay fever, and generalized dry skin (Williams et al, 1994). AD and seborrheic dermatitis share clinical features, often making correct diagnosis difficult during the neonatal period. A common feature that may distinguish one from the other form is involvement of the diaper area. This area is often dramatically spared in infants with AD and is primarily involved in infants with seborrheic dermatitis.

### Etiology

Atopic disease has been clinically recognized since 1916; however, its pathogenesis remains elusive. Recent investigations of the mechanisms and treatment of AD have focused on immune alterations. Blood eosinophilia, overproduction of immunoglobulin E (IgE), and a diminished cell-mediated delayed-type hypersensitivity response are common features. Other, in vitro immune abnormalities have been described, including alterations in monocyte cyclic AMP (cAMP) production, increased histamine release by basophils and mast cells, abnormal differentiation of antigen-presenting cells, increased serum levels of eosinophil cationic protein and interleukin-4 (IL-4), and diminished production of interferon gamma by circulating lymphocytes (Hanifin, 1991; Hanifin et al, 1993). These data support a hypothesis regarding the basic immune dysregulation causing AD. The theory assumes an imbalance of T-cell subsets, with inhibition of the cells that produce interferon-γ ($T_H1$ helper T cells) and a relative activation of the cells that produce IL-4 ($T_H2$ helper T cells). These assumed outcomes are believed to potentiate a vicious circle of enhanced production of IgE, eosinophilia, mast cell proliferation, release of histamine by basophils and mast cells, and further expansion of $T_H2$ cells (Hanifin, 1991; Hanifin et al, 1993).

*Staphylococcus aureus* plays an important role in the exacerbation of AD. Ninety percent of affected patients carry this microbe on their skin, and a course of antistaphylococcal antibiotics augments therapy during clinical flares. Staphylococcal exotoxins act as superantigens capable of stimulating a wide variety of T-cell responses (Leung et al, 1995).

Food and environmental allergens play a role in the minority of patients (Hanifin, 1991). Prolonged breastfeeding and delayed exposure to diverse solid foods may protect against AD, especially in infants with a strong family history of atopic disease (Zeiger, 1994).

### Treatment

The goal of treatment is to control signs and symptoms. A definitive cure is not yet available, but spontaneous improvement occurs before puberty in 40% of patients (Hanifin, 1991). Maintenance therapy aims to hydrate the skin, reduce inflammation, control pruritus, and eliminate inciting factors. These goals are achieved with once- or twice-daily bathing with a mild antimicrobial cleanser, sparing application of topical corticosteroids, and liberal application of a bland ointment emollient. Addition of systemic antistaphylococcal antibiotics is sometimes necessary.

Both tacrolimus 0.03% ointment and pimecrolimus 1% cream, nonsteroidal selective inhibitors of inflammatory cytokines, have been approved for the treatment of atopic dermatitis in children older than 24 months. However, studies support the safe use of both agents in infants as young as 3 months.

Infants with AD have a relative cutaneous anergy and are at increased risk for the development of cutaneous bacterial, yeast, fungal, and viral infections. A high index of suspicion for secondary infection must be maintained.

## DIAPER DERMATITIS

### Etiology

Although diaper dermatitis, described over a century ago, has been widely studied, the cause, true prevalence, and optimal treatment are still issues of debate. A majority of infants has episodes of diaper dermatitis, most commonly between 6 and 12 months of age (Jordan and Blaney, 1982). For decades, the condition was believed to be due primarily to the effects of ammonia. However, objective studies did not support this theory (Leyden et al, 1977). Many factors contribute to the pathogenesis of diaper dermatitis, but the nidus of the problem begins with occlusion, excessive hydration, friction, and maceration. Once skin barrier function has been compromised, irritants (urine, fecal lipases, proteases, bile salts) and microorganisms (urease-splitting bacteria, *S. aureus*, beta-hemolytic streptococci, *Pseudomonas* species, *Candida albicans*) exacerbate the problem. Exogenous irritants, such as soaps, commercial diaper wipes, and a myriad of over-the-counter topical products, can perpetuate the process in susceptible infants.

### Treatment

Clearly, the most important steps in preventing diaper dermatitis are maintaining skin barrier function and hygiene and preventing irritation. Traditionally, an effective but labor-intensive approach has been frequent diaper changes with gentle cleansing, thorough drying, and limited use of occlusive plastic or rubber diaper covers. This practice has been greatly simplified by the introduction of disposable diapers.

The first disposable diapers were marketed in 1963. Initially, the absorbent core was composed primarily of cellulose fluff. Subsequently, several conflicting studies were done to evaluate the incidence of diaper dermatitis in infants wearing cloth versus disposable diapers (Jordan and Blaney, 1982). In the mid-1980s, a superabsorbent core material was developed, containing a cross-linked sodium polyacrylate. Upon contact with fluid, this material undergoes a transformation to allow it to hold fluid within a gel and has the capacity to absorb many times its own weight. Several studies have concluded that superabsorbent diapers are superior to cloth diapers in preventing diaper dermatitis (Lane et al, 1990). In addition, superabsorbent diapers may prevent occult fecal contamination of clothing and fomites in daycare settings (Rory et al, 1991).

Routine use of topical preparations to prevent diaper dermatitis is not necessary in infants with normal skin. For some of these products, additional risks have been recognized. Additives have the potential to cause contact sensitization or irritation. Powders applied vigorously enough to raise a cloud pose an aspiration hazard. This is especially true for talc, which can cause irritant pneumonitis. Talc (mainly hydrous magnesium silicate) also may cause granulomatous reactions when applied to wounds.

Appropriate treatment of diaper dermatitis begins with correct diagnosis of the underlying cause. Most infants develop acute diaper dermatitis as a result of the factors described previously. However, other primary pathologic processes must be considered for any infant with chronic, severe, or recurrent diaper rash. Primary cutaneous diseases that may manifest with diaper rash include allergic contact dermatitis, seborrheic dermatitis, psoriasis, and candidiasis. Several uncommon causes of diaper dermatitis such as histiocytosis, congenital syphilis, bullous pemphigoid, and staphylococcal scalded skin syndrome have serious implications (Kazaks, 2000).

Mild to moderate, common diaper dermatitis should be treated initially with traditional frequent diaper changes and/or leaving the area exposed. A temporary switch to superabsorbent diapers may be helpful for infants diapered with cloth. All potential irritants or sensitizers should be discontinued. Commercial diaper wipes are an often-overlooked, common source of these substances. Washcloths, dampened paper towels, and mineral oil–soaked cotton balls are safe alternatives. Zinc oxide ointment and zinc paste are inexpensive, bland, protective agents with antiseptic and astringent properties. Zinc also may play a role in wound healing (Maitra and Dorani, 1992; Okada et al, 1990; Rackett et al, 1993). Some caregivers may object to the difficulty in removing zinc oxide preparations. They should be reassured that it is not necessary to remove the salve. If a parent or clinician needs to remove zinc oxide to assess the skin, this can be easily accomplished with the help of mineral oil.

If there is no objective evidence of candidiasis, a short course of a topical low-potency corticosteroid may be beneficial. A topical anticandidal agent should be used when potassium hydroxide preparation or culture suggests yeast infection. Combination products containing potent topical corticosteroids and antifungal agents are less effective than an antifungal used alone (Reynolds et al, 1991). Widespread use of one such product combining a potent, fluorinated topical corticosteroid, 0.05% betamethasone dipropionate, with 1% clotrimazole (Lotrisone), applied under the occlusion of a diaper, has resulted in reports of skin atrophy, striae, and even adrenal suppression (Barkley, 1987). Clotrimazole and a similar product combining 0.1% triamcinolone acetonide and nystatin (Mycolog II) are contraindicated for the treatment of diaper dermatitis.

## HARLEQUIN COLOR CHANGE

Harlequin color change should not be confused with an entirely different disorder called *harlequin fetus*. Harlequin color change, first described in 1952, usually occurs during the first 4 days of life (Mortensen and Stougard-Andresen, 1959). It is characterized by reddening of one half of the body and simultaneous blanching of the other half. A sharp, midline demarcation runs from the center of the forehead down the face and trunk. Occasionally, the line of demarcation may be incomplete, sparing the face and genitalia. Turning the body from one side to the other accentuates blanching of the upper half and reddening of the lower half. There is no accompanying change in respiratory rate, pupillary reflexes, muscle tone, or response to external stimuli. The total duration of these episodes may range from a few minutes to several hours. Harlequin color change occurs most frequently in low-birth-weight infants but may be seen in up to 10% of term infants. The physiologic basis of the phenomenon has not been defined. It has no pathologic significance, requires no treatment, and can be expected to disappear no later than the third week of life.

## SUBCUTANEOUS FAT NECROSIS

### Clinical Findings

Subcutaneous fat necrosis affects full-term infants who have experienced perinatal distress. Lesions usually appear within the first 2 weeks of life. They may be single or multiple, are poorly circumscribed, and often are tender nodules or plaques that are initially firm with a dusky reddish-purple hue. They are located most often in areas in which a fat pad is present: buttocks, back, arms, and thighs (Fig. 99–7). With time, subcutaneous calcification may develop, with subsequent drainage and resultant scarring. The most serious association is hypercalcemia. Infants with hypercalcemia may be asymptomatic, so the incidence and time course have not been well documented (Cook and Stone, 1992). Symptoms include irritability, vomiting, poor feeding, and failure to thrive.

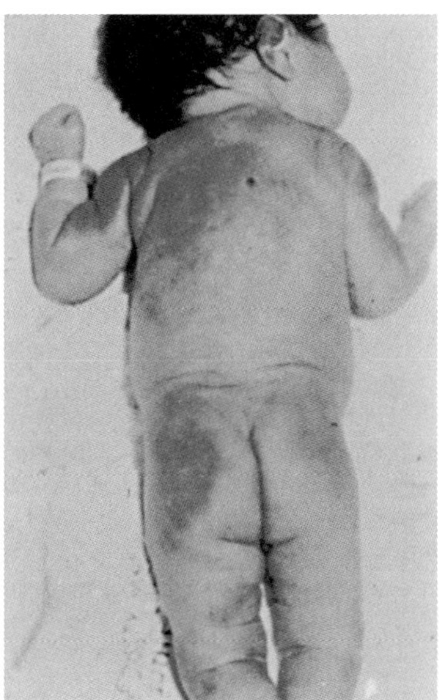

**FIGURE 99–7.** Rear view of a newborn showing several large discolored areas of subcutaneous fat necrosis. They were irregular in size and shape, felt firm to palpation, and were not hot or tender.

### Causes

The development of subcutaneous fat necrosis has been related to ischemic injury from obstetric trauma, intrauterine asphyxia (Chen et al, 1981), and hypothermia. Skin biopsy from a well developed lesion will reveal a subcutaneous granulomatous infiltrate with multinucleated giant cells. Damaged lipocytes contain characteristic needle-shaped clefts. Soft tissue necrosis and inflammation may stimulate local production of 1,25-dihydroxyvitamin $D_3$, resulting in hypercalcemia (Cook and Stone, 1992).

### Treatment

In most infants, the process is self-limited; resolution occurs over a period of weeks to months. Some experts recommend careful needle aspiration of fluctuant areas to reduce scarring (Hurwitz, 1985). Infants should be followed closely for the development of hypercalcemia for the first 6 weeks of life. Hypercalcemic infants should be managed initially with hydration and furosemide-induced diuresis. Restriction of oral calcium and vitamin D intake and the administration of systemic corticosteroids may be necessary (Cook and Stone, 1992; Norwood-Galloway et al, 1987). However, this approach may only be partially successful, and persistent hypercalcemia with its associated morbidity may ensue. Bisphosphonate agents, specifically etidronate, have recently been discussed for use as possible last resort agents to control the persistent hypercalcemia that can be secondary to subcutaneous fat necrosis. In one case report, a newborn with subcutaneous fat necrosis refractory to conservative management had etidronate added to his regimen. After initiation of the drug, the patient's urinary calcium levels soon normalized. It was postulated that the mechanism of lowering the serum and urinary calcium by etidronate was primarily a decrease in bone resorption. (Rice and Rivkees, 1999.)

Other investigators have commented on the limited use of bisphosphonates in children and question whether the hypercalcemia of subcutaneous fat necrosis is secondary to enhanced bone resorption or intestinal absorption. Controlled trials have been recommended before the use of these agents for this indication can be recommended (Bachrach and Lum, 1999). Of note, in the case study, etidronate had to be stopped because of a rash severe enough to be of clinical concern. Physicians must be aware of possible bisphosphonate-induced hypersensitivity reactions and stop the agent if suspected (Rice and Rivkees, 1999).

## SCLEREMA NEONATORUM

The lesions of subcutaneous fat necrosis are histologically similar to those of sclerema neonatorum, thereby potentially raising unnecessary concern for stable, full-term infants with localized skin lesions. Sclerema neonatorum is a diffuse, systemic process with a grave prognosis (Fretzin and Arias, 1987).

### Clinical Findings

Sclerema neonatorum occurs in debilitated or preterm neonates. It manifests with widespread, stone-hard, nonpitting cutaneous induration. The skin appears pale and waxy, shaping the face in mask-like expression (Fig. 99–8); the joints are stiff. Associated metabolic acidosis, hypoglycemia, hyperkalemia, hyponatremia, and azotemia may occur.

### Etiology

The disorder has been associated with prematurity, low birth weight, asphyxia, and hypothermia (Ji et al, 1993).

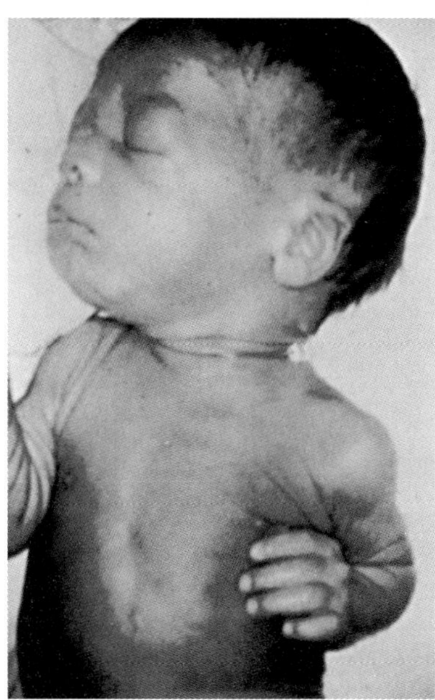

**FIGURE 99–8.** Sclerema neonatorum. Note the mask-like facial expression, "pseudotrismus" of the partially immobilized mouth, and thickening of the skin over the face, arms, and hands. *(From the Collection of the American Academy of Pediatrics. Reproduced with permission of the officers of the Academy.)*

The histologic changes of sclerema are not specific. Fat necrosis with crystallization may be seen; thinning of the epidermis and dermal and subcutaneous fibrosis with edema and thickening of the interlobular septa are more conspicuous features (Dasgupta et al, 1993).

The mechanism responsible for sclerema is unknown. Biochemical and crystalline changes in the subcutaneous fat of affected infants have suggested a decrease in the enzymatic desaturation of triglycerides (Horsefield and Yardley, 1965; Kellum et al, 1968).

### Treatment

The treatment of sclerema neonatorum is supportive care. Corticosteroid therapy has not been effective in altering the 30% to 60% mortality rate (Levin et al, 1965).

## REFERENCES


Bachrach L, Lum C: Etidronate in subcutaneous fat necrosis of the newborn [letter]. J Pediatr 135:530, 1999.

Barkley W: Strial and persistent tinea corporis related to prolonged use of betamethasone dipropionate. J Am Acad Dermatol 17:518-519, 1987.

Bassukas ID: Is erythema toxicum neonatorum a mild self-limited acute cutaneous graft-versus-host reaction from maternal-to-fetal lymphocyte transfer? Med Hypotheses 38:334-338, 1992.

Berg FJ, Solomon LM: Erythema neonatorum toxicum. Arch Dis Child 62:327, 1987.

Bergman J, Eichenfield L: Neonatal acne and cephalic pustulosis: Is *Malassezia* the whole story? [editorial]. Arch Dermatol. 138:255-257, 2002.

Bergbrant IM: Seborrhoeic dermatitis and *Pityrosporum ovale*: Cultural, immunological and clinical studies. Acta Derm Venereol Suppl (Stockh) 167(U1):7-36, 1991.

Bernier V, Weill FX, et al: Skin colonization by *Malassezia* species in neonates: A prospective study and relationship with neonatal cephalic pustulosis. Arch Dermatol 138:220-224, 2002.

Broberg A, Faergemann J: Infantile seborrhoeic dermatitis and *Pityrosporum ovale*. Br J Dermatol 120:359-362, 1989.

Carr JA, Hodgeman JE, Freedman RJ, Levan NE: Relationship between toxic erythema and infant maturity. Am J Dis Child 112:129, 1966.

Chen TH, Shewmake SW, Hansen DD, Lacey HL: Subcutaneous fat necrosis of the newborn. Arch Dermatol 117:36, 1981.

Cook JS, Stone MS: Hypercalcemia in association with subcutaneous fat necrosis of the newborn: Studies of calcium-regulating hormones. Pediatrics 90:93-96, 1992.

Cutsem J, Gerven F, Fransen J, et al: The in vitro antifungal activity of ketoconazole, zinc pyrithione, and selenium sulfide against *Pityrosporum* and their efficacy as a shampoo in the treatment of experimental pityrosporosis in guinea pigs. J Am Acad Dermatol 22:993-998, 1990.

Dasgupta A, Ghosh RN, Pal RK, Mukherjee N: Sclerema neonatorum—histopathologic study. Indian J Pathol Microbiol 36:45-47, 1993.

Faergemann J: Propylene glycol in the treatment of seborrheic dermatitis of the scalp. Cutis 42:69-71, 1988.

Ferrandiz C, Coroleu W, Ribera M, et al: Sterile transient neonatal pustulosis is a precocious form of erythema toxicum neonatorum. Dermatology 185:18-22, 1992.

Fitzpatrick JE: Inflammatory reactions of the sweat unit. In Farmer ER, Hood AF (eds): Pathology of the Skin. Norwalk, Appleton & Lange, 1990, pp 959-964.

Fitzpatrick R, Rapaport MS, Silva DG: Histiocytosis X. Arch Dermatol 117:253, 1981.

Forest MG, Cathiard AM, Bertrand GH: Evidence of testicular activity in early infancy. J Clin Endocrinol Metab 37:148, 1973.

Fretzin DF, Arias AM: Sclerema neonatorum and subcutaneous fat necrosis of the newborn. Pediatr Dermatol 4:112, 1987.

Gordon J: Miliary sebaceous cysts and blisters in the healthy newborn. Acta Obstet Gynaecol Scand 38:352, 1959.

Hanifin J: Atopic dermatitis in infants and children. Pediatr Clin North Am 38:763-789, 1991.

Hanifin J, Schneider L, Leung D, et al: Recombinant interferon gamma therapy for atopic dermatitis. J Am Acad Dermatol 28:189-197, 1993.

Hellier FF: Acneiform eruptions in infancy. Br J Dermatol 66:25, 1954.

Horsefield GJ, Yardley HJ: Sclerema neonatorum. J Invest Dermatol 44:326, 1965.

Hurwitz S: A visual guide to neonatal skin eruptions. Contemp Pediatr September:82-92, 1985.

Ji XC, Zhu CY, Pang RY: Epidemiological study on hypothermia in newborns. Chin Med J 106:428-432, 1993.

Jordan W, Blaney T: Factors influencing infant diaper dermatitis. In Maibach H, Boisits E (eds): Neonatal Skin: Predisposition, Structure and Function, vol 1. New York, Marcel Dekker, 1982, pp 205-221.

Katsambas AD et al: Acne neonatorum: A study of 22 cases. Int J Dermatol 38:128-130, 1999.

Kay J, Gawkrodger DJ, Mortimer MJ, Jaron AG: The prevalence of childhood atopic eczema in a general population. J Am Acad Dermatol 30:35-39, 1994.

Kazaks EL, Lane AT: Diaper dermatitis. Pediatr Clin North Am 47:909-919, 2000.

Kellum RE, Ray TL, Brown GR: Sclerema neonatorum: Report of case analysis of subcutaneous and epidermal-dermal lipids by chromatographic methods. Arch Dermatol 97:372, 1968.

Lane A, Rehder P, Helm K: Evaluation of diapers containing absorbent gelling material with conventional disposable diapers in newborn infants. Am J Dis Child 144:315-318, 1990.

Leung DY, Travers JB, Norris DA: The role of superantigens in skin disease. J Invest Dermatol 105 (suppl 1):37S-42S, 1995.

Levin SE, Milunsky A: Urea and electrolyte levels in the serum in sclerema neonatorum. J Pediatr 67:812, 1965.

Leyden J, Katz S, Stewart R, Kligman A: Urinary ammonia and ammonia-producing microorganisms in infants with and without diaper dermatitis. Arch Dermatol 113:1678-1680, 1977.

Maitra A, Dorani B: Role of zinc in post-injury wound healing. Arch Emerg Med 9:122-124, 1992.

Marchini G, et al. Erythema toxicum neonatorum: An immunohistochemical analysis. Pediatr Dermatol 18:177-187, 2001.

Mortensen O, Stougard-Andresen P: Harlequin color change in the newborn. Acta Obstet Gynecol Scand 38:352, 1959.

Niamba P, Weill FX, et al: Is common neonatal cephalic pustulosis (neonatal acne) triggered by *Malassezia sympodialis*? Arch Dermatol 134:995-998, 1998.

Neligan GW, Strang LB: A "harlequin" colour change in the newborn. Lancet 2:1005, 1952.

Norwood-Galloway A, Lebwohl M, Phelps RG, et al: Subcutaneous fat necrosis of the newborn and hypercalcemia. J Am Acad Dermatol 16:435, 1987.

Okada A, Takagi Y, Nezu R, Lee S: Zinc in clinical surgery—a research review. Jpn J Surg 20:635-644, 1990.

Paller AS: Childhood atopic dermatitis: Update on therapy. Clin Case Dermatol 2:9-14, 1991.

Prose NS: Mucocutaneous disease in pediatric human immunodeficiency virus infection. Pediatr Clin North Am 38:977-990, 1991.

Rackett S, Rothe M, Grant-Kels J: Diet and dermatology—the role of dietary manipulation in the prevention and treatment of cutaneous disorders. J Am Acad Dermatol 29:447-461, 1993.

Ramamurthy RS, Reveri M, Esterly NB, et al: Transient neonatal pustular melanosis. J Pediatr 88:831, 1976.

Rapelanoro R, et al: Neonatal *Malassezia furfur* pustulosis. Arch Dermatol 132:190-193, 1996.

Reynolds R, Boiko S, Lucky A: Exacerbation of tinea corporis during treatment with 1% clotrimazole/0.05% betamethasone dipropionate (Lotrisone). Am J Dis Child 145:1224-1225, 1991.

Rice A, S. Rivkees: Etidronate therapy for hypercalcemia in subcutaneous fat necrosis of the newborn. J Pediatr 134:349-351, 1999.

Rory V, Wun C, Morrow A, Pickering LK: The effect of diaper type and overclothing on fecal contamination in day-care centers. JAMA 265:1840-1844, 1991.

Ruiz-Maldonado R, Lopez-Matinez R, Chavarria E, et al: *Pityrosporum ovale* in infantile seborrheic dermatitis. Pediatr Dermatol 6:16-20, 1989.

Sharlin DN, Koblenzer P: Necrosis of subcutaneous fat with hypercalcemia: A puzzling and multifaceted disease. Clin Pediatr 9:290, 1970.

Solomon LM, Esterly NB: Eczema in Neonatal Dermatology. Philadelphia, WB Saunders, 1973, p 125.

Solomon LM, Fretzin D, Pruzansky S: Pilosebaceous dysplasia in the oral-facial-digital syndrome. Arch Dermatol 102:596, 1970.

Solomon LM, Rostenberg A Jr: Atopic dermatitis and infantile eczema. In Samter M, Talmadge DW, Rose B, et al (eds): Immunological Diseases, 3rd ed. Boston, Little, Brown, 1978, p 953.

Straka BF, Cooper PH, Greer K: Congenital miliaria crystallina. Cutis 47:103-106, 1991.

Taylor WB, Bondurant CP: Erythema neonatorum allergicum. Arch Dermatol 76:591, 1957.

Urbatsch A, Paller AS. Pustular miliaria rubra: A specific cutaneous finding of type I pseudohypoaldosteronism. Pediatr Dermatol 19:317-319, 2002.

Williams HC, Burney PG, Pembroke AC, Hay RJ: The U.K. working party's diagnostic criteria for atopic dermatitis, III: Independent hospital validation. Br J Dermatol 131:406-416, 1994.

Zeiger RS: Dietary manipulations in infants and their mothers and the natural course of atopic disease. Pediatr Allergy Immunol 5 (suppl 6):26-28, 1994.

CHAPTER

# 100

# Cutaneous Congenital Defects*

**Alison Z. Young, Bernard A. Cohen, and Elaine C. Siegfried**

The spectrum of congenital cutaneous defects can be organized by tissue of origin or location within the skin. This spectrum is summarized in Table 100–1. However, in many cases the clinical appearance is not diagnostic for the specific condition or even the tissue type. An overview of differential diagnosis by clinical appearance is included in Chapter 96.

This chapter presents information on the most common and clinically significant congenital cutaneous defects.

## VASCULAR DEFECTS

Precise diagnosis and appropriate management of the cutaneous vascular defects have been confounded by tremendous confusion in nomenclature and poor understanding of the pathogenesis of the different conditions within this group. For example, the term *hemangioma* has been used indiscriminately to refer to lesions that differ considerably in morphology, behavior, and prognosis. The classification system proposed by Mulliken and Glowacki in 1982 is accepted as the official classification scheme for congenital vascular defects by the International Society for the Study of Vascular Anomalies (Hand and Frieden, 2002). This scheme separates vascular lesions of infants and children into two major categories: hemangiomas and malformations (Mulliken and Young, 1988). A *hemangioma*, by definition, is a benign tumor of vascular endothelium, characterized by a proliferative phase and an involutional phase (Fig. 100–1A). In contrast, a *malformation* is a developmental anomaly generated from a single vascular component or from a combination of vascular components: capillary, venous, arterial, or lymphatic. These two groups can be further differentiated according to clinical, cellular, hematologic, radiologic, and skeletal characteristics (Table 100–2).

### Hemangiomas

Hemangiomas are the most common tumors of infancy; mature lesions have been noted in 10% to 12% of 1-year-old infants. They occur sporadically, most often as single lesions. For unclear reasons, hemangiomas are more common in premature infants. The male-to-female ratio in term infants is 1:3 (Esterly, 1995).

*This chapter includes material from the previous edition, to which Nancy B. Esterly, MD, contributed.

#### Clinical Findings

Typically, hemangiomas are not clinically apparent at birth but present within the first month of life as a faint blush or area of pallor, a change known as a *precursor lesion*. Most hemangiomas grow rapidly in the first 3 to 6 months; the rate and extent of growth are impossible to predict. The clinical appearance is dictated by the depth of the tumor. Superficial lesions are cherry red and sharply circumscribed. This type of hemangioma has been referred to as a "strawberry," "capillary," "plane," or "planotuberous" hemangioma. Lesions that are confined to the deep dermis and subcutis appear bluish and dome-shaped. This subset has been referred to as "cavernous" or "nodose." Most lesions have both superficial and deep components. The added descriptors have no functional or prognostic significance, with one possible exception: The superficial component may herald residual change in skin texture, whereas the deep component may leave excess fibrofatty tissue. The growth phase usually slows after 6 months and ends by 12 months of age, followed by gradual involution. Flattening occurs by age 5 in half the cases, and by age 9 in an additional 40% (Esterly, 1995). Parents are frequently concerned about the risk of hemorrhage and should be reassured that this rarely occurs. Several other complications are possible, however, and the more serious sequelae are described next.

***Obstruction.*** A hemangioma that obstructs just one eye can pose a significant threat to visual development by limiting the visual field or compressing the globe. Obstruction of both external ear canals will impair development of hearing. A lesion encompassing the beard area may indicate upper airway involvement, which should be considered life-threatening.

***Ulceration.*** This occurs in 5% of hemangiomas (Morelli et al, 1991, 1994; Mulliken et al, 1995), most often in those located in areas of friction (skin folds, diaper area), as well as in rapidly growing or involuting lesions. Ulcerated hemangiomas are painful and at risk for secondary infection.

***Disfigurement.*** During the first year of life, the presence of a prominent hemangioma can elicit a disturbing amount of unwanted attention. Many parents require emotional support through this time. In addition to the transient disfigurement, lesions of the central face, and those with a significant superficial component, predispose the affected child to permanent scarring.

***Kasabach-Merritt Syndrome.*** This syndrome was originally described as a complication of infantile hemangioma but may in fact be associated with kaposiform hemangioendothelioma (Cooper et al, 2002). The lesion consists of a rapidly expanding vascular tumor with compression and invasion of surrounding structures as well as primary platelet trapping and resultant consumptive coagulopathy. The mortality rate is 30% to 40%.

***Central Nervous System (CNS) Anomalies.*** Large facial hemangiomas may be associated with posterior fossa malformations along with arterial anomalies/hemangiomas,

**TABLE 100–1**

**Spectrum of Congenital Cutaneous Defects**

**Vascular Defects**
Hemangiomas
Malformations: lymphatic, venous, arterial, capillary, mixed

**Hypopigmented Lesions**
Ash-leaf macules, confetti-like macules
Linear and whorled hypomelanosis
Nevus depigmentosis
Nevus anemicus
Hemangioma precursor

**Melanin-Containing Lesions**
Nevocellular nevi
Melanoma
Lentigines
Café-au-lait macules
Nevus spilus
Mongolian spots
Nevus of Ota and nevus of Ito

**Tumors of Epithelial Origin**
Epidermal (keratinocytic) nevi/sebaceous nevi-nevus unius lateris, nevus verrucosis, ichthyosis hystrix
Nevus comedonicus
Pilomatrixoma
Porokeratosis of Mibelli

**Dermal Tumors**
Connective tissue nevi: collagen, elastic tissue
Digital fibroma

**Tumors of Extracutaneous Origin**
Cutaneous mastocytosis: urticaria pigmentosa, solitary mastocytoma, diffuse cutaneous mastocytosis
Juvenile xanthogranuloma
Lipoma
Osteoma cutis
Nasal glioma
Dermoid cyst
Meningioma

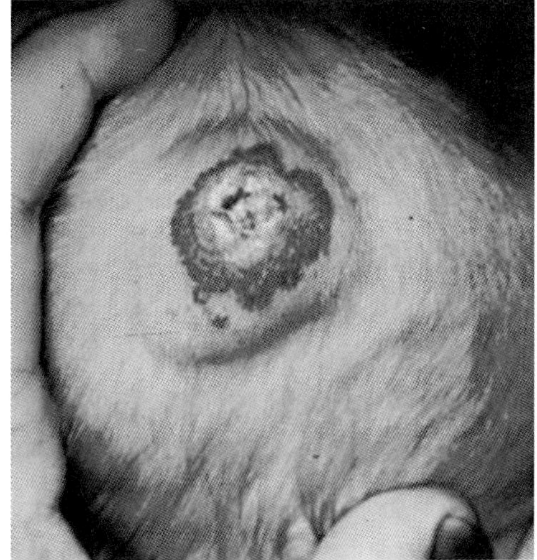

A

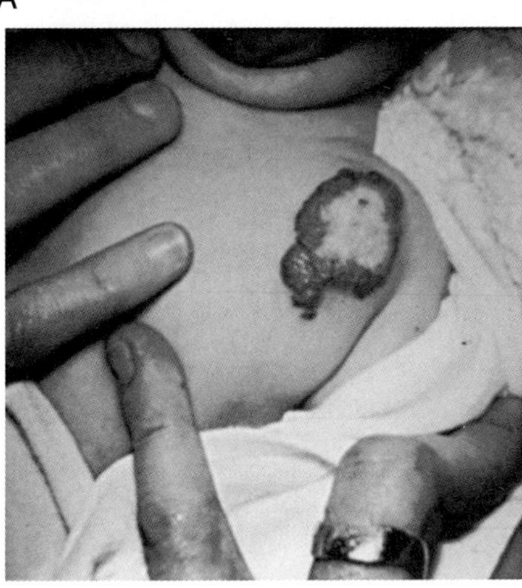

B

**FIGURE 100–1.** **A,** Hemangioma with small central ulceration on the scalp of an infant. **B,** Involuting hemangioma with central gray fibrotic area.

coarctation of the aorta and other cardiac defects, and eye abnormalities—the PHACE syndrome (Coats et al, 1999; Frieden et al, 1996; Rossi et al, 2001).

***Spinal Dysraphism.*** Sacral and lumbar hemangiomas may reveal spinal dysraphism, including tethered spinal cord and lipomyelomeningocele (Albright et al, 1989; Laurent et al, 1998; Tavafoghi et al, 1978).

***Genitourinary Abnormalities.*** Sacral hemangiomas also may be associated with imperforate anus, renal anomalies, or abnormalities of the external genitalia (Goldberg et al, 1986).

***Visceral Involvement.*** Diffuse neonatal hemangiomatosis manifests as widely scattered, small superficial hemangiomas. Infants with this pattern of cutaneous involvement may have a "benign" variant (i.e., lesions limited to skin). However, associated hemangiomatosis of the liver, gastrointestinal tract, lungs, and/or CNS can be complicated by visceral hemorrhage, hepatomegaly, high-output cardiac decompensation, or unexplained anemia or thrombocytopenia, with a significant mortality rate (Byard et al, 1991). Congestive heart failure also can occur with a large, isolated cutaneous hemangioma (Mulliken et al, 1995).

### Diagnosis

In most cases, a hemangioma can be diagnosed by its clinical appearance and pattern of evolution. A vascular lesion that is not obvious at birth, begins as a precursor noted during the first month of life, and exhibits rapid growth is undoubtedly a hemangioma. A lesion that deviates from this typical picture presents a diagnostic dilemma. Considerations in the differential diagnosis include atypical hemangioma, vascular malformation, and a nonvascular mimic. Doppler ultrasound examination is an easily performed test that may help to distinguish between a hemangioma and a high-flow malformation. Other

**TABLE 100-2**

**Characteristics of Vascular Birthmarks**

| Hemangioma | Malformation |
|---|---|
| **Clinical** | |
| Usually nothing seen at birth, 30 percent present as red macule | All present at birth; may not be evident |
| Rapid postnatal proliferation and slow involution | Commensurate growth; may expand as a result of trauma, sepsis, hormonal modulation |
| Female : male 3 : 1 | Female : male 1 : 1 |
| **Cellular** | |
| Plump endothelium, increased turnover | Flat endothelium, slow turnover |
| Increased mast cells | Normal mast cell count |
| Multilaminated basement membrane | Normal thin basement membrane |
| Capillary tubule formation in vitro | Poor endothelial growth in vitro |
| **Hematologic** | |
| Primary platelet trapping: thrombocytopenia (Kasabach-Merritt syndrome) | Primary stasis (venous); localized consumptive coagulopathy |
| **Radiologic** | |
| Angiographic findings; well-circumscribed, intense lobular-parenchymal staining with equatorial vessels | Angiographic findings: diffuse, no parenchyma<br>Low-flow: phleboliths, ectatic channels<br>High-flow: enlarged, tortuous arteries with arteriovenous shunting |
| **Skeletal** | |
| Infrequent "mass effect" on adjacent bone; hypertrophy rare | Low-flow: distortion, hypertrophy, or hypoplasia<br>High-flow: destruction, distortion, or hypertrophy |

From Mulliken JB, Young AE: Vascular Birthmarks, Hemangiomas and Malformations. Philadelphia, W. B. Saunders, 1988, p 35.

imaging modalities—magnetic resonance imaging (MRI) or angiography—may be indicated for large or obstructive lesions (e.g., ocular, upper airway) to help define the extent of involvement or associated abnormalities (Baker et al, 1993; Esterly, 1995). Skin biopsy is diagnostic for nonvascular tumors, which can mimic vascular birthmarks (e.g., pilomatrixoma, juvenile xanthogranuloma, Langerhans cell histiocytosis, infantile myofibromatosis).

### Pathogenesis

Hemangiomas in the proliferative phase are composed of syncytial aggregates of endothelial cells. These cells, like mature endothelial cells, express alkaline phosphatase, factor VIII antigen, and CD31 PECAM (platelet endothelial cell adhesion molecule), as well as Weibel-Palade bodies on electron microscopy, but $^{3}H$ labeling demonstrates active proliferation. Other histologic features that distinguish proliferating hemangiomas from malformations are the presence of multilaminate basement membranes bordering the endothelial syncytia, large numbers of mast cells (Esterly, 1995), and increased expression of other immunohistochemical markers, including proliferating cell nuclear antigen, (PCNA), vascular endothelial cell growth factor (VEGF), type IV collagenase, urokinase, and basic fibroblast growth factor (bFGF) (Takahashi et al, 1994). Elevated bFGF can be detected in urine from infants with hemangiomas, which may prove to be a useful diagnostic marker (Mulliken et al, 1995). Angiogenesis is a process that allows new blood vessel formation. It plays an important role in the growth of all vascular tumors, including hemangiomas. Identification of the basic processes that contribute to angiogenesis and effective angiogenesis inhibitors will provide insight into the pathogenesis and a more ideal therapy for hemangiomas (Morelli, 1993; Mulliken, 1991; O'Reilly et al, 1995).

It appears that hemangiomas constitute clonal expansions of endothelial cells, suggesting that these tumors are caused by somatic mutations in one or more genes regulating endothelial cell proliferation (Boye et al, 2001). Recently, it has been shown that Tie2 and its ligands angiopoietin-1 and angiopoietin-2 may be involved in the pathogenesis of hemangiomas (Yu et al, 2001).

### Treatment

Eighty percent of hemangiomas are ultimately uncomplicated, and it is impossible to predict which ones will develop problems (Mulliken et al, 1995). For a majority of lesions, the initial treatment of choice is "active nonintervention." During the phase of rapid proliferation, patients with uncomplicated hemangiomas should be examined at 2- to 4-week intervals to evaluate degree of growth and development of problems. During this phase, parents often are anxious and require ongoing, directed anticipatory guidance. A common concern is the risk of significant hemorrhage. This is rare. Minor episodes of bleeding can result from trauma and respond to short-term compression, like any superficial wound. Demonstration of before-and-after photographs of growing and involuted lesions in other children helps diminish concern. Local compression of accessible lesions (Mangus, 1973) may control growth and promote comfort. Coban dressing is a conveniently applied self-adhesive compressive wrap that easily provides compression (Kaplan and Paller, 1995).

Decades of aggressive therapy followed by suboptimal outcome from the 1940s through the 1960s were followed by a passive approach to the treatment of minimally complicated hemangiomas. The dogma has been to avoid treatment because children whose hemangiomas were allowed to involute spontaneously had less severe scarring than those subjected to cold steel excision or ionizing radiation. However, up to 20% of hemangiomas leave permanent skin changes that can be disfiguring (Enjolras and Mulliken, 1993). Psychological and social problems may result from facial or other visible deformities. Early intervention should be considered for lesions with a higher potential for complications. Such lesions include hemangiomas of the periorbital area, central face, skin folds, and hands, and those with a pattern suggestive of visceral involvement (large or multiple lesions or those encompassing the "beard area"). Newer therapeutic approaches are aimed at minimizing growth or speeding resolution without the risk of additional scarring. At present, the benefits of newer approaches to therapy outweigh the risks in many cases. Early initiation of therapy, aimed at preventing growth, is easier and probably more effective than therapy that is delayed until maximal growth has been reached. Treatment options include pulsed dye laser, corticosteroids, and α-interferon, alone or in combination.

Several small uncontrolled studies have indicated that early treatment with yellow pulsed-dye laser can prevent growth of the superficial, but not the deep, component of proliferating hemangiomas. Laser treatment of persistent hemangiomas may hasten or ensure resolution (Ashinoff and Geronemus, 1991, 1993; Barlow et al, 1996; Garden et al, 1992; Glassberg et al, 1989; Haywood et al, 2000; Poetke et al, 2000; Scheepers and Quaba, 1995; Sherwood and Tan, 1990; Waner et al, 1994; Wheeland, 1995). However, because the magnitude of growth, timing of involution, and degree of sequelae are variable and unpredictable, large, prospective, controlled studies are necessary to determine the laser's true efficacy and long-term effects. A recent prospective, randomized controlled study of 121 infants has shown that pulsed-dye laser treatment in uncomplicated hemangiomas is no better than watchful waiting (Batta et al, 2002).

Corticosteroids may be administered by topical application, intralesional injection, or enteral/parenteral dosing. Each route utilizes corticosteroid preparations of different potency and duration of action. True comparative efficacy studies would be impossible. Experience is greatest with systemic administration, considered to be the optimal regimen by some experts; the recommended regimen is oral prednisone or prednisolone, 2 to 4 mg/kg/day as a single morning dose or in divided doses (Esterly, 1995; Mulliken et al, 1995). Within 1 to 2 weeks, 30% of hemangiomas will show dramatic response; 40% will respond equivocally. In patients with slower-responding lesions, slowly tapering therapy is required through the proliferative phase. If no response is detected, the medication should be rapidly tapered after 2 weeks.

Intralesional injections may be preferred for well-localized hemangiomas, including those involving the eyelid. Colloidal suspensions of triamcinolone and dexamethasone or betamethasone in 1:1 mixtures are used. Large doses are administered, in the range of 40 mg triamcinolone plus 6 mg of betamethasone in 2 mL of suspension (Kushner, 1979). Administration of this dose to a 5-kg infant is equivalent to 20 mg/kg of prednisone given as a single dose, which may ultimately allow for a lower total systemic dose. Complications include cutaneous atrophy and skin necrosis.

The paucity of information on the treatment of hemangiomas with topical steroids suggests that this route of administration has been ineffective. However, application of newer, more potent topical preparations may prove to be beneficial (Magana et al, 1994).

Recombinant interferon alfa-2a may be an effective agent for therapy for life-threatening hemangiomas that are unresponsive to corticosteroids (Mulliken et al, 1995). Regression is not as dramatic as seen in corticosteroid-responsive lesions, making this form of therapy inadequate for vision-threatening hemangiomas; however, it is especially effective for Kasabach-Merritt syndrome. Interferon alfa-2a is administered by subcutaneous injection, in a dose in the range of 3 million units/m$^2$/day. Treatment must be continued for 6 to 10 months. Side effects include fevers of up to 39° C, reversible elevations in liver transaminases, neutropenia, and anemia (Esterly, 1995; Mulliken et al, 1995).

Angiogenesis inhibitors offer promise for more predictably effective therapy in the future. Candidates include interleukin-12 (Voest et al, 1995) and AGM-1470 (a derivative of the fungal product fumagillin) (O'Reilly et al, 1995). Interferon-α has both antitumor and antiangiogenic effects. A recent report has shown that a bFGF-overexpressing low-grade tumor can respond to interferon alfa-2b in a manner similar to that seen for life-threatening infantile hemangiomas, most likely secondary to inhibition of bFGF-mediated tumor angiogenesis by interferon alfa-2b. Measurement of urinary bFGF levels may provide an objective method for monitoring treatment response and guiding interferon-α dosage (Marler et al, 2002).

Ulceration is a therapeutic challenge that may be treated initially with the appropriate occlusive dressing. The choice of dressing and frequency of changes are dictated by the amount of exudate produced. Coban dressing is ideally suited to secure dressings over hemangiomas on the extremities (Kaplan and Paller, 1995). For sites that are difficult to dress, frequent, liberal application of zinc oxide paste is effective. To inspect the skin, zinc oxide is easily removed with mineral oil. Healing, pain relief, and involutional effects of a polyurethane film in eight cases with ulcerative hemangiomas have been reported (Oranje et al, 2000). Agents for pain control should be prescribed. Alternating doses of acetaminophen and ibuprofen usually are sufficient, but overuse of the latter may increase the risk of bleeding and cause pain from gastrointestinal upset that can be difficult to distinguish from the pain associated with ulceration. A high index of suspicion should be maintained for secondary infection, with a low threshold for use of either topical or systemic antibiotic therapy. If conservative therapy is unsuccessful, yellow light laser may relieve pain and speed reepithelialization (Achauer and Vander Kam, 1991; Morelli et al, 1991, 1994). The ulcers will heal but will inevitably leave scars.

A hemangioma that interferes with the visual axis should be treated aggressively. Evaluation by an experienced pediatric ophthalmologist is recommended. A hemangioma that limits the visual field but does not distort the globe may be treated by patching the contralateral eye. More complicated lesions may be treated initially with corticosteroids: topical, enterally administered, or intralesional. The intralesional route of administration carries the risk of embolic occlusion of the retinal arteries. This tragic adverse effect can occur ipsilaterally, contralaterally, or bilaterally (Brown et al, 1972; Fost and Esterly, 1968; Zuniga et al, 1987) (Fig. 100–2). Surgical excision should be considered for vision-threatening hemangiomas that fail to respond to corticosteroids (Mulliken et al, 1995; Walker et al, 1994).

There is no uniformly successful therapy for seriously complicated or life-threatening hemangiomas. Reported treatment options include high-dose corticosteroids, aspirin, dipyridamole, interferon-α, cold steel excision, sclerotherapy, arterial embolization, cyclophosphamide, bleomycin, and vincristine (Enjolras et al, 1990; Esterly, 1995; Mulliken et al, 1995; Payarols et al, 1995; Sarihan

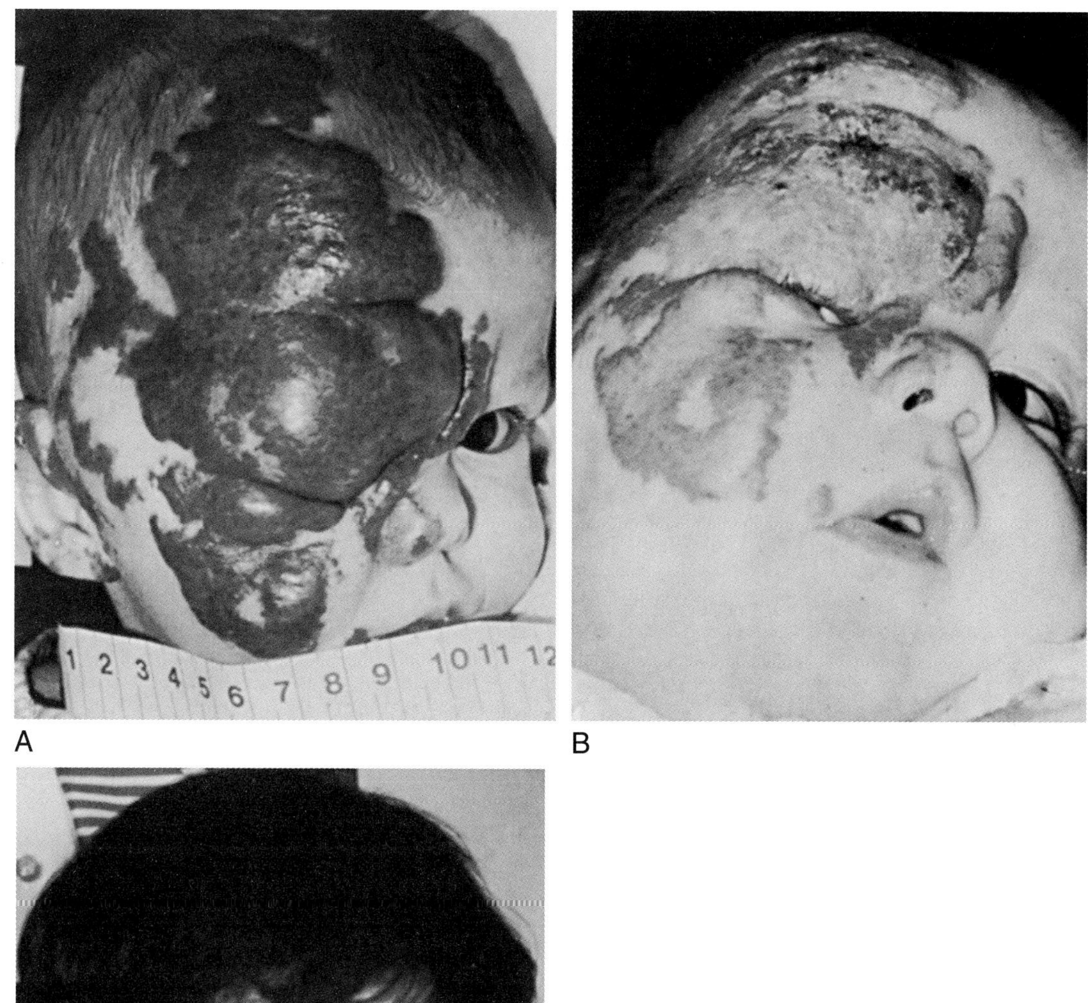


**FIGURE 100–2.** **A,** A flat hemangioma was noted at birth; by 3 weeks of age, the lesion had expanded, as shown. **B,** After 11 weeks of prednisone (20 mg/day), the lesion had regressed. **C,** Nearly complete regression is evident by age 4 years. The patient was a normally intelligent child whose only residual problem was strabismus.

et al, 1997). All carry significant risks. The use of ionizing radiation is justified for alarming-looking hemangiomas that have been unresponsive to other therapeutic modalities and are inoperable.

## Vascular Malformations

Vascular malformations may be indistinguishable from hemangiomas by clinical and light microscopic examination; however, they are biologically distinct lesions.

### Clinical Findings

Malformations are true structural anomalies, composed of one or more types of vessels—capillaries, veins, arteries, and/or lymphatics. Unlike hemangiomas, they are always present at birth. They affect males and females equally. Growth is commensurate with the child's growth, although the lesion may expand as a result of local thrombosis or inflammation. Primary platelet trapping with consumptive coagulopathy (e.g., Kasabach-Merritt syndrome) does not occur. Local skeletal or soft tissue destruction or hypertrophy is common. Spontaneous resolution is not expected except in one specific malformation, the salmon patch. Vascular malformations occur either as isolated cutaneous defects or in association with a variety of well-defined syndromes. The more common variations are described next.

***Salmon Patch.*** The glabellar salmon patch (macular stain, nevus simplex), also known as an "angel's kiss," is a bilaterally symmetrical superficial capillary defect. It is the most common vascular malformation and the only one that almost always fades spontaneously. A similar lesion in the nuchal area, the "stork bite," usually is persistent. Large lesions may also involve the eyelids and alae nasi. Prominent glabellar salmon patches are associated with dysmorphic syndromes including Beckwith-Wiedemann syndrome and fetal alcohol syndrome (Burns et al, 1991).

***Nevus Flammeus (Port-Wine Stain).*** This asymmetrical postcapillary venule malformation occurs in 0.3% of neonates. A majority are isolated cutaneous lesions. At birth they are pink, macular, and blanchable. With time, most lesions darken; papulonodular surface change and ipsilateral soft tissue or even bone hypertrophy may occur. Facial nevus flammeus is a distribution that includes the forehead or upper eyelid and may be associated with buphthalmos or glaucoma. Emergent ophthalmologic examination is indicated for affected infants.

*Sturge-Weber syndrome* (SWS) is a triad of facial nevus flammeus, leptomeningeal vascular malformation, and glaucoma that occurs sporadically. The classic finding of double-contoured (tram-line) calcifications on a skull film is not seen during infancy; this sign develops during childhood. CNS lesions are most reliably detected by MRI after 6 months of age. SWS occurs in less than 30% of infants with facial port-wine stains; the risk is increased in infants with more extensive lesions (Tallman et al, 1991). The degree of CNS involvement is variable in SWS, ranging from subclinical lesions to intractable seizures and intellectual impairment. Two national organizations have been established to serve the needs of patients and their families:

National Vascular Malformations Foundation, Inc., 8320 Nightingale, Dearborn Heights, MI 48127

The Sturge-Weber Foundation, P.O. Box 460931, Aurora, CO 80046

***Arterial/Lymph/Venous Malformation.*** This category includes a spectrum of isolated cutaneous vascular anomalies that have been given a variety of clinically descriptive names. These multifarious names do not offer insight into pathogenesis or natural history, and some experts advocate for a more simple classification based on the type of anomalous vessel (Mulliken and Young, 1988). Thus, categories would include pure lymphangiomas (e.g., "cystic hygroma," lymphangioma circumscriptum), arteriovenous malformations, and venous malformations.

These lesions do not resolve spontaneously. Corticosteroid therapy is not beneficial. Complications are related to the flow rate and extent of the lesion. Localized thrombosis and phlebitis occur in low-flow lesions; high-flow lesions can cause significant bleeding, destructive interosseous changes, and high-output cardiac failure (Mulliken and Young, 1988).

***Cutis Marmorata Telangiectatica Congenita.*** Cutis marmorata telangiectatica congenita (CMTC) is a distinct, reticulated capillary-venous malformation. CMTC can occur as a single isolated patch or involve an extensive area. With time, associated atrophy and ulceration may occur. The larger lesions may have ipsilateral hypertrophy or hypotrophy of the affected limb.

***Klippel-Trénaunay and Parkes Weber Syndromes.*** These are clinically defined, sporadic conditions consisting of extensive nevus flammeus, most often occurring unilaterally on the lower extremity, associated with venous varicosities and progressive ipsilateral limb hypertrophy. Some authors differentiate Parkes Weber syndrome, which also includes an arteriovenous fistula and its associated constellation of complications, as a discrete entity.

***Cobb Syndrome.*** This is a sporadic condition consisting of a posterior truncal nevus flammeus overlying a vascular abnormality that involves the spinal cord.

***Bonnet-Dechaume-Blanc Syndrome.*** This condition (also known as *Wyburn-Mason syndrome*) consists of a facial port-wine stain overlying a retinal and intracranial arteriovenous malformation. The retinal lesion appears as dilated, tortuous retinal vessels on routine ophthalmoscopy. Cranial bruit, mild proptosis, and conjunctival hyperemia may be present.

***Blue Rubber Bleb Nevus Syndrome.*** This condition, inherited as an autosomal dominant trait, is characterized by venous malformations of the skin and gastrointestinal tract associated with bleeding and iron deficiency anemia. Numerous lesions may be present at birth. They are blue macules or nodules that range in size from 1 mm to several centimeters, resembling the "blueberry muffin" lesions of congenital TORCH (*t*oxoplasmosis, *o*ther infections, *r*ubella, *c*ytomegalovirus, *h*erpes simplex) infection, but are easily compressible. They may be tender to palpation or surmounted by droplets of sweat.

***Maffuci Syndrome.*** This sporadic condition consists of mixed vascular malformations and characteristic enchondromas. In 25% of the cases, manifestations are present at birth or in early infancy.

***Bannayan-Riley-Ruvalcaba Syndrome.*** The abnormalities included in this category are vascular malformations, macrocephaly, and lipomas. In combination with other features, separate conditions have been described: Bannayan-Zonana, Riley-Smith, and Ruvalcaba-Myhre-Smith syndromes. The usual inheritance pattern is autosomal dominant.

***Lymphedema.*** *Lymphedema* is a term used to describe diffuse soft tissue swelling characterized by firm, pitting edema. Lymphedema can occur in the setting of anomalous lymphatic drainage. Congenital variants have been reported. Females are affected more frequently than males. The lower limbs are the most commonly affected sites, but other sites also may be involved, and rarely, chylothorax or ascites may be present. *Milroy disease* is an autosomal dominant condition that manifests with progressive lymphedema of the lower extremities. Lymphedema of the extremities occurs in Turner (XO) syndrome.

### Treatment

Treatment for an uncomplicated capillary malformation is aimed at minimizing disfigurement. With time, these lesions thicken and develop irregular surface changes, often with friable nodules. In 1986, the yellow-light pulsed-dye laser was approved by the Food and Drug Administration (FDA) for the treatment of nevus flammeus, as early as the neonatal period. The copper vapor laser and the argon-pumped tunable dye laser also are yellow light lasers. Most of the published data on laser treatment of port-wine stains in children is from studies utilizing the pulsed-dye laser. Children require an average of four or five pulsed-dye laser treatments for maximal lightening. The best results have been seen in children younger than 4 years of age. In this age group, 20% can expect 95% clearing (Goldman et al, 1993). Pulsed-dye laser therapy is less effective for facial port-wine stains that are close to midline or those on the extremities (Garden and Bakus, 1993; Renfro and Geronemus, 1993). A recent study comparing the effects of the pulsed-dye laser with those of the argon-pumped dye laser for the treatment of port-wine stains has shown that the pulsed-dye laser is clinically superior to the argon-pumped dye laser (Edstrom et al, 2002). Laser therapy can yield remarkable improvement for many port-wine stains, minimizing the emotional pain that accompanies facial disfigurement. Unfortunately, none of the currently available lasers is capable of permanently erasing port-wine stains in a majority of patients. Attempts to optimize laser treatment efficacy include using the pulsed-dye laser at higher fluences in conjunction with cryogen spray cooling, the effects of which are still unclear (Kelly et al, 2002). The range of skin conditions that may benefit from yellow-light laser therapy is expanding rapidly to include a variety of skin lesions with vascular components.

## HYPOPIGMENTED LESIONS

Localized areas of hypopigmentation on the skin of the newborn infant may be isolated phenomena, or they may be markers of extracutaneous abnormalities. The degree of hypopigmentation and the distribution of the defect help distinguish among the different conditions.

### Definition

A distinction must first be made between complete *depigmentation* and *hypopigmentation*. A depigmenting condition produces pure white lesions that are devoid of normal melanocytes. Even in fair-skinned infants, the lesions can be easily seen in ordinary daylight. This group of disorders includes tyrosinase-negative albinism and piebaldism, as well as vitiligo, which is rarely seen in infancy. A hypopigmented lesion often is subtly lighter in color than the surrounding skin. Histologic examination reveals a normal number of melanocytes. In fair-skinned children, these lesions may require Wood's lamp illumination to become obvious. This group includes anomalies with a deficient amount of either of the skin's pigments: melanin or hemoglobin. The ash-leaf macules and "confetti-like" lesions of tuberous sclerosis (Fig. 100–3), the linear and whorled patterning associated with hypomelanosis of Ito (Fig. 100–4A), and simple nevus depigmentosus are hypomelanotic lesions (see Fig. 100–4B). Nevus anemicus and hemangioma precursors are areas of pallor that result from diminished superficial blood flow.

### Ash-Leaf Macules

Ash-leaf macules are small oval areas of hypopigmentation, named for their similarity in size and shape to a leaflet from a European mountain ash tree. They are one of the few congenital markers for infants with tuberous sclerosis. Tuberous sclerosis complex (TSC) is a disorder of autosomal dominant inheritance with variable clinical manifestations characterized by the development of benign and malignant tumors in a variety of tissues: skin, CNS, and kidney. Serious complications of tuberous sclerosis include hamartomas of the lung and kidney and congenital rhabdomyomas of the heart. The diagnosis is currently made by meeting a set of diagnostic criteria, but a majority of manifestations are not present in infancy (Gomez, 1991; Janniger and Schwartz, 1993; Zvulunov and Esterly, 1995). Abnormalities at two different genetic loci have been identified in kindreds with TSC (Wienecke et al, 1995). The two genetic loci are *TSC1* on chromosome 9q and *TSC2* on chromosome 16p, and the gene products are hamartin and tuberin, respectively. Both hamartin and tuberin are expressed in neurons and astrocytes, where they physically interact (Gutmann et al, 2000).

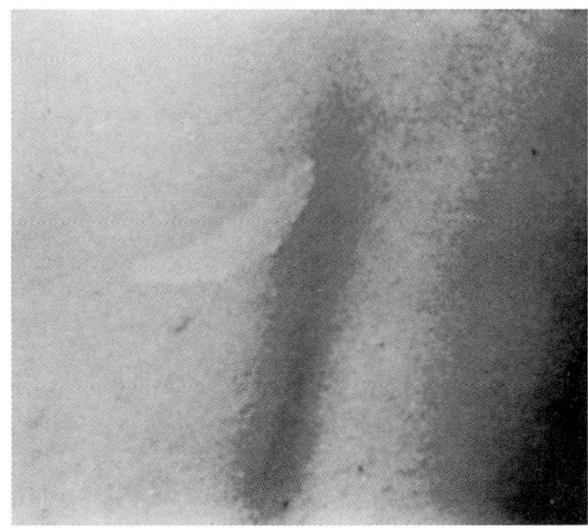

**FIGURE 100–3.** White ash-leaf macule on the back of a patient with tuberous sclerosis.

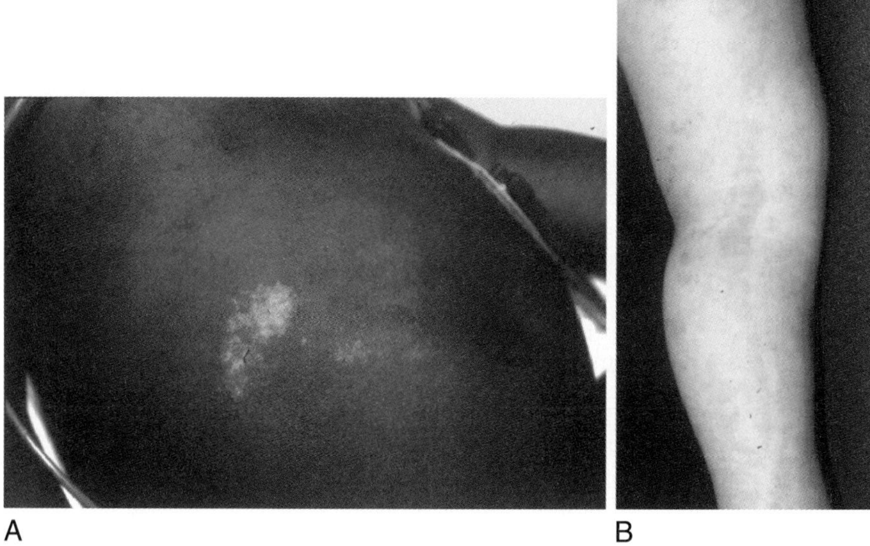


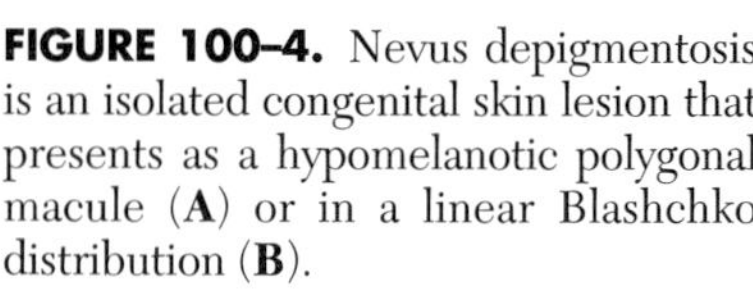
**FIGURE 100–4.** Nevus depigmentosis is an isolated congenital skin lesion that presents as a hypomelanotic polygonal macule (**A**) or in a linear Blashchko distribution (**B**).

### Hypomelanosis of Ito

The term *hypomelanosis of Ito* has been used as a diagnosis for a genetic disorder marked by a striking linear and whorled pattern of cutaneous pigment change oriented along the lines of Blaschko. Affected persons may have areas that are hyperpigmented or hypopigmented, or both. The pattern may be congenital or become apparent after birth.

This condition is a form of genetic mosaicism. In a subset of affected persons, karyotype abnormalities are demonstrable in tissue from affected sites. In a majority of reported cases, the patients have extracutaneous abnormalities (CNS, ocular, cardiac, and skeletal) (Alvarez et al, 1993; Dereser-Dennl et al, 2000; Devriendt et al, 1998; Tunca et al, 2000). Patterned pigment change confined to skin probably is a more common occurrence. For persons so affected, the term *linear and whorled nevoid melanosis* may be more appropriate. Chromosomal analysis from separate tissues (e.g., blood and skin) is indicated for children with extensive skin lesions or evidence of extracutaneous involvement (Sybert, 1994).

## MELANIN-CONTAINING LESIONS

Brown lesions usually reflect an increased number of melanocytic cells or an excess of melanin. Brown coloration also can be associated with a thickened epidermis. It may be difficult to distinguish among the lesions in this category without histopathologic examination. A majority of congenital brown lesions are isolated and benign, but it is important to recognize those that are syndrome-associated or potentially life-threatening (see Chapter 96 for a differential diagnosis).

In general, skin biopsy of a congenital pigmented lesion can be postponed until after the neonatal period. The one exception is a nodular lesion suggestive of melanoma.

### Nevocellular Nevi

The category of nevocellular nevi includes congenital or acquired nevomelanocytic neoplasms. Nevomelanocytes are dendritic cells of neural crest origin. Nevocellular nevi traditionally have been categorized by the histologic position of the tumor nests within the skin. *Junctional nevi* are the most superficial, located at the junction between the epidermis and dermis. These lesions appear clinically as macules. *Intradermal nevi* are located deep to the dermoepidermal junction and are usually papular. *"Blue" nevi* are a variant located in the deep dermis, made up of cells that have elongated, neural features. *Compound nevi* have both junctional and dermal nests of nevomelanocytes.

Melanocytic nevi can be further divided into categories based on size: small (less than 1.5 cm in greatest diameter), large (2 to 20 cm), and giant (greater than 20 cm in diameter, or 120 $cm^2$ surface area) (Zitelli et al, 1984); and time of onset: congenital, early-onset (before the age of 2 years), and acquired. Diagnostic histologic features have been described for congenital and acquired lesions, but these features may be found in both types.

Large, multiple, or congenital melanocytic nevi have been reported in association with several syndromes (Marghoob et al, 1993) (Table 100–3).

### Congenital Nevocellular Nevi

Congenital nevocytic nevi are common and generally of little or no consequence. However, the infrequent but devastating association with malignant melanoma has made management a controversial issue.

Small congenital nevi measure less than 1.5 cm in diameter at birth (Fig. 100–5). Truly congenital lesions are present in 1% of white infants and in 2% to 3% of African-American infants surveyed in the nursery (Osburn et al, 1987). There is a risk of malignancy associated with small nevi, but it may never be well defined. A distinct

**TABLE 100–3**

**Syndromes Associated with Melanocytic Nevi**

| Associated with: | Other Key Features |
|---|---|
| **Congenital Nevi** | |
| Carney syndrome (including LAMB and NAME syndromes) | Cardiac and cutaneous myxomas, endocrine abnormalities |
| Epidermal (linear sebaceous) nevus syndrome | Linear epidermal/sebaceous nevi, central nervous system and musculoskeletal defects |
| Neurocutaneous melanosis | Leptomeningeal melanocytosis and obstructive hydrocephalus |
| Neurofibromatosis type I | Cutaneous and plexiform neurofibromas, café-au-lait spots, Lisch nodules |
| Premature aging syndrome | Premature aging, short stature, bird-like facies, deafness |
| Occult spinal dysraphism/ tethered cord | Spinal cord abnormalities, lipomas, vascular malformations |
| Malformations associated with congenital melanocytic nevi | |
| **Acquired Nevi** | |
| Dysplastic nevus (atypical mole) syndrome | Increased incidence of cutaneous melanoma |
| Langer-Giedion syndrome | Distinctive facies, cone-shaped epiphyses, multiple exostoses |
| **Congenital and/or Acquired Nevi** | |
| EEC syndrome | Ectrodactyly, ectodermal dysplasia, cleft lip/palate, ocular abnormalities |
| Goeminne syndrome | Muscular torticollis, spontaneous keloids, genitourinary abnormalities |
| Kuskokwim syndrome | Skeletal abnormalities, joint contractures, muscle atrophy/hypertrophy |
| Noonan syndrome | Webbed neck, heart defects, multiple other anomalies |
| Turner syndrome | Webbed neck, heart defects, multiple other anomalies, X-chromosome defect |
| Tricho-odonto-onychial dysplasia | Hypotrichosis, enamel defects, nail dystrophy |

From Marghoob AA, Orlo SJ, Kopf AW: Syndromes associated with melanocytic nevi. J Am Acad Dermatol 29:373-388, 1993.

subset of melanocytic nevi in children, "early-onset nevi," has recently been recognized. These lesions are not necessarily congenital, appearing during the first 2 years of life. Early-onset nevi have been observed in 25% of children specifically examined for them. Twenty percent to 50% of melanomas arising in children and young adults may be associated with this type of nevus (Williams, 1993; Williams and Pennella, 1994). The frequency of congenital melanocytic nevi (CMN) is paradoxically increased in African-Americans, who have a much lower risk of melanoma (Shpall et al, 1994). The risk of melanoma associated with these very common pigmented skin lesions must be well below that in children with giant congenital nevi and possibly no higher than the 1% lifetime risk of malignant melanoma in the general white population. A decision about surgical removal of these lesions must be made on a case-by-case basis.

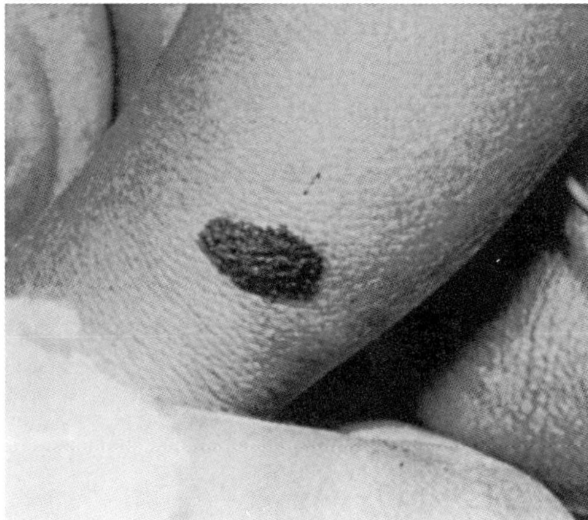

**FIGURE 100–5.** Dark brown irregular congenital nevus on the limb of an infant.

Large, giant or "garment" congenital nevi measure at least 20 cm or cover an entire body part (Fig. 100–6). These lesions are rare, occurring in less than 1 in 20,000 neonates, and have a much greater potential for malignant degeneration. The cumulative risk of malignancy is estimated to be 2% to 15% over a lifetime, with a bimodal pattern of occurrence, either before age 3 or after puberty (Kuflik and Janniger, 1994; Williams and Pennella, 1994).

Conservative management of large congenital nevi by surveillance alone is complicated by the presence of features that strongly suggest melanoma. Most of these nevi have an irregular surface appearance from birth and are variably thickened, hairy, verrucous, or nodular. Smaller, widely scattered "satellite lesions" are almost always present. Extracutaneous lesions also have been detected in several sites, including the meninges, lymph nodes, and placental villi. Often, these nevi have atypical histologic features as well. For children who develop malignant melanoma within a giant nevus, the prognosis is very poor. However, many of the lesions with an alarming appearance from birth do not exhibit malignant behavior or have widespread metastases, or cause death. In fact, congenital melanoma is very rare and is associated with congenital nevi in less than 50% of reported cases (Williams and Pennella, 1994).

The management of CMN remains controversial, with equal numbers of advocates for and against prophylactic excision. Newly published data question the rationale for routine excision. Nevertheless, case reports of melanoma arising in smaller CMN, as early as 6 months of age, continue to dramatize the issue (Ceballos et al, 1995; De Raeve et al, 1993; Ozturkcan et al, 1994). To date, the incidence of melanoma arising in small CMN remains unclear. A 3- to 21-fold increased relative risk for malignant transformation in both small and medium-sized lesions later in life has been reported, depending on the method of study (Richardson et al, 2002).

The least controversial recommendation has been for surgical excision of large or multiple CMN during

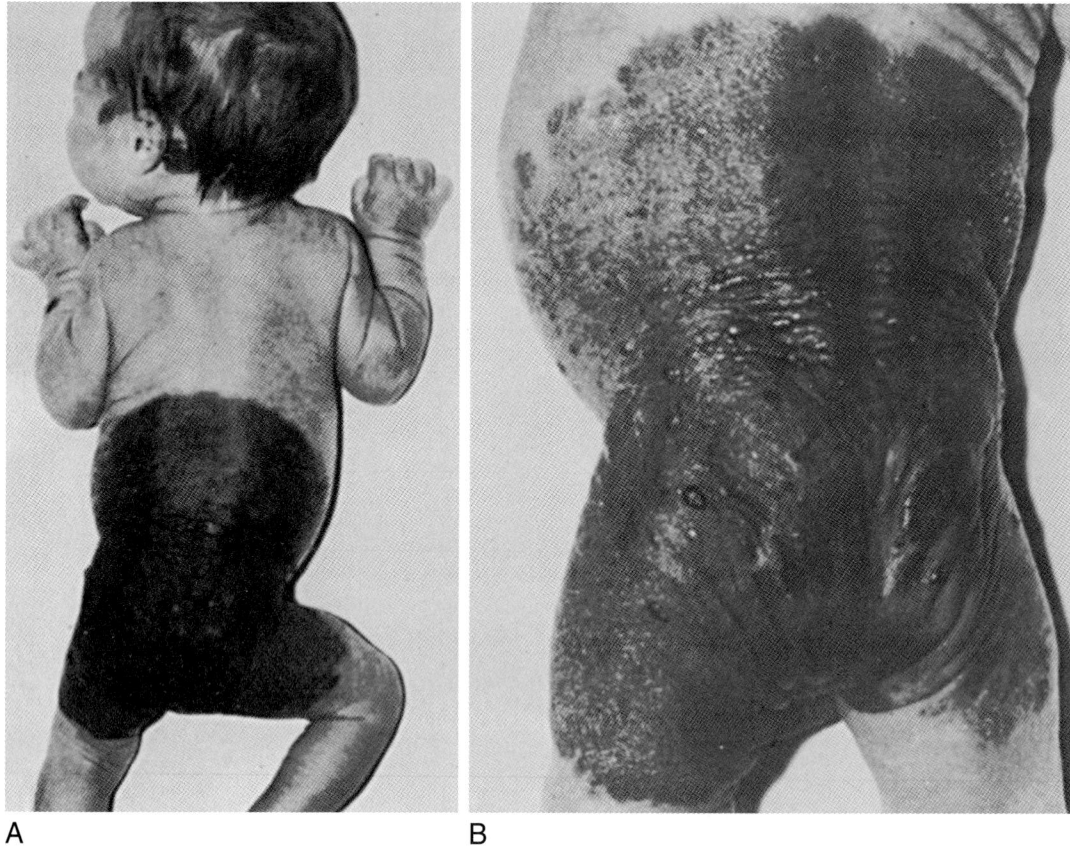


**FIGURE 100–6.** **A,** Newborn infant with large black nevus covering the "bathing trunk area." **B,** The closer view permits visualization of the nodular surface typical of giant nevi.

infancy (Casson and Colen, 1993). However, surgical removal is never an easy option. Multiple procedures usually are required, with the attendant high risks of significant morbidity, sometimes yielding results that are more disfiguring than the birthmark (Figs. 100–7 and 100–8). Newer techniques performed in early childhood, such as tissue expansion (Vergnes et al, 1993) and partial-thickness resection (Sandsmark et al, 1993), may improve the aesthetic outcome. The efficacy of this approach in the prevention of malignancy has never been documented.

A Congenital Nevocytic Nevus Registry was established at the New York University Medical Center in 1978 to prospectively study the natural history of giant CMN (Gari et al, 1988; Kopf et al, 1979). To participate by mail, clinicians should contact the Skin and Cancer Unit, Department of Dermatology, New York University Medical Center, 550 First Ave., New York, NY 10016; telephone: (212) 340-5260.

Families with an affected child may benefit from information provided by the Nevus Network, a national support group founded by Dr. Bari Joan Bett, a physician with a giant congenital nevus. To receive the organization's newsletter, families should contact the Network, c/o Bari Joan Bett, MD, 1400 S. Joyce St. #C1201, Arlington, VA 22202; telephone: (703) 920-2349 or (405) 377-3403.

Neurocutaneous melanosis (NCM) is a congenital syndrome characterized by pigment cell tumors of the leptomeninges in patients with large or multiple (at least three) CMN of the head, neck, or posterior midline (Kadonaga and Frieden, 1991). Symptomatic NCM manifests with signs or symptoms of increased intracranial pressure and carries a poor prognosis (Sandsmark et al, 1994;

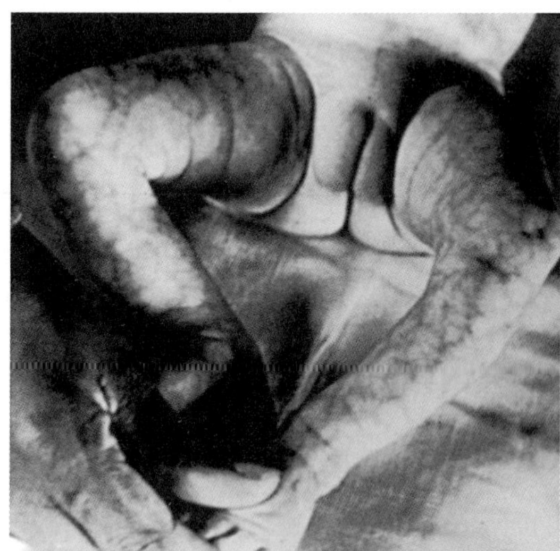

**FIGURE 100–7.** Cutis marmorata telangiectatica congenita. Note the striking network of dilated vessels, most distinct over the extremities. *(From Humphries JM: J Pediatr 40:486, 1952.)*

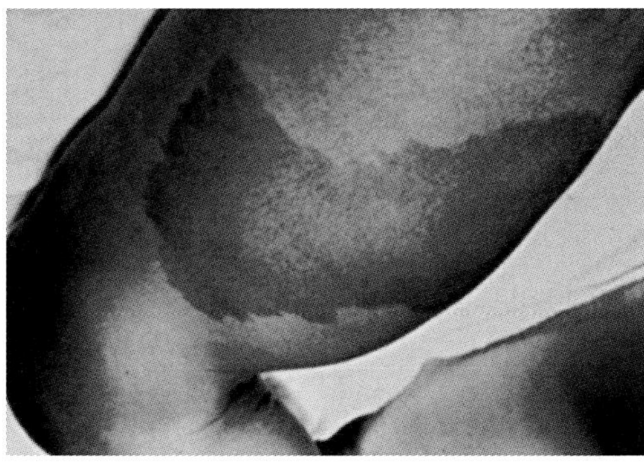

**FIGURE 100–8.** Large café-au-lait spot on the trunk of a newborn infant.

Frieden et al, 1994). MRI can aid in the diagnosis of NCM (Barkovich et al, 1994). Although initial reports emphasized thickening of the leptomeninges, the most common MRI sign of NCM is actually spin-lattice (T1) nuclear magnetic relaxation time in the parenchyma of the cerebellum or anterior temporal lobes (sometimes accompanied by spin-spin [T2] relaxation time). Radiologic identification of malignant degeneration is difficult. Roughly half of asymptomatic infants and children with giant CMN have evidence of NCM on MRI (Frieden et al, 1994), a finding suggesting that numerous and extensive operations to remove the cutaneous lesion may not be justified in these patients.

Other issues have been raised that challenge the interpretation of signs that have been accepted as ominous. The risk of melanoma in early infancy may have been overestimated by misinterpretation of the histologic findings and extent of the lesions. Neither cellular atypia nor widespread involvement, including lymph nodes and placenta, proves malignancy (Carroll et al, 1994; Hara, 1993). Attempts to further define the risk of malignant degeneration in these lesions have not been insightful (Barnhill et al, 1994; Heimann et al, 1993).

## Lentigines

Lentigines are small tan-to-dark brown macules that most commonly appear sporadically in adulthood. They are distinguished from other pigmented lesions by histologic examination that reveals elongated rete ridges, an increased number of singly dispersed melanocytes along the basal layer, and increased melanization of the basal keratinocytes. Multiple or congenital lentigines are features of several syndromes.

***Carney Syndrome (Including NAME and LAMB).*** Carney syndrome and the related phenotypes designated NAME and LAMB share the features of *a*trial *m*yxoma and pigmented skin lesions. NAME includes *n*evi and *e*phelides, while LAMB includes *l*entigines and *b*lue nevi. Pigmented lesions are present at birth.

***LEOPARD Syndrome.*** This is an autosomal dominant disorder that includes multiple *l*entigines, *e*lectrocardiographic defects, *o*cular hypertelorism, *p*ulmonic stenosis, *a*bnormal genitalia, growth *r*etardation/restriction, and sensorineural *d*eafness. Skin lesions do not appear until after the first year of life.

***Peutz-Jeghers Syndrome.*** This disorder of autosomal dominant inheritance includes mucocutaneous pigmented macules and intestinal polyposis. The pigmented lesions may be congenital and usually appear on the lips, buccal and gingival mucosae, and dorsa of the fingers and toes.

## Café-au-Lait Macules

Café-au-lait macules (CALMs) are light brown macules that vary in size, ranging from several millimeters to several centimeters in diameter. They cannot always be distinguished from nevocellular nevi on clinical grounds, but histologic examination is diagnostic, showing increased melanin within the basal keratinocytes, without melanocyte proliferation. CALMs are present in 2% of white infants and in up to 12% of African-American infants. Large or multiple CALMs in the neonatal period may be an isolated finding but should alert the physician to the possibility of an associated syndrome.

## Neurofibromatosis

Neurofibromatosis (NF) is a group of variable multisystem disorders that includes cutaneous neurofibromas and multiple CALMs. A classification that includes eight subtypes has been defined (Riccardi, 1983). The great majority of patients with NF have subtype 1 (NF-1), or von Recklinghausen disease. NF-1 is a relatively common autosomal dominant disorder with a high rate of new mutation, occurring in 1 in 3500 people. The diagnosis has traditionally been made by fulfilling a set of diagnostic criteria; the presence of six or more CALMs is the most common manifestation, occurring before age 6 years in 99% of affected persons (Zvulunov and Esterly, 1995). CALMs may be present at birth but often arise and grow during childhood. Other diagnostic cutaneous findings are axillary or inguinal freckling (Crowe sign) and cutaneous neurofibromas, which may be present at birth. Bony dysplasias (sphenoid wing dysplasia, pretibial pseudarthrosis) also can be detected at birth in a minority of patients. Symptomatic CNS involvement (developmental delay, learning disabilities, seizures) occurs in about one third of patients with NF-1. The most ominous complication of NF-1 is the development of malignant tumors (neurosarcoma, pheochromocytoma,

**TABLE 100–4**

**Syndromes that Feature Café au Lait Macules**

| | |
|---|---|
| Neurofibromatosis (NFI, II) | Turner syndrome |
| Albright syndrome | Noonan syndrome |
| Watson syndrome | Ataxia-telangiectasis |
| Ruvalcaba-Myhre-Smith syndrome | Tuberous sclerosis |
| | Basal-cell nevus syndrome |
| Bloom syndrome | Hunter syndrome |
| Russell-Silver syndrome | Gaucher syndrome |

and juvenile chronic myelogenous leukemia) (Zvulunov and Esterly, 1995). The risk of leukemia is highest among children with both NF-1 and cutaneous juvenile xanthogranuloma (see later).

The genetic defects for NF-1 have been localized to chromosome 17q11;2. Most mutations occur on the paternally derived chromosome. "Sporadic" cases may be the result of paternal transmission from a mosaic mutation of a fraction of spermatozoa from a clinically normal father (Lazaro et al, 1994). A portion of the *NF1* gene has homology with mammalian genes that code for guanosine triphosphate–activating proteins (GAPs). GAPs function to regulate cell proliferation. Therefore, a functional mutation of the *NF1* gene would result in unsuppressed cellular proliferation (i.e., tumorigenesis). Prenatal diagnosis is now available for affected families by linkage analysis (Zvulunov and Esterly, 1995). Affected families should be advised to contact the National Neurofibromatosis Foundation, 141 Fifth Ave., Suite 7-S, New York, NY 10010; telephone: (800) 323-7938 or (212) 344-6633.

Type 2 neurofibromatosis (NF-2) is an autosomal dominant disorder with an incidence of about 1/40,000. It is characterized by bilateral acoustic neuromas. CALMs are not as prominent or numerous as in NF-1, occurring in less than 40% of affected persons. The gene defect has been localized to chromosome 22q11-q13 (Zvulunov and Esterly, 1995). The deduced gene product has homology with proteins at the plasma membrane and cytoskeleton interface, a previously unknown site of action of tumor suppressor genes in humans (Rouleau et al, 1993).

### McCune-Albright Syndrome

McCune-Albright syndrome (MAS) is a sporadic disease characterized by polyostotic fibrous dysplasia, sexual precocity and other hyper functional endocrinopathies, and large café-au-lait spots (Schwindinger et al, 1992; Shenker et al, 1993). In contrast with the café-au-lait spots seen in NF-1, those in this syndrome may be unilateral with irregular borders, in a distribution that suggests the lines of Blashchko and genetic mosaicism (Rieger et al, 1994). Affected tissues from patients with MAS have been found to harbor mutations of the gene that encodes the stimulatory G protein of adenylyl cyclase (Schwindinger et al, 1992; Shenker et al, 1993).

### Nevus Spilus

Nevus spilus (speckled lentiginous nevus) is a hyperpigmented lesion that consists of focal proliferation of melanocytes along the basal layer of the epidermis (the dark spots) within a café-au-lait spot. It may be disfiguring but has no other associated abnormalities.

### Blue-Gray Macule of Infancy

More than 90% of African-American infants, 81% of Asians, and 10% of whites (Pratt, 1953) are born with blue-gray macule of infancy, formerly called *mongolian spot*. These are brown, gray, or blue macules, most commonly located on the lumbosacral area, but they can occur anywhere. Mongolian spots may be single or multiple and vary in size from a few millimeters to several centimeters in diameter. They often fade within the first few years of life. Extensive lesions have been mistakenly attributed to abuse. Histologically, blue-gray macule of infancy is a collection of spindle-shaped melanocytes located deep in the dermis. Malignant change has never been reported.

### Nevus of Ota/Ito

Nevus of Ota is a unilateral blue or gray discoloration involving the orbital and zygomatic areas, including the sclera and fundus. It is a sporadic condition, but it occurs with the highest frequency in Asians, affecting up to 1% of persons in Japan (Kopf and Weidman, 1962). The discoloration is detected at birth in 60% of cases. Glaucoma is a frequent complication. A similar lesion, located in the deltotrapezius area, is called *nevus of Ito*. Histologically, these lesions cannot be distinguished from mongolian spots. However, spontaneous resolution is not common, and association with malignant melanoma has been reported. Successful treatment has been achieved with Q-switched ruby and Q-switched yttrium-aluminum-garnet (YAG) laser surgery.

## TUMORS OF EPITHELIAL ORIGIN

### Epidermal Nevus/Nevus Sebaceus

Epidermal nevus may manifest in the newborn period as a smooth hyperpigmented patch or rough, skin-colored plaque most often on the trunk or extremities, frequently oriented along the lines of Blashchko. With time, epidermal nevi may enlarge; most become verrucous. Nevus sebaceus has a yellow hue, occurs most often on the head, and may be nodular at birth and again after puberty, flattening during childhood. A variety of neoplasms, both benign and malignant, including basal cell carcinoma, develop in up to 15% of patients with sebaceous nevi. Development of neoplasms rarely occurs before puberty.

Like other mosaic disorders, epidermal and sebaceous nevi are believed to be localized manifestations of somatic genetic mutations that would be lethal if fully expressed. A subset of patients with epidermal nevi are genetic mosaics for an autosomal dominant form of ichthyosis, called *epidermolytic hyperkeratosis* (or bullous ichthyosiform erythroderma). These persons may be at risk for having offspring with total body involvement. The striking appearance of epidermal nevi has inspired descriptive nomenclature. *Nevus verrucosus* is a solitary plaque. *Nevus unius lateris* (Fig. 100–9) is an extensive linear lesion that is unilateral, following the lines of Blashchko. Both keratinocytic and sebaceous components may occur in the same patient, the former more commonly involving the trunk and extremities and the latter more often involving the head and neck. The term *ichthyosis hystrix* refers to extensive, bilateral involvement with epidermal nevus.

Skin biopsy will rule out other conditions, distinguish between epidermal nevus and nevus sebaceus, and detect

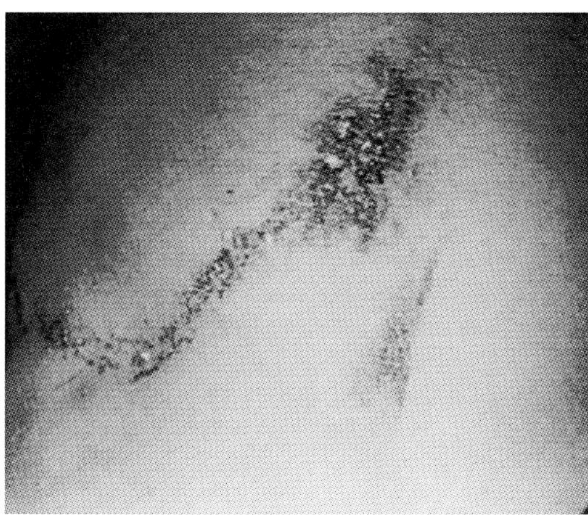

**FIGURE 100–9.** Linear hyperkeratotic epidermal nevus on the back and lateral aspect of the thorax.

the diagnostic histologic features of epidermolytic hyperkeratosis. Small epidermal nevi do not require treatment. Nevus sebaceus carries a risk of malignant degeneration and optimally is excised in adolescence using local anesthesia. Recent studies suggest that the risk of basal cell carcinoma, the most common malignancy to arise in nevus sebaceus, is closer to 1%, much lower than reported in the past (Cribier et al, 2000).

There is no optimal therapy for larger lesions or those that are disfiguring. Full-thickness excision, including the subcutaneous tissue, is recommended to decrease the risk of recurrence. Laser therapy holds promise for the future. Topically applied keratolytic agents may be palliative. Genetic counseling about the risk for offspring of fully expressed disease should be considered for persons with epidermal nevi that reveal the histologic features of epidermolytic hyperkeratosis.

### Epidermal (Linear Sebaceous) Nevus Syndrome

In less than 10% of affected people, epidermal nevi and sebaceous nevi (especially those involving the head) are associated with a variety of extracutaneous abnormalities, mainly ocular (in 33% of cases), neurologic (in 50%), and skeletal (in 70%), a condition referred to as *epidermal nevus syndrome*. Bone abnormalities include vertebral anomalies, kyphoscoliosis, limb shortening, and hemihypertrophy. CNS disorders include seizures, mental retardation, and hemiparesis; ocular abnormalities include eyelid/conjunctival nevus, coloboma, corneal opacity, and nystagmus. Malignancies also occur in this syndrome with a greater-than-expected frequency, including Wilms tumor, nephroblastoma, gastrointestinal carcinomas, and rhabdomyosarcoma (Marghoob et al, 1993).

## DERMAL TUMORS

### Juvenile Xanthogranuloma

Juvenile xanthogranuloma (JXG) is a benign, self-healing, non–Langerhans cell histiocytic tumor of infancy. JXG may be congenital; a majority of tumors manifest by 6 months of age (Nomland, 1959). Cutaneous lesions vary in color from red-brown to yellow. They occur most often on the upper half of the body (Fig. 100–10), may be solitary or multiple, and vary from several millimeters to several centimeters in diameter (see Fig. 100–4). JXG also may be localized to the eye or mucous membranes (De Raeve et al, 1994).

Skin biopsy usually is diagnostic, revealing characteristic foamy histiocytes and Touton giant cells within the dermis.

The vast majority of infants with JXG are otherwise healthy. Giant JXG can have an alarming appearance and may be confused with other types of histiocytic tumors (Magana et al, 1994). The most clinically significant associations are ocular JXG with its complications and the triad of JXG, juvenile chronic granulocytic leukemia, and NF-1. Less than 0.5% of children with skin lesions have ocular involvement, but one half of children with ocular JXG have cutaneous lesions (Giacoia and Berry, 1994). Ocular tumors may manifest as unilateral glaucoma, uveitis, heterochromia iridis, or proptosis; ocular JXG is the most common cause of hyphema in infancy (Gaynes and Cohen, 1967; Zimmerman, 1965). The iris is the most frequently affected ocular tissue (Hamdani et al, 2000). The triple association of JXG, juvenile chronic granulocytic leukemia, and NF-1 has been reported in 24 cases. The appearance of JXG usually preceded the diagnosis of leukemia; the NF, marked by multiple CALMs, was often missed (Sherer et al, 1993). Fewer than 20 patients with intracranial JXG without cutaneous manifestations have been described (Bostrom et al, 2000; Schultz et al, 1997).

The majority of cases of JXG are asymptomatic and self-limited. Giant lesions have a similar prognosis (Magana et al, 1994). Ophthalmologic evaluation is indicated for children who present in the first 2 years of life with multiple lesions. Parents should be provided with anticipatory guidance about the ocular complications (Giacoia and Berry, 1994). JXG typically involutes within 3 to 6 years (Hansen, 1992). Recurrence has been documented following surgical excision; this form of therapy is indicated only

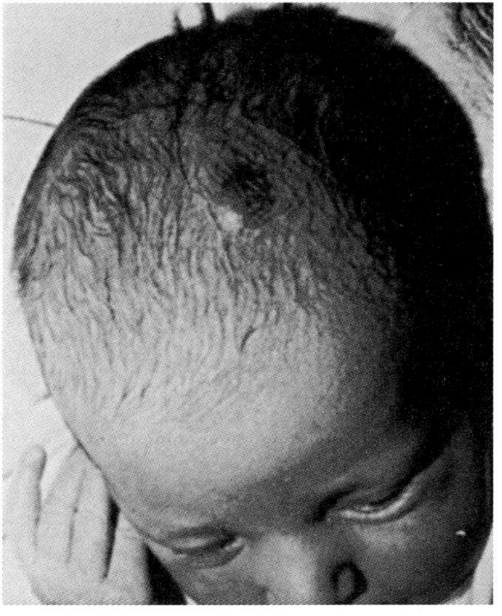

**FIGURE 100–10.** Solitary juvenile xanthogranuloma on the scalp, a typical site for these lesions.

for lesions that are frequently traumatized or are more disfiguring than the resultant scar would be.

## MASTOCYTOSIS

Mastocytosis comprises a group of disorders characterized by increased numbers of tissue mast cells. The skin is the most common site of involvement, but the lymphoreticular system, gastrointestinal tract, and bone marrow also may be affected. Symptoms result from the local or generalized effects following the release of histamine and other mast cell mediators. Pruritus, edema, blistering, and flushing are common. Abdominal pain, diarrhea, and vomiting are unusual. Hypotension is rare (Kettelhut and Metcalfe, 1991). If rubbed or traumatized, skin affected by mastocytosis will develop a diagnostic wheal (Darier sign). The site may blister or become hemorrhagic in a neonate.

*Urticaria pigmentosa* is the name given to the most common form of mastocytosis in infants, featuring multiple, small (1 to 3 cm in diameter) papules usually located on the trunk (Fig. 100–11). The disease may be congenital but usually manifests within the first 6 months of life (Kettelhut and Metcalfe, 1991). A single, localized lesion is known as a solitary mastocytoma. These tumors can vary in size from a few to several centimeters. Diffuse cutaneous mastocytosis is an unusual condition that may manifest at birth with widespread blistering or diffuse thickening of the skin (Sagher and Evan-Paz, 1967; Solomon and Esterly, 1973). Systemic mastocytosis is more commonly seen in adults and is defined by multifocal lesions in the bone marrow or other extracutaneous organs, together with signs of systemic disease. It is further divided into indolent systemic mastocytosis, systemic mastocytosis with an associated clonal hematologic non–mast cell lineage disease, aggressive systemic mastocytosis, and mast cell leukemia (Valent et al, 2001).

The diagnosis may be confirmed by a skin biopsy, which reveals mast cell hyperplasia within the dermis. Aminocaproate esterase is the most specific enzyme marker for identification of mast cells. Immunohistochemical stains for tryptase and *KIT* also are sensitive and specific markers for mast cells (Li, 2001). Mutations in c-*kit*, the gene encoding the receptor for stem cell factor, may play a significant role in the biology of mast cell malignancies (Gupta et al, 2002). Plasma histamine levels are elevated in a majority of children with mastocytosis, sometimes to remarkably high levels. Further workup for evidence of systemic involvement should be limited to pediatric patients with extracutaneous signs and symptoms, or those who require general anesthesia (Kettelhut and Metcalfe, 1991).

Caregivers should be educated to avoid exposing infants to factors that trigger mast cell degranulation, such as friction, pressure, temperature extremes, and substances that promote mast cell degranulation (aspirin, alcohol, narcotics, amphotericin B, or iodine-containing contrast media). If general anesthesia is required, perioperative administration of histamine receptor blockers is recommended (Lerno et al, 1990).

For patients with limited skin involvement, application of potent topical corticosteroids may hasten involution of lesions. Symptomatic patients may benefit from a classic histamine $H_1$ receptor blocker such as hydroxyzine or cyproheptadine. An $H_2$ blocker, such as ranitidine, or oral disodium cromoglycate may be added in the presence of gastrointestinal symptoms. Hypotension requires corticosteroids in addition to $H_1$ and $H_2$ antihistamines and intensive supportive care. Solitary mastocytomas usually involute by school age. Lesions of urticaria pigmentosa often resolve by puberty.

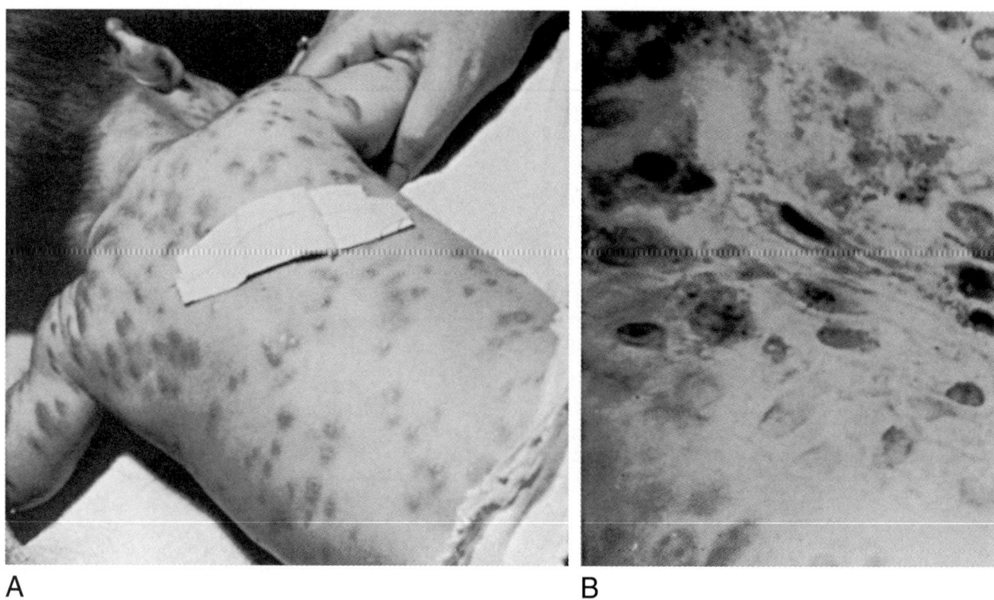


**FIGURE 100–11. A,** Deeply pigmented nodules and macules on the back of an infant with urticaria pigmentosa. A group of vesicles is visible just below the bandage that covers the biopsy site. **B,** Microscopic section from the biopsy specimen, stained with Giemsa stain. The mast cells can be identified as spindle-shaped cells containing granules that are located in the upper dermis.

## MIDLINE ANOMALIES

Congenital midline defects are a distinct group of diagnostically and therapeutically challenging conditions. These anomalies are located deep to the dermis, occurring at the cranial or caudal midline. Some of these lesions mark an underlying CNS problem or an intracranial connection. Considerations in the differential diagnosis include lesions that occasionally occur in the midline by serendipity; hemangiomas are the most common. Vascular malformations, hair tufts, dimples, and lipomas also may occur at the cranial or caudal midline and can mark a CNS or spinal malformation (Hayashi et al, 1984; Martinez-Lage et al, 1992). A midline mass in the nasal area may represent a dermoid cyst, encephalocele, or glioma (Paller et al, 1991). Occipital lesions include aplasia cutis congenita, encephalocele, and heterotopic brain tissue. The "hair collar sign" may mark ectopic neural tissue and CNS malformations (Commens et al, 1989; Drolet et al, 1995). Biopsy of a midline mass should not be performed unless an imaging study has been obtained to help clarify the nature of the lesion. If the possibility of an intracranial connection exists, referral to a neurosurgeon is indicated (Martinez-Lage et al, 1992).

## REFERENCES


Achauer BM, Vander Kam VM: Ulcerated anogenital hemangioma of infancy. Plast Reconstr Surg 87:861, 1991.

Albright AL, Gartner JC, Wiener ES: Lumbar cutaneous hemangiomas as indicators of tethered spinal cords. Pediatrics 83:977, 1989.

Alper J: Congenital nevi—the controversy rages on. Arch Dermatol 121:734, 1985.

Alper J, Holmes LB: The incidence of birthmarks in a cohort of 4, 641 newborns. Pediatr Dermatol 1:58, 1983.

Alper J, Holmes LB, Mihm MC: Birthmarks with serious medical significance: Nevocellular nevi, sebaceous nevi, and multiple cafe-au-lait spots. J Pediatr 95:696, 1979.

Alvarez J, Peteiro C, Toribio J: Linear and whorled nevoid hypermelanosis. Pediatr Dermatol 10:156-158, 1993.

Amir T, Krikler R, Metzker A, et al: Strawberry hemangioma in preterm infants. Pediatr Dermatol 3:331, 1986.

Arons MS, Hurwitz S: Congenital nevocellular nevus: A review of the treatment controversy and a report of 46 cases. Plast Reconstr Surg 72:355, 1983.

Ashinoff R, Geronemus RG: Capillary hemangiomas and treatment with the flash lamp–pumped pulsed dye laser. Arch Dermatol 127:202, 1991.

Ashinoff R, Geronemus RG: Failure of the flashlamp-pumped pulsed dye laser to prevent progression to deep hemangioma. Pediatr Dermatol 10:77, 1993.

Baker LL, Dillon WP, Hieshima GB, et al: Hemangiomas and vascular malformations of the head and neck: MR characterization. Am J Neuroradiol 14:307, 1993.

Barkovich AJ, Frieden IJ, Williams ML: MR of neurocutaneous melanosis. Am J Neuroradiol 15:859, 1994.

Barksy SH, Rosen S, Geer DE, et al: The nature and evolution of port wine stains: A computer assisted study. J Invest Dermatol 74:154, 1980.

Barlow RJ, Walker NP, Markey AC: Treatment of proliferative haemangiomas with the 585 nm pulsed dye laser. Br J Dermatol 134:700, 1996.

Barnhill RL, Aguiar M, Cohen C, et al: Congenital melanocytic nevi and DNA content: An analysis by flow and image cytometry. Cancer 74:2935, 1994.

Batta K, Goodyear HM, Moss C, et al: Randomised controlled study of early pulsed dye laser treatment of uncomplicated childhood haemangiomas: Results of a 1-year analysis. Lancet 360:502, 2002.

Berman B, Lim HWP: Concurrent cutaneous and hepatic hemangiomata in infancy: Report of a case and a review of the literature. J Cutan Surg Oncol 4:869, 1978.

Bostrom J, Janssen G, Messing-Junger M, et al: Multiple intracranial juvenile xanthogranulomas: Case report. J Neurosurg 93:335, 2000.

Boye E, Yu Y, Paranya G, et al: Clonality and altered behavior of endothelial cells from hemangiomas. J Clin Invest 107:745, 2001.

Brown SH Jr, Neerhout RC, Fonkalsrud EW: Prednisone therapy in the management of large hemangiomas in infants and children. Surgery 71:168, 1972.

Browze NL, Whimster I, Stewart G, et al: The surgical management of lymphangioma circumscriptum. Br J Surg 73:535, 1986.

Burman D, Mansell PWQ, Warin RP: Miliary hemangiomata in the newborn. Arch Dis Child 42:193, 1967.

Burns AJ, Kaplan C, Mulliken JB: Is there an association between hemangioma and syndromes with dysmorphic features? Pediatrics 88:1257, 1991.

Burrows DE, Mulliken JB, Fellows KE, et al: Childhood hemangiomas and vascular malformations: Angiographic differentiation. Am J Roentgenol 141:483, 1983.

Byard RW, Burrows PE, Izakawa T, Silver MM: Diffuse infantile haemangiomatosis: Clinicopathological features and management problems in five fatal cases. Eur J Pediatr 150:224, 1991.

Cainelli T, Marchesi L, Pasquali F, et al: Monozygotic twins discordant for cutaneous mastocytosis. Arch Dermatol 119:1021, 1983.

Carroll CB, Ceballos P, Perry AE, et al: Severe atypical medium-sized congenital nevus with widespread satellitosis and placental deposits in a neonate: The problem of congenital melanoma and its simulants. J Am Acad Dermatol 30:825, 1994.

Casson P, Colen S: Dysplastic and congenital nevi. Clin Plast Surg 20:105, 1993.

Cates CP, William ED, Ward-Booth RP, et al: Doppler ultrasound: A valuable diagnostic aid in a patient with facial hemangioma. Oral Surg 59:458, 1985.

Ceballos PI, Ruiz-Maldonado R, Mihm JMC: Melanoma in children. N Engl J Med 332:656, 1995.

Coats DK, Paysse EA, Levy ML: PHACE: A neurocutaneous syndrome with important ophthalmologic implications: Case report and literature review. Ophthalmology 106:1739, 1999.

Cribier B, Scribener Y, Groshans E: Tumors arising in nevus sebaceous: A study of 596 cases. J Am Acad Dermatol 42:263, 2000.

Cohen PR, Zalar GL: Cutis marmorata telangiectatica congenita: Clinico-pathologic characteristics and differential diagnosis. Cutis 42:418, 1988.

Commens C, Rogers M, Kan A: Heterotrophic brain tissue presenting as bald cysts with a collar of hypertrophic hair. Arch Dermatol 125:1253, 1989.

Cooper JG, Edwards SL, Holmes JD: Kaposiform haemangioendothelioma: Case report and review of the literature. Br J Plast Surg 55:163, 2002.

Crocker AL: The histiocytosis syndromes. In Fitzpatrick TB, Eisen AA, Wolff K, et al (eds): Dermatology in General Medicine, 2nd ed. New York, McGraw-Hill, 1979, p 1171.

D'Armiento M, Reda E, Camagna A, et al: McCune-Albright syndrome: Evidence for autonomous multiendocrine hyperfunction. J Pediatr 102:585, 1983.

De Raeve L, Danau W, Debacker A, Otten J: Prepubertal melanoma in a medium-sized congenital nevus. Eur J Pediatr 152:734, 1993.

De Raeve L, De Meirleir L, Ramet J, et al: Acrodermatitis enteropathica–like cutaneous lesions in organic aciduria. J Pediatr 124:416, 1994.

Dereser-Dennl M, Brude E, Konig R: Hypomelanosis Ito in translocation trisomy 9/mosaicism. Spontaneous remission in childhood. Hautarzt 9:688, 2000.

Devriendt K, Matthijs G, Meireleire J, et al: Skin pigment anomalies and mosaicism for a double autosomal trisomy. Genet Couns 9:283, 1998.

Drolet BA, Clowry L, McTigue K, Esterly NB: The hair collar sign: Marker for cranial dysraphism. Pediatrics 96:309, 1995.

Eady PAJ, Sparrow GP, Grice K: Naevoid pigmentation with giant melanosomes: Two cases. Proc R Soc Med 68:759, 1975.

Edstrom DW, Hedblad MA, Ros AM: Flashlamp pulsed dye laser and argon-pumped dye laser in the treatment of port-wine stains: A clinical and histological comparison. Br J Dermatol 146:285, 2002.

Elder DE: The blind men and the elephant—different views of small congenital nevi. Arch Dermatol 121:1263, 1985.

Elder DE, Goldman LI, Goldman SC, et al: Dysplastic nevus syndrome. Cancer 46:1787, 1980.

Enjolras O, Mulliken JB: The current management of vascular birthmarks. Pediatr Dermatol 10:311, 1993.

Enjolras O, Riche MC, Merland JJ, Escande JP: Management of alarming hemangiomas in infancy: A review of 25 cases. Pediatrics 85:491, 1990.

Enjolras O, Wassef M, Mazoyer E, et al: Infants with Kasabach-Merritt syndrome do not have "true" hemangiomas. J Pediatr 130:631-640, 1997.

Esterly NB: Cutaneous hemangiomas, vascular stains and malformations, and associated syndromes. Curr Probl Dermatol 7:65, 1995.

Esterly NB: Kasabach-Merritt syndrome in infants. J Am Acad Dermatol 8:504, 1983.

Esterly NB, Margileth AM, Kahn G, et al: The management of disseminated eruptive hemangiomata in infants: Special symposium. Pediatr Dermatol 1:312, 1984.

Esterly NB, Sahihi T, Medenica M: Juvenile xanthogranuloma: An atypical case with study of ultrastructure. Arch Dermatol 105:99, 1972.

Fienman NL, Yakovac WC: Neurofibromatosis in childhood. J Pediatr 76:339, 1970.

Fretzin DF, Potter B: Blue rubber bleb nevus. Arch Intern Med 116:924, 1965.

Frieden IJ, Reese V, Cohen D: PHACE syndrome. The association of posterior fossa brain malformations, hemangiomas, arterial anomalies, coarctation of the aorta and cardiac defects, and eye abnormalities. Arch Dermatol 132:307, 1996.

Frieden IJ, Williams ML, Barkovich AJ: Giant congenital melanocytic nevi: Brain magnetic resonance findings in neurologically asymptomatic children. J Am Acad Dermatol 31:423, 1994.

Folkman J: How is blood vessel growth regulated in normal and neoplastic tissue? Cancer Res 46:467, 1986.

Fost NC, Esterly NB: Successful treatment of juvenile hemangiomas with prednisone. J Pediatr 72:351, 1968.

Fowler JF, Porsley W, Cotter PG: Familial urticaria pigmentosa. Arch Dermatol 122:80, 1986.

Garden J, Bakus A: Clinical efficacy of the pulsed dye laser in the treatment of vascular lesions. J Dermatol Surg Oncol 19:321, 1993.

Garden JM, Bakus AD, Paller AS: Treatment of cutaneous hemangiomas by the flashlamp-pumped pulsed dye laser: Prospective analysis. J Pediatr 120:555, 1992.

Gari LM, Rivers JK, Kopf AW: Melanomas arising in large congenital nevocytic nevi: A prospective study. Pediatr Dermatol 5:151, 1988.

Gaynes PM, Cohen GS: Juvenile xanthogranuloma of the orbit. Am J Ophthalmol 63:755, 1967.

Giacoia GP, Berry GT: Acrodermatitis enteropathica–like syndrome secondary to isoleucine deficiency during treatment of maple syrup urine disease. Am J Dis Child 147:954, 1994.

Glassberg E, Lask G, Rabinowitz LG, Tunnessen JWW: Capillary hemangiomas: Case study of a novel laser treatment and a review of therapeutic options. J Dermatol Surg Oncol 15:1214, 1989.

Glovitzki P, Hallier CH, Telander RL, et al: Surgical implications of Klippel-Trenaunay syndrome. Ann Surg 192:353, 1983.

Goldberg NS, Herbert AA, Esterly NB: Sacral hemangiomas and multiple congenital abnormalities. Arch Dermatol 122:684, 1986.

Goldman M, Fitzpatrick R, Ruiz-Esparza J: Treatment of port-wine stains (capillary malformation) with the flashlamp-pumped pulsed dye laser. J Pediatr 122:71, 1993.

Golitz LE, Ruchkoff J, O'Meara P: Diffuse neonatal hemangiomatosis. Pediatr Dermatol 3:145, 1986.

Gomez MR: Phenotypes of the tuberous sclerosis complex with a revision of diagnostic criteria. Ann N Y Acad Sci 615:1, 1991.

Gordon L, Vujic I, Spicer KM: Visualization of cutaneous hemangiomas with Tc-99 m tagged red cells. Clin Nucl Med 4:468, 1981.

Greene MH, Clark WH Jr, Tucker JH, et al: Managing the dysplastic naevus syndrome. Lancet 1:166, 1984.

Greeley PW, Middleton AG, Curtain JW: Incidence of malignancy in giant pigmented nevi. Plast Reconstr Surg 36:26, 1965.

Gupta R, Bain BJ, Knight CL: Cytogenetic and molecular genetic abnormalities in systemic mastocytosis. Acta Haematol 107:123, 2002.

Gutmann DH, Zhang Y, Hasbani MJ, et al: Expression of the tuberous sclerosis complex gene products, hamartin and tuberin, in central nervous system tissues. Acta Neuropathol 99:223, 2000.

Hamdani M, El Kettani A, Rais L, et al: Juvenile xanthogranuloma with intraocular involvement. A case report. J Fr Ophtalmol 23:817, 2000.

Hand JL, Frieden IJ: Vascular birthmarks of infancy: Resolving nosologic confusion. Am J Med Genet 108:257, 2002.

Hansen RC: Dermatitis and nutritional deficiency. Arch Dermatol 128:1389, 1992.

Hara K: Melanocytic lesions in lymph nodes associated with congenital nevus. Histopathology 23:445, 1993.

Harris LE, Stayura LA, Ramirez-Talavera PF, Annegers JF: Congenital and acquired abnormalities observed in liveborn and stillborn neonates. Mayo Clin Proc 50:85, 1975.

Hayashi T, Shyojima K, Honda E, Hasimoto T: Lipoma of corpus callosum associated with frontoethmoidal lipomeningocele: CT findings. J Comput Assist Tomogr 8:795, 1984.

Haywood RM, Monk BE, Mahaffey PJ: The treatment of early cutaneous capillary haemangiomata (strawberry naevi) with the tunable dye laser. Br J Plast Surg 53:302, 2000.

Heimann P, Ogur G, Debusscher C, et al: Chromosomal findings in cultured melanocytes from a giant congenital nevus. Cancer Genet Cytogenet 68:74, 1993.

Hidano A, Nakajima S: Earliest features of the strawberry mark in the newborn. Br J Dermatol 87:138, 1972.

Hoffman HJ, Freeman A: Primary leptomeningeal melanoma in association with giant hairy nevi: Report of two cases. J Neurosurg 26:62, 1967.

Holden KR, Alexander R: Diffuse neonatal hemangiomatosis. Pediatrics 46:411, 1970.

Illig W, Weidner F, Hundeiker M, et al: Congenital nevi 10 cm precursors to melanoma: 52 cases, a review, and a new conception. Arch Dermatol 121:1274, 1985.

Janniger CK, Schwartz RA: Tuberous sclerosis: Recent advances for the clinician. Cutis 51:167, 1993.

Kadonaga JN, Frieden IJ: Neurocutaneous melanosis: Definition and review of the literature. J Am Acad Dermatol 5:747, 1991.

Kaplan M, Paller AS: Clinical pearl: Use of self-adhesive, compressive wraps in the treatment of limb hemangiomas. J Am Acad Dermatol 32:117, 1995.

Kelly KM, Nanda VS, Nelson JS: Treatment of port-wine stain birthmarks using the 1.5-msec pulsed dye laser at high fluences in conjunction with cryogen spray cooling. Dermatol Surg 28:309, 2002.

Kettelhut BV, Metcalfe DD: Pediatric mastocytosis. J Invest Dermatol 96:15, 1991.

Kopf AW, Bart RS, Hennessey P: Congenital nevocytic nevi and malignant melanomas. J Am Acad Dermatol 1:123, 1979.

Kopf AW, Weidman AJ: Nevus of ota. Arch Dermatol 85:75, 1962.

Kuflik JH, Janniger CK: Congenital melanocytic nevi. Cutis 53:112, 1994.

Kushner BJ: Local steroid therapy in adnexal hemangioma. Ann Ophthalmol 11:1005, 1979.

Laurent I, Leaute-Labreze C, Maleville J, Taieb A: Faun tail and sacral hemangioma associated with occult spinal dysraphism. Ann Dermatol Venereol 125:414, 1998.

Lazaro C, Ravella A, Gaona A, et al: Neurofibromatosis type 1 due to germ-line mosaicism in a clinically normal father. N Engl J Med 331:1403, 1994.

Lerno G, Slaats G, Coenen E, et al: Anaesthetic management of systemic mastocytosis. Br J Anaesthesia 65:254, 1990.

Lewis RA, Riccardi VM: Von Recklinghausen neurofibromatosis: Incidence of iris hamartoma. Ophthalmology 88:348, 1981.

Li CY: Diagnosis of mastocytosis: Value of cytochemistry and immunohistochemistry. Leuk Res 25:537, 2001.

Lund HA, Kraus JM: Melanotic tumors of the skin, Fascicle 3. In Atlas of Tumor Pathology. Washington, DC, Armed Forces Institute of Pathology, 1962.

Magana M, Vazquez R, Fernandez-Diez J, et al: Giant congenital juvenile xanthogranuloma. Pediatr Dermatol 11:227, 1994.

Mangus DJ: Continuous compression therapy of hemangiomas: Evaluation in two cases. Plast Reconstr Surg 49:490, 1973.

Marghoob AA, Orlow SJ, Kopf AW: Syndromes associated with melanocytic nevi. J Am Acad Dermatol 29:373, 1993.

Margileth AM: Developmental vascular abnormalities. Med Clin North Am 18:773, 1971.

Marler JJ, Rubin JB, Trede NS, et al: Successful antiangiogenic therapy of giant cell angioblastoma with interferon alfa 2b: Report of 2 cases. Pediatrics 109:E37, 2002.

Martinez-Lage J, Capel A, Costa T, et al: The child with a mass on its head: Diagnostic and surgical strategies. Child Nerv Syst 8:247, 1992.

Morelli JG: On the treatment of hemangiomas. Pediatr Dermatol 10:84, 1993.

Morelli JG, Tan OT, Weston WL: Treatment of ulcerated hemangiomas with pulsed tunable dye laser. Am J Dis Child 145:1062, 1991.

Morelli JG, Tan OT, Yohn JJ, Weston WL: Treatment of ulcerated hemangiomas infancy. Arch Pediatr Adolesc Med 148:1104, 1994.

Mulliken JB: A plea for a biologic approach to hemangiomas of infancy. Arch Dermatol 127:243, 1991.

Mulliken JB, Boon LM, Takahashi K, et al: Pharmacologic therapy for endangering hemangiomas. Curr Opin Dermatol 109, 1995.

Mulliken JB, Glowacki J: Hemangiomas and vascular malformations in infants and children: A classification based on endothelial characteristics. Plast Reconstr Surg 69:421, 1982.

Mulliken JB, Young AE: Vascular Birthmarks, Hemangiomas, and Malformations. Philadelphia, WB Saunders, 1988.

Mullins JF, Naylor D, Pedetski J: The Klippel-Trenaunay-Weber syndrome (nevus vasculosus osteohypertrophicus). Arch Dermatol 86:202, 1962.

Munkvad M: Blue rubber bleb nevus. Dermatologica 163:307, 1983.

National Institutes of Health Consensus Development Conference: Neurofibromatosis. Arch Neurol 45:575, 1988.

Nomland R: Nevoxanthoendothelioma: A benign xanthomatous disease of infants and children. J Invest Dermatol 22:207, 1959.

Oates CP, Williams ED, Ward-Booth RP, et al: Doppler ultrasound: A valuable diagnostic aid in a patient with a facial hemangioma. Oral Surg 59:958, 1985.

Oranje AP, de Waard-van der Spek FB, Devillers AC, et al: Treatment and pain relief of ulcerative hemangiomas with a polyurethane film. Dermatology 200:31, 2000.

O'Reilly MS, Brem H, Folkman J: Treatment of murine hemangioendotheliomas with the angiogenesis inhibitor AGM-1470. J Pediatr Surg 30:325, 1995.

Osburn K, Schosser RH, Everett MA: Congenital pigmented and vascular lesions in newborn infants. J Am Acad Dermatol 16:788, 1987.

Ozturkcan S, Goze F, Atakan N, Icli F: Malignant melanoma in a child. J Am Acad Dermatol 30:493, 1994.

Paller AS: The Sturge-Weber syndrome. Pediatr Dermatol 4:300, 1987.

Paller AS, Pensler JM, Tomita T: Nasal midline masses in infants and children. Arch Dermatol 127:362, 1991.

Payarols JP, Masferrer JP, Bellvert CG: Treatment of life-threatening infantile hemangiomas with vincristine. New Engl J Med 333:69, 1995.

Peachy RDG, Lim CC, Whimster JW: Lymphangioma of skin: A review of 65 cases. Br J Dermatol 83:419, 1970.

Pinkus H, Mehregan AH: A Guide to Dermatohistopathology. New York, Appleton-Century-Crofts, Inc., 1969, pp 352-354.

Poetke M, Philipp C, Berlien HP: Flashlamp-pumped pulsed dye laser for hemangiomas in infancy: Treatment of superficial vs mixed hemangiomas. Arch Dermatol 136:628, 2000.

Powell ST, Su WPD: Cutis marmorata telangiectasia congenita: Report of nine cases and review of the literature. Cutis 34:305, 1984.

Pratt AG: Birthmarks in infancy. Arch Dermatol 67:302, 1953.

Reed WB, Becker SW Sr, Becker SW Jr, Nickel WR: Giant pigmented nevi, melanoma and leptomeningeal melanocytosis. Arch Dermatol 91:100, 1965.

Reese V, Frieden IJ, Paller AS, et al: Association of facial hemangiomas with Dandy-Walker and other posterior fossa malformations. J Pediatr 122:379, 1993.

Renfro L, Geronemus RG: Anatomical differences of port-wine stains in response to treatment with the pulsed dye laser. Arch Dermatol 129:182, 1993.

Rhodes AR, Melski JW: Small congenital nevocellular nevi and the risk of cutaneous melanoma. J Pediatr 100:219, 1982.

Rhodes AR, Sober AJ, Day CL, et al: The malignant potential of small congenital nevocellular nevi: An estimate of association based on a histologic study of 234 primary cutaneous melanomas. J Am Acad Dermatol 6:620, 1982.

Riccardi VM: Early manifestations of neurofibromatosis: Diagnosis and management. Compr Ther 8:35, 1982.

Riccardi VM: Neurofibromatosis heterogeneity. J Am Acad Dermatol 8:518, 1983.

Riccardi VM: Von Recklinghausen neurofibromatosis. N Engl J Med 305:1617, 1981.

Riccardi VM, Eichner JE: Neurofibromatosis, Phenotype, Natural History and Pathogenesis. Baltimore, Johns Hopkins University Press, 1986.

Richardson SK, Tannous ZS, Mihm MC Jr: Congenital and infantile melanoma: Review of the literature and report of an uncomman variant, pigment-synthesizing melanoma. J Am Acad Dermatol 47:77, 2002.

Rieger E, Kofler R, Borkenstein M, et al: Melanotic macules following Blaschko's lines in McCune-Albright syndrome. Br J Dermatol 130:215, 1994.

Rodriguez-Erdmann F, Button L, et al: Kasabach-Merritt syndrome: Coagulo-analytical observations. Am J Med Sci 261:9, 1971.

Rogers M, McCrossin I, Commens C: Epidermal nevi and the epidermal nevus syndrome: A review of 131 cases. J Am Acad Dermatol 20:476, 1989.

Rossi A, Bava GL, Biancheri R, Tortori-Donati P: Posterior fossa and arterial abnormalities in patients with facial capillary haemangioma: Presumed incomplete phenotypic expression of PHACES syndrome. Neuroradiology 43:934, 2001.

Rouleau GA, Merel P, Lutchman M, et al: Alteration in a new gene encoding a putative membrane-organizing protein causes neurofibromatosis type 2. Nature 363:495, 1993.

Sagher F, Evan-Paz Z: Mastocytosis and the Mast Cell. Chicago, Year Book Medical Publishers, 1967.

Saijo M, Munroe IR, Mancer K: Lymphangioma: Long-term follow-up study. Plast Reconstr Surg 56:642, 1975.

Sanchez NP, Rhodes AR, Mandell F, Mihm MC: Encephalocraniocutaneous lipomatosis: A new syndrome. Br J Dermatol 104:89, 1981.

Sandsmark M, Eskeland G, Ogaard AR, et al: Treatment of large congenital nevi: A review and report of six cases. Scand J Plast Reconstr Surg Hand Surg 27:223, 1993.

Sandsmark M, Eskeland G, Skullerud K, Abyholm F: Neurocutaneous melanosis: Case report and a brief review. Scand J Plast Reconstr Surg Hand Surg 28:151, 1994.

Sarihan H, Mocan H, Yildiz K, et al: A new treatment with bleomycin for complicated cutaneous hemangioma in children Eur J Pediatr Surg 7:158, 1997.

Scheepers JH, Quaba AA: Does the pulsed tunable dye laser have a role in the management of infantile hemangiomas? Observations based on 3 years' experience. Plast Reconstr Surg 95:305, 1995.

Schultz KD Jr, Petronio J, Narad C, Hunter SB: Solitary intracerebral juvenile xanthogranuloma: Case report and review of the literature. Pediatr Neurosurg 26:315, 1997.

Schwindinger WF, Francomano CA, Levine MA: Identification of a mutation in the gene encoding the alpha subunit of the stimulatory G protein of adenylyl cyclase in McCune-Albright syndrome. Proc Natl Acad Sci U S A 89:5152, 1992.

Selmanowitz VJ, Orentreich N, Tiangco CC, Demis DJ: Uniovular twins discordant for cutaneous mastocytosis. Arch Dermatol 102:34, 1970.

Shenker A, Weinstein LS, Moran A, et al: Severe endocrine and nonendocrine manifestations of the McCune-Albright syndrome associated with activating mutations of stimulatory G protein GS. J Pediatr 123:509, 1993.

Sherer DM, Metlay LA, Sinkin RA, et al: Congenital ichthyosis with restrictive dermopathy and Gaucher disease: A new syndrome with associated prenatal diagnostic and pathology findings. Obstet Gynecol 81:842, 1993.

Sherwood KA, Tan OT: Treatment of capillary hemangioma with the flashlamp pumped-dye laser. J Am Acad Dermatol 22:136, 1990.

Shpall S, Frieden I, Chesney M, Newman T: Risk of malignant transformation of congenital melanocytic nevi in blacks. Pediatr Dermatol 11:204, 1994.

Smith JLS, Ingram RM: Juvenile oculodermal xanthogranuloma. Br J Ophthalmol 52:696, 1968.

Sober AJ: Solar exposure in the etiology of cutaneous melanoma. Photodermatology 4:23, 1987.

Solomon LM: Epidermal nevi: A study of 300 cases. In Fabrizi G, Serri F (Eds): Dermatologia Pediatrica. Transactions of a Symposium on Pediatric Dermatology. Rome, Italy, CILAG SPA, 1985.

Solomon LM: The management of congenital melanocytic nevi. Arch Dermatol 116:1017, 1980.

Solomon LM, Esterly NB: Epidermal and other congenital organoid nevi. Curr Probl Pediatr 6:1, 1975.

Solomon LM, Esterly NB: Neonatal Dermatology. Philadelphia, WB Saunders, 1973.

Solomon LM, Fretzin DF, De Wald RL: The epidermal nevus syndrome. Arch Dermatol 97:273, 1968.

Swint RB, Klaus SW: Malignant degeneration of an epithelial nevus. Arch Dermatol 101:56, 1970.

Sybert VP: Hypomelanosis of Ito: A description, not a diagnosis. J Invest Dermatol 103:141S, 1994.

Takahashi K, Mulliken JB, Kozakewich HP, et al: Cellular markers that distinguish the phases of hemangioma during infancy and childhood. J Clin Invest 93:2357, 1994.

Tallman B, Tan OT, Morelli JG, et al: Location of port-wine stains and the likelihood of ophthalmic and/or central nervous system complications. Pediatrics 87:323, 1991.

Tan KL: Nevus flammeus of the nape, glabella, and eyelids. Clin Pediatr 11:112, 1972.

Tavafoghi V, Ghandchi A, Hambrick G, Udverhelyi G: Cutaneous signs of spinal dysraphism. Arch Dermatol 114:573, 1978.

Tharapel AT: Hypomelanosis of Ito and a "mirror image" whole chromosome duplication resulting in trisomy 14 mosaicism. Ann Genet 43:39, 2000.

Tsuchida T, Oksuka H, Riimura M, et al: Biochemical study of gangliosides in neurofibroma and neurofibrosarcomas of Recklinghausen's disease. J Dermatol (Tokyo) 11:129, 1984.

Tunca Y, Wilroy RS, Kadandale JS, et al: Hypomelanosis of ito and a 'mirror image' whole chromosome duplication resulting in trisomy 14 mosaicism. Ann Genet 43:39, 2000.

Valent P, Horny HP, Escribano L, et al: Diagnostic criteria and classification of mastocytosis: A consensus proposal. Leuk Res 25:603, 2001.

Vergnes P, Taieb A, Maleville J, et al: Repeated skin expansion for excision of congenital giant nevi in infancy and childhood. Plast Reconstr Surg 91:450, 1993.

Voest EE, Kenyon BM, O'Reilly MS, et al: Inhibition of angiogenesis in vivo by interleukin 12. J Natl Cancer Inst 87:581, 1995.

Wade TR, Kamino H, Ackerman AB: A histologic atlas of vascular lesions. J Dermatol Surg Oncol 4:845, 1978.

Walker RS, Custer PL, Nerad JA: Surgical excision of periorbital capillary hemangiomas. Ophthalmology 101:1333, 1994.

Waner M, Suen JY, Dinehart S, Mallory SB: Laser photocoagulation of superficial proliferating hemangiomas. J Dermatol Surg Oncol 20:43, 1994.

Way BH, Hermana J, Gilbert EF, et al: Cutis marmorata telangiectatica congenita. J Cutan Pathol 1:10, 1974.

Wheeland RG: Advances in the surgical approach to pediatric dermatologic problems: The laser in vascular and pigmented pediatric lesions [abstract]. Paper presented at the 53rd Annual Meeting of the American Academy of Dermatology, New Orleans, February 1995.

White CW, Sondheimer HM, Crouch EC, et al: Treatment of pulmonary hemangioma tests with recombinant interferon alfa-2a. N Engl J Med 320:1197, 1989.

Whitehouse D: Diagnostic value of the café-au-lait spot in children. Arch Dis Child 41:316, 1966.

Wienecke R, Konig A, DeClue JE: Identification of tuberin, the tuberous sclerosis-2 product: Tuberin possesses specific Rap1GAP activity. J Biol Chem 270:16409, 1995.

Williams ML: Early onset nevi. Pediatr Dermatol 10:198, 1993.

Williams ML, Pennella R: Melanoma, melanocytic nevi, and other melanoma risk factors in children. J Pediatr 124:833, 1994.

Yu Y, Varughese J, Brown LF, Mulliken JB, Bischoff J: Increased Tie2 expression, enhanced response to angiopoietin-1, and dysregulated angiopoietin-2 expression in hemangioma-derived endothelial cells. Am J Pathol 159:2271, 2001.

Zimmerman LC: Ocular lesions of juvenile xanthogranuloma. Am J Ophthalmol 60:1011, 1965.

Zitelli GA, Grant MG, Abell E, et al: Histologic patterns of congenital nevocytic nevi and implications for treatment. J Am Acad Dermatol 11:402, 1984.

Zuniga S, Las Heras J, Benveviste S: Rhabdomyosarcoma arising in a congenital giant nevus associated with neurocutaneous melanosis in a neonate. J Pediatr Surg 22:1036, 1987.

Zvulunov A, Esterly NB: Neurocutaneous syndromes associated with pigmentary skin lesions. J Am Acad Dermatol 32:915, 1995.

# PART XXI

# THE EYE

Editor: H. WILLIAM TAEUSCH

CHAPTER 101

## Disorders of the Eye

Ashima Madan and William V. Good

### RETINOPATHY OF PREMATURITY

Retinopathy of prematurity (ROP) is a neovascularizing disease that, in its most severe form, can lead to retinal detachment and subsequent blindness. It is the second most common cause of blindness among children in the United States (Steinkuller et al, 1999). Although the exact number of infants who are affected by the condition is unclear, current estimates suggest that each year, ROP will lead to blindness in approximately 500 infants in the United States alone, and to visual impairment from retinal scars in another 2300 (Hunter and Mukai, 1992; Phelps, 1997; Strodtbeck et al, 1998).

#### Historical Overview

ROP, or retrolental fibroplasia (RLP), was first reported in 1942 (Terry, 1942). Before the 1940s, which witnessed an epidemic of blindness, ROP was a relatively unrecognized condition. In spite of an intense search for a specific cause, it was not until 1951 that a pediatrician in Melbourne, Australia, provided the first link between the use of oxygen and ROP (Campbell, 1951). Several reports subsequently suggested that an inspired $O_2$ concentration of less than 40% was unlikely to lead to ROP (Guy et al, 1956; Lanman, 1954; Slobody and Wasserman, 1963). The decline in the use of greater than 40% supplemental $O_2$ for premature infants in the 1950s was followed by a decline in the incidence of ROP (Cross, 1973). However, decreased $O_2$ use resulted in cerebral hypoxic changes and an increase in brain damage and death among premature infants (Avery and Oppenheimer, 1960; McDonald, 1963). These findings led to a change in practice with more liberal use of $O_2$ in premature infants. The 1960s were associated with enormous advances in the field of newborn medicine. It was now possible to resuscitate and ventilate tiny premature infants. Increased survival of these small infants together with the liberal use of oxygen led to a resurgence of ROP (James and Lanman, 1976).

#### Incidence

ROP is predominantly a disease of low-birth-weight (LBW) and premature infants. The incidence of ROP increases with decreasing gestation and birth weight. Neonatal mortality in the 1990s has been considerably lower with the advent of artificial surfactant and improved ventilation strategies for the very LBW (VLBW) infant. The current survival rate for infants weighing between 750 and 1000 g is 70%, and that for infants weighing between 1000 and 1250 g is estimated to be 90% (Hack et al, 1996; Vohr and Msall, 1997). In view of the ongoing trend for resuscitation of smaller infants at lower gestational ages, along with the increased survival of extremely LBW (ELBW) infants, an increase in the incidence of ROP is to be expected. There are no good epidemiologic data on childhood blindness in the United States. The results from local registries and from clinical trials suggest an increase in the number of infants blinded by ROP (Steinkuller et al, 1999). There is also some evidence to suggest an increased prevalence of blindness from ROP in some geographic regions (Tompkins, 2001). However, some studies have reported a decreased incidence secondary to an improvement in neonatal care (Bullard et al, 1999; Hussain et al, 1999; Keith and Doyle, 1995).

#### Development of the Retinal Vasculature

The retina is one of the last organs to be vascularized in the fetus. Retinal vascularization occurs by a process of *vasculogenesis*, de novo formation of capillaries from endothelial cells that have differentiated from spindle cell precursors (Ashton, 1966; Kretzer and Hittner, 1988), and *angiogenesis*, formation of blood vessels from existing blood vessels (Ashton, 1970). The outer layers of the retina are supplied by the choroid plexus, which lies between the outermost layer of the retina and the retinal pigment epithelium (RPE), whereas the inner layers are supplied by a superficial plexus beneath the inner limiting membrane and a deep plexus in the inner nuclear layer. The choroid vasculature is mature by 21 weeks of gestation (Gariano et al, 1994). Vascularization of the inner retina begins by vasculogenesis from spindle cell precursors at approximately 16 weeks of gestation in the posterior region around the optic disc. With advancing gestation, blood vessels by a process of angiogenesis spread across the surface of the retina in the superficial and deep plexus, following the central peripheral gradient of retinal ganglion cell maturation toward the peripheral retina (Hughes et al, 2000). Formation of the outer capillary plexus in the human fetus begins between 25 and 26 weeks of gestation, concomitant with the peak period of eye opening, when the visual evoked potential (VEP), an indication of visual function, is first detectable (Dreher and Robinson, 1988). It has been hypothesized that physiologic hypoxia, created by the increased metabolic demands of the fetal retina, is the major stimulus for the growth of the retinal blood vessels by angiogeneis in utero; retinal hypoxia leads to the release of vascular endothelial growth factor (VEGF) and subsequent growth of retinal blood vessels (Chan-Ling and Stone, 1993; Chan-Ling et al, 1990, 1995; Stone et al, 1995). However, vasculogenesis in the human retina is independent of metabolic demand and hypoxia-induced VEGF expression (Chan-Ling et al, 1995). The retinal vessels reach only 70% of the distance from the optic disc to the ora serrata at 27 weeks of gestation. Although there is considerable variation in the time course of retinal vascularization among infants, in most cases the retina is completely vascularized by 36 weeks of gestation on the nasal side and by 40 weeks on the temporal side (Palmer et al, 1991).

### Pathogenesis of Retinopathy of Prematurity

ROP is a disease of multifactorial etiology. Pathophysiology of ROP is a two-stage process: an initial phase of vasoattentuation following a second phase of abnormal proliferation. As in other ischemic retinopathies, such as sickle cell and vein occlusion retinopathy, the process probably is initiated by various environmental factors, such as hyperoxia, sepsis, or acidosis, that damage the vascular endothelium of the immature retinal blood vessels, thus leading to vaso-obliteration of existing blood vessels, as well to the arrest of new blood vessel growth. Prenatal events such as intrauterine hypoxia seen in the small-for-gestational-age (SGA) infant also may contribute to the injury. The increased susceptibility of premature infants of a lower gestational age, when compared with more mature infants, is due to the presence of a larger region of avascular retina. Given that the best maximal fetal $PO_2$ is 35 mm Hg, compared with a $PO_2$ of 60 to 80 mm Hg after birth, the process of normal retinal vascularization in the premature infant has to proceed in a relatively hyperoxic extrauterine environment.

Ashton and others have suggested that the susceptibility of the growing vessels in the retina to hyperoxia probably is related to the unique anatomic and developmental relationship between the retinal and choroidal circulations (Ashton, 1954; Dollery et al, 1969). The choroidal vasculature supplies the outer half of the retina by diffusion through the retinal pigment epithelium, while the retinal circulation supplies the inner half. The flow through the retinal circulation is far less than that through the choroidal circulation. Choroidal vessels form a honeycomb appearance, are much more permeable and have a high venous $PaO_2$. They also lack the ability to autoregulate in response to hyperoxia. Therefore, during hyperoxic conditions, $PaO_2$ levels are raised across the thickness of the retina and the retinal vessels respond by constriction.

Two hypotheses have been suggested to explain the initial mechanism that leads to retinopathy in the premature infant. The first is that hyperoxia induces vasoconstriction of developing retinal blood vessels as a regulatory response (Ashton, 1954). The other theory implicates the effect of reactive oxygen radicals in damaging cellular tight junctions in the precursor spindle cells, thereby leading to gap junction formation (Kretzer and Hittner, 1988).

Irrespective of the initial mechanism of injury, the retina then enters a quiescent phase for days or weeks, with the formation of a ridge-like structure separating the vascularized region from the peripheral avascular region. This structure, which is pathognomonic for ROP histologically, consists of mesenchymal cells and usually is seen between 33 and 36 weeks of gestation. Concomitant development of the photoreceptor retinal layer with advancing postnatal age results in increasing oxygen requirements, which cannot be met by the vaso-obliterated blood vessels, thus producing retinal hypoxia.

Some years ago, Michaelson (1948) and Ashton (1954) had suggested that retinal neovascularization occurs by release of one or more angiogenic factors from the ischemic retina. However, it was not until the 1980s that two groups of investigators identified VEGF, a glycoprotein molecule and endothelial cell–specific mitogen, as the key molecule responsible for angiogenesis (Keck et al, 1989; Senger et al, 1983). VEGF gene expression is hypoxia inducible (Forsythe et al, 1996; Levy et al, 1995). Several other lines of evidence also indicate that VEGF is the key molecule in retinal angiogenesis. VEGF levels have been shown to be increased in the vitreous and ocular fluid of patients with diabetes (Adamis et al, 1994; Aiello et al, 1994) and other neovascularizing diseases (Pe'er et al, 1995), as well as in animal models of ischemic retinopathy (Miller et al, 1994; Pierce et al, 1995). VEGF levels in the retina have been shown to be decreased in the initial phase of hyperoxic injury and increased in the hypoxic phase of retinopathy (Alon et al, 1995; Pierce et al, 1996). Inhibition of VEGF in animal models of retinopathy decreases neovascularization (Adamis et al, 1996; Aiello, 1995; Robinson et al, 1996). More recently, two separate receptors have been identified for VEGF. The one involved with new vessel growth and proliferation increases 60-fold during normal vascularization of the retina in mice. Specific activation of the other protects against vessel loss from hyperoxia without stimulating vascular proliferation and neovascularization in the mouse model, suggesting that therapies for the prevention of ROP can be targeted at this receptor (Shih et al, 2003).

Angiogenesis is a complex process that involves disruption of the basement membrane and extracellular matrix by proteolytic enzymes followed by cell proliferation and migration and subsequent formation and closure of nascent vascular tubes (Ausprunk and Folkman, 1977; Gross et al, 1982).Development of new blood vessels depends on the balance between angiogenic and angiostatic factors. Angiogenic factors implicated in retinal angiogenesis include several other growth factors besides VEGF: insulin-like growth factor (Smith et al, 1997), fibroblast growth factor (D'Amore, 1994), and platelet-derived growth factor (Andrews et al, 1999), along with interleukin 8 (IL-8), a chemotactic cytokine, and adhesion molecules VCAM-1 (vascular cell adhesion molecule-1), ICAM-1 (intercellular adhesion molecule-1), and E-selectin (Yoshida et al, 1999). Angiostatic factors include angiostatin, endostatin, and thrombospondin-1 (Folkman, 1995; O'Reilly et al, 1997). Identification of the genes involved in both normal and abnormal retinal neovascularization is the focus of intense research at the present time. Several groups of investigators are using gene chip complementary DNA (cDNA) microarray analysis to study differential gene expression in the mouse model of retinopathy. Many genes involved in vascular remodeling, such as those encoding angiopoietin-2 (Hackett et al, 2000), different isoforms of nitric oxide synthase (Brooks et al, 2001; Hangai et al, 1999; Hardy et al, 2000), angiotensin II (Lonchampt et al, 2001; Moravski et al, 2000), neuropilin-1 (Ishida et al, 2000; Oh et al, 2002), presenilin-2 (Lukiw et al, 2001), and hypoxia-inducible factor-1 (Ozaki et al, 1999), have been identified as candidates in the process of angiogenesis in cell culture studies or animal models of ischemic retinopathy.

For reasons that are at present unclear, in over 80% to 90% of cases, the ridge-like structure pathognomonic for ROP gradually regresses and mesenchymal cells differentiate into normal capillary endothelium and vascularize the avascular retina. However, in other infants, there is an increased proliferation of abnormal blood vessels from the ridge-like structure followed by progressive disease leading to exudation, hemorrhages, fibrosis, and retinal detachment.

### Animal Models of Retinopathy

Much of our knowledge regarding development of the retinal vasculature has been obtained by meticulous studies conducted in animal models of retinopathy. The kitten model has been used by some investigators because of the similarity in extent of vascularization between the kitten retina and that of a premature infant born at 5 months of gestation (Chan-Ling et al, 1990). The rat model of retinopathy involves exposure of newborn rat pups to an alternative use of a hyperoxia/hypoxia paradigm every 24 hours for 2 weeks (Penn et al, 1994). The pattern of neovascularization produced is very similar to that seen in premature infants with ROP, with peripheral avascularity and neovascularization. With the advent of transgenic mice technology there has been a gradual increase in the use of the mouse model of retinopathy. This model involves exposure of mice on day 7 of life to 75% $O_2$ for 5 days followed by a return to room air or relative hypoxia on day 12. Retinal neovascularization is seen on day 17 (Smith et al, 1994). However, none of the currently available animal models except for the beagle puppy is associated with cicatrical scarring or retinal detachment.

### Etiology

ROP is a multifactorial disease, and analysis of the risk factors associated with ROP has been the subject of several studies (Biglan et al, 1984; Brown et al, 1998; Gallo et al, 1993; Hammer et al, 1986; Seiberth et al, 2000). Many risk factors have been implicated in the development of ROP.

#### *Prematurity*

The most common causes of ROP are premature birth and low birth weight (Gunn et al, 1980; Hammer et al, 1986; Shohat et al, 1983). Incidence and severity of ROP increase with decreasing gestation. Results from the Cryotherapy for Retinopathy of Prematurity (CRYO-ROP) study (Cryotherapy for Retinopathy of Prematurity Cooperative Group, 1988) indicated that 90% of infants with a birth weight of less than 750 g and 47% of infants between 1000 and 1250 g will develop ROP. Approximately 80% of infants born at less than 28 weeks of gestation versus 30% of infants are at risk for developing ROP (Cryotherapy for Retinopathy of Prematurity Cooperative Group, 1988). In the CRYO-ROP trial, threshold ROP was noted in 10% of infants born at 27 weeks of gestation. Coats and colleagues (2000), in a retrospective study of infants born at less than 25 weeks of gestation, reported an incidence of threshold ROP of 40%.

#### *Race*

Infants of European descent are more likely to develop severe ROP than are African-American infants (Cryotherapy for Retinopathy of Prematurity Cooperative Group, 1988; Saunders et al, 1997). Data on progression of disease in Hispanic and Asian infants are not available.

#### *Oxygen*

The association between $O_2$ and ROP has been known for a long time and has been the subject of various studies (Kinsey et al, 1977; Lucey and Dangman, 1984; Patz et al, 1952). Bancalari and associates (1987) conducted a randomized prospective trial to determine whether the continuous use of transcutaneous $O_2$ ($TcPo_2$) tension monitoring could reduce the incidence of ROP. They found no protective effect of continuous versus intermittent monitoring except in infants weighing between 1100 and 1300 g. In infants weighing less than 1000 g, the severity of ROP was increased in infants with a $TcPo_2$ greater than 80 mm of Hg in the first 1 to 2 weeks of life (Flynn et al, 1987). In a retrospective study comparing the incidence of ROP between centers with two different guidelines for maintenance of $O_2$ saturation, Tin and colleagues (2001) reported a decreased incidence of ROP in patients in whom $O_2$ saturation was maintained between 70% and 90%, versus 88% to 98%. However, there are no randomized, controlled trials to show the optimal range of $O_2$ saturation or $Po_2$ at which infants should be maintained to reduce the risk of ROP. A meta-analysis by Askie and Henderson-Smart (2000) of five randomized trials conducted in preterm infants in which ambient $O_2$ concentrations were targeted to achieve either a lower or higher blood $O_2$ range was unable to determine the optimal target range for maintaining blood $Po_2$ levels in preterm infants. However, unrestricted, unmonitored $O_2$ therapy has potential harm without clear benefits. Other, smaller studies that looked at the effect of late versus early weaning of $O_2$ and the effect of gradual versus abrupt weaning of $O_2$ on the incidence of ROP were unable to find any differences between the groups (Askie and Henderson-Smart, 2001).

Although much interest has been focused on the role of oxygen in ROP, retinopathy has been known to occur without oxygen supplementation in full-term infants (Brockhurst and Chisti, 1975; Kraushar et al, 1975; Stefani and Ehalt, 1974) and in cyanotic infants (Johns et al, 1991; Kalina et al, 1972).

Frequent fluctuations of transcutaneous oxygen measurements in the first 2 weeks of life have been reported to be associated with a higher incidence of ROP (Cunningham et al, 2000). Studies in the neonatal rat model of retinopathy indicate that repeated episodes of alternating hyperoxia and hypoxia, more so than either alone, as well as the range of $PaO_2$ variation causes worse retinal vascular disease, probably as a result of increased secretion of VEGF (Penn et al, 1994, 1995).

### *Hypercapnia*

In animal studies, hypercapnia has been associated with increased retinal angiogenesis (Holmes et al, 1997). The mechanism of action appears to be either by inhibition of the normal vasoconstrictive response to hyperoxia, thus increasing retinal blood flow by vasodilation, or by decreasing the pH. A retrospective study by Bauer and Widmayer (1981) of infants weighing less than 1000 g noted that $PaCO_2$ was an important variable in predicting the development of ROP. However, other studies including a small randomized trial of permissive hypercapnea in premature infants showed no differences in the incidence of ROP between patients with $PaCO_2$ of 45 to 55 m Hg and infants with a lower $PaCO_2$ (Mariani et al, 1999).

### *Severity of Illness*

Increased severity of illness increases the odds that ROP will develop. It is a good predictor of the risk of ROP. The injury to retinal blood vessels by free radicals has been hypothesized to be the initiating insult in infants in whom development of ROP is related to severe illness (Rao and Wu, 1996; Sullivan, 1988). Sepsis (Gunn et al, 1980), particularly *Candida* sepsis, has been shown to be associated with increased severity of ROP and the need for laser surgery in premature infants (Mittal et al, 1998). It is not clear, however, if this is an independent risk factor for ROP.

### *Acidosis*

Metabolic acidosis generated by the administration of acetazolamide or ammonium chloride has been shown in studies in neonatal rats to cause preretinal neovascularization (Holmes et al, 1999). The molecular mechanism underlying the pathogenesis of this response is not known. In vitro studies in aortic endothelial cells suggest that acidosis may lead to increased VEGF expression and decreased apoptosis (D'Arcangelo et al, 2000).

### *Transfusions*

Several studies have shown that increases in the number and volume of blood transfusions are associated with an increased risk of developing of ROP (Aranda et al, 1975; Clark et al, 1981; Cooke et al, 1993; Hammer et al, 1986; Hesse et al, 1997; Inder et al, 1997; Sacks et al, 1981). However, it is not clear if the increased frequency of transfusions is indicative of the severity of illness or whether the increase directly contributes to the development of ROP. There are conflicting views on whether injury is caused by anemia or by oxidative stress from iron overload. Another hypothesis that has not been evaluated is whether transfusion of adult blood leads to an increase in retinal $Po_2$ by increased release of $O_2$ from adult hemoglobin. In contrast to the aforementioned studies, Brooks and colleagues (1999) in a randomized, prospective, masked trial in 50 patients found no association between the hematocrit and incidence or severity of ROP.

### *Light*

Lighting in the intensive care nursery has been suggested by some investigators as a potential cause of ROP and has been the subject of much debate (Glass et al, 1985; Terry, 1943). The Light Reduction in Retinopathy of Prematurity (LIGHT-ROP) trial was the first multicenter, prospective randomized study that assessed the incidence of ROP in infants who weighed less than 1250 g and were exposed to either reduced light (399 lux) or normal lighting conditions (447 lux). The incidence rates of ROP in this study were similar in both groups (Reynolds et al, 1998). A meta-analysis of five randomized trials that studied the effect of reduction of light exposure in premature infants at less than 7 days of age concluded that there was no decrease in the incidence or severity of ROP in response to light reduction (Phelps and Watts, 2000).

Other factors such as magnesium, copper, and selenium deficiencies (Caddell, 1995; Papp et al, 1993); increased incidence of chronic lung disease (Biglan et al, 1984); intraventricular hemorrhage (Brown et al, 1987; Procianoy et al, 1981); and twin gestation (Blumenfield et al, 1998) have been implicated as risk factors for ROP. The use of antenatal steroids has been suggested as being beneficial in decreasing the incidence of ROP (Higgins et al, 1998). A meta-analysis of 15 trials that analyzed the effect of early postnatal corticosteroid use in preterm infants concluded that there was no difference in the incidence of severe ROP between treated and untreated patients (Halliday and Ehrenkranz, 2001). However, late use of steroids later than 3 weeks of age has been associated with an increase in severity of ROP (Halliday and Ehrenkranz, 2001). Similar studies in the mouse model of retinopathy have suggested that the timing of steroid use may be critical to the effect on the retinal vasculature (Yossuck et al, 2000).

## Screening for ROP

In order to maximize diagnosis of ROP without subjecting patients at low risk for ROP to an eye examination, the American Academy of Pediatrics, American Association for Pediatric Ophthalmology and Strabismus, and American Academy of Ophthalmology recommend screening all infants born either at a weight of less than 1500 g or at less than 28 weeks of gestation, as well as selected infants between 1500 and 2000 g with an unstable clinical course who are therefore at risk for ROP (Screening examination, 2001). Wright and colleagues (1998), in a study of 700 infants, found that limiting screening of infants to those with a gestational age of less than 28 weeks can potentially miss the diagnosis of severe ROP in several infants. Because ROP in all infants irrespective of their gestational age is rarely seen before 34 to 36 weeks of gestation, it is recommended that infants be screened when they are physiologically stable between 4 and 6 weeks of age or within 31 to 33 weeks of postconceptional age, whichever comes later. Subhani and associates (2001) have recommended screening infants born at less than 25 weeks of gestation at 4 to 6 weeks of chronologic age, because infants of younger gestational ages can present with ROP on their first examination. Infants should undergo at least two examinations, unless the first examination shows complete retinal vascularization. A diagnosis of threshold ROP should be followed by treatment within 72 hours. A few centers are investigating the use of a new digital wide-field camera system (RetCam 120) for taking digitized images of the infant's retina and transferring the images by telemetry for reading by an experienced ophthalmologist (Roth et al, 2001; Schwartz et al, 2000; Yen et al, 2000). The examination, which involves the use of an indirect ophthalmoscope, a lid speculum, and dilating drops, is repeated every 2 weeks or weekly in the presence of prethreshold disease until discharge. The reader is encouraged to review the recent screening guidelines published by the American Academy of Pediatrics regarding timing of repeat examinations and the recommendations for ensuring timely diagnosis and treatment of ROP (Screening examination, 2001). Because the procedure could be stressful, the infant should be clinically stable at the time of examination. Parents should be informed about the diagnosis when it is first made and be given subsequent updates with following examinations.

### Staging and Classification

In 1981 ophthalmologists from eleven countries came together to adopt a uniform method of classifying ROP to enable assessment of efficacy of various modes of treatment. This led to the development of the International Classification of Retinopathy of Prematurity (ICROP) (International Classification, 1984). This classification is based on (1) staging of the disease, (2) extent of involvement along the junction of the avascular and vascular portions of the retina, (3) anterior or posterior location of the retinopathy, and (4) presence or absence of "plus disease."

Evidence of stage I disease (Table 101–1) is the earliest sign of ROP; stage I refers to a demarcation line between the vascular and avascular portions of the retina. Stage II disease is associated with the formation of a pink, ridge-like structure between the two regions. In stage III ROP, fine vessels are seen growing from the ridge-like structure into the vitreous. Stage IV is subdivided into IVA, associated with partial detachment not involving the macula, and stage IVB, associated with partial detachment involving the macula. Total retinal detachment is seen in stage V disease. Plus disease, which can be seen at any stage, refers to the presence of dilated and tortuous retinal blood vessels in the posterior pole of the eye. It is a hallmark of rapidly progressive disease.

In order to define the anterior-posterior location of the retinopathy, the retina is divided into three concentric zones. Zone I refers to the posteriormost region around the optic disc and fovea, with a radius of twice the distance from the macula to the optic disc, and is the most critical region for development of visual acuity. Zone II extends from the periphery of zone I to the ora serrata on the nasal side and to approximately the equator on the temporal side. Zone III extends from the outer edge of zone II in a crescentic fashion to the ora serrata. Location of the disease and staging are helpful in predicting the outcome of ROP. The severity of disease is defined by the stage and location of the disease as well as the number of 30-degree sectors of the retina that are involved.

Prethreshold disease is defined as any ROP in zone I, or zone II with stage III, or zone II with plus disease less than threshold, or ROP in zone II, stage III without plus disease. Threshold disease is defined as 5 or more contiguous or 8 cumulative clock hours of ROP stage III in either zone I or zone II in the presence of plus disease.

**TABLE 101–1**

**Staging of Retinopathy of Prematurity**

| Stage of Disease | Features |
|---|---|
| Stage I | Demarcation line between the vascular and avascular portions of the retina |
| Stage II | Ridge-like structure between avascular and vascular |
| Stage III | Fine vessels growing from the ridge into the vitreous |
| Stage IVA | Partial retinal detachment *not* involving the macula |
| Stage IVB | Partial retinal detachment involving the macula |
| Stage V | Total retinal detachment |
| Plus disease | Dilated and tortuous blood vessels in the posterior pole of the eye |

#### *Prediction of Risk for ROP*

Because ROP affects infants to different degrees of severity, a risk model to predict the risk of development of threshold ROP would be a useful tool for clinicians. Identification of such infants may lead to early eye examinations as well as more vigilance with respect to oxygen saturations in these infants. Risk models were developed by Hardy and colleagues (1997) from a 1986 to 1987 cohort of infants with birth weights of less than 1250 g enrolled in the CRYO-ROP trial. The model uses neonatal variables such as birth weight, gestation, gender, race, inborn/outborn status, and single/multiple birth, as well as ROP characteristics to determine the risk for progression to threshold disease for a specific eye.

### Prevention

It is difficult to prevent all cases of ROP without prevention of premature births. Close monitoring of $O_2$ saturations and prevention of repeated episodes of hyperoxia/hypoxia can possibly help decrease the incidence of severe ROP. Implementation of strict guidelines for monitoring $O_2$ saturation and prevention of repeated episodes of hypoxia that are treated with supplemental $O_2$ have been reported to reduce the incidence of ROP (Chow et al, 2001). Although bilirubin is presumed to be an antioxidant and free radical injury is hypothesized to cause ROP, there is no relationship between the incidence of ROP and hyperbilirubinemia (DeJonge et al, 1999).

Vitamin E is an antioxidant that was first reported in 1949 by Owens and Owens to have a promising effect against ROP in a group of premature infants (Owens and Owens, 1949). Lipid peroxidation has been hypothesized to be one of the mechanisms of injury that incites development of ROP. Preterm infants are relatively deficient in vitamin E (Haga et al, 1982). Of the several studies conducted to study the effect of vitamin E supplementation, only Hittner and associates (1981) demonstrated a statistically significant beneficial effect of therapy. Raju and colleagues (1997) conducted a meta-analysis of six randomized trials of vitamin E prophylaxis designed to reduce ROP. In all of these trials, vitamin E levels were above the physiologic range in the treated group and below the physiologic range in the control group. Although there was a 52% reduction in severe or stage III ROP in the treated group in comparison with the control group, there was no reduction in the incidence of ROP (Raju et al, 1997). Vitamin E use has been associated in at least two trials with an increase in incidence of necrotizing enterocolitis and sepsis (Finer et al, 1984; Johnson et al, 1985). The data indicate that the use of pharmacologic doses of vitamin E is not completely safe in newborns (Committee on Fetus and Newborn, 1985).

Gaynon and associates (1997), using a combined approach of administering supplemental $O_2$ to maintain $O_2$ saturations at 99% to 100% with exposure to ambient light in infants diagnosed with prethreshold ROP, have reported a reduction in conversion to threshold ROP and the subsequent need for laser surgery.

### Outcome

Much information about the natural history of ROP was obtained from follow-up studies of control infants who were enrolled in the multicenter CRYO-ROP trial (Cryotherapy for Retinopathy of Prematurity Cooperative Group, 1994; Schaffer et al, 1993). This randomized, blinded trial was conducted in 23 centers and included 4099 infants with birth weights of less than 1250 g who were born between January 1986 and November 1987. It was designed to evaluate the risks and benefits of transscleral cryotherapy and to describe the incidence and natural history of ROP. The "natural history" group was comprised of infants with all stages of ROP (65.8%) who did not get randomized to receive cryotherapy. The timing of appearance of ROP was at a later chronologic age but same postconceptional age (Cryotherapy for Retinopathy of Prematurity Cooperative Group, 1988) in infants of lower gestational age. ROP was found to regress in 80% of cases, with a gradual movement of the vascular shunt to the periphery (Cryotherapy for Retinopathy of Prematurity Cooperative Group, 1988). In a study of 766 infants in the "natural history" group with at least 1 clock hour of ROP between stages I and III, the mean age at regression was 38.6 weeks. ROP had involuted in 90% of infants before 44 weeks of postconceptional age (Repka et al, 2000).

Two hundred and forty-five (6%) infants developed threshold disease and were randomized to either receive cryotherapy or no treatment. Threshold ROP developed at a mean postconceptional age of 37.7 weeks, with a range of 31.9 to 50.4 weeks.

Eyes with no ROP and in which vascularization had progressed only into zone I before 35 weeks of gestation had a 1 in 3 chance of developing threshold ROP, in comparison with eyes in which vascularization had progressed into zone II. An unfavorable structural outcome was seen in infants with plus disease, zone I ROP, increased severity of ROP, increased circumferential involvement, and rapid progression from prethreshold to threshold disease.

Premature infants as a group are more likely to develop motility problems such as myopia, amblyopia, strabismus, anisometropia, and nystagmus than are full-term infants (Laws, 1992; Phelps, 1997; Quinn et al, 1992, 1998; Robinson et al, 1993). All of these problems are even more likely in premature infants with any stage of ROP. Severity of refractive errors, motility problems, and poor vision increase with increased severity of ROP (Kushner, 1982; Repka et al, 1998). Other long-term complications of ROP include distortion of the retina from contraction and dragging by scar tissue as well as acute angle glaucoma in patients with stage V disease (Michael et al, 1991; Pollard, 1980). A history of ROP predisposes the patient to late-onset detachment or retinal tears in late childhood or early adulthood. Repka and colleagues (1998), in a follow-up study of infants enrolled in the CRYO-ROP trial, found that infants with ROP required a larger number of ophthalmic interventions (0.9 per child) when compared with infants with no ROP (0.4 per child). Although no guidelines exist regarding ophthalmology examinations after discharge in premature infants, it is recommended that given the increased incidence of visual problems in premature infants, all premature infants be seen by an ophthalmologist at 1 year of age (Holmstrom et al, 1999). Infants with a history of ROP should be seen earlier, depending on the degree of ROP, and then at least yearly during childhood. A longitudinal follow-up study of premature infants enrolled in the CRYO-ROP trial showed that the severity of ROP was predictive of a poorer neurodevelopmental outcome at 5.5 years of age (Msall et al, 2000). Thus, the long-term costs of ROP are not limited to ablative surgery but involve a societal loss related to possible blindness, as well as an increased burden on parents of these infants.

### Treatment

Treatment of threshold ROP is largely surgical, although there may be a role for supplemental $O_2$ in the treatment of infants with prethreshold ROP (Mills, 2000). Surgical treatment is recommended for infants with threshold disease, the stage at which the chance that the disease will regress spontaneously is 50%. Cryosurgery and laser photocoagulation, the latter becoming more universal, are the modalities of treatment. Both of these methods involve ablation of the peripheral avascular retina, with the goal of arresting the progression of the disease by decreasing release of VEGF and other angiogenic factors from the hypoxic retina; thus, central vision is preserved at the expense of peripheral vision.

Although surgical treatment had been used in several countries as early as the 1970s, it was difficult to compare results across centers because of the small size of patient populations, as well as the absence of screening criteria until the 1980s.

Cryosurgery involves cauterization of the hypoxic avascular retina by application of a very cold probe several times to the outer surface of the eye above the avascular retina. Results at the 3-month follow-up examination of patients enrolled in the CRYO-ROP trial showed a 39.5% reduction in unfavorable anatomic outcome in treated eyes, in comparison with control eyes ($P < .00001$). Fifty-one percent of the control eyes, versus 31.1% of the treated eyes, had an unfavorable outcome (Cryotherapy for Retinopathy of Prematurity Cooperative Group, 1988). At 1 year after treatment, anatomic results were unfavorable in 26% of eyes that received cryotherapy versus 47% of eyes that did not. Functional outcome at 1 year was better in 56% of treated eyes, compared with 35% of control eyes. There was also a reduction in the incidence of total retinal detachment from 43% in the untreated eye to 21% in the treated eye as well as in the occurrence of posterior retinal folds involving the macula (Cryotherapy for Retinopathy of Prematurity Cooperative Group, 1990).

Visual acuity testing performed at the 5.5-year follow-up examination showed a 47% versus 62% rate of unfavorable visual acuity and a 27% versus 45% rate of unfavorable anatomic outcome in the treated and control groups, respectively; of the treated eyes, 32% were blind, in comparison with 48% of the control eyes (Cryotherapy for Retinopathy of Prematurity Cooperative Group, 1996). The incidence of cataracts also was lower in treated eyes. At 5.5 years, however, fewer treated eyes had a visual acuity of 20/40 (13% versus 17%), and the treated eyes had a higher chance of developing more severe myopia.

Results of the follow-up visual acuity testing at 10 years were more reassuring, with a decrease in the incidence of blindness and detachment in treated eyes and no difference between the two groups with respect to attaining a visual acuity of 20/40 (Cryotherapy for Retinopathy of Prematurity Multicenter Trial, 2001). Although the results of cryosurgery demonstrate a beneficial effect, the results are far from perfect, especially for disease in zone I. Approximately 25.7% cases had an unfavorable outcome. Andersen and Phelps (2000) reviewed the results of all trials of peripheral ablation of the retina for threshold ROP in premature infants. Peripheral retinal ablation reduced the risk of early unfavorable retinal structure from 47.9% to 26.3% and the risk of unfavorable visual acuity in early childhood from 63% to 50.6%. Visual fields in sighted eyes were slightly smaller in the pretreated group than in the control group. Complications from cryotherapy included vitreous hemorrhage, swelling of eyelids and conjunctivae, and increased intraocular pressure. In addition, the long-term effects of cauterization of the peripheral retina in infants are not known.

Laser photocoagulation therapy using newer, indirect laser delivery systems is now becoming the standard of treatment for advanced ROP (Connolly et al, 1998; Iverson et al, 1991; McNamara et al, 1991). The laser beam in this method is applied directly to retinal tissue, and because it does not pass through the entire thickness of the eye, it produces less tissue destruction and inflammation than occurs with cryotherapy. It is less painful, thereby decreasing the need for narcotics or anesthesia. Although no study as large as the CRYO-ROP trial has been conducted to compare the effects of laser with those of cryosurgery, several smaller studies have been done. McNamara and colleagues (1991) reported regression of ROP in 15 of 16 infants who received laser treatment versus 9 of 12 infants who received cryosurgical treatment. The Laser ROP Study Group (1994) conducted a meta-analysis of four trials comparing the results of cryotherapy with those of laser therapy. The investigators concluded that laser therapy is at least as effective as cryotherapy in reducing vision loss from threshold ROP.

The Early Treatment of Retinopathy of Prematurity (ETROP) was a multicenter randomized trial that compared the safety and efficacy of earlier versus conventionally timed ablation of the peripheral retina for the management of severe ROP (Early Treatment for Retinopathy of Prematurity Cooperative Group, 2003). It is hypothesized that because most of the problems associated with ROP occur in association with development of stage III disease, early treatment in carefully selected cases of infants weighing less than 1250 g may result in improved visual acuity. Infants enrolled in the trial were randomized to early treatment if they had prethreshold ROP with a 15% or greater risk of an unfavorable problem as determined by a modification of the risk analysis program described by Hardy and associates (1997). The results of this trial showed that visual acuity and structural outcome at 9 months were significantly better in the early treatment group. Thus, peripheral retinal ablation should be considered for any eye with:

- Zone I, any stage ROP with plus disease
- Zone I, stage 3 ROP without plus disease
- Zone II, stage 2 or 3 ROP with plus disease

Scleral buckling, a procedure that involves placement of a silicone band around the eye in order to reduce tension exerted by the vitreous on the scar tissue, is done in cases in which cryosurgery or laser surgery is ineffective (Chuang et al, 2000). Vitrectomy is performed in other cases of complete retinal detachment due to scar tissue (Quinn et al, 1996; Repka et al, 1998). However, the effectiveness of these procedures in preserving vision is poor at this time (Quinn et al, 1996).

### Role of Supplemental Oxygen Therapy

The rationale for the Supplemental Therapeutic $O_2$ for Prevention of ROP (STOP-ROP) study was based on results from studies performed in kittens with ROP (STOP-ROP Multicenter Study Group, 2000). Use of supplemental $O_2$ in the recovery period after exposure to hyperoxia produced a less severe degree of neovascularization in these animals (Phelps, 1984; Phelps and Rosenbaum, 1988). In addition, a few clinical case reports from the 1950s indicated an improvement in severe ROP in infants who received supplemental $O_2$ (Bedrossian et al, 1955; Szewczyk, 1953). A clinical case series reported a benefit of supplemental $O_2$ in decreasing conversion to threshold ROP (Gaynon et al, 1997). The STOP-ROP trial tested the hypothesis that administration of supplemental $O_2$ to infants with prethreshold ROP to maintain their $O_2$ saturations at 96% to 99% versus 88% to 94% would lead to a decrease in the proportion of infants with at least one eye at prethreshold who converted to threshold ROP. Infants whose $O_2$ saturations were 88% to 94% in room air were excluded from the study. Although there was a trend toward a decrease in conversion in supplemented infants (48.5% versus 40.9%), the results did not show a statistically significant difference. A statistically significant improvement (46% versus 32%) was, however, noted in a small group of infants with no plus disease. One of the surprising findings of the study was that supplemented infants tended to have more episodes of exacerbation of chronic lung disease (8.5% versus 13.2%), although there were no ill effects on the eye.

The High $O_2$ Percent in ROP (HOPE-ROP) study was designed to determine the risk of progression of prethreshold to threshold disease in infants who were excluded from the STOP-ROP study because their $O_2$ saturations were greater than 94% (McLead et al, 2000). HOPE-ROP patients progressed to threshold ROP in at least one study eye 25% of the time, compared with 46% in STOP-ROP patients. This difference was less evident in cases with plus disease.

### Antiangiogenic Agents

Pharmacologic agents that inhibit angiogenesis without destroying retinal tissue could provide newer modes of treatment of retinopathy. Because angiogenesis is a complex process, with the involvement of various growth factors and extracellular molecules, interference with progression of the disease can be achieved in several ways. Although many agents are currently undergoing trials in adult patients with neovascularization, there have been no studies in infants. One of the problems with this approach is identifying an agent that selectively destroys abnormal blood vessels without affecting the process of normal vascularization of the immature retina. Thrombospondin-1, a tumor suppressor agent and an extracellular matrix glycoprotein, has been shown to have antiangiogenic activity in a rat model of retinopathy without affecting normal intraretinal blood vessel growth (Shafiee et al, 2000). Penn and colleagues (2001) have shown anecortave acetate, an angiostatic steroid, to be effective in inhibiting angiogenesis in a neonatal rat model of retinopathy without affecting the normal retinal vasculature. Lonchampt and associates (2001), in a mouse model of retinopathy, have shown a significant decrease in angiogenesis in animals treated with perindopril (angiotensin-converting enzyme inhibitor) or angiotensin $AT_2$ receptor inhibitor (losartan) during the hyperoxic phase. Recombinant angiostatin has been used to decrease neovascularization in the mouse model of retinopathy (Meneses et al, 2001). Antiangiogenic agents hold promise for a less invasive method of treating this debilitating disease in the future

### Summary

ROP is a neovascularizing disease that affects premature and LBW newborns. It has a multifactorial etiology and is not completely preventable. There may be a role for supplemental $O_2$ in the treatment of milder forms of prethreshold disease and possibly a role for selective antiangiogenic drugs in the future. Cryosurgery or laser surgery is currently recommended for threshold disease, but the outcome is not perfect. Future trends in this area will involve changing the method and timing of treatment. An increased understanding of the molecular mechanisms underlying retinal vascular development is essential to developing better methods of prevention of ROP.

## EPIDEMIOLOGY OF VISION IMPAIRMENT IN CHILDREN

Vision impairment occurs with conditions that cause *bilateral* loss of vision. Because most of these cases occur in the perinatal period, it is appropriate to consider them in this section. Very few studies have been performed to evaluate the incidence of vision impairment in the western world, and it is also difficult to know whether there are substantial changes in the spectrum of conditions that cause vision impairment. Nevertheless, some trends can be gleaned from studies that have monitored vision impairment in children (Steinkuller et al, 1999). The incidence of vision impairment in children varies from region to region, and is economics driven. In developed regions, the incidence may be as low as 0.1/10,000, but in underserved regions of the world, the number is higher, at 1.1/10,000 (Gilbert et al, 1999).

The most common cause of vision impairment in most studies is cortical visual impairment (CVI) (Steinkuller et al, 1999). Bilateral damage to the optic radiations (e.g., periventricular leukomalacia) (Jacobson et al, 1998) or bilateral damage to the visual cortex will cause CVI. The term probably should be reserved for children who cannot see clearly—that is, have lost visual acuity (Good et al, 2001). Causes include perinatal hypoxia-ischemia, infections, infarctions, metabolic disorders, and trauma (Good et al, 1994).

Retinopathy of prematurity remains an important and leading cause of vision impairment in children (see later). The exact incidence in a modern (i.e., the past 5 years) cohort is probably unknown, although baseline data from the LIGHT-ROP study suggest that the incidence and rate of blindness have not changed from the 1980s (Reynolds et al, 1998). The Early Treatment for Retinopathy of Prematurity study will include a natural history component, and it is hoped that useful incidence data will come from this study (Good and Hardy, 2001).

Optic nerve hypoplasia, a developmental disorder of optic nerve growth and function, ranks third, followed by retinal disease (e.g., albinism). Congenital cataract, formerly a leading cause of blindness in children, is less common, owing to advances in diagnosis and management.

### Visual Development

A considerable amount of visual development occurs postnatally, with some visual functions showing improvement even as late as 12 years of age. There is more to vision than simply Snellen acuity (the ability to see small letters or numbers projected on a screen or chart). Contrast sensitivity, stereopsis (high-grade depth perception), grating acuity (ability to see finely spaced lines), and Vernier acuity (ability to judge when lines are not perfectly positioned on top of each other) are examples of visual functions that develop independently and at different rates. Different cortical mechanisms could subserve these different types of vision.

Stereopsis and contrast sensitivity probably develop to near-maturity in the first several months of life. Grating acuity is mature to half that of an adult by approximately 1 year of age, and Snellen acuity develops up to the age of 4 or 5, at which time it is near adult normal levels. Therefore, a majority of children do not have normal Snellen acuity until the age of 5. Vernier acuity develops into adolescence, a fact that makes it interesting to study in various visual disorders (Skoczenski and Norcia, 1999).

Amblyopia is loss of vision in the absence of any underlying ocular disease. At least three types of amblyopia exist, although recent evidence suggests that many overlapping varieties of amblyopia may be possible (Schor et al, 1997). Occlusion or form deprivation amblyopia, strabismic amblyopia, and anisometropic amblyopia (unequal refractive errors in the two eyes) affect visual acuity by allowing or causing lack of use of one of the visual pathways. In the neonate, occlusion amblyopia is a critical concern and must be diagnosed and treated as soon as possible. Prolonged visual development notwithstanding, diseases that involve blocking of the visual axis will permanently damage vision within 6 months of birth. Examples include corneal opacities, congenital cataracts, and complete ptosis. Prompt surgical management of these conditions is important when the visual axis is threatened. Delays in treatment affect acuity outcome such that even 20/400 visual acuity is usually impossible if treatment is rendered after 1 year of age (Birch and Stager, 1996; Birch et al, 1998).

### Physical Examination

The physical examination of the newborn should concentrate on one ophthalmologic feature: the red reflex. Ophthalmologists will perform dilated examinations when disease is suspected or in premature infants screened for retinopathy of prematurity. Conditions such as ptosis and nasolacrimal duct obstruction are easily identified. The use of the ophthalmoscope to determine that a clear visual axis is present is crucial.

Conditions that may cause leukocoria include cataracts, retinoblastoma, corneal opacity, Coats disease, detached retina due to ROP and other retinal diseases, and other, rare conditions. The neonatologist's and pediatrician's roles are to identify whether a possible problem exists and, if it does, to make a prompt referral.

Misalignment of the visual axes in the neonate, discussed next, usually is not a cause for concern in the several months following birth. Exceptions to this rule occur with suspected cranial nerve palsy (third or sixth cranial nerve). Third nerve palsy is suspected when ptosis occurs and is accompanied by deficient elevation, depression, and adduction of the eye. In many cases, the affected eye will be positioned lower (down) and abducted (out) compared with the fellow eye. Exceptions exist when third nerve palsies occur without ptosis, or without other features of motility dysfunction (Good et al, 1991).

## Congenital Disorders of Motility

### Nystagmus

Congenital nystagmus may be present at or shortly after birth, or the condition may not be noticed until 2 to 3 months of age. It is characterized by rhythmic movements of the eye or eyes occurring horizontally, vertically, or elliptically (Hertle and Dell'Osso, 1999).

Conditions that cause bilateral anterior visual pathway disease may lead to any sort of nystagmus in the first year of life. Vertical, horizontal, and elliptical nystagmic movements all have been reported. The fact that nystagmus in visually impaired childen is seldom seen in cortical blindness (termed *cortical* or *cerebral visual impairment* in children) is a helpful distinguishing feature (Good and Hoyt, 1989). Conditions that cause nystagmus include bilateral optic nerve hypoplasia, untreated congenital cataracts, and bilateral retinal detachments, occasionally seen in ROP.

Bilateral nystagmus will occasionally occur in monocular disease (Good et al, 1997), although this is not the rule. Monocular nystagmus, or dissociated nystagmus can result from monocular anterior visual pathway disease (Good et al, 1993). However, monocular or dissociated nystagmus occasionally heralds a lesion of the optic chiasm (glioma, craniopharyngioma) and should prompt a neuroimaging evaluation (Gittinger, 1988; Schulman et al, 1979). The exact incidence of glioma of the visual pathways as a cause of dissociated nystagmus is unknown, however, and some evidence suggests that gliomas may be uncommon in children with dissociated nystagmus (Arnoldi and Tychsen, 1995).

In some children with nystagmus, the anterior pathways are normal. In most of these, "motor" nystagmus is diagnosed. Genetics of this condition can be determined in some children (Kerrison et al, 1996, 1999). Again, nystagmus may be vertical, horizontal, or elliptical. Visual acuity in motor nystagmus ranges from 20/25 to 20/400 and remains stable throughout life.

Transient nystagmus can also occur in infants and may take on any waveform. Follow-up evaluation of children who had transient nystagmus shows no increased risk for central nervous system (CNS) abnormalities. There are no characteristics of transient nystagmus that identify it as such.

Periventricular leukomalacia will occasionally cause nystagmus, as will other significant diseases of the CNS (e.g., Pelizaeus-Merzbacher disease) (Jacobson and Dutton, 2000; Jacobson et al, 1998). When the etiology of nystagmus cannot otherwise be determined, a neurologic evaluation and neuroimaging investigation are warranted.

### Strabismus and Transient Motility Disorders

Newborn infants are likely to show a number of transient ocular motor signs that in older patients would indicate serious neurologic disease but that in infants are normal. Examples are skew deviations, tonic downward or upward deviation of the eyes (Ahn et al, 1989; Deonna et al, 1990; Ouvrier and Billson, 1988), and strabismus (Hoyt et al, 1980).

The significance of tonic upward deviation of the eyes, especially when it persists beyond a few months of age, has been reappraised, with some evidence that the sign may indicate more global neurologic dysfunction (Hayman et al, 1998).

Tonic downward eye deviation is not caused by serious neurologic disease, but clinicians should be careful to exclude the possibility that a child has hydrocephalus and paralysis of upgaze: the so-called setting sun sign (Chattha and Delong, 1975). With upgaze paralysis, the child exhibits the physical finding of eyes rotated down, with considerable sclera showing between the iris and upper eyelid. Periaqueductal disease probably is responsible for this important neuro-ophthalmologic finding.

Strabismus as a transient ocular motor finding also has been the subject of considerable interest and debate. Infantile esotropia and constant exotropia as abnormal findings become apparent after 2 to 4 months of age.

Before then, such strabismus-type findings are of no prognostic significance (Archer et al, 1989).

On the other hand, certain strabismus problems are characteristic and apparent at birth and persist. Cranial nerve palsies may be congenital and cause characteristic features of third, fourth, or sixth cranial nerve palsy. Fourth cranial nerve abnormalities may not become apparent until the infant gains head control, at which time a head tilt is used to adapt to the problem. Strabismus in these cases is noncomitant (i.e., changes with different directions of gaze). In the case of Möbius syndrome, a large-angle esotropia is accompanied by bilateral gaze palsies and facial paralysis.

Defects or diseases involving extraocular muscles also may cause persistent strabismus. Congenital fibrosis of the extraocular muscles will cause a large-angle hypotropia on the affected side, or esotropia that is noncomitant. As a general rule, neurologic evaluation is recommended in cases of congenital cranial nerve palsy, with the exception of isolated fourth nerve palsies.

### Nasolacrimal Duct Obstruction

Nasolacrimal duct obstruction has its onset between 2 and 6 weeks of age and is characterized by a nearly constant epiphora (tearing) and by thickened discharge from one or both eyes. The cause is an obstruction anywhere in the lacrimal system. In most children, obstruction occurs as an isolated event, although nasolacrimal duct obstruction is more common in Down syndrome (Markowitz et al, 1994), the ectodermal dysplasia–ectodactyly–clefting syndrome (EEC), and in any condition that may cause craniofacial defects (Fielding and Fryer, 1992).

In most cases the condition resolves by 6 months of age, and by 12 months of age more than 90% of cases have cleared (Paul and Shepherd, 1994). Conservative treatment with massage and topical antibiotics may help alleviate symptoms. After 8 months of age, or earlier if symptoms are severe, probing the obstructed nasolacrimal duct may be warranted.

Congenital dacryocele (Fig. 101–1) occurs when an outpouching of the lacrimal sac develops. Usually an underlying nasolacrimal duct obstruction has played a role in preventing flow of amniotic fluid or tears (postnatally). Infection can occur, resulting in dacryocystitis. The differential diagnosis should rule out anterior encephalocele, usually easily distinguished by accompanying mild telecanthus and pulsations and its location medial to the lacrimal system.

Management includes vigorous massage, probing, and, in cases in which infection is superimposed, systemic antibiotics.

## Structural Defects of the Eye

### Congenital Cataracts

Cataracts in infants occur at a frequency of approximately 2.2 per 10,000 births, with most cases presenting in the first year of life (Wirth et al, 2002). Fewer than 20% of cases are associated with a known systemic abnormality (Wirth et al, 2002). Diagnosis is based on identification of an abnormal red reflex (Fig. 101–2).

Cataracts can be classified according to morphologic appearance. Transient cataracts are known to occur and are identified by their peripheral location in the lens (McCormick, 1968).

A very long list of genetic, metabolic, and hereditary problems that may cause cataracts have been identified, but identifiable systemic causes only occasionally account for congenital cataracts (Wirth et al, 2002). When an infant is identified with a cataracts, associated abnormalities are almost always obvious, so that a lengthy workup usually is not necessary. Causes include infectious diseases, particularly rubella, metabolic disorders (e.g., galactosemia), hereditary cataracts, and trauma. Trauma is a common cause of cataracts in children, especially boys, after the age of 5, but is a very uncommon cause in those younger than 1 year.

Congenital cataracts in children is associated with a high risk for glaucoma, although this risk may be tempered somewhat by the use of an artifical intraocular lens, positioned at the time of cataract removal (Asrani et al, 2000; Parks et al, 1993). The risk for glaucoma probably lasts for decades, with glaucoma developing many years after initial surgery in some children.

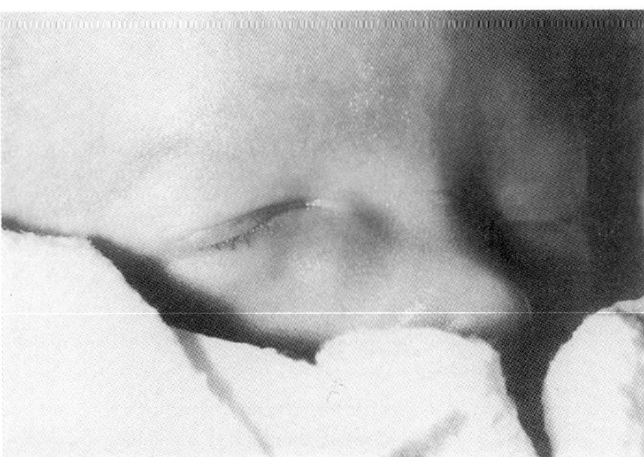

**FIGURE 101–1.** (See also Color Plate 101–1.) One-week-old infant with dacryocele. Note the bump in the area of the medial canthus.

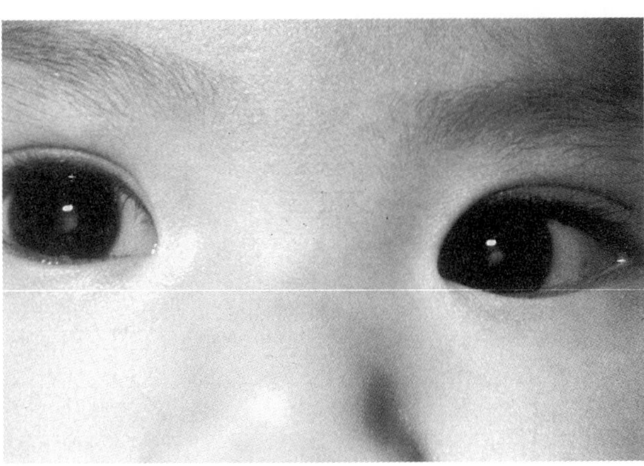

**FIGURE 101–2.** Infant with bilateral total cataracts. Note the leukocoria.

Treatment of congenital cataract usually involves surgical removal, with or without the use of an intraocular lens. Surprisingly, bilateral cases of cataract have a better prognosis than those associated with unilateral cases. In bilateral cases the prognosis for reasonable visual acuity development is good, unless diagnosis is late, or the child's eye has other ocular abnormalities (Gelbart et al, 1982). Following cataract removal, ongoing follow-up evaluation is required to treat amblyopia, strabismus, or other ocular problems that may develop (e.g., glaucoma).

### Retinoblastoma

One of the many causes of leukocoria in the newborn is retinoblastoma. This rare tumor affects 1 in 20,000 newborn children and occurs in two forms: hereditary and sporadic. Approximately 50% of cases are inherited and are due to a mutation in the *RB1* gene in the child's germ line. In most instances, inherited retinoblastoma is identified by the presence of multiple tumors, in either one or both eyes. Still, 15% of children with unilateral retinoblastoma have the inherited type, and there is a family history of retinoblastoma in only 25% (Jay et al, 1988). In unilateral cases a mutation occurs in both alleles of the *RB1* gene in a primitive somatic cell. The result is a unilateral, solitary tumor.

Retinoblastoma manifests as leukocoria in 56% of cases, followed by strabismus (20%), glaucoma (7%), and poor vision (5%). A screening examination will detect retinoblastoma in close relatives of children in whom the inherited version is present (Ellsworth, 1969). In retinoblastoma manifesting as strabismus, the affect eye is strabismic and sees poorly due to involvement of the macula.

Management includes investigation for metastases in cases in which the tumor is large. Bone marrow aspiration and lumbar puncture should be performed but may not be necessary in new cases, or with small tumors (Mohney and Robertson, 1994). After the initial evaluation, treatment may take any of several forms. Enucleation should be considered in cases of large tumors, particularly where no useful vision could be expected with local or systemic therapy. External beam irradiation is effective but can cause significant side effects, including cosmetic changes to the growing orbital bones around the eye, dry eye, cataracts, and secondary tumors in the radiation field, particularly in children with germline mutations. Chemotherapy with or without focal therapy (cryosurgery or laser applied directly to the tumor) also is used. The systemic chemotherapy often will shrink the tumor so that it is more amenable to local therapy (Gallie et al, 1992). The cure rate for retinoblastoma is 90%.

### Glaucoma

Congenital glaucoma has a nearly uniform presentation, no matter the etiology. Elevated intraocular pressure causes tearing, photophobia, enlargement of the eye (buphthalmos), and redness. Many of these signs are due to ruptures in Descemet's membrane of the cornea, as a result of elevated intraocular pressure. The cornea often appears cloudy as a result of penetration of the normally dessicated corneal stroma by intraocular fluid.

Considerations in the differential diagnosis of cloudy cornea at birth include congenital hereditary endothelial dystrophy, a rare disorder of corneal endothelial cells, and corneal infection. Neither of these conditions causes elevated intraocular pressure.

Etiologic associations include recessive inheritance and certain syndromes. The phakomatoses, Sturge-Weber syndrome and neurofibromatosis, are associated with glaucoma. Rubenstein-Taybi syndrome (Roy et al, 1968) also is commonly associated with glaucoma. Treatment is usually surgical and includes goniotomy, trabeculectomy, or other filtration surgery. Long-term follow-up evaluation is important, as in many children with glaucoma, amblyopia and refractive errors develop, even when intraocular pressure is controlled.

## Infections of the Eye

### Conjunctivitis of the Newborn

The term *conjunctivitis of the newborn* has replaced "ophthalmia neonatorum" to describe infections of the conjunctiva occurring in the first few weeks after birth (Chandler, 1989). The timing of onset may be helpful in establishing the infectious etiology, but clinical features are nonspecific. Discharge, which may be mucopurulent, and redness of the bulbar and palpebral conjunctiva are the prominent findings.

One possible exception to this rule, that physical findings are generic, occurs in gonococcal conjunctivitis, which may produce a marked purulent discharge. This type of conjunctivitis must always be carefully excluded with Gram stain and culture, because the organism has a tendency to cause keratitis and blindness from the ensuing corneal opacification. Treatment consists of a third-generation cephalosporin for 7 days, particularly in geographic areas where the organism is penicillin resistant.

Chlamydial infections occur in newborn children at a rate of 3/1000 (Schachter, 1978). Diagnosis is important, not only to prevent complications of the conjunctivitis but because the eye infection also may be accompanied by pneumonia. Pneumonia in children occurs in the first 6 weeks of life. Treatment for *Chlamydia* infection should be systemic, with erythromycin. Topical erythromycin or tetracycline also may be helpful, but neither does anything to prevent or treat concurrent pulmonary infections.

A variety of other pathogens also may cause conjunctivitis in infants, the most common of which is *Staphylococcus aureus* (Dannevig et al, 1992; Zanoni et al, 1992). Two percent silver nitrate was the mainstay of prophylaxis against neonatal conjunctivitis for more than a century, but topical erythromycin and tetracycline also are very effective, although perhaps less effective against *Chlamydia*.

### Coloboma of the Eye

A coloboma is a developmental gap that occurs as a result of failure of the fetal fissure or choroidal fissure to close. The defect is found in the inferonasal quadrant of the eye. Areas of the iris, lens, and choroid and retina may be affected, and the end result is a characteristic cleft, sometimes visible without instrumentation (Fig. 101–3).

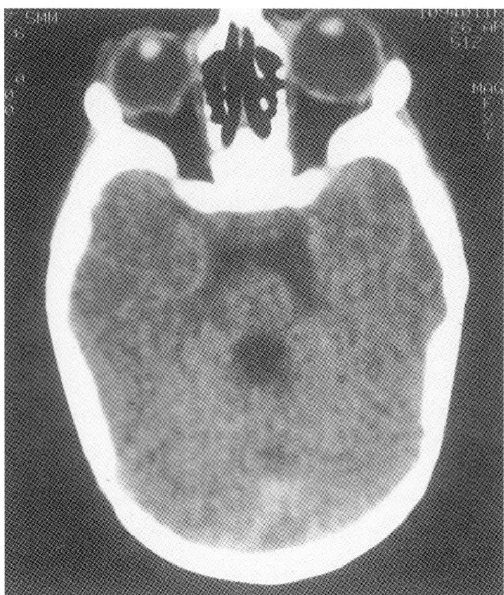

**FIGURE 101–3.** Chorioretinal coloboma.

A number of neurologic conditions can cause or be associated with colobomata, particularly CHARGE (*c*oloboma, *h*eart disease, choanal *a*tresia, *r*etarded growth/development and/or CNS anomalies, *g*enital hypoplasia, *e*ar anomalies and/or deafness) syndrome, Meckel syndrome, and linear sebaceous nevus syndrome (Onwochei et al, 2000; Pagon, 1981). The list of genetic causes is lengthy and includes trisomies 13, 18, and 22, but not trisomy 21 (Onwochei et al, 2000). Many cases are sporadic, or the defect is inherited as an autosomal dominant condition without additional systemic or neurologic abnormalities.

Diagnosis of coloboma is based on characteristic findings (see Fig. 101–3), although a careful ophthalmoscopic examination may be required to identify presence or absence in the retina. Coloboma with cyst, wherein an orbital cyst extension of the coloboma occurs, is simply an extreme manifestation of coloboma. Microphthalmia commonly accompanies severe cases of coloboma.

No treatment exists for this coloboma, although an investigation for associated anomalies and genetic tendencies is always indicated. Colobomata may be asymptomatic but may also be large enough to involve the optic disc or macula. With such involvement, visual acuity will be diminished. With bilateral colobomata of the macula, nystagmus develops and may be accompanied by an adaptation by the infant termed *overlooking*. Children literally look above objects of visual interest in order to position uninvolved areas of retina on a visual target (Good et al, 1992).

## REFERENCES

Adamis AP, Miller JW, Bernal MT, et al: Increased vascular endothelial growth factor levels in the vitreous of eyes with proliferative diabetic retinopathy. Am J Ophthalmol 118:445-450, 1994.

Adamis AP, Shima DT, Tolentino MJ, et al: Inhibition of vascular endothelial growth factor prevents retinal ischemia-associated iris neovascularization in a nonhuman primate. Arch Ophthalmol 114:66-71, 1996.

Ahn JC, Hoyt WF, Hoyt CS: Tonic upgaze in infancy. A report of three cases. Arch Ophthalmol 107:57-58, 1989.

Aiello LP, Pierce EA, Foley ED, et al: Suppression of retinal neovascularization in vivo by inhibition of vascular endothelial growth factor (VEGF) using soluble VEGF-receptor chimeric proteins. Proc Natl Acad Sci U S A 92:10457-10461, 1995.

Alon T, Hemo I, Itin A, et al: Vascular endothelial growth factor acts as a survival factor for newly formed retinal vessels and has implications for retinopathy of prematurity. Nat Med 1:1024-1028, 1995.

Andersen CC, Phelps DL: Peripheral retinal ablation for threshold retinopathy of prematurity in preterm infants. Cochrane Database Syst Rev(2):CD001693, 2000, Review.

Andrews A, Balciunaite E, Leong FL, et al: Platelet-derived growth factor plays a key role in proliferative vitreoretinopathy. Invest Ophthalmol Vis Sci 40:2683-2689, 1999.

Aranda JV, Clark TE, Maniello R, et al: Blood transfusion: Possible potentiating risk factor in retrolental fibroplasias. Pediatr Res 9:362, 1975.

Archer SM, Sondhi N, Helveston EM: Strabismus in infancy. Ophthalmology 96:133-137, 1989.

Arnoldi KA, Tychsen L: Prevalence of intracranial lesions in children initially diagnosed with disconjugate nystagmus (spasmus nutans). J Pediatr Ophthalmol Strabismus 32:296-301, 1995.

Ashton N: Animal experiments in retrolental fibroplasias. Trans Am Acad Ophthalmol Otolaryngeal 58:51-54, 1954.

Ashton N: Oxygen and the growth and development of retinal vessels. In vivo and in vitro studies. The XX Francis I. Proctor Lecture. Am J Ophthalmol 62:412-435, 1966.

Ashton N: Retinal angiogenesis in the human embryo. Br Med Bull 26:103-106, 1970.

Askie LM, Henderson-Smart DJ: Early versus late discontinuation of oxygen in preterm or low birth weight infants. Cochrane Database Syst Rev 2, 2000.

Askie LM, Henderson-Smart DJ: Gradual versus abrupt discontinuation of oxygen in preterm or low birth weight infants. Cochrane Database Syst Rev 4, 2001.

Asrani S, Freedman S, Hasselblad V, et al: Does primary intraocular lens implantation prevent "aphakic" glaucoma in children? J AAPOS 4:33-39, 2000.

Ausprunk DH, Folkman J: Migration and proliferation of endothelial cells in preformed and newly formed blood vessels during tumor angiogenesis. Microvasc Res 14:53-65, 1977.

Avery ME, Oppenheimer EH: Recent increase in mortality from hyaline membrane disease. J Pediatr 57:553-559, 1960.

Bancalari E, Flynn J, Goldberg RN, et al: Influence of transcutaneous oxygen monitoring on the incidence of retinopathy of prematurity. Pediatrics 79:663-669, 1987.

Bauer Cr, Widmayer SM: A relationship between $Pa\text{CO}_2$ and retrolental fibroplasia (RLF). Pediatr Res 15:649, 1981.

Bedrossian RH, Carmichael P, Ritter J: Effects of oxygen weaning in retrolental fibroplasias. Arch Ophthalmol 53:514-518, 1955.

Biglan AW, Brown DR, Reynolds JD, et al: Risk factors associated with retrolental fibroplasia. Ophthalmology 91:1504-1511, 1984.

Birch EE, Stager D, Leffler J, Weakley D: Early treatment of congenital unilateral cataract minimizes unequal competition. Invest Ophthalmol Vis Sci 39:1560-1566, 1998.

Birch EE, Stager DR: The critical period for surgical treatment of dense congenital unilateral cataract. Invest Ophthalmol Vis Sci 37:1532-1538, 1996.

Blumenfeld LC, Siatkowski RM, Johnson RA, et al: Retinopathy of prematurity in multiple-gestation pregnancies. Am J Ophthalmol 125:197-203, 1998.

Brockhurst RJ, Chishti MI: Cicatricial retrolental fibroplasia: Its occurrence without oxygen administration and in full term infants. Albrecht Von Graefes Arch Klin Exp Ophthalmol 195:113-128, 1975.

Brooks SE, Gu X, Samuel S, et al: Reduced severity of oxygen-induced retinopathy in eNOS-deficient mice. Invest Ophthalmol Vis Sci 42:222-228, 2001.

Brooks SE, Marcus DM, Gillis D, et al: The effect of blood transfusion protocol on retinopathy of prematurity: A prospective, randomized study. Pediatrics 104:514-518, 1999.

Brown BA, Thach AB, Song JC, et al: Retinopathy of prematurity: Evaluation of risk factors. Int Ophthalmol 22:279-283, 1998.

Brown DR, Milley JR, Ripepi UJ, et al: Retinopathy of prematurity: Risk factors in a five-year cohort of critically ill premature neonates. Am J Dis Child 141:154-160, 1987.

Bullard SR, Donahue SP, Feman SS, et al: The decreasing incidence and severity of retinopathy of prematurity. J AAPOS 3: 46-52, 1999.

Caddell JL: Hypothesis: The possible role of magnesium and copper deficiency in retinopathy of prematurity. Magnes Res 8:261-270, 1995.

Campbell K: Intensive oxygen therapy as a possible cause of retrolental fibroplasias: A clinical approach. Med J Aust 2: 48-54, 1951.

Chandler JW: Controversies in ocular prophylaxis of newborns. Arch Ophthalmol 107:814-815, 1989.

Chan-Ling T, Gock B, Stone J: The effect of oxygen on vasoformative cell division: Evidence that "physiological hypoxia" is the stimulus for normal retinal vasculogenesis. Invest Ophthalmol Vis Sci 36:1201-1214, 1995.

Chan-Ling T, Stone J: Retinopathy of prematurity: Origins in the architecture of the retina. Prog Retinal Res 12:155-177, 1993.

Chan-Ling TL, Halasz P, Stone J: Development of retinal vasculature in the cat: Processes and mechanisms. Curr Eye Res 9:459-478, 1990.

Chattha AS, Delong GR: Sylvian aqueduct syndrome as a sign of acute obstructive hydrocephalus in children. J Neurol Neurosurg Psychiatry 38:288-296, 1975.

Chow LC, Wright KW, Sola A: CSMC Oxygen Administration Study Group. Can changes in clinical practice decrease the incidence of severe retinopathy in extremely low birth weight infants? Pediatrics III:339-345, 2003.

Chuang YC, Yang CM: Scleral buckling for stage 4 retinopathy of prematurity. Ophthalmic Surg Lasers 31:374-379, 2000.

Clark C, Gibbs JA, Maniello R, et al: Blood transfusion: A possible risk factor in retrolental fibroplasia. Acta Paediatr Scand 70:537-539, 1981.

Coats DK, Paysse EA, Steinkuller PG: Threshold retinopathy of prematurity in neonates less than 25 weeks' estimated gestational age. J AAPOS 4:183-185, 2000.

Committee for the Classification of Retinopathy of Prematurity: An international classification of retinopathy of prematurity. Arch Ophthalmol 102:1130-1134, 1984.

Committee on Fetus and Newborn: Vitamin E and the prevention of retinopathy of prematurity. Pediatrics 76:315-316, 1985.

Connolly BP, McNamara JA, Sharma S, et al: A comparison of laser photocoagulation with trans-scleral cryotherapy in the treatment of threshold retinopathy of prematurity. Ophthalmology 105:1628-1631, 1998.

Cooke RW, Clark D, Hickey-Dwyer M, et al: The apparent role of blood transfusions in the development of retinopathy of prematurity. Eur J Pediatr 152:833-836, 1993.

Cross KW: Cost of preventing retrolental fibroplasia? Lancet 2:954-956, 1973.

Cryotherapy for Retinopathy of Prematurity Cooperative Group: Multicenter trial of cryotherapy for retinopathy of prematurity: Preliminary results. Arch Ophthalmol 106:471-479, 1988.

Cryotherapy for Retinopathy of Prematurity Cooperative Group: Multicenter of cryotherapy for retinopathy of prematurity: One year outcome—structure and function. Arch Ophthalmol 108: 1408-1416, 1990.

Cryotherapy for Retinopathy of Prematurity Cooperative Group: Multicenter trial of cryotherapy for retinopathy of prematurity: Snellen visual acuity and structural outcome at $5^1/_2$ years after randomization. Arch Ophthalmol 114:417-424, 1996.

Cryotherapy for Retinopathy of Prematurity Cooperative Group: The natural ocular outcome of premature birth and retinopathy: Status at 1 year. Arch Ophthalmol 112:903-912, 1994.

Cryotherapy for Retinopathy of Prematurity Multicenter Trial: Ophthalmological outcomes at 10 years. Arch Ophthalmol 119:1110-1118, 2001.

Cunningham S, McColm JR, Wade J, et al: A novel model of retinopathy of prematurity simulating preterm oxygen variability in the rat. Invest Ophthalmol Vis Sci 41:4275-4280, 2000.

D'Amore PA: Mechanisms of retinal and choroidal neovascularization. Invest Ophthalmol Vis Sci 35:3974-3979, 1994.

Dannevig L, Straume B, Melby K: Ophthalmia neonatorum in northern Norway. II. Microbiology with emphasis on *Chlamydia trachomatis*. Acta Ophthalmol (Copenh) 70:19-25, 1992.

D'Arcangelo D, Facchiano F, Barlucchi LM, et al: Acidosis inhibits endothelial cell apoptosis and function and induces basic fibroblast growth factor and vascular endothelial growth factor expression. Circ Res 86:312-318, 2000.

DeJonge MH, Khuntia A, Maisels MJ, et al: Bilirubin levels and severe retinopathy of prematurity in infants with estimated gestational ages of 23 to 26 weeks. J Pediatr 135:102-104, 1999.

Deonna T, Roulet E, Meyer HV: Benign paroxysmal tonic upgaze of childhood—a new syndrome. Neuropediatrics 21:213-214, 1990.

Dollery CT, Bulpitt CJ, Kohner EM: Oxygen supply to the retina from the retinal and choroidal circulations at normal and increased arterial oxygen tensions. Invest Ophthalmol 8:588-594, 1969.

Dreher B, Robinson SR: Development of the retinofugal pathway in birds and mammals: Evidence for a common "timetable." Brain Behav Evol 31:369-390, 1988.

Ellsworth RM: The practical management of retinoblastoma. Trans Am Ophthalmol Soc 67:462-534, 1969.

Fielding DW, Fryer AE: Recurrence of orbital cysts in the branchio-oculo-facial syndrome. J Med Genet 29:430-431, 1992.

Finer NN, Peters KL, Hayek Z, et al: Vitamin E and necrotizing enterocolitis. Pediatrics 73:387-393, 1984.

Flynn JT, Bancalari E, Bawol R, et al: Retinopathy of prematurity: A randomized, prospective trial of transcutaneous oxygen monitoring. Ophthalmology 94:630-638, 1987.

Folkman J: Seminars in Medicine of the Beth Israel Hospital, Boston. Clinical applications of research on angiogenesis. N Engl J Med 333:1757-1763, 1995.

Forsythe JA, Jiang BH, Iyer NV, et al: Activation of vascular endothelial growth factor gene transcription by hypoxia-inducible factor 1. Mol Cell Biol 16:4604-4613, 1996.

Gallie BL, Dunn JM, Hamel PA, et al: How do retinoblastoma tumours form? Eye 6:226-231, 1992.

Gallo JE, Jacobson L, Broberger U: Perinatal factors associated with retinopathy of prematurity. Acta Paediatr 82:829-834, 1993.

Gariano RF, Iruela-Arispe ML, Hendrickson AE: Vascular development in primate retina: Comparison of laminar plexus formation in monkey and human. Invest Ophthalmol Vis Sci 35:3442-3455, 1994.

Gaynon MW, Stevenson DK, Sunshine P, et al: Supplemental oxygen may decrease progression of prethreshold disease to threshold retinopathy of prematurity. J Perinatol 17:434-438, 1997.

Gelbart SS, Hoyt CS, Jastrebski G, et al: Long-term visual results in bilateral congenital cataracts. Am J Ophthalmol 93:615-621, 1982.

Gilbert CE, Anderton L, Dandona L, et al: Prevalence of visual impairment in children: A review of available data. Ophthalmic Epidemiol 6:73-82, 1999.

Gittinger JW Jr: To image or not to image. Surv Ophthalmol 32:350-356, 1988.
Glass P, Avery GB, Subramanian KN, et al: Effect of bright light in the hospital nursery on the incidence of retinopathy of prematurity. N Engl J Med 313:401-404, 1985.
Good WV, Barkovich AJ, Nickel BL, et al: Bilateral congenital oculomotor nerve palsy in a child with brain anomalies. Am J Ophthalmol 111:555-558, 1991.
Good WV, Crain LS, Quint RD, et al: Overlooking: A sign of bilateral central scotomata in children. Dev Med Child Neurol 34:69-73, 1992.
Good W, Hou C, Carden SM: Transient, idiopathic nystagmus in infants. Dev Med ChildNeurol 45:304-307, 2003.
Good WV, Hoyt CS: Behavioral correlates of poor vision in children. Int Ophthalmol Clin 29:57-60, 1989.
Good WV, Jan JE, De Sa L, et al: Cortical visual impairment in children. Surv Ophthalmol 38:351-364, 1994.
Good WV, Jan JE, Hoyt CS, et al: Monocular vision loss can cause bilateral nystagmus in young children. Dev Med Child Neurol 39: 421-424, 1997.
Good WV, Jan JE, Burden SK, et al: Recent advances in cortical visual impairment. Dev MedChild Neurol 43:56-60, 2001.
Good WV, Koch TS, Jan JE: Monocular nystagmus caused by unilateral anterior visual-pathway disease. Dev Med Child Neurol 35:1106-1110, 1993.
Gross JL, Moscatelli D, Jaffe EA, et al: Plasminogen activator and collagenase production by cultured capillary endothelial cells. J Cell Biol 95:974-981, 1982.
Gunn TR, Easdown J, Outerbridge EW, et al: Risk factors in retrolental fibroplasia. Pediatrics 65:1096-1100, 1980.
Guy LP, Lanman JT, Dancis J: The possibility of total elimination of retrolental fibroplasias by oxygen restriction. Pediatrics 17:247-251, 1956.
Hack M, Friedman H, Fanaroff AA: Outcomes of extremely low birth weight infants. Pediatrics 98:931-937, 1996.
Hackett SF, Ozaki H, Strauss RW, et al: Angiopoietin 2 expression in the retina: Upregulation during physiologic and pathologic neovascularization. J Cell Physiol 184:275-284, 2000.
Haga P, Ek J, Kran S: Plasma tocopherol levels and vitamin E/beta-lipoprotein relationships during pregnancy and in cord blood. Am J Clin Nutr 36:1200-1204, 1982.
Halliday HL, Ehrenkranz RA: Delayed (>3 weeks) postnatal corticosteroids for chronic lung disease in preterm infants. Cochrane Database Syst Rev 2, 2001.
Hammer ME, Mullen PW, Ferguson JG, et al: Logistic analysis of risk factors in acute retinopathy of prematurity. Am J Ophthalmol 102:1-6, 1986.
Hangai M, Miyamoto K, Hiroi K, et al: Roles of constitutive nitric oxide synthase in postischemic rat retina. Invest Ophthalmol Vis Sci 40:450-458, 1999.
Hardy P, Dumont I, Bhattacharya M, et al: Oxidants, nitric oxide and prostanoids in the developing ocular vasculature: A basis for ischemic retinopathy. Cardiovasc Res 47:489-509, 2000.
Hardy RJ, Palmer EA, Schaffer DB, et al: Outcome-based management of retinopathy of prematurity. Multicenter Trial of Cryotherapy for Retinopathy of Prematurity Cooperative Group. J AAPOS 1:46-54, 1997.
Hayman M, Harvey AS, Hopkins IJ, et al: Paroxysmal tonic upgaze: A reappraisal of outcome. AnnNeurol 43:514-520, 1998.
Hertle RW, Dell'Osso LF: Clinical and ocular motor analysis of congenital nystagmus in infancy. J AAPOS 3:70-79, 1999.
Hesse L, Eberl W, Schlaud M, et al: Blood transfusion: Iron load and retinopathy of prematurity. Eur J Pediatr 156:465-470, 1997.
Higgins RD, Mendelsohn AL, DeFeo MJ, et al: Antenatal dexamethasone and decreased severity of retinopathy of prematurity. Arch Ophthalmol 116:601-605, 1998.
Hittner HM, Godio LB, Rudolph AJ, et al: Retrolental fibroplasia: Efficacy of vitamin E in a double-blind clinical study of preterm infants. N Engl J Med 305:1365-1371, 1981.
Holmes JM, Leske DA, Zhang S: The effect of raised inspired carbon dioxide on normal retinal vascular development in the neonatal rat. Curr Eye Res 16:78-81, 1997.
Holmes JM, Zhang S, Leske DA, et al: Metabolic acidosis–induced retinopathy in the neonatal rat. Invest Ophthalmol Vis Sci 40:804-809, 1999.
Holmstrom G, el Azazi M, Kugelberg U: Ophthalmological follow up of preterm infants: A population based, prospective study of visual acuity and strabismus. Br J Ophthalmol 83:143-150, 1999.
Hoyt CS, Mousel DK, Weber AA: Transient supranuclear disturbances of gaze in healthy neonates. Am J Ophthalmol 89:708-713, 1980.
Hughes S, Yang H, Chan-Ling T: Vascularization of the human fetal retina: Roles of vasculogenesis and angiogenesis. Invest Ophthalmol Vis Sci 41:1217-1228, 2000.
Hunter DG, Mukai S: Retinopathy of prematurity: Pathogenesis, diagnosis, and treatment. Int Ophthalmol Clin 32:163-184, 1992.
Hussain N, Clive J, Bhandari V: Current incidence of retinopathy of prematurity, 1989-1997. Pediatrics 104:e26, 1999.
Inder TE, Clemett RS, Austin NC, et al: High iron status in very low birth weight infants is associated with an increased risk of retinopathy of prematurity. J Pediatr 131:541-544, 1997.
Ishida S, Shinoda K, Kawashima S, et al: Coexpression of VEGF receptors VEGF-R2 and neuropilin-1 in proliferative diabetic retinopathy. Invest Ophthalmol Vis Sci 41:1649-1656, 2000.
Iverson DA, Trese MT, Orgel IK, et al: Laser photocoagulation for threshold retinopathy of prematurity. Arch Ophthalmol 109:1342-1343, 1991.
Jacobson LK, Dutton GN: Periventricular leukomalacia: An important cause of visual and ocular motility dysfunction in children. Surv Ophthalmol 45:1-13, 2000.
Jacobson L, Lundin S, Flodmark O, et al: Periventricular leukomalacia causes visual impairment in preterm children. A study on the aetiologies of visual impairment in a population-based group of preterm children born 1989-95 in the county of Varmland, Sweden. Acta Ophthalmol Scand 76:593-598, 1998.
James S, Lanman JT: History of oxygen therapy and retrolental fibroplasia. Prepared by the American Academy of Pediatrics, Committee on Fetus and Newborn with the collaboration of special consultants. Pediatrics 57:591-642, 1976.
Jay M, Cowell J, Hungerford J: Register of retinoblastoma: Preliminary results. Eye 2:102-105, 1988.
Johns KJ, Johns JA, Feman SS, et al: Retinopathy of prematurity in infants with cyanotic congenital heart disease. Am J Dis Child 145:200-203, 1991.
Johnson L, Bowen FW Jr, Abbasi S, et al: Relationship of prolonged pharmacologic serum levels of vitamin E to incidence of sepsis and necrotizing enterocolitis in infants with birth weight 1,500 grams or less. Pediatrics 75:619-638, 1985.
Kalina RE, Hodson WA, Morgan BC: Retrolental fibroplasia in a cyanotic infant. Pediatrics 50:765-768, 1972.
Keck PJ, Hauser SD, Krivi G, et al: Vascular permeability factor: An endothelial cell mitogen related to PDGF. Science 246:1309-1312, 1989.
Keith CG, Doyle LW: Retinopathy of prematurity in extremely low birth weight infants. Pediatrics 95:42-45, 1995.
Kerrison JB, Arnould VJ, Barmada MM, et al: A gene for autosomal dominant congenital nystagmus localizes to 6p12. Genomics 33:523-526, 1996.
Kerrison JB, Vagefi MR, Barmada MM, et al: Congenital motor nystagmus linked to Xq26-q27. Am J Hum Genet 64:600-607, 1999.
Kinsey VE, Arnold HJ, Kalina RE, et al: $PaO_2$ levels and retrolental fibroplasia: A report of the cooperative study. Pediatrics 60:655-668, 1977.

Kraushar MF, Harper RG, Sia CG: Rentrolental fibroplasia in a full-term infant. Am J Ophthalmol 80:106-108, 1975.

Kretzer FL, Hittner HM: Spindle cells and retinopathy of prematurity: Interpretations and predictions. Birth Defects 24:147-168, 1988.

Kushner BJ: Strabismus and amblyopia associated with regressed retinopathy of prematurity. Arch Ophthalmol 100:256-261, 1982.

Lanman JT: Retrolental fibroplasias and oxygen therapy. JAMA 155:223-226, 1954.

Laser ROP Study Group: Laser therapy for retinopathy of prematurity. Arch Ophthalmol 112:154-156, 1994.

Laws D, Shaw DE, Robinson J, et al: Retinopathy of prematurity: A prospective study: Review at six months. Eye 6:477-483, 1992.

Levy AP, Levy NS, Wegner S, et al: Transcriptional regulation of the rat vascular endothelial growth factor gene by hypoxia. J Biol Chem 270:13333-13340, 1995.

Lonchampt M, Pennel L, Duhault J: Hyperoxia/normoxia-driven retinal angiogenesis in mice: A role for angiotensin II. Invest Ophthalmol Vis Sci 42:429-432, 2001.

Lucey JF, Dangman B: A reexamination of the role of oxygen in retrolental fibroplasia. Pediatrics 73:82-96, 1984.

Lukiw WJ, Gordon WC, Rogaev EI, et al: Presenilin-2 (PS2) expression up-regulation in a model of retinopathy of prematurity and pathoangiogenesis. Neuroreport 12:53-57, 2001.

Mariani G, Cifuentes J, Carlo WA: Randomized trial of permissive hypercapnia in preterm infants. Pediatrics 104:1082-1088, 1999.

Markowitz GD, Handler LF, Katowitz JA: Congenital euryblepharon and nasolacrimal anomalies in a patient with Down syndrome. J Pediatr Ophthalmol Strabismus 31:330-331, 1994.

McCormick AQ: Transient cataracts in premature infants: A new clinical entity. Can J Ophthalmol 3:202-206, 1968.

McDonald AD: Cerebral palsy in children of very low birth weight. Arch Dis Child 38:579-588, 1963.

McLead RE, McGregor ML, Bremer D, et al: The HOPE-ROP study group. Pediatr Res 47:2457a, 2000.

McNamara JA, Tasman W, Brown GC, et al: Laser photocoagulation for stage 3+ retinopathy of prematurity. Ophthalmology 98:576-580, 1991.

Meneses PI, Hajjar KA, Berns KI, et al: Recombinant angiostatin prevents retinal neovascularization in a murine proliferative retinopathy model. Gene Ther 8:646-648, 2001.

Michael AJ, Pesin SR, Katz LJ, et al: Management of late-onset angle-closure glaucoma associated with retinopathy of prematurity. Ophthalmology 98:1093-1098, 1991.

Michaelson IC: The mode of development of the vascular system of the retina: With some observation on its significance for certain diseases. Trans Ophthalmol UK 68:1347-180, 1948.

Miller JW, Adamis AP, Shima DT, et al: Vascular endothelial growth factor/vascular permeability factor is temporally and spatially correlated with ocular angiogenesis in a primate model. Am J Pathol 145:574-584, 1994.

Mills MD: STOP-ROP results suggest selective use of supplemental oxygen for prethreshold ROP. Arch Ophthalmol 118:1121-1122, 2000.

Mittal M, Dhanireddy R, Higgins RD: *Candida* sepsis and association with retinopathy of prematurity. Pediatrics 101:654-657, 1998.

Mohney BG, Robertson DM: Ancillary testing for metastasis in patients with newly diagnosed retinoblastoma. Am J Ophthalmol 118:707-711, 1994.

Moravski CJ, Kelly DJ, Cooper ME, et al: Retinal neovascularization is prevented by blockade of the renin-angiotensin system. Hypertension 36:1099-1104, 2000.

Msall ME, Phelps DL, DiGaudio KM, et al: Severity of neonatal retinopathy of prematurity is predictive of neurodevelopmental functional outcome at age 5.5 years. Behalf of the Cryotherapy for Retinopathy of Prematurity Cooperative Group. Pediatrics 106:998-1005, 2000.

Oh H, Takagi H, Otani A, et al: Selective induction of neuropilin-1 by vascular endothelial growth factor (VEGF): A mechanism contributing to VEGF-induced angiogenesis. Proc Natl Acad Sci U S A 99:383-388, 2002.

Onwochei BC, Simon JW, Bateman JB, et al: Ocular colobomata. Surv Ophthalmol 45:175-194, 2000.

O'Reilly MS, Boehm T, Shing Y, et al: Endostatin: An endogenous inhibitor of angiogenesis and tumor growth. Cell 88: 277-285, 1997.

Ouvrier RA, Billson F: Benign paroxysmal tonic upgaze of childhood. J ChildNeurol 3:177-180, 1988.

Owens WC, Owens EC: Retrolental fibroplasias in premature infants. II. Studies on the prophylaxis of the disease: The use of alpha-tocopherol acetate. Am J Ophthalmol 32:1631-1637, 1949.

Ozaki H, Yu AY, Della N, et al: Hypoxia inducible factor-1α is increased in ischemic retina: Temporal and spatial correlation with VEGF expression. Invest Ophthalmol Vis Sci 40:182-189, 1999.

Pagon RA: Ocular coloboma. Surv Ophthalmol 25:223-236, 1981.

Palmer EA, Flynn JT, Hardy RJ, et al: Incidence and early course of retinopathy of prematurity. The Cryotherapy for Retinopathy of Prematurity Cooperative Group. Ophthalmology 98:1628-1640, 1991.

Papp A, Nemeth I, Pelle Z: [Retrospective biochemical study of the preventive property of antioxidants in retinopathy of prematurity]. Orv Hetil 134:1021-1026, 1993.

Parks MM, Johnson DA, Reed GW: Long-term visual results and complications in children with aphakia: A function of cataract type. Ophthalmology 100:826-40; discussion 840-1, 1993

Patz A, Hoeck LE, De La Cruz E: Studies on the effect of high oxygen administration in retrolental fibroplasias. I. Nursery observations. Am J Ophthalmol 35:1248-1252, 1952.

Paul TO, Shepherd R: Congenital nasolacrimal duct obstruction: Natural history and the timing of optimal intervention. J Pediatr Ophthalmol Strabismus 31:362-367, 1994.

Pe'er J, Shweiki D, Itin A, et al: Hypoxia-induced expression of vascular endothelial growth factor by retinal cells is a common factor in neovascularizing ocular diseases. Lab Invest 72: 638-645, 1995.

Penn JS, Henry MM, Tolman BL: Exposure to alternating hypoxia and hyperoxia causes severe proliferative retinopathy in the newborn rat. Pediatr Res 36:724-731, 1994.

Penn JS, Henry MM, Wall PT, et al: The range of $PaO_2$ variation determines the severity of oxygen-induced retinopathy in newborn rats. Invest Ophthalmol Vis Sci 36:2063-2070, 1995.

Penn JS, Rajaratnam VS, Collier RJ, et al: The effect of an angiostatic steroid on neovascularization in a rat model of retinopathy of prematurity. Invest Ophthalmol Vis Sci 42: 283-290, 2001.

Phelps DL: Myopia of prematurity. Br J Ophthalmol 81:1021, 1997.

Phelps DL: Reduced severity of oxygen-induced retinopathy in kittens recovered in 28% oxygen. Pediatr Res 24:106-109, 1988.

Phelps DL, Rosenbaum AL: Effects of marginal hypoxemia on recovery from oxygen-induced retinopathy in the kitten model. Pediatrics 73:1-6, 1984.

Phelps DL, Watts JL: Early light reduction for preventing retinopathy of prematurity in very low birth weight infants. Cochrane Database Syst Rev 2, 2000.

Pierce EA, Avery RL, Foley ED, et al: Vascular endothelial growth factor/vascular permeability factor expression in a mouse model of retinal neovascularization. Proc Natl Acad Sci U S A 92:905-909, 1995.

Pierce EA, Foley ED, Smith LE: Regulation of vascular endothelial growth factor by oxygen in a model of retinopathy of prematurity. Arch Ophthalmol 114:1219-1228, 1996.

Pollard ZF: Secondary angle-closure glaucoma in cicatricial retrolental fibroplasia. Am J Ophthalmol 89:651-653, 1980.

Procianoy RS, Garcia-Prats JA, Hittner HM, et al: An association between retinopathy of prematurity and intraventricular hemorrhage in very low birth weight infants. Acta Paediatr Scand 70:473-477, 1981.

Quinn GE, Dobson V, Barr CC, et al: Visual acuity of eyes after vitrectomy for retinopathy of prematurity: Follow-up at 5 1/2 years. The Cryotherapy for Retinopathy of Prematurity Cooperative Group. Ophthalmology 103:595-600, 1996.

Quinn GE, Dobson V, Kivlin J, et al: Prevalence of myopia between 3 months and 5 1/2 years in preterm infants with and without retinopathy of prematurity. Cryotherapy for Retinopathy of Prematurity Cooperative Group. Ophthalmology 105:1292-1300, 1998.

Quinn GE, Dobson V, Repka MX, et al: Development of myopia in infants with birth weights less than 1251 grams. The Cryotherapy for Retinopathy of Prematurity Cooperative Group. Ophthalmology 99:329-340, 1992.

Raju TN, Langenberg P, Bhutani V, et al: Vitamin E prophylaxis to reduce retinopathy of prematurity: A reappraisal of published trials. J Pediatr 131:844-850, 1997.

Rao NA, Wu GS: Oxygen free radicals and retinopathy of prematurity. Br J Ophthalmol 80:387, 1996.

Repka MX, Palmer EA, Tung B: Involution of retinopathy of prematurity. Cryotherapy for Retinopathy of Prematurity Cooperative Group. Arch Ophthalmol 118:645-649, 2000.

Repka MX, Summers CG, Palmer EA, et al: The incidence of ophthalmologic interventions in children with birth weights less than 1251 grams. Results through 5 1/2 years. Cryotherapy for Retinopathy of Prematurity Cooperative Group. Ophthalmology 105:1621-1627, 1998.

Revised indications for the treatment of retinopathy of prematurity. Early treatment for ROP cooperative group. Arch Ophthalmol 121:1684-1696, 2003.

Reynolds JD, Hardy RJ, Kennedy KA, et al: Lack of efficacy of light reduction in preventing retinopathy of prematurity. Light Reduction in Retinopathy of Prematurity (LIGHT-ROP) Cooperative Group. N Engl J Med 338:1572-1576, 1998.

Robinson GS, Pierce EA, Rook SL, et al: Oligodeoxynucleotides inhibit retinal neovascularization in a murine model of proliferative retinopathy. Proc Natl Acad Sci U S A 93:4851-4856, 1996.

Robinson R, O'Keefe M: Follow-up study on premature infants with and without retinopathy of prematurity. Br J Ophthalmol 77:91-94, 1993.

Roth DB, Morales D, Feuer WJ, et al: Screening for retinopathy of prematurity employing the Retcam 120: Sensitivity and specificity. Arch Ophthalmol 119:268-272, 2001.

Roy FH, Summitt RL, Hiatt RL, et al: Ocular manifestations of the Rubinstein-Taybi syndrome: Case report and review of the literature. Arch Ophthalmol 79:272-278, 1968.

Sacks LM, Schaffer DB, Anday EK, et al: Retrolental fibroplasia and blood transfusion in very low-birth-weight infants. Pediatrics 68:770-774, 1981.

Saunders RA, Donahue ML, Christmann LM, et al: Racial variation in retinopathy of prematurity. The Cryotherapy for Retinopathy of Prematurity Cooperative Group. Arch Ophthalmol 115:604-608, 1997.

Schachter J: Chlamydial infections [third of three parts]. N Engl J Med 298:540-549, 178.

Schaffer DB, Palmer EA, Plotsky DF, et al: Prognostic factors in the natural course of retinopathy of prematurity. The Cryotherapy for Retinopathy of Prematurity Cooperative Group. Ophthalmology 100:230-237, 1993.

Schor CM, Fusaro RE, Wilson N, et al: Prediction of early-onset esotropia from components of the infantile squint syndrome. Invest Ophthalmol Vis Sci 38:719-740, 1997.

Schulman JA, Shults WT, et al: Monocular vertical nystagmus as an initial sign of chiasmal glioma. Am J Ophthalmol 87:87-90, 1979.

Schwartz SD, Harrison SA, Ferrone PJ, et al: Telemedical evaluation and management of retinopathy of prematurity using a fiberoptic digital fundus camera. Ophthalmology 107:25-28, 2000.

Screening examination of premature infants for retinopathy of prematurity. Pediatrics 108:809-811, 2001.

Seiberth V, Linderkamp O: Risk factors in retinopathy of prematurity: A multivariate statistical analysis. Ophthalmologica 214:131-135, 2000.

Senger DR, Galli SJ, Dvorak AM, et al: Tumor cells secrete a vascular permeability factor that promotes accumulation of ascites fluid. Science 219:983-985, 1983.

Shafiee A, Penn JS, Krutzsch HC, et al: Inhibition of retinal angiogenesis by peptides derived from thrombospondin-1. Invest Ophthalmol Vis Sci 41:2378-2388, 2000.

Shih S, Ju M, Liu N, Smith L: Selective stimulation of VEGFR-1 prevents oxygen-induced retinal vascular degeneration in retinopathy of prematurity. J Clin Invest 112:150-57, 2003

Shohat M, Reisner SH, Krikler R, et al: Retinopathy of prematurity: Incidence and risk factors. Pediatrics 72:159-163, 1983.

Skoczenski AM, Norcia AM: Development of VEP Vernier acuity and grating acuity in human infants. Invest Ophthalmol Vis Sci 40:2411-2417, 1999.

Slobody LB, Wasserman WE: Survey of Clinical Pediatrics. New York, McGraw-Hill, 1963, p 160.

Smith LE, Kopchick JJ, Chen W, et al: Essential role of growth hormone in ischemia-induced retinal neovascularization. Science 276:1706-1709, 1997.

Smith LE, Wesolowski E, McLellan A, et al: Oxygen-induced retinopathy in the mouse. Invest Ophthalmol Vis Sci 35: 101-111, 1994.

Stefani FH, Ehalt H: Non-oxygen induced retinitis proliferans and retinal detachment in full-term infants. Br J Ophthalmol 58:490-513, 1974.

Steinkuller PG, Du L, Gilbert C, et al: Childhood blindness. J AAPOS 3:26-32, 1999.

Stone J, Itin A, Alon T, et al: Development of retinal vasculature is mediated by hypoxia-induced vascular endothelial growth factor (VEGF) expression by neuroglia. J Neurosci 15:4738-4747, 1995.

STOP-ROP Multicenter Study Group: Supplemental Therapeutic Oxygen for Prethreshold Retinopathy of Prematurity (STOP-ROP): A randomized, controlled trial. I: Primary outcomes. Pediatrics 105:295-310, 2000.

Strodtbeck F: Assessment and management of ophthalmic disorders. In Kenner C, Lott JW, Flandermeyer A (eds): Comprehensive Neonatal Nursing: A Physiologic Perspective, 2nd ed. Philadelphia, WB Saunders, 1998, pp 703-712.

Subhani M, Combs A, Weber P, et al: Screening guidelines for retinopathy of prematurity: The need for revision in extremely low birth weight infants. Pediatrics 107:656-659, 2001.

Sullivan JL: Iron, plasma antioxidants, and the "oxygen radical disease of prematurity." Am J Dis Child 142:1341-1344, 1988.

Szewczyk TS: Retrolental fibroplasias and related ocular disease: Classification, etiology and prophylaxis. Am J Ophthalmology 36:1336-1361, 1953.

Terry TL: Extreme prematurity and fibroplastic overgrowth of persistent vascular sheath behind each crystalline lens. Am J Ophthalmol 24:203-204, 1942.

Terry TL: Fibroplastic overgrowth of persistent tunica vasculosa lentis in premature infants: II. Report of cases—clinical aspects. Arch Ophthalmol 29:36-53, 1943.

Tin W, Milligan DW, Pennefather P, et al: Pulse oximetry, severe retinopathy, and outcome at one year in babies of less than 28 weeks gestation. Arch Dis Child Fetal Neonatal Ed 84: F106-F110, 2001.

Tompkins C: A sudden rise in the prevalence of retinopathy of prematurity blindness? Pediatrics 108:526, 2001.

Vohr BR, Msall ME: Neuropsychological and functional outcomes of very low birth weight infants. Semin Perinatol 21:202-220, 1997.

Wirth MG, Russell-Eggitt IM, Craig JE, et al: Aetiology of congenital and paediatric cataract in an Australian population. Br J Ophthalmol 86:782-786, 2002.

Wright K, Anderson ME, Walker E, et al: Should fewer premature infants be screened for retinopathy of prematurity in the managed care era? Pediatrics 102:31-34, 1998.

Yen KG, Hess D, Burke B, et al: The optimum time to employ telephotoscreening to detect retinopathy of prematurity. Trans Am Ophthalmol Soc 98:145-150, 2000.

Yoshida A, Yoshida S, Ishibashi T, et al: Intraocular neovascularization. Histol Histopathol 14:1287-1294, 1999.

Yossuck P, Yan Y, Tadesse M, et al: Dexamethasone and critical effect of timing on retinopathy. Invest Ophthalmol Vis Sci 41:3095-3099, 2000.

Zanoni D, Isenberg SJ, Apt L: A comparison of silver nitrate with erythromycin for prophylaxis against ophthalmia neonatorum. Clin Pediatr (Phila) 31:295-298, 1992.

# PART XXII

# APPENDICES

Editor: CHRISTINE A. GLEASON

## Appendix 1

# Drugs

Robert M. Ward

**Pharmacopeia for the Newborn Period**

Dosages and comments about these drugs are based on experience, consensus among neonatologists, and the limited evidence available from studies in neonates. Other styles of treatment are often acceptable and may be superior to those listed. Newer recommendations about extended interval dosing of gentamicin for premature newborns <35 weeks of gestation have not been included because of limited safety data to date.

**ADMINISTRATION ROUTES:**
**ET**—endotracheal
**IM**—intramuscularly
**IT**—intrathecally or intratracheally
**IV**—intravenously
**PO**—by mouth
**PR**—by rectum
**SC**—subcutaneously
**TOP**—topical

| Drug | Route and Dose | Adverse Effects and Cautions |
|---|---|---|
| Acetaminophen | Loading dose: PO: 24 mg/kg; PR: 30 mg/kg<br>Maintenance: PO: 12 mg/kg; PR: 20 mg/kg; preterm: <32 wk: q12h; 32 wk: q8h; term: q6h | Divide suppositories lengthwise as drug may not be evenly distributed throughout the suppository; high doses, especially with glutathione deficiency from poor nutrition, may cause hepatic necrosis |
| Acetazolamide | IV, PO: 5 mg/kg/dose q6-8h; increase as needed to 25 mg/kg/dose (*temporarily effective*), max dose 55 mg/kg/day | Hyperchloremic metabolic acidosis, hypokalemia, drowsiness, paresthesias |
| Acyclovir | IV, PO: 15 mg/kg/dose q8h IV over 1 hr for neonatal skin, eye, or mouth infections 20 mg/kg/dose q8h IV over 1 hr for neonatal CNS or disseminated infection | Transient renal dysfunction; lengthen dose interval with renal failure |
| Adenosine | Initial: 50 μg/kg/dose IV as rapidly as possible (1-2 sec) followed by saline flush of the line<br>Increase dose by 50 μg/kg/dose IV and repeat every 1-2 min if there is no response and no AV block | Contraindicated in heart transplant patients; higher dosages needed in patients receiving methylxanthines; antidote for severe bradycardia is aminophylline 5-6 mg/kg over 5 min |
| Albumin, 5% | IV: 0.5-1 g/kg slowly | Hypovolemia, heart failure; monitor blood pressure |
| Albuterol | Aerosol: 0.5-1 mg/dose q2-6h<br>PO: 0.1-0.3 mg/kg/dose q6-8h | Tachycardia, arrhythmias, tremor, irritability |
| Amikacin | IM, IV: Postnatal age 0-4 wk, <1200 g: 7.5 mg/kg/dose q18-24h<br>≤1 week, 1200-2000 g: 7.5 mg/kg/dose q12-18h; and >2000 g 10 mg/kg/dose q12h<br>>1 week, 1200-2000 g: 7.5 mg/kg/dose q8-12h; and >2000 g 10 mg/kg/dose q8h | Nephrotoxicity; ototoxicity; blood level monitoring recommended (desirable levels: peak, 10-25 μg/mL; trough, 3-5 μg/mL) |
| Aminophylline | See Theophylline<br>*Day 1*: 0.5-1.0 mg/kg/dose infused over 4-6 hr | See Theophylline |

| Drug | Route and Dose | Adverse Effects and Cautions |
|---|---|---|
| Amiodarone | Loading dose: 5 mg/kg IV over 30-60 min, preferably by central venous catheter<br>Maintenance: infusion: 5-15 μg/kg/min; PO: 5-10 mg/kg/dose q12h | Phlebitis, hypotension, bradycardia, liver enzyme elevations, increased and decreased thyroid function, photosensitivity, optic neuritis, pulmonary fibrosis in adults |
| Amoxicillin | PO: 15 mg/kg/dose q12h; *urinary tract prophylaxis*: often dosed at 5 mg/kg/dose q day | Diarrhea, nausea, vomiting |
| Amoxicillin–clavulanic acid | PO: 15 mg/kg/dose q12h based on amoxicillin component | Diarrhea, nausea, vomiting |
| Amphotericin | *Day 1*: 0.5-1.0 mg/kg/dose infused over 4-6 hr (may start at the maximum dose on day 1 if tolerated); *do not use filters with pore size <1 μm*; 1.5 mg/kg/dose q24h may be used with resistant infections; total dosage: 30-35 mg/kg over 6 wk | Decreased renal potassium reabsorption, anemia, thrombocytopenia, fever, chills, nausea, vomiting |
| Amphotericin B liposome | IV: 1-5 mg/kg/dose q24h over 2 hr; usually start with 1 mg/kg/day and increase to higher dose for more serious infections (e.g., osteomyelitis, meningitis) | Decreased renal potassium reabsorption, anemia, thrombocytopenia, fever, chills, nausea, vomiting |
| Ampicillin | IV: 50-100 mg/kg/dose; if <7 days and <2 kg: q12h; if ≥7 days or >2 kg: q8h<br>Highest dose for meningitis<br>Maintain q12h for 4 wk for <1200 g | Diarrhea, rash, urticaria are rare in infants; candida skin infections |
| Amrinone | Initial: 0.75 mg/kg over 2-3 min; maintenance: 3-5 μg/kg/min | Fluid balance, electrolytes, renal function |
| Ascorbic acid | See Vitamin C (ascorbic acid) | |
| Atropine | IV, IM, ET, SC: 0.01-0.03 mg/kg, repeat q4-6h prn; minimum dose of 0.1 mg | Hyperthermia, tachycardia, urinary retention |
| Bacitracin | TOP: as ointment (500 units/g), q4-8h | |
| Beractant | IT: *for prophylactic treatment*: Give 4 mL/kg as soon as possible; may repeat at 6-hr intervals to a maximum of 4 doses in 48 hr<br>IT: *for rescue treatment*: Give 4 mL/kg as soon as respiratory distress syndrome is diagnosed; may repeat at 6-h intervals to a maximum of 4 doses in 48 hr | May give additional doses if infant still has respiratory distress and needs >30% $FIO_2$ to keep $PAO_2$ >50 mm Hg<br>Administer each dose as 4 doses of 1 mL/kg each, giving each dose over 2-3 sec and turning newborn to a different position after each dose |
| Bethanechol | PO: 0.1-0.2 mg/kg/dose q6-8h or 3 mg/m²/dose q8h 20 min before feeding | Diarrhea, jitteriness, tremors, sleeplessness, bronchoconstriction, increased tracheobronchial secretions |
| Bumetanide | IV, PO: 0.02-0.2 mg/kg/dose q8-12h | Loop diuretic that also acts on proximal tubule; 40 times as potent as furosemide; less ototoxicity than furosemide; hypokalemia, hyponatremia, metabolic alkalosis |
| Caffeine | PO, IV: loading dose: 10 mg/kg; maintenance dose: 2.5 mg/kg/dose q24h (*doses are for the nonsalt form of drug—caffeine base*) | Restlessness, emesis, tachycardia; therapeutic plasma concentration 5-20 μg/mL free base |
| Calcium chloride 10% (27 mg elemental $Ca^{2+}$/mL) | IV: 0.2 mL (9 mg $Ca^{2+}$)/kg/dose for acute hypocalcemia; repeat q10 min | Bradycardia if injected too quickly; necrosis from extravascular leakage |
| Calcium glubionate 6.47% (23 mg elemental $Ca^{2+}$/mL) | PO: *treatment*: 500-1000 mg/kg/day q3-4h; *supplement*: 150 mg/kg/day q3-4h | High osmotic load of syrup may cause diarrhea |
| Calcium gluconate 10% (9.3 mg elemental $Ca^{2+}$/mL) | IV: 1 mL (9 mg $Ca^{2+}$)/kg/dose for acute hypocalcemia; repeat q10 min<br>PO: 3-9 mL/kg/day in 2-4 divided doses (28-84 mg $Ca^{2+}$/kg/day) for chronic use | Bradycardia if injected too quickly; necrosis from extravascular leakage |
| Calcium lactate 13% (130 mg elemental $Ca^{2+}$/g powder) | PO: 0.5 g/kg/day in divided doses q6-8h | Same as for calcium gluconate; gastrointestinal irritation |
| Calfactant (Infasurf) | Initial: IT: 3 mL/kg divided into 2 aliquots repeated up to 3 times q12h | Do not shake or filter; ventilate for at least 30 seconds after dose until infant is stable |

| Drug | Route and Dose | Adverse Effects and Cautions |
|---|---|---|
| Captopril | PO: 0.01-0.05 mg/kg/dose q6-24h; increase dose up to 0.5 mg/kg/dose to control blood pressure | High initial doses may cause hypotension and renal insufficiency |
| Carnitine | IV: 10 mg/kg/day added to parenteral solution when not eating | Monitor serum carnitine concentrations |
| Cefotaxime | IV: 50 mg/kg/dose; <7 days: q12h; >7 days: q8h | Adjust dose for renal impairment |
| Ceftazidime | IV: 30 mg/kg/dose over 30 min; preterm <30 wk up to 4 wk age: q12h; >4 wk: q8h; 30-36 wk up to 2 wk age: q12h; >2 wk: q8h; 37-44 wk up to 1 wk age: q12h; >1 wk: q8h | Phlebitis. Cleared by glomerular filtration; increase dosing interval with renal dysfunction |
| Cefuroxime | IV, IM: 25-50 mg/kg/dose; <7 days: q12h; >7 days: q8h | Rare hypersensitivity reactions in infants; may cross-react with penicillins in older children causing rashes, eosinophilia, granulocytopenia |
| Cephalothin | IV, IM: 20 mg/kg/dose; preterm <7 days: q12h (until 4 wk for <1200 g); >7 days q8h; term: <7 days q8h; >7 days: q6h | Phlebitis, additive nephrotoxicity with gentamicin |
| Chloral hydrate | PO, PR: sedative: 10-30 mg/kg/day divided q6-8h; hypnotic: 50-100 mg/kg as single dose | Tolerance, physical dependence, and addiction may develop with seizures<br>Irritant to skin and mucous membranes; gastritis<br>Metabolism is slower in infants than in adults; metabolite half-life = 27.8 hr in term infants to 39 hr in preterm infants<br>Repeated doses may accumulate metabolites, causing hypotension and renal failure |
| Chlorothiazide | PO: 5-15 mg/kg/dose q12-24h | Hypokalemia; hyponatremia decreases calcium excretion; hyperglycemia |
| Cimetidine | PO, IV: 2.5-5 mg/kg/dose q6h according to gastric pH ≥5 | Decreases drug clearance by hepatic cytochrome P450 |
| Citric acid/sodium citrate | Dose according to degree of metabolic acidosis; each mL is equivalent to 1 mEq $HCO_3$ and contains 1 mEq sodium | Adds sodium and potassium and must be used carefully with renal dysfunction, hyperkalemia or hypernatremia |
| Clindamycin | PO, IV: 5 mg/kg/dose; preterm <1 wk: q12h; preterm >1 week or term <1 wk: q8h; term >1 wk: q6h; maintenance: q12h till 4 wk for <1200 g | Pseudomembranous colitis is rare in newborns; limited experience in newborns, hepatic metabolism |
| Colfosceril palmitate | IT: *for prophylactic treatment*: Give 5 mL/kg as soon as possible; may repeat second and third doses 12 and 24 hr later to those infants remaining on ventilators<br>IT: *for rescue treatment*: Give 5 mL/kg as soon as respiratory distress syndrome diagnosed; may repeat second dose 12 hr later | Administer each dose as 2 doses of 2.5 mL/kg each, giving each dose over 1-2 min; and turning newborn 45 degrees for 30 seconds to the right after the first dose and then similarly to the left after the second dose |
| Corticotropin | IM, IV, SC: 3-5 units/kg/day in 4 divided doses, usual maximum of 30 units/day | Hypertension, immunosuppression, electrolyte imbalance, cataracts, growth retardation, gastrointestinal ulcers or dysfunction |
| Cosyntropin | 40 μg/kg/dose as stimulation test | Check serum cortisol 1-2 hr after dose |
| Cromolyn | Nebulization: 20 mg q6-8h; metered dose inhaler: 2 puffs q6-8h | Bronchoconstriction, nasal congestion; 8%-10% of dose is absorbed from the lung |
| Cyclopentolate 0.2% (may be combined with phenylephrine 1%) | 1-2 drops each eye 10-30 min before examination | Hypertension with concentrations >0.5%; anticholinergic effects including fever, tachycardia, dry mouth, delayed gastric emptying, decreased gastrointestinal motility |
| Desoxycorticosterone acetate (DOCA) see Fludrocortisone | | |

Continued

| Drug | Route and Dose | Adverse Effects and Cautions |
|---|---|---|
| Dexamethasone | IM, IV: *for bronchopulmonary dysplasia*: 0.25 mg/kg/dose q8-12h for 3-7 days; *for severe chronic lung*: 0.05-0.25 mg/kg/dose q12h IV or PO for 3-7 days | Delayed head growth and developmental delay associated with treatment for as little as 3 days; weigh risk and benefit |
| Diazepam | PO, IV, IM: sedative: 0.02-0.3 mg/kg/dose q6-8h; seizure: 0.1-0.2 mg/kg/dose slow IV push | Diluted injection may precipitate; IM absorption is poor; respiratory depression, hypotension |
| Diazoxide | PO: 2-5 mg/kg/dose q8h for inhibition of insulin secretion | Eliminated renally; sodium and fluid retention |
| Dicloxacillin | 4-8 mg/kg/dose (PO) q6h | Diarrhea, abdominal pain, nausea, vomiting; rare pancreatitis; may decrease absorption of ketoconazole and ciprofloxacin; may increase absorption of trimethoprim-sulfamethoxazole and ganciclovir |
| Digoxin | IV: Acute digitalization*<br>Premratures — Loading dose<br><1.5 kg — 10-20 μg/kg<br>1.5-2.5 kg — 20 μg/kg<br>Term newborns — 30 μg/kg<br>Infants (1-12 mo) — 35 μg/kg<br>Maintenance dose: 1/8 loading dose q12h<br>Begin 12 h after last digitalization dose | Risk of arrhythmias is increased during digitalization; IV formulation is twice as concentrated as oral; conduction defects, emesis, ventricular arrhythmias |
| Digoxin immune Fab | IV dose: mg digoxin immune Fab = total body digoxin load × 76<br>Total body digoxin load: mg digoxin elixir ingested × 0.8 or serum digoxin concentration (ng/mL) × 0.0056 × wt (kg) | Binds digoxin in circulation before renal excretion; serum digoxin levels within 6-10 hr of treatment will be falsely high |
| Diphenhydramine | PO: 5 mg/kg/day q6h | Somnolence |
| Diphenylhydantoin | See Phenytoin | |
| Diphtheria antitoxin | IM, IV: 20,000-50,000 units/day for 2-3 successive days | Hypersensitivity reaction |
| Dobutamine | IV: 2-20 μg/kg/min by continuous infusion and titrate to desired effect | Tachycardia, hypotension |
| Dopamine | IV: 2-20 μg/kg/min by continuous infusion and titrate to desired effect | Extravasation may lead to necrosis (phentolamine is an antidote); high dose may constrict renal arteries, but the dose for this effect is uncertain in neonates |
| Edrophonium | *Tensilon test for myasthenia gravis*: SC, IM: 0.2-0.5 mg/kg; IV: preliminary test dose: 0.04 mg slow push; test dose: 0.16 mg/kg (1 min later) | Cardiac arrhythmia, diarrhea, tracheal secretions may require atropine antagonism |
| Enalapril (PO), enalaprilat (IV) | IV enalaprilat: *for hyptertension*: 5-10 μg/kg/dose q8-24h<br>PO enalapril *for CHF*: 0.1 mg/kg/day q day to maximum of 0.5 mg/kg/day | Reduce dose with renal failure; severe hypotension may occur, especially with volume depletion from diuretic treatment |
| Epinephrine | *Resuscitation*: IV, ET—1:10,000: 0.05-0.1 mL/kg q 3-5 min<br>*Hypotension*: 0.01-0.1 μg/kg/min by continuous infusion and titrate to desired effect | Tachycardia, arrhythmia |
| Ergocalciferol | See Vitamin $D_2$ | |
| Erythromycin | PO, IV: 10 mg/kg/dose; <7 days: q12h; >7 days: q8h<br>Eye prophylaxis at birth: ophthalmic ointment 0.5% in each eye | IV administration is painful; may affect theophylline serum levels |
| Erythropoietin | 200-300 units/kg/dose 3-5 times/wk<br>SC: total weekly dose: 600-1400 units/kg/wk; treat 2-6 wk | Neutropenia; cotreat with iron |
| Famotidine | IV: 0.3-0.5 mg/kg/dose q8h<br>PO: 1-2 mg/kg/day q8h | Monitor gastric pH for dosage adjustments |

| Drug | Route and Dose | Adverse Effects and Cautions |
|---|---|---|
| Fentanyl | IV, IM: 1-2 μg/kg/dose, q4-6h prn, increase as needed | 50-100 times the potency of morphine; muscle rigidity ("stiff man syndrome") may occur with rapid dose infusions; treat with muscle relaxants |
| Fibrinogen | IV: 50 mg/kg: repeated prn as determined by clotting time | |
| Fluconazole | IV or PO: loading dose: 12 mg/kg; maintenance: 6 mg/kg/dose<br><30 wk up to 2 wk age: q72h; >2 wk: q48h<br>30-36 wk up to 2 wk age: q48h; >2 wk: q24h<br>37-44 wk up to 1 wk age: q48h; >1 wk: q24h<br>45 wk: q24h | May reduce CYP3A4 metabolism of drugs, including caffeine, theophylline, midazolam; may interfere with metabolism of barbiturates, phenytoin |
| Flucytosine | PO: 20-40 mg/kg q6h | Monitor levels; effective antifungal concentration: 35-70 μg/mL; bone marrow dysfunction: >100 μg/mL; renal dysfunction decreases clearance |
| Fludrocortisone | PO: 0.025-0.2 mg/day | Mineralocorticoid replacement where 0.1 mg of fludrocortisone is equivalent to DOCA 1 mg |
| Folic acid | PO: 50 μg/day for preterm newborns after feeding is established for maintenance; 500 μg/day for therapy | Almost none in goat's milk. Rash is very rare |
| Fosphenytoin | Fosphenytoin doses are expressed as phenytoin equivalents (PE), wherein fosphenytoin 1 mg PE = 1 mg phenytoin<br>IV or IM: loading dose: 15-20 mg/kg given no faster than 0.5 mg/kg/min<br>Maintenance: PO: 4-8 mg/kg/day divided q12h, although dosages as high as 15-20 mg/kg/day may be needed to reach therapeutic levels | Rapid IV infusions may cause bradycardia, hypotension, cardiovascular collapse, arrhythmias<br>Therapeutic serum concentration range is 10-20 μg/mL, although lower levels of 6-14 μg/mL may be appropriate in premature newborns, due to reduced protein binding |
| Furosemide | IM, IV: 0.5-2 mg/kg/dose q12-24h<br>PO: 1-2 mg/kg/dose q12-24h<br>Bioavailability reduced by cor pulmonale; may require higher dosages | Hypokalemia, hyponatremia, hypochloremia; half-life prolonged in premature newborns |
| Gentamicin | IM, IV: postnatal age ≤7 days age: <1000 g and <28 wk 2.5 mg/kg/dose q24h; <1500 g and <34 wk 2.5 mg/kg/dose q18h; >1500 g and >34 wk 2.5 mg/kg/dose q12h >7-28 days age: <1200 g 2.5 mg/kg/dose q18-24h; >28 days <1200 g 2.5 mg/kg/dose q8h; *initial loading dose*: 4 mg/kg for neonates ≤32 wk EGA shortens the time to reach therapeutic concentrations | Blood level monitoring indicated for efficacy; toxicity is rare in newborn (desirable levels: trough, <2 μg/mL to avoid toxicity; peak, 5-10 μg/mL) |
| Gentian violet | TOP (skin): as 1%-2% aqueous solution, bid<br>TOP (oral): as 1% aqueous solution, bid | Stains skin |
| Glucagon | IM, IV: 30-300 μg/kg; may be repeated after 20-30 min | Maximum dose 1 mg; higher doses possibly toxic |
| Granulocyte-stimulating factor | SC: bolus injection, IV infusion over 15-30 minutes, or continuous<br>IV infusion: 5-10 μg/kg once daily for 3 to 17 days. Dilute in 5% dextrose with/without albumin. Do not dilute with saline | Monitor blood neutrophil count. Not considered useful for neutropenia from sepsis or NEC, unless it persists for more than 3 days with absolute neutrophil count <500/μL |
| Heparin | IV: initial dose: 50 units/kg; maintenance dose: 100 units/kg q4h or 20-25 units/kg/hr continuous infusion; titrate doses to $1\frac{1}{2}$-2 times baseline whole blood clotting time or activated partial thromboplastin time | Intractable bleeding (reversible with protamine); heparin half-life: prematures < term < adults |

*Continued*

| Drug | Route and Dose | Adverse Effects and Cautions |
|---|---|---|
| Hepatitis B immune globulin | IM: 0.5 mL within 7 days of birth if mother is hepatitis $B_S$ antigen positive or status is unknown. May be given with hepatitis B vaccine | Local pain and tenderness, thrombocytopenia |
| Hydralazine | PO, IM, IV: 0.1-0.5 mg/kg every 6 hr; increase as needed in 0.1-mg/kg increments up to 4 mg/kg/day | Tachycardia, lupus-like reactions |
| Hydrochlorothiazide | PO: 2.0-4.0 mg/kg/day q12h | Hypercalcemia, hypokalemia, hyperglycemia |
| Hydrocortisone | Hypotension refractory to pressors: 1 mg/kg/dose IV; acute adrenal insufficiency: 0.25 mg/kg/dose q6h IV; physiologic replacement: 0.3 mg/kg/day IM | Treatment of more than 7-10 days requires gradual dosage reduction to avoid adrenal insufficiency; immunosuppression hyperglycemia, growth delay, leukocytosis, gastric irritation |
| Ibuprofen | PO: 4-10 mg/kg/dose q6-8h to a maximum of 40 mg/kg/day | Use cautiously in patients with active bleeding or renal or hepatic dysfunction. Avoid in patients with ductal dependent cardiac malformations |
| Imipenem-Cilastatin | IV: <1.2 kg during first 4 weeks: 20 mg/kg/dose q18-24h; 1.2-2 kg = 20 mg/kg/dose q12h; >2 kg first 7 days after birth: 20 mg/kg/dose q12h; >2 kg older than 7 days: 20 mg/kg/dose q8h | Lengthen dosing interval for reduced renal function. Early report of seizures has not been confirmed in later pediatric trials |
| Immunoglobulin intravenous, human | IV: 400-750 mg/kg/dose infused over 2-6 hr | Pyrogenic reactions, BP changes, tachycardia, necrotizing enterocolitis, volume overload |
| Indomethacin | PO, IV: 0.1-0.2 mg/kg/dose q12-24h 2-7 days; 0.25 mg/kg/dose, >7 days | Transient renal dysfunction, decreased platelet aggregation; infuse over a minimum of 30-60 min to minimize reduction in CNS and mesenteric perfusion. Avoid in patients with ductal dependent cardiac malformations |
| Insulin (Regular) | IV: hyperglycemia infusion dose, 0.01-0.1 unit/kg/h; SC; intermittent dose, 0.1-0.2 unit/kg q6-12h | Hypoglycemia |
| Iron | PO: 2-6 mg/kg/day elemental iron | Avoid with hemochromatosis |
| Isoniazid | PO: 10-15 mg/kg/day, single dose or divided q12h | Newborns do not require pyridoxine supplement; monitor liver function test |
| Isoproterenol | IV: 0.05-0.5 μg/kg/min by infusion | Arrhythmias, systemic vasodilation, tachycardia, hypotension, hypoglycemia |
| Kayexalate | See Sodium polystyrene sulfonate (Kayexalate) | |
| Levothyroxine | IV, PO: starting dose 10 μg/kg/day (round off to nearest 12.5, 25.0, or 37.5 μg to coincide with pill size); increase by 12.5-25 μg/24 hr every 2 weeks to desired effect; max 500 μg/day, IV dose = 50%-75% of oral dose after initiation of therapy | Adjust dosage on 3-6 wk schedule by clinical response and $T_4$, optimal free $T_4$, TSH |
| Lidocaine | IV: 1 mg/kg infused over 5-10 min; may be repeated q 10 min 5 times, prn; infusion dose 10-50 μg/kg/min or 1 mg/kg/hr | Monitoring of blood levels useful (therapeutic range 1-5 μg/mL plasma); dilute for ET administration |
| Lorazepam | IV: 0.05-0.1 mg/kg infused over 2-5 min | Limited data in newborns, preparations may contain benzyl alcohol; dilute |
| Magnesium sulfate | IM, IV: 25-50 mg/kg q4-6h for 3-4 doses prn; use 50% solution IM, 1% solution IV | Hypotension, central nervous system depression; monitor serum concentration; calcium gluconate should be available as an antidote |
| Medium-chain triglyceride (MCT) | PO: 1-8 mL/24 h divided in feedings (7.7 cal/mL) | Diarrhea; aspiration causes lipid pneumonia; may increase blood and CSF MCT levels causing coma with excess dose |
| Meropenem | IV: 20 mg/kg/dose q8-12h | Reduce dosage with reduced renal function. Not well studied in premature neonates, but may be needed for resistant infections |

| Drug | Route and Dose | Adverse Effects and Cautions |
|---|---|---|
| Methadone | PO, IV: 0.05-0.2 mg/kg/dose q12-24h; reduce dose 10%-20% per week according to signs of withdrawal | Ileus, respiratory depression, delayed gastric emptying. Difficult to taper due to long half-life |
| Methyldopa | IV, PO: 2-3 mg/kg q6-8h; increased as needed at 2-day intervals; maximum dosage 12-15 mg/kg/dose | Sedation, fever, false-positive Coombs test, hemolysis; sudden withdrawal of methyldopa may cause rebound hypertension |
| Methylene blue | IV: 1-1.5 mg/kg of 1% solution for methemoglobinemia, infused slowly | Do not use in patients with methemoglobinemia due to G6PD or cyanide poisoning. Do not give subcutaneously due to risk of tissue necrosis |
| Methylprednisolone | IV, IM: 0.1-0.4 mg/kg/dose, q6h | Hydrocortisone preferred for physiologic replacement |
| Metoclopramide | PO, IV: 0.1-0.2 mg/kg/dose q6-8h or prior to each feeding | Dystonic reactions, irritability, diarrhea, decreases glomerular filtration rate in adults. Efficacy for GERD shown at >6 mo |
| Metronidazole | IV or PO: loading dose: 15 mg/kg; maintenance: 7.5 mg/kg; infuse doses over 60 min<br><30 wk up to 4 wk age: q48h; >4 wk: q24h<br>30-36 wk up to 2 wk: q24h; >2 wk: q12h<br>37-44 wk up to 1 wk: q24h; >1 wk: q12h<br>45 wk: q8h | Carcinogenic in rodents, not reported in humans. Prolonged treatment in adults rarely associated with seizures and sensory polyneuropathy |
| Midazolam | IV, IM, intranasal: 0.07-0.20 mg/kg/dose q2-4h prn for sedation; infusion dosing: <33 wk; 30 μg/kg hr; >33 wk; 60 μg/kg hr | Limited experience in newborns; respiratory depression, apnea. Rapid infusion doses (<10 min) may cause tonic clonic movements |
| Morphine sulfate | IV, IM, SC: 0.05-0.1 mg/kg/dose q2-6h prn<br>0.1-0.2 mg/kg/dose PO q3-6h | Respiratory depression reversible with naloxone, local urticaria from histamine release |
| Nafcillin | IV, IM: 25 mg/kg/dose, newborns 0-7 days = q12h, infants >7 days = q6-8h; double dosage for meningitis; maintenance: q12h for 4 wk for <1200 g | Agranulocytosis; granulocytopenia; hepatic dysfunction; may require dosage adjustment |
| Naloxone | IV, IM, SC: 0.1 mg/kg/dose; may be repeated as necessary; delivery room minimum, 0.5 mg for term newborn | Onset of action may be delayed 15+ min after IM or SC administration; narcotic effects may outlast naloxone antagonism; dilute for ET administration |
| Neomycin | PO: 10-25 mg/kg/dose q6h<br>Topical: 0.5% ointment, 3-4 times daily | Renal toxicity and ototoxicity if absorbed |
| Neostigmine | IV: *Test for myasthenia gravis*: 0.02 mg/kg;<br>IM: *Test for myasthenia gravis*: 0.04 mg/kg<br>PO: *Treatment for myasthenia gravis*: 0.33 mg/kg/day q3-6h | Cholinergic crisis. Atropine pretreatment is recommended |
| Nitroprusside | IV: begin in dose of 0.25 μg/kg/min and vary as needed up to 8 μg/kg/min to control blood pressure | Profound hypotension possible; requires arterial line to monitor blood pressure; thiocyanate toxicity with long-term use or renal insufficiency |
| Nystatin | PO: 100,000-200,000 units q6h<br>TOP: as 2% ointment (in petrolatum 95% polyethylene 5%) 3-4 times daily | Poorly absorbed from GI tract; diarrhea |
| Omeprazole | PO: 0.5-1.5 mg/kg/dose q day | Hypergastrinemia, diarrhea, monitor gastric pH |
| Oxacillin | IV, IM: 25 mg/kg/dose<br>Preterm <4 wk old <1200 g: q12h;<br>1200-2000 g q12h for <7 days old;<br>1200-2000 g q8h for 7 days old<br>term 25-40 mg/kg/dose <7 days old: q12h; >7 days old; q6h | Sterile abscess formation after i.m. doses, nephrotoxicity; monitor liver enzymes and complete blood count; colitis |

*Continued*

| Drug | Route and Dose | Adverse Effects and Cautions |
|---|---|---|
| Pancreatin | PO: 2000 units of lipase with each feeding PR and into colostomy: 0.3-0.5 g in sufficient liquid (for meconium ileus) | Bowel stricture associated with excessive dosages |
| Pancuronium | IV: 0.03-0.1 mg/kg/dose q1-4h prn; titrate to age and effect desired | Ensure adequate oxygenation and ventilation; tachycardia, bradycardia, hypotension, hypertension; potentiated by acidosis, hypothermia, neuromuscular disease, aminoglycoside antibiotics |
| Paraldehyde | PR: 0.3 mL/kg q4-6h | Reserve for refractory status epilepticus; local irritation, pulmonary edema, hemorrhage; hepatic dysfunction decreases clearance; avoid IM if possible; do not give by arterial catheter; avoid plastic containers |
| Penicillin G | IV, IM: *sepsis*: 25,000-50,000 units/kg/dose; *meningitis*: 75,000-100,000 units/kg/dose q8-12h: <7 days and q6-8h >7 days; *use higher doses for group B streptococcal infections*. Maintain q12h for 4 wk for <1200 g | Use for susceptible organisms such as streptococci; syphilis |
| Pentobarbital | PO, IM, IV: 2-6 mg/kg prn | Blood level monitoring helpful (sedative level 0.5-3 μg/mL); higher doses may depress respirations and cardiac contractility; monitor blood pressure |
| Phenobarbital | IV, IM, PO: anticonvulsant loading dose: 15-20 mg/kg, may repeat 10 mg/kg/dose twice for status epilepticus; maintenance dose: 3-5 mg/kg/day q12-24h, begin 12-24 h after loading dose: Sedation: 2-3 mg/kg q8-12h prn | Blood level monitoring helpful (therapeutic range 15-40 μg/mL); half-life 40-200 hr in infants, prolonged by asphyxia |
| Phentolamine | SC: dilute to 0.5 mg/mL, inject 0.2 mL at 5 sites around alpha-adrenergic drug infiltration maximum 2.5 mg total dose | Marked hypotension, tachycardia, arrhythmia. Do not treat hypotension with epinephrine, because hypotension may worsen due to alpha-adrenergic blockade |
| Phenytoin | IV: loading dose: 15-20 mg/kg, infused <0.5 mg/kg/min PO, IV: maintenance: 4-8 mg/kg/dose q24h; higher doses q8h >7 days; flush IV tubing with saline before/after dose | Therapeutic blood level monitoring indicated (desirable level 10-20 μg/mL); infant clearance may be high |
| Phosphate, sodium, or potassium | PO: 1-3 mmol/kg/day in divided doses or supplement formula phosphorus intake to 75 mg/kg/day | Large amounts may cause catharsis; increase gradually to full supplementation; monitor electrolytes. Several formulations available |
| Piperacillin | IM, IV: 50-100 mg/kg/dose; ≤29 wk postmenstrual age at 0-4 wk age: q12h; ≤29 wk postmenstrual age >4 wk age: q8h; 30-36 wk postmenstrual age 0-2 wk age: q12h; 30-36 wk postmenstrual age >2 weeks age: q8h; 37-44 wk postmenstrual age 0-1 wk age: q12h; 37-44 wk postmenstrual age >1 wk age: q8h | Elimination is 60%-70% renal, and reduced renal function may require longer dosing intervals |
| Pitressin | See Vasopressin | |
| Plasma | IV: 5-10 mL/kg; repeated prn | Volume overload, viral infection risk |
| Poractant alfa (Curosurf) | IT: 2.5 mL/kg/dose divided into 2 aliquots, followed by 1.25 mL/kg/dose q12h up to twice if needed | Do not filter or shake; suction prior to administration; administer in 2-4 aliquots with positioning of infant to improve distribution within the lungs; ventilate for at least 30 seconds after dose until infant is stable |
| Prednisone | PO: 0.5-2 mg/kg/day, q6h | See Cortisone |

| Drug | Route and Dose | Adverse Effects and Cautions |
|---|---|---|
| Procainamide | IV: 1.5-2.5 mg/kg infused over 10-30 min; may be repeated in 30 min if needed; infusion: 20-60 μg/kg/min<br>PO: 40-60 mg/kg/day q4-6h | Asystole, myocardial depression, anorexia, vomiting, nausea. Blood level monitoring helpful (therapeutic range: procainamide, 3-10 μg/mL; *N*-acetyl procainamide, 10-20 μg/mL) |
| Propranolol | IV: 0.01 mg/kg initial dose and 0.01-0.15 mg/kg infused over 10 min; may be repeated in 10 min and then q6-8h to maximum of 0.15 mg/kg/dose<br>PO: 0.05-2 mg/kg q6h | Relatively contraindicated in low-output congestive heart failure and patients with bronchospasm |
| Propylthiouracil | PO: 2-4 mg/kg q8h; increase to maximum of 10 mg/kg/dose; onset of action may be delayed days to weeks | Dose is uncertain for newborns; monitor thyroid function |
| Prostaglandin $E_1$, alprostodil | IV: 0.03-0.1 μg/kg/min; often, dose may be reduced by ½ after initial response; intra-arterial infusion offers no advantage | Apnea, seizures, fever, disseminated intravascular coagulation, diarrhea, cutaneous vasodilatation, decreased platelet aggregation, cortical bone proliferation during prolonged infusion |
| Protamine sulfate | IV: 1 mg for each 100 units of heparin in previous 30 min; 0.5-0.75 for 30-60 min; and 0.25-0.375 for heparin given >2 hr before | Excessive doses induce coagulopathy; hypotension, bradycardia, anaphylaxis |
| Pyridoxine | See Vitamin $B_6$ (pyridoxine) | |
| Quinidine gluconate | PO, IM: 2-10 mg/kg/dose q2-6h until desired effect or toxicity occurs<br>IV route not recommended in neonates (Dose is specific for the salt form) | Check electrocardiogram before each dose; discontinue if QRS interval increases 50% or more<br>Maintain level of 2-6 μg/mL; nausea, vomiting, diarrhea, fever, atrioventricular block |
| Ranitidine | PO, IV: 1-2 mg/kg q8-12h | Minimal inhibition of hepatic cytochrome P450 enzymes; monitor gastric pH |
| Ribavirin | 6 g nebulized in hood with a solution of 20 mg/mL 12-18 hr/day for 3-7 days | May precipitate in endotracheal tube; avoid exposure of pregnant staff; possible teratogenic effects |
| Silver nitrate (1% solution) | Prophylaxis: 1 or 2 drops in each eye | Chemical conjunctivitis |
| Sodium bicarbonate (0.5 mEq/mL) | IV: 1-2 mEq/kg/dose infused slowly only if infant ventilated adequately | Intravascular hemolysis may be associated with rapid infusion |
| Sodium polystyrene sulfonate (Kayexalate) | PO, PR: 1 g/kg; approximately q6h | Usually administered as a solution with 20% sorbitol to prevent intestinal obstruction; 20% sorbitol solution may injure intestinal mucosa of very low-birth-weight newborns; may decrease serum calcium or magnesium |
| Spironolactone | PO: 1-3 mg/kg/day q8-12h | Contraindicated with hyperkalemia; onset of action delayed; drowsiness; nausea; vomiting; diarrhea; androgenic effects in females; gynecomastia in males |
| Streptomycin | IM: 20-30 mg/kg/day q24h | Nephrotoxicity, ototoxicity; use in newborns as part of triple therapy for tuberculosis |
| Sulfisoxazole | PO, IV: 25 mg/kg q6h; aggressive therapy is used only in full-term neonates >2 weeks old | In prematures or in presence of jaundice, may lead to kernicterus |
| Survanta | See Beractant | |
| Tetanus immune globulin | IM: 250-500 units/dose | Optimal dosage not established for newborns |
| Theophylline | PO, IV: loading dose: 5-6 mg/kg; maintenance dose: 1-2.5 mg/kg/dose q6-12h; aminophylline (IV) dose = theophylline (IV) dose × 1.25 | Blood level monitoring indicated (therapeutic range: *apnea*: 7-12 μg/mL, *bronchospasm*: 10-20 μg/mL); tachycardia at 15-20 μg/mL, seizures at >40 μg/mL; avoid rectal dosing due to variable absorption, clearance decreased by asphyxia and prematurity; tachycardia |

*Continued*

| Drug | Route and Dose | Adverse Effects and Cautions |
|---|---|---|
| Thiamine | See Vitamin $B_1$ (thiamine) | |
| Ticarcillin | IM, IV: 75 mg/kg/dose; <7 days: q12h, >7 days: q8h; maintain q12h for 4 wk for <1200 g | Contains 5.2 mEq $Na^+$/g; may inhibit platelet function |
| Tobramycin | See Gentamicin dosing guidelines | |
| Ursodeoxycholic acid | PO: 10-15 mg/kg/day q8-24h | Nausea, vomiting, abdominal pain, constipation, flatulence |
| Vancomycin | PO: 10 mg/kg, q6h IV: postnatal age ≤7 days: <1200 g: 15 mg/kg/day q24h; 1200-2000 g: 15 mg/kg/day q12-18h; >2000 g: 30 mg/kg/day q12h; >7 days: <1200 g 15 mg/kg/day q24h; 1200-2000 g 15 mg/kg/day q8-12h; >2000 g 45 mg/kg/day q8h<br>Cerebrospinal fluid: 5-10 mg/day (cerebrospinal fluid trough, <20 μg/mL) | Ototoxicity (therapeutic levels: peak 25-40 μg/mL; trough, 5-10 μg/mL); rapid infusion may cause cutaneous vasodilatation and shock<br>Higher concentrations are recommended for resistant organisms and toxicity appears to be low |
| Vasopressin | IM, SC: 2.5-10 U 2-4 times daily | 20 units/mL aqueous injection |
| Vecuronium | IV: 0.08-0.1 mg/kg/dose, repeat prn at 0.03-0.15 mg/kg/dose q1-2h<br>Dose to effect | Neuromuscular blockade potentiated by calcium channel blockers such as verapamil and aminoglycoside antibiotics |
| Verapamil | IV: 0.1-0.2 mg/kg infused over 2 min; if response is inadequate, repeat in 30 min<br>PO: 2-5 mg/kg/day in 3 divided doses | Monitor electrocardiogram during infusion; bradycardia, atrioventricular block, asystole; contraindicated in patients with 2nd or 3rd degree atrioventricular block during treatment with beta blockers |
| Vitamin A (oleovitamin A) | PO: preventive, 600-1500 units/day<br>IM: prevention of BPD: 5000 IU 3 × /week for 4 weeks | Pseudotumor cerebri; maintain plasma vitamin A concentration of 30 to 60 μg/mL |
| Vitamin $B_1$ (thiamine) | PO: preventive, 0.5-1 mg q day;<br>PO: therapeutic, 5-10 mg q6-8h | Unstable in alkaline solution |
| Vitamin $B_6$ (pyridoxine) | PO: *preventive*: 100 μg/L of ingested formula; *therapeutic for deficiency*: 2-5 mg/day q6h; *test dose for pyridone dependency seizures*: 50-100 mg IV | May decrease serum levels of phenobarbital, phenytoin, or folic acid; hypersensitivity |
| Vitamin C (ascorbic acid) | IM, IV, PO: *preventive*: 25-50 mg/day (term infants); 100 mg/day (premature infants) | |
| Vitamin $D_2$ (ergocalciferol) | PO: *preventive*: 400-1000 IU/day (premature infants), 40-100 IU/day (term infants) | Hypercalcemia with excess dose |
| Vitamin E (*d*-alpha tocopherol) | PO: *prevention of hemolysis*: 25-50 IU/day (1 IU = 1 mg) | Some preparations are hyperosmolar |
| Vitamin $K_1$ (phytonadione) | SC, IM: *preventive*: 0.5-1.0 mg, single dose; *therapeutic*: 1-2 mg/kg/dose q6-12h according to prothrombin time | With thrombocytopenia, slow IV infusion at same dose; anaphylaxis observed with rapid injection IV, more common with vitamin $K_3$ |

REFERENCES

American Academy of Pediatrics Committee on Drugs: Drugs for pediatric emergencies. *Pediatrics* 101:e13, 1998.
Bhatt DR, Bruggman DS, Thayer-Thomas JC, et al: Neonatal Drug Formulary 2002, ed 5. Fontana, CA, Neonatal Drug Formulary, 2002.
Young TE, Mangum B: Neofax, ed 14. Raleigh, NC, Acorn Publishing, 2001.
Zenk KE, Sills JH, Koeppel RM: Neonatal Medications and Nutrition. Santa Rosa, CA, NICU INK, 1999.

*PO dose increased 20%

AV, atrioventicular; CHF, congestive heart failure; CNS, central nervous system; DOCA, deoxycorticosterone acetate; EGA, estimated gestational age; PMA, postmenstrual age; prn, *pro re nate* (as needed); $T_4$, thyroxine; TSH, thyroid-stimulating hormone.

## TRANSFER OF DRUGS AND CHEMICALS INTO HUMAN MILK

A statement on the transfer of drugs and chemicals into human milk, by the Committe on Drugs of the American Academy of Pediatrics, was first published in 1983, with revisions in 1989, 1994 and 2001. The current statement addresses the use of psychotropic drugs and other drug therapies for the lactating woman, as well as the implications of smoking and the presence of silicone implants on breast-feeding. Information in the statement is updated to identify agents transferred into human milk and to describe their possible effects on the infant or on lactation, if known; current data are presented in Tables 1 through 7. If a pharmacologic or chemical agent does not appear in the tables, it does not mean that the agent is not transferred into human milk or that it does not have an effect on the infant; omission of the agent indicates only that no reports have appeared in the literature. These tables are provided to assist the physician in counseling the nursing mother regarding breast-feeding when she has a condition for which a drug is medically indicated. The full text of this statement is available at http://aapolicy.aapublications.org.

## REFERENCE

American Academy of Pediatrics Committee on Drugs: The transfer of drugs and other chemicals into human milk. Pediatrics 108:776-789, 2001.

**TABLE 1**

**Cytotoxic Drugs that May Interfere with Cellular Metabolism in the Nursing Infant**

| Drug | Reason for Concern, Reported Sign or Symptom in Infant, or Effect on Lactation |
|---|---|
| Cyclophosphamide | Possible immune suppression; unknown effect on growth or association with carcinogenesis; neutropenia |
| Cyclosporine | Possible immune suppression; unknown effect on growth or association with carcinogenesis |
| Doxorubicin* | Possible immune suppression; unknown effect on growth or association with carcinogenesis |
| Methotrexate | Possible immune suppression; unknown effect on growth or association with carcinogenesis; neutropenia |

*Drug is concentrated in human milk.

**TABLE 2**

**Drugs of Abuse for Which Adverse Effects on the Infant During Breast-feeding Have Been Reported***

| Drug | Reported Effect or Reason for Concern |
|---|---|
| Amphetamine† | Irritability, poor sleeping pattern |
| Cocaine | Cocaine intoxication: irritability, vomiting, diarrhea, tremulousness, seizures |
| Heroin | Tremors, restlessness, vomiting, poor feeding |
| Marijuana | Only one report in literature; no effect mentioned; very long half-life for some components |
| Phencyclidine | Potent hallucinogen |

*The Committee on Drugs strongly believes that nursing mothers should not ingest drugs of abuse, because they are hazardous to the nursing infant and to the health of the mother.

†Drug is concentrated in human milk.

**TABLE 3**

**Radioactive Compounds Necessitating Temporary Cessation of Breast-feeding***

| Compound | Recommended Time for Cessation of Breast-feeding |
|---|---|
| Copper 64 ($^{64}Cu$) | Radioactivity in milk present at 50 hr |
| Gallium 67 ($^{67}Ga$) | Radioactivity in milk present for 2 wk |
| Indium 111 ($^{111}In$) | Very small amount present at 20 hr |
| Iodine 123 ($^{123}I$) | Radioactivity in milk present up to 36 hr |
| Iodine 125 ($^{125}I$) | Radioactivity in milk present for 12 days |
| Iodine 131 ($^{131}I$) | Radioactivity in milk present 2-14 days, depending on study |
| Iodine$^{131}$ | If used for treatment of thyroid cancer, high radioactivity may prolong exposure to infant |
| Radioactive sodium | Radioactivity in milk present 96 hr |
| Technetium 99 m ($^{99m}Tc$), $^{99m}Tc$ macroaggregates, $^{99m}Tc\ O_4$ | Radioactivity in milk present 15 hr to 3 days |

*Consult nuclear medicine physician before performing diagnostic study so that radionuclide that has the shortest excretion time in breast milk can be used. Before the study, the mother should pump her breast and store enough milk in the freezer for feeding the infant; after the study, the mother should pump her breast to maintain milk production but discard all milk pumped for the required time that radioactivity is present in milk. Milk samples can be screened by radiology departments for radioactivity before resumption of nursing.

**TABLE 4**

**Drugs for Which the Effect on Nursing Infants is Unknown But May Be of Concern***

| Drug | Reported or Possible Effect |
|---|---|
| **Anxiolytics** | |
| Alprazolam | None |
| Diazepam | None |
| Lorazepam | None |
| Midazolam | — |
| Perphenazine | None |

TABLE 4

**Drugs for Which the Effect on Nursing Infants is Unknown But May Be of Concern*—Cont'd**

| Drug | Reported or Possible Effect |
|---|---|
| Prazepam† | None |
| Quazepam | None |
| Temazepam | — |
| **Antidepressants** | |
| Amitriptyline | None |
| Amoxapine | None |
| Bupropion | None |
| Clomipramine | None |
| Desipramine | None |
| Dothiepin | None |
| Doxepin | None |
| Fluoxetine | Colic, irritability, feeding and sleep disorders, slow weight gain |
| Fluvoxamine | — |
| Imipramine | None |
| Nortriptyline | None |
| Paroxetine | None |
| Sertraline† | None |
| Trazodone | None |
| **Antipsychotics** | |
| Chlorpromazine | Galactorrhea in mother; drowsiness and lethargy in infant; decline in developmental scores |
| Chlorprothixene | None |
| Clozapine† | None |
| Haloperidol | Decline in developmental scores |
| Mesoridazine | None |
| Trifluoperazine | None |
| **Others** | |
| Amiodarone | Possible hypothyroidism |
| Chloramphenicol | Possible idiosyncratic bone marrow suppression |
| Clofazimine | Potential for transfer of high percentage of maternal dose; possible increase in skin pigmentation |
| Lamotrigine | Potential therapeutic serum concentrations in infant |
| Metoclopramide† | None described; dopaminergic blocking agent |
| Metronidazole | In vitro mutagen; may discontinue breast-feeding for 12-24 hr to allow excretion of dose when single-dose therapy is given to mother |
| Tinidazole | See Metronidazole |

*Psychotropic drugs, the compounds listed under the anxiolytic, antidepressant, and antipsychotic categories, are of special concern when given to nursing mothers for long periods. Although there are very few case reports of adverse effects in breast-feeding infants, these drugs do appear in human milk and thus could conceivably alter short-term and long-term central nervous system function. See discussion in the text on psychotropic drugs.

†Drug is concentrated in human milk relative to simultaneous maternal plasma concentrations.

TABLE 5

**Drugs That Have Been Associated with Significant Effects in Some Nursing Infants and Should Be Given to Nursing Mothers with Caution***

| Drug | Reported Effect |
|---|---|
| Acebutolol | Hypotension; bradycardia; tachypnea |
| 5-Aminosalicylic acid | Diarrhea (one case) |
| Atenolol | Cyanosis; bradycardia |
| Bromocriptine | Suppresses lactation; may be hazardous to the mother |
| Aspirin (salicylates) | Metabolic acidosis (one case) |
| Clemastine | Drowsiness, irritability, refusal to feed, high-pitched cry, neck stiffness (one case) |
| Ergotamine | Vomiting, diarrhea, convulsions (doses used in migraine medications) |
| Lithium | One-third to one-half therapeutic blood concentration in infants |
| Phenindione | Anticoagulant: increased prothrombin and partial thromboplastin time in one infant; not used in the United States |
| Phenobarbital | Sedation; infantile spasms after weaning from milk containing phenobarbital, methemoglobinemia (one case) |
| Primidone | Sedation, feeding problems |
| Sulfasalazine (salicylazosulfapyridine) | Bloody diarrhea (one case) |

*Blood concentration in the infant may be of clinical importance.

TABLE 6

## Maternal Medications Usually Compatible with Breast-feeding[*]

| Drug | Reported Sign/Symptom in Infant or Effect on Lactation |
|---|---|
| Acetaminophen | None |
| Acetazolamide | None |
| Acitretin | — |
| Acyclovir[†] | None |
| Alcohol (ethanol) | With large amounts, drowsiness, diaphoresis, deep sleep, weakness, decrease in linear growth, abnormal weight gain; maternal ingestion of 1 g/kg daily decreases milk ejection reflex |
| Allopurinol | — |
| Amoxicillin | None |
| Antimony | — |
| Atropine | None |
| Azapropazone (apazone) | — |
| Aztreonam | None |
| B vitamins | |
| $B_1$ (thiamin) | None |
| $B_6$ (pyridoxine) | None |
| $B_{12}$ | None |
| Baclofen | None |
| Barbiturate | See Table 5 (phenobarbital) |
| Bendroflumethiazide | Suppresses lactation |
| Bishydroxycoumarin (dicumarol) | None |
| Bromide | Rash, weakness, absence of cry with maternal intake of 5.4 g/day |
| Butorphanol | None |
| Caffeine | Irritability, poor sleeping pattern, excreted slowly; no effect with moderate intake of caffeinated beverages (2-3 cups per day) |
| Captopril | None |
| Carbamazepine | None |
| Carbetocin | None |
| Carbimazole | Goiter |
| Cascara | None |
| Cefadroxil | None |
| Cefazolin | None |
| Cefotaxime | None |
| Cefoxitin | None |
| Cefprozil | — |
| Ceftazidime | None |
| Ceftriaxone | None |
| Chloral hydrate | Sleepiness |
| Chloroform | None |
| Chloroquine | None |
| Chlorothiazide | None |
| Chlorthalidone | Excreted slowly |
| Cimetidine[†] | None |
| Ciprofloxacin | None |
| Cisapride | None |
| Cisplatin | Not found in milk |
| Clindamycin | None |
| Clogestone | None |
| Codeine | None |
| Colchicine | — |
| Contraceptive pill with estrogen/progesterone | Rare breast enlargement; decrease in milk production and protein content (not confirmed in several studies) |
| Cycloserine | None |
| D (vitamin) | None; follow-up evaluation of infant's serum calcium level if mother receives pharmacologic doses |
| Danthron | Increased bowel activity |
| Dapsone | None; sulfonamide detected in infant's urine |
| Dexbrompheniramine maleate with *d*-isoephedrine | Crying, poor sleeping patterns, irritability |
| Diatrizoate | None |
| Digoxin | None |
| Diltiazem | None |
| Dipyrone | None |
| Disopyramide | None |
| Domperidone | None |
| Dyphylline[†] | None |
| Enalapril | — |
| Erythromycin[†] | None |
| Estradiol | Withdrawal, vaginal bleeding |
| Ethambutol | None |
| Ethanol | See Alcohol |
| Ethosuximide | None, drug appears in infant serum |
| Fentanyl | — |
| Fexofenadine | None |
| Flecainide | — |
| Fleroxacin | One 400-mg dose given to nursing mothers; infants not given breast milk for 48 hr |
| Fluconazole | None |
| Flufenamic acid | None |
| Fluorescein | — |
| Folic acid | None |
| Gadopentetic acid (gadolinium) | None |
| Gentamicin | None |
| Gold salts | None |
| Halothane | None |
| Hydralazine | None |
| Hydrochlorothiazide | — |
| Hydroxychloroquine[†] | None |
| Ibuprofen | None |
| Indomethacin | Seizure (one case) |
| Iodides | May affect thyroid activity; see Iodine |
| Iodine | Goiter |
| Iodine (povidone-iodine; e.g., in a vaginal douche) | Elevated iodine levels in breast milk, odor of iodine on infant's skin |
| Iohexol | None |
| Iopanoic acid | None |
| Isoniazid | None; acetyl (hepatotoxic) metabolite secreted but no hepatotoxicity reported in infants |
| Interferon-α | — |
| Ivermectin | None |
| $K_1$ (vitamin) | None |
| Kanamycin | None |
| Ketoconazole | None |
| Ketorolac | — |
| Labetalol | None |
| Levonorgestrel | — |
| Levothyroxine | None |
| Lidocaine | None |
| Loperamide | — |
| Loratadine | None |
| Magnesium sulfate | None |
| Medroxyprogesterone | None |
| Mefenamic acid | None |
| Meperidine | None |
| Methadone | None |

**TABLE 6**

## Maternal Medication Usually Compatible with Breast-feeding*—Cont'd

| Drug | Reported Sign/Symptom in Infant or Effect on Lactation | Drug | Reported Sign/Symptom in Infant or Effect on Lactation |
|---|---|---|---|
| Methimazole (active metabolite of carbimazole) | None | Pyrimethamine | None |
| | | Quinidine | None |
| | | Quinine | None |
| Methohexital | None | Riboflavin | None |
| Methyldopa | None | Rifampin | None |
| Methyprylon | Drowsiness | Scopolamine | — |
| Metoprolol† | None | Secobarbital | None |
| Metrizamide | None | Senna | None |
| Metrizoate | None | Sotalol | — |
| Mexiletine | None | Spironolactone | None |
| Minoxidil | None | Streptomycin | None |
| Morphine | None; infant may have measurable blood concentration | Sulbactam | None |
| | | Sulfapyridine | Caution in infant with jaundice or G6PD deficiency and ill, stressed, or premature infant; appears in mother's milk and infant's urine |
| Moxalactam | None | | |
| Nadolol† | None | | |
| Nalidixic acid | Hemolysis in infant with glucose-6-phosphate dehydrogenase (G6PD) deficiency | Sulfisoxazole | Caution in infant with jaundice or G6PD deficiency and ill, stressed, or premature infant; appears in mother's milk and infant's urine |
| Naproxen | — | | |
| Nefopam | None | | |
| Nifedipine | — | Sumatriptan | None |
| Nitrofurantoin | Hemolysis in infant with G6PD deficiency | Suprofen | None |
| | | Terbutaline | None |
| Norethynodrel | None | Terfenadine | None |
| Norsteroids | None | Tetracycline | None; negligible absorption by infant |
| Noscapine | None | Theophylline | Irritability |
| Ofloxacin | None | Thiopental | None |
| Oxprenolol | None | Thiouracil | None mentioned; drug not used in the United States |
| Phenylbutazone | None | | |
| Phenytoin | Methemoglobinemia (one case) | Ticarcillin | None |
| Piroxicam | None | Timolol | None |
| Prednisolone | None | Tolbutamide | Possible jaundice |
| Prednisone | None | Tolmetin | None |
| Procainamide | None | Trimethoprim-sulfamethoxazole | None |
| Progesterone | None | | |
| Propoxyphene | None | Triprolidine | None |
| Propranolol | None | Valproic acid | None |
| Propylthiouracil | None | Verapamil | None |
| Pseudoephedrine† | None | Warfarin | None |
| Pyridostigmine | None | Zolpidem | None |

*Drugs listed have been reported in the literature as having the effects listed or no effect. "None" means that no observable change was seen in the nursing infant while the mother was ingesting the compound. Dashes indicate no mention of clinical effect on the infant. It is emphasized that many of the literature citations concern single case reports or small series of infants.

†Drug is concentrated in human milk.

**TABLE 7**

## Food and Environmental Agents: Effects on Breast-feeding

| Agent | Reported Sign/Symptom in Infant or Effect on Lactation |
|---|---|
| Aflatoxin | None |
| Aspartame | Caution if mother or infant has phenylketonuria |
| Bromide (photographic laboratory) | Potential absorption and bromide transfer into milk; see Table 6 |
| Cadmium | None reported |
| Chlordane | None reported |
| Chocolate (theobromine) | Irritability or increased bowel activity if excess amounts (≥16 oz/day) consumed by mother |
| DDT, benzene hexachlorides, dieldrin, aldrin, hepatachlorepoxide | None |
| Fava beans | Hemolysis in patient with glucose-6-phosphate dehydrogenase deficiency |
| Fluorides | None |

*Continued*

TABLE 7

**Food and Environmental Agents: Effects on Breast-feeding—Cont'd**

| Agent | Reported Sign/Symptom in Infant or Effect on Lactation |
|---|---|
| Hexachlorobenzene | Skin rash, diarrhea, vomiting, dark urine, neurotoxicity, death |
| Hexachlorophene | None; possible contamination of milk from nipple washing |
| Lead | Possible neurotoxicity |
| Mercury, methylmercury | May affect neurodevelopment |
| Methylmethacrylate | None |
| Monosodium glutamate | None |
| Polychlorinated biphenyls and polybrominated biphenyls | Lack of endurance; hypotonia; sullen, expressionless facies |
| Silicone | Esophageal dysmotility |
| Tetrachloroethylene cleaning fluid (perchloroethylene) | Obstructive jaundice, dark urine |
| Vegetarian diet | Signs of $B_{12}$ deficiency |

# Appendix 2

# Illustrative Forms and Normal Values

Christine A. Gleason

**Neuromuscular Maturity**

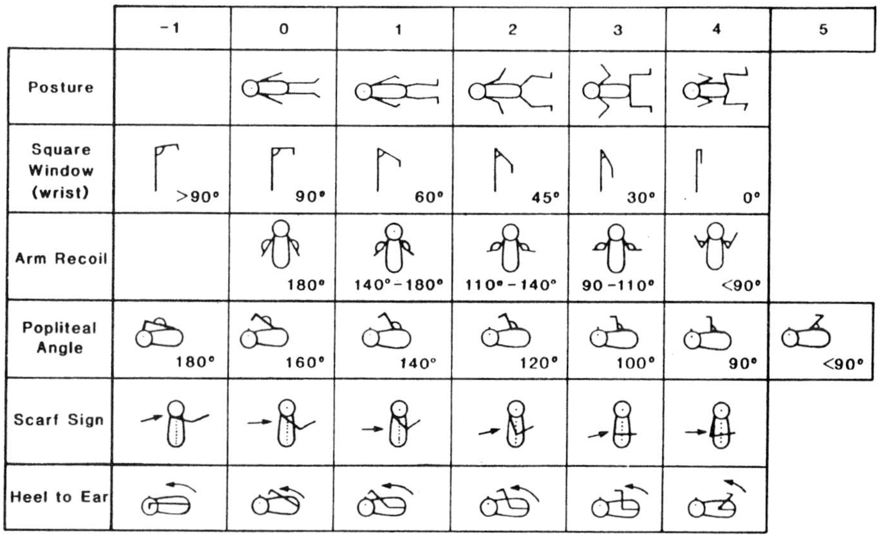

| | -1 | 0 | 1 | 2 | 3 | 4 | 5 |
|---|---|---|---|---|---|---|---|
| Posture | | | | | | | |
| Square Window (wrist) | >90° | 90° | 60° | 45° | 30° | 0° | |
| Arm Recoil | | 180° | 140°-180° | 110°-140° | 90-110° | <90° | |
| Popliteal Angle | 180° | 160° | 140° | 120° | 100° | 90° | <90° |
| Scarf Sign | | | | | | | |
| Heel to Ear | | | | | | | |

**Physical Maturity**

| | | | | | | | |
|---|---|---|---|---|---|---|---|
| Skin | sticky friable transparent | gelatinous red, translucent | smooth pink, visible veins | superficial peeling &/or rash. few veins | cracking pale areas rare veins | parchment deep cracking no vessels | leathery cracked wrinkled |
| Lanugo | none | sparse | abundant | thinning | bald areas | mostly bald | |
| Plantar Surface | heel-toe 40-50 mm: -1 <40 mm: -2 | >50mm no crease | faint red marks | anterior transverse crease only | creases ant. 2/3 | creases over entire sole | |
| Breast | imperceptible | barely perceptible | flat areola no bud | stippled areola 1-2mm bud | raised areola 3-4mm bud | full areola 5-10mm bud | |
| Eye/Ear | lids fused loosely: -1 tightly: -2 | lids open pinna flat stays folded | sl. curved pinna; soft; slow recoil | well-curved pinna; soft but ready recoil | formed & firm instant recoil | thick cartilage ear stiff | |
| Genitals male | scrotum flat, smooth | scrotum empty faint rugae | testes in upper canal rare rugae | testes descending few rugae | testes down good rugae | testes pendulous deep rugae | |
| Genitals female | clitoris prominent labia flat | prominent clitoris small labia minora | prominent clitoris enlarging minora | majora & minora equally prominent | majora large minora small | majora cover clitoris & minora | |

**Maturity Rating**

| score | weeks |
|---|---|
| -10 | 20 |
| -5 | 22 |
| 0 | 24 |
| 5 | 26 |
| 10 | 28 |
| 15 | 30 |
| 20 | 32 |
| 25 | 34 |
| 30 | 36 |
| 35 | 38 |
| 40 | 40 |
| 45 | 42 |
| 50 | 44 |

Expanded New Ballard Score includes extremely premature infants and has been refined to improve accuracy in more mature infants. *(From Ballard JL, Khoury JC, Wedig K, et al: New Ballard Score, expanded to include extremely premature infants. J Pediatr 119:417-423, 1991.)*

## Correlations Between Gestational Length and Embryonic and Fetal Body Dimensions

| Week of Gestation | Crown-Rump Length (cm) | Weight (g) | Biparietal Diameter (cm) |
|---|---|---|---|
| 6 | 0.5 | | |
| 7 | 0.8 | 0.07 | |
| 8 | 1.5 | 0.22 | |
| 9 | 2.5 | 0.88 | |
| 10 | 3.5 | 3.5 | |
| 11 | 4.6 | 6.0 | |
| 12 | 5.7 | 11.0 | |
| 13 | 6.8 | 19.0 | |
| 14 | 8.1 | 33.0 | |
| 15 | 9.4 | 55.0 | |
| 16 | 10.7 | 80.0 | |
| 17 | 12.1 | 120.0 | 3.7 |
| 18 | 13.6 | 170.0 | 4.0 |
| 19 | 15.3 | 253.0 | 4.4 |
| 20 | 16.4 | 316.0 | 4.8 |
| 21 | 17.5 | 385.0 | 5.2 |
| 22 | 18.6 | 460.0 | 5.5 |
| 23 | 19.7 | 542.0 | 5.75 |
| 24 | 20.8 | 630.0 | 5.95 |
| 25 | 21.8 | 723.0 | 6.1 |
| 26 | 22.8 | 823.0 | 6.2 |
| 27 | 23.8 | 930.0 | 6.35 |
| 28 | 24.7 | 1045.0 | 6.5 |
| 29 | 25.6 | 1174.0 | 6.65 |
| 30 | 26.5 | 1323.0 | 6.85 |
| 31 | 27.4 | 1492.0 | 7.1 |
| 32 | 28.3 | 1680.0 | 7.3 |
| 33 | 29.3 | 1876.0 | 7.6 |
| 34 | 30.2 | 2074.0 | 7.8 |
| 35 | 31.1 | 2274.0 | 8.1 |
| 36 | 32.1 | 2478.0 | 8.35 |
| 37 | 33.1 | 2690.0 | 8.6 |
| 38 | 34.1 | 2914.0 | 8.9 |
| 39 | 35.1 | 3150.0 | 9.2 |
| 40 | 36.2 | 3405.0 | 9.55 |
| 41 | | 3600.0 | 9.8 |
| 42 | | 3650.0 | 9.85 |
| | | 3750.0 | 10.0 |
| | | [illegible] | [illegible] |
| | | 4000.0 | 10.3 |
| | | 4200.0 | 10.6 |

Data based on the study of Bartolucci L: Am J Obstet Gynecol 122:439, 1975. Courtesy of Iffy L, et al: Pediatrics 56:173, 1975.

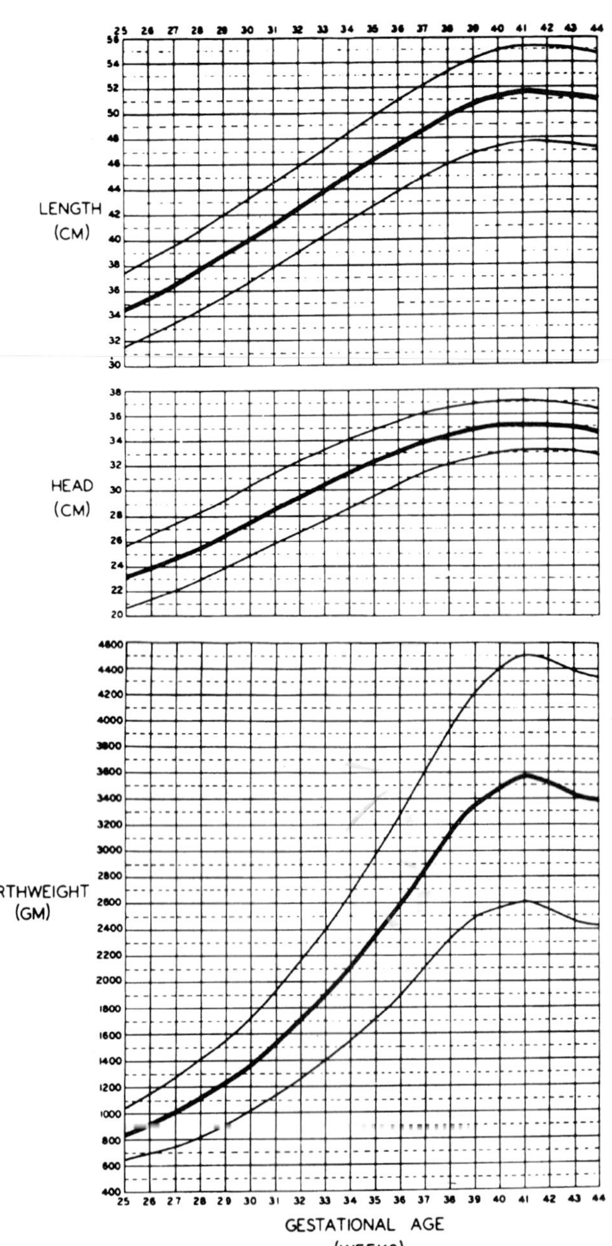


Intrauterine growth curves. *(From Usher R, McLean F: Intrauterine growth of live-born caucasian infants at sea level: Standards obtained from measurements in 7 dimensions of infants born between 25 and 44 weeks of gestation. J Pediatr 74:901, 1969.)*

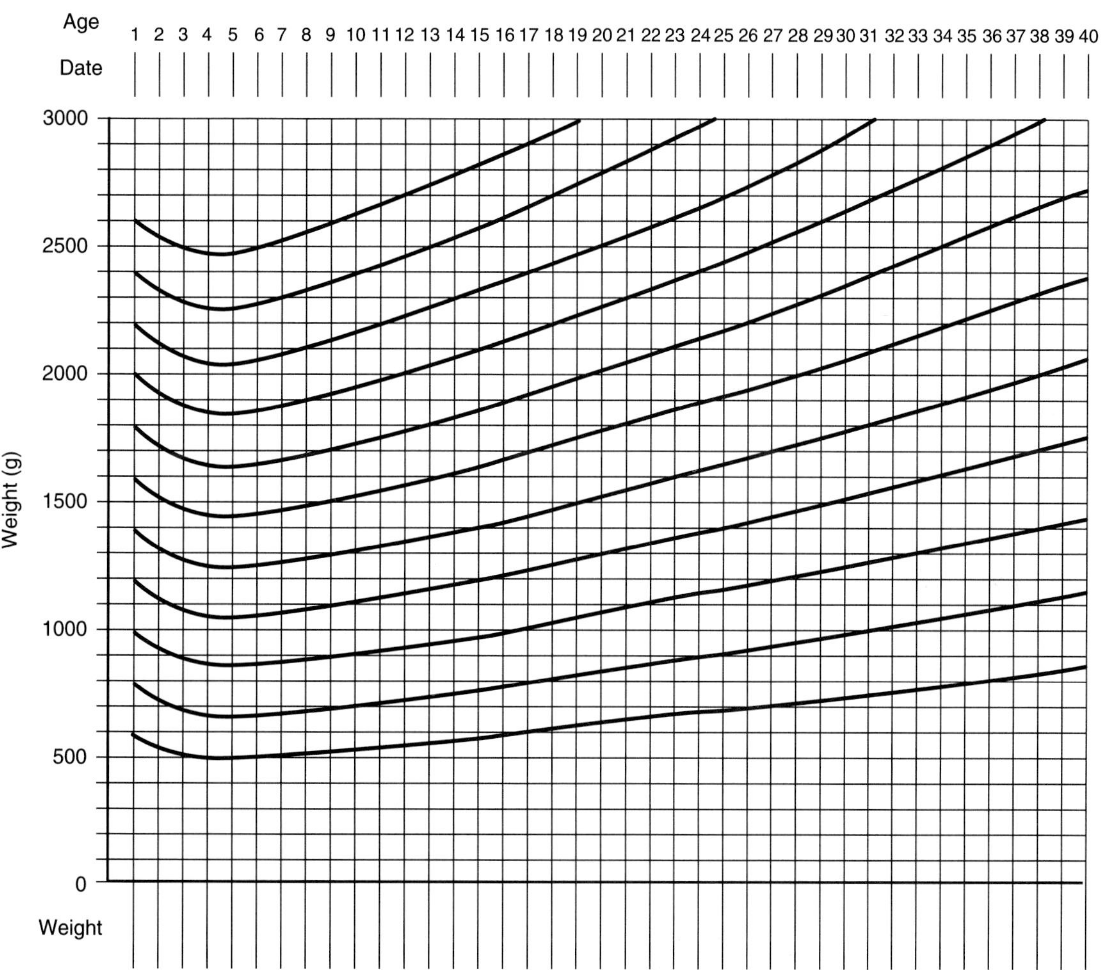


Extrauterine growth chart. *(Data from Shaffer SG, Quimiro CL, Anderson JV, et al: Postnatal weight changes in low birth weight infants. Pediatrics 79[5]: 702, 1987.)*

**Smoothed Percentiles of Birth Weight (g) for Gestational Age: U.S. 1991 Single Live Births to Resident Mothers**

| | Percentile | | | | |
|---|---|---|---|---|---|
| Gestational Age (wk) | 5th | 10th | 50th | 90th | 95th |
| 20 | 249 | 275 | 412 | 772 | 912 |
| 21 | 280 | 314 | 433 | 790 | 957 |
| 22 | 330 | 376 | 496 | 826 | 1023 |
| 23 | 385 | 440 | 582 | 882 | 1107 |
| 24 | 435 | 498 | 674 | 977 | 1223 |
| 25 | 480 | 558 | 779 | 1138 | 1397 |
| 26 | 529 | 625 | 899 | 1362 | 1640 |
| 27 | 591 | 702 | 1035 | 1635 | 1927 |
| 28 | 670 | 798 | 1196 | 1977 | 2237 |
| 29 | 772 | 925 | 1394 | 2361 | 2553 |
| 30 | 910 | 1085 | 1637 | 2710 | 2847 |
| 31 | 1088 | 1278 | 1918 | 2986 | 3108 |
| 32 | 1294 | 1495 | 2203 | 3200 | 3338 |
| 33 | 1513 | 1725 | 2458 | 3370 | 3536 |
| 34 | 1735 | 1950 | 2667 | 3502 | 3697 |
| 35 | 1950 | 2159 | 2831 | 3596 | 3812 |
| 36 | 2156 | 2354 | 2974 | 3668 | 3888 |
| 37 | 2357 | 2541 | 3117 | 3755 | 3956 |
| 38 | 2543 | 2714 | 3263 | 3867 | 4027 |
| 39 | 2685 | 2852 | 3400 | 3980 | 4107 |
| 40 | 2761 | 2929 | 3495 | 4060 | 4185 |
| 41 | 2777 | 2948 | 3527 | 4094 | 4217 |
| 42 | 2764 | 2935 | 3522 | 4098 | 4213 |
| 43 | 2741 | 2907 | 3505 | 4096 | 4178 |
| 44 | 2724 | 2885 | 3491 | 4096 | 4122 |

Data from Alexander GR, Himes JH, Kaufman RB, et al: A United States National Reference for Fetal Growth. Obstet Gynecol 87:163-168, 1996.

**Longitudinal Head Circumference of 450 Infants; Single-Point Measurements from the National Center for Health Statistics (NCHS) Norm**

| Corrected Age | Mean ± SD Birth Weight (g) | | | | | | | | NCHS Norm | |
|---|---|---|---|---|---|---|---|---|---|---|
| | 501-750 (635 ± 61) $n$ = 14 | 751-1000 (893 ± 53) $n$ = 40 | 1001-1250 (1138 ± 76) $n$ = 68 | 1251-1500 (1377 ± 70) $n$ = 84 | 1501-1750 (1633 ± 73) $n$ = 72 | 1751-2000 (1876 ± 70) $n$ = 72 | 2001-2250 (2109 ± 68) $n$ = 60 | 2251-2500 (2368 ± 93) $n$ = 40 | Boys | Girls |
| Birth | 22.3 ± 0.9 | 23.9 ± 0.8 | 25.4 ± 0.8 | 27.5 ± 0.9 | 28.2 ± 1.0 | 29.4 ± 0.8 | 30.7 ± 0.7 | 31.7 ± 0.8 | 34.6 ± 0.8 | 34.1 ± 0.6 |
| 40 wk | 31.3 ± 1.3 | 33.8 ± 1.4 | 34.7 ± 1.9 | 34.7 ± 1.3 | 36.9 ± 0.6 | 35.7 ± 1.2 | 36.1 ± 1.9 | 35.0 ± 1.2 | 34.6 ± 0.8 | 34.1 ± 0.6 |
| 1 mo | 34.3 ± 1.0 | 34.7 ± 1.2 | 36.4 ± 1.5 | 36.7 ± 2.3 | 35.1 ± 1.4 | 38.0 ± 1.8 | 37.0 ± 1.9 | 36.7 ± 0.2 | 37.3 ± 0.7 | 36.5 ± 0.6 |
| 3 mo | 39.5 ± 1.3 | 39.3 ± 1.7 | 40.7 ± 1.9 | 40.4 ± 2.2 | 40.7 ± 2.4 | 40.8 ± 1.1 | 39.7 ± 0.5 | 40.7 ± 1.2 | 40.6 ± 0.8 | 39.5 ± 0.7 |
| 6 mo | 40.3 ± 0.9 | 41.6 ± 1.4 | 41.3 ± 1.5 | 43.6 ± 1.2 | 42.6 ± 1.6 | 43.9 ± 0.8 | 44.1 ± 1.8 | 43.0 ± 1.5 | 43.7 ± 0.7 | 42.4 ± 0.7 |
| 9 mo | 42.1 ± 0.9 | 43.8 ± 1.0 | 43.9 ± 1.5 | 44.7 ± 0.8 | 45.3 ± 2.5 | 44.3 ± 0.9 | 45.7 ± 2.0 | 46.7 ± 1.5 | 45.8 ± 0.7 | 44.4 ± 0.7 |
| 12 mo | 43.7 ± 2.3 | 45.0 ± 1.9 | 44.5 ± 1.7 | 46.3 ± 2.4 | 45.0 ± 1.6 | 46.7 ± 1.6 | 46.4 ± 0.6 | 45.2 ± 0.4 | 47.1 ± 0.7 | 45.6 ± 0.7 |
| 15 mo | 45.9 ± 1.8 | 45.3 ± 1.7 | 45.9 ± 1.5 | 47.2 ± 1.1 | 47.9 ± 1.8 | 47.7 ± 1.4 | 47.0 ± 0.1 | 47.5 ± 0.9 | NA* | NA* |
| 18 mo | 45.9 ± 1.3 | 45.8 ± 1.3 | 47.0 ± 1.1 | 47.4 ± 1.0 | 47.0 ± 1.5 | 47.9 ± 1.7 | 47.2 ± 0.5 | 47.4 ± 0.7 | 48.3 ± 0.7 | 47.1 ± 0.7 |

*NA, not available.

From Sheth RD, Mullett MD, Bodensteiner JB, Hobbs GR: Longitudinal head growth in developmentally normal preterm infants. Arch Pediatr Adolesc Med 149:1360, 1995. 

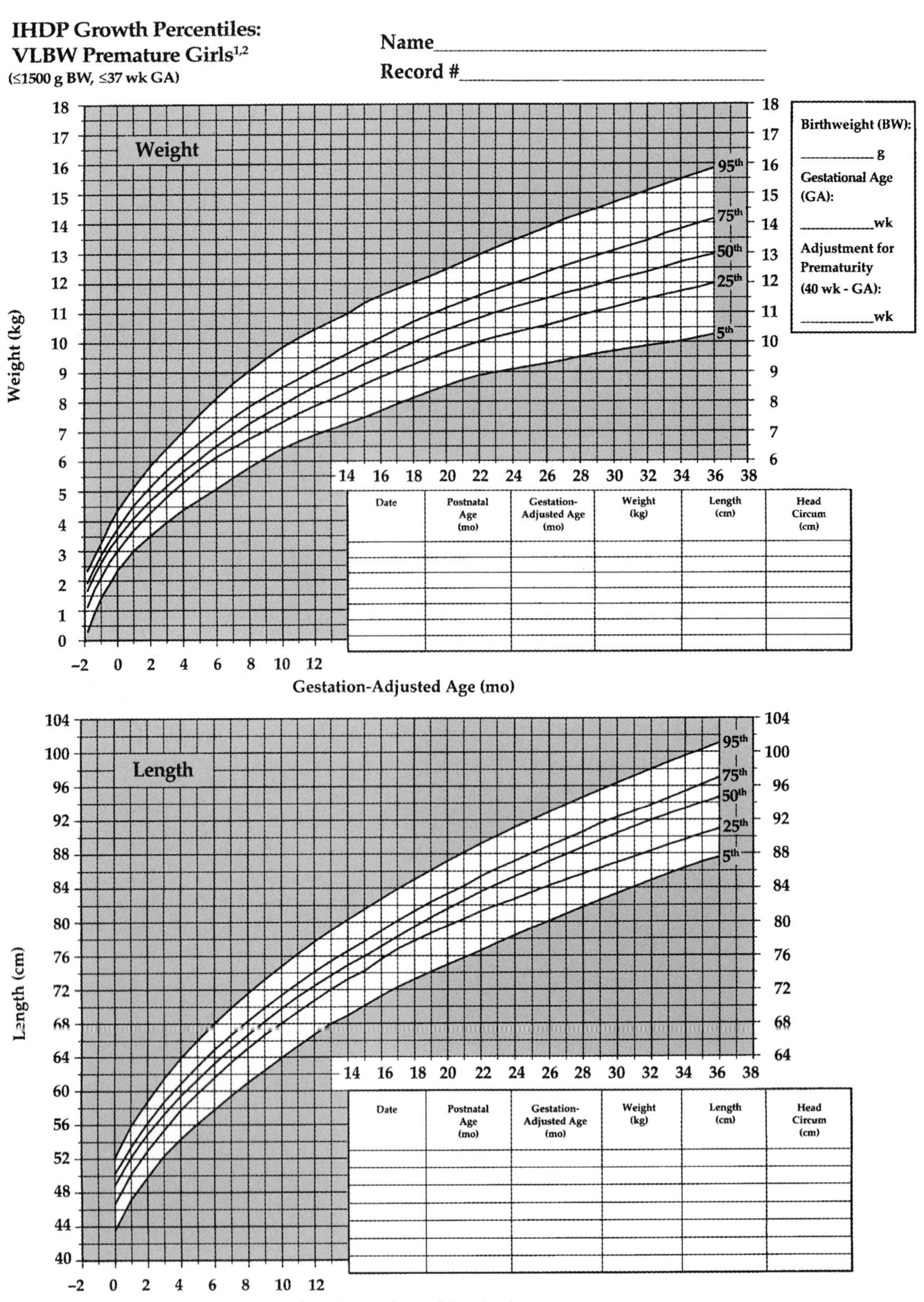
IHDP Growth Percentiles:
VLBW Premature Girls[1,2]
(≤1500 g BW, ≤37 wk GA)
Name
Record #
Weight
Weight (kg)
95th
75th
50th
25th
5th
Birthweight (BW): g
Gestational Age (GA): wk
Adjustment for Prematurity (40 wk - GA): wk
Date
Postnatal Age (mo)
Gestation-Adjusted Age (mo)
Weight (kg)
Length (cm)
Head Circum (cm)
Gestation-Adjusted Age (mo)
Length
Length (cm)
95th
75th
50th
25th
5th
Date
Postnatal Age (mo)
Gestation-Adjusted Age (mo)
Weight (kg)
Length (cm)
Head Circum (cm)
Gestation-Adjusted Age (mo)

**IHDP Growth Percentiles: VLBW Premature Girls** (cont'd)

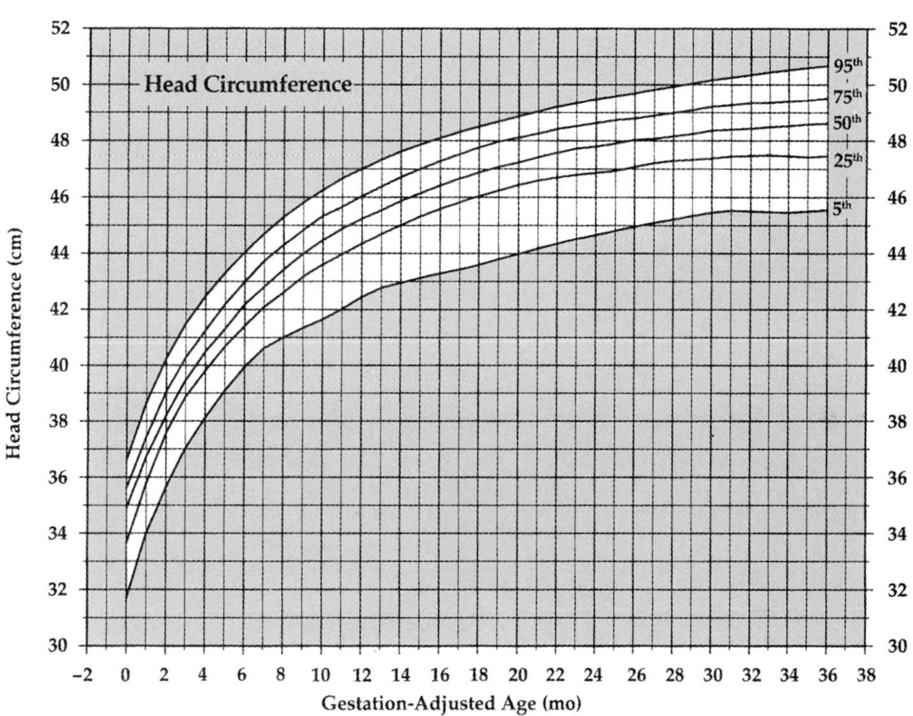

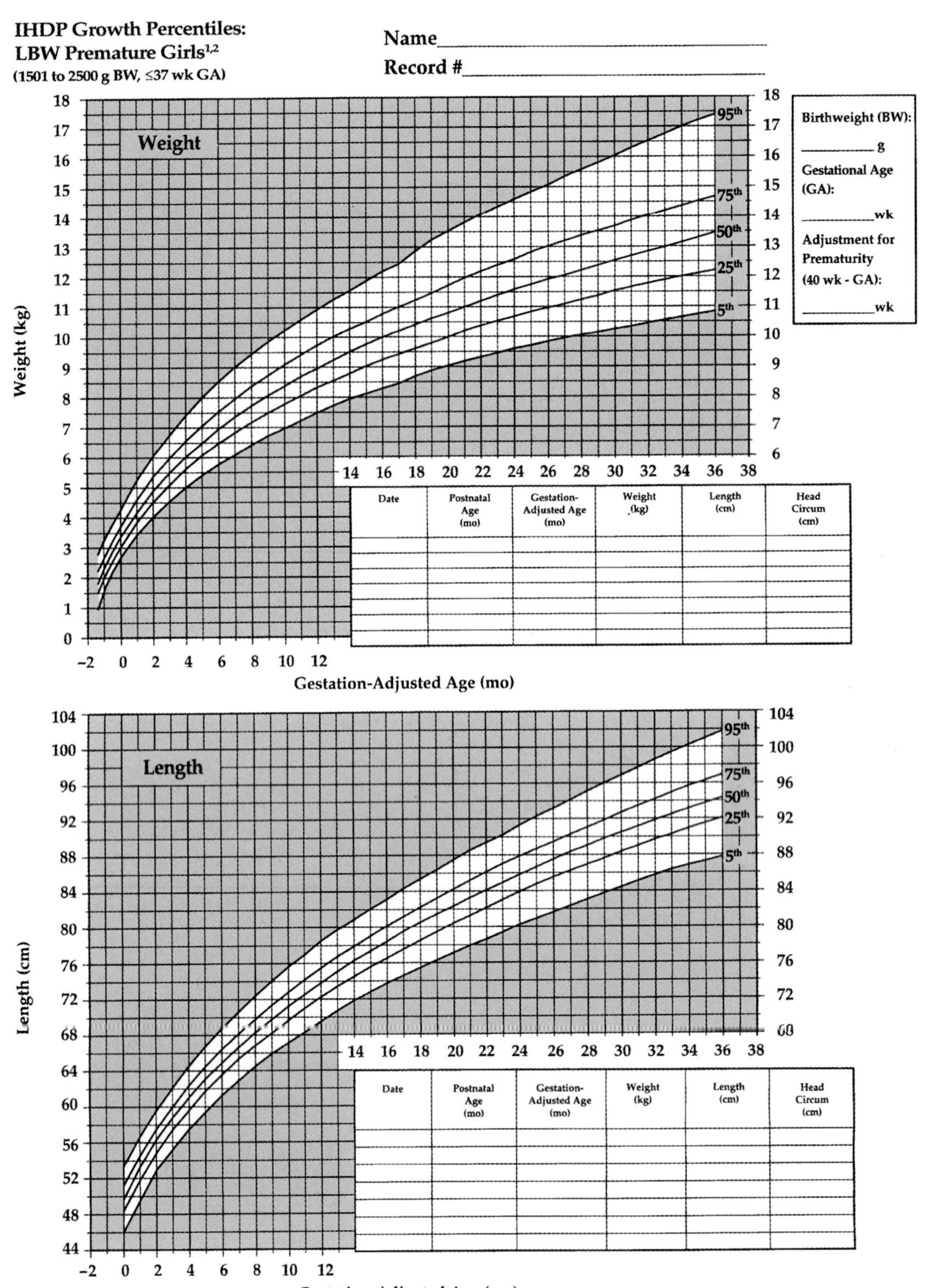
IHDP Growth Percentiles:
LBW Premature Girls[1,2]
(1501 to 2500 g BW, ≤37 wk GA)
Name
Record #
Weight
Weight (kg)
95th
75th
50th
25th
5th
Birthweight (BW):
g
Gestational Age (GA):
wk
Adjustment for Prematurity (40 wk - GA):
wk
Date
Postnatal Age (mo)
Gestation-Adjusted Age (mo)
Weight (kg)
Length (cm)
Head Circum (cm)
Gestation-Adjusted Age (mo)
Length
Length (cm)
95th
75th
50th
25th
5th
Date
Postnatal Age (mo)
Gestation-Adjusted Age (mo)
Weight (kg)
Length (cm)
Head Circum (cm)
Gestation-Adjusted Age (mo)

## IHDP Growth Percentiles: LBW Premature Girls (cont'd)

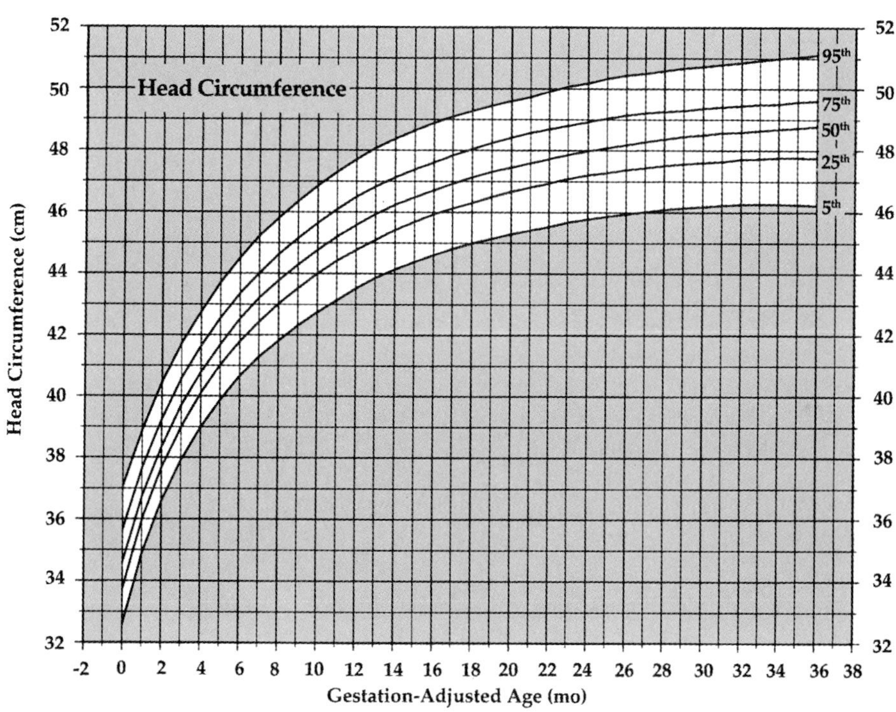

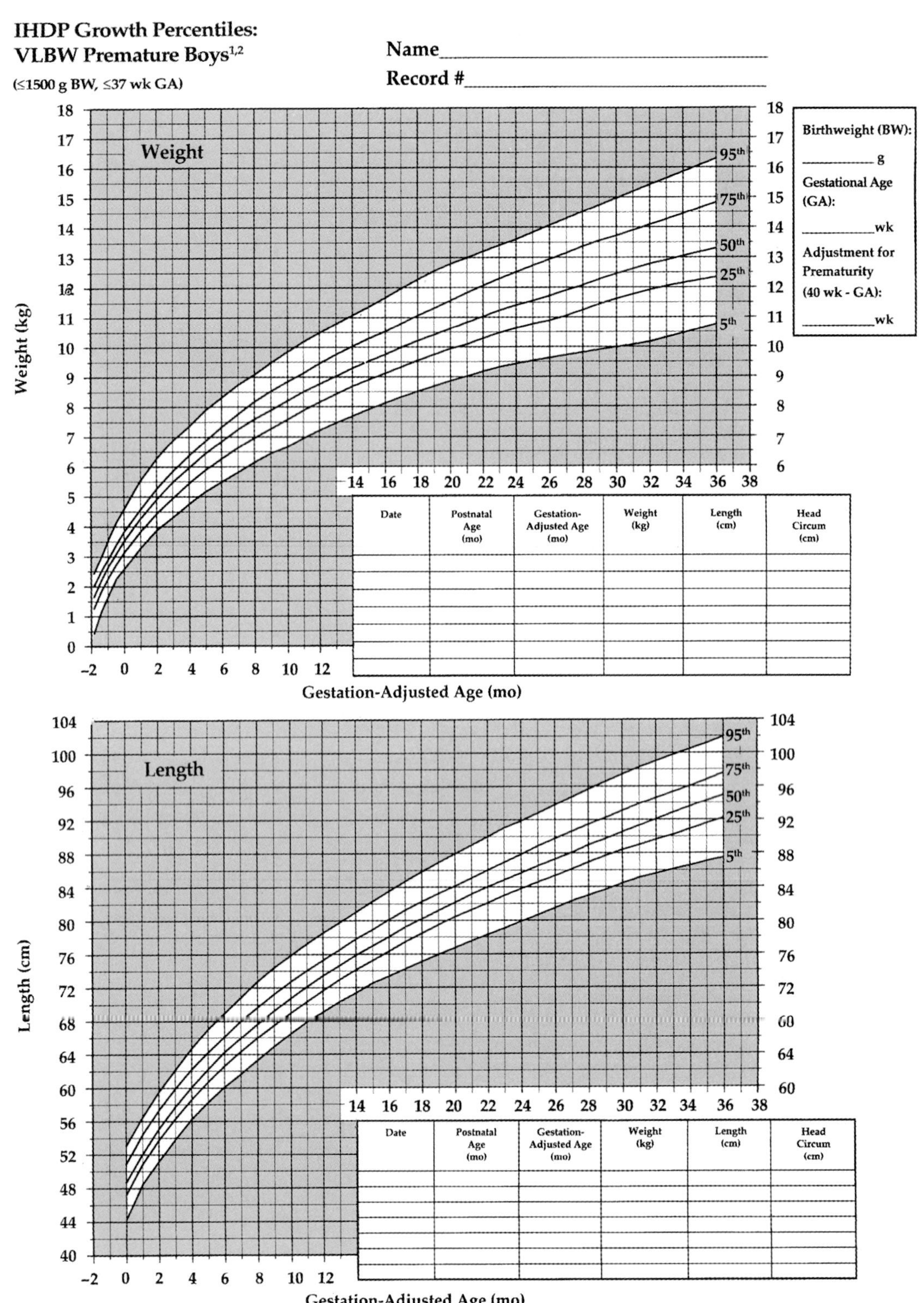
IHDP Growth Percentiles:
VLBW Premature Boys[1,2]
(≤1500 g BW, ≤37 wk GA)
Name
Record #
Weight
Weight (kg)
95th
75th
50th
25th
5th
Birthweight (BW): g
Gestational Age (GA): wk
Adjustment for Prematurity (40 wk - GA): wk
Date
Postnatal Age (mo)
Gestation-Adjusted Age (mo)
Weight (kg)
Length (cm)
Head Circum (cm)
Gestation-Adjusted Age (mo)
Length
Length (cm)
Gestation-Adjusted Age (mo)

## IHDP Growth Percentiles: VLBW Premature Boys (cont'd)

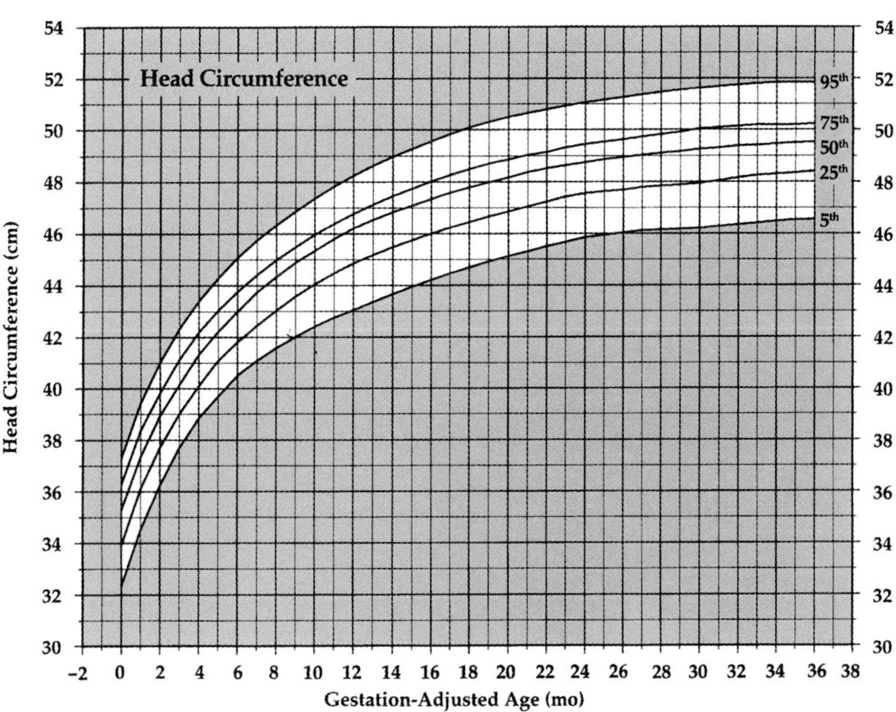

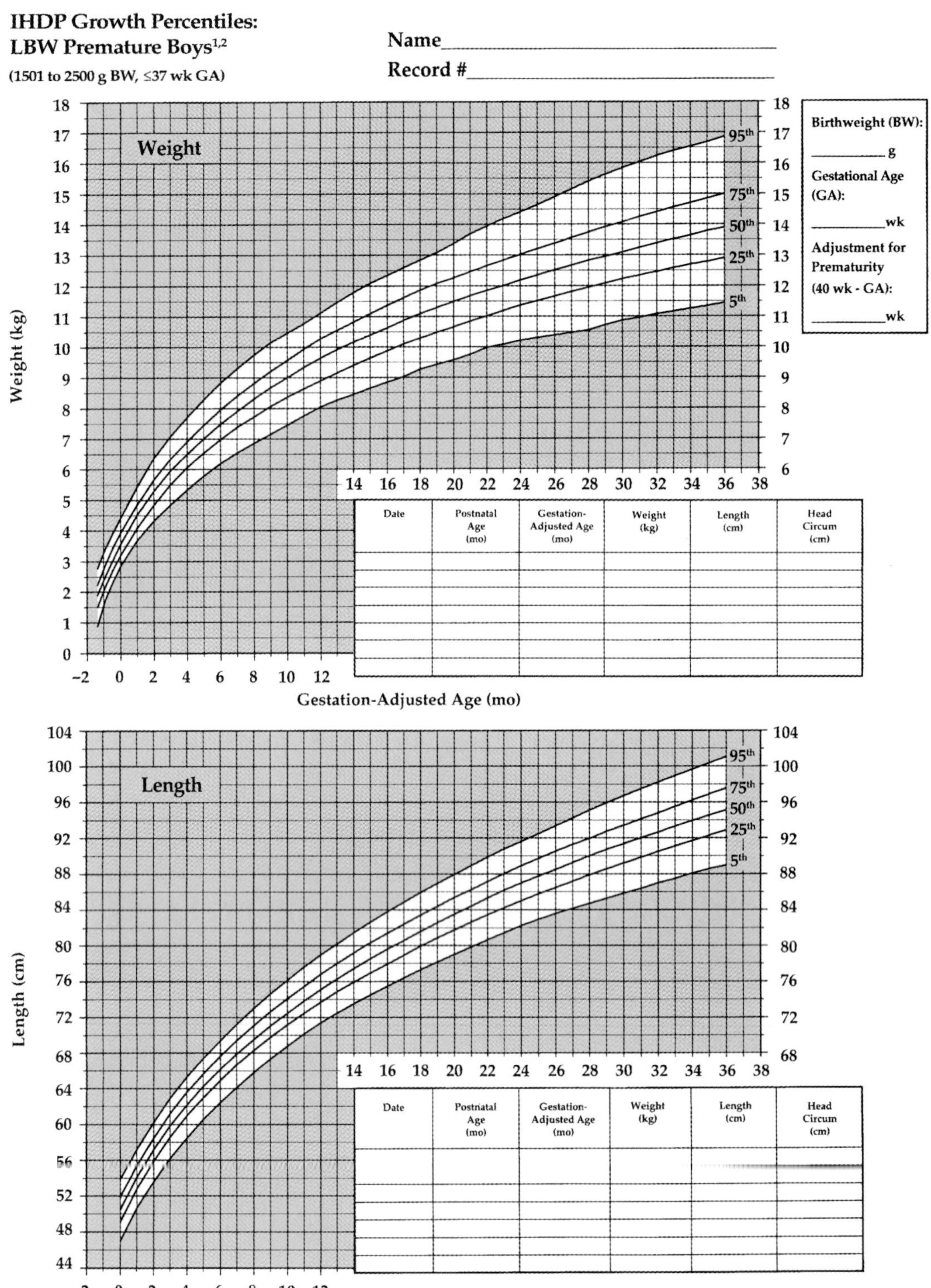
IHDP Growth Percentiles:
LBW Premature Boys[1,2]
(1501 to 2500 g BW, ≤37 wk GA)
Name
Record #
Weight
Weight (kg)
95th
75th
50th
25th
5th
Birthweight (BW): g
Gestational Age (GA): wk
Adjustment for Prematurity (40 wk - GA): wk
Date
Postnatal Age (mo)
Gestation-Adjusted Age (mo)
Weight (kg)
Length (cm)
Head Circum (cm)
Gestation-Adjusted Age (mo)
Length
Length (cm)
Gestation-Adjusted Age (mo)

**IHDP Growth Percentiles: LBW Premature Boys (cont'd)**

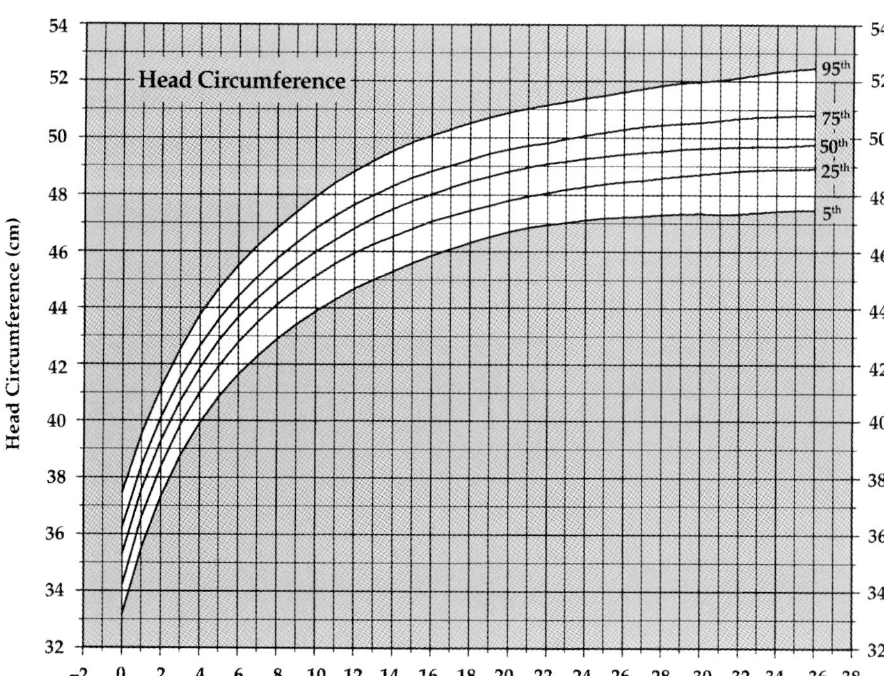


The growth of very low-birth-weight (VLBW) (≤1500 g) and low-birth-weight (LBW, 1501 to 2500 g) premature (≤37 weeks, gestational age [GA]) infants differs from that of normal-birth-weight term infants during infancy and early childhood. Because these infants may not catch up to term infants in growth during the early years, their growth should be compared with that of premature infants of similar birth weight.

The growth percentiles presented here are based on a large sample of infants enrolled in the Infant Health and Development Program (IHDP).[1,2] Some infants most likely to experience growth problems from biologic or environmental causes, premature infants with birth weight greater than 2500 g, and small-for-gestational-age term infants were excluded.[1] Study infants, however, are probably typical of premature infants who receive modern neonatal intensive care.

## REFERENCES


1. The Infant Health and Development Program: Enhancing the outcomes of low-birth-weight, premature infants. JAMA 263(22): 3035-3042, 1990.
2. Casey PH, Kraemer HC, Bernbaum J, et al: Growth status and growth rates of a varied sample of low birth weight, preterm infants: A longitudinal cohort from birth to three years of age. J Pediatr 119:599-605, 1991.


IHDP studies were supported by grants from the Robert Wood Johnson Foundation, Pew Charitable Trusts, and the Bureau of Maternal and Child Health, U.S. Department of Health and Human Services. These graphs were prepared by S.S. Guo and A.F. Roche, Wright State University, Yellow Springs, Ohio. IHDP, its sponsors, and the investigators do not endorse specific products.

Courtesy of Ross Products Division, Abbott Laboratories, Columbus, Ohio.

## Instructions for Use

1. Measure and record weight, length, and head circumference.
2. Calculate gestation-adjusted age by subtracting Adjustment for Prematurity in weeks from postnatal age in weeks. Adjustment for Prematurity equals 40 weeks minus GA. For example, at 12 weeks of postnatal age, the gestation-adjusted age for an infant born at 30 weeks of GA would be 2 weeks (0.5 month).

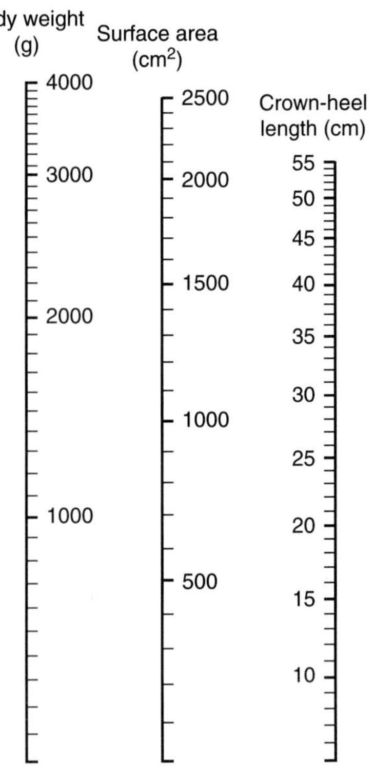


Nomogram for estimating the body surface area of human fetuses and neonates. It is based on the equation $S = 6.4954 \times W^{0.562} \times L^{0.320}$ where $S$ is the surface area in $cm^2$, $W$ is the body weight in g, and $L$ is the crown–heel length in cm. To use the nomogram, a ruler is aligned with the length and weight values on the outer axes. The point at which the central axis is intersected gives the value for body surface area. *(Data from Meban C: The surface area and volume of the human fetus. J Anat 137:271-278, 1983.)*

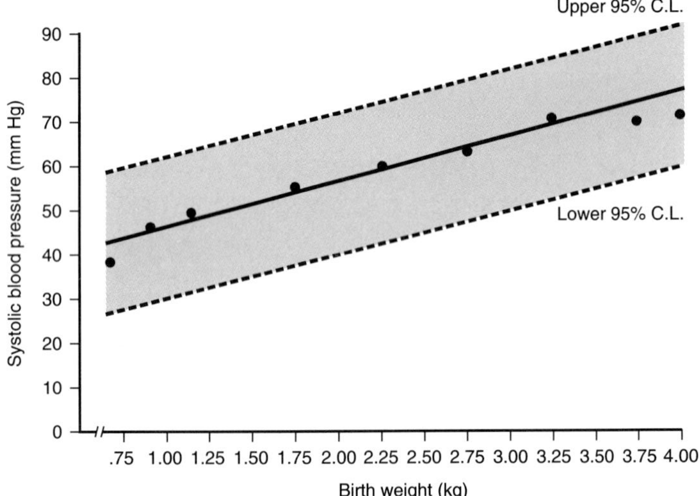


A

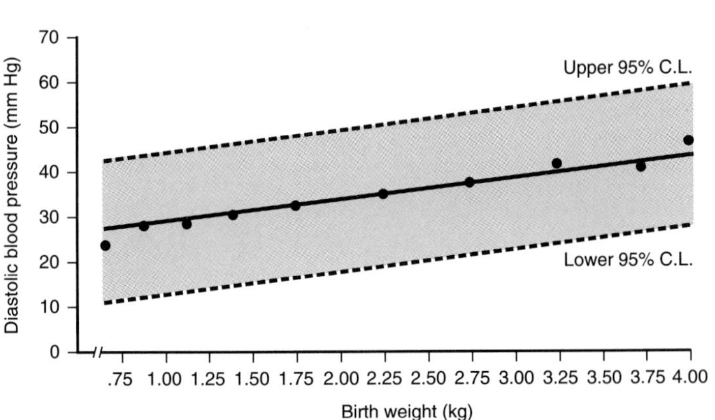


B

Linear regression of mean systolic (**A**) and diastolic (**B**) blood pressures (SBP and DBP) on birth weight in 329 infants admitted to NICU on day 1 of life is plotted. Equations are SBP = 8.52 × birth weight (kilograms) + 39.36 ($r = 0.68$, $P < 0.001$) and DBP = 5.21 × birth weight (kilograms) + 23.38 ($r = 0.48$, $P < 0.001$). Means of SBP and DBP for incremental birth weight groups are plotted about respective regression lines. The 95% confidence limits (C.L.; *shaded area surrounded by dashed lines*) is derived from standard error of regression estimate (SBP = 8.043 mm Hg, DBP = 8.370 mm Hg). This approximates mean ± 2 standard deviations. *(Data from Zubrow AB, Hulman S, Kushner H, et al: Determinants of blood pressure in infants admitted to neonatal intensive care units: A prospective multicenter study. J Perinatol 15[6]:472, 1995.)*

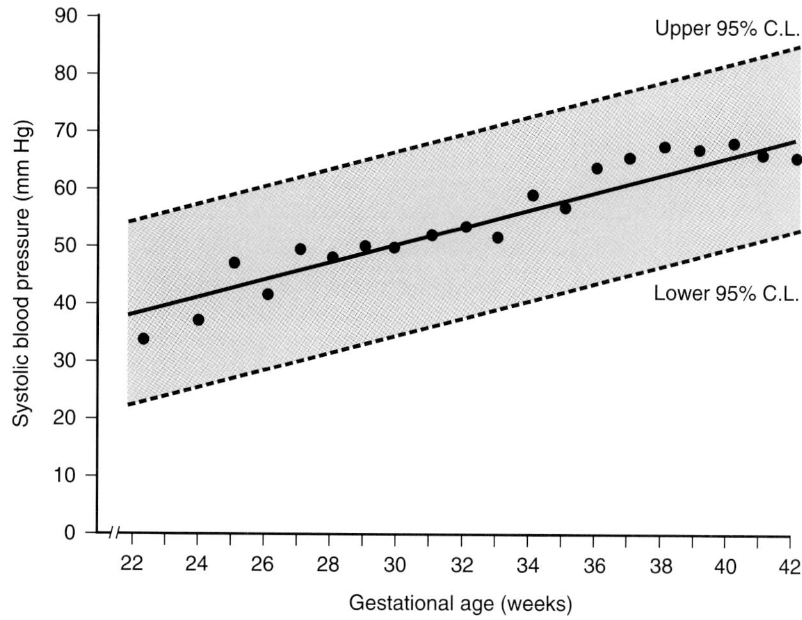


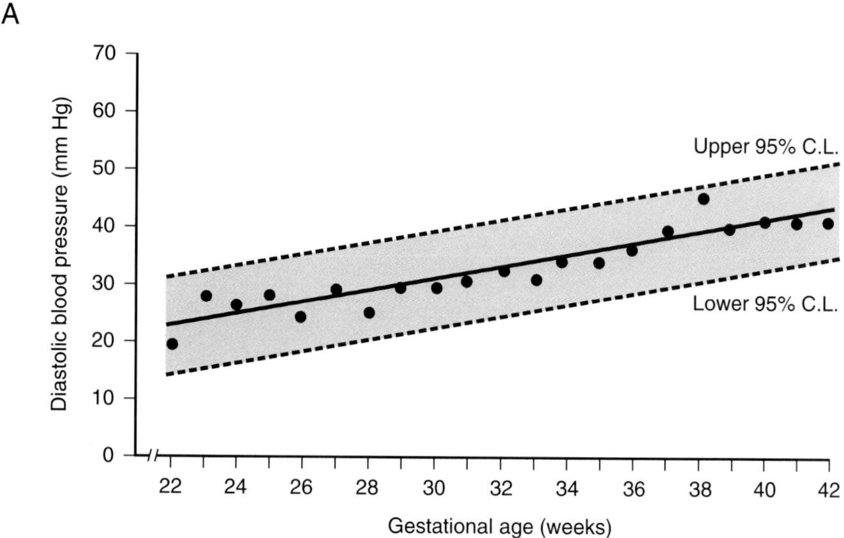


Linear regression of mean systolic (**A**) and diastolic (**B**) blood pressures (SBP and DBP) on gestational age in 329 infants admitted to the NICU on day 1 of life is plotted. Equations are SBP = 1.589 × gestational age (weeks) + 3.778 ($r$ = 0.66, $P$ < 0.0001) and DBP = 0.997 × gestational age (weeks) + 0.77 ($r$ = 0.47, $P$ < 0.0001). Computed mean values on day 1 of life are plotted for each week of gestational age at birth, from 22 to 42 weeks. The 95% confidence limits (C.L.; *shaded are surrounded by dashed lines*) is derived from standard error of regression estimate (SBP = 8.341 mm Hg, DBP = 8.474 mm Hg). This approximates mean ± 2 standard deviations. *(Data from Zubrow AB, Hulman S, Kushner H, et al: Determinants of blood pressure in infants admitted to neonatal intensive care units: A prospective multicenter study. J Perinatol 15[6]:473, 1995.)*

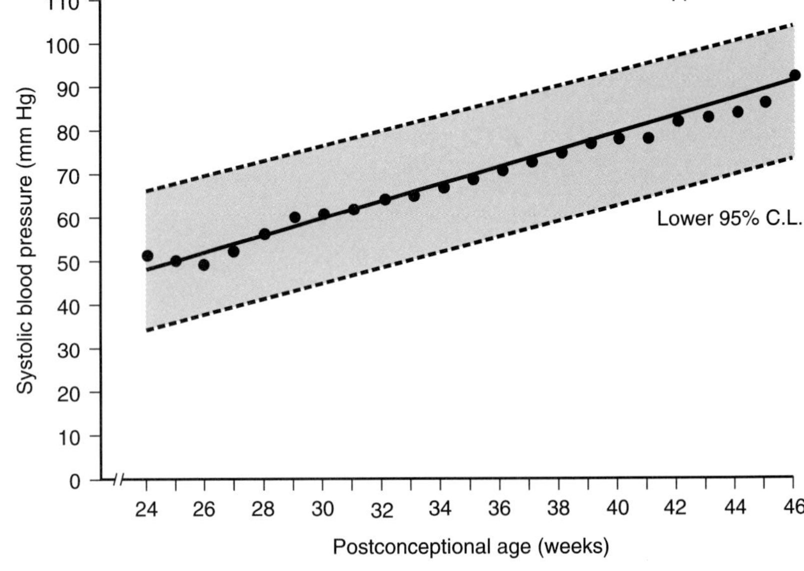


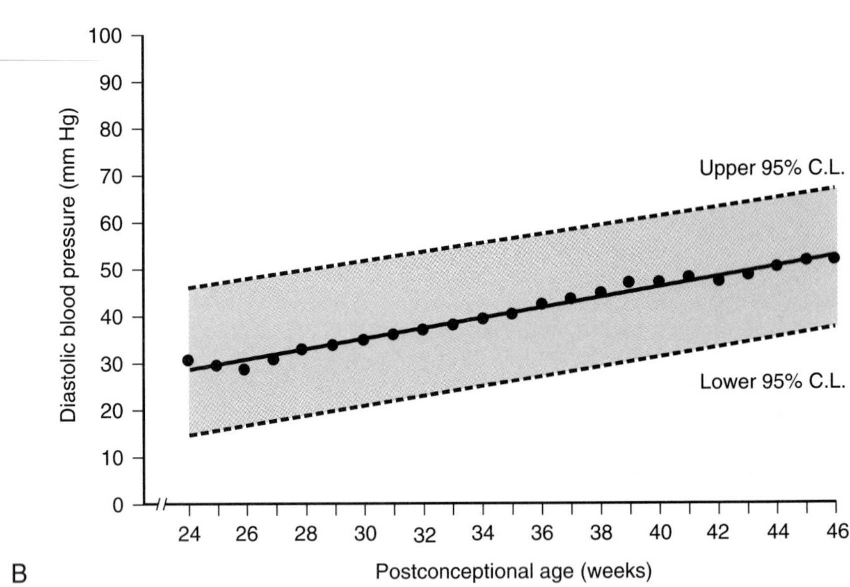


Postconceptional age (gestational age in weeks + weeks after delivery) is computed daily for each infant (8566 daily records) and regressed against mean systolic (**A**) and diastolic (**B**) blood pressures (SBP and DBP) for that day. Regression lines and equations are SBP = (0.255 × postconceptional age in weeks × 7) + 6.34, $r = 0.61$, $P < 0.0001$ and DBP = (0.151 × postconceptional age in weeks × 7) + 3.32, $r = 0.46$, $P < 0.0001$. Observed means of SBP and DBP for each postconceptional week are also plotted. C.L., confidence limit. *(Data from Zubrow AB, Hulman S, Kushner H, et al: Determinants of blood pressure in infants admitted to neonatal intensive care units: A prospective multicenter study. J Perinatol 15[6]:474, 1995.)*

**Colloid Osmotic Pressure (mm Hg) in Infants' Blood**

| | |
|---|---|
| Term, vaginal delivery | 19.5 ± 2.1 (SD) |
| Term, cesarean section | 16.1 ± 2.0 |
| Term, vaginal (sick) (sepsis, asphyxia, heart failure, abdominal surgery) | 19.5 ± 3.1 |
| Preterm (700-1980 g) (hyaline membrane disease, asphyxia, necrotizing enterocolitis, etc.) | 12.5 ± 2.5 |
| Older infants, 1-11 months | 25.1 ± 2.6 |

Data from Sola A, Gregory GA: Crit Care Med 9:568, 1981 and Sussmane JB, de Soto M, Torbati D: Plasma colloid osmotic pressure in healthy infants. Crit Care 5:261-264, 2001.

## RBC Parameters for VLBW Infants During the First 6 Weeks of Life

| | Day of Life | Valid *n* | Percentile 3 | 5 | 10 | 25 | Median | 75 | 90 | 95 | 97 |
|---|---|---|---|---|---|---|---|---|---|---|---|
| Hemoglobin (g/dL) | 3 | 559 | 11.0 | 11.6 | 12.5 | 14.0 | 15.6 | 17.1 | 18.5 | 19.3 | 19.8 |
| | 12-14 | 203 | 10.1 | 10.8 | 11.1 | 12.5 | 14.4 | 15.7 | 17.4 | 18.4 | 18.9 |
| | 24-26 | 192 | 8.5 | 8.9 | 9.7 | 10.9 | 12.4 | 14.2 | 15.6 | 16.5 | 16.8 |
| | 40-42 | 150 | 7.8 | 7.9 | 8.4 | 9.3 | 10.6 | 12.4 | 13.8 | 14.9 | 15.4 |
| Hematocrit (%) | 3 | 561 | 35 | 36 | 39 | 43 | 47 | 52 | 56 | 59 | 60 |
| | 12-14 | 205 | 30 | 32 | 34 | 39 | 44 | 48 | 53 | 55 | 56 |
| | 24-26 | 196 | 25 | 27 | 29 | 32 | 39 | 44 | 48 | 50 | 52 |
| | 40-42 | 152 | 24 | 24 | 26 | 28 | 33 | 38 | 44 | 47 | 48 |
| RBCs ($10^{12}$/L) | 3 | 364 | 3.2 | 3.3 | 3.5 | 3.8 | 4.2 | 4.6 | 4.9 | 5.1 | 5.3 |
| | 12-14 | 196 | 2.9 | 3.0 | 3.2 | 3.5 | 4.1 | 4.6 | 5.2 | 5.5 | 5.6 |
| | 24-26 | 188 | 2.6 | 2.6 | 2.8 | 3.2 | 3.8 | 4.4 | 4.8 | 5.2 | 5.3 |
| | 40-42 | 148 | 2.5 | 2.5 | 2.6 | 3.0 | 3.4 | 4.1 | 4.6 | 4.8 | 4.9 |
| Corrected reticulocytes (%) | 3 | 283 | .6 | .7 | 1.9 | 4.2 | 7.1 | 12.0 | 20.0 | 24.1 | 27.8 |
| | 12-14 | 139 | .3 | .3 | .5 | .8 | 1.7 | 2.7 | 5.7 | 7.3 | 9.6 |
| | 24-26 | 140 | .2 | .3 | .5 | .8 | 1.5 | 2.6 | 4.7 | 6.4 | 8.6 |
| | 40-42 | 114 | .3 | .4 | .6 | 1.0 | 1.8 | 3.4 | 5.6 | 8.3 | 9.5 |

On day 3, all infants are included irrespective of antenatal steroids and transfusions up to day 3. Thereafter, infants who did not receive rhEPO were studied, irrespective of the use of antibiotics and steroids.

RBC, red blood cell; rhEPO, recombinant human erythropoietin; VLBW, very low-birth-weight.

Data from Obladen M, Diepold K, Maier RF, the European Multicenter rhEPO Study Group: Venous and arterial hematologic profiles of very low birth weight infants. Pediatrics 106:707, 2000.

## Normal Blood Chemistry Values in Term Infants

| Determination | Sample Source | Cord | Age 1-12 hr | 12-24 hr | 24-48 hr | 48-72 hr |
|---|---|---|---|---|---|---|
| Sodium (mEq/L)* | Capillary | 147 (126-166) | 143 (124-156) | 145 (132-159) | 148 (134-160) | 149 (139-162) |
| Chloride (mEq/L) | | 103 (98-110) | 100.7 (90-111) | 103 (87-114) | 102 (92-114) | 103 (93-112) |
| Calcium (mg/100 dL) | | 9.3 (8.2-11.1) | 8.4 (7.3-9.2) | 7.8 (6.9-9.4) | 8.0 (6.1-9.9) | 7.9 (5.9-9.7) |
| Ionized calcium (mmol/L)** | | — | 1.24 (±0.11) | 1.19 (±0.122) | 1.21 (±0.132) | 1.22 (±0.138) |
| Phosphorus (mg/100 mL) | | 5.6 (3.7-8.1) | 6.1 (3.5-8.6) | 5.7 (2.9-8.1) | 5.9 (3.0-8.7) | 5.8 (2.8-7.6) |
| Blood urea nitrogen (mg/100 dL) | | 29 (21-40) | 27 (8-34) | 33 (9-63) | 32 (13-77) | 31 (15-68) |
| Total protein (g/100 dL) | | 6.1 (4.8-7.3) | 6.6 (5.6-8.5) | 6.6 (5.8-8.2) | 6.9 (5.9-8.2) | 7.2 (6.0-8.5) |
| Blood sugar (mg/100 dL) | | 73 (45-96) | 63 (40-97) | 63 (42-104) | 56 (30-91) | 59 (40-90) |
| Lactic acid (mg/100 dL) | | 19.5 (11-30) | 14.6 (11-24) | 14.0 (10-23) | 14.3 (9-22) | 13.5 (7-21) |
| Lactate, mm/L† | | 2.0-3.0 | 2.0 | | | |

*Data from Acharya and Payne: Arch Dis Child 40:430, 1968.

†Daniel, Adamsons, and James: Pediatrics 37:942, 1966.

‡Wandrup, Kroner, Pryds, and Kastrup: Scand J Clin Lab Invest 48:255-260, 1988.

## Serum Electrolyte Values in Preterm Infants

| | Age 1 Week | | | Age 3 Weeks | | | Age 5 Weeks | | | Age 7 Weeks | | |
|---|---|---|---|---|---|---|---|---|---|---|---|---|
| Constituent | Mean | SD | Range | Mean | SD | Range | Mean | SD | Range | Mean | SD | Range |
| Na (mEq/L) | 139.6 | ±3.2 | 133-146 | 136.3 | ±2.9 | 129-142 | 136.8 | ±2.5 | 133-148 | 137.2 | ±1.8 | 133-142 |
| K (mEq/L) | 5.6 | ±0.5 | 4.6-6.7 | 5.8 | ±0.6 | 4.5-7.1 | 5.5 | ±0.6 | 4.5-6.6 | 5.7 | ±0.5 | 4.6-7.1 |
| Cl (mEq/L) | 108.2 | ±3.7 | 100-117 | 108.3 | ±3.9 | 102-116 | 107.0 | ±3.5 | 100-115 | 107.0 | ±3.3 | 101-115 |
| $CO_2$ (mmol/L) | 20.3 | ±2.8 | 13.8-27.1 | 18.4 | ±3.5 | 12.4-26.2 | 20.4 | ±3.4 | 12.5-26.1 | 20.6 | ±3.1 | 13.7-26.9 |
| Ca (mg/dL) | 9.2 | ±1.1 | 6.1-11.6 | 9.6 | ±0.5 | 8.1-11.0 | 9.4 | ±0.5 | 8.6-10.5 | 9.5 | ±0.7 | 8.6-10.8 |
| P (mg/dL) | 7.6 | ±1.1 | 5.4-10.9 | 7.5 | ±0.7 | 6.2-8.7 | 7.0 | ±0.6 | 5.6-7.9 | 6.8 | ±0.8 | 4.2-8.2 |
| BUN (mg/dL) | 9.3 | ±5.2 | 3.1-25.5 | 13.3 | ±7.8 | 2.1-31.4 | 13.3 | ±7.1 | 2.0-26.5 | 13.4 | ±6.7 | 2.5-30.5 |

BUN, blood urea nitrogen.

From Klaus MH, Fanaroff AA: Care of the High-Risk Neonate, 3rd ed. Philadelphia, WB Saunders, 1988. Adapted from Thomas J, Reichelderfer T: Clin Chem 14:272, 1968.

## Thyroid Function in Full-Term and Preterm Infants

### Serum Thyroxine ($T_4$) Concentration

| | Estimated Gestational Age (wk) | | | | |
|---|---|---|---|---|---|
| | 30-31 | 32-33 | 34-35 | 36-37 | Term |
| Cord | | | | | |
| Mean | 6.5* | 7.5 | 6.7† | 7.5 | 8.2 |
| SD | 1.0 | 2.1 | 1.2 | 2.8 | 1.8 |
| *n* | 3 | 8 | 18 | 17 | 37 |
| 12-72 hr | | | | | |
| Mean | 11.5‡ | 12.3‡ | 12.4‡ | 15.5† | 19.0 |
| SD | 2.1 | 3.2 | 3.1 | 2.6 | 2.1 |
| *n* | 12 | 18 | 17 | 15 | 6 |
| 3-10 days | | | | | |
| Mean | 7.7‡ | 8.5‡ | 10.0‡ | 12.7† | 15.9 |
| SD | 1.8 | 1.9 | 2.4 | 2.5 | 3.0 |
| *n* | 7 | 8 | 9 | 9 | 29 |
| 11-20 days | | | | | |
| Mean | 7.5† | 8.3‡ | 10.5 | 11.2 | 12.2 |
| SD | 1.8 | 1.6 | 1.8 | 2.9 | 2.0 |
| *n* | 5 | 11 | 9 | 9 | 8 |
| 21-45 days | | | | | |
| Mean | 7.8‡ | 8.0‡ | 9.3† | 11.4 | 12.1 |
| SD | 1.5 | 1.7 | 1.3 | 4.2 | 1.5 |
| *n* | 11 | 17 | 13 | 5 | 5 |
| 46-90 days | | (30-73 weeks) | | | |
| Mean | | 9.6 | | | 10.2 |
| SD | | 1.7 | | | 1.9 |
| *n* | | 16 | | | 17 |

*$P < .05$
†$P < .005$
‡$P < .001$
for the comparison of preterm versus term infants (*t*-test).

From Cuestas RA: Thyroid function in healthy premature infants. J Pediatr 92:963, 1978.

### Serum Free Thyroxine ($T_4$) Index

| | Estimated Gestational Age (wk) | | | | |
|---|---|---|---|---|---|
| | 30-31 | 32-33 | 34-35 | 36-37 | Term |
| Cord | | | | | |
| Mean | | | 5.6 | 5.6 | 5.9 |
| SD | | | 1.3 | 2.0 | 1.1 |
| *n* | | | 12 | 10 | 14 |
| 12-72 hr | | | | | |
| Mean | 13.1* | 12.9* | 15.5† | 17.1 | 19.7 |
| SD | 2.4 | 2.7 | 3.0 | 3.5 | 3.5 |
| *n* | 12 | 14 | 14 | 14 | 6 |
| 3-10 days | | | | | |
| Mean | 8.3* | 9.0* | 12.0‡ | 15.1 | 16.2 |
| SD | 1.9 | 1.8 | 2.3 | 0.7 | 3.2 |
| *n* | 6 | 9 | 5 | 4 | 11 |
| 11-20 days | | | | | |
| Mean | 8.0§ | 9.1‡ | 11.8 | 11.3 | 12.1 |
| SD | 1.6 | 1.9 | 2.7 | 1.9 | 2.0 |
| *n* | 5 | 8 | 8 | 4 | 8 |
| 21-45 days | | | | | |
| Mean | 8.4§ | 9.0‡ | 10.9 | | 11.1 |
| SD | 1.4 | 1.6 | 2.8 | | 1.4 |
| *n* | 11 | 17 | 5 | | 5 |
| 46-90 days | | 30-35 weeks | | | |
| Mean | | 9.4 | | | 9.7 |
| SD | | 1.4 | | | 1.5 |
| *n* | | 13 | | | 10 |

*$P$ .001
†$P$ .025
‡$P$ .01
§$P$ .005
for the comparison of preterm versus term infants (*t*-test).

From Cuestas RA: J Pediatr 92:963, 1978.

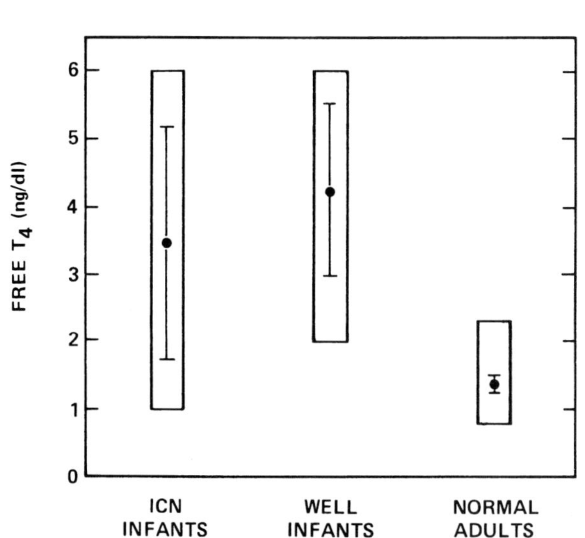


Free thyroxine ($T_4$) levels in sick intensive care nursery (ICN) infants, healthy term infants, and normal adults. The center represents the mean ± SD. *(From Wilson DM, et al: J Pediatr 101:113, 1982.)*

Thyroid-stimulating hormone (TSH) levels in healthy preterm infants. Mean, standard error of the mean, and sample size are shown. *(From Cuestas RA: J Pediatr 92:963, 1978.)*

**Results of Studies on Cerebrospinal Fluid in Noninfected Term Neonates**

| Reference | *n* | Age | WBC* (mm³) | Neutrophils* (mm³) | Glucose* (mg/dL) | Protein* (mg/dL) |
|---|---|---|---|---|---|---|
| Stewart (1928) | 6 | <8 wk | 21 (18-34) | NR | NR | 33.5 (15-45) |
| Naidoo (1968) | 135 | 1 day | 12 (0-42) | 7 (0-26) | 48 (38-64) | 73 (40-148) |
| | 20 | 7 days | 3 (0-9) | 2 (0-5) | 55 (48-62) | 47 (27-65) |
| Sarff et al (1976) | 87 | Majority <7 days | 8.2 ± 7.1<br>Median 5 (0-32) | Mean % 61 | 52 (34-119) | 90 (20-170) |
| Pappu et al (1982) | 24 | 0-32 days | 11 (1-38) | Mean % 21 (0-100) | NR | NR |
| Portnoy and Olson (1985) | 64 | <6 wk | 3.73 ± 3.4 | 1.87 ± 2.98 | NR | NR |
| Bonadio et al (1992) | 35 | 0-4 wk | 11.0 ± 10.4<br>Median 8.5 | 0.4 ± 1.4<br>Median 0.15 | 46 ± 10.3 | 84 ± 45.1 |
| | 40 | 4-8 wk | 7.1 ± 9.2<br>Median 4.5 | 0.2 ± 0.4<br>Median 0 | 46 ± 10.0 | 59 ± 25.3 |
| Ahmed et al (1996) | 108 | 0-30 days | 7.3 ± 13.9<br>Median 4 | 0.8 ± 6.2<br>Median 0 | 51.2 ± 12.9 | 64.2 ± 24.2 |

*Expressed as mean with range (number in parentheses) or ± SD unless otherwise specified.

*n*, number of patients; NR, not reported.

Data from Ahmed A, Hickey SA, Ehrett S, et al: Cerebrospinal fluid values in the term neonate. Pediatr Infect Dis 15(4):298, 1996.

**Cerebrospinal Fluid Values in Very Low-Birth-Weight Infants on the Basis of Birth Weight**

| | Group 1 (≤1000 g) ($n$ = 38*) | | Group 2 (1001-1500 g) (n = 33*) | | |
|---|---|---|---|---|---|
| | Mean ± SD | Range | Mean ± SD | Range | $P$ |
| Birth weight (g) | 763 ± 115 | 550-980 | 1278 ± 152 | 1020-1500 | |
| Gestational age (wk) | 26 ± 1.3 | 24-28 | 29 ± 1.4 | 27-33 | |
| Leukocytes/mm$^3$ | 4 ± 3 | 0-14 | 6 ± 9 | 0-44 | NS |
| Erythrocytes/mm$^3$ | 1027 ± 3270 | 0-19,050 | 786 ± 1879 | 0-9750 | |
| PMNs (%) | 6 ± 15 | 0-66 | 9 ± 17 | 0-60 | NS |
| MN leukocytes (%) | 86 ± 30 | 34-100 | 85 ± 28 | 13-100 | |
| Glucose (mg/dL) | 61 ± 34 | 29-217 | 59 ± 21 | 31-109 | NS |
| Protein (mg/dL) | 150 ± 56 | 95-370 | 132 ± 43 | 45-227 | NS |

*Number of cerebrospinal fluid specimens.

MN, mononuclear; NS, not significant ($P > .05$); PMN, polymorphonuclear leukocytes.

From Rodriguez AF, Kaplan SL, Mason EO: Cerebrospinal fluid values and the very LBW infant. J Pediatr 116:971, 1990.

**Cerebrospinal Fluid (CSF) Analysis from Previous Studies in Premature Infants with Birth Weight ≤2500 g**

| Author | No. of Infants | Postnatal Age | Mean CSF Cells/mm$^3$ (Range) | Mean Protein (mg/dL) (Range) |
|---|---|---|---|---|
| Samson (1931) | NR | Up to 1 mo | 4 | 55 |
| Otila (1948) | 46 | Up to 1 mo | 10 | 101 |
| Wolf and Hoepffner (1961) | 22 | 1-3 days | 2 (0-13) | 105 (50-180) |
| Gyllenswärd and Malmström (1962) | 36 | 1-40 days | 7 (1-37) | 115 (55-292) |
| Sarff et al (1976) | 30 | 1-6 days | 9 (0-29) | 115 (65-150) |

NR, not recorded.

From Rodriguez AF, Kaplan SL, Mason EO: Cerebrospinal fluid values and the very LBW infant. J Pediatr 116:971, 1990.

TERM NEWBORN

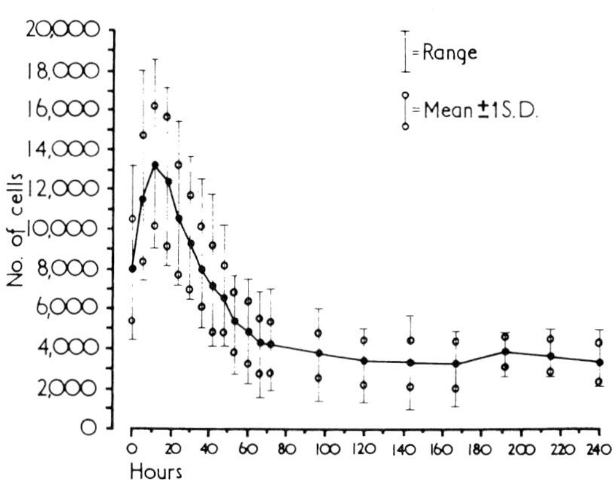


Means, ranges, and means ± 1 SD for neutrophil counts in 15 full-term healthy babies during the first 10 days of life. *(Data from Xanthou M: Arch Dis Child 45:242, 1970.)*

PREMATURES

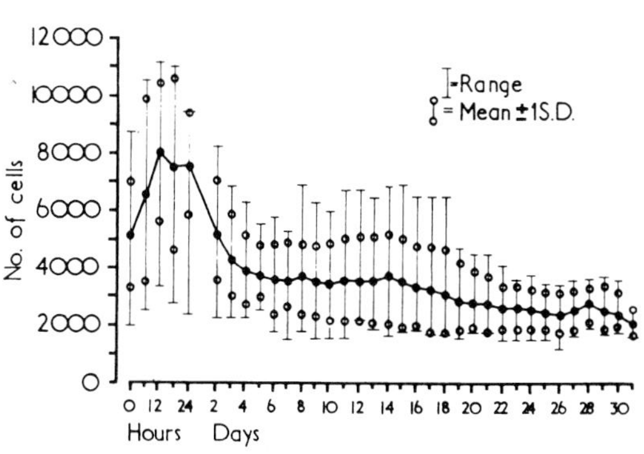


Means, ranges, and means ± 1 SD for neutrophil counts in 14 healthy babies during the first month of life (13 premature + 1 small for dates). *(Data from Xanthou M: Arch Dis Child 45:242, 1970.)*

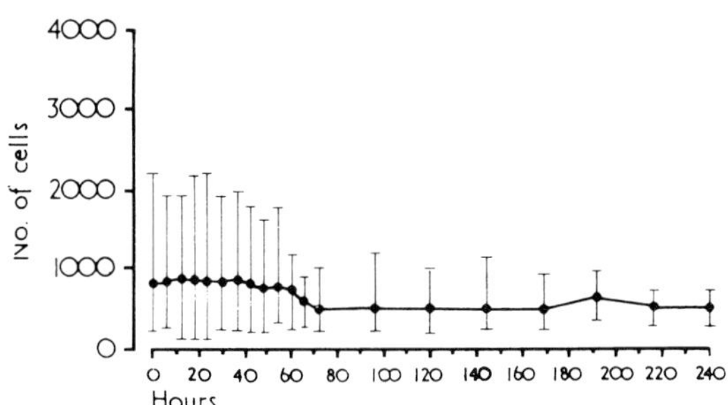


Means and ranges for eosinophil counts in full-term babies during the first 10 days of life. *(Data from Xanthou M: Arch Dis Child 45:242, 1970.)*

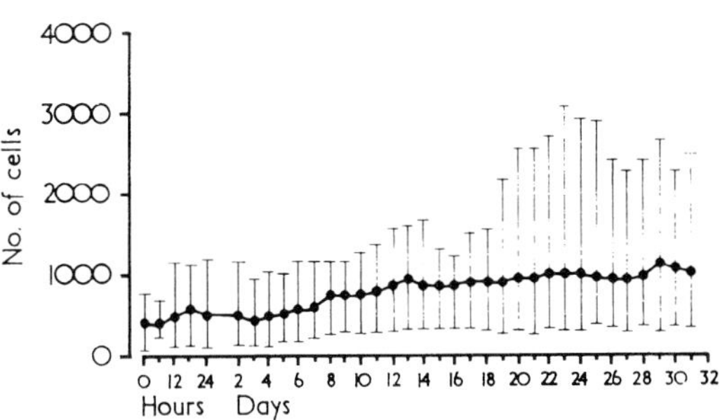


Means and ranges for eosinophil counts in low-birth-weight babies during the first month of life. *(Data from Xanthou M: Arch Dis Child 45:242, 1970.)*

## TERM NEWBORN

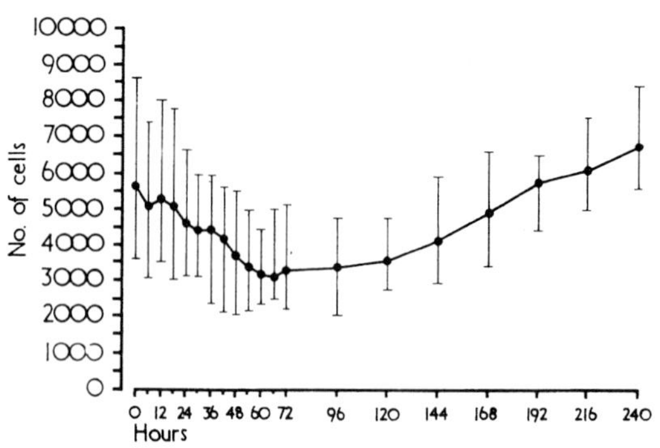


Means and ranges for lymphocyte counts in full-term babies during the first 10 days of life. *(Data from Xanthou M: Arch Dis Child 45:242, 1970.)*

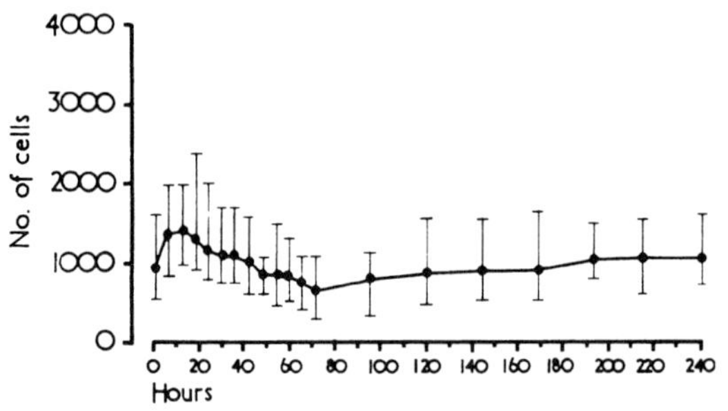


Means and ranges for monocyte counts in healthy full-term babies during the first 10 days of life. *(Data from Xanthou M: Arch Dis Child 45:242, 1970.)*

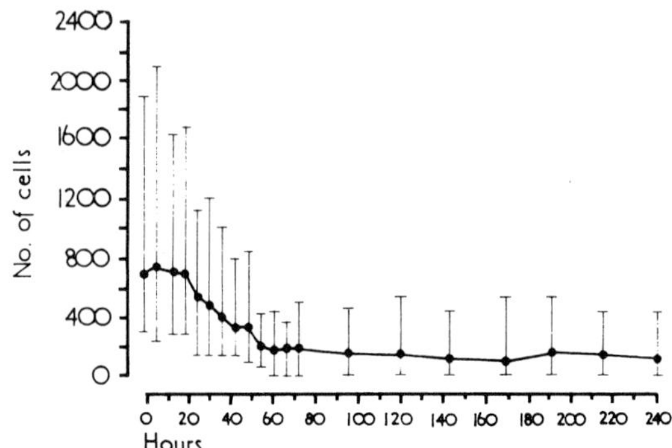


Means and ranges for metamyelocyte counts in full-term babies during the first 10 days of life. *(Data from Xanthou M: Arch Dis Child 45:242, 1970.)*

## PREMATURES

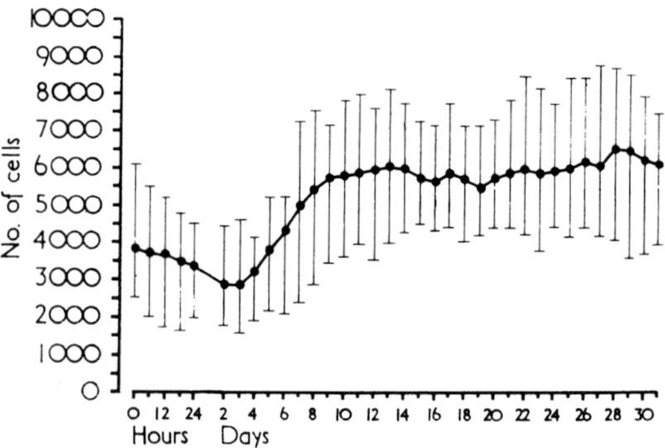


Means and ranges for lymphocyte counts in low-birth-weight babies during the first month of life. *(Data from Xanthou M: Arch Dis Child 45:242, 1970.)*

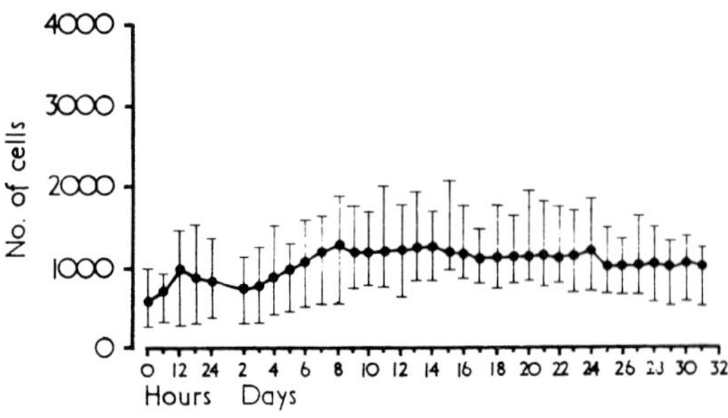


Means and ranges for monocyte counts in low-birth-weight babies during the first month of life. *(Data from Xanthou M: Arch Dis Child 45:242, 1970.)*

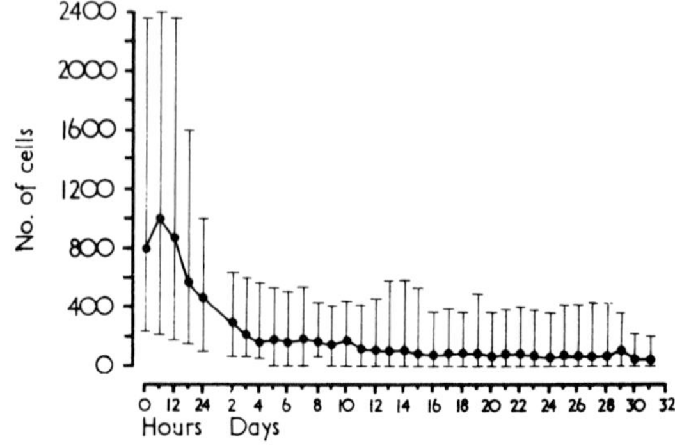


Means and ranges for metamyelocyte counts in 14 healthy babies during the first month of life. *(Data from Xanthou M: Arch Dis Child 45:242, 1970.)*

**Nucleated Red Blood Cells in Normal Infants and Infants of Diabetic Mothers**

| | | Infants of Diabetic Mothers | |
|---|---|---|---|
| Variables | Control Infants ($n$ = 102) | No Perinatal Asphyxia ($n$ = 54) | Perinatal Asphyxia ($n$ = 25) |
| Gestational age (weeks) | 39.5 ± 1.5 | 38.0 ± 1.0* | 37.9 ± 1.2* |
| Birth weight (kg) | 3.3 ± 0.3 | 3.5 ± 0.6* | 3.6 ± 0.6* |
| Leukocyte count† | 27.3 ± 9.2 | 17.1 ± 5.1* | 16.8 ± 6.1* |
| NRBCs (absolute count) | 0.4 ± 1.3 | 1.4 ± 3.1* | 1.8 ± 2.3* |
| NRBCs/100 leukocytes | 1.7 ± 6.2 | 8.3 ± 17.8* | 13.0 ± 18.9* |

*Significantly different from control infant values ($P$ at least $<.05$).

†Data are expressed as $\times 10^9$/L.

NRBC, nucleated red blood cell.

Adapted from Green DW, Mimouni F: J Pediatr 116:129, 1990.

**Umbilical Artery Cord Blood Gas Values in Healthy Term Infants**

| | | Distribution Values (Percentile) | | |
|---|---|---|---|---|
| | Range | 10th | 50th | 90th |
| pH | 7.04-7.49 | 7.21 | 7.29 | 7.37 |
| $PaCO_2$ (mm Hg) | 27.2-75.4 | 38.9 | 49.5 | 62.0 |
| $PaO_2$ (mm Hg) | 4.6-48.4 | 10.1 | 18.0 | 32.0 |
| $HCO_3$ (mmol/L) | 13.6-29.4 | 20.3 | 23.4 | 25.9 |

Data from Dudenhausen JW, Luhr C, Dimer JS: Umbilical artery blood gases in healthy term newborn infants. Intl J Gynecol Obstet 57:251-258, 1997.

**Mean Umbilical Cord Blood Gas Values in Preterm Infants**

| | Mean Value | |
|---|---|---|
| | Arterial | Venous |
| pH | 7.26 ± 0.08 | 7.33 ± 0.07 |
| $PCO_2$ (mm Hg) | 53.0 ± 10.0 | 43.4 ± 8.3 |
| $PO_2$ (mm Hg) | 19.0 ± 7.9 | 29.2 ± 9.7 |
| $HCO_3$ (mEq/L) | 24.0 ± 2.3 | 22.8 ± 2.1 |
| Base excess (mEq/L) | −3.2 ± 2.9 | −2.6 ± 2.5 |

From Dickinson JE, Eriksen NL, Meyer BA, Parisi VM: The effect of preterm birth on umbilical cord blood gases. Obstet Gynecol 79:575-578, 1992.

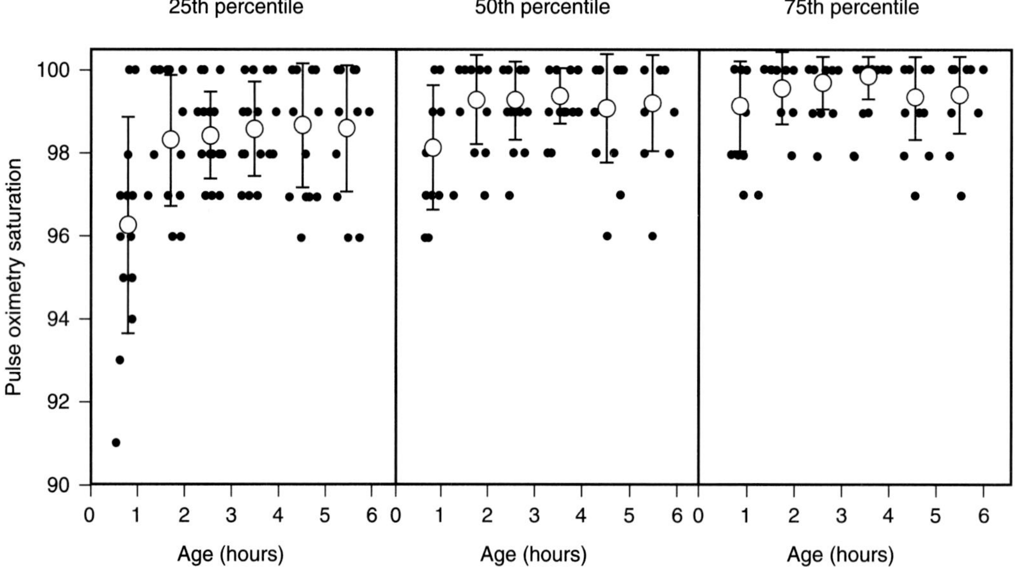


The 25th, 50th, and 75th percentile saturation values in 101 normal newborns during the first 6 hours of life. The *solid circles* represent individual saturation values. The *open circles* represent mean values for a given postnatal hour and are plotted at the mean age for the group. *Error bars* represent one standard deviation. *(Data from Reddy VK, Holzman IR, Wedgwood JF: Pulse oximetry saturations in the first 6 hours of life in normal term infants. Clin Pediatr 38:87, 1999.)*

## Body Composition of the Reference Fetus

| Gestational Age (wk) | Body Weight (g) | Units per 100 g Body Weight | | | | Units per 100 g Fat-Free Weight | | | | | | | |
|---|---|---|---|---|---|---|---|---|---|---|---|---|---|
| | | Water (g) | Protein (g) | Lipid (g) | Other (g) | Water (g) | Protein (g) | Ca (mg) | P (mg) | Mg (mg) | Na (mEq) | K (mEq) | Cl (mEq) |
| 24 | 690 | 88.6 | 8.8 | 0.1 | 2.5 | 88.6 | 8.8 | 621 | 387 | 17.8 | 9.9 | 4.0 | 7.0 |
| 25 | 770 | 87.8 | 9.0 | 0.7 | 2.5 | 88.4 | 9.1 | 615 | 385 | 17.6 | 9.8 | 4.0 | 7.0 |
| 26 | 880 | 86.8 | 9.2 | 1.5 | 2.5 | 88.1 | 9.4 | 611 | 384 | 17.5 | 9.7 | 4.1 | 7.0 |
| 27 | 1010 | 85.7 | 9.4 | 2.4 | 2.5 | 87.8 | 9.7 | 609 | 383 | 17.4 | 9.5 | 4.1 | 6.9 |
| 28 | 1160 | 84.6 | 9.6 | 3.3 | 2.4 | 87.5 | 10.0 | 610 | 385 | 17.4 | 9.4 | 4.2 | 6.9 |
| 29 | 1318 | 83.6 | 9.9 | 4.1 | 2.4 | 87.2 | 10.3 | 613 | 387 | 17.4 | 9.3 | 4.2 | 6.8 |
| 30 | 1480 | 82.6 | 10.1 | 4.9 | 2.4 | 86.8 | 10.6 | 619 | 392 | 17.4 | 9.2 | 4.3 | 6.8 |
| 31 | 1650 | 81.7 | 10.3 | 5.6 | 2.4 | 86.5 | 10.9 | 628 | 398 | 17.6 | 9.1 | 4.3 | 6.7 |
| 32 | 1830 | 80.7 | 10.6 | 6.3 | 2.4 | 86.1 | 11.3 | 640 | 406 | 17.8 | 9.1 | 4.3 | 6.6 |
| 33 | 2020 | 79.8 | 10.8 | 6.9 | 2.5 | 85.8 | 11.6 | 656 | 416 | 18.0 | 9.0 | 4.4 | 6.5 |
| 34 | 2230 | 79.0 | 11.0 | 7.5 | 2.5 | 85.4 | 11.9 | 675 | 428 | 18.3 | 8.9 | 4.4 | 6.4 |
| 35 | 2450 | 78.1 | 11.2 | 8.1 | 2.6 | 85.0 | 12.2 | 699 | 443 | 18.6 | 8.9 | 4.5 | 6.3 |
| 36 | 2690 | 77.3 | 11.4 | 8.7 | 2.6 | 84.6 | 12.5 | 726 | 460 | 19.0 | 8.8 | 4.5 | 6.1 |
| 37 | 2940 | 76.4 | 11.6 | 9.3 | 2.7 | 84.3 | 12.8 | 758 | 479 | 19.5 | 8.8 | 4.5 | 6.0 |
| 38 | 3160 | 75.6 | 11.8 | 9.9 | 2.7 | 83.9 | 13.1 | 795 | 501 | 20.0 | 8.8 | 4.5 | 5.9 |
| 39 | 3330 | 74.8 | 11.9 | 10.5 | 2.8 | 83.6 | 13.3 | 836 | 525 | 20.5 | 8.7 | 4.6 | 5.8 |
| 40 | 3450 | 74.0 | 12.0 | 11.2 | 2.8 | 83.3 | 13.5 | 882 | 551 | 21.1 | 8.7 | 4.6 | 5.7 |

Data from Ziegler EE, O'Donnell AM, Nelson SE, Fomon SJ: Body composition of the reference fetus. Growth, Dec 40(4):329-341, 1976, Table 2. PMID 1010389 (PubMed—indexed for MEDLINE), 1975.

## Plasma Immunoglobulin Concentrations in Premature Infants (25-28 weeks of gestation)

| Age (mo) | *n* | IgG* (mg/dL) | IgM* (mg/dL) | IgA* (mg/dL) |
|---|---|---|---|---|
| 0.25 | 18 | 251 (114-552)† | 7.6 (1.3-43.3) | 1.2 (0.07-20.8) |
| 0.5 | 14 | 202 (91-446) | 14.1 (3.5-56.1) | 3.1 (0.09-10.7) |
| 1.0 | 10 | 158 (57-437) | 12.7 (3.0-53.3) | 4.5 (0.65-30.9) |
| 1.5 | 14 | 134 (59-307) | 16.2 (4.4-59.2) | 4.3 (0.9-20.9) |
| 2.0 | 12 | 89 (58-136) | 16 (5.3-48.9) | 4.1 (1.5-11.1) |
| 3 | 13 | 60 (23-156) | 13.8 (5.3-36.1) | 3 (0.6-15.6) |
| 4 | 10 | 82 (32-210) | 22.2 (11.2-43.9) | 6.8 (1-47.8) |
| 6 | 11 | 159 (56-455) | 41.3 (8.3-205) | 9.7 (3-31.2) |
| 8-10 | 6 | 273 (94-794) | 41.8 (31.1-56.1) | 9.5 (0.9-98.6) |

*Geometric mean.

†The normal ranges in parentheses were determined by taking the antilog of (mean logarithm ± 2 SD of the logarithms).

From Ballow M, et al: Pediatr Res 20:899, 1986.

## Plasma Immunoglobulin Concentrations in Premature Infants (29-32 weeks of gestation)

| Age (mo) | *n* | IgG* (mg/dL) | IgM* (mg/dL) | IgA* (mg/dL) |
|---|---|---|---|---|
| 0.25 | 42 | 368 (186-728)† | 9.1 (2.1-39.4) | 0.6 (0.04-1) |
| 0.5 | 35 | 275 (119-637) | 13.9 (4.7-41) | 0.9 (0.01-7.5) |
| 1 | 26 | 209 (97-452) | 14.4 (6.3-33) | 1.9 (0.3-12) |
| 1.5 | 22 | 156 (69-352) | 15.4 (5.5-43.2) | 2.2 (0.7-6.5) |
| 2 | 11 | 123 (64-237) | 15.2 (4.9-46.7) | 3 (1.1-8.3) |
| 3 | 14 | 104 (41-268) | 16.3 (7.1-37.2) | 3.6 (0.8-15.4) |
| 4 | 21 | 128 (39-425) | 26.5 (7.7-91.2) | 9.8 (2.5-39.3) |
| 6 | 21 | 179 (51-634) | 29.3 (10.5-81.5) | 12.3 (2.7-57.1) |
| 8-10 | 16 | 280 (140-561) | 34.7 (17-70.8) | 20.9 (8.3-53) |

*Geometric mean.

†The normal ranges in parentheses were determined by taking the antilog of (mean logarithm ± 2 SD of the logarithms).

From Ballow M, et al: Pediatr Res 20:899, 1986.

## Temperature Equivalents

| Celsius | Fahrenheit | Celsius | Fahrenheit |
|---|---|---|---|
| 34.0° | 93.2° | 38.6° | 101.4° |
| 34.2 | 93.6 | 38.8 | 101.8 |
| 34.4 | 93.9 | 39.0 | 102.2 |
| 34.6 | 94.3 | 39.2 | 102.5 |
| 34.8 | 94.6 | 39.4 | 102.9 |
| 35.0 | 95.0 | 39.6 | 103.2 |
| 35.2 | 95.4 | 39.8 | 103.6 |
| 35.4 | 95.7 | 40.0 | 104.0 |
| 35.6 | 96.1 | 40.2 | 104.3 |
| 35.8 | 96.4 | 40.4 | 104.7 |
| 36.0 | 96.8 | 40.6 | 105.1 |
| 36.2 | 97.1 | 40.8 | 105.4 |
| 36.4 | 97.5 | 41.0 | 105.8 |
| 36.6 | 97.8 | 41.2 | 106.1 |
| 36.8 | 98.2 | 41.4 | 106.5 |
| 37.0 | 98.6 | 41.6 | 106.8 |
| 37.2 | 98.9 | 41.8 | 107.2 |
| 37.4 | 99.3 | 42.0 | 107.6 |
| 37.6 | 99.6 | 42.2 | 108.0 |
| 37.8 | 100.0 | 42.4 | 108.3 |
| 38.0 | 100.4 | 42.6 | 108.7 |
| 38.2 | 100.7 | 42.8 | 109.0 |
| 38.4 | 101.1 | 43.0 | 109.4 |

## Conversion of Pounds and Ounces to Grams

| Ounces | Grams | | | | | | | |
|---|---|---|---|---|---|---|---|---|
| | 1 lb | 2 lb | 3 lb | 4 lb | 5 lb | 6 lb | 7 lb | 8 lb |
| 0 | 454 | 907 | 1361 | 1814 | 2268 | 2722 | 3175 | 3629 |
| 1 | 482 | 936 | 1389 | 1843 | 2296 | 2750 | 3204 | 3657 |
| 2 | 510 | 964 | 1418 | 1871 | 2325 | 2778 | 3232 | 3686 |
| 3 | 539 | 992 | 1446 | 1899 | 2353 | 2807 | 3260 | 3714 |
| 4 | 567 | 1021 | 1474 | 1928 | 2381 | 2835 | 3289 | 3742 |
| 5 | 595 | 1049 | 1503 | 1956 | 2410 | 2863 | 3317 | 3771 |
| 6 | 624 | 1077 | 1531 | 1985 | 2438 | 2892 | 3345 | 3799 |
| 7 | 652 | 1106 | 1559 | 2013 | 2466 | 2920 | 3374 | 3827 |
| 8 | 680 | 1134 | 1588 | 2041 | 2495 | 2948 | 3402 | 3856 |
| 9 | 709 | 1162 | 1616 | 2070 | 2523 | 2977 | 3430 | 3884 |
| 10 | 737 | 1191 | 1644 | 2098 | 2552 | 3005 | 3459 | 3912 |
| 11 | 765 | 1219 | 1673 | 2126 | 2580 | 3033 | 3487 | 3941 |
| 12 | 794 | 1247 | 1701 | 2155 | 2608 | 3062 | 3515 | 3969 |
| 13 | 822 | 1276 | 1729 | 2183 | 2637 | 3090 | 3544 | 3997 |
| 14 | 851 | 1304 | 1758 | 2211 | 2665 | 3119 | 3572 | 4026 |
| 15 | 879 | 1332 | 1786 | 2240 | 2693 | 3147 | 3600 | 4054 |

## Conversion of Inches to Centimeters

| Inches | cm | Inches | cm | Inches | cm |
|---|---|---|---|---|---|
| 10 | 25.40 | 15 | 38.10 | 20 | 50.80 |
| 10½ | 26.67 | 15½ | 39.37 | 20½ | 52.07 |
| 11 | 27.94 | 16 | 40.64 | 21 | 53.34 |
| 11½ | 29.21 | 16½ | 41.91 | 21½ | 54.61 |
| 12 | 30.48 | 17 | 43.18 | 22 | 55.88 |
| 12½ | 31.75 | 17½ | 44.45 | 22½ | 57.15 |
| 13 | 33.02 | 18 | 45.72 | 23 | 58.42 |
| 13½ | 34.29 | 18½ | 46.99 | 23½ | 56.69 |
| 14 | 35.56 | 19 | 48.26 | 24 | 60.96 |
| 14½ | 36.83 | 19½ | 49.53 | | |

# Index

Note: Page numbers followed by f indicate figures; page numbers followed by t indicate tables.

## A

## B

## C

## D

## E

## F

## G

## H

# I

## O

## P

## Q



## R

## U

## V

## W



## X



## Y



## Z